UNIT 9
Renal Problems

UNIT 10
Endocrine Problems

UNIT 11
Gastrointestinal Problems

UNIT 12
Hepatic Problems

UNIT 13
Neurologic Problems

UNIT 1
Mus

UNIT 15
Reproductive Problems

UNIT 16
Eye Problems

UNIT 17
Ear Problems

UNIT 18
Skin Problems

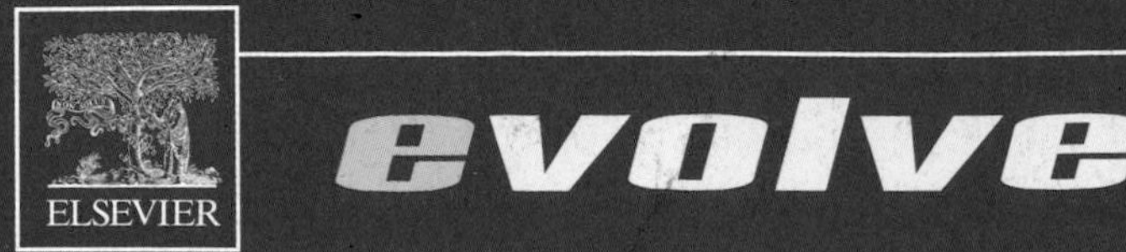

To access your Student Resources, visit the Web address below:

http://evolve.elsevier.com/Monahan/medsurg

- **Answer Guidelines for Textbook Exercises**
Gauge your comprehension and application of concepts covered in the text with answers and rationales for the *Are You Ready?* review questions and answer guidelines for the end-of-chapter critical thinking questions and *Preparing for Practice* exercises.
- **Systems Review**
Animations and video clips offer a thorough review of the anatomy and physiology of the human body.
- **Physical Examination Video**
Prepare for patient assessment in the clinical setting with this head-to-toe physical examination video.
- **Concept Map Creator**
Walks you through the thinking process of creating individualized Concept Maps, from initial diagnoses to interventions to outcomes to a complete plan of care.
- **WebLinks**
Links to hundreds of Web sites carefully chosen to supplement the content of each chapter of the textbook; regularly updated, with new ones added as they develop.
- **Content Updates**
Include the latest news and research findings related to medical-surgical nursing to keep you informed of current practice.
- **And much more!**

PHIPPS' Medical-Surgical Nursing

Health and Illness Perspectives

EIGHTH EDITION

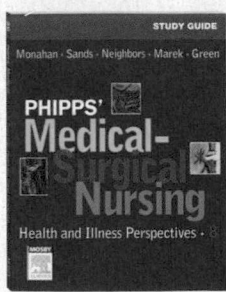

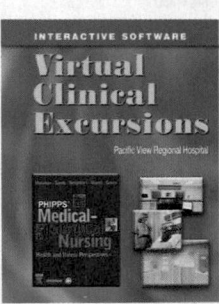

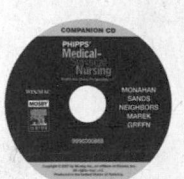

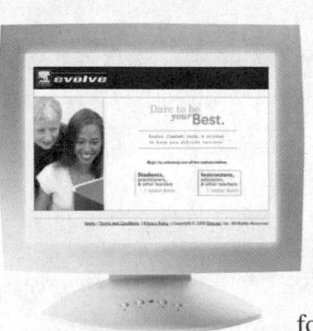

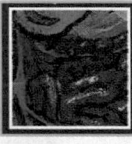

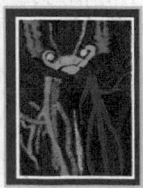

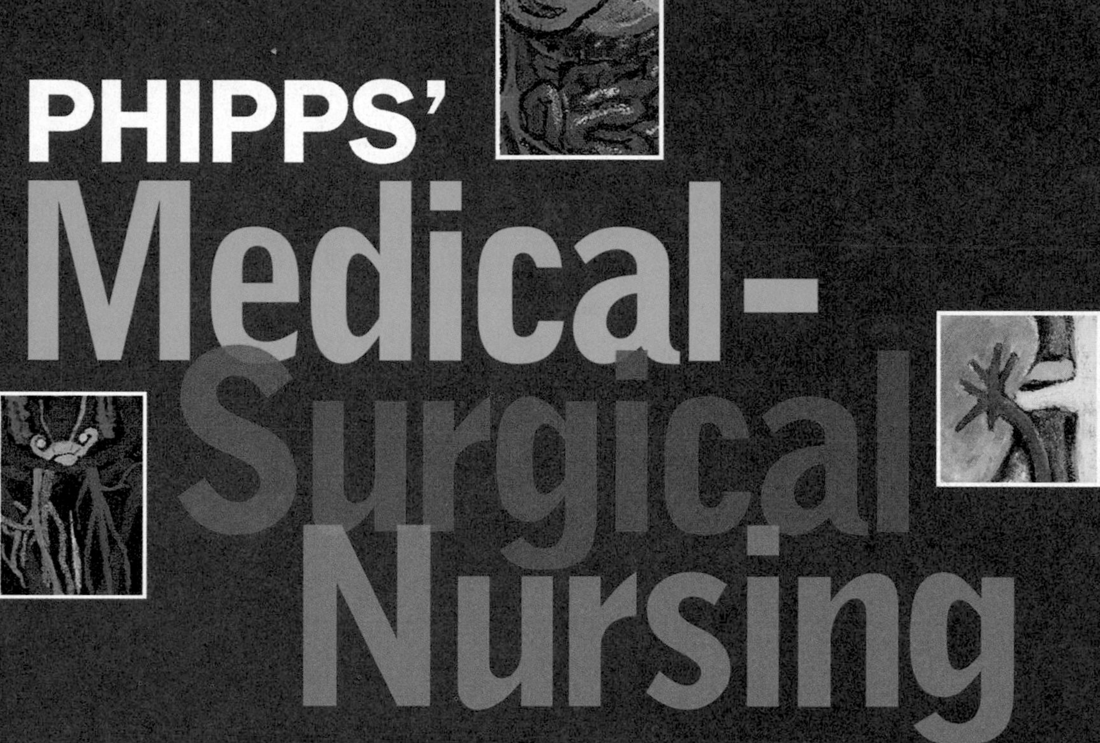

PHIPPS' Medical-Surgical Nursing

Health and Illness Perspectives

EIGHTH EDITION

FRANCES DONOVAN MONAHAN, PhD, RN
Professor of Nursing
Rockland Community College
State University of New York
Suffern, New York

JUDITH K. SANDS, EdD, RN
Associate Professor and Baccalaureate Program Director,
School of Nursing
University of Virginia
Charlottesville, Virginia

MARIANNE NEIGHBORS, EdD, RN
Professor, Eleanor Mann School of Nursing
University of Arkansas
Fayetteville, Arkansas

JANE F. MAREK, MSN, RN, APRN, BC
Instructor, Frances Payne Bolton School of Nursing
Case Western Reserve University
Cleveland, Ohio

CAROL J. GREEN, PhD, RN
Professor of Nursing
Johnson County Community College
Overland Park, Kansas;
CAPT, Nurse Corps
United States Navy

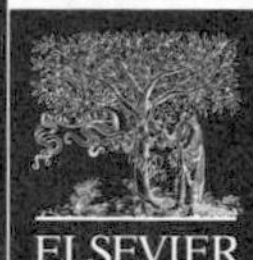

MOSBY
ELSEVIER

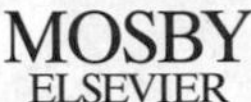

11830 Westline Industrial Drive
St. Louis, Missouri 63146

PHIPPS' MEDICAL-SURGICAL NURSING: HEALTH AND ILLNESS PERSPECTIVES, EIGHTH EDITION

ISBN-13: 978-0-323-03197-4
ISBN-10: 0-323-03197-8

ISBN-13: 978-0-323-03197-4
ISBN-10: 0-323-03197-8

Executive Editor: Michael Ledbetter, Tom Wilhelm
Senior Developmental Editor: Laurie Gower, Jill Ferguson
Publishing Services Manager: Deborah L. Vogel
Project Manager: Mary Drone, Katherine Hinkebein
Senior Book Designer: Amy Buxton
Marketing Manager: Tricia Schroeder
Multimedia Producer: Joe Selby

Printed in Canada

Last digit is the print number: 9 8 7 6 5 4 3 2 1

The first edition of Medical-Surgical Nursing *was published by Mosby in 1979, the realization of a dream for Wilma J. Phipps and her colleague and writing partner Barbara C. Long, and a result of their collaboration with Nancy Fugate Woods. They saw the need for a new textbook that would elevate the depth and completeness of coverage of both pathophysiology and medical management. Dr. Phipps devoted the next 20 years of her career to ensuring that the text underwent timely revisions and contained the most up-to-date coverage of all topics. This book was her gift to the profession she loved and the students she admired and mentored. Although she was unable to actively participate in this most recent edition, her heart will always remain with the project. We dedicate the eighth edition to her decades of leadership and contribution to the field of nursing and nursing education.*

With all my love to my aunt, Claire T. Torpey;
my daughter and son-in-law, Kerryane and Robson Diniz;
my son, Michael;
and to the memory of my husband, William T. Monahan.

FDM

To my ever-faithful supporters: my husband, Larry Butler;
my parents, Lillian and Louis Zadra;
my son, Jeremy Neighbors;
my sister, Marji Schwickrath;
and my friends Bonnie and Tommy Cooper and Gloria and Charles Fowlkes.
I have been blessed to have them in my life.

MN

To the memory of my parents,
John and Vivian Sarver,
who always encouraged me to dream big and work hard
to reach my goals.

JKS

To Ian James Frank.

JFM

To my husband and best friend, Chuck Nigro,
for his support and encouragement;
my late father, Wade Green,
who taught me to seek wisdom as well as knowledge;
and my students for their enthusiasm and caring.

CJG

Contributors

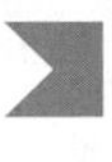

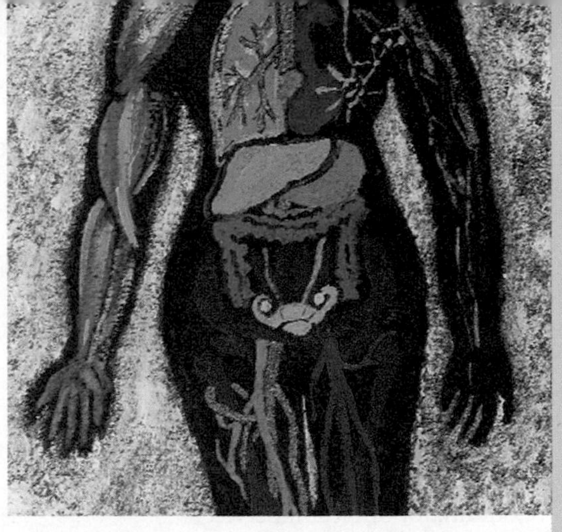

SHARON A. ARONOVITCH, PhD, APRN, BC, CWOCN
Faculty, Associate Degree Nursing Program
Excelsior College
Albany, New York

TONI O. BARNETT, PhD, APRN, BC, NP-C
Nursing Department Head
North Georgia College & State University
Dahlonega, Georgia

KATHLEEN BARTA, EdD, RN
Associate Professor, Eleanor Mann School of Nursing
University of Arkansas
Fayetteville, Arkansas

MARY JO BOEHNLEIN, MSN, RN
Program Manager, Associate Degree Nursing Program
Cuyahoga Community College
Cleveland, Ohio

HEATHER G. BOYD-MONK, SRN, BSN, CRNO
Ophthalmic Nurse Educator
Philadelphia, Pennsylvania

SALLY A. BROZENEC, PhD, RN
Complemental Faculty, College of Nursing
Rush University
Chicago, Illinois

SUSAN BULECZA, MSN, RN, CNS, APRN, BC
Registered Nursing Consultant
Florida Department of Health
Tallahassee, Florida

PAMELA D. DENNISON, MSN, RN, APRN, BC
Advanced Practice Nurse I
University of Virginia Medical Center;
Clinician/Educator
University of Virginia Health System
Charlottesville, Virginia

PEGGY ELLIS, PhD, ANP, FNP
Associate Professor, School of Nursing
St. Louis University
St. Louis, Missouri

JEANNE M. ERICKSON, MSN, RN, AOCN
General Faculty, School of Nursing
University of Virginia
Charlottesville, Virginia

ROSEMARY B. FIELD, MS, AOCN
Oncology Clinical Nurse Specialist
University of Virginia Health System
Charlottesville, Virginia

JEANNE FLANNERY, DSN, ARNP, CNRN, CRRN, CCH
Professor, School of Nursing
Florida State University
Tallahassee, Florida

LISA W. FORSYTH, MSN, RN
Clinician 4, Neuroscience
2006 President, Professional Nursing Staff Organization
University of Virginia Health System
Charlottesville, Virginia

JANET C. GARNETT, MSN, RN
Registered Nurse
University of Virginia Health System
Charlottesville, Virginia

ANN L. GARRIGUES, MSN, RN
Director of Nursing Education
NorthWest Arkansas Community College
Bentonville, Arkansas

ELIZABETH W. GOOD, MSN, RN, BC
Instructor, School of Nursing
University of Virginia;
Advanced Practice Nurse I, Surgical Care Coordinator
University of Virginia Health System
Charlottesville, Virginia

AMY E. GUTHRIE, MSN, APRN, BC, PCM, CHPN
Certified Palliative Care Nurse Practitioner
Hospice of the Western Reserve
Cleveland, Ohio

KATHY HENLEY HAUGH, PhD, RN
Assistant Professor, School of Nursing
University of Virginia
Charlottesville, Virginia

CHRISTINE HEALY, MSN, RN
Coordinator of Health Services
East Ramapo Central School District
Spring Valley, New York;
Adjunct Instructor
Rockland Community College
State University of New York
Suffern, New York

URSULA J. HEITZ, MSN, RN
Nursing Consultant
Nashville, Tennessee

JANICE HOFFMAN, MSN, RN
Instructor, School of Nursing
Johns Hopkins University
Baltimore, Maryland

KIM HUDSON, MSN, WHNP
Assistant Professor of Nursing
North Georgia College & State University
Dahlonega, Georgia

SHELLEY YERGER HUFFSTUTLER, DSN, FNP, GNP
Associate Professor and FNP Program Coordinator, School of Nursing
University of Alabama at Birmingham
Birmingham, Alabama

JEANNE LINHART, APRN, BC
Associate Professor
Department of Nursing
Rockland Community College
State University of New York
Suffern, New York

DEA MAHANES, MSN, RN, CCRN, CNRN, CCNS
Advanced Practice Nurse 1, Clinical Nurse Specialist
Nerancy Neuro Intensive Care Unit
University of Virginia Health System
Charlottesville, Virginia

PENNY L. MARSHALL, PhD, RN
Nursing Professor
Johnson County Community College
Overland Park, Kansas

MARIANNE L. MATZO, PhD, APRN, GNP-BC, FAAN
Professor and Frances E. and A. Earl Ziegler Chair in Palliative Care Nursing, College of Nursing
The University of Oklahoma Health Sciences Center
Oklahoma City, Oklahoma

CAROL LYNN MAXWELL-THOMPSON, MSN, RN, FNP-C
Assistant Professor of Nursing, School of Nursing
University of Virginia
Charlottesville, Virginia

MICHAEL H. MCGILLION, BScN, PhD(c), RN
Faculty of Nursing
University of Toronto
Toronto, Ontario, Canada

JACKIE L. MURPHREE, MNSc, EdD, RN
Assistant Professor of Nursing
University of Central Arkansas
Conway, Arkansas

GRACE NEWSOME, EdD, APRN, BC, FNP
Professor of Nursing and MS Coordinator
North Georgia College & State University
Dalhonega, Georgia

BRENDA NICHOLS, PhD, RN
Dean, College of Arts and Sciences
Lamar University
Beaumont, Texas

DENISE E. PELLEGRIN, MSN, RN
Assistant Professor of Nursing
Nicholls State University
Thibodaux, Louisiana

CYNTHIA K. POTTER, MSN, CNP
Certified Nurse Practitioner;
Instructor of Medicine
Case Western Reserve University
Cleveland, Ohio

KATHRYN B. REID, PhD, RN, CCRN, APRN, BC
Assistant Professor, School of Nursing
University of Virginia
Charlottesville, Virginia

ANGELA SAMMARCO, PhD, RN
Assistant Professor
Department of Nursing
College of Staten Island
Staten Island, New York

LEPAINE SHARP-MCHENRY, MSN
Nursing Faculty/LTC Nurse Consultant,
Eleanor Mann School of Nursing
University of Arkansas
Fayetteville, Arkansas

NAN SMITH-BLAIR, PhD, RN
Assistant Professor, Eleanor Mann School of Nursing
University of Arkansas
Fayetteville, Arkansas

AUDREY SNYDER, MSN, RN, ACNP-CS
Instructor, School of Nursing
University of Virginia
Charlottesville, Virginia

MARIANNE C. TAWA, MSN, RN, NP
Nurse Practitioner, Dermatology and Cutaneous Oncology
Center for Cutaneous Oncology
Dana-Farber Cancer Institute
Boston, Massachusetts

MARGARET M. ULCHAKER, MSN, RN, CDE, CNP, NP-C, BC-ADM
Endocrine Nurse Practitioner
North Coast Institute of Diabetes and Endocrinology, Inc.;
Clinical Instructor, School of Nursing
Case Western Reserve University
Cleveland, Ohio

MARGARET K. WARSHAW, MA, RN
Formerly Professor of Nursing
County College of Morris
Randolph, New Jersey

JUDITH H. WATT-WATSON, PhD, RN
Professor and Associate Dean, Academic Programs
University of Toronto
Toronto, Ontario, Canada

KELLY A. WEIGEL, MSN, CNP
Instructor of Medicine
Case Western Reserve University
Cleveland, Ohio

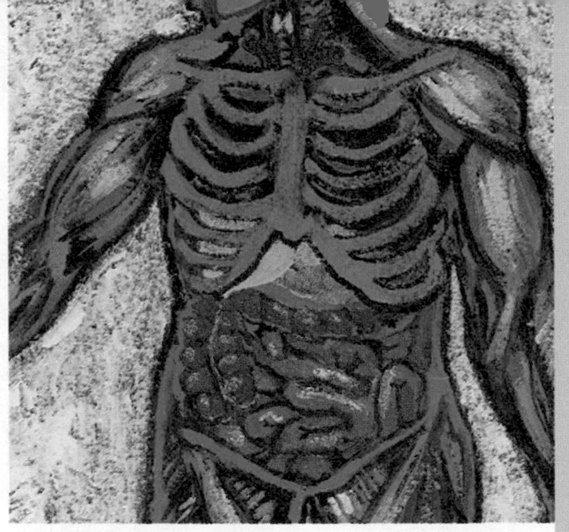

Reviewers

LUANA CATES ADAMS, MSN, RN
Associate Professor, Department of Nursing
University of Arkansas at Little Rock
Little Rock, Arkansas

CHERYL L. BITTEL, MSN, RN, CCRN
Clinical Nurse Specialist
Saint Joseph's Hospital of Atlanta
Atlanta, Georgia

MICHELLE BOTT, BScN, MN, RN
Professional Practice Coordinator
Guelph General Hospital
Guelph, Ontario

HEATHER G. BOYD-MONK, SRN, BSN, CRNO
Ophthalmic Nurse Educator
Philadelphia, Pennsylvania

LINDA M. CATER, MSN, RN
Assistant Dean
Gadsden State Community College
Anniston, Alabama

ROBIN WEBB CORBETT, PhD, RN, C
Associate Professor, School of Nursing
East Carolina University
Greenville, North Carolina

KERRYANE MONAHAN DINIZ, AB, MS
North Hutchinson Island, Florida

FRANCES R. EASON, EdD, RNC
Professor, School of Nursing
East Carolina University
Greenville, North Carolina

MARGARET GINGRICH, MSN
Associate Professor
Harrisburg Area Community College
Harrisburg, Pennsylvania

MARY E. HANSON-ZALOT, MSN, RN, AOCN
Nursing Faculty, School of Nursing
Methodist Hospital
Philadelphia, Pennsylvania

SANDRA HOFFMAN, MSN, CNS
Clinical Assistant Professor, School of Nursing
University of North Carolina at Chapel Hill
Chapel Hill, North Carolina

KATHERINE PURGATORIO HOWARD, MS, RN, BC
Instructor of Nursing, Charles E. Gregory School of Nursing
Raritan Bay Medical Center
Perth Amboy, New Jersey

PAMEULA S. JOHNSON, BSN, RN, CCRN, FNE
Clinical Coordinator
Nash Healthcare Systems, Inc.
Rocky Mount, North Carolina

JUDY KNIGHTON, MSN, RN
Clinical Nurse Specialist—Burns
Burn Resource Centre Inc.
Sharon, Ontario

NATASHA LESKOVSEK, MBA, RN, MPM, JD
Nurse Attorney
Heller Ehrman
Washington, District of Columbia

DOROTHY M. OBESTER, BSNE, MSN, PhD
Professor of Nursing
Saint Francis University
Loretto, Pennsylvania

ELDEAN PIERCE, MSN, RN, FNP
Assistant Professor, School of Nursing
East Carolina University
Greenville, North Carolina

BRUCE AUSTIN SCOTT, MSN, APRN, BC
Nursing Instructor
San Joaquin Delta College
Stockton, California;
University of California, Davis Medical Center
Sacramento, California

BELLA SMITH, MSN, RN, CCRN
B. Smith Associates, LLC
Tucson, Arizona

LINDA ULAK, EdD, RN, CS, CCRN
Associate Professor and Chair, Undergraduate Nursing/Director, RN Program
College of Nursing
Seton Hall University
South Orange, New Jersey

SUZANNE MICHELE VANET, RN, BC
Nursing Supervisor
Louis A. Johnson VA Medical Center
Clarksburg, West Virginia

Preface

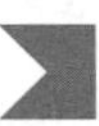

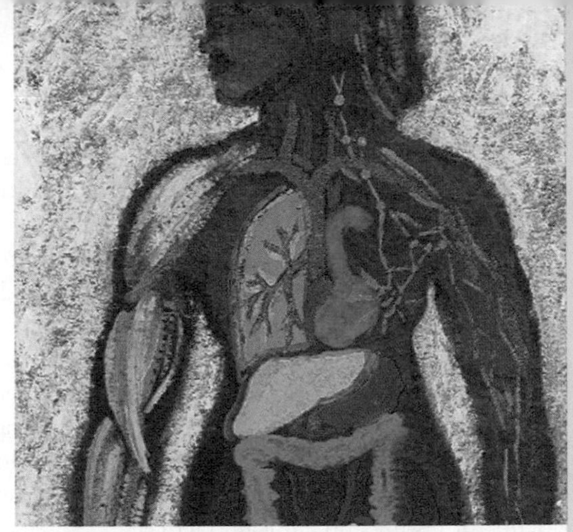

The vision for this highly respected medical-surgical nursing text as it moves, under new leadership, into its eighth edition is to maintain the quality of its content while making it relevant to the needs and abilities of today's nursing students. To realize this vision, the book has been designed and written to:

- Be understandable without being oversimplified.
- Focus clearly on major concepts while providing sufficient related information to support informed practice.
- Create an awareness of the evolving nature of health care and nursing practice.
- Emphasize the unique role of nursing in-patient care by using the format of the nursing process with references to NIC and NOC in the discussion of the care of patients with complex health problems.
- Present a clean, uncluttered text that facilitates attentive reading as opposed to distracting from it.

Content and Organization

Chapters 1 through 19 address essential aspects of practice that cross the practice lines of specific areas of medical-surgical nursing. Included are chapters that focus on varied settings such as emergency, critical, acute, long-term, and home care; specific patient populations such as the older adult, the perioperative patient, and the dying patient; and nonspecific problems related to areas such as pain, fluids and electrolytes, and shock. New content on genetics and disease, infections and bioterrorism, palliative care, and rehabilitation cover the emerging issues of today's health care environment.

The focus of the balance of the chapters is on the management of specific medical-surgical problems grouped according to body system. An assessment chapter reviews anatomy and physiology, presents comprehensive directions for obtaining health history and physical assessment data, and discusses laboratory and other diagnostic studies, orienting the student to the care of patients with problems within each body system. One or more chapters discuss specific problems of the system. In these chapters specific disorders are discussed in terms of etiology and epidemiology, pathophysiology, and collaborative care. The collaborative care section includes diagnostic and management information, concisely presenting conditions and providing a comprehensive view of treatment, regardless of which professional member of the health care team is responsible for its direct implementation. Conditions that have a major independent nursing role are presented in a Nursing Management section developed around the nursing process steps of assessment, nursing diagnosis, planning, intervention, and evaluation and include important information related to patient and family teaching.

Learning Features

Comprehensive knowledge essential to practice is highlighted in a variety of ways:

- Over 150 **Guidelines for Safe Practice** boxes provide step-by-step instructions and other considerations for providing safe and effective nursing care.
- More than 70 **Patient/Family Teaching** boxes outline information to share with patients and their families as part of comprehensive treatment.
- **Risk Factors** boxes and **Clinical Manifestations** boxes for all major disease entities make information about risk factors and signs and symptoms readily accessible.
- **Nursing Assessment** sections in each assessment chapter clearly direct the student how to perform an appropriate health assessment, and **Gerontologic Assessment** boxes in these chapters reinforce the adaptations required to care effectively for the rapidly growing aging population.
- **Common Medications** tables summarize key drug group information and nursing considerations for the most commonly administered drugs.
- **Complementary & Alternative Therapies** boxes discuss popular and emerging nontraditional therapies as they relate to traditional treatments.
- **Nursing Management** sections clearly correlate NANDA nursing diagnoses, appropriate patient outcomes, and associated interventions.
- **Nursing Care Plans** cover more than 30 patient situations to reinforce the nursing role in the management of selected problems. These are consistent in format and identify NANDA diagnoses, NIC priority interventions, and NOC suggested outcomes, placing the care plans in the forefront of contemporary practice.
- **Healthy People 2010** boxes identify national health objectives relevant to the topic of discussion.

- **Future Watch** boxes alert the reader to timely topics such as innovative procedures and potential treatments currently under investigation.
- **Research** boxes are integrated throughout to provide applications to today's nursing practice, and **Evidence-Based Practice** boxes emphasize the importance of applying relevant research to practice.
- **Critical thinking questions** at the end of each nursing management chapter challenge students to apply information they have just learned using critical thinking skills.

New features are included in this edition to better prepare students for testing and clinical practice:

- **Key terms** are listed at the beginning of the chapter with page number references and highlighted in bold in the text.
- **Ethical Alert** boxes discuss current ethical issues that nurses face in clinical practice, including decision-making, genetic testing and therapy, and forced immunization.
- **Legal Alert** boxes discuss critical legal considerations, including protocol for medical and nursing interventions, patient consent for treatment or testing, and duty to warn.
- **"Are You Ready?"** questions sprinkled throughout the text test mastery of content just covered, building a knowledge base and confidence for the NCLEX examination.
- **Preparing for Practice** boxes in select chapters are linked to a new interactive simulated hospital environment on the **Companion CD.** Exercises encourage critical thinking skills and stimulate classroom discussion based on shared clinical experiences.

Ancillaries

Learning Resources for Students

Companion CD. The Companion CD is an interactive learning tool that works with the *Preparing for Practice* exercises in the book. Students "check in" with patients in a realistic hospital setting to review patient records, conduct assessment interviews, and develop a plan of care.

Evolve Resources. Evolve is an interactive learning environment that reinforces and expands on the concepts learned in class. Valuable resources are available to accompany this text, including answers and rationales for the "Are You Ready?" questions, answer guidelines for the *Preparing for Practice* exercises and chapter-ending critical thinking questions, animations, sample clinical pathways, a concept map creator, and WebLinks.

Study Guide. This comprehensive study aid promotes a thorough understanding of the content presented in the textbook. Learning activities and case studies with critical thinking exercises are designed to enhance analytic reasoning, divergent thinking, reflection, problem solving, and decision making in the clinical setting.

Virtual Clinical Excursions. VCE is an innovative workbook/CD-ROM package that immerses students in a virtual hospital setting with hands-on activities and simulated patient interactions. Students have the opportunity to set priorities for care; collect, analyze, and interpret data; prepare and administer medications; and manage patients with complex medical conditions. It is an ideal environment for learning vital skills such as communication, documentation, assessment, critical thinking, and clinical judgment.

Teaching Resources for Instructors

Instructor's Electronic Resource. The Instructor's Electronic Resource on CD-ROM includes chapter overviews, teaching suggestions for classroom and practice applications, additional critical thinking questions, an updated test bank in ExamView, and a complete collection of PowerPoint lecture slides including full-color illustrations from the text.

Evolve Resources. Evolve provides instructors with online access to all of the learning tools available to students, all teaching resources from the Instructor's Electronic Resource on CD-ROM, and content updates as new developments in the field of medical-surgical nursing arise.

Acknowledgments

A special thanks goes to the contributors to past editions; their expertise and knowledge of current clinical practice added to the relevance and accuracy of the content and provided a strong base for this revision.

Frances Donovan Monahan
Judith K. Sands
Marianne Neighbors
Jane F. Marek
Carol J. Green

Contents

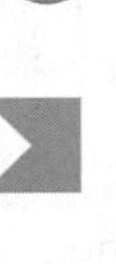

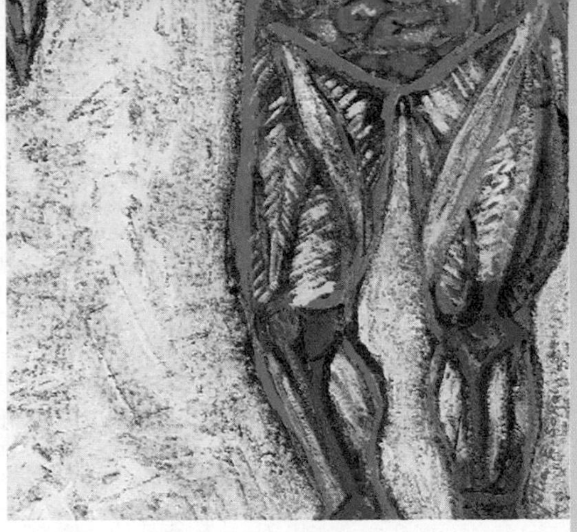

UNIT 1 Medical-Surgical Nursing Today

UNIT 5
Immunologic Problems

UNIT 6
Respiratory Problems

UNIT 7 Cardiovascular Problems

UNIT 8 Hematologic Problems

UNIT 9 Renal Problems

UNIT 10 Endocrine Problems

UNIT 11 Gastrointestinal Problems

TABLE 2-1 PRIMARY CHANGES OF AGING

Body System	Physiologic Aging Changes	Expected Physical Manifestations
Integumentary	Loss of skin elasticity	Wrinkles, folds, sagging
	Decreased subcutaneous fat and sebaceous secretions	Dry and thin, fragile skin
	Loss of melanin	Graying or white hair
	Decreased blood supply to nail bed	Thick, brittle nails
	Nerve endings decreased	Decreased sensation
Musculoskeletal	Muscle fibers decreased and atrophied	Strength and agility decreased
	Shrinkage of vertebral discs	Height decreased
	Increased flexion in joints; cartilage deterioration	Mobility decreased; range of motion limited
Pulmonary	Increased chest wall rigidity; calcification of costal cartilage; respiratory muscles atrophied	Reduced vital capacity; increased residual volume
	Decreased number of alveoli	Some shortness of breath on exertion
	Decreased ciliary action	Reduced cough reflex
Cardiovascular	Endocardial thickening; thickened heart valves	Force of contraction decreased; decreased cardiac output
	Decreased elasticity and increased rigidity of arteries	Modest increase in systolic blood pressure; cold hands and feet
Urinary	Decreased blood flow to kidneys; decreased glomerular filtration rate; reduced nephrons	Increased serum creatinine and blood urea nitrogen; decreased creatinine clearance
Gastrointestinal	Diminished saliva secretion	Dry mouth
	Decreased peristalsis	Increased tendency for indigestion and constipation
	Decreased lactase production	Lactose intolerance
Nervous	Neuron loss (brain, spine); brain size decreased	Reaction and response time decreased
	Dendrites atrophied	More time needed for cognitive processes
	Deep sleep decreased; stage IV sleep reduced	Difficulty falling and staying asleep; less sleep
Vision	Reduced lens clasticity	Presbyopia
	Lens becoming dense	Difficulty seeing in dim light
	Transparent fibers of lens beginning to yellow	Colors perceived differently
Hearing	Nerve degeneration of inner ear	Presbycusis; high frequency tone loss; auditory reaction time increased
Sexual		
Female	Hormone production diminished; vaginal pH becoming alkaline; shrinkage and atrophy of uterus, cervix, ovaries, breasts	Vaginal dryness; potential for vaginal infections increased; sagging breasts
Male	Prostate enlargement (benign); decreased testicular volume; testosterone levels decreased; penile sensation decreased	Difficulty voiding; increased refractory period; frequency of intercourse decreased; sperm count decreased; possible change in libido

Data from Ebersole P, Hess P, Luggen A: *Toward healthy aging: human needs and nursing response*, ed 6, St Louis, 2004, Mosby; and Jarvis C: *Physical examination and health assessment*, ed 4, St Louis, 2004, WB Saunders.

In addition to the primary changes of aging listed in Table 2-1, some other characteristics of organ function are important. First, the variation in organ function among individuals is much greater in older adults than in younger persons. Second, the rate of decline from one function to another varies. Basal metabolic rate and total body water of older adults decrease only minimally to about 80% of that of young adults.[22] In contrast, renal blood flow and maximum breathing capacity show a significant decline in most older persons.

A third major change related to the aging process is the response to stress. Although an older person may have adequate cardiac output at rest, stress in the form of an infection, exertion, or emotional shock will decrease cardiac output, and the person will take much longer to return to the baseline level. In addition, older persons lose reserve capacity related to a decline in coordination of brain interactions. This decline causes a slowing of reaction time and a greater susceptibility to infection and accidents.

TABLE 2-2 HOW ILLNESS CHANGES WITH AGE

Disease	Signs and Symptoms in Young Adults	Signs and Symptoms in Older Adults
Urinary tract infection	Dysuria, frequency, flank pain, fever	Many times asymptomatic Incontinence of recent onset, confusion, normal temperature
Pneumonia	Fever, cough, sputum production	May have all signs and symptoms of young adult, but more subtle Sometimes acute confusion, tachypnea, achycardia
Myocardial infarction	Severe chest pain, diaphoresis, nausea, shortness of breath	May have atypical or absent pain, confusion, tachypnea
Congestive heart failure	Dyspnea, fatigue, orthopnea, dependent edema	Same as in young adults but peripheral edema less specific as sign of congestive heart failure, plus nonspecific symptoms (e.g., confusion, weakness, failure to thrive)
Depression	Withdrawal, crying, insomnia	May have some of young adults' signs and also memory and concentration problems and increased sleep

Data from Beers MH, Berkow R, editors: *Merck manual of geriatrics,* ed 3, 2000-2004, accessed from website: www.merck.com/mrkshared/mm_geriatrics/home.jsp.

Unique Patterns of Illness Among Older Adults

A hallmark of gerontology is that diseases may have atypical presentations in older adults (Table 2-2). Often acute illnesses are superimposed on several chronic illnesses complicated by the primary changes of aging. A careful history, as well as knowledge about the unique clinical presentation in older adults, aids the nurse in performing assessments, establishing nursing diagnoses, and intervening effectively.

In assessing the health and illness of older adults, the nurse must recognize some general patterns. First, an age-related decline in immune function results in a less rapid and less effective response to infections and in an increased incidence of autoimmune and malignant disease. Second, stress situations (either physiologic or psychosocial) may produce more pronounced reactions in older persons and may require a longer time for readjustment. Third, complex functions that require multisystem coordination show the most obvious decline and require the greatest compensation and support. Fourth, older adults frequently have atypical manifestations of an illness. Confusion, restlessness, or other altered mentation, including psychiatric disorders such as depression, is common in the presence of illness. The nurse should not accept obscure or unexplained deterioration of health or function as normal aging, but must evaluate it carefully. Multiplicity and chronicity of disease are common among older adults.

▶ ARE YOU READY?

Which of the following are unique patterns in response to disease or illness in older adults?

1. Abrupt onset of clinical manifestations
2. Increased number of circulating antibodies
3. Decreased sensitivity to antibiotic therapy
4. Less effective response to infection

Functional Assessment of Older Adults: Common Concerns

Activities of Daily Living and Instrumental Activities of Daily Living

Assessment is a critical step in effective nursing care for older adults. The global aspects of health in older adults encompass three major concepts: absence of disease; performance of basic self-care activities, termed **activities of daily living** (ADLs); and performance of more complex activities, called **instrumental activities of daily living** (IADLs).

As early as the late 1800s, researchers in the United States and Europe obtained information on functional health as an estimate of morbidity. During the 1940s classifications of disability included self-care activities of dressing, toileting, and ambulation. Since that time, researchers have consistently identified three self-maintenance components: basic ADLs (e.g., bathing, eating, and toileting), more complex social activities of living (e.g., shopping, managing finances, cooking, housekeeping, transportation, managing medications, and the ability to use a telephone and cope with other aspects of one's environment—that is, IADLs.

Studies have shown that functional disability is correlated with physical illness, self-care ability, complications during hospitalization, rehabilitation potential, and even mortality. Therefore the concept of functional ability in older adults has become a valuable health indicator. Measures of functional status that examine the ability to function independently despite disease are the most useful clinical and research indicators for older adults with multiple chronic and acute illnesses. The Administration on Aging reports that 54.5% of older adults have at least one disability, 27.3% have difficulty with ADLs, and 13% have some problem with IADLs.[1]

In addition to assessing the respiratory, cardiovascular, digestive, neurologic, and other body systems of the older patient, the nurse must carefully assess functional self-care ability. Subtle changes in appetite or ambulation or even the onset of urinary incontinence may be the only clinical indicator of infections such as pneumonia, urinary tract infections, or myocardial infarctions. Several functional assessment tools and scales are widely used in a variety of clinical settings.

Risk of Falls

A major health concern that threatens the function of older adults is the risk of falls, which can result in injury and disability.[56] Even falls that do not result in serious injury may affect an older person's function and quality of life. Concern about the risk of falls is heightened when an older adult enters a hospital or long-term care facility.[52] Most health care institutions have assessment tool and protocols to assist clinicians in identifying older patients who are at risk. Care providers should assess all older patients on admission for risk of falling, and then institute a protocol to prevent falls from occurring.

Spiritual Well-Being

Spirituality focuses on the meanings one attaches to life, particularly one's own life experience. For some individuals, spirituality includes a connection to a particular religious orientation and institution. However, believing in specific religious dogma or belonging to a church may not be part of a person's spirituality. Bianchi describes aging as a "spiritual journey" that synthesizes a person's inner contemplative experience and external human concerns.[15]

Spirituality is represented by the meaning one attaches to life experiences at any age; it is a holistic integration of physical, social, psychologic, cultural, sexual, and theologic experiences. The spiritual journey of aging may be grounded in childhood and family experiences. As people age and move toward death, they understand the meaning of life in connection with other human beings and the broader society. The loss of functional abilities and disability can affect one's spirituality. The opposite is also true. Spiritual distress can result in a loss of physical, mental, and social function.[47]

Spirituality is of particular concern for persons who experience illness (see Research box).[34] The experience of physical illness and life crises can precipitate a transforming spiritual change or cause a person to become more introspective and contemplative.[20,26] The nurse can help a patient explore the meaning of a particular physical or life crisis and can provide nonjudgmental support and advocacy for patients and their families. This process helps patients find meaning in their lives through definitions of self and personhood that go beyond physical abilities.

To support older adults' spiritual well-being, nurses need to include an assessment of older adults' spirituality that goes beyond religious affiliation. Nurses should ask older adults basic questions about religious practices that comfort them, help them cope, and provide a sense of security. However, spiritual well-being has dimensions beyond religious practices. The JAREL Spiritual Well-Being Scale includes 21 questions for the older patient that the nurse scores to identify areas of spiritual concern (Box 2-2).[32] It is one of the most used scales for assessing the spiritual dimension in older adults. Care providers can use a clinical assessment and intervention protocol for spiritual well-being to assess a person's spiritual experience during an illness episode.

Research

Koenig H, George L, Titus P: Religion, spirituality and health in medically ill hospitalized older patients, *J Am Geriatr Soc* 52(4):554-562, 2004.

Researchers interviewed 834 patients, whose average age was 64.3 years, and who were admitted to a general medical service over a four-year period. The patients had a variety of medical conditions such as heart or circulatory disease, gastrointestinal disease, chronic pulmonary disease, or infectious disease. The average patient had at least five concurrent medical conditions. The study found that older adults who had strong religious or spiritual beliefs used them to cope with illness and had greater social support, fewer depressive symptoms, better cognitive function, and better physical health than those who had no religious or spiritual ties. The implications are that nurses need to assess older patients for religious and spiritual beliefs and respect and support these beliefs.

Sexuality

Both men and women maintain interest in sexual activity into late adulthood. More women cease having sexual activity after age 65 than do men. The primary reasons for the cessation are not lack of interest, but lack of an acceptable sexual partner for widows or an ailing husband for married women.

Cultural attitudes toward older adults influence both genders. Older men and women frequently are thought of as sexually unattractive and unable to engage in sex. However, Masters and Johnson found that although sexual responses are slower, older adults still have the same phases of excitement, plateau, orgasm, and resolution as younger persons.[38] Nevertheless, sexual problems occur more frequently for older adults. Women may have dyspareunia as a result of vaginal thinning and decreased lubrication caused by postmenopausal steroid starvation. Men may be affected by secondary impotence related to performance anxiety and low self-esteem. Diabetes, alcohol, and medications for hypertension are other prominent causes of impotence.

Masters and Johnson report a condition known as "widowers' syndrome."[38] After an extended period of sexual inactivity, a man cannot achieve or maintain an erection. An equivalent condition occurs in women: the vagina constricts and undergoes atrophic changes. The conclusion is that those who do not engage in sexual activity lose the ability to do so.

Sexuality is more than the physical act of intercourse. Older persons continue to need human companionship, love, and affection.[58] Nurses need to be aware of components of sexuality and how older adults may be affected by chronic illness, loss of

Box 2-2 JAREL Spiritual Well-Being Scale

Directions: Please circle the choice that *best* describes how much you agree with each statement. Circle only *one* answer for each statement. There is no right or wrong answer.

	Strongly Agree	Moderately Agree	Agree	Disagree	Moderately Disagree	Strongly Disagree
1. Prayer is an important part of my life.	SA	MA	A	D	MD	SD
2. I believe I have spiritual well-being.	SA	MA	A	D	MD	SD
3. As I grow older, I find myself more tolerant of others' beliefs.	SA	MA	A	D	MD	SD
4. I find meaning and purpose in my life.	SA	MA	A	D	MD	SD
5. I feel there is a close relationship between my spiritual beliefs and what I do.	SA	MA	A	D	MD	SD
6. I believe in an afterlife.	SA	MA	A	D	MD	SD
7. When I am sick, I have less spiritual well-being.	SA	MA	A	D	MD	SD
8. I believe in a supreme power.	SA	MA	A	D	MD	SD
9. I am able to receive and give love to others.	SA	MA	A	D	MD	SD
10. I am satisfied with my life.	SA	MA	A	D	MD	SD
11. I set goals for myself.	SA	MA	A	D	MD	SD
12. God has little meaning in my life.	SA	MA	A	D	MD	SD
13. I am satisfied with the way I am using my abilities.	SA	MA	A	D	MD	SD
14. Prayer does not help me in making decisions.	SA	MA	A	D	MD	SD
15. I am able to appreciate differences in others.	SA	MA	A	D	MD	SD
16. I am pretty well put together.	SA	MA	A	D	MD	SD
17. I prefer that others make decisions for me.	SA	MA	A	D	MD	SD
18. I find it hard to forgive others.	SA	MA	A	D	MD	SD
19. I accept my life situations.	SA	MA	A	D	MD	SD
20. Belief in a supreme being has no part in my life.	SA	MA	A	D	MD	SD
21. I cannot accept change in my life.	SA	MA	A	D	MD	SD

a partner, and the need for touch.[27] It is imperative that nurses become more knowledgeable about the specific needs of gay and lesbian older adults, groups that are often overlooked and stigmatized.[16] Sensitivity to family dynamics is just as important for a newly married couple in their seventies as for a young couple. Through counseling, the nurse can explain aging changes and suggest vaginal lubrication for women and extra physical stimulation for men. Changes in sexual position and styles of lovemaking are appropriate for those with disabling disease.

Older adults are susceptible to sexually transmitted disease, although not in the same numbers as younger adults.[24,36] Acquired immunodeficiency syndrome (AIDS) is increasingly prevalent in older adults as the epidemic spreads among all age-groups. The "at risk" categories differ for older adults (e.g., not as many are intravenous drug abusers), and the disease trajectory may progress differently. However, other risk factors are present (e.g., the immune system's declining ability to ward off infections). Women in particular are more vulnerable because of the friable vaginal lining that occurs with aging.

A final issue, often difficult for the nurse, is the need to determine whether older adults have been the victims of sexual abuse and violence. Sexual violence against older women is a growing problem and should be identified as a component of geriatric assessment.

Family

Although the media and much of society still view the institution of marriage and the family as the most acceptable lifestyle, tolerance is increasing for diversity in living patterns. Alternatives to traditional family life include cohabiting with members of the same or opposite sex, living alone, becoming a single parent, remaining a childless couple, and living communally. Other alternative family structures include homosexual couples who make a lifelong commitment and choose to raise a family. Divorce, a common occurrence today, is a highly stressful event that often creates a crisis. Most adults who are divorced, however, go on to marry again. In fact, in more than 45% of all marriages, one or both partners were married previously, with

evolve Visit the Evolve website: http://evolve.elsevier.com/Monahan/medsurg

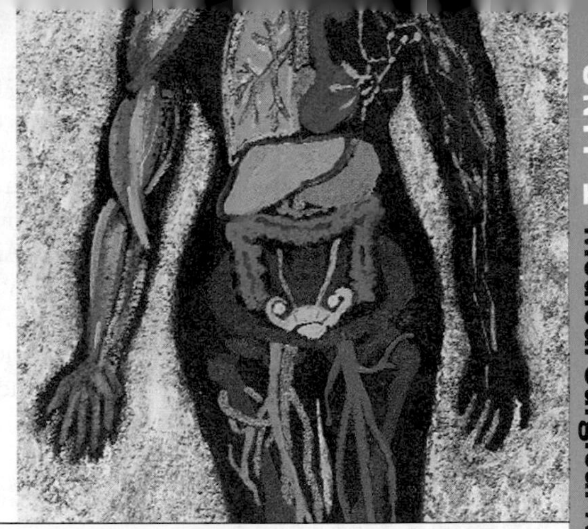

CHAPTER 1

Scope of Medical-Surgical Nursing

by Brenda Nichols, Frances D. Monahan

OBJECTIVES

After studying this chapter, the learner should be able to:

1. Define the scope and practice of medical-surgical nursing.
2. Explain the options for certification in medical-surgical nursing.
3. Identify current social and professional influences on the practice of medical-surgical nursing.
4. Differentiate *evidenced-based practice* from *research-based practice.*
5. Describe NIC, NOC, and the NANDA taxonomy and their relationship to nursing informatics.

KEY TERMS

certification, p. 2
clinical judgment, p. 6
clinical research, p. 6
cost containment, p. 4
credential, p. 3
evidence synthesis, p. 6
health maintenance organizations, p. 4
information science, p. 6
managed care, p. 4
specialty, p. 1

Medical-surgical nursing is the area of nursing practice concerned with the care of adults with predicted or existing physiologic alterations, trauma, or disability.[6] It is the backbone of modern nursing and the practice foundation of virtually all health care institutions.[2]

Traditionally medical-surgical nursing was not considered a **specialty** area. Rather, practices with a focus on a specific type of health problem within the area of medical-surgical nursing were considered specialties. These included cardiovascular, perioperative, neurologic, gynecologic, infection control, and emergency nursing, and practices limited to problems such as wound care, burns, hypertension, and diabetes. Today, this view has changed. Medical-surgical nursing is now formally recognized as a specialty in its own right,[19] and the focused practice areas are seen as subspecialties.

Formal recognition as a specialty means that a practice area meets the American Nurses Association (ANA) criteria for specialty status, which were published in the document titled *Recognition of a Specialty, Approval of Scope Statements and Acknowledgement of Nursing Practice Standards.*[11] The criteria are that the practice area must[18]:

- Be clearly defined and subscribe to the overall purposes and functions of nursing
- Define itself as nursing
- Adhere to the overall licensure requirements of the profession
- Be national or international in scope
- Be able to identify a need and demand for itself
- Have a well-derived knowledge base particular to the practice of the specialty
- Be organized and represented by a national specialty association
- Be concerned with phenomena within the discipline of nursing
- Have defined competencies for the area of specialty practice
- Have existing mechanisms for supporting, reviewing, and disseminating research to support its knowledge base
- Have continuing education programs that prepare nurses in the specialty
- Include a substantial number of nurses who devote most of their practice to the specialty

It was primarily through the work of the Academy of Medical-Surgical Nurses (AMSN) that many of these criteria were met and medical-surgical nursing attained specialty status.

Academy of Medical-Surgical Nurses

The AMSN, founded in 1991, is an international organization dedicated to fostering excellence in medical-surgical nursing practice. Its mission is to "enhance the clinical expertise, professionalism, and leadership of nurses caring for adults in hospitals, the community, and long-term care."[2] It accomplishes this through certification, education, nurturing relationships, and the promotion of high-quality nursing care and wellness. Membership is open to licensed nurses and to students at all levels of educational preparation: licensed vocational nurses/licensed practical nurses, associate degree nurses, and nurses with baccalaureate or master's degrees (see Membership section of website: http://www.medsurgnurse.org).[2] *MEDSURG Matters*, AMSN's official newsletter, contains clinical articles and news relevant to members. The official journal of AMSN is *MEDSURG Nursing, the Journal of Adult Health* (see Publications section of website).[2] AMSN has more than 20 chapters across the United States and holds an annual fall conference (see Chapters section of website).

Standards of Medical-Surgical Nursing Practice

The nursing profession has adopted standards of practice that describe the responsibilities for which practitioners are accountable. All nurses, regardless of education, use the ANA *Standards of Clinical Nursing Practice* to guide their practice.[7] This broad set of standards has two components: standards of care and standards of professional performance. The nursing process and competent level of nursing care are the foundation of the standards of care. The standards of professional performance address expected quality of care, performance appraisal, education, collegiality, ethics, collaboration, research, and resource utilization. Each standard has measurement criteria to demonstrate competent practice.

Standards of practice specific to medical-surgical nursing were developed under the auspices of AMSN. The document entitled *Scope and Standards of Medical-Surgical Nursing Practice* was first published in 1995.[1] The third edition (2005) is available through the AMSN website (see publications section).

Certification in Medical-Surgical Nursing

Certification in nursing is a mechanism for recognizing excellence in practice. Thus it is different from licensure, which recognizes a minimal level of safe practice. Certification also differs from licensure in that it is not granted by the government but by professional nursing organizations. According to the American Board of Nursing Specialties, certification is the standard by which the public recognizes high-quality nursing care.[5] The American Nurses Credentialing Center (ANCC), an arm of the ANA, is a central organization that certifies nurses in more than 40 practice areas.[31] Certification is also available through individual nursing specialty organizations. Certification in medical-surgical nursing is available through the Medical-Surgical Nursing Certification Board (MSNCB) of the AMSN and through the ANCC. Additional details on certification can be found at the AMSN and ANCC websites: http://www.medsurgnurse.org/ and http://www.ana.org/ancc/cert.html, respectively.

AMSN Certification

Certification through AMSN entitles the practitioner to use the credential Certified Medical-Surgical Registered Nurse (CMSRN). A nurse attains this certification through successful completion of AMSN's certification examination. To be eligible to take the examination, the nurse must have (see Certification section of website)[2]:

- A full and unrestricted license as a registered nurse in the United States or its territories, or equivalent registration and licensure in the country of nursing education
- Two years (within the past 5 years) of experience as a registered nurse in an adult medical-surgical clinical setting with an accrued 3000 hours of clinical practice as a staff nurse, clinical educator, manager, or supervisor

The AMSN certification test is a 4-hour examination consisting of 200 multiple-choice items, written within the framework of the nursing process. The examination focuses on the care of acutely ill, hospitalized adult patients, and each question addresses one of the patient problems and one of the domains of nursing practice shown in Box 1-1.

Once received, certification lasts for 5 years. Recertification is then required either by continuing education or by repeat examination. To be recertified, the nurse must hold a current, full, and unrestricted license to practice in the United States or its territories and have a minimum of 3000 hours of clinical practice as a staff nurse, clinical nurse specialist, clinical educator, faculty, manager, or supervisor within the previous 5 years, with 2 of the 5 years in a medical-surgical setting. For recertification through continuing education, the nurse also must have 90 approved contact hours of continuing education credits, 68 of which

Box 1-1 Patient Problems and Domains of Nursing Practice Tested on Academy of Medical-Surgical Nursing Certification Examination

Patient Problems	Domains of Nursing Practice*
Gastrointestinal	Helping role
Pulmonary	Teaching and coaching function
Cardiovascular	Diagnostic and patient monitoring function
Diabetes and other endocrine	Administering and monitoring therapeutic interventions
Genitourinary, renal, reproductive	Managing rapidly changing situations
Musculoskeletal and neurologic	Monitoring and ensuring quality of health care practices
Hematologic, immunologic, integumentary	Organizational and work-role competencies

*From Benner P: *From novice to expert: excellence and power in clinical nursing practice*, Menlo Park, Calif, 1984, Addison-Wesley, accessed from website: http://www.medsurgnurse.org/.

should be related to medical-surgical nursing. These 68 credits can be obtained through nursing programs, academic credit courses, professional publications, medical-surgical presentations, or general nursing and other health care discipline programs. When course work is used toward the 90-hour continuing education requirement, its continuing education equivalency is calculated by the formula: 1 semester hour equals 15 contact hours, and ¼ semester hour equals 10 contact hours.

Waivers of the employment eligibility requirement are available for registered nursing students in a nursing baccalaureate, master's, or doctoral degree program (see Certification Eligibility section of website).[2]

ANCC Certification

Certification in medical-surgical nursing through ANCC is based on the applicant's educational level; the **credential** awarded differs accordingly. Baccalaureate-prepared nurses can receive baccalaureate-level certification with the credential of registered nurse, board-certified (RN, BC). Associate degree or diploma nurses receive associate degree/diploma-level certification with the credential of registered nurse, certified (RN, C). Award of the credential is based on successful completion of the baccalaureate-level examination or the associate/diploma-level examination, respectively. Both examinations test the same four domains of practice, but the percentage of the total 175 questions in each domain differs according to educational level. The four domains of practice tested are biophysical and psychosocial concepts, pathophysiology of body systems, patient care issues, and issues and trends. Basic eligibility requirements for certification in medical-surgical nursing through ANCC are that the nurse must have[10]:

- A currently active registered nurse license in the United States or its territories
- The equivalent of 2 years' full-time practice as a registered nurse in the United States or its territories
- An associate degree or diploma, or baccalaureate or higher degree in nursing
- A minimum of 2000 hours of clinical practice within the past 3 years
- Thirty contact hours within the past 3 years

Once certified, a nurse remains certified for 5 years. Recertification through continuing education or by reexamination is then necessary. Recertification requires an active registered nurse license, 1000 hours of direct patient care in medical-surgical nursing during the previous 5 years, and completion of the requirements of two of the five categories of continuing education (or double the completion of one category) during the past 5 years.

Category 1 is based on continuing education credits and requires completion of 75 contact hours with at least 51% of the total in medical-surgical nursing and at least 50% of the total from courses given by an ANCC accredited or approved provider or through specifically designated organizations. Contact hours are calculated using the following equivalencies[10]:

- 1 continuing education unit (CEU) = 10 contact hours
- 1 contact hour = 0.1 CEU
- 1 contact hour = 50 minutes
- 1 academic semester hour = 15 contact hours
- 1 academic quarter hour = 12.5 contact hours
- 1 continuing medical education (CME) credit = 60 minutes or 1.2 contact hours
- 1 American Medical Association (AMA) credit = 1.2 contact hours or 60 minutes

Category 2 is based on academic credits; five semester-hour credits or six ¼-hour credits are required. For courses to be acceptable, content must be directly applicable to medical-surgical nursing. Audited courses or core courses may not be used. Academic credits may be converted to continuing education contact hours to meet category 1 requirements using the equivalency formula given above.

Category 3 is based on presenter or lecturer credits. Five different educational presentations on medical-surgical nursing are required. These may be nonapproved continuing education offerings through the nurse's place of employment or approved workshops, seminars, conferences, or guest lectures.

Category 4 relates to publishing. To meet the requirement of this category, the nurse must publish one article or book chapter, one research project, or one "other educational media" project or must complete a doctoral dissertation or master's thesis in medical-surgical nursing. To meet this requirement, published articles must be in refereed journal.

Category 5 is based on completion of a preceptorship of at least 120 hours. Strict guidelines apply as to the qualifications of the preceptor. Hours spent in a preceptorship cannot be counted toward the basic practice requirement for recertification.

Current Influences on Medical-Surgical Nursing Practice

Over the past 2 decades the practice of medical-surgical nursing, like practice in all other areas of nursing, has changed dramatically, and the change continues. Many interrelated factors are responsible for the change. The population is becoming increasingly diverse in terms of language, culture, and ethnic background. This creates new challenges for the provision of effective health care, which must be based on an understanding of individual health beliefs, values, attitudes, and practices. The population is also aging. By the year 2030, it is estimated that the over-65 population in the United States will be more than 20% of the total. Persons over age 65 are the fastest growing segment of the population; and among older adults as a whole, persons over 85 years of age represent the fastest growing age-group. As a result, the need is increasing for care related to chronic illnesses such as cancer, hypertension, heart disease, diabetes, Parkinson's disease, and Alzheimer's disease, all of which increase in frequency as people age.

Advances in medical science and technology have resulted in new options for diagnosis and treatment. These include options for health problems that were previously untreatable. The emergence of acquired immunodeficiency syndrome has created extensive needs for every level of health care. All these factors contribute to an increasing demand for high-quality health care services. Unfortunately the resources available to meet the demand are inadequate. Monetary resources are limited and stretched even further by the increasing numbers of uninsured and underinsured. The available workforce is also short in numbers and is aging.

Within this decade, the average age of the RN is predicted to be 45.4 years with more than 40% being over age 50. By 2020 the RN workforce is expected to have decreased to 20% below the expected need.[13]

The result of this complex interplay of factors is an increasing focus on **cost containment** in health care, which has been a driving force for significant changes. The **managed care** concept is one attempt to control costs. Basic elements of managed care are prenegotiated payment rates, mandatory precertification for specialty care and nonemergent hospitalization, utilization review, limited choice of providers, and fixed prices for reimbursement. Since its inception, managed care has evolved so that not every managed care program contains all these elements. **Health maintenance organizations** (HMOs), a basic form of managed care, were designed to be preventive health care organizations that actualize a holistic view of health care through a primary care provider, who might be an advanced practice nurse, a physician, or a physician's assistant. This primary care provider works with the patient to eliminate fragmentation and duplication of services, making referrals to specialists only when needed. Many variations of HMOs now exist. These include preferred provider organizations (PPOs), which are a business affiliation of physicians and hospitals that agree to care for subscribers; point-of-service plans; and Medicare+Choice plans.

As a result of these various cost-containment efforts, the locus of care is increasingly moving into the community. More patients are treated in ambulatory clinics, day surgery settings, and the home. Hospital stays are declining at the same time the acuity of hospitalized patients is increasing. The number of unlicensed assistive personnel is growing in all settings, accompanied by a movement of the registered nurse away from direct patient care to greater responsibilities in the areas of delegation and management. Practice protocols have also changed in an attempt to control costs and increase efficiency. A prime example of this change is the use of clinical pathways.

Clinical Pathways

Clinical pathways (sometimes called critical paths) are guidelines for patient care. They are best-practice standards that direct the work of all members of the health care team toward achievement of the same outcomes.

A clinical pathway begins with a medical diagnosis or major nursing diagnosis, usually one with a predictable course of treatment and recovery. The pathway describes the optimal sequencing of interventions necessary to facilitate recovery or healing. The pathway clarifies the overall plan and the role of each member of the interdisciplinary health care team (Figure 1-1). Its purpose is to ensure that the team uses the most up-to-date knowledge, skills, and research in patient care.

Agencies can purchase clinical pathways or develop their own. Effective pathways are those which maximize the quality and minimize the costs of care.

Evidence-Based Practice

The factors and trends described above are not the only determinants of change in medical-surgical nursing practice. A more recent and potentially powerful source of change is the focus on evidence-based practice (EBP).

The EBP concept appears to have originated in Canada. It grew out of efforts to improve medical education through a professional development model of problem-based learning. Its creators described it as a method of deciding on patient care based on integrating the best practices with clinical expertise that recognizes the individual's rights and situation.[27] The integration of all three sources of information made EBP unique, since until then patient care decisions were typically based on individual learning, personal experience, and clinical intuition, with or without consideration of patient circumstance. With EBP, tailoring care decisions to individuals promotes patient compliance, positive health outcomes, and optimal economic outcomes.

The EBP concept spread quickly to England, where several external factors contributed to its acceptance. The first was the need to control the rising costs of the socialized medical system. Next was the wide disparity in the costs and outcomes for medical procedures by geographic location and by practitioner. Last but not least were increasing consumer demands to understand and make informed choices about their own health care.[16] This led to creation of the Cochrane Center at Oxford. The Cochrane Collaboration is "an international non-profit and independent organization, dedicated to making up-to-date, accurate information about the effects of health care readily available worldwide. It produces and disseminates systematic reviews of health care interventions and promotes the search for evidence in the form of clinical trials and other studies of interventions."[15]

The U.S. health care system faces many of these same issues. *Cost containment* is a key phrase in virtually any discussion of health care, but no one wants to achieve it at the expense of quality. The goal, as always, is to find ways to control cost while maintaining quality. The Institute of Medicine (IOM), in 1990, defined quality in health care as the "degree to which health services to individuals and populations increase the likelihood of desired health outcomes and are consistent with current professional knowledge."[29] Irrespective of cost issues, the U.S. health care system has not attained this goal. In the words of the IOM 2001 report *Crossing the Quality Chasm: A New Health System for the 21st Century*, "Our best knowledge is not being implemented in patient care."[20] Subsequently, in its 2003 document *Health Professions Education: A Bridge to Quality*, the IOM identified a key challenge in health care as translating evidenced-based knowledge into clinical practice.[21]

Thus it is not surprising that the EBP concept soon became a part of the U.S. national health care agenda. In 1997 the Agency for Healthcare Research and Quality (AHRQ), the health services research arm of the U.S. Department of Health and Human Services (previously known as the Agency for Health Care Policy and Research [AHCPR]), created 12 Evidence-Based Practice Centers (EPCs) as part of its charge to support research focused on improving the quality of health care, reducing its cost, improving patient safety, decreasing medical errors, and broadening access to services. The purpose of these centers is to promote EBP in everyday care by developing evidence reports and technology assessments on relevant health care topics.[4]

EBP is not the same as research or research-based practice. As stated previously, a primary difference is that it integrates clinical expertise and individual patient rights and situations. However, it depends on research and its evaluation to determine its third

Patient Classification: III DATE:	PATIENT IMPRINT

TIME FRAME	TIME OF ADMISSION: 0-30 MIN	30-90 MIN	90-180 MIN	TIME OF TRANSFER: 3-6 HR
Patient Satisfaction	Pediatric support person at bedside		What can we do to enhance your stay with us?	
Discharge Planning	Identify risk factors for prolonged recovery		Plan for bed availability	Discharge to Regular Nursing Floor (RNF) or extended recovery/ICU
Airway Management	Airway Assessment Ventilator settings as ordered/O_2 as ordered Monitor O_2 Saturation Vital signs per protocol	Assess for readiness to wean	Wean ventilatory support/O_2 per protocol	Wean to room air Incentive spirometry q2h after extubation
Hemodynamic Management	Hemodynamic monitoring Hemodynamic support as necessary	Monitor need for hemodynamic support	Wean from hemodynamic support as tolerated	
Nursing and Medical Interventions	Identify patient by name and arm band Identify allergies Level of consciousness assessment Dressing assessment Systems assessment Dermatome assessment Report from anesthesia Initiate surgical-specific protocols Pain management—provide pharmacological therapies Rewarming initiated IV and arterial line management Initiate stir-up regimen (wake up) Place necessary consults Admission documentation	Review chart for patient information Pain management—provide pharmacological and nonpharmacological therapies Review orders Implement physician orders Continue stir-up regimen Emotional support Treat nausea/vomiting if necessary Monitor for potential surgical complications	Labs, x-rays complete Consults complete Wean from rewarming devices Patient repositioned Mouth care given Monitor for potential surgical complications Assess need for extended observation	Monitor for potential surgical complications Assess need for extended observation or ICU care
Patient Education	Family notified patient in PACU Orient to person, place, and time Explain activities of care while providing care	Answer patient questions Reinforce pain scale	Family called for update on patient's condition Orient to expectations of PACU discharge	Family visit for 15 minutes Instruct on postop pain management Instruct on importance of coughing, deep breathing, and exercising limbs
Outcome Criteria	Vital signs within normal parameters Oxygenation within normal range Dressing and drains intact	Vital signs within normal parameters Dressing and drains intact No excessive bleeding Pain minimized	Oriented to person and place/returned to baseline mentation Hemodynamically stable	Postanesthesia Score >8 Temp 35.5°-38.4° C Coughing and deep breathing Pain < 4 Minimal nausea/vomiting No evidence of surgical complications All appropriate physician orders initiated

Figure 1-1 Clinical pathway: postanesthesia care unit coordinated care track.

component (i.e., best practices). Sackett and colleagues described five steps essential to EBP[27]:

1. Asking the right clinical question
2. Searching the evidence to answer the question
3. Evaluating the evidence for validity and usefulness
4. Integrating findings with clinical expertise, guidelines, and patient needs and preferences
5. Implementing the change in clinical practices and evaluating performance

Asking the right clinical question requires skills in clearly identifying the problem and its characteristics, the population involved, interventions, competing interventions, and the desired outcomes. Because examination of evidence from **clinical research** is essential to EBP, the health care practitioner requires new skills, including efficient literature searching and the application of formal rules of evidence in evaluating the clinical literature.[26] The literature search involves reviewing a multitude of sources for meta-analyses, randomized clinical trials, guidelines, quasiexperimental studies, case studies, protocols, and care maps. Once identified, each research study must be evaluated for quality of questions, design, sample, measures, researcher, data collection technique, and data analysis.

Two scales for rating the quality of a research study are the American Association of Critical Care Nurses (AACN) scale and the AHRQ scale. The AACN scale has six levels. Level I is the lowest point on the scale and represents an opinion, a manufacturer's claim, or a single case. Level VI is the best evidence based on several clinical studies with a variety of subjects, in numerous settings. The AHRQ scale has five levels with level I being the best and level V being the case study or opinion.

The final step is implementing change in clinical practice. This is the most challenging aspect of EBP, as illustrated by repeated studies showing that treatment and prevention measures used in the United States are not consistent with current knowledge.

A model of the EBP process, developed by Kathleen Stevens at the Academic Center for Evidenced Based Practice, University of Texas Health Science Center San Antonio, even more clearly illustrates the differences between EBP and research.[30] This model, called the ACE Star Model of the Cycle of Knowledge Transformation, identifies five stages through which knowledge must pass as it evolves from being discovered to being incorporated into clinical practice.[28] These stages are discovery, evidence summary, translation, implementation, and evaluation. In the discovery stage, researchers uncover new knowledge by means of a traditional research study. Next, in a step unique to EBP, researchers synthesize findings of individual studies to form an evidence summary statement, which concisely and meaningfully describes the "state of the knowledge" regarding a specific clinical question. Evidence summaries are referred to as **evidence synthesis** by the AHRQ and as systematic reviews by the Cochrane Collaboration.

In the third stage, translation, practitioners translate evaluated, summarized research findings into clinical practice guidelines. In this stage the health care professional integrates research evidence with clinical judgment and knowledge of the specific care setting and patient population served. The clinical practice guidelines resulting from this process can take many different forms, including standards, protocols, care maps, or clinical pathways. Implementation follows, with a wide variety of strategies designed to change individual and organizational behaviors. The final step in the model is evaluation, which addresses the full range of parameters related to quality improvement in health care delivery. These include patient health outcomes, patient satisfaction, efficiency, and economic impact.

A variety of EBP resources are available. Perhaps the most prominent is the Cochrane Library, which has a regularly updated data base of systematic reviews that present information gathered and synthesized from original research studies.[15] These reviews examine the evidence for and against the effectiveness of health care interventions using clinical studies that meet predefined criteria of quality (The Cochrane Library: an Introduction). Cochrane systematic reviews of the literature related to specific clinical topics can be accessed at http://www.cochrane.org. A second major resource is AHRQ, which publishes evidence syntheses developed through its designated EPCs. These can be accessed at http://www.ahrq.gov. Other resources include the National Guideline Clearinghouse and the U.S. Preventive Services Task Force.

Nursing Informatics

Nursing informatics refers to a combination of computer science and **information science** as it relates to nursing practice. Nursing informatics is a specialty area of nursing but one that affects the function of all nurses in all settings. As defined by the ANA in 1994, nursing informatics is concerned with "identifying, collecting, processing, and managing data and information to support nursing practice, administration, education, research, and the expansion of nursing knowledge."[8] Information systems was one of the seven broad priorities identified in the National Nursing Research Agenda developed under the auspices of the National Institute of Nursing Research. Subsequently the Priority Expert Panel on Nursing Informatics developed six specific goals: developing nursing languages, building clinical data bases, designing information systems that would support the provision of patient care, designing patient care decision support systems, developing nurse work stations linked to an integrated information system, and designing methodologies to evaluate the impact of information systems developed on patient care.[23]

The ANA Committee for Nursing Practice Information recognizes 13 standardized languages that meet the criteria developed by ANA. These systems, each of which was designed to document and track nursing care in a specific setting,[14] are listed in Box 1-2. NANDA, NIC, and NOC are used throughout this text and so are briefly described here.

NANDA Taxonomy. A nursing diagnosis is a **clinical judgment** about an individual, family, or community response to actual or potential health problems or life processes that provides the basis for definitive therapy to achieve outcomes for which the nurse is accountable.[24] As stated by the North American Nursing Diagnosis Association International (NANDA International), nursing diagnoses are important to the profession of nursing because they[25]:

- Name client responses to actual or potential health problems, life processes, and wellness
- Document care for reimbursement of nursing services

Box 1-2 Standardized Nursing Languages and Classifications Recognized by American Nurses Association

- North American Nursing Diagnosis Association (NANDA) Taxonomy
- Omaha System
- Home Health Care Classifications (HHCC)
- Nursing Interventions Classification (NIC)
- Nursing Outcomes Classification (NOC)
- Patient Care Data Set (PCDS)
- PeriOperative Nursing Data Set (PNDS)
- Nursing Management Minimum Data Set (NMMDS)
- SNOMED CT
- Nursing Minimum Data Set (NMDS)
- International Classification for Nursing Practice (ICNP)
- ABCodes
- Logical Observation Identifiers Names and Codes (LOINC)

- Contribute to the development of informatics and information standards, ensuring the inclusion of nursing terminology in electronic health care records
- Facilitate study of the phenomena of concern to nurses for the purpose of improving patient care

The first task force to name and classify nursing diagnoses was convened in 1973 after ANA mandated the use of nursing diagnoses. This task force of the National Conference Group on the Classification of Nursing Diagnoses existed until 1982, when NANDA was formed to develop nursing diagnostic terminology. NANDA became NANDA International, which is committed to increasing the visibility of nursing's contribution to patient care by continuing to develop, refine, and classify phenomena of concern to nurses. Taxonomy II, the formal classification of nursing diagnoses developed and currently used by NANDA International, has three levels of specificity: domains, classes, and nursing diagnoses, with the last being the most specific. Thus each of the 172 accepted nursing diagnoses lies within one of the 47 classes, which in turn lie within one of the 13 domains (Figure 1-2). The taxonomy also has seven axes or dimensions of each human response[24]:

1. Diagnostic label, the most fundamental part of the nursing diagnosis
2. Time (acute, chronic, intermittent, continuous)
3. Subject of the diagnosis (individual, family, group, community)
4. Age (fetus to the old-old adult)
5. Health status (wellness, risk or actual)
6. Descriptor (limits or specifies meaning of diagnostic label; includes words such as impaired, increased, inability, effective)
7. Topology (parts or regions of the body or related functions, e.g., cerebral, renal, visual)

The taxonomy structure can be illustrated by considering the diagnostic statement *risk for impaired skin integrity related to skeletal prominence.* The diagnostic label is *skin integrity*; *impaired* refers to the descriptor axis; and *risk for* refers to the health status axis. This nursing diagnosis would be in the domain of Safety/Protection and in the class Physical Injury.

Nursing Interventions Classification. The Nursing Interventions Classification (NIC) was developed at the University of Iowa in the late 1980s. It is a comprehensive, research-based, standardized classification of nursing interventions. These include any intervention a nurse performs to enhance patient outcomes based on clinical judgment. NIC interventions are physiologic and psychosocial; they are performed for acute and chronic illnesses, as well as for health promotion, maintenance, and rehabilitation; and they are used with individuals, families, and communities. NIC is divided into seven domains: Basic Physiological, Complex Physiological, Behavioral, Safety, Family, Health System, and Community. The domains encompass 30 classes of interventions and more than 500 individual interventions. Each intervention has a unique code number to facilitate use in information systems.[17]

NIC has been adopted by information systems and accepted by the National Library of Medicine and the Joint Commission on Accreditation of Healthcare Organizations. Detailed information about NIC is available at http://www.nursing.uiowa.edu/centers/cncce/nic/nicoverview.htm.

Nursing Outcomes Classification. Nursing Outcomes Classification (NOC) is the system for describing patient status after nursing interventions. As with NIC, the standardized outcomes of NOC are used across the health-illness continuum and with all types of clients. NOC has seven domains—Functional Health, Physiological Health, Psychosocial Health, Health Knowledge and Behavior, Perceived Health, Family Health, and Community Health—with 29 outcome classes and 330 classified outcomes. NOC includes 311 individual, 10 family, and 9 community-level outcomes. To allow comparison and evaluation, each outcome is associated with a varying numbers of indicators using up to 17 indicators on a five-point Likert scale.[22]

Data about nursing care and the outcome of care are important to health care professionals, legislators, insurers, providers, and consumers. Knowing the effectiveness of an intervention is essential if we are to compare best practices and cost-effectiveness. Thus the development of a system of classification for nursing outcomes was not as controversial as the development of nursing diagnoses. Detailed information is available at http://www.nursing.uiowa.edu/centers/cncce/noc/nocoverview.htm.

▶ ARE You READY?

Which events influence the practice of medical-surgical nursing in the United States? (Choose all that apply.)

1. Aging and diversified population
2. Increasing need for care related to acute care
3. Decreasing numbers of registered nurses
4. Advances in technology
5. Decline in life expectancy after 85 years of age
6. Care needs related to acquired immunodeficiency syndrome (AIDS)

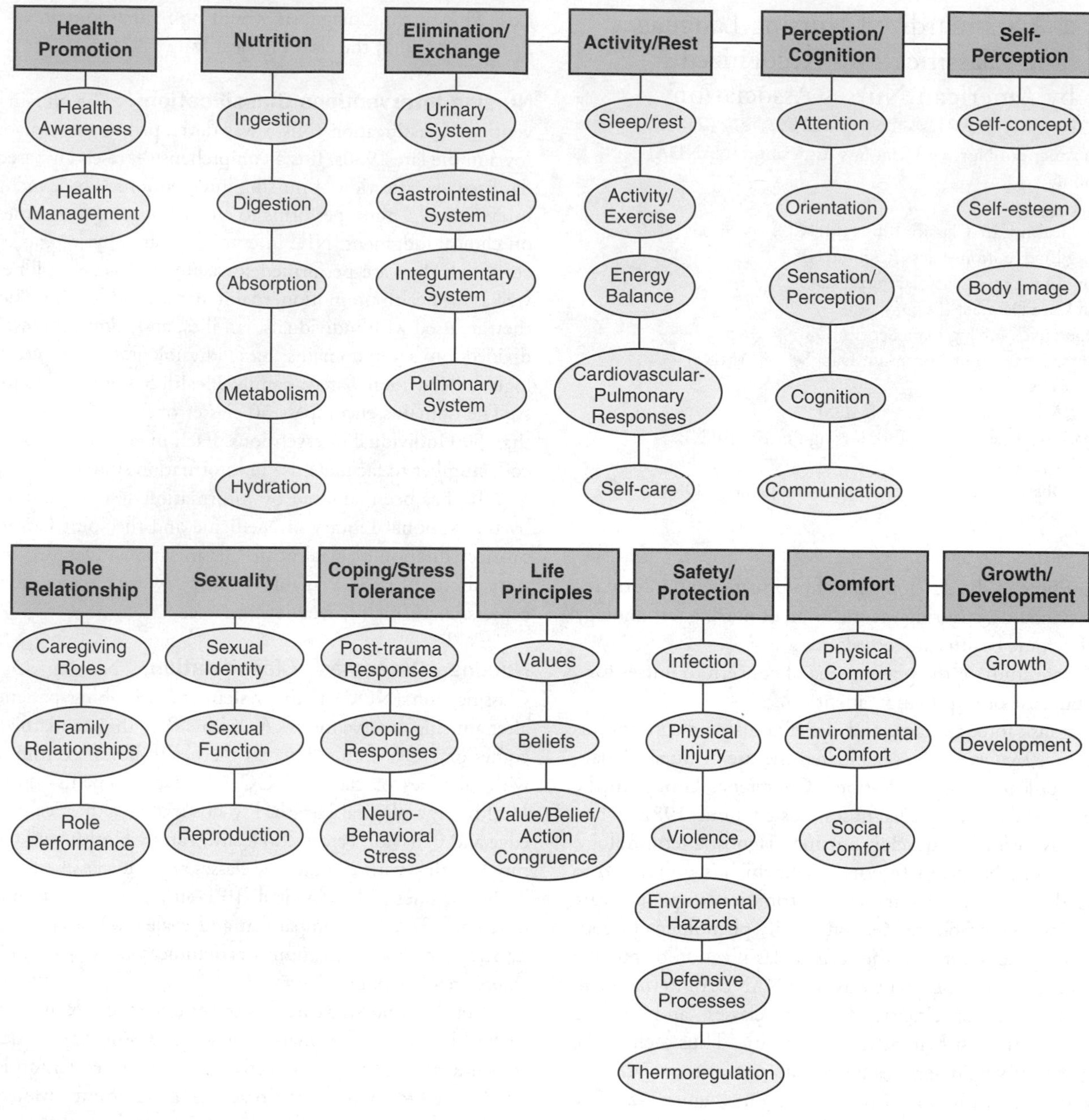

Figure 1-2 Taxonomy II domains and classes.

A new taxonomy called the NANDA, NIC, and NOC (NNN) Taxonomy of Nursing Practice is currently under development. The purpose of this endeavor is to facilitate the linkage of the three systems by creating a visible model of their relationships.[24]

Medical-Surgical Nursing Practice Skills and Abilities

Given current trends, it is clear that the traditional scope of medical-surgical practice has expanded tremendously. It is no longer sufficient to provide excellent episodic acute bedside care. High-quality care now encompasses the full range of practice activities from health promotion, disease prevention, and early detection through acute care management and rehabilitation. Because of the shift into the community setting, it is also essential that the medical-surgical nurse recognize and address the needs of the family and community, in addition to those of the patient.

AMSN has outlined the skills and abilities medical-surgical nurses need. Even beginning nurses must have the leadership and management skills to direct teams and supervise unlicensed personnel effectively. Delegation skills are critical. Nurses must have sufficient working knowledge of the financial and economic aspects of health care to manage resources effectively and articulate resource needs to administration. Nurses must understand and participate in quality assurance and improvement efforts and manage the increasing and often conflicting demands of regulatory agencies. Computer competencies, data management, and outcomes measurement must become the daily language of every nurse. Box 1-3 presents a full list of new nursing skills.

Box 1-3 Expectations for Nurses Working With Adult Populations

Expert nurses caring for adult populations must:

1. Be on the "cutting edge" of practice through continuous professional development
2. Provide high-quality patient care that is sensitive to the physical, psychologic, cultural, and socioeconomic needs of individuals, families, groups, and communities
3. Participate in outcomes measurement and program evaluation to ensure quality care
4. Be politically active regarding issues that affect the health and well-being of the American public
5. Use their knowledge of health economics to influence health resource allocations for the good of the American public
6. Test interventions that support healthier lifestyles for U.S. citizens
7. Demonstrate proficiency at patient care management through coordination of care, referrals, and resource utilization
8. Demonstrate expert communication skills with consumers, patients, families, professional colleagues, and the media

From Academy of Medical-Surgical Nursing: *Project tomorrow*, Pitman, NJ, 2000, The Academy.

Critical Thinking

1. What beliefs about nursing practice can explain the similarities and differences between AMSN and ANCC certification in medical-surgical nursing?
2. Is EBP used in the clinical agencies you are assigned to as a nursing student? Give examples.

References

1. Academy of Medical-Surgical Nursing: *Scope and standards of medical-surgical nursing practice*, ed 3, Pitman, NJ, 2005, The Academy.
2. Academy of Medical-Surgical Nursing: accessed from website: http://www.medsurgnurse.org/.
3. Academy of Medical-Surgical Nursing: *Project tomorrow*, Pitman, NJ, 2000, The Academy.
4. Agency for Healthcare Research and Quality: accessed from website: www.ahcpr.gov/clinic/cpgonline.htm.
5. American Board of Nursing Specialties (ABNS): *A position statement on the value of specialty nursing certification,* 2004, website: www.nursing certification.org.
6. American Nurses Association: *Standards of medical-surgical nursing practice,* Kansas City, Mo, 1980, The Association.
7. American Nurses Association: *Standards of clinical nursing practice,* Washington, DC, 1991, The Association.
8. American Nurses Association: *Scope of practice for nursing informatics,* Washington, DC, 1994, The Association.
9. American Nurses Association: *Standards of clinical nursing practice*, ed 2, Washington, DC, 1998, The Association.
10. American Nurses Credentialing Center: *Certification and recertification,* accessed from website: www.nursing world.org/ancc/certification/index.
11. American Nurses Association: *Recognition of a specialty, approval of scope statements and acknowledgement of nursing practice standards,* Washington, DC, 2002, ANA.
12. Buerhaus PI, Staiger DO: Trouble in the nurse labor market? Recent trends and future outlook, *Health Affairs* 18(1):214-222, 1999.
13. Buerhaus PI, Staiger DO, Auerbach D: Implications of an aging registered nurse workforce, *JAMA* 283(22):2948-2954, 2000.
14. Cherry B, Jacob SR: *Contemporary nursing: issues, trends and management,* St Louis, 2005, Mosby.
15. Cochrane Collaboration website: www.cochrane.org.
16. Courtney M: *Evidence for nursing practice*, London, 2005, Churchill Livingstone.
17. Dochterman JC, Bulechek GM, editors: *Nursing intervention classifications (NIC)*, ed 4, St Louis, 2004, Mosby.
18. Grindel CG: Medical/surgical nursing celebration of the specialty, *Nurs Spectrum,* Sept 2004, accessed from website: http://community.nursing spectrum.com.
19. Grindel C: Medical-surgical nursing: a specialty or not? *MEDSURG Nurs* 14(1):5-6, 2005.
20. Institute of Medicine: *Crossing the quality chasm: a new health system for the 21st century*, Washington, DC, 2001, National Academy Press Publisher.
21. Institute of Medicine: *Health professions education: a bridge to quality,* Washington, DC, 2003, National Academy Press Publisher.
22. Moorhead S, Johnson M, Maas M, editors: *Nursing outcomes classifications (NOC)*, ed 3, St Louis, 2004, Mosby.
23. National Institute of Nursing Research: *Nursing informatics: enhancing patient care*, Bethesda, Md, 1993, The Institute. Priority Expert Panel Report, Nursing informatics: enhancing patient care, vol 4, NIH Publication No 93-2419, website: http//ninr.nih,gov/ninr/news_info/publications.html.
24. North American Nursing Diagnosis Association International: *NANDA Nursing Diagnoses: definitions and classification, 2005-2006,* Philadelphia, 2005, The Association.
25. North American Nursing Diagnosis Association International: accessed from website: www.nanda.org.
26. Sackett DL, Rosenberg WC: Evidence-based medicine: what it is and what it isn't, *BMJ* 312:71-72, 1996.
27. Sackett DL et al: *Evidence based medicine: how to practice and teach EBM*, ed 2, London, 2000, Churchill-Livingstone.
28. Stevens KR: *ACE star model of the cycle of knowledge transformation*, July 2002.
29. Stevens KR: *Evidenced-based practice and nursing education: new competencies, new content,* preconference workshop, National League for Nursing Education Summit, Sept 18, 2003.
30. Stevens K: *Evidenced based practice workshop*, presented at SUNY Rockland Community College, March 2004.
31. Yoder-Wise PS: State and association/certifying boards: CE requirements, *J Cont Ed Nurs* 34(1):5–13, 2003.

Visit the Evolve website: http://evolve.elsevier.com/Monahan/medsurg

CHAPTER 2

The Aging Population

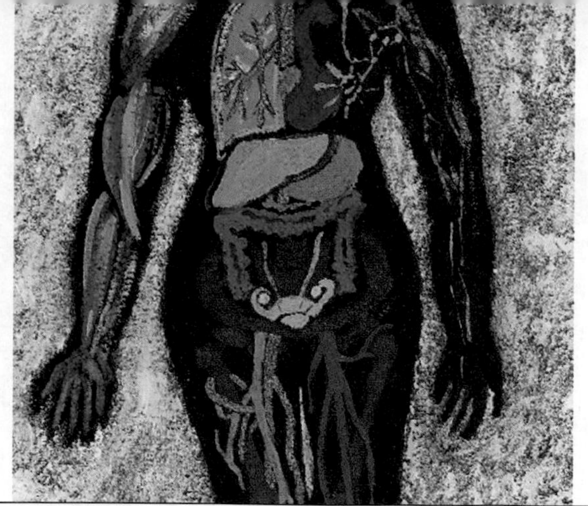

by Jackie L. Murphree, Marianne Neighbors

OBJECTIVES

After studying this chapter, the learner should be able to:

1. Describe the historical perspectives and present trends in the aging population.
2. Discuss the focus of assessment in older patients.
3. Distinguish between primary and secondary changes of aging.
4. Describe unique patterns of illness in older adults.
5. Explain domains of functional assessment to be addressed in all older patients.

KEY TERMS

activities of daily living, p. 14
Alzheimer's disease, p. 23
amyloid plaques, p. 24
cognitive function, p. 18
functional health, p. 11
geriatrics, p. 10
gerontology, p. 10
instrumental activities of daily living, p. 14
neurofibrillary tangles, p. 24
older adults, p. 11
polypharmacy, p. 21
primary changes, p. 12
secondary changes, p. 12

Historical Perspectives

Human beings have one of the longest life spans of any animal species, with the potential to live 125 years. For centuries mystery and myth have surrounded the phenomenon of aging. Aristotle believed later life to be a period of disengagement, whereas Plato described the development of wisdom in old age. As a society, the ancient Greeks believed that life force heat was gradually used up in the normal process of aging. They observed then, as has been confirmed today, that older people are subject to a host of health problems, including dyspnea, joint pains, dizzy spells, insomnia, and visual and hearing losses.

The teachings of Sir Francis Bacon (1561 to 1626) marked the beginning of the scientific approach to aging. Bacon believed that the effects of aging accounted for the physical decline of joints and vision. According to Bacon, factors slowing or accelerating the effects of aging included physical stature, temperament, environment, diet, and heredity. These factors remain important correlates for health today. Metchnikoff (1845 to 1916) regarded aging as a natural physiologic process beginning at the moment of conception, and Nasher (1863 to 1944) argued that age-related diseases were distinct from aging as a normal process.

Today we continue to emphasize the distinction between normal aging changes and secondary aging changes (diseases). In 1909 Nasher used the word **geriatrics** to refer to diseases of old age. In 1927 Rybrikov, a Russian psychologist, referred to the aging process as the study of **gerontology**. Over time, five basic patterns characteristic of aging have emerged:

1. Increased mortality
2. Changes in the body's chemical composition, including a decrease in lean body mass, an increase in fats and lipofuscins, and cross-linking of collagen tissues
3. Progressive deteriorative changes
4. Reduced ability to adapt to environmental changes
5. Increased vulnerability to multiple diseases

Nurses have cared for older adults and their family members throughout history. In 1904 the *American Journal of Nursing* published an article on old age and disease. The American Nurses Association (ANA), guided by an understanding of normal aging and the unique needs of older adults, and by a commitment to scientific care, established a division of geriatric nursing in 1966 to develop standards of nursing care for older adults. In 1995 the ANA revised the 1981 standards of care to guide generalist and advanced practice nurses caring for older adults. These standards, which apply to all settings, serve as a model for practice and for evaluation of care. Care focuses on determining the strengths of older adults and then promoting their use to maximize independence.[10] The ANA has identified seven basic considerations in providing gerontologic nursing care (Box 2-1). Three groups

Box 2-1 Factors Specific to Gerontologic Nursing

Nurses caring for older adults should consider the following important concepts related to gerontologic nursing:
- The ramifications of the aging process
- The differing rates at which people age
- The cumulative effect of the aging person's losses
- The interrelationship between social, economic, psychologic, and biologic factors
- The frequently atypical response of the elderly to disease and its treatment
- The accumulated disabling effects of multiple chronic illnesses or degenerative processes
- The cultural values and social attitudes associated with aging

Adapted from American Nurses Association: *Scope and standards of gerontological nursing practice,* Washington, DC, 1995, The Association.

constitute those collectively referred to as **older adults**: the young-old (ages 64 to 74 years), the middle-old (ages 75 to 84 years), and the old-old (ages 85 and older).

Demographic Trends

America as a nation is aging. In colonial times, half the population was younger than 16 years old. In 1900 life expectancy at birth was 49 years. From 1980 to 1990, a period described as "the graying of America," the American population of adults 85 years and older increased by 38%, whereas the numbers of persons ages 65 to 84 years increased by only 20% and those younger than 65 years old increased by only 8%.[1]

By 1990 the so-called Baby Boomers constituted one third of the population of the United States, and the number of older adults reached 30 million. Some have predicted that the number of older adults will reach 39 million by 2010 and 71.5 million by 2030. This age-group, which composed only 4% of the population in 1900, will increase 20% by the year 2030, with the largest growth occurring among ethnic minorities and those older than 85 years. The number of Hispanic-American older adults will increase by 342%, African-Americans by 164%, Asian/Pacific Islanders by 302%, American Indians/Eskimos/Aleuts by 207%, and Caucasian Americans by only 77%.[1] Four- and five-generational families are becoming common as more and more American live into their hundreds (Figure 2-1).[1]

Other dramatic demographic trends include lower rates of life expectancy for non-Caucasian persons compared with Caucasian persons, and the higher number of older women than men. In 1991 life expectancy was 72.5 years for African-American women and 79.3 years for Caucasian women. In 1986 African-American men had a life expectancy of 66 years compared with 72.6 years for Caucasian men. Although the number of both men and women over 65 will increase over the next decade, the population of women older than age 65 outnumbers that of men by about 6.1 million. The majority of noninstitutionalized older adults live with families; however, this trend is reversed for those 85 years of age and older. About 50% of persons 65 and older live in suburbs, 27% live in central cities, and 23% live in nonmetropolitan areas.[1]

The demographic trends have had a significant impact on families, the labor force, and the health care system. More older adults are living longer with chronic illnesses and functional disability and surviving catastrophic acute illnesses. Their health care needs will continue to increase. Those caring for this aging population will need increased knowledge and skills to help this group maintain health and function and avoid complications—all of which will affect the quality and cost of care for older adults.

Improving the quality of life, rather than searching for means to increase longevity, is of utmost importance (Figure 2-2). According to *Healthy People 2010,* the major goal is to increase the quality and length of healthy life for all Americans.[55] For older Americans in particular, the focus is on maintaining **functional health**, preventing disability, and reducing disparities in care and treatment.

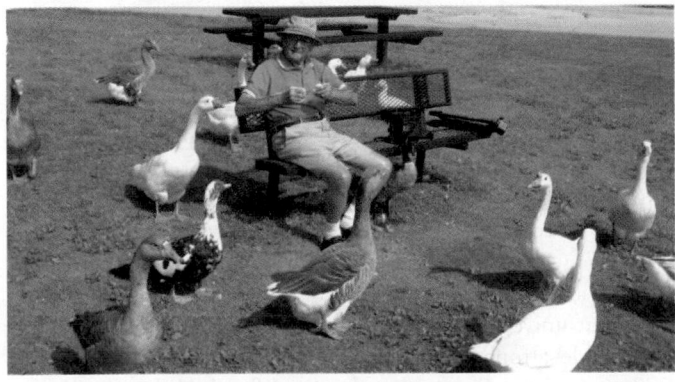

Figure 2-1 This gentleman is part of the fastest growing segment of the American population: adults over age 85.

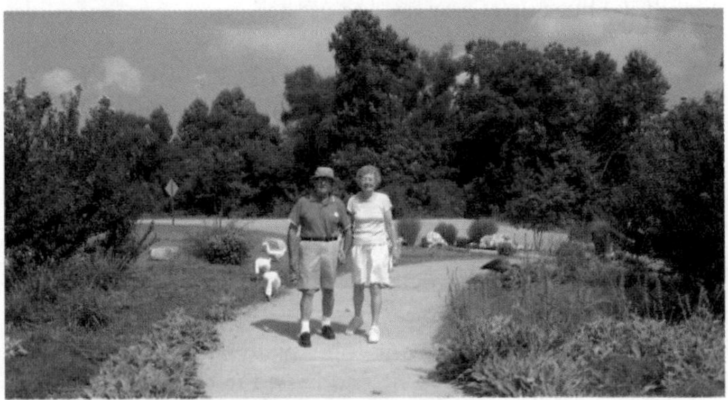

Figure 2-2 Older adults can live a happy, healthy life. Exercise is an important part of their healthy daily routine.

Significance for Nursing

The U.S. Public Health Service report *Healthy People 2010* is a guide for health professionals and consumers.[55] The document provides guidelines for nurses as they provide daily care to patients. This report will continue to provide direction for national health policies and future health care priorities and reimbursement. The publication provides a common ground for collaboration with other health care professionals and health service agencies.

The strength of *Healthy People 2010* is that it focuses on increasing the quality and years of healthy life. Thus health promotion and disease prevention strategies, traditionally emphasized in nursing practice, are incorporated into interventions to achieve health objectives. The second goal to reduce disparities in care and treatment is particularly important for aging cohorts that have increasing numbers of ethnic minorities. Many minority older adults have experienced a lack of access to health services and differential treatment by providers over their lifetimes.

Nurses can use this document to support the care and education of patients in all settings, no matter what disease process they are treating. The report also provides information about the health promotion and disease prevention needs of specific groups according to characteristics such as age, race and ethnicity, and economic status.

Assessment of Older Adults

General Issues

Skillful, knowledge-based assessment is the foundation for providing high-quality nursing care to older adults. In gerontologic care the assessment focuses on the older adult's level of function. A basic premise is that function is multidimensional and includes physical, mental, and social function. An older adult's functional health is also influenced by spiritual well-being.

People experience many commonalities in the way they age. Health concerns for aging persons are multidimensional, requiring critical evaluation of what is normative and what is the result of disease. In addition, illnesses in older adults can manifest themselves differently than in younger persons. In ethnic minority groups, secondary aging changes and chronic illnesses may appear in the late middle years, resulting in earlier functional decline and disability. Thus nurses may need to use geriatric assessment guidelines with some middle-aged adults.

Older adults who are hospitalized are at increased risk for institutionalization. Often such institutionalization results from an inability to carry out activities of daily living (ADLs) and instrumental activities of daily living (IADLs). Thus time spent on a thorough baseline assessment of an older adult's health status, with emphasis on functional abilities and periodic follow-up assessment, can potentially prevent disability and additional health care costs.

In the 1990s geriatric research focused on failure to thrive in older adults, a phenomenon first addressed in children. Failure to thrive in older persons leads to catastrophic disability and preventable deaths. In hospitalized older adults this syndrome may be seen on admission or noted for the first time during hospitalization. Failure to thrive in older adults may be multifaceted and result from factors other than disease processes, such as poor nutrition, medications, alcohol use, social isolation, losses, and depression. Nurses in acute and long-term care settings, therefore, assess for and prevent failure to thrive in older adults.[14,48]

Institutionalization and failure to thrive are extreme examples of negative health outcomes for hospitalized older adults. However, any loss of functional abilities can dramatically affect the older adults' quality of life and well-being. A holistic nursing assessment is the foundation for the care of each older patient and collaboration with other health care providers. Geriatric assessment focuses on function, with the goal of enhancing or maintaining function while preventing loss of function and subsequent disability. Health care providers should help persons maintain functional health and remain active for as long as possible. Thus gerontologic care in the new millennium emphasizes decreasing the disability curve for aging persons. Nurses play a key role in meeting this challenge through health assessment that directs primary, secondary, and tertiary intervention. Older adults and their family members are at the center of this endeavor.

The following sections present critical areas of nursing assessment when caring for older adults, no matter what the clinical setting or the acute and chronic diseases being treated. Topics include primary and secondary aging changes, differences in illness presentation, ADLs and IADLs, falls, spirituality, sexuality, family, nutrition, cognition and sensory perception, depression and suicide, alcohol and medication use, and sleep. Although the concepts are presented separately, the interaction of factors in the physical, mental, social, and spiritual domains often affects an older adult's functional health status. For example, if one has decreased physical function, one can become depressed; if one is depressed, physical function declines.

► ARE You READY?

Which of the following assessments is the priority in the older adult?

1. Sources of income
2. Family history
3. Functional ability
4. Suppport system

Primary and Secondary Aging

Critical to any approach to an integrated, functional assessment of older adults is understanding and differentiating between primary (normative) aging changes and secondary (disease related) changes. Normal aging changes are called **primary changes** (Table 2-1). Research has demonstrated that such effects of aging—for example, thinning hair and decreased pulmonary capacity—occur universally. Increasing knowledge confirms that many changes once thought to be associated with aging, such as arthritis and dementia, are actually **secondary changes** and do not occur universally as part of aging. Also, research shows that the muscle atrophy and weakened joints seen in many older adults are related more to a sedentary lifestyle than to a primary change of aging.

either or both spouses having children from previous marriages; the result is called a *blended family.*[18]

Families of older adults also reflect this diversity in family structure. Family, however defined, provides intimacy, affection, and instrumental support to older adults (Figure 2-3). Older adults may also be part of multigenerational families and households. Sometimes four or five generations live together and share resources and family tasks. For some older adults, family intimacy and support take place in groups that are unrelated (by blood) and may or may not live in the same household.

Assessment of the older adult's family as a means of social support, particularly in terms of functional health and well-being, is essential.[39] Questions include whom older adults get help from when they need it for specific activities; in whom they confide; whether the support is adequate; and, most important, whom they could really count on if they needed something. Many instruments that measure what support is needed are lengthy, but a short form is available. The Caregiver Well-Being Scale developed by Tebb includes 45 questions about caregivers' satisfaction with basic human needs and ADLs.[51] The nurse also needs to assess the older patient's role in providing support to the family. Many older adults, particularly women, are family caregivers.

Society has moved beyond the simpler caregiving model of the sandwich-generation woman who is caring for children and aging parents. Today a woman who is 70 years old and admitted for knee replacement could be caring for a 90-year-old mother, a husband, and a grandchild. A 66-year-old man could be caring for a 44-year-old mentally disabled daughter. The literature abounds with evidence of the physical, psychologic, and financial stress caregivers experience. Of particular concern are the negative health sequelae of caregiving, particularly depression.[13,20,53] Caregivers may ignore their own health and symptoms because of the demands of caregiving. Also, many caregivers experience changes in dietary habits and sleep, use psychotropic medications, and are unable to carry out their normal self-care activities. Several research instruments are available to assess caregiver stress, burden, and reward. The nurse needs to determine whether older patients are caregivers, to whom they are providing care, whether they have assistance with their caregiving, and whether they have special concerns while they are in the hospital. After identifying concerns, the nurse can refer the older adult to a clinical nurse specialist or social worker for further evaluation and monitoring.

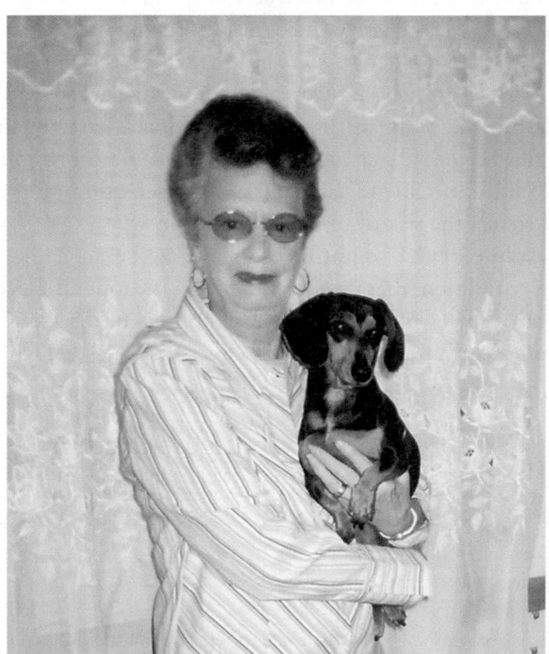

Figure 2-3 Pets are a part of the family and are particularly beneficial to older adults. They provide companionship, comfort, and caring.

Finally, an essential component of family assessment is screening for family violence. Older adults are not exempt from being victims or perpetrators.[12,35,42] For some older persons, family violence is an established pattern.[9] Older adults being cared for by a family caregiver may be at increased risk because of the stress of caregiving. The risk for violence by a family caregiver is greater when the care recipient's function declines and formal and informal support for the caregiver is lacking. Thus nurses who care for older adults need to determine if older patients are being exposed to violence and neglect in the home. The nurse needs to be aware that some states have mandatory reporting of elder abuse and neglect.

Nutrition

Nutritional requirements of older adults are essentially the same as for other adults, except that calorie needs diminish because of a decrease in lean body mass relative to fat (which burns fewer calories).[17,22] Fiber (e.g., fruits, vegetables, whole-grain bread, and cereals), although indigestible, is an important constituent in the diet. Fiber holds water in the fecal mass, which softens the stools and enhances regular evacuation. Some evidence shows that the incidence of diverticulitis, colon cancer, or gallstones is influenced by diets chronically low in fiber. Persons at or near age 65 may still have a life expectancy of 15 years or more during which dietary fiber deficiencies might play a role in development of these disorders. Because these disorders and constipation are common in older adults, moderate amounts of fiber are regularly included in the diet.

Water is vital for function and temperature regulation. A number of situations may predispose older adults to a deficiency in body water. Approximately 50% of the body's water supply is obtained from solid foods; therefore a reduction in calorie intake may mean that water intake is inadequate. Some older adults, especially those who are chronically ill, may have a defective thirst sensation mechanism, resulting in a diminished awareness of the body's signal to increase fluid intake. Finally, the older person may lose water from common conditions such as diarrhea, excessive perspiration, or polyuria or from the use of diuretics. In the event of a water deficit, older people should be encouraged to consume more fluids, particularly water (a minimum of 1500 to 2000 ml/day unless contraindicated by conditions such as congestive heart failure).

Many older adults, especially those who are ill, are malnourished. A state of malnutrition can have a significant detrimental affect on an older adult's quality of life.[57] Diets often are deficient in calcium, vitamins A and C, iron, and zinc, and a vitamin-mineral supplement may be indicated. Other than acute and chronic illnesses, possible causes of malnutrition are changes in taste, vision, smell, or dentition; limited financial resources; physical factors such as chewing and swallowing problems and gum disease; psychologic factors such as boredom and lack of companionship when eating; edentia; lifelong faulty eating patterns; fads and misconceptions regarding certain foods; lack of energy to prepare food; inability to feed oneself; and lack of sufficient knowledge of the essentials of a well-balanced diet. Living arrangements may also affect dietary patterns; a study found that older men who live alone have less adequate diets than older women living alone.[57]

Older persons often enter the hospital in a poorly nourished state because of chronic illness or other factors previously described. Trauma, surgery, or sepsis may increase nutritional demands and cause further nutritional deficiencies, particularly in protein and calories. Often, a poor state of nutrition on admission, increased nutritional needs, and decreased appetite coexist in hospitalized older adults. A nutritional assessment, including a record of food intake over several days and weight on admission with regular weight checks thereafter, should be a priority in nursing to detect deficiencies early.

Nutritional status is as important as any other nursing assessment. This is particularly true for older adults in acute care. Poor nutrition can lead to functional losses, and functional losses can lead to poor nutrition. For example, in a study of older nuns a 3% weight loss over 1 year increased the risk of an individual becoming dependent in ADLs.[54] Other researchers have reported that protein-energy undernourishment in older middle-aged patients (55 to 64 years) and older patients is a strong risk factor for mortality 1 year after discharge from a hospital.[48] The Mini Nutritional Assessment (MNA) is a screening instrument that can be used with older adults in acute care settings. The tool is a page in length and can be answered quickly. It has been widely used since its development in the late 1990s.[29] Some of the areas included in the MNA are dietary habits; medication use; and functional items such as ADLs, dental health, and depression. A simple method to monitor nutritional status used in long-term care is monthly weighing of all older adults. The entry nutrition assessment often consists of just a few questions to determine the patient's nutritional patterns (Box 2-3).

Box 2-3 Nutrition Assessment

The nurse should assess the following items related to the patient's nutritional status:

- Height, weight, and body-mass index
- Weight gain or loss in the past year
- General appearance related to nutrition (e.g., hair texture, skin turgor)
- Known nutritional problems
- Regular eating pattern: times, amount, snacks
- Water or fluid consumption and type
- Approximate daily protein, carbohydrate, fat, and calorie consumption
- Ability to self-feed; need for assistance
- Medications interfering with or supporting nutritional needs
- Food preferences and dietary restrictions

Cognition and Sensory Perception

Older adults differ from their younger counterparts in several aspects of cognitive and perceptual function. Changes occur in the central nervous system, but the function of the peripheral motor neurons and the autonomic nervous system remains relatively constant throughout the life span.

Cognitive Function. Cross-sectional studies have shown that the highest overall intelligence test performance occurs some time between the late teens and late twenties. People in their thirties, forties, and fifties tend to score somewhat lower. However, longitudinal evidence has shown that general intelligence either remains the same or increases slightly during the adult years. Certain factors such as education and other sociocultural advantages may influence intellectual development and performance.

The measure of one's intelligence is more than a score on a standardized examination. Intelligence can include a person's capacity for creativity and understanding of how systems work. Older adults do not lose the capacity for creativity as they age. Some, for the first time, have the time to pursue artistic talents that they had not fully developed because of work and family obligations. Active use of mental capacity throughout life contributes to mental productivity in old age.

Aging changes listed in Box 2-4 affect complex processes such as learning, memory, language, and mentation. Although loss of memory is not considered a primary aging change, many older persons have progressive problems with short-term memory. Older persons may need more time to take in information and can experience problems with retrieval of stored information (memory). Although persons of advancing age perform less well on neuropsychologic tests, this performance is not necessarily associated with impaired function. Therefore any change in **cognitive function** in the older adult must be taken seriously, and the etiology of the change explored. A change in cognitive function is often the first indication that an older person's health status has changed. Older adults with cognitive changes may be misdiagnosed with irreversible organic brain disease (e.g., Alzheimer's disease). At this point, the individual may not be able to make decisions about the care needed or be able to assist in self-care (see Ethical Alert box). This increases the risk of institutionalization.

The cause of the cognitive changes may be an undiagnosed medical condition that is reversible with treatment. Reversible cognitive changes may actually be symptoms of disease, depression, and delirium owing to toxic effects of drugs, dehydration,

Box 2-4 Aging Changes Affecting Cognition and Perception

- Decreased brain weight
- Diminished enzyme activity
- Slowed reflexes
- Decreased sensory receptors for temperature, pain, and tactile discrimination
- Weakening of interneuron connections
- Increased response time
- Chronic hypoxia

Ethical Alert

Decision Making

One of the most common legal and ethical issues involving older adults is related to decision making. If older adults can make their own decisions about treatment and care, end-of-life issues, and living arrangements, there is not a problem. But when they can no longer do this, issues evolve around the decision-making capacity, competence, and identification of decision makers for the individual. Older adults, especially the very old, often lack family or close friends to be their advocates. If advance directives are not in place, they may be at the mercy of decisions made by health care providers, which may or may not be in the best interest of the older adults.

fecal impaction, infection, or overstimulation. Changes in cognitive function should trigger aggressive global assessment of the older adult's health status starting with evaluation of the presence of disease or adverse drug effects.

The nurse's focus of assessment is the level of cognitive function in older patients. First the nurse performs cognitive screening. If impairment is present, then the nurse talks to family members to obtain information about the person's level of function before hospitalization. For those who have impaired function on admission, cognitive screening should continue throughout the hospital stay. A variety of cognitive screening instruments is available. The two most commonly used are the Short Portable Mental Status Questionnaire (SPMSQ), which is quick and easy to administer; and the Mini-Mental State Examination (MMSE), which includes questions that require some level of reading and writing literacy and motor function. The SPMSQ and MMSE should be used as screening tools only. If a patient's score indicates cognitive impairment, the nurse should refer the person for further evaluation.

During hospitalization, the nurse needs to assess the older patient's cognitive function on an ongoing basis. This is necessary because older patients are at risk for developing acute confusional states (Box 2-5) and may be at risk for decreased function.

Sensory-Perceptual Function. Pain, temperature, taste, and touch are all dulled to some extent as one ages. Hearing and vision also become less acute, and the older adult experiences presbyopia and presbycusis. Long-distance vision, night vision, and tolerance for glare decrease; and the older person has more difficulty hearing high tones and discriminating speech in noisy situations. These changes in hearing and vision[13] are of particular concern since they affect the older person's ability to communicate with significant others and the outside world. Older adults' ability to receive information can become compromised. For example, what appears to be recent memory loss may actually be the result of being unable to process written or spoken information. Hearing impairment can result in social isolation and depression in the older adult. In persons 70 years of age and older, 33% report hearing problems, 19% report visual impairments, and others report that they have both hearing and vision impairment.[19]

Assessment of hearing and vision should begin by asking the patients to describe (1) what problems they may be having, (2) when they were first aware of the problems, (3) whether recent changes have occurred, and (4) what they are doing to accommodate losses, including use of assistive devices. Ebersole, Hess, and Luggen describe basic, clinical observations of the older patient's behavior to assess hearing.[22] These behaviors include speaking quality and loudness, turning head toward speaker, asking that things be repeated, not being able to follow clear directions, not responding to environmental sounds, and thinking that people are talking about him or her. The nurse should also assess the patient for inappropriate anger or irritation when spoken to by staff. In addition, anytime an older adult (or the family) complains of hearing difficulties, the nurse should visually inspect the inner ear to assess for cerumen impaction. The nurse can easily assess vision using a pocket-sized Snellen chart.

Box 2-5 Some Causes of Confusion in Older Adults

- Alcohol use
- Blood glucose imbalance
- Dementia
- Electrolyte imbalance
- Elevated temperature
- Medications
- Nutritional imbalance
- Poor oxygenation

Depression and Suicide

Depression remains the major mental health problem in older adults and can lead to disability and premature death.[2,43] However, this treatable disorder goes largely unrecognized, undiagnosed, or misdiagnosed; therefore it remains untreated. Acute and primary health care providers are in the best position to assess the presence of depression in older patients.[21,26] Late-life depression may be a geriatric syndrome with multiple causes that requires interdisciplinary, multidimensional geriatric assessment. Depression in older adults results in decreased functional health in multiple domains and can lead to suicide.[44]

Evidence shows that people become more suicidal as they age, with Caucasian men ages 65 and older committing suicide at a rate six times higher than that of the general population. The highest suicide rate, among Caucasian men 85 and older, is more than five times the national U.S. rate per 100,000.[43,44] It is important for nurses to know that 75% of older adults who commit suicide have visited a primary care physician in the month before the suicide.[44] Suicidal behaviors may be aggressive and highly lethal or more covert such as refusal to eat or take necessary medication. Some older men who commit suicide commit homicide first by killing their spouses. Even if the older adult is not clinically depressed, he or she may be experiencing a level of depressive symptoms that result in functional impairment and poor health. The good news is that depression is treatable in older adults, and timely appropriate care can prevent suicidal behaviors.

Depression in older adults differs from that in younger persons. Older persons may find it less acceptable to acknowledge depression. The nurse can easily screen for depression using the

Box 2-6 Geriatric Depression Scale (Short Form)

Choose the best answer for how you felt over the past week.

The following count as one point. Scores >5 indicate probable depression.

Question			Scoring
1. Are you basically satisfied with your life?	Yes	No	1. No
2. Have you dropped many of your activities and interests?	Yes	No	2. Yes
3. Do you feel that your life is empty?	Yes	No	3. Yes
4. Do you often get bored?	Yes	No	4. Yes
5. Are you in good spirits most of the time?	Yes	No	5. No
6. Are you afraid that something bad is going to happen to you?	Yes	No	6. Yes
7. Do you feel happy most of the time?	Yes	No	7. No
8. Do you often feel helpless?	Yes	No	8. Yes
9. Do you prefer to stay at home, rather than going out and doing new things?	Yes	No	9. Yes
10. Do you feel you have more problems with memory than most?	Yes	No	10. Yes
11. Do you think it is wonderful to be alive now?	Yes	No	11. No
12. Do you feel pretty worthless the way you are now?	Yes	No	12. Yes
13. Do you feel full of energy?	Yes	No	13. No
14. Do you feel that your situation is hopeless?	Yes	No	14. Yes
15. Do you think that most people are better off than you are?	Yes	No	15. Yes

Center of Epidemiologic Studies Depression Scale (CES-D) or Geriatric Depression Scale (GDS) (Box 2-6). These instruments can be included in the nursing assessment form or used in addition to it. The questions can be asked of the older patient or read by the older patient and easily scored by the nurse. The CES-D and GDS measure the presence of depressive symptoms but are not used for differential diagnosis of major depression. The nurse can also ask standard questions for suicide assessment. If the nurse observes depressive symptoms and suicidal ideas or behaviors, he or she should refer the older person for a more complete psychiatric evaluation.

Alcohol and Medication Use and Misuse

Assessment of alcohol, medication, and drug use and abuse is an essential component of geriatric assessment. Although data about illicit drug use in older adults are minimal and the types and amount of actual use are uncertain, assessment of illicit drug use is important and may become more so, given younger cohorts' patterns of multiple substance use. Such assessments are important for many reasons. First, alcohol, medication, or drug misuse, abuse, or addiction can result in a variety of functional deficits and have negative effects on body systems. Second, even nonproblematic use of alcohol in young and middle adulthood may result in functional losses and organ damage because of normal aging changes. Third, alcohol and medications can have a variety of interactive effects that are detrimental and even life threatening. Finally, clinicians frequently mistake the clinical presentation of substance interaction, misuse, and abuse for irreversible dementia.[50]

Alcohol and the Older Adult. The true extent of alcoholism in older adults is not known. It is difficult to get physicians to accept that elderly alcoholism exists; therefore it goes unreported, undiagnosed, and ignored.[8,33] The Substance Abuse and Mental Health Services Administration reports that the need for alcohol and drug abuse treatment will triple by 2020 as Baby Boomers carry their alcohol and drug abuse into older adulthood.[22]

Researchers have identified two patterns of alcoholism in older adults. Some older alcoholics began drinking at an early age and have survived into their elder years. Other older adults are late-onset drinkers who began abusing alcohol in their later years. The abuse often begins in the fifth decade, but alcoholism and related health problems may not be detected until the sixth decade. The abuse of alcohol can occur at any time during the aging process and may actually be a symptom of other functional health problems such as depression and social isolation or may be a self-care behavior to manage insomnia or pain.

Because of the social stigma and cultural values related to alcohol use, nurses must be aware of their personal beliefs about alcohol and experiences with those who use or abuse it. An additional area to address is the professional's attitudes toward older adults

Research

Masters J: Moderate alcohol consumption and unappreciated risk for alcohol-related harm among ethnically diverse, urban-dwelling elders, *Geriatr Nurs* 24(3):155-161, 2003.

One hundred and seven older adults over age 60 from diverse ethnic backgrounds completed a survey to determine how they defined moderate alcohol consumption and interpreted the health benefits of moderate alcohol consumption. The findings concluded that 40% of the subjects had defined moderate alcohol conception as being higher than the federal guidelines. A smaller group of adults believed that alcohol consumption was good for health regardless of age or physical condition. The implication for nurses is to be aware of this interpretation to avoid overlooking alcohol misuse and abuse among the older population.

Box 2-7 The CAGE Assessment: Four Questions About Drinking

C Have you ever felt you should **C**ut down on your drinking?

A Have people **A**nnoyed you by criticizing your drinking?

G Have you ever felt bad or **G**uilty about your drinking?

E Have you ever taken a drink first thing in the morning (**E**ye opener) to steady your nerves or get rid of a hangover?

Positive answers to two or more questions suggest that you may have a problem with drinking.

One or more positive responses from an older person are significant and deserve follow-up.

who drink, including differences in attitudes related to the older person's gender. The professional's beliefs, values, and attitudes can be barriers to accurate assessment. Nurses also need to recognize that older adults may present barriers to assessment because of their own beliefs and attitudes about alcohol abuse (see Research box above).[37] Screening instruments such as the CAGE Assessment (Box 2-7) and the Elderly Alcohol Screening Test (Box 2-8) are easily integrated into multidimensional geriatric assessments.[25] One does not have to be an expert in substance abuse to effectively use alcohol-screening instruments. The role of the clinical nurse is to assess an older adult's pattern of alcohol use and screen for abuse so that appropriate referral and management can be implemented. Screening can identify the potential for problems with drug and alcohol interactions and identify those at risk for symptoms of alcohol withdrawal.

Medication and the Older Adult. The use of both prescribed and nonprescribed medications increases with age. Older Americans make up 13% of the population, but they consume an average of 30% of all prescription drugs.[40] Older adults consume disproportionately more of all kinds of drugs than do middle-aged adults, partly because they experience more chronic illness. **Polypharmacy** is the concurrent use of a large number of drugs, which can result in interactions and even dangerous adverse reactions. Medications provide tremendous benefits to older adults, but they also can create problems for the patient, family, and health care provider (Figure 2-4). The medication

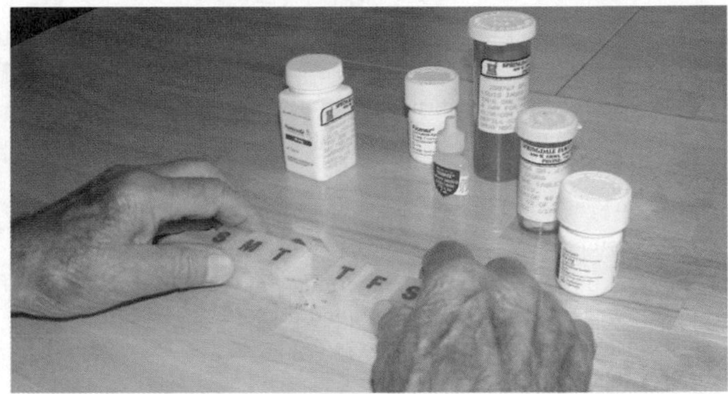

Figure 2-4 Most older adults take a variety of medications daily. Polypharmacy can be a problem if medications are not carefully monitored.

regimen may be complex and troublesome for the patient or family to administer, and as a result drug misuse can easily occur (see Research box below). Misuse is defined as overmedication, undermedication, inappropriate prescription by the professional, or errors in amount and administration.[40] Some misuse can result in drug dependency. Medications may be difficult to tolerate, cause unpleasant side effects, and interact negatively with foods. Other medications may cause adverse reactions and interactions or unpredictable responses in older adults. Misuse, dependency, and drug interactions often result in loss of physical, mental, and social function.[45]

DRUG ABSORPTION. Numerous age-related physical changes in older adults affect their response to medications. Drug absorption may be influenced by the presence or absence of nutrients or by the decrease of hydrochloric acid that normally occurs with aging; drugs that depend on an acid medium may be absorbed less efficiently. Absorption also may be altered because the rate of transit through the gastrointestinal system tends to slow with age.

Research

Spiers MV, Kutzik DM, Lamar M: Variation in medication understanding among the elderly, *Am J Health System Pharmacy* 61(4):373, 2004.

This study investigated misunderstandings elderly people in the community held about their medications. Researchers interviewed participants (375 over age 65) about their attitudes related to their medications, the dosages, timing, and what to do if a dose was missed. The results showed that 62% of the participants demonstrated excellent knowledge about their medications and the prescribed regimen. Only 7.5% of the participants with a "limited understanding" of their medications did not know what to do if a dose was missed. Some participants (7%) could not answer a variety of questions about even one of their medications. This group was deemed at high risk for noncompliance with the medication regimen. Another 23.5% of the participants had some problems answering the questions about their medications, but no definitive reason was found. The researchers concluded that the majority of individuals over age 65 had a relatively good understanding of their medication regimen.

Box 2-8 Elderly Alcohol Screening Test (EAST)

Directions: If a statement says something true about you, circle "Yes." If a statement says something not true about you, circle "No." Please answer all questions.

1. Have you ever drunk alcohol? Yes No
2. Do you feel that you are a normal drinker? Yes No
3. Have you ever awakened the morning after drinking the night before and found that you could not remember a part of the evening? Yes No
4. Does your spouse, the people you live with, or your children ever worry or complain about your drinking? Yes No
5. Can you stop drinking without a struggle after 1 or 2 drinks? Yes No
6. Do you ever feel bad about your drinking? Yes No
7. Do friends, your children, or other relatives think you are a normal drinker? Yes No
8. Have you ever used alcohol instead of prescribed medications from your doctor to treat your health problems? Yes No
9. Do you try to limit your drinking to certain prescribed times of the day or to certain places? Yes No
10. Are you always able to stop drinking when you want to? Yes No
11. Have you ever been evicted, asked to move, or been denied access to any older living accommodations or recreational facilities because of your drinking? Yes No
12. Have you ever attended a meeting of Alcoholics Anonymous (AA)? Yes No
13. Have you gotten physically or verbally aggressive when drinking? Yes No
14. Has drinking ever created problems between you and your spouse, your children, or other family members? Yes No
15. Have your children ever avoided contact with you, or not allowed you to see or visit your grandchildren, because of your drinking? Yes No
16. Has your spouse (or any other family member) ever gone to anyone for help about your drinking? Yes No
17. Have you ever lost any friends or had disagreements with neighbors because of your drinking? Yes No
18. Have you ever neglected eating, your own daily health maintenance, or your family for 2 or more days in a row because of your drinking? Yes No
19. Have you ever drunk to relieve the pain and sorrow due to the loss of or death of your spouse or other loved ones? Yes No
20. Do you drink before noon? Yes No
21. Have you ever been told by your doctor that you have liver trouble? Yes No
22. Have you ever had severe shakes, heard voices, or seen things that were not there after heavy drinking? Yes No
23. Have you ever gone to anyone for help about your drinking? Yes No
24. Have you ever been hospitalized because of your drinking? Yes No
25. Have you ever been a patient in a psychiatric hospital or on a psychiatric ward of a general hospital where drinking was part of the problem? Yes No
26. Have you ever been at a psychiatric or mental health clinic or gone to a doctor, a social worker, clergyman, or counselor for help with an emotional problem in which drinking played a part? Yes No

Elderly Alcohol Screening Testing Scoring

	Yes	No
1.	0	0
2.	0	2
3.	1	0
4.	1	0
5.	0	2
6.	1	0
7.	0	2
8.	2	0
9.	0	0
10.	0	2
11.	2	0
12.	2	0
13.	2	0
14.	2	0
15.	2	0
16.	2	0
17.	3	0
18.	3	0
19.	1	0
20.	1	0
21.	2	0
22.	5	0
23.	5	0
24.	5	0
25.	5	0
26.	5	0

Total possible score: 50
0-3 points: Probably not alcoholic
4-9 points: 80% diagnostic of alcoholism
10 points: Virtually 100% diagnostic of alcoholism

DRUG DISTRIBUTION. The loss of lean body mass and the increased proportion of body fat affect distribution of drugs within the body. Fat-soluble drugs tend to be stored in fat, thereby decreasing the intensity of the reaction while increasing the duration. Within the bloodstream the distribution of drugs is affected by the amount of serum protein, specifically albumin, available as binding sites for drugs. In aging persons the serum albumin levels tend to be lower, resulting in altered concentrations of bound (inactive) and unbound (active) drugs. Unbound drugs in the circulation are active in producing the effects of the drug. The unbound drug can be excreted by the kidneys or metabolized by the liver. A principal mechanism of drug interaction seems to be the displacement of one drug by another from these protein-binding sites. For example, warfarin may be displaced by aspirin, indomethacin, and other drugs, causing increased anticoagulation activity.

DRUG METABOLISM. The metabolism of drugs in older adults may be altered by lower levels of enzyme activity in the liver. Prolonged or incomplete metabolism increases the half-life of some drugs and allows the drug to exert its effect for a longer period.

DRUG EXCRETION. The kidney is the primary route of excretion of drugs. Changes with aging—such as decreased renal plasma flow to the kidney, decreased glomerular filtration rate, and decreased number of functional tubules—combine to result in inefficient excretion of active drug. This increases the risk of accumulation of drugs to potentially toxic levels because of decreased renal clearance. The decreased rate of excretion and the changes in binding sites in the blood prolong the elevated blood level and activity of many drugs. Digoxin, for example, has a narrow margin of safety and is critically affected by the change in renal excretion.

Medications have a definite place in the therapeutic regimen for the older adult, but they must be handled carefully. One general principle is to build the drug level up gradually, and use the lowest dose and fewest number of drugs possible. Nurses should check for untoward reactions to medications and report them to the health care provider. The basis for ongoing assessment of an older adult's response to medication is a thorough medication history. Care providers can use information from the nutritional assessment to identify possible food interactions.

Sleep-Wake Patterns

Sleep is a basic requirement for all human beings. Sufficient sleep is needed to maintain energy levels, physical appearance, and well-being. Certain changes in sleep and sleep patterns seem to occur as part of normal aging.[31] These include prolonged sleep latency (time it takes to fall asleep), increased number of awakenings during the sleep period, decreased slow-wave sleep (thought to be associated with physical restoration), and decreased rapid eye movement sleep (thought to be associated with mental restoration). These changes often result in more fragmented sleep than that experienced in earlier years. Although many older adults adapt to these normal sleep changes, others experience acute or chronic insomnia. Physical problems that cause shortness of breath, frequent urination, incontinence, impaired mobility, or confusion may disrupt sleep. Other contributing factors include certain drugs (e.g., some antihypertensive drugs) and environmental factors such as temperature, light, noise, and type of bed and location.

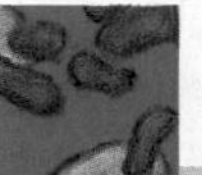

EVIDENCE-BASED PRACTICE

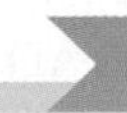

Topic Question: Is physical exercise helpful for sleep problems in adults ages 60 and older?

Evidence Base: The study reviewed random controlled trials studying physical exercise for overcoming insomnia in adults. At least 80% of the participants in the study were over age 60. The study excluded participants diagnosed with dementia or depression.

Findings: Physical exercise was effective for insomnia in one study. In this trial, sleep quality and total sleep duration significantly improved. Overall, sleep efficiency did not improve.

Conclusions: Rather than use medications for sleep enhancement, the study supports alternative methods. Although exercise might not be appropriate for many adults over age 60, it may help some reduce their sleep problems.

Montgomery P, Dennis J: Physical exercise for sleep problems in adults aged 60+, *Cochrane Review*, issue 3, 2004. In Cochrane Library, Chichester, UK, John Wiley & Sons, Ltd. Accessed July 2004 from website: www.cochrane.org.

Because quality of sleep can have far-reaching effects on the individual's well-being, the nurse's health assessment of older adults must include an evaluation of sleep. Sleep problems are of particular concern during hospitalization, which disrupts daily routines and exposes patients to new environmental stimuli. The nurse's assessment of an older person's sleep-wake pattern on admission includes a description of the sleep patterns and activities during waking periods, including periods of rest, exercise, and naps. The nurse should also ask about the patient's bedtime routines and what factors disturb or enhance sleep (see Evidence-Based Practice box). The nurse should analyze any identified sleep problem to determine its onset, subjective complaint (how the patient describes the problem), previous treatments and their effectiveness, and sleep patterns before the problem's onset. Some older adults are still working, some are retired from evening or night jobs, or some are caregivers and may have a sleep-wake pattern that differs from the hospital routine. These data are used to accommodate the older adult's normal sleep-wake cycle as closely as possible.

Alzheimer's Disease

Etiology and Epidemiology. About 4 million to 4.5 million people in the United States have **Alzheimer's disease** (AD). The number of individuals with Alzheimer's has more than doubled since the 1980s and is predicted to continue growing, possibly reaching more than 12 million by 2050.[30] About 1 in 10 individuals over age 65, and about half the individuals over age 85, have AD. Approximately 100,000 victims die each year, while 360,000 new cases are diagnosed. One of every three families in the United States is affected by the disease. Approximately half of all long-term care patients have AD. The health care costs for caring for persons with Alzheimer's are staggering, at an estimated $100 billion per year.[4] It is the most common form of dementia in the older adult population.

AD is named for Alois Alzheimer, a German physician who found the classic sign of AD, plaques in the brain, of a woman who died with a mental illness. A rare form of the disease can be inherited, but it is not known what actually causes AD in most people. The known risk factors include age and family history. Researchers believe that many more factors, including diet, environment, and viruses, may contribute to the diagnosis of AD. AD is not a normal part of growing old. Individuals diagnosed with AD have a life expectancy of 8 to 10 years, but many live 20 years or more after diagnosis.[4]

The Alzheimer's Association has developed a checklist of common symptoms found in AD patients. These include:

- Memory loss
- Difficulty performing tasks
- Problems with language
- Disorientation to place and time
- Poor or decreased judgment
- Problems with abstract thinking
- Misplacing items
- Mood and behavior shifts
- Personality changes
- Loss of initiative

Although having any or all of these symptoms does not mean a diagnosis of AD, it is important for families that recognize these symptoms in a loved one to consult a physician for further evaluation.[5]

Several other dementia-producing disorders may have similar symptoms to AD. These include Creutzfeldt-Jakob disease, Pick's disease, Huntington's disease, Parkinson's disease, Wernicke-Korsakoff syndrome, Lewy body dementia, and vascular dementias. These conditions also cause degeneration of the brain's cells. Although the pathology differs somewhat in each, a definitive diagnosis can only be made through testing and professional evaluation.[6]

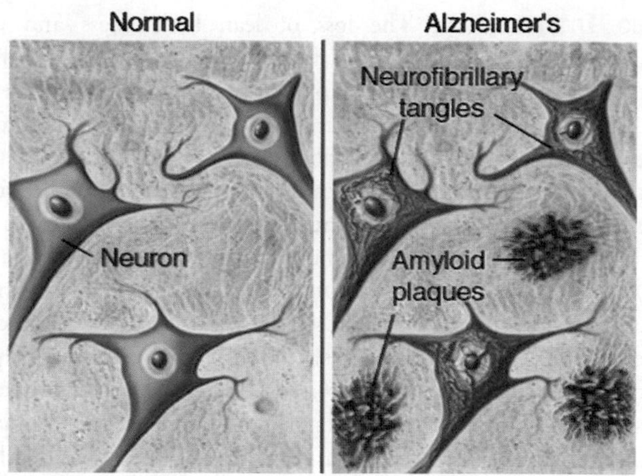

Figure 2-5 The formation of amyloid plaques and neurofibrillary tangles is thought to contribute to the degradation of the neurons (nerve cells) in the brain and the subsequent symptoms of Alzheimer's disease.

Pathophysiology. Although little is actually known about the cause of AD, research has identified the typical changes in the brain of AD patients. **Amyloid plaques** and **neurofibrillary tangles** are found in the brains of AD victims, but researchers are still studying the part these play in the disease (Figure 2-5). Other brain changes include loss of nerve cells in memory areas and

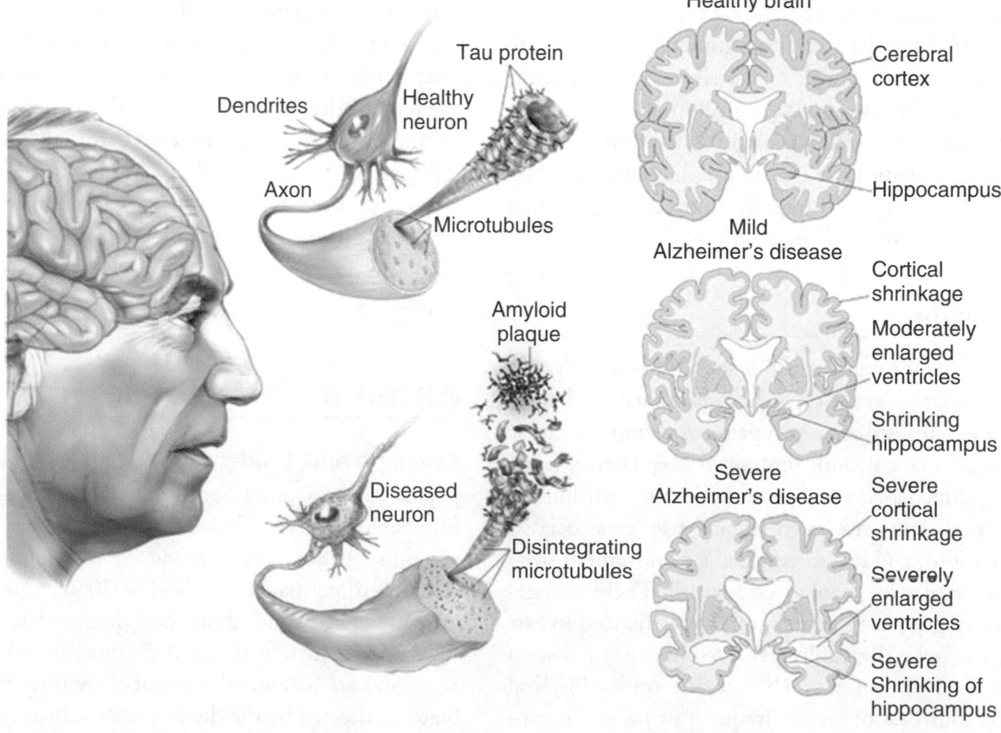

Figure 2-6 How the brain and nerve cells change during Alzheimer's disease.

lower levels of chemicals responsible for carrying messages among nerve cells (Figure 2-6).[4]

Because of these changes, symptoms of AD include memory loss, difficulty in performing ADLs, language problems, disorientation, errors in judgment, difficulty thinking, forgetfulness, mood swings, and passiveness. The disease is subtle, progressive, and often not noticed in early stages. In later stages, patients may forget how to do simple self-care activities, wander away from their residence, and become totally dependent on others for their care needs (Table 2-3).

Collaborative Care Management

DIAGNOSTIC TESTS. If an individual is experiencing symptoms of memory loss or other symptoms of AD, the patient or family should inform a physician. Treatable conditions such as depression, drug reactions, thyroid problems, and nutritional deficiencies can cause such symptoms. However, no definitive test for AD exists. A brain autopsy, searching for the plaques and cell tangles, is the only definitive way to diagnose the disease. Thus physicians use a variety of other tests to support the diagnosis of possible or probable disease (Table 2-4).

MEDICATIONS. Although AD has no cure, a variety of medications have been approved to treat the disease (Table 2-5).[49] These medications help control the changing physiologic effects of the disease in the brain, whereas other medications are used to manage the depression, agitation, and psychotic symptoms. Some of these drugs, such as the antipsychotics, have side effects such as an increased risk of cerebrovascular accident or diabetes. But, because of the behavioral symptoms—paranoia, aggression, and violent outbursts—physicians are likely to prescribe antipsychotics. This is often at the request of the family tying to care for the patient in the home. Research shows that these symptoms, rather than just memory loss, lead families to place family members with AD in nursing homes for care.[46]

A recent study shows that atorvastatin (Lipitor), used to lower cholesterol, slows the progression of AD and even reduces the deterioration. This will continue to be studied along with the actions of other statins.[11] Other drugs being studied for use in AD include (1) nonsteroidal antiinflammatory drugs, which may slow progression or lower risk of developing AD; (2) ginkgo biloba, which appears to increase blood flow to the brain, although researchers are unsure if it can delay dementia; and (3) vitamins, which may reduce the risk for AD.[7] In addition, ongoing clinical trials are testing new drugs and vaccines for AD (see Future Watch box).

TREATMENTS. Since AD has no cure, the future may seem grim for those diagnosed with the disease and their families. However,

Future Watch

New Hope for Alzheimer's Treatment

The second phase of a clinical trial for the drug Alzhemed, a new drug for the treatment of Alzheimer's disease (AD), has been completed. The drug is expected to prevent or halt the formation of amyloid fibrils in the brain by attaching to the amyloid β peptide. It is also expected to inhibit the inflammatory response in AD victims who have amyloid buildup, and to reduce the risk of fibril formation. In the first phase of the trials it was shown to be safe and tolerable in healthy volunteers. In this second phase researchers are studying the positive effects and the dose necessary to attain satisfactory results. This new AD drug directly targets the adverse effects of the disease on the brain, rather than just treating the symptoms of AD as many other drugs do. Researchers are also exploring a new synthetic vaccine to reduce the level of amyloid in the brain before the fibrils are created.

Neurochem: *Clinical development Alzheimer's disease: Alzhemed,* accessed Aug 2004 from website: www.neurochem.com/researchactivities.htm.

TABLE 2-3 STAGES OF ALZHEIMER'S DISEASE

Stage	Symptoms
1	Unimpaired
2	Beginning mild decline
3	Mild decline
4	Moderate decline
5	Moderate to severe decline
6	Severe decline
7	Continued severe decline

Data from Alzheimer's Association: *Stages of Alzheimer's disease,* accessed Aug 2004 from website: www.alz.org.

TABLE 2-4 DIAGNOSTIC TESTS FOR ALZHEIMER'S DISEASE

Test	Purpose
Brain scan	Rule out other causes of dementia
Medical history	Review present status, family history
Mental status evaluation	Assess level of comprehension, communication, memory, etc.
Laboratory tests—blood, spinal fluid, urine	Rule out other causes of dementia
Physical examination	Rule out other causes of dementia
Psychiatric evaluation	Rule out other causes of dementia Assess factors that are common to Alzheimer's disease

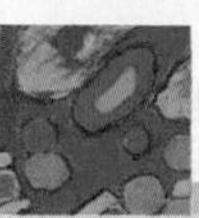

TABLE 2-5
COMMON MEDICATIONS *for Alzheimer's Disease*

Drug	Action	Nursing Intervention
Medications to slow progression of disease and control symptoms: 1. Donepezil (Aricept) 2. Galantamine (Reminyl) 3. Rivastigmine (Exelon) 4. Tacrine (Cognex)	1-4. They slow metabolic breakdown of acetylcholine and make more acetylcholine available for communication among cells.	Teach proper dosage. Tell patient to report side effects such as dizziness, headache, nausea, vomiting, or irregular pulse. Ensure adequate fluid intake.
5. Memantine (Namenda)*	5. An N-methyl-D-aspartate (NMDA) receptor antagonist, this protects brain's nerve cells against excessive glutamate, the chemical released by damaged cells in Alzheimer's disease (AD).	Identify appropriate support groups or other resources in community for increased information on drug therapy for AD.
Antipsychotics: Risperidone (Risperdal) Olanzapine (Zyprexa)	By antagonism of dopamine and serotonin receptors, they control depression, anxiety, and psychotic symptoms.	Teach proper dosage. Tell patient to avoid overheating. Be aware of potential for orthostatic hypotension. Tell patient to avoid alcohol. Tell patient to report side effects.
Vitamin E	This slows progression of AD from moderate to late stage.	Teach patient proper dosage. Tell patient to report bleeding or bruising.

*Approved for treatment of moderate to severe AD.

drug therapy may improve symptoms and lessen behavioral problems. Since AD progresses at vastly different rates in different people, treatments for specific symptoms are prescribed when necessary. Supportive therapy is instituted for problems with mobility, incontinence, and nutrition as the patient becomes less able to perform self-care activities. In advanced AD, when the patient is in the final stages of dementia and dysphagia and can no longer swallow food and fluids, artificial hydration and nutrition are necessary. At this time the family may have to make decisions about end-of-life care for their loved one.[23]

Other treatments for AD include complementary and alternative therapies such as ginkgo biloba, ubiquinone (an antioxidant also known as coenzyme Q), and huperzine A (a moss extract). None of these has yet been proven useful, but researchers continue to study their effects. Some researchers are concerned that these preparations may be promoted as effective treatments for AD, but their safety and benefits have not been established.[3]

Nursing Management
of the Patient with Alzheimer's Disease

ASSESSMENT

When caring for a patient with AD, the nurse should interact with the patient and family, since both are affected by the changes associated with the disease. If the patient cannot give an accurate history, the nurse should obtain the necessary information from the family.

Health History. Assess for:
- Memory difficulties
- Impaired judgment
- Communication difficulties
- Personality changes, delusions, paranoia, hallucinations, outbursts (may ask family)
- Ability to perform ADLs
- Eating difficulties; ability to maintain good nutrition
- Urinary and fecal incontinence
- Sleep disturbances
- Anxiety, tearfulness, nervousness
- Wandering, purposelessness, lack of energy and enthusiasm
- Appropriate use of prescribed medications and use of complementary and alternative medicine
- Safety in home and neighborhood environment

Physical Examination. Assess for:
- Changes in vital signs
- Signs of infection; fever, lesions, pain
- Signs of malnutrition, skin turgor, weight, general appearance
- Inability to swallow, chew, feed self
- Inadequate circulation, pulses, color, capillary refill
- Inappropriate verbalization during examination; ability to carry on a conversation; lapses in speech; tongue movements and body movements during conversation
- Other neurologic deficits; strength; gait; flexibility; tremors

NURSING DIAGNOSES, OUTCOMES, AND INTERVENTIONS

Nursing Diagnosis: Risk for Injury

OUTCOMES. Common examples of expected outcomes for the patient with a diagnosis of *risk for injury* are:
Patient will:
- Be free from injury in the home.
- Be protected from wandering away from home and getting lost or injured.

NURSING INTERVENTIONS. Keeping the person safe is one of the most important aspects of caregiving. The nurse can help the family identify dangerous areas or items in the home. Fall protection is important; loose carpets and clutter in pathways should be removed. The family should put medicines and other caustic and dangerous materials in a locked cabinet. Installing safety equipment in the shower or tub is helpful while the patient is still able to self-bathe. As the patient's focus and concentration on tasks decline, safety vigilance becomes even more important. Bathroom doors should not have locks so the patient cannot get accidentally locked in. Stoves are often a danger to the AD patient. Some burn safety procedures should be instituted. The nurse can refer the family to health care organizations in the community that can assist with a home safety check.

The family must ensure the AD patient carries some identification at all time. Many patients with AD wander away from home, or go out for a walk in what used to be familiar territory, but no longer is to them. The nurse should tell the family to inform friends and neighbors about the patient's condition so they will intervene if the patient is wandering in the neighborhood and cannot get back home. The family should have a recent picture of the AD patient to give to the police or a search team if necessary. They may need to keep home doors locked to prevent the patient from wandering.

RELATED NIC INTERVENTIONS. Dementia Management, Environmental Management: Safety, Risk Identification, Surveillance: Safety

Nursing Diagnosis: Risk for Caregiver Role Strain

OUTCOMES. Common examples of expected outcomes for the family with a diagnosis of *risk for caregiver role strain* are:
Caregivers will:

- Successfully balance caregiving demands with other components of lifestyle, continuing to participate in usual activities.
- Obtain routine respite services to ensure time away from caregiving.

NURSING INTERVENTIONS. Caring for an individual with AD in the home is difficult and stressful for the family. Each day can bring a variety of challenges and new demands, altering the family's everyday activities, interactions, and pattern of social contacts. Caregivers may lose familiar and meaningful family interactions and feel isolated from friends and social activities. The work can be mentally and physically exhausting for the caregivers. This may result in family members feeling overwhelmed and even angry with the patient. Eventually, depressive symptoms may become evident in the caregivers. Stress is high at this point (see Research box). This can tax the family's resources in terms of both money and time.

The nurse should provide information about the support systems available in the community. Volunteer organizations may be available to assist with transportation for physician or clinic appointments. Research has shown that support group interventions for caregivers are beneficial.[41] Local organizations may offer respite care, an essential strategy for addressing the problems associated with loneliness and isolation. Religious organizations, neighborhood associations, community centers, voluntary service groups, and professionally led support groups can all be sources of social support.

RELATED NIC INTERVENTIONS. Caregiver Support, Home Maintenance Assistance, Respite Care, Support Group

EVALUATION

To evaluate the effectiveness of nursing interventions, the nurse should compare patient and family behaviors with those in the expected patient and family outcomes.

RELATED NOC OUTCOMES. Caregiver Emotional Health,Caregiver Well-Being, Caregiving Endurance Potential, Safe Home Environment, Safety Status: Physical Injury Severity

Research

Paun O et al: Successful caregiving of persons with Alzheimer's disease, *Alzheimer's Care Q* 5(3):241, 2004.

This qualitative study examined caregiver skills over time. The study used data from 6- and 12-month group booster sessions conducted during a large clinical trial over a 5-year period. The clinical trial tested the effectiveness of a caregiver skill building treatment intervention compared with a support only intervention. Of the 272 participants in the 5-year clinical trial, 115 participated in this study. The participants were caring for a patient with Alzheimer's disease (AD) in the home. At the 6- and 12-month postintervention sessions, participants completed summaries about their caregiving experiences. The three common themes to emerge were care recipient issues, caregiver issues, and resource issues. The study revealed that caregivers for AD patients need assistance with care-related knowledge, care skill building, and self-reflection about themselves as caregivers. Caregivers who receive the appropriate information, support, and skill development are better able to accept the overwhelming task of caring for an individual with AD in the home.

Critical Thinking

1. What are the important points of a spiritual assessment for an older adult who is hospitalized?
2. An 85-year-old woman, recovering from hip replacement surgery, is being discharged from the hospital to return home, where she lives alone. She is referred to the home care agency for services. While she was in the hospital, her appetite diminished and at times she appeared confused, according to the nursing discharge sent to the home health agency. Based on this information, list the problems for which she is at risk. What specific assessments do you need to make immediately? What assessments can be delayed for a few days? What kinds of home health services can she benefit from? What resources are available in the community to assist her?

References

1. Administration on Aging: *A profile of older Americans: 2003,* Washington, DC, 2000, US Department of Health and Human Services.
2. Administration on Aging: *Older adults and mental health: issues and opportunities,* Washington, DC, 2001, US Department of Health and Human Services.
3. Alzheimer's Association: *Alternative treatments for Alzheimer's*, accessed Aug 2004 from website: www.alz.org.
4. Alzheimer's Association: *Statistics about Alzheimer's disease*, accessed Aug 2004 from website: www.alz.org.
5. Alzheimer's Association: *Ten warning signs of Alzheimer's disease*, accessed Aug 2004 from website: www.alz.org.
6. Alzheimer's Disease Education & Referral Center: *General information,* accessed Aug 2004 from website: www.alzheimers.org.
7. Alzheimer's Disease Education & Referral Center: *Treatment,* accessed Aug 2004 from website: www.alzheimers.org.
8. American Medical Association: *Alcoholism in the elderly*, accessed July 2004 from website: www.ama-assn.org/ama1/pub/upload/388/referral_treatment.pdf.
9. American Medical Association: *Diagnosis and treatment guidelines on elderly abuse and neglect,* accessed July 2004 from website: www.ama-assn.org/ama1/pub/upload/mm/386/elderabuse.pdf.
10. American Nurses Association: *Scope and standards of gerontological nursing practice,* Washington, DC, 1995, The Association.
11. Author: New study results show benefit for AD patients taking Lipitor, *Drug Week* May 21, 2004, p 26.
12. Ayres MM, Woodtli A: Concept analysis: abuse of aging caregivers by older care recipients, *J Adv Nurs* 35(3):326, 2001.
13. Beeson RA: Loneliness and depression in spousal caregivers of those with Alzheimer's disease versus non-caregiving spouses, *Arch Psychiatr Nurs* 17(3):135–143, 2003.
14. Bergland A, Kirkevold M: Thriving—a useful perspective to capture the experience of well-being among frail elderly in nursing homes, *J Adv Nurs* 36(3):426–432, 2001.
15. Bianchi EC: *Aging as a spiritual journey,* New York, 1990, Crossroad.
16. Brotman S, Ryan B, Cormier R: The health and social service needs of gay and lesbian elders and their families in Canada, *Gerontologist* 43(2):192–202, 2003.
17. Callen B: Understanding nutritional health in older adults: a pilot study, *J Gerontol Nurs* 30(1):36-43, 2004.
18. Carter B, McGoldrick M, editors: *The changing family life cycle,* Boston, 1989, Allyn & Bacon.
19. Centers for Disease Control and Prevention: *Trends in vision and hearing among older adults,* accessed July 2004 from website: www.cdc.gov/nchs/data/agingtrends/02vision.pdf.
20. Clark C: Effects of individual and family hardiness on caregiver depression and fatigue, *Res Nurs Health* 25(1):37–48, 2002.
21. Crystal S et al: Diagnosis and treatment of depression in the elderly Medicare population: predictors, disparities and trends, *J Am Geriatr Soc* 51(12):1718–1728, 2003.
22. Ebersole P, Hess P, Luggen A: *Toward healthy aging: human needs and nursing response,* ed 6, St Louis, 2004, Mosby.
23. Eggenberger SK, Nelms T: Artificial hydration and nutrition in advanced Alzheimer's disease: facilitating family decision-making, *J Clin Nurs* 13(6):661, 2004.
24. Emlet CA, Gusz SS, Dumont J: Older adults with HIV disease: challenges to integrated assessment, *J Gerontol Soc Work* 40(1/2):41–62, 2002.
25. Fioritto P, editor: *Alcoholism and aging: a matter of substance,* ed 2, Cleveland, 1997, School of Medicine, Case Western Reserve University.
26. Fischer L et al: Treatment of elderly and other adult patients for depression in adult care, *J Am Geriatr Soc* 51(11):1554–1562, 2003.
27. Fry PS: The unique contribution of key existential factors to the prediction of psychological well-being of older adults following spousal loss, *Gerontologist* 41(1):69, 2001.
28. Gottlieb S: Inappropriate drug prescribing in elderly people is common, *Br Med J* 329(7462):367, 2004.
29. Guigoz Y, Vellas B, Garry PJ: Assessing the nutritional status of the older: the Mini Nutritional Assessment as part of geriatric evaluation, *Nutr Rev* 54(1):S59, 1996.
30. Hebert LE et al: Alzheimer's disease in the U.S. population: prevalence estimates using 2000 census, *Arch Neurol* 60(8):1119, 2003.
31. Hoffman S: Sleep in the older adult: implications for nurses, *Geriatr Nurs* 24(4):211–214, 2003.
32. Hungelmann J et al: Focus on spiritual well-being: harmonious interconnectedness of mind-body-spirit—use of the JAREL Spiritual Well-Being Scale, *Geriatr Nurs* 17(6):262, 1996.
33. Knauer C: Geriatric alcohol abuse: a national epidemic, *Geriatr Nurs* 24(3):152–154, 2003.
34. Koenig H, George L, Titus P: Religion, spirituality and health in medically ill hospitalized older patients, *J Am Geriatr Soc* 52(4):554–562, 2004.
35. Levine J: Elder abuse and neglect: a primer for primary care physicians, *Geriatrics* 58(10):37–44, 2003.
36. Maes CA, Louis M: Knowledge of AIDS, perceived risk of AIDS, and at-risk sexual behaviors among older adults, *J Am Acad Nurse Pract* 15(11):509–516, 2002.
37. Masters J: Moderate alcohol consumption and unappreciated risk for alcohol-related harm among ethnically diverse, urban-dwelling elders, *Geriatr Nurs* 24(3):155–161, 2003.
38. Masters W, Johnson V: *Human sexual response,* Boston, 1966, Little, Brown & Co.
39. Meisenhelder J: Gender differences in religiosity and functional health in the elderly, *Geriatr Nurs* 24(6):343–347, 2003.
40. Miller C: Safe medication practices: nursing assessment of medications in older adults, *Geriatr Nurs* 24(5):314–315, 317, 2003.
41. Mittelman M et al: Sustained benefit of supportive intervention for depressive symptoms in caregivers of patients with Alzheimer's disease, *Am J Psychiatry* 161(5):851–857, 2004.
42. National Center on Elder Abuse: *The basics: major types of elder abuse*, accessed May 2004 from website: www.elderabusecenter.org/default.cfm?p=basics.cfm.
43. National Institute of Mental Health: *Older adults: depression and suicide facts,* accessed May 2004 from website: www.nimh.nih.gov/publicat/elderlydepsuicide.cfm.
44. National Strategy for Suicide Prevention: *Suicide among the elderly*, accessed July 2004 from website: www.mentalhealth.samhsa.gov/suicideprevention/elderly.asp.
45. Patel R: Polypharmacy and the elderly, *J Infusion Nurs* 26(3):166–169, 2003.
46. Peterson A: New treatments for Alzheimer's symptoms, *Wall Street J* 244(40):D1, 2004.
47. Powell LH, Shahabi L, Thoresen CE: Religion and spirituality: linkages to physical health, *Am Psychologist* 58(1):36–52, 2003.
48. Roth KS: Detecting "failure to thrive": a new assessment tool to identify and manage this often mystifying syndrome in elderly patients, *Nurs Homes* 50(10):60, 62, 64, 2001.
49. Standridge JB: Pharmacotherapeutic approaches to the treatment of Alzheimer's disease, *Clin Therapeutics* 26(5):615, 2004.
50. Substance Abuse and Mental Health Services Administration: *Many more older Americans will require substance abuse treatment by 2020*, accessed May 2004 from website: www.swcapt.org/samhsa_matrix/elderly_treatment_journal.pdf.
51. Tebb S: An aid to empowerment: a caregiver well-being scale, *Health Soc Work* 20(2):87, 1995.
52. Tinetti ME: Preventing falls in elderly persons, *N Engl J Med* 348(1):42–49, 2003.
53. Tsai P: A middle-range theory of caregiver stress, *Nurs Sci Q* 16(2):137–145, 2003.
54. Tully CL, Snowdon DA: Weight change and physical function in older women: findings from the nun study, *J Am Geriatr Soc* 43:1394, 1995.

55. US Department of Health and Human Services, Public Health Services: *Healthy people 2010: national health promotion and disease prevention objectives,* Washington, DC, 2000, US Government Printing Office.
56. Wallman HW: Comparison of older nonfallers and fallers on performance measures of functional reach, sensory organization, and limits of stability, *J Gerontol A Biol Sci Med Sci* 56(9):M580, 2001.
57. White JV et al: Nutrition in chronic disease: management in the elderly, *Nutr Clin Pract* 18(1):3–11, 2003.
58. Zeiss AM: Sexuality in older adults' relationships, *Generations* 25(2):18–25, 2001.

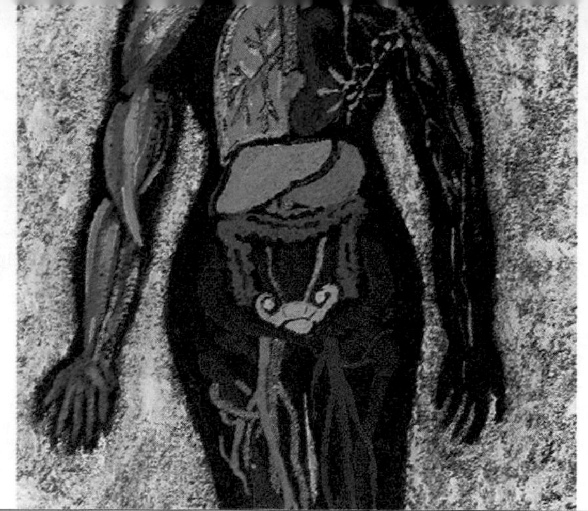

CHAPTER 3

Healthy Lifestyles

by Marianne Neighbors

OBJECTIVES

After studying this chapter, the learner should be able to:

1. Discuss the development of an agenda for health promotion in the United States.
2. Define terminology related to health promotion, risk reduction, and disease prevention.
3. Compare primary, secondary, and tertiary prevention.
4. Explain the role of physical activity, nutrition, tobacco use, substance abuse, sexual behavior, injury and violence, self-responsibility, and regimen adherence in maintaining or interfering with healthy lifestyles.
5. Describe common tools that can be used to assess the elements of a healthy lifestyle.
6. Develop strategies to help individuals adhere to a health-promoting lifestyle.

KEY TERMS

health promotion, p. 32
***Healthy People 2010*,** p. 31
injury and violence, p. 38
lifestyle choices, p. 30
nutrition, p. 34
physical activity, p. 33
primary prevention, p. 32
risk reduction, p. 32
secondary prevention, p. 33
self-responsibility, p. 39
sexual behavior, p. 37
substance abuse, p. 37
tertiary prevention, p. 33
tobacco use, p. 37

Healthy lifestyles are a key component of optimal wellness in young adults, an essential tool for minimizing the incidence and severity of chronic illnesses and their complications, and an effective strategy for controlling rising health care costs. Healthy lifestyles are the vehicle for attaining most of the goals of health promotion and disease prevention. Professional nursing has a natural connection with the promotion of healthy lifestyles. Nursing has been a strong voice for health promotion and disease prevention since Florence Nightingale first used the principles of hygiene and environmental management in the care of the wounded during the Crimean War.

Research showed the benefits of health promotion decades ago, but it has received marginal support within a health care system dominated by disease and illness management. Now a growing body of scientific evidence is increasing acceptance of health promotion programs.[9] Our knowledge about the etiology of major causes of morbidity and mortality continues to develop. Although genetics plays a crucial role in selected situations, an individual's health status is at least partially related to **lifestyle choices**, especially in the areas of nutrition, exercise, risky sexual behavior, and alcohol and tobacco use. The leading causes of death in the United States are related to modifiable behavior choices, such as smoking and overeating.[5] Preventable illnesses account for the majority of health care dollars spent annually in the United States. Thus nurses can make a significant impact on individual lives and the health of society by helping people make informed and healthful lifestyle choices.

Public health initiatives in the twentieth century began by halting the spread of infectious disease. Through sanitation, immunization, and antibiotics, the United States has virtually eliminated diseases such as typhoid, cholera, and polio and brought most childhood diseases under control. Equally impressive gains have been made through the development of sophisticated technology used for mass population screening (e.g., mammography and Pap smears). An array of pharmacologic agents and high-tech interventions has fostered the belief that eventually we will be able to control or eliminate all diseases and conditions.

Disease eradication may occur in the future, but now we are to some degree victims of our successes. Life spans continue to increase, and the elderly represent a growing proportion of the population. With the increasing incidence of chronic illness among older adults, the twofold goals of prevention and control have replaced cure. This chapter addresses the major components of healthy lifestyles and nursing interventions to help individuals make health-promoting choices.

A National Agenda for Health Promotion

The field of health promotion evolved with the holism and wellness movement of the 1970s. Its focus soon expanded to incorporate disease prevention and the optimization of health within the context of chronic illness. The first public health agenda for the United States, titled *Healthy People: The Surgeon General's Report on Health Promotion and Disease Prevention,* was released in 1979.[14] In 1980 another document, *Promoting Health/Preventing Disease: Objectives for the Nation,* targeted areas needing improvement: promoting health, increasing public awareness, decreasing risks, increasing services, and providing environmental protective measures.[15] This was the first time the surgeon general's office addressed the role of the environment in influencing health and outlined the importance of government intervention and oversight to ensure these health objectives. The report emphasized the importance of clean air and water, food safety, and occupational safety. It targeted smoking as a national health hazard.

Healthy People 2000

Healthy People 2000: National Health Promotion and Disease Prevention Objectives was the next report of national health goals.[12] This document represented the U.S. contribution to the World Health Organization's international project to achieve "health for all by the year 2000." It was also a response to evaluation data indicating that the United States had not met many of the health objectives articulated for 1990. Despite progress in a variety of areas, health promotion efforts needed to continue.

Healthy People 2010

Healthy People 2010: Understanding and Improving Health is the latest document presenting a vision for healthy people and challenging health providers and planners to achieve new national health goals. The document reflects changes in demographics; advances in medical interventions, pharmacotherapeutics, and technology; and the impact of global interactions on society's health. It identifies 10 leading health indicators as key objectives, highlighting behavioral, physical, and environmental factors that are important to the health of people (see Healthy People 2010 box below). It also identifies

Healthy People 2010

Leading Health Indicators
- Physical activity
- Overweight and obesity
- Tobacco use
- Substance abuse
- Responsible sexual behavior
- Mental health
- Injury and violence
- Environmental quality
- Immunization
- Access to health care

From US Department of Health and Human Services: *Healthy People 2010: understanding and improving health,* Washington, DC, 2000, The Department.

Healthy People 2010

Goals for Leading Health Indicators
- Improve health, fitness, and quality of life through daily physical activity.
- Promote health and reduce chronic disease associated with diet and weight.
- Reduce illness, disability, and death related to tobacco use and exposure to secondhand smoke.
- Reduce substance abuse to protect the health, safety, and quality of life for all, especially children.
- Promote responsible sexual behaviors, strengthen community capacity, and increase access to high-quality services to prevent sexually transmitted diseases and their complications.
- Improve mental health and ensure access to appropriate, high-quality mental health services.
- Reduce disabilities, injuries, and deaths resulting from unintentional injuries and violence.
- Promote health for all through a healthy environment.
- Prevent disease, disability, and death from infectious diseases, including vaccine-preventable diseases.
- Improve access to comprehensive, high-quality health care services.

From US Department of Health and Human Services: *Healthy People 2010: understanding and improving health,* Washington, DC, 2000, The Department.

goals for measuring progress relative to each health indicator (see Healthy People 2010 box above) and 467 health-related objectives in 28 focus areas (see Healthy People 2010 box, p. 32).[13]

Healthy People 2010 addresses two major changes in demographics through goals relating to our country's aging and diverse population. The document's underlying premise is that the health of individuals is integral to the health of the community. Despite declines in childhood morbidity and mortality, decreases in mortality from heart disease and stroke, and increases in longevity, our nation needs an increased focus on promoting healthy behaviors, reducing diseases, and promoting healthy communities. This chapter presents the *Healthy People 2010* objectives related to lifestyles and health promotion; other chapters throughout this text include objectives related to specific diseases and conditions.

Role of Professional Nursing

Professional nursing plays a central role in actualizing the commitment to health promotion and prevention. Nursing concepts and theories have focused on self-care, efficacy, and adaptation for decades. Nurses are acknowledged experts in health education and patient teaching, and they have long supported shifting the focus of health care from illness and cure to preventive services. Nurses in community-based settings such as schools, industry, and clinics are on the cutting edge as social and economic forces catapult health promotion into national prominence.

Increasing society's attention to healthy lifestyle choices remains a challenge. The cost of chronic illness management continues to drive the cost of health care upward. Insurers are acknowledging the cost-effectiveness of health promotion and prevention activities by offering incentives for healthy lifestyles, including discounts on

Healthy People 2010

Focus Areas

- Access to high-quality health services
- Arthritis, osteoporosis, and chronic back conditions
- Cancer
- Chronic kidney disease
- Diabetes
- Disability and secondary conditions
- Education and community-based programs
- Environmental health
- Family planning
- Food safety
- Health communication
- Heart disease and stroke
- Human immunodeficiency virus disease
- Immunization and infectious diseases
- Injury and violence prevention
- Maternal, infant, and child health
- Medical product safety
- Mental health and mental disorders
- Nutrition and overweight
- Occupational safety and health
- Oral health
- Physical activity and fitness
- Public health infrastructure
- Respiratory diseases
- Sexually transmitted diseases
- Substance abuse
- Tobacco use
- Vision and hearing

From US Department of Health and Human Services: *Healthy People 2010: understanding and improving health,* Washington, DC, 2000, The Department.

insurance for those who do not smoke or drink and who maintain a healthy body weight. Nurses are usually seen as the best-prepared health professionals to design and implement these activities.

Business and industry increasingly recognize that a healthy workforce reduces absenteeism and copayments for health care. Screening services, diet teaching, and exercise facilities are now common benefits in the workplace as companies attempt to improve their workers' health and minimize costs. Companies can estimate the benefits of risk reduction and design programs to save on their health care investment.[7] Occupational health nurses are at the center of these efforts.

Education for effective self-care is a cornerstone of management in the acute care setting as well and is again the primary domain of nursing. Today's consumers have broad access to health information via the media and Internet. Many are active in self-care interventions and lifestyle changes to preserve good health. Nurses must integrate patient education for health promotion into their practice in every setting using a variety of means (see Research box).

Overview of Health Promotion, Risk Reduction, and Prevention

Health promotion, risk reduction, and prevention are overlapping concepts, all featuring healthy lifestyles as an essential component. Health promotion is the process of increasing awareness about life activities such as eating, exercise, smoking, substance abuse, safety, and pollution. Risk reduction is the process of reducing one's risk, over time, of morbidity or mortality from chronic disease or acute events. Prevention is the broadest in scope and encompasses primary, secondary, and tertiary prevention.

Research

Oermann MH, Webb SA, Ashare JA: Outcomes of videotape instruction in clinic waiting area, *Ortho Nurs* 22(2):102, 2003.

The study examined the effectiveness of videotape instruction on health promotion and risk reduction presented to patients in a clinic waiting room. Since nurses are often too busy to educate patients about general health promotion, this method was considered a viable alternative for presenting important material. Researchers divided the clinic patients into a treatment group and a control group. The material presented was designed for a general public audience. Researchers gave the participants a pretest and posttest on the information presented and compared the group scores. They also evaluated patient satisfaction with the learning modality.

The study found (1) significant gains in knowledge about the material presented in the treatment group compared with the control group and (2) patient satisfaction with education sessions delivered in this manner. The conclusion was that education delivered via videotape in clinic waiting rooms is an effective method to get important health promotion material to patients.

Health Promotion

Health promotion is a process of fostering awareness, influencing attitudes, and identifying alternatives so that an individual can make informed lifestyle choices to help achieve or maintain optimal physical, mental, and emotional well-being. Health promotion targets personal habits, lifestyle patterns, and the environment to reduce risks and enhance health and well-being, thus strengthening the person's capacity to withstand physical and emotional stress. The concept of health promotion has expanded over the past several decades. Originally directed primarily at young healthy adults seeking optimal wellness, health promotion is now an important goal for people of all ages and health status.

Risk Reduction

Although health-promoting activities have a role in reducing risks, the term **risk reduction** is often used to emphasize strategies to prevent chronic diseases and acute events (such as some accidents and other safety-related issues) as an integral component of healthy behavior. Because many people do not make healthy choices until diagnosed with a chronic disease, it is important for nurses to educate patients at high risk for morbidity or mortality about risk reduction strategies.

Primary Prevention

Most components of health promotion fall within the parameters of **primary prevention**. Activities include those designed to prevent specific diseases. For example, asymptomatic persons receive immunizations and chemoprophylaxis with drugs and other agents to decrease their risk of developing disease. Healthy diet and exercise are also partially directed at preventing diseases such as hypertension, cancer, and coronary artery disease. Societal initiatives as diverse as water fluoridation, nutrient enrichment in foods, clean air and water, the use of seat belts, and the elimination of domestic violence are all primary prevention strategies. The scope of primary prevention is nearly limitless and is directly influenced by society's economic and political climate.

▶ ARE You READY?

Which of the following is an example of primary prevention?

1. Following guidelines for weight reduction diet
2. Ensuring compliance with required immunizations
3. Participating in blood pressure screenings
4. Adhering to prescribed regimen for treatment of diabetes

Secondary Prevention

Secondary prevention focuses on the early detection of diseases and their prompt and effective treatment, thereby limiting their seriousness and associated disability. Secondary prevention has expanded extensively as medical technology has developed. Examples include mammography; blood pressure, cholesterol, glaucoma, tuberculosis, and fecal occult blood screening; and prostate-specific antigen testing. Many other easy, low-cost screenings are under development to enable care providers to diagnose morbidity and initiate interventions sooner. Screening guidelines developed by research and service groups, such as the American Heart Association, American Cancer Society, and U.S. Preventive Services Task Force, appear throughout the text in conjunction with their associated disease processes. Secondary prevention also includes treatment modalities, which have traditionally received a majority of the health care expenditures.

Tertiary Prevention

Tertiary prevention is directed toward rehabilitation of the individual after an episode of disease or trauma. Tertiary prevention has gradually become the most significant target of health-promoting activities. People today rarely die when diagnosed with diabetes, chronic obstructive pulmonary disease, coronary artery disease, hypertension, arthritis, or human immunodeficiency virus (HIV). Instead, they often live for many years, facing the challenges of effective disease management and pursuing wellness within the context of chronic disease. After the diagnosis or exacerbation of a chronic disease, individuals may be open to education concerning risk reduction and healthier living. These readiness points are fertile areas for intervention by professional nurses. The nurse's interventions focus not only on the disease, but also on ways the patient can limit the seriousness and progression of the disease process and simultaneously improve quality of life.

Healthy Lifestyles

A healthy lifestyle encompasses behaviors that enhance the individual's health and reduce the risk of morbidity and mortality. These behaviors act in a cumulative manner to increase one's health and well-being. A healthy lifestyle is the result of choices a person makes over the course of a lifetime. Lifestyles and healthy behaviors have their foundation within the family unit and reflect the family's unique cultural, ethnic, religious, and socioeconomic heritage and beliefs. Outside influences such as peers, the media, and other life events also greatly affect one's choices related to a healthy lifestyle.[9]

Individuals practice healthy lifestyles without the supervision of a health care provider, but they can be influenced by the attitudes and interventions of health professionals. Routine screenings, prenatal and well-child visits, school health education, and public information campaigns all provide opportunities to positively influence lifestyle choices. Patient contacts during treatment of episodic illnesses are also opportunities for primary health promotion and prevention education by health professionals. These opportunities are particularly important with young adults who visit a health professional infrequently and are usually establishing lifestyle patterns that will carry them through their working years. School nurses and college health personnel can certainly have an impact at this level.

A Framework for Studying Healthy Lifestyles

The *Healthy People 2010* document, with its 10 leading health indicators and related measurable goals, provides a current, useful framework for studying healthy lifestyles. Personal behaviors and risk factors that can significantly affect morbidity and mortality are related to many of the identified health indicators. The major risk factors include age, heredity, lifestyle (e.g., diet, exercise, stress, smoking, alcohol use), environmental factors (e.g., pollution, occupational exposure, poverty), and miscellaneous personal choice elements (e.g., unprotected sex, failure to use seat belts, and drunk driving). This discussion is limited to six major categories: (1) physical activity and rest, (2) diet and nutrition, (3) tobacco use and substance abuse, (4) responsible sexual behavior, (5) injury and violence, and (6) self-responsibility and adherence to regimen.

Physical Activity and Rest. Compared with exercise, few interventions have as many proven benefits supported by major, well-constructed research studies. Active adults live longer and are less likely to experience hypertension, coronary artery disease, diabetes, osteoporosis, selected cancers, and depression. Regular exercise improves circulation, increases cardiovascular fitness and stamina, increases or maintains strength and flexibility, maintains bone mass, increases glucose tolerance, increases the proportion of high-density lipoproteins, lowers declines in oxygen use and muscle mass related to aging, and reduces the risk of coronary artery disease.[11] The benefits of exercise are particularly well established for older adults, who are more likely to sustain their independence when they integrate active exercise into their lifestyle.[2] The importance of exercise in weight control and in the prevention or delay of osteoporosis is also clearly established.

Despite this evidence, all recent reports from government studies show that American society is increasingly sedentary. This has particular significance for American children who are seriously overweight,[11] and it underscores the essential role that personal choice plays in lifestyle patterns. Participation in **physical activity** is associated with personal characteristics such as motivation, self-efficacy,

Healthy People 2010

Goal and Objectives Related to Physical Activity

Goal

Improve health, fitness, and quality of life through daily physical activity.

Objectives

Increase the proportion of persons appropriately counseled about health behaviors.
Increase the proportion of adults with high blood pressure who are taking action (e.g., losing weight, increasing physical activity, and reducing sodium intake) to help control their blood pressure.
Reduce the proportion of adults who engage in no leisure-time physical activity.
Increase the proportion of adults who engage regularly, preferably daily, in moderate physical activity for at least 30 minutes.
Increase the proportion of adults who engage in vigorous physical activity that promotes the development and maintenance of cardiorespiratory fitness 3 or more days per week for 20 or more minutes per occasion.
Increase the proportion of adults who perform physical activities that enhance and maintain muscular strength and endurance.
Increase the proportion of adults who perform physical activities that enhance and maintain flexibility.
Increase the proportion of trips made by walking.
Increase the number of trips made by bicycling.

From US Department of Health and Human Services: *Healthy People 2010: understanding and improving health,* Washington, DC, 2000, The Department.

health risk, family orientation, and education.[1] Some of the same characteristics affect choices about other health risks such as obesity and substance abuse (see Healthy People 2010 box above).

Exercise is generally classified as either aerobic or anaerobic. Aerobic exercise involves the large muscle groups and is performed in a rhythmic and continuous way, usually for at least 15 minutes. Examples include walking, bicycling, swimming, and dancing. Anaerobic exercise is characterized by bursts of energy expended in short time intervals. These activities include weight lifting, baseball, and wrestling. Although aerobic exercise contributes more directly to cardiovascular fitness and endurance, moderate strength training also plays a role in supporting muscle mass and strength, particularly for women and older adults.

Sleep and rest are often grouped together and share many purposes. The precise function of sleep is still uncertain. It is known that the amount of sleep required varies with age, activity, and health status. Modern lifestyles seem to contribute to a shortage of sleep for many adults. The hectic pace of the average person reduces the time available for restorative rest and sleep.

Physical rest plays an important role in healthy functioning. Adenosine triphosphate (ATP), which is necessary for all types of activities, is not actively stored by the body and must be continuously produced. Physical activity decreases the ATP available, and rest replenishes the supply. Rest also contributes to mental health through stress management. Activities that contribute to mental rest and relaxation vary among individuals and include such diverse strategies as participating in sports, reading, listening to music, and meditating.

Diet and Nutrition. The relationship between diet and **nutrition**, overall health, and a wide variety of disease processes receives constant attention in both professional and popular literature. Almost daily, new studies show a relationship between a dietary element and a disease process. Researchers suggest that dietary practices may be the single most important "choice" factor in determining health and longevity. However, high-quality diet research is difficult to perform and requires longitudinal approaches to yield data meaningful in relationship to long-term health and well-being. Many of the study results appear contradictory and provide insufficient guidance for making lifestyle choices. With the popularization of diets such as the Atkins diet plan, health care professionals need to remain informed about diet research to help consumers interpret and apply what they read and hear.

Diet directly affects the development of major disease processes.[4] Media attention escalated in the 1970s and 1980s as studies linked dietary practices to the development of heart disease, diabetes, and selected cancers. Research identified the effects of specific elements, including vitamins A, C, and E; beta-carotene, fiber, cholesterol, and saturated fats; nitrates and nitrites; food additives and chemicals; and even water. Now researchers are linking other elements such as zinc and antioxidants to positive health results. Even herbal products are being carefully studied for their effects on weight loss and overall well-being.

The U.S. Department of Agriculture (USDA) developed a food guide pyramid to serve as the basis for information and teaching about nutrition. The previous six-level nutritional pyramid has been changed to the MyPyramid food guidance system. Along with the new MyPyramid symbol (Figure 3-1), the system provides many options to help individuals make healthy food choices and to be active every day. One plan (as in the old food pyramid) no longer fits all individuals and lifestyles. The new pyramid assists individuals to create a food plan for daily use that incorporates their specific caloric and dietary needs. The new pyramid is still based on five food groups but focuses on a balance between food intake and physical activity and recommends limits on the use of fats, sugars, and salt. A guide is available at the website (www.mypyramid.gov) to help users navigate through the new MyPyramid system.

Americans are increasingly aware of the importance of diet choices but have not made significant changes in daily diet patterns. The average American diet still contains too much fat and is heavily skewed toward convenience and prepared foods (see Healthy People 2010 box, p. 36, left).

Current Issues in Diet and Nutrition. Nutrient research has become increasingly sophisticated and in the next decade will contribute much to our understanding of the effects of specific nutrients on such factors as immune system function, aging, and chronic disease. However, broad social issues relating to diet and nutrition remain important concerns.

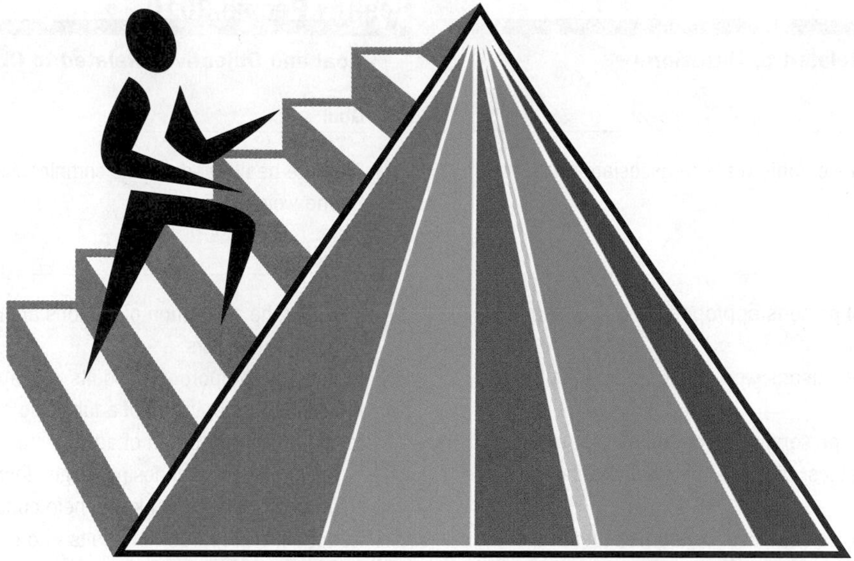

Grains
At least half should be whole-grain
Vegetables
Fresh, frozen, canned, dried, juices
Fruits
Fresh, frozen, canned, dried, juices
Oils, fats
Liquid, not solid
Milk products
Low- or no-fat, calcium-rich types
High-protein foods
Lean meat, poultry, fish; eggs; beans, nuts, seeds; tofu; peanut butter
MyPyramid.gov
STEPS TO A HEALTHIER YOU

GRAINS Make half your grains whole	VEGETABLES Vary your veggies	FRUITS Focus on fruits	MILK Get your calcium-rich foods	MEAT & BEANS Go lean with protein
Eat at least 3 oz. of whole-grain cereals, breads, crackers, rice, or pasta every day 1 oz. is about 1 slice of bread, about 1 cup of breakfast cereal, or 1/2 cup of cooked rice, cereal, or pasta	Eat more dark-green veggies like broccoli, spinach, and other dark leafy greens Eat more orange vegetables like carrots and sweet potatoes Eat more dry beans and peas like pinto beans, kidney beans, and lentils	Eat a variety of fruit Choose fresh, frozen, canned, or dried fruit Go easy on fruit juices	Go low-fat or fat-free when you choose milk, yogurt, and other milk products If you don't or can't consume milk, choose lactose-free products or other calcium sources such as fortified foods and beverages	Choose low-fat or lean meats and poultry Bake it, broil it, or grill it Vary your protein routine – choose more fish, beans, peas, nuts, and seeds
For a 2,000-calorie diet, you need the amounts below from each food group. To find the amounts that are right for you, go to MyPyramid.gov.				
Eat 6 oz. every day	Eat 2 1/2 cups every day	Eat 2 cups every day	Get 3 cups every day; for kids aged 2 to 8, it's 2	Eat 5 1/2 oz. every day

Find your balance between food and physical activity
- Be sure to stay within your daily calorie needs
- Be physically active for at least 30 minutes most days of the week.
- About 60 minutes a day of physical activity may be needed to prevent weight gain.
- For sustaining weight loss, at least 60 to 90 minutes a day of physical activity may be required.
- Children and teenagers should be physically active for 60 minutes every day, or most days.

Know the limits on fats, sugars, and salt (sodium)
- Make most of your fat sources from fish, nuts, and vegetable oils.
- Limit solid fats like butter, margarine, shortening, and lard, as well as foods that contain these.
- Check the Nutrition Facts label to keep saturated fats, *trans* fats, and sodium low.
- Choose food and beverages low in added sugars. Added sugars contribute calories with few, if any, nutrients.

Figure 3-1 MyPyramid: a guide to daily food choices and numbers of servings.

Healthy People 2010

Goal and Objectives Related to Nutrition

Goal

Promote health and reduce chronic disease associated with diet and weight.

Objectives

Increase the proportion of persons appropriately counseled about health behaviors.
Increase the proportion of persons who consume at least two daily servings of fruit.
Increase the proportion of persons who consume at least three daily servings of vegetables, with one third being dark green or orange vegetables.
Increase the proportion of persons who consume at least six daily servings of grain products, with at least three being whole grains.
Increase the proportion of persons who consume less than 10% of calories from saturated fat.
Increase the proportion of persons who consume no more than 30% of calories from total fat.
Increase the proportion of persons who consume 2400 mg or less of sodium.
Increase the proportion of persons who meet dietary recommendations for calcium.
Increase the proportion of adults with high blood pressure who are taking action (e.g., losing weight, increasing physical activity, and reducing sodium intake) to help control their blood pressure.

From US Department of Health and Human Services: *Healthy People 2010: understanding and improving health,* Washington, DC, 2000, The Department.

OVERWEIGHT AND OBESITY. Overweight and obese individuals are found in every age-group and represent a significant national health problem. About 64% of adults over age 20 and 15% of individuals under age 20 are overweight, and these numbers are rising. The percentage of overweight individuals in the Hispanic population in the United States is even higher.[3] Research has established the links between obesity and numerous chronic diseases, including coronary artery disease, hypertension, cerebrovascular accident, diabetes, arthritis, and some cancers. Some authorities consider obesity the second leading cause of preventable death in the United States, after cigarette smoking. Evidence shows that complex behavioral, genetic, and environmental factors result in obesity.

Obesity is a chronic disease requiring long-term management. At present our knowledge base does not contain many effective treatment options. Persons of the same gender and body composition have similar basal energy requirements that can be predicted from their proportion of muscle tissue and body fat. However, these data represent only a beginning understanding of how different bodies metabolize nutrients and respond to increased and decreased demands. Despite the futility of most standard treatment approaches, weight control remains an important goal, since

Healthy People 2010

Goal and Objectives Related to Obesity

Goal

Promote health and reduce chronic disease associated with diet and weight.

Objectives

Increase the proportion of persons appropriately counseled about health behaviors.
Reduce the proportion of adults who are obese.
Increase the proportion of adults who are at a healthy weight.
Increase the proportion of adults with high blood pressure who are taking action (e.g., losing weight, increasing physical activity, and reducing sodium intake) to help control their blood pressure.
Reduce the proportion of adults who engage in no leisure-time physical activity.
Increase the proportion of adults who engage regularly, preferably daily, in moderate physical activity for at least 30 minutes.

From US Department of Health and Human Services: *Healthy People 2010: understanding and improving health,* Washington, DC, 2000, The Department.

even minor losses are associated with significant declines in risks (see Healthy People 2010 box above).

MALNUTRITION. Malnutrition is still a problem in the United States despite a variety of social policy safety nets and interventions. The culture of poverty continues to expand, and poor children are extremely unlikely to eat a diet rich in fruits and vegetables. Malnutrition is endemic in the homeless and in alcohol and drug abusers and is a growing concern in the growing population of older adults. The elderly experience steady declines in taste and smell, commonly lose their natural teeth, and increasingly live alone on fixed incomes. Protein calorie malnutrition is present in a significant minority of older adults who are homebound or in long-term care facilities. Inadequate protein intake is theorized to contribute to the loss of muscle tissue, which increases the risk of falls and hampers the ability to maintain an active, independent lifestyle.

OSTEOPOROSIS. Osteoporosis is a disease characterized by low bone mass and structural deterioration of bone tissue. It primarily affects the bones of the spine, hip, and wrists, resulting in over 1 million fractures annually. Osteoporosis affects about 24 million Americans, the majority of whom are over 45 years old. About 40% of women who reach age 50 are expected to eventually suffer from osteoporosis if interventions were not started earlier. Risk factors are many but include a diet low in calcium (see Research box). (Other factors related to osteoporosis are covered in Chapter 53.) The current recommended daily calcium intake of 1500 mg requires careful diet planning or appropriate supplementation.[10]

Tobacco Use and Substance Abuse.

Smoking has been a front-page story for many years as the surgeon general's office,

Research

Sandison R, Morag G, Reid D: Lifestyle factors for promoting bone health in older women, *J Adv Nurs* 45(6):603, 2004.

The study reviewed lifestyle factors of older women who were given advice about health behaviors while they were in a research program to identify risk of osteoporosis. The researchers collected data through mailed questionnaires and telephone surveys. The study found that most of the women had not been taking calcium supplements as recommended, nor had they changed their diets even though they were diagnosed as being at risk for developing osteoporosis. However, most of the participants were taking part in a weight-bearing exercise program.

Although further research is needed, it was interesting that the women at high risk for osteoporosis were the least likely to make lifestyle behavior changes necessary to lower the risk. This finding has implications for nurses who simply inform women about osteoporosis and expect them to change their behavior. More than just education might be needed to effect change in women who are at risk for osteoporosis.

Healthy People 2010

Goal and Objectives Related to Tobacco Use

Goal

Reduce illness, disability, and death related to tobacco use and exposure to secondhand smoke.

Objectives

Increase the proportion of persons appropriately counseled about health behaviors.
Reduce tobacco use by adults.
Increase smoking cessation attempts by adult smokers.
Increase abstinence from alcohol, cigarettes, and illicit drugs among pregnant women.
Reduce the proportion of nonsmokers exposed to environmental tobacco smoke.

From US Department of Health and Human Services: *Healthy People 2010: understanding and improving health,* Washington, DC, 2000, The Department.

numerous citizens' advocacy groups, some states, and individuals battle the powerful tobacco industry over the addictive qualities and health risks associated with tobacco. Over the past 25 years research has clearly identified the health risks of smoking, but progress related to smoking cessation has been slow, and **tobacco use** remains a major social concern.

Smoking tobacco products is the main cause of preventable death in the United States. More than 400,000 Americans die each year of smoking-related illnesses. Secondhand smoke accounts for approximately 3000 deaths from lung cancer each year and has multiple adverse effects on the developing fetus. Although most Americans are aware that smoking is directly associated with lung cancer and chronic obstructive pulmonary disease, many are unaware of its contribution to cancers of the bladder, kidney, pancreas, and female reproductive organs. Smoking, combined with heavy alcohol use, dramatically increases the incidence of many gastrointestinal tract cancers. Smoking also contributes to the incidence of coronary artery disease, hypertension, peripheral vascular disease, and cerebrovascular disease.

As nicotine is inhaled into the lungs, it is absorbed into the bloodstream. Approximately 15% of the nicotine travels to the brain, where it is absorbed within 7 seconds of inhalation. Nicotine stimulates the release of catecholamines, particularly epinephrine. This release of epinephrine causes tachycardia, constricts the peripheral vessels, raises the blood pressure, and produces a feeling of euphoria. The effects of the nicotine on the blood vessels persist well after the cigarette has been smoked. Over time, many smokers are able to regulate their intake of nicotine to sustain the euphoria without the negative side effects of either overdosage or withdrawal. Nicotine is one of the most powerful known addictions, which is why efforts directed at preventing smoking are so essential (see Healthy People 2010 box at right).

Cigarette smoke also contains carbon monoxide, which binds to the hemoglobin in the blood with a binding capacity 200 times stronger than that of oxygen. As a result, the oxygen-carrying capacity of the red blood cells is significantly decreased. In high-risk individuals a decreased oxygen-carrying capacity results in hypoxia, impairs vision and thinking, and increases the incidence of atherosclerosis.

Cigarette smoking is not the only problem. Tobacco may also be chewed (snuff) or smoked in cigars and pipes. Many individuals believe these methods are "safe" because the nicotine and tar contaminants are not inhaled, but these forms of tobacco use are among the leading causes of cancers of the lips, tongue, mouth, larynx, and esophagus.

In addition to tobacco use, **substance abuse** is a lifestyle behavior with incredible consequences. It is estimated that substance abuse–related illnesses and treatments cost more than $277 billion a year.[13] Substance-related mental disorder is the diagnosis often used rather than drug addiction. Substances abused include alcohol, amphetamines, caffeine, cocaine, depressants, hallucinogens, inhalants, marijuana, nicotine, narcotics, and sedatives. The Center for Substance Abuse Treatment (under the U.S. Department of Health and Human Services) developed a National Treatment Plan Initiative that coordinates research-evaluating programs with curative measures in communities, establishes standards of care, makes effective drug treatment available, and improves public awareness and acceptance of substance abuse rehabilitation (see Healthy People 2010 box, p. 38, left). In addition, the National Partnership to Help Pregnant Smokers Quit provides community-based interventions for pregnant women.[6]

Responsible Sexual Behavior. Responsible **sexual behavior** can prevent sexually transmitted diseases (STDs) and unwanted pregnancies, both of which contribute to morbidity and even mortality, especially among young adults. STDs are among the most common and serious diseases in the public health arena in the United States. Approximately 15 million new cases occur annually. More than 20 types of STDs have been identified. They are epidemic in young adults and even teenagers. According to the Centers for Disease Control and Prevention, STDs cost the health care system more than $10 billion per year (not including treatments for HIV infection).[13] STDs affect men and women of all

Healthy People 2010

Goal and Objectives Related to Substance Abuse

Goal

Reduce substance abuse to protect the health, safety, and quality of life for all, especially children.

Objectives

Increase the proportion of persons appropriately counseled about health behaviors.
Reduce past month use of illicit substances.
Reduce the proportion of persons engaging in binge drinking of alcoholic beverages.
Reduce the proportion of adults who exceed guidelines for low-risk drinking.
Reduce the treatment gap for alcohol problems.
Reduce the treatment gap for illicit drugs in the general population.
Increase the number of admissions to substance abuse treatment for injection drug use.
Reduce drug-related hospital emergency department visits.
Increase abstinence from alcohol, cigarettes, and illicit drugs among pregnant women.
Increase the number of communities using partnerships or coalition models to conduct comprehensive substance abuse prevention efforts.

From US Department of Health and Human Services: *Healthy People 2010: understanding and improving health,* Washington, DC, 2000, The Department.

Healthy People 2010

Goal and Objectives Related to Sexually Transmitted Diseases

Goal

Promote responsible sexual behaviors, strengthen community capacity, and increase access to high-quality services to prevent sexually transmitted diseases (STDs) and their complications.

Objectives

Increase the proportion of persons appropriately counseled about health behaviors.
Increase the proportion of adults in publicly funded human immunodeficiency virus (HIV) counseling and testing sites who are screened for common bacterial STDs (chlamydia, gonorrhea, and syphilis) and are immunized against hepatitis B virus.
Reduce the proportion of adults with genital herpes infection.
Reduce acquired immunodeficiency syndrome (AIDS) among adolescents and adults.
Reduce the number of new cases of AIDS among adolescents and adult men who have sex with men.
Reduce the number of new cases of AIDS among adolescents and adult men who have sex with men and inject drugs.
Increase the proportion of adults with tuberculosis who have been tested for HIV.
Increase the proportion of HIV-infected adolescents and adults who receive testing, treatment, and prophylaxis consistent with current Public Health Service treatment guidelines.

From US Department of Health and Human Services: *Healthy People 2010: understanding and improving health,* Washington, DC, 2000, The Department.

backgrounds, ethnic groups, and economic status. The incidence is rising partly because of changing sexual practices, sexual activity beginning at earlier ages, and young people marrying later.

Health problems caused by STDs tend to be more serious in women, who often have more subtle symptoms and seek treatment only after serious problems develop. STDs in pregnant women are associated with spontaneous abortion, prematurity, low-birth-weight infants, and congenital infections.

Chlamydia infections are the most common of all bacterial STDs. Genital herpes, genital warts, and gonorrhea are also common and on the rise. The incidence of syphilis has decreased dramatically over the past 25 years, but it is increasing again in the United States.

Although the emergence of acquired immunodeficiency syndrome (AIDS) seemed to alert the public to the devastation of STDs, a large proportion of the population does not practice sexual responsibility. Despite significant progress in public education, prevention efforts still lag behind the goals set (see Healthy People 2010 box at left).

Injury and Violence. The nation's morbidity and mortality rate from **injury and violence** is excessive. Motor vehicle accidents, shootings, falls, fires, poisonings, and drownings account for most deaths in this category. Motor vehicle accidents cause most of the serious and chronic injuries. Although death rates are highest among teenagers and young adults, deaths from car accidents are common in all age-groups. Alcohol-related crashes still account for almost half the deaths from automobile accidents, but these numbers are improving slowly. Reducing the number of impaired drivers, increasing the use of safety equipment (e.g., seat belts, infant car seats), and conducting safety education programs for young adults are imperative.

Violence in the nation is an increasing problem. Homicide is one of the leading causes of death in children. Young adult males, especially African-Americans, are at high risk for being victims of homicide. Causes of violence include poverty, inadequate education, media influences, and stress.

The effects of stress have been extensively studied from both physiologic and psychologic perspectives. Chronic stress negatively affects health and is associated with an increased incidence of injury and vulnerability to infection. The incidence of chronic stress rises sharply among well-educated and highly paid individuals. Role stress in particular has received a lot of attention in the past 20 years. Many women and men face conflicts between career and family or the multiple demands of single parenthood. Although the effects of stress are difficult to predict for any individual, the nurse can help individuals and families anticipate and recognize stress, prevent it from developing into violence, and develop coping strategies to manage it (see Healthy People 2010 boxes related to injury and violence prevention in Chapter 9).

Self-Responsibility and Adherence to Regimen. Healthy lifestyles do not just happen. They are the result of conscious and unconscious choices and of commitments to specific, daily behaviors. **Self-responsibility** is perhaps the single most important element of a healthy lifestyle. Any professional involved in health promotion must understand and respect the complex personal, social, political, and economic factors that shape individual lives.

Multiple studies have shown that up to 50% of study populations do not adhere to professional recommendations concerning either disease management or health-promoting activities. This fact is reflected in the resistance associated with even "simple" regimens such as seat belt use, daily flossing, and regular exercise. Dietary changes have proven particularly resistant to change, since they involve choices that must be made several times every day. Consumers sometimes blame the food industry, particularly the fast food industry, for weight problems, but personal diet selections are the real issue for most individuals. Multiple behavioral determinants affect one's capacity to choose and stay with healthy lifestyle behaviors. Such determinants include motivation, socialization, self-efficacy, stress, and environment. Education and awareness are, of course, important influences on lifestyle choices, but they are not the sole factors. People can commonly state the rationale for lifestyle changes but may still be unable to implement this knowledge, a fact that is clearly demonstrated in smoking cessation.

Pender's model of health promotion illustrates the forces that influence behavior and lifestyle change. Pender identified factors that affect the person's perceptions of the problem, factors that modify behaviors, and factors that influence the likelihood of health-promoting actions. Participation in health-promoting behaviors is influenced by the individual's perceptions about health in general and perceptions of self, including self-concept and perceived control of the environment. Persons who do not value health, who do not see a need to improve their health status, or who are not self-motivated are less likely to engage in health-promoting activities.[8] Other models for health promotion include some of Pender's ideas and other influences, such as age, sex, and ethnicity. Although genetic factors are not modifiable, they also may affect a person's decisions about health-promoting behavior. The influence of family and friends can be another powerful factor. Research indicates that family support for health-promoting activities enhances a person's successful adaptation to a health promotion regimen.[8] Identifying an individual's specific modifying factors requires careful and sensitive assessment. Figure 3-2 portrays a health promotion model with factors that influence the individual's lifestyle choices.

Perceived barriers to health promotion and regimen adherence include concrete factors such as cost and availability, as well as personal factors such as the reactions of significant others. Box 3-1 summarizes the major barriers to regimen adherence. The complexity of the regimen, the degree of behavior change required, and the duration of the change appear to be particularly important. Simpler lifestyle changes are typically easier to make. Changes that must be implemented "for life" are particularly difficult to sustain.

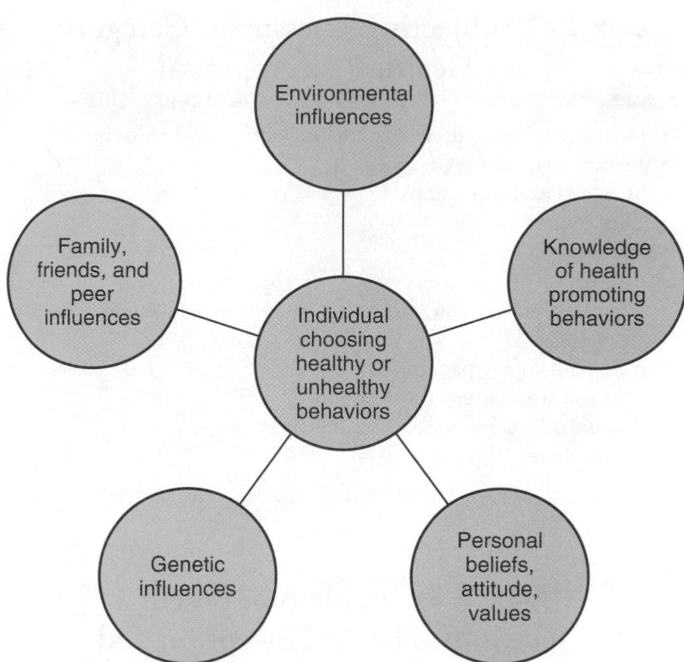

Figure 3-2 Model for health promotion. Factors affecting an individual's choices.

Box 3-1 Major Factors Affecting Regimen Adherence

- Amount of time the regimen requires
- Visibility of the regimen to others
- Amount of energy required to complete the regimen
- Difficulty of the regimen
- Amount of discomfort associated with the regimen
- Frequency of action required
- Expense of the regimen
- Duration of need for the regimen
- Amount of disruption to "normal" activities
- Perceived effectiveness of regimen in controlling or preventing the disease or condition

ARE You READY?

In completing a health history, which statement by the patient makes him at greatest risk for preventable death?

1. "My father died of a heart attack when he was 45 years old."
2. "I have been at least 20 pounds overweight since I was a teenager."
3. "My cholesterol level is too high."
4. "I have smoked a pack of cigarettes a day for the past 15 years."

Nursing Management

ASSESSMENT

The assessment challenge for the professional nurse is to understand the patient's and family's experience—their values, priorities, life circumstances, interests, intellect, situational constraints, and support network. Valid and reliable assessment tools can help gather information, but an in-depth understanding of the person's life

Box 3-2 Subjective Assessment Categories for Health Risk Appraisal

- General background information, including family history
- Preventive measures practiced
- Gender-specific questions
- Diet
- Exercise patterns
- Safety measures
- Use of over-the-counter drugs and complementary and alternative therapies
- Stress and coping patterns
- Rest and sleep patterns
- Alcohol or other substance use and abuse
- Tobacco use

Box 3-3 Sample Assessment Questions: Health Perception and Health Management

1. How has your general health been?
2. Have you had any colds in the past year? Have you had any absences from work or school?
3. What are the most important things done to keep healthy?
4. Do you use any "home remedies" to cure ailments or ease pain?
5. Have you had any accidents (home, work, driving)?
6. In the past, has it been easy to find ways to follow suggestions of doctors or nurses?
7. If appropriate: What do you think caused this illness? Action taken when symptoms perceived? Results of action?
8. If appropriate: What is important to you while you are here? How can we be most helpful?

Box 3-4 Brief Diet and Nutritional Assessment Data

- Age
- Height
- Weight
- Body mass index
- Health history
- Recent change in weight (if yes, note cause)
- Food allergies
- Food type preferences
- Cultural or religious dietary influences
- Medications, including nutritional supplements
- Usual daily nutritional intake
- Patterns of eating (e.g., time, size of meals, snacks)
- Difficulty with meals (e.g., preparing, shopping problems)
- Difficulty eating (e.g., chewing, swallowing, digesting)
- Food safety practices
- Usual meal preparer
- Other problems with diet or nutrition

circumstances emerges from skilled interviewing. A well-developed tool provides preliminary data concerning areas such as health beliefs and values, sleep and rest, and exercise. The components vary substantially according to the setting and purpose of the nurse's interactions. Although a full presentation of the range of tools is beyond the scope of this chapter, Boxes 3-2 through 3-4 provide examples of tools and questions that can be used in the initial assessment of the components of a healthy lifestyle.

Health History. Assess for:

- Family history pertinent to health risks
- Preventive screening measures practiced
- Alcohol and tobacco use
- Exercise, diet, safety, and rest patterns
- Other pertinent health practices related to the individual such as cultural or age-related factors

Physical Examination. Assess for:

- General appearance appropriate for age
- Height and weight compared with standard reference tools
- Body mass index (BMI), calculated by dividing the weight in kilograms by the height in meters squared (20 to 25 kg/m^2 is a healthy range for adults) compared with standard reference tools
- Skinfold measurements (percent body fat) compared with standard reference tools
- Range of motion of joints adequate for health status and age
- Exercise tolerance level (treadmill or other method if physician approved)
- Laboratory tests (e.g., cholesterol, lipids, hemoglobin, hematocrit) within normal limits
- Vital signs data (respiration, pulse, blood pressure) appropriate for age and health status

Nursing Diagnoses, Outcomes, and Interventions

A variety of nursing diagnoses may be applicable in any specific situation. Promotion of healthy lifestyles is a goal in working with adults of all ages, regardless of their baseline health status. The goal is to improve the health status of individuals who are basically healthy, to decrease risk factors in individuals who are asymptomatic but at risk for particular disease processes, or to improve the health of individuals already experiencing chronic diseases who need to adhere to a health regimen. The following diagnoses can serve as broad umbrellas for these situations.

Nursing Diagnosis: Ineffective Health Maintenance

Outcomes. Common examples of expected outcomes for the patient with a diagnosis of *ineffective health maintenance* are: Patient will:

- Balance food intake and energy expenditure to support a 1 pound per week weight loss and maintain an optimal body weight.
- Identify alternative coping mechanisms for dealing with life stress other than excess food intake.
- Verbalize an intent to modify dietary intake in ways that conform to the recommended food pyramid.

- Limit alcohol intake.
- Participate in a regular physical exercise program that includes weight-bearing exercise of at least 30 minutes' duration a minimum of three times per week.
- Get adequate daily rest and sleep.

NURSING INTERVENTIONS. All weight management approaches focus on establishing a lifelong balance between food intake and energy expenditure that supports gradual weight loss if needed. Diet changes are appropriate, but most exotic and highly restrictive plans have proven ineffective for long-term weight control. Diets should be individualized with the caloric intake planned at a level below the person's maintenance needs. Although "ideal" weight charts are available, the BMI is a better measurement of weight because it applies to both men and women regardless of their frame size or muscle mass (Figure 3-3). It does not work for pregnant women, competitive athletes, or frail older adults. The loss of 1 pound of fat per week requires a calorie deficit of 500 calories per day. Some persons may lose weight by eating three average balanced meals a day. Other persons are more successful with frequent small meals.

When a person severely reduces caloric intake, he or she often has a large initial weight loss through water loss. The dieter then reaches a plateau, which lasts 7 to 10 days and may be discouraging. Weight loss then continues at a slower rate as the body adapts to the decreased caloric intake by decreasing the metabolic rate. For the most effective results, weight loss programs should be integrated with moderate exercise programs. Exercise promotes the loss of fat rather than lean body tissue and positively affects serum insulin and lipid levels. Regular exercise also improves general health and well-being and allows increased flexibility in daily dietary intake.

Support from others appears to be critical. Having a weight-loss and exercise partner or belonging to a weight loss group is often beneficial. The use of appetite suppressants is controversial because of long-term inefficiency and associated health risks. Bulk-producing agents such as methylcellulose expand the stomach and provide a sense of fullness, but the same effect can be achieved by drinking two or three glasses of water before each meal. Prescription drugs such as sibutramine (Meridia) suppress the appetite but should be used in conjunction with other treatments such as exercise and diet.

The healthy eating guidelines for adults of average risk (Box 3-5) have been revised by the USDA to reflect individual needs and activity levels. Finding the balance between food intake and activity is stressed. The guidelines also emphasize distribution and variety and reflect current knowledge that good nutrition involves a balance of nutrients, fiber, fluids, vitamins, and minerals. The MyPyramid guidelines focus on the importance of vegetables, fruits, grains, and calcium-rich foods in the daily diet and encourage individuals to decrease their intake of sodium, sugars, saturated fats, and cholesterol. Individuals who are already experiencing chronic illnesses or who are assessed as being at higher risk may need more specific guidelines concerning the balance and distribution of foods. A more detailed description of the principles of healthy eating is provided in the Patient/Family Teaching box, p. 43.

The average American diet is at least 10% to 15% higher in total fats than is recommended. Fats should be used sparingly, as illustrated in the pyramid. This point is even more important for persons who have multiple risk factors or who already have heart or vascular disease. This emphasis on reducing dietary fat is reflected in the *Healthy People 2010* nutrition goal and objectives. The nurse encourages individuals to have their baseline cholesterol level determined and provides some simple strategies for reducing dietary fat and cholesterol (see Patient/Family Teaching box, p. 44). The nurse may also need to teach about the major sources of fat and cholesterol in the average diet. Reducing fat and cholesterol is often difficult because it targets foods popular in American culture such as high-fat cheeses, red meat, and cold cuts.

After identifying needed dietary changes during the initial assessment, the nurse helps the person use the MyPyramid food guidance system for effective daily meal planning. The meal plans incorporate the patient's dietary restrictions, likes and dislikes, and cultural factors. Most sedentary women and older adults need about 1600 total calories per day; this represents the lower end of the serving range on the pyramid. Men usually need about 2200 calories per day, which reflects the upper end of the serving range. Box 3-6 gives examples of standard servings for meal planning purposes. Individuals need to pay particular attention to the serving size for meat, since 2 to 3 ounces is less than most people would usually regard as a serving. The individual can use a blank pyramid to adapt the general guidelines to his or her own preferences and cultural or religious food practices.

Permanent diet changes are difficult to sustain but are more likely to succeed when modifications are made gradually. For example, the change to skim milk can be made by first switching to 2% milk and then decreasing the milk fat content again several weeks later. Altering the entire diet is rarely successful, so the nurse encourages the person to select one or two important changes to begin with. These changes can be supported through printed materials, written or pictorial, prepared at an appropriate reading level.

Whenever possible, diet discussion and teaching should include the whole family or social unit. Success is rarely possible when the family does not endorse the needed changes, particularly if the patient is not the primary food preparer. The messages given to the patient must be practical and consider financial resources and other environmental constraints such as access to food and equipment for food preparation. When the desired changes are complex, consultation with a dietitian is usually appropriate. The dietitian initiates the teaching, and the nurse reinforces it by providing additional explanations about the diet and helping the patient adapt current dietary patterns to meet the new diet prescription.

Older adults and others living alone may face additional challenges in eating a healthy diet, since food has such a strong social role in our society. Food preparation and consumption can become haphazard. Small, frequent meals and supplements can be helpful when people have difficulty sustaining an adequate intake. Meals on Wheels programs and senior center services can be viable alternatives for homebound older adults or those with limited mobility.

Food labels are an important source of information, and the nurse teaches the individual to interpret labels accurately. Recent legislation requires manufacturers to provide information about dietary supplements added and their amounts; properly label juice

Body Mass Index Chart

BMI ▶	18	19	20	21	22	23	24	25	26	27	28	29	30	31	32	33	34	35	36	37	38	39	40	41
Height ▼	Weight in Pounds ▼																							
60 ins	96	97	102	107	112	118	123	128	133	138	143	148	153	158	163	168	174	179	184	189	194	199	204	209
61 ins	98	100	106	111	116	122	127	132	137	143	148	153	158	164	169	174	180	185	190	195	201	206	211	217
62 ins	101	104	109	115	120	126	131	136	142	147	153	158	164	169	175	180	186	191	196	202	207	213	218	224
63 ins	105	107	113	118	124	130	135	141	146	152	158	163	169	175	180	186	191	197	203	208	214	220	225	231
64 ins	108	110	116	122	128	134	140	145	151	157	163	169	174	180	186	192	197	204	209	215	221	227	232	238
65 ins	110	114	120	126	132	138	144	150	156	162	168	174	180	186	192	198	204	210	216	222	228	234	240	246
66 ins	115	118	124	130	136	142	148	155	161	167	173	179	186	192	198	204	210	216	223	229	235	241	247	253
67 ins	120	121	127	134	140	146	153	159	166	172	178	185	191	198	204	211	217	223	230	236	242	249	255	261
68 ins	122	125	131	138	144	151	158	164	171	177	184	190	197	203	210	216	223	230	236	243	249	256	262	269
69 ins	125	128	135	142	149	155	162	169	176	182	189	196	203	209	216	223	230	236	243	250	257	263	270	277
70 ins	130	132	139	146	153	160	167	174	181	188	195	202	209	216	222	229	236	243	250	257	264	271	278	285
71 ins	134	136	143	150	157	165	172	179	186	193	200	208	215	222	229	236	243	250	257	265	272	279	286	293
72 ins	137	140	147	154	162	169	177	184	191	199	206	213	221	228	235	242	250	258	265	272	279	287	294	302
73 ins	140	144	151	159	166	174	182	189	197	204	212	219	227	235	242	250	257	265	272	280	288	295	302	310
74 ins	145	148	155	163	171	179	186	194	202	210	218	225	233	241	249	256	264	272	280	287	295	303	311	319
75 ins	148	152	160	168	176	184	192	200	208	216	224	232	240	248	256	264	272	279	287	295	303	311	319	327
76 ins	152	156	164	172	180	189	197	205	213	221	230	238	246	254	263	271	279	287	295	304	312	320	328	336

BMI less than 18.5, underweight; BMI 18.5-24.9, healthy weight; BMI 25-29.9, overweight; BMI 30-39.9, obese; BMI 40 and above, extremely obese.

Figure 3-3 Healthy body mass index ranges for Americans.

Box 3-5 Dietary Guidelines for Americans

Aim for Fitness

Aim for a healthy weight.
Be physically active each day.

Build a Healthy Base

Let the MyPyramid system guide your food choices.

Choose a variety of grains, consuming 3 or more ounce-equivalents of whole grains daily with the rest coming from enriched or whole grain products (at least half the grains should come from whole grains).

Choose a variety of fruits and vegetables daily from all five subgroups. Consume 2 cups of fruit and 2.5 cups of vegetables for a 2000-calorie intake, with higher or lower amounts depending on the calorie intake level.

Consume 3 cups per day of fat-free or low-fat milk or milk products.

On a 2000-calorie diet, the following weekly amounts are recommended:

Dark green vegetables	3 cups/week
Orange vegetables	2 cups/week
Legumes (dry beans)	3 cups/week
Starchy vegetables	3 cups/week
Other vegetables	6.5 cups/week

Keep food safe to eat: clean hands, food surfaces, and fruits and vegetables; keep food chilled as recommended; and cook all meat thoroughly.

Choose Sensibly

Choose a diet low in saturated fat. Less than 10% of calories should be from fat. Keep total fat between 20% and 25% of calories, with most fats coming from polyunsaturated and monounsaturated fatty acids.

Choose beverages and foods to moderate your intake of sugars; avoid products composed of simple sugars; consume fiber-rich fruits and vegetables, whole grains, and sugar-free beverages instead.

Choose and prepare foods with less salt; consume less than 2300 mg of sodium per day (about 1 tsp).

If you drink alcoholic beverages, do so in moderation: one drink per day for women and two for men. Pregnant or lactating women or individuals taking medications that might interact with alcohol should not consume any alcoholic beverages.

Key Recommendations for Specific Population Groups

People over age 50. Consume vitamin B_{12} in its crystalline form (i.e., fortified foods or supplements).

Women of childbearing age who may become pregnant. Eat foods high in heme-iron absorption such as vitamin C–rich foods.

Women of childbearing age who may become pregnant and those in the first trimester of pregnancy. Consume adequate synthetic folic acid daily (from fortified foods or supplements) in addition to food forms of folate from a varied diet.

Older adults, people with dark skin, and people exposed to insufficient ultraviolet band radiation (i.e., sunlight). Consume extra vitamin D from vitamin D–fortified foods and/or supplements.

From Center for Nutrition Policy and Promotion: *Dietary guidelines for Americans,* Washington, DC, 2005, US Department of Agriculture.

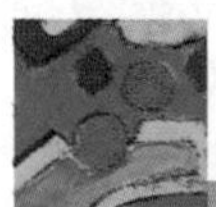

PATIENT/FAMILY TEACHING *Guidelines for Healthy Eating*

1. Always eat breakfast.
   a. Drink 100% fruit juice with breakfast or later in the day.
   b. Eat some fruit with breakfast, or take some to work with you.
2. Reduce your daily fat intake to no more than 30% of your total calories (no more than 10% should be from saturated fats), and reduce your cholesterol intake to less than 300 mg/day.
   a. Use "lite" or low-fat dairy products.
   b. Use only a tablespoon of salad dressing.
   c. Choose lean cuts of meat, trim the fat, and drain the grease.
   d. Use reduced-fat margarine or spreads.
   e. Substitute low-fat or fat-free baked goods, cookies, and ice cream.
   f. Leave the cheese off foods unless it is low fat.
3. Maintain a reasonable protein intake within the stated fat restriction.
   a. Choose lean roast beef or grilled chicken.
   b. Keep portions regular or small; do not double or "super size" portions.
4. Eat five or more servings of vegetables and fruits daily. Be sure to include green and yellow vegetables and citrus fruits.
   a. Use ready-to-eat vegetables for snacks.
   b. Use fresh fruit for snacks.
5. Increase your intake of complex carbohydrates by eating six or more servings of breads, cereals, and legumes.
   a. Choose oatmeal for breakfast and whole grain cereals.
   b. Eat beans and soy products more frequently.
6. Increase the fiber in your diet to 20 to 30 g/day. Add small amounts of fiber daily, and be sure to maintain a liberal intake of water.
   a. Choose more cruciferous vegetables for salads and side vegetables.
   b. Add fiber supplements to foods.
7. Drink five to eight 8-ounce glasses of water each day.
   a. Substitute water for sodas, tea, and coffee at least two or three times a day.
8. Limit the amount of salt you consume each day to 6 g (slightly more than 1 tsp).
   a. Refrain from adding it during cooking, and avoid adding salt at the table.
   b. Eat salty foods sparingly, especially salty snacks, which are also usually high in fat.
9. Limit or refrain from alcohol intake.

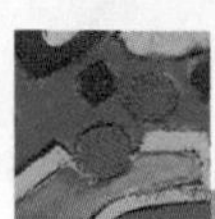

PATIENT/FAMILY TEACHING *Reducing Fat Content in the Diet*

- Eat fish or shellfish at least twice a week. Clams, scallops, and oysters contain less cholesterol than crab, shrimp, and lobster.
- Eat lean, well-trimmed meat. Trim loose fat.
- Use skinless chicken and trim loose fat. Light meat has less cholesterol than dark meat.
- Prepare foods by broiling, roasting, or baking. Avoid frying.
- Use low-fat or nonfat dairy products.
- Use tub margarine rather than stick. Stick margarine has more saturated fat, particularly the *trans*-fatty acids.
- Use low-fat or nonfat salad dressings. Read labels carefully.
- Use low-saturated-fat oils such as canola or safflower.
- Consider the use of substitutes, such as egg substitutes, cooking sprays, cream and butter powders, and products using fat substitutes.

Box 3-6 Standard Servings for Meal Planning

Each of the following counts as one serving.

Bread Group

1 slice of bread
½ English muffin or bagel
1 cup ready-to-eat cereal
½ cup cooked cereal or pasta

Fruit Group

1 medium apple, banana, or orange
¾ cup cooked or canned fruit
¾ cup fruit juice

Vegetable Group

1 cup raw leafy vegetables
½ cup cooked or chopped raw vegetables
¾ cup vegetable juice

Meat Group

2-3 ounces* cooked meat, fish, or poultry
1 cup cooked dry beans or peas
2 eggs
4 tbsp peanut butter

Milk Group

1 cup milk, yogurt, or ice cream
1-2 ounces cheese
½ cup cottage cheese

From US Department of Agriculture Center for Nutrition Policy and Promotion: *Food portions and servings,* website: www.cnpp.usda.gov, accessed June 24, 2005.

*1 ounce of meat or cheese is the size of a matchbox; 3 ounces are the size of a deck of cards; 8 ounces are the size of a paperback book.

products; clarify terms such as *low, reduced,* and *lean;* note *trans*-fatty acid content; and make appropriate nutrient content claims. The legislation attempts to facilitate consumer decision making about foods and their contents and additives; however, labels are still difficult to understand and tedious to read. The nurse attempts to ensure that individuals can understand and use the information provided on labels to make appropriate diet choices.

Complementary and alternative therapies have become popular in recent years, and dietary supplements are a major part of this booming industry. Many adults in the United States take one or more dietary supplements daily. After assessing the person's daily intake and current use of vitamins, minerals, and other supplements, the nurse can establish the need for routine, broad-spectrum supplementation. Specific supplementation of vitamins A, B, C, or E may be used as chemoprophylaxis to reduce the risk of certain cancers or to bolster immune function. The nurse explores the need for calcium supplementation with women and all older persons. If an individual does not consume dairy products, the average diet provides only about 300 mg of calcium per day, which is far below the recommended level of 1500 mg. Each milk product serving provides 300 mg. A combined calcium and vitamin D supplement is recommended for adults who are not routinely meeting their calcium needs through food.

Alcohol use must be included in any discussion of a healthy diet. Alcohol use is pervasive in American society, and the potential for abuse and addiction is tremendous. Although high in calories, alcohol has no nutrient benefits and contributes to a variety of medical disorders, including alcoholic cirrhosis. The nurse carefully explores the individual's use of alcohol and its meaning in his or her life. If a person does not currently use alcohol, there is no reason to begin. However, if alcohol use is important, the individual can safely and appropriately incorporate it into the lifestyle. Some modest health benefits have even been attributed to the occasional use of alcohol in the form of red wine. Daily alcohol intake should be limited to two cans of beer, two small glasses of wine, or two drinks containing no more than 1½ ounces of alcohol each.

The nurse tries to help the person establish and maintain a program of regular moderate exercise to enhance physical and emotional health. A variety of exercise plans can help achieve this goal, but any program should involve moderate weight-bearing exercise. The recommendations for amount, intensity, and duration of exercise have changed over the past decade. Moderate-intensity exercise that involves the large muscles and takes place at least three times per week for 30 to 60 minutes can reduce the risk for cardiovascular disease and stroke, in addition to assisting in maintaining a healthy weight. Higher levels of frequency, intensity, and duration can be established for individuals as appropriate. Regular exercise increases the person's energy and well-being; the individual should feel replenished, not depleted. Moderate-intensity exercise, with brisk walking as the classic example, carries a low risk of injury and is achievable for adults of all ages.

Consensus is lacking about who needs a physical examination or cardiac screening before beginning an exercise plan. Adults under 45 years of age who do not have significant cardiac risk factors can usually safely begin an exercise program without preliminary screening. The nurse encourages these individuals to begin slowly, increase intensity progressively, and report any unusual or unexplainable symptom promptly. Adults over age 45 or at known risk of cardiovascular problems should consult their physician before beginning an exercise program.

An exercise prescription specifically delineates the type, frequency, intensity, and duration of exercise. Intensity and duration can increase as the person's conditioning improves. In addition to this basic aerobic plan, the nurse may also advise the individual to include some strength training. Strength training has proven effective for women seeking to minimize the progression of osteoporosis and for older adults who need to maintain muscle mass, strength, balance, and flexibility.

The nurse instructs the person about the importance of both range of motion and stretching exercises before the aerobic phase of exercise, and the importance of a slow cool-down period at the conclusion of exercise so the heart rate can gradually return to its resting level. These precautions help protect the muscles and joints from injury and prevent postexercise hypotension and syncope.

Exercise is also commonly prescribed as part of tertiary prevention for persons with chronic illnesses. Exercise increases tolerance for activities of daily living, increases appetite, and decreases anxiety and depression. The exercise program is tailored to the person's needs and abilities. Exercise is begun at a low intensity, and both frequency and duration are modified as needed. Walking, cycling, and swimming are often well tolerated. When specific exercise prescriptions are indicated (e.g., after myocardial infarction or with chronic obstructive pulmonary disease), an exercise physiologist will typically perform the assessment and set the program parameters.

The nurse uses in-depth assessment to determine the patient's perceived barriers and supports for exercise. Getting started is typically the biggest barrier to establishing a regular exercise plan. Both home-based and workplace programs are effective. The nurse reminds the individual that expensive equipment and health club memberships are not necessary for a successful exercise plan. A partner to share the exercise is a strong motivator for most people. Walking remains an ideal choice for many people because the risk of injury is low, the intensity and duration are easily controlled, and the exercise requires no special training. Adherence to the plan remains a challenge, however. Some strategies to foster adherence to an exercise regimen are included in the Patient/Family Teaching box below.

The nurse helps the person plan for adequate daily rest and sleep. Most people experience sleep difficulties at some time, but can correct these problems by simple measures such as avoiding caffeine, making the environment conducive to sleep, avoiding late naps, and engaging in relaxation activities. Exercise can also increase well-being and promote sleep, and the nurse encourages the patient to engage in regular exercise for its multiple positive health benefits. Stress also negatively affects the individual's ability to achieve adequate rest and sleep. The nurse helps patients improve their overall coping abilities. People experiencing actual sleep disorders face more complex challenges and may need referral to a sleep disorders center.

The many benefits of healthy lifestyles are well documented. Most of the components of a healthy lifestyle are low tech, low cost, and seemingly simple. Yet the vast majority of adults do not integrate them into their daily lives. Simply educating people about health risks and benefits does not significantly change behavior. In interactions with patients and families, the health care professional needs to acknowledge the difficulties inherent in making lifestyle changes. The nurse needs to respect the person's right to make personal choices that conflict with recommended behaviors. The nurse must also realize that professionals cannot "force" positive changes. This does not mean, however, that intervention and teaching are either inappropriate or a waste of time. Nurses commonly encounter people at moments of readiness when health status improvement is a priority.

The nurse begins by assisting the individual in identifying supports and barriers to change and differentiating between actual and perceived barriers. Values clarification can help the person recognize and articulate his or her values related to health and personal responsibility. The nurse directly addresses the issue of self-responsibility and personal choice and helps the person recognize how his or her lifestyle behavior is either congruent or incongruent with the person's core values. The nurse then helps the person address areas of values conflict. This may provide sufficient impetus for the person to initiate needed behavior change.

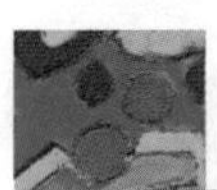

PATIENT/FAMILY TEACHING *Strategies for Establishing a Successful Exercise Plan*

- Exercise should be fun or at least pleasurable. Find an activity that you enjoy.
- Establish specific times for exercise, and schedule them into your week. You are more likely to exercise if it is a planned event.
- Start in small increments and progress slowly. Monitor your body's response to increases in intensity or duration.
- Set small, attainable goals, and reward yourself as you achieve each goal.
- Wear proper clothing, and use exercise equipment correctly.
- Be sure to warm up and cool-down thoroughly before and after exercise.
- Avoid exercising in extremes of heat, cold, or humidity.
- Avoid exercising for about 2 hours after a heavy meal. Do not eat for about 1 hour after active exercise.
- Share the activity with a friend, or consider joining a structured exercise class. Many community agencies sponsor exercise groups such as swimming, low-impact aerobics, and mall walking.

The person is next assisted in setting goals for health promotion and lifestyle change. The nurse needs to be positive and supportive of the patient's goals. Even seemingly minor changes are positive steps and can reduce health risks and improve overall health. The critical starting point is the person's commitment to take responsibility for his or her health.

The nurse then helps the individual develop and implement a plan that addresses the targeted lifestyle changes. Appropriate family and community resources and supports are identified. The nurse helps the person explore acceptable alternatives for overcoming barriers to adherence. The person must believe that the problem is solvable and that he or she is competent to solve it. The nurse needs to be enthusiastic about the person's ability to change and provide positive reinforcement for his or her efforts and accomplishments. Behavior modification principles state that positive reinforcement increases the likelihood the desired behavior will be repeated.

Other practical strategies for promoting adherence to a regimen include keeping it as simple as possible and allowing the person to adapt it as needed to. Formal contracting can occasionally be a powerful tool and underscores the importance of working collaboratively with the patient and family. The family plays a critical role in determining successful outcomes. The nurse needs to be thoroughly familiar with the community resources available to help the person integrate the regimen into his or her lifestyle. Printed materials, phone calls, and direct referrals to community support groups can help the person take that important first step. Other effective strategies for promoting adherence to a regimen are in the Guidelines for Safe Practice box.

RELATED NIC INTERVENTIONS. Anticipatory Guidance, Health Education, Health System Guidance, Risk Identification, Support System Enhancement

Nursing Diagnosis: Readiness for Enhanced Therapeutic Regimen Management

OUTCOMES. Common examples of expected outcomes for the patient with a diagnosis of *readiness for enhanced therapeutic regimen management* are:
Patient will:

- Continue to verbalize the desire to eliminate tobacco use.
- Significantly reduce the amount of tobacco used daily or quit.
- Begin a smoking cessation program.

NURSING INTERVENTIONS. The hazards of smoking are widely acknowledged in American society, but more than 46 million people continue to smoke. Nicotine is the primary addictive component of cigarettes. Becoming nicotine free is an enormous challenge that has a high risk of failure. The discouraging success rates of smoking cessation efforts reinforce the fears and hesitancies of current smokers.

Clearly, no magic programs exist that can create successful nonsmokers. But a variety of approaches can assist smokers in their efforts to quit. Hypnosis; acupuncture; aversion therapy; 12-step support programs; psychotherapy; and various forms of nicotine replacement in gums, patches, nasal sprays, and pills are all in use. The programs with the greatest success appear to be those which combine behavior modification with some form of nicotine pharmacologic support (see Research box). A significant portion of successful quitters, however, use no formal program but simply decide to quit "cold turkey." Each smoker clearly has unique needs for support throughout this process. The American Cancer Society and the American Lung Association are excellent sources of information about smoking cessation resources available in the local community.

The nurse must remember that no one can make someone else quit smoking, no matter how important it is from a health perspective. Ultimately, the motivation and effort must come from the individual. However, health care professionals need to use every opportunity to reinforce the hazards of smoking and encourage persons who are interested in smoking cessation. Patients commonly report that no health care professional has ever directly addressed the need for them to stop smoking. Approaching patients about the need to quit is clearly the most significant nursing intervention. A basic approach to smoking cessation includes the four *A*'s: ask, advise, assist, and arrange. The nurse *asks* about the patient's smoking habit and *advises* smoking cessation. If the patient agrees, the nurse *assists* the patient in developing a specific plan for smoking cessation and then *arranges* appropriate follow-up monitoring and support. Self-help materials such as brochures,

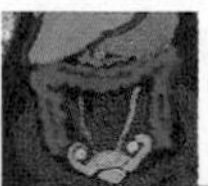

GUIDELINES FOR SAFE PRACTICE *Strategies to Increase Patient Adherence to a Therapeutic Regimen*

- Plan collaboratively with the patient. Remember, the regimen belongs to the individual, not the nurse.
- Include the family in all planning and teaching if the patient approves.
- Support the person's overall coping abilities.
- Simplify the needed regimen as much as possible.
- Help the person incorporate the regimen into his or her daily activities as much as possible. Encourage the person to tailor the regimen as needed.
- Be certain the patient and family understand the rationale for all activities. Provide appropriately written materials for them to keep as references.
- Explore the idea of contracting with the person for needed behavior change.
- Provide lots of positive feedback for efforts.
- Initiate referrals to appropriate community self-help and support groups. Provide the patient with contact phone numbers and addresses and written materials about services. Make the initial telephone contact, if appropriate.

Research

Johnson MW, Bickel WK, Kirshenbaum AP: Substitutes for tobacco smoking: a behavioral economic analysis of nicotine gum, denicotinized cigarettes, and nicotine-containing cigarettes, *Drug & Alcohol Dependence* 74(3):253, 2004.

The study used a behavioral economic design to look at the use of nicotine gum, denicotinized cigarettes, and nicotine-containing cigarettes. These products were all equally available to participants at standard retail price. The results showed that, as the retail price of the nicotine-containing cigarettes rose, the use decreased, with denicotinized cigarettes, not nicotine gum, chosen as a substitute most frequently. These results suggest that denicotinized cigarettes might be more effective than nicotine gum in smoking cessation programs. The study results also suggest that the nonpharmacologic behavioral aspects of smoking are important issues to address in cessation programs.

pamphlets, and tapes should be available in any health care setting. Some type of planned social support during the transition process is helpful for most people. This may involve the family or finding a "buddy" to make smoking cessation a joint effort. Other general behavioral strategies to support smoking cessation are given in the Guidelines for Safe Practice box.

Nicotine replacement therapy preparations minimize withdrawal symptoms while the smoker learns to live without his or her smoking-related habits. The power of these habits is reflected in yearning for a cigarette after meals or not knowing what to do with one's hands without a cigarette. Nicotine gum was the first major cessation assistant. Nicotine patches were developed next, offered first by prescription and then for over-the-counter purchase. These products slowly release sufficient nicotine into the bloodstream to minimize cravings. While no panacea for withdrawal control, these products can be useful adjuncts to a more holistic plan to stop smoking. The use of nicotine replacement therapies and the antidepressant bupropion helps some people stop smoking. Studies have shown higher long-term rates of smoking cessation using either bupropion alone or in combination with a nicotine patch.

The patches release nicotine through the skin, and skin irritation is the most common side effect. Patients are strongly cautioned not to smoke while using the patch because of the risk of nicotine overdose, particularly for patients with preexisting cardiac disease. Overdose symptoms include headache, abdominal pain, nausea, and vomiting and can progress to severe hypotension and prostration. Patients should also be aware of the predictable symptoms associated with nicotine withdrawal. These symptoms range in severity and duration but can be extremely severe. Classic withdrawal symptoms include irritability, anger, anxiety, restlessness, hunger, decreased concentration, and cravings.

For nicotine gum to be effective, patients must use it correctly. It is not a traditional gum and will not work if chewed as such. Principles of safe use are summarized in the Patient/Family Teaching box. Nicotine is now also available in nasal sprays and inhalers (Table 3-1).

RELATED NIC INTERVENTIONS. Behavior Modification, Health System Guidance, Patient Contracting, Self-Modification Assistance

EVALUATION

To evaluate the effectiveness of nursing interventions, compare patient behaviors with those stated in the expected patient outcomes.

RELATED NOC OUTCOMES. Adherence Behavior, Health Promoting Behavior, Knowledge: Health Promotion, Knowledge: Treatment Regimen, Participation in Health Care Decisions, Self-Care Status

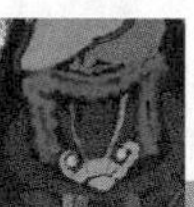

GUIDELINES FOR SAFE PRACTICE *Helping a Patient Stop Smoking*

- Help set a firm "quit" date.
- Explain available choices for nicotine replacement (e.g., gum, patches of varying concentrations, nasal sprays, pills). Teach about safe and correct use.
- Explore the advantages of a smoking cessation contract.
- Encourage using a buddy system or calling a support person when he or she experiences cravings.
- Explore effectiveness of regular gum, hard candy, and so on for use during cravings.
- Tell the individual to:
  - Avoid social activities and situations where people smoke, during the first week of abstinence.
  - Restrict the intake of caffeine if restlessness and anxiety are pronounced.
  - Incorporate daily exercise into the cessation plan.
  - Use relaxation strategies and imagery to control cravings.
- Help the person construct an image of himself or herself as a nonsmoker.
- Provide regular and enthusiastic support and encouragement for efforts. Openly express confidence that the individual can be successful in quitting.
- Encourage the individual to set aside his or her "cigarette money" and spend it on a reward for nonsmoking.
- Encourage involvement with community supports for quitting as available. Remind the family to be enthusiastic and supportive of the person's efforts.

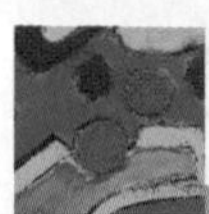

PATIENT/FAMILY TEACHING *Safe Use of Nicotine Gum*

- Remember that nicotine gum is not standard gum.
- Take a piece of nicotine gum and chew it a few times to break it down. Chewing will release a "peppery" taste. When this occurs, park the gum between the gum and cheek. Do not continue to chew it. The nicotine takes several minutes to reach the brain, so the effects are less intense than those achieved with smoke inhalation.
- Repeat at intervals, continuing the chew-and-park strategy for about 30 total minutes.
- Excessive chewing can release the nicotine too quickly. The nicotine mixes with saliva and may cause dizziness, nausea, and soreness in the mouth and throat. It is not effectively absorbed into the bloodstream and does not reduce cravings.
- Do not smoke while chewing nicotine gum.

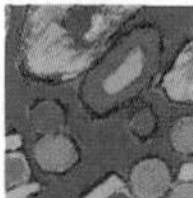

TABLE 3-1 COMMON MEDICATIONS *for Smoking Cessation Programs*

Drug	Action	Nursing Intervention
Bupropion (Wellbutrin, Wellbutrin SR, Zyban)	Inhibits reuptake of dopamine, norepinephrine, and serotonin	Assess for therapeutic effect—smoking cessation after 7 weeks; risk of seizures; withdrawal symptoms such as headache, nausea, vomiting. Teach patient to use caution when driving, to avoid alcohol ingestion, to notify provider if pregnant, and to expect effects to take 2-4 weeks and treatment to last 7-12 weeks.
Nicotine gum (Nicorette, Nicorette Plus)	Acts as antagonist at nicotinic receptors in central and peripheral nervous systems	Assess for adverse side effects such as irritation of buccal membranes. Assess for patient misuse. Teach patient to chew slowly and not to chew for more than 45 minutes.
Nicotine patch (Habitrol, NicoDerm CQ, Nicotrol)	Acts as antagonist at nicotinic receptors in central and peripheral nervous systems	Assess for therapeutic effects. Teach patient how to use properly, to cease smoking immediately when using patch treatment, to keep out of reach of children, and not to use if pregnant.
Nicotine nasal spray (Nicotrol NS)	Acts as antagonist at nicotinic receptors in central and peripheral nervous systems	Assess for therapeutic effects. Teach patient proper use of spray.
Nicotine inhaler (Nicotrol Inhaler)	Acts as antagonist at nicotinic receptors in central and peripheral nervous systems	Assess for therapeutic effects. Teach patient proper use of inhaler.

Critical Thinking

1. A 38-year-old single mother with four children between the ages of 8 and 16 works full time and finds it difficult to find time to exercise. She has been slowly gaining weight and is dissatisfied with both her appearance and fitness. Her father died in his forties of a heart attack, and she expresses concern about following in his footsteps. She has numerous barriers to establishing an exercise program. She has minimal disposable income, the children get home from school at different times and are all involved in school or community activities, and she is the only driver in the family. She states that she is always tired. What approach would you take to help her achieve her stated goal of improving her fitness, considering the constraints of her lifestyle? What other health areas of concern should you talk to her about? How important is her family history? Should she be concerned about this?
2. What is the rationale for choosing a health promotion lifestyle? How can you defend this choice to someone who states, "My dad lived to be 87 years of age but he smoked all his life and was overweight, so why should I worry about my health?"?

References

1. Barnes JB, Schoenborn CA: *Physical activity among adults: United States, 2000*, Pub No PHS 2003-1250 03-0234, Hyattsville, Md, May 14, 2003, US Department of Health and Human Services.
2. Brown DW: Associations between physical activity dose and health-related quality of life, *Med Sci Sports Exercise* 36(5):890, 2004.
3. Centers for Disease Control and Prevention National Center for Health Statistics: *Overweight prevalence,* accessed May 17, 2004, from website: www.cdc.gov/nchs/fastats/overwt.htm.
4. McInnis KJ: Diet, exercise, and the challenge of combating obesity in primary care, *J Cardiovasc Nurs* 18(2):93, 2003.

5. Mokdad AH et al: Actual causes of death in the United States, 2000, *JAMA* 291(10):293-294, 2004.
6. Orleans T et al: National action plan to reduce smoking during pregnancy: the national partnership to help pregnant smokers quit, *Nicotine Tobacco Res* Supp 2:S269, 2004.
7. Ozminkowski RJ et al: Estimating risk reduction required to break even in a health promotion program, *Am J Health Promo* 18(4):316, 2004.
8. Pender NJ et al: *Health promotion in nursing practice,* ed 4, Upper Saddle River, NJ, 2002, PrenticeHall.
9. Ratzan SC: Modernizing medicine: demonstrating a policy of prevention, *J Health Comm* 9(2):89, 2004.
10. Sandison R et al: Lifestyle factors for promoting bone health in older women, *J Adv Nurs* 45(6):603, 2004.
11. Thomas NE et al: Established and recently identified coronary heart disease risk factors in young people: the influence of physical activity and physical fitness, *Sports Med* 33(9):633, 2003.
12. US Department of Health and Human Services, Public Health Service: *Healthy People 2000: national health promotion and disease prevention objectives,* Pub No PHS 91-50212, Washington, DC, 1990, US Government Printing Office.
13. US Department of Health and Human Services: *Healthy People 2010: understanding and improving health,* Washington, DC, 2000, The Department.
14. US Surgeon General: *Healthy People: the surgeon general's report on health promotion and disease prevention,* Washington, DC, 1979, Department of Health, Education and Welfare.
15. US Surgeon General: *Promoting health/preventing disease: objectives for the nation,* Washington, DC, 1980, USDHHS.

evolve Visit the Evolve website: http://evolve.elsevier.com/Monahan/medsurg

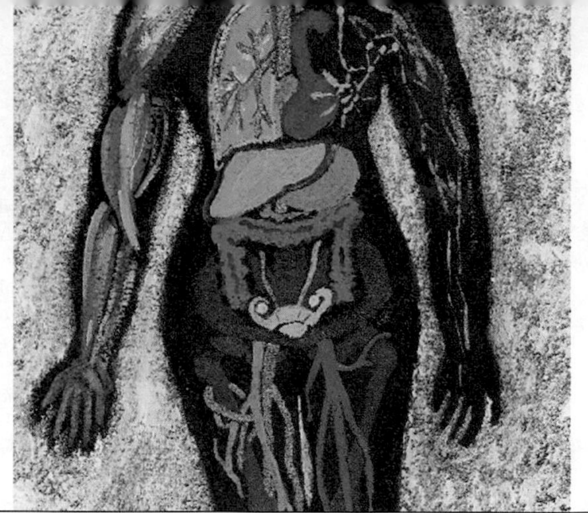

CHAPTER 4

Complementary and Alternative Therapies

by Audrey Snyder

OBJECTIVES

After studying this chapter, the learner should be able to:

1. Contrast allopathic and homeopathic philosophies.
2. Define complementary and alternative therapies.
3. Describe the theory, practice, and patterns of use associated with commonly used complementary and alternative therapies.
4. Discuss the nurse's role in advising persons about complementary and alternative therapies.

KEY TERMS

allopathy, p. 50
alternative medical systems, p. 52
alternative therapies, p. 51
biologically based therapies, p. 52
complementary therapies, p. 51
energy therapies, p. 52
homeopathy, p. 51
manipulative therapies, p. 52
mind-body therapies, p. 52

Recovery from illness is one of life's most incredible phenomena. In today's society the physician is typically viewed as the "healer," with other members of the health care team playing complementary roles in the prevention, detection, and treatment of disease. Yet for most of the human race's 2-million year history, people recovered from many illnesses without the intervention of high-technology scientific medicine. A vast array of healing practices clearly existed long before the advent of modern medicine.

In the natural course of any illness a person becomes ill, either acutely with symptoms such as pain, fever, nausea, or bleeding; or insidiously with a gradual progression of symptoms. If the illness is mild and transient, the symptoms disappear with self-treatment or even no treatment. If the illness is more severe or of longer duration, the person may seek expert help from a "healer," who is usually but not always a physician or nurse practitioner. Other choices for help include a wide range of alternative, complementary, and ethnocultural or traditional therapies. Choice of these other care options is often influenced by economic, social, and cultural factors. Many individuals move easily between more than one health care therapy.

The ill person usually recovers or expects to recover. Recovery is by and large a natural biologic phenomenon that occurs regardless of the treatment provided. This fascinating process of recovery from illness defies full understanding but has stimulated the development of numerous forms of healing that attempt to augment the natural phenomenon. Over the centuries natural healing has been attributed to all sorts of rituals, including cupping, leeching, and bleeding. Every culture has its own traditional therapies that have been passed down through generations.

The Allopathic Philosophy

The dominant health care system in the United States is allopathic and is predicated on a dualistic philosophy that sees the person as "body and mind." Allopathic practices are derived from scientific models of inquiry and involve the extensive use of technology. The word *allopathy* has two divergent origins. One origin, from a Greek root word meaning "other than disease," reflects the use of drugs that may have no consistent or logical relationship to a patient's symptoms. The second origin is from German roots that mean "all therapies." In this context **allopathy** is a "system of medicine that embraces all methods of proven value in the treatment of diseases." The American Medical Association (AMA) adopted the second definition of allopathy in 1855 and has subsequently exclusively determined who can practice medicine in the United States. For example, in the 1860s the AMA refused to admit women doctors to medical societies, practiced segregation, and demanded the purging of homeopaths from the practice of medicine.

Today allopathic physicians are becoming more accepting of other health care providers such as homeopaths, osteopaths, and chiropractors, and even such traditional healers as lay midwives and herbalists. Nursing education in the United States is firmly rooted in the domain of allopathic medicine, since traditional physicians designed the original curriculums and provided most of the instruction. However, nursing's caring ethic and holistic view of patients and illness make it easier for most nurses to accept the value and relevance of less traditional approaches. Today most nursing programs incorporate education about complementary and alternative therapies into their curriculums.

The Homeopathic Philosophy

The homeopathic health care philosophy is also practiced in the United States today, although it is less well known. Samuel C. Hahnemann developed homeopathic medicine in Germany between 1790 and 1810. Homeopathy, or homoeopathy, is derived from the Greek words *homoios* ("similar") and *pathos* ("suffering"). The practice of **homeopathy** treats the person, not the disease. The dominant allopathic system has not validated or endorsed homeopathy, yet countless people use it. Homeopathy treats illness by giving very dilute medications that are derived from plant, animal, and mineral sources. Homeopathy espouses a holistic philosophy that sees health as a "balance of the physical, mental, and spiritual whole" and encompasses a wide range of health care practices that are often referred to as "complementary" or "alternative."[18] Complementary and alternative therapies include a range of philosophies, approaches, and therapies that conventional medicine does not commonly use, accept, study, or understand. Yet many of these therapies fit comfortably into nursing's holistic philosophies.

History of Complementary and Alternative Therapies

The terms *alternative* and *complementary* therapy are often used interchangeably, but differ in their definitions and applications. **Alternative therapies** are used in place of traditional allopathic therapies, whereas **complementary therapies** are used in conjunction with traditional allopathic therapies.[12] The use of complementary and alternative therapies has grown steadily since the 1970s, when the holistic health care movement blossomed in the United States. With the growing interest in these health care options, debate has emerged concerning their usefulness in patient care. A growing body of knowledge and research and improved communication between conventional and alternative practitioners, particularly since the early 1990s, have helped bridge some of the differences, but more is left to be done. The use of the term *integrative therapies* signals a more collaborative approach to patient care. It encompasses the treatment of patients with both traditional allopathic and alternative therapies concurrently. This chapter uses the abbreviation *CAT* to indicate the broad range of complementary and alternative therapies.

Humans are complex, multidimensional beings with subtle interactions between body, mind, emotion, and spirit that connect individuals to their environment and other people. Just as the concept of wellness means more than being momentarily healthy or without disease, no illness is purely physical. The effects of illness manifest themselves physically, mentally, socially, and spiritually. Well-being in all these dimensions is the state often thought of as optimal health.

Some CATs are holistic and treat the whole person. Individuals use these holistic CATs because they foster an overall sense of well-being, offer the person a sense of control, and focus on healing the person rather than curing the disease. Many patients who desire to be active participants in diagnosis and treatment choose a CAT.[2] Other CATs are more preventive and seek to preserve or enhance the person's optimal health and thereby increase his or her resistance to disease.[4]

Although CATs have been in use in other countries for centuries, most of these therapies are just now achieving recognition and popularity in the United States. Advances in technology and communication and the evolution of our world into a "global village" have broken down some of the barriers between CATs and conventional medicine. As more research confirms the validity of specific therapies, some therapies will move from the CAT category into the realm of accepted practice. Insurance companies are increasing their coverage for certain CATs in an attempt to reduce the overall cost of health care and respond to consumer demand for services.

Research on many CATs did not take place in the past because of a lack of funding. In 1992 Congress established the Office of Alternative Medicine within the National Institutes of Health, with a budget of $2 million and a mission to evaluate CATs and communicate the results to the public. In 1998 the office expanded to become the National Center for Complementary and Alternative Medicine (NCCAM), with a $50 million budget designed to stimulate, develop, and support research on complementary and alternative medicine. More than 25 NCCAM-sponsored centers across the county are actively researching CATs.[16] Accessibility of CATs may now be a factor in an institution's ability to attract patients within a competitive health care environment.

Successful integration of CATs and traditional allopathic treatment depends on the creation of an environment of openness between health care providers and patients about the use of CATs. Despite the growing use of CATs, most patients still are reluctant to discuss their use with a primary care provider.[6] Professional education is needed to improve patient-provider communication about CATs.

Definition of CATs

CATs are interventions for improving, maintaining, and promoting health and well-being; preventing disease; or treating illness that are not a part of the standard North American system of health care or disease prevention. A more definitive definition has yet to be developed.

Many CATs alleviate symptoms, but do not cure a disease process. CATs can decrease the symptoms associated with certain chronic conditions (e.g., cancer, heart disease, diabetes, arthritis, and chronic pain syndromes) and are used to treat back pain, allergies, fatigue, arthritis, headache, neck problems, hypertension, sprain and strains, and insomnia. Most CATs incorporate the important role of mindfulness and attitude in healing. They also integrate the person's cultural background and personal beliefs into the treatment process.

In 1995 a consensus conference group evaluated the available research on CATs related to pain management and concluded that a number of well-defined complementary and alternative interventions decrease pain and increase comfort. The preponderance of the evidence supports the efficacy of cognitive-behavioral applications. At present there are insufficient data to conclude that one intervention is inherently better than another for a given condition, yet evidence does support the conclusion that one approach may be better than another for a given individual. Individual differences in response to treatment modalities have always been apparent in the practice literature.

Evaluating CATs in a familiar, scientific manner is difficult. The "gold standard" for clinical research involves the use of randomized controlled trials, but such trials cannot be the only method of evaluating safety, outcomes, effectiveness, and cost-effectiveness of CATs. CATs are based on paradigms of the person as a whole, which complicates research efforts that use a traditional scientific paradigm that looks at the impact of a therapy from just one perspective. New research strategies are needed that are capable of considering nonspecific effects, placebo responses, and individual differences in response to therapies.

Classifications of CATs

NCCAM has grouped CATs into five major domains: alternative medical systems, mind-body interventions, biologically based treatments, manipulative and body-based methods, and energy therapies.[12] Many cultures throughout the world practice **alternative medical systems**, such as Ayurvedic medicine; homeopathic or naturopathic medicine; and traditional Oriental medicine, which encompasses acupuncture, herbal medicine, Oriental massage, and qi gong.[18] **Mind-body therapies** enhance the mind's ability to affect bodily function. This domain includes meditation; hypnosis; dance, music, and art therapy; and prayer. **Biologically based therapies** include natural products such as herbal products, special diets, orthomolecular therapies, and biologic therapies. **Manipulative therapies** and body-based therapies include chiropractic and massage therapy. **Energy therapies** include biofield therapies (focusing on energy originating within the body) such as qi gong, reiki, and therapeutic touch; and electromagnetic field therapies (focusing on energy from other sources) such as pulsed fields or magnetic fields.[14]

Many therapies cross the boundaries of the domain classifications or may be used in combinations. For example, massage therapy is a body-based method, but Oriental massage is a part of traditional Oriental medicine. Qi gong is an energy therapy but is also a part of traditional Oriental medicine. Reiki is an energy therapy, and acupressure is a component of Oriental medicine. Both may be included in a massage session, which is a body-based therapy.

The following descriptions are not inclusive but are meant to increase awareness of some common CATs. Additional information about particular therapies is available from the references, organizations, and websites listed at the end of the chapter.

Alternative Medical Systems

Chinese Medicine

Chinese medicine is based on the belief that the body is pervaded with energy, or Qi, which is produced from the air and food and travels throughout the body providing nourishment and engendering movement for healthy and normal functioning. Both Qi and blood travel along the meridians, extensive pathways or channels that connect the surface of the body and the internal organs. The balance of yin and yang influences Qi. When yin and yang are balanced, they work with the natural flow of Qi to help the body achieve and maintain health. Traditional Chinese medicine includes a variety of therapies such as acupuncture, acupressure, auricular therapy, moxibustion, and qi gong.

Acupuncture. Acupuncture was developed in China and has been in use for more than 2000 years.[12] Acupuncture involves stimulating specific anatomic points in the body for therapeutic purposes such as pain reduction, healing, or physiologic changes. The body has more than 2000 acupuncture points, which connect 12 main and 8 secondary meridians.[12] Practitioners usually stimulate these points using a thin, hair-sized needle, but they may also use heat, pressure, friction, suction, laser light, or impulses of electromagnetic energy. Most states require a license, registration, or certification to practice acupuncture (Box 4-1).

Adherents believe that acupuncture balances the Qi that flows through the body's 12 major meridians. Each meridian and anatomic point are linked to internal organs and specific problems, so pathologic conditions can be accurately targeted. Basic scientific research suggests that acupuncture relieves pain through the neurologic pathways. High-threshold sensory nerves at the acupuncture points are stimulated and send messages to the spinal cord, midbrain, and pituitary to release endorphins and block pain. Cortisol levels are also elevated, which may explain the prolonged pain relief achieved by patients with arthritis.

The acupuncturist diagnoses illness by assessing the quantity and quality of Qi flowing through the channels and determining the individual's balance. After the assessment, the practitioner selects points to stimulate based on the theory that when Qi is blocked, it causes pain and dysfunction, and that restoration of flow is critical to the health of the body and mind. Treatment focuses on removing the pathogenic agents that have invaded the channels, thus relieving the stagnation of Qi and blood. Chronic conditions generally require more acupuncture sessions than acute problems.

Although our understanding of the action of acupuncture is simplistic, its effects can be profound. Acupuncture is safe and has a much lower incidence of complications than invasive surgical procedures. However, possible adverse effects, including infection and organ puncture, are possible, just as with other CATs and conventional therapies. Contraindications to acupuncture are listed in Box 4-2.

Box 4-1 Choosing a Safe Acupuncture Practitioner

- Check state laws regarding practitioner certification, licensure, and registration requirements.
- Explore a potential practitioner's training, experience, licensure, certification, and registration.
- Obtain a referral if possible.
- Ensure that the practitioner uses new, sterile needles for each acupuncture session.

Box 4-2 Contraindications to Acupuncture

- Phobias to needles
- Clotting disorders such as hemophilia
- Pregnancy
- Age less than 7 years
- The influence of alcohol or narcotic medications
- Dementia

Acupuncture is among the most researched and documented of CAT practices. However, given the pervasive skepticism in conventional medicine and the fact that acupuncture requires individualized protocols, randomized clinical trials have thus far focused on only a limited number of conditions.[17,20] At a National Institutes of Health consensus conference held in November 1997, a panel of experts scrutinized the research and literature on acupuncture to determine which conditions, based on published evidence, were best suited to acupuncture treatment.[17] They found acupuncture to be effective in treating the nausea caused by surgical anesthesia and cancer chemotherapy, as well as pain after dental surgery. Acupuncture was also found to be useful by itself or combined with conventional therapies to treat addiction, headaches, menstrual cramps, tennis elbow, fibromyalgia, myofascial pain, osteoarthritis, lower back pain, carpal tunnel syndrome, and asthma.[17] Acupuncture was also shown to assist in stroke rehabilitation. The panel asked third-party insurance carriers to reimburse for the use of acupuncture for these conditions. The Future Watch box describes the use of acupuncture points for the injection of bee venom in a unique blend of therapies.

Acupressure. Acupressure is a combination of acupuncture and massage in which the thumbs and fingertips apply pressure to stimulate pressure points along the acupuncture meridians. Acupressure may be incorporated into a massage therapy session. The Research box summarizes a review of the literature on the use of acupuncture and acupressure for relieving chemotherapy-associated nausea and vomiting.

Auricular Therapy. Auricular therapy is the diagnosis and treatment of pain and disease using the auricle, or pinna, of the ear. Points on the ear, which represent different parts of the body and its structure, are stimulated with needles, magnets, lasers, massage, or electricity. The technique has been found to be useful in smoking cessation and addiction control therapy.

Future Watch

Bee Venom Acupuncture

This study compared injection of bee venom into acupuncture points and non-acupuncture points in rats with induced arthritis. Bee venom injected into a non-acupuncture point inhibited paw edema and reduced nociceptive behaviors in comparison to the control group ($p < 0.05$). Injection into an acupuncture point produced a greater analgesic effect on arthritic pain than injection into a non-acupuncture point ($p < 0.05$). Bee venom acupuncture may become an alternative therapy for long-term arthritis treatment.

Kwon Y-B et al: Bee venom injection into an acupuncture point reduces arthritis associated with edema and nociceptive responses, *Pain* 90:271-280, 2001.

Research

Collins KB, Thomas DJ: Acupuncture and acupressure for the management of chemotherapy induced nauseas and vomiting, *J Am Acad Nurse Pract* 16(2):76-80, 2004.

This study reviewed the available research regarding the use and effectiveness of acupuncture and acupressure for chemotherapy-induced nausea and vomiting. Researchers investigated both Internet and printed scientific sources. They concluded that research supports the effectiveness of both acupuncture and acupressure for the treatment of chemotherapy-induced nausea and vomiting and that both treatments are safe and effective. Since it is estimated that even with the best antiemetic protocols about 60% of chemotherapy patients continue to experience associated nausea and vomiting, the National Institutes of Health endorses the concurrent use of these alternative therapies to improve symptom management. When used along with antiemetic medications, acupuncture and acupressure are safe and effective in relieving chemotherapy-induced nausea and vomiting.

Moxibustion. Moxibustion uses the powdered leaves of moxa herb or mugwort *(Artemisia vulgaris)*. The herb is burned above the skin or on an already inserted needle at the acupuncture points to apply heat and alleviate a variety of symptoms.

Qi Gong, Chi Kung, and T'ai Chi'. Qi gong, chi kung, and t'ai chi' all have their roots in Chinese martial arts. *T'ai chi'* means "meditation in motion." Practice may involve vigorous exercise or slow movements and postures that focus on Qi, performed in a continuous chain of movement. The technique demands mindfulness of movement and breathing and can increase circulation. The routine is usually practiced daily as a part of an overall health maintenance program.

Homeopathy

The American Institute of Homeopathy, founded in the United States in 1845, was the first national medical society. Two years later the AMA was founded, which slowed the growth of homeopathy. Homeopathy experienced a resurgence in the 1970s with the growth of the holistic health movement. Many current homeopathy practitioners have also been educated as allopathic medical doctors.

Homeopathy is based on the law of similar—like cures like. The similar principle "suggests that any state of disturbance that is not corrected spontaneously (and leads to a state of 'disease') can be corrected by minute doses of a compound which at a higher dose can produce effects closely resembling the symptoms of the disease being treated; or by minute amounts of the compound actually causing the disease."[13] This theory was the basis for early vaccine development. The immune system is strengthened when it is exposed to a small amount of a disease component. The component is too weak to cause the disease but allows the body to fight off the related disease. Currently allergies are treated in the same manner with the introduction of the allergen in small doses.

The dose is progressively increased, and an antibody response or resistance to the allergen develops.

The homeopathic practitioner gives small doses of a compound, derived from plant, animal, or mineral sources, which in large doses may produce symptoms of a disease in a healthy person. Frequently homeopathic remedies are prepared with tinctures of plants in ethyl alcohol or water. The mixture is shaken and strained over a 2- to 4-week period. Potentization is the combination of diluting and shaking of a substance. The higher potencies (meaning more dilute) are more powerful than lower potencies. Homeopathic medicines may be so dilute that no molecules of the original substance remain, but adherents believe that a pattern of the substance remains. Preparations are given in tablet, granule, ointment, liquid, or suppository form, and more than one remedy can be used to treat the same problem. Determination of a specific remedy is based on a person's unique pattern of symptoms.

Homeopathy is one of the most difficult forms of CAT for most people to accept. Individuals simply do not expect it to work. Clinical trials, however, have shown positive effects, which cannot be explained by the placebo effect alone. A foundational metaanalysis that compared the results of homeopathic treatment with placebo is reported in the Research box. More research is clearly needed.

Consumers can purchase homeopathic remedies over the counter without a prescription. Health food stores also stock homeopathic preparations containing minute amounts of several remedies believed to be beneficial in treating the symptoms indicated on the label. The use of multiple substances is based on the premise that each substance has been beneficial in some patients, so one of them should work. Homeopathy has few documented adverse effects.

▶ ARE You READY?

In discussing the use of acupuncture with a patient experiencing chemotherapy-induced nausea and vomiting, the nurse includes which of the following statements?

1. "This treatment will prevent the nausea and vomiting."
2. "This treatment works by distracting you from the nausea and vomiting."
3. "Many people believe that their nausea and vomiting are successfully controlled with this treatment."
4. "You will experience less nausea and vomiting as the duration of treatment increases."

Research

Linde K et al: Are the clinical effects of homeopathy placebo effects? A meta-analysis of placebo-controlled trials, *Lancet* 350:834, 1997.

In a review of 186 studies of homeopathy treatment, 89 of which fit predefined criteria for metaanalysis double blind or randomized placebo-controlled clinical trials, the clinical effects of homeopathy could not be explained solely by the placebo effect. Homeopathic medicine treatment was found to have a 2.24 times greater positive effect on patients than placebo alone.

Mind-Body and Spiritual Therapies

Mind-body medicine involves psychologic (behavioral), social, and spiritual approaches, with a great deal of overlap among the categories (Box 4-3). Options include art therapy, biofeedback, color therapy, hypnosis, imagery, prayer and spiritual healing, relaxation techniques, and sound therapy, including binaural beat technology.

Hypnosis

Hypnosis is a state of attentive, focused concentration with suspension of some peripheral awareness. A hypnotic state has four components: absorption or deep contemplation of a theme or focus, controlled alteration of attention, dissociation or compartmentalization of one's experience, and suggestibility or capacity for heightened responsiveness to instructions. Hypnosis has been used to treat pain, duodenal ulcers, irritable bowel syndrome, and nausea, as well as for smoking cessation. Some people are more susceptible than others to hypnosis.

Imagery

Imagery is an ancient healing technique that uses pictures and symbols to open communication among perception, emotion, and bodily changes. Guided imagery can help reduce pain, alter the course of a disease, and improve a patient's outlook concerning illness. Imagery can help the person feel more in control of his or her health or recovery process. It has been used to treat anxiety, enhance the immune response, help children cope with the stress of illness, help cancer patients cope with pain, support the dying process, and provide support during stressful procedures[11] (Box 4-4). It can also be used in conjunction with music to enhance healing, support coping, promote relaxation, and enhance postoperative recovery. Imagery in psychotherapeutic settings can deepen patients' ability to reach therapeutic levels of insight and growth. Imagery is a strategy that nurses can easily integrate into their clinical practice.

Imagery involves mental processes (as in imagining) that encourage attitude, behavior, or physiologic reactions. It attempts to cause an internal representation of events that involves the senses (vision, smell, touch, hearing, taste, and proprioception). It is believed to be the natural language of the unconscious mind and involves "thinking with one's senses." Physiologically, imagery communicates information between the mind, the senses, and the emotions so that psychologic insight or bodily responses can become agents of therapeutic change. The technique has also been effectively adapted to help athletes prepare for competitive events.

Guided imagery uses cognitive techniques: simple visualization or direct suggestions, metaphor and storytelling, dream interpretation, drawing, and active imagination. The clinician actively engages the patient's capacity for imagery to affect a specific outcome (Box 4-5). Imagery is a factor in the biofeedback process, in which subjects learn how to alter their physiologic responses. The practice of imagery can contribute to insight and understanding into current concerns, support symptom management (e.g., pain, depression, difficulty breathing), and improve the patients' functional status (e.g., self-soothing to decrease bingeing and vomiting in bulimia nervosa).

Box 4-3 Categories of Mind-Body Therapies

Behavioral (Psychologic)

Psychotherapy
Meditation
Imagery
Hypnosis
Biofeedback
Relaxation techniques
Support groups

Spiritual

Prayer and mental healing
Cross-cultural aspects

Overlapping

Art therapy
Music therapy
Dance therapy
Journaling
Humor
Body psychology
Color therapy
Sound therapy (binaural beat)

Box 4-4 Clinical Applications of Imagery

- Perioperative pain and anxiety
- Control of nausea and vomiting in chemotherapy
- Pain management in cancer
- Psychotherapy and depression
- Restoration of physical function
- Enhancement of the immune system
- Wound healing
- Control of anxiety and pain for those with human immunodeficiency virus or acquired immunodeficiency syndrome
- Asthma management
- Stress management
- Control of burnout
- Bulimia nervosa treatment

Box 4-5 Types of Imagery

- *diagnostic imagery:* Patients describe how they feel in sensory and emotional terms to guide the therapist in designing interventions.
- *mental rehearsal imagery:* Clinicians prepare patients for medical procedures by teaching a relaxation strategy and guiding them through the procedure.
- *end-stage imagery:* Imagery is used to produce a specific physiologic or biologic change in the body such as enhancing immunity.

Training in imagery facilitates its use. Interested clinicians can educate themselves, pursue personal growth work through imagery, practice on themselves, practice with colleagues, and take training programs (see Guidelines for Safe Practice box on p. 56). Empiric research on the effectiveness of imagery is difficult to conduct but is sorely needed. There is also a dearth of well-qualified imagery practitioners.

Spirituality

Spirituality is one's inward sense of something greater than the individual self, a personal awareness of dimensions of existence that extend beyond the physical domain. Spirituality encompasses a variety of perspectives, and personal biases and terminology can be confusing. Spirituality frequently involves but is different from religion. Religion is the outward, concrete experience of believing in something greater than the individual self. Religious care involves helping people maintain their belief systems and worship practices. Spiritual care, on the other hand, involves helping people to maintain their personal relationship to a higher authority as defined by that person, and to identify meaning and purpose in life. Both spirituality and religion have therapeutic potential.

All cultures incorporate spirituality, although many in today's Western culture value material pursuits more highly than spiritual ones. Many people are dismissive of spiritual therapies, since they are not physical or verifiable through the five senses. Material things can be quantified, analyzed, and manipulated. Spiritual understanding depends on a basic faith, and it has no tangible or physical benefit or value.

The healing component of spirituality involves the intentional influence of one or more persons on a living system without using known physical means of interaction. Quieting the mind is usually a prelude to spiritual healing, which is predominantly an activity of the mind as it impinges on matter. The planned use of spirituality includes the laying on of hands, intent, prayer, psychic healing, spiritual healing, faith healing, mental healing, and transpersonal healing. It can also involve the energy of heat, tingling, vibration, and color, although it remains unclear whether an unidentified exchange of energy or energy fields actually occurs during the healing interaction.

Spiritual healing has two main types. In the first the healer enters a prayerful altered state of consciousness and views the patient and self as a single entity. In the second the healer touches the person, and energy flows through the healer's hand to the patient's area of disease. Many cultures accept the laying on of hands as a powerful means of healing. Reports have been published

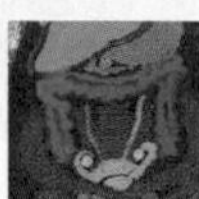

GUIDELINES FOR SAFE PRACTICE *The Use of Imagery*

- Imagery techniques can alter blood glucose levels. Blood glucose should be monitored with the use of imagery in diabetic patients. Imagery may be contraindicated in patients with unstable diabetes.
- Imagery can induce seizures in susceptible patients as it alters brain wave activity.
- It is inadvisable to use imagery for patients with a history of psychosis. Imagery is generally a safe technique, but it can evoke intense latent feelings and inner conflicts, and caution is necessary.
- Imagery should not produce harmful physical or psychologic effects in patients. Imagery is an adjunct, a support system, and not a replacement for clinical care.

of healers being able to influence a variety of cellular and other biologic systems through mental means. Physiologic function can be affected from a distance.

Nurses need to explore spiritual and religious issues with patients as consistently as they do physical ones. The experience of illness has the potential to transform a person. People may reexamine goals and values, clarify priorities, mend broken relationships, and discover inner resources. Reports of spontaneous healing indicate that patients may occasionally heal themselves. The belief that life-threatening diseases such as cancer can disappear suddenly and completely, and that radical healing is somehow connected with one's state of mind, is more common than is generally acknowledged. The belief that "miracles do happen" may help restore hope and a fighting spirit, which are important to recovery from illness.

Prayer

Prayer is a universal spiritual practice, a conscious relationship with the force of the universe, or God. It may take the form of intercessory prayer, confession, gratitude, or silent communion. Prayer involves no direct physical contact and no attempt to do anything or give anything. The only goal is to become one with the person and his or her god. Seeking medical care and using prayer are not mutually exclusive activities.

Meditation

Meditation creates a state of deep, quiet contemplation that filters out distractions and seeks to refine consciousness so that thought and being are in tune with the universal plan. Quiet centering or meditation for just 20 minutes each day can redirect energies for healing and decrease stress (see Research box). Meditation decreases oxygen consumption and cardiac and respiratory rates and is a component of some types of yoga. Meditation is contraindicated for persons who fear loss of control such as those with a history of schizophrenia or psychosis.

Yoga

Yoga is a philosophy that integrates the spiritual, mental, emotional, and physical aspects of life. The word *yoga* means the union of different aspects of the individual. Yoga has several different forms, but they all involve self-improvement through focused breathing, stretching, and meditation. Yoga emphasizes breath as the link connecting mind, body, spirit, and emotions. *Prana,* or life force energy, is taken in through the nose with breathing. Principles of the Alexander technique (discussed later in this chapter) are derived from yoga. Yoga techniques are used to improve a wide variety of problems (e.g., hypertension, depression, osteoporosis, and the discomforts associated with menopause).

Group Therapy

Group therapy provides mutual support, encouragement, and socialization. It can be used for psychologic therapy, to work through grief and loss, to lose weight, or to work on self-improvement. Group therapy usually centers around a common theme, for example, a breast cancer survivors support group.

Art and Color Therapy

Art, light, color, and environment affect mood and attitude. Art and color allow a person to express inner needs and desires and record dreams and meditations. Art and color therapy may be used along with other mind-body therapies.

Music Therapy

Music is part of everyday life. Different parts of the body resonate to different sounds and pitches. The controlled use of music can influence a person during illness or injury treatment. Some music is specifically recorded at 60 beats/min, the rate of the resting heartbeat, to promote relaxation and decrease heart rate. This music has been used effectively in coronary care units, neonatal nurseries, and cancer units. Music therapy can also decrease stress

Research

Gross C et al: Mindfulness meditation to reduce symptoms after organ transplant: a pilot study, *Alt Ther* 10(3):58-66, 2004.

This longitudinal study evaluated the effect of a Mindfulness-Based Stress Reduction (MBSR) program on symptoms of depression, anxiety, sleep disturbance, and quality of life at baseline, postcourse, and 3 months later for solid organ transplant patients. Participants completed an MBSR program for 2.5 hours a week for 8 weeks and were asked to practice meditation at least five times a week for 45 minutes. Scores for depression ($p=0.006$) and sleep disturbance ($p=0.011$) improved at completion of the course. At 3 months scores for sleep disturbance ($p=0.002$) and anxiety ($p=0.043$) improved over baseline. Quality of life ratings were not improved.

and anxiety. Binaural beat tapes use a combination of rhythm and beat, delivering it asynchronously and separately to each ear through headphones. Voice-guided imagery with voice over music or music over voice can also be used. Music chosen for relaxation must meet the individual's needs and preferences, since individual responses can vary.

Biofeedback

Biofeedback involves the self-regulation or voluntary control of an internal state. Patients learn to regulate their physiologic functions in subtle ways through the use of noninvasive electronic monitoring equipment involving blood pressure, heart rate, skin temperature, electroencephalogram, or electromyogram recordings. The technique allows patients to participate in their own healing. It has been particularly helpful in treating hypertension, Raynaud's disease, migraines, and lower back pain.

Relaxation Therapy

Stress erodes health and well-being. It affects the nervous and immune systems, emotions, and how we relate to others. Stress management techniques may reverse disease and lower blood pressure and heart rate. Virtually all the mind-body therapies can also be effectively used as part of a stress management program.

Relaxation therapy can be somatic or cognitive. Somatic relaxation therapy uses observation to purposefully relax muscles, whereas cognitive relaxation therapy uses a mental device such as a word, sound, or breathing to relax the body and mind. Relaxation techniques are effective in reducing chronic pain such as headache, back pain, menstrual pain, orthopedic postoperative pain, and rheumatic pain. They are easy to teach and learn, and a nurse can use them effectively at the bedside. Relaxation is the foundation of widely used techniques for prepared childbirth such as Lamaze.

Psychoneuroimmunology

Psychoneuroimmunology is the study of mechanisms that turn thoughts and feelings into chemical and neurologic sequelae. It explores the interaction between behavior, neural and endocrine activity, and the immune process. Psychologic distress can suppress the immune system and increase the risk of illness. At the same time a person can work with mind and emotions to increase resistance to disease or to influence recovery. It has been used effectively to treat headaches; moderate blood pressure, heart rate, and rhythm; heal ulcers and irritable bowel syndrome; manage pain, anger, anxiety, and panic; and reduce muscle spasms.

▶ ARE You READY?

Imagery is inadvisable in patients with a history of which of the following?

1. Chronic pain
2. Psychosis
3. Chemotherapy-induced nausea and vomiting
4. Diabetes mellitus

Biologically Based Therapies

Biologically based therapies include the use of natural products, both botanical and herbal, and nutritional supplements. Natural products represent one of the fastest growing consumer markets in the United States. This section discusses some commonly used nutritional supplements and herbal therapies.

Herbal Medicine

Phytomedicine, the use of plant material for medicinal purposes, has been used by every known culture. In the United States the Frontier Nursing Service nurses used herbs in addition to pharmaceuticals to treat a variety of health problems. They made tea from ginseng leaves to treat colic and menstrual pain, made arrowwood bark into cough syrup, and used cloves to treat toothaches. Many of these early herbal remedies are still used today.[8] Table 4-1 presents common accessory nutrients.

Unlike pharmaceuticals, herbal and dietary supplements are not regulated and lack quality standards. Different parts of plants yield different things, and a variety of different herbal preparations may be produced (Box 4-6). Herbal elements and content vary depending on the part of the plant harvested, time of year harvested, and soil content. Herbal products often are not as potent as commercially prepared medicines and may take several weeks to build up blood levels of the active ingredient and produce their effects. Box 4-7 summarizes general principles governing the use of herbal products.

People often assume that herbal products are safe because they are natural; but natural does not always guarantee safety, and they are not inherently a better option. A new drug goes through a lengthy clinical trials process to attempt to ensure its safety and efficacy. Pharmaceuticals that are derived from plants (e.g., aspirin, digitoxin, atropine, and morphine) are the chemically isolated constituents of plants. Prescription drugs are purified, standardized, and thoroughly researched; and their pharmacokinetics

Box 4-6 Preparations of Herbal Products

- *infusions (tea):* Steeping herb is added to hot water.
- *decoctions:* Preparations are made from bark and roots.
- *juicing:* Parts are chopped and pressed to get the water-soluble parts.
- *powder:* Dried plant is ground.
- *syrup:* Herb is added to honey and brown sugar in water, then boiled and strained.
- *tincture:* Herb is added to 5% alcohol; it stands 2 weeks, is shaken daily, and then is strained and bottled.
- *ointment:* Herb is added to hot petroleum jelly.
- *poultice:* Crushed plant is mixed with hot moist flour or corn meal to make a warm paste, which is applied to the skin.
- *cold compress:* A cloth is soaked in a cooled infusion and applied to the affected part.
- *herb baths:* Herbs are crushed; bath water is run over the crushed herbs.

TABLE 4-1 ACCESSORY NUTRIENTS

Accessory Nutrient	Effect	Uses and Contraindications
Alpha-lipoic acid	Naturally occurs in the body; taken for its additional antioxidant effect; regenerates glutathione, vitamin E, vitamin C, and other antioxidants in the body	Used for treatment of diabetes, HIV, and age-related diseases; use may alter dose of diabetic medication; long-term effects unknown
Chromium	Necessary nutrient; deficiency contributes to adult diabetes and atherosclerosis; chromium levels decrease with age	Chromium picolinate, the only active form, improves glucose transport across cells, lowers cholesterol, improves lipid profiles
Creatine	Increases muscle power and performance; storage reservoir for quick energy	Used by athletes to increase energy and endurance; GI problems common with high doses
DHEA	Precursor to testosterone in males and progesterone in females; builds muscle mass	Should have laboratory work to see if DHEA level is low; enhances mood and memory; improves immune system; can aid in prevention of heart disease *Caution: hormone precursors are as potent as hormones bought by prescription.*
Glucosamine	Key component in synthesis of proteins found in joint cartilage. These proteins are negatively charged and attract water for production of synovial fluid in joints. Glucosamine used as a supplement is thought to help the body replenish synovial fluid and produce new cartilage.	Frequently recommended in treatment of osteoarthritis, rheumatoid arthritis, tendonitis, gout, and bursitis; in Europe, nonsteroidals are used less, and glucosamine is used more; used frequently in combination with chondroitin or MSM
Melatonin	Hormone that regulates body's circadian rhythms and sleep patterns	Useful for jet lag; helps reset body clock with changing time zones if taken in new time zone at bedtime
NADH	Involved in Krebs cycle and production of energy	May play role in treatment of Parkinson's disease, depression and dementia, and chronic fatigue syndrome; expensive
SAMe	Found in all living cells; a naturally occurring molecule; precursor to certain essential amino acids; supports mood and emotional well-being, as well as joint mobility	Used in treatment of depressive disorders, osteoarthritis, migraine headaches, fibromyalgia, liver disease, and sleep disorders
Omega-3 fatty acids	Lower hyperlipidemia and prevent lowering of HDL	Used in treatment of hypertriglyceridemia
Niacin	Raises HDL cholesterol and lowers triglycerides	Used in treatment of dyslipidemia; reduces cardiovascular risk
Coenzyme Q-10 (ubiquinone)	Used by cells to produce energy needed for cell growth and maintenance; also used as an antioxidant or substance that protects cells from free radicals; may function in tissues as a free radical scavenger, membrane stabilizer, or both	Useful in stabilizing blood pressure, reducing shortness of breath and palpitations, and lessening heart muscle hypertrophy; may have uses in treating ischemic heart disease, in heart failure, and in protecting ischemic myocardium during surgery
MSM	Organic sulfur that exists in all living things; has antioxidant antiinflammatory and analgesic effects	Used in treatment of muscle and joint pain, including arthritis; can interfere with action of arthritis drugs
Probiotics	Live bacteria; restore and improve balance of normal bacterial flora in the GI tract	Useful in regulating microbes in gastrointestinal tract; may be used to improve digestion, prevent infections, or treat diarrheal illnesses

HDL, High-density lipoprotein; *HIV,* human immunodeficiency virus; *DHEA,* dehydroepiandrosterone mesylate; *MSM,* methylsufonylmethane; *NADH,* reduced form of nicotinamide adenine dinucleotide; *SAMe, S*-adenosylmethionine.

Box 4-7 General Principles Concerning Herbal Products

- Herbal products are relatively safe because of the lower concentration of active ingredients.
- A desired therapeutic effect takes time to develop.
- Pharmacologic actions of herbal products are not well understood.
- Herbal products are not usually appropriate in emergency or acute care situations.
- Herbal products are most often used for patients with chronic illnesses with mild, ambiguous symptoms.
- Herbal products have the potential for drug interactions with prescribed drugs and each other, and there are contraindications to use.
- Herbal products have the potential for multiple effects.

and pharmacodynamics are well known. In contrast, herbal or natural products are regulated as foods rather than drugs and are not subject to the clinical trials process. All the chemical ingredients of an herb may not even be known, and the presence of multiple ingredients may create unplanned synergistic effects or potential adverse interactions with prescribed drugs and foods.

Most available information on natural products and associated drug interactions is based on case reports rather than clinical trials. Knowledge concerning drug-herbal interactions is limited by the lack of herbal product standardization: variations in purity and potency, the presence of multiple ingredients, product adulteration, misidentification of ingredients, and batch-to-batch and manufacturer variations related to crop conditions and yield.[5] The pharmacokinetic and physiologic effects of most herbal products are poorly or incompletely understood, and caution must guide the use of any herbal product or nutritional supplement, especially during pregnancy and lactation (Box 4-8).

The 1994 U.S. Dietary Supplement Health and Education Act regulates herbs and herbal products as dietary supplements. Herbal products must now be labeled with side effects, contraindications, potential safety problems, and special warnings. The Food and Drug Administration (FDA) allows manufacturers to make certain health, nutrient content, and structure or function claims on the labels, but the FDA must now review the claims before marketing.[15] For example, companies can make limited structure or function claims such as "promotes healthy prostate." Product labels may also contain statements such as, "This product has not been evaluated by the Food and Drug Administration. This product is not intended to diagnose, treat, cure, or prevent disease." Therapeutic drug effect claims are not allowed. Manufacturers of herbal products and dietary supplements are expected to voluntarily comply with good manufacturing practices. The 1997 Federal Commission on Dietary Supplements recommended that manufacturers provide scientific evidence about their products to consumers. The Guidelines for Safe Practice and Patient/Family Teaching boxes summarize important information about the safe use of herbal products.

Box 4-8 Herbs Contraindicated During Pregnancy and Lactation

Pregnancy

Aloe
Autumn crocus
Black cohosh root
Buckthorn bark and berry
Cascara sagrada bark
Chaste tree fruit
Chinchona bark
Cinnamon bark
Coltsfoot leaf
Combinations of licorice, peppermint, and chamomile
Combinations of senna, peppermint oil, and caraway oil
Combinations of licorice, primrose, marshmallow, and anise
Echinacea purpurea herb
Fennel oil
Ginger root
Indian snakeroot
Juniper berry
Kava kava root
Licorice root
Marsh tea
Mayapple root
Petasite (butterbur)
Rhubarb root
Sage leaf
Senna

Lactation

Aloe
Basil
Buckthorn bark and berry
Cascara sagrada
Coltsfoot leaf
Combinations of senna, peppermint oil, and caraway oil
Indian snakeroot
Kava kava root
Petasite (butterbur)
Rhubarb root
Senna

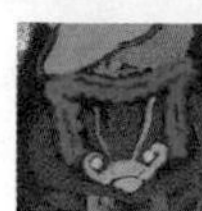

GUIDELINES FOR SAFE PRACTICE *Cautions for the Use of Herbal Products*

- Herbs that should be used cautiously with concurrent anticoagulant use include dong quai *(Angelica sinensis)*, feverfew *(Tanacetum parthenium)*, garlic *(Allium sativum)*, ginseng *(Panax ginseng)*, ginger *(Zingiber officinale)*, and gingko *(Gingko biloba)*. A general rule is that patients on anticoagulants should not use natural products.
- Milkvetch (locoweed, *Astragalus* species) is an immune system enhancer. Its use is contraindicated in patients with autoimmune diseases.
- Chamomile may create a cross-sensitivity in persons allergic to ragweed, asters, and chrysanthemums.
- When stinging nettles are used for allergy treatment, the freeze-dried preparation is needed.
- Ephedra is now being marketed in weight loss products and sports drinks. It has both bronchodilator and stimulant effects and can produce adverse cardiovascular side effects. It interacts with caffeine, decongestants, and stimulants. Deaths have been reported with its use in large quantities. The Food and Drug Administration (FDA) has removed it from U.S. markets as a dietary supplement.
- Senna, when used for colonic stimulation, can potentiate cardiac glycosides, possibly by increasing the loss of potassium.
- Products containing comfrey have been found to cause hepatotoxicity in animal studies.
- Any patient who experiences an adverse reaction to a medication should be questioned about the use of herbal products. Potential herb-drug interactions should be reported according to institution policy or directly to the FDA MedWatch at https://www.accessdata.fda.gov/scripts/medwatch.

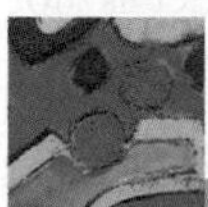

PATIENT/FAMILY TEACHING *Using Herbal Products*

- Discuss herbal products with your health care practitioner.
- Evaluate the available research on the use of the product.
- Research effective herbal dosages.
- Take note of all cautions listed.
- Consider herb-drug interactions.
- Investigate companies that market the herbs. What are their standards?
- Choose a name brand company with quality control.
- Purchase the same brand each time.
- Take herbal products at the same time each day.
- Follow the manufacturer's recommendations (e.g., "drink with 8 oz of water").
- Keep a log of any adverse reactions, and report these to the health care practitioner.

Licensed health care practitioners cannot prescribe natural substances to treat disease, although glucosamine handouts in orthopedic offices have somewhat changed this standard of practice. Many orthopedic physicians routinely recommend the use of glucosamine for joint cartilage regeneration. At present no official mechanism exists for licensing or certifying herbalists in the United States. In Germany, in contrast, herbs are available on the open market, but are thoroughly evaluated by an expert panel of pharmacists, physicians, toxicologists, epidemiologists, and other professionals.[1,3] The rapid globalization of markets for all products underscores the importance of achieving some degree of standardization and uniformity in product preparation around the world.

Research

Schellenberg R: Treatment for premenstrual syndrome with agnus castus fruit extract: prospective, randomized, placebo controlled study, *Brit Med J* 322 (7279):134, 2001.

This placebo-controlled study evaluated the effect of chaste tree berry extract on premenstrual syndrome over three consecutive menstrual cycles. Participants receiving chaste tree berry daily reported less irritability, mood swings, headaches, anger, breast fullness, and bloating than those in the control group. Physicians who were blinded to the group assignments also reported clinical improvement in the treatment group.

Commonly Used Herbal Products. A multitude of herbal preparations are currently on the market. The following section provides an overview of several commonly used herbal products. See the Research box for a study that has validated the usefulness of an herbal product in patient care.

BLACK COHOSH *(CIMICIFUGA RACEMOSA)*. Black cohosh root is a Native American therapy. It is used primarily for treatment of menopausal symptoms and menstrual irregularities and to stimulate uterine contraction. The mechanism of action is unknown. It does exert some estrogenic activity.

BUTTERBUR *(PETASITES HYBRIDUS)*. Butterbur extract is made from the rhizomes, roots, and leaves of this perennial shrub. It is frequently used in the treatment of migraines, chronic cough, asthma, and bladder spasms and in the prevention of gastric ulcers. There may be cross reactivity in patients allergic to daisies and ragweed.

ECHINACEA (AMERICAN CONEFLOWER, PURPLE CONE FLOWER). Echinacea is widely used as an immune system enhancer. Although its efficacy has been challenged by the conclusions of a new series of research studies. It is believed to have antiseptic, antiviral, and peripheral vasodilatory properties and can be used as supportive therapy for colds and flu. Many persons use it for prevention, which is inappropriate use. It is most effective when used at the onset of cold symptoms to reduce the duration and severity of upper respiratory tract infections, both viral and bacterial (Figure 4-1, Patient/Family Teaching box, p. 61).

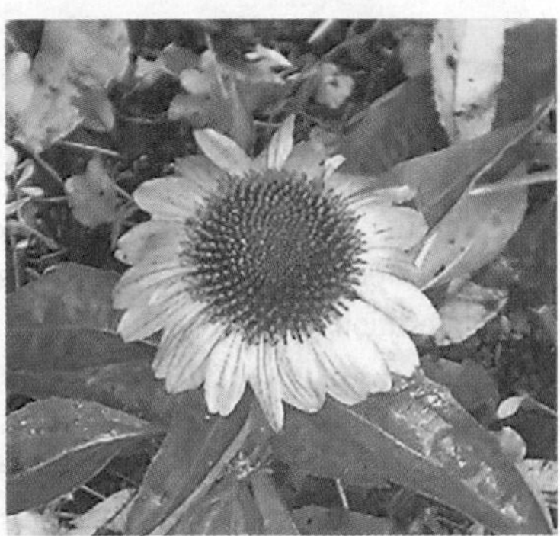

Figure 4-1 Echinacea, a member of the daisy family, bears a single flower with a cone-shaped center and purple rays. It is commonly seen in gardens in the United States.

ELDERBERRY *(SAMBUCUS NIGRA)*. Elderberry is a small tree that grows to heights of 12 feet. All parts of the plant have been used for centuries in traditional folk medicine. The berries contain vitamins A, B, and C; flavonoids; carotenoids; and amino acids. Today it is used topically for infections and to decrease inflammation and swelling. Elderberry tea can help speed recovery from cold and flu symptoms.

FEVERFEW *(TANACETUM PARTHENIUM)*. Feverfew is a member of the sunflower family. It has antipyretic properties and acts like nonsteroidal antiinflammatory medications. It is used to treat arthritis and to reduce fever and inflammation. It also inhibits platelets and should be used with caution by persons concurrently taking anticoagulants. Feverfew should be stopped two weeks before surgical procedures. Feverfew can be effective in preventing migraine headaches, but it must be taken continually and is not useful once a headache has started.

GARLIC *(ALLIUM SATIVUM)*. Garlic has been valued throughout history, at times even used as currency. It is often thought of as a cure-all with antioxidant properties. It lowers cholesterol (lowers low-density lipoprotein cholesterol and triglycerides and raises high-density lipoprotein cholesterol), regulates blood sugar, decreases blood pressure and platelet adhesiveness, prevents age-related vascular changes, and has antibacterial properties. It is believed to be helpful in avoiding heart disease, although it may take months of use before its cholesterol-lowering and hypotensive effects are seen. It is not used with anticoagulants because it can prolong bleeding.

GINGER *(ZINGIBER OFFICINALE)*. Sailors historically chewed ginger root to alleviate seasickness. Today it is used to prevent the nausea and vomiting associated with motion sickness, as a digestive aid, and as a peripheral circulatory stimulant. It is used cautiously with anticoagulants, since it can potentiate bleeding.

GINGKO (KEW TREE, MAIDENHAIR TREE). Gingko is the oldest living plant on earth. In China it is a sacred tree, and Buddhists use it as a temple decoration. It increases general circulation, improves microcirculation, inhibits platelet aggregation, and inactivates oxygen free radicals. It is therefore useful for intermittent claudication and dementia syndromes. It does not appear to improve memory in healthy people but is effective with age-related changes. Gingko may slow the progress of Alzheimer's disease, but it is not a cure. Because gingko inhibits platelet aggregation, it should be used with caution after trauma or surgery. Bleeding is a potential side effect of use. Gingko must be commercially prepared to decrease its toxin content.

GINSENG *(PANAX GINSENG)*. Ginseng has been used since colonial days. It increases resistance to stress and excessive activity and has an invigorating and fortifying effect in times of fatigue or disability. Americans tend to use ginseng out of its proper context. The Chinese have a saying that "if you can feel your ginseng, you've used too much." Ginseng can interact with anticoagulants and potentiate bleeding.

HORSE CHESTNUT *(BASCULES HIPPOCASTANUM)*. Horse chestnut decreases capillary permeability. It has been used to treat symptoms of venous insufficiency and to prevent varicose veins, but it cannot reverse them. Its effects seem to be equivalent to the use of compression stockings.

KAVA KAVA *(PIPER METHYSTICUM)*. Kava kava acts as a sedative and sleep enhancer. It has been used for conditions of nervous anxiety, stress, and restlessness. It should not be combined with alcohol or central nervous system depressants (e.g., antipsychotics, sedatives, sleeping pills). The skin can turn yellow with excessive use. The preparation should not be used for more than 3 months. In some countries kava kava is used as a recreational drug.

ST. JOHN'S WORT *(HYPERICUM PERFORATUM)*. St. John's wort has been used since medieval times as a treatment for mild to moderate depression. It is thought to work like a monoamine oxidase (MAO) inhibitor, and concurrent use with MAO inhibitors should be avoided.[14] Increased evidence shows that St. John's wort interacts with many medications. Reported side effects include hypertension, headache, insomnia, arrhythmias, nervousness, tremors, seizures, stroke, and myocardial infarction.

SAW PALMETTO *(SABAL SERRULATA)*. Saw palmetto has both antiinflammatory and antiedema effects. It is used to treat the urination

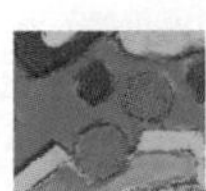

PATIENT/FAMILY TEACHING *Safe and Effective Use of Echinacea*

- Echinacea is contraindicated for patients with autoimmune diseases or those undergoing immunosuppressive therapy.
- Echinacea should be taken at onset of cold symptoms and not used as a preventive therapy.
- Echinacea has no known toxicity, but its effectiveness declines with prolonged use. Many practitioners recommend that a person use echinacea for 10 days and then discontinue use. It should definitely not be used for longer than 8 consecutive weeks without a break.

problems associated with stage 1 and 2 benign prostatic hyperplasia (BPH). Saw palmetto decreases levels of dihydrotestosterone, a hormone believed to be responsible for some of the prostate tissue enlargement associated with BPH.[10] It may produce fewer side effects than common related pharmaceuticals.

TEA TREE OIL *(MELALEUCA ALTERNIFOLIA)*. Tea tree oil has been used for centuries as a topical antiseptic. It is also used for a multitude of skin conditions (e.g., athlete's foot, acne).

VALERIAN ROOT *(VALERIANA OFFICINALIS)*. Valerian root works on gamma-aminobutyric acid receptors, acting like the benzodiazepines. It is used for restlessness, sleeping disorders resulting from nervous conditions, and insomnia. Its effects are immediate, but it does not work for everybody and is not recommended for chronic use.

▶ ARE YOU READY?

In teaching a patient taking Echinacea, the nurse includes which of the following? (Choose all that apply.)

1. "It is most effective in the prevention of cold symptoms."
2. "It should be stopped after 10 days of use."
3. "It is contraindicated for patients on immunosuppressive therapy."
4. "It is not effective with bacterial infections."
5. "It supports the immune system."
6. "It should be started at the onset of cold symptoms."

Nutrition

Nutrition is the science that studies the use of food to promote health and avoid disease; it is one of the most commonly used CATs. Patients recovering from trauma or major illness benefit from nutritional support, but nutrition also plays a major role in the prevention and treatment of chronic disease. Maintaining good nutrition in the face of chronic illness is challenging. Certain foods are associated with improvement of certain symptoms, and laboratory findings can guide nutritional supplementation. For example, instead of using hormone replacements to control menopausal symptoms, a patient can use soy products because of their phytoestrogen content and can supplement the diet with whole grain cereals, vitamin E, vitamin C, beta-carotene, fish oil, calcium, folate, and vitamin B_6. Researchers are evaluating green tea for a variety of positive benefits for the cardiovascular system and for reducing the risk of certain forms of cancer (see Research box). The role of nutrition in health promotion is discussed in more depth in Chapter 3.

Research

Maron DJ et al: Cholesterol-lowering effect of theaflavin-enriched green tea extract, *Arch Intern Med* 163(12):1448-1453, 2003.

This study attempted to determine the effect of green tea extract on high- and low-density lipoprotein cholesterol levels in patients with mild to moderate elevations in cholesterol. The study involved 242 men and women from six urban hospital hypertension clinics in China. All participants were consuming a low-fat diet. Participants were randomized to receive a placebo or a theaflavin-enriched green tea extract capsule taken once daily. Cholesterol levels were evaluated at 4, 8, and 12 weeks. Participants in the treatment group experienced a significant reduction in their total cholesterol ($p=0.01$) and low-density lipoprotein ($p=0.01$) cholesterol levels after 12 weeks. The researchers concluded that green tea extract was a safe and effective adjunct to a low-fat diet for managing mild to moderate cholesterol elevations.

Aromatherapy

Aromatherapy involves the use of essential oils and hydrosols to promote personal health and balance and heal the mind, body, and spirit. The use of aromatherapy dates back 5000 years. Distillation devices to extract oils were found in the ruins of Mesopotamia. Egyptians embalmed the dead with oil from frankincense and myrrh. More recently, soldiers in World Wars I and II carried lavender oil with them on the battlefield to disinfect wounds. In the 1930s Dr. René-Maurice Gattefosse coined the term *aromatherapy* and published a book that earned him the title of "father of modern aromatherapy." Chemically produced medications began to replace essential oils and herbs in medical treatment during the nineteenth century.

Essential oils are applied or inhaled to achieve physical, emotional, and spiritual balance and harmony. Odors are transmitted to the brain via the olfactory nerve and stimulate the limbic system of the brain, which controls primitive needs such as hunger, thirst, and emotion. Odors also act on the hypothalamus, which controls the secretion of hormones in the endocrine system. Smells can affect intuition, emotion, and creativity. A person's reaction to an odor occurs on an emotional and largely subconscious level. Smell is connected with memory; some smells, like a loved one's perfume or home-baked bread, can evoke happy memories; other smells are unpleasant (e.g., antiseptic smells of hospitals) or even painful if the memories are associated with a loved one who has died.

Oils contain hormones, vitamins, natural antibiotics, and antiseptics. Oils are obtained by the process of distillation, in which roots, leaves, flowers, seeds, resins, and gums from plants, flowers, shrubs, or trees are heated with water to release oils in a vaporized form. The steam and vapor are then condensed to a liquid state, and the essential oil floats to the top of the water. The remaining water and micromolecules of essential oil are termed the *hydrosol.*

Aromatherapy may be used with or without touch therapies. Aromatherapy hydrosols are mixed with a base oil of lotion and applied to the skin. They can be used in massage lotions, baths, compresses, steam inhalation, and hair and skin care products. They also may be used in aroma lamps or rings on light bulbs. Small quantities are therapeutic, but larger quantities could be toxic. Internal use is rarely recommended (Table 4-2, Guidelines for Safe Practice box).

Bach Flower Remedies

Bach flower remedies are combinations of flower essences discovered by Edward Bach, a British physician. The combinations are selected from among 38 common, nontoxic flowers. His book, *The Bach Flower Remedies,*[1a] is a reference guide used to help select the appropriate remedy for an individual state of mind. For example, rescue remedy is a combination of five flowers—star of Bethlehem, rock rose, impatiens, cherry plum, and clematis—used to

TABLE 4-2 ESSENTIAL OILS AND REPORTED EFFECTS

Essential Oil	Reported Effect	Medicinal Uses
Cinnamon	Increases appetite	Promotes oral intake
Lavender	A natural antibacterial, antiseptic, and antiinflammatory agent	Headaches, muscular aches, insomnia, hypertension, heart palpitations
Clary sage	Muscle relaxant and digestive stimulant	Respiratory distress, premenstrual syndrome (PMS), headaches *Contraindicated in pregnancy*
Rosemary	Antiseptic and antidepressant; lowers blood pressure; lowers blood glucose	Hypertension, hyperglycemia, colds, flu, asthma, rheumatism
Geranium	Stimulates adrenal cortex; functions as diuretic, astringent, and antiseptic	Balances hormones; menopause, PMS, diabetes, kidney stones, sore throats, skin problems
Peppermint	Stimulates digestion and settles stomach	Used as aid in quitting smoking; may relieve nausea and headaches; topically used as insect repellent and antiseptic *Caution: too strong for use with infants*
Eucalyptus	Promotes respiration and open bronchioles; functions as antiseptic, fever reducer, pain reliever, and diuretic	Used for asthma, bronchitis, sinus infections, sore throat, kidney infections, and rheumatism
Chamomile	Antiinflammatory, pain reliever, fever reducer, and wound healer	Fever, wounds, pain
Rose	Antiseptic; relieves cramps; promotes menstruation	Fever, migraines, PMS
Sandalwood	Antiseptic, diuretic, and expectorant	Fertility problems and imbalances in urinary and reproductive systems
Myrrh	Soothes inflammation, clears congestion and secretions, antiseptic properties, and fungicidal agent	Wound healing and ulcers
Frankincense	Antiseptic, disinfectant, astringent, and wound healer	Bronchitis, colds, sinusitis, stomach and intestinal discomfort, wound healing
Vanilla	Increases appetite	Promotes oral intake

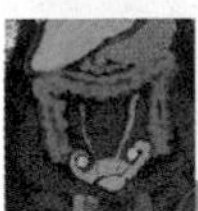

GUIDELINES FOR SAFE PRACTICE *Cautions With the Use of Aromatherapy*

- Many people are allergic to certain fragrances. Never suggest or use an aromatherapy with a patient without inquiring into allergies and the patient's preferences.
- Oils to avoid because of risk of toxicity or skin irritation include bitter almond, boldo leaf, calamus, jaborandi leaf, mugwort, mustard, pennyroyal, rue, sage, sassafras, savin, southernwood, tansy, thuja, wintergreen, wormseed, and yellow camphor.
- Oils to avoid during pregnancy include all of the above plus basil, clary sage, cypress, fennel, jasmine, juniper, marjoram, myrrh, peppermint, rose, rosemary, and thyme.
- Before using aromatherapy clinically, a health professional should complete a course in the medicinal uses of oils.

deal with everyday emergencies. It is benign and produces no unpleasant reaction. It is preserved using brandy, which can be omitted, but the essence will not stay preserved as long. Patients place two to four drops of an essence under the tongue or in a glass of water that they sip throughout the day. Patients using Bach flower remedies may have a faint odor of alcohol on their breath. Hydrotherapy baths, douches, and packs can also be made with Bach flower remedies.

Manipulative and Body-Based Therapies

Manipulative and body-based therapies integrate the structural and functional integrity of the body using manual methods. They may involve reeducation about movement and structured exercise. "Bodywork" and manipulative therapies with a structural focus include chiropractic, craniosacral, Trager, and Alexander technique. Neuromuscular therapies include reflexology and Trager. Structural and postural reintegration therapies include Rolfing and Alexander technique.

Massage

Massage therapy, perhaps the best known of the manipulative therapies, involves the manipulation of tissues to enhance healing and health. Massage manipulates the soft tissues (skin, muscles, tendons, ligaments, fascia) and structures within the soft tissue to normalize these tissues.[7] Massage therapists may use their hands, forearms, or elbows to apply pressure and move the body tissues. Techniques include touch, stroking (effleurage), friction, vibration, percussion (tapotement), kneading (petrissage), stretching, compression, and passive and active joint movements.[7] Massage modalities include European massage, Swedish massage, deep tissue therapy, sports massage, manual lymph draining, and Esalen massage.

The origins of massage can be found in Chinese folk medicine; the India yoga cult; and Egyptian, Persian, and Japanese literature. After the Middle Ages the use of massage in the West was relegated to an obscure place in folk culture. In 1900 Albert Hoffa published *Technik Der Massage*, which became the basis of all modern massage techniques. The polio epidemic of 1918 triggered a renewed interest in massage therapy in the United States and Europe, but its use again waned until the 1970s holistic health movement. Massage therapy is now the second most commonly used practitioner-based therapy in the United States, after chiropractic care.[18]

Massage integrates mechanical, physiologic, reflexive, mind-body, and energetic mechanisms. Massage affects the musculoskeletal, circulatory, lymphatic, nervous, and other body systems. It can reduce muscle tension, improve circulation, decrease blood pressure, reduce acute and chronic pain, and increase joint mobility and range of motion. It increases oxygen delivery to the tissues and improves the removal of lactic acid and other waste products from the cells. The levels of beta-endorphins increase moderately after connective tissue massage, which decreases pain perception.

Massage also creates a state of relaxation that relieves anxiety and enhances the individual's sense of well-being. Mental centering can also occur. Deep massage can create a meditative state that recharges energy and activates the parasympathetic nervous system for restoration and rejuvenation.[7]

Touch is the fundamental medium of massage therapy. A therapist works with the patient to determine sensitivity to touch and the optimal degree of pressure. Massage establishes a mind-body connection between the therapist and patient in a safe, nonsexual environment. Used correctly, touch conveys caring as well.

Many hospitals employ massage therapists in settings such as cancer clinics, obstetrics and gynecology, postsurgical units, and rehabilitation units. Massage therapies may also be helpful in hospice settings or nursing homes. Nursing staff and family members may find massage helps reduce stress (Figure 4-2). Treatment may also include other bodywork and touch therapies. Massage therapists frequently receive additional training in medical massage to understand disease processes and indications and contraindications to therapy.

Historically, nursing programs taught back massage as a part of nighttime care and to help patients relax. It is unfortunate that the move to high-technology care erased this therapy from common use in nursing just as massage was achieving prominence as an alternative therapy.

Chiropractic

Chiropractic means "hand work" and refers to manual therapy that focuses on the spine and its effect on the nervous system. The practitioner analyzes structural relationships and manipulates them to restore proper alignment and function. Chiropractic practitioners are the third largest medical specialty after medicine and dentistry, and practitioners are licensed in all 50 states. Chiropractic is an ancient healing art, but the position of chiropractic practitioners in health care has been ambiguous. Today Chiropractic care is really more a mainstream than an alternative therapy. Chiropractors use the patient history, physical examination, neuromuscular examination, radiographic examination, and laboratory or special studies to determine the appropriateness of chiropractic care for the individual patient.

Chiropractic care is used to treat shoulder pain, lower back pain, and temporomandibular joint disorders. Chiropractors use mobilization and manipulation as a treatment modality for spinal disorders, pain, altered musculoskeletal function, altered flexibility, and disturbed physical performance. Many studies have shown that chiropractic care for lower back pain is more effective and less costly than conventional medical care. Chiropractic care also has demonstrated effectiveness in the treatment of headaches and neck pain, although more research is needed.

Chiropractic care focuses on a strong patient-practitioner relationship. Chiropractic treatment does carry a risk of adverse outcomes such as brainstem or cerebellar infarction, spinal cord injury, vertebral fracture, tracheal rupture, diaphragm paralysis, and even death. Case reports are published in the literature, but hard data about complication rates are not readily available.

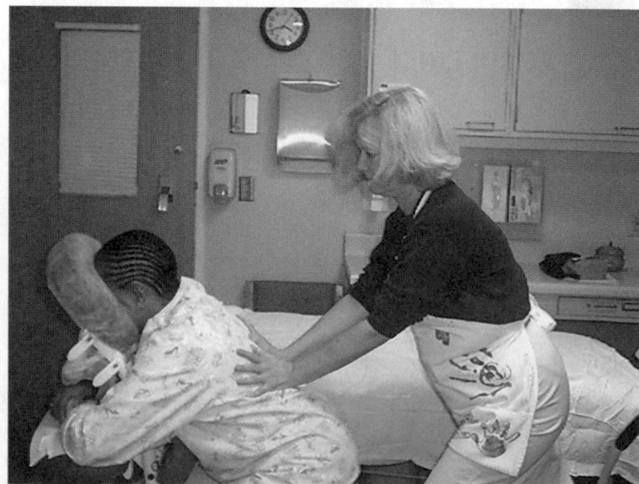

Figure 4-2 Many hospitals use massage therapists to work along service lines providing massage therapy for specific types of patients. The massage therapist may also provide seated massages for hospital staff and family members.

Craniosacral Therapy

Craniosacral therapy focuses on normalization of the craniosacral system. John Upledger, an osteopathic physician, developed craniosacral therapy in the 1970s. The therapy is based on the theory that a craniosacral rhythm or pulse motion reflects the rise and fall of the cerebrospinal fluid within the dura mater compartment and occurs 6 to 12 times per minute in a healthy person. Upledger believed that the skull sutures are not entirely fused, as is commonly believed, but can be used to access the flow of cerebrospinal fluid through the dural membranes. The therapist works with the patient to identify where this pulsing rhythm is obstructed. The therapist monitors the rhythm using light, gentle touch, no heavier than 5 g (weight of a nickel). After identifying an obstruction, the practitioner assists the natural flow of fluid to help the body self-correct. Work in this area can increase energy flow and break up restrictions. Craniosacral therapy is used to manage chronic fatigue syndrome, chronic headaches, joint problems, and head injury and as part of stroke rehabilitation.

Trager

Trager uses gentle rhythmic movements or rocking to give the mind sensory information about where body parts are and how they feel and move. The technique was developed by Milton Trager in the 1920s (Box 4-9). Trager connects a person to his or her body, stimulates deep relaxation, and focuses on a model of optimal functioning. This approach provides a background for physical therapy, occupational therapy, massage therapy, chiropractic care, physical rehabilitation, and psychotherapy. Movement education can also involve Mentastics, a program of do-it-yourself exercises, designed to release blocked areas in both the mind and body.

Alexander Technique

Alexander technique is a system of posture and movement that capitalizes on the body's natural grace and poise. The technique focuses on postural reflexes or antigravity reflexes, "the use of ourselves." At the end of the nineteenth century an Australian, Frederick Mathius Alexander, a Shakespearean reciter who consistently lost his voice after performances, developed the technique and permanently cured his vocal problems. Since then his technique has been used for two main purposes: performing arts and physical therapy.

Alexander technique involves kinesthetic reeducation. Children have excellent use of their body from birth. A young child walks with an erect spine, free joints, and a large head that is balanced easily on the neck. Over time, through environmental socialization, the person loses this poise; the Alexander technique reteaches it. Through one-on-one lessons with a teacher, a person learns to move the body with minimal strain and maximum balance for optimal functional mobility and decreased pain. Over time a person acquires a sense of postural awareness, which enables him or her to automatically modify muscular responses to stress.

Alexander technique has been clinically beneficial to persons with chronic pain conditions; traumatic injuries; back, hip, and neck dysfunction; repetitive stress injuries; neurologic dysfunctions; respiratory dysfunction; and posture or balance disorders.

Box 4-9 Principles of Trager

- Finding elongation: Length creates freedom of movement, which takes less effort.
- Finding width: Taking up our full space gives way to feeling.
- Presence in relationships does matter.
- Giving up weight makes one feel lighter.
- Movements increase sensation.
- Repetition is the way we learn, and we learn our entire lives.
- Assessment is treatment.

Reflexology

Reflexology involves applying pressure with the thumb and fingers to stimulate the reflex areas in the feet and hands that correspond to all the glands, organs, and parts of the body. It can improve the function of the whole body or a specific targeted area that may be distant from the area being stimulated. Reflexology encourages energy flow and removes impurities to promote healing.

Some form of reflexology has been practiced by many cultures throughout the ages, but its roots are in the ancient art of Oriental pressure therapy or acupuncture. All these approaches are based on the theory that blockages of the body's energy pathways can lead to energy loss, discomfort, and illness. Reflexologists work each reflex, triggering release of stress and tension in the corresponding area or body zone and promoting an overall relaxation response. Patients express relief from tension and pain, greater well-being, and increased energy.

Exercise

Exercise is movement that promotes health and fitness, including cardiovascular endurance, muscle strength, and body flexibility. Appropriate physical activity and exercise condition the heart and other muscles and provide a sense of well-being. Stretching relaxes and loosens muscles, releases toxins, and increases blood flow. Lymph movement in the body depends on stretching and breathing. Exercise decreases stress hormones, improves relaxation, and helps the body deal with stress more effectively. Exercise can improve cardiovascular and pulmonary function, hypertension, diabetes, osteoporosis, and depression (see Research box). Exercise has achieved such a prominent place in health and wellness programs in the United States that most people do not consider it a CAT. Exercise and its important role in health promotion are discussed in Chapter 3.

Energy Therapies

All living systems are based on energy and vibration, and all forms of bodywork interact with this energy in some way. Energy therapies include therapeutic touch, reiki, physioacoustics, and bioelectromagnetics.

Therapeutic Touch

Therapeutic touch was developed in 1972 by Delores Kreiger, a nurse and professor at New York University, and Dora Kunz, a natural healer. Contrary to what the name implies, the therapeutic touch practitioner modulates the patient's energy field without physically touching the patient. The technique is based on Rogers' theory of the unitary human being, which theorizes that the body is an open energy field that interacts with the environment. The practitioner consciously directs and sensitively modulates human energies. The therapist *centers* and then assesses the energy fields, *unruffles* or clears and immobilizes the energy field, directs energy, and balances the energy field.

Practitioners use therapeutic touch to decrease pain perception and anxiety, to improve wound healing, and to promote relaxation. Many nurses learn therapeutic touch techniques and use them with consenting patients. It is one of the more controversial CATs among nurses.

Healing Touch

With healing touch the practitioner uses the hands to clear, energize, and balance the human energy field, thus mobilizing the person's own ability to heal. Healing touch was offered in the 1980s as a continuing education program for nurses, endorsed by the American Holistic Nurses Association, and is now taught through Healing Touch International. Healing touch is widely used in conjunction with allopathic treatments (see Research box).

Reiki

Reiki involves the use of intentional touch with a receptive patient to promote healing. The term *reiki* means "universal life force energy." Reiki practitioners draw energy into their bodies through the crown of their heads. This energy then passes through the body and out of their hands to the patient. Practitioners use specific hand placements to cover the major human organs, focusing on the body's seven major energy centers, or chakras. Healing can occur as energy passes to the patient (Box 4-10). Reiki practitioners may also perform self-healing techniques and can teach them to patients.

Vibrational Medicine

All matter is believed to vibrate to a precise frequency. Vibrational medicine uses the fluctuating energy fields from electronic devices, the human voice, or musical instruments to promote health. The use of resonant vibration through music and sound can produce changes in heart rate, blood pressure, brain waves, and muscle contractions and restore this balance in the body.

Physioacoustics. Physioacoustics specifically applies low-frequency stimulation to the human body to obtain desired effects. It uses sine waves in the range of 20 to 120 Hz. The subject may sit in a special chair or lie on a special mattress. Preselected frequencies or sounds are played through simple speakers and are more felt than heard. A contraindication for vibrational therapy is an acutely herniated disk. Potential uses include stress, anxiety, and pain reduction.

Bioelectromagnetics

Bioelectromagnetics explores the interactions of electromagnetic fields and radiation with living tissues. Everything in our world is magnetic at some level, and all physical bodies have magnetic fields. The earth itself has a geomagnetic field of 0.5 gauss. Exogenous static and electromagnetic fields influence and moderate the properties of biologic systems, yet there is no consensus about how they operate.

In Western culture people usually think of magnetic fields as manufactured (e.g., the current in an electrical outlet), even though the use of electromagnetic fields in health care is well known. Electrocardiograms and electroencephalograms have been used to measure electrical activity in the heart and brain for many years. Electricity and magnetism are frequently used in diagnosis (e.g., magnetic

Research

Cook CA et al: Healing touch and quality of life in women receiving radiation treatment for cancer: a randomized controlled trial, *Alt Therap* 10(3):34-40, 2004.

This two-arm single-blind randomized clinical trial was conducted in a convenience sample of 62 women over age 17 with newly diagnosed gynecologic or breast cancer. All patients received radiation treatment for their cancer. Patients were chosen at random to receive six healing touch or mock therapy treatments. The healing touch group had significantly different scores ($p < 0.05$) on three subscales (pain, vitality, and physical functioning) on the quality of life outcome tool than the mock therapy treatment group. Patients in the healing touch group reported improved vitality, improved physical functioning, and decreased pain.

Research

Ishikawa-Takata K et al: How much exercise is required to reduce blood pressure in essential hypertension: a dose-response study, *Am J Hypertens* 16:629-633, 2003.

This randomized study evaluated the effect of exercise on blood pressure in sedentary, healthy adults with essential hypertension. Subjects were randomized to nonexercise or exercise groups for 8 weeks. During analysis the exercise group was subdivided according to amount of weekly exercise. Subjects in the nonexercise group had no change in systolic and diastolic blood pressure. Those in the 61 to 90 minutes per week group had an average 11.8 mm Hg reduction in systolic blood pressure, compared with those in the 30 to 60 minute group, who achieved an average reduction of 6.9 mm Hg ($p < 0.05$). There was no significant change in diastolic blood pressure across groups.

Box 4-10 Principles of Reiki

Just for today I will live the attitude of gratitude.

Just for today I will not worry.

Just for today I will not anger.

Just for today I will do my work honestly.

Just for today I will show love and respect for everyone.

resonance imaging). Other common examples are eye magnets used to remove shrapnel, a magnetic technique used to treat retinal tears, and external cardiac defibrillators and pacemakers.

Researchers are currently studying the use of magnets for a variety of purposes, including wound healing and the treatment of bone, muscle, and joint pain. No proven protocol yet exists that sets out the optimal dosage for therapeutic effects, maximal magnetic flux density, frequency of change in density, duration of exposure, or frequency of exposure. The therapeutic mechanism remains unclear. Theories include gene expression and an increase in blood flow.

One of the difficulties with blinded research in this area is how to effectively use magnetized versus sham magnets. In addition to considering the variables of dose, field strength, and duration, magnetic research must also take into account competing effects, side effects, and cultural influences. Women with bladder incontinence and men who have had prostatectomies are using chairs with pulsed magnetic fields to improve continence. Questions about the effectiveness of these interventions will gradually be resolved through clinical trials. Researchers are also continuing to evaluate the potential dangers of low-frequency fields. Individual case reports speculate about the potential role of weak magnetic energies from cellular phones, high-tension power lines, and household appliances in the development of cancer, birth defects, and other health problems (see Chapter 23).

Nursing Management

The United States' demographic composition is undergoing rapid and profound changes. Nurses frequently come from different social, ethnic, cultural, and religious backgrounds than their patients. To provide nursing care to persons using CATs, nurses must be aware of and sensitive to the patient's unique sociocultural background, interpretations of health and illness, and health promotion and disease prevention traditions. Unique health beliefs and practices must be identified and respected, not challenged or disparaged.

Patients from different cultures may have used alternative therapies as their primary approach to health and illness care, and they may be extremely uncomfortable with and suspicious of mainstream Western medicine. Nurses need to be knowledgeable about varied cultural beliefs and alternative practices. Some nurses believe they should treat all patients the same. This attitude conveys a sense of equality but fails to acknowledge that real cultural differences exist between people. It is not possible to act exactly the same with all patients and still deliver effective, individualized holistic care. Blending divergent viewpoints is difficult but not impossible, and nurses are important advocates for patients within the health care system.

Nursing was one of the first health professions to facilitate the use of CATs. Nursing deals with individuals as whole persons, and CATs complement this philosophy. Many nursing programs formally incorporate complementary health practices into the curriculum, which prepares the nurse to select interventions that are compatible with the patient's belief system and lifestyle. It is not important to consumers of CATs that the nurse believe a therapy is effective. Patients will still use them. Nurses need to be able to speak knowledgeably about CATs and their application, contraindications, and potential beneficial and adverse effects.

A variety of tools are available to assist the nurse in assessing the patient and family from a CATs perspective. However, it is equally important for the nurse to carefully assess his or her own sociocultural heritage, health and illness beliefs, and how they may affect a patient's care. As representatives of the dominant allopathic health care philosophy, nurses need to work carefully to communicate an openness to CATs as well as traditional practices of health and healing.

The nurse should ask the patient or family members about the cause of the illness or problem in a manner that suggests a familiarity with traditional health beliefs, as well as mainstream medical care. The patient and family may not believe in the epidemiologic or medical model of disease causation. Therefore they may not understand the rationale for modern treatment modalities and may choose not to follow the recommended treatment regimen. The nurse's acknowledgment of and respect for diverse health beliefs can prevent an impending cultural collision. A compromise solution that recognizes the values of both sides is usually possible. One approach is to assume that all patients are using some type of traditional therapy or CAT and state, "Tell me about the complementary or alternative treatments or products you are using." The nurse can identify conflicts between the patient's health beliefs and practices and the medical care plan. Box 4-11 outlines some elements for the nurse to consider in assessing a patient concerning CATs.

The nurse may act as a broker between the patient's traditional practices and the allopathic health care system, or may attempt to introduce CAT therapies to a patient who has never considered their use. Both roles require sensitivity and excellent communication skills. Health beliefs and practices, such as the use of special prayers, amulets, or special foods, are integrated into the plan of care whenever possible. Successes may be small, such as facilitating patient access to cultural food items or convincing an anxious patient to participate in a relaxation exercise, but their cumulative effect can be powerful. As the care coordinator, the nurse is invaluable in interpreting the patient's beliefs and needs to the entire multidisciplinary care team.

It is especially important to consider the patient's heritage, educational level, and language skills when planning patient education. The assistance of a qualified interpreter may be appropriate. When patients are not comfortable speaking English, the nurse should allow additional time to orient the patient to the hospital's routines and equipment. The nurse anticipates that the patient will be unfamiliar with most of the hospital environment, which can be overwhelming when language barriers make it difficult to ask questions.

CATs may be used as interventions for a variety of nursing diagnoses (Box 4-12) and are well represented in the Nursing Interventions Classification (NIC) (Box 4-13). When introducing CATs, the nurse should provide information on indications, contraindications, potential benefits, and adverse side effects (Box 4-14). The nurse may suggest that the patient keep a daily log of therapies used and document symptom improvement and side effects. Nurses help patients explore CAT therapies that are suitable for them. As the popularity of CATs continues to expand, it is increasingly important for patients to know how to

Box 4-11 Assessment Considerations Related to CATs

Native Language

Patient and family skills in English:

Speaking, understanding, reading, and writing

Availability of family, friends, or others to interpret

Availability of institutional interpreters

Cultural Heritage

Patient and family's cultural background

Health beliefs

Use of traditional health practices

Use of and Knowledge About CATs

Beliefs about CATs and their role in managing disease or supporting health

Experience with CATs

Use of traditional healers

CATs in current use and their effectiveness

Box 4-12 Nursing Diagnoses That May Incorporate CATs Into the Care Plan

- Acute pain
- Chronic pain
- Constipation
- Disturbed energy field
- Health-seeking behaviors
- Imbalanced nutrition: less than body requirements
- Impaired comfort
- Impaired memory
- Ineffective coping
- Ineffective health maintenance
- Ineffective therapeutic regimen management
- Readiness for enhanced spiritual well-being
- Risk for infection
- Risk for injury
- Risk for spiritual distress
- Spiritual distress

Box 4-13 Common NIC Interventions That Incorporate CATs

- Acupressure
- Anxiety Reduction
- Aromatherapy
- Biofeedback
- Calming Technique
- Culture Brokerage
- Cutaneous Stimulation
- Exercise Therapy
- Heat/Cold Application
- Hypnosis
- Music Therapy
- Progressive Muscle Relaxation
- Simple Guided Imagery
- Simple Massage
- Simple Relaxation Therapy
- Therapeutic Touch
- Touch

Box 4-14 Strategies for Introducing CATs to Clients

- Identify the patient's goals for treatment (e.g., symptom management).
- Assess the patient's knowledge, beliefs, and interest in CATs.
- Educate the patient on CAT options.
- Offer options that may be beneficial to the patient.
- Share current research outcomes.
- Discuss expected outcomes of therapy.
- Obtain clinical informed consent.
- Ask the patient to evaluate the therapy following treatment.

Box 4-16 CAT Resources

- American Academy of Medical Acupuncture: www.medicalacupuncture.org
- American Association of Oriental Medicine: www.aaom.org
- American Botanical Council: www.herbalgram.org
- American Holistic Medical Association: www.holisticmedicine.org
- American Holistic Nurses Association: www.ahna.org
- American Massage Therapy Association: www.amtamassage.org
- American Society for the Alexander Technique: www.alexandertech.com
- American Yoga Association: www.americanyogaassociation.org
- Association for Applied Psychophysiology and Biofeedback: www.aapb.org
- Healing Touch International: www.healingtouch.net
- Homeopathic Educational Services: www.homeopathic.com
- National Center for Homeopathy: www.homeopathic.org
- National Certification Board for Therapeutic Massage and Bodywork: www.ncbtmb.com
- National Certification Commission for Acupuncture and Oriental Medicine: www.nccaom.org
- National Institutes of Health: National Center for Complementary and Alternative Medicine: http://nccam.nih.gov
- Trager International: www.trager.com
- The Upledger Institute (craniosacral therapy): www.upledger.com
- U.S. Food and Drug Administration: Center for Food Safety and Applied Nutrition: http://vm.cfsan.fda.gov

Box 4-15 Evaluating CAT Therapies and Practitioners

Locate a CAT Practitioner

Speak to your primary health care provider.

Get recommendations from friends.

Check with your doctor's office or health center.

Ask at a natural health center or health food store.

Look on the Internet.

Go to national organization referral programs.

Assess a Therapy's Safety and Effectiveness

Do the benefits outweigh the risks of treatment?

Is a benefit likely for the typical patient from the average practitioner?

Discuss the therapy with the health care provider.

Tell the practitioner of all CATs currently being used.

Make a list of questions to ask at your first visit.

Examine the Practitioner's Expertise and Credentials

Talk to state or local regulatory agencies with authority over practitioners in the therapy you seek. Does the practitioner meet their qualifications?

Ask for references and talk with people who have experience with this practitioner. How was their experience?

Talk with the practitioner in person to find out about education, additional training, licenses, and certifications. Is there a code of ethics for the professional organization?

Consider Service Delivery

How is the therapy given and under what conditions?

Visit the practice setting. Are the conditions of the office or clinic acceptable?

Does the service delivery adhere to regulated standards for medical safety and care?

Consider Costs

What therapies will your health insurance carrier cover or reimburse? Compare cost among several practitioners.

Consult Your Health Care Provider

Discuss all issues of treatment and therapies with your health care provider.

Adapted from National Center for Complementary and Alternative Medicine: *Selecting a complementary and alternative medicine practitioner,* Pub No D168, accessed Sept 2004 from website: http://nccam.nih.gov/health/practitioner/index.htm.

access and evaluate safe and competent practitioners (Box 4-15). Information resources on CATs also continue to expand, and a partial listing of sources is included in Box 4-16.

? Critical Thinking

1. A 40-year-old woman who lives in a commune settlement has been suffering from severe lower back pain and was admitted for a disk procedure. After visits from friends she tells you she thinks that a reiki practitioner might be able to help her, and she asks you to help her discuss this with her physician.
   a. How would you proceed?
   b. What would change, if anything, if you knew her physician considered CATs to be "completely worthless"?
2. What CATs are currently practiced in your family?

References

1. American Botanical Council: *Popular herbs in the US market: therapeutic monographs,* Austin, Tex, 1997, The Council.

1a. Bach E, Wheeler EJ: *The Bach flower remedies,* New York, 1998, McGraw Hill.

2. Berra K: Clinical update on the use of niacin for the treatment of dyslipidemia, *J Am Acad Nurse Pract* 16(12):526-534, 2004.
3. Blumenthal M, Brinckmann J, Wollschlaeger B, editors: *The ABC clinical guide to herbs,* New York, NY, 2003, Thieme Medical Publishers.
4. Committee on the Use of Complementary and Alternative Medicine by the American Public, Board on Health Promotion and Disease Prevention: *Complementary and alternative medicine in the United States,* Washington, DC, 2005, National Academies of Sciences.
5. DerMarderosian A: *Review of natural products,* St Louis, 2005, Facts & Comparisons.
6. Eisenberg DM et al: Perceptions about complementary therapies relative to conventional therapies among adults who use both: results of a national survey, *Ann Intern Med* 135(5):344, 2001.
7. Fritz S: *Mosby's fundamentals of therapeutic massage,* St Louis, 2005, Mosby Lifeline.
8. Keeling A: Herbal medicine in the Kentucky mountains: the Frontier Nursing Service, 1925-1950, *Windows in Time* 11(2):6–8, 2003.
9. Reference deleted in proofs.
10. Marks LS, Hess DL, Dore FJ: Tissue effects of saw palmetto and finasteride: use of biopsy cores for in situ quantification of prostatic androgens, *Urology* 57:999, 2001.
11. Menzies V: *Guided imagery as a clinical intervention.* Paper presented at Graduate Nursing Seminar in Complementary and Alternative Therapies, University of Virginia, Charlottesville, Va, April 2001.
12. National Center for Complementary and Alternative Medicine, National Institutes of Health: *What is complementary and alternative medicine (CAM)?,* Pub No D156, accessed May 2002 from website: http://nccam.nih.gov/health/whatiscam.
13. National Center for Complementary and Alternative Medicine, National Institutes of Health: *Research report: questions and answers about homeopathy,* Pub No D183, accessed April 2003 from website: http://nccam.nih.gov/health/homeopathy/index.htm.
14. National Center for Complementary and Alternative Medicine, National Institutes of Health: *St. John's wort and the treatment of depression,* Pub No

D005, accessed March 2004 from website: http://nccam.nih.gov/health/stjohnswort.

15. National Center for Complementary and Alternative Medicine, National Institutes of Health: *Biologically based practices: an overview,* Pub No D237, accessed Oct 2004, http://nccam.nih.gov/health/backgrounds/biobased-prac.htm.
16. National Center for Complementary and Alternative Medicine, National Institutes of Health: *NCCAM Research Centers Program,* accessed Nov 2004 from website: www.nccam.nih.gov/training/centers/index.htm.
17. National Center for Complementary and Alternative Medicine, National Institutes of Health: *Acupuncture,* Pub No D003, accessed Dec 2004 from website: http://nccam.nih.gov/health/acupuncture.
18. National Center for Complementary and Alternative Medicine, National Institutes of Health: *The use of complementary and alternative medicine in the United States,* Pub No D234, Washington, DC, 2004, The Center.
19. Reference deleted in proofs.
20. Smith ME, Lopez-Bushnell K: Acupuncture as complementary therapy for back pain, *Holistic Nurs Pract* 15(3):35–44, 2001.

evolve Visit the Evolve website: http://evolve.elsevier.com/Monahan/medsurg

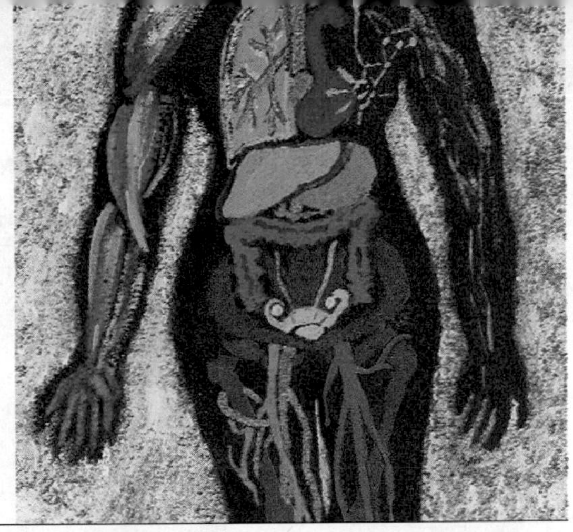

CHAPTER 5

Genetics and Disease

by Kathleen Barta

OBJECTIVES

After studying this chapter, the learner should be able to:

1. Identify the basic concepts of molecular biology relevant to understanding genetic influences on health and illness.
2. Describe examples of genetic influences on health and illness.
3. Describe use of genetic information in diagnosis, treatment, and prevention of disease.
4. Explain the role of the generalist nurse in helping people use genetic information.
5. Explain the indications for and process of genetic counseling.
6. Outline the key ethical issues related to emerging genetic technology.
7. Describe misuses of genetic information.

KEY TERMS

autosomal-dominant inheritance, p. 75
autosomal-recessive inheritance, p. 75
carrier, p. 80
ethics, p. 81
gene therapies, p. 81
genetic counseling, p. 85
genetic testing, p. 80
Human Genome Project, p. 71
pharmacogenetics, p. 81
recombinant DNA, p. 81
sex-linked inheritance, p. 75

Genetics is called the new central science of health care. Knowledge about molecular biology is necessary for future health care professionals to understand innovations in diagnosis, treatment, and prevention of disease based on genetic information. Nursing, with its tradition of holistic care, offers a unique contribution to patients and families trying to make sense of new genetic information for making health decisions.

Because nurses serve people throughout the life span and across settings, they are in a key position to integrate knowledge of genetic influences into health care. The National Coalition of Health Professional Education in Genetics provides a model of interdisciplinary preparation through the identification of shared professional competencies and principles. This model provides the framework for this chapter.[23,24]

Future students in health care professions will be exposed to concepts of molecular biology and genetics in high school as the impact of mapping the human genome reaches public education. Meanwhile current health care professionals and students need to revise their understanding of disease prevention and treatment in light of new genetic knowledge. Several sources are available, including many online, that highlight basic concepts needed to appreciate the future development of genetic testing and genetic-based treatments. Table 5-1 lists Internet-based educational sources. Such sources illustrate the latest information on the structure and function of the double helix located in the cell nucleus. Scientists have long been able to see the coiled strands of deoxyribonucleic acid (DNA) that comprise each of the 23 pairs of chromosomes in human cells (Figure 5-1). The **Human Genome Project** identified the exact sequence of all the nitrogenous base pairs of guanine, cytosine, adenine, and thymine that make up each strand of DNA (Figure 5-2). Proteins are considered gene products and are the basic component of all cells, organs, and subsequent metabolic functioning. Current research efforts are examining which segments code for which proteins and how the proteins work together for specialized cellular functioning. Such efforts will increase understanding of individual variation and adaptation in health and disease[35] (see Healthy People 2010 box).

Advances in genetic science raise questions as to what is normal and abnormal; when variation is called disease; and when variation should be treated, prevented, or both. Cultural perspectives on when to consider a variation a disease are a source of potential conflict among population groups in a diverse world. As knowledge of human variation increases, care must be taken to ensure that human rights are not violated.

Basic Concepts of Molecular Biology

The Department of Energy initiated the Human Genome Project in 1986 to map the entire sequence of base pairs in human DNA. Work was completed in 2003. The genetic map may be viewed from various perspectives, down to the molecular level.[33] Knowing the sequence of base pairs is the first step in identifying specific

TABLE 5-1 INTERNET RESOURCES ON GENETICS

Sponsor	Address	Highlights
National Human Genome Research Institute	http://www.genome.gov	Information on research, grants, genetic health, policy and ethics, educational resources, and careers
International Society of Nurses in Genetics	http://www.isong.org	Position statements, scope of practice, and nursing research projects related to genetics
U.S. Department of Energy Office of Science	http://www.doegenomes.org	Details on Human Genome Project; educational resources, including multimedia and text-based sources
Genetics Education Center at University of Kansas Medical Center	http://www.kumc.edu/gec	Extensive links to resources for all types of students and practitioners; frequent additions highlighted
National Conference of State Legislatures	http://www.ncsl.org/programs/health/genetics.htm	Genetic Technologies Project, tracking genetic news stories of interest to policymakers
Dolan DNA Learning Center, Cold Spring Harbor Laboratory	http://www.eugenicsarchive.org	Archive with text and graphics materials from center of eugenics in early 19th century
Access Excellence @ The National Health Museum	http://www.accessexcellence.org	Resources for education health and bioscience, including genetics
Dartmouth Medical School: Genetics in Clinical Practice	http://iml.Dartmouth.edu/education/cme/Genetics/	Virtual genetics clinic patients; emphasizes team approach
Online Mendelian Inheritance in Man (OMIM)	http://www.ncbi.nlm.nih.gov/entrez/query.fcgi?db=OMIM	Data base and catalog of human genes and disorders
U.S. National Library of Medicine Genetics Home Reference	http://ghr.nlm.nih.gov	Genetic information in easy-to-understand formats
University of Washington: GeneTests	http://www.genetests.org	Medical genetics information resource (data base online); includes illustrated glossary with strong graphics and case studies
University of Iowa: Virtual Hospital	http://www.vh.org	Includes self-study on genetics under resources for providers
Howard Hughes Medical Institute	http://www.hhmi.org	Multimedia resources on genetics, including a virtual laboratory

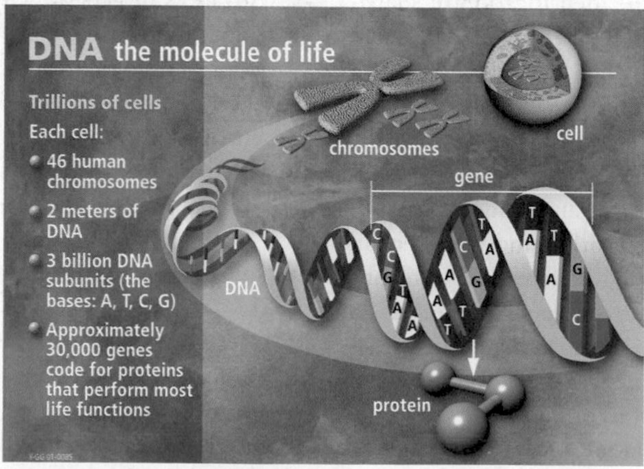

Figure 5-1 DNA: the molecule of life. Illustrates the embedding of protein codes in base pair sequences of genes on DNA strands of chromosomes in the nucleus of the cell.

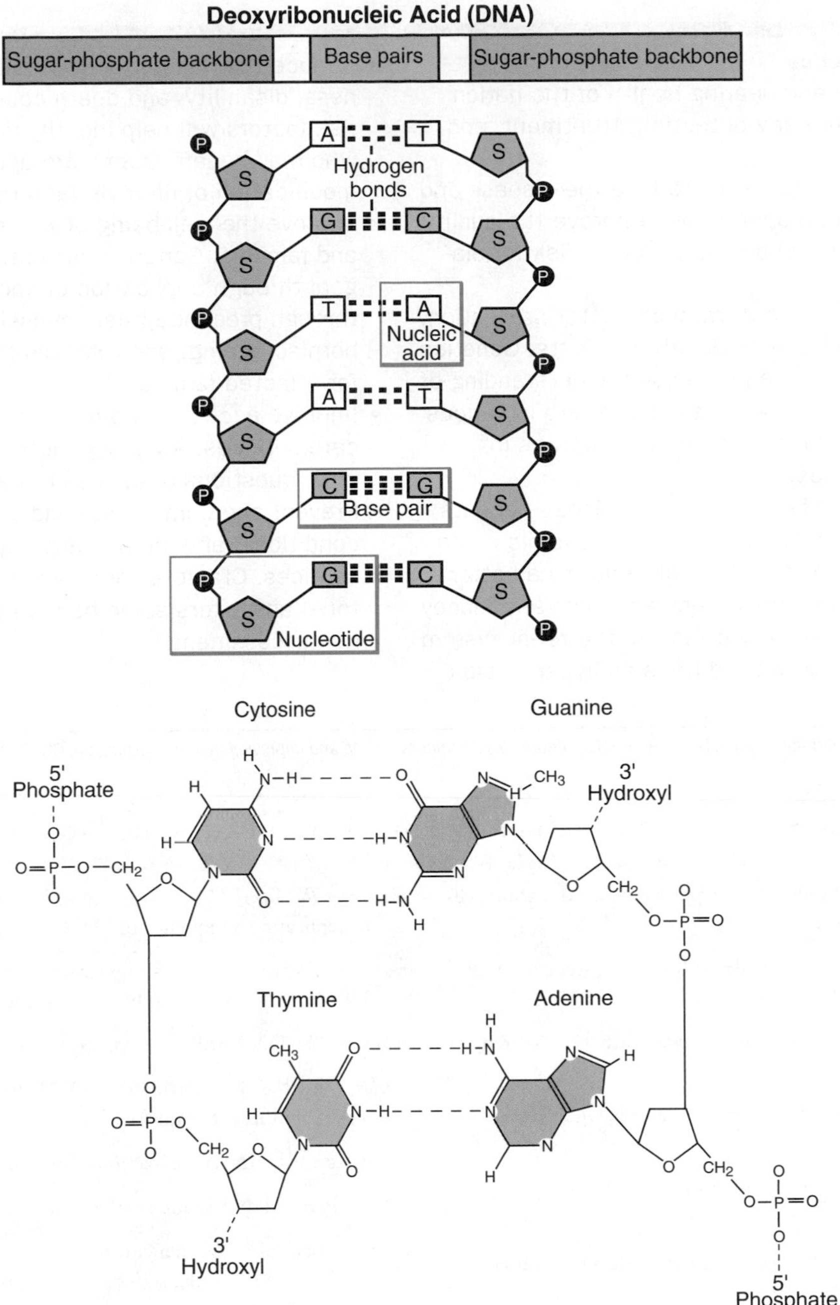

Figure 5-2 Base pairs of DNA include *A*, adenine, pairs with *T*, thymine; *G*, guanine, pairs with *C*, cytosine. *P*, Phosphate; *S*, sugar.

genes and their functions relative to protein production. Work continues on clarifying the functions of various proteins produced by DNA sequences and their interactions. Several key terms describe the structure and function of genetic expression in living organisms (Box 5-1).[2,12,34] An understanding of the following key concepts in molecular biology will help the nurse educate patients regarding the influence of genetics on health status, the rationale for genetic disease prevention and treatment, and the implications for future generations:

- Genes are located on chromosomes and carry significant sequences of base pairs that direct the production of amino acids within a cell (Figures 5-3 and 5-4).
- Messenger RNA (mRNA) copies the sequence and carries it to the cell ribosome, where it is translated into amino acids (Figure 5-5).
- Amino acid molecules link into chains that are used to create thousands of different types of proteins used for cell structure and function (Figure 5-6).
- Genes determine differences in protein structure and function and, along with environmental influences, are a major source of human variation in health and disease (Figure 5-7).
- Some characteristics are the result of single genes; however, most are the result of multiple gene products responding in a given environment.

Healthy People 2010

Goals Related to Genetics

- Improve the visual and hearing health of the nation through prevention, early detection, treatment, and rehabilitation.
- Through prevention programs, reduce the disease and economic burden of diabetes, and improve the quality of life for all persons who have or are at risk for diabetes.
- Promote respiratory health through better prevention, detection, treatment, and education efforts. Genetics will likely contribute to an increased understanding of individual risks and sensitivities to triggers in various environments, as well as individual variations in response to therapies.
- Reduce new cases of chronic kidney disease and its complications, disability, death, and economic costs. Genetic contributions to this goal relate to a better understanding of such conditions as polycystic kidney disease and the secondary effect on the renal system from such multifactorial conditions as hypertension and diabetes.[3]
- Reduce the number of new cancers, as well as the illness, disability, and death caused by cancer. Genetic risk factors will help identify individuals and families who may benefit from more aggressive screening and modification of lifestyle factors.
- Improve the well-being of women, infants, children, and families. Genetics currently contributes to this goal through application of knowledge of inheritance through preconceptual counseling, prenatal and newborn screening, and referrals for genetic counseling for affected families.
- Improve access to comprehensive, high-quality health care services. As new genetic services become available, questions of access to care become important.
- Prevent and control oral and craniofacial diseases, conditions, and injuries and improve access to related services. Craniofacial disease is considered multifactorial and offers some hope of prevention as well as risk assessment.

From US Department of Health and Human Services: *Healthy People 2010: understanding and improving health,* Washington, DC, 2000, The Department.

Box 5-1 Basic Terminology From Human Genome Project

mitosis: Process of nuclear cell division that results in two daughter cells identical to each other and to the parent cell.

meiosis: Process of cell division that results in four daughter cells each with half of the parent cell chromosomes.

guanine (G): Nitrogenous base that forms a nucleotide when paired with cytosine.

cytosine (C): Nitrogenous base that forms a nucleotide when paired with guanine.

thymine (T): Nitrogenous base that forms a nucleotide when paired with adenine.

adenine (A): Nitrogenous base that forms a nucleotide when paired with thymine.

DNA double-stranded helix: Deoxyribonucleic acid, a double-stranded molecule consisting of base pairs of nucleotides adenine (A) and thymine (T) or guanine (G) and cytosine (C) held together by weak bonds.

nucleotide: Segment of DNA that includes a nitrogenous base (adenine, guanine, thymine, or cytosine) or in RNA (adenine, guanine, uracil, or cytosine) along with a phosphate molecule and a sugar molecule.

deoxyribose: The sugar molecule found in the DNA nucleotide.

ribose: The sugar molecule found in the RNA nucleotide.

base pairs: Combinations of nucleotides that are attracted to one another and held together by weak bonds; abbreviated as CG (cytosine/guanine) and AT (adenine/thymine).

ribonucleic acid (RNA): A structure in the cell nucleus and cytoplasm that assists with protein synthesis and chemical activities.

messenger RNA (mRNA): A segment of base pairs that acts as a template for replicating a sequence of DNA to make amino acids.

ribosome: Protein manufacturing structure in cells; "reads" messenger RNA and creates protein based on sequence of base pairs.

kilobase (kb): DNA unit of length equal to 1000 nucleotides.

cordon: The three bases (triplet) in DNA that specify directions for one of the 20 different amino acids.

exons: Part of DNA with directions for creating a specific protein.

introns: Part of DNA sequence that interrupts protein production.

gene: Segment of DNA in a chromosome that provides directions for heredity; made up of a series of base pairs that encode for a protein, RNA molecule, or enzyme.

amino acid: One of 20 different molecules used to form proteins.

proteins: Substances used to regulate body structure and functioning; made up of amino acids determined by the DNA in genes that code for specific proteins.

gene expression: Conversion of genetic information of DNA into protein; not all genes are expressed.

transcription: Synthesis of RNA from DNA, the first step in gene expression.

translation: Process of directing protein synthesis based on the code contained in messenger RNA.

From US Department of Energy: *Genomics and its impact on science and society,* accessed July 2004 from website: www.ornl.gov/hgmis/publicat/primer/; and National Human Genome Research Institute: *Talking glossary of genetic terms,* accessed July 2004 from website: www.genome.gov/glossary.cfm.

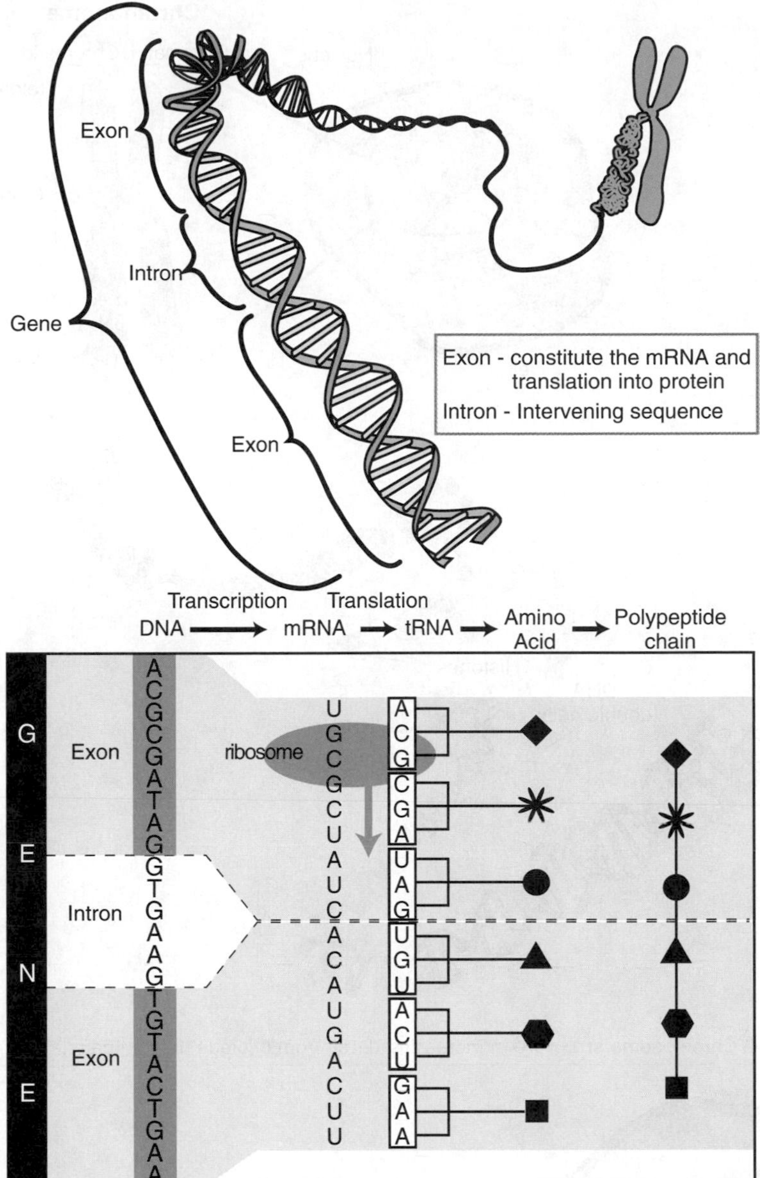

Figure 5-3 Diagram of genetic components that produce amino acid chains using the script from the DNA base pairs. Messenger RNA carries directions from part of the gene to cell ribosomes, where one of 20 possible amino acids are created. Amino acids form proteins. *nRNA*, Messenger ribonucleic acid; *tRNA*, transfer RNA; *A*, adenine; *G*, guanine; *C*, cytosine; *T*, thymine; *U*, uracil.

The next phase of research is proteomics, which is the study of how various proteins and their combinations function within cells to promote health or result in disease in a given individual in a specific environment (Figure 5-8).

The Role of Genetics in Health and Illness

Inheritance and Variation

Individuals inherit specific genetic information from their parents through the combination of genetic material in the egg and the sperm. The individual receives 23 chromosomes from the mother in the nucleus of the egg and 23 chromosomes from the father in the nucleus of the sperm. An individual's chromosomes consist of 22 pairs of autosomes and one pair of sex chromosomes. Each chromosome carries a different number of genes with different purposes. A visual display of the chromosomes in pairs is called a karyotype (Figure 5-9).

The three main mechanisms of genetic inheritance are autosomal-recessive, autosomal-dominant, and sex-linked (Figure 5-10). **Autosomal-recessive inheritance** requires an individual to have an affected gene from each parent for the characteristic or disease to be manifested; cystic fibrosis is an example of a genetic condition resulting from autosomal recessive inheritance from two carrier parents. **Autosomal-dominant inheritance** requires a person to receive an affected gene from only one parent for the characteristic or disease to be manifested; Huntington's disease is an example. **Sex-linked inheritance** can be dominant or recessive and includes conditions associated with the X chromosome that usually

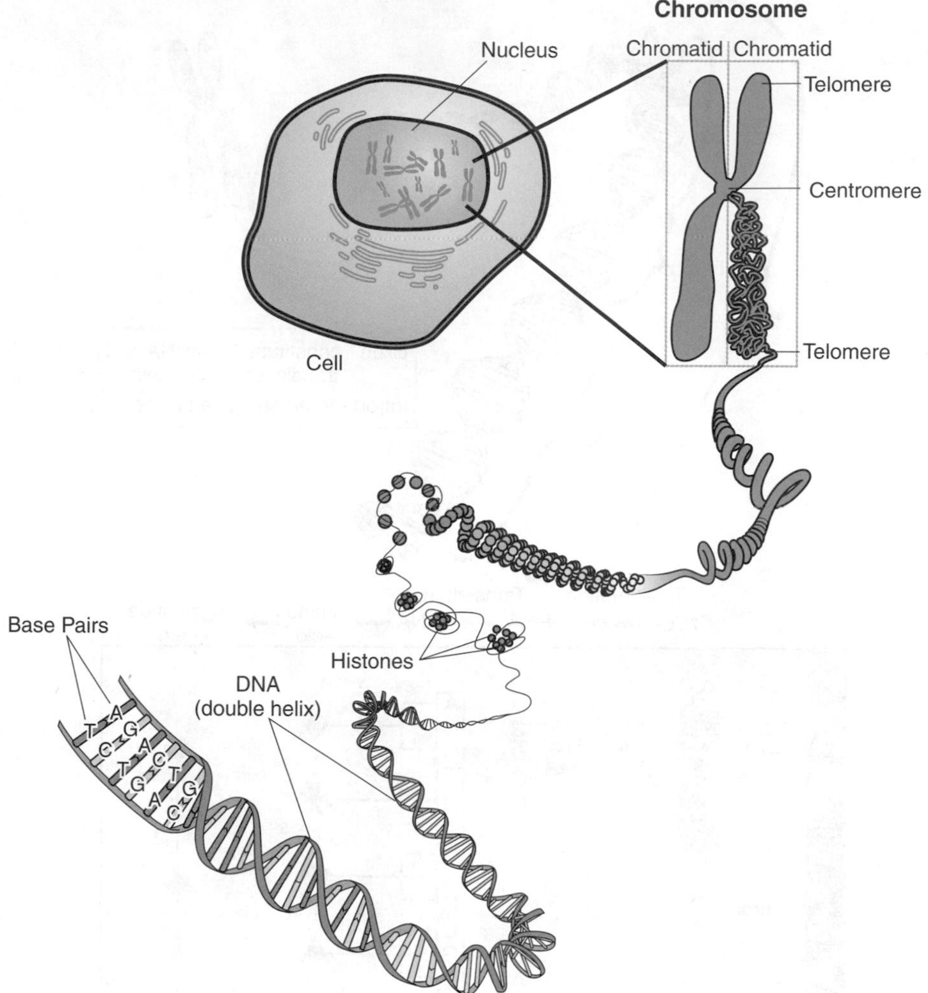

Figure 5-4 Chromosome structure in increasing detail from nucleus to base pairs.

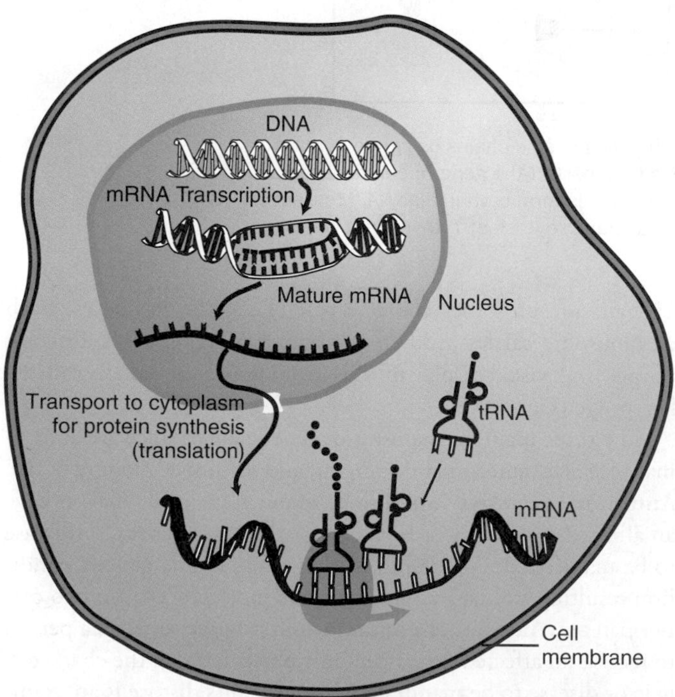

Figure 5-5 Messenger ribonucleic acid (mRNA). *tRNA*, Transfer RNA.

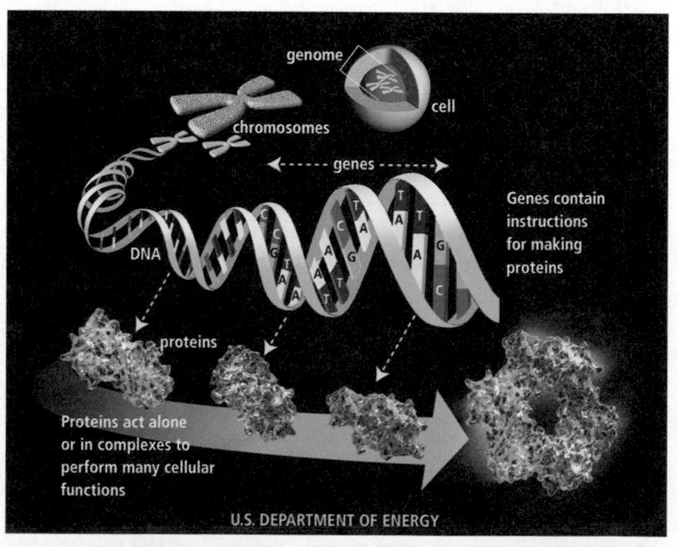

Figure 5-6 Molecular machine. Illustrates the relationship of base pairs to proteins. Base pairs include *A*, adenine, pairs with *T*, thymine; *G*, guanine, pairs with *C*, cytosine.

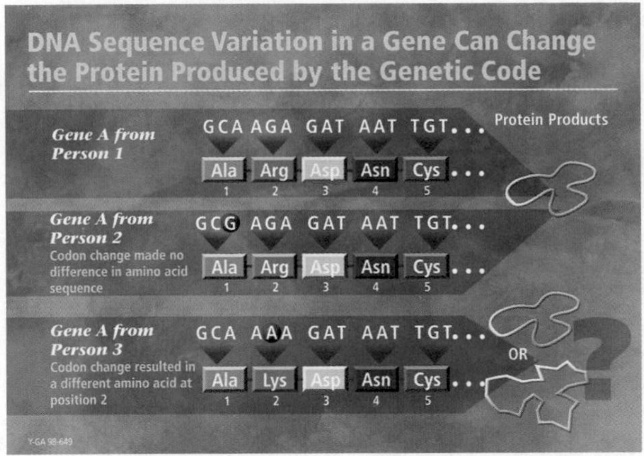

Figure 5-7 DNA sequence variation. Base pairs include *A*, adenine, pairs with *T*, thymine; *G*, guanine, pairs with *C*, cytosine. Amino acids illustrated include *Ala*, alanine; *Arg*, arginine; *Asp*, aspartic acid; *Asn*, asparagines; *Cys*, cysteine; *Lys*, lysine.

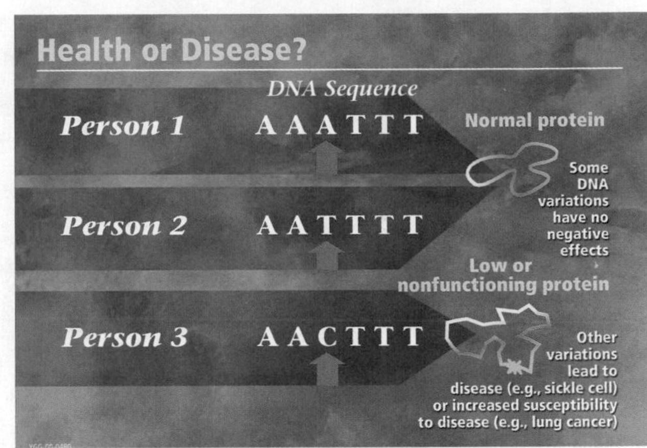

Figure 5-8 Health or disease. *A*, adenine, pairs with *T*, thymine; *G*, guanine, pairs with *C*, cytosine. The substitution of one base pair can change the protein produced and lead to disease.

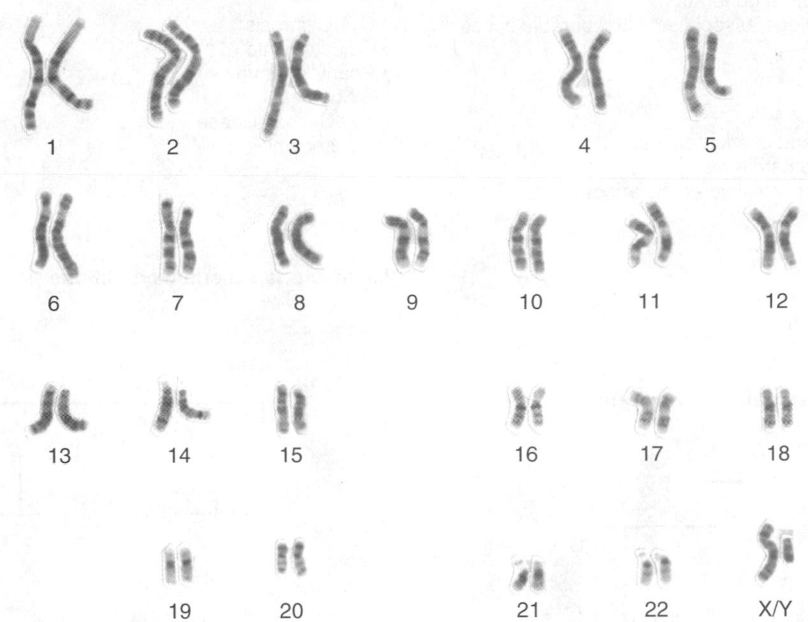

Figure 5-9 Karyotype. Visual display of the 22 pairs of chromosomes and male sex chromosomes.

result in carrier states in females and expression of the characteristic or disease in males; hemophilia A and Duchenne's muscular dystrophy are two examples.

Chromosomal disorders are another explanation for human variation. Examining the karyotype of an individual can reveal significant chromosomal variations. Variations include duplication of chromosomes; deletion of parts or all of a chromosome; exchange of segments of two chromosomes, as in translocations; inversions, when parts of a chromosome are reattached in a different location; and insertions, when a part of one chromosome is inserted into another chromosome[25] (Figure 5-11). Boxes 5-2 and 5-3 define terms related to chromosomes and inheritance patterns.[9,12,33]

Many diseases are multifactorial in etiology, the result of the interaction of gene products and environmental factors that differ in "kind, duration, and intensity" of exposure.[24] Examples include alcoholism, diabetes, and heart disease. The relative contribution of genetics and environment for such illnesses is not fully known. One way of understanding disease is to view it as the failure of an individual's genetic predisposition to adapt to his or her unique environmental experiences since birth.[5] Our understanding of genetic influences and unique environments shifts the focus from the disease manifestation to the person with the disease, a frame of reference deeply rooted in the discipline of nursing.

Population Genetics

The Human Genome Project is uncovering both similarities and differences in the human population. Scientists estimate that 99.9% of the human genome is the same for all people.[28] Distinct differences occur as a result of mutations in the other 0.1%. Identifying mutations involves looking for differences in chromosome number and structure and variations in base pairs and genes. Even

■ male ● female ■● affected person ◨◑ carrier

Autosomal dominant inherited conditions

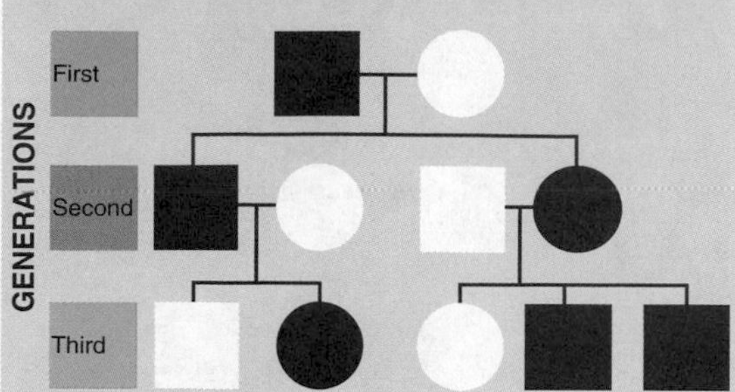

Features

- Vertical transmission in families
- Males and females equally affected
- Variable expression among family members and others with the condition
- Reduced penetrance in some conditions (the condition doesn't affect everyone who has the gene mutation and appears to "skip" a generation)
- Advanced paternal age associated with sporadic cases

Examples

- Hereditary breast and ovarian cancer
- Familial hypercholesterolemia
- Hereditary nonpolyposis colorectal cancer
- Huntington's disease
- Marfan syndrome
- Neurofibromatosis

X-linked recessive inherited conditions

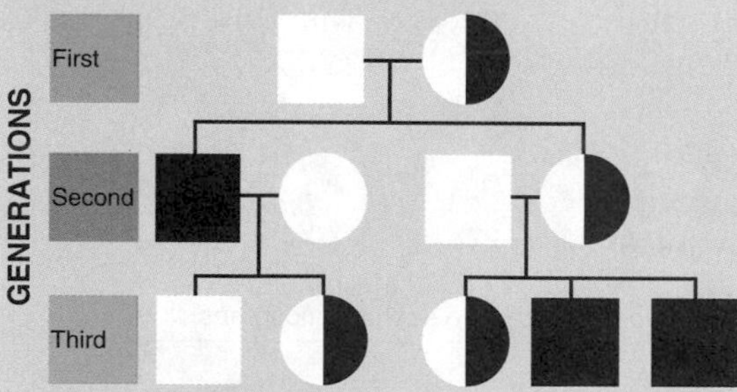

Features

- Vertical transmission in families
- Predominantly males affected

Examples

- Duchenne muscular dystrophy
- Hemophilia
- Wiskott-Aldrich syndrome
- Protan and Deutran forms of color blindness

Autosomal recessive inherited conditions

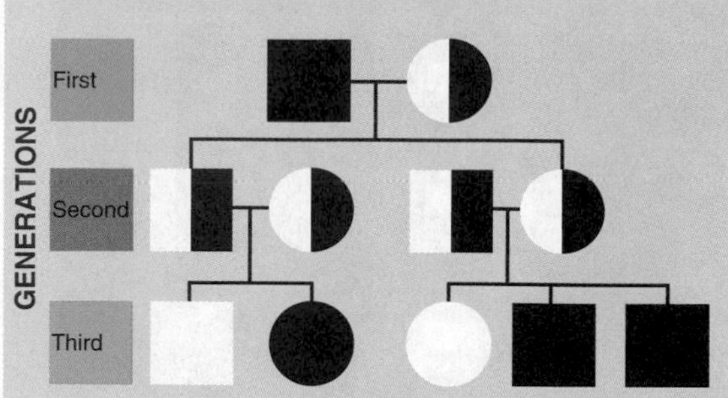

Features

- Horizontal occurrence in families
- Males and females equally affected
- Associated with genetic relatedness (consanguinity)
- Associated with particular ethnic groups

Examples

- Cystic fibrosis
- Galactosemia
- Phenylketonuria
- Sickle-cell disease
- Tay-Sachs disease
- Thalassemia

Multifactorial inherited conditions

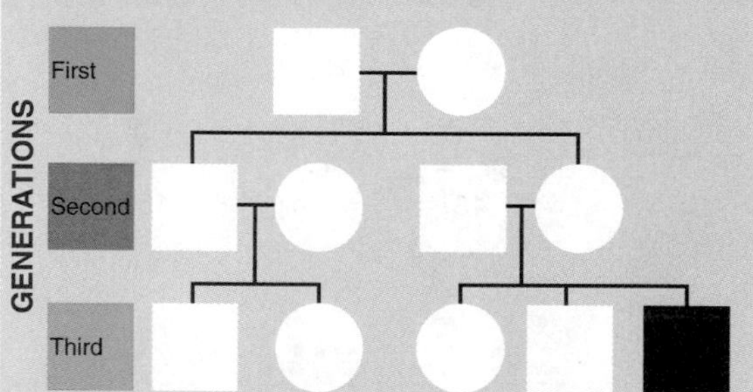

Features

- Caused by a combination of genetic and enviromental factors
- Conditions may recur in families
- Inheritance pattern may appear random and doesn't demonstrate the characteristic pattern seen with Mendelian inherited conditions

Examples

- Congenital heart defects
- Cleft lip (with or without cleft palate)
- Congenital hip dislocation
- Neural tube defects such as anencephaly and spina bifida

Figure 5-10 Mapping out hereditary conditions.

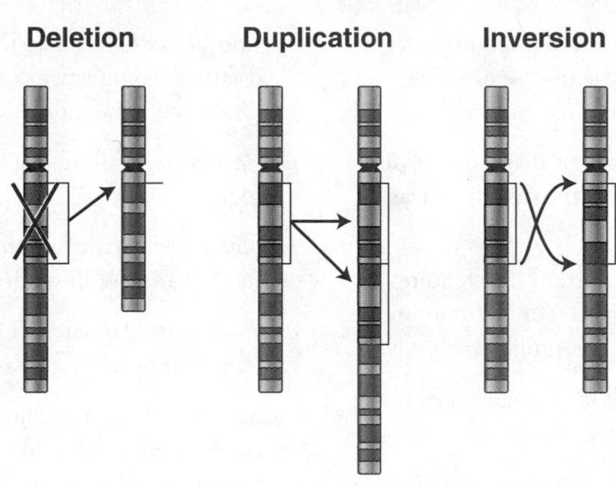

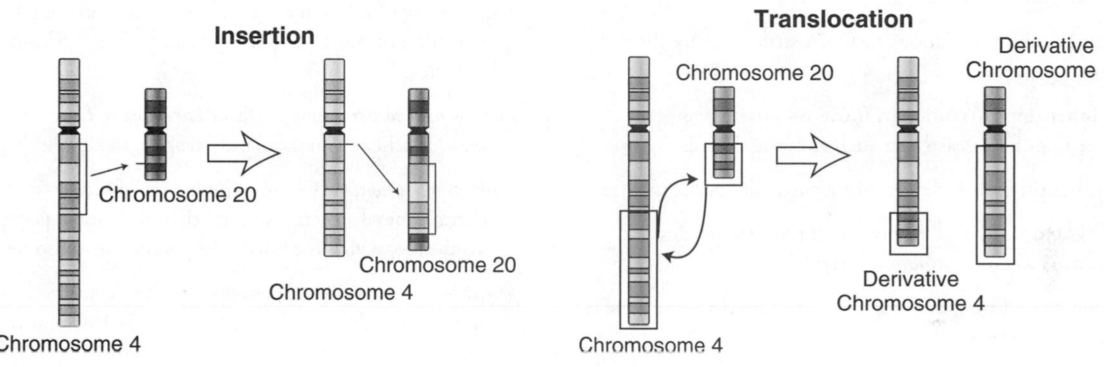

Figure 5-11 Main types of chromosome mutation.

Box 5-2 Terms Related to Chromosomes and Inheritance

chromosome: A collection of genes arranged in the nucleus of the cell.

autosome: A nonsex chromosome composed of deoxyribonucleic acid (DNA) base pairs. Human beings have 22 pairs of autosomes.

sex chromosomes: Pair of chromosomes that is usually found as either two X chromosomes (female) or an XY combination (male), which determines the sex of the fetus.

centromere: Central region of a chromosome between p and q arms.

chromatids: Areas above and below a chromosome's centromere.

p arm of a chromosome: Short segment of a chromosome; used to define the location of a particular gene.

q arm of a chromosome: Long segment of a chromosome; used to define the location of a particular gene.

locus: Position or location of a gene (segment of DNA) on a particular chromosome.

allele: Alternative form of gene's locus or location. A person can inherit different alleles from each parent.

linkage: Tendency of certain markers to be located near one another on a chromosome. Close proximity results in more frequent inheritance together.

genotype: Genetic profile of an individual represented by base pair sequences.

karyotype: The map of paired chromosomes from a cell nucleus; allows visual inspection of the number, size, and shape of each chromosome.

phenotype: Visible expression of the genetic makeup of an individual evident in physical appearance.

mutations: Change in DNA structure limited to certain individuals.

polymorphisms: Common variations in DNA structure.

From Human Genome Project, US Department of Energy: *Genomics and its impact on science and society: a 2003 primer,* accessed July 2004 from website: www.ornl.gov/hgmis/publicat/primer/; and National Human Genome Research Institute: *Talking glossary of genetic terms,* accessed July 2004 from website: www.genome.gov/glossary.cfm.

Box 5-3 Terms Related to Inheritance Patterns

autosomal recessive: Mendelian inheritance pattern that requires two affected genes for an individual to express the disease or trait (e.g., cystic fibrosis).

autosomal dominant: Mendelian inheritance pattern that requires only one affected gene for an individual to express the disease or trait (e.g., Huntington's disease).

sex-linked transmission: Mendelian inheritance pattern that requires an affected gene on one of the sex chromosomes (X or Y) for an individual to express the disease or trait (e.g., hemophilia).

mutations: Changes in deoxyribonucleic acid (DNA) that can be either harmful or harmless (e.g., BRCA 1).

variable expressivity: Differences in severity of a disorder among people (e.g., in neurofibromatosis).

polymorphisms: Common variations in DNA structure (not disease causing).

heterozygous: Inheriting two different forms of a particular gene (can be a carrier of a disease trait such as cystic fibrosis).

homozygous: Inheriting the same form of a particular gene.

multifactorial: Conditions that involve multiple gene products (i.e., proteins) and environmental interaction.

polygenic: Genetic conditions that result from more than one gene (e.g., Alzheimer's disease).

mitochondrial DNA: Genetic material found in the mitochondria (organelles that generate energy for the cell).

trinucleotide repeats: Non-Mendelian inheritance evidenced by copies of the same three nucleotides (e.g., fragile X syndrome).

anticipation: Worsening of a genetic condition in each succeeding generation (e.g., Kennedy's syndrome).

imprinting: Non-Mendelian inheritance mechanism that results in a disease phenotype in a child that varies depending on which parent (mother or father) had the affected gene (e.g., Prader-Willi syndrome if father's complement of chromosome 15 missing; Angelman's syndrome if the mother's is missing).

nondisjunction: Failure of a segment of chromosome to separate during meiosis.

translocations: Parts of a chromosome being interchanged (e.g., Prader-Willi syndrome).

deletions: Loss of a part of DNA possibly leading to disease (e.g., early-onset familial Alzheimer's disease).

mosaicism: Different cell lines within an individual that are passed on through cell division and may eventually cause disease (e.g., neurofibromatosis).

polygenic disorder: Complex genetic disorder resulting from more than one allele or more than one gene (e.g., heart disease, diabetes, some cancers).

single gene disorder: Genetic disorder resulting from one allele (e.g., Duchenne's muscular dystrophy, sickle cell disease).

chromosome disorders: Clinical conditions resulting from variations in chromosomal structures rather than individual genes (e.g., Down syndrome, which is caused by an extra chromosome 21).

penetrance: Proportion of people with an affected gene who show symptoms (e.g., achondroplasia penetrance is 100%, meaning all persons with the affected gene will show symptoms).

From GeneTests: *Medical genetics information resource, educational materials: glossary,* copyright University of Washington, Seattle, 1993-2004, accessed Sept 2004 from website: http://www.genetests.org/; Human Genome Project, US Department of Energy: *Basic terminology,* in *Genomics and its impact on science and society: a 2003 primer,* accessed from website: http://www.ornl.gov/hgmis/publicat/primer/; and National Human Genome Research Institute: *Talking glossary of genetic terms,* accessed July 2004 from website: www.genome.gov/glossary.cfm.

mutations can be common across populations. Such variations are called *polymorphisms*.

The ability to identify an individual's genetic profile allows for increasingly detailed information about potential risks and susceptibility to disease. Individuals and families can use genetic information to reduce their risk by altering modifiable factors such as nutrition and exercise. In the future scientists may use genetic technologies to alter genes that place the individual at risk and thus prevent the onset of illness (see Future Watch box).[6]

Use of Genetic Technologies for Diagnosis and Treatment of Disease

Diagnosis

Genetic testing is done to determine whether a fetus is affected by a genetic condition; to screen the newborn for conditions such as phenylketonuria; to assess **carrier** status for cystic fibrosis to help couples make decisions about parenting; to diagnose presymptomatic genetic conditions such as Huntington's disease; and to provide risk assessment for certain diseases such as breast cancer.[9]

Tests are now available to identify the presence of affected genes for selected diseases. Prenatal determination of sex and some chromosomal disorders such as trisomy 21, or Down syndrome, is possible through examination of the karyotype of a fetal cell. Prenatal screening for such conditions as neural tube defects, chromosomal anomalies, and cystic fibrosis provides parents with information about their developing fetus. The parents can use such information to decide whether to continue the pregnancy, thus raising difficult ethical issues for both patients and providers. Newborns are screened for a least two disorders, phenylketonuria and galactosemia, which can be treated and would result in serious health consequences if left undetected.

Predispositional testing provides an individual with information about the likelihood of developing a genetic disorder later in life. For example, hemochromatosis is an adult-onset disease with currently available treatment.[29] Tests for adult-onset diseases for which there is no effective clinical treatment are also available. An example is Huntington's disease, an autosomal dominant disorder,

Future Watch

Genomics in Health Care

Knowing the sequence of base pairs is only the first step in understanding the structure and function of genes. The Human Genome Project continues its work to increase knowledge about the structure and function of genes and proteins and the use of new knowledge in preventing and treating disease. Future efforts of the Human Genome Project focus on three areas.

Relationship of Genome to Life Sciences

Identify all the functional sequences that produce proteins.

Identify the interactions of proteins (proteomics).

Catalog the variety of human inheritable conditions.

Compare gene sequences of different species.

Develop policies on intellectual property rights to new information.

Relationship of Genome to Health and Illness

Identify how genes influence disease.

Identify how genes influence human response to medications.

Identify how genes affect resistance to disease.

Create a list of diseases based on molecular characteristics.

Develop new treatments targeting biologic pathways.

Use genetic information in the clinical setting for clinical decision making for improved outcomes.

Ensure the benefits of genomic research are widely accessible.

Relationship of Genome to Society

Develop public policies that address issues of access and discrimination.

Examine human variation and its relationship to race and ethnicity.

Examine the potential use and misuse of genetic information.

From Collins FS et al: A vision for the future of genomics research, *Nature* 422: 1-13, 2003, accessed Sept 2004 from website: http://www.nature.com/nature.

whose symptoms manifest in the third and fourth decades of life. Tests are also available for adult-onset diseases whose impact can be minimized through early intervention, including some forms of breast cancer and familial adenomatous polyposis.

A growing trend is the development of tests to identify whether a person is a carrier for a gene mutation known to cause a disorder that could be passed onto the next generation. Examples include tests for cystic fibrosis, sickle cell anemia, and Duchenne's muscular dystrophy. Individuals can use information about their carrier status to make decisions about childbearing. The National Institutes of Health funds a website that provides information for health care providers and patients about genetic disorders, tests, and clinics.[9] Primary care providers are often the first people to identify the need for further genetic evaluation and make the referral. Most genetic tests are offered within the context of a genetic counseling relationship so the patient and family can be educated about the risks and benefits of obtaining genetic information. Table 5-2 describes types of genetic tests.

Treatment

Most genetic disorders are treated symptomatically using current medical therapies such as surgery and pharmacotherapy. Gene therapy is primarily in the experimental testing phase and includes clinical trials to replace, change, or assist affected genes. The National Institutes of Health defines **recombinant DNA** as "molecules that are constructed outside living cells by joining natural or synthetic DNA segments to DNA molecules that can replicate in a living cell" or the by-products of such molecules.[26]

Gene therapies are divided into two categories: somatic and germline. Somatic gene therapies target genes in affected cells other than in the reproductive or germline cells in the ovaries or sperm. Germline gene therapies target the affected genes in the person's eggs or sperm or in the zygote before implantation.[25] Changes in germline cells affect all of a person's future offspring. The research community recognizes the potential for unintended consequences of altering affected genes for all future generations and is concerned about the **ethics** of such research. At present, germline therapies are not approved for clinical trials (see Ethical Alert box).

Somatic gene therapies may use viruses as vectors to carry the replacement or modified gene to cells with the affected gene. Normal genetic material is inserted into the virus vector and then injected into the affected cells. The normal genetic material provides information required for the cell to produce the correct protein. Alternatives to using virus vectors include packaging the correct DNA in a liposome coated in polyethylene glycol that can cross the cell membrane and correct the defective DNA. Another avenue of research is the development of an artificial therapeutic 47th chromosome that would carry corrected DNA information into the cell nucleus of affected tissue.[11] Examples of clinical trials investigating the potential of gene therapy include protocols for experimental treatment of melanoma, ovarian and breast cancers, Alzheimer's disease, and muscular dystrophy.

Pharmacogenetics

Traditionally, physicians prescribe medications used to treat disease based on the patient's diagnosis, signs, and symptoms.[28] In the future, more health care providers will tailor prescriptions based on genetic tests that predict an individual's response and, it is hoped, avoid serious side effects and nonresponse.[36] Genetic differences (mutations or polymorphisms) in how people metabolize medications may help explain why certain people have toxic reactions to or no therapeutic effect from commonly prescribed medications.[30] An example of an identified variation that affects an individual's response to medications is the differences in cytochrome P-450 (CYP) liver enzymes that metabolize certain drug classes. People whose CYP enzymes are weak may develop drug overdoses. Researchers are developing tests that will allow clinicians to identify individuals with CYP variations and establish more frequent monitoring protocols for them while they are undergoing drug therapy.[13]

A major goal of **pharmacogenetics** is to reduce adverse drug reactions.[10] Genetic testing can provide a genotype profile of all of an individual's single-nucleotide polymorphisms, which are thought to

TABLE 5-2 TYPES OF GENETIC TESTS

Type of Genetic Tests	Description	Examples of Genetic Conditions
Molecular Genetic Tests		
Direct deoxyribonucleic acid (DNA) testing	Tests for presence of genes known to cause disease	Hemophilia Huntington's disease Polycystic kidney disease
Linkage testing	Tests genetic material from several family members for presence of genetic markers believed to be located near affected gene	Familial adenomatous polyposis Huntington's disease Malignant hyperthermia susceptibility Neurofibromatosis Polycystic kidney disease
Methylation studies	Examines attachment of methyl groups to DNA molecule	Angelman's syndrome Beckwith-Wiedemann syndrome Prader-Willi syndrome Rett syndrome
Protein truncation test (PTT)	Tests for proteins that have been shortened and whose function has been altered	Breast cancer Familial adenomatous polyposis
Uniparental disomy (UPD)	Tests for two chromosomes from same parent rather than one from each	Angelman's syndrome Prader-Willi syndrome
X-inactivation studies	Tests for carrier status in women with some X-linked disorders	Fragile X syndrome Rett syndrome X-linked severe combined immunodeficiency
Cytogenic Test		
FISH (fluorescence in situ hybridization)	Identifies presence or absence of chromosome segments using fluorescein-tagged DNA probes	Angelman's syndrome Aniridia Williams syndrome
Chemical Genetic Tests		
Analyte testing	Assesses presence of substance in body indicative of genetic disorder	Hemocystinuria
Enzyme assay	Measures rate of chemical reaction of an enzyme in presence of a particular protein associated with genetic disorder; can identify affected individual or carrier	Gaucher's disease Lowe syndrome Galactosemia
Protein analysis	Tests for structure of proteins known to be associated with genetic disorders	Marfan syndrome Spinocerebellar ataxia

From GeneTests: *Medical genetics information resource, educational materials: glossary.* Copyright, University of Washington, Seattle, 1993-2004, accessed Sept 2004 from website: http://www.genetests.org/.

Ethical Alert

Germline Gene Therapy

Current research on curing genetic disorders has focused on somatic cell interventions. In somatic cell gene therapy, individuals who receive the therapy are the only ones affected by the treatment. Germline interventions that target the reproductive cells are considered off limits until science has a better idea of the potential for unintended consequences. It is also not possible to obtain the consent of future generations for interventions that will influence them. The National Institutes of Health currently does not fund clinical trials that would introduce changes in the genetic makeup of sperm or oocytes.

affect how an individual might respond to certain drugs.[30] With this knowledge, the care provider can select or withhold medications based on predicted response. For nurses, one practical issue is how to explain to patients why two people with the same diagnosis receive different medications based on genotype differences that cannot be "seen" but only tested for in the laboratory.[30]

Prevention

As previously stated, most disease is multifactorial; that is, a person is born with certain genetic predispositions and lives within specific challenging environments. Although individuals cannot

Research

West DS et al: The impact of a family history of breast cancer on screening practices and attitudes in low-income, rural, African American women, *J Women's Health* 12(8):779-787, 2003.

In this study, West and colleagues conducted telephone interviews with 320 African-American women who had not had a mammogram within the past 2 years. They asked women about any family history of breast cancer, their perceived risk of developing breast cancer, screening behaviors (mammography and self-breast examination), and attitudes and knowledge about mammography. Researchers also calculated the participants' relative risk of developing breast cancer using the Gail model, which takes into consideration known risk factors for breast cancer, including age and childbearing status. The researchers found that women with a positive family history for breast cancer were no more likely to engage in screening behaviors than women without a family history. Also, many women were not aware that a positive family history for breast cancer increased their risk of getting breast cancer. The findings support the need to help women understand their risks and increase their use of screening behaviors, since early detection is associated with higher cure rates.

change their genetic predispositions, they can use information about their genetic makeup to modify their environments (internal and external) through lifestyle choices. Knowledge of increased risk may motivate some individuals, families, or communities to adjust lifestyle risks.

As understanding of the structure and function of different proteins and their interactions increases, estimates of risk for disease will be more accurate. Interventions that target modifiable risk factors may reduce the chance of developing certain genetically influenced illnesses such as cancer, heart disease, and alcoholism. Potentially life-threatening diseases with genetic components and modifiable factors include coronary heart disease (CHD), asthma, diabetes, and melanoma. The nurse should advise at-risk patients on how to limit their risk through lifestyle modifications such as good nutrition, physical activity, and environmental management (e.g., avoiding triggers in the case of asthma or limiting sun exposure in the case of melanoma). People with genetic risk factors for breast cancer and familial adenomatous polyposis may benefit from more aggressive screening schedules (mammogram and colonoscopy) to ensure early detection and treatment before metastasis. Early detection and treatment can maximize survival rates[31] (see Research box).

CHD provides an example of using genetic predisposition information for primary prevention through modification of risk factors. Review of a family pedigree may reveal one or more first-degree relatives who developed CHD at an early age.[22] Families with a positive history for CHD also show the following characteristics: dyslipidemia, high blood pressure, diabetes, tobacco use, lack of exercise, dietary excesses, alcohol use, and obesity.[2] Lifestyle modification in the form of increased activity, improved nutritional intake, smoking cessation, and management of high blood pressure may reduce or delay an individual's risk of developing CHD despite genetic predisposition.

Until genetic interventions are safe and effective, people who are identified as genetically at risk for cancer, heart disease, and other disorders should focus on prevention strategies based on modifiable risk factors. Nurses are in a unique position to identify

Gerontologic Assessment

Traditionally genetic disorders were considered a childhood or young adult issue; however, recent advances in genetic testing and therapies provide tools for assisting older adults with genetic conditions through identification, referral, and support. Examples of conditions with genetic influences that affect older adults include Huntington's disease, Alzheimer's disease, breast and prostate cancer, familial adenomatous polyposis, hemochromatosis, and Parkinson's disease.

Important assessment factors include family history displayed in pedigree format; ethnicity; reproductive history, including pregnancy losses; presence of adult-onset disorders in any of the generations; and psychosocial resources (current knowledge, family communication, willingness to explore impact of genetic factors on family health).

Once a potential genetic condition is identified in a family, the nurse provides referrals to local and regional genetic services. Such specialty services supplement care provided by the health care team.

From Schutte DL: Evidence-based protocol: identification, referral, and support of older adults with genetic conditions, *J Gerontol Nurs* 28(2):6, 2002.

family members who might benefit from primary prevention. As more tests become available for determining genetic risk factors, individuals will be faced with deciding whether to be tested and what to do with the results.

Many genetically related conditions do not manifest until adulthood (see Gerontologic Assessment box).[31] Individuals with such conditions as Huntington's disease, Alzheimer's disease, and cancer may live long productive lives before the onset of debilitating symptoms. Deciding whether to be tested when no treatments exist will continue to be an issue for some. Helping couples use the information for preconceptual decision making will be important. Genetic testing of children for the presence of adult-onset disorders is controversial, since the individual does not get to choose whether to find out if he or she is predisposed to the "adult" genetic disorders. Nurses can assist patients and families in considering the disadvantages and benefits of new knowledge.

▶ ARE You READY?

Predispositional genetic testing is indicated for which of the following disorders?

1. Huntington's disease
2. Cystic fibrosis
3. Sickle cell anemia
4. Phenylketonuria

Nursing Management

of the Patient with a Potential Genetic Condition

ASSESSMENT

Family History. Blood relatives share the most similar genetic information and are thus at risk for acquiring characteristics or disease present in family members. Preparing a family pedigree is useful in identifying classic inheritance patterns and potential conditions for referral. A family pedigree using standardized documentation symbols indicating familial relationships, gender, and living or dead status should be part of the patient's medical record.[1] Notes from the interview relevant to particular family members can be added to the pedigree. A three-generation display including the patient, parents, and grandparents is most useful in identifying patterns of inheritance (Figure 5-12). Pedigree symbols indicate whether the members are male or female, affected or unaffected by the disease of concern, and living or dead; lines denote relationship to the patient. A pedigree should also include marginal notes regarding current health status or diseases, age of onset for serious conditions, age of death, cause of death, consanguinity, reproductive history, age of pregnant women, and ethnicity.[20]

Additional areas to assess include:

- Environmental factors (exposure to teratogens, triggers, radiation, and toxic substances)
- Lifestyle factors (substance use and abuse, prescription drug use, and complementary therapies)
- Nutrition
- Psychosocial factors (emotional state, coping mechanisms, social support)
- Family system (cohesion, communication styles, resources)

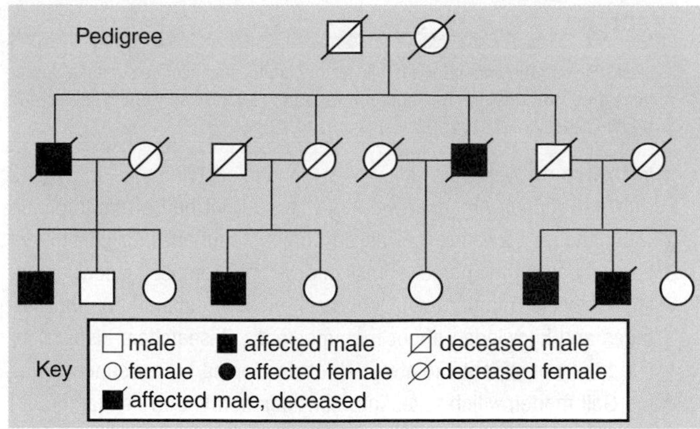

Figure 5-12 Three-generation family pedigree using standard symbols for male/female, affected/unaffected, living/deceased.

NURSING DIAGNOSES, OUTCOMES, AND INTERVENTIONS

Nursing Diagnosis: Decisional Conflict: Genetic Testing

Outcomes. Common examples of expected outcomes for the person faced with *decisional conflict* related to genetic testing are all associated with decision making (the ability to make judgments and choose between two or more alternatives[19,21]).

The person will:

- Identify relevant information about the genetic condition and associated genetic tests.
- Identify the alternatives of testing and not testing as a choice.
- Identify the consequences of having the genetic information and not having it.
- Identify where and how to obtain specialized support.
- Recognize potential family resistance to pursuing genetic testing.
- Acknowledge the potential impact of genetic information on other family members.
- Acknowledge the risks of having genetic information in one's health record.
- Weigh alternatives.
- Choose whether to pursue genetic testing.

Nursing Interventions. Nursing interventions for persons faced with a choice related to genetic testing include:

Active listening:

- Attend closely to the verbal and nonverbal messages conveyed by the patient; clarify messages with follow-up questions.

Risk identification—genetic:

- Provide for privacy and confidentiality during assessments and conferences.
- Review relevant diagnostic procedures.

Decision-making support:

- Provide information about alternatives.
- Assist patient in identifying advantages and disadvantages of options.
- Facilitate discussions with other family members.

Emotional support:

- Provide reassurance, acceptance, and encouragement during the decision-making process; be nonjudgmental and convey empathy.

Referrals:

- Arrange for services of a genetic counselor if desired; contact provider.

Documentation:

- Record details of conferences and include relevant patient quotes.
- Prepare referral forms.

Generalist nurses come in contact with many people who could benefit from genetic counseling. Nurse generalists can help patients and families obtain specialized care. For people with conditions listed in Box 5-4, the nurse should discuss referral to specialists who can help them identify, understand, and use personal and family genetic information.

Interpreting genetic tests is a primary responsibility of genetic nurse specialists. Awareness of the implications of testing is important for all nurses. Testing positive for a genetic disorder without a cure can be devastating to an individual and family. Loss of hope may affect the quality of life and at the extreme may result in despair and suicide. Nurses can help people consider the possible impact of information before they seek testing. Recognizing the current limits of therapy in healing the potentially devastating results of genetic disorders may assist persons in weighing the risks and benefits of genetic knowledge. It is not possible to "unknow" one's risks, and such knowledge can be a brutal reminder of a bleak future.

RELATED NIC INTERVENTIONS. Coping Enhancement, Health System Guidance, Mutual Goal Setting, Patient Rights Protection, Support System Enhancement, Teaching: Individual, Values Clarification

Box 5-4 Indications for Referral for Genetic Counseling

Preconceptual and Prenatal

Maternal age of 35 years or greater

History of chromosomal abnormality

Abnormal alpha-fetoprotein tests

History of birth defects or mental retardation in a previous child

Unexplained pregnancy loss

Exposure to teratogens

Pediatric

Abnormal screening tests such as phenylketonuria or hearing

Birth defects such as cleft lip and palate or neural tube defect

Unusual appearance (dysmorphic features)

Growth abnormalities

Chromosomal abnormality such as Down syndrome

Adult

Multiple unexplained miscarriages

Adult-onset hemochromatosis or neurodegenerative disorder

Family history of genetically related disorders (cystic fibrosis, diabetes, cancer, heart disease)

Data from Lea DH: Look back to move forward: how genetics changes daily practice, *Nurs Manag* 34(11), 2003 (electronic version); and Nussbaum MD, McInnes RR, Willard HF: *Thompson and Thompson genetics in medicine*, ed 6, rev. reprint, Philadelphia, 2004, WB Saunders.

EVALUATION

To evaluate the effectiveness of nursing interventions, compare patient behaviors with those stated in the expected patient outcomes.

RELATED NOC OUTCOMES. Health Beliefs, Personal Autonomy, Participation in Health Care Decisions

Follow-up Management and Counseling. Considering the newness of genetic information and the potential for future interventions, individuals must stay connected to a reliable source of information as they gain knowledge of their own genetic risks and determine how to use it. Although the ability to identify risk will precede the ability to treat conditions, new therapies on the horizon may affect the quality of life for individuals and their families.

Individuals at risk for genetically influenced disease can be counseled to address modifiable factors such as lifestyle (nutrition, diet, exercise), use preventive therapies, and maintain more stringent screening schedules. Management of adults with "childhood" genetic disorders will become increasingly common as early intervention extends life. Former pediatric patients with cystic fibrosis, sickle cell anemia, and hemophilia will need care by adult health practitioners. Current technologies allow children with once life-limiting genetic conditions to survive into adulthood, where they need continued management and help in deciding whether to have children of their own.

Genetic Counseling

Genetic counseling is a specialty with national standards and certification requirements for practitioners. Both nurses and non-nurses work as genetic counselors and may choose to specialize with certain populations. Genetic counseling is the "use of an interactive helping process focusing on assisting an individual, family, or group, manifesting or at risk for developing or transmitting a birth defect or genetic condition, to cope."[7]

The International Society of Nurses in Genetics (ISONG) developed a scope of practice statement for nurses, which was approved and published by the American Nurses Association in 1998.[14,18] The scope of practice identifies various levels of competencies from nurse generalist to nurse specialist. Nurse generalists identify, refer, and support persons, families, and communities at risk for genetic conditions. According to ISONG, genetic clinical nurse specialists are prepared to:

1. Obtain a detailed family history and construct a pedigree
2. Assess and analyze hereditary and nonhereditary disease risk factors
3. Identify potential genetic conditions or genetic predispositions to disease
4. Provide genetic information and psychosocial support to individuals and families
5. Provide nursing care for patients and families at risk for or affected by diseases with a genetic component

In addition, advanced practice nurses in genetics are prepared to provide genetic counseling and to facilitate and interpret genetic test results and laboratory reports.[18] Goals of genetic counseling are to help people understand the genetic aspects of their medical conditions including the impact on other family members; identify their values; recognize the risks and benefits of diagnostic and treatment choices, including costs; and maximize adjustment to living with genetic disorders.[29]

The National Society of Genetic Counselors (NSGC) is the professional association for a variety of health care providers, including nurses, who specialize in genetic counseling.[27] NSGC was instrumental in standardizing symbols used to record human pedigree diagrams. Members of NSGC see individuals and families for genetic counseling before testing to discuss potential implications of the results. Historically, genetic counselors used a nondirective counseling approach to shield patients from personal bias and assist them in making their own decisions.

▶ ARE YOU READY?

The generalist nurse's scope of practice includes which of the following?

1. Providing genetic counseling
2. Constructing a family history and pedigree
3. Interpreting genetic results
4. Referring a patient at risk for a genetic condition

Ethical Issues

Ethical issues are an important element of the national research agenda. The Ethical, Legal, and Social Implications program of the Human Genome Project receives funds to examine the impact of the genetics, new "central science" on clinical practice. Past projects have focused on genetic discrimination and health insurance, genetic testing, conduct of genetic research, and underrepresented minorities.

Informed Consent for Genetic Testing

Nurses are key advocates in ensuring informed consent for both standard and experimental testing and treatment of patients and families. Such efforts become even more important as the long-term implications of genetic knowledge are uncovered. Providing biologic material (blood or tissue samples) for testing is the easy part. Having and using knowledge from the test is more complicated.[30] For example, a person may have a genotype that is later linked to a life-limiting disease without known treatment. Will the person want this new information? Will the person's family want the information? Who is responsible for deciding when to tell? How will information about predisposition to disease affect the childbearing decisions of future generations? Should parents avoid childbearing if their children have the potential or likelihood of developing an adult-onset disorder such as Alzheimer's or Huntington's disease? Who is to say that someone who lives only 40 years has any less satisfying or productive a life than someone with an average life expectancy? Why deny the world the next Einstein?

ISONG outlines the professional nurse's responsibilities in ensuring informed consent. Responsibilities include alerting patients of their right to informed consent before testing and treatment; advocating for client autonomy, privacy, and confidentiality; ensuring clear discussion of the benefits and risks of testing or treatment, including physical, psychologic, and social risks; providing care within the context of the client's unique circumstances; adhering to professional ethical guidelines; engaging in professional development to remain updated on the latest information; and collaborating with the health care team to ensure informed decision making.[15]

A special case of informed consent relates to participation in clinical trials that will collect genetic information or provide gene therapy. The National Institutes of Health has strict guidelines on full disclosure to potential participants. These requirement include the usual human subject requirements related to purpose; procedures; alternatives; voluntary nature of participation; potential benefits; possible risks, discomforts, and side effects; and costs. They also include special provisions describing reproductive considerations, long-term follow-up, request for autopsy, interest of the media, and privacy.

Privacy and Confidentiality

Genetic information about individuals comes from a variety of sources, including family history, biologic samples, physical examination, and the medical record. As more of an individual's genetic information is analyzed and stored in medical records, issues arise as to who has access to the information and for what purposes. An individual's genetic information also reveals information about family members, thus widening the sphere of privacy. ISONG reiterates the importance of maintaining the patient's trust through assurances of privacy and confidentiality of genetic information.[16] Professional nurses are charged with ensuring professional practice that maintains privacy and confidentiality, as well as ensuring that institutional policies and procedures are in place that highly value privacy and confidentiality.[4]

Discrimination

The development of genetic testing raises many issues about how knowledge gained from such tests will be used. A major barrier to widespread genetic testing is the concern that employers could use information about personal risk to discriminate against individuals in hiring and benefits decisions (see Legal Alert box). Risk factors for a condition do not necessarily guarantee that a person will develop the disease. Still, being labeled as someone who is "cancer-prone" or likely to develop a mentally disabling condition could harm a person's reputation and create social and economic barriers.

Access to Genetic Services

Gene therapy will likely be very expensive once it is shown to be clinically effective. A major ethical issue for society will be access to such interventions. Will they be limited to those who can afford health insurance? ISONG calls on professional nurses to act as advocates for individuals in their right to choose to use or not use genomic health care services and to ensure that access to such services is not based on economic factors.[17]

Legal Alert

Preventing Discrimination

To establish a "national and uniform basic standard" to prevent discrimination of individuals based on genetic information, the U.S. Senate passed the Genetic Information Nondiscrimination Act of 2003. It prevents insurance companies from (1) denying coverage or charging higher premiums for individuals based on genetic information, and (2) requiring genetic testing to receive coverage. It prevents employers from discriminating against employees based on genetic information in hiring and firing decisions and also prevents employers from seeking out genetic information about employees or their family members. Several provisions also apply to labor organizations and their membership criteria. Special provisions highlight the standards for confidentiality of medical records of employees. The act also spells out "remedies" for a person who is discriminated against. A similar bill, H.R. 3636, was under consideration in the U.S. House of Representatives, but was referred to the House Subcommittee on health.

U.S. Senate, 108th Congress. S. 1053, 2004.

Misuse of Genetic Information

History provides vivid examples of how dominant social and political groups have used genetic information to try to manipulate future populations based on preferences for certain traits in the phenotype, or what people look like. Starting in the late nineteenth century, eugenics was a social and scientific movement whose purpose was to shape future populations by limiting the reproductive capacity of individuals whom the influential class deemed less desirable. Based on what is now considered "faulty science," 33 states passed sterilization laws to prevent people with certain characteristics from reproducing and continued to do so into the 1970s.[8]

The misuse of genetic information is most profoundly illustrated by the events in Germany in the 1930s, which had a well-orchestrated plan to limit reproduction of people with mental illness and other conditions. What followed was the eventual extermination of millions of men, women, and children who did not meet the criteria for the master race established by the Hitler's Nazi Party.[32]

Unfortunately the past is present; there is no shortage of groups who seek to influence the population genome. This is illustrated by policies in China that support gender preference and tolerate abandonment and infanticide of female children. Vigilance by all is required to see that new genetic knowledge is used with respect for human rights.

? Critical Thinking

1. Construct a three-generation pedigree from the following information: your patient is Sally Steiner, a 51-year-old woman seen in the clinic with a diagnosis of hypertension. She is a pack-a-day smoker who is overweight with a body mass index of 27. She has two siblings: a brother, age 48, a former smoker with hypertension; and a sister, age 53, who is overweight and smokes a pack a day. Ms. Steiner's mother died at age 55 of a stroke. Her mother's sister died at age 58 of a stroke. Her mother's brother died at age 42 from a motor vehicle accident. Her father, age 75, is alive and has high blood pressure treated with diuretics. His brother died at age 50 from a work-related accident. His sister is 70 and has Alzheimer's disease. Ms. Steiner's maternal grandmother died at age 60 of a stroke. Her maternal grandfather died at age 48 of a myocardial infarction. Her paternal grandmother is alive with a history of osteoarthritis and high blood pressure. Her paternal grandfather died at age 59 from a myocardial infarction.
2. You are caring for a 25-year-old woman whose father died of Huntington's disease. She asks you what her chances of having the same disease are. How would you explain her risks?

References

1. Bennett RL et al: Recommendations for standardized human pedigree nomenclature, Pedigree Standardization Task Force of the National Society of Genetic Counselors, *Am J Human Genetics* 56(3):745–752, 1995.
2. Burke LE: Primary prevention in patients with a strong family history of coronary heart disease, *J Cardiovasc Nurs* 18(2):139–143, 2003.
3. Cashion AK, Driscoll CJ: Genetics and kidney dysfunction, *Nephrol Nurs J* 31(1):14–18, 2004.
4. Cassells JM et al: An ethical assessment framework for addressing global genetic issues in clinical practice, *Oncol Nurs Forum* 30(3):383-390, 2003.
5. Childs B: Medicine through a genetic lens. In Hager M, editor: *The implications of genetics for health professional education*, New York, 1999, Josiah Macy, Jr. Foundation.
6. Collins FS et al: A vision for the future of genomics research, *Nature* 422: 1-13, 2003, accessed Sept 2004 from website: www.nature.com/nature.
7. Dochterman JM, Bulechek GM, editors: *Nursing intervention classification (NIC)*, ed 4, St Louis, 2004, Mosby.
8. Dolan DNA Learning Center, Cold Spring Harbor Laboratory: *Image archive on the American eugenics movement*, accessed July 2004 from website: www.eugenicsarchive.org.
9. GeneTests: *Medical genetics information resource, educational materials: glossary*, accessed Sept 2004 from website: http://www.genetests.org.
10. Haga SB, Burke W: Using pharmacogenetics to improve drug safety and efficacy, *JAMA* 291(23):2869-2871, 2004.
11. Human Genome Project, US Department of Energy: *Gene therapy*, accessed Sept 2004 from website: www.ornl.gov/sci/techresources/Human_Genome/medicine/genetherapy.shtml/.
12. Human Genome Project, US Department of Energy: *Genomics and its impact on science and society*: a *2003 primer*, accessed July 2004 from website: www.ornl.gov/hgmis/publicat/primer/.
13. Human Genome Project, US Department of Energy: *Pharmacogenetics*, accessed Sept 2004 from website: www.ornl.gov/sci/techresources/Human_Genome/medicine/pharma.shtml/.
14. International Society of Nurses in Genetics: *Statement on the scope and standards of genetics clinical nursing practice*, Washington, DC, 1998, American Nurses Publishing.
15. International Society of Nurses in Genetics: *Position statement: informed decision-making and consent: the role of the nurse*, 2000, accessed July 2004 from website: www.isong.org/about/position_statements/genetics_healthcare .html.
16. International Society of Nurses in Genetics: *Position statement: privacy and confidentiality of genetic information: the role of the nurse*, 2001, accessed July 2004 from website: www.isong.org/about/position_statements/genetics_healthcare.html.
17. International Society of Nurses in Genetics: *Position statement: access to genomic healthcare: the role of the nurse*, 2003, accessed July 2004 from website: www.isong.org/about/position_statements/genetics_healthcare.html.
18. International Society of Nurses in Genetics: *What is a genetic nurse?* 2003, accessed July 2004 from website: www.isong.org.
19. Johnson M et al: *Nursing diagnosis, outcomes, and interventions: NANDA, NOC, and NIC linkages*, St Louis, 2001, Mosby.
20. Lea DH: Look back to move forward: how genetics changes daily practice, *Nurs Manage* 34(11), 2003 (electronic version).
21. Moorhead S, Johnson M, Maas M, editors: *Nursing outcomes classification (NOC)*, ed 3, St Louis, 2004, Mosby.
22. National Coalition for Health Professions Education in Genetics: Not just for geneticists, *Genetic Fam History Practice* 1(1):1, 2003.
23. National Coalition for Health Professions Education in Genetics: *Core competencies in genetics essential for all health-care professionals*, accessed July 2004 from website: www.nchpeg.org/.
24. National Coalition for Health Professions Education in Genetics: *Principles of genetics for health professionals*, accessed July 2004 from website: www.nchpeg.org/.
25. National Human Genome Research Institute: *Talking glossary of genetic terms*, accessed July 2004 from website: www.genome.gov/glossary.cfm.
26. National Institutes of Health: *NIH guidelines for recombinant DNA and gene transfer*, accessed Sept 2004 from website: http://www4.od.nih.gov/oba/rac/guidelines/guidelines.html.
27. National Society of Genetic Counselors: *Position statement*, accessed July 2004 from website: www.nsgc.org/about/position.asp/.
28. Nicol MJ: The variation in response to pharmacotherapy: pharmacogenetics—a new perspective to "the right drug, for the right person," *MEDSURG Nurs* 12(4):242–249, 2003.

29. Nussbaum MD, McInnes RR, Willard HF: *Thompson and Thompson genetics in medicine*, ed 6, rev reprint, Philadelphia, 2004, WB Saunders.
30. Prows CA, Prows DR: Medication selection by genotype, *Am J Nurs* 104(5):60-71, 2004.
31. Schutte DL: Evidence-based protocol: identification, referral, and support of older adults with genetic conditions, *J Gerontol Nurs* 28(2):6, 2002.
32. Bachrach S, Kuntz D, editors: *US Holocaust Memorial Museum: Deadly medicine: creating the master race,* exhibition catalog, Washington, DC, 2004, University of North Carolina Press.
33. US Department of Energy: *Primer on molecular genetics,* accessed Feb 2004 from website: www.ornl.gov/hgmis/publicat/publications.html#primer.
34. US Department of Energy: *Genomics and its impact on science and society,* accessed July 2004 from website: www.ornl.gov/hgmis/publicat/primer/.
35. US Department of Health and Human Services: *Healthy people 2010: understanding and improving health,* ed 2, Washington, DC, 2000, US Government Printing Office.
36. Yetter-Read C: Pharmacogenomics: an evolving paradigm for drug therapy, *MEDSURG Nurs* 11(3):122-124, 2002.

Visit the Evolve website: http://evolve.elsevier.com/Monahan/medsurg

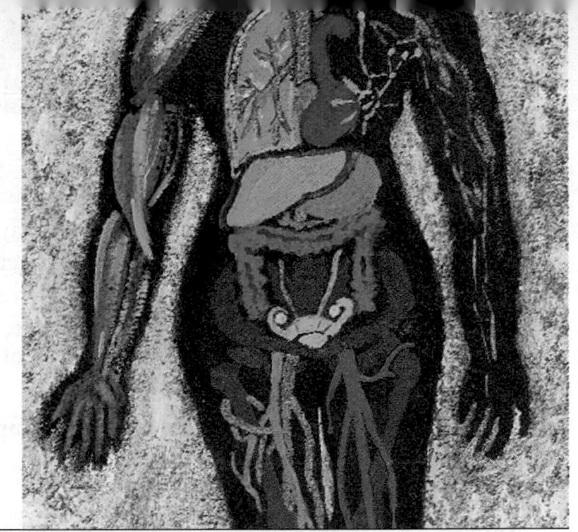

CHAPTER 6

Infectious Diseases and Bioterrorism

by Carol J. Green

OBJECTIVES

After studying this chapter, the learner should be able to:

1. Explain the chain of infection.
2. Discuss the characteristics of common infectious agents.
3. Identify factors contributing to the emergence and reemergence of infectious diseases.
4. Identify factors contributing to microbial resistance.
5. Describe measures to prevent and control nosocomial infections.
6. Cite the major components of the Centers for Disease Control and Prevention guidelines for Standard and Transmission-Based Precautions used in hospitals.
7. Describe nursing care for the patient with an infection.
8. Identify agents considered to be ideal biologic warfare agents.
9. Discuss preparations necessary for potential bioterrorist events.
10. Discuss chemical agents that may be used by terrorists.
11. Describe emergency care of persons exposed to chemical agents.
12. Discuss injuries that may be caused by exposure to radiation.
13. Describe emergency care of persons exposed to radiation.

KEY TERMS

carrier, p. 91
colonization, p. 90
endogenous, p. 89
endotoxin, p. 90
exogenous, p. 89
exotoxin, p. 90
herd immunity, p. 107
pathogenicity, p. 90
prion, p. 93
retroviruses, p. 93
susceptibility, p. 91
vectorborne, p. 100
virulence, p. 91
zoonotic, p. 100

Infectious Diseases

Infectious diseases have plagued people throughout history. Archeologists have documented evidence of fungal infections and parasitic roundworms in prehistoric humans. Millions of people died of smallpox before immunizations and eradication of the disease. Bubonic plague killed more than 20 million people as it spread throughout Asia, Europe, and the Middle East in the fourteenth century. A worldwide pandemic of influenza killed between 20 million and 40 million people from 1918 to 1919. In 2000 the mortality from human immunodeficiency virus (HIV) was greater than 36.1 million.[36]

With effort, infectious diseases can be controlled. Nurses and other health care providers play key roles in preventing transmission of infections in health care settings and educating patients and the public about disease prevention, transmission, and control. To intervene effectively, nurses must have a working knowledge of the infectious disease process, agents that cause infections, diseases that threaten society, and methods to control their spread.

Infectious Disease Process

Microorganisms are a necessary part of everyday life. Many, known as *resident* or *normal flora*, adapt and live peacefully with the human body, providing benefits such as vitamin production or cellulose digestion in the intestines, and protection from disease-producing pathogens.[22] *Transient flora* may stay for weeks to months but do not remain permanently because of fierce competition from resident flora. When the delicate balance between the host and normal flora is disturbed, *infection* occurs. **Endogenous** infections arise when normal flora contaminate tissues or body areas not usually occupied by the organism, such as skin bacteria entering tissues through wounds or insect bites. **Exogenous** infections arise from outside sources such as soil, water, animals, or the hands of health care workers.

Pathogens are nonbeneficial microbes capable of harming the host. Bacteria, viruses, mycoplasma, fungi, prions (proteins), and parasites (worms, protozoa, and arthropods) may serve as pathogens (Table 6-1). Infection results when pathogens multiply and spread, interfere with cellular function, destroy cells, or produce poisonous substances called *toxins.* **Endotoxins,** present in the cell walls of gram-negative bacteria, are released when the cell wall is disrupted. **Exotoxins** are soluble protein substances secreted by bacteria. Toxins alter host cell physiology and compromise cellular defenses, which can result in tissue necrosis, fever, bleeding, clotting, or shock syndromes.[31]

Pathogens have varying degrees of pathogenicity and invasiveness. **Pathogenicity** refers to the pathogen's ability to cause disease or damage. *Invasiveness* is the pathogen's ability to penetrate target tissues. For example, pneumococci are highly invasive but only moderately pathogenic. *Clostridium tetani,* on the other hand, is highly pathogenic but not very invasive. An infection is *symptomatic* if it causes clinical signs and symptoms, and *asymptomatic* if no perceivable clinical or subclinical signs or symptoms are present. When pathogens collect in cells or tissues such as the nasal passages or skin surfaces without causing injury, they are colonized. **Colonization** can be a significant source of infection to the host and others. Several microbial and host interactions are involved in the onset and spread of infection and are known collectively as the *chain of infection.*

Chain of Infection

A common sequence of events underlies the development of all infectious diseases (Figure 6-1). The links in this chain are the:

- *Causative agent:* The infectious or pathogenic agent must first exist. It may be a bacterium, virus, fungus, prion, protozoa, or helminth (worm).
- *Reservoir:* The reservoir is the place where the agent lives, receives nourishment, and multiplies. It can be animate (human or animal) or inanimate (e.g., soil, water, intra-

TABLE 6-1 COMMON PATHOGENS AND ASSOCIATED INFECTIONS

Organism	Major Reservoir(s)	Major Infections and Diseases
Bacteria		
Escherichia coli	Colon	Gastroenteritis, urinary tract infection
Staphylococcus aureus	Skin, hair, anterior nares	Wound infection, pneumonia, food poisoning, cellulitis
Streptococcus (beta-hemolytic group A) organisms	Oropharynx, skin, perianal area	Strep throat, rheumatic fever, scarlet fever, impetigo, wound infection
Streptococcus (beta-hemolytic group B) organisms	Adult genitalia	Urinary tract infection, wound infection, postpartum sepsis, neonatal sepsis
Mycobacterium tuberculosis	Droplet nuclei from lungs	Tuberculosis
Neisseria gonorrhoeae	Genitourinary tract, rectum, mouth	Gonorrhea, pelvic inflammatory disease, infectious arthritis, conjunctivitis
Rickettsia rickettsii	Wood tick	Rocky Mountain spotted fever
Staphylococcus epidermidis	Skin	Wound infection, bacteremia
Viruses		
Hepatitis A virus	Feces	Hepatitis A
Hepatitis B virus	Blood and body fluids	Hepatitis B
Hepatitis C virus	Blood	Hepatitis C
Herpes simplex virus (type I)	Lesions of mouth or skin, saliva, genitalia	Cold sores, aseptic meningitis, sexually transmitted disease, herpetic whitlow
Human immunodeficiency virus (HIV)	Blood, semen, vaginal secretions (also isolated in saliva, tears, urine, and breast milk, but not proved to be sources of transmission)	Acquired immunodeficiency syndrome (AIDS)
Fungi		
Aspergillus organisms	Soil, dust, mouth, skin, colon, genital tract	Aspergillosis, pneumonia, sepsis
Candida albicans	Mouth, skin, colon, genital tract	Candidiasis, pneumonia, sepsis
Protozoa		
Plasmodium falciparum	Blood	Malaria

From Potter PA, Perry AG: *Fundamentals of nursing*, ed 6, St Louis, 2005, Elsevier.

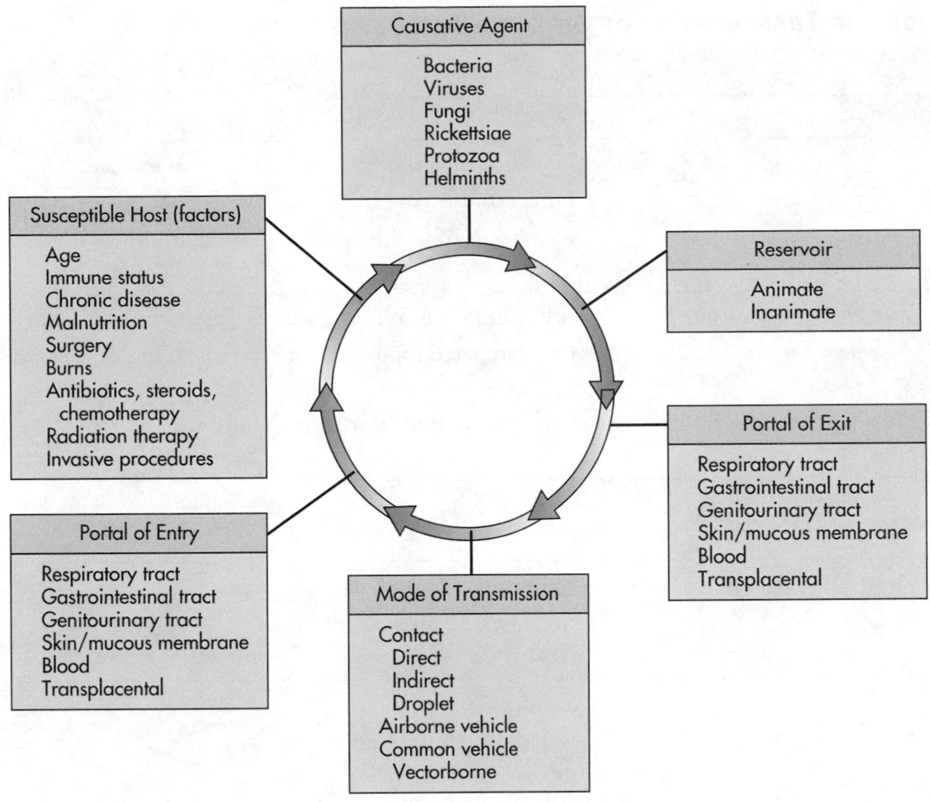

Figure 6-1 The infectious disease process.

venous solutions, equipment). Human reservoirs can be persons with acute clinical infection, persons who are colonized, or asymptomatic carriers. **Carriers** are persons or animals infected with the pathogen that have no clinical signs or symptoms of infection, but are capable of transmitting it to others.

- *Portal of exit:* The portal of exit is the means by which the agent leaves the reservoir. Common exit sites are the respiratory tract, the gastrointestinal tract, the genitourinary tract, open lesions on the skin, and across the placenta and blood.
- *Mode of transmission:* After exit from a reservoir, the agent requires a mode of transport to its next host. Transmission can occur by contact (direct, indirect, or droplet), air, vehicles, or vectors (Table 6-2).
- *Portal of entry:* After being transmitted to a host, the microorganisms must gain entry. Portals of entry are similar to portals of exit and include the respiratory tract, the gastrointestinal tract, the genitourinary tract, breaks in the skin or mucous membranes, the placenta, and blood. Portals of entry are usually the first areas colonized by infecting microorganisms (Figure 6-2).
- *Susceptible host:* Entry of an infectious agent into a host does not mean that infection will occur. The host's **susceptibility**, dose of the infecting agent received, and **virulence** of the organism are factors that determine whether the agent will proliferate and cause infection. The healthy human body is extremely resistant to infection; however, when basic biologic defense mechanisms are compromised, infectious agents have increased potential for causing infections. Chapter 20 discusses immune defenses that prevent host infection and injury.

Pathophysiology

Once a pathogen gains access to a susceptible host, an *incubation period* occurs before the appearance of clinical manifestations. During incubation the organism establishes itself, spreads to target organs or tissues, and proliferates within various areas of the body. Incubation periods vary from hours to years, depending on the organism and the host's condition, but they are often predictable and diagnostically significant. The second period of infection is the *prodromal period* characterized by the onset of nonspecific symptoms such as malaise, anorexia, headache, muscle aches, and joint pain. As the pathogen rapidly multiplies and spreads, the *acute period* ensues. Infections during the acute period may be *localized* (having a focal point of symptoms or injury) or *systemic* (affecting the entire body). A localized acute infection produces an inflammatory response with classic signs and symptoms: redness, heat, swelling, pain, and varying degrees of dysfunction.

Systemic acute infections increase the metabolic demand and result in manifestations such as fever and chills, tachycardia, and tachypnea. Other specific symptoms depend on the type of injury caused by the virulent pathogen and its site within the body. The final phase of the infectious process is the *convalescent period*. During this stage healing occurs and symptoms disappear (Box 6-1).

The course of infection may be acute or chronic. An *acute infection* often incites an immediate violent host response. The

TABLE 6-2 MODES OF TRANSMISSION OF SELECTED PATHOGENS

Pathogen	Common Reservoir
Gram-Positive Cocci	
Staphylococcus aureus	Contaminated objects, hands, and nasal tracts of health care workers, air, self
Group A streptococci	Direct contact, air, hands, rarely objects
Enterococcus group	Self, hands of health care workers, environmental surfaces
Gram-Negative Rods	
Escherichia, Klebsiella, Enterobacter organisms	Self, hands of health care workers, contaminated solutions
Proteus, Salmonella, Providencia, Serratia, Citrobacter organisms	Contaminated food and water, hands of health care workers, self
Pseudomonas organisms	Contaminated environment, hands, self
Anaerobic Bacteria	
Clostridium, Bacteroides organisms	Self, contaminated environment, hands
Fungal Organisms	
Yeasts	Self, hands of health care workers
Fungi	Air, contaminated environment
Viruses	
Varicella	Air, direct contact
Herpes	Self, direct contact, air
Rubella	Direct contact, air
Hepatitis B and C	Contaminated instruments, sharps, direct contact

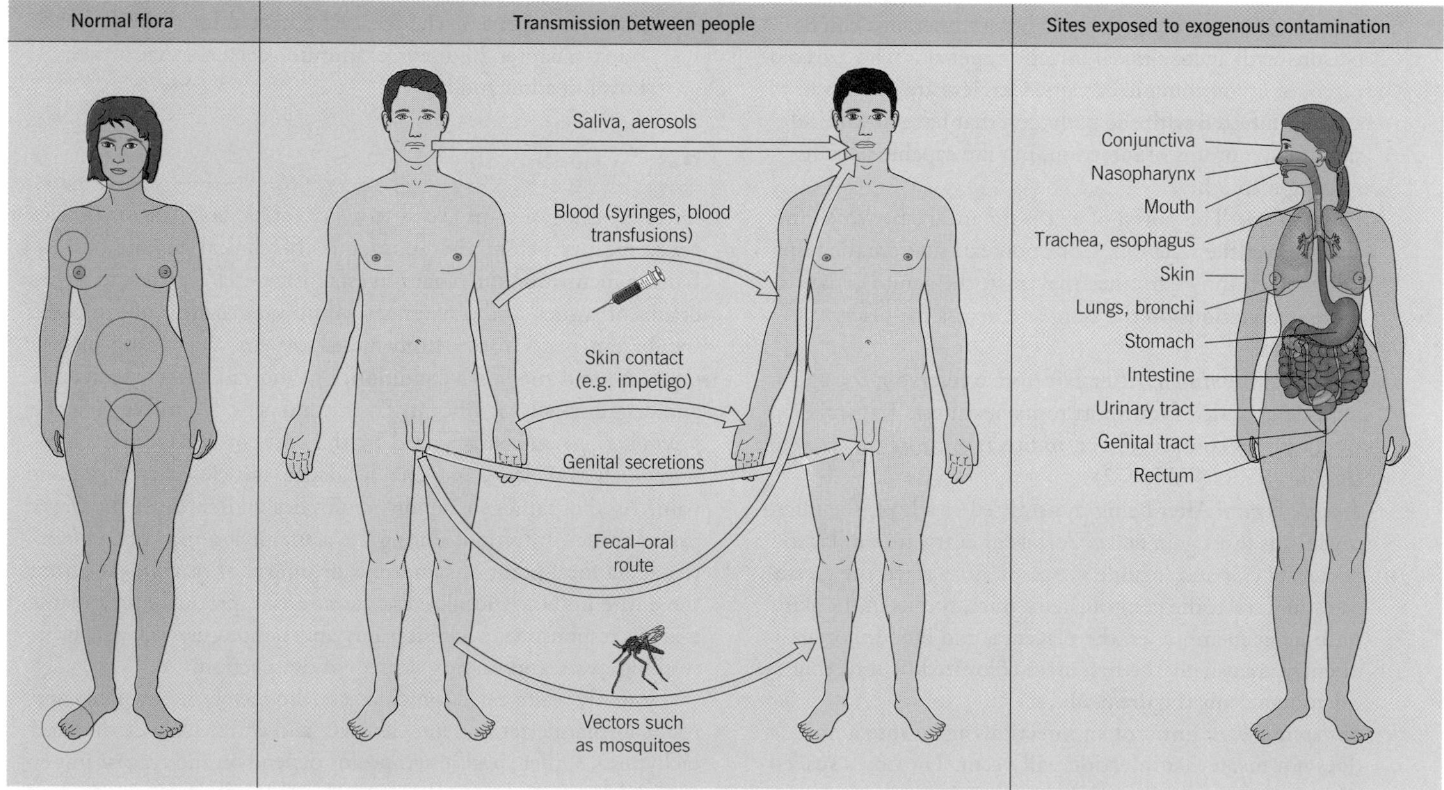

Figure 6-2 Contamination of humans by microbes. Many parts of the body are colonized by normal flora, which can be the source of endogenous infection. Large numbers of microbes are found in moist areas of the skin, the upper respiratory tract, the digestive tract, the ileum and large intestine, the anterior parts of the urethra, and the vagina. Other routes are from human transmission of infections and exposure to exogenous contamination.

Box 6-1 Stages of Infection

Incubation Period

From the time the organism gains entrance into the host and:
- Establishes itself
- Spreads to target organs or tissues
- Proliferates within various areas of the body

Prodromal Stage

From the onset of nonspecific clinical manifestations (e.g., malaise, anorexia, headache):
- Pathogen rapidly multiplying and spreading
- Onset of specific clinical manifestations (e.g., sore throat, high fever)
- Primary period of contagion

Acute Stage

Interval of maximum clinical illness:
- Localized—specific focal point of infection
- Systemic—involves entire body

Convalescence

Interval during which manifestations of infection resolve and disappear, which may take days, weeks, or months

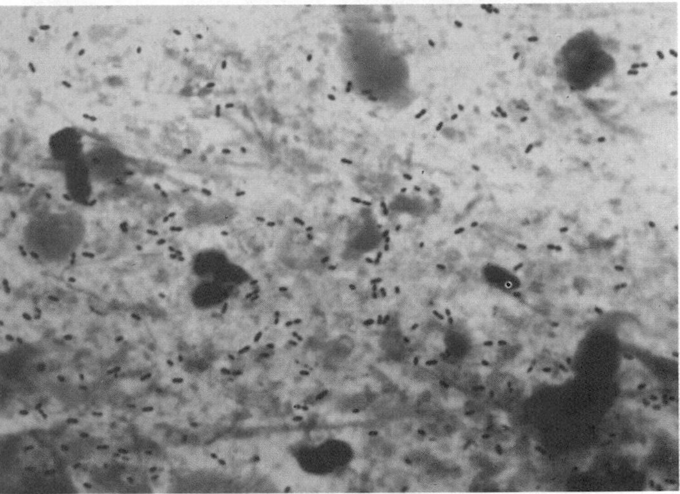

Figure 6-3 Gram stain of a sputum sample infected with *Streptococcus pneumoniae.*

outcome of the infection, pathogen over host or host over pathogen, is determined within a relatively short time, as in mumps, plague, or smallpox. With *chronic infection* the pathogen establishes itself more subtly within the host, does not cause immediate damage, and tends to provoke less of a host response. Tuberculosis and aspergillosis are typical chronic infections. Acute infections may become chronic, and vice versa.

Pathogens producing infections are varied and produce disease and injury by different mechanisms. The major pathogens affecting humans are bacteria, viruses, fungi, prions, and parasites.

Bacteria. Thousands of species of bacteria exist, but all are made up of a single cell. Some are as small as viruses, whereas others are considerably larger. They are classified by their shape (rod, cocci, helical, or spiral), by their staining reactions (gram positive or gram negative), by the presence of endospores, and by their oxygen requirements (Figure 6-3). *Aerobic* bacteria require oxygen to live and grow. *Anaerobic* bacteria do not require oxygen. Relatively few bacteria cause disease. In fact, less than 1% are pathogenic.[22] Without bacteria, humans could not live. They help digest food, fight cancer cells, break down wastes, and destroy pathogens. However, the 1% of bacteria that are pathogenic can exert considerable havoc on humans and animals alike. New strains of pathogenic bacteria are emerging, many of which are resistant to antibiotics.[42]

Viruses. A *virion* is a complete and fully developed viral particle that is composed of single- or double-stranded ribonucleic acid (RNA) or deoxyribonucleic acid (DNA) and nucleic acid that contains only a few genes (Figure 6-4). Most virions have a protein coat called the *capsid,* and some have a second covering, or *envelope*. These coverings protect the virions and aid in their transmission from one host cell to another. Virions by themselves are metabolically inactive and require the host cell to activate their nucleic acid to synthesize new viruses. Once the virion gains entrance into the host cell and establishes an environment that supports replication, it transforms the host cell's metabolic machinery into a virus-producing cell. Once assembled, the new virions are released from the host cell and are free to infect other cells. The process of viral replication can cause significant injury or death to host cells.

Retroviruses are a subset of viruses that require the enzyme reverse transcriptase to integrate themselves into host cell RNA and reproduce. HIV is a retrovirus. Unlike bacteria, most viruses are pathogenic, even though they are among the smallest of the microbial organisms. Human viruses target specific cells and tissues; for example, HIV specifically targets T4 helper lymphocytes.[22,28] When a host is infected by a virus, his or her immune system produces antibodies against it in an attempt to inactivate the virus. (See Chapter 20 for a discussion of immune responses to foreign antigens.)

Fungi. Molds and yeasts are known as fungi. Many fungi are beneficial, such as those used to produce penicillin and other antibiotics. Only about 100 of the known 100,000 species of fungi cause disease in humans or animals. Reproduction of fungi occurs via the formation of *spores* that detach from the parent cell and germinate into new fungi elsewhere. Localized fungal infections, known as *mycoses,* typically occur on the hair, skin, or nails. Systemic infections can affect any organ or tissue but generally begin in the lungs from the inhalation of spores. Mycoses occur more frequently in immunosuppressed persons and as nosocomial infections (Figure 6-5).

Prions. **Prions**, also known as transmissible spongiform encephalopathy agents (TSEs), are a group of infectious protein particles first recognized in the late 1970s. They differ significantly

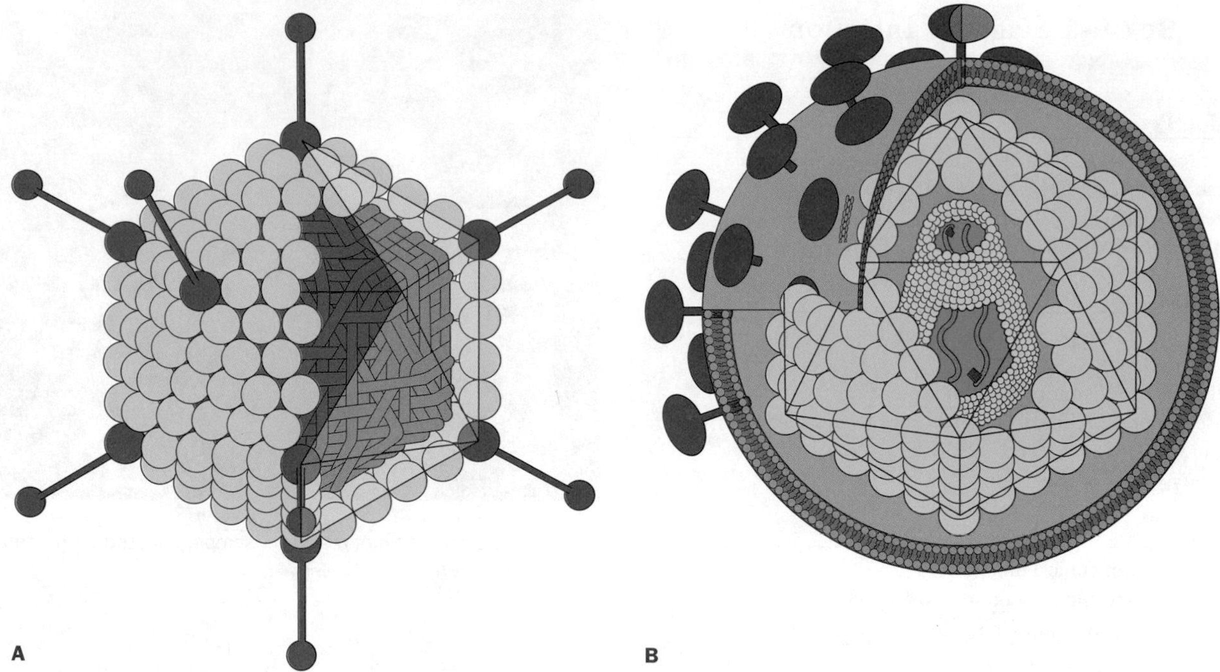

Figure 6-4 Examples of virions. **A,** Adenovirus. **B,** HIV-1.

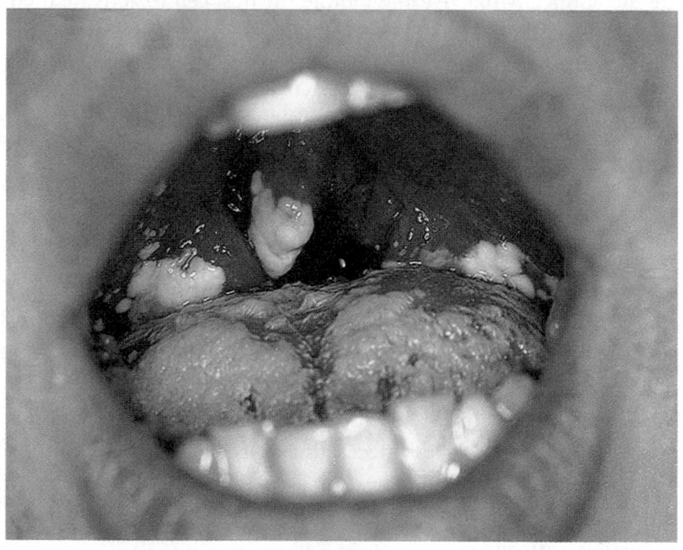

Figure 6-5 *Candida albicans* fungal infection of the mouth.

from other organisms because they cannot be destroyed or inactivated by conventional sterilization methods. Prions are transmissible among and between species, but routes of transmission remain in question. Person-to-person transmission is thought to be unlikely. There have been reports, however, of bloodborne transmission via surgical instruments sterilized by traditional methods, transplanted organs, and blood transfusions.[31] Some countries recommend blood donor exclusions to prevent the transmission of prion diseases. Currently there are nine known animal TSEs and four human TSEs. All these diseases are characterized by the accumulation of the abnormal prion proteins within the central nervous system, which alter normal cellular protein folding. Prions are believed to cause scrapie in sheep, bovine spongiform encephalopathy (BSE) in cattle, chronic wasting disease in deer and elk, and new variant Creutzfeldt-Jakob disease (nvCJD) in humans (discussed later in the chapter).

Parasites. Protozoa and helminths are the primary parasites that infect humans. Protozoa are one-celled animals that are generally pathogenic to humans. They move as ameboids or by cilia or flagella. Protozoa are found in animal reservoirs or as free-form parasites in the environment and are frequently transmitted by mosquitoes or flies. They invade deep tissues and reside within the host cell until excreted. Many produce *cysts*, which are protective capsules that allow the organism to survive outside the host until a new host is found.[40]

Helminths (worms and flukes) are parasites that live inside and absorb nutrients from their host. Their life cycle requires a succession of intermediate hosts to complete their larval stages. Humans may serve as intermediate hosts for larvae or definitive hosts for adult worms such as *Taenia solium*, the pork tapeworm. Parasitic infections are important emerging and reemerging infections throughout the world.

Emerging Infectious Diseases

After World War II scientists commonly believed that the war against infectious diseases had been won. Death rates from wound infections, pneumonia, and tuberculosis plummeted as a result of antibiotics. Vaccines conquered diseases such as polio, measles, diphtheria, and polio. Improved sanitation and water quality decreased infections from bacterial contamination. Overall, the future looked bright as the incidence of infectious diseases declined throughout the United States and other developed countries. For the first time in history, many infections could be prevented or cured.

In spite of the gains, the next 50 years proved that the war on microbes was far from over. As early as the 1950s the drug penicillin, used extensively for pneumonia and wound infections, began to lose its effectiveness against common bacteria such as *Staphylococcus aureus, Staphylococcus penumoniae,* and gonorrhea.[17] The 1970s and 1980s brought even more evidence of the growing threat from microbes. Scientists identified new or previously unrecognized infections such as legionnaires' disease, toxic shock syndrome, Lyme disease, new strains of influenza, and acquired immunodeficiency syndrome (AIDS). Older infections, once thought to be well controlled, began to resurface in forms that were more virulent or resistant to previously effective antimicrobial agents (Table 6-3). In the early 1990s the Institute of Medicine (IOM) concluded that emerging infectious diseases were a major threat to U.S. health. Today infections continue to be a major threat as diseases such a West Nile fever, severe acute respiratory syndrome (SARS), and hantavirus pulmonary syndrome emerge and spread throughout the world.[28]

Infections cause significant illness, disability, and death. In the United States the mortality rates from infectious diseases increased 58% between 1980 and 1992; they are now the third leading cause of death. Worldwide, infectious diseases are the first leading cause of death, with an estimated 177 million deaths per year, 90% of which are from respiratory infections, AIDS, tuberculosis, malaria, and measles.[4] The World Health Organization (WHO) estimates that an average of 1500 people die each hour, with half of those deaths occurring in children under the age of 5.[25]

In addition to being a major health threat, infectious diseases have a profound negative impact on human life and economic development. Cost estimates for treating infections in the United States alone reach $120 billion annually, with $6.7 billion of the total attributed to hospital-acquired infections.[36] As a whole, infectious diseases create huge financial burdens, tax first responders and medical personnel, challenge the government's ability to respond, and contribute to political instability.[4,26]

In spite of important advances in prevention and treatment, infectious diseases continue to pose a growing health threat to people throughout the world. Recent behavioral, environmental, demographic, and medical trends have led to the emergence of new diseases, the reemergence of well-known but previously controlled diseases, increased resistance to effective microbial agents, and chemical and biologic weapons. Taken together, infectious diseases are a global problem that will require global solutions, ideally directed at prevention.[26,29]

Factors Affecting the Emergence of Infections

New diseases are emerging throughout the world in both developed and developing countries. The Centers for Disease Control and Prevention (CDC) defines new infections as "those that have not previously occurred in humans, those that have previously occurred but affected very few people in isolated areas, or infections that occurred previously but were not recognized as infections until the infectious agent was identified." Over the past 25 years, on average, one new or newly recognized infection has been reported each year[5] (Table 6-4).

Infections that were once considered controlled are now reemerging. The CDC defines reemerging infection as "the

TABLE 6-3 SELECTED WORLDWIDE REEMERGING INFECTIONS OVER PAST 20 YEARS

Disease	Possible Contributing Factors
Bacterial Infections	
Cholera	Travel, contaminated food and water
Diphtheria	Decreased immunizations
Escherichia coli 0157:H7	Food processing and distribution
Group A streptococci	Unknown
Pertussis	Social behaviors (fear of immunization)
Plague	Demographics, land use
Pneumococci	Demographics, microbial resistance, travel
Salmonella	Demographics, microbial resistance, food handling
Viral Infections	
Dengue	Travel, demographics
Rabies	Travel, demographics, breakdown of public health
Yellow fever	Microbial resistance
Parasitic Infections	
Acanthamebiasis	Social behaviors (soft contact lens)
Echinococcosis	Climatologic changes and environmental alterations
Giardiasis	Social behaviors (child care centers)
Malaria	Climatologic changes (favor mosquito vectors)
Schistosomiasis	Climatologic changes and environmental alterations
Toxoplasmosis	Immunodeficiency, immunosuppression

reappearance of a known disease after a significant reduction in incidence."[5] Malaria, tuberculosis, salmonella, diphtheria, *Escherichia coli*, toxic-producing strains of *S. aureus,* and sexually transmitted infections are examples. Reemerging infectious organisms are often more virulent and resistant to antimicrobial agents than the original strains.

Numerous factors contribute to the emergence of new and reemergence of previously known infectious diseases throughout the world (Box 6-2):

- *Human behavior:* Changing sexual mores, intravenous drug use, and other high-risk behaviors are associated with the spread of HIV infection, hepatitis, and sexually transmitted

TABLE 6-4 NEW MICROBES

	Microbe	Type	Disease
1973	Rotavirus	Virus	Major cause of infantile diarrhea worldwide
1975	Parvovirus B19	Virus	Aplastic crisis in chronic hemolytic anemia
1976	*Cryptosporidium parvum*	Parasite	Acute and chronic diarrhea
1977	Ebola virus	Virus	Ebola hemorrhagic fever
1977	Hantaan virus	Virus	Hemorrhagic fever with renal syndrome
1977	*Legionella pneumophila*	Bacterium	Legionnaires' disease
1977	*Campylobacter jejuni*	Bacterium	Enteric pathogens distributed globally
1980	Human T-lymphotropic virus 1 (HLTV-1)	Virus	T lymphocyte lymphoma-leukemia
1981	Toxin-producing strains of *Staphylococcus aureus*	Bacterium	Toxic shock syndrome
1982	*Escherichia coli* O157:H7	Bacterium	Hemorrhagic colitis; hemolytic uremic syndrome
1982	Human T-lymphotropic virus 2 (HTLV-2)	Virus	Hairy cell leukemia
1982	*Borrelia burgdorferi*	Bacterium	Lyme disease
1983	Human immunodeficiency virus (HIV)	Virus	Acquired immunodeficiency syndrome (AIDS)
1985	*Helicobacter pylori*	Bacterium	Peptic ulcer disease
1985	*Enterocytozoon bieneusi*	Parasite	Persistent diarrhea
1986	*Cyclospora cayetanensis*	Parasite	Persistent diarrhea
1988	Human herpesvirus 6 (HHV-6)	Virus	Exanthema subitum
1988	Hepatitis E	Virus	Enterically transmitted non-A, non-B hepatitis
1989	*Ehrlichia chaffeensis*	Bacterium	Human monocytic ehrlichiosis
1989	Hepatitis C	Virus	Parenterally transmitted non-A, non-B hepatitis
1991	Guanarito virus	Virus	Venezuelan hemorrhagic fever
1991	*Encephalitozoon hellem*	Parasite	Conjunctivitis, disseminated disease
1991	New species of *Babesia*	Parasite	Atypical babesiosis
1992	*Bartonella henselae*	Bacterium	Cat-scratch disease; bacillary angiomatosis
1993	Sin Nombre *(Bunyaviridae)* virus	Virus	Hantavirus pulmonary syndrome (HPS)
1993	*Encephalitozoon cuniculi*	Parasite	Disseminated disease
1994	Sabia virus	Virus	Brazilian hemorrhagic fever
1994	Hendra virus	Virus	Encephalitic disease transmitted from horses to humans
1995	Human herpesvirus 8 (HHV-8)	Virus	Associated with Kaposi's sarcoma in AIDS patients
1996	New variant Creutzfeldt-Jakob disease agent	Prion	Progressive degenerative neurologic disease
1997	H5N1 strain of avian influenza	Virus	Influenza transmitted from chickens to humans; often fatal
1999	Nipah virus	Virus	Encephalitic disease transmitted from pigs to humans
2001	Human metapneumovirus	Virus	Acute respiratory infections
2002	Vancomycin-resistant *Staphylococcus aureus*	Bacterium	First vancomycin-resistant *S. aureus* identified in the United States
2003	Coronavirus	Virus	Severe acute respiratory syndrome (SARS)

Updated from World Health Organization: *World health report, 1996: fighting disease: fostering development,* Geneva, 1996, The Organization. From Cohen J, Powderly G, editors: *Infectious diseases,* ed 2, St Louis, 2004, Elsevier.

Box 6-2 Factors Affecting Emergence of Infections

- Microbial change and adaptation
- Human vulnerability because of genetics or altered defense mechanisms
- Climate and weather changes upsetting ecologic balance
- Centralized food processing and globalization of food supply
- Population growth
- Urbanization and crowding
- Migration of human populations into previously uninhabited areas, such as rain forests or other wildernesses
- Irrigation and deforestation, which alters the habitat of disease-carrying insects and animals
- Increased global travel and commerce
- Risky human behaviors such as intravenous drug use and unprotected sex
- Increased use and overuse of antimicrobial agents and pesticides
- Inadequate public health measures
- Poverty

infections. Increased use of child care facilities exposes children to more infections because of the generally poor hygiene habits of children. A growing number of people are seeking outdoor leisure activities, which brings them in close proximity with animal habitats and insect vectors that carry disease.

- *Demographics:* Economics prompts people to move from rural to urban areas, which allows infections that were once isolated to reach larger populations. Overcrowding, poor hygiene, inadequate sanitation, and unclean drinking water often accompany urban population growth and result in increased person-to-person transmission of infectious diseases such as tuberculosis, influenza, and other vaccine-preventable diseases.[42,48] Conversely, overpopulation causes expansion of suburbs into previously uninhabited areas, resulting in increased human contact with disease-carrying animals and insects. Lyme disease has been linked to humans moving into reforested areas that are rich with deer, deer ticks, and mice that carry the bacteria (Figure 6-6).
- *Economic development:* Land developments near watershed areas, increased logging in tropical rain forests and other wilderness habitats, and the widespread use of irrigation programs that enhance vector breeding place humans in closer contact with known and unknown infectious agents.
- *Global travel:* The ability to readily travel throughout the world has allowed infectious agents to move at a steady and rapid pace without being noticed until an outbreak occurs. Microbes can be transmitted by food, animals, insects, or unsuspecting travelers. West Nile virus, which was introduced into the United States in 1999 via air transport, is now well established and spreading throughout the continent. Malaria was imported into the United Kingdom by travelers in 2000 and SARS to Canada in 2003. With the ease and affordable cost of international travel, a person incubating an infection can board a plane in one country and infect many people in another country before the infection is even detected.[4,31]
- *Food distribution:* Centralized food processing and international food shipments allow for quick and widespread distribution of contaminated food sources (see discussion on waterborne and foodborne illnesses).
- *Medical technology:* Humans have become more susceptible to microbial invasion because they are living longer. During the past 50 years the number of people in the United States

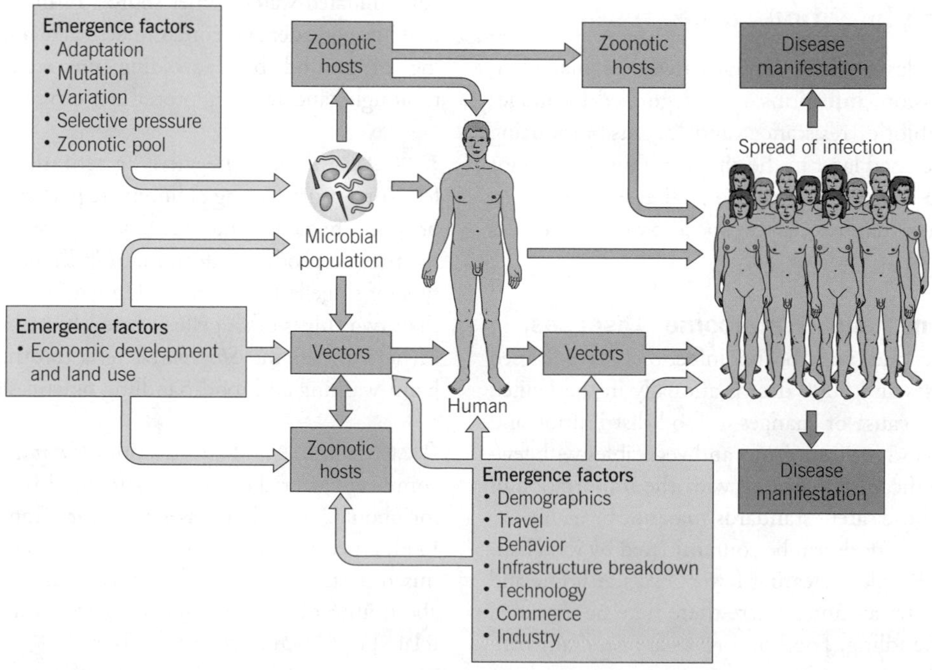

Figure 6-6 Interactions among humans, vectors, and the environment that contribute to disease emergence.

more than doubled and the number of 65-year-olds increased from 25.5 million to about 34 million. With advancing age the immune system slows and is less responsive to bacterial and viral infections. The commonplace use of immunosuppressive therapy as treatment for many chronic diseases, cancer, and solid-organ transplants has prolonged life but contributed to increased infection susceptibility, since these drugs blunt normal immune responses. Additionally, medical science has extended the lives of many people who have compromised immune systems from diseases such as AIDS and are incapable of combating infections. Another source of potential infection is invasive diagnostic and treatment procedures that are generally performed on those who are most vulnerable to microorganisms because of illness or injury.[31]
- *Ecologic change:* Recent environmental and climate changes have provided the opportunity for microbial organisms to appear from obscurity and infect humans directly or through carriers. Weather conditions that favored the proliferation of mice and subsequent contact with agricultural workers have been linked to Sin Nombre virus, which causes hantavirus pulmonary syndrome (HPS).[31] Many scientists believe that global warming could increase the incidence of insect-borne infections such as yellow fever, dengue, St. Louis encephalitis, and malaria as warmer climates provide suitable habitats for their vectors. If natural disasters increase in response to ecologic changes, increased infections will follow due to loss of sanitation, effective communications, and governmental ability to respond.[4,31]
- *Microbial evolution:* Bacteria, viruses, and parasites have evolved and adapted as needed, spreading rapidly, mutating, jumping species, and building resistance to antimicrobial agents.

Specific Emerging Infectious Diseases

Emerging diseases are classified by several categories that often overlap. For this discussion, infections are categorized by modes of transmission. Antibiotic resistance and agents producing chronic diseases are discussed later in the chapter. This text cannot present all the new and reemerging infectious diseases, but examples are given here; other chapters discuss specific diseases such as tuberculosis and AIDS.

Emerging Foodborne and Waterborne Diseases. In recent years foodborne and waterborne infections have caused about 76 million illnesses and 5000 deaths annually in the United States alone, primarily because of changes in food distribution and eating habits.[5] The demand for fresh fruits and vegetables with fewer preservatives has significantly increased with the importation of foods from countries whose safety standards may not be as high as those in the United States. Foods can be contaminated by food handlers or during transit. People are eating fewer meals at home and relying on take-out and restaurants, where there may be increased risk of improper food handling. Food outbreaks are generally connected to undercooked meat, poultry, and seafood; unpasteurized milk; or foods that were previously thought to be safe such as sprouts, lettuce, tomatoes, eggs, or juices.[31]

Disinfected drinking water and improvement in sewage treatment has nearly eliminated the threat from waterborne pathogens such as typhoid fever. However, cryptosporidiosis, which was first identified in humans in 1975, has appeared sporadically following water filtration procedure breakdowns and is a significant cause of opportunistic infection in AIDS patients. Public swimming pools, lettuce, and apple cider have been implicated in isolated outbreaks. Waterborne and foodborne infections, commonly known as diarrheal illnesses, of growing concern are connected to *Salmonella* organisms; *E. coli* O157:H7; *Shigella, Campylobacter, Cyclospora,* and *Cryptosporidium* organisms; and avian influenza (Table 6-5).

SALMONELLA. Several strains of gram-negative salmonellae exist. The most serious type is *Salmonella typhi*, which causes the life-threatening illness typhoid fever. Typhoid fever affects about 12.5 million people annually in developing countries. In the United States it affects about 400 people annually. Of those, about 70% acquired the disease during international travel. People acquire typhoid by contact with infected animals or people or by ingestion of food or water contaminated with fecal matter. Typhoid fever is preventable by vaccines and can be successfully treated with antibiotics. A more common infection, salmonella, is an important public health problem in the United States and several European countries. *Salmonella enteritidis* can be transmitted via raw or undercooked eggs, beef, poultry, or milk, although eggs are the most common source of transmission.[11]

ESCHERICHIA COLI. Hundreds of strains of *E. coli* live in the intestines as nonpathogenic residents. However, *E. coli* O157:H7, a strain recognized in 1982, is an emerging foodborne infection that produces a powerful toxin, which results in serious illness. *E. coli* O157:H7 is transmitted by eating undercooked ground beef that has been contaminated during slaughtering and packaging, drinking raw milk from cows with contaminated udders, or drinking sewage-contaminated water. Other sources of infection include unpasteurized juice or cider and contaminated alfalfa sprouts. Thorough cooking of ground beef, avoiding unpasteurized milk, and using thorough hand-washing procedures can prevent the infection.[18]

SHIGELLA. A gram-negative bacterium, shigella is spread by the fecal-oral route. Young children are particularly susceptible because of poor hygiene practices and the small amount of bacteria required to produce infection. *Shigella sonnei* is the most common type of shigella found in the United States and accounts for more than two thirds of shigellosis cases. It is possible for asymptomatic carriers to pass the *Shigella* bacteria to others; consequently, good hand-washing and food-handling practices are essential.[12]

CAMPYLOBACTER. The bacterium *Campylobacter jejuni* is the most common bacterial cause of gastroenteritis in the world, accounting for about 2.4 million cases per year. Transmission is via infected food, especially poultry, or animals. Infection in immunocompromised hosts can produce life-threatening sepsis. It is estimated that about 40% of cases of Guillain-Barré syndrome in this country are related to *Campylobacter* infections.[15]

CYCLOSPORA. *Cyclospora cayetanensis* causes cyclosporiasis, a parasitic infection first identified in humans in 1979. Oocysts, which are excreted in feces from infected persons, require days to sporulate; thus direct person-to-person transmission of the infection is unlikely. Indirect transmission occurs from the ingestion of fresh produce or water contaminated with oocysts. It is not known if animals can be infected or if they serve as sources of infection for humans. Untreated illnesses may continue for weeks to months and assume a remitting-relapsing course.[43]

CRYPTOSPORIDIUM. During the past 20 years, cryptosporidiosis has become one of the most common causes of waterborne diarrhea in the world. The pathogenic organism is a parasite, *Cryptosporidium parvum*, which lives in the intestines of immunocompetent humans and animals without causing disease. It is transmitted by the fecal-oral route and may be acquired from contaminated drinking, ground, or recreational water; contaminated food; pets; farm animals; or person-to-person contact. The parasite can live outside the body for prolonged periods because its outer shell is resistant to chlorine disinfection. Although the disease occasionally produces symptoms for up to 3 months, it is usually self-limiting in immunocompetent individuals and does not require treatment.

The disease accounts for about 20% of diarrheal infections in patients who have severe immunodeficiency from HIV, especially in the presence of other infections. Cryptosporidiosis has no cure but does improve if the patient's immune system stabilizes from antiretroviral therapy.[22]

AVIAN INFLUENZA. The avian influenza virus (H5N1) generally affects only poultry. However, since 1997 more than 200 confirmed or suspected human cases of avian influenza A have occurred in Vietnam, Hong Kong, China, the Netherlands, Thailand, Canada, and New York.[51] The virus is thought to be transmitted to humans via infected poultry or contaminated surfaces. To date, no infections have been transmitted from human to human. Although the number of human infections throughout the world is not significant at this time, public health authorities are carefully monitoring the virus because of concerns over the possibility of more widespread infections.[20]

Avian influenza produces influenza-like manifestations such as fever, cough, sore throat, and muscle aches, as well as pneumonia, acute respiratory distress, and life-threatening complications. The mortality rate has ranged between 33% and 50% depending on

TABLE 6-5 EMERGING FOODBORNE AND WATERBORNE INFECTIOUS DISEASES

Agent	Incubation Period	Clinical Manifestations	Treatment
Salmonella enteritidis	12-72 hr after ingestion of bacterium	Fever, abdominal cramps, diarrhea	Most people recover without treatment within 4-7 days, although illness can be severe enough to warrant hospitalization. Those with impaired immunity (infants, elderly, or those with chronic or severe illnesses) are at increased risk for more serious infection and can die without adequate and prompt antibiotic treatment.
Escherichia coli O157:H7	24-72 hr	Severe bloody diarrhea, abdominal cramping	Generally resolves within 5-10 days without treatment. Antibiotics do not help course of disease and may increase risk for renal complications such as hemolytic uremic syndrome, which may be life threatening. Antidiarrheal medications may exacerbate symptoms and are thus avoided.
Shigella sonnei	16-72 hr	Fever; abdominal cramping; diarrhea, which may be bloody; within 24-48 days after infection	Mild infection generally resolves within 5-7 days. Antibiotic treatment for mild infections is discouraged, since some *Shigella* bacteria are developing drug resistance. Hospitalization may be required for persons with severe diarrhea or high fever, in which case antibiotic therapy with ampicillin or trimethoprim and sulfamethoxazole may be necessary. Antidiarrheal medications should be avoided because they make symptoms worse.

Continued

TABLE 6-5 EMERGING FOODBORNE AND WATERBORNE INFECTIOUS DISEASES—CONT'D

Agent	Incubation Period	Clinical Manifestations	Treatment
Campylobacter jejuni	2-5 days	Abdominal pain; cramping; fever; diarrhea, which may be bloody and accompanied by nausea and vomiting; lasting for about a week	Majority of patients recover without treatment. Erythromycin or fluoroquinolone may be prescribed for those with severe illness, although about 14% of cases are known to be caused by fluoroquinolone-resistant organisms.
Cyclospora cayetanensis	About 7 days	May be asymptomatic or cause frequent, sometimes explosive, watery diarrhea; anorexia; weight loss; flatulence; abdominal cramping; nausea; vomiting; low-grade fever; fatigue; and muscle aches	Treat with trimethoprim and sulfamethoxazole.
Cryptosporidium parvum	5-28 days	Variable clinical course: (1) immunocompetent persons—asymptomatic or seen with watery diarrhea, abdominal pain, nausea, vomiting, anorexia, flatulence, fatigue, and low-grade fever lasting 10-14 days; (2) immunocompromised persons—severe, chronic, and potentially life-threatening illness; watery diarrhea leading to serious fluid and electrolyte depletions, malnutrition, wasting, cachexia, and death	Paromomycin and nitazoxanide are being investigated as potential control agents, but to date this infection has no consistently effective treatments.
Avian influenza A (H5N1)	Within 10 days of infection	Fever, cough, sore throat, muscle aches, pneumonia, dyspnea, acute respiratory distress	Amantadine, rimantadine, oseltamivir, and zanamivir may be effective treatments.

the geographic location. Antiviral therapy may be useful in treatment of avian influenza. The U.S. Food and Drug Administration (FDA) has approved the drugs amantadine, zanamivir, oseltamivir, and rimantadine for avian influenza. Some strains of the virus, however, are resistant to amantadine and rimantadine, and monitoring for drug resistance is ongoing.[20]

Emerging Vectorborne and Zoonotic Diseases. The vast majority of new and reemerging diseases are acquired from animals and insect vectors. An infection directly acquired from an animal is a **zoonotic** infection. One acquired indirectly from insect vectors is a **vectorborne** infection. Zoonotic and vectorborne infections are important because more than 75% of the 150 pathogens linked to emerging infections come from animal reservoirs.[31] This process is known as *species jumping* and occurs when the microbe gains access to a new host or new condition that fosters its growth (Table 6-6).

HANTAVIRUS PULMONARY SYNDROME. HPS was first recognized in 1993 and is currently seen throughout the United States. The disease is caused by one of several *Bunyaviridae* viruses that are found worldwide. The microbe is transmitted to humans through inhalation of aerosolized urine, droppings, and saliva from infected rodents (Figure 6-7). Although rare, HPS is a deadly febrile disease carrying a 50% mortality rate. Currently HPS has no drug therapy or vaccine. Prevention focuses on reducing contact with rodents and their excretions by eliminating them from homes, preventing them from living around homes, and taking precautions when cleaning areas that may be rodent infested.[31]

WEST NILE VIRUS. West Nile fever is caused by one strain of flavivirus that is transmitted by blood-feeding arthropods such as mosquitoes and by sand flies (Figure 6-8). Birds and animals can serve as reservoirs for the virus. Although direct human-to-human transmission of West Nile has not been identified, cases of transmission have been reported in persons receiving organ transplants or blood transfusions from infected donors.[36] Recognized in the United States in 1999, the virus has now spread throughout the country. It has also been identified in Canada, but is thought to have been contracted by travelers visiting the United States. There is no drug therapy or vaccine for West Nile virus.

LYME DISEASE. Lyme disease is caused by the spirochete *Borrelia burgdorferi,* which affects about 23,000 people per year

(Figure 6-9). Deer ticks that feed on infected deer, mice, or chipmunks transmit the disease to humans by inserting their mouths into host skin (Figure 6-10). The risk for disease transmission is significantly increased when the tick feeds for more than 2 days. *B. burgdorferi* can produce localized or disseminated disease. Serologic testing may be done to detect antibodies when disseminated disease is suspected. Fortunately, effective antibiotic treatments for Lyme disease exist.

TABLE 6-6 EMERGING VECTORBORNE AND ZOONOTIC DISEASES

Disease	Agent	Incubation Period	Clinical Manifestations	Treatment
Hantavirus pulmonary syndrome (HPS)	*Bunyaviridae* virus	14-17 days	Disease progresses through three phases. *Prodromal* stage lasts 3-4 days and consists of fever, chills, myalgia, headache, and gastrointestinal symptoms, which are often mistaken for influenza. During *shock* stage, patient experiences cardiac and respiratory compromise similar to acute respiratory distress syndrome and requires intubation and mechanical ventilation. If the patient survives, *recovery* occurs within several days, although residual cognitive and respiratory sequelae have been identified.	HPS has no drug treatment or vaccine. Care is supportive with treatment for shock and hypoxia. Early treatment with the antiviral agent ribavirin may reduce mortality in some patients, although it does not specifically target HPS.
West Nile fever	West Nile virus (flavivirus)	3-14 days	Majority of people contracting West Nile are asymptomatic; 20% develop West Nile fever with swollen lymph nodes, fever, headache, fatigue, body aches, and occasional skin rash. About 1% of people infected develop severe encephalitis or meningitis with high fever, stiff neck, headache, confusion, coma, muscle weakness, convulsions, and paralysis.	Care is supportive and includes intravenous fluids, respiratory management if needed, and prevention of secondary infections. West Nile virus has no drug therapy or vaccine.
Lyme disease	*Borrelia burgdorferi*	7-14 days	Infected persons may be asymptomatic or have characteristic bull's eye rash, headache, fever, fatigue, myalgia, and arthralgia. Disseminated disease causes multiple erythema migrans lesions, meningitis, cranial neuropathy such as facial nerve palsy, joint pain, myocarditis, and transient atrioventricular heart blocks. While rarely fatal, untreated disseminated disease can cause chronic joint inflammation, cognitive disorders, sleep disturbances, lethargy, and personality changes.	Doxycyline and amoxicillin are effective treatments when given for 3-4 wk. Cefuroxime and erythromycin are effective alternatives for people allergic to tetracycline drugs.

Continued

TABLE 6-6 EMERGING VECTORBORNE AND ZOONOTIC DISEASES—CONT'D

Disease	Agent	Incubation Period	Clinical Manifestations	Treatment
Severe acute respiratory syndrome (SARS)	A coronavirus	2-7 days	Patients have high fever greater than 100.4° F (38.0° C), chills, headache, body aches, and generalized discomfort. Diarrhea and/or mild respiratory symptoms may also be present. Dry cough and pneumonia develop within 2-7 days after initial onset of symptoms and may be accompanied by hypoxia requiring mechanical ventilation.	Supportive care is only treatment for SARS, although antiviral agents are being tested.
Dengue or dengue hemorrhagic fever	Flavivirus	2-7 days	Dengue virus may produce asymptomatic infection or a mild febrile illness that is indistinguishable from other common viral infections. Classic dengue manifests with sudden onset of acute fever, frontal headache, muscle and joint pain, nausea, vomiting, maculopapular rash, and leukopenia. Acute phase of illness lasts about 1 wk and is followed by a 2-wk period of convalescence. Dengue hemorrhagic fever is life threatening and occurs 2-7 days from onset of acute illness. It begins with severe abdominal pain, vomiting, hypothermia, mental status changes, and signs of shock, known as dengue shock syndrome. Without treatment, shock progresses to circulatory failure, hemorrhage, and death in 44% of cases.	Acetaminophen can be administered for pain and fever, but aspirin is avoided because of its anticoagulant effects. Fluid replacement therapy is essential.

SEVERE ACUTE RESPIRATORY SYNDROME. SARS, first reported in Asia in 2003, is a viral respiratory illness caused by a coronavirus, the virus associated with the common cold. The virus rapidly spread from Asia to Canada, South America, and Europe before being contained. Transmission of the virus to humans has been linked to the slaughtering and consumption of palm civet cats, which are native Asian tree-dwelling animals. Transmission between people occurs primarily via respiratory droplets from close contact with an infected person exhibiting symptoms. Asymptomatic persons have not been shown to transmit the virus. Other potential routes of transmission are fecal droplets, blood, and body fluids.[50] About 10% of patients died during the 2003 outbreak of SARS. SARS has no treatment, but transmission can be contained by use of Contact Precautions, airborne infection isolation, and Standard Precautions.

DENGUE. Dengue is caused by one strain of flavivirus that is transmitted to humans via the *Aedes aegypti* mosquito, which also transmits yellow fever. Generally a disease of the tropics, dengue has become an important mosquito-borne disease because of its increasing global distribution. Worldwide, dengue is estimated to affect about 20 million people, with 250,000 cases occurring in

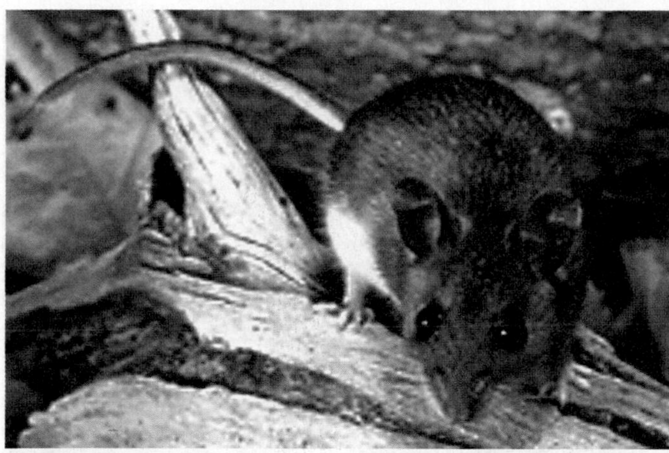

Figure 6-7 Rodent vector for *Hantavirus* organisms.

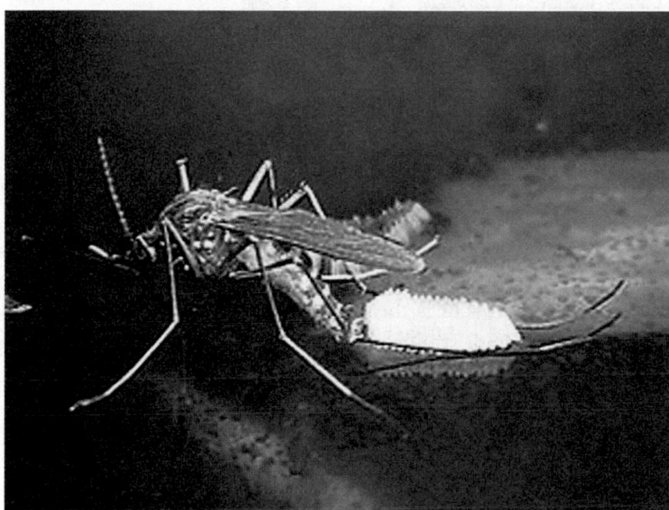

Figure 6-8 Mosquito vector for West Nile virus. Culex mosquito laying eggs.

the United States annually.[49] The mortality rate from dengue reaches 44% without early diagnosis and treatment. Early treatment may limit mortality to less than 1%. The course of dengue illness depends on the patient's age, immunocompetence, and strain of infecting virus. Infection from one strain does not provide immunity to other flavivirus strains, such as West Nile virus.

Emerging Bloodborne Diseases. Blood remains a potential source of infection for disease agents, even though numerous safeguards are in place to protect public safety. Screening of blood and organ donors, newly implemented transfusion standards, and serologic testing protect the nation's blood supply, which is among the safest in the world. The greatest risk for transmission of bloodborne pathogens is during the incubation period, when the person is unaware of the infection, has no clinical indications of infection, and has not yet produced antibodies to the infectious agent. Therefore persons with risk factors for bloodborne diseases are excluded from donating blood or organs (see Box 21-5).

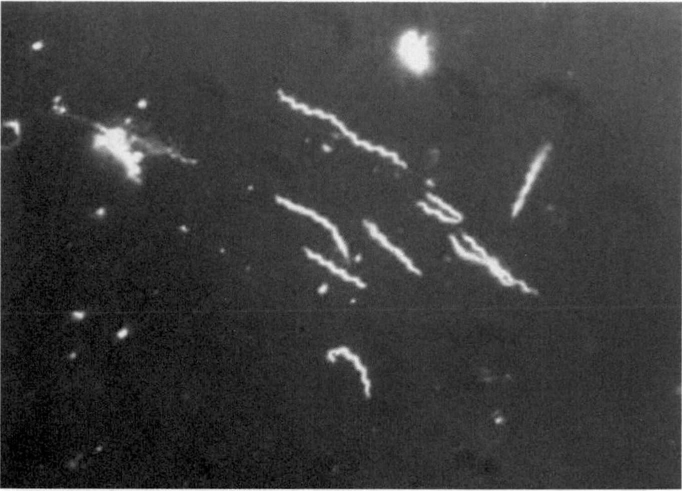

Figure 6-9 *Borrelia burgdorferi*, the causative agent of Lyme disease.

HUMAN IMMUNODEFICIENCY VIRUS. HIV disease was first noted in the United States in the late 1970s. The virus, initially referred to as the lymphadenopathy virus, was identified in 1983. Scientists believe that the virus became established in humans through cross-species transmission from chimpanzees either through bites, butchering, or ingestion of the animals for food. A complete discussion of HIV and AIDS is found in Chapter 22.

NEW VARIANT CREUTZFELDT-JAKOB DISEASE. New variant Creutzfeldt-Jakob disease (nvCJD) was first described in 1996 in the United Kingdom after the deaths of several young people from a fatal neurodegenerative disorder similar to mad cow disease, or bovine spongiform encephalitis (BSE). BSE was identified in the UK in 1986 after a livestock epidemic of the disease. Two theories of beef contamination are proposed. Until 1988 cattle were fed a meat and bonemeal product produced from rendered sheep and other livestock carcasses. Since sheep that died from scrapie, the sheep version of BSE, were included in the rendering process, transmission may have occurred from ingestion of contaminated feed. The second theory is that beef may have been contaminated by exposure to nervous system tissues during meat processing.[3,31]

Human consumption of beef products containing BSE has been linked to the disease in humans, called new variant CJD or nvCJD because it is similar to the known human disease, Creutzfeldt-Jakob disease. nvCJD is transmitted via prion proteins, which produce neuronal death by altering the way cellular proteins are folded. These changes produce a "Swiss cheese" effect in brain tissue from degeneration of neurons, which causes rapidly progressive dementia and death. Of the 153 cases of nvCJD reported as of December 2003, 143 cases originated in the United Kingdom and one in the United States. nvCJD has a long incubation period and no known treatment or cure. In response to the BSE epidemic in the United Kingdom, the United States and several European countries have established surveillance centers to monitor the occurrence of prion diseases and spongiform encephalopathies in an effort to protect public safety.[3,31]

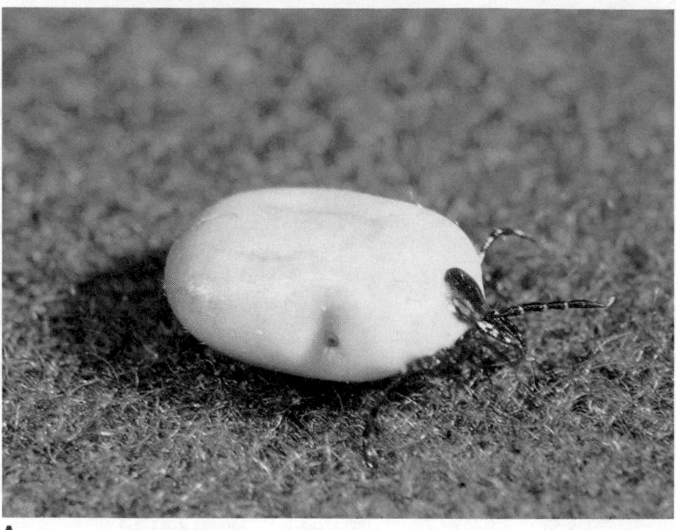
A

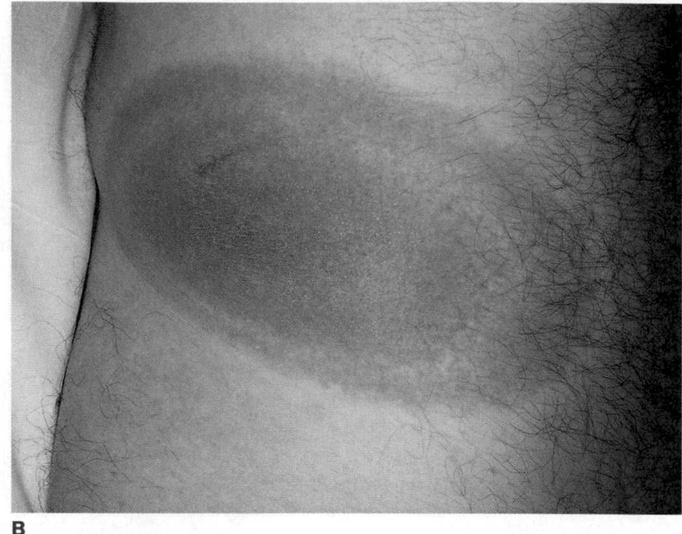
B

Figure 6-10 **A,** Tick vector of Lyme disease. **B,** Classic bull's eye rash caused by *Borrelia burgdorferi* after tick bite.

Emerging Microbial Resistance

Drug resistance is one of the most important factors contributing to the reemergence of bacterial diseases, and one of the most serious health threats today. Antibiotics either kill bacteria (bactericidal) or prevent their growth (bacteriostatic). They have been improved over time to provide increased effectiveness, broader spectrums of coverage, and decreased toxicity to host cells. Nevertheless, many diseases such as tuberculosis, HIV, malaria, and salmonella are developing drug resistance and becoming more virulent. Crowding, nonadherence to prescribed antibiotic therapies, and overuse of antibiotics by humans and agriculture are factors contributing to microbial mutation and subsequent resistance.[32] This growing trend may lead to corresponding increases in the incidence of and mortality from untreatable infectious diseases, frequency and length of hospital stays, health care costs, research costs, and global spread of untreatable pathogens.[32]

Antibiotic resistance is particularly troublesome in today's hospitals, where bacteria are responsible for an increasing number of nosocomial, or hospital-acquired, infections. The CDC estimates that about 80,000 hospitalized patients are infected with methicillin-resistant *S. aureus* (MRSA) annually, and the incidence of vancomycin-resistant enterococci (VRE) is on the rise.[16] The use of vaccines, prudent use of antibiotics for humans and animals, and effective infection control measures may limit the spread of antibiotic resistance.

Methicillin-Resistant *Staphylococcus aureus.* *S. aureus* generally resides on the skin or within nasal passages without causing disease in healthy persons. However, it can cause boils, skin or bone infections, wound infections, pneumonia, or septicemia in susceptible individuals. MRSA is a resistant strain of *S. aureus* that may develop in hospitalized patients who are cared for in intensive care or burn units; are receiving broad-spectrum antibiotics; are elderly or immunocompromised; have open wounds, urinary catheters, or invasive lines; or undergo prolonged hospitalization. MRSA infections are more likely to occur in hospitals and long-term care facilities, but community-acquired infections also occur. They are associated with active skin diseases, recent antibiotic use, overcrowding, and sharing of contaminated articles.[38] People who are colonized with MRSA do not have symptoms of infection, whereas those who are infected do have clinical manifestations of infection. Vancomycin is the primary treatment for *S. aureus* and MRSA, but resistant strains have been reported in recent years (see Evidence-Based Practice box).

Vancomycin-Resistant *Enterococcus.* There are several strains of enterococci, which are bacteria found in the feces of humans and animals. Enterococci are a leading cause of nosocomial bacteremia, urinary tract infections, surgical wound in-

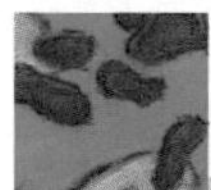

EVIDENCE-BASED PRACTICE

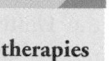

Topic Question: Do topical or systemic antimicrobial therapies eradicate nasal or extranasal methicillin-resistant *Staphylococcus aureus* (MRSA)?

Evidence Base: Four studies, involving six trials and 384 patients colonized with MRSA, were conducted to determine the effectiveness of topical or systemic antimicrobials in eradicating the organisms. Studies compared topicals, systemic antimicrobials, and combinations of topicals and systemic antimicrobials with placebo, no treatment, and topical or systemic antimicrobials alone.

Findings: Twenty percent of participants developed drug side effects, and all agents used were reported to develop drug resistance.

Conclusions: The evidence was not sufficient to conclude that either topical or systemic antimicrobials eradicate colonized MRSA. Side effects are serious, and resistance can result from antimicrobial therapy.

Loeb M et al: Antimicrobial drugs for treating methicillin-resistant *Staphylococcus aureus* colonization, *The Cochrane Library* Issue 2, Chichester, UK, 2005, John Wiley & Sons.

fections, and occasionally endocarditis or meningitis. As with MRSA, colonized bacteria do not cause illness in the patient but can be a source of infection for others. Transmission within the hospital most likely occurs on the hands of health care providers or equipment. VRE is consistently associated with prior treatment with vancomycin and other antibiotics such as clindamycin, cephalosporin, ciprofloxacin, and aminoglycosides. Patients at increased risk for VRE are those with prolonged hospitalizations, abdominal surgeries, enteral tube feedings, renal insufficiency, or acute illnesses. VRE tends to be resistant to many antibiotics, including ampicillin and the aminoglycosides. Quinupristin/dalfopristin and linezolid are the primary drugs effective for VRE infections at this time.[35]

Mycobacterium *tuberculosis*. Once well controlled by effective antituberculosis drugs, a resurgence of tuberculosis was seen in the 1980s. In 2000, 3% to 4% of the 8.7 million new cases of tuberculosis in the United States were identified as multidrug resistant.[28] Decreased focus on tuberculosis, increased immigration, homelessness, drug abuse, the HIV epidemic, and poor compliance with medication regimens are factors that favored the development of tuberculin drug resistance in this country. In developing countries, inadequate laboratory resources and inappropriate treatment of tuberculosis compound the spread of the resistant organism.[36] Chapter 26 discusses tuberculosis in greater detail.

Penicillin-Resistant *Streptococcus pneumoniae*. *Streptococcus pneumoniae* is a community-acquired pathogen commonly associated with ear infections and pneumonia. It is also an important cause of secondary infections in persons with influenza, resulting in bronchitis, sinusitis, pneumonia, and meningitis. Those at increased risk for streptococcus infections include older adults; people with HIV, diabetes mellitus, or blood disorders; people with renal, cardiac, or lung disease; chronic smokers; and those who are immunosuppressed from steroid drugs. Over the past 50 years the organism has evolved from being highly sensitive to penicillin to being highly resistant to penicillin and numerous other antibiotics. *S. pneumoniae* resistance has been traced to the increased and indiscriminate use of antibiotics. Fortunately, infections from the organism have decreased since the introduction of the pneumococcal conjugate vaccine.[17]

▶ ARE You READY?

Methicillin-resistant *Staphylococcus aureus* (MRSA) is most prevalent in which of the following populations?

1. Daycare workers
2. Immigrants from impoverished countries
3. Patients in long-term care facilities
4. Patients in ambulatory surgery centers

Infections and Chronic Disease

Only recently has the association between microbial agents and cancer or chronic disease been established (Table 6-7). For some diseases the causative agent is known. For others the association is strong or evidence suggests a link (Box 6-3). The difficulty in establishing an infectious cause of diseases that have no known etiology has several explanations, including[22,31]:

- Scientists may fail to consider the possibility that the disease is caused by an infectious agent. Such was the case with *Helicobacter pylori*, now known to cause peptic ulcer disease.
- The infectious agent may elicit an inflammatory response but be absent when the disease is clinically apparent. Rheumatic fever is good example. Antibodies produced against throat infections from *Streptococcus pyogenes* bound to myocardial tissues producing myocarditis and valve disease. By the time myocarditis developed, the agent was no longer infecting the throat.
- The link between the causative agent and the disease may be obscured. For example, many people are infected with the Epstein-Barr virus, but few develop the associated malignancies. The agent may be necessary, but other factors must serve as triggering factors for development of malignancy.
- Copathogens, as opposed to one causative agent, may be needed to produce a disease. For example, hepatitis D virus requires the hepatitis B surface antigen to produce disease.
- Some microbes may not possess the properties necessary to be detected by current technologic methods. They may be too small, do not stain, cannot be cultured using customary media, or do not occur in large enough numbers to be detected.
- The disease is, in fact, not caused by a microbial agent.

Since 1980, scientists have identified 24 agents, most of which are newly emergent, that are responsible for chronic diseases. Many other diseases with unknown causes may be caused by infectious agents. If so, the treatment and nursing care of persons with those chronic diseases may change significantly. Research is ongoing in this important area of disease pathogenesis. It is important that nurses understand the possibilities and remain informed of ongoing research that may improve the prevention, diagnosis, and treatment of chronic diseases[22] (see Future Watch box).

Collaborative Care Management

Infection Control in the Community

A *communicable disease* is any disease that is highly transmissible to other persons. Communicable diseases acquired outside of the hospital setting are known as *community-acquired* infections. Efforts to recognize and control communicable diseases are the responsibility of national, state, and local agencies. On the national level, the CDC provides epidemiologic and laboratory services to state health facilities on request. It enforces quarantine regulations and conducts foreign quarantine activities; administers international programs for the control of malaria, smallpox, and measles; and provides consultation to other nations on the control of preventable diseases. It also collects, tabulates, and assesses data on reportable diseases from state health departments and publishes the findings in the *Morbidity and Mortality Weekly Report*. Through its continuous surveillance, the CDC detects new cases of disease and intervenes to control disease outbreaks. In addition, the CDC is instrumental in providing guidelines and recommendations for infection control.

TABLE 6-7 INFECTIOUS AGENTS IDENTIFIED SINCE 1980 AND THE DISEASES THEY CAUSE

Microbe	Disease
Helicobacter pylori	Peptic ulcer disease, gastric adenocarcinoma
Borrelia burgdorferi	Lyme disease
Tropheryma whippelei	Whipple's disease
Helicobacter cinaedi	Proctitis
Streptococcus iniae	Cellulitis
Bartonella henselae	Cat-scratch disease, bacillary angiomatosis
Escherichia coli O157:H7	Hemolytic uremic syndrome
Campylobacter organisms	Guillain-Barré syndrome
Anaplasma phagocytophaga	Human granulocytic ehrlichiosis
Ehrlichia chaffeensis	Human monocytic ehrlichiosis
Rickettsia japonica	Spotted fever
Mycoplasma fermentans	Arthritis
Mycobacterium genavense	Disseminated mycobacteriosis in acquired immunodeficiency syndrome (AIDS)
Human immunodeficiency virus (HIV)	AIDS
Human herpesvirus 6	Roseola infantum
Human herpesvirus 8	Kaposi's sarcoma
Human metapneumovirus	Respiratory tract infection
Nipah virus	Encephalitis
Hendra virus	Encephalitis
Hepatitis C virus	Hepatitis, hepatocellular carcinoma
Hepatitis E virus	Hepatitis
Cyclospora cayetanensis	Diarrhea
SARS coronavirus	Severe acute respiratory syndrome (SARS)

From Cohen J, Powderly G, editors: *Infectious diseases*, ed 2, St Louis, 2004, Elsevier.

BOX 6-3 Diseases of Unknown Etiology Suspected To Be Caused by Infectious Agents

- Crohn's disease
- Ulcerative colitis
- Sprue
- Necrotizing enterocolitis of newborns
- Sclerosing cholangitis
- Primary biliary cirrhosis
- Cholelithiasis
- Brainerd diarrhea
- Scleroderma
- Ankylosing spondylitis
- Seal finger
- Polymyositis
- Polyarteritis nodosa
- Rheumatoid arthritis
- Systemic lupus erythematosus
- Wegener's granulomatosis
- Behçet's syndrome
- Goodpasture's syndrome
- Takayasu's arteritis
- Eosinophilic pustular folliculitis
- Sweet's syndrome
- Psoriasis
- Kawasaki disease
- Sarcoidosis
- Kikuchi's lymphadenitis
- Multiple sclerosis
- Schizophrenia
- Obsessive-compulsive personality disorder
- Diabetes mellitus
- Cancer
- Chronic fatigue syndrome
- Atherosclerosis
- Idiopathic pulmonary fibrosis
- Bronchiolitis obliterans with organizing pneumonia
- Idiopathic pneumonia syndrome
- Still's disease
- Malacoplakia
- Bacterial vaginosis
- Nephrolithiasis
- Chronic culture-negative prostatitis

From Cohen J, Powderly G, editors: *Infectious diseases*, ed 2, St Louis, 2004, Elsevier.

Future Watch

Is an Infectious Agent Responsible for Atherosclerosis?

Risk factors such as smoking and hyperlipidemia account for about 50% of cases of atherosclerosis. Infectious agents may be responsible for the remaining cases. Studies have shown that patients with coronary artery disease have circulating markers of inflammation. Currently research is ongoing to determine whether microbes are responsible for that inflammation. Although *Chlamydia pneumoniae* is the most likely, cytomegalovirus and *Helicobacter pylori* are also under investigation. Some small studies have demonstrated reductions in coronary artery events when patients are treated with antibiotics, but further research is needed.

Cohen J, Powderly G, editors: *Infectious diseases,* ed 2, St Louis, 2004, Elsevier.

Legal Alert

Legal Reasons for Exemption from Required Immunizations

Medical Exemptions

Licensed physician must sign certificate indicating a medical contraindication to the vaccine.

Adverse reaction must fall within specific parameters within a vaccine injury chart.

Exemptions may be temporary and apply only to the vaccine believed to have caused the reaction.

Religious Exemptions

Requires an affidavit from the person stating that the immunization conflicts with the teachings and practices of their church or religious organization.

Philosophic Exemptions

Requires a written certification from persons that they have either a philosophic or personal objection to the immunization.

Control of infectious diseases in the United States is primarily the responsibility of each state. State health officers usually delegate this responsibility to a division of communicable diseases in which a staff of physicians, nurses, veterinarians, and sanitary engineers works closely with a state epidemiologist in the detection, assessment, and control of specific reportable diseases. Local public health departments work in conjunction with state health departments in this effort.

Physicians and health care facilities have a responsibility to report communicable diseases promptly to the health department. Health agencies in the community use the reported data to determine potential or real problems, identify the causative agent and if possible its source, and identify the population at risk. These agencies then devise and implement a plan to control the problem, care for those exposed, and protect the population at risk.

Prevention and Control Measures. Prevention and control measures are many and varied in that they address each of the different links in the chain of infection. Environmental measures eliminate or reduce the number of infectious agents directly or by targeting reservoirs, vectors, fomites, and common vehicle transmitters. Thus the prevention and control of disease in the community involve control measures such as ensuring proper sanitation; monitoring the health practices in institutions that handle, package, and prepare foods; implementing environmental controls such as spraying to kill mosquitoes in areas of disease outbreaks; offering immunization programs; and monitoring for new cases of infections. Public education is a key component of all these efforts.

IMMUNIZATION PROGRAMS. The goal of immunization programs is to prevent infectious diseases and thus inhibit their spread. A pathogen can be virtually eliminated if 90% of the population is immunized and thus protected against the organism, since there are too few susceptible hosts to allow transmission of the pathogen. This type of protection is called **herd immunity**.

Immunizations provide artificially active immunity. They work by inducing an immune response and synthesis of antibodies against the offending organism, such as measles or poliovirus. Immunity to some infections, such as chickenpox or hepatitis, may require more than one vaccination to challenge the immune system to make a sufficient number of antibodies and memory cells to provide permanent immunity (see Chapter 20). Other organisms that are not transmitted from person to person, such as tetanus, which is found in the soil, require periodic immunizations throughout life to maintain immunity, since contact with the pathogen is rare. These periodic vaccinations are called *booster injections.*

PRIMARY IMMUNIZATIONS. The National Immunization Program (NIP) is a disease-prevention program sponsored by the CDC. NIP provides leadership for the planning, coordination, and conduct of immunization activities throughout the United States. This resource, found at http://www.cdc.gov/nip, provides information when questions arise about immunization recommendations, proper immunization practices, prophylaxis, interruption in immunization schedules, or adverse reactions and side effects.

In America, primary immunizations are initiated at birth, with the administration of the hepatitis B vaccine, and continued at various intervals throughout life. Recommended childhood and adolescent immunization schedules for the current year are available on the CDC website (www.cdc.gov). Children are required to receive immunizations before attending public school unless they meet certain exemption criteria (see Legal Alert box).

The most successful immunization program in the world occurred with smallpox, which was officially eradicated in 1977. Although adverse reactions are rare, immunizations are not completely without risks. Nurses need to be able to recognize and differentiate between common and serious immunization reactions (Table 6-8) and intervene as necessary to protect the patient's safety. Several precautions can help eliminate potential problems with vaccine administration (Box 6-4). Nurses also need to educate parents about the importance of monitoring for serious reactions so that early treatment can be initiated when warranted (see Patient/Family Teaching box, p. 109).

ADULT IMMUNIZATIONS. Proper protection against certain diseases is as important for adults as it is for children. If not already protected, adults should be vaccinated against measles, mumps, rubella, and varicella. Hepatitis A vaccine is administered only to

TABLE 6-8 COMMON AND SERIOUS IMMUNIZATION REACTIONS

Immunization	Common, Harmless Reactions	Serious Reactions
DTaP	Pain, tenderness, swelling, or redness at injection site for 24-48 hr (51%) Fever for 24-48 hr (47%) Painless lump (or nodule) at injection site 1-2 wk later Mild drowsiness (32%), fretfulness (54%), or poor appetite (21%) for 24-48 hr	Fever over 105° F (40.5° C) (0.3%) Crying for more than 3 hr (1%) High-pitched, unusual cry (0.1%) Convulsions (0.06%) Any other unusual reaction
MMR	Fever of 101°-103° F (38.3°-39.5° C) for 2-3 days Measles vaccine rash: mild pink rash mainly on the trunk; nonpruritic, lasting less than 3 days (5%)	Anaphylactic reaction (to egg in vaccine) Hives, shock, wheezing, stridor, and swelling of mouth or throat beginning within 2 hr of time child received vaccine
Polio	None	Paralytic polio (symptoms include stiff neck, muscle tenderness, and weakness); very rare, occurs mainly in immunocompromised children or adults who care for them, usually within 30 days of when vaccine was given
HIB	Sore injection site or mild fever (1.5%)	None reported
Hep B	Sore injection site (30%) or mild fever (3%)	None reported
Influenza	Pain, tenderness, or swelling at injection site within 6-8 hr (10%) Fever of 101°-103° F (38.3°-39.5° C) (18%); mainly occurs in young children	Anaphylactic reaction if allergic to egg in vaccine; common symptoms of severe allergic reaction, including hives, shock, wheezing, stridor, and swelling of mouth or throat, within 2 hr of time vaccine was administered
Chickenpox (varicella)	Pain or swelling at injection site for 1-2 days Fever that begins 2-4 wk after vaccination and lasts 1-3 days Mild rash at injection site or elsewhere on body, beginning 5-26 days after vaccine; looks like a few chickenpox lesions, and usually lasts a few days	None reported

From Schmitt BD: *Immunization reactions, clinical reference systems annual,* San Francisco, updated 2003, McKesson Health Solutions.

NOTE: Never give aspirin for any symptom within 6 weeks of giving a vaccine (Reye's syndrome has been linked with use of aspirin to treat fever or pain caused by a virus). For fever or pain, give acetaminophen.

adults who are at high risk. The recommended adult immunization schedule for the current year is available on the CDC website. Important information about commonly used vaccines is summarized in Table 6-9.

A marked reduction in vaccine-preventable diseases has occurred in the United States and throughout developed countries. However, the number of U.S. children being immunized has declined due to inaccessibility, cost, and growing concerns about the safety of immunizations. Free immunizations are no longer equally available in all 50 states because of the reduction in federal money used to support local immunization efforts. Infections formerly seen only in children are now occurring more frequently in adults because of lack of immunizations and resulting failure of the population to develop acquired immunity during early childhood (see Ethical Alert box, p. 111).

PASSIVE IMMUNIZATIONS. Antibodies produced by other persons or by animals such as the horse, cow, and rabbit can be introduced into a person's bloodstream for protection against pathogens (Table 6-10). This protection is temporary, usually lasting only a few weeks, and stimulates no production of antibodies by the recipient. It is called *artificial passive immunity.* Artificial passive immunization is given to a person who has been exposed to a disease and has no natural or artificial active immunity. It usually is administered before the disease develops but may be given to modify disease symptoms. To be effective after the disease has developed, however, it must be administered early, before extensive damage to body tissue.

Passive immunization is usually reserved for persons to whom the disease would be detrimental. For example, it rarely is given to prevent a disease such as chickenpox or mumps in healthy chil-

Box 6-4 Vaccine Precautions

Potential Allergic Reactions

Vaccines prepared from chicken or duck embryos may cause reactions in persons allergic to eggs.

Do not administer products containing horse serum (tetanus antitoxin) to people with horse serum allergies unless they have undergone intradermal (sensitivity) testing and no reaction has occurred after 20 minutes.

Additional Considerations

Do not give active immunologic products to persons with acute febrile illnesses to avoid an excessive inflammatory reaction from the vaccine.

Do not give live attenuated virus vaccines to persons with immunodeficiency, since uncontrolled viral replication is possible.

Do not administer live attenuated virus vaccines at the same time as passive immunization, since passively acquired antibodies can interfere with the desired active immune response.

In general, inactivated vaccines and live vaccines (except cholera and yellow fever) can be administered simultaneously in separate sites.

When possible, administer live vaccines on the same day or at least 30 days apart.

Do not give pregnant women live attenuated vaccines because of theoretic risk to the fetus.

When receiving antitoxins, antisera, or antivenins, patients remain for observation for 20 to 30 minutes, since most severe allergic reactions occur within that time frame.

Have epinephrine 1:1000 available for immediate intramuscular administration to counter allergic reactions when vaccines are administered.

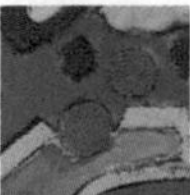

PATIENT/FAMILY TEACHING
Vaccines

Teaching for the patient and family receiving a vaccine should include information about:

- Expected effects of vaccine
- Possible side effects of vaccine (local and systemic).
- Manifestations that they need to report (severe local or systemic reactions).
- Time frame for any needed booster injections.

And the following instructions:

- Avoid scratching the area to prevent infection.
- Apply hot, wet dressing to reduce localized reactions.
- Avoid aspirin for fever related to viral vaccines.

dren because they are at an optimal age for the body to respond immunologically with minimal adverse effects. Because of occasional side effects, it is recommended that the use of antibodies be limited to those disorders in which its efficacy has been definitely established.

Infection Control in Health Care Facilities

The underlying principle of infection control is the establishment and maintenance of a safe environment for patients, visitors, and health care providers.[30] Agencies have specialized departments and committees that develop specific policies and procedures, monitor for infections and conditions that favor the development of infections, collect and analyze data, and educate personnel about effective infection control measures. An infection control team or person who is certified in infection control generally addresses the day-to-day issues of prevention and control and provides advice to staff carrying out infection control procedures. However, it is essential that every staff member accept responsibility for and maintain infection control standards.

Nosocomial Infections. Nosocomial infections are those that patients did not have before their hospitalization but acquired after admission. Persons admitted to the hospital with community-acquired infections may develop a *superinfection* from another organism while hospitalized. The superinfection may be a more virulent or drug-resistant organism. For example, a patient admitted with a leg ulcer infected with *S. aureus* may develop an MRSA wound infection.

Nosocomial infections are a major problem in that they increase patient morbidity, mortality, and hospital costs. Approximately 5% of hospitalized patients contract nosocomial infections, which amounts to greater than 2 million patient hospitalizations per year. They increase the average length of stay by 7.4 to 9.4 days and the cost for caring for patients by an average of $15,275 per patient.[39]

Some patients are at greater risk for nosocomial infections than others for a variety of reasons (Box 6-5). Seventy-five percent of all nosocomial infections occur in the urinary tract from catheterizations, indwelling urinary catheters, and urologic procedures. The next most frequently encountered sites are infected surgical wounds, followed by lower respiratory tract infections, cutaneous infections, and bloodstream infections, some associated with the use of intravascular lines.[21] Pathogens that are typically responsible for nosocomial infections and their related infection sites are listed in Table 6-11.

Patients, personnel, visitors, equipment, and lines are all potential sources of infection in hospitals and long-term care facilities. Specific control measures for containing exogenous and endogenous sources of infection are important. However, in many instances health care providers could prevent nosocomial infections simply by consistently using appropriate hand-washing

TABLE 6-9 DESCRIPTION OF SELECTED VACCINES

Vaccine	Description	Comments
DPT		
Diphtheria	Toxoid Inactivated Diphtheria toxin	Booster dose every 10 yr
Tetanus	Inactivated Tetanus toxoid	Booster dose every 10 yr For contaminated wound management, additional booster given if more than 5 yr since last booster dose
Pertussis	Killed whole *Bordetella pertussis*	Not recommended for persons older than 7 yr, since risk of pertussis low and reaction possibly severe
MMR		
Measles	Live attenuated virus vaccine	Contraindications: pregnancy, immunocompromised state, history of anaphylactic reaction to eggs
Mumps	Live attenuated virus vaccine	Contraindications: pregnancy, immunocompromised state, history of anaphylactic reaction to eggs
Rubella	Live attenuated rubella virus grown in human diploid cells	Contraindications: pregnancy, immunocompromised state
Polio		
OPV	Live attenuated oral poliovirus vaccine	Contraindications: pregnancy, immunocompromised state
IPV	Inactivated poliovirus vaccine	Administered by subcutaneous injection; contraindicated in pregnancy
Influenza	Inactivated whole or disrupted (split) influenza viruses	Antigenic content annually changed to reflect influenza A and B virus strains in circulation; administered annually; contraindication: history of anaphylactic hypersensitivity to eggs
Pneumococcal	Purified preparation of 23 different types of pneumococcal capsular polysaccharide	Should be given to persons 2 yr and older who have chronic illnesses specifically associated with increased risk for pneumococcal disease and to all healthy adults over 65 years
Hepatitis A	Killed whole virus grown in human diploid cells	Administered by intramuscular injection with booster in 6-12 mo
Hepatitis B		
Recombinant deoxyribonucleic acid (DNA)	Purified surface antigen of virus produced by recombinant yeast cells	Given in series of 3 injections, with the latter ones given 1 and 6 mo after the first; indicated for persons who have routine or frequent contact with blood and body fluids; contraindicated for persons allergic to yeast
Human serum	Purified, inactivated surface antigen of virus from plasma of human carriers	Administration schedule same as for recombinant DNA form; recommended for hemodialysis patients
***Haemophilus influenzae* b (Hib)**	Bacterial polysaccharide conjugated to protein	Administration schedule may vary depending on brand of vaccine used
Varicella	Live attenuated virus vaccine	Administered by intramuscular injection; transmission of virus to susceptible persons can occur; contraindications: pregnancy, immunocompromised state

techniques, strict aseptic technique when giving care, and greater restraint in the use of invasive procedures and antibiotics.

Controlling Exogenous Sources of Infection

HAND WASHING. Hand washing is the most important measure for controlling the transmission of infections. Hand washing decreases transient and resident flora on the hands and thus acts as a deterrent to cross-infection. Ample washing facilities are necessary throughout the facility and all personnel should use them before and after patient contact; after contact with excretions, secretions, wound drainage, or any contaminated articles; and before any clean or sterile procedure or contact with clean or sterile equipment (see Research box, p. 112). Friction and rinsing are the two most important components of good hand washing.

Ethical Alert

Forced Immunizations

As part of the larger Homeland Security bill, H.R. 5710, the secretary of defense would be able to declare an actual or potential bioterrorist event and order smallpox treatment that could include forced immunizations and quarantine. Congress passed the bill on the premise it was necessary to protect the population from bioterrorism threats. The bill also provides protection for vaccine manufacturers should vaccines cause harm. Many organizations and individuals oppose this section of the bill because they believe it interferes with their basic right of choice. Twenty-two states have rejected or stalled the law, and 16 others have passed all or parts of it. In states where the law was passed, citizens could be charged with a crime if they refuse vaccinations. The issue of forced immunizations creates an ethical dilemma for those who believe the government has no right to force individuals to be immunized and that such decisions should be by individual choice.

Unfortunately, consistent hand washing continues to be a problem in health care facilities (see Research box, p. 113, top). Alcohol-based and other antiseptic solutions facilitate hand hygiene in clinical settings and have been proven effective in preventing the transmission of many organisms when used consistently (see Research box, p. 113, bottom left).

ARTIFICIAL NAILS AND JEWELRY. A growing body of evidence supports the transmission of pathogens, especially gram-negative bacilli and yeast, by artificial nails, since they are more likely to harbor microbes than native nails. As a result, the CDC recommends that health care workers not wear artificial fingernails or extenders when providing patient care and that they keep native nails less than ¼ inch long. No recommendations regarding use of nail polish have been made.

HOUSEKEEPING AND SANITATION. Hospitals need to strictly enforce practices to reduce dust and environmental reservoirs of organisms, especially in high-risk areas such as nurseries, operating rooms, and intensive care units. Health care workers should promptly clean up blood or body fluid spills with an approved hospital disinfectant or a 1:10 dilution of 5.25% sodium hypochlorite (household bleach and water). They should change linens with as little contact with the nurse's uniform as possible. They should not throw linens on the floor or shake them in the air because it further contaminates the linens and stirs up dust particles that can transmit pathogens.

Health care workers should dispose of waste products in the appropriate receptacle. State and federal laws regulate the disposal of infectious waste from health care institutions. Items such as needles and syringes, laboratory cultures and tissue specimens, and other disposable items that are saturated with blood or body substances are considered regulated infectious waste. Regulated infectious waste must be incinerated or treated to render it noninfectious before disposal. Other waste materials from patient rooms may be disposed of as regular trash. Proper cleaning and sterilization of contaminated reusable articles and equipment are essential. Reusable items, such as stethoscopes, are often overlooked but are potential sources of infection in the health care setting.

Air is generally not considered an important factor in nosocomial cross-infection. However, in the case of *Aspergillus* spores and *M. tuberculosis,* adequate air exchanges are necessary to reduce the number of organisms. Minimal standards for air exchanges in patient care areas are published by the U.S. Department of Health and Human Services (USDHHS) (see Guidelines for Safe Practice box, p. 113).

Controlling Endogenous Sources of Infection. Reducing endogenous sources of infection is more difficult than controlling exogenous sources because the source is often the patient's normal flora. Preventive measures are directed at decreasing risk by increasing the patient's defense mechanisms. Basic care includes teaching patients the importance of adequate nutrition, hydration, and personal hygiene. Maintaining the patient's normal flora and preventing colonization with pathogens that can serve as a source of infection are other effective measures, but these are not always possible when patients are receiving antibiotics or undergoing chemotherapy, which disrupt the normal flora and promote colonization. Appropriate use of antibiotics for prophylaxis and treatment helps prevent colonization with pathogens and decreases the incidence of infection with drug-resistant organisms. A summary of major prevention and control measures is provided in the Guidelines for Safe Practice box, p. 114.

TABLE 6-10 PRODUCTS THAT PROVIDE PASSIVE IMMUNITY

Products	Mechanism	Protects Against
Antitoxins Whole blood Animal or human sera	Detoxify and inactivate bacteria and neutralize viruses	Diphtheria Tetanus Botulism Gas gangrene Snake venom Black widow spider venom
Immune serum globulin (ISG) Gamma-globulin	Preformed antibodies that attack and destroy antigen (pathogens)	Measles (prophylaxis or modification) Viral hepatitis type A (prophylaxis or modification) Immunodeficiency diseases

Box 6-5 Factors That Predispose a Person to Nosocomial Infections

- Severe or prolonged illness that alters natural defenses
- Age, the very young and the very old being the most susceptible
- Impaired immunity caused by chronic disease (cancer, renal failure, chronic lung disease, diabetes, acquired immunodeficiency syndrome)
- Immunosuppression (from radiation, steroids, or chemotherapy)
- Antibiotics, which can eliminate the patient's normal flora, providing opportunity for colonization with pathogenic and drug-resistant organisms
- Invasive diagnostic and therapeutic procedures and devices (indwelling urinary catheters, monitoring devices, intravenous catheters, and respiratory assistive devices)
- Surgery
- Burns
- Lengthy hospitalization with prolonged exposure to others with infections

Protective Precautions. Protective precautions, which include specific types of patient isolation procedures, are intended to decrease the risk of transmission of microorganisms within hospitals and long-term care facilities. Some general principles apply regardless of the type of isolation. Health care workers should use barriers such as gowns, gloves, and masks only once and then discard them in an appropriate receptacle before leaving the patient's room. These barriers should be conveniently available for each patient room. Employees must wash hands before and after each patient contact even when gloves are worn.

In 1996 the CDC and the Healthcare Infectious Control Practices Advisory Committee (HICPAC) published revised guidelines for isolation precautions in hospitals (Box 6-6). The precautions are two tiered. The first tier, Standard Precautions, is used with all patients regardless of whether the diagnosis is known. The second tier, Transmission-Based Precautions, is designed to reduce the risk of airborne, droplet, and contact transmission. It is used when caring for patients with documented or suspected infection with highly transmissible or epidemiologically important pathogens for which Standard Precautions may be insufficient. Standard Precautions are used in combination with one or more of the Transmission-Based Precautions, depending on the disease identified.

Standard Precautions apply to (1) blood; (2) all other body fluids and secretions except sweat, regardless of whether they contain visible blood; (3) nonintact skin; and (4) mucous membranes. Table 6-12 lists the techniques used for Standard Precautions.

Airborne Precautions are used to prevent airborne transmission of organisms contained in dust particles or the droplet nuclei of evaporated droplets. Special air handling may include negative pressure, frequent air exchanges, direct-to-the-outside exhaust, high-efficiency particulate air (HEPA) filters, or ultraviolet light. Patients with actual or suspected airborne infections are placed in private rooms with negative pressure room air and 12 air exchanges per hour. Staff entering the room use HEPA filter respirators. Patients must stay in the room with the door closed until they are no longer infectious. Tuberculosis, measles, and varicella are airborne infections.

Droplet Precautions are used when the patient's cough, sneeze, or talking or procedures such as suctioning or bronchoscopy can transmit the infective agent. Organisms transmitted by this method travel about 3 feet from the patient but quickly settle onto surfaces and can no longer be inhaled by an uninfected person. Wearing a mask while working within 3 feet of patients protects workers from droplet infections, including diseases such as influenza and *Neisseria meningitidis* pneumonia.

Research

Trick WE et al: Impact of ring wearing on hand contamination and comparison of hand hygiene agents in a hospital, *Clin Infect Dis* 36:1383–1390, 2003.

Researchers identified risk factors for hand contamination (number of rings, presence of cuts on the hand, fingernail length, artificial fingernails) and compared the efficacy of three hand hygiene agents: alcohol-based hand rub, plain soap and water, and medicated hand wipes. In their analysis of surgical intensive care nurses, they found that rings on nurses' hands resulted in an increased frequency of hand carriage of *Staphylococcus aureus*, gram-negative bacilli, or *Candida* species and that the incidence of any transient organism increased when the nurses wore several rings. The study also demonstrated that hand contamination with any transient organism was significantly less likely to occur after use of an alcohol-based hand rub when compared with plain soap and water or medicated hand wipes. Researchers concluded that ring wearing increases the frequency of hand contamination with potential nosocomial pathogens and that use of an alcohol-based hand rub resulted in significantly less frequent hand contamination.

Table 6-11 Common Agents Responsible for Nosocomial Infections

Pathogen	Common Infection, Site, or Risk Factor
Escherichia coli	Urinary tract infection
Coagulase-negative staphylococci	Wound infection, bacteremia
Staphylococcus aureus	Wound infection, pneumonia
Pseudomonas aeruginosa	Pneumonia, infections secondary to burns, leukemia, cystic fibrosis, immunodeficiency states, prolonged course of antibiotics, immune suppressive agents, inhalation therapy, tracheostomy, urinary catheterization, renal transplants
Candida albicans	Infections secondary to antibiotic therapy, immunodeficiency, immunosuppression, organ transplants

Research

Centers for Disease Control and Prevention: CDC guidelines for hand hygiene in health-care settings, *MMWR* 51(RR16):1-44, 2002, accessed from website: http://www.cdc.gov/mmwr/preview/mmwrhtml/rr5116a1.htm.

In a study of surgical intensive care unit nurses, researchers found that of the 2824 opportunities for hand washing, only 48% of health care workers washed their hands. Nonadherence was lowest among nurses (compared with other health care workers) and highest in intensive care units compared with medical units. Self-reported barriers to hand washing included irritation caused by "hand-hygiene agents, inaccessible hand-hygiene supplies, interference with priority of care, wearing of gloves, forgetfulness, lack of knowledge of the guidelines, insufficient time for hand hygiene, high workload and understaffing, and the lack of scientific information indicating a definitive impact of improved hand hygiene on health-care associated rates."

Research

Parienti JJ et al: Hand-rubbing with an aqueous alcoholic solution vs traditional surgical hand-scrubbing and 30-day surgical site infection rates: a randomized equivalence study, *JAMA* 288(6):722-727, 2002.

This study evaluated the effectiveness of performing a surgical scrub with an aqueous alcohol solution versus antiseptic soap in preventing surgical site infections. Nurses on three surgery units scrubbed their hands with antiseptic soap, and nurses on three other surgery units scrubbed with an aqueous alcohol solution, both according to Centers for Disease Control and Prevention guidelines for surgical scrubbing. Researchers concluded that the routine surgical practice of scrubbing hands with an aqueous alcohol solution was as effective as hand scrubbing with antiseptic soap. The incidence of surgical site infections did not differ for patients at the end of 30 days.

Contact Precautions are used to interrupt transmission of organisms by direct (skin-to-skin) or indirect (skin-to-contaminated item) contact. Patients with infectious diarrhea, herpes simplex virus, or MRSA-infected wounds, for example, require contact isolation when hospitalized. Contact isolation is used in conjunction with Standard Precautions, with each institution adapting the HICPAC recommendations based on its particular circumstances and endemic rate. Table 6-13 summarizes types of precautions and patients requiring the precautions. Additional information about various types of protective precautions can be found on the CDC website http://www.cdc.gov/ncidod/hip/.

▶ ARE You READY?

Which of the following patients is at greatest risk for development of a nosocomial infection?

1. 38-year-old female with indwelling catheter for 10 days
2. 42-year-old male post operative lung resection
3. 55-year-old female with active hepatitis
4. 62-year-old male with gastroenteritis

National Goals

On the national level, the USDHHS publishes an ongoing document that lists goals for all Americans designed to improve the health of the nation as a whole. Goals related to this chapter from the most recent document, *Healthy People 2010,* may be found in the Healthy People 2010 box.

Diagnostic Tests

Diagnostic tests are an important adjunct in the diagnosis of infection. Chapter 20 discusses common diagnostic tests for immune function.

White Blood Cell Count. The white blood cell (WBC) count with differential provides information about the type of infection and the body's response to it. A WBC count less than 5000/mm^3 generally signifies a viral infection, whereas a WBC count greater than 10,000/mm^3 indicates an inflammatory response to a pathogen. The differential count (neutrophils, basophils, eosinophils, lymphocytes, or monocytes) increases or decreases based on the type and acuity of infection (see Chapter 20 for a discussion of WBC response to infection).

Culture and Sensitivity Testing. The primary purpose for culturing is to ensure that the patient receives the correct antibiotic for the organism causing the infection. *Sensitivity* refers to the antibiotic's ability to kill the pathogen producing an infection. Laboratories generally assess sensitivity by placing paper disks impregnated with antibiotics into a culture that contains the

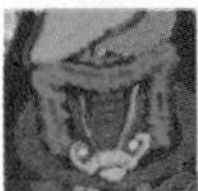

GUIDELINES FOR SAFE PRACTICE *Prevention and Control of Exogenous Sources of Infection*

Health Care Providers

Do not care for patients when you are ill.

Stay current with immunizations.

Practice approved hand hygiene.

—Seek attention for dry, broken skin.

—Do not give direct patient care if herpes lesions are present.

Use personal protective equipment (e.g., gloves, mask, face shield) as appropriate.

Housekeeping and Sanitation

Do not shake or place linens on floor.

Dispose of liquids and solids in appropriate containers.

Properly clean and sterilize contaminated articles.

Place patients in rooms with proper ventilation.

Mop and damp dust to remove dust and other environmental reservoirs for infection.

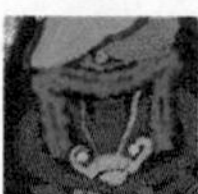

GUIDELINES FOR SAFE PRACTICE *Prevention and Control of Endogenous Sources of Infection*

Measures to increase patient's defenses and decrease risk for infection include:

- Teach patient the importance of good nutrition.
- Encourage personal hygiene, especially hand washing.

Measures to decrease risk of development of resistant organisms in patients receiving antibiotics include:

- Administer antibiotics on time to maintain blood levels.
- Teach patients to take all of prescribed antibiotics.
- Teach patients regarding the dangers of taking antibiotics when not prescribed.

Box 6-6 Types of Precautions

Standard Precautions

Use Standard Precautions for the care of all patients.

Airborne Precautions

In addition to Standard Precautions, use Airborne Precautions for patients known or suspected to have serious illnesses transmitted by airborne droplet nuclei. Examples of such illnesses include:

- Measles
- Varicella (including disseminated zoster)*
- Tuberculosis

Droplet Precautions

In addition to Standard Precautions, use Droplet Precautions for patients known or suspected to have serious illnesses transmitted by large particle droplets. Examples of such illnesses include:

- Invasive *Haemophilus influenzae* type b disease, including meningitis, pneumonia, epiglottitis, and sepsis
- Invasive *Neisseria meningitidis* disease, including meningitis, pneumonia, and sepsis
- Other serious bacterial respiratory infections spread by droplet transmission, including:
  —Diphtheria (pharyngeal)
  —Mycoplasma pneumonia
  —Pertussis
  —Pneumonic plague
  —Streptococcal pharyngitis, pneumonia, or scarlet fever in infants and young children
- Serious viral infections spread by droplet transmission, including:
  —Adenovirus*
  —Influenza
  —Mumps
  —Parvovirus B19
  —Rubella

Contact Precautions

In addition to Standard Precautions, use Contact Precautions for patients known or suspected to have serious illness easily transmitted by direct patient contact or by contact with items in the patient's environment. Examples of such illnesses may include:

- Gastrointestinal, respiratory, skin, or wound infections or colonization with multidrug-resistant bacteria judged by the infection control program, based on current state, regional, or national recommendations, to have special clinical and epidemiologic significance
- Enteric infections with a low infectious dose or prolonged environmental survival, including:
  Clostridium difficile

For diapered or incontinent patients: enterohemorrhagic *Escherichia coli* 0157:H7, shigella, hepatitis A, or rotavirus

- Respiratory syncytial virus, parainfluenza virus, or enteroviral infections in infants and young children
- Skin infections that are highly contagious or that may occur on dry skin, including:
  —Diphtheria (cutaneous)
  —Herpes simplex virus (neonatal or mucocutaneous)
  —Impetigo
  —Major (noncontained) abscesses, cellulitis, or decubiti
  —Pediculosis
  —Scabies
  —*Staphylococcal furunculosis* in infants and young children
  —Zoster (disseminated or in the immunocompromised host)*
- Viral hemorrhagic conjunctivitis
- Viral hemorrhagic infections (Ebola, Lassa, or Marburg)

From Garner JS and Hospital Infection Control Practices Advisory Committee: Guidelines for isolation precautions in hospitals, part 2, Recommendations for isolation precautions in hospitals, *Am J Infect Control* 22:24–52, 1996.
*Certain infections require more than one type of precaution.

microbe. If the disk retards growth, the organism is susceptible to that particular antibiotic. If growth is not retarded, the organism is resistant. Prescribed antibiotics are often based on sensitivity results.

Medications

The principle treatment for infectious diseases is *antimicrobial therapy*, which includes antibacterial, antiviral, and antifungal agents.

Antibacterial Agents. Antibacterial agents, commonly referred to as antibiotics, are classified according to their chemical structure and further differentiated based on their antibacterial spectrum, mechanism of action, toxicity, potency, and pharmacokinetic properties. The main classes of antibiotics are the penicillins, cephalosporins, sulfonamides, aminoglycosides, tetracyclines, and macrolides. Antibiotics work by either inhibiting the growth of organisms (bacteriostatic) or killing organisms (bactericidal). Before initiating antibiotic therapy, the health care provider should attempt to identify the causative organism and

TABLE 6-12 STANDARD PRECAUTIONS TECHNIQUES

Item	Precautions
Hand washing	After touching blood, body fluids, secretions, excretions, contaminated items, whether or not gloves are worn
Gloves	When touching blood, body fluids, secretions, excretions, and contaminated items and when performing invasive procedures; remove gloves promptly after use and wash hands
Mask, eye protection, face shield	To protect mucous membranes of eyes, nose, and mouth during activities likely to generate splashes or sprays of blood, body fluids, secretions, or excretions
Private room	Indicated if personal hygiene is poor or if body substances contaminate the environment
Needles	Uncapped and unbent needles disposed of at point of use in puncture-resistant container; one-handed or device-assisted recapping if necessary
Soiled linen	Placed in leak-proof bags; laundry workers sorting all soiled linen wear gown and gloves
Reusable equipment	Bagged for transport to decontamination area; decontamination personnel wear gowns, gloves, masks, and eye protection

Modified from Garner JS and Hospital Infection Control Practices Advisory Committee: Guidelines for isolation precautions in hospitals, part 2, Recommendations for isolation precautions in hospitals, *Am J Infect Control* 22:24–52, 1996.

determine antibiotic susceptibilities through culture and sensitivity testing so that the most effective antibiotic can be administered. Antibiotics can have many side effects, including hypersensitivity reactions, gastrointestinal tract disturbances, and bone marrow suppression. The health care provider should always assess patients for allergies before administering antibiotics.[33] A growing problem associated with antibiotic therapy is microbial resistance (see discussion above).

Antiviral Agents. Medications that kill viruses are known as *antiviral agents*. Viruses use host cells for replication. They attach to and enter a cell, and then use the host cell's RNA or DNA to copy their genetic information and make new viral particles. Antiviral agents interfere with steps of the replication process so that replication does not take place. Antiviral agents are effective only against a few viruses, including cytomegalovirus, herpes simplex virus, influenza A, respiratory syncytial virus, and HIV. Antivirals are ineffective against most viruses primarily because the virus has usually replicated and infected most cells before clinical manifestations are present. Side effects of antiviral agents can be more profound than for antibiotics because viral-infected host cells are also killed by these agents[33] (Table 6-14).

Antifungal Agents. Fungi are difficult to kill because they require drug dosages that humans cannot tolerate well. Therefore few antifungal agents are available. Antifungals may be topical, oral, or parenteral and act by (1) binding to sterols in the fungal cell membrane, causing loss of intracellular ions, altered cellular metabolism, and death; (2) inhibiting an enzyme needed by the fungi to produce sterols, again resulting in loss of intracellular ions; or (3) preventing fungal reproduction[33] (Table 6-15).

Antitubercular Agents. Antitubercular agents are used to treat diseases caused by various *Mycobacterium* organisms, such as *M. tuberculosis*. A discussion of these drugs and tuberculosis is found in Chapter 26.

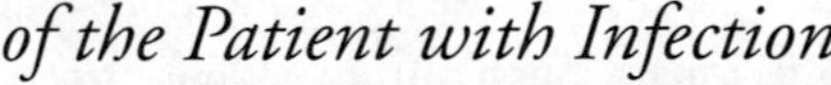

Nursing Management *of the Patient with Infection*

ASSESSMENT

Health History. Assess for:

- Recent known exposure to infectious agents (e.g., influenza, strep throat)
- Length of time since onset of symptoms
- History of fever, chills, enlarged lymph nodes, headache, fatigue, loss of appetite, muscle aches, cough, sore throat, pain on urination, nausea, diarrhea, or joint pain
- History of localized areas of pain or itching
- Understanding of disease process

Physical Examination. Assess for:

- Localized infection (swelling, warmth, erythema, drainage)
- Systemic infection (fever, elevated WBC, hypotension, tachycardia, altered mental status)
- Respiratory infection (crackles, thick green or yellow sputum)
- Gastrointestinal tract infection (vomiting, diarrhea)
- Urinary tract infection (foul-smelling urine, concentrated or cloudy urine)
- Enlarged lymph nodes

NURSING DIAGNOSES, OUTCOMES, AND INTERVENTIONS

Nursing Diagnosis: Risk for Infection

OUTCOMES. Common examples of expected outcomes for the patient with the diagnosis of *risk for infection* are:

Patient will:

- Remain free from infection.
- Remain free from fever, chilling, and malaise.
- Maintain WBC count within normal limits.
- Use measures to protect self from exposure to infections.

TABLE 6-13 CLINICAL SYNDROMES OR CONDITIONS WARRANTING ADDITIONAL EMPIRICAL PRECAUTIONS TO PREVENT TRANSMISSION OF EPIDEMIOLOGICALLY IMPORTANT PATHOGENS PENDING CONFIRMATION OF DIAGNOSIS

Clinical Syndrome or Condition	Potential Pathogens	Empirical Precautions
Diarrhea		
Acute diarrhea with likely infectious cause in incontinent or diapered patient	Enteric pathogens	Contact
Diarrhea in adult with history of recent antibiotic use	*Clostridium difficile*	Contact
Meningitis		
	Neisseria meningitidis	Droplet
Rash or Exanthems, Generalized, Cause Unknown		
Petechial or ecchymotic with fever	*N. meningitidis*	Droplet
Vesicular	Varicella	Airborne and Contact
Maculopapular with coryza and fever	Rubeola (measles)	Airborne
Respiratory Infections		
Cough, fever, upper lobe pulmonary infiltrate in human immunodeficiency virus (HIV)—seronegative patient and/or patient at low risk for HIV infection	*Mycobacterium tuberculosis*	Airborne
Cough, fever, pulmonary infiltrate in any lung location in HIV-infected patient and/or patient at high risk for HIV infection	*M. tuberculosis*	Airborne
Paroxysmal or severe persistent cough during periods of pertussis activity	*Bordetella pertussis*	Droplet
Respiratory infections, particularly bronchiolitis and croup, in infants and young children	Respiratory syncytial or parainfluenza virus	Contact
Risk of Multidrug-Resistant Microorganisms		
History of infection or colonization with multidrug-resistant organism	Resistant bacteria	Contact
Skin, wound, or urinary tract infection in patient with recent hospital or nursing home stay in facility where multidrug-resistant organisms are prevalent	Resistant bacteria	Contact
Skin or Wound Infection		
Abscess or draining wound that cannot be covered	*Staphylococcus aureus*, group A streptococcus	Contact

From Garner JS and Hospital Infection Control Practices Advisory Committee: Guidelines for isolation precautions in hospitals, part 2, Recommendations for isolation precautions in hospital, *Am J Infect Control* 22:24–52, 1996.

NURSING INTERVENTIONS. Prevention of infection begins with educating uninfected persons who are at increased risk for contracting infections, such as those who are immunosuppressed or immunodeficient, have chronic illnesses, or work or live in close contact with infected persons. The nurse consistently monitors vital signs, skin integrity, mucous membranes, respiratory status, gastrointestinal function, and mental status for signs of possible infection. The nurse monitors WBC levels when signs of infection are present.

Health care personnel as a whole are at increased risk for exposure to various infections. Consequently, institutions have developed procedures for the effective management of such exposures depending on the type of infectious agent.

RELATED NIC INTERVENTIONS. Infection Control, Infection Protection, Surveillance, Teaching: Disease Process

Nursing Diagnosis: Ineffective Protection

OUTCOMES. Common examples of expected outcomes for the patient with a diagnosis of *ineffective protection* are:
Patient will:

- Achieve normal WBC count and differential.
- Remain free from secondary infections.
- Verbalize understanding of need to avoid other persons with infections until infection has subsided.
- Verbalize understanding of need to complete course of prescribed medications.

NURSING INTERVENTIONS. The patient with an active infection is at risk for secondary infections, since the immune system can become overwhelmed. Therefore the patient is protected from potential sources of infection and monitored for treatment effectiveness and potential complications. The nurse monitors the

Healthy People 2010

Goals Related to Infection Control

Although the past 100 years have seen a reduction in the incidence of infectious diseases (e.g., smallpox, diphtheria, and polio) through development of vaccines, underimmunized groups still exist. The persistence of many vaccine-preventable infections remains a threat to public health. Without prevention of disease and the promotion of a healthy lifestyle, many consumers demand antibiotics for a cure. This leads to the increasing problem of antibiotic resistance. *Healthy People 2010* goals related to control of infection are:

- Reduce or eliminate indigenous cases of vaccine-preventable disease.
- Increase the proportion of providers who have measured the vaccination coverage levels among children in their practice population within the past 2 years.
- Increase the proportion of children who participate in fully operational population-based immunization registries.
- Reduce chronic hepatitis B virus infections in infants and young children (perinatal infections).
- Achieve and maintain effective vaccination coverage levels for universally recommended vaccines among young children.
- Maintain vaccination coverage levels for children in licensed day care facilities and children in kindergarten through first grade.
- Increase the proportion of young children and adolescents who receive all vaccines that have been recommended for universal administration for at least 5 years.
- Increase routine vaccination coverage levels for adolescents.
- Increase hepatitis B vaccine coverage among high-risk groups.
- Reduce hepatitis A.
- Reduce hepatitis C.
- Increase the proportion of persons with chronic hepatitis C infection identified by state and local health departments.
- Reduce hospitalization rates for immunization-preventable pneumonia and influenza.
- Increase the proportion of international travelers who receive recommended preventive services when traveling in areas at risk for selected infectious diseases: hepatitis A, malaria, and typhoid.
- Increase the proportion of local health departments that have established culturally appropriate and linguistically competent community health promotion and disease prevention programs.
- Reduce invasive early onset group B streptococcal disease.
- Reduce the number of courses of antibiotics for ear infections for young children.
- Reduce the number of courses of antibiotics prescribed for the sole diagnosis of the common cold.
- Reduce hospital-acquired infections in patients in intensive care units.
- Reduce vaccine-associated adverse events.

By attaining these goals, the American public should be able to make significant progress in meeting the two overarching goals—increase quality and years of healthy life, and eliminate health disparities—by the year 2010.

From US Department of Health and Human Services: *Healthy People 2010: understanding and improving health,* Washington, DC, 2000, The Department.

TABLE 6-14 SELECTED ANTIVIRAL AGENTS

Agent	Common Uses
Acyclovir	Herpes simplex Viral encephalitis Other herpes infections
Amantadine	Influenza A Influenza B
Ganciclovir	Cytomegalovirus (CMV) retinitis CMV gastritis
Nevirapine	Human immunodeficiency virus (HIV) infection
Didanosine	HIV infection
Indinavir	HIV infection
Ribavirin	Severe respiratory syncytial virus bronchopneumonia Influenza A Influenza B Lassa fever *Hantavirus* infection

patient's vital signs and WBC and differential to determine changes from baseline and evaluate effectiveness of medications and other treatments. The nurse also monitors the patient for therapeutic and adverse effects of prescribed antibiotics. The nurse informs the patient and family about the purpose of prescribed medication and treatment modalities. When discharged home, the patient and family members need to understand the importance of the patient completing the entire course of antibiotic therapy to prevent reinfection and potential drug resistance.

Depending on the severity of illness, persons with infections are frequently cared for at home. Consequently, the nurse stresses health promotion techniques such as washing hands and avoiding potential sources of infection. The nurse also teaches family members how to protect themselves and visitors from contracting the patient's infection. Many of the same principles of infection control apply in the home as in the hospital. Hand washing is the most effective measure in preventing the spread of infection in the home. Caregivers should wash hands before care and after contact with body substances (blood, urine, feces, sputum, vomitus, or wound drainage). Caregivers should wear a smock or coverall to protect their clothes. They should wear gloves when handling body substances.

Caregivers should put soiled dressings, used disposable gloves, and other disposable items that contain body substances in plastic bags before discarding them in the trash. All liquid waste can be flushed down the toilet. Used needles and syringes should be put in a puncture-resistant plastic container or can, which is tightly closed before discarding them in the trash.

Disposable dishes are not required. Dishes and linen should be washed in hot soapy water. A cup of bleach should be added to the detergent to disinfect laundry soiled with blood. Blood and body substance spills should be cleaned using an effective household disinfectant. If gloves are not available, the caregiver can

TABLE 6-15 SELECTED ANTIFUNGAL AGENTS

Agent	Common Uses
Amphotericin B	Severe systemic infections Topical candidiasis
Fluconazole	Severe systemic infections Mouth and throat infections Vaginal infections Oral candidiasis
Flucytosine	Severe systemic infections
Grieseofulvin	Skin infections (athlete's foot, ringworm) Scalp, fingernail, and toenail infections
Itraconazole	Systemic infections (lungs, blood) Toenail infections
Ketoconazole	Skin infections (jock itch, athlete's foot, ringworm) Fingernail and toenail infections Mouth (thrush) infection Lung and blood infections Vaginal infections
Miconazole	Skin infections (athlete's foot, jock itch) Vaginal infections
Nystatin	Skin infections Mouth infections Vaginal infections Intestinal tract infections
Terbinafine	Toenail and fingernail infections

wear plastic bags to protect the hands. All persons should be taught to cover the nose and mouth when coughing. In general, the caregiver does not need to wear a mask in the home.

RELATED NIC INTERVENTIONS. Infection Control, Infection Protection, Surveillance

Nursing Diagnosis: Hyperthermia

OUTCOMES. Common examples of expected outcomes for the patient with the diagnosis of *hyperthermia* are:
Patient will:

- Achieve body temperature within normal range.
- Achieve heart and respiratory rates within baseline range.
- Verbalize methods to control or reduce body temperature.
- Demonstrate correct method of taking temperature.

NURSING INTERVENTIONS. Fever is a protective response to pathogens. Treatment focuses on eradicating the causative organism by administering antibiotics and allowing for natural thermoregulation. If fever in adults exceeds 104° F orally (40° C), antipyretics and other interventions to reduce fever are necessary. Hypothermia blankets, ice packs, and tepid water baths may be used. The nurse must avoid cooling the patient too quickly, since rapid cooling produces shivering, which increases heat production and oxygen consumption and contributes to fever. The use of hypothermia blankets should be discontinued when the patient's temperature is within 1° to 3° of the desired temperature.

The nurse monitors vital signs, which includes an accurate assessment of core temperature. Seizures and a decreased level of consciousness are potential complications of fever. Patients with fever need to be bathed and given dry linen when the fever breaks (defervescence) and sweating occurs.

During the acute phase of illness when fever is present, the patient needs between 2500 and 3000 ml of fluid per day to prevent fluid volume deficits. Fever causes fluid loss from evaporation of body fluids and increased perspiration. Signs of dehydration include increased thirst, dry mucous membranes, and decreased skin turgor. The nurse needs to encourage intake of oral fluids and possibly administer intravenous fluids to support circulating volume and tissue perfusion. As the body attempts to increase heat loss by evaporation, conduction, and diffusion, diaphoresis occurs. An accurate record of intake and output, including an estimate of diaphoresis, is necessary to assess all sources of fluid loss and calculate fluid replacement.

RELATED NIC INTERVENTIONS. Fever Treatment, Fluid Management, Temperature Regulation, Medication Management, Vital Signs Monitoring

Nursing Diagnosis: Impaired Comfort

OUTCOMES. Common examples of expected outcomes for the patient with the diagnosis of *impaired comfort* are:
Patient will:

- Verbalize relief of discomfort following implementation of comfort measures.

- Report relief of discomfort from malaise, myalgia, and fever.
- Verbalize understanding of treatment measures to increase comfort.

NURSING INTERVENTIONS. Both pharmacologic and nonpharmacologic methods of pain relief are indicated (see Chapter 16). Analgesics such as acetaminophen or nonsteroidal antiinflammatory agents (NSAIDs) are effective in reducing discomfort related to fever. NSAIDs decrease the inflammatory response. Both acetaminophen and NSAIDs may be used as antipyretics.

Rest is encouraged during the acute phase of infection to allow healing and to promote comfort. The nurse should encourage the patient to be as independent as possible without becoming overly fatigued. When possible, tests and activities should be scheduled when the patient is fully rested. Other hygienic measures such as a warm bath, soft music, and relaxation techniques may enhance the patient's comfort until the infection subsides.

RELATED NIC INTERVENTIONS. Coping Enhancement, Distraction, Medication Administration, Positioning, Simple Massage

EVALUATION

To evaluate the effectiveness of nursing interventions, compare patient behaviors with those stated in the expected patient outcomes.

RELATED NOC OUTCOMES. Comfort Level, Hydration, Immune Status, Infection Severity, Thermoregulation

GERONTOLOGIC CONSIDERATIONS

Older adults are at significantly increased risk for nosocomial infections and infections in general because of their increased incidence of chronic diseases, increased hospitalizations, potentially poor nutritional and hydrational status, and slowing immune response. Nurses in acute and long-term care facilities need to be vigilant in protecting older adults from infection by maintaining excellent hand-washing techniques, limiting the use of invasive lines, and intervening should nutrition become compromised. They also need to be astute in their initial and ongoing assessments of older adults to identify infections and initiate appropriate treatments early in the infectious process.

Bioterrorism

The use of crude biologic weapons has occurred for centuries. The Mongols catapulted plague-infested corpses over the walls of enemies in the 1300s. The British army is thought to have given smallpox-contaminated blankets to the Indians in the mid-1700s, producing a smallpox epidemic among immunologically unprotected tribes. But most Americans did not realize that intentional harm could occur on their own soil until after an actual terrorist event took place on September 11, 2001. In response to those events, local, state, and national agencies are undertaking numerous efforts to improve preparation for and response to biologic agents in case of another attack.[45]

Biologic Weapons

Agents considered to be ideal biologic weapons are those which produce panic, fear, and dread in the targeted society. Attacks could involve the dissemination of aerosolized anthrax spores, botulism or other toxins, food or water supply contamination, aerial spays, or direct contact with infected individuals. Specific agents may be plant or animal diseases that are readily available, highly virulent or lethal, and easy to aerosolize and disseminate without harming the terrorists themselves. Chemical weapons could also be used during terrorist attacks. Although many agents fit the criteria for biologic weapons (Box 6-7), smallpox, plague, and anthrax are the three that promote the greatest fear because they are the best known (Table 6-16).

Variola (Smallpox)

Recognized throughout history, smallpox is a highly contagious and potentially fatal disease caused by the variola virus. Smallpox occurs in two forms. Variola minor is mild and uncommon. Variola major occurs in 90% of cases and carries a 30% mortality rate. Infection occurs from inhaling a very small amount of virus that travels from the lungs to regional lymph nodes where it replicates (Figure 6-11).

Smallpox is vaccine preventable. Patients who have been immunized can contract smallpox, known as modified smallpox,

Box 6-7 Possible Microbial Agents of Bioterrorism

Bacteria

Bacillus anthracis (anthrax)

Brucella organisms (brucellosis)

Burkholderia mallei (glanders)

Burkholderia pseudomallei (melioidosis)

Yersinia pestis (plague)

Francisella tularensis (tularemia)

Coxiella burnetii (Q fever)

Viruses

Smallpox

Venezuelan equine encephalitis

Viral hemorrhagic fevers:

—Lassa fever

—Rift Valley fever

—Ebola

—*Hantavirus* organisms

—Marburg

TABLE 6-16 AGENTS OF BIOTERRORISM

Disease	Agent	Incubation Period	Clinical Manifestations	Treatment	Required Precautions
Smallpox	Variola major	7-17 days	High fever, chills, severe fatigue, headache, backache, vomiting, and characteristic maculopapular rash. Rash occurs in oropharyngeal area first and appears as small red lesions. During this time the virus is expelled via respiratory secretions and patients are most contagious (Lashley).[31] Rash progresses in downward fashion from face to limbs and then to all parts of body in about 24 hr, although trunk usually has fewer lesions than limbs. Initially lesions are red and raised, but pustules form as lesions fill with opaque fluid and produce a depression in the center, a distinguishing characteristic of the disease. Fever often subsides when rash appears but returns when lesions become pustules. All lesions usually scab over by end of second week following appearance of rash and fall off by end of third week, leaving a pitted scar. Patients are considered contagious until lesions are healed and all scabs have fallen off.	Supportive Vaccinate within 2-3 days of exposure	Standard Precautions Contact Precautions Droplet Precautions Airborne Precautions

which produces a mild form of the disease.[7] The United States ceased its immunization program for citizens in the 1980s and for those in the military in 1989. Although some people may have retained a degree of immunity, the population as a whole is susceptible to smallpox. Currently, the Advisory Committee on Immunization Practices recommends that states establish and maintain immunized smallpox response teams and that acute care facilities identify and vaccinate designated health care workers who would provide screening for or direct medical care to suspected smallpox patients in the event of a terrorist attack.

Bacillus anthracis (Anthrax)

Anthrax may be seen as one of three different clinical entities in humans: cutaneous, inhalation, and gastrointestinal disease

TABLE 6-16 AGENTS OF BIOTERRORISM—CONT'D

Disease	Agent	Incubation Period	Clinical Manifestations	Treatment	Required Precautions
Anthrax	*Bacillus anthracis*	1-7 days	*Cutaneous:* Pustular lesions on hands or forearms that form a black scab (eschar) on drying *Gastrointestinal*: Nausea, vomiting, bloody diarrhea, fever *Inhalation*: Fever, malaise, cough, and mild chest discomfort that progresses to diaphoresis, dyspnea, respiratory distress, cyanosis, and death within about 24-36 hr	Treat suspected exposure to anthrax spores with oral doxycycline or ciprofloxin. Once symptoms are present, administer high-dose antibiotics, although their effectiveness may be limited.	Standard Precautions Contact Precautions (until after decontamination) Disinfect instruments from invasive procedures with sporicidal agents
Bubonic or pneumonic plague	*Yersinia pestis*	1-6 days	Chills, high fever, headache, fatigue, and cough, which may be bloody Rapidly progresses to dyspnea, cyanosis, respiratory failure and death	Doxycycline is the drug of choice for exposure to *Y. pestis*, although ciprofloxacin, tetracycline, or chloramphenicol can be used. Streptomycin, gentamicin are effective treatments for disease.	*Bubonic:* Standard Precautions *Pneumonic:* Droplet Precautions
Tularemia	*Francisella tularensis*	3-14 days	*Ulceroglandular*: Local ulcer followed by fever, chills, headache, malaise, and regional lymphadenopathy *Typhoidal:* Fever, chills, headache, malaise, chest discomfort, nonproductive cough, anorexia, and weight loss	Gentamicin, ciprofloxacin, streptomycin, or doxycycline	Standard Precautions

(Figure 6-12). Cutaneous anthrax is most often seen in persons who work with infected livestock. Although rare in humans, gastrointestinal anthrax is acquired by eating undercooked meat from infected animals. Inhalation anthrax occurs when the spores are inhaled. Without treatment the mortality rate from inhalation anthrax is close to 100%. An FDA-approved vaccine is available for anthrax; however, it is not recommended for civilians unless they have repeated exposures to aerosolized *Bacillus anthracis* spores through their occupation. At-risk military personnel do receive anthrax immunizations.[6]

Yersinia pestis (Plague)

Plague is a zoonotic disease of rodents. The bacterium is transmitted via fleas to humans who develop bubonic plague, which is manifested by high fever, malaise, and painful lymph nodes.

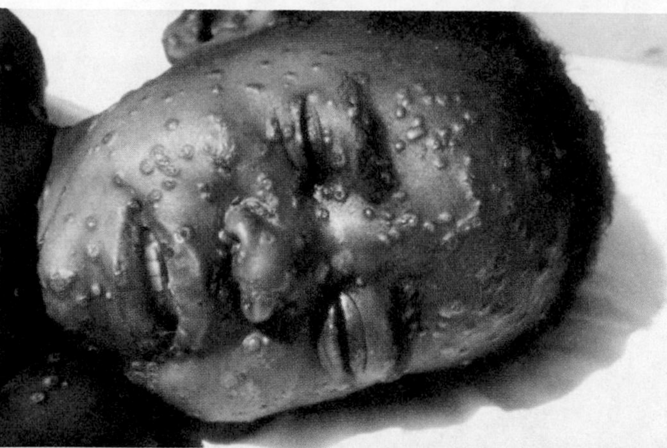

Figure 6-11 Face lesions on child with smallpox.

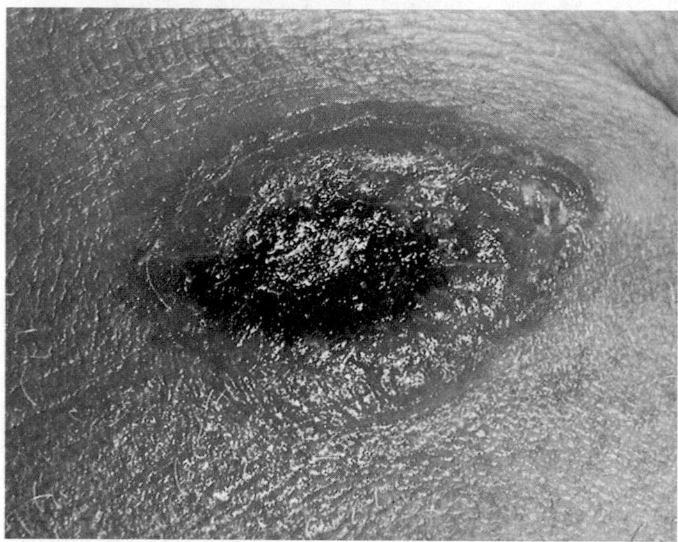

Figure 6-12 Cutaneous anthrax.

Bubonic plague can progress to septicemia, shock, and death or pneumonic plague. Pneumonic plague results in death if antibiotic treatment is not initiated within 24 hours after the onset of symptoms. Currently, scientists are developing an oral vaccine to protect against plague and anthrax, but it will not be available for several years (see Future Watch box).[47]

Future Watch

Will There Be a New Vaccine for Plague and Anthrax?

Avant Immunotherapeutics is developing an oral vaccine to protect against anthrax, plague, and cholera infections. Military personnel will be the first to receive the vaccine if and when it is available. It would provide protection in a matter of days instead of months and could be used to protect health care workers and civilians from terrorist attacks. Although the vaccine looks promising, it will be years before it is ready for distribution.

UCLA Department of Epidemiology: *Avant works on oral vaccine for plague, anthrax,* accessed 2003 from website: http://www.ph.ucla.edu/epi/bioter/avantoralvaccine.html.

Francisella tularensis (Tularemia)

Tularemia, also known as rabbit fever, is a zoonotic disease contracted by humans after exposure to the tissues or body fluids of infected animals or from infected tick, deerfly, or mosquito bites. Tularemia occurs in several forms, the most common of which are ulceroglandular and typhoidal. A vaccine is available but is not in widespread use in the United States. Human-to-human transmission of tularemia has not been identified; therefore isolation is not required.[47]

Biologic Toxins

Toxins are damaging substances produced by animals, plants, or microbial agents. They are stable, generally more toxic than chemical agents, and easy to produce (Table 6-17).

Clostridium botulinum produces potent neurotoxins, which are used therapeutically and cosmetically. If the spores of *C. botulinum* are ingested or inhaled, they produce a paralytic illness that constitutes a medical emergency. An antitoxin is available that may prevent respiratory failure if administered early in the disease process. A vaccine is available but is administered only to people who are at high risk for exposure. Botulism is not transmitted from person to person, and Standard Precautions are adequate for health care personnel.

Ricinus communis (ricin) is a potent protein cytotoxin easily extracted from castor beans. It is highly toxic by several routes of exposure, including inhalation, ingestion, and injection. When aerosolized and inhaled, the toxin can produce respiratory failure within 36 to 74 hours. Ingestion of ricin produces severe gastrointestinal effects. Ricin is not transmitted from person to person; thus Standard Precautions are appropriate.[44]

Collaborative Care Management

Recognition

An increased number of people with similar clinical manifestations will most likely be the first indicator that a biologic attack has taken place. Consequently, public health authorities and health care systems alike must have surveillance systems in place so they can readily identify and report unusual diseases patterns. First responders and other health care workers must have a heightened awareness of trends that suggest covert dissemination of a disease agent and be prepared to respond rapidly. Some of the factors consistent with a biologic attack include[45]:

- A large epidemic with similar disease clinical manifestations in a discrete population
- Multiple epidemics of the same disease in different geographic locations
- Unexplained disease or death among many people
- Failure of standard treatment or increased severity for a specific pathogen
- Variation in or unusual route of exposure for a pathogen
- Disease occurring in an unusual geographic location
- Unusual strains or patterns of drug resistance
- Unusual disease outbreak among animals
- Threats or claims by aggressors of a potential attack

TABLE 6-17 BIOLOGIC TOXINS

Disease	Agent	Incubation Period	Clinical Manifestations	Treatment and Implications
Botulism	*Clostridium botulinum*	6 hr to 10 days	Cranial nerve palsies, blurred vision, dysphagia, and slurred speech, followed by descending flaccid paralysis, generalized weakness, and progressive respiratory failure	Intubation or tracheostomy and mechanical ventilation may be necessary to prevent death.
Ricinism	*Ricinus communis*	4-8 hr	*Ingestion:* Severe gastrointestinal distress, vascular collapse, and death *Inhalation:* Fever, cough, and dyspnea within 8 hr and acute hypoxia and respiratory failure within 36-72 hr	Ricin ingestion or inhalation has no specific treatment, vaccine, or antitoxin. Patients are treated supportively for pulmonary edema.

Early recognition of unusual events will help save lives and contain the disease. Health care workers who are alert and knowledgeable about the differences between natural events and intentionally caused events are more likely to recognize terrorist attacks. A delay in response until classic disease manifestations appear delays containment and places many more lives at risk.[41]

Early Treatment

A thorough history and physical assessment may help health care providers identify the suspected agent so that early treatment with antibiotics, immunizations, or antisera can begin. The initial assessment is similar to that for other emergency situations and focuses on airway, breathing, and circulation. While waiting for definitive laboratory results, health care providers can make a diagnosis based on clinical indicators. For example, plague and tularemia initially appear as pneumonias, whereas botulism is first seen with neuromuscular changes. Unfortunately, to be effective, treatment for many diseases must be initiated during the prodromal phase. Consequently, not all lives will be saved, since many patients will not recognize the seriousness of their illness and report for care until the prodromal phase has passed. Antibiotics, fluid resuscitation, and supportive care are the primary treatments for biologic warfare agents.[27]

Immunizations against organisms such as smallpox or anthrax are one method of protection from biologic agents. The federal government does not recommend that members of the general public be vaccinated at this point, since the vaccines carry significant side effects and risks. However, some health care workers and first responders have received immunizations on a voluntary basis. The vaccine will be made available to people within an affected community should an attack take place. The CDC also has nine stockpiles of antibiotics, antidotes, and other medical supplies located around the country. They can be mobilized to any region in less than 12 hours and used to help with disease treatment and containment.[34]

Chemical Agents

Chemical agents are highly toxic, act rapidly, and have widespread effects on organs and tissues. They are commonly used in insecticides but not at the potency levels used by the military or terrorists. Chemical agents are classified as nerve, blister or vesicant, pulmonary, or blood agents.

Nerve Agents

Among the most toxic of known chemical agents are tabun, sarin, soman, cyclohexyl methylphosphonofluoridate (GF), methylphosphonothioic acid (VX), phosphonofluoridic acid (GE), phosphonothioic acid (VE), amiton (VG), and phosphonothioic acid (VM). As a group, they are known as nerve agents. In medicine, similar acetylcholinesterase compounds are either carbamates or organophosphorus compounds. The carbamates, neostigmine (Prostigmin), ambenonium, and pyridostigmine bromide (Mestinon), have been used for decades in the United States to treat myasthenia gravis (see Chapter 49) and glaucoma. Commonly used insecticides contain either an organophosphorus compound (malathion) or a carbamate (Sevin).

Nerve agents disable the transmission of nerve impulses by inhibiting cholinesterase (ChE), which can then not hydrolyze acetylcholine (ACh). They also inhibit other enzymes that directly affect neuromuscular receptor sites. The overall toxic effects of nerve agents are due, then, to the accumulation of ACh, which continues to produce postsynaptic action potentials and activity in organs or tissues that require ACh, such as the mouth; glands; and muscles of the respiratory, skeletal, and gastrointestinal systems and the heart via the vagus nerve (see Chapter 47).

Nerve agents are considered ideal weapons of terrorism because they are clear, colorless, and tasteless and some, such as Sarin and VX, are odorless. They are inexpensive, readily dispersed, absorbed through inhalation or skin exposure, and effective in small quantities. The actions of nerve agents on various organs and systems are summarized in the Clinical Manifestations

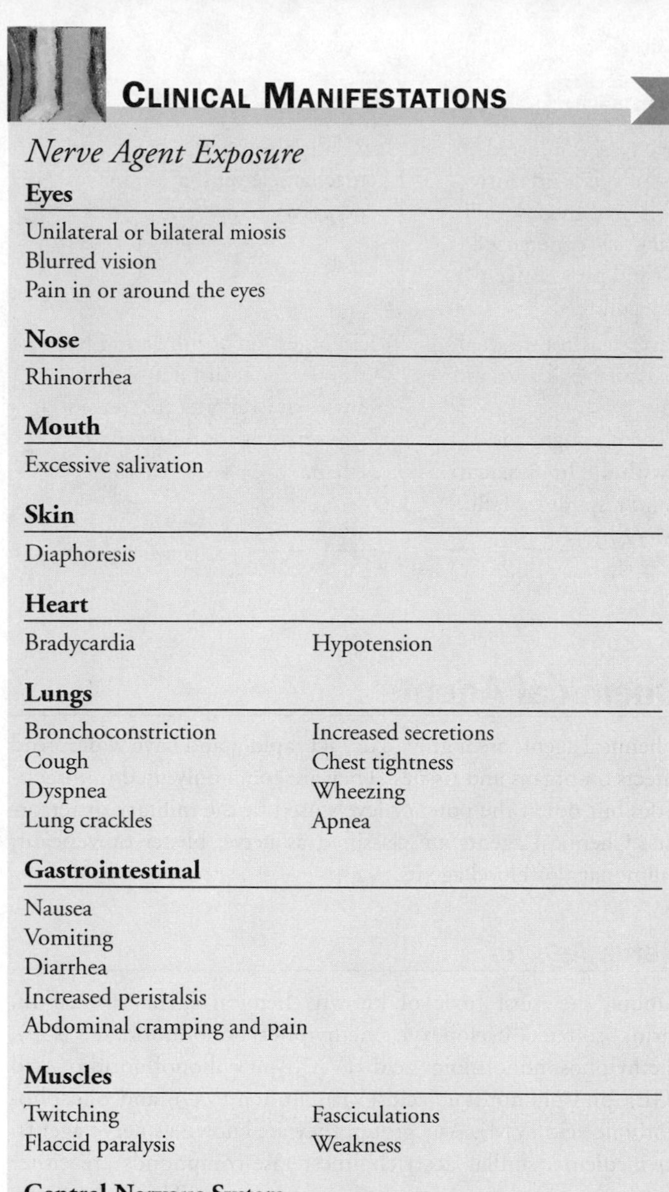

CLINICAL MANIFESTATIONS

Nerve Agent Exposure

Eyes

Unilateral or bilateral miosis
Blurred vision
Pain in or around the eyes

Nose

Rhinorrhea

Mouth

Excessive salivation

Skin

Diaphoresis

Heart

Bradycardia	Hypotension

Lungs

Bronchoconstriction	Increased secretions
Cough	Chest tightness
Dyspnea	Wheezing
Lung crackles	Apnea

Gastrointestinal

Nausea
Vomiting
Diarrhea
Increased peristalsis
Abdominal cramping and pain

Muscles

Twitching	Fasciculations
Flaccid paralysis	Weakness

Central Nervous System

Altered consciousness	Seizures (following paralysis)

box above. Mild-to-moderate exposure to nerve gases can produce symptoms for days to weeks, including irritability, impaired judgment, forgetfulness, decreased concentration and comprehension, anxiety, depression, insomnia, or nightmares.[47]

Treatment. Nerve agents act rapidly and can cause respiratory arrest within minutes following absorption; therefore immediate treatment is essential. The exposed person must undergo decontamination before medical intervention can safely occur. Those assisting with decontamination must be careful not to become exposed themselves; protective clothing and chemical masks are essential. The victim's clothing is removed, which may remove as much as 85% of the chemical agent, and placed in leak-proof containers. Residual from the skin is then removed by water rinses or showers, detergent scrubs, or rinsing with a 10% bleach solution.[47]

Drug therapy is aimed at relieving symptoms and preventing complications such as seizures or respiratory arrest. Atropine is the mainstay of treatment for nerve agents. It may be administered intravenously or intramuscularly, although the intravenous route is preferred due to faster action. Doses range from 2 to 4 mg and may be given as often as every 3 minutes for 24 hours or until symptoms are controlled.[47]

Pralidoxime, a drug used in medicine to treat organic phosphorus pesticide poisoning or as an antidote to neostigmine, pyridostigmine, or ambenonium, may also be used to treat nerve agent exposure. The drug reactivates ChE, which removes ACh from the synaptic cleft, allowing muscles to return to a resting state. Pralidoxime is administered intramuscularly and is used as an adjunct to atropine.

Another drug, primarily used by the military as a nerve agent antidote, is 2-PAM chloride. This drug breaks the bond between the acetylcholinesterase enzyme and nerve agent in order to restore normal nerve function. Military personnel and first responders carry nerve agent antidote kits that contain atropine and 2-PAM chloride in automatic injectors for emergency use.[47]

Vesicants

Vesicants, also known as blister agents, are caustic chemicals that are commonly used in warfare. They produce incapacitating injuries among large numbers of people but infrequently result in death. Nitrogen mustard, sulfur mustard, distilled mustard, lewisite, phosgene, sesqui mustard, and mustard-lewisite are all vesicant agents.

Vesicants produce cellular damage by reacting with proteins and other cellular components. Phosgene oxime and lewisite produce immediate injury, whereas the mustards produce delayed reactions within 2 to 24 hours after exposure. Symptoms and the degree of injury from vesicants depend on the amount and route of exposure, the specific vesicant, and the presence of any preexisting medical conditions.[14] The vesicants' effects on organs and systems are summarized in the Clinical Manifestations box, p. 125, top left.

Treatment. Treatment for vesicant exposure involves decontamination by removing contaminated clothing and washing the skin with soap and water as soon as possible following exposure. Other cleaning agents are avoided because they can further damage contaminated skin. Eyes are flushed with copious amounts of water. As with nerve agents, contaminated clothing is placed in plastic bags to avoid contaminating health care personnel. Vomiting and oral fluids are contraindicated for persons who have ingested vesicants, since both may produce further injury. Dimercaprol (BAL in Oil) is an antidote for lewisite exposure. It binds with lewisite to form a chelate, which is excreted in the urine and feces. It is given by deep intramuscular injection and must be administered as soon as possible after exposure to the chemical to decrease the degree of injury.[2]

Pulmonary Agents

Pulmonary agents such as phosgene, chlorine, and bromine are liquid irritants that can damage the eyes, nose, throat, and lungs. The extent of damage depends on the amount and route of chemical exposure, and length of chemical contact before decontamination. These agents prevent the exchange of oxygen and carbon

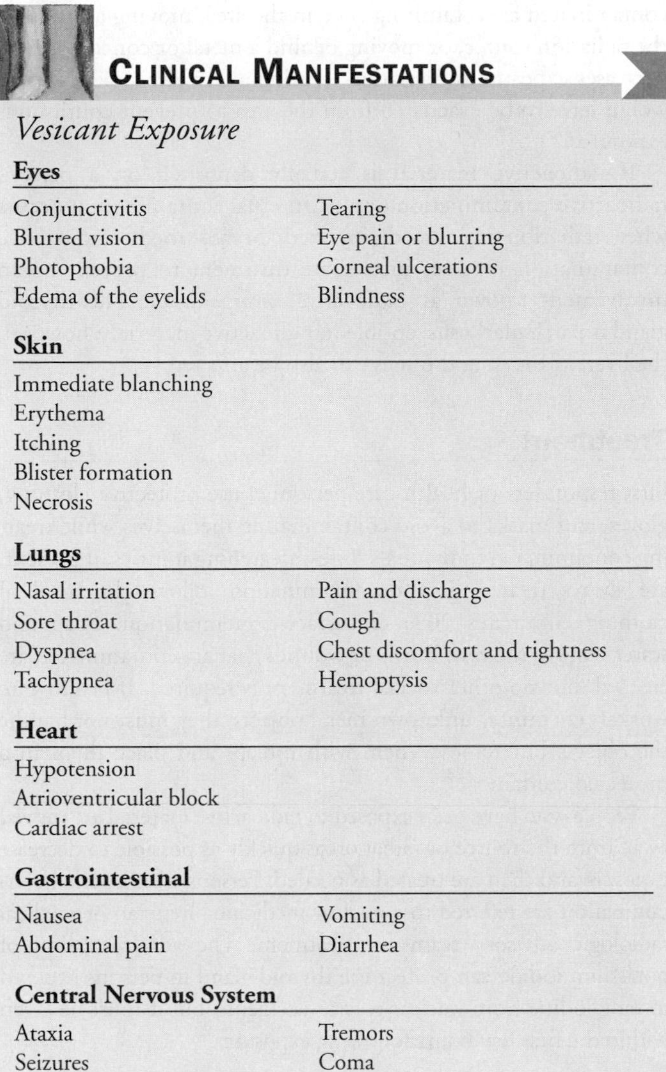

CLINICAL MANIFESTATIONS

Vesicant Exposure

Eyes

Conjunctivitis
Blurred vision
Photophobia
Edema of the eyelids
Tearing
Eye pain or blurring
Corneal ulcerations
Blindness

Skin

Immediate blanching
Erythema
Itching
Blister formation
Necrosis

Lungs

Nasal irritation
Sore throat
Dyspnea
Tachypnea
Pain and discharge
Cough
Chest discomfort and tightness
Hemoptysis

Heart

Hypotension
Atrioventricular block
Cardiac arrest

Gastrointestinal

Nausea
Abdominal pain
Vomiting
Diarrhea

Central Nervous System

Ataxia
Seizures
Tremors
Coma

dioxide in the lungs because they damage the pulmonary membrane between the alveolus and capillary bed. Clinical manifestations of exposure to pulmonary agents are summarized in the Clinical Manifestations box at right.

Treatment. Treatment for pulmonary agent exposure consists of removing contaminated clothing, decontaminating exposed skin with soap and water, and providing supportive care in an acute care facility. Victims need to be observed for at least 48 hours after exposure because symptoms may be delayed or redevelop. These chemical agents have no antidotes.[10]

Blood Agents

Cyanogen chloride and hydrogen chloride are important examples of chemical agents known as blood agents because they affect red blood cells. Both agents are potentially deadly gases that are colorless. Cyanide, which smells like peach kernels or bitter almonds, is found in cigarette smoke and is released from burning synthetic materials such as plastic, furniture textiles, and rugs.

Blood agents are absorbed from the skin and mucous membranes and are most dangerous when inhaled. They penetrate the bronchial mucosa and alveoli and interfere with oxygen utilization at the cellular level. The respiratory center is especially susceptible to cyanide, and respiratory failure is the usual cause of death. A few breaths of highly concentrated cyanide may be enough to cause immediate death. Lower concentrations of cyanide produce small areas of hemorrhage in the brain, which are associated with delayed death.[19]

Cyanogen chloride produces systemic effects similar to those of cyanide and also causes local irritant effects to the eyes, upper respiratory tract, and lungs. It damages the respiratory tract by producing severe inflammation of the bronchioles and pulmonary edema.[19] Clinical manifestations of blood agents are summarized in the Clinical Manifestations box, p. 126.

Treatment. Poisoning from blood agents is treated by first removing the victim from the contaminated environment. If respirations are compromised or have ceased, intubation and mechanical ventilation are essential. Sodium nitrite is immediately administered intravenously, followed by intravenous sodium thiosulfate. Sodium nitrite sequesters cyanide, which is bound to methemoglobin. Sodium thiosulfate combines with the sequestered cyanide to form sodium thiocyanate, which is eliminated by the kidneys. An alternative treatment for cyanide poisoning in persons with smoke inhalation, who have increased levels of carboxyhemoglobin, is the administration of hydroxycobalamin, which is vitamin B_{12a}. Hydroxycobalamin binds with cyanide to form vitamin B_{12}.[47]

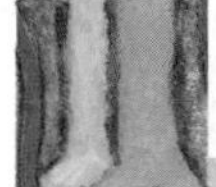

CLINICAL MANIFESTATIONS

Pulmonary Agent Exposure

Eyes

Watery eyes
Blurred vision
Burning sensation

Skin

Burn- or frostbite-appearing lesions with skin contact

Lungs

Cough
Burning sensation in throat
Dyspnea
Pulmonary edema
Bloody and frothy sputum

Heart

Cardiac failure
Hypotension

Gastrointestinal

Nausea
Vomiting

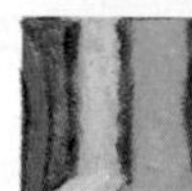

CLINICAL MANIFESTATIONS

Blood Agent Exposure

Lungs

Dyspnea
Respiratory failure
Respiratory arrest

Heart

Palpitations
Atrial fibrillation
Ventricular ectopic beats
Abnormal QRS and T wave changes
Sinus bradycardia
Cardiac arrest

Gastrointestinal

Nausea
Vomiting

Central Nervous System

Headache
Altered level of consciousness
Central nervous system depression
Ataxia
Seizures
Coma
Death

Skin

Bright pink coloration caused by high concentrations of oxyhemoglobin in the venous return (similar to carbon monoxide poisoning)

Radiation Agents

When planning for possible terrorist attacks, public health officials must consider radiation from devices such as dirty bombs or attacks on nuclear reactors. Dirty bombs serve two purposes. They combine explosives with radioactive material so the material can be easily dispersed over a small area. People are contaminated with radioactive material, and buildings and land are left unusable for a long time. These bombs are quite different from nuclear fission weapons such as the atomic bomb used during World War II to cause widespread and devastating destruction.[9]

Nuclear power plants and nuclear weapons sites have the most harmful radioactive materials; consequently, security at these facilities has been significantly increased to prevent terrorists from obtaining such materials. Low-level radioactive materials are found in hospitals, construction sites, and irradiation plants, but dirty bombs made from these materials are not sufficient to produce serious illness from radiation; therefore they are not considered a significant risk to the public.[9]

Radioactive material can cause injury from *external radiation exposure* or from *radioactive contamination*. Exposure to a radiation source can cause tissue damage such as skin burns or bone marrow depression if the radiation source has a high level of energy and intensity. Exposure increases the longer the person stays in the contaminated area. Limiting time in the area, moving away from the radiation source, or moving behind a metal or concrete shield decreases exposure to radiation. During a terrorist attack, people would have to be evacuated from the area to prevent continuous exposure.[37]

If radioactive material is actually deposited on a person, radioactive contamination occurs. Internal contamination occurs when radiation is inhaled, ingested, or absorbed. Radioactive contamination requires immediate treatment to prevent organ involvement known as radioactive *incorporation*. The thyroid gland is particularly susceptible to radioactive materials; however, the liver, kidneys, and bones can also be affected.

Treatment

First responders or health care personnel use protective clothing, gloves, and masks to avoid contaminating themselves while treating contaminated individuals. Life-threatening injuries, if present, are always treated first; decontamination follows. Removal of clothing eliminates 90% of surface contamination. Soap and water remove the rest. Burns or wounds that are contaminated are cleaned, but no other special treatment is required. If health care workers encounter unknown metal objects, they must not handle the objects but remove them with forceps and place them in a protected container.[23]

People who have been exposed to radioactive material are moved away from the source of radiation as quickly as possible to decrease exposure and then are treated as needed. Persons with internal contamination are referred to a nuclear medicine physician or medical radiologic advisory team for treatment. The administration of potassium iodide can protect the thyroid gland in persons exposed to radioiodine from nuclear reactor accidents, but it must be given within the first few hours following exposure.[23]

Acute Radiation Syndrome

Acute radiation syndrome (ARS) develops after a very high dose of rapidly received radiation. Risk factors for ARS include exposure to a penetrating type of radiation that reaches internal organs, is high dose (greater than 100 rad), and is rapidly received, with a large percentage of the body exposed. ARS may be complicated by serious trauma that occurs at the time of radiation exposure or by preexisting conditions that delay or hamper healing or otherwise complicate the injury.[8]

ARS follows a predicable course, divided into phases (Table 6-18). Symptoms begin within minutes after exposure, may last for several days, and then subside. After a symptom-free period, symptoms again occur. Serious illness can last for several months. Recovery can take weeks to years. Mortality from ARS is directly related to the radiation dose, with increased doses leading to increased mortality. Death generally occurs within a few months of initial exposure from bone marrow suppression, which ultimately leads to infections and bleeding.[37]

Treatment. If the victim has life-threatening injuries, those are treated first, followed by decontamination (see discussion above). Wounds are cleaned and dressed to prevent infection. Further treatment for ARS depends on the dose of radiation received. For exposures less than 200 rad, treatment involves close observation of the patient and frequent monitoring of the complete blood count and differential to detect bone marrow depression. Most patients can be treated and monitored on an outpatient basis.[37]

Infection and bleeding from bone marrow suppression are the primary concerns following radiation exposure greater than 200 rad. Health care providers place patients on protective precautions; initiate supportive care; and frequently assess for erythema, hair loss, fever, skin injury, and other signs of ARS. Specific treatment for bone marrow suppression may include growth factors such as interleukin-11, granulocyte colony-stimulating factor, or granulocyte-macrophage colony-stimulating factor to simulate hematopoiesis or stem cell transfusion. Platelets are administered if bleeding occurs from low platelet counts.[27]

The FDA recently approved the drugs pentetate calcium trisodium (Ca-DTPA) and pentetate zinc trisodium (Zn-DTPA) for treatment of radiation emergencies from plutonium, americium, or curium. Contamination from these agents is most likely to occur from industrial accidents or terrorist use of dirty bombs. Either drug may be administered when radiation contamination occurs; however, Ca-DTPA is more effective than Zn-DTPA in the 24-hour period after contamination. After that time period, both drugs have similar effectiveness. Administering the drugs simultaneously is contraindicated. If both drugs are available, Ca-DTPA is administered initially. Zn-DTPA may be administered if follow-up treatment is needed. Both drugs are safe, have few side effects, and speed the elimination of radiation from the body.[46]

▶ ARE You READY?

In assessing a client with suspected exposure to a nerve agent, the nurse focuses on which of the following as consistent with this exposure?

1. Elevated blood pressure
2. Dry mucous membranes
3. Elevated body temperature
4. Bronchoconstriction

Terrorism Prevention Programs

In 2004 the USDHHS, the CDC, and the Agency for Toxic Substances and Disease Registry released the *National Public Health Strategy for Terrorism Preparedness and Response*. The imperatives listed in the document are designed to help national, state, and local governments and health care agencies prepare for and respond to terror-related public health emergencies and to prevent death, disability, disease, and injury. The 11 imperatives address issues such as effective and integrated detection and investigation; sustained prevention and consequence management; coordinated public health emergency preparedness and response; and innovative, relevant, and applied research and evaluation. Many of the imperative outcomes have been achieved, including the National Smallpox Program and the Enhanced Laboratory Response Network (Box 6-8).

Since September 11, 2001, the USDHHS has invested more than $3.7 billion dollars to strengthen the nation's public health infrastructure. The department has awarded money to states, territories, and major metropolitan areas to strengthen their ability to respond to bioterrorism attacks, infectious diseases, and natural disasters. Specifically, funds were allocated for ongoing surveillance programs in areas such as human health, hospital preparedness, state and local preparedness, vaccine research and procurement, animal health, food and agriculture safety, and environmental monitoring.[45]

The nation receives protection from many other organizations, including the National Incident Management System, which coordinates and standardizes homeland security preparations and communications when an actual event takes place. The Association of Professionals in Infection Control and Epidemiology developed a bioterrorism readiness plan template that focuses on prophylaxis and infection control procedures in health care institutions.

Health Care Facility Emergency Preparedness Plans

The Joint Commission on the Accreditation of Healthcare Organizations sets standards to ensure that health care facilities provide a safe environment for patients and workers. Disaster planning falls under the standards titled Environment of Care (EC). The EC standards require that health care agencies develop, implement, and exercise emergency operation plans that are integrated and consistent with community emergency plans.

Developing a disaster plan begins with an assessment of risks, capabilities, and capacity. *Risk assessment* includes determining the potential risk factors for that community, such as proximity to nuclear power plants, military bases, schools, or high-density areas of population. The plan also calls for evaluating vulnerability to natural disasters such as flooding, earthquakes, hurricanes, or tornados. *Capability* and *capacity* pertain to the facility's ability to respond to a natural disaster or terrorist attack, which depends on its resources such as supplies, equipment, personnel, and finances. Capability also entails the facility's policies, procedures, and guidelines that direct its overall response and how it interfaces with the community disaster and bioterrorism plan.[41]

After the initial risk assessment, the facility develops an emergency operations plan (EOP) that addresses mitigation, preparedness, response, and recovery. Specific components of the plan include[41]:

- *Activation and notification:* The EOP defines procedures for when to activate a response and who to notify. Notification guidelines include departments within the facility, community agencies such as the police department, and public health entities.
- *Facility protection:* Protection of the hospital environment takes priority after activation of the emergency plan. Security is necessary to control crowds and limit access to the facility. Personnel and patients need protection from infected or contaminated individuals, who may need to be sequestered until triage and further evaluations can occur. For bioterrorism attacks, Standard Precautions are instituted, as well as disease-specific precautions once the agent is identified.
- *Decontamination:* Decontamination involves guidelines for receiving contaminated patients, facilities available for

TABLE 6-18 PHASES OF ACUTE RADIATION SYNDROME

Exposure	Prodromal	Latent	Acute Illness	Mortality
100-200 rad	Nausea and vomiting within 3-6 hr postexposure Absence of central nervous system impairment	Symptoms abate Occurs within 7-15 days	Moderate leukopenia Occurs after 12 weeks	Minimal
200-800 rad	Nausea and vomiting within 1-4 hr Decreased lymphocyte count Cognitive impairment after 24 hr postexposure	Symptoms abate Occurs within 2-7 days	Severe leukopenia, purpura, hemorrhage, pneumonia, hair loss Occurs between 2 days and 2 wk Treatment most effective 4–6 wk after exposure	Low with aggressive treatment
Lethal dose	Nausea and vomiting within minutes to 1 hr Lymphocyte count decreased within hours Rapid incapacitation following lucid period	None occurs	Diarrhea, fever, electrolyte imbalance, lethargy, seizures, ataxia, tremor Occurs within 1–3 days	Very high

From Centers for Disease Control and Prevention: *Acute radiation syndrome, fact sheet for physicians,* accessed March 2003 from website: http://www.cdc.gov/nceh/radiation/factsheets/AcuteRadSyndrome.pdf.

Box 6-8 Preparing Public Health Agencies for Biologic and Chemical Attacks

Biologic Attacks

Enhance epidemiologic capacity to detect and respond to biologic attacks.

Supply diagnostic reagents to state and local public health agencies.

Establish communication programs to ensure delivery of accurate information.

Enhance bioterrorism-related education and training for health care professionals.

Prepare educational materials that will inform and reassure the public during and after a biologic attack.

Stockpile appropriate vaccines and drugs.

Establish molecular surveillance for microbial strains, including unusual or drug-resistant strains.

Support the development of diagnostic tests.

Encourage research on antiviral drugs and vaccines.

Chemical Attacks

Enhance epidemiologic capacity for detecting and responding to chemical attacks.

Enhance awareness of chemical terrorism among emergency medical service personnel, police officers, fire fighters, physicians, and nurses.

Stockpile chemical antidotes.

Develop and provide bioassays for detection and diagnosis of chemical injuries.

Prepare educational materials to inform the public during and after a chemical attack.

From Centers for Disease Control and Prevention Strategic Planning Work-group: Biological and chemical terrorism: strategic plan for preparedness and response, *MMWR* 49:1-14, 2000.

decontamination, and specific measures for decontamination based on the type of contamination (biologic, chemical, radiologic).

- *Expansion of services and alternate care sites:* Part of the EOP pertains to plans for expanding facility capacity when possible or the use of alternate sites within the community should the facility become taxed beyond its ability to accommodate victims. The Department of Defense has formulated a template for use by hospitals and other health care facilities to help them plan for use of alternate sites when needed. The plan also involves priorities for securing additional personnel, which may include pulling personnel

Box 6-9 Personal Protective Equipment

Before approaching a person suspected of having been exposed to biologic agents, health care workers must protect themselves. Personal protective equipment, such as protective suits, gloves, boots, and respirators, are available to first-line responders and emergency personnel. However, such devices have risks and limitations and should not be used without appropriate training and practice.[23] Protective clothing is divided into four categories:

1. Level A protection provides the highest level of skin and respiratory protection. The user is fully enclosed in a chemically impervious environment with a self-contained breathing apparatus (SCBA). Level A protection is not intended for use by frontline health care providers.
2. Level B protection includes a splash protective suit and SCBA. It is the minimal level of protection that the Occupational Safety and Health Administration requires for first responders and frontline health care providers. It provides the same degree of respiratory protection as level A, but less skin and eye protection.
3. Level C protection involves the use of a full or half-face air purifying respirator, which is used after the contaminant has been identified.
4. Level D protection is the lowest level of protection. It provides no respiratory protection and only minimal skin protection. The user avoids the contaminant, but takes no clothing precautions other than ordinary work clothes and safety shoes. Standard Precautions are adequate in hospitals and other health care facilities.

from outpatient settings, surgical areas, or nearby nursing or medicals schools.

- *Supplies and logistics:* Regardless of the plan, it will fail when supplies are exhausted. Few facilities maintain an abundance of supplies, and shortages may quickly occur during a disaster or terrorist attack. Therefore the National Pharmaceutical Stockpile program provides supplies and antibiotics within 12 hours of release by the director of USDHHS. The facility's EOP contains guidelines for securing additional supplies or antibiotics from neighboring hospitals or health care facilities until the stockpile arrives.
- *Staff education and training:* Personnel cannot function unless adequately educated. Education programs vary depending on the anticipated level of participation by various staff members. Minimally, staff education should include an orientation to the facility's disaster response plan, mass casualty triage protocols, use of personal protective equipment (Box 6-9), isolation techniques, decontamination guidelines, and terrorism awareness. Periodic assessment of skill performance is necessary to maintain knowledge retention until it is actually needed.
- *Coordination and communication:* This aspect of the EOP addresses guidelines for interfacing and communicating with various community agencies such as the police department, fire department, and public health agencies.
- *Recovery:* Recovery involves guidelines and policies for decontaminating equipment, restocking supplies, fumigating the building, obtaining financial reimbursement from the Federal Emergency Management Agency or other governmental agencies, and providing psychologic support for staff.

The hospital or facility's EOP also defines the roles of individuals who are likely to be involved when a disaster or terrorist event occurs. An incident control system is a management tool for coordinating security, emergency personnel teams, decontamination efforts, communication with other agencies and the media, and procurement of needed supplies. The EOP is essential to eliminate chaos and expedite effective patient care.

Community Emergency Medical Services Systems

The aim of a community emergency medical services system is to halt the events occurring after a terrorist attack using a chemical, biologic, or radiologic agent (Box 6-10). Doing so requires that the event be recognized and confirmed as an abnormal event, so that the response plan can be set into motion. Abnormal events may be classified based on the anticipated necessary response (Box 6-11). Components of the community emergency system include[27]:

- *Surveillance and event discovery:* Recognizing an abnormal event early
- *Epidemiologic surveillance:* Using current systems to identify the specific agent
- *Syndromic surveillance:* Recognizing a group of clinical manifestations or series of events that cause suspicion about a particular disease or cause
- *Data mining:* Identifying disease markers such as an increased incidence of animal diseases or large segments of absenteeism from work or school (see earlier discussion on recognition of bioterrorism events)
- *Clinical suspicion and diagnostic studies:* Recognizing and confirming the clinical disease during the early phase of attack and disease process
- *Response, activation, and notification:* Setting into motion the what, why, and when of the terrorist event, which is described in the above section on hospital preparedness

Box 6-10 Local Public Health Agency Preparedness

Because the initial detection of a covert biologic or chemical attack will probably occur at the local level:

- Disease surveillance systems at state and local health agencies must be capable of detecting unusual patterns of disease or injury, including those caused by unusual or unknown threat agents.
- Epidemiologists at state and local health agencies must have expertise and resources for responding to reports of clusters of rare, unusual, or unexplained illnesses.

Adapted from Centers for Disease Control and Prevention Strategic Planning Work-group: Biological and chemical terrorism: strategic plan for preparedness and response, *MMWR* 49:1–14, 2000.

Box 6-11 Disaster Classifications

- *Level I:* Disaster can be managed and contained by local emergency responders and agencies.
- *Level II:* Disaster can be managed and contained by regional emergency responders and agencies.
- *Level III:* Disaster requires assistance of state or national agencies to manage and control the disaster.

- *Containment and protection of personnel:* Preventing the spread of the event to unaffected populations; using physical, immunologic, and pharmacologic measures to protect personnel who may be exposed during emergency response
- *Managing health consequences of event:* Decontaminating personnel, equipment, or facilities; providing postexposure immunization or pharmacologic treatment to reduce the impact of a biologic attack
- *Mass patient care and fatality management:* Using triage systems to divert patients to alternate facilities and following plans to secure additional staff as needed; establishing temporary morgues
- *Coordination of response groups:* Managing communications and cooperation among community and government responders
- *Recovery and rehabilitation:* Providing long-term care for victims if needed, and counseling for responders and survivors

Most communities have disaster plans, but they may not be fully developed for all-hazards events. The process is ongoing as communities and government agencies work together to assess the potential risks and plan for the possibility of hazardous events.

Nursing Implications

Nurses, along with first responders and other health care workers, need to understand the importance of being prepared for the possible health consequences of all hazards, including natural disasters, bioterrorism, and chemical or radiologic attacks. Depending on the magnitude of the attack, hundreds to thousands could be injured or killed. Additionally, such an attack could bring about widespread fear, anger, and panic, resulting in chaotic conditions.

In response to concerns of nurses and the public, in 2002 the American Nurses Association established the National Nurses Response Team (NNRT) in cooperation with the USDHHS. The organization's goal is to ensure that nurses have a role in the nation's preparedness. When fully implemented, the NNRT will consist of 10 regionally based teams of 200 registered nurses who can be called on to assist with mass immunization or chemoprophylaxis campaigns for approximately 2 weeks.[1]

Nurses at all levels of heath care need to become involved in disaster planning and disaster awareness programs in their communities and work settings. To do so, they must become familiar with the types of agents that can be used, the effects of those agents, emergency management of victims, and methods for protecting themselves. They need to practice necessary response skills so that they can function without hesitation. Numerous websites are available through the CDC, USDHHS, and other specialty groups that provide information and guidance about biologic warfare and preparation for bioterrorism.

Preparing for Practice

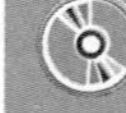

CD-Rom Activity Select Exercise One: Infectious Diseases and Bioterrorism on the Companion CD.

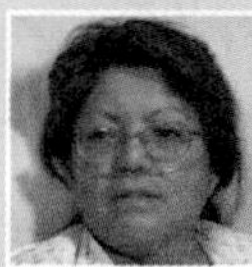

Patient: *Sally Begay,* **Room 304**

Sally Begay, a 58-year-old Navajo woman was admitted with a rule out diagnosis of Hantavirus that was subsequently changed to pneumonia. Ms. Begay has a history of hypertension, coronary heart disease, and myocardial infarction.

Assessment

View the patient's **Report.**

Review the patient's **Medical Record.** Focus on the History & Physical, noting the diagnosis of Hantavirus.

Conduct a **Patient Interview.** As you conduct your interview, focus primarily on data that will be helpful in planning care for this patient. Record the data you collect.

Nursing Diagnoses, Outcomes, and Interventions

1. Identify the specific and the nonspecific defenses that the body uses to prevent and combat infection.
2. What may have contributed to the failure Sally Begay's body to prevent this infection?
3. In addition to communicable infections, hospitalized patients are also at risk for nosocomial, or hospital-acquired, infections. List the factors that increase Sally Begay's risk of contracting a nosocomial infection. *Hint:* Refer to p. 109 if needed for descriptions of risk factors.
4. Which risk factor(s) identified in Question 3 is (are) applicable to this patient's condition?
5. Use your assessment findings and responses to Questions 1 through 4 above to formulate an appropriate nursing diagnosis for Ms. Begay. What outcome do you expect?
6. This chapter describes general interventions for patients with infection. Write specific interventions that could be used when caring for Sally Begay. In addition, for each intervention, include a plan for patient teaching.

The possibility for global biologic, chemical, or nuclear warfare is serious, and the potential for devastating casualties is high for many of the weapons. Nurses will play an integral role in care of victims during and after such an event if it occurs. However, with appropriate interventions currently available or being developed, many of the casualties can be minimized or prevented.

Critical Thinking

1. A 65-year-old patient with type 2 diabetes is admitted for a femoral popliteal bypass graft for impaired circulation to his left lower extremity. Two months before this admission, he was discharged after treatment for an infected left foot ulcer, which grew MRSA and was colonized with VRE. What precautions would you take in planning care for this patient?
2. A patient arrives at the emergency department complaining of flulike symptoms for several days and a rash that began this morning. Within the next hour two more people arrive at the same emergency department with similar complaints and physical findings. What should the nurse do?

References

1. American Nurses Association: *National nurses response team prepared to respond*, accessed 2004 from website: http://nursingworld.org/news/disaster/response.htm.
2. Armada M, Mendelson M: Chemical terrorism update: vesicants, *Emerg Med* 34(9):51, 2001.
3. Belay ED et al: Chronic wasting disease and potential transmission to humans, *Emerg Infect Dis* 6(10), 2004, accessed from website: http://www.cdc.gov/ncidod/EID/vol10no6/03-1082.htm.
4. Brower J, Chalk P: *The global threat of new and reemerging infectious diseases*, Santa Monica, Calif, 2003, RAND.
5. Centers for Disease Control and Prevention (CDC): *Preventing emerging infectious diseases: a strategy for the 21st century*, Atlanta, 2001, US Department of Health and Human Services.
6. CDC: Anthrax vaccine recommendations, *MMWR*, accessed 2002 from website: http://www.cdc.gov/mmwr/preview/mmwrhtml/mm5145a4.htm.
7. CDC: *Smallpox disease overview*, accessed 2002 from website: http://www.bt.cdc.gov/agent/smallpox/overview/disease-facts.asp.
8. CDC: *Acute radiation syndrome*, accessed April 2003 from website: http://www.bt.cdc.gov/radiation/ars.asp.
9. CDC: *Dirty bombs*, accessed July 2003 from website: http://www.bt.cdc.gov/radiation/dirtybombs.asp.
10. CDC: *Facts about phosgene*, accessed March 2003 from website: http://www.bt.cdc.gov/agent/phosgene/basics/facts.asp.
11. CDC: *Salmonella enteritidis,* accessed 2003 from website: http://www.cdc.gov/ncidod/dbmd/diseaseinfo/salment_g.htm.
12. CDC: *Shigellosis*, accessed 2003 from website: http://www.cdc.gov/ncidod/dbmd/diseaseinfo/shigellosis_g.htm.
13. CDC: Smallpox vaccine recommendations, *MMWR*, accessed 2003 from website: http://www.cdc.gov/mmwr/preview/mmwrhtml/rr5207a1.htm.
14. CDC: *Vesicant/blister agent poisoning*, accessed Dec 2003 from website: http://www.bt.cdc.gov/agent/vesicants/tsd.asp.
15. CDC: *Campylobacter infections*, accessed 2004 from website: http://www.cdc.gov/ncidod/dbmd/diseaseinfo/campylobacter_g.htm.
16. CDC: Consequences of bacterial resistance to antimicrobial agents, *Emerg Infect Dis,* accessed 2004 from website: http://www.cdc.gov/ncidod/EID/index.htm.
17. CDC: *Drug-resistant* Streptococcus pneumoniae *disease*, accessed 2004 from website: http://www.cdc.gov/ncidod/dbmd/diseaseinfo/drugresisstreppneum_t.htm.
18. CDC: Escherichia coli *O157:H7*, accessed 2004 from website: http://www.cdc.gov/ncidod/dbmd/diseaseinfo/escherichiacoli_g.htm.
19. CDC: *Facts about cyanide*, accessed Jan 2004 from website: http://www.bt.cdc.gov/agent/cyanide/basics/facts.asp.
20. CDC*: Avian influenza infections in humans*, accessed 2005 from website: http://www.cdc.gov/flu/avian/gen-info/avian-flu-humans.htm.
21. Clark A: Nosocomial infections: an issue of patient safety, part 2, *Clin Nurse Spec* 18(2):62–64, 2004.
22. Cohen J, Powderly G, editors: *Infectious diseases,* ed 2, St Louis, 2004, Elsevier.
23. Department of Homeland Security: *Radiological dispersal device preparedness*, accessed May 2003 from website: http://www1.va.gov/emshg/docs/Radiologic_Medical_Countermeasures_051403.pdf.
24. Reference deleted in proofs.
25. Fauci AS: *NIAID targets four major areas*, National Institute of Allergy and Infectious Diseases, accessed from website: http://www.niaid.nih.gov/director/usmed/2001/usmed01text.htm.
26. Flower J: Plague century, *Health Forum J* 46(3):10, 2003.
27. Flowers LK, Mothershead JL, Blackwell TH: Bioterrorism preparedness, part 2, The community and emergency medical services systems, *Emerg Med Clin North Am* 20(2):457–476, 2002.
28. Gardner M: *Emerging and re-emerging infectious diseases: an update,* accessed 2003 from website: http://www.infectioncontroltoday.com/articles/241feat2.html.
29. Heymann D: *Strengthening global preparedness for defense against infectious disease threats,* World Health Organization, accessed Sept 2001 from website: http://www.who.int/emc/pdfs/hearing.pdf.
30. Horton R, Parker L: *Informed infection control practice*, Edinburgh, 2002, Churchill Livingstone.
31. Lashley FR, Durham JD: *Emerging infectious diseases trends and issues*, New York, 2002, Springer.
32. Lewis R: The rise of antibiotic resistant infections, *FDA Consum* 29(7): 11–15, 1995.
33. Lilley LL, Aucker RS: *Pharmacology and the nursing process*, ed 4, St Louis, 2004, Mosby.
34. Lillibridge S: New developments in health and medical preparedness related to the threat of terrorism, *Prehospital Emergency Care* 17(1):56–59, Jan-March 2003.
35. Muder RR: Treatment of infections caused by vancomycin-resistant enterococci, *Curr Treat Options Infect Dis*, accessed 2003 from website: http://www.biomedcentral.com/content/pdf/cto-id5524.pdf.
36. National Institute of Allergy and Infectious Diseases, National Institutes of Health: *Microbes in sickness and health*, accessed 2001 from website: http://www.niaid.nih.gov/publications/microbes.htm.
37. Radiation Emergency Assistance Center: *Managing radiation emergencies*, accessed March 2002 from website: http://www.orau.gov/reacts/manage.htm.
38. Rayner D: MRSA: an infection control review, *Nurs Stand* 17(45):47, 2003.
39. Roberts RR et al: The use of economic modeling to determine the hospital costs associated with nosocomial infections, *Clin Infect Dis* 36:1424–1432, 2003.
40. Sande M, Ronald A: Update in infectious diseases, *Ann Intern Med* 140(4):290–295, 2004.
41. Schultz CH, Mothershead JL, Field M: Bioterrorism preparedness, part 1, The emergency department and hospital, *Emerg Med Clin North Am* 20(2):450–457, 2002.
42. Smolinski M, Hamburg M, Lederberg J, editors: *Microbial threats to health: emergence, detection and response,* Washington, DC, 2003, Institute of Medicine Committee on Emerging Microbial Threats, US National Academy of Sciences.
43. Tortora G, Funke R, Case C: *Microbiology*, San Francisco, 2002, Prentice Hall.
44. US Army Medical Research Institute of Infectious Diseases: *USAMRIID's medical management of biological casualties handbook*, ed 4, Fort Detrick, Md, 2001, US Army.
45. US Department of Health and Human Services: *HHS awards $849 million to improve public health preparedness*, accessed 2004 from website: http://www.dhhs.gov/news/press/2004pres/20040617.html.
46. US Food and Drug Administration: *Calcium-DTPA and zinc-DTPA*, accessed Aug 2004 from website: http://www.fda.gov/cder/drug/infopage/DTPA/default.htm.

47. US Government: *21st century complete guide to bioterrorism, biological and chemical weapons, germs and germ warfare, nuclear and radiation terrorism,* Washington, DC, 2001, Progressive Management.
48. Wilson J: Risks from microbes on the rise: reasons why and ways to prevent future epidemics, *Ann Intern Med* 140:497-501, 2004.
49. World Health Organization: *Dengue and dengue hemorrhagic fever*, accessed 2002 from website: http://www.who.int/mediacentre/factsheets/fs117/en/.
50. World Health Organization: *SARS: breaking the chains of transmission*, accessed 2003 from website: http://www.who.int/features/2003/07/en/.
51. World Health Organization: *Influenza: situation in Viet Nam*, accessed 2005 from website: http://www.who.int/csr/don/2005_03_11/en/.

evolve Visit the Evolve website: http://evolve.elsevier.com/Monahan/medsurg

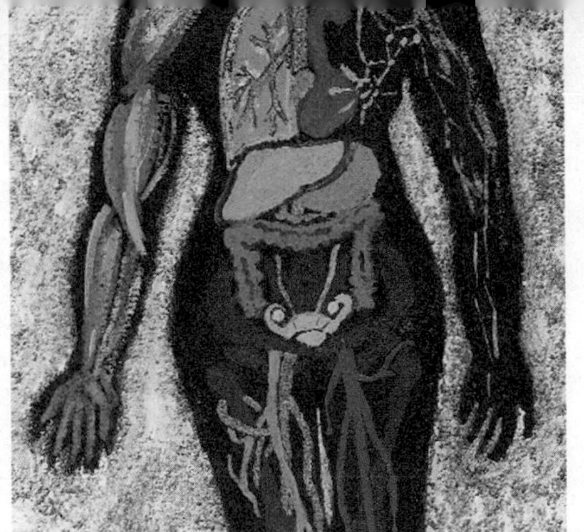

CHAPTER 7
Rehabilitation and Chronic Illness

by Christine Healy, Frances D. Monahan

OBJECTIVES

After studying this chapter, the learner should be able to:

1. Explain the philosophy and process of rehabilitation.
2. Describe the role of the rehabilitation nurse and other members of the rehabilitation team.
3. Differentiate between acute and chronic illness.
4. Describe factors that influence chronic illness.
5. Identify areas of assessment for the chronically ill person.
6. Identify the role of the nurse caring for the chronically ill.

KEY TERMS

adaptive devices, p. 133
Americans With Disabilities Act, p. 153
disability, p. 138
epidemiology, p. 140
exacerbation, p. 138
functional ability, p. 133
impairment, p. 133
incidence, p. 138
patient advocacy, p. 134
prevalence, p. 138
remission, p. 138
shifting perspective model, p. 149
trajectory, p. 149

Rehabilitation

Rehabilitation is the area of patient care that focuses on helping patients achieve maximal independence and an acceptable quality of life in physical, emotional, psychologic, social, and vocational function. Rehabilitation is not directed at cure but at enabling patients to live as fully as possible. The need for rehabilitation can result from any type of **impairment** (problem in body function or structure), including those associated with trauma and acute or chronic disease. Shorter hospital stays for acute problems and the aging of the population with its growing incidence of chronic disease have greatly increased the need for rehabilitation programs and facilities.

Rehabilitation Settings

Impairments requiring rehabilitation may be temporary or permanent; intermittent or continuous; slight or severe; and progressive, regressive, or static. As a result, rehabilitation programs differ in type, length, and setting. Types of rehabilitation programs include musculoskeletal, cardiac, respiratory, and oncologic. Rehabilitation settings include inpatient units, outpatient units, day treatment centers, and the home. Inpatient settings may be acute or subacute. Acute rehabilitation may take place in a rehabilitation hospital or on a dedicated unit in a general hospital; subacute settings may be either a dedicated unit in a rehabilitation hospital or a unit in a long-term care facility.

Philosophy of Rehabilitation

Regardless of type or setting, rehabilitation is based on a philosophy centered on a wellness perspective, with an individualized, patient-centered, goal-oriented approach to care. Rehabilitation focuses on abilities, not disabilities. It uses an interdisciplinary approach to meet the patient's unique needs and aims to support or develop the patient's **functional ability** through training, retraining, and the use of **adaptive devices** (Box 7-1). The members of each interdisciplinary rehabilitation team vary depending on the individual patient's needs. In all cases, however, the patient is the center of the team, and family members or significant others play a key role. Box 7-2 lists professionals that commonly function as part of a rehabilitation team.

Rehabilitation Process

The rehabilitation process begins with assessment of the patient's ability to benefit from rehabilitation and, if positive, selection of an appropriate facility. This selection is based on a number of factors,

Box 7-1 Adaptive Devices

Adaptive devices, also called assistive or self-care support devices, are any items that allow a person to perform an activity with greater independence. The variety of adaptive devices is extensive and growing daily. Devices are available to aid mobility, hygiene, dressing, eating, working in the kitchen, writing, seeing, and participating in recreational activities. Examples of adaptive devices that meet the needs of persons with a variety of impairments are:

- Raised toilet seat with arms for support
- Shower chair
- Hand-held shower attachment
- Straight canes, quadripod canes, and canes with a curved shape that provides a lower hand grip for leverage getting up from a seat
- Walkers with or without a basket or a seat mechanism
- Portable hydraulic seat lift to lower a patient into a chair and raise him or her out of the chair
- Long-handled reachers with a "jaw" controlled by a trigger mechanism for grasping hard-to-reach objects, often with a magnetic tip for picking up small metal items
- Buttonhook for buttoning clothing
- Extended "tall" shoe horn to eliminate bending
- Dressing stick
- Shoes and clothing with Velcro fasteners
- Nonskid feet for dishes to prevent slipping
- Foam buildups or EasyGrips on eating and other utensils that compensate for limitations in grip
- Forks and spoons whose handles bend to any angle and can be used in the right or left hand
- Two-handled mugs
- Plate guard (clear plastic "wall"), which surrounds plate and prevents food from falling off plate onto table

Box 7-2 Rehabilitation Team

- *Physiatrist:* Physician specializing in rehabilitation medicine
- *Rehabilitation nurse:* Often the case manager responsible for coordinating the work of the team
- *Physical therapist:* Promotes mobility and performance of selected activities of daily living (ADLs)
- *Occupational therapist:* Promotes development of coordination and fine motor skills used in ADLs
- *Speech-language pathologist:* Provides retraining for the management of speech, language, and swallowing problems
- *Recreational therapist:* Facilitates participation in hobbies and development of interests
- *Cognitive therapist:* Works with brain-injured patients with cognitive impairments
- *Social worker:* Identifies available support services and resources, including financial assistance
- *Psychologist:* Provides counseling and assistance with coping
- *Vocational counselor:* Assists with job placement, job training, or education

including the patient's medical needs, type of rehabilitation therapy needed, financial resources, and facility location. Once this selection is made, the rehabilitation nurse completes an in-depth assessment of the patient's physical, psychologic, emotional, and social functional ability. This assessment provides the basis for planning the rehabilitation program. A variety of standardized tools for assessing the various areas of function are available (Boxes 7-3 and 7-4). After completing the assessment, the nurse sets goals and designs a care plan.

Nurse's Role in Rehabilitation

The nurse's role in rehabilitation is a challenging one that requires skills in individual assessment, community assessment, teaching, modeling, **patient advocacy**, initiating change, and reevaluation. The rehabilitation nurse case manager assesses the patient's needs, establishes a care plan with cooperation of the patient and family, coordinates the care plan, and evaluates the outcome, with the goal of coordinating care from admission to discharge.

Unlike other specialty nursing fields, rehabilitation nursing encompasses patients of all ages and conditions and therefore requires a broad knowledge base to tailor care appropriately to both age and diagnosis. The rehabilitation nurse must have excellent interpersonal skills to establish a therapeutic trusting relationship with the patient and family. Initially, the patient may accept the nurse because of the information and assistance the nurse provides in managing the disability. However, this acceptance and trust may decrease over time, especially if the patient's expectations are not met and the patient and family are discouraged because a cure is impossible. Working through such changes to build and maintain a partnership with the patient is essential for the patient to remain an active participant in setting goals and planning the steps necessary to achieve them. Successful achievement of goals is fostered when patients and families take ownership of the goals of management and the patient accepts the level of independence he or she is able to achieve.

Goals should be both short and long term and specific so that progress can be objectively evaluated. Goal achievement depends in large part on the patient's motivation to learn, which in turn is largely determined by the patient's confidence in his or her ability to achieve a goal. The nurse can build confidence in the ability to meet a goal by:

- Breaking down the goal into smaller steps so it does not seem too large or overwhelming
- Allowing the patient to master a skill a little at a time
- Modeling or demonstrating the task to help the patient understand the process
- Encouraging the patient to perform a task after it has been demonstrated
- Coaching and providing positive feedback as appropriate each time the patient performs the task
- Working with the patient to set priorities among activities of daily living (ADLs) or tasks to be mastered and to decide on a reasonable time frame for their accomplishment

Box 7-3 Standardized Tools for Functional Assessment

- *Functional Independence Measure (FIM):* Indicates severity of disability regardless of type; useful in monitoring the effects of rehabilitation programs. Consists of a minimum data set measuring 18 items in 5 categories: self-care, sphincter control, mobility and locomotion, communication, and cognition.
- *Katz Index of Independence in Activities of Daily Living (Katz ADLs):* Rates patient as dependent or independent in six functional categories: bathing, dressing, toileting, achieving transfers, continence, and feeding. Patient's overall functional status can range from a grade of A (independent in all six areas) to a grade of G (dependent in all six areas). Can be used for tracking the effects of care or the progression of disability over time.
- *PULSES Profile:* Assigns patient a score of 1 to 4 representing degree of dependency related to each of six areas: basic physical condition, upper limb functions, lower limb functions, sensory status, excretory functions, and social and financial support factors. The closer to the maximum score of 24, the lower is the patient's functional ability and the higher the patient's dependency.
- *Level of Rehabilitation Scale (LORS):* Rates patient as 0 to 4 on 11 items related to ADLs, mobility, cognition, home and outside-the-home activities, and communication and social interaction to yield a general assessment of the patient's function for use in rehabilitation program evaluation.
- *Barthel Index:* Measures level of independence in ADLs; does not rate cognition or communication (see Box 7-4).
- *Patient Evaluation Conference System (PECS):* Is more encompassing than many other instruments in that it includes in its 15 categories areas such as medications, nutrition, recreation, and vocation.

Box 7-4 Barthel Index

Feeding

0 = unable
5 = needs help cutting, spreading butter, etc., or requires modified diet
10 = independent

Bathing

0 = dependent
5 = independent (or in shower)

Grooming

0 = needs help with personal care
5 = independent face/hair/teeth/shaving (implements provided)

Dressing

0 = dependent
5 = needs help but can do about half unaided
10 = independent (e.g, including buttons, zippers, laces)

Bowels

0 = incontinent (or needs to be given enemas)
5 = occasional accident
10 = continent

Bladder

0 = incontinent, or catheterized and unable to manage alone
5 = occasional accident
10 = continent

Toilet Use

0 = dependent
5 = needs some help, but can do some things alone
10 = independent (on and off, dressing, wiping)

Transfers (bed to chair, and back)

0 = unable, no sitting balance
5 = major help (one or two people, physical), can sit
10 = minor help (verbal or physical)
15 = independent

Mobility (on level surfaces)

0 = immobile or < 50 yards
5 = wheelchair independent, including corners, >50 yards
10 = walks with help of one person (verbal or physical) >50 yards
15 = independent (but may use any aid such as a stick) >50 yards

Stairs

0 = unable
5 = needs help (verbal, physical, carrying aid)
10 = independent

TOTAL (0–100):

The Barthel ADL Index: Guidelines

1. The index should be used as a record of what a patient does, not as a record of what a patient could do.
2. The main aim is to establish degree of independence from any help, physical or verbal, however minor and for whatever reason.
3. The need for supervision renders the patient not independent.
4. A patient's performance should be established using the best available evidence. The patient, friends, relatives, and nurses are the usual sources of information, but direct observation and common sense are also important. However, direct testing is not needed.
5. Usually the patient's performance over the preceding 24-48 hours is important, but occasionally longer periods will be relevant.
6. Middle categories imply that the patient supplies more than 50% of the effort.
7. Use of aids to be independent is allowed.

From Mahoney FI, Barthel D: Functional evaluation: the Barthel Index, *Maryland State Med J* 14:56–61, 1965.

- Never rushing the patient or trying to teach more than time will allow
- Redefining goals as necessary

Throughout the rehabilitation process, the nurse must support the patient in maintaining his or her sense of identity and control of his or her life. The nurse should support effective coping strategies used in the past and assist the patient in developing or maintaining a positive self-image.

Helping patients relearn to perform ADLs independently or with the aid of an assistive person or device is integral to the rehabilitation process. Ability to perform ADLs is a major determinant of the patient's independence and ultimately the patient's ability to live in the community. Specific problems encountered in the rehabilitation setting relate to self-care deficits, impaired mobility, altered bowel and bladder function, and impaired skin integrity.

Success in developing self-care abilities depends on a number of factors. The environment must support the patients' willingness to learn. Patients must be comfortable with taking the time needed to perform a self-care activity. They cannot be rushed or made to feel they are taking too long as they work to perform basic movements and actions. Patients also must know what is safe to attempt alone and must feel comfortable asking for help. Health care providers must tailor instructions and guidance to the individual patient's abilities and care plan to ensure consistency. Receiving different instructions from shift to shift, day to day, or person to person creates frustration and dampens motivation. When guiding patients in the performance of a task, the nurse must identify component actions, so patients focus first on developing the necessary gross movements and then on the finer movements. Nurses must take care not to push patients beyond their tolerance, to praise effort and accomplishments, and to provide practice in real as opposed to simulated situations when possible. When patients are incapable of learning or resuming self-care, the nursing focus is on enabling them to direct their care.

Impaired mobility often occurs in patients in rehabilitation as an effect of underlying disease or trauma. It may also be a result of prescribed bed rest. Because mobility status is a major influence on quality of life, a primary goal of nursing care is to maximize the patient's mobility. The plan to achieve this goal is typically designed and implemented in conjunction with physical therapy. Depending on individual patient needs, the plan may include interventions to enable the patient to sit or stand up; to transfer from bed to chair, to commode or toilet, or to shower or tub chair; or to walk and use crutches, a walker, or a cane if needed. In all cases, care is designed to prevent musculoskeletal complications of immobility such as muscle weakness, foot drop, and contractures, which limit mobility potential (see Guidelines for Safe Practice box and Figure 7-1).

Patients in rehabilitation settings frequently have alterations in bladder and bowel elimination, including urinary incontinence, fecal incontinence, urinary retention, and constipation and impaction. These problems can be a source of discomfort and embarrassment and lead to social withdrawal. Thus bladder training and establishment of a routine of bowel evacuation are important goals of care. (Types of incontinence and details of bladder and bowel training routines are found in Chapters 35 and 43, respectively.)

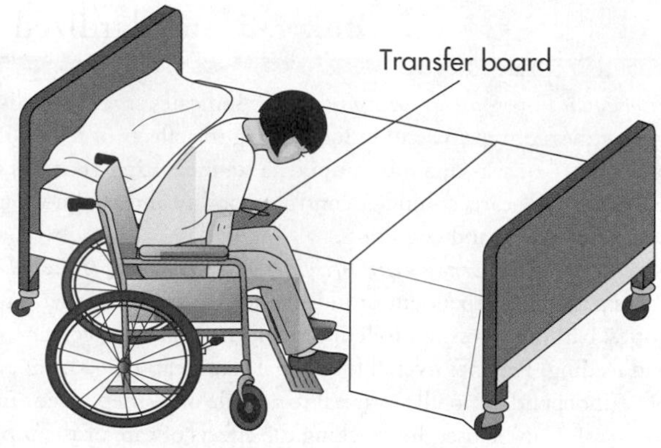

Figure 7-1 Patient using a sliding board to transfer. One end of the board is placed under the patient's buttocks, and the other end is placed on the surface to which the person is transferring. Wheelchairs and beds are locked for transfer; the patient slides or is assisted to slide across the board onto the seat of the wheelchair.

All these problems—impaired mobility, bowel and bladder incontinence, and inability to perform self-care—contribute to impaired skin integrity, which is a major nursing challenge in rehabilitation settings. Detailed information on the prevention and management of pressure ulcers is found in Chapter 65.

Working with patients who are chronically ill is a challenge. The nurse works with individuals with actual or potential health problems to help them achieve and maintain their highest level of function. To achieve this goal, the nurse works with the patient, family, health team, and community to adapt situations to meet patient needs.

ARE You READY?

In evaluating a patient in a rehabilitation setting, the nurse uses the Barthel Index for assessment of which of the following? (Choose all that apply.)

1. Memory
2. Feeding
3. Bathing
4. Dressing
5. Bowel control
6. Speech
7. Mobility

Chronic Disease

The prevention and management of chronic disease are major challenges facing the health care system today. Awareness of unmet needs among persons with long-term health problems is increasing. Individuals have needs that extend beyond the strictly medical. Their problems demand the use of multiple sources of help and care, especially since the coping abilities of chronically ill persons often are reduced because of advancing age; serious functional impairment and disability; and limited personal, social, and financial resources.

Chronic disease is not an entity in itself but an umbrella term that encompasses long-lasting diseases, which often are associated

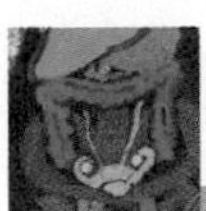

GUIDELINES FOR SAFE PRACTICE *Promoting Maximum Mobility*

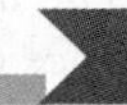

Preventing Musculoskeletal Complications

Maintain correct body alignment.

—Use pillows to support arms, legs, and back in good alignment as needed when in bed.

—Use a trochanter roll to prevent external hip rotation.

—Prevent foot drop by maintaining feet at right angles to the legs through the use of protective boots or by placing feet flat on floor or on wheelchair foot rests when sitting up.

—Use splints to prevent wrist drop or maintain hand alignment.

Perform range-of-motion (ROM) exercises to maintain joint movement.

—Perform active, assistive, or passive ROM exercises (each movement three times) twice every day.

—Support the part being exercised: stabilize the bone above the joint while moving the part below.

—Stop when resistance is encountered or at point of pain.

Perform therapeutic exercises (passive, active-assistive, active, resistive, isometric) as ordered to maintain or increase muscle strength, maintain joint motion, prevent deformity, stimulate circulation, develop endurance, and induce relaxation and a sense of well-being.

Assisting the Patient to Sit or Stand

Have patient change position in relationship to gravity slowly.

Observe for signs (drop in blood pressure, pallor, nausea, dizziness, diaphoresis, and tachycardia) of orthostatic hypotension and resultant cerebral anoxia when patient sits or stands up.

Lie the patient down and elevate the patient's legs if signs of orthostatic hypotension occur.

Use a reclining wheelchair with elevated leg rests, a tilt table that can be moved 5 to 10 degrees at a time from horizontal to vertical, and compression stockings or a compression garment for patients who need assistance in maintaining adequate blood pressure with position changes.

Assisting the Patient During Transfers

Guide the patient in doing push-up exercises in bed to strengthen arm and shoulder muscles in preparation for learning to transfer. Use a small board or book to provide a hard surface for the patient's hands to push down on.

Begin teaching and reinforcing transfer techniques as soon as the patient is allowed out of bed.

Use appropriate equipment to facilitate transfers: raised, padded commode or toilet seats, wheelchairs with removable arm and leg rests, tub or shower seats or chairs, sliding boards, chairs raised to an easier height by blocks under legs or extra cushions on the seat, grab bars for toilet and tub (see Figure 7-1).

Protect patient safety:

—Lock bed and wheelchair before beginning transfer.

—Remove environmental obstacles to transfer.

—Help patient move to stronger side.

—Support but do not pull on an impaired extremity.

Helping the Patient Walk or Use Assistive Mobility Devices

In conjunction with physical therapy, guide the patient in exercises to strengthen the quadriceps and gluteal muscles, which are essential to ambulation:

—Quadriceps setting: Instruct the patient to contract quadriceps muscles, which stabilize the knee, by trying to push the back of knee area flat to mattress while raising the heel; hold for a count of 5, then relax for a count of 5; repeat 10 to 15 times per hour while awake.

—Gluteal setting: Instruct the patient to squeeze the buttocks together for a count of 5, then relax for a count of 5; repeat 10 to 15 times per hour while awake.

Guide the patient in exercises designed by physical therapy to develop balance, stability, and coordination and to strengthen upper extremity muscles, which are essential to using any needed ambulation aids.

Make certain the patient understands any restrictions on weight bearing.

Reinforce teaching on the correct use of any ambulatory aids: crutches, walker, cane. (Consult a fundamentals of nursing text for details of procedure.)

Be certain the patient wears sturdy shoes and is aware of falling hazards such as slippery floors, inclines, and scatter rugs.

Teach patients with an orthesis (external appliance such as a brace, splint, collar, corset, or other device that provides support, combats deformity, or improves function) how to apply it, remove it, and care for the underlying skin. The latter involves inspecting and cleaning the skin daily; wearing a cotton protector garment free of seams or rough, uneven areas under the orthesis; and checking that padding is evenly distributed and fit is neither too tight nor too loose.

Provide appropriate care and teaching for patients with a prosthesis (artificial body part). See specific sections in this text such as care of the patient with an amputation, a knee or hip replacement, etc.

with some degree of disability. Although each chronic illness is unique and has a different impact on the individual, family, and community, there is a common core of problems and complications that the nurse must understand to competently care for any person with a long-term illness. The Robert Wood Johnson Foundation defines chronic conditions as medical conditions or health problems with associated symptoms or disabilities that require long-term management (3 months or longer).[8]

Incidence and Prevalence

The incidence and prevalence of chronic diseases have increased since the beginning of the twentieth century. **Incidence** refers to the number of cases of illness that had their onset during a specified period, typically a calendar year. **Prevalence** refers to the total number of cases at a given time. Thus prevalence rates are higher than incidence rates because they include all persons (cases) with a specified condition—that is, old cases plus those who acquired the condition during a specified time (new cases).

Both the incidence and prevalence of chronic diseases are increasing because fewer persons are dying from acute diseases. Mortality from infectious diseases such as whooping cough and chickenpox in children and pneumonia in persons of all ages has decreased. Improved sanitation, the introduction of effective vaccines and mass immunizations, and the discovery of antibiotics have all contributed to this decrease in deaths from infectious diseases.

An estimated 110 million Americans have one or more chronic conditions, and the number is expected to increase annually. By the year 2010, 120 million persons will be affected; and by 2030 148 million will be affected (Figure 7-2).

Disability

According to the National Health Interview Survey (NHIS), a **disability** is a limitation in social or other activity that is caused by a chronic mental or physical disorder, injury, or impairment. Impairment includes congenital, acquired, or secondary deficits of physical structure or function, sensory impairments, loss of limb, or problems in orthopedic or neuromuscular function.[3] Estimates are that 1 in 8 to 10 persons throughout the world have a limitation that is severe enough to limit activity. Heart diseases lead all conditions, followed by orthopedic and arthritis-like conditions.

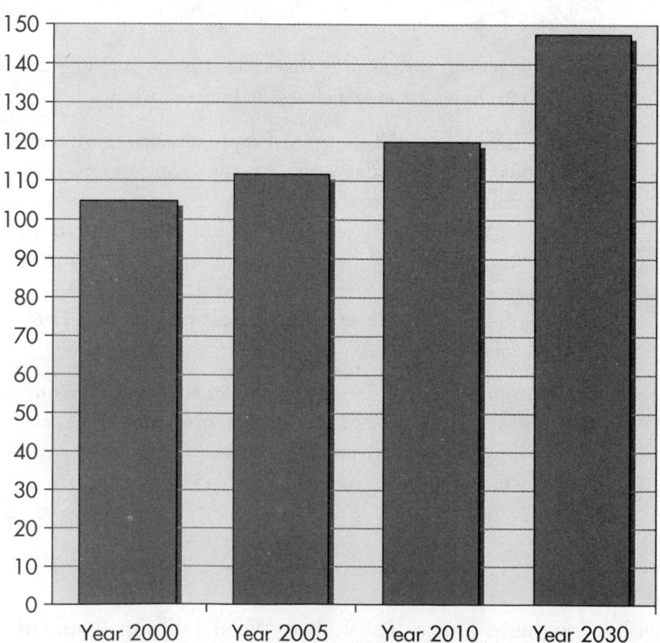

Figure 7-2 Estimated number of people with chronic conditions (in millions).

Acute Versus Chronic Illness

An acute illness is one caused by a disease that produces symptoms and signs soon after exposure to the cause, that runs a short course, and from which there is usually a full recovery or an abrupt termination in death. An acute illness may become chronic. For example, a common cold may develop into chronic sinusitis. A chronic illness is one caused by disease that produces symptoms and signs within a variable period, that runs a long course, and from which there is only partial recovery. Criteria used to define chronic conditions on the NHIS are as follows: (1) the conditions were first noticed 3 months or more before the interview, or (2) they belong to a group of conditions (including heart disease and diabetes) that are considered chronic, regardless of when they began. These criteria are in accordance with the definition of the Commission on Chronic Illness, which states that chronic illness is any impairment or deviation from normal that has one or more of the following characteristics:

- The illness or impairment is permanent.
- The illness or impairment leaves residual disability.
- The illness or impairment is caused by nonreversible pathologic alteration.
- The illness or impairment requires a long period of supervision, observation, or care.

The symptoms and general reactions caused by chronic disease may subside with proper treatment and care. The period during which the disease is controlled and symptoms are not obvious is known as **remission**. However, at a future time the disease may become active again with recurrence of pronounced symptoms. This is known as an **exacerbation** of the disease.

Exacerbations of chronic disease often cause the patient to seek medical attention and may lead to hospitalization. The needs of a patient who has an acute illness may differ from those of the patient with an acute exacerbation of a chronic disease. For example, a young person may enter the hospital with complaints of fever, chest pain, shortness of breath, fatigue, and a productive cough. If the diagnosis is pneumonia, the patient usually can be assured of recovery after a period of rest and antibiotic treatment. If, however, a patient has rheumatic heart disease and is admitted to the hospital for the third, fourth, or fifth time, reassurance is not so easy to give. In such a case it is necessary to begin planning care that will extend beyond the period of hospitalization, taking into consideration many aspects of the patient's total life situation. The concerns of the patient who has repeated attacks of illness are different from those of one who has a short-term illness.

Furthermore, the needs of patients who are admitted to the hospital with an acute illness but who also have an underlying chronic condition must not be overlooked. For example, older patients who enter the hospital with pneumonia may receive treatment for the pneumonia and recover from this illness. However, they may still be hampered by the arteriosclerotic heart disease and arthritis that they have had for years. Also, the acute infection may have aggravated these two chronic conditions, or joint stiffness resulting from bed rest and inactivity may hinder the return to former activity. Consideration of a patient's multiple diagnoses is essential to prevent new problems associated with the chronic illness.

The NHIS classifies chronic physical conditions as (1) selected skin and musculoskeletal conditions; (2) impairments (visual, hearing, speech, paralysis, deformity, or orthopedic impairment); (3) selected digestive conditions; (4) selected conditions of the genitourinary, nervous, endocrine, metabolic, and blood and blood-forming systems; (5) selected circulatory conditions; and (6) selected respiratory conditions.

Many chronic conditions cause a limitation of activity, which affects the patient's lifestyle. Although the impact of acute illness has diminished, the burden of chronic health problems and related disability has increased. Approximately 12% of the population (34.3 million people) experiences some activity limitations. Some activity limitations are associated with mental disabilities, but most are the result of physical handicaps caused by heart conditions and arthritis. Because chronic disability increases in direct proportion to age, persons older than 65 years of age are most prone to severe chronic disability.

The inability to work or move about greatly influences the kind of medical treatment and health supervision needed by persons who have a chronic illness. Some persons need only periodic medical examinations and perhaps continuing treatment with medications; others may require complete physical care. Some have a disease that progresses slowly without remissions, whereas others have episodes of acute illness and then seem comparatively well for a time. Each person requires a thorough assessment to determine the stage of the illness, the course the illness is likely to take, the type of care needed, and the method by which that care will be delivered.

Financing Chronic Illness Care

As the number of persons with chronic conditions increases, so do the direct medical costs. Table 7-1 shows the estimated medical costs for people with chronic illness from 1995 to 2050.[8] The cost of the care of persons with chronic conditions includes hospital care, physician care, and nursing home care. Other costs include prescriptions, dental care, various health and home care providers, and medical equipment. Health care costs will continue to rise as long as the incidence of chronic conditions rises.

Factors Influencing Occurrence and Management of Chronic Illness

Age

Different age-groups have different experiences with acute and chronic diseases. The young are more likely to experience intense, acute conditions that are over quickly. Older persons are more likely to have long, drawn-out chronic diseases. Nevertheless, anyone can have either an acute or a chronic disease at any age. Chronic illness and disability may date from birth (e.g., spina bifida with neurologic damage), or it may originate in childhood, adolescence, or early adult life (e.g., multiple sclerosis or rheumatoid arthritis). The major chronic illnesses among those 65 years and older identified in the NHIS are arthritis, diabetes, heart disease, and hypertension.

Because of strides in pediatric medicine, children who 30 years ago would have died of diseases such as cystic fibrosis are living longer. The reduction in death rates among the younger age-groups has allowed a higher percentage of the population to reach the age of greatest risk for chronic diseases. Cancer develops far more frequently in older than in younger persons. Because the average age of our population continues to rise, about 30% of persons now alive will eventually develop cancer.[1]

A common question is, What distinguishes the changes of normal aging from chronic illness? Differences found within age-groups or changes found in individuals as they age represent normal aging (i.e., a universal, intrinsic process of growth and development that is inevitable and irreversible). Remissions and exacerbations are possibilities with chronic illness; with aging, they are not. Even though aging, a normal process, is distinct from chronic disease, a pathologic process, chronic illness often accompanies aging. The problems of aging and chronic disease influence each other in major ways; for example, the social problems confronting older adults are strongly influenced by the presence and severity of chronic disabilities.

Race, Ethnicity, and Culture

The prevalence of specific types of chronic illness varies among populations. For example, diabetes is more than twice as prevalent among Native Americans and Alaskan Natives compared with the

TABLE 7-1 ESTIMATED NUMBER OF PEOPLE AND DIRECT MEDICAL COSTS FOR PEOPLE WITH CHRONIC CONDITIONS, SELECTED YEARS, 1995-2050

Year	Number of People (in millions)	Cost (in billions)
1995	99	$470
2000	105	$503
2005	112	$539
2010	120	$582
2020	134	$685
2030	148	$798
2040	158	$864
2050	167	$906

From Robert Wood Johnson Foundation: *Chronic care in America: a 21st century challenge,* Princeton, NJ, 1996, The Foundation.

total population. Hypertension occurs more often among African-Americans and Hispanics than Caucasians.

Responses to illness also vary among people of different race, ethnicity, and culture. Each culture has symbolic meanings, beliefs, and values that health professionals need to understand to meet individual health needs. Some persons may view their chronic disease as a form of punishment and may experience guilt. Those who view their chronic disease as a leper phenomenon may experience a sense of social rejection. Others may see their chronic illness as a destructive force without meaning or simply as a physical response of the body. Appreciation of the person's beliefs and behavior in the context of his or her cultural heritage enables the health care professional to deliver care in a manner congruent with an individual's cultural values, thus increasing the patient's compliance.

Nursing care needs to be tailored to the population served. Many potential barriers exist to competent and culturally sensitive care. Physical handicaps, obesity, skin color, speech or language patterns, style of dress, and body language can induce anxiety and negative feelings in patients, families, or caregivers.[2] The nurse must be aware of this potential and also recognize his or her own preconceived ideas and responses.

The patient's ethnic heritage may produce different responses to the same phenomenon. Individual responses to catastrophic illness are filtered through differing belief systems and practices. Consequently nurses need to consider the influence of family culture on the selection of coping strategies.

Western culture tends to be cure oriented, valuing health care for acute conditions more than health care for chronic ones. Compared with the excitement of sophisticated technology, caring for chronically ill persons is often considered boring. The continual struggle to cope with day-to-day living soon becomes tedious for chronically ill persons, their families, and health professionals. The rewards of treating chronic illness cannot be measured by a cure but by the degree to which the nurse can prevent complications and help persons function at their optimal level.

Personal Cost of Disability

Chronically ill persons and their families must deal with great personal and emotional losses. Loss of self-esteem, loss of status within the family, loss of independence, feelings of rejection, and feelings of helplessness can be more devastating than economic deprivation. However, the economic cost to the patient and family can be considerable. The cost of hospitalization rises yearly. Frequent or extended hospitalization and medical expenses can be ruinous if patients are inadequately insured or if they cannot afford medical insurance or have been dropped by an insurance company because of their chronic condition.

Many persons with chronic illness are forced to seek public assistance to survive. Placement in high-quality nursing homes often is financially impossible. The cost of medications to control or maintain a patient's health status may deplete a major part of the family budget. Additional expenses may include special diets and equipment; home modifications (e.g., installing ramps or widening doors for wheelchairs); transportation; and support services provided by homemakers, day or live-in attendants, or nurses.

A family's ability to afford this care is determined in part by which family member becomes chronically ill or disabled, their income, and their health insurance status. Sometimes a family member can retain the predisability socioeconomic status through disability insurance policies, substantial savings, workers' compensation, paid sick leave, retirement funds, and the like. Individuals may also have supplemental health insurance that complements the Medicare program. Too often, however, the individual dealing with chronic illness is also living with insufficient income and inadequate or no health insurance. This decrease in income can affect the entire family, especially if the sick person was the primary wage earner.

Medicare, a federally administered program, provides hospital and medical insurance protection for persons 65 years of age and older, as well as for those younger than 65 years who are disabled and eligible for Social Security benefits. Persons under age 65 who are medically indigent because of health problems may be eligible for assistance through the Medicaid program. Medicaid is regulated by individual states, and individuals qualify based on the value of assets. Before becoming eligible for Medicaid, individuals are usually required to "spend down," or decrease the asset value, through private payment for health care. Many individuals use the services of elder law attorneys to place their assets into a living trust. A formula based on geographic location is applied to the asset value, allowing individuals to retain certain assets and still qualify for Medicaid.

Epidemiology and Etiology

Epidemiology examines the distribution of chronic disease and the measurement of health status in the general population. It is both a body of knowledge and a method for obtaining knowledge. As a methodology, epidemiology can assist in explaining the multifactorial causal patterns of chronic diseases.

Problems in Determining Causality of Chronic Diseases

The etiology of many chronic diseases is difficult to identify. Factors that contribute to this difficulty are:

- *Multifactorial nature of etiologic factors:* Multiple factors operate in chronic diseases. The interaction of factors may be purely additive or synergistic (i.e., the combined potential for harm of many risk factors is more than the sum of the individual factors). They interact, reinforce, and even multiply each other. Asbestos workers, for example, have increased lung cancer risk. Asbestos workers who smoke have 30 times greater risk than co-workers who do not smoke and 90 times greater risk than persons who neither smoke nor work with asbestos.
- *Absence of a known agent:* Because no specific diagnostic test exists for many chronic diseases, the distinction between persons with a disease and those free of disease can be more difficult to establish than with most infectious diseases.
- *Long latency period:* Many chronic diseases have a long latency period. The latency period is the equivalent of the incubation period in infectious disease, except that it is generally longer. Because of the extended latency, it is often difficult to link antecedent events with outcomes. However, increasing evidence links the onset of ill health to the physi-

cal, social, economic, and family environments. It is easy to identify the common exposure to chickenpox at school, but it is much more difficult to identify the impact of drastic alterations in family circumstances caused by mental disorders or slow-onset physical illnesses.

- *Indefinite onset:* With many chronic conditions such as degenerative diseases and mental illnesses, it is difficult to pinpoint the initial occurrence of the disease. The vague onset of chronic illnesses makes it is difficult to collect statistics on the number of new cases in any given year.
- *Differential effect of factors on incidence and course of disease:* Factors in the socioeconomic environment that affect health include income, housing, employment status, culture, and lifestyle. For example, Mormons who abstain from smoking and alcohol have lower cancer rates than the general population as a whole.
- *Disease-specific mortality rates:* These rates are difficult to determine with chronic illness because death may result from factors other than the chronic disease itself.

One approach for studying chronic illness from an epidemiologic viewpoint is to emphasize that interrelated factors—biologic, cultural, economic, emotional, and social—determine illness. The multiple interactions involving the host, the environment, and the agent sometimes are described as the web of causation. Until the web of causation of a disease is understood, rational decisions regarding therapeutic interventions are difficult to make, and identification of preventive actions is even more difficult. To develop a chain of causation, one must identify first the natural history of disease by systematic studies of groups of people.

Natural History of Chronic Disease

All diseases have a natural history. For example, chronic diseases extend over time and develop through a sequence of stages. The epidemiology of a disease refers to its natural history (i.e., observations of the outcomes of a particular disease, and the numbers of affected persons developing each outcome). This information is used to predict an individual's possible future health. Knowledge of the natural history of diseases allows intervention to prevent or limit the effects of the diseases. The stages involved in the natural history of a disease are:

- *Stage of susceptibility:* The disease has not yet developed, but the groundwork has been laid by factors that favor its occurrence. These may be referred to as *risk factors*. The need to identify risk factors is increasing along with incidence of chronic diseases. Some major risk factors are environmental and behavioral and therefore are amenable to change (e.g., smokers can be persuaded to give up smoking).
- *Stage of presymptomatic disease:* No manifestation of disease is present, but pathologic changes have begun. An example is atherosclerotic changes in coronary vessels before any overt signs or symptoms of illness appear.
- *Stage of clinical disease:* By this stage sufficient anatomic or functional changes have occurred so that recognizable signs of disease exist.
- *Stage of disability:* Disability, which can result from an acute or a chronic condition, reduces a person's activity. The extent of long-term disability resulting from chronic disease is significant to the person and society because of the person's reduced income, the impact on his or her psychosocial roles, and the burden on community resources.

The subtlety of the natural history of chronic diseases often leaves the person unaware of a disease process for an extended period. Recently, researchers have extensively studied predisposing characteristics or habits that help identify the person at risk for developing a particular chronic disease. By altering habits of eating, rest, activity, or smoking, people may be able to change the course of certain chronic illnesses such as emphysema, hypertension, diabetes, or heart disease.

Prevention

Because chronic disease evolves over time and pathologic changes may become irreversible, the goal is to detect risk factors as early as possible. Although these diseases differ from their infectious disease predecessors, many are preventable through the adoption of healthy lifestyles and compliance with recommended screening protocols. The National Center for Chronic Disease Prevention and Health Promotion, a division of the Centers for Disease Control and Prevention, leads the work in the United States aimed at preventing and controlling chronic diseases. It studies the causes of chronic diseases, supports health promotion programs, and monitors the nation's health through surveys (for more information, visit its website at www.cdc.gov/nccdphp).

Chronically Ill Persons and Their Families

Chronic illness affects patients and family members in numerous and varied ways. The first impact of the disability may nearly immobilize them. Time must be provided for them to talk through their concerns and fears before they can begin coping with their new situation.

Significant changes are often required in family living as a result of chronic illness. Some families may find themselves drawn more closely together. Other families may drift apart, with individual members incapable of helping one another. At times, chronic illness may threaten a person's basic emotional stability, and the whole situation may be unbearable to others. Sometimes family members may be unaware of the person's emotional needs early in the illness, and then feel unable to cope when the needs grow obvious. The length of illness; periodic hospitalizations; and increased financial, emotional, and social burdens are stressors that threaten the family's integrity.

Chronic illness imposes additional problems of learning how to cope with restrictions on ADLs, how to prevent or identify medical crises, and how to carry out treatment regimens as delineated by the health care provider. Family members also need to learn about the patient's restrictions, not only to be of assistance but also to adjust to resultant disruptions in their own activity patterns.

Because chronic illness may have periods of exacerbation when symptoms become more acute and medical crises occur, patients and family members need to know which symptoms to report to the health care provider, as well as the time interval for reporting these symptoms. They also need to know how to contact the provider and what measures to take if a medical crisis occurs. For example, if a person has a history of myocardial infarction, family members must know what to do if the person experiences severe chest pain. Should they call 911? Should they immediately take the person to a hospital emergency department? Should they contact the physician first? Patient and family members should plan the sequence of actions to take during a medical crisis, depending on the presenting symptoms.

To address the complex needs of patients and families affected by chronic illness, the nurse must understand family characteristics and function. Thus a discussion of family and family systems theory follows to provide a basis for planning nursing care, not only for chronically ill patients but for almost all others as well.

Definition of Family

The definition of family has changed over time. In the past the extended family was considered the societal norm. With urbanization, the norm became the nuclear family (mother, father, and children). Today the concept of family includes the single-parent family, the reconstituted family, and the gay or lesbian couple, among others. Family may be defined according to geographic proximity, as in shared households or residential retirement homes. Family also may be defined by shared emotional bonds between individuals or within a support network. From the perspective of nursing, family is regarded as those people whom the ill individual or spokesperson identifies as family. Any long-term rehabilitation of a chronically ill patient is a joint effort between the patient, family, and health care providers. It is important that the nurse find ways to involve both patient and family as full participants in the patient's care. The nurse must recognize the many differences among families, including gender, stages of development, culture, environment, communication patterns, and economics.

Models of Family Function

Models of family function provide ways of thinking about the family that allow one to understand and predict behavior. Models suggest ways that families may be helped. The model described here is useful to nurses when they think about how families cope with illness. When selecting a theoretic framework of family function to address an ethnically diverse population, the nurse needs to determine whether it reflects changes in today's family compositions. For example, family systems theory assumes that family members must be together to have relationships. However, family members who live at a distance may be just as intimate as those who live together. Anthropologic and developmental perspectives suggest that family must be legally sanctioned or that all families go through the same developmental stages at the same time. Because these two perspectives fail to address nonblood relationships or the earlier ages at which many minority families go through some of the developmental stages, they provide less guidance to the nurse for planning interventions. Despite these limitations, family systems theory is still frequently used because it focuses on the interaction of the family members with the external environment.

Family Systems Theory. Family systems theory, credited to L. von Bertalanffy, conceptualizes the family as an open system that functions within a broader environmental context.[9] The more open the family system, the greater is the exchange of information with the environment. Within the family's boundary, dynamic interactions between the members or subsystems (such as the subsystem of parents or children) are governed by the family organization. The organization of the family system is characterized by roles, relationships, expectations, and rules.

Family members occupy and function in roles in relationship to one another. They seem to function in these roles according to the expectations of the whole family. Thus one family member may take on the role of breadwinner, whereas another may take on the role of homemaker. One family member may be the decision maker, another the primary caregiver for small children, and another the caregiver for a chronically ill adult.

The term *rules* applies to the family expectations about how each person in his or her role relates to other family members; this becomes a standard for behavior over time. Whether spoken or implicit, these rules result in patterns of relating that characterize the family's interpersonal relationships and their attempts to maintain equilibrium.

The family organization governs the dynamic interactions that take place within the family. According to family systems theory, these interactions are directed toward achieving and maintaining equilibrium within the system. Homeostasis reflects the family's striving to maintain equilibrium in the face of internal or external changes. Other family theorists refined this thinking with development of the concepts of morphostasis, or maintenance of the status quo within the family system, and morphogenesis, which reflects the family's ability to change its basic structure and organization to survive. Morphogenesis and morphostasis describe the family system as existing in a dynamic balance between change and stability in response to the environment.

Principles that describe these characteristics of the family system are circular causality, nonsummativity, and equifinality. The principle of circular causality describes family as a group of individuals who are interrelated such that changes in one member evoke changes in another, which in turn affect the first individual. That is to say, individuals living in a family do not exist in a vacuum. They are constantly affected by the behavior of others in the family, which in turn affects their own behavior.

The principle of nonsummativity holds that the family as a whole is more than the sum of the individuals who make up that family. A family cannot be described by the characteristics of its individuals alone because this does not allow for the interaction among them.

Understood within the framework of family systems theory is the idea that the organism of the family is constantly moving toward goals. The principle of equifinality states that different outcomes may have the same beginnings and that different beginnings may lead to the same outcomes. Because families are open systems, they are constantly exchanging information with the larger environment. Thus the system's outcome is affected by more than just its initial conditions.

The family systems framework suggests several key assessment areas for the nurse (Box 7-5).

Box 7-5 Family Systems Theory: Key Assessment Areas

- What are the family rules related to the patient, caregiver, and all other identified family member roles?
- How flexible is each family member in creating and adapting roles to accommodate changes in the patient's health?
- What are the patient and family goals related to the illness?
- What environmental sources of information and support are known and unknown to the family?

Adaptability and Cohesion

Family adaptability is its ability to reorganize and change roles, rules, and patterns of interaction in response to either situational or developmental stress. To the extent that family members can be flexible in their roles, rules, and patterns of interaction, the family can successfully manage changes brought about by having a chronically ill member. Families who cannot make the necessary changes in their role structure and who have difficulty changing family rules are described as being rigid. Families at the opposite end of the adaptability continuum are described as being chaotic; they experience such dramatic role shifts and rule changes that family members often do not know what rules apply.

Family cohesion describes the extent to which family members feel bonded to one another and concerned and committed to the family. Cohesion is conceptualized as being on a continuum. Extreme cases of cohesion are (1) enmeshment, an overinvolvement of family members in each other's lives, and, at the other end, (2) disengagement, in which family members are detached from the family and have little commitment to it. Healthy families lie somewhere between these two extremes. A sense of commitment in family members is vital if the ill member is to be cared for and the family is to continue.

Chronic illness increases stress for both patient and family. The goal of stress management is to work toward stress reduction and increased coping techniques. The nurse needs to identify how the family and its individual members view the chronic illness. Do they all view the chronic illness in the same way, or is there a difference? What are their coping mannerisms? Is the family more together or more apart since the patient's chronic illness? Do cultural or religious beliefs or practices need to be included in the care plan?

In 1951 Lewin suggested that for successful change to happen, three steps need to occur: unfreezing, moving, and refreezing (Figure 7-3). In the first step the nurse collects data and may identify various barriers that impede the change process. Barriers can include financial concerns, lack of family support, physical barriers in the home, and emotional denial. During the moving step the nurse establishes interventions and strategies to help the patient and family overcome obstacles and move toward a goal. Movement toward goal achievement is a cooperative journey between patient, family, and nurse. After attaining the goal, the patient will maintain these new behaviors through the refreezing process.[2]

Family Characteristics

Family composition also affects the family response. The nurse may need to view the entire family as the patient when assessing the needs of the individual with chronic illness. The family may be large, with several persons who can share in the caregiving, or it may be a single-parent household already pressed to care for its members. The nurse must assess not only the actual participation of household members in caregiving activities, but also the caregiver's and care receiver's perceptions about the helpfulness of these activities. A large household does not always mean shared caregiving, and a small household does not always mean more limited support. Remember that family is a group of individuals with whom the patient has a relationship and defines as his or her family.

Family Health. Family health is also important. The caregiver may also have a chronic illness, particularly if the patient is elderly. Families have different structures, health practices, and health or illness beliefs. Table 7-2 lists several cultures and describes family structure, health practices, and beliefs.

Problem Solving. Family members may or may not have the knowledge and ability to do the problem solving required to care for an ill member and also meet the family's demands. The perceived caregiver costs and rewards and the helpfulness of available social support are major factors in the ability to cope.

Social Support and Support Network. A support network composed of persons external to the family who can help the members carry out their tasks and give them emotional support is important for coping. The nurse should determine whether the family receives help with the patient's care needs, the family's emotional needs, and activities outside the household. Can the family identify persons who visit them, call them, provide respite to them, or assist them with decision making? The caregiver's perception of positive social support decreases the feelings of burden and social isolation.

Religion. The nurse should never overlook the role of the patient and family's religion during an illness, hospitalization, and rehabilitation. Nursing staff members should assess the patient's spiritual and religious needs and arrange for the times the patient will need privacy for prayer. Failure to integrate prayer times into

Text continued on page 149.

Unfreezing (L1) ------►	*Moving (L2)* -------►	*Refreezing (L3)*
1. Data collection 2. Assessment of factors that facilitate and/or resist change	1. Planning strategies 2. Execution of interventions	1. Maintenance 2. Evaluation/renewal

Figure 7-3 Steps in the process of planned change.

TABLE 7-2 Cultural Family Structure, Health Practices, and Health Beliefs

Culture	Geographic Patterns	Family Structure	Health Practices	Health and Illness Beliefs
Prevailing U.S. culture	Members live in all regions of United States.	Great value is placed on nuclear family. Family is individual centered; members believe in individual, self-determination, and empowerment.	Physician is gateway to health and to treatment of illness. Human body is divided according to specialists. Members try to get best medical care by best physician specialist and in best hospital possible. Members use medical model—scientific investigation and problem solving based on symptoms being diagnosed and cured by "the doctor." Members are confident in ability of technology and science to cure disease. There has been little emphasis on prevention and preventive practices until recently. Recent trend within dominant society is to use herbs, certain foods, special dietary prescriptions, and natural curative measures to gain sense of well-being outside the boundary of modern medicine. Nursing can be narrowly conceived of as carrying out medical orders.	Disease process is a result of germs, micro-organisms. Disease creates structural and functional changes. Symptoms are diagnosed and treated. There is a split between mind and body. Emphasis is on disease rather than illness. Integration of mind and body to maintain health is a recent belief about health. Emphasis on self-determination and empowerment in maintaining health is a phenomenon of the 1960s that has only recently generalized to the public.
African-American	50% live in the South; majority live in 11 large cities: Atlanta; Washington, DC; Baltimore; Jackson, Miss.; Gary, Ind.; Newark, N.J.; Detroit; Memphis; Birmingham, Ala.; Richmond, Va.; and New Orleans. Members represent a large segment of blue-collar workers. Jamaicans tend to locate in New York or Miami.	Family has egalitarian structure, with shared economic responsibility. There are a large number of female-headed households. Close relationship may exist between women and their mothers. Grandmother has central role in economic contribution and child rearing. Because informal "adopting" is an accepted practice,	Evil spirit or a hex is put on person by someone; needs to be taken off by a root doctor to cast out or contain the evil. Members may consult with a root doctor who is born with gift for healing. Many times the root doctor is described as being born with a "veil." Folk medicine healers also include spiritualists or fortune tellers who	Health is being in balance spiritually, emotionally, and physically; health hinges on leading good Christian life, having strong faith in God and Jesus, and oneness with God. Wellness is related to being productive and absence of pain. Each event, including health and illness, has socioreligious significance.

TABLE 7-2 CULTURAL FAMILY STRUCTURE, HEALTH PRACTICES, AND HEALTH BELIEFS—CONT'D

Culture	Geographic Patterns	Family Structure	Health Practices	Health and Illness Beliefs
African-American—cont'd	Members constitute about 12% of the population of United States.	family may include non-blood relatives; children are taken into households when a relative or neighbor dies or is unable to function as a parent for a time because of crises. Family system supports adult children as they meet career goals after early parenthood.	combine reading or telling the future with herbs and special oils to ward off evil. Folk practices are usually combined with Western medicine. There is tendency to take medication on as-needed basis, when there are signs of illness such as pain or headaches; medication stops when symptom disappears. God remains important source of coping and healing. Prayer and touching are believed helpful in curing and illness. Process of healing is relationship with God. When in physical and emotional pain, talk to God. To purge body of "evil spirits," some may use potions, including sugar and turpentine, herbal drinks, and hot drinks with tea and honey. Poultices may be used to treat variety of illnesses. Belly band around abdomen of newborn is thought to prevent umbilical hernia. Garlic placed on person or in room is believed to rid area of evil spirits. By turning black, copper or silver bracelets are believed to protect the wearer when illness is about to occur. There is a tolerant attitude toward obesity.	Illness is disharmony with nature resulting from natural or unnatural causes. Natural illnesses are caused by nature's forces such as weather, bad food, or bad water. Unnatural illnesses are brought about by evil forces such as hoodoo, voodoo, witchcraft, rootwork, or hexes.
Jewish-American	Members are found in every large city, with a greater prevalence in California, New York, Texas, Pennsylvania, Illinois, New Jersey,	Care of Jewish society is emphasized. Marriage is ideal state. In terms of life transitions, Jews may give particular attention to bar mitzvah	Emphasis is on keeping mind and body clean.	Body is the temple of God and must be protected from harm.

Continued

TABLE 7-2 CULTURAL FAMILY STRUCTURE, HEALTH PRACTICES, AND HEALTH BELIEFS—CONT'D

Culture	Geographic Patterns	Family Structure	Health Practices	Health and Illness Beliefs
Jewish-American—cont'd	Massachusetts, Maryland, and Ohio; 49% live in Northeast.	(for boys) or bat mitzvah (for girls), religious rites of passage and recognition of adulthood. Maximization of individual potential is emphasized.		
South-Asian	Members live in New York; Washington, DC; Massachusetts; Pennsylvania; Michigan; Ohio; Illinois; Texas; and California.	Extended family is norm; married sons, along with their wives and children, live with their parents and are subject to parental authority. Self-determination and empowerment have little value. Decisions are made by family elders or head of household based on good of the family; daughters, whose marriages are usually arranged by their parents, live with their in-laws. Filial piety refers to duty and obligation of son to care for elderly parents. Perception of self is in relation to family. A woman in the household may expect husband or other male to speak for her.	Oldest woman is considered authority on health and healing matters. Family is expected to be involved in all health care decisions. Often women are reluctant to seek care because of emphasis on modesty and shyness about disrobing; families object to female family members being examined by men. Members may delay seeking care because of fear that medical diagnosis may decrease marriage prospect. Health problems and solutions are viewed as concern of entire family; husbands and fathers are spokesmen about all family matters, including health; if the patient is the wife, she expects her husband to answer all the questions. Husband's mother is perceived as family expert on health and nutrition and is frequently consulted on these matters.	Familism and fatalism influence health pattern. Some believe in faith healing, and others believe illness is punishment for one's sins or actions in previous or present life. There is strong belief in fate—individual has little control over what happens.
Asian-American	Large communities are located in cities, mostly in Western United States, with small groupings of inhabitants evident in almost all communities. Largest Chinese community in United States is in New York City, and	Kinship is traditionally organized around male lines; fathers, sons, and uncles are important, recognized relationships between and among families. There are strong family ties; family comes first, individual last.	Oriental medicine encompasses meditation, nutrition, martial arts, herbology, acumassage, acupressure, moxibustion, acupuncture, and spiritual healing. Acupressure, acumassage, and moxibustion apply to focal points to re-	Oriental medicine is based on theoretic concept of energy with emphasis on mind--body integration, health, and prevention. Concept of energy is derived from Taoist religion, which holds that nature maintains

TABLE 7-2 CULTURAL FAMILY STRUCTURE, HEALTH PRACTICES, AND HEALTH BELIEFS—CONT'D

Culture	Geographic Patterns	Family Structure	Health Practices	Health and Illness Beliefs
Asian-American—cont'd	second largest in San Francisco. 70% of Japanese live in Hawaii and California.	Daughter-in-law is submissive to mother-in-law. For Japanese Issei (first-generation immigrant), family obligations may take precedence over own needs, including health needs. Role is to nurture husband and children and care for in-laws. Age is important for prestige. Obedience to parents and preservation of family's good name are highly regarded.	establish balance between yin and yang. Spiritual healing is carried out by temple healers in Chinese culture, called *espiritas* in Filipino culture; this involves healing by using auras and psychic energies within and surrounding human body. Acupuncture is most visible demonstration of energy system; it involves insertion of hairlike needles into special acupuncture points on skin; these points are located on meridians, pathways of energy (or qi), leading to various organs of body. Herbal therapy falls into four categories of energy (cold, hot, warm, cool), five categories of taste, and a neutral group. Shiastsu is Japanese style of massage, involving intense pressure to specific areas of foot or hand to treat various ailments.	energy balance in humans by dual polarities of yin and yang; yin is negative, dark, cold, and feminine; yang is positive, light, warm, and masculine. Members believe that most imbalances in energy are caused by wrong diet or by strong emotional feelings; self-restraint, healing techniques, and herbs can restore balance. Japanese health beliefs are rooted in Shinto religion, which holds that humans are inherently good; evil is caused by outside spirits that punish humans who have succumbed to temptation; health is achieved through balance, prevention, and cleanliness.
Hispanics	Majority of the population lives in Los Angeles and San Diego, Calif; Texas; New York; Phoenix, Ariz; Denver; and New Mexico. Large number of Puerto Ricans live in north central United States. Nicaraguans and Cubans live in Miami. Dominicans live in New York and New Jersey. Columbians live in New York and Florida. Guatemalans live in Los Angeles, and Salvadorans in Los Angeles,	The family is the main focus of social identification; familism is extended to third and fourth cousins and often includes best friends; extended family provides safety and security for the individual and in turn expects loyalty. Members have *compadre* system or one who will assume the parenting role should anything happen to the natural parents. Older daughters and sons do as their parents	Members use home remedies *(remedies casero);* degree of reliance on folk practices is related to class. Members consult folk healers *(curanderos* and *espiritualista),* as well as Western health professionals. Curandero is consulted by family; he assesses the situation and symptoms, followed by an individualized care plan using touch, talking, herbs, etc. A hot disease is treated	Members view disease as having a spiritual and social context and use people, artifacts, and materials to combat illness. Members believe in hot-cold theory of four humors in the body: black bile, blood, phlegm, and yellow bile; black bile is dry and cold; blood is wet and hot; phlegm is wet and cold; yellow bile is dry and hot; disease occurs when there is excess of hot, cold, wet,

Continued

TABLE 7-2 CULTURAL FAMILY STRUCTURE, HEALTH PRACTICES, AND HEALTH BELIEFS—CONT'D

Culture	Geographic Patterns	Family Structure	Health Practices	Health and Illness Beliefs
Hispanics—cont'd	Washington, D.C., and Houston. Mexicans live in California, Arizona, and Texas.	suggest and live in close proximity to families of procreation. Families are usually large, with five or more children; children cement the marital relationship between parents and are considered to be more important than the marital relationship. Emotional intimacy is not expected; children are the center of the family. Hierarchic organization is usual and the older male is in the central position and given much respect. There are pronounced differences in gender roles; females may not leave home until married. *Machismo* is an important value for men; term denotes aggressiveness, sexual experience, manliness, courage, and being protective of females. *Marianismo* is the complementary role that implies a self-sacrificing mother, nurturer, and manager of the household.	with cold treatments (e.g., an earache is thought to be caused by cold air and is treated with heat such as hot soups and broths); a hot disease such as a kidney infection is treated with cold fluids such as juices. Common herbs used to treat illnesses are garlic for fever, anorexia, bronchitis, or toothache; rose water for fever, cold sweats, or infant diarrhea; oregano for fever, dry cough, or asthma; mint for indigestion, stomach pains, or nausea; aloe for burns or sunburn. *Mal de ojo* is an illness resulting from the influence of an intruder outside the family who, as a result of envy, creates imbalance by sickness; victim usually seeks out an espiritualista who had special powers while still in his mother's womb, has the ability to see the future and can institute magical protection through prayer, medals, and certain rituals. If a client is being treated for infection with symptoms of diarrhea, which is considered hot, members may be reluctant to use a hot medicine such as penicillin; the hot effect of penicillin can be neutralized by mixing with fruit juices.	or dry conditions, which upsets one of the humors. Members have strong belief in magic and witchcraft; diseases are attributed to a spell or hex or poor relationships or to evil eye (*mal de ojo*).

Modified from Derstine JB, Hargrove SD: *Comprehensive rehabilitation nursing*, Philadelphia, 2001, Saunders.

the patient treatment plan may result in tension between the family and health care professionals.

At other times a patient's religion may forbid the acceptance of a treatment. For example, Jehovah Witnesses refuse blood transfusions, and Orthodox Jews refuse the use of anything electrical on the Sabbath.

Sometimes patients wear religious symbols, which the nurse must treat respectfully. These include rosaries for Catholics, sacred threads around necks or arms of Hindus, medicine bundles for Native Americans, red ribbons for Mexican children, and mustard seeds worn by some Mediterranean people to ward off the evil eye. When a medical procedure needs to be performed, removal of these religious symbols may be a problem. After explaining the rationale for removing the symbol in a calm, soothing tone, the nurse should gently place the symbol in close contact with or at least within eyesight of the patient.

These are just a few cultural characteristics of families that can affect the family experience with chronic illness. As positive attributes, they can be indicators of family resources. As negative attributes, they may be predictors of deficits in family coping.

Conceptual Frameworks for Chronic Illness

Trajectory of Chronic Illness

In the 1960s social scientists began developing a conceptual framework for examining chronic illness. Anselm Strauss, a sociologist, was responsible for some of the earliest work. He and fellow sociologist Barney Glazer developed a Chronic Illness Trajectory Framework, with the term *trajectory* borrowed from the physical sciences. A **trajectory** is defined as a course of illness over time plus the actions taken by patients, families, and health professionals to manage or shape the course. When nurses and nurse researchers began to use the trajectory framework, they adapted it to fit their understanding of chronic illness based on experience. Over time the dynamic and changing character of chronic illnesses resulted in the delineation of nine phases: pretrajectory, trajectory onset, stable, unstable, acute, crisis, comeback, downward, and dying. Table 7-3 defines these phases and identifies appropriate management goals for each. The following paragraphs discuss selected aspects of the trajectory and its phases.

Stable Phase. In the stable phase symptoms are under control. In some chronic diseases such as multiple sclerosis, when symptoms are under control, the disease is considered to be in remission. Maintaining health-promoting behaviors that often conflict with ADLs may be tiresome and demanding. Fatigue, inconvenience, disabilities, lack of time and money, and conflicting role responsibilities are frequent reasons given for not exercising regularly. However, when the person does not maintain health-promoting behaviors, complications and destabilization are probable. Thus contact with nurses for ongoing monitoring and reinforcement of healthy lifestyles is essential, even during stable periods, to minimize relapses and complications.[8]

Unstable Phase. An unstable trajectory denotes a period when the person is not acutely ill and yet symptoms are not under control and direct medical intervention is indicated to stabilize the condition. This period is marked by uncertainty and patient questions such as, Is it possible to bring the symptoms under control? Will the disabilities increase? Was the condition discovered early enough? With diseases such as cancer the uncertainty is even greater because one can never be certain of the outcome.[8] Because medical management is frequently done on an outpatient basis, patients and families often have to cope on their own when the support of nurses could be very helpful.[8] By reaching out into the community and maintaining contact with persons during unstable periods, nurses can help patients develop strategies for managing the uncertainties that illness brings into their lives.[5]

Comeback Phase. *Comeback* refers to returning to a satisfactory way of life after a crisis, within any physical or psychosocial limits imposed by the chronic condition. The work of comeback is threefold: physical recovery, limitations stretching, and psychosocial reintegration.[4] *Physical recovery* refers to the healing process that occurs after major body trauma. *Limitations stretching* refers to the formal rehabilitation process and to what patients discover about their body once at home and on their own. Some patients discover they can stretch their limitation through repeated attempts and reach higher levels of activity than originally expected. Eventually, however, patients encounter limits in how far they can stretch and must accept the remaining disabilities.

Psychosocial reintegration refers to the psychologic and social aspects of learning to live with the disabilities that remain, plus the identity reconstitution that occurs as the person incorporates an illness and its ramifications into his or her life. Comeback is a gradual process, and it is difficult to say whether it is ever fully achieved.[8]

Promoting comeback is complicated. It involves understanding individuals and their families within the total framework of their lives, including their physical condition and psychologic and social contexts, and using this information to help patients remain on the comeback trail until they reach their potential.

Downward Phase. In this phase the patient experiences progressive bodily deterioration. Symptoms of disabilities intensify despite efforts to contain them. The patient may deteriorate until death occurs, or the disease can be arrested for a period of time. Chronic sorrow may develop as patients experience symptoms and disability. The nursing goal is to stay on top of the chronic disease and slow the rate of decline.

Dying Phase. This phase involves profound physiologic and psychosocial changes. The need for a nursing presence during the difficult weeks or months of dying cannot be overemphasized.[8] This phase is characterized by decreases in the body functions necessary for life. The nurse provides direct care to the patient and support to the family. This may be accomplished through hospice programs.

Shifting Perspective Model of Chronic Illness

A second model of chronic illness is the **shifting perspective model,** derived from a metasynthesis of 292 qualitative rese[illegible] studies about the reported experiences of adults with chı

TABLE 7-3 TRAJECTORY PHASES

Phase	Definition	Goal of Management
Pretrajectory	Genetic factors or lifestyle behaviors that place an individual or community at risk for development of chronic condition	Prevent onset of chronic illness
Trajectory onset	Appearance of noticeable symptoms; includes period of diagnostic workup and may be accompanied by biographic limbo as person begins to discover and cope with implications of diagnosis	Form appropriate trajectory projection and scheme
Stable	Illness course and symptoms under control; biography* and everyday life activities† being managed within limitations of illness; illness management centering in the home	Maintain stability of illness, biography, and everyday life activities
Unstable	Period of inability to keep symptoms under control or reactivation of illness; biographic disruption and difficulty in carrying out everyday life activities; adjustments being made in regimen, with care usually taking place at home	Return to stable
Acute	Severe and unrelieved symptoms or development of illness complications necessitating hospitalization or bed rest to bring illness course under control; biography and everyday life activities temporarily placed on hold or drastically cut back	Bring illness under control and resume normal biography and everyday life activities
Crisis	Critical or life-threatening situation requiring emergency treatment or care; biography and everyday life activities suspended until crisis passes	Remove life threat
Comeback	A gradual return to an acceptable way of life within limits imposed by disability or illness; involves physical healing, limitations stretching through rehabilitative procedures, psychosocial coming to terms,‡ and biographic reengagement with adjustments in everyday life activities	Set in motion and continue to move trajectory projection and scheme forward
Downward	Rapid or gradual physical decline accompanied by increasing disability or difficulty in controlling symptoms; requires biographic adjustment and alterations in everyday life activities with each major downward step	Adapt to increasing disability with each major downward turn
Dying	Final days or weeks before death; gradual or rapid shutting down of body processes, biographic disengagement and closure, and relinquishment of everyday life interests and activities	Bring closure, let go, and die peacefully

From Hyman RB, Corbin JM: *Chronic illness: research and theory for nursing practice*, New York, 2001, Springer.

**Biography*, Life course made up of the many aspects of the self. It is the temporal dimension of identity. Together biography and self constitute identity. *Biographic impact* refers to the manner in which these many aspects of self-care can be affected by illness or its management.[10]

†*Everyday life activities*, Actions of daily living through which persons live out the many aspects of their selves.[10]

‡*Coming to terms*, The process of making identity adaptations that are necessary to live with chronic conditions.[10]

illness[7] (see Research box). The metastudy reviewed research on the chronic illness experience from nursing, medicine, and allied health reported from January 1986 to January 1996.

In contrast with the trajectory model phases, the shifting perspective model acknowledges that the chronically ill live in the dual kingdoms of well and sick.[8] Sometimes the person's illness is in the foreground, and at other times wellness is in the foreground (Figure 7-4). Persons with chronic illness select people with whom they can share their experiences in ways that will not be detrimental to their preferred perspective. Those with illness in the foreground perspective may choose practitioners who emphasize symptoms of the disease. Those with a wellness in the foreground perspective will look

Research

Paterson BL: The shifting perspectives model of chronic illness, *J Nurs Scholarship* 33:21-26, 2001.

This study, a metasynthesis, analyzed and synthesized 292 qualitative research reports that investigated the experience of living with a chronic illness from the perspective of the person with the disease. "Perspectives of chronic illness determine how people respond to the disease, themselves, caregivers, and situations that are affected by the illness such as employment" (p. 23). Two perspectives emerged in this analysis. The "illness in the foreground" perspective is characterized by a focus on sickness, suffering, loss, and burden associated with a chronic illness. This perspective is commonly seen in persons newly diagnosed with chronic illness, but it also may reappear in response to new symptoms. The "wellness in the foreground" perspective is characterized by seeing the chronic illness as an opportunity for change in several life realms. This perspective is gained by learning about the disease, creating supportive environments, developing personal skills needed to manage the disease, and sharing knowledge of the disease with others. It allows the person to focus on other aspects of life. Perceived threats to control may initiate a shift from a wellness to an illness perspective; the study also identified processes involved in moving back to a wellness perspective. Health care professionals can help persons with chronic illness identify and understand their perspectives and the fluctuations to expect. Some evidence exists to support the notion that health care professionals can assist with shifts to wellness perspectives. Changes in approach to the care of a person with a chronic illness to fit the perspective at hand may also be necessary.

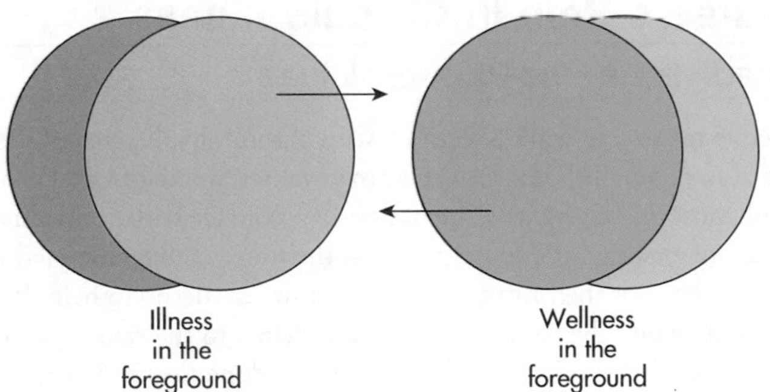

Figure 7-4 The shifting perspectives model of chronic illness.

for practitioners who suggest ways and techniques to manage ADLs in spite of the chronic illness or disability.

Illness in the Foreground. When illness is in the foreground, the focus is on the sickness, loss, and burden associated with living with a chronic illness. The patient and family view the chronic illness as a condition that can destroy them. People in this phase are self-absorbed in their illness perspective and often have difficulty attending to the needs of significant others. This phase occurs most often in the newly diagnosed individual who is overwhelmed by the disease. It can be protective, allowing time for the person to deal with changes in the body caused by the chronic illness. The sick person can also use it to develop coping behaviors such as conserving energy.

Shifting From Wellness to Illness in the Foreground. The major factor that causes a shift from wellness to illness in the foreground is the perception of threat to control. These threats are personally defined and may not be seen as threats by observers. Any threat to control that exceeds the person's threshold of tolerance will cause a shift in perspective from wellness to illness in the foreground.[8]

Wellness in the Foreground. When wellness is in the foreground, the self, not the diseased body, becomes the source of identity. The body becomes something to which things are done, not what controls the person.[8] People acquire this perspective and shift from being a victim of circumstances to a creator of circumstances by:

- Learning as much as they can about their disease
- Creating supportive environments
- Developing personal skills such as negotiating
- Identifying their body's unique patterns of response
- Sharing knowledge with others

Distancing from the illness allows the person to focus on the emotional, spiritual, and social aspects of life rather than on the diseased body. Persons reporting this change have a greater appreciation of life and loved ones and give greater attention to others, often acting as an advocate for other people with the disease.[8]

Assessment of the Person With a Chronic Illness

Before devising a care plan for the chronically ill person, health care providers carry out a thorough assessment of needs and capabilities, as discussed earlier under the rehabilitation process. Included in such an assessment is the individual's physical, psychologic, social, and financial status.

Physical Status

Because medical diagnoses do not accurately reflect the chronically ill person's physical status and function, the use of a profile system or assessment tool may be instituted as a guide for those working with the patient (see Box 7-3). Components of the assessment include (1) overall physical condition: cardiovascular, pulmonary, gastrointestinal, genitourinary, endocrine, and cerebrovascular; (2) upper extremity structure and function, including that of the shoulder girdle and cervical and upper dorsal spine; (3) lower extremity structure and function, including that of the pelvis and lower dorsal and lumbar sacral spine; (4) speech, vision, and hearing; and (5) bowel and bladder function. The completed assessment should indicate any difficulties, and their extent, in carrying out ADLs (e.g., dressing, feeding, bathing, brushing teeth, combing hair, using the toilet, and moving from place to place). Such a guide can be used in planning goals for care, both immediate and long term, and can help the individual and family make realistic plans for care. Because a chronic condition is not static, reassessment is carried out at regular intervals to identify improvement or regression.

Psychologic Status

Assessment of the person's psychologic needs and capabilities includes determining attitudes and stage of adaptation to the illness, feelings concerning how the illness affects the family or significant others, and the person's own goals in regard to living with an illness. For example, those who are almost totally helpless as a result of a long-term chronic condition may seem to have no interest in learning ways to help themselves. Family members may react in the same manner and be of little assistance. Both the affected person and family need interest and support from nurses and other professionals as they learn to cope with changes in their life situations.

Some chronically ill persons who face unending pain and loss of economic and social security may express anxiety, frustration, irritability, bitterness, and guilt. Some persons become obsessed with their health problems and spend much of each day thinking about what will happen and what to do. Guilt may result from being unable to work and support oneself or from the belief that one must deserve the suffering. Depression is common among chronically ill persons, especially those who feel powerless because they cannot control or overcome what has happened to them. Patients who are depressed may be suicidal, and the nurse should be alert to cues that the patient may be contemplating suicide.

Coping skills may be challenged by persistent problems such as chronic pain, medical expenses, or difficulties in carrying out ADLs. Usual coping methods, such as expending energy in physical activity, may become impossible. The person who usually copes by discussing problems with family members will need to find an alternative method if family communication patterns break down. The nurse should help the person identify usual coping methods and to explore alternative approaches when necessary.

Chronically ill persons or their families may suffer from unresolved sadness known as chronic grief. Chronic grief is accumulated or prolonged grief. It extends over long periods, with permanent characteristics developing in many persons, and carries with it a potential for decreased function. The causes are varied, and new waves of grief are constantly triggered. One example is grief caused by the losses associated with aging: youth, dreams, jobs, hair, friends, family, health, visual acuity, social role, money, body parts, and mobility. Each loss is accompanied by grief, which builds on previous grief, just as individual bricks create a wall. In chronic grief the person may face repeated acute episodes. These episodes may coincide with exacerbation of the condition, new limitations, or new indignities. Each new episode requires a renewed struggle back and forth through the various stages of grief.

The nurse can assist by listening and helping the person explore feelings and related issues. Because the grief is ongoing, the nurse can also help family members identify their feelings and strengthen the communication patterns within the family structure for normal support of its members.

Social and Financial Status

The assessment must consider social and financial status, since both relate specifically to the support and resources available to meet the person's goals. For example, it would be unrealistic to plan for a hydraulic bathtub chair if the patient cannot afford it, if family members are unavailable to help operate it, or if the patient's apartment manager will not allow it to be installed. Alternative methods of helping the patient take a tub bath would have to be explored.

The social assessment includes living arrangements, family roles, support of significant others, cultural and social group memberships, education, and vocational and avocational activities. The data collected through this kind of thorough assessment should make it possible to devise a care plan to accomplish attainable goals that are mutually acceptable to the patient, the family, and the caregivers.

Compliance

Health care providers often label persons with chronic illness as compliant or noncompliant in carrying out their prescribed regimens. Many factors influence the person's ability or motivation to carry out the regimen. If the person does not carry out the regimen (noncompliant), it does not necessarily mean that he or she is refusing to do so deliberately, although sometimes this is the case. The nurse needs to assess whether the individual understands why the regimen was prescribed, is able to learn the task, and is able to complete the task. Is a financial barrier impeding the process? Does the individual lack necessary support or find the regimen embarrassing?

The nurse also must assess the patient's readiness to learn. Patients must be psychologically capable of participating in a learning experience. They must find the learning experience relevant to their needs and emotionally appealing so they are motivated to learn.[3]

Nurse's Role in Chronic Illness

Clarifying Nurse-Patient Values

Before nurses can work effectively with chronically ill persons, they need to distinguish between their own values, standards, and goals and those of the patient. In day-to-day contact with individuals who are making little or no progress, the nurse may be tempted to make plans for their future because of a sincere desire to help. Particularly when the patient and nurse are close to the same age, the nurse may believe that something must be done to speed progress. However, he or she must recognize that care management for a chronically ill person requires a slow-moving, persistent pace with possibly little or no change for a long time. The person's physical and mental condition must be maintained at its present level or improved, as efforts are made to encourage the family's adaptation to the patient's condition. Eagerness and readiness to progress are determining factors for the future. The nurse's role in the care of the chronically ill person is not always a physical action with the hands. Often maintaining a positive approach and attitude and demonstrating real interest are the greatest help to the patient.

Promoting Self-Care

Asking the person to identify what is meaningful is a primary step toward fostering self-care. Physical needs are of paramount importance for chronically ill persons. Meeting these physical needs provides a way to convey an interest in their progress and welfare. Chronically ill persons who are hospitalized should be allowed to perform as much of their own care as possible. Persons who have been independent in self-care before hospitalization should not be allowed to regress in these abilities if at all possible. Helping patients take their own baths or showers, attend to toilet needs, and groom themselves can give some sense of accomplishment and self-respect. Helping them dress appropriately promotes a sense of wellness. The nurse should encourage persons who are in their homes or in substitute homes to dress in regular, comfortable street clothing rather than pajamas or gowns. Visitors to the home and family members who constantly see such individuals dressed in bedclothes think of them as sick and are reminded of their illness. Seeing them dressed as usual helps maintain normal attitudes, relationships, and expectations.

Patient teaching is an inherent component of self-care promotion. However, traditional teaching, which focuses on sharing information and modeling skills, is not sufficient. Self-care requires self-management ability. This means that the nurse must teach the patient to solve problems and make decisions about his or her needs. For example, it is not enough for a patient with diabetes to understand basic information about blood sugar measurement and dietary requirements. For self-care, he or she must be able to decide when to test blood sugar and make dietary choices based on the results.

Promoting Self-Esteem

Care of chronically ill persons requires alertness in feeling, seeing, and hearing. Continued warmth and interest help bolster the self-esteem of any chronically ill person. Often a relationship based on an understanding of these requirements promotes self-esteem and helps motivate the individual. It may be taxing for the nurse to listen to the same questions and say the same things day after day, but the nature of chronic illness may require this attention, and the manner in which responses are given will convey warmth and interest. The world of chronically ill persons, whether they are in the hospital or elsewhere, becomes narrowed and circumscribed. Their conversations may be largely about themselves, their immediate environment, a few close objects, and the persons around them. Although they may be confined to their bed or room, others can update them on outside news. Depending on their adaptation to their illness, they may welcome hearing about outside events, or they may not be able to think beyond themselves. When they reach the stage of being able to look beyond themselves, newspapers, magazines, radio, television, computer, or crafts or other activities may interest them in others and in outside events.

Supporting the Person With a Progressive Disability

Health care personnel must be prepared to care for patients whose disease will follow a course of progressive disability, as with multiple sclerosis, rheumatoid arthritis, or Alzheimer's disease. In these instances goals of care are to retard the downhill progression of disability rather than to maintain or improve physical status. Helping the patient and family cope with progressive deterioration and in some cases eventual death is a demanding task.

Providing Community Resources

Health care providers have shown an increasing interest in providing programs for chronically ill persons and in helping them and disabled persons assume a more active role in their communities. Volunteer workers may act as readers both in hospitals and in homes or may assist with other diversional activities. Institutions receiving federal funds are required to make aids such as ramps available to persons who are unable to climb stairs or who are in wheelchairs. With the development of structural changes that facilitate mobility, some persons with physical limitations are more involved in local activities and associations.

Nurses can assist by supporting structural changes in all community buildings and by encouraging chronically ill persons to participate in community activities of interest. Information is available from national organizations involved with chronic illness and disability, many of which offer services in local communities (Box 7-6). Programs, facilities, and legislation of this nature reflect the public's increasing awareness of the difficulties faced by chronically ill and disabled persons.

Advocating for the Chronically Ill

Nurses have a responsibility to inform the disabled about their rights under the law. Therefore nurses should be aware of provisions of the **Americans With Disabilities Act**, which was passed by Congress in 1990 and is called by some the Civil Rights Act for the disabled. It provides protection to the estimated 48 million Americans with disabilities. Its four main components address employment, public services, public accommodations and services operated by private entities, and telecommunication services (Box 7-7). A copy of the Americans With Disabilities Act, Public Law 101-239, can be obtained free from the U.S. Government Documents Office in Washington, DC, or from one's congressional representative.

As citizens, all nurses can advocate for the disabled and chronically ill by helping articulate their needs to the general public. Nurses can be active in their own communities to ensure that the public accommodations and public service provisions are carried out.

▶ ARE You READY?

The nurse reviews discharge instructions with a patient diagnosed with a chronic neurologic disorder. Which statement indicates that the nurse's teaching was effective?

1. "I will have to learn how to live with these limitations."
2. "I cannot wait to get back to my regular activities."
3. "I will have to go on permanent disability from my work."
4. "I know that I can beat this disease."

Box 7-6 Community Resources for Chronic Health Problems

Various types of information may be obtained by contacting these national organizations. In addition, services of the various agencies are usually available at the local level.

General

AARP (American Association of Retired Persons): www.aarp.org
Alzheimer's Association: www.alz.org
American Association of Diabetes Educators: www.aadenet.org
American Cancer Society: www.cancer.org
American Diabetes Association: www.diabetes.org
American Heart Association: www.americanheart.org
American Lung Association: www.lungusa.org
American Parkinson Disease Association: www.apdaparkinson.org
The Arc of the United States: www.thearc.org
Arthritis Foundation: www.arthritis.org
Brain Injury Association of America: www.biausa.org
Cystic Fibrosis Foundation: www.cff.org
Easter Seals Disability Services: www.easterseals.com
Epilepsy Foundation: www.epilepsyfoundation.org
ILSI North America: www.ilsina.org
Juvenile Diabetes Research Foundation International: www.jdf.org
Leukemia and Lymphoma Society: www.leukemia-lymphoma.org
March of Dimes Birth Defects Foundation: www.marchofdimes.com
Muscular Dystrophy Association: www.mdausa.org
National Association for Down Syndrome: www.nads.org
National Association for Visually Handicapped: www.navh.org
National Council on the Aging: www.ncoa.org
National Hemophilia Foundation: www.hemophilia.org
National Jewish Medical and Research Center: www.njc.org
National Kidney Foundation: www.kidney.org
National Mental Health Association: www.nmha.org
National Multiple Sclerosis Society: www.nmss.org
Parents of Children with Down Syndrome: www.arcmontmd.org/pods.html
Shriners Hospitals for Children: www.shrinershq.org
Sickle Cell Disease Association of America: www.sicklecelldisease.org
United Cerebral Palsy: www.ucp.org
United Ostomy Association, Inc.: www.uoa.org

Rehabilitation

Mainstream: www.mainstream-mag.com
National Dissemination Center for Children with Disabilities: www.nichcy.org
National Spinal Cord Injury Association: www.spinalcord.org
Paralyzed Veterans of America: www.pva.org
United States Access Board: www.access-board.gov

Box 7-7 Provisions of Americans With Disabilities Act

Employment

1. Employers may not discriminate against a qualified person with a disability in hiring or promotion.
2. Employers can ask about the person's ability to perform a job but may not ask if someone has a disability or use tests that tend to screen out persons with disabilities.
3. Employers need to provide "reasonable accommodation" to individuals with disabilities, including job restructuring and modification of equipment.
4. Employers do not need to provide accommodations that impose an "undue hardship" on business operations.
5. Employers with 25 or more employees were to comply by July 1992.
6. Employers with 15 to 24 employees were to comply by July 1994.

Transportation

1. New public transit buses must be accessible to persons with disabilities.
2. Transit authorities must provide comparable paratransit or other special transportation services to persons with disabilities who cannot use fixed route bus service, unless an undue burden would result.
3. Existing rail systems were required to have an accessible car per train by July 1995.
4. New rail cars must be accessible.
5. New bus and train stations must be accessible.
6. Key stations in rapid, light, and commuter rail systems had to be made accessible by July 1993, with extensions up to 20 years for commuter rail (30 years for rapid and light rail).
7. All existing Amtrak stations must be accessible by July 2010.

Public Accommodations

1. Restaurants, hotels, and retail stores may not discriminate against persons with disabilities.
2. Auxiliary aids and services must be provided to persons with hearing or vision impairments or other persons with disabilities, unless an undue burden would result.
3. Physical barriers in existing facilities must be removed, if removal is readily achievable. If not, alternative methods of providing the service must be offered, if they are readily achievable.
4. All new construction and alterations of facilities must be accessible.

Telecommunications

Companies offering telephone service must offer telephone relay services to persons who use telecommunication devices for the deaf (TTDs) or similar devices.

State and Local Governments

State and local governments may not discriminate against qualified persons with disabilities.

Critical Thinking

1. C.D. is a 62-year-old woman who has had multiple sclerosis for the past 18 years. She is about to be discharged from the hospital after treatment for a urinary tract infection. This is her third admission in the past 2 years. In the past year she has had progressive neurologic deterioration. She is alert and oriented. She has become more dependent on her husband to assist her at home. Her husband is self-employed and works from home. As the nurse assigned to C.D.'s home care:
   a. Identify the assessment factors necessary to develop a plan of care.
   b. List three goals with interventions to meet the goal in priority order.
   c. Identify community resources that can assist the patient and the family.
2. How may the care of one person with a chronic illness be generalized to the care of other persons with chronic illnesses?

References

1. American Cancer Society: *2001 cancer facts and figures*, Atlanta, 2001, The Society.
2. Derstine J, Hargrove S: *Comprehensive rehabilitation nursing,* Philadelphia, 2001, WB Saunders.
3. Hoeman S: *Rehabilitation nursing: process, application and outcomes*, St Louis, 2002, Mosby.
4. Hoffman C, Rice D, Sung H: Persons with chronic conditions: their prevalence and costs, *JAMA* 276(18):1473–1479, 1996.
5. Hyman RB, Corbin JM, editors: *Chronic illness research and theory for nursing practice*, New York, 2001, Springer.
6. Reference deleted in proofs.
7. Paterson BL: The shifting perspectives model of chronic illness, *J Nurs Scholarship* 33(1):21–26, 2001.
8. Robert Wood Johnson Foundation: Chronic care in America: the system that isn't, *Adv Issue* 4:1, 9–10, 1996.
9. Von Bertalanffy L: General systems theory and psychiatry. In Ariti S, editor: *American handbook of psychiatry*, ed 2, New York, 1974, Basic Books.
10. Woog P, editor: *The chronic illness trajectory framework: the Corbin and Strauss nursing model,* New York, 1992, Springer.

evolve Visit the Evolve website: http://evolve.elsevier.com/Monahan/medsurg

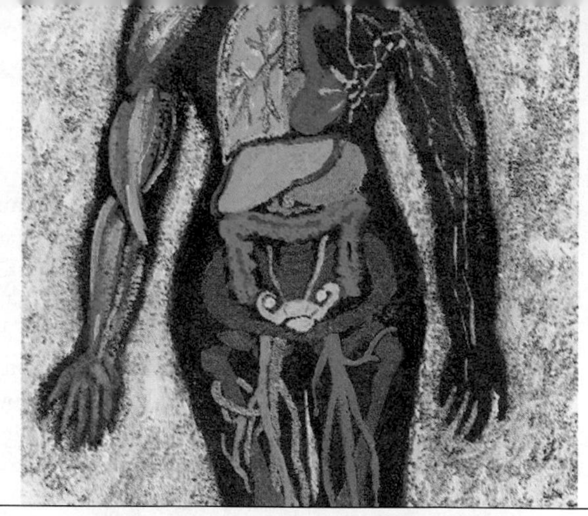

CHAPTER 8

Palliative and End-of-Life Care

by Amy E. Guthrie, Carol J. Green, Marianne L. Matzo

OBJECTIVES

After studying this chapter, the learner should be able to:

1. Describe the philosophy and working model of palliative care.
2. Identify individuals who may benefit the most from palliative care treatment.
3. Identify societal trends and gaps in health care that precipitated the need for palliative care.
4. Identify nursing strategies for assessment and treatment of pain and other undesirable symptoms associated with chronic, serious, and terminal illness.
5. Describe ethical issues surrounding end-of-life care.
6. Describe the three phases of the perideath period.
7. Discuss bereavement theory, and apply it to a generalist's practice.
8. Describe self-care strategies for nurses in managing the demands of caring for a dying patient and grieving family.
9. Differentiate between withholding/withdrawing treatment and euthanasia.

KEY TERMS

bereavement, p. 169
brain dead, p. 175
euthanasia, p. 174
grief, p. 169
hospice, p. 156
intractable symptoms, p. 165
off-label, p. 160
palliative care, p. 156
religiosity, p. 169
spirituality, p. 169

The World Health Organization (WHO) defines **palliative care** as "an approach which improves the quality of life of patients and their families facing life-threatening illness, through the prevention, assessment, and treatment of pain and other physical, psychosocial, and spiritual problems"[53] (Box 8-1).

Palliative Care

Palliative care is whole-person care provided by an interdisciplinary team of physicians, nurses, social workers, chaplains, and other health care professionals. The interdisciplinary care model aims to relieve suffering and improve quality of life for patients with chronic, serious, and advanced disease and their families. Palliative treatments can consist of many different interventions, including aggressive interventions to control pain and other distressing symptoms. Palliative care is offered along with all other appropriate medical treatments.[19,22,51,54]

Palliative care is developing into a nursing and medical specialty because of the unique knowledge and skills necessary to alleviate the patient's and family's suffering and enhance the quality of life. What started as a philosophy of care is evolving into a care delivery system. The traditional disease cure-care model focused on medical treatments (Figure 8-1). When cure was not possible, health care providers told the patient there was "nothing else to be done" and then referred the patient for palliative care. The new model for palliative care offers services and interventions from the time of diagnosis[8,19,21,51,54] (Figure 8-2).

Palliative care principles enhance the effectiveness of nursing care by providing nurses with research and guidance in pain and symptom management. Palliative care is interdisciplinary care and makes use of complementary therapies and psychosocial support to facilitate the dying individuals' goals throughout their life, illness, and impending death[36,37] (see Complementary & Alternative Therapies box).

Palliative care began as a philosophy of caring for the terminally ill within the **hospice** movement, which continues as an integral component of end-of-life care. In the United States the hospice movement with the palliative care philosophy became firmly established when Medicare hospice benefits (MHBs) were established in 1983. The MHBs' original goal was to support families caring for

Box 8-1 The World Health Organization Definition of Palliative Care

Palliative care is a model of care that improves the quality of life of patients and their families facing problems associated with life-threatening illness, through the prevention and relief of suffering by means of early identification and treatment of pain and other distressing symptoms (physical, psychosocial, and spiritual).

Palliative Care

Provides relief from pain and other distressing symptoms

Affirms life and regards dying as a normal process

Intends to neither hasten nor postpone death

Integrates the psychologic and spiritual aspects of patient care

Offers a support system to help patients live as actively as possible until death

Offers a support system to help the family cope during the patient's illness and in their own bereavement

Uses a team approach to address the needs of patients and their families, including bereavement counseling

Enhances quality of life, positively influences the course of illness, and supports death with dignity

Is applicable early in the course of illness, offered simultaneously with other therapies that are intended to prolong life, such as chemotherapy or radiation therapy, and includes those investigations needed to better understand and manage distressing clinical complications

From Storey P, Knight C, Schonwetter R: *Pocket guide to hospice/palliative medicine*, Glenview, Ill, 2003, American Academy of Hospice and Palliative Medicine.

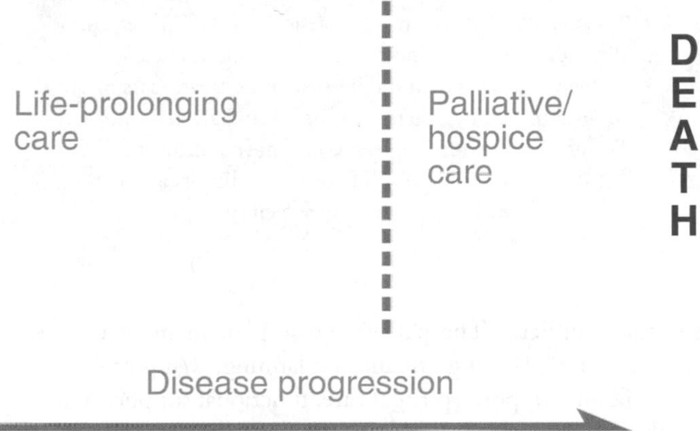

Figure 8-1 The cure-care model: the old system.

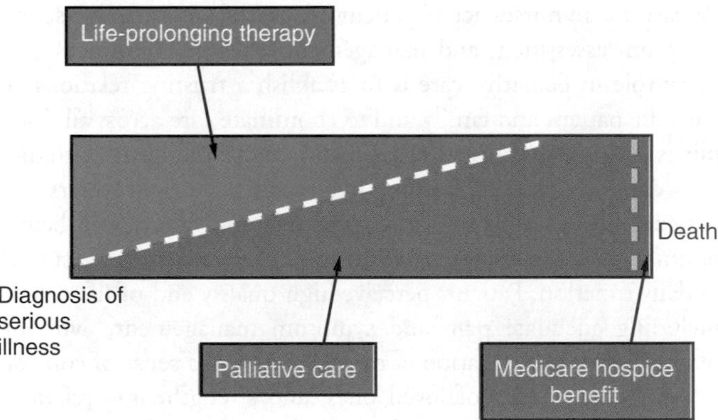

Figure 8-2 Palliative care's place in the course of illness.

dying loved ones at home. Now, hospice services under the MHB can be provided in a nursing home or an acute care setting for respite care or intense symptom management. Referral for hospice care is appropriate when the overall care plan is directed toward comfort rather than reversing or eradicating the disease. Services provided by MHB require medical care oversight (Box 8-2). MHB eligibility requirements are[5]:

1. The patient must be entitled to Medicare Part A (hospital payments). When the patient signs on (elects) to receive hospice care, he or she signs off of Part A. This process is reversible when the goal of care changes to curative or the patient travels outside the local hospice's service area.
2. The hospice medical director, along with the primary physician, must certify that the patient has a life expectancy of less than 6 months. Patients continue to receive care after 6 months as long as the primary physician and hospice medical director continue to believe death is likely within 6 months.
3. Under Medicare, do-not-resuscitate status cannot be used as a requirement for admission.

Complementary & Alternative Therapies

Complementary Therapies Used in Palliative Care

Complementary therapies, also called complementary medicine, offer nonpharmacologic options for symptom control. As used in palliative care, many of these therapies provide an opportunity for the individual to learn new skills and gain control. This in turn reduces hopelessness. Complementary therapies are designed to move the individual into an active role while shifting the power base from the disease and medical technology to the patient.

Complementary therapies used in palliative care include:

- Relaxation and guided imagery
- Massage and other touch-based therapies
  - —Incidental to nursing actions
  - —Expressive—as in caring
- Acupuncture
- Aromatherapy
- Pet therapy
- Music therapy
- Art therapy

Box 8-2 Services Provided by Medicare Hospice Benefit

With medical care oversight, Medicare hospice benefits provide:

- Nursing care for symptom assessment
- Skilled services, treatments, and case management
- Routine nursing visits with 24-hour, 7-day a week emergency contact
- Medical social work for counseling and planning
- Counseling services for spiritual or bereavement care
- Durable medical equipment
- Medication and supplies pertaining to the terminal illness
- Home health aide and homemaker services
- Speech, nutrition, physical, and occupational therapies when medically necessary
- Bereavement support to families after the death
- Short-term inpatient care for problems that cannot be managed at home
- Short-term respite care up to 5 days to give family or caregivers a break
- Continuous care at home for short episodes of acute need

From Centers for Medicare and Medicaid Services: http://cms.hhs.gov/manuals/21_hospice/hs200.asp.

The hospice team works together to maximize quality of life by jointly developing the patient's care plan. The care plan is based on the patient's health care wishes, diagnosis, symptoms, and other needs. The hospice philosophy supports the long-term objective of creating a personalized experience for each patient at the end of life. This care is referred to as *palliative care* and provides an opportunity for growth, quality of life, and death with dignity. Palliative care emphasizes that the patient and family live each day as fully as possible.[6]

Palliative care is necessary due to advances in technology that may mask or delay recognition of the need for human compassion for the dying and their loved ones. The need is reflected in the growing public demand for a more holistic, integrated approach toward health, illness, and death.[8,45] Because hospice is a Medicare model requiring participants to have a life expectancy of 6 months or less and to forego curative treatment, many hospices are creating expanded care delivery models to offer the same interdisciplinary holistic care to individuals with a longer life expectancy and to those receiving curative treatment.[20]

Palliative care practice typically takes on the characteristics of the community it serves. Box 8-3 describes palliative care delivery models. Box 8-4 lists populations most commonly served by palliative care.

The Palliative Care Plan

Care provided by all team members is holistic and directed by the patient and family. Best practice in palliative care uses the strengths of the interdisciplinary team. The leader of the team is the person, regardless of discipline, who knows the most about the issue at hand. This is strategic, since not all symptoms arise from a physical need. Dyspnea may occur due to anxiety, pain can be exacerbated by depression, and restlessness may be a result of spiritual conflict.[43] The palliative care plan includes care goals, advance care planning, financial planning, symptom management, family support, spiritual care, functional support status and rehabilitation, and comorbid disease management.

Box 8-3 Palliative Care Delivery Models

- Consultation service team consisting of physician, advanced practice nurse, nurse, and social work evaluations
- Dedicated inpatient unit in an acute or long-term care setting or combined with a freestanding inpatient hospice
- Combined consultative team within an inpatient unit
- Combined hospice program and palliative care program
- Hospital- or private practice-based outpatient palliative care clinic
- Hospice-based palliative care at home
- Hospice-based consultation in outpatient settings
- Community network with home visits

Box 8-4 Populations Commonly Served by Palliative Care Specialists

- Persons of any age with acute, serious, and life-threatening illnesses where the condition is potentially reversible
- Individuals dependent on life-sustaining treatments or long-term care by others for support in daily activities
- Persons living with progressive chronic conditions
- Seriously and terminally ill patients requiring care in a hospital, home, or long-term care facility

Role of the Nurse

Palliative care nurses act as patient advocates, case managers, and symptom assessment and management experts. The nurses' primary role in palliative care is to establish a trusting relationship with the patient and family and to coordinate care across all disciplines and health care settings. Quality of life and death with dignity can be achieved with a treatment plan that fosters the patient's physical, psychosocial, spiritual, and family well-being; optimal patient and family perception of care; and the highest level of daily function. Patients perceive high-quality end-of-life care as including adequate pain and symptom management, avoiding inappropriate prolongation of dying, achieving a sense of control, relieving the burden of loved ones, and strengthening relationships with loved ones and a higher power. Other factors important to high-quality end-of-life care vary by role, developmental stage, and personal preferences.[7] Table 8-1 summarizes how people view death at various developmental stages.

Palliative Care Goals

The nurse ascertains the patient's understanding of and desire to know about the diagnosis and prognosis so that the palliative care interdisciplinary team can construct the most effective plan to

TABLE 8-1 DEVELOPMENTAL VIEWS OF DEATH

Age	Developmental Stage	Task or Area of Resolution
Birth to 2 yr	Infancy	Sense of separation with no concept of death
2–5 yr	Early childhood	Death perceived as temporary
6–12 yr	Late childhood	Beginning awareness of the reality of death
13–25 yr	Adolescence Young adulthood	Realization of mortality and eventual death Death anxiety more prevalent Death perceived as a future event
26–65 yr	Middle age Older adulthood	More awareness and accepting of death

From Potter M: Loss, suffering, bereavement, and grief. In Matzo M, Sherman D, editors: *Palliative care nursing: quality care to the end of life*, New York, 2001, Springer.

manage the disease and its symptoms. Family meetings are an effective forum to discuss the patient and family's goals, hopes, and expectations of treatment. The meeting occurs in a private area large enough to accommodate as many individuals as the patient feels necessary to include. The nurse invites other members of the palliative care team to provide additional support and education. Not everyone in the meeting will necessarily agree on treatment goals initially. Acting as facilitator, the nurse provides information on benefits versus burdens of treatments and allows everyone to express concerns. The nurse plans for additional education and follow-up meetings as needed. He or she continually reviews the goals of care with the patient and family throughout the course of the illness and treatment. When decisions need to be made, ethical standards of decision making provide guidance. They involve considering what is known of the patient's wishes and preferences given the current condition, balancing the burdens and benefits of each option in terms of the patient's quality of life, and achieving a consensus among decision makers (family, friends, and health care professionals).

Communication is essential for achieving consensus on a course of action. To the extent possible, communication includes all who are emotionally invested in the outcome and who provide information about the patient's wishes and best interest regarding quality of life.[22,38]

Advance Care Planning

Advance care planning is an important part of palliative medicine and end-of-life care. Exploration of a patient's life and treatment goals are the foundation for future health care decision making. Advance care planning discussions should occur with healthy, competent, adult patients in the primary care setting. Such discussions include living wills, durable power of attorney for health care, an advance medical care directive, and a patient-completed values history, which serves as a foundation for advance care decisions.[15,47]

An advance medical care directive combines the living will and the durable power of attorney for health care, providing specific instructions for various medical situations. Like the durable power of attorney, an advance medical care directive may appoint a health care proxy to aid in treatment decision making when the patient is no longer able to communicate medical wishes.[15]

A values history reveals the patient's values and beliefs and directs health care clinicians, proxies, and family members through difficult treatment decisions. A values history should be part of the initial assessment and revisited frequently, preferably yearly. When the clinicians and health care proxy are aware of the patient's treatment choices and the values that support those decisions, medical treatment efficacy increases. This, in turn, enhances the patient's and family's quality of life by preserving autonomy. Nurses in all settings provide opportunities for the patient to discuss medical wishes. Advance directives can be in verbal or written form. Any verbal statements made by the patient regarding treatment choices should be documented in the patient's medical file and brought to the attention of other interdisciplinary team members.[15] Advance directives are not recognized for dying children; however, allowing a child to share in his or her own medical care decisions is critical.

According to surveys, many patients prefer health care professionals to initiate advance care planning discussions; more important, they request that these discussions occur during times of good health. Enhancing communication between health care professionals and their patients increases not only the number of completed advance directives, but also the possibility of medical and nursing care matching the patient's wishes.[15] Box 8-5 summarizes the nurse's role in advance care planning.

Box 8-5 Nurse's Role in Advance Care Planning

- Determine the patient's chosen surrogate health care decision maker.
- Stress the importance of choosing someone the individual trusts to carry out medical treatment decisions that the individual has clearly stated are important.
- Determine the surrogate decision maker's comfort in accepting this responsibility.
- Encourage the individual to complete the legal documents required in the state in which treatment occurs and to have ongoing conversations regarding medical treatment values with the surrogate decision maker, other friends and family, and all other clinicians involved in care.

Financial Planning

When considering the patient's ability to adhere to a treatment plan, the nurse must assess the resources available. For example, if the patient is unable to pay for pain medications, then it is likely that pain will not be managed at home and hospitalization will be routinely required. The nurse can work with the social worker on the interdisciplinary team to obtain assistance for the patient and family with estate planning, long-term care, other insurance options, and community medication reimbursement programs. The care providers assess the patient's understanding of health care coverage (medical, home care, prescription, long-term care, and family support needs) and make referrals as needed. Referrals may include other medical assistance programs such as Medicare-covered hospice care, Medicaid, and Passport, if personal resources are inadequate to cover the patient's needs.[38]

Collaborative Care Management

Functional Status Support and Rehabilitation

The nurse assesses patients' ability to perform activities of daily living (ADLs) and instrumental activities of daily living (IADLs), then refers patients for rehabilitation evaluation and conditioning exercises as appropriate. The nurse also assesses the home for safety and provides referrals for IADL support, fall risk reduction, and gait-assist devices if needed. Physical, occupational, and complementary therapies are useful for assessing, optimizing, and maintaining functional status. However, underlying, reversible causes of functional impairment must be ruled out. The nurse ascertains the patient's functional ability 1 year before the initial visit and clarifies activity goals for the patient and family. At times, family members may have conflicting goals regarding the patient's activity level. The nurse provides time during the family meeting for family members to expresses their ideas, then holds separate, private meetings with the patient and family to assess their coping and behavioral habits. Allowing family members to express their fears about the patient's irreversible decline sometimes is sufficient to alleviate any conflict.[38]

Comorbid Disease Management

The nurse must monitor for coexisting illnesses and coordinate with other health care specialists. This is necessary to provide high-quality, coordinated care and services that agree with the individual's health care wishes and achieve the goal of maintaining health and function.[39] The nurse reviews medications on an ongoing basis to identify potential drug interactions and make changes as needed. The nurse also reviews treatment options offered by specialists and helps the patient understand the benefit versus burden of treatment in terms of quality and length of life. When the patient can no longer benefit from treatment, the nurse recommends that it be discontinued. At that point all the members of the palliative care team are involved in providing emotional support.

The palliative care nurse often experiences firsthand the milestones that indicate the patient and family are moving through the process of letting go. That process includes a willingness to admit recovery is not likely or possible; acknowledging what quality of life really means to the patient; and vacillating about whether or not the right decisions were made and whether or not those decisions will negatively impact the relationships between the patient, nurse, and family.[39,42]

Symptom Management

Symptom management is the cornerstone to ensuring a high quality of life and death with dignity. Nurses caring for individuals with chronic, serious, and terminal illness must monitor symptoms such as pain, dyspnea, nausea and vomiting, anorexia, constipation, and changes in level of consciousness. A whole-patient assessment is a comprehensive assessment of the physical, social, emotional, and spiritual aspects of the patient, family members, and caregiver, examining a range of issues that may cause suffering.

Routine symptom assessment using validated instruments such as the Edmonton Symptom Assessment Scale, the Brief Pain Inventory, and other validated tools helps the nurse identify and treat symptom distress, manage side effects of medical treatment, and monitor condition changes.[4,11,16,31,46]

Occasionally physicians prescribe **off-label** drugs, meaning that they are approved for one problem but are prescribed because of beneficial side effects rather than intended use. Any drug that is administered to a different age-group, by a different route, or for a purpose other than the FDA-approved purpose is considered "off-label." For example, the drug olanzapine is an FDA-approved drug for the treatment of psychiatric disorders. However, the drug is also useful in controlling nausea and vomiting, since it binds to receptors that modulate physical responses. The symptoms of palliative care patients are often resistant to control by traditional measures, so a growing number of clinically sanctioned off-label drugs are being used. Table 8-2 lists commonly prescribed, clinically sanctioned off-label medications for palliative care patients.

Pain. Studies indicate that roughly 25% of hospitalized patients are in moderate to severe pain for the majority of their hospital stay.[18] Pain assessment tools allow for accurate assessments when used consistently. Box 8-6 lists selected pain assessment tools. Pain is highly subjective, and the patient's report is the gold standard for assessment.

It is imperative for nurses to understand the pathophysiology of pain. Somatic nociceptive pain involves direct stimulation of intact mechanical, chemical, or thermal nociceptors and transmission of electrical signals along normally functioning nerves. It is associated with tissue damage caused by bone metastasis, mucositis, skin lesions, fracture, etc., and is sometimes referred to as *somatic or body pain syndrome.* Somatic pain is partially responsive to opioid therapy but may require antiinflammatory agents, steroids, or radiotherapy.[4,11,16,31,46] Descriptive words that patients use to describe somatic pain include dull, aching or gnawing, throbbing pain that is localized, constant, or intermittent.

Visceral nociceptive pain results from stimulation of the autonomic nervous system, which innervates viscera. Visceral pain is also referred to as *visceral gut pain syndrome.* Descriptive words commonly used for visceral pain are sharp, aching or squeezing,

TABLE 8-2 PALLIATIVE MEDICINE OFF-LABEL MEDICATION PARAMETERS

Medication	Common FDA-Approved Use	Clinically Sanctioned Off-Label Use
Gabapentin (Neurontin)	Seizures	Neuropathic pain*
Trazodone	Depression	Sleep disorder*
Transdermal scopolamine	Motion sickness	Terminal secretions†
Atropine ophthalmic	Ocular disorder	Terminal secretions†
Hyoscyamine (Levsin)	Irritable bowel syndrome	Terminal secretions‡ Gastrointestinal benefits§
Imipramine	Depression	Neuropathic pain¶
Amitriptyline	Depression	Neuropathic pain¶
Nortriptyline	Depression	Neuropathic pain¶
Haloperidol (Haldol)	Psychosis	Nausea and vomiting¶
Metronidazole (Flagyl powder)	Infection	Malodorous odor‡

FDA, U.S. Food and Drug Administration.

*Turkosi B, Lance B, Bonfiglio M: *Drug information handbook for advanced practice nursing,* ed 3, Hudson, 2001-2002, Lexi-Comp.

†Palliative Care Consultant Group: *Preferred drug list,* Hospice of Wayne County Ohio, Wooster, NY, 2001, Palliative Care Consultant Group.

‡*Oxford textbook of palliative medicine,* ed 2, Oxford, 1998, Oxford University Press.

§Dickerson E et al: *Palliative care pocket consultant,* ed 2, Dubuque, Iowa, 2001, Kendall-Hunt Publishing.

¶Kaye P: *Symptom control in hospice and palliative care,* rev ed 1, Victoria, Australia, 1995, Hospice Education Institute.

cramping, pulling pain, which is more difficult to describe and localize than somatic pain.[4,11,16,31,46] Opioids are the drug class of choice for visceral pain, although it may require adjuvants such as anticholinergics or octreotide.

Neuropathic pain is believed to result from disordered function of the peripheral and central nervous system and may be due to many causes (e.g., postherpetic neuropathy or shingles pain, diabetic neuropathy, human immunodeficiency virus, chemotherapy). Descriptive words linked to neuropathic pain include burning, tingling, numbness, shooting, stabbing, radiating, or electric-like feelings.[4,11,16,31,46] Primary drug therapy for neuropathic pain is opioid therapy with or without tricyclic antidepressants or anticonvulsants.

Clinical considerations for pain syndromes include acute versus chronic, noncancer versus cancer, and nociceptive versus neuropathic versus mixed syndromes. Regardless of the causes and characteristics of pain, the WHO's analgesic ladders make treatment planning comprehensible (Figure 8-3). Steps are:

1. Determine the type of pain: nociceptive (somatic/bone, visceral) or neuropathic.[53]
2. Assess for descriptive words, intensity, location, duration, and alleviating factors.
3. Treat underlying causes.
4. Using the WHO analgesic ladders for cancer and noncancer pain, add adjuvant medications and nonpharmacologic interventions to the opioids, as appropriate.[4,11,16,31,46,53]

Dyspnea. Dyspnea is an uncomfortable awareness of breathing. It is highly subjective and involves both the perception of breathlessness and the patient's reaction to it. Because of its subjective nature, effective assessment requires the nurse to ask the patient specifically about shortness of breath. Some may be tachypneic and yet deny feeling short of breath. Other patients not visibly in respiratory distress may report feeling short of breath. In any case, the patient's report is the gold standard for assessment. The nurse must consider many possible causes of dyspnea and make an attempt to treat the cause, since it is responsible for the distressing symptom. Low-dose, immediate-release opioids are often effective for the treatment of dyspnea.

Box 8-6 Selected Comprehensive Pain Assessment Tools

- Brief Pain Inventory
- Examination of psychosocial and physical effects of pain
- Numeric Rating Scale
- 0 to 10 scale evaluating the intensity of each pain site
- Functional Pain Scale

Nausea and Vomiting. Like pain and dyspnea, nausea is highly subjective; therefore the nurse makes a thorough assessment to identify all the potential causes. Effective treatment geared to the specific emetic pathways can be accomplished after identification of all the relative assessment data and completion of a physical examination, including a gastrointestinal history (Box 8-7). The history and physical examination should focus on the oral cavity, abdomen, rectum, and neurologic system. Laboratory tests are used to rule out electrolyte, fluid, and chemical

The World Health Organization (WHO) Analgesic Ladder for **Treatment of Cancer Pain**

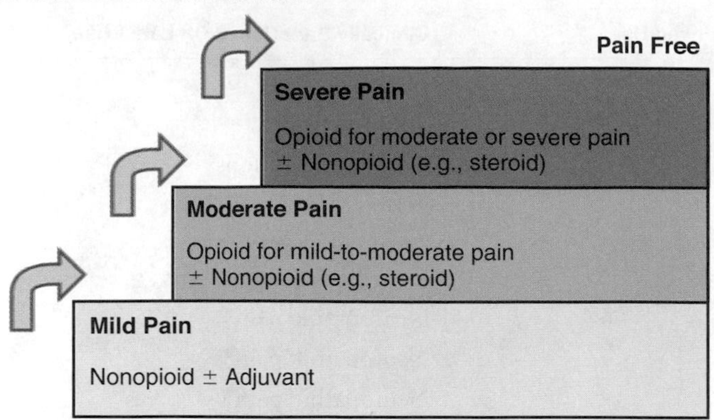

Treatment of Noncancer Pain

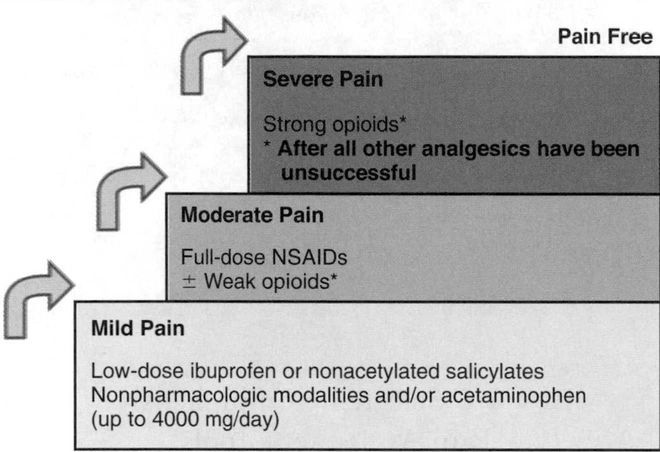

Figure 8-3 Comparison of treatment of noncancer pain with the World Health Organization's analgesic ladder for treatment of cancer pain. *NSAID*, Nonsteroidal antiinflammatory drugs.

imbalances, with a focus on calcium levels, sodium levels, kidney function, and liver function.[10,14,46,51]

The first-line treatment for nausea and vomiting is to reverse any underlying causes. The Education for Physicians on End-of-life Care Project simplifies the major causes of nausea and vomiting to "11 M's of emesis": metastases, meningeal irritation, movement, mentation, medications, mucosal irritation, mechanical obstruction, motility, metabolic, microbes, and myocardial.[48]

Selection of the most effective antiemetic treatment involves identifying the suspected causes of nausea and vomiting and identifying the pathways causing nausea and vomiting triggers. Initial concerns are choosing the antagonist most responsive to that receptor and the route of administration that will ensure the drug reaches the site of action. Routine administration of the antiemetic, symptom reassessment, and medication titration are important in optimal treatment.[10,14,46,51]

Intractable Nausea and Vomiting. Even with the identification of triggers and the implementation of receptor-specific antiemetics, intractable nausea and vomiting affect a minority of patients. Younger patients with pelvic malignancies, patients experiencing anxiety because of treatment or disease unknowns, and those identified with autonomic failure have a high incidence of intractable nausea and vomiting. If symptoms persist and a single agent has been titrated to the maximum recommended dose, adding treatments that are specific to other receptors is frequently effective, since more than one emetic pathway is often involved.

An effective treatment for nausea and vomiting is lorazepam (Ativan), 1 mg; diphenhydramine (Benadryl), 25 mg; metoclopramide, 10 mg; and haloperidol, 1 mg per suppository (see Table 8-3 for dosing schedules). This combination is more cost-effective than ondansetron (Zofran) or other alternatives. Each of the drugs suppresses the chemoreceptor sites that are trigger points for nausea and vomiting. Dexamethasone (Decadron) is an effective adjuvant to suppress tumor growth, or if the cause of intractable nausea and vomiting is unknown. Dexamethasone also gives the patient a feeling of well-being.[25] See Table 8-3 for medications used in palliative care.

Anorexia. Anorexia and cachexia are common in many advanced illnesses and may result in significant distress, especially for caregivers. Caregivers are often concerned that lack of eating and weight loss are contributing to the underlying illness, but the reverse is typically the case. Adequate feeding, even artificial feeding, rarely reverses the course of advanced disease in patients with poor functional status and limited prognosis. However, feeding may be beneficial for selected patients such as those with good functional status, malabsorption, temporary unconsciousness, and sepsis. It also helps with symptom control when true hunger exists. The decision not to use an artificial feeding tube may be considered ethical if the burdens outweigh the benefits, the

Box 8-7 Gastrointestinal Assessment for Nausea and Vomiting

An initial gastrointestinal assessment for nausea and vomiting includes questions such as:

- Do nausea and vomiting occur before or after meals?
- Does vomiting occur after nausea, after coughing, or without warning?
- Are the nausea and vomiting associated with colicky pain, diarrhea, fever, or chills?
- Is there a pattern or specific times of the day that nausea and vomiting occur?
- Are they intermittent or continuous?
- Have there been recent changes in bowel habits or medication regimen?
- Is there pain or burning sensations related to nausea and vomiting?
- Are there any other causes that you suspect are triggering the nausea and vomiting?

From Davis M, Walsh D: Treatment of nausea and vomiting in advanced cancer, *AAHPM Bull* Fall 2001, pp 4, 5, 9, 15; Engel G: A life setting conducive to illness: the giving-up-given-up complex, *Ann Intern Med* 69(2):293-300, 1968; SUPPORT: A controlled trial to improve care for seriously ill hospitalized patients, *JAMA* 22/29(274):20, 1591–1598, 1995; and Tyler L: Nausea and vomiting in palliative care. In Lipman A, Jackson K, Tyler L, editors: *Evidence based symptom control in palliative care,* New York, 2000, Pharmaceutical Products Press.

TABLE 8-3 MEDICATIONS USED IN PALLIATIVE CARE

Symptom	Drug	Dose	Implications
Pain	Morphine	Titrate to relief	Cramping pain: increase dose
	Hydromorphone	Adjust for route changes	May add hyoscyamine (Levsin) 0.125 mg SL q4-8hr
			If unrelieved: celiac plexus block
Nausea	Haloperidol	5-15 mg/day SC, PO, or IV	Mix in 5% dextrose for SC infusion
	Metoclopramide	60-240 mg/day SC, PO, or IV	May cause colic if opioid dose low
	Hydroxyzine	100-200 mg/day SC, PO, or IV	Add to haloperidol if necessary
	Chlorpromazine	25-100 mg/tid PO, PR, or IV	Suppositories useful if SC infusion of above agents is unavailable
			Sedating
	Diphenhydramine (Benadryl)	25-50 mg/q6h PO, IV	Sedative, anticholinergic effects
	Lorazepam (Ativan)	1-10 mg/day in divided doses, PO, IM, IV	Sedative, hypnotic
Persistent vomiting (despite above measures)	Octreotide	0.1-0.6 mg/day by continuous SC infusion or bolus bid-tid	Expensive
			Effective in decreasing secretions
Constipation	Docusate	100 mg PO bid q4hr	Reduces colic more than stimulant laxatives
Incomplete obstruction	Dexamethasone	4 mg PO or SC bid-qid	May relieve obstruction caused by bowel wall edema; discontinue in 5 days if ineffective

SL, Sublingual; *q*, every; *SC*, subcutaneous; *PO*, by mouth; *IV*, intravenous; *tid*, 3 times a day; *PR*, by rectum; *bid*, twice a day; *qid*, 4 times a day.

options have been discussed with the patient and/or family, and they agree with the plan. When planning care, the nurse must consider and address conditions that may exacerbate loss of appetite and weight (Table 8-4).

Constipation. Constipation is an uncomfortable and distressing symptom that often accompanies abdominal tumors, chronic illness, malnutrition, dehydration, hypokalemia, hypercalcemia, and use of opioids for pain management.[40,46,51] The nurse encourages patients and caregivers to monitor bowel routine with a 24-hour diary of bowel activity, including changes in physical activity and intake, and bowel management agents taken. If bowel obstruction is suspected, a plain abdominal x-ray examination may be useful. Signs and symptoms of bowel obstruction include nausea and vomiting, which occur in almost all patients with complete obstruction; abdominal (visceral) pain; abdominal distention; high-pitched or absent bowel sounds; tympanic sounds on percussion of abdomen; history of infrequent bowel movements; and absence of flatus. Patients with bowel obstructions are assessed for surgical suitability based on general physical condition, evidence of mechanical obstruction, and reasonable expectation of survival and quality of life.[46,50,51].

Medical management of inoperable bowel obstruction begins with a determination of partial or complete obstruction. A prokinetic agent may be appropriate in the presence of an incomplete obstruction, but not for a complete obstruction. Hypodermoclysis—hydration through a subcutaneous infusion of 1 to 2 L/day—is often used in the inpatient setting to relieve dehydration. The subcutaneous route is less invasive and causes less physical distress than intravenous therapy.

Corticosteroids can be used to reduce swelling and inflammation related to peritumor edema (see Table 8-3). Nausea and vomiting are controlled and gastrointestinal secretions and severe abdominal cramping reduced with octreotide. For short-term treatment, use of an nasogastric tube provides significant relief until the obstruction is overcome or until a percutaneous endoscopic gastrostomy (PEG) tube is inserted. Mouth care is provided if the patient is to take nothing by mouth.[40,46,51]

TABLE 8-4 EXACERBATING FACTORS FOR NAUSEA, VOMITING, AND LOSS OF APPETITE

Cause	Treatment
A: Aches and pains	Improve pain management.
N: Nausea and gastrointestinal dysfunction (dysphagia, odynophagia)	Evaluate whether invasive diagnostics are appropriate. Treat according to guidelines.
O: Oral candidiasis/oral lesions	For candidiasis, give nystatin 5 ml (500,000 unit), swish and swallow qid; hold in mouth 2-5 min. Evaluate for herpes simplex, etc.
R: Reactive or organic depression, anticipatory grief	Administer antidepressants. Refer to social worker. Offer spiritual intervention.
E: Evacuation problems (constipation)	Treat according to guidelines.
X: Xerostomia (dry mouth)	Provide artificial saliva with mucin.
I: Iatrogenic: chemotherapy, radiation	Reevaluate risks and benefits of treatment.
Medications	Stop if unnecessary, especially anticholinergics.
Feeding problems	Ensure that caregivers are adequately helping with feeding if necessary and that desirable foods are offered.
Infections	Evaluate risks and benefits of treatment, patient goals.
A: Acid: gastroesophageal reflux disease, peptic ulcer disease	Administer antacids. Give histamine$_2$ blockers.

qid, 4 times a day.

Mental Status Changes. One of the most devastating symptoms occurring at the end of life is a change in the patient's mental status. This change not only undermines the patient's quality of life, but also complicates the family's grief response in facing a loved one in a confused, agitated, and at times violent condition before death. *Impaired mental status* (IMS) is the term used to describe cognitive changes that frequently occur in advanced disease, especially at the end of life.

IMS manifests as confusion, agitation, delirium, nervousness, excessive worry, cognitive failure, fluctuating levels of consciousness, altered sleep-wake cycles, erratic psychomotor function, and perceptual alterations such as hallucinations and delusions. It is one of the most recurrent and most underdiagnosed neuropsychiatric complications affecting the medically ill, terminally ill, and geriatric populations. The frequency of IMS ranges from 14% to 56%, and even higher in those with cancer.[40,46,51]

IMS has several characteristics. *Hypoactive IMS* involves social withdrawal, somnolence, and psychomotor retardation, making it difficult for health care providers to recognize the subtle changes that are early signs of delirium and confusion. *Hyperactive IMS* is seen as severe agitation, anger, and possibly combative behavior. *Restlessness* manifests as myoclonus, delirium, or pure motor restlessness, without mental disturbance. *Delirium* is associated with hallucinations, paranoia, agitation, or hyperactiveness or hypoactiveness.

MEASUREMENT SCALES. Restlessness and confusion both fluctuate based on alterations in attention. The detection of inattention is the primary requirement for the positive diagnosis of confusion and delirium. The Bedside Confusion Scale (BSCS) is a simple, sensitive, and valid diagnostic tool for confusion and delirium (Table 8-5). The first step in the BSCS is to assess the level of alertness, which is classified as normal (0 points), hyperactive (1 point), or hypoactive (1 point). A hypoactive level of alertness is characterized by drowsiness, stupor, or coma. A hyperactive state includes agitation, pressured speech, and possibly aggressive behavior. The second part, the test of attention, is a timed recitation of the months of the year in reverse order beginning with December. Scores from the alertness and attention tests are added. The scores range from 0 to 5, with 0 considered normal, 1 considered borderline, and 2 to 5 considered abnormal and diagnostic of confusion.

Treatment for IMS involves nonpharmacologic interventions when possible, such as providing the patient with a quiet, safe, and supportive environment. Opiates with a low metabolite profile are used when pain is the primary problem, since morphine metabolites are a primary cause of IMS. These initial steps are followed by an investigation of the underlying cause (Box 8-8). One of the causes, hepatorenal failure, may not be reversible. However, medication changes and most metabolic abnormalities are easily reversed.[31,47,48] Patients receiving three or more medications are at increased risk for IMS.

When dehydration is the cause of IMS, a trial of hydration with a small amount of solution (1 L/day) is enough hydration to reduce, if not, resolve, the problem. Hypodermoclysis is often used as a short-term procedure, since subcutaneous administration is less invasive than intravenous.

When pharmacologic interventions are necessary, neuroleptics (e.g., haloperidol and chlorpromazine) are first-line agents for delirium and agitated restlessness. The benzodiazepines lorazepam,

TABLE 8-5 BEDSIDE CONFUSION SCALE

Parameter	Scoring	
I. Assess level of alertness	Normal	0
	Hypoactive	1
	Hyperactive	1
II. Test of attention: a timed recitation of months of the year in reverse order beginning with December	Delay greater than 30 sec	Add 1
	1 omission	Add 1
	2 omissions	Add 2
	≥3 omissions, reversal of task, or termination of task	Add 3
	Inability to perform	Add 4

To score: Total the score from I and II. The score range is from 0 to 5. A score of 0 is considered normal, 1 is considered borderline, and 2-5 is abnormal and diagnostic of confusion.

Box 8-8 Causes of Impaired Mental Status

- Drug side effects—related to build up of drug metabolites in the blood as a result of impaired renal function; can occur with drugs such as opioids, anticholinergic agents, corticosteroids and antineoplastic agents
- Drug-drug interactions (e.g., ranitidine [a histamine$_2$ blocker], hydroxyzine [an antiemetic])
- Drug withdrawal (e.g., nicotine, narcotics)
- Underlying pathologic condition (e.g., brain malignancy)
- Terminal multiorgan failure (e.g., hepatorenal dysfunction)
- Fluid imbalance (e.g., prerenal azotemia, hyperosmolarity, dehydration)
- Electrolyte imbalance (e.g., hypernatremia, hyponatremia, hypercalcemia)
- Blood gas imbalance (e.g., hypoxia, hypercapnia)
- Hematologic disturbance (e.g., anemia)
- Blood glucose disturbance (hyperglycemia or hypoglycemia)
- Infection
- Emotional and physical pain

midazolam, and diazepam are indicated for mild restlessness (Table 8-6). If needed, a palliative sedation regimen with temporary sedative intent may be implemented.[34,46,51]

Palliative Sedation. **Intractable symptoms** associated with the dying process include pain, nausea and vomiting, confusion, respiratory distress, muscle twitching, anguish, and agitation. Terminally ill patients often experience more than one of these symptoms at a time.[9] The presence of refractory symptoms should be considered a palliative care emergency. It has a profound impact on the physical and emotional comfort of the patient, family, and health care staff and also interferes with life review, family closure, and meaningful good-byes.[27] Symptoms that are not adequately controlled despite aggressive efforts are considered intractable, and sedation is recommended.[23]

Patients who are appropriate candidates for sedative therapy (1) are terminally ill with advanced and incurable illness; (2) are actively dying with a prognosis of hours to days as judged by vital signs, urine output, and level of consciousness; 3) are experiencing acute or refractory symptoms, including pain, nausea, myoclonus, restlessness, or respiratory distress; and (4) are not responsive to conventional symptom management, or require prompt intervention to relieve distress because of the severity of symptoms and natural history of the disease. It is important that the nurse establish with the patient and family that when distressing symptoms become intolerable and all underlying pathologic conditions have been investigated, intermittent sedation can be administered to relieve those symptoms without hastening the patient's death.[9,33]

Ethical concerns surrounding palliative sedation therapy include the principle of double effect and the societal confusion about issues of assisted death. The principle of double effect holds that an act is ethical if its primary goal is to relieve pain and suffering, even though the patient may die as an unintended consequence of the act. This doctrine emphasizes that an act to secure a desired effect can be justified even if it has an expected, but excessive outcome. In many cases, sedation can be achieved without hastening death.[34] The difference between palliative sedation and assisted death lies in the intent of the person carrying out the action. In sedation, death is not intended, yet often foreseen. Assisted death, on the other hand, has the direct intent of ending the patient's life. In addition, a sedative dose is not a killing dose, but a dose given in recognition of the patient's right to find relief from distressing, intractable symptoms.[21] The aim to sedate only to the level that relief of suffering occurs is within established medical standards. Sedation may last for hours or days, yet the death is a result of the terminal illness. Hydration and food intake is not an issue at this time, since the patient has probably reached the point that oral intake has diminished or ceased.[12]

▶ ARE YOU READY?

In discussing palliative care with a patient who has an inoperable lung mass, which statement by the patient indicates the need for further teaching?

1. "I will no longer receive any type of treatment for my disease."
2. "It is very important to me that my family be involved in my care."
3. "I hope that my pain will be controlled."
4. "I understand that there is no cure for this disease."

Perideath Nursing

The perideath period encompasses the symptoms and experiences right before death, the actual death, and the care of the body after death.[30] At this time in patients' lives they rely on the nurse's skills to help them, and their families, through uncharted waters.

Phase 1: Preparation for Death

The signs and symptoms summarized in the Clinical Manifestations box are indicative of the first phase of the perideath period as the body prepares itself for death.

Coolness. The person's hands, arms, feet, and legs may be increasingly cool. At the same time, the skin color may change. The underside of the body may become darker and the skin

TABLE 8-6 MEDICATION FOR IMPAIRED MENTAL STATUS

Drug	Implications
Neuroleptics	
First-line agents for delirium and agitated restlessness	
Haloperidol	For severe restlessness, 5-20 mg q30min until settled (PO, SC, IV)
Chlorpromazine	25-100 mg q4-12hr PR
Benzodiazepines	
May be effective for mild restlessness before delirium. Increased adverse effects in delirium. If needed, benzodiazepine may be added to neuroleptic regimen.	
Lorazepam	0.5-2 mg q1-4hr (PO, SL, IV, IM)
Midazolam	Single dose 2.5-10 mg; 30-60 mg in 24 hr (IV, IM, SC) for short-term anxiety treatment in older adults. Close monitoring required in inpatient setting.
Diazepam	For severe restlessness with delirium, paranoia, confusion, aggression, 5-10 mg q4-12hr (PO, PR, IV) or q4hr until settled

q, Every; *PO*, by mouth; *SC*, subcutaneous; *IV*, intravenous; *PR*, by rectum; *SL*, sublingual; *IM*, intramuscular.

mottled or discolored. This is a normal indication that blood circulation is decreasing to the body's extremities and being reserved for the most vital organs.

Sleeping. The person may spend an increasing amount of time sleeping and appear uncommunicative or unresponsive, at times difficult to arouse. This normal change is due in part to changes in metabolism. The nurse should encourage family members to stay with the patient even if he or she is asleep. Although no evidence exists to support this, many believe that hearing is the last sense to be lost. Families should talk to the patient as though they can be heard, even though they may not get a response.

Fluid and Food Decrease. The person may have a decrease in appetite and thirst, wanting little or no food or fluid. The body will naturally begin to conserve energy that would be expended to digest them. Food or drink should not be forced. Small chips of ice, frozen Gatorade, or juice may be refreshing in the mouth if the patient is still able to swallow. Glycerine swabs may help keep the mouth and lips moist and comfortable. A cool, moist washcloth on the forehead may also increase physical comfort. Withholding fluid and food may pose an ethical dilemma for family members who feel they are abandoning their loved one (see Ethical Alert box).

Incontinence. Control of urine and bowels may be lost as the muscles begin to relax. If urinary incontinence is a problem, a catheter may be inserted so the patient does not need to expend precious energy getting to the bathroom. The urine may decrease in volume and become dark because of the decreased circulation through the kidneys.

Congestion. The person may have gurgling sounds (at times loud) coming from the chest as though marbles were rolling around inside. This normal change is due to the decreased fluid intake and the inability to cough up normal secretions. The sound of the congestion does not indicate the onset of severe or new pain. Suctioning usually increases the secretions and is therefore not recommended. Scopolamine transdermal patches can be used to decrease secretion production and alleviate the "death rattle," which does not distress the patient, but can upset the family. Medications like atropine or hyoscyamine (Levsin) can also be used to dry the secretions.

Breathing Pattern Change. The person's regular breathing pattern may become irregular; for example, shallow breaths with periods of no breathing for 5 to 30 seconds or 1 minute. This is called *Cheyne-Stokes respiration*. The person may also experience periods of rapid shallow panting, a classic sign that death is near. Elevating the head or turning the person on one side may bring comfort.

Disorientation. The person may seem confused about the time, place, and identity of people, including those close and familiar. This is due in part to changes in metabolism and in part to either medications or terminal illness.

Restlessness. The person may make restless and repetitive motions, such as pulling at bed linen or clothing. This is due to the decrease in oxygen circulation to the brain and to metabolism changes. The nurse should not interfere with or try to restrain such motions. Occasionally the person may twitch or make jerking motions, which may have to do with medication or the disease itself. Antianxiety medications like lorazepam are often prescribed to help with this terminal restlessness. Family members should be encouraged to speak in a quiet, natural way; lightly massage the forehead, back, or arms; read to the person; or play soothing music. The number of persons around the patient should be minimized. Asking many questions may increase the person's agitation.

Withdrawal. The person may seem unresponsive, withdrawn, or in a comatose-like state. This indicates preparation for death, a detaching from surroundings and relationships, and a beginning of "letting go." Since hearing is thought to be one of the last

CLINICAL MANIFESTATIONS
Symptoms Common at the End of Life

Gastrointestinal Function

Anorexia	Nausea and vomiting
Dysphagia	Weight loss
Unpleasant taste	Ascites

Bowel Function

Constipation
Diarrhea
Loss of function or control

Mood

Depression
Anxiety

Bladder Function

Incontinence
Changes in function or control
Bladder spasms

Cognition

Insomnia
Confusion, dementia, or delirium
Memory changes

Skin Integrity Issues

Pressure ulcer	Mucositis
Candidiasis	Pruritus
Edema	Ascites
Hemorrhage or blood loss	Herpes zoster

Breathing

Dyspnea	Cough, congestion, or rattles
Hiccups	Altered breathing patterns

Functional Ability

Fatigue	Immobility
Pathologic fractures, spinal cord compression	Weakness

Other

Fever
Diaphoresis

From Ferrell BR, Virani R, Grant M: Hope: home care outreach for palliative care education, *Cancer Pract* 6(2):79-85, 1998.

remaining senses, encourage family members to say whatever they need to say. The patient may want to be with only a few or just one person. If family members or friends are not part of this "inner circle" at the end, reinforce that this does not mean they are not loved or are unimportant. It likely indicates that they have already fulfilled their tasks, and it is time to say good-bye.

Visionlike Experiences. The patient may speak or claim to have spoken to persons who have already died, or seen places not visible to others. This does not indicate hallucinations or a drug reaction. The patient is beginning to detach from this life and is preparing for death. It is best not to contradict, explain, belittle, or argue with the patient about what he or she claims to have seen or heard. Rather, affirm the experiences; they are normal and natural.

Ethical Alert

Artificial Hydration and Nutrition at the End of Life

Withholding artificial hydration and nutrition at the end of life is difficult to address because family members, or the patient, may perceive it as abuse, neglect, or a means of hastening death. Family members may also fear that withholding food and fluid will increase pain or discomfort during the final hours of life. No clear answer exists to the question of withholding or giving artificial fluid and nutrition. Patients with prolonged debilitating diseases, such as cancer, may benefit from artificial hydration and nutrition, although enhanced quality of life has not been proven. In other instances, artificial hydration and nutrition contribute to pulmonary secretions, dyspnea, and edema.

To prevent this ethical dilemma at the end of life, the nurse should address both the indications and contraindications associated with feeding and hydrating the patient before such decisions have to be made. When family members have their misconceptions corrected and understand the benefits as well as the unwanted effects of artificial feeding and hydration, they are better able to make such difficult decisions.

Letting Go. The patient may continue to perform repetitive and restless tasks, which may indicate that something is still unresolved or unfinished and preventing the letting go. Sometimes people important to the patient may need to say that they will be okay and give the patient "permission" to let go.

Saying Good-bye. When the patient is ready to die, saying good-bye is a final gift of life and helps achieve closure. The nurse may encourage family and friends to hold or touch the patient and to say the things they want to say. These sentiments may be as simple (or as complicated) as, "I love you" or "Thank you." Or family may want to recount favorite memories, places, and activities they have shared. They may say, "I'm sorry for whatever I've done to cause any tensions or difficulty." Tears are a normal part of saying good-bye and a natural expression of sadness and loss.

Phase 2: Death

The signs of death include no heartbeat, release of bowel and bladder, no response, eyelids slightly open, pupils enlarged, eyes fixed on a certain spot, no blinking, jaw relaxed, and mouth slightly open.

Throughout the dying process, and particularly at the very end of life, the nurse must be aware of cultural and religious values, practices, and traditions of the patient and the family.[30] Religious and ethnic group practices regarding postmortem care vary widely in the United States. Although it is possible to generalize about the practices of various groups or religions, the nurse must avoid stereotyping. The deceased's family may have strong affiliations with their religious or ethnic group, or they may not identify with it all. The best approach is for the nurse to ask the family how they would like postmortem care to be done and whether any rituals are important to follow. Customs and rituals have tremendous significance in the healing process after death and often structure the grief response. The nurse's role is to help the family carry out the rites and practices that provide solace and support.[30]

Phase 3: After Death

Once the patient has died, the family has many decisions to make or plans to carry out, depending on whether the patient has already arranged the funeral. Choices include organ donation, cremation, traditional burial, and internment of the body. For some families the wake, or visitation, is the first component of postdeath ritual. It may be one of the few times the entire family reassembles. It is a time for family and friends to view the dead body and to pay their final respects. Seeing the dead body emphasizes that the person is dead; declining to see the body may delay grieving.[30]

The second component of postdeath rituals is the funeral. It is a ceremonial service that typically includes music, prayers, poetry, and eulogies. This may take place as part of a funeral mass where communion is celebrated. Some people plan their funeral before they die, which can be comforting to both the dying person and family. The last ritual is the committal service, the concluding funeral rite. It is the final act of caring for the deceased and is celebrated at the grave, tomb, or crematorium.[30]

Nurses may occasionally attend funerals, especially when they have been in close contact with the family for a long time. Physicians do not generally attend funerals, although research indicates they are interested in providing support to family members (see Research box).

Family Support

In palliative care the family is whomever the patient calls family; another term is *family of choice*. The nurse asks the patient and family about practical support needs such as transportation, prescription drug coverage, respite care, and personal care. They are assisted with investigating resources in the facility and the community that can meet their practical support needs.

Research

Ellison N, Ptacek JT: Physician interaction with families and caregivers after a patient's death: current practices and proposed changes, *J Palliative Med* 5(1):49-55, 2002.

Investigators surveyed 143 physicians regarding their practices in attending former patients' funerals, making family condolence visits, and sending letters or telephoning, and their desire to participate in such activities. One hundred nineteen of the respondents had experienced patient deaths in their practices. Most of the 119 did not participate in such activities. They made telephone calls 39% of the time for inpatient deaths, and approximately 40% of the physicians sent condolence notes. No correlations existed between the physicians' actions and the number of deaths experienced or the setting the deaths occurred in. Physicians have a significant desire to find an easy way to identify and contact family members grieving the loss of a loved one. The physicians agreed that if such a service were available, they would use it.

Counseling can help patients and family reconnect and build relationships. The nurse should establish relationships with all significant family and friends so that he or she can provide follow-up bereavement support after the patient's death. The patient should be assured that bereavement follow-up will occur and that loved ones' concerns will be addressed.

The nurse encourages family and friends to assist in care if they desire. The patient and the family together are considered the unit of care. Caregivers are prone to negative physical, social, and emotional effects of caring for individuals with chronic and serious conditions. They tend to ignore their own health maintenance because of the demands of their roles and, as a result, may have health conditions that require treatment. By including the caregivers in the unit of care, the nurse can ensure all benefit from the positive outcomes of palliative care.[20]

Cultural Care

It is assumed in Western culture that the patient is the best person to make health care decisions. In non-Western cultures the family or community has a vital role in receiving, organizing, and disclosing information needed to make a decision regarding care. Establishing rapport with the patient and family allows the nurse to foster an individualized care plan addressing personal beliefs, wishes, and needs.[45]

Spiritual Care

Nurses are not expected to be experts in spiritual assessment and care giving, yet they may assist the patient in acknowledging the meaning and last effects of a life lived. Nurses are pivotal in the process of spiritual assessment because of their frontline health care position, role as coordinator, intimacy with the patient, and holistic perspective on care. The nurse can establish a trusting relationship with the patient and family through active listening and acceptance. Individuals who live with an irreversible disease often consider aspects of spirituality a major contributing factor to quality of life and death with dignity.

After assessing for the desire for spiritual counseling and support, the nurse obtains information regarding religious rituals, beliefs, and practices that are significant to the patient and family. Spiritual support at the end of life may not include religious faith and its expression. Individuals may be more concerned with finding a purpose and meaning of life. Other concepts associated with spiritual support involve forgiveness of self and others, love and relatedness, hope, and creativity. When confronted by a life-threatening illness, many people realize traits that have been hidden and place a priority on being true to self. The nurse can foster these insights by leading the patient through a life review and values history.

The nurse also encourages patient and family to verbalize values and beliefs that affect health. Caregivers of the seriously ill find comfort, strength, and direction from their own spirituality. The nurse identifies religious rituals important to the patient and family and encourages their practice to the extent possible. If the patient does not participate in religious rituals, the nurse can explore other customs or traditions that the patient finds meaningful.[3,18]

According to a Gallup Poll on spiritual beliefs and the dying process, more than half of those questioned stated that their greatest fears regarding their own deaths related to the absence of God's forgiveness, the lack of reconciliation with others, and dying while feeling cut off from God or a higher power. People facing serious physical illness need help to overcome fears, find hope, find meaning in life, find peace of mind, and find spiritual resources. Including patients, family, friends, and caregivers in developing the care plan enables the patient to sustain relationships that might be overburdened by a serious illness.[3,18] Each member of the interdisciplinary team should establish a relationship with the patient and family.[3,18]

One of the many strengths of palliative care is the expanded focus beyond pain and physical symptom control to psychiatric, psychosocial, existential, and spiritual domains of supportive care. In the Gallup Poll mentioned earlier, 40% of the respondents said that if they were dying it would be "very important" to have a physician who is spiritually attuned to them. This may be difficult to obtain because of differences in belief, coupled with confusion regarding spirituality and how it relates to religious beliefs.

Spirituality and religiosity are two different concepts. **Spirituality** refers to the experience of transcendent meaning in life. The word *transcendence* derives from the Latin *transcendere* (trans, meaning "over," and scendere, meaning "climbing" or "surmount"). Viktor Frankl's "will to meaning" theory describes self-transcendence as an inherent desire to connect with that which is greater than one's own individual concerns and needs. Through this connection, one finds or makes meaning of one's life. Other definitions describe the word as surpassing the ordinary.

Religiosity, on the other hand, refers to religious rituals and doctrine. Religious rituals and doctrine are instrumental in spiritual support, but do not measure the level of transcendence. For example, many older adults with chronic illness do not have the strength to attend church services, study scripture regularly, or even pray. Evaluating spirituality based on rituals would deplete the patient's sense of meaning and purpose of life. Optimal spiritual supportive care sustains, or even heightens, the patient's sense of meaning, purpose, and peace. This, in turn, enables the patient to value the time remaining even more intensely and to make a positive appraisal of a life lived.[3,6,18] This is important in preventing the patient from becoming demoralized, which might lead to the triad of hopelessness, loss of meaning, and a desire for death.[3,18]

During the initial assessment, the nurse obtains a spiritual history to determine which faith and beliefs are meaningful to the patient, the importance of those beliefs, the influence of circumstances (past and present), and religious community involvement.[3] A spiritual assessment tool commonly used in palliative care is represented by the acronym FICA[46]:

F: What is your faith or belief?
I: Is it important in your life?
C: Are you part of a spiritual or religious community?
A: How would you like me, your health care provider, to address these issues in your health care?

Spirituality is an important component of many patients' physical well-being and mental health. The nurse addresses it at each visit, since spirituality is an ongoing issue. The nurse portrays an attitude of acceptance by respecting the patient's right to privacy regarding spiritual beliefs, not imposing personal beliefs on others, and referring the patient to the clergy of choice or palliative care clergy for additional spiritual support as needed. Personal spiritual beliefs overflow in encounters with patients. When health care providers understand their own values and beliefs, it allows the nurse-patient encounter to become more humanistic and effective.[46]

Grief, Bereavement, and Life Review

Grief is the response to the perception of loss and is transitional in the overall process of mourning. Grief has also been described as (1) deep mental anguish; (2) a normal reaction to the perception of loss; and (3) a transitory, acute state in response to loss, often with temporary disruption of the individual's ability to function.

Bereavement is the state of having suffered a loss and the condition of being left desolate or alone, especially by death. Simply put, bereavement is an overall reaction or a process. Mourning, a process initiated by loss, represents sociocultural and religious beliefs and values related to customs and rituals.[41]

Bereavement, grief, and mourning are all expected throughout our lives. Personally and professionally, nurses routinely confront death. Individual and societal attitudes toward dying and bereavement are formed by one's culture and responses to life experience. Individuals working with the bereaved need inspect their own attitudes and understand how these attitudes influence care. Reactions to grief, for professionals and laypersons, are highly variably and individualized. A person who has many experiences with death may still have difficulty coping, whereas a person inexperienced with death may face few problems. To understand how to provide palliative care bereavement, the nurse should understand the theories pertaining to bereavement.[1,41]

Phase Model of Grief

Bowlby developed the phase model of grief by exploring the instinctive attachment bonds between mother and child. He identified three phases of grief: the angry and longing phase, the disorganization and despair phase, and the reorganization phase. As the theory was adapted and applied to adults in research, a new first phase was added labeled numbness. Elisabeth Kübler-Ross applied this phase approach to the individual's psychologic adjustment to the diagnosis of life-threatening illness. Bowlby's theory recognized that it was not possible to develop a predictable course of events for grief. That being said, his model has been inaccurately used as a template for grieving by disregarding the individuality of the experience.[1] Table 8-7 summarizes the stages of grief proposed by various theorists.

Medical Model of Grief

Lindemann constructed a medical model of grief proposing that grief is similar to a disease that exhibits symptoms. This theory presents grief as a physiologic stressor that contributes to the manifestations of physical and emotional symptoms and acknowledges that symptoms are normal and should be expected in bereavement. A criticism of Lindemann's theory is that it categorizes some people who are grieving as mentally ill. However, research has shown that a small number of people experience complicated grief and do, therefore, have a potential for mental imbalance.[1,41]

TABLE 8-7 COMPARISON OF GRIEF THEORIES

Author	Initial Stage	Acute Grief	Recovery
Lindemann	Shock and disbelief	Acute mourning	Resolution
Kübler-Ross	Shock and denial	Anger Bargaining Depression	Acceptance
Bowlby	Numbing	Yearning and longing Disorganization and despair	Reorganization
Worden	Accepting reality	Experiencing the pain Withdrawing	Reinvesting Reacting to separation Recollecting and reexperiencing
Rando	Recognizing loss		Relinquishing old bonds Readjusting Reinvesting

Descriptive Model of Grief

Freud identified a descriptive model of grief as work, which is hard, painful, and time consuming. Freud theorized that since grief work is hard work, many people avoid dealing with their loss and hide their thoughts, feelings, and emotions. He recommended grieving on the surface, especially within the first few weeks. Freud's model laid the foundation for multiple modern day theories related to the tasks of mourning (Worden) and the stages of response (Kübler-Ross). Freud's theory falls short in acknowledging difficulties that some individuals have in openly showing their feelings and does not consider cultural variations in expression. This theory has, however, generated further study into the importance of the bereaved taking time in private for emotional release, and advocating for not forcing people to grieve.[1,41]

Bereavement Care

Bereavement care involves care of the family, information giving and receiving, care of the body (when appropriate), supporting mourning customs, legal and medical interventions, and ongoing support. Care is linked to the bereaved being ensured of the dying person's comfort. This assurance is also linked to facilitating the expression of emotions and understanding the individualized and private nature of grief. Palliative bereavement care is based on ongoing support, risk identification (see Risk Factors box), and levels of bereavement intervention (generalist support, intermediate care, and specialist counseling).[1,41]

Risk Factors

Bereavement
- Younger age
- Poor social support
- Sudden death
- Previous poor physical and mental health
- Limited coping strategies
- Multiple losses with unresolved grief
- Stigmatized death
- Financial difficulties
- Personality variables
- Learning disabilities

Data from Anstey S, Lewis M: Bereavement, grief, and mourning. In Kinghorn S, Gamlin R, editors: *Palliative nursing: bringing comfort and hope*, United Kingdom, 2001, Baillière Tindall.

Nursing Management

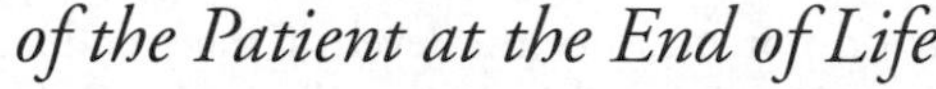

of the Patient at the End of Life

ASSESSMENT

Health History. Assess for:
- Awareness of clinical diagnosis and prognosis
- Perception of losses
- Fears (suffering, abandonment, loss of control, helplessness)
- Past experiences with major illnesses or crises
- Verbalizations of negative feelings ("Why me?" "I'm going crazy," "I'm lonely," "Life is empty")
- Comments regarding blame or guilt
- Suicidal ideation
- Verbalizations of doubts about past religious belief, faith, and fairness of the world
- Changes in eating, sleeping, or elimination
- Pain, headaches, fatigue, anorexia, constipation, abdominal pain, etc.
- Spiritual and cultural beliefs or preferences
- Presence (or absence) of personal support systems
- Coping mechanisms

Physical Examination. Assess for:
- Changes in respiratory system (tachypnea, Cheyne-Stokes respiration, dyspnea, lung crackles, airway obstruction, thick secretions)
- Changes in cardiac status (tachycardia, weak thready pulse, pallor, mottling)
- Decreased urine output; concentrated urine
- Increased, decreased, or absent bowel sounds

- Changes in mental status (confusion, disorientation, delirium, lethargy, apathy, surges of energy, stupor, absence of response to painful stimuli, coma)
- Restlessness, agitation, withdrawal, speaking to someone who is not there
- Cool, clammy skin; diaphoresis
- Oral lesions, skin lesions

NURSING DIAGNOSES, OUTCOMES, AND INTERVENTIONS

Nursing Diagnosis: Pain

OUTCOMES. Common examples of expected outcomes for the patient with a diagnosis of *pain* are:
Patient will:

- Identify pain as the body's means to protect itself.
- Identify tolerable level of pain using a scale of 0 (no pain) to 10 (too much to bear).
- Request prescribed analgesics or initiate appropriate noninvasive relief modalities before pain becomes intolerable.
- Report pain within stated tolerable level using descriptive words like sharp, dull, moving, or localized and a scale of 0 (no pain) to 10 (too much to bear).

NURSING INTERVENTIONS. Pain management is most effective when teaching is accomplished before the painful event. The nurse should discuss preventive measures such as deep breathing, oxygen use, and pharmacologic and nonpharmacologic measures at the onset of pain. The nurse needs to believe the patient's report of pain and act on it quickly. The nurse informs the patient that pain is best treated before it gets past the tolerable level and that pain is often coupled with anxiety. Remember that unresolved emotional and spiritual issues can exacerbate physical pain.

Pharmacologic agents are often prescribed on an as-needed basis for homebound patients. The nurse helps the patient develop a plan for noninvasive pain relief modalities such as distraction and relaxation to be used routinely to prevent episodes of pain.

Oral administration is the preferred route of analgesia in palliative care. If the patient is unable to take oral medications, subcutaneous, rectal, transdermal, or intravenous routes are considered. The initial occurrence of moderate to severe pain is treated with immediate-release opioids administered every 1 to 4 hours and as needed until the pain is controlled, then a sustained-release medication is used. Initial doses of pain medication are based on the number of 24-hour pain medication requirements plus the number of breakthrough doses (BTDs), divided by the appropriate dosing intervals. BTD is calculated as 10% of total 24-hour dose (or 1/2 the every 4-hour dose). To convert oral to subcutaneous dose, divide by 2.

BTDs should be available to the individual every hour as needed for oral medications and every 20 minutes as needed for subcutaneous medications. All BTD medications should be immediate release. If BTD medications are required in 24 hours for several days continuously, the regular dosage of pain medication is increased. Pain medication dosages are recalculated as needed to control pain. BTDs and stool softener or laxatives are ordered on initiation of opioids.[31,35,40,46]

RELATED NIC INTERVENTIONS. Analgesic Administration, Anxiety Reduction, Environmental Management: Comfort, Pain Management, Sedation Management

Nursing Diagnosis: Ineffective Breathing Pattern

OUTCOMES. Common examples of expected outcomes for the patient with a diagnosis of *ineffective breathing pattern* are:
Patient will:

- Describe breathing pattern based on self-perception of respiratory effort.
- Report that the feeling of respiratory demand has decreased.

NURSING INTERVENTIONS. The nurse assess patients with breathing difficulties for underlying cause(s), which are then treated. The mnemonic BREATH AIR explains specific causes:

- **B**ronchospasm
- **R**ales
- **E**ffusions
- **A**irway obstruction
- **T**hick secretions
- **H**emoglobin (low)
- **A**nxiety
- **I**nterpersonal issues
- **R**eligious concerns

Interventions for difficult breathing include reducing the need for exertion and arranging for help. The nurse helps the patient into an upright position to facilitate air intake and exchange. To improve air circulation in the room, the nurse opens a window or provides a fan. Humidity is adjusted with a humidifier or air conditioner. The nurse addresses anxiety by encouraging relaxation techniques and providing reassurance.

A balance between rest periods and breathing exercises and other physical activities helps the patient conserve energy. The nurse discusses home management with patient and caregiver regarding oxygen use and safety. And the nurses arranges ongoing monitoring within the home setting.

General symptomatic measures for dyspnea include administering supplemental oxygen at a rate to maintain O_2 saturation above 90% (with caution in patients with congestive obstructive pulmonary disease [COPD]). If O_2 saturation is less than 90% while the patient is breathing room air, oxygen is administered per nasal cannula at 1 to 3 L/min. Oxygen may be titrated up to 6 L/min depending on the patient's response and resolution of feelings of shortness of breath. An oxygen mask may be used if the nasal cannula is not effective. Oxygen is then titrated the same as with a nasal cannula. Both modes require patients to be reassessed every 20 minutes.

The extent of breathlessness may or may not correlate with O_2 saturation levels. For example, in patients with COPD, CO_2 may be chronically elevated and, therefore, fail to provide stimulus to breathe as it does in healthy people. Breathing is stimulated by low O_2 levels; therefore O_2 saturations are kept at around 90%.

In spite of concerns regarding the use of opioids for dyspnea, especially in older adults, morphine is the treatment of choice for breathlessness at the end of life. Opioids decrease the perception of dyspnea and consequently enhance comfort. BTDs may be ordered for those patients using opioids for pain management. If the patient is not taking opioids, immediate-release morphine at doses of 5 to 10 mg by mouth, or 2.5 to 5 mg subcutaneously, may be administered every 4 hours. Morphine may be titrated to control breakthrough dyspnea and administered every hour until dyspnea is relieved or sedation becomes problematic.

Expectorants are effective only if the cough reflex is present. Atropine ophthalmic drops (1 to 3 sublingual every 4 to 6 hours as needed) are effective if cough reflex is absent. Atropine is not recommended for cardiac patients unless death is imminent. Diuretics (furosemide, 20 to 40 mg subcutaneously) are used occasionally for patients with pulmonary congestion. Diuretics are not used routinely with patients for dyspnea or hypoalbuminemia-induced edema unless a concurrent heart condition requires diuretic use. Other medications that may control dyspnea are corticosteroids, bronchodilators, or anesthetics. Suctioning is generally not indicated for patients with dyspnea because secretions are generally below the larynx and inaccessible. Nebulized opioids are questionable or no benefit (no clear scientific or clinical basis to justify their use).[40,46,51]

The nurse informs the patient and family about the pathologic process involved with dyspnea and the intended goals of treatment, which are to modify the pathologic process, reduce the need for exertion, arrange for readily available help, and provide comfort.

RELATED NIC INTERVENTIONS. Airway Management, Anxiety Reduction, Respiratory Monitoring, Medication Administration, Oxygen Therapy

Nursing Diagnosis: Imbalanced Nutrition: Less Than Body Requirements

OUTCOMES. Common examples of expected outcomes for the patient with a diagnosis of *imbalanced nutrition: less than body requirements* are:

Patient (or family) will:

- Report control of nausea and vomiting.
- Identify foods of interest.
- Express feelings regarding lack of appetite and inability to eat.
- Discuss belief system surrounding nourishment through food and express feelings regarding loved one's inability to eat.

NURSING INTERVENTIONS. Treatment for nutritional deficit begins by assessing the patient's eating habits over the past 24 hours, 2 weeks, and 6 months; ability to swallow; presence or absence of bowel sounds; bowel habits; and mucous membranes in the mouth. The nurse also identifies smells that appear to be noxious to the patient.[40,46,51]

The nurse discusses dietary management strategies with the patient and family and provides information about anorexia, cachexia, and treatment limitations. For example, forcing patients to eat has no positive effect on well-being or survival. Parenteral nutrition is associated with morbidity and lack of benefit. It produces serious side effects in 15% of patients, and the financial cost is high. The nurse encourages intake of favorite foods for comfort and enjoyment, but cautions that their nutritional value is of limited importance. The nurse sets realistic goals that meet the patient's and family's needs.

If possible, the health care team tries to improve the patient's quality of life by relieving the underlying cause of imbalanced nutrition and treating exacerbating conditions such as constipation, oral candidiasis, nausea, pain, or depression. Gastrointestinal motility agents, such as metoclopramide, may be useful in relieving nausea so that patients can eat. Corticosteroids, such as dexamethasone (3 to 8 mg/day) may be administered to boost appetite on a trial basis. If the trial is successful, steroids are tapered slowly over a 3-week period. If the trial is unsuccessful, steroids are tapered more rapidly. Improvement is temporary, and side effects from steroids can be significant. Progestational agents such as megestrol acetate (Megace) or medroxyprogesterone acetate may be helpful in stimulating appetite when anorexia is present. Dronabinol (Marinol) has demonstrated effectiveness in stimulating appetite in patients with acquired immunodeficiency syndrome; however, the drug can cause mental disturbances and is cost prohibitive. Alcohol with meals may also increase appetite.[40,46,51]

RELATED NIC INTERVENTIONS. Diet Staging, Medication Management, Nutrition Management, Self-Care Assistance: Feeding

Nursing Diagnosis: Anxiety

OUTCOMES. Common examples of expected outcomes for the patient with a diagnosis of *anxiety* are:

Patient will:

- Report a tolerable level of anxiety, or no anxiety, using a 0 (no anxiety) to 10 (unable to cope with anxiety) scale.

NURSING INTERVENTIONS. The nurse establishes a therapeutic and trusting relationship with patient and tries to identify the underlying type and cause of anxiety. *Situational anxiety* generally occurs when the patient worries about family, finances, physical condition, isolation, abandonment, role loss, or an uncertain future. *Drug-related anxiety* may occur when the patient worries about therapies commonly used in palliative care, or experiences drug-induced hallucinations or medication withdrawal from benzodiazepines or opioids. *Organic anxiety* occurs from uncontrolled pain, dyspnea, hypoxia, weakness, hypoglycemia, or insomnia. Causes of *psychologic anxiety* may be related to patient's inner world, such as existential distress, hopelessness, fear of mental impairment, fear of pain, thoughts about death, or regrets about the past.

Treatment begins with nonpharmacologic therapy that involves a multidisciplinary assessment, treatment of reversible causes, spiritual support, and short-term psychotherapy. If nonpharmacologic therapies are ineffective, benzodiazepine for simple anxiety or tranquilizers for severe anxiety with hallucinations need to be considered.

RELATED NIC INTERVENTIONS. Anxiety Reduction, Calming Technique, Coping Enhancement, Distraction Presence, Simple Guided Imagery, Simple Relaxation Therapy

Nursing Diagnosis: Constipation

OUTCOMES. Common examples of expected outcomes for the patient with a diagnosis of *constipation* are:

Patient will:

- Verbalize measures to promote bowel movements and prevent constipation.
- Have a bowel movement at least every 3 days.

NURSING INTERVENTIONS. Prevention is considered first-line treatment for constipation. The nurse encourages generous fluid intake (8 to10 glasses per day). Dietary fiber intake is gradually increased. Metamucil, which requires a greater increase in fluid intake, is avoided. The nurse encourages the patient to exercise as tolerated. Stool softeners or laxatives are started simultaneously with opiates (senna, 1 to 2 tablets at bedtime, plus docusate, 100 mg twice a day by mouth). They are titrated upward until bowel movements occur regularly (every 1 or 2 days). If no bowel movement occurs in 3 days, a Fleet enema or bisacodyl suppository is administered. For patients who are not taking opiates, laxatives or softeners are started while the stool is soft. If stool becomes hard, laxatives or stool softeners are increased until regular bowel movements return. Senna may be increased up to 2 to 4 tablets four times a day, and docusate may be increased up to 240 mg four times a day as needed.[40,46,51]

If the patient does not have a bowel movement following a Fleet enema or bisacodyl, an oil retention enema is administered followed by a soapsuds enema several hours later (a high phosphosoda enema may be substituted for a soapsuds enema for frail, debilitated patients). If impaction occurs in the proximal colon, magnesium citrate up to 250 ml by mouth may be ordered.

RELATED NIC INTERVENTIONS. Bowel Management, Constipation/Impaction Management, Fluid Management, Nutrition Management

EVALUATION

To evaluate the effectiveness of nursing interventions, compare patient behaviors with those stated in the expected patient outcomes.

RELATED NOC OUTCOMES. Anxiety Level, Bowel Elimination, Comfort Level, Coping, Fear Level, Fluid Balance, Nutritional Status, Pain Control, Pain Level, Sleep, Symptom Control

GERONTOLOGIC CONSIDERATIONS

Gerontologic palliative care includes the palliation of symptoms related to chronic illness. Older adults may have multiple chronic conditions (e.g., heart disease, COPD) that can worsen at any time. Although these older adults, their families, and their primary care providers may not think of these diseases as terminal, they are, and the older patient would greatly benefit from palliative care services. Symptomatic congestive heart failure, chronic lung disease, dementia, stroke, recurrent infection accompanying cancer, and degenerative joint disease causing functional impairment and chronic pain are disease-specific reasons to initiate palliative care.[36]

The nursing home is an appropriate environment in which to offer palliative care services. Federal policies from the 1980s resulted in shorter hospital stays and increased use of nursing homes. On a given day, 1.5 million Americans are in a nursing home. Nearly one in two persons who lives to his or her eighties will spend time in a nursing home before death. By 2020, it is estimated that 40% of Americans will die in nursing homes.[4a] Already, in some states nearly 40% of Americans die in nursing homes. The question remains, though, whether nursing homes are prepared to care for increasingly sick, old, and dying residents.

A 1998 *JAMA* study found that 40% of cancer patients discharged to a nursing home had daily pain. Of those in pain, one in four did not have any analgesic prescribed, not even acetaminophen. This study found that 41.2% of persons who had pain at their first assessment also had either moderate daily pain or an excruciating level of pain at their next assessment (completed 60 to 180 days later).[4a] Of those persons with two Minimum Data Set assessments, one in seven was in persistent severe pain.

Nurse's Grief

Nurses also experience loss when a patient dies. It is important for nurses to recognize the universal experience, as well as signs of their own grieving. Losing a patient can remind nurses of other losses of patients, family, or friends. Nurses may view a patient's death as a personal failure, with a corresponding loss of control or self-esteem. If the nurse is unable to help prevent suffering or resolve a family's conflict before a patient's death, the nurse may feel inadequate. It is crucial for nurses to evaluate the differences they have made for their patients and their families, even in the face of death. Recognition of specific successes and contributions leads to feelings of achievement and helps nurses cope with the loss. Cumulative loss over time can challenge nurses' well-being and professional satisfaction.[50]

Like patients and their families, nurses need a supportive environment in which to express their grief. Many institutions establish bereavement resources for health care workers, ranging from on-call employee assistance programs, to walk-in pastoral care, to group debriefing sessions with a trained facilitator. Peer support is an important source of validation and grief support. Peer support can be accomplished through formal or informal sharing of common experiences in a group setting. One-on-one interactions with a trusted peer or significant other may alleviate some of the stress related to working with dying persons.[50] Although potentially stressful, caring for patients and their families at the end of life offers nurses countless opportunities to make a difference in promoting quality of living and dying.

Ethical Considerations

Historically the profession and activities of nursing have been concerned with life and based on two fundamental principles: all people should live as whole persons, and all people should live long and healthy lives. The expectation has been that nurses and physicians will help fulfill these principles.[50]

In the past, when death was often caused by infection and communicable disease, nurses and physicians fulfilled their obligations by striving to save lives. Our capacity to prolong life and to ease the pain and suffering of seriously ill persons has greatly improved, but not without consequences. Increasingly, deaths occur in institutions, often in critical care units to the sound of monitors. More and more often, death is a result of someone's decision rather than the failure of the body systems. Death becomes impersonal when the body and the tubes and machines become one and there is only a deteriorating organ system present. The situation becomes so confusing that those involved have conferences to determine whether life or death is being prolonged.[32]

Discussions of issues such as "quality of life," "right to die," "death with dignity," "living wills," and "informed consent" in lay and professional literature demonstrate the public's awareness of the conflicts associated with modern therapies that extend life, but at great cost.[50] Concern over decisions regarding life-and-death issues has led to the development of organizations that represent differing views, such as the Hemlock Society, the Society for the Right to Die, and the Americans United for Life.

The question of who should decide under what circumstances is important. Other important questions include: What is death? What constitutes informed consent? When are therapies ordinary, and when are they extraordinary? Should all life be preserved, regardless of quality? Should pain be treated, even though the medication may shorten the life span? What is euthanasia? Is there a distinction between active and passive euthanasia? Is suicide a person's right? All these questions create ethical issues that can make coping with death and dying overwhelming for patients, family members, and the health care team.[30]

Many ethical issues revolve around indications for nursing and medical interventions. These issues arise from questions such as: When should medical therapies be started or stopped? When should life supports be discontinued? What constitutes death? In the 1980s hospitals began establishing ethics committees as mechanism to deal with such clinical dilemmas and develop policies regarding the appropriate use of medical technology. Generally ethics committees provide consultation for difficult cases and make policy recommendations. Although individual ethics committees vary in their membership, most are composed of physicians, nurses, allied health professionals, clergy, social workers, and various ethicists.

Withholding or Withdrawing Treatment

It is appropriate to consider withholding or withdrawing specific therapy when the therapy offers no reasonable expectation of helping the patient attain any human awareness; the therapy is proving medically ineffective and useless after sufficient trial; or the patient (or decision-making representative) has expressed the view that the therapy is cumulatively a greater burden than a benefit.

When decisions are made to withhold or withdraw life-sustaining treatment, the goal of medical and nursing care focuses on keeping the patient comfortable; preventing suffering and pain; and providing support, comfort, and care on physical, emotional, and spiritual levels. Identifying those procedures not directed to supportive care becomes more difficult once medical procedures designed to prolong life are withheld or withdrawn. Perhaps the most controversial area is that of determining the proportionate benefit and burden of medical (artificial) nutrition and hydration.[50] The issue of withdrawing treatment, once it is started, is also difficult.

Euthanasia

The term *euthanasia* comes from the Greek words meaning "good or pleasant death." It implies that under some circumstances a person may prefer death to life. **Euthanasia**, or "mercy killing," is a topic surrounded by controversy. There is no agreement on whether death is ever preferable to life or on what constitutes euthanasia.[44]

The more common distinctions made when discussing euthanasia are those of active, passive, voluntary, and involuntary. *Active euthanasia* refers to an act that directly and intentionally shortens a person's life. It is an act of commission. *Passive euthanasia* usually refers to an act of omission—letting death occur by either withholding or withdrawing treatment that might prolong a person's life.[44] In questions related to euthanasia, a continuum ranges from a strict belief in the sanctity of life (antieuthanasia, treatment at all costs) to passive euthanasia (letting die) to active euthanasia (ending life, killing).

A persistent moral issue is the question of whether letting death occur is morally equivalent to killing, or whether omission is equivalent to commission. No action is an action. Both active and passive euthanasia are intentional choices. The distinction seems to be that of the intent. The 2002 statement from the American Medical Association Council on Ethical and Judicial Affairs holds that the patient or immediate family can decide to "discontinue all means of life-prolonging medical treatment" even "if death is not imminent but a patient's coma is beyond doubt irreversible."[8] Some ethicists distinguish ordinary treatment from extraordinary treatment by stating that ordinary treatment offers a reasonable prospect of benefit for the patient without excessive pain, expense, or inconvenience.[24,44] Extraordinary treatment refers to measures such as artificial nutrition or hydration or mechanical ventilation.

In more direct terms, killing is wrong, but letting someone die in the sense of not instituting extraordinary efforts or by discontinuing extraordinary treatments is morally permissible. In fact, most physicians accept that killing a patient is morally wrong and thus not permissible, but in some circumstances, it may become morally required to let a patient die. Nurses generally accept the same view.

Laws provide the framework for decision making in regard to many end-of-life issues, whereas ethical principles offer guidelines about what "should" be done in a given situation (see Legal Alert box).

Legal Alert

Is It a Legal or Ethical Issue?

Sometimes determining whether an end-of-life issue is a legal or ethical issue can be difficult. Ethics involves principles that are weighed and balanced to determine what "ought" to be done in a given situation. Law, on the other hand, is based on the values of society and reflects that society's consensus on a particular issue such as informed consent. In some situations something may be permissible based on ethical principles, but illegal under the law. The converse may also be true. Laws vary among societies and states. Laws are helpful because they provide the framework for decision making when ethical principles are inadequate. Common law guides decision making for end-of-life issues such as informed consent or withholding or withdrawing treatment. Statutory law guides decision making for issues such as do-not-resuscitate orders, physician-assisted suicide, and the Uniform Definition of Death Act.

Suicide

Quality of living and quality of dying may be closely associated. A person with a terminal illness may assess the situation and decide that living with pain, disability, or despair is not living. He or she may ask the question, Is it better to take measures to bring about a peaceful death than to continue in such a state?

Suicide, or voluntary euthanasia carried out by the individual on his or her own behalf, has been seen variously as an affirmation of life, a denial of life, and a questioning of life. The traditional religious teachings of the Western world condemn all forms of self-destruction. Some people consider suicide to be a sin and an interference with God's will.[44] Many assert that human beings do not have the right to dispose of their bodies. They can only treat their bodies as they choose in relation to self-preservation. These views have been challenged in the past and are challenged today.[13] Some physicians believe that under certain circumstances, when death is imminent, persons who are severely ill have the right to be helped by their physician to commit suicide. However, few laws exist in the United States to cover physician participation in assisted suicide. Oregon is an exception; the state does have such laws. Other countries, such as the Netherlands, Uruguay, Switzerland, Peru, Japan, and Germany, do have such laws.

Suicide is of particular concern to health care professionals who may be in a position to offer alternatives and thus prevent it. It is difficult to evaluate what constitutes suicide. Is refusal to eat or to continue with prescribed therapies a form of suicide, or must there be an overt act, such as an overdose of medications? Is suicide always a voluntary act, or is a person driven to suicide by rejection of others or by pain that might have been controlled? When is suicide justifiable for a person known to be dying? What do you do when a patient who is dying slowly and painfully asks for your assistance in ending it all?

Nurses and physicians are committed to another imperative: never abandon care. Never abandoning care includes ensuring that a dying person is not alone, that others are aware of his or her dying, and that he or she is free of pain and anxiety. It is not an obligation to assist in ending life. In fact, the ethical basis for suicide prevention is the psychologic thesis that a suicide attempt is often a cry for help rather than a firm decision to end one's life.[44,50] Thus nurses and physicians have a legal and ethical obligation to assess and recognize patients' suicidal risk and depression and to make efforts to help them receive counseling.[44]

The impact of pain is really a quality-of-life question that can best be evaluated by the dying individual experiencing the pain. If quality of life is determined by the person living the life, is suicide a purely personal decision? It seems that the quality of life of survivors also should be considered. When the survivors have had no warning or part in the decision, and when they do not see the suicide as an action to achieve comfort, their anguish may be great. For some the anguish never ends; grief is compounded by guilt, shame, and even anger.[17]

Suicide may be a form of control by the dying person, or it may be a form of escape. Some dying people seek an escape from loss of control over the event of dying; others seek an end to suffering.[49] Nurses can be influential in providing dying persons and their families with a sense of control by assisting with problems such as pain, bowel and bladder control, and depression. They can decrease the uncertainty of the situation by explaining what the dying person and family can anticipate over the coming days.

Nurses can also involve other members of the interdisciplinary team in offering the dying patient and family tangible support through referrals.[17] Music, art therapy, and imagery can help patients and their family express and work through the process of grieving, as well as provide relaxation and diversion from symptom distress.[28] Pastoral care can offer opportunities for dying patients and their families to make sense of their experience in terms of their religious beliefs.[2,44] Social workers can facilitate family communication and end-of-life planning when conflicts are present. By coordinating involvement of the interdisciplinary team, nurses can further enhance quality of life.

Definitions of Death

Much controversy surrounds the question, What is death? Is death the irreversible cessation of respiration and circulation, or is death the irreversible cessation of all functions of the brain, including the brainstem?

The term **brain dead**, in use for some time, still causes much confusion. Originally, it referred to a person whose lungs were activated by a ventilator but whose centers in the brainstem were destroyed. Removal from the support system would result in death because of the patient's inability to resume spontaneous breathing. *Brain dead* also means that the person is dead in the sense that a functioning brain is the seat of identity. How does this apply to persons in a persistent vegetative state? They show no evidence of cortical functioning but have sustained capacity for spontaneous breathing and heartbeat.[2,44]

Advocates use definitions that reflect their values and provide them with a rationale to act. Each appeal or action has its own consequences. For example, some definitions of brain death provide more latitude for organ transplantation and experimentation. The rationale for this latitude is that the removal of organs from the person who is brain dead aids the living. This is a worthy endeavor, but does retrieving organs constitute violation of the dead? What are the constraints? Who gives consent for donation? There are no clear rules that dictate decisions in these matters. Decisions are accompanied by conflict, insecurity, and discomfort—entirely appropriate emotions, since the decisions are irreversible.[24,44]

The important factor in any ethical issue, regardless of whether it is dealing with euthanasia, suicide, or treatment decisions, is to be aware of the values or forces that lead us to make the decisions we do. An understanding of one's own values and perspectives, as well as of formal ethical systems, does not give explicit answers to dilemmas. However, it does help with consistency and the ability to understandably communicate with others. This does not ensure agreement, but it does facilitate discussion and attention to different perspectives and to the consequences of actions.

? Critical Thinking

1. You are the night nurse at a small community hospital. You are caring for an 81-year-old woman with congestive heart failure, type 1 diabetes mellitus, and anemia. She has needed

multiple hospitalizations in the past 6 months and suffers from extreme fatigue and dyspnea at rest. Her status is full code. She calls you into her room asking for help repositioning in bed. While you help her, she confides in you that she does not want any more aggressive treatment and feels she has lived a blessed life full of happiness. She wants to change her code status to do-not-resuscitate, but has not discussed it with her family. What do you do next?

2. You are caring for an older man in the first stage of senile dementia who was recently diagnosed with metastatic lung cancer. The physician has told the family that no curative treatments are available and that comfort care is the only option. The family asks you and the rest of the nursing staff not to tell the patient that he has cancer. What do you do?

References

1. Anstey S, Lewis M: Bereavement, grief, and mourning. In Kinghorn S, Gamlin R, editors: *Palliative nursing: bringing comfort and hope,* United Kingdom, 2001, Baillière Tindall.
2. Berry P, Griffe J: Planning the actual death. In Ferrell B, Coyle N, editors: *Palliative nursing,* New York, 2001, Oxford University Press
3. Breitbart W: Spirituality and meaning in supportive care: spirituality-and meaning-centered group psychotherapy interventions in advanced cancer, *Support Care Cancer* 10(4):272–280, 2001.
4. Brennan M et al: *Pharmacologic management of breakthrough or incident pain,* Feb 26, 2003, accessed May 2003 from website: medscape.com.

4a. Brock DB, Foley DJ: Demography and epidemiology of dying in the United States with emphasis on death of older persons, *Hospice J* 13(1):49–60, 1998.

5. Centers for Medicare and Medicaid Services: *Hospice manual, Chapter 2, Coverage of services,* accessed Oct 2002 from website: http://cms.hhs.gov/manuals/21_hospice/hs200.asp.
6. Chochinov M: Dignity-conserving care: a new model for palliative care, *JAMA* 287(17):2253–2259, 2002.
7. Commonwealth Fund: *Findings from the Commonwealth Fund 2002 International Health Policy Survey, The United States Health Care System: Views and Experiences of Adults with Health Problems,* 2003, accessed from website: http://www.cmwf.org.
8. Council on Ethical and Judicial Affairs, American Medical Association: *Withholding or withdrawing life-sustaining medical treatment,* 2002, accessed from website: http://www.ama-assn.org/ama/pub/category/8457.html.
9. Cowan J, Walsh D: Terminal sedation in palliative medicine—definition and review of literature, *Support Care Cancer* 9:403–407, 2001.
10. Davis M, Walsh D: Treatment of nausea and vomiting in advanced cancer, *AAHPM Bull* Fall 2001, pp 4, 5, 9, 15.
11. Duquette C: *Improving function and quality of life for older adults through pain assessment and management,* presented to National Conference of Gerontological Nurse Practitioners, 2002, accessed Sept 2003 from website: medscape.com.
12. Emanuel L: Ethics and pain management: an introductory overview, *Pain Med* 2(2):112–116, 2001.
13. Engel G: A life setting conducive to illness: the giving-up-given-up complex, *Ann Intern Med* 69(2):293–300, 1968.
14. Ross DD, Alexander CS: Management of common symptoms in terminally ill patients, Part I, *Am Fam Physician* 64(5):807–814, 2001.
15. Fagerlin A, Schneider C: Enough: the failure of the living will, *Hastings Center Rep* 34(2):30–42, 2004.
16. Ferris F, von Gunten C, Emanuel L: Ensuring competency in end-of-life care: controlling symptoms, *BMC Palliative Care* 1:15, 2002, accessed from website: http.//www.biomedcentral.com/1472–684X/1/5.
17. Fine C, Myers M: Suicide survivors: tips for health professionals, *Medscape Gen Med* 5(3), 2003, accessed from website: http://www.medscape.com/viewarticle/460958.
18. Haes H, Koedoot N: Patient centered decision-making in palliative cancer treatment: a world of paradoxes, *Pat Educ Counsel* 50:43–49, 2003.
19. Hopper S: *Moving palliative care into the community: new services, new strategies,* New York, 2004, United Hospital Fund.
20. Hudson P, Sanchia A, Kristjanson L: Meeting the supportive needs of family caregivers in palliative care: challenges for health professionals, *J Palliative Med* 7(1):19–25, 2004.
21. Jevine RF, Miller JE: *Finding hope: ways to see life in a brighter light,* Fort Wayne, Ind, 1999, Willogreen Publishing.
22. Karloawish J, Quill T, Meier D: A consensus-based approach to providing palliative care to patients who lack decision-making capacity, *Ann Intern Med* 130:435–440, 1999.
23. Kingsbury R: *Palliative sedation: may we sleep before we die?* Center for Bioethics and Human Dignity, 2001, accessed Nov 2001 from website: www.cbhd.org/newletter/012/01kingsbury.htm.
24. Kramer L et al: The nurse's role in interdisciplinary and palliative care. In Ferrell B, Coyle N, editors: *Palliative nursing,* New York, 2001, Springer.
25. Lenz K: The pharmacology of symptom control. In Taylor G, Kurent J, editors: *A clinician's guide to palliative care,* Malden, Mass, 2003, Blackwell Publishing.
26. Reference deleted in proofs.
27. Maluso-Bolton T: Terminal agitation, *J Hospice Palliative Nurs* 2(1):9–20, 2000.
28. Mariano C: Holistic integrative therapies in palliative care. In Matzo M, Sherman D, editors: *Palliative care nursing: quality care to the end of life,* New York, 2001, Springer.
29. Reference deleted in proofs.
30. Matzo M: Peri-death nursing care. In Matzo M, Sherman D, editors: *Palliative care nursing education: toward quality care at the end of life,* New York, 2001, Springer.
31. National Pain Eduction Council: *Progress in chronic pain management: chronic pain syndromes: cancer, chronic lower back pain, osteoarthritis, fibromyalgia,* 2002, http://www.npecweb.org/default.asp.
32. Metzer M, Kaplan K: *Transforming death in America: a state of the nation report,* Washington, DC, 2001, Last Acts.
33. Morita T, Tsuneto S, Shima Y: Proposed definitions for terminal sedation, *Lancet* 358:335–336, 2001.
34. Morita T et al: Underlying pathologies and their associations with clinical features in terminal delirium of cancer patients, *J Pain Symptom Manage* 22(6):997–1006, 2001.
35. Morley JS, Makin MK: The use of methadone in cancer pain poorly responsive to other opioids, *Pain Rev* 5:51–58, 1998.
36. Morrison RS, Meier D: Introduction. In Morrison RS, Meier D, editors: *Geriatric palliative care,* New York. 2003, Oxford University Press.
37. National Consensus Project for Quality Palliative Care: *Clinical practice guidelines for quality palliative care,* 2004, accessed from website: www.nationalconsensusproject.org.
38. Pan C et al: How prevalent are hospital-based palliative care programs? Status report and future directions, *J Palliative Med* 4(3):315–324, 2001.
39. Partnership for Solutions, Johns Hopkins University: *Chronic conditions: making the case for ongoing care,* Baltimore, 2002, Johns Hopkins University Press.
40. Pereira J, Bruera E: *The Alberta palliative care resource,* Edmonton, 2001, Division of Palliative Care Medicine University of Alberta.
41. Potter M: Loss, suffering, bereavement, and grief. In Matzo M, Sherman D, editors: *Palliative care nursing: quality care to the end of life,* New York, 2001, Springer.
42. Prendergast TJ, Puntillo KA: Withdrawal of life support, *JAMA* 288(21):2732–2740, 2002.
43. Rushton C, Spencer K, Johanson W: Bringing end-of-life care out of the shadows, *Nurs Manage* 35(3):34–40, 2004.
44. Schwarz J: Ethical aspects of palliative care. In Matzo M, Sherman D, editors: *Palliative care nursing: quality care to the end of life,* New York, 2001, Springer.
45. Singer P, Bowman K: Quality of end-of-life care: a global perspective, *BMC Palliative Care* 1(4), 2002, accessed from website: http://www.biomedcentral.com/I472-684X/I/4.

46. Storey P, Knight C, Schonwetter R: *Pocket guide to hospice/palliative medicine*, Glenview, Ill, 2003, American Academy of Hospice and Palliative Medicine.
47. SUPPORT: A controlled trial to improve care for seriously ill hospitalized patients, *JAMA* 22/29(274):20, 1591–1598, 1995.
48. Tyler L: Nausea and vomiting in palliative care. In Lipman A, Jackson K, Tyler L, editors: *Evidence based symptom control in palliative care,* New York, 2000, Pharmaceutical Products Press.
49. University of Michigan Health System: *Suicide: what is suicide?* Accessed 2003 from website: http://www.med.umich.edu/1libr/aha/aha_suicide_bha.htm.
50. Vachon M: The nurse's role: the world of palliative care nursing. In Ferrell B, Coyle N, editors: *Palliative nursing*, New York, 2001, Oxford University Press.
51. Vancouver Island Health Authority: *Palliative care symptom management guidelines,* Victoria, 2003, Seniors Community & Home Community Care Central Island.
52. Reference deleted in proofs.
53. World Health Organization: *Definition of palliative care*, accessed June 2004 from website: http://www.who.int/cancer/palliative/definition/en/.
54. Zhukovsky D: A model of palliative care: the palliative medicine program of the Cleveland Clinic Foundation, *Support Care Cancer* 27(8):268–277, 2000.

evolve Visit the Evolve website: http://evolve.elsevier.com/Monahan/medsurg

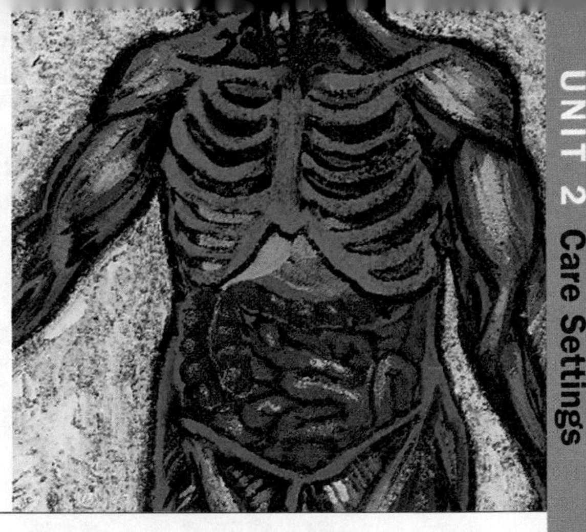

CHAPTER 9

Emergency Care

by Marianne Neighbors

OBJECTIVES

After studying this chapter, the learner should be able to:

1. Discuss the unique challenges of nursing practice in an emergency care setting.
2. List the most common types of trauma and interventions to prevent trauma.
3. Identify the components of an initial trauma assessment.
4. Describe the principles of collaborative management of the trauma patient.
5. Discuss the role of the emergency department nurse in caring for a person who was sexually assaulted.
6. Outline the guidelines for care of victims of intimate partner violence.

KEY TERMS

critical pathways, p. 181
emergency department, p. 179
Emergency Medical Treatment and Active Labor Act, p. 181
emergent condition, p. 180
Good Samaritan statute, p. 184
level I, level II, or level III trauma centers, p. 185
multiple trauma, p. 186
rape trauma syndrome, p. 188
sexual assault, p. 187
standardized four color–coded triage system, p. 180
trauma, p. 183
triage, p. 180

Emergency nursing is a diverse and multidimensional specialty area of professional nursing. It includes care for all age-groups that ranges from disease management and injury prevention to lifesaving resuscitative measures. Astute decision-making abilities, analytic and scientific inquiry, and critical thinking skills are very much a part of the practice of the nurse in the **emergency department** (ED).

More than 39 million people seek assistance in hospital EDs each year.[4] These patients come to the ED with a variety of problems, some of which are life threatening (Table 9-1). The demands on ED nurses continue to grow and become more challenging as health care changes, with an increased incidence of violence, greater numbers of uninsured, and the advent of managed care. Managed care, one of the primary financing mechanisms for health care, is of great importance in current ED practice as insurance programs increasingly dictate who receives care, what care can be provided, and which care settings may be used. The challenge of providing health care to the large numbers of uninsured and underinsured individuals and families falls heavily on departments of emergency services, which are commonly used in lieu of a primary care provider. Combined market forces and legislation seem to indicate that managed care payment mechanisms will continue to be a major force in health care for the near future.

This chapter on emergency care provides an overview of the unique environment of emergency nursing, triage practice, trauma assessment, and the impact of violence on emergency nursing practice.

Scope of Practice for Emergency Nursing

The scope of emergency nursing practice encompasses assessment, analysis, nursing diagnosis, outcome identification, planning, implementation of interventions, and evaluation. The problems addressed may be perceived, actual, or potential; sudden or urgent; physical or psychosocial; and primarily episodic or acute.[8] Treatment of these problems may require minimal care or lifesaving measures, patient and family education, appropriate referral, and discharge planning. The quality of practice depends on the nurse's psychomotor, interpersonal, and decision-making skills. Nurses deliver this care in a variety of settings, including acute care facilities; prehospital and military settings; clinics and health maintenance organizations; ambulatory care centers; and business, educational, industrial, and correctional institutions. Box 9-1 lists some of the unique characteristics of emergency nursing practice. The Emergency Nurses Association developed the standards of practice for emergency nurses.[7]

TABLE 9-1 INJURY-RELATED VISITS TO HOSPITAL EMERGENCY DEPARTMENTS

	Injury-Related Visits Per 10,000 Persons	
Type of Injury	**Male**	**Female**
Falls	1377.0	1636.7
Struck by or against objects or persons	1083.1	529.2
Motor vehicle accident	906.2	874.8
Cut or piercing	768.4	359.6
Other unintentional injuries	6132.5	4873.8

Data from Centers for Disease Control and Prevention, National Center for Health Statistics: *Fast stats A to Z: all injuries, injury-related visits to hospital emergency departments by sex, age, and intent and mechanism of injury: United States, 2000-2001,* accessed Aug 2004 from website: www.cdc.gov.

Box 9-1 Characteristics of Emergency Nursing Practice

- Assessment, analysis, nursing diagnosis, planning, implementation of interventions, outcome identification, and evaluation of human responses of individuals in all age-groups
- Care that is complicated by the limited access to medical history and the episodic nature of the health care
- Triage and prioritization
- Emergency operations preparedness
- Stabilization and resuscitation
- Crisis intervention for unique patient populations, such as sexual assault survivors
- Provision of care in uncontrolled or unpredictable environments
- Consistency as much as possible across the continuum of care

From Emergency Nurses Association: *Scope of emergency nursing practice,* 1999, accessed March 2005 from website: www.ena.org.

Emergency nursing activities occur in a sequential arrangement or flow pattern based on the acuity of the person's condition. Most persons who request ED service are ambulatory and have nonacute conditions; many EDs have developed a specific care area, often termed *fast track* or *urgent care,* to identify a designated area in or near the ED for persons with nonacute conditions. These areas may be open only after physicians' offices have closed, or they may provide quick service 12 to 24 hours a day. Fast-track or urgent care areas are less expensive treatment areas than the ED. Persons treated in these areas require less time with the health care staff compared with the typical ED patient because of the nature of their signs and symptoms. Regardless of whether EDs are designed to separate the nonacute from the acutely ill person, and regardless of ability to pay, a nurse must evaluate every person requesting care on arrival.

Triage

All patients coming to the ED need to be accurately triaged. The word **triage** means to sort or sift out. It is a systematic method health care personnel use in both prehospital situations and EDs.

Box 9-2 Four Color–Coded Disaster Triage System

0—Black: Dead

I—Red: Critical or Life Threatening

These victims have a reasonable chance of survival only if they receive immediate treatment. Emergency treatment is initiated immediately and continued during transportation. This category includes victims with respiratory insufficiency, cardiac arrest, hemorrhage, and severe abdominal injury.

II—Yellow: Serious

These victims can wait for transportation after they receive initial emergency treatment. They include victims with immobilized closed fractures, soft-tissue injuries without hemorrhage, and burns on less than 40% of the body.

III—Green: Minimal

Victims in this category are ambulatory, have minor tissue injuries, and may be dazed. They can be treated by nonprofessionals and held for observation if necessary.

In the ED a registered nurse uses the triage system to identify those patients whose condition is most seriously compromised so that they are the first to receive medical intervention. This method of placing priorities on care has been practiced since patient care began and has been used extensively in disasters and wars. A **standardized four color–coded triage system** (used during disasters) quietly communicates to all health care providers the priority of treatment (Box 9-2 and Figure 9-1).

The most important function of triage is to provide an initial assessment of patients, assign a triage urgency category, and direct each person to the right place at the right time. Persons who need to be seen immediately have an **emergent condition,** or life-threatening situation; persons who need to be seen as soon as possible have an urgent condition that has the potential of becoming life threatening; and persons who can be seen as time allows have nonurgent conditions, with no life-threatening symptoms at the time of presentation and no symptoms that typically become life

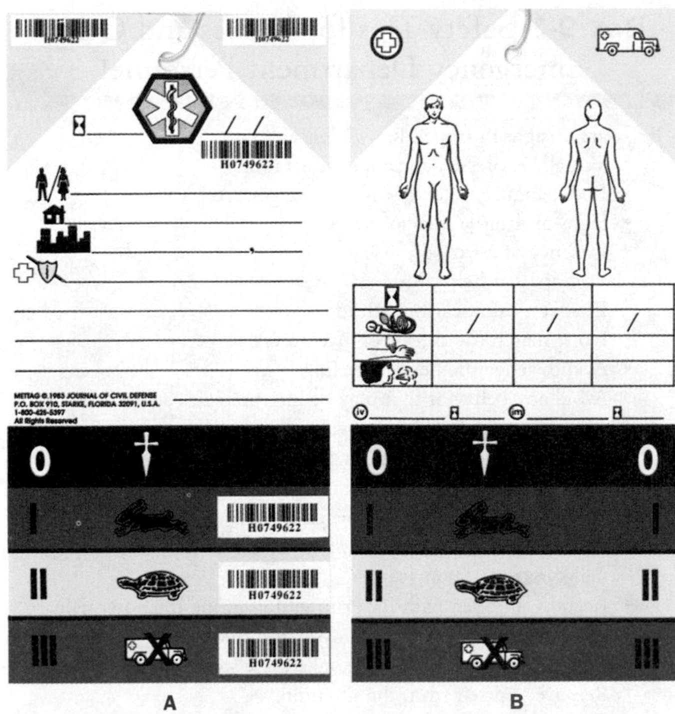

Figure 9-1 Medical emergency field triage tag. A, Front. B, Back. The color-coded triage tag system is used to denote the victim's status at the initial assessment point in the field. This assessment may change as the victim is more thoroughly assessed at another time or if the victim's status changes. The tag is attached to the victim and the layers torn off up to the color matching the assessment by the triage person. Notes or a name can also be added to the tag (if time permits).

threatening. The emergency medical service (EMS) system uses this system of prioritization of patients. The use of common terms helps staff understand the situation and communicate uniformly for both prehospital and in-hospital care.

Fast-track or urgent care areas treat patients with urgent or nonurgent conditions. Persons with emergent conditions are seen in the main ED area. To increase efficiency and improve patient outcome, many EDs have developed a chest pain center (CPC) within their department to immediately diagnose and treat acute myocardial infarctions. Patients are triaged directly into the CPC with a triage category of emergent.

Triage, Managed Care, and the Uninsured. All ED health care providers must be well informed about provisions of the Consolidated Omnibus Reconciliation Acts (COBRA) and the **Emergency Medical Treatment and Active Labor Act (EMTALA)**, which outline guidelines for service provision and reimbursement in EDs. The EMTALA provisions require that each patient who comes to the ED receive a screening examination to determine whether an emergency condition exists. Many patients who belong to a managed care organization come to the ED without the required preauthorization. The responsibility for providing a medical screening examination and securing preauthorization then falls on the ED staff. Approximately 3 of 10 emergency room patients are uninsured. This has become a national emergency of its own. About three fourths of the cost of caring for this group in the ED is paid by the government, private insurers, and self-pay patients.[12] Health care stakeholders will need to address this problem in the near future.

Triage and Computerized Tracking. A universal concern in all EDs is patient flow. Computerized tracking provides clinicians with an automated patient locator board. Patient name, arrival time, chief complaint, and caregiver names are available on the screen. Registration and triage personnel are always aware of open beds and the location of patients via the patient tracking systems.

Tracking systems take advantage of abbreviations, symbols, color codes, and icons to note current patient status. Many systems also use color codes to identify which caregivers have already seen a patient, as well as admission or discharge pending information. The tracking system can also improve efficiency in gathering triage information during initial patient assessment and is an excellent tool for research and analysis of department utilization. Computerized tracking also improves communication among department personnel.

Critical Pathways in Emergency Departments

Time tracking of patients in the ED is essential to ensure the provision of high-quality care for many reasons. It allows quality assurance teams to track workload activity, identify trends, and determine appropriate staffing. Many hospitals use **critical pathways** (also called *clinical paths*) to achieve these goals. Use of critical pathways in the ED increases the consistency and rapidity of diagnosis and treatment, with earlier initiation of intervention being key to effectiveness.[5] For example, a person with an arm injury and signs of a fracture will have an x-ray examination to determine the type of fracture. A critical pathway for this type of patient identifies the x-ray examination as the major diagnostic activity to be accomplished and a period for completion, such as 20 minutes after the assessment and evaluation by the ED physician and the ED nurse. Once the hospital has identified interventions, outcomes, and times for a particular patient population or diagnosis, the nurse can assume that the interventions should be completed and outcomes addressed within the time period. Critical pathways are tools and guidelines that provide standardization of care, consistency with interventions, and a means to evaluate effectiveness of care. Thus critical pathways promote quality of care, increase its effectiveness, improve staff communication, and increase staff and patient satisfaction.

Communication

Maintaining effective communication in any clinical setting is a challenge; however, in the ED the challenge is compounded by the number of health care personnel involved and by the emergent situation. All health care providers should keep in mind that communication is the process through which the patient-clinician relationship develops. The patient may base his or her perception of care provided on the communication and interpersonal skills demonstrated by the nurse, as much as by the nurse's clinical competence.

Regardless of the type or location of the emergent incident, one extremely important communication need is the ability to access emergency help. All agencies and communities that provide health care have a code or system that activates a call for help within a short period. Most communities in the United States have a 911 access number for activating the EMS system. The chain of survival following emergent injuries requires excellent communication skills to access care and initiate appropriate emergency services.

Managing violent situations in the ED also requires excellent communication skills. Nurses need to be able to deescalate a pattern of violent behavior before it is out of control. Appropriate techniques to deescalate such a situation include a calm and interested demeanor, a low and controlled voice, and a willingness to avoid interrupting the verbal responses of those involved. If a nurse finds it impossible to apply these communication skills in a particular situation, another nurse may be asked to take over or assist.

Environment

Noise. The nurse working in the emergency arena focuses on controlling environmental factors that can infringe on the quality of care. Noise is a major environmental factor and a significant stressor in the ED. Nurses must make an effort to work quietly and to identify this approach (quiet work) as a standard for the ED. As hospitals construct new EDs, they are including soundproofing whenever possible. Other noise-controlling behaviors include:

- Setting all telephones on soft ring
- Equipping all dispatch radios with telecommunication devices that limit the broadcast to one person (e.g., earphones, telephones)
- Setting alarms on monitors as low as safely possible
- Closing doors quietly and as appropriate
- Using personal pagers (on vibrate mode) to locate staff, rather than overhead paging

Implementation of these guidelines greatly enhances the quality of the caregiving environment.

Violence. Treating critically ill and injured patients is stressful enough without the addition of violent acts. It is estimated that 1.5 million workplace assaults occur annually in the United States, and approximately half of these occur in health care institutions. Health care workers are not at elevated risk of workplace homicide, but they are at greatly increased risk of nonfatal assaults.[3] Box 9-3 lists safety tips for nurses and other ED personnel.

Violence is often triggered by stressors that patients and families are unable to cope with effectively. Stress, pain, fear, long waits, and noxious stimuli are environmental variables that may trigger a violent act. Other environmental triggers are unpleasant waiting areas, lack of access to refreshments, insufficient and uncomfortable seating, and lack of feedback to patients and significant others about a patient's condition or progress. Attention to these details deescalates the potential for violent behavior and provides a safer working environment.

External violence in the ED setting has increased in association with escalations in street violence, family violence, and drug and alcohol abuse. Nurses are often called on to manage both the victim and the victimizer in the health care setting. Health care providers always need to be extremely aware of their environment and its potential for violence. Triage nurses and registration staff are at greater risk because they are often situated at the entrance of the ED and in a more isolated location. Box 9-4 reviews steps to increase security within the ED.

Box 9-3 Safety Tips for Nurses and Other Emergency Department Personnel

Be aware of signs of impending violence:
- Verbally expressed anger and frustration
- Body language such as threatening gestures
- Signs of drug or alcohol abuse
- Presence of a weapon

Use behaviors that help diffuse anger:
- Present a calm, caring attitude.
- Don't match the threats or give orders.
- Acknowledge the person's feelings.
- Avoid any behavior that may be interpreted as aggressive.

Be safe from potential problems by:
- Evaluating each situation for potential violence when you enter a room or begin to relate to a patient or visitor
- Being vigilant throughout the encounter
- Having someone with you when you are caring for a potentially violent person
- Keeping an open path for exiting; not letting the potentially violent person stand between you and the door

If the situation cannot be diffused, take these steps:
- Remove yourself from the situation.
- Call security for help.
- Report any violent incidents.

Adapted from Centers for Disease Control and Prevention, National Institute for Occupational Safety and Health: *Violence occupational hazards in hospitals,* DHHS (NIOSH) Pub No 202-101, April 2002, accessed Aug 2004 from website: www.cdc.gov/niosh.

Legal and Forensic Considerations

Nurses must be aware of state and local regulations that require mandatory reporting of cases of suspected child and elder abuse, accidental deaths, and suicides. Each ED has written policies and procedures to assist nurses and other health care providers in making appropriate reports.

Physical evidence is real, tangible, or latent matter that can be visualized, measured, or analyzed. ED nurses are often called on

Box 9-4 Measures to Increase Security in the Emergency Department

- Limited access (as few entrances to the emergency department treatment area as possible)
- Metal detectors
- Security personnel at entrances
- Secure triage areas
- Placement of panic buttons
- Video cameras
- Enforcement of visitor control measures
- Protective glass

to collect evidence, and all hospitals should have policies governing the collection of forensic evidence.[9] It is of utmost importance that the chain of custody be followed to ensure the integrity and credibility of the evidence. The chain of custody is the pathway that evidence follows from the time it is collected until it has served its purpose in the legal investigation of an incident.

Topics of Concern in Emergency Care

Trauma

Trauma is the most common cause of death in persons younger than 44 years old and is the fifth leading cause of death in persons of all age-groups. More than 400 Americans die each day from injuries resulting primarily from motor vehicle crashes, firearms, poisonings, suffocation, falls, fires, and drowning. Unintentional injuries are a major source of morbidity and mortality in the United States; therefore accident prevention is a major public health goal.[14] The U.S. Public Health Service and the American Public Health Association actively promote accident prevention. National health care objectives for the year 2010 related to accidents (unintentional injuries), formulated under the direction of the U.S. Department of Health and Human Services, are listed in the Healthy People 2010 box.[14]

Prevention of Trauma. Accidents are the underlying cause of trauma. Although accidents have no single cause, human error is a predominant factor. Onset of illness such as a cerebrovascular accident or myocardial infarction accounts for only a small percentage of accidents. Motor vehicle accidents (MVAs) account for more deaths than all natural disasters combined. Males are twice as likely to die in an MVA as females. More than half of all MVAs are the result of improper driving practices or human error. A much smaller percentage of accidents are caused by vehicle defects or poor road conditions. Between ages 16 and 62, alcohol consumption contributes to 20% of MVA fatalities, and between ages 21 and 44, it contributes to about 50% of MVA fatalities.[4] Young drivers are significantly overrepresented in alcohol- and drug-related crashes. Illegal drugs, as well as many legally prescribed medications, can slow reaction time and contribute to the occurrence of accidents. About 15% of the MVA fatalities are pedestrians, bicyclists, or walkers.[4]

The home can be a dangerous place. Falls account for about half of the deaths that result from trauma in the home, and they are usually preventable. ED visits because of falls are most common in individuals over age 64. Older women suffer injuries from falls more often than older men.[4] Falls commonly occur as persons, particularly the elderly, walk from room to room. Some falls are caused by heavily waxed floors, loose rugs, poor lighting, scattered toys, and other preventable conditions (Box 9-5). People fall from roofs, windows, high ladders, and steps, often because they have not used proper equipment or taken appropriate precautions.

Burns and other injuries result from improper use of solvents and cleaning agents. The number of electrical appliances used in the home has increased the danger of electrical shock and fire from overloaded circuits. Many persons die in fires caused by cigarette ashes dropped on furniture or rugs or discarded in waste containers, or by cigarettes dropped when the smoker falls asleep. Homeowners with older heating systems need to be encouraged to have these systems checked for gas leaks or other unsafe features. Members of a household should hold fire drills and know what to do if a fire occurs. Smoke alarms in kitchens, bedrooms, hallways, and basements should be considered essential.

More than 2 million poisonings occur each year. Three fourths of these involve ingestion of a poisonous substance. Others include inhalation of a poisonous gas, poisonous bites and stings, and poisonous substance in the eye. Fifty-two percent of the victims of accidental poisonings are children under the age of 6, although older children and adults also are at risk. Adults over 60 years of age account for only 4% of the poison exposure cases, but they account for 14.4% of fatalities.[1] All poisonous substances should be kept in original containers; tightly capped; and *never* placed in containers such as soft-drink bottles, drinking glasses, or cups. Medications should never be removed from the source bottle and placed in an unmarked bottle. Likewise, medications should not be used if they are in unmarked or poorly marked containers.[8] Even some herbal preparations may result in poison exposure if not taken correctly or if produced improperly (see Complementary & Alternative Therapies box).

Head injuries are the most serious type of injury sustained by bicyclists of all ages. More than 85 million people ride bikes in the United States. About 540,000 bicyclists each year sustain injuries serious enough for an ED visit. Male bicyclists are more likely to suffer a serious injury than female bicyclists. One of eight cyclists with

Healthy People 2010

Objectives Related to Unintentional Injury Prevention

- Reduce deaths caused by unintentional injuries.
- Reduce nonfatal unintentional injuries.
- Reduce deaths caused by motor vehicle crashes.
- Reduce pedestrian deaths on public roads.
- Reduce nonfatal injuries caused by motor vehicle crashes.
- Reduce nonfatal pedestrian injuries on public roads.
- Increase use of safety belts.
- Increase use of child restraints.
- Increase proportion of motorcyclists using helmets.
- Increase number of states and the District of Columbia that have adopted a graduated driver licensing model law.
- Increase use of helmets by bicyclists.
- Increase number of states and the District of Columbia with laws requiring bicycle helmets for bicycle riders.
- Reduce residential fire deaths.
- Increase functioning residential smoke alarms.
- Reduce deaths from falls.
- Reduce hip fractures among older adults.
- Reduce drownings.
- Reduce hospital emergency department visits for nonfatal dog bite injuries.
- Increase the proportion of public and private schools that require use of appropriate head, face, eye, and mouth protection for students participating in school-sponsored physical activities.

From US Department of Health and Human Services: *Healthy people 2010: understanding and improving health,* Washington, DC, 2000, The Department.

Box 9-5 Measures to Increase Home Safety

Floors

Anchor large rugs and carpets.

Use nonskid backing on small rugs.

Avoid floor wax unless nonskid.

Stairs

Ensure uniform height.

Use nonskid treads.

Mark risers with contrasting color.

Have strong hand rails at appropriate heights.

Have adequate lighting.

Bathroom

Have hand rails in tub or shower and by toilet.

Use skid-proof bath mats.

Apply treads in tub or shower floor.

Have shower seat for elderly or unstable persons.

Other

Have smoke alarms on every level.

Have working fire extinguisher in kitchen.

Have escape ladder if home is more than one story.

Secure all medications and cleaning products out of reach of children.

a reported injury sustains a head injury.[2] Bicycle helmets are effective in decreasing bicycle-related head injuries. Emergency nurses are in a unique position to teach children proper bicycle safety.

Scooters are more popular now than ever. Injuries from accidents on scooters, particularly the lightweight scooters popular among young teens, are increasing rapidly. More than 4000 scooter-related injuries were treated in EDs in 1 month in 2003. Sixty percent of the injuries could have been prevented if the rider had worn protective gear. Proper safety gear, such as, helmets, wrist guards, and knee and elbow pads, is effective in decreasing scooter injuries.[13] Additional safety measures nurses should teach scooter riders include:

- Ride the scooter on smooth, paved surfaces.
- Avoid high-traffic areas, wet surfaces, and loose gravel.
- Ride only during daylight.
- Ride alone on the scooter; do not ride double or triple.

Complementary & Alternative Therapies

Toxic Contaminants in Herbal Medicines

About three fourths of the world's population rely on herbal medicines for treating a variety of ailments. Although much of this occurs in developing countries, the use of over-the-counter herbal products has increased in developed countries as well. Some of these over-the-counter products may be contaminated with pesticides, heavy metals, or chemical toxins, or they may have been altered with other drugs. The contaminants may come from the source of the products. If they were grown in a contaminated environment or contaminated during processing, they can be dangerous to the user. Chemical toxins may come from improper storage or chemical treatment for preserving the product. Drugs may have been added by an unprofessional producer or supplier. Some herbal products are safe, but the public's belief that herbal products are safer and better for you than pharmacologic products may be incorrect in many circumstances. The consumer should be careful of products not produced by well-known, reputable manufacturers.

From Chan K: Some aspects of toxic contaminants in herbal medicines, *Chemosphere* 52(9):1361, 2003.

Nurses should also alert the public to the importance of accident prevention. As participants in legislative activities, community committees, and community education, nurses must continually emphasize the role of human error and violence in trauma. Legislative initiatives focus on prevention as the primary method for decreasing the incidence, effects, and related costs of trauma to society.

Good Samaritan Statute. Nurses may encounter trauma situations as bystanders or within their family. When an off-duty nurse happens on an accident, he or she has an ethical and moral, if not a legal, duty to stop and render assistance. To encourage professionals to help accident victims, all state legislatures have passed statutes that grant health care professionals immunity from liability when assisting in an emergency situation. The **Good Samaritan statute**, named after the biblical "Good Samaritan," states that a health care professional who stops and aids accident victims without compensation will not be liable for untoward results related to his or her acts.

The Good Samaritan statute has an exception. The law does not exempt a nurse from acts that constitute gross negligence. The statute states that if care was rendered in good faith and an emergency existed, the nurse will be free from liability. The situation is reviewed, asking the question: Is this what any reasonably competent nurse would do in the same situation? However, if the nurse does not act as "a reasonably competent nurse would," but instead, acts willfully, with gross negligence, a judgment of liability is possible.

Trauma Centers. Trauma centers are classified as **level I, level II, or level III trauma centers** according to national designations implemented by state rules and regulations. Level I–designated facilities are usually tertiary referral centers in large metropolitan areas and have a strong commitment to manage all types of trauma and emergencies. To offset the cost of the trauma service, as well as to ensure that clinical skills are maintained at a high level, the centers treat at least 1000 trauma patients per year. A level I trauma center must have clinicians and specialists immediately available 24 hours a day. Level II trauma facilities have similar characteristics, with the exception of in-house availability of specialists. Specialists in this case are on call and must be available within an established time frame, usually 20 to 30 minutes. Level III facilities are usually located in smaller institutions in communities in which a level I or II facility is unavailable. Level III centers have a responsibility to adequately stabilize trauma patients and follow clear and concise protocols for transfer to level I or II facilities. Facilities may also elect to have a nontrauma ED. This designation needs to be clearly communicated to the local community and EMS systems.

▶ ARE You READY?

In preparing a presentation for a high school conference, the nurse includes which of the following statements about accidents and trauma? (Choose all that apply.)

1. Trauma is the leading cause of death in persons younger than 44 years old.
2. The majority of automobile accidents result from mechanical problems.
3. Alcohol consumption contributes to more accidents in drivers 21 to 44 years old.
4. Males are twice as likely to die in motor vehicle accidents as females.
5. Older males suffer more fall injuries than females.
6. Over 50% of all accidental poisonings occur in children under age 6.

Collaborative Care Management of Trauma

Emergency nurses and trauma systems can have an impact on patient outcomes by taking into account the trimodal distribution of trauma deaths. The trimodal distribution illustrates the time frame in which the highest incidences of death occur after injury. The first peak occurs within minutes of injury, and death usually results from severe injury to the brain, upper spinal cord, heart, aorta, and other major blood vessels. The second peak occurs within 2 hours of injury, and death is related to subdural or epidural hematomas, hemopneumothorax, ruptured spleen, lacerated liver, fractured femurs, or other injuries causing major blood loss. The third peak occurs days to weeks after the injury, and death usually results from complications such as sepsis and multiple organ failure.

In the prehospital care setting, nurses and paramedics (e.g., flight crews, rescue squad) can possibly reduce the first death peak with rapid and accurate lifesaving interventions. The second death peak usually occurs in EDs. All members of the trauma team must work together efficiently and effectively to deliver optimal and comprehensive trauma care. The emergency nurse is an important member of the trauma team. Although he or she may provide trauma care in a variety of settings, certain nursing functions are common to trauma patient care, regardless of the setting (Box 9-6).

Assessment. In trauma care a systematic process for initial assessment of the trauma patient is crucial for recognizing life-threatening conditions and initiating appropriate interventions. Box 9-7 summarizes this process in order of priority.

Box 9-6 Nursing Trauma Care Activities

- Triage patient initially, getting the patient to the appropriate room and personnel for care.
- Perform a rapid, initial assessment of the trauma patient to identify injuries and care needs (see Box 9-7).
- Institute any necessary lifesaving interventions.
- Monitor the patient's responses to treatment interventions.
- Communicate with other health professionals.
- Perform as the patient advocate, and communicate with family and friends in attendance as appropriate.
- Document all assessments and interventions performed, and communicate with the unit receiving the patient as needed.

The initial assessment of all trauma patients (prehospital or ED) is based on specific priorities of care. The initial assessment is divided into primary and secondary surveys and should be completed within minutes unless resuscitative measures are needed. If life-threatening conditions exist, the assessment should not proceed until the trauma team has instituted appropriate interventions to manage these problems.[5]

The primary survey is an assessment of airway, breathing, and circulation. Controlling for a potential cervical spine injury is essential. Disability, deficit, and dysfunction (brief neurologic assessment) is also part of the primary survey, as is exposing the patient to ensure assessment of all body areas. The nurse may decide to include a brief assessment of the environment and initiate control measures if family or friends are with the patient. The secondary survey is a systematic head-to-toe assessment, with the objective of recognizing all injuries. It is always important to check cervical stability before moving the patient. If possible, at this time the nurse gathers additional information, such as mechanism of injury, medical history information, allergies, last meal eaten, and current medications.[5]

Box 9-7 Trauma Assessment

Primary Survey

Airway (with cervical spine management)

Breathing

Circulation

Disability, deficit, and dysfunction

Exposure and environment control

Secondary Survey

Rapid head-to-toe assessment to determine all injuries

If possible, a brief history: allergies, medications, medical history, last time of ingestion of fluid or food, events leading up to the injury

From Cole E: Assessment and management of the trauma patient, *Nurs Standard* 18(41):45, 2004.

The primary and secondary surveys begin the initial cycle of trauma care:

- Cycle I: field stabilization and resuscitation
- Cycle II: in-house resuscitation and operative phase
- Cycle III: critical care
- Cycle IV: intermediate care
- Cycle V: rehabilitation

Assessment, analysis, and action are ongoing in the trauma situation. The trauma flow record varies in format and is specific to each institution. However, it generally contains ongoing data about the patient and may contain data from the primary and secondary surveys that are combined to identify a trauma score. Other information being collected and recorded includes fluids, medications, blood, or blood components administered and the patient's response; urine, blood, nasogastric, and other secretion loss; and cardiac rate and rhythm strips.

Analysis of data occurs concurrently with data collection. Some of the major judgments demanded of the nurse caring for the patient who has experienced trauma are presented next.

MULTIPLE TRAUMA. Many trauma patients sustain **multiple trauma**, or injury to two or more body systems (Box 9-8). Motor vehicle crashes and falls, two major causes of trauma, may involve injury to the head or neck, an extremity, or the chest or abdominal area. Penetrating wounds to the chest wall may also affect the abdomen.

Persons with severe injuries require administration of intravenous fluids as soon as possible to prevent or control shock. In the field or ED, health care personnel place two or three large-bore intravenous catheters to administer fluids and drugs. They may insert a central line. They also insert an indwelling bladder catheter to monitor urinary output and core body temperature.

In multiple trauma, the trauma team first focuses on the patient's highest priority problem and then moves to the next highest pri-ority problem. Some problems such as penetrating wounds of the heart and aorta require immediate surgery. In other types of injury, if bleeding is controlled, surgery can be delayed while the team focuses on other problems. Although the trauma team has priorities, they must remain focused on the needs of the total patient.

The trauma team must always consider that treatment of one system may add to the problems of another injured system. For example, large amounts of fluid given to prevent or alter renal problems may compromise an inadequate ventilatory system, leading to failure of both systems. Assessment, analysis, and action in trauma require focusing on these multiple-system problems.

Box 9-8 Severe Injuries Often Seen in Multiple Trauma

- Crushing and penetrating chest injuries
- Crushing pelvic injuries
- Head injuries with decreasing levels of consciousness
- Injuries causing hemorrhage with shock
- Multiple bone or soft-tissue injuries
- Spinal cord injuries

AIRWAY AND BREATHING. The rate, depth, and character of respirations provide clues to the presence of ventilatory, central nervous system (CNS), or metabolic problems. Most trauma victims breathe a little faster than normal (18 to 24 respirations/min). In the presence of abnormal respiratory effort (nasal flaring; suprasternal, intercostal, or substernal retractions), the airway may be partially obstructed. The following respiratory findings suggest specific emergency care problems:

- Rate:
  —Slow (below 10 respirations/min): ventilatory or CNS problems
  —Rapid (above 26 respirations/min): hypoxia, acidosis, shock
- Depth:
  —Shallow: shock, chest pain, chest injuries
  —Deep: hypoxia, hypoglycemia, metabolic acidosis
- Sounds:
  —Inspiratory stridor: upper airway obstruction (above tracheal bifurcation)
  —Expiratory wheezes or stridor: lower airway obstruction
- Frothy, blood-tinged sputum: lung injury, pulmonary edema, pulmonary embolus

CIRCULATION. The trauma team assesses pulse quality, locations, and rate. They also assess skin color and any obvious sources of bleeding. Life-threatening conditions that may be found when assessing circulation include uncontrolled external bleeding, shock, and pericardial tamponade. Persons who sustain major trauma or a major stressor to the body usually develop shock (hypovolemic, neurogenic, or multisystem failure shock). Signs of shock vary depending on the type and severity of the shock (see Chapter 19).

DISABILITY, DEFICITS, DYSFUNCTION: NEUROLOGIC ASSESSMENT. After completing the primary survey, the trauma team performs a more detailed neurologic assessment. Level of consciousness may be altered in trauma from a variety of causes (Box 9-9). Refer to Chapter 47 for further information regarding neurologic assessment.

General Trauma Interventions. Some general principles of management for accidental injuries or sudden illnesses serve as guidelines in giving first aid at a scene:

- Remain calm and think before acting.
- Summon assistance or ensure that EMS has been contacted.
- Identify yourself as a nurse to victim and bystanders.
- Do a primary survey for *priority* data (cessation of breathing or heartbeat, interference with breathing, hemorrhage, coma).
- Carry out measures as indicated by the primary survey (see Box 9-7).
- Do a secondary survey.
- Keep the victim lying down or in the position found (unless cardiopulmonary resuscitation is necessary), protected from dampness or cold. Position the person to support airway management and some degree of comfort, but maintain cervical spine management.
- Avoid unnecessary handling or moving of the victim; move the victim only if danger is present.

BOX 9-9 Possible Causes of Changes in Level of Consciousness

Hypoxia (Decreased Oxygen to Brain)

Respiratory insufficiency:
- Airway obstruction from foreign body, secretions
- Pneumothorax
- Spinal cord injury

Shock:
- Cardiogenic cardiac arrest
- Hypovolemic hemorrhage
- Multisystem failure shock

Metabolic (Chemical Brain Depressants)

Extrinsic:
- Drugs: alcohol, narcotics, barbiturates, antihistamines, tranquilizers
- Poisons: carbon monoxide, carbon tetrachloride, hydrocarbons, methane gas

Intrinsic:
- Ketones: diabetic ketoacidosis, starvation
- Glucose: hypoglycemia, hyperglycemia
- Ammonia: liver failure
- Urea: kidney failure
- Hormonal hypofunction: hypothyroidism, adrenocortical insufficiency
- Electrolyte imbalance: sodium, potassium, calcium, hydrogen ions

Brain Pathologic Conditions

Trauma: concussion, brainstem contusion, intracranial hematoma

Seizures: epilepsy, tumors, idiopathologic condition

Cerebrovascular accident: cerebral hemorrhage, thrombosis

Tumors: benign, malignant

Infections: meningitis, encephalitis

- If the victim is conscious, explain what is occurring and provide assurance that help is on the way.
- Do not give oral fluids if there is a possibility of abdominal injury or if anesthesia will be necessary within a short time.

The nurse implements lifesaving measures when the primary survey indicates the presence of breathing or circulatory difficulties. Once breathing has been reestablished and excessive bleeding controlled, other interventions wait until the secondary survey is completed.

Rescue squad and ED personnel are trained to detect and respond to the patient's physical life-threatening conditions (see Evidence-Based Practice box). Because these needs assume priority, it is easy to overlook the psychologic needs of the patient and significant others. The impact of severe trauma or critical illness can be devastating not only for the patient, but also for the patient's family and significant others. Care of the emergency patient always extends beyond the patient to the psychosocial care of the patient's family and friends. In times of crisis families need support but may not be able to provide it for each other. Emergency nurses must be there to provide empathy, support, and direction, as well as act as resource persons. A calm, interested approach that conveys concern for the victim as a person is helpful.

Giving information frequently during all phases of emergency care to both patient and significant others helps them understand what is occurring, thereby decreasing some of the anxiety. During resuscitation attempts, it is imperative that personnel contact the family. The family needs clear information regarding the patient's prognosis and condition. The nurse contacts chaplains, social workers, or family friends who can stay with the family. Some hospitals have volunteers who can stay with patients or families during crisis periods. The nurse is honest and does not offer false hope about the patient's condition or expected outcome.

The nurse offers family and friends the option of seeing the patient, if only for a moment, before the patient is rushed to surgery or an intensive care unit. This contact is crucial for the family. If the patient has injuries or multiple tubes, the nurse prepares the family members for what they will see before taking them into the room.

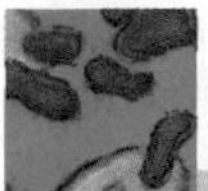

EVIDENCE-BASED PRACTICE

Topic Question: Is advanced trauma life support training necessary for hospital staff?

Evidence Base: The trauma care model, advanced trauma life support (ATLS), has been touted as an important intervention to improve trauma patients' outcomes. The studies reviewed compared the effectiveness of this model with that of hospitals not using ATLS, based on patients' morbidity and mortality after trauma.

Findings: In the limited amount of literature comparing hospitals whose staff was trained with ATLS and those whose staff was not, no significant data were found to confirm that the patient outcomes improved in hospitals with ATLS-trained staff.

Conclusions: The evidence does not support the need for ATLS training for hospital staff. However, emergency personnel need to stay abreast of research on care of the trauma victim. Continued study is needed in this area to determine whether ATLS training significantly affects the outcomes for trauma patients treated at hospitals.

Habibula S, Sethi D, Maree-Kelly A: Advanced trauma life support training for hospital staff, *Cochrane Rev*, issue 3, 2004. In Cochrane Library, Chichester, UK, John Wiley & Sons, accessed July 2004 from website: www.cochrane.org.

ARE YOU READY?

The patient with which of the following injuries is at greatest risk of death within minutes of their injury?

1. Subdural hematoma
2. Hemothorax
3. Ruptured spleen
4. Upper spinal chord

Sexual Assault: Rape

Sexual assault is a horrifying, even life-threatening, experience. Rape is defined as forced sexual intercourse, which can be oral, vaginal, or anal. This includes penetration by foreign objects, psychologic coercion, and physical force.[10] The number of reported rapes has been steadily increasing, but it is still estimated that two to three times that number of rapes go unreported. Approximately 876,000 rapes and almost 6 million assaults against women occur in the United States annually. Of these, about 800,000 result in the victim seeking medical intervention. Many of these women are under 18 years of age.[10] Accurate statistics about rape, rapists, and victims of rape are difficult to compile because of the large number of unreported cases. There are also many misconceptions concerning rape. Some facts are:

- Rape occurs among persons of all social classes.
- Rape occurs mostly between persons of the same race.
- Most rapes are committed by someone the victim knows.
- Males, especially young boys, may be rape victims; the attacker usually is a heterosexual male.
- During the rape the victim may be unable to resist the attack.

Care of Sexual Assault Victims in the Emergency Department. Most hospitals have developed protocols for care of the sexual assault survivor in the ED. The protocols include the following measures:

- High priority in triage
- Provision for privacy without leaving the victim alone
- Provision of a victim advocate (such as a worker from the sexual assault resource agency)
- Development of sexual assault nurse examiner (SANE) programs
- Routines to ensure the victim's protection and comfort (if the hospital does not have a SANE program)
- Designation of:
  - Person(s) to have primary contact with the victim
  - Authority of the primary contact person to make the decision about the victim's readiness for medical examination or police interview (if no life-threatening injury is present)
  - Procedures to ensure evidence is protected and maintained (i.e., clear documentation of injuries and collection and storage of)

In a rape case the ED's documentation is important, since it may become evidence in a trial at a later date. The nurse should record his or her own assessment; the victim's statements, including a description of the sexual act, areas affected, and number of participants (with a description); and objective information provided by others. Other information to document for a female victim is the date of her last menstrual period, obstetric/gynecologic history, and whether she bathed or douched before coming to the ED. Include a list of injuries, treatment given, and list of photographs (if taken). The nurse should also document any support and education provided.[6]

Sexual Assault Resource Agencies. Sexual assault resource agencies are available in many cities. The services of these centers differ but usually include one or more of the following:

- Direct service and counseling to the survivor
- Service to professional agencies (health, law)
- Community education

Service to health professionals and community education are efforts to help change the system for the rape victim. Many victim services agencies are staffed by volunteers who serve as victim advocates throughout the medical examination and police interview. Some form of follow-up service, such as counseling, may be available (see Research box). Some resource agencies also have attorney volunteers who offer the victim legal advice or representation.

Rape Trauma Syndrome. Rape is a traumatic event for the victim physically, psychologically, and socially. **Rape trauma syndrome** refers to the emotional state of discomfort and stress resulting from memories of an extraordinarily catastrophic experience. Patients show a wide range of emotions and various physical responses, including gastrointestinal irritability; genitourinary disturbance; and sleeping, eating, and sexual disruption.

Rape is an act of physical violence, and force often is used. The rapist may use a weapon to threaten or injure the victim, or use the hands or fists to beat or choke the victim. Injury also can occur if the victim struggles or attempts to defend himself or herself. The vagina and perineum may be injured by the force of the sexual attack, and the rectum also may be lacerated if anal sex has been attempted. The victim may contract sexually transmitted diseases, including human immunodeficiency virus (HIV).

The psychologic trauma of rape usually is severe; the rape victim is in a state of crisis. Fear is an overwhelming emotion because the victim perceives the rape as life threatening. Other feelings expressed by victims are depersonalization, shame, degradation, defilement, violation, guilt, humiliation, and anger. The victim not only has been harmed or threatened with harm but also may have been subjected to multiple sexual assaults by one or more persons. Fellatio (oral sex) commonly is demanded, and some rapists will urinate on the victim before leaving. The victim may also fear pregnancy or contracting a sexually transmitted disease.

The person who has been raped goes through the same phases as any person facing a crisis situation. The initial phase is one of shock, disbelief, and disorganization. After the initial acute phase,

Research

Smith ME, Kelly, LM: The journey of recovery after a rape experience, *Issues Mental Health Nurs* 22(4):337, 2001.

The study was an existential-phenomenologic investigation of seven women's rape experiences. The purpose was to discover the meaning of the recovery experience from the victim's perspective, and to determine what contributed to their healing process. The interviews of the women were transcribed and analyzed for themes. Three main themes emerged: (1) reaching out, (2) reframing the rape experience, and (3) redefining the person (self). The researchers found that women recovering from a rape experience need to reach out to others for emotional and spiritual help. They also need to reevaluate the experience with the help of professional caregivers who are supportive and empathetic. They need assistance and support to rebuild their lives, and they need to forgive and search for inner peace. The study is important to practitioners who have contact with rape victims. It gives nurses a better understanding of the rape victim's needs as he or she goes through the journey of recovery.

Healthy People 2010

Objectives Related to Violence and Abuse Prevention

- Reduce homicides.
- Reduce maltreatment and maltreatment fatalities of children.
- Reduce the rate of physical assault by current or former intimate partners.
- Reduce the annual rate of rape or attempted rape.
- Reduce sexual assault other than rape.
- Reduce physical assaults.
- Reduce physical fighting among adolescents.
- Reduce weapon carrying by adolescents on school campuses.

From US Department of Health and Human Services: *Healthy people 2010: understanding and improving health,* Washington, DC, 2000, The Department.

a period of pseudoequilibrium ensues, when the victim rationalizes the event or attempts to suppress thoughts concerning the rape. Later, as the survivor tries to reorganize his or her life, there may be periods of depression, phobic reactions, and nightmares.

The rape victim also experiences sociologic crisis. If the victim is married, the marital relationship may be affected. If single, the victim often fears repeated occurrences and may feel the need to relocate, especially if the attack occurred in the victim's home. The victim needs to make decisions about the incident, since needed support from family and friends may be lost. Job security or relationships with co-workers may be threatened. Sociologic problems may emerge during the initial emergency period and may take considerable time to resolve. The social importance of rape in the overall context of violence is reflected in its inclusion in the *Healthy People 2010* objectives presented in the Healthy People 2010 box.[14]

Prevention. All individuals need to know basic rape prevention measures (Box 9-10). Some communities include issues of rape and self-defense in secondary school curriculums. College campuses, a somewhat vulnerable area, usually offer sexual assault awareness programs and self-defense classes. Sexual assault agencies and police stations may provide information about other self-defense classes in the local community.

Persons who are raped may seek medical help directly or call the police, who will then take the person to the appropriate facility for medical examination. Some survivors fear reprisal by the rapist or are unwilling to let others know about the rape and therefore do not seek medical attention. Rape survivors need to be encouraged to report the incident.

Sexual Assault Nurse Examiners. Providing care to survivors of sexual assault involves unique challenges. The victim requires skilled and empathetic care to begin the process of emotional recovery; at the same time, professional, thorough, and accurate examination is essential to gather evidence for successful prosecution of the rapist. Health care providers recognized the need for better services to provide complete, comprehensive, and sensitive care to the rape victims in the ED. The sexual assault nurse examiner (SANE) role was developed to respond to the multiple challenges of caring for survivors of sexual assault.[11]

The first SANE program was developed in Memphis in 1976, and the role has rapidly spread throughout the country. The SANE provides a more time-efficient evidentiary examination process by eliminating the victim's wait for a physician or resident to be available to complete the examination. The forensic quality of the examination is improved as well, since the nurse examiner knows exactly what forensic evidence to collect and how to meet the survivor's crisis intervention needs.[11]

Nursing Management

of the Victim of Sexual Assault

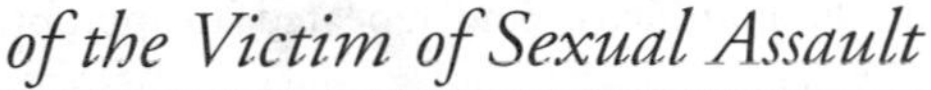

ASSESSMENT

The SANE asks the victim many questions to determine the details of the assault and the nature and extent of all injuries. Depending on the extent of injuries, the nurse might address physical needs before continuing the assessment or collecting evidence. Life-threatening injuries take priority over the victim's other needs.

Box 9-10 Rape Prevention Measures

Prevention of Attack	If Attacked
Set house lights to go on and off by timer.	Run toward a lighted house; yell "Fire!"
Keep light on at all entrances.	Spit in rapist's face; act bizarre; vomit.
Install safety locks on windows and doors.	Rip off rapist's glasses.
Have key ready before reaching door of house or car.	Step hard on rapist's foot (instep).
Look in car before entering.	Aim at eyes; try to gouge eyes, scrape face.
Never let strangers enter the house; insist on identification from all service personnel; check identity with agency if suspicious.	Hit throat at Adam's apple (larynx).
Do not list first name on mailbox or in telephone directory.	Use fighting and screaming with caution; this may scare some rapists, encourage others.
Be alert when walking; stay in lighted areas.	Try talking to avoid rape.
Walk down center of street if possible.	Make close observations about rapist, car, location.
Avoid lonely or enclosed areas.	

Health History. Assess for:

- Length of time since the assault, location, and any other information the victim remembers (description of perpetrator, etc.)
- Medical history, including last menstrual period

Physical Examination. Assess for:

- Alterations in victim's demeanor and emotional state
- Feelings of degradation, shame, guilt, and anger
- Vital sign alterations
- Pain or discomfort: localized, generalized, or diffuse
- Sore throat if choking or oral sex occurred
- Nausea
- Signs of physical trauma: head-to-toe assessment

Evidence Collection. After explaining the procedure to the survivor and obtaining permission, the SANE begins collecting evidence. This process is both time consuming and difficult for the survivor. Most states have standardized kits for evidence collection and storage. The SANE collects scrapings from beneath the victim's fingernails, pulls head and pubic hairs, obtains saliva samples, swabs the genitalia and vagina, and conducts a vaginal examination. Some SANE protocols also include colposcopy, or examination with a movable microscope positioned outside an inserted speculum. The colposcope is used to assess microtrauma and internal injuries that are difficult to visualize without magnification and has a camera attached to photograph the injuries.

The SANE performs a pregnancy test in women of childbearing age and tests for HIV antibody. Tests for other sexually transmitted diseases may be conducted and repeated at appropriate intervals.

Nursing Diagnoses, Outcomes, and Interventions

Nursing Diagnosis: Rape-Trauma Syndrome

Outcomes. Common examples of expected outcomes for the patient with a diagnosis of *rape trauma syndrome* are:

Patient will:

- Acknowledge the traumatic effect of the rape.
- Express feelings and responses to the rape.
- State rationale for treatment and evidence collection procedures.
- Identify available rape counseling and support resources in the community.

Nursing Interventions. Most victims need to talk with someone who cares about what is happening to them and who is nonjudgmental. The nurse uses crisis intervention theory to decide how best to help the survivor. Many hospitals have contacts with sexual assault agencies, and the nurse offers the victim the choice of having a victim advocate from the center be present during the entire examination period, both medical and legal. Interviews by the police are often done as a team interview with the SANE.

Having a pelvic examination after a sexual assault can be a traumatic experience, especially if the survivor has never had a pelvic examination, so the nurse prepares the victim for the physical examination before starting.

The survivor often has concerns related to sexuality. Time is needed to work through these concerns, and long-term counseling is helpful for many victims.

Concerns about possible pregnancy depend on the circumstances: whether the victim is a woman in the childbearing years, whether birth control was used during the assault, and at what point in the menstrual period the rape occurred.

Concern about sexually transmitted diseases is common. The nurse gives the victim antibiotic therapy after the initial examination as a preventive measure. The victim needs to know that medical follow-up assessment is important and that he or she should be retested for sexually transmitted diseases and screened for HIV infection at appropriate intervals. In addition, women may experience vaginal discharge, itching, and a burning sensation caused by an acute vaginal infection (vaginitis).

Clean clothes need to be provided, and no survivor of sexual assault should ever be sent home alone. Every ED should maintain a current list of battered women's shelters. Social workers may be called on to help the victim secure a safe place to stay. The survivor needs to know about the availability of follow-up medical and counseling services. Some medical centers have psychiatrists who are expert in counseling rape survivors. The survivor may go to the police station to follow up with the police report after medical care is completed (see Guidelines for Safe Practice box).

Related NIC Interventions. Counseling, Crisis Intervention, Rape-Trauma Treatment

Evaluation

To evaluate effectiveness of nursing interventions, compare patient behaviors with those stated in the expected patient outcomes.

Related NOC Outcomes. Abuse Protection, Abuse Recovery Status, Abuse Recovery: Emotional, Abuse Recovery: Sexual, Coping

Intimate Partner Violence. Intimate partner violence (IPV) is usually associated with short- and long-term problems between the couple. Alcohol or drug abuse are frequent contributing factors. Female victims are more likely to need medical attention than male victims. Government studies estimate that 10% to 15% of all women who come to the ED are victims of IPV. The health care costs of IPV exceed $5.8 billion per year. One out of four women has been assaulted by an intimate partner, and about one out of 14 men report having been assaulted also.[4] The link between IPV and sexual assault is striking: as many as a third or more women who have been physically abused by their partners were also sexually assaulted.

For many of the 1.5 million women who are abused each year, the ED is their primary source of medical care after abusive episodes.[4] Although the battered woman may come to the ED, opportunities for IPV intervention are often lost because health care providers do not ask the right questions. Physicians and nurses should directly ask all injured women if they are in an abusive relationship. Partner abuse cannot be predicted based on socioeconomic status, race, profession, or educational level. Battering is an equal-opportunity problem.

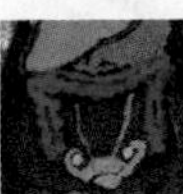

GUIDELINES FOR SAFE PRACTICE *Caring for the Sexual Assault Survivor*

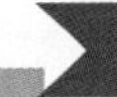

- Assess severity of all injuries and treat accordingly.
- Provide a safe environment.
- Obtain consent for evidence collection.
- Document chief complaint and history of assault.
- Complete assessment of vital signs, history of medications, allergies, and pertinent health history.
- Observe and document emotional status.
- Observe and document physical injuries (written, diagrams, and photographs).
- Observe and document genital injuries (using tolonium chloride dye, Wood's light, and colposcopy).
- Complete evidence collection.
- Order laboratory studies per protocol.
- Order additional testing based on results of the examination.
- Plan for the patient's discharge, including referrals, prescriptions, and follow-up care.

The ED staff follows several principles in caring for patients suspected of sustaining physical abuse. First, nurses incorporate questions and observations into the initial patient assessment. Historical questions and examination techniques may elicit information or evidence about IPV. Victims may not readily provide this information if it is not solicited; however, if given the opportunity, the victim often shares the information. Second, nurses must know the resources available for victims of IPV. Financial help and safe housing are often priority concerns. Victims, once placed in safe environments, can be helped to use the legal system to maintain their safety. Long-term counseling, vocational rehabilitation, and other support are necessary to promote total health. Finally, the ED staff must have clear procedures on how to handle victims of IPV and must define the process used to notify local authorities.

Critical Thinking

1. While working in the ED, you receive a call stating that paramedics will be bringing in at least nine victims from a motor vehicle accident. Some are listed in critical condition. Two of the victims are infants, four are older adults, and three are young adults. One of the adults is 6 months' pregnant. How will you prepare for this event? What type of triage will be necessary? How will you ensure that there is effective and appropriate communication among the ED personnel, patients, families, paramedics, and media? What preparations are needed based on the ages and status of the victims?
2. What colors are used to tag victims in disaster triage before bringing them to the ED? What do the colors indicate related to nursing and medical interventions needed?

References

1. American Association of Poison Control Centers: *Quick facts on poison exposures in the United States,* accessed Aug 2004 from website: www.1-800-222-1212.info.
2. Bicycle Helmet Safety Institute: *Statistics from the Consumer Product Safety Commission October 2003,* accessed Aug 2004 from website: www.bhsi.org.
3. Centers for Disease Control and Prevention, National Institute for Occupational Safety and Health: *Violence occupational hazards in hospitals,* DHHS (NIOSH) Pub No 202-101, April 2002, accessed Aug 2004 from website: www.cdc.gov/niosh.
4. Centers for Disease Control and Prevention, National Center for Health Statistics, *Fast stats A to Z: all injuries,* accessed Aug 2004 from website: www.cdc.gov.
5. Cole E: Assessment and management of the trauma patient, *Nurs Standard* 18(41):45, 2004.
6. Documenting rape trauma, *Nursing* 33(2):74, 2003.
7. Emergency Nurses Association: *Standards of emergency nursing practice,* 1999, accessed July 2004 from website: www.ena.org.
8. Meyers JW, Neighbors M, Tannehill-Jones R: *Principles of pathophysiology and emergency medical care,* New York, 2002, Delmar Thomson Learning.
9. Ort JA: The sexual assault nurse examiner, *Am J Nurs* 102(9):24, 2002.
10. Sommers MS, Buschur C: Injury in women who are raped, *Dimensions Crit Care Nurs* 23(2):62, 2004.
11. Taylor WK: Collecting evidence for sexual assault: the role of the sexual assault nurse examiner (SANE), *Int J Gynecol Obstet* 78(2):S91, 2002.
12. Uninsured deserve better, *USA Today* June 15, 2004, p 11a.
13. US Consumer Product Safety Commission: *CPSC reports as scooter sales skyrocket, injuries soar,* news from CPSC Sept 5, 2003, accessed Aug 2004 from website: www.cpsc.gov.
14. US Department of Health and Human Services: *Healthy People 2010: understanding and improving health,* Washington, DC, 2000, The Department.

evolve Visit the Evolve website: http://evolve.elsevier.com/Monahan/medsurg

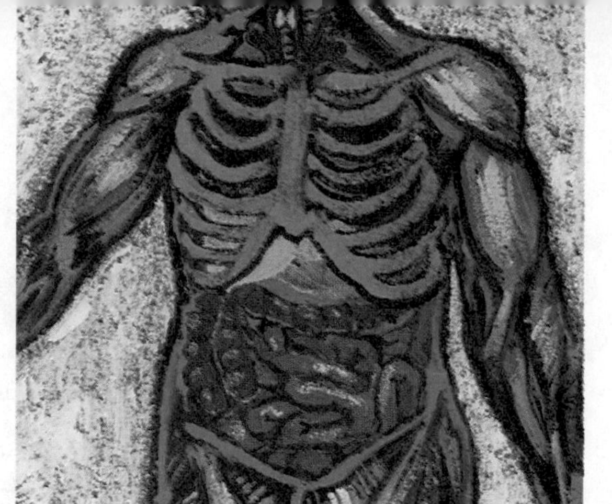

CHAPTER 10
Critical Care

by Nan Smith-Blair

OBJECTIVES

After studying this chapter, the learner should be able to:

1. Describe the role of the critical care nurse.
2. Describe how the critical care nurse affects the quality of care patients and families receive.
3. Describe the physical and psychologic environment of critical care units.
4. Identify the types of data needed for care of critically ill patients.
5. Identify essential assessment parameters required in care of critically ill patients.
6. Develop interventions to alleviate physiologic stressors that are specific to the critical care setting.
7. Explain the rationale for interventions to prevent and alleviate physiologic, psychologic, and social stressors for the critically ill patient and family.

KEY TERMS

acute confusion, p. 195
cardiac monitoring, p. 198
central venous pressure, p. 199
continuous airway pressure monitoring, p. 199
critical care, p. 192
critical care unit, p. 192
hemodynamic monitoring, p. 198
intraarterial monitoring, p. 199
intracranial pressure, p. 199
pulmonary artery monitoring, p. 199
sensory deprivation, p. 194
sensory overload, p. 194
sleep deprivation, p. 194

The delivery of **critical care** as we know it today originated from the need to centralize specially trained personnel and equipment in a separate area of the hospital to optimize the care of critically ill and injured patients. The concept of gathering patients together for care can be traced back to Florence Nightingale, who wrote[12]:

> It is not uncommon, in small country hospitals, to have a recess or small room leading from the operating theatre in which the patients remain until they have recovered, or at least recovered from the immediate effects of the operation.

Nurses began to group their most unstable patients closer to the nurses' station so they could provide "watchful vigilance" or intensive observation. As Louisa May Alcott noted [1]:

> I had managed to sort out the patients in such a way that I had what I called "my duty room, my pleasure room, and my pathetic room," and worked for each in a different way. One, I visited, armed with a dressing tray, full of rollers, plasters, and pin; another, with books, flowers, games, and gossip; a third, with teapots, lullabies, consolation, and, sometimes, a shroud.

Since the earliest days of nursing, the sickest patients have been placed near the nurses' station, underlining the importance of frequent assessment and rapid intervention. From the development of postoperative wards and polio centers to triage centers during various wars, to the evolution of the coronary care unit, this concentration of highly specialized caregivers with access to unique technology has remained the guiding principle for the evolution of critical care environments.

Today's **critical care unit** continues to be a unique, high-paced environment in which the most sophisticated medical, nursing, and technical interventions are integrated to combat life-threatening illness. These units are referred to as intensive care units (ICUs), critical care units, coronary care units, and other names that identify the type and intensity of patient care. The one constant is that the role of nursing is critical to success. Through vigilant observation of a patient's ever-changing condition, the critical care nurse monitors the complex treatment regimen, quickly identifies problems and initiates appropriate therapies, and intervenes to prevent or correct life-threatening situations. However, the focus of critical care nursing practice is no longer only on the patient's critical illness or injury. Critical care nurses have broadened their focus to include preventive care and risk modification to decrease future patient hospitalizations.

This chapter provides an overview of some common aspects of critical care nursing and the critical care environment. It discusses effects of this environment on patient, family, and staff; assessment of the critically ill patient; and selected interventions to alleviate physiologic, psychologic, and social stressors experienced by critically ill patients, their families, and the clinicians who staff the units.

Critical Care Nursing Practice

Critical care nursing is concerned with human responses to life-threatening problems, such as major surgery, trauma, infection, and shock, as well as prevention of potential life-threatening conditions. The critical care nurse is a patient advocate responsible for ensuring that all critically ill patients and families receive optimal care through a process of establishing goals for patient care and providing mechanisms to assess the patient's progress toward the goals. Clinical competencies for critical care nurses include clinical judgment and reasoning skills coupled with the ability to think critically and make decisions. The critical care nurse relies on specialized skills and knowledge to monitor and support the patient's physiologic stability of patients and provides an interface between the patient and technology. The nurse tailors clinical practices to the needs of each individual patient and family through collaboration with the health care team members to meet desired patient outcomes. Today's critical care is provided by a multidisciplinary team of health care professionals, including physicians, nurses, advanced practice nurses, case managers, pharmacists, respiratory therapists, social workers, and clergy. The critical care nurse is an integral part of this team in coordinating care activities for patients and families.

The Critical Care Environment

Physical Environment

Many of the early critical care units were small spaces carved out of existing recovery rooms or other areas in the hospital. Soon, however, the ICU emerged as a distinct area for care of complex patients, different from the recovery room in that patients were also admitted from outside the hospital and from other units. The units were staffed 24 hours a day, 7 days a week.

Today's critical care unit is designed, equipped, and staffed to meet the anticipated needs of patients in life-threatening situations. The physical layout is frequently a modified circle that allows for direct visualization of all patients at all times. Patients may be separated into cubicles with glass windows or situated in a large open area with curtains for partitions. The advantage of direct nurse-patient visualization is accompanied by the disadvantages of limited privacy and patient exposure to frequent crisis interventions.

Although direct visualization of patients facilitates patient monitoring, maximizes the use of available staff, and is required by some hospital accrediting organizations, the cost to the patient in terms of sensory overload and loss of control can be significant. Optimal patient care requires maintaining a sensitive balance between the needs of patients and those of caregivers.

The central nurse's station contains sophisticated monitoring and even video equipment that enables nurses to continuously monitor vital data for each patient. Certain technologies are available for constant use at each bedside (e.g., cardiac monitor, oxygen, hemodynamic monitoring equipment, and suction equipment), whereas others must be available within seconds (e.g., defibrillator, ventilator, 12-lead electrocardiogram [ECG] machine, emergency medications). Still other technologies must be available for constant or intermittent use with certain patient populations (e.g., intraaortic balloon pumps, continuous venovenous hemofiltration or hemodialysis, extracorporeal membrane oxygenator, temporary or permanent pacemakers, ventricular assist devices, intermittent conventional hemodialysis, and a variety of pumps for infusion of intravenous fluids or enteral feedings).

The concentration of complex technologic equipment creates a unique hazard in the critical care environment: the risk of electrical microshock. The invasive monitoring and therapeutic interventions used with critically ill patients (e.g., central venous pressure lines, pulmonary artery catheters, and temporary pacemakers) often create a direct pathway to the heart. Direct contact with stray or leaked current could prove fatal, particularly to critically ill patients whose resistance may be further decreased by other breaks in skin integrity or electrolyte imbalances. Critical care nurses are responsible for using electrical equipment properly and safely.

As the need for more specialized and sophisticated critical care equipment grows, the patient often becomes surrounded by a sea of machinery for monitoring and care delivery (Figure 10-1). A popular feature of newer or remodeled critical care environments is the centralized or headwall power columns, designed to support the complex power needs for monitoring equipment, oxygen, suction equipment, and electrical outlets; to store equipment; and to provide a workspace at each patient's bedside. With the advent of microprocessing and digital processing, continued research and development of critical care equipment focus on how to provide the most service in the smallest available space.

Psychologic Environment

The critical care environment confronts patients with advanced forms of medical and nursing therapies. Although the patient and family are partially aware of the dynamics of critical care, their attention primarily focuses on the confusing and frightening environment: flashing lights, buzzing machines, painful procedures, bright lights, noise, and hyperactivity. The stressors on the patient and family are immense. The recovery period from psychologic stressors experienced in critical care may extend well past discharge from the hospital.[11] Some factors that precipitate stress, especially in the ICU, are sensory deprivation and overload, sleep deprivation, and acute confusion.

Sensory Deprivation and Overload. To interact optimally with the environment, an individual requires the stimulation of all five senses. The optimal level and variety of this stimulation vary significantly among individuals. Patients in a critical care unit have little or no control over the amount or frequency of stimuli they receive. Too much stimuli can be as undesirable as too little. Critical care environments rarely contain the type of sensory stimuli that are familiar or understandable to patients.

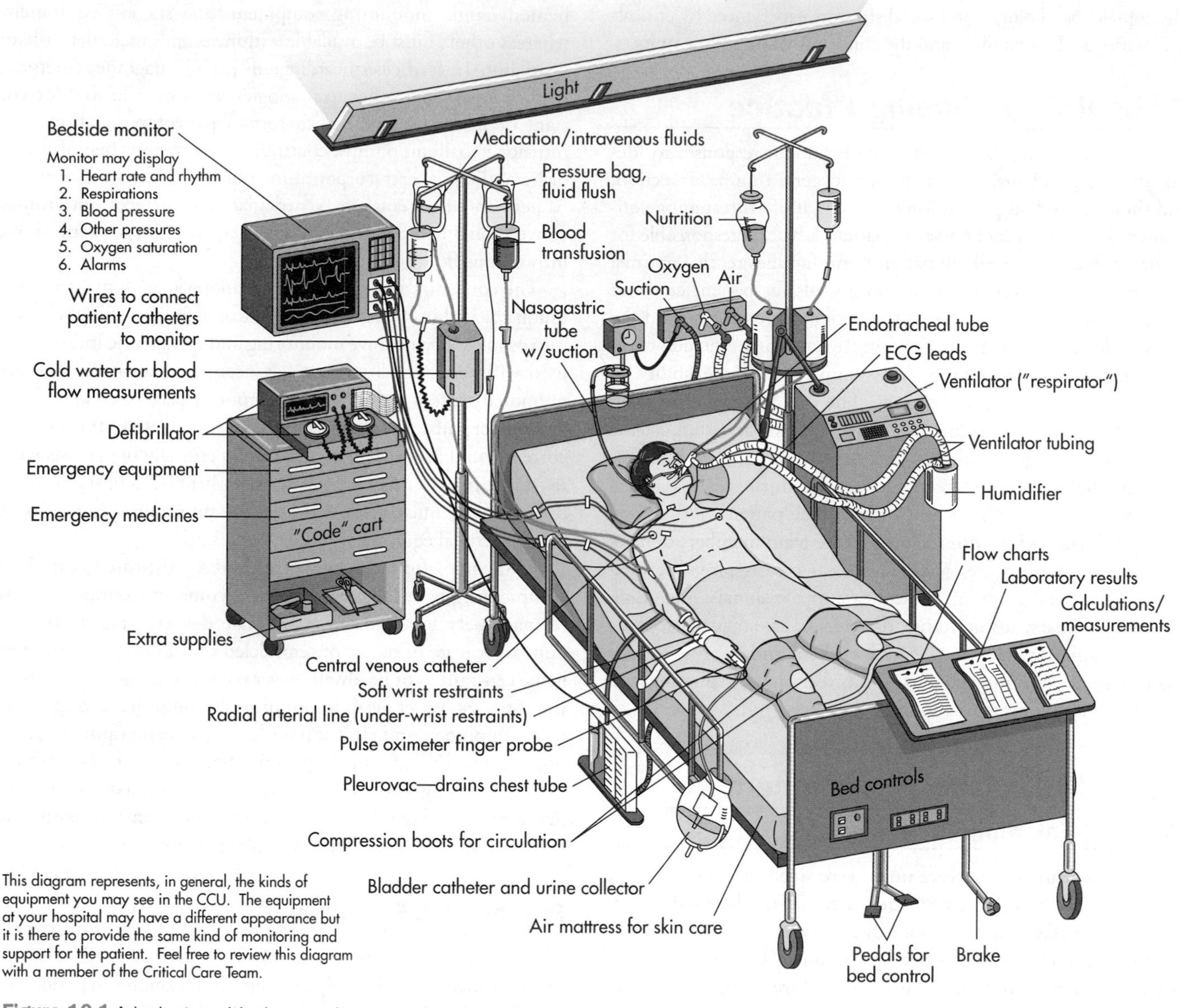

Figure 10-1 A look at a critical care unit room and equipment.

Unfamiliar voices, equipment noise, continuous bright lights, and frequent assessment interventions all add to the patient's stress level. This level of stimulation does not disappear during the night and is in fact minimally diminished.[17] Years of research indicate that **sensory overload** and **sensory deprivation** in the critical care environment frequently result in perceptual distortion, hallucinations, and paranoia.

Staff members may not realize the impact of this level of stimuli and frequently perpetuate it. Staff, of course, is also able to leave the high-energy critical care environment at the end of their shift, whereas the patient is unable to escape it. The nurse needs to be constantly aware of the type and amount of stimuli directed toward the patient and must help maintain the level of stimulation within tolerable limits.[2] Research has found that a concentrated effort by staff to reduce environmental stimuli increases the likelihood of patients being able to sleep[13] (see Research box). Staff should make every effort to reduce noise and other controllable variables and to help the patient understand this complex environment, thereby reducing the stress of the unknown.

Sleep Deprivation. An essential part of the 24-hour cycle, sleep accounts for approximately one third of a person's life. An adequate amount of uninterrupted sleep is essential to prevent exhaustion or illness and maintain physiologic and psychologic well-being. Rapid eye movement (REM) sleep, important for mental restoration, occurs primarily in the last cycles of uninterrupted sleep and is the most likely form of sleep to be affected by **sleep deprivation** in the ICU.[16,18]

Hourly intervention is frequently necessary in the critical care unit to maintain physiologic homeostasis. This recurrent disruption in the sleep cycle quickly leads to a lack of REM sleep.[8] Adverse effects of REM sleep deprivation include irritability, anxiety, physical exhaustion, disruption of metabolic functions, and respiratory distress.[7]

Research

Tamburri LM et al: Nocturnal care interactions with patients in critical care units, *Am J Crit Care* 13(2):102-112, 2004.

This randomized retrospective study reviewed the medical records of 50 patients admitted to four critical care units. Researchers reviewed interactions during 147 nights to analyze the frequency, pattern, and types of nocturnal care interactions experienced and the relationship between the interactions and patient variables (age, sex, and acuity). The mean number of care interactions per night was 42.6 (SD 11.3), with the most frequent interactions occurring at midnight and the least frequent interactions occurring at 3 AM. There were only nine uninterrupted periods of 2 to 3 hours available for patients to sleep. In addition, the frequency of interactions significantly correlated with the patient's acuity score. The study also found that 62% of baths were given to patients between 9 PM and 6 AM. Only one sleep-promoting intervention was documented on 1 of the 147 nights. Researchers concluded that interventions to expand uninterrupted periods available for patients to sleep could be implemented around 3 AM, when interactions are least common.

The critical care nurse must assess the patient and determine whether adequate periods of uninterrupted time have been provided to promote all stages of sleep. Sleep periods should be included in the care plan and adhered to as much as possible.[13] Consideration must be given to the importance of interventions versus the necessity of uninterrupted sleep periods. Health care personnel should not subject patients to activity or stressful procedures during the early morning hours unless they are imperative. Visiting times should balance the needs of the patient and family while supporting adequate rest. Recent studies suggest that longer but less frequent visits may be more desirable than the traditional plan of a few minutes each hour.[10]

Acute Confusion. The risk of developing **acute confusion** is high in the critical care setting. The high-technology environment is overwhelming and can be frightening for the patient. The presence of serious or traumatic illness adds additional psychologic and physiologic stress. Confusion is common among all patients in ICUs but especially older patients. It has a rapid onset and is generally reversible but can be distressing for both patient and family.[6] Symptoms of acute confusion include hallucinations (both visual and auditory), restlessness, memory impairment, and fluctuations in the patient's level of awareness.[9]

Initial patient assessment should include information about the patient's mental status before admission. If the patient was able to adequately perform activities of daily living, it is reasonable to expect that he or she can return to that level of function once the acute confusion resolves.

Overwhelming stress is a frequent contributor to acute confusion, and the nurse must try to make the critical care environment therapeutic rather than stressful. In the past patients were physically restrained to protect them from harm. This type of intervention controls the patient's behavior but frequently increases confusion and leads to combativeness, which may necessitate chemical sedation. Interventions ideally focus on removing stressors rather than adding to the problem. Current thinking focuses on alternatives to physical restraints. Fostering reality orientation by spending time with the patient and encouraging interaction with family and significant others should be a priority with the confused patient.[2] Reality orientation is an ongoing regimen of providing information to the patient at regular intervals as needed. This intervention is initiated immediately after admission to the ICU and is maintained until the patient can repeat the information on request.[14]

The Critical Care Nurse

The critical care environment is exceptionally stressful for the nursing staff. The nurses' stress stems partially from high expectations: advanced knowledge of physiology related to all body systems, astute observational and physical assessment skills, ability to quickly prioritize and make decisions regarding patient care, and technical proficiency in operating the highly sophisticated equipment.[4] Nurses also increasingly face complex ethical issues that consume their time and emotional energy. In addition, the constant vigilance and emergency-ready atmosphere may promote an uneasy sense of impending crisis. Critical care nurses must be able to remain and communicate effectively with the patient and family during crisis situations.

Most critical care nurses select this area of practice at least in part because they feel stimulated by a fast-paced environment that requires them to effectively integrate a detailed knowledge base, excellent assessment skills, and significant technologic proficiency. Manageable stress levels can promote creativity and productivity. However, continuous high-level stress can be as detrimental to the nurse as to the patient. Box 10-1 summarizes some of the stressors in the critical care environment.

In addition to understanding how stressors affect the patient and family, critical care nurses must guard their own physical and psychologic health by recognizing and decreasing their own stress levels. They must develop an ability to understand and respond appropriately to their own needs for support in the daily work environment, as well as the needs of their colleagues. Failure to develop self-care strategies may hamper the nurse's ability to respond appropriately to patient needs and ultimately leads to nurse burnout and exit from the health care field.

Long-term involvement with patients in a critical care environment is a relatively new phenomenon and is accompanied by significant new stressors. Technology currently enables medical science to extend the life of some critically ill patients, such as those awaiting organ transplantation, who may have critical care hospitalizations that extend weeks to months. Consistent nurse caregivers can develop a strong therapeutic relationship with the patient and family and help them cope with the stressors of the critical care environment. Nurses caring for patients on an ongoing basis may even be able to more quickly assess and respond to changes in the patient's condition. However, they may become so close to the circumstances of the patient's illness that their own psychologic health suffers. It is important for clinicians to recognize when ongoing care for a patient results in undue stress and to develop strategies for protecting their mental health. Strategies include:

- Development of support networks among nursing peers.
- Use of employee assistance personnel (counselors, social services personnel, and chaplains; critical stress debriefing) to cope with stressful circumstances.

Box 10-1 Stressors on Patients, Families, and Staff in Critical Care Environment

Patients and Family	Staff
Unfamiliar environment, new faces	Expectations of self
Noise, light levels	Expectations of peers, clinical supervisors, other health care team members, hospital administrators
Sensory deprivation or overload	Intricate machinery and techniques
Interruption of sleep-wake cycles	Closed, crowded work area
Inaccessibility of family, friends	Constant contact with seriously ill or dying patients
Lack of privacy	Continual vigilance over multiple patients
Lack of information or understanding of prognosis and care plan	Constant emergency readiness
Lack of information or understanding of policies and procedures	Sustained high activity level
Anticipation of painful interventions	Limited breaks from high-stress unit
Confusion or disorientation related to physiologic factors	Limited communication with many patients because of intubation or altered level of consciousness
Impaired communication related to intubation	Limited opportunity to communicate with families
Observation of crisis interventions in other patients	Isolation from other nurses in hospital
Fear related to diagnosis	Ethical conflicts related to resuscitation and use of life-support equipment
Fear of death	Legal issues
Conflict between patient or family goals and staff goals	Exposure to infectious diseases
Pain	

- Development of interests outside the critical care environment to help keep personal and professional worlds separate.
- Careful self-evaluation of the values, beliefs, and feelings associated with the critical care milieu.
- Use of a multidisciplinary team approach to nursing care, in collaboration with direct caregivers such as physicians; respiratory, speech, and physical therapists; and other care providers such as nutritionists, pharmacists, clergy, social workers, radiology technicians, clerical assistants, and hospital volunteers.
- Acknowledgment of the need to occasionally change assignments to provide respite for the clinician.
- Scheduling of regular clinical care conferences with the patient, significant others, and other multidisciplinary team members to help the patient feel less dependent on the nursing staff. Conferences allow the patient and family to provide important input into the overall care plan and to feel the tangible involvement of various members of the multidisciplinary team. This approach is particularly important for the long-term critical care patient. Care goals can be reevaluated, modifications agreed on, or new goals established.

Experience has demonstrated that new graduate nurses can succeed in a critical care environment, but the hiring of novice nurses requires careful attention to both their orientation and mentoring.[5,15] Particular emphasis needs to be placed on the novice's development of the clinical expertise and emotional maturity needed for handling the stresses of the critical care environment. The experienced clinician more quickly identifies the subtle changes in the condition of a critical care patient. Without adequate time, support, and supervision, the novice will simply escalate the stress experienced by other critical care clinicians. Ultimately patient care can suffer.

Caring for a Dying Patient in Critical Care

The death of a critically ill patient can be the source of tremendous emotional stress to the nurse. To help protect against overwhelming stress, when caring for a dying patient the nurse should:

- Examine his or her own feelings about death.
- Listen attentively to the expressed needs of the patient and family.
- Remain available to the patient and family both physically and emotionally.
- Use touch, if culturally acceptable, in caring for the patient and family.
- Reassure the patient and family that the patient will continue to receive skilled and compassionate care even if a do-not-resuscitate decision has been made.
- Attempt to remain nonjudgmental about family or hospital issues.
- Respect the strengths and limitations of the patient-family relationship, which existed long before the patient-hospital relationship.
- Include the family in care.
- Provide for patient and family privacy.
- Provide the opportunity for the family to exercise religious or cultural traditions.

Providing comprehensive care to critically ill patients and their families is a challenging opportunity. The critical care nurse combines the technologic sophistication of this unique setting with a personal, individualized care approach to maximize the positive potential outcomes for the patient.

Ethical Decision Making in Critical Care

In many ways technologic advances in health care have evolved faster than society's ability to understand the associated ethical dilemmas. Life can be prolonged in ways that were previously impossible, sometimes beyond all known hope of recovery. Tremendous emotional, financial, legal, and social ramifications exist as patients are stabilized in conditions for which long-term health care options are limited. For example, few families and even fewer skilled care facilities have the resources to care for a patient who requires continuous mechanical ventilation.

With the advent of advance directives, nurses frequently assume responsibility for gathering information about the patients' wishes concerning the extent of their care or treatment. Patients frequently have not prepared advance directives or are incompetent to render such a decision, leaving the family and significant others to determine the type and extent of medical care the patient would or would not want in this situation. Critical care nurses frequently assist families with highly emotional decisions such as forgoing resuscitation or withdrawing life support systems. Assisting families with these decisions is painfully complex.

All health care professionals must examine their own beliefs about life and death, termination of life, organ and tissue donation, and use of limited resources. Education and support for the nurse are available from formal classes, support groups, peers, and hospital ethics committees. Ethics committees are also available to patients, families, and staff members who wish consultation and support in difficult or divisive situations.

Biomedical advances at times seem to challenge the compassionate aspects of care giving. The critical care nurse is the professional caregiver best qualified to play a pivotal role in identifying and supporting the patient's wishes.

Nursing Management *of the Critically Ill Patient*

The nursing process is the same in critical care situations as in any other patient setting. Management of critically ill patients requires establishment of a database, identification of actual and potential nursing diagnoses and collaborative problems, delineation of priorities, definition of outcome criteria, execution of planned interventions, and modification of future interventions and plans on the basis of current outcomes. Management of critically ill patients differs from management of other patients because of an ever-changing database, a larger number of complex and interrelated problems, frequent priority reorganization, a greater variety of equipment and methods for measuring changes in patient status, and time limitations imposed by the patient's rapidly changing condition.

ASSESSMENT

The assessment process for the critically ill patient differs from the assessment of other patients only in terms of the technologies used. The cardiac monitor, hemodynamic monitoring lines, and laboratory analyses provide data that the nurse must incorporate into the total patient assessment. Technologies provide adjuncts to the data the nurse gathers through observation, history taking, and physical examination. Monitored data are useless unless correlated with physical findings and integrated into meaningful analysis by the critical care nurse.

The importance of accurate, thorough initial information cannot be overemphasized. However, the multiple sources of data and fluctuating condition of critically ill patients make constant priority reorganization a necessity. The critical care nurse continually updates the database to reformulate short-term goals and interventions.

Patient assessment must be thorough, yet rapid. The nurse must consider the physical and psychologic reactions of an entire organism under stress, while remaining open to the unusual or unexpected. Patient assessment also must be organized and repetitive so that small alterations or deviations from previous findings will be apparent. Finally, the assessment must be individualized, with time and attention given to significant aspects.

Health History. The patient may be admitted to critical care as either a direct admission (usually through the emergency department), as a transfer from another patient care division in the same or a different hospital, or as a postoperative admission after certain operations. The critical care nurse integrates data from the patient and family, written history, and the transfer report of other nurses into the patient's initial treatment plan. Consultation between transferring and receiving nursing unit staffs is essential to accomplish this process effectively. These data sources help ensure continuity of care and communication of all issues important to the patient or family. The nurse carefully explores the patient's and family's response to the need for critical care placement. A full patient profile may be deferred until later in the hospitalization, as hemodynamic stabilization is always the first priority of care. The initial contact with the critical care personnel sets the tone for all future interactions and is an invaluable opportunity for the nurse to demonstrate competence and caring and begin to establish a foundation of trust.

Physical Examination. The physical assessment of the patient, while augmented by the technology of the intensive care unit, still uses the skills of inspection, palpation, percussion, and auscultation to determine the patient's care needs and evaluate responses to interventions. The critical care nurse combines these physical assessment skills with information received from the patient and appropriate monitoring data to establish an initial care plan and set priorities. In the critical care setting physical assessment may take place hourly or even more frequently as patient status dictates. All disciplines involved in the patient's care participate in the ongoing assessment process. The dynamic and collaborative nature of critical care assessment allows for rapid responses to any changes in patient status, but it may also contribute to the patient's sensory overload. The need to evaluate status changes frequently may leave the patient with little time for rest and privacy. Significant nursing skill is required to balance information gathering and patient rest. It may take years of experience for the nurse to gather and synthesize several pieces of data simultaneously, thoroughly, and rapidly, with the least disruption to the patient.

Monitored Data. Nurses in all clinical settings use tools such as stethoscopes, sphygmomanometers, thermometers, and scales to collect patient data. Critical care nurses also have access to tools that are capable of continuous data collection, such as cardiac monitors, hemodynamic pressure lines, intracranial pressure monitoring devices, and airway pressure monitoring devices. The explosion in critical care technology since the 1970s provides the critical care nurse with amazing quantities of objective data. Digital computerized monitoring systems occupy less space and provide more capabilities than ever before. The most sophisticated patient data management systems take information from all the monitored parameters (ECG, respirations, intraarterial pressure, pulmonary artery pressure, venous oxygen saturation, central venous pressure, intracranial pressure, and body temperature), combine it with manually entered data (such as weight, height, intake and output, and times of drug administration), and produce a wide array of hemodynamic and pulmonary calculations and patient response trends for analysis by critical care practitioners.

Technologic adjuncts to critical care assessment are continuously changing, combining older and well-tested monitoring systems with newer advances. Certain types of monitoring equipment are used in all critical care environments. Waveforms and other data produced by these devices may be viewed continuously on a video screen or be graphed for a permanent record.

Many monitoring systems involve use of fluid, tubing, and transducer equipment, which acts as portals of entry for microorganisms. Strict aseptic technique is essential to prevent complications associated with nosocomial infections.

CARDIAC MONITORING. **Cardiac monitoring** is a noninvasive procedure that poses minimal risk to the patient. It consists of placing conductive electrodes on the patient's chest that recognize the electrical activity of the heart and relay it to a video display screen. Depending on the sophistication of the monitoring equipment, the clinician may be able to view the patient's ECG and heart rate at the bedside and at remote locations in the critical care unit, monitor changes during activity (with mobile equipment), and set flexible monitoring parameters as changes in cardiac status occur. Parameters may include changes in heart rate and rhythm; in respiratory rate and rhythm; in analysis of dysrhythmias; and in specific ECG segments, such as the ST segment for ischemia recognition. Alarms notify the clinician when preset limits have been reached. Most monitors default to preset limits if the clinician does not set specific alarm parameters and only allow clinicians to silence the alarms for a limited time.

HEMODYNAMIC MONITORING. **Hemodynamic monitoring** refers to invasive monitoring of the arterial or venous system. Monitoring is accomplished through catheters that measure changes in air and fluid pressures and can also be used to administer intravenous fluids and obtain arterial or venous blood for laboratory analysis. Transducers connected to the system interpret the air and fluid pressure readings and display the results as waveforms on cardiac monitoring equipment (Figure 10-2). The two most commonly used hemody-

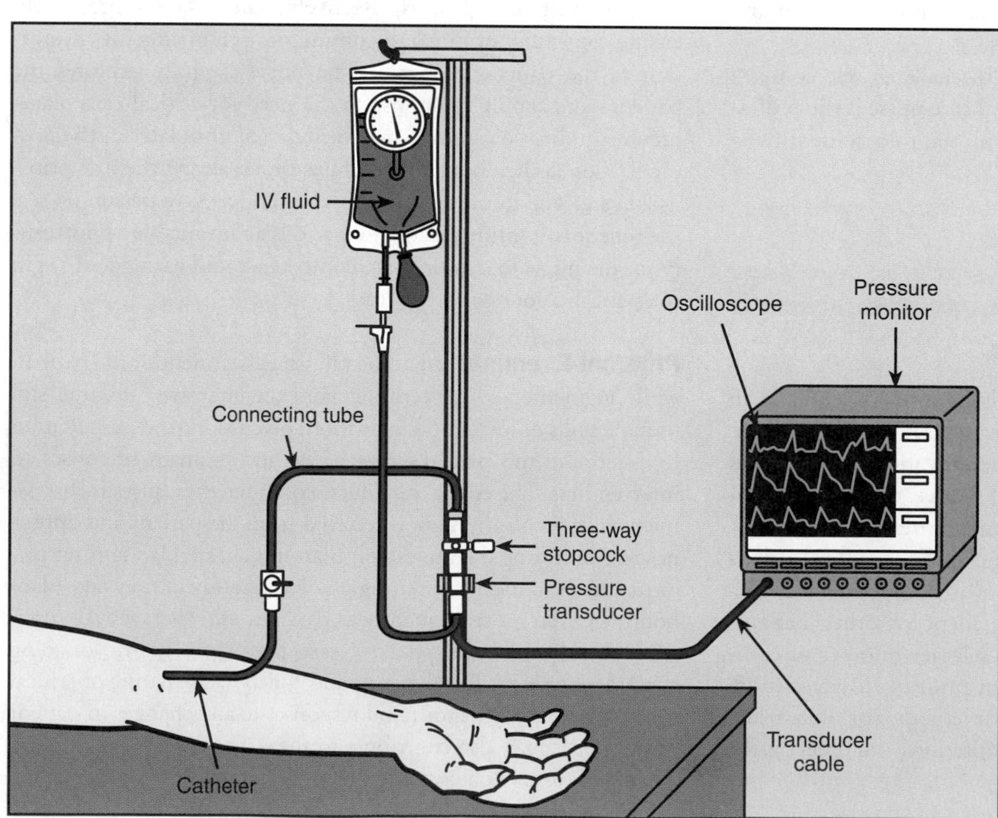

Figure 10-2 Components of a pressure monitoring system. The cannula, shown entering the brachial artery, is connected via pressure tubing to the transducer. The transducer converts the pressure wave into an electronic signal. The transducer is wired to the electrical monitoring system, which amplifies, conditions, displays, and records the signal.

namic monitoring systems are intraarterial monitoring and pulmonary artery monitoring.

It is important for the nurse to verify the digital display of waveform values with a manual sphygmomanometer, regularly calibrate the transducer equipment with the transducer positioned at specific landmarks on the patient's body, and assess the entire system for patency and accuracy. The nurse can obtain measurements with the patient in an up to 30-degree lateral or supine position if the patient is hemodynamically stable. The nurse requires a thorough knowledge of waveform interpretation to appropriately interpret and respond to the values displayed on the screen or on a manual printout. Even minor errors in reading and interpreting values or small problems in the patency of the system, such as a tiny air bubble in the transducer system, can result in inaccurate data and may cause profound complications for the patient.

Aseptic technique is critical to the maintenance of these systems with the least possible risk to the patient. Ongoing assessment of the patient's response to the equipment is also critical to avoid dangerous complications such as air emboli, bleeding, malposition of catheters, tissue damage, or hemodynamic compromise as a result of foreign body insertion or malposition.

INTRAARTERIAL MONITORING. **Intraarterial monitoring** involves inserting a catheter into an artery, usually the radial or femoral artery, and connecting the catheter to a high-pressure flush system filled with either a heparinized or nonheparinized saline solution. The high-pressure flush counterbalances arterial resistance to maintain patency of the system. Intraarterial systems display a continuous reading of the patient's blood pressure and provide ready access to obtain arterial blood gas or other laboratory specimens.

PULMONARY ARTERY MONITORING. **Pulmonary artery monitoring** involves inserting a catheter through the subclavian or internal jugular vein and advancing it into the pulmonary artery, usually under fluoroscopic guidance. These catheters have several lumens encased within a larger lumen, and each opens at a different point along the length of the catheter. Each lumen may be used for fluid administration, and specific lumens may be used to attach monitoring and transducer equipment. The large bore of the lumens and placement of the catheter in large arteries permit administration of caustic intravenous solutions that could damage peripheral veins.

A balloon at the distal tip of the catheter is filled with approximately 1 ml of air when the natural flow of blood through the patient's heart pulls the balloon into place in the pulmonary artery.[16] When the catheter is correctly placed, the balloon is deflated. Monitoring and transducer equipment is attached to the catheter.

The catheter and monitoring equipment are used to obtain significant data about the patient's hemodynamic and cardiac function. Available data include pulmonary artery and central venous pressure recordings and cardiac output measurements. Combining these values with parameters such as blood pressure and body surface area make it possible to calculate additional information that is not directly available from catheter readings. Newer monitoring equipment calculates these values automatically when data are entered into the database, decreasing the chance for error from manual calculation. The pulmonary artery catheter rapidly provides valuable information to evaluate the patient's response to vasoactive drugs by providing data about left- and right-sided heart function. It is also a significant tool for managing severe cardiac failure and cardiogenic shock.

CENTRAL VENOUS PRESSURE MONITORING. A **central venous pressure** (CVP) catheter may be used in lieu of a pulmonary artery catheter when evaluation of pulmonary artery pressure and left-sided heart function are not required. CVP catheters may be connected to a transducer and used to measure right-sided heart pressures and deliver intravenous fluids, but they are more limited than pulmonary artery catheters in the scope of data they provide. A newer type of central line is called a peripherally inserted central venous catheter (PICC). The nurse assesses and maintains the external portion of the PICC and may instruct patients and families in these techniques for home use. PICC lines are long-dwell catheters that require the same aseptic care as other central lines. They can be used for long-term fluid and medication administration but at present have no monitoring capabilities.

INTRACRANIAL PRESSURE MONITORING. Monitoring **intracranial pressure** (ICP) involves placing a catheter through the skull into either the subarachnoid space or the cerebral ventricle to monitor changes in pressure within the cranial cavity. A transducer and tubing system gather the data, which are displayed on monitoring screens. Newer monitoring systems have the capacity to sense changes in intracranial pressure and display pressure readings on a bedside monitor without the use of fluid-filled pressure tubing and transducer systems. Although insertion through the skull into the cranial cavity is still required, these newer systems reduce the risk of contamination by microorganisms.

Patients with unstable intracranial pressure may be sensitive to routine nursing interventions such as turning, suctioning, and changing bed position. Continuous display of ICP readings allows the nurse to constantly evaluate the patient's responses to all interventions and take prompt action if the patient's pressure reaches unsafe levels. The catheter also can be used to aspirate cerebrospinal fluid for analysis or culture and to relieve elevated ICP. The nurse is responsible for identifying changes in pressure readings, analyzing trends, evaluating patient responses to interventions or therapies, and preventing complications.

CONTINUOUS AIRWAY PRESSURE MONITORING. **Continuous airway pressure monitoring** (CAPM) is a simple, noninvasive technique that uses a transducer cable, high-pressure tubing (as used for measuring pulmonary and arterial pressures), and a display monitor. The monitoring equipment is connected to a ventilator circuit at the Y connector near the airway. Standard calibration procedures are used, but the monitoring tubing is filled with air, not fluid, and the transducer can be at any level while calibration is performed. The absence of fluid in the transducer system minimizes the risk of infection. The waveforms produced by CAPM may be continuously displayed, graphed, and compared with hemodynamic waveforms.

The waveforms produced by the system enable the clinician to continuously monitor the patient's response to various modes of mechanical ventilation and therapeutic interventions. CAPM is also useful in identifying one of the most common complications of mechanical ventilation: patient-ventilator asynchrony or intolerance. Asynchrony can result from mechanical malfunction, inappropriate ventilator mode selection and inadequate inspiratory flow rate, airway obstruction from excessive secretions, or patient anxiety or agitation. Asynchrony increases the work of breathing and can result in inadequate gas exchange. When a patient experiences asynchrony, the CAPM waveforms deviate from the expected patterns, alerting the nurse to the need for prompt intervention. CAPM can be especially helpful in monitoring sedated, very ill, or chemically relaxed patients who may be unable to communicate patient-ventilator intolerance. CAPM provides the bedside nurse with continuous visual assurance that the patient is receiving adequate ventilation and that chemical relaxation is being delivered at an appropriate dose. Any interruption of ventilation is immediately apparent by waveform absence.[3]

Analysis of the patient's waveforms and comparison with expected waveforms allow the care team to evaluate the patient's response to mechanical ventilation and modify the plan if necessary. Hemodynamic pressure data frequently serve as the foundation of treatment for critically ill patients. However, both real and artificial changes in the hemodynamic waveforms occur in response to pressure gradients produced by the pulmonary and systemic circulation. True pressures can be further obscured by tachypnea and underlying cardiac pathologic conditions. CAPM may be used in these situations to help standardize measurements. Simultaneous graphing of CAPM and pulmonary artery pressures provides a clear visual picture of end expiration. CAPM has thus been shown to be a simple, cost-efficient, and effective adjunct to critical care monitoring.

SUMMARY OF MONITORING. In using any invasive or noninvasive monitoring tools, the nurse must be knowledgeable about the proper use and maintenance of the equipment, including the normal appearance of the waveform associated with each line, standard interventions used to prevent complications, signs and symptoms of complications, and troubleshooting techniques for when problems develop. The patient risk associated with invasive monitoring lines is significantly reduced when knowledgeable personnel manage the lines. In addition to the various invasive lines used for monitoring, critical care nurses also must be skillful in using central lines for medication, fluid, and nutrition administration.

As monitoring techniques become increasingly sophisticated, the health care provider may be tempted to treat patients solely based on the numbers and waveforms produced by the equipment. It is essential for the clinician to remember that these data must always be combined with data from routine physical assessment, including the patient's general appearance and subjective response to all therapeutic measures. A flat line on a waveform may be the result of a disconnected wire or tubing rather than a change in the patient's condition. The nurse must remain vigilant and keep one eye on the monitor and one eye on the patient to avoid treating the equipment instead of the patient. The nurse must also tailor the use of each monitoring technique to each unique patient situation.

▶ ARE YOU READY?

The critical care nurse depends on information from which of the following systems to most accurately evaluate a patient's response to vasoactive medications?

1. Cardiac monitor
2. Central venous pressure monitor
3. Intraarterial monitor
4. Pulmonary artery monitor

NURSING DIAGNOSES, OUTCOMES, AND INTERVENTIONS

Nursing Diagnosis: Impaired Gas Exchange

OUTCOMES. Common examples of expected outcomes for the patient with a diagnosis of *impaired gas exchange* are:

Patient will:

- Demonstrate satisfactory pulmonary function: adequate blood oxygenation, hemoglobin saturation, and forced expiratory volume in 1 second.
- Maintain a satisfactory respiratory rate and pattern.

NURSING INTERVENTIONS. In a critical care setting the immediate goal of ensuring a patient's survival determines the priorities for intervention; physiologic problems must be addressed first. Once the critical care team has alleviated life-threatening stressors, they can reevaluate priorities and address other problems. Physiologic priorities are determined by the degree of threat to the person's survival. Certain body systems are more prone to disorders requiring intensive therapeutic interventions that are frequently encountered in the critical care unit. At the most basic level, these priorities can be organized in the same "ABC" framework as basic cardiac life support. Establishment of airway, breathing, and circulation remains the foundation for therapeutic management of the critical care patient. By applying the ABCs of basic life support, the critical care nurse is able to move from the most pressing to least pressing patient problems. When a patient's physiologic status begins to deteriorate, clinicians take immediate actions to reverse the problem. Correct positioning of the endotracheal tube with suctioning as needed ensures airway patency. The nurse then assesses the patient's ability to breathe and the effect of physical restraints or physiologic conditions such as acute respiratory failure. The patient's pulse oximetry and blood gases are also monitored for normalcy and early signs of distress.

RELATED NIC INTERVENTIONS. Airway Management, Oxygen Therapy, Respiratory Monitoring

Nursing Diagnosis: Decreased Cardiac Output

OUTCOMES. Common examples of expected outcomes for the patient with a diagnosis of *decreased cardiac output* are:

Patient will:

- Maintain systolic blood pressure above 100 mm Hg, urine output greater than 30 ml/hr, and cardiac rate and rhythm within acceptable limits.
- Maintain good tissue perfusion.
- Maintain stable vital signs.

NURSING INTERVENTIONS. After initially focusing on airway and breathing management, the nurse addresses circulatory needs, such as the establishment of normal cardiac rhythm, intravenous access for administration of medications, and adequate cardiopulmonary perfusion of vital organs. The critical care clinician may continue to use this basic ABC principle in ongoing assessments to ensure that problems are recognized before complications develop. The nurse improves cardiac output by reducing workload on the heart and increasing venous return. The patient is placed in the semi-Fowler's position. Rest and quiet are important. The nurse continues to assess the blood pressure, capillary refill, urine output, presence of edema, and laboratory values. Maintaining intravenous accesses is important, since most medications and fluids are delivered intravenously.

RELATED NIC INTERVENTIONS. Cardiac Care: Acute, Hemodynamic Regulation, Medication Administration

Nursing Diagnosis: Anxiety

OUTCOMES. Common examples of expected outcomes for the patient with a diagnosis of *anxiety* are:
Patient will:

- Report an increase in psychologic comfort.
- Report a decrease in restless and other behavioral manifestations of anxiety.

NURSING INTERVENTIONS. The initial step in preventing or alleviating psychologic stress is to identify the patient's and family's perception of the critical event. Their perceptions will be affected by their individual personalities, current psychologic health, general understanding of the situation and its projected outcome, tolerance for ambiguity, and normal patterns of coping. Initial perceptions are often significantly affected by previous exposure to similar events, either positive or negative, and general level of familiarity with medical interventions and the hospital environment. The critically ill person, separated from familiar surroundings and dependent on others to meet the most basic needs, becomes partially or totally isolated from usual support systems. Feelings of helplessness, loneliness, and depersonalization, as well as disturbances in body image, are common. Modes of expressing and thereby relieving frustration, anger, hostility, fear, or depression are limited by the physical constraints of the critical care environment. Anger and hostility are often indications of fear and anxiety. Depression and withdrawal may be normal signs of hopelessness, loneliness, powerlessness, or loss.

Consistently assigned caregivers can be an effective way to establish a therapeutic relationship with the patient and family. An atmosphere of openness and acceptance that encourages expression of feelings can help patients cope. The nurse talks openly and honestly with the patient to decrease feelings of depersonalization, isolation, and alienation. The nurse encourages the patient and family to express their feelings and assists the patient in identifying the fears and concerns that may be causing unusual or inappropriate behavior. The nurse or other health care team members who help patients talk about feelings must be ready to accept whatever emotionally laden information might be expressed. Nonjudgmental recognition and acceptance of the patient's feelings help reinforce the patient's right to the feelings.

Intubated patients are unable to express their feelings freely even when alert and oriented and are therefore particularly vulnerable to psychologic stressors. The nurse must guard against the normal inclination to communicate less with persons who cannot talk easily. Strategies such as keeping a letter board, paper and pencil, or "magic slate" within the patient's reach and providing assistance to the patient help reduce the sense of isolation. However, such methods do not allow the patient to truly express feelings and concerns. The nurse carefully assesses the patient for cues concerning his or her emotional state and anticipates common concerns among critically ill patients. The nurse can verbalize the potential concerns and allow the patient to validate them as appropriate. The direct expression of empathy for the patient and family conveys acceptance and understanding.

RELATED NIC INTERVENTIONS. Anxiety Reduction, Calming Technique, Coping Enhancement

Nursing Diagnosis: Interrupted Family Processes

OUTCOMES. Common examples of expected outcomes for the patient with a diagnosis of *interrupted family processes* are:
Patient and family will:

- Identify the stress of having a family member admitted to a critical care unit.
- State community and personal resources available to enhance coping abilities.

NURSING INTERVENTIONS. The essence of crisis intervention is helping persons cope with a major life crisis that a critical illness may precipitate. Critical care nursing is far broader in scope and more future oriented than crisis intervention alone, but specific situations frequently require the immediacy and limited focus of crisis intervention. At the time of crisis the nurse helps the patient and family establish short-term goals and minimizes the number and scope of decisions they must make. As the crisis situation stabilizes, the nurse provides the patient and family with more information and helps them accept additional responsibility for decision making and goal setting. When the patient and family are knowledgeable about the goals of therapy and understand the patient's diagnosis, current status, and prognosis, they can be involved in many aspects of care planning and can make decisions consistent with the treatment regimen.

Involvement of significant others decreases the patient's feelings of powerlessness, frustration, and anxiety. The family is likely to be involved in caregiving at some point in the patient's recovery, and the multidisciplinary team must begin including them in care planning as soon as possible. The patient is reassured by having a loving advocate represent his or her wishes and concerns. Even when a patient is unconscious, visits by key support figures who talk to and touch the patient may have positive, if unmeasurable, effects on the patient while ameliorating the family's feelings of helplessness.

The nurse actively involves all alert patients in goal setting and care planning. The nurse seeks to increase the patient's feeling of personal control in structuring the daily schedule of activities.

The knowledge that nursing staff values the patient's preferences and views the patient as capable of making decisions reinforces the importance of the patient's role in recovery.

The environment of the critical care unit presents multiple stresses to the patient and family. Narcotics and sedatives, anxiety, hypoxia, sleep deprivation, and multiple metabolic derangements all contribute to acute confusion, disturbed thought processes, and perceptual distortions. The nurse uses reality orientation on an ongoing basis to help patients regain their mental stability. Although some environmental factors cannot be altered, the nurse can use a variety of strategies to control the sensory level of the critical care unit.

Critical care units increasingly recognize the importance of visits by the patient's significant others in minimizing psychologic stressors. The practice of restrictive and minimal visitation is being replaced by varying degrees of open visitation. Open visitation policies range from longer and more frequent visitation hours to true open visitation, where the patient and family participate fully in care activities and care team rounds. Although these policies appear to improve the patient's and family's trust and therapeutic relationship with the care team, the nurse must be careful to avoid overwhelming the family with the daily stress and sensory overload of the critical care unit. The nurse should encourage significant others to meet their own needs for rest, nutrition, psychosocial support, relaxation, and spiritual renewal. Many significant others need support in their decision to leave the critical care environment at regular intervals, even when visitation policies would allow them to remain.

In the critical care setting the patient's physiologic needs often assume priority, and care providers may ignore the patient's needs as a social being. Limited visiting hours, the strange technical environment, and the aura of danger in the critical care unit isolate patients from their supportive family and friends and prevent them from participating in their usual social roles. For the most part, staff members view a person who is critically ill primarily in the patient role. The more significant roles of spouse, parent, child, lover, sibling, friend, or provider may go virtually unrecognized unless staff members initiate interventions to provide continuity in these relationships.

The nurse can foster continuity in social roles through the same types of interventions used to reduce psychologic stress: increasing visits between patient and family; including the family in discussions of disease process, prognosis, and care plans; and encouraging the family to report events and activities occurring in other significant spheres of the patient's life. Relaying telephone messages between the patient and distant friends is another way the nurse can help the patient maintain contact with his or her broader external world.

One effective way to prevent disruption in relationships is for the nurse to carefully explain the patient's physical appearance and the critical care environment to family or friends before their first visit with the patient in the critical care unit. Visitors need to understand the patient's level of consciousness, ability to communicate, and comprehension. They need to understand the importance of their presence to the patient and the patient's need for their support. When visitors approach the bedside, the nurse remains with them if possible to facilitate their initial interaction with the patient. Family frequently needs to be encouraged to touch the patient and offer other physical expressions of their love and support. Fear of hurting the patient or disrupting the multiple monitoring devices can virtually immobilize the family member. The nurse can help family members find safe places to stand and explain the basic purpose of the various lines and tubes. The nurse also encourages the family to speak with the patient, especially unconscious or intubated patients. At each subsequent visit the nurse caring for the patient meets with the family to answer questions and apprise them of the patient's progress.

The critical care nurse also must recognize the inevitability of role changes for some patients and families during a critical illness. Roles of provider, decision maker, employer, and employee may be altered, reversed, or eliminated. Family and friends may need to assume some or all of the patient's responsibilities at this time.

During the critical phase of illness, family members trying to cope with significant role changes and additional responsibilities may need help in working through problems. The nurse needs to be sensitive to these problems and provide the family with professional guidance, such as from a social worker, to assist in reorganizing themselves and their resources. The nurse may help the family appoint a temporary family representative, someone who knows and is able to represent the wishes of the family as a whole and who can be contacted in an emergency. The nurse also may help the family plan visiting schedules that meet the patient's needs without preventing family members from fulfilling their own responsibilities. This is a period of great emotional stress for both patient and family.

Patient and family teaching is an integral part of nursing care for the patient in the critical care unit (see Patient/Family Teaching box).

RELATED NIC INTERVENTIONS. Emotional Support, Family Process Maintenance, Family Support.

EVALUATION

To evaluate the effectiveness of nursing interventions, compare patient behaviors with those stated in the expected patient outcomes.

RELATED NOC OUTCOMES. Cardiac Pump Effectiveness, Circulation Status, Coping, Family Functioning, Family Resiliency, Respiratory Status: Ventilation, Vital Signs

GERONTOLOGIC CONSIDERATIONS

Older adults in a critical care unit may have more complex problems, since they often have other chronic diseases. In addition, older adults may not recuperate as quickly as younger patients (see Ethical Alert box).

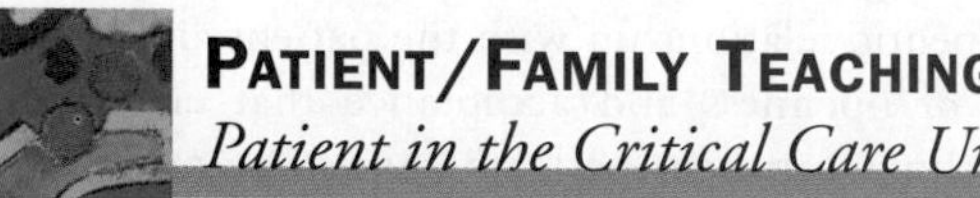

PATIENT/FAMILY TEACHING *The Patient in the Critical Care Unit*

Teaching in the critical care unit is focused on the short term. The nurse communicates to the patient and family:

- Rationale for all treatments, procedures, medications, etc.
- Plans for ongoing care
- Goals for treatments
- Interpretations of the diagnosis, diagnostic tests, and expectations
- Resources available for financial, coping, support, and other personal needs

▶ ARE You READY?

Which of the following statements by the spouse of a patient in the critical care unit requires follow-up by the nurse?

1. "I would like to hold his hand while I visit."
2. "I will stay in the waiting room until he gets better."
3. "I need to talk to him because he may hear me even if he does not open his eyes."
4. "I should tell my family that I will keep them updated on his condition."

Ethical Alert

Elderly Patients in Intensive Care Unit

Critical care units account for up to a third of hospital expenditures, and caring for the critically ill elderly consumes a disproportionate amount of intensive care unit resources. Despite the push to base practice on evidence-based approaches to treatment, models of care for elderly patients have been limited and not validated. Estimations of elderly patients' quality of life may significantly influence physicians' and nurses' attitudes in regard to futility of care issues, thresholds for continuing life-sustaining treatment, and even admission to the critical care unit. In the future, vital decisions concerning critical illness in the elderly will be subjected to many ethical, legal, and socioeconomic pressures that will influence clinical practice.

? Critical Thinking

1. In a fast-paced critical care unit in which patient care is highly complex, the critical care nurse must provide competent care and be constantly vigilant for changes in the patient's condition. How can the nurse reduce stress associated with working in the critical care environment?
2. How can the nurse promote adequate periods of sleep for the critically ill patient?

References

1. Alcott LM: *Hospital sketches,* Boston, 1863, James Redpath.
2. Bennun I: Critical care: the effects of a high technology environment, *Care Crit Ill* 19(3):88-91, 2003.
3. Burns SM: Protocols for practice: applying research at the bedside-continuous airway pressure monitoring, *Crit Care Nurse* 21:66, 2001.
4. Currey J, Worrall CL: Making decisions: nursing practices in critical care, *Aust Crit Care* 14:127, 2001.
5. Everhart B, Slate M: New graduates in the burn unit, *Crit Care Nurs Clin North Am* 16(1):51-59, 2004.
6. Foreman MD et al: Delirium in elderly patients: an overview of the state of the science, *J Gerontol Nurs* 27:12, 2001.
7. Freedman NS et al: Abnormal sleep/wake cycles and the effect of environmental noise on sleep disruption in the intensive care unit, *Am J Respir Crit Care Med* 163:451, 2001.
8. Goodwin M, Truman B, Ely EW: Potentiating the problem of delirium? Monitoring delirium in critically ill patients: using the confusion assessment method for the intensive care unit, *Crit Care Nurse* 23(4):13-14, 2003.
9. Granberg-Axell A, Bergbom I, Lundberg D: Clinical signs of ICU syndrome/delirium: an observational study, *Intensive Crit Care Nurs* 17:72, 2001.
10. Lee KA: Sleep and fatigue, *Ann Rev Nurs Res* 19:249, 2001.
11. Maddox M, Dunn SV, Pretty LE: Psychosocial recovery following ICU: experiences and influences upon discharge to the community, *Intensive Crit Care Nurs* 17:6, 2001.
12. Nightingale F: *Notes on hospitals,* ed 3, London, 1863, Longman, Green, Longman, Roberts & Green.
13. Olson DM et al: Quiet time: a nursing intervention to promote sleep in neurocritical care units, *Am J Crit Care* 10:74, 2001.
14. Rapp CG: Acute confusion/delirium protocol, *J Gerontol Nurs* 27:21, 2001.
15. Seago JA, Bar SJ: New graduates in critical care: the success of one hospital, *J Nurses Staff Dev* 19(6):297-304, 2003.
16. Shaffer RB: Arterial catheter insertion (assist), care, and removal. In Lynn-McHale DJ, Carlson KK, editors: *AACN procedure manual for critical care,* ed 4, Philadelphia, 2001, WB Saunders.
17. Solsona JF et al: Are auditory warnings in the intensive care unit properly adjusted? *J Adv Nurs* 35:402, 2001.
18. Topf M, Thompson S: Interactive relationships between hospital patients' noise-induced stress and other stress with sleep, *Heart Lung J Acute Crit Care* 30:237, 2001.

evolve Visit the Evolve website: http://evolve.elsevier.com/Monahan/medsurg

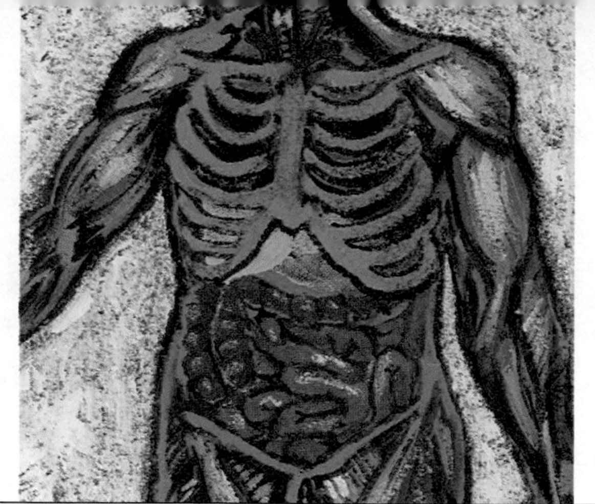

CHAPTER 11
Community-Based Care

by Marianne Neighbors

OBJECTIVES

After studying this chapter, the learner should be able to:

1. Discuss the trends in community-based care for medical-surgical patients.
2. Describe the agencies delivering care in the community for medical-surgical patients.
3. Explain the nursing responsibilities related to managing the transition from acute care to community-based care.
4. Apply the nursing process in planning care for patients and their families in community settings.
5. Discuss the unique challenges of the community as an environment for providing nursing care.
6. Identify current social, ethical, and economic issues related to community-based care.
7. Describe the unique factors related to nursing care of patients in the home.

KEY TERMS

adult day care centers, p. 205
ambulatory clinic, p. 205
case managers, p. 207
community-based medical-surgical care, p. 204
correctional facility, p. 206
discharge planning, p. 207
home health care, p. 207
hospice care center, p. 206
long-term care facilities, p. 205
nurse-managed health centers, p. 205
occupational health office, p. 206
outpatient surgical centers, p. 205
parish health office, p. 206
public health unit, p. 206
rehabilitation centers, p. 205
school health offices, p. 205

Traditionally, in the Western medical model of health care, medical-surgical nursing practice was associated with acute care agencies such as hospitals and surgery centers. Most nurses were employed by hospitals in general medical-surgical units. With the onset of the diagnosis-related group system, the influx of managed care organizations, expanded technology, and the need to reduce expenditures for inpatient services, health care services underwent a major shift to community-based settings. A variety of factors triggered this movement. These included cost-containment policies, consumers' increased knowledge of health care, demographic changes, advances in technology and nursing education, and the growth of home care agencies.

Community-based medical-surgical care is defined as the delivery of health services to patients and families where they live, work, or go to school. The focus of the care is on acute and chronic conditions that require interventions and, at times, continuous services and follow-up monitoring. The nurse's role in the delivery of care in these settings is diverse.[17]

Trends in Community-Based Care

As the cost for in-hospital care increases, as technology advances, and as the health care consumer becomes more knowledgeable and takes on greater responsibility for self-care, health care services will continue to move to the community as the base for the delivery of care. An increasing number of surgeries that previously required hospitalization are now routinely performed in outpatient settings. More care is being delivered in the home, in schools, and at the worksite. With the resources given to health promotion and risk reduction, an even greater number of services will be offered in community-based settings. Some experts have predicted that 75% of all health care will be delivered in community settings by the year 2025, opening up new opportunities for nurses. In the past years the American Nurses Association has defined and approved several new specialties in community health nursing, such as parish nursing and correctional nursing.[1,2]

Practice Roles and Settings in Community-Based Care

Health care in community-based settings is often managed by a multidisciplinary team, including the physician, registered nurse, dietitian, social worker, physical or occupational therapist, respiratory therapist, clergy, and nursing care assistants. The medical-surgical nurse of today must be knowledgeable, highly skilled, and increasingly independent to handle the health care needs of patients in community-based settings. Care delivered by medical-surgical nurses in nonhospital settings is based on the nursing process. Assessment skills are crucial in defining the patients' needs. Setting goals for the patient and determining appropriate interventions that can be delivered in the community setting may require the expertise and ingenuity of the health care team. Services may be delivered by the nurse or may be delegated to other appropriate health care personnel. Evaluating the patient's status and continued need for care is an ongoing process.

The setting for delivery of health care in the community may be an ambulatory clinic, outpatient surgery center, adult day care center, school health office, nurse-managed center, long-term care facility, rehabilitation center, hospice care facility, public health unit, occupational health office, correctional facility, or home. The nurse's roles and responsibilities vary with the setting, job description, and particular agency. Nurses may have many colleagues to support and assist them in an ambulatory surgery or clinic setting, but they are usually independent in industrial, school, or home environments. Components of the nursing roles include providing care to patients at various points on the wellness-illness continuum, working with multidisciplinary teams of health care professionals, and meeting the needs of diverse populations in the community.

Ambulatory Clinic

Medical-surgical care in the community is commonly provided in an **ambulatory clinic**. Patients are familiar with visiting the physician's office or other clinic for many of their acute health care needs. Nurses employed in these clinics may work with physicians or may be nurse practitioners who retain autonomy in their practice. This is common in "free clinics," community support clinics, and some government-run clinics in indigent areas.

Outpatient Surgery Center

Freestanding **outpatient surgical centers** have become commonplace in the past few years. With improved surgical techniques and advanced technology, a variety of surgical procedures can be performed safely and the patient discharged after a short recovery period. Many eye and dental outpatient surgery centers also employ nurses. Medical-surgical nurses in outpatient centers usually do preoperative assessments and education for patients, assist with the surgical procedures in the operating suite, and care for patients after the surgery. In some cases they may be responsible for postoperative teaching and even follow-up care at home.

Adult Day Care Center

Adult day care centers provide supervision, meals, and some health care for elderly patients during the daytime. Nurses in these settings do assessments and care planning, provide treatments and health education, and supervise other assistive personnel at the center. They work with families and the multidisciplinary health care team to develop and implement the care plans for the patients served.

School Health Office

School health offices are established to provide services for students. In kindergarten through grade 12 (K-12), school nurses assess and treat acute conditions, respond to emergencies, administer medications, maintain health records, and deliver ongoing care for students with chronic health problems. The school nurse monitors the school environment for health and safety issues and engages in health education for students, staff, and parents. Nurses in this setting require an in-depth knowledge of state mandates for school health, growth and development, health promotion and education, first-aid, and usual childhood problems and diseases. The school nurse has become an integral component of the K-12 school environment.

School nurses are also employed at the university or community college level to care for the student population. Nurses in this setting often focus on recurring medical-surgical problems such as respiratory diseases, nutritional disorders, and acute emergencies. Health centers on college campuses may be nurse-managed centers or ambulatory clinics with physicians, nurses, and laboratory and pharmacy services. One of the major roles of the nurse in this setting is health promotion and education.

The National Association of School Nurses and the American Nurses Association publish scope and standards of practice for the school nurse and the college health nurse.

Nurse-Managed Health Center

Nurse-managed health centers are facilities controlled by nurses. Nurse practitioners, as primary care providers; other nurses; and health service personnel provide the care. Physicians are usually not employed by the centers but may be on advisory boards. Nurse-managed clinics are especially common on university campuses. Health promotion and education are integral components of the practice at nurse-managed health centers.

Long-Term Care Facility

Long-term care facilities in the community provide services to elderly and medically frail patients who cannot be cared for at home. The nurse's role in long-term care usually focuses on medical-surgical care needed to preserve function, restore health, treat chronic disease, and support patients and families during the dying process. See Chapter 12 for detailed information on the long-term care setting.

Rehabilitation Center

Rehabilitation centers provide special services to patients with complex problems that require extensive professional intervention. Subacute rehabilitation centers deliver care to patients who require some medical monitoring during the rehabilitation period. Nurses in these facilities may perform interventions just as in hospitals, or they may care for and treat patients with disabilities. The most frequent medical-surgical problems seen in rehabilitation nursing include cerebrovascular accident (stroke), amputation, paralysis from back or brain injuries, and postsurgical cases such as total hip or knee replacements. The nurse in this setting must be familiar with the pathophysiology, prognosis, and recovery period of these disorders. Because some patients in rehabilitation settings have minimal recovery ability, the nurse should also have skills in psychologic interventions and communication. Progress for some patients may be extremely slow, and both the patient and family can become easily frustrated. The nurse also works with families or other care providers to assist them in learning to care for the patient at home.

Hospice Care Center

The **hospice care center** is a facility that cares for terminally ill patients. The medical-surgical nurse working in a hospice care center usually delivers palliative care to patients. Care focuses on preservation of dignity, comfort, and emotional and spiritual support. In addition, the nurse provides ongoing consultation for the hospice team and support for family and significant others. Hospice care may also be delivered in the home or in long-term care facilities. See Chapter 8 for additional information on end-of-life care.

Public Health Unit

The county **public health unit** is the facility responsible for the health of the community as a whole. The nurse in this facility provides a variety of services to patients such as immunizations, maternity services, assessment of children, treatment of communicable diseases, birth control, and interventions for other acute and chronic medical problems. The most common adult medical-surgical problems seen at the health unit are chronic respiratory disorders such as asthma, tuberculosis and emphysema, diabetes, cardiovascular diseases, sexually transmitted diseases, and nutritional disorders such as iron-deficiency anemia. The public heath nurse is instrumental in providing education programs to help patients understand their disease processes, medications, treatments, and how to prevent complications. The nurse may be actively involved in case finding (tracking contacts) when a person is diagnosed with tuberculosis, hepatitis, or any other communicable disease; distributing medications to the patient and contacts for prevention; monitoring adherence to the prescribed regimen; and performing follow-up testing and education. The nurses are also involved with epidemiology, education, and environmental safety.

Because sexually transmitted diseases continue to plague society, public health nurses play an important role in prevention, counseling, and treatment of these diseases.

Occupational Health Office

Occupational health is concerned with preserving and protecting the health of employees. The nurse in an **occupational health office** is usually involved with employee physical examinations, environmental health and safety, workplace initiatives, acute assessment and intervention, and health promotion (Figure 11-1). The Occupational Safety and Health Administration has standards for workplace health and safety that the nurse implements in cooperation with other assigned personnel. The *Healthy People 2010* document has a goal and objectives specifically addressing occupational health issues (see Healthy People 2010 box).

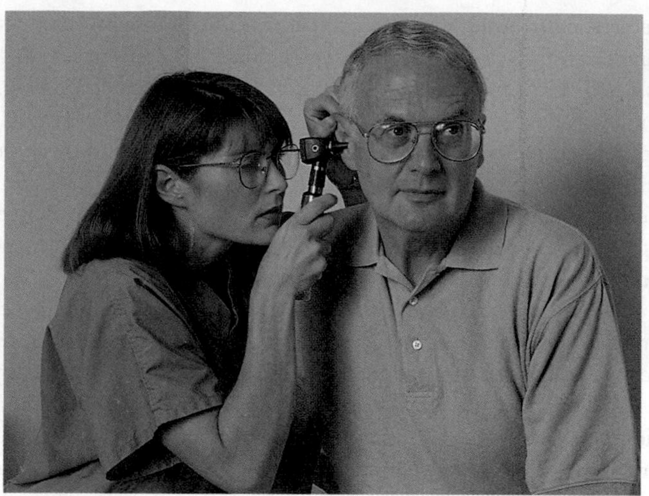

Figure 11-1 Occupational health nurse checks ears of industrial employee. Hearing loss can be a significant problem in industrial plants if preventive measures are not in place. Reducing work-related hearing loss is an objective related to occupational health in *Healthy People 2010.*

Correctional Facility

Nursing in a **correctional facility** focuses on primary and secondary preventive services and some treatment interventions. The facility may be a local jail, a youth detention center, or a state or federal prison. The medical-surgical nurse in this community-based setting is involved with assessments, triage, counseling, and treatment of common recurring illnesses. Health promotion and health education may be another major aspect of the nurse's role. The American Nurses Association has developed standards of practice for this specialty.[1]

Parish Health Office

The faith community nurse (previously known as parish nurse) is a relatively recent addition to community-based practice roles. The faith community nurse role focuses on the interrelationship of the spiritual dimension with the physical and emotional dimensions. Faith community nurses are usually employed by a church and provide services for its parishioners. The American Nurses Association publishes standards of practice for faith community nursing. The **parish health office** is usually on the church grounds, but nurses also make home visits as needed. Health promotion education is a major component of this role[2] (see Research box).

The Home

Home care for patients has become an increasingly important part of the health care system. The ongoing changes in managed care organizations and Medicare have decreased hospital admissions and increased early discharges. As a result, admissions to home health services have increased. The American Nurses Association recognizes home health nursing as a specialty with its own standards of practice. Home health nursing requires the competencies of the acute medical-surgical nurse with enhanced proficiency in case

Healthy People 2010

Goal and Objectives Related to Occupational Safety and Health

Goal

Promote the health and safety of people at work through prevention and early intervention.

Objectives

Reduce deaths from work-related injuries.
Reduce work-related injuries resulting in medical treatment, lost time from work, or restricted work activity.
Reduce the rate of injury and illness cases involving days away from work caused by overexertion or repetitive motion.
Reduce pneumoconiosis deaths.
Reduce deaths from work-related homicides.
Reduce work-related assaults.
Reduce the number of people who have elevated blood lead concentrations from work exposure.
Reduce occupational skin diseases or disorders among full-time workers.
Increase the proportion of worksites employing 50 or more persons that provide programs to prevent or reduce employee stress.
Reduce occupational needlestick injuries among health care workers.
Reduce new cases of work-related, noise-induced hearing loss.

From US Department of Health and Human Services: *Healthy people 2010: understanding and improving health,* Washington, DC, 2000, The Department.

finding, screening, assessment, critical thinking, teaching, collaboration, and health promotion. Home health nurses often work with children, families, and older adults, so the nurses must have knowledge of health care needs and interventions across the life span.

Transition From Acute Care to Community-Based Settings

Efficient **discharge planning** can facilitate the transition from acute care to community-based settings. Whether the patient is being discharged to a long-term care facility, to the home, or to another community-based care agency, discharge planning includes assessing patient needs at discharge, making arrangements and referrals for follow-up care and assistance, and coordinating the various professional and volunteer services in the community.

Hospital discharge planning takes a wide variety of forms. It may be a cursory assessment done by an assigned staff nurse on the day of discharge, or a multidisciplinary planning process conducted under the guidance of an experienced discharge planner. The discharge planner is usually a professional nurse, but social workers also fulfill this responsibility in some institutions.

Effective discharge planning is a multidisciplinary group process that should begin with admission and continue throughout the hospital stay. Planning complex discharges usually necessitates a team conference in which professionals from a variety of disciplines discuss the patient's discharge needs and plans with the patient and, if possible, the family. However, the luxury of team conferences for discharge planning is not feasible for most patients, and the nurse planner often must work individually with

Research

Wallace DC et al: Patient perceptions of parish nursing, *Pub Health Nurs* 19(2): 128, 2002.

Since parish nursing is a relatively new concept of health care delivery, little research is available on its success and patients' satisfaction and understanding of this nursing role and service. This study examined patient perspectives about parish nursing. The participants were members of two congregations located in a southeast Appalachia area that are served by a parish nurse. The researchers collected data through direct interviews with the participants and used an ethnographic approach to data analysis.

Five themes emerged from the interviews, focusing on participants' understanding of parish nursing, their relationship and contact with the nurse, and the care and services provided. The authors concluded that, for the participants, "the important characteristics of parish nursing were: (1) being available, (2) combining health and spirituality, (3) helping participants help themselves, (4) explaining and defining parish nursing, and (5) evaluating the role of parish nursing." The study found the participants liked the concept of parish nursing, found it useful and beneficial, and thought parish nurses were effective health care service providers.

each discipline to determine the patient's needs for service and support after discharge. Keeping the patient and family fully involved in the planning process is challenging but essential.

Nurses working in discharge planning may be expected to serve as **case managers** in a managed care environment. This role can take a variety of forms. Private industries and the federal government support case management as a means of reducing insurance costs and making early hospital discharge to a community setting safe. The nurse case manager may be employed by a home health agency, a hospital, a health maintenance organization discharge program, or an insurance company. Some nurse entrepreneurs have established their own companies that provide case-managed services for major insurance carriers or large corporations. Their responsibility is to meet patient needs in the best manner possible while maintaining cost-effective care delivery.

The nurse case manager may provide direct care to patients or coordinate the efforts of other personnel. In either role the case manager conducts a detailed assessment of the patient's needs, discusses options with the patient and family, coordinates selected services with the home care agency staff, and ensures high-quality care by evaluating patient outcomes on a regular basis. Open communication among the patient, family, and nurse case manager is essential for successful transition to the home or other community-based setting.

Home Health Care

Home health care focuses on acute and chronic problems and delivers specific care to the patient in the home. Nursing services provided in the home include skilled nursing care, ventilator care, pediatric or newborn care, psychiatric care, parenteral nutrition, and chemotherapy (Box 11-1). Home care agencies may also offer services such as personal care, homemaker assistance,

Box 11-1 Common Home Care Service Lines

- Intermittent skilled services
- Hospice services
- Home medical equipment (e.g., beds, wheelchairs, ventilators)
- Psychiatric program
- Early obstetrics discharge
- Parenteral therapy program (hydration, antibiotics, total parenteral nutrition, chemotherapy)
- Respite program
- Rehabilitation program (occupational therapy, physical therapy, speech therapy)
- Personal care services (activities of daily living)
- Supplies
- Private-duty nursing
- Pediatric home care
- Ventilator care
- Newborn home care
- Oncology program
- Prenatal monitoring

light housekeeping, yard work, pick-up and delivery of goods and supplies, respite care, and personal home management.

Agencies providing home care services may be private for profit or not for profit; public, associated with the county heath department; or associated with hospitals. Some private agencies are also associated with larger institutions or health care corporations, or they may be freestanding, independent agencies in the community. Freestanding agencies account for about 68 percent of the total home health agencies in the United States. The rest are facility-based home health agencies, affiliated with a hospital or skilled nursing facility[11] (Table 11-1).

Trends in Home Health Care

The number of homebound patients with complex medical needs is rising rapidly because of economic trends in health care, technologic innovations, and population demographics. Simultaneously giant mergers in health care agencies, budget constraints, advancing technology, and the Outcome Assessment Information Set (OASIS) have significantly affected home health care agencies and home health nursing practice.

The OASIS is a core set of screening and assessment elements, including standardized definitions and coding categories, that form the foundation of the comprehensive assessment for all patients of home health agencies certified to participate in the Medicare or Medicaid program (see Research box). More than 7000 Medicare-certified agencies currently provide home care services, but the numbers are declining. This is attributed to the changes in Medicare reimbursement since 1997.[11] More than 2200 Medicare-certified hospices also exist.[12] Noncertified home care agencies and hospices are also numerous but remain outside Medicare for several reasons. Many of them do not provide the kinds of services that Medicare covers, or they do not provide skilled nursing care and are not eligible to participate in Medicare. The number of registered nurses practicing in the home care setting has increased in spite of the overall decline in numbers of agencies.

Expenditures for home care in 2004 were 10.5% of the total Medicare spending for health care. This was an increase of 4% over the previous year's expenditures. The economic predication was that Medicare home health care spending would increase through the early twenty-first century and so would private spending for home care.[11] With legislative changes in reimbursements, home care expenditures decreased in 1999 and 2000 but have steadily increased since then.

Home care has been documented as cost-effective, and cost considerations were clearly a driving force behind the dramatic

TABLE 11-1 HOME HEALTH AGENCIES IN THE UNITED STATES, 2003

Type	Definition	Number
Freestanding		
Visiting nurse associations	Voluntary, not-for-profit organizations; governed by board of directors; financed by contributors and earnings	439
Public agencies	Government agencies operated by state, county, or city	888
Proprietary agencies	For-profit home care agencies	3402
Private not-for-profit	Privately governed and owned not-for-profit agencies	546
Other	Freestanding agencies that do not fit the above categories	74
Facility Based		
Hospital agencies	Hospital-based agencies operating as a department of the hospital	1776
Rehabilitation agencies	Agencies based in rehabilitation facilities	0
Skilled nursing facility agencies	Agencies based in skilled nursing facilities	113

Data from National Association for Home Care: *Basic statistics about home care,* accessed July 2005 from website: http//www.nahc.org.

Research

Brown EL et al: Recognition of late-life depression in home care: accuracy of the outcome and assessment information set, *J Am Geriatr Soc* 52(6):995, 2004.

The study evaluated the accuracy of home health nurses' use of the Outcome Assessment Information Set (OASIS) depression assessment items. The study was conducted in a Medicare-certified voluntary home health agency. The participants included 64 home health nurses. The nurses assessed 220 patients over age 65 using the OASIS items and a diagnostic assessment based on the Structured Interview for Axis I Diagnostic and Statistical Manual of Mental Disorders (SCID). Using the SCID assessment, the nurses diagnosed 35 cases of depression, but they found only 13 cases using OASIS. With the OASIS assessments they diagnosed an absence of depression in 175 cases, whereas with the SCID assessments they found 185 cases with no depression. The results of the study demonstrate that nurses do not always accurately rate OASIS depression items for older adult patients. Further investigation of the use of OASIS by home health nurses is warranted.

growth of home care in the past. Health personnel and consumers seem to agree that the privacy and safety of the home environment make it the preferred site of care for most patients and families. Other advantages of home care over institutional care include decreased nosocomial infection and improved nutritional status.[7] Home care allows for the resumption of more normal interactions and routines. Care can be more easily personalized to the unique needs of the patient and family, and patients experience a greater sense of control and higher morale when they are cared for in their home environments.

Technologic progress has influenced home care greatly. Patients can now be monitored at home through computer linkages to sophisticated diagnostic systems. Technologic innovations such as small, easily programmed intravenous infusion pumps have made parenteral home therapies safe and affordable. A variety of respiratory therapies, ranging from oxygen compression tanks to mechanical ventilators, are used widely today with older adults or patients with multiple chronic illnesses. Infusion of blood, home defibrillators, and home monitoring of patients at risk for cardiac dysrhythmias are common today.

The changing demographics of our population also have influenced the need for more home health care. The numbers of older adults will more than double by the year 2030, whereas the younger generation is decreasing in numbers. Home care is delivered to patients of all ages, but increasing age and functional disability are two major predictors of the need for home care. Home care has helped many elderly people in the community live on their own for a much longer period.[7]

Family involvement is integral to the success of home care. Often health care professionals convey to families, in direct or unspoken messages, an expectation that they will assume the caregiving role regardless of the cost. The family's interest, willingness, or capability is rarely seriously considered. The burden of caregiving can be extensive yet difficult to formally quantify. Not all homes are suitable for caregiving, especially when high-technology care is required, and the demands of monitoring and implementing high-technology care can overwhelm the caregiver. Patients and families also need to investigate the local agencies delivering care in the

Box 11-2 Medical-Surgical Problems Commonly Managed by Home Health Nurses and Home Care Agencies

- Neoplasms and palliative care for terminal cancer patients
- Chronic pain
- Peripheral vascular disorders
- Metabolic or endocrine disorders, especially diabetes mellitus
- Chronic obstructive pulmonary disorders
- Nutritional and digestive disorders
- Musculoskeletal and neurologic disorders
- Acute injuries and infections
- Genitourinary disorders
- Chronic pediatric disorders
- Hematologic disorders

home to find one suitable for their particular needs and financial status. The Centers for Medicare and Medicaid Services (CMS), a division of the federal government, provides information about the quality of care provided by home health care agencies on the Home Health Compare website.[4] Home health agencies can also apply for "magnet status" from the American Nurses Association Credentialing Center. An agency's magnet recognition reassures the patient and family that it has met specific quality standards.[5]

The needs of home care patients vary significantly. Needs range from assistance with personal care and activities of daily living (ADLs), to long-term technology support, to short-term skilled interventions after surgery. One or two home visits or around-the-clock nursing care may be required.[15] Patients diagnosed with cancer make up the largest group of patients treated in the home environment. Patients with peripheral vascular disorders and diabetes are the second and third most frequently seen patients by home health care agencies. Other major types of disorders that are treated in the home are listed in Box 11-2.

The home as the environment for nursing care offers a particular challenge to the nurse. Working in home care is an autonomous practice. Over time, nurses delivering care in the home must adapt to each patient's individual needs, resources, and health beliefs. Home care practice requires organizational skills, good communication, creativity, flexibility, and increased knowledge.[6] Nurses use many standard medical-surgical nursing skills, but also need special skills to work effectively with patients in their homes. The caseload routinely includes patients with diverse illnesses such as cardiac disease, respiratory disease, diabetes, cancer, and neurologic problems. The home care nurse may provide or direct nursing services to assist with ADLs, manage wound care and high-technology interventions, and teach families self-management skills. The home health nurse works with patients and families to promote self-care and independence and to improve the patient's quality of life.[6]

Discharge Planning in Home Health

Discharge planning needs to be initiated at admission and then continued throughout the hospitalization. Short hospital stays necessitate prompt initiation of the planning process to avoid a gap in services. It is not uncommon for patients with complex needs to be discharged and then wait for 24 to 48 hours before

▶ ARE You READY?

In assessing the need for home care, which of the following is one of the major predictors for this level of care?

1. Financial resources
2. Functional ability
3. Location of nearest medical center
4. Interest in remaining in home setting

being contacted by the home care agency. Families are left alone to cope with the patient's needs during the most vulnerable portion of the transition home and may not have the necessary skills, equipment, or support. This service gap can have serious consequences for both the patient's care and the family members' confidence in their ability to successfully manage care at home. The arrival of the home care nurse becomes not support but family rescue.

Ideally, the home health nurse responsible for planning the patient's home care should visit the patient before discharge and assess the medical needs, special equipment requirements, physical and financial restrictions, and family's ability to provide care and emotional support. Unfortunately this first contact is usually viewed as a luxury, and families take patients home without knowing who will be providing needed care and support.

The goal of effective discharge planning is to provide the patient and family with (1) information about what to expect after discharge; (2) instruction in appropriate self-care; (3) identification of family and community resources; (4) awareness of procedures to follow for emergencies; (5) information about follow-up care; (6) teaching specific to the patient's concerns; and (7) an explanation of home care services, telephone numbers, and, when possible, introductions to home care personnel.

The plan for discharge from home care services begins with the initial visit to the patient (in the hospital or the home) and focuses on setting realistic, achievable outcomes. The home health nurse in the discharge planning role follows up with an evaluation visit and completes the discharge summary for the home health agency.

Determining Discharge Planning Needs. Discharge planning for home care includes a careful assessment of the patient's home environment. The unique demands of the patient's physical care are compared with the resources available in the home (e.g., running water, refrigeration, and dry storage space). The nurse also assesses the patient and family's resources and support systems, including the immediate and extended family, neighbors, friends, and religious supports. Box 11-3 presents a basic discharge planning assessment.

The nurse needs to determine whether the patient and family have adequate coping mechanisms to manage the illness and the common stressors of home care. The patient's attitude toward discharge to home, family members' reactions to the caregiver role, and the family's ability to accept help from the home care team are important determinants of successful home management. The patient and family's perceptions and concerns about recovery influence acceptance of home care.

Financial Assessment. The nurse must undertake a financial assessment before discharge, since home care can be expensive and is usually not completely reimbursable. After Medicare, patient and family self-payments are the second-largest source of payments for home care services. Cost analyses indicate that home care expenses vary in relation to the type, intensity, and length of services needed. Medicare, Blue Cross-Blue Shield, and an increasing number of private insurance companies pay for acute, posthospital

Box 11-3 Discharge Planning Needs Assessment

Home Environment

Living arrangements

House or apartment

One floor or multilevel

Stairs—how many to reach bedrooms, bathrooms, kitchen

Adequacy of heating, cooling, electricity, plumbing, telephone service, etc.

Care Needs

Equipment and supplies

Adequacy of storage facilities

Support Systems

Persons present in the home

Family roles

Extended family, kinship network

Family coping strategies

Knowledge of and willingness to use external supports from community

Friendship, neighborhood, community, and church supports available

Learning Needs

Knowledge base

Skill acquisition

Comfort with caregiver role

Emotional Responses

Feelings about diagnosis, discharge, and home care expectations

Potential role conflicts and burdens for caregivers

Financial Assessment

Family resources

Insurance coverage

Supplemental care expenses

Box 11-4 Financial Resources Screening Checklist

1. Check the governmental or private resources available to the patient (benefits vary with each plan):
   - ________ Medicaid
   - ________ Medicare Part A (home care services)
   - ________ Medicare Part B (home care equipment)
   - ________ Health insurance, including health maintenance organizations and preferred provider organizations
   - ________ Employer insurance
   - ________ Social Security
   - ________ American Cancer Society (free equipment, bandages)
   - ________ Multiple Sclerosis Society (wheelchair loans)
   - ________ Volunteer or charitable organization resources
   - ________ Old-age assistance
   - ________ Supplemental Security Income
   - ________ Financial help (family)
   - ________ Disability payments
   - ________ Retirement pensions
   - ________ Welfare programs
   - ________ Meals-on-Wheels
   - ________ United Way agencies
   - ________ Private insurance
   - ________ Savings accounts
   - ________ Veterans Administration
   - ________ Military retirement
2. Do you think that your total income for this year was enough to meet your (the patient and other family members') usual monthly expenses and bills?
   ________ Yes ________ No
3. In the past 6 months, has money been spent on the patient's physician, hospital, nursing home, or medication bills that has not been reimbursed by insurance?
   ________ Yes ________ No

home care services to reduce the length of hospital stay. For such coverage, however, the care required must be defined as intermittent rather than ongoing.[10] Medicaid and a few insurers will pay for longer term home care services for those whose condition is chronic. Supplemental coverage can be obtained in some cases from agencies that provide old-age assistance, workers' compensation, disability, Medicaid, or other financial aid programs.

Financial assessment is often difficult for nurses to undertake, and in larger hospitals this aspect of discharge planning is usually the responsibility of a social worker. However, nurses need access to financial data to ensure that patients receive the full benefits for which they are eligible under government or private insurance. Nurses need to understand the services that are reimbursed by different insurers. With the high costs of health care, even middle-income families may need assistance, since they may be ineligible for governmental or other programs. Box 11-4 lists financial resources that may be available to patients requiring home care. The involvement of a social worker or financial discharge planner who is aware of the current eligibility and reimbursement criteria is essential, especially for older adults.

Case Management in Home Health

The unique charge of the nurse case manager in home health includes early identification of patients who are high risk or need high-cost services.[14] The nurse case manager organizes the treatments, choosing treatment alternatives that control the overall cost to the health care provider agency or third-party payer. The case manager performs ongoing assessments of patient needs and finds resources to meet the identified needs. The nurse also identifies expected outcomes for the services delivered and time frames for completion of the goals and evaluation of the outcomes. The use of nurse case managers in home health has proven to be cost-effective and successful over time.

The clinical outcome manager is a relatively new title and role for nurses in home care case management. The clinical outcome manager may replace the case manager or be an addition to the patient care team. The clinical outcome manager's goal also is to improve the quality of care while decreasing its costs.[13] Advanced practice nurses are finding success in this role. With their increased knowledge and skills, they can evaluate outcomes; create safe, effective care plans; and develop cost-saving strategies to meet the patient and family needs.[3] They are also important in care delivery for homebound patients with complex needs and multisystem problems.[16]

Reimbursement Issues for Home Health Services

Medicare is the single largest reimbursement source for home care services. The serious concern over Medicare's level of reimbursement for home care is reflected in the decline in Medicare-certified home health agencies since 1997.[11] Most other insurers use Medicare's service and reimbursement guidelines as models. Home care cannot be initiated without a physician's order, and it cannot proceed without a physician-approved care plan (Box 11-5).[11] Box 11-6 summarizes the basic requirements for service and scope of reimbursable services for Medicare and Medicaid.

Box 11-5 Medicare's Required Data for Care Plan

- All pertinent diagnoses
- A notation of the beneficiary's mental status
- Types of services, supplies, and equipment ordered
- Frequency of visits to be made
- Patient's prognosis
- Patient's rehabilitation potential
- Patient's functional limitations
- Activities permitted
- Patient's nutritional requirements
- Patient's medications and treatments
- Safety measures to protect against injuries
- Discharge plans
- Any other items the home health agency or physician wishes to include

Box 11-6 Eligibility Requirements for Medicare and Medicaid Home Care Services

Medicare

Medicare covers skilled nursing, physical therapy, occupational therapy, and speech therapy; medical supplies and equipment; and home health aide or social services if delivered in conjunction with skilled service. Persons covered are:

- 65 years or older and entitled to Social Security benefits
- Under 65 years and qualified for Social Security disability benefits
- Patients with end-stage renal disease

Requirements

1. Patient must be homebound.
2. Services must be "medically necessary" and be prescribed in a physician care plan.
3. Patient must require skilled nursing, physical therapy, or speech and language therapy.

NOTE: The skilled provider is authorized to (1) assess an acute process or change in condition; (2) teach about a new or acute situation; and (3) perform a skilled procedure or hands-on service that requires the skill, knowledge, and judgment of a registered nurse.

Medicaid

Medicaid must cover intermittent nursing service, a home health aide, and medical supplies and equipment. It may cover physical therapy, occupational therapy, speech and language therapy, private-duty nursing, or personal care services. Persons covered are:

- Recipients of Temporary Assistance for Needy Families
- Recipients of Aid to the Aged, Blind, or Disabled with income criteria
- Others who meet federal or state income guidelines

NOTE: States have some discretion in determining which groups their Medicaid programs will cover and the financial criteria for Medicaid eligibility. To be eligible for federal funds, states are required to provide Medicaid coverage for most individuals who receive federally assisted income maintenance payments, as well as for related groups not receiving cash payments. States also have the option to provide Medicaid coverage for other "categorically needy" groups. These optional groups share characteristics of the mandatory groups, but the eligibility criteria are somewhat more liberally defined.

Requirements

1. Patient must be homebound.
2. Services must be "medically necessary" and be prescribed by a physician.
3. Additional requirements vary by state; participation in case management may be required.

Home care reimbursement may also come from the Veterans Administration, the Civilian Health and Medical Program of the Uniformed Services (CHAMPUS), the Older American Act, and Title XX Social Services Block Grant. Most insurers cover skilled care, assessment and monitoring of unstable conditions, and initial teaching for self-care.[11] The home health nurse should have knowledge of the reimbursement methods and eligibility requirements and review them frequently, since the guidelines often change. The continued medical dominance of the health care system and its persistent focus on illness are reflected in the fact that general health maintenance, health promotion, and interventions such as psychoemotional support are not covered services, despite the complexities of most home care situations. Covered services do not consider the full range of nursing practice or the realities of the lives of most patients and caregivers. This creates problems for the nurse who identifies needs for services that cannot be delivered because of reimbursement limitations.

▶ ARE You READY?

Which of the following information is needed to meet Medicare requirements for the plan of care? (Choose all that apply.)

1. Mental status
2. Financial resources
3. Prognosis
4. Resuscitation status
5. Nutritional requirements
6. Medication and treatments

Cultural Issues in Home Health Care

Effective home care acknowledges and incorporates the patient's cultural background and religious beliefs. The plurality of American society necessitates that the nurse know and respect the patient's cultural beliefs. Cultural or religious conflicts may arise between the patient's, family's, and health care professional's approaches to patient care. The nurse must remember to maintain professional boundaries: the patient is in control and the home health nurse is a guest in this setting.[9] Patients and families may ignore the health care team's advice and teachings and elect not to follow the prescribed regimen. Control over the patient's care is clearly in the hands of the patient and family.

Family Issues in Home Health Care

The home health nurse may also need to explore the dynamics of the extended family, and to empower the patient and family to participate more fully in decision making and caregiving. This promotion of patient and family involvement in care is fundamental, especially if self-care will be the only option once insurance and other benefits are depleted.

Families can easily become overwhelmed by the demands of caregiving. Typical problems include the burden of providing daily physical care, steady financial drain, and lack of support or resources. Many family members are employed full time and cannot arrange their schedules to meet the patient's care needs. Other problems include the stress of learning the skills needed to perform the care or to handle the necessary equipment. They may also face ethical dilemmas such as end-of-life issues. Long-term caregiving may also require structural remodeling of the home and result in social isolation for the caregivers. The greatest challenge for the home care nurse is helping families find solutions that work within the context of their own lifestyle.

It may also be apparent that there is a need for custodial or respite care. Care of dying patients in the home has increased significantly with the success of the hospice movement.[12] Home care nurses must be open to discussion of spiritual concerns, life review, and reconciliation. Families may also wrestle with decisions about long-term care placement for the home patient and seek the nurse's advice. The home health nurse may refer the family to a social worker, directly to a long-term care facility, or the Home Health Care Compare website mentioned earlier.[4]

Nursing Management *of the Patient in the Home*

The family home is a unique environment for providing care to the adult patient and must be taken into account in developing the patient's care plan. The combined influences of the physical and psychologic environments of the home affect the outcomes of care provided. The nurse assesses the home's physical environment and the psychologic factors affecting home care in light of the effects on patient and family.

The concept of self-care is extremely important in home care. It does not mean the patient or family is able to take care of all of the patient's needs; rather it reflects the complex interaction between the home health nurse and the household members. It implies the belief that patients can maintain a level of independence, while receiving some assistance from family and professional health care workers. Growing numbers of patients and their families successfully manage home care with mechanical ventilators, parenteral nutrition infusions, home hemodialysis, intravenous antibiotics or chemotherapy, and other life-sustaining interventions.

ASSESSMENT

The home care nurse must be skillful in conducting patient and environmental assessments. During the discharge planning process, hospital or home care agency personnel should have carefully assessed the patient's needs, but the home care nurse needs to promptly and efficiently verify the accuracy of the predischarge assessment and determine whether the patient has any additional needs for equipment, care, or support.

Assessment of Expectations. The nurse must assess both the patient's and family's willingness, motivation, and expectations for home care. The nurse should also assess their knowledge of the treatment plan, equipment management, and patient's needs. The nurse may need to clarify roles and responsibilities of family caregivers versus those of the nurse or home health aide. It is important to ensure that family caregivers have thoughtfully considered the changes in their daily lives and schedules that will result from assuming the challenges of caregiving.

Cultural values may make it extremely difficult for some families to accept the prescribed treatment regimen. Fear of exposing personal lifestyles and information might affect their acceptance of having the nurse in the home. Sensitivity to cultural beliefs and family values is important to the success of the overall treatment plan. Cultural network resources can also be explored as an additional source of support for the family. The success of home care depends to a large extent on the ability and willingness of family members or significant others to draw on internal and external resources. Internal resources include the family's or individual's positive attitudes toward home care, ability to problem solve or seek advice, and willingness to accept help or assistance from external resources. Accepting help from friends, neighbors, and church or community groups often is difficult for families. The home health care nurse can determine the availability of these and other external resources and then assess the family's willingness to accept such help.

Each family member's reactions to his or her role in home care influences the family's internal resources. The home care nurse may need to periodically assess family members' role responsibilities, since these change over time. Also, individual reactions to responsibilities and the energy required to carry them out vary with the length of time that caregiving continues. Situational depression in both patients and caregivers is not uncommon. Families also react to changes, whether improvement, decline, or stabilization, in the patient's condition. Box 11-7 lists interview questions used to assess caregiver roles and reactions.

When the nurse regularly assesses family responses, he or she may be able to promptly intervene with assistance in occasional or regular respite care so that caregivers can spend some worry-free time away from the caregiving situation. The nurse must realize that as home care continues, the resources, motivation, and emotional reactions of the family and patient will change and must be taken into account in revising the home care plan.

Assessment of the Home. The home is the physical environment for delivery of nursing care. Criteria used to assess the home's safety depend to some extent on the patient's abilities and needs. The home of a patient who is discharged with special equipment may require alterations to provide a safe environment for care.

Box 11-7 Caregiver Role Assessment

1. How have the responsibilities of family members changed since the patient has been at home?
2. How do you and other family members feel about these changes in responsibility?
3. Has your health changed since you have been caring for the patient at home? If so, describe how.
4. Family members tell us they have emotional reactions to the changes in the person they are caring for. What has your experience been with these emotional reactions?
5. Family members often state that responsibilities of home care can be overwhelming and difficult. Do you find this true or not true?
6. Family members also have found they have gained strengths or a sense they are successful in caring for the patient at home. Do you find this to be true or not true?
7. Tell me the successes you have experienced.
8. Tell me about when you have not felt successful.

Assessment of the environment should always include basic information about the location of the home in relation to necessary home care services, durable medical equipment companies, and care sites for emergencies. Another factor is the availability of transportation to and from needed resources such as a pharmacy or physician's office.

The nurse must assess the home's physical environment for basic factors that affect the patient's health and adjustment to home care. The nurse should determine the adequacy of heating, cooling, electrical outlets, plumbing, refrigeration, and telephone service. Lack of these basic resources does not preclude home care, however, unless they are necessary for safety.

The nurse also assesses the home for infestation by insects or rodents, which can compromise the patient's safety and ability to maintain cleanliness for needed care supplies. Plumbing and toilet facilities are assessed in light of the patient's needs, as is the actual physical layout of the home, particularly the patient's bedroom. Assessment of the physical layout is important because the patient may be bedridden, unable to climb stairs, or restricted to one area because of medical equipment.

Assessment of the Patient. Assessment of the adult patient in the home environment encompasses many of the same data-collection procedures used in the acute care setting, but the patient and family caregivers are the major data collectors. The nurse asks them to describe the patient's condition and discuss any concerns. The nurse may never have seen the patient before the initial home visit and may have only the limited data provided on the home care referral form. The nurse depends on the family's observations and monitoring for ongoing, specific data.

Assessment proceeds in an orderly fashion. The nurse asks the patient and family members about their concerns and gathers specific data about each identified medical problem, nursing diagnosis, or symptom. Because several days or more may elapse between visits, detailed assessment is necessary to provide a solid basis for comparison on follow-up visits.

Assessment also includes the patient and primary caregiver's responses to home management. The primary caregiver is the person who provides most of the physical or daily care for the patient. This may be a spouse, parent, sibling, significant other, grown child, or friend. Multiple persons may be involved in the patient's home care. The responsibility of providing care can be both physically and psychologically demanding, and the nurse needs to openly assess the severity of the burden being experienced by the caregivers.

Assessment of the Treatment Plan. The treatment plan outlines the general care the patient needs and any special skills the patient and family must master. General areas for assessment include basic care needs, medications, nutrition, home environment, emergency procedures, specific patient needs, and equipment checks. General care assessment includes needs for assistance with hygiene, elimination, communication, transportation, and socialization; rest and activity schedules; and continued contact with health care professionals.

The treatment plan includes prescriptions for medication, diet, exercise, and physical or psychologic care. The nurse discusses with the patient the specific therapy and exactly how it is being carried out. In addition, the nurse asks the patient and family about any difficulties with treatments and solicits their opinions about the benefits or drawbacks of the therapy.

The nurse also identifies all prescription and over-the-counter medications in use and the patient's and caregivers' knowledge of their purpose, desired effects, proper administration, and possible side effects. Specific mention of herbal products and therapies is important. Many patients do not consider these medications. These therapies are commonly used by older adults, especially women (see Research box). The nurse must carefully consider the possibility of adverse drug interactions involving multiple medications and herbal products. The nurse should provide written patient education materials about all medications and review these carefully with the patient and caregiver to ensure understanding.

Confusion over multiple medications is a common problem. Patients may resume taking medications they took before hospitalization that no longer are prescribed. The nurse asks about what is taken daily and when it is taken and asks the patient to count the remaining in the prescription to determine how many were taken. Assessing actual dosage taken versus prescribed dosage is critical, since patients and families might change the dosage for a variety of reasons, including finances and forgetfulness. Drug-sorting boxes can be another useful way to assist the family in medication administration and allow the nurse to more accurately monitor the patient's adherence to the medication regimen. Regular assessment of the supply of medications also helps ensure that necessary prescriptions are refilled before they run out.

The nurse also regularly assesses the patient's nutritional status. The ability to follow through on diet prescriptions is affected by food costs, accessibility, and lifelong eating patterns. Objective data about nutritional status obtained through interval measure-

Research

Gozum S, Unsal A: Use of herbal therapies by older, community-dwelling women, *J Adv Nurs* 46(2):171, 2004.

The study assessed the use of herbal therapies by older women in the community. The 385 participants were drawn from a cross-sectional random sample of women over age 65 who lived independently in the community. The researchers interviewed participants about their use of herbal therapies. The results showed that 48.3% of the sample used herbal therapy within the past 12 months. No significant differences were found in demographic data for the users and the nonusers. The use of herbal therapies was significantly higher in women who perceived their health status to be poor, had problems with daily activities, sought physician consultation frequently, or had a diagnosed chronic disease such as diabetes or cancer.

Since herbal products are frequently used by women and patients with chronic health problems worldwide, the study, although done in Turkey, has implications for many community health nurses. Herbal remedies may have adverse interactions with prescription medications, cause the patient to delay seeking medical treatment, or be seen as a less expensive treatment for a serious medical problem. Community health nurses need to be knowledgeable about herbal preparations and to assess patients for their use of these products.

ments of body weight, intake and output, or calorie counts can be useful.

Assessment of Learning Needs. To promote high-quality, cost-effective care, education of patients and families is extremely important. The nurse must be skillful in assessing readiness to learn, providing information, and evaluating outcomes of teaching. The nurse should be familiar with the general principles of teaching and learning and adult learning theory. The education process begins with assessment and diagnosis of learning needs. Assessing the patient's and family's understanding of the illness and its treatment establishes a baseline for teaching. The nurse also must assess the family members' desire for information. In addition to information about the patient's biologic condition, family members have personal knowledge and skills needs.

The nurse must assess any barriers to learning that the patient and family may have. Learning is influenced by attitudes, beliefs, and values and varies for each person through the various stages of home health care. The nurse should reinforce positive behavior changes. Patients and families who are in a stage of denial have difficulty learning.

The nurse should also assess the family's and patient's knowledge of emergency procedures. Each family member should know how to use the community's emergency telephone system and how to contact the home health care nurse for less serious situations. Family members can be taught cardiopulmonary resuscitation. An exit plan should be made in case of fire, especially when the patient is unable to walk or has difficulty with mobility. Equipment checks are a specific and important part of home care assessment. Typically, each piece of equipment comes with written materials that outline the safety checks, cleaning procedures, and routine maintenance. The family must understand the manuals and incorporate safety checks into everyday schedules.

NURSING DIAGNOSES, OUTCOMES, AND INTERVENTIONS

Nursing diagnoses are based on the assessment data collected in the home and on the data gathered through discharge planning. The nursing diagnoses should reflect each family's actual and potential strengths, problems, and responses to the condition, treatment plan, and rigors of home care. By diagnosing strengths, the nurse identifies abilities family members can use in dealing with the actual and potential problems they face. The nurse also analyzes the data to determine the coping skills, external resources, and other family strengths essential for managing the home care alone.

A wide variety of diagnoses may be applicable in any particular situation. These include all of the specific disorder-related diagnoses identified throughout the text. A few diagnoses are more specifically applicable to the unique home care situation. One example relates to the problem of *relocation stress syndrome,* in which patients and family members experience stress and anxiety when they leave the acute care setting. This problem needs to be acknowledged and planned for before the patient's discharge from the acute care setting. Relocation stress is reduced through extensive preparation, through teaching and involving the patient and family in coordinating resources that are readily accessible and economically feasible.

Nursing Diagnosis: Impaired Home Maintenance

OUTCOMES. Common examples of expected outcomes for the patient and caregivers with a diagnosis of *impaired home maintenance* are:

Patient and caregivers will:

- Demonstrate the ability to perform necessary patient care skills.
- Identify needs for further skills or knowledge to effectively manage the patient's home care regimen.
- Adapt the home environment successfully to ensure patient safety.

NURSING INTERVENTIONS. The nurse must first gain access to the patient's home. Home care services may be crucial to the patient's successful discharge and home maintenance, but patients and families may still view the process as an invasion of privacy. Providing nursing care in a person's home cannot be undertaken without developing a successful approach to home care services. Preferably, the nurse and other professionals in the acute care setting initiate discharge planning, and family members accept the need for the home care nurse and possibly other professionals in their home.

Ideally the first visit with the patient and family should be conducted in the hospital before discharge, but often the first visit is to the home. Therefore the initial contact with the patient is almost always by telephone. The nurse clearly identifies herself or himself and the home care agency and arranges for the initial home visit, which should take place as soon as possible to confirm the patient's individual care needs. The nurse sets up a specific appointment and asks the family members how they prefer the nurse to enter the home. The nurse gives the family an agency contact telephone number for use in changing appointments or obtaining assistance in case of an abrupt change in the patient's status. This initial phone contact sets the tone for the nurse's working relationship with the patient and family and begins the process of rapport and trust building. When timely and appropriate discharge planning has been performed, the transition to home care can be smooth.

Safety concerns for the nurse working in the community setting are always important, especially on the first home visit. The nurse always needs to be aware of the environment and be sensitive to environmental cues that would indicate an unsafe situation. The nurse can ask family members questions about safe places to park, walk, and use phones in their neighborhood (see Guidelines for Safe Practice box).

Families are often unsure of the nurse's exact role in the home and need to clearly understand the scope and boundaries of the nurse's practice. At the first visit the nurse assesses patient's needs and discusses available home care options. Control of the home care situation clearly rests with the patient and family, a fact that the nurse must recognize and respect. The nurse is often welcomed to the home in a social manner on the first home visit. The nurse is a guest in the home and should not address any personal beliefs or feelings about the patient's lifestyle. The nurse uses this visit to establish trust, rapport, and a working relationship with the patient and the primary caregiver. The nurse emphasizes the collaborative nature of their partnership in the patient's care. The nurse also sets clear expectations about the time limits for the initial visit and future ones.

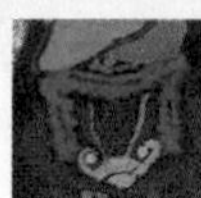

GUIDELINES FOR SAFE PRACTICE *Safety Precautions for Home Visiting*

- Let the agency know your schedule in advance and phone numbers of the patients to be visited.
- Have accurate information about the exact location of the patient's home and parking availability. Always carry a detailed street map.
- Park in a well-lighted, busy area near the patient's home. If possible, schedule visits only during daylight hours.
- Reconfirm appointments with the family before arrival.
- Maintain your car in good working order. Keep the car free of personal belongings. Keep any needed supplies in the trunk, and always keep the car locked.
- Avoid carrying a purse or wearing jewelry.
- Be alert at all times. If you do not feel safe, leave the area. Visit high-crime areas only with a second nurse, never alone.
- If a patient, family member, or visitor is drunk or hostile, leave the home and then reschedule the visit.
- If a serious argument, fight, or abuse is occurring in or around the home, leave and then report the incident to the proper authorities.
- Always carry agency identification and emergency phone numbers. A cellular phone provides added security.

The patient and family also require clear information about the costs of home care services, insurance reimbursement, and other economic details. Options to reduce home care expenditures safely, such as family members providing wound dressing changes 3 days a week or the nurse reducing visits to twice weekly, should be explored. The nurse should note that most insurers have restrictions on the lifetime number of visits that the patient can receive. Insurers also have limits on how much they will pay for selected patient conditions. Discussing the economics of the health care situation with families can be difficult, but helps them understand that cost-effective use of their insurance will maintain coverage for a later date. The initial visit concludes with mutual agreement about the patient's care needs, the distribution of care responsibilities between the family and home care agency, and the frequency and nature of future visits.

The knowledge and skills that the patient and family must have to manage the patient's care safely and effectively are specifically related to the patient's unique diagnosis and treatment plan. Patient and family teaching is directed at (1) understanding the illness and treatment plan, (2) developing competence in managing the patient's care, and (3) fostering effective coping with the lifestyle implications of home care. Understanding the patient's and family's lifestyle helps the nurse plan with them how to make necessary changes with the least disruption. When a care regimen causes minimal disruptions in lifestyle, the patient is more likely to comply with it. Teaching is more effective when it includes not only knowledge of treatment but also assistance in tailoring the care regimen to the family's circumstances and preferences. Flexibility and creative problem solving are essential.

Implementation of teaching plans can take many forms, including the use of computer-assisted instruction and videotapes in the home. Demonstrating a technique and having the caregiver or patient perform a "return demonstration" helps ensure the individual understands the correct way to perform the procedure. Methods of teaching that incorporate the whole family and emphasize the need to change behavior are most likely to have positive results. Using praise and reinforcement and providing an opportunity for questions and to evaluate learning effectiveness are important parts of implementation.

Establishing cues as reminders for new behaviors enhances adjustment to home care. For example, encouraging patients with many treatments to try to schedule these with meals or other regular activities helps them remember the treatments.

The nurse must remember to bring teaching materials for the home visit even if the patient has received handouts before discharge. Duplication of materials and information reinforces previous teaching. The nurse builds on teaching materials already given to the patient so that it does not appear that only new content is being taught. However, home care workers must avoid covering the same information. For example, the nurse and physical therapist should decide who will be responsible for teaching range-of-motion exercises.

The nurse should be aware of the patient's and family member's ability to read and understand the information provided. If English is a second language in the household, it is imperative that the nurse determine whether caregivers understand the material. Sometimes using fewer written words and more descriptive pictures is helpful in households where the literacy is poor or English is not the primary language. Written materials and the nurse's vocabulary should be at an appropriate level for the patient. Patients may not understand "medical words." Using the patient's own terms is usually most effective. Even for functionally literate patients, the stress associated with illness may reduce their comprehension of spoken words, written materials, and even visual teaching resources.

Cultural factors such as beliefs related to health practices also affect the patient's response to teaching. The nurse should adapt to the cultural practices of the patient and caregivers if the particular practice is not harmful to the patient.

Documentation of specific teaching activities is also crucial. Although patient education is clearly one of the most essential professional interventions in home care, it remains a struggle to secure reimbursement for education services. Reteaching patients is usually not reimbursable, regardless of learning or need, and thus must be included in other reimbursable care or charged directly to the family. Medicare considers teaching to be a skilled care activity and reimburses for it if the need is justified. Box 11-8 summarizes the guidelines for teaching activities for home health services.

Patients and families often state that procedures they were taught or that they observed in the hospital seem more complicated at home. Procedures can be adapted for use in the home when health care personnel are not available to provide assistance. The caregivers' confidence in their ability to successfully and safely manage care may falter. Scheduling the total care, including bathing, feeding, and technical treatments, may be difficult. The varied aspects of transferring learning into the home situation ide-

BOX 11-8 Medicare Guidelines for Teaching

The activities that require the skills of a licensed nurse and are reimbursable by Medicare include (but are not limited to) teaching about:

- Self-administration of injectable medications
- Bowel or bladder training if dysfunction exists
- Maintenance of peripheral and central venous lines
- Administration of intravenous medications
- Diabetic management
- Wound care if complex
- Self-catheterization
- Gastrostomy or enteral feedings
- Ostomy care
- Application of specialized dressings
- Ambulation with assistive devices
- Use of prosthesis, braces, crutches, walker, cane
- Preparation of a therapeutic diet
- Performance of activities of daily living if special equipment is necessary

ally are discussed with the family before the patient's discharge. An emphasis on problem solving that incorporates the patient and family environment, including daily routines, is helpful. The nurse reassures family members that they can contact the home health agency if they have questions at any time.

Physical problems of the patient and caregiver may make learning the self-care regimen more difficult, especially for older adults. Pain, electrolyte imbalances, or the primary disease process can alter the patient's cognitive function and prevent the patient from being an active partner in the learning process. The patient may also simply lack sufficient mental or physical energy for learning. Arthritic problems may compromise an elderly caregiver's ability to master psychomotor tasks. The effort to manipulate small objects such as needles and syringes can be frustrating. Nurses must identify any physical changes that might hamper learning and take steps to alleviate these barriers when teaching patients and families.

Another personal factor that can make a difference in the patient and family's learning is mental or psychologic state. Nurses may need to use methods to reduce anxiety so the patient and family can attend to learning. For some patients, complex equipment may be overwhelming and increase their anxiety. The nurse initially may need to perform the technical care and gradually teach self-care as the patient or family is able to manage it.

The physical environment may need to be adapted to ensure the patient's safety. Modifications in the home environment for safety also may be based on the patient's disabilities or physical condition, such as using high-rise toilet seats, installing grab bars in the bathroom, or changing a living room into a bedroom. Throw rugs may need to be removed, a ramp added, or a doorway widened to accommodate a patient using a walker or wheelchair. Creative problem solving may be necessary to ensure that family members can use the space in their home without medical equipment causing too much noise or interference. Physical modifications are often necessary to support long-term care provision.

RELATED NIC INTERVENTIONS. Health Education, Health System Guidance, Referral, Self-Responsibility Facilitation

Nursing Diagnosis: Risk for Caregiver Role Strain

OUTCOMES. Common examples of expected outcomes for the family with a diagnosis of *risk for caregiver role strain* are:
Caregivers will:

- Successfully balance caregiving demands with other components of lifestyle.
- Obtain routine respite services to ensure time away from caregiving.
- Identify ways to increase social interactions and relationships beyond the caregiving role.

NURSING INTERVENTIONS. Families and other caregivers undergo stress when their schedules change because of a patient's health care needs. Home care management requires adaptations to new routines, responsibilities, and learning requirements. The work can be mentally and physically taxing for the caregivers, who may become overwhelmed and even angry with the patient. The changes tax the family's resources in terms of both money and time.

Home care alters communication patterns and generally disorganizes a family, at least temporarily. The length of home care affects coping within the family. The longer that home care is required, the more the family's coping skills can become depleted. More situational crises arise during prolonged home care, further challenging the family's coping abilities. Other contributing factors include experiences and expectations of home care. Families with positive experiences who can accurately predict the length of home care and who have realistic expectations about the daily schedule are better able to cope with prolonged home care.

The home care nurse must assess and address family members' fatigue and stress. The nurse can assist family members in adjusting to disruptions. Although the family may be reluctant to accept outside help, the nurse should provide information and strategies to find outside assistance with care or financial support when necessary. Social support in the form of help with everyday care, contacts with a network of peers, acceptance of caregiving by family members, and expressions of emotional concern or praise seems to ease the caregiver's perception of burden.

The nurse also ensures that the family is aware of and appropriately using all support systems available in the community. Volunteer organizations may be available to assist with transportation for physician or clinic appointments, and charitable organizations such as the American Cancer Society can be a source of supplies and equipment to offset the costs of care. Respite care is available through several organizations in some communities. Local communities typically have a variety of specific social support resources that can be mobilized to assist the family.

Religious denominations, neighborhood associations, community centers, voluntary service groups, and professionally led support groups can all be sources of social support. These groups can help ensure that the patient or family caregiver does not become isolated and overburdened with care. In addition, if the family has an adequate financial resource base, the part-time involvement of a compatible home health aide to assist with daily care demands can release the primary caregiver to devote some time to his or her own needs.

Caring for a family member in the home may alter individual members' everyday activities, interactions, and pattern of social contacts. Participation in religious, leisure, and school activities may be affected. Caregivers may lose familiar and meaningful family interactions such as intimate talks, humorous exchanges, the comfort of physical contact through hugs, and the joy of intimate sexual contact. The caregiver can feel increasingly isolated from normal social contact. The possibility of acute loneliness in both patient and caregiver in the context of overwhelming daily care demands is a real concern.

The nurse can help the family explore how home care has changed family function. Family members' own descriptions will clarify the alterations in communications and personal exchanges they are experiencing. The patient and family need assistance to anticipate these problems and suggestions on how to deal with such reactions. Respite care can be an essential strategy for addressing the problems associated with loneliness and isolation.

RELATED NIC INTERVENTIONS. Caregiver Support, Home Maintenance Assistance, Respite Care, Support Group

Nursing Diagnosis: Decisional Conflict

OUTCOMES. Common examples of expected outcomes for the patient and family with a diagnosis of *decisional conflict* are: Patient and family will:

- Discuss advantages and disadvantages of options for long-term care management.
- Share fears and concerns regarding choices for long-term care and reactions of others.

NURSING INTERVENTIONS. Dealing with a patient's chronic disability and home care management places constraints on family members' daily schedules and use of the home for activities. The family must make many decisions each day about the patient's home care. These decisions may result in conflicts between family members. The patient and family members have direct responsibility for managing such conflicts.

Insufficient financial resources are a common problem reported by families at home. Reimbursements from insurance companies or Medicare vary widely and are constantly changing. The home care nurse must be skilled in understanding governmental regulations and advocating for the patient's eligibility for coverage. The nurse may enlist the help of a social worker familiar with home care coverage regulations to ensure the family has information on the costs of home care covered by insurers. In addition, the nurse (with the assistance of the social worker) needs to identify any voluntary sources of financial support for families.

The nurse also must be concerned about specialty services available to the family. In some instances, the patient may need technical support services that are so far away, safety is a concern. When this occurs, the nurse must ensure that the family recognizes and can readily manage emergencies such as equipment failure or lack of supplies.

The physical and financial burdens of caregiving may eventually overwhelm the family's coping abilities and necessitate a decision about placement of the patient for long-term care. The home care nurse can help caregivers realistically evaluate their situation, explore alternatives, and achieve a degree of comfort with their ultimate decision. This is usually an exceedingly stressful decision for everyone concerned. The collaborative involvement of a social worker to explore realistic placement options and associated costs can be helpful.

Box 11-9 Home Care Documentation

- Whatever form the documentation takes, it should clearly indicate:
  - Why the service was initiated
  - What skilled interventions are needed and why
  - Expected outcomes for the patient
  - What plans exist for preparing the patient to manage without home visits
- The nurse needs to regularly reaffirm the patient's basic homebound status, since this is the primary criterion for care. The limitations that keep the patient homebound need to be reiterated (e.g., fracture, paralysis, shortness of breath, pain).
- Documentation needs to reflect the patient's ongoing need for care. Entries focus on the patient's limitations rather than strengths and progress.
- Entries should provide specific factual information about the exact services provided.
- Each reimbursable service needs to be reflected in the documentation. The need for every visit must be clearly indicated.
- Entries should clearly indicate in what way the care has been tailored to meet the unique needs of the patient or home situation.

RELATED NIC INTERVENTIONS. Counseling, Decision-Making Support, Support System Enhancement

EVALUATION

To evaluate the effectiveness of nursing interventions, compare patient and family behaviors with those in the expected patient or family outcomes.

RELATED NOC OUTCOMES. Caregiver Emotional Health, Caregiving Endurance Potential, Decision-Making, Family Functioning, Participation in Health Care Decisions, Role Performance, Safe Home Environment

GERONTOLOGIC CONSIDERATIONS

Since the majority of patients receiving home health care are older adults, the assessment and interventions noted on the previous pages are particularly applicable.

Documentation

Documentation plays an essential role in nursing practice in any setting, and home care is no exception. The patient's home health service record establishes a legal record of the care provided, demonstrates that established standards of care have been met, and serves as the basis for cost reimbursement. Agencies are more dependent on third-party reimbursement, and appropriate documentation is the key to cost recovery.

Documentation takes an increasing amount of time for the home health nurse, as Medicare and Medicaid reimbursement guidelines dictate the exact and narrow nature of reimbursable services. The documentation of each home visit must reflect these elements. Standardized forms are typically used for documentation, especially for Medicare reimbursement. The patient should understand the need for the detailed documentation and that confidentiality is maintained.[8] The nurse may use a combination of written notes, tape-recorded notes, or a laptop or hand-held computer, and the reason for using these tools should be shared with the family.

Each agency uses its own unique documentation forms and procedures, but common elements characterize effective documentation. The nurse completes documentation as soon as possible after providing care; time is scheduled into the visit to allow for this task. Laptop computers enable the nurse to promptly record data and transmit it to the agency in a timely way. The nurse documents details of assessment, care delivered, and health teaching, including all attempted or completed telephone contacts with the patient and family. Box 11-9 contains some tips for accurate and appropriate home care documentation.

The Omaha System of documentation is popular in home health agencies. It is a standardized language for documentation and care planning that is coded for ease of reimbursement.[8] Clinical pathways are also being used in the home setting to establish the nature and goals of nursing interventions. They provide a solid framework from which to construct accurate documentation.

Critical Thinking

1. A 59-year-old woman was discharged from the acute care hospital, after having bilateral total knee surgery, to a community-based rehabilitation center for continued physical therapy. She will return home after a week in the center. As her case manager, you will be finding resources in the community for her ongoing care needs, implementing the treatment plan, and monitoring the outcomes of the interventions for her health maintenance organization. While hospitalized, she was also diagnosed with type 2 diabetes mellitus. Develop a care plan for her ongoing care needs. What referrals will need to be made? How will you evaluate her progress? How can you monitor the costs of her care and institute cost-saving strategies? What other community resources might be available?
2. List the places in your community where nurses are employed. Which of these sites appeals to you? Why does that particular community setting seem interesting? What unique nursing skills are needed at that site? How is the role of the nurse at that community site different from the medical-surgical nursing role in the hospital?

References

1. Bacheimer K: Correctional nursing practice: what makes this practice different? *Corrections Today* 63(4):84, 2001.
2. Brudenell I: Parish nursing: nurturing body, mind, spirit, and community, *Pub Health Nurs* 20(2):85, 2003.
3. DePalma JA: Advance practice nurses as outcomes managers: a successful example, *Home Health Care Manage Pract* 15(6):513, 2003.
4. Fermazin M: Home health care compare: web site offers critical information to consumers and professionals, *Home Healthcare Nurse* 22(6):408, 2004.
5. Frazier SC: Magnet home care agencies: a professional way to impact quality and retention, *Home Health Care Manage Pract* 21(9):603, 2003.
6. Giese DJ: Community-oriented nurse in home health and hospice. In Stanhope M, Lancaster J, editors: *Community and public health nursing*, ed 6, St Louis, 2004, Mosby.
7. Kohn C, Henderson CW: Project aims to help nursing home residents live on their own, *Man Care Weekly Digest* April 12, 2004, p 49.
8. Monsen KA, Kerr MJ: Mining quality documentation data for golden outcomes, *Home Health Care Manage Pract* 16(3):192, 2004.
9. Morton S: Revitalizing professional boundaries policy into meaningful practice improvement, *Home Health Care Manage Pract* 16(4):255, 2004.
10. Nathanson M, Cuervo AM: *Home care compliance manual*, ed 2, Gaithersburg, Md, 2002, Aspen.
11. National Association for Home Care: *Basic statistics about home care*, accessed July 2005 from website: http//www.nahc.org.
12. National Association for Home Care: *Hospice facts and statistics*, accessed June 2004 from website: http//www.nahc.org.
13. Olmstead BJ, Cooke JM: The role of clinical outcome manager in home care, *Home Health Care Manage Pract* 15(6):486, 2003.
14. Smith AP: Case management: key to access, quality, and financial success, *Nurs Econ* 21(5):237, 2003.
15. Tinetti ME et al: Evaluation of restorative care vs usual care for older adults receiving an acute episode of home care, *JAMA* 287(16):2098, 2002.
16. Tull KB, Carroll RM: Advanced practice nursing in home health, *Home Health Care Manage Pract* 16(2):81, 2004.
17. Williams-Barnard CL et al: The clinical home community: a model for community-based education, *Intern Nurs Rev* 51(2):104, 2004.

Visit the Evolve website: http://evolve.elsevier.com/Monahan/medsurg

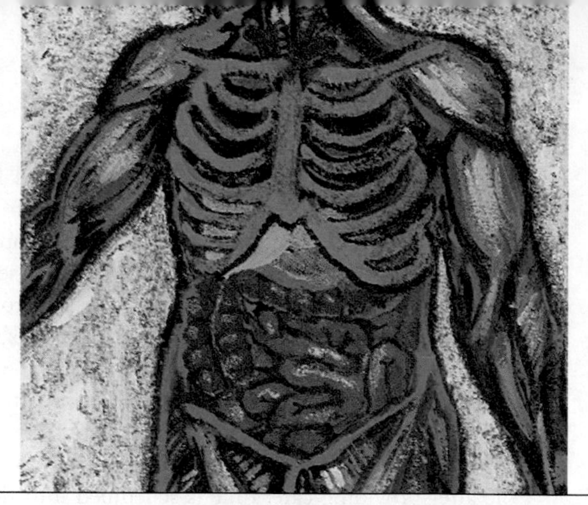

CHAPTER 12 Long-Term Care

by Lepaine Sharp-McHenry

OBJECTIVES

After studying this chapter, the learner should be able to:

1. Describe the trends of health care needs in the long-term care setting.
2. Discuss the regulatory process and its impact on care provided in nursing facilities.
3. Identify challenges facing long-term care.
4. Implement the nursing process using the Resident Assessment Instrument.
5. Differentiate between factors that enhance and those which inhibit the delivery of high-quality care in the long-term care setting.

KEY TERMS

Centers for Medicare and Medicaid Services, p. 224
Eden Alternative, p. 228
Green House Project, p. 228
intermediate care facilities, p. 224
long-term care, p. 220
Medicaid, p. 221
Medicare, p. 221
Minimum Data Set, p. 232
Resident Assessment Instrument, p. 231
Resident Assessment Protocols, p. 232
skilled nursing facilities, p. 220
Utilization Guidelines, p. 232

Until the mid-1960s long-term care (LTC) was provided mostly by families, sometimes with hired help, or by purchased care in private institutions. Dependent people with no family care options or financial resources had little choice aside from charity-sponsored or county homes (occasionally called almshouses and poor farms) where they might get housing and meals. States also established chronic illness hospitals for people with mental illness, dementia, developmental disabilities, and severe physical disabilities, but public funding and standards of care suffered from little public visibility or accountability for the use of funds. Exposure of adverse conditions might prompt temporary public attention, but problems would often recur.

Today **long-term care** refers to services provided to individuals who need ongoing health care or assistance with activities of daily living (ADLs). It includes subacute, rehabilitative, medical, skilled nursing, and supportive social services for those with functional limitations or chronic health conditions. The nurse's role in LTC is multifaceted, but depends heavily on knowledge of medical-surgical conditions, nutrition, pathophysiology, pharmacology, growth and development, and psychoemotional and spiritual needs of individuals with chronic disorders. Although LTC primarily meets the needs of the elderly, other population groups, such as individuals with disabilities or acquired immunodeficiency syndrome (AIDS), also benefit from it.

During the mid-1990s the American Nurses Association reframed its definition of LTC to reflect this broader scope, encompassing all population groups and allowing for more varied care settings. Whereas in years past LTC often referred only to nursing homes, now LTC services are provided in nursing facilities, **skilled nursing facilities** (SNFs), residential care and assisted living facilities, congregate day cares, homes, and other community-based settings. Box 12-1 lists common terminology relating to LTC.

Approximately 3.5 million people live in the nation's 16,291 nursing facilities over the course of a year.[24] Nursing facilities have 1.8 million beds.[2,6] In 2004 126,400 of these were special care beds. The breakdown of special care beds are Alzheimer's, rehabilitation (see Evidence-Based Practice box), ventilator, hospice, AIDS, and other.[5] Individuals ages 85 and older are the most common users of LTC. Between 1994 and 2020 America's 85 and older population is projected to double to 7 million; by 2050 it will swell to between 18 million and 27 million, making these seniors the fastest growing segment of the population. Figure 12-1 illustrates the dramatic upsurge in the 85 and over population. From 2010 to 2030, the number of "Baby Boomers" ages 65 to 84 will grow an estimated 80%, while the population ages 85 and older will grow 48%.[32]

Despite the development of noninstitutional LTC services, the need and demand for nursing home care will continue to increase

Box 12-1 Common Terminology Used in Long-Term Care

- *long-term care (LTC):* A continuum of medical and social services designed to help people who have disabilities or chronic care needs.
- *intermediate care facility (ICF):* Medicaid-certified facility.
- *skilled nursing facility (SNF):* A skilled unit that cares for patients with skilled needs as determined by Medicare.
- *prospective payment system (PPS):* A system of predetermined reimbursement rates for Medicare LTC services.
- *intermediate care facility for mentally retarded (ICF/MR):* A facility that cares for individuals who are developmentally disabled.
- *interim payment system (IPS) (Medicare):* A system implemented through Balanced Budget Act of 1997 to incorporate limits based on historical spending levels that are applied to cost-based spending payments to constrain program outlays. Interim limits vary for each provider to reflect the substantial home health spending across agencies and geographic areas.
- *Resident Assessment Instrument (RAI):* An instrument consisting of three basic components: the Minimum Data Set (MDS), Resident Assessment Protocols (RAPs), and Utilization Guidelines.
- *Resident Assessment Protocols (RAPs):* A component of the Utilization Guidelines; structured, problem-oriented frameworks for organizing MDS information and examining additional clinically relevant information about an individual; help to identify social, medical, and psychologic problems and form the basis for individualized care planning.
- *Minimum Data Set (MDS):* Federally mandated standardized assessment tool used in nursing facilities that participate in the Medicare and Medicaid programs.
- *provider:* Facility or owner of the facility who provides long-term care services.
- *nursing facility (NF):* Nursing home that provides Medicare or Medicaid services or both.

over the next several decades. The major factors contributing to this growth are an increasing population of frail older adults with greater functional disabilities, fewer available and qualified caregivers, and lack of consistent access to community services. The increasing need for LTC will affect not only how services are delivered but also their affordability within the current system.

Reimbursement

During the 1940s and 1950s health insurance emerged as an employment benefit in large companies. Pricing and cost of health services rose along with insurance coverage, and the problem of insuring those at greatest risk of needing care became increasingly apparent. For older individuals and those with disabilities or chronic illness, commercial insurance was generally unavailable or unaffordable. As families shouldered the high cost of caring for elderly and disabled people without insurance, pressure grew for establishing a public system of health care financing to cover "uninsurable" people. The situation was exacerbated by closure of psychiatric hospitals when new medications made it possible to stabilize mental illness. Many frail individuals of all ages with profound disabilities and no financial resources still needed residential care. Reimbursement concerns became a major national issue in health care.

Medicare and Medicaid

After years of debate, in 1965 Congress enacted **Medicare** (Title XVIII), establishing a federal system of financing acute care and posthospital care for older adults on a short-term basis (100 institutional days or 100 home visits). Later it was expanded to cover people with disabilities and end-stage renal disease, and home care benefits were liberalized.

Medicaid (Title XIX) was enacted in 1966, making both acute care and institutional LTC available to people who were financially destitute, through combined state and federal funding. This is a "safety net" for those least able to purchase health care. Together Medicare and Medicaid brought substantial funds to the LTC marketplace, extending access to care to millions. The programs also helped finance construction of buildings and the purchase of medical equipment. A boom in construction of nursing facilities and establishment of home health agencies followed enactment of these programs.

Medicare and Medicaid operated heavily on trust, reimbursing providers of services without effective mechanisms to control how the funds were used. Providers could manipulate essentials such as

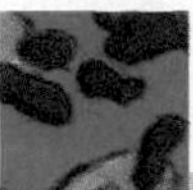

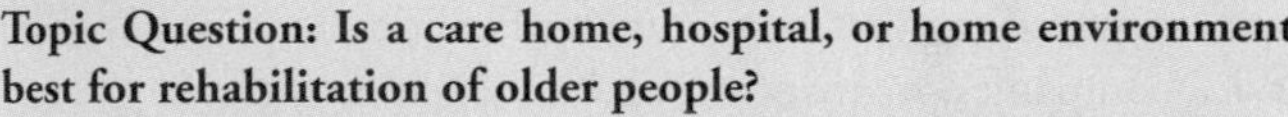

EVIDENCE-BASED PRACTICE

Topic Question: Is a care home, hospital, or home environment best for rehabilitation of older people?

Evidence Base: This review looked at the effects of care homes (long-term care facilities), hospitals, and home environments on the rehabilitation of older adults. All databases containing health-related journal articles were included in the search for randomized trials and other studies comparing rehabilitation outcomes for individuals ages 60 and older in these environments. Outcomes included ability to perform activities of daily living, health status, quality of life, return to place of residence, readmission to acute care, satisfaction, and number of days of rehabilitation.

Findings: Despite the extensive literature, not enough evidence existed to compare the three environments and their impact on the rehabilitation of older adults. Three problems appeared: the description of the environment in the studies was not always specific, the rehabilitation program used was not clearly defined, or the methodology was not comparable among the studies.

Conclusions: Not enough evidence exists to conclude which environment is best for rehabilitation of older adults.

Ward D et al: Care home versus hospital and own home environments for rehabilitation of older people, *Cochrane Review.* In Cochrane Library, issue 3, 2004, John Wiley & Sons, Chichester, UK, accessed July 2004 from website: www.cochrane.org.

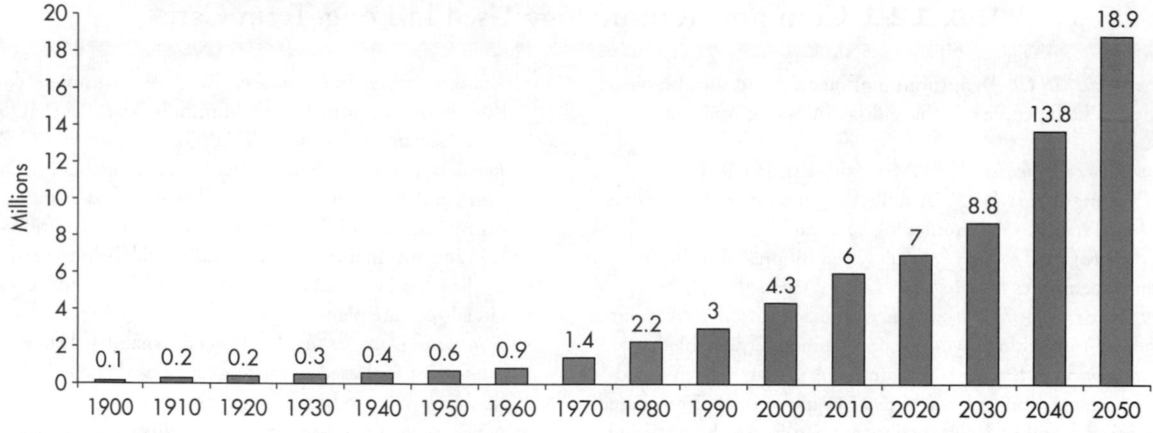

Figure 12-1 Population 85 years and over: 1900 to 2050.

nursing services and food services (counted as "routine services") to cut costs, while diverting funds to other uses such as transportation, administrative salaries, marketing, interior design, and profits. Ancillary service charges, paid on the basis of "allowable cost" without limit or much challenge, grew in size and number. Some corporations that own nursing facilities acquired ancillary service companies, many of which have been profitable.

By 1980 Medicare expenditures in cost-based reimbursement to hospitals were escalating. Congress reacted by instituting a prospective payment system (PPS), which established rates of payment for care in advance according to the diagnosis or procedure. The system identified more than 400 diagnosis-related groups and assigned a payment rate to each. Hospitals now had the incentive to treat and discharge a patient as soon as possible so the cost of care did not exceed the fixed payment.

By 1984 patients were being diverted in greater numbers to home health agencies, SNFs, rehabilitation hospitals, and LTC facilities after short hospital stays. Many were in unstable condition and needed skilled services with rehabilitation. Facilities and agencies needed more personnel, equipment, and staff with specialized skills. An ensuing boom in Medicare spending for postacute care services did not necessarily relieve the stress on facility staff. Staff was not always increased in proportion to the responsibilities in many LTC facilities with SNF units. Medicaid and private-pay residents who also required a great deal of personal and skilled care primarily populated many of these facilities.

With generous public funding, LTC became big business after the mid-1960s. For-profit companies dominate the nursing home industry (65.4%) and set standards that affect competing not-for-profit companies (28.4%)[5] (Figure 12-2).

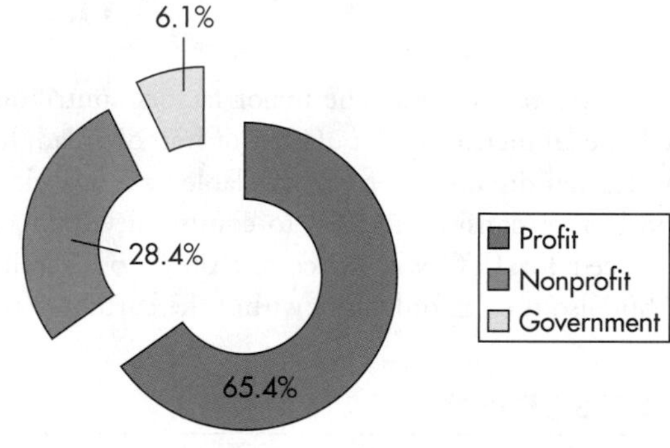

Figure 12-2 Nursing facility ownership.

Many multifacility companies have acquired individually owned facilities and small group chains. Less than 7% of certified facilities are government owned. Beyond maintaining financial viability of an agency or institution, a provider company has the responsibility to deliver the care that has been purchased by resident or their family or the government program paying for the care. For-profit companies also want to produce earnings for owners. Nursing professionals are key players in assessments that determine payment for care and in the delivery of care. The quality of nursing care enhances a company's reputation and attracts new business where competition exists in the market. However, the nurse's role as company "team player" in meeting financial goals must be consistent with professional commitment to advocate for residents and ensure that their needs drive the delivery of care.

Long-Term Care Reform

In the 1960s, when Medicare was passed, government became a major purchaser of health care services for one segment of the American people: older adults. As this group grew, so did the amount of money the government paid out (Box 12-2). At the same time, federal and state governments were paying for additional health care services for the poor through the Medicaid program. The number of people served by Medicaid had also grown, adding to the percentage of federal dollars purchasing health care for certain groups of Americans.

The growth of managed care health insurance plans throughout the 1990s has exacerbated the trend of early hospital discharges to SNFs, home health agencies, rehabilitation hospitals, and LTC facilities. Insurers (including Medicare and health maintenance organizations) limit their costs in hospital contracts, and the hospitals in turn limit patient days. More patients requiring technical support (e.g., intravenous lines, respirators) have been transferred to SNFs and home health agencies. The total expenditures for nursing facility care continue to rise. In recent years it has accounted for 6.9% of total health care spending.[9] The profile of nursing facilities certified by Medicaid and Medicare continues

Box 12-2 Medicaid Prescription Drug Benefit

The new Medicaid prescription drug benefit, enacted as part of the Medicare Prescription Drug, Improvement, and Modernization Act of 2003, will have a significant impact on the practice of medicine for geriatric and long-term care patients. Implementation was January 1, 2006. The drug benefit is mandatory for Medicare beneficiaries who are also on Medicaid ("dual-eligibles"), because Medicaid coverage for drugs for dual-eligibles ended January 1, 2006. The drug benefit is optional for other Medicare beneficiaries. There is no cost-sharing for dual-eligibles who are institutionalized.

Covered drugs and biologicals must be available only by prescription, approved by the Food and Drug Administration, used and sold in the United States, and used for a medically accepted indication. The definition includes insulin and related medical supplies, as well as vaccines. Compounded drugs are covered under most circumstances. Excluded drugs include those for weight loss or gain, barbiturates, benzodiazepines, outpatient drugs for which the manufacturer seeks to require associated tests purchased exclusively from the manufacturer, and over-the-counter drugs. Drugs are not covered under Part D if they can be paid for under Parts A or B (including the drugs furnished "incident to" a physician's service, pneumococcal pneumonia vaccines, hepatitis B vaccines, and influenza virus vaccines). State Medicaid programs may elect to cover drugs that are not covered under Part D.

From American Medical Directors Association: *Final Medicare Part D Drug Benefit Regulation.* http://www.amda.com/federalaffairs/mma/summary.htm, June 5, 2005.

to change. According to the latest data, 72.8% are doubly certified, 18.5% are Medicaid only, 3.7% are Medicare, and 5% are noncertified[2] (Figure 12-3).

The 1997 Balanced Budget Act mandated significant cuts in anticipated Medicare spending by instituting PPS in home health agencies and SNFs. Early anecdotal reports indicated a negative impact on nursing services staffing. Within a year home health agency closures and reductions in nursing staff were attributed to sharp revenue cuts under Medicare's interim payment system. In some SNFs, despite greater responsibilities, nursing staff was reduced. When the PPS for SNFs began phasing in on July 1, 1998, Medicare began reimbursement for skilled nursing care in LTC facilities based on residents' clinical needs and the nursing resources necessary to meet those needs.

Medicare residents of LTC facilities are classified into a case mix group associated with the Resource Utilization Group Version III (RUG-III) case mix classification system to determine the payment the nursing home will receive for providing care. The classification is based on a nationally mandated standardized assessment instrument called the Resident Assessment Instrument, which identifies functional deficits and care needs by reference to Resident Assessment Protocols, and documents them in a Minimum Data Set (MDS). These instruments are discussed in more detail later in the chapter.

Computerized analysis of the MDS classifies each resident into one of the 44 homogeneous case-mix groups in the RUG-III system, which is the basis for reimbursement. This system is also used for Medicaid reimbursement in some states. Registered nurses (RNs) coordinate frequent assessments and related care plans during a resident's Medicare SNF benefit stay. These assessments determine the classification of residents for reimbursement purposes.

The primary payer source for nursing facility residents continues to be Medicaid. In 2003 Medicaid paid the largest portion of nursing home expenditures at 48%, compared with the private sector at 38%, Medicare at 12%, and other Federal sources at 2%[6] (Figure12-4).

According to the American Health Care Association, our nation's LTC financing system steers people toward impoverishment and reliance on Medicaid, a government welfare program. However, Medicaid will not withstand the demographic tidal wave of aging Baby Boomers. Proposed cuts in Medicaid will present tremendous problems unless the nation makes a fundamental shift to a system that relies more heavily on private LTC insurance, which can help protect Americans from financial ruin as they grow older and ease the fiscal burden on state and federal governments. Currently LTC insurance generates a small portion of nursing facility revenue. Few Americans buy private LTC health insurance, and when they do, it is often at an advanced age, which defeats the purpose of the insurance design. Unless this trend is reversed, likely through changes in tax policy, the growing financing burden will remain on the taxpayer base and present

Noncertified 5%
Medicare and Medicaid 72.8%
Medicaid 18.5%
Medicare 3.7%
0% 20% 40% 60% 80%

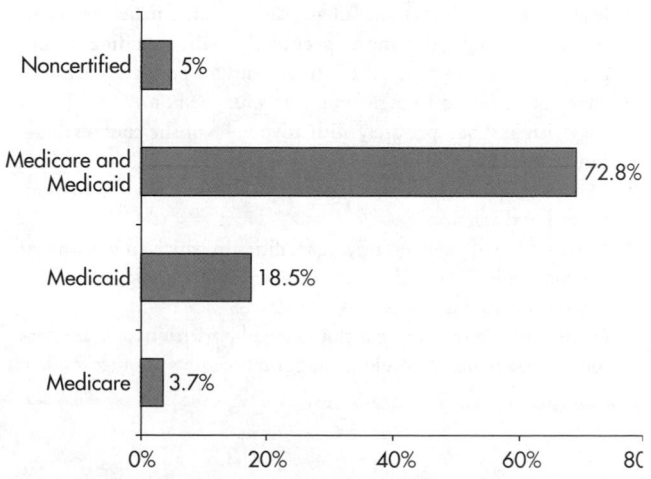

Figure 12-3 Nursing facility certification.

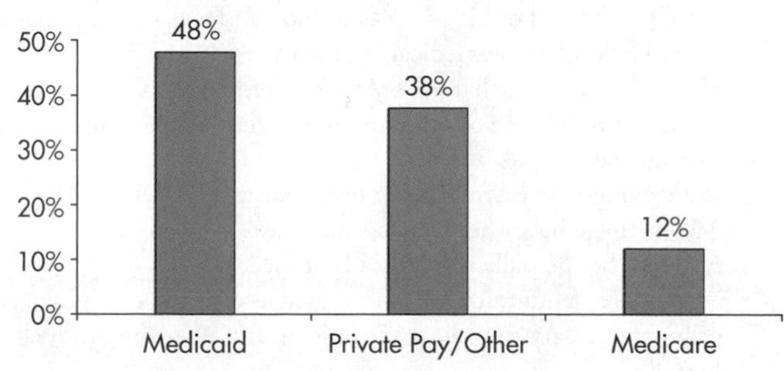

Figure 12-4 Percentage of nursing facility by payer source.

rapidly increasing fiscal pressures on the Medicare and Medicaid programs.[9]

As the population ages, more resources are needed to cover the rising costs of LTC. Numerous federal efforts have attempted to reduce the Medicare budget, with much opposition from consumers. As federal and state tax dollars continue to be the primary source of funding for LTC services, regulatory accountability becomes essential to ensure that high standards of care are maintained.

Regulations

Before 1965 most nursing home regulation was the responsibility of the state; however, with enactment of Medicare and Medicaid in 1965, federal involvement in payment for nursing home services increased substantially, as did involvement in regulating services provided with federal funds.

Nursing homes that provide services to Medicare and Medicaid beneficiaries enter into provider agreements with the **Centers for Medicare and Medicaid Services** (CMS) for Medicare and the individual state Medicaid agencies for Medicaid. To obtain and sustain the agreements (and thereby establish eligibility to receive payment for services rendered to beneficiaries), nursing homes must meet certain requirements set forth in the Social Security Act and implementing regulations in the Code of Federal Regulations (CFR) 483, Subpart B. Nursing homes have the option of participating in Medicare, Medicaid, both, or neither.

In the 1970s investigations conducted by the U.S. Public Health Service's Division of Nursing, state legislative commissions, and congressional committees revealed widespread poor care, deplorable conditions, and harmful neglect in nursing homes. Inadequate staffing for good care was repeatedly cited. Ineffective regulation by state and federal governments was seen as part of the problem. These revelations led to temporary tightening of enforcement but not enough systemic improvement to ensure provision of sufficient nursing services. No substantial staffing requirements were enacted because of industry opposition and government reluctance to commit to paying the cost of good staffing.

In 1982 the Health Care Financing Administration (HCFA) (precursor to CMS) proposed changes in regulation of SNFs and Medicaid nursing homes, termed **intermediate care facilities** (ICFs), that would have reduced government oversight of nursing homes. This was countered by Congress requiring HCFA to fund a study of nursing home regulation by the Institute of Medicine (IOM) at the National Academy of Sciences. The IOM's Committee on Nursing Home Regulation issued a report, "Improving the Quality of Care in Nursing Homes," based on both objective information and a consensus of professional opinions.[12,14] This led to HCFA's enactment of the 1987 Nursing Home Reform Act, commonly referred to as Omnibus Budget Reconciliation Act (OBRA '87).[27]

Nursing Home Reform Act

The Nursing Home Reform Act discontinued the Medicaid intermediate care facility (ICF) designation, except for facilities caring for people with mental retardation (ICF/MR). It replaced ICF designation with nursing facility (NF) designation and extended skilled nursing facility (SNF)–licensed nurse-staffing requirements to Medicaid NFs. It did not establish staffing requirements for direct caregivers and licensed nurses in proportion to number of residents.

This law set new requirements for resident assessments, resident rights, nurse aide training, monitoring of psychiatric medications and restraints, and medical direction. These new regulations dramatically changed the delivery of LTC, turning it into one of the most regulated industries in the country. Resident rights were a significant aspect of OBRA '87. Residents were guaranteed the right to a dignified existence, self-determination, and communication with and access to persons and services inside and outside the facility (Box 12-3).

OBRA '87 instituted minimal quality-of-care standards that established the least acceptable care that can be provided to resi-

Box 12-3 Resident Rights

Nurses should inform new residents and their families that the nursing facility must guarantee that each resident:

- Is informed of all rules and regulations before or at the time of admission.
- Is told of all services available and the cost.
- Is informed of the right to complete an advance directive.
- Is fully informed of his or her condition and is given an opportunity to help plan the medical treatment.
- If transferred or discharged only for medical reasons, nonpayment, or the welfare of other residents, must be given notice and may appeal.
- Is encouraged to exercise his or her rights as a resident and citizen.
- May manage his or her personal affairs.
- May not be mentally or physically abused.
- Will be free from restraints unless used as directed by a physician only as necessary to protect the resident from harming himself or herself.
- Is assured of confidentiality of all personal and medical records.
- Is treated with dignity and respect by the staff, including having privacy for certain types of treatment and for personal needs.
- May not be forced to perform services for the home.
- May visit and talk privately with anyone he or she chooses, and can send and receive mail unopened.
- May participate in social, religious, and community activities at his or her discretion.
- If married, will be given private facilities in which to meet his or her spouse; if a married couple is together in a home, must be allowed to share a room.
- May retain and use personal clothing and possessions as space permits, unless doing so would infringe on the rights of other residents.

dents in LTC facilities. Failures to meet these minimal standards indicate the delivery of substandard care. These standards apply to every SNF and nursing facility in the United States that participates in Medicare and Medicaid. States may have additional regulations, but they must meet the minimal requirements set forth by CMS guidelines, which are organized into 15 categories (Box 12-4).

Standard Survey

CMS requires each state to have a plan for survey and certification of LTC facilities. This plan must comply with federal guidelines to determine whether LTC facilities meet requirements for participation in Medicare and Medicaid. State survey agencies are required to conduct unannounced annual surveys by a multidisciplinary team of professionals, including an RN. Other professionals who may be included in the survey team are physicians, physical therapists, speech therapists, occupational therapists, dietitians, sanitarians, engineers, licensed practical nurses, pharmacists, or social workers.

A standard survey must include (1) a case mix stratified sample; (2) a survey of the quality of care furnished, as measured by indicators of medical, nursing, rehabilitative care; dietary and nutrition services; activities and social participation; sanitation; infection control; and the physical environment; (3) an audit of written care plans and residents' assessments to determine the accuracy of such assessments and the adequacy of such care plans; and (4) a review of compliance with residents' rights requirements. When an SNF or nursing facility is found to be in violation of requirements for participation in Medicare and Medicaid, the government may impose remedies to ensure prompt compliance (Box 12-5).

Enforcement Initiatives

In July 1998, March 1999, and July 1999, reports by the U.S. General Accounting Office noted that enforcement of Medicare and Medicaid regulations by both federal and state authorities had been ineffective.[27-29] Insufficient staffing was repeatedly cited by witnesses at hearings convened by the U.S. Senate Special Committee on Aging, echoing a theme heard in state and congressional hearings since the 1970s. As a result, CMS conducted investigations of nursing home care and imposed more stringent enforcement procedures on LTC facilities.

In early 1999 legislators in as many as 21 states drafted bills to improve staffing in nursing homes across the country. A number of these bills were based on the Consumers Minimum Staffing Standard for Nursing Homes developed by experienced LTC nurses and recommended by the National Citizens' Coalition for Nursing Home Reform (website: www.nccnhr.org).

In 2003 the GAO was charged to complete a follow-up investigation on the quality of care in nursing homes. Its findings revealed that the magnitude of documented serious deficiencies that harmed nursing home residents remains unacceptably high, despite some improvements.[26,31]

Box 12-4 Long-Term Care Regulatory Categories

- Resident rights
- Admission, transfer, and discharge rights
- Behavior and facility practices
- Quality of life
- Resident assessment
- Quality of care
- Nursing services
- Dietary services
- Physician services
- Special rehabilitative services
- Dental services
- Pharmacy services
- Infection control
- Physical environment
- Administration

From Regulations: 42 CFR Part 483, Subpart B—Requirements for Long Term Care Facilities.

Box 12-5 Remedies for Failure to Comply with Medicaid and Medicare Requirements

- Termination of agreement
- Temporary management
- Denial of payment, including:
  Denial of payment for all individuals, imposed by Centers for Medicare and Medicaid Services (CMS), to a:
  —Skilled nursing facility (for Medicare)
  —State (for Medicaid)
  Denial of payment for all new admissions
- Civil money penalties
- State monitoring
- Transfer of residents
- Closure of the facility and transfer of residents
- Directed plan of correction
- Directed in-service training
- Alternative or additional state remedies approved by CMS

From Health Care Financing Administration, HHS 488.406 42 CFR Ch IV (10-1-99).

Nurse Staffing

Until 1999 Medicare SNF staffing requirements were minimal. The law required that SNF services be authorized by a licensed physician and that a licensed nurse (RN or licensed practical or vocational nurse [LPN/LVN]) be on duty at all times, including an RN for 8 consecutive hours each day. Implementing this regulation required that each SNF employ a full-time RN as director of nursing. ICFs were required to have a licensed nurse (RN or LPN/LVN) on duty on the day shift 7 days a week as charge nurse. If the charge nurse was not an RN, at least 3 hours of weekly consultation with an RN was required.

On the federal level, neither Medicare nor Medicaid set a standard for the number of nursing personnel in proportion to the number of residents being cared for in the nursing home. Neither program set standards for nurse aide training. States often set additional staffing requirements for facility licensure, but these were still minimal and in many cases were more protective of state funds than of beneficiaries.

The 1986 IOM report cited widespread inadequate care in U.S. nursing homes and related this to too few professional nurses, inadequate training and supervision of nursing assistants, excessive workloads for these direct caregivers, and inadequate government oversight of the care. The report called for more professional nurse staffing; required assessment and documentation of each resident's care needs; required nurse aide training; and improved regulation, oversight, and enforcement. The IOM report was the impetus for the implementation of OBRA '87; however, it did not establish staffing requirements for direct caregivers and licensed nurses in proportion to number of residents, but did require 75 hours of training of nurse aides with 12 hours of continuing education yearly.

OBRA '87 required that facilities certified by Medicare and Medicaid have a nursing services department headed by an RN director of nursing, who is a full-time employee. Except in facilities of 60 or fewer beds, the director of nursing may not be counted as direct care staff. A staff RN must be on duty 8 consecutive hours of each day, and a licensed nurse (RN or LPN/LVN) must be on duty at all other times. Waivers of these requirements are allowed in certain situations. For Medicare SNFs, the secretary of Health and Human Services can waive 2 days a week of the 8-hour RN requirement if the facility made a diligent effort to obtain the nurses at prevailing nursing home compensation but was unsuccessful, a physician ensures it will not harm residents, and a physician or RN is on call. For Medicaid nursing facilities, the state can waive any of the licensed nurse requirements if the facility makes diligent but unsuccessful efforts to obtain the nurses at prevailing nursing home compensation, a physician ensures it will not harm residents, and a physician or RN is on call.

In 1996 the IOM was again charged with studying the adequacy of nurse staffing in hospitals and nursing homes. This committee concluded there was a need for increased funding of research related to staffing levels, skill mix, and studies focused on quality of care and outcomes in nursing homes. The committee recommended that "Congress require a 24-hour presence of RN coverage by the year 2000 in nursing facilities as an enhancement of the current 8-hour requirement specified under OBRA '87." The committee recommended the use of geriatric nurse specialists and geriatric nurse practitioners, along with an increased emphasis on the educational preparation of directors of nursing.[15]

In 1998 consumer advocates persuaded President Bill Clinton and the CMS to develop a consumer information system to inform the public about current staffing levels in each nursing facility. CMS established an online consumer information system for all 16,000 certified nursing facilities. In 1999 nurse-staffing information was added to the information system. This website, http://www.medicare.gov/nhcompare/home.asp, allows the public to compare nursing facilities across the United States.

Another attempt to increase monitoring of staffing levels in nursing facilities came through new legislation passed in the federal budget act (Benefits Improvement and Protection Act of 2000). This regulation requires nursing facilities that receive Medicare or Medicaid funding to post daily "the number of licensed and unlicensed nursing staff directly responsible for resident care in the facility. This information shall be displayed in a uniform manner (as specified by the Secretary) and in a clearly visible place."[4]

In an effort to explore the need for a national minimal staffing standard for nursing facilities, an expert panel of nurse researchers, educators, and administrators in LTC; consumer advocates; health economists; and health services researchers convened at the John A. Hartford Institute for Geriatric Nursing Division of Nursing at New York University in 1999. The panel found that the average nursing staff level in some nursing homes is too low to ensure high-quality care. The panel recommended 24-hour RN supervision, additional education and training, and minimal staffing standards for nursing administration. The panel also recommended establishment of minimum ratios of caregivers and licensed nurses to residents, depending on the time of day and resident needs, and recommended that residents receive at least 4.5 hours of direct care each day.[13] In an effort to ease the staffing crunch, CMS issued a rule in September 2003 to permit LTC facilities for the first time to hire workers specifically for the purpose of feeding residents. Because the function is a "single task," the feeding assistants need only 8 hours of training instead of the 75 hours required for certified nurse aides.[3]

Since 1997 nurse staffing levels have not significantly improved. Today, the average U.S. nursing facility provides each resident a total of 3.32 hours of care each day by RNs, LVN/LPNs, and certified nursing assistants (CNAs). Of the 3.32 hours of care, 2.29 hours are given by CNAs, 0.70 hours by LPN/LVNs, and 0.33 hours by RNs.[5] These figures reflect only averages. In fact, half of US nursing facilities provide fewer staff hours per resident per day.[32] Studies have shown that inadequate nurse staffing and poorly trained staff contribute to negative resident outcomes.

Today a critical concern is the growing demand for qualified nurses in LTC. Another important challenge facing LTC is the recruitment and retention of staff who provide direct care for older adults. Heavy workloads, inadequate training, and lack of respect continue to be cited as factors hindering the recruitment and retention of high-quality nursing staff in LTC. CNAs and LPNs make up the majority of direct care staff in LTC settings, with CNAs providing 80% to 90% of direct care.[22] Experts anticipate that the need for qualified caregivers in nursing homes will increase. It is projected that by 2020, nursing homes will need 184,400 RNs, 338,500 LPNs, and 1,121,700 CNAs.[10]

At the beginning of the twenty-first century, when nursing facility care should have improved, many nursing facility residents continue to experience worsening outcomes. With nursing homes caring for more cognitively impaired, frail elderly residents with chronic conditions, the failure to increase nursing facility staffing will have a negative impact on the health and well-being of these individuals. Unless federal and state regulatory agencies are willing to establish mandated staffing levels and provide the resources to support it, securing more professional nurse staffing will continue to be a challenge.

Long-Term Care Facility

The LTC nursing facility is a fascinating, complex microcosm. It is a temporary place of recovery and rehabilitation for posthospital, short-term residents. It provides respite and support for families and is the home and community for residents. The LTC facility is an employer and place of career development for health care personnel. It is also a business, competing with others for customers. One LTC facility may be part of a larger business, or a group of facilities, which may own other companies supplying medical equipment and services.

The nursing facility is a system of interacting departments that offers all basic services for supporting and sustaining life for dependent people. By law and regulation, it must provide a safe environment for residents and staff. To function well, it must have clear lines of responsibility and authority. Each facility is unique because of its location, the residents who live there, and the people who manage and work in the home. However, there are many similarities, especially among the more than 16,000 facilities certified for Medicare or Medicaid participation.

CMS requires LTC facilities to have a governing body. The board has fiduciary responsibility for the company's financial viability. The board is accountable for conforming to all relevant laws and regulations. The board selects and delegates responsibility to an administrator or a management company, who reports back to the board. Although each LTC facility is different, the following discussion outlines elements of facility organization that are common to many (Figure 12-5).

All departments, even those with just a few employees, are essential to the organization. The nursing services department has by far the biggest staff. It is responsible for ensuring that direct and individualized personal care is available to each resident 24 hours a day.

The administrator is chief executive of the facility, with authority delegated from the board or chief executive of the corporation. The administrator must be licensed as a nursing home administrator in the state where the facility is located. He or she is responsible for compliance with all local, state, and federal laws and regulation, keeping the facility ready for inspection at all times. The administrator must ensure that the facility obtains required licenses, permits, and approvals in a timely manner and maintains Medicare and Medicaid certification (if the facility participates in those programs). Business and financial management is a primary responsibility.

Each facility participating in Medicare and Medicaid must have a licensed physician as medical director, who is responsible for implementing resident care policies and the overall coordination of medical care. The medical director may be on staff part time or full time. The medical director must ensure that each Medicare and Medicaid resident has an admitting order from a physician and is seen by a physician whenever needed and at least every 30 days for 3 months after admission and every 60 days thereafter. Attending physicians may delegate routine medical visits and orders to a clinical nurse specialist, nurse practitioner, or physician assistant if state law permits.

Nursing services must be sufficient to provide supportive, restorative care that allows each resident to attain the highest

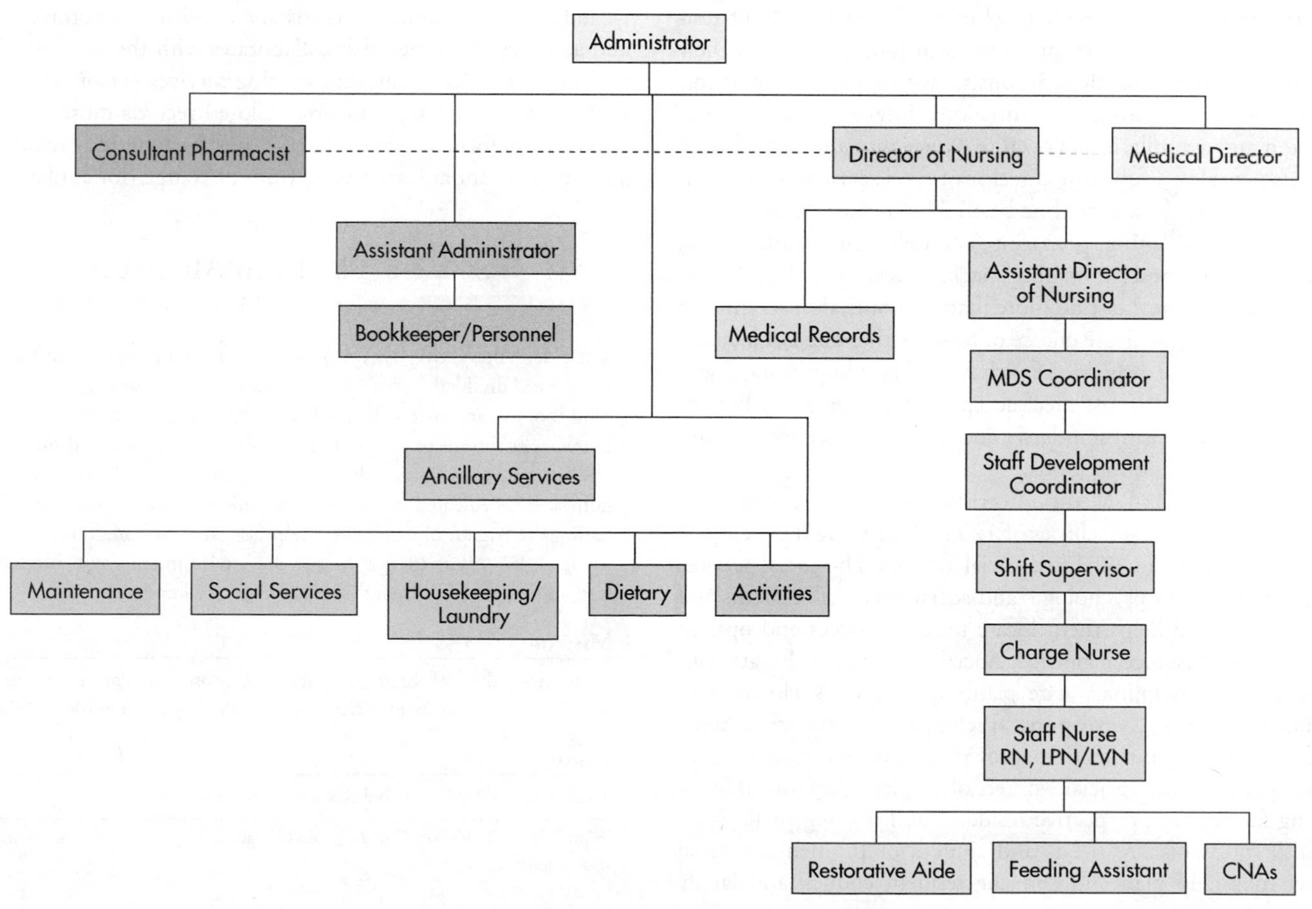

Figure 12-5 Nursing facility organizational chart.

practicable level of physical, mental, and psychosocial well-being. Nursing services must be able to meet special needs of residents for medication and treatments, including injections; ostomy care; urinary catheter care; enteral and parenteral feeding; respiratory care (including tracheotomy care, suction, and oxygen administration); foot care; and assistance with use of prostheses, hearing aids, glasses, and dentures. Basic nursing care must ensure that the resident has adequate nutrition, hydration, and assistance as needed with ADLs such as eating, bathing, dressing, personal hygiene, toileting, transferring, and mobility. Restorative care, which can help residents regain lost function, recover strength, and heal wounds, is integral to good nursing care. To avoid complications in dependent residents, nursing services must emphasize preventive care such as ensuring adequate nourishment and fluid intake, range of motion, frequent turning and supportive positioning to relieve pressure, mouth care, and cleansing and lubrication of skin. The continuing challenge for nursing services is to organize the care so that all elements are provided consistently.

In addition to direct care staff, nursing facilities employ an MDS coordinator, whose primary responsibility is to coordinate the interdisciplinary care plan process. A staff development coordinator may also be employed to coordinate in-service education and orientation training.

The facility must employ a qualified dietitian either full time, part time, or on a consultant basis. The dietitian assesses each resident's nutritional needs, participates in interdisciplinary care planning, and plans therapeutic diets. The dietitian must interact with the nursing department to obtain information about residents' acceptance of meals, preferences in foods, ability to chew and swallow, need for altered consistency or content of foods, need for assistance with meals, nutritional intake, and evidence of retention and assimilation of food (e.g., weight gain). The facility must also employ a full-time director of food services if the dietitian is employed on a part-time basis. The dietary department is responsible for planning, preparing, and delivering regular meals, therapeutic diets, and nourishing snacks to residents. The department must serve breakfast no more than 14 hours after serving the evening meal. A substitute choice of foods with comparable nutritious value must be available at each meal. Handling, storage, and preparation of foods must meet accepted state standards. Personnel must meet health standards and observe infection control requirements in handling foods.

All Medicare- and Medicaid-certified facilities must provide medical social services; facilities of 120 beds or more must employ at least one full-time, qualified social worker. The social services department assesses psychologic and social needs of residents and their families and helps them locate needed services and options for payment assistance if needed. Social workers collaborate with nurses in interdisciplinary care planning and work closely with families in planning admissions, discharges, and transfers. Some social workers are qualified to provide individual counseling or therapy for a resident. Social workers often play a key role in interviewing families of prospective residents and making preliminary determinations of care needs and sources of payment. A social worker may help plan and convene resident council and family council meetings.

Federal law requires an activities program to enhance residents' quality of life. The facility must employ an activities professional or recreational therapist. Ideally, the program involves a plan for individualized activities of interest to each resident, whether bed bound, chair bound, or ambulatory. Often only one professional and an activities aide carry out the program, so collaboration with nursing is needed. Cooperative planning between nursing and the activities department can do much to ensure that the program reaches all residents, even if some stay in their rooms. Nursing personnel need to schedule resident care to allow time for, and transport to, activities each day. Unit conferences and care planning in collaboration with families allow staff to identify diversions and activities related to each resident's individual interests and tastes, and plan for incorporating these into the resident's day.

In recent years new approaches have brought more interest, sense of community participation, and personal autonomy to the lives of nursing home residents. William Thomas, MD, pioneered a concept called the **Eden Alternative**, which allows live animals, growing plants, and visiting children to be a regular part of daily life in nursing facilities (Box 12-6). Another Thomas concept, the **Green House Project**, is founded on the idea that the physical and social environments in which LTC is delivered should be warm, smart, and green. The concept comes from the Eden Alternative method of empowering staff by making the resident the center of the community and enlivening the nursing home environment with plants, animals, and children (Box 12-7).

For quality assurance, a medical records specialist may routinely audit resident clinical records for consistency, completeness, and accuracy. This specialist collaborates with the medical director, attending physicians, and nursing services personnel to promote compliance with standards. Closed records must be maintained in conformance with state law and in an orderly manner in a secure place for at least 5 years from discharge (for adults).

Box 12-6 The Eden Alternative

The Eden Alternative has introduced a refreshing experience for the elderly and disabled across America and around the world. It is a powerful tool for improving the quality of life of nursing home residents. It creates coalitions of people and organizations that are committed to creating better social and physical environments for elders in nursing homes. It is dedicated to creating enlivening environments and eliminating the pagues of loneliness, helplessness, and boredom. The key to the Eden Alternative is to see the environments as habitats for human beings rather than facilities for the frail and elderly.

Mission

To improve the well-being of elders and those who care for them by transforming the communities in which they live and work

Vision

To eliminate loneliness, helplessness, and boredom

From Eden Alternative: *Our 10 principles*, accessed June 2004 from website: www.edenalt.com.

Box 12-7 The Green House Project

The Green House Project, founded by William Thomas, is an attempt to design, build, and test a radically new approach to residential long-term care for the elderly. It is predicated on the idea that the physical and social environment in which we deliver long-term care can and should be warm, smart, and green. The Green Houses themselves will be small (8 to 10 person) community homes where people requiring skilled nursing services can live and receive the care they need. The Green House is a group home for elders built to a residential scale that situates necessary clinical care within a habilitative, social model that gives primacy to the older person's quality of life.

The Green House meets typical regulatory requirements for skilled nursing, assisted living, and adult homes. The goal is to provide the frail older adult with an environment that promotes autonomy, dignity, privacy, and choice. The Green House Project includes changes in:

- Facility size
- Interior design
- Staffing patterns
- Job descriptions
- Patterns of clinical care delivery

From Green House Project, accessed June 2004 from website: www.thegreenhouseproject.com.

Housekeeping, maintenance, and laundry are essential ancillary services to ensure a clean, comfortable environment; safe and well-maintained equipment and facility; and proper cleaning and storage of linens and personal clothing. Nursing works closely with ancillary service providers by arranging schedules to coordinate with their services; ensuring appropriate documentation in the residents' clinical records; and ordering necessary supplies.

A licensed consultant pharmacist must review the medication regimen for each Medicare and Medicaid resident at least once a month to confirm the appropriateness of prescriptions, dosages, and combinations of drugs. The pharmacist also inspects the labeling, expiration dates, and storage conditions of medications and biologicals, as well as records of receipts and disposition of all controlled substances.

A LTC nursing facility is also required to have the following services available to its residents:

- Physical therapy, occupational therapy, and speech or language therapy professionals retained on staff or by contract with outside providers
- Respiratory therapy services (often arranged through hospitals with which the facility has a transfer agreement)
- Laboratory, radiology, and other diagnostic services provided by agreement with providers of these services if they are not available at the facility
- Transportation provided in insured company cars with approved drivers, or by contract with outside taxi and ambulance services
- Agreements for service provision with one or more licensed dentists and providers of foot care (licensed podiatrist or physician)
- Access to religious services and spiritual counseling

In the facility, many departments must function as one unit to meet residents' needs. Admission to a nursing facility is often a difficult decision affecting numerous aspects of a person's life. Ensuring that the facility functions properly and according to mandated standards is essential to the physical, emotional, social, psychologic, and spiritual well-being of each resident. When the facility meets all requirements, it can meet its objective of enhancing each resident's quality of life.

Nursing Home Admission

As individuals age, the likelihood of using a nursing facility increases. During their lifetime, 20% of all men and 34% of all women can expect to be admitted to a nursing facility at least once. Single persons (widowed, divorced, or never married) are likely to spend significantly more days in a nursing facility than their married counterparts. The U.S. Census Bureau estimates that, with the growing elderly population in the United States, the number of nursing facility residents will increase to 2.9 million by the year 2020.[1]

Of the 1.8 million nursing facility beds, 88.4% are occupied.[5] The typical nursing facility resident is a white woman. Women have historically accounted for largest percentage of residents in nursing homes. Many factors affect family members' decision to place a loved one in a nursing facility. Loss of functional status plays a major role in nursing home admissions. Diseases of the circulatory and respiratory system continue to be primary diagnoses at the time of admission.[1] Other contributing conditions are dementia, falls, arthritis, stroke, osteoporosis, and visual impairment. Pain and depression are often conditions that go undetected. The Last Acts study of end-of-life care in America reported that more than 40% of nursing homes residents who were in pain at their first pain assessment were still in severe pain 60 to 180 days later[16] (see Research box).

The facility can take several steps to ensure a better transition for residents and families into the nursing home environment (Box 12-8).

Research

Mezinskis PM et al: Assessment of pain in the cognitively impaired older adult in long term care, *Geriatr Nurs* 25:107-112, 2004.

This study's objectives were twofold: to identify pain assessment methods used by caregivers of cognitively impaired older adults in long-term care, and to identify medications ordered and administered to the older adults. More than 60% of registered nurses, with fewer licensed practical nurses and certified nurse assistants, used formal pain assessment tools. Patient records revealed that 77.5% of cognitively impaired patients had a regularly ordered pain medication, and 91% had a pain medication order prn (as needed). Thirty percent of patients received at least one prn medication in a 1-week period. No one diagnosis was significantly associated with a greater tendency for prn pain medications to be administered, with cancer a possible exception. Eighty-two percent of cognitively impaired patients had a prn order for acetaminophen. Using Minimum Data Set criteria, this study found that patients with greater communication impairments received fewer pain medications.

Box 12-8 Keys to Resident and Family Satisfaction

- Communicate openly; keep family informed of health status and any changes.
- View family as ally.
- Encourage family involvement in care; clarify scope of participation through facility policies.
- Encourage participation in care planning process and meetings.
- Promote and support an active resident council.
- Promote and support an active family council.
- Ensure that staff understands and respects resident rights.

Common Problems in Nursing Homes

Nursing home abuse and neglect are increasing concerns. A 2001 report was the first investigation to assess the incidence of physical, sexual, and verbal abuse in nursing homes; it comprehensively evaluated the results of state inspections or complaint investigations in 1999 and 2000.[19] The study found that 5283 nursing homes—almost one out of every three U.S. nursing homes—were cited for an abuse violation in the 2-year period studied. All these violations had at least the potential to harm nursing home residents. In more than 1600 of these nursing homes, the abuse violations were serious enough to cause actual harm to residents or to place the residents in immediate jeopardy of death or serious injury (see Legal Alert box).

Legal Alert

Having a strong prevention program in a nursing facility is necessary for resident safety and to reduce litigation. Strategies for a prevention program include:

- Ensure *coordination* between law enforcement, regulatory, adult protection, and nursing home advocacy groups.
- Support *education and training* in interpersonal caregiver skills, managing difficult resident care situations, problem solving, cultural issues that affect staff-resident relationships, conflict resolution, stress reduction techniques, information about dementia, and witnessing and reporting abuse.
- Improve *work conditions*, through adequate staffing; enhanced communication between direct care and administrative staff; more time to nurture relationships between staff and residents; humane salaries; opportunities for upward mobility; and greater recognition, respect, and understanding for the difficult lives many workers lead.
- Ensure *compliance* with federal requirements concerning hiring of abusive nurse aides.
- Promote *environments conducive to good care.*
- Ensure strict *enforcement* of mandatory reporting, and educate professionals and the public (nonmandatory reporters).
- Improve *support for nurse aides* (support groups).
- Support and strengthen *resident councils.*
- Ensure that *hiring practices* include screening of prospective employees for criminal backgrounds, history of substance abuse and domestic violence, their feelings about caring for the elderly, reactions to abusive residents, work ethics, and their ability to manage anger and stress.

From National Center on Elder Abuse: *Nursing home abuse,* accessed July 2004 from website: http://www.elderabusecenter.org.

Pressure ulcers are another common problem among nursing home residents. Pressure ulcers are expensive to treat, and their development is associated with a twofold to sixfold independent increase in mortality. Pressure ulcers have become a proxy measure for quality of care and one of the five most common subjects of malpractice lawsuits filed against nursing homes and professional staff.[21] As a result of the efforts of the National Pressure Ulcer Advisory Panel, one objective of *Healthy People 2010* is to reduce the incidence of pressure ulcers by 50%[25] (see Healthy People 2010 box).

In 2004 nursing facilities reported that their residents (on average) require assistance with or are dependent on nursing staff for 3.91 of the five ADLs (eating, bathing, dressing, toileting, and transferring). ADL dependence is a measure of resident acuity that helps facilities gauge the needs of their resident population. The area of greatest dependency identified was bathing; 95% of all nursing facility residents depended on staff or require assistance with bathing. Nearly 88% are either dependent or require assistance to dress, 51% require some assistance with eating, 76% are dependent on staff for transferring, and 81% require assistance with or are dependent on staff for toileting.[5]

Polypharmacy, the concurrent use of several drugs, is a growing problem for older adults, who consume more medications than any other patient group. In 1991 the first Beers list was released, which listed potentially inappropriate medications used in adults ages 65 and older. This list has been updated twice since its inception, with the latest version being released in 2003[11] (see Research box).

Improving the outcomes and quality of life for nursing facility residents is a primary concern for consumers, nurses, administrators, and regulatory agencies. Proper nurse staffing is paramount to ensure accurate and thorough assessment of each resident to prevent deterioration and promote the highest practicable level of physical, mental, and psychosocial well-being.

Nursing Management

Resident Assessment Instrument

The Nursing Home Case-Mix and Quality Demonstration refined case mix methodology for nursing homes. This project can trace its origins to a 1986 IOM study on nursing home quality[12] and from there to reforms in OBRA '87. This legislation mandated a resident-specific MDS. After several generations of revision, this data set has become the primary source of information for both monitoring quality and establishing payment. Data collected in this standardized assessment tool are electronically transmitted to CMS to establish an information database. A second source of data on nursing facilities is from OSCAR, the federal On-Line Survey Certification and Reporting System. This information is used to identify items such as care trends, resident profiles, reimbursement, staffing, admissions, and discharges. The data allow CMS to compare LTC facilities within each state, regionally, and nationally.

OBRA '87 gave nurses significant mandated responsibility within the nursing home industry. An RN must coordinate the

Healthy People 2010

Pressure Ulcers

Objective

Reduce the proportion of nursing home residents with a current diagnosis of pressure ulcers.

Target

8 diagnoses per 1000 residents

Baseline

Sixteen diagnoses of pressure ulcers per 1000 nursing home residents were made in 1997.

Pressure ulcers in all settings are sufficiently common to warrant concern, particularly as a quality-of-care issue. A significant number of people are at risk for pressure ulcers in nursing homes. Older adults are particularly prone to pressure ulcers as a result of decreased mobility, multiple contributing diagnoses, loss of muscle mass, and poor nutrition. About 24% of the nation's 1.4 million nursing home residents require the assistance of another person to transfer from bed to chair.

According to studies of the treatment of pressure ulcers, it is difficult to determine the exact extent of the problem, including the number of new cases and the number of people who have pressure ulcers. Pressure ulcers have long been recognized as a serious quality-of-care problem in both acute care facilities and nursing homes. The prevention of pressure ulcers depends on close observation, appropriate nutrition, and effective nursing care. The number of new cases of pressure ulcers could indicate the overall quality of care provided to nursing home residents. Evidence-based guidelines have been issued on the prevention and treatment of pressure ulcers.

From US Department of Health and Human Services: *Healthy people 2010: understanding and improving health,* Washington, DC, 2000, The Department.

Research

Fick DM et al: Updating the Beers criteria for potentially inappropriate medication use in older adults, *Arch Intern Med* 163:2716-2724, 2003.

Medicated toxic effects and drug-related problems can have profound medical and safety consequences for older adults and economically affect the health care system. The purpose of this initiative was to revise and update the Beers criteria for potentially inappropriate medication use in adults age 65 and older in the United States.

This study used a modified Delphi method, a set of procedures for formulating a group judgment for a subject matter in which precise information is lacking. The criteria reviewed covered two types of statement: (1) medications or medication classes that should generally be avoided in persons 65 years or older because they are either ineffective or they pose unnecessarily high risk for older person and a safer alternative is available, and (2) medications that should not be used in older persons known to have specified medical conditions.

The study identified 48 individual medications or classes of medications to avoid in older adults, and 20 diseases or conditions and medications to avoid in older adults with these conditions. Of these potentially inappropriate drugs, the panel considered 66 panel to have adverse outcomes of high severity.

This study is an important update of previously established criteria that have been widely used and cited. The application of the Beers criteria and other tools for identifying potentially inappropriate medication use will continue to enable providers to plan interventions for decreasing both drug-related costs and overall costs and thus minimize drug-related problems.

interdisciplinary assessment of each resident's care needs at least four times a year and with each significant change in health and functional status. The care plan for each resident must reflect the needs identified in the assessment. The **Resident Assessment Instrument** (RAI) provides a regulatory framework that promotes good clinical practice. Federal requirements state that facilities must use the RAI specified by the state. This assessment system provides a comprehensive, accurate, standardized, reproducible assessment of each LTC facility resident's functional capabilities and helps staff identify health problems (Figure 12-6).

The four types of federally mandated assessments are as follows:

1. Admission (Initial) Assessment must be completed by the fourteenth day of the resident's stay in the facility [(483.20(b)(2) (F 273)].

MDS + Triggers + RAPs → Comprehensive Assessment
Utilization Guidelines

Figure 12-6 Resident Assessment Instrument (RAI) framework.

2. Annual Reassessment must be completed within 12 months of the most recent full assessment [(483.20 (b)(4)(iii) (F 275)].
3. Significant Change in Status Assessment must be completed by the end of the fourteenth calendar day following determination that a significant change has occurred [(483.20 (b)(2)(ii) (F 274)].
4. Quarterly Assessment, a set of MDS items mandated by the state (containing at least the CMS-established subset of MDS item), must be completed at least once every 3 months [(483.20(c) (F 276)].

The RAI provides a structured, standardized process for identifying problems in LTC facilities. Figure 12-7 depicts how the problem identification process would look as a pathway.

Assessment (MDS/Other) → Decision Making (RAPs/Other) → Care Plan Development → Care Plan Implementation → Evaluation

Figure 12-7 Problem identification process.

Minimum Data Set, Resident Assessment Protocols, and Utilization Guidelines. The RAI consists of three basic components: the **Minimum Data Set** (MDS), **Resident Assessment Protocols** (RAPs), and **Utilization Guidelines** specified in state operations manuals. Use of these three components yields information about a resident's functional status, strengths, weaknesses, and preferences and offers guidance for further assessment after problems have been identified. Each component flows naturally into the next.

MINIMUM DATA SET. The MDS is a core of screening, clinical, and functional status elements, including common definitions and coding categories, that form the foundation of the comprehensive assessment for all residents of LTC facilities certified to participate in Medicare or Medicaid. The items in the MDS standardize communication about resident problems and conditions within facilities, between facilities, and between facilities and outside agencies. The triggers are specific resident responses for one or a combination of MDS elements. The triggers identify residents who either have or are at risk for developing specific functional problems and require further evaluation using RAPs designated within the state-specified RAI. Currently, the MDS is in its second version. It is a lengthy assessment and care screening tool, available on the Internet at http://www.cms.hhs.gov/quality/ mds20/MDSAllForms.pdf.

RESIDENT ASSESSMENT PROTOCOLS. A component of the utilization guidelines, the RAPs are structured, problem-oriented frameworks for organizing MDS information and examining additional clinically relevant information. RAPs help identify social, medical, and psychologic problems and form the basis for individualized care planning. There are 18 problem-oriented RAPs, each of which includes MDS-based "trigger" conditions that signal the need for additional assessment and review (Box 12-9).

Box 12-9 Resident Assessment Protocols

- Delirium
- Cognitive loss/dementia
- Visual function
- Communication
- Activities of daily living functional/rehabilitation
- Urinary incontinence and indwelling catheter
- Psychosocial well-being
- Mood state
- Behavioral symptoms
- Activities
- Falls
- Nutritional status
- Feeding tubes
- Dehydration/fluid maintenance
- Dental care
- Pressure ulcers
- Psychotropic drug use
- Physical restraints

From *Long-term care facility Resident Assessment Instrument (RAI) user manual,* Dec 2002.

RAPs are a helpful tool for facilities that choose to use them. They take the form of a worksheet, not a required form. The triggered conditions are indicated in the appropriate column on the RAP Summary Form. Based on the review of assessment information, the interdisciplinary team decides whether the triggered condition affects the resident's functional status or well-being and warrants a care plan intervention. The team indicates a decision to proceed to care planning on the RAP Summary Form.

UTILIZATION GUIDELINES. Utilization Guidelines provide instructions concerning when and how to use the RAI. Version 3.0 of the MDS is currently under development. The new MDS will include new and modified items based on input from professional groups and a technical expert panel (see Future Watch box).

The use of the MDS has expanded to include the quality indicators (QIs) and quality measures (QMs). A team of researchers at the Center Systems Research and Analysis at University of Wisconsin developed the QIs as part of a national demonstration to develop and test both a payment system and a quality monitoring system based on the resident-level data in the MDS; the QIs were implemented in 1999. The final version includes 24 QIs, representing 11 domains of care, based on resident-level data from the MDS (Table 12-1).

The QIs provide information on the presence (or absence) of selected care processes and outcomes, capture both processes and outcomes of care, and address questions of how the resident fared as a consequence of the provision of care (i.e., whether the resident

Future Watch

Minimum Data Set 3.0

The following items are being evaluated for the Minimum Data Set (MDS) 3.0:

- Section A: Identification Information
  Rationale: Reduce tracking forms, serve multiple users, and add important information
- Section B: Cognitive/Behavior Patterns
  Rationale: Improve clinical relevance, use standardized instrument, and better organize items
- Section E: Mood
  Rationale: Improve clinical relevance, obtain resident's voice, use standardized instrument, and better organize items
- Section F: Quality of Life (QoL)
  Rationale: Collect QoL information that is built on evidence-based research to improve choices for residents, and to hear resident voice in direct responses
- Section G: Functional Status
  Rationale: Build on research and clinical advances, and improve item organization.
- Section I: Disease Diagnoses
  Rationale: Improve accuracy of coding information, build on research, and improve form design
- Section J: J2 & J3 Pain
  Rationale: Improve pain items, build on evidence-based research, and strengthen public reporting

From Anderson A et al: *MDS 3.0 development process,* Centers for Medicare and Medicaid Services, accessed June 2004 from website: http://www.cms.hhs.gov/quality/mds30/.

TABLE 12-1 QUALITY INDICATORS

Domain	Quality Indicators	Process or Outcome	Risk Adjustment
Accident	Incidence of new fractures	Outcome	No
	Prevalence of falls	Outcome	No
Behavioral and emotional patterns	Prevalence of behavioral symptoms affecting others	Outcome	Yes
	Prevalence of symptoms of depression	Outcome	No
	Prevalence of symptoms of depression without antidepressant therapy	Both	No
Clinical management	Use of 9 or more different medications	Process	No
Cognitive patterns	Incidence of cognitive impairment	Outcome	No
Elimination continence	Prevalence of bladder or bowel incontinence	Outcome	Yes
	Prevalence of occasional bladder or bowel incontinence without a toileting plan	Both	No
	Prevalence of indwelling catheters	Process	No
	Prevalence of fecal impaction	Outcome	No
Infection control	Prevalence of urinary tract infections	Outcome	No
Nutrition and eating	Prevalence of weight loss	Outcome	No
	Prevalence of tube feeding	Process	No
	Prevalence of dehydration	Outcome	No
Physical functioning	Prevalence of bedfast residents	Outcome	No
	Incidence of decline in late loss activities of daily living	Outcome	No
	Incidence of decline in range of motion	Outcome	No
Psychotropic drug use	Prevalence of antipsychotic use in absence of psychotic and related conditions	Process	Yes
	Prevalence of antianxiety and hypnotic drug use	Process	No
	Prevalence of hypnotic use more than 2 times in last week	Process	No
Quality of life	Prevalence of daily physical restraints	Process	No
	Prevalence of little or no activity	Outcome	No
Skin care	Prevalence of stage 1-4 pressure ulcers	Outcome	Yes

From AHCA Long-Term Care Survey, Center for Health Systems Research and Analysis, Jan 19, 1999, University of Wisconsin, Madison.

improved, remained the same, or declined). They can be used as an external or internal quality assessment or review process; as part of a provider's quality improvement activities; as the basis of research into care practices; as a source of consumer information; and as a guide for policymakers. Surveyors use QI reports before inspections to identify potential areas of concern for the on-site survey process.[9,33]

In 2002 CMS conducted a six-state pilot project before implementing Nursing Home Quality Measures in November of 2002. Originally, 10 QMs were selected. An enhanced set of 15 QMs was implemented in January 2004[17] (Table 12-2). These QMs are posted on the Medicare Nursing Home Compare website for public review. The nursing home QMs, calculated from the MDS, provide another public source of information about how well nursing homes are caring for their residents' physical and clinical needs. The QMs have four intended purposes[7]:

1. To give information about the care at nursing homes to help consumers choose a nursing home
2. To give information about the care at nursing homes where a family member may reside
3. To encourage people to talk to nursing home staff about quality of care
4. To provide data to nursing homes to assist them with quality improvement efforts[8]

Because RNs have the primary responsibility for completing the MDS, it behooves nursing facilities to ensure that RNs not only possess the skills to accurately complete the assessment but also are knowledgeable about its purpose and key role in the LTC setting.

Interdisciplinary Care Plan

Once completed, the comprehensive assessment provides the foundation for formulating the care plan. Facilities are mandated to develop a comprehensive care plan for each resident that includes measurable objectives and timetables to meet the medical, nursing, mental, and psychosocial needs identified in the

TABLE 12-2 QUALITY MEASURES

Quality Measures	Minimum Data Set Observation Time Frame*
Long-Term Measures	
Percentage of residents whose need for help with daily activities has increased	Looks back 7 days
Percentage of residents who have moderate to severe pain	Looks back 7 days
Percentage of high-risk residents who have pressure ulcers	Looks back 7 days
Percentage of low-risk residents who have pressure ulcers	Looks back 7 days
Percentage of residents who were physically restrained	Looks back 7 days
Percentage of residents who are more depressed or anxious	Looks back 30 days
Percentage of low-risk residents who lose control of their bowels or bladder	Looks back 14 days
Percentage of residents who have/had a catheter inserted and left in their bladder	Looks back 14 days
Percentage of residents who spent most of their time in bed or in a chair	Looks back 7 days
Percentage of residents whose ability to move about in and around their room got worse	Looks back 7 days
Percentage of residents with a urinary tract infection	Looks back 30 days
Percentage of residents who lose too much weight	Looks back 30 days
Short-Stay Measures	
Percentage of short-stay residents with delirium	Looks back 7 days
Percentage of short-stay residents who had moderate to severe pain	Looks back 7 days
Percentage of short-stay residents with pressure ulcers	Looks back 7 days

From Centers for Medicare and Medicaid Services: *Nursing home compare: what are quality measures?* accessed Jan 2004 from website: www.medicare.gov/NHCompare.

*When multiple MDS items with more than one "look back" time frame are used to calculate the measure, this table displays the longest "look back" time frame.

comprehensive assessment. The care plan is a living, breathing document that provides all staff with a guide of the resident's care needs. As the resident's condition changes, so should the care plan. It is designed to prevent a decline in the resident's condition. If a potential decline is expected, this should be identified on completion of the initial assessment. The focus should not only be on resolution of clinical problems but also on prevention of further decline.

The care plan must describe:

- The services that will be furnished to attain or maintain the resident's highest practicable physical, mental, and psychosocial well-being
- Any services that would not be provided to attain or maintain the resident's highest practicable physical, mental, and psychosocial well-being due to the resident's exercise of rights, including the right to refuse treatment

The interdisciplinary team must develop a comprehensive care plan within 7 days after completion of the comprehensive assessment. The team must include the attending physician; an RN with responsibility for the resident; other appropriate staff as determined by the resident's needs; and, to the extent practicable, the resident, the resident's family, or the resident's legal representative. A team of qualified professionals must periodically review and revise the care plan after each assessment. The services provided or arranged by the facility must meet professional quality standards and be provided by qualified persons in accordance with each resident's written care plan.

Most nursing facilities analyze the MDS using a computer program, which then produces a standardized care plan. The facility then individualizes the care plan to address the resident's needs, strengths, and preferences as reflected in the comprehensive assessment. The plan should focus on prevention and include steps for managing real and potential risk factors. Objectives should reflect realistic measurable outcomes with time frames. Interventions must be appropriate for the resident's identified needs and may involve disciplines outside nursing. A clear mechanism should be in place to ensure that all disciplines complete and document their interventions, the effect, and results. Progress notes are often used to accomplish this.

Care plans are not static documents and should reflect changes in the resident's condition. The care plans must be translated into instructions or checklists for the caregivers of each resident. Unit charge nurses (LPNs or RNs) assign resident care responsibilities to CNAs. CNAs should be able to describe the care, services, and expected outcomes of the care they provide. Also, they should possess a general knowledge of the care plan and services being provided by other therapists and understand the expected outcomes of this care and the relationship of these expected outcomes to the care they provide. This process helps the staff attain the objective of improving each resident's quality of life.

ARE You READY?

In coordinating care for a resident in a long-term care facility, the nurse ensures that the interdisciplinary care plan is developed within ____________ of the comprehensive assessment.

1. 24 hours
2. 48 hours
3. 5 days
4. 7 days

Documentation

Federal guidelines require LTC facilities to maintain clinical records on each resident in accordance with professional standards and practices. The records must be complete, accurate, readily accessible, and systematically organized. The clinical record must include sufficient information to identify the resident, a record of the assessments, the care plan, services provided, and progress notes. Documentation should provide a picture of the resident's progress, including response to treatment, change in condition, and changes in treatment. Medicare requires documentation, including a nursing assessment, to be completed on each shift for residents receiving skilled services. Medicaid documentation frequency and content requirements vary from state to state. In addition to Medicare and Medicaid requirements, nursing facilities may have additional facility-specific documentation requirements.

As a legal document, the clinical record should contain an accurate chronologic representation of the resident's experiences in the facility. Documentation should include sufficient information to demonstrate the facility is aware of the resident's status. The documentation should also show that staff is assessing and addressing the effects of care provided and response to treatments. Effective documentation portrays a picture of the resident's progress, change in condition, and changes in treatment. The record should show progress toward achieving care plan goals. This allows clinicians access to accurate information that aids in making good clinical judgments for treatment interventions. Failure to maintain accurate objective and subjective data obtained from assessments, residents, family, or caregivers can result in negative outcomes, inappropriate treatment, or no treatment at all. As in all clinical settings, proper documentation is key to effective communication among disciplines and staff.

Critical Thinking

1. An 87-year-old woman is admitted to an LTC facility with osteoarthritis and osteoporosis. She weighs 80 pounds. She is malnourished, frail, weak, and in a lot of pain. Her skin is in good condition except for two small skin tears on her right lower leg. She has an advance directive that indicates she wants all measures taken except the use of tube feedings. She is taking ibuprofen for pain as needed. Discuss alternatives to improve her nutritional status and pain management.
2. How do you compare one LTC facility with another? What are some resources available to assist families in finding an appropriate LTC facility?

References

1. American Health Care Association Health Services Research and Evaluation Group: *Facts and trends: the nursing facility sourcebook,* Washington, DC, 2001, The Association.
2. American Health Care Association Health Services Research and Evaluation Group: *The long term care sector 2003: nursing homes, ICFs/MR, and government funding,* Washington, DC, 2004, The Association.
3. Andrews J: Feeding assistants hired despite legal challenge, *McKnight's Long-Term Care News,* accessed June 2004 from website: www.mcknightsonline.com/news/.
4. Benefits Improvement and Protection Act of 2000, 42 U.S.C. 139995I-3(b)§1919(b), 2000.
5. Centers for Medicare and Medicaid Services: OSCAR Form 671: F15-22, F41-43; L18, L37-39; 672: F78-93, accessed June 2004 from website: http://ahca.org/research/index.html.
6. Centers for Medicare and Medicaid Services: *Health care industry market update, nursing facilities,* accessed May 2003 from website: http://ahca.org/research/cms_market_update_030520.pdf.
7. Centers for Medicare and Medicaid Services: *Nursing home compare: what are quality measures?* January 2004, accessed June 2004 from website: www.medicare.gov/NHCompare.
8. Compas C, Golden WE: New federal initiative features public reporting of nursing home data, *Closer Look Quality* 99(6), 2002.
9. Cornacchione M: Quality indicators in long term care, *ElderCare* 1(4):4-6, 2001.
10. Decker FH et al: Staffing of nursing services in nursing homes: present issues and prospects for the future, *Seniors Housing Care J* 9(1):3-26, 2001.
11. Fick DM et al: Updating the Beers criteria for potentially inappropriate medication use in older adults, *Arch Intern Med* 163:2716-2724, 2003.
12. Harrington C: Nursing home staffing: a need for humane policy, nursing facility staffing policy: a case study for political change, *Policy Politics Nurs Pract* 2(2), 2001.
13. Harrington C et al: Experts recommend minimum nurse staffing standards for nursing facilities in the United States, *Gerontologist* 40(1), 2000.
14. Institute of Medicine: *Improving the quality of care in nursing homes,* Washington, DC, 1986, National Academy Press.
15. Institute of Medicine: *Nursing staff in hospitals and nursing homes: is it adequate?* Washington, DC, 1996, National Academy Press.
16. Last Acts: *Means to a better end: a report on dying in America today,* Nov 2002, accessed June 2004 from website: www.lastacts.org/scripts/.
17. Medicare Quality Improvement Community: *Nursing home project description,* accessed June 2004 from website: http://www.medqic.com/content/nationalpriorities/topics/projectdes.jsp?topicID=413&pageID=3.
18. Mezinskis PM et al: Assessment of pain in the cognitively impaired older adult in long term care, *Geriatric Nurs* 25:107-112, 2004.
19. Minority Staff Special Investigations Division Committee on Government Reform, US House of Representatives: *Abuse of residents is a major problem in U.S. nursing homes,* July 2001, accessed June 2004 from website: www.house.gov/reform/min/pdfs/pdf.
20. National Center on Elder Abuse: *Nursing home abuse,* Oct 2003, accessed June 2004 from website: www.elderabusecenter.
21. Riggs A: Pressure ulcers lead to increased mortality, liability, *Closer Look Quality* 100(5), 2003.
22. Stolley JM: Recruiting and retaining nursing staff, part 2, *ElderCare* 4(1): 8-10, 2004.
23. US Bureau of the Census: *1996, current population reports special studies,* Washington, DC, 1996, US Government Printing Office.
24. US Bureau of the Census: *Statistical abstract of the United States: 1998, we the American elderly,* Washington, DC, 1998, US Government Printing Office.
25. US Department of Health and Human Services: *Healthy People 2010: understanding and improving health,* Washington, DC, 2000, The Department.
26. US Department of Health and Human Services: *An overview of nursing home facilities: data from 1997 national nursing home survey,* Pub No DHHS (PHS)

2000-1250 0-0169 (2/00), Hyattsville, Md, 2000, The Department, Centers for Disease Control and Prevention, National Center for Health Statistics.

27. US General Accounting Office: *Nursing home care: the unfinished agenda, 1987 Omnibus Budget Reconciliation Act (OBRA '87),* report to Special Committee on Aging, US Senate, Washington, DC, 1986.
28. US General Accounting Office: *California nursing homes: care problems persist despite federal and state oversight,* report to Special Committee on Aging, US Senate (GAO/HEHS 98-202), Washington, DC, 1998.
29. US General Accounting Office, *Nursing homes: additional steps needed to strengthen enforcement of federal quality standards,* report to Special Committee on Aging, US Senate, (GAO/HEHS 99-46), Washington, DC, 1999.
30. US General Accounting Office: *Nursing homes: complaints investigation processes often inadequate to protect residents,* report to Special Committee on Aging, US Senate, Washington, DC, 1999.
31. US General Accounting Office: *Nursing homes: prevalence of serious quality problems remains unacceptably high, despite some decline,* testimony before Committee on Finance, US Senate (GAO-03-1016T), Washington, DC, 2003.
32. Wunderlich GS, Kohler P, Institute of Medicine: *Improving the quality of care in nursing homes,* Washington, DC, 2001, National Academy Press.
33. Zimmerman D: Improving nursing home quality of care through outcomes data: the MDS quality indicators, *Stride* Aug 2002, accessed June 2004 from website: www.stridemagazine.com.

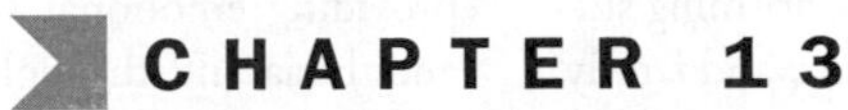

Visit the Evolve website: http://evolve.elsevier.com/Monahan/medsurg

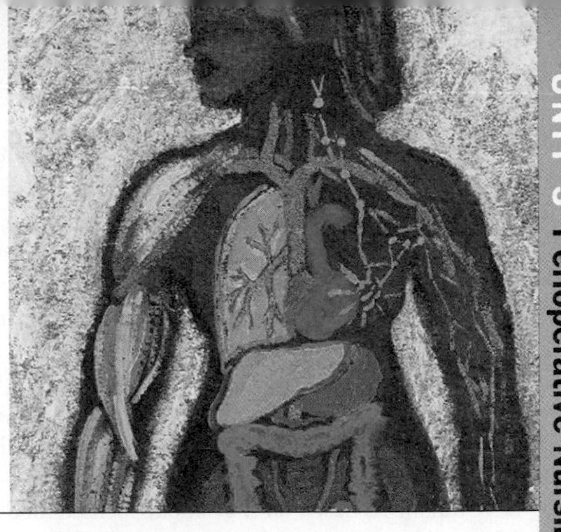

UNIT 3 Perioperative Nursing

CHAPTER 13

Preoperative Nursing

by Jane F. Marek, Mary Jo Boehnlein

OBJECTIVES

After studying this chapter, the learner should be able to:

1. Identify the major influences on the emergence of perioperative nursing.
2. Describe the preoperative phase as a component of the surgical experience.
3. Identify different classifications of surgeries.
4. Identify the biopsychosocial responses of patients to surgery.
5. Discuss the components and significance of the preoperative patient assessment.
6. Explain the potential for postoperative complications.
7. Identify preoperative nursing diagnoses.
8. Discuss expected patient outcomes for the preoperative phase.
9. Discuss nursing interventions in the preoperative phase.
10. Discuss final preparations for the preoperative patient.

KEY TERMS

ambulatory surgery, p. 240
endoscopic procedures, p. 239
informed consent, p. 241
minimally invasive surgery, p. 238
perioperative nursing, p. 238

Historical Perspective

History of Surgery

Surgery is defined as "the branch of medicine dealing with manual and operative procedures for correction of deformities and defects, repair of injuries, and diagnosis and cure of certain diseases."[35] The word *surgery* comes from the Greek *kheirurgos,* which means working by hand. Hippocrates, the father of surgery, reportedly used wine or boiled water for wound irrigation as early as 450 BC. By AD 130 to 200 surgery became a specific medical discipline. At that time, the Greek physician Galen was said to have boiled his instruments before use. A variety of surgical techniques were practiced throughout the following years. During the 1500s ligatures were used to control bleeding. Morton's use of ether at Massachusetts General Hospital in 1846 heralded the advent of anesthesia as an adjunct to surgery. Use of anesthesia permitted the physician to perform slower, more precise, and pain-free procedures. Despite these advances, wound infection and mortality rates were high. In the mid to late 1800s, the mortality rate for patients undergoing amputation reportedly was as high as 40%.[33]

Not until the middle of the nineteenth century did surgery emerge as a true medical specialty. Ignaz Semmelweis's work in 1847 showed the importance of hand washing between procedures and patients in decreasing the incidence of puerperal fever after childbirth. In 1867 Joseph Lister advocated the use of antiseptics such as carbolic acid sprays during surgery to kill microorganisms. However, Semmelweis and Lister's methods were not adopted until the 1880s with the introduction of the principles of aseptic technique. The late 1890s brought improvements in diagnostic tools, including the discovery of x-rays and advancements in surgical instrumentation. At the turn of the century most surgical procedures were limited to the abdomen. William and Charles Mayo published an article in 1904 describing the results of 1000 abdominal procedures.[33] Surgical techniques continued to develop as thoracic, neurologic, and cardiovascular procedures were introduced. Throughout the twentieth century advances in anesthesia, the surgical environment, and technology have allowed more predictable and safer outcomes for patients.

Perioperative Nursing: Past and Present

In the early 1900s many surgical procedures were performed in the patient's home. Nursing's role focused on preparing the environment and supporting the patient. Increasingly complex procedures and greater demands on the physician's time made performing surgery in the home inconvenient for the surgeon, patient, and family. Thus physicians began performing surgery in private medical boarding houses, which provided both hotel and nursing services.[33] By the 1920s and 1930s most physicians were affiliated with hospitals. Nursing's primary role was providing technical assistance to the surgeon.

Perioperative nursing is an outgrowth of operating room (OR) nursing as it was practiced in its early years and encompasses the preoperative, intraoperative, and postoperative phases of the patient's surgical experience. The professional practice of perioperative nursing is based on the patient-focused model, which consists of four domains: patient safety, the health system, and physiologic and behavioral responses. Perioperative nursing practice is directed toward helping patients and their families achieve a level of wellness equal to or greater than that which they had before the surgical or invasive procedure.[8]

The role of the registered nurse in the OR has been expanded, defined, and standardized by the members of the perioperative nurses' professional organization, the Association of periOperative Registered Nurses (AORN). The AORN defines the perioperative nurse as:

The registered nurse who, using the nursing process, develops a plan of nursing care and then coordinates and delivers care to patients undergoing operative or other invasive procedures. Perioperative nurses have the requisite skills and knowledge to assess, diagnose, plan, intervene, and evaluate the outcomes of interventions. The perioperative nurse addresses the physiologic, psychologic, sociocultural, and spiritual responses of surgical patients.[8]

Using the American Nurses Association (ANA) Code for Nurses with Interpretive Statements, the AORN developed perioperative nursing explications of the Code for Nurses. The explications provide perioperative nurses with a framework to relate the ANA code to their own practice. Members of the AORN developed the Perioperative Nursing Data Set (PNDS) in 2000. Approved by the ANA, the PNDS is a specific, standardized nursing vocabulary that addresses the perioperative patient experience. Clinical applications of the PNDS include:

- A framework for standardized documentation and universal language
- The measurement and evaluation of patient care outcomes
- A basis for perioperative nursing research
- Validation of the contributions of perioperative nurses to patient outcomes

The preoperative phase begins when the decision for surgical intervention is made. The scope of nursing activities includes preoperative assessment of the patient's physical, psychologic, and social states; the planning of nursing care to prepare the patient for surgery; and the implementation of nursing interventions. This phase ends when the patient is safely transported to the OR and transferred to the OR nurse for care.

Movement of the patient onto the OR bed begins the intraoperative phase; this period lasts until the patient is admitted to the postanesthesia care unit. During this phase nursing responsibilities focus on continuing assessment of the patient's physiologic and psychologic status and planning and implementation of effective nursing interventions to promote safety and privacy, prevent wound infection, and promote healing. Specific nursing activities include providing emotional support to the patient during induction of anesthesia and throughout the procedure, establishing and maintaining functional positioning, maintaining asepsis, protecting the patient from electrical hazards, assisting in fluid balance, ensuring accurate sponge and instrument counts, assisting the surgeon, and communicating with the patient's family and other health care team members. Other nursing roles include the registered nurse first assistant and certified registered nurse anesthetist (see Chapter 14).

The postoperative phase "begins with admission to the postanesthesia care area and ends with a resolution of surgical sequelae."[8] Nursing activities include ongoing assessment of changes in the patient's physical and psychologic status, along with appropriate planning, implementation, and evaluation of care. Nursing interventions include monitoring airway patency, vital signs, and neurologic status; assessing and maintaining fluid and electrolyte balance; managing pain; managing the surgical site; and providing a thorough summary report of the patient's status to the nurse receiving the patient on the unit and to the patient's family or friends.

Surgical Procedures

Most surgical procedures are given names that describe the site of surgery and the type of surgery performed. For example, appendectomy refers to removal (-ectomy) of the appendix. Box 13-1 lists common surgical suffixes. Some surgeries carry the name of the surgeon who developed the technique, such as Billroth's operation (partial gastrectomy). Surgeries may be classified according to the degree of risk, extent, purpose, anatomic site, timing, or physical setting.

Degree of Risk

The degree of risk involved in the surgical procedure is classified as either minor or major. *Minor surgery* is simple surgery that presents little risk to life. Many minor surgeries are performed with the use of local anesthesia, although general anesthesia may be used (see Chapter 14). *Major surgery* is more extensive than minor surgery and may involve risk to life. Major surgery usually is performed with use of general or regional anesthesia.

Extent

The extent of the surgical procedure can be classified as minimally invasive, open, simple, or radical. **Minimally invasive surgery** (MIS) is usually performed with the use of fiberoptic endoscopes

Box 13-1 Common Surgical Suffixes

- -ectomy: Removal of an organ or gland
- -rrhaphy: Repair
- -ostomy: Providing an opening (stoma)
- -otomy: Cutting into
- -plasty: Formation or plastic repair
- -scopy: Looking into

and does not require traditional or extensive incisions. MIS involves the use of smaller incisions, customized instrumentation, specialized imaging, computerized global navigation systems, and robotics (Figure 13-1). Minimally invasive procedures usually result in improved patient outcomes, including fewer postoperative complications, decreased blood loss, less scarring, decreased length of hospital stay, reduced postoperative pain, and earlier resumption of normal activities.

Endoscopic procedures have both diagnostic and therapeutic purposes and can be used alone or in conjunction with open techniques. Endoscopic procedures can be performed on a variety of anatomic sites. Endoscopes may be introduced through natural openings in the body or through porthole incisions, which also permit passage of surgical instruments. Table 13-1 gives examples of endoscopic, endoscopically assisted, and minimally invasive procedures.

Open procedures involve the traditional opening of a body cavity or body part to perform the surgery. Because of the more extensive surgical approach, the patient may experience more postoperative pain and a longer recovery period. The extent and length of the procedure may also influence postoperative infection rates.

Simple procedures are generally limited to a defined anatomic location and do not require extensive exposure and dissection of adjacent tissue. In contrast, *radical procedures,* which are usually associated with malignancies, involve dissection of tissue and structures beyond the immediate operative site. In most cases the surgeon excises adjacent lymph nodes, muscle, and fascia that have been invaded by tumor.

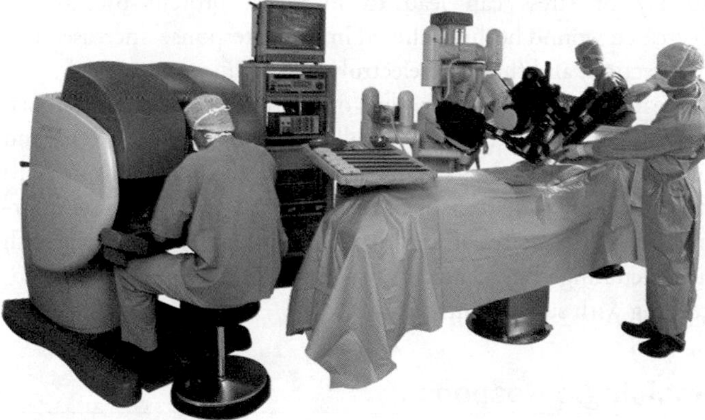

Figure 13-1 Minimally invasive surgery (MIS) is a general term for procedures that reduce trauma by using small ports rather than large incisions for the operation. Robotic surgery, a computer-enhanced, advanced form of MIS, allows complex procedures such as prostatectomy, mitral valve and atrial septal defect repair, and gastric bypass procedures to be done because it allows for greater vision, dexterity, and precision than does standard MIS. Advantages are reduced bleeding, less pain, fewer complications, smaller risk of internal scarring, shorter hospital stay, and faster recovery. This photograph shows the da Vinci Surgical System, which consists of three parts: endoscope, instrument tips, and viewer. The surgeon sits in the console of the surgical system several feet from the patient. He or she looks through the vision system—like a pair of binoculars—and gets three-dimensional view of the patient's body and area of the operation. While watching through the vision system, the surgeon moves the handles on the console. The robotic system translates and transmits these precise hand and wrist movements to tiny instruments that have been inserted into the patient through small access incisions.

TABLE 13-1 TYPES OF ENDOSCOPIC, ENDOSCOPICALLY ASSISTED, AND MINIMALLY INVASIVE SURGICAL PROCEDURES

Surgical Specialty	Procedure
General	Adrenalectomy Cholecystectomy Colectomy Appendectomy Herniorrhaphy Modified Whipple procedure Nissen fundoplication Gastric bypass
Orthopedic	Anterior cruciate ligament repair Carpal tunnel release Acromioplasty Diskectomy Total hip and total knee arthroplasty
Gynecologic	Tubal ligation Laparoscopic assisted vaginal hysterectomy Hysteroscopy
Ear, nose, throat	Temporomandibular joint repair Nasal polypectomy Ethmoidectomy Frontal antrostomy
Urology	Prostatectomy Nephrectomy Bladder neck suspension
Cardiothoracic	Mediastinoscopy Lymph node dissection Coronary artery bypass Repair of atrial septal defect Valve surgery
Neurosurgical	Pituitary surgery Optic nerve decompression

Purpose

Surgical procedures may be classified according to their indications. Breast biopsy is an example of a *diagnostic* procedure performed to determine the cause of symptoms or origin of the problem. The goal of *curative* surgery, such as an appendectomy, is to resolve a health problem or disease state by removing the involved tissue. *Restorative* or *reconstructive* surgical procedures are performed to correct deformity, repair injury, or improve functional status. Procedures done to relieve symptoms without the intent to cure are termed *palliative. Ablative* surgery is performed to excise tissue that may contribute to the patient's existing medical condition (e.g., an orchiectomy performed for a patient with prostate cancer). *Cosmetic* surgery is performed for aesthetic purposes.

Anatomic Site

Another way of classifying surgical procedures is by location of body parts or systems, such as cardiovascular surgery, chest surgery, intestinal surgery, or neurologic surgery. Information specific to these types of surgery is found in appropriate chapters elsewhere in the text.

Timing or Physical Setting

The timing of surgical intervention may be classified as *elective, urgent,* or *emergent.* Planned, nonessential surgical procedures are elective. Urgent procedures are unplanned and require timely intervention but do not pose an immediate threat to life. Emergent procedures must be performed immediately to preserve life and limb. The same principles related to preoperative care apply to all types of surgery, although modifications are made for emergent surgical intervention because of the limited preoperative time.

Ambulatory surgery does not require inpatient admission and may be performed with the patient under general, local, or regional anesthesia. The patient is admitted to the facility on the day of surgery, remains for postoperative care, and is discharged within 23 hours. Rapid-acting anesthetic agents, MIS techniques, technologic advances, and changes in reimbursement policies by the federal government and third-party payers all contributed to the emergence of ambulatory surgery as a safe and cost-effective method of providing surgical services. Ambulatory surgical care facilities include hospital-based centers, hospital-affiliated satellite centers, freestanding facilities, and physicians' offices.

Most patients who remain hospitalized after surgery are admitted the day of the procedure. Terms associated with this type of admission include *to be admitted* (TBA), *same day admit* (SDA), and *to come in* (TCI). Health care professionals conduct patient assessment and preoperative teaching on an outpatient basis before admission. Some patients may require admission to the hospital one or more days before surgery because of health status or type of procedure.

Special Considerations for Patients in Surgical Setting

Surgery is a unique experience for each patient, depending on underlying psychosocial and physiologic factors. Although hospital personnel consider some operations minor procedures, surgery is always a major experience for the patient and family. Surgery produces both physiologic stress reactions (neuroendocrine responses) and psychologic stress reactions (anxiety, fear). Surgery is also a social stressor, requiring family adaptation to temporary or permanent role changes.

Neuroendocrine Response

Impending surgery evokes the physiologic stress response, coordinated by the central nervous system. The central nervous system activates the hypothalamus, the sympathetic nervous system, the anterior and posterior pituitary glands, and the adrenal medulla and cortex. This activation results in the release of catecholamines and hormones, which are responsible for the physiologic events that occur in response to stress.

Systemic effects of the neuroendocrine response are manifested by many complex changes, including increased heart rate and blood pressure, increased blood flow to the brain and vital organs, decreased motility and blood flow to the gastrointestinal tract, increased gastric acid production, elevated blood glucose, increased respiratory rate, increased perspiration and piloerection, dilation of pupils, and platelet aggregation. The nurse's knowledge of the patient's physiologic response to stress is vital for planning and implementing care throughout the perioperative experience.

Psychologic Response

Anxiety is a normal adaptive response to the stress of surgery and can occur at any time throughout the perioperative period. Potential sources of anxiety include anticipation of impending surgery, pain and discomfort, changes in body image or function, role changes, loss of control, family concerns, or potential alterations in lifestyle. Previous surgical experiences may positively or negatively affect the patient's level of anxiety. Anxiety may be decreased if the patient anticipates the surgery will have positive results, such as curing disease, relieving discomfort, or creating a more attractive physical appearance. In contrast, anxiety usually is increased when the underlying pathologic condition is, or is perceived to be, life threatening.

Physiologic manifestations of anxiety include increased pulse and respiratory rate, increased blood pressure, abdominal distress, and increased urinary frequency. Mild levels of anxiety are known to enhance learning and performance; however, moderate to high levels of anxiety may interfere with the individual's ability to make informed decisions and may decrease effective coping mechanisms. In the surgical patient, extended or excessive periods of anxiety or stress can lead to increased protein breakdown, decreased wound healing, altered immune response, increased risk of infection, and fluid and electrolyte imbalance.

Fear of the unknown and loss of control are common responses to surgery. Other fears specifically relate to the type, extent, and purpose of surgery. Fears concerning pain, disfigurement, disability, or death may be realistic or may be influenced by lack of information or the personal experiences of others. The patient with incapacitating fear or anxiety warrants intervention before proceeding with surgical intervention.

Sociologic Response

The usual role of a person hospitalized even for 1 day is disrupted. This disruption inevitably necessitates role adaptation on the part of other family members and friends as they help with transporting the patient to and from the hospital, psychologic support of the patient, child care, and other family responsibilities. Inability to work may also be a problem for both patient and family. Job security may be threatened, and financial stress may result.

Family members often experience more anxiety than the patient because they feel helpless concerning the surgery. Family and friends may be anxious for a variety of reasons, including concern about prognosis and potential changes in lifestyle or routines. Providing emotional support for the patient may place an added burden on the family or caregiver. Personal experiences with surgery and anesthesia may influence the family's perception of the current situation.

▶ ARE You READY?

Which of the following is characteristic of physiologic manifestations of anxiety during the preoperative period?

1. Decreased urinary output
2. Decreased respiratory rate
3. Increased heart rate
4. Increased bowel sounds

Legal and Ethical Issues

Informed Consent

The **informed consent** process protects a patient's right to self-determination and autonomy regarding surgical intervention. Before surgery the physician asks the patient to sign a statement consenting to the operative procedure. The consent implies that the patient has been given the information necessary to understand the nature of the procedure and its known and possible consequences. The physician is responsible for providing the patient with sufficient information to weigh the risks and benefits of the proposed surgery (disclosure duty). This information usually includes the disease process and diagnosis; the nature of the surgery with its benefits, risks, and prognosis if treatment is withheld; and alternative treatment modalities. Legal responsibility for obtaining informed consent from the patient resides with the physician. Failure of the surgeon to provide the patient or legal guardian with full disclosure can result in litigation for negligence. Although nurses may be named in litigation, legal precedence holds that the sole responsibility for obtaining informed consent lies with the physician.[30]

The perioperative nurse's role is that of patient advocate. The nurse assesses the patient's decision-making capacity, confirms that the patient has been given the necessary information to give informed consent, and clarifies any misconceptions. The AORN's explications of the ANA Code of Ethics underscore the nurse's ethical obligation to confirm that the physician has obtained appropriate consent for surgery.[8] In addition to the surgeon, the anesthesia provider also has the legal responsibility to provide the patient or legal guardian full disclosure regarding the risks and benefits of any anesthetic agents or medications that may be administered during the procedure. The Joint Commission on Accreditation of Healthcare Organizations (JCAHO) requires the anesthesia provider to attest that informed consent regarding the risks of anesthesia has been obtained.

The necessary components of the consent document include the patient's full legal name; surgeon's name; specific procedure(s) to be performed; signature of the patient, next of kin, or legal guardian; witness(es); and date. Witnessing the informed consent does not ensure that the patient has a complete understanding of the surgical procedure and its consequences. By signing the consent form, the witness validates *only* the identification of the patient or legal substitute, the patient's mental status at time of signature (alert and competent and not under the effects of mind-altering substances), and the patient's voluntary signature.

Signing of the official consent form primarily provides evidence that the consent process occurred and that the patient is aware of the concept of informed consent. It is imperative that this process occur before the patient receives any sedation. If an adult is incapable of giving informed consent, the physician must obtain consent from the next of kin. The order of kin relationship for an adult, as determined from legal interstate succession, is usually spouse, adult child, parent, and sibling. A parent or legal guardian usually provides consent for a minor child. Emancipated minors, that is, minors who are married or earning their own livelihood and retaining the earnings, can sign their own consent forms. The signature of the husband or wife of a married minor is also acceptable. In an emergency the surgeon may operate without written permission of the patient or family, although every effort is made to contact a family member or guardian if time permits. Consent in the form of a telephone call is permissible in this situation. Two persons must witness the call.

If no family member or legal guardian can be contacted, two physicians who are not associated with the procedure may make the decision for surgical intervention. In this circumstance a relative must sign an operative consent as soon as possible. Patients who are illiterate must understand the verbal explanation of the consent process and may sign the form with an *X*. This process must be witnessed by two persons. The healthcare facility must provide translators for patients with language barriers. The legal guardian may sign the consent form for mentally incompetent persons; in the guardian's absence, a court of competent jurisdiction may legalize the procedure.

It should also be noted that the patient has the right to refuse surgical intervention. A patient has the right to withdraw informed consent at any time before the procedure if that decision is reached voluntarily and rationally. The nurse's responsibility is to support the patient's decision.

Advance Directives

Patients' rights of autonomy and self-determination are protected by the Patient Self-Determination Act of 1991 (PSDA). The law requires health care providers to inform patients of their rights in decision making regarding health care choices. *Advance directives* are developed in accord with state law and allow an individual to indicate his or her preferences for treatment if he or she becomes unable to make independent health care decisions.

A *living will* and *durable power of attorney for health care* are common examples of advance directives. The patient completes both documents while still competent. A living will outlines the patient's wishes regarding medical care, artificially supplied nourishment, life support, and resuscitation measures. The durable power of attorney identifies the person who is authorized to make decisions on the patient's behalf if the patient becomes incapacitated. The PSDA does not apply to all health care settings. Any institution receiving Medicare or Medicaid funds is required by the PSDA to inform patients about their states' advance directives and inquire whether such the patient has such documents. The perioperative nurse must be aware of a patient's decisions regarding advance directives.

Do-Not-Resuscitate Orders

As discussed in the preceding paragraphs, advance directives concern decisions regarding end-of-life treatments. The decision not to initiate cardiopulmonary resuscitation is written as a specific directive by a physician, which is termed a *do-not-resuscitate (DNR) order.* Perioperative nurses may encounter patients with DNR orders who are undergoing surgical procedures for improving the quality of life or for palliative care. DNR orders are not automatically suspended when the patient enters the OR. The AORN's position statement on perioperative care of patients with DNR orders is supported by the PSDA, JCAHO, the ANA Code for Nurses, and "A Patient's Bill of Rights." The AORN position statement asserts that "required reconsideration of DNR decisions with patients is an integral component of the care of patients undergoing surgery."[8] Reviewing DNR status ensures that the risks and benefits of anesthesia and surgery are discussed with the patient or family before surgery. Discussion should include goals of surgical treatment, potential for and nature of resuscitative measures, and possible outcomes with and without resuscitative efforts. The patient or the individual with durable power of attorney will decide whether to maintain, suspend, or modify the DNR orders during anesthesia and surgery. If the DNR order is suspended during the intraoperative period, documentation must indicate when it is to be reinstated. The perioperative nurse has the responsibility to support the patient's end-of-life treatment choices and right to refuse treatment.

ARE You READY?

The registered nurse's primary responsibility in the process of informed consent is to:

1. Provide the patient with details of proposed surgical procedure.
2. Advocate for the patient to ensure understanding of proposed procedure.
3. Discuss possible complications of proposed procedure.
4. Ensure that the anesthetist/anesthesiologist has met with patient before procedure.

Nursing Management
of the Patient in the Preoperative Period

ASSESSMENT

Health History. Assessment of the patient during the preoperative phase begins with the initial contact between patient and nurse and continues throughout the perioperative period. Patient assessment occurs in a variety of settings. JCAHO guidelines mandate that the history and physical examination be completed within 30 days of the surgical date.[36] On the day of surgery the nurse evaluates the patient for any changes to the initial history and physical examination. Allowing sufficient time between the interview and surgery date permits treatment of identified problems and further consultation if needed, thus avoiding surgical cancellation. Researchers in the Netherlands concluded that conducting the preoperative evaluation up to 3 weeks before surgery resulted in fewer cancelled cases.[29]

The nurse's initial contact with the patient may be in the physician's office, preadmission testing area, inpatient hospital unit, or ambulatory surgery facility or over the telephone. The nurse compiles a complete health history to identify factors that may increase surgical risk or contribute to postoperative complications. The goal of preoperative assessment is to identify individuals at risk for intraoperative and postoperative complications and implement interventions to decrease risk and improve surgical outcomes.

Assess for:

- Allergies
- Medications and substance abuse
- Herbs and nutritional supplements use
- Cultural and religious preferences
- Availability of social support
- Ability to perform activities of daily living (ADLs) (functional assessment)
- Anxiety
- Presence of preexisting or systemic disease
- Previous surgical and anesthetic experience
- Pain
- Degree of surgical risk
- Actual knowledge and understanding of perioperative experience

ALLERGIES. The nurse should assess the patient for allergies to iodine, medications, latex, cleansing solutions, and adhesive tape, since many of these products are used throughout the surgical procedure. The nurse should document the type of reaction in the patient's record. Povidone-iodine is commonly used during surgery for cleansing the patient's skin. Iodine is also a component of many contrast media that may be used during surgery. If the patient is unsure whether he or she has an allergy to iodine, the nurse should ask about allergies to shellfish, which has a high iodine content. Patients with latex allergies require special latex-free supplies and equipment (see Chapter 14).

MEDICATIONS AND SUBSTANCE ABUSE. The nurse collects data regarding history of smoking, substance abuse, and prescribed and over-the-counter (OTC) medications. These data are important because of the potential adverse interactions of these substances with some anesthetic agents and increased risk for perioperative complications.

Smoking, first identified as a risk factor for postoperative pulmonary complications in 1944, increases intraoperative and postoperative risks even in individuals without chronic lung disease. Smokers have a higher risk of cardiopulmonary and wound complications than do nonsmokers. Four to eight weeks of smoking cessation is effective in reducing postoperative morbidity.[21,22,36] During the preadmission interview, the nurse should inform patients about the benefits of smoking cessation and smoking cessation techniques.

Drug and alcohol use can alter the effects of anesthetic and analgesic agents, necessitating adjustments of the recommended dosages. In addition to an accurate history of recreational drug use, the nurse should elicit an accurate history of alcohol consumption. Unidentified alcohol use may result in withdrawal symptoms in the surgical patient whose regular alcohol intake is decreased or discontinued. An accepted screening tool for potentially problematic alcohol consumption is the CAGE questionnaire (see Box 2-7) developed by Ewing in 1984.[31]

A thorough history of medication use is essential. Many types of prescription and OTC medications may affect reactions to anesthetics or surgery (Table 13-2). Medication history is of particular importance in the preoperative assessment of older adults, who use 31% of prescription drugs in the United States.[17] The typical older adult has multiple medical illnesses and receives multiple medications,[2] which significantly increases the potential for drug interactions, adverse side effects, and interactions with anesthetic agents.

In addition to prescribed medications, the nurse must also assess the patient for use of OTC medications. Many drugs that previously required a prescription are now available without one. Self-administered OTC medications may interact with the patient's prescription medications, anesthetic, and drugs prescribed during the perioperative period. A complete medication history is necessary to decrease the risk of perioperative adverse drug reactions; as many as 30% of hospitalized patients experience an adverse drug reaction.[27]

HERBS AND NUTRITIONAL SUPPLEMENTS. Used extensively in Europe and Asia for years, dietary supplements, vitamins, minerals, and homeopathic and herbal products are nontraditional therapies that are becoming increasingly popular in the United States. In the past decade the use of herbal products has increased as much as 380%. Internationally, approximately 1200 to 1800 herbal products are available. An estimated 32% of perioperative patients report the use of herbal products or dietary supplements.[11,18]

The terminology for these products is often confusing; herbs, also known as botanicals, nutraceuticals, or phytomedicines, are medicinal plants and possess pharmacologic properties. In the United States herbs are classified as dietary supplements, not medications, and hence are under control of the Federal Trade Commission rather than the U.S. Food and Drug Administration (FDA).[32] Herbal products lack the rigorous control and approval process required by the FDA for medications. In 1994 the Dietary Supplement Health and Education Act established regulations for dietary supplements. Under these regulations, the FDA can restrict use of a dietary supplement only if proven unsafe. Currently no regulations address purity, identification of ingredients, or manufacturing processes for herbals and dietary supplements[18]; however, the FDA does issue warnings and responds to medical complaints regarding dietary supplements.

Media exposure, marketing, and accessibility of herbal products contribute to the increased use of these products among Americans. Many consumers mistakenly assume that all herbal products are safe and do not realize the implications of their use, including side effects and potential drug-herb interactions. Some herbal products, when taken with prescribed medication, may cause serious interactions. However, as many as 70% of patients taking herbal products or other supplements do not disclose the use of these products to the health care provider.[11] Furthermore, many providers do not specifically question patients regarding the use of alternative therapies during the assessment interview. Therefore it is essential that the preoperative assessment include specific questions regarding the use of herbal products and other complementary and alternative therapies.

There is a paucity of data regarding the use of herbal products and anesthetic interactions and the benefit of discontinuing these products before surgery. Currently the American Society of Anesthesiologists (ASA) has no formal standard of care for phytomedicines. Information released by the ASA, however, advises clinicians that patients discontinue herbal medications at least 2 to 3 weeks before surgery.[2] In practice, this may be impossible, since most patients are not seen that far in advance for elective surgery. The perioperative nurse may see many patients who are still taking herbal medications at the time of surgery; therefore the perioperative nurse must be aware of the common names, actions, side effects, drug-herb interactions, and perioperative implications of commonly used herbal products (Table 13-3). The nurse also must ask about vitamin usage, since vitamin E may increase the risk of bleeding, particularly in patients already taking anticoagulants. Until the ASA establishes standards, the perioperative nurse needs to know the institutional policies regarding discontinuation of these products before surgery.

CULTURAL AND RELIGIOUS PREFERENCES. Cultural and ethnic background influences an individual's response to health, illness, surgery, pain, and death. An awareness of cultural differences may enhance the nurse's knowledge of how the patient and family may perceive the surgical experience. If a patient has a language barrier, the nurse should arrange for an interpreter to be present throughout the perioperative process.

Like cultural beliefs, religious beliefs influence individual and family responses to health, illness, pain, surgery, and death. Religion can be a source of support and comfort for the patient. Some religions allow for little individual control over the environment and therefore may dictate the medical interventions a patient chooses. Awareness of a patient's individual religious beliefs enables the nurse to appropriately support the patient's decisions regarding care throughout the perioperative period. For example, the nurse would support a Jehovah's Witness's refusal to receive blood transfusions.

SOCIAL SUPPORT. Assessment of the social situation of the patient, the patient's family, and significant others is necessary to coordinate postoperative care, discharge, and follow-up care. During the preoperative interview the nurse should evaluate the patient's role in the family and social support network. The primary source of psychologic support for the patient is usually the family or significant others. Knowledge of the patient's and family's coping mechanisms enables the nurse to assist them in coping effectively with the impending events. The nurse should also assess the patient's financial status and insurance coverage, since these factors may have considerable implications for the immediate surgical intervention, hospitalization, and follow-up care.

FUNCTIONAL ASSESSMENT. To assess the patient's ability to perform ADLs, the nurse can interview the patient or use a standardized tool such as the Sickness Impact Profile. The patient's preoperative level of function provides a baseline and can be used in projecting the capacity for postoperative self-care. An important consideration is whether the proposed surgery will result in a decline in the person's functional status. The nurse should assess potential discharge needs during the preoperative evaluation. If the patient is likely to need assistance with ADLs, a caregiver(s) should be identified. If the patient is expected to

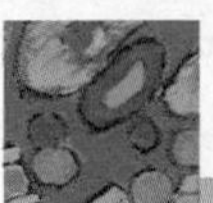

TABLE 13-2
COMMON MEDICATIONS *and Their Effects on Anesthesia and Surgery*

Drug	Action	Nursing Intervention
Anticoagulants, antiplatelets		
Aspirin	Inhibits platelet aggregation	Discontinue 7 days before surgery.
Heparin	Inhibits action of antithrombin	Monitor for bleeding. May discontinue before surgery.
Clopidogrel	Inhibits platelet aggregation	May discontinue 5-7 days before surgery.
Low-molecular-weight heparins	Inhibit factor Xa	Monitor for bleeding. Be aware of increased bleeding risks when used with other anticoagulants. May give before surgery for prophylaxis for deep venous thrombosis.
Warfarin	Interferes with vitamin K–dependent coagulation factors	Monitor coagulation studies, international normalized ratio, prothrombin time. Usually discontinue 2-4 days before elective surgery. It is highly protein bound; drug interactions may potentiate anticoagulant effects.
Nonsteroidal antiinflammatory drugs	Block prostaglandin synthesis Inhibit platelet aggregation Prolong bleeding time Have significant analgesic and antipyretic properties	Use cautiously in patients with impaired renal and hepatic function. Monitor for bleeding. Be aware of increased risk of bleeding with concomitant use of anticoagulants. May increase blood pressure in normotensive and hypertensive individuals. Drugs will decrease hypotensive response to thiazides, beta-blockers, and vasodilators. May discontinue before surgery.
Steroids	Decrease neuroendocrine response, antiinflammatory and immunosuppressive action Delayed wound healing	Maintain drug therapy perioperatively (dosages may need to be temporarily increased). May give intravenously intraoperatively. Monitor for bleeding. Monitor closely for signs and symptoms of infection.
Antihypertensives	May cause possible perioperative cardiac complications, including myocardial infarction and congestive heart failure	Maintain antihypertensive therapy before and day of surgery. Monitor blood pressure and pulse.

experience a significant change in role or loss of independence, both the patient and family may need counseling and support. Social service referrals can be initiated at this time. The case manager or discharge coordinator is the primary facilitator for discharge needs, including medical equipment and supplies, home care, and therapy.

LEVEL OF ANXIETY. Anxiety is a common response to the stressors of surgical intervention. Signs of anxiety in the presurgical patient are no different from those in another person. Anxiety results in elevated levels of cortisol and adrenaline, which are normal physiologic responses to stress. If unmanaged or prolonged, anxiety may lead to increased protein breakdown, decreased wound healing, increased risk of infection, altered immune response, and fluid and electrolyte imbalances. Changes in sleep patterns also provide clues about increased anxiety.

The nurse needs to determine how family members or significant others affect the patient's level of anxiety. Before surgery and throughout the perioperative experience, family members may be more anxious than the patient, perhaps because of feelings of powerlessness and helplessness.

MEDICAL HISTORY. The medical history should focus on preexisting medical conditions that contribute to increased perioperative risk. A nurse should also elicit a family history to identify risk factors for cardiac disease. The nurse takes a thorough review of systems to collect data on all body systems. The nurse should inquire about any past hospitalizations and illnesses and collect data to determine the presence of systemic or chronic disease, which may place the patient at higher risk for surgical or anesthetic complications. However, the mere presence of chronic disease does not always increase surgical risk. The nature and extent of the disease or diseases and the degree to which they are under control are important variables. Nursing assessment and documentation of these factors are critical in the preoperative period.

CARDIAC STATUS. Intraoperative cardiac events, including myocardial infarction, unstable angina, congestive heart failure,

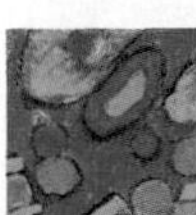

TABLE 13-2
COMMON MEDICATIONS *and Their Effects on Anesthesia and Surgery—cont'd*

Drug	Action	Nursing Intervention
Diuretics	Lower blood pressure Used in treatment of edema	Monitor for fluid and electrolyte imbalance. May withhold on day of surgery.
Insulin	Lowers blood glucose	Stress response will increase dosage requirements. Since nothing-by-mouth status and decreased intake will decrease dosage requirements, consider withholding or reducing PM dose (if taken) and AM dose day of surgery.
Oral diabetic medications	Aid in glycemic control	May hold or reduce evening dose day before surgery and AM dose day of surgery. Discontinue metformin 48 hours before surgery or procedures using iodinated contrast material to decrease risk of lactic acidosis. May resume metformin 48 hours after surgery, with return of normal renal functioning and adequate oral intake.[27]
Analgesics (opiate agonists)	Depress central nervous system	Monitor for respiratory depression and suppression of cough reflex. Monitor for drug tolerance. Be aware of synergistic effects with other central nervous system depressants.
Antihistamines	H_1-receptor antagonist Have anticholinergic properties	Be aware that they potentiate central nervous system depressant effects of benzodiazepines, barbiturates, phenothiazines, and opioids. Monitor for tachycardia. Use cautiously in patients with hypertension.
Decongestants	Sympathomimetics	Use cautiously in patients with hypertension and cardiac disease. Monitor for increased pressor effects and toxicity with other sympathomimctics (epinephrine).
Monoamine oxidase (MAO) inhibitors	Antidepressants	Discontinue several weeks before elective surgery. Newer MAO may have shorter half-lives. Avoid known triggering medications, including meperedine and indirect-acting sympathomimetic agents, which cause release of norepinephrine.[36]

dysrhythmias, and sudden cardiac death, are leading causes of mortality and morbidity in the operative patient. After surgery cardiac complications continue to be a leading cause of morbidity and mortality. Thirty percent of the population is estimated to be at risk for perioperative cardiac mortality.[29] The American College of Cardiology and American Heart Association have developed guidelines to identify patients at risk for perioperative cardiac complications. Major clinical predictors include angina, history of myocardial infarction, congestive heart failure (CHF), hypertension, and symptomatic arrhythmias.[1] Patients with a questionable or positive history of cardiac disease may need a cardiac consultation before undergoing elective surgery.

The patient with coronary artery disease has a significantly higher risk of perioperative complications. A standardized tool such as the Canadian Cardiovascular Society Angina Classification System or the Goldman index (which identifies clinical risk factors for adverse cardiac outcomes after noncardiac surgery) can be used for preoperative assessment. The health history should include questions regarding the presence and severity of chest pain or angina at rest, during physical activity, and with exercise. The nurse should question patients about a history of excessive or unexplained fatigue, palpitations, and syncope. Patients with unstable angina should be referred for cardiac clearance before surgery. A history of myocardial infarction increases cardiac risk up to 20%. If the patient had a myocardial infarction within the past 6 months, surgery may be delayed or cancelled.[29]

Persons with CHF are at increased risk for perioperative pulmonary and cardiac arrest. If digoxin is used to manage left ventricular dysfunction, these patients may also be at risk for perioperative dysrhythmias. Patients with known dysrhythmias should be stabilized and controlled before surgery to reduce the risk for perioperative complications.

Hypertension is a common comorbid condition among preoperative patients. Perioperative complications of hypertension include myocardial infarction, CHF, cerebrovascular accident, and death. The highest risk of death is in persons with systolic arterial pressure higher than 180 mm Hg.[15] Elective surgery should be delayed until severe hypertension is under control.

TABLE 13-3 COMMONLY USED HERBS AND PERIOPERATIVE IMPLICATIONS

Herb	Common Name	Common Uses	Perioperative Implications
Echinacea angustifolia	Purple coneflower	Immune stimulant Antiinfective	Possible allergic reactions Risk of hepatotoxicity with other hepatotoxic drugs or long-term use May decrease effectiveness of corticosteroids Contraindicated in patients with immune disorders
Tanacetum parthenium	Feverfew Midsummer daisy	Migraine prophylaxis Antipyretic Antiarthritic Menstrual irregularity	May inhibit platelet activity and increased bleeding time Avoid concomitant use with aspirin, warfarin, other anticoagulants, and thrombolytics
Allilum sativum	Garlic	Hyperlipidemic Antibiotic Antihypertensive Antiplatelet and antithrombolytic Antioxidant	Inhibits platelet aggregation May potentiate warfarin May increase international normalized ratio (INR) and prothrombin time (PT) May cause gastrointestinal upset May decrease blood glucose levels
Zingiber officinale	Ginger	Prevention of motion sickness Analgesic and antiinflammatory, particularly for treatment of rheumatoid arthritis and osteoarthritis	Anticoagulant action In large doses increases risk of bleeding and dysrhythmias
Panax ginseng *P. quinquefolius*	Ginseng root	Decreases fatigue and stress Enhances well-being and energy level	May cause tachycardia and hypertension, especially with use of cardiac stimulants Inhibits platelet aggregation May decrease effectiveness of warfarin May decrease INR and PT Lowers blood glucose May potentiate effects of digoxin May cause electrocardiogram changes Assess for ginseng abuse syndrome (insomnia, hypotonia, and edema)

The nurse should question the patient for a history of prosthetic heart valves, valvular disease, cardiomyopathy, and bacterial endocarditis. These persons may need antibiotics perioperatively to prevent bacterial endocarditis.

PULMONARY STATUS. Identification of patients at risk for pulmonary complications is an important component of the preoperative assessment. Postoperative pulmonary complications occur almost as frequently as postoperative cardiac complications and may prolong the patient's hospital stay.

Perioperative pulmonary complications include aspiration, pneumonia, respiratory failure, bronchospasm, atelectasis, hypoxemia, and exacerbation of chronic lung disease. Risk factors known to contribute to postoperative pulmonary complications include smoking, advanced age, cough, dyspnea, chronic obstructive pulmonary disease (COPD), asthma, morbid obesity, obstructive sleep apnea-hypopnea syndrome (OSAHS), and type of surgery (thoracic, cardiac, and upper abdominal procedures).[16,36] Persons receiving inhalant anesthetics are also at risk for pulmonary complications, particularly atelectasis and pneumonia. Pulmonary aspiration of gastric contents is a serious complication of general anesthesia. Aspiration may lead to pneumonia and respiratory failure. Box 13-2 outlines risk factors for pulmonary aspiration.[25,36] Table 13-4 summarizes the major risk factors for postoperative pulmonary complications.

Severe or untreated OSAHS may cause hypoxia, hypertension, and pulmonary hypertension. Perioperatively patients are at risk for hypoxia, prolonged apnea, and cardiac complications. Many patients may not know they have sleep apnea. It is important for the nurse to question the patient regarding a history of sleeping problems or loud snoring and to identify persons at risk. Risk factors for sleep apnea include obesity, male gender, a history of snor-

TABLE 13-3 Commonly Used Herbs and Perioperative Implications—cont'd

Herb	Common Name	Common Uses	Perioperative Implications
Gingko biloba	Gingko	Increases cerebral blood flow Improves memory and mental functioning Antioxidant Decreases symptoms of peripheral vascular disease, vertigo, and tinnitus	Inhibits platelet-activating factor, increases risk of bleeding Prolongs bleeding time Increases effects of anticoagulants Side effects include subconjuctival hemorrhage and spontaneous subdural hematoma
Piper methysticum	Kava-kava Kawa	Anxiolytic	Potentiates effects of central nervous system depressants, anesthetics, and alcohol
Glycyrrhiza glabra	Licorice	Antiulcer agent (gastric and duodenal ulcers) Expectorant	Contraindicated in chronic hepatic disease, renal disease, and hypokalemia May increase hypertension and edema May cause electrolyte imbalance (particularly hypokalemia) Neutralizes antibiotics May potentiate corticosteroids
Hypericum perforatum	St. John's wort	Antidepressant Anxiolytic	May prolong sedative effects of anesthesia and opioids Contraindicated with use of selective-serotonin reuptake inhibitors and ephedra Possible interactions with warfarin, steroids, benzodiazepines, calcium channel blockers, and protease inhibitors
Valeriana officinalis	Valerian	Mild sedative Hypnotic Anxiolytic Muscle relaxant	Risk of hepatotoxicity with other herbs (particularly skullcap and mistletoe) Long-term users may require increased dosage of anesthetics Prolongs sedative effects of anesthesia Potentiates action of barbiturates and alcohol Avoid concomitant use with sedatives and anxiolytics

ing, impaired daytime functioning, thick neck (circumference greater than 17 inches), and craniofacial and upper airway structural abnormalities.[24,29] Persons with known or suspected OSAHS will require additional monitoring and may have a longer length of stay in the recovery room. If the patient uses a continuous positive airway pressure device at home, the nurse may ask him or her to bring the machine to the hospital on the day of surgery.[14]

Box 13-2 Risk Factors for Pulmonary Aspiration

- Emergent procedure
- Full stomach
- High gastric pressure and incompetent lower esophageal sphincter
- Gastric esophageal reflux disease (GERD)
- Hiatal hernia
- Gastric motility disorders
- Pregnancy
- Bowel obstruction
- Diabetes
- Obesity

Any condition that restricts movement of the chest wall places the person at risk for perioperative respiratory complications. Persons with morbid obesity may have difficulty with chest wall expansion owing to excessive weight on the thoracic cavity. Obese persons may also be dyspneic when lying supine.

The patient should be questioned for a history of neuromuscular disease, including muscular dystrophy, myasthenia gravis, and polio. Neuromuscular disease impairs respiratory muscle function and may result in hypoventilation, decreased ability to remove secretions, and hypoxemia.

Surgical procedures lasting longer than 3 hours have been associated with a higher risk of pulmonary complications. The type of anesthesia also influences development of pulmonary complications; persons who receive epidural or spinal anesthetics have fewer respiratory complications than those receiving general anesthetics.

Smoking causes blood vessel constriction and increased secretions. The carbon monoxide in smoke binds with hemoglobin, decreasing tissue oxygenation. The increased lung compliance, increased airway resistance, and chronic mucus hypersecretion found in COPD may lead to inadequate ventilation, severe hypoxemia, dysrhythmias, and respiratory failure. Cessation of smoking 8 weeks before the surgery date is beneficial, since it allows recovery of the mucociliary apparatus, a decrease in carboxyhemoglobin

TABLE 13-4 RISK FACTORS FOR POSTOPERATIVE PULMONARY COMPLICATIONS

Risk Factor	Effect
Smoking	Irritation of lining of bronchial passages
Chronic obstructive pulmonary disease	Airway obstruction, increased mucus, decreased ciliary action to remove secretions, bronchoconstriction, bronchospasm, decreased ventilatory capacity, hypoxemia
Respiratory infection	Increased secretions, blockage of bronchial passages and alveoli
Skeletal deformities	Impaired ventilation, susceptibility to infection (kyphoscoliosis, rheumatoid arthritis of spine)

levels, and decreased cardiac effects of nicotine.[16,36] Patients with asthma are at an increased risk for bronchospasm during intubation, extubation, and after surgery. If the patient uses an inhaler at home, he or she should bring it to the hospital the day of surgery.

Assessment of the patient's respiratory status should include questions regarding exercise intolerance, dyspnea on exertion, unexplained dyspnea, cough, and increased sputum production. The nurse should specifically ask the patient about his or her ability to climb stairs and the number of stairs that cause dyspnea.

To reduce the risk and severity of perioperative pulmonary complications, the patient's pulmonary status should be optimized before surgery. The presence of respiratory infection may delay elective surgery.

RENAL STATUS. Decreased renal function is another factor associated with increased surgical risk. A decline in kidney function can impair the body's ability to excrete waste products, medications, and anesthetic agents. Patients over age 70 have some impairment in renal function as a result of the aging process. Persons with chronic renal insufficiency are at risk for adverse events in the perioperative period because of alterations in electrolyte balance, acid-base balance, platelet function, fluid balance, and immune function. A number of patients with renal disease have concomitant diabetes and hypertension and thus are at increased risk for complications from coexisting illness.

During the perioperative period, acute kidney failure (AKF) can develop in the patient with preexisting renal insufficiency and also in the patient without renal disease. Factors contributing to AKF include intraoperative hypotension, sepsis, and certain types of surgical procedures. Administration of nephrotoxic drugs or of contrast media can also result in postoperative AKF.

The presence of preexisting renal disease (serum creatinine level of 1.4 to 2 mg/dl and higher) is associated with an increased risk for postoperative renal dysfunction and increased morbidity and mortality. Azotemia is associated with an increased risk of cardiovascular complications.[1]

HEPATIC FUNCTION. Because of the metabolic functions of the liver, assessment of hepatic functioning is an important component of the patient's preoperative evaluation. Patients with liver dysfunction are at risk for perioperative complications, including hemorrhage, altered pharmacokinetics, liver and kidney failure, encephalopathy, hepatitis, and infection.

The patient with liver disease who receives general anesthetic agents, mechanical ventilation, or spinal or epidural anesthesia experiences a decrease in hepatic blood flow during surgery, which may lead to ischemic injury. Volatile anesthetic agents such as halothane and enflurane depress cardiac output and systemic pressure, resulting in decreased hepatic blood flow. If assessment reveals the presence of acute, viral, or alcoholic hepatitis or cirrhosis, elective surgery may need to be postponed.

NEUROLOGIC STATUS. Assessment of neurologic status establishes baseline function and identifies patients at risk for perioperative neurologic complications. Perioperative stroke and acute delirium are the most common neurologic complications.

The biggest risk factor associated with perioperative ischemic stroke is a history of stroke. The incidence of perioperative stroke ranges from 1.5% to 2% in patients undergoing cardiac procedures and less than 1% in patients undergoing noncardiac procedures. A history of previous stroke or transient ischemic attack (TIA) increases the risk of perioperative stroke following cardiac surgery to as high as 8% to 13%. The presence of hypoperfusion, thromboembolism, carotid stenosis, aortic arch stenosis in older persons, recent myocardial infarction, and atrial fibrillation are additional risk factors.[9]

Symptomatic carotid stenosis poses a significant risk for patients undergoing cardiac surgery. Patients with symptomatic carotid stenosis may be candidates for carotid endarterectomy or carotid angiography and stenting and should be evaluated before undergoing any general or cardiac surgery. No guidelines exist regarding the length of time elective surgery should be delayed following acute stroke.[9] Any patient with a history of stroke or TIA should be thoroughly evaluated before undergoing any surgical procedure. Delaying surgery at least 1 month after an ischemic stroke is recommended to allow the brain to recover before being subjected to the hemodynamic stressors associated with anesthesia and surgery.

Delirium is an acute, reversible state of agitated confusion characterized by hallucinations; disorientation; distractibility; insomnia; and emotional, physical, and autonomic overactivity. Risk factors for delirium include advanced age, drug and alcohol withdrawal, medication side effects, sepsis, pain, electrolyte and acid-base imbalance, sensory deprivation and sensory overload, cardiac dysrhythmias, myocardial infarction, and stroke. Medications are frequently cited as the most common causes of delirium.[28] Although almost any medication can cause delirium, certain medications have been identified as high risk (Box 13-3). If preoperative assessment reveals the presence of risk factors, medications such as meperidine and benzodiazepines should be avoided, since they increase the risk of postoperative delirium.[4,26,28] Early identification of patients at risk enables the nurse to be alert for signs of emerging delirium in the postoperative period. Refer to Chapter 15 for further discussion of delirium.

BOX 13-3 High-Risk Medications for Causing Delirium

- Diuretics
- Calcium channel blockers
- Anticholinergics (antihistamines, antispasmotics, tricyclics)
- Opioids
- Antiinflammatories
- Antiparkinsonians
- Corticosteroids
- Theophylline
- Barbiturate premedications
- Benzodiazepines
- Anesthetics
- Immunosuppressants
- Oral hypoglycemics
- Antimicrobials

HEMATOLOGIC STATUS. Hematologic assessment of the patient is essential, especially in procedures with an expected blood loss. The nurse should question patients regarding a history of anemia, bleeding disorders, and hematologic malignancies. The nurse should elicit a history of blood transfusions and any adverse reactions to blood or blood products. It is also important to ask whether the patient has donated his or her own blood (autologous donation) for the surgical procedure. A thorough medication history is important, with particular attention to medications that inhibit platelet function, such as anticoagulants, nonsteroidal antiinflammatory drugs, aspirin, tricyclic antidepressants, alcohol, and beta-blockers. The nurse should consult with the anesthesiologist or surgeon to determine if and when these medications need to be discontinued before surgery.

Persons with a history of atrial fibrillation, venous thromboses, and mechanical heart valves are often treated with the oral anticoagulant warfarin. Warfarin therapy increases the patient's risk for bleeding and hemorrhage. Preoperative management of these patients is a challenge, since discontinuing anticoagulant therapy increases the risk for thromboembolism. The literature has no evidence to support the best practice for managing patients on long-term anticoagulant therapy. The nurse needs to consult with the surgeon and anesthesiologist regarding perioperative management of anticoagulation therapy.

Another cornerstone of the preoperative assessment is questioning the patient about a history of deep venous thrombosis (DVT) and pulmonary embolism. Persons with polycythemia, thrombocytosis, and other conditions that increase blood viscosity are at risk for hemorrhage and thromboembolism. Risk factors for DVT include age over 40 years, prior history of DVT, decreased mobility, pelvic or cardiovascular surgery, total hip and total knee surgery, fracture or trauma, history of smoking, use of estrogen, and obesity. Refer to Chapter 31 for a full discussion of DVT.

ENDOCRINE FUNCTION. Diabetes mellitus is a common condition, whose perioperative management depends on the type of diabetes and treatment modality. Patients with diabetic gastroparesis are also at risk for pulmonary aspiration of gastric contents. Patients with diabetes mellitus are at risk for delayed wound healing and infection. The presence of obesity, advanced age, and complications resulting from diabetes places the patient at additional risk. Many patients with diabetes also have cardiovascular and renal disease and are at an increased risk for negative perioperative outcomes from these problems.

The goal of managing patients with diabetes in the perioperative period is stabilization of blood glucose levels. The trauma of surgery and accompanying factors such as stress, nothing-by-mouth (NPO) status, anesthesia, tissue trauma, and reduced postoperative activity all affect the regulation of blood glucose levels. Refer to Chapter 39 for further discussion of diabetes.

Thyroid disorders are common conditions that affect the outcomes of surgical patients. Hypothyroidism commonly occurs in older patients and is often undiagnosed. The signs and symptoms of decreased thyroid function may be confused with normal signs of aging. Myxedema coma, an extreme form of hypothyroidism, may occur perioperatively as a result of the stress of the surgery itself. Severe hypofunction of the thyroid gland places the patient at risk for intraoperative hypotension, CHF, cardiac arrest, and death.

Persons with increased thyroid function are also at risk for perioperative complications, such as cardiac dysrhythmias, ischemia, and thyroid storm. Thyroid storm may also be precipitated by the stress of surgery or severe illness. The nurse should consult with the anesthesiologist regarding perioperative pharmacologic management of the patient with thyroid dysfunction.

IMMUNOLOGIC STATUS. Assessment of the surgical patient's immunologic status is important because of the immune system's role in the body's physiologic response to stress and trauma. A decrease in immune function can lead to impaired wound healing and infection. As a result of the normal aging process, the older patient has decreased immune function. The nurse should question the patient about any history of risk factors for immunosuppression such as cancer, diabetes mellitus, chemotherapy, radiotherapy, and long-term steroid use.

Oral steroids are commonly prescribed to treat a variety of conditions. Persons taking exogenous steroids continue to require steroids throughout the perioperative period. The perioperative nurse should consult with the anesthesiologist for dosage recommendations. Patients on long-term steroid therapy are at risk for adrenal insufficiency. Refer to Chapter 38 for further discussion of adrenal insufficiency.

NUTRITIONAL STATUS. Patients with impaired nutritional status are at high risk for complications from surgery or anesthesia. Patients most likely to have nutritional deficiencies are older adults and those who are chronically ill, particularly persons with gastrointestinal tract conditions or malignant tumors. As a result of malnutrition, the patient has an increased risk of morbidity and mortality and may experience negative nitrogen balance, failure of blood clotting mechanisms, alterations in wound healing, infection, and electrolyte imbalance.

The nurse should gather data on the patient's nutritional status, including any changes in appetite, fluctuations in weight (intentional and unexplained weight loss or gain), and special dietary requirements. These data are relevant in predicting postoperative outcomes and determining nutritional requirements in the postoperative period. A nutritional consult may be indicated at the time of the preoperative evaluation.

The person who is emaciated or cachectic or who has lost weight below an acceptable level usually has a prolonged postoperative recovery. The malnourished person already has diminished reserves of carbohydrates and fats, so body proteins are used to provide the necessary energy to maintain metabolic functioning of cells. Nitrogen imbalances are greater than normal, and less protein is available for healing. Collagen, the connective tissue that is the substance of scar tissue, is a protein. Wound healing therefore becomes considerably delayed, and wound separation and infection may occur.

If the surgery is not emergent and can be delayed for several weeks, the malnourished patient is placed on a high-protein, high-carbohydrate diet before surgery. Nutritional supplementation is necessary for at least 2 weeks before clinical outcomes are improved.[16] In the preoperative or postoperative period, total parenteral nutrition may be given until the patient is able to tolerate a high-protein, high-carbohydrate diet by mouth. High protein intake does not result in increased body protein unless sufficient carbohydrate is available to provide the necessary energy. Activity or exercise is also required for protein synthesis.

Nutritionally depleted patients usually have a deficiency of vitamins. Vitamins B_1, C, and K are necessary for wound healing and clot formation, and supplemental vitamins may be prescribed for malnourished patients. Box 13-4 identifies common causes of malnutrition that may affect perioperative outcomes and delay postoperative recovery.

Patients who are 10% over their ideal weight are considered obese and are at risk for increased morbidity and mortality from concomitant systemic disease. The obese patient is often malnourished from lack of appropriate nutrient intake. Obesity is known as a risk factor for a number of chronic diseases and also presents a risk factor for surgery, including enlarged organs such as heart, kidneys, and liver.

During induction, intubation, and maintenance of anesthesia, there are additional concerns while caring for the obese patient.

Box 13-4 Common Causes of Malnutrition

- Chronic infection
- Inflammatory bowel disease
- Immune disorders
- Chronic pancreatitis
- Carcinoma (increased with stomach or colon cancer)
- Liver disease
- Renal disease
- Congestive heart failure
- Weight loss (10% of body weight in 3 months before surgery)
- Abdominal trauma
- Severe multiple trauma (especially pelvic, hip, and leg fracture)
- Major burns
- Wound sepsis
- Acute pancreatitis
- Small bowel fistulas
- Severe peritonitis

Increased abdominal pressure while in the supine position may reduce ventilation capacity, and inefficient ventilation may prolong induction time. Higher doses of anesthetic agents are required for maintenance of anesthesia because of continuous uptake by adipose tissue. After surgery the adipose tissue retains fat-soluble anesthetic agents, resulting in slow elimination and a prolonged recovery.

During surgery, fluctuations of vital signs are more common in the obese person because of the excessive demands on the cardiovascular system. Operating time may be increased because of difficulties in exposing the surgical site. The surgeon incising through layers of fatty tissue has to exert more traction on the tissues to expose the surgical site, which increases trauma to the tissues. Incisional hernias may occur at a later date.

During the immediate postoperative period obese patients often require more assistance with turning, coughing, and deep breathing. Excess fat deposits often limit movement of the diaphragm, thereby decreasing ventilation. It is also more difficult for obese persons to move about, and they may require additional assistance. Both decreased activity and decreased diaphragmatic expansion contribute to postoperative pulmonary complications. In addition, obesity and decreased activity increase the risk for thrombophlebitis.

Although weight reduction usually cannot be accomplished before surgery, during the preoperative evaluation the nurse can offer the patient information on the benefits of maintaining an ideal body weight, nutritional guidelines, and methods of weight reduction. Persons over 300 pounds require special equipment (OR beds, surgical instrumentation, wheelchairs, etc.) during the perioperative period. The nurse performing the preoperative assessment can initiate plans for perioperative management of these patients.

Surgical and Anesthetic History. The nurse assesses the patient's previous experiences with surgery and anesthesia. These data provide the surgical team with information regarding any reactions or complications to surgical procedures or anesthetics. The patient's and family's previous surgical experiences can affect the upcoming event and influence physical and psychologic responses to the procedure.

To determine potential problems with airway maintenance and endotracheal intubation, the nurse should ask the patient about any problems with cervical mobility, mouth opening, dentures or loose teeth, and the temporomandibular joint. In addition, the nurse should assess the patient for a history of adverse reactions, such as nausea and vomiting, to anesthetic agents or medications used perioperatively. Knowledge of the patient's previous problems with postoperative nausea and vomiting can influence the choice of medications used for anesthesia and analgesia.

Assessing the patient's anesthetic history also helps determine the risk for serious complications such as malignant hyperthermia. The nurse should elicit a family history of anesthetic complications, since malignant hyperthermia is an autosomal-dominant inherited syndrome. A positive family history for malignant hyperthermia may include a sudden or unexplained death while the patient is under anesthesia (see Chapter 14).

The nurse should question the patient for any problems with incisions or wound healing. African-Americans and persons with darkly pigmented skin are prone to formation of keloids, an increased growth of collagen fibers and fibroblasts that form at the site of tissue injury, including surgical incisions. If the patient is prone to keloid formation, the surgeon may inject a corticosteroid during the surgical procedure to reduce scar tissue formation.

PERCEPTION OF SURGICAL PROCEDURE. The nurse must determine the patient's understanding of the proposed surgical procedure, postoperative routine, and expected outcomes. The nurse should also assess the patient's informed consent. Knowing the level of the patient's understanding of the surgical event is required before any teaching can take place. It is important to find out exactly how the patient perceives the surgery, since persons respond on the basis of their perceptions. If possible, the nurse should clarify any misunderstandings or misconceptions; however, the nurse may need to refer the patient to the surgeon for further information, particularly when the lack of information influences informed consent.

PERCEPTION OF PAIN. JCAHO mandates that all patients have their pain assessed and appropriately managed. This includes providing postoperative discharge pain management instructions. Preoperative assessment of the patient's perception of pain is necessary for effective postoperative pain management. The nurse should perform a complete assessment for pain (see Chapter 16) and for the patient's expectations for pain management after surgery. It is important to include the family in the assessment and pain management plan. A preoperative pain assessment provides a baseline and allows for comparison of the patient's level of postoperative pain.

ASSESSMENT OF SURGICAL RISK. Every person responds to the surgical experience in a unique way. A number of variables influence psychologic and physiologic responses throughout the entire surgical experience. Some of these include age, the presence of chronic disease or disabilities, impaired nutritional status, and type of surgical procedure. The type of procedure performed influences the degree of risk involved. Surgical mortality is higher in thoracic and abdominal procedures. Regardless of the type of procedure being performed, it is important to consider the individual's preoperative health status.

AGE. Although other demographic data are collected, age is particularly relevant in the patient assessment. Age affects surgical and postoperative outcomes. Between the ages of 30 and 40, the functional capacity of each organ system begins to decrease. The surgical patient's age identifies those individuals at increased risk for surgical and postoperative complications. Refer to the section on gerontologic considerations for further discussion.

AMERICAN SOCIETY OF ANESTHESIOLOGISTS STATUS. Surgical risk can be assessed by different methods. In 1963 the ASA developed an objective method of determining the degree of risk for a particular patient based on the number and severity of preexisting medical conditions independent of the proposed surgical procedure (Table 13-5). Higher ASA scores indicate a greater risk of perioperative complications and death. The anesthesiologist or anesthetist performs the patient assessment and classification before surgery. The scale is easy to use and requires no special testing; a disadvantage is that it relies on subjective clinical judgment.

▶ ARE You READY?

For a patient scheduled for cardiac surgery, history of which of the following is the greatest risk factor for perioperative ischemic stroke?

1. Stroke
2. Carotid stenosis
3. Recent MI
4. Hypertension

Physical Examination. The patient's physical examination is performed by the preadmission staff (physician or advanced practice nurse), anesthesia provider, and nurse. The physical examination focuses on risk factors for cardiovascular, pulmonary, and infectious complications. The health care professionals evaluate the patient specifically for signs of cardiopulmonary dysfunction, which has been strongly associated with major perioperative complications.[16] The care providers also assess the patient's functional capacity, specifically the ability to perform ADLs, and general mobility status. The anesthesia provider's assessment includes minimally a physical examination of the airway, respiratory status (including auscultation of the lungs), and cardiovascular status.[6]

The nurse performs a complete head-to-toe physical assessment. Objective data are collected and recorded in the preoperative phase for two reasons: (1) to obtain baseline data for comparison during the intraoperative and postoperative phases and (2) to identify potential problems that may require preventive nursing interventions before surgery. If the patient has been hospitalized, the admission history and physical assessment should contain much of the pertinent data that can serve as baseline data before surgery. The nurse assesses and documents preoperative vital signs. The nurse documents any abnormalities in the patient's physical assessment and reports them to the attending surgeon and anesthesiologist for further evaluation. The surgical procedure may be canceled based on the severity of the abnormal findings. Refer to individual assessment chapters for a complete discussion of each body system.

Much information can be obtained from the initial contact with the patient. The patient may have special needs such as visual impairment, hearing deficit, cognitive impairment, or language barrier. The general survey should include an assessment of the patient's mood, affect, and level of anxiety. A general overview of the patient's functional status can be obtained by observing the individual's gait, ability to transfer, and performance of ADLs. The nurse should also assess the patient's use of any prostheses such as artificial limbs or eyes, dentures, or hearing aids.

Preoperative assessment of cardiovascular status is essential to identify patients at risk for perioperative cardiac complications. Elevated blood pressure at the presurgical assessment requires further evaluation. The nurse auscultates heart sounds and notes the presence of extra sounds, irregular rate and rhythm, or murmurs. The nurse auscultates the carotids for bruits; looks for evidence of jugular venous distention and edema, indicative of heart failure or fluid volume imbalance; and evaluates the extremities for the

TABLE 13-5 PHYSICAL (P) STATUS CLASSIFICATIONS OF AMERICAN SOCIETY OF ANESTHESIOLOGISTS

Status*†	Definition	Description and Examples
P1	A normal healthy patient	No physiologic, psychologic, biochemical, or organic disturbance
P2	A patient with mild systemic disease	Cardiovascular disease with minimal restriction on activity, hypertension, asthma, chronic bronchitis, obesity, or diabetes mellitus
P3	A patient with severe systemic disease that limits activity, but is not incapacitating	Cardiovascular or pulmonary disease that limits activity; severe diabetes with systemic complications; history of myocardial infarction, angina pectoris, or poorly controlled hypertension
P4	A patient with severe systemic disease that is constant threat to life	Severe cardiac, pulmonary, renal, hepatic, or endocrine dysfunction
P5	A moribund patient who is not expected to survive 24 hours with or without operation	Surgery done as last recourse or resuscitative effort; major multisystem or cerebral trauma, ruptured aneurysm, or large pulmonary embolus
P6	A patient declared brain dead whose organs are being removed for donor purposes	

Modified from American Society of Anesthesiologists (ASA), 520 N. Northwest Highway, Park Ridge, IL 60068–2573.
*In status P2, P3, P4 the systemic disease may or may not be related to the cause for surgery.
†For any patient (P1 through P5) requiring emergency surgery, an E is added to the physical status (e.g., P1E, P2E). ASA 1 through ASA 6 is often used for physical status.

presence and quality of peripheral pulses, capillary refill, warmth, color, and edema.

A preoperative baseline assessment of respiratory status is important for early identification of patients at high risk for postoperative respiratory complications. Respiratory assessment should include respiratory rate, effort, and rhythm; chest excursion; use of accessory muscles; auscultation of breath sounds; and pulse oximetry.

The nurse evaluates the patient's neurologic status, including level of consciousness, orientation, and motor and sensory function. This information is necessary to detect any deviations from baseline function that may occur during the perioperative period. The nurse also evaluates the patient for sensory deficits such as problems with vision, hearing, and sensation.

The nurse assesses the patient's musculoskeletal status for abnormalities in joint structure and function. Limitation in range of motion or arthritis may interfere with intraoperative patient positioning. It is important to assess range of motion of the cervical spine because of the positioning required for endotracheal intubation. Persons with alterations in musculoskeletal function may be predisposed to postoperative complications associated with immobility.

The patient's integumentary system is assessed for integrity and areas prone to pressure ulcers. Breaks in the skin, decreased subcutaneous tissue, and other pathologic changes in the skin will affect intraoperative patient positioning and placement of monitoring devices, skin preparation, and placement of surgical drapes and other surgical equipment.

An assessment of the hydration status of the patient is important because of potential alterations in fluid volume balance resulting from NPO status, administration of intravenous fluids, intraoperative and postoperative hemorrhage, and excessive wound drainage. Physical examination findings that suggest alterations in hydration status may include weight outside of ideal range, decreased muscle tone, lack of subcutaneous tissue, dry and flaky skin, brittle nails, decreased skin turgor, dry mucous membranes, edema, and adventitious breath sounds.

An assessment of the patient's nutritional status should include height, weight, and body mass index (BMI). BMI is an important prognostic indicator for chronic disease. The World Health Organization defines overweight as a BMI of 25 to 29.9 kg/m^2; obesity as a BMI of 30 to 39.9 kg/m^2; and morbid obesity as a BMI of 40 kg/m^2 or greater.[24] Other factors affecting nutritional status include loose teeth, improperly fitting dentures, and poor dentition.

Diagnostics. Laboratory and diagnostic testing is performed before the patient is cleared for surgery. Patient age and physical condition, type of procedure and anesthetic, and institutional requirements determine the extent of laboratory testing. Laboratory and diagnostic testing may take place in a variety of settings and at varying times before the procedure depending on institutional protocol and reimbursement regulations. Admission panel testing protocols are based on patient history and age and type of procedure. Because of the high incidence of coronary artery disease, male patients over 40 years old and female patients over 50 years old generally require an electrocardiogram. Chest radiography is not relevant as a routine preoperative screening test but may be indicated for patients at high risk for pulmonary complications. Other tests may be indicated based on the patient's medical history, risk factors, and the proposed surgical procedure. Table 13-6 provides examples of common preoperative tests.

If surgical blood loss is anticipated, a blood sample is sent for type and screen or type and cross-matching so that packed red blood cells are available for transfusion during and after surgery. Ideally the patient should have a preoperative hematocrit of at least 30% to 45% and hemoglobin of at least 10 g/dl. Hematocrit

TABLE 13-6 COMMON PREOPERATIVE DIAGNOSTIC TESTS

Test	Indications	Possible Findings
Complete blood count with differential	Procedures with anticipated significant blood loss Chronic illness or disease History of infection	Baseline hematologic function Anemia Infection Blood dyscrasias
Basic metabolic panel (blood urea nitrogen, creatinine, glucose, potassium, chloride, sodium, and CO_2)	Age over 60 years (age may vary with institutional protocol) Cardiac disease Chronic disease Renal disease Liver disease Use of diuretics	Electrolyte imbalance Acid-base imbalance Hydration status Renal function Hepatic function Hypoglycemia Hyperglycemia (with fasting glucose)
Coagulation studies (prothrombin time, partial thromboplastin time, international normalized ratio)	Bleeding disorders Anticoagulant use Procedures with anticipated significant blood loss Liver disease	Baseline coagulation status Risk of perioperative bleeding Response to anticoagulant therapy Liver disease
Liver enzymes	History of liver disease History of or current alcohol abuse	Hepatic function
Beta-human chorionic gonadatropin	Women of childbearing years	Pregnancy status
12-lead electrocardiogram	Men over 40 years old Women over 50 years old History of cardiac disease Abnormal cardiac examination	Cardiac rhythm Dysrhythmias Ischemia Infarct
Chest radiograph	History of pulmonary disease Thoracic surgical procedures Significant smoking history (per institutional protocol) Abnormal findings on auscultation Acute respiratory symptoms	Heart size Chronic obstructive pulmonary disease Pneumonia Structural abnormalities Heart failure
Pulmonary function tests	Establish baseline pulmonary function Evaluate or predict risk for perioperative complications History of pulmonary disease Significant smoking history (per institutional policy)	Obstructive or restrictive lung disease
Urinalysis	Procedures involving instrumentation of urinary tract Urologic symptoms	Urinary tract infection Kidney disease

levels of less than 28% are associated with a greater incidence of perioperative ischemia and complications in persons undergoing vascular and prostate surgery.[1] In the case of elective surgery, the patient may choose to do autologous donation. Use of the patient's blood eliminates the risk of contracting hepatitis or human immunodeficiency virus from blood transfusions. According to the guidelines of the American Association of Blood Banks, the patient's hematocrit must be at least 34% and the white blood cell count must be below 12,000/mm^3 for autologous donation. Donations must be completed at least 72 hours before surgery, and the blood may be used up to 36 days after donation. The patient may be advised to take an iron supplement after donation, depending on the number of units donated and baseline hematocrit. The surgeon should inform the patient about autologous donation at the time the decision is made for surgical intervention to allow sufficient time for donation.

NURSING DIAGNOSES, OUTCOMES, AND INTERVENTIONS

Nursing Diagnosis: Anxiety

OUTCOMES. Common examples of expected outcomes for the patient with a diagnosis of *anxiety* are:

Patient will:

- Describe techniques to control anxiety.
- Report an increase in psychologic and physiologic comfort.
- Verbalize an understanding of perioperative routines.

NURSING INTERVENTIONS. Impending surgery may result in anxiety because of unfamiliarity with perioperative routines, fear of the unknown, pain, the wait for surgery, body image changes, treatments, fear of not being asleep during the surgical procedure, altered function, loss of control, and fear of death. It is the registered nurse's responsibility to assist the patient and his or her family and significant others in identifying sources of anxiety and implementing effective coping mechanisms.

The key nursing intervention in the preoperative period is patient and family education regarding the perioperative experience. Preoperative teaching provides information that addresses individual learning needs, promotes safety, enhances psychologic comfort, involves the patient and family in care, and promotes compliance with instructions. Given changes in health care delivery, the perioperative nurse must implement preoperative patient education programs in shortened time frames, in alternative settings, and with a variety of methods, including online resources. For example, the nurse may conduct a preoperative teaching and learning assessment online and refer the patient to websites that contain instructional information regarding the surgical procedure and hospital stay.

Structured preoperative teaching results in improved patient outcomes.[23] Most patients are less anxious and participate more effectively if they know the reasons for tests and perioperative activities. The nurse must allow time to answer questions and address patient and family concerns. However, giving the patient or family more information than they want may increase their anxiety and stress, so the nurse must assess how much information they want.

The preoperative education plan should begin with an assessment, including the patient and family's baseline knowledge, readiness to learn, barriers to learning, concerns, and learning styles and preferences. Another important intervention is to ensure the patient's physical comfort before initiating teaching. For an in-depth discussion of the principles of teaching and learning, refer to a fundamentals of nursing textbook.

The content of preoperative teaching includes information to increase patients' familiarity with procedural events, thus decreasing anxiety, and activities to enhance physiologic healing and prevent postoperative complications.

The patient's anxiety level affects the receptiveness and ability to comprehend preoperative instructions. Mild anxiety enhances learning. However, moderate levels of anxiety are characterized by selective inattention, and severe levels of anxiety may completely impede the individual's ability to comprehend information, thus making learning impossible. When the level of anxiety has decreased sufficiently, the nurse should instruct the patient using appropriate methods to facilitate learning and enhance problem solving. The nurse also can help the patient recall effective coping mechanisms or explore alternative methods of coping with the current situation.

Empowering patients by increasing their sense of control before surgery is essential for decreasing anxiety. Loss of control is one of the fears associated with surgery. Involving patients in decision making concerning their care allows them to maintain some control over events. The nurse can also teach patients activities that help decrease anxiety and regain control, such as deep breathing, relaxation exercises, music therapy (see Research box), and guided imagery. More recent interventions incorporating holistic nursing include humor, touch therapy, aromatherapy, acupressure, massage, and animal-assisted therapy.

Research

Ikonomidou E, Rehnstrom A, Naes O: Effect of music on vital signs and postoperative pain, *AORN J* 80(2):269-279, 2004.

Pharmacologic methods to decrease postoperative pain and anxiety are well studied. Previous studies suggest that music may have a direct effect on reducing patients' postoperative pain. This study examined the effects of relaxation music before and after surgery on the patients' experiences of well-being, pain, nausea, and vital signs.

Participants were women between 25 and 45 years of age undergoing gynecologic laparoscopy under general anesthesia. All participants received a compact disk (CD) with headphones and listened to the CDs undisturbed for 30 minutes before and after surgery. The experimental group listened to flute music; the control group listened to a blank CD. Pain, nausea, and well-being were all measured using visual analog scales.

Music was an effective intervention in lowering the participants' respiratory rates before surgery and decreasing opioid use after surgery. The results of the study suggest that a period of uninterrupted rest before and after surgery has a positive impact on well-being. This study supports the effectiveness of a quiet perioperative environment and the use of music to improve patient comfort.

The nurse must consider the patient's family and friends when planning psychologic support. The patient's family members or close friends are usually as anxious as the patient. This anxiety can be transmitted to patients, increasing their anxiety levels. The same principles for exploring concerns and giving information to the patient hold true for significant others. Family involvement in preoperative education decreases the anxiety of both the patient and family, with resultant increased satisfaction with care and increased patient cooperation with routines.

An important source of anxiety for the presurgical patient is fear of pain. The nurse should initiate the topic of postoperative pain control at the preoperative interview. Understanding that pain will be present but controlled may help relieve this anxiety and add to the patient's sense of control. Dispelling myths about pain and pain management can allay fears and decrease anxiety. Common myths include that (1) pain is necessary, (2) taking pain medication will cause addiction, and (3) women experience less pain than men. Education regarding pain management should include medications used, potential side effects, alternative pain relief measures, methods to assess pain, expected course of pain, and, most important, the patient's role in the pain management plan. A relatively recent method of controlling postoperative pain, as well as the anticipatory anxiety associated with the pain experience, is preemptive analgesia (see Chapter 16).

The anxious preoperative patient may require medication to relieve anxiety and promote comfort during this stressful time. If the nurse's assessment reveals the need for medication to reduce anxiety, the anesthesiologist should be consulted.

RELATED NIC INTERVENTIONS. Active Listening, Anxiety Reduction, Emotional Support, Music Therapy, Preoperative Coordination, Surgical Preparation, Teaching: Preoperative

Nursing Diagnosis: Risk for Ineffective Airway Clearance

OUTCOMES. Common examples of expected outcomes for the patient with a diagnosis of *risk for ineffective airway clearance* are:
Patient will:

- Demonstrate effective coughing.
- Demonstrate satisfactory performance of postoperative respiratory exercises.

NURSING INTERVENTIONS. Teaching the patient about the necessity of deep breathing and coughing after surgery is a common component of preoperative education. Deep breathing facilitates oxygenation and removal of residual inhalant anesthetics and also prevents alveolar collapse, which may lead to atelectasis. Effective coughing removes secretions that may block the airways. All patients potentially at risk for postoperative pulmonary complications are taught deep breathing and coughing exercises before surgery to enhance performance and increase patient participation in postoperative recovery routines.

All patients need to know how to correctly perform diaphragmatic breathing, which increases lung expansion by permitting the diaphragm to descend fully. With diaphragmatic breathing, the abdomen rises with inspiration and falls with expiration. The nurse assesses the patient's normal breathing pattern by placing a hand lightly on the patient's abdomen and asking the patient to take a deep breath. If diaphragmatic breathing does not occur naturally, the nurse can teach the patient to inspire deeply while pushing the abdomen up against the hand.

The patient performs deep breathing and coughing exercises in a sitting position. The nurse instructs the patient in deep breathing, as outlined in Box 13-5. The nurse also instructs the patient in how to cough. It is important for the patient to hold the breath for 3 seconds to promote alveolar expansion. If the patient has difficulty with a deep cough, the nurse can encourage the patient to do a "huff" cough. Repeated huff coughs often stimulate a deep cough. The nurse also shows the patient how to splint an incision with a pillow, a towel, or his or her hands to help decrease pain while coughing.

Box 13-5 Deep Breathing and Coughing Exercise

Deep Breathing

1. Lie in semi-Fowler's or high Fowler's position with knees flexed to relax abdomen and allow full chest expansion.
2. Place a hand lightly on the abdomen.
3. Breathe in slowly through the nose, letting chest expand and feeling abdomen rise against hand.
4. Hold breath for 3 seconds.
5. Exhale slowly through pursed lips (abdomen contracts).
6. Repeat deep breathing three times, then cough (see next).

Coughing

1. Breathe in as described previously.
2. Count to 3.
3. On "3," cough *deeply* three times.
4. If unable to cough deeply, do repeated "huff" coughs (forced expiration with glottis open).

An additional method of promoting lung expansion is with the use of an incentive spirometry device. Various models are commercially available. The nurse teaches the patient to seal the lips around the mouthpiece and inhale. After achieving maximal inhalation, the patient should hold his or her breath for 3 seconds and then exhale slowly. The patient should not exceed 10 to 12 breaths per minute. The device can be set to a predetermined volume to achieve maximal lung expansion (Figure 13-2).

RELATED NIC INTERVENTIONS. Cough Enhancement, Teaching: Preoperative

Nursing Diagnosis: Risk for Ineffective Peripheral Tissue Perfusion

OUTCOMES. Common examples of expected outcomes for the patient with a diagnosis of *risk for ineffective peripheral tissue perfusion* are:
Patient will:

- Verbalize knowledge of treatment regimen.
- Demonstrate correct performance of postoperative exercises.

NURSING INTERVENTIONS. A variety of nursing interventions are directed toward promoting adequate peripheral circulation. Measures to decrease venous stasis include antiembolism hose, pneumatic compression devices, leg exercises, early ambulation, adequate hydration, and deep breathing. Venous stasis in the postoperative period may lead to DVT, thrombophlebitis, and pulmonary emboli.

Antiembolism stockings, alone or in combination with pneumatic compression devices (also known as intermittent pulsatile

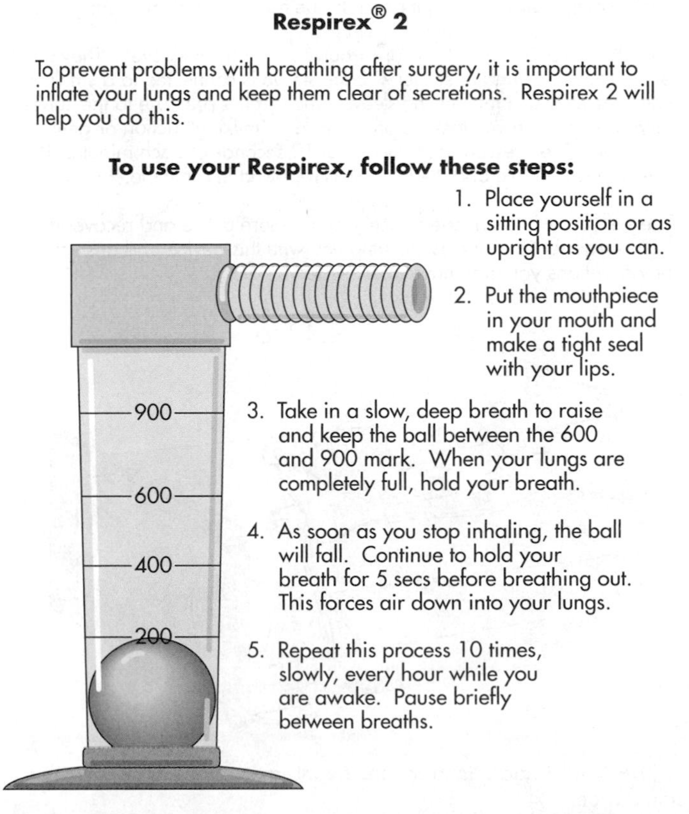

Respirex® 2

To prevent problems with breathing after surgery, it is important to inflate your lungs and keep them clear of secretions. Respirex 2 will help you do this.

To use your Respirex, follow these steps:

1. Place yourself in a sitting position or as upright as you can.
2. Put the mouthpiece in your mouth and make a tight seal with your lips.
3. Take in a slow, deep breath to raise and keep the ball between the 600 and 900 mark. When your lungs are completely full, hold your breath.
4. As soon as you stop inhaling, the ball will fall. Continue to hold your breath for 5 secs before breathing out. This forces air down into your lungs.
5. Repeat this process 10 times, slowly, every hour while you are awake. Pause briefly between breaths.

Figure 13-2 Patient instructions for using incentive spirometer.

compression devices or sequential compression devices), are often used perioperatively to enhance venous return in the lower extremities. The pneumatic compression device provides intermittent periods of compression starting from the ankle and progressing proximally to promote venous return. The nurse must measure the patient's lower extremities to obtain the appropriate size of sleeves and stockings. These devices are applied in the OR and continued until the patient is ambulatory (Figure 13-3).

Leg exercises help prevent venous congestion and promote peripheral tissue perfusion. The nurse teaches the patient leg exercises before surgery and has the patient perform a return demonstration using proper technique (Figure 13-4). The nurse also informs the patient about the usual postoperative routines to decrease venous stasis, including early ambulation, frequent turning, and active or passive range-of-motion exercises. Early mobilization prevents pulmonary and circulatory complications, prevents pressure ulcers, stimulates intestinal motility, and decreases pain.

Related NIC Interventions. Embolus Precautions, Teaching: Preoperative

Patient/Family Teaching. Patient and family teaching, as presented in the accompanying Patient/Family Teaching box, is an integral part of nursing care for the preoperative patient. The content of preoperative teaching includes information about events that will occur during the surgical experience (procedural), what the patient may experience during the perioperative period (sensory), and what actions may help decrease anxiety (behavioral).

Intermittent Pulsatile Compression Device (IPC)

The intermittent pulsatile compression device (IPC) gives a regular, gentle massage (or compression) to both legs. This action helps you avoid complications brought about by being less active after surgery.

The IPC is a pair of plastic wrap-around stockings or sleeves. They are put on both legs before surgery. Each sleeve is connected to a small compressor which inflates the sleeves and applies pressure to the calves of your legs. You will feel the pressure as a "milking" action or gentle massage. The pressure lasts for about 10 seconds of each minute. The sleeves then deflate and the process is repeated in a minute.

The sleeves will be removed once you are more active and recovering from surgery. Your nurses will help you with this device and answer any questions you may have after surgery.

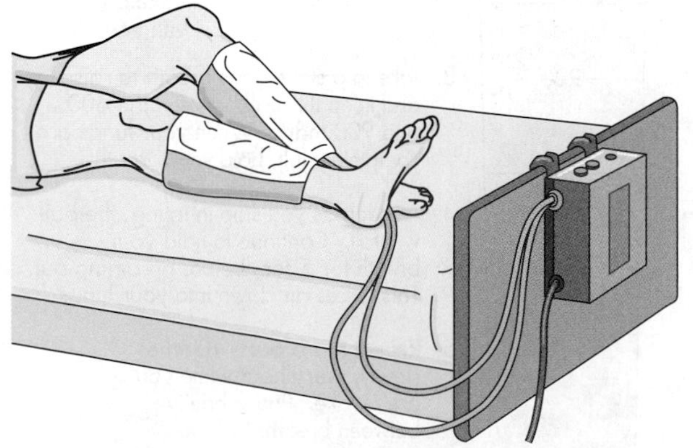

Figure 13-3 Patient instructions for intermittent pulsatile compression device.

Evaluation

To evaluate the effectiveness of nursing interventions, compare patient behaviors with those stated in the expected patient outcomes.

Related NIC Outcomes. Anxiety Level, Anxiety Self-Control, Coping, Knowledge: Treatment Procedure(s)

Gerontologic Considerations

By the year 2030, an estimated 20% of Americans will be over the age of 65 years. The number of older persons continues to increase; individuals 85 years and older are the fastest growing segment of the elderly population. Individuals over the age of 80 account for more than 3% of the population; it is estimated that the average 80 year old will live another 8 years.[13]

The perioperative nurse must be aware of special considerations for assessment of the older patient. Regardless of the setting, the perioperative nurse will encounter older patients. Fifty percent of Americans over 65 will undergo a surgical procedure, compared with 12% of those ages 45 to 60 years.[3,5] The older patient is at high risk for perioperative complications regardless of the presence of concomitant disease. Compounding this fact, an estimated 80% of older adults have multiple health problems. The presence of comorbid conditions and emergency procedures increases morbidity and mortality.[5] The increased incidence of death and postoperative complications are associated with cardiac disease, pulmonary complications, sepsis, and kidney failure.

The older patient's ability to tolerate surgery depends on the extent of the physiologic changes that have occurred with the aging process, the duration of the surgical procedure, and the presence of chronic illness. Surgical procedures that present an increased risk for older patients include abdominal, thoracic, neurosurgical, and emergency procedures. The normal aging process produces a general decline in organ function, alterations in pharmacokinetics, and alterations in thermoregulatory ability. The nurse's knowledge of the normal aging process is essential for planning perioperative interventions for the geriatric patient (Table 13-7).

The nurse also needs to be aware that physiologic and psychologic stressors may cause confusion in older patients. It is important to determine the reason for confusion. Common causes include hypoxia, electrolyte imbalance, cerebral hemorrhage, diabetes, infection, dehydration, medications, Alzheimer's disease, and unfamiliar surroundings.

Depression and alcohol abuse are common in older persons but often go undiagnosed. Both can affect postoperative patient outcomes and therefore need to be assessed in the preoperative period.

While performing the preoperative assessment, the nurse should remember that older persons vary in the extent to which the physiologic changes associated with aging occur. The greater the number of physiologic changes, the greater the patient's potential for developing perioperative complications.

Postoperative Leg Exercises

After surgery you will need to do some leg exercises. These exercises will help the blood circulation in your legs and keep your muscles in shape for walking. Before surgery, your nurse will help you practice the exercises you need to know. Your nurse will check or mark the exercises below that you need to practice.

☐ **Ankle Pumps**
(See Figure 1)

- Move both ankles by pointing toes up, then down, then in circles to stimulate circulation.
- Repeat at least 10 times every hour.
- You may do this while lying on your back or when sitting and dangling your feet over the side of your bed.

☐ **Quad Sets**
(See Figure 2)

- Lying on your back with both legs straight, tighten your thigh muscles so that the backs of your knees press down into the bed.
- Hold your muscles tight for 5 seconds.
- Exhale slowly while holding your muscles tight. Relax.
- Repeat at least 5 times every hour.

Figure 1: Ankle Pumps

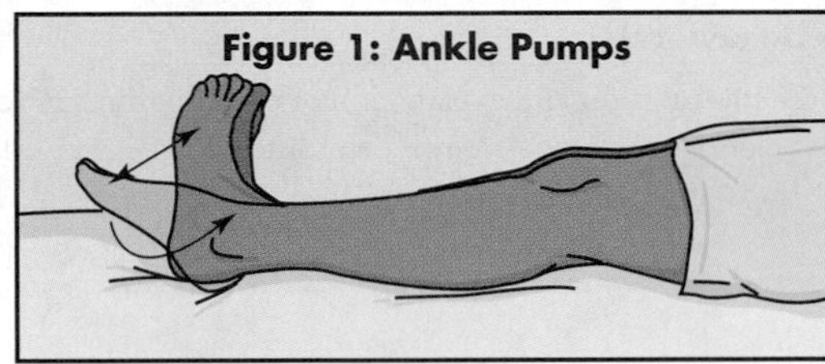

Figure 2: Quad Sets

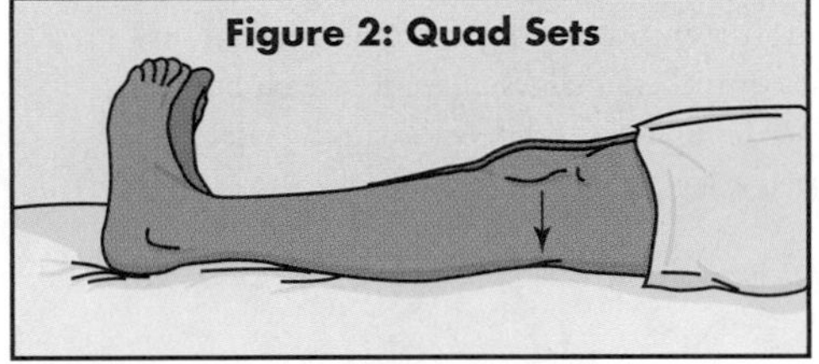

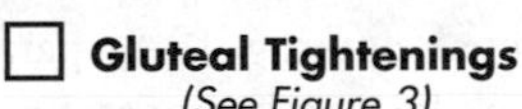

☐ **Gluteal Tightenings**
(See Figure 3)

- Lying on your back, tense your buttocks muscles tightly as if holding back a bowel movement.
- Hold these muscles tight for 5 seconds.
- Exhale slowly while holding your buttocks tight. Relax.
- Repeat at least 5 times every hour.

☐ **Straight Leg Raises***
(See Figure 4)

- Lying on your back, bend your right hip and knee so your foot rests flat on the bed. This helps to take the strain off your lower back.
- Keeping your left knee straight, point your toes toward the ceiling and lift the leg a few inches off the bed. Exhale slowly while lifting your leg.
- Slowly lower your leg to the bed. Rest.
- Repeat at least 5 times. Then do the same exercise 5 times with your right leg. Do straight leg raises 4 times a day.

** DO NOT do this exercise if you are having abdominal surgery, or if you have back problems.*

Figure 3: Gluteal Tightenings

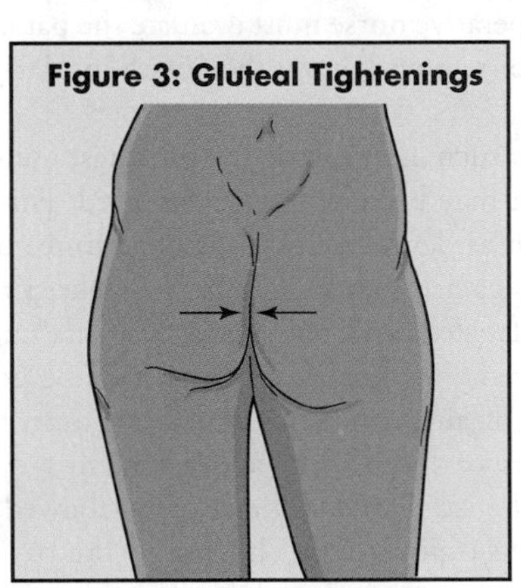

Figure 4: Straight Leg Raises

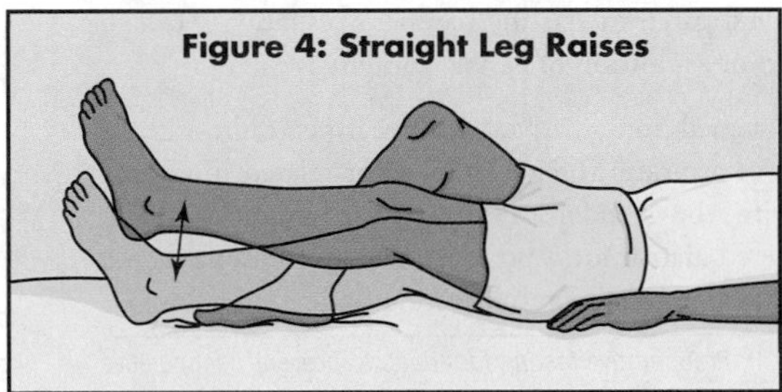

Figure 13-4 Patient instructions for postoperative leg exercises.

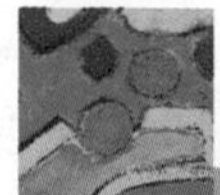

PATIENT/FAMILY TEACHING *Preoperative Teaching Content*

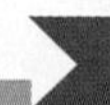

Procedural

Informed consent
Site marking procedure
Preoperative screening (laboratory, diagnostic tests, history, physical assessment)
Arrival time
Preoperative routines (bowel prep, antimicrobial shower, skin prep, vital signs, clothing, personal belongings)
Nothing-by-mouth status (see Evidence-Based Practice box)
Preoperative medication
Transfer to surgical suite (timing, holding area, surgical waiting room, visiting hours, duration of procedure)
Postanesthesia care unit routines
Presence of intravenous lines, surgical drains, surgical incision, catheters
Pain control methods (preemptive analgesia, oral intravenous epidural, patient-controlled analgesia [see Research box])
Postoperative routines (coughing and deep breathing exercises, incentive spirometry, leg exercises, antiembolism stockings, pneumatic compression devices, ambulation, diet advancement, expected discharge date, home care needs)

Sensory

Needle insertion
Medication effects (drowsiness, dry mouth, amnesia)
Operating room environment (cold, monochromatic, surgical attire, warm blankets, hard narrow bed, bright lights, noise, face mask for gaseous inhalation)
Pain (incisional, muscular, sore throat)
Dizziness when standing or walking for the first time
Sensations associated with invasive devices (e.g., pneumatic compression devices, antiembolism hose)

Behavioral

Demonstration and explanation of exercise routines (coughing, deep breathing, incentive spirometry, leg exercises)
Transfer techniques, splinting of incision, progressive ambulation

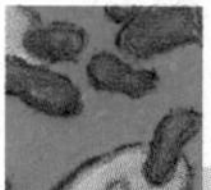

EVIDENCE-BASED PRACTICE

Topic Question: What is the effect of preoperative fasting regimens on perioperative complications and patient well being?

Evidence Base: Thirty-eight randomized controlled comparisons made with 22 trials on healthy adult participants. Participants were not at increased risk for regurgitation or aspiration during anesthesia. Studies compared the standard nothing-by-mouth (NPO) past-midnight fast with a shortened preoperative fluid fast, which included water, coffee, fruit juice, clear liquids, and isotonic drinks.

Findings: The volume of fluid permitted during the preoperative period did not result in different perioperative outcomes. Few studies reported the incidence of aspiration or regurgitation but measured intraoperative gastric volume and pH. No differences were found in the volume or pH of gastric contents in the shortened fast and the standard fast groups. Patients allowed a drink of water before surgery had lower gastric volumes than participants in the standard fast group. Few trials investigated the fasting regimens of patients at high risk for regurgitation or aspiration of gastric contents.

Conclusions: A shortened preoperative fasting regimen did not result in an increased risk of aspiration, regurgitation, or related morbidity when compared with the standard NPO past-midnight regimen. Patients not considered at risk for aspiration or regurgitation should be evaluated for a shortened preoperative fasting period.

Brady M, Kinn S, Stuart P: *Preoperative fasting for adults to prevent perioperative complications (Cochrane Review). In Cochrane Library, Issue 3, 2004, Chichester, UK, John Wiley & Sons.*

Final Preparations for Surgery

In the final phase of preoperative nursing care the nurse is responsible for ensuring the patient is ready to be safely transferred to the surgical suite. All the patient's personal belongings are identified and secured. The patient dons a hospital gown and removes all personal clothing. If the patient is wearing nail polish or artificial nails, one or more fingernails or toenails are exposed to allow for accurate assessment of capillary refill and pulse oximetry.

Jewelry is usually removed; however, rings may be taped according to institutional policy. The AORN has no guidelines regarding the removal of body piercing jewelry. Body piercings can be potential foreign bodies, sources of infection, and electrical conductors. In addition, the body piercing jewelry may disrupt skin integrity by tearing or putting pressure on surrounding tissues. Tongue and nasal piercing may compromise the airway, and or piercings near the surgical site may be sources of infection. The perioperative nurse must evaluate the patient piercing and, if they are not removed, cover them with insulated surgical tape for protection.[19]

Objects such as eyeglasses or prostheses sent to the OR with the patient may become lost or damaged. For this reason, prostheses such as dentures and prosthetic limbs or eyes are usually removed, labeled, and placed in safekeeping. Dentures are removed, labeled, and placed in a denture cup. If dentures are not removed, the patient's airway may be compromised with induction of anesthesia. The nurse documents the presence of dental caps or loose teeth and relays this information to the anesthesiologist. Patients are usually allowed to wear hearing aids to the surgical suite. This allows the patient to communicate with the surgical team throughout the perioperative period. The nurse must document the presence of the hearing aid to prevent loss or damage. Patients who want to take religious items or jewelry to the OR are usually permitted to do so. To prevent loss of the item, a paper emblem obtained from a religious representative is sometimes substituted.

To ensure patient safety, it is necessary to verify the surgical site, particularly when laterality is involved (e.g., right or left eye for cataract extraction). The nurse must thoroughly review the

Research

Chumbley GM: Pre-operative information and patient-controlled analgesia: much ado about nothing, *Anaesthesia* 59(4):354-358, 2004.

Patient-controlled analgesia (PCA) is a widely used method of postoperative pain control. In a previous study the authors found that patients received effective pain control with PCA but reported fears of addiction and overdose, which decreased their use of it. Participants in the previous study did not receive any preoperative information regarding the PCA regimen.

This study examined the effects of preoperative information on patients' use of PCA, quality of pain relief, knowledge of side effects, and concerns about addiction and safety. The control group received routine information provided by the anesthetist or staff nurse; the experimental groups received either an information brochure or a preoperative interview, which included a demonstration of a PCA pump. Participants who received the brochure were better informed about the PCA than the control group; however, there were no differences in pain relief, concerns about addiction and safety, and knowledge of side effects among the three groups. Patients who received the brochure were able to use the PCA pump more readily than the other two groups. The information brochure, based on the findings of the authors' previous study, was developed to reflect patients' concerns and needs.

This exploratory study failed to demonstrate the effectiveness of a preoperative interview or brochure in changing patients' beliefs about addiction and safety of PCA. The brochure was more effective in increasing patients' knowledge about PCA. More research is warranted to address patients' concerns about addiction and the safety of PCA regimens.

medical record and operative consent to validate the type of surgical procedure and the surgical site. JCAHO's Universal Protocol adopted in 2004 outlines criteria to prevent wrong site, wrong procedure, wrong person surgery (see Legal Alert). The patient's role is to verbally confirm the surgical procedure; the surgeon should mark the operative site, if applicable, with the patient's involvement. The nurse documents the verification process on the preoperative checklist in the medical record.

In addition to the surgical consent form, the nurse is responsible for verifying the need for any special consent forms. A special consent form would be indicated for refusal of blood transfusions or blood products, patients undergoing an amputation, and in some circumstances sterilization procedures.

Premedication

Before administering any premedication, the nurse must ascertain that the consent form has been completed, signed, and placed in the chart. The purposes of premedication are to decrease anxiety and provide sedation, to decrease secretion of saliva and gastric juices, to decrease gastric volume and acidity, to prevent or decrease nausea and vomiting, and to relieve pain and discomfort (Table 13-8). These medications commonly are given "on call to the OR" but also may be given just before anesthesia induction in the OR suite. Premedications may be omitted altogether, depending on the anesthesiologist's preference. Once premedications have been administered, it is essential that the patient be kept in bed with the side rails up to ensure safety.

Preoperative Checklist

A preoperative checklist is a method of summarizing patient data and the final preparations for surgery (Figure 13-5). The patient is transferred to a stretcher and transported to the OR. The patient's chart and archival records, if any, accompany the patient.

Documentation

The nursing report serves as a concise evaluation of the care given during the preoperative phase. The nurse records biopsychosocial assessment data and communicates all pertinent data to the OR nurse. The nurse records preoperative teaching content and the patient's and family's responses, and reports any relevant social factors that need to be considered while the patient is in surgery. Vital signs, preoperative medications, and laboratory and diagnostic results are recorded on the patient's medical record.

Legal Alert

JCAHO Universal Protocol for Preventing Wrong Site, Wrong Procedure, and Wrong Person Surgery

Preoperative Patient Verification

At least two patient identifiers must be used to verify patient identity. Examples include asking the patient to state his or her full name and date of birth or Social Security number. Each institution determines which identifiers will be used and the number required.

- Confirm and verify the following:
  - Patient's name on identification (ID) band
  - Date of birth
  - Medical record number
  - Consent forms
  - Availability of implant if needed
  - Availability of blood
  - Radiologic examinations
- Patient responses must match:
  - Marked site
  - ID band
  - Consent forms
  - Radiologic examinations
  - Scheduled procedure

Site Marking

Site verification is required for all procedures that involve laterality, multiple structures, or multiple levels.

- Site is marked with a permanent marker that is visible after the skin is prepped and draped.
- Operating surgeon marks the site with his or her initials before the patient enters the OR suite.
- Site is marked with patient participation (i.e., verbal confirmation or pointing).
- A patient has the right to refuse to mark the site. Each institution will determine the policy for these situations.

TABLE 13-7 AGE-RELATED PHYSIOLOGIC CHANGES AND ASSOCIATED PERIOPERATIVE COMPLICATIONS

Physiologic Changes	Potential Perioperative Complications
Cardiovascular	
Decreased elasticity of blood vessels	Shock (hypotension), fluctuations in blood pressure, dysrhythmias, congestive heart failure, thrombosis with pulmonary emboli, delayed wound healing, postoperative confusion, hypervolemia, decreased response to stress
Reduced cardiac output	
Reduced stroke volume	
Increased peripheral vascular resistance	
Fibrosis of electrical conduction system	
Decreased sensitivity to baroreceptors	
Respiratory	
Decreased elasticity of lungs	Loss of laryngeal reflexes, aspiration, atelectasis, pneumonia, postoperative confusion
Chest wall rigidity	Decreased gas exchange, ineffective cough, difficulty maintaining airway
Increased residual lung volume	
Decreased forced expiratory volume	
Decreased vital capacity	
Decreased alveolar volume	
Decreased ciliary action	
Thoracic kyphosis	
Arthritic changes of cervical spine	Difficult intubation
Costochondral calcification	
Tenacious sputum	
Renal	
Decreased renal blood flow	Prolonged response to anesthesia and drugs, overhydration with intravenous fluids, hyperkalemia, renal failure
Decreased glomerular filtration rate	Delirium, drug toxicity, electrolyte and acid-base imbalance, edema
Decreased muscle tone in ureters, bladder, urethra	Incomplete bladder emptying, urinary tract infection, urinary incontinence, urinary retention, urinary frequency
Decreased bladder tone	
Decreased bladder capacity	
Benign prostatic hypertrophy	
Gastrointestinal	
Decreased intestinal motility	Aspiration, paralytic ileus
Delayed gastric emptying	Constipation, fecal impaction
Decreased liver mass	
Decreased hepatic blood flow	Altered drug metabolism

Table 13-7 AGE-RELATED PHYSIOLOGIC CHANGES AND ASSOCIATED PERIOPERATIVE COMPLICATIONS—CONT'D

Physiologic Changes	Potential Perioperative Complications
Neurologic	
Reduced number of brain cells	Cognitive deficits, confusion, delirium, misinterpretation of stimuli, injury, falls, increased anxiety
Decreased neurons	
Decreased cerebral blood flow	
Presbycusis	
Presbyopia	
Decreased proprioception	
Changes in sleep pattern	
Musculoskeletal	
Decreased muscle mass, tone, and strength	Immobility, deep venous thrombosis, atelectasis, pulmonary embolism, pneumonia
Loss of bone mass	Positioning difficulty, pathologic fracture
Reduced bone density	Falls
Degenerative joint disease	
Integumentary	
Decreased elasticity	Pressure ulcers, bruising
Small vessel fragility	Delayed wound healing
Reduced lean body mass, increase in overall body fat	Delayed recovery from anesthetics because of storage in adipose tissue
Decreased subcutaneous fat	Hypothermia
Immunologic	
Fewer killer T cells	Reduced ability to protect against invasion by pathogenic microorganisms
Decreased response to foreign antigens	Delayed wound healing, wound infection
Metabolic	
Reduced gamma-globulin level	Decreased inflammatory response
Decreased plasma proteins	Delayed wound healing, wound dehiscence or evisceration
Decreased serum albumins	Altered fluid dynamics, edema, decreased binding capacity with potential for ineffective drug dosing
Benign hypothermia (temperature < 98.6° F)	
Reduced basal metabolic rate	Increased cardiac workload, hypoxia, intraoperative and postoperative hypothermia
Impaired thermoregulatory ability	Delayed shivering, delayed recovery from anesthetics

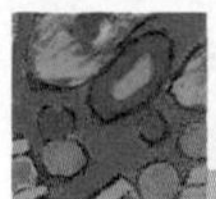

TABLE 13-8 COMMON MEDICATIONS *Administered Before Surgery*

Drug	Action	Nursing Intervention
Midazolam (Versed)	Short-acting parenteral benzodiazepine Central nervous system (CNS) depressant Muscle relaxant Anxiolytic Anticonvulsant Anterograde amnesic effects (impairs memory of perioperative events) Used in conscious sedation and short surgical procedures	Monitor for CNS depression; effects potentiated with other CNS depressants. Monitor respiratory status and vital signs closely. Avoid rapid injection, which increases risk of respiratory depression. Hypotension may occur if used with opioid agonist analgesic. Be aware of prolonged half-life in obese patients. Inform patients of amnesic effects.
Diazepam (Valium)	Anxiolytic Anticonvulsant Transient analgesia with intravenous administration	Monitor for CNS depression; effects potentiated with other CNS depressants. Monitor respiratory status and vital signs closely. Monitor patient for hypotension, muscular weakness, tachycardia, and respiratory depression when administered parenterally. Monitor patient for adverse reactions, including drowsiness, ataxia, and urinary retention (more common in older adults).
Lorazepam (Ativan)	Most potent benzodiazepine Skeletal muscle relaxant Anxiolytic Sedative Hypnotic Impairs memory of perioperative events	Monitor for CNS depression; effects potentiated with other CNS depressants. Monitor respiratory status and vital signs closely. Monitor patient for drowsiness and sedation. Inform patient of amnesic effects. Be aware of additive effects with other CNS depressants.
Morphine sulfate	Opium alkaloid Opiate agonist Produces analgesia, sedation, euphoria, and miosis	Monitor for CNS depression; effects potentiated with other CNS depressants. Monitor respiratory status and vital signs closely; respirations ≤12/min may indicate toxicity. Sedation and dizziness are common side effects; ensure patient safety after administration. Nausea and pruritus are common side effects. Promote coughing and deep breathing after surgery, since cough and sigh reflexes are depressed with opiate analgesics.
Fentanyl citrate (Sublimaze, Duragesic)	CNS depressant Opiate agonist Sedative Analgesic Supplement to general and regional anesthesia	Monitor for CNS depression; effects potentiated with other CNS depressants. Monitor respiratory status and vital signs closely. Respiratory depressant effect may persist longer than analgesic effect; have opioid antagonist (naloxone) and resuscitative equipment available.
Atropine sulfate	Autonomic nervous system agent Anticholinergic Antimuscarinic Sympatholytic Mydriatic and cycloplegic Antisecretory and vagolytic effects (suppresses salivation, perspiration, and respiratory tract secretions) Used before surgery to reduce incidence of laryngospasm, reflex bradycardia, and hypotension during general anesthesia	Monitor vital signs closely, especially pulse. May cause urinary retention. In general, use smaller doses for older patients. Older patients may exhibit CNS stimulation or drowsiness; ensure patient safety after administration.
Glycopyrrolate (Robinul)	Effects similar to atropine Reduces saliva secretion	Monitor vital signs closely. Monitor for urinary retention, particularly in older patients. Dizziness and blurred vision may occur; ensure patient safety after administration.

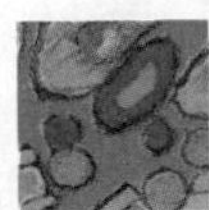

TABLE 13-8
COMMON MEDICATIONS *Administered Before Surgery—cont'd*

Drug	Action	Nursing Intervention
Scopolamine hydrobromide (Hyoscine)	Autonomic nervous system agent Anticholinergic Parasympatholytic Antimuscarinic Produces amnesia and sedation	Monitor respiratory status and vital signs closely. Monitor for excitement and disorientation shortly after administration; ensure patient safety after administration.
Hydroxyzine hydrochloride (Vistaril, Atarax)	CNS depressant Anticholinergic Antihistamine Bronchodilator Relieves anxiety May be given to reduce analgesic requirements before or after surgery	Monitor for CNS depression; effects potentiated with other CNS depressants. Drowsiness and dizziness are common side effects; ensure patient safety after administration.
Ranitidine	H_2 antagonist Prophylaxis for aspiration Decreases gastric acid production	Use cautiously in patients with hepatic or renal impairment.
Metoclopramide	Prophylaxis for aspiration Gastrointestinal stimulant Antiemetic	Monitor for drowsiness, extrapyramidal symptoms. CNS depression is increased with other CNS depressants. May exaggerate hypotension during general anesthesia. May increase neuromuscular blockade with succinlycholine. Opioids and anticholinergics may antagonize gastrointestinal effects.

Preoperative Checklist	Yes	No	N/A
Patient identity confirmed (method: ____________)			
ID Band			
Allergies (if Yes, band applied and chart labeled) • Type ____________ • Reaction ____________			
Operative procedure, surgical site, and laterality verified with patient and surgeon			
Surgical site is marked by surgeon and patient			
Surgical consent signed, dated, and witnessed			
Special consents signed, dated, and witnessed (if Yes, identify specific consents(s) • Special consent(s) ____________			
Advanced directives			
History and physical examination completed, reviewed, and verified no changes • Date of preoperative assessment ____________			
Surgical prep completed • Voided • Catheterized			
I & O flowsheet on chart			
Vital signs flowsheet on chart			
Medication record on chart			

Figure 13-5 Preoperative checklist.

Continued

Valuables

Circle if applicable:	**Disposition**
Dentures/partial plates	
Hearing aid	
Wigs/hairpins/hairpieces	
Jewelry/body piercings	
Glasses/contact lenses	
Prosthesis	
Acrylic nails/nailpolish removed	
Other ______________________	

Level of Consciousness

	Yes	**No**	**N/A**
Alert and oriented × 3			
Confused			
Lethargic			
Awake			
Unresponsive			
Other • Comments ______________________			

Functional Status

ROM or physical limitations (specify) ______________________

Sensory function

- Visual ______________________
- Auditory ______________________
- Tactile ______________________

Language barrier ______________________

Comments ______________________

Figure 13-5 Preoperative checklist (cont'd).

Diagnostic	**On Chart WNL**	**ABNL: Physician Notified**	**N/A**
CBC			
K			
Glucose			
bHcg			
Sickle prep			
ECG			
Blood products T&S ____ # of units ________ T&C____ # of units ________ autologous donation ____ # of units ________			
Other ________________________			

Assessment

Skin: Intact __________ Rash __________ Bruises __________ Ostomy __________ Color __________

Ht. ____________________ Wt. ____________________

Vital signs: T ___ P ___ R ___ BP ___ Pulse oximetry ____________________

Pain rating (0-10) ____________________ Anxiety rating (0-10) ____________________

NPO status ____________________

IV Fluids:

IV Site ____________________ Catheter size, type ____________________

Solution ____________________

Rate ____________________ Site assessment ____________________

Premedications:

Drug: ____________ Dosage: ____________ Route: ____________ Time Given: ____________

Drug: ____________ Dosage: ____________ Route: ____________ Time Given: ____________

Other medications taken by patient day of surgery:

Drug: ____________ Dosage: ____________ Route: ____________ Time Taken: ____________

Drug: ____________ Dosage: ____________ Route: ____________ Time Taken: ____________

Preoperative teaching completed: Yes ____ No ____

Patient accompanied by: ____________________

Comments: ____

Signature: ________________________ Date: ____________ Time: ____________

Review of preoperative checklist by operating room nurse:

Signature: ________________________ Date: ____________ Time: ____________

Figure 13-5 Preoperative checklist (cont'd).

Critical Thinking

1. A 45-year-old man is scheduled for a gastric stapling surgery for morbid obesity. He is seen in the preadmission testing for preoperative evaluation. The history reveals the patient is single and lives alone; his elderly parents live nearby and are supportive; he has a history of smoking, obstructive sleep apnea, and sedentary lifestyle; and he is employed as a computer programmer. Physical assessment data include weight of 177 kg (390 pounds), BMI of 52 kg/m^2, blood pressure of 188/100 mm Hg, pulse of 96 beats/min, and respirations of 18 breaths/min. What other assessment data are needed to complete the patient's preoperative evaluation? What possible psychosocial needs should be addressed? What laboratory and diagnostic tests are indicated for this patient? What pertinent data and special care needs should the preoperative nurse communicate to the OR nurse and anesthesia provider? Describe the content of preoperative teaching for the patient and his family.
2. An 85-year-old widow residing in an assisted living facility is admitted for repair of a pathologic hip fracture. Medical history includes breast cancer and degenerative joint disease. She has a daughter who lives out of state and a few friends at her residence. Her advance directive includes a durable power of attorney for health care and a wish for no life-sustaining treatment and resuscitation measures. During the preoperative interview she appears anxious, is disoriented to time, and is unaware of the type of surgery to be performed, although she expresses concerns about not waking up after surgery. Describe potential perioperative complications for this patient. Describe interventions to help manage her anxiety and address her concerns. Discuss the care plan, including collaboration with the patient, surgeon, anesthesiologist, and OR staff concerning her advance directive and surgical consent.

References

1. American College of Cardiology/American Heart Association: *ACC/AHA guideline update on perioperative cardiovascular evaluation for noncardiac surgery*, 2002, accessed from website: www.acc.org/clinical/guidelines/perio/clean/pdf/perio_pdf .
2. American Society of Anesthesiologists: *Considerations for anesthesiologists: what you should know about your patients' use of herbal medicines*, accessed June 2004 from website: www.asahq.org/patientEducation/herbPhysician.pdf.
3. American Society of Anesthesiologists, Barnett SR: *Preanesthetic evaluation for the elderly patient,* accessed June 2004 from website: www.asahq.org/clinical/geriatrics/prean_eval.htm.
4. American Society of Anesthesiologists, Chung FF: *Postoperative delirium in the elderly*, accessed June 2004 from website: www.asahq.org/clinical/geriatrics/posto.htm.
5. American Society of Anesthesiologists, Liu LL: *Perioperative complications in elderly patients*, accessed June 2004 from website: www.asahq.org/clinical/geriatrics/posto.htm.
6. American Society of Anesthesiologists Task Force on Preanesthesia Evaluation: *Practice advisory for preanesthesia evaluation*, approved Oct 17, 2001, and amended Oct 15, 2003.
7. American Society of Anesthesiologists, Warner DO: *Anesthetic risk and the elderly*, accessed June 2004 from website: www.asahq.org/clinical/geriatrics/posto.htm.
8. Association of periOperative Registered Nurses: *2004 standards and recommended practices*, Denver, 2004, AORN Publications.
9. Blacker DJ: The preoperative cerebrovascular consultation: common cerebrovascular questions before general or cardiac surgery, *Mayo Clinic Proceed* 79(2):223-229, 2004.
10. Reference deleted in proofs.
11. Crock RD: Herbal medicines: top 5 herbs your patients take . . . but don't tell you, *Consultant* 43(10):1199-1210, 2003.
12. Reference deleted in proofs.
13. Gatti G et al: Predictors of postoperative complications in high-risk octogenarians undergoing cardiac operations, *Ann Thorac Surg* 74:671-677, 2002.
14. Guido BA: The role of a nurse practitioner in an ambulatory surgery unit, *AORN J* 79(3):606-615, 2004.
15. Howell SJ et al: Hypertension, hypertensive heart disease and perioperative cardiac risk, *Brit J Anaesthes* 92(4):570-583, 2004.
16. Kiran RP et al: Preoperative evaluation and risk assessment scoring, *Clin Colon Rectal Surg* 16(2):75–84, 2003.
17. Lehne RA: *Pharmacology for nursing care,* ed 5, Philadelphia, 2004, Saunders.
18. MacKichan C, Ruthman J: Herbal product use and perioperative patients, *AORN J* 79(5):947-964, 2004.
19. Marenzi B: Body piercing: a patient safety issue, *J PeriAnesthesia Nurs* 19(1):4-10, 2004.
20. Reference deleted in proofs.
21. Moller A, Villebro N, Pedersen T: Interventions for preoperative smoking cessation, *Cochrane Database Syst Rev* (4):CD002294, 2001.
22. Moller AM et al: Effect of preoperative smoking intervention on postoperative complications: a randomised clinical trial, *Lancet* 359:114-117, 2002.
23. Mordiffi SZ, Tan SP, Wong MK: Information provided to surgical patients versus information needed, *AORN J* 77(3):546-562, 2003.
24. Murray D: Morbid obesity: psychosocial aspects and surgical interventions, *AORN J* 78(6):990-994, 2003.
25. Nagelhout JJ: Aspiration prophylaxis: is it time for changes in our practice? *AANA J* 71(4):229-303, 2003.
26. O'Brien D: Acute postoperative delirium: definitions, incidence, recognition, and interventions, *J PeriAnesthesia Nurs* 17(6):384-392, 2002.
27. Pribisko AL: Preventing perioperative adverse drug reactions, *AORN J* 77(1):106-120, 2003.
28. Richardson S: Delirium: assessment and treatment of the elderly patient, *Am J Nurse Pract* 7(1):9–15, 2003.
29. Scales BA: Screening high-risk patients for the ambulatory setting, *J PeriAnesthesia Nurs* 18(5):307-316, 2003.
30. Schroeter K: Informed consent, *Surg Serv Manage* 9(6):52-54, 2004.
31. Seidel HM et al: *Mosby's guide to physical examination,* ed 5, St Louis, 2003, Mosby.
32. Skidmore-Roth L: *Mosby's handbook of herbs and natural supplements,* ed 2, St. Louis, 2004, Mosby.
33. Starr P: *The social transformation of American medicine*, New York, 1982, Basic Books.
34. Reference deleted in proofs.
35. Venes D, editor: *Taber's cyclopedic medical dictionary*, ed 19, Philadelphia, 2001, FA Davis.
36. Ziolkowski L, Strzyzewski N: Perianesthesia assessment: foundation of care, *J PeriAnesthesia Nurs* 16(5):359-370, 2001.

evolve Visit the Evolve website: http://evolve.elsevier.com/Monahan/medsurg

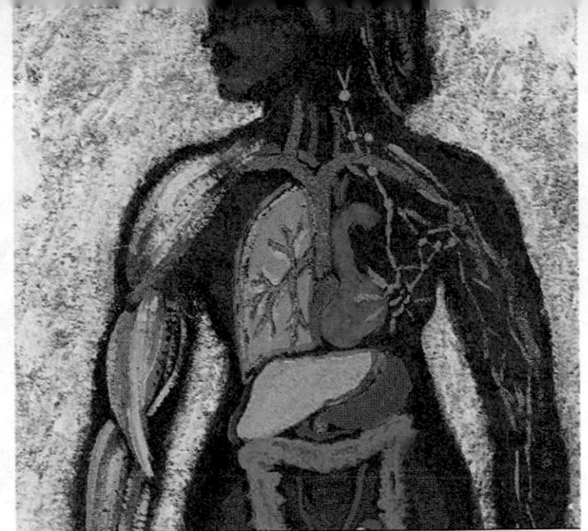

CHAPTER 14

Intraoperative Nursing

by Mary Jo Boehnlein, Jane F. Marek

OBJECTIVES

After studying this chapter, the learner should be able to:

1. Describe the intraoperative phase as a component of the surgical experience.
2. Describe the roles of each member of the surgical health care team.
3. Discuss the significance of aseptic technique.
4. Explain the purpose of appropriate attire in the surgical suite.
5. Compare and contrast the different types of anesthesia.
6. Describe the physiologic stress responses to anesthesia and surgery.
7. Describe the components of the intraoperative patient assessment.
8. Formulate appropriate nursing diagnoses for the intraoperative patient.
9. Explain the potential for the development of intraoperative complications.
10. Identify desired patient outcomes for the intraoperative phase.
11. Discuss nursing interventions to minimize intraoperative risks.
12. Explain the basis for evaluation of nursing interventions during the intraoperative period.

KEY TERMS

anesthesia, p. 275
asepsis, p. 270
emergence, p. 280
hyperthermia, p. 284
hypothermia, p. 281
induction, p. 279
maintenance, p. 280
sterility, p. 267
surgical conscience, p. 270

Intraoperative Phase

The intraoperative phase begins with the transfer of the patient onto the operating room (OR) bed and continues until the patient is admitted to the postanesthesia care unit (PACU). The intraoperative nursing care plan is designed to address individual patient needs and safely facilitate the surgical procedure.

Surgical Specialties

Surgery emerged as a true medical specialty in the mid-nineteenth century. The work of Ignaz Semmelweis, Louis Pasteur, and Joseph Lister laid the foundation for current aseptic practices used in the OR.

General surgery is the basis for all surgical specialties. Surgical specialties emerged as a result of understanding the etiology of various disease processes and using specific treatments for various parts of the body. Each specialty involves surgical procedures performed on a specific system or anatomic region (Table 14-1).

Intraoperative Patient Care Team

The coordinated efforts of the surgical team are required to deliver safe and effective intraoperative patient care. Each member of the surgical team must be familiar with the specific surgical procedure, adhere to policies and procedures, and adjust quickly to alterations in the patient's condition and the surgical procedure.

The OR team is divided into categories based on its members' responsibilities. Members of the scrubbed sterile team scrub their hands and arms, don sterile gowns and gloves, maintain **sterility**, and work in the sterile field. Members of this team consist of the primary or operating surgeon, assistants to the surgeon, and the scrub nurse.

Members of the nonscrubbed, nonsterile surgical team function outside the sterile field. Team members are responsible for ensuring patient safety, positioning the patient, monitoring the patient, maintaining sterile technique, handling nonsterile supplies and equipment, and providing items for the sterile team. Members of the nonsterile team include the circulating nurse, anesthesiologist and anesthetists, and other allied personnel.

TABLE 14-1 SURGICAL SPECIALTIES BY ANATOMIC REGION OR BODY SYSTEM

Specialty	Representative Surgical Procedures
General surgery: digestive organs, abdominal wall, thyroid, breast	Intestinal resection—surgical removal of part of intestine Gastric resection—surgical removal of part or all of stomach Thyroidectomy—surgical removal of thyroid gland Mastectomy—surgical removal of breast Herniorrhaphy—repair of hernia
Colon and rectal surgery: large bowel, rectum, anus	Abdominal perineal resection Colostomy—surgical creation of artificial colon Colectomy—surgical removal of colon
Genitourinary surgery: male reproductive organs, male and female renal system	Orchiectomy—surgical removal of one or both testicles Prostatectomy—surgical removal of prostate gland Nephrectomy—removal of kidney Cystectomy—removal of part or all of urinary bladder
Gynecology and obstetrics: female reproductive system	Oophorectomy—surgical removal of one or both ovaries Hysterectomy—surgical removal of uterus
Neurosurgery: brain, spinal cord, nerves	Craniotomy—creation of opening in skull to allow access to brain Cerebral aneurysm clipping Laminectomy—removal of all or part of vertebral lamina Microdiskectomy—excision of herniated disk using microscope
Ophthalmic surgery: eye	Cataract removal Corneal transplant Enucleation—surgical removal of eyeball
Orthopedic surgery: bones, muscles, tendons, ligaments	Hip replacement Spinal fusion Tendon repair
Otorhinolaryngology, head, and neck surgery: ear, nose, throat, sinus, trachea, esophagus	Stapedectomy—removal of stapes bone from middle ear and replacement with prosthesis Tonsillectomy—surgical removal of tonsils Esophageal resection
Plastic and reconstructive surgery: congenital anomalies, trauma-related disfigurements, cosmetic corrections	Cleft palate repair Skin grafting Rhinoplasty—surgical reconstruction of nose
Thoracic and cardiovascular surgery: lungs, heart, great vessels, peripheral veins and arteries	Pneumonectomy—removal of lungs Mitral valve repair Femoral-popliteal bypass Coronary artery bypass graft

Primary Surgeon and Assistants

The primary or operating surgeon has the knowledge, skill, and expertise to successfully perform the identified surgical procedure. The surgeon is responsible for determining the preoperative diagnosis, identifying and performing the appropriate surgical procedure, explaining the risks and benefits of the surgical procedure to the patient, obtaining informed patient consent for the surgical procedure, identifying and marking the surgical site, and managing postoperative care.

Under the direction of the operating surgeon, the surgeon's assistant is responsible for exposing the surgical site, providing hemostasis to prevent blood from obscuring the anatomy, and assisting with suturing throughout the operative procedure. The first assistant may be a surgeon, resident, registered nurse first assistant (RNFA), advanced practice nurse, surgical assistant, or physician's assistant.

The Association of periOperative Registered Nurses (AORN) acknowledged the role of the registered nurse (RN) as a first assistant to the surgeon and adopted an official statement recognizing the RNFA in 1984. The association defined the scope of practice, requirements, education, and clinical privileges that are required for the RNFA. Some state boards of nursing have accepted the AORN statement and incorporated RNFA functions into the scope of nursing practice.[17]

Scrub Nurse

The scrub nurse role may be performed by an RN, licensed practical nurse (LPN), or OR scrub technologist. The scrub nurse must understand the specific surgical procedure and the anatomy and physiology of the involved system. Some of the scrub nurse's responsibilities include preparing supplies and equipment on the sterile field; ensuring patient safety; maintaining the integrity of the sterile field; monitoring the scrubbed team members for breaks in sterile technique; providing appropriate sterile instrumentation, sutures, and supplies to the operating surgeon; and adhering to established policies and procedures for sponge, instrument, and sharps counts.

To perform this role effectively, the scrub nurse must possess manual skills and dexterity and strictly adhere to the principles of aseptic technique. The nurse needs to perform all duties consistently and with precision and accuracy to ensure the patient's safety throughout the surgical procedure.

Circulating Nurse

The circulating nurse is an RN whose responsibility is to serve as the patient advocate while coordinating events before, during, and after the surgical procedure. The circulating nurse is responsible for creating a safe environment for the patient, managing the activities outside the sterile field, and providing nursing care to the patient. Some state boards of nursing allow LPNs and surgical technologists to perform some circulating duties under the direct supervision of the RN.[18]

Before and during administration of the anesthetic the circulating nurse provides emotional support to the patient and assists the anesthesia team during the induction period. Throughout the surgical procedure the circulating nurse implements measures to ensure patient safety, obtains supplies and equipment for the sterile team members, and enforces policies and procedures. The circulating nurse is also responsible for documenting intraoperative nursing care and ensuring that surgical specimens are identified and placed in the appropriate media. The circulating nurse also enforces the principles of aseptic technique; recognizes and implements actions to resolve possible environmental hazards that involve the patient or surgical team members; ensures that sponge, instrument, and sharps counts are completed and appropriately documented; and communicates relevant information to individuals outside the OR, such as family members and other health care workers.

Anesthesiologist and Anesthetist

An anesthesiologist is a physician who specializes in administering anesthetic agents and monitoring the patient's response to the agents. An anesthetist administers anesthetics under the direct supervision of an anesthesiologist or surgeon. Anesthetists may be resident physicians or a certified registered nurse anesthetist.

In the preoperative period the anesthesiologist and anesthetist evaluate the patient and determine the appropriate anesthetic to administer. Intraoperative responsibilities include anesthetizing the patient, providing appropriate levels of pain relief, monitoring the patient's physiologic status, and providing the best operative conditions for the surgeon. In the immediate postoperative period the anesthesiologist assumes medical responsibility for the patient.

Other Personnel

A number of allied personnel also contribute to meeting the needs of the surgical patient. Pathologists, radiologists, radiology technicians, perfusionists, environmental services personnel, and clerical staff are a few of the many individuals whose skills and expertise provide assistance to the surgical team and ultimately to the patient.

The Surgical Environment

A surgical suite is designed to provide a safe therapeutic environment for the patient. The design of the suite addresses issues of traffic patterns, infection control, safety, and efficiency.

Traffic Control

Traffic in and out of the operating suite is kept to a minimum. Only essential personnel are allowed inside the OR. As the number of persons increases, potential contamination from bacterial shedding and air turbulence increases.

Traffic control patterns are designed to address activity and movement into and out of the surgical suite, as well as within the suite. The floor plan of a surgical suite is divided into three zones according to the types of activities that occur within each area. The three zones are known as the unrestricted area, the semirestricted area, and the restricted area. The unrestricted area provides an entrance to and exit from the surgical suite. The holding area, PACU, lounges, dressing rooms, and offices are located in the unrestricted area. In this area people may wear street clothes, and traffic is not restricted. The semirestricted area provides access to restricted zones and peripheral support areas within the surgical suite. Peripheral support areas consist of storage for clean and sterile supplies, work areas for processing supplies and equipment, and corridors to the individual ORs. Scrub attire and hair covering must be worn in the semirestricted area. The restricted area includes the individual ORs, scrub areas, substerile rooms, and clean core areas. In this area scrub attire, hair covering, and masks must be worn.

Environmental Conditions

The design of the OR and the materials used within it are chosen to address issues of infection control, safety, and environmental control. Ceiling and walls are constructed of nonporous, smooth, fire-resistant materials that are easy to clean with antimicrobial agents. Tile wall covering is not advocated because microorganisms could grow in porous grout lines. Materials used for floor coverings have the same specifications as for walls and ceiling, but are highly wear resistant with slip-proof surfaces to prevent injury. Sliding doors prevent air turbulence in the OR. Fire regulations dictate that doors should be able to swing open if needed.

Temperature and humidity are environmental conditions that need to be controlled to reduce the incidence of infection. Temperature within an OR is maintained between 68° and 75° F (20° and 22° C). Most pathogenic bacteria metabolize and reproduce at or near normal body temperature. Bacterial growth may be inhibited by keeping room temperature below body temperature. The lower room temperature also helps decrease the surgical patient's metabolic demands. The relative humidity in the OR is maintained within the range of 40% to 60%. This level of humidity diminishes bacterial growth and restricts static electricity.

Many ORs have high-efficiency particulate air filters in the air systems to assist with infection control. Inlet air is dispersed from vents in the ceiling and exhausted through vents at floor level. Slightly less air is exhausted than is introduced, creating a positive pressure gradient that prevents potentially contaminated air from entering the room. This is why all doors to individual ORs remain closed except for patient and team members' entry and exit. Each OR should have at least 15 room air exchanges per hour. Three of the exchanges should be fresh air exchanges.[28]

Infection Control

Surgical site infections (SSIs) are the second most common hospital-acquired infection, accounting for 17% of all nosocomial infections. Each year an estimated 27 million persons have surgery and approximately 500,000 develop a nosocomial infection; 40% to 60% of these infections are considered preventable.[12,26] Postoperative bloodstream infections are the most serious and costly medical injury, increasing hospital stays up to 11 additional days with more than $57,000 in associated costs and a 21.9% increased risk of postoperative death.[26] Additional sources of nosocomial infection for the surgical patient include postoperative pneumonia, pneumonia related to ventilator use, and bacteremia related to the surgical procedure or intravenous catheter insertion.

As a result of these problems, the Centers for Medicaid and Medicare Services (CMS) and the Centers for Disease Control and Prevention (CDC) developed the CMS/CDC Surgical Intervention Project (SIP). Goals for the SIP include reducing morbidity and mortality associated with postoperative infections in the Medicare patient population and reducing preventable SSIs by 90%.[12] Interventions to achieve these outcomes include guidelines for the use of prophylactic antibiotics, hair removal at the surgical site, and normothermia. SSIs are considered a sentinel event, and prevention of SSI is a major focus of the Joint Commission on Accreditation of Healthcare Organizations (JCAHO) National Patient Safety goals.[21]

Asepsis is defined as the absence of microorganisms that cause disease. Surgical asepsis promotes tissue healing by deterring pathogens from coming into contact with the surgical wound. Practices that suppress, reduce, and inhibit infectious processes are known as *aseptic technique*. Infection control policies and procedures, based on principles of microbiology and bacteriology, guide the practice of aseptic technique in the OR. Infection control policies are guided by AORN-recommended practices for perioperative nursing. These recommended practices address aseptic technique, surgical attire, environmental services activities, sterilization of supplies and equipment, surgical hand scrub, and skin cleansing.

All members of the OR team are responsible for strict adherence to aseptic technique. It is essential that OR nurses acquire a **surgical conscience**, or vigilant adherence to aseptic technique throughout the entire perioperative period. This involves constant examination and observation of the patient, OR environment, and personnel. A surgical conscience is completely developed when the nurse automatically attends to sterile technique; the nurse understands the principles of asepsis and sterile technique, acquires self-discipline in managing nursing practice, and develops good communication and assertiveness skills to identify patient needs and communicate breaks in sterile technique.

Basic Rules of Surgical Asepsis. Strict adherence to aseptic technique minimizes the potential for contamination of the sterile field and wound infection. The AORN has developed protocols and recommended practices for creating and maintaining a sterile field; six of the practices are briefly discussed below. The seventh practice addresses the administrative function of establishing and reviewing policies and procedures for aseptic technique.

The first recommended practice states that "scrubbed persons function within a sterile field."[8] Scrubbed personnel wear sterile gowns and gloves at the surgical field. Gowns and gloves provide a barrier to the transfer of microorganisms from the scrubbed person's hands and clothing to the surgical wound. The gown of a scrubbed team member is considered sterile in front from the chest to the level of the sterile field, and the sleeves are sterile from 2 inches above the elbow to the stockinette cuff. The stockinette cuff portion of the gown is nonsterile and needs to be completely covered by a sterile glove. The nonsterile areas of the surgical gown include the neckline, shoulder, axillary region, and back. Articles dropped below the waist or table level are considered contaminated.

The second practice states that sterile drapes are used to create a sterile field.[8] Surgical drapes provide a barrier that impedes the movement of microorganisms from a nonsterile area to a sterile area. Sterile drapes are placed on the patient, equipment, and furniture used within the sterile field. Draped tables are sterile only at the table level; items extending over the table edge are contaminated. Handling of drapes should be minimized. When placing sterile drapes, gloved hands are protected by a cuff of the drape.

The third practice states that all items used in the sterile field are sterile.[8] If the sterility of an item is questioned, it must be considered nonsterile. Packaging materials must guarantee that items will remain sterile until removed. Before opening a sterile package, health care personnel must inspect it for seal integrity, tears, pinholes, the presence of a sterilization indicator, and the expiration date as indicated.

The fourth practice states that supplies introduced into the sterile field are to be delivered in a manner that ensures the sterility of the item and maintains the integrity of the sterile field.[8] The nurse opens a sterile package from the far side first and the near side last, and holds the wrapper tails when the item is presented to the sterile field (Figure 14-1). The nurse pours solutions carefully to avoid splashing liquids onto the field. After opening a bottle of sterile solution, the nurse must present the entire contents to the sterile field or discard it. The edges of a bottle cap are considered nonsterile after the cap is removed. If the cap is replaced, the sterility of the bottle contents cannot be ensured; therefore the remaining contents must be discarded.

The fifth recommended practice addresses maintenance and monitoring of the sterile field. The possibility for contamination increases with time; therefore the sterile field should be estab-

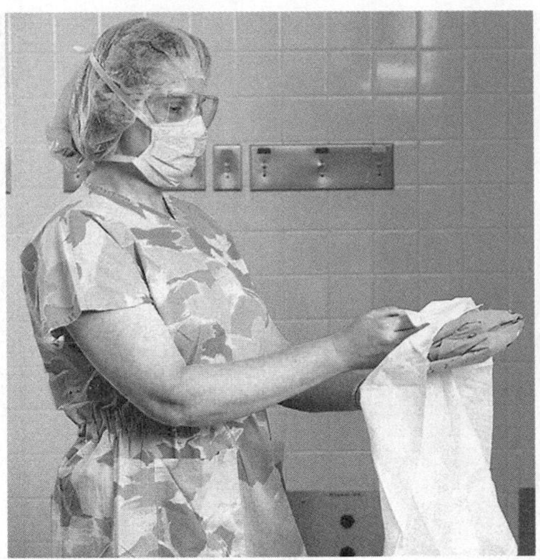

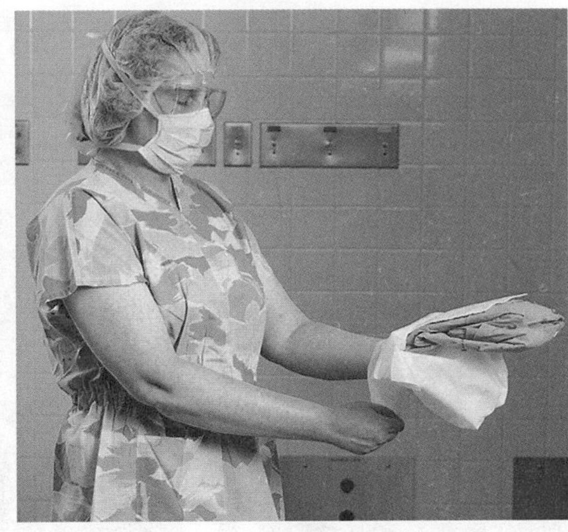

A B

Figure 14-1 **A**, When opening sterile package, scrub nurse opens corner nearest body last to avoid potential contamination of inner pack. **B**, To prevent nonsterile corners of outer wrapper from touching scrub nurse or sterile field, scrub nurse draws back corners of opened wrapper when presenting inner package.

lished as close to the time of use as possible. Unattended sterile fields are considered contaminated.[8]

The sixth practice states that the integrity of the sterile field must be maintained by individuals moving within or around the sterile field.[8] Only scrubbed personnel touch and reach over sterile areas. Sterile persons remain close to the sterile field and never turn their backs to it. Sterile individuals change positions by passing back-to-back or face-to-face. Unscrubbed personnel only touch and reach over nonsterile areas, do not walk between sterile fields, and approach sterile fields by facing them.

Infection Control Practices for Operating Room Personnel. All individuals working in the OR serve as a major source of microbial contamination to the environment because of the large quantities of bacteria in the respiratory tract and on the skin, hair, and attire. To reduce the risks of OR personnel serving as sources of infection for the patient, everyone must wear surgical attire in the semirestricted and restricted areas of the OR. Surgical attire also protects personnel from exposure to infectious microorganisms and hazardous substances. Surgical attire includes a scrub suit, hat or hood, and face mask or shield.

Dressing in OR attire proceeds from head to toe. Personnel put the surgical hat on first to prevent contamination of the scrub clothes with hair or dandruff. The hat must be clean and free of lint and must completely cover all head and facial hair. If the hat does not provide sufficient coverage of facial hair, the person should wear a hood.

Scrub suits are put on after the hair is covered. The suits, which are laundered daily, should be made of material that meet the requirements of the National Fire Protection Agency and should be closely woven to minimize bacterial shedding. Scrub shirts are either tied at the waist or tucked into scrub pants to decrease bacterial shedding and prevent contamination of the sterile field by a loose shirt. Unscrubbed personnel should wear long-sleeved warm-up jackets to prevent possible shedding of microorganisms from bare arms (Figure 14-2).

Footwear should be comfortable. In the interest of safety, clogs, open-toe, and cloth athletic shoes are not recommended. Shoe covers are a part of personnel protective equipment and are to be worn whenever splashes or spills are expected. If worn, they should be changed when torn, soiled, or wet and removed when leaving the surgical suite.

Masks are necessary to prevent contamination of the surgical environment by respiratory droplets. A mask is worn where sterile supplies are open and in areas where scrubbed persons are present. The mask must totally cover the nose and mouth and must be secured to prevent ventilation from the sides of the face. It is either on or off; it should not be saved by being hung around the neck, placed on the forehead, or placed in a pocket. When removing a mask, the person must take care to prevent contamination of the hands. The filter portion of the mask should not be touched. The mask should be removed only by touching its strings; once removed, it should be immediately discarded (Figure 14-3).

All personnel who are in close proximity to the operative site should wear face shields and protective eyewear to decrease the risk of splash or spraying of fluids into the mucous membranes of the mouth, nose, and eyes.

Lead aprons and thyroid shields protect OR personnel from radiologic exposure. These items are worn when personnel must be present during fluoroscopic procedures or when x-rays are used intraoperatively.

The use of cover gowns or laboratory coats when leaving the OR suite is controversial, mainly because of practicality and cost. Although cover apparel may be effective in reducing bacterial contamination from the waist up, it has not been shown to decrease the rate of surgical wound infection.[8]

Standard Precautions. Uncontained blood and body fluids—an inevitable part of surgery—present a great hazard to OR personnel. Because routine medical history and examination cannot identify all patients with human immunodeficiency virus, hepatitis, or other bloodborne pathogens, Standard Precautions are used for all

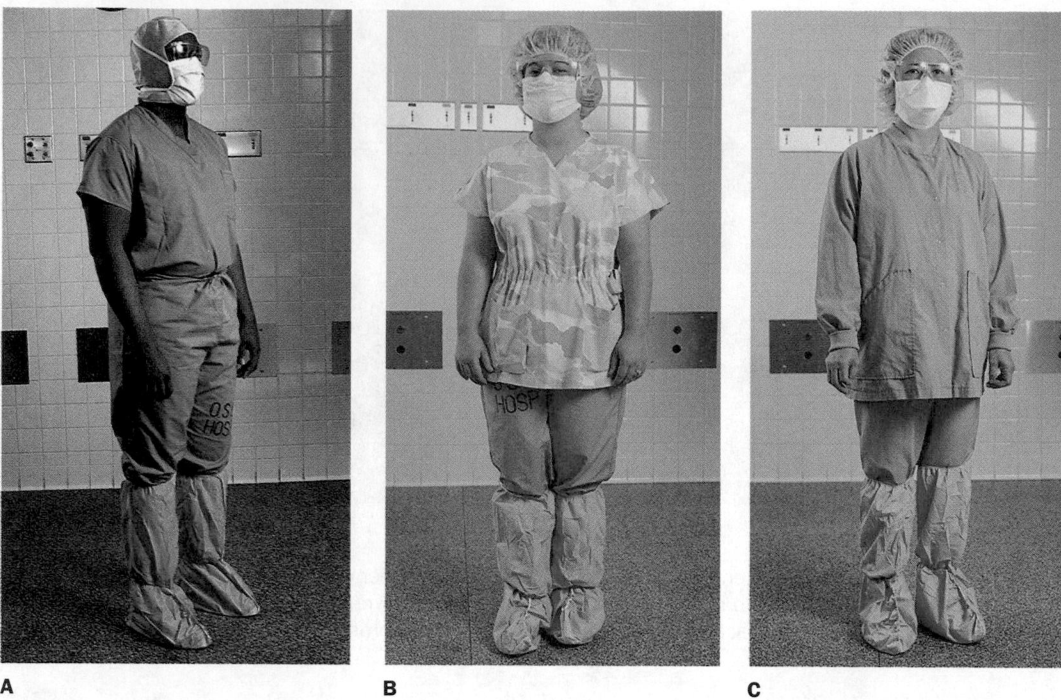

Figure 14-2 Proper surgical attire. **A**, Two-piece scrub suit with shirt tucked in. **B**, Tunic top. **C**, Nonscrubbed personnel with long-sleeved jacket.

patients. Table 14-2 provides some examples of intraoperative applications of Standard Precautions.

The proper handling and disposition of needles, knife blades, and sharp instruments, along with strict compliance with the CDC's Standard Precautions, protects OR personnel. The Occupational Safety and Health Administration's (OSHA's) bloodborne pathogen standard and federal legislation provide guidelines to protect health care workers from exposure to body fluids and needlestick and sharps injuries. Provisions require the use of engineering controls, including safer medical devices such as needleless systems and sharps with built-in injury protectors. Other requirements include an exposure control plan and sharps injury log for documenting and tracking exposure. Adhering to these practices and strictly maintaining aseptic technique minimizes the chance of transmitting pathogens between patients and personnel.

Sterilization of Supplies. Microorganisms that do not normally invade healthy tissue are capable of causing infection if introduced directly into the body. For this reason all supplies and instruments used for the surgical procedure must be properly sterilized. Sterilization renders items safe for contact with tissue without transmission of infection as long as their sterility is maintained.

Sterilization processes for instruments and products used in the surgical suite must be performed according to guidelines established by the regulatory agencies that conduct research and set guidelines for the methods, products, and equipment used in sterilization processes. These agencies include the CDC, OSHA, AORN, Food and Drug Administration (FDA), and American Association for Medical Instrumentation. Table 14-3 summarizes methods of sterilization.

Although the sterilization process prevents the potential spread of disease via surgical instruments and other supplies used during the surgery, data indicate that some pathogens are not susceptible to the normal sterilization processes. *Prions,* abnormal isoforms of cellular proteins, are unlike all other known pathogens and do not contain genetic material. Prions are responsible for the transmission of Creutzfeldt-Jakob disease and other encephalopathies, including "mad cow" disease (bovine spongiform encephalopathy). These highly resistant pathogens can survive routine sterilization and disinfection processes, including steam sterilization, dry heat, ethylene oxide, and plasma sterilization.

Items used during anesthesia induction, such as laryngoscope blades and laryngeal mask airway devices, are capable of transmitting prions unless properly decontaminated. Tissues with a high risk for prion infection include brain, spinal cord, and eye. Tissues considered at medium risk for infection are cerebrospinal fluid, lymph node, spleen, pituitary gland, and tonsils.[8,9] The CDC, World Health Organization, AORN, and JCAHO have developed protocols for decontamination and sterilization of instruments and supplies that come in contact with prions and thus prevent transmission of these virulent pathogens.

Surgical Hand Antisepsis. In the surgical environment the skin is a major source of potential microbial contamination. The single most effective and least expensive intervention to prevent infection is hand hygiene. The following are important considerations for the perioperative nurse:

- *General hand hygiene* consists of decontamination by hand washing with an antimicrobial or plain soap and water, or with an antiseptic hand rub.

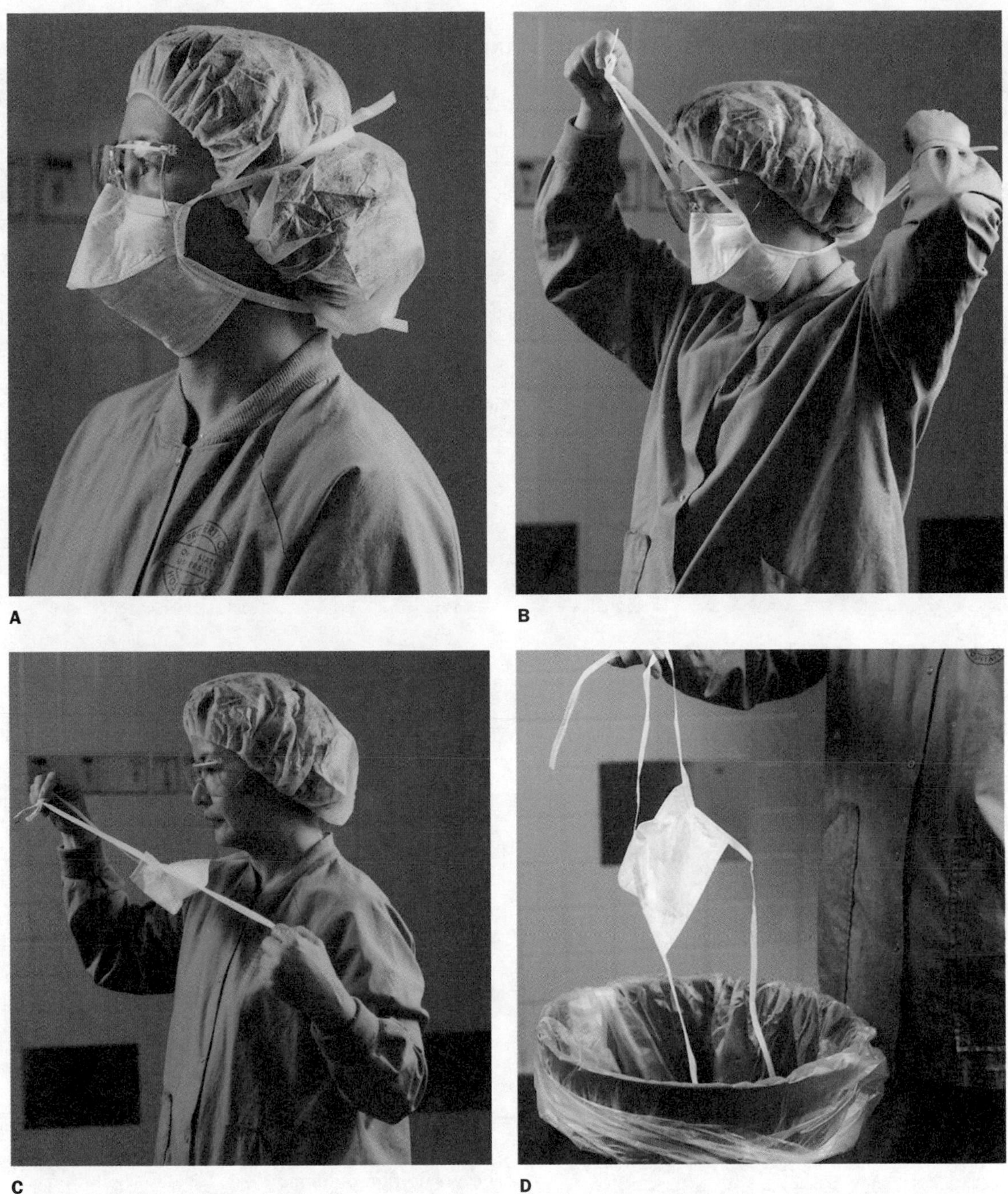

Figure 14-3 Proper handling of mask. **A**, Edges of properly worn mask conform to facial contours when mask is applied and tied correctly. **B** and **C**, Personnel should avoid touching filter portion of mask when removing it. **D**, Masks should be discarded on removal.

- *Surgical hand antisepsis/hand scrub* consists of the antiseptic surgical scrub or antiseptic hand rub before donning sterile attire. The purpose is to:
  - Remove dirt and microorganisms from the hands, fingernails, and forearms
  - Decrease the resident microbial count to minimum levels
  - Retard the regrowth of microorganisms

The microbial skin flora are classified as transient and resident bacteria. Transient flora are acquired by contact and loosely adhere to the skin. The majority of transient microorganisms are removed by chemical and mechanical methods. Resident flora are found deep in the skin in hair follicles and sebaceous glands. These microorganisms are shed from the body as old cells move from the dermal to the epidermal layer of the skin with perspiration and other skin secretions. Because of these actions, resident flora are potential sources of contamination. Resident bacteria are decreased but not completely removed during the surgical scrub.

The skin cannot be sterilized; however, it can be made surgically clean. Obtaining surgically clean skin involves a mechanical

TABLE 14-2 INTRAOPERATIVE APPLICATIONS OF STANDARD PRECAUTIONS

Nursing Action	Potential Contaminant	Precautions
Changing blood-filled suction liner at end of procedure	Blood splashing out of suction liner	Goggles or face shield, nonsterile gloves
Transferring actively bleeding trauma patient to operating room bed	Direct contact with blood	Goggles or face shield, nonsterile gloves, fluid-resistant apron or gown
Organizing blood-filled sponges for sponge count	Direct contact with blood-contaminated sponges	Goggles or face shield, nonsterile gloves
Removing or changing surgical knife blade	Cuts and direct contact with blood	Manufacturer's safety device, instrument, or surgical clamp to disassemble knife blade and handle
Sharps handling and disposal	Needlestick injury, contaminated sharps	Needleless systems; hands-free technique for passing sutures, knife blades, and other sharp instruments; one-handed recapping technique; blunt suture needles; resheathing needle; written exposure control plan and sharps injury log

TABLE 14-3 MAJOR METHODS OF STERILIZATION

Method	Manner of Sterilization	Advantages	Disadvantages
Steam	Steam under pressure infiltrates permeable materials with moist heat, causing denaturation and coagulation of cellular protein system, leading to death of microbe or spore.	Safe Easy Economic Permeates porous substances Leaves no film on items	Does not work with items sensitive to heat Items corroded by steam and moisture Ineffective against prions
Dry heat	Dry heat in form of hot air destroys microbes by coagulating cellular protein.	Safe Easy Economic Noncorrosive to delicate or fine instruments	Requires long exposure period Uneven penetration of some surfaces Time and temperature dependent on materials being sterilized
Chemical (ethylene oxide gas)	Chemical disrupts cellular protein metabolism and reproduction, leading to death of microbe or spore.	Effective for heat-sensitive items Noncorrosive Permeates dry substances Leaves no film on items	Time consuming Expensive Toxic byproducts can formulate
Peracetic acid	Acetic plus extra oxygen atom inactivates microbe's cellular functions.	Noncorrosive Nonabsorbable	Requires rinsing Prolonged exposure necessary for some items Hazardous effects associated with exposure
Plasma	Low-temperature hydrogen peroxide creates gas plasma, consisting of ions, electrons, and neutral atomic particles. Free radicals in gas interact with cellular membranes, enzymes, or nucleic acids, leading to death of microbe or spore.	Faster than ethylene oxide gas Dry nontoxic method Environmentally safe byproducts (water and oxygen) No aeration Safe for heat-sensitive items Noncorrosive to metal	Ineffective against prions Incompatible with cotton-woven fabric and paper Ineffective on small-diameter cannulae

process that removes transient flora with friction, along with a chemical process using an antimicrobial detergent to decrease the number of flora on the epidermis.

The procedure and types of material used for the surgical scrub vary among institutions. Agents should be limited to those that are FDA compliant with a documented ability to kill microorganisms immediately on contact and demonstrated persistence and cumulative activity.[7,15,25]

In 2002 the CDC guidelines stated that the use of a brush or sponge was no longer necessary to reduce the microbial count on hands provided an alcohol-base scrub product was used.[10] Use of an alcohol-based hand rub or brushless scrubbing is thought to be less irritating to the skin than traditional scrubbing and may promote skin integrity even after repeated use. Solutions containing between 60% and 95% demonstrate the greatest ability to decrease bacterial counts; most antiseptic hand rubs are alcohol based either with or without emollients.[10] The hands and arms must be washed and dried before applying an alcohol-based hand rub because these agents do not remove dirt and debris.[15]

Two accepted methods exist for performing the traditional surgical hand scrub: the timed scrub procedure and the brush-stroke procedure. Both are effective and follow an anatomic pattern of scrub, beginning at the fingertips and ending with the elbows. Evidence to support the best practice for length of scrub time is inconclusive. In the timed scrub each anatomic area of the hands and forearms is scrubbed for an identified length of time with special attention given to the fingers and hands. At the conclusion of the timed scrub, the hands and arms are rinsed. The brush stroke scrub differs from the timed scrub method only in that there is a defined number of brush strokes used for each area of the fingers, hands, and arms. Methods of rinsing and entering the operating room are the same as for the timed scrub process.

Only individuals who are free of skin problems and upper respiratory tract infections should scrub. Skin cuts and abrasions can discharge serum, which can provide an environment for microbial growth and thereby increase the potential for infection. Fingernails must be kept short to prevent tearing of surgical gloves and clean to prevent harboring of microorganisms. Nail polish that is chipped or worn for more than 4 days appears to foster larger amounts of bacteria. If nail polish is worn, it should be freshly applied and free of chips. Artificial nails prevent effective hand washing by harboring gram-negative microorganisms and should not be worn.[7]

Patient Skin Preparation. The recommended practices developed by the AORN provide guidance for preoperative skin preparation of the operative site. The goal of skin preparation is to reduce the risk of postoperative wound infection by (1) removing soil and transient microbes from the skin, (2) reducing the resident microbial count to subpathogenic amounts in a short time and with minimal tissue irritation, and (3) inhibiting rapid rebound growth of microbes.

Skin preparation can be performed before the induction of anesthesia. If the preparation is done when the patient is awake, the circulating nurse needs to explain the purpose of the procedure, attend to the patient's privacy by avoiding unnecessary exposure, and provide for the patient's comfort and safety.

Hair is removed from the surgical site only when necessary. Methods for hair removal include wet shaving, use of clippers, and use of a depilatory. The incidence of wound infection is increased in patients who are shaved before surgery.[2] If a shave prep is necessary, the nurse must avoid nicks, scratches, or cuts, since any breaks in the skin surface provide a medium for the growth of microorganisms and a resultant infection.

The preparation begins with mechanical scrubbing at the incision site, extending in a circular fashion away from the site to the periphery. At the periphery the preparation sponge is considered contaminated and is discarded. The soiled sponge is never brought back over the area previously scrubbed. Each time the area is scrubbed, a new sponge is used.

When it is necessary to prepare an area that includes an open draining wound or a body orifice, the practice of cleansing from the incision site to the periphery is modified so that cleaning proceeds from clean to dirty areas. The most contaminated area is scrubbed last, even if it is the site of the surgical incision.

Anesthesia

The field of anesthesiology is acknowledged as a major contributor to medicine and has enabled the growth and scientific development of modern surgery. The term **anesthesia** is derived from the Greek word *anaisthesis,* meaning "no sensation."[28]

In the early nineteenth century patients were given alcohol or opium for pain relief or for muscle relaxation during surgical procedures. Surgeons had to work rapidly to complete the surgical procedure because these drugs were unable to provide sufficient pain relief or relaxation. In 1842 the surgeon Crawford Long began using ether as an anesthetic for surgical patients. In 1846 dentists Horace Wells and William Morton used nitrous oxide for dental extractions. Later that year William Morton demonstrated the use of ether as an effective method for rendering a surgical patient unconscious. Morton's work provided the foundation for the modern practice of anesthesia.[16]

Anesthesia is the limited or total loss of feeling with or without loss of consciousness. The two broad classifications of anesthesia are general and local. General anesthesia produces unconsciousness; local anesthesia creates a loss of sensation in a particular area. The anesthesiologist determines the method of administering the anesthesia and the choice of anesthetic agent (Table 14-4). Factors that influence the decision include the patient's preference, age, physical status, and emotional status; coexisting disease; type and length of the surgical procedure; patient's position during the surgical procedure; postoperative recovery from specific anesthetic agents; and any requirements of the surgeon. The American Society of Anesthesiologists (ASA) developed a classification system to identify risk factors based on the patient's health status (see Chapter 13). As part of the preoperative evaluation, the anesthesiologist classifies the patient according to physical status.

OR nurses do not administer anesthetic agents, but they must understand the various anesthetics used in surgery, the methods of administration, and the potential side effects and complications. This knowledge enables the nurse to plan intraoperative nursing care and to assist the anesthesia team.

TABLE 14-4 TYPES OF ANESTHESIA

Type	Expected Result	Method of Administration	Risks
Local	Depressed peripheral nerves Blocked conduction of pain impulses	Administration of anesthetic agent by surgeon to specific area of body by topical application or local infiltration	Allergic reaction Toxicity Cardiac or respiratory arrest Anxiety resulting from patient's "awake" state Infection
Regional			
Spinal	Analgesia Anesthesia Muscle relaxation	Anesthetic agent injected into cerebrospinal fluid (CSF) in subarachnoid space	Hypotension Total spinal anesthesia (inadvertent high level of spinal anesthesia, causing respiratory arrest and complete paralysis) Neurologic complications (tinnitus, arachnoiditis, meningitis, paresthesias, bowel/bladder dysfunction, paralysis) Headache Infection
Epidural	Analgesia Anesthesia Muscle relaxation	Anesthetic agent injected into epidural space and CSF	Dural puncture Intravascular injection with possible convulsions, hypotension, cardiac arrest Hypotension Total spinal anesthesia Neurologic complications Hematoma Infection
Nerve block	Anesthesia of selected nerve	Local anesthetic injected around peripheral nerve	Inadvertent intravascular injection Nerve damage
Bier block	Anesthesia of extremity (usually used on upper extremity)	Anesthetic agent injected into veins of arm or leg while using pneumatic tourniquet	Infection Pain from tourniquet Overdose or toxicity of anesthetic agent

Types of Anesthesia

Local. Local anesthetic agents (Table 14-5) can be used alone or in conjunction with other types of anesthesia, including inhalation and intravenous agents. The patient's condition, the procedure performed, and the use of other agents determine whether an anesthesia provider will be present to monitor the patient. In some instances the RN is responsible for patient monitoring. To ensure patient safety and quality of care, the AORN has developed recommended practices for nurses who monitor patients receiving local anesthetics.

Local anesthesia interferes with the initiation and transmission of nerve impulses by the use of medications administered topically or injected by local infiltration, regional block, or field block (where an anesthetic agent is injected into a wide area surrounding the surgical site). Motor and sensory nerves are affected, resulting in paralysis of both voluntary and involuntary muscles. The action of the local anesthetic and systemic absorption are affected by local blood flow and vascular supply to the region. Medications may be given to either increase or decrease the rate of absorption; for instance, epinephrine added to the local agent causes vasoconstriction and increased anesthesia time. Another advantage of adding epinephrine to the local anesthetic is decreased bleeding at the surgical site.

The patient may experience a burning and stinging sensation with injection of the local agent. Side effects include allergic and toxic reactions. Although the physician administers the local anesthetic, it is important for the nurse to monitor the amount of medication the patient receives, since toxic reactions are dose related. The addition of epinephrine may also lead to toxic reactions because of increased catecholamine response. Signs of toxicity include tachypnea, bradycardia or tachycardia, perioral numbness, tinnitus, drowsiness, metallic taste, paresthesias, tremors, seizures, and coma.

Regional. Regional anesthesia causes a temporary loss of sensation in a particular portion of the body (dermatome) by the use of local anesthetics. The use of local anesthesia agents temporarily prevents generation and conduction of nerve impulses and may or may not affect motor functions.

TABLE 14-4 TYPES OF ANESTHESIA—CONT'D

Type	Expected Result	Method of Administration	Risks
Minimal sedation	Sedation Anxiolysis Respiratory and cardiac function unaffected	Intravenous	Potential for impaired cognitive function and coordination Potential for injury
Moderate sedation and analgesia	Ability to maintain independent cardiorespiratory function Decreased level of consciousness Ability for purposeful responses to verbal and tactile stimuli Sedation Analgesia Amnesia Anxiolysis Rapid, safe return to activities of daily living	Intravenous May or may not have anesthesia provider in attendance Registered nurse often responsible for patient monitoring	Oversedation Respiratory depression, apnea Airway obstruction Hypotension Aspiration
Deep sedation and analgesia	Depressed consciousness Ability to respond purposefully after repeated or painful stimulation	Intravenous	Airway obstruction Inability to maintain spontaneous ventilation May require ventilatory support
General	Reversible unconsciousness Analgesia Anesthesia Amnesia Muscle relaxation (immobility) Depression of reflexes	Inhalation Intravenous	Oral or dental injury Cardiac or respiratory arrest Residual muscle paralysis Hypertension Hypotension Hypothermia Hyperthermia Renal dysfunction Neurologic dysfunction

Regional anesthetics are used with patients for whom general anesthesia is contraindicated. The choice of regional agent depends on the type and anticipated length of procedure, the patient's position during the procedure, and the patient's physical and psychologic status. Box 14-1 outlines the advantages and disadvantages of regional anesthesia. The types of regional anesthesia include spinal, epidural, nerve block, and Bier block.

SPINAL. Spinal anesthesia is usually administered for surgical procedures performed on the lower abdomen, inguinal region, perineum, or lower extremities. With the patient lying on one side curled into a fetal position or in a sitting position, the physician injects a local anesthetic agent into the cerebrospinal fluid in the subarachnoid space (Figure 14-4). After injection, there is an almost immediate onset of anesthesia at the site.

The duration and level of spinal anesthesia are determined by the site and speed of injection, body height or length of the vertebral column, specific gravity of the anesthetic agent, intraabdominal pressure, and position of the patient immediately after injection. Patient position is extremely important when using hyperbaric agents (agents with a specific gravity heavier than that of the spinal fluid), since gravity moves the anesthetic agents to the lowest point of the vertebral column. Altering the patient's position causes the hyperbaric agent to be directed up, down, or to a particular side of the spinal cord.

Hypotension is a potential complication associated with high-level spinal anesthesia; it is important to monitor the patient's vital signs and level of consciousness. Anesthesia extending above the T4 dermatome may cause cardiorespiratory arrest as a result of sympathetic block. Venous stasis in the lower extremities as a result of paralysis is an important consideration. Sudden changes in the patient's position may result in a sudden drop in blood pressure; elevating the legs may increase venous return to the heart.[16] Other complications of spinal anesthesia include infection and transient or permanent neurologic symptoms such as paresthesias, paralysis, tinnitus, arachnoiditis, meningitis, and auditory or ocular disturbances.[35]

Spinal headache may occur as a result of a cerebrospinal fluid leak from the dural needle puncture. A persistent leak leads to

TABLE 14-5 COMMONLY USED LOCAL ANESTHETIC AGENTS

Agent	Indication	Advantages	Disadvantages
Bupivacaine (Marcaine, Sensorcaine)	Epidural, spinal, peripheral nerve block, local	Minimal cardiovascular effects Addition of epinephrine to decrease rate of absorption also lowers risk of systemic toxic reaction, prolongs anesthetic effects	Older adults more at risk for systemic toxic reaction Potential for overdose causing cardiac arrest
Lidocaine (Xylocaine)	Epidural, spinal, peripheral, intravenous blocks, local	Short acting Low toxicity	Potential for overdose leading to cardiac and respiratory arrest and convulsions Cautious use in patients with family history of malignant hyperthermia
Procaine hydrochloride (Novocain)	Spinal, peripheral nerve block, local	Rapidly absorbed from injection site Low toxicity No local irritation	Low potency Possible anaphylaxis
Tetracaine (Pontocaine)	Spinal; topical	Long duration 10 times more potent than procaine	Slow onset Possible anaphylaxis 10 times more toxic than procaine Higher risk for systemic toxicity

decreased pressure within the spinal cord, which causes the headache when the patient assumes an upright position. Treatment modalities include strict bed rest in the supine position for 24 to 48 hours, hydration, analgesia, and epidural blood patch (5 to 20 ml of the patient's blood injected at the puncture site).

Box 14-1 Advantages and Disadvantages of Regional Anesthesia

Advantages

- Simplicity
- Reasonable cost
- Easily induced
- Minimal equipment required
- Reduced postoperative care requirements
- Fewer systemic effects on body functions
- Avoidance of adverse effects of general anesthesia
- Decreased nausea and vomiting
- Useful for a variety of patients in circumstances where general anesthesia is contraindicated

Disadvantages

- Lack of patient acceptance—patient's fear of being awake during the surgical procedure
- Impracticality of anesthetizing certain areas of the body
- Insufficient duration of anesthesia—patient's fear anesthetic will wear off prematurely
- Rapid absorption of agent into circulation, leading to cardiac arrest

EPIDURAL. Epidural anesthesia is achieved by injecting a local anesthetic agent through the intervertebral space into the space surrounding the dura mater in the spinal column (see Figure 14-4). Anesthetic may be delivered at the thoracic, lumbar, or caudal levels. The anesthesia, administered either through a single dose or intermittently through an epidural catheter, diffuses slowly into the cerebrospinal fluid. Epinephrine may be added to slow absorption. Epidural analgesia may be used after surgery for pain control or via an implanted pump for control of chronic pain.

Common indications for epidural anesthesia include abdominal, genitourinary, and lower extremity procedures. In contrast to spinal anesthesia, epidural anesthesia requires greater doses of local anesthetics, has a slower onset, and is not dependent on the patient's position for the level of anesthesia. Epidural anesthesia also allows the provider to titrate dosing throughout the procedure.

Hypotension, headache, respiratory depression, and neurologic complications are not as common as with the use of spinal anesthesia. Other complications include infection and a higher potential for failure than with spinal anesthesia.

NERVE BLOCK. A nerve block is achieved with the injection of a local anesthetic into or around a nerve or group of nerves that innervates the operative site. Either continuous or intermittent infusion may be used. Examples include intercostal, axillary, and digital blocks. Nerve blocks interfere with sensory, motor, or sympathetic transmissions. Onset and length of the block depend on the amount and concentration of the anesthetic. Besides intraoperative use, nerve blocks are also used to relieve chronic pain.

BIER BLOCK. Bier block, a type of intravenous regional anesthesia, is achieved by administering local anesthetic agents into the

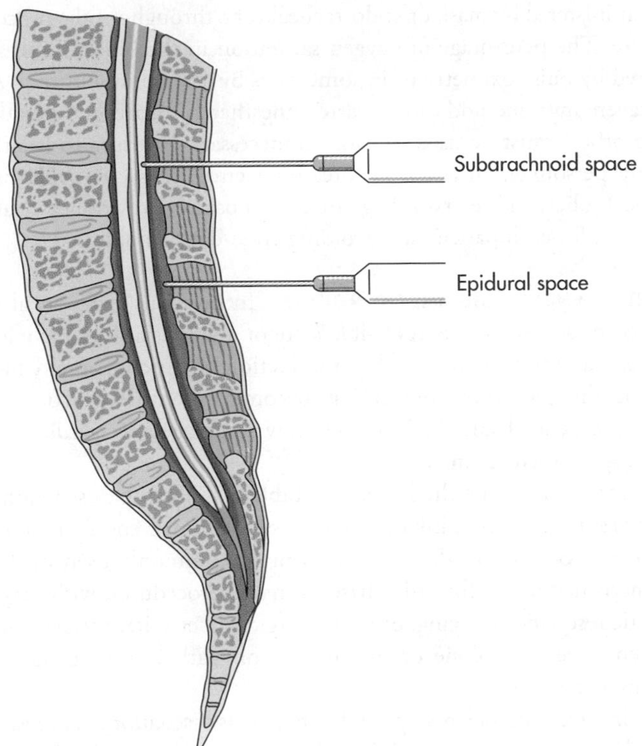

Figure 14-4 Agent is injected into subarachnoid space for spinal anesthesia or into epidural space for epidural anesthesia.

venous system of an exsanguinated extremity. A tourniquet is used to prevent the agent from entering the systemic circulation. When the tourniquet is deflated at the end of the procedure, the patient is monitored for systemic effects of the local anesthetic, which may cause cardiovascular or central nervous system complications. Advantages of this technique are a quick onset of anesthesia and a short recovery time. The major disadvantage is that this technique is limited to procedures lasting 2 hours or less. If the tourniquet is inflated longer than 2 hours, tissue damage can occur.

Minimal Sedation. Minimal sedation uses sedatives and anxiolytics that allow the patient to remain responsive and breathe independently. Indications are for minor surgeries or as a supplement to local or regional anesthesia. Advantages for the patient include anxiety relief, amnesia, analgesia, comfort, and safety.

Moderate Sedation and Analgesia. The ASA in conjunction with JCAHO[20] has developed standards and definitions for levels of sedation and anesthesia. Moderate sedation and analgesia, formerly known as *conscious sedation*, is a drug-induced depression of consciousness in which the patient is able to respond purposefully to verbal commands and tactile stimulation. Cardiovascular function is usually maintained, and the patient independently maintains an airway and spontaneous ventilation.[8] Moderate sedation and analgesia are commonly administered to patients undergoing ambulatory surgical procedures and short surgical or diagnostic procedures that require sedation and amnesia. Advantages for the patient include relief of fear and anxiety, elevation of pain threshold, maintenance of consciousness and protective reflexes, amnesia, and a quick return to normal activities.

Orders for medications used during sedation and analgesia must be written by the physician performing the procedure or by the anesthesia provider. The American Nurses Association and AORN have determined that RNs may administer these medications, assess the patient's response, and monitor the patient during the procedure. Qualifications of nurses administering medications and protocols for patient care during sedation and analgesia vary by state and institution.[8]

Monitored Anesthesia Care. Monitored anesthesia care (MAC) is a technique used when the patient's status necessitates the presence of an anesthesia provider. A variety of anesthetic techniques, including local, moderate sedation and analgesia, regional, or intravenous nerve blocks, may be used, depending on the procedure and patient status. A member of the anesthesia team is present to monitor the patient's vital signs, respiratory status, and cardiac status and administer oxygen as needed. In addition to monitoring the patient's physical status, the anesthesia provider can administer intravenous analgesics, sedatives, or amnesic agents as necessary for patient comfort. MAC is used with patients who are too unstable to withstand a general anesthetic or lengthy local procedures.

General Anesthesia. General anesthesia is the depression of the central nervous system by administration of drugs or inhalation agents. Patients are not arousable even with painful stimuli; cardiovascular and respiratory functions are often impaired. Patients under general anesthesia often require ventilatory assistance and positive pressure ventilation because of medication-induced depression of neurologic function or decreased or absent spontaneous ventilation.[15] The exact methods by which general anesthetic agents produce unconsciousness, analgesia, and muscle relaxation are unknown. It is thought that each anesthetic affects the central nervous and musculoskeletal systems in unique ways and works with multiple sites and areas.[28]

DEPTH OF ANESTHESIA. For anesthesia to be safe, the anesthesiologist must monitor its depth or level. Guidelines to estimate the depth or level of anesthesia used to be based on clearly delineated physiologic changes and reflex responses that were seen with the administration of ether (Box 14-2). Because ether is no longer used, physiologic responses may vary with the agents and techniques used today. However, these guidelines can still be used to estimate the depth of anesthesia.

The depth of anesthesia and sedation can be monitored with a bispectral index (BIS) monitor. The BIS is a simple monitoring device that uses the electroencephalogram wave form providing a number representing the depth of anesthesia. The number ranges from 100 (fully conscious) to 0 (absence of brain activity); 40 represents profound coma. BIS monitoring may be used to decrease patients' awareness during general anesthesia, titrate drug dosages, decrease recovery time, and reduce the incidence of nausea and vomiting.[5,28]

PHASES OF GENERAL ANESTHESIA. The three phases of general anesthesia are induction, maintenance, and emergence. **Induction** begins with the administration of intravenous agents or with the inhalation of a combination of anesthetic gases and oxygen. Endotracheal intubation is performed during this phase. This

Box 14-2 Stages of General Anesthesia

- Stage I begins with the administration of anesthetic agents and ends with the loss of consciousness. This is also known as the relaxation stage.
- Stage II begins with the loss of consciousness and ends with the onset of regular breathing and loss of eyelid reflexes. This stage is referred to as the excitement or delirium phase because it is often accompanied by involuntary motor activity. The patient must not receive any auditory or physical stimulation during this period.
- Stage III begins with the onset of regular breathing and ends with the cessation of respirations. This stage is known as the operative or surgical phase.
- Stage IV begins with the cessation of respiration and leads to death.

phase is completed when the patient is ready for positioning, skin preparation, or the incision.

Once it is safe for any of these activities to commence, the patient has entered the **maintenance** phase of anesthesia. During this phase the anesthesiologist maintains the appropriate levels of anesthesia with inhalation agents and intravenous medications. The anesthesiologist pays close attention to the surgical field and anticipates the surgeon's actions in order to alter the depth of anesthesia whenever necessary.

The **emergence** period begins when the anesthesiologist decreases the anesthetic agents and the patient begins to awaken. Extubation usually occurs during this period. Potential complications during this period include laryngospasm, vomiting, slow spontaneous respirations, and uncontrolled reflex movement.

Balanced Anesthesia. Balanced anesthesia is one of the most commonly used methods of administering general anesthesia. This method combines various agents to produce hypnosis, analgesia, and muscle relaxation with minimal physiologic disturbance. Each agent is administered for a specific purpose. Intravenous barbiturates are used for induction, regional anesthetics for muscle relaxation and analgesia, and inhalation agents for maintenance. Variations of this technique are used depending on the patient's physical status and the requirements of the surgical procedure.

Inhalation Anesthesia. Inhalation anesthesia involves administering a mixture of anesthetic gases and oxygen directly to the lungs. The gases are passed into pulmonary circulation, delivered to the brain and other body tissues, and readily eliminated through the respiratory system. Table 14-6 describes some of the more common inhalation anesthetics in use.

These agents are administered to the patient by a face mask or directly into the lungs through an endotracheal tube (Figure 14-5). The endotracheal tube may have a balloon that is inflated after insertion; the balloon fills the tracheal space, reducing the chance of aspiration of gastric contents. Regardless of the anesthesiologist's skill, an endotracheal tube may cause some irritation to the trachea and subsequent edema. After surgery patients commonly report a sore, irritated throat.

Several measures used during inhalation anesthesia promote the safety of both patient and health care workers. Oxygen is administered by mask or endotracheal tube throughout the procedure. The percentage of oxygen saturation in the blood is measured by pulse oximetry or in some cases by arterial monitoring. A scavenging method for waste anesthetics (carbon dioxide absorber) must be used to avoid unnecessary exposure to health care personnel. In addition, breathing circuits, masks, endotracheal tubes, and reservoir bags are all disposable, providing a clean circuit for each patient and avoiding cross-contamination.

Intravenous Anesthetic Agents. Intravenous drugs are also used to achieve a safe, reversible state of anesthesia. Patients may prefer an intravenous anesthesia induction because it is rapid and generally pleasant. Thus it has become a routine practice to induce general anesthesia with intravenous agents regardless of the agent used for maintenance.

Intravenous anesthetic agents (Table 14-7) can be used alone or as supplements to inhalation agents. Total intravenous anesthesia may be used in the OR but is more commonly used in the emergency room, for office-based surgical procedures, with magnetic resonance imaging, or in the surgical laser suite. Intravenous agents are used alone or in conjunction with nitrous oxide or muscle relaxants.

Intravenous agents provide hypnosis, sedation, amnesia, and/or analgesia and are injected into a peripheral vein. Unlike inhalation agents, which are reversed by discontinuing the drug and ventilating the lungs with 100% oxygen, intravenous drugs must be metabolized by the liver and excreted by the kidneys.

Opioid Analgesics. Opioids provide analgesia and sedation and can be used in high doses as anesthetics for short surgical procedures (Table 14-8). These drugs are administered either in bolus doses or by continuous intravenous infusion. The opioids do not produce muscle relaxation; in fact they may increase muscle tone. Neuromuscular blocking agents are used during surgery to counteract this action.

After surgery patients who receive high-dose opioid anesthesia are susceptible to respiratory depression. Patients may hypoventilate and become hypoxic; therefore careful monitoring of vital signs is necessary in the postoperative period. Opioid-induced respiratory depression can be reversed with the administration of an opioid antagonist such as naloxone (Narcan).

Neuromuscular Blocking Agents. Neuromuscular blocking agents are used as adjuncts to anesthetic agents. The major action of neuromuscular blocking agents is the relaxation of voluntary muscles. These agents are used to facilitate the passage of endotracheal tubes, prevent laryngospasm, control muscle tone throughout the surgical procedure, and decrease the amount of general anesthesia used. Neuromuscular blocking agents interfere with the transfer of impulses from the motor nerves to the voluntary muscle cells.

The two categories of neuromuscular blocking agents are depolarizing and nondepolarizing agents (Table 14-9). Depolarizing agents react with receptors at the end plate region of the muscle and begin depolarization of the muscle membrane, which causes muscle contraction. The muscle contraction is uncoordinated and is referred to as *muscle fasciculation*. After surgery patients may complain of muscle stiffness and soreness resulting from muscle fasciculation.

TABLE 14-6 COMMONLY USED INHALATION ANESTHETIC AGENTS

Agent	Indication	Advantages	Disadvantages
Nitrous oxide (N_2O)	Maintenance; sometimes for induction	Rapid induction and emergence Additive effects to other anesthetics	Poor muscle relaxation Can depress myocardium Risk of hypoxia with high dose or faulty anesthesia machine
Desflurane (Suprane)	Induction; used in ambulatory surgery and shorter procedures	Rapid induction and emergence Low lipid-solubility; good choice for obese patients	Can cause coughing with induction Increased heart rate and decreased blood pressure
Enflurane (Ethrane)	Maintenance; sometimes for induction	Good relaxation Permits larger amounts of epinephrine to be used than with halothane	Can increase heart rate and decrease blood pressure Risk of nephrotoxicity Slightly irritating odor
Halothane (Fluothane)	Maintenance; sometimes for induction	Rapid induction and emergence Pleasant, nonirritating odor	Sensitizes myocardium to epinephrine Decreases heart rate and arterial blood pressure Risk for arrhythmias Risk for hepatotoxicity Delayed emergence in obese patients
Isoflurane (Forane)	Maintenance; sometimes for induction	Good relaxation Rapid induction and emergence Little myocardial depression Safe for patients with hepatic and renal disease	Increased heart rate Slightly irritating odor
Sevoflurane (Ultane)	Induction (often with mask); maintenance	Rapid induction and emergence Pleasant odor	Possible risk of nephrotoxicity Costly

Nondepolarizing agents cause paralysis of the voluntary muscles, are slower acting, and have a longer duration than depolarizing agents. These agents vary in rate of onset and duration and may interact with other drugs such as antibiotics and lead to prolonged muscle relaxation.

Other Types of Anesthesia. *Planned perioperative hypothermia* or *induced hypothermia* may be used as an adjunct to other anesthetic agents. **Hypothermia** refers to the reduction of body temperature below normal to reduce oxygen and metabolic requirements. Extracorporeal cooling, a method of bloodstream cooling, consists of removing the blood from a major vessel, circulating it through coils immersed in a refrigerant, and returning it to the body through another vessel. Bloodstream cooling is the fastest method for producing hypothermia and is used primarily for patients undergoing open-heart or brain surgery.

Monitoring the Patient

Any surgical procedure subjects the patient to many stressors. Potent anesthetic agents, tissue trauma, blood loss, and positioning can interfere with and alter the patient's respiratory and cardiovascular status. Continuous monitoring and assessment are necessary to detect changes in the patient's physiologic status and to initiate necessary treatment in a timely manner.

The ASA developed basic intraoperative monitoring standards. The AORN developed standards of care to guide the practice of nurses working in the perioperative setting. Both organizations have determined that the basic standards include performing electrocardiograms (ECGs); monitoring blood pressure, heart rate, and temperature; and continuously monitoring ventilation, circulation, and level of consciousness. The nurse uses both invasive and noninvasive methods for monitoring the patient. Automatic devices also assist in the monitoring processes (Table 14-10). It is imperative that the anesthesiologist and nurse be familiar with the functions and uses of the specialized equipment and ensure that it is in proper working order. Even with the availability of automatic monitoring equipment, the anesthesiologist or nurse must remain in close contact with the patient to immediately observe any significant physiologic changes.

During the procedure, monitoring the anesthetized patient's vital functions is primarily the responsibility of the anesthesiologist. The circulating nurse assists in patient monitoring by estimating and reporting blood loss, measuring urine output, and

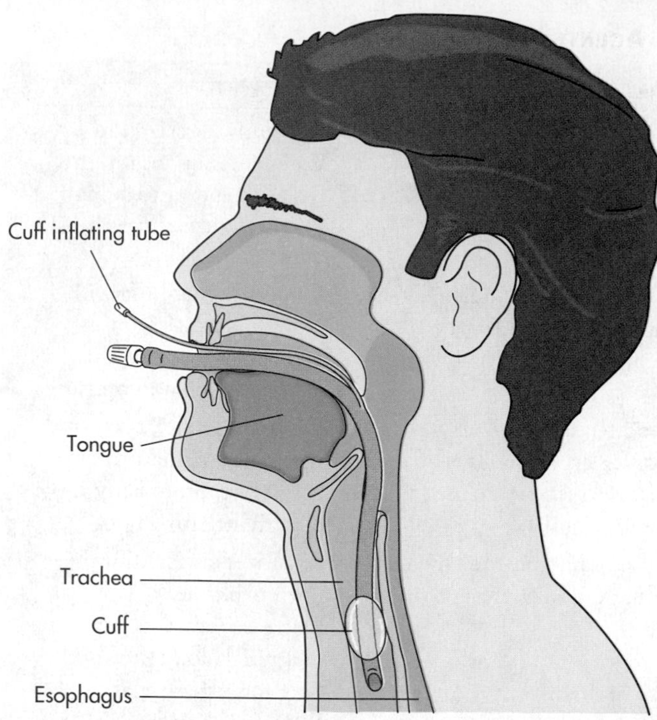

Figure 14-5 Endotracheal tube in position.

assessing the patient's overall status. In emergent situations the circulating nurse assists the anesthesia team.

Nurse's Role During Induction and Emergence

The induction of and emergence from general anesthesia are critical points in the intraoperative care of the patient. During induction the circulating nurse should remain at the bedside to provide the patient with physical and psychologic support and to assist the anesthesia provider. The circulating nurse should ensure a quiet, calm atmosphere, avoiding excessive noise and movement of the patient. The circulating nurse may be asked to assist the anesthesia provider by providing pressure to the cricoid cartilage before intubation. This technique, known as Sellick maneuver, prevents aspiration and regurgitation of stomach contents by obstructing the esophagus and is commonly performed for patients at risk for pulmonary aspiration.

Similar concerns for patient care occur during emergence from general anesthesia. Maintenance of a patent airway and ventilation is the primary responsibility of the anesthesia provider; however, the nurse needs to be available to assist as necessary. Safety and comfort are primary nursing concerns, since the patient may exhibit retching, vomiting, shivering, or restlessness during emergence.

Anesthesia Complications

Anesthetic-related operative mortality rate is relatively low. For a healthy person the risk is about 0.01%. Some of the more common complications of anesthesia are related to untoward reactions to the anesthetic agent. The major complication is cardiac arrest. Laryngospasm and inhalation of gastric contents are serious potential complications that may occur during the emergence or induction phase of general anesthesia.

As discussed in Chapter 13, evidence does not support the traditional nothing-by-mouth (NPO) past-midnight fasting guidelines. The ASA's revised guidelines for healthy patients undergoing elective procedures recommend the following minimal fasting periods: clear liquids 2 to 4 hours, a light meal 6 hours, and meat and fatty foods 8 hours.[3] It is important to remember that these are recommendations only and clinical practice may vary.

Both general and regional anesthesia causes dilation of peripheral blood vessels and a drop in blood pressure. Venous blood pools in dependent areas, reducing blood return to the heart and lungs for oxygenation and redistribution. General anesthesia depresses the medulla, which maintains cardiac output and peripheral vascular constriction. Muscle relaxants reduce the milking action of normal muscles that assists in venous return. The anesthesiologist constantly monitors the patient and is prepared to compensate for complications of these changes. The circulating nurse, knowledgeable about anesthesia methods, patient risk factors, complications, and preventive interventions, provides efficient and appropriate assistance to the anesthesia team members. Chapter 15 discusses common postoperative complications and interventions used to prevent or treat them.

▶ ARE You READY?

Which of the following is the major complication of anesthesia?
1. Laryngospasm
2. Gastric aspiration
3. Cardiac arrest
4. Hypertension

Physiologic Stress Responses to Surgery and Anesthesia

Surgery affects all body systems and stimulates the physiologic response to stress. The physiologic components involved in the stress response include the central nervous system, hypothalamus, sympathetic nervous system, anterior and posterior pituitary glands, adrenal medulla, and adrenal cortex. Not all these components are necessarily involved in the response to surgery. Refer to a physiology text for a thorough discussion of the stress response.

Neuroendocrine Responses

Neuroendocrine responses play a major role in the patient's reaction to the stress of surgery. Responses include stimulation of the autonomic nervous system (primarily the sympathetic nervous system) and stimulation of selected hormones (primarily aldosterone and glucocorticoid hormones from the adrenal cortex and antidiuretic hormone [ADH] from the posterior pituitary). Table 14-11 summarizes the endocrine stress responses to surgery.

Stimulation of the sympathetic nervous system protects the body from further damage. Vasoconstriction of peripheral blood vessels enables the body to compensate for blood loss and redirect blood flow to critical areas such as the heart and brain. Increased

TABLE 14-7 COMMONLY USED INTRAVENOUS ANESTHETIC AGENTS

Agent	Indication	Advantages	Disadvantages
Diazepam (Valium)	Amnesia; hypnotic; sedation; analgesia	Good sedation	Prolonged duration Irritating to vein
Etomidate (Amidate)	Induction	Rapid induction and emergence Fewer cardiovascular and respiratory effects than thiopental	Pain with injection May cause spontaneous muscle movements Increased incidence of nausea and vomiting after induction Costly
Ketamine (Ketalar)	Induction; occasional maintenance; good for dressing changes, wound debridement, and short diagnostic procedures; may be administered intravenously, intramuscularly, orally, or rectally	Short acting Patient maintains airway Produces amnesia Good choice for patients with reactive airway disease	May cause emergence reactions, including confusion, hallucinations, euphoria May increase heart rate, blood pressure, and intracranial pressure No muscle relaxation
Methohexital sodium (Brevitol)	Induction	Rapid onset and very short duration of action	May cause hiccups, respiratory depression, apnea, laryngospasm, hypotension Pain with injection
Midazolam (Versed)	Hypnotic; sedation; analgesia; amnesic; anxiolytic	Rapid onset and short duration No pain with injection	Respiratory depressant Prolonged effect with obese patients
Propofol (Diprivan)	Induction; maintenance; good choice for short procedures and ambulatory surgery	Rapid onset and short duration Antiemetic Antipruritic Anxiolytic	Respiratory depression, may cause apnea after induction Bradycardia Decreased blood pressure May cause tremors, dystonia, and spontaneous muscle movement during induction and emergence Pain at injection site
Thiopental sodium (Pentothal)	Induction; brief anesthesia without analgesia	Rapid induction and emergence Anticonvulsant	Respiratory depression, apnea Laryngospasm Hypotension

cardiac output also helps maintain blood flow. However, severe trauma or excessive blood loss will overwhelm the compensatory mechanisms, and blood pressure will fall. Certain types of anesthetics or high spinal anesthesia also may interfere with the compensatory vasoconstriction, producing hypotension.

Another sympathetic response is decreased gastrointestinal activity, which may have an adverse effect on the patient. Before surgery psychologic stress may result in anorexia and constipation; after surgery the patient may experience anorexia, gas pains, and constipation from decreased peristalsis in the gastrointestinal tract.

Adrenocortical activity is increased in response to the trauma of surgery, producing greater amounts of aldosterone and cortisol. Aldosterone is released primarily from the adrenal cortex in response to activation of the renin-angiotensin system. Aldosterone acts on the distal kidney tubule cells, causing sodium and water resorption and excretion of potassium and hydrogen ions. Aldosterone helps maintain vascular volume and blood pressure, which may compensate for blood and fluid loss during surgery.

During the first 24 to 48 hours after surgery increased aldosterone secretion is accompanied by an increase in ADH secretion by the posterior pituitary gland. Water is resorbed by the

TABLE 14-8 COMMONLY USED OPIOID ANALGESICS

Agent	Indication	Advantages	Disadvantages
Alfentanil (Alfenta)	Induction; balanced anesthesia	Rapid onset and short duration	Respiratory depression, apnea Half-life prolonged in patients with cirrhosis Nausea
Fentanyl (Sublimase, Duragesic)	Surgical analgesia; supplement to other anesthetic agents	Rapid onset and short duration	Circulatory and respiratory depression
Remifentanil (Ultiva)	Induction and maintenance; surgical analgesia	Rapid action Easily titrated	Respiratory depression Nausea Costly
Sufentanil (Sufenta)	Balanced anesthesia; surgical analgesia; supplement to other anesthetic agents	Rapid onset and recovery 7 times more potent than fentanyl	Respiratory depression, apnea Skeletal muscle rigidity Pruritus

kidney, resulting in decreased urine output. Spontaneous diuresis occurs as the amount of ADH is decreased, usually in about 2 to 4 days.

Cortisol is released from the adrenal cortex and has major effects on glucose, protein, fat metabolism, and fluid and electrolyte balance; it also has antiinflammatory and immunosuppressant effects. Glucocorticoids also play a major role in the maintenance of blood pressure and cardiac output. Increased levels of cortisol in response to stress may stimulate gastric acid secretion, possibly resulting in ulceration of the gastric mucosa. Excessive cortisol may also result in poor wound healing, increased risk of infection, and decreased inflammatory response.

The stress response to surgery varies in intensity depending on the type and duration of surgery and the patient's health. Understanding the body's physiologic response to stress is critical to understanding the effects of prolonged or unresolved stress and the impact of surgical intervention on the patient's overall health and well-being.

Metabolic Responses

After surgery the patient is in a relative state of starvation; metabolism is increased, and fluid and nutrient intake is decreased. Carbohydrate metabolism increases as a result of the increased production of glucocorticoid hormones. Usually for a time the patient is not permitted to eat and receives only intravenous fluids. The patient without oral intake experiences a daily fluid loss of more than 1200 ml. The nurse should administer maintenance fluids on the basis of body weight and at a rate sufficient to maintain urine output. Additional fluids may be needed to replace intraoperative blood or other fluid loss.

Anorexia also may occur as part of the stress response, compounding the problem of inadequate carbohydrate intake even if food is permitted by mouth. The body must meet its glucose needs by the breakdown of stored liver glycogen or by the synthesis of glucose from noncarbohydrate sources.

Fat metabolism increases to allow mobilization of fat from the cells as an energy source. With the decreased intake of carbohydrates and fats after surgery, body fats are metabolized for energy and the patient may lose weight. Protein metabolism is increased after surgery to supply essential amino acids necessary for tissue healing. The net effect of these metabolic processes depends on the patient's preoperative nutritional state.

Thermoregulatory Reponses

The narrow range of normal body temperature is maintained by both physiologic and behavioral responses. The physiologic thermoregulatory control center in conscious adults is in the hypothalamus. Normothermia (96.8° to 100.4° F [36° to 38° C]) is maintained by regulating heat loss with heat production. Most of the body's heat is produced by the basal metabolic rate, and under normal conditions the body's core temperature remains relatively constant. Heat loss in the OR can occur through a variety of mechanisms, including radiation, convection, conduction, and evaporation. General anesthetic agents, muscle relaxants, and opioids all contribute to a decrease in body temperature.

Almost any patient undergoing general anesthesia will become hypothermic unless active measures are taken for warming. After surgery, return to normothermia occurs when anesthetic concentration decreases sufficiently to allow the return of normal thermoregulatory responses. A return to normothermia may take 2 to 5 hours depending on the individual patient, anesthetic technique, and degree of hypothermia.

Intraoperative **hyperthermia,** or an increase in body temperature of 3.6° F (2° C) per hour, occurs less often than hypothermia in the perioperative setting. Common causes include sepsis and infection and less commonly malignant hyperthermia.

Unplanned Perioperative Hypothermia. Unplanned perioperative hypothermia (UPH), a drop in core temperature to below 96.8° F (36° C), is classified as mild (89.6° to 95° F [32° to 35° C]), moderate (80.6° to 89.6° F [27° to 32° C]), or severe (less than 80.6° F [27° C]). The physiologic effects depend on the degree of hypothermia. Untreated or severe hypothermia can lead to coma and death; ventricular fibrillation is likely at 86° F (30° C); below 68° F (20° C) brain activity ceases. UPH occurs in approximately 60% of surgical patients and is associated with such adverse effects as shivering, patient discomfort, decreased drug metabolism, coagulopathy, increased catecholamine production,

TABLE 14-9 COMMONLY USED NEUROMUSCULAR BLOCKING AGENTS

Agent	Indication	Advantages	Disadvantages
Depolarizing Muscle Relaxant			
Succinylcholine (Anectine)	Intubation; short procedures	Rapid onset Short duration	Bradycardia Respiratory depression Increased intracranial pressure Causes muscle fasciculation and release of potassium Avoid in patients with kidney failure, burns, neuromuscular disease; increased intracranial pressure (ICP) Postoperative dysrhythmias
Nondepolarizing Muscle Relaxants			
Atracurium (Tracrium)	Intubation; maintenance	Good choice for patients with renal and hepatic disease Minimal cardiovascular effects	Respiratory depression Cautious use in patients with cardiovascular disease and asthma because of histamine release
d-Tubocurarine chloride (curare)	Maintenance; may be given before depolarizing agent (succinylcholine)	No effect on intellectual functions or consciousness	Decreased blood pressure, circulatory collapse Respiratory depression, apnea, bronchospasm May cause histamine release No anesthetic or analgesic properties
Pancuronium (Pavulon)	Maintenance	Rapid action 5 times as potent as tubocurarine with less histamine release	May increase heart rate and blood pressure in high doses Respiratory depression Primarily renal excretion
Rocuronium (Zemuron)	Intubation; maintenance	Rapid onset	Increased heart rate Prolonged effects in patients with renal or hepatic dysfunction
Vecuronium (Norcuron)	Intubation; maintenance	Minimal cardiovascular effects Little histamine release	Prolonged effects in patients with renal or hepatic dysfunction
Mivacuronium (Mivacron)	Intubation; maintenance	Short acting Used as bolus or infusion Rapid metabolism Minimal cardiovascular effect Reversal agents not usually required	Expensive

and postoperative myocardial infarction.[29] Because of decreased metabolism, the patient may have delayed recovery from anesthesia and increased postoperative morbidity and mortality.

Anesthesia inhibits the reflexes that generate heat and depresses the thermoregulatory center in the hypothalamus, decreases the basal metabolic rate, and increases vasodilation. Anesthesia also causes the loss of normal protective reflexes such as shivering. In the OR the body may lose core heat by exposure to a cool environment; infusion of intravenous fluids; skin preparation with cool solutions; cold, dry anesthetic gases; and escape through the surgical incision. Patients receiving general anesthesia commonly experience 0.5° to 1.5° C loss in core temperature; the loss is greatest during the first hour of anesthesia.[16] General anesthesia causes a decrease in the metabolic rate by 15% to 40%.[19] Preoperative sedation, the length of the procedure, and blood and fluid losses add to the heat loss.

TABLE 14-10 PATIENT MONITORING METHODS DURING ANESTHESIA

Parameter	Methods
Arterial blood pressure	Auscultation using blood pressure cuff and stethoscope Direct measurement with arterial cannulation and connection to pressure transducer (arterial line) Automatic device that measures systolic, diastolic, and mean blood pressure and heart rate
Heart rate	Palpation of superficial artery Auscultation of heart with precordial or esophageal stethoscope Doppler monitoring probe applied to radial pulse Electrocardiogram with continuous display
Respiratory status	Direct observation of chest movements Auscultation of chest with stethoscope or esophageal stethoscope
Body temperature	Skin surface probes or strips applied to body to monitor surface temperature Core temperature probe inserted into nasopharynx, esophagus, bladder, or rectum*
Urinary output	Indwelling urinary catheter
Pulse oximetry	Noninvasive measurement of arterial oxyhemoglobin saturation
Capnography—end tidal carbon dioxide	Noninvasive measurements of end tidal concentration of carbon dioxide Detects changes in respiratory, circulatory, or metabolic status Useful to detect onset of inadvertent hypothermia, malignant hyperthermia, and anesthesia equipment problems
Bispectral index monitor (BIS)	Use of electroencephalogram technology to monitor depth of anesthesia

*Note that core temperature is best measured via esophageal or pulmonary artery probes. Bladder and rectal temperatures are not universally accepted as a true measurement of core temperature.

TABLE 14-11 ENDOCRINE STRESS RESPONSES

Physiologic Changes	Results	Effect
Increased norepinephrine secretion	Peripheral vasoconstriction Decreased gastrointestinal activity	Helps maintain blood pressure when circulating volume is decreased May lead to anorexia or constipation
Increased aldosterone secretion	Sodium retention	Maintains circulating blood volume Increases susceptibility to fluid overload Decreases urinary output
Increased glucocorticoid secretion	Gluconeogenesis Increased protein catabolism Ketogenic effect Antiinflammatory effect Increased platelet production Increased gastric acid secretion	Provides energy to meet stress of surgery Provides additional energy source Provides amino acids for cell synthesis after tissue destruction Provides fat as energy source Increases susceptibility to infection Promotes clotting to prevent bleeding Contributes to development of thrombophlebitis
Increased antidiuretic hormone secretion	Sodium and water resorption in kidney tubules	Maintains circulating blood volume Increases susceptibility to fluid overload Decreases urinary output Potential for hypokalemia

Inadvertent hypothermia may result in cardiac dysrhythmias, metabolic acidosis, hyperglycemia, coagulopathy, decreased platelet aggregation, and coma. The usual signs of hypothermia are often masked by administration of anesthetic agents, and symptoms may not be evident until the postoperative period. Symptoms include shivering, speech impairment, cyanosis, decreased blood pressure, weak pulse, and dilated pupils. Shivering occurs as a hypothalamic response to a drop in core temperature and as result of some anesthetic agents. Untreated shivering can lead to increased oxygen consumption (as much as 400%), increased cardiac workload, cardiac ischemia, decreased cerebral blood flow, and hypoxia.[28]

Hypothermia also decreases the body's immunologic function. The incidence of surgical wound infection is increased in hypothermic patients possibly because of nitrogen loss and hyperkalemia.[28] Intraoperative interventions to prevent and treat heat loss include humidification and warming of anesthetic gases; warming of blood products, intravenous fluids, and irrigation fluids; and various warming devices.

Malignant Hyperthermia. Malignant hyperthermia (MH), first identified in the 1960s, is a serious and potentially fatal complication of general anesthesia. Even though MH occurs most commonly during induction or surgical procedure, it can occur or recur in the PACU or on the nursing unit 24 to 72 hours after surgery. MH reportedly occurs in 1 in 50,000 adults and 1 in 15,000 children.[32] More common in males and adolescents, the incidence of MH decreases after age 50.[33] Other syndromes associated with an increased incidence of MH include central core disease and Duchenne's muscular dystrophy.[28] With prompt recognition and treatment, the mortality rate is less than 10%.[8]

MH is a genetic autosomal-dominant defect resulting in altered muscle metabolism. It is triggered by certain anesthetic agents (Box 14-3) and extreme physiologic and emotional stress. A genetic defect in the muscle cell membrane permits anesthetic agents to trigger a sudden increase of calcium ions within the muscle cells. The rapid increase of calcium starts a series of biochemical reactions that elevate the metabolic rate, causing hyperthermia (with temperatures rising to 109.4° F [43° C]), muscle rigidity, respiratory and metabolic acidosis, hypercapnia, and cell breakdown. Muscle rigidity occurs in approximately 75% of patients with MH.[14] Diagnostic findings include hypercalcemia, metabolic and respiratory acidosis, hyperkalemia, hypermagnesemia, hypercapnea, and elevated serum creatine phosphokinase (CPK).

Masseter muscle spasms or fasciculations after administration of succinylcholine during induction should alert the anesthesiologist to the potential for an MH episode. The earliest and most consistent clinical sign of MH is unexplained ventricular dysrhythmia, specifically tachycardia or premature ventricular contractions, associated with an increase in end tidal carbon dioxide. Additional clinical symptoms include tachypnea, cyanosis, other dysrhythmias, skin mottling, unstable blood pressure, elevated levels of CPK, and elevated levels of myoglobin. As a result of desaturation, blood at the surgical field may appear dark. The patient's temperature may rise 1.8° to 3.6° F (1° to 2° C) every 5 minutes and may exceed 109.4° F (43° C). Because it occurs in the late stages, an elevated temperature is not a reliable indicator of MH. The patient's urine may appear dark due to rhabdomyolysis (breakdown of striated muscle with excretion of myoglobin in urine). Other late clinical manifestations of MH include hyperkalemia, acute renal failure, left-sided heart failure, disseminated intravascular coagulation, pulmonary embolus, and neurologic deficits.

Treatment of the patient experiencing MH includes immediately ceasing the inhalation agent or muscle relaxant, hyperventilating with 100% oxygen, cooling with ice packs or cooling blankets, lavaging body cavities with iced saline, restoring acid-base balance, treating hyperkalemia, and providing rapid intravenous infusion of dantrolene. Cooling measures should be discontinued when the patient's temperature reaches 100.4° F (38° C).

Dantrolene is the only known treatment able to stop an MH crisis. Dantrolene relaxes skeletal muscle and retards the biochemical actions that cause muscle contractions. Dosage recommendations by the Malignant Hyperthermia Association of the United States (MHAUS) include an initial bolus of 2 to 3 mg/kg with subsequent dosing of up to10 mg/kg.[22] Dantrolene should be continued for at least 24 hours after initial treatment.

All perioperative personnel should be aware of the protocol for patients who develop MH. Many institutions have an MH kit or cart containing necessary supplies for treatment. More information is available from MHAUS at www.mhaus.org. The MH hotline number for physician consultation in emergencies is 800-MH-HYPER.

Identification of patients at risk is the primary method for prevention of MH. The preoperative history should include an assessment of the patient's previous experience with surgery, a history of heatstroke in the patient or family, or known muscular abnormalities. The CPK level may also be elevated, but this is not specific to MH, since elevations may also occur as a result of alcoholism or muscle disease. The key assessment finding is familial history of unexplained death under general anesthesia. For persons with suspected MH, diagnosis is confirmed by preoperative muscle biopsy. Prophylactic administration of dantrolene for MH-susceptible patients is no longer recommended.[22] Anesthetic agents known to trigger MH should not be administered to persons who are at significant risk for developing MH. Family members of individuals with known MH should undergo diagnostic testing as a prophylactic measure.

Box 14-3 Anesthetic Agents Triggering Malignant Hyperthermia

Inhalation Agents

Halothane
Enflurane
Isoflurane
Desflurane
Sevoflurane

Neuromuscular Blocking Agent

Succinylcholine

Nondepolarizing Muscle Relaxant

d-Tubocurarine chloride

▶ ARE You READY?

In monitoring a patient for malignant hyperthermia, which of the following is the earliest clinical sign?

1. Hyperventilation
2. Ventricular dysrhythmias
3. Muscle spasms
4. Cyanosis

Other Considerations

Bloodless Surgery

Bloodless surgery reduces or eliminates the need for transfusions, thus avoiding the use of allogenic blood products. Initially intended for Jehovah's Witnesses and other patients with objections to receiving blood products, bloodless surgery can be used for any surgical patient. The concern regarding the risks of allogenic transfusion and blood shortages have resulted in more widespread application of bloodless techniques.

Techniques to decrease the need for blood transfusion include preoperative autologous blood donation, intraoperative techniques to improve hemostasis, minimally invasive procedures, and the use of regional instead of general anesthesia. Medications such as erythropoietin and iron can be given before surgery to increase preoperative hemoglobin levels.

Surgical techniques to improve hemostasis include the use of gamma Knife radiosurgery, electrocautery, radiofrequency ablation, and laser beam coagulation. Intraoperative methods to conserve blood include hypotensive anesthesia, which lowers the mean arterial blood pressure and decreases the risk for bleeding; moderate levels of hypothermia; hemodilution; cell salvage; and the use of volume expanders and topical and systemic hemostatic agents.

Latex Allergy

Allergic reactions to latex were reported as early as the 1930s; however, the number of reported cases has increased since the introduction of Standard Precautions and the use of latex gloves in the 1980s. Among health care workers the incidence of latex allergy may be as high as 10% to 17%, in contrast to an estimated 1% incidence in the general population.[27,34]

Latex allergy is an immune reaction to one or more proteins in natural rubber latex. Surgical gloves and many of the supplies used in the perioperative area contain latex, which can cause an allergic response in latex-sensitive individuals (Box 14-4). The allergic response can be life threatening; therefore it is essential for perioperative nurses to be able to deal with patients and other health care workers who develop a reaction to latex.

Natural Rubber Latex. Natural rubber latex originates from the white, milky sap of the *Hevea brasiliensis* plant, more commonly known as the rubber tree. During the refinement process many accelerators, antioxidants, emulsifiers, stabilizers, extenders, colorants, retardants, ultraviolet light absorbers, and fragrances are added to the sap. Because of manufacturing techniques, the level of latex allergen in latex gloves varies considerably among brands. Less than 5% of the proteins found in latex have immunoglobulin E (IgE)–binding activity.[34] Manufacturing techniques allow the amount of latex protein to be reduced to less than 50 mcg/g of glove, thus reducing the potential for latex sensitivity.[34]

Box 14-4 Examples of Medical Supplies Containing Latex

- Adhesive tape
- Airways
  - —Nasal
  - —Oral
- Breathing bags
- Breathing circuits
- Bulb syringes
- Catheters
  - —Foley
  - —Straight
  - —Central venous
  - —Pulmonary artery
- Elastic bandages
- Electrode pads
- Fluid-warming blankets
- Gloves
- Intravenous ports
- Rubber stoppers on multi-dose vials
- Stethoscope tubing
- Syringe plungers
- Ventilator bags
- Wound drains

Reactions to Latex. Latex reactions are classified as irritant, type IV, and type I reactions (Table 14-12). Irritant reaction, or nonallergic contact dermatitis, occurs in 75% of cases and is a reaction to nonprotein irritants.[31,34] An irritant reaction to latex gloves may cause symptoms such as flaking skin, inflammation, blisters, or a dry pruritic rash on the hands.[27] Type IV sensitivity, or allergic contact dermatitis, produces a delayed response and comprises 25% of cases.[31] The reaction is caused by the residual chemicals used in the manufacturing of the latex product. Each exposure increases sensitivity; mild sensitivity may progress to anaphylaxis after multiple or continued exposures.[31]

Type I, or immediate hypersensitivity, is the only type of reaction that is a reaction to the latex protein. Type I sensitivity is systemic and produces an immediate reaction. IgE antibodies are produced in response to inhalation of or contact with the latex protein. The IgE binds onto receptors on mast cells and basophils. Subsequent exposure to the latex protein causes mast cell proliferation, the release of basophil histamine, and anaphylaxis. The reactions occur suddenly and range from a skin flare response to wheezing, bronchospasm, angioedema, and anaphylaxis.

In contrast, no antibody formation occurs with a type IV or cell-mediated reaction. Macrophages and T lymphocytes are activated in response to the allergen and cause tissue inflammation and contact dermatitis. The onset of the reaction is slow and usually requires hours of contact before the appearance of symptoms. However, symptoms may occur years after continued exposure.

Routes of Exposure. Five routes of exposure to the latex protein can cause severe reactions in latex-sensitized individuals. Cutaneous exposure to medical supplies such as anesthesia masks, tourniquets, ECG electrodes, adhesive tape, fluid warming blankets, and elastic bandages can trigger reactions in susceptible patients.

Many of the severe reactions to latex occur as a result of the latex protein coming in contact with the mucous membranes of the mouth, vagina, urethra, or rectum. Oral mucosal reactions may occur in response to the products used in dentistry, as well as to other medical products such as nasogastric tubes. Serious reac-

TABLE 14-12 REACTIONS TO LATEX PRODUCTS

Type I Reactions	Type IV Reactions
Immunoglobulin E activated (antibody formation)	T lymphocyte activated (no antibody formation)
Systemic responses Cutaneous: flushing, diaphoresis, pruritus Gastrointestinal: nausea, vomiting, cramping, diarrhea Cardiovascular: hypotension, tachycardia, dysrhythmias Respiratory: dyspnea, bronchospasm, laryngeal edema	Localized responses Symptoms resolve in 72-96 hr Individual remains sensitized and will react with every contact
Rapid onset of reactions Immediate response	Delayed onset of reactions Primary reaction occurs within 18-24 hr Subsequent reactions can develop sooner
Can be life threatening	Causes discomfort but is not life threatening

tions have also been reported as a result of exposure of the vaginal mucosa to latex during examinations, sexual intercourse, deliveries, and abortions. Although contact of examination gloves, enema kits, and rectal pressure catheters with the rectal mucosa has precipitated reactions, the most severe mucous membrane reactions occur as a result of contact of the rectal mucosa with catheters used during barium enemas.

Inhalation of the latex proteins also causes severe reactions. Inhalation reactions are associated with anesthesia equipment and endotracheal tubes; however, the most common source is inhalation of aerosolized glove powder.[8] The latex protein binds to the powder used in the gloves; as gloves are removed from the box or from the hands, the powder is aerosolized and the particles dissipate onto surgical drapes and sponges. Aerosolization increases the risk of exposure for all sensitized individuals.

During the surgical procedure internal tissue absorbs the latex protein. A reaction is triggered when internal organs come in contact with surgical gloves and other products such as irrigation syringes, instruments, and catheters used throughout the surgical procedure.

The intravascular administration of latex proteins is not well understood. It is postulated that reactions occur from the use of disposable syringes, medications stored in vials with latex plugs, and intravenous tubing with latex ports.

Individuals at Risk for Latex Allergy. A number of groups of individuals are at risk for a latex allergy. Individuals at greatest risk are those with neural tube defects. This patient population undergoes multiple surgeries, uses rubber catheters for urinary or bowel programs, and has multiple exposures to latex gloves in daily care. Other at-risk populations include individuals who have urinary conditions requiring continuous or intermittent catheterization; a history of allergies and asthma; a history of reactions to latex products; a history of multiple surgical procedures, especially bowel procedures; food allergies to bananas, avocados, tropical fruits, kiwis, potatoes, and chestnuts (possible cross-reaction between the food and the latex allergens); and jobs in health care with daily exposure to latex products. The AORN recommends the use of low-allergen and powder-free latex products. Because of the increased incidence of latex allergy among perioperative staff, nonlatex surgical gloves are used in many settings (see Research box).

Research

Korniewicz DM et al: Failure rates in nonlatex surgical gloves, *Am J Infect Control* 32(5):268-273, 2004.

Latex-free gloves are widely used in the surgical environment because of concerns about latex hypersensitivity. Multiple studies have examined failure of latex surgical gloves. However, few have compared failure rates of latex to nonlatex gloves.

Investigators studied the failure rates and surgeon satisfaction with latex and nonlatex gloves while performing surgery. The study included multiple surgical specialties and evaluated barrier integrity using Food and Drug Administration requirements. The researchers concluded that both intact latex and nonlatex sterile gloves provide adequate barrier protection; however, nonlatex gloves tear more frequently during surgery than latex gloves. Nonlatex gloves were more likely to have visible defects than latex gloves. Glove tears were more common in oral, plastic, dental, and cardiac surgical specialties. Both latex and nonlatex gloves developed tears with lengthier surgical procedures. Overall, surgeons preferred to use latex rather than nonlatex gloves.

The authors recommend that a standard be developed for the length of time a pair of gloves should be worn during a surgical procedure. Current standards state that gloves should be changed when a defect occurs or when gloves are worn from 1 to 4 hours.

Intraoperative Patient Management. The nurse must obtain a thorough history before surgery to provide safe intraoperative patient care for individuals who are at high risk for a systemic reaction to latex. Once the nurse identifies a patient as having a latex allergy, the information must be documented and relayed to all other health care workers who provide care. The nurse should mark the chart and give the patient an allergy band. The nurse should reassure the patient and patient's family that the team is aware of the latex allergy and explain the perioperative care plan for protective measures.

During the surgical procedure the circulating nurse ensures that only latex-free products are used. Traffic flow is restricted before and during the procedure. The anesthesia team ensures that the breathing circuit, face mask, and ventilator bag are latex free. If possible, medications are drawn from a latex-free vial.

Removal of the rubber stopper is controversial, since latex may actually leach from the stopper. The AORN does not recommend removing the stopper unless there are no other options.[8] Medications are injected through three-way stopcocks instead of through rubber ports. Latex-free tape is used when applying the dressing. Most institutions have designed latex-free supply carts for use when caring for latex-sensitive individuals.

Education and Prevention. Patient and family education should include instructions regarding management of symptoms and prevention of further allergic reactions. Patients allergic to latex are encouraged to wear an identity bracelet and carry an epinephrine pen.

Because of the prevalence of latex allergy, education and prevention are concerns for health care workers. Standards are in place that limit the amount of powder and residual powder in gloves and also protein levels in latex products.[6] The National Institute for Occupational Safety and Health (NIOSH) has mandated that powder-free and nonlatex gloves be provided to employees who are allergic to latex. The FDA requires manufacturers of medical devices to clearly label items containing latex. NIOSH also recommends environmental measures to decrease latex dust particles through cleaning of furniture, carpeting, and ventilation systems. When latex gloves are necessary, health care workers should use powder-free gloves and avoid wearing oil-based lotions.

A national objective of *Healthy People 2010* is to increase the number of health care facilities that use prevention strategies to protect employees from latex allergies. Education of employees should include strategies to decrease exposure in high-risk and sensitive individuals, alternatives to natural latex products, management of symptoms and treatment of latex allergy, and mandatory annual review of latex allergy protocols.

Nursing Management

of the Patient in the Intraoperative Environment

Providing nursing care in the intraoperative environment involves many technical activities required to facilitate the surgical procedure and maintain patient safety. However, the perioperative nurse is also responsible for meeting the patient's psychosocial needs.

The operative phase of the perioperative experience is short, and the patient may be sedated or unconscious most of the time. Nonetheless, the nurse has a significant impact on the patient's response to the surgical experience. The experience is almost universally stressful for patients. Allowing patients to participate as much as possible in their perioperative care is believed to improve the quality of care. Explanations of procedures and events are critical, since patients may not know what questions to ask. These interventions promote a sense of security and effective coping.

ASSESSMENT

When a patient is admitted to the OR suite, the perioperative nurse must assess his or her physical and emotional status, paying particular attention to any factors increasing intraoperative risk. A preoperative interview should take place on the patient's arrival to the OR admission suite. Psychosocial assessment should include the patient's family or significant other if possible. Assessment continues during the patient's transfer to the OR, positioning on the OR bed, and induction of anesthesia, and during and immediately after the surgical procedure.

Health History and Physical Examination. The circulating nurse reviews the preoperative health history and physical examination, validates the data, and assesses the patient for any changes. During this interview the circulating nurse reviews the chart and preoperative checklist, and assesses and verifies the patient's physical and psychologic readiness for surgery. Perioperative assessment data include:

- Identification of the patient
- Verification of procedure, surgical site, and surgeon by patient; consent form
- Preprocedural vital signs and pain rating
- NPO status
- Allergy and medication history
- Presence of prostheses, implants, jewelry
- Religious, cultural, and philosophic beliefs
- Expectations of treatment
- Laboratory and diagnostic findings
- Need for blood products
- Need for implants
- Neurologic status
- Mobility and functional status
- Pulmonary status
- Cardiovascular status
- Renal and hydration status
- Skin integrity
- Nutritional status

NURSING DIAGNOSES, OUTCOMES, AND INTERVENTIONS

The nursing diagnoses discussed in this chapter focus on high-incidence problem areas for patients during a surgical intervention. The North American Nursing Diagnosis Association does not recommend the routine use of the *risk for infection* diagnosis for patients undergoing surgery. The use of this diagnosis should be limited to high-risk patients. This diagnosis is included to familiarize the learner with routine standards of care and aseptic practices used in the OR. Note that the nursing diagnoses *risk for latex allergy response* and *latex allergy response* can be used to guide nursing care for patients with latex allergy.

Nursing Diagnosis: Risk for Perioperative-Positioning Injury

OUTCOMES. Common examples of expected outcomes for the patient with a diagnosis of *risk for perioperative-positioning injury* are: Patient will:

- Remain free from neuromuscular and neurovascular deficits or injury related to surgical positioning.
- Remain free from injury and signs of skin and tissue injury for at least 24 to 48 hours after the procedure.

NURSING INTERVENTIONS. Injury may occur to tissues and neurovascular structures as a result of positioning required for the surgical procedure. Positioning affects the cardiovascular, respiratory, neurologic, and integumentary systems. Prolonged pressure on the bony prominences, pressure on the peripheral nervous or vascular systems, or the shearing force of sheets and drapes during patient movement may be responsible for pressure ulcers. Several risk factors have been identified as contributing to the development of pressure ulcers in the surgical patient (see Risk Factors box). The circulating nurse should assess the patient for risk factors during the preoperative interview.

A pressure ulcer, as defined by the Agency for Healthcare Research and Quality, is a lesion caused by unrelieved pressure that results in damage to the underlying tissues.[1] The incidence of pressure ulcers in hospitalized patients ranges from 1% to 11%, while the incidence in surgical patients ranges from 4.7% to 66%.[29] During surgery patients are immobile and unable to feel pain caused by pressure and shearing forces. Researchers concluded that 23% of the total number of pressure ulcers that develop in hospitalized patients are acquired intraoperatively.[29,30] The most significant risk factor for acquiring a pressure ulcer during surgery is the length of surgery. Patients undergoing surgery lasting more than 4 hours are at greatest risk; for every 30 minutes past 4 hours, the risk of pressure ulcers increases by 33%.[29] Other risk factors include the use of warming blankets, extracorporeal circulation, age, and vascular disease.[29] Patients undergoing cardiac surgery are at high risk for pressure ulcers (see Research box).

Tissue perfusion is a critical factor in the development of pressure ulcers. Normal capillary interface pressure is 23 to 32 mm Hg. Pressures in excess of normal can alter tissue perfusion and cause ischemia.[4] However, much lower pressures may occlude blood flow in older patients and those with hemiplegia and peripheral vascular disease. Gravity forces patients against the

Risk Factors

Development of Pressure Ulcers in Surgical Patients

- Surgical position
- Type of surgical exposure and method of retracting tissues
- Length of procedure (over 2½ to 3 hours)
- Standard operating room mattress
- Positioning devices
- Warming blankets
- Anesthetic agents
- Vasoactive drugs
- Shearing forces
- Friction
- Moisture from preparation and irrigating solutions
- Advanced age
- Body weight (obesity and malnourishment)
- Comorbid disease (diabetes, cardiovascular disease, peripheral vascular disease, pulmonary disease, paralysis)
- Decreased immune functioning
- Compromised tissue perfusion
- Decreased range of motion
- Immobility
- Compromised skin condition before surgery
- Low preoperative albumin level
- Low score on Braden scale

Research

Pokorny ME, Koldjeski D, Swanson M: Skin care intervention for patients having cardiac surgery, *Am J Crit Care* 12(6):535-544, 2003.

The incidence of pressure ulcers in cardiovascular surgical patients ranges from 9.2% to 38%. Nonsurgical risk factors associated with the development of pressure ulcers include age, comorbid disease, nutritional status, body size, activity level, and body temperature. Surgical risk factors include heat, shearing forces, friction, and moisture. This study examined the effects of a skin care intervention in patients having open-chest cardiac surgery.

Interventions included a skin assessment and risk factor score (Braden scale), done before surgery and twice daily while hospitalized, and patient education. Patients at higher risk for developing pressure ulcers and those with altered skin integrity also received treatment by an enterostomal therapist.

The prevalence of pressure ulcers decreased from 11.7% to 6.8% after implementing the study protocol. In the experimental group 7% of the patients developed pressure ulcers; the majority were stage I. Most pressure ulcers developed by postoperative day 4. Risk factors identified in the group with skin breakdown included hypertension, diabetes, obesity, and heart failure. Admission Braden scores were not reliable predictors for the development of pressure ulcers. Measures effective in identifying and treating effects of pressure were frequent risk assessment and consistently applied nursing interventions to promote skin integrity done on the day of surgery and the first 5 postoperative days.

hard surface of the OR bed; compresses skin, muscle, and bone; and increases capillary interface pressures. Compression of vessels, external pressure, uneven body weight distribution, and constant pressure on bony prominences can result in pressure ulcers. Compounding this, anesthetic agents lower blood pressure and alter tissue perfusion, which may also result in tissue damage.

Most pressure ulcers develop within 48 hours after surgery, although it may take 3 to 5 days for visible signs to appear in some individuals.[29] Pressure ulcers that originate in the OR develop outwardly from the muscle and subcutaneous tissue and progress to the dermis and epidermis. Reddened skin areas that appear 1 to 2 days after surgery may be mistaken for burns. These incorrectly diagnosed reddened areas may then progress to stage III or IV pressure ulcers.

Pressure injuries commonly occur over bony prominences, such as the occiput, spine, scapulae, coccyx, sacrum, or calcaneus. Figure 14-6 illustrates common surgical positions and the associated pressure points. Table 14-13 describes commonly used operative patient positions.

The respiratory system is influenced greatly by positioning. The thoracic cage normally expands in all directions except posteriorly. The respiratory system is most vulnerable in the prone and the lithotomy positions because of the mechanical restriction of lung expansion at the ribs or sternum. The diaphragm is unable to fully descend against the abdominal musculature, and respiratory function is impaired.

Several changes in the cardiovascular system that occur with positioning may also result in complications. A tight restraint, crossed legs, or limb hyperextension can compromise blood flow by compressing a vessel against a bony structure and may result in

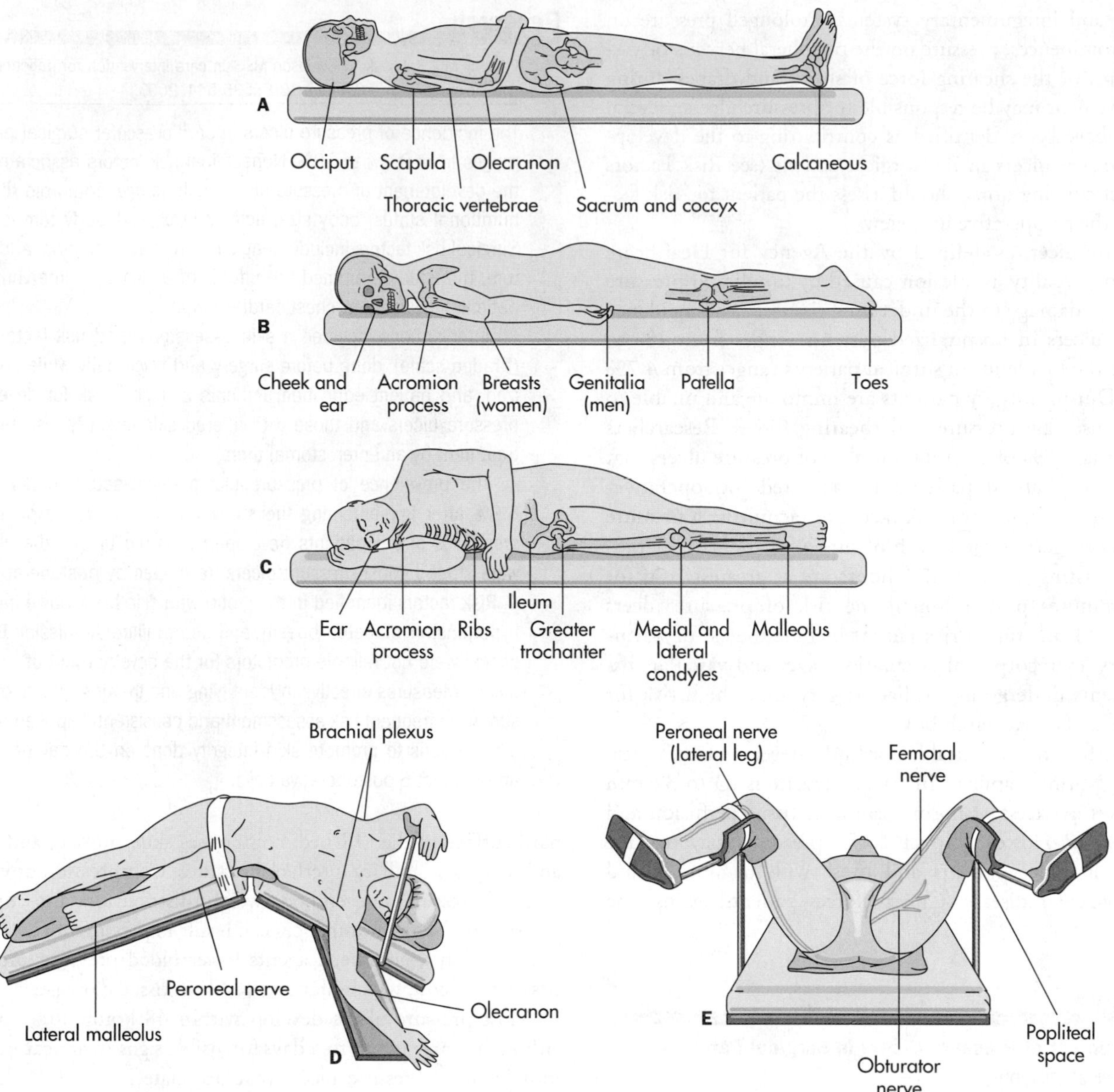

Figure 14-6 Examples of common surgical positions and their associated potential pressure points. **A**, Supine (dorsal recumbent) position. **B**, Prone position. **C**, Lateral position. **D**, Lateral (kidney) position. **E**, Lithotomy position.

venous stasis or ischemia. Rapid changes of position, such as when legs are lowered quickly from the lithotomy position, may cause sudden hypotension. The lithotomy position also may lead to circulatory pooling in the lumbar region and compression of abdominal contents onto the inferior vena cava and abdominal aorta. In both situations, venous return decreases, which affects cardiac output.

Most of the problems associated with the neurologic system are not discovered until recovery from anesthesia is complete. Postoperative sedation may mask symptoms of peripheral nerve damage. Most postoperative peripheral neuropathies result from an inappropriate positioning on the operating bed, usually as the result of direct mechanical pressure. Ischemia and insufficient blood supply caused by stretching or compression are chief factors in nerve injuries. The lithotomy position is especially likely to cause injury to the saphenous and common peroneal nerves. These injuries result from either misplaced stirrups or acute flexion of the thighs. In all positions in which the arms are extended on armboards, hyperextension of the arms may damage the brachial plexus.

The circulating nurse assists the surgeon and the anesthesia care provider in safely and comfortably positioning the patient for the surgical procedure, using appropriate devices to minimize complications (see Table 14-13). Distribution of body weight should be as even as possible, with the patient maintained in correct alignment.

The type of positioning device used depends on the patient, procedure, and surgeon's preference. Positioning devices come in a wide variety of shapes, styles, and materials. Some examples are foam pads and mattresses, face guards, sand bags, bean bags, air

TABLE 14-13 COMMONLY USED OPERATIVE PATIENT POSITIONS

Description	Comments
Supine: flat on back with arms at side, palms down, legs straight with feet slightly separated	Most commonly used position; venous pooling in legs may result from reduction of venous pressure
Prone: patient lying on abdomen with face turned to one side, arms at sides with palms pronated, elbows slightly flexed; feet elevated to prevent plantar flexion	Patient anesthetized in supine position and then placed prone; chest rolls or frame used for support; respiratory excursion decreased; risk for injury to head, eyes, nose, facial nerve, genitalia, and breasts
Trendelenburg's: patient supine; head and body lowered into a head-down position; knees are flexed by "breaking" table	Respiratory excursion decreased from upward movement of abdominal viscera; cerebral edema or venous thrombosis possible because of congestion of cerebral vessels
Lithotomy: patient lying on back with buttocks to edge of table; thighs and legs placed in stirrups simultaneously to prevent muscle injury; head and arms secured to prevent injury	Elastic wraps or antiembolism stockings possibly used on legs to prevent thrombus formation; risk for vein compression in legs, increased intraabdominal pressure, injury to obturator and femoral nerves because of flexion of thighs; injury to common peroneal nerve caused by fibular neck resting against stirrups; risk for acute hypotension when legs are lowered; avoid abduction greater than 90 degrees of arms
Lateral: patient lying on side; table may be bent in middle	Risk for injury to dependent brachial plexus and dependent common peroneal nerve, pressure ulcer development over dependent greater trochanter of femur; potential interference with cardiac action because of possible shift in heart position

mattresses, gel pads, frames, and rolls. The device chosen should maintain the desired intraoperative position and minimize the potential for injury by redistributing pressure and preventing excessive stretching. The device must have the documented ability to reduce capillary interface pressure to 32 mm Hg or less. Ideally, the device should be durable, nonallergenic, radiolucent, easily stored, resistant to moisture and microorganisms, able to be disinfected or disposed of, and cost-effective. The standard OR mattress is less effective than foam and gel mattresses in reducing pressure, although none has been shown to be effective in reducing pressure below 32 mm Hg. Bath blankets, turn sheets, and heating blankets, all commonly used in positioning, actually increase pressure.

To avoid stretching and compressing nerve and muscle tissue, positioning of extremities must not exceed a 90-degree angle to the body. Bony prominences such as heels, elbows, and sacrum are vulnerable pressure points and should be well padded. The safety strap should be applied 2 inches above the knees to avoid pressure on the popliteal nerve. Compression of the popliteal nerve from stirrups or knee braces also should be avoided.

Surgical equipment, such as pneumatic saws and drills and retractors, placed directly on the patient may lead to pressure injuries. The circulating nurse monitors members of the team in the field to ensure they do not lean on the patient during the procedure. Antiembolism stockings or intermittent pneumatic compression devices may be used to decrease venous pooling in the lower extremities.

Changing positions gradually is important to prevent drastic shifts in blood volume from one area of the body to another. Foam-filled cushions can be used to maintain adequate respiratory excursion and to prevent pressure on the chest, breasts, genitalia, and abdominal structures. Refer to the Guidelines for Safe Practice box for nursing interventions associated with intraoperative patient positioning.

A detailed procedure for each surgical position should be written and available for OR personnel who are responsible for or assist with positioning of patients. Detailed documentation by the circulating nurse should include the preoperative skin condition, type of position, any intraoperative changes in positioning, placement of extremities, type and placement of positioning aids and supplemental padding, and the site of placement of the electrosurgical conduction pad.

RELATED NIC INTERVENTIONS. Positioning: Intraoperative, Skin Surveillance, Surgical Precautions

Nursing Diagnosis: Risk for Injury

OUTCOMES. Common examples of expected outcomes for the patient with a diagnosis of *risk for injury* are:

Patient will:

- Remain free from injury or trauma related to electrical, chemical, physical, and environmental factors.

NURSING INTERVENTIONS. The OR contains many potentially life-threatening and mechanically injurious situations related to electrical shock, burn, fire, and explosions. Many nursing activities are focused on protecting the patient from electrical, chemical, physical, and environmental hazards. It is imperative that all members of the surgical health care team have current knowledge of the equipment and supplies used in the operative suite. The most significant hazards are inadequately trained personnel, malfunctioning equipment as a result of improper maintenance,

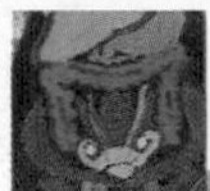

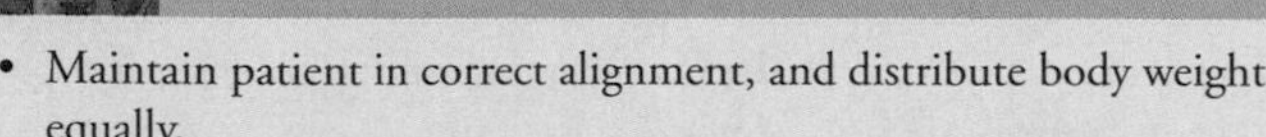

GUIDELINES FOR SAFE PRACTICE *Preventing Complications of Surgical Positioning*

- Maintain patient in correct alignment, and distribute body weight equally.
- Any positioning devices should maintain normal intracapillary pressure of 32 mm Hg or less.
- If foam overlays are used, they should be constructed of thick, dense foam that resists compression.
- Towels, blanket rolls, and pillows are not effective in reducing pressure and may cause injury due to friction.[8]
- Gel pads are effective in reducing overall pressure in a large surface area.
- Pad all bony prominences.
- Use antiembolism hose and intermittent pneumatic compression devices to decrease venous pooling as indicated.
- Change patient positions gradually to avoid drastic shifts in blood volume.
- Avoid local compression from safety straps, knee braces, stirrups, equipment, or personnel.
- Avoid stretching and compression of neuromuscular and vascular structures.
- Position extremities at no more than a 90-degree angle to the body.
- After positioning the patient's body, reassess alignment and tissue integrity.
- Documentation of positioning should include preoperative assessment; position, type, and location of devices; names and titles of personnel; and postoperative assessment.

inappropriate design of OR suites, and inappropriate surveillance by team members.

Federal regulations mandate the marketing and safety standards of electronic devices used in the operating room. Hazards can be minimized or prevented by the following nursing interventions:

- Use only electrical equipment designed for OR use.
- Use cords of adequate length.
- Ground the patient correctly.
- Test equipment before use.
- Establish and follow sound clinical engineering testing and maintenance programs.
- Participate in in-service sessions for new equipment, and maintain an adequate knowledge base for correct use of all electrical equipment.
- Adhere to manufacturer's guidelines for use.
- Report faulty equipment immediately.
- Maintain humidity levels at 50% or higher to minimize static electricity.
- Prevent pooling of fluids under the patient.

The use of electricity introduces hazards of electric shock, power failure, and fire to patients. If a voltage differential exists between any two electrical conductors touching the patient, the flow of current can result in electric shock or electrocution. If the voltage is high enough, ventricular fibrillation and sudden death may result.

Laser (light amplification by stimulated emission of radiation) technology is an effective treatment modality; however, it presents hazards for patients and members of the surgical team. As the high-powered beams of light are directed into tissue, the resultant intense heat vaporizes the tissue and causes a rapid coagulation of blood vessels. When lasers are used, special equipment is necessary to protect both the patient and surgical team members. Eye protection specific to the type of laser (e.g., argon, carbon dioxide) prevents retinal damage from misdirected beams of light. If aberrant light beams land on surgical drapes, they can cause fire. Improperly functioning surgical instruments can deflect light to other tissue. Measures such as the use of coated instruments, wet towels on the field, smoke evacuation methods, and warning signs on the door of the operative suite are routinely taken to protect the patient and OR team members.

Chemical hazards in the operating room include exposure to solutions used for cleaning, cementing bone, gas sterilization of instruments, and skin preparation. Iodine and iodophors are two of the most effective bactericidal agents for preoperative skin scrubbing but are irritants to the skin if the concentration is too high. Alcohol, which sometimes is used in incision site preparation, is flammable. Precautions are necessary for prevention of injury from any hazardous chemicals. All personnel must follow safe chemical usage recommendations set by the hospital's safety department and the manufacturer. It is imperative that the circulating nurse determine or verify any patient allergies that may increase risk of injury from certain solutions used during the surgical procedure. To prevent skin irritation and electrical shock or burn, solutions used for skin preparation should not be allowed to pool under the patient.

The circulating nurse is responsible for protecting the patient from injury from physical hazards. Prevention of injury includes careful movement during positioning, use of appropriate positioning methods, and use of protective devices such as side rails and safety straps. Personnel can safely transfer the patient to or from the OR bed by using lift devices or a minimum of four people, obtaining sufficient support help, ensuring that all tubes are visible and protected from inadvertent removal, and coordinating the movement among all team members.

To ensure that injury does not occur from misidentification of the patient or the correct operative site, the circulating nurse must verify the patient's identity and operative site (see Chapter 13). The circulating nurse brings any discrepancy or concerns to the attention of the surgeon, anesthesiologist, patient, and, when necessary, hospital administrator. Before the incision is made, a "time out" occurs that involves the entire surgical team (see Future Watch box and Legal Alert box).

PREVENTION OF FOREIGN OBJECT RETENTION. Because of the risk to the patient related to foreign object retention in the surgical wound, counting materials used during a surgical procedure is an important intraoperative nursing intervention. The nurse counts sponges, sharps, and instruments before the procedure, as additional items are added, at initial closure, and finally at skin closure. An additional count is necessary when either the scrub or

Future Watch

New Technology To Help Reduce Surgical Error

JCAHO reports that the most common surgical errors involve surgery on the wrong patient, the wrong surgical procedure, or the wrong site. Methods to reduce surgical error include "time out" and marking the extremity or surgical site. SurgChip is an FDA-approved procedure that uses radio frequency identification technology (RFID) to help prevent wrong-site, wrong-procedure, and wrong-patient surgery.

The SurgiChip is a small computer chip that is secured to the patient's skin with adhesive and is removed before making the incision. The chip is programmed with the following information:

- Patient's full name
- Surgical site
- Description of the procedure to be performed
- Surgeon's name

The information is encoded and printed on a SurgiChip smart label. The chip can be prgrammed at the preoperative evaluation, in the emergency department, or on the hospital unit. After entering the information, the chip is scanned by the nurse or physician, using an RFID reader and then validated by the patient.

On the day of surgery the chip is rescanned, and the information reviewed and validated with the patient before any sedatives are given. The chip is then affixed to the skin at the incision site. In the operating room the chip is scanned with a hand-held reader, and the information is reviewed by the operating team. The information on the chip must match the data in the chart and the patient's identity bracelet. After validating the information, the chip is removed and placed in the patient's chart. The SurgiChip was developed by an orthopedic surgeon to be used in addition to JCAHO's Universal Protocol to reduce surgical error.

Legal Alert

Time Out

"Time out" occurs in the operating room after the patient has been prepped and draped. The entire team must verbally verify their agreement on the following:

- Patient's name
- Procedure to be performed
- Surgical site
- Laterality, implants, radiologic examinations, if applicable

Documentation of "time out" should indicate the following was verified:

- Correct patient
- Correct site and side
- Agreement to proceed
- Correct patient position
- Availability of implants or special equipment

circulating nurse leaves the case. Facilities must have written policies and procedures with specific guidelines for counting items during each surgical procedure. Both the circulating and scrub nurse should perform the surgical count.

AORN-recommended practices state that sharps should be counted on all procedures. Sponges and instruments should be counted on procedures in which there is a possibility that such items could be retained,[8] such as procedures in which a major body cavity is opened or a deep incision is made.

Sponges and other products have radiopaque markings, so in the event of an incorrect count, an x-ray film can be obtained to determine the presence of the missing item in the patient. The nurse documents all counts performed and places it in the patient's record. Any corrective action taken in the event of a discrepancy and the resultant outcome are also recorded.

RELATED NIC INTERVENTIONS. Laser Precautions, Positioning: Intraoperative, Surgical Precautions, Surgical Preparation, Technology Management

Nursing Diagnosis: Risk for Imbalanced Body Temperature

OUTCOMES. Common examples of expected outcomes for the patient with a diagnosis of *risk for imbalanced body temperature* are: Patient will:

- Maintain desired intraoperative body temperature.
- Maintain body temperature within normal range in the immediate postoperative period.

NURSING INTERVENTIONS

HYPOTHERMIA. Factors that put patients at risk for alterations in body temperature are trauma, advanced age, malnutrition, prolonged preoperative inactivity, and sedation. The greatest heat loss occurs in the first hour of surgery; therefore the perioperative nurse should initiate heat-conservation methods early.

Prevention is the best treatment of hypothermia. An intervention that can be initiated immediately after admission to the OR is the application of warm blankets. Before surgery begins, the patient should remain covered as much as possible. An ample supply of blankets should be available in warming cabinets at all times. Blankets should be warmed to 105° F (40.5° C) and changed every 15 minutes. Radiant heat lamps are also effective in providing warmth. Applying thermal coverings, particularly to the head, is recommended to reduce radiant heat loss. During surgery an automatic thermal blanket is often placed under the patient.

The temperature and humidity of the room should be controlled. The nurse should ensure that the patient's skin is exposed as little as possible during positioning, prepping, and draping. Skin prep solutions can be warmed before use. The nurse should ensure that the sheets and drapes on and under the patient are dry, both to prevent heat loss and skin irritation and to maintain asepsis. A forced-air warming device (Bair Hugger) is commonly used during surgery to conserve body temperature. The ambient room temperature may be increased at the end of the procedure to increase patient comfort.

The core body temperature should be monitored throughout the procedure. Sites for measurement of body temperature are chosen based on accessibility, comfort, and safety. Pulmonary artery monitoring provides the most accurate measurement but is an invasive technique. Tympanic membrane measurement correlates closely to core temperature because of the proximity of the carotid arteries that supply blood both to the tympanic membrane and the hypothalamus. Body temperature can also be measured by probes inserted into the esophagus, rectum, or urinary bladder, although rectal and bladder readings may overestimate core temperature. If the patient is intubated, an esophageal probe may be inserted for continuous temperature monitoring. Temperature probes placed in the distal third of the esophagus are closely correlated with core temperature. Temperatures measured in the middle or proximal esophagus are affected by inhaled gases and are not reliable.

During most surgical procedures a large amount of fluid is administered intravenously and topically for wound irrigation. The circulating nurse ensures that all fluids presented to the anesthesiologist or added to the surgical field are warm. In the immediate postoperative period the nurse applies warm blankets as soon as surgical patient drapes are removed.

HYPERTHERMIA. Hyperthermia occurs less frequently than hypothermia in the surgical patient. MH generally occurs in response to certain anesthetics. Other risk factors for hyperthermia include dehydration, fever, vasoconstriction from medication, endocrine disorders such as thyroid disease, and intracranial infection or injury to the hypothalamus.

During surgery nursing interventions for cooling include removing excessive drapes, applying alcohol or cool water to the patient's skin, assisting with monitoring vital signs, using an automatic cooling blanket, and assisting with the preparation and administration of cool intravenous fluids and emergency medications. The nurse should record the patient's preoperative baseline temperature and monitor core body temperature throughout the procedure.

As with all nursing interventions, documentation includes all measures taken, equipment used (including serial numbers and temperature settings), and patient responses to treatment. Communication with the postoperative receiving unit is imperative for the continuity of patient care. This is especially important in cases in which an alteration in normothermia resulted in an emergent situation.

RELATED NIC INTERVENTIONS. Malignant Hyperthermia Precautions, Temperature Regulation: Intraoperative

Nursing Diagnosis: Risk for Imbalanced Fluid Volume

OUTCOMES. Common examples of expected outcomes for the patient with a diagnosis of *risk for imbalanced fluid volume* are:
Patient will:

- Demonstrate fluid balance.

NURSING INTERVENTIONS. Intraoperative monitoring of fluid loss and adequate replacement are high priorities throughout the procedure for both anesthesiologist and circulating nurse. The nurse assists the anesthesiologist in monitoring the patient during surgery.

In the surgical patient alterations in fluid balance carry the risk for both hypovolemia and hypervolemia. Hypovolemia can be defined as isotonic fluid loss from the extracellular space. An excess of isotonic fluid in the extracellular (interstitial or intravascular) compartment results in hypervolemia. Untreated hypovolemia (loss of 40% or more of intravascular volume) can lead to hypovolemic shock. Hypervolemia may result from excessive isotonic fluid replacement or excessive blood or plasma replacement. Fluid shifts into the intravascular space may be caused by administration of albumin and hypertonic intravenous fluids. Hypervolemia, if not corrected, can result in pulmonary edema and congestive heart failure. Electrolyte imbalance may also occur as a result of preexisting disease, surgical stress, preoperative steroid or diuretic use, preoperative regimens such as enemas or laxatives, and gastric suction and lavage.

Nursing interventions to promote fluid volume balance include monitoring vital signs, particularly pulse and blood pressure, and accurately monitoring intake and output of all fluids, including irrigation and blood loss. The nurse inserts an indwelling urethral catheter before the start of surgery if the patient is at risk for fluid volume imbalance, critically ill, or having a lengthy procedure or if significant blood loss is anticipated. The nurse records urine output hourly and monitors blood loss by keeping an accurate record of the fluids administered into the wound, the amount of fluid suctioned from the operative site, and the amount of saturation of all sponges (sponges may be weighed for a more accurate estimation).

Common causes of fluid volume deficit include bleeding, decreased intake because of NPO status, inadequate intravenous fluid replacement, excessive gastrointestinal losses, evaporation of fluid from exposed cavities during surgery, inhalation of dry anesthetic gases, and third-spacing of fluid. Third-spacing occurs when fluid moves out of the intravascular space, but not into the intracellular space, as a result of increased capillary membrane permeability or decreased plasma colloid osmotic pressure. The fluid may shift into the surgical site such as the abdominal or pleural cavity. Third-space fluid losses may be significant after extensive tissue dissection; other causes include peritonitis, bowel obstruction, ascites, and hypoalbuminemia.

Treatment goals related to hypovolemia include replacement of lost fluids, maintenance of normal blood pressure, and restoration of blood volume. To increase blood volume, the nurse administers isotonic fluids such as normal saline or lactated Ringer's solution. Blood replacement may be necessary if blood loss exceeds 1200 ml or the hematocrit drops below 30%. Blood or blood products may be transfused to compensate for the loss or to prevent shock. Transfusions may be homologous or autologous. Blood products include whole blood, packed red cells, fresh frozen plasma, platelets, serum albumin, and blood substitutes. The nurse must continually assess the available blood and order additional blood to remain ahead of anticipated needs. Before administering any blood product, the nurse must follow the necessary identification and safety precautions.

During the procedure blood may be recovered from the field for autotransfusion. Blood can be suctioned from the wound, body cavity, or drapes and sponges. All blood recovery devices must be approved by the FDA. If a microfibrillar collagen has been used for hemostasis, blood may not be salvaged because of the risk of diffuse intravascular coagulation or adult respiratory distress syndrome. Persons with known systemic infections or open trauma are not candidates for autotransfusion.

The nurse must be familiar with the use of autotransfusion devices if intraoperative cell salvage is used. Three basic systems available for autotransfusions are cell salvage processors, canister collection systems, and salvage collection bags. All components of the system are sterile and disposable. If not used intraoperatively, the blood collected may be processed and bagged for transfusion after surgery. Alternative methods include salvaging blood from reinfusion drains. The blood is anticoagulated and may be collected for a maximum of 6 hours; the red cells are reinfused intravenously. The anesthesiologist records all blood products given, the amount of solutions used by the surgeon, the estimated blood loss, and all intraoperative events concerning fluid imbalances.

RELATED NIC INTERVENTIONS. Autotransfusion, Blood Products Administration, Electrolyte Management, Fluid Management, Fluid Monitoring, Vital Signs Monitoring

Nursing Diagnosis: Risk for Infection

OUTCOMES. Common examples of expected outcomes for the patient with a diagnosis of *risk for infection* are:

Patient will:

- Remain free from postoperative wound infection.

NURSING INTERVENTIONS. All patients who undergo surgery have the potential to acquire an infection. Surgical intervention breaks down some of the body's primary defenses against infection. Infection can prolong the hospital stay and even endanger the patient's life. Protecting the patient from infection is a major focus of intraoperative nursing care. The goal of nursing interventions is to control the number and types of microorganisms present during surgery, primarily by monitoring and controlling the environment. The most important measure in preventing postoperative wound infection is adhering to meticulous aseptic technique principles and to Transmission-Based Precautions. The entire surgical team has a responsibility to uphold principles of aseptic technique and follow the policies and procedures established to protect the patient from unnecessary risks and breaks in technique.

Each year, approximately 780,000 people develop an infection from surgery.[26] The patient's own organisms are responsible for most surgical site infections.[11,24] Despite strict aseptic technique, *Staphylococcus aureus* has been found at clean surgical sites.[11,24] Of particular concern is the emergence of antibiotic-resistant strains of both gram-negative and gram-positive organisms, including methicillin-resistant *S. aureus* and vancomycin-resistant enterococci.

The CDC recommends the classification of surgical wounds to predict the probability of postoperative infection. The circulating nurse is responsible for assigning and documenting the classification. Wounds are classified as clean, clean contaminated, contaminated, or dirty (Table 14-14). Documentation of the appropriate wound classification assists the infection control nurse with follow-up planning and nosocomial wound infection reporting.

Because of antibiotic resistance, surgical antimicrobial prophylaxis (AMP) should be used judiciously. Surgical prophylaxis refers to a brief course of antibiotic therapy administered just before an operation begins.[24] Intravenous infusion is the most common route of antibiotic administration. The goal of surgical antimicrobial prophylaxis is to reduce the number of pathogens resulting from intraoperative contamination; it is not intended to prevent postoperative contamination.[23] If antimicrobial prophylaxis is not initiated within 2 hours before the incision is made, the surgical site infection rate increases two to six times.[26] Antibiotics are chosen based on which microorganisms are most likely to be found at the surgical site.

Procedures considered by the CDC as high risk for potential infection include coronary artery bypass graft, cardiac and colon surgery, hip and knee joint replacement, abdominal and vaginal hysterectomies, and some vascular procedures.[26] The surgical wound classification described earlier can be helpful in estimating postoperative infection rates and the need for antibiotic therapy.

Cefazolin, a first-generation cephalosporin, is effective against many gram-positive and gram-negative organisms and is generally regarded as the antimicrobial agent of choice for surgical prophylaxis in clean operations. If the patient has a penicillin allergy, alternatives are clindamycin and vancomycin. However, vancomycin should not be used routinely for antimicrobial prophylaxis. To achieve maximum effectiveness, 1 to 2 g of cefazolin should be administered to patients at least 30 minutes before incision time.[23] Antibiotics are most effective when they are present in

TABLE 14-14 CENTERS FOR DISEASE CONTROL AND PREVENTION SURGICAL WOUND CLASSIFICATION

Classification	Definition	Examples
I. Clean wound	Uninfected, primary closure Closed wound drainage system No inflammation present	Total knee arthroplasty Mitral valve replacement Breast biopsy
II. Clean contaminated wound	Respiratory, alimentary, or genitourinary tract entered without spillage No sign of infection, minor break in sterile technique	Total abdominal hysterectomy Radical prostatectomy Pneumonectomy
III. Contaminated wound	Major break in aseptic technique Signs of infection Contamination from gastrointestinal tract Open fresh traumatic wound	Appendectomy for ruptured appendix Laparotomy for perforated bowel
IV. Dirty or infected wound	Old trauma with necrotic tissue Preexisting infection Perforated viscera Acute inflammation	Incision and drainage of abscess

tissues before bacteria enter the surgical site. A single dose of antibiotics is sufficient for most surgical procedures. However, more research is needed to determine the needs of patients undergoing lengthy surgical procedures. Nursing responsibilities include assessing the patient for drug allergies, administering the correct drug at the correct time, and monitoring the patient for therapeutic and adverse effects of the drug. Maintaining sterile technique during venipuncture and fluid administration is also essential to prevent any further sources of infection.

The etiology of wound infection is diverse and may be related to the environment, host, or pathogen (wound healing is discussed in Chapter 15). Appropriate closure and drainage of dead space facilitate wound healing. Wound healing by *primary intention* occurs in most surgical incisions. After completing the operation, the surgeon closes the wound edges. Wound closure is usually done in layers, with the type and method of closure dependent on the size, location, and type of surgical wound and the patient's condition and age. Primary closure is indicated for clean straight incision lines with all layers of the wound able to be well approximated.

The goal of wound closure is to promote healing with minimal scarring. Wound closure options include sutures, clips, staples, tapes, tissue adhesives, and wound zippers. Although suturing allows precise closure, sutures usually require removal, have a potential for needlestick injury to the surgical staff, and may cause tissue reactivity in the patient. Tissue adhesives do not require removal, have no risk of needlestick injury, and are easily applied. No significant differences exist between tissue adhesives and sutures in terms of dehiscence, infection, and cosmetic appearance.[13]

Regardless of the method of closure, wound edges must be closely approximated to achieve an anatomically secure wound; wound edges will not heal readily if not in close contact. A dead space may occur from separation of wound edges or from air trapped between layers of tissue. Serum, blood, or other fluid may accumulate in a dead space and prevent healing. Sutures, staples, drains, or any foreign body at the surgical site may promote inflammation and increase the risk of a surgical site infection.[23] Suture materials are either absorbable or nonabsorbable. Monofilament sutures have been shown to produce the least amount of inflammation.[23] Surgical stapling is believed to cause less reaction than suturing.

If it is anticipated that fluid may collect in a body area near the wound after surgery, the surgeon usually inserts a tube or drain to permit the fluid to escape. Drains are usually made of latex or silicone. The surgeon places one end of the tube or drain in or near the organ or cavity to be drained, and passes the other end through the body wall, usually through a separate small incision near the operative site. A closed suction drain placed through a separate incision distant from the operative incision reduces the risk of infection. Suction drains create a negative pressure in a reservoir. The negative pressure gently suctions fluid from the wound into the attached reservoir. The Hemovac and Jackson-Pratt drains (Figures 14-7 and 14-8) are examples of closed-suction drainage systems. Closed drains also may be attached to wall or portable suction devices for a greater range of suction capacity. The level of suction is based on the amount and area to be evacuated. Some suction drains, such as Gish and Solcotrans drains, contain filters and have the capacity for reinfusion of blood products. In some cases, drainage is by gravity through a tube, such as a T tube

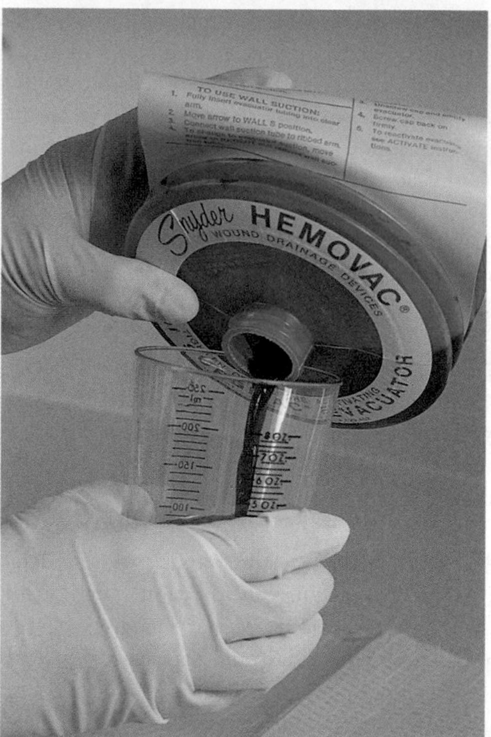

Figure 14-7 Hemovac drain.

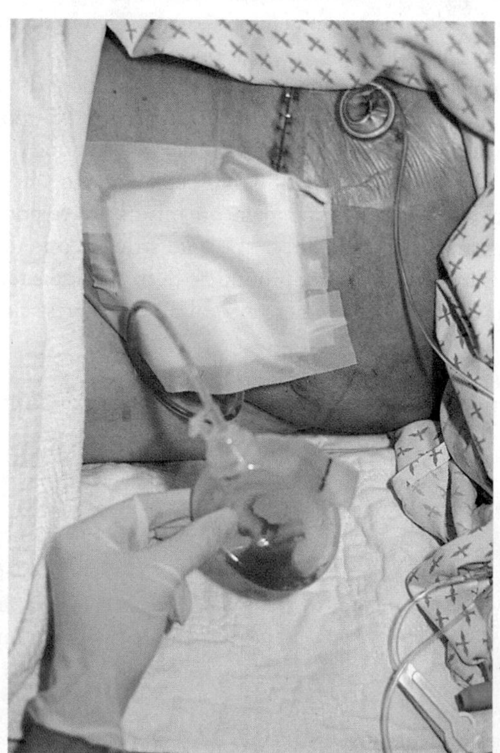

Figure 14-8 Jackson-Pratt drain.

(Figure 14-9) or Penrose drain. Colonization of drain tracts increases with time; therefore drains should be left in place the shortest time possible to evacuate hematomas or seromas.

Nursing interventions related to drains focus on preparation of the drainage system components, assessment of patency and

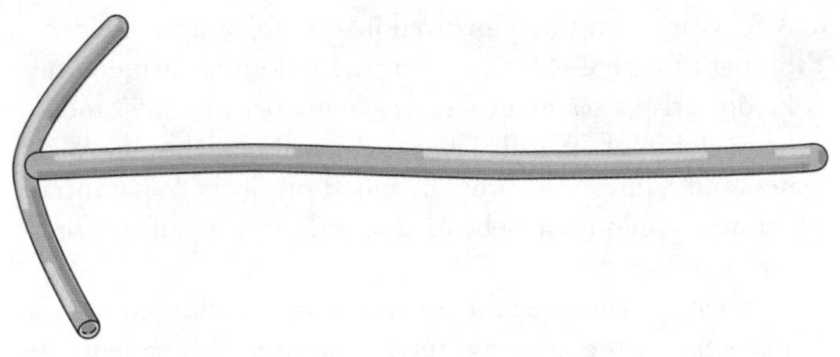

Figure 14-9 T tube drain.

drainage, and accurate documentation. After the surgeon places the tubing, the nurse assembles the drain using sterile technique. The nurse assesses patency of the system and the amount, type, color, and consistency of the drainage. The nurse records the type and location of drainage and the drainage assessment and reports this to the nurse in the postoperative receiving unit.

Protecting the incision site from contamination minimizes risk for postoperative wound infection. After the surgeon closes the wound, the nurse applies a sterile dressing, which is maintained for 24 to 48 hours.[23] Data are inconclusive to support maintaining a dressing beyond 48 hours to prevent infection and promote healing.[23] Dressings also absorb drainage, protect the incision from trauma, and support the incision and surrounding skin. The circulating nurse is responsible for ensuring dressing security and documenting the condition of the dressing before the patient is transferred to the postoperative unit.

RELATED NIC INTERVENTIONS. Infection Control: Intraoperative, Surgical Assistance

Patient/Family Teaching. Patient and family teaching, as presented in the accompanying Patient/Family Teaching box, is an important part of nursing care for the intraoperative patient.

EVALUATION

To evaluate the effectiveness of nursing interventions, compare patient behaviors with those stated in the expected patient outcomes.

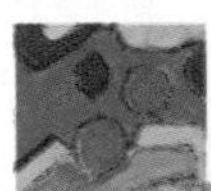

PATIENT/FAMILY TEACHING
Preoperative Routines

The nurse should instruct the patient and family about perioperative routines on arrival in the operating room suite. Although this information was covered in a preoperative teaching session (location will vary depending on circumstances), reinforcement is beneficial because of the anxiety the patient may be experiencing. Anticipating both the patient and family's questions helps allay their concerns. The teaching should include information about:

- The holding area
- Anesthesia induction
- Monitoring techniques
- Length of procedure
- Waiting area
- Postanesthesia care
- Surgeon follow-up

RELATED NOC OUTCOMES. Hydration, Knowledge: Infection Control, Neurologic Status: Spinal Sensory/Motor Function, Risk Control, Thermoregulation, Wound Healing: Primary Intention, Wound Healing: Secondary Intention

GERONTOLOGIC CONSIDERATIONS

As discussed in Chapter 13, many elderly patients have multiple chronic health problems that affect recovery from surgical intervention. Morbidity associated with geriatric surgical patients is usually a result of preexisting medical problems.

The perioperative nurse needs to understand the effects of aging and chronic disease on the outcome of surgery for older patients. This knowledge allows the nurse to use the nursing process to ensure safe patient care throughout the perioperative experience. Although many of the intraoperative interventions are the same for any patient undergoing anesthesia and surgery, to meet the special care needs of the geriatric patient, the circulating nurse recognizes the patient's increased risk for unplanned perioperative hypothermia, cardiovascular complications, and potential complications related to intraoperative positioning.

Unplanned Perioperative Hypothermia. Body temperature is regulated when cutaneous thermoreceptors detect alterations in ambient temperatures and signal the anterior hypothalamus. The sensors in the anterior hypothalamus monitor the temperature of cerebral blood flow. The difference between those temperatures and a set point determined by the hypothalamus triggers the heat-generating response. This response is influenced by age, exercise, medications, and anesthetics.

The body's normal response to heat loss and cold is shivering to generate heat. Because of impaired thermoregulatory ability, the shivering response to cold is less sensitive in older adults than in younger patients. A slower metabolic rate, decreased cardiovascular reserve, thinning of skin, loss of subcutaneous tissue, and diminished muscle mass affect the geriatric patient's ability to produce and conserve body heat. The stress of surgery and anesthesia, intraoperative routines, environmental factors, and anesthesia-related factors can also affect perioperative thermoregulation in the geriatric patient (Box 14-5).

The nurse assesses the patient for risk of hypothermia. This includes assessment of physiologic status and body size. Knowledge of the extent of the surgical procedure along with the type of anesthesia planned assists the circulating nurse in formulating a plan of patient care that will decrease intraoperative body heat loss. Increasing the temperature in the OR; covering the patient with warm blankets; warming anesthetic gases, intravenous fluids, irrigation solutions, and skin preparation fluids; covering the patient's head; and limiting exposure of body surface are measures to prevent inadvertent hypothermia in the older patient.

Positioning. The potential for postoperative skin problems presents a significant risk for the geriatric patient. Decreased adipose tissue, poor skin turgor, decreased peripheral circulation, and tissue fragility can cause postoperative skin problems. Arthritis, deceased range of motion, and skin fragility make patient positioning one of the most important aspects of intraoperative patient care. In addition to the threat of skin problems, improper positioning can also cause joint pain unrelated to the surgical procedure.

Box 14-5 Factors Affecting Perioperative Thermoregulation in Geriatric Patients

Procedural

Intravenous infusion of cool solutions
Irrigation of incision sites with cool solutions
Lengthy surgical procedures
Surgical procedures involving large body surfaces or open cavities

Environmental

Cool air temperature in the operating room
Air currents related to air exchanges within the operating room

Anesthetic

Inhalation of cool, nonhumidified gaseous agents

Anesthesia Considerations. The normal aging process causes a variety of physiologic changes that affect the geriatric patient's response to anesthesia. The patient's response to anesthesia may be unpredictable and significant. Diminished physiologic reserves, preexisting medical conditions, and the physical stress caused by anesthesia and surgical intervention pose increased risks. Thorough preoperative assessment and careful anesthesia management can improve patient outcomes.

The geriatric patient is more susceptible to the action of medications. Decreased liver and kidney function and reduced cardiac output affect the metabolism and excretion of drugs from the body. Therefore geriatric patients generally require lower doses of anesthetic agents and take longer to eliminate them.

The presence of pulmonary disease or pulmonary insufficiency may pose ventilatory difficulties. Alterations in the airway of older patients also cause ventilatory difficulties. Loss of teeth and alterations in jaw contours can cause an inadequate fit of the anesthesia mask. Decreased range of motion in the jaw, head, and neck presents difficulties for intubation.

Critical Thinking

1. A 68-year-old woman is scheduled for coronary artery bypass surgery. On arrival in the holding room, she has an oral temperature of 97° F (36.1° C). She is oriented to person only. Her history includes hypertension, congestive heart failure, and type 2 diabetes. What elements of her history will influence her intraoperative management? What nursing interventions should be included in her care plan to prevent complications?
2. A 46-year-old woman is scheduled for a right mastectomy. During the immediate preoperative interview the circulating nurse notes that the patient's perception of the procedure is not congruent with the scheduled surgical procedure and informed consent. What actions by the circulating nurse are appropriate? What documentation is required?
3. A 28-year-old man with paraplegia is scheduled for a skin graft for a stage IV pressure ulcer. He has a documented history of type I allergic response to latex. Devise an intraoperative care plan for the patient.
4. A 35-year-old woman involved in a motor vehicle accident is brought to the OR for an emergent abdominal exploration. Preoperative assessment reveals a hematocrit of 32% and hemoglobin of 10 g/dl. The patient is also a Jehovah's Witness and refuses receipt of any blood products. What intraoperative techniques may be used to reduce this patient's risk for bleeding?
5. A patient is scheduled for cosmetic surgery with sedation and analgesia. As the nurse assigned to monitor this patient, develop an intraoperative care plan.

References

1. Agency for HealthCare Research and Quality, Treatment of Pressure Ulcers Guideline Panel: *Treatment of pressure ulcers*, AHCPR Pub No 9509652 (clinical practice guideline No15), Rockville, Md, 1994, Department of Health and Human Services.
2. Allen G: Evidence for practice hair removal and surgical site infection rates, *AORN J* 78(3):496-497, 2003.
3. American Society of Anesthesiologists Task Force on Preanesthesia Evaluation: *Practice advisory for preanesthesia evaluation*, approved Oct 17, 2001, and amended Oct 15, 2003.
4. Angle DA, Leafgreen P: Reducing the incidence of pressure ulcer development in the ICU, *AJN* 101(5):24EE-24JJ, 2001.
5. Association of periOperative Registered Nurses: BIS monitoring reduces awareness, *AORN Connections* 2(6):8, 2004.
6. Association of periOperative Registered Nurses: Latex guideline, *AORN J* 78(3):653-673, 2004.
7. Association of periOperative Registered Nurses: Recommended practices for surgical hand antisepsis/hand scrubs, *AORN J* 79(2):416–430, 2004.
8. Association of periOperative Registered Nurses: *2001 standards and recommended practices,* Denver, 2004, AORN Publications.
9. Belkin NL: Creutzfeldt-Jakob disease identifying prions and carriers, *AORN J* 78(2):204-210, 2003.
10. Berman M: One hospital's clinical evaluation of brushless scrubbing, *AORN J* 79(2):349-358, 2004.
11. Blanchard J: Clinical issues, *AORN J* 79(2):405-408, 2004.
12. Blanchard J: Clinical issues: surgical site infections, *AORN J* 79(7):1301, 2004.
13. Coulthard P et al: Tissue adhesive for closure of surgical incisions, *Cochrane Database of Systemic Reviews*, issue 2, 2004.
14. Drain CB: Care of the patient with thermal imbalance. In Drain CB, editor: *Perianesthesia nursing: a critical care approach*, ed 4, St Louis, 2003, Saunders.
15. Fogg D: Clinical issues, *AORN J* 73(3):654-652, 2003.
16. Fortunato NH: *Berry and Kohn's operating room technique,* ed 10, St Louis, 2004, Mosby.
17. Franko FP: Regulating first assistants, *AORN J* 80(2):327-331, 2004.
18. Franko FP: The RN in the circulator role—a proactive approach, *AORN J* 79(3):683-689, 2004.
19. Hooper VD: Thermoregulation. In DeFazio Quinn DM, Shick M, editors: *Perianesthesia nursing core curriculum preoperative, phase I and phase II PACU nursing*, Philadelphia, 2004, WB Saunders.
20. Joint Commission on Accreditation of Healthcare Organizations: Standards and intents for sedation and anesthesia care, *Comprehensive Accreditation Manual for Hospitals,* 2001, accessed from website: http://www. jcaho.org/standard/aneshap.html.
21. Joint Commission on Accreditation of Healthcare Organizations: *2004 national patient safety goals-FAQ's,* accessed Dec 2003 from website: http://www.jcho.org/accredited+organizations/patient+safety/04+npsg/04_faqs.htm#7.
22. Krause T et al: Dantrolene—a review of its pharmacology, therapeutic use and new developments, *Anaesthesia* 59:364-373, 2004.
23. Mangram AJ et al: Guidelines for prevention of surgical site infection, *Infect Control Hospital Epidemiol* 20(4):247-269, 1999.

24. Nichols RL: Preventing surgical site infections: a surgeon's perspective, *Emerg Infect Dis* 7(2):220-224, 2001.
25. Pugliese G, Bartley JM: Can we build a safer OR? *AORN J* 79(4):763–779, 2004.
26. Reed D: Update on latex allergy among healthcare personnel, *AORN J* 78(3):407-428, 2003.
27. Rothrock JC, Smith DA, McEwen DR: *Alexander's care of the patient in surgery,* ed 12, St Louis, 2003, Mosby.
28. Schoonhoven L, Defloor T, Grypdonck MHF: Incidence of pressure ulcers due to surgery, *J Clin Nurs* 11:479-487, 2002.
29. Schoonhoven L et al: Risk indicators for pressure ulcers during surgery, *Applied Nurs Res* 16(2):163-173, 2002.
30. Tesiorowski CC: Latex allergies in the healthcare worker, *J PeriAnesthesia Nurs* 18(1):18-31, 2003.
31. Weiss L: Malignant hyperthermia. In Duke J: *Anesthesia secrets,* ed 2, Philadelphia, 2000, Hanley & Belfus.
32. Weppler F: Malignant hyperthermia, *European J Anaesthesiol* 18:632-652, 2001.
33. Yip ES: Accommodating latex allergy concerns in surgical settings, *AORN J* 78(4):595-603, 2003.
34. Zaric et al: Transient neurologic symptoms following spinal anaesthesia with lidocaine versus other local anesthetics, *Cochrane Library,* Issue 3, 2004, Chichester, UK, John Wiley & Sons.

evolve Visit the Evolve website: http://evolve.elsevier.com/Monahan/medsurg

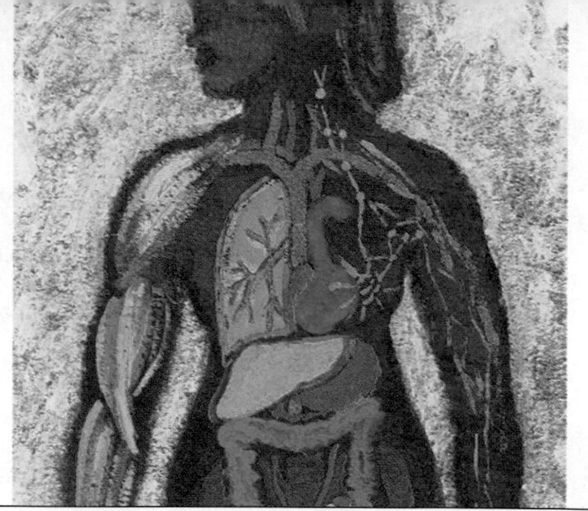

CHAPTER 15 Postoperative Nursing

by Jane F. Marek, Mary Jo Boehnlein

OBJECTIVES

After studying this chapter, the learner should be able to:

1. Describe the postoperative phase as a component of the surgical experience.
2. Compare and contrast nursing care of the patient in postanesthesia phase I and phase II.
3. Identify postoperative complications that may compromise a patient's safety and stability after anesthesia and surgical intervention.
4. Discuss patient risk factors for postoperative complications.
5. Formulate relevant postoperative nursing diagnoses.
6. Describe nursing interventions to prevent or treat postoperative complications.

KEY TERMS

analgesics, p. 321
aspiration, p. 307
atelectasis, p. 310
dehiscence, p. 319
delirium, p. 330
evisceration, p. 319
hypoxemia, p. 306
laryngospasm, p. 307
preemptive analgesia, p. 322
venous stasis, p. 314

The postoperative phase begins with the transfer of the patient from the operating room (OR) to the appropriate postoperative unit and ends with the discharge of the patient from the surgical facility or the hospital. The focus of postoperative nursing care is to assist the patient in returning to optimal functioning as quickly as possible.

The primary focus of this chapter is the nursing care of the patient in the postanesthesia care unit (PACU). Postoperative nursing care on the patient care unit is reviewed in lesser detail. The nursing diagnoses and interventions address the postoperative patient care needs in both the PACU and the patient care unit.

The immediate postanesthesia phase presents multifaceted challenges in patient care. Anesthesia and surgical interventions place great stress on all body systems (see Chapter 14). The postanesthesia nurse must understand the patient's risks for postoperative complications and be prepared to quickly implement appropriate interventions should an acute change in the patient's status occur.

To meet the criteria for transfer from the PACU to the clinical unit or to the home, the patient must be stable and free from symptoms of complications. However, the potential for developing complications continues beyond the immediate postoperative phase. Ongoing nursing assessment is essential after the patient is transferred to a specific clinical unit. Nursing interventions focus on minimizing the potential for postoperative complications and planning for recovery and discharge. Effective preoperative patient teaching (see Chapter 13) prepares the patient for an active role in the recovery course; the nurse reinforces this information in the postoperative period.

It is common practice to discharge patients the day of surgery or after a short hospital stay. In addition to economic incentives, improvements in surgical and anesthetic techniques have made ambulatory and short-stay surgery both safe and efficient. Minimally invasive surgical techniques have contributed significantly to the increase in ambulatory and short-stay surgery. As a result, the patient and family have greater responsibility for self-care and more complex teaching and discharge needs. Assessing the patient's needs and providing relevant information are crucial responsibilities for nurses who care for patients in the early postoperative period.

Historical Background

General anesthesia has been used since the late 1890s, and surgical procedures date back to ancient Egypt. A specially designated area for the recovery of postsurgical patients is comparatively new, dating to the 1860s when Florence Nightingale described the use of a small room adjacent to the operating theater where the patient recovered from the immediate effects of the operation.[11] World War II had the greatest impact on the development of the modern-day PACU. Because of the shortage of nurses, patients and equipments were centralized to efficiently deliver care.

Many PACUs opened in the 1940s after the discovery that a specialized unit decreased patient morbidity and mortality and shortened length of stay.[36] Postoperative mortality within the first 24 hours after administration of anesthesia and surgical intervention was caused by airway obstruction, laryngospasm, hemorrhage, cardiac arrest, or medication error. Other factors that contributed to mortality included a lack of standardized patient care and an absence of medical and nursing supervision.[11] As a result of these findings, many hospitals opened specialized units for the care of patients recovering from anesthesia staffed with specially trained nurses. Most patients recovering from general or regional anesthesia are transferred from the OR to the PACU before discharge or transfer to a nursing division. Critically ill patients may be directly transferred from the OR to an intensive care unit (ICU).

Postanesthesia Care

The PACU is usually located adjacent to the operating rooms. It is a large open room divided into individual patient care spaces. The number of spaces depends on the number of individual ORs in the surgical suite. In general, PACUs have 1.5 to 2 patient care spaces per OR.[38] Each individual patient care space is supplied with a cardiac monitor, blood pressure monitoring device, pulse oximeter, airway management equipment, suction, and oxygen. Emergency medications and equipment are centrally located. Isolation rooms are available if needed.

The length of stay in the PACU is generally less than 24 hours. Traditional care mandated a minimum stay requirement in the PACU. American Society of Anesthesiologists (ASA) practice guidelines for postanesthetic care state that length of stay should be determined on a case-by-case basis, not a time-based discharge. The American Society of PeriAnesthesia Nurses (ASPAN) recommends that critically ill patients do not recover in the same area as ambulatory surgery patients. Many ambulatory surgical units incorporate a wellness-focused approach, with noninstitutional décor such as wallpaper, greenery, and modern cabinets to hide the clinical look of the PACU.[9]

Personnel

Registered nurses in the PACU have an in-depth knowledge of anesthetic agents and patient responses to these agents, pain management techniques, surgical procedures, and potential complications. The PACU nurse demonstrates competence in physical assessment and management of emergency situations.

ASPAN offers specialty certification for registered nurses working in the PACU. Certification in ambulatory postanesthesia is available for nurses working in ambulatory surgical settings.[11] Other staff assisting the nurse in the PACU include licensed practical nurses and unlicensed assistive personnel.

Phases of Postanesthesia Care

ASPAN identified three phases of perianesthesia care and three phases of postanesthesia care. Perianesthesia nursing is similar to perioperative nursing and includes preanesthesia, intraoperative and intraprocedural, and postanesthesia patient care. The three phases of postanesthesia care are:

- Phase I, immediate postanesthesia period: prepare patient for transfer to phase II, inpatient nursing unit, or ICU
- Phase II, continued recovery: transfer to phase III, home, or extended care facility
- Phase III, ongoing care for patients needing extended observation and intervention after phase I or phase II: preparing patients for self-care

Postanesthesia phase I encompasses the care of the patient emerging from anesthesia until the patient is physiologically stable and does not require one-on-one care. Protective reflexes and motor function return during this phase. The PACU nurse makes a preliminary assessment of breath sounds, respiratory effort, oxygen saturation, blood pressure, cardiac rhythm, level of consciousness, and muscle strength.

Postanesthesia phase II begins when the patient's consciousness returns to baseline and the patient has a patent airway; intact upper airway reflexes; manageable pain; and stable pulmonary, cardiac, and renal functioning. During this phase the patient is transferred to the nursing division or short-stay unit. Phase II practice settings include those adjacent to or located within the phase I PACU or in another area of the facility.

Because of the increased volume of ambulatory surgical procedures, advances in surgical and anesthetic techniques, and improved pain management, many ambulatory surgery patients are transferred from the OR to phase II PACU, bypassing phase I. This process, known as *fast-tracking,* can improve patient outcomes after ambulatory surgery through earlier discharge from both freestanding and hospital-based units and increased patient satisfaction.[38,40]

The length of stay in the recovery area for ambulatory surgery patients is under consideration. The Aldrete score (discussed later in this chapter) is a commonly used tool to assess a patient's recovery from anesthesia. Aldrete's criteria have been modified to determine which patients are eligible to bypass the PACU (Table 15-1). Scoring systems allow patients to be safely discharged from the PACU or the phase II recovery area.

Postanesthesia phase III practice settings include 23-hour observation suites, in-hospital units, and recovery care centers within the hospital or community. Nursing care continues until the patient completely recovers from anesthesia and surgery and is ready to resume activities of daily living (ADLs).

ASPAN has recommended staffing ratios for each phase of postanesthesia care.[9] The nurse/patient ratio depends on the phase of anesthesia, the surgery performed, and patient stability. Critically ill, unstable patients on mechanical life support may require two nurses, whereas the nurse caring for patients in phase III may be assigned three to five patients.

Anxiety in PACU Environment

The environment of a postanesthesia unit is sometimes noisy and hectic. Florence Nightingale first noted that unnecessary noise is detrimental to patients.[11] Patient care needs change swiftly and

TABLE 15-1 SCORING SYSTEM TO DETERMINE ELIGIBILITY FOR FAST-TRACKING*

Criterion	Score
Level of Consciousness	
Awake and oriented	2
Arousable with minimal stimulation	1
Responsive only to tactile stimulation	0
Physical Activity	
Able to move all extremities on command	2
Some weakness in movement of extremities	1
Unable to voluntarily move extremities	0
Hemodynamic Stability	
Mean arterial pressure <15% of baseline value	2
Mean arterial pressure 15%-30% of baseline value	1
Mean arterial pressure >30% below baseline value	0
Respiratory Stability	
Able to breathe deeply	2
Tachypneic with good cough	1
Dyspneic with weak cough	0
Oxygen Saturation Status	
Maintains value >90% on room air	2
Requires supplemental oxygen (nasal cannula)	1
Saturation <90% with supplemental oxygen	0
Postoperative Pain Assessment	
None or mild discomfort	2
Moderate to severe pain controlled with intravenous analgesics	1
Persistent severe pain	0
Postoperative Emetic Symptoms	
None to mild nausea with no active vomiting	2
Transient vomiting or retching	1
Persistent moderate to severe nausea and vomiting	0

From Joshi GP: New concepts in recovery after ambulatory surgery, *J Ambulatory Surg* 10:167–170, 2003.

*Score ≥12 for fast-tracking.

sometimes dramatically. A balance of caring and technologic skills provides a safe and supportive approach to patient care that can help relieve patient anxiety.

On awakening from anesthesia, the patient needs frequent reorientation and reassurance of not being alone. The patient also needs to know that the operation is over and that recovery from anesthesia is satisfactory. The nurse should provide careful explanations of procedures even when it appears the patient is not alert. The nurse should reassure the patient who has had regional anesthesia that sensation and movement in the extremities will return.

The nurse also needs to reassure the patient that family or significant others have been notified of the patient's safe arrival in the recovery room. Traditionally, visitors are not allowed in PACUs, but some institutions may allow it.

Most surgeons discuss the results of the operation with the patient and family immediately after the surgery. Family members are often anxious about the patient's condition and may not hear or understand all that the surgeon tells them. Patients often experience periods of amnesia when they first regain consciousness and may not remember what they have been told. To provide satisfactory answers to the patient's and family's questions, the nurse needs to know what information was given. The family also needs to know what to expect when the patient returns to the unit and when the patient is ready for discharge.

Some of the concerns that were present in the preoperative period (see Chapter 13) may continue into the postoperative period. These concerns generally focus on the performed surgery, the results of the surgery, and the temporary or permanent effects that may change a patient's lifestyle. The patient may have concerns about changes in roles, body image, return to work, lifestyle, emotional status, economic implications of the surgery, or prognosis.

Nursing Management *of the Postoperative Patient*

ASSESSMENT

Transfer to Postanesthesia Care Unit. The circulating nurse informs the PACU of the patient's estimated time of arrival in the unit and also of any special care or equipment needs. The nurse gives a detailed report when the patient is admitted to the unit.

The PACU nurse must emphasize patient safety until the patient is fully awake or has complete return of sensation after regional blocks. The unconscious patient must be protected from falling and injury as a result of improper positioning. The nurse should put the patient's call light within reach and implement interventions to prevent falls, such as maintaining side rails in the upright position.

While connecting the monitoring equipment, applying oxygen, and making an immediate physiologic assessment, the PACU nurse receives reports from the anesthesiologist, surgeon, and circulating nurse. The verbal report includes data regarding the surgical procedure and intraoperative patient responses. Data in the report are based on recommendations made by ASPAN (Box 15-1).[1,36] ASA standards require that a member of the anesthesia care team remain in the PACU until the PACU nurse accepts responsibility for the patient.[36]

BOX 15-1 Patient Status Report on Admission to Postanesthesia Care Unit

- Patient demographics
- Need for life support equipment
- Allergies
- Pertinent medical history
- ASA (American Society of Anesthesiologists) status
- Baseline vital signs
- Surgical procedure performed
- Skin preparation
- Intraoperative positioning
- Intraoperative complications
- Type and length of anesthetic
- Time and type of reversal agents given
- Estimated blood loss
- Amount of intraoperative fluid replacement
- Urinary output
- Intravenous and invasive lines
- Medications administered
- Laboratory and diagnostic data
- Vital signs
- Presence of implants
- Dressings
- Drainage tubes and locations with recorded output
- Skin condition
- Orders to be initiated in postanesthesia care unit
- Presence of family in waiting area
- Preoperative anxiety level

Immediate Postanesthesia Assessment. After the verbal reports and immediate assessment of the patient's airway, respiratory, and circulatory status, the PACU nurse performs a more thorough patient assessment (Box 15-2). Nursing units differ in the method of organizing patient assessment data. Some use a head-to-toe approach; others use a major body systems approach (Figure 15-1).

Preventing complications as the patient recovers from anesthesia is an important aspect of nursing care. The *stir-up regimen* consists of interventions to prevent atelectasis and venous stasis.[30] These interventions are deep breathing exercises, coughing, positioning, mobilization, and pain management.

Nursing care in the immediate postoperative phase focuses on maintaining ventilation and circulation, monitoring oxygenation and level of consciousness, preventing shock, and managing pain. The nurse assesses and documents respiratory, circulatory, and neurologic functions at frequent intervals. The nurse notes response to verbal or noxious stimuli, the pupils' responsiveness to light and accommodation, and the ability to move all extremities. Equality and strength of handgrip also are assessed. A handgrip sustained for 5 seconds indicates that neuromuscular function is returning.

Laboratory and diagnostic data are also used for patient assessment in the PACU. Objective assessment of the patient's respiratory status may include pulse oximetry, arterial blood gases, and chest x-ray examination. The patient's heart rate and rhythm are continuously monitored via electrocardiogram. Frequent assessment of the patient's hematologic and renal status may be indicated, especially if there were significant intraoperative blood and fluid losses.

RESPIRATORY. Respiratory complications are the leading cause of morbidity and mortality in the immediate postoperative period.[8] Although respiratory complications are more common in patients with known respiratory disease or other risk factors, the potential for complications exists for all patients (see Chapter 13). Immediate respiratory complications that may occur include airway obstruction, hypoxemia, hypoventilation, aspiration, and laryngospasm. The nurse should ascertain whether the patient has a patent airway and adequate respiratory function.

AIRWAY OBSTRUCTION. The amount of airway support required depends on the individual patient, anesthetic technique, and type of surgery. Patients may be admitted to the PACU with an endotracheal tube or laryngeal mask airway in place. However, anesthesia techniques often allow extubation or airway removal in the OR as the patient emerges from general anesthesia, recovers reflexes, and responds to verbal stimuli. Box 15-3 outlines extubation criteria.[9]

A serious complication for patients recovering from general anesthesia is airway obstruction, commonly a result of movement of the tongue (relaxed from anesthesia) into the posterior pharynx (Figure 15-2); anesthetic-induced changes in pharyngeal and laryngeal muscle tone; and laryngospasm, edema, and secretions

Box 15-2 Nursing Assessment in Postanesthesia Care Unit

Vital Signs

- Oxygen saturation
- Blood pressure (cuff or arterial line)
- Pulse (apical, peripheral)
- Temperature (method of measurement)

Respiratory

- Presence of artificial airway
- Ventilator settings as needed
- Rate
- Rhythm
- Breath sounds
- Skin and mucous membrane color
- Oxygen delivery system

Cardiovascular

- Monitored cardiac rhythm
- Peripheral pulse
- Skin temperature

Neurologic

- Level of consciousness
- Orientation
- Ability to follow commands
- Ability to move all extremities and lift head
- Papillary response
- Sensation

Urinary Output

Skin Integrity

Pain

- Location
- Presence
- Severity
- Character
- Pain scale rating

Patient-Controlled Analgesia

Dressings

Condition of Surgical Wound

Drainage Tubes

- Type
- Location
- Amount and character of drainage
- Patency

Presence of Intravenous Lines

- Type and location of site
- Type, amount, and rate of solution infusing

Additional Monitoring Parameters (as Appropriate)

- Intracranial
- Central venous
- Arterial line
- Pulmonary artery

Position of Patient

Patient Safety Needs

- Side rails

Level of Psychosocial Support

Anxiety

Numeric Score (as Applicable)

Adapted from Rothrock JC: *Alexander's care of the patient in surgery,* ed 12, St Louis, 2003, Mosby.

or other fluid collecting in the pharynx, bronchial tree, or trachea. Clinical manifestations include gurgling, wheezing, stridor, sternal and intercostal retractions, hypoxemia, and hypercarbia. Initial treatment consists of administration of 100% oxygen, physical maneuvers to maintain airway (jaw-thrust maneuver), suctioning of secretions, and insertion of an oral or nasal airway. Insertion of an oral airway must be accompanied by the jaw-thrust maneuver. If these interventions are unsuccessful, endotracheal intubation, cricothyroidotomy, or tracheostomy may be necessary.

Another population at risk for airway obstruction is patients with a history of obstructive sleep apnea syndrome (OSAS). OSAS is caused by complete or partial collapse of the pharynx during inspiration, resulting in airway obstruction, and is associated with hypoxemia, apnea, and interrupted sleep. The effects of anesthesia increase the risk for airway obstruction. Patients with OSAS are also at risk for hypoxemia because of the residual effects of anesthetic agents. The nurse should monitor the patient for periods of apnea and dysrhythmias and continuously monitor oxygen saturation.

HYPOXEMIA. Hypoxemia (pulse oximetry less than 90% and PO_2 less than 60 mm Hg per arterial blood gas) is a common complication that occurs in the immediate postoperative period. Hypoxemia may occur as a result of hypoventilation, which diminishes the exchange of oxygen between the alveoli and the atmosphere. The risk for hypoventilation and hypoxemia is related to:

- Opioids (respiratory center depression)
- Insufficient reversal of neuromuscular blocking agents (residual muscle paralysis)
- Increased tissue resistance (emphysema, infections)
- Decreased lung and chest wall compliance (pneumonia, restrictive diseases)
- Obesity; gastric and abdominal distention

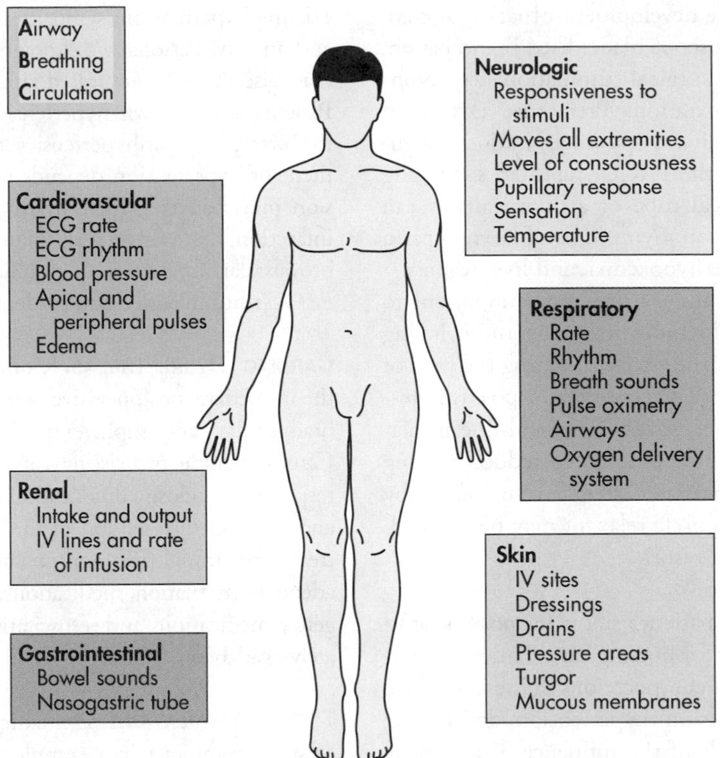

Figure 15-1 Body system approach to assessment. *ECG,* Electrocardiogram; *IV,* intravenous.

Box 15-3 Extubation Criteria

- Return of muscle strength
- Equal hand grasps
- Ability to lift head for at least 5 seconds
- Open eyes
- Ability to protrude tongue
- Appropriate responses to questions (yes/no head movements, picture board)
- Intact swallow and cough reflex
- Respiratory rate greater than 10 breaths/min
- Respiratory parameters:
  Tidal volume at least 5 ml/kg
  Vital capacity at least 15 to 20 ml/kg
  Negative inspiratory force of 20 to 25 cm H_2O

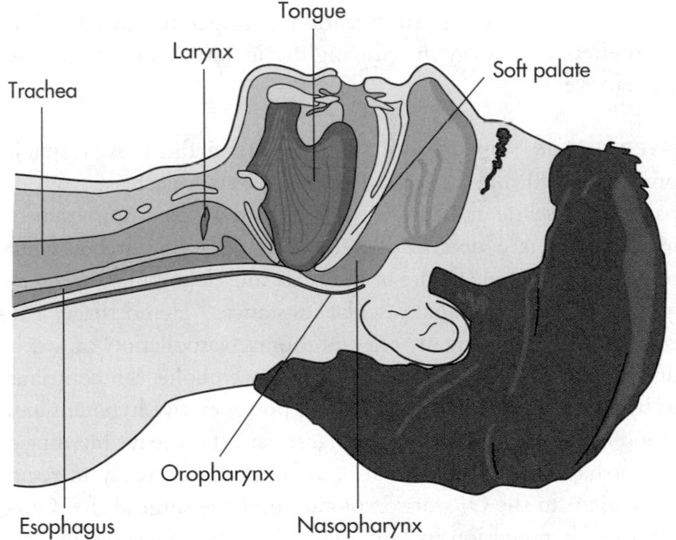

Figure 15-2 Obstruction of airway by tongue blocking oropharynx in unconscious person lying supine.

- Constrictive dressings
- Incision site close to the diaphragm
- General anesthesia
- Postoperative pain

ASPIRATION. Aspiration is the inhalation of gastric contents or blood into the tracheobronchial system. Aspiration usually is caused by regurgitation; however, aspiration of blood may result from trauma or surgical manipulation (e.g., tonsillectomy). Aspiration of gastric contents can cause chemical irritation, pneumonitis, destruction of tracheobronchial mucosa, and secondary infection. Risk factors for aspiration include decreased level of consciousness, dysphagia, delayed gastric emptying, head and neck surgery, obesity, history of hiatal hernia, and emergent intubation of a patient with a full stomach.

LARYNGOSPASM. Laryngospasm, a spasm of laryngeal muscle tissue, may manifest as complete or partial closure of the vocal cords, resulting in airway obstruction. Untreated, laryngospasm can cause hypoxia, cerebral damage, and death. Airway irritation is a major causative factor for the development of laryngospasm. Certain anesthetic agents, laryngoscope blades used in intubation, endotracheal tube placement, or surgical stimulation (e.g., bronchoscope passage) can cause irritation. Premature extubation may place the patient at risk for airway spasm, aspiration, coughing, and airway obstruction. In the PACU, repeated suctioning and irritation by the endotracheal tube or artificial airway can cause laryngospasm after extubation. Symptoms of laryngospasm include dyspnea, crowing sounds, hypoxemia, and hypercapnia.

The nurse's presence and calming attitude are important to reassure the patient. Treatment includes removing the irritating stimulus, hyperextending the patient's neck, elevating the head of the bed, oxygenation, suctioning if necessary, and positive pressure ventilation by mask and bag. Racemic epinephrine inhalation, lidocaine, and steroids may be ordered to reduce swelling and airway irritation.[3] If symptoms persist or are unrelieved by ventilation, administration of a muscle relaxant may be required. Reintubation is used only as a last resort.

CARDIOVASCULAR. Assessing the patient's status for postoperative cardiac complications is a priority for nursing care. The most commonly encountered cardiovascular complications in the immediate postanesthesia period are hypotension, hypertension, and cardiac dysrhythmias occurring as a result of the influence of anesthetic agents on the central nervous system (CNS), myocardium, and peripheral vascular system.

Perioperative myocardial infarction is a serious complication whose incidence is expected to increase as the population ages and more surgical procedures are performed on older persons. In addition to preoperative risk stratification, perioperative beta blockade is an effective strategy in reducing the incidence of perioperative cardiac events.[13,18,32]

HYPOTENSION. Hypotension is generally defined as a systolic pressure of 90 mm Hg or below or as a 20% decrease from the patient's baseline measurement.[36] The most common cause of hypotension is a decreased preload secondary to hypovolemia; other causes include failure of the heart muscle to pump adequately and reduced peripheral vascular resistance.[36] Hemorrhage, inadequate fluid replacement, pneumothorax, vasodilation caused by drugs or anesthetic agents, or pulmonary embolus can contribute to hypovolemia. A common cause of postoperative hypotension is blood loss or inadequate fluid replacement. If excessive bleeding or hemorrhage occurs, the PACU nurses should be ready to return the patient to the OR for reexploration of the surgical site. Other causes of hypotension include shock, ischemia, hypoxia, myocardial infarction, dysrhythmias, third-space fluid loss, and congestive heart failure. Clinical manifestations of hypotension and hypovolemia include increased heart rate, decreased urinary output, pallor of extremities, confusion, and restlessness.

HYPERTENSION. Stage I hypertension is defined as systolic blood pressure of 140 to 159 mm Hg or diastolic blood pressure of 90 to 99 mm Hg.[26] In the perioperative area hypertension is defined as a 20% to 30% increase from the patient's preoperative or baseline level. Common causes of hypertension include pain; reflex vasoconstriction in response to hypoxia, hypercarbia, or hyperthermia; preexisting hypertension; sympathetic stimulation; bladder distention; and anxiety. Persons with known hypertension or a history of cardiac disease are at increased risk for postoperative complications. Patients with known hypertension should be encouraged to take the prescribed antihypertensive medication before surgery. Treatment of hypertension depends on the cause. Untreated hypertension may lead to cardiac dysrhythmias, myocardial ischemia and infarction, left ventricular failure, pulmonary edema, and cerebrovascular accident. Patients should not be discharged from the PACU until hypertension is adequately treated.

CARDIAC DYSRHYTHMIAS. Common dysrhythmias occurring in the immediate postoperative period include sinus tachycardia, sinus bradycardia, and supraventricular and ventricular dysrhythmias. Causes include preexisting cardiac disease, hypoxia, hypercarbia, respiratory acidosis, fluid and electrolyte imbalance, hypothermia, and pain. Determination of the cause is essential before initiating treatment. Initial treatment includes assessment of airway patency, adequate ventilation, medications, and supplemental oxygen. Emergency medications and resuscitative equipment should be immediately available.

THERMOREGULATION. Premedication, anesthesia, and the stress of surgery interact in a complex fashion to disrupt normal thermoregulation (see Chapter 14). Both hypothermia and hyperthermia are associated with physiologic alterations that may interfere with recovery. Patients at the age extremes and those who are extremely debilitated are at even greater risk for developing postoperative temperature abnormalities.

HYPOTHERMIA. Prevention of abnormalities in thermoregulatory responses begins preoperatively with the nursing admission history (see Chapter 14). As many as 60% of patients admitted to the PACU experience some degree of hypothermia,[7] which can extend recovery, delay wound healing, and increase postoperative morbidity. Delayed recovery time results from prolonged elimination of muscle relaxants and delayed drug metabolism by the liver and kidneys.

Anesthetic gases trigger heat loss by causing peripheral vasodilation. After induction of anesthesia, the body's homeostatic mechanisms in response to cold are decreased and the core temperature drops lower than normal before the body is able to begin adaptive responses.

Shivering, an involuntary skeletal muscular activity initiated by the hypothalamus to produce heat, is a compensatory mechanism in response to hypothermia and normally occurs with a 1.8° F (1° C) drop in temperature. As the body temperature decreases, the basal metabolic rate drops 5% per degree Celsius heat loss.[17] Shivering, the normal response to cold, increases oxygen demands up to 400%, resulting in an increased metabolic rate and myocardial workload. The patient without cardiac disease usually has no significant sequelae; however, the patient with coronary artery disease or cardiac myopathy may decompensate. Some inhalation agents and muscle relaxants given during surgery decrease heat production and impede the shivering response.

Hypothermia also impairs coagulation and causes disseminated intravascular coagulation. Blood viscosity increases 2% for every 1.8° F (1° C) drop in core temperature.[17] Hypothermia directly inhibits enzyme reactions in the coagulation cascade. Thrombocytopenia and increased fibrinolysis occur as the body temperature drops, thus increasing the risk of bleeding. Lower intraoperative core temperatures are associated with increased bleeding.

Hypothermia also causes decreased cerebral blood flow, resulting in CNS depression. Cerebral blood flow decreases 6% to 7% per degree Celsius of heat loss.[17] The hypothermic patient may exhibit dilated pupils, slowed reactions and thought processes, and decreased coordination.

Vasoconstriction occurs in hypothermic patients and may cause a fluid shift from the extracellular space, resulting in intravascular volume loss. Vasodilation occurs as the patient rewarms and approaches normothermia. To avoid hypovolemia during rewarming, the patient may require large amounts of intravenous fluids. Hypothermia also affects acid-base balance; acidosis occurs in approximately 30% of hypothermic patients.[16] After rewarming, hypokalemia may develop.

Objective signs of hypothermia include tachypnea, shivering, and tachycardia, but these signs may be difficult to detect in the anesthetized patient. Inadvertent perioperative hypothermia is often not detected until the immediate postoperative period as the effects of anesthesia wear off.

Rewarming is essential in the immediate postoperative care of the patient in the PACU. Unrecognized or untreated hypothermia can pose a significant risk for patients during postoperative recovery.

HYPERTHERMIA. Hyperthermia is defined as core temperature above 102.2° F (39° C). In the early postoperative period hyperthermia may be caused by an infectious process, sepsis, or malignant hyperthermia. Although malignant hyperthermia is most often associated with the intraoperative period, it may occur or recur 24 to 72 hours after surgery. If unrecognized or untreated, malignant hyperthermia results in death (see Chapter 14).

FLUID VOLUME. Fluids are lost during surgery through blood loss and increased insensible fluid loss as a result of hyperventilation and exposed skin surfaces. Because of fluid retention at the surgical site, fluids also may be "lost" to the circulation after major surgery involving extensive tissue dissection.

Excessive blood volume lost during surgery requires intraoperative and postoperative replacement therapy. Blood, blood products, colloids, and crystalloids may be ordered as replacement. In addition, volume may be replaced with intravenous fluids such as normal saline or lactated Ringer's solutions. Postoperative parenteral fluid requirements vary with the patient's preoperative status and the surgical procedure.

The normal body response to the stress of surgery is renal retention of water and sodium. For at least 24 to 48 hours after surgery, the body retains fluids because of the stimulation of antidiuretic hormone as part of the stress response to trauma and the effects of anesthesia. During surgery, renal vasoconstriction and increased aldosterone activity also occur, leading to increased sodium retention with subsequent water retention. Overhydration can occur with vigorous fluid replacement, especially in the small, older patient. Both water intoxication and pulmonary edema can occur, depending on the type and amount of fluids given.

Electrolyte disturbances also may be seen in the postoperative period. Although these disturbances are more common in patients with diabetes and kidney failure, they also may occur in the young, the elderly, and the debilitated patient. Such electrolyte disturbances should be treated promptly (see Chapter 17).

The patient receiving fluids intravenously is monitored for signs of pulmonary edema (dyspnea, cough, adventitious lung sounds, bounding pulse, jugular vein distention) or water intoxication (change in behavior, confusion, warm moist skin, sodium deficit). The patient also is monitored for fluid and electrolyte imbalances. Extra potassium may be necessary to replace losses from gastric suctioning.

If hydration is adequate, a patient usually voids within 6 to 8 hours after surgery. Fluid intake exceeds fluid output during the first 24 to 48 hours. Although 2000 to 3000 ml of intravenous fluid usually are given on the operative day, the first voiding may not be more than 200 ml, and the total urinary output for the operative day may be less than 1500 ml. As body functions stabilize, fluid and electrolyte balance returns to normal within 48 hours.

GASTROINTESTINAL. Nausea and vomiting are common postoperative problems affecting many patients in the PACU. These disturbing occurrences are often associated with general anesthesia, obesity (which results in decreased elimination of anesthetic agents), abdominal surgery, the use of opiate analgesics, history of motion sickness, and psychologic factors. Postoperative vomiting can lead to fluid and electrolyte imbalance, dehydration, stress on abdominal incisions, aspiration, and increased intracranial pressure. Vomiting, diarrhea, and prolonged nasogastric intubation may result in the loss of gastrointestinal secretions high in sodium and potassium (see Chapter 17).

► ARE You READY?

The nurse in the PACU suspects laryngospasm in the patient who develops which of the following symptoms?

1. Crowing sounds
2. Hypocapnia
3. Increased oral secretions
4. Sternal retraction

Anesthetic Complications

COMPLICATIONS OF GENERAL ANESTHESIA. Common side effects after inhalation anesthesia include muscle weakness, sore throat, nausea and vomiting; the incidence of sore throat is significantly higher in intubated patients.[39] Prolonged somnolence and muscle weakness are major nervous system complications that may occur immediately after general anesthesia has been achieved. Failure to awaken promptly or completely is usually the result of the anesthetic's residual effect. Other causes of stupor include severe hypoxia, hypothermia, metabolic imbalances, hyponatremia, hyperglycemia, and severe hypercapnia. Muscle weakness is associated with inflammatory mediators, postoperative sleep disturbances, inhalation anesthetics, muscle relaxants, and opioids.

Postoperative muscle weakness is more common in patients who receive inhalation anesthesia than those who receive total intravenous anesthesia.

Emergence delirium is another alteration that may occur during the immediate postanesthesia phase. Emergence delirium is more common in children, the elderly, and persons with a history of drug dependence or psychiatric disorders. Patients who are anxious at anesthesia induction or who awaken restrained are also at an increased risk for delirium. Medications administered preoperatively or intraoperatively may precipitate delirium. These include ketamine, droperidol, opioids, benzodiazepines, large doses of metoclopramide, and atropine. In this short-lived state, the patient exhibits increased motor activity, disorientation, and vocalizations.

Complications of Regional Anesthesia. Complications, although rare, can occur if a patient has received spinal or epidural anesthesia. These complications are the result of neurologic injury caused by local anesthetic toxicity, needle trauma, or cord ischemia. Symptoms include hypoxia, agitation, hypotension, nausea, and motor or sensory loss.

Discharge From Postanesthesia Care Unit. The PACU nurse documents all assessments and interventions for the duration of the patient's stay in the unit (Figure 15-3). Patients usually remain in the PACU until their vital signs are stable and they are capable of reasonable self-care. Discharge from the PACU is determined by physician order or a numeric scoring system (postanesthesia recovery score [PAR]) approved by the department of anesthesia.

The Aldrete score is the most common tool in use. There are two Aldrete recovery scores, one for phase I recovery and one for phase II. The phase I Aldrete score (Table 15-2) measures activity, respiration, circulation, consciousness, and oxygen saturation (or color). Each criterion is scored from 0 to 2, with a total score of 9 or 10 warranting discharge from the PACU. The anesthesiologist is usually responsible for discharging the patient from phase I. The phase II Aldrete score (Table 15-3) is used for patients who have progressed from phase I and are now conscious or those who have received local or regional anesthesia.

Depending on admission status, the patient may be discharged to a short-stay unit, home, or an inpatient unit. The postanesthesia discharge scoring system (PADS) is commonly used to evaluate the patient's eligibility for discharge to home (Table 15-4).

If the patient remains hospitalized, the PACU nurse telephones the report to a nurse on the inpatient unit who will assume responsibility for care. The report includes information regarding the patient's preoperative history, surgical procedure and recovery, type of anesthetic and medications administered, and physician orders.

Admission to Surgical Unit. A patient who is to remain hospitalized is transferred from the PACU to the surgical division. The nurse orients the patient to the room, ensures the call light is within reach, and keeps side rails up until the patient is completely oriented. The nurse on the surgical division completes a head-to-toe patient assessment and reviews all perioperative documentation.

Assessment for Complications

Respiratory. Risk factors for respiratory complications include chronic obstructive pulmonary disease, smoking, advanced age, thoracic and upper abdominal surgical procedures, marked obesity, and acute respiratory infections (see Chapter 13).[2,24] Only 2% to 5% of patients without significant risk factors experience significant pulmonary complications.[24] The most common respiratory complications are atelectasis, pneumonia, and pulmonary embolus. The majority of postoperative respiratory complications are the result of anesthesia, decreased lung volumes, and poor postoperative pain control. Decreased lung volumes in PACU patients are caused by shallow, sighless breathing patterns related to general anesthesia, pain, and opioids.

Atelectasis. **Atelectasis**, the collapse or incomplete expansion of the lung, usually occurs within 36 hours after surgery. Common presenting symptoms are dyspnea and hypoxia, which may be accompanied by fever, crackles, or diminished or absent breath sounds. Inadequate lung expansion is a primary cause of postoperative atelectasis. The effects of anesthesia, reluctance to cough and deep breathe resulting from inadequate pain control or location of the surgical incision, and immobility contribute to inadequate lung expansion.

Pneumonia. Pneumonia is an inflammation of one or more lobes of the lung resulting from infection. In the surgical patient pneumonia often develops in the dependent lower lobes as a result of inadequate lung expansion and retained secretions. Postoperative pneumonia generally occurs after the third postoperative day. Common presenting symptoms are dyspnea, fever, chills, productive cough, and pleuritic chest pain.

Pulmonary Embolism. A clot or part of a clot may break away and flow through the heart into the pulmonary circulation until it occludes a pulmonary vessel (pulmonary embolism). Emboli alter the pulmonary circulation and decrease the function of the right and left sides of the heart. Pulmonary embolism (see Chapter 26) is a complication of deep venous thrombosis (DVT); the risk of pulmonary embolism from untreated proximal DVT is 50% to 80%.[6] Pulmonary embolism is a serious postoperative complication; 30% to 40% of untreated patients will die.[6]

Assessment for pulmonary embolism is challenging; symptoms are often vague and nonspecific, depending on the size of the blood vessel that has been occluded. Common signs and symptoms are tachypnea, anxiety, tachycardia, dyspnea, pleuritic chest pain, cyanosis, and hypoxia. In some patients, pulmonary embolism causes sudden death. Any complaints of sudden sharp thoracic or upper abdominal pain or dyspnea, as well as any signs of shock, should be reported immediately to the physician.

Cardiovascular. Immediate complications of hypotension and dysrhythmias were previously discussed. Later complications include venous thrombosis and pulmonary embolism. Early recognition and management of cardiovascular complications before they become serious are critical.

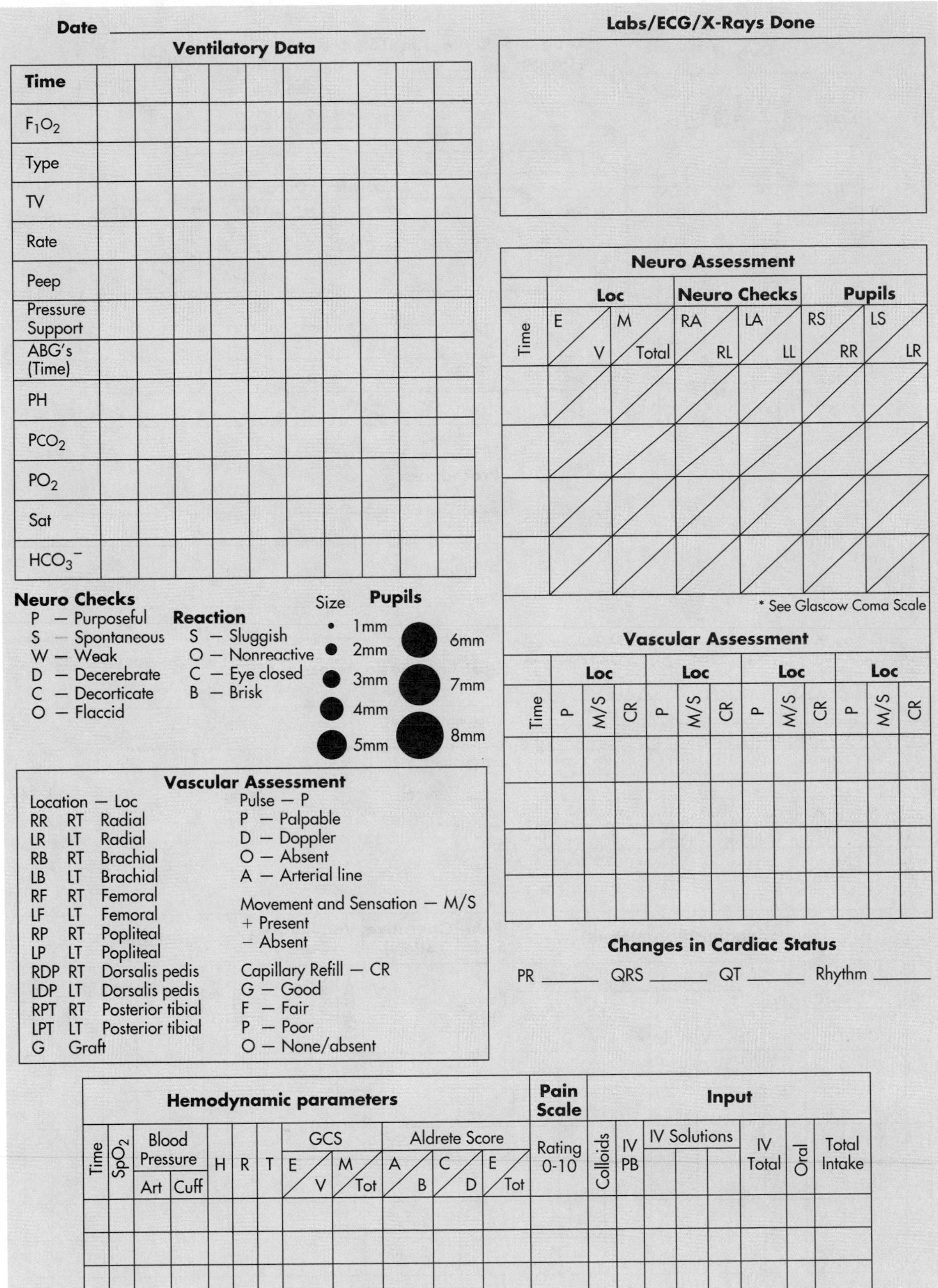

Date ____________________

Ventilatory Data

Time										
F_1O_2										
Type										
TV										
Rate										
Peep										
Pressure Support										
ABG's (Time)										
PH										
PCO_2										
PO_2										
Sat										
HCO_3^-										

Labs/ECG/X-Rays Done

Neuro Assessment

	Loc		Neuro Checks		Pupils	
Time	E / V	M / Total	RA / RL	LA / LL	RS / RR	LS / LR

* See Glascow Coma Scale

Neuro Checks
P — Purposeful
S — Spontaneous
W — Weak
D — Decerebrate
C — Decorticate
O — Flaccid

Reaction
S — Sluggish
O — Nonreactive
C — Eye closed
B — Brisk

Pupils
Size
1mm
2mm
3mm
4mm
5mm
6mm
7mm
8mm

Vascular Assessment

	Loc			Loc			Loc			Loc		
Time	P	M/S	CR	P	M/S	CR	P	M/S	CR	P	M/S	CR

Vascular Assessment

Location — Loc
RR RT Radial
LR LT Radial
RB RT Brachial
LB LT Brachial
RF RT Femoral
LF LT Femoral
RP RT Popliteal
LP LT Popliteal
RDP RT Dorsalis pedis
LDP LT Dorsalis pedis
RPT RT Posterior tibial
LPT LT Posterior tibial
G Graft

Pulse — P
P — Palpable
D — Doppler
O — Absent
A — Arterial line

Movement and Sensation — M/S
+ Present
– Absent

Capillary Refill — CR
G — Good
F — Fair
P — Poor
O — None/absent

Changes in Cardiac Status

PR ______ QRS ______ QT ______ Rhythm ______

Hemodynamic parameters													Pain Scale	Input							
Time	SpO_2	Blood Pressure		H	R	T	GCS		Aldrete Score				Rating 0-10	Colloids	IV PB	IV Solutions			IV Total	Oral	Total Intake
		Art	Cuff				E / V	M / Tot	A / B	C / D	E / Tot										

Figure 15-3 Postanesthesia care unit record.

Output					
Total Output	Emesis	NG	Urine Foley	Urine Void	Irrigation

Drug and Dosage	Route	Time	Signature

Blood Sugar	Insulin	Time

Laboratory Data							
Na / K	Cl / CO_2	Glu / BUN	Cr / WBC	RBC / Hgb	Hct / Plat	PT pt. / cont.	PTT pt. / cont.

Procedures: ______________________

____

Allergies ______________________

PMH ______________________

Meds __________ **EBL/IVF** __________

Post Anesthesia Assessment

____

Anesthesiologist

____

Surgeon

____ General ____ Spinal ____ Epidural

____ AMC ____ Local ____ Other

Drug & Dosage	Route	Time	Signature

Hemodynamic Parameters													Pain Scale	Operative Site(s)	Ventilatory Data		Input							
Time	SpO_2	Blood Pressure		H	R	T	GCS		Aldrete Score				Rating 0-10		Airway	O_2 Percent	Colloids	IV PB	IV Solutions			IV Total	Oral	Total Intake
		Art	Cuff				E / V	M / Tot	A / B	C / D	E / Tot													

Figure 15-3 (cont'd)

Glascow Coma Scale (GCS)

	≥ 2 yrs.	≤ 2 yrs.
E	— Eyes	
4	— Open spontaneously	Open spontaneously
3	— Open to speech	Open to speech
2	— Opens to pain	Opens to pain
1	— No response	No response
V	— Verbal	
5	— Oriented	Coos and babbles
4	— Confused	Irritable cry
3	— Inappropriate words	Cries to pain
2	— Incomprehensible words	Moans to pain
1	— No response	No response
T	— Intubated or TRACH	
M	— Motor	
6	— Obeys commands	Spontaneous movements
5	— Localizes pain	Withdraws to touch
4	— Withdraws to pain	Withdraws to pain
3	— Flexion	Flexion (decorticate)
2	— Extension	Extension (decerebrate)
1	— No response	No response

Activity (A)
2 — Able to move 4 extremities voluntarily
1 — Able to move 2 extremities voluntarily
0 — Unable to move any extremities

Discharge summary Time ______
Level of consciousness ______
BP: ___ P: ___ R: ___ T: ___
Breath sounds: ______
Bowel sounds: ______
Dressings: ______
______
Neurovascular checks: ______
______
Pt. belongings: ______
PO intake ______ Urine: ______
IV intake: ______ Emesis/NG ______
Other: ______ Drains: ______
Total in: ______ Total out: ______
Discharge IV and site: ______
Other: ______

Plan of Care

Standard Care Statement Initiated:

____ Post/Anesthesia Patient ____ Other ______

Evaluation of Goals: By discharge patient will:

Met	Not Met	N/A	
____	____	____	1. Achieve/Maintain pre-anesthetic and optimal level of respiratory function.
____	____	____	2. Achieve (pre-anesthetic) normal fluid and electrolyte balance.
____	____	____	3. Express a decrease or improvement in discomfort as evidence by verbal/non-verbal communication.
____	____	____	4. Acknowledge understanding of recovery procedures.

Additional Protocols Initiated

______
______
______
______

Output								Progress Notes
Total Output	Emesis	NG	Urine Foley	Urine Void	Irrigation			**Admission Assessment** IV Site ______ Breath Sounds ______ Drains ______ Bowel Sounds ______

The patient has met the criteria for discharge:

Anesthesiologist signature: ______

Recovery RN ______ Transferred to: ______

Transported by: ______ Report given to: ______

Written discharge instruction given ______
Title

Figure 15-3 (cont'd)

TABLE 15-2 ALDRETE'S MODIFIED PHASE I POSTANESTHETIC RECOVERY SCORE*

Patient Sign	Criterion	Score
Activity	Able to move 4 extremities†	2
	Able to move 2 extremities†	1
	Able to move 0 extremities†	0
Respiration	Able to deep-breathe and cough	2
	Dyspnea or limited breathing	1
	Apneic, obstructed airway	0
Circulation	BP ± 20% of preanesthesia value	2
	BP ± 20%-49% of preanesthesia value	1
	BP ± 50% of preanesthesia value	0
Consciousness	Fully awake	2
	Arousable (by name)	1
	Nonresponsive	0
Oxygen saturation	Spo_2 >92% on room air	2
	Requires supplemental O_2 to maintain Spo_2 >90%	1
	Spo_2 <90% even with O_2 supplement	0
Color	Pink or normal	2
	Pale or dusky, mottled, or flushed	1
	Cyanotic	0

From Aldrete JA: Discharge criteria. In Thomson D, Frost E, editors: *Baillierе's clinical anesthesiology: postanesthesia care,* London, 1994, Balliere-Tindall.

BP, Blood pressure; *Spo_2,* oxyhemoglobin saturation determination via pulse oximetry.

*A score of 9 or 10 is necessary before patient discharge.

†Voluntarily or on command.

VENOUS THROMBOSIS. The formation of clots (DVT) in the veins of the pelvis and the lower extremities impairs circulation and is a potentially serious postoperative complication. DVT may also develop into pulmonary embolism.

Three factors (Virchow's triad) contribute to the formation of DVT: damage to the endothelial lining of the vein, **venous stasis** (slowing of blood flow), and hypercoagulability. Platelets adhere to the vessel wall, with the resulting inflammatory response stimulating blood coagulation and fibrin development, resulting in a blood clot on the vessel wall (thrombophlebitis). Postoperative clots often form in a vein of the foot, calf, thigh, or pelvis. The clot grows, usually in the direction of the slow-moving blood. Clots can occur in either a deep or superficial vein (Figure 15-4).

Postoperative venous stasis occurs for a number of reasons. A major contribution to venous stasis is immobility. Every time the leg is moved, the muscle compresses the vein, pushing the blood toward the heart (venous pump); valves prevent the blood from moving backward. Ambulation and mobility promote return of venous blood to the heart and prevention of venous stasis.

Risk factors include a history of DVT, clotting abnormalities, immobility, obesity, type of surgery (lower extremity, pelvic, and abdominal), trauma, malignancy, and oral contraceptive use. Other factors include prolonged sitting with the legs dependent, decreased mobility, intestinal distention, pressure on the popliteal area, anesthetic effects, and tight dressings or casts on lower extremities. Typical signs and symptoms of DVT include pain, edema, erythema, local tenderness, palpable cord, and calf circumference inequality. A positive Homans's sign (calf pain on dorsiflexion of the foot) is often associated with DVT but is not a reliable indicator. See Chapter 31 for further discussion of DVT.

GASTROINTESTINAL. Postoperative gastrointestinal complications include hiccups, nausea and vomiting, abdominal distention, paralytic ileus, stress ulcer, and abdominal compartment syndrome. These gastrointestinal disturbances can cause a great deal of discomfort.

HICCUPS. Hiccups (singultus) are produced by involuntary contraction of the diaphragm and rapid closure of the glottis. This annoying postoperative complication interferes with eating and sleeping, and is among the most exhausting postoperative complications. The exact cause of hiccups is unknown, but postoperative hiccups are associated with abdominal distention, irritation of the diaphragm or phrenic nerve, and peritonitis. Fortunately, hiccups usually resolve within a few hours.

NAUSEA AND VOMITING. Postoperative nausea and vomiting (PONV) is one of the most common complications after general anesthesia, occurring in 25% to 30% of surgical patients.[14,28] PONV usually occurs in the first 24 hours; the highest incidence

TABLE 15-3 ALDRETE'S PHASE II POSTANESTHETIC RECOVERY SCORE*

Patient Sign	Criterion	Score
Activity	Able to move 4 extremities†	2
	Able to move 2 extremities†	1
	Able to move 0 extremities†	0
Respiration	Able to deep-breathe and cough	2
	Dyspnea, limited breathing, or tachypnea	1
	Apneic or on mechanical ventilator	0
Circulation	BP ± 20% of preanesthesia value	2
	BP ± 20%-49% of preanesthesia value	1
	BP ± 50% of preanesthesia value	0
Consciousness	Fully awake	2
	Arousable on calling	1
	Not responding	0
Oxygen saturation	Spo_2 >92% on room air	2
	Requires supplemental O_2 to maintain Spo_2 >90%	1
	Spo_2 <90% even with O_2 supplement	0
Dressing	Dry and clean	2
	Wet but stationary or marked	1
	Growing area of wetness	0
Pain	Pain free	2
	Mild pain handled by oral meds	1
	Severe pain requiring IV or IM meds	0
Ambulation	Can stand up and walk straight‡	2
	Vertigo when erect	1
	Dizziness when supine	0
Fasting-feeding	Able to drink fluids	2
	Nauseated	1
	Nauseated and vomiting	0
Urinary output	Has voided	2
	Unable to void but comfortable	1
	Unable to void and uncomfortable	0

From Aldrete JA: Discharge criteria. In Thomson D, Frost E, editors: *Baillière's clinical anesthesiology: postanesthesia care,* London, 1994, Balliere-Tindall.

BP, Blood pressure; *Spo_2*, oxyhemoglobin saturation determination via pulse oximetry; *IV,* intravenous; *IM,* intramuscular.

*Total possible score is 20. A score of 18 or more is required before patient discharge.

†Voluntarily or on command.

‡May be substituted by Romberg's test, or picking up 12 clips in 1 hand.

is within the first 2 hours.[28] Particularly distressing to the patient, nausea and vomiting prolong recovery time, increase length of stay and hospital costs, and increase postoperative morbidity. PONV may result in unplanned hospital admission for an ambulatory surgery patient.

Factors associated with PONV include the use of inhalation agents, particularly nitrous oxide; opioid use before or during anesthesia; type of surgical procedure (abdominal, gynecologic, plastic, laparoscopic, oral, and eye and ear); duration of surgical procedure; intraoperative hypotension; dehydration; obesity; history of motion sickness; delayed gastric emptying; history of PONV; paralytic ileus; pain; and anxiety. Both the anesthetic type and method of delivery have an effect on the development of PONV. The incidence of nausea and vomiting following spinal and epidural anesthesia is lower than with general anesthesia. Gastric distention as a result of ventilation with an anesthesia face mask increases the risk of PONV. Propofol (Diprivan) is less emetogenic than other intravenous induction agents. PONV occurs three times more frequently in women than men; there is also a higher incidence in children.[14,28] Nausea and vomiting may result in fluid and electrolyte imbalance and increased risk of aspiration, wound dehiscence, and esophageal tears.[28]

TABLE 15-4 MODIFIED POSTANESTHESIA DISCHARGE SCORING SYSTEM FOR EVALUATING DISCHARGE TO HOME*

Criterion	Score
Vital Signs	
Blood pressure and pulse within 20% of preoperative value	2
Blood pressure and pulse 20%-40% of preoperative value	1
Blood pressure and pulse >40% of preoperative value	0
Activity Level	
Steady gait, no dizziness, or meets preoperative level	2
Requires assistance	1
Unable to ambulate	0
Nausea and/or Vomiting	
Minimal: successfully treated with oral medication	2
Moderate: successfully treated with intramuscular medication	1
Severe: continues after repeated treatment	0
Pain	
Acceptable	2
Not acceptable	1
Surgical Bleeding	
Minimal: does not require dressing change	2
Moderate: up to 2 dressing changes required	1
Severe: more than 3 dressing changes required	0

From Joshi GP: New concepts in recovery after ambulatory surgery, *J Ambulatory Surg* 10:167-170, 2003.

*Score greater than or equal to 9 required for discharge.

ABDOMINAL DISTENTION. Postoperative abdominal distention is a result of an accumulation of nonabsorbable gas in the intestines caused by manipulating the bowel during surgery, swallowing air during recovery from anesthesia, and passing gases from the bloodstream to the atonic portion of the bowel. Distention persists until normal bowel tone and peristalsis resume, usually within 24 hours. Most patients experience distention to some degree after abdominal and renal surgery.

Patients with abdominal distention may report diffuse abdominal pain. Gas pains in the intestinal tract, which usually occur as peristalsis returns, can be extremely painful. Distention may cause dyspnea by pressure on the diaphragm and may lead to atelectasis. Abdominal girth is increased because of the collection of gas. Acute gastric dilation may produce signs of shock (restlessness; rapid, weak, thready pulse; hypotension) and overflow vomiting.

PARALYTIC ILEUS. Paralytic ileus, a decrease or absence of peristalsis, may occur after abdominal surgery or peritoneal injury. This condition is characterized by diffuse abdominal discomfort, hypoactive or absent bowel sounds, distention, vomiting, and lack of flatus. Fever, decreased urinary output, and respiratory distress may accompany this condition. Untreated or unrecognized paralytic ileus may lead to hypovolemia, fluid and electrolyte imbalance, shock, and death (see Chapter 43).

STRESS ULCER. Erosion of the gastric or duodenal mucosa that occurs in previously unaffected individuals as a result of the physiologic and psychologic stressors of surgery is known as a stress ulcer. Epigastric pain and bleeding are common presenting symptoms. H_2-receptor antagonistic agents (famotidine) and proton pump inhibitors (omeprazole) are effective in reducing gastric acidity and volume during the perioperative period. Antacids (sodium bicarbonate or sodium citrate) are also effective in reducing gastric acidity, but not gastric volume. These agents may be prescribed as prophylaxis for the development of stress ulcers.

ABDOMINAL COMPARTMENT SYNDROME. A compartment is an anatomic space consisting of muscles, nerves, and blood vessels surrounded by a nonelastic covering. Compartment syndrome occurs when increased pressure causes ischemia and compromises the viability of the tissues within the space. Although compartment syndrome most often occurs in the extremities, abdominal compartment syndrome (ACS) occurs in association with abdominal surgery or trauma.

ACS results from increased intraabdominal pressure and intraabdominal hypertension, which may be caused by an accumulation of fluid or gas, trauma, coagulopathy, abdominal packing after emergency laparotomy, hemorrhage, intestinal obstruction, ascites, severe intraabdominal infection, and liver transplantation.

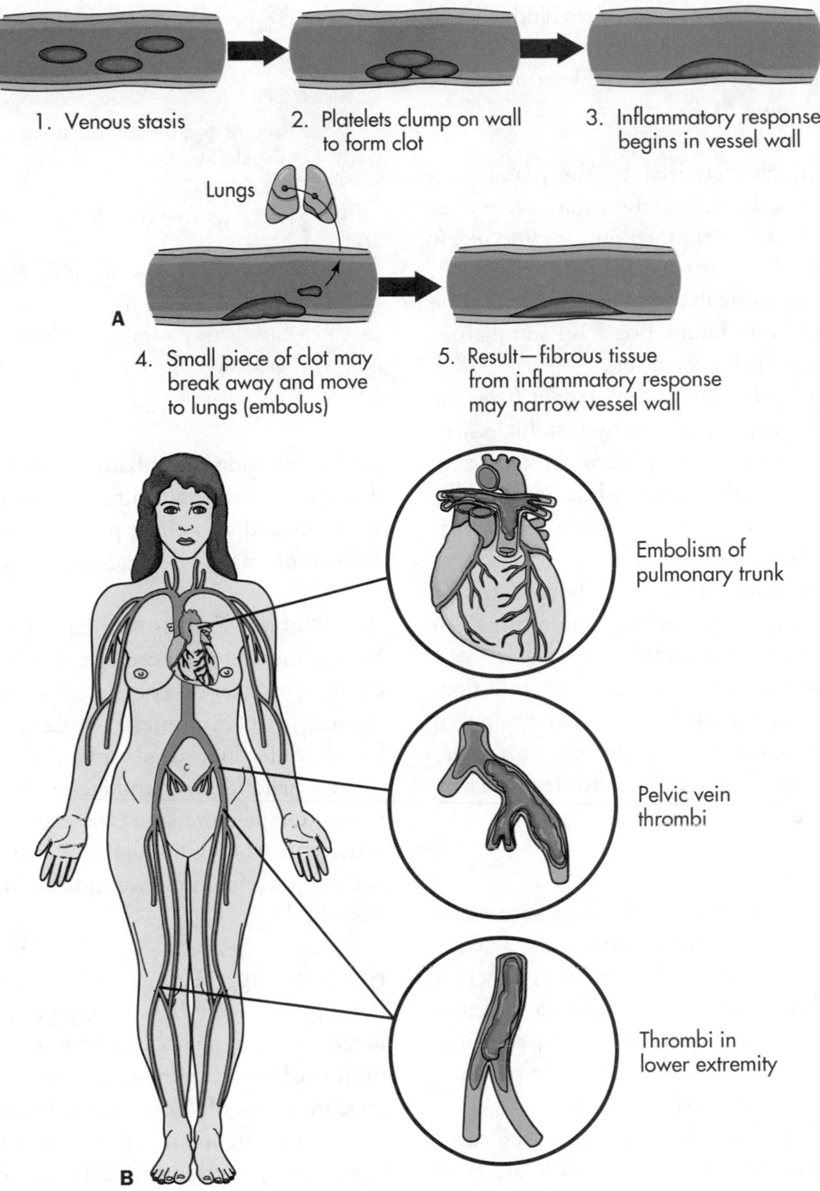
1. Venous stasis
2. Platelets clump on wall to form clot
3. Inflammatory response begins in vessel wall
Lungs
A
4. Small piece of clot may break away and move to lungs (embolus)
5. Result—fibrous tissue from inflammatory response may narrow vessel wall
Embolism of pulmonary trunk
Pelvic vein thrombi
Thrombi in lower extremity
B

Figure 15-4 A, Formation of thrombus on wall of vein after venous stasis, resulting in narrowing of blood vessels. **B,** Common locations of venous thrombi.

Increased pressure within the compartment causes decreased tissue perfusion, acidosis, and eventually tissue necrosis. Signs and symptoms include abdominal distention, decreased urinary output, increased intracranial pressure, decreased cardiac output, tachycardia, hypercapnia, and tachypnea.

Normal intraabdominal pressure varies with the respiratory cycle and ranges from slightly subatmospheric to 6.5 mm Hg. After abdominal surgery or trauma, pressure may increase. Intraabdominal pressure greater than 20 mm Hg causes significant dysfunction of all body systems. Cardiac output is significantly decreased with pressures of 20 mm Hg and greater, hypotension and oliguria occur at pressures of 15 to 20 mm Hg, and anuria occurs at pressures in excess of 30 mm Hg.[19] Diagnosis of ACS is based on intraabdominal pressure greater than 25 mm Hg and adverse effects on organ function, including decreased cardiac output, oliguria, hypoxia, hypercapnia, and acidosis.[19]

Although intraperitoneal monitoring is the most accurate method of measuring intraabdominal pressure, this method requires placement of a tube in the abdomen, which increases the patient's risk for infection or bowel injury. A more commonly used method of measuring intraabdominal pressure is by monitoring bladder pressure via a Foley catheter. Changes in intraabdominal pressure are reflected by changes in bladder pressure. Measurement of intraabdominal pressure is recommended every 8 hours in at-risk patients.[19]

Although ACS is associated with high mortality, many of the adverse effects on organ systems are reversible with early recognition and treatment. Identification of patients at risk also improves outcomes. Treatment goals are immediate release of intraabdominal pressure and preservation of cardiac, respiratory, neurologic, and renal function. The type of treatment depends on the cause of the increased pressure. The decision to perform decompressive laparotomy is based on intraabdominal pressures and clinical signs and symptoms. More evidence is needed to support the practice of temporary abdominal closure after laparotomy in patients at high risk for developing ACS.[19]

URINARY. Urine retention is characterized by the inability to void over a 6- to 8-hour period. Urine retention may occur after spinal anesthesia or surgery of the rectum, colon, or gynecologic structures as a result of local edema or temporary disturbance of the innervation of the bladder musculature. Postoperative urine retention usually resolves within 48 hours. Box 15-4 summarizes common causes of postoperative urine retention.

With urine retention, light palpation of the bladder (over the lower part of the abdomen just above the symphysis pubis) usually elicits discomfort, and distention may be present. In some cases the patient voids frequently in small amounts, but without discomfort, to relieve pressure in the overdistended bladder. This pattern is called retention with overflow.

If the patient is unable to void after 6 to 8 hours, straight catheterization may be necessary until bladder tone returns. An indwelling Foley catheter is not recommended.

Another postoperative complication is urinary tract infection. Causes include urine retention, catheterization, and prolonged immobility leading to urinary stasis. Signs of urinary tract infection include frequency, dysuria, hematuria, and fever. These symptoms usually are observed 24 to 48 hours after surgery.

WOUND STATUS

TYPES OF HEALING. Tissues may heal by primary, secondary, or tertiary intention (Figure 15-5). Wound healing by *primary intention* occurs in most surgical incisions. The incision is a clean straight line with all layers of the wound (muscle, fascia, subcutaneous tissue, and epithelial tissue) well approximated by suturing. If these wounds remain free from infection and do not separate, healing occurs rapidly with minimal scarring.

Wound healing by *secondary intention* occurs when the edges of the wound cannot be approximated, such as with ulcers or contaminated or infected wounds whose management requires they be left open. Healing by secondary intention occurs from the inside out by a filling in of the wound with granulation tissue. Usually extensive scar tissue formation results. Healing time is longer than by primary intention, with a greater possibility for infection.

Tertiary intention, or delayed primary closure, occurs when a delay of 3 to 5 days or more occurs between injury and suturing. These wounds are initially left open because of possible contamination, allowing the inflammatory process in the wound bed to decrease the bacterial count and risk of infection. Tissue edges are approximated as well as possible after the wound is clean. The amount of scarring depends on the type of wound.

Box 15-4 Causes of Postoperative Urine Retention

- Effects of anesthetics that interfere with bladder sensation and the ability to void
- Epidural analgesia
- Medications (opioids and anticholinergics)
- Recumbent position
- Pelvic, perineal, bowel surgery
- Prolonged immobility
- Sympathetic nervous stimulation resulting from pain, fear, or anxiety

INFLUENCING FACTORS. Major factors that can delay wound healing include advanced age, nutritional status (malnutrition or obesity), vascular disease, decreased immune status, diabetes, corticosteroid use (suppresses inflammation), presence of foreign bodies, infection, dead space, irradiation (affects fibroblastic activity), and local wound factors (vascular supply to the wound, wound temperature, and type and method of closure). Enzymatic activity in wounds is highest during the early stages of wound healing; therefore new wounds are more sensitive to factors that delay healing.

HEMORRHAGE. Hemorrhage is most likely to occur within 48 hours after surgery. The slipping of a ligature (suture) or the dislodging of a clot may cause hemorrhage. During surgery bleeding from small vessels may go unnoticed because of decreased blood pressure or use of a tourniquet. Hemorrhage may occur with the reestablishment of blood flow. Careful assessment of wound dressings, drainage systems, and blood counts (hemoglobin and hematocrit) is required.

WOUND INFECTION. After surgery the patient remains at risk for wound infection, a major nosocomial infection. Excessive body cavity exposure and decreased body defense mechanisms are among the contributing factors to postoperative wound infection. A wound may become infected as a result of factors intrinsic to the patient, factors that delay healing, or a lapse in aseptic technique by health care personnel. Factors associated with an

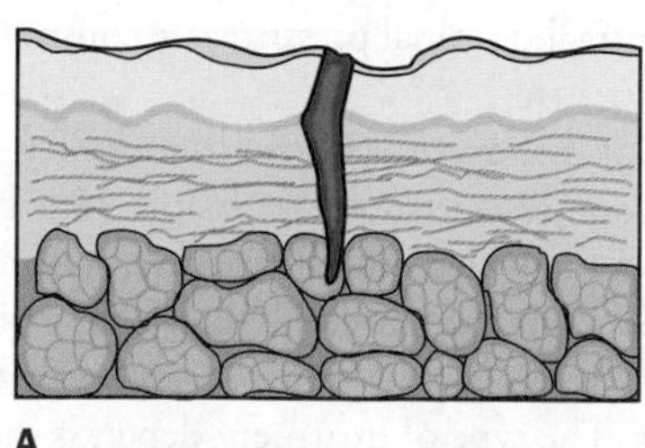
A

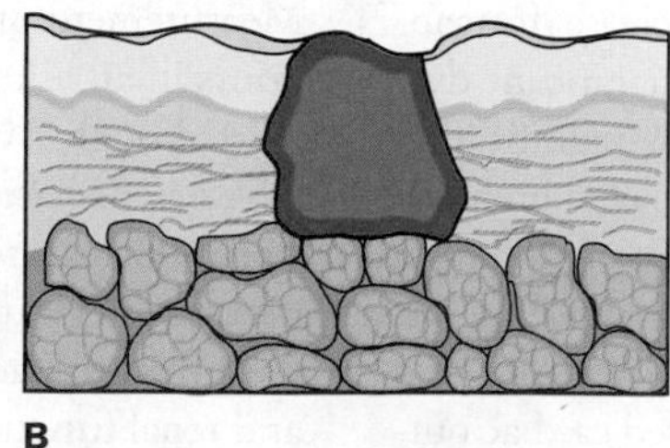
B

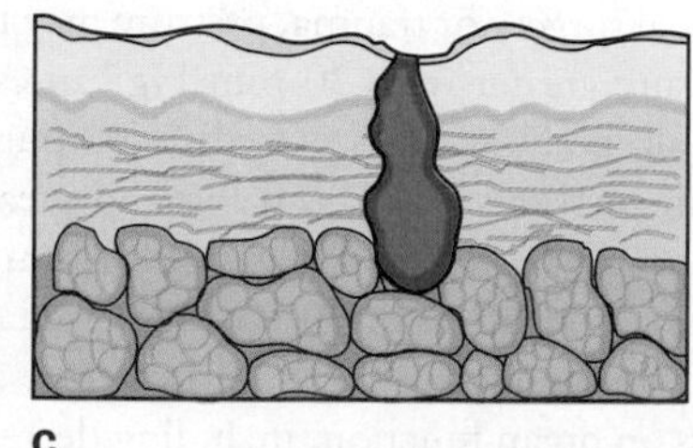
C

Figure 15-5 Types of wound healing. **A,** Primary. **B,** Secondary. **C,** Tertiary.

increased incidence of surgical site infection (SSI) include hematoma, foreign body, excessive use of electrocautery, and dead space in the wound.[12] Mild hypothermia also increases the risk of SSI by causing vasoconstriction and decreased oxygenation to the wound space, impairing the action of local phagocytes (neutrophils).

Objective signs of infection include pain, fever, edema, erythema, purulent discharge, and leukocytosis. Understanding the principles of Standard Precautions, wound healing, and wound care is imperative when caring for the surgical patient.

WOUND DEHISCENCE AND EVISCERATION. Wound **dehiscence** is a partial to complete separation of the surgical incision. Wound **evisceration** is protrusion of an internal organ through the incision and onto the skin. Both wound dehiscence and evisceration typically occur in the abdomen (Figure 15-6). Dehiscence most commonly occurs 3 to 10 days after surgery, before the formation of collagen.

Wound separation that occurs during the first 3 postoperative days usually is related to technical factors, such as wound closure technique. Dehiscence usually is associated with obesity, abdominal distention, vomiting, coughing, or infection. Factors such as cachexia, hypoproteinemia, avitaminosis, increased age, decreased resistance to infection, malignant tumor, multiple trauma, chronic steroid use, and hypothermia can also contribute to separation. Many of these complications can be prevented by identification of persons at risk and preventive nursing interventions (such as patient instruction regarding respiratory exercises, early ambulation, splinting the incision, and aseptic technique).

On a subjective level, the patient may report a "giving" sensation at the incision or a feeling of wetness. If evisceration has occurred and a loop of bowel is obstructed, the patient will report severe localized pain at the incision. The dressing will be saturated with clear pink drainage. The wound edges may be partially or entirely separated, and loops of intestine may be lying on the abdominal wall. Signs of shock may occur. Both dehiscence and evisceration are surgical emergencies and require immediate repair.

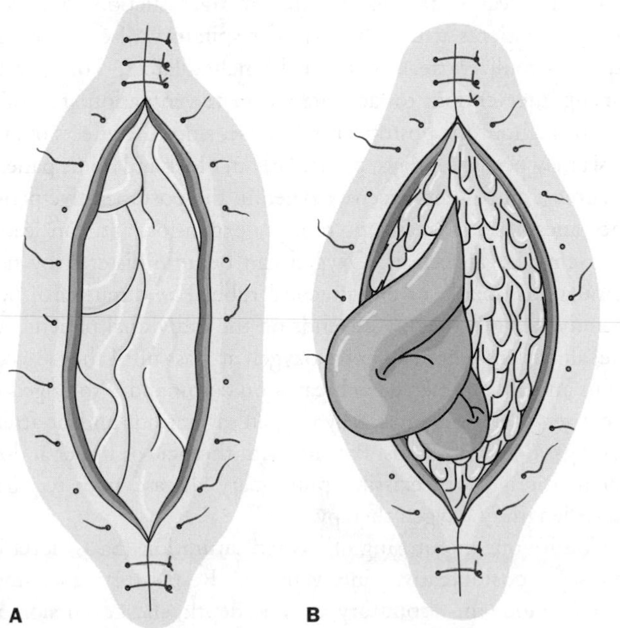

Figure 15-6 **A,** Wound dehiscence. **B,** Wound evisceration.

NURSING DIAGNOSES, OUTCOMES, AND INTERVENTIONS

Nursing Diagnosis: Ineffective Airway Clearance

OUTCOMES. Common examples of expected outcomes for the patient with a diagnosis of *ineffective airway clearance* are:
Patient will:

- Maintain a patent airway with lungs clear on auscultation.
- Maintain effective breathing pattern, with regular respiratory rate.
- Remain free from aspiration of secretions, fluids, or vomitus.
- Demonstrate effective coughing and deep breathing techniques and correct use of incentive spirometer.

NURSING INTERVENTIONS. The goals of respiratory care for the postanesthesia patient are to maintain airway patency and to promote adequate ventilation, thereby preventing hypoxemia and hypercapnia. Nursing management plays a critical role in preventing respiratory complications.

Promoting optimal respiratory function begins in the PACU and continues throughout the patient's hospital stay. The effects of neuromuscular blocking agents used in general anesthesia to facilitate endotracheal intubation and relaxation during the surgical procedure may need to be reversed. Barbiturates, opioids, muscle relaxants, and inhalation anesthetic agents depress respirations; naloxone (Narcan) may be used for reversal of postoperative opioid depression. Nondepolarizing muscle relaxants may be reversed with antagonists such as anticholinesterases. The anesthesiologist determines if it is necessary to administer drugs to reverse anesthetic effects.

The patient may arrive in the PACU with an oral, nasal, or pharyngeal airway or an endotracheal tube. The airway or endotracheal tube remains in place until the patient is able to breathe independently and maintain his or her own airway.

If airway obstruction occurs, it may be necessary to insert an airway or intubate the patient. The insertion of an oral airway alone may be insufficient to relieve airway obstruction caused by anesthetic-induced changes in the pharynx and larynx and may need to be accompanied by the jaw-thrust maneuver and positive-pressure ventilation.

The pharyngeal airway is most commonly used (Figure 15-7) and keeps the air passage open and the tongue forward until pharyngeal reflexes have returned. The airway should be removed as soon as the patient begins to awaken and has regained cough and gag reflexes. After this time, the presence of an airway can be irritating and can stimulate gagging, vomiting, or laryngospasm.

An endotracheal tube allows mechanical ventilation, prevents the tongue from falling back, and prevents airway obstruction resulting from laryngospasm. A cuffed endotracheal tube also helps prevent aspiration. The tube should be left in place until spontaneous and adequate respirations are ensured. The patient is extubated when he or she is awake, maintains the airway, and maintains spontaneous and adequate respirations, as evidenced by

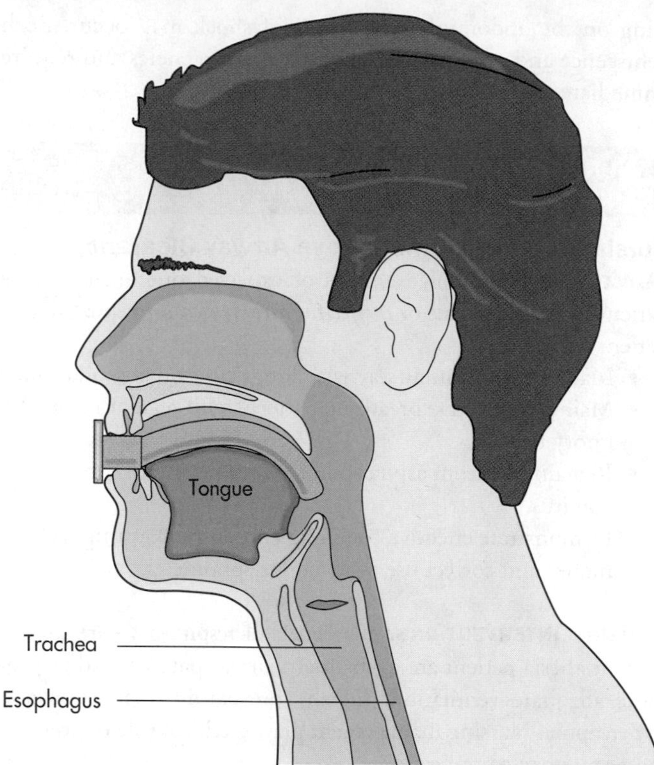

Figure 15-7 Pharyngeal airway in place to prevent tongue from blocking oropharynx.

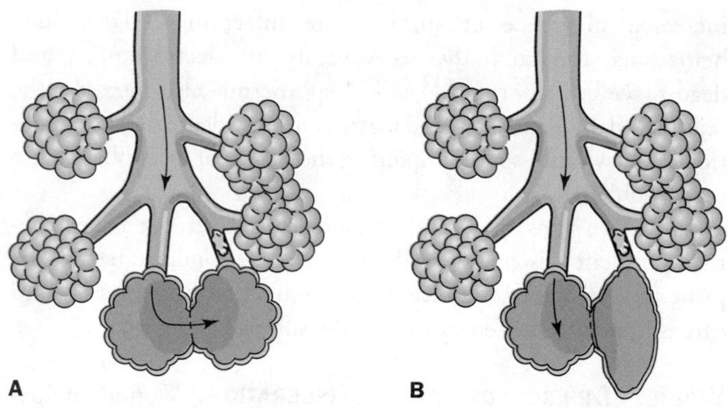

Figure 15-8 Mucous plug blocking alveolar duct in obstructive atelectasis. **A,** Aeration of blocked alveolus through intraalveolar duct with deep inspiration. **B,** Collapse of blocked alveolus with shallow inspiration.

the patient's ability to raise the head and grip a hand, as well as by normal blood gas or oxygen saturation levels.

Excessive secretions from the nasopharynx or tracheobronchial mucosa can lead to partial or complete airway obstruction (Figure 15-8). Pooled secretions in the lower airways as a result of inadequate inspiration and immobility after surgery may result in hypostatic pneumonia. Removal of these secretions in the early postoperative period can prevent airway obstruction and infection. If the patient is unable to effectively clear secretions, the nurse must remove the secretions by suctioning. Often pharyngeal suctioning is all that is required. If endotracheal suctioning (see Chapter 26) is necessary, the patient should be hyperventilated with 100% oxygen before and after each introduction of the catheter into the trachea. When thick secretions are a problem, humidification is increased to keep secretions as thin as possible and to prevent dry air from further irritating the respiratory passages.

Airway obstruction may also occur as a result of aspiration. Secretions aspirated into the tracheobronchial tree can cause pneumonia. The patient may require suctioning until the cough and gag reflexes are present. Until protective reflexes are regained, the patient is at risk for aspiration.

Patients should have received preoperative instructions regarding deep breathing, cough (huff coughing), and the use of incentive spirometry (see Chapter 13). The patient should perform deep breathing, coughing, and incentive spirometry every hour while awake. The nurse should also encourage the patient to turn and move about in bed, if able, or should reposition the patient at least every 2 hours. The patient should sit in a chair if permitted, since maintaining an upright position promotes optimal lung expansion. If fluids are not contraindicated, an intake of at least 2500 ml should be encouraged to thin secretions and reduce drying of mucous membranes.

The postsurgical patient may be reluctant to cough and breathe deeply because of pain, particularly after thoracic or abdominal procedures. The nurse ensures the patient's pain is adequately controlled before beginning respiratory exercises; however, it is important to remember that opioids depress respirations and the cough reflex.

Teaching the patient to splint the incision with a folded sheet or small pillow may help promote coughing. Splinting prevents excessive muscular strain around the incision and reduces acute pain. Family members should be included in the demonstration and teaching. The nurse can instruct them to remind the patient to perform breathing exercises and coughing at regular intervals.

The nurse auscultates the lungs before and after ventilatory measures to determine effectiveness. If the patient is unable to effectively clear secretions, respiratory tract suctioning may be required. Patients with a history of respiratory disease may also require nebulizer treatments or bronchodilators. Postoperative nursing interventions to facilitate adequate ventilation are continued throughout the postoperative course, since the effects of anesthesia may persist for days, particularly in older and obese patients.

Almost all patients receive oxygen in the postoperative period, since anesthesia decreases pulmonary expansion and can lead to hypoxemia or atelectasis. Oxygen can be administered by nasal cannula, face mask, or endotracheal tube. The duration of postoperative oxygen therapy depends on the individual patient. As a rule, all patients should receive oxygen at least until they are conscious and able to take deep breaths on command. Prolonged use of oxygen therapy is guided by oxygen saturations and/or arterial blood gas determinations. Patients with thoracic or upper abdominal incisions or preexisting pulmonary disease may require a longer length of oxygen therapy.

Continuous monitoring of oxygen saturation (SaO_2) level is a necessary postoperative intervention. Respiratory assessment should include the respiratory rate and depth, chest excursion, use of accessory muscles, and presence of dyspnea. Symptoms of hypoxemia include restlessness, anxiety, change of mental status, and a decrease in SaO_2.

Pain management and positioning are important interventions to promote effective breathing patterns and optimal respiratory function. Anxiety may affect respiratory function, causing the patient to hyperventilate or take shallow breaths. Nursing interventions to decrease anxiety may help promote effective breathing.

RELATED NIC INTERVENTIONS. Airway Insertion and Stabilization, Airway Management, Airway Suctioning, Aspiration Precautions, Cough Enhancement, Oxygen Therapy, Respiratory Monitoring

Nursing Diagnosis: Acute Pain

OUTCOMES. Common examples of expected outcomes for the patient with a diagnosis of *acute pain* are:

Patient will:

- Demonstrate decreased pain by absence of facial grimacing, guarding, or diaphoresis.
- Report pain intensity at 4 or less on a scale of 0 to 10.

NURSING INTERVENTIONS. Pain is a complex process that involves sensory stimuli, neural processes, individual experiences, cultural background, and anxiety. Pain results in the stress response with accompanying changes in the cardiovascular system, hormonal release, anxiety, tension, and muscle contraction. From the patient's point of view, the distress of pain is probably the most significant postoperative problem.

Pain (see Chapter 16) is a common occurrence after nearly all types of surgical procedures. Postoperative pain is most severe after intrathoracic, intraabdominal, and major orthopedic surgeries. After laparoscopic abdominal surgery, pain results from residual pneumoperitoneum, irritating the diaphragm and chest and from shoulder pain.[21] Surgical pain is usually acute and is classified as nociceptive pain. Nociceptive pain results from tissue trauma during surgery, from cutting, pulling, and manipulating tissues and organs and positioning and pressure areas. Stimulation of nerve endings by chemical substances released at the time of surgery or from tissue ischemia caused by interference of blood supply to tissues also contributes to pain. Reduced blood supply may be caused by pressure, muscle spasm, or edema.

Pain can be further classified as either somatic or visceral. Somatic pain occurs as a result of trauma to bone, joint, muscle, connective tissue, or skin. The quality of somatic pain is usually aching or throbbing and localized. Extensive tissue dissection and prolonged retraction of muscle and fascia contribute to the development of somatic pain. Visceral pain occurs as a result of trauma to the visceral organs. Visceral pain occurring as a result of tumor involvement is usually described as localized and aching. Obstruction of hollow visceral organs usually results in intermittent cramping and poorly localized pain.

After surgery other factors can contribute to the pain sensation: distended bladder, gas used for insufflation during endoscopic procedures, infection, distention, muscle spasms surrounding the incisional area, tight dressings or casts, and the patient's pain threshold and response to pain. The presence of pain can prolong recovery by interfering with return to activity.

Postoperative pain is inadequately managed, and many patients report moderate to severe pain after surgery.[22] Of the 79 million surgical procedures performed in the United States annually, as many as 60% are ambulatory procedures. Despite the use of analgesics, as many of 80% of ambulatory surgery patients report moderate to severe pain after discharge.[37]

Many negative effects are associated with unresolved acute pain: more complications, longer hospital stays, greater disabilities, and the potential for chronic pain. An association exists between high pain scores and nausea, respiratory complications, slower return of gastrointestinal function, and increased risk of DVT.[22]

Adequate and prompt pain relief is a critical nursing intervention. Effective management of pain (see Chapter 16) begins with a trusting nurse-patient relationship. Active participation and empowerment of the patient can increase the effectiveness of a pain management program. ASPAN has developed clinical guidelines for pain and comfort management of the surgical patient (see Guidelines for Safe Practice box).

In the immediate postanesthesia period it is important to remember that opioid **analgesics** may produce respiratory depression, nausea, and vomiting. It is a challenge to find the proper medication, dosage, and timing of administration that produces the least amount of adverse side effects. The goal is to keep the patient comfortable without overmedication and intolerable side effects. The nurse should adjust the dose and interval of medication until satisfactory pain relief is achieved. It is usually necessary to administer opioids during the first 12 hours after major surgery. If severe pain is expected, the nurse should offer the patient medication at regular intervals around the clock to maintain effective blood levels.

Two goals of effective pain management are preventing pain and maintaining a pain intensity rating that is tolerable for the patient. Methods to provide effective postoperative pain relief include preemptive analgesia, around-the-clock administration of analgesics, patient-controlled analgesia (PCA), as needed (or prn) dosing, management of breakthrough pain, and nonpharmacologic interventions. Nonopioids, opioids, and adjuvant medications can be used to manage postoperative pain. Balanced or multimodal analgesia, which combines opioid, nonsteroidal antiinflammatory, and local anesthetics, has been shown to be effective in relieving postoperative pain and reducing analgesic use.[25,37]

Routes of administration include intravenous, epidural, spinal, perineural, and oral. Perineural local anesthetic infusion provides longer duration of analgesia than does traditional nerve block. This therapy is ordinarily used for ambulatory surgery patients. The surgeon or anesthesiologist inserts a catheter subcutaneously near the operative site. A continuous perineural infusion of local anesthetic near the nerves innervating the surgical area can provide continuous pain relief. The catheter is not usually sutured in place, allowing easy removal by the clinician, patient, or family member at the end of therapy. Medications used for perineural anesthesia include long-acting local anesthetics such as bupivacaine or ropivacaine, opioids, and clonidine.[31]

Other techniques more commonly used in ambulatory surgery include wound infiltration and intraarticular anesthetics or opioids following general anesthesia. Because of shortened lengths of hospital stay and the volume of ambulatory surgery patients, oral

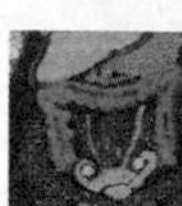

Guidelines for Safe Practice *ASPAN Pain and Comfort Clinical Guideline*

Preoperative Phase

Assessment

Pain and comfort goals
Pain and comfort history
Pain behaviors
Analgesic history
Patient's preferences for pain and comfort measures
Acceptable levels of pain and comfort

Interventions

Discuss pain and comfort assessment.
Discuss use of pain assessment tools.
Dispel myths and misconceptions of pain and pain management.
Provide patient and family education regarding pain management strategies (as-needed medications, patient-controlled analgesia [PCA], nonpharmacologic methods).
Determine pain and comfort goals.

Postanesthesia Phase I

Assessment

Review of preoperative assessment data, surgery performed, anesthetic techniques and agents
Pain and comfort levels
Complete pain assessment
Other sources of discomfort
Physiologic status, response to medications

Interventions

Identify patient, five rights, type of surgery, surgical site.
For mild to moderate pain, administer nonopioids; may consider opioids.
For moderate to severe pain, offer multimodal therapy (nonopioids, mu-agonist opioids, and adjuvants).
Provide intravenous and regional PCA.
Use nonpharmacologic interventions to complement pharmacologic interventions.
Offer comfort measures (positioning, heat/cold, antiemetics).

Postanesthesia Phase II and III

Assessment

Review of preoperative and phase I data and outcomes
Pain and comfort goals, patient satisfaction with pain management strategies
Pain and comfort management plan for discharge

Interventions

Identify patient, validate order, five rights.
Use pharmacologic interventions as ordered: nonopioid, mu-agonist opioids, adjuvant analgesics.
Continue nonpharmacologic interventions initiated in phase I.
Provide patient/family teaching regarding pain and comfort measures, side effects, complications.
Address need for treatment for nausea, using antiemetics or other techniques.
Address patient satisfaction.

From American Society of PeriAnesthesia Nurses: ASPAN pain and comfort clinical guideline, *J PeriAnesthesia Nurs* 18(4):232–236, 2003.

routes may become more common choices for treatment of acute postoperative pain. Intrathecal blockade is another technique used in ambulatory surgery, using local anesthetics, opioids, combinations of both, or adjuvants such as ketamine or epinephrine. Intrathecal blockade is preferred over epidural or caudal block because of its faster onset of action and greater reliability.[37] The use of a short-acting opioid such as fentanyl allows an easier transition to oral analgesics in the postoperative phase.

Preemptive analgesia, first described in 1986, blocks the painful (nociceptive) stimuli from entering the CNS before the surgical procedure. This method results in less pain and lower pain intensity in the postoperative period. Controversy exists regarding when this intervention should be implemented: before the surgical incision, before the onset of pain, or during the postoperative period. Some clinicians recommend that preemptive analgesia include preoperative, intraoperative, and postoperative administration of analgesics such as nonsteroidal antiinflammatory drugs (NSAIDs) to reduce nociceptive input, local anesthetics to block sensory input, and opioid administration.[25]

Analgesics have greater effect if they are administered before pain becomes severe. Assessment of the patient's pain is the first priority. The patient's report is the most reliable indicator of pain intensity. The visual analog scale or numeric rating scales are reliable, valid tools to measure pain intensity. The faces rating scale can be used for nonverbal patients or those with language barriers.

Around-the-clock dosing provides stable serum levels of analgesics. Another advantage is the assurance that analgesia is provided to patients who may be hesitant to ask for pain medication or to report their pain. Around-the-clock dosing may be given by the oral or intravenous route. A provision for treating breakthrough pain (see Chapter 16) should accompany around-the-clock dosing.

PCA (see Chapter 16) involves patients in their pain management and avoids delay between the patient's request for and administration of analgesia. The effective use of PCA is based on the assumption that patients can best evaluate and manage their own pain. The patient must be evaluated before surgery to determine whether PCA is an appropriate choice for postoperative pain management.

PCA is usually administered by the intravenous or epidural route and uses an infusion control device for medication delivery. The infusion control device can be set to administer a basal rate of medication, or the patient can receive a predetermined bolus of opioid by activating a hand control when pain relief is desired, or both methods can be used. It is important to remember that no one but the patient may push the PCA button. Assessing and documenting the patient's response to the PCA therapy are nursing responsibilities. Other nursing interventions include assessing for side effects such as respiratory depression, excessive sedation, nausea, vomiting, and pruritus.

Epidural analgesia usually combines the use of opioids and local anesthetics. Drugs most commonly used include morphine, fentanyl, hydromorphone, and bupivacaine. Using both an opioid and local anesthetic reduces opioid side effects and may help prevent paralytic ileus and reduce respiratory and cardiovascular complications.[25] The addition of local anesthetics also produces an opioid-sparing effect, allowing a significant reduction in the opioid dose, which in turn may eliminate or decrease the severity of adverse effects. If medications are administered epidurally, smaller doses are required than if they are administered systemically because the medication is delivered near its action site on the opioid receptors in the spinal cord. Because of the vasculature in the epidural space, opioids given epidurally are also absorbed systemically. Lipid-soluble opioids such as fentanyl are absorbed quickly through epidural fat, cerebrospinal fluid, and spinal tissue and have a rapid onset of action. Morphine and hydromorphone are hydrophilic and have a slower onset of action. Lipid-soluble opioids are most effective when administered by continuous infusion.[31]

Epidural catheters should be well secured with tape, with great care taken to prevent displacement of the catheter. The nurse should assess the catheter site for signs of infection. In addition to the assessment associated with intravenous PCA, the nurse should assess the patient for hypotension, headache, motor and sensory deficits, urine retention, and local anesthetic toxicity (tinnitus, metallic taste, irritability, dysrhythmias, and seizures). A pain management team or anesthesiologist usually coordinates management of patients with PCA.

The amount of analgesic medication required by patients varies according to their age, type of surgery, and numerous individual variables that determine pain perception and reaction. In general, after the first 48 to 72 postoperative hours, pain decreases in severity and may be controlled by a less potent analgesic. Physicians commonly write prn orders for different analgesics and doses, thus permitting the nurse to select the combination that best meets the patient's immediate needs.

Pain is often accompanied by anxiety. The PACU environment, which is usually busy and sometimes noisy, may contribute to anxiety and pain. Dimming the lights, providing privacy, playing soothing music, and involving family when feasible may alleviate some stress associated with the environment.

Nonpharmacologic methods for managing pain and anxiety are helpful adjuncts to traditional methods of pain management (see Complementary & Alternative Therapies box). Comfort measures such as positioning or the use of heat or cold may help alleviate the patient's pain. Relaxation techniques are another strategy to control stress, anxiety, and the muscle tension associated with pain. The patient should be in a quiet environment, have an object to contemplate, and assume a comfortable position. Music therapy is effective in reducing postoperative pain and may be used throughout the perioperative experience (see Research box). The Agency for Healthcare Research and Quality guidelines for managing pain, which use a holistic and interdisciplinary approach, are a useful reference for clinicians.

Complementary & Alternative Therapies

Postoperative Pain

Pain management strategies should incorporate nonpharmacologic interventions for patients who are receptive to alternative therapies. Effective interventions for postoperative pain control include[21,37]:

- Guided imagery
- Music
- Acupuncture
- Transcutaneous electrical nerve stimulation at acupuncture points
- Relaxation
- Massage therapy
- Hypnosis

Pain may also influence other aspects of the patient's recovery. To increase patient cooperation in postoperative ambulation, the nurse should first ensure that the patient's pain is under control. Uncontrolled pain can limit transfer ability and tolerance of ambulation (see Research box). Pain can also cause rapid, shallow breathing and a hesitancy to cough, which may lead to stasis of pulmonary secretions, atelectasis, and pneumonia.

RELATED NIC INTERVENTIONS. Analgesic Administration, Anxiety Reduction, Music Therapy, Pain Management, Patient-Controlled Analgesia (PCA) Assistance

Nursing Diagnosis: Risk for Imbalanced Fluid Volume

OUTCOMES. Common examples of expected outcomes for the patient with a diagnosis of *risk for imbalanced fluid volume* are:
Patient will:

- Demonstrate fluid balance as evidenced by balanced intake and output, elastic skin turgor, moist mucous membranes, and absence of edema.
- Demonstrate vital signs within baseline range.
- Void within 6 to 8 hours after surgery.

NURSING INTERVENTIONS. Fluid volume deficits require fluid replacement after major surgery. The nurse should expect the patient's urinary output to be less than intake for the first 48 hours after surgery because of increased secretion of antidiuretic hormone and intraoperative blood loss. Intake and output should be balanced after 48 hours.

Most patients receive intravenous fluids to maintain fluid and electrolyte balance. The exact amount and type of fluid administered depend on the surgical procedure; estimated intraoperative blood loss; and the patient's age, weight, body surface area, preoperative status, intraoperative course, and individual response to stress. A solution of 5% dextrose in 0.9% sodium chloride commonly is given. Alternatively, lactated Ringer's solution may be given for prolonged periods to supply the necessary electrolytes. Potassium may be added to the base solution to prevent hypokalemia. In some instances intravenous replacement therapy may be ordered for excessive gastrointestinal fluid losses from nasogastric suctioning or surgical drains.

Nursing interventions associated with intravenous therapy include assessing the site for correct placement and signs of

Research

Nilsson U, Rawal N, Unosson M: A comparison of intra-operative or postoperative exposure to music—a controlled trial of the effects on postoperative pain, *Anesthesia* 58:684–711, 2003.

Postoperative pain control should be safe and effective, facilitate recovery, and be easily managed by the nurse and the patient. Music therapy is a nonpharmacologic modality that has been shown to decrease postoperative pain.

The purpose of the study was to determine the effects of music in decreasing patients' perception of pain. The researchers randomly assigned patients to one of three groups: intraoperative music, postoperative music, and control. Intraoperative anesthetic and postoperative pain techniques were standardized. The researchers assessed pain using a numeric scale, and documented patients' postoperative requirements for morphine, acetaminophen, and ibuprofen.

The authors state that patients exposed to music intraoperatively or postoperatively reported lower pain scores 1 to 2 hours postoperatively than those in the control group. Timing of the music did not make a difference in pain scores. There were no differences between all 3 groups in pain scores at time of discharge. The results suggest that music therapy can produce short-term pain-reducing effects for patients who listen to music in the intraoperative or postoperative periods. Music can be a safe and cost-effective adjunct to multimodal analgesic regimens used in the postoperative period.

infection, ensuring patency of the lines, assessing the patient's fluid balance, and monitoring the flow rate, at least hourly. Infusion rates vary, but the average for an adult patient in the PACU ranges from 80 to 150 ml/hr. An infusion control device is usually used. The Joint Commission on Accreditation of Healthcare Organization's 2004 patient safety goals recommend free-flow protection on all general-use and PCA intravenous infusion pumps.

Evaluation of hydration status includes assessing the patient's intake and output, skin turgor, mucous membranes, weight, level of consciousness, and vital signs. The nurse should carefully monitor output, including urine and that from nasogastric tubes and drainage devices. The nurse should also assess the patient for edema. Adventitious lung sounds, dyspnea, orthopnea, and jugular vein distention are signs of fluid overload, which the nurse should report to the physician. Laboratory values, including serum electrolytes, albumin, complete blood count, creatinine, and blood urea nitrogen, also reflect the patient's fluid balance.

Oral administration of fluids begins as soon as bowel sounds are positive and cough and gag reflexes are present. Ice chips or sips of water are offered first. The nurse should offer oral care frequently for patients recovering from general anesthesia and those who cannot take food or liquids by mouth.

The nurse closely monitors urinary output after surgery until normal urinary tract function is reestablished. A urinary output of at least 30 ml/hr is required to maintain adequate kidney function. Urinary output typically is less than fluid intake during the first 24 to 48 hours because of the fluid shifts that occur in response to the stress of surgery. If urinary output is decreased or the patient is unable to void, the nurse palpates the bladder to identify possible urine retention. Urine retention may occur as a result of sympathetic stimulation associated with pain, anxiety, or the depressant effects of anesthesia or opioid analgesics. Signs of urine retention include a report of bladder fullness, frequent voiding of small amounts (25 to 60 ml), bladder distention, and dribbling of urine.

Initial postoperative voiding may be facilitated by measures such as offering fluids, getting the patient up to the bathroom or commode as permitted, providing interventions to stimulate the micturation reflex (running water in the bathroom and pouring water over the perineum), and ensuring adequate time and privacy. Measures to decrease pain and anxiety may help by blocking stimulation of the sympathetic nervous system. To avoid adverse side

Research

Roykulcharoen V, Good M: Systematic relaxation to relieve postoperative pain, *J Adv Nurs* 48(2):140–148, 2004.

Unrelieved pain can lead to postoperative complications and increase recovery time and length of stay. Opioids are a mainstay of pain management, but have adverse effects. In addition to opioids, nonpharmacologic methods of pain control are important nursing interventions to relieve postoperative pain.

The purpose of this study was to examine the effects of systematic relaxation on postoperative pain, anxiety, and opioid use after ambulation in persons recovering from abdominal surgery. After abdominal surgery, patients' pain increases 31% after ambulation and may not return to preambulation levels for 10 minutes after returning to bed. Because of the increased pain, patients may be reluctant to walk and be at risk for complications associated with immobility. Relaxation has been shown to decrease postoperative pain and allows patients to be actively involved in their care. The authors used Orem's theory of self-care as the conceptual framework for the study.

The convenience sample consisted of 102 adults who had undergone abdominal surgery; participants were divided into relaxation (intervention) and control groups. The systematic relaxation technique was developed specifically for postoperative patients. Participants in the intervention group were taught the relaxation technique before surgery using a tape and earphones. Pain was measured using the Visual Analogue Sensation of Pain and Distress Scale, which measures the sensory and affective components of pain.

After walking for the first time, participants were given the relaxation tape in bed for 15 minutes, and then rated their pain, distress, and anxiety. The researchers recorded opioid use for 6 hours after ambulation. The intervention group experienced less pain than the control group. Relaxation decreased pain from severe to mild levels, and almost all the intervention group reported an increase in their sense of control.

Relaxation is noninvasive, is easy to learn, and can be used independently, promoting self-care. It is an effective intervention and should be integrated into pain management of postoperative patients. The study was conducted in Thailand with a primarily female sample, which limits generalization. More studies are needed to support these findings.

effects of opioid use, the patient should be switched to a nonopioid once severe pain is adequately controlled.

If the patient is unable to void within 6 to 8 hours after surgery, straight catheterization may be ordered. The catheter may be left in for continuous drainage, depending on the volume of urine obtained. If signs of urine retention are present, the physician may order the residual volume to be checked postvoiding. Urinary residuals greater than 100 ml or 25% of the bladder capacity may require an indwelling catheter and further evaluation.

An indwelling urinary catheter is usually inserted in the OR before major surgical procedures and is removed after surgery as soon as possible. Patients receiving epidural anesthesia have an indwelling urinary catheter while the epidural catheter is in place. Meticulous catheter care is imperative. Fluids by mouth are encouraged as soon as they can be tolerated. Increasing the patient's fluid volume aids in flushing the bladder. The nurse should ensure patency of the catheter and perform catheter irrigation as ordered. Patients with indwelling catheters should also be monitored for signs of infection.

RELATED NIC INTERVENTIONS. Fluid Management, Fluid Monitoring, Fluid/Electrolyte Management, Intravenous (IV) Therapy, Tube Care: Urinary, Urinary Catheterization

Nursing Diagnosis: Nausea

OUTCOMES. Common examples of expected outcomes for the patient with a diagnosis of *nausea* are:

Patient will:

- Be free from nausea and vomiting.
- Be free from abdominal distention.

NURSING INTERVENTIONS. PONV is a distressing complication for patients and the most common reasons for poor patient satisfaction in the postoperative period.[15] Traditional methods of treating PONV include using anesthetic agents with fewer emetogenic properties (such as propofol) and postoperative antiemetics. Nontraditional methods such as acupressure (see Evidence-Based Practice box) and complementary therapy (see Research box) may be used to supplement traditional approaches of treating PONV. Since PONV has multiple causes, treatment strategies are multimodal[15] (Box 15-5). No one drug is completely effective in eliminating PONV; thus combination therapy using antiemetics from different pharmacologic classes may be more effective than single-agent therapy (Table 15-5).

Vomiting can result in aspiration of stomach contents. To prevent possible aspiration, the nurse should place the patient in a side-lying position. The nurse provides frequent oral care, removes offensive odors from the environment, and provides distraction with music or relaxation techniques. When vomiting has subsided, and unless contraindicated, ice chips, sips of clear liquids, or small amounts of dry, solid food may relieve the patient's nausea. Excessive vomiting may result in fluid and electrolyte imbalance, particularly hypokalemia. Adequate hydration up to 2000 ml has been shown to be an effective strategy in decreasing PONV.[3] Accurate recording of intake and output and monitoring of serum electrolytes and chemistry results are important interventions.

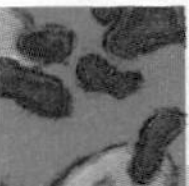

EVIDENCE-BASED PRACTICE

Topic Question: Is wrist acupuncture an effective treatment strategy for postoperative nausea and vomiting (PONV)?

Evidence Base: PONV is a common complication after anesthesia and surgery. Pharmacologic therapy is not completely effective in treating PONV. Acupuncture using the P6 acupuncture point in the wrist is an alternative therapy, but results of trials are inconclusive. The study reviewed 26 randomized trials comparing the effectiveness of stimulating the P6 acupuncture point with either sham treatment or antiemetic drug therapy. Techniques for stimulating the wrist point were acupuncture, electroacupuncture, transcutaneous nerve stimulation, laser stimulation, acustimulation, and acupressure.

Findings: The incidence of nausea, vomiting, and the need for antiemetics was significantly reduced in the P6 acupuncture point stimulation group when compared with the sham treatment, although many of the trials were heterogeneous. There was a significant decrease in the incidence of nausea, but not vomiting, in the P6 acupuncture point group compared with the antiemetic group.

Conclusions: Evidence supports the use of P6 acupuncture point stimulation for the prevention of PONV in patients not receiving antiemetic prophylaxis. When compared with antiemetic prophylaxis, P6 acupuncture point stimulation reduces the incidence of nausea, but not vomiting.

Lee A, Done ML: Stimulation of the wrist acupuncture point P6 for preventing postoperative nausea and vomiting (*Cochrane Review*). Cochrane Library, Issue 3, 2004, Chichester, UK, John Wiley & Sons.

Abdominal distention may lead to nausea and vomiting. Ambulation is one of the most effective means for stimulating peristalsis and expelling flatus. Ambulation usually begins as early as permissible. Dilation of the stomach can be relieved by aspiration of fluid or gas with a nasogastric tube. Before the patient resumes oral intake, the nurse should assess the abdomen for the presence of bowel sounds. When appropriate, the diet should be resumed gradually and advanced as tolerated. Hot or cold liquids and carbonated beverages tend to cause excess gas and should be avoided when peristalsis is sluggish; ice chips do not have the same effect because the water warms before it reaches the stomach. The nurse should encourage the patient not to use a straw to sip fluids to avoid excess intake of air into the stomach.

RELATED NIC INTERVENTIONS. Acupressure, Aromatherapy, Medication Management, Nausea Management, Vomiting Management

Nursing Diagnosis: Risk for Activity Intolerance

OUTCOMES. Common examples of expected outcomes for the patient with a diagnosis of *risk for activity intolerance* are:

Patient will:

- Ambulate and perform activity without dyspnea, fatigue, or significant change in vital signs.
- Display pulse and blood pressure at or near preoperative baseline.

Research

Anderson LA, Gross JB: Aromatherapy with peppermint, isopropyl alcohol, or placebo is equally effective in relieving postoperative nausea, *J PeriAnesthesia Nurs* 19(1):29-35, 2004.

Postoperative nausea and vomiting (PONV) is a common complication following ambulatory surgery, resulting in increased length of stay in the postanesthesia care unit (PACU) and patient dissatisfaction. Pharmacologic therapy to relieve PONV is expensive and associated with side effects, including drowsiness and cardiac dysrhythmias. Aromatherapy with alcohol or peppermint has been an effective therapy for postoperative nausea in other settings. It is easy to use, is inexpensive, acts quickly, and has no known side effects. Complementary therapies are becoming widely accepted in Western culture.

After rating their nausea on a visual analog scale (VAS), patients reporting postoperative nausea in the PACU randomly received aromatherapy with alcohol, oil of peppermint, or saline (placebo). Patients inhaled the vapors deeply through the nostrils from gauze pads, and then slowly exhaled through the mouth. After therapy, they rated their nausea at 2- and 5-minute intervals using the VAS.

Patients' nausea scores decreased significantly after aromatherapy, but did not differ among the treatment groups. Only 52% of the patients required traditional intravenous antiemetic therapy while in the PACU. Patient satisfaction scores with their nausea management were positive. The researchers concluded that aromatherapy reduces patients' subjective perception of nausea and antiemetic use in the PACU. A limitation of the study was the small sample size (n=33). Future research is needed to explore the effectiveness of deep breathing as a treatment strategy, given the effectiveness of the saline placebo in reducing nausea scores. Aromatherapy with alcohol should be considered as a treatment strategy for PONV in the PACU.

Box 15-5 Treatment Strategies to Reduce Postoperative Nausea and Vomiting

- Anxiolytic premedication
- Propofol for induction and maintenance of anesthesia
- Avoidance of:
  - —Nitrous oxide
  - —Reversal of neuromuscular blockade
  - —Perioperative opioids
  - —Hypotension
  - —Overuse of oral airways and oral pharyngeal suctioning
- Adequate intravenous hydration
- Adequate pain relief
- Use of a nasogastric tube in gastrointestinal surgery
- Prophylactic antiemetics using a combination of drugs (balanced antiemesis) for high-risk patients

Nursing Interventions. Encouraging early activity and mobility in the postoperative period can reduce the risk and severity of cardiovascular, pulmonary, gastrointestinal, and urinary complications. The nurse should assess the patient's ability to tolerate activity by monitoring the patient's vital signs and respiratory and circulatory status before and after initiating activity. In addition, the nurse should assess the patient's motor and sensory function and ability to perform ADLs.

Early ambulation is especially important in the older postoperative patient. Cardiovascular deconditioning can manifest as fluid imbalance, decreased cardiac output, and increased resting heart rate. Signs of cardiac decompensation may occur in response to activity; these include fatigue, confusion, dizziness, nausea, pallor, palpitations, angina, bradycardia (decrease in heart rate greater than 10 beats/min), decreased systolic blood pressure, and increased diastolic blood pressure. If these symptoms occur, the activity should be stopped immediately. Other signs of activity intolerance include excessive dyspnea or tachypnea after activity or failure to return to the resting pulse rate within 3 to 4 minutes.[4]

The effects of cardiovascular deconditioning can be minimized by having patients sitting or in an upright position as soon as possible several times a day. The nurse should teach the patient to change positions slowly, gradually increase activity, and allow for adequate rest periods. The nurse should encourage range-of-motion activities once a shift for patients who are unable to walk or tolerate activity. If the patient is unable to perform active range of motion, the nurse can perform passive range-of-motion exercises. A physical therapy referral may be needed for muscle strengthening activities and progressive ambulation.

To avoid the multisystemic complications of immobility, nurses begin ambulation with patients as soon as permitted by the surgeon. After the patient demonstrates the ability to assume the upright position without orthostatic changes or syncope, activity is advanced as tolerated. Before getting out of bed for the first time, the patient is dangled. Most patients are dangled the evening of surgery or the next day. Dangling allows the nurse to assess the patient's activity tolerance and ability to withstand progressive ambulation. When a patient stands, blood shifts from the thorax to the pelvis and lower extremities because of the effects of gravity. This redistribution of blood is accompanied by a drop in arterial pressure, which then activates compensatory mechanisms to maintain blood pressure.

Several interventions can prevent orthostatic changes in blood pressure when dangling or ambulating for the first time. Isometric leg exercises help prevent muscle deconditioning; these along with the use of with antiembolism hose help promote venous return. Before surgery the nurse should have instructed the patient regarding the proper technique of isometric leg exercises (see Chapter 13). Until fully ambulatory, the patient should perform these exercises at least every 2 hours.

The nurse should teach patients to take slow, deep breaths to promote venous return and to prevent vagal stimulation. To maintain spatial orientation, the nurse should remind patients to keep their eyes open and look ahead. To maintain venous flow while standing, the nurse instructs patients to wiggle their feet and contract the leg muscles. Contracting the muscles of the lower extremities generates a 90 mm Hg force, propelling blood back to the heart. The nurse should assist the patient in changing positions gradually and avoiding passive standing for more than 3 minutes to avoid pooling of blood in the lower extremities. Assessing the patient's heart rate, blood pressure, color, and level of consciousness is essential throughout the procedure.

Ambulation should be gradual and progressive: sitting in bed to dangling, sitting in a chair, standing, and then walking. Slowly increasing activity helps to maintain muscle tone, strength, and endurance. To increase patient cooperation in postoperative ambulation, the nurse should ensure that the patient's pain is under control before ambulation. Uncontrolled pain can limit transfer ability and tolerance of ambulation.

RELATED NIC INTERVENTIONS. Energy Management, Exercise Therapy: Ambulation, Exercise Therapy: Joint Mobility

Nursing Diagnosis: Risk for Ineffective Tissue Perfusion (Peripheral)

OUTCOMES. Common examples of expected outcomes for the patient with a diagnosis of *risk for ineffective tissue perfusion (peripheral)* are:

Patient will:

- Demonstrate adequate peripheral tissue perfusion as evidenced by warm, dry skin; strong peripheral pulses; and prompt capillary refill.
- Experience adequate venous return and absence of DVT and pulmonary embolism.

NURSING INTERVENTIONS. Adequate tissue perfusion is important in the postoperative period to provide oxygenation to all tissues, especially to the traumatized tissue to aid in wound healing. Pallor in light-skinned patients and a dullness or decrease in red tones in dark-skinned patients indicates decreased circulation. In dark-skinned persons, examining the oral mucous membranes is another way to assess for pallor. Vasoconstriction may result from cold temperatures or a decrease in the amount of circulating blood as a result of blood loss or from the neuroendocrine response to stress. The nurse can assess nail beds for prompt capillary refill.

The nurse should report to the physician any significant changes from baseline vital signs or output from drains. A weak, thready pulse with a significant drop in blood pressure may indicate hemorrhage or circulatory failure. The nurse notifies the surgeon, anesthesiologist, or both at once if any of these signs occurs, especially if signs of shock are present. Oxygen therapy is initiated to increase the oxygen saturation of the circulating blood. Treatment for shock may be necessary (see Chapter 19).

Trauma to vein walls during surgery, hypercoagulability as a result of surgical trauma, and venous stasis associated with decreased activity or positioning during surgery all contribute to the potential for development of thromboembolism. Nursing management often can prevent postoperative thrombophlebitis and pulmonary embolism.

Nursing interventions begin with assessment of peripheral pulses; skin integrity, temperature, color, and texture; capillary refill; edema; pain; and motor and sensory function of the lower extremities. The nurse should also assess the calves for symmetry, pain, tenderness, redness, and a palpable venous cord. Homans' sign is not a reliable indicator for presence of DVT. Not all patients with DVT will exhibit a positive Homans' sign; false-positive results are also common. Baseline and ongoing assessment of calf and thigh circumference is important for patients at risk for DVT; the nurse should report an increase or asymmetry to the physician. Isometric leg exercises should be initiated as soon as the patient is able. Leg exercises increase venous return, strengthen calf muscles, and encourage collateral circulation. These exercises should be performed hourly while awake until the patient is ambulatory.

Antiembolism stockings to facilitate blood return from the lower extremities to the heart may be applied during the preoperative period and remain in place until the patient is ambulatory. Positioning should not compromise circulation; no pressure should be permitted on the popliteal area. Restrictive dressings should be avoided. Elevating the legs increases venous return and decreases edema. If legs are supported on pillows, pressure should be equally distributed along the entire leg. When sitting, the patient should cross legs only at the ankles. Intermittent external pneumatic compression devices may be used, either alone or in combination with antiembolism hose on the lower extremities. They should also remain in place continuously until the patient is ambulatory.

Pharmacologic therapy may also be indicated to prevent thrombus formation. Unfractionated heparin and low-molecular-weight heparin (LMWH) both inhibit platelet function and are options for prophylaxis for DVT in postoperative patients. The risks of heparin therapy in the surgical patient include bleeding, wound disruption, and thrombocytopenia. The usual prophylactic dose of unfractionated heparin is 5000 units subcutaneously every 8 to 12 hours; the first dose should be administered within 6 to 12 hours after surgery. Enoxaparin, an LMWH, is usually given in 30- to 40-mg doses every 12 hours for DVT prophylaxis after total knee or hip replacement or abdominal surgery. Patients receiving LMWH and epidural analgesia have an increased risk of epidural hematoma. After epidural catheter removal, the dose of LMWH should be held for at least 2 hours; the nurse should assess the patient for neurologic function and bleeding.

Before initiating therapy, the nurse should assess the patient for bleeding disorders, pregnancy, peptic ulcer disease, and use of aspirin or other anticoagulants. During anticoagulation therapy, laboratory data to be assessed include complete blood count and clotting studies. Bleeding precautions should be maintained while the patient is receiving anticoagulants.

RELATED NIC INTERVENTIONS. Embolus Precautions, Exercise Therapy: Ambulation

Nursing Diagnosis: Risk for Infection

OUTCOMES. Common examples of expected outcomes for the patient with a diagnosis of *risk for infection* are:

Patient will:

- Display timely healing of surgical wound.
- Be free from signs of infection, including fever, erythema, and purulent drainage.
- Have laboratory values within normal range.

NURSING INTERVENTIONS. Adhering to Standard Precautions and meticulous wound care are major components of nursing interventions to prevent infection. Such interventions are necessary throughout the postoperative course. Frequent assessment of the surgical site and accurate recording of findings are vital in the immediate postoperative period. Laboratory data to be assessed include the complete blood count for an elevation in white blood cell count and wound culture results for the growth of organisms. The nurse should notify the surgeon if signs of infection or complications are noted. The nurse should encourage the patient to consume adequate calories, protein, and vitamin C to aid in wound healing. Diet instructions are included in the discharge teaching as well.

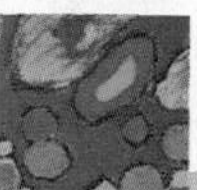

TABLE 15-5
COMMON MEDICATIONS *for Postoperative Nausea and Vomiting*

Drug	Action	Nursing Intervention
Phenothiazines (promethazine, prochlorperazine)	Block dopaminergic receptors in CTZ No effect on gastric emptying Anticholinergic and antihistamine properties	Monitor for: Sedation Prolonged recovery from anesthesia Hypotension Extrapyramidal symptoms Anticholinergic effects Neuroleptic malignant syndrome
Butyrophenones (haloperidol, droperidol)	Dopaminergic receptor antagonist	Monitor for: Sedation and drowsiness Hypotension Urinary retention Extrapyramidal symptoms Tachycardia Additive CNS depression with other CNS depressants Use with caution in ambulatory surgery patients, since restlessness and anxiety may occur with use of droperidol.
Antihistamines (hydroxyzine, diphenhydramine)	Block H_1- and acetylcholine receptors	Monitor for: Sedation and drowsiness Additive CNS depression with other CNS depressants Extrapyramidal symptoms Provide frequent oral hygiene to reduce side effects of dry mouth.
Anticholinergics (transdermal scopolamine, atropine)	Block CNS emetic receptors May be used as premedication	Monitor for: Sedation Dry mouth Blurred vision Memory loss Mental confusion Disorientation Hallucinations Urinary retention

Meticulous care of the surgical incision is an important nursing measure to promote wound healing. Strict aseptic technique is used for dressing changes. Wounds treated with primary closure should be covered with a sterile dressing for 24 to 48 hours. There is inconclusive evidence to support the use of dressings beyond 48 hours.[23] Wounds healing by secondary intention or delayed primary closure are usually packed and covered with a sterile dressing.

If drains are present, the nurse should assess the insertion sites for signs of infection. A closed drainage system should be maintained and tubing secured to avoid displacing the drain. Accurate recording regarding the amount and character of output from drains is critical. The nurse should report immediately to the surgeon any excessive or abnormal drainage. Commonly used drains are discussed in Chapter 14.

Antibiotics may be ordered as prophylaxis against infection; the first dose is usually administered in the OR (see Chapter 14). Administration of antibiotics must take place at the scheduled times to maintain adequate blood levels.

Hemorrhage can interfere with wound healing. When bloody drainage is noted on a dressing, the nurse can outline the amount with a pen and reassess it at 10- to 15-minute intervals. If necessary, the nurse can apply a pressure dressing over an existing dressing. Constant monitoring of vital signs is required. It may be necessary for the patient to return to surgery for ligation of the bleeding vessel.

If wound dehiscence or evisceration occurs, the nurse notifies the surgeon immediately. The patient is placed in a low Fowler's position, kept quiet, instructed not to cough, and provided emotional support. The nurse covers protruding viscera with a warm, sterile saline dressing. Interventions to treat shock are initiated if signs and symptoms of shock are present (see Chapter 19). A minor wound dehiscence may be either resutured or allowed to remain open and heal by secondary intention. In the presence of infection or drainage, the wound usually is left open. The treatment for evisceration is immediate closure of the wound under local or general anesthesia.

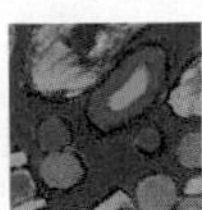

TABLE 15-5
COMMON MEDICATIONS *for Postoperative Nausea and Vomiting—cont'd*

Drug	Action	Nursing Intervention
Benzamides (metoclopramide, domperidone)	Block receptors at CTZ Block dopamine receptors in GI tract Increase lower esophageal sphincter tone Enhance gastric and small bowel motility	Monitor for: Sedation Extrapyramidal symptoms Agitation Dysphoria Rapid IV administration of metoclopramide may produce hypotension, bradycardia, or tachycardia. Administer metoclopramide at end of surgery or in PACU because of short duration of action.
Serotonin antagonists (ondansetron, dolasetron, granisetron)	Selective serotonin antagonist (5-HT_3) in CTZ and GI tract May be used as prophylaxis at induction or end of procedure Also used postoperatively	Monitor for: Constipation Diarrhea Headache Dizziness May cause elevated liver enzymes; use with caution in patients with liver impairment.
Corticosteriods (dexamethasone, betamethasone)	Precise mechanism of action unknown Antiemetic action may be due to antiinflammatory membrane stabilizing or release of endorphins	Side effects are more common with long-term or high-dose therapy. Adverse effects include: DVT Hypertension Mood alterations Hyperglycemia GI bleed Decreased wound healing Adrenal suppression

CNS, Central nervous system; *CTZ,* chemoreceptor trigger zone; *DVT,* deep venous thrombosis; *GI,* gastrointestinal; *IV,* intravenous; *NMS,* neuroleptic malignant syndrome; *PACU,* postanesthesia care unit.

RELATED NIC INTERVENTIONS. Infection Control, Infection Protection, Wound Care, Wound Care: Closed Drainage

Patient/Family Teaching. Patient and family teaching, as presented in the accompanying Patient/Family Teaching box, is an important part of nursing care for the postoperative patient.

EVALUATION

To evaluate the effectiveness of interventions, compare patient behaviors with those stated in the expected patient outcomes.

RELATED NOC OUTCOMES. Activity Tolerance, Aspiration Prevention, Circulation Status, Comfort Level, Electrolyte & Acid/Base Balance, Fluid Balance, Hydration, Kidney Function, Nausea & Vomiting Control, Pain Control, Pain Level, Post Procedure Recovery Status, Respiratory Status: Airway Patency, Stress Level, Respiratory Status: Gas Exchange, Ventilation, Tissue Perfusion: Peripheral, Urinary Elimination, Wound Healing: Primary Intention

GERONTOLOGIC CONSIDERATIONS

Because of the changes associated with the aging process, the prevalence of chronic diseases, alteration in fluid and nutrition status, and the increased use of medications, older patient have special care requirements in the postoperative period. Older patients commonly have a slower recovery from anesthesia because of the increased time required to eliminate sedatives and anesthetic agents.

Respiratory complications are more common in the older patient with a history of pulmonary disease and with abdominal procedures because of the proximity of the surgical site to the diaphragm. The older patient is at a higher risk for aspiration, postoperative atelectasis, and pneumonia because of diminished airway reflexes and less efficient coughing. The physiologic changes in the

PATIENT/FAMILY TEACHING
Planning for Discharge

Patient and family education in the postoperative period begins with what was taught in the preoperative period (see Chapter 13). Explanations regarding rationales for treatment may increase patient cooperation and compliance with postoperative routines. Teaching should include postoperative routines and planning for discharge. The specific information taught will vary depending on the procedure performed, type of anesthesia, and length of stay. Written materials are helpful to reinforce what was covered in the teaching session.

Discharge teaching includes:

- Procedure performed
- Home-going medications (dose, frequency, administration techniques, adverse effects)
- Diet
- Activity restrictions
- Wound care
- Signs and symptoms of infection
- Signs and symptoms of complications
- Return to work or usual activities
- Follow-up appointment
- Contact information for questions
- Referrals if needed

It is important for the nurse to recognize that the patient who is discharged directly to home after surgery may be unable to absorb a great deal of information. Therefore nursing personnel should make a follow-up telephone call to complete both the education and evaluation.

pulmonary system alter lung function, causing a decrease in partial pressure of arterial oxygen tension (PaO_2). The physiologic changes in conjunction with the effects of opioids, muscle relaxants, and anesthetic agents increase the older patient's risk for developing hypoxia. Hypoxia in the older adult may be exhibited as combativeness or restlessness.

Older patients are also at risk for hypertension, myocardial ischemia, and congestive heart failure. As discussed in Chapter 14, the older patient is also susceptible to inadvertent perioperative hypothermia.

Mental Status. Older patients often experience changes in mental status in the perioperative period. Changes in mental status may be attributed to medications, pain, anxiety, depression, or confusion. Although the severity of symptoms may vary, depression, delirium, and dementia often have similar symptoms. Some evidence supports a relationship between delirium and depression; both conditions are difficult to recognize and often poorly managed.[27] Patients may also be affected by a combination of these disorders, which poses a challenge in identifying the cause of the change in mental status.

Delirium and dementia are the two most common cognitive disorders and negatively affect elderly patients' hospitalization and postdischarge outcomes. Both can result in increased length of stay and higher health care costs.[27]

DELIRIUM. **Delirium** is a temporary, usually reversible, altered state of consciousness. This often overlooked disorder is characterized by an acute change in mental status, inattention, disorientation, and altered perception, which fluctuates throughout the day.[5] The incidence of postoperative delirium may be as high as 73%; patients undergoing orthopedic surgery have an increased risk of delirium.[30,35] In addition to increased length of stay and cost, the mortality rate for patients with delirium is 10% to 65% higher than those patients without delirium.[29] Negative outcomes associated with delirium include cardiac arrest, ventricular tachycardia or fibrillation, myocardial infarction, pulmonary embolism, respiratory failure, renal failure, and stroke.[29]

Risk factors for developing delirium in the postoperative period include advanced age; preexisting cognitive impairment; myocardial infarction; acute infection, particularly renal or respiratory; stroke; hypotension; fractures; metabolic or electrolyte imbalance; use of indwelling Foley catheter; dehydration; and nutritional deficiencies. Other factors associated with delirium include use of restraints, sleep deprivation, sensory impairment, and medications. Medications commonly cited as a cause of delirium include CNS depressants and anticholinergics (see Box 13-3). The addition of three or more new medications may precipitate the onset of delirium.

Symptoms are vague and vary with the individual; common symptoms include difficulties with social interactions, restlessness, agitation, disrupted sleep-wake cycles, lethargy, and memory loss. In most cases delirium can be resolved by treating the underlying physiologic cause. According to the American Psychological Association, early recognition of the symptoms of delirium and correction of the underlying cause are more likely to result in complete recovery and fewer adverse outcomes.[29] In extreme cases, however, permanent brain damage may occur.

Assessing the patient's baseline mental status and closely monitoring for early alterations and changes in cognition are important nursing interventions. Mental status instruments such as the Mini-Mental State Examination or the Confusion Assessment Model (Box 15-6) are reliable methods of monitoring changes in cognition and mental status and can alert caregivers to potential problems.

DEMENTIA. Dementia is characterized by memory and cognitive impairment, including language disturbance, changes in behavior and personality, decreased ability to perform ADLs, and memory loss. Alzheimer's disease is the most common type of dementia; other disorders that cause dementia include Parkinson's disease, multiple sclerosis, stroke, drug or alcohol toxicity, acquired immunodeficiency syndrome, and hydrocephalus.

Box 15-6 Confusion Assessment Model

1. Acute onset and fluctuating course
2. Inattention
3. Disorganized thinking
4. Altered level of consciousness

Both numbers 1 and 2 and either 3 or 4 must be present to make the diagnosis of delirium.

This tool has a sensitivity of 94% to 100%, and a specificity of 90% to 95%.

Dementia is caused by destruction of brain tissue and is usually not reversible. In general, the onset is insidious and symptoms are progressive. Patients with chronic dementia may experience delirium as a result of hospitalization, medications, or acute illness. Knowledge of the baseline mental status of patients with dementia enables the nurse to recognize acute changes in function that may indicate the onset of delirium. It is important to elicit the family's input, since they may be able to recognize subtle changes in cognitive function that go unnoticed by staff.

Older hospitalized patients may exhibit symptoms of increased agitation and confusion in the late afternoon, a phenomenon known as *sundowning.* Sundowning may occur in patients with or without dementia. Factors thought to contribute to sundowning include sleep disturbances, sleep apnea, decreased functioning of the hypothalamus, decreased visual acuity, and lack of structure in the afternoon or early evening.[34]

Pain. A common misconception is that pain perception or sensitivity decreases with age. Pain management in the older adult should be based on the assumption that the neurophysiologic processes involved in nociception are not affected by age.[25] Acute pain in the older patient may be inadequately treated, perhaps as a result of underreporting the presence or level of pain. However, the older adult is more likely to have atypical acute pain.[25]

Older patients are frequently given lower dosages of analgesics than younger patients.[33] Research indicates that older postoperative patients received only 24% to 27% of prescribed analgesics.[25] In addition to undermedicating, nurses do not always follow recommended guidelines for managing acute pain in older adults.[10]

Untreated pain can negatively affect patient outcomes and result in depression, anxiety, delayed ambulation, increased respiratory complications, falls, sleep disruption, increased length of stay, and increased health care costs.[33] Patient factors contributing to inadequate pain assessment in older adults include hearing and vision impairment, cognitive impairment, and self-report of pain. Some patients with cognitive impairment may be unable to give a reliable self-report of pain or use a pain-intensity scale.[16,33] Although pain is known to be a multidimensional concept, pain intensity is thought to be the most important component of pain assessment in the postoperative period. When reliable self-report cannot be obtained, the nurse can observe the patient for behaviors associated with pain, including guarding; facial expressions; and changes in interpersonal reaction, activity patterns, and mental status. It is important to remember that patients with mental status changes may exhibit behaviors that are difficult to interpret and may seem unrelated to pain.[16]

The principles of pain management that apply to the younger population are also appropriate for older adults. Analgesics with the fewest side effects and shortest half-lives should be used. The first-line treatment is morphine; hydromorphone, fentanyl, and controlled-release oxycodone are also effective.[25]

Although opioids have no analgesic ceiling, dosages should be reduced for older patients. Because older adults experience a higher peak effect and longer duration of analgesia, they may be more sensitive to the analgesic effects of opioids.[25] The initial dose of an opioid should be 25% to 50% of the suggested adult dosage; it should be slowly increased to achieve satisfactory pain control.[25,33] Because of altered distribution and excretion of drugs, the potential for side effects is greater for the older population. For patients with adequate pain control, reducing the dose of the opioid by 25% to 50% may be an effective method to manage side effects. For patients without adequate pain control, decreasing the opioid dose and adding an NSAID may both reduce the incidence of side effects and provide adequate pain control. Nonpharmacologic methods may also be effective adjuncts.

Patients generally develop tolerance to the respiratory depressant effects of opioids 72 hours after administration. Tolerance to most opioid side effects, except constipation, develops over time.[25] Because of the increased incidence of constipation in older adults, a laxative or stool softener should be prescribed while the patient is receiving opioids and until regular bowel habits resume.

Because of the quick onset and ease of titration, the intravenous route of opioid administration is the best route for severe pain control for older postoperative patients. Intramuscular injections should be avoided because of the decreased muscle mass in older persons. Hypothermia often occurs in older patients recovering from anesthesia; until the patient is normothermic, drug absorption may be delayed because of injection into a cold muscle.

Although clinicians may be reluctant to prescribe intravenous PCA for older patients, this is an effective method of pain control as long as the patient has been screened for the cognitive and physical ability to use the PCA. It may be possible to modify the PCA equipment for patients who are physically unable to use it. During the preoperative interview the nurse should spend time explaining the use of the PCA; this information should be reinforced in the postoperative period. Monitoring of sedation and respiratory status is an important assessment for older patients with PCAs.

For older patients unable to tolerate PCA, lower doses of pain medications administered on a routine basis rather than prn provide more effective pain control. Other options include short-term use of NSAIDs for management of postoperative pain. Although NSAIDs are effective in managing moderate levels of pain and avoid opioid-induced side effects, the risk of gastrointestinal irritation, renal insufficiency, and platelet dysfunction may outweigh their benefits. These medications must be used with caution and only on a short-term basis. Intravenous ketorolac is an option for the older patient; contraindications include renal disease, cirrhosis, heart failure, or dehydration. For patients older than 65 years, the usual dose must be decreased by 50% and the daily dose should not exceed 60 mg.[25] Use of ketorolac should not exceed 5 days.

Critical Thinking

1. An 81-year-old woman has been transferred to your unit from the PACU. She has undergone an exploratory laparotomy for bowel obstruction. She received general anesthesia and 1 unit of packed red blood cells during the operation. She has a history of congestive heart failure and hypertension. She has a Jackson-Pratt drain to self-suction and a nasogastric tube to continuous suction. Five percent dextrose in 0.45% saline is being infused via a central venous catheter at 100 ml/hr. Medication history includes digoxin, 0.125 mg orally daily; furosemide, 40 mg orally daily; and lisinopril, 20

mg orally daily. Describe the assessments you would make in priority order and the rationale for each. What laboratory tests would you expect to be ordered for the next few days? Provide the rationale for each. What complications is this patient most at risk of developing and why? Develop a postoperative care plan for this patient.

2. A 25-year-old woman is being discharged after major abdominal surgery. Her postoperative course has been complicated by wound dehiscence and infection. She is scheduled for delayed closure after resolution of the infection. Discuss the discharge needs of this patient.
3. A 54-year-old man is being discharged after a split-thickness skin graft to a sacral pressure ulcer. His medical history includes paraplegia resulting from a motor vehicle accident. He is married with two teenage boys, is employed as a sales manager, and will have to be off work for at least 2 months. How might his medical condition and prolonged recovery time affect his role performance within his family and job? Describe how normal wound healing might be altered for this patient. What assessments must be made before his discharge? What information would you give him as homegoing instructions?
4. You are caring for a 45-year-old woman who has undergone a total abdominal hysterectomy. She is obese and smokes 1½ packs of cigarettes a day. She has an intravenous PCA and rates her pain at an 8. You observe her repeatedly pressing the button of the PCA device, and she is reluctant to perform respiratory exercises or get out of bed because of her severe pain. Describe appropriate nursing interventions and rationales for this patient.

References

1. Ball K: Transition from the operating room to the PACU. In DeFazio Quinn DM, Schick L, editors: *Perianesthesia nursing core curriculum: preoperative, phase I and phase II PACU nursing,* Philadelphia, 2004, Saunders.
2. Burnaugh RL, Brice JW: The respiratory system. In Rakel RE, Bope ET, editors: *Conn's current therapy*, Philadelphia, 2004, Saunders.
3. Carlson K: Perianesthesia complications. In DeFazio Quinn DM, Schick L, editors: *Perianesthesia nursing core curriculum: preoperative, phase I and phase II PACU nursing,* Philadelphia, 2004, Saunders.
4. Carpenito LJ: *Nursing diagnosis application to clinical practice*, ed 10, Philadelphia, 2004, JB Lippincott Williams & Wilkins.
5. Chung FF: Postoperative delirium in the elderly, *Syllabus on Geriatric Anesthesiology*, accessed from website: www.asahq.org/clinical/geriatircs/pdfsyllabus5-011002.pdf.
6. Deloughery TG: Venous thrombosis. In Rakel RE, Bope ET, editors: *Conn's current therapy*, Philadelphia, 2004, Saunders.
7. Drain CB: Care of the patient with thermal imbalance. In Drain CB, editor: *Perianesthesia nursing: a critical care approach*, ed 4, St Louis, 2003, Saunders.
8. Drain CB: The respiratory system. In Drain CB, editor: *Perianesthesia nursing: a critical care approach,* ed 4, St Louis, 2003, Saunders.
9. Ferrara-Love R: Immediate post-operative assessment. In DeFazio Quinn DM, Schick L, editors: *Perianesthesia nursing core curriculum: preoperative, phase I and phase II PACU nursing,* Philadelphia, 2004, Saunders.
10. Ferri RS, Sofer D: Pain management in older adults, *AJN* 104(2):19, 2004.
11. Fortunato NH: *Berry and Kohn's operating room technique*, ed 10, St Louis, 2004, Mosby.
12. Fry DE: *Preventing surgical site infections*, 8th Conference on Infectious Diseases, *AORN J* 80(2):307, 2004.
13. Giles JW, Sear JW, Foex P: Effect of chronic B-blockade on peri-operative outcome in patients undergoing non-cardiac surgery: an analysis of observational and case control studies, *Anaesthesia* 59(6):574–583, 2004.
14. Golembiewski JA, O'Brien D: A systematic approach to the management of postoperative nausea and vomiting, *J PeriAnesthesia Nurs* 17(6):364–376, 2002.
15. Habib AS, Gan TJ: Combination therapy for postoperative nausea and vomiting—a more effective prophylaxis? *Ambulatory Surgery* 9:59–71, 2001.
16. Herr K: Pain assessment in cognitively impaired older adults, *AJN* 102(12):65-68, 2002.
17. Hildebrand F et al: Pathophysiologic changes and effects of hypothermia on outcome in elective surgery and trauma patients, *Am J Surg* 187:363–371, 2004.
18. Howell SJ, Sear JW, Foex P: Hypertension, hypertensive heart disease and perioperative cardiac risk, *Brit J Anaesthesia* 92(4):570–583, 2004.
19. Hunter JD, Damani Z: Intra-abdominal hypertension and the abdominal compartment syndrome, *Anaesthesia* 59(9):899–907, 2004.
20. Reference deleted in proofs.
21. Laurion S, Fetzer SJ: The effect of two nursing interventions on the postoperative outcomes of gynecologic laparoscopic patients, *J PeriAnesthesia Nurs* 18(4):254–261, 2003.
22. MacLellan K: Postoperative pain: strategy for improving patient experiences, *J Adv Nurs* 46(2):179–185, 2004.
23. Mangram AJ et al: Guideline for prevention of surgical site infection, 1999, *Infect Control Hosp Epidemiol* 20(4):247, 1999.
24. Mason JE, Freeman B: Perioperative medical care. In Dorherty GM et al, editors: *The Washington manual of surgery*, ed 3, Philadelphia, 2002, JB Lippincott Williams & Wilkins.
25. McCaffery M, Pasero C: *Pain clinical manual,* ed 2, St Louis, 1999, Mosby.
26. National Institute of Health: *Seventh report of the Joint National Committee on Prevention, Detection, Evaluation, and Treatment of High Blood Pressure,* US Department of Health and Human Services National Heart, Lung, and Blood Institute, NIH Pub No 03–5231, May 2003.
27. Naylor M: Delirium, depression often overlooked, *AJN* 103(5):116, 2003.
28. Nelson TP: Postoperative nausea and vomiting: understanding the enigma, *J PeriAnesthesia Nurs* 17(3):78–189, 2002.
29. O'Brien D: Acute postoperative delirium: definitions, incidence, recognition, and interventions, *J PeriAnesthesia Nurs* 17(6):384–392, 2002.
30. O'Brien D: Care of the perianesthesia patient. In Drain CB, editor: *Perianesthesia nursing: a critical care approach,* ed 4, St Louis, 2003, Saunders.
31. Pasero C: Perineural local anesthetic infusion, *AJN* 104(7):89–93, 2004.
32. Price DJ, Kluger MT, Fletcher K: The management of patients with ischaemic heart disease undergoing non-cardiac elective surgery: a survey of Australian and New Zealand clinical practice, *Anaesthesia* 59(5):428–434, 2004.
33. Rakel B, Herr K: Assessment and treatment of postoperative pain in older adults, *J PeriAnesthesia Nurs* 19(3):104–208, 2004.
34. Ratchford J: Confusion in the elderly. In Ratchford J, editor: *Continuing education for nurses 2001*, Lakeway, Tex, 2001, National Center for Continuing Education.
35. Richardson S: Delirium: assessment and treatment of the elderly patient, *Am J Nurse Pract* 7(1):9–15, 2003.
36. Rothrock JC, Smith DA, McEwen DR: *Alexander's care of the patient in surgery*, ed 12, St Louis, 2003, Mosby.
37. Shang AB, Gan TJ: Optimising postoperative pain management in the ambulatory patient, *Drugs* 63(9):855–867, 2003.
38. Smith B, O'Brien D: Space planning and basic equipment systems. In Drain CB, editor: *Perianesthesia nursing: a critical care approach*, ed 4, St Louis, 2003, Saunders.
39. Ture H et al: The incidence of side effect and their relation with anesthetic techniques after ambulatory surgery, *J Ambulatory Surg* 10:155–159, 2003.
40. White PF et al: PACU fast-tracking: an alternative to "bypassing" the PACU for facilitating the recovery process after ambulatory surgery, *J PeriAnesthesia Nurs* 1(4):247–253, 2003.

evolve Visit the Evolve website: http://evolve.elsevier.com/Monahan/medsurg

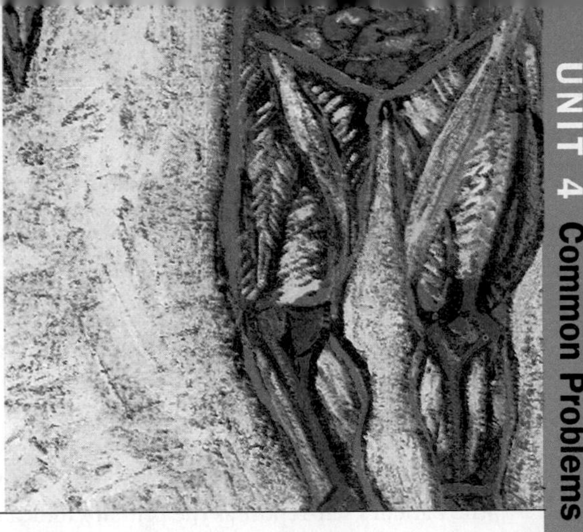

CHAPTER 16
Pain

by Michael H. McGillion, Judith H. Watt-Watson

OBJECTIVES

After studying this chapter, the learner should be able to:

1. Describe some common misbeliefs about pain management.
2. Describe the physiology of pain and related theories of pain transmission.
3. Compare factors that influence perception of and response to pain.
4. Differentiate between acute and chronic pain.
5. Compare pain assessment tools used in clinical practice.
6. Describe pharmacologic and nonpharmacologic approaches to pain management.
7. Identify five nursing interventions for pain management.
8. Explain the purpose and methods of the team approach for chronic pain management.

KEY TERMS

acute pain, p. 334
addiction, p. 342
adjuvant medications, p. 341
agonist, p. 341
antagonist, p. 341
chronic pain, p. 334
endorphins, p. 337
equianalgesic dose, p. 341
neuropathic pain, p. 340
nociceptors, p. 336
nonopioid analgesics, p. 341
opioid analgesics, p. 341
physical dependence, p. 342
referred pain, p. 340
somatic pain, p. 340
tolerance, p. 342
visceral pain, p. 340

Nature of the Problem

Pain relief is a management problem for many patients, their families, and the health professionals caring for them. Although everyone experiences pain to some degree, responses to it are different for each person. Difficulties in recognizing and understanding someone else's pain are clinically well known. The International Association for the Study of Pain has defined pain as an unpleasant sensory and emotional experience associated with actual or potential tissue damage or described in terms of such damage.[49] Pain therefore is multidimensional and entirely subjective. With verbal children or adults, only the person experiencing the pain can describe or evaluate it. Pain can be evoked by a multiplicity of stimuli, but the reaction to it cannot be measured objectively. Pain is a learned experience that is influenced by the entire life situation.

McCaffery and Pasero's definition, that pain is "whatever and whenever the person says it is,"[42] has changed practice by focusing health professionals' attention on the subjectivity of pain. Patients' self-reports about their pain are the key to effective management. However, we now realize that interpreting this definition at the simplest level may cause problems. Patients do not always admit to pain. They do not necessarily know how and when to tell us they are hurting. Sometimes they expect to have severe pain, so they do not complain. Patients also may not differentiate between pain and what the pain means to them, that is, suffering.[44] Therefore the focus on the individuality of pain in both of these definitions underlines the importance of careful listening and valuing of patient information to understand the patient's pain experience as completely as possible.

Pain accompanies many disorders, as well as some therapies. It is a sensation frequently feared by persons undergoing surgery. Although some persons with cancer do not experience pain, it is one of the major concerns people have about cancer.

Relief of pain and discomfort is a major nursing objective. Knowledge about concepts related to pain, data collection, and useful therapies is essential. Sensitivity and empathy, and trying to understand what the person is experiencing, are important components of a systematic approach to the patient in pain. Too often management decisions are made without valid assessment and evaluation, including sufficient input from patients. Consequently, pain management is ineffective.

Pain is referred to as the fifth vital sign. The pain management standards from the Joint Commission on Accreditation of Healthcare

Organizations[28] (JCAHO) (http://www.jcaho.org) and the Canadian Pain Society (CPS) (http://www.canadianpainsociety.ca). Position Statement on Pain Relief[80] both emphasize that patients have a right to the best pain relief possible and that measures to prevent or reduce acute pain are a priority. The JCAHO Statement on Pain Management includes the following directives:

1. Inform patients at the time of their initial evaluation that relief of pain is an important part of their care and that health providers need to respond quickly to reports of pain.
2. Ask patients on initial evaluation and as part of regular assessments about presence, quality, and intensity of pain, and use the patient's self-report as the primary indicator of pain.
3. Work together with the patient and other health care providers to establish a goal for pain relief and develop and implement a plan to achieve that goal.
4. Review and modify the care plan for patients who have unrelieved pain.

The Canadian Pain Society's management principles in its position paper are similar[80]:

1. Unrelieved acute pain complicates recovery.
   Unrelieved pain after surgery or injury results in more complications, longer hospital stay, greater disability, and potentially long-term pain.
2. Routine assessment is essential for effective management, including patient's self-report where possible, to minimize or prevent pain.
   Pain is a subjective and highly variable experience. Therefore patients' self-report of pain should be used whenever possible. For patients unable to report pain, a nonverbal assessment method must be used. Health professionals have a responsibility to assess pain routinely, to believe patients' pain reports, to document pain reports, and to intervene to prevent pain.
3. The best pain management involves patients, families, and health professionals, where patient-families are encouraged to communicate the severity of pain and health professionals are knowledgeable about pain relief options.
   Patients and families must be informed that they have a right to the best pain relief possible and are encouraged to communicate the severity of their pain.

Patients, families, and health professionals need to understand pain management strategies, including nonpharmacologic techniques and the appropriate use of opioids.

Etiology

Pain results from a variety of causes and its trajectories have different patterns. Some patients may experience both acute and persistent pain, depending on the complexity of the problem. **Acute pain** is usually short-lived with a known cause or pathologic process. Trauma, infection, inflammation, diagnostic tests, surgeries, and treatments are common sources of acute pain. Acute pain can recur in people who experience headaches, dysmenorrhea, arthritis, sickle cell anemia, cancer, or inflammatory bowel disease. **Chronic pain** is defined as pain that persists beyond the usual time for healing to occur,[49] generally more than 3 months. Chronic pain may occur with progressive diseases such as cancer, acquired immunodeficiency syndrome, sickle cell anemia, and multiple sclerosis and with neuropathic pain syndromes such as postherpetic neuralgia (shingles). Some patients have idiopathic chronic pain, whose cause is unknown.

Unnecessary pain can result from incomplete pain assessments or treatments based on assumptions rather than on patient data. Regardless of the etiology of pain, the foundation for effective pain management is to believe that all pain is real and that malingerers (people who deliberately lie about their pain) are rare (fewer than 2%). Patients' self-reports of their pain are critical to the choice of strategies and the evaluation of the effectiveness of interventions. It is important to recognize that patients in pain will not necessarily ask for help until they are in severe pain,[81] and they may use words such as *pressure* or *soreness* instead of *pain.*

Both children and older adults frequently experience unrelieved pain because health professionals incorrectly assume that their age minimizes the pain experience.[76] Careful observation, especially of facial expressions at rest and during movement, is particularly important with infants and with cognitively impaired older adults. Instruments that are clinically easy to use are available to help assess pain in vulnerable populations unable to verbally communicate pain.[25,51]

Unrelieved acute pain has numerous negative consequences. Postoperative pain can cause cardiovascular, pulmonary, gastrointestinal (GI), and immunologic complications.[5,15,33,35,57,78,79] Unrelieved pain after surgery may increase heart rate, blood pressure, peripheral resistance, risk for arrhythmias, and cardiac output via sympathetic response. These changes increase myocardial demand and oxygen consumption, potentially leading to myocardial oxygen demand and supply mismatch, particularly for those with preexisting coronary artery disease.[79] Risk for atelectasis after surgery is greater in patients with higher pain intensity.[62] Unrelieved pain after surgery elevates the stress response, thereby weakening the immune system and delaying healing.[11,15] Moreover, in a major study, early unrelieved postoperative pain for thoracotomy patients was the only factor that significantly predicted pain 18 months later.[32] In addition to physiologic consequences, unrelieved postoperative pain is associated with delayed ambulation and discharge and long-term functional impairment.[53] Accordingly, both the CPS and JCAHO have emphasized the importance of effective pain management to meet managed care demands for earlier patient mobilization, reduced hospital stays, and reduced costs. Most important, research suggests that early treatment of acute pain before it begins, when possible, may prevent future long-term pain.[19,31]

Significant numbers of hospitalized patients experience moderate to severe pain unrelieved by treatment.[40,81,84] Unrelieved pain; inadequate pain management; and the related physiologic, psychologic, and economic consequences remain a problem.[47] A major contributing factor to this problem is knowledge gaps or misbeliefs about pain among health professional groups.[9,12,83] Although health professionals more recently have supported the principle of pain relief, this goal does not appear to have significantly altered practice. Health professionals either have not recognized unrelieved pain or have tolerated poor pain relief as the norm.[52] Many health care professionals do not ask patients about their pain, and discrepancies have been documented between patients' pain ratings and ratings by health professionals.[41,81] This problematic communication is compounded if patients expect to have pain while hospitalized or are reluctant to ask staff members for help.[81] Some commonly held misbeliefs influence our practice and may contribute to ineffective pain management (Box 16-1).[76] These misbeliefs are crucial to recognize and correct because they influence our approaches to both the assessment and management of pain.

Epidemiology

Eleven percent to twelve percent of Canadians ages 12 and over report moderate to severe pain interfering with daily activities.[65] In the United States, 42% of households report one or more persons with persistent pain, affecting various aspects of life or employment status.[60] The total cost of lost work time from common pain conditions (e.g., headache, arthritis, musculoskeletal pain) among active workers in the United States was estimated at $61.2 billion per year.[66] Pain is a common reason for seeking help from health care professionals. Despite seeking help, patients may only experience partial relief of pain.[37] Millions of patients have surgery every year, and the majority continue to report unrelieved pain after surgery. Inadequate assessment of patients' postoperative pain contributes to this problem.[38] Older, female, and minority cultural groups have been found most at risk for inaccurate assessment.[47] Although 90% of cancer pain can be controlled, about 40% to 80% of cancer patients report moderate to severe pain.[59] The prevalence of unrelieved pain in the older persons living in the community is almost 50%, and 70% to 80% of older residents of nursing homes report pain.[27] Unfortunately, cumulative evidence supports that people across the life span in a variety of settings continue to experience considerable acute and persistent pain in spite of the availability of effective treatment options.

Minimal or no pain should be the goal of acute pain management. A hospital admission should not automatically mean a pain experience for any patient, including older adults, children, and infants. Patterns of pain intensity vary, and the diagnosis or type of surgery is not an effective basis for determining the amount of pain experienced or the analgesic required. Although not all pain can be eliminated, the use of multiple modalities usually can decrease the intensity to at least the minimal range.

Pain is a complex experience, and multiple strategies are often more effective than single-modality treatment to alleviate pain. Incorrect beliefs about analgesic administration (particularly opioids), inadequate assessment, and assumptions and judgments about the patient's pain experience contribute to the undertreatment of pain.[61,81,82]

It can be difficult to understand and recognize another person's pain.[56] Therefore it is crucial to gain as much information about the patient as possible rather than making assumptions about what may be happening.[73] The nurse must be vigilant about personal expectations, biases, and factors that may interfere with the delivery of individualized nursing care. For example, in one study of 180 patients who underwent an appendectomy, older patients and ethnic minorities (Asian, African-American, or Hispanic) received significantly smaller doses of opioids postoperatively than did Caucasian patients.[43]

Physiology

Theories of Pain

Various theorists through the centuries have tried to explain pain[48] (Box 16-2). Aristotle's perception of pain as an emotion or "passion of the soul" was rejected by specificity theorists who accepted Descartes' separation of mind and body. Specificity theorists believed pain messages were carried via specific straight-line

Box 16-1 Misbeliefs About Pain

Misbeliefs are incorrect beliefs that are accepted as truths and frequently used to guide practice.

Misbeliefs About the Pain Experience

Patients should expect to have pain in the hospital.
Obvious pathologic conditions, test results, and type of surgery determine the existence and intensity of pain.
People who are in pain always have observable signs.
Chronic pain is not as serious a problem for people as acute pain.
Patient self-reports of pain are not accurate.
All patients will tell us when they are in pain and will use the term *pain*.

Misbeliefs About Pain Management

One pain treatment or strategy is all that is needed.
Addiction is a major problem with people taking opioids for pain.
Patient-controlled analgesia is not appropriate for oral analgesia.
Patients must demonstrate pain before receiving analgesic medication.
People who respond to placebos do not have real pain.
Injectable opioids are the most effective.
Respiratory depression is a common and severe side effect of opioids in all patients.

Misbeliefs About Pain and Age

Children, Including Infants

Children do not experience pain.
Children cannot accurately describe their pain.
Children should not be given opioids for pain.
Opioids are best given by the intramuscular route.
Children forget painful experiences.
Children who are playing or sleeping do not have pain.
Parents should not stay with children during painful procedures.

The Older Adult

Pain is a normal part of getting older; pain sensation decreases with age and therefore can never be very intense.
Opioids are too potent for older patients.
Pain cannot be assessed with older patients who are cognitively impaired.

From Watt-Watson J: Misbeliefs about pain. In Watt-Watson J, Donovan M, editors: *Pain management: nursing perspective*, St Louis, 1992, Mosby.

transmission from specialized pain receptors in the periphery to a central pain center in the brain; therefore pain was considered always equal to the degree of injury. Pattern theorists questioned this premise because it was evident that people responded differently to the same stimulus. This observation challenged the underlying premise of specificity theory that noxious stimuli are transmitted via straight-line pathways.[48] Instead, they proposed that patterns of impulses were more important than specificity in explaining pain. Although these theories contributed to understanding pain mechanisms, all had major limitations. Melzack and Wall[48] built on the relationships between these theories in proposing their gate control theory (GCT) in 1965, which contributed considerably to our current understanding of the pain process.[23]

According to the GCT,[70] pain is not a simple, sensory experience but a complex integration of sensory, affective, and cognitive dimensions. Pain involves dynamic interactions between ascending and descending neural systems along with ongoing balancing of inhibitory-excitatory mechanisms. Pain perception and responses to pain are not predictable but vary with each person and experience. This variability results from the modulation of noxious input at several levels of the central nervous system (CNS).

Excitatory stimuli, both painful and innocuous, are converted into an action potential that stimulates the primary afferent neurons in the periphery. The message is then transmitted by these neurons to converge onto common second-order neurons in the dorsal horn of the spinal cord. The substantia gelatinosa (SG) in the dorsal horn is the major site where modulation of painful stimuli results from complex excitatory and inhibitory processes acting as a "gate." The GCT postulates that increased activity in the large, nonnociceptive primary afferent neurons (A-beta), such as that produced with massage or transcutaneous electrical nerve stimulation (TENS), can reduce pain messages carried by the small, nociceptive afferent neurons (A-delta and C) to cells in the SG.[70,86] As a result, further transmission of the pain message is inhibited. However, if pain impulses reach a critical level without being blocked, they will be transmitted to second-order neurons in the SG. Pain impulses then are transmitted by nociceptive pathways, which ascend from the second-order neurons to the thalamus and cerebral cortex. These ascending tracts transmit sensory-discriminative data about the quality and intensity of pain, contribute to the motivational-affective dimension about the meaning of pain, and activate descending inhibitory systems. Pain transmission can be blocked by descending inhibition involving neurotransmitters such as enkephalin, serotonin, and norepinephrine.

Impulses sent to the brainstem, the center for motivational-affective and sensory-discriminative actions, can influence cognition or evaluation in the cortex. Impulses are then sent from the cortex back to the SG via corticospinal pathways to inhibit or permit passage of pain impulses. Table 16-1 describes the various factors that can open or close the gate.

Melzack and Wall emphasized that noxious stimuli enter an already active nervous system that is a substrate of past experience, culture, anticipation, and emotion.[48] Cognitive processes related to the meaning of pain act selectively on sensory input in the midbrain and cerebral cortex to influence pain transmission via the descending tracts to the dorsal horn. As a result, the amount and quality of pain are influenced by factors such as previous pain experiences and one's concept of the cause of pain and its consequences. Cultural values can influence how one feels and responds to pain. Therefore pain is a highly personal experience and more than just a painful stimulus.[55] For example, there is no one standard response to surgery, and the same pain-relieving intervention may not be effective for all patients.

Box 16-2 Theories of Pain Transmission

Affect Theory

Pain is an emotion, and its intensity depends on the meaning of the part involved.
Limitations: Does not include physiologic aspects

Specific Theory

Specific pain receptors project impulses over neural pain pathways to the brain.
Limitations: Does not account for psychologic aspects of pain perception and variability of response

Pattern Theory

Pain results from combined effects of stimulus intensity and summations of impulse in the dorsal horn of the spinal cord.
Limitations: Does not account for psychologic aspects

Gate Control Theory

Pain impulses can be controlled by a gating mechanism in the substantia gelatinosa of the dorsal horn of the spinal cord to permit or inhibit transmission. Gating factors include effect of impulses transmitted over fast- or slow-conducting nerve fibers and effects of descending impulses from the brainstem and cortex.

The Pain Process

The process by which a painful stimulus is perceived involves four steps: transduction, transmission, modulation, and perception.[22] Transduction and transmission involve processing the pain message from the nociceptors to the spinal cord. Modulation in the spinal cord will determine whether the stimuli will be perceived as pain.

Transduction. The pain receptors, or **nociceptors**, are free nerve endings of unmyelinated or lightly myelinated afferent neurons. Nociceptors are located extensively in the skin and mucosa and less frequently in selected deeper structures, such as viscera, joints, arterial walls, and bile ducts. Nociceptors possess an array of molecular receptors, enabling them to respond to a wide range of harmful or potentially harmful stimuli. Transduction, or receptor activation, involves converting a painful stimulus into an electrochemical impulse (i.e., action potential) that is carried from the periphery to the CNS. Noxious stimuli in the peripheral microenvironment of nociceptors are converted to an action potential. Resultant ionic transfer activates the nerve fiber to send the impulse to the CNS. Noxious stimuli may be chemical, thermal, or mechanical.[30] Chemical stimuli for pain (which activates noci-

TABLE 16-1 **FACTORS AFFECTING PAIN TRANSMISSION BASED ON GATE CONTROL THEORY**

Site	Close Gate (Block Transmission)	Open Gate (Permit Transmission)
Fibers	Impulses transmitted by large, fast, myelinated A-beta and A-alpha fibers Stimulation of unaffected skin areas (e.g., massage)	Impulses transmitted by slow, small A-delta and C fibers Stimulation of affected skin areas (e.g., sunburned skin)
Brainstem (descending pathway)	Endorphin effect Sufficient or maximal sensory input (e.g., distraction)	No endorphin effect Insufficient sensory input (e.g., monotony)
Cortex	Past experiences Feelings of pain control	Past experiences Anxiety

ceptors) include histamines, bradykinin, prostaglandins, and acids, some of which are released by damaged tissues. Anoxic tissue also releases chemicals that lead to pain. Tissue swelling may cause pain by creating pressure (mechanical stimulation) on nociceptors in adjoining tissues.

Transmission. Pain impulses are transmitted to the spinal cord by two types of fibers: thinly myelinated, faster-conducting A-delta fibers and slower-conducting unmyelinated C fibers. The A-delta fibers transmit easily localized pain that may be described as "sharp" or "pricking," such as the pain of a needle prick. C fibers transmit more diffuse pain that may be described as "burning," "dull," or "aching." Impulses transmitted on the larger diameter myelinated A-beta and A-alpha fibers have an inhibitory effect on those transmitted over A-delta and C fibers.

The primary afferent nerve fibers enter the spinal cord through the dorsal root and synapse onto second-order neurons within six interconnected levels, or laminae, in the dorsal horn, specifically, the SG (Figure 16-1). The SG is the major site for modulation of nociceptive input. Substance P, an amino acid peptide, is released at synapses in the SG by primary afferent fibers. Substance P is thought to be a major neurotransmitter of pain impulses, activating second-order neurons at the dorsal horn.[3]

Secondary neurons synapse with projection neurons in the dorsal horn of the spinal cord. The pain impulses then cross the spinal cord over interneurons and connect with ascending spinal pathways. The most important ascending pathways for nociceptive impulses located in the ventral half of the spinal cord are the spinothalamic tract (STT) and the spinoreticular tract (SRT). The STT is a discriminative system and conveys information about the nature and location of the stimulus to the thalamus and then to the cortex for interpretation. Impulses transmitted over the SRT, which goes to the brainstem and part of the thalamus, activate the autonomic and limbic (motivational-affective) responses. The ultimate perception of pain depends on modulation of neuronal impulses in ascending pathways in relation to the activation of descending inhibitory systems.

Modulation. Discovery of receptors in the brain to which opiate compounds bind led to the discovery of two naturally occurring endogenous morphine-like pentapeptides (five-amino acid compounds): met-enkephalin and leu-enkephalin. These enkephalins

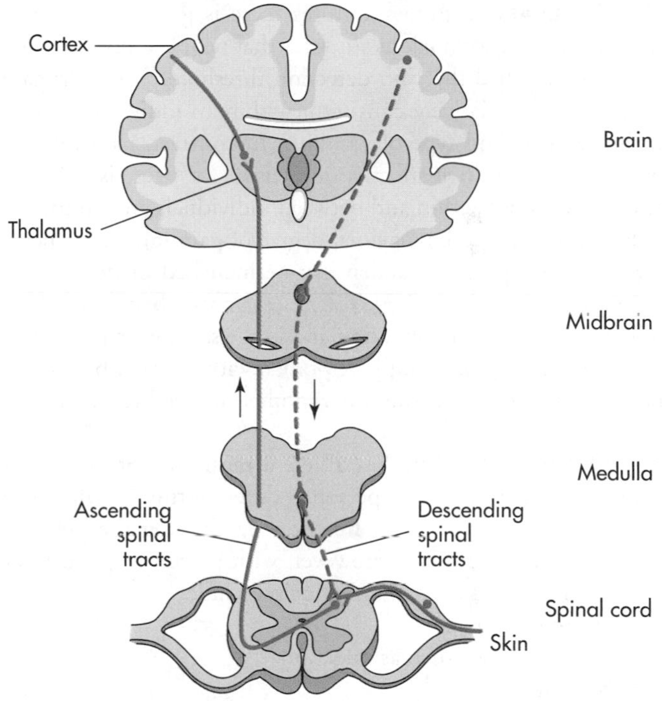

Figure 16-1 Pathways of pain transmission to and from cortex.

are classified as **endorphins** (from the terms *endogenous* and *morphine*). Other endorphins, such as beta-endorphin, also have been identified. The endorphins are thought to suppress pain by acting presynaptically to inhibit release of the neurotransmitter substance P or acting postsynaptically to inhibit conduction of pain impulses.[48] The endorphins are found in high concentration in the basal ganglia of the brain, thalamus, midbrain, and dorsal horn of the spinal cord.

Descending spinal pathways, from the thalamus through the midbrain and medulla to the dorsal horns of the spinal cord, conduct nociceptive inhibitory impulses. Serotonin, norepinephrine, and endorphins are released by descending fibers and inhibit the release of neurotransmitters presynaptically. Therefore nociceptive stimuli will not be transmitted to second-order neurons. Gamma-aminobutyric acid and glycine, inhibitory amino acids found in the spinal cord, also act presynaptically to inhibit neurotransmitter release. These amino acids are also thought to hyperpolarize second-order neurons, thereby decreasing the evoked response to stimuli from primary afferents.[14] Treatment modalities such as TENS can activate endogenous opioid analgesia. Acupuncture is also thought to act via the opioid pathways.

Perception. Four main regions of the cerebral cortex are known to be activated by pain signals from the ascending pathways. These include the insular cortex, the anterior cingulate cortex, and the primary and secondary somatosensory cortices.[14] These regions, along with other areas of the forebrain, interact to produce the sensory-discriminative, motivational-affective, and cognitive aspects of pain, as well as motoric integration of pain stimuli and memory of pain.[3,4,14] In particular, the insular cortex is thought to be key for the integration of sensory, affective, and cognitive components of pain.

Pain Tolerance. Across cultures there is great uniformity in the minimal level of noxious stimulus that people report as pain.[13] This level is called the pain detection threshold.[48] It is primarily biologic and is relatively consistent within an individual, relative to the location and type of stimulus. In contrast, pain tolerance involves the cognitive-affective dimension of pain, is subjective and varies widely within and between individuals and cultures.

Pain tolerance is the maximal degree of pain intensity a person is willing to experience, and it can be increased or decreased by numerous factors (Box 16-3). Tolerance can vary between different individuals in the same situation and in the same individual in differing situations. For example, a woman with a tender breast lump may complain of more pain if her mother died of breast cancer.

Meaning of Pain. Pain has different meanings for each person and may differ for the same person at different times. Pain initially has an important protective function by warning the person of impending tissue damage. However, with persistent pain, meanings can change. The meanings of pain include:

- Harm or damage
- Complication, such as infection
- New illness
- Recurrence of illness
- Fatal disease
- Increasing disability
- Loss of mobility
- Aging
- Healing
- A necessity for cure
- Punishment for sins
- Challenge
- Appreciation for suffering of others
- Something to be tolerated

Numerous factors influence the meaning of pain for an individual. These include age, gender, sociocultural background, environment, and past or present experience.[10,69] For example, two women may be experiencing pain from a fractured leg. The 75-year-old woman living alone with few social contacts may interpret pain in terms of fear of aging and inability to maintain her independent living status. The 28-year-old lawyer might interpret the pain as an expected nuisance, with the realization that healing will occur and she can soon get back to work.

Box 16-3 Factors That Influence Pain Tolerance

Increase Tolerance	Decrease Tolerance
Alcohol	Fatigue
Drugs	Anger
Hypnosis	Boredom
Warmth	Anxiety
Rubbing	Persistent pain
Distraction	Stress
Faith	Depression
Strong beliefs	

Response to Pain. People respond to pain in different ways, depending on their perception of the pain, including what it means to them. Some may be fearful, apprehensive, and anxious, whereas others are tolerant and optimistic. Some people in severe pain weep, moan, scream, beg for relief or help, threaten to destroy themselves, thrash about in bed, or move about aimlessly; others lie quietly and may only close their eyes, grit their teeth, bite their lips, clench their hands, or perspire profusely.

On the basis of their cultural beliefs, some persons are taught to endure severe pain without reacting outwardly, whereas others are taught to be expressive when experiencing any degree of pain. People whose health beliefs and education emphasize prevention tend to accept pain as a warning to seek help, expecting that the cause of pain will be found and cured.

For many years researchers have examined how ethnicity influences patients' pain behavior.[54] Research has been inconclusive because of methodology issues concerning existing differences and how they affect pain perception and response.[32,51] Cleeland and colleagues examined the relationship between standardized self-report numerical scales of pain intensity and pain interference for cancer patients from several countries.[13] Their findings indicated cross-cultural similarity in the self-report ratings. All samples used activity and affect to report how patients reacted to pain. What differed was the focus of interference (e.g., work and activities versus mood and relationships). Therefore it is important to recognize that ethnic groups may differ in their perception and response to pain, including whether they will approach the caregiver for help. However, many variations also occur within groups, and it is important not to stereotype.

Numerous factors influence individuals' responses to pain (Box 16-4). One cannot predict how any given person will respond, and value judgments should not be made. It is important for health professionals to recognize misbeliefs about expected pain responses that prevent effective pain management.

Pathophysiology

The pathophysiology of pain includes processes that are thought to contribute to pathophysiologic or persistent pain, that is, how the nervous system is changed with repeated noxious stimuli. The duration and site of pain determine its clinical manifestations.

Box 16-4 Factors That Influence Responses to Pain

- Meaning of pain to individual person
- Degree of pain perception
- Past experience
- Cultural values
- Social expectations
- Physical and mental health
- Parental attitudes toward pain
- Setting in which pain occurs
- Fear, anxiety
- Usual way of responding to stressors
- Age
- Preparation for pain context
- Health professionals' responses

Prolonged Pain

Acute pain results when the sensory endings of primary afferent nerve fibers are activated by strong noxious stimuli, and the brain interprets the input carried by them as painful. This pain is called *nociceptive,* since it results from the activity of healthy, intact nociceptive afferent fibers that are aroused only by intense stimuli. Prolonged pain that is evoked by repeated or sustained noxious stimuli that sensitize and change the nervous system is called *neuropathic* pain.[16] Three key processes help explain persistent pain.[16]

Neural plasticity is the capacity of neurons to change their function, chemical profile, or structure in the presence of damaging stimuli.[85] Primary sensitization occurs peripherally when tissue trauma or infection lowers the response threshold of intact nociceptors to nonnoxious or weak stimuli.[3] Hyperalgesia describes pain that is exacerbated by a noxious stimulus such as slapping sunburned skin. Allodynia describes pain from a stimulus that is not painful, such as wearing a shirt over sunburned skin. Inflammatory mediators around the peripheral terminals of the nociceptors such as bradykinins and prostaglandins (which lower the pain threshold of primary afferents) contribute to this sensitization. Intervention strategies to decrease the inflammatory response, such as ice, nonsteroidal antiinflammatory drugs (NSAIDs), and sometimes immobilization of the area using a splint or cast, are essential.

Peripheral neuropathic pain can arise when otherwise intact sensory neurons become hyperexcitable and begin to discharge at abnormal (ectopic) locations along their course. The most important locations of this discharge are the sites of nerve injury and the associated dorsal root ganglion. Postherpetic neuralgia after shingles is an example. Prevention using early diagnosis of acute herpes zoster, vaccination to prevent chickenpox, and antiviral therapy for acute zoster are standard practices.

Central sensitization involves a progressively increased response to repeated noxious stimuli and hyperexcitability in the dorsal horn (windup). Continued stimuli from hyperexcitable afferents result in postsynaptic biochemical changes. These changes render second-order neurons in the dorsal horn hyperresponsive.[14] As a result, weak, nonpainful stimuli can cause pain by central amplification (allodynia). For example, surgery without adequate preemptive analgesia can cause central sensitization that increases postoperative pain intensity and the need for analgesia. Therefore perioperative analgesic strategies, including opioids, regional anesthesia, and preemptive analgesia (see Chapter 14), are essential.[68] Patient-controlled analgesia (PCA) after surgery helps patients prevent or maintain minimal pain levels and also prevents this sensitization. Central amplification is thought to involve *N*-methyl-D-aspartate (NMDA) receptors, and NMDA antagonist drugs such as ketamine and dextromethorphan may help reduce this.[6]

Longevity of Pain

Two types of pain may occur separately or together: acute and chronic. Unfortunately, many health care professionals do not make this differentiation and provide care for the person experiencing chronic pain as though it were acute pain. Acute and chronic pain are different (Table 16-2), as are the approaches to pain relief, although some of the same techniques may be used.

Acute Pain. Acute pain is essentially a transient episode and informs the person that something is wrong. The onset is usually sudden from a perceived cause, and the painful areas can generally be well identified.

Sudden severe pain activates the autonomic nervous system, which may produce signs of sympathetic overactivity, including tachycardia, increased blood pressure, pupillary dilation, diaphoresis, and stimulation of adrenal medullary secretion. In some situations, such as with severe visceral pain of sudden onset, vasodilation may occur with a subsequent fall in blood pressure and shock. Continuous painful stimulation can also produce a steadily maintained reflex contraction of adjacent or distant muscles, such as abdominal rigidity in persons with intraabdominal pain.

Acute pain is commonly accompanied by increased muscle tension and anxiety, both of which may contribute to increased perception of pain (Figure 16-2). If the pain is moderate or severe, overt physiologic and behavioral signs facilitate assessment of the pain. The person usually seeks pain relief.

Chronic Pain. Chronic pain persists beyond the usual time for healing, usually 3 to 6 months. Chronic pain may begin as acute pain but then persists[49] (e.g., full-thickness burns), or the onset may be so insidious that the person cannot pinpoint when it first occurred. The source of the pain may be unknown or impossible to determine, such as intractable pain associated with some cancers. The pain sensation can be more diffuse than acute pain so the person is unable to identify a specific pain site.

Responses to chronic pain can vary, and health care providers need to consider the unique pattern for each person and family. Often, however, chronic pain is characterized by irritability (often compounded by insomnia), which leads to decreasing interests and isolation from friends and family[77] (Figure 16-3). These patients undergo tremendous disruptions in many aspects of their usual activities, including work, family roles, socialization, sleep, and leisure.[77] The person's life may center on ways to modify the pain experience. Some patients go from one physician to another seeking pain relief, expending time, effort, and money but often losing faith in the ability of anyone to help them. The lack of continuity of care exacerbates the problem.

TABLE 16-2 COMPARISON OF ACUTE AND CHRONIC PAIN

Characteristic	Acute Pain	Chronic Pain
Onset	Usually sudden	May be sudden or insidious
Duration	Transient (up to 3 months)	Prolonged (months to years)
Pain localization	Pain versus nonpain areas generally well identified	Pain versus nonpain areas less well identified; intensity more difficult to evaluate (change in sensation)
Clinical signs	Signs of sympathetic overactivity (such as increased blood pressure)	Usually no change in vital signs (adaptation)
Purpose	Warning that something is wrong	Meaningless; no purpose
Pattern	Self-limiting or readily corrected	Continuous or intermittent; intensity may vary or remain constant
Prognosis	Likelihood of eventual complete relief	Complete relief usually not possible

Physicians often feel helpless when the patient continues to report pain. The development of pain clinics and inpatient pain teams has led to successful control of chronic pain for some (but not all) persons. Box 16-5 presents information about pain centers in the United States and Canada.

Specific Types of Pain

Somatic vs. Visceral Pain. Pain may originate in the skin and subcutaneous tissue (superficial pain), in the muscles and bones (deep **somatic pain**), or in the body organs (**visceral pain**). Somatic and visceral pain differ in their characteristics, particularly in the quality of pain, localization, causes, and accompanying symptoms (Table 16-3).

Referred Pain. **Referred pain** is felt in areas other than those stimulated by injury or disease. For example, the person having a myocardial infarction (MI) may report pain radiating down the left arm and neck, when in fact the tissue damage is occurring in the myocardium because of ischemia.

Referred pain occurs most often with damage or injury to the visceral organs, and the pain is referred to cutaneous surfaces (Figure 16-4). The origin of referred pain is complex and not clearly understood. Mechanisms of referred pain are thought to relate to spatial organization of the grey matter of the spinal column into five distinct laminae, or layers. Cell bodies of primary afferent nociceptors are located in the marginal layer of the dorsal horn (lamina I), the SG (lamina II), and ventral to the SG (laminae III and IV). Lamina V cells, or wide-dynamic-range neurons, respond to noxious stimuli from superficial and deep somatic structures, as well as visceral structures.[4] One theory postulates that convergence of noxious stimuli from somatic and visceral structures via lamina V neurons may account for referred pain.[4] Because a single lamina V neuron receives input from somatic and visceral regions, higher brain centers may not be able to accurately discriminate the source of the pain. Hence, the person having an MI reports pain to the left arm or neck.

Neuropathic Pain. **Neuropathic pain** arises from injury to the nervous system and can occur in different forms. Sharp, spasmlike pain can occur along the course of one or more nerves, such as the trigeminal nerve in the face (trigeminal neuralgia, or tic douloureux) or the sciatic nerve in the lower back and extremity (sciatica). Severe, burning pain can be associated with injury to a peripheral nerve in the extremities. As a result, the patient may go to great lengths to protect against irritating stimuli, which may be something as simple as the noise of a plane overhead.

Phantom limb pain is experienced in an amputated extremity. This problem is more likely to develop in those who had signifi-

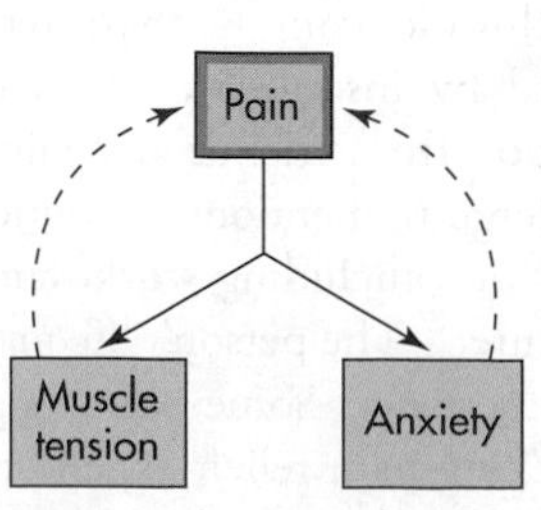

Figure 16-2 Acute pain.

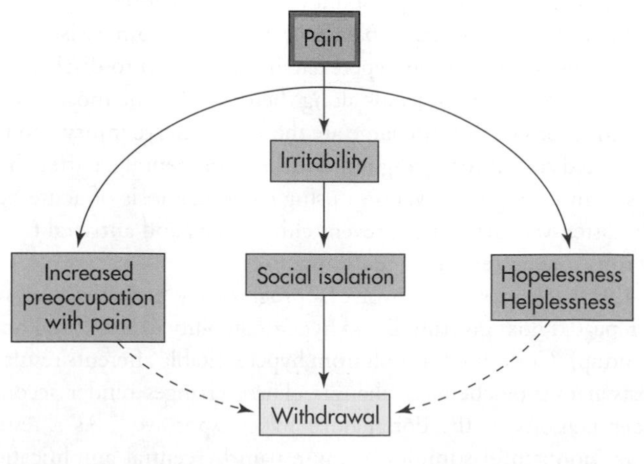

Figure 16-3 Chronic pain.

BOX 16-5 Organizations Providing Information on Pain in the United States and Canada

- American Chronic Pain Association: www.theacpa.org
- American Council for Headache Education: www.achenet.org
- National Chronic Pain Outreach Association: www.chronicpain.org
- Canadian Pain Society: www.canadianpainsociety.ca
- Chronic Pain Association of Canada: www.chronicpaincanada.com
- Commission on Accreditation of Rehabilitation Facilities: www.carf.org
- International Association for the Study of Pain: www.iasp-pain.org

cant pain before amputation, and it may persist long after healing has occurred. This phenomenon has been successfully prevented in the postoperative period by the administration of effective preemptive analgesia before surgery. Refer to Chapter 31 for a discussion of the management of amputation.

Pharmacologic management of neuropathic pain may require an ongoing multimodal approach, including use of opioids, tricyclic antidepressants, and anticonvulsants.

ARE You READY?

The nurse assesses for which of the following clinical manifestations to substantiate acute pain?

1. Hot, dry skin
2. Decreased level of consciousness
3. Elevated heart rate
4. Irregular breathing pattern

Collaborative Care Management

Pharmacologic Approaches

Analgesics. Two groups of analgesics, as well as adjuvant medications, are important components of effective pain management. **Opioid analgesics**, such as morphine, act mainly on the CNS to alter the perception of pain. **Nonopioid analgesics**, such as aspirin, block impulses mainly in the periphery and decrease inflammation-related pain by inhibiting the synthesis of prostaglandins. For some types of pain, such as pain with bone cancer, analgesics from both groups are necessary. **Adjuvant medications** such as amitriptyline (Elavil) help relieve some types of neuropathic pain such as that with postherpetic neuralgia.[74]

Standard doses are helpful guidelines for analgesic prescription and administration, but dosages need to be evaluated for each patient. Although most nurses do not prescribe analgesics, they do make administration choices about the type, dose, and frequency when drug options are given.[21] Nurses are also responsible for evaluating the patient's response to analgesic and adjuvant medications. This includes evaluating the effectiveness of the medication, monitoring for side effects and side effects management, and advocating for change when needed.

Common side effects from opioids include constipation, nausea, and vomiting, which need to be preempted. Side effects may also include pruritus, myoclonus, sedation, and delirium. Respiratory depression may also occur, but this side effect is rare with appropriate drug dosing and titration to effect.

Equianalgesic dosing is an important concept in pharmacologic management. An **equianalgesic dose** is the dose of one analgesic that has the same pain-relieving effect as a specific dose of another drug. This concept makes it possible to change one analgesic for another, or to change the route of administration, for example, from parenteral to oral. Equianalgesic dosing also allows comparisons between weak analgesics such as codeine for mild pain, and stronger analgesics such as morphine for moderate to severe pain. Table 16-4 presents equianalgesic doses of common opioids.

OPIOID ANALGESICS. Opioid analgesics can be classified according to the strength of their effect; for example, codeine is a weak opioid and morphine is a strong opioid. Opioids are also classified as agonist, antagonist, or mixed agonist-antagonist opioids, depending on their effect at mu, delta, and kappa receptor sites. For example, morphine is an **agonist** as it binds to and activates the receptors, mainly mu, to produce analgesia. **Antagonist** opioids, such as naloxone, bind to a receptor without activating it; they also block and displace agonist opioids such as morphine and prevent their analgesic effect. Butorphanol (Stadol) is an example of a

TABLE 16-3 COMPARISON OF SUPERFICIAL, SOMATIC, AND VISCERAL PAIN

	Superficial Pain	Somatic Pain	Visceral Pain
Characteristic	Skin and subcutaneous tissue	Deep muscles and bones	Internal organs
Quality	Sharp, pricking, burning	Sharp or dull and aching	Sharp or dull and aching, cramping
Localization	Good	Poor	Poor
Referred pain	No	No	Yes
Provoking stimuli	Cut, abrasion, excessive heat or cold, chemicals	Cut, pressure, heat, ischemia, displacement (bone)	Distention, ischemia, spasms, chemical irritants (no cutting)
Autonomic reactions	No	Yes	Yes
Reflex muscle contractions	No	Yes	Yes

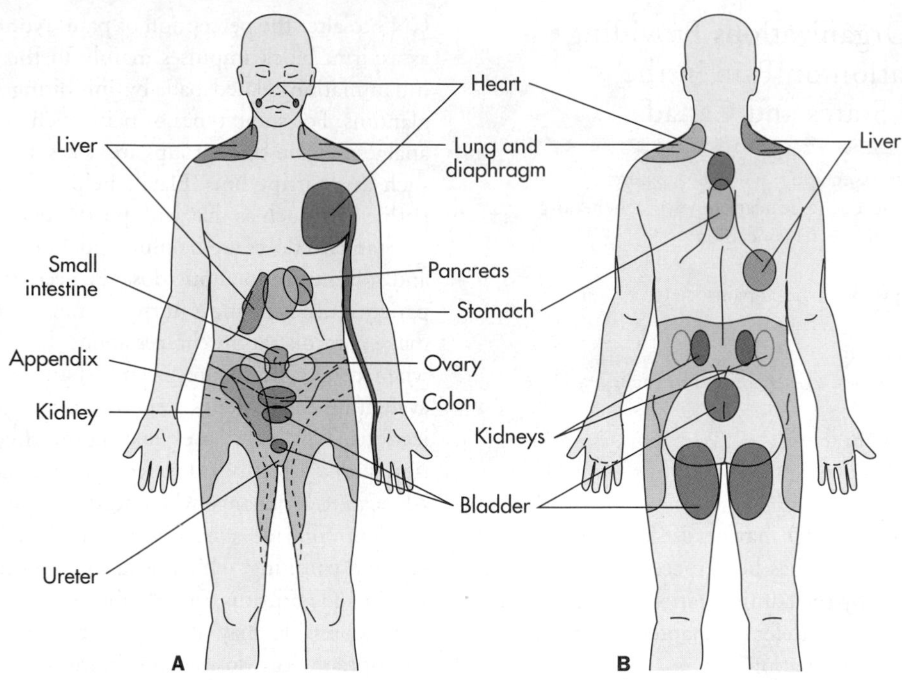

Figure 16-4 Usual sites of referred pain. **A,** Front. **B,** Back.

mixed agonist-antagonist that acts like naloxone when given to someone who is taking an agonist such as morphine on a regular basis. Therefore people receiving agonist opioids should not be given concurrent agonist-antagonist opioids, or a state of withdrawal will result.

Opioids are the most effective analgesic for the relief of moderate to severe pain and must be given on a regular basis to prevent pain from recurring. Side effects of opioids vary with the patient's physiologic state. Constipation is the most common side effect. Naloxone (Narcan) will reverse any depressive effect.

When administering opioids, it is important to distinguish between the effects of tolerance, physical dependence, and addiction[29]:

- **Tolerance**: Progressively larger doses are needed to produce the same analgesic effects.
- **Physical dependence**: Continuing drug use is required to prevent symptoms of withdrawal.
- **Addiction**: Adverse behavioral pattern features compulsion for drug and preoccupation with drug use predominantly for psychologic effect, despite actual or potential harm.

Drug tolerance occurs with some patients and with some conditions, usually when the patient's pain is first being controlled or when the pain increases. It is important to note that the reason for dose escalation may often be disease or pain progression, rather than tolerance.[29] Drug tolerance is a physiologic response and requires increasing the dose until pain relief is attained. Because there is no ceiling or maximal amount of opioid that can be given, drug tolerance should not preclude achievement of adequate analgesia.

Physical dependence is characterized by withdrawal symptoms concomitant with sudden decrease or abrupt termination of opioid use, or administration of an opioid antagonist.[29] Withdrawal symptoms may include vomiting, diarrhea, abdominal cramping, tremors, chills, diaphoresis, myalgia, arthralgia, and coryza. Physical dependence and drug tolerance are involuntary behaviors and are the physiologic result of frequent, ongoing opioid administration. Even when physical dependence and tolerance develop, symptoms of withdrawal rarely occur because, as pain decreases, the dosage is gradually tapered and no symptoms are experienced.

Physical dependence and drug tolerance do not represent addiction. Determination of opioid addiction requires expert assessment of risk factors for addiction and potential biopsychologic factors. Clinicians should not presume that patients' persistence or expression of the urgent need for pain relief is "drug-seeking" or addictive behavior. Opioid addiction is rare if medications are appropriately prescribed.[29] With expert care and supervision, opioids can be effective for those with a history of chemical dependency on opioids.[75] Guidelines for safe administration of opioids are available from a number of pain societies (see Box 16-5), as well as the practice setting.

Administration Routes. Opioids can be administered by a variety of routes. The oral route is preferred unless the patient is vomiting, is unable or not permitted to swallow, or is in acute pain. Oral opioids are generally available in immediate-release and sustained-release formulations. Immediate-release formulations typically achieve peak concentration in the blood within 30 to 60 minutes. Sustained-release preparations, such as morphine ER (MS Contin), are typically given every 8 to 12 hours, allowing less focus on the pain and better pain control with fewer side effects. Range of therapeutic effectiveness of sustained-release formulations varies (from 8 to 24 hours), depending on efficacy of biochemical mechanisms used to control drug absorption.[24]

TABLE 16-4 EQUIANALGESIC DOSES OF OPIOIDS COMMONLY USED FOR SEVERE PAIN

Name	Equianalgesic Dose (mg) Oral	Equianalgesic Dose (mg) Parenteral*	Comments
Morphinelike Agonists			
Morphine	30†	10	Standard of comparison for opioid analgesics; sustained-release preparations (MS Contin, Oramorph-SR) release drug over 3-12 hr
Hydromorphone (Dilaudid)	7.5	1.5	Slightly shorter duration than morphine
Oxycodone	30	—	
Methadone (Dolophine)	20	10	Good oral potency; long plasma half-life (24-36 hr) Accumulates with repetitive dosing, causing excessive sedation (on days 2-5)
Levorphanol (Levo-Dromoran)	4	2	Long plasma half-life (12-16 hr) Accumulates on days 2-3
Fentanyl	—	0.1	Transdermal fentanyl (Duragesic), 25-50 mcg/hr, roughly equivalent to 30 mg sustained-release morphine every 8 hr Because of skin reservoir of drug, 12-hr delay in onset and offset of transdermal patch; fever increases dose rate
Oxymorphone (Numorphan)	—	1	5 mg rectal suppository = 5 mg morphine intramuscularly
Meperidine (Demerol)	300	75	Slightly shorter acting than morphine Normeperidine (toxic metabolite) accumulates with repetitive dosing, causing central nervous system excitation; avoid in patients with impaired renal function or those receiving monoamine oxidase inhibitors
Mixed Agonist-Antagonists			
Nalbuphine (Nubain)	—	10	Not available orally; not scheduled under Controlled Substances Act Incidence of psychotomimetic effects lower than with pentazocine; may precipitate withdrawal in opioid-dependent patients
Butorphanol (Stadol)	—	2	Like nalbuphine
Dezocine (Dalgan)	—	10	Like nalbuphine May precipitate withdrawal in opioid-dependent patients; subcutaneous injection irritating
Partial Agonists			
Buprenorphine (Buprenex)	Sublingual	0.3	Used for treatment of opiod addiction (sublingual route for dependence); less abuse potential than morphine; does not produce psychotomimetic effects May precipitate withdrawal in opioid-dependent patients; not readily reversed by naloxone; avoid for women in labor

Adapted from American Pain Society Quality of Care Committee: Quality improvement guidelines for the treatment of acute and cancer pain, *JAMA* 274:1874, 1995.

*These are standard intramuscular (IM) doses for acute pain in adults and also may be used to convert doses for intravenous (IV) infusions and repeated small IV boluses. For single IV boluses, use half the IM dose.

†Some experts argue that 60 mg of oral morphine is the more accurate equivalent dose and suggest caution in converting patients from high doses of oral morphine to other drugs if the 30 mg equivalent is used.

Intravenous infusion and subcutaneous injections are also common administration routes. Injectable meperidine (Demerol) is given via intramuscular injection, but is *not recommended* because of its neurotoxic metabolite, normeperidine. Opioids may also be administered buccally, rectally, transdermally, sublingually, epidurally, or intranasally, as well as via the respiratory tract.[42] When intravenous access is not possible, sublingual, rectal, and buccal routes should be considered as alternatives to opioid injection. Selection of appropriate administration route depends on a thorough pain assessment and the nature of the pain problem.

Epidural infusions of opioids such as morphine or fentanyl can be administered through a catheter placed in the epidural or intrathecal space by the physician (Figure 16-5). An infusion device attached to the line provides a continuous supply of the opioid. This method relieves pain without diminishing CNS function. Patients with intractable pain can be well managed at home using this route.[42] Epidural administration is extremely effective and can help prevent perioperative complications such as myocardial ischemia, atelectasis, and infection. Epidural analgesia can also reduce dynamic pain after surgery caused by movement and deep breathing and coughing.[7]

With all administration routes, health care providers need to anticipate and manage common side effects of opioid administration. See the Guidelines for Safe Practice box for a summary of side effect management. Side effects of epidural administration include respiratory depression, postural hypotension, and urinary retention. The nurse should monitor patients for postural hypotension while transferring and ambulating, particularly when getting out of bed for the first time after surgery. Hypotension may be accompanied by nausea. Urinary retention is related to the opioid's effect on the detrusor muscle in the bladder. Most patients with epidural PCA have a Foley catheter for continuous drainage. The nurse should monitor the patient for neurologic deficits, including sensation and motor function in the lower extremities, and assess muscle strength before ambulation. The catheter site must be assessed for signs of infection. In addition, patients frequently report pruritus (itching), which can be severe. Antihistamines and comfort measures are effective for many patients, but occasionally it is necessary to reduce the opioid dosage or administer low-dose naloxone (Narcan), which generally controls the itching without reversing the analgesic effect.

PCA is a method that allows patients to administer their own opioids whenever they feel it is necessary. PCA may involve oral medications or an infusion system with a pump. With a PCA pump, the patient pushes a button to release a set amount of opioid by bolus intravenously, subcutaneously, or epidurally. A basal rate of infusion may be ordered in addition to the on-demand dosage. A refractory period prevents delivery of another bolus before a preset time interval. The device also records the patient's attempts to receive the opioid in a given period. A suggested protocol for intravenous PCA includes loading doses such as 3 to 5 mg of morphine, repeated every 5 minutes until the pain is decreased.[18,42] On-demand doses are usually 0.5 to 1.5 mg of morphine every 6 minutes to a maximum of 10 mg/hr. With shorter hospital stays, patients need to be given oral analgesics as soon as possible and have their pain well managed before discharge. Equianalgesic oral opioids can be started before or when the last PCA dose is given.

People using PCA tend to take less total analgesia than those receiving intermittent injections.[22,42] PCA is used for the management of postoperative pain, other types of acute pain such as sickle cell crisis, and cancer pain.[18,22] A major advantage to PCA is that it can meet pain relief needs of patients in a flexible manner compared with conventional analgesic methods.[46]

The nurse needs to assess patient concerns about addiction and side effects and to provide health teaching about addiction and side effects management before initiation of PCA.

Regional Anesthesia. Regional anesthesia is anesthesia of a part of the body using a plexus block, nerve block, subarachnoid or epidural block, or cryotherapy. A nerve block involves the injection of substances such as local anesthetics (e.g., bupivacaine, ropivacaine) or neurolytic agents (e.g., alcohol, phenol) near the nerve(s) to block conduction of impulses and provide symptomatic relief of pain. Nerve blocks are used to treat chronic pain associated with peripheral vascular disease, trigeminal neuralgia, causalgia, and cancer. Key nursing considerations for regional anesthesia include perfusion of the involved extremity, safety precautions with respect to ambulation and movement, and protection of the extremity(ies) with decreased sensation from harm.

Sedation and Analgesia. Sedation and analgesia (previously known as conscious sedation) involves the administration of drugs to produce a state of sedation and analgesia (see Chapter 14 for additional discussion). This medically controlled state of depressed consciousness allows the patient to (1) maintain protective reflexes, (2) maintain a patent airway independently and continuously, and

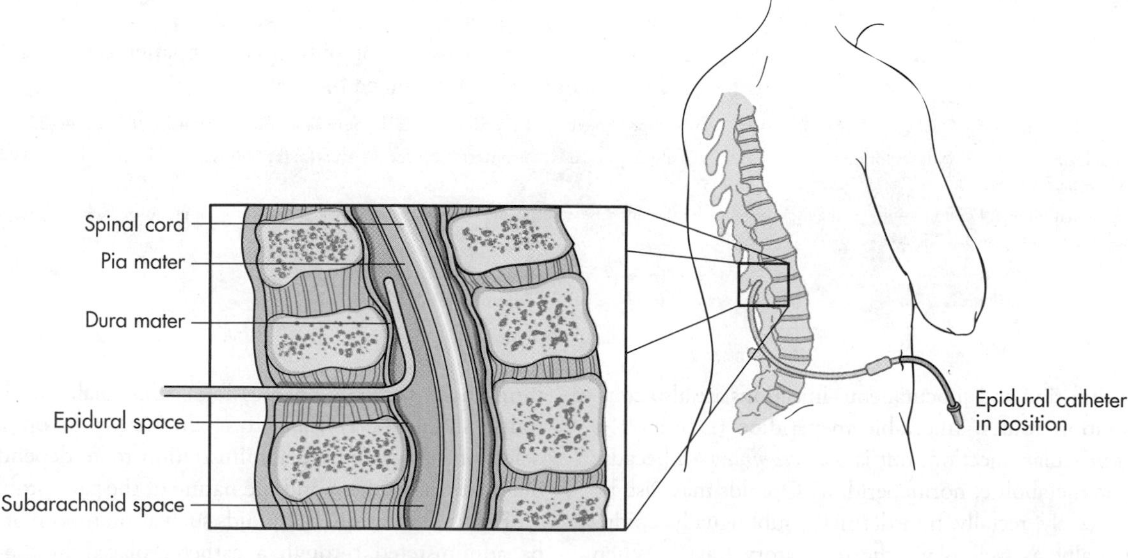

Figure 16-5 Site of epidural catheter placement.

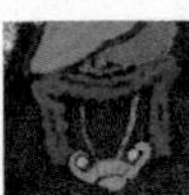

GUIDELINES FOR SAFE PRACTICE *Managing Opioid Side Effects*

Opioid Side Effects

Hypotension (particularly postural hypotension)
Decreased respirations and decreased cough
Dizziness and sedation
Constipation
Nausea

Preventing Constipation

Opioids bind to receptor sites in the gastrointestinal (GI) tract and slow GI motility. The resultant constipation is best managed by administering a stool softener or stimulant as soon as the opioid is started. Monitor the patient's bowel pattern carefully and ensure adequate fluids.

Managing Sedation

The sedative effects of opioids on the central nervous system last from 1 to 3 days and then the patient builds up tolerance. Initially it may be beneficial to allow the patient to catch up on needed sleep. If problematic:

—Reduce the opioid dose, add a nonsteroidal antiinflammatory drug if possible, or administer more frequently.
—Change the opioid and evaluate the patient's response.
—Monitor respiratory rate and track the patient's sedation level using a sedation scale.
—Have a reversal agent available for use if needed (e.g., naloxone [Narcan]).

Managing Nausea

Nausea is believed to result from stimulation of the chemoreceptor trigger zone in the brain and decreased GI motility. Tolerance to the effects usually develops within a few days. If problematic:

—Administer an antiemetic such as prochlorperazine (Compazine). Administer on a scheduled basis, not as needed.
—Add metoclopramide (Reglan) if antiemetics are initially ineffective.
—Change the opioid if nausea persists.

Preventing Respiratory Depression

Effective pain relief allows the patient to be more active in self-care, get out of bed, and ambulate more freely, which counter the effects of respiratory depression. In addition:

—Encourage deep breathing and the use of incentive spirometry.
—Monitor the patient's sedation level. Respiratory depression is usually only a problem when sedation becomes excessive.

Ensuring Safety

Orthostatic hypotension and dizziness cause an increased risk for injury. Teach patients to change positions slowly, and monitor their early attempts to be out of bed.

(3) respond to physical stimulation or verbal command (e.g., "open your eyes"). Nurses involved in the administration of these drugs must understand the sedation continuum. Under the direction of a physician, the nurse may be responsible for the medication and monitoring of persons receiving sedation and analgesia.

Nursing care of the patient under conscious sedation requires expert knowledge of the agents being used and continuous one-on-one monitoring. Thus special training within a well-equipped clinical setting is required. This training involves learning institution-specific protocols for preparing and administering the sedative agents, continuous assessment, maintaining and supporting the patient's airway until recovery, and strategies for emergency management of adverse events such as respiratory arrest (e.g., administration of reversal agent as ordered, emergency airway support).

NONOPIOID ANALGESICS. Mild to moderate pain generally can be controlled by nonopioid analgesics, most commonly NSAIDs such as aspirin, and by acetaminophen. Acetaminophen (Tylenol, Datril) is comparable to aspirin in analgesic effect, but, unlike aspirin, lacks any antiinflammatory action. Although acetaminophen does not alter the prothrombin level and has fewer side effects, overdoses can cause severe liver damage. This analgesic is useful for persons who are allergic to aspirin or for whom aspirin is contraindicated, such as persons with peptic ulcers.

The NSAIDs are the most widely used analgesics because of their general lack of serious side effects and their effectiveness in pain relief.[42] These drugs act primarily by inhibiting the synthesis of prostaglandins, which "sensitize" nerve endings and trigger pain. In lower doses NSAIDs have analgesic properties; in higher doses there is antiinflammatory action in addition to analgesia. NSAIDs are used to control the moderate pain of dysmenorrhea, arthritis, and other musculoskeletal disorders (see Chapter 53), postoperative pain, and migraine headaches. Other indications include analgesia for patients with bone cancer. Table 16-5 lists NSAIDs commonly used for pain management.

NSAIDs, particularly acetylsalicylic acid (aspirin), inhibit platelet aggregation and increase bleeding time. Common side effects include GI disturbances, dizziness, tinnitus, and headache. Persons who are hypersensitive to aspirin may be hypersensitive to other NSAIDs. In addition to blocking prostaglandin synthesis, salicylates also produce analgesia by blocking pain impulses peripherally or centrally, possibly in the hypothalamus. Aspirin is also a weak vitamin K antagonist and prolongs prothrombin time when given in large doses. Therefore aspirin is contraindicated for persons receiving anticoagulants or other NSAIDs. Aspirin should be avoided by persons with a history of bleeding disorders or peptic ulcer and by children and teenagers because of the risk of Reye's syndrome.

Two classifications of NSAIDs are available: the traditional COX-1 inhibitory agents that block prostaglandins in gastric mucosa and hemostasis, and newer COX-2 inhibitory agents that are thought to be selective to pain, inflammation, and fever.[67] COX NSAIDS inactivate cyclooxygenases, enzymes involved in inflammation. Irritation of the gastric mucosa is a common side effect of COX-1 NSAIDs, and dyspepsia can occur with COX-2 formulations.[8] Therefore these drugs should be taken with meals or with a snack such as a glass of milk. The protein structure of COX-2 is larger than that of COX-1, allowing for its selective inhibition via COX-2 agents.

TABLE 16-5
COMMON MEDICATIONS *for Mild-to-Moderate Pain: NSAIDs*

Drug	Action	Nursing Intervention
Acetylsalicylic acid (aspirin)	Inhibits formation of prostaglandins, which are involved in production of pain and inflammation Blocks pain impulses peripherally and/or centrally, possibly in hypothalamus Is weak vitamin K antagonist and prolongs prothrombin time Powerfully inhibits platelet aggregation	Teach patient to: Minimize gastric irritation by taking with food, full glass of liquid, or antacid Consider enteric-coated preparations if GI upset persists Immediately report any bleeding (e.g., bruising, gums, nose bleed, urine, stool)
Ibuprofen (Advil, Motrin) Naproxen, naproxen sodium (Anaprox, Naprosyn, Aleve) Ketoprofen (Orudis) Fenoprofen (Nalfon) Mefenamic acid (Ponstel) Ketorolac tromethamine (Toradol)	As above, inhibits prostaglandin synthesis Inhibits platelet aggregation	Teach patient to: Take on empty stomach with full glass of water unless GI upset occurs As above, report any bleeding Avoid concurrent use of aspirin, alcohol, other NSAIDs Monitor renal and hepatic function When given intramuscularly, must be administered deeply into large muscle

GI, Gastrointestinal, *NSAID*, nonsteroidal antiinflammatory drug.

ADJUVANT MEDICATIONS. Adjuvant drugs may be given with analgesics to augment pain relief.[42] These drugs are also an option for pain relief when other analgesics are not effective.

Sedatives and antianxiety agents sometimes are prescribed for persons with pain. These drugs do not have any analgesic effects, but may permit relaxation and sleep, decrease anxiety, prevent an increase in pain, or enable the person to cope more effectively with the pain.

Phenothiazines such as promethazine (Phenergan) do not potentiate the analgesic effect of opioids. However, they do increase opioid-related sedation, hypotension, and respiratory depression and should not be used for pain relief.[26] In some persons sedatives and antianxiety agents may lead to disorientation and agitation, which can increase the pain and decrease the person's ability to cope. Treating pain with analgesics is the more effective and preferred method.

Tricyclic antidepressants such as amitriptyline produce analgesia at doses lower than those used for depression (an average of 50 to 75 mg/day).[74] These drugs are useful in nerve injury pain, such as with postherpetic neuralgia. They are believed to prevent the uptake of serotonin and norepinephrine in the descending inhibitory modulation in the spinal cord and reduce sensitization mechanisms.

A variety of other medications may be used as adjuvants for pain relief. Anticonvulsants such as carbamazepine (Tegretol), phenytoin (Dilantin), and gabapentin (Neurontin) are used to suppress abnormal (ectopic) nerve discharges that occur in nerve injury pain such as trigeminal neuralgia.[26] Dexamethasone (Decadron), a corticosteroid, is helpful in relieving pain from increased intracranial pressure, nerve compression, spinal cord compression, bowel obstruction, and bone metastases. Corticosteroids block the production of arachidonic acid, which is necessary for the synthesis of prostaglandins and other inflammatory chemicals that cause pain.[26] These drugs also stimulate appetite and may elevate mood. Counterirritants are over-the-counter drugs that relieve local pain by producing counterirritation (stimulation of the large A-beta fibers). Examples of counterirritants include ointments containing methylsalicylate (oil of wintergreen) or ethyl aminobenzoate and oil of cloves (for toothaches).

▶ ARE YOU READY?

Which of the following statements by the patient about the ordered patient-controlled analgesia pump indicates the need for further teaching?

1. "I can push the button when I need more medication."
2. "I am relieved that I cannot overdose myself."
3. "I should not let the pain get too severe before pushing the button."
4. "I have instructed my spouse to push the button every 20 minutes if I fall asleep."

Nonpharmacologic Approaches

Nonpharmacologic approaches can be used with analgesics for effective pain management.[42] This type of intervention can alter pain transmission, modify the response to pain, and modify the pain stimulus. This section discusses physical strategies that are invasive or nonnursing interventions. Nursing measures are discussed under Nursing Management.

Altering Pain Transmission

ELECTRICAL STIMULATORS. The purpose of an electrical stimulator is to modify the pain stimulus by blocking or changing the painful stimulus with another perceived as less painful. The GCT suggests that stimulating large myelinated A-beta fibers "closes the gate" to pain stimuli.[48] Selected forms of electrical stimulation may activate the descending inhibitory system.

TENS uses a battery-powered stimulator worn externally. This is a convenient, nonintrusive, adjunctive pain therapy that the patient can easily learn. Success is variable, and the device is typically used with other pain therapies.

A number of TENS devices are available; all consist of a battery-powered portable pulse generator about the size of a pocket pager. Control knobs on the generator permit adjustment of the impulse. The generator is connected by a pair of cables to electrically conductive adhesive electrodes placed at appropriate sites on the skin. TENS delivers a balanced biphasic potential in a waveform, typically in frequencies from 10 to 50 Hz; intensity is determined by patient response.

TENS may be effective for postoperative pain, posttraumatic pain, phantom limb pain, peripheral neuralgias, lower back pain, and muscle pain. Although it can be effective for mild or moderate pain, it is less effective for severe pain. Analgesia from TENS is widely debated, since few clinical trials have been done to support its effectiveness for pain relief.[63] Despite equivocal evidence, TENS has few contraindications and may be effective for some people. Nurses are responsible for monitoring the effectiveness of treatments and for patient teaching concerning the safe use of TENS (see the Patient/Family Teaching box).

TENS electrodes should not be placed over hair, irritated or open skin, sutures, the carotid sinus (may produce bradycardia), laryngeal or pharyngeal muscles (may trigger spasms), or the uterus of a pregnant woman. A cardiac pacemaker may interfere with TENS effects. Suggested electrode placement may include (1) directly over the painful area, (2) at trigger points along the nerve pathways, or (3) at trigger points in the same dermatome as the pain.

Spinal cord stimulators are similar to TENS except that they require an invasive procedure to place electrodes on or near the spinal cord. This is achieved either surgically over the ventral surface of the spinal cord or percutaneously through the back into the epidural space. Because the percutaneously inserted spinal cord electrical stimulator can be inserted under local anesthesia, it is preferred over surgical placement of dorsal column stimulator electrodes. Postoperative care after dorsal column stimulator implantation includes the same care that follows laminectomy (see Chapter 53), with monitoring for infection and leakage of cerebrospinal fluid.

ACUPUNCTURE. Acupuncture is an ancient form of disease treatment that can be used for pain relief. Developed in Asia, this method has become more popular in Western countries. The practitioner skillfully inserts small needles and manipulates them at specific body points, depending on the type and location of pain. The GCT provides the best explanation for the effectiveness of acupuncture. The local stimulation of large-diameter fibers by the needles "closes the gate" to pain. It is not known to what extent the psyche and the power of suggestion contribute to the effectiveness of this therapy.

NEUROSURGICAL PROCEDURES. Neurosurgical procedures do not play a major role in management of chronic pain.[25] Major limitations include short duration of relief, occurrence of dysesthesia (pain induced by gentle touch of the skin), central pain syndrome (burning sensations in skin areas lacking sensation from surgical afferent interruptions), and possible further neurologic dysfunction.[42] However, for relentless chronic pain that cannot be controlled by analgesics (intractable pain), various neurosurgical procedures may reduce or eliminate the pain (Box 16-6). Other forms of pain control usually are attempted before neurosurgical intervention.

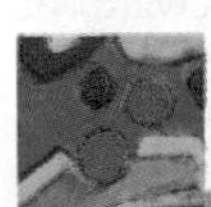

PATIENT/FAMILY TEACHING *The Use of Transcutaneous Electrical Nerve Stimulation*

Teach the patient to:

- Remove and clean electrodes daily.
- Wash skin with soap and water.
- Allow skin to air dry.
- Wipe skin with a prep pad before reapplying the conductor pad.
- Check the battery if numbness or tingling is not felt during treatments.
- Report if sensation is either absent or uncomfortable.

Modifying Pain Response. A wide range of strategies are available for modifying the pain response. Many of these strategies are within the realm of independent nursing practice and are discussed in the next section. Others may be used by nurses with special training but are frequently used by other members of the collaborative care team.

BEHAVIOR MODIFICATION. Behavior modification consists of a planned change in the way a person behaves by means of rewarding desired behavior and ignoring undesirable behavior. Forms of behavior modification are used unconsciously all the time: a young child "throwing a tantrum" may be ignored, but as the behavior becomes more appropriate, the child's mother may reward him or her with time and attention.

Behavior modification may be useful for persons with chronic pain. For example, one protocol for patients with chronic lower back pain is to set a limit of 10 minutes daily for discussion of their pain experiences (with the exception of data-gathering interviews). Pain medications are prescribed on a regular schedule to

BOX 16-6 Neurosurgical Procedures for Pain Control

- *Neurectomy:* severing of nerve fibers from the cell body
- *Rhizotomy:* resection of posterior nerve root before it enters spinal cord
- *Cordotomy:* severing of ascending anterolateral pain-conducting pathways of spinal cord
- *Sympathectomy:* excision or destruction of one or more sympathetic ganglia or nerves

dissociate the feelings of pain with inappropriate use (reward) of analgesics or other unhealthy behaviors.

In using behavioral methods to alter pain-associated behavior or to encourage patient activities, the health care team can achieve success only with a consistent approach. Although the nurse should always praise patients for their efforts to comply or assist with treatment regimens, a true behavior modification program requires careful analysis of patient behavior and development of a specific and comprehensive treatment plan.

Biofeedback and Autogenic Training. Some persons are able to alter their body functions through mental concentration. Biofeedback training uses an electroencephalograph to monitor brain wave activity. The individual concentrates on slowing his or her brain wave activity to rates at which pain and distress are unlikely to cause discomfort (i.e., complete relaxation). It may take months of practice to achieve the desired level of control. The nurse should encourage and praise the person's efforts.

In autogenic training the same type of self-regulation is used to alter various autonomic nervous system functions, such as pulse, blood pressure, and muscle tension. The use of transcendental meditation and other methods of concentration and self-control may achieve the same degree of autoregulation without the use of sophisticated physiologic monitoring equipment.

Psychoeducation. Increasing attention is being given to psychoeducation as an adjunctive means to manage the impact of chronic pain on health-related quality of life and disability[36,45] (see Research box). Psychoeducation interventions are group self-management education programs delivered by a trained facilitator. Participants may be accompanied by family members or friends. The focus is to help participants increase their potential for self-care. Through rehearsal and application of various cognitive and behavioral self-management techniques, participants learn to set realistic self-management goals. The goal-setting process allows the individual to take control in managing symptoms, thereby improving the patient's perceived self-efficacy. Nurses facilitating psychoeducation programs require expertise in group process and assessment of participants' readiness to engage in self-management.

Hypnosis. Hypnosis may be used in the treatment of various conditions, particularly those aggravated by tension and stress. The practitioner helps patients alter their perception of pain through the acceptance of positive suggestions made to the subconscious. Many persons are able to learn self-hypnosis. Individuals vary widely in their suggestibility and readiness to try this approach. The nurse's most helpful role may be to support the patient's desire to make hypnosis work.

Nursing Management

of the Patient experiencing Pain

Assessment

Effective pain management can occur only with systematic, regular assessments. An important nursing intervention is assessing subjective and objective data at least once a shift and often more

Research

LeFort SM et al: Randomized controlled trial of a community-based psychoeducation program for the self-management of chronic pain, *Pain* 74(2-3):297-306, 1998.

This study examined the effectiveness of a low-cost, community-based, nurse-run group psychoeducation program for improving pain-related and other quality-of-life outcomes for those living with chronic musculoskeletal pain problems. One hundred and ten participants were randomized to either (1) a 12-hour chronic pain self-management program, or (2) a 3-month wait-list control. At 3 months the treatment group showed significantly improved scores in pain, dependency, vitality, aspects of role functioning, life satisfaction, self-efficacy to manage pain, and resourcefulness compared with controls. This research demonstrated short-term effectiveness of psychoeducation for key pain-related outcomes and has provided preliminary data for evaluation of the long-term effectiveness of a standard nursing psychoeducation intervention for the self-management of chronic musculoskeletal pain.

frequently when pain is anticipated.[34] Patient input is important, since health professionals and patients assess pain differently.[13,81] It is crucial to gather as much information as possible from the patient to avoid making incorrect assumptions about pain. To aid in data collection and to evaluate the effectiveness of interventions, a variety of pain assessment tools are available.[17,20,42,50]

Although many patients continue to experience postoperative pain, many will not ask for help[72,81,84] (see Research box). For this reason, it is best to use a numeric rating scale (e.g., 0 to 10 scale, where 0 is no pain and 10 is the worst possible pain) to validate the pain the patient is experiencing. The numeric rating scale is valid and easy to use. The frequency of assessment varies depending on the intensity of the patient's pain and the pharmacokinetics of the analgesic given. If the pain intensity does not decrease after analgesic administration, further assessment is indicated, including drug choice and dosage.

Health History. Most patients have previously experienced severe pain and continue to expect severe pain after surgery.[81,84] The nurse needs to ask patients on admission about their expectations, knowledge, and concerns about pain.[71] Many persons are unaware they are expected to speak out when they have pain or discomfort. Some patients think they will be considered "complainers" or "bad patients" if they state that they are in pain. Then the nurse should teach them how and when to verbalize their discomfort and the various methods available for pain relief. As already mentioned, the best assessment of pain is the patient's own evaluation.

Data to be collected by the nurse include the location, intensity, quality, timing (onset, duration, frequency, cause), and aggravating and relieving factors. One approach for evaluating these characteristics is the use of the mnemonic PQRST:

P: Provoking factors: what makes the pain worse or relieves it
Q: Quality: dull, sharp, crushing
R: Region or radiation: site and radiation to other areas
S: Severity or intensity
T: Time: onset, duration, frequency, cause

Research

Watt-Watson J et al: The impact of nurses' empathic responses on patients' pain management in acute care, *Nurs Res* 49:4, 2000.

In this study researchers interviewed 225 patients on their third day after coronary bypass graft surgery, along with their assigned nurses (n=94), to examine the relationship between nurses' empathic responses and their patients' pain intensity and analgesic administration after surgery. Most patients reported moderate to severe pain, yet received only 47% of their prescribed analgesia. Two thirds of patients did not see their nurse as a resource for their pain management. Although most patients said they would not ask for help with pain, their nurses expected them to. Nurses' responses to pain intensity were moderately empathic and did not influence their patients' pain intensity or analgesic use. Deficits in knowledge and misbeliefs about pain management, which would have limited empathic responses, were evident.

Diagrams of the body can help patients point out the sites of their pain (Figure 16-6). Pain intensity can be assessed using several measures, as outlined in Box 16-7. The nurse documents the patient's numeric rating of pain intensity and discusses intervention options for ratings greater than 3. Ratings can be recorded on a vital sign sheet similar to temperature and blood pressure data. More detailed flow sheets are also helpful for ongoing assessment of progression of the pain and responses to various interventions (Figure 16-7). The nurse should assess pain intensity at least once a shift or more often if the patient rated his or her pain at 4 or greater (on a 0 to 10 scale) and is receiving interventions for pain (such as analgesics, relaxation exercises, or TENS). When acute pain has subsided, the nurse can collect further data about the meaning of pain for the person. Long-term pain requires a more in-depth assessment. Hospitals or pain clinics using a team approach for chronic pain often develop their own pain history form or questionnaire. One or more health team members may collect this history.

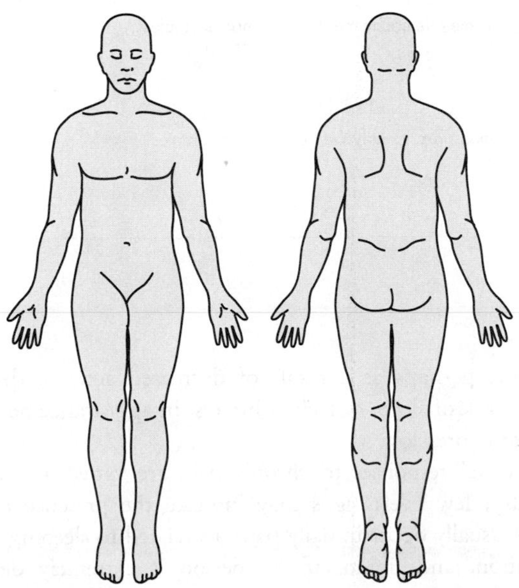

Figure 16-6 Body diagrams for pointing out sites of pain.

Box 16-7 Examples of Pain Intensity Rating Scales

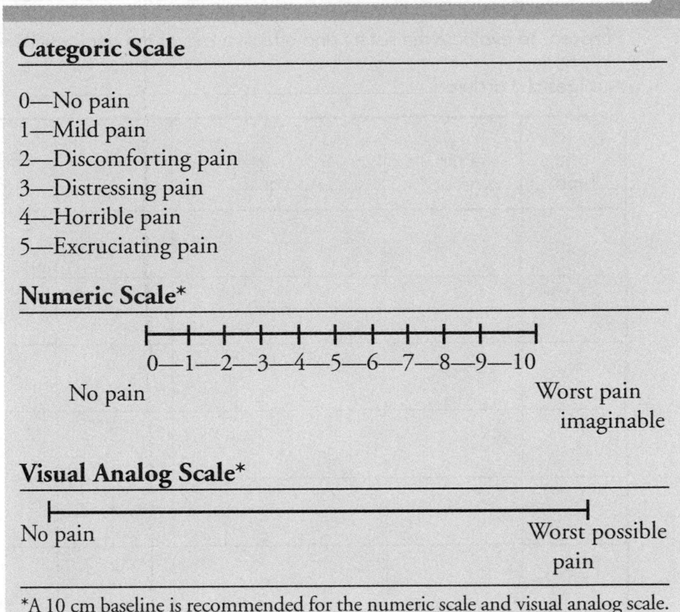

Categoric Scale

0—No pain
1—Mild pain
2—Discomforting pain
3—Distressing pain
4—Horrible pain
5—Excruciating pain

Numeric Scale*

0—1—2—3—4—5—6—7—8—9—10

No pain / Worst pain imaginable

Visual Analog Scale*

No pain / Worst possible pain

*A 10 cm baseline is recommended for the numeric scale and visual analog scale.

Assess for:

- History of the pain pattern from time of onset
- Factors perceived to increase or decrease the pain
- Effects of the pain on the person's lifestyle, including work, family responsibilities, sexuality, leisure, sleep, nutrition, and activity
- Meaning of the pain for the person
- Effects of the patient's pain on other family members or friends
- Methods used for pain control and their effectiveness

Physical Examination. Physiologic and behavioral data help the nurse identify possible pain or discomfort in a person who has not reported pain or is unable to do so (see Clinical Manifestations box). Physiologic signs of pain result from activation of the sympathetic nervous system. With severe pain, neurogenic shock may result from the stress to the system. The behavioral signs are not specific to pain; therefore, if the observable data suggest that pain may be present, the nurse must elicit subjective data to validate the assumption where possible.

Assess for:

- Appearance (grimacing, gritting teeth, clenching fists, lying rigidly as if afraid to move)
- Motor behavior
- Affective and verbal responses
- Vital signs
- Skin moisture and color
- Tenderness of painful area
- Presence of trigger points that initiate pain

Sometimes the patient's behavior does not seem to match his or her verbalization of pain. For example, the patient may request an analgesic, a back rub, or other measure to relieve pain; but when the nurse arrives to carry out the request, the patient is asleep. However, the patient who is sleeping or lying quietly is not necessarily pain

Patient ______________________________ Date ______________

*Pain rating scale used ______________________________

Purpose: To evaluate the safety and effectiveness of the analgesic(s).

Analgesic(s) ordered: ______________________________

Time	Pain rating*	Analgesic	R	P	BP	Level of arousal†	Other‡	Plan and comments

* Pain rating: A number of different scales may be used. Indicate which scale is used and use the same one each time. Two common examples:
- 0 to 10 with 0 being no pain and 10 being as bad as it can be.
- Melzack's scale:
0 = no pain; 1 = mild; 2 = discomforting; 3 = distressing; 4 = horrible; 5 = excruciating

† Possible arousal scale: 1 = wide awake; 2 = drowsy; 3 = sleeping; 4 = difficult to arouse

‡ Possibilities for other columns: bowel function, activities, nausea and vomiting, other pain relief measures. Identify the side effects of greatest concern to patient, family, physician, nurses, etc.

Figure 16-7 Flow sheet for monitoring patient's response to pain.

free. The patient may be exhausted from the pain, and sleeping is a coping mechanism. Patients may also use distraction such as talking and joking with visitors to manage unrelieved pain. The person's self-report of pain is the key to effective management.

Physiologic signs of pain can disappear quickly for the person with acute pain and are typically not present with chronic pain because of the body's compensatory mechanisms. Although the person adapts to the pain stimuli, the pain persists. The absence of physiologic signs, therefore, does not indicate absence of pain. Prolonged pain, however, may change the person's appearance over time, perhaps as a result of decreased activity, decreased appetite, lack of sleep, or lack of interest in appearance because of fatigue or depression.

Behavioral responses to chronic pain are varied and unique. Here, also, few overt signs may indicate the presence of pain. Changes usually occur in daily patterns related to sleeping, eating, socialization, and libido. If the person is extremely depressed because of ongoing pain, the nurse may note withdrawal behaviors.

Pain assessment is particularly complex when the person is unable to describe what he or she is experiencing, as in patients with developmental issues or cognitive impairment. Older people with normal to moderately impaired cognitive function, as well as some severely impaired older adults, have been found capable of rating their pain using self-report scales.[39] Research is ongoing to develop valid behavioral measures to help assess pain more accurately in this population (see Research box).

NURSING DIAGNOSES, OUTCOMES, AND INTERVENTIONS

Nursing Diagnosis: Acute Pain

OUTCOMES. Common examples of expected outcomes for the patient with a diagnosis of *acute pain* are:

Patient will:

- State pain intensity as mild or less (e.g., 4) on a scale of 0 to 10 (0, no pain; 10, most severe pain imaginable), and describe quality, location, and aggravating or alleviating factors of pain.
- Demonstrate relaxed facial expression and body position and participates in activities.
- Discuss concerns about asking for help and taking analgesics.

NURSING INTERVENTIONS. The nurse's role in planning and monitoring outcomes of care is critical for effective pain management. The initial thorough assessment serves as the foundation for establishing priorities and devising treatment strategies. The Guidelines for Safe Practice box contains some basic principles of pain management for guidance in the planning period.[1] The patient's ability and desire to play an active role in using pain relief measures needs to be considered. Decreased ability results from severe pain, fatigue, sedation, depression, or unconsciousness. Decreased desire or will occurs in some persons with chronic pain who have experienced numerous failures in pain relief. The nurse is able to function independently with many interventions, but careful planning with other members of the health care team is essential to ensure that all have the same patient outcomes or goals in mind. The patient and family are included in all planning activities if possible.

One aspect of the treatment plan that often is neglected is incorporating measures the *patient* thinks may help relieve the pain, even if these measures differ from those usually carried out in that institution. Without encouragement, the patient may hesitate to mention these remedies (e.g., nonprescription liniments, special applications of heat and cold, unusual positioning, favorite homemade foods or drinks, the use of music, humor, or t'ai chi). If the remedy the patient wishes to try has no contraindications, the health care team may consider using it before trying other relief measures.

Time constraints can make planning difficult. However, arranging for the same group of health care providers to care for the patient helps ensure a more consistent approach and care plan. The small group of health care team members and the patient can develop a care plan that honors the patient's decisions, and they can develop a daily routine that reduces anxiety and frustration. The plan should include, if appropriate, premedication before uncomfortable procedures, specified blocks of time for rest or napping, and coordination between various departments such as physical therapy and occupational therapy. For some patients fatigue is a significant problem, and regular visits to off-unit departments should be interspersed with rest periods; for other patients the most beneficial plan includes going directly from one department to the next so that time is not wasted getting in and out of bed or performing other painful maneuvers.

Pain is a complex experience involving sensory, affective, and behavioral components that require a multimodal treatment approach. Pain such as muscle spasms in the lower back may be relieved more effectively by heat and ultrasound than by medications. Strategies such as breathing exercises, muscle relaxation, imagery, and distraction do not replace analgesics for patients who need pharmacologic management, but can be useful adjuncts in treatment. Nonpharmacologic interventions can be effective in reducing the dose of medication required and in decreasing the pain while the patient waits for pain medication to work.

Guided imagery is a term that describes the use of guidance-invoked images to improve physiologic status, mental state, self-image, or behavior. Imagery techniques require practice to be

Research

Feldt K: The checklist of nonverbal pain indicators (CNPI), *Pain Manage Nurs* 1:1, 2000.

The checklist of nonverbal pain indicators (CNPI) was designed to measure pain behaviors in cognitively impaired older adults. Pilot testing of the instrument with people over 65 years old (X=83 years) with hip fractures demonstrated that pain was poorly tolerated in older patients, particularly those who were very elderly and those who were cognitively impaired. Nurses in both acute and long-term care settings have indicated a need for a measure to assess pain in cognitively impaired elders. The CNPI is a simple, dichotomous measure of six observed pain behaviors, including verbal and nonverbal vocalizations, grimacing, bracing, rubbing, and restlessness. The CNPI has preliminary reliability and validity; further testing is in progress.

CLINICAL MANIFESTATIONS
Acute Pain

Physiologic Signs

Pulse: increased rate
Respirations: increased depth and frequency
Blood pressure: increased systolic and diastolic
Diaphoresis, pallor
Dilated pupils
Muscle tension (face, body)
Nausea and vomiting (if pain is severe)

Behavioral Signs

Rigid body position
Restlessness
Frowning
Clenched teeth
Clenched fists
Crying
Moaning

GUIDELINES FOR SAFE PRACTICE
ABC Principles of Pain Assessment and Planning

A Ask about pain regularly.
Assess pain systematically.
B Believe the patient and family in their reports of pain and what relieves it.
C Choose pain control options appropriate for the patient, family, and setting.
D Deliver interventions in a timely, logical, and coordinated fashion.
E Empower patients and their families.
Enable them to control their course to the greatest extent possible.

Complementary & Alternative Therapies

Therapeutic Touch

The rationale for the success of therapeutic touch is not clearly understood, and related research is limited. Many health care professionals reject therapeutic touch, but it has been shown to be helpful for some patients and some types of pain. Before implementing this technique, the nurse requires special education and training. The nurse undergoes a brief period of meditation before deliberately moving his or her hands over the patient's body to assess, direct, or modulate body energy patterns. The nurse does not touch the patient's skin. In theory, the nurse is focusing his or her own internal energy and then transmitting this healing energy to the patient.

effective, and the level of concentration required may be unattainable for patients who are fatigued from acute or chronic pain. Imagery can be used simply to support mental relaxation by visualizing oneself in a favorite setting such as a quiet beach, or it can be a more active part of the pain management plan. Patients can consciously control the pain experience by using complex images of their pain such as fire that is gradually extinguished. The technique works best when the patient selects the image and decides how it is to be used. Guided imagery audiotapes are also widely available.

Complementary and alternative therapies are well suited as adjuncts to the management of acute and chronic pain. Relaxation techniques and massage are commonly used for the treatment of back and chronic pain.[42] Music has been successful in decreasing postoperative pain levels. The use of companion animals may help some patients relax.[42] For patients who are unable to actively engage in relaxation techniques, superficial massage can reduce muscle tension and anxiety.[42] By relaxing muscles, massage may also reduce pain. The most easily accessible areas of the body to massage are the back and shoulders, but the hands and feet may also be massaged. Therapeutic touch may be helpful to patients in pain[42,64] (see the Complementary & Alternative Therapies box).

Cutaneous (dermal) stimulation is thought to innervate the large A-beta fibers, closing the gate to impulses from the periphery.[63,86] The physician may order TENS (previously discussed). Strategies that nurses can use include massage, light rubbing of the area involved or of a contralateral site, whirlpool baths, heat, or cold. These interventions are effective, simple, low risk, not time consuming, and inexpensive. Patients may need to try several to find which ones have the best effects. Box 16-8 lists various alternatives for the application of heat. The Guidelines for Safe Practice box, p. 353, top, reviews the basic principles for the safe use of these interventions.

Patients who are immobilized or who splint (guard) a body part to minimize pain need to be encouraged to perform passive or active exercises when possible to prevent complications. Premedication may be necessary to prevent or reduce pain. For example, when the body or an extremity is moved, supporting the trunk or extremity prevents an increase in pain by unilateral pulling on muscles, joints, and ligaments. The Guidelines for Safe Practice box, p. 353, middle, summarizes interventions for nurses and home caregivers to reduce the pain associated with positioning.

Box 16-8 Types of Heat Application

Superficial Heat

Dry heat: heating pad, hot-water bottle, lamp, sun
Moist heat: whirlpool baths, soaks, hydrocollator packs

Deep Heat

Short-wave diathermy
Ultrasound vibration
Microwave diathermy (contraindicated if patient has implanted cardiac pacemaker)

The patient's physical environment can create sensory overload and potentiate the pain stimuli. If nurses would stand still for 5 minutes in the patient's environment and watch and listen, they might understand that some patients are continuously bombarded with noise and visual stimulation. Modifying the environment may be helpful, but not all patients respond positively to the same environment. Some patients may benefit from a quiet room with minimal lighting, whereas others prefer a bright environment with distractions such as television or music. The nurse can explore possible changes with the patient and implement any acceptable suggestions. The Guidelines for Safe Practice box on p. 353, bottom, lists potential environmental modifications.

The American Pain Society (APS) quality improvement guidelines[1,2] identify assessment and treatment with analgesics as the two most important components of care for patients with acute pain or cancer pain. Monitoring outcomes is an important component of the APS guidelines (Box 16-9). When health professionals are more knowledgeable about pain assessment and management, they are better prepared to clarify patient concerns and help them with management. Patients may have concerns about being a "good" patient or fears about analgesics that interfere with their reporting pain[73] (Box 16-10). Nurses need to ask patients about these concerns. Addiction from taking opioids continues to be a concern for both health professionals and patients. However, the incidence of opioid addiction in hospitalized patients is less than 1%.[29] Nurses can ask patients who are concerned about

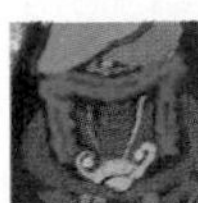

GUIDELINES FOR SAFE PRACTICE *Using Heat and Cold Effectively*

- Explain the options available, and involve the patient in choosing which options to use. Ice is rarely the patient's first choice, but it probably is a more effective pain reliever than heat.
- Apply heat and cold directly to the site of pain; if this is not possible, use them:
  —Around the painful site
  —Between the pain and the brain
  —On the opposite side of the body from the pain site
  —Over acupuncture or trigger point sites
- Use heat and cold at a comfortable intensity. They should not cause pain.
- Apply heat and cold for 20 to 30 minutes at a time. The minimal effective time is about 10 minutes. Ice should not be applied for longer than 10 minutes to minimize the chance of tissue damage.
- Encourage the patient to explore options for frequency of application. Alternating heat and cold can be effective in some situations.
- Do not apply heat or cold directly to the skin. Cover the heat source or cold pack with a towel before applying to skin. Assess the skin after every application.
- Use heat and cold before pain becomes severe whenever possible.

Adapted from McCaffery M, Pasero C: *Pain: clinical manual,* ed 2, St Louis, 1999, Mosby.

becoming addicted, "Would you take this medication if you were not in pain?" Unfortunately, health professionals are also overly concerned about addiction, and opioids are underprescribed by physicians and underadministered by nurses.[81,84]

Patients can also refuse to take opioid analgesics because of side effects such as constipation and nausea. Nurses should give laxatives and stool softeners to any patient receiving opioids on a regular basis. Some patients experience nausea and vomiting, but they usually respond well to antiemetics. Sedation and drowsiness may occur for the first 48 to 72 hours, but the nurse needs to consider that the patient may be catching up on sleep lost because of the pain. Nurses can use a sedation scale to monitor level of arousal (Box 16-11). Respiratory depression is rarely a problem with standardized doses and careful titration. Strategies for managing opioid side effects are summarized in the Guidelines for Safe Practice box on p. 345.

Nursing activities related to PCA include educating patients, maintaining the system, assessing the effectiveness of and patient response to analgesia, monitoring for side effects, and recording the number of times the patient activates the system. The patient and family members need to know how to monitor the patient's response to the medication and how to care for the PCA system if the patient is at home. Patients need to understand how and when to push the button to get a medication dose. They need to be encouraged to take the next dose when pain increases above mild intensity or above the desired level identified by the patient. In the hospital the medication button should be clearly differentiated from the call button for help, such as by color or shape. *No one but the patient should press the PCA button.*

Patients, families, and health professionals need to understand how to assess pain and the importance of giving analgesic medication regularly to prevent or reduce pain to a mild level

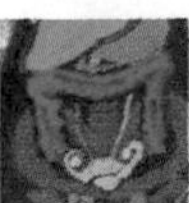

GUIDELINES FOR SAFE PRACTICE *Reducing Pain With Positioning*

- Give analgesics to prevent or minimize pain before care is given if pain is anticipated.
- Use a turning sheet for patients with severe neck, back, or general trunk pain.
- Place a pillow under a painful joint when helping a patient change position.
- Support limbs at the joints rather than the muscle bellies when handling an extremity.
- Use special beds (RotoRest, water bed) for patients with severe general or trunk pain.
- Avoid bumping the bed or moving it suddenly.
- Use bed cradles to support linens off painful extremities.
- Assist with range of motion and evaluate joint flexibility.

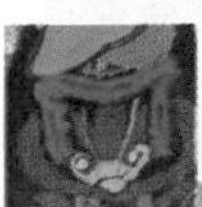

GUIDELINES FOR SAFE PRACTICE *Modifying the Environment*

- Move the patient to a quieter room away from the center of activity.
- Dim bright lights; pull shades if sunlight is intense.
- Minimize verbal interactions when pain is severe.
- Encourage other patients to use headphones or keep television or radio at a reasonable level.
- Control the number of persons entering the patient's room according to patient's wishes.
- Explore the effect of soft music or nature sound tapes.

when possible. Patients have the right to determine their analgesic intake, but they must have adequate knowledge for making this decision. Refer to the Guidelines for Safe Practice box below for a summary of basic principles of effective opioid analgesic administration.

Box 16-9 American Pain Society Guidelines for Managing Acute Pain

- Recognize and treat pain promptly.
  - —Chart and display patients' self-report of pain.
  - —Commit to continuous improvement of one or several outcome variables.
  - —Document outcomes based on data and provide prompt feedback.
- Make information about analgesics readily available.
- Promise patients attentive analgesic care.
- Define explicit policies for use of advanced analgesic technologies.
- Examine the process and outcomes of pain management with the goal of continuous improvement.

Box 16-10 Patient Concerns About Reporting Pain and Using Analgesics

- *Addiction:* Believe it occurs if they take frequent medication
- *Tolerance:* Believe they need to "save" medication for later pain
- *Side effects:* Fear constipation, nausea, mental confusion
- *Fatalism:* Expect pain to be inevitable and not treatable
- *Being a good patient:* Means not complaining
- *Distract physician:* Pain management wastes time that could be spent on treatment
- *Progress:* Reporting pain means acknowledging disease progression
- *Injections:* Believe major route is by injection, which is not wanted

From Ward S et al: Patient-related barriers to management of cancer pain, *Pain* 52:319, 1993.

The *placebo response* occurs when people experience pain relief from an intervention that may not be directly related to the applied pain relief method. Health professionals can cause a positive placebo response by the ways in which they interact with patients. If a person expects relief from pain, anxiety and muscle tension decrease, and less pain is experienced. The nurse's empathic approach toward the patient such as listening without judgment, providing ways to express pain and the right to do so, and recognizing the person's unique responses indirectly facilitate pain relief. Medication placebos, such as giving saline injections instead of an opioid or giving oral doses of inappropriate drugs such as 50 mg of meperedine, are unethical.

There are some special considerations for analgesic use with older patients. Unrelieved pain in this population has been shown to result in problems after surgery such as confusion. Older people usually tolerate opioids as long as the nurse closely monitors them for response to the analgesic prescribed.[26,58] The Guidelines for Safe Practice boxes, p. 355, discuss ways to minimize the risk of side effects from the use of opioids and NSAIDs in older patients.

RELATED NIC INTERVENTIONS. Analgesic Administration, Anxiety Reduction, Environmental Management: Comfort, Heat/Cold Application, Medication Management, Pain Manage-

Box 16-11 Sample Sedation Scale for Monitoring Opioid Side Effects

S = Sleep, easy to arouse
1 = Awake and alert
2 = Slightly drowsy, easily aroused
3 = Frequently drowsy, arousable, drifts off to sleep during conversation
4 = Somnolent, minimal or no response to physical stimulation

From McCaffery M, Pasero C: *Pain: clinical manual,* ed 2, St Louis, 1999, Mosby.

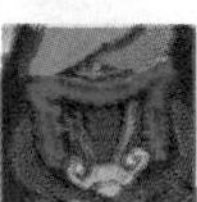

GUIDELINES FOR SAFE PRACTICE *Using Opioid Analgesics Effectively*

- Base all analgesic decisions on thorough and ongoing patient assessment.
- Individualize the route, dosage, and schedule, using the oral route wherever possible.
- Administer opioid analgesics regularly around the clock if pain is present most of the day. Give analgesics to prevent or minimize pain.
  - —As-needed (prn) dosing may be used late in the postoperative course when continuous pain is no longer present or expected. Ask the patient regularly for pain ratings to ensure adequate control.
- Become familiar with the dose and duration of the major strong opioids such as morphine, hydromorphone, oxycodone (OxyContin), and fentanyl.
  - —Morphine is the standard strong opioid. However, individuals respond differently, and other opioid analgesics maybe be necessary because of idiosyncratic side effects.
  - —Several types of analgesics may be used together to maximize effects (e.g., adding nonsteroidal antiinflammatory drugs).
  - —Titrate the dose and administration interval to ensure adequate analgesia and minimize side effects.
  - —Reserve meperidine (Demerol) for brief courses in patients who have allergies or intolerance to morphine and morphine derivatives.
- Monitor patients closely for pain relief, particularly when beginning or changing analgesic regimens. Change the regimen as needed.
- Recognize and treat side effects as soon as possible.
- Use cognitive, behavioral, and nonpharmacologic interventions appropriately to augment analgesic pain management.

Adapted from American Pain Society: *Principles of analgesic use in the treatment of acute pain and cancer pain,* ed 4, Glenview, Ill, 1999, The Society.

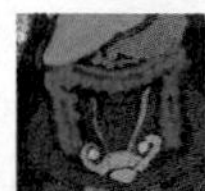

GUIDELINES FOR SAFE PRACTICE *Use of Opioids With Elderly Patients*

- Height, weight, and body surface are not accurate measures for determining drug dosages in older patients.
- Analgesics usually last longer in older patients because their renal and hepatic clearance rates are slower.
- Age is not significant in determining dose, but it is important in determining frequency of dose.
- Dose is based on the therapeutic response and undesirable side effects (confusion, untoward central nervous system effects, respiratory depression).
- Older patients may be hesitant to ask for pain relief. Monitor patients closely for nonverbal signs of pain. The stress of unrelieved pain leads to fatigue, anxiety, and confusion, which are physically and psychologically debilitating.
- Review other medications the patient is taking to avoid drugs that may interact unfavorably with the analgesic.

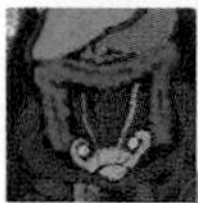

GUIDELINES FOR SAFE PRACTICE *Use of NSAIDs With Elderly Patients*

Precautions to be observed with the use of nonsteroidal antiinflammatory drugs (NSAIDs) in older adults include:
—NSAIDs cause more ulcers and bleeding episodes in older adults than they do in younger adults.
—Older adults with renal impairment are at increased risk for liver and renal toxicity and need to be monitored closely for signs of toxicity, including serum levels of the NSAID.

Gastrointestinal disturbances from decreased prostaglandin production can be reduced by the administration of misoprostol (see Chapter 42). The NSAIDs should also be buffered by food and liquid.

ment, Patient-Controlled Analgesia Assistance, Cutaneous Stimulation, Positioning

Nursing Diagnosis: Chronic Pain

OUTCOMES. Common examples of expected outcomes for the patient with a diagnosis of *chronic pain* are:

Patient will:

- Select preferences for ongoing therapies.
- Identify self-management goals and plans for increasing independence in activities in daily living.
- Identify and mobilize supports for encouragement and help.
- Verbalize factors that alter the pain and effective control measures.

NURSING INTERVENTIONS. Nurses can teach patients to control pain by modifying their sensory input through activities that promote relaxation or distraction. Because anxiety increases pain, measures taken to decrease anxiety may help decrease pain. Distraction interferes with the pain stimulus, thereby modifying the patient's awareness of the pain. The patient can reduce mild or moderate pain by focusing on activity in the environment. A quiet environment providing little or no sensory input actually can intensify the pain experience because the person has nothing else to focus on. The Guidelines for Safe Practice box, p. 356 presents strategies to reduce anxiety and pain.

Distraction requires the individual's active participation in an effort to block out the painful stimulus. This can be enhanced by involving two or more sensory modalities, such as vision, hearing, touch, or movement. The distractors must be powerful enough to involve the person's total interest without resulting in fatigue. Pain of long duration requires a variety of meaningful distractions. Box 16-12 gives examples of easily used distractors.

Full relaxation decreases the muscle tension and fatigue that usually accompany pain; it also helps decrease anxiety, thereby preventing augmentation of the pain stimulus. In addition, relaxation techniques can be an effective form of distraction. The use of relaxation techniques has been shown to be effective in treating chronic pain and insomnia.[42] Relaxation exercises may be especially beneficial for persons with chronic pain to help reduce stress that may exacerbate the pain and to help the person achieve a sense of control and more effectively cope with the pain. There is less evidence validating relaxation as an effective intervention for reducing acute pain.[42]

Among the numerous forms of relaxation techniques, most tend to focus on the repetition of a word, sound, or phrase or repetition of an activity, such as deep breathing, jaw relaxation, or yawning. Progressive muscle relaxation (PMR) is a structured relaxation exercise wherein participants focus on tensing and relaxing major muscle groups to ease overall muscle tension. Some patients may not like PMR. Success with any relaxation technique requires selection of the appropriate strategy, active patient involvement, practice, and encouragement.

Increased understanding of the nature of chronic pain and the need for collaborative care has resulted in the establishment of pain clinics and inpatient pain teams for control of chronic pain. Persons with chronic, persistent pain sometimes are admitted to a hospital for evaluation or initiation of treatment, such as for chronic back pain or substance abuse. Each team member evaluates the patient separately and shares his or her assessment in a team conference during which they develop a specific treatment plan with protocols for controlling the pain. All persons providing patient care during the hospitalization need to become familiar with the protocols so that they use a consistent approach.

Nursing responsibilities include patient assessment, documentation of observations, patient teaching, and coordination of a patient-centered, multiprofessional approach to pain management. Collaboration among health care professionals is essential. For example, the nurse should work with the physical therapist to coordinate visits so that optimal analgesia can be planned to minimize dynamic pain. The culmination of the hospitalization is a discharge conference with the patient, family, and team to discuss future treatment plans and recommendations.

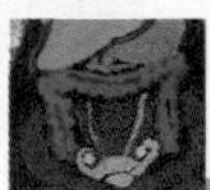

GUIDELINES FOR SAFE PRACTICE *Reducing Anxiety and Pain*

- Help the patient explore concerns related to the pain (meaning of pain for the patient).
- Emphasize the importance of the patient's role in communicating pain to the nurse (e.g., 0 to 10 pain intensity).
- Respect the patient's response to pain, even if it differs considerably from what the nurse expects.
- Teach the family and close friends ways in which they can help the patient, such as massage, encouraging the patient to use distraction or relaxation techniques, or supporting painful parts when moving or changing the patient's position. People often feel helpless when observing a loved one in pain and may need help themselves to cope.
- Arrange for someone to be with the patient if the person fears being alone.
- Talk with family or close friends and help allay their anxieties so that these are not transmitted to the patient.
- Use gentle touch in patient interactions if it is acceptable to the patient.

Box 16-12 Common Simple Modes of Distraction

- Playing games, watching television
- Talking with someone
- Listening to favorite music
- Rhythmic breathing.
- Focusing on an object

Most pain clinics also use a team approach that includes physicians (internists, anesthesiologists, surgeons, and psychiatrists), nurses, physical and occupational therapists, social workers, psychologists, vocational rehabilitation counselors, and pharmacists. Each pain clinic is organized differently and emphasizes different aspects of pain relief. Common approaches to the management of chronic pain include:

- Medications: NSAIDs, tricyclic antidepressants, and opioids
- Behavior modification
- Exercise and activity prescriptions
- Psychoeducation (self-management goal setting)
- Family education to support planned goals and activities
- Hypnosis, acupuncture, or other cognitive and behavioral strategies

The nurse's responsibility varies depending on the available team members and may include patient assessment, documentation of observations, creating and maintaining a therapeutic milieu, providing emotional support for patient and family, and patient teaching.

RELATED NIC INTERVENTIONS. Analgesic Administration, Behavior Modification, Distraction, Pain Management

EVALUATION

To evaluate the effectiveness of nursing interventions, compare patient behaviors with those stated in the expected patient outcomes.

RELATED NOC OUTCOMES. Comfort Level, Pain Control, Pain: Disruptive Effects, Pain Level, Pain: Adverse Psychological Response

Critical Thinking

1. If you were a scientist who wanted to develop an ideal analgesic, which properties would you borrow from opioids and NSAIDs if you could select only two properties from each? What side effects would you eliminate if you could eliminate one from each group? Why did you make these choices?
2. How does the assessment of acute pain differ from the assessment of chronic pain? Think about two patients for whom you have provided care—one with acute pain and one with chronic pain. In what ways did their responses to pain differ, and how did these responses influence management approaches?
3. Your 45-year-old male patient says he can be strong and stand his pain, which he rates as 8 (on a scale from 0 to 10). From your understanding of pain pathophysiology and analgesics, how would you respond?
4. A 65-year-old woman is admitted to your unit with metastatic lung cancer. She speaks very little English; her primary language is Spanish. How would you assess and manage her pain?

References

1. American Pain Society: *Principles of analgesic use in the treatment of acute pain and cancer pain*, ed 5, Glenview, Ill, 2004, The Society.
2. American Pain Society Quality of Care Committee: Quality improvement guidelines for the treatment of acute and cancer pain, *JAMA* 274:1874, 1995.
3. Basbaum A, Bushnell MC: Pain: basic mechanisms. In Giamberardino MA, editor: *Pain 2002—an updated review: refresher course syllabus*, Seattle, 2002, IASP Press.
4. Basbaum AI, Jessell TM: Perception of pain. In Kandel E, Schurtz J, Jessell TM, editors: *Principles of neuroscience,* ed 4, New York, 2000, McGraw-Hill.
5. Benedetti C, Bonica J, Belluci G: Pathophysiology and therapy of postoperative pain: a review. In Benedetti C, Chapman C, Moricca G, editors: *Recent advances in the management of pain*, New York, 1984, Raven Press.
6. Bennett G: Update on the neurophysiology of pain transmission and modulation: focus on the NMDA-receptor, *J Pain Symptom Manage* 19(1)(suppl):2–6, 2000.
7. Breivik H: Postoperative pain: toward optimal pharmacological and epidural analgesia. In Giamberardino MA, editor: *Pain 2002—an updated review: refresher course syllabus*, Seattle, 2002, IASP Press.

8. Brune K: Non-opioid (antipyretic) analgesics. In Giamberardino MA, editor: *Pain 2002—an updated review: refresher course syllabus*, Seattle, 2002, IASP Press.
9. Brunier G, Carson G, Harrison D: What do nurses know and believe about patients in pain? Results of a hospital survey, *J Pain Symptom Manage* 10:436, 1995.
10. Carter EL et al: Effects of emotion on pain reports, tolerance and physiology, *Pain Res Manage* 7(1):21–30, 2002.
11. Charlton JE: Treatment of postoperative pain. In Giamberardino MA, editor: *Pain 2002—an updated review: refresher course syllabus*, Seattle, 2002, IASP Press.
12. Clarke E et al: Pain management knowledge, attitudes and clinical practice: the impact of nurses' characteristics and education, *J Pain Symptom Manage* 11(1):18, 1996.
13. Cleeland C et al: Effects of culture and language on ratings of cancer pain and patterns of functional interference. In Jensen T, Turner J, Wiesenfeld-Hallin Z, editors: *Proceedings of the 8th World Congress on Pain*, vol 8, Seattle, 1997, IASP Press.
14. Craig AD, Sorkin LS: Encyclopedia of life sciences: *Pain and analgesia*, accessed Aug 2004 from website: www.els.net.
15. Dahl JL et al: Institutionalizing pain management: the post-operative pain management quality improvement project, *J Pain* 4(7):361–371, 2003.
16. Devor M: Pain mechanisms and pain syndromes. In Campbell J, editor: *Pain 1996—an updated review, IASP refresher course syllabus*, Seattle, 1996, IASP Press.
17. Donovan MI: A practical approach to pain assessment. In Watt-Watson JH, Donovan MI, editors: *Pain management: nursing perspective*, St Louis, 1992, Mosby.
18. Dunbar P et al: Clinical analgesic equivalence for morphine and hydromorphone with prolonged PCA, *Pain* 68:265, 1996.
19. Farris DA, Fiedler MA: Preemptive analgesia applied to postoperative pain management, *AANA J* 69(3):223-228, 2001.
20. Feldt K: The checklist of nonverbal pain indicators (CNPI), *Pain Manage Nurs* 1(1):13, 2000.
21. Ferrell B, McCaffery M, Grant M: Clinical decision making and pain, *Cancer Nurs* 14:289, 1991.
22. Ferrell B, Nash C, Warfield C: The role of patient-controlled analgesia in the management of cancer pain, *J Pain Symptom Manage* 7:149, 1992.
23. Fields H: *Pain*, Toronto, 1987, McGraw-Hill.
24. Gourlay GK: Clinical pharmacology of opioids in the treatment of pain. In Giamberardino MA, editor: *Pain 2002—an updated review: refresher course syllabus*, Seattle, 2002, IASP Press.
25. Gylbels J, Tasker R: Central neurosurgery. In Wall P, Melzack R, editors: *Textbook of pain*, London, 1999, Churchill Livingstone.
26. Hardman J, Limbird L: *Goodman and Gilman's the pharmacological basis of therapeutics*, ed 9, New York, 1996, McGraw-Hill.
27. Herr K: Chronic pain: challenges and assessment strategies, *J Gerontol Nurs* 28(1):20–27, 2002.
28. Joint Commission on Accreditation of Healthcare Organizations: website: http://www.jcaho.org.
29. Jovey RD et al: Use of opioid analgesics for the treatment of chronic noncancer pain: a consensus statement and guidelines from the Canadian Pain Society, 2002, *Pain Res Manage* 8(suppl A): 3A–28A, 2003.
30. Julius D, Basbaum AI: Molecular mechanisms of nociception, *Nature* 413:203–210, 2001.
31. Kalso E: Prevention of chronicity. In Jensen T, Turner J, Wiesenfeld-Hallin Z, editors: *Proceedings of the 8th World Congress on Pain*, vol 8, Seattle, 1997, IASP Press.
32. Katz J: Perioperative predictors of long-term pain following surgery. In Jensen T, Turner J, Wiesenfeld-Hallin Z, editors: *Proceedings of the 8th World Congress on Pain*, vol 8, Seattle, 1997, IASP Press.
33. Kehlet H: Pain relief and modification of the stress response. In Cousins M, Phillips G, editors: *Acute pain management*, New York, 1986, Churchill Livingstone.
34. Kessenich K: Cyclo-oxygenase 2 inhibitors: an important new drug classification, *Pain Manage Nurs* 2(1):13, 2001.
35. Kollef M: Trapped-lung syndrome after cardiac surgery: a potentially preventable complication of pleural injury, *Heart Lung* 19(6):671, 1990.
36. LeFort SM et al: Randomized controlled trial of a community-based psychoeducation program for the self-management of chronic pain, *Pain* 74(2–3):297–306, 1998.
37. Loveridge N: Ethical implications of achieving pain management, *Emerg Nurs* 8(3):16–21, 2000.
38. Manias E: Medication trends and documentation of pain management after surgery, *Nurs Health Sci* 5(1):85–94, 2003.
39. Manz B et al: Pain assessment in the cognitively impaired and unimpaired elderly, *Pain Manage Nurs* 1(4):106, 2000.
40. Marks RM, Sachar EJ: Undertreatment of medical inpatients with narcotic analgesics, *Ann Intern Med* 78:173, 1973.
41. Marquié L et al: Pain rating by patients and physicians: evidence of systematic pain miscalibration, *Pain* 102(3):289-296, 2003.
42. McCaffery M, Pasero C: *Pain: clinical manual*, ed 2, St Louis, 1999, Mosby.
43. McDonald D: Gender and ethic stereotyping and narcotic analgesic administration, *Res Nurs Health* 17:45, 1994.
44. McGillion M et al: Learning by heart: a focused group study to determine the self-management learning needs of chronic stable angina patients, *Can J Cardio Nurs* 14(2):12–22, 2004.
45. McGillion M et al: A systematic review of psychoeducational intervention trials for the management of chronic stable angina, *J Nurs Manage* 12(3):174–182, 2004.
46. McIntyre PE: Safety and efficacy of patient controlled analgesia, *Brit J Anaesth* 87:36–46, 2001.
47. McNeil J, Sherwood G, Starck P: The hidden error of mismanaged pain: a systems approach, *J Pain Symptom Manage* 28(1):47-58, 2004.
48. Melzack R, Wall PD: *The challenge of pain*, New York, 1996, Penguin Books.
49. Merskey H, Bogduk N: *Classification of chronic pain: descriptions of chronic pain syndromes and definitions of pain terms*, ed 2, Seattle, 1994, IASP Press.
50. Miaskowski C et al: Assessment of patient satisfaction utilizing the American Pain Society's quality assurance standards on acute and cancer-related pain, *J Pain Symptom Manage* 9(1):5, 1994.
51. Mitchell A, Brooks S, Roane D: The premature infant and painful procedures, *Pain Manage Nurs* 1(2):58, 2000.
52. Morley-Forster PK et al: Attitude toward opioid use for chronic pain: a Canadian physician survey, *Pain Res Manage* 8(4):189–194, 2003.
53. Morrison RS et al: The impact of post-operative pain on outcomes following hip fracture, *Pain* 103:303–311, 2003.
54. Neill K: Ethnic pain styles in acute myocardial infarction, *Western J Nurs Res* 15(2):531, 1993.
55. Ng D: Pain: a culturally informed experience, *Pain Res Manage* 7(2):109–111, 2002.
56. Oberle K: Pain, anxiety and analgesics: a comparative study of elderly and younger surgical patients, *Can J Aging* 9(1):13, 1990.
57. O'Gara P: The hemodynamic consequences of pain and its management, *J Intensive Care Med* 3:3, 1988.
58. Pasero C, McCaffery M: Postoperative pain management in the elderly. In Ferrell B, Ferrell B, editors: *Pain in the elderly*, Seattle, 1996, IASP Press.
59. Payne R, Paice J: Cancer pain clinical practice guidelines for clinicians and patients: rationale, barriers to implementation, and future directions. In Payne R, Pratt R, Hil C, editors: *Assessment and treatment of cancer pain*, vol 12, Seattle, 1998, IASP Press.
60. Peter D Hart Research Associates: *Americans talk about pain*, accessed Aug 2004 from website: www.researchamerica.org/polldata/Pain_Poll_report.pdf.
61. Prkachin KM et al: Does experience influence judgments of pain behaviour? Evidence from relatives of pain patients and therapists, *Pain Res Manage* 6(2):105–112, 2001.
62. Puntillo K, Weiss S: Pain: its mediators and associated morbidity in critically ill cardiovascular surgical patients, *Nurs Res* 43(1):31, 1994.
63. Sluka KA, Walsh D: Transcutaneous electrical nerve stimulation: basic science mechanisms and clinical effectiveness, *J Pain* 4(3):109–121, 2003.
64. Spross J, Burke M: Nonpharmacological management of cancer pain. In McGuire D, Yarbro C, Ferrell B, editors: *Cancer pain management*, Boston, 1995, Jones & Bartlett.
65. Statistics Canada: *Pain or discomfort by severity*, accessed July 2004 from website: www.statcan.ca/english/freepub/82-221-XIE/00502?high/region/hsever.htm.

66. Stewart WF et al: Lost productive time and cost due to common pain conditions in the US workforce, *JAMA* 290(18):2443-2454, 2003.
67. Sunshine A: A comparison of the newer COX-2 drugs and older nonopioid oral analgesics, *J Pain* 1(3)(suppl 1):10, 2000.
68. Taylor B, Brennan T: Preemptive analgesia: moving beyond conventional strategies and confusing terminology, *J Pain* 1(2):77, 2000.
69. Turk DC: A diathesis-stress model of chronic pain and disability following traumatic injury, *Pain Res Manage* 7(1):9–19, 2002.
70. Wall P: Comments after 30 years of the gate control theory, *Pain Forum* 1:12–22, 1996.
71. Ward S, Gordon D: Application of the American Pain Society quality assurance standards, *Pain* 56:266, 1994.
72. Ward S, Gordon D: Patient satisfaction and pain severity as outcomes in pain management: a longitudinal view of one setting's experience, *J Pain Symptom Manage* 11(4):242, 1996.
73. Ward S et al: Patient-related barriers to management of cancer pain, *Pain* 52:319, 1993.
74. Watson CPN, Watt-Watson J: Treatment of neuropathic pain: antidepressants and opioids, *Pain Res Manage* 4:168:2000.
75. Watson CPN, Watt-Watson J, Chipman ML: Chronic noncancer pain and the long term utility of opioids, *Pain Res Manage* 9(1):19–24, 2004.
76. Watt-Watson J: Misbeliefs. In Watt-Watson J, Donovan M, editors: *Pain management: nursing perspective*, St Louis, 1992, Mosby.
77. Watt-Watson J, Evans R, Watson CP: Relationships among coping responses and perceptions of pain intensity, depression and family functioning, *Clin J Pain* 4(2):101, 1988.
78. Watt-Watson J, Graydon J: Impact of surgery on head and neck cancer patients and their caregivers, *Nurs Clin North Am* 30:659, 1995.
79. Watt-Watson J, Stevens B: Managing pain after coronary artery bypass surgery, *J Cardiovasc Nurs* 12(3):39–51, 1998.
80. Watt-Watson J et al: Canadian Pain Society position statement on pain relief, *Pain Res Manage* 4(2):75, 1999.
81. Watt-Watson J et al: The impact of nurses' empathic responses on patients' pain management in acute care, *Nurs Res* 49:4, 2000.
82. Watt-Watson J et al: Relationship between nurses' pain knowledge and pain management outcomes for their postoperative cardiac patients, *JAN* 36(4):535–545, 2001.
83. Wattt-Watson J et al: An integrated undergraduate pain curriculum, based on IASP curricula, for six health science faculties, *Pain* 110:140–148, 2004.
84. Watt-Watson J et al: Pain management following discharge after ambulatory same-day surgery, *J Nurs Manage* 12:153–161, 2004.
85. Woolf CJ, Salter M: Neuronal plasticity: increasing the gain in pain, *Science* 288(5472):1765–1769, 2000.
86. Woolf C, Thompson J: Stimulation-induced analgesia: transcutaneous electrical nerve stimulation (TENS) and vibration. In Wall P, Melzack R, editors: *Textbook of pain,* London, 1994, Churchill Livingstone.

evolve Visit the Evolve website: http://evolve.elsevier.com/Monahan/medsurg

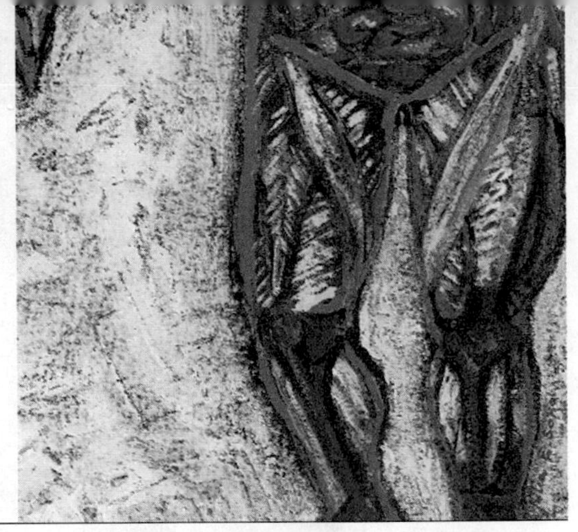

CHAPTER 17

Fluid and Electrolyte Imbalance

by Penny L. Marshall

OBJECTIVES

After studying this chapter, the learner should be able to:

1. Describe the mechanisms that maintain fluid and electrolyte balance.
2. Compare the mechanisms and effects of fluid deficit and excess.
3. Discuss the mechanisms and effects of deficits and excesses of sodium, potassium, calcium, and magnesium.
4. Describe the management of patients with a fluid or electrolyte imbalance.

KEY TERMS

colloid oncotic pressure, p. 361
diffusion, p. 360
electrolytes, p. 359
extracellular, p. 359
intracellular, p. 359
isotonic, p. 361
hydrostatic pressure, p. 361
osmolality, p. 360
osmosis, p. 360
tonicity, p. 361

Fluid and electrolyte balance is fundamental to the process of life. Abnormal fluid volume and electrolyte concentrations can seriously alter physiologic homeostasis and can be life threatening. Although medical therapy to prevent and treat fluid and electrolyte disturbances is the physician's responsibility, nurses play a major role in all aspects of patient care. Understanding how fluid and electrolyte disturbances occur and how the body compensates serves as a foundation for understanding many diseases and associated nursing management.

Body Fluid and Electrolyte Compartments, Distribution, and Function

Fluid and electrolytes in the body are found in the cell **(intracellular)** or outside the cell **(extracellular)**. The extracellular fluid (ECF) compartment is further subdivided into the interstitial fluid (fluid between the cells), intravascular fluid (fluid in the blood vessels), and transcellular fluid (within special body cavities) compartments. Transcellular fluid makes up only 1% to 3% of body weight and includes digestive, pleural, synovial, lymphatic, intraocular, and cerebrospinal fluids.[4] Large amounts of transcellular fluid can become sequestered in a transcellular compartment; this is referred to as a *third space,* since the fluid is not available for exchange with the remainder of the ECF.[9]

Water is the largest constituent of the body, accounting for 45% to 75% of body weight. The volume and distribution of body water vary with age and gender (Figure 17-1). In the newborn, almost 75% of body weight is water, with the greatest percentage found in the extracellular compartment. In the adult man, 60% of body weight is water, with two thirds being in the intracellular compartment. In the adult woman, approximately 50% of body weight is water because women in general have a higher ratio of fat, which holds less water than skeletal muscle.

Water has many important functions: (1) maintenance of blood volume, (2) cellular transport of vital substances such as oxygen and glucose, (3) transport of cellular waste products to the lungs and kidneys for removal, (4) lubrication and cushioning, (5) hydrolysis of food in the digestive system, (6) reactant and medium for the chemical reactions in cells, and (7) maintenance of body temperature.

Electrolytes carry an electrical charge and have the ability to combine with other ions. The most prominent positively charged ions (cations) are hydrogen, sodium, potassium, magnesium, and calcium. The negatively charged ions (anions) are chloride, bicarbonate, sulfate, and phosphate. Electrolyte concentration in the body is expressed in milliequivalents (mEq) per liter—a measure of combining power rather than a measure of weight (such as milligrams). Precise concentrations of electrolytes are vital to osmolarity, body pH, and overall homeostasis. Each electrolyte has specific functions, which are addressed later.

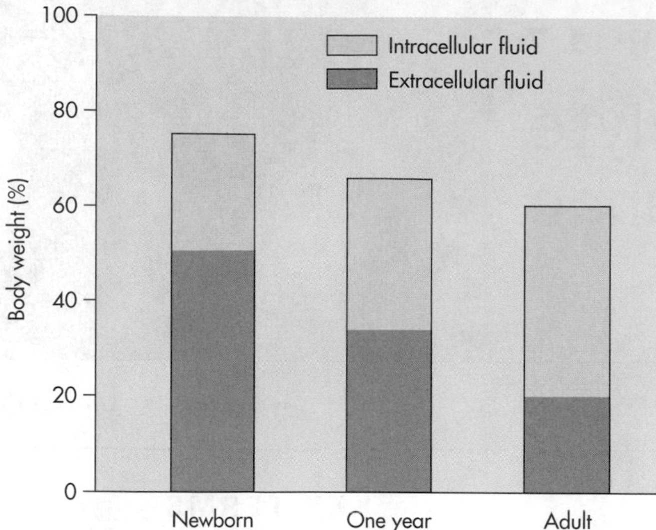

Figure 17-1 In the newborn infant more than half of total body fluid is extracellular. As the child grows, proportions gradually approximate adult levels.

The concentration of electrolytes in the intracellular fluid (ICF) differs significantly from that in the ECF (Table 17-1). The serum level of any given electrolyte indirectly represents the total body level, since a blood sample only measures the concentration of electrolytes in the ECF.[8] For example, serum potassium ranges from 3.5 to 5 mEq/L but is approximately 28 times more concentrated inside the cell than outside.[9]

Movement of Fluid and Solutes Between Compartments

The constant dynamic interchange of body fluids is a product of several essential processes that help regulate fluid volume, composition, and distribution between compartments.

Fluid and Solute Transport Between Extracellular and Intracellular Compartments

Solutes flow across cell membranes by passive or active processes. Passive transport of solute across a membrane is called **diffusion** and is influenced by concentration and electrical charge. The increased motion of solutes in a concentrated solution causes movement of the solutes to the less concentrated solution until both sides of the membrane are equal. The exchange of oxygen and carbon dioxide between the pulmonary capillaries and alveoli is an example of diffusion.

The tendency of sodium to diffuse into the cell down its concentration gradient, and for potassium to exit the cell, is offset by active transport via the *sodium-potassium pump* located in the cell membrane. This *active* process requires energy in the form of adenosine triphosphate (ATP). Since the ECF can tolerate only small amounts of potassium, the body expends a great deal of energy moving potassium back into the cell.

Osmotic forces control the movement of water between the ECF and ICF. **Osmosis** is the movement of water across a semipermeable membrane from an area of low solute to an area of high solute concentration until the solutions are of equal concentration. The rate at which water moves depends on the concentration of the solutes in the solution (osmolality) and the subsequent osmotic pressure exerted by that solution.

The term **osmolality** expresses the concentration of a solution in terms of how strongly it can attract water across a membrane. Expressed in osmoles (the amount of molecules/ions in solution) or milliosmoles per kilogram (mOsm/kg) of the solution, plasma osmolality averages 290 ± 5 mOsm/kg and is relatively constant from day to day. Osmolality can be indirectly estimated by doubling the serum sodium level, since sodium is the major determinant of serum osmolarity.[4] The difference in the terms *osmolality* and *osmolarity* (Box 17-1) is of practical interest to a research chemist who uses electrolytes dissolved in different types of solutions. In clinical practice the difference in these terms is negligible

TABLE 17-1 NORMAL ELECTROLYTE CONTENT OF BODY FLUIDS

	Extracellular		
Electrolytes* (Anions and Cations)	**Intravascular (mEq/L)**	**Interstitial (mEq/L)**	**Intracellular (mEq/L)**
Sodium (Na^+)	142	146	15
Potassium (K^+)	5	5	150
Calcium (Ca^{++})	5	3	2
Magnesium (Mg^{++})	2	1	27
Chloride (Cl^-)	102	114	1
Bicarbonate (HCO_3^-)	27	30	10
Protein ($Prot^-$)	16	1	63
Phosphate (HPO_4^{-2})	2	2	100
Sulfate (SO_4^{-2})	1	1	20
Organic acid	5	8	0

*Note that electrolyte level of intravascular and interstitial fluids (extracellular fluids) is approximately the same and that sodium and chloride contents are significantly higher in these fluids, whereas potassium, phosphate, and protein contents are significantly higher in intracellular fluid.

Box 17-1 Comparison of Osmolarity and Osmolality

- *Osmolarity* refers to the osmolar concentration in 1 L of solution (mOsm/L).
- *Osmolality* refers to the osmolar concentration in 1 kg of water (mOsm/kg H_2O).

Note that both are measured in milliosmoles (one-thousandth of an osmole) in clinical practice.

because of the low solute concentrations in body fluids, all of which are basically water. Osmolality is the measure used to evaluate serum and urine in the clinical setting.[9]

Measuring plasma and urine osmolality is useful in assessing fluid and electrolyte imbalances and monitoring treatment regimens. The significance of plasma osmolality is that it is the main regulator of the release of antidiuretic hormone (ADH), which plays a major role in water regulation. Symptoms resulting from increased osmolality usually occur at levels greater than 350 mOsm. Various pathologic states can affect osmolality and cell membrane permeability, causing cellular edema or cellular dehydration.

Tonicity refers to the ability of the combined effect of *all of the solutes* (e.g., glucose, mannitol, sodium) in a compartment to create the osmotic force that drives water from one compartment to another.[10] Sodium, glucose, and mannitol do not readily cross the cell membrane and therefore produce an osmotic force that affects the movement of water. Glucose alone does not contribute significantly to either osmolality or tonicity unless grossly elevated, in which case it can cause hypertonicity and pull water out of the cell. An abrupt increase in ECF tonicity will cause cells to shrink from water movement outward, and an abrupt decrease in ECF tonicity will cause cells to swell from water movement inward.

Isotonic solutions have the same osmolality as body fluids and expand the ECF volume without causing a fluid shift from one compartment to another. If the ECF space were to become *hypotonic,* with a solution of lower osmolality, the ICF compartment would swell as water moves inward. Conversely, cells surrounded by a *hypertonic* solution would shrink as water is pulled out of the cell to achieve equal osmolality.

Fluid and Solute Transport Between Vascular and Interstitial Spaces

Colloid oncotic pressure is the pressure created by the pull of proteins (colloids), especially albumin, in the blood. The colloid oncotic pressure within the vascular space serves to pull or absorb fluid from the interstitial space. If a large amount of protein leaves the capillary (e.g., secondary to burns), vascular oncotic pressure drops, further reducing the ability of the vascular space to retain fluid.

The control of fluid movement *between the vascular and interstitial spaces* is a function of filtration. In the process of filtration, **hydrostatic pressure**, created by the weight of fluid pressing against the walls of blood vessels, forces molecules through the capillary membrane. The difference between the hydrostatic pressure and the colloid osmotic pressure at the arteriole end of the capillary favors the movement of fluid out of the vascular compartment. The difference between the hydrostatic pressure and the colloid osmotic pressure at the venule end of the capillary favors the movement of fluid into the vascular compartment (Figure 17-2).

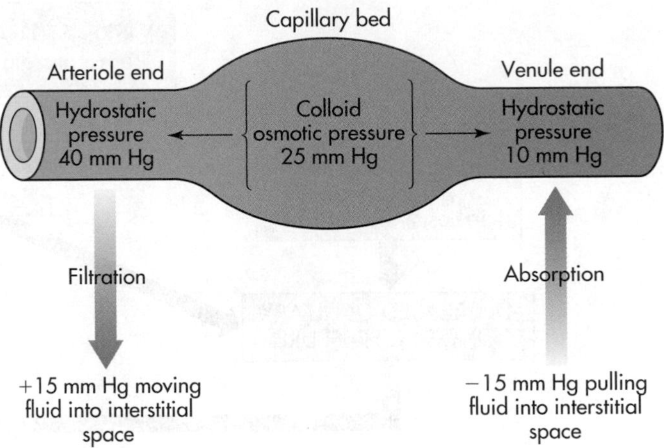

Figure 17-2 Movement of fluids between capillary and interstitial space.

Edema

Disease processes can interfere with fluid regulatory mechanisms and result in edema, a collection of excess fluid in body tissue. Edema is not the same as overhydration, although the two can occur together. The distinction is important, since edema does not always indicate fluid volume overload and treatment depends on causation. The nurse assesses the patient for potential causes such as inflammation, vascular impairment, tissue injury, and volume excess. Nursing management of persons with edema is discussed later along with fluid imbalances.

Etiology. *Intracellular edema* may occur as a result of severe cellular malnutrition that impairs the ability of the sodium-potassium pump to remove sodium from the cell. The relative hypertonicity of the intracellular space results in the osmotic intrusion of water. This usually heralds tissue death and may be seen in severe peripheral vascular disease or hypothermic injury. Cellular swelling may also develop as a result of the altered cellular membrane permeability that occurs in inflammation, allowing sodium and other ions to leak into the cell interior and osmotically attract fluid. Intracellular edema is part of the complex response to endotoxins seen in septic shock.

Extracellular edema is much more common than intracellular edema and is associated with several pathologic processes. The four physiologic mechanisms that contribute to the formation of interstitial edema are illustrated in Figure 17-3 and outlined in Box 17-2.

Pathophysiology. *Increased capillary hydrostatic pressure* can be caused by administering too much fluid to a patient who cannot eliminate the surplus. As the pressure gradient increases, fluid moves into the interstitium and gravity causes the fluid to accumulate (edema) in dependent parts of the body (i.e., ankles and

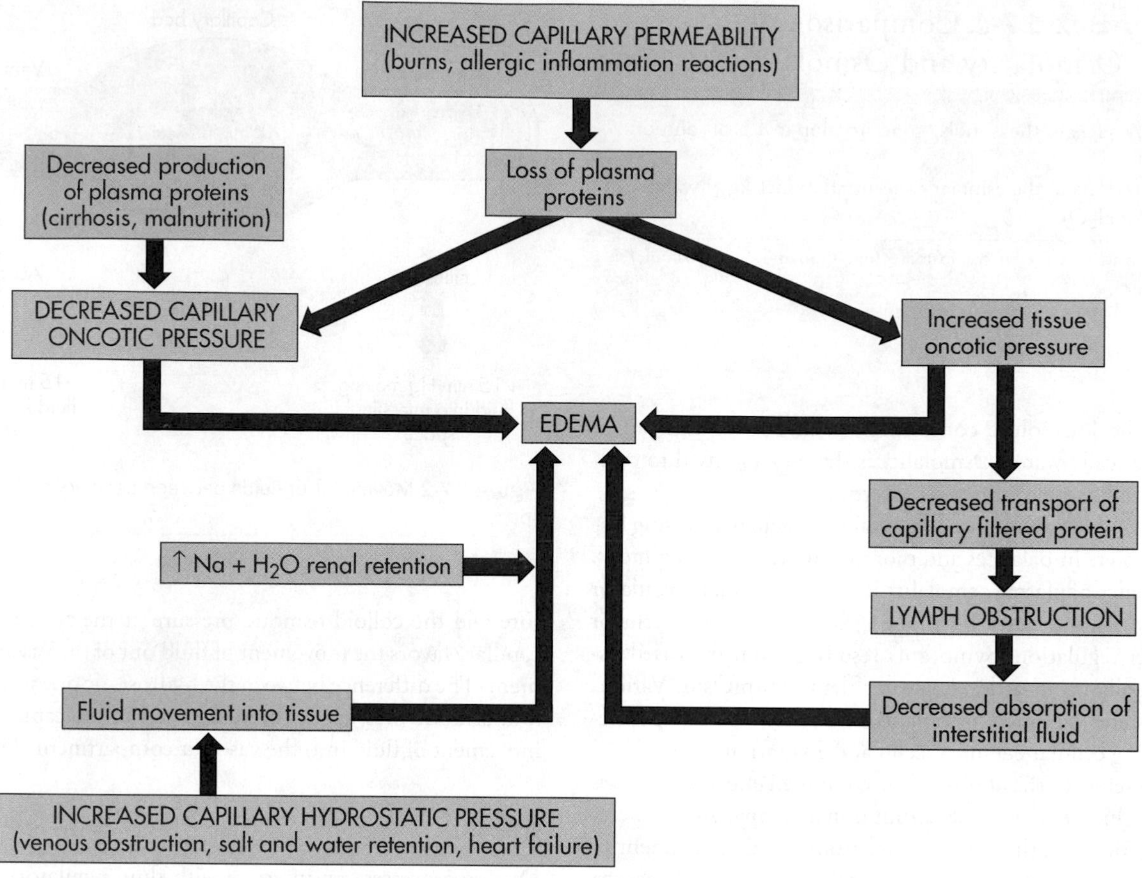

Figure 17-3 Mechanisms of edema formation. *Na^+*, Sodium; *H_2O*, water.

Box 17-2 Causes of Edema According to Underlying Physiologic Mechanism

Increased Capillary Hydrostatic Pressure

Increased venous pressure
Vein obstruction
Varicose veins
Thrombophlebitis
Pressure on veins from casts, tight bandages, or clothing
Increased total volume with decreased cardiac output
Congestive heart failure
Fluid overloading
Sodium and water retention, increased aldosterone
Decreased renal blood flow
Renal failure
Cushing's syndrome
Aldosterone added to system
Corticosteroid therapy
Inability to destroy aldosterone
Cirrhosis of liver

Decreased Capillary Oncotic Pressure

Loss of serum protein
Burns, draining wounds, fistulas
Hemorrhage
Nephrotic syndrome
Chronic diarrhea
Decreased intake of protein
Malnutrition
Kwashiorkor
Decreased production of albumin
Liver disease

Increased Capillary Permeability

Increased capillary permeability to protein
Burns
Inflammatory reactions
Trauma
Infections
Allergic reactions (hives)

Lymph Obstruction

Blocked lymphatics: decreased removal of tissue fluid and protein
Malignant diseases
Surgical removal of lymph nodes
Elephantiasis
Infectious states
Occlusive tumors
Surgical node excision

feet). Other factors that increase capillary fluid pressure include localized inflammation from histamine and other inflammatory mediators that cause dilation of the arterioles.

Decreased capillary oncotic pressure allows fluid to move out of the vascular compartment into the interstitial space. Loss of serum proteins can occur with inadequate intake, loss through denuded skin (burns and wounds), renal disease, or decreased production by the liver. The edema associated with decreased capillary colloidal oncotic pressure affects all tissues of the body regardless of gravitational forces.

Increased capillary permeability allows plasma protein to leak into the interstitial space where the protein exerts its pulling effect, causing interstitial edema. This process occurs in burns and many inflammatory and infectious states.

Lymphatic obstruction can quickly result in significant fluid accumulation or lymphedema as proteins leak into the interstitial space, colloid osmotic pressure rises, and fluid moves into the interstitium. Lymphatic blockage may occur in infections or as a result of an occlusive tumor or surgical node excision.

Internal Regulation of Body Water and Sodium

The human body uses a number of operations to closely regulate the volume and composition of body fluids. Changes in fluid volume are sensed by special receptors in the carotid sinuses, aortic arch, atria, and renal vessels. A change in sympathetic tone provides the initial compensatory response to rapid changes in ECF volume. If fluid volume decreases, cardiac rate and contractility increase to improve cardiac output, vasoconstriction of the arteries enhances blood pressure, and renin release by the kidney prompts release of aldosterone. Aldosterone controls sodium resorption, and ADH controls water resorption.[11]

Mechanisms of Sodium Regulation

Sodium ingestion and excretion control the total volume of plasma sodium, while the degree of its dilution in water determines its concentration or osmolality. Factors regulating plasma sodium include (1) the renin-angiotensin-aldosterone system and (2) atrial natriuretic peptide (ANP).[10]

Renin-Angiotensin-Aldosterone System. Renal excretion or conservation of sodium is coordinated by the sympathetic nervous system and the renin-angiotensin-aldosterone system. The sympathetic nervous system adjusts the glomerular filtration rate (GFR) and rate of sodium filtration from the blood in response to changes in arterial pressure and blood volume. When the blood volume decreases, the juxtaglomerular cells in the kidney secrete renin, a protein that precipitates a cascade of events that produce potent vasoconstrictors (angiotensin), which increase systemic blood pressure, restore renal perfusion, and stimulate the adrenal cortex to secrete aldosterone, which increases renal resorption of sodium and water.[9] Figure 17-4 depicts the renin-angiotensin-aldosterone system.

Atrial Natriuretic Peptide. ANP, also called atrial natriuretic factor, is a hormone produced in response to fluid overload detected by special cells in the atria in such conditions as heart failure, renal failure, hypertension, and certain dysrhythmias. ANP opposes the sodium-retaining action of the plasma renin-angiotensin-aldosterone system and inhibits ADH release.[5] The main effects of ANP are direct arterial vasodilation, increased renal blood flow and GFR, decreased sodium resorption, and diuresis.

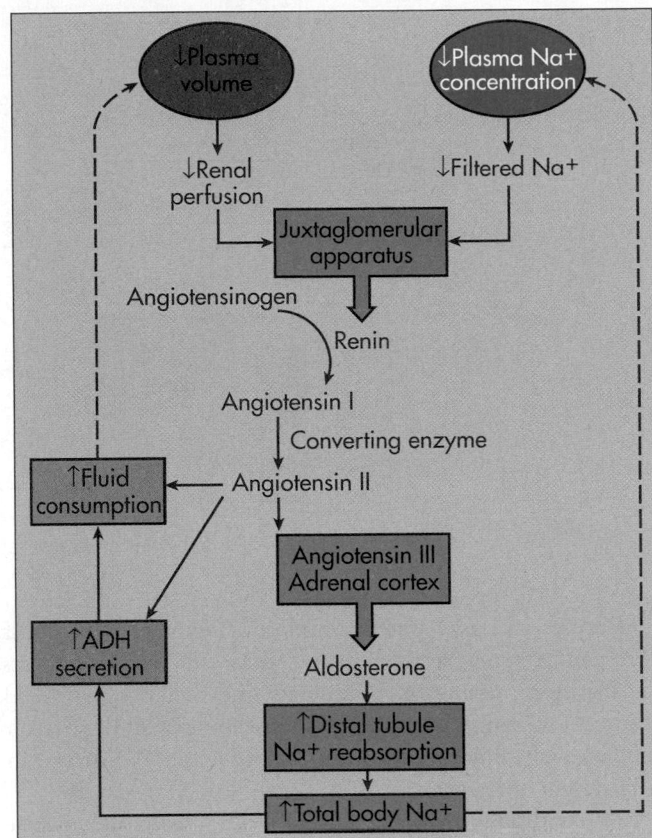

Figure 17-4 The renin-angiotensin-aldosterone system. *ADH*, Antidiuretic hormone; *Na^+*, sodium.

Mechanisms of Water Regulation

The two primary factors regulating water in the body are the thirst mechanism and ADH.

Thirst. The major control of fluid intake is thirst. Osmoreceptors located in the hypothalamus respond to changes in extracellular osmolarity by stimulating the sensation of thirst.[9] The thirst center itself is stimulated by hypertonic body fluid, decreased blood pressure, decreased cardiac output, and angiotensin. Water losses associated with diarrhea, vomiting, diabetes mellitus, and diabetes insipidus are some of the common causes of true thirst.

Antidiuretic Hormone. The resorption of water by the kidneys is regulated by ADH, also known as vasopressin, which is synthesized by the hypothalamus and stored in the posterior pituitary gland. Decreased blood volume or increased serum osmolality stimulates volume receptors located in the left atrium and great veins, and is sensed by osmoreceptors in the hypothalamus, which causes the production and release of ADH. In the kidney,

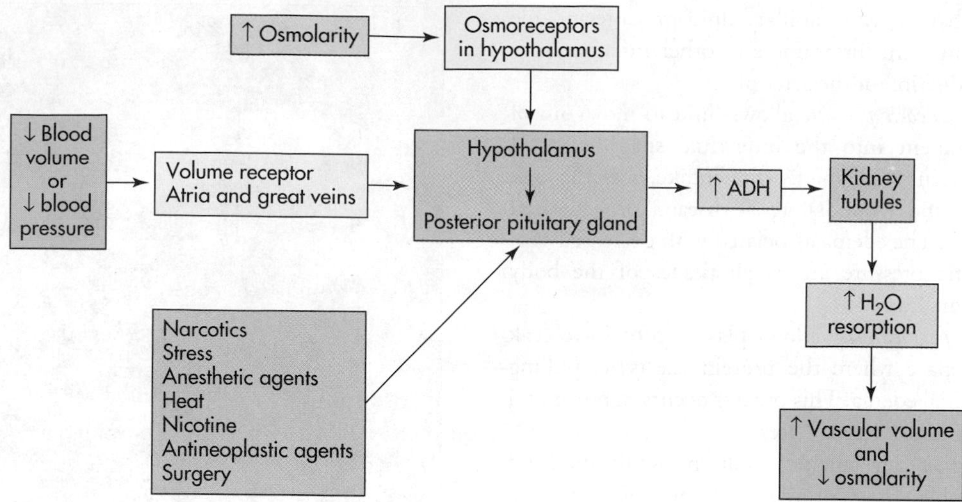

Figure 17-5 Mechanisms regulating antidiuretic hormone (ADH) secretion. *H_2O*, Water.

ADH causes increased water resorption. Angiotensin, narcotics, severe pain, trauma, stress, heat, nicotine, antineoplastic agents, and anesthetic agents also stimulate the secretion of ADH. Because ADH can be secreted in response to many of these factors simultaneously, fluid overload can occur. Figure 17-5 depicts the ADH system of regulation.

Two conditions involving altered ADH levels are diabetes insipidus and inappropriate secretion of ADH. *Syndrome of inappropriate ADH* (SIADH) occurs when the normal physiologic stimuli for ADH release are absent. The secretion of ADH is "inappropriate" in that it continues despite the decreased osmolarity of the plasma. In contrast, *diabetes insipidus* involves a deficiency of ADH leading to polyuria and polydipsia. The kidneys excrete large volumes of urine, sometimes 3 to 20 L/day depending on the degree of ADH deficiency (central or neurogenic diabetes insipidus) or renal insensitivity to ADH (nephrogenic diabetes insipidus).[9] Table 17-2 compares the two conditions. Nursing care is discussed in the section on sodium imbalances.

▶ ARE You READY?

In caring for a patient with fluid volume disturbances, the nurse correlates which of the following to the release of renin and aldosterone?

1. Increased urine pH
2. Decreased blood pressure
3. Decreased urine output
4. Increased sodium excretion

Normal Gains and Losses of Fluid and Electrolytes

In the healthy person, body fluids are constantly being lost and replaced. Fluid intake varies greatly from person to person because of social, cultural, emotional, and physiologic factors. In addition to liquids, a large amount of normal fluid intake is obtained from water in food. Table 17-3 summarizes the normal routes of gains and losses of fluid in an adult consuming approximately 2500 calories/day.

Under normal conditions, the average urinary output is 1500 ml. A minimum of 400 ml of urine must be produced to excrete the daily load of metabolic wastes.[4] Control of body heat also demands continual water expenditure. The volume of fluid expended depends on external temperature, humidity, metabolic rate, and physical activity. Insensible losses (through the skin, respiratory tract, and gastrointestinal [GI] tract) account for approximately two fifths of the fluid lost daily. Insensible loss through the skin is evaporative and considered pure water. When perspiration is visible, the loss of water through the skin is greater than the normal 500 ml/day.

The GI tract accounts for a relatively small amount of fluid lost each day under normal conditions. With illness, however, the GI tract can be a major site of profound fluid loss, especially in children and infants, who have a greater proportion of fluid in the ECF space. Fluid losses from both the upper and lower GI tract contain sodium and potassium. Bicarbonate losses can occur with loss of lower GI fluids (e.g., diarrhea), and chloride with loss from the upper GI tract (e.g., vomiting).

Water and Sodium Imbalance

The tonicity or osmolality of the ECF compartment is largely determined by the ECF sodium concentration. Because sodium is the major extracellular cation and osmotic driving force, the intake or excretion of sodium plays a significant role in determining ECF volume. Although the concentration of sodium in the ECF can be altered by sodium intake or excretion, the mechanisms that control water intake and output are far more significant in determining the ECF sodium concentration. The homeostatic controls that add or remove water from the body respond to changes in tonicity of the ECF. Thus alteration in fluid volume often are created by problems with sodium control mechanisms, and alterations in sodium concentration are often due to malfunction of water control mechanisms.[10] Fluid imbalances may occur as isotonic, hypotonic, or hypertonic alterations. Table 17-4 outlines the different combinations of sodium and water imbalances based on tonicity.

A proportionate change in both sodium and water is referred to as an isotonic alteration and represents either an expansion (excess) or contraction (deficit) of the ECF.

TABLE 17-2 DIABETES INSIPIDUS VERSUS SYNDROME OF INAPPROPRIATE ANTIDIURETIC HORMONE (SIADH)

	Diabetes Insipidus	SIADH
Causes	Hypothalamic tumors, leukemia, lymphoma, sarcoidosis, head trauma or hypoxic brain injury, hypophysectomy, pyelonephritis, polycystic disease, lithium carbonate, general anesthetics, demeclocycline, vinblastine	Oat-cell carcinoma of the lung, leukemia, head injury, brain tumor, pneumonia, acute respiratory failure, tuberculosis, release of vasopressin after surgery, psychogenic polydipsia, excess administration of hypotonic solutions during periods of stress, stroke, spinal surgery[1]
Pathophysiology	ADH deficiency leading to polyuria and polydipsia; excretion of large volumes of dilute urine	Inappropriate secretion of ADH with water retention creating hypotonic ECF and water movement inside cells, causing neurologic symptoms
Laboratory findings	Normal serum sodium and osmolarity if thirst mechanisms intact; if not, excessive urinary output leading to severe fluid volume deficit and high serum sodium and osmolarity; low urine specific gravity	Low serum sodium and osmolarity, low BUN and creatinine, increased urine osmolarity and specific gravity, normal adrenal and thyroid function
Signs and symptoms	Polyuria, nocturia, continuous thirst, polydipsia, craving ice water	Weight gain, fingerprinting edema (cellular edema), no peripheral edema Sodium 130-140 mEq/L Æ thirst, anorexia, fatigue, dulled sensorium Sodium 120-130 Æ nausea, vomiting, abdominal cramps Sodium < 115 mEq/L Æ lethargy, confusion, headaches, personality changes, diminished deep tendon reflexes, seizures, coma
Treatment	Oral hydration; may require ADH replacement with vasopressin	Mild hyponatremia Æ fluid restriction and increased salt intake Severe hyponatremia and CNS symptoms (e.g., seizures) Æ saline (3% or 5% NaCl) in addition to fluid restriction and furosemide Demeclocycline and lithium carbonate interfere with effects of ADH on kidney; reserved for patients who cannot comply with water restriction and oral salt intake[1]

ADH, Antidiuretic hormone; ECF, extracellular fluid; *BUN,* blood urea nitrogen; CNS, central nervous system; *NaCl,* sodium chloride.

TABLE 17-3 NORMAL FLUID INTAKE AND LOSS IN ADULT CONSUMING 2500 CALORIES/DAY (APPROXIMATE VALUES)

Intake Route	Amount of Gain (ml)	Output Route	Amount of Loss (ml)
Water in food	1000	Skin	500
Water from oxidation	300	Lungs	350
Water as liquid	1200	Feces	150
		Kidneys	1500
Total	2500	**Total**	2500

Isotonic Fluid Deficit (Hypovolemia)

An isotonic loss of fluid from the ECF is referred to as isotonic fluid deficit, or hypovolemia. Many clinicians and texts refer to this imbalance as isotonic dehydration or isotonic contraction. Since the loss of both is proportional, osmolarity does not change and fluid does not shift between compartments.

Etiology. An isotonic ECF deficit may occur from the direct loss or sequestration (compartmentalization) of body fluids. In either case the contraction of the ECF space is primarily a problem of sodium control, although serum sodium does not measurably change. Persons at risk are those with (1) a compromised mental state who may not recognize or respond appropriately to

TABLE 17-4 TYPES OF SODIUM AND WATER IMBALANCE

Imbalance	Total Body Water/ Sodium Ratio	Sodium/Osmolarity	Common Causes	Treatment Focus
Isotonic Imbalances				
Fluid volume deficit with normal serum sodium	Proportionate loss in both water and sodium; decreased total body sodium	Decreased total body sodium Decreased fluid volume Normal serum sodium Normal osmolarity	Hemorrhage, vomiting, diarrhea, loop diuretics, profuse diaphoresis	Isotonic IV fluids, colloid solutions, oral rehydration
Fluid volume excess with normal serum sodium	Proportionate gain in both water and sodium; increased total body sodium	Increased total body sodium Increased fluid volume Normal serum sodium Normal osmolarity	CHF, cirrhosis, renal failure, steroids	Restriction of sodium and water; loop diuretics
Hypotonic Imbalances				
Fluid volume deficit with hyponatremia	Sodium loss greater than water loss; too much water relative to sodium, too little sodium	Decreased total body sodium Decreased fluid volume Decreased serum sodium Decreased osmolarity	Vomiting, thiazide diuretics, diarrhea, prolonged sweating	0.9% sodium chloride
Fluid volume excess with hyponatremia	Water gain greater than sodium gain; too much water relative to sodium, and too much sodium	Increased total body sodium Increased fluid volume Decreased serum sodium Decreased osmolarity	CHF, cirrhosis, renal failure	Water restriction for hyponatremia; sodium restriction and loop diuretics to remove edematous fluid
Normal fluid volume with hyponatremia	Pure water gain; abnormal water control (too much water in relation to sodium)	Normal total body sodium Normal fluid volume Decreased serum sodium Decreased osmolarity	SIADH	Water restriction and treat underlying cause
Hypertonic Imbalances				
Fluid volume deficit with hypernatremia	Water loss greater than sodium loss; decreased total body sodium; too little water relative to sodium, and too little sodium	Decreased total body sodium Decreased fluid volume Increased serum sodium Increased osmolarity	Excess solute intake with osmotic diuresis (e.g., diabetic ketoacidosis, high protein intake), severe diarrhea	Oral water replacement; 0.9% saline with severe ECF depletion then hypotonic IV solution(s)
Fluid volume deficit with hypernatremia	Pure water loss; too little water relative to sodium	Normal total body sodium Decreased fluid volume Increased serum sodium Increased osmolarity	Diabetes insipidus	Desmopressin acetate (DDAVP)
Fluid volume excess with hypernatremia	Sodium gain	Increased total body sodium Increased fluid volume Increased serum sodium Increased osmolarity	Administration of hypertonic sodium solutions	Diuretics in combination with oral or IV water replacement; sodium restriction

Adapted from Preston RA: *Acid-base, fluids and electrolytes made ridiculously simple,* Miami, 2002, MedMaster.

CHF, Congestive heart failure; *ECF,* extracellular fluid; *IV,* intravenous; *SIADH,* syndrome of inappropriate antidiuretic hormone.

thirst; (2) physical limitations that impair the ability to obtain adequate fluids and nutrition; (3) disease states that may cause sodium and water loss; or (4) limited access to adequate food and fluids because of social, environmental, recreational, or occupational circumstances.

Sodium and water loss through the GI tract is the most common source of fluid loss. Table 17-5 shows approximate amounts of GI fluids. Losses from vomiting, GI suctioning, and bleeding may result in significant isotonic fluid deficit. Severe diarrhea can cause liters of fluid to be lost, quickly leading to *hypotonic* imbalances (discussed later in the chapter). Significant isotonic fluid losses can also occur from hyperventilation, diaphoresis, and excessive tracheostomy secretions.

Sequestration of body fluids in third-spaces is associated with an intravascular volume deficit. Although not lost from the body, the fluid is lost from the vascular space, and symptoms are consistent with volume deficit. Abnormal amounts of fluid can collect in the intrapleural cavity between the lung and chest (pleural effusion), and between the heart and pericardial sac (pericardial effusion). Fluid can also accumulate between the intestines and the abdominal wall (ascites). Fluid shifts may occur during the postoperative period after major abdominal surgery, pancreatitis, hepatic failure, burns, and intestinal obstruction.[6]

Pathophysiology. Fluid volume deficit stimulates the thirst center to increase water consumption, the production of ADH to promote water resorption from the renal tubule, and the renin-angiotensin-aldosterone system to increase both *sodium and water retention.* Thirst and weight loss are early signs of water deficit and become more pronounced as the deficit increases. Weight loss is not present with third-spacing phenomena because fluid is not lost from the body. As a fluid deficit evolves, body temperature begins to rise and fever may develop. In severe ECF volume deficit, such as acute hemorrhage, signs of circulatory collapse may ensue. The Clinical Manifestations box lists signs of ECF volume deficit.

Collaborative Care Management. Nurses play a critical role in preventing fluid volume deficit, identifying vulnerable patients, preventing complications, and reducing hospital stays. People who are mildly dehydrated may only notice symptoms of increased thirst or dry mouth. A profound fluid deficit, however, may be associated with circulatory collapse and death. Severe fluid depletion is an emergency requiring rapid fluid replacement, restoration of electrolyte balance, and circulatory support.

An evaluation of serum electrolytes is essential to identify changes in serum osmolality and cellular involvement. The nurse reviews serum and urine electrolytes and reports abnormalities so that appropriate adjustments in therapy can be initiated. Factors that may alter fluid and electrolyte status include certain medications (particularly diuretics), hyperventilation, fever, burns, diarrhea, and diabetes. For review of a method to prevent dehydration by decreasing diarrhea, see the Evidence-Based Practice box.

PARENTERAL FLUIDS. Under most circumstances, fluids are replaced at the speed with which they are lost. Fluid replacement needs are often calculated according to weight. Because 1 L weighs 1 kg, the amount of weight (in kilograms) lost during the period of fluid depletion approximates the volume of water deficit. Replacement requires administration of the volume lost plus an additional 1.5 L to fulfill daily needs.[7] Fluid replacement may require several days of therapy to avoid complications associated with rapid volume infusion such as intercompartmental fluid shifts and pulmonary edema.

Oral fluid resuscitation is preferable, but if the patient is unable to tolerate oral fluids, intravenous therapy may be required. The type of intravenous solution is based on the

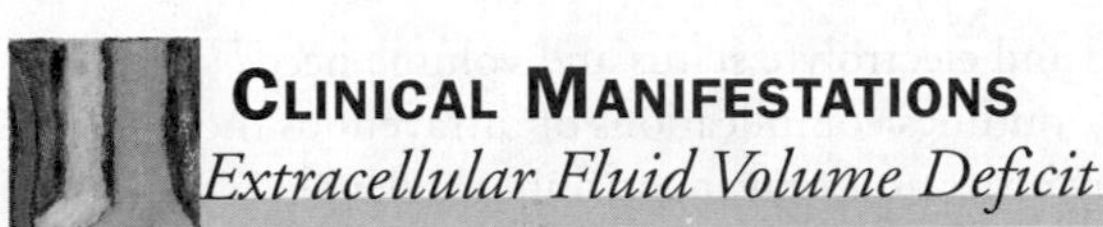

CLINICAL MANIFESTATIONS
Extracellular Fluid Volume Deficit

- Thirst, dry mucous membranes
- Poor turgor, low-grade temperature
- Postural hypotension, slow vein filling
- Tachycardia, postural hypotension, rapid respirations
- Weight loss
- Low urinary output, increased specific gravity

TABLE 17-5 GASTROINTESTINAL FLUID VOLUMES

Type of Fluid	Approximate Amount of Fluid (ml/day)
Saliva	1500
Gastric juice	2500
Intestinal juice	2000
Pancreatic juice	1500
Bile	500
Total	8000 ml/day

Note that approximately 8 L of fluid are used daily for digestive purposes. Normally most of this fluid is resorbed. Some of each of the ions found in blood plasma is present in each of the fluids listed, but individual concentration varies with each fluid.

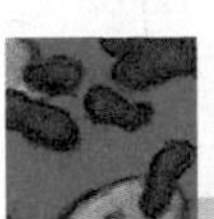

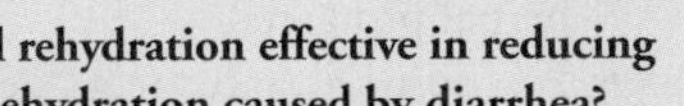

EVIDENCE-BASED PRACTICE

Topic Question: Is rice-based oral rehydration effective in reducing stool output when used to treat dehydration caused by diarrhea?

Evidence Base: Twenty-two trials compared standard oral rehydration salts solution containing glucose to a rice powder solution containing the same electrolytes. Subjects were people with cholera and people with noncholera diarrhea.

Findings: People with cholera who were given the rice solution had substantially lower rates of stool loss than those rehydrated with salts solution. Infants and children with noncholera diarrhea had little reduction in stool loss from the rice solution.

Conclusion: Rice-containing solutions appear to be effective in reducing stool output when cholera is the cause of diarrhea but not when diarrhea is from causes other than cholera.

Fontaine O, Gore SM, Pierce NF: Rice-based oral rehydration solution for treating diarrhea, *Cochrane Library,* Issue 1, 2005.

patient's fluid and electrolyte status and volume needs (Table 17-6). Table 17-7 outlines complications of intravenous therapy. The physician may order an intravenous fluid challenge to determine whether low urinary output is caused by reduced renal blood flow secondary to severe volume deficit or acute renal failure. A bolus of isotonic intravenous fluid is administered over a short period. If volume depletion is the primary problem, urinary output will increase to 20 ml/hr within a few hours. If urinary output does not increase, acute renal failure may be present.[8] Ideally fluid challenges take place in the critical care setting. Frequent nursing assessments of lung sounds, central venous pressure, and blood pressure are essential during this period to prevent severe fluid volume overload.

Particular care must be taken when delivering fluids to (1) infants, (2) older patients with circulatory or renal impairments, (3) patients (such as those with burns) at risk for potential plasma shifts, and (4) those with extensive tissue trauma. Burns, for example, can initially cause massive shifts of fluid into the interstitial space, and then after several days fluid moves back into the vascular space, increasing blood volume. The nurse must closely monitor patients for signs of pulmonary edema.

Health Promotion and Prevention. Prevention for the normal person means learning about the importance of adequate fluid and food intake, especially when under physiologic or thermal stress. The nurse should encourage individuals who engage in strenuous activities to replace both water and electrolytes, and caution them that sport drinks, if consumed too rapidly, can cause osmotic diarrhea.

Nursing Management

of the Patient with Isotonic Fluid Deficit

ASSESSMENT

Health History. Assess for:

- History of fever, sweating, vomiting, diarrhea, reduced fluid intake, diuretic therapy, changes in food or fluid intake, blood loss, renal or cardiac disease, bowel obstruction
- History of weight change, dizziness, lethargy
- Medications (e.g., diuretics, laxatives, narcotics, alcohol, herbal products)
- Psychosocial status (e.g., depression, social support, living conditions)

Physical Examination. Assess for:

- Postural hypotension, tachycardia, weak pulse, and cool skin if hypovolemia is severe
- Poor skin turgor (not reliable in the older adult because of decreased skin elasticity); slow vein filling in hands or neck
- Dry mucous membranes (Note that mouth breathing, other evaporative processes, and medications can cause oral dryness. The area where the cheek and gum meet should be moist with normal fluid volume, even in mouth breathers.)
- Acute weight loss (weight gain with third-spacing)
- Decreased urine volume, elevated specific gravity, alterations in hematocrit and blood urea nitrogen (BUN)

NURSING DIAGNOSES, OUTCOMES, AND INTERVENTIONS

Nursing Diagnosis: Deficient Fluid Volume

OUTCOMES. Common examples of expected outcomes for the patient with a diagnosis of *deficient fluid volume* are:

Patient will:

- Have a balanced intake and output over 24 hours.
- Exhibit signs of adequate hydration.
- Exhibit hematocrit, urine specific gravity, and BUN within patient's normal range.

NURSING INTERVENTIONS. The nurse should monitor vital signs every 4 hours or more often depending on the severity of the fluid loss. The nurse weighs the patient daily, since weight is the single best indicator of fluid volume status in the adult. Trends in weight gains or losses help determine fluid loss, generalized edema, or "hidden" fluid in body cavities. Note that patients who are not eating and are being maintained on intravenous fluids other than those specifically designed for parenteral nutrition are expected to lose approximately 0.2 to 0.25 kg/day. The health care provider calculates the specific amount of free water to be administered to patients receiving enteral feedings (e.g., generally 30 ml/kg of body weight).[3] The nurse should urge caution in drinking coffee, tea, and colas with caffeine, which has a diuretic effect.

RELATED NIC INTERVENTIONS. Electrolyte Management, Fall Prevention, Fluid Management, Fluid Monitoring, Hypovolemia Management, Intravenous (IV) Therapy, Shock Management

Nursing Diagnosis: Ineffective Tissue Perfusion (Cerebral, Renal, Peripheral)

OUTCOMES. Common examples of expected outcomes for the patient with ineffective tissue perfusion are:

Patient will:

- Maintain a systolic and diastolic blood pressure in expected ranges, and a heart rate less than 100 beats/min.
- Exhibit urinary output within normal volume limits (> 0.5 mg/kg/hr or > 30 ml/hr).
- Demonstrate fluid balance, as evidenced by a balanced 24-hour intake and output, with hematocrit, BUN, and serum electrolytes within normal range.

NURSING INTERVENTIONS. The nurse assesses vital signs regularly. Postural (orthostatic) hypotension is common with fluid volume deficit. A drop in the systolic blood pressure of more than 15 mm Hg or heart rate increase of more than 15 beats/min is consistent with intravascular volume depletion.[7] The nurse must implement safety precautions, since significant reductions in standing blood pressure can result in dizziness and falls. The nurse assesses the patient for signs of decreased cerebral perfusion, including syncope, confusion, anxiety, and agitation. Body temperature and weight are accurately recorded in a timely manner because health care practitioners use daily weights to calculate fluid replacement. High fever and rapid breathing can account for as much as 2500 ml of fluid loss per day. The nurse maintains an accurate record of intake and output, including irri-

TABLE 17-6 TYPES OF INTRAVENOUS SOLUTIONS

Tonicity in Bag or Bottle	Intravenous Solutions	Common Use
Isotonic	0.9% NaCl (308 mOsm/L) [Na^+ 154 mEq/L, Cl^- 154 mEq/L]	Expands ECF; beneficial in providing fluid replacement when chloride and sodium loss has occurred (e.g., profuse vomiting). However, may provide more sodium and chloride than needed; thus not desirable for routine maintenance. Patient may also need potassium replacement. Watch for circulatory overload. Only solution used with blood products.
	D_5W (5% dextrose in water) (252 mOsm/L)*	*Hypotonic* in body; distributed evenly throughout body compartments. Can lead to water intoxication and dilutional hyponatremia. Used in treating hypernatremia when it is desired to replace H_2O *without* sodium. Provides 170 calories.
	Lactated Ringer's solution (274 mOsm/L) [Na^+ 130 mEq/L, Cl^- 109 mEq/L, K^+ 4 mEq/L, Ca^{++} 3 mEq/L, lactate 28 mEq/L]	Often used for replacement fluid because of multiple electrolytes and isotonic expansion of plasma volume. Used frequently for GI losses. Do not provide calories unless dextrose is added. Not given for >48 hr because of risk of calorie depletion and/or electrolyte excesses. Should not be used in patients with lactic acidosis.
	Dextran 70 (6% solution of polysaccharide combined with saline or dextrose and water)[9]	Rapidly expands plasma volume. Low-molecular-weight dextran decreases blood viscosity and allows greater flow of blood through capillaries.
	Hetastarch (310 mOsm/L)	Used for rapid volume expansion. Like dextran, may cause bleeding and circulatory overload. Both are useful in cardiogenic, hemorrhagic, or septic shock. May cause prolonged bleeding time and is contraindicated in patients with renal failure, severe bleeding disorders, and severe heart failure.
Hypotonic	0.45% NaCl (½ strength) (154 mOsm/L) [½ normal saline, ½ water] 0.33% NaCl (⅓ strength) (103 mOsm/L) [⅓ normal saline, ⅔ water]	Both 0.33% and 0.45% NaCl are hypotonic fluids that help hydrate the cell. Do not provide calories. Useful in treating hypernatremia when it is desired to replace water *and* sodium.
Hypertonic	5% dextrose in 0.45% NaCl* (406 mOsm/L)	Good maintenance solution if potassium is added (provides calories, free water, and sodium chloride). Promotes hydration and diuresis in dehydrated patients. Used as a replacement solution for GI losses.
	50% dextrose in water (2525 mOsm/L)	Very hypertonic; used to treat hypoglycemia and provide long-term nutritional replacement. Can cause osmotic diuresis.
	3% or 5% NaCl (grossly hypertonic)	Dangerously hypertonic solutions used to treat severe symptomatic hyponatremia as with SIADH. Pulling fluid from ICF to ECF can cause fluid overload (hypervolemia) and increased intracranial pressure.
	Albumin (25% [1500 mOsm/L]) given in 50 or 100 ml units	Expands plasma volume and increases plasma oncotic pressure, pulling fluid out of interstitial spaces. Use with caution in patients with cardiac or renal failure (risk of fluid overload).

Ca^{++}, Calcium; *Cl^-*, chloride; *ECF,* extracellular fluid; *GI,* gastrointestinal; *H_2O,* water; *ICF,* intracellular fluid; *K^+*, potassium; *Na^+*, sodium; *NaCl,* Sodium chloride.

**Solution tonicity*—adding dextrose to any electrolyte solution renders the solution hypertonic in the bag. However, within a short time after administration, dextrose is metabolized, and tonicity of infused solution decreases in proportion to tonicity of nondextrose components (electrolytes) within the solution. Any initial effect on cell is temporary. For example, 5% dextrose in 0.45% NaCl is hypertonic in container but becomes hypotonic once dextrose is metabolized by body. Similarly, 5% dextrose in Ringer's lactate is hypertonic in container but isotonic once dextrose is used.

TABLE 17-7 COMPLICATIONS OF INTRAVENOUS FLUID THERAPY

Observations	Nursing Actions
Circulatory Overload	
Bounding pulse, venous distention, hoarseness, dyspnea, cough, pulmonary rales, restlessness	Notify physician. Reduce flow to "keep open" rate. Raise head of bed to facilitate breathing.
Local Infiltration	
Decreased rate or cessation of fluid flow Tissue around needle or catheter site cold, pale, swollen, hard Complaint of local pain	Stop infusion. Arrange to restart infusion at another site. Apply moist heat. Elevate lower arm.
Thrombophlebitis	
Pain, redness, warmth, edema along vein	Same as for local infiltration. Cold compress may be applied initially.
Pyrogenic Reaction	
Fever, chills, general malaise, nausea, and vomiting 30 min after infusion started Hypotension (if severe)	Switch to another infusion solution and run at "keep open" rate. Notify physician. Monitor vital signs. Save infusion fluid for culture.
Anaphylactic Reaction (With Proteins)	
Apprehension, dyspnea, wheezing, tightness of chest, itching, hypotension	Switch infusion to nonprotein solution and run at "keep open" rate. Notify physician. Monitor vital signs.

gating solutions, drainage from body orifices, and excessive wound drainage. Serum osmolarity and urine specific gravity, which normally ranges between 1.010 and 1.030 in healthy adults, are monitored for variations so that interventions can be implemented as needed.

RELATED NIC INTERVENTIONS. Fluid/Electrolyte Management, Fluid Management, Hemodialysis Therapy, Peritoneal Dialysis Therapy

EVALUATION

To evaluate the effectiveness of nursing interventions, compare patient behaviors with those stated in the expected patient outcomes.

RELATED NOC OUTCOMES. Circulation Status, Electrolyte & Acid/Base Balance, Fluid Balance, Hydration, Nutritional Status: Food & Fluid Intake

Isotonic Fluid Excess (Hypervolemia)

An isotonic gain of fluid in the ECF, referred to as isotonic fluid excess or hypervolemia, is characterized by a proportional gain of water *and* sodium.

Etiology. An isotonic ECF excess occurs from a gain of both sodium and water, or failure of the kidneys to eliminate sodium and water. In either case the expansion of the ECF space is primarily a problem of sodium control, although serum sodium does not measurably change. *Sodium and water gain* may occur as a result of intravenous or nasogastric administration of isotonic fluid(s). Isotonic intravenous fluids such as 0.9% sodium chloride and lactated Ringer's solution can lead to ECF excess if given in large volumes or administered to patients with renal or cardiac compromise. *Impaired renal regulatory and excretory function* accounts for sodium and water retention in many disease processes such as heart or liver failure. Long-term corticosteroid use can also contribute to sodium and water retention.

Pathophysiology. Fluid volume excess is associated with weight gain that develops over a short time (i.e., several pounds in a 24-hour period). If fluid excess is severe or cardiac function is compromised, pulmonary edema and respiratory failure can occur. Serum sodium stays within normal range unless hypervolemia occurs from excessive water retention, in which case the ECF becomes hypotonic.

A common condition that alters renal sodium and water regulation is heart failure, which reduces cardiac output and subsequent glomerular filtration, which chronically stimulates the kidneys to conserve sodium and water. Initially sodium and water retention is isotonic, but as heart failure worsens and renal mechanisms are stressed, hypotonic fluid imbalances occur (greater water gain than sodium gain).[9] The Clinical Manifestations box lists signs of ECF volume excess.

Collaborative Care Management. The goals of treatment are to restore normal fluid balance, provide symptomatic care until balance is achieved, and prevent future fluid volume excess. Mild volume overload may be corrected with sodium and water restriction. Severe volume overload, particularly in persons with compromised renal or cardiac function, may be associated with pulmonary edema, a potentially life-threatening condition that requires emergency care.

Long-term dietary modifications may be necessary to control fluid volume. Patients are taught to read product labels and to avoid high-sodium foods. Patients and family members are educated about food preparation techniques, including seasoning options that minimize sodium use. Loop diuretics (e.g., furosemide) are often used in severe ECF excess or renal failure. Sometimes it is necessary to limit fluid intake to avoid overhydration. However, sodium and fluid restrictions are not generally ordered in conjunction with diuretics, since the patient could become dehydrated.

Nursing Management

of the Patient with Isotonic Fluid Volume Excess

ASSESSMENT

Health History. Assess for:

- History of heart failure, cirrhosis, acute or chronic renal failure with oliguria
- Medication that may contribute to sodium and water retention (e.g., glucocorticosteroids)
- Complaints of shortness of breath or orthopnea

Physical Examination. Assess for:

- Peripheral edema, neck vein distention, pulmonary edema: crackles, dyspnea, cough, acute weight gain
- Increased blood pressure, bounding pulses (gallop rhythm with heart failure)

CLINICAL MANIFESTATIONS
Extracellular Fluid Volume Excess

- Sudden weight gain
- Decreased hematocrit, decreased urine specific gravity
- Distended neck veins, increased central venous pressure
- Bounding pulse, increased blood pressure
- Peripheral edema, usually not marked
- Crackles, shortness of breath
- Signs of pulmonary edema

NURSING DIAGNOSES, OUTCOMES, AND INTERVENTIONS

Nursing Diagnosis: Excess Fluid Volume

OUTCOMES. Common examples of expected outcomes for the patient with a diagnosis of *excess fluid volume* are:

Patient will:

- Achieve fluid balance as evidenced by adequate urine output, specific gravity within normal range, stable weight, absence of edema, blood pressure within patient's normal range, clear lung sounds.
- Verbalize understanding of fluid and dietary restrictions and prescribed medications.
- Maintain skin integrity as evidenced by absence of pressure areas.

NURSING INTERVENTIONS. Patients at risk for fluid volume excess include those with altered renal, cardiac, hypothalamic, or adrenal function. The nurse monitors plasma volume by assessing jugular neck veins and hand veins, which will appear distended. The nurse monitors and documents the patient's response to diuretic therapy, assesses and incorporates cultural dietary and fluid patterns into dietary plans, and encourages patients to maintain prescribed sodium restrictions.[4] The nurse assesses circulation to extremities at least every 8 hours, noting capillary refill, pulse amplitude, and color (edematous skin appears pale). Pitting edema is differentiated from lymphedema, which is characterized by a brawny as opposed to a more pliant feel associated with interstitial edema. The extremities are elevated to reduce dependent edema except when significant heart failure or pulmonary edema is present, since it increases venous return and cardiac workload. The nurse turns and repositions patients at least every 2 hours to protect edematous parts of the body from prolonged pressure, injury, and temperature extremes. Excess fluid in the tissues results in poor cellular nutrition, increased risk for trauma and infection, and reduced healing.

RELATED NIC INTERVENTIONS. Fluid Monitoring, Fluid Management, Electrolyte Monitoring, Skin Surveillance, Positioning

EVALUATION

To evaluate the effectiveness of nursing interventions, compare patient behaviors with those stated in the expected patient outcomes.

RELATED NOC OUTCOMES. Electrolyte & Acid/Base Balance, Fluid Balance, Hydration, Tissue Perfusion: Peripheral, Vital Signs Status, Respiratory Status: Ventilation

HYPOTONIC FLUID VOLUME ALTERATIONS AND HYPONATREMIA

Sodium is the predominant electrolyte in ECF. Normal sodium concentration in the plasma is 135 to 145 mEq/L. Disorders of sodium balance are commonly seen in clinical practice and generally *occur in association with fluid imbalance.* Hyponatremia (serum sodium concentration less than 135 mEq/L) can occur with a fluid volume deficit or fluid volume excess. Impaired water regulation manifests as an alteration in serum sodium concentration (high serum sodium with water loss, low serum sodium with water gain).

Etiology. *Fluid volume deficit with hyponatremia* results from a disproportionate loss of water and sodium. Thiazide diuretics commonly cause a greater loss of sodium in relation to water, which lowers the ECF sodium concentration.[10] Although diuretic-provoked hyponatremia is generally mild, it can become severe if it occurs with other factors that cause sodium wasting, or if sodium intake is markedly restricted, as often occurs in patients with severe heart failure. Postoperative hyponatremia is common and is most likely due to loss of GI fluids that are high in sodium content. Some endocrine problems, such as adrenal insufficiency, may result in aldosterone and cortisol deficiency, which promote renal sodium loss and increased release of ADH, respectively.[8]

Fluid volume excess with hyponatremia is the most common form of hyponatremia. It results from continued water intake in the presence of impaired renal excretion of water, which leads to dilutional hyponatremia. The impaired renal excretion may be due to decompensated heart failure, cirrhosis, or nephrotic syndrome. Postoperative patients may become hyponatremic from overhydration with nonelectrolyte solutions.

Normal fluid volume with hyponatremia can result from a *gain in pure water* associated with SIADH. The pure water gain is distributed throughout body compartments in normal proportion; thus symptoms of volume excess are not usually evident even though total body water increases.

Pathophysiology. Sodium imbalances are usually associated with parallel changes in osmolarity with either a net gain of water or loss of sodium-rich fluids.[4] In either situation the patient may exhibit clinical manifestations of cellular edema (water intoxication). Because brain cells are particularly sensitive to the increase in intracellular water, the most common signs of hypoosmolar overhydration are changes in mental status associated with cerebral edema and increased intracranial pressure. Seizures, coma, and permanent neurologic damage may occur with plasma sodium levels under 115 mEq/L. Chronic hyponatremia, however, may not be manifested by acute symptoms, since the brain can blunt the movement of water into the cells by releasing intracellular solutes and lowering osmolarity inside the cell.[4]

Hyponatremia with decreased ECF volume is also manifested by typical low-volume hemodynamic measures. *Hyponatremia with increased ECF volume* may be manifested by weight gain and elevated blood pressure. The Clinical Manifestations box presents signs and symptoms of hyponatremia. A comparison of clinical conditions, serum sodium, and actual total body sodium levels are listed in Table 17-4.

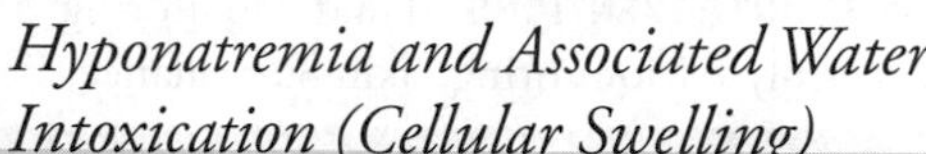

CLINICAL MANIFESTATIONS
Hyponatremia and Associated Water Intoxication (Cellular Swelling)

Headache
Muscle cramps, weakness, fatigue
Irritability, apprehension
Tachycardia, postural hypotension
Anorexia, nausea, vomiting
Abdominal cramps, diarrhea
Weight loss or gain depending on fluid volume disturbance
Signs of extracellular fluid (ECF) volume excess with water excess
Signs of ECF volume deficit with sodium loss
Serum sodium less than 135 mEq/L
Serum osmolality less than 280 mOsm/kg

Severe

Fingerprint edema
Mental confusion
Delirium
Shock
Convulsions, coma

Collaborative Care Management. Management of hyponatremia includes educating those at risk such as athletes, persons working in hot environments, and older adults to recognize signs of sodium depletion, and to replace insensible fluid losses with sufficient sodium and water. Specific interventions are guided by how quickly the condition develops, the severity of the hyponatremia, and the clinical presentation.[10] *Acute* symptomatic hyponatremia (i.e., seizures, coma, and respiratory arrest) requires aggressive intervention. Gradual return of serum sodium to a normal level occurs within the context of the patient's fluid volume (replacement or restriction of water). Overly rapid or aggressive treatment of *chronic* hyponatremia may result in permanent neurologic damage.

Hyponatremia with ECF deficit requires volume replacement to interrupt the physiologic stimulus to ADH release.[4] Normalization of sodium concentration is achieved by administering isotonic fluids orally, gastric feeding, and/or intravenous fluids. Hypertonic sodium solutions are given *only* in emergency situations with *severely symptomatic patients*, and with judicious monitoring to avoid cellular dehydration. *Hyponatremia with ECF excess* is treated with loop diuretics and/or sodium restriction. Water restriction may be initiated if the serum sodium level is low and edema is absent; if edema is present *and* the serum sodium level is within normal range, sodium is restricted. If both edema and a low serum sodium level are present, then both water and sodium are restricted.[10]

Nursing Management
of the Patient with Hypotonic Fluid Volume Alterations (Hyponatremia)

ASSESSMENT

Health History. Assess for:

- Dietary history, especially of protein and salt intake
- History of vomiting, diarrhea, renal failure, heart failure, thiazide diuretics, risk factors for SIADH, lung or pancreatic cancer, head injury or stroke, recent surgery

Physical Examination. Assess for:

- Signs of ECF volume deficit or fluid volume excess
- Alterations in level of consciousness and neurologic status
- Abnormalities in serum sodium, serum osmolarity, urine specific gravity

NURSING DIAGNOSES, OUTCOMES, AND INTERVENTIONS

Nursing Diagnosis: Ineffective Protection

OUTCOMES. Common examples of expected outcomes for the patient with a diagnosis of *ineffective protection* are:

Patient will:

- Verbalize orientation to person, place, and time.
- Remain free from physical injury.

NURSING INTERVENTIONS. The nurse advises the patient and family that altered sensorium may occur and will improve with treatment. Disoriented patients are at increased risk for injury and must be closely monitored. The bed is placed in the lowest position with side rails up and wheels locked in case the patient attempts to get out of bed without assistance. The nurse closely monitors serum sodium levels throughout the treatment period. The patient and family members need to be informed about the importance of maintaining fluid or sodium restrictions. Family members may be particularly helpful in monitoring patients who are experiencing mental status changes and may not understand the need for restriction.

RELATED NIC INTERVENTIONS. Behavior Management, Delirium Management, Environmental Management: Safety, Fall Prevention, Family Support, Reality Orientation, Surveillance

EVALUATION

To evaluate the effectiveness of nursing interventions, compare patient behaviors with those stated in the expected patient outcomes.

RELATED NOC OUTCOMES. Cognition, Cognitive Orientation, Fall Prevention Behavior, Risk Control

Hypertonic Fluid Volume Alterations and Hypernatremia

Hypernatremia (serum sodium level above 145 mEq/L) may result from fluid deficit or sodium excess. Thirst is the primary defense against hypernatremia; therefore sodium excess usually occurs as a result of water deprivation rather than the lack of desire to drink. The kidneys also protect the body from hypernatremia by excreting excess sodium. Any condition interfering with renal sodium excretion or concentrating ability (e.g., diabetes insipidus) in conjunction with impaired water intake can contribute to hypernatremia.[4] People most vulnerable to hypernatremia are infants, the elderly, and those with chronic renal disease or impaired thirst mechanism.

Etiology. *Fluid volume deficit with hypernatremia* occurs when there is a *loss of water* and failure to adequately replace it.[10] Diabetes mellitus, which causes osmotic diuresis, is a common cause of renal water loss. Large amounts of glucose and ketone bodies collect in the blood, creating a hyperosmolar state and pulling water out of the cell into the plasma (initially diluting the serum sodium). As water is excreted (osmotic diuresis), hypernatremia develops. Similarly, osmotic diarrhea can occur from enteral tube feedings when high osmolar solutions are given without sufficient water. Impaired or inadequate water intake further compounds renal or extrarenal water loss. Patients who are unable to (1) ask for fluids, (2) identify their need for fluid, or (3) swallow easily may develop fluid deficits.

Fluid volume excess with hypernatremia secondary to increased exogenous sodium may lead to hyperosmolarity of the ECF, which promotes renal conservation of fluid. As the ECF volume expands to restore normal osmolarity, signs of extracellular volume excess develop. Other sources of sodium gain include intravenous administration of hypertonic saline, primary aldosteronism, saltwater near-drowning, or certain drugs (e.g., sodium bicarbonate).[4]

Pathophysiology. When an excess of sodium occurs without a proportional increase in body fluid, or when water loss occurs without proportional loss of sodium, osmolarity changes and water shifts out of the cells, causing *cellular dehydration*. As both intracellular and ECF volumes decrease, cell function is impaired due to inadequate diffusion of food, oxygen, and waste products. In addition to signs and symptoms of volume alteration, patients exhibit clinical manifestations of cellular dehydration. The Clinical Manifestations box lists signs and symptoms of hypernatremia.

Collaborative Care Management. Very young, elderly, and debilitated patients require careful monitoring and need to be offered fluids at least every 2 hours. Water content in hypertonic feeding solutions should be increased when (1) the patient complains of thirst, (2) the protein or electrolyte content of the solution is high, (3) the patient has a fever or a disease causing an increased metabolic rate, (4) the urinary output is concentrated, or (5) signs of water deficit develop.

Usually osmolar balance can be restored with oral fluids. A pure water deficit, exhibited by a serum sodium level of 160 mEq/L or higher, is treated with 5% dextrose in water (D_5W) or hypotonic saline. The nurse carefully monitors patients for their response to fluids and indications of fluid overload. Sodium gain

CLINICAL MANIFESTATIONS
Hypernatremia and Associated Cellular Dehydration

Thirst
Warm, flushed skin, fever
Dry, sticky mucous membranes
Signs of extracellular fluid (ECF) volume excess with true sodium gain
Signs of ECF volume deficit with water loss
Firm, rubbery subcutaneous tissue
Rough, fissured tongue
Concentrated urine (except with diabetes insipidus)
Serum sodium greater than 145 mEq/L
Serum osmolality greater than 295 mOsm/kg
Increased hematocrit, blood urea nitrogen

Severe

Manic excitement
Decreased reflexes
Seizures, coma
Death

is treated with diuretics in combination with oral or intravenous water replacement. People with kidney failure, congestive heart failure, or endocrine (adrenal or thyroid) conditions may require dietary sodium alterations.

Nursing Management

of the Patient with Hypertonic Fluid Volume Alterations (Hypernatremia)

ASSESSMENT

Health History. Assess for:

- Risk factors, including excessive sweating, vomiting, diarrhea, diuretic therapy, decreased water intake, confusion, hyperglycemia, osmotic enteral feedings, total parenteral nutrition (TPN) therapy
- Central nervous system effects of cellular dehydration (restlessness, irritability, mental status changes, seizures)
- Factors that affect safety needs (e.g., altered mental status, potential seizure activity)

Physical Examination. Assess for:

- Signs and symptoms of fluid volume excess or deficit (see discussion above)
- Clinical manifestations of cellular dehydration (e.g., dry, sticky mucous membranes; red, swollen tongue; avid thirst)
- Alterations in serum sodium and osmolarity

NURSING DIAGNOSES, OUTCOMES, AND INTERVENTIONS

Nursing Diagnosis: Risk for Injury

OUTCOMES. Common examples of expected outcomes for the patient with a diagnosis of *risk for injury* are:

Patient will:

- Reduce risk for injury by adhering to nursing interventions for a safe environment.
- Recognize early signs of fluid imbalance and follow strategies to prevent physical injury.

NURSING INTERVENTIONS. An accurate record of intake and output is essential to facilitate quick recognition of a negative fluid balance. The nurse assesses level of consciousness at least every 4 hours and reorients the patient as necessary. Side rails are padded and an airway is placed at the bedside if seizures are anticipated. The nurse administers comfort measures such as mouthwash or oral swabs to decrease thirst. Water replacement is administered within the prescribed time frame to avoid rapid reduction in plasma sodium and subsequent cerebral edema.

RELATED NIC INTERVENTIONS. Environmental Management: Safety, Fall Prevention, Reality Orientation, Seizure Precautions, Surveillance

EVALUATION

To evaluate the effectiveness of nursing interventions, compare patient behaviors with those stated in the expected patient outcomes.

RELATED NOC OUTCOMES. Cognition, Cognitive Orientation, Risk Control, Fall Prevention Behavior

GERONTOLOGIC CONSIDERATIONS

One of the most common diagnoses reported for hospital admissions in older adults is dehydration. Fluid volume deficits and sodium imbalances in the older adult population can be caused by impaired renal function and reduced ability to concentrate urine, voluntary fluid restriction to minimize incontinence, reduced mobility, dulled thirst mechanism, and medications that cause water and electrolyte losses.[3] For these reasons, older adults must be educated regarding sufficient water replacement and observed closely during periods of illness. Classic indicators may not be reliable unless volume loss is profound because of decreased skin elasticity and comorbid cardiac conditions. Angiotensin-converting enzyme (ACE) inhibitors and the nonsteroidal antiinflammatory drugs (NSAIDs) commonly prescribed for older adults reduce blood pressure, diminish filtration, and increase the risk for volume deficit.[13] Other medications that directly influence fluid loss include diuretics and laxatives; indirect contributors include analgesics, sedatives, and tranquilizers that impair physical or cognitive ability.

Potassium

Potassium (K^+) is the major intracellular cation and regulator of intracellular osmolarity. Because most of the potassium in the body is intracellular (150 to 160 mEq/L), the serum potassium level (3.5 to 5.0 mEq/L) does not necessarily indicate the total body potassium content. A 24-hour urinary potassium excretion must be measured to obtain accurate information about total body potassium.[2] Potassium is important in the control of acid-base balance, conduction of nerve impulses, and promotion of proper skeletal and cardiac muscle activity.

Potassium is filtered by the kidneys, where approximately 90% is reabsorbed in the proximal tubules and loop of Henle. Unlike sodium, the body conserves potassium *less effectively*. However, acute increases in serum potassium are handled quickly through increased cellular uptake and renal excretion of potassium excesses in response to aldosterone secretion.[5]

Hypokalemia

Hypokalemia exists when the serum potassium falls below 3.5 mEq/L. Potassium deficit is rarely caused by inadequate intake, but rather a combination of factors. Since potassium is not stored well in body cells, a daily intake of 40 to 60 mEq is needed.[6] Figure 17-6 summarizes the causes and effects of hypokalemia.

Etiology. *Dietary restrictions* (e.g., during diagnostic testing) may lead to hypokalemia especially if large amounts of potassium-free parenteral fluids are given. The parenteral administration of 5% dextrose in water without the addition of potassium tends to dilute serum potassium. *GI losses* often lead to hypokalemia, since GI fluids are rich in potassium. Severe hypokalemia may be seen in patients with eating disorders involving vomiting or laxative abuse, draining fistulas, or acute or chronic diarrhea.

Potassium shifts can occur during the formation of new tissues (e.g., during the recovery phase of burns); during the conversion of

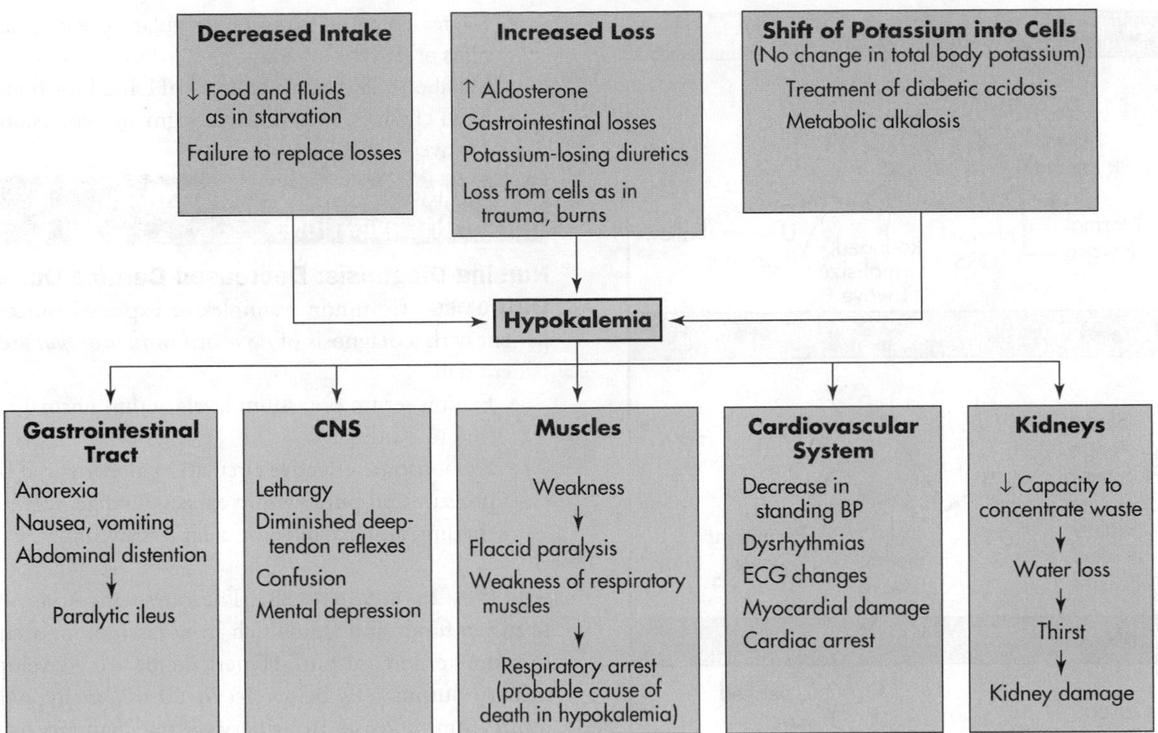

Figure 17-6 Causes and effects of hypokalemia. *CNS,* Central nervous system; *BP,* blood pressure; *ECG,* electrocardiogram.

glucose to glycogen; or after insulin administration, which promotes the movement of glucose and potassium into the cells. In addition, alkalosis causes movement of potassium into cells in exchange for hydrogen ions; potassium excretion increases as hydrogen ions are retained.

Renal losses from increases in tubular potassium excretion occur from osmotic diuretics and disease states that produce osmotic diuresis. Potassium excretion is also increased by tubular diuretics (e.g., hydrochlorothiazide and furosemide); primary or secondary hyperaldosteronism; and other antibiotics such as amphotericin B, some penicillins, and gentamycin.[8]

Pathophysiology. Chronic hypokalemia allows time for the body to compensate for the loss of potassium through intracellular shifting, which explains why the severely depleted person may not show signs of marked hypokalemia.[5] However, acute potassium loss causes profound alterations in neuromuscular excitability, with smooth muscle weakness and decreased GI tone, decreased reflexes, and weakness in the larger muscles of the legs and arms and ultimately the diaphragm and respiratory muscles.

The cardiac effects of low serum potassium can be manifested by potentially life-threatening ventricular dysrhythmias. Figure 17-7 shows the effects of potassium on the electrocardiogram (ECG). Patients receiving digitalis preparations are at particular risk for cardiac rhythm disturbance, since hypokalemia potentiates the effects of digitalis.

Collaborative Care Management. Persons who are receiving potassium-wasting diuretics are instructed to include foods high in potassium in their diet (Box 17-3). Older adults are educated about the hazards of laxative and enema abuse. If cleansing enema regimens are ordered, no more than three should be given to the patient without consulting the health care provider, since enemas cause potassium loss.

The safest way to administer supplemental potassium is orally. Tablets or capsules require 24 hours to metabolize and are the best way to prevent potassium loss in patients receiving diuretics. Liquid potassium supplements are superior to tablets because liquids act more quickly. Potassium supplements are irritating to the GI tract; therefore they are taken with at least 8 ounces of water. Intravenous potassium is given when prompt reversal of life-threatening hypokalemia is necessary. Potassium must be diluted before administration and preferably given through a central line rather than a peripheral line because it is caustic to veins. An intravenous infusion pump is essential to safely control the flow rate (10 to 20 mEq/hr). Rapid infusion of intravenous potassium can precipitate lethal cardiac dysrhythmias. Cardiac monitoring is essential for patients who already have cardiac disturbances. In some instances of severe depletion, potassium may be gi concentrated solution (40 mEq/dl) over 4 h *never* be administered by intraveno

Nursing Manage *of the Patient wit*

ASSESSMENT

Health History. Assess for:
- High-risk factors, including deficiency, gastric losses, pu

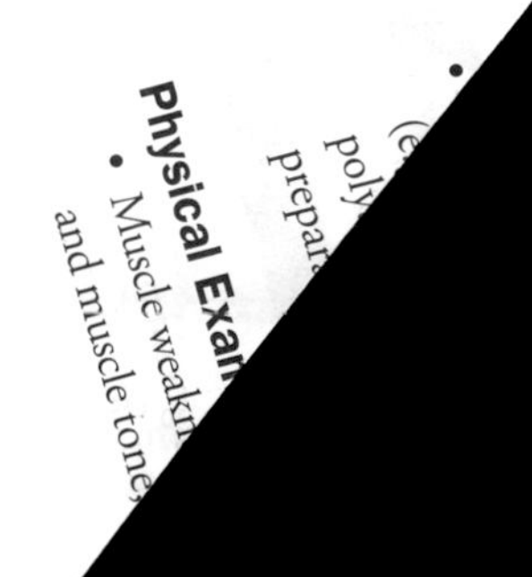

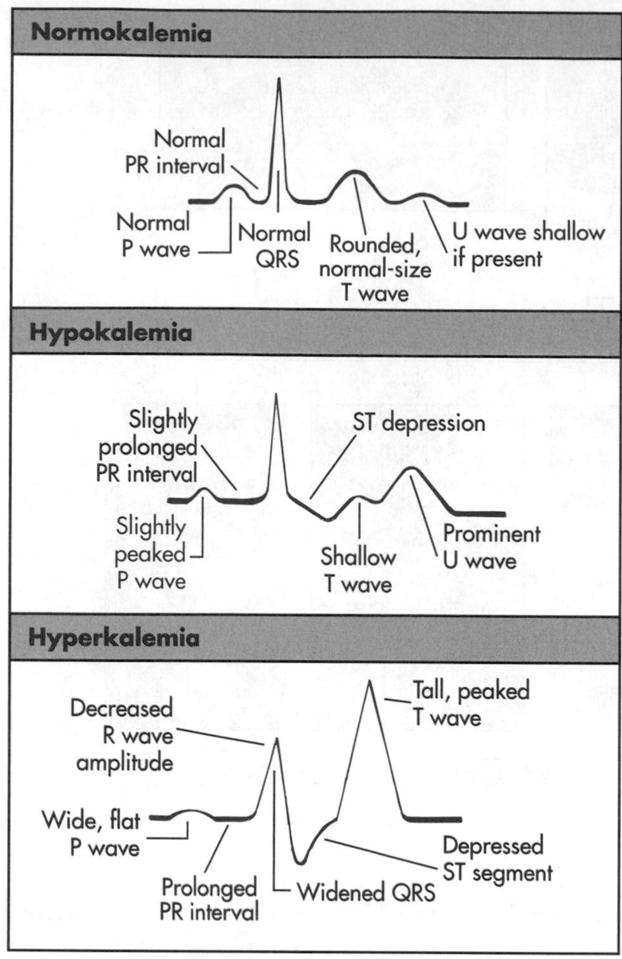

Figure 17-7 Effects of potassium on the electrocardiogram.

Box 17-3 Foods High in Potassium*

- Apricots
- Bananas
- Beans
- Cantaloupe
- Carrots
- Chocolate
- Honeydew
- Meats
- Milk
- Mushrooms
- Nuts
- Oranges
- Peas
- Potatoes
- Salt substitute
- Spinach
- Squash
- Tomatoes

*Most raw vegetables contain potassium, much of which is lost during cooking.

diets, diaphoresis, alkalosis, tissue repair (burns, trauma), osmotic diuresis

- Fatigue, muscle cramps, nausea, constipation, paresthesias
- Medication history of potential potassium-wasting agents (e.g., thiazide and loop diuretics), insulin, TPN, sodium ...styrene (Kayexalate) or other laxatives, enemas, digitalis ...ations

...mination. Assess for:

- ...ess (first seen in quadriceps), decreased reflexes
- ... vomiting, constipation (ileus)
- Decreased blood pressure, irregular pulse or pulse deficit, signs of digoxin toxicity
- Metabolic alkalosis (increased pH and bicarbonate)
- ECG changes, including ST-segment depression, flattened T wave, U wave

Nursing Diagnoses, Outcomes, and Interventions

Nursing Diagnosis: Decreased Cardiac Output

Outcomes. Common examples of expected outcomes for the patient with a diagnosis of *decreased cardiac output* are:
Patient will:

- Exhibit serum potassium levels within normal range (3.5 to 5 mEq/L).
- Demonstrate effective circulation as evidenced by blood pressure and pulse within expected range, regular pulse rhythm, absence of ventricular dysrhythmias.

Nursing Interventions. The nurse encourages the patient to ingest foods and fluids rich in potassium, and closely monitors intake and output. Hyperkalemia can develop rapidly if urinary output falls below 15 to 20 ml/hr; hypokalemia may result from increases in urinary output. Patients receiving digitalis preparations are monitored for cardiac dysrhythmias. Potassium chloride is not added to intravenous containers already hanging, since doing so can create the possibility for administering a bolus of medication.[4] The nurse frequently monitors the patient's intravenous site for erythema, heat, or pain, which are signs of venous irritation. Potassium is administered cautiously to patients receiving potassium-sparing diuretics or ACE inhibitors (e.g., captropril), since the potential for hyperkalemia is enhanced.[12] The patient and family members need to learn how to assess apical heart rates so they can report heart irregularities if they develop.

Related NIC Interventions. Cardiac Care, Dysrhythmia Management, Electrolyte Management: Hypokalemia, Medication Management

Nursing Diagnosis: Ineffective Breathing Pattern

Outcomes. Common examples of expected outcomes for the patient with a diagnosis of *ineffective breathing pattern* are:
Patient will:

- Demonstrate effective breathing patterns as evidenced by symmetric chest expansion, absent adventitious breath sounds, respiratory rate and rhythm and pulmonary function within normal limits for the patient.

Nursing Interventions. The nurse monitors the patient's respirations for rate, rhythm, depth, effort, chest movement, and use of accessory muscles. The nurse notifies the health care provider if respirations become shallow or rapid, since these changes indicate worsening hypokalemia, which can lead to respiratory arrest. The nurse auscultates breath sounds, noting areas of diminished ventilation or adventitious sounds. The nurse monitors SaO_2 and arterial blood gases and reports them as appropriate. Increased restlessness, anxiety, air hunger, or dyspnea may also indicate that hypokalemia is worsening.

RELATED NIC INTERVENTIONS. Acid-Base Monitoring, Airway Management, Anxiety Reduction, Positioning, Respiratory Monitoring, Vital Signs Monitoring

EVALUATION

To evaluate the effectiveness of nursing interventions, compare patient behaviors with those stated in the expected patient outcomes.

RELATED NOC OUTCOMES. Cardiac Pump Effectiveness, Circulation Status, Respiratory Status: Ventilation, Tissue Perfusion: Peripheral, Vital Signs

Hyperkalemia

Hyperkalemia (serum potassium level greater than 5.5 mEq/L) may be acute or chronic. The severity of symptoms depends on the rate of gain or loss as well as the overall total body potassium level.[4] Figure 17-8 presents the causes and effects of hyperkalemia.

Etiology. *Excessive potassium because of intake* rarely occurs unless accompanied by reduced renal function. Intake exceeding excretion can occur from excessive intravenous potassium administration, and when salt substitutes, which are rich in potassium, are generously used. Some herbal juices are high in potassium.[6] *Decreased renal function* can cause hyperkalemia in older adults, especially in conjunction with drugs that promote potassium retention (e.g., ACE inhibitors, beta-blockers, cyclosporine, NSAIDs, lithium).

Potassium shifts out of the cell during severe tissue damage from trauma or surgery, sepsis, fever, dehydration, starvation, acidosis, and insulin deficiency or hyperglycemia. Cell lysis and a false serum potassium elevation may result from drawing a blood sample using a small needle or from drawing the sample after prolonged tourniquet application.[8] Care must be taken to avoid drawing blood samples from a site proximal to an intravenous infusion containing potassium.

Pathophysiology. A rapid increase in serum potassium of only 1 to 3 mEq/L can be lethal. On the other hand, some persons with renal failure develop severe hyperkalemia slowly and adjust to the potassium excess with few symptoms. Acute elevations of extracellular potassium affect neuromuscular irritability as the ECF and ICF potassium ratio is disrupted, whereas long-term increases in ECF potassium result in potassium shifts into the cell to help reestablish a normal ratio.[10]

Alterations in the stimulation properties of muscle and rate of repolarization may cause weakness or even paralysis. Generally, these problems do not occur until the serum potassium exceeds 8 mEq/L.[12] Hyperkalemia causes decreased cardiac conduction, leading to ventricular fibrillation or cardiac arrest.

Patients with heart failure are at risk for hyperkalemia and hypokalemia, which can be life threatening.[12] Early stages of heart failure are associated with hypokalemia from compensatory mechanisms to conserve sodium. In the advanced stages of heart failure, hyperkalemia occurs from renal insufficiency and potassium retention. The problem is confounded when patients are advised to consume potassium-rich foods or supplements to offset diuretic losses of potassium. As heart failure worsens and renal function declines, diuretics generally become less effective and potassium excretion declines. ACE inhibitors, aldosterone receptor antagonists like spironolactone, and angiotensin-receptor blockers (e.g., eplerenone) reduce potassium excretion and need to be monitored in patients who are at risk for hyperkalemia.

Collaborative Care Management. Prevention of excess serum potassium is the best approach to the condition. People with impaired renal function are cautioned about the possibility of potassium retention and advised to avoid salt substitutes high in potassium and over-the-counter medications that can

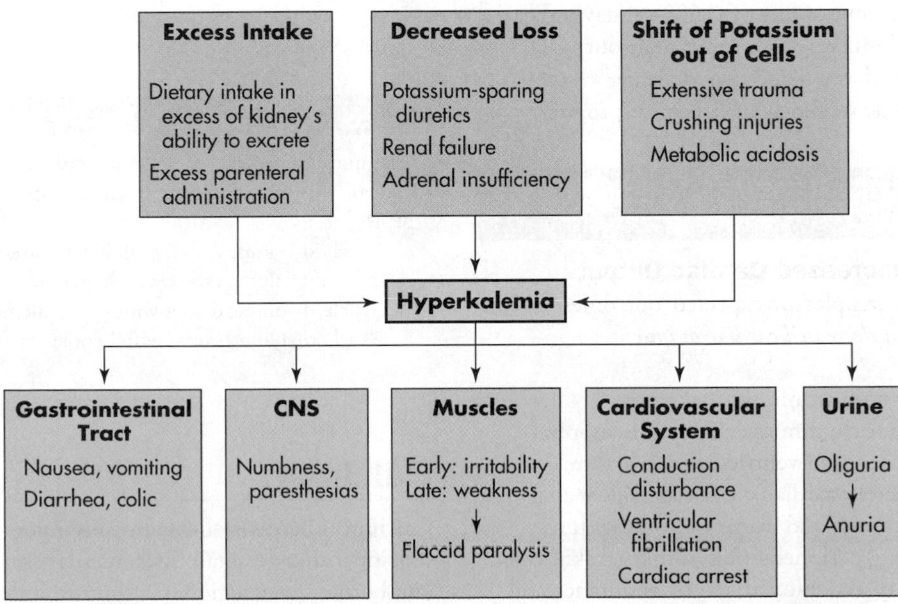

Figure 17-8 Causes and effects of hyperkalemia. *CNS*, Central nervous system.

cause hyperkalemia. The severity of the hyperkalemia guides therapy. Withholding the causative agent (e.g., potassium supplement) may be the only intervention required. Potassium-wasting diuretics may be prescribed to promote excretion, or a cation-exchange resin, such as Kayexalate, may be ordered. Bowel function must be maintained for this therapy to be effective, since the resin is exchanged for the potassium and excreted in the stool.

Severe hyperkalemia (generally greater than 6 mEq/L) is a medical emergency that requires continuous cardiac monitoring. Aggressive treatment is indicated if tall, peaked T waves, wide QRS complexes, or ventricular dysrhythmias are present on 12-lead ECG. Intravenous calcium gluconate counteracts the neuromuscular and cardiac effects of hyperkalemia. Intravenous insulin and sodium bicarbonate promote intracellular movement of potassium; these interventions are temporary and require further therapy that actually removes excess potassium from the body (e.g., dialysis, exchange resins).

Nursing Management *of the Patient with Hyperkalemia*

ASSESSMENT

Health History. Assess for:

- Health problems or procedures placing the patient at high risk for potassium excess
- Hidden sources of potassium: medications (e.g., potassium-sparing diuretics, ACE inhibitors, NSAIDs, beta-blocking agents), banked blood, salt substitutes, GI bleeding
- Irritability, anxiety, abdominal cramps, diarrhea, weakness, paresthesias, numbness

Physical Examination. Assess for:

- Serum potassium level greater than 5 mEq/L
- Signs of metabolic acidosis (decreased pH and bicarbonate)
- Decreased urinary output of less than 600 ml/day indicative of reduced fluid intake, decreased cardiac output, or renal insufficiency and associated hyperkalemia[6]
- Irregular pulse, muscle weakness or flaccidity, progressive ECG changes

NURSING DIAGNOSES, OUTCOMES, AND INTERVENTIONS

Nursing Diagnosis: Decreased Cardiac Output

OUTCOMES. Common examples of expected outcomes for the patient with a diagnosis of *decreased cardiac output* are:

Patient will:

- Exhibit serum potassium within normal range.
- Exhibit regular cardiac rhythm as evidenced by normal ECG wave strips, absence of ventricular dysrhythmias.
- Demonstrate satisfactory cardiac output as evidenced by blood pressure, heart rate, and urinary output within expected range; strong peripheral pulses; normal skin color.
- Tolerate usual activity as demonstrated by endurance and completion of self-care activities.

NURSING INTERVENTIONS. The nurse monitors at-risk patients for signs of hyperkalemia. ECG assessment can be helpful, since the physical signs and symptoms of abnormal potassium are difficult to identify in critically ill patients. Prescribed treatments are administered cautiously to prevent rapid changes in serum potassium. Electrolyte-binding resins are administered as prescribed. Kayexalate can contribute to hypomagnesemia or hypocalcemia by binding with other cations in the GI tract.[4] The nurse monitors cardiorespiratory response to activity and helps plan adequate rest periods.

Patient and family teaching, as presented in the accompanying Patient/Family Teaching box, p. 379, is an important part of nursing care for the patient with hyperkalemia.

RELATED NIC INTERVENTIONS. Cardiac Care, Dysrhythmia Management, Electrolyte Management: Hyperkalemia, Energy Management, Fluid/Electrolyte Management, Medication Management, Self-Care Assistance

EVALUATION

To evaluate the effectiveness of nursing interventions, compare patient behaviors with those stated in the expected patient outcomes.

RELATED NOC OUTCOMES. Cardiac Pump Effectiveness, Circulation Status, Endurance, Energy Conservation, Respiratory Status: Ventilation, Self-Care: Activities of Daily Living (ADL)

GERONTOLOGIC CONSIDERATIONS

Both potassium deficiency and excess are concerns in older adults. Potassium losses often occur in correlation with excessive laxative or enema use and diuretic therapy. Potassium excess from salt substitutes may be a more frequent contributing factor in this population in which heart failure is more common and sodium restrictions are prescribed. Older adults or their caregivers need to be educated about foods and beverages that contain high levels of potassium so that they use those products sparingly.

▶ ARE You READY?

The nurse caring for the patient with hyperglycemia secondary to diabetic mellitus incorporates which nursing diagnosis into the care plan?

1. Fluid volume deficit with hypernatremia
2. Fluid volume excess with hypernatremia
3. Fluid volume deficit with hyperkalemia
4. Fluid volume excess with hypokalemia

Calcium

Calcium is necessary for many physiologic activities: nerve transmission, cardiac excitability, muscular contraction, blood clotting, and hormone regulation. Calcium is excreted principally through the GI tract.

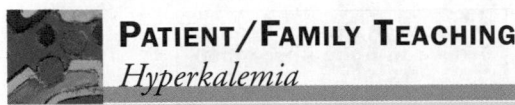

PATIENT/FAMILY TEACHING
Hyperkalemia

Teaching for the patient with hyperkalemia and his or her family includes instruction to:

- Listen to apical rate and assess for heart irregularities.
- Report heart irregularities to health care provider.
- Consume high-energy foods that are low in potassium.
- Increase fluid intake to increase urinary output and potassium excretion.
- Use strategies that minimize oxygen consumption and maximize energy conservation.

Calcium Distribution

Calcium (Ca^{++}) and phosphorus are found primarily in the bones and teeth (99%), with a very small amount dissolved in the blood (1%). Of that 1%, approximately 40% is bound to plasma proteins, mainly albumin; 10% is combined with other anions such as citrate, phosphate, and sulfate; and the remaining 50% is ionized (free). Only the ionized form is able to leave the vascular compartment and be physiologically active in cellular functions, whereas the bound calcium cannot diffuse through the capillary.[9] The serum levels usually reported are measures of total dissolved calcium (both bound and ionized), with normal values ranging from 8.5 to 10.5 mg/dl. The ionized fraction can be measured separately, but this is not done routinely.

Regulation of Calcium

The serum level of calcium depends on parathyroid hormone (PTH), vitamin D, and calcitonin. The body produces PTH in response to decreased serum calcium levels, causing increased movement of calcium from the bone to plasma, increased absorption of calcium from the GI tract, and increased resorption of calcium from the renal tubules. PTH cannot increase the absorption of calcium from the GI tract and bone resorption unless activated vitamin D is present. Calcitonin, a hormone produced by the thyroid gland, opposes the effects of PTH and vitamin D on bones. High calcium levels stimulate the thyroid gland to release calcitonin, which inhibits the release of calcium from the bone, thus lowering serum calcium levels.

Hypocalcemia

Hypocalcemia is defined as a total serum calcium concentration of less than 8.5 mg/dl or an ionized calcium concentration of less than 4 mg/dl. Figure 17-9 shows the causes and effects of hypocalcemia.

Etiology. A reduction in serum albumin can create a pseudohypocalcemia without symptoms, since there is a decrease in the percentage of protein-bound rather than ionized calcium. Patients who have *actually lost ionized calcium* will be symptomatic.

Decreased ionized calcium can be affected by pH. Acidosis causes more calcium to be ionized (less protein bound), whereas alkalosis causes more of the ionized fraction to become bound to protein (a compensatory effect to reduce protein buffers). The proportionate reduction in ionized calcium can cause tetany in patients who already have low serum calcium levels from other causes. Increased chelation (binding) of calcium to nonprotein substances such as phosphorus or citrate can also cause a proportionate loss of ionized calcium. Because citrate is commonly used as an anticoagulant in stored blood, patients rapidly receiving a large number of transfusions are carefully monitored for signs of hypocalcemia.[4]

Hormonal and electrolyte alterations can lead to potassium loss. Suppression of PTH by hypoparathyroidism, elevated vitamin D levels, and hypomagnesemia can impair the movement of calcium from bone. *Absorptive alterations* commonly play a role in hypocalcemia. Reduced oral calcium intake exerts its primary effects on bone stores rather than plasma calcium levels.[17] However, vitamin D deficiency, the inability of the kidney to change provitamin D to functional vitamin D, and diseases of the small intestine or pancreas can alter the normal absorption of calcium from the GI tract.

Pathophysiology. Calcium is important for normal cardiac muscle function and impulse propagation. Hypocalcemia may be associated with myocardial pump dysfunction, hypotension, and potentially life-threatening cardiac dysrhythmias.[9] When serum calcium levels are low, sodium moves more easily into the cell, and depolarization of neurons takes place more readily. Skeletal, smooth, and cardiac muscle functions are all affected by overstimulation. The severity of clinical manifestations depends on rate of onset, pH, and other electrolyte disorders.

Patients with hypocalcemia often complain initially of numbness and tingling of the nose, ears, fingertips, or toes. Painful muscular spasms, especially of the feet and hands (carpopedal spasms), muscle twitching, and convulsions may follow. Severe hypocalcemia can lead to tetany, laryngeal spasm, seizures, and death. Two classic indicators of tetany are (1) Trousseau's sign, elicited by inflating a blood pressure cuff on the upper arm for 2 minutes; a positive response is palmar flexion and carpal spasm; and (2) Chvostek's sign, elicited by tapping the patient's face lightly over the facial nerve (just below the temple); facial muscle twitching is a positive response. However, a person may have hypocalcemia in the absence of these signs or not have hypocalcemia in the presence of these signs.

Collaborative Care Management. For patients with mild hypocalcemia, a high-calcium diet or oral calcium salts may be sufficient. Vitamin D therapy may be necessary to enhance absorption of calcium from the GI tract. For patients with chronic renal failure, the high serum phosphorus level must be treated before the secondary hypocalcemia is treated. Aluminum hydroxide gel or calcium carbonate antacids bind with phosphorus and remove excesses from the GI tract. Hypocalcemia often coexists with hypomagnesemia and is difficult to resolve until the magnesium deficiency is corrected.

Acute hypocalcemia is a medical emergency. An intravenous solution of calcium gluconate is administered slowly when acute signs such as tetany are present. Continuous cardiac monitoring is necessary for patients receiving intravenous calcium replacements. Patients undergoing thyroid, parathyroid, and radical neck surgery

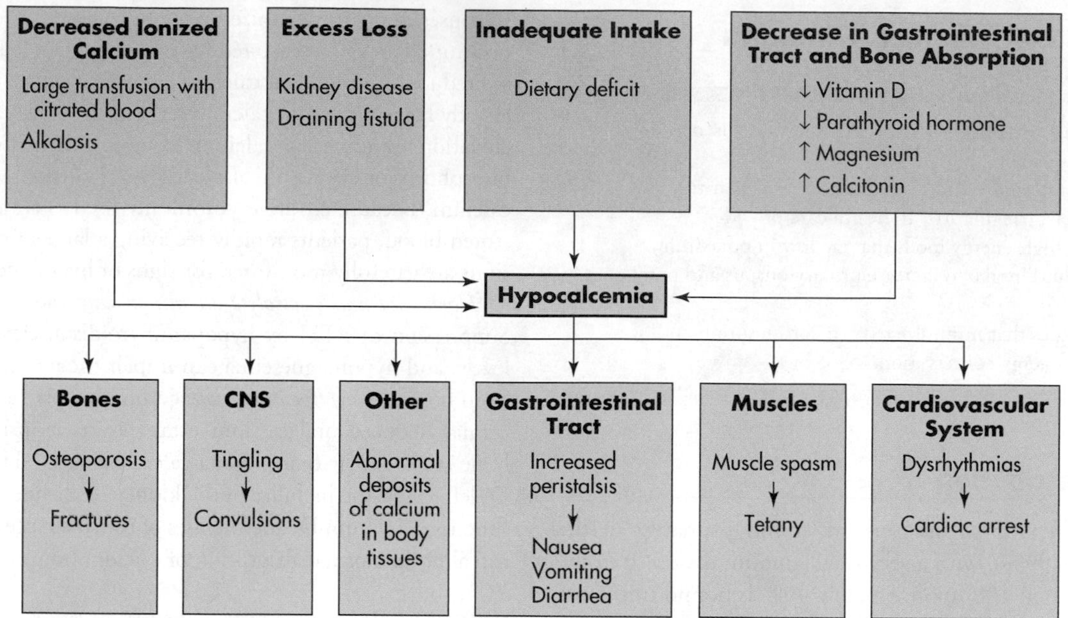

Figure 17-9 Causes and effects of hypocalcemia. *CNS,* Central nervous system.

are particularly vulnerable to hypocalcemia secondary to inadvertent removal or temporary suppression of the parathyroid glands by localized edema. Intravenous calcium gluconate must always be available for emergency use during the postoperative period.

▶ ARE You READY?

A decrease in which of the following may be correlated to serum electrolyte abnormality in a patient with hypocalcemia?

1. Sodium
2. Potassium
3. Albumin
4. Phosphorus

Nursing Management

of the Patient with Hypocalcemia

ASSESSMENT

Health History. Assess for:

- History of risk factors, including recent blood transfusions, loop diuretics, chronic diarrhea, thyroid surgery, alcoholism, acute alkalosis, malnutrition
- Lethargy, anxiety, depression, numbness, tingling, muscle cramps

Physical Examination. Assess for:

- Positive Trousseau's or Chvostek's signs, hyperactive reflexes
- ECG changes, including prolonged QT interval

NURSING DIAGNOSES, OUTCOMES, AND INTERVENTIONS

Nursing Diagnosis: Risk for Injury

OUTCOMES. Common examples of expected outcomes for the patient with a diagnosis of *risk for injury* are:

Patient will:

- Be free from injury caused by complications of severe hypocalcemia (e.g., tetany and seizures).
- Exhibit serum calcium levels within normal range.

NURSING INTERVENTIONS. The nurse removes environmental hazards and educates the patient and family about the risk for seizures. Patients are encouraged to ingest foods that are high in calcium and calcium supplements, which may include vitamin D. Intravenous calcium is cautiously administered at a rate no faster than 0.5 to 1 ml/min.[4] The correct type of intravenous calcium must be identified before administration (calcium chloride and calcium gluconate are both provided in 10 ml ampules but contain *different* amounts of calcium—13.6 mEq of calcium chloride, 4.5 mEq of calcium gluconate). The nurse frequently monitors the intravenous site, since calcium solutions can cause tissue sloughing if infiltration occurs.

RELATED NIC INTERVENTIONS. Environmental Management: Safety, Intravenous (IV) Therapy, Medication Management, Seizure Management, Seizure Precautions

EVALUATION

To evaluate the effectiveness of nursing interventions, compare patient behaviors with those stated in the expected patient outcomes.

RELATED NOC OUTCOMES. Fall Prevention Behavior, Risk Control

Hypercalcemia

Hypercalcemia (serum calcium concentration greater than 10.5 mg/dl) can result from conditions that promote release of calcium from bone, excess intake, and decreased urinary excretion. Figure 17-10 shows the causes and their effects.

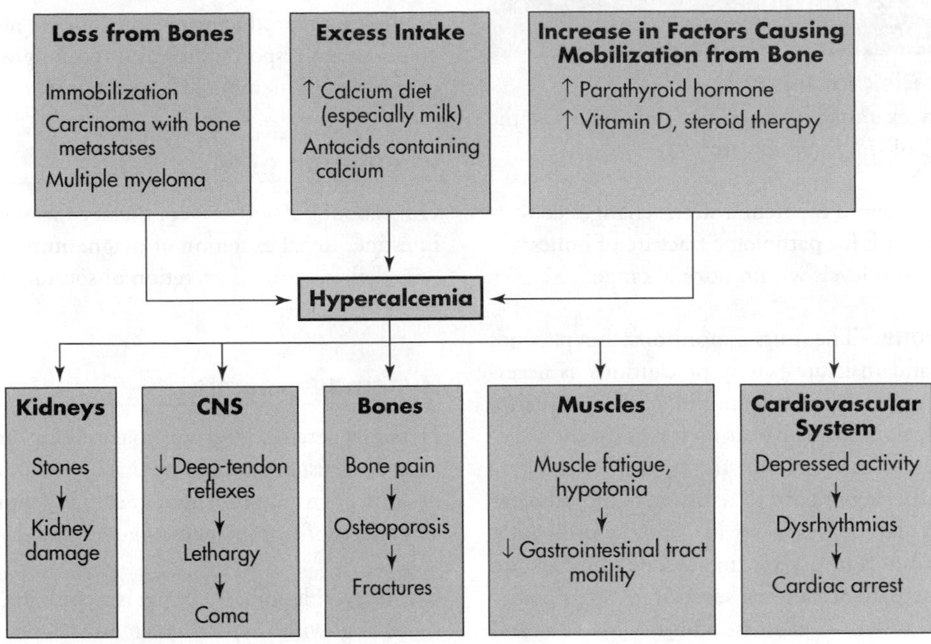

Figure 17-10 Causes and effects of hypercalcemia. *CNS,* Central nervous system.

Etiology. Hypercalcemia can result from excessive intake of calcium, especially from milk and calcium-containing antacids (milk-alkali syndrome) and excessive vitamin D intake. Renal failure decreases urinary excretion of calcium, and thiazide diuretics cause resorption in the distal tubules. The most common causes of hypercalcemia are conditions that cause loss of calcium from the bone. Some malignant tumors destroy the bone, whereas others secrete parathyroid-like hormones or agents that stimulate osteoclastic activity, releasing calcium salts into the blood. Fractures and prolonged immobilization also cause demineralization of bone and release of calcium into the plasma.

Pathophysiology. Immobilization causes calcium to leave the bone and concentrate in the ECF. Subsequent high calcium levels in urine impair the concentrating ability of the kidneys by interfering with ADH and causing diuresis. Excess calcium excreted in the urine predisposes the person to calcium precipitation and stone formation. When calcium and phosphorus retention occur together, crystals may precipitate in the blood and deposit throughout soft tissue.[4]

Excess calcium decreases excitability of nerve tissue and muscle, producing generalized muscle weakness and flaccidity and decreased or absent deep tendon reflexes. Constipation, nausea, and vomiting are common due to decreased smooth muscle activity in the GI tract. The cardiac effects of elevated serum calcium levels include ventricular dysrhythmias and increased risk for digitalis toxicity.

Malignant disease and hyperparathyroidism can cause hypercalcemic crisis when the increase in serum calcium is acute. Clinical manifestations include polyuria, excessive thirst, volume depletion, altered levels of consciousness, and cardiac arrest. Symptomatic hypercalcemia is associated with a high mortality rate.[9]

Collaborative Care Management. Severe hypercalcemia is a medical emergency. Continuous cardiac monitoring is necessary, and emergency equipment should be readily available. Initial treatment consists of hydration. The nurse assesses cardiac and renal status before and at least every 2 hours during fluid therapy. After ECF volume is restored, sodium chloride and diuretics may be prescribed by the physician to increase urinary elimination of calcium. Thiazide diuretics are avoided because they cause resorption of calcium, whereas loop diuretics promote calcium excretion. Measures to inhibit bone breakdown or resorption include biphosphonates (e.g., etidronate disodium) and calcitonin. Administration of glucocorticosteroids reduces intestinal absorption of calcium by competing with vitamin D and is given for cancer-related hypercalcemia.

Nursing Management

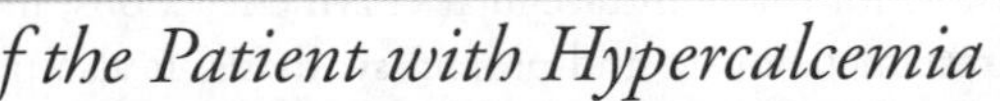

of the Patient with Hypercalcemia

ASSESSMENT

Health History. Assess for:

- Signs and symptoms of hypercalcemia, including altered level of consciousness (e.g., confusion, stupor), personality changes, hallucinations, paranoia, constipation, nausea, anorexia, thirst
- High-risk factors, including cancer history, prolonged immobilization, thiazide diuretic therapy, steroid therapy, multiple fractures

Physical Examination. Assess for:

- Flabby muscles, reduced deep tendon reflexes, dysuria (renal calculi), bone-related pain (pathologic fractures)
- ECG changes, including shortened QT interval and cardiac dysrhythmias

Nursing Diagnoses, Outcomes, and Interventions

Nursing Diagnosis: Risk for Injury

Outcomes. Common examples of expected outcomes for the patient with a diagnosis of *risk for injury* are:

Patient will:

- Be free from injury caused by mental status changes coupled with increased risk for pathologic fracture of bones.
- Exhibit serum calcium levels within normal range.

Nursing Interventions. The nurse monitors the patient's level of consciousness and institutes safety precautions as necessary. The nurse encourages the patient to ambulate with assistance to minimize bone resorption. Weight-bearing forces on the skeleton promote movement of calcium into the bones. Patients are handled gently and set their own pace to reduce risk of pathologic fracture. Neuromuscular depression with poor coordination and impaired gait contributes to risk for injury. The nurse assures family members that the patient's altered sensorium is temporary and will subside with treatment. The nurse administers saline and loop diuretics and evaluates patient response. Patients are encouraged to remain well hydrated to help dilute serum calcium and prevent renal calculi formation. Unless contraindicated, 3000 to 4000 ml of fluid per day is desirable.

Related NIC Interventions. Delirium Management, Exercise Therapy: Ambulation, Fall Prevention, Fluid Management, Hallucination Management

Evaluation

To evaluate the effectiveness of nursing interventions, compare patient behaviors with those stated in the expected patient outcomes.

Related NOC Outcomes. Cognition, Cognitive Orientation, Fall Prevention Behavior, Neurological Status: Consciousness, Risk Control

Magnesium

Magnesium is a major intracellular cation second only to potassium and is responsible for many intracellular enzyme reactions, including carbohydrate metabolism and protein synthesis. It also plays a role in neuromuscular excitability and calcium absorption through its effect on PTH. Magnesium affects the release of acetylcholine at neuromuscular junctions, promoting normal neural and muscular excitability. Magnesium also triggers the sodium-potassium pump and is necessary for movement of potassium into the cell.

Magnesium Distribution

Approximately 50% to 60% of magnesium is found in bone, and only a small amount (1%) in the ECF with the remainder inside the cell. The normal serum magnesium level is 1.5 to 2.5 mEq/L. Like calcium, a significant amount of magnesium (20% to 30%) is protein bound. A low albumin level decreases the total magnesium level in the body, although ionized magnesium remains unchanged. Magnesium may compete with calcium for protein binding sites, producing the appropriate response, no response, or an undesired response such as interfering with calcium movement across the cell membrane.[9]

Regulation of Magnesium

Only about 30% to 40% of dietary magnesium is absorbed in the intestine. Renal excretion of magnesium is inhibited by fluid volume deficit, reduced excretion of sodium or calcium, or increased PTH.

Hypomagnesemia

Hypomagnesemia (serum magnesium level of less than 1.5 mEq/L) is usually caused by urinary loss, reduced GI absorption, or shift of magnesium into the ICF. Figure 17-11 shows causes and effects of hypomagnesemia.

Etiology. Hypomagnesemia is a common clinical problem often coexisting with hypokalemia and hypocalcemia. Factors contributing to decreased magnesium levels include (1) loss of GI fluids or decreased intestinal absorption; (2) prolonged malnutrition; (3) renal disorders; (4) drug therapies increasing urinary losses (e.g., aminoglycosides, loop diuretics); and (5) endocrine disorders altering secretion of ADH, aldosterone, or calcium. A relative hypomagnesemia can develop secondary to intracellular shifts with alkalosis and rapid administration of parenteral fluids containing glucose, insulin, or both.

Pathophysiology. Magnesium deficiency frequently occurs in combination with calcium and potassium deficits, all producing related neurologic and cardiovascular symptoms. Tetany-like muscle contractions may be present, especially when hypocalcemia occurs in conjunction with hypomagnesemia. Although symptoms are not generally evident until serum levels fall below 1 mEq/dl, the characteristic manifestations are muscle weakness and tremors.

Cardiovascular manifestations include tachycardia, ventricular dysrhythmias, and torsades de pointes (variant of ventricular tachycardia that causes blackouts or sudden death). ECG indications of magnesium deficiency include a widening QRS complex, flattened or inverted T waves, and prolongation of the PR interval. These findings may reflect magnesium, calcium, and potassium deficiencies. Low magnesium levels potentiate the action of digitalis.

Collaborative Care Management. Treatment of the cause of hypomagnesemia is the first consideration, since the underlying magnesium deficit may be refractory to treatment until the associated calcium and potassium deficits are corrected. If hypokalemia does not respond to potassium replacement, low serum magnesium should be suspected.[9]

If the deficit is severe, intravenous magnesium replacement is indicated using continuous cardiac monitoring by infusion pump to ensure accurate dosing. Cardiac or respiratory arrest can occur with too-rapid administration of magnesium. Caution is used when checking the health care provider's order, and at least 100 ml/hr of urinary output needs to be established before administration. The nurse monitors patients for hypotension, flushing, sweating, depressed reflexes (knee jerk), and res-

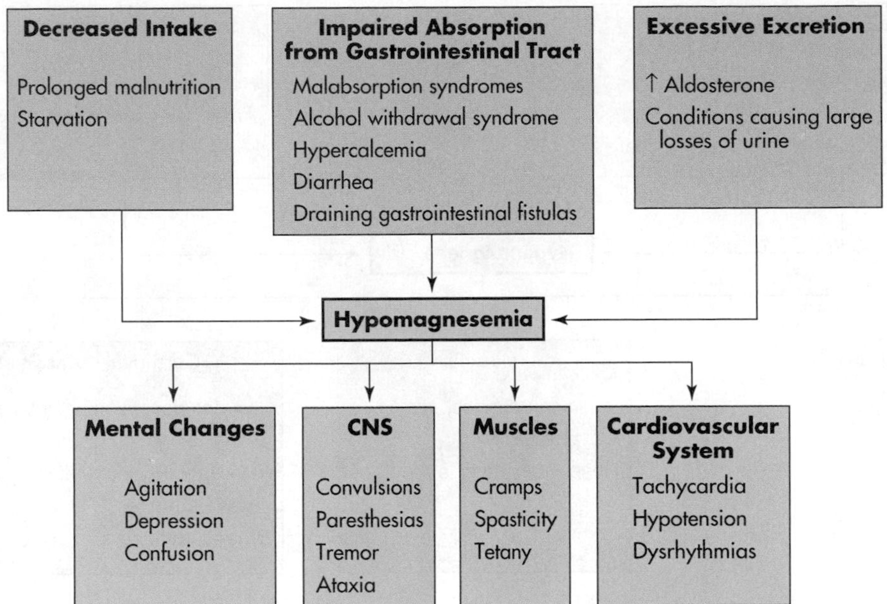

Figure 17-11 Causes and effects of hypomagnesemia. *CNS,* Central nervous system.

piratory depression, since they indicate too much magnesium. Significant depression of deep tendon reflexes signals hypermagnesemia and is a precursor to respiratory depression and cardiac arrest. Calcium gluconate must be available in case of sudden hypermagnesemia and hypocalcemic tetany.[4]

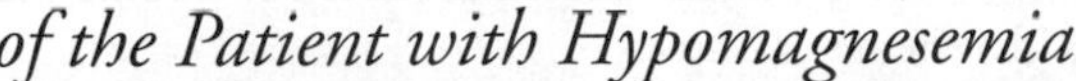

Nursing Management of the Patient with Hypomagnesemia

ASSESSMENT

Health History. Assess for:

- High-risk factors, including alcoholism, protein-calorie malnutrition, medications that promote urinary excretion of magnesium, GI losses
- Clinical manifestations, including lethargy, weakness, fatigue, insomnia, mood changes, confusion, anorexia, paresthesias, tremors, chest pain, dysphagia

Physical Examination. Assess for:

- Physical signs, including hyperactive reflexes, convulsions, tetany, positive Chvostek's and Trousseau's signs, tachycardia, hypertension, angina
- Decreased serum albumin, magnesium, potassium, and calcium levels
- ECG changes, multifocal or bigeminal premature ventricular contractions

NURSING DIAGNOSES, OUTCOMES, AND INTERVENTIONS

Nursing Diagnosis: Ineffective Protection

OUTCOMES. Common examples of expected outcomes for the patient with a diagnosis of *ineffective protection* are:

Patient will:

- Remain free from injury potential related to hypomagnesemia and related seizures, fatigue, muscle weakness, confusion.
- Verbalize an understanding of safety risks associated with altered sensorium.

NURSING INTERVENTIONS. The nurse administers oral magnesium salts as prescribed. They are given cautiously to patients with reduced renal function to prevent hypermagnesemia. The nurse monitors patients for diarrhea, which is a common side effect of magnesium. Patients are encouraged to ingest foods that are high in magnesium, including green, leafy vegetables, meats, nuts, bran, legumes, and fruits. Patients receiving digitalis preparations are closely monitored for digitalis toxicity. The nurse institutes seizure precautions for patients with severe, symptomatic hypomagnesemia. The gag reflex and swallowing capability is assessed before the patient is allowed food or medications, since dysphagia can occur. Intravenous magnesium sulfate must be administered slowly and always on an infusion pump to prevent rapid administration.

RELATED NIC INTERVENTIONS. Aspiration Precautions, Delirium Management, Neurologic Monitoring, Positioning, Seizure Precautions

EVALUATION

To evaluate the effectiveness of nursing interventions, compare patient behaviors with those stated in the expected patient outcomes.

RELATED NOC OUTCOMES. Airway Management, Cognitive Orientation, Fall Prevention Behavior, Neurological Status: Consciousness, Risk Control

Hypermagnesemia

Hypermagnesemia (serum magnesium level greater than 2.5 mEq/L) is rare, since the kidney is efficient at eliminating excess

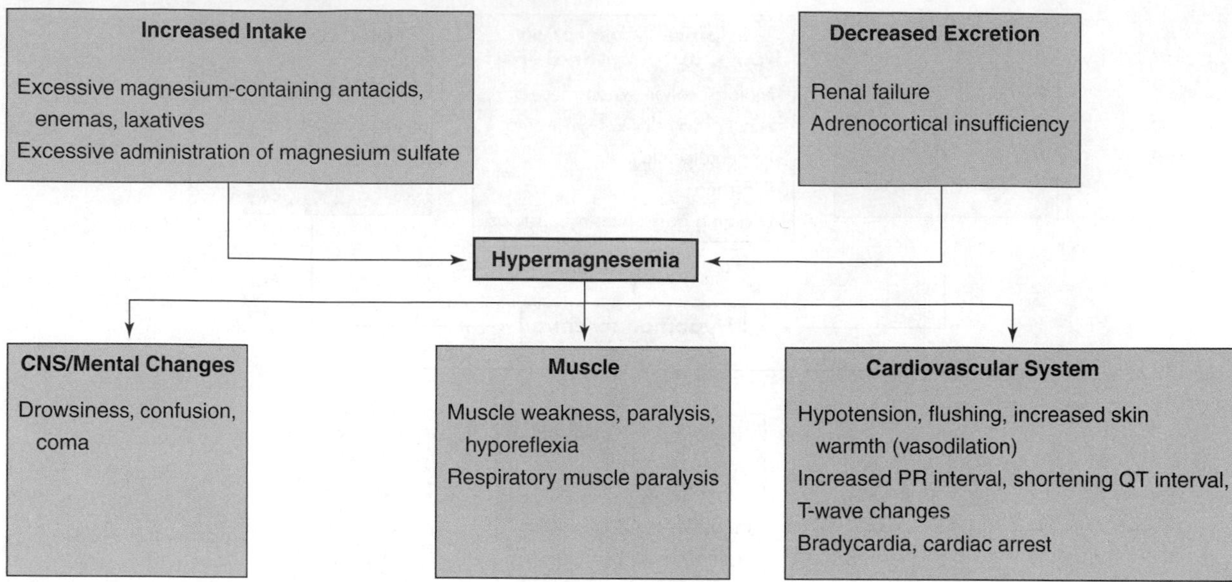

Figure 17-12 Causes and effects of hypermagnesemia. *CNS,* Central nervous system.

magnesium from the body. Figure 17-12 shows causes and effects of hypermagnesemia.

Etiology. Hypermagnesemia is usually a result of renal insufficiency or failure and excess ingestion of magnesium-containing medications such as antacids or laxatives. Excess serum magnesium may occur after the administration of magnesium sulfate to prevent seizures resulting from eclampsia.

Pathophysiology. Signs and symptoms are not generally evident unless the serum magnesium level exceeds 4 mEq/L. The characteristic manifestations of hypermagnesemia are due to depressed neuromuscular impulse transmission. As the magnesium level rises, the patient becomes drowsy and lethargic with diminished reflexes. Periodic assessment of reflexes during magnesium administration is essential, since loss of deep tendon reflexes occurs before severe respiratory problems. Hypotension, flushing, and increased skin warmth may be noted. Cardiac effects of hypermagnesemia include slow heart rate, atrioventricular conduction block, and cardiac arrest.

Collaborative Care Management. Patients with impaired renal function are cautioned to avoid over-the-counter medications that contain magnesium (e.g., Milk of Magnesia, Mylanta). Any patient receiving parenteral magnesium therapy is assessed frequently for signs of hypermagnesemia. Withholding magnesium-containing medications may correct mild hypermagnesemia. Diuretics and 0.45% sodium chloride are given to promote excretion of magnesium in patients with adequate renal function.4 Severe hypermagnesemia may require treatment with intravenous calcium gluconate to offset the neuromuscular effects. Dialysis may be required for patients in renal failure or with acute, life-threatening hypermagnesemia.

Nursing Management *of the Patient with Hypermagnesemia*

Assessment

Health History. Assess for:

- Risk factors (e.g., diminished renal function, chronic use of antacids, enemas, laxatives)
- Nausea, confusion, drowsiness, muscular weakness, use of accessory muscles for breathing

Physical Examination. Assess for:

- Peripheral vasodilation, hypotension, bradycardia, diminished deep tendon reflexes, dyspnea, diaphoresis, flushing, dysrhythmias
- Serum magnesium level greater than 2.5 mEq/L
- ECG alterations, including prolonged QT interval

Nursing Diagnoses, Outcomes, and Interventions

Nursing Diagnosis: Imbalanced Nutrition: More Than Body Requirements (Magnesium)

Outcomes. Common examples of expected outcomes for the patient with a diagnosis of *imbalanced nutrition: more than body requirements* for magnesium are:

Patient will:

- Recognize sources of magnesium that can contribute to body excess.
- Explain the importance of avoiding excessive use of laxatives and enemas, and identify alternative bowel management strategies.

NURSING INTERVENTIONS. The nurse advises patients to avoid foods that are rich in magnesium and medications that contain magnesium (e.g., Riopan, Mylanta, Maalox). The nurse encourages patients and caregivers to read drug labels and review all over-the-counter medications with their health care provider. Patients, in particular those with renal compromise, are cautioned about the hazards of excess use of laxatives and enemas that contain magnesium. The nurse reviews signs and symptoms that need to be reported so that patients understand when to contact their health care provider.

RELATED NIC INTERVENTIONS. Bowel Management, Nutrition Management, Nutritional Counseling, Nutritional Monitoring

EVALUATION

To evaluate the effectiveness of nursing interventions, compare patient behaviors with those stated in the expected patient outcomes.

RELATED NOC OUTCOMES. Knowledge: Medication, Nutritional Status: Food & Fluid Intake, Nutritional Status: Nutrient Intake

? Critical Thinking

1. A 72-year-old patient with chronic congestive heart failure takes laxatives at least twice a week. His prescribed medications include 20 mg furosemide and 0.125 mg of lanoxin daily. Assess the patient's risk for fluid and electrolyte imbalance. Describe measures the nurse should anticipate implementing for this patient.
2. A well-trained 30-year-old is planning to participate in a bicycle marathon that involves 2 days of riding for a total of 150 miles. It is mid-July and temperatures are expected to be in the high eighties to mid-nineties. How can the biker prepare for the marathon? What are the risks given the temperature and her expected level of physical activity? Which fluid or electrolyte imbalances, if any, is the biker at risk for developing?

References

1. Amini A, Schmidt M: Syndrome of inappropriate secretion of antidiuretic hormone and hyponatremia after spinal surgery, *Neurosurg Focus* 16(4), 2004.
2. Cohn JN et al: New guidelines for potassium replacement in clinical practice: a contemporary review by the National Council on Potassium in Clinical Practice, *Arch Intern Med* 160(16):2429, 2000.
3. Grandjean, AC, Reimers KG, Buyckx ME: Hydration: issues for the 21st century, *Nutrition Rev* 61(8):261, 2003.
4. Heitz UE, Horne MM: *Pocket guide to fluid, electrolyte, and acid-base balance*, ed 4, St Louis, 2001, Mosby.
5. Huether SE, McCance KL: *Understanding pathophysiology*, ed 4, St Louis, 2004, Mosby.
6. Kee JL, Paluanka BJ, Purnell LD: *Fluids and electrolytes with clinical applications: a programmed approach*, ed 7, New York, 2004, Delmar Learning.
7. Larson K: Fluid balance in the elderly: assessment and intervention—important role in community health and home care nursing, *Geriatr Nurs* 24(5):306–309, 2003.
8. Metheny NM: *Fluid and electrolyte balance nursing considerations*, ed 4, Philadelphia, 2000, JB Lippincott.
9. Porth CM: *Essentials of pathophysiology: concepts of altered health states*, Philadelphia, 2004, JB Lippincott.
10. Preston RA: *Acid-base, fluids, and electrolytes made ridiculously simple*, Miami, 2002, MedMaster, Inc.
11. Shier D, Butler J, Lewis R: *Hole's human anatomy and physiology*, ed 10, Boston, 2004, McGraw-Hill.
12. Sica DA, Gehr WB, Yancy C: Hyperkalemia, congestive heart failure and aldosterone receptor antagonism, *Congestive Heart Failure* 9(4):224–229, 2003.
13. Skidmore-Roth L: *Mosby's 2004 nursing drug reference*, St Louis, 2004, Mosby.
14. Speakman E, Weldy NJ: *Body fluids and electrolytes: a programmed presentation*, ed 8, St Louis, 2002, Mosby.
15. Swearingen PL, Keen JK: *Manual of critical care nursing: nursing interventions and collaborative management*, ed 4, St Louis, 2001, Mosby

evolve **Visit the Evolve website:** http://evolve.elsevier.com/Monahan/medsurg

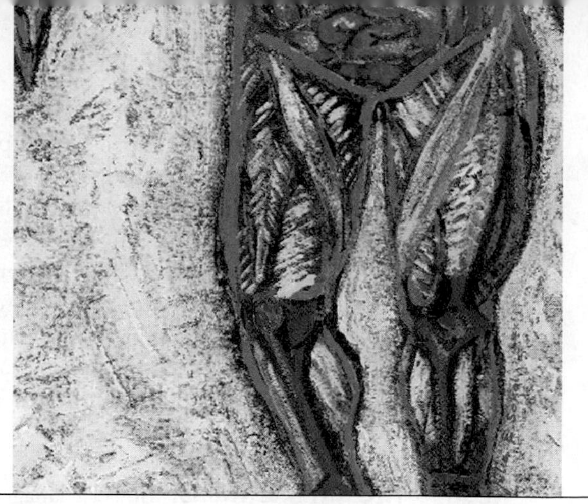

CHAPTER 18
Acid-Base Imbalance

by Ursula J. Heitz

OBJECTIVES

After studying this chapter, the learner should be able to:

1. Describe the mechanisms that maintain acid-base balance.
2. Differentiate between respiratory and metabolic acidosis and alkalosis.
3. Apply the principles of acid-base balance to the interpretation of arterial blood gas (ABG) measurements.
4. Analyze components of ABGs to identify type of acid-base disturbance.
5. Describe the causes and effects of each type of acid-base imbalance.
6. Formulate a care plan for the patient with an acid-base imbalance based on ABG findings.

KEY TERMS

acidemia, p. 387
acids, p. 386
alkalemia, p. 387
bases, p. 386
chemical buffers, p. 387
compensation, p. 388
hypercapnia, p. 389
hypocapnia, p. 389
hypoxia, p. 389
hypoxemia, p. 389

Nature of the Problem

Alterations in acid-base balance can affect cellular metabolism and enzymatic processes. Consequently acid-base balance is critical in the maintenance of homeostasis. Understanding the basic terms, principles, and concepts of acid-base aids in patient assessment and helps determine the need for specific interventions.

Acids and Bases

Acids are substances that can give up a hydrogen ion (H^+). **Bases** are substances that can accept a hydrogen ion (H^+). A common acid is hydrochloric acid (HCl), which can separate into hydrogen (H^+) and chloride (Cl^-). Bicarbonate (HCO_3^-) is a common base that can accept a hydrogen ion to form carbonic acid ($H_2CO_3^-$), a weak acid. In acid-base balance and regulation, the weak acid, carbonic acid ($H_2CO_3^-$) and the base bicarbonate (HCO_3^-) are the most important.[1] While carbonic acid plays a critical role in acid-base, balance, it is difficult to measure directly because it dissolves in plasma to form carbon dioxide (CO_2) and water (H_2O):

$$H_2CO_3^- \rightleftharpoons CO_2 + H_2O$$

Carbonic acid + Carbon dioxide = Water

Because carbon dioxide is in balance with carbonic acid and is easier to measure directly, carbon dioxide is used to express the acid component of acid-base. By definition, carbon dioxide is not an acid, since it does not have a hydrogen ion to donate. It is referred to as an acid because of its relationship to carbonic acid. Carbon dioxide is referred to as PCO_2 when discussing acid-base balance. The "P" represents the partial pressure of carbon dioxide. $PaCO_2$ is used when referring to carbon dioxide in arterial blood.

Carbon dioxide is a volatile acid because it is eliminated by the lungs. Both carbon dioxide and water are generated by the metabolism of food. In health the amount of carbon dioxide generated daily equals the amount that is excreted daily, thus maintaining a constant state. Other acids that are generated by metabolism but cannot be eliminated by the lungs are called *nonvolatile acids* and are excreted by the kidneys.

The base bicarbonate is added to the body in small amounts from dietary intake. The gain of bicarbonate is offset by the normal loss of bicarbonate through the stool. Bicarbonate has a critical role in acid-base regulation, since it accepts a hydrogen ion to neutralize acids.

In health the acid-base ratio is 1:20. In other words, there is 1 part acid for every 20 parts base.[5] If this ratio is altered, derangements occur in the acid-base environment (Figure 18-1).

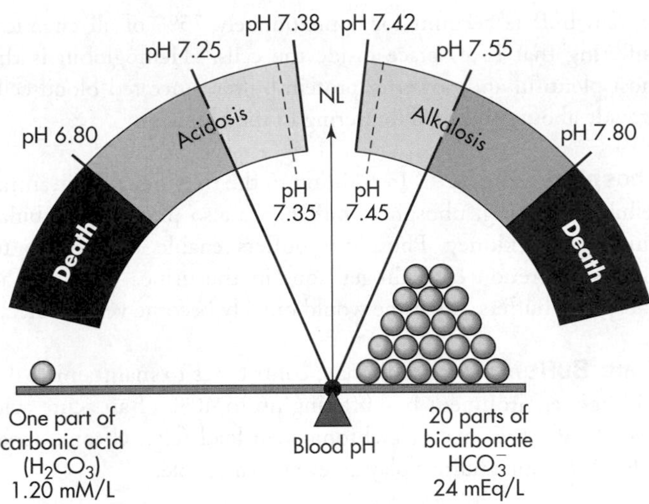

Figure 18-1 Note that the relationship of 1 part carbonic acid (H_2CO_3) to 20 parts bicarbonate (HCO_3^-) maintains hydrogen ion concentration (pH) within normal limits. Changes in this ratio will alter pH. *NL,* Normal limits.

pH

Acidity or alkalinity of body fluids is expressed in terms of the concentration of hydrogen ions. The body regulates hydrogen ion concentration in a narrow range because minute changes in this concentration can have a dramatic influence on cellular functions.[5] The normal concentration of hydrogen ions is so small it is difficult to work with in the clinical setting, so the concentration of hydrogen ions is expressed as pH. The pH has an inverse relationship to hydrogen ions. The more hydrogen ions present, the lower the pH (acidic); the fewer hydrogen ions present, the higher the pH (alkaline).

Numerous terms describe the ratio of acid to base within the body fluids. *Acidosis* is the process leading to the accumulation of acid or loss of base with or without a change of pH. **Acidemia** refers to an actual decrease in pH of arterial blood to less then 7.40. *Alkalosis* is the process leading to the accumulation of base or loss of acid with or without a change in pH. **Alkalemia** refers to an actual increase in arterial pH to greater then 7.40.

Respiratory acidosis results from the retention of the volatile acid carbon dioxide, whereas *metabolic acidosis* occurs because of the retention of fixed or nonvolatile acids or loss of base. Similarly, the reduction in the level of carbon dioxide is termed *respiratory alkalosis,* and *metabolic alkalosis* is the result of retention of bases or loss of nonvolatile acids.

Physiology

The normal acid-base environment is achieved and maintained by three primary mechanisms: (1) chemical buffering (neutralizing) by extracellular and intracellular buffers, (2) respiratory control of carbon dioxide via changes in rate and depth of respiration, and (3) renal regulation of bicarbonate concentration and secretion of hydrogen (Table 18-1 and Figure 18-2).

Chemical Buffering

The presence of **chemical buffers** in body fluids and tissue allows the pH to remain in a narrow range.[1] Chemical buffers are substances that act as sponges to soak up or release free hydrogen ions so that the pH is not greatly altered. Chemical buffers do not change the absolute number of hydrogen ions liberated by a strong acid or removed by a strong base, but buffers do limit the number of free hydrogen ions, thus lessening the effect a strong acid or base would have on the pH.[5] Buffers are present in all body fluids (e.g., plasma, intracellular, interstitial fluid), tissue, and bone, and their response is instantaneous. The primary chemical buffers include bicarbonate, organic phosphate, protein, and bones.

Bicarbonate Buffers. This is the most important buffer in the plasma and interstitial fluid and is responsible for 80% of the buffering in extracellular fluid. Inorganic phosphates and plasma proteins play a small role in extracellular buffering. As a weak base, bicarbonate buffers by accepting a hydrogen ion and forming the weak acid carbonic acid. The carbonic acid then separates into carbon dioxide and water, which are eliminated by the lungs. Carbon dioxide can also combine with water to form carbonic

TABLE 18-1 MECHANISMS REGULATING ACID-BASE BALANCE

Action Time	Effect
Chemical Buffers in Cells and Extracellular Fluid	
Instantaneous	Combine with acids or bases added to system to prevent marked changes in pH
Respiratory System	
Minutes to hours	Controls carbon dioxide concentration in ECF by changes in rate and depth of respiration
Kidneys	
Hours to days	Increases or decreases quantity of sodium bicarbonate in ECF Combines bicarbonate or hydrogen with other substances and excretes them in urine

ECF, Extracellular fluid.

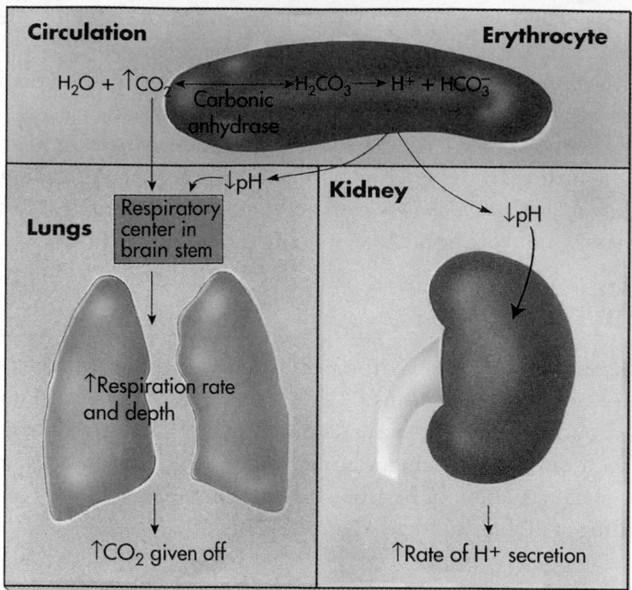

Figure 18-2 Integration of pH control mechanisms. Elevated carbon dioxide (CO_2) levels result in increased formation of carbonic acid (H_2CO_3) in red blood cells. The resulting increase in hydrogen ions (H^+), coupled with elevated CO_2 levels, results in an increase in respiratory rate and secretion of H^+ by the kidneys, thus helping regulate the pH of body fluids.

acid, which can then separate into bicarbonate and water. This buffering system is shown in the equation:

Bicarbonate		Hydrogen ion		Carbonic acid		Carbon dioxide		Water
HCO_3^-	+	H^+	⇌	H_2CO_3	⇌	CO_2	+	H_2O
(base)		(strong acid)		(weak acid)		(eliminated by lungs)		

Bicarbonate can be depleted quickly when buffering large acid loads, but in the short term it is effective in maintaining a life-sustaining pH (Figure 18-3).

Intracellular Buffers. Although not as important or powerful as the bicarbonate-carbonic acid buffering system, intracellular buffers play an important role in maintaining acid-base balance.

Protein buffers account for approximately 75% of all chemical buffering that takes place inside the cells.[5] Hemoglobin is the most plentiful and powerful protein buffer, since red blood cells provide about 70% of all buffering in the blood.

Phosphate Buffers. In addition to the role they play in intracellular buffering, phosphate buffers are also present in tubular fluid in the kidney. Phosphate buffers enable the kidney to increase excretion of hydrogen ions in the urine. Without the phosphate buffers, the urine would quickly become very acidic.

Bone Buffers. Bone carbonate contributes to maintaining the acid-base environment by buffering up to 40% of an acute acid load. In the presence of a chronic acid load (e.g., chronic renal failure) the bone buffers play an even greater role.

Respiratory Regulation

The role of the lungs in acid-base balance involves the regulation of carbon dioxide. The rate and depth of alveolar ventilation determines how much carbon dioxide is eliminated or retained. Normally the amount of carbon dioxide eliminated equals the amount produced by metabolic processes. When this balance is not maintained, either respiratory acidosis (too little carbon dioxide eliminated for amount produced) or respiratory alkalosis (too much carbon dioxide eliminated for amount produced) occurs. The respiratory center of the medulla controls ventilation. When changes occur in PCO_2 or in the pH of the cerebrospinal fluid, the respiratory rate and depth are almost instantly altered accordingly. Respiratory **compensation** does occur with metabolic disturbances, but since the lungs are only able to eliminate volatile acids, compensation is limited when a fixed acid load occurs. A normal pH cannot be maintained, although compensation usually keeps the pH in a life-sustaining range. Maximal respiratory compensation can take up to 12 to 24 hours.[2]

Renal Regulation

Every day, as fixed acids are generated, they are buffered by bicarbonate. Without renal regulation of acid and base, a progressive metabolic acidosis would occur as buffers are used up. Normally functioning kidneys are able to prevent this through their role in

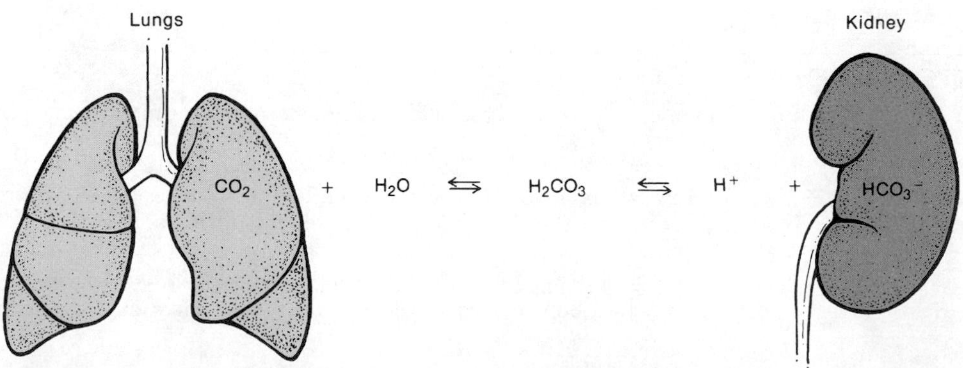

Figure 18-3 The lungs help control acid-base balance by blowing off or retaining carbon dioxide (CO_2). The kidneys help regulate acid-base balance by excreting or retaining bicarbonate (HCO_3^-).

resorption and regeneration of bicarbonate and excretion of hydrogen ions. The kidneys regulate the acid-base environment through a series of complex reactions that involve hydrogen, sodium (Na^+), and bicarbonate secretion, resorption, and conservation.

Bicarbonate resorption depends on the secretion of hydrogen ions by the kidney. When hydrogen is secreted in tubular fluid, it combines with bicarbonate and forms carbonic acid, which quickly separates into carbon dioxide and water. The water is excreted and the carbon dioxide is resorbed, converted back to bicarbonate, and returned to body fluids. In addition to resorbing the bicarbonate, the kidneys can actually regenerate bicarbonate, thus replacing the bicarbonate lost to buffering. In the presence of alkalosis, less bicarbonate is generated because fewer hydrogen ions are secreted. Conversely in acidosis, an increased amount of bicarbonate is generated because of the increase in hydrogen ion secretion.

The kidneys help maintain a 1:20 ratio of acids to bases by excreting excess hydrogen ions depending on pH. Other factors influencing hydrogen ion secretion are PCO_2 levels, plasma potassium (K^+) levels, effective circulating volume, and aldosterone levels. Increased PCO_2 causes increased hydrogen ion secretion, whereas a decrease in PCO_2 causes a decrease in hydrogen ion secretion. Elevated plasma potassium (hyperkalemia) causes a decrease in hydrogen ion secretion, whereas diminished plasma potassium (hypokalemia) causes an increase in hydrogen ion secretion. Hydrogen ion secretion increases with a decrease in effective circulating volume, whereas volume expansion leads to a decrease in hydrogen ion secretion. Last, elevated aldosterone levels promote increased hydrogen ion secretion.

Renal compensation for respiratory acidosis or alkalosis can return the pH to near normal. Renal compensation is much more effective for respiratory disturbances than respiratory compensation is for metabolic disorders. However, the initial renal compensatory response takes up to 24 hours, with a maximal response taking 3 to 4 days. It is important to note that the body never overcompensates for an acid-base disturbance. If it appears as though overcompensation has occurred, more then one disorder may be present.

Arterial Blood Gases

Valuable information is provided about the acid-base status through the measurement of arterial pH, $PaCO_2$, bicarbonate, PaO_2, oxygen saturation, and base excess. Arterial blood is used because venous blood is not suitable for the assessment of oxygen tension and pH. The nurse draws arterial blood without exposure to air in a heparinized syringe using the appropriate artery (radial, brachial, or femoral). Institutions generally have specific guidelines for obtaining arterial blood gases (ABGs).

pH. The most important component of ABG analysis when assessing acid-base status is the pH (Box 18-1). It is a direct reflection of H^+ concentration and thus the acid/base ratio. Changes in pH signal the presence and severity of the disorder, although not the cause. The perfect pH is 7.40, with a normal range of 7.35 to 7.45. A normal pH may exist with a mixed acid-base disturbance (e.g., respiratory acidosis and metabolic alkalosis), or when compensation has returned the pH to normal or near normal.

$PaCO_2$. $PaCO_2$ reflects alveolar function. **Hypercapnia** ($PaCO_2$ greater than 45 mm Hg) signals alveolar hypoventilation and respiratory acidosis or compensation for metabolic alkalosis. **Hypocapnia** ($PaCO_2$ less than 35 mm Hg) is the result of alveolar hyperventilation causing respiratory alkalosis or compensation for metabolic acidosis.

Bicarbonate. As the major base component, bicarbonate is frequently calculated from the pH and $PaCO_2$. Serum bicarbonate can also be obtained from venous blood drawn at the same time as the ABG and included in the chemistry profile. The terminology maybe confusing, but serum carbon dioxide, serum bicarbonate, and total carbon dioxide content all refer to the total concentration of bicarbonate in the blood. Normal values of bicarbonate are 22 to 26 mEq/L.

PaO_2. The partial pressure of arterial oxygen is referred to as PaO_2. A PaO_2 within normal limits has no primary role in acid-base regulation; however, a low PaO_2 (hypoxemia) indicates an alteration in respiratory function or breathing air with a low level of oxygen (high altitude). **Hypoxemia** is defined as a PaO_2 below the normal range for the individual's age (normal values vary slightly with age). **Hypoxia,** which refers to inadequate oxygenation at the tissue level, can occur as the result of hypoxemia. Hypoxia is most common when the PaO_2 drops below 50 to 60 mm Hg. Mild hypoxemia exists when the PaO_2 is between 60 and 80 mm Hg; moderate hypoxemia when PaO_2 is between 40 and 60 mm Hg; and severe hypoxemia when PaO_2 is 40 mm Hg or less. Hypoxemia is determined by the PaO_2, whereas hypoxia is inferred from signs and symptoms (increased heart rate, increased respiratory rate, decreased blood pressure, diaphoresis, and breathlessness) and supporting data (e.g., lactate level).

Saturation. The degree to which hemoglobin is saturated with oxygen is called saturation. It can be affected by changes in temperature, pH, and $PaCO_2$.

Base Excess. Base excess is the measurement of an excess or deficit of buffer base for a specific patient based on pH, bicarbonate, and hemoglobin concentration. The normal base excess is ±2. An increase in base excess indicates metabolic alkalosis; a decrease indicates metabolic acidosis.

Other Important Laboratory Values

Serum Electrolytes. Electrolytes affect and are affected by the acid-base status. Acute changes in pH are accompanied by changes in serum potassium concentration. In acidemia the potassium shifts out of the cell and excess hydrogen moves into the cell to be buffered. The opposite occurs with alkalemia. Electrolyte values are necessary to calculate the anion gap. Anion gap is the difference between measured cations (sodium and potassium) and measured anions (chloride and bicarbonate). Because potassium has a low value, it is not used in calculating anion gap.

$$\text{Anion gap} = Na^+ - (Cl^- + HCO_3^-)$$

Box 18-1 Guidelines for Analysis of Acid-Base Status

Normal Acid-Base Parameters

pH: 7.40 (range 7.35 to 7.45)
$PaCO_2$: 40 mm Hg (range 35 to 45 mm Hg)

Cations
Sodium (Na^+): 140 to 44 mEq/L
Potassium (K^+): 3.8 to 4.4 mEq/L

Anions
Bicarbonate (HCO_3^-): 22 to 26 mEq/L
Chloride (Cl^-): 99 to104 mEq/L
Anion gap: 12 (±2)
Albumin: 4 g/dl

Acid-Base Analysis

1. Determine pH status:
   Acidemia: < 7.40
   Alkalemia: > 7.40
2. Determine if change in pH is related to respiratory or metabolic process or both:
   Acidemia
   —Respiratory: $PaCO_2 > 40$ mm Hg
   —Metabolic: $HCO_3^- < 25$ mEq/L
   Alkalemia
   —Respiratory: $PaCO_2 < 40$ mm Hg
   —Metabolic: $HCO_3^- > 25$ mEq/L
3. Check for degree of compensation:
   Respiratory acidemia
   —Acute: For every $PaCO_2$ increase of 10 mm Hg, bicarbonate increases by 1 mEq/L.
   —Chronic: For every $PaCO_2$ increase of 10 mm Hg, bicarbonate increases by 4 mEq/L.
   Respiratory alkalemia
   —Acute: For every $PaCO_2$ decrease of 10 mm Hg, bicarbonate decreases by 2 mEq/L.
   —Chronic: For every $PaCO_2$ decrease of 10 mm Hg, bicarbonate decreases by 5 mEq/L.
   Metabolic acidemia
   —1 decrease in $PaCO_2$ = 1.3 decrease in bicarbonate
   Metabolic alkalemia
   —1 increase in $PaCO_2$ = 0.6 increase in bicarbonate
4. Calculate serum anion gap (AG)
   $AG = Na^+ - (Cl^- + HCO_3^-)$
   —AG increased > 12 mEq/L can indicate metabolic acidosis.
   —AG increased beyond 20 mEq/L *always* indicates metabolic acidosis.
   —For every 1 g/dl albumin is less than normal (4.5 g/dl), add 2.5 to calculated AG.
   —Every point increase in AG should have 1 mEq/L decrease in HCO_3^-. If HCO_3^- is higher, metabolic alkalosis is also present. If HCO_3^- is lower than expected, a normal AG acidosis is also present.

Modified from Whittier WL, Rutecki GW: Primer on clinical acid-base problem solving, *Dis Month* 50(3):122–162, 2004.

The normal anion gap is 12 ±2. A gap greater then 14 usually indicates the presence of unmeasured anions such as the organic acids lactate or ketoacids. Anion gap is helpful in determining the causes of metabolic acidosis and is usually calculated and analyzed with ABG results.

Albumin. Albumin is a measurable anion and important buffer that can affect anion gap when decreased (e.g., in nephrotic syndrome).

▶ ARE You READY?

The nurse reviews the following laboratory results:

Na^+	154
K^+	3.2
Cl^-	100
HCO_3^-	24

Using these values, calculate the anion gap.

Acid-Base Disturbances

Disturbances of acid-base balance can be respiratory or metabolic in origin and cause either an acidosis or alkalosis. Based on the duration of the disorder, it can also be classified as acute or chronic. The primary acid-base disorders are discussed here, but it is important to note that more than one disorder can be present at the same time. The only two acid-base disorders that cannot occur simultaneously are respiratory acidosis and respiratory alkalosis (Table 18-2).

Respiratory Acidosis

Respiratory acidosis, whether acute or chronic, is the result of alveolar hypoventilation and results in hypercapnia ($PaCO_2$ greater than 40 mm Hg). The degree to which the increased PCO_2 alters the pH depends on how rapidly the increase occurs and the body's ability to compensate with the blood buffer system and renal regulation.[3] Because of the limitations of the blood buffer system and the delay in renal regulation, a rapid decrease in pH is usually seen with acute increases in PCO_2 (Figure 18-4).

The most common causes of acute respiratory failure leading to respiratory acidosis are depression of the respiratory center by drugs, cerebral injury or disease, and sudden cardiac arrest.[3] Other causes include structural abnormalities (flail chest), neuromuscular abnormalities (hypokalemia), systemic problems (acute respiratory distress syndrome [ARDS]), metabolic factors (high-carbohydrate diet), airway obstruction (aspiration), and lung disorders (pneumonia) (Boxes 18-2 and 18-3). With acute lung disorders, hypoxemia develops before hypercapnia.[3] Small increases in $PaCO_2$ in a previously healthy person are a serious sign of respiratory muscle fatigue and may indicate impending respiratory failure (see Clinical Manifestations box, p. 392). This situation requires careful monitoring and assessment.

TABLE 18-2 SIMPLE ACID-BASE DISTURBANCES AND COMPENSATORY RESPONSES

Disturbance	pH	$PaCO_2$	Bicarbonate (HCO_3^-)	Compensatory Response
Respiratory Acidosis				
Acute	↓ 0.08 for every 10 mm Hg ↑ in $PaCO_2$	↑	Very slight increase or no change	Immediate release of tissue buffers
Chronic	Slight decrease	↑	↑	Increased renal resorption of HCO_3^-; renal compensation starts in 8 hr; maximal effect 3-5 days
Respiratory Alkalosis				
Acute	1 ↑ 0.08 for every 100 mm Hg decrease in $PaCO_2$	↓	No change or very slight decrease	Immediate release of tissue buffers
Chronic	Normal or slight increase*	↓	↓	Decreased renal resorption of HCO_3^-; initial effect 8 hr; maximal effect 3-5 days
Metabolic Acidosis and Alkalosis				
Metabolic acidosis	↓ 0.15 for every 10 mEq/L decrease in HCO_3^-	↓	↓	Chemical buffering and hyperventilation occurs immediately; maximal respiratory compensation 12-24 hr
Metabolic alkalosis	↑ 0.15 for every 10 mEq/L increase in HCO_3^-	↑	↑	Chemical buffering and hypoventilation occur immediately

*The only acid-base disturbance in which compensation can return pH to normal.

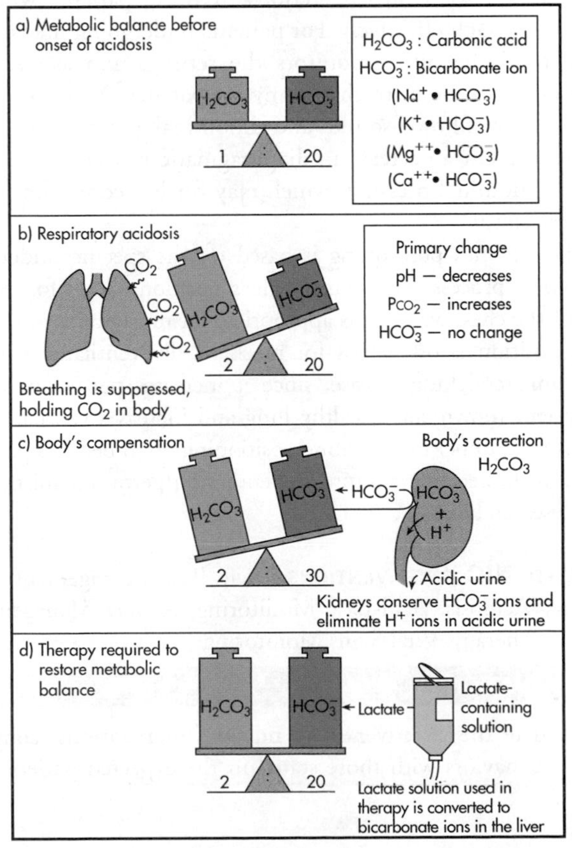

Figure 18-4 Respiratory acidosis.

Collaborative Care Management. Identification and treatment of the underlying disorder is necessary to restore respiratory function. Assessment of airway and lung fields for adequate movement of air and analysis of ABGs are critical. Patients may require suctioning to ensure open airway, and chest physiotherapy may be ordered. (Chest physiotherapy or clapping may be contraindicated in some patient populations.) If $PaCO_2$ is greater than 50 to 60 mm Hg, the patient may require intubation and mechanical ventilation. In patients with chronic respiratory acidosis, treatment with supplemental oxygen must be approached cautiously.[3] It is usually administered at only 1 to 3 L/min, with careful, ongoing monitoring. Changes in oxygen concentration or ventilator parameters are evaluated by monitoring ABGs. Permissive hypercapnea, allowing the $PaCO_2$ to rise above normal limits, in mechanically ventilated patients has been shown to help protect lung tissue in some patients with ARDS.[7] Antibiotics are prescribed if infection is causing or contributing to respiratory acidosis.

Nursing Management

of the Patient with Respiratory Acidosis

ASSESSMENT

Health History. Assess for:

- Length of time since onset of symptoms
- Presence of dyspnea
- Complaints of anxiety or restlessness
- Changes in level of consciousness-confusion or lethargy

Box 18-2 Causes of Acute Respiratory Acidosis

Pulmonary/Thoracic

Severe pneumonia
Acute respiratory distress syndrome (ARDS)
Flail chest
Pneumothorax
Smoke inhalation

Neuromuscular Abnormalities

Hypokalemia
Guillain-Barré syndrome
High cervical injury
Drugs, toxins

Airway Obstruction

Aspiration
Laryngospasm

Systemic Causes

Cardiac arrest
Massive pulmonary emboli
Severe pulmonary edema

Central Nervous System Depression

Sedative overdose
Anesthesia
Cerebral trauma
Cerebral infarct

Metabolic Causes

High-carbohydrate feedings

Box 18-3 Causes of Chronic Respiratory Acidosis

Obstructive Diseases

Emphysema
Chronic bronchitis
Cystic fibrosis
Obstructive sleep apnea

Restriction of Ventilation

Kyphoscoliosis
Severe chronic pneumonitis
Obesity-hypoventilation syndrome (pickwickian syndrome)

Neuromuscular Abnormalities

Polio
Muscular dystrophy
Multiple sclerosis
Amyotrophic lateral sclerosis

Depression of Respiratory Center

Brain tumor
Chronic sedative overdose

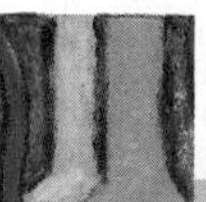

Clinical Manifestations
Respiratory Acidosis

Dyspnea
Tachypnea
Restlessness
Confusion
Diaphoresis

Severe

Lethargy
Ventricular dysrhythmias
Dilated conjunctival and facial blood vessels
Cyanosis
Coma

Physical Examination. Assess for:

- Increased heart rate and respiratory rate
- Signs of diaphoresis
- Asterixis
- Dilated conjunctival and facial blood vessels
- Ventricular dysrhythmias
- Cyanosis (late sign)

Nursing Diagnoses, Outcomes, and Interventions

Nursing Diagnosis: Impaired Gas Exchange

Outcomes. Common examples of expected outcomes for the patient with a diagnosis of *impaired gas exchange* are:

Patient will:

- Return to baseline ABGs or achieve ABG values of $PaCO_2$, less than 45 mm Hg; PaO_2, greater than 60 mm Hg; and pH, between 7.35 and 7.45.
- Achieve a respiratory rate of 12 to 20 breaths/min with a normal pattern and depth.
- Be free from signs of anxiety, restlessness, and confusion depending on preillness baseline.

Nursing Interventions. To assess the patient's response to therapy, the nurse closely monitors and documents serial ABGs and respiratory status, including rate, depth, rhythm, and effort of respirations. Subtle changes in level of consciousness, such as anxiety, restlessness, confusion, lethargy, somnolence, or coma, may indicate progression of respiratory acidosis. The patient's airway is maintained by encouraging coughing. Suctioning may be necessary to remove secretions in those patients who are unable to cough effectively. For patients undergoing mechanical ventilation, the nurse monitors the settings and assesses the endotracheal tube or tracheostomy for patency. Monitoring for the presence of bowel sounds and abdominal distention is necessary to prevent a decrease in diaphragmatic movement secondary to abdominal pressure, which may further compromise respiratory status.

The patient's positioning is based on the specific underlying pathologic process. The semi-Fowler's position allows for expansion of the chest wall and is appropriate for most patients. A side-lying position is often best for mechanically ventilated patients with unilateral lung disease, since it increases perfusion to the dependent (down side) healthy lung and increases ventilation to the diseased upper lung.[7] Prone positioning often benefits patients with ARDS because it improves ventilation/perfusion mismatch[8] (see Research box).

Related NIC Interventions. Acid-Base Management: Respiratory Acidosis, Acid-Base Monitoring, Airway Management, Oxygen Therapy, Vital Signs Monitoring

Evaluation

To evaluate the effectiveness of nursing interventions, compare patient behaviors with those stated in the expected patient outcomes.

Related NOC Outcomes. Electrolyte & Acid/Base Balance, Respiratory Status: Gas Exchange, Respiratory Status: Ventilation

Research

Murray T, Patterson L: Prone positioning of trauma patients with acute respiratory distress syndrome and open abdominal incisions, *Crit Care Nurse* 22(3):52-56, 2002.

Research has shown most patients with acute respiratory distress syndrome benefit from prone positioning, which improves oxygenation through several mechanisms, including changes in diaphragm motion and redistribution of lung water and exudates. Prone positioning can even benefit patients with trauma, including open abdominal incisions. The authors discuss and reference various methodologies describing prone placement.

Respiratory Alkalosis

Respiratory alkalosis is the result of hyperventilation leading to hypocapnia ($PaCO_2$ less than 40 mm Hg). The acute decrease in PCO_2 causes a mild but rapid decrease in serum bicarbonate, occurring within minutes and reaching a constant state in approximately 10 minutes. If respiratory alkalosis persists beyond 6 hours, it is classified as chronic, and renal compensatory changes cause a further decrease in bicarbonate concentration and an increase in pH toward normal levels (Figure 18-5).

Acute respiratory alkalosis is most commonly associated with hyperventilation related to anxiety (see Clinical Manifestations box). It also occurs with pain, gram-negative sepsis, high altitude sickness, and some pulmonary disorders with or without coexisting hypoxemia.[4] Salicylate overdose and intracerebral trauma both exert direct stimulation on the respiratory center leading to hyperventilation. Hyperventilation secondary to hypoxemia is limited because, as the pH increases, the respiratory center is no longer stimulated and the respiratory rate decreases. Chronic respiratory alkalosis occurs with high altitude residence, hepatic insufficiency, pregnancy (because of the effects of progesterone), cerebral trauma, and restrictive pulmonary disease (pulmonary fibrosis secondary to cystic fibrosis). Respiratory alkalosis persists throughout the course of pulmonary fibrosis. A normal $PaCO_2$ followed by hypercapnia indicates the terminal stages of this disease. Chronic respiratory alkalosis is the only simple acid-base disorder in which the pH returns to normal range because of renal compensation.[4] Box 18-4 lists causes for respiratory alkalosis.

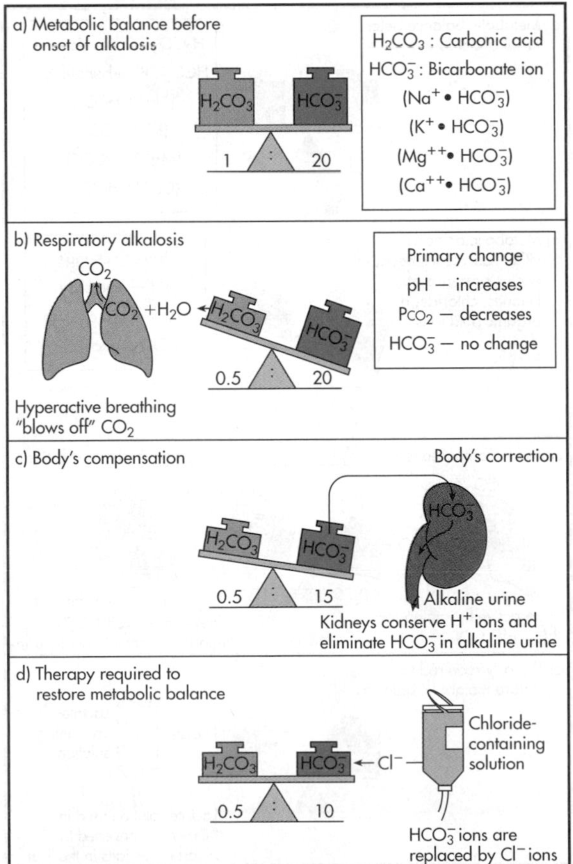

Figure 18-5 Respiratory alkalosis.

Collaborative Care Management. Treatment for respiratory alkalosis involves identifying and treating the underlying disorder. The physician may order sedatives and tranquilizers to treat anxiety-induced respiratory alkalosis. If symptoms are severe, rebreathing into a paper bag or an oxygen mask with a carbon dioxide reservoir may be useful. Pulse oximetry may be used to assess oxygenation before and during treatment. Adequate pain management is important if the alkalosis is related to patients' response to pain. If hypoxemia is the cause, oxygen therapy may

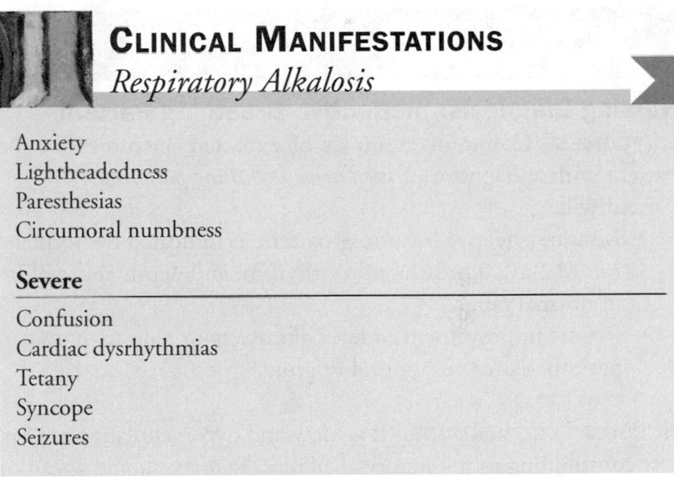

CLINICAL MANIFESTATIONS
Respiratory Alkalosis

Anxiety
Lightheadedness
Paresthesias
Circumoral numbness

Severe

Confusion
Cardiac dysrhythmias
Tetany
Syncope
Seizures

BOX 18-4 Causes of Respiratory Alkalosis

Direct Stimulation of Respiratory Center

Anxiety
Fever
Pain
Salicylates
Voluntary or mechanical hyperventilation
Intracerebral trauma
Gram-negative sepsis
Pregnancy
Hepatic insufficiency

Hypoxemia

Pneumonia
High altitude (over 6500 feet)
Hypotension
Severe anemia
Congestive heart failure

Pulmonary Disorders

Pulmonary emboli
Pulmonary edema
Asthma (initially)
Inhalation of irritants
Interstitial fibrosis

be necessary; if the patient is being mechanically ventilated, adjustments to respiratory rate and volume, and assessment of dead space may be needed.

Nursing Management of the Patient with Respiratory Alkalosis

Health History. Assess for:

- Length of time since onset of symptoms
- Complaints of anxiety or pain
- Complaints of shortness of breath, dyspnea, lightheadedness
- Presence of paresthesias or circumoral numbness
- Current history of intentional or unintentional overdose of salicylates
- History of asthma, other pulmonary disorders, and central nervous system trauma and related information

Physical Examination. Assess for:

- Increased rate and depth of respiration
- Confusion
- Tetany, syncope, and seizures
- Cardiac dysrhythmias and ST-T wave changes

Nursing Diagnoses, Outcomes, and Interventions

Nursing Diagnosis: Ineffective Breathing Pattern

Outcomes. Common examples of expected outcomes for the patient with a diagnosis of *ineffective breathing pattern* are:

Patient will:

- Resume effective breathing pattern as indicated by normal rate (12 to 20 breaths/min), rhythm, and depth and ABGs in normal range.
- Report improvement in level of anxiety or pain with no paresthesias or circumoral tingling.

Nursing Interventions. If anxiety and hyperventilation are factors contributing to respiratory alkalosis, the nurse should assess for the degree of anxiety and offer reassurance or stay with the patient during the acute episode. The nurse assesses and treats pain as ordered; reassesses 30 minutes after pain treatment to determine effectiveness of interventions; and documents level of pain, treatment, and response to treatment for later comparisons. The nurse should encourage a normal breathing pattern by pacing the patient's breathing or having the patient mimic staff's breathing pattern. It also may help to encourage the patient to rebreathe into a paper bag or oxygen mask with an attached carbon dioxide reservoir (if prescribed) to increase the P_{CO_2} in inspired air. The nurse should monitor pulse oximetry before and during this treatment. Modest alkalosis can cause dysrhythmias in patients with preexisting heart disease who are taking cardiotropic medications; therefore the nurse monitors cardiac rhythm and notifies the physician of any dysrhythmias.

Related NIC Interventions. Airway Management, Anxiety Reduction, Progressive Muscle Relaxation, Respiratory Monitoring, Vital Signs Monitoring

Evaluation

To evaluate the effectiveness of nursing interventions, compare patient behaviors with those stated in the expected patient outcomes.

Related NOC Outcomes. Respiratory Status: Airway Patency, Respiratory Status: Gas Exchange, Respiratory Status: Ventilation

Metabolic Acidosis

Metabolic acidosis exists when there is a primary decrease in serum bicarbonate concentration (to less than 24 mEq/L) with acidemia (pH less than 7.40). The decrease in serum bicarbonate can be caused by one or more of the following: loss of base (HCO_3^-) from the body via gastrointestinal or renal routes, excess fixed acid (hydrogen ion) production (ketoacidosis, lactic acidosis), and the kidney's inability kidneys to excrete the fixed acid load (acute or chronic renal failure) (Figure 18-6).

Acute metabolic acidosis causes numerous serious alterations in cellular and organ function.[9] Although chemical and respiratory compensation occurs immediately, these responses can easily be overwhelmed by the rapid accumulation of acids or loss of bicarbonate. Renal compensation is limited because of the rapid onset of the acidosis and the delay in the renal compensatory response. Anion gap analysis helps identify the nature of the metabolic acidosis, and further testing (e.g., toxin screens, lactate

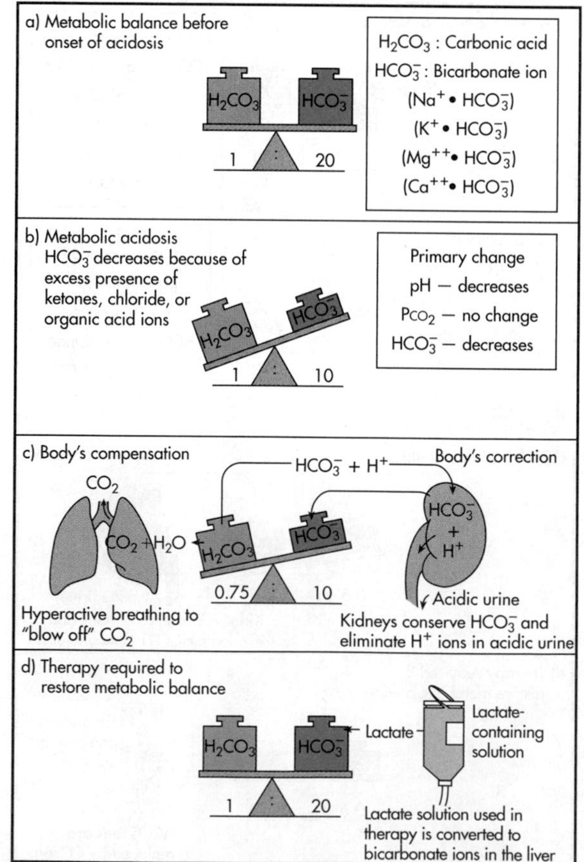

Figure 18-6 Metabolic acidosis.

and ketone levels) helps clarify specific causes. Normal anion gap (12 ±2) indicates a loss of bicarbonate or decreased renal secretion of hydrogen, whereas a high anion gap points to the addition and accumulation of organic acids faster than the body can metabolize or excrete them.[9]

Chronic renal failure is the most common cause of chronic metabolic acidosis. The inability of the kidney to adequately excrete hydrogen ion leads to a persistent acidemia (pH less than 7.40). In most instances chronic metabolic acidosis develops slowly with a gradual decrease in bicarbonate. Patients with chronic renal failure and chronic metabolic acidosis develop renal bone disease secondary to the leeching of calcium from bone to buffer the accumulated hydrogen. Box 18-5 lists causes of metabolic acidosis. The Clinical Manifestations box summarizes common clinical findings in persons with metabolic acidosis.

Collaborative Care Management. Treatment of metabolic acidosis is directed at the underlying disorder and the restoration of acid-base, fluid, and electrolyte balances. In diabetic ketoacidosis, fluids and insulin are required, whereas with alcohol-related ketosis, glucose and saline are necessary. The causes of lactic acidosis must be identified and treated, although mortality can remain high even with appropriate treatment.[9] Acute and chronic renal failure requires hemodialysis or peritoneal dialysis to restore acid-base balance. Poisonings and drug toxicity may also demand hemodialysis. Moderate amounts of bicarbonate may be given orally every day to patients with renal tubular acidosis. If acute metabolic acidosis is severe (pH less than 7.20, or bicarbonate of 6 to 8 mEq/L), it may be necessary to treat patient with sodium bicarbonate ($NaHCO_3$). The administration of intravenous sodium bicarbonate, even for severe acidosis, is controversial because it can often cause a profound metabolic alkalosis as the underlying disease is corrected.[9] Sodium bicarbonate must be used with extreme caution in patients with congestive heart failure or pulmonary edema because of the risk of fluid overload.

Box 18-5 Causes of Metabolic Acidosis

Loss of Bicarbonate

Gastrointestinal
- Diarrhea
- Biliary and pancreatic drainage
- Ileostomy

Renal
- Renal tubular acidosis type 2
- Acetazolamide

Excess Acid Production
- Ketoacidosis
- Diabetes
- Alcohol-induced starvation
- Lactic acidosis
- Rhabdomyolysis

Excess Acid Ingestion
- Salicylates
- Cocaine
- 3,4-Methylenedioxymethamphetamine (Ecstasy)
- Methamphetamine

Inability of Kidney to Excrete Hydrogen Ion Load
- Renal failure
- Renal tubular acidosis type 1
- Hyperaldosteronism
- Potassium-sparing diuretics

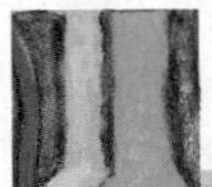

CLINICAL MANIFESTATIONS
Metabolic Acidosis

	Severe
Hypotension	Kussmaul's respirations
Tachypnea	Flushed, warm, dry skin
"Fruity" breath	Dysrhythmias
Cold, clammy skin	Stupor
Nausea, vomiting	Coma
Diarrhea	
Confusion	

Nursing Management
of the Patient with Metabolic Acidosis

ASSESSMENT

Health History. Assess for:
- Length of time since onset of symptoms
- History of headache, anorexia, nausea, vomiting, diarrhea, abdominal pain
- Polyuria
- Polydipsia

Physical Examination. Assess for:
- Hypotension
- Tachypnea or Kussmaul's respirations
- Cold, clammy skin progressing to flushed, warm, and dry skin
- "Fruity" breath
- Changes in level of consciousness
- Ventricular dysrhythmias

NURSING DIAGNOSES, OUTCOMES, AND INTERVENTIONS

Nursing Diagnosis: Decreased Cardiac Output

OUTCOMES. Common examples of expected outcomes for the patient with a diagnosis of *decreased cardiac output* are:

Patient will:
- Achieve a pH of greater than 7.20.
- Achieve a return to baseline on electrocardiogram.
- Remain free from cardiac dysrhythmias.

NURSING INTERVENTIONS. Decreased cardiac output related to dysrhythmias and decreased myocardial function are potential consequences of metabolic acidosis. Therefore the nurse monitors patients for cardiac dysrhythmias, especially ventricular dysrhythmias, and follows established protocols or prescribed treatments. The nurse monitors apical and radial pulses for pulse deficits, which may indicate weak cardiac contractions or heart failure. ABGs and other laboratory data are monitored to assess for effectiveness of treatment measures.

RELATED NIC INTERVENTIONS. Acid-Base Management, Acid-Base Management: Metabolic Acidosis, Acid-Base Monitoring, Cardiac Care, Vital Signs Monitoring

EVALUATION

To evaluate the effectiveness of nursing interventions, compare patient behaviors with those stated in the expected patient outcomes.

RELATED NOC OUTCOMES. Cardiac Pump Effectiveness, Electrolyte & Acid/Base Balance

Metabolic Alkalosis

Metabolic alkalosis occurs when there is excess serum bicarbonate from either a gain of bicarbonate or a loss of hydrogen, resulting in a pH of greater than 7.40. The increase in serum bicarbonate can result from (1) loss of hydrogen ions from the gastrointestinal tract via vomiting or nasogastric suctioning; (2) an increase in hydrogen ion secretion by the kidneys in amounts greater then necessary to eliminate the normal acid load (as with diuretic use); (3) loss of fluid that contains more chloride than bicarbonate, causing a contraction alkalosis (as with diuretic use or cystic fibrosis); and (4) administration or ingestion of large quantities of bicarbonate or its precursors (citrate in blood products).

Rapid correction of chronically elevated P_{CO_2} levels can cause a serious metabolic alkalosis, referred to as postchronic hypercapneic metabolic alkalosis. This occurs because renal compensation (elevated bicarbonate), even though no longer necessary, remains in place until the kidneys can respond to the new P_{CO_2} level, which can take days (Figure 18-7). Metabolic alkalosis is a common acid-base disorder in hospitalized patients, with 90% of all cases resulting from nasogastric suctioning or use of diuretics, especially thiazide diuretics.[6] Hypokalemia often coexists with alkalosis as potassium shifts into the cells in exchange for hydrogen. Respiratory compensation occurs as the pH increases and the respiratory center responds by decreasing ventilation, resulting in an increase in P_{CO_2}. This response is limited by the hypoxemia caused by the decreased ventilation. Patients with metabolic alkalosis should have a Pa_{CO_2} of greater than 40 mm Hg from compensation, but the Pa_{CO_2} rarely increases above 55 mm Hg. A Pa_{CO_2} greater than 55 mm Hg indicates a coexisting respiratory acidosis.[6]

Chronic metabolic alkalosis is related to long-term diuretic use or mineralcorticoid excess (Cushing's disease, primary hyperaldosteronism). Box 18-6 lists causes of metabolic alkalosis. The Clinical Manifestations box summarizes clinical findings in persons with metabolic alkalosis.

Collaborative Care Management. Mild or moderate metabolic alkalosis does not usually require specific therapeutic intervention. Treatment of the underlying disorder is the goal. Testing of urine electrolytes, specifically chloride, before beginning treatment may help differentiate among causes of the alkalosis.[6] Serum potassium is usually decreased. Hypokalemia is responsible for muscle weakness, and cardiac rhythm disturbances frequently

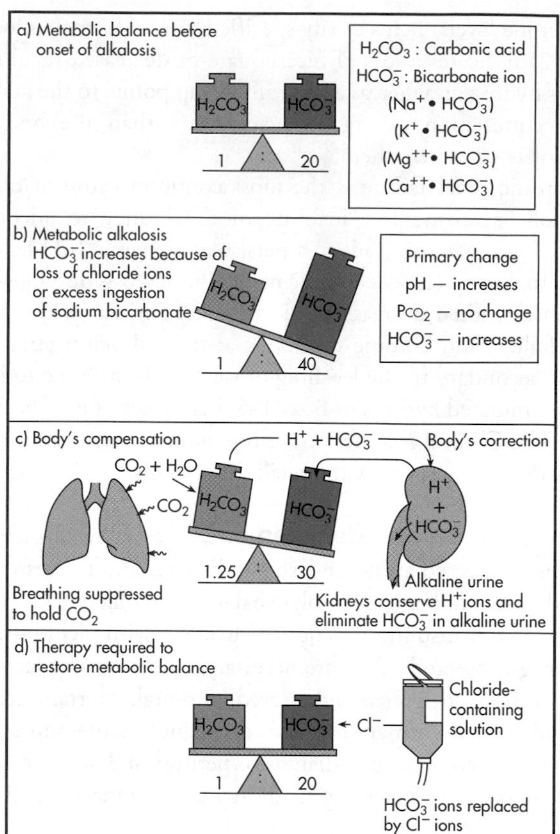

Figure 18-7 Metabolic alkalosis.

Box 18-6 Causes of Metabolic Alkalosis

Hydrogen Ion Losses

Gastrointestinal
- Vomiting
- Nasogastric suctioning

Renal
- Diuretics (thiazides especially)
- Mineralcorticoid excess
- Postchronic hypercapnia
- Hypercalcemia, hypoparathyroidism

Hydrogen Ion Shift Into Cells
- Hypokalemia
- Carbohydrate refeeding after starvation

Bicarbonate Retention
- Administration or ingestion of bicarbonate
- Massive blood transfusion

Contraction Alkalosis
- Diuretics
- Cystic fibrosis

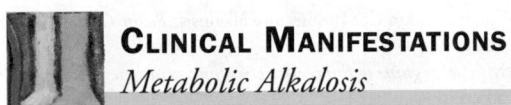

CLINICAL MANIFESTATIONS
Metabolic Alkalosis

	Severe
Muscle weakness	Neuromuscular excitability (tetany)
Hyporeflexia	Apathy
Polyuria or polydipsia (related to hypokalemia)	Confusion
Cardiac rhythm disturbances	Stupor

seen. Severe hypokalemia may cause tetany. Hypokalemia is treated with either oral or intravenous potassium salts. (See Chapter 17 for guidelines on administering potassium.) Isotonic saline infusion may be necessary to correct volume deficits related to metabolic alkalosis caused by diuretics or loss of gastric secretions. Metabolic alkalosis is difficult to resolve if hypovolemia and chloride losses are not corrected. Acetazolamide (Diamox) may be used in patients with congestive heart failure who cannot tolerate rapid volume expansion. Acetazolamide can cause large losses of potassium and bicarbonate; therefore potassium supplementation may be necessary before starting treatment.[2]

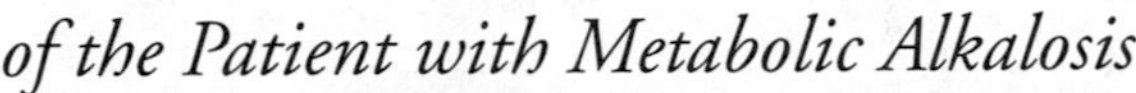

Nursing Management
of the Patient with Metabolic Alkalosis

ASSESSMENT

Health History. Assess for:

- Length of time since onset of symptoms
- History of vomiting, nasogastric suctioning, bulimia, diuretic use or abuse
- Presence of muscle weakness
- History of polyuria
- History of polydipsia

Physical Examination. Assess for:

- Postural hypotension
- Neuromuscular excitability associated with tetany
- Changes in level of consciousness—apathy, confusion, stupor

NURSING DIAGNOSES, OUTCOMES, AND INTERVENTIONS

Nursing Diagnosis: Decreased Cardiac Output

OUTCOMES. Common examples of expected outcomes for the patient with a diagnosis of *decreased cardiac output* are:

Patient will:

- Achieve a pH of less than 7.45.
- Maintain an electrocardiogram within normal limits.

NURSING INTERVENTIONS. Vomiting, gastric suctioning, or potassium-wasting diuretics may precipitate metabolic alkalosis and trigger electrical conduction abnormalities and decreased cardiac output. Therefore the nurse must monitor the electrocardiogram for the presence of dysrhythmias. The nurse assesses apical and radial pulses simultaneously when evaluating cardiac rate and rhythm to detect pulse deficit. Abnormalities are documented for future comparison and reported to the physician so appropriate treatment may be initiated. The nurse monitors laboratory data, especially pH and serum bicarbonate, to determine the patient's response to therapy. Serum potassium levels are particularly important to monitor, especially in patients receiving digitalis preparations, since hypokalemia sensitizes patients to the cardiotoxic effect of digitalis. The nurse notifies the physician if potassium levels drop to less than 3.5 mEq/L. The nurse weighs patients daily and records intake and output to determine volume status so that fluid replacement can be administered if needed. Gastric contents removed by suction are measured and the amount of fluid removed is documented. If gastric irrigation is required, isotonic saline is used to prevent electrolyte washout.

RELATED NIC INTERVENTIONS. Acid-Base Management, Acid-Base Management: Metabolic Alkalosis, Acid-Base Monitoring, Cardiac Care, Vital Signs Monitoring

EVALUATION

To evaluate the effectiveness of nursing interventions, compare patient behaviors with those stated in the expected patient outcomes.

RELATED NOC OUTCOMES. Cardiac Pump Effectiveness, Electrolyte & Acid/Base Balance

GERONTOLOGIC CONSIDERATIONS

Preexisting or underlying conditions such as renal, cardiac, pulmonary, and endocrine disorders increase the risk for acid-base disturbances among older adults.[10] In addition to underlying disease states affecting acid-base balance, older adults often take numerous medications that may alter the body's ability to compensate for changes in acid-base status. Once an acid-base disorder develops, the older patient is less able to compensate for imbalance because of age-related changes in the kidneys.

▶ ARE You READY?

The nurse is reviewing a patient's arterial blood gas results:

pH	7.29
Pao_2	84
$Paco_2$	50
Hco_3	26
O_2 Sat	95%

These results indicate which of the following?

1. Respiratory acidosis
2. Metabolic acidosis
3. Respiratory alkalosis
4. Metabolic alkalosis

? Critical Thinking

1. If a patient has a low pH and a high $PaCO_2$, what primary disorder do you know is present?
2. If the patient has a high pH and a high bicarbonate, what primary disorder must be present?
3. A patient has a 3-day history of nausea and vomiting. ABGs are pH, 7.51; $PaCO_2$, 42 mm Hg; and bicarbonate, 34 mEq/L. What acid-base disorder, acidemia or alkalemia, is indicated by the pH? Is it respiratory or metabolic in nature? Has compensation occurred? To the expected degree? What treatment is indicated?

References

1. Adrogue HE, Adrogue HJ: Acid-base physiology, *Respir Care* 46(4):328–341, 2001.
2. DuBose T, Hamm L: *Acid-base and electrolyte disorders*, Philadelphia, 2002, Saunders.
3. Epstein SK, Singh N: Respiratory acidosis, *Respir Care* 46(4):366–383, 2001.
4. Foster GT, Vaziri ND, Sassoon CS: Respiratory alkalosis, *Respir Care* 46(4):384–391, 2001.
5. Heitz U, Horne M: *Pocket guide to fluid, electrolyte, and acid-base balance*, ed 5, St Louis, 2005, Elsevier.
6. Khanna A, Kurtzman NA: Metabolic alkalosis, *Respir Care* 46(4):354–365, 2001.
7. Marion B: A turn for the better: prone positioning of patients with ARDS, *AJN* 101(5):26–34, 2001.
8. Murray TA, Patterson LA: Prone positioning of trauma patients with acute respiratory distress syndrome and open abdominal incisions, *Crit Care Nurs* 22(3):2–56, 2002.
9. Swenson ER: Metabolic acidosis, *Respir Care* 46(4):342–353, 2001.
10. Whittier WL, Rutecki GW: Primer on clinical acid-base problem solving, *Dis Month* 50(3):122–162, 2004.

Visit the Evolve website: http://evolve.elsevier.com/Monahan/medsurg

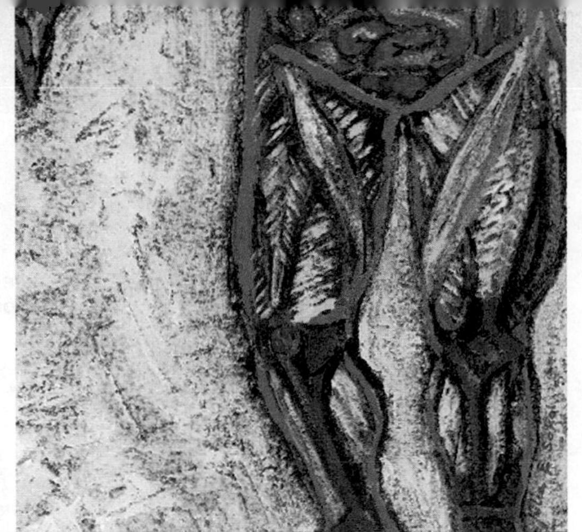

CHAPTER 19
Shock

by Nan Smith-Blair

OBJECTIVES

After studying this chapter, the learner should be able to:

1. Define physiologic shock.
2. Correlate the four classifications of shock with their pathophysiology.
3. Discuss the progression of clinical manifestations through the three stages of shock.
4. Identify assessment findings related to each type of shock.
5. Identify medical and nursing management strategies in the treatment of shock.
6. Describe methods of fluid replacement during shock.
7. Correlate effects of pharmacologic agents used to treat shock with nursing measures for patients receiving drug therapy.

KEY TERMS

afterload, p. 401
anaphylactic shock, p. 407
cardiogenic shock, p. 402
compensatory stage, p. 408
contractility, p. 401
distributive shock, p. 404
hypovolemic shock, p. 402
neurogenic shock, p. 406
oxygen transport, p. 401
preload, p. 401
progressive stage, p. 411
refractory stage, p. 411
septic shock, p. 404

Nature of the Problem

Shock is a complex physiologic entity representing a diverse group of life-threatening circulatory conditions. Mortality rates from uncomplicated hemorrhagic shock are low, provided adequate replacement of blood volume is instituted early. However, despite advances in the assessment and treatment of this complex physiologic syndrome, mortality rates from other forms of shock continue to range from 65% to 80%. Shock may develop in any patient, in any setting. Mortality from shock depends on the patient's physiologic state before the initial incident, the duration of the shock state, and response to therapy. Early recognition of clinical manifestations and initiation of therapeutic measures may halt the progression of shock and prevent death.

Physiology

Every cell in the body needs adequate tissue perfusion to provide the necessary supply of oxygen and nutrients and to remove metabolic byproducts. In shock, blood flow to vital organs becomes inadequate, or the cells become unable to extract and use oxygen and substrates. If left untreated, this functional impairment of cells, tissues, organs, and body systems progresses to multiple organ dysfunction and death.

Hemodynamic Principles

The circulatory system is composed of the heart, large blood vessels, and microcirculation (also called the peripheral or capillary circulation). These three components function interdependently to maintain an adequate cardiac output and tissue perfusion. Adequate blood flow depends on:

- Adequate amounts of blood for the heart to pump
- Effective pumping by the heart
- Constriction and dilation of blood vessels to maintain normal blood pressure

Shock results when one or more of these functions is disrupted.

Patients in shock may require placement of an arterial catheter and an indwelling balloon-flotation pulmonary artery catheter and use of sophisticated bedside monitors to evaluate cardiac function, circulating blood volume, and physiologic response to treatment (Figure 19-1). From these measured pressures, health care providers can obtain various hemodynamic parameters to assess the mechanisms that support normal cardiovascular function: cardiac output, cardiac index, central venous pressure, stroke volume, and systemic and pulmonary vascular resistance (Table 19-1).

Cardiac Output. Cardiac output reflects the amount of blood the heart pumps from the ventricles in 1 minute. Determinants of

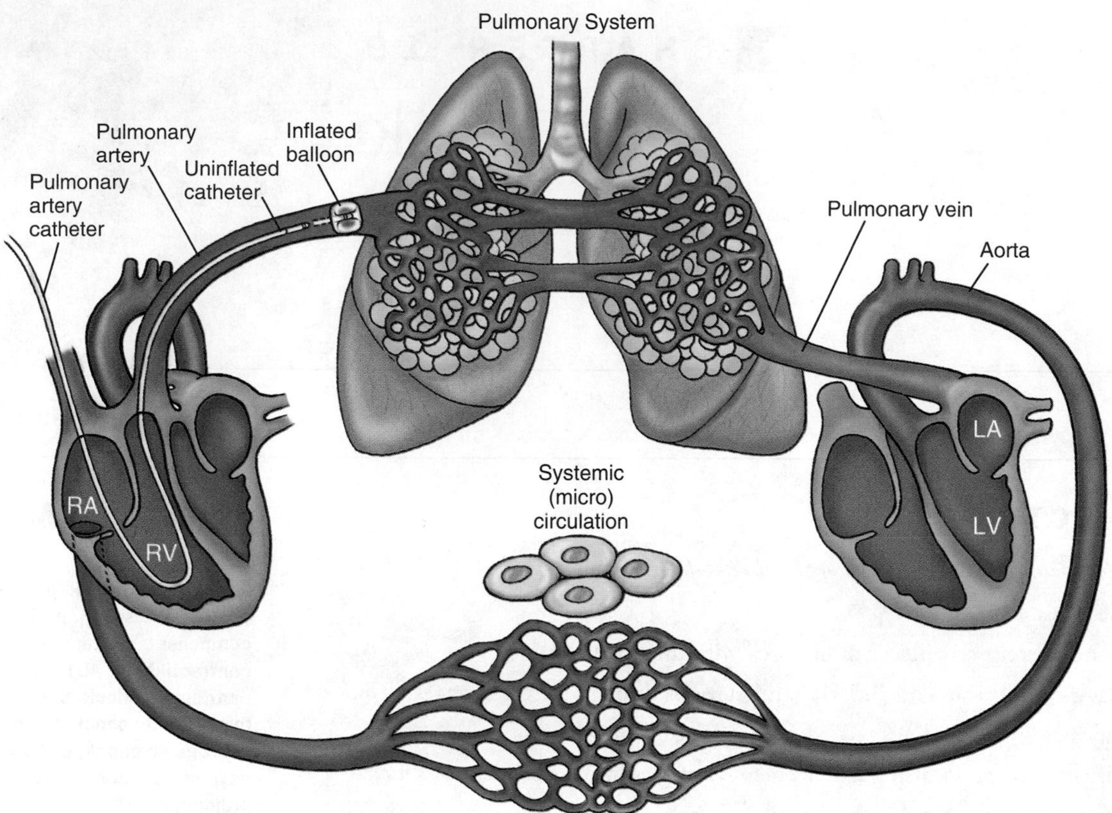

Figure 19-1 Pulmonary artery catheter position. When balloon is deflated, pressures in pulmonary artery can be measured. When balloon is inflated, blood flow propels catheter until tip "wedges" in a small arterial branch. Pressure is normally transmitted from left side of heart through pulmonary artery wedge pressure. *LA,* Left atrium; *LV,* left ventricle; *RA,* right atrium, *RV,* right ventricle.

TABLE 19-1 HEMODYNAMIC PARAMETERS AND NORMAL VALUES

Parameter	Acronym	Normal Range	Definition
Cardiac output	CO	4-6 L/min	Volume of blood pumped by each ventricle each minute
Cardiac index	CI	2.4-4.0 L/min/m^2	CO divided by body surface area; indexed to body surface area to adjust for difference in body size
Central venous pressure	CVP	2-4 mm Hg	Pressure created by volume in right side of heart
Stroke volume	SV	60-70 ml	Amount of blood ejected by ventricle with each heartbeat
Systemic vascular resistance	SVR	900-1400 dynes/sec/cm^{-5}	Resistance to blood flow created by systemic vasculature (arteries and arterioles) against which left ventricle must pump to eject its volume; as SVR increases, CO decreases
Pulmonary vascular resistance	PVR	30-100 dynes/sec/cm^{-5}	Resistance to blood flow created by pulmonary arteries and arterioles against which right ventricle must pump to eject its volume

cardiac output include heart rate and stroke volume. Stroke volume is defined as the amount of blood ejected by the ventricle with each heartbeat. It is influenced by three factors: preload, afterload, and contractility. Changes in either heart rate or stroke volume can change cardiac output. As the body's metabolic needs change, the heart adjusts cardiac output by altering either heart rate or stroke volume.

Heart Rate. Heart rate is influenced by the autonomic nervous system. Sympathetic innervation results in an increase in heart rate, whereas parasympathetic innervation results in a decrease in heart rate. Healthy individuals can increase cardiac output up to three times the normal levels for short periods by increasing the heart rate. Increases in heart rate decrease diastolic filling time, allowing less time for perfusion of the coronary arteries. In individuals with reduced cardiac reserve, as in ischemic heart disease, increasing heart rate may actually decrease cardiac output, since myocardial oxygen demand becomes greater than myocardial oxygen supply.

Preload. **Preload** is the amount of stretch in the ventricle at the end of diastole. As blood returns to the ventricle, the ventricle distends, myocardial fibers stretch, and the force of contraction increases. The amount of ventricular stretch at end of diastole determines the pressure on the walls of the ventricle. End-diastolic pressure refers to the amount of pressure in the ventricle. The fundamental control mechanism, Starling's law of the heart, states that as the normal left ventricle accepts increases in volume, it distends and cardiac output increases until a critical point is reached. After that critical point, further increases in filling volume beyond the maximal length-tension relationship will result in a decrease in stroke volume and cardiac output. Thus preload is a function of the volume of blood presented to the ventricle and compliance (ability of the ventricle to stretch) of the ventricle at the end of diastole. Factors affecting volume include changes in venous return, total blood volume, and the amount of blood ejected from the atrium during contraction, termed *atrial kick*. Factors affecting ventricular compliance include the "stiffness" and thickness of the muscular wall.

Afterload. **Afterload** is the ventricular wall tension or stress during systolic ejection. Systemic vascular resistance influences left ventricular afterload. Pulmonary vascular resistance affects right ventricular afterload. Increased afterload usually results in an increase in the work of the heart. Factors that oppose ejection of blood from the ventricle increase afterload. Afterload may be increased in conditions that impede aortic or pulmonary outflow (aortic stenosis or pulmonary stenosis), obstruction in the outflow tract (septal hypertrophy), increased systemic or pulmonary vascular resistance (vasoconstriction), or an increased blood volume or viscosity. As resistance to left ventricular ejection increases, stroke volume decreases. Conversely, as systemic resistance falls, stroke volume from the left ventricle increases. The heart's ability to contract and respond to alterations in preload and afterload significantly affects cardiac output.

Contractility. **Contractility** refers to the heart's contractile force or inotropy (from *ino,* strength; *tropy,* enhancing). Inotropy can be either positive (stronger contraction) or negative (weaker contraction). Contractility is negatively influenced by myocardial ischemia and underlying heart disease. Contractility can also be altered by a variety of pharmacologic agents, especially those mimicking the sympathetic nervous system (sympathomimetics, adrenergics).

Control of Peripheral Circulation. Intrinsic control of blood flow mechanisms to individual vascular beds occurs through response of arteriolar smooth muscle to products of metabolism, causing either vasodilation or vasoconstriction. Other factors influencing this balance include local release of catecholamines, histamine, acetylcholine, serotonin, angiotensin, adenosine, and prostaglandins. These factors are released in response to tissue injury, hypoxemia, or hormones. Local circulation is also influenced by temperature and carbon dioxide.

The central nervous system mediates extrinsic control of peripheral blood flow. The autonomic nervous system exerts dual antagonistic control over organ systems via sympathetic and parasympathetic fibers. Stimulation of the vasoconstrictor region in the medulla causes an increase in mean arterial pressure and heart rate by enhancing sympathetic nervous system outflow and inhibiting parasympathetic nervous system outflow. Sympathetic outflow targets resistance vessels, causing vasoconstriction. Inhibition of these areas causes the opposite effect, vasodilation. Sympathetic fibers causing vasoconstriction supply arteries, arterioles, and veins. Capacitance vessels (veins) are also responsive to sympathetic stimulation, but the effects are not as easily seen as on the arterial side.

Oxygen Transport Principles

All forms of shock involve impaired delivery of oxygen to the tissues. Variables that influence **oxygen transport** include the amount of oxygen delivered to the tissues, oxygen consumption by the tissues, and the oxygen extraction ratio (Table 19-2).

Oxygen delivery depends on blood flow (cardiac output), the amount of hemoglobin available to carry oxygen, and the percentage of arterial oxygen hemoglobin saturation. The body normally delivers three to four times more oxygen to the tissues than they need for normal metabolism. Any condition that reduces cardiac output, hemoglobin availability, or hemoglobin saturation has an impact on the amount of oxygen delivered to tissues.

Oxygen consumption represents the body's demand for oxygen and is a reflection of tissue metabolism. Reduced oxygen consumption is common in all forms of shock and may be due to a reduction in blood flow (delivery) as in hypovolemic or cardiogenic shock, or may be due to an uneven distribution of blood as in septic shock. The magnitude of the oxygen consumption deficit in patients experiencing shock has been correlated with mortality rates.

Oxygen consumption and delivery can be measured using a specialized pulmonary artery catheter. The oxygen extraction ratio (VO_2/DO_2) provides an estimate of the balance between tissue oxygen demand (consumption) and oxygen supply (delivery). It also indicates the tissues' ability to extract and use the oxygen delivered.

TABLE 19-2 OXYGEN TRANSPORT VARIABLES

Variable	Acronym	Definition
Oxygen delivery	DO_2	Amount of oxygen delivered to tissues each minute; reflects ability of circulatory system to supply oxygen to tissues
Oxygen consumption	VO_2	Amount of oxygen used by tissues each minute; reflects body's total metabolism
Oxygen extraction ratio	VO_2/DO_2	Ratio of oxygen consumption to oxygen delivery; indicates ability of tissues to extract and use oxygen delivered

Etiology

Shock may be classified as hypovolemic, cardiogenic, or distributive depending on the pathophysiologic cause.

Hypovolemic Shock

Hypovolemic shock is the most common type of shock. It is caused by a loss of whole blood, plasma, or interstitial fluid in quantities such that the body's metabolic needs can no longer be met. Box 19-1 lists the etiologic factors in hypovolemic shock.

Hypovolemic shock develops from an absolute or relative hypovolemia. Absolute hypovolemia results from an external loss of fluid from the body, as in hemorrhage. Relative hypovolemia results from an internal shift of fluid from the intravascular space to the extravascular space. It may occur as the result of increased capillary permeability, decreased colloidal osmotic pressure, or loss of intravascular integrity. Reduced intravascular blood volume leads to a decreased amount of blood returning to the heart (venous return). This, in turn, decreases the amount of blood received by the ventricles during diastolic filling (preload) and decreases the amount of blood available for ejection from the ventricle (stroke volume). As compensatory mechanisms begin to fail and can no longer maintain cardiac output, tissue perfusion to organ systems significantly decreases (Figure 19-2).

Clinical manifestations of hypovolemic shock depend on the severity of fluid loss and the person's ability to compensate for the loss. Disease processes, age, amount of blood loss, rate of loss, and length of time over which the loss occurs all affect the speed with which clinical manifestations of hypovolemic shock appear. Hemorrhagic shock is divided into four classes: early, moderate, progressing, and profound. Table 19-3 lists assessment findings for each of these classes. The clinical presentations of the various types of hypovolemic shock are all similar to the presentation of hemorrhagic shock.

Class I hemorrhagic shock represents a fluid loss of up to 15% and may be tolerated without any symptoms if compensatory mechanisms are effective in maintaining cardiac output.

Box 19-1 Etiologic Factors of Hypovolemic Shock

Loss of Blood Volume	Gastrointestinal
External	Severe vomiting
Trauma	Severe diarrhea
Gastrointestinal bleeding	**Renal**
Surgery	Diabetic ketoacidosis
Internal	Hyperosmolar nonketotic diabetes
Hemothorax	Diabetes insipidus
Ruptured aortic aneurysm	High-output renal failure
Hemoperitoneum	Adrenal insufficiency
Retroperitoneal hemorrhage	Diuretic therapy
Loss of plasma volume	
Burns	
Desquamated-exudated lesions	
Loss of other body fluids	

Class II hemorrhagic shock represents more significant volume losses of 15% to 30%. The body tries to initiate compensatory mechanisms to return to homeostasis. The heart rate increases to between 100 and 120 beats/min in response to sympathetic nervous system stimulation. The patient's blood pressure remains normal or is slightly decreased, but the pulse pressure is narrowed. Urinary output ranges from 20 to 30 ml/hr. Capillary refill time is prolonged.

Class III hemorrhagic shock occurs with major blood losses of 30% to 40% of total volume. The patient becomes increasingly anxious and progressively confused. Systolic blood pressure drops below 80 mm Hg and pulse pressure is narrowed. Respirations increase in rate and depth. Urinary output falls to 5 to 15 ml/hr. Capillary refill continues to be prolonged.

Class IV hemorrhagic shock represents a severe blood loss of greater than 40% of the total volume. The patient develops severe hypotension. Heart rate may exceed 140 beats/min, and respirations may exceed 35 breaths/min. Urinary output decreases to only negligible amounts. Peripheral capillary refill time is significantly longer than 3 seconds.

▶ ARE You READY?

Which of the following clinical manifestations relate to the client in class II (moderate) hemorrhagic shock? (Choose all that apply.)

1. Blood loss of 2000 ml
2. Loss of 25% blood volume
3. Stuporous
4. Heart rate of 110
5. Slight decrease in blood pressure
6. Cold, moist skin
7. 15 ml/hr urine output

Cardiogenic Shock

Cardiogenic shock refers to a shock response generated when the heart's ability to pump blood becomes impaired, decreasing cardiac output. If peripheral vascular resistance is not adequate to compensate for a decrease in tissue perfusion, shock may develop. Cardiogenic shock can be caused by dysfunction of the left ventricle, right ventricle, or both. It may result from primary ventricular ischemia, structural problems, or dysrhythmias. Box 19-2 lists etiologic factors in cardiogenic shock.

The most common cause of cardiogenic shock is a loss of contractile elements of the myocardial muscle owing to ischemia. This usually results from ischemia related to acute myocardial infarction (AMI). Cardiogenic shock develops when 40% or more of the functional myocardium has been damaged by either a massive AMI or several smaller AMIs. Massive damage usually occurs in the anterior wall of the left ventricle.

Structural problems may cause cardiogenic shock if forward motion of blood is disrupted. Causes include papillary muscle rupture and septal rupture. Regurgitant or stenotic valve lesions also interrupt forward flow of blood through the heart and may result in abrupt onset of congestive heart failure progressing to shock.

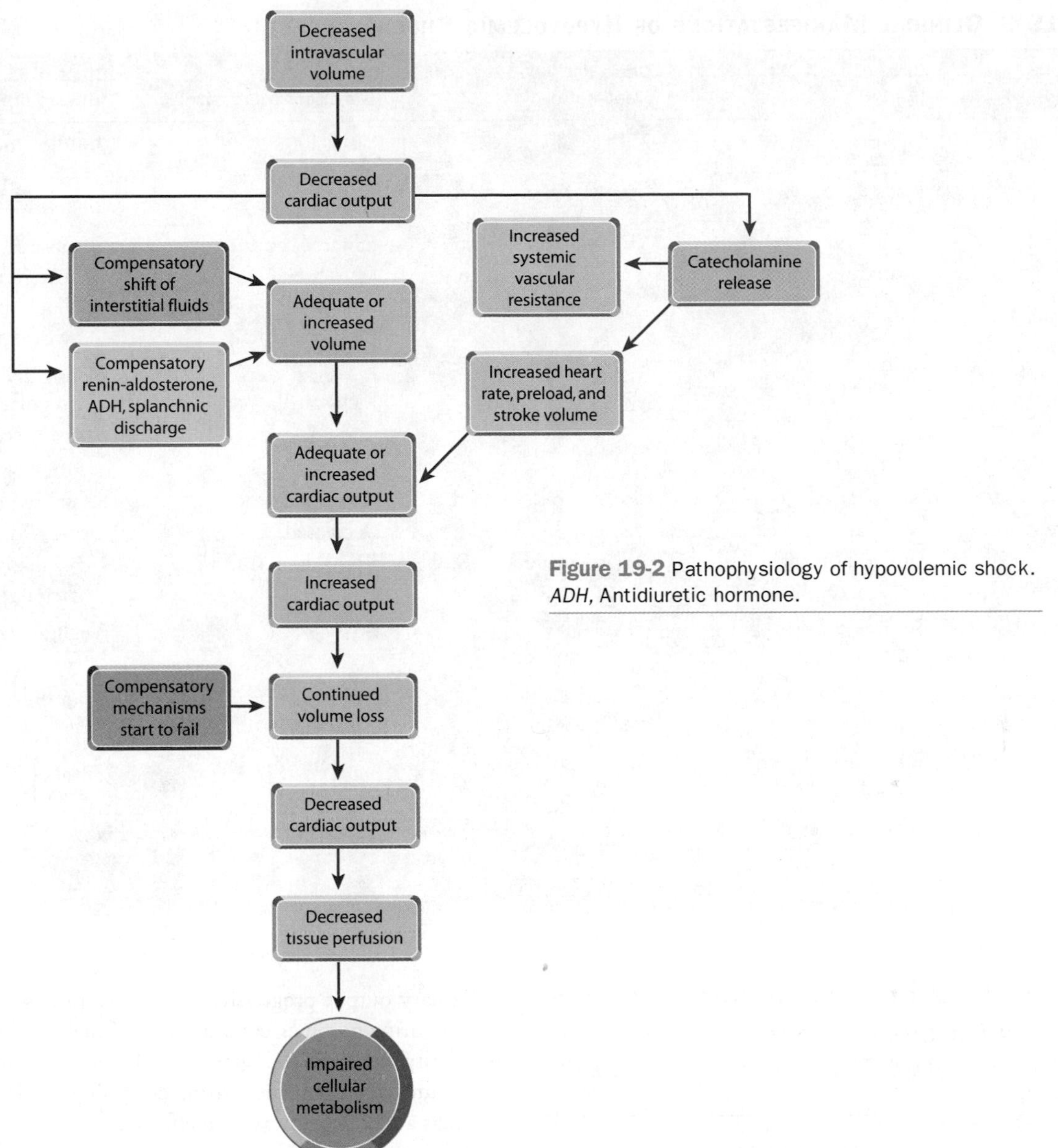

Figure 19-2 Pathophysiology of hypovolemic shock. *ADH*, Antidiuretic hormone.

Dysrhythmias affecting heart rate can disrupt pump function and cause cardiogenic shock. Bradydysrhythmias can lower cardiac output, especially in patients unable to compensate by increasing stroke volume. Conversely, in tachydysrhythmias, as the heart rate increases, diastolic filling time decreases, reducing stroke volume because the filling time is too short.

When the left ventricle is unable to pump blood forward adequately, three primary problems result. First, the amount of blood ejected from the ventricle with each heartbeat (stroke volume) decreases. This subsequently decreases cardiac output, blood pressure, and tissue perfusion. Second, as blood pressure falls, coronary artery perfusion decreases, which in turn decreases myocardial muscle perfusion. The increased workload and oxygen demand of the myocardium exacerbates myocardial ischemia and predisposes the patient to further muscle damage, creating a vicious cycle. Third, the amount of blood remaining in the left ventricle at the end of systole increases. If the primary problem involves the left ventricle, this increased end-systolic volume eventually leads to increased ventricular filling pressure. Increased filling pressures are transmitted back to the left atrium and then to the pulmonary circulation. This increases pulmonary vascular pressure, causing fluid to move into the interstitial space and alveolar spaces, resulting in pulmonary congestion, hypoxia, and deteriorating blood gases. Increased pulmonary pressures are eventually reflected backward to the right ventricle, causing both left and right ventricular failure. As the ventricular pressures remain elevated, systemic manifestations of right-sided heart failure become evident (Figure 19-3).

Compensatory mechanisms initially may be able to maintain blood pressure and adequate tissue perfusion to vital organs. However, as the left ventricle fails to effectively pump blood out to the circulatory system, compensatory mechanisms begin to fail and clinical manifestations develop. The patient shows a decline in sensorium; systolic blood pressure falls to less than 90 mm Hg; and diastolic pressure increases, narrowing the pulse pressure. Heart rate increases to more than 100 beats/min. A weak, thready pulse develops, and heart sounds reveal a diminished S1 and S2

TABLE 19-3 CLINICAL MANIFESTATIONS OF HYPOVOLEMIC SHOCK

Parameter (for 70 kg man)	Class I (Early)	Class II (Moderate)	Class III (Major or Progressive)	Class IV (Severe or Profound)
Approximate blood volume loss (ml)	Up to 750	750-1500	1500-2000	2000 or more
Blood volume loss (%)	Up to 15%	15%-30%	30%-40%	40% or more
Neurologic and behavioral status	Slightly anxious or anxious	Mildly anxious, restless; muscle fatigue and weakness evident	Agitated, confused, progressive decrease in activity; progressive thirst evident	Stuporous, lethargic, unresponsive; dilated pupils may be evident
Heart rate (beats/min)	<100	>100 Mild tachycardia	>120 Tachycardia	140 or higher; irregular pulse; decreased pulse, amplitude
Blood pressure	Normal	Normal to decreased	Decreased	Severe hypotension
Pulse pressure	Normal to increased	Decreased	Decreased	Decreased
Respirations (breaths/min)	14-20, normal	20-30, normal	30-40, hyperpnea	>35, shallow, irregular
Urinary output (ml/hr)	30 or more	20-30	5-15	Negligible
Capillary refill (blanch test)	Normal	Slight delay	Defined delay	No refilling observed
Skin	Pale, flushed, slightly cool	Slightly cold, pale	Cold and moist	Cold, cyanotic, mottled

From McQuillian KA, Wiles CE: Initial management of traumatic shock. In Cardona DV et al: *Trauma nursing from resuscitation through rehabilitation,* Philadelphia, 1988, Saunders.

Box 19-2 Etiologic Factors in Cardiogenic Shock

Ventricular Ischemia

Myocardial infarction
Open heart surgery
Cardiac arrest

Structural Problems

Valvular dysfunction
Septal rupture
Papillary muscle rupture
Ventricular aneurysm
Cardiomyopathies
Intracardiac tumors

Dysrhythmias

Bradydysrhythmias
Tachydysrhythmias

caused by decreased contractility. A summation gallop may be audible over the left apex from increased pressure in the left ventricle and decreased compliance. Skin becomes pale, cool, and moist from peripheral vasoconstriction. A variety of dysrhythmias may occur, depending on the underlying problem.

Urinary output progressively decreases to less than 30 ml/hr, and the urine becomes concentrated. Urinalysis shows increased osmolarity and specific gravity and decreased urine sodium. Blood urea nitrogen and serum creatinine levels rise as waste products are no longer excreted effectively.

Respiratory rate and depth increase in an attempt to improve oxygenation. Arterial blood gases initially demonstrate respiratory alkalosis, but this progresses quickly to respiratory and metabolic acidosis with hypoxemia from alveolar hypoventilation. Auscultation of the lungs reveals crackles and wheezes.

Distributive Shock

Distributive shock results from inadequate vascular tone that leads to massive vasodilation. Although vascular volume remains normal during distributive shock and the heart pumps blood adequately, the size of the vascular space increases. The result is a maldistribution of blood within the circulatory system. This disproportion between blood volume and capillary vessel size effectively decreases blood pressure. Distributive shock is frequently subdivided into three types: septic, neurogenic, and anaphylactic.

Septic Shock. Septic shock is a multisystem response to infection in which, unlike other forms of shock, the fall in blood pressure and resultant insufficient perfusion of vital organs does not respond to fluid administration. The incidence of severe sep-

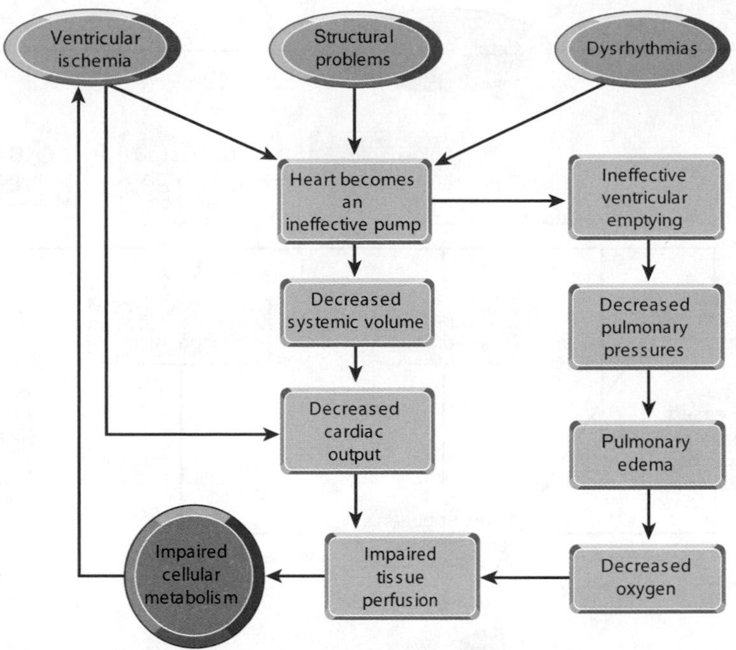

Figure 19-3 Pathophysiology of cardiogenic shock.

sis appears to be on the rise due to the aging population, increasing resistance to antibiotics among pathogens, and increasing numbers of immunocompromised patients.[4] Each year severe sepsis affects an estimated 750,000 people in the United States. This rate is expected to rise to 1 million cases a year by 2010 as the population ages. The incidence rate of sepsis has increased 91.3% over the last 10 years. It is the leading cause of death in intensive care units (noncardiac units). About one third of those affected will die of septic shock.[8]

Septic shock generally occurs in immunocompromised patients, infants, older adults, or patients undergoing procedures with risk of significant bacterial contamination. Box 19-3 lists microorganisms implicated in sepsis and septic shock. The initial infection produces an overwhelming systemic inflammatory response triggered by release of endotoxins, formyl peptides, exotoxins, and proteases from gram-negative organisms; or exotoxins, enterotoxins, hemolysins, peptidoglycans, and lipoteichoic acid from gram-positive organisms. These substances exert a harmful effect on the vascular, coagulation, and immune systems. Bacterial toxins stimulate release of macrophage-derived cytokines that intensify the inflammatory response. Nitric oxide is released from endothelial cells, vascular smooth muscle cells, and macrophages and is postulated to be a major mediator of vasodilation, hypotension, and myocardial depression seen in septic shock. The immune system becomes so overwhelmed that the system designed initially to protect the body now works against it. The antiinflammatory substances released to modulate the inflammatory response produce a period of immune depression after the initial shock episode, placing the patient at an additional risk of nosocomial infection and death.[6]

Four primary pathophysiologic changes occur in septic shock: myocardial depression, massive vasodilation, maldistribution of the intravascular volume, and formation of microemboli. Myocardial depression occurs when the ventricular force of contraction decreases from biochemical mediators, including myocardial depressant factor, endotoxins, tumor necrosis factor, endorphins, complement products, and leukotrienes. Massive vasodilation and increased capillary permeability reduce the amount of blood returning to the heart (decreased preload). Afterload decreases as well from massive vasodilation that occurs secondary to the release of such mediators as bradykinin, endorphins, complement products, histamine, and prostaglandins. Although plasma volume is normal in the early phases of septic shock, it becomes maldistributed as shock progresses because of increased capillary permeability, selective vasoconstriction, and vascular occlusion. Increased capillary permeability allows protein and fluid to shift to the interstitial and intracellular compartments. However, not all vascular beds vasodilate. Stimulation of the sympathetic nervous system and prostaglandin and other biochemical mediators cause selective vasoconstriction in the pulmonary, renal, and splanchnic circulations.

Box 19-3 Causative Microorganisms Implicated in Septic Shock

- Gram-negative bacteria
  - —*Bacteroides* organisms
  - —*Escherichia coli*
  - —*Enterobacter* organisms
  - —*Klebsiella pneumoniae*
  - —*Pseudomonas aeruginosa*
  - —*Serratia marcescens*
  - —*Haemophilus influenzae*
- Gram-positive bacteria
  - —*Staphylococcus aureus*
  - —*Staphylococcus epidermidis*
  - —*Streptococcus pneumoniae*
  - —*Clostridium* organisms
- Fungi
- Protozoa
- Parasites
- Rickettsiae
- *Spirochaeta* organisms
- Viruses

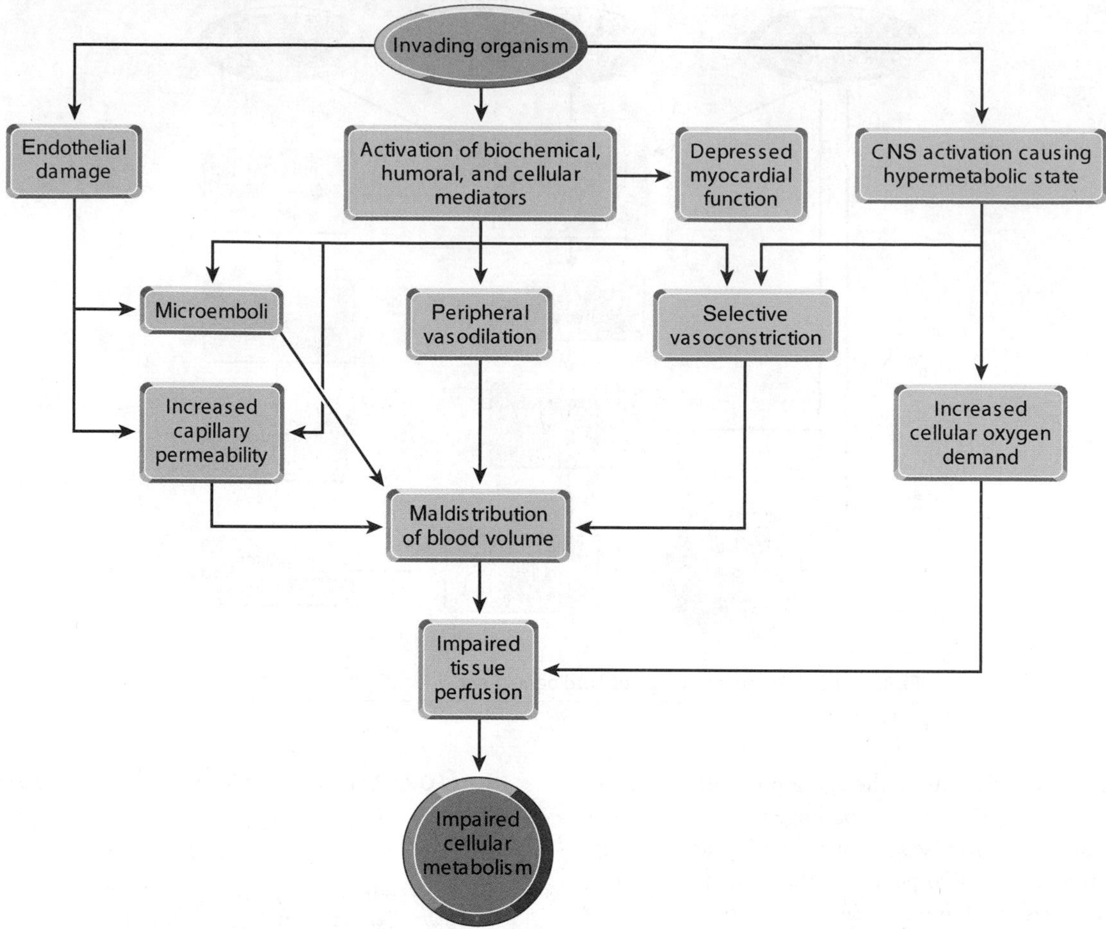

Figure 19-4 Pathophysiology of septic shock. *CNS*, Central nervous system.

Activation of the clotting system and aggregation of neutrophils cause formation of microemboli that become lodged in the small blood vessels, causing some vascular beds to receive more blood than they need, whereas others receive too little. This maldistribution of blood leads to hypoxia and a lack of nutritional support to some areas, causing cellular dysfunction that ultimately ends in cell death (Figure 19-4).

The early stage of septic shock is characterized by a hyperdynamic or warm phase as compensatory mechanisms are activated (Table 19-4). During this phase, massive vasodilation occurs in venous and arterial beds, causing a decrease in systemic vascular resistance. Venous dilation decreases venous return to the heart and decreases preload. Dilation of the arterial beds decreases afterload. The patient's blood pressure declines in response to reduced preload and afterload. The vasodilation leads to decreased blood pressure; widened pulse pressure; and warm, flushed skin. The heart rate increases to compensate for the hypotension, increased metabolic acidosis, sympathetic nervous system stimulation, and adrenal stimulation. A ventilation/perfusion mismatch occurs in the lungs as a result of pulmonary vasoconstriction. The respiratory rate increases to compensate for the hypoxemia. Crackles develop as increased pulmonary capillary membrane permeability leads to pulmonary edema. Arterial blood gas values reveal respiratory alkalosis, metabolic acidosis, and hypoxemia. Level of consciousness is altered, with the patient becoming disoriented, confused, combative, or lethargic. The patient's temperature rises in response to the pyrogens released from invading microorganisms.

As septic shock progresses, the patient's condition deteriorates to a hypodynamic phase, with a fall in cardiac output and profound hypotension. This phase results from ventricular failure caused by myocardial hypoxemia, release of myocardial depressant factor, and acidosis, producing an increase in afterload. Tachycardia occurs as the body attempts to compensate for the decline in cardiac output and hypotension. Peripheral vasoconstriction causes increased systemic vascular resistance to compensate for the falling blood pressure. The patient's skin now is pale, cold, and clammy.

Neurogenic Shock. **Neurogenic shock** is characterized by massive vasodilation from loss or suppression of sympathetic tone. It is a temporary condition associated with injury or disease of the upper spinal cord or brainstem or with administration of general or spinal anesthesia. Neurogenic shock can be caused by any condition that interrupts sympathetic nerve impulse transmission or blocks sympathetic outflow from the vasomotor center in the brain. Interruption of sympathetic activity occurs with trauma to the spinal cord or medulla, conditions that disrupt the supply of oxygen to the medulla, or conditions that deprive the medulla of glucose (such as an insulin reaction). Other causes of neurogenic shock include high-level spinal anesthesia, ganglionic- and adrenergic-blocking

TABLE 19-4 CLINICAL MANIFESTATIONS OF SEPTIC SHOCK

	Hyperdynamic Phase	Hypodynamic Phase
Cardiac output and cardiac index	Increased	Decreased
Systemic vascular resistance	Decreased	Increased
Right atrial pressure	Decreased	Increased
Pulmonary capillary wedge pressure	Decreased	Increased
Heart rate	Increased	Increased
Respiratory rate	Increased	Decreased
Blood pressure	Decreased	Decreased
Pulse pressure	Wide	Narrow
Skin	Warm, pink, flushed	Cool, pale, clammy
Level of consciousness	Decreased	No response to painful stimuli
Urinary output	Decreased	Anuria
Temperature	Increased	Increased or decreased

drugs, severe emotional stress, pain, depressive drugs, and drug overdoses.

The onset of neurogenic shock may occur within minutes of the injury, and the condition may last for days, weeks, or months depending on the precipitating cause. Lack of sympathetic tone leaves a dominant parasympathetic nervous system, which results in massive vasodilation. Neurogenic shock creates a relative hypovolemia in which the blood volume is distributed inappropriately. Vasodilation decreases venous return and cardiac output, resulting in hypotension. Inhibition of the baroreceptor response results in the loss of compensatory reflex tachycardia so that the heart rate cannot increase in response to the reduction in blood pressure. Loss of vasomotor tone in cutaneous blood vessels disrupts thermoregulation, so the patient must depend on the environment for temperature regulation (Figure 19-5).

Anaphylactic Shock. **Anaphylactic shock** (also referred to as *anaphylaxis*) is a sudden, life-threatening hypersensitivity reaction to an antigen. It is characterized by massive vasodilation and increased capillary permeability. Unless treatment begins immediately, the patient quickly develops shock.

Anaphylactic reactions can be either immunoglobulin E (IgE)-mediated or non-IgE-mediated responses. In IgE-mediated anaphylaxis, IgE is produced after the first exposure to an antigen. It binds to the surface of mast cells and basophils. During subsequent exposures, the antigen binds to and cross-links antigen-specific IgE molecules on the surface of tissue mast cells, initiating mast cell degranulation and release of vasoactive, chemotactic, and enzymatic mediators, including histamine, eosinophil chemotactic factor of anaphylaxis, neutrophil chemotactic factor of anaphylaxis, proteinases, heparin, serotonin, leukotrienes, prostaglandins, and platelet-activating factor.[7]

These chemical mediators cause vasodilation, increased capillary membrane permeability, bronchoconstriction, and coronary capillary permeability. Shock develops as a consequence of hypotension from profound vasodilation and low cardiac output. Increased capillary permeability and peripheral pooling of blood cause the relative fluid volume deficit. As a result of the rapid and profound development of shock, normal compensatory mechanisms are unable to reverse or retard it. Death can result because of severe hypoxemia secondary to bronchoconstriction or cardiovascular collapse (Figure 19-6).

Non-IgE-mediated anaphylactic reactions occur as a result of direct activation of mast cells to release biochemical mediators and are not due to IgE antibody production. This type of reaction, called an *anaphylactoid reaction*, can occur with the first exposure to an antigen.

Early recognition of anaphylaxis is crucial because, within minutes, it can progress to shock, respiratory arrest, and cardiovascular collapse. The earliest signs of systemic anaphylaxis include feelings of anxiety and uneasiness, flushing, diaphoresis, sneezing, and weakness. Nausea, dizziness, itching, and sometimes edema quickly follow these; and severe hypotension from vasodilation and increased capillary permeability rapidly develop.

ARE You READY?

The nurse is monitoring a patient in the early (hyperdynamic) stage of septic shock. Which of the following clinical manifestations would indicate a worsening of the patient's condition?

1. Increased cardiac output
2. Increased systemic vascular resistance
3. Decreased pulmonary capillary wedge pressure
4. Decreased right atrial pressure

Pathophysiology

The clinical syndrome of shock results from sustained, inadequate tissue perfusion leading to alterations in tissue metabolism and function at the cellular and organ system level. Untreated, the patient progresses through a continuum of shock stages manifested by specific signs and symptoms that vary according to the patient's individual response and ability to compensate.

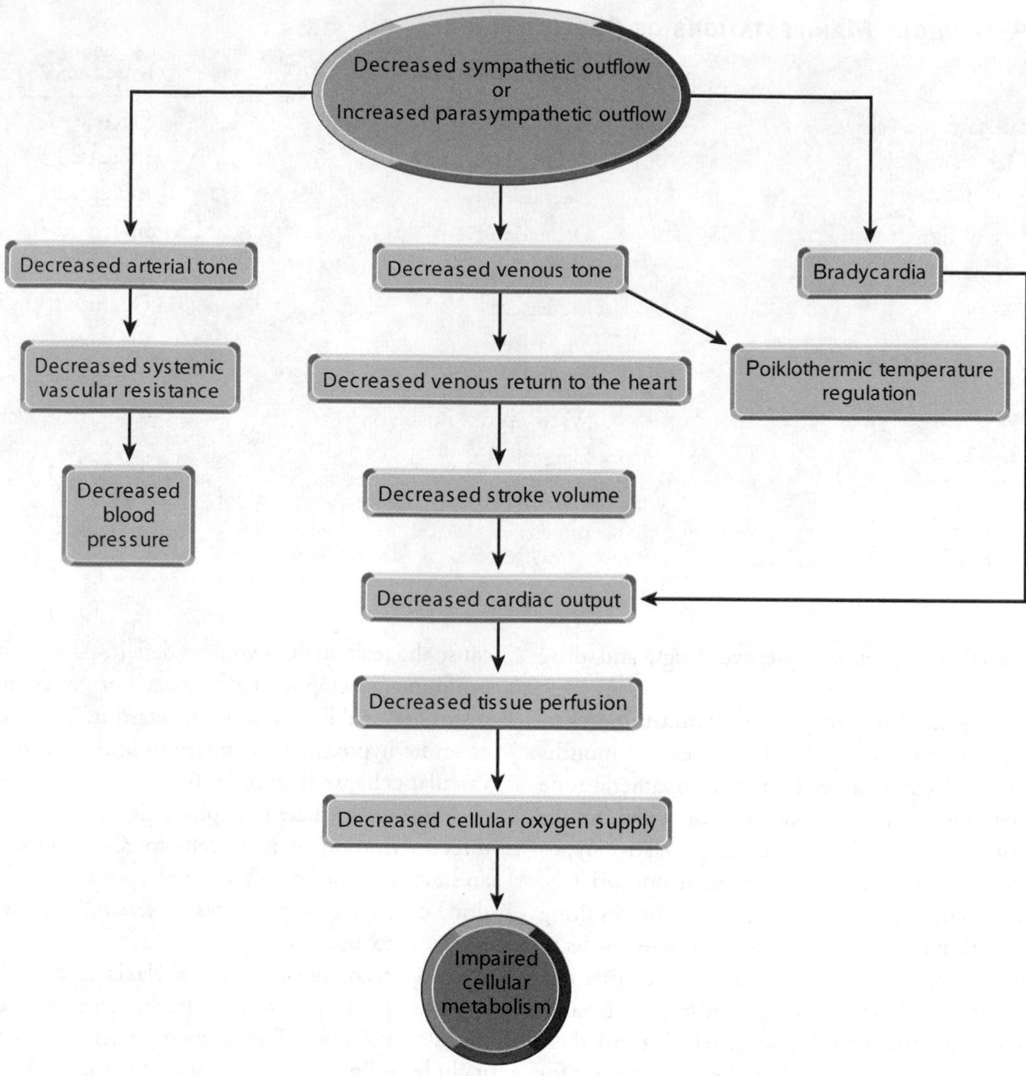

Figure 19-5 Pathophysiology of neurogenic shock.

Shock stages are compensatory, progressive, and refractory (or irreversible). Table 19-5 summarizes manifestations of the shock stages.

Compensatory Stage

The **compensatory stage** of shock is characterized by an initial decrease in cardiac output and tissue perfusion. The resulting reduction in delivery of oxygen and nutrients at the cellular level decreases aerobic metabolism and increases anaerobic metabolism, resulting in the production of lactic acid. Compensatory mechanisms begin and, at least initially, maintain adequate cardiac output and tissue perfusion. No clinical manifestations are evident during this early stage of shock.

Initial compensatory mechanisms are complex, widespread, and aimed largely at maintaining blood pressure within a low normal to normal range with adequate perfusion to vital organs. The sympathetic nervous system is quickly activated when arterial blood pressure falls. Pressoreceptors in the arterial walls of the aorta and carotid sinuses sense a decrease in pressure and transmit signals to the vasomotor center in the medulla. The autonomic nervous system signals sympathetic nerve fibers throughout the body to discharge norepinephrine. This release causes arterioles to constrict, which assists in increasing arterial pressure. The adrenal medulla is stimulated to release the catecholamines epinephrine and norepinephrine into the bloodstream. Stimulation of beta$_1$-adrenergic receptors in the heart increases the rate and force of contraction. Stimulation of beta$_2$-adrenergic receptors causes coronary artery vasodilation and increased blood flow to the myocardium to meet the heart's increased oxygen demand. Alpha-adrenergic receptor stimulation causes vasoconstriction. This results in blood being shunted away from organs, including skeletal muscles, fat, and skin. Arterioles in vital organs, such as the heart and brain, remain open and continue to receive blood flow.

Chemoreceptors in the aorta and carotid arteries respond to decreased arterial oxygen tension by sending signals to the respiratory center in the brain. The respiratory center responds by

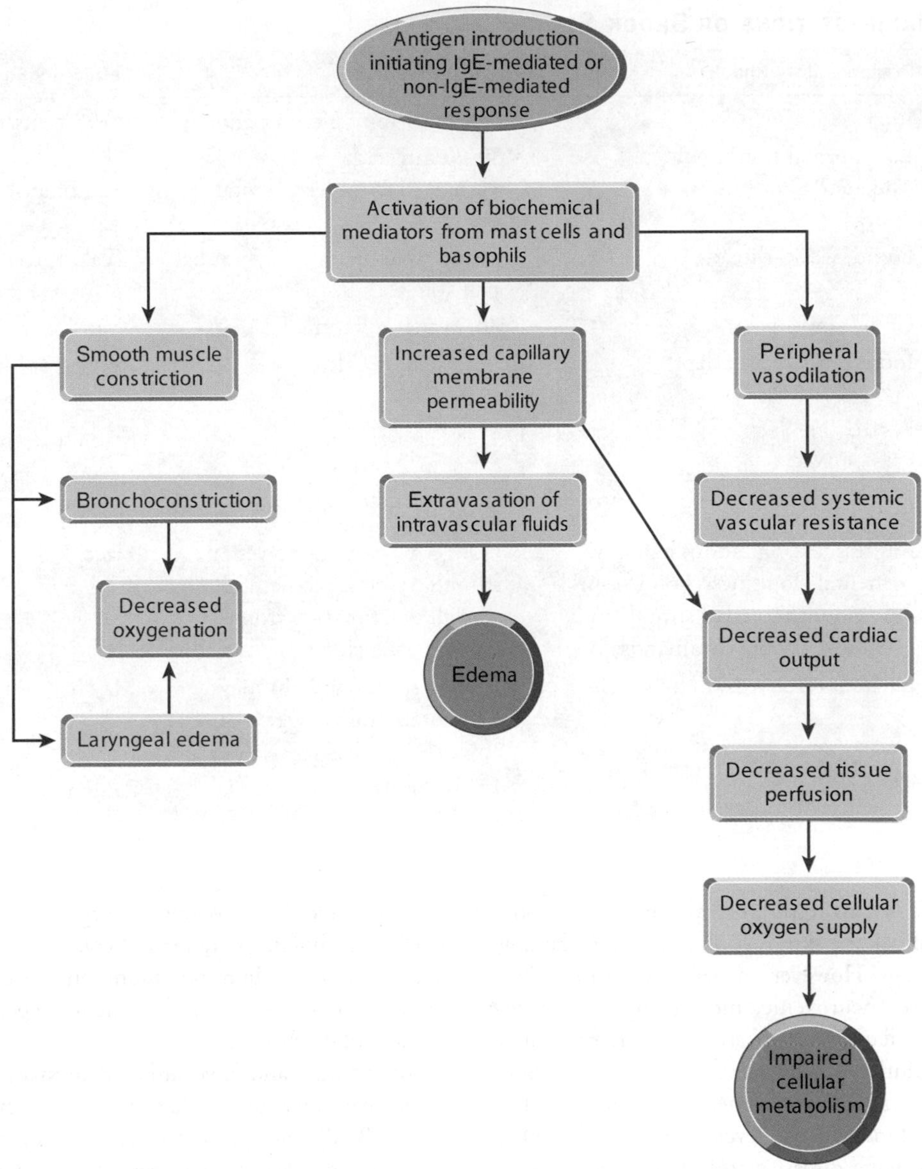

Figure 19-6 Pathophysiology of anaphylactic shock.

increasing the rate and depth of respirations, which results in a respiratory alkalosis.

Decreased cardiac output and vasoconstriction in the kidneys result in decreased renal perfusion. Resultant renal ischemia stimulates the release of renin by the juxtaglomerular apparatus. Circulating renin reacts with angiotensinogen produced in the liver, resulting in production of angiotensin I. A converting enzyme in the lungs converts angiotensin I to angiotensin II. Angiotensin II, a potent vasoconstrictor, helps increase blood pressure and venous return. It also stimulates release of aldosterone from the adrenal cortex, causing reabsorption of sodium and water and increased venous return to the heart. Reduced renal perfusion results in oliguria, with urinary output falling below 0.5 ml/kg/hr. Further reductions in cardiac output result in additional decreases in urinary output.

Catecholamine stimulation also causes contraction of the radial muscle of the iris, causing pupillary dilation. Vasoconstriction of the vessels in the skin and stimulation of the sweat glands cause the skin to be cool, pale, and moist. Decreased tissue perfusion in the liver stimulates breakdown of glycogen stores to increase availability of glucose for energy production. This results in increased blood glucose levels. The body's cells (with the exception of the liver, kidneys, and muscles) have limited stores of glycogen.

How long the body can maintain tissue perfusion and homeostasis depends on the patient's general health and reserves. Compensatory mechanisms may be able to maintain arterial blood pressure and tissue perfusion only briefly. If the underlying cause of shock is not managed, the patient progresses to the next stage of shock.

Many of the clinical manifestations of compensated shock result from an excess of catecholamines and other vasoconstricting hormones and from increased sympathetic neural activity to the heart and vasculature. Sinus tachycardia is present; with heart rates exceeding 100 beats/min. Respirations become deep and

TABLE 19-5 MANIFESTATIONS OF SHOCK STAGES

Parameter	Compensatory Shock	Progressive Shock	Refractory Shock
Heart rate	Increased	>150 beats/min; often irregular	>150 beats/min; irregular
Blood pressure	Low normal to normal Adequate to perfuse vital organs	<80-90 mm Hg No longer able to perfuse vital organs	<80 mm Hg; may not be audible
Arterial pulses	Rapid, weak, thready	Thready, weak, rapid; may not be palpable	Weak, thready, or nonpalpable
Skin	Cool, moist, pale	Cold, cyanotic, mottled	Cyanotic, mottled
Respirations	Increased rate and depth	Rapid, shallow, rales	Respiratory failure
Arterial blood gases			
PaO_2	Decreased	Decreased	Severely decreased
$PaCO_2$	Decreased	Increased	Increased
pH	Increased	Decreased	Severely decreased
Level of consciousness	Restlessness, agitation, lethargy, mental cloudiness, confusion; responds to verbal stimuli and follows simple commands	No longer responding to verbal stimuli; response to painful stimuli deteriorating from flexion, extension to flaccid	Flaccid
Pupils	Dilated; reactive to light	Dilated; response to light may deteriorate from sluggish to absent	May be fixed, dilated
Urinary output	<0.5 ml/kg/hr	<0.5 ml/kg/hr	Anuria or negligible

rapid. Blood gas analysis reveals respiratory alkalosis and hypoxemia. In most forms of shock the skin is cool, moist, and clammy, especially in the extremities. However, in patients with distributive forms of shock (septic, neurogenic, and anaphylactic), inappropriate peripheral vasodilation occurs and the extremities may remain warm. Urine volume is reduced. An altered sensorium may be present, characterized by restlessness and agitation. The pupils are dilated, and blood glucose levels increase. The nurse must be aware that underlying disease states, such as diabetes, or the effects of such drugs as beta-blockers or vasodilators may mask the compensatory responses of tachycardia and vasoconstriction.

Progressive Stage

As shock progresses, compensatory mechanisms can no longer make up for decreased cardiac output and fail to maintain blood pressure sufficient to perfuse vital organs. Physiologic changes that initially helped shunt blood to vital organs become ineffective, and organs begin to malfunction. The primary cause of the shock disorder must be corrected quickly, or severe hypoperfusion of organs will lead to multisystem organ failure.

As cellular metabolism shifts from aerobic to anaerobic as a result of prolonged cellular hypoxia, production of adenosine triphosphate decreases, reducing metabolic cellular processes. The net result is decreased oxygen consumption. Glycolysis results in conversion of pyruvate to lactate. Increased lactate levels cause metabolic acidemia and promote cardiac dysrhythmias. The decreased adenosine triphosphate availability also causes the sodium-potassium pump to malfunction. Active transport of sodium and potassium across the cell membrane diminishes. Sodium ions accumulate inside the cell, causing intracellular swelling. As organelles inside the cell begin to swell, their function deteriorates. Potassium collects outside the cell. Changes in the sodium-potassium ion concentration cause the resting membrane potential to become more positive, leading to development of dysrhythmias.

Bradykinin and myocardial depressant factor are important vasoactive polypeptides that appear to play a significant role in shock. Bradykinin produces vasodilation, increased capillary permeability, smooth muscle relaxation, and infiltration of an area with leukocytes. Bradykinin is thought to have a major impact in later stages of shock and may be a factor in the development of associated pulmonary insufficiency. Myocardial depressant factor is released in response to splanchnic ischemia and appears to depress cardiac muscle contraction, further contributing to a decreased cardiac output.

Metabolic acidosis worsens and causes precapillary sphincters to relax. Postcapillary vasoconstriction continues, creating increased resistance and decreased capillary flow rates. Capillary hydrostatic pressure increases, causing fluid to move out of the capillary beds into the interstitial space. Interstitial edema further decreases blood return to the heart. As capillary flow rates decrease, microemboli can form, placing the patient at risk of disseminated intravascular coagulation.

As pulmonary capillary bed hypoperfusion persists, alveolar cells become ischemic and unable to produce surfactant. This causes alveoli to collapse, producing massive microatelectasis and reduced pulmonary compliance. Ischemia also increases pulmonary capillary permeability, allowing fluid to leave pulmonary capillaries, producing interstitial and intraalveolar edema. Pulmonary edema drastically reduces diffusion of oxygen and intensifies hypoxemia. Respiratory insufficiency and failure commonly occur with persistent shock states.

Prolonged kidney hypoperfusion potentiates development of acute tubular necrosis, progressing to renal insufficiency and acute renal failure. Toxic waste products cannot be excreted, resulting in an increase in blood urea nitrogen and serum creatinine levels.

Prolonged hypoperfusion of the liver impairs the organ's ability to perform important functions, including metabolism of drugs and hormones and conjugation of bilirubin. As a result, bilirubin accumulates in the blood and causes jaundice. The liver loses its ability to metabolize waste products such as ammonia and lactic acid. As cellular damage occurs and cellular death approaches, intracellular enzymes are released into the blood and can be observed as increases in serum glutamicoxaloacetic transaminase, serum glutamicpyruvic transaminase, and lactic dehydrogenase. Pancreatic hypoperfusion and ischemia result in release of pancreatic enzymes amylase and lipase.

Clinical manifestations associated with the **progressive stage** of shock include decreased blood pressure with a narrow pulse pressure, decreased heart rate, decreased urine production, increased urine specific gravity, decreased creatinine clearance, increased serum creatinine, and increased blood urea nitrogen. Peripheral edema develops from altered capillary fluid dynamics.

Decreased cerebral blood flow causes further decreases in the level of consciousness. As the persistent hypoperfusion state continues, more stimulation is required to elicit a response from the patient. Response to painful stimuli progressively decreases until the patient becomes flaccid (no response to painful stimuli).

Respiratory rate increases and the patient develops audible crackles as a result of interstitial pulmonary edema. Arterial blood gases show metabolic and respiratory acidosis with hypoxemia.

Refractory Stage

The irreversible or **refractory stage** is the final stage of shock. The body becomes refractory to all therapeutic measures attempted. Multiple organ failure develops and produces signs and symptoms of cardiac, respiratory, neurologic, hepatic, gastrointestinal, pancreatic, and hematologic failure. Intractable circulatory failure develops as blood pressure and heart rate continue to decrease. The shock state is so profound and the degree of cellular destruction so severe that death is imminent.

Collaborative Care Management

Therapeutic management of the patient in shock is determined by the stage of shock and the patient's signs and symptoms. Collaborative care in the management of patients in shock is essential to improve their chances of survival. Therapy to maintain tissue perfusion in the shock patient may be simple, involving only volume replacement; or complex, involving volume replacement, pharmacologic manipulation, and mechanical support. The nurse's role is vital in identifying subtle parameters of inadequate perfusion and the effectiveness of medical interventions. The nurse plans, implements, and evaluates appropriate nursing interventions to limit effects of inadequate perfusion while concurrently collaborating with the physician and other health care professionals to implement medical therapies to reverse the shock state.

Patient Positioning

Traditionally the patient in shock has been placed in Trendelenburg's position. However, this position should be avoided if possible because it causes fluid to rapidly shift to the upper thorax, activating baroreceptors in the aortic arch and carotid arteries. Activation of these receptors sends misleading signals that blood pressure is elevated, shutting off the body's sympathetic nervous system response to the shock state. Instead, placing the patient in a supine position with the legs slightly elevated above the level of the heart promotes venous return from the legs to the heart and improves cardiac output and organ perfusion. If this type of position impairs the patient's ventilation, elevation of the patient's head 30 to 45 degrees should aid breathing.

Fluid Therapy

Fluid resuscitation has been a mainstay in the management of patients in hypovolemic shock. Benefits of fluid administration include increased intravascular volume, increased venous return to the heart (preload), improved cardiac contractility, and increased cardiac output. The goal of fluid therapy is to improve tissue perfusion. The nurse should collaborate with the physician regarding the administration of fluid and accurately monitor the patient's intake, output, and daily weights. Nursing intervention also includes minimizing fluid loss by limiting blood sampling and applying pressure to bleeding sites.

Patients in severe hypovolemic shock may require immediate and rapid volume replacement. A minimum of two large-bore intravenous catheters (no. 14 or 16) should be inserted into the patient to provide routes for immediate and rapid administration of large volumes of fluids and medications. The large peripheral veins in the antecubital fossa are recommended. Severe vasoconstriction and venous collapse may require the physician to perform a venous cutdown for vascular access. A multilumen central venous catheter or pulmonary artery catheter can also be used to administer large fluid volumes and to measure hemodynamic status. In patients not responding to fluid infusion or those with underlying cardiac or renal disease, the insertion of a pulmonary artery catheter should be considered.

The major goals in treating hypovolemic shock are to find and aggressively control the source of blood loss and to reverse that loss with administration of appropriate fluids to restore tissue perfusion. At times, fluid replacement is the only therapy needed in hypovolemic shock. Distributive and septic shock are accompanied by hypovolemia because fluid is leaking out of the capillaries and because the vascular space has increased with vasodilation. Patients in cardiogenic shock may also require fluid therapy, although many may require fluid restriction or removal of fluid. The nurse must closely monitor fluid administration in these patients. Before institution of fluid therapy, a pulmonary artery catheter is inserted, and the pulmonary end-diastolic pressure is measured. If the pressure is less than 18 mm Hg and the cardiac index is less than 2.2 L/min, volume replacement should be given.

Fluid Challenge. Once intravenous access has been established, the nurse infuses an intravenous fluid challenge of 200 ml to 2 L of crystalloid solution to see if fluid administration improves circulation and therefore oxygen delivery. Nursing responsibilities include obtaining baseline hemodynamic measurements, administering the fluid challenge, and assessing the patient response. The nurse should carefully monitor the patient's hemodynamic status during such fluid challenges, especially in patients suspected of having impaired left ventricular function. Patient response to this initial bolus of fluid determines further treatment with additional fluids or other therapeutic modalities.

Fluid Selection. The selection of resuscitation fluid remains controversial. The physician's choice of fluid or fluids is determined by the cause of the volume deficit and the patient's clinical status. The goal of fluid therapy is to return laboratory and hemodynamic values to the patient's normal baseline levels. The nurse should carefully monitor the patient's response to fluid therapy. Fluids are generally classified as either crystalloid or colloid solutions (Table 19-6).

Crystalloids are inexpensive and readily available solutions. These fluids move freely from the intravascular space into the tissues. Lactated Ringer's solution closely resembles plasma and is commonly used to expand intravascular volume; the amount infused is usually 3 ml for each 1 ml of blood loss. If large volumes of crystalloids are required, the potential exists for hemodilution of red blood cells (RBCs) and plasma proteins. Hemodilution of RBCs may impair delivery of oxygen to tissues. Hemodilution of plasma proteins decreases colloidal osmotic pressure and places the patient at risk for pulmonary edema.

Colloids contain proteins that increase osmotic pressure and remain in the vascular system longer than crystalloids. The improved osmotic pressure holds and attracts fluid into vascular compartment. The patient may require smaller volumes of colloids infused.

Current research indicates that colloids are effective in expanding the circulation, but no evidence exists that this improves the outcome of patients in shock. Additionally, colloids did not reduce the risk of death when compared with crystalloids in patients with trauma, with burns, and after surgery.[3] Fluid resuscitation with colloid solutions is considerably more expensive than with crystalloids and therefore should be used only if their effect can be shown to be clearly superior (see Evidence-Based Practice box).

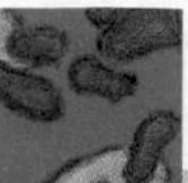

EVIDENCE-BASED PRACTICE

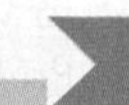

Topic Question: Are colloids or crystalloids more effective for fluid resuscitation in critically ill patients?

Evidence Base: The researchers used a meta-analysis to synthesize evidence of the effects on mortality from 36 randomized or quasirandomized controlled trials comparing colloid and crystalloid fluid resuscitation in critically ill patients. The studies' participants were placed in treatment groups (receiving colloids of dextran 70, hydroxyethyl starches, modified gelatins, albumin, or plasma protein fraction) or a control group (receiving either isotonic or hypertonic crystalloids). All participants were adults who were critically ill as a result of conditions such as trauma, burns, or surgery, or who had other critical conditions such as complications of sepsis.

Findings: Results of albumin or plasma protein fraction (18 trials with a total of 641 patients) demonstrated a pooled relative risk factor (RRF) of 1.34; hydroxyethyl starch (7 trials with a total of 197 patients) a RRF of 1.16; modified gelatin (4 trials with 95 patients) a RRF of 0.50; dextran (8 trials with 668 patients) a RRF of 1.24; and dextran in hypertonic crystalloid with isotonic crystalloid (8 trials with 1283 patients) an RRF of 0.88.

Conclusions: The researchers concluded there was no evidence that resuscitation with colloids reduces risk of death compared with crystalloids in patients with trauma, with burns, and after surgery.

Alderson P et al: *Colloids versus crystalloids for fluid resuscitation in critically ill patients,* Cochrane Review. In *Cochrane Library*, Issue 2, 2001, Chichester, UK, John Wiley & Sons, accessed Aug 2004 from website: www.cochrane.org.

Blood Administration. Whole blood, packed RBCs, washed RBCs, fresh frozen plasma, and platelets are administered for the treatment of major blood loss. Patients are typed and crossmatched to identify their blood type, to determine presence of Rh factor, and to ensure compatibility with the donor blood to prevent blood transfusion reactions. In extreme emergencies the patient may be transfused with O-negative blood (universal donor blood type).

Blood and blood products are given until the hemoglobin is 10 g/dl or greater. Packed RBCs increase blood volume and oxygen-carrying capacity without placing the patient at risk of volume overload associated with whole blood. One unit of packed RBCs can increase the hematocrit by 3% and the hemoglobin by 1 g/dl.

Administration of blood products in the treatment of shock is not free of risks, especially when massive transfusions are required. Because blood for transfusion contains an anticoagulant to prevent clotting while the blood is stored, the patient who receives large amounts of blood may develop clotting defects. Stored blood is also deficient in platelets and other clotting factors. When massive transfusions are required, fresh frozen plasma, which contains all clotting factors except platelets, is administered to restore coagulation factors. One unit of fresh frozen plasma is given for every 4 to 5 units of blood transfused.

Massive transfusion of cold blood can result in hypothermia, which can cause cardiac dysrhythmias. If blood is to be rapidly infused, it should be warmed before administration using approved blood warmer devices (see Guidelines for Safe Practice box).

Although all blood is transfused through a standard blood filter, when several units are administered, some debris resulting from aggregation of platelets, leukocytes, and fibrin can pass through the filter. This debris is eventually filtered out of the blood by the pulmonary capillaries, and causes little difficulty in patients who receive only a few units of blood. Microfilters may be used when massive transfusions (10 units of whole blood or packed cells in less than 24 hours) are given.

The pH value of stored blood is lower than that of normal blood. The added anticoagulant makes the blood more acidic. In addition, because blood is stored in an airtight bag, the metabolism that continues is anaerobic, and the end products are lactic and pyruvic acids.

BLOOD SUBSTITUTES. Currently three types of red cell substitutes are under investigation but are not yet part of conventional volume replacement therapy. These agents are perfluorocarbon emulsions, cell-free hemoglobin, and liposome-encapsulated hemoglobin.[5] Red cell substitutes do not require type and cross-matching, can act as

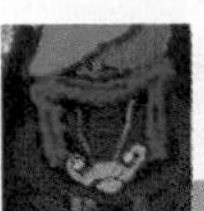

GUIDELINES FOR SAFE PRACTICE
Safe Administration of Multiple Units of Blood

- Ensure typing and cross-matching for blood type, Rh factor, and compatibility with donor blood is performed before administration of each unit.
- Administer blood products through at least a 20-gauge, preferably an 18-gauge or larger, catheter.
- Do not infuse intravenous medications into the same port with blood.
- Administer all transfusions with a blood filter to trap debris and tiny clots.
- Use approved blood warmers when massive transfusions are required to prevent hypothermia.
- Monitor closely for signs of transfusion reaction, fluid overload, acidosis, hyperkalemia, and coagulation disorders.

potent plasma volume expanders, and have significant capacity for carrying oxygen. Because these substances do not transmit viral or bacterial infection and do not cause immunosuppression, they offer considerable promise for the future.

Pharmacologic Management

The major treatment goals are to enhance the effectiveness of the heart's pumping action and to improve tissue perfusion. Pharmacologic management of shock is based on manipulation of contractility, preload, afterload, and heart rate (Table 19-7).

Improving Contractility. Positively inotropic drugs are used to increase contractility, cardiac output, and tissue perfusion in cardiogenic and distributive shock. They also increase myocardial oxygen demand by increasing the workload of the heart. Therefore these agents must be used with caution in patients with ischemic heart disease or cardiogenic shock.

Drugs such as dopamine, dobutamine, and low doses of epinephrine stimulate beta-receptor sites in the heart, causing improved myocardial contractility and improved cardiac output.

Altering Preload. The primary treatment to improve preload is the administration of fluids. Pharmacologic agents may also be given to improve preload in hypovolemic and distributive shock. Vasopressors, such as epinephrine and norepinephrine, cause vasoconstriction and increase venous return to the heart. Vasopressors should be used with caution in hypovolemic shock patients, since their primary need is fluid replacement. In patients in cardiogenic shock, preload reduction may be required to decrease the heart's workload. Vasodilators such as nitroglycerin and nitroprusside decrease the heart's workload by reducing peripheral vascular resistance. Continuous blood pressure monitoring during administration of nitroglycerin or nitroprusside is essential, since either drug can cause hypotension.

Altering Afterload. Afterload reflects the force the heart must overcome to eject blood. In distributive shock, systemic vascular resistance is low. To increase vascular tone and improve venous return to the heart (preload), drugs that increase afterload such as norepinephrine, phenylephrine, or high doses of dopamine may be required (see Research box). In patients in cardiogenic shock, reducing afterload may be necessary to reduce the heart's workload. Because of their vasodilation actions, nitroglycerin and nitroprusside are commonly used afterload-reducing agents.

Research

Malay MB: Heterogeneity of the vasoconstrictor effect of vasopressin in septic shock, *Crit Care Med* 32(6):1327, 2004.

This study attempted to determine whether graded doses of vasopressin or phenylephrine would adversely affect organ blood flow in septic shock. The study was completed in a university hospital research laboratory. The graded doses, starting at the clinically recommended dose level, were given intravenously to pigs. The researcher measured mean arterial pressure, cardiac output, heart rate, arterial blood flow, and pulmonary artery occlusion pressure. The results showed that low doses of vasopressin, which is ordinarily used in the management of patients in septic shock, raised arterial pressure. Graduated higher doses had a vasoconstrictive action and decreased renal and mesenteric blood flow.

The researcher concluded that low-dose vasopressin does not impair blood flow in toxic shock, but moderately higher doses may cause ischemia in renal and mesenteric vessels. The recommendation is to continue the practice of using low-dose (0.04 units/min) administration of vasopressin in septic shock and to not exceed 0.1 unit/min.

Other Drugs. Early coverage with appropriate intravenous antibiotics is important for successful treatment of septic shock. Broad-spectrum antibiotics to cover gram-positive, gram-negative, and anaerobic organisms are ordered until culture and sensitivity reports are obtained. Once the organism is identified, coverage should be tailored according to the organism's susceptibility.

ARE YOU READY?

What is the rationale for administering nitroglycerin to the patient in cardiogenic shock?

1. Increase heart rate
2. Increase systemic vascular resistance
3. Decrease contractility
4. Decrease afterload

Mechanical Management

Intraaortic balloon counterpulsation (IABP) may be indicated for temporary circulatory assistance to restore hemodynamic stability in patients in cardiogenic shock. The physician inserts a polyurethane balloon percutaneously through the femoral artery and positions it just distal to the left subclavian artery (Figure 19-7). The balloon is inflated during diastole and deflated in systole. The overall effects of counterpulsation are to increase coronary perfusion and cardiac output, and decrease preload and afterload. IABP is an effective means of decreasing the work of the myocardium and

TABLE 19-6 FLUIDS USED FOR REPLACEMENT THERAPY IN SHOCK

Type	Uses or Indications	Special Considerations
CRYSTALLOID SOLUTIONS		
Isotonic		
Normal saline	Increases plasma volume Replaces body fluid	Improves plasma volume without changing normal sodium concentration or serum osmolality RBC mass adequate if large volumes are infused to prevent decrease in oxygen-carrying capacity Potential fluid overload because of sodium content Does not improve oncotic pressure
Lactated Ringer's solution	Increases body fluid Buffers acidosis	Lactate converted to bicarbonate in liver and buffers acidosis Increased lactic acidosis in shock conditions caused by lactate Potential fluid overload because of sodium content Added potassium may cause problems in patients with renal failure or adrenal insufficiency Use with caution in patients in shock or with hypoperfusion, since lactate conversion requires aerobic metabolism
Ringer's solution	Replaces body fluid Provides additional potassium and calcium	Does not contain lactate so may be used in treatment of shock Potential fluid overload because of sodium content High-chloride concentration may cause hyperchloremic metabolic acidosis
Hypotonic		
½ normal saline	Raises total body fluid volume	Potential for interstitial and intracellular edema from rapid movement of this fluid from vascular space Dilution of plasma proteins and electrolytes
5% dextrose in water (D_5W)	Raises total fluid volume Provides 0.2 kcal/ml	Acts as free water and is distributed throughout all body compartments Prevents hyperosmolar states Dilution of plasma proteins and electrolytes possible from rapid metabolism of glucose and free water
COLLOID SOLUTIONS		
Plasma protein fraction	Expands plasma volume Increases serum colloid osmotic pressure	Prepared from pooled plasma Reduced risk of hepatitis because of processing procedure Osmotically equivalent to plasma Low risk of hepatitis Deficient in clotting factors Can cause hypotension with rapid infusion (>10 ml/min) Does not protect against HIV transmission risk Use with caution in patients with CHF and renal failure
5% or 25% (salt poor) albumin	Increases plasma colloid osmotic pressure Expands plasma volume 25% albumin used in patients with pulmonary edema, peripheral edema, and hypoproteinemia	Administration rate <2-4 ml/min with 5%; <1 ml/min with 25 % Diuretic may be administered with 25% albumin to ensure diuresis May precipitate CHF after rapid infusion in patients with circulatory overload and compromised cardiovascular function Rare transmission of hepatitis virus Albumin important protein for drug and ion transport

TABLE 19-6 FLUIDS USED FOR REPLACEMENT THERAPY IN SHOCK—CONT'D

Type	Uses or Indications	Special Considerations
PLASMA EXPANDERS		
Hetastarch (Hespan)	Expands plasma volume	Similar volume expansion characteristic as 5% albumin but effects last up to 36 hr; maximum infusion rate 20 ml/kg/hr Low risk of allergic and anaphylactic reactions Cost is about half that of albumin or plasma protein fraction No danger of hepatitis transmission Possible dilution of clotting factors (monitor clotting and platelet counts), plasma proteins, and decreased osmotic pressure Causes a rise in serum amylase level (>200 ml/dl) persisting up to 4 days because of action of amylase in hetastarch degradation Infuse through separate line if possible
BLOOD AND BLOOD PRODUCTS		
Whole blood	Replaces blood volume Provides intravascular volume	Increases oxygen-carrying capacity of blood Risk of hepatitis and HIV transmission, and allergic reactions Requires type and cross-matching Should be stored at 1°-6° C but must be warmed 20-30 min before use or use approved blood warmer device Administered via Y-connector tubing with normal saline; must use blood filter
Packed RBCs (packed concentrate, fresh frozen [leukocyte poor])	Increases hematocrit Improves oxygen-carrying capacity of blood	Used to prevent excess fluid administration in patients in cardiogenic shock Fewer risks of metabolic complications than stored bank whole blood Risk of hepatitis and HIV transmission, and allergic reactions Type and cross-matching required Does not provide adequate volume alone for volume replacement in hypovolemic shock Monitor for clotting derangements when more than 20 units are administered; give 1 unit fresh frozen plasma for each 4 units of RBCs to replenish clotting factors
Human plasma (fresh frozen, dried)	Increases osmotic pressure to improve circulating volume Restores plasma volume Restores clotting factors (except platelets)	Effective for rapid volume replacement Contains clotting factors Risk of hepatitis and HIV transmission, and allergic reactions Administer as soon as possible after thawing to prevent deterioration of clotting factors V and VIII

CHF, Congestive heart failure; *HIV*, human immunodeficiency virus; *RBCs*, red blood cells.

TABLE 19-7
COMMON MEDICATIONS *for Shock*

Drug	Action	Nursing Intervention
Positive Inotropic Drugs		
Dopamine (Intropin) Dobutamine (Dobutrex) Amrinone (Inocor) Norepinephrine (Levophed)	Increases contractile force of heart	Used in management of cardiogenic and distributive shock. These agents increase heart's workload and myocardial oxygen demand. Use with caution in patients with ischemic heart disease and cardiogenic shock. Administer into large veins of antecubital fossa or through central line whenever possible. Correct hypovolemia before administering drugs.
Drugs That Affect Preload		
Increasing Preload		
Epinephrine Norepinephrine	Causes vasoconstriction and increases venous return to heart	Used in treatment of distributive shock. Use with caution with patients in hypovolemic shock.
Decreasing Preload		
Nitroprusside	Decreases venous return to heart by vasodilation of arterioles and venules	Monitor hemodynamic parameters closely to prevent extreme loss of volume, and hypoperfusion to cells.
Drugs That Affect Afterload		
Increasing Afterload		
Dopamine (in high doses) Norepinephrine Phenylephrine	Increases vascular tone, venous return, and consequently cardiac output	Increased afterload may increase myocardial oxygen demand; monitor respiratory pattern.
Decreasing Afterload		
Nitroprusside Nitroglycerine	Increases cardiac output by decreasing left ventricular afterload	Monitor hemodynamic parameters carefully to prevent hypoperfusion to cells. Venous effects of nitroglycerine predominate and decrease myocardial oxygen consumption.
Positive Chronotropic Drugs		
Atropine	Increases heart rate by inhibiting muscarinic actions of acetylcholine in postganglionic parasympathetic neuroeffector sites	As heart rate increases, myocardial oxygen consumption also increases. Correct hypovolemia before administering these drugs.
Isoproterenol	Increases heart rate and force of contraction by mediation of $beta_1$- and $beta_2$-adrenergic receptors	

decreasing oxygen consumption. The nurse needs to closely monitor patients who require IABP therapy for development of complications, including emboli formation, thrombocytopenia, improper balloon placement, bleeding, balloon rupture, and circulatory compromise of the cannulated extremity.

A *ventricular assist device* is used to temporarily support the failing ventricle not responding to IABP and pharmacologic therapy. These devices can support the function of a single ventricle or the whole heart. They divert blood from the failing ventricle or ventricles and pump it back into the aorta (left ventricular assist device), the pulmonary artery (right ventricular assist device), or both arteries.

Pneumatic antishock garments (PASGs), also known as military antishock trousers, external counter-pressure devices, and G suits, raise blood pressure by increasing systemic peripheral resistance and possibly cardiac output (Figure 19-8). These inflatable garments also put direct pressure on bleeding sites, helping to control bleeding in pelvic and long-bone fractures and abdominal and extremity vascular injuries. The PASG is usually instituted in emergency situations in the field. In addition, PASG may be beneficial in hypotension resulting from ruptured abdominal aortic aneurysm, suspected pelvic fracture, anaphylactic shock unresponsive to standard therapy, uncontrollable lower extremity hemorrhage, and severe traumatic hypotension (when a palpable pulse is present, but blood pressure is unobtainable). Use of PASG is contraindicated for patients with pulmonary edema, pregnancy, impaled objects, evisceration of the abdomen, and thoracic and diaphragmatic trauma.

If a patient is admitted with a PASG in place, the nurse monitors the circulatory status of the lower extremities and assesses for the reappearance of shock symptoms. As the patient stabilizes, the PASG is removed by gradual reduction in the pressure in the garment compartments. The abdominal section is deflated first, allowing gradual redistribution of blood volume, followed by deflation of the lower extremities. The nurse monitors the patient's vital signs closely and reapplies pressure if shock symptoms appear until other stabilization measures can be implemented.

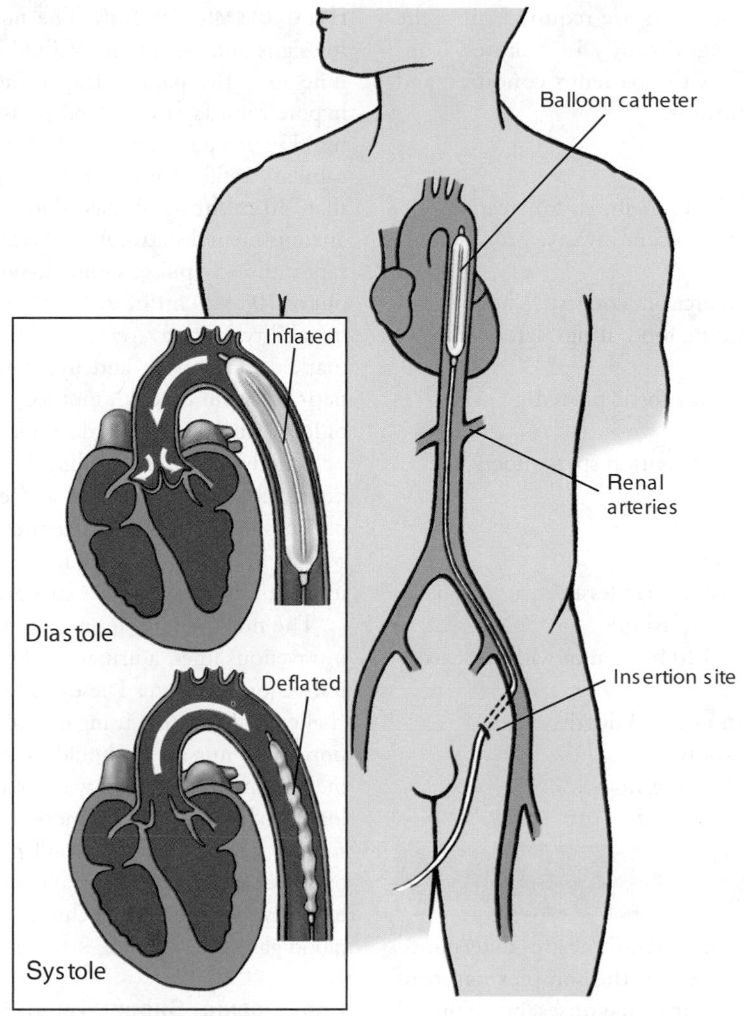

Figure 19-7 Placement of intraaortic balloon pump catheter.

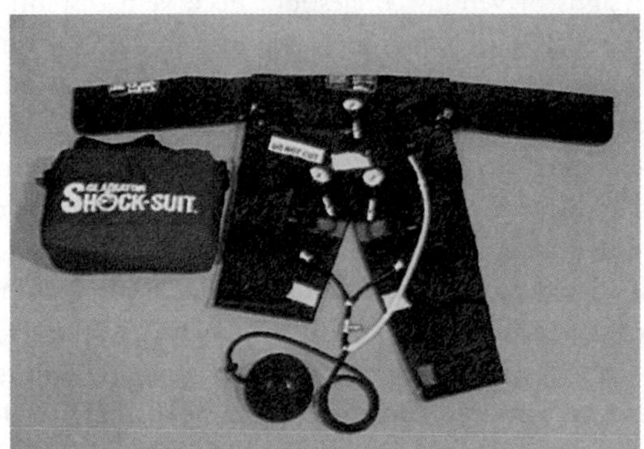

Figure 19-8 Pneumatic antishock garment with abdominal and leg compartments, valves, and foot pump.

Surgical Interventions

Invasive cardiac procedures, such as percutaneous transluminal coronary angioplasty, thrombolytic therapy, stent placement, rotoblade therapy, and laser therapy, are used to attempt early revascularization of an occluded coronary artery after an AMI complicated by cardiogenic shock. Early use of these procedures has resulted in greater survival rates in patients less than 75 years old.[2] Heart transplantation may be an option for a small percentage of patients with severe myocardial damage and cardiogenic shock.[1]

Nursing Management

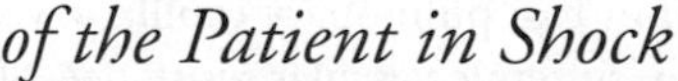

of the Patient in Shock

ASSESSMENT

Nursing management of a patient in shock is both complex and challenging. By remaining aware of the risk of shock in susceptible patients, the nurse may be able to recognize signs and symptoms that signal the onset of shock and correct them before they can progress. Assessment must be accomplished quickly, almost simultaneously with initiation of treatment. Assessment steps include watching for changes in clinical manifestations and monitoring hemodynamic parameters and laboratory values to detect subtle changes warning of progression of the shock state. Some early manifestations of shock include difficulty focusing on questions being asked; expression of a sense of restlessness; and changes in mood, mental status, or behavior. Frequent nursing assessments are required, since the patient's condition can change significantly in minutes. Concise documentation should reflect the patient's condition and response to therapeutic interventions.

Health History. Assess for:

- Recent illness; history of diabetes mellitus, pancreatitis, or compromised immune system; recent invasive procedure, surgery, trauma, or burns
- Hypertension, myocardial infarction, congestive heart failure
- Exposure to allergens, including food, drugs, latex, venom from insect bite or sting
- Recent blood transfusion or diagnostic procedure using contrast media
- Patient response to questions, attention span, mood, and behavior

Physical Examination. Assess for:

- Changes in level of consciousness (restlessness, agitation, lethargy, mental cloudiness, confusion)
- Heart rate more than 100 to 120 beats/min with widened pulse pressure, thready pulse
- Respiratory rate increased in rate and depth
- Skin cool, moist, pale or cyanotic
- Urinary output less than 0.5 ml/kg/hr
- Capillary refill greater than 3 seconds

NURSING DIAGNOSES, OUTCOMES, AND INTERVENTIONS

Nursing diagnoses and their prioritization are determined from analysis of patient data. Because of the complex nature of shock, it is essential that all nursing diagnoses be managed simultaneously.

Nursing Diagnosis: Decreased Cardiac Output

OUTCOMES. Common examples of expected outcomes for the patient with a diagnosis of *decreased cardiac output* are:
Patient will:

- Demonstrate signs of hemodynamic stability as evidenced by the following values: heart rate, less than 100 beats/min; systolic blood pressure, greater than 110 mm Hg or within 10 mm Hg of baseline; cardiac output, 4 to 8 L/min, and/or cardiac index, greater than 2 L/min/m^2; central venous pressure, 0 to 8 mm Hg; pulmonary capillary wedge pressure, 8 to 12 mm Hg; systemic vascular resistance, 800 to 1400 dynes/sec/cm^{-5}; warm extremities with capillary refill time of less than 3 seconds; absence of dysrhythmias or presence of hemodynamically stable dysrhythmias; normal sensorium.
- Remain free from side effects from medication used to achieve adequate cardiac output.

NURSING INTERVENTIONS. Treatment of shock varies depending on the cause of the shock, the organ systems affected, and the patient's condition. As with all life-threatening conditions, care priorities follow the basic principles of airway, breathing, and circulation. However, shock is treated most effectively if the underlying cause can be determined quickly and treated.

HYPOVOLEMIC SHOCK. The nurse should observe the patient for signs and symptoms of fluid loss. With a *minimal* fluid volume loss, the patient may exhibit slight tachycardia; postural hypotension (systolic blood pressure decreased by more than 10 mm Hg or a pulse pressure decreased by more than 20 beats/min); capillary refill of more than 3 seconds; urinary output of more than 30 ml/hr; cool, pale skin, especially in arms and legs; and anxious mental status. A *moderate* fluid volume loss manifests as a rapid, thready pulse; supine hypotension; cool skin; urinary output of 10 to 20 ml/hr; severe thirst; and restlessness, confusion, or irritability. With a *severe* fluid volume loss, the patient will exhibit marked tachycardia and hypotension; weak, thready, or absent peripheral pulses; cold, mottled, or cyanotic skin; urinary output of less than 10 ml/hr; and stupor or nonresponsiveness.

If active external bleeding is present, the nurse should apply direct, continuous pressure and elevate the area if possible. The patient's legs should be elevated above heart level, unless the patient has active bleeding from the head or neck, suspected head injury, or increased intracranial pressure or is in cardiogenic shock.

The nurse should insert and maintain two or more large-bore intravenous lines, a urinary catheter, and a setup to monitor central venous pressure. These enable the nurse to administer a fluid challenge if ordered, using crystalloid or colloid intravenous solutions. The nurse also should monitor the trend of hemodynamic measurements and urinary output; observe for signs of fluid overload, including crackles, neck-vein distention, or a third heart sound; monitor arterial blood pressure and mean arterial blood pressure via arterial line; and obtain a complete blood count, blood type and cross-matching, and serum electrolyte and arterial blood gas values.

CARDIOGENIC SHOCK. For patients in cardiogenic shock, the nurse observes for signs and symptoms of poor arterial perfusion, including tachycardia, hypotension, dysrhythmias, poor peripheral pulses, oliguria, or decreased level of consciousness. The nurse also looks for signs of venous congestion: neck vein distention, lung crackles, S_3 heart sound, and increased liver margin measurement.

The nurse monitors the electrocardiogram (ECG) continually for new or worsening signs of ischemia or infarction (T-wave inversion, ST-segment displacement, or Q-wave development) or significant dysrhythmia (premature ventricular contractions, severe sinus bradycardia or tachycardia). The nurse also assists with insertion of a flow-directed catheter for hemodynamic pressure monitoring. Inotropic or vasodilator drugs or both may be administered to improve cardiac output (see Future Watch box). The nurse assists with insertion of an intraaortic balloon pump catheter, if used, and maintains optimal timing of balloon inflation and deflation.

DISTRIBUTIVE SHOCK. With distributive shock, the nurse observes for signs and symptoms of vasogenic shock: hypotension and decreased systemic vascular resistance (peripheral vasodilation), and for signs of specific types of distributive shock:

- *Septic shock:* history of exposure to infectious agent or immunocompromised state

  Early stage (hyperdynamic or warm shock): warm, dry, or flushed skin; fever; tachycardia; decreased filling pressures; decreased systemic vascular resistance; increased cardiac output; confusion, restlessness, hyperventilation

Future Watch

New Treatment in Cardiogenic Shock on Horizon?

Nitric oxide synthase inhibitors may be beneficial in the treatment of refractory cardiogenic shock. Thirty patients with refractory cardiogenic shock following maximal percutaneous coronary revascularization were treated with supportive care, including intraaortic balloon pump, intravenous (IV) dopamine, furosemide, and fluids. Patients were randomized to a control group receiving supportive care only (n=15) or to supportive care plus administration of L-NAME, a nitric oxide synthase inhibitor (1 mg/kg bolus and 1 mg/kg/hr continuous IV drip). At 24 hours after entry into the study, the L-NAME group demonstrated a significant increase in mean arterial blood pressure and urinary output compared with the control group; the time on the intraaortic balloon pump and mechanical ventilation was also significantly lower in the L-NAME group. Death rates at 1 month were 27% in the L-NAME group versus 67% in the control group.

Cotter G et al: LINCS: L-NAME (a NO synthase inhibitor) in the treatment of refractory cardiogenic shock: a prospective randomized study, *Europ Heart J* 24(14):1287-1295, 2003.

Late stage (hypodynamic or cold shock): increased systemic vascular resistance; decreased cardiac output; cold, clammy skin; oliguria; generalized edema; pulmonary crackles; hypothermia

- *Neurogenic shock:* history of spinal cord injury, head injury, drug overdose; normal or increased cardiac output, decreased filling pressure
- *Anaphylactic shock:* history of allergen exposure, itching, hives, stridor, wheezing, or angioneurotic edema

The nurse administers intravenous fluids as ordered (typically isotonic saline solution) and pharmacologic agents. Epinephrine and antihistamines are given to patients in anaphylactic shock; antibiotics and antipyretics to patients in septic shock; and norepinephrine or phenylephrine to patients with decreased systemic vascular resistance.

RELATED NIC INTERVENTIONS. Cardiac Care, Hemodynamic Regulation, Shock Management

Nursing Diagnosis: Ineffective Tissue Perfusion

OUTCOMES. Common examples of expected outcomes for the patient with a diagnosis of *ineffective tissue perfusion* are:

Patient will:

- Have increased tissue perfusion as evidenced by signs of hemodynamic stability (as listed previously); alertness and orientation to time, place, and person; adequate peripheral tissue perfusion (skin warm and dry, absence of cyanosis, capillary refill greater than 3 seconds); urinary output of more than 30 ml/hr; no dysrhythmias present; arterial blood gases within normal limits.

NURSING INTERVENTIONS. In caring for the patient with ineffective tissue perfusion, the nurse monitors neurologic status, noting subtle changes in sensorium, which are early signs of decreased circulation and oxygen to cerebral tissues. The nurse checks the dorsalis pedis and posterior tibial pulses bilaterally. If unable to palpate them, the nurse uses a Doppler stethoscope and notifies the physician. Diminished or absent pulses are indicative of a low flow state and poor tissue perfusion. The nurse also checks capillary refill, which should occur within 3 seconds; and notes the color and temperature of skin. Cool skin, pallor, or mottling can signal a low flow state and poor tissue perfusion.

RELATED NIC INTERVENTIONS. Circulatory Care: Arterial Insufficiency, Circulatory Care: Venous Insufficiency, Neurologic Monitoring

Nursing Diagnosis: Deficient Fluid Volume

OUTCOMES. Common examples of expected outcomes for the patient with a diagnosis of *deficient fluid volume* are:

Patient will:

- Have an intravascular volume within normal limits as evidenced by stable hemodynamic variables (as listed previously); body weight within 5% of baseline; balanced fluid intake and output; urinary output of more than 30 ml/hr; fluid and electrolyte balance within normal limits as demonstrated by laboratory data (electrolytes, hematocrit, hemoglobin, blood urea nitrogen, and serum creatinine); normal body temperature; adequate peripheral perfusion (skin warm and dry, absence of cyanosis).

NURSING INTERVENTIONS. The nurse assesses the patient to identify factors causing deficient fluid volume (e.g., burns, vomiting, diarrhea, diabetic ketoacidosis, diuretic therapy). Early intervention can decrease the occurrence and severity of shock. The nurse also monitors for early signs of hypovolemia (e.g., weakness, postural hypotension, muscle cramps). Note that late signs of hypovolemia include oliguria; cold, clammy skin; confusion; and thready pulses.

The nurse monitors intake and output hourly until urinary output averages 30 ml/hr, and monitors daily weights for sudden decreases. Weights should be taken on same scale with the same type of clothing and at the same time of day. Change in body weight is one of the best indicators of changes in body fluid volume.

The nurse also needs to monitor vital signs for decreased pulse pressure, hypertension, tachycardia, decreased pulse volume, and decreased core temperature. A decreased pulse pressure is an early indicator of shock and occurs before a drop in blood pressure.

The nurse maintains patent intravenous access and monitors infusion types and amounts. When ordered, the nurse initiates a fluid challenge of crystalloids and notes response of vital signs, urinary output, and lung sounds. Hemodynamic parameters (central venous pressure, pulmonary artery pressure, pulmonary wedge pressure) are monitored, since they are sensitive indicators of intravascular fluid volume.

The patient is positioned flat with legs elevated above the level of the heart (if not contraindicated). This position enhances venous blood return to the heart and improved cardiac output, but it should be used with caution in patients suspected of being in cardiogenic shock.

RELATED NIC INTERVENTIONS. Electrolyte Monitoring, Fluid Management, Hypovolemia Management

Nursing Diagnosis: Impaired Gas Exchange

OUTCOMES. Common examples of expected outcomes for the patient with a diagnosis of *impaired gas exchange* are:
Patient will:

- Have improved gas exchange and adequate oxygenation as evidenced by an airway that is patent and clear of secretions; arterial blood gas values within normal limits (pH, 7.35 to 7.45; PaO_2, at least 80 mm Hg; $PaCO_2$, 35 to 45 mm Hg; SaO_2, at least 95%); respiratory rate of 12 to 20 breaths/min; breath sounds clear to auscultation; absence of cyanosis; capillary refill of no more than 3 seconds.

NURSING INTERVENTIONS. The nurse monitors respiratory rate, depth, and effort and observes the patient's breathing, since use of accessory muscles, nasal flaring, abdominal breathing, and increased respiratory rate may be seen with hypoxia. The nurse also monitors the client's mental status for onset of restlessness, agitation, confusion, or lethargy. Changes in behavior and mental status can be early signs of impaired gas exchange. In late stages the patient becomes lethargic, progressing to somnolence and coma.

The nurse monitors for cyanosis, especially of the tongue and oral mucous membranes, which is indicative of serious hypoxia. Blood gas results and continuous oxygen saturation are monitored. A PaO_2 of less than 80 mm Hg or an oxygen saturation of 90% indicates significant oxygenation problems. In such cases, nursing measures are implemented to prevent desaturation of oxygen during nursing care.

The nurse administers humidified oxygen through an appropriate device (e.g., nasal cannula, face mask, endotracheal tube) and auscultates breath sounds frequently, noting the development of crackles. The major complication is acute respiratory distress syndrome (ARDS), which occurs secondary to reduced pulmonary blood flow and increased pulmonary vascular resistance. Pulmonary capillary permeability increases, leading to noncardiogenic pulmonary edema. Surfactant production is reduced, resulting in decreased pulmonary compliance and hypoxemia that becomes refractory to oxygen therapy. If symptoms of ARDS develop, the patient may require intubation and mechanical ventilation using positive end-expiratory pressure. Positive pressure at the end of expiration prevents surfactant-deficient alveoli from collapsing, resulting in atelectasis.

RELATED NIC INTERVENTIONS. Airway Management, Oxygen Therapy, Respiratory Monitoring

EVALUATION

To evaluate the effectiveness of nursing interventions, compare patient behaviors with those stated in the expected patient outcomes.

RELATED NOC OUTCOMES. Cardiac Pump Effectiveness, Circulation Status, Fluid Balance, Respiratory Status: Gas Exchange, Respiratory Status: Ventilation, Tissue Perfusion: Peripheral, Vital Signs

Critical Thinking

1. Compare and contrast assessment findings of a patient in cardiogenic shock and a patient in hypovolemic shock.
2. Mr. Jones is a patient in the critical care unit who has experienced some shock episodes in recent days. While assessing the 48-hour intravenous flow rates, you note that each shift has been infusing the drug at a different rate. What are some possible explanations for the variation in the flow rates?

References

1. Entwistle JW III et al: Improved survival with ventricular assist device support in cardiogenic shock after myocardial infarction, *Heart Surg Forum* 6(5):316-319, 2003.
2. Hochman JS et al: One-year survival following early revascularization for cardiogenic shock, *JAMA* 285(2):190-192, 2001.
3. Kwan I, Bunn F, Roberts I, WHO Pre-Hospital Trauma Care Steering Committee: Timing and volume of fluid administration for patients with bleeding (Cochrane Review). In *Cochrane Library*, Issue 3, 2004, Chichester, UK, John Wiley & Sons.
4. Riedemann NC, Ren-Feng G, Ward PA: Novel strategies for the treatment of sepsis, *Nat Med* 9(5):517–524, 2003.
5. Sarteschi LM et al: Rationale for the development of red-cell substitutes and status of the research, *Int Med* 9:36-44, 2001.
6. Sharma S, Jumar A: Septic shock, multiple organ failure, and acute respiratory distress syndrome, *Cur Opinion Pulmon Med* 9(3):199–209, 2003.
7. Tang AW: A practical guide to anaphylaxis, *Am Fam Phys* 68(7):1325-1332, 1339-1340, 2003.
8. US National Library of Medicine and Institutes of Health: *Sepsis: what you should know;* website: www.nlm.nih.gov, accessed July 2005.

evolve Visit the Evolve website: http://evolve.elsevier.com/Monahan/medsurg

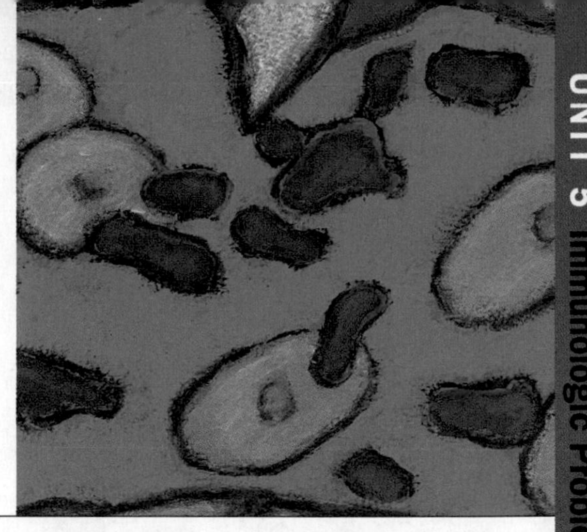

CHAPTER 20

Assessment of the Immune System

by Carol J. Green

OBJECTIVES

After studying this chapter, the learner should be able to:

1. Recall the structure and function of the immune system.
2. Differentiate between innate and adaptive immunity.
3. Describe the internal and external components of defense.
4. Describe the process and clinical manifestations of inflammation.
5. Discuss the components and function of adaptive immunity.
6. Discuss immune system changes that occur with normal aging.
7. Identify immune assessment parameters.
8. Describe common diagnostic tests used to assess immune function.
9. Explain the nursing implications of immune-related diagnostic tests.

KEY TERMS

adaptive immunity, p. 421
antibodies, p. 423
antigens, p. 421
cell-mediated immunity, p. 433
complement, p. 426
degranulation, p. 426
immunocompetent, p. 421
inflammation, p. 424
innate immunity, p. 421
interferons, p. 427
humoral immunity, p. 434
opsonization, p. 426
self-cells, p. 421
tolerance, p. 441

This chapter provides an overview of innate immunity, the inflammatory response, adaptive immunity, related assessment data, and diagnostic tests for immune function. Immune disorders are presented in Chapters 21 and 22.

Anatomy and Physiology

The immune system is a unique network of specialized cells, tissues, and organs that protect the body from invading microorganisms, neutralize foreign substances, destroy malignant cells, and dispose of cellular debris. Such functions are possible because the immune system is able to recognize proteins that protrude through cell membranes. These proteins are unique to each individual and allow the immune system to distinguish between "self" and "nonself" cells. **Self-cells** are protected. Substances without self-markers are identified as nonself and are neutralized or destroyed. Foreign particles and microorganisms, infected or weakened body cells, self-cells that have undergone malignant transformation, pollens, foods, drugs, transplanted organs or tissues, and venoms are examples of nonself cells. Collectively, foreign substances that are capable of eliciting an immune response are known as **antigens.**

The immune system provides two lines of defense. **Innate immunity**, also known as natural or native immunity, provides initial immune protection by blocking the entry of foreign substances. If antigens do gain host entry, the *inflammatory response* reacts to isolate, destroy, and eliminate them. The second line of defense is **adaptive immunity**, also known as acquired or specific immunity. Adaptive immunity develops over time and in response to exposure to various antigens. It is highly specific for each invading pathogen, remembers the infectious agent so that future protection is provided, and improves with each subsequent exposure to the offending antigen[9] (Figure 20-1). These basic responses are meshed together to give individuals their own unique immunologic reaction to antigens. Variations in immunologic response occur because each person has a different genetic background, is exposed to different environmental conditions, and responds differently to antigenic stimulation.

Specialized cells and organs that make up the immune system are located throughout the body. Immune organs are called lymphoid organs because they are involved with the growth, development, and function of lymphocytes (white blood cells, or WBCs). The primary lymphoid organs are the bone marrow and thymus gland. Lymphocytes mature in these organs and become **immunocompetent** cells

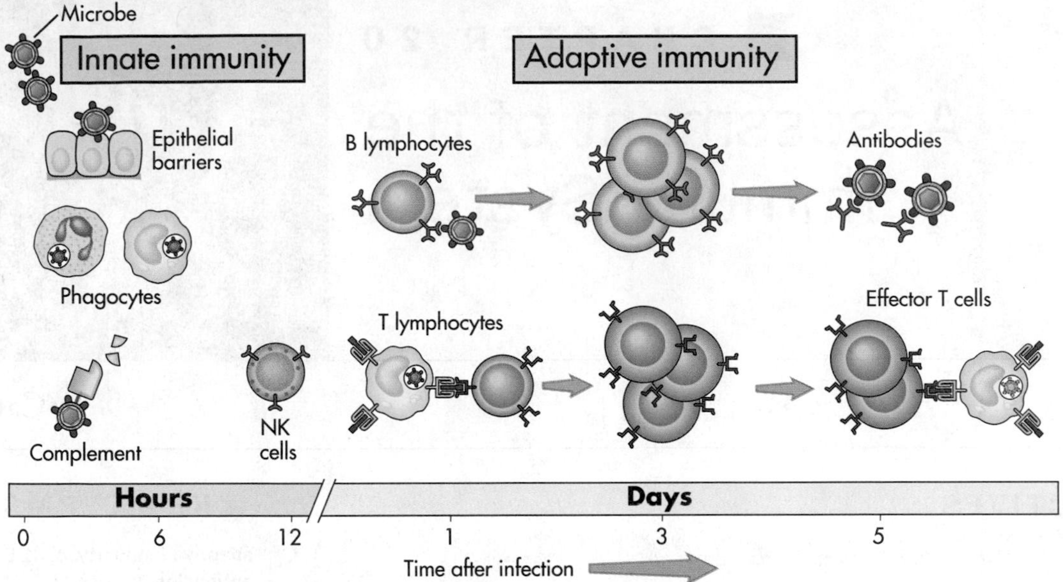

Figure 20-1 Principal mechanisms of innate and adaptive immunity. Innate immunity provides initial defense against infections, which may involve prevention of infection or elimination of microbes (e.g., phagocytes, natural killer [NK] cells, complement). Adaptive immunity develops later and involves production of lymphocytes and antibodies that specifically target invading antigens.

capable of producing an immune response. Lymphocytes maturing in the bone marrow are called B lymphocytes. Those which migrate and mature in the thymus gland are called T lymphocytes.

The thymus gland is believed to regulate the overall immune system. Its activity reaches its peak in childhood, and the gland begins to shrink in size after puberty. Research has shown that if the thymus is removed (thymectomy) early in life, a severe state of immunodeficiency is induced and T cell–mediated immunity never develops.

The lymph nodes; spleen; tonsils and adenoids; appendix; and patches of specialized lymphoid tissues that lie beneath the mucous membrane layer of the respiratory, gastrointestinal (GI), and genitourinary tracts are the secondary lymphoid organs (Figure 20-2). Mature immune cells concentrate within these secondary lymphoid organs. Lymph nodes are small, bean-shaped structures that occur along lymphatic vessels. They consist of an inner medullary and paracortical region made up primarily of T cells, and an outer cortex composed of clusters of B cells. Lymph nodes (Figure 20-3) filter foreign substances from lymph. When stimulated, macrophages and B cells in the lymph nodes can rapidly proliferate and differentiate into immunoglobulin-producing cells, which results in lymph node enlargement (lymphadenopathy).

The spleen lies inferiorly and posteriorly to the stomach in the upper left quadrant of the abdomen. The spleen is a major storage depot for macrophages and lymphocytes, both of which can launch an immune response when stimulated by foreign cells. Patches of specialized lymphoid tissue block submucosal entry of antigens into the area where the patches are located (e.g., the respiratory, GI, and genitourinary tracts or skin). Collectively, the tonsils, the patches of specialized lymphoid tissue in the GI tract known as *Peyer's patches*, and the appendix are known as gut-associated lymphoid tissues. The tonsils screen airborne and ingested antigens. The appendix and Peyer's patches specifically protect against alimentary antigens. The lymphoid cells and organs act in concert to protect skin surfaces, mucous membranes, blood, lymph, and internal organs from foreign invasion.

Innate Immunity

Innate immunity is present at birth and does not require exposure to an antigen for its development. It consists of anatomic and chemical barriers that recognize and respond to damaged self-cells or nonself, foreign antigens. Once believed to be nonspecific, innate immunity is now known to provide a powerful and specific initial defense mechanism that targets, controls, and even eradicates microbes before adaptive immunity is activated. The specificity of innate immunity differs from that of adaptive immunity. Innate immune components have receptors, known as pattern recognition receptors, that recognize cell markers common to various types of microbes that are not present on host cells. For example, host phagocytes recognize and respond to double-stranded ribonucleic acid (RNA), which is common to viruses but not to human cells. Another characteristic that makes innate immunity highly effective is its ability to recognize microbial properties that are essential to their infectivity and survival. Thus microbes cannot escape detection even when they mutate or do not express their cell markers.[1]

The response from innate immunity is always the same, regardless of the type of offending antigen or the number of encounters with the same antigen. The response is produced within hours of contact with an offending antigen, but no memory of the immunologic event is produced for future protection; therefore innate immunity is short term and temporary. Innate and adaptive immunity communicate with one another and act synergistically to prevent and eliminate infections.[1]

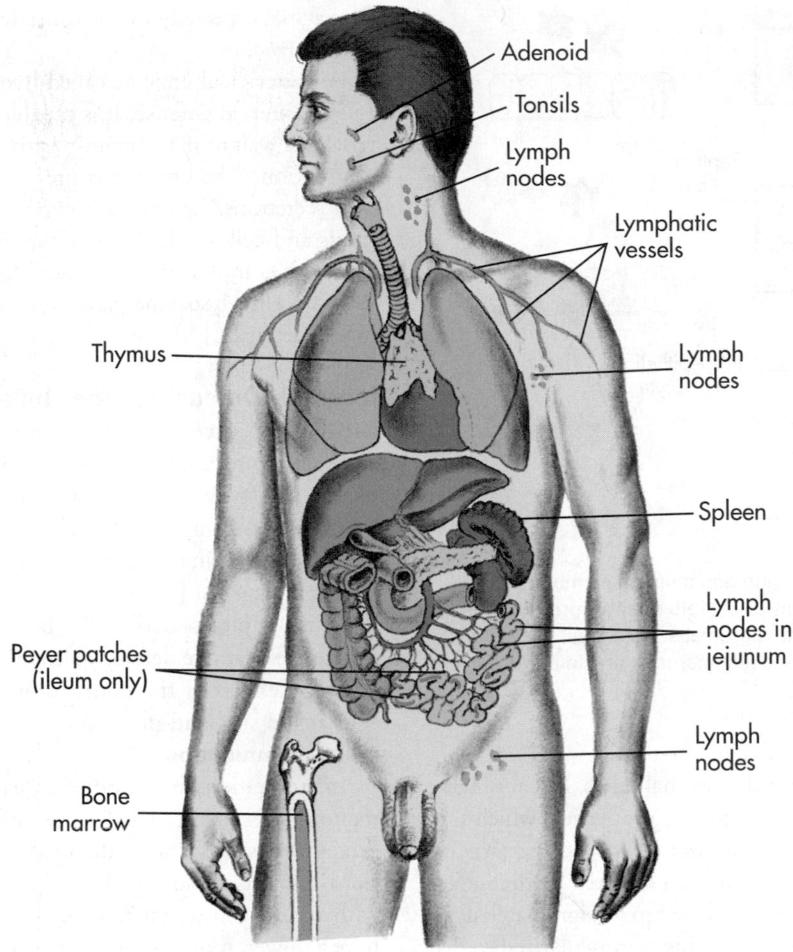

Figure 20-2 Lymphoid tissues and structures of immune system.

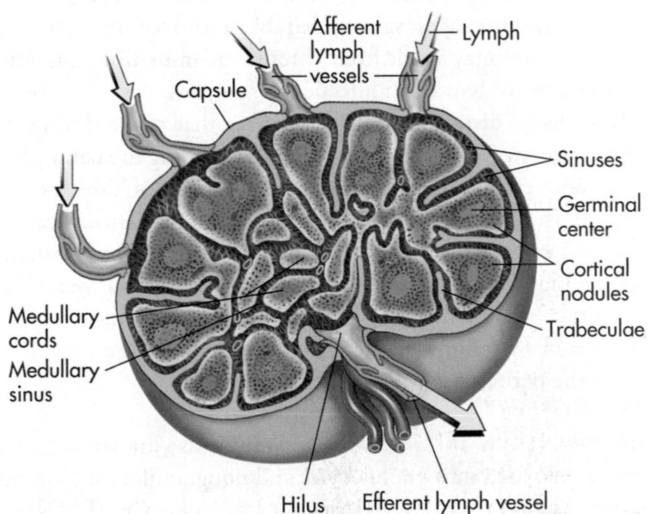

Figure 20-3 Structure of a lymph node. Lymph nodes are organized into three main areas: outer cortex, where B cells proliferate and mature; deeper paracortex, populated mainly by macrophages and T cells; and inner medulla, containing both B and T cells. Macrophages, B cells, and T cells interact with one another, often in the presence of antigen being filtered through the node, resulting in inductive phase of immune response.

External Defenses. The skin, mucous membranes, protective secretions, enzymes, phagocytic cells, and protective proteins provide the body with its innate immunity. The most basic of these defenses is the external barrier protection composed of the skin and mucous membranes, which prevents entry of harmful agents into the body. Intact skin is an extremely efficient physical barrier to harmful agents and environmental forces such as heat, cold, and trauma. The keratinized surface cells of the skin provide a tough, dense, waterproof covering. Some of the fatty acids released to the skin surface by the sebaceous glands have antimicrobial activity and inhibit the growth of selected microorganisms. Acetic acid and salt in perspiration is toxic to many pathogenic microorganisms. Resident floras compete for nutrients and space with transient, potential pathogens, and some release antimicrobial substances that retard the growth of transient organisms seeking to colonize the same site (Figure 20-4).

Mucous membranes protect the eye and line all body tracts that have external openings. When intact, mucous membranes, like the skin, are basically impervious to foreign materials and microorganisms. A viscous secretion covers the surface of mucous membranes that tends to trap and inactivate microorganisms. A specific class of immunoglobulins **(antibodies)** known as immunoglobulin A (IgA) is found in mucosal secretions and within the secretory

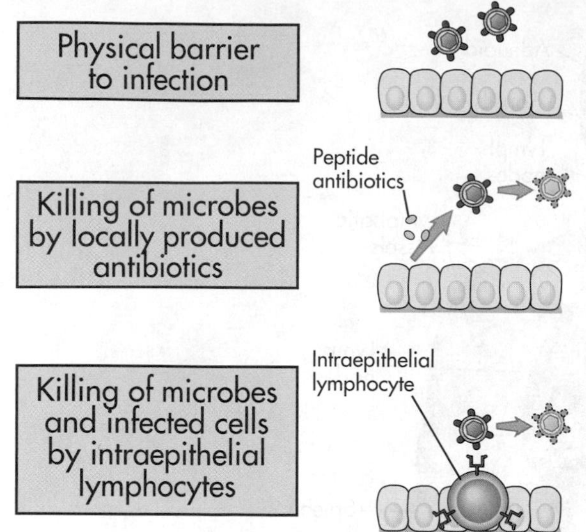

Figure 20-4 Functions of intact skin and mucous membranes in innate immunity. Epithelia present at portals of entry provide physical barriers to microbes, produce antimicrobial substances, and harbor lymphocytes, which are believed to kill microbes and infected cells.

mucosal cells of the respiratory and intestinal tracts. IgA antibodies have antibacterial, antiviral, and antitoxic properties, which prevent microbial adherence and colonization of body tracts by pathogens. The respiratory tract is further protected by the surface activity of ciliated epithelial cells, which sweep foreign material out of the airways. Mucous membranes are highly vascularized so that the internal defense mechanisms are readily available to attack any microorganisms that do gain internal access.

Many other structures and functions of the body also contribute to external defense. The nasal hairs have a unique filtration action that traps particles and microorganisms. The flushing action of saliva and urine prevents the buildup of organisms. The eyelids and lashes protect the eyes from dirt particles and organisms. Foreign material that does gain entrance to the eye tends to be washed out by tears. In the stomach, the acidity (approximately pH 2) of gastric secretions kills many organisms and detoxifies certain potentially toxic substances. For this reason, when gastric pH is increased, special precautions must be taken to avoid introduction of organisms through the nose and mouth. The action of bile and proteolytic enzymes generally keeps the upper intestine free of organisms. The constant movement of foods through the stomach and intestines also prevents the buildup of organisms and toxic waste products. Even vomiting and the watery stools of diarrhea are active modes of removal of harmful products from the GI tract.

In the vagina, secretions support the colonization of lactobacilli, which are harmless, acid-producing bacteria. This colonization results in an acid environment and reduces the chance of pathogens colonizing the vagina. When either the amount or the acidity of vaginal secretions is reduced, the risk of vaginal infection increases. Because vaginal secretions are not present before puberty and are greatly reduced after menopause, both young girls and older women are more prone to vaginitis. Some oral contraceptives may cause a shift in the composition and pH of the vaginal secretions, thereby increasing the possibility of colonization of the vagina, especially by the causative agent of gonorrhea, *Neisseria gonorrhoeae.*

A bactericidal enzyme called lysozyme also plays a significant role in external defense. It is capable of lysing (splitting) the bacterial cell wall of many gram-positive organisms and causing their destruction. The enzyme is present in mucus, tears, saliva, and skin secretions. Lysozyme is also found in many of the internal fluids and cells of the body, where it tends to work in combination with complement and other blood factors to destroy bacteria directly. Thus lysozyme plays a role in both external and internal innate defense.

Internal Defenses: The Inflammatory Response. If antigens are successful in penetrating external protective barriers, an even more complex array of internal defense mechanisms comes into play. The cells and molecules of the mononuclear phagocyte system, blood, complement, and interferons, all of which take part in the inflammatory response, provide immediate protection against invading antigens and tissue injury.

When injury occurs in the body, all the innate and to some degree the adaptive defense mechanisms are directed toward localizing the effects of the injury, protecting against microbial invasion at the site, and preparing the site for repair. This process is called **inflammation**.

Inflammations are classified as acute or chronic. Acute inflammations are characterized by a sudden onset, a marked fluid exudative response, and a duration of 1 to 2 weeks. After the injurious agent is removed, the inflammation resolves, and healing with return of normal function ensues. Chronic inflammations have a slower, more insidious onset (over weeks, months, or years) and are characterized by increased cellular exudation. Scarring and loss of functional tissue may occur. Chronic inflammation can occur when acute inflammation remains unresolved or when persistent irritation exists. A granuloma is a lesion composed of modified macrophages surrounded by a rim of mononuclear leukocytes that may result from chronic inflammation. Granulomas can effectively wall off infectious organisms.

Knowledge of the physiologic changes that occur during the inflammatory process is essential to understanding the pathophysiology and clinical manifestations of a variety of diseases. For example, the death of heart muscle that occurs with myocardial infarction causes an inflammatory response. Fat deposits (atheromas) on blood vessel walls that injure the lining of the vessel wall also initiate an inflammatory response. Similarly, irritation of the peritoneum by trauma or bacterial invasion can cause inflammation of the peritoneum (peritonitis).

Components of Inflammation. WBCs, also known as leukocytes, are divided into granulocytes and nongranulocytes. Granulocytes, also known as polymorphonuclear leukocytes (PMNs) or polys, are further divided on the basis of their structure and function into neutrophils, eosinophils, and basophils. The "granules" found within these cells represent discrete packets of enzymes used to digest the engulfed microbes or foreign materials. Lymphocytes and monocytes are nongranulocytes. Lymphocytes are further divided into two subsets: T cells and B cells, which are primarily involved in adaptive immunity and are discussed later in the chapter. WBCs provide internal defense by differing mechanisms. Neutrophils and monocytes are *phagocytic* cells, whereas eosinophils and basophils protect by releasing vasoactive chemicals (Table 20-1).

PHAGOCYTES. Neutrophils and monocytes are circulating WBCs that are summoned to sites of infection, where they recognize, ingest, and kill invading microbes via detection of surface markers. They are attracted to the scene by chemicals released during infection or injury. This cellular response to chemical attractants is known as *chemotaxis*, and the substances released are called *chemotactic substances*. The process of phagocytosis is carried out in several discrete steps (Figure 20-5).

Most infecting microbes are quickly and efficiently destroyed by phagocytosis; however, some pathogens can escape this destruction. Some strains of streptococci and staphylococci and *Bacillus anthracis* (anthrax) produce factors that kill phagocytic cells. A few microbes are capable of resisting ingestion and may survive within the phagocyte itself. This allows for transport of the organism to other sites in the body or may serve as the focus for continued infection.

Neutrophils, which comprise between 55% and 70% of the total leukocyte count, are the most efficient and responsive of the phagocytic cells involved in the inflammatory response. Neutrophil production is stimulated by colony-stimulating factors known as cytokines, which are produced by different cell types in response to infection. New cells, segmented neutrophils, require between 7 and 14 days to mature. Consequently, when there is significant, ongoing inflammation, immature cells known as *bands* or *stabs* become more prevalent in the peripheral circulation. The condition sometimes is referred to as a "shift to the left," a clinical phrase derived from the past clinical laboratory method of counting the less mature cells and tabulating them in the left-hand columns of differential count forms.

Once an inflammatory response is initiated, neutrophils are the first cells to migrate to the site of infection or injury, provided the region has adequate blood supply. They are constantly available to

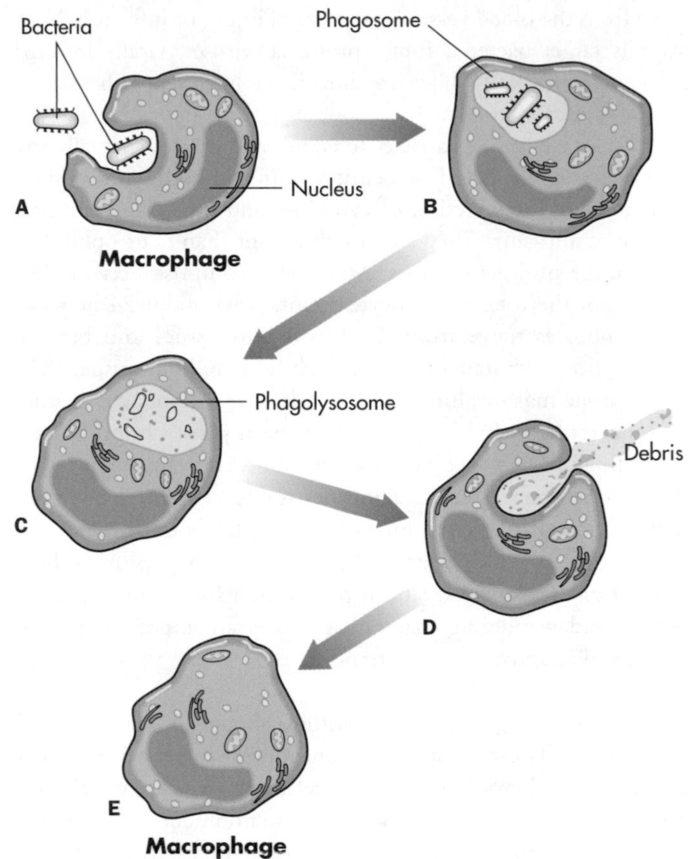

Figure 20-5 Phagocytosis. **A,** Opsonized bacteria engulfed by phagocyte (macrophage). **B,** Phagosome formed. **C,** Phagosome becomes phagolysosome; bacteria digested. **D,** Debris is ejected (neutrophil dies here). **E,** Macrophage returns to resting state.

TABLE 20-1 WHITE BLOOD CELL RESPONSE TO INFECTIONS

Leukocyte Response	Associated Infectious Process
Increase in neutrophils (neutrophilia)	Typical in many acute local and systemic infections cause by bacteria (especially pyogenic bacteria), rickettsia, some viruses, and a few protozoa
Decrease in neutrophils (neutropenia)	Frequent in salmonellosis, brucellosis, whooping cough, overwhelming bacterial infections, influenza, infectious mononucleosis, hepatitis A infection, mumps, rubella, rubeola, and some rickettsial and protozoan diseases
Increase in eosinophils (eosinophilia)	Frequent in allergic reactions, chronic skin disease, helminthic infections, and scarlet fever
Increase in lymphocytes (lymphocytosis)	Frequent in chickenpox, mumps, measles, infectious mononucleosis, influenza, whooping cough, syphilis, tuberculosis, salmonellosis, viral hepatitis, and viral pneumonia; sometimes seen in convalescent phase of acute bacterial infection
Increase in monocytes (monocytosis)	Common in tuberculosis, chickenpox, brucellosis, mumps, syphilis, and certain rickettsial diseases; may occur in certain viral and protozoan diseases and in convalescent phase of acute bacterial infections
Decrease in lymphocytes (lymphocytopenia)	Human immunodeficiency virus

move from the blood vessels to the site of injury or infection. Neutrophils target bacteria, fungi, protozoa, viruses, virally infected cells, and tumor cells. They are short lived, however, with an average life of 4 to 10 hours.

Monocytes have the capacity to engulf and destroy virtually any type of foreign material or debris within the body. Other functions include the secretion of cytokines and processing and presenting of antigens. They are less abundant than neutrophils but can live for months to years. Monocytes comprise between 2% and 8% of the total lymphocyte count. After about 24 hours of life monocytes move from the blood into tissues and become fixed. Once anchored in tissues such as lymphoid tissue, liver, spleen, bone marrow, lungs, and blood vessels, monocytes mature into macrophages. Macrophages have been given unique names, depending on their specific tissue location within the body (Table 20-2). Macrophages capture and destroy foreign antigens found in the fluids of their environment. Macrophages that are not stationary are called *wandering macrophages.* They provide final cleanup of the damaged site in preparation for repair. Both stationary and wandering macrophages play an important role in innate and adaptive immune responses.

EOSINOPHILS. Eosinophils constitute about 4% of the total WBC count. They are capable of phagocytosis, but it is not their primary role. They kill microbes by releasing granules, which contain enzymes, into the extracellular environment by a process known as **degranulation**. They actively defend against pathogens such as parasitic worms, protozoa, and fungi that are too large to be ingested by phagocytic cells. Eosinophils also play a major role in allergic reactions. They release substances, one of which is histaminase, which inactivates histamine to dampen the inflammation occurring during an allergic response.[9]

BASOPHILS. Basophils make up less than 1% of the total WBC count. They play an important role in the inflammatory process by their actions on blood vessels. Basophils are similar to mast cells. Mast cells are leukocytes that store inflammatory mediators. Both cells degranulate and release vasoactive mediators that act on smooth muscle and blood vessel walls. Allergens often serve as the stimulus for basophil or mast cell degranulation and release of histamine, heparin, leukotrienes, and eosinophil chemotactic factor of anaphylaxis. These mediators, especially histamine, are responsible for the adverse symptoms produced by allergens. Histamine narrows the lumens of the respiratory system and restricts breathing, produces vasoconstriction that decreases venous blood flow while increasing blood flow in the small arteries and capillaries, and enhances capillary permeability. Increased capillary permeability is thought to be protective in that it enhances the antimicrobial properties of the blood at sites of inflammation and infection. Vasoactive mediators are also protective in that they assist with immunity against parasites by increasing the inflammatory response.

TABLE 20-2 DISTRIBUTION OF MACROPHAGES IN VARIOUS TISSUE SITES

Tissue	Name
Peripheral blood	Monocyte
Loose connective tissue	Histiocyte
Liver	Kupffer's cells
Spleen	Wandering or fixed macrophage
Lung	Alveolar macrophage or dust cell
Granulomatous tissue	Epithelioid and giant cells
Peritoneal cavity, pleural cavity, bone	Macrophages

BLOOD. Blood is a primary source of elements that protect against injurious agents. It contains granulocytes, lymphocytes, monocytes, thrombocytes (platelets), and plasma. The fluid portion of uncoagulated blood is called plasma. Plasma transports immunoglobulins, which are produced as part of adaptive immunity, throughout the body so they can attach to invading antigens. Receptor sites on the surface of phagocytic cells can easily recognize the immunoglobulin-bound antigens, thereby greatly enhancing the phagocytic cell's ability to engulf the antigen. This process of enhanced phagocytosis is known as **opsonization**. Through this process, adaptive immune mechanisms contribute to innate immunity, making it significantly more efficient.

Another plasma constituent, fibrin, participates in the inflammatory process by creating a meshwork around the injured area and sealing it off. Microorganisms become trapped within this meshwork, where phagocytic cells can more easily capture them. Platelets also play an important role in internal defense by participating in the inflammatory response. They collect at and adhere to injured endothelial cells. They then release serotonin and fibrinogen, which increase capillary permeability, activate complement, and enhance chemotaxis of leukocytes.[9]

NATURAL KILLER CELLS. About 10% of blood and peripheral lymphoid organ lymphocytes are natural killer (NK) cells that provide internal protection by enhancing macrophage function and directly killing infected cells. Their ability to protect is enhanced by macrophages coming into contact with microbes and secreting the NK-activating cytokine interleukin-12. Once activated, NK cells are able to recognize host cells that have been altered by viral infection and phagocytic cells that harbor intracellular bacteria or viruses. NK cells directly kill infected host cells by releasing from their cytoplasmic granules proteins and other substances that produce holes in plasma membranes of infected cells and activate enzymes that induce cellular death. NK cells also protect by producing a macrophage-activating cytokine called interferon gamma (Figure 20-6). Just as macrophages augment NK cellular function, NK cells augment macrophage function by secreting interferon gamma, which enhances macrophage ability to kill phagocytosed microbes. NK cells work in concert with macrophages to effectively kill infected host cells and eliminate cellular reservoirs of infection and intracellular viruses[1] (Figure 20-7).

COMPLEMENT SYSTEM. One of the most important constituents of plasma is a complex collection of circulating and membrane-associated proteins known by the singular name of **complement**. Complement has as many as 20 different protein components, many of which are proteolytic enzymes. The liver is the predominant site for synthesis of complement components,

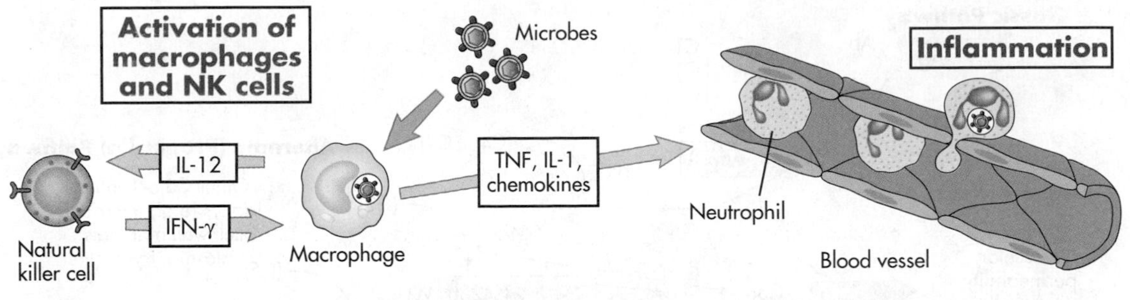

Figure 20-6 Cytokines in innate immunity. Macrophages responding to microbes produce cytokines that stimulate inflammation (leukocyte recruitment) and activate natural killer (NK) cells to produce the macrophage-activating cytokine interferon gamma (IFN-γ). *TNF,* Tumor necrosis factor; *IL-12,* interleukin-12; *IL-1,* interleukin-1.

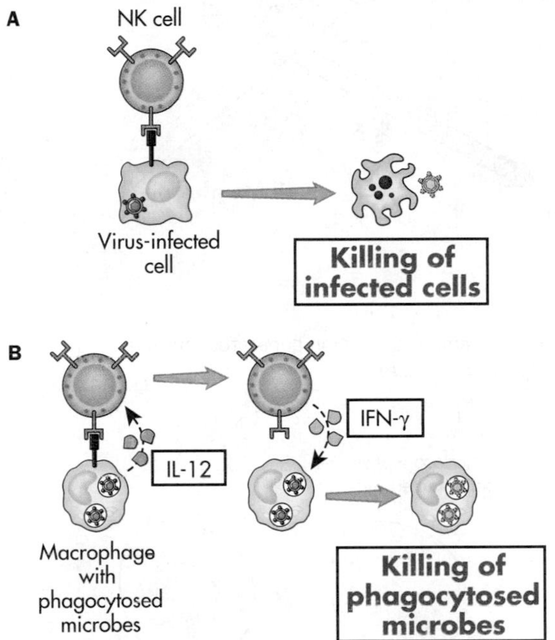

Figure 20-7 Functions of natural killer (NK) cells. **A,** NK cells kill host cells infected by intracellular microbes, thus eliminating reservoirs of infection. **B,** NK cells respond to interleukin-12 (IL-12) produced by macrophages and secrete interferon gamma (IFN-γ), which activates the macrophages to kill phagocytosed microbes.

whose primary role is the lysis (rupturing) of cell membranes. Complement is considered nonspecific because it is not increased by immunization or antigenic challenge.

Different pathways may activate the complement cascade, which is a sequential interaction of protein subunits. The *classic pathway* is part of adaptive immunity and is triggered by an antibody binding to a microbe or other antigen, forming an antigen-antibody complex. The *alternate pathway* is part of innate immunity. It is triggered when complement proteins are activated on microbial surfaces that do not contain regulatory proteins.

Regardless of the activation pathway, complement accentuates or completes the action of an immunoglobulin. An immunoglobulin by itself cannot produce cell lysis, but with the addition of complement in the reaction, the cell may be ruptured. When an antigen-antibody complex on the surface of a cell binds the first component, C1, it acquires the enzymatic ability to activate many molecules of the next components in the sequence, C4 and C2, to form an active C42 complex. (Unfortunately, the numbering system of the complement components reflects their order of discovery and not their sequential additive pattern.) Each of the activated C42 complexes (the activation units) is then able to act on multiple molecules of the next components and so on, producing a cascade effect and a greatly amplified reaction. As each component is added, new enzymatic activity is created to initiate the next step, similar to that of the clotting process[8] (Figure 20-8).

The final component is able to create a lesion in the antigen cell membrane; if enough lesions are created, cell death results. The intermediate stages in the complement sequence give rise to complexes and fragments that produce significant biologic activities as well. These include leukocyte chemotaxis, release of histamines, enhancement of phagocytosis, viral neutralization, and bactericidal actions.

INTERFERONS. Interferons are a group of proteins produced by various cells when viruses invade them. Interferon is produced almost immediately following viral entrance into the cell. It is released into its surrounding environment, where it prompts healthy cells to manufacture an enzyme that counters infection. This antiviral action is exerted before the synthesis of immunoglobulins specific for the virus reaches protective levels. The elaboration of interferons from virally infected cells continues for a few hours (up to about 24 hours) after infection, thereby playing a significant role in isolating the infective foci in many, but not all, viral infections.

Although viruses seem to be the most potent agents for the induction of interferon, other intracellular parasites such as rickettsia, bacteria, and parasites may also trigger its formation. Even bacterial and fungal extracts, as well as materials such as double-stranded RNA, synthetic polymers, and plant extracts, may serve as signals.

Different cell types in the human body produce three distinct types of interferons, and each type appears to exert different protective effects. *Interferon alpha* is produced by lymphocytes and has antiviral activity. Fibroblasts, epithelial cells, and macrophages form *interferon beta,* which is definitely antiviral. *Interferon gamma* is produced by T lymphocytes and has an immunoregulatory effect (Figure 20-9).

In addition to their antiviral activities, the interferons are capable of inhibiting cell growth by slowing down cell replication and enhancing NK cell activity. Therefore they are considered an important medical resource as antitumor agents.

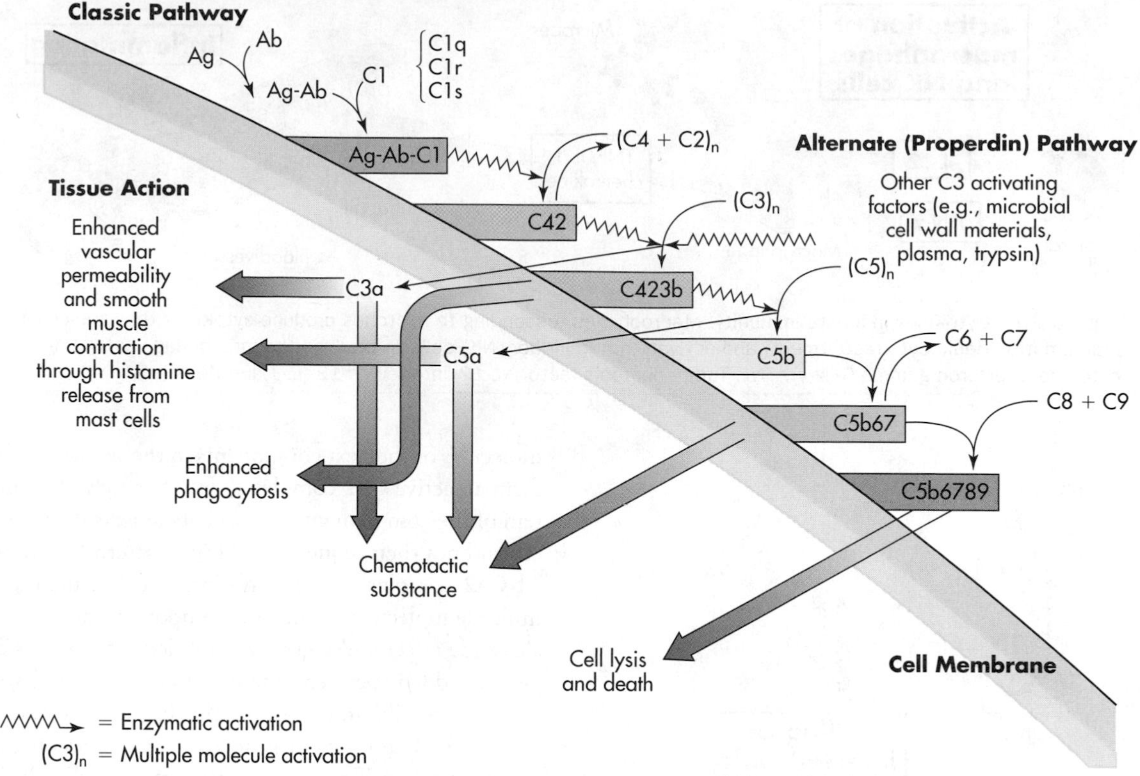

Figure 20-8 Classic and alternate complement cascade. Sequence of complement activation generates multiple biologically active intermediate molecules, which are active in inflammatory response.

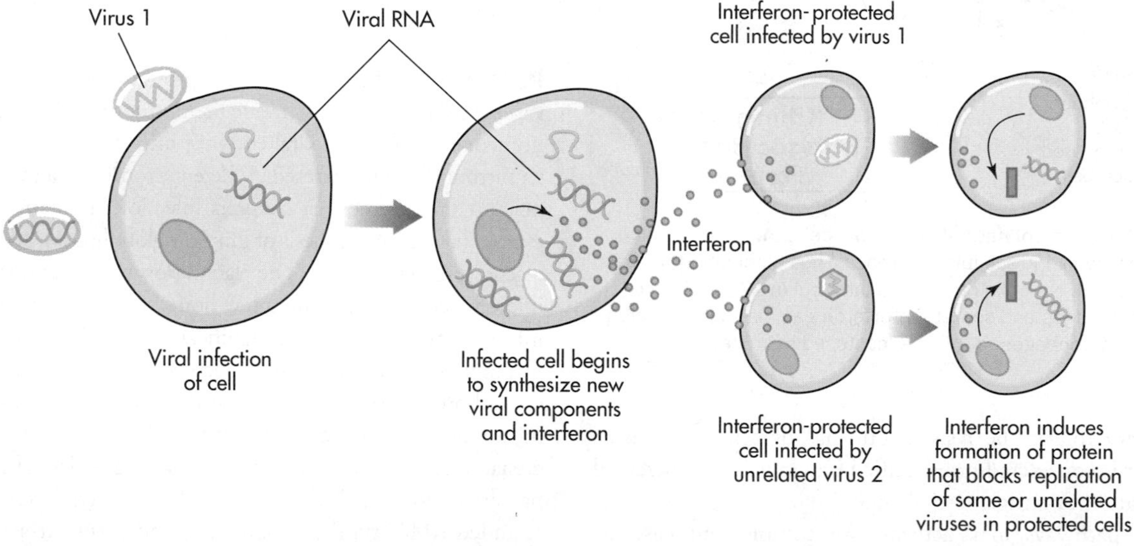

Figure 20-9 Mechanisms of interferon action. *RNA*, Ribonucleic acid.

> **ARE YOU READY?**
>
> During change of shift, the off-going nurse states that a patient has a "shift to the left" when describing the complete blood count. The oncoming nurse interprets this as which of the following?
>
> 1. There is an increased number of immature neutrophils.
> 2. The patient's infection is resolving.
> 3. There is a decreased number of basophils.
> 4. The patient is showing signs of immunosuppression.

STAGES OF INFLAMMATION. Inflammation is divided into five stages: injury, vascular response, fluid exudation, cellular exudation, and repair or healing (Table 20-3).

INJURY. Any type of exogenous (outside the body) or endogenous (inside the body) injury can initiate the inflammatory response: heat; cold; irradiation; chemical (toxin or poison); trauma, including surgery; infection; immunologic injury (hypersensitivity reaction); ischemic damage; or neoplasia. Whatever the

TABLE 20-3 STEPS IN INFLAMMATORY RESPONSE

Steps	Mediators	Outcome
1. Injury	Physical, chemical, biologic, immunologic stimulus	Cell and tissue injury
2. Vascular response		
a. Vascular dilation	Histamine, plasmin, serotonin, kinins, prostaglandins released or activated by injury	Dilation of vessels, causing stasis of blood and margination of leukocytes
b. Fibrin clot formation	Activation of clotting mechanism	Containment of irritants
3. Fluid exudation	Histamine, kinins, prostaglandins causing opening of venule-endothelial cell junction	Fluid exudation into tissues
4. Cellular exudation		
a. Leukocyte exudation	Chemotactic substances released by complement activation, clot formation, injured cells	Passage of leukocytes from blood to site of injury and accumulation there
b. Attack and engulfment of foreign materials	Neutrophils, macrophages	Removal and digestion of bacteria, foreign particles, damaged tissues
5. Healing	Fibroblasts producing collagen fibers, tissue regeneration	Resolution of inflammation; formation of scar tissue

stimulus, the response itself is the same, but the degree of response varies with the type and severity of the injury.

VASCULAR RESPONSE. The vascular response consists of transitory vasoconstriction followed by immediate vasodilation. This reaction is due to vasoactive chemical mediators such as histamine, serotonin, or kinins being released at the site of injury or invasion. The mediators cause an increase in blood flow to the area *(hyperemia)*, causing redness and heat. They also cause increased permeability of the capillary walls, which, along with the increased hydrostatic pressure secondary to increased blood flow, results in the exudation of fluid out of the capillaries and into the interstitial spaces. The extra fluid dilutes toxins and microorganisms in the area and serves as the vehicle by which phagocytes and nutrients needed for healing reach the injured site.[8]

FLUID EXUDATION. Fluid exudation from the capillaries into the interstitial spaces begins immediately and is most active during the first 24 hours after injury or invasion. Initially the fluid exudate is primarily serous fluid, but as the capillary wall becomes more permeable, protein (albumin) is lost into the interstitial spaces. This increases the colloid osmotic pressure in these spaces, which encourages more fluid exudation, producing tissue swelling, or edema.

CELLULAR EXUDATION. Cellular exudation occurs when WBCs are summoned to the vessels in the affected area as a result of the release of chemotactic substances from injured cells and activation of complement. The WBCs adhere to the capillary wall and then migrate through the wall by way of widened endothelial junctions. Neutrophils (polymorphonuclear leukocytes, PMNs) are the first leukocytes to respond, usually within the first few hours. Neutrophils ingest the bacteria and dead tissue cells and then die, releasing proteolytic enzymes that liquefy the dead neutrophils, dead bacteria, and other dead cells, forming *pus*. Monocytes, which continue the phagocytosis, and lymphocytes, which play a role in the antigen-antibody response at the site, appear later (see discussion later in chapter).

HEALING. The inflammatory response contains the spread of bacteria and prepares tissues for healing by two overlapping processes: reconstruction and maturation. For repair to proceed, acute inflammation must subside and pus and dead tissue must be removed. Pus is the local accumulation of dead phagocytes, dead bacteria, and dead tissue. The bacteria most frequently causing this reaction are staphylococci, streptococci, *Neisseria* organisms, and *Pseudomonas aeruginosa (Pseudomonas pyocyanea)*. A collection of pus that is localized by a zone of inflamed tissue is called an *abscess* (Figure 20-10). When pus collects in a preexisting cavity such as the pleura or gallbladder, it is called *empyema*. An abscess that develops a suppurating channel that ruptures onto the surface or into a body cavity is called a *sinus*. A tubelike passage forming from an epithelium-lined organ or normal body cavity to the surface or to another organ or cavity is called a *fistula*.

Repair of a wound involves three processes: (1) filling in the wound, (2) sealing the wound, and (3) shrinking the wound. Injuries that involve little or no tissue loss and require little sealing or shrinking, such as a surgical incision, heal by *primary intention*. When the injury produces a large amount of tissue loss, as in a gouging wound or pressure ulcer, more tissue repair is required and healing occurs from the bottom of the wound to the top by *secondary intention*[5] (Figure 20-11).

Reconstruction. Once the inflamed area is clean or debrided, reconstruction begins and new cells are produced to fill in the space left by the injury. To prevent the spread of bacteria, fibroblasts are attracted to the area and secrete fibrin, a threadlike substance that encircles the affected area to wall it off from healthy tissue. If anything interferes with this walling-off process, bacteria can spread into the surrounding tissues. Thus abscesses should not

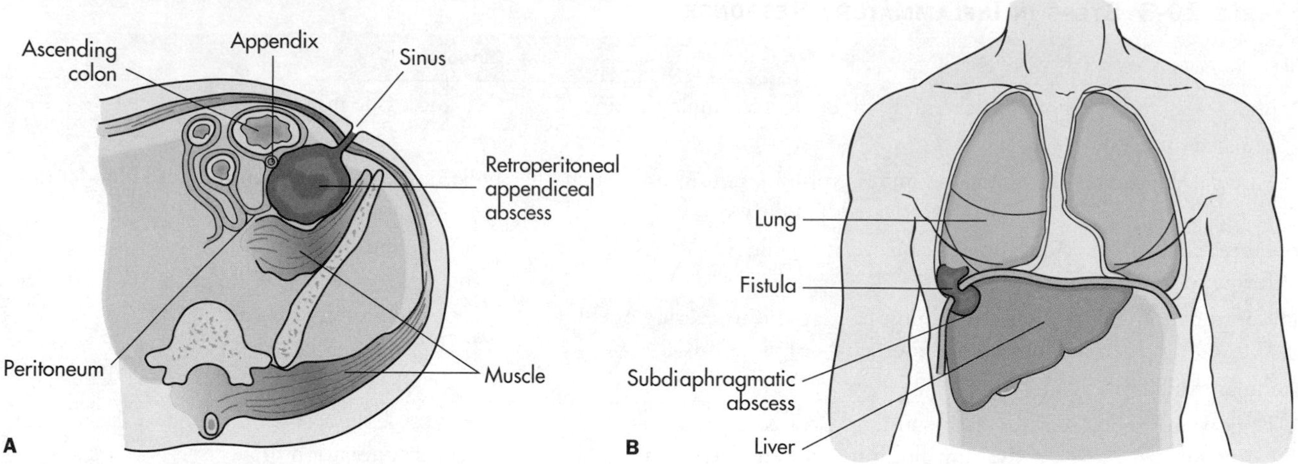

Figure 20-10 **A,** Cross-section of torso showing appendiceal abscess with sinus that has developed through abdominal wall. **B,** Subdiaphragmatic abscess that has developed fistula opening into pleural cavity.

be incised and drained until they have localized or "come to a head," which indicates the walling-off process has been completed.

New cells may be normal and functional (parenchymal) or nonfunctional fibrotic cells, which are scar tissue. Some body tissues readily regenerate, whereas others do not. Bone marrow; the epithelial layer of the skin; and mucous membranes of the respiratory, GI, and genitourinary tracts consist of labile cells that continually regenerate over the life span. Hence their regeneration is rapid and effective. Bone, liver, pancreas, and kidney cells have parenchyma composed of stable cells that normally stop regenerating when full growth is attained. These cells are capable of regeneration, but it takes longer than for tissues composed of labile cells. Nerve cells, skeletal muscle cells, and cardiac muscle cells are permanent or fixed cells and are unable to regenerate. These cells are always replaced with fibrous tissue.

Maturation. Maturation follows the reconstructive phase. During maturation, which can last months to years, scar tissue is remodeled; capillaries contract, leaving an avascular scar; and structure and function of damaged tissue are restored.[5] If a large amount of tissue is destroyed, replacement with parenchymal cells may not be possible, regardless of the type of tissue, and abnormalities of healing such as keloids or adhesions may form.

MANIFESTATIONS OF INFLAMMATION. The five cardinal symptoms of inflammation, first identified many centuries ago, are (1) redness (rubor), (2) heat (calor) caused by the hyperemia, (3) swelling (tumor) caused by the fluid exudate, (4) pain (dolor) caused by the pressure of the fluid exudate and by chemical (bradykinin and prostaglandins) irritation of the nerve endings, and (5) loss of function of the affected part caused by the swelling and pain. The amount of pain and related loss of function depend on the location and extent of injury (Figure 20-12).

REGIONAL MANIFESTATIONS: LYMPH NODES. If bacteria cannot be contained locally, they may spread to other parts of the body by means of the lymph system or bloodstream. If picked up by the lymph stream, bacteria are carried to the nearest lymph node where they can be ingested and destroyed. If the bacteria are virulent enough to resist the action of the lymph nodes, leukocytes are brought in by the bloodstream to attack and engulf the bacteria in the node. The node then becomes swollen and tender because of the accumulation of phagocytes, bacteria, and destroyed lymphoid tissue. This process is known as *lymphadenitis.* Swollen lymph nodes can be palpated primarily in the neck, axilla, and groin (Figure 20-13).

SYSTEMIC MANIFESTATIONS. Moderate-to-severe inflammatory responses can produce systemic manifestations. The three major systemic manifestations are (1) increased body temperature (fever), (2) increased WBCs in peripheral circulation (leukocytosis), and (3) increased erythrocyte sedimentation rate.

Generalized fever is produced by the release of substances known as endogenous pyrogens at the inflammatory site. Pyrogens are substances released from injured cells, materials released by WBCs that accumulate at the site, and components of the cell wall of invading bacteria. Prostaglandins, leukotrienes, bacterial endotoxins, and interleukin-1 are all pyrogens. These substances are carried to the temperature-regulating center in the hypothalamic region of the brain, where they signal a resetting of the body temperature set-point. The body responds by increasing heat production and decreasing heat loss. As long as the pyrogens remain in circulation, the set-point stays elevated. The fever response is part of the defense mechanism and helps increase production of antimicrobial agents such as interferon. It also tends to support increased phagocytic activity of some cells, including macrophages.

Leukocytosis develops when leukopoietins, agents released from damaged cells and from WBCs accumulating at the inflammatory site, are carried by the circulation to the bone marrow, where WBCs are produced. When leukopoietins reach the bone marrow, they signal the release of mature neutrophils held in reserve there. This leads to an immediate increase in the WBC count in the peripheral circulation to more than $10,000/mm^3$. Chemotactic agents draw these cells to the inflammatory site. Leukopoietins also increase the production of WBCs in the bone marrow. During prolonged inflammation the bone marrow stores

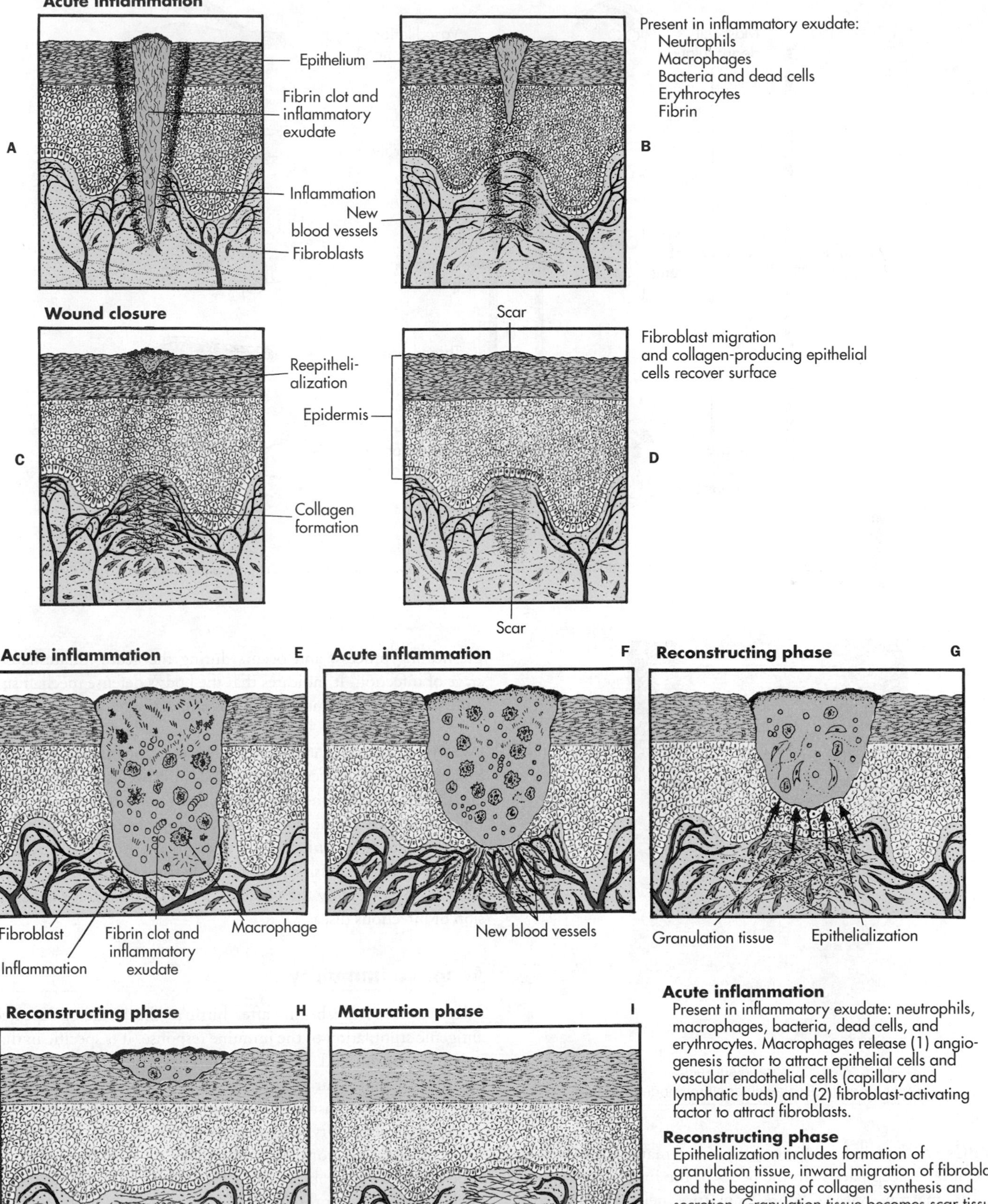
Acute inflammation
A
Epithelium
Fibrin clot and inflammatory exudate
Inflammation
New blood vessels
Fibroblasts
B
Present in inflammatory exudate:
Neutrophils
Macrophages
Bacteria and dead cells
Erythrocytes
Fibrin
Wound closure
C
Reepitheli-alization
Epidermis
Collagen formation
Scar
D
Fibroblast migration and collagen-producing epithelial cells recover surface
Scar
Acute inflammation
E
Fibroblast
Inflammation
Fibrin clot and inflammatory exudate
Macrophage
Acute inflammation
F
New blood vessels
Reconstructing phase
G
Granulation tissue
Epithelialization
Reconstructing phase
H
Collagen fibers
Maturation phase
I
Scar tissue
Acute inflammation
Present in inflammatory exudate: neutrophils, macrophages, bacteria, dead cells, and erythrocytes. Macrophages release (1) angiogenesis factor to attract epithelial cells and vascular endothelial cells (capillary and lymphatic buds) and (2) fibroblast-activating factor to attract fibroblasts.
Reconstructing phase
Epithelialization includes formation of granulation tissue, inward migration of fibroblasts, and the beginning of collagen synthesis and secretion. Granulation tissue becomes scar tissue, contraction begins, and differentiation begins.
Maturation phase
This phase includes completion of contraction, differentiation and remodeling of scar tissue, and disappearance of capillaries from scar tissue.

Figure 20-11 Wound repair by primary or secondary intention. **A** to **D,** Healing by primary intention. **E** to **I,** Healing by secondary intention.

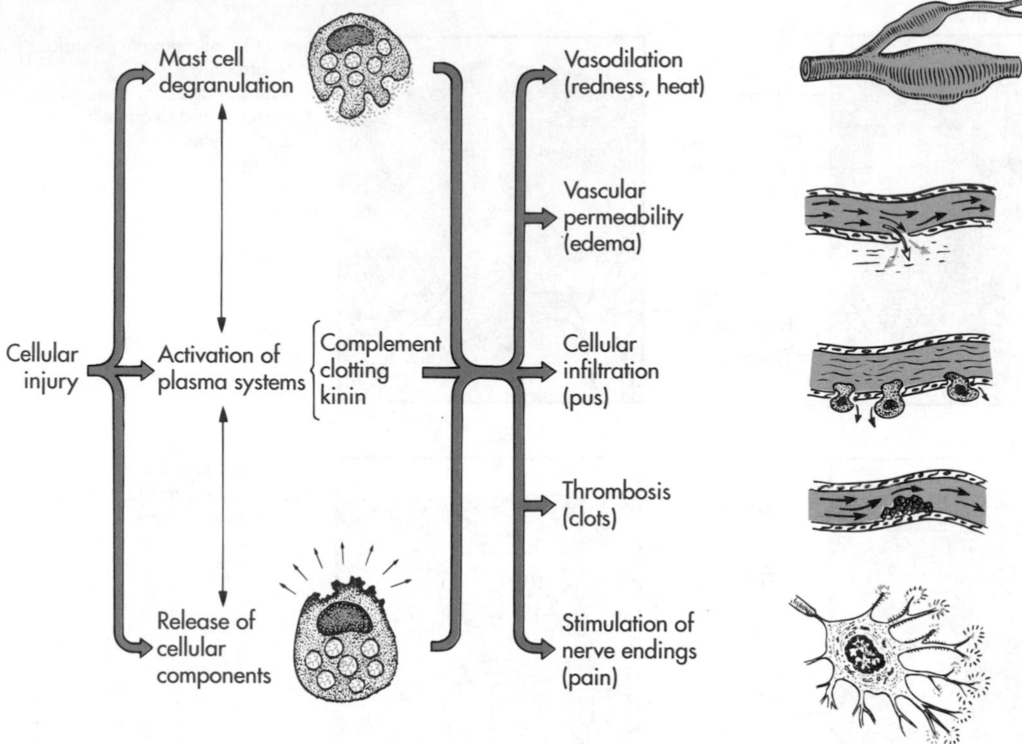

Figure 20-12 Sequence of events producing clinical manifestations associated with acute inflammatory response.

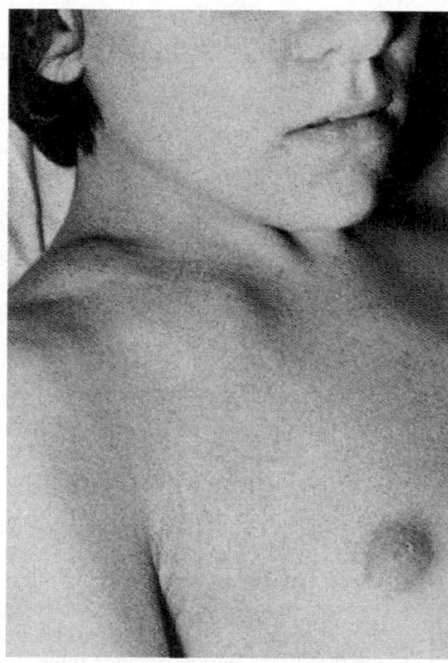

Figure 20-13 Enlarged supraclavicular and infraclavicular lymph nodes.

of WBCs are depleted, and the synthesis of mature WBCs may not be able to keep pace with the needs of the inflammatory site; thus the marrow releases more immature neutrophils as the inflammation continues.

When an anticoagulant is added to blood in the laboratory, the red blood cells (RBCs or erythrocytes) settle to the bottom of a test tube more rapidly than normal. This diagnostic test is called the erythrocyte sedimentation rate (ESR). An elevated ESR is related to an increase in fibrinogen, a blood protein essential to the healing process, and occurs during the acute inflammatory stage of infection. It indicates that the body's defense mechanisms aimed at repair of damaged tissue are operating.

Infection vs. Inflammation. The concepts of infection and inflammation are sometimes confused. Infection is the presence of a pathogenic organism in the body that multiplies and produces injurious effects to the host. Inflammation occurs in response to infection and tissue injury. Injury may occur from the spread of the pathogenic organisms through body tissues or from the effects of toxins produced by the pathogens. See Chapter 6 for a discussion of infectious diseases.

Adaptive Immunity

Adaptive immunity begins after birth as the result of repeated antigenic stimulation of the immune response. It is specific in that it is initiated by and targeted against specific antigens such as microbes or molecular entities. Adaptive immunity provides lifelong protection against many diseases.

Adaptive immunity follows exposure to antigens or the transfer of antibodies from one individual to another. Antigens, which may be microbes or other substances (polysaccharides, nucleoproteins, lipoproteins, and glycoproteins), are recognized as nonself and elicit the formation of antibodies (reactive proteins), or specifically sensitized cells called cytotoxic lymphocytes, or both. Particularly small molecules cannot induce the formation of antibodies unless they are coupled with a high-molecular-weight carrier. These molecules are known as incomplete antigens or *haptens*.

Immune cells recognize a part of the antigen molecule known as the *antigenic determinant,* which elicits the formation and proliferation of antibodies and cytotoxic lymphocytes. These antibodies and lymphocytes subsequently bind to the antigenic determinant. Binding can have direct beneficial effects such as detoxification of toxins; inactivation of viruses; or, when coupled with complement, the direct lysis of cells. In most cases, however, the antigen-antibody combination initiates and facilitates innate defense mechanisms such as phagocytosis, the complement cascade, and the inflammatory response. The specific type of immune response—that is, synthesis of antibodies, development of antigen-reactive lymphocytes, or a combination of the two—varies with the characteristics of each individual antigen.

Adaptive immunity possesses memory, which allows it to remember prior contact with antigenic material. It takes days to weeks for the immune system to produce a sufficient response to be protective after initial exposure to the antigen. However, the immune system is able to respond faster and more vigorously to subsequent encounters with the same antigen.

Types of Immunity. Immunity acquired from exposure to antigens such as measles is *active* immunity. It is active because the host's immune system recognizes the antigen and actively responds to it. Active immunity provides permanent protection against many diseases. *Artificially acquired active immunity* occurs from vaccines that prompt the same immune reaction as the actual antigen. Sometimes periodic booster vaccines are required to maintain permanent immunity.

Adaptive immunity that is transferred from one person to another is known as *passively acquired* immunity. It is passive because the host's immune system is not involved in production of the protective antibodies. Antibodies may be received through a natural pathway, such as infants who receive antibodies from their mother in utero and through breast milk. This type of immunity is known as *naturally acquired passive immunity.* Immunoglobulins acquired through injections of gamma globulin, antiserum, and immune serum provide passive immunity that is artificially acquired, since it is not transferred via natural pathways. Naturally and artificially acquired passive immunity provides short-term, temporary protection against diseases such as hepatitis, tetanus, rabies, and snake bites. Table 20-4 summarizes the types of adaptive specific immunity.

Functional Components of Adaptive Immunity. Adaptive immunity has two complex functional components. One is a **cell-mediated immunity** that provides cytotoxic lymphocytes.

TABLE 20-4 TYPES OF ADAPTIVE SPECIFIC IMMUNITY

Type of Immunity	Acquisition of Immunity	Protection	Examples
ACTIVE			
Antibodies synthesized by body in response to antigenic stimulation	*Natural:* natural contact with antigen through clinical or subclinical case	*Development:* develops slowly; protective levels reached in few weeks *Duration:* long term; often lifetime *Spectrum:* specific to antigen contacted	Recovery from childhood diseases (e.g., chickenpox, measles, mumps)
	Artificial: immunization with antigen	*Development:* develops slowly; protective levels reached in few weeks *Duration:* several years; extended protection with "booster" doses *Spectrum:* specific to antigen immunized against	Immunization with live or killed vaccines; toxoid immunization
PASSIVE			
Antibodies produced in one individual transferred to another	*Natural:* transplacental and colostrum transfer from mother to child	*Development:* immediate *Duration:* temporary; several months *Spectrum:* all antigens that mother has immunity to	Maternal immunoglobulins passed to neonate
	Artificial: injection of serum from immune human or animal	*Development:* immediate *Duration:* temporary; several weeks *Spectrum:* all antigens that source has immunity to	Injection of pooled human gamma globulin; injection of animal hyperimmune sera

The other is a **humoral immunity** that provides circulating antibodies. Cells of both components are derived from undifferentiated stem cells of the bone marrow. The primary cells of the immune system develop from lymphocytic cells (Figure 20-14). One population of lymphocytes differentiates under the influence of the thymus gland and become thymus-dependent lymphocytes, or T cells. These cells are responsible for facilitating cell-mediated immunity. The second population of lymphocytes matures in a site other than the thymus and is known as thymus-independent lymphocytes, or B cells. B cells are responsible for producing immunoglobulins and providing humoral immunity. B and T lymphocytes are distinguished from one another by the specific markers (membrane-bound proteins) on their surfaces.

Cell-Mediated Immunity. Cell-mediated adaptive immunity offers protection from (1) chronic bacterial infections (e.g., syphilis, tuberculosis, leprosy), (2) many viral infections (e.g., measles, herpesvirus infections, chickenpox), (3) fungal infections (e.g., candidiasis, histoplasmosis, cryptococcosis), (4) parasitic infections (e.g., leishmaniasis, toxoplasmosis, and *Pseudomonas carinii*), and (5) transplanted or transformed cells (e.g., tissue transplants and some cancer cells).

T cells, which are part of cellular immunity, make two important contributions to internal defense. They are vital to the coordination of cellular and humoral immunity, and they directly attack and kill antigens. T cells are produced in the bone marrow and mature in the thymus gland. From the thymus gland they migrate to regional lymph nodes and the spleen, where they populate the medullary regions. Each mature immunosensitive T cell is capable of responding to a specific antigen. On exposure to its specific antigen, T cells proliferate and enter the circulation where they are transported throughout the body. Several T lymphocyte subsets act to regulate T cell function and augment production of antibodies by B cells. Helper or inducer T cells (also called TH, T4, or CD4 cells) are essential for activating other T lymphocytes, B lymphocytes, NK cells, and macrophages. Without the helper T cell, B cells are unable to make sufficient antibodies to protect against most invading antigens.

Cytotoxic T cells (T_c) attack and destroy antigen or antigenically labeled cells on site. Specifically they attack infected, tumor, and foreign graft cells.[7] Suppressor T cells (T_S or T8) prevent or modify the functions of the two adaptive immunity systems. It is thought that they turn off the specific immune reaction when it is no longer needed. Delayed cells (TD) are involved in delayed

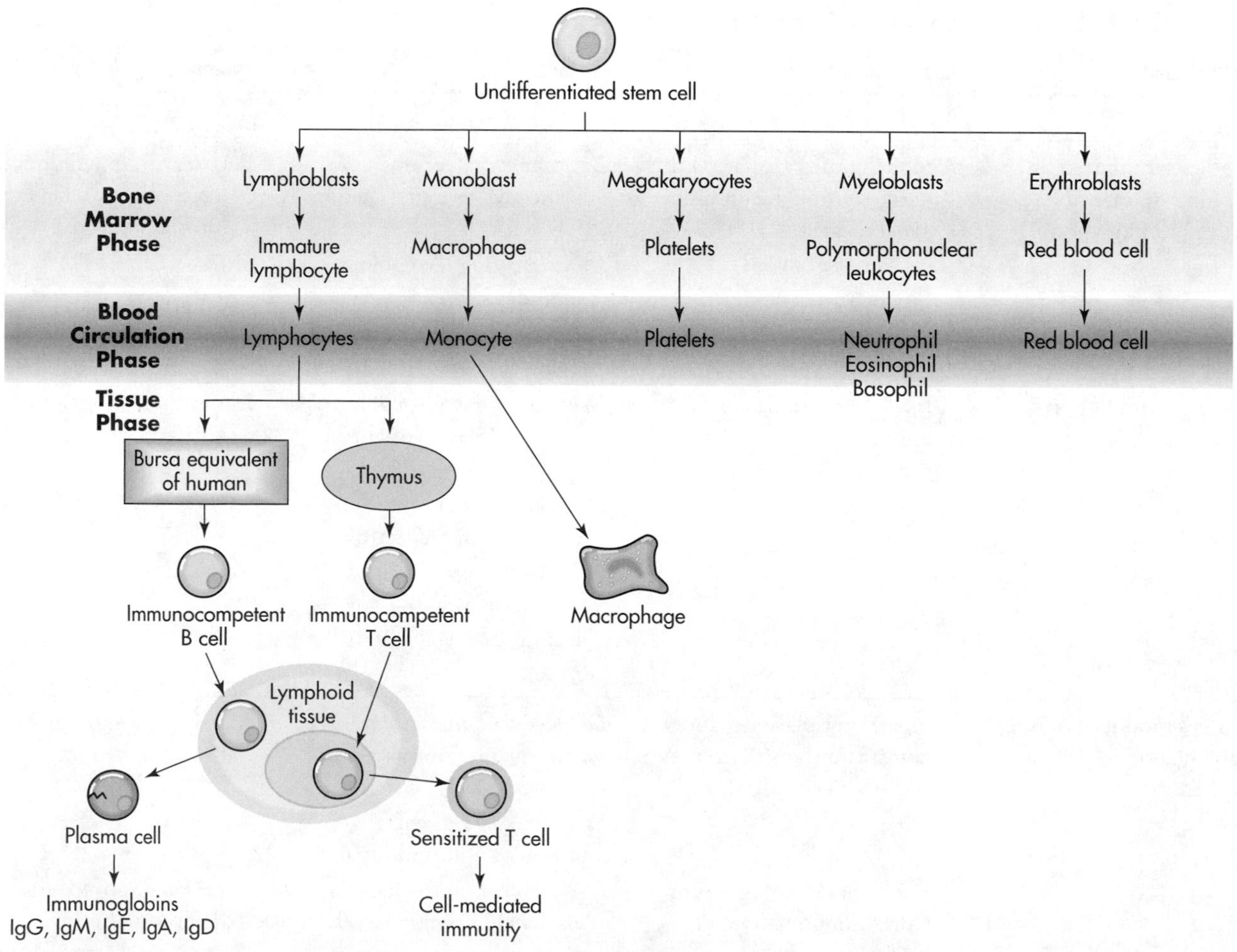

Figure 20-14 Development of B and T lymphocytes. Undifferentiated stem cells move from bone marrow to either thymus gland or bursa-equivalent, where they are transformed into T cells or B cells. They then move to one of secondary lymphoid organs, where they may contact an antigen and become activated.

hypersensitivity involving fungi and mycobacteria allergic responses. The last subset of T lymphocytes is the memory T cell (TM), which remembers contact with specific antigens and immediately responds on subsequent exposure (Figure 20-15).

T lymphocytes work primarily by secreting potent chemical messengers known as cytokines, or specifically lymphokines. Lymphokines are soluble substances that recruit and activate phagocytic cells, components of the inflammatory response, and lymphokine-activated killer cells.[5] Helper T cells produce a lymphokine known as interleukin-2, which stimulates the production of NK cells that target tumor cells and virally infected cells. NK cells are similar to the cytotoxic T cell subset, but do not need to recognize a specific antigen to attack. Once activated by interleukin-2, NK cells release potent chemicals that kill on contact.[9] Table 20-5 summarizes the functions of the various T cell subsets.

HUMORAL IMMUNITY. The humorally mediated system provides major immunity against (1) bacteria that produce acute infection (such as *Staphylococcus, Streptococcus,* and *Haemophilus* organisms), (2) bacterial exotoxins (diphtheria, botulinum, and tetanus toxins), (3) viruses that must enter the bloodstream to reach their target tissues (e.g., poliomyelitis and hepatitis virus), and (4) organisms that enter the body from the mucosal tissues (e.g., cold viruses, enteroviruses, and influenza viruses). Even though circulating antibodies may be produced against other organisms (such as tuberculosis, human immunodeficiency virus [HIV], and fungi), these antibodies do not protect the body from infection.

B lymphocytes, which are part of humoral immunity, are produced and primarily mature in the bone marrow. After maturing, B lymphocytes migrate to the spleen and lymphoid tissues located along the gut, bronchus, and tonsils, since these are strategic locations that are continuously exposed to antigens.[7] Immunosensitive B lymphocytes are programmed to respond to a single antigen. When the antigen is present, B cells proliferate and differentiate into plasma cells. Plasma cells are designed to synthesize and release large amounts of immunoglobulin (antibody) into the circulation, where they become part of the gamma-globulin fraction of the serum. From there, they attach to the antigen prompting their production.

Immunoglobulin-producing B cells remain in the lymphoid tissue and continue to synthesize additional molecules of the specific antibody. This process differs from the T cell response in which cytotoxic T cells are released from lymphoid tissue. B cells remain, and their product is released. Hence the level of active specific antibodies begins to rise in the serum fraction (antibody titer), as well as in the level of the gamma-globulin fraction in general. Antibodies bind to their specific antigen after being carried by the blood and other body fluids to the site where needed. On binding, the antibody may inactivate the antigen or activate

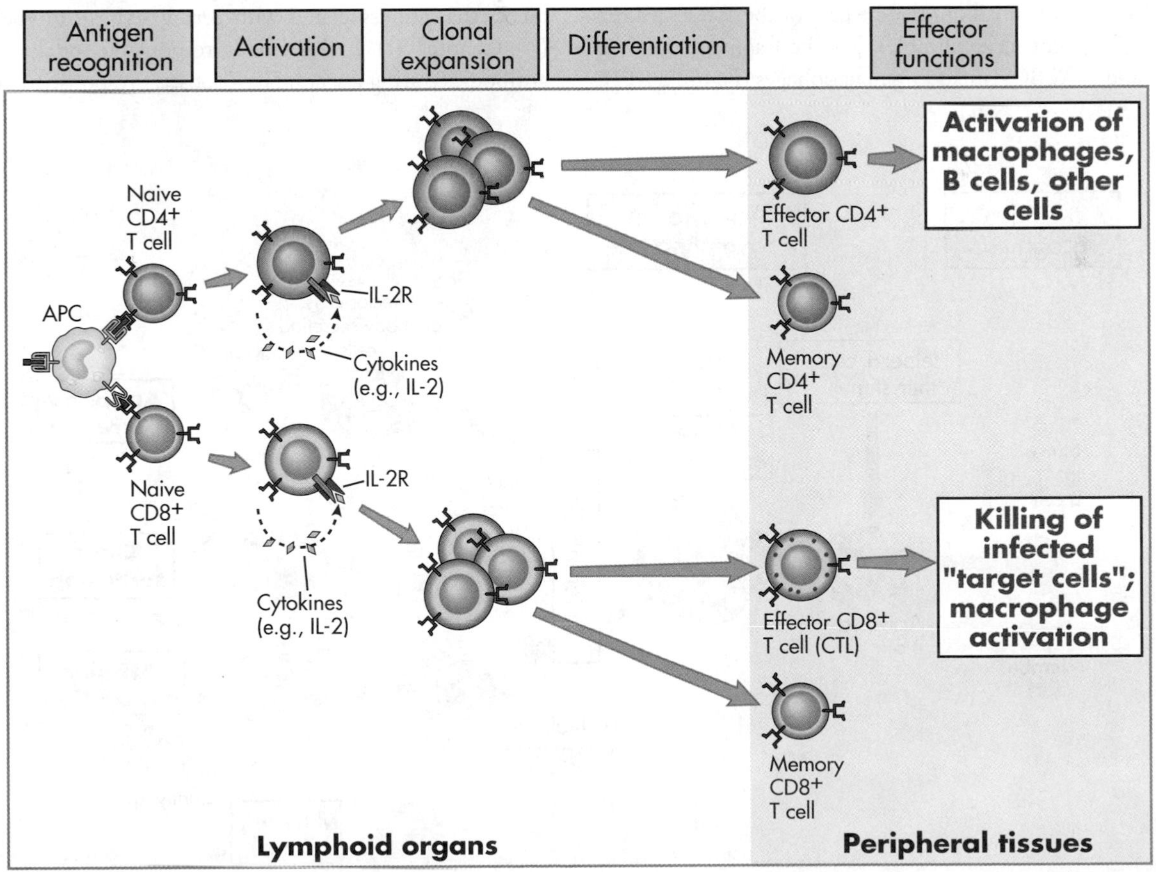

Figure 20-15 Cell-mediated immune response. T cells recognize foreign antigens and respond by producing cytokines and proliferating. Progeny cells differentiate into CD4 helper cells, CD8 suppressor cells, and memory cells that serve various functions in cell-mediated immunity. *APC,* Antigen-processing cell; *IL-2,* interleukin-2.

TABLE 20-5 FUNCTIONS OF VARIOUS T-CELL SUBSETS

T-Cell Subsets	Function(s)
Helper T cells (T4, T_H, CD4)	Release lymphokines that: Regulate antibody production by B cells Activate other T cells Activate macrophages Activate natural killer cells
Suppressor T cells (T8, T_S)	Prevent or modify functions of T cells and B cells May suppress immune reaction when no longer needed
Cytotoxic T cells (T_c)	Kill virus-infected cells, tumor cells, and foreign graft cells
Delayed T cells (T_d)	Cause delayed hypersensitivity Induce inflammatory response
Memory T cells (T_M)	Induce secondary immune response

other antigen-damaging processes, such as the complement cascade, to destroy it (Figure 20-16).

The immunoglobulins are subdivided into different classes on the basis of molecular structure and function (Table 20-6). The generic symbol for immunoglobulins is Ig, and each class is designated by a letter of the alphabet: IgG, IgM, IgA, IgE, and IgD. The basic structural pattern for all immunoglobulins is four-peptide chains arranged in a Y shape. At the ends of the two arms of the Y are the sites where antigen is bound. The base of the Y is called the Fc region (for fragment, crystallizable). The Fc fragment binds to complement and to WBCs, including macrophages (Figure 20-17).

The predominant class of immunoglobulins in normal adult serum is IgG, which makes up about 75% to 85% of the immunoglobulin fraction. IgG, which is capable of crossing the placenta to provide the newborn with temporary natural passive immunity to those diseases against which the mother has circulating antibodies, is also found in extravascular fluids. Its primary functions are to neutralize toxins and inactivate viruses and bacteria. It also forms antigen-antibody complement immune complexes that are associated with certain types of hypersensitivities (see Chapter 21). IgG is chiefly responsible for the rise in serum antibodies during a secondary (booster) response to an antigen.

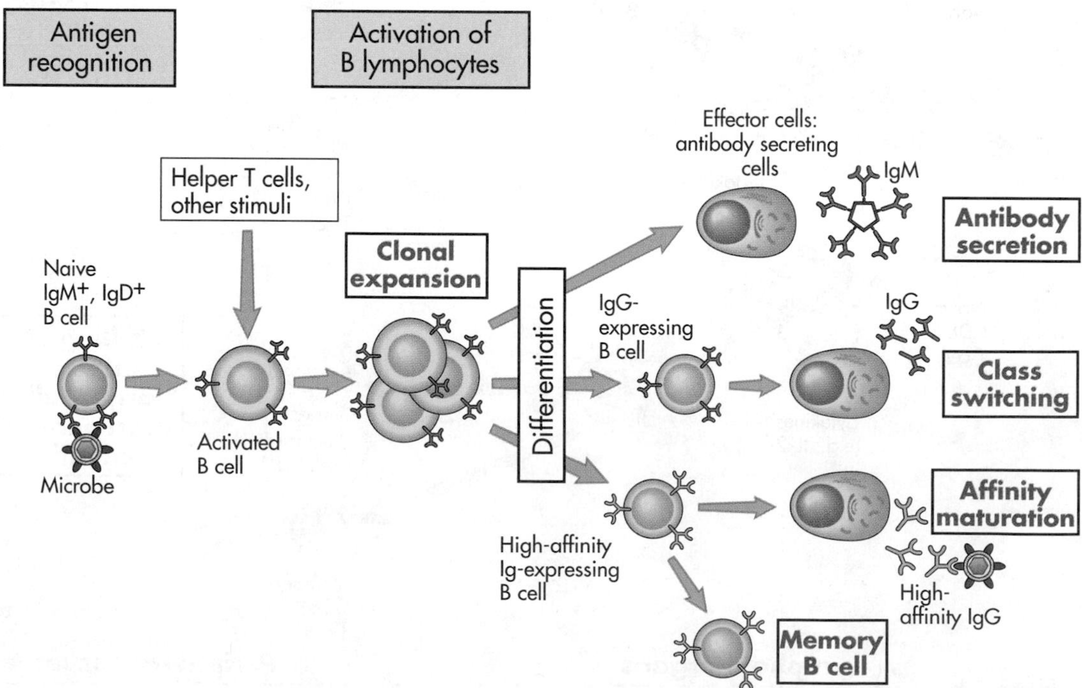

Figure 20-16 Humoral immune response. B lymphocytes recognize antigens, and under influence of helper T cells and other stimuli, B cells are activated, proliferate, and differentiate into antibody-secreting cells, some of which become memory cells.

TABLE 20-6 CHARACTERISTICS OF IMMUNOGLOBULINS

Class	Properties	Estimated Serum Concentration*	Location
IgG subtypes:	Major antibody found in blood	13.5 mg/ml	Interstitial fluids
	Coats microbes to facilitate destruction		Plasma
IgG 1-4	Complement activation		
	Neonatal immunity		
	Feedback inhibition of B cells		
IgA	Lines mucous membranes	3.5 mg/ml	Body secretions
	Protects against mucous membrane, bronchial, and digestive tract infections		Breast milk
	Neonatal passive immunity		
IgM	Primary immune response	1.5 mg/ml	Plasma
	Forms antibodies to ABO blood antigens		
	Complement activation		
IgD	Present on surface of B lymphocytes	Trace	Plasma
	Assists with B lymphocyte differentiation		
IgE	Mast cell activation (immediate hypersensitivity)	0.05 mg/ml	Interstitial fluids
	Defends against parasitic infections		Plasma
			Exocrine secretions

From Abbas AK, Lichtmann AH: *Basic immunology*, ed 2, Philadelphia, 2005, Saunders.

*Values are laboratory specific and age variable.

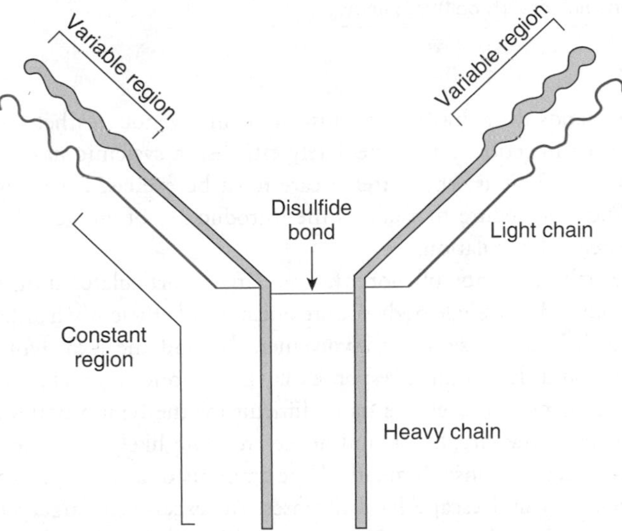

Figure 20-17 Basic antibody molecule is Y-shaped unit composed of two heavy chains and two light chains. Each chain has a constant region and a variable region that contains specific antigen-binding site.

IgM is primarily found in intravascular fluids and constitutes about 7% of the immunoglobulins in serum. Also called macroglobulin because of its molecular size, IgM, like IgG, is capable of initiating the complement cascade. In each antigenic stimulation, IgM antibodies are the first to appear, but they neither reach the levels of IgG nor exhibit a booster response on subsequent antigen contact. The chief function of IgM is to protect against viral and bacterial invaders in the blood. IgM, as a result of its ability to bind complement, is also involved in certain immune complex hypersensitivities and autoimmune diseases, such as rheumatoid arthritis.

About 10% of the total immunoglobulin in serum is IgA. IgA is termed the *secretory immunoglobulin* because it is found in the exocrine secretions of the body (milk, mucus, saliva, and tears). IgA specifically protects the mucosal surfaces of the respiratory, digestive, and genital tracts from pathogenic invasion by preventing the attachment of bacteria to epithelial surfaces.

IgD makes up only about 1% of the immunoglobulin fraction of serum, but its function is uncertain. Because most IgD is found on the surface of B cells, it is thought to play a role in activating or suppressing their function.

IgE is present in the serum in extremely small amounts (0.002%), since it selectively attaches to the surface of mast cells and basophils. When bound to the surface of these cells, which are rich in the potent, physiologically active vasoactive substances, IgE mediates hypersensitivity reactions such as hayfever, allergic asthma, and anaphylactic shock (see Chapter 21). The protective role of this immunoglobulin is unclear.

The humorally mediated B cell system is similar to the T cell system in that it is controlled by helper and suppressor T cells, produces memory cells, and is rendered self-tolerant by the same mechanisms. Figure 20-18 depicts the relationships and functions of macrophages, T cells, and B cells.

Cell-mediated or humoral immunity or both can be or become immunodeficient (see Chapter 21). When one system is not functioning properly, the person becomes susceptible to infection. For example, infection with HIV reduces the protection afforded by

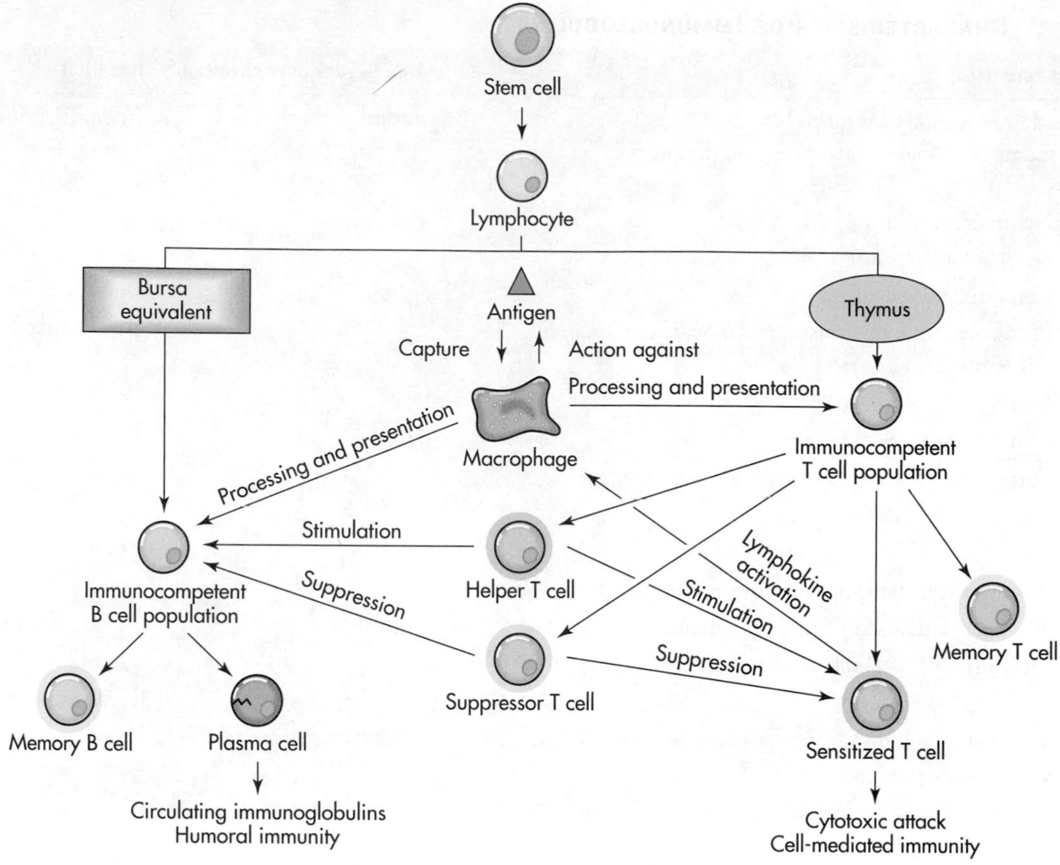

Figure 20-18 Combined response of cell-mediated (T cell) and humoral (B cell) immunity.

the cell-mediated system, making the individual susceptible to fungal infections (candidiasis), protozoan infections (*P. carinii* pneumonia), viral infections (herpesvirus infection), and cancers (Kaposi's sarcoma or lymphoma). Alternatively, the loss of the humoral immunity that occurs in X-linked (Bruton's) agammaglobulinemia is accompanied by increased acute bacterial infections, respiratory tract infections, and GI tract problems. If both systems are lost or compromised, the individual is fully susceptible to infectious agents and cannot survive in an unprotected, nonsterile environment.

▶ ARE You READY?

Which of the following immunoglobulins is primarily responsible for newborn temporary passive immunity?

1. IgA
2. IgE
3. IgD
4. IgG

Immune Response Sequence: Antigenic Challenge. When an antigen is introduced into the body (antigenic challenge), it triggers a spectrum of response mechanisms. The specific pattern of response depends on (1) the type of antigen introduced, (2) the site of introduction, and (3) the amount of antigen introduced. Highly invasive antigens (e.g., bacteria such as *S. aureus* or *Streptococcus pyogenes*) or those introduced directly into the bloodstream by blood transfusion, intravenous catheterization, or injection can immediately establish a systemic immune response. This is why extreme care must be exercised with any medical procedure that allows the introduction of antigens into the general circulation.

Small amounts of noninvasive, large, particulate antigens introduced at a single body site are quickly and efficiently handled with little or no systemic involvement beyond the local lymph nodes, and the immune response may go unnoticed. Small, soluble antigens, however, are more difficult for the lymph nodes to clear from the circulation and hence are more likely to induce a widespread response. Similarly, large amounts of any antigen can overwhelm and escape local defenses. An excessively large, sustained antigen dose can exhaust not only the local site but also the entire system. This greatly reduces the body's ability to respond to even minor invasive challenges and renders the host vulnerable to secondary infections.

When an antigenic substance is introduced into the body, it is engulfed by an antigen-processing cell (APC). There the antigen is degraded, and the antigenic determinants are attached to one of the cell membrane proteins on the surface of the APC, known as a major histocompatibility complex (MHC) antigen. These same MHC antigens are the markers on the cell's surface that allow recognition of self- versus nonself-cells. The APC, with the concentrated antigenic determinants, then presents the antigenic signal to specifically reactive B or T cells in the regional lymph node via cell-to-cell contact. From this interaction the specific B or T

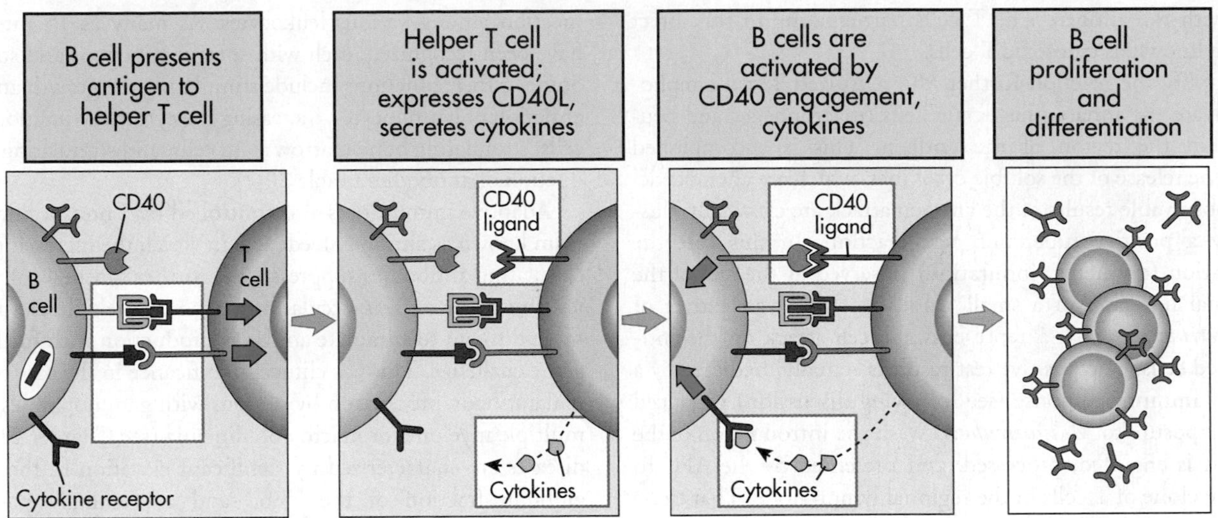

Figure 20-19 Activation of B cells by helper T cells. Helper T cells recognize and are activated by foreign antigens presented by B cells. They bind to receptors on the same B cells, activating B cell to produce specific antibodies against the antigen.

cell is stimulated to undergo proliferation (cell division) and differentiation (change in structure and function). The release of interleukin 1 from the APC signals the lymphocytes to divide and differentiate.[1]

The progeny of the stimulated cell increase in number within the lymph node, forming clones of specifically adapted lymphocytes. If a B cell is stimulated, each new generation of lymphocytes becomes more differentiated toward a cell population ideally suited for the synthesis and release of immunoglobulins. This occurs most effectively when influenced by helper $CD4^+$ (TH) cells (Figure 20-19).

Several days after the introduction of the antigen, antibodies to the antigen can be detected in the lymph node. It is not until about 7 days after the antigenic challenge, however, that detectable levels of specific antibodies appear in the serum. The plasma cell population of the lymph node and the levels of antibody in the blood continue to increase for another 2 to 3 weeks, and then both begin to retreat. Some of the B cell lymphocytes of the activated clone become memory cells, which are much more responsive, both in time of reaction and efficiency of antibody synthesis, to subsequent contact with the antigen (Figure 20-20).

T cell lymphocyte activation is similar to that of B cell activation. When an antigen comes in contact with a T cell, it sensitizes the T cell, causing it to proliferate and enter the circulation. Sensitized T cells migrate to the site where the antigen entered the body and where the invading agent or residual antigen is located. These activated T cell lymphocytes, along with macrophages, infiltrate the region and directly attack the antigen or tissue cells

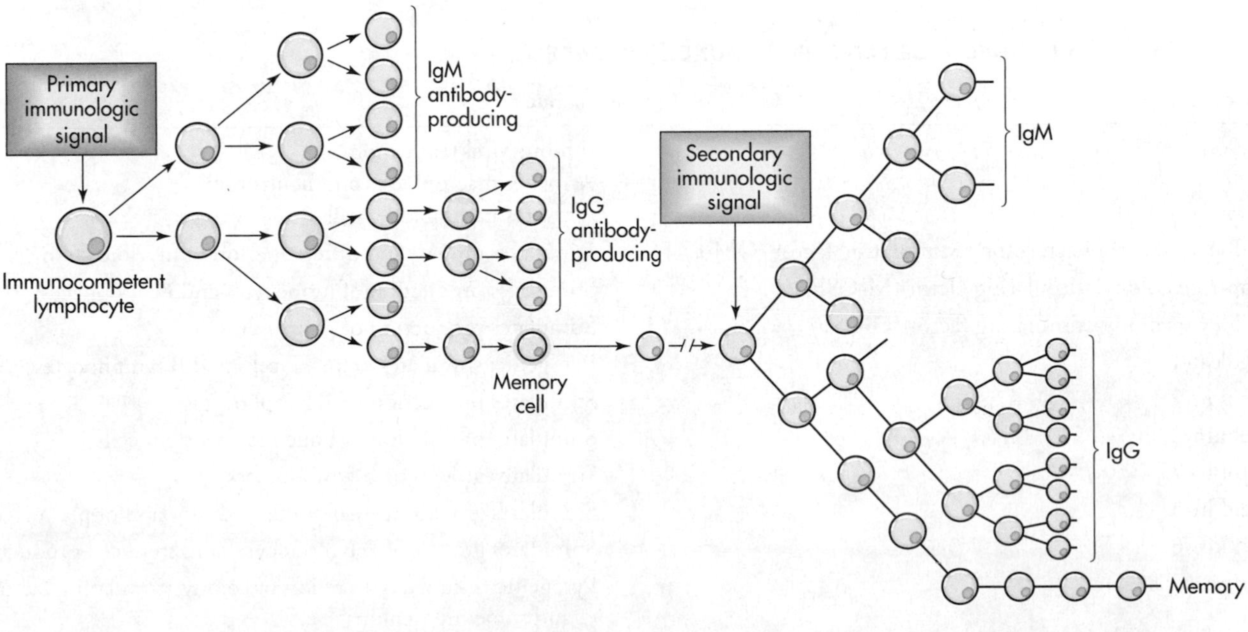

Figure 20-20 Response of memory cells to antigen challenge.

labeled with the antigen. The T cells participating in this direct attack are known as cytotoxic T cells.

To amplify the reaction further, the sensitized T cell lymphocytes activate the innate phagocytic cells (macrophages and neutrophils) in the region of the antigen. This is accomplished through the release of the soluble cytokines, which are chemotaxic.

The observable results of the antigen attack are classically illustrated by a positive tuberculin test reaction. In this case the inflammation (erythema, induration) observed at the site of the intradermal injection of a small amount of cell wall extract of *Mycobacterium tuberculosis* represents a T cell attack on the antigen-labeled cells. The positive test result is actually mediated by a secondary immune response (see following discussion) produced by prior exposure to *M. tuberculosis.* With the introduction of the antigen, it is engulfed, processed, and presented by the APC to responsive clone of T cells in the regional lymph node. That clone of cells is stimulated to undergo proliferation, and activated T cells are released into circulation. They seek out the antigen (at the site of injection) and begin to accumulate at the site and release cytokines (lymphokines) that stimulate neutrophils and macrophages to attack the antigens at the focal site. The lag time (24 to 48 hours) required for the development of inflammation at the site is consistent with the time needed to trigger the release of the responsive cells from the regional lymph node and for them to accumulate at the site of the antigen-labeled tissues.

Control of Adaptive Immunity. Cytokines are soluble protein mediators that induce and control various aspects of immunity. They act as hormones and are synthesized by a variety of cells: macrophages, neutrophils, eosinophils, monocytes, and T lymphocytes. These protein mediators have been called by various names. Initially they were termed *lymphokines* because many of them were produced by activated T cell lymphocytes. When it was generally acknowledged that other cells secreted them as well, they were termed *cytokines*. An even more specific name, *interleukins*, recognizes that the major function of many of the cytokines is communication among various leukocytes. As many as 15 interleukins have been recognized, each with specific functions and structures. Some of their functions include stimulating the growth and differentiation of lymphocytes, increasing the cytotoxic functions of NK cells, stimulating bone marrow stem cells, and stimulating the production of antibodies (Table 20-7).

Adaptive immunity is also controlled by a nonspecific mechanism known as antibody feedback, in which the increasing level of circulating antibodies suppresses the further synthesis of antibodies. In other words, if circulating antibody levels are elevated, it is more difficult to stimulate antibody production with further antigenic challenge. This has clinical significance in the case of abnormal antibody production by persons with gammopathies, such as multiple myeloma or macroglobulinemia (see Chapter 21). These diseases are characterized by significant elevation in the gammaglobulin fraction of the blood and a seemingly paradoxical increase in susceptibility to infection. The high levels of nonspecific gamma globulin exert an immunosuppressive effect on further specific antibody synthesis when the host is challenged by a pathogen.

The presence of the helper T cells, which cooperate with the B cells and other T cells to allow the full expression of a B cell or T cell response, further controls adaptive immunity. If a B cell requires the aid of a helper T cell that is missing, the B cell will not undergo proliferation and differentiation to form plasma cells that produce the specific immunoglobulin. On the other hand, the presence of suppressor T cells prevents or suppresses the full development of immunoresponsive lymphocytes. If the normal balance between immunoresponsive T or B cells and suppressor and helper T cells is disrupted, control over proper immune response reactions may be lost. The classic example of this problem is acquired immunodeficiency syndrome (AIDS), in which a disproportionate ratio occurs in the number of suppressor T cells compared with helper T cells in peripheral circulation; this results from destruction of the helper T cells caused by HIV infection. In other conditions, such as some autoimmune diseases, the loss of

TABLE 20-7 CYTOKINES LIBERATED IN IMMUNE RESPONSE

Cytokine	Function
Interferon	Inhibits viral replication Activates macrophages and neutrophils Activates natural killer cells
Granulocyte-macrophage colony-stimulating factor (GM-CSF)	Stimulates growth and differentiation of myeloid stem cells
Macrophage colony-stimulating factor (M-CSF)	Stimulates production of monocytes and macrophages
Granulocyte colony-stimulating factor (G-CSF)	Stimulates production of neutrophils
Interleukin-1	Pyrogenic; stimulates helper T cells and B lymphocytes
Interleukin-2	Stimulates production of T lymphocytes
Interleukin-3	Stimulates production of bone marrow stem cells
Interleukin-4	Stimulates growth of B lymphocytes
Interleukin-5	Stimulates growth of eosinophils and function of plasma cells
Interleukin-6	Stimulates growth of B lymphocytes and stem cell production
Tumor necrosis factor	Pyrogenic; stimulates secretion of colony-stimulating factors and some interleukins

certain suppressor T cells may allow the production of antibodies against self-antigens.

In addition to these "in system" controls, immune cells are influenced by, and in turn influence, other regulatory systems in the body, specifically, the endocrine and neural systems. The immune response cells have receptors on their surfaces to receive modifying input from hormones, such as insulin, growth hormone, glucocorticoids, estrogen, and testosterone. Some of these hormone signals (glucocorticosteroids, testosterone, estrogen, and progesterone) have been shown to depress immune function. Other hormones (growth hormone, thyroxine, and insulin) tend to improve immune function. Other neurotransmitters and hormones found in lower doses in the body also influence immune response cell function. The negative effects of the corticosteroids are so great that they are widely used as pharmacologic agents to suppress immune function (see Chapters 21 and 22).

Primary and Secondary Immune Responses. The primary immune response occurs after the initial host exposure to a specific foreign antigen. Immune cells capture and decode the antigen for future recognition. After a significant lag time, antibodies formed against the antigen appear in the circulation. Immunoglobulins of the IgM class are the first to appear, but they maintain protective levels for only a short period. Specific IgG antibodies follow and reach protective levels within 12 to 14 days, but they also fall off fairly quickly after the initial exposure. Even so, the antigen has been "recognized" and the immune system "primed" for future encounters with the same antigen.[1]

On subsequent host exposure to the same antigen, the primed immune system generates a secondary response, which is more rapid, more intense, and longer lasting than the primary response. The secondary response is a characteristic of both the B and T cell systems. The initial contact with the antigen is stored in special memory cells of both cell lines. As illustrated in Figure 20-21, the memory cells respond immediately to the antigenic signal, so the lag time between the subsequent exposure to the antigen and production of protective antibody levels is greatly reduced. This phenomenon provides the basis for active immunization and "booster" doses that maintain protective levels of immunity. In the immunized person, memory cells elicit the rapid response in time for the immune system to overwhelm the pathogen or toxin before it can produce its damage. Memory cells are long-living lymphocytes, able to respond for many years after their development.

Immune Tolerance. Immune **tolerance** is the state of immunologic nonresponsiveness. Normally the body is immune tolerant toward self while maintaining responsiveness to foreign antigens. Research has established that self-tolerance is acquired primarily during embryonic development, though the exact mechanism is unclear.

Physiologic Changes With Aging

The extent of immunologic change that occurs with aging varies among individuals, depending on factors such as genetics, nutritional status, and disorders that deplete the immune system. In general, however, with aging the thymus gland atrophies, and some aspects of the immune response decrease. There is a decline in T cell responsiveness and proliferation, even though the number of T cells is not reduced overall. Helper and suppressor T cell proportions are decreased, which results in increased numbers of circulating autoantibodies. Leukocyte migration ability slows, and cytotoxic (killer) T cells decrease, which diminishes antigen-specific cytotoxicity. Helper T cells produce less interleukin-2, which further diminishes stimulation of T cell lymphocytes and NK cells. T cells respond more slowly to certain viral antigens, allografts (transplants from other persons), and tumor cells.

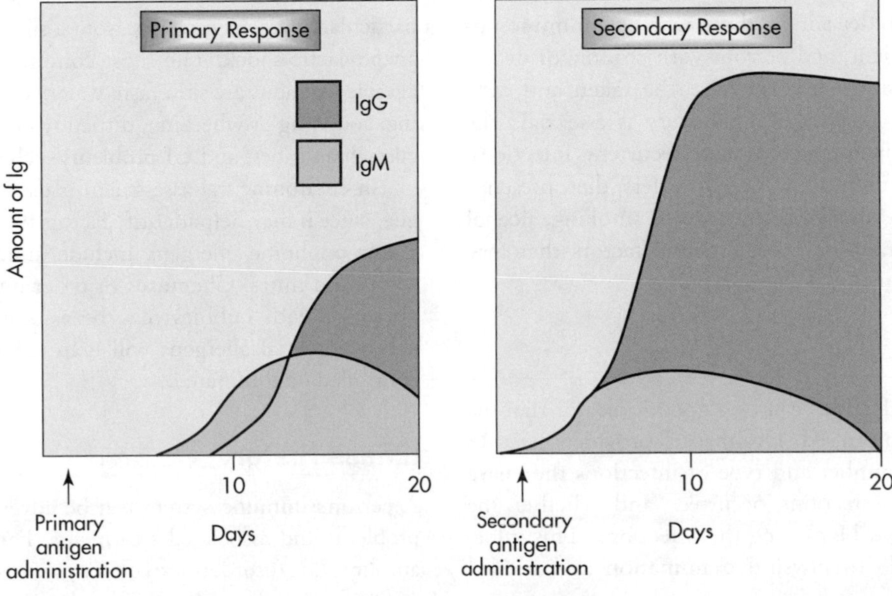

Figure 20-21 Primary and secondary humoral immune responses.

B cell function is thought to remain relatively stable, even though autoantibody production is increased.[2]

Other physiologic changes affect older adults' immunocompetence and place them at increased risk for infection. Decreased epidermal and dermal skin thickness and decreased elasticity make older adults more vulnerable to trauma and environmental injuries. Once the skin is broken, the healing process occurs more slowly because of decreased vascularity. Chemical barriers within many organs decrease, increasing older adults' susceptibility to pathogenic invasion. Estrogen loss in women, urinary retention, bladder muscle weakness, and prostatic disease place older adults at increased risk for urinary tract infections. Decreased ciliary action of the respiratory tract and decreased cough reflex can lead to aspiration or pneumonia. Decreased gastric acid and emptying predispose older adults to gastroenteritis or diarrhea. These changes in biologic processes can cause poor removal of organisms and an increase in microbial flora.[5]

Older adults experience multiple chronic illnesses, are hospitalized more frequently than younger persons, and undergo treatments that put them at risk for infection. Chronic illness may cause older adults to be less mobile, and immobility coupled with altered immune responses increases the risk of complications such as pneumonia and skin breakdown. The end result of immune system changes in older adults is an increased risk for and incidence of infections, increased number of tumors, and increased incidence of autoimmune disorders. Common infections tend to be more severe, with slower recovery and less probability of developing effective immunity after an infection. Older adults are not, however, immunocompromised to the same degree or in the same manner as a person with immunodeficiency diseases such as AIDS or those receiving immunosuppressive drugs. Assessment measures and variations in normal findings relevant to the care of older adults are presented in the Gerontologic Assessment box.

Gerontologic Assessment

- Assess for decreased skin thickness, elasticity, and neurosensory function.
  - –Decreased awareness of injury makes aging skin more vulnerable to trauma.
  - –Torn skin provides a portal of entry for microorganisms.
- Assess for signs of infection (fever, increased heart rate, increased respirations, fatigue) and for decreased breath sounds or crackles, which may indicate pneumonia.
  - –Increased risk for respiratory infections comes from decreased ciliary action, reduced respiratory muscle strength, and decreased gag and cough reflexes, which reduces the ability to expel inhaled microorganisms.
- Assess skin for evidence of adequate circulation.
  - –Increased risk for altered circulation is caused by decreased cardiac output and increased peripheral resistance. Altered circulation delays inflammation and increases the risk for ischemic injury.
- Assess for indigestion, nausea.
  - –Decreased gastric emptying, secretion of hydrochloric acid, and selected dietary enzymes result in less efficient digestion and decreased production of serum proteins.
- Assess for signs of infection.
  - –Increased risk for infection is caused by decreased number and size of lymph nodes, decline in T cell proliferation and responsiveness, and decreased number of circulation antibodies.

Health History

Health care personnel need to identify persons at increased risk for infection (children, older adults, those who are immunosuppressed or immunodeficient, and persons with chronic or debilitating illnesses) so preventive measures can be taken and early treatment initiated. An accurate health history is essential. The health history should include recent and recurrent infections, known allergies, history of autoimmune disorders, diet, prescription and over-the-counter medications, cigarette smoking, alcohol use, and any other therapy or environmental factors that may affect the immune system.

Infection History

A history of recurrent infections can be a good indicator that the immune system is compromised. Health care providers need to ask patients about the number and type of infections they have experienced, when the infections occurred, and whether the patient knows what might be causing the infections. This information provides a guide to physical examination and needed teaching.

Allergy History

Allergic symptoms are triggered by a variety of allergens; therefore the health care team collects data regarding allergens such as food, contrast media, medications, or other substances. The reactions to particular allergens can vary from a slight rash to life-threatening anaphylactic shock. The most common signs and symptoms of allergic reactions are skin rash, watery eyes, nasal discharge, sneezing, coughing or wheezing, difficulty hearing from obstruction of eustachian tubes, and GI problems such as diarrhea or colic.[6]

An environmental assessment is useful for patients with allergies, since it may help identify factors that precipitate the allergies. Common home allergens include animal dander, house dust, mold, and mites. Chemicals or other items used at work, in the home, or with hobbies may be associated with allergies. Data about potential allergens will help identify sources that can be controlled or eliminated.

Illness History

A person's immune system can be adversely affected by medical problems and associated treatments. For example, patients with autoimmune disorders are often treated with steroids or immunosuppressant drugs such as prednisone. Patients with cancer undergo treatments with radiation or chemotherapy, which may cause bone marrow destruction and further immunodeficiency. Patients with diabetes mellitus or renal failure may undergo systemic changes that depress the immune response. Medical treatments, such as surgery, or invasive diagnostic tests can interrupt the integrity of immune defense mechanisms. Because all these conditions place the patient at increased risk for infection, it is important to collect data about their presence and any prescribed, alternative, or over-the-counter treatments or medications.

Immune disorders such as AIDS and systemic lupus erythematosus (SLE) may produce dementia from inflammation and cellular destruction. Patients with multiple sclerosis often experience personality changes, varying from inappropriate euphoria to severe depression, which can alter behavioral patterns. Cognitive dysfunction, disorientation, and confusion need to be investigated, since they may indicate an immune alteration.

Risk factors for HIV infection (blood transfusions, illicit intravenous drug use, high-risk occupations such as nursing and medical technology, homosexuality, unprotected sexual intercourse, or multiple sexual partners) need to be identified during the assessment, since HIV infection is associated with immunodeficiency (see Chapter 22).

Travel History

With the ease of global travel, a travel history is now an essential part of any assessment. Persons who travel outside their home country are at increased risk for infections to which they have not been previously exposed. Even though immunizations are required before traveling to some countries, for many infections immunizations are not available. See Chapter 6 for a discussion of infectious diseases.

Psychosocial History

The psychosocial history includes information about the patient's family; interests; daily activities and habits; home, school or work environments; finances; religious and cultural practices; and relationships within and outside the family. This information helps the care providers identify risks for infection, potential or missing sources of support, and any factors that may affect the patient's response to treatment.[10]

Stress, which increases the production of cortisol, can compromise immune function. If the patient has experienced recent stressors, such as the death of a loved one, divorce, or negative relationships, it is important to examine this aspect completely and determine how the patient is coping with the stressor, how it has changed the patient's relationships with others, and whether it has affected the patient's health status.

Lack of financial resources may lead to delayed diagnosis and treatment for infections and produce considerable stress for the patient and family. Days or weeks away from work and actual or potential loss of income may compound the financial burden of prolonged infections.

Infection itself can be anxiety provoking. Even minor infections can produce fatigue, which may negatively affect the person's ability to function within family or social structures. Severe or prolonged infections can result in debilitating fatigue, inability to carry out daily activities, fear of death, fear of transmission of the infection to others, or social isolation.

Physical Examination

Disorders of the immune system are difficult to assess objectively because of subtle physical markers. However, observations of the patient's general behavior, as well as the skin, lymph nodes, lungs, ears, eyes, nose, throat, and other body systems, may provide clues about immune dysfunction.

Skin, Hair, and Nails

The nurse inspects the skin carefully for color, turgor, texture, temperature, and moisture. Skin changes provide information about altered immune processes. For example, jaundice of the skin may indicate an autoimmune disorder such as hemolytic anemia. Systemic sclerosis (scleroderma) is associated with thick, smooth, taut, shiny skin, whereas patients with Sjögren's syndrome have scaly skin and decreased sweating. Increased skin temperature may indicate an inflammation, whereas coldness suggests arterial insufficiency as seen with Raynaud's disease (see Chapter 31).

Various skin lesions are often associated with immune alterations. People with allergic reactions often have a maculopapular rash at the site where they were exposed to the allergen or over the whole body if the allergy is systemic. Persons with SLE have a characteristic erythemic rash across the bridge of the nose and cheek in a butterfly pattern. Patients with AIDS often have malignant skin lesions called Kaposi's sarcoma, which are typically maculopapular and range in color from pink to bluish purple (see Chapter 22). Patients with rheumatoid arthritis experience bony spurs primarily over the knuckles and finger joints (see Chapter 54). Some autoimmune processes cause notable alopecia (patchy hair loss) or dry, brittle, and broken hair. The nails may show changes in color, configuration, or brittleness.

Ears, Eyes, Nose, and Throat

Assessment of patients with allergies may reveal serous otitis media with retracted tympanic membranes, which indicates obstruction of the eustachian tubes and fluid collection within the ear. The patient may repeat questions many times because of difficulty with hearing.

Patients with autoimmune disorders or hypersensitivity reactions may have periorbital edema. The nurse may note dark circles under the eyes of patients with allergy because of chronic nasal obstruction that results in venous stasis.[6] Autoimmune disorders may cause changes in the conjunctiva, such as discoloration and vascular hemorrhage.

Nasal obstruction may cause the patient to breathe through the mouth and to speak in a nasal tone. Examination of the mouth and throat reveals any lesions in the mucous membrane or changes in mucosal color. Many autoimmune disorders cause oral lesions, and immunosuppressed or immunodeficient patients may experience thrush, a *Candida albicans* infection that produces white exudate over the tongue and mucous membranes.

Fever

Fever may be caused by an inflammatory response, an impaired immune system, or rapid proliferation of WBCs. The pattern of the fever often provides clues to the type of infective process involved; therefore the onset, range, and duration of the fever, and the presence of night sweats or chills, are important data to collect. High fevers may be associated with viral or bacterial infections or serum sickness, whereas low-grade fevers may indicate allergies or autoimmune processes. Fever may also be a sign of transplant rejection.

Lymph Nodes

Assessment of the lymph nodes includes inspection and palpation, beginning at the neck and extending to the entire body. The nurse documents the lymph nodes' location, size, surface characteristics, consistency, symmetry, mobility, and discomfort with palpation. Inflamed, tender, or fixed nodes indicate the need for further investigation. The location of enlarged lymph nodes helps identify possible sources of infection by the pattern of node involvement and usual drainage route (Figure 20-22). Enlarged lymph nodes (lymphadenopathy) usually accompany inflammation and infection, but may also be seen with Hodgkin's disease or non-Hodgkin's lymphoma, or may occur from transplant rejection.

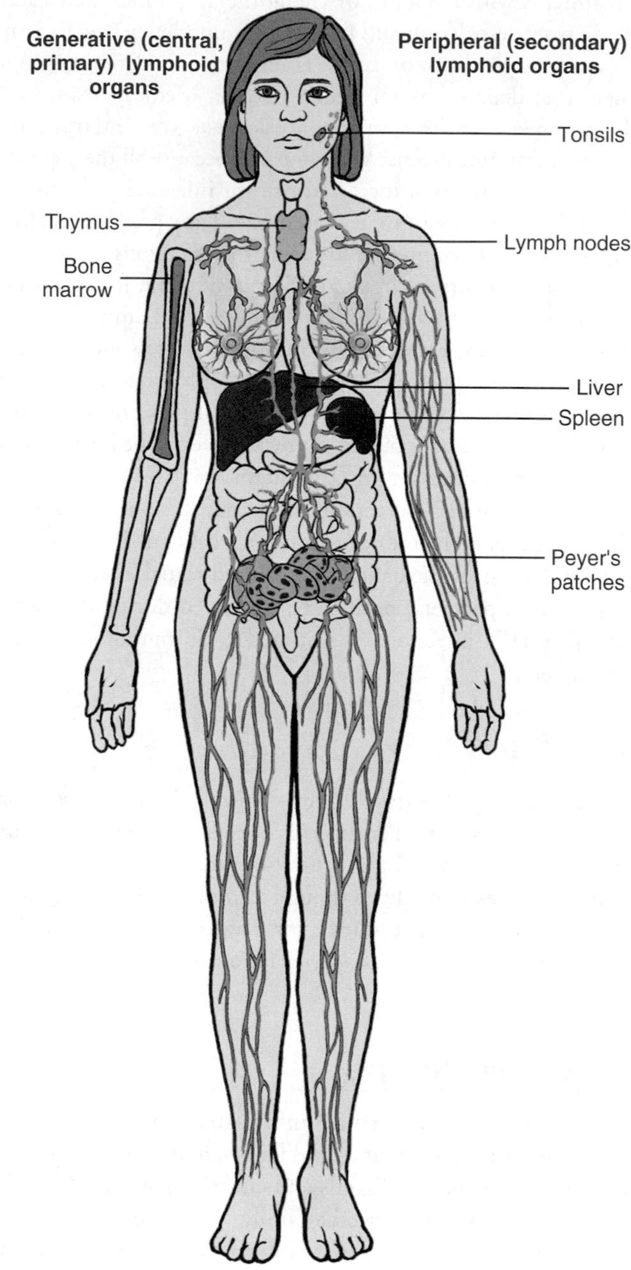

Figure 20-22 Primary and secondary lymphoid organs and tissues.

Respiratory System

Because persons with allergies typically show respiratory symptoms and immunosuppressed patients are particularly prone to pneumonia, it is critical to perform a complete respiratory assessment. Cough pattern, sputum color, skin color, the work of breathing, and lung sounds need to be given special attention. Patients with pneumonia display tachypnea and thick yellow or green sputum. They use accessory muscles for breathing. Allergic patients typically wheeze and cough, but experience little or no dyspnea. An allergic cough is characteristically hacking and nonproductive.

Diagnostic Tests

Laboratory tests, skin tests, and biopsies are the main sources of diagnostic evaluation of the immune system.

Laboratory Tests

Health care providers use laboratory tests to assess the patient's immune status, identify offending antigens, and monitor the effectiveness of treatments. The WBC count with differential, ESR, C-reactive protein, total complement activity test, and phagocytic cell function tests measure natural, innate immunity and phagocytosis. Protein electrophoresis, immunoglobulin electrophoresis, autoantibody tests, and antigen tests measure specific, adaptive immune processes.

White Blood Cell Count With Differential. The WBC count with differential provides information about the type of infection and the body's response to it. Normally a healthy adult has a WBC count between 4300 and 10,800/mm^3; the healthy older adult range is typically 3000 to 9000/mm^3. Leukopenia, a WBC count of less than 4300/mm^3, often signifies a compromised inflammatory response or a viral infection. Leukocytosis, a WBC count greater than 10,800/mm^3, indicates an inflammatory response to a pathogen or a disease process.[4]

If the WBC count is elevated, the clinician examines the differential count to determine which specific group of WBCs (neutrophils, basophils, eosinophils, lymphocytes, or monocytes) is increased or decreased. The differential is listed in such a way that the percentages of cells total 100%. This means that if the bone marrow proliferates one type of cell, it increases the percentage of this cell and conversely decreases the percentages of

TABLE 20-8 COMPARISON OF NORMAL AND ABNORMAL WHITE BLOOD CELL COUNT AND DIFFERENTIAL

	Bands (Stabs)* (%)	Neutrophils (segs) (%)	Eosinophils (%)	Basophils (%)	Lymphocytes (%)	Monocytes (%)
Normal WBC (5000/mm^3) and differential	1	49	1	1	38	10
Bacterial infection: 23,000/mm^3 (with "shift to left")	15	65	2	1	13	4

*Note shift from mature to immature neutrophils, called stabs or bands. Absolute neutrophil count has increased from 2500 to 18,400 (derived by multiplying total WBC count by combined percentage of bands and segmented neutrophils).

the other cell types. Neutrophils are among the first cells to migrate to the site of a bacterial infection, so an increase in the total neutrophil percentage greater than 70% usually indicates the presence of bacterial infections. The phrase *shift to the left* refers to the decrease in number of mature neutrophils (segmented neutrophils) and corresponding increase in number of immature neutrophils (bands or stabs) that occurs during acute bacterial infections (Table 20-8).

Lymphocytes are some of the first cells to respond to viral infections. Lymphocytes are the second most commonly occurring WBC. An elevated lymphocyte count is generally associated with viral infections, mononucleosis, tuberculosis, or some tumors. Increased eosinophil counts are associated with allergic reactions and parasitic infestations.[4]

Erythrocyte Sedimentation Rate. The ESR or sedimentation rate (sed rate) is the rate at which RBCs settle and is expressed in ml/hr. An increased ESR indicates increased globulins, fibrinogen, or other substances in the blood, which make it clump faster than normal, usually because of infection, malignancy, or collagen vascular disease. The ESR is frequently higher in healthy older adults.

C-Reactive Protein. C-reactive protein (CRP) measures an abnormal protein found 18 to 24 hours after certain inflammatory processes. It is commonly used to distinguish inflammatory from noninflammatory diseases, such as osteoarthritis from rheumatoid arthritis. A positive test result indicates the presence of an acute inflammatory reaction. CRP is frequently monitored in patients with acute inflammatory disorders to determine the effectiveness of treatments.

Total Hemolytic Complement. Total hemolytic complement (CH50) is a group of nine major protein components and some inhibitor proteins that assist with the inflammatory and immune responses. Once activated, complement facilitates chemotaxis, phagocytosis, and immune destruction of antigen. In healthy adults the CH50 ranges from 75 to 160 units/ml. During active antibody-antigen reactions or acute inflammation, complement is consumed and serum levels fall. As these conditions are treated and reversed, serum complement levels return to normal. As with the CRP, clinicians monitor complement levels in patients with acute inflammatory conditions such as SLE to determine the effectiveness of treatment. Low serum complement levels are associated with autoimmune diseases, glomerulonephritis, renal transplant rejection, and serum sickness. Elevated total complement levels are associated with acute rheumatic fever. Older adults typically show higher values for these proteins than younger adults, since they have a higher incidence of inflammatory conditions.[5]

Phagocytic Cell Function Tests. Tests can be performed to evaluate the phagocytic ability of PMNs and macrophages. One method is observing the absolute and relative numbers of monocytes and PMNs on the WBC count. The neutrophil functional assay is a primary test to evaluate the motility, recognition and adhesion, ingestion, degranulation, and killing ability of leukocytes and macrophages.

Protein Electrophoresis. Protein electrophoresis analyzes blood for protein content, specifically albumin and the globulins (alpha globulin, beta globulin, and gamma globulin). These measurements are helpful in assessing immune function and in identifying various disease states such as hypogammaglobulinemia, macroglobulinemia, inflammatory disorders, neoplastic disorders, and dysproteinemia.[4] Immunoglobulins can be either increased or decreased, depending on the specific immune disorder present (Figure 20-23).

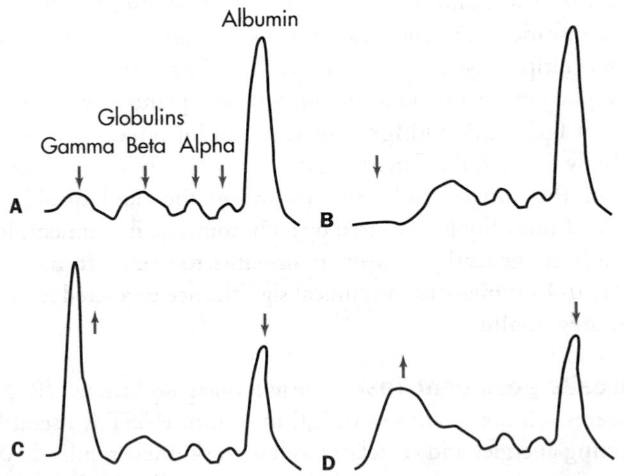

Figure 20-23 Electrophoretic patterns. **A,** Normal. **B,** Hypogammaglobulinemia. **C,** Monoclonal gammopathy. **D,** Polyclonal gammopathy.

TABLE 20-9 CLINICAL SIGNIFICANCE OF ALTERED LEVELS OF IMMUNOGLOBULIN

Class of Immunoglobulin	Increased Level	Decreased Level
IgG	IgG myeloma bacterial infection, hepatitis A, glomerulonephritis, rheumatoid arthritis, SLE, AIDS	Agammaglobulinemia, IgA myeloma, IgA deficiency, chronic lymphocytic leukemia, type I dysgammaglobulinemia, lymphoid aplasia, combined immunodeficiency, common variable immunodeficiency, X-linked hypogammaglobulinemia
IgM	Hepatitis A and B, Waldenström's macroglobulinemia, trypanosomiasis, chronic infections, type I dysgammaglobulinemia, hepatitis, SLE, rheumatoid arthritis, Sjögren's syndrome, AIDS	Lymphoid aplasia, hypogammaglobulinemia, chronic lymphocytic leukemia, IgG myeloma, IgA myeloma, agammaglobulinemia
IgA	SLE, rheumatoid arthritis, IgA myeloma, glomerulonephritis, chronic liver disease	Ataxia telangiectasia (AT), hypogammaglobulinemia, acute and chronic lymphocytic leukemia, IgA deficiency, combined immunodeficiency, common variable immunodeficiency, X-linked hypogammaglobulinemia, agammaglobulinemia, IgG myeloma, chronic infections (especially upper respiratory type)
IgE	Atopic disorders: allergic rhinitis, allergic asthma, atopic dermatitis, Wiskott-Aldrich syndrome with eczema, parasitic infestation, hyperimmunoglobulin E	Associated with IgA deficiency, intrinsic (nonallergic) asthma
IgD	Eczema, skin disorders	Unknown

From Mudge-Grout CL: *Immunologic disorders,* St Louis, 1993, Mosby.

SLE, Systemic lupus erythematosus; *AIDS,* acquired immunodeficiency syndrome.

Immunoglobulin Electrophoresis. Immunoglobulin electrophoresis separates serum immunoglobulins from one another based on their quantity and electrical charge. The separated immunoglobulins are compared with specific antisera to determine which immunoglobulins are present. The test shows relative but imprecise quantities of immunoglobulins. Normal adult IgG levels are 600 to 1800 mg/dl, IgA levels are 100 to 400 mg/dl, and IgM levels are 60 to 150 mg/dl. Immunoglobulin electrophoresis is used to detect and monitor hypersensitivity disorders, autoimmune disorders, chronic viral infections, immunodeficiency diseases, multiple myeloma, and intrauterine infections.

Nephelometry provides a rapid, accurate quantitative measurement of IgG, IgM, and IgA. The clinician introduces the specific antibody into a fluid containing the specific antigen. The interaction of the antigen and antibody makes the fluid turbid; the degree of turbidity is measured by a photometric instrument. IgD and IgE are generally present in amounts too small to measure. Table 20-9 summarizes the clinical significance of altered levels of immunoglobulins.

Radioallergosorbent Test. The radioallergosorbent test (RAST) measures minute quantities of IgE in serum. RAST is useful for detecting allergies and correlates well with skin test results. RAST testing is expensive, but useful in testing for allergies in patients taking antihistamines that suppress skin reactions.

Antibody Screening Tests. Numerous tests are available to detect antibodies formed against specific bacteria, viruses, fungi, or parasites Antibody screening tests confirm the presence of antibodies toward a particular antigenic source. A positive test implies that the person has been exposed to an antigen and produced antibodies against it, but does not necessarily mean that the person has the disease. Medications, infections, or chronic diseases can influence test results.

Autoantibody Tests. Abnormal antibodies that the body produces against itself are termed *autoantibodies.* Autoantibodies injure self-tissues and produce the symptoms associated with autoimmune conditions. Several tests are useful in confirming the presence of autoantibodies. Rheumatoid factor (RF) is an abnormal protein consisting of IgM antibodies found in the serum of persons with rheumatoid arthritis and other autoimmune diseases. Antinuclear antibodies (ANAs) or anti–deoxyribonucleic acid (DNA) antibodies are gamma globulins formed against properties of the cell nucleus. Tests for ANAs are positive in a large number of patients with autoimmune disorders such as SLE or systemic sclerosis. Healthy older adults have increased antibodies (ANAs and RF), but the clinical relevance of these increases is unclear.[2]

Antigen Tests. Laboratory tests are useful for isolating and identifying specific invading antigens. For example, a positive result for HBsAg indicates the presence of the hepatitis B surface antigen, a specific antigenic determinant of the hepatitis B virus. Other tests isolate the antigenic properties of the antibodies toward RBCs. The indirect Coombs' test indicates serum antibodies to RBCs, which are not connected to the cell. It can identify a patient's Rh factor. ABO and Rh typing help determine blood type compatibility and thereby reduce the possibility of transfusion reactions. The direct Coombs' test detects antibodies coating the RBCs that are not detected by ABO typing. A positive test facilitates diagnosis of hemolytic disease and autoimmune disorders.[9]

The lupus erythematosus (LE) cell test is used to help confirm the diagnosis of SLE, a classic autoimmune disorder. LE cells are neutrophils that contain large groups of abnormal DNA in their cytoplasms. Such cells are seen in 70% to 80% of patients with SLE. Cryoglobulins are abnormal serum globulin proteins found in the blood of patients with various diseases. Cryoglobulins can precipitate within blood vessels of the fingers when exposed to low temperatures, producing arthralgia or Raynaud's phenomenon (coldness, pain, cyanosis).[8]

Certain subsets of T-lymphocyte cells called clusters of differentiation (CD) provide information about the extent of immunodeficiency present in patients with AIDS. When the $CD4^+$ (TH) levels fall below certain parameters, therapy is initiated to help restore immune function. Infection and autoimmune disorders can also result in reduced CD4 levels. Other T-cell subsets are used to detect T-cell leukemias, T-cell lymphoma, or B-cell tumors.

Human Immunodeficiency Virus Tests. The enzyme-linked immunosorbent assay (ELISA) and Western blot tests are used to detect the presence of HIV antibodies. The ELISA is positive when blood or body fluid reacts with the surface antigen of a killed HIV virus. The test is highly sensitive and is the primary test used for mass screening for HIV infection. The Western blot, another immunoassay, is used to confirm the presence of HIV antibodies in persons who test positive on the ELISA test. It identifies HIV protein antigen–specific antibodies. When used in combination, these tests have a specificity for HIV antibodies greater than 99.9%.

The OraQuick Rapid HIV-1 Antibody Test detects HIV-1 antibodies in serum. The test uses less than a drop of fingerstick blood (venipuncture whole blood can also be used), and the result is available in about 20 minutes. In clinical trials the test demonstrated 99.6% accuracy in HIV-1–infected persons and 100% accuracy in noninfected persons. Since it is a screening test, a positive result requires confirmation by another, more specific test.[3] A version of this test called Home Test HIV Antibody Detection Kit is available for purchase from a Canadian company over the Internet.

The OraSure HIV-1, HIV-2, and HIV 1/2 tests detect HIV antibodies to HIV-1, HIV-2, and HIV-1/HIV-2, respectively. The HIV type 2 is a second but far less common cause of AIDS than HIV-1. Both of these tests use the enzyme-linked immunosorbent assay to detect HIV antibodies in oral fluid called oral mucosal transudate, which is different from saliva. The sample is collected using a cotton fiber pad attached to a nylon stick. The pad is placed between the cheek and the lower gum, rubbed gently back and forth until wet, and then left in place for 2 to 5 minutes. The pad, which extracts IgG antibodies out of the cheek and gum tissues, is then deposited in a transport vial and sent to a laboratory for testing. Because it takes about 3 months (or up to 6 months) for antibodies to develop, repeat testing of patients with negative results is needed if they may have been exposed to HIV within these time frames.

The absolute $CD4^+$ cell count is used to test the progressive depletion of $CD4^+$ T cell lymphocytes in persons with HIV infection. The risk for disease progression and development of opportunistic infections increases as the number of $CD4^+$ T cell lymphocytes declines. Another test that predicts HIV disease progression is the plasma viral load. This test measures the amount or concentration of HIV in the circulation and is a reflection of viral replication. As viral load increases, the risk for disease progression increases. Both of these tests are used to monitor treatment effectiveness and determine the need for more or less aggressive HIV therapy. See Chapter 22 for other HIV/AIDS-related diagnostic studies.

Special Tests

Gallium Scan. A gallium scan is a nuclear scan in which the radioactive substance gallium citrate is injected intravenously though a peripheral vein. Within a few days the gallium collects in "hot" spots, which are areas where WBCs have accumulated or inflammation is present. It is useful for diagnosing infections or inflammatory diseases, such as abscess formation, osteomyelitis, and tumors such as lymphomas, or for diagnosing the cause of fevers of unknown origin.

Biopsy. A lymph node biopsy may be performed in patients with enlarged lymph nodes (lymphadenopathy) to determine whether inflammation or malignancy is present. A synovial biopsy may be performed to obtain synovial fluid from a joint to differentiate among various types of arthritis or bone malignancies.

The nurse's role in biopsy procedures includes teaching the patient about the procedure and assisting the physician. Most biopsies are completed with the patient under local anesthesia in an ambulatory setting. After anesthesia is effective, the patient should perceive only a pressure sensation; pain generally indicates insufficient anesthesia. After biopsy, the nurse covers the area with a sterile bandage and instructs the patient to monitor for bleeding and infection. Postbiopsy discomfort can be relieved by analgesics.

Skin Tests. Skin tests are a simple, relatively painless, and inexpensive means to diagnose particular IgE-mediated allergies. The suspected allergen is delivered by intradermal injection or a scratch, prick, or puncture of the skin. Skin tests are influenced by skin reactivity to the allergen, amount of allergen administered, and degree of host mast cell sensitivity. Older persons tend to have a poorer response to skin testing because of changes in their mast cell reactivity. Although intradermal skin tests are the most sensitive, they can also produce systemic reactions, anaphylaxis, or false-positive results. The scratch test is difficult to standardize and has the highest probability of producing a systemic reaction, anaphylaxis, or a false-positive result. The prick test enables the clinician to test more substances at one time, but bleeding can cause false-positive results. Closely placed sites can also interfere with accurate interpretation of results. The puncture method is used more than the other skin testing methods because of greater reliability, safer administration, and ease of use with children.

Anergy Tests. Skin testing is used to screen patients for T cell immunodeficiency. Specific antigens, including purified protein derivative, *Candida* antigens, mumps antigen, streptokinase-streptodornase, coccidiodin, histoplasmin, and *Trichophyton* antigens, are injected intradermally. Reactions are read at 24-, 48-, and 72-hour intervals. The reactions determine hypersensitivity to the antigen, not the presence of disease. More than 90% of healthy persons show a response to one of these antigens within 48 hours. Areas of induration are carefully measured. An induration of 5 mm or greater indicates a positive result. A person who does not react to any of these antigens is said to be *anergic*. Anergy is associated with immunodeficiency disorders.

Nurses frequently administer skin tests. The nurse must administer the correct amount of allergen by the correct method to ensure patient safety and test reliability. Emergency equipment should be available before skin tests are administered because of the risk of anaphylaxis, and the nurse should monitor the patient for at least 30 minutes after allergen administration.

Nursing Implications for Laboratory Testing

Many of the tests presented in this chapter require little patient preparation or nursing intervention other than teaching. In addition, they require little or no observation after the test. Even so, a clear understanding of the various tests allows the nurse to conduct routine teaching, answer patient questions accurately, and recognize abnormal data that need to be monitored and reported.

References

1. Abbas AK, Lichtmann AH: *Basic immunology*, ed 2, Philadelphia, 2005, Saunders.
2. American Federation for Aging Research: *How does the immune system change with age?*, accessed 2002 from website: http://www.infoaging.org/b-immune-home.html.
3. Centers for Disease Control and Prevention: *Frequently asked questions about the OraQuick Rapid HIV-1 antibody test*, accessed 2003 from website: http://www.cdc.gov/hiv/PUBS/faq/oraqckfaq.htm.
4. Chernecky CC, Berger BJ: *Laboratory tests and diagnostic procedures*, ed 4, Philadelphia, 2004, Saunders.
5. Huether S, McCance K: *Understanding pathophysiology*, ed 3, St Louis, 2004, Mosby.
6. Jarvis C: *Physical examination and health assessment*, ed 4, Philadelphia, 2004, Saunders.
7. National Cancer Institute: *Understanding the immune system*, accessed 2001 from website: http://rex.nci.nih.gov/.
8. Price SA, Wilson LM: *Pathophysiology: clinical concepts of disease processes*, ed 6, St Louis, 2003, Mosby.
9. Roitt I, Brostoff J, Male D: *Immunology*, ed 6, St Louis, 2001, Mosby.
10. Shaw JK, Mahoney EA: *HIV/AIDS nursing secrets*, Philadelphia, 2003, Saunders.

Visit the Evolve website: http://evolve.elsevier.com/Monahan/medsurg

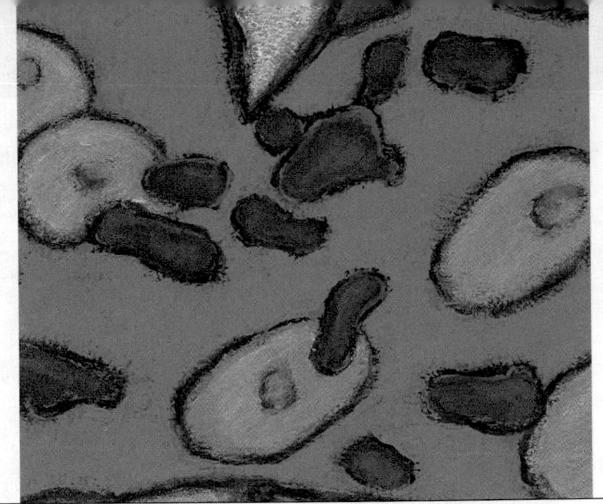

CHAPTER 21 Immunologic Problems

by Carol J. Green

OBJECTIVES

After studying this chapter, the learner should be able to:

1. Compare primary and secondary immunodeficiency disorders.
2. Describe the pathophysiologic changes that occur from monoclonal gammopathies.
3. Explain the differences between the five classifications of hypersensitivity disorders.
4. List conditions associated with each of the five hypersensitivity disorders.
5. Describe the pathologic changes that occur from immunologic blood reactions.
6. Discuss the theories of autoimmunity.
7. Describe nursing management for the person with immune disorders.
8. Describe nursing management for the person with chronic fatigue syndrome.

KEY TERMS

allergy, p. 458
atopy, p. 458
autoimmunity, p. 449
gammopathy, p. 449
hemolytic, p. 468
hypersensitivity, p. 449
immunodeficiency, p. 449
immunosuppression, p. 451
immunotherapy, p. 462
monoclonal antibodies, p. 452
systemic anaphylaxis, p. 458

The immune response is protective in healthy individuals; however, that protection depends on an intact immune system. Four primary immune aberrations can lead to disease: (1) a deficiency of one or more immune components **(immunodeficiency)**, (2) an abnormal production of antibodies **(gammopathy)**, (3) an exaggerated or inappropriate immune response **(hypersensitivity)**, and (4) immunologic attacks on host cells **(autoimmunity)**.

Immunodeficiences

The four components of the immune system—humoral (B cell mediated) immunity, cellular (T cell) immunity, phagocytosis, and complement—act together and independently to protect the host from infection and disease. Both primary (congenital) and secondary (acquired) immunodeficiencies produce chronic or recurring infections that can, without effective treatment, lead to death.

Etiology and Epidemiology. Primary immunodeficiencies (PIs) are a group of disorders that occur from congenital genetic defects that block or prevent the maturation or function of immune cells. More than 100 different PIs have been identified, although an estimated 20 of them are responsible for 90% of cases. Most PIs are autosomal, or X linked, and have both dominant and recessive inheritance patterns. They commonly occur in persons under the age of 20 and, because of inheritance patterns, affect males in 70% of cases.[5] PIs are grouped according to the immune components that are defective or lacking (Table 21-1).

The actual frequency of PI disease in the general population is unknown due to factors such as lack of recognition or reporting and death before diagnosis.[5] One in 10,000 persons is diagnosed with PIs annually, with between 25,000 and 50,000 of those being severely affected. However, estimates place the possible incidence of varying degrees of PI disease as high as one in five persons in the United States and Europe.[15]

The most common immunodeficiencies are secondary or acquired. Most people are born with a normal immune response, but secondary factors or occurrences affect the immune system, causing dysfunction. Immunosuppressive agents; malignancies; chronic diseases; nutritional deficits; age; and some viral infections, such as human immunodeficiency virus (HIV), can cause secondary immunodeficiency.

Pathophysiology

PRIMARY IMMUNODEFICIENCIES. PI disorders are characterized by defects in immunologic cell development or function that result in B-lymphocyte (also known as B cell), T cell, complement, or phagocytic cell deficiency (Figure 21-1). Recurrent infections or

TABLE 21-1 SELECTED PRIMARY IMMUNODEFICIENCIES

Disorder	Basis of Deficiency
B-CELL DEFICIENCIES	
X-linked (Bruton's) agammaglobulinemia	Sex-linked depression of all immunoglobulin classes; failure of prelymphocytes to mature into B lymphocytes; all serum immunoglobulins decreased
Common variable immunodeficiency	Variable degree of ability to synthesize primarily IgA or IgM in adults; high concentrations of autoantibodies and abnormal immunoglobulins
Selective IgA deficiency	Total absence or severe deficiency of IgA; B lymphocytes that normally produce IgA unable to convert to IgA-producing plasma cells
T-CELL DEFICIENCIES	
DiGeorge syndrome (thymic hypoplasia)	Nongenetic failure of thymic development related to abnormal embryonic development of head and neck tissues and cells; normal or increased serum immunoglobulins; decreased T cells
MIXED T-CELL AND B-CELL DEFICIENCIES	
Severe combined immunodeficiency disease	Defect in stem cell differentiation and maturation of T and B cells; T and B cells decreased or absent
Wiskott-Aldrich syndrome	Sex-linked IgM and T-cell deficiency in males; tendency toward bleeding because of low numbers of platelets
Ataxia-telangiectasia	Autosomal recessive deficit in IgA and IgE; decreased normal T cells
Nezlof syndrome	Congenital failure of embryonic thymic development; normal or increased serum immunoglobulins; lymphopenia
PHAGOCYTIC CELL DEFICIENCIES	
Chronic granulomatous disease	Sex-linked genetic disease in males that results in failure to destroy phagocytized organisms and particles
Chédiak-Higashi syndrome	Autosomal recessive disorder with abnormal granule formation, neutrophil chemotactic response, and intracellular killing of microorganisms
COMPLEMENT DEFICIENCIES	
C1, C3, and C4	Development of bacterial infections; tendency to autoimmune process (systemic lupus erythematosus, glomerulonephritis, Sjögren's syndrome)
Hereditary angioedema	Autosomal dominant disorder associated with C1 inhibitor deficiency; results in large amount of vasoactive peptides and increased vascular permeability

IgA, Immunoglobulin A; *IgM,* immunoglobulin M; *IgE,* immunoglobulin E.

repeated infection treatment failures generally prompt the clinician to suspect the presence of immunodeficiency. Without treatment, most individuals suffering from these deficiencies die of overwhelming infections early in life.[5] See the Clinical Manifestations box related to immunodeficiencies.

ANTIBODY DEFICIENCIES. Selective immunoglobulin A (IgA) deficiency is the most common PI and has both autosomal dominant and recessive inheritance traits. The exact defect that leads to low serum IgA levels is unknown, but may be related to impaired B cell differentiation and subsequent loss of immunoglobulin-secreting ability. The disorder is associated with increased incidence of infections, autoimmunity, allergies, gastrointestinal disorders, and cancer.[7]

B lymphocytes produce *antibodies* that recognize and mark foreign antigens so that other immune components will react and destroy them. X-linked agammaglobulinemia is an example of an inherited, B cell immunodeficiency that results from failure of pre-B cells to differentiate into mature B cells. This disorder occurs exclusively in males and is usually diagnosed within the first 3 years of life. Individuals with agammaglobulinemia are particularly susceptible to infections from pyrogenic bacteria such as streptococci, staphylococci, *Pseudomonas* organisms, and *Haemophilus influenzae;* infections of the eyes, sinuses, ears, nose, and lungs; and viruses such as hepatitis and polio.[7]

COMBINED B AND T CELL DEFICIENCIES. Stem cell immunodeficiency (severe combined immunodeficiency, or SCID) refers to the complete absence of both T cell (cellular) and B cell (humoral) immunity. This disorder has many variants. In the most severe form the common stem cell for white blood cells is absent, resulting in subsequent loss of B cells, T cells, and phagocytic cells. Infants with this condition generally die in utero or soon after birth. A less severe form of SCID results from impaired stem cell maturation, which interferes with T and B cell development. T and B cells are significantly reduced or absent even though other

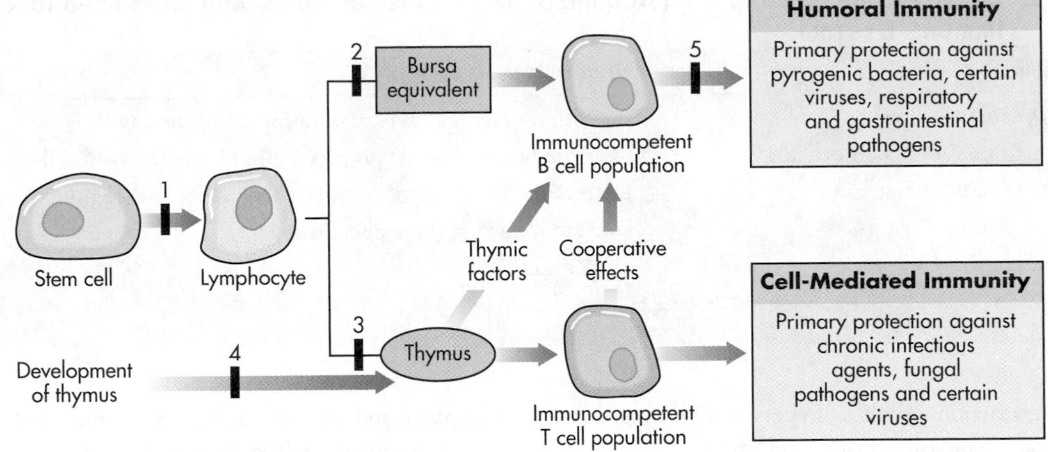

Figure 21-1 Causes of immunodeficiencies. Abnormalities at *1* result in combined humoral and cell-mediated immunodeficiency. Blockage at *2* produces agammaglobulinemia. Blockage at *3* or *4* results in drastic reduction in T cell–mediated function and subsequent reduction in humoral response. Abnormalities in synthesis of specific immunoglobulin classes are reflected by blockage at *5*. Some blockages result in complete deficiency; others show up as reduction in response.

CLINICAL MANIFESTATIONS
Immunodeficiencies

Immunodeficiencies produce a variety of clinical manifestations based on the type of deficiency. Not all patients experience all manifestations listed. Common manifestations include:

- Frequent bacterial and viral infections
- Infection with unusual or opportunistic organisms
- Associated autoimmune disease
- Painful, swollen wrist, elbow, ankle, or knee joints
- Digestive problems, nausea, or vomiting
- Chronic skin or mucous membrane infections
- Blood disorders
- Diarrhea
- Fever
- Fatigue
- Weakness
- Enlarged lymph nodes or spleen

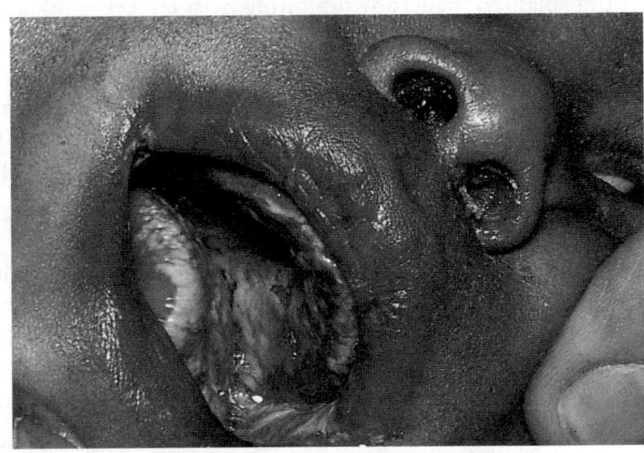

Figure 21-2 *Candida albicans* in mouth of patient with severe combined immunodeficiency. The organism grows abundantly when immune function is compromised.

white blood cells are present in normal numbers.[6] People with SCID are at high risk for developing nearly every type of infection because of pancytopenia (Figure 21-2).

Thymic hypoplasia (DiGeorge syndrome) is a cellular immunodeficiency resulting from thymus gland hypoplasia and inability to assist in the maturation of T cells. Even though B cells are normal, children with total loss of thymic function are at increased risk for infection and may not live more than 5 or 6 years without treatment.[17]

PHAGOCYTIC DEFECTS. Phagocytes (neutrophils and macrophages) are white blood cells that engulf and destroy antibody-coated antigens. Phagocytic defects may interfere with their ability to move to the site of an infection or destroy pathogens. Chronic granulomatous disease is the most severe form of phagocytic cell deficiency. It involves a deficiency in the molecules needed by neutrophils to destroy foreign antigens.[7] Individuals with phagocytic disorders are at risk for developing mild to severe bacterial infections. Signs and symptoms depend on the site of infection and type of infecting organism.

COMPLEMENT SYSTEM DEFECTS. The complement system is composed of proteins that attach themselves to antibody-coated antigens and facilitate destruction of the antigen. Persons with complement deficiency have a diminished ability to destroy invading pathogens and are at increased risk for infection. A common complement deficiency, C2 deficiency, is associated with an increased incidence of autoimmune disease, such as glomerulonephritis or rheumatoid arthritis, and severe infection such as meningitis.[17]

SECONDARY IMMUNODEFICIENCIES

IMMUNOSUPPRESSIVE THERAPIES. Secondary immunodeficiencies result from numerous factors (Table 21-2). Generalized **immunosuppression** is often induced therapeutically to decrease

TABLE 21-2 EXAMPLES OF SECONDARY (ACQUIRED) IMMUNODEFICIENCIES AND CORRESPONDING DEFECTS IN IMMUNE SYSTEM

Disease or Condition	Effect on Immune System
Malnutrition (protein, caloric)	Inhibition of lymphocyte maturation and function
Cancer treatments (radiation, chemotherapy)	Decreased bone marrow precursors for all white blood cells (leukocytes)
Metastases of cancer to bone marrow	Decreased leukocyte development because of reduced site (bone marrow)
Spleen removal	Decreased microbial phagocytosis
Human immunodeficiency virus	Depletion of CD4+ helper cells

Data from Abbas AK, Lichtmann AH: *Basic immunology*, ed 2, Philadelphia, 2005, Saunders.

unwanted immune reactions, such as hypersensitivity reactions, autoimmune diseases, neoplasia, or organ rejection.

Corticosteroids have both antiinflammatory and immunosuppressive properties. They inhibit movement of leukocytes and alter cellular and humoral immunity. When infection is present in a person receiving corticosteroids, the severity of the infection may increase despite the induced minimization of symptoms. Cyclosporine, a primary immunosuppressant drug used after organ transplantation, acts by inhibiting helper T cells and facilitating development of suppressor T cells.

Cytotoxic drugs and other cancer chemotherapeutic agents (alkylating agents, antifolates, and antimetabolites) destroy replicating cells. Consequently, they produce immunosuppression by destroying rapidly dividing immunologically stimulated cells. They also interfere with basic cellular metabolic processes in which B and T cell numbers are reduced.

Specific immunosuppression may be induced in people with hypersensitivities by administration of antigens in small amounts over time. This antigenic stimulation forms circulating immunoglobulin G (IgG) antibodies (immunoglobulins) that combine with the offending antigen to block contact with immunocompetent cells or immunoglobulin E (IgE)-coated mast cells, thus suppressing the immune response and preventing hypersensitivity reactions. Allergists use an adaptation of this method to desensitize persons who are allergic to antigens such as pollens or dust mites. A slightly different method of immunosuppression involves administration of a specific antibody, which then combines with the antigen to block contact with the immunocompetent cell. This method is used successfully in obstetrics in preventing the sensitive Rh-negative mother from reacting to an Rh-positive fetus during pregnancy.

Antilymphocytic globulin and antithymocytic globulin are antisera prepared by isolating the active globulin fraction from the serum of horses, goats, or rabbits that have been immunized with human lymphocytes or thymocytes. These antisera produce immunosuppression by decreasing all lymphocytes, although T cells are more affected than B cells. Because these globulins are xenogeneic (from another species), serum sickness may occur, and this limits their use to short-term therapy.

Monoclonal antibodies (MoAbs) are also used to suppress immunity. Because they are derived from a single cell line (monoclonal), they are very specific and can be targeted against subpopulations of lymphocytes, such as helper T cells. Monoclonal antibodies are useful in treating cancers, autoimmune disorders, and renal allograft rejection.[4] (See Chapter 36 for a discussion of renal transplant and allograft rejection.) Table 21-3 describes major immunosuppressive drug categories.

Many chemicals have immunosuppressive effects in exposed humans. T lymphocytes seem to be affected more severely than other immune cells. Examples of potentially damaging environmental chemicals are asbestos, dioxin, insecticides, and heavy metals. Irradiation also suppresses immunity by suppressing both primary and secondary immune responses, although primary suppression is more effective. Irradiation destroys lymphocytes either directly or through depletion of precursor stem cells.

OTHER FACTORS. Prolonged physical and psychosocial stress stimulates the production of corticosteroids, which suppress immunity and increase the risk for infections and tumors. T and B cells are reduced for up to a month after surgery, most likely because of stress. Chronic conditions such as diabetes mellitus are common causes of secondary immunodeficiency. Malnutrition and subsequent protein and calorie deficiencies result in reduced T cell numbers.[17] The immune systems of older adults are less efficient, with decreased T cell function, variable ability to respond to antigenic stimulation, and decreased proliferation of immune cells. HIV causes a serious secondary immunodeficiency, acquired immunodeficiency syndrome (AIDS) (discussed in detail in Chapter 22). Table 21-4 presents specific conditions that can suppress immunity.

COMPLICATIONS. Frequent acute and chronic bacterial, viral, and fungal infections and repeated infection treatment failures are the complications of primary and secondary immunodeficiencies. Without adequate treatment, these complications can lead to weight loss, fatigue, poor quality of life, sepsis, septic shock, and death. Refer to the Clinical Manifestations box related to immunodeficiency, p. 451.

Collaborative Care Management. The primary goals of collaborative management for patients with suspected immunodeficiency disorders are to (1) identify those at risk for the disorder, (2) prevent infection or effectively treat existing infections, and (3) replace missing humoral or cellular immunologic factors as possible.

DIAGNOSTIC TESTS. Diagnosis is based on patient history, physical examination, and laboratory findings; however, there is no one specific test for all diseases. Box 21-1 lists common diagnostic tests to confirm and monitor immunodeficiencies. Chapter 20 contains more information regarding diagnostic tests for immune function.

TABLE 21-3 MAJOR IMMUNOSUPPRESSIVE DRUG CATEGORIES

Immunologic Action	Indications for Use
CORTICOSTEROIDS (E.G., PREDNISONE)	
Inhibit T cell proliferation	Disease in which immune disorder is unknown
Decrease interleukin-2 production	Autoimmune diseases (e.g., systemic lupus erythematosus)
Decrease macrophage and neutrophil function	Allergic disorders (e.g., asthma)
Inhibit helper T and suppressor T cell activity	Transplant rejection (e.g., kidney transplant)
CYTOTOXIC DRUGS	
Alkylating Agents (e.g., Cyclophosphamide)	
Interfere with DNA, RNA, and protein synthesis	Autoimmune diseases (e.g., systemic sclerosis)
Lymphocytolytic	Lymphomas
Depress B cell, macrophage, and monocyte function	Leukemias Granulomatous diseases (e.g., thyroiditis)
Antimetabolites (e.g., Azathioprine)	
Interfere with RNA, DNA, and protein synthesis	Autoimmune disease (e.g., multiple sclerosis, systemic lupus erythematosus)
Depress bone marrow and antibody production	Organ transplantation
Depress T cell, macrophage, and monocyte function	Pemphigus (e.g., skin disease) Neoplasia (e.g., cancers)
Antifolates (e.g., Methotrexate)	
Cause deficiency of folate coenzymes, preventing synthesis of thymine and purines	Autoimmune disease (e.g., rheumatoid arthritis) Neoplasia (e.g., cancers)
TRANSPLANT IMMUNOSUPPRESSANTS (E.G., CYCLOSPORINE [SANDIMMUNE])	
Inhibits helper T cell, lymphokine, and interleukin-2 production	Allograft rejection
Facilitates suppressor T cell development	Graft-versus-host disease

DNA, Deoxyribonucleic acid; *RNA,* ribonucleic acid.

TABLE 21-4 CONDITIONS THAT CAN SUPPRESS IMMUNITY

Condition	Effect on Immune System
Nephrotic syndrome Burns Protein-losing enteropathy	Loss of serum protein
Severe liver disease	Decreased protein synthesis
Cancer Alcoholism Malabsorption	Severe malnutrition; decreased protein synthesis
Uremia Diabetes mellitus Infections (especially viral) Autoimmune disorders	Decreased T cell function
Lymphomas Leukemias	Alterations in B cell and T cell numbers and function

BOX 21-1 Diagnostic Tests for Immunodeficiency

- Complete blood cell count
- Tests for cellular immunity
  —Lymphocyte or mononuclear cell quantity and function assays
  —Complement components and function
  —Phagocytic cell function
- Tests for humoral immunity
  —Immunoglobulin protein assays
  —Specific antibody assays
- Genetic testing
  —Deoxyribonucleic acid
  —Ribonucleic acid
  —Chromosomes
  —Proteins and metabolites

From Centers for Disease Control and Prevention: Applying public health strategies to primary immunodeficiency diseases, *MMWR*, accessed 2004 from website: http://www.cdc.gov/mmwr/preview/mmwrhtml/rr5301a1.htm.

MEDICATIONS. Antimicrobial agents to treat existing and prevent new infections are key to the successful management of both primary and secondary immunodeficiencies. Immunoglobulin replacement therapy, which contains intravenous immunoglobulin (IVIG), is accepted treatment for patients with antibody deficiencies. The optimal dose of immunoglobulin, which is usually between 400 and 500 mg/dl, is maintained by monitoring the trough of immunoglobulin levels in the blood. Immunoglobulins are usually given intramuscularly or intravenously on a monthly basis. Reactions to immunoglobulins can include back or abdominal pain, nausea and vomiting, chills and fever, headache, myalgia, or fatigue. Fortunately, anaphylactic reactions to immunoglobulins are rare.

Other chemotherapeutic treatments for immunodeficiency include (1) injections of interferon gamma, a cytokine that activates phagocytes; (2) injections of growth factors, which increase neutrophil production; and (3) granulocyte-macrophage colony-stimulating factor or granulocyte colony-stimulating factor, both of which stimulate the production of granulocytes (white blood cells).[7]

TREATMENTS. Bone marrow transplantation may be used for patients with T cell deficiencies. The major risk of this therapy is graft-versus-host disease, which is discussed later in the chapter. Bone marrow cells from family members with identical human leukocyte antigens have been used successfully in treating patients with combined immunodeficiencies.[5]

DIET. Patients with immunodeficiency diseases have no specific dietary restrictions. A well-balanced, nutritious diet that includes all food groups and has adequate calories and protein to support tissue healing and growth is recommended, since it helps support immunity. Efforts should be made to prevent the transfer of food-borne microbes that may be potential sources of infection by thoroughly washing or cooking fruits and vegetables, thoroughly cooking meat products, and avoiding placing cooked foods on surfaces where raw meat was prepared.

Nursing Management

of the Patient with Immunodeficiency Disorder

ASSESSMENT

Health History. Assess for:

- Frequency and length of any chronic bacterial or viral infections
- Bacterial infections of the ears, sinuses, lungs, bronchi
- Painful joints of the wrist, elbows, ankles, or knees
- Digestive problems, nausea, or vomiting
- Frequent bouts of diarrhea
- Chronic skin infections
- Blood disorders

Physical Examination. Assess for:

- Enlarged lymph nodes or spleen
- Fever
- Poor skin turgor, bruising, lesions on the skin or mucous membranes
- Swollen joints
- Decreased weight for height

NURSING DIAGNOSES, OUTCOMES, AND INTERVENTIONS

Nursing Diagnosis: Risk for Infection

OUTCOMES. Common examples of expected outcomes for the patient with a diagnosis of *risk for infection* are:

Patient will:

- Recognize signs of new infections and report for treatment early.
- Use precautions to prevent new infections.
- Maintain treatment regimens for treatment or prevention of infections.

NURSING INTERVENTIONS. The nurse consistently monitors patients who have immunodeficiencies or are undergoing immunosuppression therapy for indications of systemic infection, such as fever, changes in vital sign pattern, irritability, fatigue, or cough (see Chapter 20). Meticulous skin and perineal care and a clean environment reduce the patient's potential for contact with infectious organisms. Injections are avoided and invasive lines kept to a minimum to prevent a portal of entry for microbes. When invasive lines are necessary, the nurse carefully monitors insertion sites for signs of localized infection. The nurse cultures suspicious drainage and monitors laboratory data to detect new infections and to determine the effectiveness of medications and other treatments. Live immunizations and oral polio vaccines are avoided in immunocompromised patients because of the risk of contracting infections via the immunization.

Immunodeficient or immunosuppressed patients and their families need to know the nature of the immunodeficiency and how to avoid infection. Many patients do not require hospitalization, but they do need to be taught about infection control measures to follow at home. They need to be able to recognize the signs and symptoms of infection and which symptoms to report to the health care provider. Teaching includes information about the use of protective strategies such as hand washing techniques and asking people with infections such as colds or chickenpox not to visit. Frequent turning and deep breathing exercises are encouraged to prevent atelectasis and pneumonia. Careful attention should be given to older adults because of their increased risk for infection resulting from a decline in T cell function and immune response efficiency (see Patient/Family Teaching box).

There are no specific activity restrictions; however, the nurse counsels patients about the need to avoid becoming overly fatigued. Patients with immunodeficiency disorders need to understand the importance of ongoing follow-up care. Referrals to community or home health nurses for continued assessment and treatment of infections may be necessary. Hospice care may be appropriate for patients with terminal primary or secondary immunodeficiency disorders.

RELATED NIC INTERVENTIONS. Infection Control, Infection Protection, Medication Management, Skin Surveillance, Surveillance

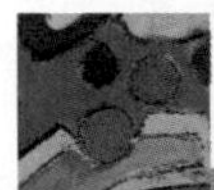

PATIENT/FAMILY TEACHING *The Patient With Immunodeficiency*

Patient teaching should include information about the nature of immunodeficiency and prescribed medications, as well as the following instructions regarding the prevention and management of infection:

- Avoid persons with infections (especially colds).
- Inspect skin daily for lesions or breaks.
- Avoid bumping, breaking, or tearing skin.
- Eat a well-balanced diet with sufficient calories to maintain ideal weight.
- Drink at least six glasses of fluid daily.
- Avoid becoming overly fatigued.
- Try to get sufficient sleep every night.
- Decrease environmental contaminants:
  —Avoid stagnant water (e.g., in vases) to prevent bacterial growth.
  —Keep indoor pets clean by bathing frequently.
  —Avoid cold-mist humidifiers that can harbor bacteria.
- Take prophylactic antibiotics before any manipulative or invasive procedures (dental procedures, biopsies, endoscopies, arteriograms).
- Keep scheduled follow-up appointments with health care provider.
- Report signs of infection immediately (increased temperature, redness or swelling of skin or mucous membranes, change in color of sputum, unusual drainage, diarrhea).

EVALUATION

To evaluate the effectiveness of nursing interventions, compare patient behaviors with those stated in the expected patient outcomes.

RELATED NOC OUTCOMES. Immune Status, Infection Severity, Knowledge: Infection Control, Risk Control, Risk Detection

GERONTOLOGIC CONSIDERATIONS

Older adults are at significantly increased risk for the development of secondary immunodeficiencies because of a number of factors. They experience a slowing of the immune response; have an increased incidence of chronic illnesses, such as diabetes mellitus and cancer; are more likely to be taking medications that alter immunity; may be immobile, which places them at risk for skin breakdown; and may not be able to meet their own nutritional needs, which places them at risk for malnutrition.

Gammopathies

Gammopathies, also known as hypergammaglobulinemias, refer to elevated levels of serum gamma globulin resulting from overproduction. The blood normally contains a large number of different proteins collectively called plasma proteins. One type of protein, gamma globulin, combines to make varying types of antibodies for fighting different infections. When the majority of protein produced is an identical type of gamma globulin, the abnormally produced protein is called *monoclonal gammopathy* or *plasma cell dyscrasia.* Multiple myeloma and macroglobulinemia are plasma cell dyscrasias that have distinctive clinical patterns.

When a monoclonal gammopathy occurs in the absence of disease such as myeloma or lymphoma, the disorder is called monoclonal gammopathy of unknown significance (MGUS). The incidence of MGUS varies with age, occurring in about 2% of adults over age 50 and 3% to 4% over age 70. The abnormal protein of MGUS is found in both sexes and all races.[10] The clinical importance of the condition is not well understood. The majority of patients have a low level of monoclonal proteins, remain symptom free, and lead normal lives. It is estimated that about 0.03% of patients over age 50 develop multiple myeloma each year.[8]

Polyclonal gammopathies involve the overproduction of virtually all classes of immunoglobulins in response to inappropriate antigenic stimulation. High levels of dysfunctional immunoglobulins depress the synthesis of normal immunoglobulins, leaving the patient susceptible to infection. IgG and IgM are most commonly involved. The immunoglobulin levels reflect the severity of disease produced. Polyclonal gammopathies are associated with chronic bacterial infections and connective tissue diseases such as lupus erythematosus and rheumatoid arthritis. Table 21-5 summarizes the polyclonal gammopathies.

Multiple Myeloma

Etiology and Epidemiology. Multiple myeloma, which is plasma cell cancer, is the most serious and prevalent of the monoclonal gammopathies. It affects approximately 45,000 people in the United States, with about 14,600 new cases appearing each year, primarily in people between the ages of 65 and 70 years. It occurs in slightly more males than females and twice as often in African-Americans as in Caucasians. The cause of multiple myeloma is unknown, but research has shown possible associations with genetic factors, a decline in immune function, exposure to chemicals or radiation, and more recently a viral origin.[11]

Pathophysiology. Multiple myeloma is a type of bone marrow cancer, which occurs from uncontrolled growth of plasma cells. Normally the bone marrow contains less than 5% plasma cells. Patients with multiple myeloma have bone marrow that contains between 10% and 90% plasma cells. The malignant plasma cells are most often monoclonal, originating from one single defective cell.[11] The cancerous plasma cells collect in many bones, where they may form tumors, weaken bones, and cause pain and fractures. Calcium is released from damaged bones, causing hypercalcemia and resultant fatigue, muscle weakness, or confusion (see Chapter 17). The increased numbers of myeloma cells within bone marrow prevent the formation of white blood cells, erythrocytes, and normal plasma cells, leading to anemia and increased

TABLE 21-5 POLYCLONAL GAMMOPATHIES (HYPERGAMMAGLOBULINEMIA)

Causes	Characteristics
Infectious diseases: chronic bacterial infections (lung abscess and osteomyelitis)	Diffuse increase in antibody synthesis results from inappropriate antigen stimulation. IgG and IgM are most commonly involved immunoglobulins.
Connective tissue disease: Systemic lupus erythematosus Rheumatoid arthritis Chronic active liver disease	Immunoglobulin levels correlate with severity of disease. High levels of dysfunctional immunoglobulins depress synthesis of normal immunoglobulins, leaving person susceptible to infection.

IgG, Immunoglobulin G; *IgM,* immunoglobulin M.

susceptibility to infections. The kidneys are also affected and at increased risk for damage because of the excretion of excess antibodies and calcium.[12]

Patients with multiple myeloma are staged to determine treatment options and prognosis. Staging is based on the estimated number of myeloma cells calculated from the amount of abnormal monoclonal immunoglobulin in the urine and blood; the amount of calcium in the blood; the degree of bone destruction noted on x-ray examination; and the amount of hemoglobin in the blood. Table 21-6 summarizes the three stages of multiple myeloma.

Early in the disease process patients may be symptom free. When manifestations do occur, they may consist of back or rib pain, weight loss, fatigue, weakness, or repeated infections. Later stages of the diseases are associated with nausea, vomiting, anemia, renal damage, or extremity weakness.[9] By the time of diagnosis, bone lesions are typically present in the skull, spine, and pelvis (see Clinical Manifestations box). The major problems encountered by patients with multiple myeloma are related to the complications of pathologic fractures, renal failure, and infection.

Collaborative Care Management. Collaborative management of multiple myeloma is directed at improving the quality of the patient's life by controlling symptoms, reducing tumor cell burden, and preventing complications. Chemotherapy prolongs the survival for patients with stage I disease for 40 to 46 months, stage II disease for 35 to 40 months, and stage III disease for 24 to 30 months.

DIAGNOSTIC TESTS. Various laboratory and other diagnostic tests are completed when patients are symptomatic. Box 21-2 summarizes common diagnostic tests for multiple myeloma.

MEDICATIONS. Combination drug therapy has proven to be a more effective treatment for multiple myeloma than single chemotherapeutic agents. Oral melphalan combined with prednisone is the treatment of choice to reduce tumor load. Other chemotherapy combinations are (1) vincristine sulfate, doxorubicin, cyclophosphamide, and carmustine; (2) vincristine, doxorubicin, and dexamethasone; and (3) thalidomide and dexamethasone. Interferon-alpha therapy has been shown to prolong

TABLE 21-6 STAGING OF MULTIPLE MYELOMA

Stage*	Criteria
Stage I: Relatively small number of myeloma cells are found.	All features must be present: Hemoglobin level only slightly below normal (above 10 g/dl) Bone x-rays normal or show only 1 area of bone damage Normal blood calcium levels (<12 mg/dl) Relatively small amount of monoclonal immunoglobulin in blood or urine
Stage II: Moderate number of myeloma cells are found.	Features between stage I and stage III
Stage III: Large number of myeloma cells are found.	1 or more features must be present: Hemoglobin level reduced significantly (<8.5 g/dl) High blood calcium level (>12 mg/dl) Three or more areas of bone destroyed by cancer Large amount of monoclonal immunoglobulin in blood or urine

Adapted from Multiple Myeloma Research Foundation: *Staging of multiple myeloma,* accessed 2002 from website: http://www.multiplemyeloma.org/about_myeloma/2.06.asp.

*Stage I indicates the least amount of tumor. Stage III indicates the greatest amount of tumor.

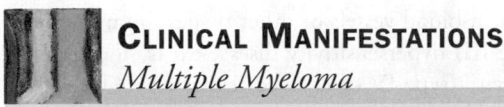

CLINICAL MANIFESTATIONS *Multiple Myeloma*

- *Pain (an early symptom):* Plasma cells accumulate within the bone marrow, causing destruction of bone, which results in fractures.
- *Renal compromise:* Excessive amounts of protein excreted in the urine and hypercalcemia adversely affect renal function.
- *Infections:* Abnormal plasma cells accumulate in the bone marrow, decreasing the production of normal white blood cells (WBCs). Decreased WBCs result in increased bacterial infections.
- *Weakness:* The accumulation of abnormal plasma cells in the bone marrow prevents red blood cell production and results in anemia.

the duration of initial remission once achieved. Glucocorticoids and calcitonin reduce the lytic bone destruction of hypercalcemia. Erythropoietin stimulates the production of red blood cells and helps correct anemia.

The type of combination therapy or other agents used depends on several factors, including the patient's age, the stage of the disease, and the patient's kidney function. If cell transplantation is being considered, drugs with increased risk for bone marrow damage are avoided.

TREATMENTS. For patients who have a solitary skeletal lesion (plasmacytoma) but are otherwise asymptomatic and have fewer than 5% plasma cells in their bone marrow, radiotherapy has been shown to increase survival rates. When bone damage to the spine is extensive, orthopedic fixation devices may be used for stabilization and to prevent cord compression. For patients in renal failure, dialysis may be necessary to correct azotemia and hypercalcemia. Plasmapheresis, a process that filters the blood, may be useful in removing accumulated myeloma proteins that thicken blood and impede circulation to the brain.[3]

DIET. Adequate hydration is necessary to prevent renal complications related to the excretion of increased amounts of urates and calcium in the urine. Fluid intake needs to be sufficient to ensure a minimal urinary output of 1500 ml/day to maintain renal function. If the patient is unable to maintain adequate fluid intake orally or requires nothing-by-mouth status for diagnostic or surgical procedures, intravenous fluids need to be administered. The nurse weighs the patient daily to assess for fluid retention, and monitors the patient's blood urea nitrogen and serum creatinine levels to evaluate renal function. A well-balanced diet is encouraged, but there are no specific dietary restrictions unless renal failure occurs. See Chapter 36 for a discussion of dietary restrictions for patients in renal failure.

Box 21-2 Diagnostic Tests for Multiple Myeloma

- Urine and serum protein electrophoresis to determine the presence of abnormal proteins, and number of normal immunoglobulins
- Bone marrow biopsy to determine the presence and number of cancerous plasma cells
- Computed tomography scans and radiography that show a "punched-out" type of bone lesion or generalized osteoporosis of the axial skeleton
- Complete blood count to determine the presence of anemia, leukopenia, or thrombocytopenia
- Magnetic resonance imaging to detect the presence of bone abnormalities and fractures
- Blood chemistries to detect the presence of hypercalcemia and elevated uric acid levels
- Estimated myeloma cell mass to estimate the tumor burden

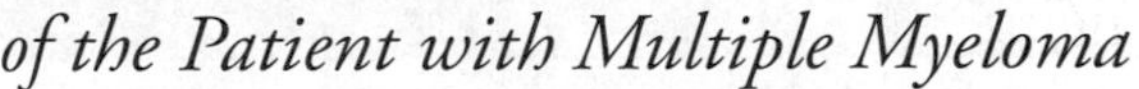

ARE You READY?

Which of the following laboratory results is related to stage III multiple myeloma?

1. Elevated hemoglobin
2. Elevated serum calcium
3. Decreased red blood cell count
4. Decreased serum albumin

Nursing Management *of the Patient with Multiple Myeloma*

ASSESSMENT

Health History. Assess for:

- Back or rib pain
- Excessive fatigue or weakness
- Increased incidence of bacterial infections, urinary tract infections, or shingles
- Changes in urinary pattern or output
- Recent or frequent fractures
- Increased thirst, nausea, loss of appetite

Physical Examination. Assess for:

- Weight gain and edema
- Pale skin or mucous membranes
- Cough
- Abnormal lung sounds

NURSING DIAGNOSES, OUTCOMES, AND INTERVENTIONS

Nursing Diagnosis: Pain (Acute or Chronic)

OUTCOMES. Common examples of expected outcomes for the patient with a diagnosis of *pain* are:

Patient will:

- Use nonanalgesic measures to control pain (e.g., relaxation).
- Rate pain as 3 or less on a scale of 1 (no pain) to 10 (severe pain).
- Verbalize satisfactory control of pain.

NURSING INTERVENTIONS. In the early stages of multiple myeloma, patients may experience little pain or discomfort. During the advanced stage of disease, pain is likely due to fragile bones and fractures. General comfort measures, such as back care, fresh linens, or a quiet environment, may reduce the patient's discomfort. Analgesic medications may include nonsteroidal antiinflammatory agents or narcotic analgesics. Ambulation is encouraged to prevent further bone demineralization associated with immobility, but skeletal pain may be a deterrent to ambulation. A lightweight spinal brace, analgesics, local radiotherapy, and nonanalgesic pain control methods such as distraction may be of benefit.

Safety is of vital importance because of the risk of fractures. Area rugs should be removed from the home to eliminate a potential source of falls. If the patient is completely immobile, careful turning is important. Even a tug on the arm or a turn toward the bed rail can cause a fracture. A lift sheet and the assistance of several people are necessary to facilitate moving the patient gently and safely without causing extensive pain.

RELATED NIC INTERVENTIONS. Analgesic Administration, Coping Enhancement, Distraction, Environmental Management, Pain Management, Patient-Controlled Analgesia (PCA) Assistance, Positioning

Nursing Diagnosis: Risk for Infection

OUTCOMES AND NURSING INTERVENTIONS. See outcomes and interventions in the above discussion on PIs.

EVALUATION

To evaluate the effectiveness of nursing interventions, compare patient behaviors with those stated in the expected patient outcomes.

RELATED NOC OUTCOMES. Comfort Level, Infection Severity, Knowledge: Infection Control, Pain Control, Pain Level, Risk Control, Risk Detection, Symptom Control

GERONTOLOGIC CONSIDERATIONS

Plasma cell cancer (myeloma) is a disease of older adults, with the average age of diagnosis being 68 years. In fact, only 1% of cases occur in persons under the age of 40. The death rate from multiple myeloma is about 11,070 Americans per year, the majority of whom are older adults.[3] Consequently, older adult patients with bone pain, hypercalcemia, or fractures need to be carefully evaluated for myeloma so that management can be initiated early in the disease process.

Hypersensitivities

The immune system is always ready to respond to foreign antigens. Under certain circumstances, however, this response may bring harm as well as protection. Hypersensitivity diseases may be related to two abnormalities: the immune response to antigens may be unrestrained, producing tissue injury; or the immune response may be directed toward self-antigens because of a loss of self-tolerance, which is known as autoimmunity.

Hypersensitivity diseases are broadly divided into five categories based on the immunologic mechanisms involved in the reaction. Immediate hypersensitivity (type I) is mediated by IgE and causes injury from the release of histamine from mast cells. Antibody-mediated (type II) hypersensitivity exists when antibodies are directed against self-antigens. When antigen-antibody complexes collect in blood vessels or other tissues, immune complex disease (type III) hypersensitivity disease exists. T cell mediated hypersensitivity (type IV or delayed) exists when T cells are directed against self-antigens in tissues.[1] Another relatively new hypersensitivity, known as stimulatory (type V), involves the binding of autoantibodies to hormone receptors that mimic the hormone itself, which stimulates target cells (Table 21-7).

Immediate Hypersensitivity

Immediate or type I hypersensitivity is an exaggerated immune response occurring in persons who have been previously sensitized to the specific antigen. The antigen producing the reaction is referred to as an *allergen,* and the reaction itself is called **allergy** or **atopy.** Immediate hypersensitivities are characterized by inappropriate, rapid, and exaggerated responses mediated by IgE antibodies and mast cells. People who tend to produce IgE in response to antigens such as pollen or dust mites are said to be *atopic.* A severe, potentially lethal systemic form of immediate hypersensitivity reaction is known as **systemic anaphylaxis** or *anaphylactic shock.*

Etiology and Epidemiology. The onset of allergic diseases generally occurs between the ages of 2 and 15 years, although they can begin at any age. More than 50 million Americans suffer from allergies, which are the sixth leading cause of chronic disease in the United States. Atopic dermatitis is the most common skin disease, but allergic rhinitis accounts for the majority of visits to health care providers each year. It is estimated that 8% of children under the age of 6 and 1% to 2% of adults have food allergies. Approximately 3 million Americans are allergic to peanut or nut tree allergens, which produce the most severe food-induced reactions. Allergic reactions account for 5% to 10% of all adverse drug reactions. Penicillin, which is the most common drug allergen, causes about 400 deaths annually, making it a more common cause of death than food allergens.[14]

The tendency to become hypersensitive and produce IgE antibodies in response to inhaled or ingested substances is inherited as a dominant trait. If both parents have allergies, their children have a 50% probability of also having allergies.[17] The specific substances that an individual develops hypersensitivity to, however, are determined by the allergens to which that individual is exposed. A person does not inherit a specific allergy, only the predisposition to develop allergies. No association has been found between gender, race, or geographic area and an increased risk of anaphylaxis.

Allergens are primarily characterized by their route of exposure. Inhaled allergens such as pollens, dust mite fecal matter, fungal hyphae or spores, and animal dander are main causal agents of hayfever, chronic rhinitis, and asthma. Common food allergens, such as peanuts, eggs, milk, soy, chicken, and shellfish, are thought to trigger mast cell degranulation in the gut after entering the circulation (see Future Watch box, p. 460). Whether an allergic response occurs and to what degree depends on a combination of interrelated factors (Box 21-3).

Pathophysiology. Immediate hypersensitivities are mediated by the IgE class of immunoglobulins. In genetically predisposed people, initial exposure to an allergen prompts the activation of

TABLE 21-7 HYPERSENSITIVITY REACTIONS

Type	Immune System Mediators	Allergens	Response to Intradermal Skin Test	Pathophysiologic Effects	Examples
HUMORAL (IMMEDIATE)					
I—Anaphylactic	IgE bound to mast cells	Exogenous antigens	Wheal and flare within 30 min, edema	Release of histamines, kinins, chemotactic factors, and active products of arachidonic acid metabolism (leukotrienes, prostaglandins, and thromboxanes) from mast cells, which affect smooth muscle, mucous glands	Systemic anaphylaxis, atopic allergies, hayfever, insect sting reactions
TISSUE SPECIFIC					
II—Antibody mediated (cytotoxic)	IgG or IgM (plus complement)	Foreign cells or alteration of cell surface antigens	Not done	Direct cytotoxic destruction of cells	Hemolytic disease of the newborn (Rh), transfusion reactions
III—Antigen-antibody complex (immune complex)	IgG or IgM (plus complement)	Soluble antigens	Erythema and edema within 3-8 hr	Acute inflammatory reaction; primarily polymorphonuclear neutrophil leukocytes	Serum sickness, Arthus reaction, glomerulonephritis
CELLULAR (DELAYED)					
IV—T cell mediated	T cells, macrophages	Infectious agent, contact allergens, foreign tissues, cancer cells	Erythema and induration within 24-48 hr	Tissue destruction; primarily lymphocytes and macrophages	Tuberculin reaction, skin graft rejection, poison ivy
STIMULATORY					
V—B cell mediated	B cells, auto-antibodies	Unknown	Not done	Inappropriate stimulation of target cell with uncontrolled secretion of hormone	Graves' disease (hyperthyroidism)

IgG, Immunoglobulin G; *IgM,* immunoglobulin M.

T_H2 cells, which are not produced by normal individuals. T_H2 cells stimulate the production of IgE antibodies that sensitize the person to the allergen. This initial contact with the allergen is known as the *sensitizing dose.* In some cases it may take several doses of allergen before the person's immune system is fully sensitized. Once sensitization is complete, subsequent exposure (termed the *challenging dose*) results in the allergen combining with IgE and binding to receptor sites on mast cells and basophils. This antigen-antibody reaction results in a rapid release of potent vasoactive mediators such as histamine, kinins, chemotactic factors, and active products of arachidonic acid metabolism (leukotrienes, prostaglandins, and thromboxanes)[1] (Figure 21-3).

Vasoactive mediators produce the clinical manifestations associated with immediate hypersensitivity, which includes smooth muscle contraction, increased vascular permeability, and increased mucous gland secretion. These changes may occur locally or at the site of the antigen-antibody reaction. Atopic allergens generally

Future Watch

Is a New Drug To Prevent Peanut Allergy on the Way?

Researchers have estimated that about 1.5 million Americans have peanut allergies and that 50 to 100 of them die annually from severe anaphylactic reactions. In clinical trials, researchers found that monthly injections of TNX-901, an engineered antibody that blocks the allergy-causing antibody (immunoglobulin E), reduces the risk of an allergic reaction to peanuts in sensitive persons. Study participants who reacted to as few as one half to two peanuts were able to tolerate an average of nine peanuts, and about a fourth of the participants were able to tolerate as many as 24 peanuts, without suffering severe reactions.

While promising, this drug is only available to study participants. Even if further clinical trials validate current findings, the treatment is not likely to be available to the public for several years.

Food Allergy and Anaphylaxis Network: *New peanut allergy drug shows great promise,* accessed 2003 from website: http://www.foodallergy.org/press_releases/statement.html.

produce *localized* tissue reactions that remain confined to a specific area such as the skin, nasal passages, or lungs. Hives (urticaria) are pruritic lesions characterized by a pale pink elevated edge (wheal) on an erythematous background (Figure 21-4). Skin exposed to latex can precipitate contact urticaria. Chronic urticaria that occurs in response to heat, cold, or various light waves is not an IgE-mediated hypersensitivity. Angioedema is a form of urticaria that involves the subcutaneous tissue rather than the skin. It can affect an entire anatomic part, such as the eyelid, thumb, or lip. Swelling is present, but not pruritus. Atopic diseases are not usually life threatening, but the symptoms can be uncomfortable and may cause the individual to miss school or work. A mosquito bite is a classic example of this type of reaction; the intradermal injection of the mosquito anticoagulants produces a wheal-flare type of reaction within minutes. The Clinical Manifestations box on p. 461 summarizes other symptoms associated with immediate hypersensitivity.

Anaphylaxis may be localized or widespread. Localized anaphylaxis produces hives and angioedema (Figure 21-5). If widespread mast cell degranulation occurs, producing systemic effects such as decreased blood pressure, bronchial obstruction, and edema in many tissues, systemic anaphylaxis or anaphylactic shock is said to exist (Figure 21-6). It is the most severe form of immediate hypersensitivity in humans. Apprehension and sneezing are two of the earliest symptoms of systemic anaphylaxis. Edema and itching may also occur at the site of antigen entrance. These mild reactions are rapidly followed, sometimes in a matter of seconds or minutes, by severe manifestations that lead to vascular collapse, shock, and death unless rapid action is taken (see Clinical Manifestations box, p. 462). Chapter 19 contains a discussion of shock. Insect or snake venoms; foods; and drugs such as penicillin, streptokinase, or amphotericin B are most often associated with anaphylaxis, although almost any antigen to which a person is hypersensitive has the potential for producing a systemic reaction.

Latex hypersensitivity, which has a high potential for producing anaphylaxis, has become a universal concern among health

Box 21-3 Factors That Determine a Hypersensitivity Response

- *Responsiveness of the host to the allergen:* If the host is highly sensitive to the antigen, a greater than normal chance exists that a tissue-damaging reaction will occur.
- *Amount of allergen:* Generally the greater the amount of allergen contacted, the more severe the reaction.
- *Nature of the allergen:* Any foreign protein or protein-containing component can serve as an allergen when coupled with a normal tissue protein carrier. Examples include pollens, foods, animal dander, house dust, and feathers.
- *Route of entrance of the allergen:* Allergens may gain host entry via the respiratory tract, through epidermal or mucosal surfaces, by injection, or through the digestive tract.
- *Timing of exposure to the allergen:* If the host's contacts with the allergen are widely separated by time, the immunologic mediators may be so dilute that little response occurs. Conversely, if frequent contact is made with the allergen, reactions are more likely to occur.
- *Site of the allergen–immune mediator reaction:* A reaction can occur in the tissues with little consequence; however, the same reaction occurring in the bloodstream can lead to a severe reaction.
- *Host's threshold of reactivity:* The host's immune system can be changed by factors such as stress, fatigue, or infection, all of which can decrease the immune system's responsiveness to potential allergens.

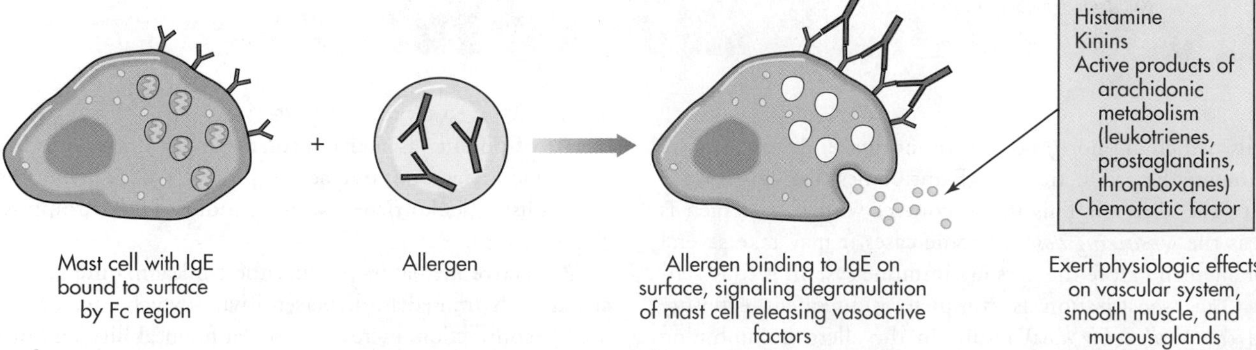

Figure 21-3 Mediators of immediate (type I) hypersensitivity. *Fc*, fragment, crystallizable; *IgE*, Immunoglobulin E.

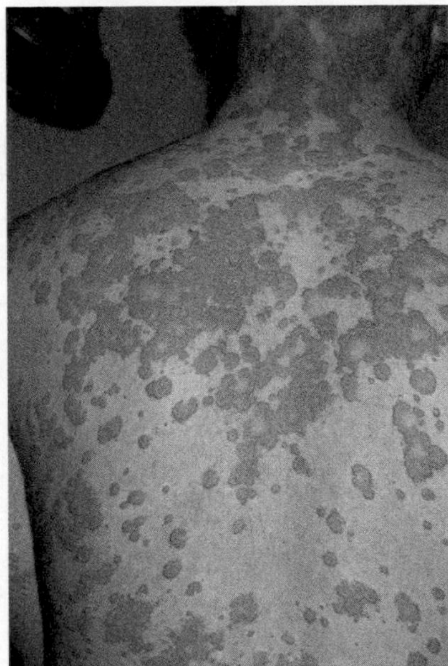

Figure 21-4 Diffuse urticaria. Lesions have raised edges and appear within minutes to hours. They almost always resolve within 12 hours, leaving no trace on skin.

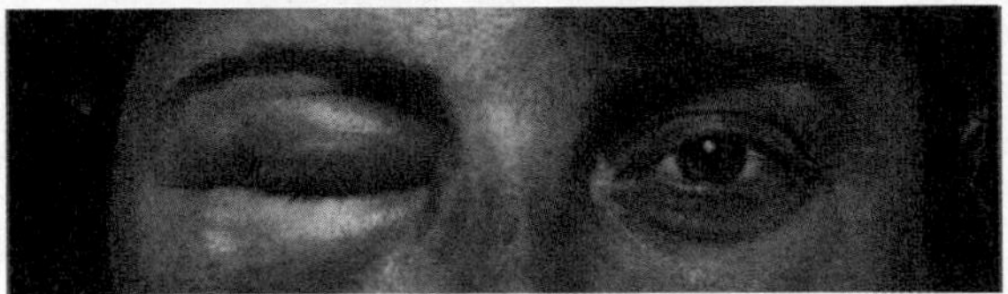

Figure 21-5 Localized anaphylactic response to bee sting. Immediate reaction occurs within 20 minutes and is mediated by release of histamine and other mediators from mast cells. Although this reaction is localized, it can become systemic, producing systemic anaphylaxis and shock.

care workers, since numerous medical products such as gloves, catheters, and tubes contain latex and about 200 cases of anaphylaxis and three deaths from latex are reported annually. In 1997 the National Institute for Occupational Safety and Health (NIOSH) issued an alert titled *Preventing Allergic Reactions to Natural Latex in the Workplace.* The prevalence of latex allergy is estimated at about 6% for the general population.[14] Signs of latex allergy depend largely on the route of exposure. When latex particles are aerosolized, wheezing, rhinitis, and conjunctivitis may occur. Mucosal exposure frequently results in angioedema. There is no cure for latex hypersensitivity, and avoidance is the principal treatment.

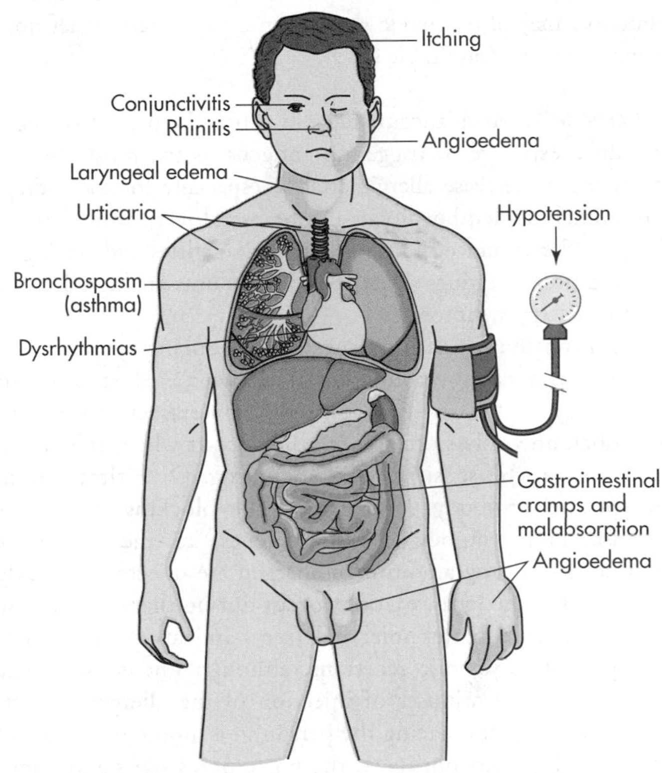

Figure 21-6 Clinical manifestations of systemic anaphylaxis.

CLINICAL MANIFESTATIONS *Immediate (Type I) Hypersensitivity*

Respiratory
- Rhinorrhea
- Watery, itching eyes
- Obstruction of eustachian tubes
- Sneezing
- Sinusitis
- Headache
- Facial pain
- Bronchospasm
- Dyspnea
- Stridor
- Tachypnea
- Wheezing
- Cyanosis
- Use of accessory muscles for breathing
- Flaring of nare

Dermal
- Hives
- Rash
- Angioedema

Abdominal
- Nausea
- Vomiting
- Cramping
- Diarrhea

General
- Fever
- Diaphoresis
- Malaise
- Joint pain
- Hematopoietic suppression
- Anxiety
- Anaphylaxis

Collaborative Care Management

DIAGNOSTIC TESTS. The health history, including an environmental assessment, is one of the most valuable diagnostic tools for the health care provider evaluating the patient for immediate hypersensitivities. Intradermal skin testing and the radioallergosorbent test (RAST) may be helpful in identifying antigens and determining therapy for persons with allergies (Table 21-8, Figure 21-7). Eosinophilia (increased eosinophil count) is associated with antigen-antibody reactions and occurs in persons with allergies, hayfever, and drug hypersensitivity.[6]

MEDICATIONS. Symptom relief is the primary aim of drug therapy for allergies. Urticaria and angioedema are usually self-limiting; therefore treatment is often not required. Anaphylaxis is treated with epinephrine to shorten its duration and prevent relapse. When intravenous access is not available, epinephrine is administered by intramuscular injection to provide the highest level of absorption (see Research box). Antihistamines, such as diphenhydramine (Benadryl), are given to block histamine receptors. Short-term corticosteroid therapy, either oral or inhaled (cromolyn sodium), may be useful for decreasing the inflammation associated with allergic responses. Leukotriene-mediated bronchoconstriction is treated with leukotriene receptor blocking agents such as montelukast (Singulair) or zafirlukast (Accolate). Aminophylline or inhalants such as isoproterenol (terbutaline, albuterol) may also provide short-term symptomatic relief from bronchoconstriction (Table 21-9).

TREATMENTS. Avoidance therapy, in which the patient is taught to reduce exposure to triggering antigens, is the most effective treatment to decrease allergic attacks, especially for food, drug, and animal dander, but it can also be useful in treating seasonal allergies. For instance, limiting outdoor activities and staying in air-conditioned settings when the pollen counts are high decrease seasonal allergy symptoms.

Immunotherapy is often useful in reducing symptoms in patients who cannot avoid antigens such as dust mites or pollen. The health care provider injects an extract of the allergen subcutaneously starting with the dose at which the person was found to be sensitive by skin testing. Over time, serum IgE-specific antibody levels fall, IgG blocking antibodies increase, and lymphocyte responsiveness to the antigen is reduced. Increasing amounts of allergen are injected at weekly intervals. If large local reactions occur during therapy, the dose is lowered until better tolerated (see Clinical Manifestations box, p. 464). Systemic reactions, although uncommon, may occur within 30 minutes of injection of the allergen extract. Treatment includes placing the person in a supine position and administering epinephrine. If the nurse notes signs and symptoms of systemic anaphylactic shock, oxygen is administered and intravenous fluids infused rapidly to support blood pressure (see Chapter 19 for treatment of shock). Because of its potential for anaphylaxis and death, the patient and primary caregiver must be certain that the symptoms warrant the risk, expense, and inconvenience of immunotherapy.

The future of immediate hypersensitivity treatment appears to lie in learning how to more effectively modulate the immune response. Possible therapies include manipulating IgE response by using IgE-specific suppressor T cells; using antibodies against IgE idiotopes; or using cytokines to suppress IgE synthesis (see Future Watch box, p. 466).

DIET. The diet may be altered in patients with food allergies to avoid those foods precipitating the response. Suspected foods are eliminated to see if allergy symptoms disappear. They may be reintroduced to see if they again cause symptoms. Foods suspected of causing systemic anaphylaxis are not reintroduced or only reintroduced under supervision in a hospital setting (see Complementary & Alternative Therapies box, p. 466).

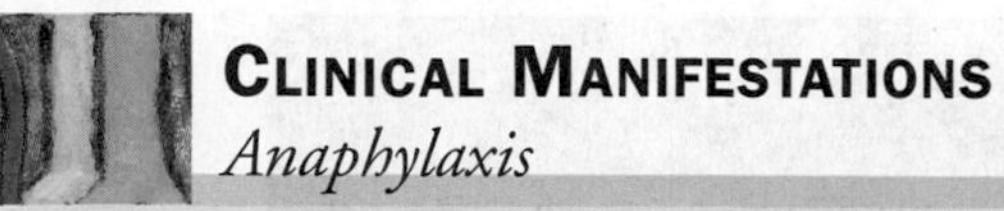

CLINICAL MANIFESTATIONS
Anaphylaxis

Localized

Hives
Angioedema

Systemic

Apprehension
Edema of the face, hands, or other parts of the body
Wheezing
Dyspnea
Respiratory collapse
Vascular collapse with shock
—Rapid, weak pulse
—Falling blood pressure
—Cyanosis
Death

ARE You READY?

The nurse suspects systemic anaphylaxis when a patient demonstrates which of the following clinical manifestations?

1. Hyperventilation
2. Elevated blood pressure
3. Elevated temperature
4. Rapid, weak pulse

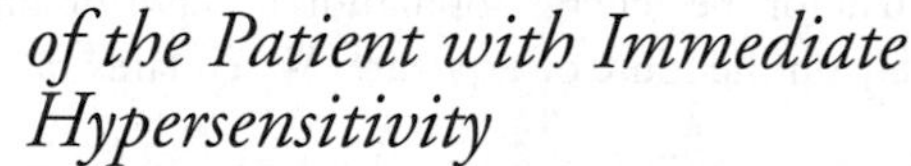

Nursing Management
of the Patient with Immediate Hypersensitivity

ASSESSMENT

Health History. Assess for:
- History of allergic reactions (type, frequency, or perceived causes)
- Familial history of allergies
- Recent exposure to sensitizing substances (chemicals, drugs)
- Changes in living, working, or environmental conditions
- Characteristics of present environment (house, clothing, plants, trees, or animals)
- Symptoms experienced: respiratory, dermal, gastrointestinal, or general
- Alleviating factors, either prescribed, herbal, or over the counter

Physical Examination. Assess for:
- Rashes (location, color)
- Mouth breathing (nasal obstruction)
- Flaring nares
- Difficulty hearing (plugged eustachian tubes)
- Pale bluish turbinates that are edematous with clear secretions
- Tearing or dark areas under eyes (venous dilation of skin)
- Scleral or conjunctival infections
- Increased respiratory rate

TABLE 21-8 DIAGNOSTIC TESTS FOR ALLERGENS

Test	Implications
Skin prick test	Tiny amount of suspected antigen is placed onto skin (forearm, upper arm, or back), then several small scratches or pricks are made to provide portal of entry for antigen. Skin is observed for signs of reaction to allergen, which generally occurs within 20 min. Swelling and redness at site indicates positive reaction. This is best test for immediate hypersensitivity reactions (type I). Positive test only indicates sensitization to a particular allergen; it does not predict clinical significance.
Intradermal test	Tiny amount of suspected allergen is injected intradermally. Injection site is then observed for signs of reaction, which generally occur in about 20 min. Positive reaction is similar to hives with swelling and redness. Intradermal test generally provides more reliable results than prick test because it is more sensitive.
Radioallergosorbent testing (RAST)	RAST is performed by withdrawing blood and testing for specific immunoglobulin E antibodies to suspected antigen. It is less sensitive than skin testing and more expensive. It is generally done when patients have skin problems that prevent skin testing, or they are taking medications (histamines, antidepressants) that make skin testing difficult, or anaphylactic shock could result from skin test.
Provocation testing	Patient breathes in air or uses nasal spray containing suspected allergen to see if it produces allergic reaction. These tests are performed under supervised conditions in case serious reactions occur.
Eosinophil count	Eosinophil count is part of white blood cell count differential. Eosinophil are generally elevated in presence of allergic responses.

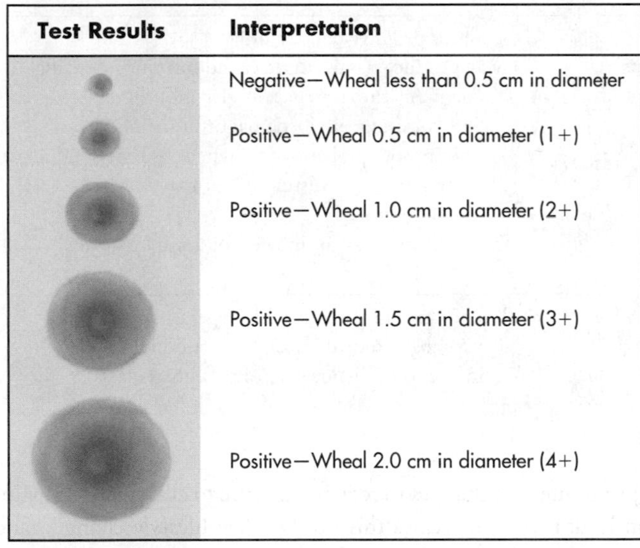

Figure 21-7 Interpretation of intradermal allergy test results based on size of wheal after 15 to 30 minutes.

- Use of accessory muscles for breathing
- Audible wheezing
- Anxious expression

NURSING DIAGNOSES, OUTCOMES, AND INTERVENTIONS

Nursing Diagnosis: Risk for Latex Allergy Response

OUTCOMES. Common examples of expected outcomes for the patient with a diagnosis of *risk for latex allergy response* (or other allergy responses) are:

Research

American Academy of Allergy Asthma and Immunology, *Pediatricians and food-induced anaphylaxis*, accessed 2004 from website: http://allergies.about.com/gi/dynamic/offsite.htm?zi=1/XJ&sdn=allergies&zu=http%3A%2F%2Fwww.aaaai.org%2Fmedia%2Fnews_releases%2F2004%2F03%2F031904.stm.

Researchers at Mount Sinai School of Medicine surveyed 61 pediatricians regarding treatment of food-induced anaphylaxis using a simulated case in which a 12-year-old child suffers an anaphylactic reaction. As part of the study, physicians were asked about the initial treatment for anaphylaxis. Ninety-one percent of study participants stated that the initial treatment should be with epinephrine. However, only 48% would have administered the medication intramuscularly, which would have resulted in the highest level of absorption. Even though epinephrine is recognized as the gold standard of treatment, many of the pediatricians selected the incorrect dose and route of administration. The researchers concluded that the study results indicate the need for further education about the importance of administering epinephrine intramuscularly when treating food-induced anaphylaxis.

Patient will:

- Verbalize understanding of approaches for avoiding allergen (all latex-containing products).
- Plan to alter habits or environment to reduce exposure to antigens.
- Verbalize understanding of prescribed and alternative approaches to symptom relief.

NURSING INTERVENTIONS. An important aspect of nursing care for the patient with allergies is helping the patient identify and

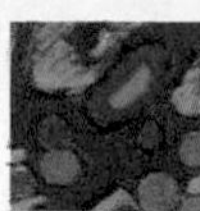

TABLE 21-9
COMMON MEDICATIONS *for Type I Hypersensitivities*

Drug	Action	Nursing Intervention
Antihistamines		
Diphenhydramine (Benadryl) Chlorpheniramine (Chlor-Trimeton) Brompheniramine (Dimetane) Astemizole (Hismanal) Loratadine (Claritin) Clemastine (Tavist) Fexofenadine hydrochloride (Allegra)	Antihistamine; compete with histamine for effector cell H_1-receptor sites, thus preventing action of histamine	May produce significant drowsiness (Benadryl) or central nervous system stimulation (Chlor-Trimeton); causes dry mouth; may produce blurred vision. Do not use for patients with hypersensitivity, narrow-angle glaucoma, lower respiratory tract disease, or acute asthma attacks; patients who are pregnant or breastfeeding; or patients who took monoamine oxidase inhibitors within past 14 days. Advise patient to take 1 hr before or 1 hr after meals to facilitate drug absorption.
Decongestants		
Phenylephrine (Neo-Synephrine) Pseudoephedrine (Sudafed)	Stimulate alpha-adrenergic receptors to shrink respiratory mucous membranes	May produce nausea, vomiting, headache, anxiety, tremors, dizziness, seizures, tachycardia, hypertension, dysrhythmias, mucous membrane irritation, or dry mouth. Monitor blood pressure and pulse; give several hours before bedtime if drug produces sleeplessness. Do not use for patients with hypertension. Teach patient to stop drug if tremors or restlessness occurs.
Mast Cell Degranulator Inhibitor		
Cromolyn sodium inhaler (Intal) Cromolyn sodium nasal spray (Nasalcrom)	Inhibit mast cell release of histamine and slow-reacting substance of anaphylaxis, thus preventing allergic response	Give for prophylactic use only. May produce nasal irritation and burning, sneezing, cough, or throat irritation; dry mouth; nausea and vomiting; angioedema; or bronchospasm. Do not give to patients with hypersensitivity, acute asthma, or history of coronary artery disease or dysrhythmias. Teach effective use of inhaler for accurate dosing.
Corticosteroids		
Prednisone Methylprednisone Dexamethasone (Decadron)	Suppress migration of polymorphonuclear leukocytes and fibroblasts, thereby reducing inflammation	Do not give to patients with hypersensitivity, psychoses, fungal infections, acquired immunodeficiency syndrome, tuberculosis.

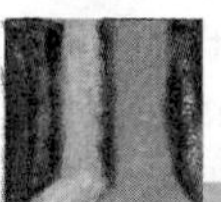

CLINICAL MANIFESTATIONS
Immunotherapy Reactions

Localized	
Redness	Edema
Pruritus	Tenderness
Systemic	
Nasal stuffiness	Sneezing
Reddening of conjunctiva	Chest tightness
Wheezing	Fainting
Apprehension	Anaphylactic shock

adjust to lifestyle changes to reduce exposure to allergens and maintain health. In many cases this involves few lifestyle changes, and the patient and family readily adjust. In other cases the patient may need to adjust to a complex medication schedule, give up a beloved pet, or move to another climate. Patients may have to change employment to avoid allergens such as chemicals, molds, or fibers. These changes may place emotional or financial burdens on the patient and family, especially if the job market or patient's skills are limited. The nurse's role is to help the patient explore alternative solutions and make the best choices possible to maintain health.

Teaching the patient and family about the disorder and methods to avoid the allergen is another important nursing intervention for the patient with allergies. The nurse reviews results of allergy testing, assessment findings, and patient history so the patient and family understand which allergens need to be controlled or avoided. The nurse teaches patients the importance of controlling their liv-

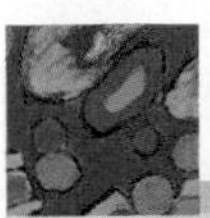

TABLE 21-9
COMMON MEDICATIONS *for Type I Hypersensitivities—cont'd*

Drug	Action	Nursing Intervention
Corticosteroids (cont'd)		
Beclomethasone (Vancenase, Beconase)		Monitor for thrombocytopenia, increased intraocular pressure, poor wound healing, nausea, diarrhea, headache, mood changes. Monitor daily weight, serum potassium levels, blood glucose levels, blood pressure, signs of infection, mood changes. Tell patients to take with food or milk to decrease gastrointestinal irritation. Caution patient not to stop taking drug abruptly and to notify health care provider if infection develops.
Adrenalin		
Epinephrine	Opposes action of histamine through vasoconstriction to raise blood pressure; promotes bronchiole relaxation to facilitate breathing; stimulates both alpha and beta receptors to reproduce effects of sympathetic nervous system	Use for temporary relief from anaphylaxis, hypersensitivity reactions, bronchospasm, and acute asthma attacks. Do not use for patients with hypersensitivity, narrow-angle glaucoma, dysrhythmias. Monitor for anxiety, tremors, palpitations, tachydysrhythmias, hypertension, pulmonary edema. Use intramuscular route when intravenous access is not available, since it provides highest level of absorption during systemic anaphylaxis.
Aminophylline		
Theophylline (Theo-Dur)	Xanthine blocks phosphodiesterase, thus increasing cyclic adenosine monophosphate, which alters intracellular calcium and ion movement, produces respiratory tract relaxation and bronchodilation, and increases pulmonary blood flow	Monitor for central nervous system stimulation, dizziness, anxiety, restlessness, seizures, tachycardia, dysrhythmias, nausea, vomiting, insomnia. Do not give to patients with hypersensitivity to xanthine or history of tachydysrhythmias. Instruct patient to avoid intake of stimulant foods such as coffee, tea, and colas. Monitor theophylline blood levels. Instruct patient to avoid smoking because it interferes with absorption.

ing and working environments to reduce exposure to antigens and, hence, the risk of reactions (see Patient/Family Teaching box, p. 467, left). If animal dander is a source of allergy and removal of a family pet is unacceptable to the patient or family, they may explore ways to decrease the pet's impact on the allergic patient, such as keeping the pet outdoors or away from the room where the patient sleeps or spends large amounts of time (see Research box, p. 467).

The nurse emphasizes the need for total avoidance for patients who are latex sensitive. Patients are taught about prescribed medications, including desired actions, dosage schedules, and potential side effects. The nurse stresses the importance of maintaining drug schedules for prophylactic drugs, such as cromolyn, and reminds the patient and family that these drugs are of no value during an acute allergic attack.

Anaphylaxis can occur after exposure to offending antigens or from immunotherapy; consequently, the nurse teaches the patient and family about symptoms that need to be reported, potential reactions that necessitate emergency measures, and use of emergency care kits. If the patient chooses to undergo immunotherapy, the nurse discusses the risks and benefits, schedules, and costs. The nurse informs the patient that immunotherapy can be reinstituted if symptoms recur (see Nursing Care Plan, p. 468).

Patients with immediate hypersensitivities need to be aware of situations in which their specific allergens are likely to be present. The nurse gives those with insect sting sensitivity information about where to obtain and how to use emergency kits for insect stings. The nurse teaches both the patient and family how to use the self-injecting syringe to administer epinephrine. If the patient is unable to use the syringe, an inhalation of high-dose epinephrine may be taken from a metered-dose aerosol, which is found in some emergency kits (see Patient/Family Teaching box, p. 467, right).

Future Watch

Will Pets Lead to New Developments in Allergy Therapy?

According to a study supported by the National Institute of Allergy and Infectious Diseases and the National Institute of Environmental Health Sciences, children raised in a house with two or more dogs or cats during the first year of life may be less likely to develop allergic diseases compared with children raised without pets. The researchers monitored 474 children from birth to 6 or 7 years of age. When children were age 1, the researchers contacted parents to determine the number of pets in the house. At age 2, researchers measured the level of dust mite allergen in the children's bedrooms. At age 6 or 7, the researchers tested the children for allergic antibodies to common allergens by skin prick test and blood measurement.

Researchers found that children exposed to two or more dogs or cats during the first year of life were on the average 66% to 77% less likely to have any allergic antibodies to common allergens (dogs, cats, dust mites, ragweed, grass), compared with children exposed to only one or no pets during their first year. According to the researchers, study findings suggest that bacteria carried by pets may be responsible for suppressing the immune system's allergic response by shifting it away from responding antigens through a class of lymphocytes called T_H2 cells, which are associated with allergic reactions. They further concluded that if it could be determined exactly what it is about pets or the bacteria they carry that prevents the allergic response, it could lead to new developments in allergy therapy.

Ownby DR et al: Exposure to dogs and cats in the first year of life and risk of allergic sensitization at 6 to 7 years of age, *JAMA* 288(8):963-972, 2002.

RELATED NIC INTERVENTIONS. Allergy Management, Risk Identification, Surveillance, Teaching: Disease Process

Nursing Diagnosis: Ineffective Airway Clearance

OUTCOMES. Common examples of expected outcomes for the patient with a diagnosis of *ineffective airway clearance* are:

Patient will:

- Maintain a patent airway.
- Correctly demonstrate the use of emergency anaphylactic equipment.
- Verbalize the need to have emergency anaphylactic equipment available at all times.
- Verbalize the need to inform all health care providers regarding his or her latex sensitivity.

NURSING INTERVENTIONS. Death from anaphylaxis occurs from asphyxiation because of upper airway edema and congestion, irreversible shock, or a combination of these factors (see the section on clinical manifestations of systemic anaphylaxis). The primary concern during an anaphylactic reaction is ensuring that the patient's airway is patent. The nurse positions the patient in a high Fowler's position to maximize ventilation; inserts an oral airway if necessary; and removes secretions by suction or by encouraging the patient to cough. Oxygen therapy is initiated in accordance with facility protocols. The nurse encourages slow, deep breathing to facilitate the intake of oxygen and decrease anxiety. The administration of epinephrine or bronchodilators such as aminophylline may be necessary to decrease bronchospasm. In severe cases, tracheostomy may be necessary to maintain a patent airway. The nurse closely monitors the patient both during and after anaphylaxis, since recurrence is possible.

Respiratory compromise can lead to impaired cardiac function and death within minutes. At the first sign of anaphylaxis, the nurse gives the patient epinephrine, 1:1000 solution, 0.3 to 0.5 ml subcutaneously or intramuscularly. If shock continues, the nurse may administer albuterol (Ventolin) or epinephrine through aerosol treatments. Vasopressors such as dopamine may be prescribed for severe shock to assist in maintaining blood pressure and cardiac output (see Chapter 19 for a discussion of the treatment of shock).

Since drug allergies are a significant cause of anaphylaxis, the nurse questions all patients about allergies and drug sensitivities before initiating drug therapy. High-risk persons are instructed to wear an identification bracelet or necklace at all times that indicates the known allergy. Such devices may be obtained from MedicAlert or other commercial sources. Persons with known drug allergies are advised to alert health care workers of their allergies when animal sera, allergenic extracts, or contrast media containing iodide need to be given for any reason, so that epinephrine can be readily available. The nurse monitors the patient for at least 30 minutes after administration of such substances. Any reaction that occurs within a few minutes forewarns of an impending emergency.

Nurses need to recognize the potential for drug cross-sensitivity when administering alternative drugs to allergic patients. For example, cephalosporins are frequently administered to patients who are sensitive to penicillin. A small percentage of patients will, however, also be sensitive to cephalosporin because it has a cross-sensitivity with penicillin. The yellow dye contained in some tablets has a cross-sensitivity with aspirin and may cause anaphylaxis in aspirin-sensitive patients.

RELATED NIC INTERVENTIONS. Airway Management, Airway Suctioning, Allergy Management, Anaphylaxis Management, Risk Identification, Shock Management: Vasogenic, Surveillance

Complementary & Alternative Therapies

Green Tea Could Block Allergic Reactions

For years, people have been drinking tea to fight the sneezing, coughing, and watery eyes that are characteristic of colds and allergies. Now a new study suggests that drinking green tea may also block allergic reactions. Researchers in Japan have identified a compound, methylated epigallocatechin gallate (EGCG), in green tea that blocks the production of histamine and immunoglobulin E, two compounds in the body that are chiefly involved in triggering and sustaining allergic reactions. Although similar compounds in green tea have previously been shown to be antiallergenic, this particular compound appears to be the most potent. According to Tachibana, the principal researcher, this new study adds to a small but growing body of scientific evidence that green tea may actually work. If it does, green tea may be useful against a wide range of allergens, including pollen, dust, pet dander, and certain chemicals.

Warner J: Antioxidant in tea may prevent allergic reactions, *Consumer Health Rev,* accessed September 2002 from website: http://www.consumerhealthreviews.com/articles/ChineseHerbs/GreenTeaHelpsAllergies.htm.

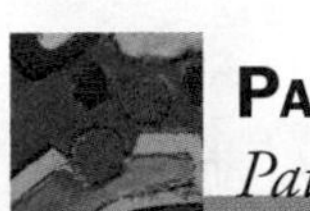

PATIENT/FAMILY TEACHING *The Patient With Allergies*

Patient teaching should include information about the allergy and prescribed medications, as well as the following instructions on avoiding allergens.

Animal Dander

Avoid fur-bearing pets if possible, or keep pets outdoors.
Avoid furniture stuffed with horsehair or feathers.

Pollen Spores

Use air conditioning if possible; keep windows closed at night; if using air conditioner in car, start car, roll down windows, and allow air conditioner to run for 10 to 15 minutes before entering car.
Limit time outdoors between sunset and sunrise, especially when windy.
Do not hang wash outside to dry. (Pollen and molds stick to wet wash.)
Avoid gardening, raking leaves, mowing lawn, or being near freshly cut grass.
Keep car windows closed when driving.
Minimize number of indoor plants.
Vacation in selected geographic areas, such as beach or sea, that are free of specific allergen during seasonal height, if possible.

House Dust

Use synthetic materials; avoid wool and cotton.
Use a minimum of lint-producing articles.
Put away items that are difficult to dust.
Dust with damp cloth daily.
Use air conditioner if possible.
Change furnace filter every month when in use.

Research

National Institute of Environmental Health Sciences: *National survey examines factors related to high level of dust mite and cockroach allergen in beds,* accessed from website: http://allergies.about.com/gi/dynamic/offsite.htm?site=http://www.nih.gov/news/pr/may2001/niehs%2D22.htm.

Researchers from the National Institute of Environmental Health Sciences undertook a study to determine whether the level of dust mite and cockroach allergens in bedding was high enough to induce allergies or asthma. Antigen levels greater than 2 mcg per gram of dust are considered allergic. Taking dust samples from 831 homes in different regions throughout the United States, researchers found that 45% of homes have greater than 2 mcg per gram of dust, and that 45% of those had levels greater than 10 mcg/g. The study concluded that a large number of homes have dust mite antigen levels sufficient to pose a significant risk for development of allergies and asthma, and that housekeeping practices and antigen-proof bedding are necessary to reduce exposure to high levels of allergens.

PATIENT/FAMILY TEACHING *The Patient With Immediate Hypersensitivity: Sting*

Patient teaching should include:

- Emergency care for the specific allergy
- Availability and use of commercially prepared emergency kit
- Concentration and route of emergency use epinephrine (1:1000 epinephrine injection)
- Use of self-injection syringe of epinephrine supplied with kit (spring loaded; can be given through clothing)

Also include the following instructions about the emergency procedure if sting occurs:

- Immediately swallow the uncoated antihistamine tablet.
- Inject the epinephrine.
- If unable to self-inject, inhale high-dose epinephrine from metered-does aerosol* (if included in kit).

*Epinephrine is rapidly absorbed through respiratory tract and will help relieve bronchoconstriction and bronchospasms; not recommended as primary treatment because it does not correct hypotension.

EVALUATION

To evaluate the effectiveness of nursing interventions, compare patient behaviors with those stated in the expected patient outcomes.

RELATED NOC OUTCOMES. Allergic Response: Localized, Allergic Response: Systemic, Respiratory Status: Airway Patency, Risk Control, Symptom Control

GERONTOLOGIC CONSIDERATIONS

Older adults undergo changes in their patterns of immunologic response that leave them with a decreased ability to respond to immunologic events, including allergens; thus their allergies may actually improve or cease to exist. Even so, between 27% and 38% of adults with a history of childhood allergic asthma have a recurrence of the disease in later life. Therefore the nurse assesses older adults for allergies and teaches them the same emergency interventions as younger adults. If older adults are unable to care for themselves, it is particularly important that the family or caregiver be taught how to deal with potential and actual hypersensitivities.

Tissue-Specific Antibody Hypersensitivities

In antibody-mediated hypersensitivity, also known as cytotoxic hypersensitivity, antibodies are directed against specific target cells or tissues; thus the damage is restricted to those cells or tissues that bear the specific surface antigen, such as platelets. These reactions differ from immune-complex (type III) reactions in that type III reactions involve circulating antigen-antibody complexes.

Etiology and Epidemiology. A classic example of a specific antibody-mediated (type II) hypersensitivity reaction occurs with

Nursing Care Plan

Patient With Type I Hypersensitivity Reaction

Data A 48-year-old woman with pneumonia and no known allergies is receiving intravenous piperacillin, which is an antibiotic. After the third dose of medication the patient develops apprehension, wheezing, and difficulty breathing.

Recognizing that the patient is experiencing an anaphylactic reaction and the need for immediate action, the nurse stops the antibiotic infusion, raises the head of the bed, assesses the patient's airway for patency, and initiates oxygen by mask. Since the patient has intravenous (IV) access, the nurse administers 0.5 mg of 1:10,000 solution of epinephrine IV. Five minutes later the nurse administers a second dose of epinephrine. The patient responds to treatment and begins to breathe with less difficulty.

Nursing Diagnosis

Ineffective airway clearance related to bronchoconstriction secondary to allergic reaction to antibiotic

Outcomes

- Patient will maintain patent airway.
- Respiratory rate returns to normal range for patient.
- Patient demonstrates an absence of wheezing.

Related NOC Outcomes

- Allergic Response: Systemic
- Respiratory Status: Airway Patency
- Respiratory Status: Ventilation

Related NIC Interventions

- Airway Management
- Anaphylaxis Management
- Respiratory Monitoring

Nursing Interventions/Rationales

- Assess for airway patency. *Anaphylaxis can result in respiratory collapse within minutes if the patient cannot move air into and out of the lungs. Intubation or tracheostomy may be needed to establish and maintain a patent airway during anaphylaxis.*
- Elevate the head of the bed. *Placing the patient upright relieves pressure on the diaphragm and allows the patient to maximize ventilation.*
- Administer oxygen. *Since the patient is unable to breathe oxygen in effectively, the concentration of oxygen delivered must be increased. A rebreather mask delivers a higher concentration of oxygen and should be used when available.*
- Administer epinephrine. *Epinephrine is a sympathomimetic drug that produces bronchial dilation. It may be given intramuscularly (IM) when IV access is not available. The IM dose is 0.3 to 0.5 ml of 1:1000 solution (0.3 to 0.5 mg). IM epinephrine is preferred over subcutaneous doses because of increased absorption rate from muscle. When IV access is available, 0.5 to 1.0 mg (5 to 10 ml) of 1:10,000 solution is administered.*
- Assess respiratory status and lung sounds. *Wheezing and dyspnea are directly related to the release of vasoactive mediators from mast cell degranulation during a type I hypersensitivity reaction (allergy). Bronchoconstriction, bronchiolar inflammation, and decreased oxygen intake increase respiratory workload. Tachypnea occurs as a compensatory mechanism to deliver more oxygen to the lungs.*
- Monitor vital signs. *Anaphylaxis can recur within 24 hours after the initial reaction even though treatments have alleviated symptoms. The nurse monitors vital signs to detect changes from baseline that indicate a change in the patient's status and possible recurrence of anaphylaxis.*

Nursing Diagnosis

Anxiety related to inability to breathe with ease

Outcomes

- Patient will report relief from fear and anxiety.
- Patient will rest calmly without signs of apprehension.
- Vital signs will remain within normal parameters for patient before the event.

Related NOC Outcomes

- Anxiety Control
- Coping

the infusion of mismatched blood. *Acute hemolytic transfusion reaction* (ABO incompatibility) is the most serious adverse reaction to blood transfusions and results in approximately 1 death per 100,000 units of blood infused. The reaction occurs within the first 30 minutes of blood administration. Studies of **hemolytic** reactions have shown that mistakes in specimen collection and labeling or inadequate patient identification are the primary errors responsible[18] (Table 21-10).

Another type of antibody-mediated hypersensitivity occurs when the mother is sensitized to antigens on the infant's erythrocytes and makes antibodies against those antigens. This condition is known as *hemolytic disease of the newborn.* The Rhesus D (RhD) factor is the most commonly involved antigen of the 27 known antigens within this system. The term *Rh positive* means that the antigen RhD is present; the term *Rh negative* means that the RhD antigen is absent. Approximately 85% of the population has Rh-positive blood. Between 10% and 15% of Caucasian infants and approximately 5% of African-American infants experience Rh incompatability.[17]

Pathophysiology. Tissue-specific hypersensitivities injure host cells by binding IgG or IgM to an antigen on the surface of a target cell, such as a platelet. Once binding occurs, the cell is destroyed by phagocytic attack, nonspecific lymphocytic attack, or lysis of the cell through the activation of the full complement cascade (see Chapter 20). Figure 21-8 illustrates the mechanism of tissue-specific antibody reactions.

Immunologic Transfusion Reactions. *Acute hemolytic reactions* are caused by antigen-antibody complexes on the erythrocyte membrane. These complexes activate Hageman factor (coagulation factor XII) and the complement cascade. The Hageman fac-

Related NIC Interventions
- Anaphylaxis Management
- Anxiety Reduction
- Presence

Nursing Interventions/Rationales
- Stay with the patient until airway is ensured and allergic reaction subsides. *Patients experience apprehension and a "feeling of doom" when bronchoconstriction interferes with their ability to breathe. Remaining with the patient provides a sense of security and decreases anxiety. Anxiety increases heart rate and respirations and contributes to oxygen consumption and dyspnea. Patients with hyperactive airways from hypersensitivity are at greatly increased risk for respiratory collapse; therefore they must be continually monitored until the risk for compromised airway is over.*
- Approach the patient calmly. *When nurses are apprehensive, patients detect and often mirror that apprehension. A calm manner reassures the patient and provides a sense of security.*
- Explain all care and procedures. *Patients who understand what is happening and what is expected of them are better able to deal with the situation. Fear of the unknown creates apprehension and anxiety.*

Nursing Diagnosis
Deficient knowledge related to lack of experience with anaphylactic reaction

Outcomes
- Patient verbalizes understanding of cause of hypersensitivity reaction, signs of reaction, and emergency treatment.
- Patient participates in self-care (e.g., notifying health care providers of allergies, avoiding known allergens).

Related NOC Outcomes
- Knowledge: Disease Process
- Knowledge: Medication
- Risk Detection

Related NIC Interventions
- Allergy Management
- Medication Administration
- Teaching: Disease Process

Nursing Interventions/Rationales
- Teach patient about the need to avoid allergens when possible. *Avoidance of the allergen is the best way to eliminate the risk for hypersensitivity reactions. Most serious hypersensitivities are present throughout life, and patients are cautioned to permanently avoid the allergen unless advised otherwise by an allergist.*
- Teach patient the signs and symptoms of localized and systemic hypersensitivity reactions. *Early recognition of clinical manifestations allows for early treatment and possible elimination of severe reactions.*
- Encourage use of medical alert jewelry. *Patients suffering from systemic anaphylaxis may not be able to communicate their allergens to emergency or health care providers. Wearing an alert tag fosters early recognition of the problem and appropriate treatment.*
- Teach use of prescribed emergency medication, such as self-injections with epinephrine. *The nurse teaches patients with serious systemic allergies how to self-administer epinephrine to prevent severe bronchoconstriction and possible respiratory collapse. They are taught how to use the equipment and allowed to practice so that, if the need arises, they can self-administer the medication without hesitation or fear.*
- Discuss allergen control methods for the home. *If patients are allergic to medications, the nurse teaches them to avoid the medication. However, if the allergen is an environmental allergen, such as dust mites or molds, the nurse teaches methods for decreasing their exposure to the allergen, such as removing carpets, moving pets away from the patient's sleeping area, and covering mattresses and pillows with protective coverings.*

Evaluation
Evaluation is based on comparing the patient's outcomes with desired outcomes.

tor initiates the kinin system, causing increased capillary permeability, arteriole vasodilation, and hypotension. The complement system initiates intravascular hemolysis, as well as histamine and serotonin release from the mast cells. Hageman factor also combines with free incompatible erythrocytes, activating the intrinsic clotting cascade, which causes disseminated intravascular coagulation (DIC).

Febrile nonhemolytic reactions are among the most common transfusion reactions. They occur when the recipient becomes sensitized to the donor's white blood cells, platelets, or plasma. Symptoms usually begin 30 minutes after the start of the infusion. Although this reaction is not usually serious, it is uncomfortable.

Allergic transfusion reactions are due to the recipient's sensitivity to foreign plasma proteins. Common symptoms include hives, rash, and urticaria. If the symptoms are mild, the patient is treated with antihistamines and the transfusion is restarted slowly. Anaphylaxis can occur but fortunately is rare.

Delayed hemolytic reactions occur 7 to 14 days after the transfusion and are thought to be the result of sensitization of the recipient's immune system to the transfused erythrocyte antigens. The recipient may also have been previously sensitized but have antibody titers that are undetectable at the time of transfusion.

Posttransfusion graft-versus-host disease, which was once relatively rare, is occurring more frequently because of increased use of purposeful immunosuppression as treatment (e.g., bone marrow transplantation). The donor lymphocytes begin to reject the patient's host cells 4 to 30 days after the infusion of blood.

Noncardiac pulmonary edema is thought to be caused by a high titer of leukocyte antibodies in either the donor or recipient plasma. These antibody-to-granulocyte reactions cause granulocyte

TABLE 21-10 IMMUNOLOGIC REACTIONS TO BLOOD TRANSFUSION

Reaction	Clinical Manifestations	Management	Prevention
Acute hemolytic*	Chills, fever, lower back pain, flushing, tachycardia, tachypnea, hypotension, vascular collapse, hemoglobinuria, hemoglobinemia, bleeding, acute renal failure, shock, cardiac arrest, death	Treat shock. Draw blood samples for serologic testing. To avoid hemolysis from procedure, use new venipuncture (not existing central line) and avoid small-gauge needles. Send urine specimen to laboratory. Maintain blood pressure with intravenous (IV) colloid solutions. Give diuretics as prescribed to maintain urine flow. Insert indwelling catheter or measure voided amounts to monitor hourly urine output. Dialysis may be required if renal failure occurs. Do not transfuse additional red blood cell–containing components until transfusion service has provided newly cross-matched units.	Meticulously verify and document patient identification from sample collection to component infusion. Transfuse blood slowly for first 15-20 min with nurse at patient's side.
Febrile, nonhemolytic (most common)*	Sudden chills and fever (rise in temperature of greater than 2° F [1° C]), headache, flushing, anxiety, muscle pain	Give antipyretics as prescribed. Do not give aspirin to thrombocytopenic patients. *Do not restart transfusion.*	Consider leukocyte-poor blood products (filtered, washed, or frozen).
Mild allergic*	Flushing, itching, urticaria (hives)	Give antihistamines as directed. If symptoms are mild and transient, restart transfusion slowly.	Treat prophylactically with glucocorticosteroids or antihistamines (dexamethasone

aggregates that are filtered out by the lung. The antibodies attached to the granulocytes initiate the complement cascade and promote histamine release, causing an influx of inflammatory cells into the lung.

HEMOLYTIC DISEASE. Hemolytic disease, most commonly seen in newborns, occurs when the Rh-negative mother is first exposed to the fetus's Rh-positive blood. Rh antibodies are formed against the Rh-positive blood. On subsequent exposures to Rh-positive blood, such as a second pregnancy, the Rh antibody binds to its corresponding antigen on the surface of the erythrocyte containing Rh factor. The Rh antibodies do not usually fix complement; therefore hemolysis does not occur immediately as it does in the ABO system. Instead, the Rh factor erythrocytes are rapidly broken down by macrophages in the spleen, with conversion of hemoglobin to bilirubin, resulting in jaundice.

NONIMMUNOGENIC TRANSFUSION REACTIONS. The administration of blood can cause reactions that are not immunologic. These include circulatory overload, sepsis, and transmission of disease (Box 21-4). The Clinical Manifestations box, p. 472, presents clinical manifestations of nonimmunogenic transfusion reactions.

Collaborative Care Management. Prevention is the key to management of transfusion reactions. Blood received from volunteer donors through the American Red Cross Blood Service or hospital blood banks is carefully screened and labeled (Box 21-5). Most of the serious reactions that occur from transfusions are the result of human error. Typing, screening, and cross-matching of blood in the laboratory must be accurate. Typing is established by testing the recipient's serum against commercial A and B cells to detect isoagglutinins. The recipient's serum is then screened for all antibodies that were not found in the typing. The goal of cross-matching is to ensure the recipient's blood does not contain antibodies that will attack and destroy the transfused erythrocytes (see Legal Alert box).

One method for preventing immunologic blood transfusion reactions and disease transmission is planned autologous transfusion, which involves using the person's own blood for replacement. Health care providers collect blood at regular intervals before anticipated use, such as forthcoming surgery, and store and freeze the blood until needed. This method is especially useful for persons with rare blood types, for those whose religious beliefs preclude receiving donor blood, or for those expected to need several units of blood during surgery (e.g., selected heart surgeries or joint replacements).

TABLE 21-10 IMMUNOLOGIC REACTIONS TO BLOOD TRANSFUSION—CONT'D

Reaction	Clinical Manifestations	Management	Prevention
Mild allergic* *(cont'd)*		Do not restart transfusion if fever or pulmonary symptoms develop.	[Decadron], diphenhydramine [Benadryl]) given 30-60 min before transfusion.
Anaphylactic*	Anxiety, urticaria, wheezing, tightness and pain in chest, difficulty swallowing, progressing to cyanosis, shock, and possible cardiac arrest	Initiate cardiopulmonary resuscitation if indicated. Have epinephrine ready for injection (0.4 ml of a 1:1000 solution diluted to 10 ml with saline for IV use). *Do not restart transfusion.*	Transfuse extensively washed red blood cell products from which all plasma has been removed. Alternatively, use blood from IgA-deficient donor.
Delayed hemolytic	Fever, chills, back pain, jaundice, anemia, hemoglobinuria	Monitor adequacy of urinary output and degree of anemia. Treat fever with acetaminophen (Tylenol). May need further blood transfusion.	Do more specific type and cross-match when giving patient blood.
Posttransfusion graft-versus-host disease	Anorexia, nausea, diarrhea, high fever, rash, stomatitis, liver dysfunction	No effective treatment. Administer steroids.	Give irradiated blood products.
Noncardiac pulmonary edema	Fever, chills, hypotension, cough, orthopnea, cyanosis, shock	Stop transfusion. Continue IV saline. Give oxygen prn. Administer steroids as directed. Give furosemide (Lasix) and epinephrine as ordered.	

*Modified from National Blood Resource Education Program's transfusion therapy guidelines for nurses, NIH Pub No 90–2668, 1990.
IgA, Immunoglobulin A; *prn,* as needed.

Autotransfusion, which consists of collecting, filtering, and immediately reinfusing the person's own blood, may be performed in the emergency department, the operating room suite during surgery, the postanesthesia care unit, or the critical care unit. Blood draining from the surgical site is suctioned into a bag and passed through a filter to remove microaggregates. When the bag is full, it is disconnected from the system and the blood is infused into the patient with an administration set, using a standard or microembolic filter.

Blood components are often administered rather than whole blood. Blood can be fractionated into red blood cells, platelets, and plasma (Table 21-11) either by centrifuge or automated cell separators. Blood can also be withdrawn from a donor, a portion separated out, and the remainder returned to the donor (apheresis). Using blood components rather than whole blood is a more efficient use of a scarce commodity for more recipients, prevents fluid overload, and decreases the risk of adverse effects.

The nurse administering blood or blood products carefully monitors it and follows strict institutional protocols (see Guidelines for Safe Practice box, p. 473). If a patient reports any of the symptoms associated with transfusion reaction, the nurse stops the transfusion immediately, maintains venous patency by administering normal saline, and notifies the primary care provider immediately. Patients who exhibit any sign of anaphylaxis or hemolytic reaction receive frequent vital sign monitoring and are assessed for signs of impending shock, renal failure, or DIC. The blood and tubing are returned to the laboratory for analysis, and a first-voided urine specimen is collected to analyze for signs of hemolysis. The patient's hemoglobin and hematocrit levels are carefully monitored to determine the extent of the reaction. Patients who experience mild allergic reactions to blood may receive premedication with an antihistamine if they should need transfusion in the future.

Treatment for hemolytic disease of the newborn involves the administration of Rh-immunoglobulin (RhoGAM) to mothers who have not been sensitized by a former pregnancy. The immunoglobulin is given by injection at about 28 weeks of pregnancy or within 72 hours after birth, amniocentesis, or interrupted pregnancy because of miscarriage or abortion. The immunoglobulin contains antibodies that destroy any of the fetus's red blood cells that have entered the mother's blood, preventing sensitization and Rh incompatibility during the next pregnancy.

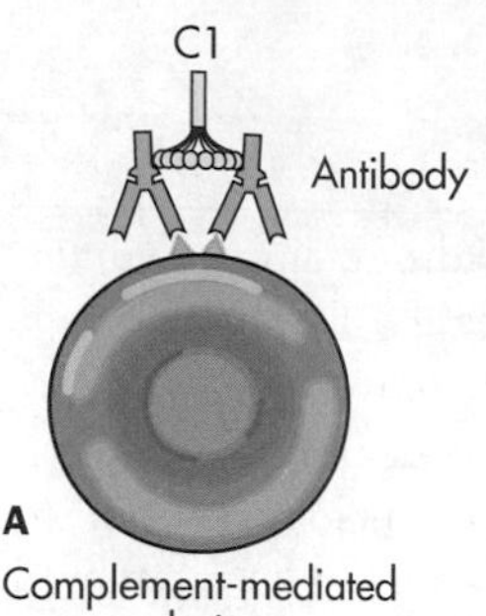

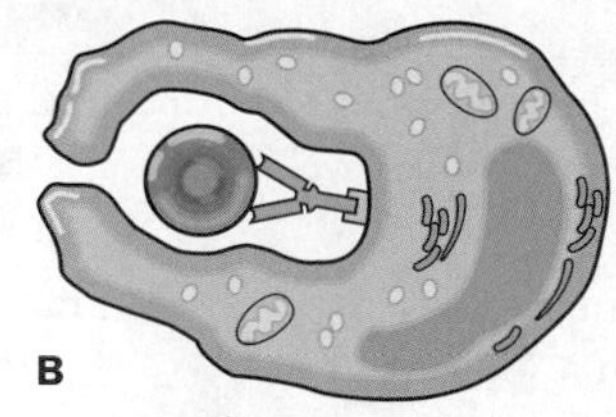

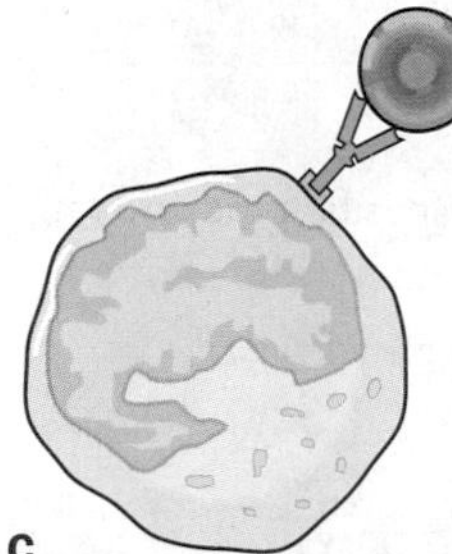

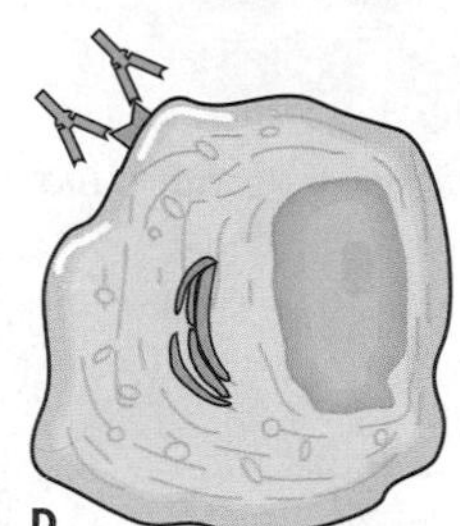

Figure 21-8 Mechanisms of tissue-specific (type II) hypersensitivity reactions. Antigens on target cell bind with antibody and are destroyed or prevented from functioning by, **A,** complement-mediated lysis; **B,** clearance by macrophages in tissues; **C,** antibody-dependent cell-mediated cytotoxicity; or **D,** modulation or blockage of receptors on target cell.

Box 21-4 Major Nonimmunologic Transfusion Reactions

- *Circulatory overload:* This can occur when blood is given too rapidly or in large quantities. Older adults are particularly vulnerable. Patients develop signs of fluid overload and pulmonary congestion. The transfusion is stopped and oxygen and diuretics may be administered.
- *Sepsis:* Bacterial contamination can occur at any time during the collection or handling of blood. Signs of sepsis begin almost immediately. The transfusion is stopped, and the patient receives antibiotics and treatment for shock if it occurs.
- *Disease transmission:* Hepatitis, cytomegalovirus, and human immunodeficiency virus are the most common diseases transmitted by blood transfusions. Hepatitis A and B are effectively identified with current screening capabilities, but hepatitis C is still readily transmissible.

Antigen-Antibody Complex Hypersensitivities

Antigen-antibody complex (type III) (also known as immune-complex) hypersensitivities are caused by the formation or deposition of antigen-antibody complexes in various tissues, which results in complement activation and inflammation. These reactions generally occur several hours after exposure to the antigen. Unlike antibody-mediated (type II) responses, these reactions tend to be systemic and characterized by widespread vasculitis, arthritis, or nephritis. Systemic lupus erythematosus (see Chapter 53), post-streptococcal immune complex glomerulonephritis (see Chapter 35), and serum sickness are examples of antigen-antibody hypersensitivity diseases.

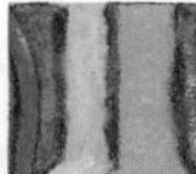

CLINICAL MANIFESTATIONS
Nonimmunologic Transfusion Reactions

Circulatory Overload	Sepsis
Dyspnea	Fever over 104° F (40° C)
Chest tightness	Abdominal cramps
Headache	Nausea
Hypertension	Vomiting
Tachypnea	Diarrhea
Cough	Septic shock
Cyanosis	
Peripheral edema	
Jugular vein distention	
Crackles (rales)	
Abnormal heart sounds	

Box 21-5 Screening Guidelines for Blood Donors

Persons with any of the following are not permitted to donate blood:

- History of infectious diseases such as hepatitis, human immunodeficiency virus infection, acquired immunodeficiency syndrome (AIDS), tuberculosis, syphilis, or malaria
- Malignant diseases
- Allergies or asthma
- Polycythemia vera
- Abnormal bleeding tendencies
- Hypotension (current)
- Anemia (current)
- Recent pregnancy or major surgery
- Men with at least one homosexual or bisexual contact since 1975 (concern for AIDS)
- International travel to malarial areas or high-risk countries (concern for AIDS)
- Blood transfusion during past 6 months
- History of jaundice
- Diseases of the heart, lung, or liver
- Immunizations or vaccinations with attenuated viral vaccine rubella or rabies vaccine
- Hemoglobin level below 13.5 g/dl for men or 12.4 g/dl for women
- Abnormalities in vital signs, particularly fever
- History of residence for greater than 6 months in the United Kingdom between 1980 and 1996

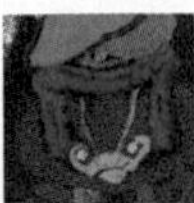

GUIDELINES FOR SAFE PRACTICE
Patient Receiving Blood Transfusion

1. Carefully check all of the following:
   a. Identity of patient to receive transfusion
   b. The label of the unit of blood for the name of the person for whom it is intended to ensure that it matches the patient's wristband before administering the blood
   c. Expiration date of the blood
   d. Color and consistency of blood (If the bag appears to have clots, gas, or a dark purple color, it could be contaminated and should not be infused.)
2. Obtain baseline vital signs and check at frequent intervals throughout the procedure.
3. Administer all blood products through micron mesh filters.
4. Assess patient for any unusual sensations felt throughout the transfusion. (This information may help with early identification of any reactions.)
5. Infuse blood within 4 hours after it is taken from the blood bank (to prevent bacterial growth).
6. If blood cannot be infused within 4 hours, return it to the blood bank for proper refrigeration.
7. Follow facility guidelines for proper disposal of empty blood bag and tubing.
8. Record patient's response to the infusion.
9. Report any adverse effect to the primary care provider immediately.
10. Return the blood bag and tubing to the laboratory for testing if a reaction occurs.

Serum Sickness

Etiology and Epidemiology. Serum sickness develops within 1 to 3 weeks after administration of a foreign serum, such as horse or rabbit serum. It may also occur after administration of certain drugs (e.g., antimicrobials such as penicillin and sulfonamides). Classic serum sickness is rarely encountered today because large doses of foreign sera are rarely administered.

Pathophysiology. The pathogenesis of serum sickness involves the attachment of foreign serum proteins to IgM and IgG. These antigen-antibody complexes bind to complement, initiating the complement cascade and resulting in chemotaxis, vasodilation, and cell lysis. These chemotactic factors lead to an influx of phagocytes, which tend to intensify the inflammatory response (Figure 21-9).

The antigen-antibody reactions of serum sickness occur in many organs, but the kidneys, choroid plexus, joints, skin, and lungs are primarily affected. Itching and discomfort at the injection site are usually the first symptoms, followed by lymphadenopathy, fever, urticaria or erythematous rash, angioedema of the face, and joint pain. Splenomegaly, abdominal pain, headache, nausea, and vomiting may also occur.

Collaborative Care Management. Treatment of antigen-antibody hypersensitivity depends on the cause. Serum sickness is a self-limiting disease. Mild symptoms respond well to antihistamines and salicylates. More severe symptoms are treated with steroids such as prednisone, and symptom relief is often achieved within hours. Epinephrine is given if an anaphylactic reaction occurs.

Legal Alert

Blood Transfusions

Health care personnel must obtain informed consent before administering blood or blood products. Informed consent must include:

- Type of blood or blood product being administered
- Expected benefits and outcomes of administering the blood product
- Potential risks of the transfusion and blood product
- Alternative therapies and their risks and benefits
- Risks of not receiving the blood or blood product

Informed consent must be in the patient's native language, or a translator must be provided to read the consent form to the patient.

T Cell–Mediated Hypersensitivity

T cell–mediated (type IV) hypersensitivity, also known as delayed hypersensitivity, is mediated by T cells rather than antibodies. Graft rejection, contact dermatitis, and hypersensitivity induced by chronic infection (e.g., tuberculosis) are examples of T cell–mediated hypersensitivity reactions.

Etiology and Epidemiology. T cell–mediated hypersensitivity generally occurs within 12 to 72 hours after a sensitized individual comes in contact with the offending antigen. The reaction occurring from an inactivated or purified protein derivative (PPD) tuberculin test is a classic example. People who have undergone sufficient exposure to *Mycobacterium tuberculosis* to be sensitized to the organism, whether or not they have the disease, develop redness and induration in response to the injection within 8 to 12 hours.

Allergic contact dermatitis is an inflammatory response confined to the skin that results from repeated exposure of a sensitized person to an allergen. Environmental substances such as cosmetics, hair dyes, detergents, poison ivy or oak, or latex may serve as the offending antigen in these reactions.

Another important T cell–mediated hypersensitivity reaction occurs when organs or tissues are transferred from one person to another. Transplantations have been performed for many years, but they remain limited because of the rejection process resulting from this type of hypersensitivity.

Pathophysiology. T cell–mediated hypersensitivities do not involve antibodies such as IgE. Rather, macrophages identify the antigen as foreign, encode it, and present it to T cell lymphocytes, which become sensitized to the specific antigen. On subsequent exposure to the same antigen, the sensitized lymphocyte forms cytotoxic T cells or activates nonspecific phagocytic cells (macrophages and polymorphonuclear leukocytes) through release of lymphokines. The cytotoxic T cell lymphocytes destroy the antigen directly by breaking down the cell membrane, causing lysis and cell death.

Allergic contact dermatitis is one of the most commonly encountered T cell–mediated hypersensitivities and type of allergic disease. Dermal contact with the antigen produces sensitization and the clinical manifestations associated with the reaction. The allergen attaches to skin proteins, which function as haptens

TABLE 21-11 TYPES OF BLOOD COMPONENTS

Blood Component	Description	Usage	Comments
RED BLOOD CELLS (RBCS)			
Packed RBCs (PRBCs)	RBCs separated from plasma and platelets	Anemia Moderate blood loss	Decreased risk of fluid overload compared with whole blood
Autologous PRBCs	Same as PRBCs	Elective surgery for which blood replacement is expected	Units may be stored for up to 35 days
Washed RBCs	RBCs washed with sterile isotonic saline before transfusion	Previous allergic reactions to transfusions	Increased removal of immunoglobulins and protein
Frozen RBCs	RBCs frozen in a glycerol solution; cells washed after thawing to remove glycerol	Storage of rare blood type Storage of autologous blood for future use	Relatively free of leukocytes and microemboli Expensive
Leukocyte-poor RBCs	RBCs from which most leukocytes have been removed	Previous sensitivity to leukocyte antigens from prior transfusions or from pregnancy	Fewer RBCs than PRBCs; washed leukocyte-poor RBC units have more RBCs than nonwashed
Neocytes	RBC units with high number of reticulocytes (young RBCs)	Transfusion-dependent anemias	Fewer problems with iron overload Expensive
OTHER CELLULAR COMPONENTS			
Platelets			
Random donor packs	Platelets separated from RBCs by centrifuge; given in 50 ml of plasma	Thrombocytopenia Disseminated intravascular coagulation	Plasma base rich in coagulation factors Can also be packed, washed, or made leukocyte poor
Pheresis packs	Platelets from a human leukocyte antigen–matched donor, separated by apheresis	Allosensitized persons with thrombocytopenia	Requires specialized techniques
Granulocytes	Granular leukocytes separated by apheresis	Granulocytopenia from malignancy or chemotherapy	Allergen sensitization may occur with chills and fever
PLASMA COMPONENTS			
Fresh frozen plasma (FFP)	Freezing of plasma within 4 hr of collection	Clotting deficiencies Liver disease Hemophilia Defibrination	Preserves factors V, VII, VIII, IX, and X and prothrombin Minimizes hepatitis risk Administered through a filter
Factor concentrates VIII and IX	Prepared from large donor pools Heated to inactivate human immunodeficiency virus	VIII: hemophilia A IX: hemophilia B	Increased risk of hepatitis (VIII, IX) and thromboembolism (IX) Given in small volumes
Cryoprecipitate	Precipitated material obtained from FFP when thawed	Hemophilia A Infection of burns Hypofibrinogenemia Uremic bleeding	Contains factors VIII, XIII, and fibrinogen
Serum albumin Normal serum albumin Plasma protein fraction (PPF)	Albumin chemically processed from pooled plasma	Hypovolemic shock Hypoalbuminemia Burns Hemorrhagic shock	No risk of hepatitis Does not require ABO compatibility Lacks clotting factors Hypotension possible if PPF is given faster than 10 ml/min
Immune serum globulin	Obtained from plasma of preselected donors with specific antibodies	Hypogammaglobulinemia Prophylaxis for hepatitis A, tetanus	Given intramuscularly

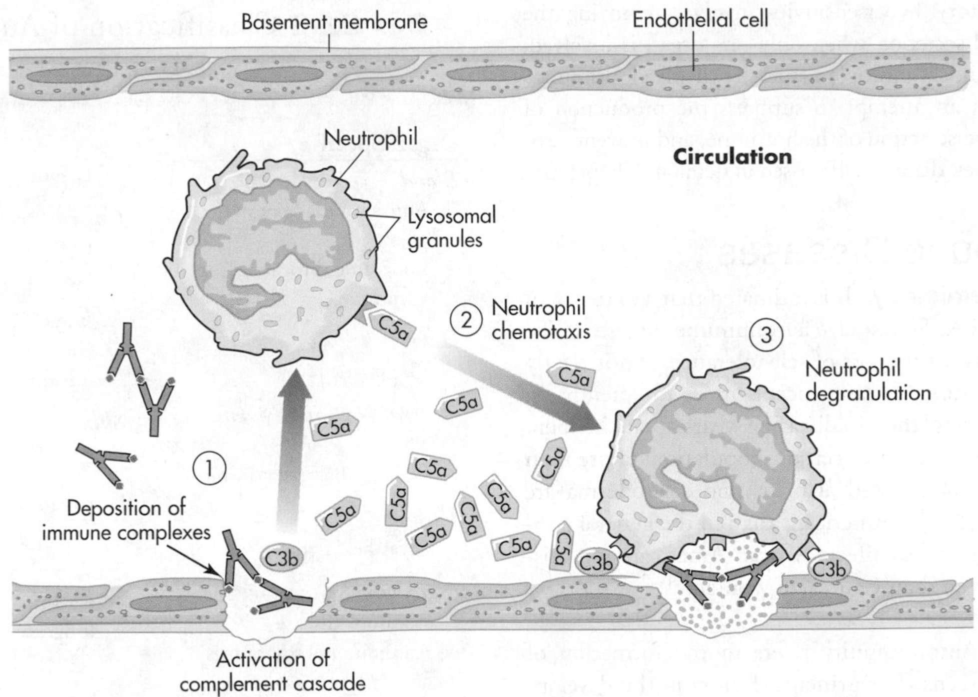

Figure 21-9 Mechanism of immune complex (type III) hypersensitivity reactions. Immune complexes are deposited in vessels of other healthy tissue, where they activate complement cascade *(1)*. Complement attaches to IgG in immune complexes and pulls neutrophils to area *(2)*. Neutrophils degranulate and release a variety of destructive enzymes that destroy healthy tissues *(3)*.

to stimulate the proliferation of a T cell population sensitized to the allergen. After sensitization, subsequent exposure to the contact allergen leads to formation of an erythematous, vesiculated (blistered) lesion. The inflamed area is red, swollen, and warm and may itch, burn, or sting. The location of the lesions often provides data about the causative allergic agent.

The tubercle bacillus *(M. tuberculosis)* itself is not directly toxic to human cells or tissues. The organism invades the tissues of a nonsensitized host and establishes residence in the host tissues, causing virtually no damage. However, in time, as the organism sheds antigenic material, the T cell–mediated response is triggered. The sensitized lymphocytes and activated macrophages attack not only the organism but also the tissues surrounding the organism. This process is aimed at destroying the foreign organism, but tissue destruction may result. The lesions associated with tuberculosis (such as caseation necrosis cavitation) and general toxemia are results of the hypersensitivity. After the initial sensitization with the infectious organism, subsequent contact with the tuberculosis organism or an extract of a purified protein from the organism elicits a hypersensitivity reaction. This is the basis of the Mantoux tuberculin skin test. The skin rashes of smallpox and measles and the lesions of herpes simplex virus are all examples of microbially induced T cell hypersensitivities.

In organ transplantation the foreign tissue or organ serves as the allergen against which the cell-mediated response is directed. Cytotoxic T lymphocytes attack and destroy the tissues directly, resulting in destruction of transplanted tissues. Discussions of specific types of transplants are found in chapters dealing with the disorders for which they are used as treatment.

Collaborative Care Management. Treatment for contact dermatitis includes elimination of known allergens, decreased exposure, or both. Topical antiinflammatory agents such as corticosteroid creams may be useful in reducing the discomfort associated with itching and in decreasing healing time. For severe reactions, systemic corticosteroids and antihistamines may be necessary.

There is no specific treatment, other than treatment of the underlying infection, for hypersensitivity reactions to infective agents. If secondary infection develops as a result of the patient scratching the area, antibiotics may be prescribed. Immunosuppression therapy is used to control transplant rejection.

Stimulatory Hypersensitivity

Etiology, Epidemiology, and Pathophysiology. Stimulatory hypersensitivity is a B cell–mediated response that occurs when autoantibodies bind to target cell surface receptors and cause inappropriate stimulation of the cell, such as the thyroid gland. The usual feedback mechanism is lost; consequently the cell continuously secretes its hormone in an uncontrolled manner. Thyrotoxicosis (Graves' disease) is thought to be induced by this mechanism. It is believed that thyroid-stimulating immunoglobulin and thyroid-stimulating hormone–binding inhibitory immunoglobulin stimulate the secretion of thyroid hormone. Signs and symptoms of hyperthyroidism are produced even though the actual condition is not present and the thyroid gland itself is completely normal.[17]

Collaborative Care Management. The causes of stimulatory reactions are unknown but may be related to loss of self-tolerance.

Treatment of stimulatory hypersensitivity involves removing the focus of the abnormal secretion when only one organ is involved, such as the thyroid gland. If multiple tissues are involved, immunosuppression is used in an attempt to suppress the production of autoantibodies, halt oversecretion of the hormone, and prevent associated symptoms. Graves' disease is discussed in detail in Chapter 38.

Autoimmune Diseases

Etiology and Epidemiology. It is estimated that 1% to 2% of individuals in the United States have autoimmune diseases.[1] The cause of autoimmunity, or the loss of self-tolerance, is not clearly understood. Autoimmune diseases occur more frequently in women, especially during the childbearing years, than in men. Some autoimmune diseases affect certain populations more than others. For example, rheumatoid arthritis and scleroderma are more common among Native Americans than in the general population. Lupus erythematosus affects African-American and Hispanic women more often than Caucasian women.[16]

Pathophysiology. Autoimmunity refers to the formation of antibodies against self-cells. The principal factors in the development of autoimmunity are genetic predisposition, environment, and viral infections. Antibodies produced against one's own cells are referred to as *autoantibodies.* When produced against deoxyribonucleic acid (DNA), they are called anti-DNA antibodies. These self-reactive immunoglobulins are often associated with pathologic states in the body; however, they can also be isolated from the serum of disease-free individuals and are present in about half of adults over the age of 70 years.

Several theories exist about the mechanism of autoimmunity:

- *Release of sequestered antigens:* If an antigen does not come into contact with the immune system during fetal development when self-tolerance normally develops, the antigen remains antigenic. Later, as a result of trauma or infection, the antigen may be exposed to the immune system, eliciting an autoimmune response (e.g., autoantibodies against heart muscle after acute myocardial infarction).
- *Defective suppressor T cells:* Suppressor T cell function may be lost or altered so that autoantibodies are allowed to proliferate without control.
- *Synthesis of cross-reactive antibodies:* Antibodies synthesized in response to certain foreign antigens may have cross-reactivity with similar antigenic components within human tissues.
- *Alteration of self-antigens:* Normal body proteins may be altered by chemicals, infectious organisms, or therapeutic drugs and present new antigenically active groups to the immune system. Autoimmune hemolytic anemia may result from alteration of the Rh antigens of the red blood cells, rendering it antigenic. Certain antibiotics can have a similar effect.

Autoimmune disorders are grouped into categories according to the body part or tissues involved (Box 21-6). *Organ-specific* diseases produce chronic inflammatory changes in a specific organ, such as the kidney or heart. *Nonorgan-specific* autoimmune disorders are characterized by chronic inflammatory changes in many different organs and tissues throughout the body.

Box 21-6 Classification of Autoimmune Disorders

Organ Specific

Blood
- Autoimmune hemolytic anemia
- Idiopathic thrombocytopenic purpura

Heart
- Rheumatic fever

Central Nervous System
- Multiple sclerosis
- Guillain-Barré syndrome

Muscles
- Myasthenia gravis

Endocrine System
- Addison's disease
- Autoimmune thyroiditis (Hashimoto's disease)
- Graves' disease
- Hypothyroidism

Eye
- Uveitis

Gastrointestinal System
- Pernicious anemia
- Ulcerative colitis

Kidneys
- Glomerulonephritis
- Goodpasture's syndrome

Skin
- Pemphigus vulgaris

Nonorgan Specific
- Systemic lupus erythematosus
- Rheumatoid arthritis
- Progressive systemic sclerosis

Collaborative Care Management. Treatment for autoimmune disorders consists of immunosuppression and control of clinical manifestations, primarily through systemic corticosteroid therapy. Initial doses of 60 mg of oral prednisone often bring about a noticeable decrease in symptoms. Once symptoms are controlled, dosages are slowly decreased and then discontinued until the next exacerbation. Cytotoxic drugs such as cyclophosphamide, azathioprine, and methotrexate are sometimes prescribed for patients with severe or persistent manifestations. Treatment of specific autoimmune disorders is discussed elsewhere in this textbook.

Patients with autoimmune disorders are encouraged to eat well-balanced diets, maintain daily exercise patterns without becoming excessively fatigued, and get adequate rest and sleep. The nurse explains the anticipated benefit of prescribed medications, dosage schedules, and adverse effects, especially when patients are taking corticosteroids or other immunosuppressive drugs. The nurse cautions patients against abruptly withdrawing steroid medications, since abrupt cessation can result in adrenal insufficiency or crisis. Close follow-up care is emphasized for all patients taking immunosuppressive agents.

Chronic Fatigue Syndrome

Chronic fatigue syndrome (CFS) is a condition of unexplained fatigue that lasts 6 months or longer and eventually leads to disability. CFS may follow a cold, influenza, bronchitis, or mononucleosis. In other instances CFS develops gradually, with no clear initiating event.[13] Accompanying manifestations, such as muscle and joint discomfort, headache, loss of concentration, weakness, and tender lymph nodes, may go unnoticed because they are similar to the flu. Unlike the flu, however, the fatigue and other symptoms remain or reappear frequently.

Etiology and Epidemiology. It is estimated that CFS or a CFS-like condition affects as many as half a million people in the United States alone. Early studies of CFS patients indicated that 98% were Caucasian and 85% were female, with an average age of onset of 30 years. More than 80% of the women in these studies were well educated and from upper-income families, which may be one reason why CFS was originally mislabeled as "yuppie flu." The earlier incidence studies only included patients receiving medical care; thus the numbers were underestimated. CFS is now recognized in people of all ages, races, and socioeconomic groups.[13]

The Centers for Disease Control and Prevention published a revised case definition of CFS in 2001 (Box 21-7). The primary clinical manifestation of CFS is prolonged, debilitating fatigue accompanied by any or all of the symptoms listed in the box.

Pathophysiology. The exact cause of CFS remains unknown despite intensive research. Conditions that may trigger its development are genetic and environmental factors, viral infection, transient traumatic conditions, toxins, or stress. The clinical course of CFS varies considerably among patients, and it is difficult to diagnose because the same symptoms occur with many other conditions and diseases. CFS often follows a cyclic course, alternating between illness and relatively symptom-free intervals, which is similar to that of autoimmune disorders such as lupus erythematosus or multiple sclerosis. About 50% of patients recover within the first 5 years after onset. No characteristics of the disease or persons with the disease have been identified to show that one person is more likely to recover than another.[13]

Research

Wallman KE et al: Randomised controlled trial of graded exercise in chronic fatigue, *Med J Aust* 5(180), 2004.

Sixty-one patients between ages 16 and 74 years with the diagnoses chronic fatigue syndrome participated in a 12-week graded exercise program or relaxation and flexibility therapy to see if it would improve their physiologic, psychologic, and cognitive functioning. They performed exercises twice daily over the 12-week period. The researchers used several different scales and physical assessments to assess changes. Results demonstrated that graded exercise was associated with improvements in physical work capacity and in specific psychologic and cognitive variables and minimized deconditioning, which can result in increased symptoms. No changes were observed in the relaxation and flexibility therapy group. Researchers concluded that improvements in the exercise group might have occurred from patient abandonment of avoidance behaviors.

Collaborative Care Management. Treatments for CFS have included antiviral agents, antidepressants, and immune modulators, but none have proven effective (see Research box). Consequently, treatments are aimed at controlling symptoms and helping patients return to a normal or near-normal lifestyle. Nonsteroidal antiinflammatory drugs may be beneficial in reducing body aches or fever, and nonsedating antihistamines have been useful for relieving allergy symptoms. No cure for this disease exists at this time.

Patient care focuses on self-management of fatigue to improve function and quality of life. The nurse helps the patient identify potential triggers to fatigue and encourages them to avoid situations or activities that adversely affect their energy levels. Periods

Box 21-7 CDC Case Definition of Chronic Fatigue Syndrome

1. Clinically evaluated, unexplained, persistent or relapsing chronic fatigue that is of new or definite onset (i.e., not lifelong), is not the result of ongoing exertion, is not substantially alleviated by rest, and results in substantial reduction in previous levels of occupational, educational, social, or personal activities.
2. The concurrent occurrence of four or more of the following symptoms:
   - Substantial impairment in short-term memory or concentration
   - Sore throat
   - Tender lymph nodes
   - Muscle pain
   - Multijoint pain without swelling or redness
   - Headaches of a new type, pattern, or severity
   - Unrefreshing sleep
   - Postexertional malaise lasting more than 24 hours

   These symptoms must have persisted or recurred during 6 or more consecutive months of illness and must not have predated the fatigue.

Conditions That Exclude a Diagnosis of Chronic Fatigue Syndrome

1. Any active medical condition that may explain the presence of chronic fatigue, such as untreated hypothyroidism, sleep apnea and narcolepsy, and iatrogenic conditions such as side effects of medication.
2. Some diagnosable illnesses that may relapse or may not have completely resolved during treatment. If the persistence of such a condition could explain the presence of chronic fatigue, and if it cannot be clearly established that the original condition has completely resolved with treatment, then such patients should not be classified as having chronic fatigue syndrome. Examples of illnesses that can present such a picture include some types of malignancies and chronic cases of hepatitis B or C virus infection.
3. Any past or current diagnosis of a major depressive disorder with psychotic or melancholic features; bipolar affective disorders; schizophrenia of any subtype; delusional disorders of any subtype; dementias of any subtype; anorexia nervosa; or bulimia nervosa.
4. Alcohol or other substance abuse, occurring within 2 years of the onset of chronic fatigue and any time afterward.
5. Severe obesity as defined by a body mass index [body mass index = weight (kg)/height $(m)^2$] equal to or greater than 45. (NOTE: Body mass index values vary considerably among different age groups and populations. No "normal" or "average" range of values is meaningful. The range of 45 or greater was selected because it clearly falls within the range of severe obesity.)

From Centers for Disease Control and Prevention: *CFS case definition,* accessed 2003 from website: http://www.cdc.gov/ncidod/diseases/cfs/info.htm.

of activity are scheduled at times when patients feel better and are alternated with rest periods. Exercise may seem contradictory in the presence of fatigue, but exercise improves conditioning and can restore energy. Patients are assisted with developing individualized exercise programs that incorporate a gradual increase in exercise intensity and duration. Exercise needs to be incorporated in a manner that does not exacerbate fatigue, yet promotes regular participation.

A well-balanced diet is essential to promote adequate energy stores. Nighttime sleep should be as free of interruption as possible, and daytime naps are avoided if they interfere with nighttime sleep. The patient may also benefit from relaxation, meditation, massage, imagery, therapeutic touch, music, or biofeedback.

Chronic fatigue syndrome is a disease with overwhelming subjective symptoms, and health care providers commonly treat patients experiencing persistent debilitating fatigue with overt skepticism, if not direct accusations of malingering. Symptoms of CFS may be attributed to life stress, unhappiness, female hormone imbalances, or simply psychosomaticism. The nurse plays an important role in reassuring the patient about both the validity and severity of the symptoms. Family members should be included in discussions and teaching sessions about disease etiology and management. Family support is critical to the patient because many occupational and family roles may have to be reduced or eliminated in the face of overwhelming fatigue. Patients and families may be encouraged to contact local or national CFS support groups to establish networks of information and support for dealing with this debilitating chronic disease.

? Critical Thinking

1. A patient lived in a warm, humid climate for 30 years. After moving to another climate, she developed an upper respiratory tract infection for which her physician gave her an injection of penicillin. She stated that she had taken penicillin and, to her knowledge, had no allergies. Within 20 minutes after receiving the penicillin, she developed symptoms of anaphylaxis. What explanation can be given for her reaction? What actions need to be taken immediately?
2. A patient is to receive a unit of packed red blood cells at 3 PM. It is now 10 AM. What actions are essential to ensure the safe administration of the packed red blood cells to the patient?

References

1. Abbas AK, Lichtmann AH: *Basic immunology,* ed 2, Philadelphia, 2005, Saunders.
2. Reference deleted in proofs.
3. American Cancer Institute: *Detailed guide: multiple myeloma,* accessed 2003 from website: http://www.cancer.org/docroot/cri/content/cri_2_4_3x_how_is_multiple_myeloma_diagnosed_30.asp.
4. American Cancer Society: *Monoclonal antibody therapy (passive immunotherapy),* accessed 2004 from website: http://www.cancer.org/docroot/ETO/content/ETO_1_4X_Monoclonal_Antibody_Therapy_PassivI mmunotherapy.asp?sitearea=ETO.
5. Centers for Disease Control and Prevention: Applying public health strategies to primary immunodeficiency diseases, *MMWR,* accessed 2004 from website: http://www.cdc.gov/mmwr/preview/mmwrhtml/rr5301a1.htm.
6. Chernecky CC, Berger BJ: *Laboratory tests and diagnostic procedures,* ed 4, Philadelphia, 2004, Saunders.
7. Department of Health and Human Resources: *Primary immune deficiency, fact sheet,* accessed 2003 from website: http://www.niaid.nih.gov/factsheets/pid.htm.
8. Gertz M: *What is monoclonal gammopathy of undetermined significance (MGUS)?* International Myeloma Foundation, accessed 2003 from website: http://www.myeloma.org/myeloma/faq.jsp?type=detail&id=879.
9. Huether S, McCance K: *Understanding pathophysiology,* ed 3, St Louis, 2004, Mosby.
10. International Myeloma Foundation (UK): *MGUS and myeloma,* accessed 2003 from website: http://www.myeloma.org.uk/pdf/MGUS.PDF.
11. Multiple Myeloma Research Foundation: *Introduction to multiple myeloma,* accessed 2002 from website: http://www.multiplemyeloma.org/about_myeloma/.
12. National Cancer Institute: *What you need to know about multiple myeloma,* accessed 2002 from website: http://www.cancer.gov/cancertopics/wyntk/myeloma/page6.
13. National Center for Infectious Diseases: *Chronic fatigue syndrome,* accessed 2003 from website: http://www.cdc.gov/ncidod/diseases/cfs/.
14. National Institute of Allergy and Infectious Diseases: *Allergy statistics,* US Department of Health and Human Services, accessed 2002 from website: http://www.niaid.nih.gov/factsheets/allergystat.htm.
15. National Institute of Allergy and Infectious Diseases: NIAID initiative addresses primary immune deficiency diseases, *NIAID News,* accessed 2003 from website: http://www2.niaid.nih.gov/newsroom/releases/pirc.htm.
16. National Institutes of Health: *Understanding autoimmune diseases,* accessed 2003 from website: http://www.niaid.nih.gov/publications/autoimmune/default.htm.
17. Roitt I, Brostoff J, Male D: *Immunology,* ed 6, St Louis, 2001, Mosby.
18. Sandler SG, Sandler, DA: *Transfusion reactions,* accessed from website: http://www.emedicine.com/med/topic2297.htm.

Visit the Evolve website: http://evolve.elsevier.com/Monahan/medsurg

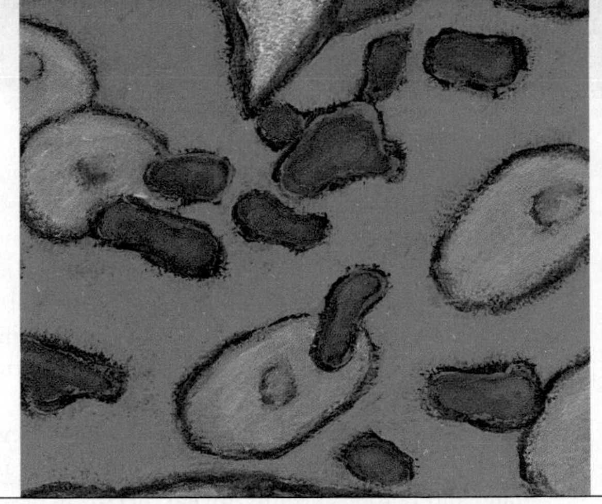

CHAPTER 22 HIV Infection and AIDS

by Carol J. Green

OBJECTIVES

After studying this chapter, the learner should be able to:

1. Describe the epidemiology of HIV infection.
2. Identify the causative agent of HIV infection.
3. Describe the continuum of HIV infection.
4. Discuss the infection and replication process of HIV.
5. Describe measures to prevent the transmission of HIV.
6. Compare nursing care for the person with HIV infection and AIDS.
7. Discuss drug therapy for the patient with AIDS.
8. Describe the clinical manifestations and collaborative management of common opportunistic infections that occur with AIDS.

KEY TERMS

antibody assay, p. 482
asymptomatic, p. 481
CD4 lymphocyte, p. 481
cofactor, p. 481
highly active antiretroviral therapy, p. 487
opportunistic, p. 482
retrovirus, p. 479
viral load, p. 484

Human Immunodeficiency Virus Infection

Human immunodeficiency virus (HIV) infection is an acquired infection in which the HIV integrates itself into CD4 (helper T4) cells, causing severe immune dysfunction. HIV infection renders the person unusually susceptible to other life-threatening infections and malignancies. In its most serious form, HIV results in acquired immunodeficiency syndrome (AIDS).

Etiology. The origin of HIV is still largely unknown. Evidence suggests an African origin, since an AIDS-like illness in Central Africa has been known to exist since the early 1960s. Some researchers hypothesize that the most likely source of human infection was from nonhuman primates.

The causative agent of HIV infection is HIV, a **retrovirus** belonging to the *Lentivirus* subfamily. Several human retroviruses have been identified. Two of them, HIV-1 and HIV-2, are associated with depletion of helper T4 cells and subsequent loss of cellular immunity. HIV-1 is the predominant cause of HIV infections, accounting for more than 80% of cases worldwide. HIV-2 is most prevalent in West Africa and is, so far, limited in geographic distribution.[12] Despite significant scientific and clinical progress in developing new treatments and models of care, HIV disease remains incurable.

Epidemiology. Worldwide, more than 20 million people have died from AIDS since the first case was identified in 1981. In 2003 close to 5 million people contracted HIV, the largest number since the epidemic began. Currently it is estimated that between 34.6 and 42.3 million people are living with HIV, with the largest number, 25 million, residing in sub-Saharan Africa. HIV infection is rapidly expanding, with 7.4 million cases in Asia, 1.6 million in Latin American, and 1.3 million in Eastern Europe and Central Asia.[12]

Infections are on the rise in the United States and Western Europe. The Centers for Disease Control and Prevention (CDC) estimates that 950,000 people are living with HIV in the United States, and approximately 40,000 new HIV infections occur each year.[6,7] In Western Europe, 580,000 people are living with AIDS.[12]

By gender, approximately 70% of HIV infections in the United States are among men, although the incidence among women has been steadily increasing.[6] Worldwide, 50% of people living with HIV are female.[12] In the U.S. population, African-Americans and Hispanics are disproportionately affected by HIV.

More than half (64%) of HIV infections occur among African-Americans, and 18% among Hispanics, even though these groups represent 13% and 12% of the population, respectively[7] (Figure 22-1). Forty-two percent of new HIV infections occur among men who have sex with men, 33% among heterosexuals, and 25% among intravenous (IV) drug users.[5] Perinatal transmission is another source of HIV infection, with rates varying between 13% and 48%. To date, more than 457,667 reported deaths from AIDS have occurred in the United States.[7]

In spite of an increase in the number of new cases of HIV, mortality from AIDS has leveled off in recent years in the United States and Europe.[12] Antiretroviral therapy in developed countries has slowed the progression of HIV to AIDS, allowing those infected to live longer.

HIV is a bloodborne, sexually transmitted disease (STD). The routes of viral transmission are well documented: (1) direct transmission from person to person by sexual contact, (2) direct inoculation with contaminated blood products, needles, or syringes, and (3) infection from mother to her fetus or newborn. Sexual practices, including vaginal or anal penetration without a condom and oral sexual practices, are associated with a high risk for infection. The use of contaminated needles for subcutaneous, intramuscular, or IV injection is another source of infection. Women who are HIV infected may pass the virus onto their newborns via three potential routes: gestation, delivery, and, rarely, breast milk.[2,8]

Blood, semen, and vaginal secretions are primary sources for infection, and epidemiologic studies indicate that transmission via saliva, tears, and breast milk is inefficient and unlikely to produce infection. HIV is not transmitted by casual contact, including sneezing; coughing; spitting; hand shaking; and contacting potential secretions on toilet seats, bathtubs, showers, swimming pools, utensils, dishes, or linens used by infected persons. HIV is not transmitted by biting or blood-sucking insects.[3]

Blood transfusions are not a significant source of HIV infection today. In the United States each unit of donated blood is tested for HIV infection, as well as several other bloodborne infections, such as hepatitis B. HIV screening of blood products has been conducted since 1985; only recipients of transfusions before that time were at significant risk for infection via the blood supply. It is possible for a contaminated unit of blood to test negative for HIV if the donor has not yet formed antibodies to the virus at the time of donation. As a result, the risk of exposure to HIV via the U.S. blood supply is estimated to be 1 in 1.4 to 1.8 million units of blood.[9] Since 1985, seven cases have been reported of organ transplant recipients contracting HIV. In all cases, problems prevented the identification of the donor's HIV status before harvesting of organs[9] (see Risk Factors box).

The risk for HIV transmission to health care workers prompted the CDC to implement Universal Precautions. Those precautions, now known as Standard Precautions, apply to all patients regardless of their medical diagnosis. The Standard Precautions protocol acknowledges that recognized and unrecognized microorganisms can exist in any body fluid, and the use of appro-

Risk Factors

HIV

- Sexual practices*
  - Unprotected sex
  - Multiple sexual partners
  - Anal or oral sexual activity
  - Improper condom use or condom breakage
  - Open sores, lesions, or irritation in the genital area
- Contaminated blood
- Contaminated needles
- Occupational exposure
  - All health care workers—acute care, long-term care, and home care
  - Dental workers
  - Corrections officers and law enforcement personnel
- Perinatal exposure (during pregnancy, birth, or breastfeeding)
  NOTE: Approximately 25% of children of HIV-positive mothers are infected with the virus.

*An individual's sexual practices, not sexual preferences, create the HIV risk. The only true "safe sex" involves two seronegative partners in a monogamous relationship.

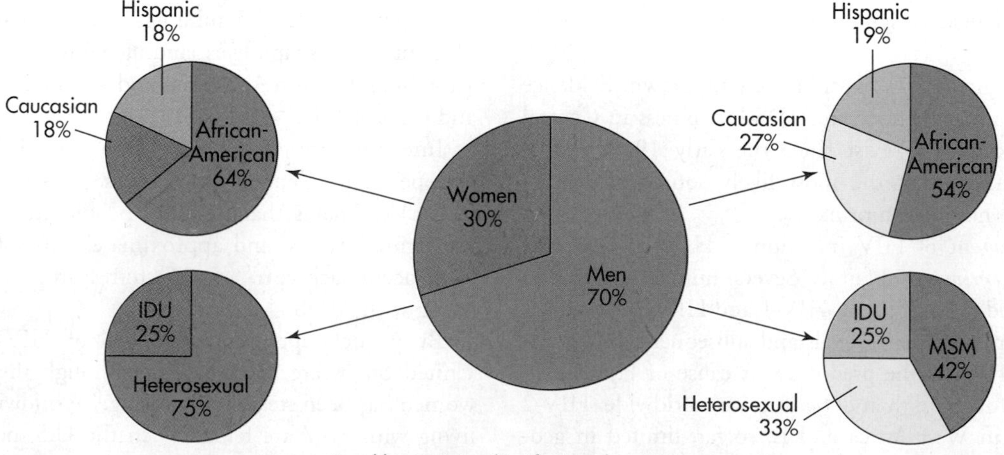

Figure 22-1 National estimates of annual new HIV infections among men and women by race/ethnicity and risk, 2002. *IDU*, Injection drug users; *MSM*, men who have sex with men.

priate precautions reduces the risk for transmission within the hospital environment (see Chapter 6 for a discussion of Standard Precautions).

Pathophysiology. The natural history of HIV infection is associated with an unpredictable course of disease progression. Patients may undergo a prolonged period of clinically silent infection, often lasting more than 10 years, during which the virus remains dormant. Although the virus is consistently detected throughout this time, patients may exhibit only subtle immunologic alterations. Once viral replication begins, which can occur rapidly, **CD4 lymphocytes** are destroyed and the patient becomes symptomatic.

The life cycle of HIV is similar to that of the other retroviruses. HIV interacts with a CD4 glycoprotein found on the membrane of CD4 lymphocytes. CD4 refers to the particular protein expressed on the surface of the helper T4 lymphocyte. The CD4 glycoprotein is also found on the surface of several other cells, including some monocytes, macrophages, glial cells, and gastrointestinal (GI) cells. Presence of the CD4 glycoprotein allows the virus to fuse to the host cell. Once fused, the virus is injected into the cell cytoplasm, where it sheds its two outer coats, releasing two ribonucleic acid (RNA) copies, which are subsequently transcribed into proviral deoxyribonucleic acids (DNA). The proviral DNA is then integrated into the CD4 cell by the retroviral enzyme reverse transcriptase.

The virus may remain dormant in the CD4 cells, or replicate by using the host cell's genetic machinery to assemble and release new viral particles. Viral replication eventually depletes the host's CD4 cells, resulting in a dramatic loss of immune protection (Figure 22-2). Infections that were once disarmed by the healthy immune system are eventually able to cause serious and potentially life-threatening diseases.

It is unclear why HIV escapes the host's immune system. It is thought that viral entry into host cells occurs before the host's virus-specific immune response is initiated. Once HIV gains entry into T cells, the virus reshapes the host's immune system, impairing antigen-processing function, humoral neutralizing response, the production of new CD4 cells, and HIV-specific CD8 cells.[8]

Several potential **cofactors**, which may be viral, host, or environmental, are thought to directly influence the replication of HIV or the severity of its pathogenic effects. Viral cofactors may include herpes simplex virus, cytomegalovirus (CMV), and Epstein-Barr virus. Host cofactors may include a variety of cytokines and intracellular mediators. Environmental cofactors may include repeated exposure to HIV, which may induce hyperactivation of the immune system, resulting in an expansion of the pool of HIV-replicating cells.

The spectrum of HIV infection ranges from asymptomatic primary infection to overt AIDS, which is characterized by potentially life-threatening opportunistic infections. Early in the AIDS epidemic, it was believed that HIV infection could be divided into four separate processes: acute HIV infection, latent infection, AIDS-related complex, and AIDS. It is now known that the infection is one continuous disease process with three stages: primary HIV infection, chronic asymptomatic disease, and AIDS (Figure 22-3). The CDC uses a case definition for AIDS surveillance and reporting, which has evolved over time and incorporates both

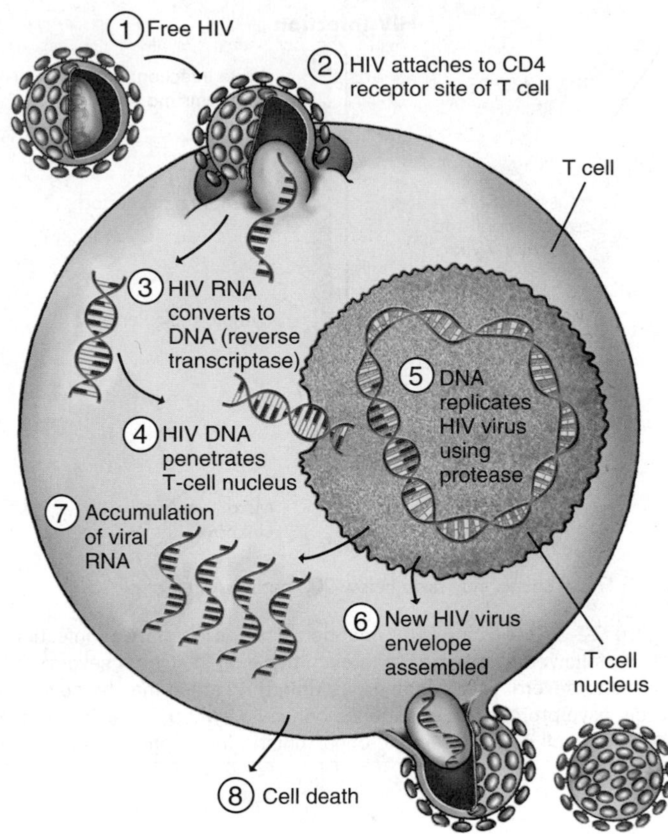

Figure 22-2 Life cycle of HIV.

laboratory and clinical stages (Box 22-1). However, it is more useful to discuss the disease in terms of staging.

PRIMARY HIV-1 INFECTION. Symptoms of primary HIV infection generally occur within 2 to 4 weeks after HIV exposure and last between 2 and 10 weeks. Symptoms are similar to the flu or mononucleosis, consisting of fever, sore throat, fatigue, nausea, vomiting, headache, rash, or lymphadenopathy. Most of these manifestations go away without intervention; however, the lymphadenopathy usually persists throughout the course of the disease. During this time there is a corresponding rapid rise in serum HIV RNA copies, which may reach 1 million copies/ml or more; a decrease in CD4 cell numbers; and a large increase in CD8 cell numbers.[8] The decline in viral copies coincides with the resolution of clinical manifestations. Antibodies to HIV-1 are usually negative during the primary HIV-1 phase of infection.

CHRONIC ASYMPTOMATIC INFECTION. The initial phase of infection may be followed by a period of latency that can last from several months to 10 years or more. During this time the person may be completely **asymptomatic** or experience only mild symptoms such as fatigue, headache, or lymphadenopathy. Over time, however, active viral replication begins. As viral load increases, CD4 cell counts gradually decline. The actual rate of decline varies among individuals and can be altered by antiretroviral therapy. Generally, by 12 weeks after infection, anti-HIV antibodies have been produced and can be detected by immunoassay even when the patient is asymptomatic.

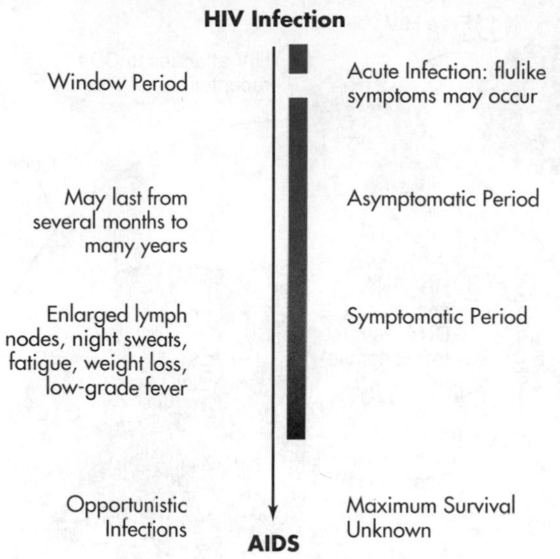

Figure 22-3 Spectrum of HIV infection. The initial phase of infection may be followed by a period of latency that may last from several months to several years. During this time the person may be completely asymptomatic or experience only mild symptoms. AIDS exists when CD4 cell counts drop and opportunistic infections occur.

AIDS. As viral replication continues and more CD4 cells are destroyed, the immune system becomes further compromised. Clinical manifestations associated with AIDS are primarily those of opportunistic infections, which are discussed later in this chapter. The Clinical Manifestations box summarizes other manifestations. Figure 22-4 illustrates the scope of HIV infection in the body and the range of organs and tissues that can be affected. AIDS is the end stage of HIV infection. Without treatment death occurs within 3 to 5 years.

COMPLICATIONS. AIDS and its associated opportunistic infections can affect every organ and body system. **Opportunistic** infections are those pathogens that take advantage of decreased immunity to produce disease. Pulmonary infection from a variety of organisms is a constant threat and is often the first manifestation of AIDS. Such infections can rapidly lead to severe hypoxemia. Numerous GI problems are associated with opportunistic infections or antiretroviral therapy. Other common problems include granulomatous hepatitis, drug toxicity hepatitis, or coinfection with a hepatitis virus; masses or lesions from lymphomas and Kaposi's sarcoma; cholangitis or cholestasis; and pancreatic lesions. Patients may have difficulty eating or swallowing or may experience dyspepsia, diarrhea, and weight loss. Loss of lean muscle mass is common.

HIV crosses the blood-brain and blood–cerebrospinal fluid (CSF) barriers and infects microglia and possibly other cells, resulting in encephalopathy. This process results in loss of cognitive and motor function. Many of the opportunistic infections also can affect the central nervous system. Peripheral neuropathy with loss of motor function often occurs. The eyes are vulnerable to CMV, which can result in blurred vision and decreased acuity. The lesions are progressive and may lead to total blindness unless early and aggressive treatment is instituted.

Thrombocytopenia, anemia, and neutropenia may be present with AIDS. The causes of these problems are not precisely known, but it is thought that HIV decreases red blood cell production. Drug side effects also affect the hematologic system and can cause impaired production and increased destruction of red blood cells.

Opportunistic infections can affect the heart by producing pericarditis or myocarditis. Severe pulmonary hypertension associated with multiple episodes of *Pneumocystis carinii* pneumonia can cause right ventricular failure.

Although not as common as other system dysfunctions, all endocrine glands can be infiltrated with HIV. The adrenal gland is most commonly affected. Adrenal insufficiency may result from invasion by infective organisms, tumor growth, or drug therapy.

Musculoskeletal manifestations of HIV are common and may be mild or severe. Arthralgia is seen with acute infection and may also result from drug therapy. Myalgia, weakness, and wasting may also occur secondary to decreased appetite.

Fluid and electrolyte and acid-base imbalances occur from a variety of causes, including renal, GI, or endocrine changes or drug therapy. Renal dysfunction may occur from acute kidney failure secondary to hypovolemia, interstitial nephritis caused by invasion of renal tissue by tumors or infective organisms, or glomerulosclerosis from HIV-associated nephropathy. Specific opportunistic infections are discussed later in the chapter.

CLINICAL MANIFESTATIONS
HIV/AIDS

- Chills and fever
- Night sweats
- Dry, productive cough
- Dyspnea
- Lethargy
- Confusion
- Stiff neck
- Seizures
- Headache
- Malaise
- Fatigue
- Oral lesions
- Skin rash
- Abdominal discomfort
- Diarrhea
- Weight loss
- Lymphadenopathy
- Progressive generalized edema

Collaborative Care Management

DIAGNOSTIC TESTS

ANTIBODY ASSAYS. Antibody assays measure the immune system's response from exposure to a specific antigen. When an antigen enters the host, the immune system recognizes the antigen and produces specific antibodies against it (see Chapter 20). Antibody assay tests depend on antibody formation, but a patient's serum may not have detectable levels of antibody during the initial stage of infection. Approximately 90% of the population forms antibodies in response to HIV within 3 weeks to 3 months after exposure, although this period can be as long as 6 months. The time lag between exposure to HIV and the production of detectable antibodies is known as the "window period." Newborns maintain maternal antibodies for as long as 18 months;

Box 22-1 CDC Surveillance Case Definition for AIDS

I. HIV status of patient is unknown or inconclusive
If laboratory tests for HIV infection were not performed or gave inconclusive results and the patient had no other cause of immunodeficiency listed in IA (see below), a definitive diagnosis of any disease listed in IB (see below) indicates AIDS.
- A. Causes of immunodeficiency that disqualify a disease as an indication of AIDS in the absence of laboratory evidence of HIV infection
  1. The use of high-dose or long-term systemic corticosteroid therapy or other immunosuppressive/cytotoxic therapy within 3 months before the onset of the indicator disease
  2. A diagnosis of any of the following diseases within 3 months after diagnosis of the indicator disease: Hodgkin's disease, non-Hodgkin's lymphoma (other than primary brain lymphoma), lymphocytic leukemia, multiple myeloma, any other cancer of lymphoreticular or histiocytic tissue, or angioimmunoblastic lymphadenopathy
  3. A genetic (congenital) immunodeficiency syndrome or an acquired immunodeficiency syndrome that is atypical of HIV infection, such as one involving hypogammaglobulinemia
- B. Diseases that indicate AIDS (requires definitive diagnosis)
  1. Candidiasis of the esophagus, trachea, bronchi, or lungs
  2. Cryptococcosis, extrapulmonary
  3. Cryptosporidiosis with diarrhea persisting for more than 1 month
  4. Cytomegalovirus disease of an organ other than the liver, spleen, or lymph nodes in a patient older than 1 month
  5. Herpes simplex virus infection causing a mucocutaneous ulcer that persists longer than 1 month; or herpes simplex virus infection causing bronchitis, pneumonitis, or esophagitis for any duration in a patient older than 1 month
  6. Kaposi's sarcoma in a patient younger than 60 years
  7. Lymphoid interstitial pneumonia or pulmonary lymphoid hyperplasia (LIP/PLH complex) in a patient younger than 13 years
  8. Lymphoma of the brain (primary) affecting a patient younger than 60 years
  9. *Mycobacterium avium* complex or *M. kansasii* disease, disseminated (at a site other than or in addition to the lungs, skin, or cervical or hilar lymph nodes)
  10. *Pneumocystis carinii* pneumonia
  11. Progressive multifocal leukoencephalopathy
  12. Toxoplasmosis of the brain in a patient older than 1 month

II. Patient is HIV positive
Regardless of the presence of other causes of immunodeficiency (see IA, above), in the presence of laboratory evidence of HIV infection, any disease listed in IB (see above) or in IIA or IIB (see below) indicates a diagnosis of AIDS. In addition, beginning in 1993, all HIV-positive adults and adolescents with CD4 T cell counts less than 200/mm^3 or with pulmonary tuberculosis, recurrent pneumonia, or invasive cervical carcinoma should also be included in the AIDS case definition.
- A. Diseases that indicate AIDS (requires definitive diagnosis)
  1. Bacterial infections, multiple or recurrent (any combination of at least two within a 2- to 4-year period), of the following types in a patient younger than 13 years: septicemia, pneumonia, meningitis, bone or joint infection, or abscess of an internal organ or body cavity (excluding otitis media or superficial skin or mucosal abscesses) caused by *Haemophilus, Streptococcus* (including pneumococcus), or other pyogenic bacteria
  2. Coccidioidomycosis, disseminated (at a site other than or in addition to the lungs or cervical or hilar lymph nodes)
  3. Histoplasmosis, disseminated (at a site other than or in addition to the lungs or cervical or hilar lymph nodes)
  4. HIV encephalopathy
  5. HIV wasting syndrome
  6. Isosporiasis with diarrhea persisting for more than 1 month
  7. Kaposi's sarcoma at any age
  8. Lymphoma of the brain (primary) at any age
  9. *M. tuberculosis* disease, extrapulmonary (involving at least one site outside the lungs, regardless of whether there is concurrent pulmonary involvement)
  10. Mycobacterial disease caused by mycobacteria other than *M. tuberculosis,* disseminated (at a site other than or in addition to the lungs, skin, or cervical or hilar lymph nodes)
  11. Non-Hodgkin's lymphoma of B cell or unknown immunologic phenotype and the following histologic types: small noncleaved lymphoma (Burkitt's or non-Burkitt's) or immunoblastic sarcoma
  12. *Salmonella* (nontyphoidal) septicemia, recurrent
- B. Diseases that indicate AIDS (presumptive diagnosis)
  1. Candidiasis of the esophagus
  2. Cytomegalovirus retinitis, with loss of vision
  3. Kaposi's sarcoma
  4. Lymphoid interstitial pneumonia or pulmonary lymphoid hyperplasia (LIP/PLH complex) in a patient younger than 13 years
  5. Mycobacterial disease (acid-fast bacilli with species not identified by culture), disseminated (involving at least one site other than or in addition to the lungs, skin, or cervical or hilar lymph nodes)
  6. *P. carinii* pneumonia
  7. Toxoplasmosis of the brain in a patient older than 1 month

III. Patient is HIV negative
With laboratory test results negative for HIV infection, a diagnosis of AIDS for surveillance purposes is ruled out unless
- A. All the other causes of immunodeficiency listed in IA (see above) are excluded; and
- B. The patient has had either of the following:
  1. *P. carinii* pneumonia diagnosed by a definitive method
  2. A definitive diagnosis of any of the other diseases indicative of AIDS listed in IB (see above) and a CD4 helper-inducer T-cell count of less than 400/mm^3

CDC, Centers for Disease Control and Prevention.
CDC: Appendix: revised surveillance case definition for HIV infection, *MMWR* 48(RR–13):29–31, 1999.

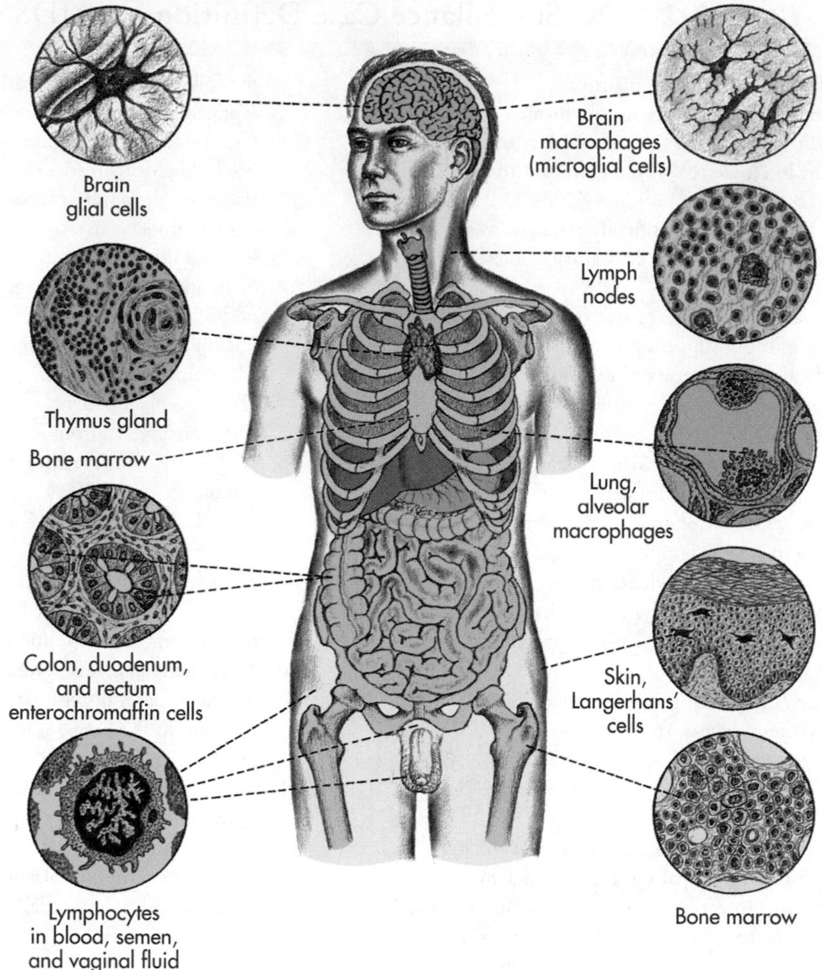

Figure 22-4 Distribution of tissues that can be infected by HIV. Infection is closely linked to presence of CD4 receptors on host tissue, with possible exceptions of glial cells in brain and chromaffin cells in colon, duodenum, and rectum.

therefore antibody testing is unreliable until the infant is 18 months of age.

Enzyme-Linked Immunosorbent Assay (ELISA). The ELISA is a highly specific test that is close to 99.6% sensitive for HIV-1 antibodies. If the patients' serum is reactive, the patient is considered seropositive for HIV antibodies. False-positive tests are possible and may occur from recent influenza or hepatitis B vaccines; in multiparous women; after multiple blood transfusions; or with multiple myeloma, alcoholic hepatitis, or biliary cirrhosis.

Western Blot. If a patient has a positive ELISA, is it confirmed by the Western blot technique, another more sensitive test for HIV-1 antibodies. The Western blot tests for antibodies to four major HIV antigens, two of which must be present for a positive result. Like the ELISA, the Western blot test relies on the production of antibodies and, therefore, may not detect antibodies during the early stages of infection.

Rapid Tests. The ELISA and Western blot tests have been the most widely used tests to determine the presence of antibodies to HIV-1. However, these tests are technically demanding and require sophisticated equipment. Rapid HIV antibody tests are being more widely used today because of ease of use and convenience. Many have comparable sensitivities to the ELISA and Western blot.[1] Table 22-1 describes rapid HIV antibody tests.

Viral Load. Plasma HIV RNA levels indicate the amount of virus in the person's serum, which is a reflection of active viral replication, or **viral load**. The steeper the rate of increase in plasma HIV RNA, the greater the risk of disease progression unless antiretroviral therapy is started.[10] HIV RNA viral load is measured by one of three assays: quantitative RNA-PCR, branched DNA (bDNA) assay, or nucleic acid sequence–based amplification (NASBA). These tests are greater than 98% sensitive and can detect as few as 40 HIV RNA copies/ml. Another test, the p24 antigen assay, detects the viral protein p24 in the blood of HIV-infected patients. Since the assay is only about 50% sensitive, it is used less often than the quantitative tests for HIV RNA.

Viral load is measured periodically in HIV-positive persons to assess their disease progression and to monitor the effectiveness of antiretroviral therapy. Therapy is aimed at reducing plasma HIV RNA levels to below the limit of detection by assay. For accuracy, two HIV RNA assays are completed within 1 to 2 weeks, and

TABLE 22-1 RAPID HIV ASSAY TESTS

Diagnostic Test	Uses and Characteristics
Particle agglutination assay	Test for HIV antibodies Performed on serum or plasma Some tests available for whole blood Latex particles coated with HIV antigen cause agglutination of HIV antibodies Results interpreted visually (readers are available) Results available in 10 to 60 min Reagents require refrigeration Some tests detect HIV-1 and HIV-2 Costs \$2 to \$4 per test
Immunoconcentration flow-through device	Tests for HIV antigens Performed on serum or plasma Flow-through technique captures HIV antigens that form visible line on a membrane for reading Requires several procedural steps Results available in 5 to 15 min Reagents require refrigeration Cost \$4 to \$12 per test
Immunochromatographic (lateral flow) strips	Tests for HIV antigen Performed on serum, plasma, or whole blood Specimen applied to absorbent pad along with buffer and inserted into test device Positive reaction results in visual line on pad where antigen was applied Some tests detect HIV-1 and HIV-2 Results available in less than 20 min No refrigeration of reagent required Costs less than \$10 per test
Oral fluid HIV-1 antibody test	Tests for HIV-1 antibodies Performed on plasma or oral fluid obtained by swabbing around upper and lower outer gums (Oral test has lower sensitivity and specificity than plasma test.) Specimen placed into developer solution Positive result determined if 2 reddish purple lines appear in small window of devices Results available in 20 to 40 min Store at room temperature Costs \$8 to \$20 per test

both values are used to establish a baseline for the infected person. It is important for nurses to understand that suppression of HIV RNA levels to below the limits of detection does not mean that HIV infection has been eliminated or that viral replication has been halted completely. It simply means that HIV levels have been reduced to such a degree that they cannot be measured by present methods.

CD4 CELL COUNTS. CD4 cell counts are used to measure the extent of immune damage that has occurred as a result of HIV infection and its complications, and to monitor the immunologic benefit of antiretroviral therapy. CD4 cell counts are obtained on all newly diagnosed patients to establish a baseline and every 3 to 4 months thereafter if counts are above 350/mm^3 and the patient is asymptomatic and not receiving drug therapy. Once drug therapy is initiated, counts are monitored every 2 to 4 weeks initially and then every 3 to 4 months if the patient stabilizes.

CD4 cell counts are used in conjunction with viral load to predict the possibility of disease progression, determine when to start antiretroviral therapy, and monitor the effectiveness of treatment. Patients with plasma HIV RNA levels of less than 7000 copies/ml and CD4 counts of greater than 350/mm^3 have less than a 2% likelihood of progressing to AIDS within 3 years without treatment. Conversely, those with viral loads greater than 55,000 copies/ml and CD4 counts of less than 200/mm^3 have an 85% likelihood of progressing to AIDS within 3 years (Table 22-2). Figure 22-5 illustrates the relationship among HIV viral load, CD4 cell counts, and HIV antibody levels at various points along the HIV continuum.

OTHER TESTS. Other diagnostic studies are obtained to establish baselines, monitor patient progress, and identify possible coinfections (Table 22-3).

MEDICATIONS. Recent drug developments have decreased the speed of disease progression in many HIV-infected individuals and increased the life span of those living with AIDS. In 1995 the U.S. Food and Drug Administration approved a class of drugs

TABLE 22-2 LIKELIHOOD OF PROGRESSING TO AIDS WITHIN 3 YEARS WITHOUT DRUG THERAPY

	HIV RNA Viral Load (copies/ml)			
CD4 count (cells/mm^3)	>55,000	20,000-55,000	7,000-20,000	1,500-7,000
>750	32.6%	9.5%	3.2%	2.0%
501-750	32.6%	16.1%	8.1%	2.0%
351-500	42.9%	16.1%	8.1%	2.0%
201-350	64.4%	40.1%	8.1%	—
<200	85.5%	40.1%	—	—

Data from Viral Load Testing by Panel on Clinical Practices for Treatment of HIV Infection: *Guidelines for the use of antiretroviral agents in HIV-1-infected adults and adolescents*, Washington, DC, 2004, US Department of Health and Human Services.
RNA, Ribonucleic acid.

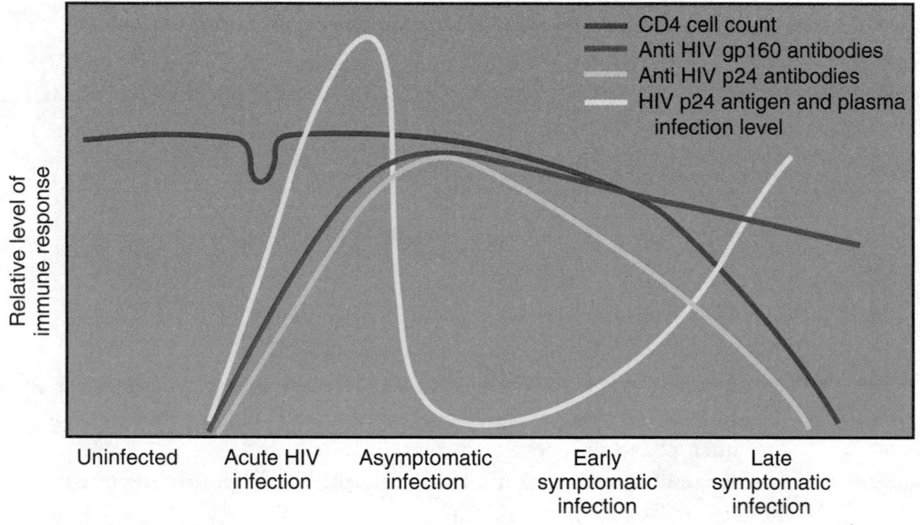

Figure 22-5 Relative levels of immune response to HIV infection.

TABLE 22-3 DIAGNOSTIC TESTS FOR HIV/AIDS

Test	Implications
T cell subset (CD4 and CD8 counts and ratios)	Used to stage HIV infection and prognosis. Repeat every 6 months if CD4 count above 500/mm^3. Repeat every 3 months for CD4 count below 500/mm^3 or if patient is symptomatic.
Plasma HIV-1 RNA	Estimates risk for disease progression; determines need for antiretroviral therapy.
CBC with differential and platelets	Detects anemia, thrombocytopenia, leukopenia. Repeat every 6-12 mo.
Biochemical profile	Detects hepatic enzyme elevations, electrolyte abnormalities, hyperglycemia, renal insufficiency, drug toxicity. Repeat yearly and as needed during antiretroviral therapy.
Lipid profile	Provides baseline before initiating HAART. Repeat every 4-6 wk until desired LDL level reached, then every 4-6 mo.

Adapted from Initial and Interim Labs: Panel on Clinical Practices for Treatment of HIV Infection: *Guidelines for the use of antiretroviral agents in HIV-1-infected adults and adolescents*, Washington, DC, 2004, US Department of Health and Human Services.
CBC, Complete blood count; *HAART,* highly active antiretroviral therapy; *LDL,* low-density lipoprotein; *RNA,* ribonucleic acid.

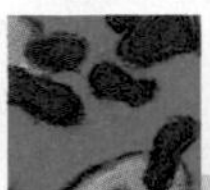

EVIDENCE-BASED PRACTICE

Topic Question: Are two antiretroviral agents as effective as three or four antiviral agent combinations in maintaining HIV viral loads?

Evidence Base: Four trials involving HIV-infected adults compared two, three, and four combinations of antiretroviral drugs as maintenance therapy following initially successful treatment for HIV. Before the study, participants had plasma viral loads of less than 500 copies/ml.

Findings: Maintenance therapies with two drugs (zidovudine and lamivudine) were associated with loss of HIV suppression and significantly higher levels of virologic failure. When protease inhibitors were discontinued after use in initial therapy, similar results were noted.

Conclusions: Reducing the number of antiretroviral agents for maintenance therapy to decrease toxicity and increase compliance significantly increases the risk for resistance and loss of viral suppression.

Rutherford GW, Sangani PR, Kennedy GE: Three- or four- versus two-drug antiretroviral maintenance regimens for HIV infection, *Cochrane Review*, Cochrane Library, Issue 2, 2004.

named protease inhibitors. When a protease inhibitor is combined with two other drugs (reverse transcriptase inhibitors), a **highly active antiretroviral therapy** (HAART) "cocktail" is created that reduces HIV viral load to undetectable levels. Those drug combinations are the mainstay of HIV treatment[17] (see Evidence-Based Practice box).

HAART works by disrupting HIV at different stages during its replication process (Figure 22-6). The nucleoside and nucleotide reverse transcriptase inhibitors (NRTIs), abacavir (ABC), zidovudine (AZT), didanosine (ddl), stavudine (d4T), lamivudine (3TC), zalcitabine (ddC), and tenofovir, act through two mechanisms. They competitively bind to reverse transcriptase, and they block the elongation of the DNA chain, both of which interfere with the early stages of HIV viral replication. The nonnucleoside reverse transcriptase inhibitors (NNRTIs, or nucleoside analogs), nevirapine (NVP), efavirenz (EFV), and delavirdine (DLV), prevent viral replication through competitive binding of reverse transcriptase, but they do not terminate DNA chains.[8]

The protease inhibitors (PIs) indinavir (IDV), ritonavir (RTV), amprenavir (APV), saquinavir (SAQ), lopinavir (LPV), and nelfinavir (NFV) prevent HIV from making the long protein molecules necessary to create new viruses, thus halting replication toward the end of viral replication.[8] Enfuvirtide is a class of drugs known as a fusion inhibitor. It is the first agent of its class to be approved for treatment of HIV. It binds the glucoprotein region of the HIV envelope and prevents viral fusion with the CD4 target cell membrane.

The goals of HAART treatment are to maximally suppress plasma HIV RNA levels to below detectable levels on assay, restore or preserve immunologic function by preventing the destruction of CD4 cells for as long as possible, improve the quality of life, and reduce mortality.[17] Clinical trials are ongoing to find more effective drug therapies with fewer side effects. Table 22-4 summarizes the medications commonly used to treat HIV infection and AIDS.

In 2004 the CDC revised their guidelines for use of antiretroviral agents in HIV-infected adults and adolescents. The guidelines include recommendations for initiating antiretroviral therapy in persons who are asymptomatic, as well as those with established disease. The recommendations were derived from studies designed to identify the risks versus benefits of treatment. Clinical trials indicated that patients whose CD4 T cell counts fell below 200 cells/mm^3 were at significantly increased risk for opportunistic infections and should be offered antiretroviral therapy.[17] Table 22-5 describes indications for initiating antiretroviral therapy.

No optimal time to initiate antiretroviral therapy has been identified for HIV-infected patients with CD4 cell counts greater than 200 cells/mm^3 who are asymptomatic, although many clinicians offer therapy when CD4 counts are less than 350 cells/mm^3. The available drug regimens are potent, complex, and challenging for adherence. Thus the decision to initiate therapy must be a joint decision between the patient and practitioner.

Patients are likely to experience drug toxicity and numerous side effects. They must be compliant with large pill burdens and tightly prescribed administration regimens; be able to financially withstand the cost of therapy; and be prepared for the possibility of drug resistance, which may limit future therapy options. Drug resistance can develop if viral replication is not sufficiently suppressed or the person is already infected with a resistant strain of HIV. On the other hand, patients who delay therapy run the risk of permanent immune system damage, inability to effectively inhibit viral replication at a later stage in the disease, and increased risk of HIV transmission. Table 22-6 summarizes risks versus benefits of early and delayed retroviral therapy for asymptomatic HIV-infected persons.[11,17]

At present HIV infection and AIDS have no vaccine or cure, although the number of potential HIV vaccines in clinical trails supported by the International AIDS Vaccine Initiative and other agencies has doubled since 2000 (see Future Watch box). Although many trials show promise, more research and funding are needed. In addition, ethical questions regarding testing of potential vaccines on healthy subjects must be addressed as trials go forward (see Ethical Alert box).

Future Watch

Is a new vaccine that reduces viral load the answer to prevention of AIDS?

Researchers at the Wistar Institute and University of Philadelphia reported promising results from an innovative HIV triple vaccine in monkeys. The triple vaccine was successful in dramatically stimulating the production of CD8 T cells that remained stable over time. The researchers believe that augmenting the production of these cells is an important step in producing an effective vaccine. The vaccine will not prevent HIV infection but may be successful in reducing viral loads. This approach is different from the traditional approach of generating antibodies that neutralize HIV. This vaccine, if successful in humans, could become part of an effective anti-HIV vaccine regimen.

Wistar Institute: *Triple-vaccine strategy stimulates strong HIV-specific immune response in monkeys*, accessed 2004 from website: http://www.wistar.upenn.edu/news_info/pressreleases/pr_07.12.04.html.

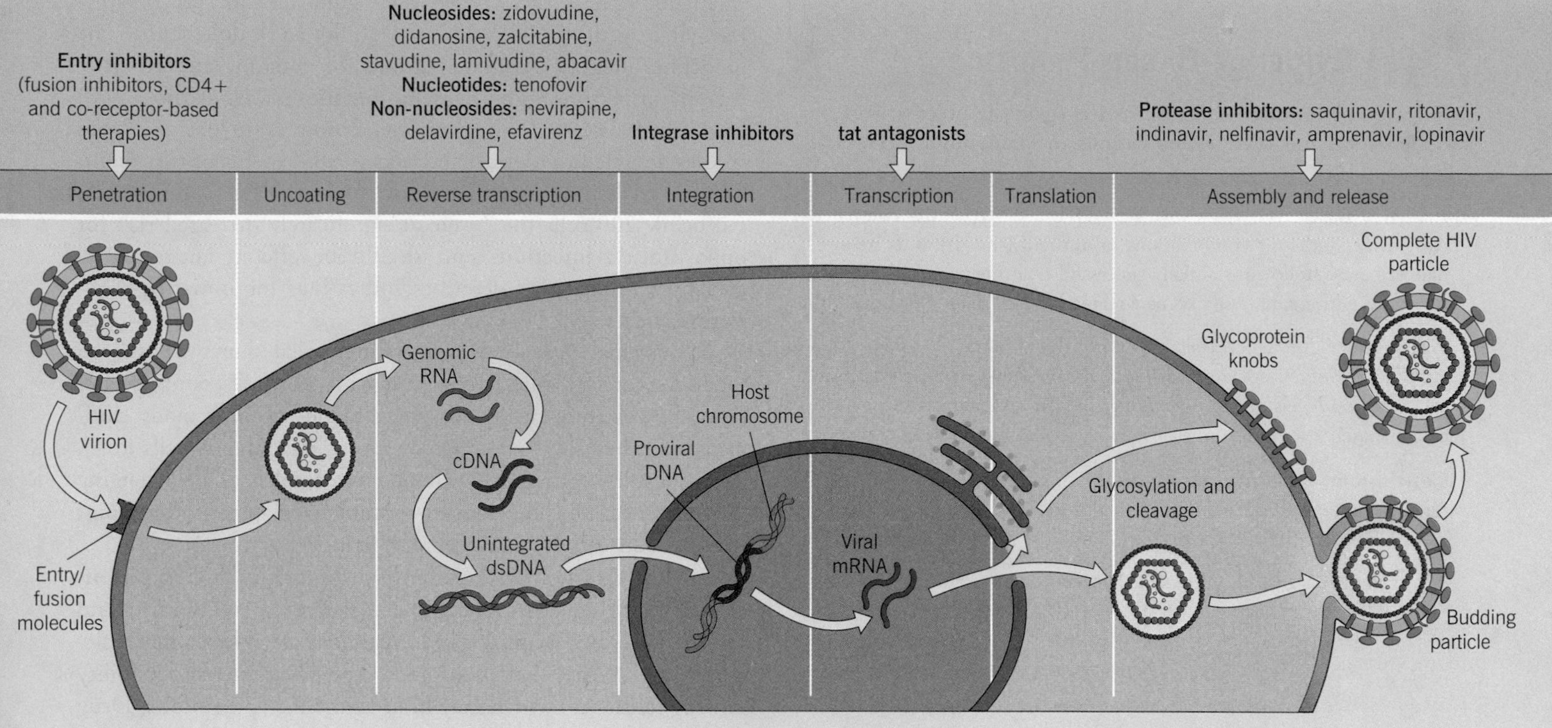

Figure 22-6 Possible sites of intervention in the inhibition of HIV replication.

Treatments. No special treatments exist for the early stages of HIV infection. Respiratory treatments may become necessary as the patient's disease progresses. Standard Precautions are necessary during hospitalization and at home. Treatments associated with maintenance and improvement of nutritional status usually become necessary. Specific treatments related to opportunistic infections are discussed later in this chapter.

Surgical Management. Surgery does not play a role in the standard management of HIV. Patients may undergo surgical biopsy of skin lesions, surgical treatment of internal Kaposi's sarcoma lesions that do not respond to chemotherapy, or drainage of abscesses or other sites of infection. These all represent management of AIDS complications, however, and are not primary therapies for HIV disease.

Diet. Although no particular diet is indicated for persons with HIV, nutritional deficits commonly develop from both the disease itself and the opportunistic infections associated with the disease. Anorexia, nausea, and diarrhea are commonly associated with antiretroviral therapy, further contributing to nutritional alterations. Many persons with AIDS develop wasting syndrome, especially late in the disease. Wasting syndrome involves involuntary weight loss in excess of 10% to 15% of normal baseline weight. It is related to decreased nutrient intake, decreased nutrient absorption, and metabolic disturbances.

Patients must be carefully monitored to evaluate the adequacy of intake and food intolerances. A high-calorie, high-protein diet is encouraged to prevent weight loss and potential cachexia. In the later stages of disease, when infections and muscle wasting prevent adequate food intake, IV nutritional support may be necessary.

Health Promotion and Prevention. Because HIV is a multifaceted problem, the first priority of care is to halt the spread of infection. To achieve this goal, the U.S. Department of Health and Human Services and U.S. Public Health Service developed Healthy People 2010 objectives related to HIV infection (see Healthy People 2010 box).[21] To meet the goals, education efforts have primarily focused on protecting persons who are not infected with the virus. In spite of abundant educational programs, the incidence of new HIV infections in the United States has remained steady rather than decreasing as was intended. Consequently, new efforts are under way to implement strategies that emphasize the prevention of transmission by HIV-infected persons in the hope of achieving previously set goals.[13] See the Evidence-Based Practice box, p. 493, for information on the effectiveness of interventions designed to prevent HIV infection through modifications of sexual risk behaviors.

In 2003 the CDC, the Health Resources and Services Administration, the National Institutes of Health, and the HIV Medicine Association of the Infectious Diseases Society of America issued evidence-based recommendations to facilitate the incorporation of HIV prevention strategies into the care of all persons. The recommendations are categorized into three major components (Figure 22-7) that encompass specific recommendations for screening HIV-infected patients for risk behaviors; communicating prevention messages; discussing sexual and drug-use behavior; positively reinforcing changes to safer behavior; referring patients for services such as substance abuse treatment; facilitating partner notification (see Legal Alert box, p. 493), counseling, and testing; and identifying and treating other STDs. Although primarily intended for health care providers, the recommendations are appropriate for anyone involved in educating or counseling the public about HIV disease.[13]

Ethical Alert

HIV Vaccine

As science continues to search for a vaccine against HIV-1, many ethical issues require consideration regarding testing of the vaccine on humans:

- Is there an imbalance of power if a vaccine is developed by one country but tested on humans in another country?
- Do the participants in HIV-related trials suffer from social or psychologic harm?
- Which populations will be selected to participate in clinical trials, and will those selections be fair?
- What level of care will be afforded to those who suffer adverse reactions to an experimental HIV vaccine?
- What level of care and treatment for HIV/AIDS will be given to participants who become infected through risky behavior during the trial?

These and many other questions are being considered as vaccine trials continue in this and other developed countries.

The prevention of HIV transmission is a health care priority not only in the United States but throughout the world. The Joint United Nations Programme on HIV/AIDS is similarly involved in HIV prevention and included key elements for a comprehensive, worldwide HIV prevention program in its 2004 report on the global AIDS epidemic.[12] Funds for new programs aimed at prevention are needed. An estimated $5 billion was made available through various international agencies, yet it was estimated to be less than half of what actually would be needed by 2005.[12]

ARE You READY?

Which of the following statements by a patient with wasting syndrome secondary to AIDS indicates the effectiveness of dietary teaching?

1. "I need to get most of my calories from carbohydrates."
2. "It is important that I eat foods high in protein."
3. "I need to limit fat in my diet."
4. "I should avoid alcoholic beverages."

Nursing Management *of the Patient with HIV/AIDS*

ASSESSMENT

Health History. Assess for:

- Risk factors (unprotected sex, exposure to blood or blood products, needle exposure, use of mood-altering drugs), which cause loss of inhibitions and risky behavior
- Sexual history, including past and present sexual activities (see Chapter 55)
- Clinical manifestations (weight loss, low-grade fever, night sweats, painful lymph nodes, fatigue, nausea, headache)
- Factors that exacerbate or relieve symptoms
- Allergies
- Medications and alternative remedies
- Ability to perform activities of daily living (ADLs)
- Concurrent medical problems (diabetes mellitus, tuberculosis)

Healthy People 2010

Objectives Related to HIV/AIDS

- Reduce the prevalence of HIV infection to no more than 1 new case per 100,000 people.
- Reduce the number of new cases of HIV infection among men who have sex with men to no more than 13,385 cases per year.
- Reduce the number of new AIDS cases among women and men who inject drugs to no more than 9075 cases per year.
- Reduce the number of new cases of HIV infection among men who have sex with men and inject drugs to no more than 1592 per year.
- Increase to 85% the proportion of adults with tuberculosis who have been tested for HIV.
- Increase to 50% the proportion of sexually active persons who use condoms.
- Increase the proportion of adults in publicly funded HIV counseling and testing sites who are screened for common bacterial sexually transmitted diseases (chlamydia, gonorrhea, and syphilis) and are immunized against hepatitis B virus.
- Increase the proportion of HIV-infected adolescents and adults who receive testing, treatment, and prophylaxis consistent with current U.S. Public Health Service treatment guidelines.
- Increase the number of HIV-positive persons who know their serostatus.
- Increase by 70% the proportion of substance abuse treatment facilities that offer HIV/AIDS education, counseling, and support.
- Increase the number of state prison systems that provide comprehensive HIV/AIDS, sexually transmitted diseases, and tuberculosis education.
- Increase the proportion of inmates in state prison systems who receive voluntary HIV counseling and testing during incarceration.
- Reduce deaths from HIV infection to no more than 0.7 deaths per 100,000 persons.
- Extend the interval of time between an initial diagnosis of HIV infection and AIDS diagnosis to increase years of life of an individual infected with HIV.
- Increase years of life of an HIV-infected person by extending the interval of time between an AIDS diagnosis and death.
- Reduce new cases of perinatally acquired HIV infection.
- Reduce HIV infections in adolescent and young adult women ages 13 to 24 years that are associated with heterosexual contact.
- Increase the proportion of pregnant women screened for sexually transmitted diseases (including HIV infection and bacterial vaginosis) during prenatal health care visits, according to recognized standards.

From US Department of Health and Human Services: *Healthy people 2010: understanding and improving health,* Washington, DC, 2000, The Department.

- Presence of family or other support systems
- Advance directive

Physical Examination. Assess for:

- Weight below ideal for height
- Abnormal vital signs (fever, increased heart rate)
- Nonelastic skin turgor, excoriated mucous membranes, lesions

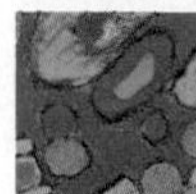

TABLE 22-4
COMMON MEDICATIONS *for HIV/AIDS*

Drug	Action	Nursing Intervention
Nucleoside Reverse Transcriptase Inhibitors (NRTIs)		
Zidovudine (AZT, ZDV, Retrovir)	Nucleoside analog Prevents initial step in which HIV turns its RNA into DNA and integrates itself into human genes Drug acts as decoy preventing replication of HIV.	Monitor for bone marrow suppression: anemia or neutropenia. Monitor for gastrointestinal (GI) intolerance, headache, insomnia, asthenia. Monitor for drug effectiveness. Teach patient and significant other about drug dose, schedule, and possible adverse effects.
Didanosine (ddl, Videx)	Nucleoside analog Prevents replication of HIV	Monitor for drug-associated pancreatitis, peripheral neuropathy, nausea, diarrhea. Monitor CD4 cell counts for drug effectiveness. Teach patient and significant other about drug dose, schedule, and possible adverse effects.
Zalcitabine (ddC, Hivid)	Nucleoside analog Prevents replication of HIV	Monitor for peripheral neuropathy, stomatitis. Monitor for drug effectiveness. Teach patient and significant other about drug dose, schedule, and possible adverse effects.
Stavudine (d4T, Zerit)	Nucleoside analog Prevents replication of HIV	Monitor for peripheral neuropathy. Monitor for drug effectiveness. Teach patient and significant other about drug dose, schedule, and possible adverse effects.
Lamivudine (3TC, Epivir)	Nucleoside analog Prevents replication of HIV	Minimal toxicity noted. Monitor for drug effectiveness. Teach patient and significant other about drug dose, schedule, and possible adverse effects.
Abacavir (ABC, Ziagen)	Nucleoside analog Prevents replication of HIV	Monitor for drug effectiveness, toxicity, and side effects (hypersensitivity, fever, rash, nausea, vomiting, malaise, loss of appetite). Hypersensitivity and lactic acidosis may be life threatening. Do not restart drug when hypersensitivity is suspected. Be aware of numerous drug interactions.
Nucleotide Reverse Transcriptase Inhibitors (NtRTIs)		
Tenofovir disoproxil (Fumarate, Viread)	Nucleotide analog Inhibits reverse transcriptase and prevents replication of HIV	Monitor for drug effectiveness, toxicity, and side effects (asthenia, headache, diarrhea, nausea, vomiting, flatulence, and rarely renal insufficiency). May be taken with or without food.
Emtricitabine (Emtriva)	Nucleotide analog Inhibits viral DNA synthesis and terminates DNA chain at point of incorporation, preventing replication of HIV	Monitor for drug effectiveness, toxicity, and side effects (headache; nausea; skin rash; discoloration of skin on palms and soles; lactic acidosis and severe hepatomegaly with steatosis, which can be fatal; exacerbation of hepatitis in coinfected patients; redistribution of body fat; peripheral wasting; facial wasting; breast enlargement; and cushingoid appearance). May be taken with or without food. Do not use in patients with hypersensitivity to drug components.

- Cough, dyspnea, crackles, wheezing
- Diarrhea, abdominal distention or tenderness
- Enlarged lymph nodes
- Concentrated, foul-smelling urine
- Mental confusion; lack of orientation to person, place, time
- Tachycardia
- Dehydration
- Electrolyte imbalances
- Acid-base imbalances

NURSING DIAGNOSES, OUTCOMES, AND INTERVENTIONS

Nursing Diagnosis: Risk for Infection

OUTCOMES. Common examples of expected outcomes for the patient with a diagnosis of *risk for infection* are:

Patient will:

- Remain free from infection.
- Remain free from fever, chilling, and malaise.
- Maintain white blood cell count within normal limits.

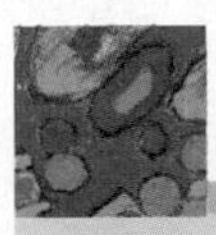

TABLE 22-4
COMMON MEDICATIONS *for HIV/AIDS—cont'd*

Drug	Action	Nursing Intervention
Nonnucleoside Reverse Transcriptase Inhibitors (NNRTIs)		
Nevirapine (Viramune)	Blocks HIV replication by protecting non-HIV-infected cells	Monitor for rash. Monitor for drug effectiveness. Be aware of drug interactions: rifampin, rifabutin, oral contraceptives, protease inhibitors.
Delavirdine (Rescriptor)	Blocks HIV replication	Monitor for rash. Do not administer within 1 hr of antacids.
Efavirenz (Sustiva)	Blocks HIV replication	Be aware of drug interactions: terfenadine, astemizole, alprazolam, midazolam, cisapride, rifabutin, rifampin. Be aware of drugs that decrease drug effectiveness: phenytoin, carbamazepine, phenobarbital. Increases drug levels of clarithromycin, dapsone, rifabutin, ergot alkaloids, dihydropyridines, quinidine, warfarin, indinavir, saquinavir. Monitor for adverse effects: rash, CNS symptoms, increased transaminase levels.
Protease Inhibitors		
Indinavir (Crixivan)	Protease inhibitors interfere with step of HIV replication in which virus makes long protein chains necessary to reproduce itself from DNA. Long protein chains must be cut by protease enzyme to turn proteins into the correct length to create HIV. Protease inhibitors prevent this action and render virus noninfectious.	Monitor CD4 cells and viral load for drug effectiveness. Teach patient and significant other about drug dose, schedule, and potential side effects. Monitor for nephrolithiasis, GI intolerance, headache, asthenia, blurred vision, dizziness, rash, metallic taste, thrombocytopenia. Be aware of drug interactions: rifampin, terfenadine, astemizole, cisapride, triazolam, ergot alkaloids, ketoconazole, rifabutin, midazolam.
Ritonavir (Norvir)	Protease inhibitor	Monitor CD4 cells and viral load for drug effectiveness. Teach patient and significant other about drug dose, schedule, and potential side effects. Monitor for GI intolerance, nausea, vomiting, diarrhea. Keep refrigerated. Be aware of drug interactions: meperidine, piroxicam, flecainide, quinidine, rifampin, bepridil, terfenadine, cisapride, bupropion, clozapine, diazepam, alprazolam, dihydroergotamine, ergotamine.
Saquinavir (Invirase)	Protease inhibitor	Monitor CD4 cells and viral load for drug effectiveness. Teach patient and significant other about drug dose, schedule, and potential side effects. Monitor for GI intolerance, nausea, diarrhea, headache, elevated transaminase enzymes. Be aware of drug interactions: rifampin, rifabutin, astemizole, terfenadine, cisapride.

Continued

- Maintain CD4 cells above 350 cells/mm^3.
- Maintain HIV RNA viral load levels below 7000 copies/ml.

NURSING INTERVENTIONS. Prevention of infection begins with educating noninfected persons who are at increased risk for contracting the virus and preventing HIV-infected persons from transmitting the virus to others. For those already infected, opportunistic infections are the major complications of HIV disease. Patients with AIDS must be protected from further infectious insults. The nurse consistently monitors vital signs, skin integrity, mucous membranes, respiratory status, GI function, and mental status for signs of possible infection. The nurse monitors white blood cell levels when signs of infection are present.[4] At least one study has shown that the antioxidant effects of vitamins C and E reduces the incidence of both oral infections and diarrhea (see Complementary & Alternative Therapies box, p. 494).

The need to control infections does not mean that the person with HIV disease should be socially isolated. It is important that

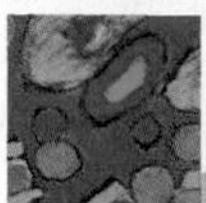

TABLE 22-4 COMMON MEDICATIONS *for HIV/AIDS—cont'd*

Drug	Action	Nursing Intervention
Nelfinavir (Viracept)	Protease inhibitor	Monitor for diarrhea. Monitor CD4 cells and viral load for drug effectiveness. Teach patient and significant other about drug dose, schedule, and potential side effects. Be aware of drug interactions: rifampin, astemizole, terfenadine, cisapride, midazolam, triazolam.
Amprenavir (Agenerase)	Protease inhibitor	High-fat meal can decrease effectiveness. Monitor for adverse effects: GI intolerance, rash, oral paresthesias, hyperglycemia, fat redistribution. Alters liver function tests. Watch for numerous drug interactions.
Lopinavir and ritonavir (Kaletra)	Protease inhibitor	Monitor for adverse effects: GI intolerance, nausea, vomiting, asthenia, elevated transaminase enzymes, hyperglycemia, fat redistribution, increased bleeding in hemophilia. Watch for numerous drug interactions.
Atazanavir (Reyataz)	Protease inhibitor	Must be taken with food to ensure absorption into bloodstream. Monitor for adverse effects: jaundice of skin, nails, and whites of eyes; cardiac dysrhythmias; headache; pain or tingling of arms and legs; nausea; diarrhea; abdominal discomfort; rash. Produces significant beneficial elevations in HDL cholesterol levels. Watch for numerous drug interactions.
Fosamprenavir (Lexiva)	Protease inhibitor	Monitor for adverse effects: rash, anorexia, headache, malaise, diarrhea, nausea, vomiting, increased cholesterol and triglycerides, lipodystrophy, diabetes. Watch for numerous drug interactions.
Fusion Inhibitors		
Enfuvirtide (Fuzeon)	Prevents viral replication by binding to region on HIV envelope and preventing viral fusion with CD4 target cell membrane	Administer by subcutaneous injection. Monitor for adverse effects: itching, pain, redness, swelling, or tenderness at injection site; pain or numbness of legs or feet; muscle pain; insomnia; depression; anorexia; constipation; peripheral neuropathy; eosinophilia; hypersensitivity characterized by rash, fever, nausea, vomiting. Watch for numerous drug interactions.

Data from Panel on Clinical Practices for Treatment of HIV Infection: *Guidelines for the use of antiretroviral agents in HIV-1-infected adults and adolescents,* Washington, DC, 2004, US Department of Health and Human Services.
CNS, Central nervous system; *DNA,* deoxyribonucleic acid; *HDL,* high-density lipoprotein; *RNA,* ribonucleic acid.

TABLE 22-5 INDICATIONS FOR INITIATION OF ANTIRETROVIRAL THERAPY IN HIV-INFECTED PERSONS

Clinical Category	CD4 Count (cells/mm³)	HIV RNA Viral Load (copies/ml)	Recommendations
Asymptomatic	>350	<55,000 (bDNA)	Most experienced clinicians recommend deferring HAART and monitoring CD4 counts, recognizing that 3-yr risk for developing AIDS is less than 15% in untreated patients.
Asymptomatic	>350	>55,000 (bDNA)	Some experienced clinicians recommend initiating therapy; others do not. The 3-yr risk for developing AIDS is greater than 30% in untreated patients.
Asymptomatic	200-350	Any value	Treatment is generally offered.
Symptomatic, AIDS	<200	Any value	Treat
Symptomatic, AIDS or severe symptoms	Any value	Any value	Treat

Adapted from *Guidelines for the use of antiretroviral agents in HIV-1-infected adults and adolescents,* Washington, DC, 2004, US Department of Health and Human Services.
bDNA, Branched deoxyribonucleic acid; *HAART,* highly active antiretroviral therapy; *RNA,* ribonucleic acid.

TABLE 22-6 RISKS AND BENEFITS OF DELAYED AND EARLY THERAPY IN ASYMPTOMATIC HIV-INFECTED PERSONS

	Risks	Benefits
Early therapy	Reduced quality of life because of drug side effects Greater cumulative drug-related adverse effects Earlier development of drug resistance (if viral suppression is suboptimal) Risk for transmission of virus resistant to antiretroviral drugs because of suboptimal suppression Limited future antiretroviral treatment options	Control of viral replication easier to achieve and maintain Delay or prevention of immune system compromise Lower risk of resistance with complete viral suppression Possible decreased risk of HIV transmission
Late therapy	Possible risk of irreversible immune system depletion Possible greater difficulty with suppressing viral replication Possible increased risk of HIV transmission	Avoids negative effects on quality of life (side effects and inconvenience) Avoids drug-related adverse effects Delay in development of drug resistance Preserves maximal number of available future treatment options

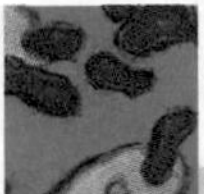

EVIDENCE-BASED PRACTICE

Topic Question: Do interventions modify sexual risk behaviors for preventing HIV infection in men who have sex with men (MSM)?

Evidence Base: Thirteen randomized studies examined the effects of behavioral interventions on the reduction of risky sexual behaviors among MSM to prevent the transmission of HIV and other sexually transmitted diseases. Studies compared interpersonal skills and individual, small group, and community interventions.

Findings: Intervention effects resulted in a 23% reduction in the number of men engaging in unprotected sex. Community-level interventions and those which promoted interpersonal skills were slightly more effective among men in their twenties than other interventions.

Conclusions: Interventions can promote reduction of risk behaviors in MSM. However, more controlled intervention trials are needed to substantiate the effects of specific behavior interventions.

Johnson WD, Hedges LV, Diaz RM: Interventions to modify sexual risk behaviors for preventing HIV infection in men who have sex with men, *Cochrane Review*, Cochrane Library, Issue 2, 2004.

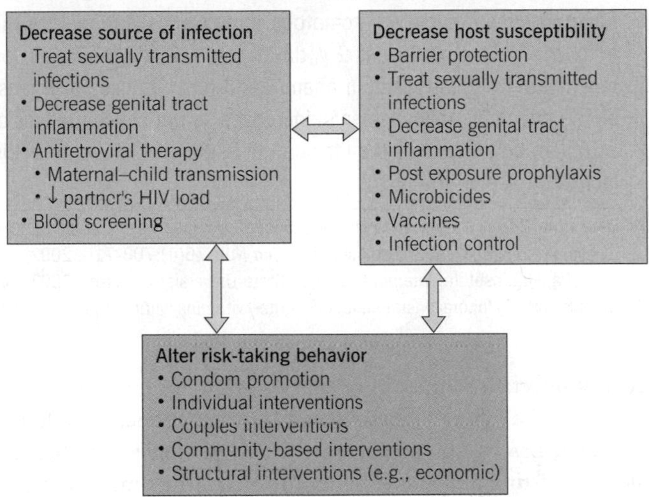

Figure 22-7 Approaches to preventing HIV transmission.

patients maintain their usual social relationships. Many communities have support groups with volunteers who are willing to make routine visits or become the patient's "buddy" or "ally." This can be of particular benefit to those who have no nearby relatives or significant others (see Nursing Care Plan, p. 496).

Health care personnel as a whole are at increased risk for exposure to HIV. Consequently, institutions have developed procedures for the effective management of such exposures. Health care personnel must be diligent about reporting needlesticks and other exposures to prevent, to the extent possible, infection with HIV. Their confidentiality is ensured, which fosters reporting of such incidents.

Although postexposure policies vary at different facilities, some basic procedures are common to all. Facility policies must, however, be consistent with local and state laws. Initially, the infected health care worker's wounds are cleaned with soap and water and irrigated

Legal Alert

Duty To Warn

The majority of states and some cities or localities have laws and regulations related to informing partners that they have been exposed to HIV:

- Clinicians may be required to report to the state partners of HIV-infected persons, even if the patient refuses to report the partner.
- Clinicians may be required to disclose to third parties a high risk for future HIV transmission from patients known to be infected (duty to warn).

Nurses and other clinicians need to know and comply with local and state requirements in the areas where they practice. Clinicians also need to be aware of and adhere to all laws and regulations related to providing services to minors.

Complementary & Alternative Therapies

Vitamins C and E

Patients with HIV and AIDS often take vitamins for their antioxidant effect and to counter weight loss, fatigue, muscle cramps, or nerve pain. The antioxidant effects of vitamins C and E in particular may slow the progression of HIV to AIDS and reduce the number of mouth infections and diarrhea. One 5-year study conducted by American and Tanzanian researchers supported this finding in pregnant women.

Vitamin E is thought to augment components of the immune system and to be one of the most potent antidotes to free radicals, chemically deactivating them before they can destroy cells. Vitamin E is found in vegetable oils, margarine, green leafy vegetables, whole grains, soybeans, eggs, nuts, and many fruits. Supplements are available. A dose of 400 IU/day is optimal; doses greater than 1000 IU/day can be detrimental. Large doses can contribute to blood clot formation. Vitamin E potentiates the effects of anticoagulants.

Vitamin C is a potent antioxidant. It is thought to positively affect the thymus and lymph nodes, which are primary immune organs. Vitamin C may help promote antibody production. It is found in citrus fruits, green vegetables, tomatoes, strawberries, and melons. The optimal supplement dose is 2 g/day; 4 g/day is the maximum. Too much vitamin C can result in anemia and renal stones. It decreases the effects of anticoagulants; increases serum concentrations of estrogen; and increases the life span of aspirin, which can result in increased aspirin toxicity.

Data from Brigelius-Flohe R et al: The European perspective on vitamin E: current knowledge and future research, *Am J Clin Nutr* 76(4):703-716, 2002; and Linus Pauling Institute: *Vitamin C*, Oregon State University, accessed 2003 from website: http://lpi.oregonstate.edu/infocenter/vitamins/vitaminC/.

with a disinfectant solution. Eyes are vigorously irrigated with clean water or sterile saline. Contaminated mucosal surfaces are flushed with water. Baseline blood chemistries and serologies are obtained. Follow-up testing occurs every 3 months from the time of exposure for a year. If the worker develops signs of acute, primary HIV infection, more aggressive diagnostic testing takes place.

The U.S. Public Health Service published guidelines that recommend antiretroviral agents for postoccupational exposure to HIV (Table 22-7). Chemoprophylaxis is initiated as early as possible after exposure and continues for at least 4 weeks if tolerated. The use of these agents in healthy persons is not without problems. Side effects are substantial and often result in noncompletion of the course of therapy. The risks of antiretroviral therapy to pregnant health care workers who are exposed to HIV are largely unknown; therefore pregnant employees who decide to take chemoprophylaxis are closely monitored for fetal and maternal signs of toxicity.[8]

Nonoccupational exposure to HIV can also occur from sexual abuse, rape, consensual sex, and parenteral exposure in the community. Similar to recommendations for health care workers, the U.S. Public Health Service has issued chemoprophylactic recommendations for nonoccupational exposure to HIV (Table 22-8).[8]

Related NIC Interventions. Infection Control, Infection Protection, Surveillance, Teaching: Disease Process

Nursing Diagnosis: Imbalanced Nutrition: Less Than Body Requirements

Outcomes. Common examples of expected outcomes for the patient with a diagnosis of *imbalanced nutrition: less than body requirements* are:

Patient will:

- Maintain present weight, not lose weight, or gain weight to within 0.5 kg of preillness weight.
- Verbalize need to increase caloric and protein intake in the presence of weight loss.
- Maintain fluid hydration.

Nursing Interventions. The nutritional status of patients with HIV disease may range from normal early in the disease process to extreme cachexia and wasting syndrome from progressive disease and opportunistic infections. Therefore the nurse monitors nutritional status and implements strategies to promote enough food intake to maintain maximal health and functioning. After identifying current dietary intake, likes and dislikes, dietary restrictions, food tolerances and intolerances, height, and weight, the nurse monitors the patient for signs of altered nutrition or factors that may alter nutritional status, such as a pattern of decreasing weight, decreased muscle strength and tone, decreased energy levels, anorexia, nausea, stomatitis, impaired swallowing, or self-care deficits.

Side effects of drug therapy may impair the patient's desire to eat or cause nausea and vomiting. Eating toast or dry crackers and

Table 22-7 Current U.S. Public Health Service Recommendations for Chemoprophylaxis of Occupational Exposures to HIV

Exposure	Regimen	Drugs
HIV exposures with recognized transmission risk	"Basic regimen"	Zidovudine (ZDV) plus lamivudine (3TC)
	Alternative	Stavudine (D4T) plus lamivudine
	"Basic regimen"	Stavudine plus didanosine (ddl)*
HIV exposures for which nature of exposure suggests elevated transmission risk†	"Basic regimen" plus 1 of following agents	Indinavir*
		Nelfinavir
		Abacavir
		Efavirenz*

From Cohen J, Powderly G, editors: *Infectious diseases*, ed 2, St Louis, 2004, Mosby.

*Agents not advisable for use in pregnancy and increasingly not recommended in practice.

†Elevated risk is associated with "larger" volume of blood and/or blood containing a high titer of HIV.

TABLE 22-8 SUGGESTED BASIC AND EXPANDED POSTEXPOSURE PROPHYLAXIS REGIMENS FOR CHEMOPROPHYLAXIS AFTER NONOCCUPATIONAL EXPOSURES TO HIV

Exposure	Regimen	Drugs
HIV exposures with recognized transmission risk	"Basic regimen"	Zidovudine (ZDV) plus lamivudine (3TC)
	Alternative "basic regimens"	Stavudine (D4T) plus lamivudine
		Stavudine plus didanosine (ddl)*
HIV exposures for which nature of exposure suggests elevated transmission risk†	"Basic regimen" plus 1 of following agents	Indinavir*
		Nelfinavir
		Abacavir
		Efavirenz*

Data from Cohen J, Powderly G, editors: *Infectious diseases*, ed 2, St Louis, 2004, Mosby.
*Agent(s) and regimens not advisable for use in pregnancy.
†Elevated risk is associated with exposures associated with increased risks for transmission (e.g., sexual assault, trauma, blood exposure, concomitant sexually transmitted disease, source patient with high circulating viral burden).

drinking beverages 30 minutes before meals may be effective in reducing nausea. Antiemetics may be necessary for severe nausea and vomiting. Acupuncture has also been shown to be helpful (see Complementary & Alternative Therapies box, p. 498). Cannabinoid drugs (marijuana) may offer broad-spectrum relief for some patients with AIDS, especially those with wasting syndrome. Nausea, anorexia, anxiety, and pain are associated with wasting and can be diminished by marijuana. Because marijuana is a schedule I drug and remains controversial, it is rarely recommended until all other practical options have failed.[12a]

Oral analgesics and topical anesthetics can often aid in reducing mouth pain. Mouth care before meals, sitting in a chair to eat, eating with others, and taking meals in pleasant surroundings are measures that may successfully promote adequate oral intake.[18]

A high-calorie, high-protein diet divided into six small meals per day is recommended, since fatigued patients with little appetite may feel overwhelmed by the sight of a large meal. Specific food likes and dislikes are incorporated into meal planning to enhance intake. If the patient is losing weight, he or she can keep a calorie and protein count or food diary for 1 week to determine the presence of deficits. The patient may need to be assisted with eating if fatigue or weakness is a problem. Impaired swallowing is reported promptly to the physician. Family members, friends, or community agencies can be an important source of support and can be contacted to provide meals, visit during mealtimes, or assist with feeding.

RELATED NIC INTERVENTIONS. Nutrition Management, Nutrition Therapy, Nutritional Counseling, Nutritional Monitoring, Weight Management

Nursing Diagnosis: Fatigue

OUTCOMES. Common examples of expected outcomes for the patient with a diagnosis of *fatigue* are:
Patient will:

- Perform ADLs independently without fatigue.
- Report satisfactory energy level.
- Report sufficient sleep to meet energy needs.

NURSING INTERVENTIONS. Fatigue is a primary complaint of persons with HIV infection or disease; therefore energy management is important. The nurse assesses the patient's ability to perform ADLs, including weakness, gait, endurance, strength, and motor and sensory deficits, to determine changes from baseline. The patient balances activities with rest periods to maintain normal or near-normal activity levels as long as possible. The nurse encourages the patient to respect the signs of fatigue and reduce activities when required. The use of assistive devices, such as wheelchairs, canes, or walkers, can help conserve energy.

The environment is arranged so that items used daily are conveniently located and readily accessible. The nurse can help the patient identify creative ways to conserve energy in a home environment that may be less than optimal. Attention is given to conditions that may jeopardize patient safety, such as stairs, area rugs, or lack of hand rails on bathtubs. The nurse can solicit the support of family members or significant others to assist with home maintenance tasks to mitigate the patient's fatigue.

Environmental stimuli can be adjusted so that the patient achieves at least 6 to 8 hours of sleep per night. Although the person with AIDS has no specific activity restrictions, a pattern of rest and activity is encouraged to help maintain lean body mass and prevent deconditioning. Activity also provides a sense of control for the individual. During acute infections, activity may need to be restricted. Increasing the amount of sleep and reducing sleep interruptions may be effective in combating fatigue. The nurse can arrange for visits from a home health aide or community support group to assist with physical care when necessary.

RELATED NIC INTERVENTIONS. Energy Management, Exercise Promotion, Simple Relaxation Therapy, Sleep Enhancement

Nursing Diagnosis: Ineffective Coping

OUTCOMES. Common examples of expected outcomes for the patient with a diagnosis of *ineffective coping* are:
Patient will:

- Verbalize own anxiety and fears.
- Engage in communication that leads to sharing of feelings, decision making, and problem resolution as appropriate.
- Verbalize unresolved feelings or concerns.
- Verbalize decreased anxiety or increased satisfaction with resolution of problems or concerns.

Nursing Care Plan

Patient With HIV/AIDS

Data A 41-year-old woman was diagnosed with HIV infection 8 years ago. She has been divorced for 14 years and has one adult son who attends college in another state. Currently she lives with her 70-year-old mother who is her primary caregiver. Three years before her diagnosis the woman was involved in an automobile accident. She received several blood transfusions for multiple traumas. Her current medications include a protease inhibitor combined with two nucleotide reverse transcriptase inhibitors. She has been able to work full time until recently. During the past 3 months she has experienced increased fatigue and a 10-pound weight loss. She was admitted to the hospital 2 days ago with complaints of fever, night sweats, myalgia, malaise, chest discomfort, dry nonproductive cough, abdominal discomfort, and diarrhea. Vital signs are temperature, 101.8° F orally; heart rate, 92 beats/min and regular; and respiratory rate, 28 breaths/min and mildly labored. Her abdomen is firm and tender with hyperactive bowel sounds. Her CD4 count is 200/mm^3, and her HIV ribonucleic acid (RNA) count is 18,000 cells/ml (bDNA). After diagnostic bronchoscopy and stool specimen examination, the health care provider diagnosed *Pneumocystis carinii* pneumonia and *Cryptosporidium* infections.

Nursing Diagnosis

Ineffective airway clearance related to excessive secretions secondary to opportunistic infection *(P. carinii)*

Outcomes

- Patient will maintain a patent airway.
- Patient will achieve respiratory rate and rhythm within normal limits based on baseline.

Related NOC Outcomes

- Respiratory Status: Airway Patency
- Respiratory Status: Gas Exchange
- Respiratory Status: Ventilation
- Vital Signs

Related NIC Interventions

- Airway Management
- Chest Physiotherapy
- Cough Enhancement
- Respiratory Monitoring
- Vital Signs Monitoring

Nursing Interventions/Rationales

- Monitor respiratory rate, rhythm, and effort. *To detect respiratory compromise and determine effectiveness of treatment.*
- Monitor lung sounds. *To detect breathing pattern abnormalities and determine effectiveness of treatment.*
- Encourage slow, deep breathing. *To alleviate dyspnea while allowing for maximum oxygenation. Slow respirations prevent collapse of airways that are hypersensitive because of inflammation and infection.*
- Teach patient how to cough effectively. *To prevent stasis of secretions without expending excessive respiratory energy.*
- Encourage increased fluid intake. *To promote liquefaction of secretions for easy expectoration.*
- Administer prescribed supplemental oxygen. *To enhance oxygenation, prevent hypoxia, and decrease dyspnea.*

Nursing Diagnosis

Imbalanced nutrition: less than body requirements related to diarrhea secondary to opportunistic infection

Outcomes

- Patient will cease to lose weight.
- Patient will describe meal plan with adequate calories and fluids.
- Patient will maintain electrolyte balance.

Related NOC Outcomes

- Nutritional Status: Food & Fluid Intake
- Nutritional Status: Nutrient Intake
- Weight Control

Related NIC Interventions

- Fluid/Electrolyte Management
- Fluid Management
- Fluid Monitoring
- Nutrition Management
- Nutrition Monitoring
- Weight Management

Nursing Interventions/Rationales

- Monitor intake and output. *To determine if fluid output is excessive when compared with fluid intake so that fluid deficits can be avoided or treated early.*
- Monitor hydration status (skin turgor, mucous membranes). *To determine adequacy of fluid intake. To initiate fluid replacement early if needed.*
- Obtain daily weights and monitor trends. *Weight is a clinical indicator of adequate nutrition and fluid balance. To determine need for nutritional supplements or total parenteral nutrition.*

Nursing Interventions. HIV-infected persons have many fears and concerns, such as fear of losing their jobs and independence, fear of becoming debilitated, fear of bodily changes, and fear of death. The persistent threat of disease progression can easily create a state of chronic fear that makes it difficult to enjoy the present. Fear produces anxiety, which can result in ineffective coping patterns.

The recognition of fear is often the first step in alleviating it. The nurse assesses the patient's psychologic response to the situation and availability of support systems and helps the patient identify additional sources of financial and physical support. The nurse encourages patients to talk about their concerns and helps them identify means for dealing with those concerns. Patients are encouraged to maintain social and community activities with persons who have common interests and goals and use support groups because they offer a safe place for individuals to express themselves. Uncontrolled fear may interfere with care.

As part of the coping process, the nurse encourages patients to consider and discuss their feelings about the disease progression and the potential for further physical and mental deterioration. The nurse assesses the patient-caregiver relationship and attempts to anticipate how the stressors of disease progression may affect that relationship.

A therapeutic nursing relationship built with empathy, acceptance, and support is essential. People with AIDS often feel stig-

- Monitor laboratory data (blood urea nitrogen, serum protein, hemoglobin, hematocrit, transferrin levels). *Provides objective data regarding nutritional status so that corrective actions can be initiated early. To evaluate effectiveness of treatments.*
- Encourage six small meals, excluding dairy products and raw fruits and vegetables. *Small meals prevent gastric distention and nausea. Lactose in dairy products may enhance diarrhea. Raw foods contain naturally occurring microorganisms that may cause infection in the immunocompromised host.*
- Administer intravenous fluids as prescribed. *To prevent fluid volume deficits, hypovolemia, and cellular dehydration.*
- Teach patient to increase intake of high-calorie, protein-rich, high-carbohydrate foods. *To provide calories, aid healing, and prevent wasting.*
- Assess and monitor for factors that impede intake (e.g., oral lesions, pain). *To prevent nutritional deficits related to inability to intake food or fluids.*

Nursing Diagnosis

Risk for deficient fluid volume related to diarrhea secondary to cryptosporidiosis

Outcomes

- Patient will maintain (or regain) fluid volume balance.
- Patient will maintain (or regain) electrolyte balance.

Outcomes

- Electrolyte & Acid/Base Balance
- Fluid Balance
- Hydration

Related NIC Interventions

- Fluid Management
- Fluid Monitoring
- Intravenous (IV) Therapy

Nursing Interventions/Rationales

- Monitor skin turgor and mucous membranes. *Poor skin turgor and sticky mucous membranes are indications of fluid volume deficit.*
- Monitor weight daily. *Weight is a good indicator of hydration status. Rapid changes in weight are usually due to changes in fluid volume.*
- Monitor consistency and amount of stools. *Fluid lost in stool must be replaced, since diarrhea is a significant source of fluid loss.*
- Monitor vital signs. *To detect changes associated with fluid deficit. Tachycardia, hypotension, and low-grade fever are associated with fluid volume deficit.*
- Monitor intake and output. *To determine if deficits between intake and output exist. To determine fluid deficiency effect on renal function. To evaluate effectiveness of treatments.*
- Encourage fluid intake when tolerated. *To replace fluid losses.*
- Administer prescribed intravenous fluids. *To replace fluid losses and prevent hypovolemia.*
- Administer prescribed antidiarrheal medications. *To correct the cause of the fluid loss.*

Nursing Diagnosis

Anxiety related to fear of unknown outcome of disease

Outcomes

- Patient will report decreased anxiety.
- Patient will be able to participate in decision making.

Related NOC Outcomes

- Anxiety Level
- Coping
- Fear Level

Related NIC Interventions

- Anxiety Reduction
- Calming Technique
- Coping Enhancement

Nursing Interventions/Rationales

- Explain all care and procedures. *To decrease fear, which is manifested as anxiety. Anxiety often occurs when unfamiliar procedures are scheduled.*
- Encourage verbalization of fears and concerns. *Venting of feelings often allows patient to put fears into perspective and may decrease anxiety.*
- Discourage decision making while under extreme stress. *Stress inhibits the ability to problem solve and approach decisions in a rational manner.*
- Discourage decision making until outcomes are known. *Decisions based on inadequate information may cause greater stress in the future.*
- Explore past effective coping strategies that were successful. *Patterns of past successful coping are indicators of present resources and strengths.*

Evaluation

Evaluation is based on comparing the patient's outcomes with desired outcomes.

matized by their disease. An empathetic nurse can support individuals simply by talking to them at times other than when providing physical care. The nurse encourages patients and caregivers to express their feelings and fears, to identify past and current coping strategies, and to explore effective and ineffective aspects of their relationship. The nurse reinforces the use of effective coping strategies.

A vital resource for the person with HIV disease is the assistance and support of a competent and dependable caregiver. That person may be a spouse, partner, friend, or relative. During the early stages of disease, the patient may rely on the caregiver to help diminish mood fluctuations, provide encouragement, foster motivation, and assist with some aspects of daily care. As the condition of the person with HIV deteriorates, however, the caregiver's role is significantly increased to include physical, psychologic, and financial support. Consequently, caregiver burden can become an important issue. It is important for the nurse to help caregivers find suitable outlets for their own emotions. The nurse encourages caregiver to get adequate rest and nutrition so they will have the physical stamina to meet the demands placed on them. Use of community resources, family members, or friends is encouraged to provide time away from the physically ill individual for the purpose of shopping, work, or recreation.

Complementary & Alternative Therapies

Acupuncture

Research on acupuncture shows that it is effective in treating pain and nausea. It is also believed to reduce many other unpleasant body sensations by improving the flow and balance of energy. Acupuncture is not a cure for HIV infection or AIDS. However, many people with AIDS believe it improves their overall energy, helps them tolerate the side effects of highly active antiretroviral therapy, reduces nausea and diarrhea, and helps them tolerate the pain associated with HIV-induced neuropathies.

Acupuncture is a traditional Chinese healing method that uses very thin needles to stimulate specific points in the body. They are left in place for 30 to 45 minutes and may be stimulated with mild electrical current. Many people sleep during the procedure.

Acupuncture has only mild side effects, including mild pain, numbness, tingling, or a decrease in blood pressure when the needles are removed. Some points should not be stimulated in pregnant women. Acupuncture has been found to be useful in the treatment of more than 40 different conditions.

Data from New Mexico AIDS Infonet: *Chinese acupuncture*, accessed 2004 from website: http://www.aidsinfonet.org/articles.php?articleID=703&newLang=en.

Persons with HIV/AIDS who do not have a dependable support system are at a considerable disadvantage. Not only do they require earlier referrals for home care and other community services, but they lack the day-to-day comfort and encouragement offered by a close personal companion. Patients without support systems are at risk for suicide; in many cases the nurse must fill part of the void by being a compassionate listener, offering encouragement, and fostering hope.

Social services personnel are valuable assets and may need to be consulted early in the patient's disease process, whether the person is being cared for at home or in the hospital. They can assist with solving financial problems; help the patient apply for Medicare or Medicaid; and facilitate contact with a variety of other services, including food pantries, housing assistance, community AIDS services, and support groups. For hospitalized persons, social services can assist with discharge planning and arranging home care.

Related NIC Interventions. Anxiety Reduction, Coping Enhancement, Crisis Intervention, Decision-Making Support, Emotional Support, Support System Enhancement

Nursing Diagnosis: Ineffective Therapeutic Regimen Management

Outcomes. Common examples of expected outcomes for the patient with a diagnosis of *ineffective therapeutic regimen management* are:

Patient will:

- Report the ability to manage and adhere to prescribed treatment regimen.
- Develop and follow a plan to achieve treatment regimen.
- Avoid risk-taking behaviors.
- Recognize and report changes in disease status.

Nursing Interventions. A wide range of knowledge, skills, and resources may be needed to carry out the complex therapeutic regimen at home during the various stages of HIV and AIDS. Additionally, HIV disease places heavy physical, psychologic, and financial burdens on both the patient and caregiver. The nurse assesses the patient for functional abilities, disabilities, and extent of illness, and the caregiver for ability and willingness to assist with or perform needed care. The nurse encourages the patient to maintain self-care to the extent possible, without incurring injury.

The nurse reviews treatment protocols, particularly drug regimens, with the patient and assesses the patient's understanding of the drug dosages, administration schedules, and side effects. The patient is encouraged to anticipate some unpleasant drug side effects and plan strategies for addressing them, such as using a cool cloth on the head or napping to relieve nausea. Patients are encouraged to report their use of complementary or alternative medications so that they can avoid drug interactions.

The early success of drug cocktail protocols has added new uncertainties to the lives of persons with HIV. Dramatic successes have been widely reported, with some patients experiencing a drop in their viral load to undetectable levels. It may be difficult for patients to know how to use this newfound well-being, especially if their lives have been fully consumed with disease management. Even if returning to work is not a possibility because of ongoing fatigue, the person may no longer be overtly sick. This creates new and unexpected challenges for patients and caregivers, who must find new ways to relate and effectively use this gift of time.

Some people with AIDS may be able to continue to work as their disease progresses, whereas others find it necessary to quit because they can no longer meet the physical requirements of their job. Inadequate health insurance coverage forces some patients to stop working prematurely and seek disability assistance to cover the costs of drug therapy. This step makes it nearly impossible for patients to return to work even if their health status allows it. Loss of work generally means loss of income and eventual loss of independence.

The impact of lost income and the psychologic impact of inability to work both need to be explored. The nurse should provide information about how and where to apply for financial assistance for medical care before it becomes a crisis. Multiple resources, including social services, clergy, public and private mental health resources, and special funding initiatives such as the Ryan White funds, are available to assist patients in their efforts to effectively self-manage AIDS in their home environment.

Related NIC Interventions. Coping Enhancement, Counseling, Emotional Support, Teaching: Prescribed Medication

Patient/Family Teaching. Patient and family teaching, as presented in the accompanying Patient/Family Teaching box, is an integral part of nursing care for the patient with HIV/AIDS.

Evaluation

To evaluate the effectiveness of nursing interventions, compare patient behaviors with those stated in the expected patient outcomes.

Related NOC Outcomes. Acceptance: Health Status, Activity Tolerance, Compliance Behavior, Coping, Decision-

PATIENT/FAMILY TEACHING
HIV/AIDS

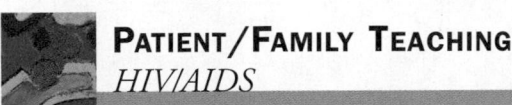

Teaching for the patient with HIV/AIDS and his or her caregiver should include information about the disease and prescribed medications, as well as the following instructions:

- Monitor for and report signs of infection, which may indicate disease progression:
  —Fever, vomiting, diarrhea, abdominal pain
  —Changes in health status from baseline
- Use strategies to prevent infections:
  —Wash hands thoroughly and frequently; maintain scrupulous personal hygiene.
  —Take meticulous care of all invasive lines.
  —Thoroughly cook meat products and wash fruits and vegetables before eating.
  —Avoid foods that may be contaminated or harbor bacteria (raw fruits, vegetables, fish, or seafood) especially when absolute neutrophil counts are less than 500 cells/cm^3.
  —Remove fresh plants and flowers from the patient's bedroom that may harbor bacteria.
  —Keep inside pets clean.
  —Avoid cleaning cat litter boxes.
  —Ask visitors to wear masks during their visits if the patient's condition warrants it. People with infections such as colds or chickenpox are requested not to visit until they are well.
- Implement measures to maintain nutrition and prevent weight loss by intaking sufficient calories to maintain or gain weight as needed.
- Implement measures to prevent transmission of infection to others.
- Take medications as prescribed and monitor for and report side effects.
- Keep emergency telephone numbers and telephone numbers for community agencies in a location where they can be readily found.

Making, Endurance, Energy Conservation, Knowledge: Medication, Knowledge: Treatment Regimen, Nutritional Status: Food & Fluid Intake, Nutritional Status: Nutrient Intake

GERONTOLOGIC CONSIDERATIONS

Between 11% and 15% of people with AIDS in the United States are 50 years of age or older, with older women affected more frequently than older men.[14] This percentage is expected to rise steadily as adults being treated with HAART live longer. Recognition of HIV infection in older adults may be difficult for several reasons. A diagnosis of AIDS may be missed, since this group commonly experiences symptoms such as pneumonia, dementia, shortness of breath, weakness, fatigue, poor nutritional intake, and weight loss. In addition, caregivers may fail to evaluate thoroughly such risk factors as IV drug use or unprotected sex in this age-group.[14]

Care and counseling of the older adult with HIV/AIDS are similar to those of younger adults, except that age-related changes need to be incorporated into the care plan. Older adults with compromised immune functions or chronic illnesses often have little reserve to resist or fight the multiple infections that accompany HIV infection. In general, this age-group is less tolerant of aggressive drug therapies that fight infections as a whole, which makes them particularly susceptible to the side effects associated with aggressive HIV drug therapy.

Because older adults are not generally targeted as an at-risk group for HIV infection, they are often neglected when it comes to AIDS outreach and teaching. Nurses must keep in mind that older adults are sexually active and be prepared to provide health teaching about HIV infection and transmission when appropriate.

AIDS-Related Opportunistic Infections

The infections associated with HIV disease are called opportunistic, since the organisms producing infection are not ordinarily pathogenic because an intact immune system renders them harmless. In patients with HIV, whose immune regulators are severely compromised, these organisms thrive, multiply, and produce disease. When CD4 cell counts fall below 400/mm^3, signs and symptoms of immunodeficiency are likely to occur; when counts fall below 200/mm^3, more than one opportunistic infection is encountered (Figure 22-8). Opportunistic infections are not limited to persons with AIDS, but may affect any person who is immunodeficient or immunosuppressed as a result of chronic illness or chemotherapy.

Persons with AIDS may experience one or more infections at the same time, producing a challenge for nurses, physicians, and other health care providers. Patients may receive several antibiotics for extended periods, causing an increased incidence of side effects and the potential for drug resistance. Opportunistic infections often return when antibiotics are reduced or discontinued.

In 2001 the U.S. Public Health Service and the Infectious Disease Society of America updated their earlier guidelines for preventing opportunistic infections in AIDS patients (Table 22-9). HAART is the most effective means of preventing opportunistic infections in AIDS patients. For those who cannot or will not undergo HAART, prophylaxis against opportunistic infections is recommended. Prophylaxis has been shown to provide survival benefits even among those who are receiving HAART.[17] The goal of treatment is to prevent infection or reduce its severity.

Bacterial Infections

Mycobacterium avium Complex

Etiology and Epidemiology. *Mycobacterium avium* and *Mycobacterium intracellulare* are closely related nontuberculous or atypical mycobacteria that are usually grouped together as *M. avium* complex (MAC). These organisms are widespread in the environment, with high concentrations in water, soil, unpasteurized dairy products, and aerosol droplets. There is a low incidence of clinical disease in the normal host because of the low pathogenicity of the organism, but MAC is the most common bacterial infection in AIDS, occurring in up to 50% of patients late in the course of HIV infection.

Pathophysiology. MAC is generally manifested as a tuberculosis-like pulmonary process. The majority of people who are colonized with MAC are not HIV infected and are asymptomatic. HIV-infected persons with MAC may be asymptomatic or have a persistent fever as high as 104° F (40° C), night sweats, fatigue,

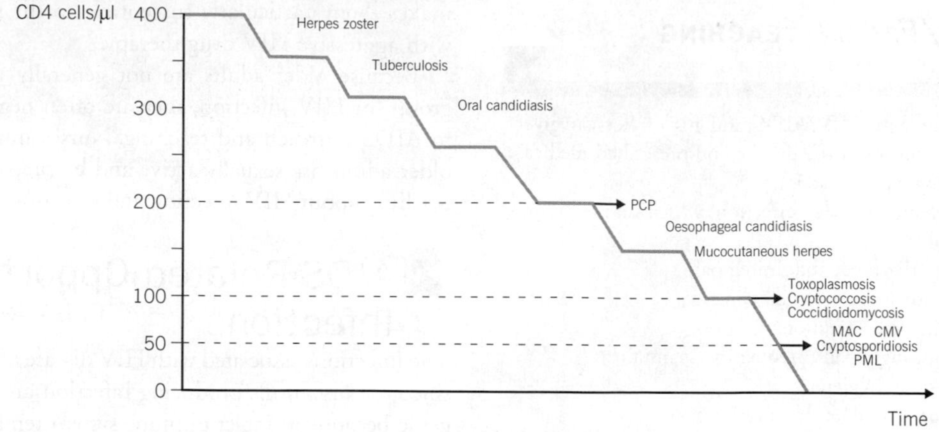

Figure 22-8 Association between opportunistic infections and CD4 cell counts. *CMV,* Cytomegalovirus; *MAC, Mycobacterium avium* complex; *PCP, Pneumocystis carinii* pneumonia; *PML,* progressive multifocal leukoencephalopathy.

anorexia, weight loss, abdominal pain, or diarrhea. MAC most often produces disseminated disease and may be found in every organ. Physical examination reveals lymphadenopathy or hepatosplenomegaly. The infection is thought to be a major contributing factor to the development of wasting syndrome.

Collaborative Care Management. Most people with MAC have high-grade bacteremia; consequently, a single blood culture is usually sufficient for diagnosis. Diagnosis can also be confirmed by culturing MAC from normally sterile body sites such as the liver, bone, or lymph nodes. The most common laboratory abnormality associated with MAC is anemia. A sudden fall in hematocrit or the need for repeat transfusions may be associated with disseminated MAC. An elevated alkaline phosphatase level may indicate direct liver involvement.

Disseminated MAC is associated with significant morbidity and mortality; therefore preventing it is a significant part of therapy for patients at risk. The preferred prophylactic agents for HIV-infected adults with CD4 cell counts of less than 50 cells/mm^3 are clarithromycin or azithromycin, which are similar drugs. Use of drugs to prevent MAC, such as azithromycin or clarithromycin combined with ethambutol, clofazimine, or rifabutin, is particularly advantageous because they also confer protection against other respiratory bacterial infections.[20]

Combining drugs may prevent drug resistance but is also associated with increased incidence of drug side effects. Table 22-10 lists medications used to treat MAC. Persons who have been diagnosed with MAC infection continued to receive full therapeutic doses of antimycobacterial agents for life.[20] See Patient/Family Teaching box.

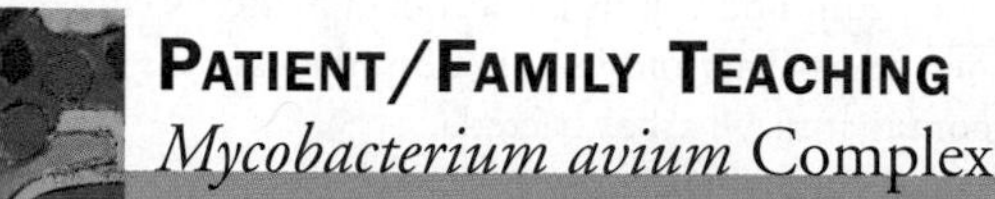

PATIENT/FAMILY TEACHING
Mycobacterium avium Complex

Teaching for the patient with *Mycobacterium avium* complex (MAC) is similar to teaching for HIV disease in general:

- No special diet is required; however, weight loss is a common problem. Oral, enteral, or parenteral supplementation may be necessary if weight loss is excessive or does not return toward preillness weight.
- There are no specific activities or activity restrictions. Fatigue is usually present and may be a limiting factor in activity levels. Maintain activities without becoming overly fatigued.
- Supplemental oxygen may be necessary to prevent hypoxia if breathing difficulties are encountered. Use oxygen as directed.
- Maintain drug and treatment schedules as prescribed. Monitor for and report drug side effects.
- A respiratory care consultation may be necessary if respiratory difficulties cannot be adequately managed.

Mycobacterium tuberculosis

Mycobacterium tuberculosis is affecting increasing numbers of immunodeficient or immunosuppressed individuals. HIV is thought to be one of the most important factors responsible for the increased incidence of *M. tuberculosis* in the United States. U.S. Public Health Service guidelines recommend that all HIV-positive persons be skin tested annually for tuberculosis, and those with positive results placed on prophylactic isoniazid daily (or twice weekly) for 9 months, or either rifampin or pyrazinamide therapy for 2 months.[15] This respiratory disease represents a complex community health illness and is discussed in detail in Chapter 26.

All HIV-infected persons who have a positive tuberculin skin test (more than 5 mm induration) should be suspected of having active tuberculosis and should undergo diagnostic evaluation. HIV-infected persons who are symptomatic should undergo diagnosis even if their tuberculin skin test is negative.[20] Definitive diagnosis of tuberculosis is made when acid-fast *M. tuberculosis* bacilli are identified in sputum or tissue samples.

Five primary drugs are used to treat tuberculosis: isoniazid, rifampin, pyrazinamide, streptomycin, and ethambutol. HIV-infected persons with active tuberculosis are placed on a multidrug treatment regimen and kept on respiratory isolation while chemotherapy is initiated until sputum specimens are free of the bacillus. Chronic suppressive therapy for the HIV-infected person who has completed chemotherapy for active tuberculosis is not necessary or recommended. HIV-infected persons who are in close contact with people who have active, infectious tuberculosis are started on prophylactic therapy regardless of their tuberculin skin test result, age, or prior courses of chemotherapy after active

TABLE 22-9 PROPHYLACTIC TREATMENT FOR SELECTED OPPORTUNISTIC INFECTIONS

Infection	Prophylactic Interventions	Comments
Pneumococcal pneumonia	Administer pneumococcal vaccine.	Provide as soon as possible during course of infection; antibody response is optimal when CD4 cells are >350/mm^3.
Hepatitis B virus (HBV)	Administer hepatitis B vaccine series; screen and vaccinate those who show no evidence of previous HBV infection.	Provide as soon as possible during course of infection; encourage vaccine in injecting drug users, sexually active gay men, and sex partners or household contacts of HBV-infected individuals.
Herpes simplex virus (HSV) types 1 and 2	Low-dose acyclovir therapy may be initiated if prompt treatment of outbreaks is not sufficient for control.	Provide ongoing assessment and intervention.
Pulmonary tuberculosis	Treat if PPD is >5 mm reactive or if patient is anergic or at risk; administer isoniazid (INH) for 12 mo; consider directly observed therapy (clinical disease requires treatment with 4 or more drugs).	Rule out active or extrapulmonary disease, which requires multidrug therapy; remember that a negative PPD in presence of HIV does not exclude diagnosis of tuberculosis; provide ongoing assessment and intervention.
Pneumocystis carinii pneumonia (PCP)	Give trimethoprim-sulfamethoxazole (TMP-SMX) (drug of choice) or dapsone or pentamidine by inhalation.	Initiate when CD4 cells go below 200/mm^3; offer TMP-SMX to any patient with a history of PCP, regardless of CD4 cell count; oral drugs that provide systemic effect are preferred.
Mycobacterium avium complex (MAC)	Treat with rifabutin.	Initiate when CD4 cells go below 100/mm^3; rifabutin has caused dose-related uveitis (above 600 mg/day), which is reversible with drug withdrawal or dose reduction.
Toxoplasmosis	Treat with TMP-SMX or dapsone with pyrimethamine and folinic acid.	Initiate when CD4 cells go below 100/mm^3.

Adapted from US Public Health Service, Infectious Disease Society of America: Guidelines for the prevention of opportunistic infections in persons infected with human immunodeficiency virus, *MMWR* 51(RR08):1–46, 2002.
PPD, Purified protein derivative.

tuberculosis has been ruled out.[20] Chapter 26 discusses nursing implications for the patient with tuberculosis.

▶ ARE You READY?

In the patient with AIDS, which of the following laboratory values is related to *Mycobacterium avium* complex?

1. Elevated white blood cell count
2. Elevated erythrocyte sedimentation rate
3. Decreased serum albumin
4. Decreased hematocrit

Fungal Infections

Fungal infections are a common problem among people with AIDS. The three most commonly encountered fungal diseases are candidiasis, cryptococcosis, and histoplasmosis.

Candidiasis

Etiology and Epidemiology. Thrush (candidiasis), caused by *Candida albicans,* may be one of the earliest signs of HIV infection and is often the first opportunistic infection. It is normally found in the mouth, GI tract (throat, esophagus, stomach, or bowel), vagina, and skin. Not usually pathogenic in immunocompetent individuals, *C. albicans* can become pathogenic when the immune system is altered by disease, diabetes, cancer, or immunosuppressant drugs. In people with AIDS, mucocutaneous *Candida* infections of the mouth are most common, followed by infections of the esophagus, skin, rectum, and vagina. Although annoying, oral or vaginal candidiasis presents no significant risk of mortality. Disseminated infections, however, are associated with significant morbidity and mortality. There are no known measures to reduce exposure to this fungus.

Pathophysiology. *C. albicans* infection is characterized by the formation of white, curdlike patches; erythema; and ulcers on mucous membranes. The patches are painful and often bleed when disturbed or removed. Oral lesions occur as thrush. Esophageal lesions produce irritation and dysphagia. Vaginal infections are associated with itching, irritation, and discharge (often described as thick and cheesy). Rectal lesions also produce itching and irritation. Disseminated infections are characterized by high fever, chills, and hypotension.

Candida infections are generally diagnosed by their characteristic appearance of glistening white patches on the tongue or oral mucosal surfaces or creamy white vaginal discharge. Scrapings of the lesions and examination under a microscope allow identification of the

TABLE 22-10 COMMON MEDICATIONS *for Mycobacterium avium Complex*

Drug	Action	Nursing Intervention
Rifampin (Rifadin)	Bacteriostatic and bactericidal Inhibits DNA-dependent polymerase activity, thereby decreasing replication	Monitor for rash, hepatotoxicity, neutropenia. Assess skin integrity. Monitor liver function studies, CBC. Institute neutropenic precautions if necessary. Drug may turn urine orange.
Clarithromycin (Biaxin) Azithromycin (Zithromax)	Inhibit protein synthesis by binding to 50S ribosomal subunit of susceptible bacteria	Monitor for nausea, abdominal pain, diarrhea, hepatotoxicity. Assess nutritional status. Monitor intake and output. Monitor liver function studies.
Amikacin (Amikin)	Bactericidal Inhibits protein synthesis in susceptible organisms	Monitor for ototoxicity, nephrotoxicity. Obtain peak and trough as ordered. Monitor renal studies.
Streptomycin	Bactericidal Interferes with bacterial protein synthesis	Same as amikacin
Ciprofloxacin (Cipro)	Bactericidal Interferes with conversion of intermediate DNA into high-molecular DNA	Monitor for nausea, abdominal pain, diarrhea, rash. Monitor nutritional status. Assess hydration status. Assess skin integrity.
Ethambutol (Myambutol)	Inhibits RNA synthesis, decreasing organism replication	Monitor for nausea, abdominal pain, changes in visual acuity. Monitor nutritional status. Assess visual acuity and monitor for changes.
Clofazimine (Lamprene)	Binds to mycobacterial DNA, inhibiting growth of organism	Monitor for nausea, abdominal pain. Assess and monitor nutritional status. Educate patient that drug may cause hyperpigmentation.

DNA, Deoxyribonucleic acid; *CBC*, complete blood count; *RNA*, ribonucleic acid.

yeast organism. *Candida* infections can progress to other mucocutaneous sites as well. Oral infections, when left untreated, can progress into the esophagus and stomach. Diagnostic scraping of these lesions may then require an endoscopic procedure to obtain the sample and assess the extent of infection.

Collaborative Care Management. The current recommended treatment and maintenance therapy for mouth and esophageal candidiasis is oral fluconazole or ketoconazole. However, fluconazole-resistant strains of *C. albicans* are emerging. Alternative treatments include itraconazole, clotrimazole, and nystatin. Vaginal yeast infections may be treated with nystatin cream, ointments, or suppositories. For persistent or systemic infections, amphotericin B may be required.[20] Table 22-11 presents an overview of these medications.

Although candidiasis is a common complication of HIV infection, primary prophylactic drug therapy is not recommended because the mortality rate is low and therapy for acute infections is highly effective. Persons with repeated episodes of esophageal candidiasis, however, are considered candidates for chronic suppression therapy with fluconazole.[20] See Patient/Family Teaching box.

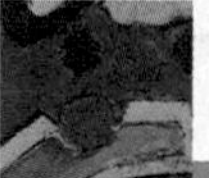

PATIENT/FAMILY TEACHING *Candida albicans*

Teaching for the patient with *Candida albicans* infection (candidiasis) includes:

- No specific diet is required, and there are no dietary restrictions. Any foods that can be tolerated are allowable.
- Oral *Candida* lesions make it difficult to tolerate temperature extremes and spicy foods. Soft foods may be better tolerated.
- A soft-bristled toothbrush for oral hygiene will decrease the risk of pain and bleeding. A referral to a dietitian may be necessary if nutrition maintenance is difficult because of pain from oral lesions.
- If the patient is receiving amphotericin therapy for disseminated disease, fatigue may occur, which greatly reduces activity tolerance. Seek assistance as needed and establish an activity regimen that can be tolerated.
- A gynecologic referral (for females) will be needed if vaginal yeast infections recur.

Cryptococcosis

Etiology and Epidemiology. *Cryptococcus neoformans* is a yeastlike fungus that is ubiquitous worldwide. The organism is found in pigeon droppings and can be contracted from nesting places, soil, fruit, and fruit juices. *C. neoformans* can remain viable for up to 2 years even in desiccated pigeon feces. Neither person-to-person nor animal-to-person transmission has been documented. The disease is naturally acquired from the environment, where the organism is aerosolized and inhaled. In patients with pro-

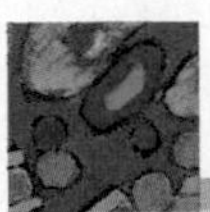

TABLE 22-11 COMMON MEDICATIONS *for Candida Infections*

Drug	Action	Nursing Intervention
Fluconazole (Diflucan)	Fungistatic, fungicidal Inhibits ergosterol biosynthesis, damaging fungal cell wall	Monitor for headache, nausea, vomiting, hepatotoxicity, gynecomastia. Monitor liver function studies, CBC. Monitor nutritional status.
Ketoconazole (Nizoral)	Fungistatic, fungicidal Inhibits fungal enzymes Alters cell membrane Prevents fungal metabolism	Same as fluconazole
Clotrimazole (Mycelex)	Fungistatic, fungicidal Changes integrity of cell membrane, allowing leakage of cell nutrients and halting fungal replication	Monitor for nausea and vomiting. Monitor for liver function studies. Monitor nutritional status.
Nystatin (Mycostatin)	Same as clotrimazole	Monitor for nausea, vomiting, epigastric pain, diarrhea. Assess nutritional status. Educate patient about swish-and-swallow procedure.
Amphotericin B (Fungizone)	Fungistatic Increases cell membrane permeability, thus inhibiting replication Decreases potassium, sodium, and nutrients in fungal cell	Monitor for fever with shaking chills, headache, anorexia, malaise, generalized pain. Treat symptoms of discomfort during therapy.

CBC, Complete blood count.

longed, severe immunodeficiency caused by HIV, the immune system may not be competent against *C. neoformans,* and cryptococcosis can develop. Cryptococcal infection usually manifests as meningitis in AIDS patients.

Pathophysiology. *C. neoformans* primarily affects the central nervous system and lungs, but it can also affect the skin, mouth, bones, liver, and kidneys. Pulmonary cryptococcal infection is generally asymptomatic, although it can cause dyspnea, cough, and chest discomfort. Central nervous system findings include low-grade fever, headache, blurred vision, dizziness, memory changes, irritability, nausea or vomiting, lassitude, fatigue, and convulsions. If untreated, cryptococcal infection can cause coma and death as a result of cerebral edema or hydrocephalus. Cryptococcal skin lesions are painless, red papules that may be similar in appearance to Kaposi's sarcoma (Figure 22-9).

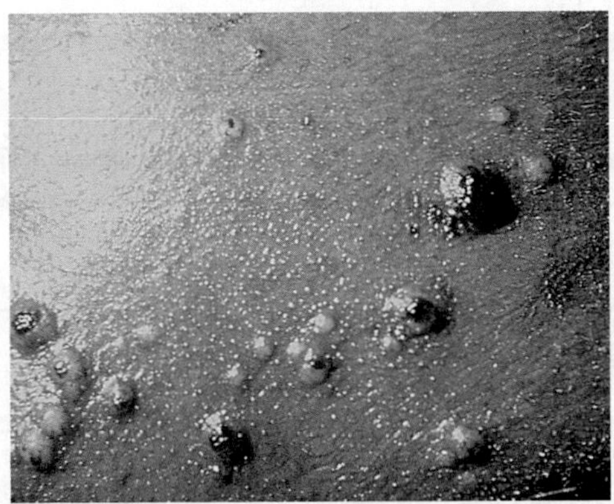

Figure 22-9 Cutaneous cryptococcosis in patient with AIDS.

Collaborative Care Management. Diagnosis of cryptococcosis is achieved by identifying the fungus in the CSF. The organism can also be detected by antigen testing in urine or serum. Cryptococcal antigen titers and cultures of blood or CSF are the most reliable diagnostic measures. Computed tomography of the head may be performed to rule out hydrocephalus and to look for focal lesions. Chest radiographs are helpful if cryptococcal pneumonia is suspected.

Central nervous system infection can be fatal if appropriate therapy is not instituted in a timely manner. The primary drug used to treat an initial cryptococcal infection is amphotericin B; however, studies have shown that fluconazole and itraconazole can also reduce the frequency of cryptococcal infections in AIDS patients. When CD4 cell counts are less than 50 cells/mm^3, prophylactic treatment with fluconazole is usually considered. Patients who have had an episode of cryptococcal infection generally receive lifelong suppressive therapy. In addition to the usual IV infusion of amphotericin B, intrathecal administration has been used in patients failing to respond to IV infusion.[20]

Flucytosine and fluconazole are also used to treat cryptococcosis. Flucytosine is an oral agent that is given in combination with amphotericin B. Fluconazole is less toxic than amphotericin and is better tolerated but may not be as effective in some patients. Table 22-12 summarizes the side effects and nursing implications of drug therapies for cryptococcosis.

As with many of the opportunistic infections associated with AIDS, the successful treatment of the initial acute infection does not cure the patient. Long-term suppressive therapy is necessary to prevent recurrence. Primary prophylaxis (instituted before the patient develops an initial infection) and long-term suppressive therapy may be accomplished with oral fluconazole.

TABLE 22-12
COMMON MEDICATIONS *for Cryptococcosis*

Drug	Action	Nursing Intervention
Flucytosine	Antiinfective Antibiotic Antifungal Converted to fluorouracil within fungal cell, inhibiting fungal cell metabolism	Monitor for anemia, jaundice, skin rash, itching, sore throat, fever, unusual bleeding or bruising, confusion, diarrhea, nausea, vomiting, headache, lightheadedness, drowsiness. Assess for signs of unusual bleeding. Monitor nutritional status.
Fluconazole (Diflucan)	Fungistatic, fungicidal Inhibits ergosterol biosynthesis, damaging fungal cell wall	Monitor for headache, nausea, vomiting, hepatotoxicity, gynecomastia. Monitor liver function studies, CBC. Monitor nutritional status.
Amphotericin B (Fungizone)	Fungistatic Increases cell membrane permeability, thus inhibiting replication Decreases potassium, sodium, and nutrients in fungal cell	Monitor for fever with shaking chills, headache, anorexia, malaise, generalized pain. Treat symptoms of discomfort during therapy.

CBC, Complete blood count.

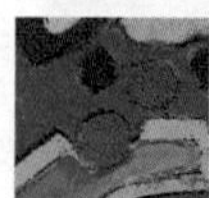

PATIENT/FAMILY TEACHING
Cryptococcal Infection

Teaching for the patient with cryptococcal infection includes:

- No special dietary considerations are required for this infection. A healthy, well-balanced diet is encouraged.
- Activity restrictions are based on the degree of fatigue. If meningitis is present, somnolence or confusion may occur, in which case activities must be limited to prevent injury.
- Avoid contact with infected animals, human or animal feces, and soil.
- Avoid sexual practices that may result in oral exposure to feces.

As with other serious opportunistic infections that occur in late-stage disease, patients with cryptococcal infections may require multiple referrals. Social services, home nursing services, physical or occupational therapy, and psychiatry or counseling may be appropriate. See Patient/Family Teaching box above.

Histoplasmosis

Histoplasma capsulatum causes the common, usually benign, fungal infection histoplasmosis, which occurs primarily in the lungs. Histoplasmosis in HIV-infected persons may manifest as acute pulmonary infection or, more often, as disseminated disease. Because chest radiographs are normal in up to 30% of individuals with disseminated histoplasmosis, bone marrow biopsy and cultures, examination and culture of pulmonary tissue and secretions, and blood cultures are the most common means of establishing a diagnosis in patients with AIDS.

Disseminated histoplasmosis is invariably fatal if not treated aggressively with antifungal therapy. Amphotericin B and fluconazole are the drugs of choice in induction therapy for acute infection. Patients who have candidiasis and histoplasmosis require lifelong suppressive treatment with itraconazole. AIDS patients with CD4+ cell counts below 100 cells/mm^3 are considered for prophylactic therapy with itraconazole; however, concerns over drug toxicities, interactions, resistance, and cost may delay prophylactic treatment.[20]

Patients receiving prophylactic therapy are taught the signs and symptoms of drug toxicity and informed about potential drug interactions. As with other serious opportunistic infections that occur in late-stage disease, patients with histoplasmosis may require multiple referrals. Dietary services, social services, home nursing services, physical or occupational therapy, and psychiatry or counseling may be appropriate. See Patient/Family Teaching box below.

Protozoal Infections

Protozoal infections are caused by a variety of organisms, many of which are parasitic. *Cryptosporidium* organisms, *P. carinii,* and *Toxoplasma gondii* are commonly encountered opportunistic protozoal infections in patients with AIDS.

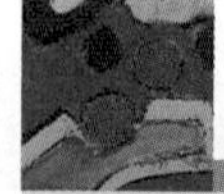

PATIENT/FAMILY TEACHING
Histoplasmosis

Teaching for the patient with histoplasmosis includes:

- No specific dietary or activity restrictions are required.
- Maintain follow-up visits to monitor CD4 counts. When counts are below 200 cells/mm^3, activities that are known to pose increased risk for infection must be avoided:
  - Creating dust when working with surface soil
  - Cleaning chicken coops that are heavily contaminated with droppings
  - Disturbing soil beneath bird-roosting sites
  - Cleaning, remodeling, or demolishing old buildings
  - Exploring caves
- Adhere to prescribed drug dosages and schedules.
- Monitor for and report drug side effects.

Cryptosporidium Organisms

Etiology and Epidemiology. *Cryptosporidium* organism is a parasite present in a variety of animal species, including birds, reptiles, fish, cattle, sheep, and humans. It is a well-recognized pathogen in both immunologically intact individuals and immunocompromised hosts, such as persons with HIV disease. In addition to animal-to-human transmission, person-to-person transmission has also been documented among persons at day care centers, household contacts, hospitalized patients, and health care workers. Waterborne transmission has also been documented. Chlorination of water does not kill *Cryptosporidium* organisms.

Pathophysiology. The most common site of *Cryptosporidium* infection is the small intestine. It is a self-limiting disease in immunocompetent individuals; however, it is extremely pathogenic in immunocompromised persons. It can affect the entire GI tract, producing fever, nausea, vomiting, abdominal pain and cramping, and severe watery diarrhea. Death from profound malabsorption, electrolyte imbalances, malnutrition, and dehydration can occur.

Collaborative Care Management. Diagnosis is made by identifying *Cryptosporidium* oocytes in fresh or formalin-preserved stool specimens. No effective anticryptosporidial therapy currently exists for either treatment or prevention. The drugs paromomycin and azithromycin may help suppress the infection in some people, but they are not always effective. Octreotide may be used to reduce the volume of stool. Otherwise therapy is aimed at controlling pain and decreasing peristalsis.[20] See Patient/Family Teaching box below.

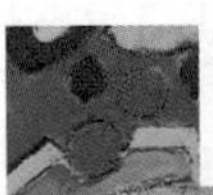

PATIENT/FAMILY TEACHING
Cryptosporidium Infection

Teaching for the patient with *Cryptosporidium* infection includes:

- Avoid contact with infected animals, contaminated drinking water, lake water, diaper-age infants and children, and human and animal feces.
- Dietary needs:
  - —Intravenous therapy for fluid replacement may be required for excessive fluid losses.
  - —Nutritional supplements or total parenteral nutrition may be required to replace fluids, calories, and nutrients lost through the massive volumes of diarrhea.
  - —Reducing bulk in the diet may reduce stool volume.
- Drug effects and side effects:
  - —Side effects of the drug octreotide can include hyperglycemia, hypoglycemia, abdominal pain, nausea, vomiting, pain at the injection site, headache, fatigue, dizziness, edema, facial flushing, and hepatic dysfunction.
  - —Self-monitoring of stool volume is needed to assess the drug's effectiveness.
- Frequent perineal care is essential due to frequent diarrhea. Use nondrying soaps, and keep the skin clean and dry. Apply protective topical creams or lotions to prevent skin cracking and excoriation.

Pneumocystis carinii

Etiology and Epidemiology. *P. carinii* pneumonia (PCP) is a common, severe opportunistic infection among AIDS patients. *P. carinii* is a ubiquitous organism with worldwide distribution. It is found in the air, on food, and in water, although most transmission appears to be via airborne routes. Most healthy children have acquired *P. carinii* infection by 4 years of age. It is not highly virulent, and infection in a normal host is usually asymptomatic. In the immunocompromised host, however, *P. carinii* can cause fulminant disease.

Pathophysiology. *P. carinii* is generally confined to the lungs, although extrapulmonary infection can occur. The infection causes increased permeability of alveolar capillary membranes, degenerative lung cell changes, and diffuse alveolar injury, resulting in impaired gas exchange and altered lung compliance. Without treatment, the infection leads to respiratory insufficiency and death. Clinical manifestations include dyspnea, nonproductive cough, intermittent fever, fatigue, anorexia, weight loss, and tachypnea. Persons with advanced disease may exhibit crackles, decreased breath sounds, and cyanosis.

Collaborative Care Management. Bronchoalveolar and transbronchial biopsies are usually performed to identify *P. carinii* in patients with pneumonia. Chest radiography may reveal pneumonia, although 5% to 10% of chest radiographs in AIDS patients with PCP appear normal. Pulmonary function studies usually reveal decreased vital capacity, decreased total lung capacity, and decreased single-breath diffusing capacity of carbon monoxide. Arterial blood gas studies may reveal hypoxemia, hypocarbia, and an increase in the alveolar-arterial oxygen gradient, particularly with exercise.

Presumptive diagnosis of PCP is often made based on CDC guidelines: (1) history of dyspnea on exertion or nonproductive cough of recent onset; (2) chest radiographic evidence of diffuse bilateral interstitial infiltrates or gallium scan evidence of diffuse bilateral pulmonary disease; (3) arterial blood gas analysis showing an arterial oxygen tension of less than 70 mm Hg, a low respiratory diffusing capacity, or an increase in the alveolar-arterial oxygen tension gradient; and (4) no evidence of bacterial pneumonia.[20]

The most effective treatments for PCP are IV pentamidine isethionate or either IV or oral trimethoprim-sulfamethoxazole (TMP-SMX, Co-trimoxazole). TMP-SMX is the preferred therapy because it is better tolerated. However, many patients are sensitive to sulfa drugs such as TMP-SMX, which may limit the medication options. Other therapies that may be used include aerosolized pentamidine, trimetrexate, clindamycin, primaquine, or atovaquone. Table 22-13 summarizes information about pentamidine and TMP-SMX.

Significant progress has been made in controlling PCP. Prophylactic therapy is recommended for patients who have not yet developed PCP but have CD4 cell counts below 200 cells/mm^3, exhibit unexplained fever for 2 weeks or longer, or have a history of oropharyngeal candidiasis. TMP-SMZ is the recommended prophylactic agent. One double-strength tablet per day is preferred if it can be tolerated, otherwise one single-strength tablet is administered. If the patient cannot tolerate TMP-SMX, dapsone, dapsone

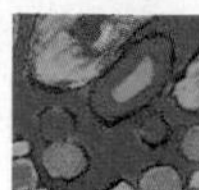

TABLE 22-13
COMMON MEDICATIONS *for Pneumocystis carinii Pneumonia*

Drug	Action	Nursing Intervention
Pentamidine isethionate (Pentam 300)	Interferes with protozoan DNA and RNA synthesis, thus interfering with parasite reproduction	
Intravenous		Monitor for blood dyscrasias; rapid, irregular pulse; hyperglycemia; hypoglycemia; diabetes mellitus; skin rash; hypotension; pain at injection site. Monitor blood and renal studies. Rotate injection sites.
Inhalation		Implement respirator therapy precautions. Administer bronchodilators as indicated. Monitor for chest pain, congestion, cough, dyspnea, pharyngitis, wheezing, skin rash, metallic taste, pneumothorax.
Sulfamethoxazole and trimethoprim (Co-trimoxazole, Bactrim, Septra)	Trimethoprim: antiinfective and folic acid antagonist; interferes with bacterial cell growth Sulfamethoxazole: bacteriostatic sulfonamide; halts multiplication of bacteria	Monitor for hemolytic, megaloblastic, or aplastic anemia; agranulocytosis; skin rash; Stevens-Johnson syndrome; dysphagia; nausea; vomiting; stomatitis; headache; convulsions. Do not give to patients with hypersensitivity to sulfa agents. Give oral preparation with full glass of water. Monitor intake and output.

DNA, Deoxyribonucleic acid; *RNA,* ribonucleic acid.

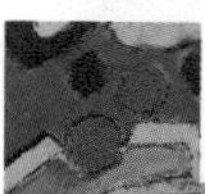

PATIENT/FAMILY TEACHING
Pneumocystis Pneumonia

Teaching for the patient with *Pneumocystis carinii* pneumonia includes:

- Maintain prescribed medication dosages and schedules.
- Monitor for and report signs of adverse drug effects to the health care provider. Severe adverse effects may include fever, nausea and vomiting, and liver tenderness or pain.
- Follow recommended procedures for use of inhaled drugs so that drugs reach the lung bases.
- Supplemental oxygen can be used as needed when dyspnea is severe. Mechanical ventilation may be required if respiratory failure develops.
- There are no special diet or activity recommendations. Eat a well-balanced, nutritional diet with adequate fluid intake.
- Activity depends on the degree of illness. Dyspnea often results in fatigue; therefore activities should be alternated with rest periods.

plus pyrimethamine plus leucovorin, aerosolized pentamidine, or atovaquone are alternative drugs. An advantage of dapsone is that it also protects against toxoplasmosis. Secondary prophylaxis is often recommended after the first episode of PCP.[20] The use of prophylactic therapy has significantly reduced the number of PCP recurrences, ultimately reducing the mortality rate. See Patient/Family Teaching box above.

Toxoplasma gondii

Etiology and Epidemiology. *T. gondii* is a protozoan that occurs worldwide and infects both humans and domestic animals. The definitive hosts are members of the cat family, although not all cats are infected, and toxoplasmosis has been documented in locales without cats. Transmission of *T. gondii* in humans is primarily through ingestion of meats and vegetables containing oocysts. The prevalence of *Toxoplasma* tissue cysts in meat consumed by humans may be as high as 25%. Cockroaches, earthworms, snails, and slugs may serve as transport hosts for the oocysts. It is estimated that as many as 67% of adults in the United States are seropositive for toxoplasma, with the incidence increasing with age.[19] Human-to-human transmission is from mother to fetus, by blood transfusion, or by organ transplantation.

Pathophysiology. *Toxoplasma* infection does not generally cause significant illness in healthy hosts. It is, however, a major cause of encephalitis in persons with AIDS. Toxoplasmosis produces localized and disseminated infections. Localized infections may be mild with symptoms similar to those of mononucleosis. Disseminated infections are serious and include manifestations such as headache, confusion or delirium, fever, encephalitis, vomiting, hemiparesis, seizures, and loss of vision.

Collaborative Care Management. Persons newly diagnosed with HIV infection are tested for *Toxoplasma* antibodies to detect latent toxoplasmosis infection.[20] Because *T. gondii* causes encephalitis, definitive diagnosis generally requires brain biopsy. Presumptive diagnosis is most often accomplished by (1) brain-imaging evidence of a lesion with a mass effect, (2) recent onset of focal neurologic abnormality, (3) serum antibody to toxoplasmosis, or (4) successful response to therapy for toxoplasmosis.

HIV-infected persons who are seropositive for toxoplasmosis and who have CD4 cell counts below 100/mm^3 are started on

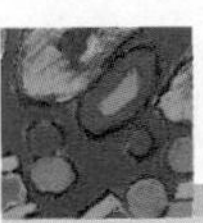

TABLE 22-14
COMMON MEDICATIONS *for Toxoplasmosis*

Drug	Action	Nursing Intervention
Sulfadiazine (PO)	Bacteriostatic sulfonamide Halts multiplication of bacteria but does not fully kill mature microorganism	Maintain fluid intake of 1500 ml/day. Educate patient about importance of maintaining drug dosage and schedules. Monitor for fever, blood dyscrasias. Monitor liver and renal studies.
Pyrimethamine (PO)	Inhibits folic acid metabolism in organism Stops growth of fertilized gametes to inhibit parasitic transmission	Do not give if hypersensitivity exists. Monitor for CNS stimulation, convulsions, tremors, fatigue, nausea, vomiting, anorexia, diarrhea, gastritis, thrombocytopenia, leukopenia, megaloblastic anemia, agranulocytosis. Monitor liver and renal studies.
Clindamycin (Cleocin) (PO, IM, IV)	Antibacterial agent that suppresses protein synthesis Binds to 50S subunit of bacterial ribosomes	Monitor for rash, urticaria, nausea, vomiting, diarrhea, pseudomembranous colitis, vaginitis, leukopenia, eosinophilia, agranulocytosis. Monitor liver studies. Do not give if hypersensitivity exists. Competes with chloramphenicol and erythromycin.

PO, By mouth; *CNS,* central nervous system; *IM,* intramuscular; *IV,* intravenous.

prophylactic drug therapy with TMP-SMX. Dapsone with pyrimethamine is alternate therapy for patients who are unable to tolerate TMP-SMX. HIV-infected persons who have been diagnosed with toxoplasmosis receive suppressive drug therapy for the remainder of their lives.

The primary therapy for toxoplasmosis in persons with AIDS is a combination of sulfadiazine and pyrimethamine (Table 22-14). Adjunctive therapy includes dexamethasone (Decadron) for cerebral inflammation associated with abscesses, and phenytoin (Dilantin) for infection-induced seizures. Approximately 40% to 60% of patients may have severe adverse reactions during the initial treatment phase, and alternative regimens, including cessation of sulfadiazine or addition of clindamycin, may be required.[20] See Patient/Family Teaching box.

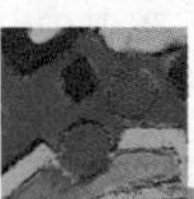

PATIENT/FAMILY TEACHING
Toxoplasmosis

Teaching for the patient with toxoplasmosis includes:

- Avoid sources of infection by:
  —Washing hands after handling raw meat
  —Avoiding the ingestion of raw or undercooked meat
  —Avoiding contact with soil
  —Washing raw fruits and vegetables before eating them
  —Avoiding changing cat litter, or thoroughly washing hands afterward
- There are no specific dietary or activity restrictions.
- Safety precautions are required if mental status changes or seizures occur.
- Maintain follow-up monitoring to detect side effects of drug therapy, since blood dyscrasias are possible.

Viral Infections

CMV and herpes simplex virus (HSV) types 1 and 2, which are widespread in the general population, are viruses that can significantly affect AIDS patients.

Etiology and Epidemiology. CMV infection is caused by cytomegalovirus, a virus belonging to the herpesvirus family. Seroprevalence of CMV ranges from 30% to 100% in the United States. It is found in breast milk, saliva, cervical secretions, semen, feces, urine, and blood.[20]

Herpes simplex virus is caused by *Herpesvirus hominis.* HSV type 1 is transmitted via oral and respiratory secretions. HSV type 2 is transmitted by sexual contact. Both CMV and HSV remain dormant in tissues after initial infection and are reactivated in the presence of HIV and immunodeficiency.

Pathophysiology. CMV is thought to spread throughout the body via lymphocytes or mononuclear cells. The infection is usually asymptomatic in the immunocompetent host but can exist as a latent or chronic infection. In the immunocompromised host, CMV is pathogenic and produces symptoms. Disseminated infection can produce inflammatory reactions in the lungs, GI tract, liver, central nervous system, and eyes, leading to chorioretinitis, pneumonitis, encephalitis, adrenalitis, colitis, esophagitis, cholangitis, and hepatitis. CMV is a significant cause of blindness in persons with HIV disease.

HSV type 1 affects the skin and mucous membranes, producing painful vesicular lesions. HSV type 2 produces similar lesions but in the genital or perianal regions. Disseminated herpes infections affect the brain, liver, and lungs, producing blindness, seizures, deafness, and death.

Collaborative Care Management. CMV and HSV types 1 and 2 are diagnosed by identification of antibodies in the serum. The drugs approved for treatment of CMV retinitis are oral and

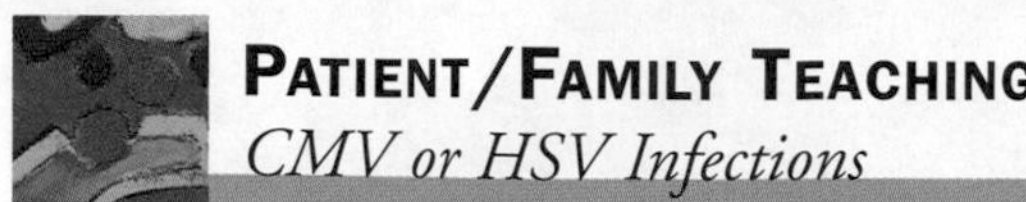

PATIENT/FAMILY TEACHING
CMV or HSV Infections

Teaching for the patient with cytomegalovirus (CMV) or herpes simplex virus (HSV) infections includes:

- Avoid sources of infection:
  —CMV is shed in saliva, semen, and cervical secretions.
  —HSV is spread by oral and sexual contact.
  —Use latex condoms during sexual contact to reduce the risk of viral transmission.
  —Use of excellent hygienic practices, such as hand washing, can significantly reduce the risk of infection.
- There are no specific dietary or activity restrictions for CMV or HSV.
- Follow-up care must be maintained to determine effectiveness and drug toxicity of prescribed antiviral medications.
- Home screening tools are used to identify early CMV-related visual changes.
- Regular professional eye screening is encouraged, since CMV retinitis can rapidly progress toward blindness.

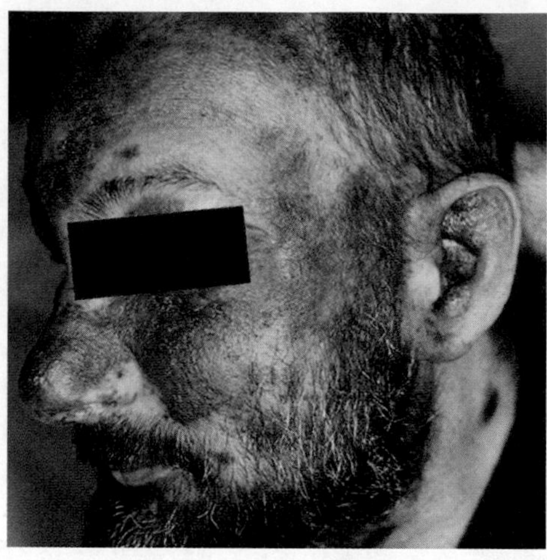

Figure 22-10 Kaposi's sarcoma in patient with AIDS.

IV ganciclovir, IV foscarnet, IV cidofovir, and an intravitreal ganciclovir implant. The implant provides the longest period of localized retinitis suppression but does not prevent systemic infection.[16] Parenteral or oral ganciclovir, parenteral foscarnet, and parenteral cidofovir are the drugs of choice for treatment of systemic CMV infections. Prophylaxis with oral ganciclovir may be considered for HIV-infected adults with CD4 cell counts below 50 cells/mm^3. It is not always recommended, however, because of cost, limited effectiveness, and side effects. Chronic suppressive therapy or maintenance therapy is recommended for persons with recurrent disease.[20]

HSV is treated effectively with acyclovir. Prophylaxis is not generally recommended because acyclovir is an effective treatment for acute episodes. Persons who tend to have chronic herpes lesions are candidates for daily suppressive therapy with acyclovir. IV foscarnet and cidofovir are alternative drugs that can be used when acyclovir is not effective.[20] See Patient/Family Teaching box above.

HIV-Related Cancer

Etiology and Epidemiology. Kaposi's sarcoma is by far the most common neoplasm found in AIDS patients. It is a rare cancer that most commonly occurs in older non-HIV-infected persons. It is most commonly associated with AIDS but may affect any person who is immunosuppressed or immunodeficient. The incidence of unexplained cases of Kaposi's sarcoma was one of the initial manifestations that led to the identification of HIV infection in this country.

Pathophysiology. The exact cause of Kaposi's sarcoma is unknown. The lesions may appear on the skin, mucous membranes, mouth, tongue, tonsils, sclera, or conjunctiva and may also affect the internal organs. Lesions extend from the mid dermis upward into the epidermis and appear as dark blue, purple, or red papules (Figure 22-10). They may ulcerate and are associated with pain and itching. Systemic manifestations include lymphatic obstruction with resulting edema, dyspnea or respiratory distress when the lungs are affected, and digestive problems when the GI tract is involved.

Collaborative Care Management. Kaposi's sarcoma is diagnosed by skin biopsy, but high suspicion exists when persons with lesions are immunocompromised. Local lesions can be surgically removed, but systemic lesions are treated with radiation or chemotherapy. Doxorubicin, vinblastine, vincristine, and etoposide are agents of choice for treatment of Kaposi's sarcoma.[20] Kaposi's sarcoma is not a major cause of death in persons with AIDS; however, systemic disease can result in the need for medical or surgical intervention (see Patient/Family Teaching box below).

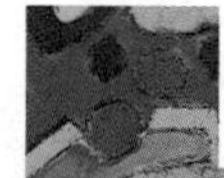

PATIENT/FAMILY TEACHING
Kaposi's Sarcoma

Teaching for the patient with Kaposi's sarcoma includes:

- Keep any draining lesions covered, avoid scratching or picking at lesions, and keep them clean and dry. Implement skin care protocols for ulcerated areas.
- If drug therapy is elected, follow-up appointments need to be maintained to determine drug effectiveness and side effects. Report symptoms of drug side effects to the health care provider.
- Verbalize feelings about the changes in appearance produced by Kaposi's sarcoma so that strategies can be identified to lessen the appearance of obvious lesions.

Preparing for Practice

CD-ROM Activity Select Exercise Two: HIV Infection and AIDS on the Companion CD.

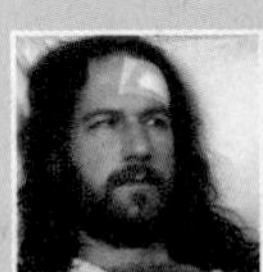

Patient: *Ira Bradley,* **Room 309**

Ira Bradley, a 43-year-old Caucasian male, is diagnosed with AIDS, dehydration, *Pneumocystis carinii* pneumonia, candidiasis, and Kaposi's sarcoma.

Assessment

View the patient's **Report.**

Review the patient's **Medical Record.** Focus on the following records: Physician's Orders—review the initial admission order for Ira Bradley; History & Physical—read the entire report, including the Emergency Department Report.

Conduct a **Patient Interview.** As you conduct your interview, focus primarily on data that will be helpful in planning care for this patient. Record the data you collect.

Nursing Diagnoses, Outcomes, and Interventions

1. How does the textbook discriminate between HIV infection and AIDS?
2. What are the three major modes of transmission for the HIV virus that are identified in the textbook? *Hint*: Refer to p. 480 if needed.
3. According to the information found in the **Medical Record,** what is the route of transmission by which Ira Bradley contracted the HIV virus? To what degree does his gender and race fit the demographics for HIV as described in the Epidemiology section in your textbook?
4. How many years ago did Ira Bradley contract the HIV virus?
5. What four conditions does Ira Bradley have that are listed in Box 22-1 that clearly indicate that he has AIDS rather than positive HIV status?
6. What laboratory tests are used to diagnose HIV infection? In which order are they done? Once it is known that a person is infected with HIV, what laboratory tests will help track the status of the patient's immune system?
7. You are the nurse caring for Ira during this admission. Formulate a plan of care to support Ira in coping effectively with the diagnosis of AIDS.

Critical Thinking

1. A woman engaged in unprotected sex 2 weeks ago. Concerned, she decided to have her blood drawn to determine her HIV status. Four days later she learns that her ELISA is negative. What conclusions can be drawn about her ELISA findings at this time? What information should be provided to the woman? What follow-up care, if any, is necessary?
2. A patient who is HIV infected has a CD4 T cell count of 250 cells/mm^3. She asks for advice about initiating antiretroviral therapy. How should you answer her question?

References

1. Branson BM: *Point-of-care rapid tests for HIV antibody*, Centers for Disease Control and Prevention Division of HIV/AIDS Prevention, accessed March 2004 from website: http://www.cdc.gov/hiv/rapid_testing/materials/J_Lab_Med_20031.htm.
2. Centers for Disease Control and Prevention (CDC): Recommendations to help patients avoid exposure to or infection from opportunistic pathogens, *MMWR* 51(RR08):47-52, 2002.
3. CDC: *HIV and its transmission*, accessed Sept 2003 from website: http://www.cdc.gov/hiv/pubs/facts/transmission.htm.
4. CDC Division of HIV/AIDS Prevention: Advancing HIV prevention: new strategies for a changing epidemic, accessed Sept 2003 from website http://www.cdc.gov/hiv/partners/AHP-brochure.htm.
5. CDC Division of HIV/AIDS Prevention: AHP initiative quick facts, accessed Jan 2004 from website: http://www.cdc.gov/hiv/partners/QuickFacts.htm.
6. CDC Division of HIV/AIDS Prevention: *Basic statistics*, accessed July 2004 from website: http://www.cdc.gov/hiv/stats.htm.
7. CDC National Center for HIV, STD and TB prevention: *HIV/AIDS update: a glance at the HIV epidemic*, accessed April 2004 from website: http://www.cdc.gov/nchstp/od/news/At-a-Glance.htm.
8. Cohen J, Powderly G, editors: *Infectious diseases*, ed 2, St Louis, 2004, Mosby.
9. Donagan E: Transmission of HIV by blood, blood products, tissue transplantation, and artificial insemination, *HIV InSite*, accessed Oct 2003 from website: http://hivinsite.ucsf.edu/InSite?page=kb-07-02-09#S2X.
10. Gupta V, Gupta S: Laboratory markers associated with progression of HIV infection, *Indian J Med Microbiol* 22(1), accessed Jan 2004 from website: http://www.ijmm.org/issues/jan04/reviewarticle1.htm.
11. Health Resources and Services Administration: *Clinical management of the HIV-infected adult*, Washington, DC, 2003, US Department of Health and Human Services.
12. Joint United Nations Programme on HIV/AIDS: *2004 Report on the global AIDS epidemic*, accessed June 2004 from website: http://www.unaids.org/bangkok2004/GAR2004_pdf/GAR2004_Execsumm_en.pdf.

12a. Joy JE, Watson SJ, Benson JA: *Marijuana and medicine: assessing the science*, Institute of Medicine, Washington, DC, 1999, National Academy Press.

13. Mylonakis E, Paliou M, Rich JD: Plasma viral load testing in the management of HIV infection, *Am Fam Phys*, accessed Feb 2001 from website: http://www.aafp.org/afp/20010201/483.html.
14. National Association on HIV Over Fifty: *HIV and older adults*, accessed March 2004 from website: http://www.hivoverfifty.org/tip.html.
15. National Center for HIV, STD and TB Prevention: Incorporating HIV prevention into the medical care of persons living with HIV, *MMWR* 52(RR12):1-24, 2003.
16. National Institutes of Health: *CMV retinitis*, US National Library of Medicine, accessed Feb 2004 from website: http://www.nlm.nih.gov/medlineplus/print/ency/article/000665.htm.
17. Panel on Clinical Practices for Treatment of HIV Infection: *Guidelines for the use of antiretroviral agents in HIV-1-infected adults and adolescents*, Washington, DC, US Department of Health and Human Services, accessed March 2004 from website: http://aidsinfo.nih.gov/guidelines/adult/AA_032304.pdf.
18. Shaw JK, Mahoney EA: *HIV/AIDS nursing secrets*, Philadelphia, 2003, Hanley & Belfus.
19. Subauste CS: Toxoplasmosis and HIV, *HIV InSite*, accessed Jan 2004 from website: http://hivinsite.org/InSite?page=kb-05-04-03.
20. US Department of Health and Human Services: *Guidelines for the prevention of opportunistic infections in persons infected with human immunodeficiency virus*, accessed Nov 2001 from website: http://aidsinfo.nih.gov/guidelines/op_infections/OI_112801.pdf.
21. US Department of Health and Human Services, US Public Health Service: *Healthy people 2010,* Washington, DC, 2001, The Department.

Visit the Evolve website: http://evolve.elsevier.com/Monahan/medsurg

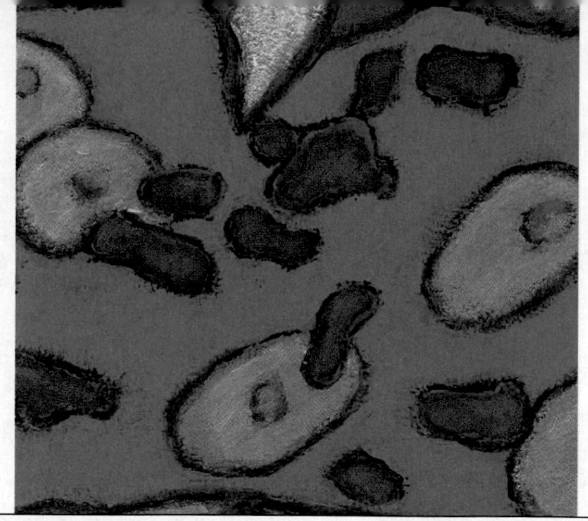

CHAPTER 23
Cancer

by Jeanne M. Erickson, Rosemary B. Field

OBJECTIVES

After studying this chapter, the learner should be able to:

1. Describe epidemiologic trends in the incidence of cancer.
2. Identify factors related to carcinogenesis.
3. Describe the pathophysiology of cancer, including the characteristics of malignant cells, growth of neoplasms, and nature of metastases.
4. Relate the pathophysiologic changes of cancer to common clinical manifestations.
5. Identify the nurse's role in the prevention and early detection of cancer.
6. Apply the nursing process to the care of patients in the diagnostic and treatment phases of cancer.
7. Explain the rationale for the major types of cancer therapy.
8. Discuss the nursing care for patients undergoing surgery, radiotherapy, chemotherapy, or biotherapy for treatment of cancer.

KEY TERMS

alopecia, p. 540
anaplasia, p. 519
angiogenesis, p. 519
biotherapy, p. 527
brachytherapy, p. 537
carcinogens, p. 513
carcinogenesis, p. 513
cell-kill hypothesis, p. 544
cytokines, p. 527
dysplasia, p. 519
gene therapy, p. 529
grading, p. 521
growth factors, p. 527
interferons, p. 527
interleukins, p. 527
ionizing radiation, p. 516
metastasis, p. 519
monoclonal antibodies, p. 528
oncogenes, p. 513
radiosensitivity, p. 535
staging, p. 521
venous access device, p. 549

Cancer was recognized in ancient times by skilled observers who gave it the name *cancer* (L. *cancri*, crab) because it stretched out in many directions like the legs of a crab. The term *cancer* is an "umbrella" word used to describe a group of more than 100 diseases in which cells multiply and spread without restraint, interrupting normal body physiology and causing life-threatening complications. Although mainly a disease associated with aging, cancer is diagnosed in people of all ages.

Few diseases cause greater anxiety and apprehension than cancer. Its physiologic and psychologic impact on patients and their families causes profound changes in their lives. Cancer treatments may last a lifetime and too often do not result in the cure for which patients hope. Myths still surround malignant disease, often focusing on its incurability, and may foster feelings of hopelessness and dread. Yet much progress has been made in the prevention, early detection, and treatment of cancer, improving survival rates and quality of life for those undergoing treatment. Today, more than 10 million Americans can be classified as cancer survivors.

Cancer nursing has been recognized as a subspecialty in the nursing profession since 1975. The Oncology Nursing Society (ONS) has more than 30,000 members and is the largest organization of oncology professionals in the world. Oncology nurses care for patients of all ages in a variety of settings, from acute care hospitals to ambulatory care clinics, home care agencies, and hospices. Oncology nurses fill the roles of direct care provider, case manager, genetic counselor, researcher, educator, and consultant. Outside the clinical setting, oncology nurses provide important cancer education to the public in industry, schools, and community forums. Oncology nursing care requires a broad base of knowledge in both pathophysiology and psychosocial areas and frequently involves complex technical and psychomotor skills. Patients and their families look to oncology nurses for assistance and guidance in all phases of the illness; during prevention and screening programs; from diagnosis, through therapy and terminal care. Cancer nursing challenges the nurse's skill, commitment, creativity, and compassion.

Etiology and Epidemiology

Cancer affects human beings wherever they live, whatever their race, color, cultural background, or economic status. Overall cancer incidence peaked in 1992 and has now stabilized.[1] More than 1,370,000 new cases of cancer were diagnosed in the United States in 2004, proving that cancer remains a major health problem. More important, cancer incidence is expected to increase again as the American population ages. Currently, the lifetime risk of developing cancer at any site is 1 in 2 for men and 1 in 3 for women.

Cancer is now the leading cause of death in the United States for persons younger than 85 years, exceeding heart disease. The death rate from cancer decreased in the last decade but has now stabilized with an overall 5-year survival rate of 63 percent. This trend compares poorly with other leading chronic illnesses such as heart disease and cerebrovascular illness, where death rates have dramatically decreased over the past 50 years. Nevertheless, great improvements in survival have been made over the past 30 years, particularly for the common cancers such as breast, colon, and prostate, largely because of earlier detection and improvements in therapy.

Despite these advances, more than 500,000 Americans—more than 1500 a day—die from cancer each year. The actual number of cancer deaths continues to increase because of an aging and expanding population. Unfortunately, large disparities in cancer incidence and mortality also occur across racial and ethnic boundaries.

Gender and Site

Basal and squamous cell skin cancers are the most prevalent cancers, with more than 1 million cases diagnosed each year. Luckily these skin cancers are highly curable and are usually not included in the analysis of the more invasive cancers. For men the most common sites of cancer are the prostate, lung, colon, and rectum. Lung cancer incidence in men continues to decline, and rates of prostate, colorectal, and bladder cancer have stabilized. Prostate cancer accounts for about 33% of new cancers in men each year. For women the top three cancer sites are the breast, lung, colon, and rectum. The incidences of breast and lung cancer in women continue to increase, but these increases have slowed in recent years. Rates of female cases of colon cancer and uterine cancer have stabilized, whereas ovarian cancer incidence has shown a recent decline. Breast cancer accounts for 31% of new cancers in women.

Deaths from lung, prostate, and colorectal cancers cause 52% of cancer-related deaths in men. In women, lung, breast, and colorectal cancer cause 50% of cancer-related deaths. Lung cancer has been the leading cause of death in women since 1987 and now accounts for 25% of all cancer deaths in women. Figure 23-1 shows the estimated cancer deaths and new cancer cases for men and women in 2004.

Age

Cancer is a disease of aging. At age 20 the risk of developing cancer is less than 1%. By age 50, however, the risk of developing cancer in the next 10 years is 7%; and by age 60, it is more than 16% for men and more than 10% for women.[36] The three most prevalent malignancies in women (breast, lung, colorectal) peak in incidence between ages 55 and 74 years. In men this same age span reflects the years in which the most deaths occur from prostate, lung, and colorectal cancer.

Today the average life expectancy is 74.4 years for men and 79.8 years for women. The population over age 65 has been steadily growing and now makes up about 13% of the population. By 2030 this population will represent 20% of the U.S. population.[2] In addition, Hispanic, African-American, Native-American, and Asian-Pacific ethnicities make up a growing percentage of the older population. This "graying of America" has an immense impact on the health care system and health care policies (see Chapter 2).

The quality of health for many older adults is influenced by a variety of factors. The older population may be limited by the financial constraints of a fixed income and inadequate health insurance; limited transportation; and established cultural, ethnic, or religious practices that may conflict with health care recommendations. These factors may help explain why older persons are diagnosed with more advanced cancers and do not participate as frequently in prevention and screening programs. In addition, older adults have more chronic diseases, with symptoms that may mask a malignancy, thereby preventing early detection. Disparities may also exist in cancer treatment offered to older patients because of questions related to their ability to withstand aggressive cancer therapy. Older patients may be inadequately represented in clinical trials, limiting the evidence about the efficacy of cancer therapy in this population.

Race and Ethnicity

The National Cancer Institute defines cancer health disparities as differences in the incidence, mortality, and burden of cancer among specific population groups in the United States. Racial and ethnic minorities experience a greater cancer burden compared with the general population, mainly because of delayed diagnosis, unequal socioeconomic status, and unequal access to care. African-American men have a higher cancer incidence than men of other races and a lower survival rate than Caucasian men for many cancers. Among women Caucasians have the highest cancer incidence, although African-American women have a higher cancer mortality. These disparities reflect both the diagnosis of cancer at later disease stages and the presence of comorbid diseases. With the exception of breast cancer, the incidence and mortality rates for the most common cancers are higher in African-Americans than in Caucasian Americans. The 5-year survival rate for African-Americans diagnosed with cancer is only 49% compared with 62% for Caucasian Americans. Lower survival rates result from diagnosis at later stages of the disease, as well as lower survival rates at each stage, suggesting possible differences in treatment, tumor characteristics, or other factors.

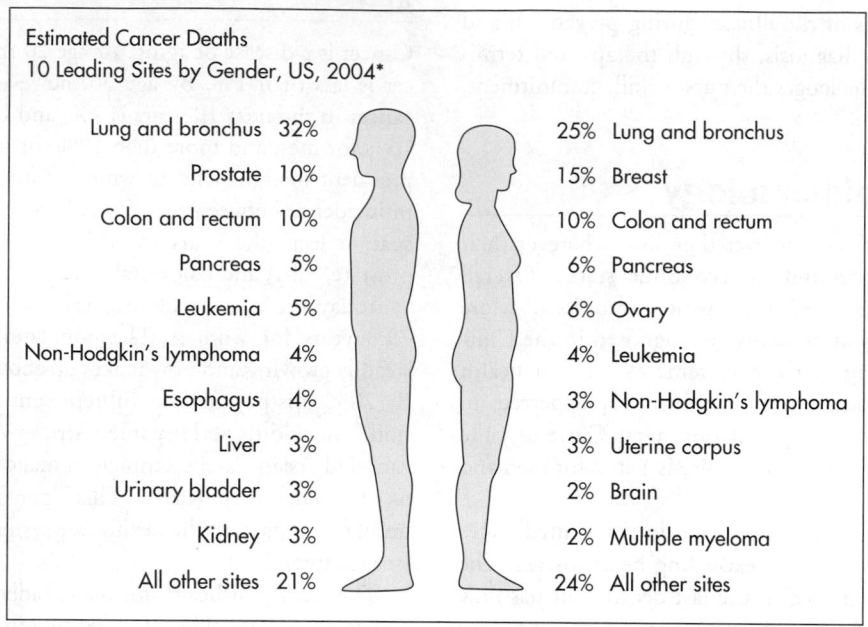

Estimated Cancer Deaths
10 Leading Sites by Gender, US, 2004*

Site	%	%	Site
Lung and bronchus	32%	25%	Lung and bronchus
Prostate	10%	15%	Breast
Colon and rectum	10%	10%	Colon and rectum
Pancreas	5%	6%	Pancreas
Leukemia	5%	6%	Ovary
Non-Hodgkin's lymphoma	4%	4%	Leukemia
Esophagus	4%	3%	Non-Hodgkin's lymphoma
Liver	3%	3%	Uterine corpus
Urinary bladder	3%	2%	Brain
Kidney	3%	2%	Multiple myeloma
All other sites	21%	24%	All other sites

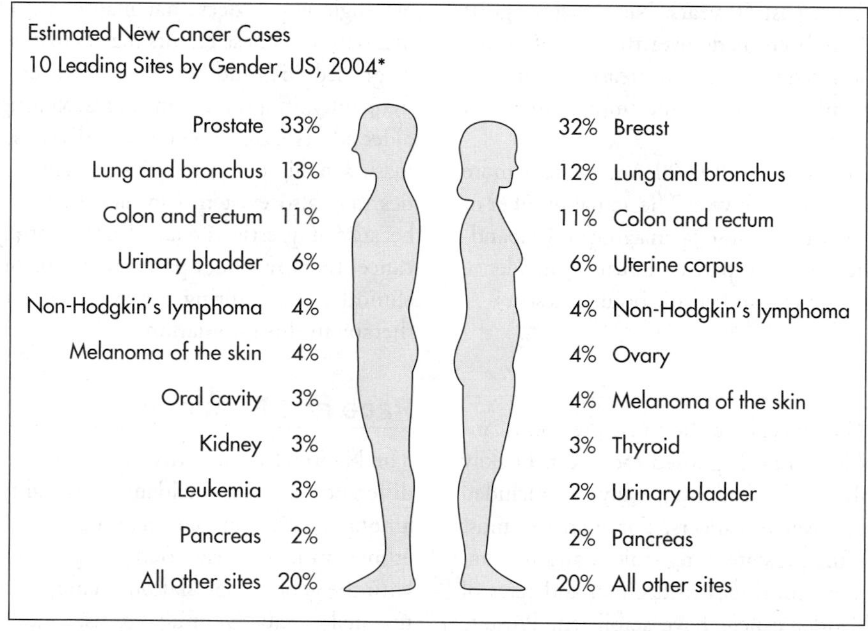

Figure 23-1 Estimated U.S. cancer deaths and hew cancer cases by gender, 2004.
*Most recent available statistics.

Hispanic-Americans, Asian-Americans/Pacific Islanders, and Native Americans have lower incidence and mortality rates for cancers than do either African-Americans or Caucasian Americans. Yet an American Cancer Society (ACS) survey showed that Hispanic-Americans are not adequately aware of cancer warning signs and ways to reduce cancer risk, participate less frequently in screening, and tend not to seek treatment as readily.

Cultural and ethnic behaviors and beliefs, as well as socioeconomic factors such as poverty and access to health care, play important roles in how quickly a person seeks health care and treatment. Health care insurance is also often unavailable or too expensive for members of minority groups.

Geographic Factors

The worldwide distribution of cancer reveals significant differences among different populations. For example, primary cancer of the liver is common in Indonesia and parts of Africa and Asia but rare in other regions. Breast cancer is more common in the United States and Western Europe than it is in Japan. Ugandans, Nigerians, and South African blacks experience a low incidence of cancer of the lung, stomach, large intestine, uterus, and kidney compared with the incidence rates in Western countries. Genetic differences among populations may contribute to international variations but are unlikely to explain all variations encountered, since migration from one country to another frequently results in major changes in the cancer incidence pattern.

Multistep Process of Carcinogenesis

The development of cancer (**carcinogenesis**) is a dynamic and multistep process that is influenced by many independent variables. A mutation in the deoxyribonucleic acid (DNA) that controls cellular growth and replication is the basic cause of many types of cancer. These mutations disrupt the orderly, controlled events of the cell cycle, which are regulated by specific genes and their production of various proteins and growth factors. Proto-oncogenes are the normal genes that regulate cell growth. When mutations occur in proto-oncogenes, they become **oncogenes** and can allow uncontrolled cell growth to occur. Tumor suppressor genes inhibit cell growth and program cell death, or apoptosis. A third type of gene is the DNA mismatch or repair gene, which identifies a mismatched nucleotide in DNA and orchestrates the necessary repairs. A mutation to this gene prevents recognition and repair of such errors.[35]

A growing number of gene mutations, growth factors, and growth factor receptors have been linked to specific cancers. Clinicians are now able to screen for the presence of these markers, which provides important diagnostic and prognostic information. Overexpression of the growth factor receptor HER-2/neu, for example, is linked to a more aggressive breast cancer in younger women. Mutations of the tumor suppressor gene, p53, are associated with more aggressive tumors and early metastasis in several solid tumors.[20]

Several mechanisms, occurring one at a time or together over a number of years, cause the cellular mutations that result in a malignancy. Although it is difficult to integrate all mechanisms into a single theory of how cancer develops, several pathways are probably involved. The first mechanism is the genetic abnormality that causes a malignant transformation. The second mechanism is linked to endogenous factors, such as hormones, and the third mechanism involves the influence of exogenous **carcinogens**. Exogenous factors include environmental influences, such as tobacco, radiation, and chemicals known to cause cellular damage.

The complex process of carcinogenesis involves three overlapping and multistep stages: initiation, promotion, and progression (Figure 23-2). In initiation a single genetic change occurs in a normal cell, altering cellular growth, function, or both. During promotion the altered cell undergoes additional malignant changes. Progression involves the continued growth of the cell population containing the malignant phenotype. In both the initiation and promotion stages the carcinogenic process can be stabilized or reversed if the cell is able to repair or control the genetic alteration. In the final stage of progression, however, reversal of carcinogenesis is no longer possible.

Risk Factors

A cancer risk factor is a characteristic that raises a person's chance of developing cancer. Some risk factors are endogenous and not amenable to change, such as age and genetic heritage. Other risk factors are exogenous and modifiable, such as the lifestyle habits of tobacco use and physical inactivity. Common risk factors are listed in the Risk Factors box. Risk factors may cause cancer either by damaging the genes that regulate normal cellular growth or by enhancing the growth of abnormal cells already present (e.g., by accelerating cell division). The presence of one or more risk factors does not guarantee the development of cancer, but knowledge about a person's cancer risk factors can help clinicians individualize the most effective plan for prevention and early detection of the disease.

Risk Factors

Cancer

Endogenous

Age: Cancer incidence increases with age.
Genetic factors: Some cancers exhibit a clear inheritance pattern.
Hormonal factors: Hormones are not primary carcinogens, but appear to influence the process of carcinogenesis.

External

Tobacco: Tobacco is the single most lethal known carcinogen.
Radiation: Both ionizing and ultraviolet radiation can cause cancer.
Nutrition: Excess energy intake leading to obesity is associated with a higher incidence of cancer.
Inactivity and obesity: Physical inactivity associated with obesity is associated with a higher incidence of cancer.
Infectious organisms: Several viruses, including sexually transmitted disease organisms, increase the risk of cancer.

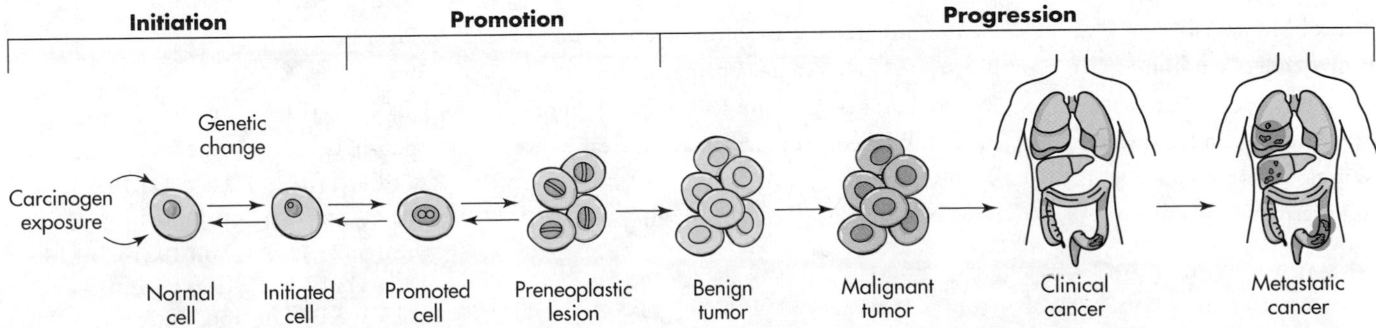

Figure 23-2 Multistage process of carcinogenesis.

Age. Age is a major risk factor associated with cancer development; 60% of all diagnosed cases and 70% of all deaths occur in persons 65 years and older.[36] The median age at cancer diagnosis is 67 years. Several theories have been proposed to explain this increase in cancer that accompanies aging. First, older people have been exposed to a greater cumulative number of carcinogens over a longer period, increasing the chances for malignant transformations. Second, older cells may be less capable of repairing the genetic abnormalities that result in cancer. And finally, a weakened immune system in older persons may allow the abnormal cell growth of cancer.[29]

Based on current projections regarding cancer incidence and the aging population, new cases of cancer in the United States are estimated to increase by 29% by the year 2010. This increase in cancer incidence, as well as the complex care needs of older patients with cancer, demands that increased efforts and resources be directed to prevent and manage the burden of cancer in this segment of the population. Geriatric oncology is a rapidly growing subspecialty in the area of cancer care.

Genetic Factors. Most cancers are not inherited, but occur because of random genetic mutations in people with little or no relevant family history. Nevertheless, 5% to 10% of all cancers are inherited and create a significant predisposition to cancer in offspring (Table 23-1). The patterns of transmission are autosomal dominant inheritance, where inheritance of only one altered copy of a gene produces cancer susceptibility; autosomal recessive inheritance, which requires two altered copies of a gene (one from each parent) to cause cancer susceptibility; and X-linked recessive inheritance, where males inherit an altered X chromosome–linked gene from their mothers.[24]

Hereditary cancer syndromes are usually autosomal dominant and are associated with an altered tumor suppressor gene, which is unable to suppress cellular mutations that ultimately lead to a malignancy. Examples of these hereditary cancer syndromes include hereditary breast and ovarian cancer, associated with the BRCA1 and BRCA2 genes; and hereditary nonpolyposis colon cancer. A few other hereditary cancer syndromes are associated with oncogenes, mutated genes that lead to the uncontrolled cell

TABLE 23-1 HEREDITARY CANCER SYNDROMES AND ASSOCIATED GENES

Syndrome or Condition	Associated Cancer	Gene Location
Ataxia-telangiectasia	Leukemia, lymphoma, breast	ATM at 11q22.3
Breast-ovarian syndrome	Breast, ovarian, prostate, colon	BRCA1 on 17q21
Breast–other cancer syndrome	Breast (male and female), pancreatic, colon, prostate	BRCA2 on 13q12-q13
Cowden disease	Breast, thyroid	PTEN at 10q23
Familial adenomatous polyposis (Gardner's syndrome)	Colon, thyroid, gastric	APC on 5q32-22
Familial melanoma, with or without dysplastic nevi	Melanoma, pancreatic	CMM1 at 1p36; CMM2 at 9p21; 12q14
Familial prostate cancer	Prostate	PRCA1 on 10q25; HPC1 on 1q24-q25
Fanconi's anemia	Leukemia, liver, head and neck, esophageal	FA-A on 16q24.3; FA-C at 9q22.3; FA-D at 3p26-p22
Hereditary nonpolyposis colorectal cancer (Lynch syndrome and Muir-Torre's syndrome)	Colon, endometrial, ovarian, stomach	HMLH1 at 3p21.3; hMSH2 at 2p22-p21; hPMS1 at 2q31-q33; hPMS2 at 7p22; hMSH6 at 2p16
Li-Fraumeni syndrome	Sarcoma, breast, brain, leukemia, adrenal	17p13.1
Multiple endocrine neoplasia type 1	Carcinoid, lung, ovarian, pancreatic	11q13
Multiple endocrine neoplasia types 2A and 2B	Thyroid, pheochromocytoma	RET at 10q11.2
Neurofibromatosis type 1	Neurofibrosarcoma, astrocytoma, carcinoid	17q11.2
Peutz-Jeghers syndrome	Breast, cervical, testicular, pancreatic	19p13.3
Retinoblastoma	Retinoblastoma, sarcoma, leukemia, lymphoma	RB1 at 13q14
Von Hippel–Lindau disease	Renal cell, pheochromocytoma, pancreatic	3p25-p26
Wilms' tumor	Wilms' tumor	WT1 at 11p13; WT2 at 11p15.5
Xeroderma pigmentosum	Basal cell, squamous cell, brain, lung, gastric	XP-A on 9q34.1; XP-B on 2q21; XP-C on 3p25.1; XP-D on 19q13.2; XP-E on 11p12-p11; XP-F on 16p13.2;-13.1; XP-G on 13q32-q33

Adapted from Lindor NM, Greene MH: The concise handbook of family cancer syndromes, *J Nat Cancer Inst* 90:1039, 1998.

division of a malignancy. These syndromes are hereditary papillary renal cancer, multiple endocrine neoplasia type II, and familial melanoma.[15]

A group of genetic disorders with primarily nonmalignant manifestations is also associated with a predisposition to malignant disease. Ataxia-telangiectasia is a genetic syndrome associated with childhood leukemia. Muir-Torre's syndrome is associated with colorectal and endometrial cancers.

Finally, cancer seems to "cluster" in some families at a higher than statistically expected incidence, but the associated genetic factors have not been clearly identified. Familial cancer refers to the presence of at least one relative with the same cancer but no clear inheritance pattern or known mutation. Many patients in these families voice concern about their increased susceptibility to cancer. These cancers probably result from multiple genetic mutations and other specific and nonspecific promoting factors.

Hormonal Factors. Evidence suggests that both endogenous and exogenous hormones may be connected with the development of certain cancers. Hormones, such as estrogen, do not appear to be primary carcinogens but seem to influence carcinogenesis in three ways: (1) through a preparatory action on the target tissues, making them susceptible to the carcinogenic agent; (2) through a "permissive" influence on carcinogenesis, allowing the process to progress; and (3) by a conditioning effect on the tumor.

Carcinogenesis may also be influenced by the duration of the hormonal effect. In breast cancer, for example, risk factors related to endogenous estrogen include early age at menarche and nulliparity or later age at first live birth, whereas breastfeeding appears to have a protective effect. These facts suggest that the development of breast cancer may be associated with a woman's cumulative exposure to estrogen; that is, the longer the exposure to the hormone, the greater the chance of cancer development.

Recent evidence points to the need to carefully balance the risks and benefits of exogenous hormone therapy, such as estrogen replacement therapy for the treatment of menopausal symptoms, especially with respect to cancer risk. Four large randomized controlled trials have raised doubts about the purported benefits of estrogen and progestin therapy in preventing coronary heart disease, stroke, and dementia in postmenopausal women. The increased risks for breast and endometrial cancers associated with estrogen therapy, therefore, may outweigh the benefits of hormone therapy, especially in women with other cancer risk factors.[32] More research is still needed to guide both physician and patient decisions regarding the use of hormone replacement therapy to alleviate postmenopausal symptoms and prevent chronic illnesses.

Precancerous Lesions. Certain benign lesions and tumors exhibit a tendency toward malignant change. The resulting cancers may be preventable if minor precursor conditions can be located and treated early. Precancerous lesions belong to a large and heterogeneous group; in some the progression to cancer is inevitable, whereas in others the risk is so low that medical intervention is unnecessary. Precancerous conditions include polyps of the colon and rectum, certain pigmented moles, dysplasias of the cervical epithelium, Paget's disease of the bone, senile keratoses, and leukoplakias of the oral mucous membranes.

Immunologic Factors. Scientists have become increasingly aware of the role of the immune system in the natural history of malignant disease. They believe that the presence of an immune surveillance system to control cancer is suggested by the following examples: (1) the high incidence of cancer in older persons who may have a weakened immune system, (2) an increased incidence of cancer in persons who have immunodeficiency diseases associated with a defect in cellular immunity, and (3) the increased incidence of neoplasia (e.g., non-Hodgkin's lymphoma) in persons who receive immunosuppressive drugs such as cyclosporine or azathioprine to prevent organ transplant rejection.

In the presence of an immune surveillance system, mutated cells that become malignant and are antigenically different from normal cells should be recognized as foreign and destroyed by the body's cell-mediated immune system. Research continues to explore how and why the initial tumor cells are able to progress to clinical cancer when an intact immune surveillance system exists. Scientists believe that some tumors arise in areas that are poorly served by the immune system, such as the central nervous system or the retrobulbar aspect of the eye. Some tumors may fail to stimulate antibody formation because they are so similar to normal cells. In other cases the normal control system for the immune response may become overactive and suppress the function of the immune system. Finally, some persons may lack the genetic ability to mount an effective immune response.

The normal immune system is capable of detecting and destroying as many as 10 million cancer cells at a time. However, when a tumor grows faster than this, it will continue to grow unchecked. Typically, a tumor must measure at least 1 cm in diameter before it can be detected by conventional diagnostic methods.[40] Unfortunately a tumor 1 cm in diameter already contains more than 1 billion cells. The role of the immune system is discussed further in Chapter 20.

Drugs and Chemicals. Many chemicals, drugs, and products in the environment are known to be carcinogenic; hundreds more are suspected to be associated with the development of cancer. Scientists have identified important links between cancer and the environment by studying patterns of incidence and mortality. As people move from place to place throughout the world, however, the baseline incidence and mortality rates for each type of cancer change. It is theorized that up to two thirds of all cancers may be related to environmental factors.

The National Toxicology Program publishes the *Report on Carcinogens* every 2 years, which lists agents known to be human carcinogens and those reasonably anticipated to be human carcinogens.[33] Box 23-1 provides a partial list of these substances. The Occupational Safety and Health Administration (OSHA) of the U.S. Department of Labor enforces regulations related to maximal allowable concentrations of exposure to known carcinogens (threshold limit values) in the workplace and environment.

Certain drugs have been shown to be carcinogenic. Oral contraceptives were first recognized as having carcinogenic potential for breast cancer, but are now known to also exhibit a protective effect against ovarian and endometrial cancers. In 1971 a rare form of vaginal cancer in women was linked to the ingestion by their mothers of diethylstilbestrol, a drug prescribed to prevent spontaneous abortion.

Box 23-1 Substances Known to Be Carcinogens in Humans[33]

- Aflatoxins
- Alcoholic beverages
- Analgesic mixtures containing phenacetin
- Arsenic compounds
- Asbestos
- Azathioprine
- Benzene
- Benzidine
- Beryllium
- Bis(chloromethyl)ether
- Broad-spectrum ultraviolet irradiation
- Busalfan (Myleran)
- 1,3-Butadiene
- Cadmium and cadmium compounds
- Chlorambucil
- Chloromethyl methyl ether
- Coal tar
- Coke oven emissions
- Creosote (coal and wood)
- Cristobalite
- Cyclophosphamide
- Cyclosporin A
- Diethylstilbestrol
- Dyes that metabolize to benzidine
- Environmental tobacco smoke
- Erionite
- Ethylene oxide
- Melphalan
- Methoxsalen with ultraviolet A therapy
- Methyl CCNU (lomustine)
- Mineral oils
- Mustard gas
- 2-Naphthylamine
- Nickel compounds
- Radon
- Silica
- Smokeless tobacco
- Soot
- Steroidal estrogens
- Strong inorganic acid mists containing sulfuric acid
- Tamoxifen
- Thiotepa
- Thorium dioxide
- Tobacco smoke
- Vinyl chloride
- Wood dust

From *Report on carcinogens,* ed 10, Washington, DC, December 2002, US Department of Health and Human Services, Public Health Service, National Toxicology Program.

Cancer therapy itself may increase the risk for other cancers. The use of alkylating agent chemotherapy, such as chlorambucil, cyclophosphamide, and thiotepa, is accompanied by a significant subsequent risk of acute leukemia and other malignancies. Consequently, decisions to use these drugs are carefully made after weighing their risks and benefits.

Radiation. **Ionizing radiation** consists of electromagnetic waves or material particles that have sufficient energy to ionize atoms or molecules (i.e., remove electrons from them) and thereby alter their biochemical behavior. Large amounts of radiation can be lethal to living cells. Ultraviolet radiation (UVR) is composed of lower energy electromagnetic waves, but it is still capable of causing carcinogenic changes. Various forms of radiation, both waves and particles of energy, can cause cancer.

Ionizing Radiation. Every living thing is exposed to small amounts of radiation from natural elements in the earth, such as uranium, a condition known as natural background radiation. Other sources of radiation exposure include medical radiation, in the form of diagnostic or therapeutic x-rays examinations; and synthetic radiation from nuclear energy sources or nuclear weapons. Problems related to radiation exposure were first recognized when the roentgen-ray (x-ray) machine was developed and became widely used in the diagnosis of disease. This was followed by the discovery of radium, which was used for the treatment of cancer. Scientists working with this technology were found to have an abnormally high incidence of skin cancer, and workers employed to paint radium on watch dials experienced high rates of oral and sinus carcinomas and osteosarcomas. High levels of radiation exposure also affected the survivors of the bombings of Hiroshima and Nagasaki, and the incidence of cancer in this population was extremely high, confirming the causative link between the radiation exposure and cancer development.

Radiation exposure results in breakage of either a single or double strand of the DNA helix.[31] The damage is permanent and cumulative with each additional radiation exposure. Exposure of the entire body significantly increases the amount of radiation received. For this reason all of the body except the part being treated is protected from exposure when radiation is administered for therapeutic purposes.

High-dose radiation exposure can cause leukopenia, leukemia, bone cancer, and sterility or damage to the reproductive cells. Because of this risk, persons whose daily work exposes them to radiation wear film badges that contain photographic film capable of absorbing radiation. The film badge is developed each month to measure cumulative radiation exposure, and any personnel who are becoming overexposed are temporarily reassigned.

Because radiation poses a danger to a fetus, particularly during the early weeks of gestation, pregnant women are advised not to work in radiology departments or to care for patients receiving radioactive materials.

Ultraviolet Radiation. UVR is produced by the sun, by artificial sources such as tanning beds, and in industry. This radiation can act as an initiator, a promoter, a cocarcinogen, and an immunosuppressive agent. Broad-spectrum UVR, whether from the sun or an artificial source, is a known human carcinogen that can cause skin cancer, cancer of the lip, and melanoma of the eye. Skin cancer occurs most commonly on areas of the body most exposed to sunlight. Sunburn and an increased duration of exposure increase the risk of skin cancer.

Radon. Radon is a colorless, odorless, radioactive gas that results from the decay of uranium found in soil and rocks. Prolonged breathing of radon gas at high levels has been linked to an increased incidence of lung cancer. The cancer risk from radon occurs indoors where concentrations may be high, especially in underground mines or in buildings that are poorly ventilated and near radon emission sites.[22] Improving ventilation of the building or mine can lower radon levels. Home monitoring kits are available, and the Environmental Protection Agency has established guidelines for detecting and controlling radon levels.

Electromagnetic Radiation. The effect of living or working near electromagnetic fields (EMFs) is a more recent environmental concern. EMFs are extremely low-frequency energy fields, and exposure can come from household appliances, electrical power lines, and electricity-generating facilities. Electrical power lines generate both electric and magnetic fields that can easily pass through body tissue and most materials. The intensity of the EMF is in proportion to the electrical energy running through the lines. The nearer one is to the source (within 50 m), the greater the exposure. Studies have shown a minimal increase in the incidence of leukemia and brain tumors in electric utility workers and a possible association between electromagnetic radiation and childhood leukemia.[33] More research is needed in this area, and efforts to reduce exposure to EMFs are continuing.

Questions have arisen about the safety of cellular phones, which emit small amounts of low-frequency electromagnetic radiation. Recent epidemiologic evidence, however, shows no connection between cellular phone use and cancer, particularly brain cancer. More long-term studies are needed, however, especially as the number of cellular phone users continues to grow and the cumulative exposure increases.

Lifestyle Practices

SMOKING AND TOBACCO USE. Tobacco smoke is the single most lethal cause of cancer in the United States, associated with at least 10 different cancers and responsible for up to 30% of all cancer deaths.[23] Cigarette smoking is the most important risk factor for all types of lung cancer, the leading cause of cancer death among both women and men in America. Cigarette smoking is also linked to cancers of the mouth, pharynx, larynx, esophagus, pancreas, kidney, bladder, colon, and rectum. Cigarette smoking is also associated with cardiovascular disease; acute and chronic respiratory diseases; and other detrimental effects on fertility, bone mass, and dentition. Nevertheless, about one in four adults still smokes cigarettes, and more than 3000 children and adolescents begin smoking each day.[10]

Tobacco smoke contains more than 60 known carcinogens, which are present in both mainstream smoke (directly inhaled by smokers) and sidestream, or second-hand, smoke (inhaled by smokers and nonsmokers). Cancer mortality bears a correlation with the number of cigarettes smoked daily, the number of years a person has smoked, and the age at which the person began to smoke. Smokers have a lung cancer risk more than 20 times greater than that of a lifetime nonsmoker.[28] Stopping smoking has immediate and long-term health benefits. People who stop smoking live longer and can cut their risk of dying from lung cancer by at least 50%. They also reduce their risk of heart disease and pregnancy-associated problems.

Many smokers switch to filtered cigarettes, pipe smoking, or smokeless tobacco (plug, leaf, snuff) in the misguided belief that their cancer risk will be lessened or eliminated. Evidence is strong that there is no "safe" cigarette and that smokeless tobacco products still contain high levels of carcinogens.

Since 1971, cigarette advertising has been banned from television and radio. Cigarette packages contain definitive warnings that cigarette smoking causes cancer, heart disease, and emphysema. In 1990 federal law prohibited the sale of tobacco products to minors. Legislation limiting public smoking and the advertisement and sale of tobacco products, especially legislation targeted at adolescents, will continue to be important interventions in the effort to reduce smoking-related diseases and cancers.

NUTRITION. Diet is the second most significant lifestyle factor contributing to cancer, with nutritional factors accounting for about 30 percent of cancers in developed countries.[43] Nutrition research has increased steadily over the past decade, but still little is known about how specific nutritional factors cause or protect against cancer. Research has focused on the effects of energy balance and obesity as cancer risk factors.

The consumption of a high-fat diet has been researched as a risk factor in many common cancers, including cancers of the colon, prostate, and breast. These studies found no strong evidence that decreasing total fat intake can prevent cancer, but suggest that additional research focus on the type of fat (animal versus vegetable) and fat as a component of total energy intake. A higher intake of red meat, for example, appears to be associated with higher incidences of colon and prostate cancers.[43]

The consumption of fruits and vegetables is associated with a lower incidence of many cancers, including lung cancer, several gastrointestinal and genitourinary cancers, and breast cancer. Fruits, vegetables, and whole grain foods, which are good sources of vitamins C and D, beta-carotene, and selenium, appear to deter cancer. These vitamins and minerals, known as antioxidants, assist in repairing cellular damage caused by free radicals. Free radicals damage the genetic makeup of the cell and its natural ability to resist cancer. The roles of other micronutrients, including beta-carotene, calcium, and folate, are also being studied. Although diets high in fiber initially appeared to offer some protection against colon cancer, prospective studies have not consistently supported this premise.

A significant association exists between high alcohol intake and cancer of the mouth, larynx, esophagus, and liver. Alcohol consumption may also increase the risk of breast cancer and colorectal cancer. The effects are frequently compounded by cigarette smoking and a variety of vitamin and dietary deficiencies. It is speculated that alcohol and nutritional deficiencies may enhance carcinogenesis by increasing the metabolic activity of specific tobacco carcinogens. These alcohol- and smoking-related tumors occur with greater frequency in men, African-Americans, older adults, and persons from lower socioeconomic groups and urban settings.

OBESITY. Obesity, characterized by an excess of body fat, results from long-term excess energy intake and is a problem reaching epidemic proportions in the United States. Obesity is considered a risk factor for colon, breast, endometrial, renal, and esophageal cancers (see Research box). One theory relates excess energy intake, increased body mass, physical inactivity, and levels of insulin and insulin-like growth factors, which play important roles in regulating cellular proliferation and apoptosis.[16] Physical activity may have an effect on circulating estrogen and thereby provide some protection against breast cancer. It is believed that overweight individuals can decrease their risks of cancer with a program of regular recreational exercise.

SEXUAL AND REPRODUCTIVE FACTORS. Sexual practices play a role in the incidence of certain cancers because several sexually transmitted diseases have been linked to cancer, including human papillomavirus (HPV), hepatitis, and human immunodeficiency virus (HIV). (See the discussion on the role of viruses below.) Although age at first coitus and multiple sex partners were once considered risk factors for cervical cancer, these lifestyle factors are primarily related to a greater exposure to sexually transmitted diseases, and hence an increased incidence of cancer. The risk may also be related to the length of time in which a woman is exposed to her own endogenous estrogen. A woman's age at menarche, the

Research

Calle EE et al: Overweight, obesity, and mortality from cancer in a prospectively studied cohort of US adults, *N Engl J Med* 348:1625, 2003.

The Cancer Prevention Study II began in 1982 and monitored more than 900,000 men and women in the United States and Puerto Rico for up to 16 years. The average age of subjects was 57 years at the time of enrollment. Over the study period, 57,145 subjects died from cancer. The study examined the relationship between body mass index, a measure of body fat in 1982, and the risk of death from cancer. The most overweight male subjects had cancer death rates 52% higher than men of normal weight, whereas the cancer death rate for overweight women was 62% higher than for women of normal weight. Higher body mass index values were associated with higher rates of death from 12 types of cancer, including cancers of the esophagus, colon, liver, gallbladder, pancreas, and kidney, and for non-Hodgkin's lymphoma and multiple myeloma. Findings from this study provided evidence that obesity is a cancer risk factor. As a result, efforts to reduce the risk of cancer should include maintaining a normal body weight or losing weight for those who are overweight, eating a healthy diet, and exercising regularly.

birth of her first child, and menopause are relevant factors in assessing for the risk of breast cancer. Women who give birth to their first child early in life have a lower incidence of breast cancer than those who do so later in life or never have children. Early menarche and late menopause are also considered to be factors that raise a women's risk of breast cancer.

Viruses and Other Microorganisms. The number of cancers linked to viruses is small, and the prevalence and spread of these viruses are more common in developing countries, where communicable disease rates are higher. Almost all cases of cervical cancer are associated with the presence of HPV. Although more than 100 different types of HPV have been identified, most HPV infections in women are transient and low risk. HPV-16 and HPV-18 are responsible for the majority of cases of cervical cancer. Other cofactors that increase the risk of cervical cancer in women with HPV infections include older age, use of oral contraceptives, smoking, and HIV infection.[3] Hepatitis B and C viruses can cause chronic infections that are associated with hepatocellular cancer. The Epstein-Barr virus, which causes mononucleosis, is associated with cancer of the upper pharynx and non-Hodgkin's lymphoma. HIV is also linked to Kaposi's sarcoma and lymphoma.

Helicobacter pylori, a bacterium, causes chronic inflammation of the stomach mucosa, and stomach ulcers. These conditions may be associated with a higher incidence of carcinoma and lymphoma of the stomach. Current research focuses on how theses conditions produce carcinogenic changes.

Psychosocial Factors. Stress that results from psychosocial trauma, loss of a significant other, and personality variables, such as helplessness and repression, have been suggested as etiologic factors in the development of cancer. How a person's state of mind affects the immune and hormonal systems is not easily explained. One hypothesis suggests that sustained activation of the hypothalamic-pituitary axis may impair the immune response and the individual's ability to fight cancer. Most reports of the occurrence of cancer in these instances are anecdotal, however, and prospective studies have not confirmed the role of psychologic factors in the development of cancer.[14] Ongoing studies in psychoneuroimmunology will contribute to this discussion.

▶ ARE You READY?

In preparing an educational session about nutrition and cancer, the nurse recommends a diet high in which of the following to lower chances of cancer?

1. Fiber
2. Vegetables
3. Low-fat milk products
4. Vitamin-enriched processed foods

Physiology

The knowledge of cell kinetics, or how cells grow and divide, is necessary to understand the process of cancer development and the principles of cancer treatment. Much of what is now known about cancer cells is the result of research in which normal cells were transformed into malignant cells in a controlled laboratory setting. Transformation to a malignant cell is recognized as a multistep process that originates in a single proliferating cell. The transformed cell then has an altered ability to differentiate and proliferate.

Normal Cellular Proliferation

In normal tissue, cellular growth takes place in an orderly process that responds to a need such as trauma, surgery, or an inflammatory event. Once the need is met, cell multiplication stops. Normal cells recognize the presence of other cells near them by means of the process of contact inhibition. When cells are in close contact with other cells, they normally adhere closely together. This contact inhibits overlap of cells and disorganized growth. In normal cells these restraints on growth are maintained until the need for new cells arises because of cell death. Some cell turnover rates are rapid, as in the bone marrow, skin, and gastrointestinal tract, because the need for cell replacement in these areas is greater than in slower growing tissue. Finally, with the exception of certain blood cells, normal cells do not migrate but have a designated location.

Cell Cycle. Mitosis refers to the splitting of one cell into two cells during the cell cycle. The concept of cell cycle time is pertinent to understanding normal cell replication and has implications for drug use in cancer therapy. Cell cycle time may be described as the interval from mitosis of a cell to its mitosis into daughter cells. There is a stationary period (G_0) of apparent rest after mitosis takes place. The cells are not in the cycle but are viable and capable of undergoing mitosis if necessary. The cell cycle is divided into four phases (Figure 23-3): (1) a quiescent phase consisting of G_1 (G denotes a gap) in which ribonucleic acid (RNA) and protein synthesis begins; (2) S, a period of DNA synthesis; (3) G_2, further RNA and protein synthesis and the development of the mitotic spindle; and (4) mitosis (M). The cell cycle is controlled by the cell nucleus, which receives signals from growth-regulating proteins that stimulate or suppress cell division. As described earlier, certain

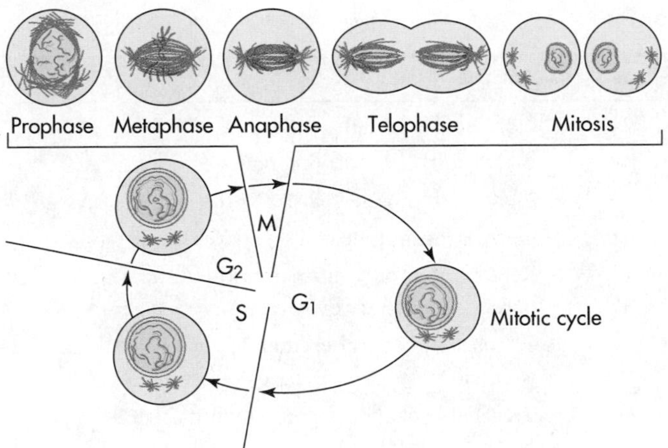

Figure 23-3 Cell cycle. G_1, RNA/protein synthesis; G_2, RNA/protein synthesis and interphase; *M*, mitosis; *S*, DNA synthesis.

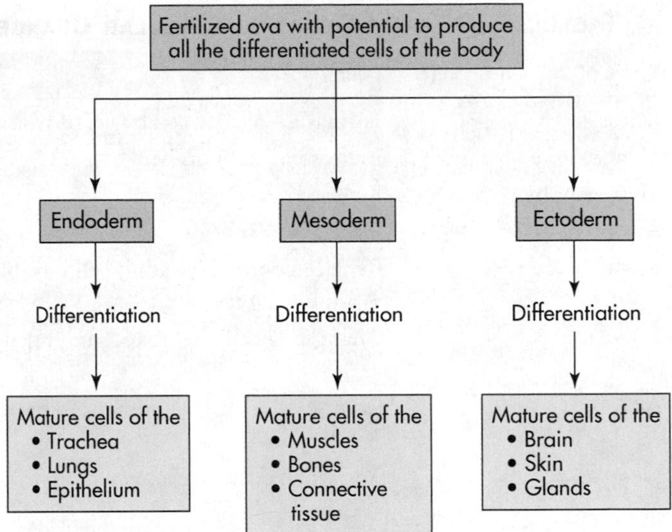

Figure 23-4 Normal cellular differentiation.

genes, including proto-oncogenes and tumor suppressor genes, code for these proteins.

Differentiation. All body tissue is derived from stem cells, which are immature cells with no specific cell lineage. These cells have the ability to proliferate rapidly and renew themselves as needed and to develop specialized functions as they grow and mature. The process of cellular differentiation causes the cells to resemble their normal forebears and have fully mature, specialized function and morphology. For example, all kidney cells are similar to each other but different from muscle cells, and each type has its specialized function.

The method by which differentiation takes place is unknown. One theory is that all cells carry the same genetic material but that selective repression of different genetic characteristics occurs because of buildup of different repressor substances in the cytoplasm. Different cells repress different genetic characteristics. Cell differentiation, once begun, proceeds along a path toward specialized function that cannot then revert to a previous immature state. Figure 23-4 shows the normal cellular differentiation process.

Pathophysiology

Alterations in Cell Growth

Malignant or cancerous growths represent one form of abnormal cell growth. Other types of cellular growths are benign and include hyperplasia and hypertrophy. Hyperplasia is an increase in cell number, whereas hypertrophy is an increase in cell size but not number. Although many neoplasms are characterized by hyperplasia, normal tissues also may undergo hyperplasia. Wound healing, callus formation, and growth in embryonic tissue are all normal forms of hyperplasia.

Metaplasia is a reversible process in which one adult cell type in an organ is replaced by another adult cell type. The new cell type usually is not one normally seen in the area in which metaplasia occurs. The change of columnar or pseudostratified columnar epithelium of the respiratory tract to squamous epithelium, or squamous metaplasia, represents the most common type of metaplasia. **Dysplasia** is an alteration in adult cells characterized by changes in their size, shape, and organization. Neoplasia represents abnormal cellular division not necessary for normal cell growth and development. Table 23-2 summarizes these terms.

Benign tumors show normal cell growth patterns, even though the new tissue growth is not needed. Benign tumors closely resemble the tissue from which they arose and often perform the same function, such as moles on the skin. Benign tissues usually bind closely together and do not invade other tissues. Once removed, benign tumors usually do not recur.

Malignant cells, by contrast, do not show normal growth patterns, and they divide almost continuously. Cancer cells gradually lose the appearance of the cells from which they arose, often becoming smaller and rounder with a larger nucleus. The grading system for cancer reflects how much the cancer cells resemble the tissue of origin. Generally cancer with more poorly differentiated cells has a poorer prognosis because of a higher degree of malignancy. The total loss of differentiation is termed **anaplasia**. Cancer cells do not serve any useful function, do not exhibit contact inhibition, and migrate through blood vessels and tissues, spreading to and growing in other body locations, a process called **metastasis**. Table 23-3 summarizes the differences between benign and malignant tissue growth.

Metastasis. Metastasis is the major cause of cancer death.[17] The presence of metastases is an important prognostic factor for many cancers, and research continues to uncover important details of this malignant process. Mechanisms that contribute to metastasis include **angiogenesis**, or formation of a new blood supply; motility; alterations in cell adhesion; and mechanisms to escape immune detection.

Angiogenesis involves the migration and proliferation of endothelial cells from existing blood vessels near the tumor. Both positive and negative regulators of angiogenesis influence the formation of a new blood supply to nourish the metastatic tumor. Tumor cells produce motility factors, which enable them to circulate through blood vessels and lymphatics. Cell adhesion molecules

TABLE 23-2 Terms Denoting Cellular Changes

Types of Cellular Change	Definition	Example
Mitosis	Formation of new cell by cell division	Normal cell growth
Hyperplasia	Increase in cell number	Breast epithelium in pregnancy
Hypertrophy	Increase in cell size	Increase in muscle cell size with exercise
Atrophy	Decrease in cell size	Decrease in muscle cell size with disuse
Metaplasia	Replacement of one adult cell type by different adult cell type	Replacement of columnar epithelium of respiratory tract by squamous epithelium
Dysplasia	Changes in cell size, shape, and organization	Changes in cervical epithelium in longstanding cervicitis
Anaplasia	Reverse cellular development to more primitive cell type	Irreversible change accompanying cancer
Neoplasia	Abnormal cellular changes and growth of new tissues	Malignancies

TABLE 23-3 Difference Between Benign and Malignant Neoplasms

Benign	Malignant
Limited growth potential	May proliferate rapidly or grow slowly
Localized	Spread (metastasize) throughout the body
Fibrous capsule	No enclosing capsule
Rarely recur after removal	May recur even after treatment
Usually regular in shape	Irregular shape with poorly defined border
Cells similar to cell of parent tissue (well differentiated)	Cells much different from parent cells (poorly differentiated)
Expansive growth	Infiltrative growth

on the cell surface are important mediators that allow detachment of tumor cells from the primary tumor site. Finally, tumor cells escape the immune system in a variety of ways, including secretion of immunosuppressive factors and cellular proteins that have no antigenic structure. With better understanding of the metastatic cascade, a greater potential exists for development of therapies that can interrupt this invasive process.

Cancer spreads in several different ways (Figure 23-5). Cancer cells differ from normal cells in their unique ability to move without restraint into surrounding tissue. Tumor cells lack adhesiveness (the ability to stay in contact with other cells), so they can easily break away from the tumor mass of which they are a part and directly invade surrounding tissues. This is referred to as *local invasion*. Local spread may cause skin changes and ulcerations of the involved tissues. Infection may accompany the local infiltration.

Cancer cells tend to spread along the path of least resistance, such as in tissue clefts, along blood vessels, or along the perineural spaces. The fibrous capsule that covers some organs may limit tumor growth. For example, primary tumors of the kidney, liver, or testes may increase the size of the organ without destroying the capsule. Local spread is not an orderly process but one that occurs unequally and haphazardly. Because of local spread, any surgical attempt to remove the cancer must include a margin of surrounding tissues to ensure removal of all malignant cells.

Cancer also spreads by lymphatic permeation and embolization. Once cells have invaded the lymph vessels, they may detach and become emboli, which lodge in the lymph nodes, forming a metastatic lesion. Spread then continues to the next group of nodes and into other organs. The presence of cancer in the lymph nodes is certain evidence of spread, but even if lymph node metastasis does not occur, malignant cells may still disseminate through the blood. Lymphatic and vascular dissemination may take place concurrently. Vascular spread can result in more widely disseminated disease because of the tumor cells' ability to move freely through both the lymphatic and venous systems. Bloodborne cancer cells escape from the bloodstream by a process of attachment and invasion through endothelial cells lining the blood vessel.

Finally, cancer can spread by diffusion, the spread of clumps of cancer cells from the surface of the tumor by mechanical means. This type of spread is particularly prevalent in serous cavities such as the abdominal or pleural cavity. In the peritoneal cavity, cells tend to gravitate to the pelvis. Cancer cells also can be implanted, or "seeded," during a surgical procedure, causing metastatic lesions. Metastasis may also regress or disappear without apparent cause and remain dormant for many years, only to resume growth years later.

Sites of Metastases. The site of metastatic spread depends on the venous or lymphatic drainage of the organ involved, the type of cancer, and tissue factors in potential metastatic sites. Various body tissues seem to have different attractions for metastases. Common sites for metastasis are, in order, the liver, lungs, bone, brain, and adrenal glands. The spleen, muscle, and skin are rarely

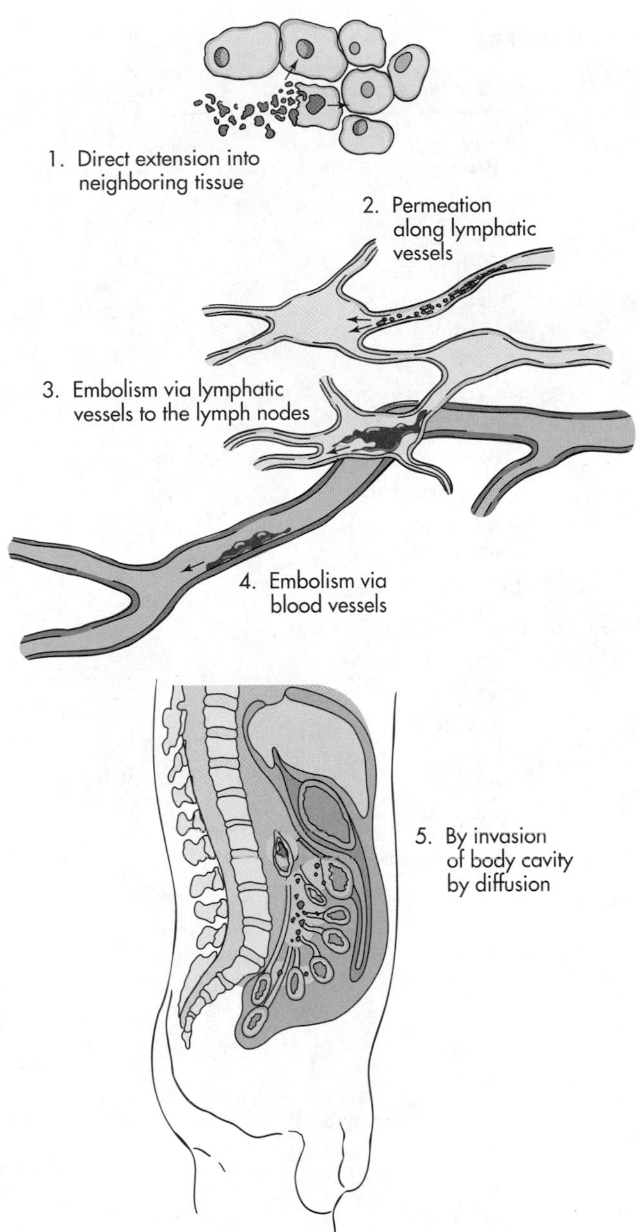

Figure 23-5 Modes of dissemination of cancer.

involved. Table 23-4 shows the pattern of metastasis of some common primary tumors.

▶ ARE YOU READY?

Which of the following is the leading site for cancer metastasis?

1. Spleen
2. Brain
3. Bone
4. Liver

Classifying and Naming Neoplasms

Tumors derive their names from the type of tissue involved (Table 23-5). In general, the names of benign tumors carry the suffix *-oma* after the name of the parent tissue (e.g., neuroma, fibroma). Some tumors are known by the names of the scientists who first described them (e.g., Hodgkin's lymphoma, Wilms' tumor). Other tumors are named after the organ from which they arise (e.g., hepatoma, thymoma).

Cell type of origin can also be used to classify cancers. Two main cell types are epithelial and mesenchymal (connective tissue). The term *carcinoma* denotes a malignant tumor of epithelial cells, and the term *sarcoma* denotes a malignant tumor of connective tissue cells. Carcinomas may be further classified as arising from glandular epithelium with the prefix *adeno–*, or arising from squamous epithelium with the word *squamous*. When a malignant tumor contains all three types of embryonal tissue, it is termed a *teratoma*. Tumors that originate during the primitive blastula embryonic phase have the suffix *-blastoma*. Other terms may be added to describe the histology, or tissue structure, within the tumor, such as follicular or cystic. In a small percentage of cases the tissue of origin may never be identified, despite aggressive investigation, including postmortem examination.

Classification systems are used to describe the type and extent of cancer. In the process of **grading**, the cancer is examined for its cellular maturity and characteristics. Tumors are graded by Arabic numerals into four grades. A higher grade means the tissue appears more abnormal and generally is more aggressive (Box 23-2). When identity with the tissue of origin is completely lost, the tumor is called *undifferentiated* or *anaplastic*. The grade of a tumor can guide decisions about treatment and provide prognostic information, although tissue differentiation may vary within a tumor and change over time. Classification of malignant tumors is difficult because many cancers contain several different types of cells, including benign tissue.

Staging is a form of classification that describes the extent of the tumor throughout the body. This classification is critical in planning the appropriate treatment and giving prognostic information. Three types of staging can be performed: (1) clinical staging, using the patient's clinical signs and symptoms and information obtained through imaging; (2) surgical staging, based on a surgical inspection; and (3) pathologic staging, which uses information about the tumor obtained through microscopic examination of involved tissue. Pathologic staging is the most definitive type of staging.

The International Union Against Cancer and the American Joint Committee on Cancer (AJCC) use the TNM system of classification, where T refers to primary tumor, N to regional lymph

Box 23-2 Classification of Malignant Lesions by Grade

- Grade 0: Normal tissue
- Grade 1: Well differentiated, with minimal deviation from tissue of origin
- Grade 2: Moderately well differentiated, with evidence of structural changes from normal tissue of origin
- Grade 3: Poorly differentiated, with extensive structural changes from normal tissue of origin
- Grade 4: Very anaplastic, with no resemblance to tissue of origin

TABLE 23-4 COMMON SITES OF METASTASES IN SELECTED CANCERS

Cancer	Sites of Metastasis
Bladder	Bone Bone marrow Brain Liver Lung Skin
Breast	Adrenal glands Bone Brain Liver Lung Lymph nodes —Axillary —Internal mammary —Supraclavicular Skin
Lung	Adrenal glands Bone Brain Liver Lung (ipsilateral) Lymph nodes —Hilar —Mediastinal
Prostate	Bone Kidney Liver Lung Lymph nodes —Perineural —Sacral —External iliac —Lumbar region —Pelvic Seminal vesicles
Cervical	Bone Liver Lung Lymph nodes —Femoral —Iliac —Hypogastric
Endometrial	Lymph nodes —Femoral —Iliac —Hypogastric
Ovarian	Lymph nodes —Iliac —Inguinal —Paraaortic —Retroperitoneal Peritoneal surfaces —Bladder —Diaphragm —Intestines —Liver Retroperitoneal region
Testicular	Bone Brain Liver Lymph nodes —Paraaortic region —Pelvic —Supraclavicular
Colorectal	Adrenal glands Bone Brain Liver Lung Lymph nodes —Inguinal —Perineal
Leukemia	Central nervous system Skin Testes
Melanoma	Liver Lung Lymph nodes —Regional
Head and neck	Bone Liver Lung Lymph nodes —Regional
CNS tumors	Rarely metastasize Seeding to distant CNS structure (e.g., spinal cord)

From Hawkins R: Mastering the maze of metastasis, *Oncol Nurs Forum* 28:959, 2001.

nodes, and M to metastases. The TNM system is a uniform system used worldwide for describing the anatomic extent of most solid cancers (Box 23-3). The purpose of the TNM system is to create categories for site-specific cancers that can be used to guide treatment decisions and give prognostic information. The AJCC frequently modifies the TNM staging categories for specific cancers to incorporate new prognostic evidence.

Other cancer-specific classification systems are in use, especially for hematologic malignancies. Leukemias are classified using categories developed by the World Health Organization,

TABLE 23-5 CLASSIFICATION OF NEOPLASMS

Parent Tissue	Benign Tumor	Malignant Tumor
EPITHELIUM		
Skin and mucous membrane	Papilloma Polyp	Squamous cell carcinoma Basal cell carcinoma Transitional cell carcinoma
Glands	Adenoma Cystadenoma	Adenocarcinoma
ENDOTHELIUM		
Blood vessels	Hemangioma	Hemangiosarcoma Angiosarcoma
Lymph vessels	Lymphangioma	Lymphangiosarcoma
Bone marrow		Multiple myeloma Ewing's sarcoma Leukemia Lymphosarcoma Lymphangioendothelioma
Lymphoid tissue		Reticular cell sarcoma (difficult to classify because of cell embryology) Lymphatic leukemia Malignant lymphoma
CONNECTIVE TISSUE		
Embryonic fibrous tissue	Myxoma	Myxosarcoma
Fibrous tissue	Fibroma	Fibrosarcoma
Adipose tissue	Lipoma	Liposarcoma
Cartilage	Chondroma	Chondrosarcoma
Bone	Osteoma	Osteogenic sarcoma
Synovial membrane	Synovioma	Synovial sarcoma
MUSCLE TISSUE		
Smooth muscle	Leiomyoma	Leiomyosarcoma
Striated muscle	Rhabdomyoma	Rhabdomyosarcoma
NERVE TISSUE		
Nerve fibers and sheaths	Neuroma Neurinoma (neurilemoma)	Neurogenic sarcoma Neurofibrosarcoma
Ganglion cells	Neurofibroma	Neuroblastoma
Glial cells	Ganglioneuroma Glioma	Glioblastoma Spongioblastoma
Meninges	Meningioma	
PIGMENTED NEOPLASMS		
Melanoblasts	Pigmented nevus	Malignant melanoma Melanocarcinoma
MISCELLANEOUS		
Placenta	Hydatidiform mole Dermoid cyst	Choriocarcinoma (chorioepithelioma) Embryonal carcinoma Embryonal sarcoma Teratocarcinoma

Box 23-3 TNM Staging Classification System

Tumor	
T0	No evidence of primary tumor
Tis	Carcinoma in situ
T1, T2, T3, T4	Ascending degrees of tumor size and involvement
Tx	Tumor cannot be measured or found
Nodes	
N0	No evidence of disease in lymph nodes
N1a, N2a	Disease found in regional lymph nodes; metastasis not suspected
N1b, N2b, N3	Disease found in regional lymph nodes; metastasis suspected
Nx	Regional nodes cannot be assessed clinically
Metastasis	
M0	No evidence of distant metastasis
M1, M2, M3	Ascending degrees of metastatic involvement
Mx	Metastasis cannot be measured or found

which incorporate white blood cell morphology, cytogenetics, and immunologic markers that provide the most valid prognostic information. For non-Hodgkin's lymphoma, the Ann Arbor staging system is used, which reflects the location of involved lymph node groups and organs and the presence of "B" symptoms such as weight loss, fever, and night sweats.

Clinical Manifestations of Cancer

The clinical manifestations of cancer may be diverse and affect multiple systems, depending on the site and size of the tumor. Tumors can cause obstructive problems if they occur within tubular structures such as the trachea, ureter, or gastrointestinal tract. Tumors may also cause ulceration and infection of epithelial tissue. Intraspinal and intracranial tumors cause symptoms of increased pressure when they grow within a closed structure. Immunologic, hormonal, and neuromuscular changes may result from a malignant process. Systemic symptoms, such as fatigue, loss of appetite, and weight loss, may occur early in the disease process or accompany progressive disease.

Nurses need to be aware of the signs and symptoms of the most common cancers to aid in their early detection. Early warning signs for lung cancer include persistent cough and hemoptysis. A change in bowel habits or blood in the stool can be early signs of colon cancer. Changes in the appearance or texture of breast tissue or breast lumps are suspicious for breast cancer. Nurses can encourage and support patients to take the important step of seeking medical attention when symptoms raise the possibility of a cancer diagnosis.

Collaborative Care Management

Diagnostic Tests

Diagnostic tests can provide critical information about the primary tumor, extent of the disease, and its stage. When looking for evidence of the tumor throughout the body, the clinician considers the natural course of each specific cancer and its pattern of spread. Table 23-6 outlines some common malignancies and the diagnostic tests used in their evaluation.

Patients and families often experience a great deal of anxiety about the possibility of a cancer diagnosis. Diagnostic tests and procedures can cause anxiety and apprehension even when the rationale for their use is clearly explained. Nurses offer support to the patient and the entire family at this critical time.

Laboratory Tests. Laboratory tests can be used to diagnose a specific organ malfunction or metabolic aberration that may be caused by a malignant condition. Common tests used in cancer detection include a complete blood count; a serum chemistry profile; and examination of body fluids, such as sputum and urine, for blood. More specific laboratory tests measure for the presence of tumor markers, or proteins associated with specific cancers. For example, a serum prostate-specific antigen (PSA) test may be done if prostate cancer is suspected, or a carcinoembryonic antigen test may be performed as follow-up testing for suspicious lesions of the gastrointestinal tract or to monitor for disease progression after treatment. Tumor markers can also be used to monitor the patient's response to cancer therapy (Table 23-7). Newer laboratory techniques used in the diagnosis of cancer include radioimmunoassays and flow cytometry. Radioimmunoassay techniques measure tumor antigen in the serum using radiolabeled antigens. Flow cytometry identifies cellular and DNA characteristics of the tissue that may yield important diagnostic and prognostic information (e.g., to differentiate the types of leukemia).

Cytology. In 1942 Dr. George Papanicolaou showed that the diagnosis of cancer could be made from the study of cells that have sloughed or exfoliated from a tumor. These cells are found in body secretions such as cervical discharges, sputum, gastric washings, pleural fluid, and urinary washings. The secretion is spread on a slide, stained, and examined by a pathologist, who can classify the tissue as benign, dysplastic ("suspicious"), or malignant. The main use of the Pap smear, as it is often called, is to diagnose cancer in an asymptomatic person and to identify precancerous lesions or noninvasive cancer. If suspicious cells are found, a biopsy is performed to confirm the diagnosis of cancer. The Pap smear is most widely used for examining cervical washings.

Tumor Imaging. Radiographs, or x-ray studies, are commonly obtained to provide two-dimensional views of organs. Because air, bone, and soft tissue absorb x rays differently, their structure and function can be distinguished on the film. Chest x-ray studies and mammograms are common radiographic examinations used in the diagnosis of cancer. Computed tomography (CT) scans provide three-dimensional views of internal structures and are some of the most useful and widely used tests in the diagnosis of cancer because they can detect smaller lesions than x-rays studies. Positron emission tomography (PET) studies glucose metabolism in body tissues and is proving useful in differentiating varying rates of tissue metabolism. Because tumors have a high rate of glycolysis, malignant tissues accumulate higher concentrations of radioactive glucose compounds, which are detected with gamma camera tomography.

TABLE 23-6 COMMON MALIGNANT CONDITIONS AND COMMONLY USED DIAGNOSTIC TESTS AND PROCEDURES*

Malignancy	Laboratory Tests and Procedures Used
GASTROINTESTINAL CANCERS	
Esophagus	Chest x-ray examination Computed tomography (CT scan) Magnetic resonance imaging (MRI) Esophagoscopy and biopsy Barium contrast studies (barium swallow)
Stomach	Gastric secretion analysis Carcinoembryonic antigen Gastroscopy and biopsy Baruim contrast studies
Colorectal	CT scan MRI Stool guaiac Barium enema Colonoscopy and biopsy Cancer antigen [CA] 19-9
Liver	Liver biopsy Liver enzyme studies, alpha-fetoprotein Ultrasound CT scan MRI Angiography
GENITOURINARY CANCERS	
Prostate	Digital rectal examination Bone scan Biopsy Urinalysis Laboratory: prostate-specific antigen, serum acid phosphatase
Bladder	Cytology Cystoscopy Intravenous pyelogram (IVP) Urinalysis
Kidney	CT scan Renal angiogram, sonogram X-ray studies of kidney, ureters, and bladder Urinalysis IVP
GYNECOLOGIC CANCERS	
Cervix	Colposcopy Biopsy Papanicolaou test (Pap smear)
Ovary	Pelvic physical examination IVP Barium enema Urinalysis
Uterus	Endometrial biopsy and aspiration
OTHER CANCERS	
Breast	Breast physical examination Ultrasound Mammography Tissue and lymph node biopsy Estrogen receptor and progesterone receptor status
Lung	Chest x-ray examination CT scan Sputum cytology Fiberoptic bronchoscopy with biopsy and bronchial washings Mediastinography (endoscopic examination of mediastinum and nodes) Thoracentesis

*Diagnostic tests cited are not a comprehensive list of tests and procedures used to detect specific cancers, but are only a representative sample.

Other radiographic tests, such as the barium enema, use contrast media to better outline and distinguish structures. Nuclear medicine procedures involve scanning organs such as the liver, thyroid, or bones after the ingestion or instillation of a radiolabeled material. Diseased organs often show increased or abnormal uptake of the radioisotope. Table 23-8 lists some common scanning procedures used to diagnose cancer.

Invasive Diagnostic Techniques

BIOPSY. A biopsy is the only definitive way to diagnose cancer. It is essential to obtain and accurately identify an adequate tissue sample before any cancer therapy is prescribed. When possible, an aspiration biopsy (needle biopsy), which removes a small plug of tumor by a needle or syringe, is used to avoid the larger incisional or excisional biopsy. However, needle biopsy, although it is inexpensive

TABLE 23-7 MARKERS USED TO DETECT AND MONITOR CANCER

Markers	Associated Tumor
Human chorionic gonadotropin, beta subunit (B-HCG)	Testicular cancer, choriocarcinoma
Bence Jones protein	Multiple myeloma
Alpha-fetoprotein (AFP)	Testicular, choriocarcinoma, pancreas, colon, lung, stomach, liver
Carcinoembryonic antigen (CEA)	Lung, gastrointestinal, breast, pancreas
Prostate-specific antigen (PSA)	Prostate
Cancer antigen (CA) 125	Ovarian, pancreas, breast, colon, lung, liver
CA 19-9	Ovarian, pancreas, colorectal
CA 15-3	Breast

TABLE 23-8 COMMON IMAGING PROCEDURES TO DIAGNOSE CANCER

Study	Procedure	Comment
X-ray	Two-dimensional image on plate of selenium-coated metal	Provides picture of soft tissue and bone
Computed tomography (CT) scan	Three-dimensional image using computerized x-ray films	Produces images of plane sections of body; identifies size and location of tumors
Magnetic resonance imaging (MRI)	Uses radio waves and magnetic field to image tissue	May be more sensitive than CT to image soft tissue
Ultrasound	Uses sound waves to provide images	May be used to direct biopsy needle
Positive emission tomography (PET)	Uses a sugar and radioactive substance to image chemical changes in tissues	Effective to diagnose larger malignant tumors when other scans are normal
Single-photon emission computed tomography (SPECT)	Images of uptake of radioactive substance that may be linked to monoclonal antibody	Provides information about blood flow to tumors

and relatively simple to perform in an outpatient setting, has the potential of missing the malignant focus and "seeding" tumor cells along the needle track as it is inserted and withdrawn. An incisional biopsy involves the surgical removal of a section of the neoplasm. If the tumor is small and can be removed in its entirety, an excisional biopsy is performed.

The biopsy specimen is examined to establish a histologic diagnosis and identify important cytologic features of the tumor. A growing number of cancers are now associated with cytogenetic abnormalities, such as chromosomal translocations and deletions. Chronic myelogenous leukemia (CML) has long been associated with the Philadelphia chromosome that features a translocation between chromosomes 9 and 22, forming the BCR-ABL oncogenic protein that has high tyrosine kinase activity. This oncogene is now the target of a new genetic therapy, Gleevec. Other cytogenetic changes can be used as tumor markers and yield prognostic information. In acute myelogenous leukemia the presence of chromosomal translocations such as t(15;17) and t(8;21) indicates a good prognosis. The HER-2/neu growth factor receptor is an important marker in breast cancer.

ENDOSCOPY. Fiberoptic tubes equipped with a light source are commonly used to illuminate various body cavities, permitting visual inspection of the interior of the cavity being examined. Other abdominal structures can be examined by laparoscopy and the insertion of an instrument into the abdominal space. The laparoscope can be used to inspect the liver, diaphragm, and peritoneum, as well as gastrointestinal, gynecologic, and genitourinary structures, thus avoiding a major surgical procedure. Biopsy specimens of a mass or secretions from the organ can be obtained during any of these endoscopic procedures.

Medications

Once a diagnosis of cancer is confirmed and the extent of the disease defined, the patient and health care team begin the complex process of determining the most effective and appropriate therapy. The choice of treatment is based on patient characteristics, information about the specific cancer, and factors related to both quantity and quality of life. Cancers can be treated with surgery, radiotherapy, chemotherapy, and biologic therapy. Today most patients with cancer are treated with a combination of therapies referred to as multimodality therapy.

A wide variety of medications are routinely used in the management of cancer and its symptoms. Chemotherapy, the use of drugs in the primary treatment of cancer, is one of the major cancer treatment modalities and is discussed later in the chapter.

Treatments

Radiotherapy, a primary treatment modality for cancer for many years, is discussed later in the chapter. A variety of other treatments are emerging for the treatment of specific forms of cancer. Biotherapy is the most commonly used of these newer treatments.

Biotherapy. The immune system and the immune response to cancer have been studied for many years. The link between cancer and the immune system is illustrated when (1) some tumors spontaneously regress, (2) cancer incidence increases in persons who are immunosuppressed (such as posttransplant patients or older adults), (3) metastatic tumor size decreases after surgical removal of the primary tumor, and (4) metastatic disease becomes dormant after successful local treatment of a tumor. These observations have stimulated continuing research on the role of the immune system and how the immune response can be enhanced to fight cancer growth.

The focus of **biotherapy**, or immunotherapy, is manipulation of the immune system through the use of naturally occurring biologic substances (cells, cell products) or genetically engineered agents and drugs that modify the body's immune response to cancer or cancer therapy. Biotherapy is now an established component of cancer therapy and is effective both alone and in conjunction with surgery, chemotherapy, and radiotherapy. A number of biologic agents have been developed that function as regulators and messengers of immune function.

The use of biotherapy is expensive because of the complex technology required to produce these products. Continued research to attach anticancer drugs and radioisotopes to tumor-specific immune cells may provide therapies that are able to seek out and destroy only cancer cells, thus protecting normal cells and decreasing side effects. Greater understanding of the genetic errors that result in cancer at a cellular level continues to provide new avenues for research and treatment.[8]

TYPES OF BIOTHERAPY. Biotherapy agents can be classified into five categories: cytokines, monoclonal antibodies (MABs), cellular therapies, immunomodulators, and retinoids. **Cytokines** are proteins that mediate and regulate various immune functions. The most common cytokines are the interferons (IFNs), interleukins (ILs), and hematopoietic growth factors (HGFs). MABs are antibodies produced by hybridoma techniques for specific antigens on tumor cell surfaces.[9] Cellular therapy uses activated immune cells such as lymphokine-activated killer cells and tumor-infiltrating lymphocytes. Immunomodulators include vaccine therapy, where the patient is vaccinated with a variety of antigens to stimulate either a nonspecific immune response or a tumor-specific immune response. Finally, retinoids are natural derivatives of retinol, or vitamin A, and stimulate cellular differentiation. Table 23-9 presents the common biotherapy agents and their clinical applications.

INTERFERONS. **Interferons** are a group of glycoproteins produced by T lymphocytes in response to viral infections or other stimuli. IFNs bind to receptors on nearly all the cells in the body, and all nucleated cells are capable of IFN production. IFNs can be induced by natural agents and can also be synthetically produced by recombinant DNA technology by the insertion of genes for an IFN into *Escherichia coli.*

IFNs have the ability to alter cellular metabolism in both normal and cancer cells. IFNs produce changes in viral RNA and protein synthesis and inhibit the function of several oncogenes. IFNs also can activate natural killer cells, mediators that can identify and destroy some tumor cells.[34]

Three types of IFNs are manufactured: alpha, beta, and gamma. Each type has unique dosing parameters, administration guidelines, and side effects. Interferon-alpha first received Federal Drug Administration approval for the treatment of hairy cell leukemia and has since been approved for the treatment of CML and Kaposi's sarcoma and as adjuvant therapy for melanoma. Flu-like symptoms are common side effects of IFN administration.

INTERLEUKINS. **Interleukins** are a group of biologic factors that stimulate and increase a number of other immune cells and other cytokines, including lymphocytes, macrophages, complement factors, and monocytes. They are produced by thymus cells and are involved in cell-mediated immunity. Of the 17 interleukins identified, IL-2 has been most thoroughly studied. IL-2 is produced by recombinant technology and is used in the treatment of renal cell cancer and melanoma. In addition to flulike symptoms, IL-2 can cause a capillary leak syndrome, which causes tachycardia, hypotension, edema, and pulmonary side effects such as dyspnea and pulmonary edema. Neurologic, renal, and hepatic toxicities can also occur.

GROWTH FACTORS. Hematopoietic **growth factors** are glycoproteins that stimulate the development of hematopoietic cell lines. The proteins attach to the surface of a stem cell and stimulate the cell to proliferate, differentiate, and mature. Some HGFs stimulate a single cell type, whereas others stimulate multiple cell lines. Granulocyte colony-stimulating factor (G-CSF) stimulates the growth and activation of neutrophils. Granulocyte-macrophage colony-stimulating factor (GM-CSF) stimulates the production of neutrophils, eosinophils, and macrophages.[5] Both G-CSF and GM-CSF have shown the ability to accelerate bone marrow recovery of neutrophil counts after myelosuppressive therapy. The use of these factors has dramatically decreased the sepsis-related morbidity and mortality that often follow aggressive chemotherapy and bone marrow transplant. With decreased bone marrow suppression, patients can receive their full course of chemotherapy without delays or toxicity. G-CSF and GM-CSF are usually given as subcutaneous injections but may also be given by the intravenous route.

Erythropoietin (EPO) is a recombinant growth factor approved for the treatment of anemia associated with end-stage renal disease and myelosuppressive cancer therapy. EPO can effectively decrease the transfusion requirements for anemic patients and improve their quality of life. EPO is most commonly given as subcutaneous injections but may also be given as an intravenous infusion.

IL-11 is the newest HGF and is used to stimulate platelet production in patients who are at high risk for severe thrombocytopenia. Although the other HGFs have generally mild side effects, IL-11 is associated with mild to moderate toxicity, especially fluid imbalance and cardiac arrhythmias, and its use must be carefully evaluated in the clinical setting. IL-11 is administered as a subcutaneous injection.

TABLE 23-9 SELECTED BIOTHERAPY AGENTS WITH FDA-APPROVED APPLICATIONS

Agent	Category	Definition and Biologic Actions	Approved Indications
INTERFERONS			
Interferon-alpha	Cytokine	Family of glycoprotein hormones with antiviral, immunomodulatory, and antiproliferative effects Derived primarily from leukocytes	Hairy cell leukemia Kaposi's sarcoma Condyloma acuminatum Chronic hepatitis B Chronic hepatitis C Chronic myelogenous leukemia Adjuvant therapy for melanoma
Interferon-beta		Derived primarily from fibroblasts	Multiple sclerosis
Interferon-gamma		Derived from activated T lymphocytes	Chronic granulomatous disease
INTERLEUKINS			
Interleukin-2	Cytokine	Molecular messengers between cells of immune system; activate cells of immune system and stimulate production of other cytokines; 17 interleukins currently identified	Melanoma, renal cell carcinoma
MONOCLONAL ANTIBODIES			
	Antibodies	Pure immunoglobulins derived from single cell (hybridoma); bind to target antigens on tumor cells and signal other cells of immune system to destroy tumor through phagocytosis or by complement-mediated lysis	
Satumomab pendetide			Detection of colon and ovarian cancer
Capromab pendetide			Detection of prostate cancer
Rituximab (Rituxan)			CD 20^+ B-cell non-Hodgkin's lymphoma

MONOCLONAL ANTIBODIES. **Monoclonal antibodies** are produced by hybridoma techniques that involve immunizing animals (usually mice) with an antigen, and then fusing B cells from the mouse's spleen with tumor cells to make hybrid cells. MABs can be produced to bind with almost any antigen. They are effective in the serologic detection of tumors, since malignant cells often express antigens that are not usually found on the surfaces of normal cells. These markers may be sensitive enough to detect early cancer and can be used to monitor the progress of disease in patients undergoing therapy.

Rituximab is an MAB used in the treatment of B-cell lymphomas whose cells express the CD20 surface antigen. Rituximab binds with the CD20 antigen on the malignant B cells, causing cell-mediated cytotoxicity. Trastuzumab (Herceptin) is another MAB used in the treatment of breast cancers that express the HER-2 antigen on their cells.[9] Herceptin binds to the HER-2 antigen and causes cell death. MABs are usually administered as intravenous infusions and can be used alone or in combination with chemotherapy. The most common adverse effect of MAB use is a symptom complex in which patients experience fever, chills, and rigors during administration of the drug. The syndrome usually occurs with the initial but not with subsequent treatments and is usually not serious enough to discontinue treatment.

ADVERSE EFFECTS OF BIOTHERAPY. Flulike side effects are associated with several biotherapy agents, including the IFNs and ILs, and can include fever, chills, rigors, headache, and malaise. Fevers and myalgias can be prevented or alleviated by the use of acetaminophen as a premedication or as needed to promote comfort.[38] Nonsteroidal antiinflammatory drugs (NSAIDs) may also be used, but aspirin and aspirin-containing products are avoided because of the risk of bleeding in myelosuppressed patients. Meperidine may be administered to relieve chills and rigors. Flulike symptoms are generally worse with initial doses of the biotherapy agents and diminish over time, an adaptation called *tachyphylaxis.*

An infusion-related complex of symptoms can also occur, especially during the initial administration of an MAB. This symptom complex includes fever, chills, and urticaria and can, in rare cases, progress to bronchospasm, hypotension, and angioedema. Patients may be premedicated with acetaminophen and diphenhydramine; the rate of the MAB infusion is slowly increased according to patient tolerance, and the patient is closely monitored throughout the infusion. Skin rashes and local injection site reactions may also occur.

TABLE 23-9 SELECTED BIOTHERAPY AGENTS WITH FDA-APPROVED APPLICATIONS—CONT'D

Agent	Category	Definition and Biologic Actions	Approved Indications
MONOCLONAL ANTIBODIES—CONT'D			
Trastuzumab (Herceptin)			Breast cancer with HER-2 protein overexpression
Gemtuzumab (Mylotarg)			CD 33^{+} acute myelogenous leukemia
GROWTH FACTORS			
Granulocyte-macrophage colony-stimulating factor (GM-CSF)	Hematopoietic growth factor	Natural hormonelike protein produced by variety of immune cells that stimulates maturation, differentiation, and proliferation of granulocytes and monocytes or macrophages	Accelerate myeloid recovery in lymphoid malignancies and after bone marrow transplant; mobilize stem cells for transplantation
Granulocyte colony-stimulating factor (G-CSF)	Hematopoietic growth factor	Natural hormonelike protein produced by variety of cells, mainly monocytes and macrophages, as well as endothelial cells, fibroblasts, and stromal cells that stimulate growth and activation of granulocyte precursor cells	Reduce severity, duration, and sequelae of neutropenia; mobilize stem cells for transplantation
Erythropoietin	Hematopoietic growth factor	Natural hormone produced by kidney that regulates and controls red blood cell production and maturation	Chemotherapy-related anemia Anemia related to chronic renal failure and zidovudine administration in patients with HIV
RETINOIDS			
	Vitamin A derivatives	Class of agents that perform significant role in vision, growth, reproduction, epithelial cell differentiation, and immune function	All-*trans*-retinoic acid in treatment of acute promyelocytic leukemia Bexarotene for cutaneous T-cell lymphoma

Adapted from Rieger PT: Biotherapy: an overview. In Rieger PT, editor: *Biotherapy: a comprehensive review,* Boston, 2001, Jones & Bartlett.
FDA, US Food and Drug Administration; *HIV,* human immunodeficiency virus.

Fatigue is reported by almost all patients receiving biotherapy, and its cumulative effect is a common reason for reducing dosage or discontinuing therapy. Other factors contributing to fatigue include anemia, poor nutrition, and disease status. Nurses help patients identify strategies to conserve energy and establish priorities for activities that require energy. Patients are encouraged to seek a balance between rest and activity and incorporate rest periods into each day's activities. Nurses also encourage the use of relaxation and stress-reducing activities such as listening to music or reading.

Neurologic toxicities associated with biotherapy include somnolence, anxiety, depression, and mental status changes. Nurses must be skilled in mental status examination and complete baseline and ongoing assessments. Antidepressants and behavioral therapy are prescribed, but in severe cases, doses of the MAB may need to be reduced or discontinued to relieve these side effects.

Cardiovascular and pulmonary toxicities are most commonly associated with high-dose IL-2 therapy. Potential cardiotoxicities include arrhythmias and hypotension. IL-2 increases capillary permeability and allows fluid to leak from the vessels to interstitial spaces. Fluid retention can result in weight gain, as well as peripheral and pulmonary edema from vascular leak syndrome. Fluid balance is carefully monitored.

Severe gastrointestinal toxicity from biotherapy is not common, but patients may experience anorexia, nausea, and diarrhea. Nurses help patients optimize their nutritional intake and use appropriate antiemetic and antidiarrheal medications.

Patients receiving biotherapy need a basic understanding of how the immune system functions in relation to cancer, why biotherapy is being prescribed, and common side effects (Table 23-10). The intensity and duration of toxicity depend on the agent used, dose, route, and schedule. The nurse provides a printed instruction sheet that addresses prevention, management, and reporting of side effects. Patients need to understand the level of monitoring required during therapy. Most side effects occur shortly after administration and are reversible when the drug is discontinued. If the patient is self-administering the biotherapy agent, the nurse teaches the patient proper drug preparation and storage, techniques for subcutaneous injections, and safe handling and disposal of all equipment and drug materials.

Gene Therapy. Advances in the understanding of cancer as a genetic disease have led to new therapies directed toward the genetic mutation of cancer itself. **Gene therapy** involves the identification and treatment of the defective gene function underlying

TABLE 23-10 COMMON SIDE EFFECTS OF BIOTHERAPY AGENTS

Biotherapy Agent	Common Side Effects	Occasional Side Effects
Interferon	Myelosuppression Anorexia Fever and chills Fatigue Headache and myalgias Hepatotoxicity	Mental status changes Bone pain Diarrhea Flushing Nausea Skin rash
Granulocyte colony-stimulating factor (G-CSF)	Increased WBC count	Bone pain Injection site reactions Headache
Erythropoietin	Increased RBC count	Headache
Interleukin-11 (oprelvekin)	Increased platelet count	Fluid retention Peripheral edema Tachycardia
Monoclonal antibodies	Fever and chills Flushing Fatigue	Anorexia Bronchospasm Diarrhea Headache Hypotension Hepatotoxicity Mucositis Myalgias Myelosuppression Nausea Skin rashes Infusion-related hypersensitivity reaction
Interleukin-2	Anorexia Capillary leak syndrome Fever, chills, flushing Fluid retention and peripheral edema Fatigue Headache and myalgias Diarrhea Hypersensitivity Hepatotoxicity	Mental status changes Skin rash Pulmonary edema Mucositis

Adapted from Rieger PT: Patient management. In Rieger PT, editor: *Biotherapy: a comprehensive overview,* ed 2, Boston, 2001, Jones & Bartlett.
RBC, red blood cell; *WBC,* white blood cell.

the patient's cancer. Treatment may involve the transfer of a new gene that compensates for the genetic alteration in the cancer cells. A retroviral agent may be used to insert the desired gene into the cell's genome.

Two examples of gene therapy already in use are the biotherapy agent all-*trans*-retinoic acid (ATRA), used for the treatment of acute promyelocytic leukemia (APL), and STI 571 (Gleevec) for CML and gastrointestinal stromal tumor. In APL a chromosomal translocation, t(15;17), results in the production of a protein that causes abnormal myeloid differentiation. ATRA binds to altered retinoic acid receptors on the abnormal gene and halts production of the carcinogenic protein. In CML the target for gene therapy is the Philadelphia chromosome, t(9;22), a reciprocal translocation that occurs between chromosome 9 and 22 in the bone marrow. The result of this chromosomal abnormality is production of an abnormal enzyme that instructs cells to reproduce uncontrollably. Gleevec inhibits the activity of the mutant enzyme.

As more specific cancer genes and gene products are identified, further therapies will be developed that can halt abnormal cell growth at the molecular level. New treatments might include therapies that restore normal p53 function and cell death, inhibit DNA and RNA coding for abnormal proteins, or interfere with cellular signals that allow uncontrolled cell growth.

Molecular Targeted Therapies. A variety of new agents stop tumor growth by inhibiting specific molecular targets in tumors. Target therapies inhibit receptors such as epidermal growth factor receptor-tyrosine kinase (EGFR-TK), and vascular endothelial growth factor. Inhibitors of EGFR-TK have demonstrated an anticancer effect on a variety of common solid tumors. Gefitinib (Iressa) has a positive effect on advanced non–small cell cancer, head and neck cancer, breast cancer, colorectal cancer, and other solid tumors. Erlotinib (Tarceva) has an effect on pancreatic cancer. Side effects have been generally mild, reversible, and noncumulative.[34]

Another group of compounds, called angiogenesis inhibitors, blocks the development of new blood vessels, thereby cutting off the tumor's supply of oxygen and nutrients. This helps slow tumor growth and spread to other parts of the body. Thalidomide is an example of one such agent. It is being studied for the treatment of multiple myeloma and other cancers.

Bone Marrow and Peripheral Stem Cell Transplantation. Bone marrow transplantation and peripheral stem cell transplantation are most commonly used in the treatment of leukemia and lymphoma. The goals are to replace diseased bone marrow with healthy bone marrow, rescue healthy bone marrow and protect it from the effects of intensive therapy for a solid tumor, or replace diseased stem cells with healthy stem cells. These treatments are most effective when the leukemia or lymphoma is in remission. They may also be used to treat other malignant conditions, including preleukemic states, multiple myeloma, and neuroblastoma. Other applications are being researched in clinical trials.[26]

There are three types of bone marrow transplants: syngeneic, in which the bone marrow donor is an identical twin and tissue is a perfect human leukocyte antigen (HLA) match; allogeneic, in which bone marrow comes from a related or unrelated donor and may or may not be HLA matched; and autologous, in which the patient's own bone marrow cells are used. Bone marrow stem cells can be harvested from the posterior iliac crests during a surgical procedure, or blood stem cells designated to become bone marrow cells can be harvested from the patient's peripheral blood using plasmapheresis. Collection of stem cells in the peripheral blood through plasmapheresis is much easier than harvesting marrow cells, and stem cells also engraft more rapidly than transplanted marrow cells. Chemotherapy and the administration of growth factors "mobilize" the patient's stem cells, and they can then be collected with less possibility of tumor cell contamination. Autologous peripheral stem cell transplantation has become the most common type of marrow transplant because most patients do not have a donor for HLA-matched bone marrow.

In every marrow transplant regimen the patient is treated with high doses of chemotherapy, radiotherapy, or both. The therapies carry significant toxicity, and the patient requires intensive support with blood products, antibiotics, and growth factors during the period of engraftment, which may last several weeks. In addition to mucositis, myelosuppression, and various organ toxicities, allogeneic transplants also carry the risk of acute and chronic graft-versus-host disease, which can cause skin, liver, and gastrointestinal abnormalities. The transplant process is complex and requires interdisciplinary coordination of care during every phase.

Surgical Management

Of the four major forms of cancer therapy (chemotherapy, radiotherapy, biotherapy, and surgery), surgery is the oldest and most widely used option. Surgery may be used for cancer diagnosis and staging, cure, adjuvant treatment, control of oncologic emergencies, or palliation of symptoms (Table 23-11). Trends in cancer surgery include the use of more ambulatory procedures, minimally invasive approaches, and multimodality treatment plans. The operative procedures used to treat various types of cancer are discussed in later chapters under the specific organ systems.

The initial role of surgery in cancer therapy is in the diagnosis and staging of the disease. Surgical biopsy, as described under diagnostic tests, confirms the diagnosis of cancer, defines the histologic features of the tumor cells, and ascertains the presence of metastatic disease.

When surgery is used in an effort to cure the disease, the malignant lesion must be small, localized, and amenable to complete surgical removal. It is standard procedure to remove a wide margin of tissue surrounding the involved organ and to dissect the regional lymph nodes at the time of surgery. This technique can greatly reduce the incidence of local recurrence and increase survival rates, especially in tumors that disseminate through the lymphatics. However, the benefits of extensive surgery must be weighed against the prolonged recovery period and the disfigurement caused by radical resections. Newer and more potent cytotoxic agents, improved radiotherapy, and surgical techniques such as cryosurgery and laparoscopic approaches support the use of more conservative surgical approaches, which result in better functional and cosmetic outcomes. Adjuvant (meaning *aiding* or *assisting*) chemotherapy or radiotherapy can be given before or after surgery to eliminate any microscopic cancer not removed by the surgery.

TABLE 23-11 SURGICAL APPROACHES TO CANCER CARE

Intervention	Example
Diagnosis	Breast biopsy
Staging	Staging laparotomy Second-look laparotomy
Treatment of primary tumor	Curative resection (abdominal perineal resection)
Reconstruction, rehabilitation	Breast reconstruction Continent urostomy or ileostomy
Palliation	Endocrine ablation Pericardial window
Adjuvant therapy	Paraaortic node dissection Hickman catheter insertion
Complications of other methods	Excision of bowel stricture Excision of radionecrotic tissue
Resection of metastases	Partial hepatectomy Pulmonary resection
Cytoreductive surgery	Abdominal soft tissue sarcomas Ovarian peritoneal carcinoma
Emergencies	Obstruction Hemorrhage
Cancer prevention	Colectomy (familial poylposis) Orchidopexy (testicular tumors)

From McCorkle R et al: *Cancer nursing*, ed 2, Philadelphia, 1996, Saunders.

Surgical approaches for early stage breast cancer illustrate the use of less invasive therapy. Breast conservation techniques, such as lumpectomy followed by radiotherapy, have replaced the radical mastectomy. Lymphatic mapping and sentinel node biopsy are now performed rather than full axillary node dissections in some patients with early breast cancer. In this approach, a radiocolloid dye is injected into the tumor site and scanned with a gamma probe. The primary lymph node drainage site, or sentinel node, is identified, excised, and examined. If the sentinel node has no evidence of tumor, theoretically the cancer has not spread further down the lymph node chain and a full axillary dissection is not performed. The patient can be spared the additional surgery and the potential pain, immobility, and lymphedema associated with axillary node dissections.

Surgery may also be used as a palliative intervention for patients with more advanced disease. Palliative surgery can reduce the bulk of an unresectable tumor or stabilize a pathologic fracture. Examples of other palliative procedures include the placement of a jejunostomy tube for nutritional support or the creation of a tracheostomy to relieve tracheal obstruction. The formation of a colostomy to relieve bowel obstruction and a laminectomy to reduce spinal cord compression are examples of surgical procedures that improve the patient's quality of life but do not affect the cancer itself. Surgery can also improve pain control through a variety of surgical blocks.

Surgical interventions can also be used to support other treatment modalities such as radiotherapy and chemotherapy. Surgical placement of a vascular access device enables safer chemotherapy administration. Applicators, which hold internal sources of radiotherapy, are commonly placed in the operating room with the patient under general anesthesia. Finally, reconstructive surgical procedures play an important role in improving body function and appearance for the patient with cancer. Breast reconstruction after mastectomy and facial reconstruction after head and neck surgery are commonly performed.

Before surgery the health care team assesses the patient's physical and emotional status to predict how well the patient can withstand the proposed surgical procedure. Important factors to consider include age, nutritional status, the results of diagnostic tests, performance status, and any comorbid medical problems. The health care provider informs patients about all postoperative care routines and answers specific questions and concerns as honestly and promptly as possible. Discussion of care during the immediate postoperative period includes explanation about any special equipment that may be needed, such as catheters, monitors, infusion lines, or chest tubes.

The focus of care after cancer surgery is on preventing complications, since many patients are already physically compromised or immunodeficient before surgery. Immunocompromised patients are at increased risk for infection and problems with wound healing and maintenance of strict asepsis. The nurse teaches the patient and other caregivers the signs of infection and how to prevent, detect, and manage infectious complications. Visitors with an infectious process are advised to refrain from physical contact with the patient during this vulnerable period. Patients with cancer are also at risk for developing postoperative complications like hyperacoagulability, thrombosis, and thrombophlebitis because of elevated levels of clotting factors and shortened partial thromboplastin and prothrombin times.[19] See Chapter 15 for a detailed discussion of standard postoperative care.

One of the first questions the patient may ask when awakening from anesthesia after surgery is, "Was it cancer?" or "Did they get it all?" The family often asks the same questions. Fear that the tumor was malignant or unresectable is normal. The nurse anticipates these questions and is prepared to respond appropriately. The nurse needs to be cognizant of what the surgeon has communicated to the patient and family so that the information conveyed is clear and consistent.

After cancer surgery the patient faces the prospect of changes in lifestyle, role, and self-concept. Patients who have had a mastectomy, colostomy, or gynecologic surgery may be especially troubled by body changes that make them feel less attractive and less functional. Depression may manifest as mood disturbances; changes in activity, appetite, or sleep; or sexual dysfunction for many months after surgery. Patients need to know that grieving a lost body part or function is natural. Support groups are helpful to many people, and the nurse ensures that the patient receives the name and phone number of appropriate groups in the local community, or initiates contact directly with the patient's permission.

Diet

The role of diet in the incidence of cancer in specific populations has been under intensive investigation for many years. Diet clearly plays a protective role against certain types of cancer and is implicated in promoting the incidence of others. Wide variations in cancer incidence are found worldwide, a phenomenon that is at least partially attributable to diet. Current research focuses on the role of a high-fat diet and obesity in cancer development. Diet also plays a role in certain approaches to cancer treatment, but largely in the realm of unproven remedies. A great deal of anecdotal information is available about individuals who seem to have responded positively to all kinds of elimination diets, including macrobiotics. But at present diet has no proven role in the treatment of most cancer except for maintaining optimal nutrition during treatment and managing treatment-related side effects.

Health Promotion and Prevention

Nurses play a major role in educating the public about primary and secondary cancer prevention. The government's health initiative, *Healthy People 2010*, outlines multiple objectives related to cancer prevention and control[39] (see Healthy People 2010 box). Nurses have many opportunities to promote these initiatives through public education.

Even though the public has a greater knowledge of cancer than ever before, positive attitudes about cancer and its therapy are essential if persons are to follow good health practices. Many factors play a role in determining whether or not a person will change an unhealthy or undesirable behavior after receiving health teaching. What individuals believe about their susceptibility, the costs of changing the behavior, and the health message all influence their behavior. In addition, successful cancer screening programs face many barriers, including health care providers' lack of time and expertise to integrate comprehensive cancer screen-

Healthy People 2010

Objectives Related to Cancer

- Reduce the overall cancer death rate to 159.9 deaths per 100,000 population or by 21%.
- Reduce the lung cancer death rate to 44.9 deaths per 100,000 population or by 22%.
  –Target risk factors of cigarette smoking, occupational exposures, and air pollution.
- Reduce the breast cancer death rate to 27.9 deaths per 100,000 population or by 20%.
  –Encourage mammography screening.
  –Target risk factor of obesity.
- Reduce the death rate for cancer of the uterine cervix to 2.0 deaths per 100,000 females.
  –Encourage screening with a Pap test.
  –Encourage protection against sexually transmitted diseases.
- Reduce the colorectal cancer death rate to 13.9 deaths per 100,000 population or by 34%.
  –Target risk factors of obesity, diet, and alcohol intake.
  –Encourage screening and early detection tests.
- Reduce the oropharyngeal cancer death rate to 2.7 deaths per 100,000 population or by 10%.
  –Target risk factors of alcohol and tobacco use.
- Reduce the prostate cancer death rate to 28.8 deaths per 100,000 males or by 10%.
  –Encourage participation in trials to identify benefits of screening and treatments.
- Reduce the rate of melanoma cancer deaths to 2.5 deaths per 100,000 population or by 11%.
  –Target risk factor of sun exposure.
- Increase to 75% the proportion of persons who limit sun exposure, use sunscreens and protective clothing when exposed to sunlight, and avoid artificial sources of ultraviolet light.
- Increase to 85% the proportion of physicians and dentists who counsel their at-risk patients about tobacco use cessation, physical activity, and cancer screening.
- Increase to 97% of women ages 18 years and older who have ever received a Pap test, and to 90% of women ages 18 years and older who received a Pap test within the preceding 3 years.
- Increase to 50% the proportion of adults who receive a colorectal cancer screening examination.
- Increase to 67% the proportion of women ages 40 years and older who have received a mammogram within the preceding 2 years.
- Increase the number of states to 45 that have a statewide population-based cancer registry that captures case information on at least 95% of the expected number of reported cancers.
- Increase to 70% the proportion of cancer survivors who are living 5 years or longer after diagnosis.

From US Department of Health and Human Services: *Healthy People 2010: understanding and improving health,* Washington, DC, 2000, The Department.

ing; patients' lack of funds, transportation, or support to access the screening program; and the health care system's inadequate resources to offer comprehensive screening. A population with increasing cultural diversity also presents challenges to effective screening. For example, certain minority groups, the uninsured and economically disadvantaged, those who live in rural areas, and those who are less educated are less likely to use screening programs. Nurses need to consider a wide range of issues when designing and participating in cancer prevention and screening activities.

Anxiety and fear about cancer may prevent an individual from learning about his or her cancer risk. A cancer diagnosis, aspects of treatment, and uncertainty about prognosis can be frightening. People may view cancer as meaning the inevitable loss of a job, income, and an enjoyable lifestyle, as well as premature death. All nurses can emphasize the positive aspects of the early diagnosis of cancer, including a greater chance for cure and a normal lifestyle. An estimated one third of persons diagnosed with cancer are cured. Another one third could perhaps be cured by medical treatment if the cancer were diagnosed early enough. The 5-year survival rate for all cancers is 63% and continues to increase with ongoing discoveries that improve diagnosis and treatment methods.

Primary Prevention. Primary prevention attempts to reduce a person's exposure to known cancer risk factors that might lead to disease. This is a virtually impossible task in cancer prevention, inasmuch as all risk factors are not known or have not yet been proved as specific factors in cancer development. However, substantial evidence supports a direct link between certain environmental and lifestyle factors and cancer development. Examples include smoking and lung cancer, excessive sun exposure and skin cancer, and low dietary fiber content and colon cancer.

Nurses with knowledge of these cancer risk factors can be effective in educating the public and supporting healthy lifestyles. Nurses can teach in clinical settings, where cancer care may not be the primary health problem, and in the community, where health promotion and counseling are routine components of a primary care practice. Nurses can also participate in community health fairs and health education events in schools and businesses to educate the public about cancer prevention.

Every nurse has the responsibility to promote a tobacco-free and smoke-free lifestyle. Tobacco is the leading cause of disease and death in the United States, and effective treatments for tobacco dependence are available. In 2000 the U.S. Public Health Service, in collaboration with a multidisciplinary panel of consultants, published a reference guide, *Treating Tobacco Use and Dependence*, to assist all clinicians in incorporating tobacco dependence interventions into their practice (Box 23-4). The interventions include identifying and assessing tobacco use in every patient, providing patients who are willing to quit with the appropriate interventions, treating patients who are not willing to quit at this time with motivational interventions, and, finally, providing relapse prevention treatment to patients who have recently quit using tobacco. Counseling and behavioral therapies are effective interventions for tobacco cessation, as are numerous pharmacotherapies, such as nicotine replacement products (gum, patch, inhalers) and bupropion (Zyban).

Primary prevention for skin cancer involves avoiding excessive and prolonged exposure to the sun and other sources of UVR, such as tanning beds. Nurses should discourage these practices,

Box 23-4 Treating Tobacco Use and Dependence: A Guide for All Clinicians

- Identify tobacco use and assess willingness to quit.
- For tobacco users willing to quit, implement the "5 As":
  —*Ask* about tobacco use.
  —*Advise* all users to quit.
  —*Assess* willingness to make a quit attempt.
  —*Assist* the patient with a plan to quit:
    —Set a date.
    —Give practical counseling.
    —Identify social supports.
    —Recommend the use of approved pharmacotherapy.
    —Provide supplemental materials.
  Arrange scheduled follow-up.
- For tobacco users unwilling to quit, implement the "5 Rs":
  —Explain why quitting is personally *relevant.*
  —Highlight the *risks* of tobacco use.
  —Identify the potential *rewards* of stopping.
  —Identify the *roadblocks* to quitting.
  —*Repeat* at every opportunity.
- For former smokers, implement relapse prevention strategies:
  —Discuss benefits from cessation.
  —Emphasize their success in quitting.
  —Discuss any problems or threats encountered.

Adapted from Fiore MC et al: *Treating tobacco use and dependence: quick reference guide for clinicians,* Rockville, Md, October 2000, US Department of Health and Human Services, Public Health Service.

especially among children and adolescents, who are developing lifelong habits. Nurses can emphasize to patients that skin damage from the sun occurs even without sunburns, and that regular use of a sunscreen with a sun protection factor of 15 or higher can significantly reduce the lifetime incidence of skin cancer.

Strategies to prevent colon cancer include nutritional interventions, maintenance of a healthy weight, and removal of precancerous adenomatous polyps. One dietary risk factor for colon cancer is a diet high in animal fat. Other risk factors may include alcohol consumption and lack of physical activity. Nurses need to counsel all patients about nutrition and physical activity to reduce their risks of cancer (Box 23-5).

Chemoprevention involves the use of chemical agents to reduce the risk of developing cancer. Chemoprevention trials have identified many agents with potential benefit for use with individuals at increased risk for certain cancers. In 1998 studies showed the drug tamoxifen reduced the chance of developing breast cancer by 49% in women at high risk for breast cancer. The STAR trial is currently evaluating whether raloxifene is as effective as tamoxifen in reducing breast cancer incidence but with fewer side effects.[25] Additional chemoprevention trials are under way to determine whether finasteride can prevent prostate cancer and whether NSAIDs and calcium compounds have a preventive effect against colon cancer. Vaccination against common oncogenic forms of HPV may also significantly reduce the incidence of cervical cancer in the future (see Future Watch box).

The importance of identifying cancer risk through genetic counseling is becoming increasingly evident as more genetic mutations are directly linked to cancer development. Patients with and without family histories of cancer seek information about their unique cancer risks. A number of risk assessment models and genetic tests are available to answer these questions, but numerous ethical and legal issues are associated with identifying individuals and families at high risk for cancer, including informed consent, confidentiality, and employment and insurance discrimination. Nurses play a key role in many aspects of care.

Patients whose family or health history indicates a genetic predisposition to cancer may be referred for cancer genetic risk assessment and counseling. Nurses in a variety of settings may encounter patients seeking information about their genetic risk, and nurses need to know how and when to refer patients for genetic counseling. Patients and families who test positive for a genetic risk factor need intensive education and support to make decisions about interventions that may reduce their risk of cancer. Oncology nurses have the opportunity to specialize as genet-

Box 23-5 Guidelines on Nutrition and Physical Activity for Cancer Prevention

- Choose most of the foods you eat from plant sources.
  —Eat five or more servings of fruits and vegetables every day.
  —Choose whole grains over processed grains and sugars.
  —Limit your intake of red meat and high-fat meats.
- Adopt a physically active lifestyle.
  —Be at least moderately active for 30 minutes on 5 or more days of each week.
  —Activity for more than 45 minutes on 5 or more days can further reduce the risks of breast and colon cancers.
  —Children should exercise for 60 minutes on 5 or more days of each week.
- Maintain a healthful weight throughout your life.
  —Balance your intake of food with physical activity.
  —Lose weight if you are overweight.
- Limit your consumption of alcoholic beverages, if you drink at all.

Modified from American Cancer Society: *Cancer prevention and early detection: facts and figures 2004,* Atlanta, 2004, The Society.

Future Watch

Vaccination Against HPV Could Prevent Cancer

Human papillomavirus (HPV) is one of the most common causes of cervical dysplasia, which can lead to invasive cervical cancer. Vaccines have been made against HPV-16 and HPV-18, two of the most common oncogenic HPV types. In several large clinical trials the vaccines were effective in reducing the incidence and persistence of HPV 16/18 infections. Prevention of HPV 16/18 infections could lead to a significant reduction in cervical cancer, in both developed and developing countries around the world. The vaccines were found to be safe and well tolerated, but more research is needed to determine their long-term safety and effectiveness, particularly with international population-based studies.

Data from Harper D et al: Efficacy of a bivalent L1 virus like particle vaccine in prevention of infection with human papillomavirus types 16 and 18 in young women: a randomized controlled trial, *Lancet* 364(9447):1757-1765, 2004.

ic counselors who perform risk assessments, educate about risk and risk reduction options, and coordinate individualized cancer surveillance plans.

Secondary Prevention. Secondary prevention efforts are aimed at early diagnosis and prompt treatment for persons without clinical signs or symptoms of cancer. Once the diagnosis is established, definitive treatment can be initiated. Successful secondary prevention requires a means to detect and cure the cancer at an early stage. Most cancer screening programs are examples of secondary prevention activities.

At present, early detection methods are not available for all cancers. Screening tools that have enabled the detection of early asymptomatic cancers and are known to reduce cancer mortality include mammograms and Pap smears. Use of PSA to detect early stage prostate cancer has also caused dramatic declines in the mortality rates for prostate cancer. The use of chest x-ray examinations to screen for lung cancer has been largely unsuccessful because of their low sensitivity in detecting early lesions. Clinical trials are investigating the feasibility of low–radiation dose CT as a screening tool for lung cancer. The ACS has developed guidelines for early detection of common cancers for average-risk individuals with no symptoms (Table 23-12). In addition, the ACS recommends that individuals with higher risks for particular cancers have more frequent or additional examinations. Health care professionals can help patients choose the most appropriate early-detection protocol. The goal is to discover early cancers before patients develop symptoms.

The nurse's role in screening and early detection begins with a sound knowledge of cancer, known risk factors, and the treatment modalities available. Cancer risk assessment must be an integral part of every interaction the nurse has with the public. Data obtained from interviews, the nursing history, physical examinations, social and family histories, health surveys and questionnaires, and employment records help the nurse determine the person's individual cancer risk factors.

Nurses can inform women that the breast, lung, gastrointestinal tract, and uterus are the most common sites of cancer in women. Women should be taught to examine their breasts each month immediately after the menstrual period or, after menopause, on a designated day each month and to have mammography at regular intervals. Even though the value of breast self-evaluation (BSE) in early detection has not been confirmed through research, nurses should still encourage BSE until conclusive evidence is found. Women of all ages should know the importance of reporting any abnormal vaginal bleeding or discharge that occurs between menstrual periods or after menopause. Women are encouraged to have routine gastrointestinal screening and gynecologic examinations and to take precautions against sexually transmitted diseases. (See Chapter 56 for information about early symptoms of cancer of the female reproductive system.)

Nurses should ensure that men are aware that their risk is greatest for cancers of the prostate, lung, and gastrointestinal tract. They should encourage men to have regular screening for colorectal cancer with routine fecal occult blood testing and colonoscopy, and screening for prostate cancer with the digital rectal examination and PSA test. The incidence of testicular cancer overall is small; however, it is most prevalent in young men between the ages of 15 and 40 years. Regular testicular self-examination, like BSE in women, is important for this age group.

Older adults as a group require more individualized health teaching about cancer risk and detection methods. This population may already have other chronic illnesses and take various medications. New symptoms, therefore, may be difficult to recognize as early warning signs of cancer. Older adults may also be reluctant to undergo routine screening or to report new physical complaints because of their fears of cancer, a tenuous financial state, or feelings of hopelessness if cancer is diagnosed. Health care professionals need to encourage older patients to participate in health education and screening programs and tailor these programs to the unique needs of this population. Nurses in all settings need to incorporate cancer assessment and teaching about early detection into the care of older patients.

Radiotherapy

Radiotherapy, or the use of radiation in the treatment of disease, has been used since the discovery of x rays in 1895 and radium in 1898. Today, radiotherapy is used for more than half of patients with cancer at some point. Radiotherapy can be prescribed as a single, curative modality; used as a palliative measure to relieve the symptoms of metastatic disease; or combined in a multitude of ways with chemotherapy and surgery.

Radiation Physics

Ionizing radiation, either natural or manufactured, contains energy that is capable of breaking the chemical bonds in molecules, which can lead to cellular damage or cell death. Therapeutic ionizing radiation is classified into two types: electromagnetic and particulate. Electromagnetic radiation includes x rays and gamma rays—energy rays that have no mass. Special machines produce x rays, and radioactive materials emit gamma rays. Both x rays and gamma rays penetrate deep into tissue before releasing their energy and causing cellular changes. Particulate radiation has mass and includes particles of radiation such as electrons, neutrons, and alpha particles. Because of their mass, these particles cannot penetrate deeply into tissues and instead release their energy into cells close to the surface (Figure 23-6). Radiotherapy is prescribed in units called grays (Gy) or in centigrays (cGy). In the past the dosage was measured by the amount of radiant energy absorbed by tissues, expressed in the unit rad.[22]

Radiation Biology

Ionizing radiation causes cell death either through direct damage to the double strands of DNA or as a consequence of biochemical changes that interfere with cellular repair and reproduction. Before prescribing radiotherapy, the radiation oncologist determines the radiosensitivity of the target tissue. **Radiosensitivity** is a measure of the potential susceptibility of cells to injury from ionizing radiation and the speed at which damage will occur. All body tissue has a known degree of radiosensitivity (Table 23-13). The radiation oncologist calculates the maximal treatment dosage that can be administered without compromising the normal tissues surrounding the tumor. Other considerations include the

TABLE 23-12 AMERICAN CANCER SOCIETY RECOMMENDATIONS FOR EARLY DETECTION OF CANCER IN AVERAGE-RISK ASYMPTOMATIC PEOPLE

Cancer Site	Population	Test or Procedure	Frequency
Breast	Women, ages 20+	Breast self-examination (BSE)	Monthly self BSE is an option for women starting in their 20s. Any changes should be promptly reported to their health professional.
		Clinical breast examination (CBE)	CBE should be part of periodic health examination, preferably at least every 3 years for women in their 20s and 30s and every year for women age 40 and over.
		Mammography	Begin annual mammography at age 40.* Women at increased risk should consult with their health care professional about the benefits and risks of additional or more frequent screening.
Colorectal	Men and women, ages 50+	Fecal occult blood test (FOBT),†or fecal immunochemical test (FIT)	Annual, starting at age 50 *or*
		Flexible sigmoidoscopy	Every 5 years, starting at age 50 *or*
		FOBT or FIT, and flexible sigmoidoscopy‡	Annual FOBT or FIT, and flexible sigmoidoscopy, every 5 years, starting at age 50 *or*
		Colonoscopy	Every 10 years starting at age 50 *or*
		Double-contrast barium enema	Every 5 years starting at age 50.
Prostate	Men, ages 50+	Digital rectal examination (DRE) and prostate-specific antigen test (PSA)	Both PSA test and DRE should be offered annually, starting at age 50, for men who have a life expectancy of at least 10 yr.¶ Men at higher risk should begin testing at age 45 or even age 40.
Cervix	Women, ages 18+	Pap test	Cervical cancer screening should begin approximately 3 years after woman begins having vaginal intercourse but no later than 21 years of age. —Annually with conventional Pap tests or every 2 years with liquid-based tests —Every 2-4 years for women over 30 who have three normal tests in a row; women at higher risk should continue annual screening —Women over 70 with no abnormal tests in 10 years may stop screening; women who have had a total hysterectomy may also stop screening.
Endometrial	Women, at menopause	Women at average risk should be informed about risks and symptoms of endometrial cancer and strongly encouraged to report any unexpected bleeding or spotting to their physicians.	
Cancer-related checkup	Men and women, ages 20+	At periodic health examination, cancer-related checkup should include health counseling and screening for cancers of thyroid, testicles, ovaries, lymph nodes, oral cavity, and skin.	

From Smith RA, Cokkinides V, Eyre HJ: American Cancer Society guidelines for the early detection of cancer, *CA* 55:31–44, 2005.
*Beginning at age 40, annual CBE should be performed before mammography.
†The take-home multiple sample method of FOBT should be used.
‡Flexible sigmoidoscopy together with FOBT or FIT is preferred compared with FOBT or FIT or flexible sigmoidoscopy alone.
¶Information should be provided to men about benefits and limitations of testing so that they can make an informed decision about testing with the clinician's assistance.

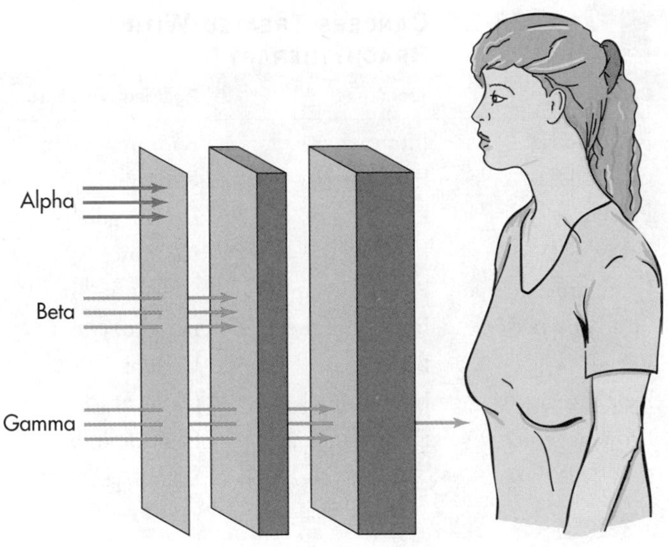

Figure 23-6 Relative penetrating power of three types of radiation.

patient's age, tumor size and stage, degree of spread, and overall prognosis if radiation is used to treat the tumor.

Cells that are in the mitosis (M) phase of the cell cycle are the most sensitive to the effects of radiation; however, damage also may occur during DNA synthesis (S phase). Tissues that have high proliferative rates, such as the bone marrow, skin, and gastrointestinal tract, are most affected by radiation. Tumor resistance to radiation can be a major problem that is usually related to tissue hypoxia. Hypoxic cells are known to be radioresistant and require about three times as much radiation as a well-oxygenated cell to achieve the same degree of cell kill.[31] Cell kill refers to the number of tumor cells expected to be destroyed after a radiation treatment. Tumor cells become hypoxic when they outgrow the nearest capillary blood supply during their growth. The mechanism of how hypoxia makes a cell radioresistant is not fully understood.

TABLE 23-13 RADIOSENSITIVITY OF SELECTED BODY ORGANS

Organ	Radiosensitivity
Bone marrow	High
Ovaries	
Testes	
Intestine	
Skin	Medium high
Oral cavity and esophagus	
Vagina, cervix	
Growing bone and cartilage	Medium
Fine vasculature	
Mature bone and cartilage	Medium low
Kidney	
Liver	
Thyroid	
Muscle	Low
Brain and spinal cord	

Although the goal of radiotherapy is to achieve maximal tumor cell kill while sparing normal tissue, it is impossible to completely avoid injury. The total dose of radiation is divided into multiple small doses and is typically delivered daily over a period of weeks, a process called fractionization. This theoretically allows the normal cells time to repair themselves. Cancer cells do not have the same ability as normal cells to repair and reverse the changes caused by radiation and are more likely to die. Hyper or accelerated fractionization, two or more treatments per day, may be used in selected cases. Radiotherapy may also be delivered as a "split course" of therapy, where the patient receives part of the total dose followed by a rest of 1 to 2 weeks until the final cumulative dose is given. This plan is advantageous for several reasons. Normal cells that received a sublethal dose of radiation have time to repair the damage. Tumor cells that were in a nonsensitive cell cycle phase may progress to a more radiosensitive phase; therefore a larger cell kill can be attained when treatment is resumed.

Types of Radiotherapy

Radiotherapy can be delivered to the patient in two ways. External radiation, or teletherapy, directs radiation from an external source toward the body. External sources of radiotherapy are usually megavoltage machines, such as the linear accelerator, which produce gamma and electron radiation. An external radiation treatment can range from 1 minute to a few minutes. The exact duration depends on the dose delivered, the energy, type of radiation beam, and depth of the tumor.

Brachytherapy, or internal radiation, places a radioactive source directly inside the body. The radioactive source may be sealed in a needle, seed, or wire and temporarily implanted in the tumor. The radioactive source may also be unsealed and administered in the form of a systemic intravenous or oral preparation.

External Radiotherapy. External radiation may be used alone or in conjunction with surgery. Used alone, radiotherapy can cure cancer of the skin, oral cavity, larynx, uterine cervix, prostate, pelvis, and early stages of Hodgkin's disease. When radiation is used in conjunction with surgery, it is used either for cure or palliation of symptoms. Cancers of the head and neck, lung, breast, uterus, bladder, bone, and testes can be cured with combined surgery and radiation.

Radiation may be administered before or after surgery. Preoperative treatment decreases tumor size, increases the potential for removal of the entire tumor during surgery, eradicates subclinical disease that might be present beyond the intended surgical field, and eradicates lymph nodes where disease could form or support metastasis. The major disadvantage of preoperative radiation is a delay in wound healing in normal tissues that were within the treatment field.

Postoperative radiotherapy is usually performed to eradicate any residual tumor and subclinical disease. Higher doses can be administered than could have been used before surgery. The most cited disadvantage of postoperative radiotherapy is the need to delay the treatment until postoperative wound healing is complete. Stereotactic radiosurgery is a specialized technique that delivers a single dose of radiation directly to intracranial lesions (gamma knife) and small tumors in extracranial sites. External radiotherapy also is frequently combined with chemotherapy.

A number of medications, called radiosensitizers, can be used to enhance the effect of radiotherapy. These drugs act in a variety of ways such as changing the oxygenation of the targeted tissue. Other medications are radioprotectors, which help protect tissue against the damage caused by radiotherapy.

Pretreatment Preparation. Before administering any external radiotherapy, the radiation oncologist thoroughly examines the patient and initiates a simulation, or planning, phase. The oncologist defines the precise target area where the tumor is located; the anatomic area that will receive the radiation, called a port, is outlined with either ink markings or small permanent tattoo markings. These outlines are essential so that only the small, defined area receives the radiation.

Different ports may be used on different days, or the port position may be changed at intervals so that an optimal yet safe dose of radiation can be given through each port. The patient may need to assume difficult or uncomfortable positions during the treatment, and immobilization is critical for accurate delivery of the radiation. Immobilizing or positioning devices made specifically for the patient can help maintain proper positioning during the treatment. Pediatric and elderly patients often require casts or molds, special boards, or safety belts to help them maintain the correct position. The need for organ-shielding devices also is determined during simulation.

The pretreatment phase may require several sessions in the radiation oncology department. A picture of the patient in the exact desired position, with immobilizing devices and shields in place, is kept in the patient's treatment file. The photograph helps the technicians who administer the radiation to correctly position the patient for each treatment. The technician documents the treatment number, cumulative dose, patient position, immobilizing devices, and any specific patient concerns or problems.

Brachytherapy (Internal Radiotherapy). A number of cancers can be successfully treated with brachytherapy (Table 23-14). Internal radiation may be delivered by sealed or unsealed techniques. In either type of brachytherapy, special precautions are necessary because care providers can be exposed to the radioactive source. The radiation safety measures employed are based on the radioisotope used, its location, and the radiation emitted.

Sealed Internal Radiotherapy. Sealed internal radiotherapy is used to deliver a concentrated dose of radiation directly to the malignant lesion or tumor area at a low-dose rate (LDR) or a high-dose rate (HDR). LDR brachytherapy usually involves insertion of radioactive substances within hollow cavities or within tissues. Table 23-15 lists radioisotopes commonly used in brachytherapy. These radioactive substances may be placed in molds, plaques, needles, wires, special applicators, or ribbons.

Placement of the sealed container is carried out in the operating room, radiation department, or a treatment room. Exact positioning of the container is essential so the tumor receives the maximal dose of radiation while exposure of normal tissues and organs is minimized. X-ray films are taken to verify appropriate placement. The patient then returns to a private hospital room where the

Table 23-14 Cancers Treated With Brachytherapy

Cancer	Technique	Radioactive Source
Endometrial	Intracavitary	Radium, cesium
Cervical	Intracavitary	Radium, cesium
Prostate	Interstitial	Iodine, gold
Breast	Interstitial	Iridium
Ocular melanoma	Plaque therapy	Cobalt, iodine
Head and neck	Interstitial thermal	Iridium, cesium
Rectal	Interstitial	Cesium
Esophageal	Intraluminal	Cesium
Bronchogenic	Endobronchial	Iridium, iodine

From Dow KH et al: *Nursing care in radiation oncology,* ed 2, Philadelphia, 1997, Saunders.

Table 23-15 Radioisotopes and Their Properties

Radioisotope	Symbols	Half-Life	Type
Cesium 137	^{137}Cs	30 yr	Beta, gamma
Gold 198	^{198}Au	2.7 days	Beta, gamma
Iodine 125	^{125}I	60 days	Beta, gamma
Iodine 131	^{131}I	8 days	Beta, gamma
Iridium 192	^{192}Ir	74.4 days	Beta, gamma
Phosphorus 32	^{32}P	14.3 days	Beta
Radium 226	^{226}Ra	1620 yr	Alpha, gamma
Strontium 90	^{90}Sr	28.1 yr	Beta

From Dow KH et al: *Nursing care in radiation oncology,* ed 2, Philadelphia, 1997, Saunders.

radioactive substance is inserted. This technique is called afterloading and is used to prevent unnecessary exposure of staff members in various departments to the radiation source.[31] The length of time the radiation material is left in place depends on the element used and the dose prescribed. Time ranges from a few hours to several days, and the patient remains hospitalized for this period.

HDR brachytherapy is a second technique for positioning an applicator in the tumor cavity. The radiation source, in the form of pellets or tubes, is loaded into the applicator through wires by remote control and then unloaded at the end of the treatment, which typically lasts several minutes. HDR treatments may be scheduled weekly for several weeks. HDR brachytherapy can be completed in an outpatient setting and does not require hospitalization.

Unsealed Internal Radiotherapy. Unsealed internal radiation is delivered to the patient by mouth or as an intravenous solution. An example is the radioisotope iodine 131, which is used to treat thyroid cancer. Because the isotope is excreted in body fluids, persons caring for the patient can be exposed to the radiation from the patient (external exposure) or from contact with the patient's discharges, which contain the radioactive substance (internal exposure). It may be inhaled, ingested, or absorbed through the skin. The mode of elimination from the body varies with the specific isotope, but generally traces are found in urine, feces, emesis, sputum, wound drainage, and perspiration. The exposure risk varies with each of the substances used, and safety for the staff members caring for the patient depends on a thorough knowledge of the substance and its action within the body. Caregivers need to follow specific instructions from radiation oncology personnel to minimize radiation exposure when working with these patients. Special precautions are not needed with the trace doses used for diagnostic procedures.

Other radioisotopes commonly used for unsealed brachytherapy include radioactive phosphorus (^{32}P) and gold (^{198}Au). These substances may be administered orally, intravenously, or by direct instillation into a body cavity. Each isotope is a potential source of radiation exposure for health care personnel.

Protection of Health Care Professionals From Radiation Hazards

Radiation treatment rooms are shielded with concrete and lead walls, and no one enters the room during the treatment. Patients with internal radiation sources that emit gamma rays expose caregivers to radiation for varying periods, and the length of time that a staff member can be safely exposed is an important consideration in planning care.

Exposure to radiation can be controlled in three ways: time, distance, and shielding. Caregivers should both minimize the total time spent with the patient and maximize their distance from the patient. Radiation is subject to the inverse-square law: a person who stands 2 m away from the source of radiation receives only one fourth as much exposure as when standing only 1 m away. At 4 m only one sixteenth of the exposure is received (Figure 23-7). Lead gloves and aprons are used during x-ray and fluoroscopy procedures, but lead is insufficient to block gamma rays during brachytherapy.[41] Shields, however, may be effective reminders to caregivers to more safely manage the time spent with the patient. Some hospitals have single, lead-lined rooms designated for implant patients. Radiation safety guidelines require that personnel who deliver radiotherapy or care for brachytherapy patients wear dosimetry badges to measure their radiation exposure. Care for brachytherapy patients is rotated among a team of nurses, and no pregnant caregiver is assigned to deliver care.

Staff education is important to ensure compliance with the safety and monitoring procedures involved with radiotherapy. Hospitals in which therapeutic doses of radioactive isotopes are administered are required to designate a radiation safety officer. The radiation safety officer, often a physicist, determines the precautions to be observed in each situation, and nurses consult the safety officer to address questions and concerns. Most hospitals post printed instruction sheets on the door of the patient's room that detail the precautions to be followed and warn all staff of the radiation risk. Health care personnel should be fully acquainted with all precautions and meticulous in carrying them out.

Side Effects of Radiotherapy

Because radiotherapy is a local treatment, most side effects are site specific, depending on which organs and tissues are within or close to the treatment field. Side effects can be classified as acute or late (Table 23-16). Acute toxicities occur within days and affect tissues with a rapid renewal rate, such as the skin, bone marrow, and mucosal lining of the gastrointestinal tract and vagina. Late toxicities occur months or years after treatment and may be due to injury to the blood vessels and connective tissue that surround the treatment field. Late effects include cataracts, pulmonary fibrosis, and strictures.

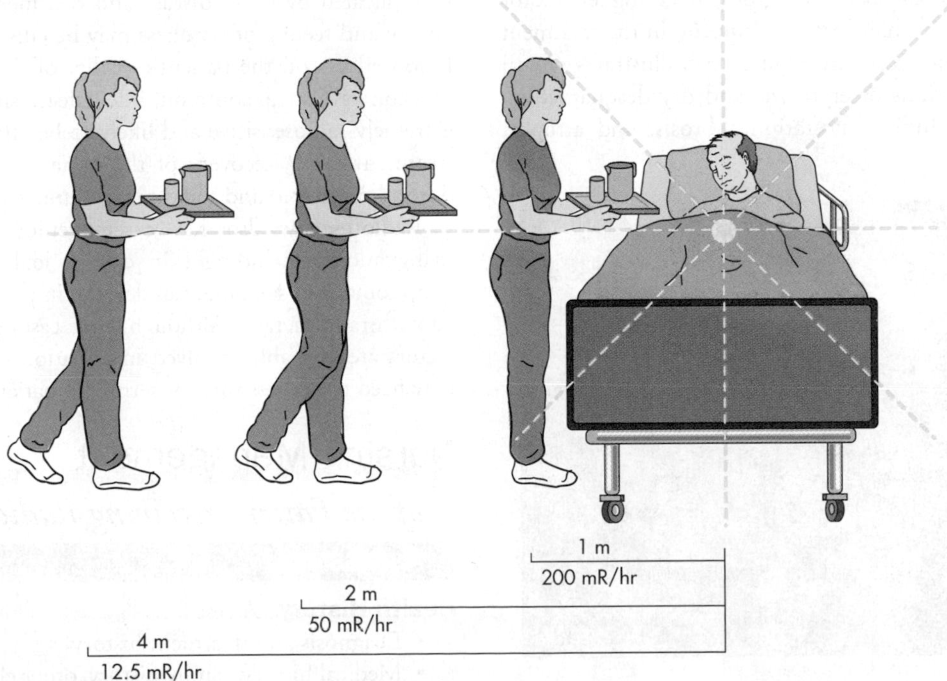

Figure 23-7 Nurse nearest source of radioactivity (patient) is exposed to more radioactivity.

TABLE 23-16 POSSIBLE SEQUELAE OF RADIOTHERAPY

Anatomic Site	Acute Sequelae (Early)	Late Sequelae
Brain	Earache, headache, dizziness, hair loss, erythema	Hearing loss, damage to middle or inner ear, pituitary gland dysfunction, cataracts, brain necrosis
Head and neck	Odynophagia, dysphagia, hoarseness, xerostomia, parageusia, weight loss	Subcutaneous fibrosis, skin ulceration, necrosis, thyroid dysfunction, dental decay, osteoradionecrosis of mandible, delayed wound healing, damage to middle and inner ear
Lung and mediastinum or esophagus	Odynophagia, dysphagia, cough, hoarseness pneumonitis, carditis	Progressive fibrosis of lung, dyspnea, chronic cough; esophageal stricture Rare: chronic pericarditis, myelopathy
Breast or chest wall	Odynophagia, dysphagia, hoarseness, cough; pneumonitis (asymptomatic); carditis; cytopenia	Fibrosis, retraction of breast; lung fibrosis; arm edema; chronic endocarditis, myocardial infarction Rare: osteoradionecrosis of ribs
Abdomen or pelvis	Nausea, vomiting, abdominal pain, diarrhea; urinary frequency, dysuria, nocturia; cytopenia	Proctitis, sigmoiditis; rectal or sigmoid stricture; colonic perforation or obstruction; contracted bladder, urinary incontinence, hematuria, vesicovaginal fistula; rectovaginal fistula; leg edema; scrotal edema, sexual impotency; vaginal retraction or scarring; sterilization Rare: damage to liver or kidneys
Extremities	Erythema, dry or moist desquamation	Subcutaneous fibrosis: ankylosis, edema; bone and soft tissue necrosis

From Perez CA, Brady LW: *Principles and practices of radiation oncology,* ed 3, Philadelphia, 1998, Lippincott.

Most patients receiving radiotherapy experience skin reactions in the treatment port. Slight initial erythema, from the effect of radiation on capillary blood flow, progresses to pronounced erythema in 2 to 3 weeks and then fades. The skin reaction may progress further to dry desquamation and then moist desquamation. Skin folds, such as the axilla and groin, are at higher risk for skin reactions. Temporary hair loss, or **alopecia**, in the treatment area also occurs in about 3 weeks. Figure 23-8 illustrates typical radiotherapy skin reactions of erythema and dry desquamation. Long-term effects, including ulceration, fibrosis, and atrophy, may occur months after irradiation is completed and are attributed to changes in endothelial permeability, edema, and increased skin temperature. Scoring systems are available to evaluate skin toxicity (Table 23-17).

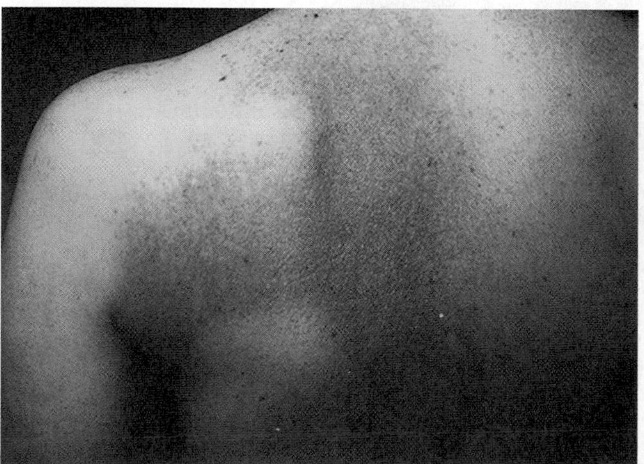

Figure 23-8 Erythema and dry desquamation of skin in response to external radiotherapy.

Nearly all patients receiving radiotherapy experience fatigue. Complicated by other disease and treatment factors, the loss of energy and feeling of tiredness may be cumulative and have profound effects on the patient's quality of life. Bone marrow suppression is also a common side effect, since bone marrow is extremely radiosensitive and likely to be affected in almost every treatment port. Recovery of the bone marrow depends on the dose administered and the tumor volume treated.

Radiotherapy also has carcinogenic potential. Secondary malignancies, including skin cancer, leukemia, non-Hodgkin's lymphoma, and sarcoma, can develop in patients previously treated with radiotherapy. Although these cases are rare and multiple factors are probably involved in radiation carcinogenesis, nurses may need to address this concern with patients.

Nursing Management

of the Patient receiving Radiotherapy

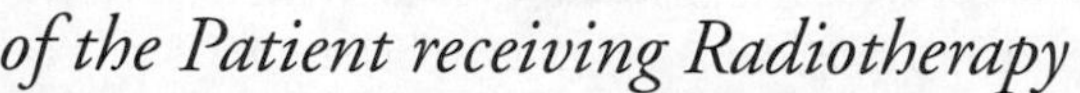

ASSESSMENT

Health History. Assess for:

- Diagnosis and treatment history
- Medical history, family history, other chronic illnesses and treatment
- Medications in use: prescription, over the counter, herbal

TABLE 23-17 ACUTE RADIATION MORBIDITY SCORING CRITERIA (RTOG) AND LATE RADIATION MORBIDITY SCORING SCHEME (RTOG, EORTC) FOR SKIN

0	Grade 1	Grade 2	Grade 3	Grade 4	Grade 5
ACUTE MORBIDITY					
No change over baseline	Follicular, faint or dull erythema, epilation, dry desquamation, decreased sweating	Tender or bright erythema, patchy moist desquamation, moderate edema	Confluent, moist desquamation, other than skin folds; pitting edema	Ulceration, hemorrhage, necrosis	
LATE MORBIDITY					
None	Slight atrophy, pigmentation change, some hair loss	Patchy atrophy, moderate telangiectasia, total hair loss	Marked atrophy, gross telangiectasia	Ulceration	Death directly related to radiation late effect

- Allergies to foods, drugs, other
- Social support, availability of transportation services
- Financial resources, insurance coverage for planned treatment
- Knowledge of treatment plan, goals of therapy, number and schedule of treatments planned
- Knowledge of expected treatment side effects, restrictions
- Fears and concerns related to radiation treatment

Physical Examination. Assess for:

- Performance status, self-care abilities or limitations
- Nutritional status, weight gain or loss, appetite
- Elimination pattern, concerns
- Mobility status, limitations
- Skin and mucous membrane integrity, treatment port and markings

NURSING DIAGNOSES, OUTCOMES, AND INTERVENTIONS

Nursing Diagnosis: Risk for Impaired Skin Integrity

OUTCOMES. Common examples of expected outcomes for the patient with a diagnosis of *risk for impaired skin integrity* are:

Patient will:

- Implement appropriate skin protection interventions.
- Maintain intact skin over the radiation ports.

NURSING INTERVENTIONS. Skin care measures vary among institutions, but generally include measures to keep the skin clean, dry, and protected from irritants (see the Guidelines for Safe Practice box). The nurse provides the patient with written instructions about skin care and verifies that the patient understands. The nurse also provides support and interventions for patients who have lost scalp hair, since this side effect may be particularly distressing. Specific skin care measures are warranted if moist desquamation occurs. Various ointments and dressings may be prescribed for skin protection and comfort.

RELATED NIC INTERVENTIONS. Radiation Therapy Management, Skin Surveillance, Teaching: Procedure/Treatment

Nursing Diagnosis: Fatigue

OUTCOMES. A common example of an expected outcome for the patient with a diagnosis of *fatigue* is:

Patient will:

- Exhibit sufficient energy to complete daily self-care activities.

NURSING INTERVENTIONS. Decreased energy levels and fatigue are common symptoms during radiotherapy, especially when daily treatments are given over several months. Concurrent problems such as anemia, malnutrition, and recovery from surgery may worsen the fatigue from radiotherapy. The nurse

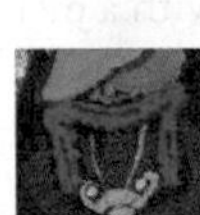

GUIDELINES FOR SAFE PRACTICE
Preventing Skin Irritation During Radiotherapy

- Cleanse radiation field (area within ink markings or inside tattoo outline) daily with mild soap and water. *Do not* erase ink markings if present.
- Clean and keep dry any skin folds that overlap and places where moisture collects (abdominal skin folds, under and between pendulous breasts, between buttocks or perineum).
- Avoid use of perfumed soaps, lotions, or deodorant on involved skin surface.
- Guard against irritation from belts, bras, and rough clothing on treatment field. Cotton clothing is least irritating.
- Do not use heating pads, hot water bottles, or ices packs on treatment field.
- Avoid exposure to sunlight. If unavoidable, use sunscreen for protection.
- Use an electric razor only to shave within treatment area.
- Avoid scratching, vigorous rubbing, or massage of the treatment field.
- Do not apply any lotions, powders, or ointments to treated area unless advised to do so by radiologist.

assesses for the severity and impact of fatigue on the patient's quality of life. Several performance scales, such as the Karnofsky Scale (Box 23-6), are available to help evaluate the patient's functional status. Other useful tools are the Eastern Cooperative Oncology Group (ECOG) scale and the World Health Organization scale, which gives the patient a score of 0 (bedridden or totally disabled) to 4 (asymptomatic and independent). The availability of support systems is another important consideration, since the patient may be unable to meet all of his or her work and family obligations.

Treatable factors that contribute to fatigue, such as anemia and pain, are addressed as thoroughly as possible. The nurse encourages patients to incorporate rest periods throughout the day and ensure adequate sleep at night. The nurse may need to counsel patients about reducing activities that demand too much energy, incorporating a mild exercise or activity plan into the daily routine, and using distraction or relaxation techniques. These strategies are all known to help with fatigue. It is difficult to overestimate how debilitating fatigue can be for the patient, and nurses make every effort to provide support and encouragement with this difficult symptom.

RELATED NIC INTERVENTIONS. Energy Management, Sleep Enhancement, Support System Enhancement

Nursing Diagnosis: Risk for Imbalanced Nutrition: Less Than Body Requirements

OUTCOMES. Common examples of expected outcomes for the patient with a diagnosis of *risk for imbalanced nutrition: less than body requirements* are:

Patient will:

- Maintain adequate nutritional intake and desired weight.
- Experience a normal bowel elimination pattern.
- Maintain moist, intact oral mucous membranes.

NURSING INTERVENTIONS. Maintaining good nutrition with a diet high in carbohydrates, protein, and calories supplies the necessary energy for daily activities. The cancer's catabolic activity may combine with treatment side effects such as anorexia to make maintenance of good nutrition difficult. The nurse incorporates nutritional assessment into routine care. The patient may experience compromised nutrition before treatment, with moderate to severe weight loss, decreased muscle mass, and loss of adipose tissue. The nurse and dietary support team are challenged to devise a plan for nutritional support that the patient can accept and follow. The nurse checks weight at least weekly to determine whether the patient's dietary intake is sufficient or additional supplements are needed.

Patients receiving radiotherapy to abdominal ports are at risk for both nausea and diarrhea, and the nurses assesses regularly for these symptoms. Nausea can usually be controlled with the regular use of an antiemetic. The nurse encourages the patient to consume a low-residue diet and use antidiarrheal agents as needed. Assessment of fluid and electrolyte status is imperative when these side effects are severe to prevent dehydration and electrolyte abnormalities.

Mucositis, or inflammation of the mucosal membranes of the gastrointestinal or genitourinary tract, occurs when this tissue is included in the radiation port. The inflammation can be severe, causing pain, ulceration, and bleeding. When mucositis occurs in the mouth and throat, the nurse implements measures to keep the mouth and throat clean. Mouth rinses, such as salt and peroxide solutions, are usually recommended for cleansing. Patients should avoid spicy and acidic foods, alcohol, and tobacco. Patients may have difficulty swallowing and complain of heartburnlike pain. Local anesthetics and systemic analgesics may be necessary to relieve pain. Radiotherapy to mouth and throat ports causes a severe dry mouth, called xerostomia, as well as taste changes, called parageusia. The nurse educates patients about dietary strategies to deal with these symptoms (e.g., the use of artificial saliva solutions) and stresses the importance of mouth care measures (see the Guidelines for Safe Practice box). Patients receiving therapy through head and neck ports may require aggressive nutritional support (e.g., placement of a percutaneous feeding tube and the use of enteral feedings).

RELATED NIC INTERVENTIONS. Nutrition Management, Oral Health Maintenance, Radiation Therapy Management, Weight Management

Box 23-6 Karnofsky Performance Scale*

Normal; no complaints; no evidence of disease	100
Able to carry on normal activity; minor signs or symptoms of disease	90
Normal activity with effort; some signs or symptoms of disease	80
Cares for self; unable to carry on normal activity or to do active work	70
Requires occasional assistance but is able to care for most needs	60
Requires considerable assistance and frequent medical care	50
Disabled; requires special care and assistance	40
Severely disabled; hospitalization is indicated, although death is not imminent	30
Hospitalization is necessary; very sick; active supportive treatment necessary	20
Moribund; fatal processes progressing rapidly	10
Dead	0

*A subjective assessment tool to assess and compare the patient's activity and performance ability.

Nursing Diagnosis: Risk for Infection

OUTCOMES. Common examples of expected outcomes for the patient with a diagnosis of *risk for infection* are:

Patient will:

- Maintain a normal body temperature.
- Exhibit no signs of infection.

NURSING INTERVENTIONS. The nurse monitors laboratory studies at intervals during treatment to determine the effects of therapy on bone marrow production of white blood cells (WBCs), red blood cells (RBCs), and platelets. The nurse also assesses patients for early signs of infection, anemia, and bleeding, which can result from bone marrow suppression, especially in patients receiving concurrent chemotherapy. Interventions to manage these serious complications, such as antibiotic therapy, blood transfusions, and growth factor support, may be necessary to complete the course of radiotherapy. Myelosuppression is discussed in more detail on p. 545. The nurse instructs patients about the importance of basic

GUIDELINES FOR SAFE PRACTICE
Mouth Care for the Patient receiving Radiotherapy or Chemotherapy

- Brush teeth with a soft toothbrush after meals, after snacks, and at bedtime.
- Rinse mouth after brushing with salt solution (½ tsp of salt in 8 oz of water) or with mouthwash containing less than 6% alcohol.
- Remove and clean dentures after meals, after snacks, and at bedtime. Do not wear dentures that do not fit well or when the mouth is sore.
- Floss teeth at least daily. Omit flossing if it causes pain or if at high risk for infection or bleeding.
- Apply protective lubrication to lips.
- Avoid irritants, such as tobacco and alcohol.
- If mouth dryness occurs:
  —Increase mouth rinses to every 2 to 4 hours.
  —Increase fluid intake.
  —Consider use of artificial saliva.
- If mouth soreness develops:
  —Use topical anesthetics.
  —Implement dietary strategies to avoid foods that are spicy, hard, coarse, or acidic.
  —Consider use of systemic analgesics.
- If infection develops, use local or systemic antimicrobial medications.
- Consult with health care providers before having any dental procedures.

measures such as meticulous personal hygiene, frequent mouth care, and hand washing as primary strategies for avoiding infection. Patients are also encouraged to avoid exposure to individuals with active viral infections.

Cystitis, urethritis, and vaginitis may occur when radiotherapy is given through a pelvic port. The nurse needs to encourage specific hygiene measures and a high fluid intake to relieve discomfort and assess for and treat any local infections.

RELATED NIC INTERVENTIONS. Environmental Management, Infection Protection, Surveillance, Vital Signs Monitoring

Patient/Family Teaching. The nurse plays a vital role in teaching the patient and family about radiotherapy and dispelling common fears. The nurse clarifies and reinforces information about the number of treatments planned, the body area to be irradiated, and the preliminary planning and treatment sessions. During the initial phases of treatment, the patient needs the nurse's support to adjust to the reality of a new diagnosis of cancer, accept prognostic information, and understand therapy goals. When outpatient radiotherapy is planned, the nurse assesses the type and availability of the patient's support system, financial concerns, and transportation issues. The nurse arranges additional support for any area of need.

Some patients receiving external radiotherapy fear that they will be "radioactive" after treatment and a danger to others around them. Others are anxious that radiation will be painful. Both are misconceptions. No sensation is felt during treatment. The patient is informed that he or she will be alone in the treatment room but continuously monitored on television and able to talk to the radiation technician at all times. Immobilizing devices, such as special molds or casts, may be used to maintain proper body position during treatment. Treatments are generally completed in a matter of minutes. Patients who are anxious or unable to lie still during the treatment period may require sedation. Visiting the radiotherapy facility may allay some common fears.

The nurse teaches the patient about common side effects that may be anticipated with radiotherapy. Because many patients receive radiotherapy on an outpatient basis, teaching about self-care measures to prevent and manage side effects is critical. Radiotherapy also has carcinogenic potential and may lead to secondary malignancies such as skin cancer, leukemia, non-Hodgkin's lymphoma, and sarcoma. Although these cases are rare and multiple factors are probably involved in radiation carcinogenesis, nurses may need to address this concern with patients.

EVALUATION

To evaluate the effectiveness of nursing interventions, compare patient behaviors with those stated in the expected patient outcomes.

RELATED NOC OUTCOMES. Activity Tolerance, Appetite, Energy Conservation, Knowledge: Infection Control, Nutritional Status: Food & Fluid Intake, Self-Care: Hygiene, Self-Care: Instrumental Activities of Daily Living (IADL), Tissue Integrity: Skin & Mucous Membranes, Weight: Body Mass

GERONTOLOGIC CONSIDERATIONS

The patient's age may influence his or her response to the treatment and its success. Immune system function declines with age, regeneration of the bone marrow takes longer, and the effects of fatigue are more pronounced. The skin and mucosa are less elastic and take longer to repair after injury. Consequently, older adults have less tolerance to radiation than younger persons with the same cancer. Finally, older persons may be more fearful and anxious about therapy, especially if they recall experiences with the early days of radiotherapy or have confusion or memory loss related to other illnesses.

Chemotherapy

Advances in knowledge concerning cancer growth and the development of a vast array of chemotherapeutic agents have led to concomitant advances in cancer treatment. Improvement in overall survival and longer disease-free intervals can be directly attributed to the use of chemotherapeutic agents, particularly in combination chemotherapy regimens and as adjuvant therapy. The past 50 years, particularly the past decade, have brought rapid change and excitement into clinical practice.

Chemotherapy, like other treatment modalities, may be used for cure, for long-term control of cancer growth, or for palliation to temporarily shrink a tumor mass. If chemotherapy is used when the malignant cell population is small and likely to be susceptible, complete tumor cell eradication is possible. Table 23-18 shows the responsiveness of various neoplastic diseases to chemotherapy.

TABLE 23-18 NEOPLASTIC DISEASE RESPONSE TO CHEMOTHERAPY

Response	Neoplastic Disease
Cures in advanced cancer	Gestational trophoblastic tumor Acute lymphoblastic leukemia Acute myeloblastic leukemia Hodgkin's disease Non-Hodgkin's lymphoma (children) Diffuse histiocytic lymphoma Burkitt's lymphoma Testicular tumors
Cures with adjuvant chemotherapy	Wilms' tumor Osteogenic sarcoma Rhabdomyosarcoma
Complete remissions and increased survival with chemotherapy or adjuvant chemotherapy	Breast cancer Small cell lung carcinoma Acute myeloblastic leukemia Non-Hodgkin's lymphoma Prostate cancer Chronic myelocytic leukemia Hairy cell leukemia
Complete and partial remissions with uncertain prolongation of survival with chemotherapy or adjuvant chemotherapy	Multiple myeloma Ovarian cancer Endometrial cancer Neuroblastoma Colorectal cancer Liver cancer
Minor responses with chemotherapy or adjuvant chemotherapy; no demonstrable prolongation of life	Non-small cell lung carcinoma Head and neck cancer Stomach cancer Cervical cancer Melanoma Cancer of adrenal cortex Soft tissue sarcoma

Adjuvant chemotherapy refers to chemotherapy administered in conjunction with either surgery or radiotherapy. It is aimed at the destruction of micrometastases believed to be present but too small to be detected by current diagnostic techniques. Left untreated, micrometastases have a high potential for tumor growth and cancer recurrence.

Chemotherapeutic drugs are carefully tested before being approved for use as cancer treatment. The National Cancer Institute coordinates a rigorous drug-screening process for potential new agents. This process identifies compounds with antitumor activity; demonstrates the activity in animal studies; determines the pharmacokinetic characteristics of the drug; and defines dosing levels, adverse effects, and toxicity. Drugs then go through the four phases of clinical trials outlined in Table 23-19. Patients can volunteer to participate in various aspects of clinical trials at cancer treatment centers across the country. Patients receiving cutting-edge treatments need extensive support and education throughout the treatment period.

TABLE 23-19 PHASES OF CLINICAL TRIALS FOR CHEMOTHERAPEUTIC DRUGS

Phase	Purpose
I	Identify toxic reactions; determine optimal dose within safe limits and set schedule
II	Determine extent of antineoplastic activity
III	Compare action of new drug with standard antineoplastic drugs
IV	Determine effect on advanced cancer, effect of combined therapy with other antineoplastic drugs, and effect with adjuvant therapy

Principles of Chemotherapy

Normal and malignant cells progress through various phases in the cell cycle as they replicate. Most chemotherapy agents cause cell death by interrupting cell growth and replication at some point in the cell cycle (Figure 23-9). Drugs are classified by their mechanism of action. Drugs that act during a particular point of the cell cycle are termed *cell cycle phase–specific drugs*, whereas drugs that are active throughout the cell cycle are called *phase-nonspecific drugs* (Figure 23-10). Chemotherapy drugs are selected for use with a particular tumor based on tumor characteristics, such as the fraction of tumor cells in replication at a given time, tumor size, and location.

Cell Population Growth. Chemotherapy is most effective when the tumor is small and growing rapidly, a time when a relatively high proportion of cells are undergoing division. At this time, tumor cells are more sensitive to drugs that are toxic to dividing cells (phase-specific drugs). Larger, slower growing tumors respond better to drugs that act regardless of whether a cell is dividing (phase-nonspecific drugs).

Cell-Kill Hypothesis. Chemotherapy is thought to kill a fixed percentage of the total number of cancer cells. Theoretically, if a drug had a 90% cell-kill rate and 1 million cells were present, the first treatment course would kill 900,000 cancer cells, leaving 100,000. The second treatment would again destroy 90% of the cells, leaving 10,000. Again, theoretically, after a number of chemotherapy treatments, only one cell would remain and that would be killed by the body's immune system (Figure 23-11). The **cell-kill hypothesis** provides the rationale for scheduling chemotherapy in multiple courses over time.[27]

Combination Chemotherapy. Most chemotherapy agents are given as a combination regimen. Combination chemotherapy has a therapeutic effect superior to single-agent therapy for many cancers, since drugs that attack the tumor cells in various ways can produce maximal tumor kill. The use of multiple drugs also decreases the likelihood of the tumor becoming resistant to a specific therapy, a process similar to antibiotic resistance. Drugs included in combination chemotherapy protocols typically:

- Are active when used alone
- Have different mechanisms of action

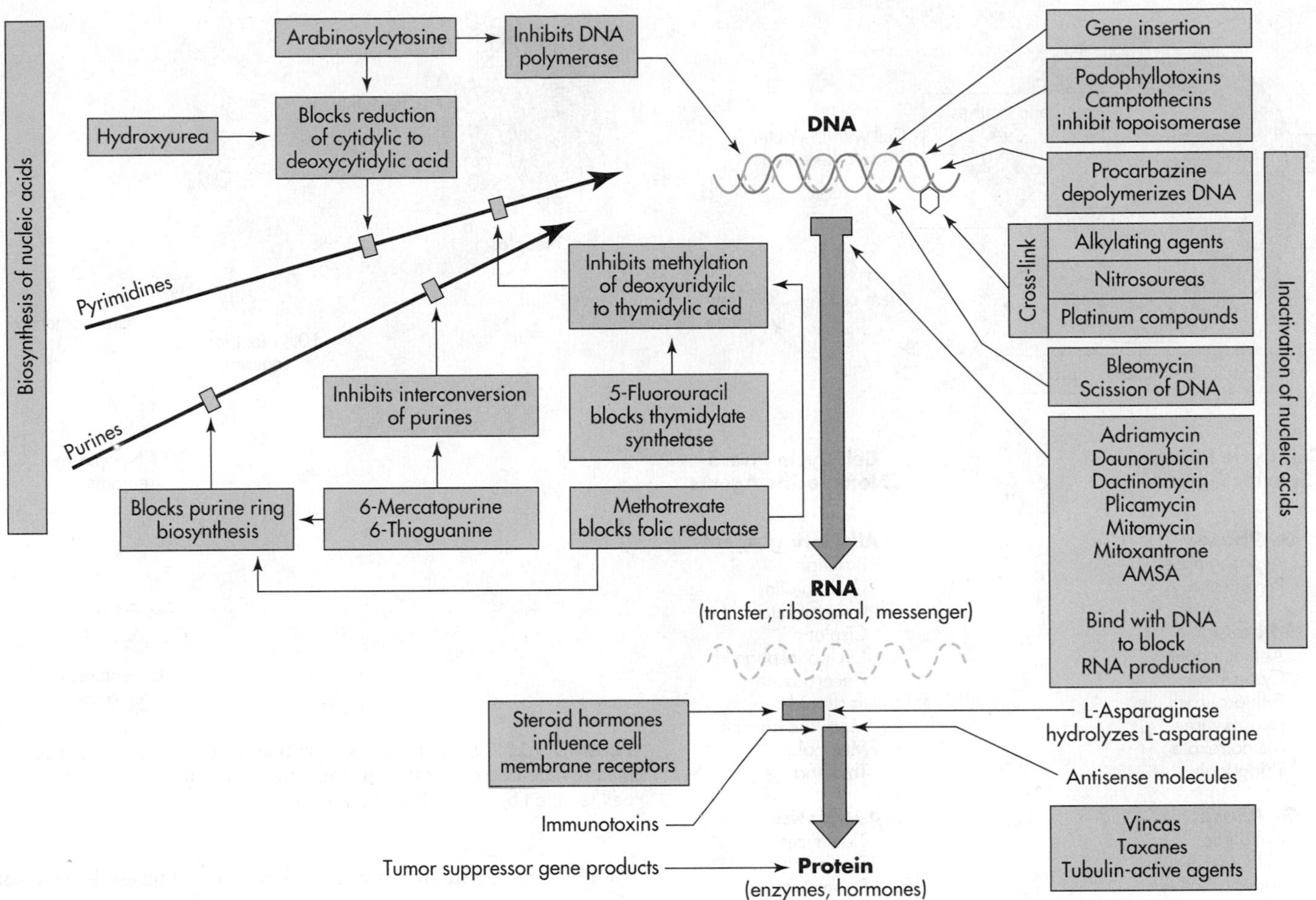

Figure 23-9 Mechanism of action for chemotherapeutic and biologic agents. *DNA*, Deoxyribonucleic acid; *RNA*, ribonucleic acid.

- Have a biochemical basis for possible synergism
- Do not produce toxicity in the same organs
- Produce toxicity at different times after administration

Dose Intensity. Chemotherapy is most effective when sufficient doses of the drugs are delivered within a specified period to achieve maximal tumor kill. Many factors, however, can disrupt the treatment plan, particularly toxicity, which may necessitate dose reductions or delays. Dose reductions often result in a significant reduction in clinical response when highly active cancers are treated. Many options are now available to ensure the dose intensity of curative regimens, including the use of hematopoietic growth factor support.

Tumor Resistance to Chemotherapy. Malignant neoplasms can become resistant to both single and multiple chemotherapeutic agents. This resistance may be present before any treatment has begun, termed *primary resistance*, as a result of a specific genetic trait. Secondary resistance may be acquired during treatment, probably as a result of spontaneous genetic alterations such as mutations, translocations, and deletions, which occur as the cell divides. These genetic alterations then change the drug's mechanism of action or metabolism within the cell. A tumor that initially responded to chemotherapy with shrinkage or decreased growth begins to increase in size or metastasize. Multiple-drug resistance (MDR) can occur when several agents are used in combination, and acquired MDR is documented for many chemotherapeutic drugs.[12] Research into MDR is aimed at identifying the molecular and biochemical changes that lead to resistance.

Chemotherapeutic Agents

Drugs used for chemotherapy may be classified as alkylating agents, antimetabolites, plant (vinca) alkaloids, antitumor antibiotics, and steroids. Table 23-20, pp. 548 to 550, lists chemotherapeutic agents by classification, action, toxicities, and nursing interventions. Chemotherapy injures normal cells as well as cancer cells. The bone marrow, gastrointestinal epithelium, and hair follicles are the most sensitive to chemotherapy because of their high rate of growth. Other side effects include fatigue and organ toxicities that are unique to the particular drug.

Bone Marrow Effects. Many chemotherapeutic agents are toxic to the bone marrow and produce myelosuppression, which results in neutropenia, thrombocytopenia, and anemia. Myelosuppression can be the dose-limiting factor for many drugs, and life-threatening complications of infection and bleeding can result. Each drug has a predictable nadir, or the time when

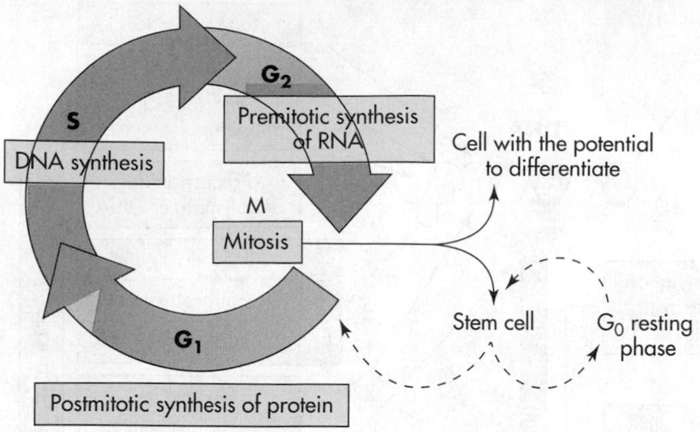

G_2
Premitotic synthesis of RNA
S
DNA synthesis
M
Mitosis
Cell with the potential to differentiate
Stem cell
G_0 resting phase
G_1
Postmitotic synthesis of protein

Cell Cycle Phase–Specific Agents

G_1 Phase
Asparaginase
Prednisone

S Phase
Antimetabolites
Cytarabine
5-fluorouracil
Hydroxyurea
Methotrexate
Thioguanine

G_2 Phase
Antibiotic
Bleomycin
Podophyllotoxin
Etoposide

Mitosis
Vinca alkaloids
Vinblastine
Vincristine
Vindesine
Paclitaxel

Cell Cycle Phase–Nonspecific Agents

Alkylating Agents
Busulfan
Carboplatin
Chlorambucil
Cisplatin
Cyclophosphamide
Dacarbazine
Ifosfamide
Mechlorethamine
Melphalan
Thiotepa

Antibiotics
Bleomycin
Dactinomycin
Daunorubicin
Doxorubicin
Mitomycin

Nitrosoureas
Carmustine (BiCNU)
Lomustine (CCNU)
Semustine (MeCCNU)

Miscellaneous
Mitoxantrone
Navelbine
Procarbazine

Figure 23-10 Common cancer chemotherapeutic agents and their activity within the cell cycle.

WBCs, RBCs, and platelets are at their lowest point. For many drugs, the nadir occurs 7 to 10 days after drug administration.[42] Blood counts are obtained before chemotherapy administration and at regular intervals to identify the nadir and monitor the bone marrow recovery.

The most serious complication of myelosuppression is infection, which is the leading cause of morbidity and mortality in patients with cancer. Neutropenia, or a neutrophil count of less than $1000/mm^3$, is a critical risk factor for infection, since neutrophils form the primary defense against bacterial invasion.[7] A minor infection in a person with neutropenia can result in septic shock within a few hours. Common sites for infections in myelosuppressed persons are the oropharynx, lungs, urinary tract, and skin.

Stomatitis, an inflammation of the oral mucous membranes, is a common side effect of many chemotherapeutic drugs (Box 23-7). Effects range from mild erythema to severe and painful ulcerations

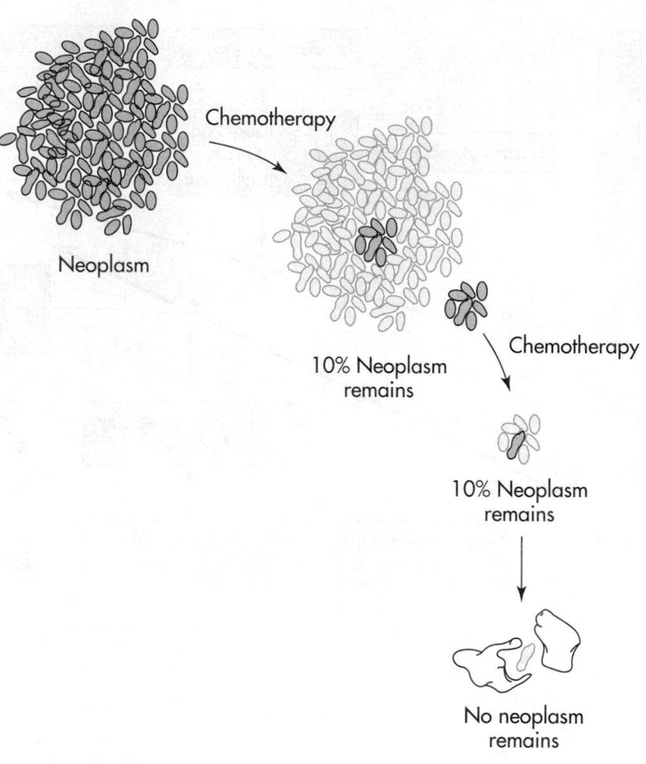

Figure 23-11 Cell-kill theory. Chemotherapy destroys 90% of neoplasm; repeated chemotherapy repeats process until last neoplastic cell is killed by body's immune response.

on the lips and in the mouth and throat.[21] The peak effect of chemotherapy on the mucosal cells occurs 7 to 10 days after treatment and typically parallels the drug's myelosuppressive effects.[4]

The patient is also at a significant risk for bleeding when the platelet count is less than $50,000/mm^3$. Bleeding may be minor, such as bruising or a nosebleed, or can be serious hemorrhage in the brain or gastrointestinal tract.

Patients with anemia exhibit signs of altered tissue perfusion, which can affect every organ system and cause a variety of symptoms, ranging from fatigue, decreased endurance, and headache to tachycardia, angina, dizziness, and dyspnea at rest.

Gastrointestinal Effects. Patients with cancer often identify nausea and vomiting as the most uncomfortable and distressing side effects of chemotherapy. Much progress has been made in understanding how chemotherapy causes nausea and vomiting, and new treatments have dramatically improved the management of these symptoms. In addition to the many chemotherapeutic

Box 23-7 Drugs Causing Stomatitis

- Bleomycin (Blenoxane)
- Doxorubicin (Adriamycin)
- Cytarabine (Ara-C)
- Cyclophosphamide (Cytoxan)
- Daunorubicin (Cerubidine)
- Methotrexate
- 5-Fluorouracil (5-FU)

drugs that can cause severe nausea and vomiting, other physical and emotional factors may also complicate the problem.

Chemotherapy may act as a direct chemical trigger in the chemoreceptor trigger zone (Figure 23-12, p. 551), or may cause secretion of serotonin antagonists (5HT3) by the gastrointestinal tract, which in turn stimulate the vomiting center. Visceral triggers of nausea occur when physical or emotional factors stimulate the vagus nerve. Central nervous system factors, such as psychologic distress, and vestibular mechanisms, which cause vertigo or imbalance, may also play a role. Chemotherapeutic agents vary greatly in their potential to cause nausea (Table 23-21, p. 551). Chemotherapy typically causes a predictable pattern of nausea that peaks within the first 12 hours and may be followed by delayed nausea that lasts 2 to 5 days. Patients may also experience anticipatory nausea, which is a conditioned response that develops after initial courses of chemotherapy.

Patients receiving chemotherapy also commonly experience constipation and diarrhea. These symptoms may be a direct side effect of a particular chemotherapeutic drug and can be exacerbated by factors such as altered dietary intake and activity, other medications such as opioids, or surgical procedures. The gastrointestinal tract is also susceptible to complications of infection and bleeding.

Alopecia. Not all chemotherapeutic drugs cause alopecia, and the degree of hair loss depends on the dose of the drug and method of administration. When it does occur, hair loss ranges from mild thinning on the scalp to complete loss of all body hair. Hair loss usually begins 2 to 3 weeks after the start of therapy and is reversible, with regrowth usually occurring 1 to 2 months after treatment is completed. New hair growth may take up to a year and may have a different thickness and texture.

Fatigue. Fatigue is a common side effect for patients receiving chemotherapy and may seriously compromise the patient's quality of life. Many factors play a role in causing fatigue, including the physical, psychologic, and social changes that result from cancer and cancer therapy, and the anemia that may result from bone marrow suppression. Chemotherapy causes fatigue when cellular metabolism is altered and the end products of cellular destruction accumulate in the body. Fatigue is a subjective experience but does have objective consequences. Fatigued patients complain of feeling weak and having no energy, feelings that are not relieved with adequate rest. They may be unable to complete normal activities of daily living without feeling exhausted.

Sexual Dysfunction. Cancer chemotherapy affects the germinal epithelium of the ovary and testes, and many patients experience reproductive dysfunction during and after chemotherapy. Cycle-nonspecific agents such as the alkylating agents are most commonly associated with altered fertility. For female patients, age is an important predictor of whether these changes will be permanent. Women less than 30 years old are more likely to regain ovarian function because they have more oocytes that are not undergoing constant mitosis. Women may become amenorrheic during chemotherapy, followed by a period of irregular menstrual cycles. Perimenopausal women receiving chemotherapy are likely to become menopausal and develop the short- and long-term symptoms and complications of estrogen depletion. The testes are extremely susceptible to the effects of chemotherapy because of the constant mitosis necessary for sperm production. Testicular damage results in decreased sperm production and sperm and semen abnormalities. The incidence and length of time for recovery depend on the particular drug and dose the patient has received, but both men and women can regain the ability to conceive children after chemotherapy.

Hypersensitivity Reactions. A number of chemotherapeutic drugs are associated with hypersensitivity reactions (Box 23-8, p. 552), and nurses administering or caring for patients receiving these drugs must institute specific precautions. Administration protocols outline specific interventions for the administration of these medications such as the use of premedication, frequent monitoring, and standing orders for emergency care.

Specific Organ Toxicities. Certain chemotherapeutic agents cause specific organ toxicity, affecting the heart, lungs, liver, kidneys, and bladder. The organ damage may be permanent. The anthracycline agents directly damage the cardiac cells. Short-term side effects include electrocardiogram changes; heart failure may develop over time. Pulmonary fibrosis may develop with the use of bleomycin, and other lung toxicities may occur with cytarabine, cyclosphosphamide, and a number of other drugs.[29] Liver toxicity can develop, especially with higher doses of drugs. Nephrotoxicity is a dose-limiting side effect of cisplatin and is also associated with high-dose methotrexate. Hemorrhagic cystitis is a bladder complication seen with cyclophosphamide and ifosfamide use. Drugs that are known to cause irreversible organ damage are administered within cumulative lifetime dose limits.

Some organ toxicity may be prevented or minimized with the use of medications that protect normal tissue, called cryoprotectants. Three cryoprotective agents are currently available for use, but others are under investigation. Dexrazoxane (Zinecard) is used to decrease the cardiotoxicity associated with doxorubicin, and mesna (Mesnex) is used to decrease the hemorrhagic cystitis caused by ifosfamide. The third agent, amifostine (Ethyol), may protect a broad range of normal tissues, including the kidneys, gastrointestinal tract, lungs, and nerves, from the effects of many chemotherapeutic agents. Because cryoprotective agents have a side-effect profile of their own, the risks and benefits of their use must be considered in the treatment plan.

▶ ARE You READY?

In caring for a patient receiving chemotherapy for cancer, the nurse recognizes which of the following as most indicative of myelosuppression?

1. Thrombocytosis
2. Neutropenia
3. Leukocytosis
4. Anemia

Chemotherapy Administration

Chemotherapy administration is primarily the responsibility of a registered nurse who has specific knowledge about the pharmacology and dosing of the drug, as well as competence in drug

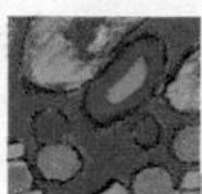

TABLE 23-20
COMMON CHEMOTHERAPEUTIC AGENTS *for Treating Cancer*

Drug	Action	Nursing Intervention
Alkylating Agents*		
Nitrogen Muszards		
Busulfan (Myleran) Cyclophosphamide (Cytoxan) Chlorambucil (Leukeran) Dacarbazine (DTIC) Ifosfamide (Ifex) Melphalan (Alkeran) Nitrogen mustard (mechlorethamine) Thiotepa (Thioplex)	Cell cycle nonspecific and act against already formed nucleic acids by cross-linking DNA strands, thereby preventing DNA replication and transcription of RNA	Monitor for major toxicities: Hematopoietic: Anemia Leukopenia Thrombocytopenia Gastrointestinal: Nausea and vomiting Diarrhea Reproductive: Infertility Change in libido Ovarian and sperm suppression Genitourinary: Cystitis and renal toxicity
Nitrosoureas		
Carmustine (BiCNU) Lomustine (CCNU) Streptozocin (Zanosar)	Alkylating agents that cross blood-brain barrier Also alter functions of cell membrane and mitochondria	Drug specific: Hemorrhagic cystitis (cyclophosphamide and ifosfamide) SIADH (cyclophosphamide)
Platinum-Containing Compounds		
Carboplatin (Paraplatin) Cisplatin (Platinol)		Nephrotoxicity Ototoxicity
Antimetabolites		
Capecitabine (Xeloda) Cytarabine (Ara-C, Cytosar-U) Pentostatin (deoxycoformycin) Floxuridine (FUDR) Fludarabine phosphate Gemcitabine (Gemzar) Methotrexate 6-Mercaptopurine (6-MP) 6-Thioguanine (6-TG) 5-Fluorouracil (5-FU)	Act by interfering with synthesis of chromosomal nucleic acid; antimetabolites are analogs of normal metabolites and block enzyme necessary for synthesis of essential factors or are incorporated into DNA or RNA and thus prevent replication; are cycle specific	Monitor for major toxicities (depends on specific drug): Hematopoietic: Bone marrow suppression Anemia Leukopenia Thrombocytopenia Gastrointestinal: Mucositis, stomatitis Diarrhea Nausea and vomiting Alopecia Photosensitivity (5-fluorouracil, floxuridine, methotrexate)

preparation, administration, and management of toxicity. The ONS recommends, and various state boards of nursing and many health care institutions require, that nurses who administer chemotherapy complete formal chemotherapy education or certification programs to ensure competent practice.

Chemotherapeutic drugs are associated with serious side effects, including carcinogenicity and teratogenicity. Health care workers who handle antineoplastic drugs can be exposed to low doses of the drug by direct contact, inhalation, and injection and can be at risk for some of the same side effects associated with therapeutic use. Because the long-term effects of chronic exposure are not completely known, OSHA and other health care institutions have developed guidelines for safe handling of chemotherapeutic drugs (see Guidelines for Safe Practice box, p. 553). It is essential that any health care provider working with cytotoxic drugs follow these guidelines to prevent injury to self and others.

Chemotherapy doses are usually based on the individual's body surface area (BSA), which is calculated using the patient's height and weight. Both high- and low-dose regimens can be prescribed for many commonly used drugs.[12] It is critical that the drug prescription be accurate and complete to avoid dosing or administration errors. The method of administration for each drug is based on its pharmacokinetic properties and characteristics of the patient and cancer. The route of choice is the one that delivers the optimal

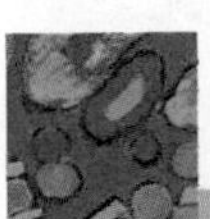

TABLE 23-20
COMMON CHEMOTHERAPEUTIC AGENTS *for Treating Cancer—cont'd*

Drug	Action	Nursing Intervention
Antitumor Antibiotics		
Bleomycin (Blenoxane) Dactinomycin (Actinomycin D, Cosmegen) Daunorubicin (daunamycin) Doxorubicin (Adriamycin) Idarubicin (Idamycin) Mitomycin (Mutamycin) Mitoxantrone (Novantrone) Plicamycin (Mithramycin, Mithracin)	Interfere with synthesis and function of nucleic acids and inhibit RNA and DNA synthesis; are cycle nonspecific	Monitor for major toxicities: Hematopoietic: Bone marrow suppression Gastrointestinal: Mucositis, stomatitis Anorexia, nausea, vomiting Alopecia Tissue necrosis if extravasation of vesicant drugs Cardiac and pulmonary toxicity (doxorubicin, daunorubicin, idarubicin) Pulmonary fibrosis (bleomycin)
Hormonal Agents		
Androgens		
Testosterone propionate Fluoxymesterone (Halotestin)	Alter pituitary function and directly affect malignant cell	Monitor for major toxicities: Fluid retention Masculinization
Corticosteroids		
Dexamethasone (Decadron) Hydrocortisone sodium succinate (Solu-Cortef) Methylprednisolone sodium (Solu-Medrol) Prednisone (Meticorten)	Lyse lymphoid malignancies and have indirect effects on malignant cells	Monitor for major toxicities: Fluid retention Hypertension Diabetes Increased susceptibility to infection
Estrogens		
Diethylstilbestrol Estradiol	Suppress testosterone production in males and alter response of breast cancers to prolactin	Monitor for major toxicities: Fluid retention Feminization Uterine bleeding
Progestins		
Estramustine (Emcyt) Megestrol (Megace) Medroxyprogesterone (Provera)	Promote differentiation of malignant cells	
Estrogen Antagonists		
Leuprolide (Lupron) Tamoxifen (Nolvadex)	Compete with estrogens for binding with estrogen receptor sites on malignant cells	Monitor for side effects: Minimal with occasional headache Hot flashes

Continued

amount of drug to the tumor. Chemotherapeutic agents can be given orally, subcutaneously, intramuscularly, intravenously, and topically and can also be directly instilled into the bladder, peritoneum, cerebrospinal fluid or tumor bed. These latter routes allow the delivery of high-dose concentrations to the tumor site without undue systemic effects and may be used when a malignant organ or tissue cannot be treated surgically. Administration of chemotherapy into the cerebrospinal fluid, called the intrathecal route, can be done either by a lumbar puncture or by using a cerebrospinal (Ommaya) reservoir (Figure 23-13).

Intravenous Drug Administration. The intravenous route is the most common route for chemotherapy administration. Chemotherapy can be administered through standard peripheral intravenous lines, but patients who require long-term, repeated venous access; receive intensive chemotherapy regimens; or have poor peripheral vein access will usually receive chemotherapy through a centrally placed **venous access device** (VAD). A central VAD is an intravenous catheter located in a central vessel, usually positioned in the superior vena cava with its tip at the entrance to the right atrium. The type of VAD depends on treatment variables and the patient's general condition and preference.

Centrally located catheters allow for intermittent or continuous administration of chemotherapeutic agents, blood and blood products, other medications, and total parenteral nutrition. These catheters may have single, double, or triple lumens for multidrug administration. Central VADs can be short term, such as percutaneous subclavian catheters, which are

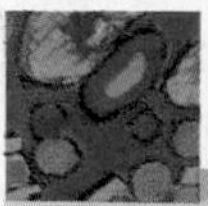

TABLE 23-20
COMMON CHEMOTHERAPEUTIC AGENTS *for Treating Cancer—cont'd*

Drug	Action	Nursing Intervention
Antiadrenal		
Aminoglutethimide	Produces equivalent of medical adrenalectomy, thereby inhibiting formation of estrogens and androgenesis and function of nucleic acids and inhibiting RNA and DNA synthesis; are cycle nonspecific	Monitor for side effects: Adrenal insufficiency
Vinca Alkaloids		
Vinblastine (Velban) Vincristine (Oncovin) Vindesine sulfate Vinorelbine (Navelbine)	Bind to proteins within cells, causing metaphase arrest and thus inhibiting RNA and protein synthesis; act in M phase	Monitor for major toxicities: Myelosuppression (except vincristine) Peripheral neuropathy Constipation Extravasation Alopecia
Epipodophyllotoxins		
Etoposide (VP-16) Teniposide (VM-26)	Act in late G_2 and S phase; cause breaks in DNA strands; interfere with topoisomerase II enzyme reaction	Monitor for major toxicities: Myelosuppression Nausea and vomiting Alopecia Hypotension
Taxanes		
Paclitaxel (Taxol) Docetaxel (Taxotere)	Act in G_2 and M phase; stabilize microtubule to inhibit cell division	Monitor for major toxicities: Myelosuppression Hypersensitivity Alopecia Peripheral neuropathy (paclitaxel) Fluid retention (docetaxel)
Camptothecins		
Irinotecan (Camptosar) Topotecan (Hycamtin)	Act in S phase; inhibit topoisomerase I enzyme reaction	Monitor for major toxicities: Myelosuppression Diarrhea Alopecia Flulike syndrome (topotecan)
Other		
Hydroxyurea (Hydrea)	S-phase antimetabolite	Monitor for major toxicities: Myelosuppression Nausea and vomiting Stomatitis
L-Asparaginase (Elspar)	Inhibits protein synthesis	Monitor for major toxicities: Nausea and vomiting Hypersensitivity
Thalidomide	Inhibits angiogenesis	Monitor for major toxicities: Sedation Peripheral neuropathy Constipation Skin rash

DNA, Deoxyribonucleic acid; *RNA,* ribonucleic acid; *SIADH,* syndrome of inappropriate antidiuretic hormone.
*Be aware of potential to develop second malignancy later in life (e.g., leukemia) when taking alkylating agents.

nontunneled, sutured catheters, usually used when immediate central access is needed (Figure 23-14). Long-term VADs are tunneled and cuffed and made out of softer silicone, so that they may stay in place for years. The technique of "tunneling" the catheter beneath the skin helps to prevent bacterial entry and growth along the catheter tract. All tunneled catheters have a small "cuff" around which fibroblasts form and help secure the catheter in place.[6] Figure 23-15 shows positioning of a tunneled and cuffed central VAD. The exit site of central catheters requires a sterile dressing change, and each catheter lumen must be flushed to maintain patency when it is not being used. Protocols for dressing changes and flushing vary among institutions.

Implanted VADs, or ports, are tunneled and cuffed catheters attached to a reservoir made out of titanium or steel with a self-sealing septum (Figure 23-16). The port is placed in a subcuta-

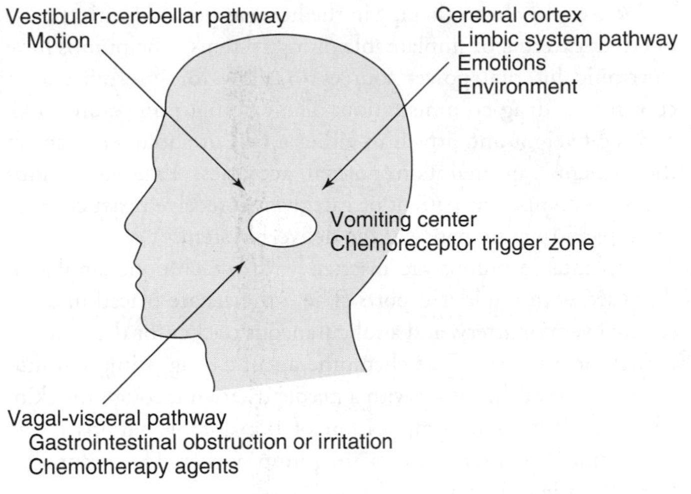

Figure 23-12 Pathways of nausea and vomiting.

neous pocket in the upper chest, and the catheter does not have an external segment. The catheter is accessed by inserting a noncoring needle through the skin and into the reservoir. When the catheter is not in use, no external dressing is used, and flushing is required only once a month.

Peripherally inserted central catheters (PICCs) are catheters inserted into a peripheral vein and advanced into a central vein. Access is usually obtained via the cephalic or basilic vein in the upper

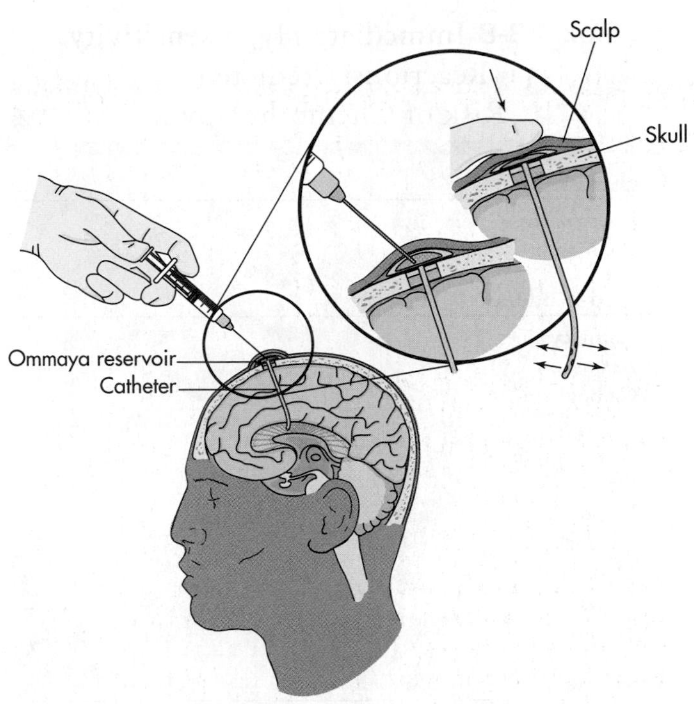

Figure 23-13 Ommaya reservoir for administration of chemotherapeutic agents directly into central nervous system. NOTE: Medication is administered into reservoir and moves through catheter into lateral ventricle.

TABLE 23-21 EMETOGENIC POTENTIAL OF COMMON CHEMOTHERAPEUTIC AGENTS

Incidence	Agent	Onset (hr)	Duration (hr)
High	Cisplatin	1–6	24–48
	Dacarbazine	1–3	1–12
	Cyclophosphamide	4–12	12–24
	Cytarabine (high dose)	1–4	12–48
	Etoposide (high dose)	4–6	24
	Methotrexate (high dose)	1–12	24–72
Moderate	Doxorubicin	4–6	6
	5-Fluorouracil	3–6	24
	Carboplatin	4–6	12–24
	Daunorubicin	2–6	24
	Topotecan	6–12	24–72
	Ifosfamide	3–6	24–72
	Irinotecan	6–12	24
Low	Bleomycin	3–6	—
	Cytarabine (low-dose)	6–12	3-12
	Etoposide (low-dose)	3–8	—
	Methotrexate(low-dose)	4–12	3–12
	Vinblastine	4–8	—
	Gemcitabine	—	—
	Vinorelbine	—	—
	Fludarabine	—	—
	Vincristine	4–8	—
	Paclitaxel	4–8	—
	Docetaxel	—	—
	Hydroxyurea	—	—

Adapted from Camp-Sorrell D: Chemotherapy: toxicity management. In Yarbro CH et al, editors: *Cancer nursing: principles and practice,* ed 5, Boston, 2000, Jones & Bartlett.

Box 23-8 Immediate Hypersensitivity Reactions: Predicted Risk of Chemotherapy

High Risk

l-Asparaginase*
Paclitaxel

Low-to-Moderate Risk

Anthracyclines
Bleomycin
Carboplatin
Cisplatin
Cyclosporine
Docetaxel
Etoposide
Melphalan*
Methotrexate
Procarbazine
Teniposide

Rare Risk

Chlorambucil
Cyclophosphamide
Cytarabine
Dacarbazine
5-Fluorouracil
Ifosfamide
Mitoxantrone

From Oncology Nursing Society: *Cancer chemotherapy guidelines and recommendations for practice*, Pittsburgh, 1999, Oncology Nursing Press.
*Significantly increased risk with intravenous route.

arm. This technique allows for easier insertion. External dressing and daily flushing procedures are necessary to maintain the patency of the catheter. Table 23-22, p. 555, presents a comparison of VADs.

Complications with all VADs include local and systemic infection, thrombosis, occlusion, and air embolism. Local infection can occur at the exit site of the catheter, along the tunnel, or at the pocket of a port. Thromboses can occur around and along the catheter, preventing blood flow in the vessel around the catheter. Compromised circulation can affect the extremity, face, and neck. Thromboses can also occur within the catheter, causing difficulty with infusion of fluids and withdrawal of blood.

A number of chemotherapeutic agents cause tissue damage if they extravasate, or leak out of the vein and infiltrate soft tissue. These drugs, termed *vesicants*, cause severe tissue ulceration and necrosis when extravasated in significant amounts (Box 23-9, p. 555). Nurses who administer chemotherapy institute specific safety protocols for vesicant administration. The nurse monitors for possible intravenous infiltration and immediately institutes appropriate treatment to minimize tissue damage, including the application of heat and cold and the administration of specific antidotes. Although infrequent, extravasation injuries do occur with central VADs.

Delivery of chemotherapy in the home is possible with the use of either external or implantable pump systems. The pumps have electronic internal power sources to allow for intermittent or continuous drug administration. The external pumps are small and lightweight and attach to either a belt or shoulder strap, so the patient can maintain normal activities. External pumps require a competent patient or caregiver to receive instruction in the care and maintenance of the delivery system.

Implantable pumps are inserted with a technique similar to that used with implanted ports. The catheters are placed into the selected vein or artery, and a subcutaneous pocket for the pump is created near the site. The chemotherapeutic drug is injected into the chamber of the pump with a needle inserted through the skin. The most common complication of implantable pumps is the development of a seroma over the pump pocket. This accumulation of sterile fluid may require aspiration.

Nursing Management

of the Patient receiving Chemotherapy

Assessment

Health History. Assess for:

- Age
- Comorbid health problems, current treatment
- Medical history, family history
- Medications in use: prescribed, over the counter, and herbal
- Allergies to food, drugs
- Social support, family composition
- Learning ability, education level, occupation
- Financial status, insurance coverage

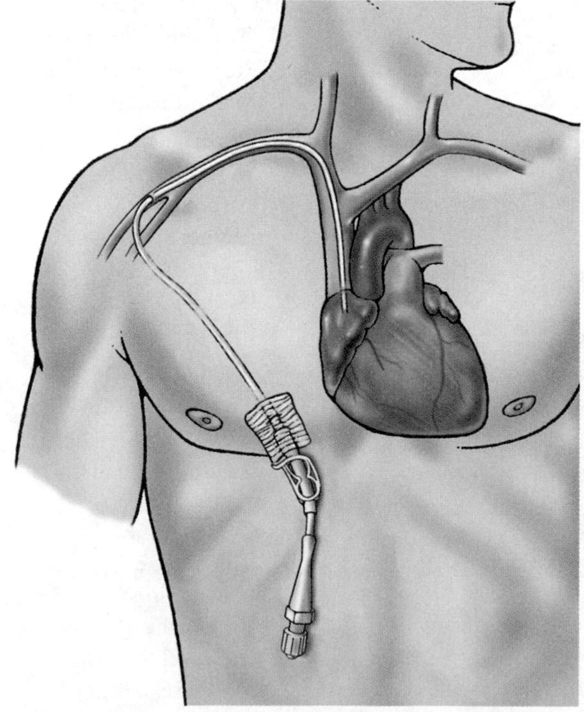

Figure 23-14 Central venous catheter in place.

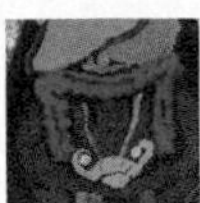

GUIDELINES FOR SAFE PRACTICE *Safety in Handling Chemotherapeutic Agents*

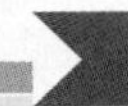

Prevention of Inhalation of Aerosols

Mix all drugs in an approved class II or III vertical airflow biologic safety cabinet (BSC), wearing gloves made of latex or nitrile at all times. Surgical masks do not prevent aerosol inhalation and should not be used. Wear eye and face barriers if splashes are likely to occur or sprays or aerosols are used.

Prime all intravenous (IV) bags within the BSC before adding the drug. Use a maintenance bag of normal saline or 5% dextrose in water (D_5W) to prime the tubing and all the chemotherapy bags afterward.

Break ampules by wrapping a sterile gauze pad or alcohol wipe around the neck (decreases chance of droplet contamination).

Vent vials with only enough air to allow the drug to be aspirated easily using a hydrophobic filter needle.

Syringes and needles used in cytotoxic drug preparation should not be crushed, clipped, or recapped. They should immediately be placed in a sharps container labeled "cytotoxic waste" for disposal.

Use a gauze pad when removing syringes and needles from IV injection ports or spikes from IV bags.

Prevention of Drug Absorption Through Skin

Wear latex or nitrile gloves and a gown of nonpermeable fabric with a closed front and cuffed, long sleeves.

Change gloves every 60 minutes.

Remove gloves immediately after spilling drug solution on them or puncturing or tearing them.

Wash hands before putting on gloves and after removing them.

Cover the work surface with a plastic-backed absorbent pad; change pad when cabinet is cleaned or after a spill.

Clean all surfaces of the BSC before and after drug preparation in accordance with manufacturer's instructions. Discard equipment used in a leakproof, puncture-proof, chemical-waste container.

Use syringes and IV sets with Luer-Lok fittings.

Place an absorbent pad under injection sites to catch accidental spillage.

Label all antineoplastic drugs with a chemotherapy warning label.

Wash skin thoroughly with soap and water as soon as possible in the event of skin contact with drugs.

Flush eyes with eye solution or clean water in the event of eye contact; seek medical attention.

Prevention of Ingestion

Do not eat, drink, chew gum, apply cosmetics, store food, or smoke in drug preparation areas.

Wash hands before and after preparing or giving drugs.

Avoid hand-to-mouth or hand-to-eye contact when handling the drugs.

Safe Disposal

Discard nonsharp cytotoxic waste products in a leakproof, puncture-proof, sealable plastic bag of a different color than regular trash bags. Label "cytotoxic waste."

Use a leakproof, puncture-proof container labeled "cytotoxic waste" for needles and sharp, breakable items.

Keep waste containers in labeled, covered waste containers for disposal.

Ensure housekeeping personnel are instructed in safe procedures and wear latex or nitrile gloves and gowns of nonpermeable fabric.

All waste produced by cytotoxic drug administration in the home should be placed in a sealed receptacle and transported in the non-passenger area of a vehicle to the home agency for disposal.

Prevention of Contamination by Body Fluids

Wear latex or nitrile gloves and disposable, nonpermeable fabric when handling any body fluids.

Empty waste products into the toilet by pouring close to the water to avoid splashing. Close the lid and flush two or three times (in the home).

Wear gloves and gown when handling linen soiled with body fluids; place in isolation linen bag for separate laundry.

Place soiled linens in separate, washable pillow cases and wash twice, separately from other household linens (in the home).

A standard duration of 48 hours is accepted as the time after which most cytotoxic drugs will have been metabolized or excreted. For most cytotoxic agents, urinary excretion is complete within 48 hours after administration (range of 1 to 6 days) and stool excretion is complete within 7 days (range of 5 to 7 days).

- Understanding of chemotherapy and its use in cancer treatment
- Knowledge of planned treatment and expected side effects

Physical Examination. Assess for:

- Performance status, self-care abilities
- BSA (height and weight)
- Nutritional status, recent weight gain or loss
- Venous access, availability, patency
- Elimination patterns, current problems with constipation or diarrhea
- Mobility, activities of daily living
- Skin and oral mucous membrane integrity
- Level of consciousness, cognitive status
- Vital signs, peripheral pulses, pulse oximetry
- Airway patency, breath sounds

NURSING DIAGNOSES, OUTCOMES, AND INTERVENTIONS

Nursing Diagnosis: Risk for Infection

OUTCOMES. Common examples of expected outcomes for the patient with a diagnosis of *risk for infection* are:

Patient will:

- Maintain a normal body temperature.
- Exhibit no signs of infection.
- Maintain optimal personal hygiene.
- Maintain intact oral mucous membranes.

NURSING INTERVENTIONS. Nursing interventions to prevent infection include measures to maximize the patient's own defenses against infection, minimize sources of infection, and aggressively identify and treat infection. The nurse teaches the patient about the

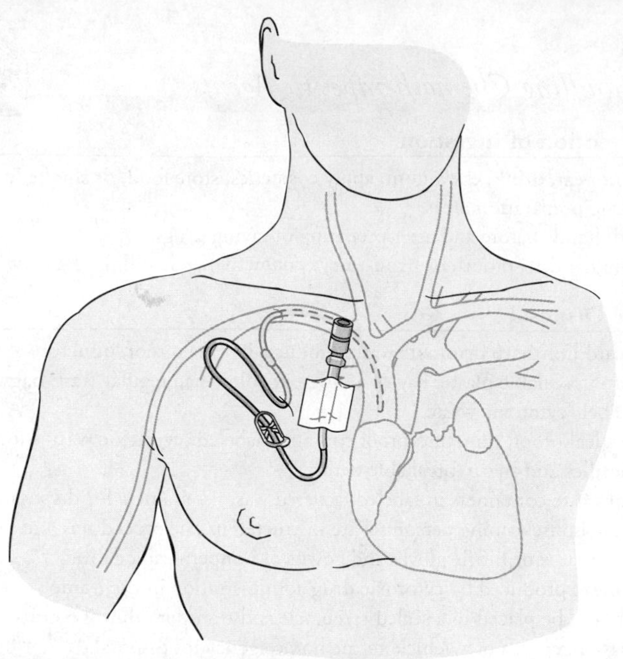

Figure 23-15 Tunneled catheter.

risk for infection, specific signs and symptoms of infection, and how infections can be prevented and treated. Patients who will be at home need to have a thermometer and know how to use it. Patients are taught to report any fever and any new sign of infection, and need specific instructions about whom to notify and when.

The patient needs to maintain good personal hygiene, particularly skin and mouth care. The nurse emphasizes protocols for specific VAD, wound, or tube care. The patient should avoid contact with family, staff, or visitors who have an infection. Caregivers should wash their hands thoroughly before any patient contact. The frequency of patient assessments depends on the degree of myelosuppression expected with the regimen. Patients undergoing induction chemotherapy for leukemia, for example, may require assessment and measurement of vital signs every 4 hours with daily monitoring of blood counts.[42] Patients on a monthly outpatient regimen may have blood counts checked weekly with a physical assessment before each treatment.

Signs of early infection may be absent or diminished in neutropenic patients. Without neutrophils, patients do not develop the classic signs of infection such as redness, swelling, and pus formation. Mild localized tenderness and fever, defined as a temperature over 101° F (38.5° C), may be the only indications of a potentially dangerous infection. Any sign of infection in a neutropenic patient is considered a medical emergency that requires immediate treatment. Physical and laboratory examinations are performed to determine the site of infection, and aggressive antimicrobial therapy is instituted to control the infection. Colony-stimulating factors are increasingly being used to reduce the severity and duration of neutropenia after chemotherapy. G-CSF and GM-CSF are WBC growth factors given as subcutaneous injections after chemotherapy administration (see p. 527). Infection precautions are summarized in the Guidelines for Safe Practice box, p. 556.

Chemotherapeutic agents also disrupt the integrity of mucous membranes, causing dryness, painful ulcerations, and infections. Although this inflammation can affect mucosal cells throughout the gastrointestinal, genitourinary, and respiratory tracts, oral problems are the most common. The nurse closely inspects the patient's mouth, including lips, teeth, gums, tongue, palate, and throat, to identify any lesions or abnormalities. Patients may report the early signs of mouth dryness and increased sensitivity. A cleansing and hydrating mouth care regimen started at the

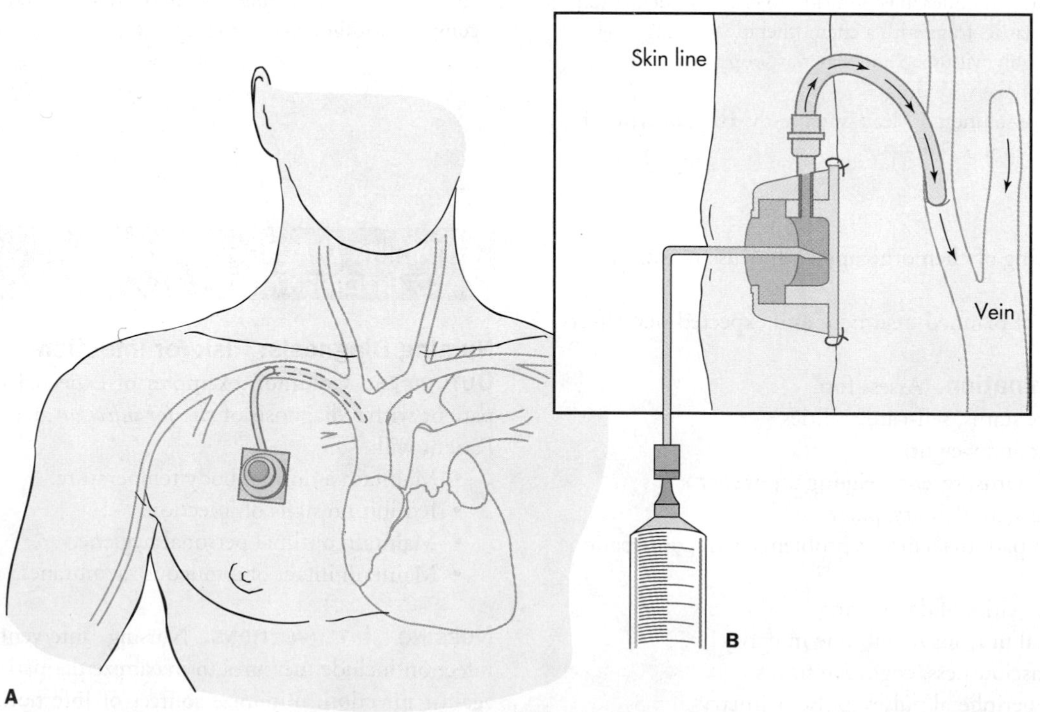

Figure 23-16 A, Implanted port. B, Cross-section of port with needle access.

TABLE 23-22 COMPARISON OF VENOUS ACCESS DEVICES

Type of Device	Advantage	Disadvantage
Peripheral catheter	Easy and quick to insert at bedside No major complications No self-care	Short life span (3 days) Discomfort and difficult insertion for some Not safe for certain drugs and infusions
Not-tunneled central venous catheter	Inserted at bedside Safe for all fluids and blood drawing	Short term Not for outpatient use
Peripherally inserted central catheter (PICC)	Can remain for 6 mo or longer Easier to insert and less expensive than other central catheters Safe for all fluids and blood drawing	Inserted in angiography suite May limit arm mobility and activities Requires self-care for dressing changes and flushes Blood drawing may be difficult
Tunneled central venous catheter	Can remain for years Good for long-term, intensive, frequent intravenous therapy Safe for all fluids and blood drawing	Inserted in angiography suite Causes minor insertion discomfort Requires self-care for dressing changes and flushes Higher risk of infection
Implanted port	Can remain for years Requires no self-care Maintains body image and mobility Low infection rate Safe for all fluids and blood drawing	More difficult and expensive insertion in angiography suite Causes minor insertion discomfort More difficult removal Minor discomfort with needle access

beginning of chemotherapy can reduce the severity of mucositis. The Guidelines for Safe Practice box on p. 543 outlines a mouth care program for chemotherapy patients.[37] Patients may develop infections, such as the raised blisters of herpes and the white patchy lesions of candidiasis, and antibiotics may be prescribed. Analgesics and local anesthetics are prescribed to treat the pain that accompanies severe mucositis. Nutritional therapy may be prescribed when mucositis significantly limits oral intake.

RELATED NIC INTERVENTIONS. Environmental Management, Infection Protection, Oral Health Maintenance, Surveillance, Venous Access Device (VAD) Maintenance, Vital Signs Monitoring

Nursing Diagnosis: Risk for Injury

OUTCOMES. Common examples of expected outcomes for the patient with a diagnosis of *risk for injury* related to bleeding are:
Patient will:

- Experience minimal bruising.
- Not experience spontaneous bleeding.

Box 23-9 Vesicant Chemotherapeutic Agents

- Dactinomycin
- Daunorubicin
- Doxorubicin
- Epirubicin
- Idarubicin
- Mechlorethamine
- Mitomycin
- Vinblastine
- Vincristine
- Vindesine
- Vinorelbine

NURSING INTERVENTIONS. The myelosuppressed patient is at risk for bleeding because of an inadequate number of platelets. The nurse institutes bleeding precautions to maintain the integrity of the skin and mucous membranes. The nurse assesses the patient for signs and symptoms of bleeding, including testing for occult blood in body fluids and excretions, and monitors the platelet count as indicated by the degree of bleeding risk. A platelet count below 10,000/mm^3 or the presence of active bleeding in a thrombocytopenic patient indicates the need for prompt supportive platelet transfusion. Nurses need to be knowledgeable about the safe administration of platelet transfusions, including how to prevent and control transfusion reactions. The Guidelines for Safe Practice box, p. 557, outlines specific nursing interventions designed to prevent bleeding in thrombocytopenic patients.

RELATED NIC INTERVENTIONS. Bleeding Precautions, Blood Products Administration, Risk Identification, Surveillance

Nursing Diagnosis: Fatigue

OUTCOMES. Common examples of expected outcomes for the patient with a diagnosis of *fatigue* are:
Patient will:

- Maintain independence in self care.
- Maintain stable vital signs without dyspnea, chest pain, or dizziness.

NURSING INTERVENTIONS. The myelosuppressed patient may experience severe anemia and profound treatment-related fatigue that makes it extremely difficult to participate in the normal activities of daily living. The nurse works with the patient to develop energy-conserving strategies and a plan for needed rest periods, and he or she encourages the patient to balance activity and rest throughout the day. The focus is on maintaining the patient's ability to be independent in self-care and continue participation in important family, work-related, and social activities as much as possible. The nurse engages the family in seeking ways to reduce energy demands on the patient and encourages them to explore new strategies for support and assistance.

The patient with anemia experiences other symptoms related to poor tissue perfusion, such as dyspnea, tachycardia, and headaches. Patients who are symptomatic or who experience severe anemia may require RBC transfusions to temporarily restore RBC levels during treatment. Nurses are responsible for the safe administration of blood products and the identification and management of RBC transfusion reactions. Therapy with EPO, an RBC growth factor, can prevent severe anemia related to chemotherapy, reducing the need for transfusions and preventing the common symptoms. EPO is given as a subcutaneous injection, usually on a weekly schedule.

RELATED NIC INTERVENTIONS. Energy Management, Sleep Enhancement, Support System Enhancement

Nursing Diagnosis: Risk for Imbalanced Nutrition: Less Than Body Requirements

OUTCOMES. Common examples of expected outcomes for the patient with a diagnosis of *risk for imbalanced nutrition: less than body requirements* are:

Patient will:

- Maintain optimal desired body weight.
- Ingest sufficient balanced nutrients to meet body energy needs.
- Experience minimal nausea and no uncontrolled vomiting.

NURSING INTERVENTIONS. The gastrointestinal tract is highly sensitive to the effects of chemotherapy. Anorexia, nausea, and vomiting are common problems. Diarrhea or constipation can also occur. The outcome can be weight loss and fluid volume deficit, which can lead to serious malnutrition and dehydration. For the outpatient, nausea may interfere with the ability to continue work. Persistent vomiting can result in fluid and electrolyte imbalance, general weakness, and weight loss. A decline in nutritional status makes the person more susceptible to infection and less able to tolerate therapy. The onset and duration of both nausea and vomiting vary greatly from patient to patient and with the drugs given.

Nausea and vomiting are two of the more dreaded side effects of chemotherapy. Although nausea and vomiting are expected with many chemotherapeutic agents, advances in the use of antiemetics have successfully reduced their incidence and severity. A variety of antiemetic agents with different mechanisms of action are available, and agents are prescribed based on the severity of the problem (Table 23-23). Both premedication with antiemetics before treatment and scheduled coverage during chemotherapy are essential. Antiemetics should also be available in case patients experience delayed nausea several days after therapy.[18] The nurse evaluates the effectiveness of the antiemetic regimen and makes adjustments as needed for subsequent courses of treatment. If diarrhea or constipation occurs, the nurse uses dietary strategies in addition to pharmacologic agents to promote regular bowel function. When fluid losses are moderate, the nurse encourages a higher fluid intake and monitors fluid balance. Intravenous rehydration may be necessary when fluid losses are severe.

Anorexia, nausea, vomiting, and stomatitis can also put the patient at risk for altered nutrition. The nurse emphasizes that eating a nourishing diet helps maintain energy and meet body nutrient and repair needs. A comprehensive care plan needs to address all the contributing factors that may compromise dietary

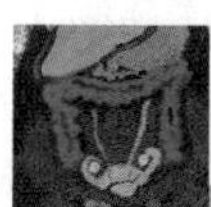

GUIDELINES FOR SAFE PRACTICE *The Patient With Neutropenia*

- Maximize the patient's own defenses against infection.
  - —Implement skin care regimen to maintain skin integrity.
  - —Implement oral hygiene regimen to maintain integrity of the mouth.
  - —Avoid intramuscular and subcutaneous injections, rectal thermometers, and rectal medication administration.
  - —Avoid invasive procedures, such as urinary catheterizations.
  - —Avoid medications likely to mask a fever, such as aspirin, acetaminophen, and steroids.
- Minimize the patient's exposure to sources of infection.
  - —Emphasize the need for thorough hand washing for all persons who have physical contact with the patient.
  - —Restrict persons with colds and infections from physical contact with the patient.
  - —Limit dietary intake of fresh fruits and vegetables, or wash them thoroughly.
  - —Limit patient contact with obviously infected items, such as cat litter and bird cages.
- Assess for signs and symptoms of infection.
  - —Monitor vital signs as indicated.
  - —Monitor total white blood cell count and neutrophil count as indicated.
  - —Examine potential sites of infection, including lungs, skin, intravenous sites, mouth, and perirectum.
- Implement a plan for aggressive antimicrobial therapy.
  - —Immediately report temperature greater than 101° F (38.5° C) or any new sign of infection.
  - —Obtain bacterial and fungal cultures of body fluids before starting initial antibiotic therapy.
  - —Administer broad-spectrum antimicrobial therapy as soon as possible and adjust coverage as necessary. Check drug allergies and monitor for side effects.
- Administer granulocyte colony-stimulating factor or granulocyte-macrophage colony-stimulating factor therapy as prescribed.
  - —Teach patient self-administration technique if necessary.
- Educate patient and family about the risk of infection.
  - —Inform the patient about the relative risk of infection.
  - —Implement a teaching plan that includes:
    - —Symptoms of infection
    - —Self-care measures to prevent infection
    - —When and how to report symptoms of infection
    - —How potential infections will be treated

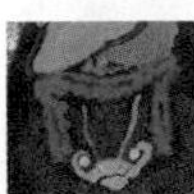

GUIDELINES FOR SAFE PRACTICE

The Patient With Thrombocytopenia

- Minimize trauma and other sources as cause of bleeding.
  - —Avoid intramuscular and subcutaneous injections, rectal thermometers, and rectal medication administration.
  - —Avoid aspirin, aspirin-containing products, and nonsteroidal antiinflammatory drugs, which may increase bleeding.
  - —Minimize venipunctures and other invasive procedures, such as urinary catheterization.
  - —Apply pressure to venipuncture sites for at least 5 minutes.
  - —Implement mouth care regimen with soft toothbrush. Avoid flossing and other dental procedures.
  - —Use only electric shavers for hair removal.
  - —Provide assistance with activity as necessary to prevent falls.
  - —Limit activities likely to cause trauma, such as contact sports.
- Assess for signs and symptoms of bleeding.
  - —Inspect potential sites of bleeding, such as skin, nose, and mouth.
  - —Check sputum, urine, stool, emesis, and other body fluids for occult blood.
  - —Monitor platelet count as indicated.
- Administer platelet transfusions when platelet count is below 10,000/mm^3, when there is active bleeding, or before an invasive procedure.
- Educate patient and family about the risk of bleeding.
  - —Inform the patient about the relative risk of bleeding.
  - —Implement a teaching plan that includes:
    - —Symptoms of bleeding, such as bruises; petechiae; nose bleeds; blood in urine, stool, sputum, or emesis
    - —Self-care measures to prevent bleeding
    - —When and how to report symptoms of bleeding
    - —How potential episodes of bleeding would be treated

intake. The nurse carefully assesses the patient's nutritional status before and throughout treatment. Signs of poor nutrition may already be present before a definitive diagnosis and treatment plan are established. Oral care that relieves mouth and throat dryness or discomfort is instituted. The patient may need to rest before meals to help conserve energy for eating. Patients with anorexia often are hungrier at breakfast than other meals, especially when they have had an uninterrupted night of sleep. The nurse encourages a diet high in calories and proteins, and suggests the consumption of multiple small meals and snacks throughout the day. Intake may also be enhanced by creative strategies that make mealtimes more pleasant, such as the company of others, a comfortable position, and an environment free from noxious smells and stimuli. The nurse monitors body weight frequently to evaluate the effectiveness of nutritional interventions. Additional interventions include a diet history, anthropometric measurements, and laboratory data evaluation. Oral supplements or enteral feedings may be ordered if the patient has a severely limited intake but maintains a functional gastrointestinal tract. Total parenteral nutrition is used with patients who are at severe risk of malnutrition and unable to tolerate gastrointestinal feedings.

RELATED NIC INTERVENTIONS. Medication Administration, Nutrition Management, Oral Health Maintenance, Weight Management

Nursing Diagnosis: Disturbed Body Image

OUTCOMES. Common examples of expected outcomes for the patient with a diagnosis of *disturbed body image* are:

Patient will:

- Acknowledge changes in physical appearance and body image.
- Demonstrate positive coping strategies.

NURSING INTERVENTIONS. The alopecia that results from cancer therapy is one of the most traumatic side effects. Hair loss is a constant reminder of cancer and makes the illness visible to others. Alopecia, weight loss, changes in body function and appearance, and altered social roles can all affect the patient's body image or feelings about himself or herself. Chemotherapy treatments can cause all these changes, and the nurse needs to assess their impact on each individual.

The nurse informs patients scheduled for chemotherapy that causes hair loss of this likelihood early in the course of therapy so they are prepared when hair loss occurs. Some patients shave their heads or cut their hair short in preparation for hair loss. Others choose to use wigs, head scarves, or caps to disguise hair loss, and the nurse provides counseling and information about acquiring these resources early in the therapy, before hair loss occurs. At present, no intervention is available that prevents hair loss, although basic research is showing promise in this area. Hair dyes, permanents, and vigorous hair brushing are avoided to minimize thinning. The patient is reassured that hair loss is temporary and hair will grow back, possibly with a different shade and texture, after chemotherapy is discontinued.

Patients receiving chemotherapy face changes in lifestyle, roles, self-concept, and body image that may make them feel less attractive. Patients who experience alterations in sexuality or sexual function need specific counseling and interventions. The nurse provides information on the expected side effects of chemotherapy related to sexual function, such as amenorrhea, decreased sperm function, infertility, and risk to a fetus. Patients of reproductive age are advised to use birth control measures during the treatment period to avoid conception; sperm banking may be appropriate for some men. Treatment side effects such as nausea, fatigue, and anxiety may also affect sexual desire. The nurse addresses these side effects and answers questions about sexual concerns. The nurse can make appropriate referrals when more intensive counseling and interventions are necessary. It is important to include the patient's partner in all discussions related to sexuality and reproduction if possible and to support effective, open partner communication. Alternative methods of sexual expression may be appropriate during the most intensive treatment, and the nurse encourages both partners to make physical touching and intimacy a priority means of communication and support.

RELATED NIC INTERVENTIONS. Coping Enhancement, Emotional Support, Fertility Preservation, Self-Esteem Enhancement, Teaching: Sexuality

Patient/Family Teaching. Patient and family teaching is a critical part of the nursing care provided to patients undergoing chemotherapy. The nurse first clarifies the goal of chemotherapy for the patient, whether chemotherapy is used for cure, palliation

TABLE 23-23 EXAMPLES OF ANTIEMETIC REGIMENS FOR CHEMOTHERAPY-RELATED NAUSEA AND VOMITING

Type of Nausea	Agents	Examples of Regimen
Nonemetogenic	Bleomycin Busulfan Chlorambucil Cladribine Fludarabine Melphalan Mercaptopurine Methotrexate Vinca alkaloids	Same as for low, if needed
Low	Asparaginase Cytarabine <1 g/m^2 Docetaxel Etopside 5-Fluorouracil <1000 mg/m^2 Gemcitabine Methotrexate 50-250 mg/m^2 Paclitaxel Teniposide Thiotepa	Dexamethasone (Decadron), 8 mg po/IV *or* Prochlorperazine (Compazine), 10 mg IV *or* po 30 min before chemotherapy
Moderate	Altretamine Cyclophosphamide <750 mg/m^2 Daunorubicin Doxorubicin 20-60 mg/m^2 Epirubicin <90 mg/m^2 Idarubicin Ifosfamide Irinotecan Methotrexate 250-1000 mg/m^2 Mitomycin Mitoxantrone <15 mg/m^2 Pentostatin Plicamycin	Ondansetron (Zofran), 16 mg po *or* 8 mg IV Dexamethasone, 8-20 mg po *or* 10 mg IV 30 min before chemotherapy Methylprednisolone (Depo-Medrol), 40-125 mg IV, may be given in place of dexamethasone
Moderately high	Carboplatin (AUC <7.5) Carmustine <250 mg/m^2 Cisplatin <50 mg/m^2 Cyclophosphamide 750-1500 mg/m^2 Cytarabine >1 g/m^2 Dactinomycin Doxorubicin >60 mg/m^2 Melphalan Methotrexate >1 g/m^2 Mitoxantrone >15 mg/m^2 Procarbazine	Ondansetron, 24 mg po *or* 8-16 mg IV Dexamethasone, 8-20 mg po *or* 10-20 mg IV 30 min before chemotherapy Methylprednisolone, 40-125 mg IV, may be given in place of dexamethasone
High	Carboplatin (AUC ≥7.5) Carmustine >250 mg/m^2 Cisplatin >50 mg/m^2 Cyclophosphamide ≥1500 mg/m^2 Dacarbazine Lomustine >60 mg/m^2 Mechlorethamine Streptozocin Combination chemotherapy regimens	Ondansetron, 24 mg po *or* 8 mg IV Dexamethasone, 20 mg po *or* IV 30 min before chemotherapy Methylprednisolone, 125 mg IV, may be given in place of dexamethasone
Delayed		Same as regimens outlined above as necessary

po, By mouth; *IV*, intravenous.

of symptoms, or as adjuvant therapy. The nurse needs accurate and detailed information about the patient's cancer, its stage and extent, and the proposed chemotherapy regimen and may play a role in any interdisciplinary team conference to plan the most appropriate treatment regimen.

Information about the planned chemotherapy protocol includes the major side effects to be expected and what supportive interventions are indicated. The nurse then develops an individualized patient teaching and care plan.

The assessment interview clarifies the patient's expectations of therapy and explores the patient's fears or anxieties about the treatment. Patients facing chemotherapy for the first time usually know of someone who has been treated with chemotherapy and can often recite its many negative aspects. They wonder whether they will face the same discomforts, such as nausea and vomiting, weight loss, and hair loss. Patients who have previously undergone chemotherapy may fear resumption of therapy and express doubts regarding its effectiveness and the wisdom of subjecting themselves once again to its adverse side effects. It is important for the nurse to respect and support the unique response of each patient. Each patient is reassured that every effort will be made to prevent and control undesirable side effects. The nurse provides honest, detailed, and realistic information at a level that meets the patient's needs.

Patients commonly express concern related to the cost of a lengthy course of chemotherapy, especially if they have inadequate health insurance. They may fear becoming a financial drain on family resources, since most treatment regimens require frequent clinic visits and repeated hospitalizations. Transportation, child care, and work responsibilities are other possible areas of concern. The nurse attempts to understand each patient's unique situation and plan collaboratively to address individual concerns.

EVALUATION

To evaluate the effectiveness of nursing interventions, compare patient behaviors with those stated in the expected patient outcomes.

RELATED NOC OUTCOMES. Activity Tolerance, Appetite, Energy Conservation, Knowledge: Infection Control, Nutritional Status: Food & Fluid Intake, Risk Control, Self-Care: Instrumental Activities of Daily Living (IADL), Self-Care: Hygiene, Self-Esteem, Sexual Functioning, Tissue Integrity: Skin & Mucous Membranes, Weight: Body Mass

GERONTOLOGIC CONSIDERATIONS

Chemotherapy is increasingly being used as a treatment option for older persons with cancer. Cancer clinicians were once reluctant to use chemotherapy with older patients out of concern for their ability to safely tolerate this rigorous treatment. This reluctance is based on real concerns about the unpredictable response of older adults to chemotherapy and their reduced immunocompetence at baseline. But, as cancer becomes an ever greater challenge to a rapidly aging population, experience with chemotherapy has dramatically improved. Older patients should be provided with careful and accurate information about the risks and benefits of chemotherapy and then supported in making an informed choice that is respected and honored by family and professionals. The individual's goals and wishes are paramount.

Careful consideration is given to the type of tumor being treated, its stage of growth, and its aggressiveness. The toxicities of preferred treatment options are carefully evaluated. The patient's functional status is a critical component in decision making. Healthy older adults can and do respond extremely well and tolerate the rigors of aggressive chemotherapy, whereas frail older patients may respond less positively and experience more complications. Closer monitoring is required, and responses are more unpredictable overall than with younger patients. The entire care team needs to be prepared to shift treatment plans rapidly in response to changes in the patient's condition and tolerance. The nurse's role in teaching, assessment, and support of the patient during each stage of treatment is critical.

Cancer Pain

Pain is one of the most feared symptoms of cancer, although contrary to popular belief, it is usually one of the last symptoms to appear. Pain is generally not a problem in the early, localized stage of disease. About 30% of patients with cancer experience pain while undergoing treatment. As the cancer progresses and metastasizes, more than 90% of patients experience pain. The ONS developed a position paper on cancer pain because pain management is a significant clinical problem faced by the nurse caring for cancer patients and because cancer pain has been poorly managed in the past. The ONS statement makes the nurse responsible for coordinating pain management, including effective assessment, intervention, and evaluation of the pain.

Patients with cancer experience pain from three sources. First, tumors directly cause pain of three types: somatic, visceral, or neuropathic. Somatic pain is caused by tumors that infiltrate cutaneous or connective tissue, such as muscle, bone, and blood vessels. One common example is the pain from bone metastases. Visceral pain results from organ involvement, such as pancreatic cancer.[30] Neuropathic pain results from involved nerve fibers or central nervous system tissue, such as a peripheral neuropathy. These pain syndromes each have distinct characteristics (Table 23-24). Patients can also experience pain from cancer therapy. Examples include acute pain related to diagnostic procedures, postoperative pain, or pain that results from the mucositis caused by chemotherapy. Finally, as many as 10% of patients experience significant pain from a condition or disease unrelated to their cancer, such as migraine headaches or arthritis.

The goal of pain management is to provide pain relief that enables the patient to carry on with normal activities of daily living without discomfort. Pain management for patients with cancer includes the use of appropriate therapies to control the cancer, pharmacologic measures to manage the patients' perception of pain, and a variety of nonpharmacologic measures to provide additional relief. Surgery, chemotherapy, and radiotherapy may all be appropriate treatments for pain (Table 23-25). Pharmacologic therapy with several classes of drugs is the foundation of pain control. Patients may be prescribed nonopioid analgesics; opioids; or other agents that contribute to pain relief, such as antidepressants or anticonvulsants. Principles of pain management include using the least invasive route possible and ensuring around-the-clock administration to maintain therapeutic blood levels. Mild pain is treated with nonopioid medications, such as NSAIDs or adjuvant

TABLE 23-24 PATHOPHYSIOLOGY OF CANCER PAIN

Cause	Type of Pain
Bone destruction with infraction (fracture without displacement)	Increased sensitivity over area or sharp, continuous pain
Obstruction of a viscus (gastrointestinal or genitourinary tract)	Severe, colicky, crampy type of pain; may be dull, diffuse, poorly localized
Obstruction of artery, vein, or lymphatic	Dull, diffuse, aching (caused by arterial ischemia, venous engorgement, edema)
Infiltration, compression of peripheral nerves or nerve plexus	Continuous, sharp, or stabbing pain; sometimes hyperesthesia or paresthesia
Infiltration or distention of integument, fascia, or tissue (e.g., ascites)	Localized, dull aching pain
Inflammation, infection, and necrosis of tissue	Varied pain caused by pressure or ischemia

TABLE 23-25 ROLES OF PRIMARY THERAPIES IN MANAGEMENT OF CANCER PAIN

Primary Therapy	Major Pain Indications
Radiotherapy	Painful bony metastases Epidural spinal cord compression Cerebral metastases Tumor-related compression or infiltration of peripheral neural structures
Chemotherapy	Nociceptive or neuropathic pain syndromes caused by tumors likely to respond to chemotherapy
Surgery	Stabilization of pathologic fractures Spinal cord decompression Relief of bowel obstructions Drainage of symptomatic ascites
Antibiotic therapy	Overt infections (e.g., pelvic abscess or pyonephrosis) Occult infections (e.g., in head and neck tumors or ulcerating tumors)

From Cherny NJ, Portenoy RK: The management of cancer pain, *CA Cancer J Clin* 44(5):272, 1994.

drugs. As pain increases, opioids are used, increasing in potency and dose as necessary. Opioids can also be combined with nonopioids and adjuvant drugs for improved pain relief. Nonpharmacologic measures for pain include behavioral techniques, such as relaxation or diversional activities; meditation, hypnosis, or imagery; and the use of heat and cold, cutaneous stimulation, and massage. See Chapter 16 for a discussion of pain assessment and management. The Guidelines for Safe Practice box lists nursing strategies for dealing with the cancer patient's pain.

Cancer pain may not be effectively managed for a variety of reasons, including fear of addiction, inadequate understanding of the regimen, a belief that nothing can be done to relieve the pain, or lack of financial and supportive resources to obtain appropriate analgesics. The nurse discusses pain management with the patient and family and emphasizes the importance of promptly reporting pain, using adequate doses of analgesics to control the pain, and regular dosing to sustain effective analgesic blood levels. The nurse also teaches the patient about the physiologic phenomena of tolerance and dependence and reassures the patient that regular use of an opioid is both safe and appropriate and does not constitute addiction. In hospice or palliative care settings, issues related to euthanasia and assisted suicide may enter into discussions about pain management, necessitating careful ethical reasoning, education, and interventions.

Complementary and Alternative Therapies for Cancer

Complementary therapies are often used to better manage cancer-associated pain, but they may also be used to improve the patient's functional status and sense of well-being. Examples of complementary therapies are massage, aromatherapy, relaxation therapy, meditation, and yoga. Alternative therapies include practices that were once considered outside of Western medicine, such as acupuncture, herbal remedies, and homeopathy.

Nurses need to know what complementary and alternative therapies their patients may be using, and should include this question in all patient assessments. The popularity of many of these therapies continues to grow, and more than half of patients with cancer may be using these therapies in addition to their prescribed treatments. Some of these therapies are widely recognized as helpful and can be incorporated into the patient's treatment regimen. Other therapies may have undesirable or harmful effects. For example, some herbs

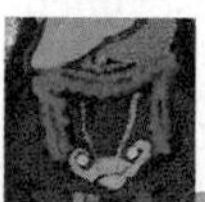

GUIDELINES FOR SAFE PRACTICE

Dealing Effectively With Cancer Pain

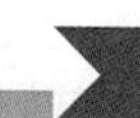

- Know the patient and the pattern of pain experienced. Document findings.
- Use an organized pain assessment method that is easy to use and provides sufficient data to assist in selecting the most appropriate intervention for relief.
- Understand the pharmacology of the drugs being used, including classification, probable side effects, route of administration, and expected outcomes in terms of when to expect pain relief to occur.
- Understand the difference between addiction, dependence, and tolerance.
- Use appropriate drug combinations.
- Advocate for effective analgesic regimens.
- Become familiar with equianalgesic doses of common analgesics.
- Provide patient and family teaching related to pain control.

Box 23-10 Herbs That Increase Risk of Bleeding or Sedation

Increased Sedation		Increased Risk of Bleeding	
Calamus	Lemon balm	Alfalfa	Gingko
Calendula plants	Sage	Angelica	Horse chestnut
California poppy	St. John's wort	Anise	Horseradish
Capsicum	Sassafras	Arnica	Licorice
Catnip	Siberian ginseng	Asafetida	Meadowsweet
Celery	Skullcap	Bogbean	Onion
Couch grass	Shepherd's purse	Boldo	Papain
Elecampane	Stinging nettle	Capsicum	Passionflower
German chamomile	Valerian	Celery	Poplar
Goldenseal	Wild carrot	Chamomile	Prickly ash
Gotu kola	Wild lettuce	Clove	Quassia
Hops	*Withania* root	Danshen	Red clover
Jamaican dogwood	*Yerba mansa*	Fenugreek	Tumeric
Kava		Feverfew	Wild carrot
		Garlic	Wild lettuce
		Ginger	Willow

From Decker GM, Myers J: Commonly used herbs: implications for practice, *Clin J Oncol Nurs,* vol 5 (suppl), 2001.

can increase the patient's risk of bleeding or increase sedation (Box 23-10). Patients may also reveal that they are pursuing the use of unconventional or unproven therapies instead of standard treatment. This may be especially true for patients with limited treatment options and poor prognoses or patients with unrealistic fears about the side effects of radiation or chemotherapy.

Nurses need to answer questions and provide information about alternative and complementary therapies in a nonjudgmental way to help patients make informed decisions about their therapy and support their right to pursue therapies that deviate from mainstream approaches.[13]

Oncologic Emergencies

Oncologic emergencies include a variety of complications associated with cancer or its treatment. These syndromes may signal a new diagnosis of cancer or occur as the cancer progresses. Obstructive emergencies include spinal cord compression, superior vena cava syndrome, tracheal or bowel obstruction, and increased intracranial pressure caused by tumor growth in and around the brain. Metabolic crises include hypercalcemia, tumor lysis syndrome, syndrome of inappropriate antidiuretic hormone secretion (SIADH), hyperviscosity, and disseminated intravascular coagulation. In some cases, such as SIADH, the cancer cells secrete a hormonelike substance that causes abnormal chemical and metabolic processes.[11] In other cases, cancer treatment can precipitate the crisis, as in tumor lysis syndrome. Table 23-26 lists some common oncologic emergencies.

Nurses need to be alert to patient populations at risk for oncologic emergencies. Nursing assessments often detect signs and symptoms that indicate an impending crisis. Early diagnosis and immediate treatment of these life-threatening conditions are critical. During these crises the patient may require transfer to an intensive care unit for hemodynamic monitoring and cardiopulmonary support. Continuity of care and emotional support for the patient and family are essential. In most cases successful treatment of the emergency requires control of the underlying cancer process in addition to supportive therapy.

Resources for Cancer Education, Detection, and Treatment

A variety of oncology-related organizations provide free information about cancer care to consumers and health care providers (Box 23-11). This information is available in print and on websites. With rapid advances in informatics, consumers and health professionals have immediate access to the most current information about even the rarest medical conditions. As a result, consumers of cancer care today are more educated than ever before.

Box 23-11 Oncology-Related Organizations

- American Brain Tumor Association: www.abta.org
- American Cancer Society: www.cancer.org
- American Lung Association: www.lungusa.org
- American Society of Clinical Oncology: www.asco.org
- Leukemia & Lymphoma Society: www.leukemia-lymphoma.org
- Lung Cancer Alliance: www.lungcanceralliance.org
- National Cancer Institute: www.nci.nih.gov
- National Coalition for Cancer Survivorship: www.cansearch.org
- National Marrow Donor Program: www.marrow.org
- National Ovarian Cancer Coalition: www.ovarian.org
- National Prostate Cancer Coalition: www.4npcc.org
- Oncology Nursing Society: www.ons.org
- Susan G. Komen Breast Cancer Foundation: www.komen.org
- United Ostomy Association: www.uoa.org

TABLE 23-26 ONCOLOGIC EMERGENCIES

Type	Pathophysiology	Clinical Manifestations
OBSTRUCTIVE		
Increased intracranial pressure	Increased brain mass from tumor, hemorrhage, or edema; alteration in internal jugular vein flow caused by head or neck tumor or by surgical resection—results in alteration in function	Change in mental status, vomiting, headache, dizziness, seizures (see Chapter 48)
Spinal cord compression	Primary or metastatic lesions causing disruption of reflexes and motor function because of neuron impairment and interruption of motor or sensory nerve fibers; symptoms depend on location	Flaccid paralysis, paresthesias, locomotion difficulties, respiratory impairment at C5 level (see Chapter 50)
Superior vena cava (SVC) syndrome	Obstruction of SVC caused by primary (usually lung cancer) or metastatic tumors in mediastinal or paratracheal nodes	Dyspnea, facial and neck swelling, chest pain, cough, dysphagia, ruddy edematous face
Tracheal obstruction	Reduction in lumen from tracheal stenosis, extrinsic compression, or mass in lumen	Signs and symptoms of inadequate gas exchange and respiratory dysfunction (see Chapter 26)
METABOLIC		
Hypercalcemia	Bone disease or metastasis increasing bone resorption with bone destruction and release of calcium in extracellular fluid; tumor producing (1) substance that enables bone resorption of calcium or (2) ectopic parathyroid hormone that increases serum calcium levels	Nausea and vomiting, constipation, muscle weakness, coma, dysrhythmias, polyuria, nephrolithiasis (see Chapter 17)
Tumor lysis syndrome	Rapid tumor cell destruction after cytotoxic chemotherapy resulting in release of intracellular electrolytes; may occur in cancers characterized by rapid cell growth (leukemia and lymphomas)	Hyperphosphatemia (oliguria, azotemia), hyperkalemia, hyperuricemia (nausea and vomiting, lethargy, anuria, azotemia), hypocalcemia (see Chapter 17)
Syndrome of inappropriate antidiuretic hormone secretion	Increase in antidiuretic hormone seen in cancers such as lung carcinoma (especially small cell), duodenal and pancreatic carcinoma, thymoma, lymphomas, uterine carcinoma, and central nervous system tumors; may also occur with some chemotherapeutic agents (cyclophosphamide)	Fluid and electrolyte and neurologic changes (see Chapter 48)

Nurses are challenged to know and use the same technology to be able to answer the questions of well-informed patients.

Critical Thinking

1. You are speaking to a group of senior citizens at a local retirement center about the three most common cancers for men and women. What are the three most common cancers? What information would you give this audience about risk factors, prevention, and early detection strategies for these cancers?
2. A 69-year-old retired man with squamous cell carcinoma of the tonsil will begin a 6-week course of radiotherapy to ports that include the primary tumor site and lymph nodes in the neck. What side effects will you expect with this radiotherapy plan? What assessments and interventions will be important to include in his care?

References

1. American Cancer Society: *Cancer facts and figures 2004,* Atlanta, 2004, The Society.
2. Administration on Aging, US Department of Health and Human Services: *Older Americans 2004: key indicators of well-being,* accessed 2004 from website: http://aoa/dhhs.gov.
3. Anhang R et al: HPV communication: review of existing research and recommendations for patient education, *CA-Cancer J Clin* 54:248, 2004.
4. Beck SL: Mucositis. In Yarbro CH, Frogge MH, Goodman M, editors: *Cancer symptom management,* ed 3, Boston, 2004, Jones & Bartlett.
5. Bedell C: Pegfilgrastim for chemotherapy induced neutropenia, *Clin J Oncol Nurs* 7:55-56, 63-64, 2003.
6. Camp-Sorrell D: *Access device guidelines: recommendations for nursing practice and education,* Pittsburgh, 2004, Oncology Nursing Society.
7. Crighton MH: Dimensions of neutropenia in adult cancer patients, *Cancer Nurs* 27(4):275-284, 2004.
8. Cuaron L, Thompson J: The interferons. In Rieger PT, editor: *Biotherapy, a comprehensive overview,* ed 2, Boston, 2001, Jones & Bartlett.
9. DeJulio JE: Monoclonal antibodies: overview and use in hematologic malignancies. In Rieger PT, editor: *Biotherapy, a comprehensive overview,* ed 2, Boston, 2001, Jones & Bartlett.

TABLE 23-26 ONCOLOGIC EMERGENCIES—CONT'D

Type	Pathophysiology	Clinical Manifestations
METABOLIC—CONT'D		
Hyperviscosity	Increased blood viscosity from increase in cell number, loss of flexibility of cells, or overproduction of serum proteins; causes increased resistance to blood flow	Bleeding from gastrointestinal or urinary tracts or puncture sites, visual disturbance, headache, dizziness, weakness, dyspnea, distended neck veins
Anaphylaxis	Hypersensitivity responses (I, II, III, IV) caused by chemotherapeutic agents (asparaginase, cisplatin, etoposide, paclitaxel, docetaxel, bleomycin, melphalan)	Signs of anaphylactic reactions (see Chapter 21)
Septic shock	Increased susceptibility to infection from impaired immune system or effect of immunosuppressive agents, leading to bacterial septicemia	Signs and symptoms of septic shock (see Chapter 19)
Disseminated intravascular coagulation	Chronic bleeding consuming all clotting factors; may also result from sepsis	Thrombocytopenia, bleeding of mucous membranes and tissues (see Chapter 33)
CARDIAC TOXICITIES		
Cardiac tamponade	Intrapericardial pressure increase from accumulation of fluid from direct tumor invasion, metastatic lesion, or infection or from pericardial thickening after radiation; results in decreased diastolic ventricular filling, decreased stroke volume and cardiac output	Dyspnea, cough, chest pain, muffled heart sounds, cyanosis, edema, decreased systolic pressure, decreased central venous pressure (see Chapter 30)
Cardiomyopathy with congestive heart failure	Chemotherapeutic drugs (such as anthracyclines, mithramycin, plicamycin, and cyclophosphamide) apparently damage cardiac myofibrils, causing sarcoplasmic reticular swelling that leads to destruction of myofibril; hypertrophy of heart muscle with decreased function results	Acute: tachycardia, dysrhythmias Chronic: signs of congestive heart failure (see Chapter 30)

10. Fiore MC et al: *Treating tobacco use and dependence: a quick reference guide for clinicians,* Rockville, Md, 2000, US Department of Health and Human Service, US Public Health Service.
11. Fisch J, Bruera E: *Handbook of advanced cancer care,* New York, 2003, Cambridge Press.
12. Fischer DS: *The cancer chemotherapy handbook,* ed 6, Philadelphia, 2003, Mosby.
13. Fitzpatrick JJ, Montgomery KS: *Internet resources for nurses,* ed 2, New York, 2003, Springer.
14. Garssen G: Psychological factors and cancer development: evidence after 30 years of research, *Clin Psych Rev* 24:315, 2004.
15. Greco KE, Mahon S: Common hereditary cancer syndromes, *Semin Oncol Nurs* 20:164, 2004.
16. Hardman AE: Physical activity and cancer risk, *Proc Nutr Soc* 60:107, 2001.
17. Hawkins R: Mastering the maze of metastasis, *Oncol Nurs Forum* 28:959, 2001.
18. Henke CY: Advanced cancer care. In Yarbro CH, Frogge MH, Goodman M, editors, *Cancer symptom management,* ed 3, Boston, 2004, Jones & Bartlett.
19. Hodgson NA, Given CW: Determinants of functional recovery in older adults surgically treated for cancer, *Cancer Nurs* 27(1):10-16, 2004.
20. Kwitkowski VE, Daub JR: Clinical applications of genetics in sporadic cancers, *Semin Oncol Nurs* 20:155, 2004.
21. Kwong KKF: Prevention and treatment of oropharyngeal mucositis following cancer therapy, *Cancer Nurs* 27(3):183-205, 2004.
22. Leibel SA, Phillips TL: *Textbook of radiation oncology,* ed 2, Philadelphia, 2004, Saunders.
23. Levitz JS et al: Overview of smoking and all cancers, *Med Clin North Am* 88:1655, 2004.
24. Lindor NM, Greene MH: The concise handbook of family cancer syndromes, *J Nat Cancer Inst* 90:1039, 1998.
25. Mahon SM, Jennings-Dozier K: *Cancer prevention, detection and control: a nursing perspective,* Pittsburgh, 2002, Oncology Nursing Society.
26. McCarthy PL et al: Stem cell transplantation: past, present and future. In Buchsel PC, Kapustay PM, editors: *Stem cell transplantation: a clinical handbook,* Pittsburgh, 2004, Oncology Nursing Press.
27. Nagle T: Help patients cope with chemo, *RN* 67(10):25-31, 2004.
28. Office of US Surgeon General: *The health consequences of smoking: a report of the surgeon general,* Centers for Disease Control and Prevention, Office on Smoking and Health, 2004, accessed from website: http://www.surgeongeneral.gov/library/smoking consequences/.
29. Overcash J, Balducci L: *The older cancer patient,* New York, 2003, Springer.
30. Paice JA: Pain. In Yarbro CH, Frogge MH, Goodman M, editors: *Cancer symptom management,* ed 3, Boston, 2004, Jones & Bartlett.

31. Perez CA et al: *Principles and practice of radiation oncology,* ed 4, Philadelphia, 2004, Lippincott, Williams & Wilkins.
32. Peterson HB et al: Hormone therapy: making decisions in the face of uncertainty, *Arch Intern Med* 164:2308, 2004.
33. *Report on carcinogens,* ed 10, US Department of Health and Human Services, Public Health Service, National Toxicology Program, December 2002.
34. Rieger PT: Biotherapy: an overview. In Rieger PT, editor: *Biotherapy: a comprehensive overview,* ed 2, Boston, 2001, Jones & Bartlett.
35. Rieger PT: The biology of cancer genetics, *Semin Oncol Nurs* 20:145, 2004.
36. Ries LAG et al: *SEER cancer statistics review, 1973-1997,* Bethesda, Md, 2000, National Cancer Institute.
37. Sadler GR et al: Managing oral sequelae of cancer therapy, *Medsurg Nurs* 12(1):28, 2003.
38. Skelton BK: Flu-like syndrome. In Yarbro CH, Frogge MH, Goodman M, editors: *Cancer symptom management,* ed 3, Boston, 2004, Jones & Bartlett.
39. US Department of Health and Human Services: *Healthy people 2010: understanding and improving health,* Washington, DC, 2000, The Department.
40. Varricchio CG: *A cancer source book for nurses,* Sudbury, Mass, 2004, Jones & Bartlett.
41. Veenena TG, Karam PA: Radiation: clinical response to radiologic incidents and emergencies, *Am J Nurs* 103(5):32-40, 2003.
42. White N et al: Protocols for managing chemotherapy induced neutropenia in clinical oncology practices, *Cancer Nurs* 28(1):62-69, 2005.
43. Willett WC: Diet and cancer, *Oncologist* 5:393, 2005.

evolve Visit the Evolve website: http://evolve.elsevier.com/Monahan/medsurg

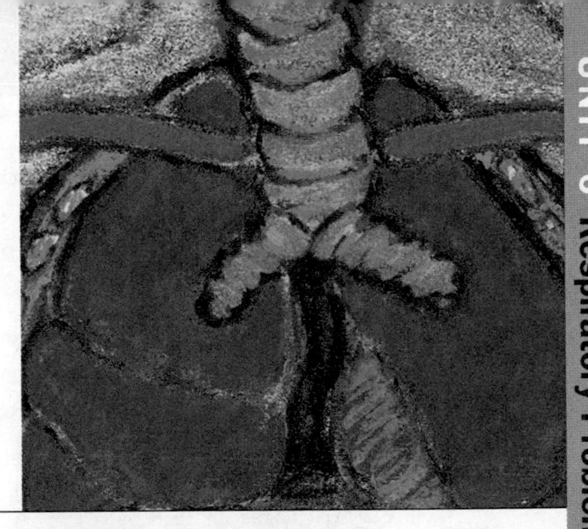

CHAPTER 24

Assessment of the Respiratory System

by Shelley Yerger Huffstutler

OBJECTIVES

After studying this chapter, the learner should be able to:

1. Identify the structural components of the respiratory system.
2. Differentiate ventilation from respiration.
3. Explain the respiratory system's primary function of gas exchange.
4. Describe the mechanisms that control ventilation.
5. Discuss the defense mechanisms of the lungs.
6. Explain age-related changes in the respiratory system.
7. Identify subjective and objective data needed to obtain a complete respiratory assessment.
8. Describe common diagnostic tests and related nursing care used to evaluate respiratory conditions.

KEY TERMS

arterial blood gas, p. 578
bronchoscopy, p. 585
chemoreceptors, p. 570
dyspnea, p. 571
environmental irritants, p. 571
perfusion, p. 569
pulmonary function tests, p. 583
pulse oximetry, p. 574
respiration, p. 565
risk factors, p. 573
thoracentesis, p. 584
ventilation, p. 565
V/Q ratio, p. 569
wheezing, p. 573

A daily activity that most of us rarely think about is breathing air in and out of our lungs. However, the ease or discomfort of breathing has a major impact on the quality of our daily activities. The act of breathing involves two interrelated processes: ventilation and respiration. **Ventilation** is the movement of air into and out of the lungs. **Respiration** refers to the exchange of oxygen and carbon dioxide across cell membranes.

This chapter reviews the anatomy and physiology of the respiratory system, discusses the subjective and objective data essential to the health assessment of a patient experiencing a respiratory problem, and describes tests commonly used to diagnose and monitor patients with respiratory dysfunction.

Anatomy and Physiology

Upper Airway

Nose and Sinuses. The nose functions primarily as the organ of smell and as a passage through which air travels on its way in and out of the lungs. The upper part of the nose is supported by bone, and the lower part is supported by cartilage. The external openings to the nose are the nostrils, or nares. These lead into the two nasal cavities, which are separated by the nasal septum.

Mucus-lined, curved, bony projections, called turbinates, form the lateral walls of the nasal cavities (Figure 24-1) and provide a large surface area for warming, humidifying, and filtering the inspired air. Because the turbinates have a rich blood supply, air that is inhaled is heated almost to body temperature by the time it reaches the posterior nasopharynx. The inspired air is also humidified by the nose and is 100% saturated with water vapor by the time the air reaches the alveoli. This humidification results in an insensible fluid loss of 250 ml/day. Filtration of large particles of dust and other matter is accomplished by nasal hairs trapping the particulates. These irritants can trigger the sneeze reflex to remove the foreign particles. In addition, the mucous membrane of the turbinate bones entraps small particles, and they are propelled by cilia (hairlike projections that beat in a wavelike motion) to the pharynx for swallowing or expectoration.

Each turbinate has an opening for draining the nasolacrimal ducts and four paranasal sinuses (Figure 24-2). The sinuses are air-filled spaces lined with mucous membrane that is continuous with that of the nose. Their primary purpose is to produce mucus for the nasal cavity and promote vocal resonance and timber.

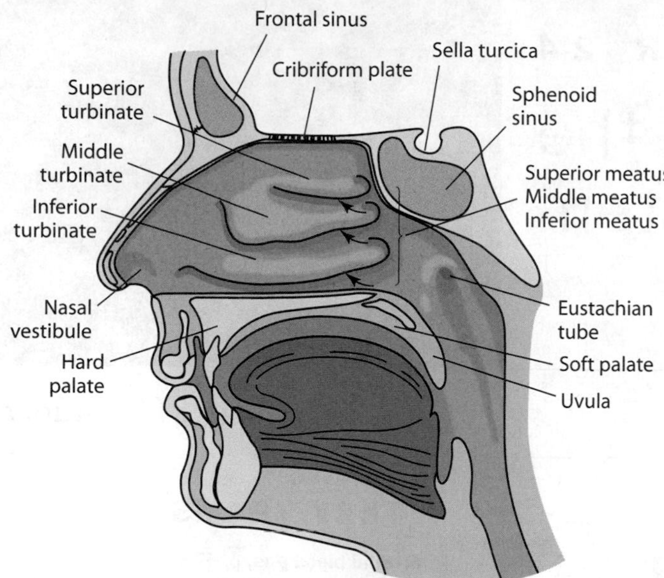

Figure 24-1 Lateral wall of nose, showing superior, middle, and inferior turbinates.

Pharynx. The pharynx, or throat, is divided into the nasopharynx, oropharynx, and laryngopharynx (Figure 24-3). Because it is the only opening between the nose and mouth and the lungs, any obstruction of the pharynx (e.g., tissue swelling, foreign body, or the tongue falling back into the pharynx) can lead to cessation of ventilation. The nasopharynx is posterior to the nose and above the soft palate and contains the adenoids and openings of the eustachian tubes. The oropharynx is located in the posterior portion of the mouth and contains the tonsils. The adenoids and tonsils are made up of lymphoid tissue that helps filter bacteria or other foreign matter that enters the nose and throat. The laryngopharynx opens into the larynx and esophagus.

Larynx. The larynx, also known as the *voice box,* connects the pharynx to the trachea. It is made up of cartilage, muscle, and ligaments (Figure 24-4) and houses the vocal cords, which form the V-shaped opening of the glottis or entrance to the larynx. Sound is produced as exhaled air is forced through a closed glottis, causing the vocal cords to vibrate. The closing of the glottis also allows for an increase in intrathoracic pressure, which is needed when a person coughs or lifts. The entrance to the larynx is protected by

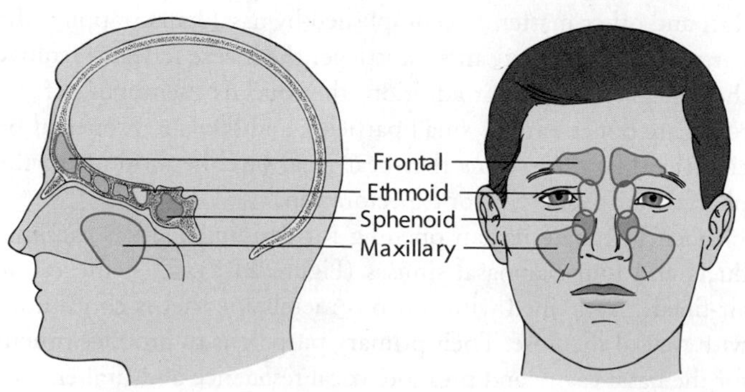

Figure 24-2 Location of sinuses.

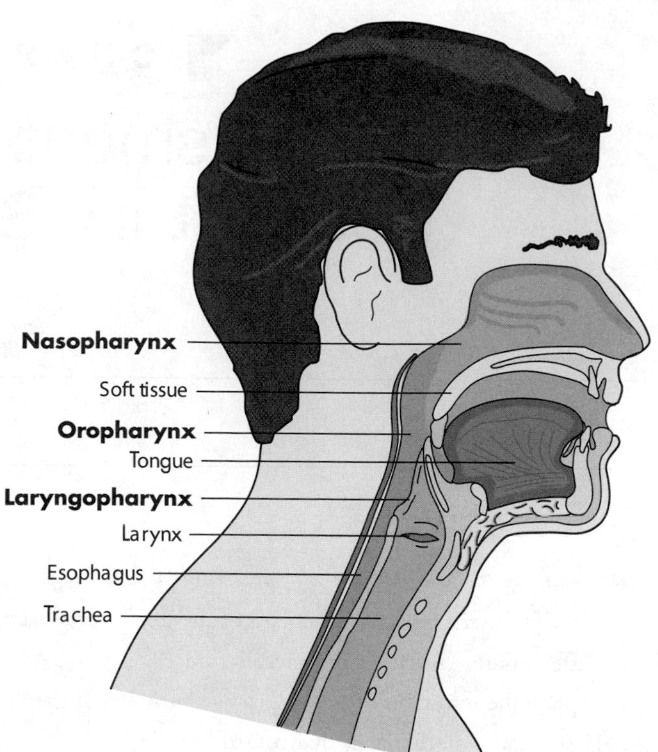

Figure 24-3 Sagittal section of head showing pharynx and larynx.

the epiglottis. This leaf-shaped lid of fibrocartilage covers the glottis during swallowing to prevent aspiration of food or fluids into the lungs. The larynx is innervated by the laryngeal nerve, which initiates the cough reflex in response to stimulation by foreign particles, dry mucous membranes, and other irritants. Damage to the laryngeal nerve results in paralysis of the laryngeal muscles and allows foreign materials to enter the lungs.

Lower Airway

Trachea, Bronchi, and Bronchioles. As inhaled air passes through the larynx, it enters the lower airway, which consists of the trachea, bronchi, bronchioles, and terminal respiratory units (Figure 24-5). The trachea, commonly known as the windpipe, connects the larynx to the right and left main-stem bronchi. The point at which the trachea bifurcates into the right and left bronchi is called the *carina.* The carina contains cough receptors that can be easily stimulated, for example, by tubes such as suction catheters or endotracheal tubes. The landmark used to locate the carina is the manubriosternal junction, often called *Louis' angle.*

The trachea and bronchi are supported by incomplete cartilaginous rings that prevent airway collapse when the pressure in the thorax becomes negative. The trachea shares a small muscle with the esophagus at the point where the cartilaginous rings do not meet. This is a potential site for a tracheoesophageal (T-E) fistula. Cuffed tubes, such as endotracheal or tracheostomy tubes, may lead to T-E fistulas as a result of high pressures within the cuffs.

These lower airways are lined with goblet cells that produce mucus, which traps debris, and ciliated epithelium, which propels foreign particles toward the pharynx for removal. Mucus and particles are removed from the airway by swallowing, coughing, or

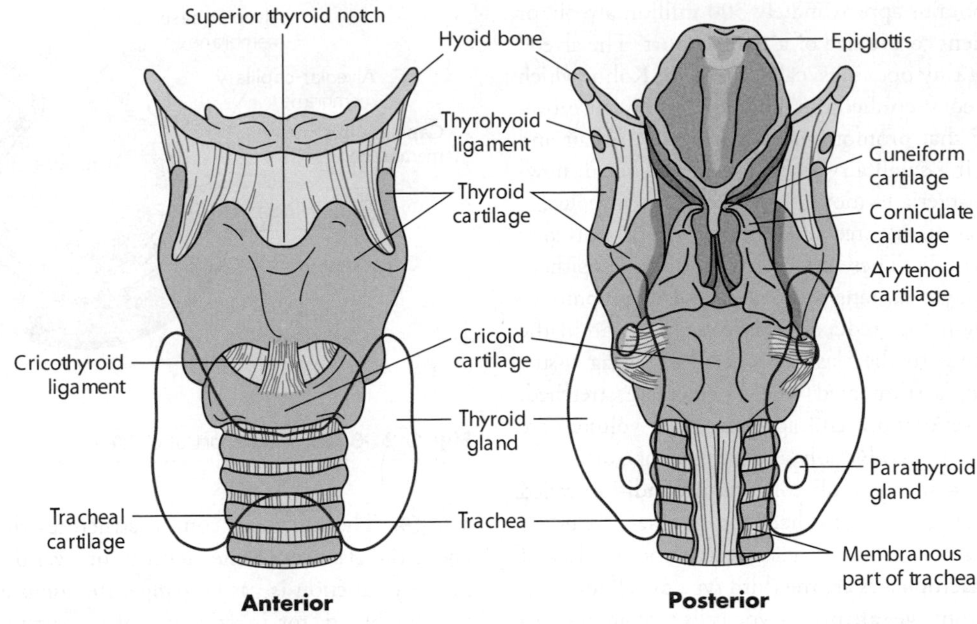

Figure 24-4 Larynx.

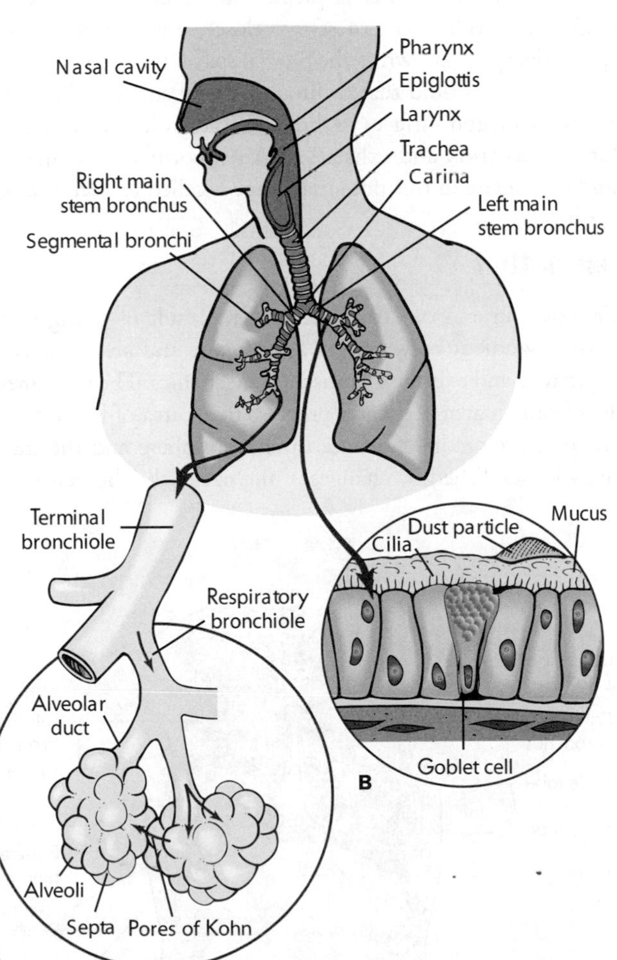

Figure 24-5 Respiratory system. **Inset A,** Acinus, or pulmonary functional unit. **Inset B,** Ciliated mucous membrane.

sneezing. See the following sections for a complete discussion of pulmonary defense mechanisms.

The bronchi enter the lungs through an opening called the hilum. The right bronchus is wider and shorter than the left bronchus, extending nearly vertically from the trachea. Aspiration or misplaced intubation is more likely to occur with the right lung because of this anatomic feature. Thus it is important to secure an endotracheal tube so that proper ventilation can be maintained. If the tube is misplaced or slips into the right bronchus, air will not be able to enter the left lung. The left bronchus is narrower and extends at more of an acute angle off the trachea, making it more difficult to pass a catheter into it for removal of secretions from the left lung.

The right and left main-stem bronchi divide into smaller branches: the left bronchus divides into two lobar branches, and the right bronchus divides into three lobar branches. The lobar branches divide into segments that further subdivide into subsegmental bronchi, terminal bronchi, bronchioles, terminal bronchioles, and respiratory bronchioles. Respiratory bronchioles divide further into respiratory terminal bronchioles, alveolar ducts, alveolar sacs, and alveoli.

The bronchioles contain no cartilage for support. The patency of these airways is determined by smooth muscle, which relaxes or contracts, thus affecting their diameter. The diameter of the airway determines the amount of airway resistance. For example, if the radius of the airway was cut in half, the resistance would increase 16 times. Mucous plugs, bronchoconstriction, airway edema, and external compression of the airway are conditions that increase airway resistance and impair airflow into the lungs. Cilia and secretory gland cells that aid in the removal of dust and particles are absent at the level of the terminal bronchioles (see Figure 24-5, *B*).

Terminal Respiratory Unit. The structures distal to the terminal bronchioles are collectively referred to as *acini,* or terminal respiratory units (see Figure 24-5, *A*). The acini include the respiratory bronchioles, alveolar ducts, alveolar sacs, and alveoli.

The adult lung contains approximately 300 million alveoli, or a surface area equivalent to the size of a tennis court. The alveoli are interconnected by tiny openings, called pores of Kohn, which are present in the alveolar epithelium. The pores allow air movement between alveoli that promotes even distribution of air and collateral ventilation if a small airway becomes obstructed; however, they also allow bacteria to move from alveolus to alveolus.

The alveolar sacs contain three types of cells. Type I alveolar cells are flat squamous cells. These cells form the alveolar epithelium, which is the site of gas exchange. Type II alveolar cells produce surfactant, a lipoprotein that reduces surface tension within the alveolus and contributes to the elastic properties of lung tissue. Surfactant production is stimulated when alveoli are stretched. Thus sighing, active ventilation, and adequate tidal volumes are important factors in the production and release of surfactant. Without adequate surfactant, alveoli collapse (a condition called *atelactasis)* can occur. A number of other lung diseases, including acute respiratory distress syndrome, can also result from the lack of surfactant. Alveolar macrophages are the third type of cell found in the alveolar sacs. Macrophages are phagocytic cells that are responsible for ingesting and removing bacteria and other foreign particles from the alveolar surface. The macrophages transport the microorganisms to the lymphatics or bronchioles for removal via the mucociliary escalator. The alveolar macrophage is one of the most important defense mechanisms against lung infection.

Lung Circulation

The lungs receive blood from both the pulmonary and bronchial circulation. Bronchial circulation provides nutrients to the tissues of the tracheobronchial tree and warms and moistens inspired air but does not participate in gas exchange. The bronchial arteries originate from the thoracic aorta. Blood is returned from the bronchial system to the left atrium by the azygos vein.

Pulmonary circulation is a high-volume, low-pressure circuit by means of which blood received from the right ventricle of the heart interacts with the airway at the terminal bronchioles. The deoxygenated blood from the right ventricle is transported through the main pulmonary artery that branches into smaller arteries and arterioles and finally to the alveolar capillaries of the acini. Once the blood is oxygenated and carbon dioxide is removed, the blood is returned to the left atrium of the heart via the pulmonary veins. The oxygenated blood then enters the left ventricle where it is pumped out of the aorta into the systemic circulation.

The alveoli are surrounded by a pulmonary capillary network. Each alveolus is separated from the pulmonary capillary by an interstitial space (Figure 24-6), a distance of less than 1 mm. At this site, oxygen travels from the alveolus into the capillary blood for distribution to the cells of the body, and carbon dioxide passes out of the blood into the alveolus for passage to the external environment.

Lungs and Thoracic Cage

Thoracic Cage. The thoracic cage is composed of the ribs, sternum, scapulae, and vertebral column. The thoracic cage houses the lungs, heart, great vessels, lymph nodes, thymus gland, and esophagus. Intercostal muscles lie between the ribs, and the diaphragm forms the floor of the thoracic cage. Figure 24-7 depicts the anatomy of the thorax and lungs.

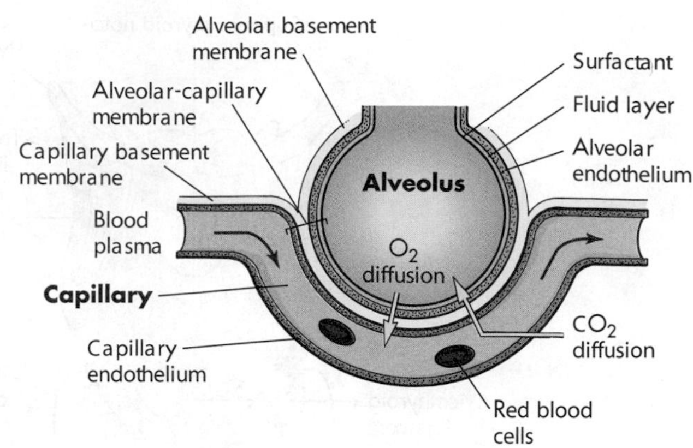

Figure 24-6 Blood transport of oxygen.

Lungs. The lungs are conical structures that extend from just above the clavicles to the eleventh or twelfth rib. Although their primary function is gas exchange, the lungs also serve as a reservoir for blood, for inactivation of vasoactive substances such as bradykinin, and for conversion of angiotensin I into angiotensin II. The right lung has three lobes (upper, middle, and lower); the left lung has two lobes (upper and lower). A serous membrane called the parietal pleura lines the inside of the thoracic cavity. It is continuous with the visceral pleura that covers the surface of the lungs. The area between these two closely opposed pleurae forms a potential space known as the pleural space. It contains a few milliliters of serous fluid that facilitates pleural surface adhesion and allows the pleural surfaces to slide over each other without friction during inhalation and exhalation. An abnormal accumulation of fluid or exudate in this potential space is called *pleural effusion.*

Ventilation

Air moves in and out of the lungs as a result of changes in the pressure gradient between the atmosphere and alveoli caused by inspiratory and expiratory muscular mechanics. The movement of air is from an area of greater pressure to an area of lesser pressure. The pressure gradient between the atmosphere and the thoracic cavity is established by changes in the size of the thoracic cavity.

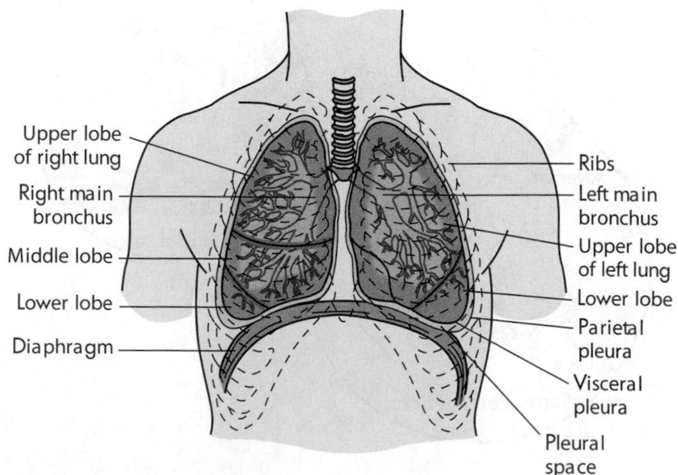

Figure 24-7 Anatomy of thorax and lungs.

Inspiratory Muscles. Inhalation is an active process that requires contraction of the inspiratory muscles, including the diaphragm, external intercostal muscles, and scalene muscles. The diaphragm is a large dome-shaped muscle that flattens during contraction, initiating inspiration. It is the primary muscle of breathing and is innervated by the right and left phrenic nerves. Injury or damage to the phrenic nerves causes paralysis of the diaphragm, adversely affecting lung movement on the affected side. The chest moves upward instead of downward on the side of the paralysis during inspiration. This is known as *paradoxic movement.* Contraction of the external intercostal and scalene muscles causes the anterior part of the thoracic cage to rise during inspiration, increasing the chest dimensions. During exercise or in diseased states the sternocleidomastoid muscles, accessory muscles used to assist in inhalation, raise the sternum, resulting in an increased diameter of the thoracic cage. Because of the thorax's change in size, the resultant increase in volume causes a change in pressure such that the intrapleural pressure, as well as the intrapulmonary pressure or airway pressure, decreases in relation to atmospheric pressure. This pressure gradient causes air to move into the lungs.

Expiratory Muscles. Exhalation is normally a passive process produced by elastic recoil of the chest wall and the lungs. Relaxation of the diaphragm and intercostal muscles decreases the size of the thoracic cage. Active exhalation that results from disease, exercise, or coughing causes the internal intercostal and abdominal muscles to contract. Contraction of these accessory muscles causes the ribs to move upward, abdominal contents to rise, and diaphragm to move upward. The resultant decrease in volume leads to an increase in the intrapulmonary and intrapleural pressures. The pressure gradient that is created between the atmosphere and the airways causes the air to flow out of the lungs.

Compliance and Elasticity. Two properties that permit the lungs to expand and return to their resting state are compliance and elasticity. Compliance is a quality of yielding to pressure and represents the ease with which the lungs can be stretched while consuming a volume of air. Determinants of compliance include the elastic recoil of the lung and chest wall, along with the alveolar surface tension. An increase in compliance means that the lungs are abnormally easy to inflate; a decrease in compliance indicates stiffness or difficulty in inflating the lungs.

Elasticity of the chest wall is determined by the musculature and bones of the thoracic cage and is reduced in patients with bony deformities, abdominal distention, and obesity. Elastic recoil of the lungs is the tendency of the lungs to return to the resting state. The elasticity of the lungs is determined by the elastic and collagen fibers of the lungs. The fibers are stretched out when the lungs are inflated and contract when the lungs are deflated. Conditions in which lung tissue stiffens, such as pulmonary fibrosis or interstitial lung disease, decrease compliance.

Gas Exchange: Diffusion

Gas movement across the alveolar-capillary membrane occurs by the process of diffusion. Once the inspired oxygen reaches the alveoli, oxygen diffuses into the pulmonary capillary because of the greater partial pressure of oxygen in alveolar air in contrast to the partial pressure of oxygen in venous blood. Carbon dioxide diffuses in the opposite direction because the partial pressure of carbon dioxide in venous blood is greater than the partial pressure of carbon dioxide in alveolar air (Figure 24-8). Diffusion of oxygen is decreased by (1) a decrease in atmospheric oxygen, (2) a decrease in alveolar ventilation, (3) a decrease in alveolar-capillary surface area, and (4) an increase in thickness of the alveolar capillary membrane.[2]

Ventilation-Perfusion Ratio

Efficient gas exchange depends on a balance between ventilation or air flow (V) and **perfusion** or blood flow (Q). In other words, areas that receive ventilation should be well perfused with blood, and areas that receive blood flow should be capable of ventilation.

In the normal lung, alveolar ventilation is about 4 L/min and pulmonary capillary blood flow is about 5 L/min. Gravity causes greater blood flow to the lower portion of the lungs. Thus, in an upright person, the bases of the lungs receive a greater volume of blood than the apices. If a patient is supine, the dependent portions of the lungs receive more blood flow than the upper parts. Similarly, ventilation is not uniformly distributed. In an upright person, the upper parts of the lungs contain a greater residual volume of gas and the alveoli are less compliant than in the lower parts of the lungs; thus more gas is distributed to the bases of the lungs. These slight imbalances in ventilation and perfusion have little effect on overall gas exchange in normal lungs. The overall **V/Q ratio** of normal lungs is 0.8.[1]

Mismatched ventilation and perfusion may occur as a result of dead air space and shunting of blood. Dead air space refers to those areas of the respiratory tract that are ventilated but not perfused by

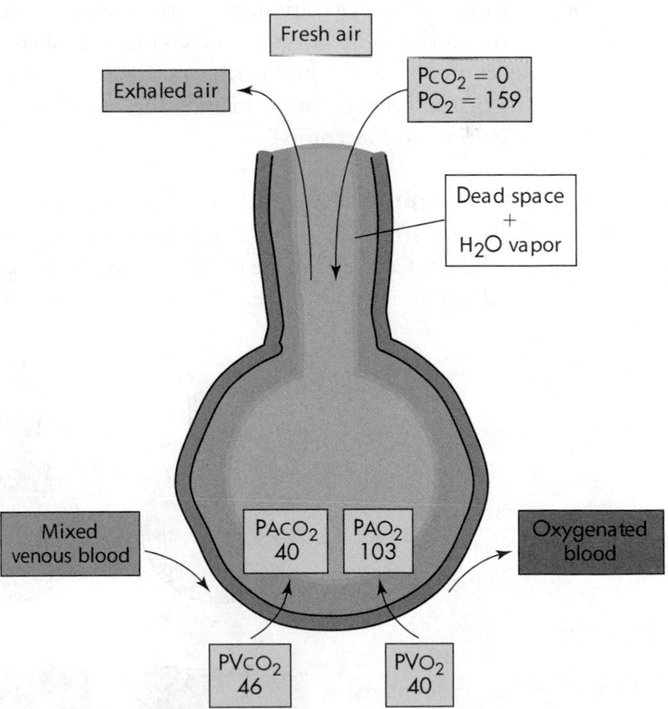

Figure 24-8 Diffusion of gases across the alveolar-capillary membrane. *Pco_2 and PO_2*, Partial pressure of carbon dioxide and oxygen; *$Paco_2$ and Pao_2*, alveolar Pco_2 and PO_2; *$Pvco_2$ and Pvo_2*, mixed venous Pco_2 and PO_2.

the pulmonary circulation and therefore do not allow gas exchange. There are two types of dead space: anatomic and alveolar. Anatomic dead space consists of the conducting airways above the level of the alveolus. Alveolar dead space consists of alveoli that are not perfused. Alveolar dead air space may be the result of normal factors such as gravity or may be due to disease. Impaired blood flow in relation to the amount of ventilation to the alveoli or excessive ventilation relative to blood flow results in mismatch. For example, blood flow (perfusion) to the alveoli may be blocked by a pulmonary embolus, yet the alveoli may be well ventilated. Perfusion also may be blocked when gas pressure within the alveolus is greater than within the capillary, causing the capillary to collapse. These are both examples of high V/Q ratios resulting in dead-space ventilation or "wasted" ventilation. The air does not participate in gas exchange but does contribute to the work of breathing.[3]

Low V/Q ratios indicate that the lungs are poorly ventilated in relation to the amount of blood flow. For example, blood flow to the alveolus may be normal, but fluid in the alveolus, bronchospasm, or mucous plugs increase airway resistance and may prevent adequate ventilation. As a result, V/Q inequality, or shunting, now exists. The blood perfuses the area of the lung that is not ventilated; thus blood is "shunted" past the area and no gas exchange occurs. This is known as wasted perfusion. Figure 24-9 shows examples of V/Q relationships.

Control of Respiration

Breathing can be viewed as an automatic loop process in which **chemoreceptors** (sensors) continuously feed data to a central processor (medulla oblongata and pons). Subsequently, the respiratory muscles are directed to adjust ventilation to meet the needs of the body (Figure 24-10). In addition, an override feature (cerebral cortex) exists, so that ventilation can be consciously altered. The major sensors are the central and peripheral chemoreceptors. Other receptors that affect ventilation include the neural receptors (stretch receptors and J receptors).

Central Chemoreceptors. Central chemoreceptors, located near the medulla, are sensitive to hydrogen ion concentration (pH) in the spinal fluid. Carbon dioxide readily crosses the blood-brain barrier and combines with water to form carbonic acid, which dissociates into hydrogen ions. A change in arterial carbon dioxide levels affects the pH of the cerebrospinal fluid, which in turn stimulates the chemoreceptors. Ventilation increases in depth and rate when carbon dioxide levels increase, and ventilation decreases in depth and rate when carbon dioxide levels decrease.

Ventilation is regulated primarily by the central chemoreceptor response to changes in arterial carbon dioxide levels and its effect on the pH of the cerebrospinal fluid. However, the central chemoreceptors become less sensitive in patients with chronically high carbon dioxide levels and low oxygen levels. In these patients the peripheral chemoreceptors are the primary stimuli for ventilation.

Peripheral Chemoreceptors. Peripheral chemoreceptors, located in the carotid bodies and aortic arch, primarily respond to low arterial blood oxygen levels (a PaO_2 of 60 mm Hg) and signal the respiratory center in the medulla. Efferent signals are then sent to the respiratory muscles to increase the ventilatory rate. Patients who rely on their hypoxic drive for breathing (e.g., those with chronic obstructive pulmonary disease [COPD]) depend on the peripheral chemoreceptors for control of ventilation. Administration of an uncontrolled amount of oxygen or failure to monitor arterial PaO_2 levels with oxygen administration in these patients can depress or abolish their hypoxic ventilatory drive, and death may result.

Neural Receptors. The stretch receptors located in the conducting airways respond to changes in the pressure within the airways. Inspiration is inhibited once the lungs are inflated, an effect known as the Hering-Breuer inflation reflex, which acts to prevent overinflation of the lungs. J receptors, located in the alveolar walls, respond with rapid, shallow breathing in conditions associated with an increase in interstitial fluid volume such as pulmonary edema and pneumonia.

▶ ARE You READY?

Which of the following is a physiologic response to elevated carbon dioxide levels?

1. Increased respiratory rate
2. Increased inspiratory response
3. Increased expiratory effort
4. Increased functional residual capacity

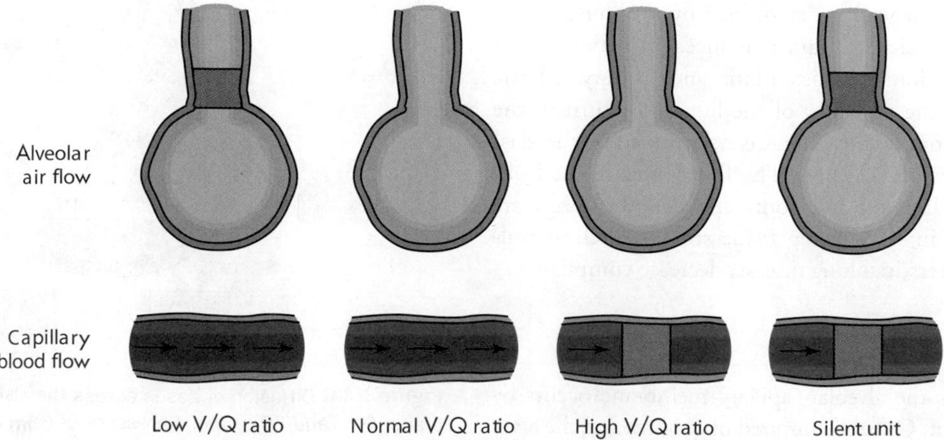

Figure 24-9 Range of ventilation to perfusion (V/Q) ratios from 0 to infinity.

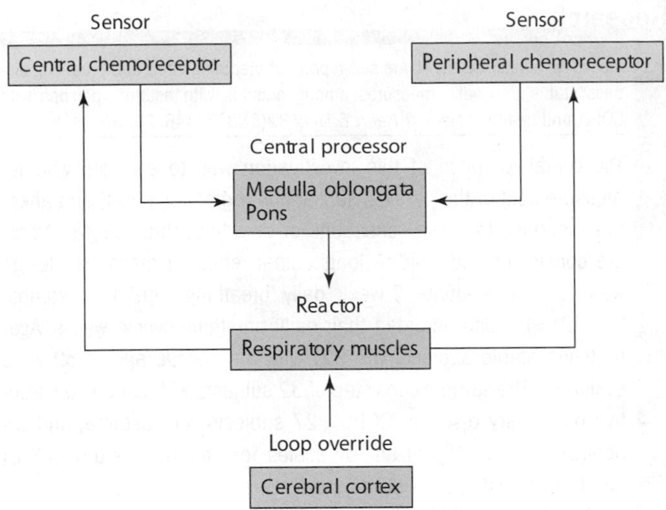

Figure 24-10 Respiratory control loop.

Physiologic Changes With Aging

Changes in respiratory anatomy and physiology with aging can produce variations in clinical findings. This section discusses some of the changes more commonly detected during assessment of the older adult.

The thoracic cage becomes rigid from cartilage calcification, osteoporosis of the ribs, and arthritic changes in the joints of the ribs. Kyphosis, or accentuated dorsal curvature of the thoracic spine (hunch back), may also occur with aging. An increase in the anteroposterior diameter of the chest occurs in older adults. Chest wall compliance is reduced because of stiffening of the chest wall and a loss in elastic recoil of the lungs associated with advanced age. This results in increased work of breathing. Muscle strength also decreases with aging, affecting lung volumes and pressures; however, exercise may enhance respiratory muscle strength.

Structural changes within the lungs include calcification of bronchial cartilages, increased anatomic dead space, decreased diameter of noncartilaginous bronchioles, increased size of the pores of Kohn, and enlarged alveolar ducts. Pulmonary diffusion capacity decreases because of a loss in the surface area of the alveolar-capillary membrane and inequalities in the distribution of air or blood. The room air alveolar-arterial oxygen gradient (PAO_2-PaO_2) increases with aging. Arterial oxygen pressure (PaO_2) levels are lower, but carbon dioxide levels and pH are not affected by age. Ventilatory and heart rate responses to brief periods of hypoxia or hypercarbia are blunted. Sleep apnea may be observed in older adults but has not been reported to be clinically significant. Although total lung capacity is relatively unchanged, the effects of aging on lung volumes and spirometry include an increase in residual volume, a decrease in forced vital capacity, a decrease in forced expiratory volume, a decrease in maximum voluntary ventilation, and a decrease in peak expiratory airflow.

Health History

Respiratory assessment should be tailored to the patient's health status. If the patient exhibits signs of respiratory distress such as increased restlessness, paradoxic breathing pattern, increased ventilatory rate, complaints of dyspnea, or use of accessory muscles, the nurse should defer gathering subjective information and perform an abbreviated physical assessment. Once the patient is physiologically stable, data collection can resume. Information can also be obtained from a significant other, if available.

Common Symptoms

The most common pulmonary symptoms for which persons seek health care include dyspnea, cough, increased sputum production, hemoptysis, wheezing, and chest pain. Upper airway symptoms include nasal obstruction, nasal discharge, sinus pain, sore throat, and hoarseness.

Dyspnea. **Dyspnea,** which is defined as difficult breathing, is one of the most common clinical manifestations of respiratory disease. The term describes both difficult or labored breathing observed by another and a patient's subjective experience of breathlessness or breathing discomfort. A defining attribute of dyspnea is that it is a distinctly distressful sensation, described by terms such as *chest tightness, suffocation, not getting enough air, choking,* and *smothering.* Dyspnea is distinct from tachypnea (an increased respiratory rate) or hyperpnea (an increased depth of respiration) because of the associated discomfort.

As for any symptom, the nurse needs to collect comprehensive data about the timing and characteristics of dyspnea as part of the assessment. Pertinent data related to timing include whether the problem is acute or chronic (persisting over time with only the intensity of the symptom changing), whether it is episodic or paroxysmal, the date and type of onset (sudden or gradual), duration, and frequency. Characteristics to be explored include perceived severity; phase of the respiratory cycle affected (inspiratory, expiratory, or both); and associated factors such as time of day, seasonal or weather changes, exposure to **environmental irritants**, anxiety, activity, and body position.

Body position is important, since two distinct types of dyspnea are orthopnea, which is breathlessness on assuming the recumbent position, and paroxysmal nocturnal dyspnea (PND), which is the sudden onset of difficult breathing while sleeping in the recumbent position. The nurse needs to identify symptoms such as use of respiratory accessory muscles, dilated nostrils, tachycardia, and cyanosis, which are commonly associated with dyspnea. Some studies reveal that the qualitative characteristics vary by disease category.[7] Persons with asthma report severe but episodic dyspnea and may have complete resolution of symptoms between episodes. Persons with emphysema, chronic bronchitis, and pulmonary vascular disease report constant dyspnea. Additional studies[5,6] have tried unsuccessfully to link the worsening of dyspnea with the degree of deterioration of lung function.

Assessing the severity of dyspnea, particularly when referencing the subjective experience of breathlessness, is particularly challenging but critical for patient evaluation and management decisions. One method to objectify and quantify the subjective sense of breathlessness is use of a self-report visual analog scale (Figure 24-11). This scale can be used to evaluate the effectiveness of interventions and to monitor the patient's response to therapy. Another approach to assessing dyspnea is to determine its effect on activities of daily living (ADLs). This approach is valuable

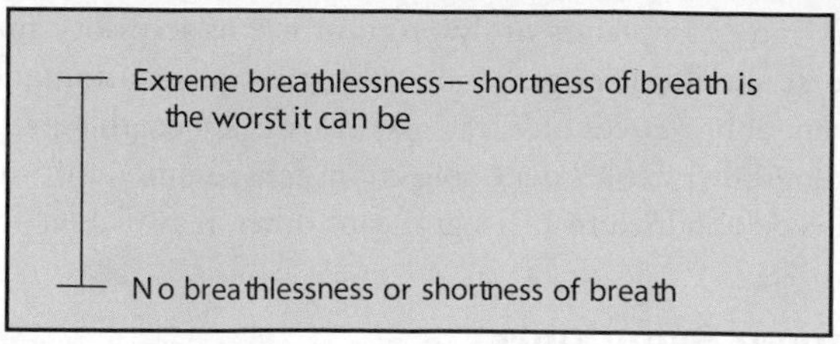

Extreme breathlessness—shortness of breath is the worst it can be

No breathlessness or shortness of breath

Figure 24-11 Breathlessness visual analog scale. The patient is asked to place a mark on the line between "no breathlessness" and "extreme breathlessness" at the place that corresponds with severity of breathlessness.

because chronic dyspnea can lead to a reduction in physical activity and may affect the person's ability to work, socialize, and perform usual ADLs. Fatigue frequently accompanies dyspnea. Dyspnea during moderate exertion causes a reduction of physical activities and results in physical deconditioning. Physical deconditioning then results in dyspnea with only mild exertion and eventually with ADLs. To determine the effect of dyspnea on ADLs, the nurse asks, "How does your breathing difficulty affect your ability to bathe, dress, and groom yourself; walk or exercise; prepare meals and eat; get about your home; climb stairs; sleep; perform chores and hobbies; get to the bathroom; maintain family and social relationships; maintain employment; perform sexually; and attend activities away from home?"

Chronic dyspnea, chronic fatigue, and the reduction of physical activities lead to loss of previous role identification, inability to earn a living, social isolation, and, often, depression. People with chronic dyspnea need preventive and therapeutic plans for dealing with both acute and chronic distress. It is essential that nurses assess the level of dyspnea experienced, understand its effects on health, and offer tools to help with its management. The Research box presents a report of a study that looked at the nurse's intervention for patients with breathlessness.

Cough. Coughing has two main functions. It protects the lungs from aspiration, and it helps propel foreign matter and excess mucus up through the airways. Receptors for the cough reflex are located in the tracheal and bronchial mucosa, with the largest concentration found in the larynx, carina, and bifurcations of the large and medium-sized bronchi. When these receptors are stimulated, impulses are transmitted primarily via the afferent nervous pathways (vagus, phrenic, and spinal motor nerves) to expiratory musculature (larynx, tracheobronchial tree, diaphragm, and abdominal wall). Cough is a common symptom of airway disease.

Cough is described as acute, chronic, or paroxysmal (periodic forceful episodes that are difficult to control), and as productive, nonproductive, or dry progressing to productive. Productive refers to the production of sputum. Not all patients with a productive cough expectorate sputum; sometimes, they swallow it. However, the term *productive cough* is used when sputum is produced regardless of the patient's ability to expectorate it. Coughs can also be described as barking, hoarse, or hacking.

Cough must be analyzed in terms of onset (gradual or sudden), duration and frequency, pattern (occasional, on arising, with activity), perceived severity (effect on ADLs, e.g., inability to eat, talk, or sleep), aggravating factors (hot or cold weather or exercise), associated symptoms (sputum production, chest tightness, fever, or choking), and alleviating factors (medications, treatments, and folk remedies). Even though cough is an important defense mechanism, cough lasting longer than 2 to 3 weeks may indicate serious respiratory dysfunction and should be evaluated.

Research

Meek PM, Lareau SC, Jie H: Are self-reports of breathing effort and breathing distress stable and valid measures among persons with asthma, persons with COPD, and healthy persons? *Heart & Lung* 32(5):335-346, 2003.

The overall purpose of this investigation was to evaluate whether measurement of the physical sensations (breathing effort) and affective response to these sensations of breathing (breathing distress) are consistent and valid. A longitudinal repeated measures design was used to evaluate 2-week daily breathing with a subsample (n=43) who also recorded their daily breathing over 4 weeks. Age-matched stable subjects (n=92) with an average age of 62 were evaluated. The sample consisted of 32 subjects with chronic obstructive pulmonary disease (COPD), 27 subjects with asthma, and 33 healthy subjects. Visual analog scales for breathing effort (VAS-E) and breathing distress (VAS-D) were scored daily.

The VAS-E and VAS-D mean, highest, and lowest scores were found to be stable over time in the subsample, with a significant difference ($F=2.56$, $p<0.05$) between VAS-E and VAS-D. Differences were found in mean and highest VAS-E and VAS-D by group, with the COPD group reporting the highest values. This investigation provided initial evidence of the stability and validity of daily VAS-E and VAS-D measures and preliminary support for the use of daily VAS logs to evaluate differences in breathing effort and breathing distress.

Changes in Sputum Production. As described previously, a mucous blanket lines the epithelial layer of the tracheobronchial tree and cleanses it of inhaled particles and debris. The goblet cells and submucosal glands produce mucus. The cilia propel the mucus (which contains foreign particles, pus, blood, and debris) upward toward the pharynx where it is coughed up, suctioned, or swallowed. Normal sputum is clear and thin and averages 100 ml/day. With pulmonary disease sputum can change in amount and characteristics, and the type of change can reflect the specific pathologic condition present. Thus it is important to assess baseline sputum characteristics.

Sputum is described in terms of color, consistency, and amount. Color varies widely. It can be clear as with noninfectious processes, creamy yellow or rusty as seen in staphylococcal pneumonia, green as seen in *Pseudomonas* pneumonia, "currant jelly" as seen in *Klebsiella* pneumonia, or pink and frothy as seen with pulmonary edema. Consistency may be thick, viscous (gelatinous), or watery. Sputum may also be described as mucoid or mucopurulent. Amount of sputum is assessed using objective measurements such as teaspoons, tablespoons, or cups rather than subjective terms such as "scant" or "moderate." Sputum is most accurately assessed by seeing it as opposed to accepting the patient's description.

Hemoptysis. Hemoptysis is the coughing up of blood or blood-tinged sputum. The sputum is usually frothy with air bubbles, alkaline in pH, and bright red. The source of bleeding may be anywhere in the upper or lower airways or the lung parenchyma. Hemoptysis must be distinguished from hematemesis, which is vomiting blood that originates in the gastrointestinal tract. Hematemesis is never frothy, has an acid pH, and may be mixed with food particles. If it has been in the stomach long enough to be acted on by the digestive enzymes, it is dark red (mahogany) or looks like coffee grounds. Epistaxis must be considered as a potential cause of hemoptysis. The amount of hemoptysis should be quantified in milliliters or teaspoons, tablespoons, or cups. The coughing up of 400 to 600 ml of blood in a 24-hour period is considered a massive amount and requires immediate evaluation.[3]

Wheezing. **Wheezing** is a continuous, high-pitched, whistling sound produced when air passes through narrowed or obstructed airways. It generally occurs during expiration but can be heard throughout the respiratory cycle. Wheezing is usually heard with a stethoscope; however, it may be audible to the patient or heard by others in close proximity. Information to be collected includes presence of factors that can cause bronchospasm and produce wheezing, such as asthma, exposure to physiologic irritants, stress, or anxiety. *Stridor* or loud snoring may also be reported with an airway obstruction. Patients who awaken frequently because of loud snoring may be experiencing sleep apnea syndrome.

Chest Pain. Chest pain can result from several conditions. A detailed investigation is required to differentiate chest pain of cardiac origin from that of other causes. Chapter 28 describes chest pain of cardiac origin. Chest pain of pulmonary origin can originate from the chest wall, parietal pleura, or lung parenchyma. Table 24-1 summarizes the characteristics of pulmonary chest pain.

Upper Airway Symptoms. Symptoms to be explored related to the upper airway include difficulty breathing through the nose, nasal discharge, sinus pain, or vocal change. Changes in voice can be caused by obstruction or congestion of nasal passages or by inflammation of the vocal cords (hoarseness). Hoarseness may be associated with tumors, recurrent laryngeal nerve damage, or laryngitis. Patients may experience hoarseness after removal of an endotracheal tube.

Respiratory Risk Factors

In addition to reviewing the symptoms or reasons the patient is seeking health care, the nurse should interview the patient about risk factors associated with respiratory dysfunction. The most important **risk factors** to explore include smoking, past pulmonary illnesses or exposure to respiratory infections, predisposition to genetic disorders, and exposure to environmental irritants. The nurse also needs to explore with the patient the psychosocial effects of any respiratory disorder.

Smoking. Smoking has been implicated as a major cause of lung disease. A strong relationship exists between smoking and the development or exacerbation of chronic bronchitis, emphysema, asthma, lung cancer, and respiratory infections. Passive smoke has also been implicated in increasing the risk for nonsmokers. The *Healthy People 2010* document has a goal and objectives for smoking reduction and cessation (see Chapter 3). The nurse must assess the patient's current and past history of tobacco use, including the type of tobacco (cigars, cigarettes, or pipe) and the number of packs and number of years smoked. Pack-years (for cigarette use) can be determined with the following equation: Pack-year = Number of years smoked × Number of packs smoked per day (e.g., 20 years of 2 packs/day = 540 pack-years). The nurse should also ask about any attempts to quit smoking and exposure to second-hand smoking (in the home or at work). If the patient has quit smoking, pack-years are still determined in addition to the length of time since the patient stopped smoking. The use of cigars, pipes, marijuana, and smokeless tobacco is measured as amount used per day.

Respiratory Disorders. The nurse should obtain a history of respiratory illnesses and hospitalizations for lung diseases or disorders (e.g., childhood allergies, frequent respiratory infections, influenza, frequent colds, pneumonia, pleurisy, emphysema, asthma, chronic sinusitis, chest surgery or trauma, tuberculosis, and adult-onset allergies). The nurse should explore any exposure to tuberculosis or other respiratory infections such as severe acute respiratory syndrome (SARS), or travel to areas with risk for respiratory infections such as histoplasmosis (Southwest United States) or coccidioidomycosis (Southwest United States, Central America, or Mexico).

TABLE 24-1 CHARACTERISTICS OF PULMONARY CHEST PAIN

Origin	Characteristics	Possible Cause
Chest wall	Well localized, constant ache increasing with movement	Trauma, cough, herpes zoster
Pleura	Sharp, abrupt onset, increasing with inspiration or with sudden ventilatory effort (cough, sneeze), unilateral	Pleural inflammation (pleurisy) Autoimmune and connective tissue disease
Lung parenchyma	Dull, constant ache, poorly localized	Benign pulmonary tumors Carcinoma
	Well localized, sharp, sudden onset	Pneumothorax
	Sudden onset, increasing stabbing pain on inspiration, may radiate	Pulmonary embolus and infarction

Family History. Some respiratory diseases have a genetic component, so the nurse must ask the patient if there is a family history of allergy, asthma, atopic dermatitis, or lung cancer. Also the nurse should obtain a family history of documented alpha$_1$-antitrypsin inhibitor deficiency or cystic fibrosis. A strong family history of emphysema or the development of respiratory symptoms at an early age could prove helpful in identifying patients who are candidates for genetic testing and counseling. Panlobular emphysema is a disease that usually affects young adults and is caused by an alpha$_1$-antitrypsin inhibitor deficiency. Cystic fibrosis is a disease that involves mucus-secreting and eccrine sweat glands. The overproduction of secretions affects the lungs by obstructing respiratory passages, impairing oxygenation, and impairing mucociliary clearance.

Environmental Irritants. The nurse should assess the patient's exposure to pollutants and irritants such as dust, fumes, gases, coal dust, and other allergens. It is important to ask about the workplace and type of work the patient does, the home environment and adjacent area, and hobbies to check for exposure to irritants, allergens, or pollutants such as pets, glues, and paints. Also, the nurse should gather information about family members' occupations because this may help determine the source of the patient's respiratory complaint.

Psychosocial History. Respiratory problems can affect a patient's functional status; therefore it is important to ascertain the patient's perception of the situation, coping skills, and resources. Patients with respiratory disorders may believe their quality of life has been diminished.

Need satisfaction is important to understanding the patient's functional performance. The nurse should assess the patient's sense of self, sense of control, satisfaction with family life, safety-security needs, leisure activities, financial resources, and social support. Although symptoms may affect psychosocial functioning, psychosocial effects of a respiratory disorder may also impair cognitive functioning and adaptation to the disorder. This may be manifested as sleeping difficulties, irritability, helplessness or hopelessness, tension, anxiety, depression, and isolation.

An assessment of emotional responses that occur with dyspnea and other respiratory symptoms is important to understanding the patient's experiences and selecting successful interventions. Patients frequently experience anxiety, depression, hostility, fear, or panic. Inquiring about the degree of emotional response and the extent of physical or psychologic impairment yields a more complete assessment of the patient. These data are relevant for the health care provider to incorporate in the care plan.

Review of Other Systems. The nurse should ask the patient about problems with swallowing and walking, as well as any history of neurologic or muscular disease. Factors that may adversely affect respiratory function include immobility, dysphagia, and diseases affecting muscular strength (e.g., amyotrophic lateral sclerosis, myasthenia gravis, stroke). Assessing sleep patterns may also be crucial in determining nursing care for the patient with respiratory problems (see Research box). It is helpful to perform a general review of all body systems to assist the patient in recalling all signs and symptoms.

Research

Carlson BW, Mascarella JJ: Changes in sleep patterns in COPD: a new vital sign in the management of people with chronic obstructive pulmonary disease, *Am J Nurs 103*(12):71-74, 2003.

When evaluating older adults who have chronic obstructive pulmonary disease (COPD), nurses routinely ask questions about activities of daily living while measuring temperature, pulse, respiration, and blood pressure, as well as oxygen saturation, which many consider the sixth vital sign. The assessment typically does not include questions pertaining to changes in sleep patterns. Without an assessment of sleep patterns, nurses may have an incomplete understanding of the patient's health. New research is suggesting that taking a sleep history and following up on changes in sleep patterns may be crucial in monitoring patients with COPD.

Nurses should routinely incorporate sleep as the seventh vital sign by asking about changes in sleep patterns and breathing patterns when assessing vital functions in patients with COPD. Questions to ask are:

- How long does it typically take for you to fall asleep?
- How often do you awaken during the course of the night?
- Do you awaken from sleep coughing, wheezing, short of breath, and/or gasping? If so, how often?
- If you awaken during the night, what time does this usually happen?
- If you awaken during the night, how long does it take to fall back to sleep?
- Do you take a nap during the day, and if so, for how long?
- If you have a bed partner, does he or she ever report noticing your sleep disturbances such as restlessness, apnea, or abrupt awakening?

ARE You READY?

During a health assessment, a 64-year-old patient states that he has been smoking approximately 1½ packs of cigarettes since he was 14 years old. What is this patient's pack-year smoking history?

Physical Examination

The nurse collects objective data on the patient during the physical examination, assessing vital signs and upper and lower airways to identify any deviations from the normal for the patient's age and health problems.

Respiratory Vital Signs

Respiratory Rate and Ventilation. The nurse counts the respiratory rate and assesses the depth and rhythm of the breathing pattern. The expansion of the chest should be bilaterally symmetric. See Figure 24-12 and Table 24-2 for normal and abnormal breathing patterns.

Pulse Oximetry. **Pulse oximetry** is a noninvasive procedure that provides continuous readings of arterial blood oxygen saturation (Spo_2) using a sensor site (earlobe or fingertip). The Spo_2 equals the ratio of the amount of oxygen contained in the hemoglobin to the maximum amount of oxygen contained in hemoglobin, expressed as a percent. The device used is a clip or probe that produces a light beam with two different wavelengths. A sensor measures the absorption of each of the wavelengths of light to determine the oxygen saturation reading. Normal findings are greater than or equal to 95%.

Mixed Venous Oxygen Saturation (Svo_2). Svo_2 measurement is a valuable tool used to assess oxygenation status in the critically ill person. It can be measured continuously or periodically with a specialized pulmonary artery catheter (see Chapter 26). Svo_2 provides information about the amount of oxygen that is supplied to the tissues relative to the oxygen demand at the tissue level. Oxygen demand reflects the amount of oxygen extracted for use at the tissue level. Normal Svo_2 is 60% to 80% and indicates adequate tissue perfusion. A decrease in Svo_2 (to less than 60%) signifies that the oxygen demand is greater than the supply. An increase in Svo_2 (to more than 80%) signifies that the oxygen supply is greater than the oxygen demand. A value of less than 60%, or a change of +10% from the patient's baseline, is significant.[3]

Upper Airway

Examination of the upper airway includes inspection of the nose and nasal septum for deformities and asymmetry. Some septal deviation is common in adults and is usually asymptomatic. To assess the patency of the nares, the health care provider presses each naris closed while asking the person to sniff inward through the other naris. The examiner also observes the nares for flaring, which is a sign of respiratory distress. The nasal mucosa and turbinates are observed for color, edema, exudate, or polyps. Excessive redness, edema, exudate, or bleeding is an abnormal finding. Red, swollen nasal mucous membranes accompanied by watery to mucopurulent nasal discharge indicates acute rhinitis. Nasal mucosa that is swollen, pale, boggy, and usually gray to dull red indicates allergic rhinitis.

The health care provider palpates the sinuses for signs of tenderness over the frontal and maxillary areas. Transillumination can be performed if infection is suspected. Normally, the sinuses demonstrate differing degrees of a red glow. When disease is present, however, the light does not penetrate the sinuses and the red glow is not seen through the hard palate or above the eyebrow.

The oropharynx is examined with a tongue blade and a light source. The anterior and posterior tonsillar pillars, uvula, tonsils, and posterior pharynx are inspected for color, symmetry, exudate, edema, ulcerations, and tonsillar enlargement. Some tonsils are enlarged without being infected, especially in the younger population. The uvula should be midline and rise with phonation. The gag reflex is also tested. Absence of a gag reflex affects the patient's ability to manage the airway.

Chest and Lungs

Inspection. The examiner inspects the patient's thorax for shape and symmetry. The anteroposterior diameter should be less than the transverse diameter (1:2 to 5:7). The spine should be straight and the scapulae on the same level. The patient is also observed for indicators of respiratory distress, including use of the accessory muscles of respiration. Table 24-2 summarizes normal and abnormal findings related to respiratory function.

Palpation. The examiner palpates the chest and spinal column for tenderness, bulges, and abnormalities; palpates the trachea for position; palpates the chest for symmetry of expansion; and palpates all areas of the chest for fremitus. To do this, the examiner

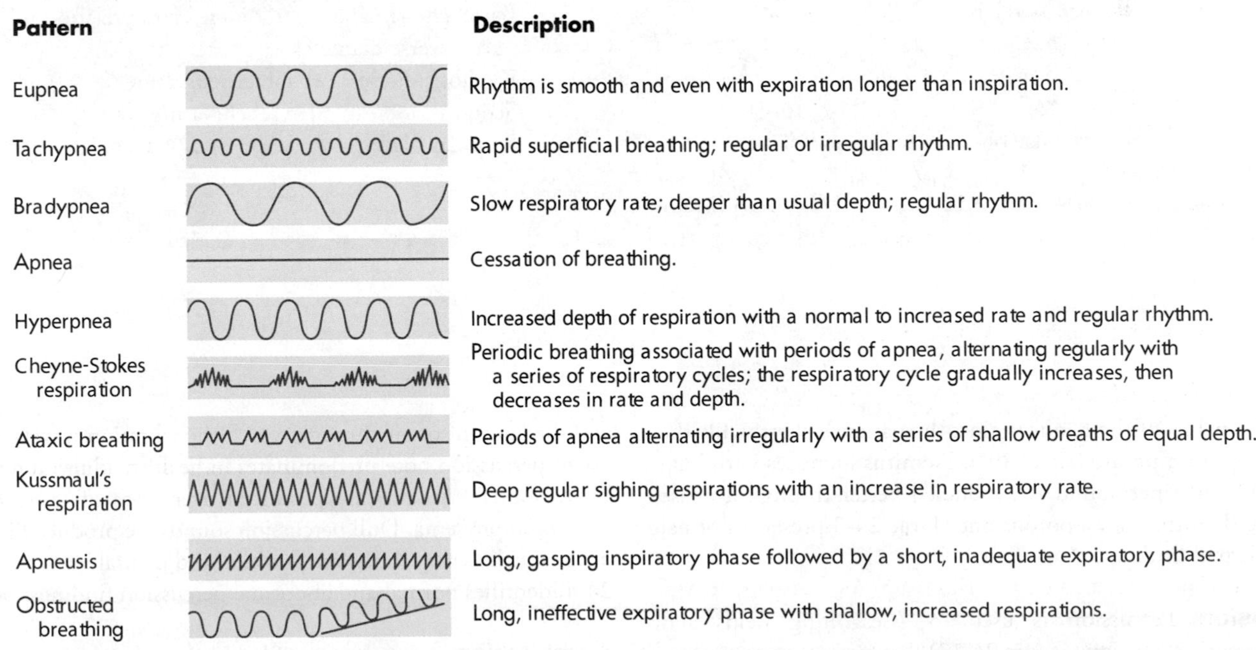

Pattern
Description
Eupnea
Rhythm is smooth and even with expiration longer than inspiration.
Tachypnea
Rapid superficial breathing; regular or irregular rhythm.
Bradypnea
Slow respiratory rate; deeper than usual depth; regular rhythm.
Apnea
Cessation of breathing.
Hyperpnea
Increased depth of respiration with a normal to increased rate and regular rhythm.
Cheyne-Stokes respiration
Periodic breathing associated with periods of apnea, alternating regularly with a series of respiratory cycles; the respiratory cycle gradually increases, then decreases in rate and depth.
Ataxic breathing
Periods of apnea alternating irregularly with a series of shallow breaths of equal depth.
Kussmaul's respiration
Deep regular sighing respirations with an increase in respiratory rate.
Apneusis
Long, gasping inspiratory phase followed by a short, inadequate expiratory phase.
Obstructed breathing
Long, ineffective expiratory phase with shallow, increased respirations.

Figure 24-12 Respiratory patterns.

TABLE 24-2 POSSIBLE FINDINGS BY INSPECTION IN PULMONARY EXAMINATION

Observe	Normal	Abnormal
General appearance	Quiet respiration Sitting or reclining without difficulty Skin translucent, appears dry Nail beds pink Mucous membranes pink and moist*	Lips puckered when exhaling (pursed-lip breathing) Nasal flaring Audible wheezing Restless and apprehensive Leaning forward with hands or elbows on knees (tripod position) Skin: diaphoretic, dull pale, or ruddy Cyanosis: bluish cast on skin or mucous membranes Central cyanosis: results from decreased oxygenation of blood† Peripheral cyanosis: result of local vasoconstriction or decreased cardiac output Digital clubbing: painless enlargement of terminal phalanges related to chronic tissue hypoxia
Trachea	Midline in neck	Tracheal deviation; displacement either lateral, anterior, or posterior Jugular venous distention Cough: strong or weak, dry or wet, productive or nonproductive Sputum production: amount, color, odor, and consistency
Rate	Eupnea: 12-20 breaths/min	Tachypnea: rate >20 breaths/min Bradypnea: rate <10 breaths/min
Breathing pattern	Minimal effort with inspiration; passive, quiet expiration Inspiration/expiration ratio: 1:2 Male: diaphragmatic breathing Female: thoracic breathing	Accessory muscle breathing Paradoxic: part of chest wall moves in during inhalation and out during exhalation Stridorous: audible, loud, low-pitched sound with inhalation and exhalation
Thoracic configuration	Symmetric appearance Anteroposterior (AP) diameter less than transverse diameter Spine straight Scapulae on same horizontal plane	Chest expanding unevenly Muscular development asymmetric Barrel chest: AP diameter increased in relation to transverse diameter Kyphosis: increased thoracic curvature Scoliosis: increased lateral curvature Scapular placement asymmetric

*Dark-skinned people might have normal bluish mucous membranes.
†Central cyanosis is relevant to respiratory status. Observe nail beds, mucous membrane, and lips.

places the palms of the hands against the patient's chest while the patient repeats a phrase (e.g., "99"). Fremitus increases with lung consolidation, since sound is conducted better through a dense structure than through a porous one. Table 24-3 presents normal and abnormal findings.

Percussion. Percussion is used to assess lung fields and diaphragmatic excursion (Figure 24-13). Percussion tones are produced from vibration created by tapping the chest wall. The type of percussion note depends on the density of the underlying tissue and the amount of air through which the vibration travels. A resonant percussion note predominates in healthy, adult lung tissue. Hyperresonant sounds are produced over areas of trapped gas, such as emphysema. Dull percussion sounds are produced in conditions such as atelectasis, pneumonia, and pleural effusion. Table 24-4 identifies normal and abnormal percussion findings.

Auscultation. Auscultation of breath sounds and voice sounds provides valuable information about the lungs and pleura. The examiner instructs the patient to take slow, deep breaths through

TABLE 24-3 POSSIBLE FINDINGS BY PALPATION IN PULMONARY EXAMINATION

Palpate	Normal	Abnormal
Skin and chest wall	Skin nontender, smooth, warm, and dry Skin moist or exceedingly dry	Crepitation—"crackling" when skin palpated—caused by air leak from lung into subcutaneous tissue
Fremitus*	Spine and ribs nontender Symmetric, mild vibrations felt on chest wall during vocalization	Localized tenderness Increased fremitus—a result of vibration through more solid medium, such as lung tumors, pneumonia Decreased fremitus—a result of vibration through increased space (excess air) in chest, such as pneumothorax or chronic obstructive pulmonary disease Asymmetric fremitus—always abnormal
Lateral chest expansion	Symmetric 3-8 cm expansion†	Expansion less than 3 cm, painful or asymmetric†

*Normal fremitus varies from person to person. A patient's baseline must be established.
†Reduced expansion can result from either overexpanded chest (barrel chest) or restricted chest.

the mouth during the examination. Using a stethoscope, the examiner listens systematically to all lung fields and compares breath sounds of the right and left sides during inspiration and expiration (Figure 24-14). Three normal and distinct breath sounds are produced based on the specific area of the respiratory tract (Table 24-5).

Adventitious breath sounds (Table 24-6) are caused by moving air colliding with secretions in the tracheobronchial passageways, or by the inflation of previously deflated airways. They can be caused by any pathologic condition that is associated with excess mucus or fluid, tissue inflammation, bronchospasm, or airway obstruction. These are "added" sounds that are not normally auscultated in the lungs. Another abnormal auscultatory finding is diminished or absent breath sounds. This finding indicates either obstruction or changes in the elasticity of lung fibers. Conditions that lead to alveolar hypoventilation include COPD, pleurisy, and pneumothorax.

Normal voice sounds are usually muffled and indistinct while listening with the stethoscope. Pathologic conditions that increases lung density enhance transmission of voice sounds (Table 24-7). Assessment of voice sounds is not part of the routine examination; it is done when a pathologic condition is suspected.

The Gerontologic Assessment box, p. 580, presents assessment measures and variations in normal findings relevant to the care of older adults. Also identified are disorders common in older adults, which may be responsible for abnormal assessment findings.

Diagnostic Tests

Laboratory Tests

Complete Blood Count. The complete blood count provides information about red blood cells (RBCs), hemoglobin, hematocrit, and white blood cells (WBCs). The RBC count is valuable in assessing overall oxygen-carrying capacity. Normally each cubic millimeter of blood contains 4 million (female) to 5 million (male) RBCs, and each RBC contains an estimated 280 million hemoglobin molecules. Oxygen that diffuses into the pulmonary

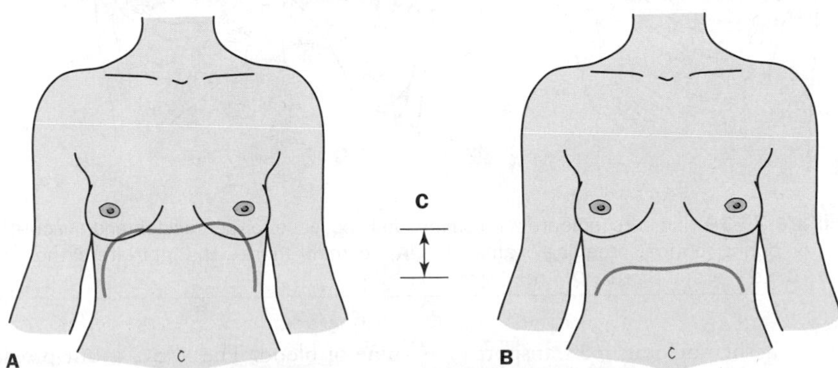

Figure 24-13 Diaphragmatic excursion. **A,** Position of diaphragm at full-end expiration. **B,** Position of diaphragm at full-end inspiration. **C,** Range of diaphragmatic movement—distance from expiration to inspiration.

TABLE 24-4 POSSIBLE FINDINGS BY PERCUSSION IN PULMONARY EXAMINATION

Percussion	Normal	Abnormal
Lung fields	Resonance: low-pitched, hollow, easily heard sounds; equal quality bilaterally	Hyperresonant: heard with air trapping (emphysema or pneumothorax) Dull or flat: results from decreased air in lungs (tumor, atelectasis, fluid)
Diaphragm position and movement	Resting diaphragm at 10th thoracic vertebra Each hemidiaphragm moves 3-6 cm	High position—stomach distention or phrenic nerve damage Decreased or no movement in either hemidiaphragm*

*Decreased excursion can result from hyperinflated lungs pushing down on diaphragm, diaphragmatic disorders, or loss of diaphragmatic innervation.

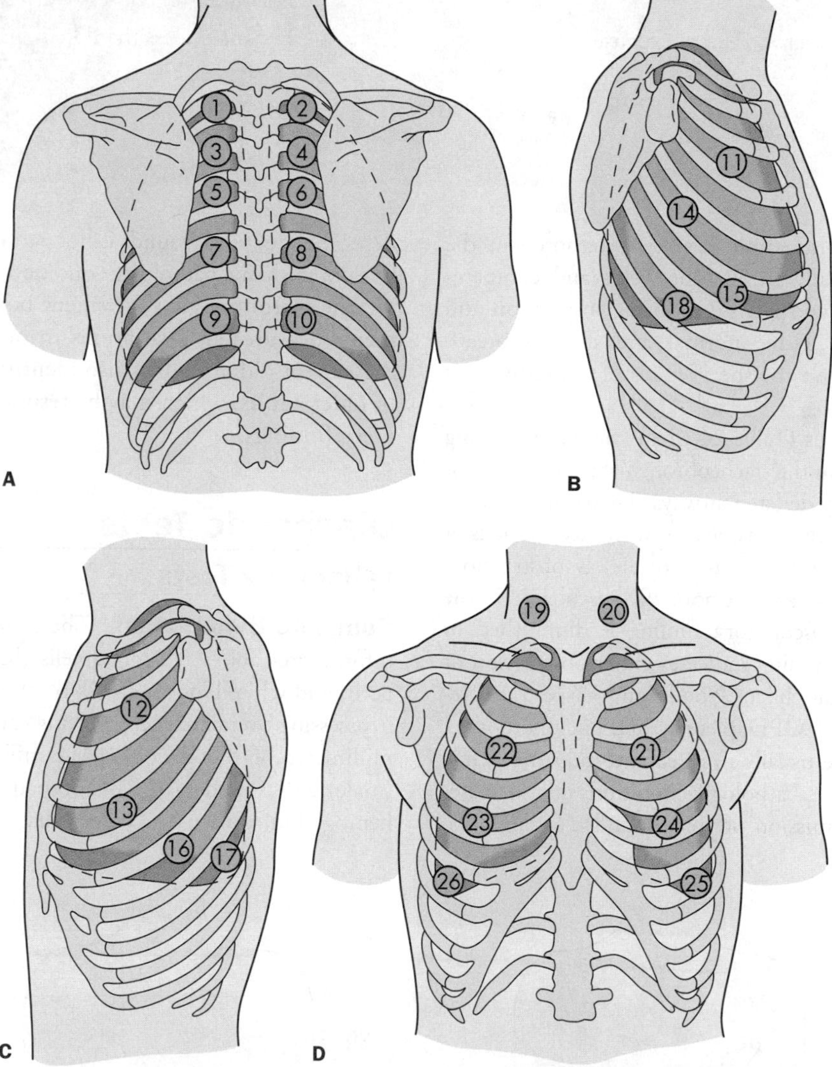

Figure 24-14 Numbers indicate a recommended sequence for percussion and auscultation during routine screening examination. **A,** Posterior thorax. **B,** Right lateral thorax. **C,** Left lateral thorax. **D,** Anterior thorax.

capillary chemically attaches to the hemoglobin for transport to the tissues. An abnormally low hemoglobin level can adversely affect the body's ability to carry oxygen to the cells to meet metabolic needs. Hemoglobin is the iron-containing pigment of the RBCs, and hematocrit is the volume of RBCs within a given volume of blood. The WBC count provides information regarding infection or immune system dysfunction.

Arterial Blood Gases and Acid-Base Balance. Arterial **blood gas** analysis provides information about oxygenation, ven-

TABLE 24-5 CHARACTERISTICS OF BREATH SOUNDS

Sound	Duration of Inspiration and Expiration	Diagram of Sound	Pitch	Intensity	Normal Location	Abnormal Location
Vesicular	Inspiration > expiration, 5:2	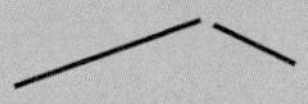	Low	Soft	Peripheral lung	Not applicable
Bronchovesicular	Inspiration = expiration, 1:1	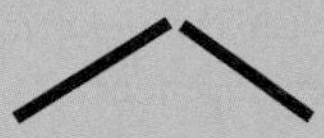	Medium	Medium	First and second intercostal spaces at sternal border anteriorly; posteriorly at T4 medial to scapulae	Peripheral lung
Bronchial (tubular)	Inspiration < expiration, 1:2	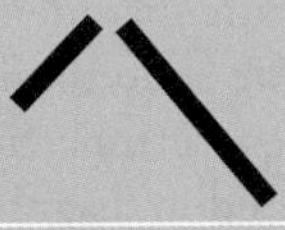	High	Loud	Over trachea	Lung area

From Malasanos L et al: *Health assessment*, ed 4, St Louis, 1990, Mosby.

TABLE 24-6 ABNORMAL (ADVENTITIOUS) BREATH SOUNDS

Type	Physiology	Auscultation	Sound	Possible Condition
Crackles	Air passing through fluid in small airways, or sudden opening of deflated, weakened airways	More commonly heard during inspiration	Fine high-pitched or coarse low-pitched popping sounds that are short and discontinuous	Pneumonia, heart failure, atelectasis, emphysema
Rhonchi	Large airway obstructed by fluid	Heard commonly during expiration	Low-pitched, continuous snoring sound	Chronic obstructive pulmonary disease (COPD), bronchospasm, pneumonia
Wheezes	Air passing through narrowed airways	Can be heard throughout inspiration and expiration	High-pitched, whistling sound	Airway obstruction, bronchospasm as in asthma, COPD
Pleural friction rub	Rubbing of inflamed pleura	May occur throughout respiratory cycle; heard best at base of lung at end of expiration	Scratching, grating, rubbing, creaking	Inflamed pleura, pulmonary infarction

TABLE 24-7 VOICE SOUNDS*

Type	Instruction to Patient	Sound	Abnormal
Egophony	Say prolonged "e"	Muffled "e"	"a"
Whispered pectoriloquy	Whisper "1, 2, 3"	Muffled "1, 2, 3"	Loud, clear "1, 2, 3"
Bronchophony	Say "1, 2, 3"	Muffled "1, 2, 3"	Loud, clear "1, 2, 3"

*Examiner auscultates for characteristic changes when voice sounds are transmitted through chest wall.

Gerontologic Assessment

- Inspect the chest. Increased chest diameter and kyphosis occur with aging and result in decreased chest expansion.
- Check ability to breathe deeply and cough forcefully. Decreased muscular strength and reduced chest wall compliance with decreased chest expansion impair the ability to deep breathe and cough, increasing the risk of low arterial oxygen levels and atelectasis. Decreased ability to handle secretions increases the risk of aspiration.
- Auscultate breath sounds. Crackles may be heard and breath sounds decreased because of shallow breathing or atelectasis related to the factors cited above.
- Observe carefully for signs of respiratory infection. Overall, respiratory defenses function less effectively with age, increasing the risk of infection.
- When reviewing the results of pulmonary function tests, expect the following:
  - —Increased residual volume
  - —Decreased forced vital capacity
  - —Decreased forced expiratory volume
  - —Decreased maximum voluntary ventilation

Common Disorders in Older Adults

Emphysema
Chronic bronchitis
Asthma
Pneumonia

tilation, and acid-base balance, as explained in Chapter 18. It is valuable in assessing the efficiency of pulmonary gas exchange and the presence of an acid-base disorder. Table 24-8 shows the arterial blood gas parameters. The examiner obtains a blood sample by direct puncture of a radial, brachial, or femoral artery. If the radial artery is to be used, the examiner performs an Allen's test first to ensure the hand has adequate collateral blood flow (Figure 24-15). To prevent clotting of the sample, the examiner uses a preheparinized syringe to collect the blood. Once 2 ml of blood is obtained, air bubbles are expelled, and the syringe is sealed with an impermeable cap to prevent contact with room air. The blood sample is placed on ice until analyzed. Arterial punctures are contraindicated in patients receiving thrombolytic agents.

An indwelling arterial catheter is commonly used to obtain blood samples in the critically ill; the catheter should be flushed according to hospital protocol to prevent clotting. Continuous arterial blood gas monitoring is also performed in certain instances.

NURSING CARE. The nurse explains the purpose of the test and its procedure. If the patient is receiving supplemental oxygen, the nurse notes the amount of oxygen and does not change or remove the oxygen (unless ordered) before the test. Other interventions in the care plan should be withheld for 20 minutes before the test. No other preparation is necessary. After making the arterial puncture, the nurse applies constant, firm, direct pressure to the puncture site for 5 minutes, or longer for patients with blood-clotting abnormalities. Subsequently, the nurse observes the site for bleeding and hematoma formation. The nurse also monitors the involved extremity for circulatory impairment, which must be reported immediately.

Alpha$_1$-Antitrypsin Assay. Alpha$_1$-antitrypsin is a globulin that inhibits certain enzymes from destroying the alveolar walls. Alpha$_1$-antitrypsin deficiencies are inherited; patients with this deficiency are highly susceptible to lung tissue destruction at an early age. This blood test is valuable in the identification of patients with the genetic abnormality that greatly increases their risk for development of emphysema without the usual predisposing factors.

Sputum Analysis. A sputum sample may be ordered for microbiologic and cytologic testing. Sputum examination can be helpful in evaluating patients suspected of having tuberculosis, pneumonia, or lung cancer. Gram stains and cultures define a causative organism. Sensitivity is a test ordered in conjunction with the culture that identifies antibiotics to which the organisms present in the sputum are sensitive. An acid-fast bacilli stain is used to diagnose tuberculosis. Cytologic examination identifies cell types to aid in diagnosis, such as in lung cancer. However, an absence of malignant cells in the specimen cannot be interpreted as an absence of cancer. Sputum examination may also reveal the presence of parasites, macrophages, or other cells that aid in the evaluation of lung disease.

To produce a sputum sample, the patient rinses the mouth with water, takes a series of deep breaths, and then coughs to raise sputum and expectorate it into a sterile container. To do this correctly, the patient needs to understand the difference between saliva and sputum, and may need to practice deep breathing and coughing. The nurse should instruct patients to notify the staff as soon as a specimen is collected.

Sputum specimens are best collected as the patient awakens in the morning. A bronchodilator or inhalation of a hypertonic solution may be ordered for patients who have difficulty raising secretions. Patients who are intubated, or have a tracheostomy, require suctioning via the artificial airway with a catheter and special collection container. Sputum specimens can also be obtained by invasive methods such as transtracheal aspiration or fiberoptic bronchoscopy.

Throat Culture. A throat culture helps identify microorganisms so that appropriate treatment can be initiated. To obtain the throat culture, the examiner asks the patient to tilt the head back and open the mouth. A tongue depressor is used so that the swab is less likely to come in contact with the normal flora of the mouth. Both tonsillar pillars and the posterior pharynx should be swabbed. The swab is placed in the culture tube, labeled, and transported to the laboratory.

Radiologic Tests

Chest Roentgenograms. Chest radiographs are obtained to diagnose disorders of the lung; to evaluate effectiveness of treatment; and to determine the extent, location, and progression of lung disease. In addition, they can be used to evaluate proper placement of catheters and tubes. Chest radiographs are usually performed in the radiology department, where the patient stands

TABLE 24-8 ARTERIAL BLOOD GASES

Parameter	Measurement	Value
Acid-base balance	pH: hydrogen ion concentration	Normal: 7.35-7.45 Alkalemia: >7.45 Acidemia: <7.35
Oxygenation	PaO_2: partial pressure of dissolved O_2 in blood	Normal: 80-100 mm Hg Hyperoxia: >100 mm Hg Hypoxemia: <80 mm Hg, 95%-98%
Ventilation	SaO_2: percentage of O_2 bound to hemoglobin $PaCO_2$: partial pressure of CO_2 dissolved in blood	Normal: 35-45 mm Hg Hypercapnia: >45 mm Hg Hypocapnia: <35 mm Hg

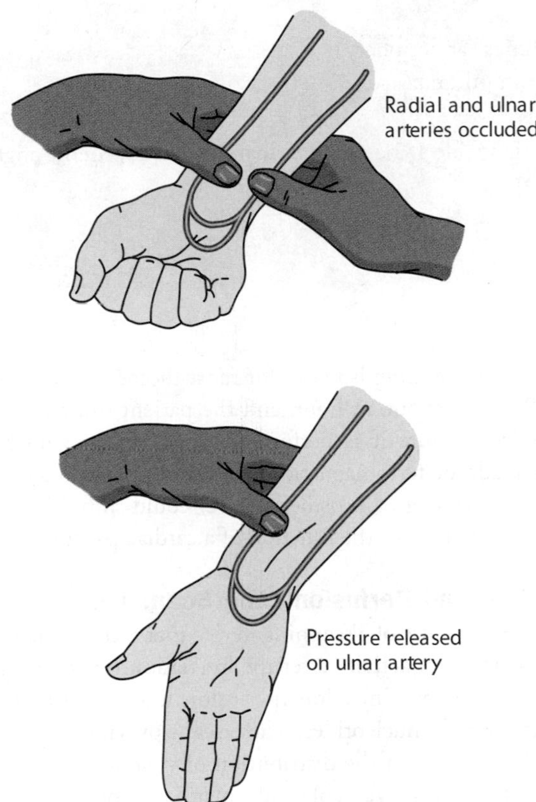

Figure 24-15 Allen's test. Hold patient's hand with palm up. Have patient clench and unclench hand while occluding radial and ulnar arteries. The hand will become pale. Lower the hand and have patient relax the hand. While continuing to hold radial artery, release pressure on ulnar artery. Brisk return of color (5 to 7 seconds) demonstrates adequate ulnar blood flow. If pallor persists for more than 15 seconds, ulnar flow is inadequate and radial artery cannulation should not be attempted.

in an upright position with the anterior side of the chest pressed against the film cassette holder. This produces a posteroanterior (PA) radiograph in which the x-ray beam travels through the posterior side of the patient's chest to the x-ray film. However, if the patient is acutely ill, the x-ray can be taken at the bedside with a portable x-ray machine. If the patient can sit up, the x-ray camera is positioned toward the anterior side of the chest, and the x-ray beam travels through the anterior side of the chest to the x-ray film placed behind the patient's back. This is referred to as an anteroposterior view.

A lateral radiograph is generally taken along with a PA radiograph. Generally, the left side of the chest is pressed against the film cassette, and the x-ray beam travels through the side of the body. Figure 24-16 shows PA and lateral chest radiographs. Special views such as the oblique, lordotic, or decubitus may be obtained to visualize specific parts of the chest.

In preparation for the radiograph, the patient removes all metal objects above the waist. During the test the patient is asked to take a deep breath and hold it. There is no discomfort, although the

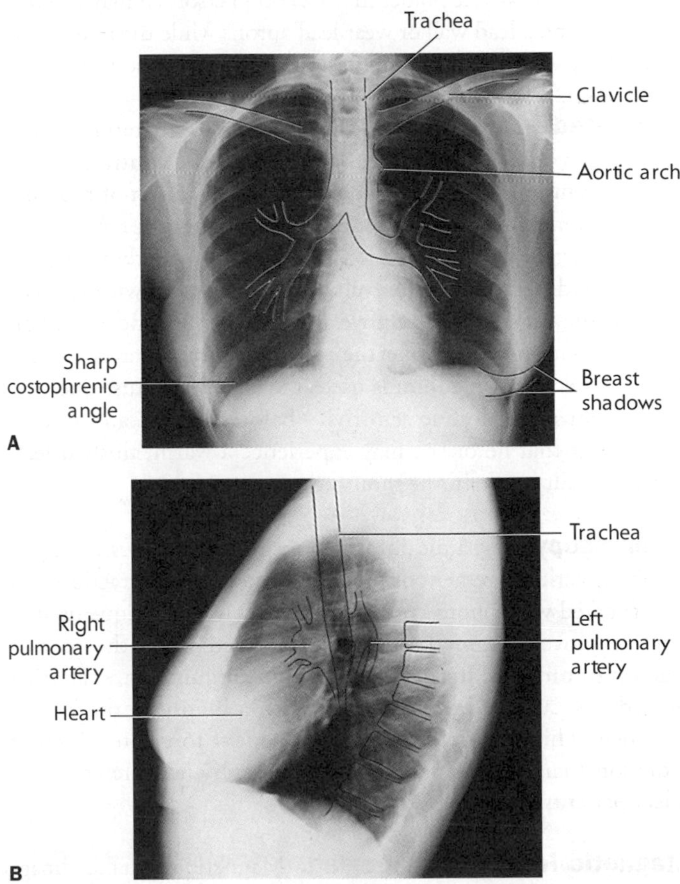

Figure 24-16 Location of structures on a chest radiograph. **A,** Anterior view. **B,** Lateral view.

TABLE 24-9 RADIOGRAPHIC FINDINGS

Structure	Findings
Trachea	Midline, translucent, tubelike structure found in anterior mediastinal cavity
Clavicles	Equally distant from sternum
Ribs	Thoracic cavity encasement
Mediastinum	Shadowy space between lungs that widens at hilum
Heart	Solid-appearing structure with clear edges visible in left anterior mediastinal cavity; cardiothoracic ratio should be less than half the width of chest wall on posteroanterior (PA) film; cardiac shadow appears larger on anteroposterior (AP) film
Carina	Lowest tracheal cartilage at bifurcation
Main-stem bronchus	Translucent, tubelike structure visible approximately 2.5 cm from hilum
Hilum	Small, white, bilateral densities present where bronchi join lungs; left bronchus should be 2-3 cm higher than right
Bronchi	Not usually visible
Lung fields	Usually not completely visible except for "lung markings" at periphery Blackened area without tissue markings suggests pneumothorax Patchy infiltrates suggest pneumonia, atelectasis
Diaphragm	Rounded structures visible at bottom of lung fields; right side 1-2 cm higher than left; costophrenic angles should be clear and sharp Loss of costophrenic angle sharpness suggests pleural effusion Flattened diaphragm suggests emphysema

room and film cassette holder may be cool. Personnel may be positioned behind a lead wall or wear lead aprons while the radiograph is taken. Possible radiographic findings are listed in Table 24-9.

Computed Tomography. Computed tomography (CT) scanning, with or without the use of radiopaque contrast media, uses computer programming to permit visualization of multiple cross-sectional "slices" of the lung. Each tomogram represents a specific part of the lung. Lesions that are not clearly visualized on chest radiography can be evaluated more clearly with CT. For this test the patient must remove all metal articles and lie still on an examination table while the x-ray machine rotates to take films. If a contrast medium is used, the examiner must question the patient about iodine sensitivity before the test and inform the patient that he or she may experience a warm, flushed feeling and a salty taste in the mouth.

Fluoroscopy. Dynamic information about the chest, such as diaphragmatic movement or lung expansion and contraction, can be evaluated with fluoroscopy. Fluoroscopy is a technique used to observe movement in the area being filmed while the specific study is in progress. It can also be used in conjunction with other procedures, such as bronchoscopy, when a biopsy of the lung is obtained. This technique exposes the patient to greater doses of radiation than the standard chest radiograph and is reserved for select patients.

Magnetic Resonance Imaging. Magnetic resonance imaging (MRI) produces cross-sectional images of the body that are helpful in detecting subtle lesions. It is superior to CT scanning in detecting lesions of the chest wall and congenital heart disease. However, CT scanning is better for most thoracic abnormalities. The MRI takes about an hour, and the patient must remove all metal objects before it is performed. Any patient who has an implant made of ferromagnetic material cannot undergo MRI, since the device (e.g., a prosthetic valve) could shift. The imager may also interfere with the function of a cardiac pacemaker.

Ventilation and Perfusion Lung Scan. Lung scan procedures involve the use of a scanning device that records the pattern of pulmonary radioactivity after the inhalation (ventilation lung scan) or intravenous injection (perfusion lung scan) of gamma ray–emitting radionucleotides. These scans provide the clinician with a visual image of the distribution of ventilation and perfusion in the lungs. Valuable information about ventilation-perfusion patterns can aid in the diagnosis of parenchymal lung disease and vascular disorders, such as pulmonary embolism. For the ventilation scan the patient is required to breathe a small amount of radioactive gas through a ventilation system. During the procedure the patient must be able to take a breath and hold it. For a perfusion lung scan the patient receives an injection of a radioactive agent, and the camera takes a series of images. An accurate preprocedure weight is needed to calculate the dosage of radioactive agent, and the patient must be assessed for allergies. No special care is needed after the test.

Pulmonary Angiography. Pulmonary angiography visualizes the pulmonary vascular system and is used to detect pulmonary emboli and a variety of congenital and acquired lesions of the pulmonary vessels. Additional data obtained in conjunction with this test include measures of pulmonary pressures, cardiac output, and pulmonary vascular resistance. A radiopaque material is injected into a catheter that has been introduced into a peripheral vein and advanced through the right side of the heart to the pulmonary artery. A series of radiographic films are then taken to follow the distribution of the contrast material throughout the pulmonary vascular system. The catheter is removed at the completion of the test, and a pressure dressing applied (see Guidelines for Safe Practice box).

Special Tests

Pulmonary Function Tests. Pulmonary function testing is a noninvasive method of assessing the functional capacity of the lungs. These tests cannot be used in isolation to diagnose specific disease but are integral to the diagnostic process. **Pulmonary function tests** (PFTs) are used to evaluate pulmonary disability, to evaluate pulmonary function in patients before surgery, to evaluate the patient's disease progression and response to therapy, and to differentiate obstructive lung disease from restrictive lung disease. The patient is asked to breathe into a mouthpiece that is connected to a spirometer. Nose clips are applied to permit mouth breathing only; the patient is required to inhale deeply, hold his or her breath, and then quickly and forcefully exhale. It may take the patient several attempts to perform this successfully. Shortness of breath or lightheadedness may be experienced.

NURSING CARE. The nurse explains the purpose of the test and its procedure to the patient. Food and fluids are not restricted; however, the test should not be scheduled after a meal, since the diaphragm will be exerted during the test. Medications that may affect respiration are omitted before the PFTs, unless specifically ordered. Height and weight measurements are obtained before the test. After the PFTs the nurse assesses the patient's respiratory status.

SPIROMETRY. Spirometry, the most common pulmonary function test, is a test to determine lung capacities (the sum of two or more lung volumes), lung volumes, and flow rates. The patient breathes through a mouthpiece connected to a spirometer that measures the air moving through the apparatus and records a graphic tracing of the lung volumes and capacities (Figure 24-17).

Tidal volume (TV) periodically increases in spontaneously breathing, healthy patients. This is referred to as sighing. Patients whose breathing pattern is shallow without sighing are at risk for atelectasis and pneumonia. TV is monitored closely in critically ill patients who are mechanically ventilated.

Vital capacity (VC) reflects the muscle strength and volume capacity of the lung. It is important to maintain an effective cough, to take a deep breath, and to clear the airways of secretions. In addition to its use in evaluating respiratory function before surgery, VC is used to monitor and diagnose pulmonary disorders. VC provides information about airway resistance when measured as forced vital capacity (FVC).

One of the most meaningful clinical measurements is the forced expiratory volume (FEV). The FEV measures the amount of air in liters that is forcefully expired over a specified time, generally 1, 2, or 3 seconds. When compared with the FVC, the FEV can identify the pulmonary impairment as restrictive or obstructive. In obstructive disease blocked airways interfere with expiration more than inspiration. When airway obstruction (resistance) increases, air flow rates decrease. The amount of time necessary to forcefully exhale an amount of air after full inspiration is increased in obstructive disease. The FEV/FVC ratio is low. In restrictive disease air can be expelled rapidly, and the FEV/FVC ratio is usually high. Most patients should be able to exhale approximately 75% of their VC in 1 second.[4]

Functional residual capacity (FRC) reflects the volume of gas remaining in the lungs at the end of a normal passive exhalation; this gas is in continuous contact with pulmonary capillary blood. If FRC is decreased, alveoli collapse, and gas exchange is adversely affected.

PFTs can also be performed during bronchial provocation and while a patient is exercising to identify triggers to bronchospasm, to determine if the obstruction (bronchospasm) is reversible with bronchodilator therapy, and to determine the extent of exercise limitation. Bronchodilators are generally withheld before the bronchial provocation test.

FLOW-VOLUME LOOPS. Flow-volume loops aid in distinguishing obstructive from restrictive lung disorders and intrathoracic from

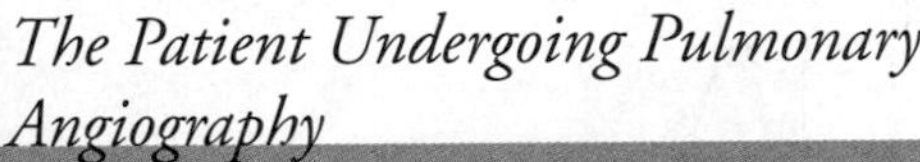

GUIDELINES FOR SAFE PRACTICE
The Patient Undergoing Pulmonary Angiography

Before Angiography

- Explain the purpose of the test and its procedure.
- Give the patient nothing by mouth for 4 to 6 hours before the test.
- Check the signed consent form.
- Check laboratory data: electrolytes, complete blood count, blood urea nitrogen, creatinine, and clotting studies should be within normal limits.
- Assess the patient for allergies to contrast media.
- Obtain baseline vital signs before the procedure.
- Inform the patient that the dye may cause flushing, coughing, and a warm sensation.

Immediately After Angiography

- Monitor vital signs every 15 minutes.
- Observe dressing and site for bleeding or hematoma development every 15 minutes.
- Assess site for infection or thrombophlebitis (swelling, warmth, redness, or pain).
- Maintain bed rest for 4 to 6 hours.

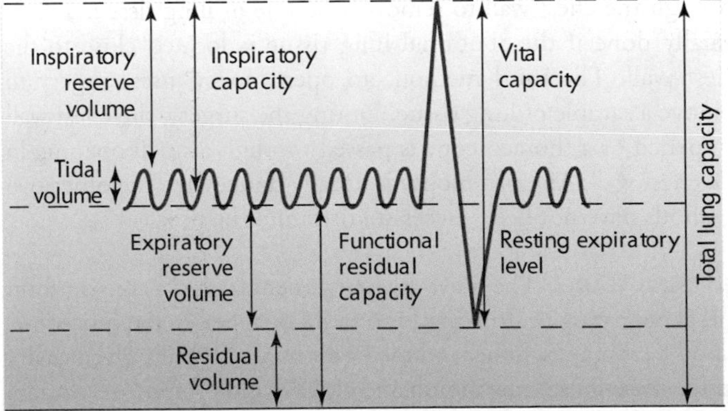

Figure 24-17 Lung volumes and capacities illustrated by spirography tracing.

extrathoracic disorders. Inspiratory and expiratory volumes are plotted against flow rates to produce a flow-volume loop (Figure 24-18). Typically a patient with obstructive airway disease has a "scooped out" appearance in the expiratory flow curve. In restrictive disease there is a symmetric reduction in volume and flow; it appears as a smaller version of a normal flow-volume loop.

PULMONARY DIFFUSION CAPACITY. The ability of gas to diffuse across the alveolar-capillary membrane is measured by a test called diffusing capacity of the lung for carbon monoxide (D_{LCO}). One method involves the patient breathing in a known amount of carbon monoxide and exhaling it after 10 seconds of breath holding (to allow the gas to diffuse across the alveolar-capillary membrane). The carbon monoxide concentration in the blood is estimated from the amount of carbon monoxide exhaled. A normal value is approximately 25 ml/min/mm Hg; however, predicted values are based on age, height, and gender. The D_{LCO} is decreased in patients with lung disorders that involve the alveolar-capillary membrane such as emphysema and interstitial lung disease.

Thoracentesis. **Thoracentesis** involves the insertion of a needle into the pleural space to instill medications into the pleural space, biopsy the pleura, or remove pleural fluid (Figure 24-19). Aspiration of pleural fluid may be done for gross or microscopic examination or to relieve respiratory distress. Therefore thoracentesis may be performed for diagnostic or therapeutic purposes. The procedure is usually performed at the bedside or in a treatment room with the patient under local anesthesia (see Guidelines for Safe Practice box).

Lung Biopsy. A lung biopsy is performed to diagnose certain lung conditions such as sarcoidosis, pulmonary fibrosis, or lung cancer or to confirm results of other tests such as a chest x-ray or a CT scan. The surgeon removes a small sample of lung tissue for examination under a microscope using one of three methods: (1) bronchoscopic, (2) needle, or (3) open. The method chosen often depends on where the tissue is located, the patient's health and age, and whether the patient has underlying lung diseases. A bronchoscopic biopsy uses a bronchoscope inserted through the mouth or nose to remove a lung tissue sample. This is usually done if an infectious disease is suspected, the abnormal lung tissue is located next to the bronchi, or more invasive procedures will also be performed. A needle biopsy uses a lengthy needle inserted through the chest wall to remove a sample of lung tissue. This is usually done if the abnormal lung tissue is located close to the chest wall. The third method, an open biopsy, uses surgery to remove a sample of lung tissue. During the surgery, the chest wall is opened or a thoracoscope is passed through a small opening in the chest wall. An open biopsy is usually done when the other two methods have not been successful or cannot be used.

NURSING CARE. The nurse asks the patient to sign a consent form and avoid eating or drinking for 6 to 8 hours before the procedure. Blood tests may be done, and medications are typically given to dry up the secretions in the mouth and airways and promote relaxation. Both the bronchoscopic and needle biopsies are usually done on an outpatient basis, whereas an open biopsy requires hospitalization. The procedure usually takes 30 to 60 minutes. Patients are instruct-

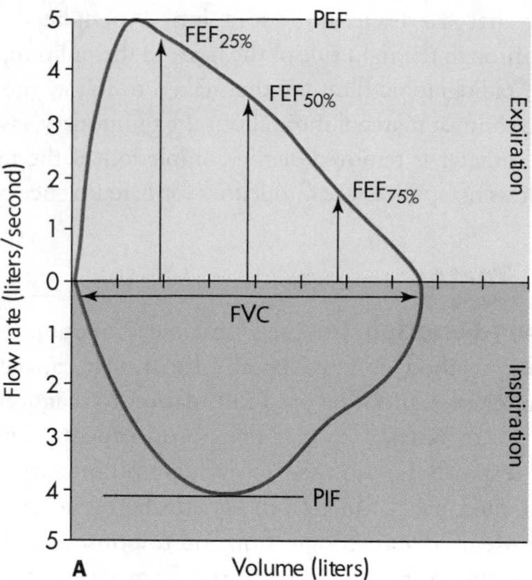

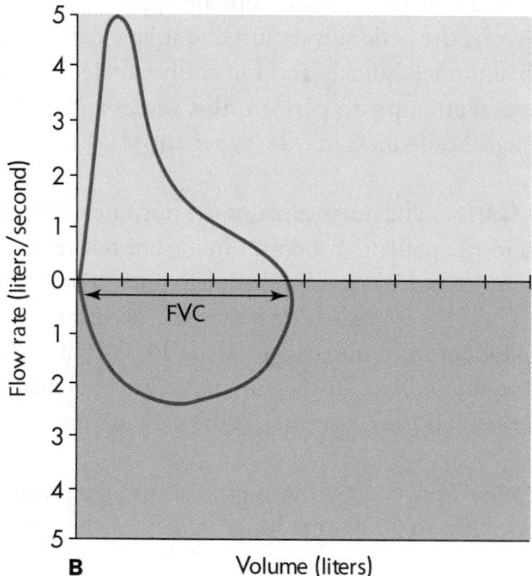

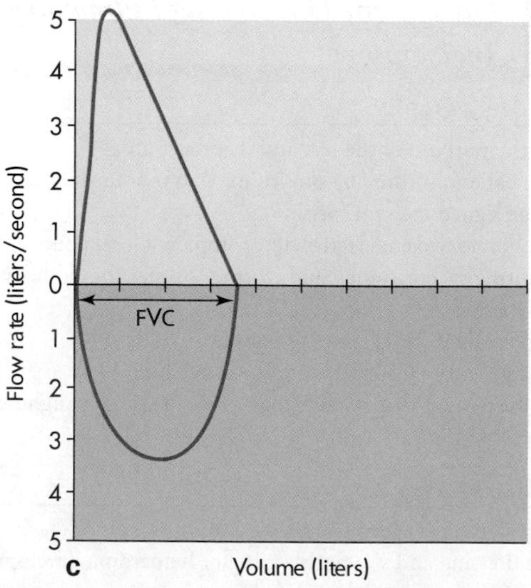

Figure 24-18 Flow-volume loops. **A,** Peak expiratory flow (*PEF*); peak inspiratory flow (*PIF*); forced expiratory flow at X% (*FEF%*) of forced vital capacity (*FVC*). **B,** Obstructive disorder. **C,** Restrictive disorder.

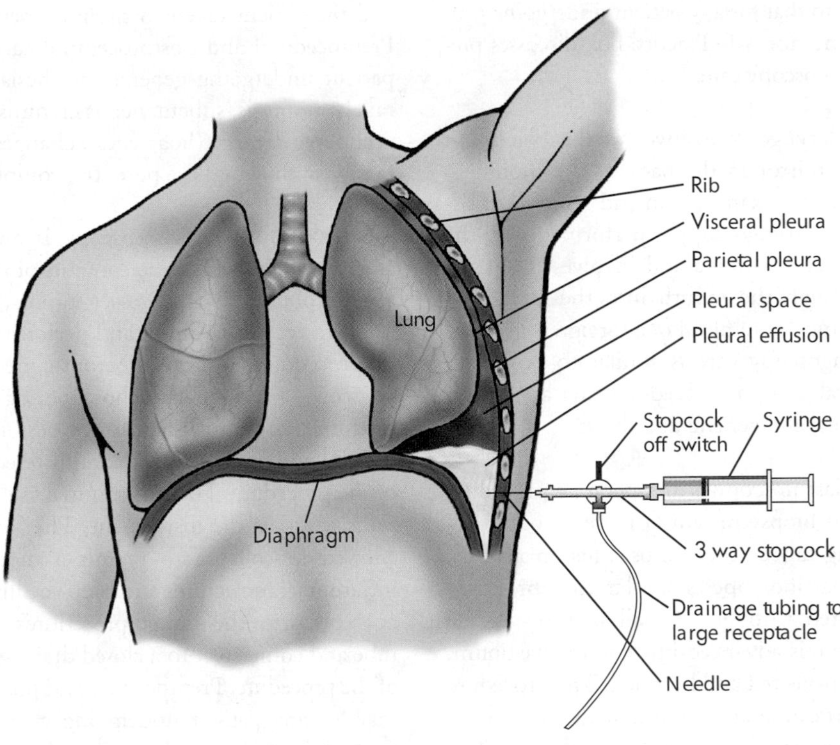

Figure 24-19 Thoracentesis.

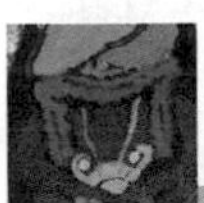

GUIDELINES FOR SAFE PRACTICE
The Patient Undergoing Thoracentesis

- Explain the procedure, and obtain a signed consent form. Emphasize the importance of not moving, breathing quietly, and not coughing during the procedure to avoid damage to the pleura and lung. Explain that the local anesthetic may cause a slight burning sensation and pressure may be felt when the needle is inserted.
- Assess the patient's respiratory status and vital signs before the procedure. Pulse oximetry may be monitored. Do not discontinue supplemental oxygen.
- If possible, help the patient sit on the edge of the bed with the affected side closest to the foot of the bed. Support the patient's feet with a footstool. Raise the bedside table and put pillows on the table so the patient can lean forward and rest his or her head and crossed arms comfortably on the pillows. If the patient is unable to sit up, place him or her in the position indicated by physician.
- Reassure the patient and provide physical support, such as holding the patient's hand, as needed.
- Monitor vital signs, general appearance, and respiratory status throughout the procedure. Up to 1 L of fluid may be removed at one time. If the patient develops pernicious coughing, reexpansion pulmonary edema should be suspected and the procedure terminated. Other signs and symptoms to monitor include hypotension, increased shortness of breath, bloody sputum, tracheal deviation, vasovagal reflex, and hypoxemia.
- Assist the patient to a position of comfort after the needle is withdrawn and a sterile occlusive dressing is applied.
- Prepare the patient for a postprocedural chest radiograph to check for a possible pneumothorax.
- Manage postprocedural pain.

ed to notify the physician or nurse immediately if they experience chest pain, lightheadedness, dyspnea, cyanosis, fever, or continuous seepage of blood through the bandage (open biopsy only). Lung biopsy results are usually available in 2 to 4 days.

Endoscopy

Bronchoscopy. **Bronchoscopy** is used to diagnose and treat airway and lung disorders. It is used to examine vocal cord movement; to obtain specimens by biopsy, bronchial brushing, bronchoalveolar lavage; and to remove foreign bodies or mucous plugs. Specimens can be examined for cytology or bacteriology and cultured for fungi, acid-fast bacilli, *Legionella pneumophila,* and *Pneumocystis carinii.* Localization of bleeding or tumor sites can also be detected by bronchoscopy.

Fiberoptic bronchoscopy is frequently performed because of the instrument's small size and ability to visualize the segmental and subsegmental bronchi. The fiberoptic scope has two channels: one channel for the clinician to visualize the structures and one channel to accommodate equipment such as biopsy forceps, suction, cytology brush, or oxygen. The clinician sprays or swabs a local anesthetic on the tongue and oropharynx, then introduces the scope into the nose (the mouth or an endotracheal tube or tracheostomy tube can also be used). The anesthetic is also applied to the scope; additional anesthetic may be applied through the scope as it advances toward the vocal cords and carina.

Bronchoscopy with the rigid bronchoscope is generally performed in the operating room because general anesthesia is required. It is usually reserved for removing foreign objects, controlling massive hemoptysis, placing airway stents, and dilating tracheobronchial strictures. The care is similar to that for any patient undergoing general anesthesia. The Guidelines for Safe Practice box discusses prebronchoscopy and postbronchoscopy care.

Laryngoscopy. Indirect laryngoscopy involves the placement and rotation of a laryngeal mirror in the back of the mouth to visualize the larynx. It is used for examination and removal of tissue or foreign objects. Direct laryngoscopy is performed with the patient under local or general anesthesia and involves the insertion of a laryngoscope through the mouth into the larynx for examination. Biopsy of a tumor or removal of a foreign object can be accomplished. Postlaryngoscopy care is similar to postbronchoscopy care. Preprocedural and postprocedural care are similar to that for any patient undergoing general anesthesia.

Mediastinoscopy. Mediastinoscopy is an operative procedure that allows visualization and biopsy of lymph nodes. The procedure is helpful in diagnosing cancer, tuberculosis, histoplasmosis, and other diseases. A mediastinoscope is similar to a bronchoscope; however, it is inserted through a small incision in the suprasternal notch. The scope is advanced into the mediastinum, where lymph nodes can be inspected and biopsied. The procedure is generally performed in the operating room with the patient under general anesthesia. A small incision is made to allow entrance of the scope. After the procedure, the incision is sutured and the patient taken to the postanesthesia care unit to recover. Preprocedural and postprocedural care is similar to that for any patient undergoing general anesthesia and surgery. Pneumothorax, hemoptysis, subcutaneous crepitus of neck or face, and laryngeal nerve damage (hoarseness, changes in vocal patterns, and difficulty swallowing) are potential complications.

Thoracoscopy. Thoracoscopy is an operative procedure that allows visualization of the contents of the thoracic cavity. It can be used to obtain biopsies, resect tumors, perform esophageal operations, resect pericardium, and perform many other thoracic surgical procedures. A simple fiberoptic mediastinoscope, a rigid bronchoscope, a flexible bronchoscope, or video-assisted laparoscopic instrumentation may be used to perform thoracoscopy. A general or local anesthetic may be administered, depending on the extent of the procedure. The surgeon makes two to four small chest incisions to insert the instrument. The lung on the operative side is allowed to collapse to permit a more panoramic view of the intrathoracic structures and keep the lung immobile while the surgeon performs the desired procedures. The surgeon inserts a chest tube and connects it to a closed drainage system at the completion of the procedure. Preprocedure and postprocedure care is similar to that for any patient undergoing general anesthesia and surgery. Care of the patient with a chest tube is discussed in Chapter 26.

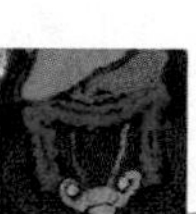

GUIDELINES FOR SAFE PRACTICE
The Patient Undergoing Flexible Bronchoscopy

- Monitor respiratory rate and pattern and auscultate lungs. Observe for changes in breathing pattern and breath sounds. Oxygen saturation may be monitored with pulse oximetry.
- Give the patient nothing by mouth until cough and gag reflexes return.
- Position the patient in a semi-Fowler's or side-lying position.
- Monitor the patient for bleeding, laryngeal edema, or laryngospasm (stridor) and increasing shortness of breath.
- Explain to the patient that sputum may be blood streaked if a biopsy was performed.
- Manage throat discomfort with warm saline gargles or throat lozenges.

References

1. Barkauskas VH et al: *Health and physical assessment,* St Louis, 2002, Mosby.
2. Finesilver C: *Perfecting your skills: respiratory assessment,* accessed June 2004 from website: http://www.nursing.drexel.edu/nlc/courses/ce/ce905/start.htm?coursekey=74815.
3. Nettina SM: *The Lippincott manual of nursing practice,* ed 7, Philadelphia, 2001, Lippincott.
4. Schnell ZB, Van Leeuwen AM, Kranpitz TR: *Davis's comprehensive handbook of laboratory and diagnostic tests with nursing implications,* Philadelphia, 2003, Davis.
5. Thomas M: Breathing dysfunction in asthma, *Update* 70(5):58–64, 2005.
6. van Schayck CP et al: Comparison of existing symptom-based questionnaires for identifying COPD in the general practice setting, *Respirology* 10(3):323–333, 2005.
7. Vickers K, McNally RJ: Respiratory symptoms and panic in the National Comorbidity Survey: a test of Klein's suffocation false alarm theory, *Behav Res Ther* 43(8):1011–1018, 2005.

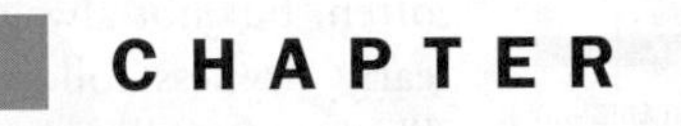 Visit the Evolve website: http://evolve.elsevier.com/Monahan/medsurg

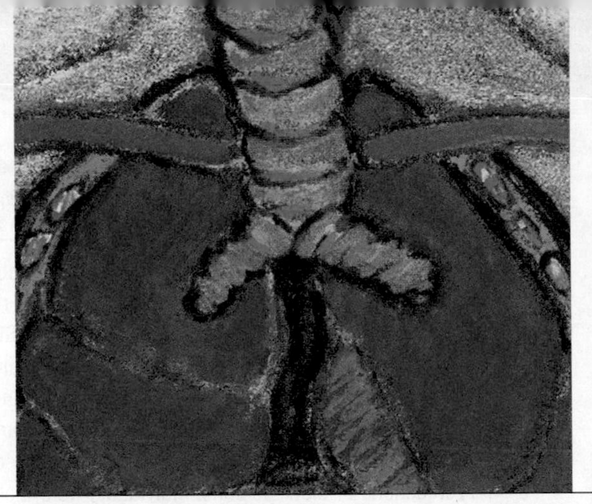

CHAPTER 25

Upper Airway Problems

by Shelley Yerger Huffstutler, Frances D. Monahan

OBJECTIVES

After studying this chapter, the learner should be able to:

1. Compare the etiology, pathophysiology, clinical manifestations, and management of infections of the upper airway.
2. Discuss conditions that cause obstructions of the upper airway and their management.
3. Describe clinical manifestations and management of the patient experiencing epistaxis.
4. Contrast the nursing care of the patient after various surgical procedures of the upper airway.
5. Describe the home care interventions and patient teaching necessary for the patient with a permanent tracheostomy tube.

KEY TERMS

apnea, p. 602
artificial airway, p. 615
epistaxis, p. 603
esophageal speech, p. 613
laryngeal edema, p. 599
laryngectomy, p. 606
nasal septum, p. 600
sinuses, p. 587
tracheoesophageal speech, p. 612
tracheostomy, p. 599
tracheostomy tube, p. 607

The upper airway includes the nose and **sinuses**, upper throat (nasopharynx and oropharynx), and lower throat (laryngopharynx and larynx). Disorders of the upper airway are common, and patients often ask nurses to give them advice about these kinds of disorders. Disorders range from the common cold and sore throat to life-threatening infections, obstructions, and cancers.

Infections of Nose and Sinuses

The skin around the external nose is easily irritated during acute attacks of rhinitis or sinusitis. Furunculosis (boils) and cellulitis occasionally develop. Infections around the nose are extremely dangerous because the venous blood supply from this area drains directly into the cerebral venous sinuses. Septicemia therefore can occur easily, so pimples or lesions in the area should not be squeezed. If any infection in or around the nose persists or shows even a slight tendency to spread or increase in severity, a physician should be consulted. Herpetic lesions, often referred to as fever blisters, may develop around the nose and mucous membranes. These lesions are commonly associated with viral infections and, when scratched, may spread to other areas of the body or to other persons. Other infections that involve the upper airway as a portal of entry and site of symptoms are anthrax and smallpox.

Rhinitis

Etiology and Epidemiology. The term *rhinitis* refers to inflammation of the mucous membrane of the nose. Rhinitis may be acute or chronic. Acute rhinitis, also known as coryza or the common cold, is an inflammatory condition of the mucous membranes of the nose and accessory sinuses caused by a filterable virus. It affects almost everyone at some time and occurs most often in the winter, with additional high incidences in early fall and spring. The known causes of the common cold include 100 serotypes of rhinoviruses, coronoviruses, adenoviruses, echoviruses, influenza and parainfluenza viruses, and coxsackievirus. The common cold is contagious for the first 2 or 3 days and is spread by droplet nuclei from sneezing.

Colds may also be spread by the contaminated hands of persons who are frequently sneezing and blowing their noses or by fomites, such as a telephone used by these persons. Secondary invasion by bacteria may cause pneumonia, acute bronchitis, sinusitis, and otitis media. Older adults, especially those living in long-term care facilities, are particularly susceptible to colds (see Research box).

Allergic rhinitis (hayfever) is a type I hypersensitivity reaction that develops as a result of inhaled allergens. More than 35 million

Research

Graat JM et al: Effect of daily vitamin E and multivitamin-mineral supplementation on acute respiratory tract infections in elderly persons, *JAMA* 288:715-721, 2002.

Vitamin supplements are widely used by older patients, and studies demonstrate that multivitamins (MVIs), MVIs plus minerals, and vitamin E are the most commonly used supplements. Studies have shown that such supplements improve some cellular immune parameters, but evidence about the actual clinical effects is inconclusive. A randomized controlled study was conducted to determine the effect of various supplements on the incidence and severity of acute respiratory infections in older persons. Individuals were included if they were 60 years of age or older; had no history of cancer, liver disease, or fat malabsorption; and had not used supplements, immunosuppressive treatments, or certain anticoagulants in the previous 2 months.

Participants were monitored for 15 months and were randomized to a placebo, vitamin E, MVI with minerals, or MVI with minerals and vitamin E. The main outcomes measured were acute respiratory infection incidence and severity. The analysis included 547 subjects, 98% of whom were noninstitutionalized.

In the group that took the MVIs with minerals, 71% had at least one acute respiratory tract infection. In the group that received vitamin E, 68% had an infection, whereas of those in the group that received MVI with minerals and vitamin E, 66% had an infection. Only 67% of the placebo group had an infection. Patients given vitamin E who had a respiratory tract infection had longer illnesses and statistically and significantly more symptoms than other patients.

The authors concluded that neither MVIs with minerals or with vitamin E are associated with a lower incidence of acute respiratory tract infection in older patients. Vitamin E was associated with longer duration and increases in symptoms. Older persons should be cautious about supplementing their diet with vitamin E, at least as a means of improving immune function.

Americans have allergic rhinitis. Inhaled allergens are classified as outdoor (seasonal; also classified as acute) or indoor (perennial; also classified as chronic). The outdoor allergens are pollens of trees, grasses, or weeds. The indoor allergens are mold spores, dust mites, and animal dander. Although some persons believe they are allergic to flowers, this is often not so; many flowers such as roses are insect pollinated, and only flowers that are pollinated by pollen in the air can cause an allergic reaction. Table 25-1 lists the medications commonly used to treat allergic rhinitis.

Chronic rhinitis is a chronic inflammation of the mucous membrane characterized by increased nasal mucus. Chronic rhinitis may be the result of repeated acute infection; allergy; or vasomotor rhinitis, which is thought to be associated with instability of the autonomic nervous system caused by stress, tension, or some endocrine disorder. Often it manifests as a nasal allergy, but an allergen cannot be identified.

Rhinitis can also be caused by the overuse of nosedrops or medication via nasal sprays. This is a rebound phenomenon that usually disappears within 1 to 2 weeks after the nasal medication is discontinued.

Pathophysiology. All types of rhinitis cause sneezing, nasal discharge with nasal obstruction, and headache, but the pattern of these symptoms varies with each (Table 25-2). A sore throat often, but not always, accompanies these symptoms because of early dryness followed by irritation from postnasal drainage. With acute rhinitis, signs of acute inflammation such as early chilliness followed by feverishness and malaise also are present. If uncomplicated, a cold is usually self-limiting and lasts for about 1 week.

In chronic rhinitis, acute symptoms are absent. The chief complaint is nasal obstruction accompanied by a feeling of stuffiness and pressure in the nose. Polyp formation may occur, and vertigo may be present.

Collaborative Care Management. No specific treatment exists for the common cold. The goals of treatment are to (1) relieve symptoms, (2) inhibit spread of the infection, and (3) reduce the risk of bacterial complications such as sinusitis and otitis media. Decongestants (sympathomimetic amines) are the recommended treatment for relieving nasal congestion and enhancing eustachian tube function. Decongestants can be purchased over the counter (OTC) and are administered as nasal drops or sprays two or three times a day for no more than 3 days (see Patient/Family Teaching box). Topical decongestants include oxymetazoline (Afrin) and phenylephrine (Neo-Synephrine) nasal sprays. In persons with severe congestion, these medications facilitate the uptake of other topical drugs such as nasal cromolyn (Nasalcrom) and corticosteroid sprays.[4]

The side effects of decongestants include rebound nasal congestion (with chronic use), nervousness, and transient increases in blood pressure. Decongestants are contraindicated in patients receiving tricyclic antidepressants or monoamine oxidase inhibitors. Room humidifiers are helpful in liquefying secretions, thereby promoting drainage and decreasing congestion. Antihistamines are not recommended because studies have indicated that oral antihistamines are not effective in treating viral upper respiratory tract infections.

For allergic rhinitis the basic treatment is maintenance of an allergen-free environment. Hyposensitization or desensitization (administering the allergen in gradually increasing doses to establish immunity) may be helpful. Antihistamines give relief

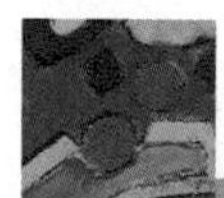

Patient/Family Teaching
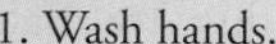
Self-Administration of Nosedrops

1. Wash hands.
2. Assume a position that will facilitate the flow of medication, such as one of the following:
   - Sit in chair and tip head well backward.
   - Lie down with head extended over edge of bed.
   - Lie down with pillow under shoulders and head tipped backward.
3. Turn head to the side that will receive the drops.
4. Place no more than three drops of solution into each nostril at one time (unless otherwise prescribed).
5. Remain in position with head tilted backward for 3 to 5 minutes to permit solution to reach posterior nares.
6. If marked congestion is still present 10 minutes after nosedrop insertion, administer another drop or two of solution (nasal constriction from first insertion may facilitate additional drops reaching posterior nares).

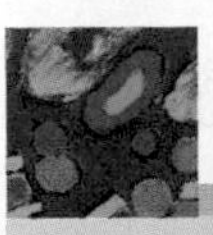

TABLE 25-1 COMMON MEDICATIONS *for Allergic Rhinitis*

Drug	Action	Nursing Intervention
Nonsedating Antihistamines		
Fexofenadine (Allegra) Cetirizine (Zyrtec) Loratadine (Claritin) Desloratadine (Clarinex) Astemizole (Hismanal)	Prevents release of histamine and other substances causing symptoms	Evaluate effectiveness.
Sedating Antihistamines		
Diphenhydramine (Benadryl) Chlorpheniramine (Chlor-Trimeton) Hydroxyzine (Vistaril)	Prevents release of histamine and other substances causing symptoms	Evaluate effectiveness. Warn patient about potential for drowsiness.
Low-Dose Steroid Nasal Sprays		
Beclomethasone (Vancenase, Beconase) Flunisolide (Nasalide, AEROBID) Fluticasone (Flonase) Triamcinolone (Nasacort) Budesonide (Rhinocort, Rhinocort Aqua) Mometasone (Nasonex) Dexamethasone (Dexacort, Decadron)	Depresses inflammatory reactions	Evaluate effectiveness. Ask patient to demonstrate use of nasal spray.
Other Nasal Sprays		
Cromolyn sodium (Nasalcrom) Ipratopium (Atrovent)	Reduces mucus production and swelling Blocks ability of nervous system to stimulate nasal mucous glands	Evaluate effectiveness. Ask patient to demonstrate use of nasal spray. Assess for allergy to atropine; may cause sensitivity to the decongestant.

to most persons, but their effectiveness often decreases as the "hayfever season" continues. In addition, side effects such as sleepiness or dribbling of urine can sometimes affect activities of daily living.

For chronic rhinitis, careful medical follow-up monitoring is indicated. When nasal obstruction persists, surgery may be necessary to remove polyps (polypectomy) or to revise septal tissue (septoplasty).

If the nasal passages are dry, a nasal spray of normal saline can be purchased OTC, or made by mixing 1 teaspoon of salt in 1 quart of boiling water. The homemade solution should be made fresh daily. The solution is best administered from a spray bottle with both nostrils open. Guidelines for instructing the patient and family about rhinitis can be found in the Patient/Family Teaching box.

Sinusitis

The sinuses are air-filled cavities lined with mucous membranes. The term *sinusitis* refers to any inflammation of the mucous membranes. Sinusitis is a common disorder that may be acute or chronic. The most common types of acute sinusitis are allergic and viral. It is often difficult to distinguish between these two types, although the patient's history may be helpful. Allergic sinusitis is usually seasonal, and redness and itching of the eyes may be present. Viral sinusitis is usually accompanied by fever, malaise, and systemic symptoms such as achiness. The patient may also have a history of recent exposure to an infected person. Common viral causes of sinusitis are rhinovirus, influenza virus, adenovirus, and parainfluenza virus. Of all the patients who consult an otolaryngologist because of "sinus trouble," few actually have sinusitis.

TABLE 25-2 SYMPTOMS OF RHINITIS

Symptom	Acute Rhinitis	Allergic Rhinitis	Chronic Rhinitis
Nasal discharge	Initially watery, then mucoid	Thin, watery	Serous, mucopurulent, or purulent
Eyes	Tearing during early phase	Tearing, itching	No tearing
Turbinates	Edematous	Pale, edematous, mucoid	Enlarged
Nasal polyps	No	Sometimes	Sometimes
Headache	Generalized	Generalized	Generalized

PATIENT/FAMILY TEACHING
The Patient With Rhinitis

- Obtain additional rest.
- Drink at least 2 to 3 L of fluid daily.
- Use nasal spray or nosedrops two or three times per day as ordered.
- Prevent further infection:
  —Blow nose with both nostrils open to prevent infected matter from being forced into arytenoid tube.
  —Cover mouth with disposable tissues when coughing and sneezing to prevent droplet nuclei from contaminating the air.
  —Dispose of used tissues carefully.
  —Avoid exposure when possible (i.e., avoid crowds, people with colds, specific allergens).
  —Older adults and those with chronic lung disease are particularly vulnerable and should have a flu shot yearly.
  —Wash hands frequently, especially after coughing, blowing the nose, sneezing, and so on. Evidence suggests that many colds are transmitted from person to person by hand contact and from touching objects handled by a person with a cold.
- Seek medical attention for:
  —High fever, severe chest pain, earache
  —Symptoms lasting longer than 2 weeks
  —Recurrent colds

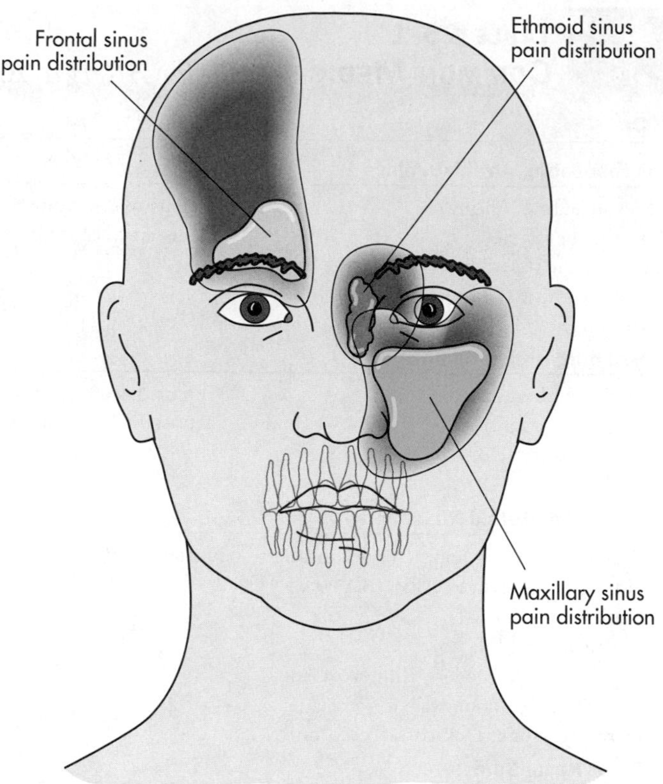

Figure 25-1 Sinus pain: area of local tenderness and pain referral. Maxillary sinus pain often is referred to teeth. Frontal pain is generally localized to supraorbital area. Ethmoid pain is generally deep to the eye.

Acute Bacterial Sinusitis

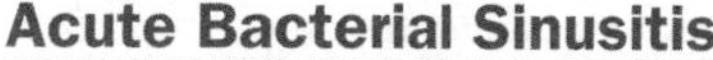

Etiology and Epidemiology. The most common form of sinusitis, after allergic and viral, is acute bacterial sinusitis. Pathogens most often causing acute bacterial sinusitis include *Streptococcus pneumoniae, Haemophilus influenzae,* beta-hemolytic streptococci, *Klebsiella pneumoniae,* and various anaerobic organisms.

Pathophysiology. The first symptom of acute bacterial sinusitis is usually a stuffy nose followed by slowly developing pressure over the involved sinus. Other signs and symptoms include malaise, persistent cough, postnasal drip, headache, slightly elevated temperature, and mild leukopenia. Symptoms worsen over 48 to 72 hours, culminating in severe localized pain and tenderness over the involved sinus (Table 25-3 and Figures 25-1 and 25-2). The patient often believes the pain is due to an infected tooth.

In acute frontal and maxillary sinusitis, pain usually does not appear until 1 to 2 hours after awakening. It increases for 3 to 4 hours and then becomes less severe in the afternoon and evening. Usually this is due to increased drainage as a result of gravity from standing during the day. There may be bloody or blood-tinged discharge from the nose in the first 24 to 48 hours. The discharge

TABLE 25-3 LOCATION OF PAIN WITH SINUSITIS

Sinus	Pain Location
Maxillary	Over cheek and upper teeth (see Figure 25-1)
Frontal	Above eyebrow (see Figure 25-1)
Ethmoid	Medial and deep in eye (see Figure 25-2)
Sphenoid	Deep behind eye, over occiput, or top of head

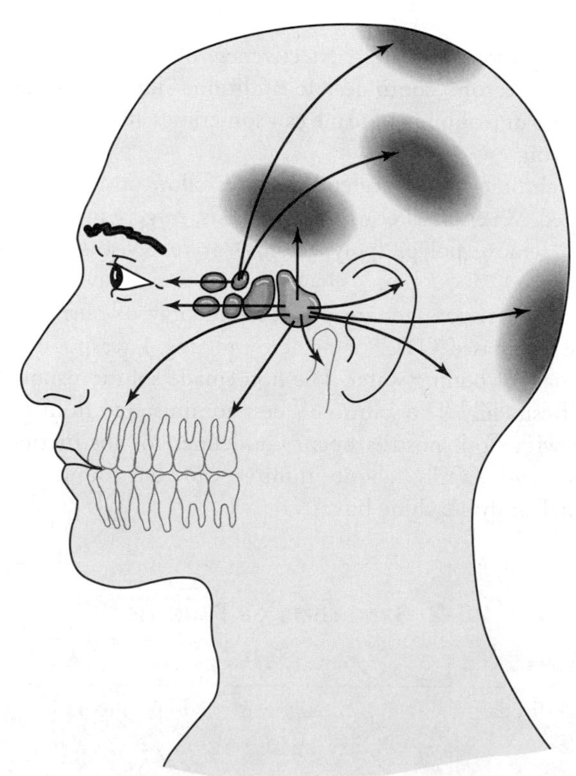

Figure 25-2 Pain from anterior ethmoid is deep to the eye. Pain from posterior ethmoid cells and sphenoid is referred to eyes, teeth, ears, or temporal area of occiput.

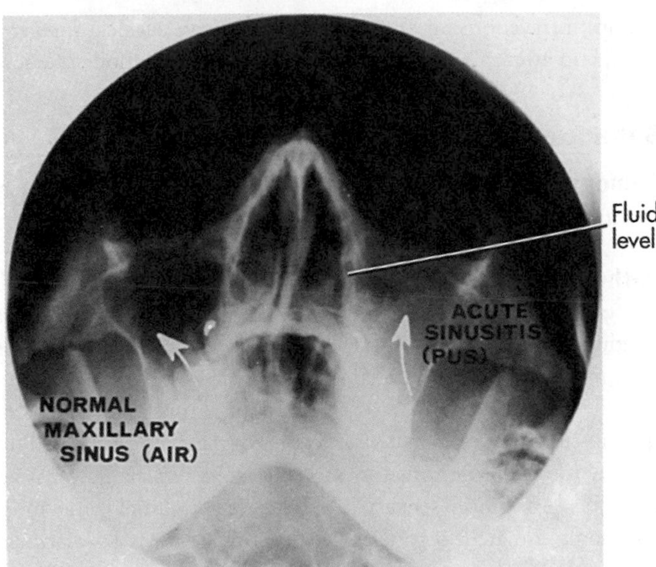

Figure 25-3 X-ray film of maxillary sinus showing normal sinus on left and acute sinusitis with clouding and visible fluid level on right.

rapidly becomes thick, green, and copious, blocking the nose. The throat may become inflamed and sore on one side because of the purulent discharge. On examination, the involved nasal mucosa is hyperemic and edematous, and the turbinates are enlarged. X-ray films show that the involved sinus is clouded, and a fluid level is visible (Figure 25-3).

Collaborative Care Management. Diagnostic tests include transillumination of the sinuses, conventional sinus x-ray films, computed tomography (CT), and magnetic resonance imaging (MRI). Fiberoptic examination of the nose (rhinoscopy) may also be used. For the majority of patients, however, a diagnosis of sinusitis is made without radiographic studies.

Management of acute bacterial sinusitis centers on relief of pain and shrinkage of the nasal mucosa. Ibuprofen (Advil) and an oral decongestant such as pseudoephedrine (Sudafed) are commonly prescribed. The decongestant is given orally or by nasal spray for 2 to 3 days. In some patients, codeine (usually acetaminophen and codeine, or Tylenol No. 3) may be required for pain relief for several days. Giving Tylenol No. 3 and ibuprofen at alternate times assists in managing fever.

The antibiotic of choice is amoxicillin for 10 to 14 days. Failure of the infection to respond to amoxicillin in 5 to 7 days is an indication for aspiration of the maxillary sinus to obtain a specimen for culture and sensitivity and for a possible change in antibiotic. A new antibiotic, telithromycin (Ketek), has recently been approved for the treatment of drug-resistant sinusitis. Box 25-1 lists the antimicrobial agents used to treat acute sinusitis. Also see the Future Watch and Complementary & Alternative Therapies boxes.

Patients may obtain relief from saline nasal sprays, steam from a shower, or a humidifier. Hot wet packs applied to the face over the infected sinus(es), either continuously or for 1 to 2 hours at a time four times a day, may provide symptomatic relief. A washcloth wrung out in hot water is a convenient way to provide wet packs, as are wet cloth towels slightly warmed in a microwave.

Box 25-1 Antimicrobial Therapy for Acute Bacterial Sinusitis

- Amoxicillin (Amoxil, Trimox, Wymox)
- Loracarbef (Lorabid)
- Amoxicillin and clavulanate potassium (Augmentin)
- Cefaclor (Ceclor)
- Cefprozil (Cefzil)
- Cefuroxime axetil (Zinacef IV, Ceftin PO)
- Doxycycline (Vibramycin, Monodox)
- Trimethoprim and sulfamethoxazole (Bactrim, Septra)
- Clarithromycin (Biaxin)
- Azithromycin (Zithromax)
- Telithromycin (Ketek)

Complementary & Alternative Therapies

Homeopathy vs. Antibiotic Resistance

Antibiotic resistance is a global public health problem. Once confined primarily to hospitals, antibiotic resistance is now increasingly common in primary care. The prevalence of resistant bacteria has risen considerably, and organisms resistant to almost all antibiotics continue to increase. The main causes are indiscriminate prescribing and the use of antibiotics in animal feeds and other agricultural applications. Policies to restrict use of antibiotics have had limited success.

Homeopathy may have a role to play in combating the development of antibiotic resistance. Clinical research suggests that homeopathy is effective in the treatment of upper respiratory tract infections, a frequent cause of inappropriate antibiotic prescribing. More research is needed to determine the extent that homeopathy can prevent further antibiotic resistance.

Viksveen P: Antibiotics and the development of resistant microorganisms: can homeopathy be an alternative? *Homeopathy* 92(2):99-107, 2003.

Acute frontal sinusitis with pain, tenderness, and edema of the frontal or sphenoid sinus may require hospitalization because of the risk of intracranial complications or osteomyelitis. The physician usually orders high-dose intravenous antibiotics and nasal decongestants given orally or by spray. When the infection has subsided, the physician prescribes an oral antibiotic and discharges the patient home. In some cases osteomyelitis of the frontal bone occurs; *Staphylococcus aureus* is the most common causative organism.

Teaching is an important component of nursing care for the patient with acute bacterial sinusitis (see Patient/Family Teaching box).

Fungal Sinusitis

Sinusitis of fungal origin ranges from a mild infection resembling chronic sinusitis to a severe, life-threatening, invasive infection. Noninvasive fungal sinusitis caused by *Aspergillus* and *Candida* organisms is often found in patients after other infections or prolonged administration of antibiotics. Treatment may require surgical drainage of the sinuses.

Future Watch

Trends in Antibiotic Prescribing

According to recent research, the rate of antibiotic prescribing has slowed in the United States. Given the growing problem of antimicrobial resistance partially attributable to the overprescribing of antibiotics for upper respiratory tract infections, primary care providers may be altering their decision-making process.

Of the 421 patients who completed a survey in this study, 16% of the patients strongly agreed that they wanted an antibiotic for their illness, whereas 22% agreed, 47% had no opinion, 9% disagreed, and 5% strongly disagreed. More than one fourth of the patients agreed or strongly agreed with the statement, "I plan on asking the doctor for an antibiotic today." The proportion of patients who wanted antibiotics was lower than the proportion in previous studies. It is unknown whether this finding represents an overall decline in desire for antibiotics or was particular to the specific clinic in which the study was conducted. Nonetheless, an association between desire for antibiotics and antibiotic prescribing persists even after adjusting for physical examination findings predictive of antibiotic prescribing. It will be interesting to discern whether trends will continue in this direction in the future.

Linder JA, Singer DE: Desire for antibiotics and antibiotic prescribing for adults with upper respiratory tract infections, *J Gen Intern Med* 18:795-801, 2003.

Invasive fungal sinusitis is most likely to occur in transplant patients, patients receiving chemotherapy, patients with acquired immunodeficiency syndrome, or persons with poorly controlled diabetes. *Aspergillus* and *Mucor* fungi are the two types most likely to cause invasive disease. Symptoms include facial fullness, cranial neuropathies, and pain. Exophthalmos, facial swelling, and blood-tinged nasal discharge may be present. On examination the nasal mucosa appears gray or black. The diagnosis is confirmed by biopsy of the affected membranes. Treatment consists of hospitalization, intravenous amphotericin B, aggressive surgical management, and attempts to correct the underlying immunodeficiency.

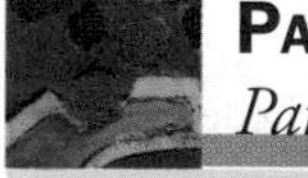

PATIENT/FAMILY TEACHING *The Patient With Acute Bacterial Sinusitis*

Instruct the patient to:

- Get plenty of rest.
- Increase fluid intake to 2 to 3 L per day.
- Use a nasal spray or steam from the shower to keep nasal mucosa moist.
- Seek medical attention if any of the following occur:
  —Increase in bloody drainage from the nose
  —Severe headache or increased pain in the face, teeth, or ears
  —Elevation of temperature above 99° F (37° C) or persistent elevated temperature
  —Increase in fatigue or general achiness
  —Increased nasal stuffiness and inability to clear secretions from the nose
  —Purulent or foul-smelling nasal discharge

Explain the medication regimen and give a written copy to the patient and family. For patients taking antibiotics, stress the importance of taking the antibiotics as prescribed and tell them to contact a health care provider if no change in symptoms occurs after 5 to 7 days. Explain that ibuprofen and any decongestant need to be taken as prescribed.

Subacute Bacterial Sinusitis

Etiology and Epidemiology. A subacute bacterial sinusitis persists in a few patients after an episode of acute bacterial sinusitis.

Pathophysiology. Persistent, purulent nasal discharge is the only constant symptom. A sinus x-ray film or CT scan determines whether one or more than one sinus is involved. Because it is uncommon for acute bacterial sinusitis to persist, when an infection lingers, an unusual causative organism must be suspected. Special culture and sensitivity techniques may be required to identify the particular organism to be treated, especially if it is an anaerobe. Antibiotic sensitivity studies are essential. The most commonly isolated organisms are *H. influenzae, Streptococcus pneumoniae,* and *Branhamella catarrhalis.*[5]

Collaborative Care Management. Infections are treated with antibiotics to which the causative organisms are sensitive, usually penicillin or amoxicillin, unless the patient is allergic to them. Systemic sulfonamide therapy or erythromycin with a sulfonamide is used for infections caused by *B. catarrhalis,* which is resistant to penicillin and amoxicillin. Other treatment consists of nasal vasoconstriction, moist heat applied to the sinus(es), and irrigation of the involved sinus(es). No pain medication is required, since pain is not severe. An antral puncture, which can be repeated several times without damaging the nose or maxillary sinus, is commonly used for irrigation of the maxillary sinus. Anesthesia for antral puncture is achieved by placing a cotton applicator moistened with 5% cocaine solution high under the inferior turbinate against the lateral wall of the nose. A second applicator is placed under the middle turbinate. After the anesthesia takes effect (in about 5 to 10 minutes), the physician inserts a 16- to 18-gauge needle under the turbinate until the needle pierces the medial wall of the antrum and enters the sinus cavity (Figure 25-4). The physician attaches a syringe to the needle and aspirates purulent material or air, which is sent to the laboratory for culture and sensitivity testing. Saline solution is instilled to wash out the sinus. Antibiotic solutions may be used, but mechanical cleansing is more important than the solution used.[4]

It is impossible to irrigate the ethmoid sinuses directly; thus ethmoiditis is treated systemically. Antibiotics are usually prescribed for 10 to 14 days. Treatment of subacute bacterial sinusitis focuses on preventing chronic bacterial sinusitis.

Chronic Bacterial Sinusitis

Etiology and Epidemiology. Chronic bacterial sinusitis develops when irreversible mucosal damage occurs. Damage can result from recurrent attacks of sinusitis or from suppurative sinusitis being untreated or inadequately treated during the acute or subacute phase.

Pathophysiology. The major symptom of chronic bacterial sinusitis is nasal congestion with thick, green, purulent discharge, present for at least 3 months. Fever and facial pain also may be

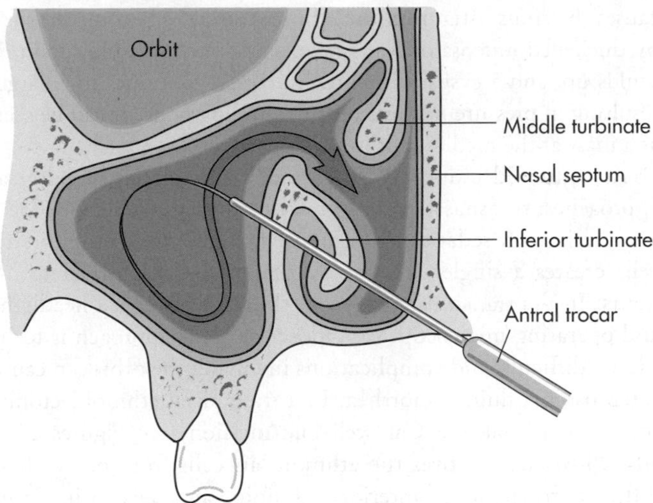

Figure 25-4 Antral puncture. Trocar inserted under inferior turbinate (through medial wall of antrum). Contents of sinus are washed into nose through natural ostium.

present. Usually the patient does not have a headache but may experience symptoms such as lightheadedness. Chronic bacterial sinusitis is often polymicrobial, with anaerobes present in most cases. The most commonly involved organisms are *S. aureus, H. influenzae,* and anaerobes. Complications of sinusitis usually are the result of either inadequate therapy during the acute stage or a delay in treatment. The nurse should observe for:

- Generalized persistent headache
- Vomiting
- Convulsions
- Chills or high fever
- Edema or increasing swelling of the forehead or eyelids
- Blurring of vision, diplopia, or persistent retroocular pain
- Signs of increased intracranial pressure
- Personality changes or dulling of the sensorium
- Increase in white blood cell count above $20,000/mm^3$

Serious complications that may develop from untreated chronic sinusitis include cavernous sinus thrombosis, bacteremia or septicemia, and osteomyelitis. Orbital infections may also occur. Seventy-five percent of orbital infections are caused by extension from paranasal sinusitis, usually involving the ethmoid sinuses. Orbital infection can cause inflammatory edema, orbital cellulitis, subperiosteal abscess, orbital abscess, and cavernous sinus thrombosis. Complications are treated vigorously with intravenous antibiotics and, in the case of abscess, incision and drainage.[2]

Cavernous sinus thrombosis is a particularly serious complication that occurs when infection extends through the venous pathways (usually the angular vein) to the cavernous sinus. The patient is very ill, with chills and a temperature as high as 106° F (41° C). The patient has deep pain behind the eye and becomes toxic and sometimes semicomatose. The primary treatment of cavernous sinus thrombosis is intravenous antibiotics, without which death can occur in 48 to 72 hours.

Collaborative Care Management

DIAGNOSTIC TESTS. The sinuses can be aspirated to obtain organisms for culture and sensitivity. A CT scan of the sinuses is used to determine if there is blockage of the nasal sinus drainage system, polyps, mucous plugs, or other findings that would require endoscopic sinus surgery. Before endoscopic sinus surgery is used to treat chronic sinusitis, the patient is also evaluated with nasal endoscopy and coronal CT scans. The nasal endoscopy reveals subtle changes that cannot be seen in an anterior rhinoscopy using a nasal speculum, and the coronal CT scan determines the underlying cause of sinusitis. The coronal CT scan is best performed after acute inflammation has subsided and medical treatment has been attempted.

MEDICATIONS. Decongestants are usually sufficient treatment. Patients who are not experiencing fever, facial pain, or tenderness usually obtain no benefit from antibiotics. When antibiotics are necessary, the results of the culture and sensitivity test are used to determine the appropriate antibiotic. Antibiotics are usually prescribed for 2 to 3 weeks.

TREATMENTS. Nasal saline irrigations and surgery are the major treatments.

SURGICAL MANAGEMENT. Treatment of chronic sinusitis involves surgery to remove all diseased soft tissue and bone, provide adequate postoperative drainage, and obliterate the sinus cavity when necessary. The goal of surgery is to eradicate infection and leave contiguous structures intact. Several types of surgical procedures are used to treat patients with chronic sinusitis.

FUNCTIONAL ENDOSCOPIC SINUS SURGERY. In functional endoscopic sinus surgery (FESS), also known as endoscopic sinus surgery, the physician uses a fiberoptic endoscope that illuminates and magnifies to enter the sinus. Diseased tissue, located by CT scan, can be dissected. A major advantage of this approach is that, because the actual pathologic site can be identified, there is minimum loss of healthy tissue and thus better preservation of sinus function. In early sinus disease the air cells are opened to allow for ventilation and drainage. In advanced disease the air cells may need to be removed. The procedure can be performed with the patient under local or general anesthesia. If local anesthesia is used, the procedure is performed in an ambulatory surgery center, where the patient is kept for 2 to 3 hours postoperatively and then discharged. Thus FESS allows patients with sinus disease to be treated without hospitalization and prevents facial scarring and extended recovery periods.

Although the main use of FESS is to treat recurrent or chronic sinus disease by improving sinus ventilation, promoting sinus drainage, and removing diseased tissue, it also can be used for the removal of polyps, foreign bodies, or other growths; treatment of recurrent or chronic pain caused by nasal or sinus blockage; or examination with the patient under anesthesia, usually with a biopsy.

CALDWELL-LUC SINUS OPERATION. The Caldwell-Luc operation, also known as a radical antrum operation, is the generally accepted operative procedure for chronic maxillary sinusitis that cannot be cured with antibiotics and other medical therapy. Local or general anesthesia may be used.

The procedure is performed through an incision under the upper lip (Figure 25-5). The surgeon removes part of the anterior

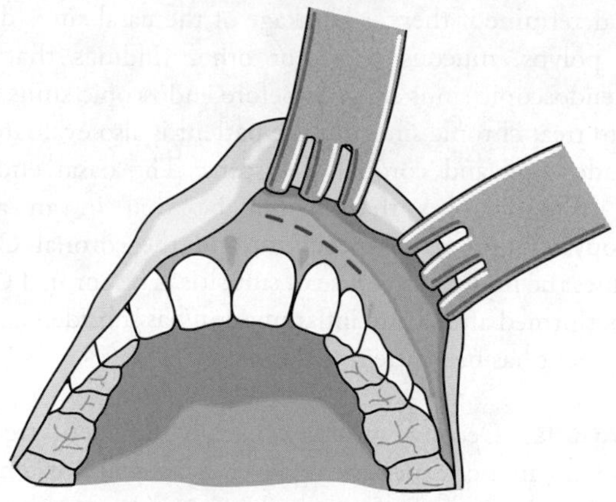

Figure 25-5 Incision into maxillary sinus (Caldwell-Luc operation) is made under upper lip.

bony wall of the antrum, producing a permanent window (Figure 25-6), and removes all the diseased mucosa and periosteum through the window. The bone of the lateral wall of the nose in the inferior meatus, which divides the nose from the antrum, is also removed. The mucous membrane and periosteum of the lateral wall of the nose are preserved and fashioned into a hinged flap.

The antrum may be packed to prevent bleeding. Packing is removed through the nose 24 to 48 hours after surgery. As the maxillary sinus heals, the exposed bone is covered by mucosa. Numbness of the upper lip and upper teeth may be present for several months after a Caldwell-Luc operation because some nerves to these structures pass through the incision site.

ETHMOIDECTOMY. An ethmoidectomy, which entails removal of ethmoid air cells, is performed to remove diseased mucosa, nasal polyps (which commonly originate in the ethmoid cells), or mucoceles from the ethmoid sinus. A mucocele is a mucous cyst that is a consequence of repeated infection. Repeated infection causes the sinus ostia from the ethmoid sinus to become blocked by thickened mucosa or scar tissue. Thus mucus cannot drain, it builds up, and a cyst forms. The mucocele continues to enlarge, resulting in pressure necrosis on surrounding bone. It can be seen as a mass at the medial canthus.[2]

An ethmoidectomy is performed through three surgical approaches: transnasal, transantral, or external. General or local anesthesia with sedation may be used. Removal of ethmoid air cells creates a single large cavity that is packed for 24 to 48 hours. In the transnasal approach, the surgeon uses a headlight and operating microscope or endoscope. This approach is technically difficult, and complications involving the orbit can cause cerebrospinal fluid rhinorrhea. In a transantral ethmoidectomy, the surgeon makes a Caldwell-Luc incision (see Figures 25-5 and 25-6) and removes the ethmoid air cells from below. It is difficult to remove anterior ethmoid air cells using this approach, and a combined intranasal and transantral approach may be necessary. Complications of the transantral approach include damage to the infraorbital nerve, which causes numbness of the lip or upper teeth. The external approach (Figure 25-7) is preferred because it allows better visualization and reduces the risks of complications such as damage to the optic nerve and cerebrospinal fluid leak. A pressure dressing is usually applied over the operative eye to prevent postoperative edema.

SPHENOID SINUS SURGERY. Surgery of the sphenoid sinus can be accomplished using an endoscopic technique, through an external or transantral ethmoidectomy approach, or through a transseptal approach. The surgeon usually removes the ethmoid sinus and opens the anterior wall of the sphenoid sinus. Diseased tissue is removed, along with the mucous membrane lining the sinus. To facilitate drainage directly into the nasopharynx, the sinus ostium is opened wide.

FRONTAL SINUSECTOMY. The use of the osteoplastic flap operation makes frontal sinus surgery different from that performed on the other sinuses. Surgery of the other sinuses basically provides for an open, well-drained cavity, which in the past proved inadequate for the frontal sinuses because recurrence of disease

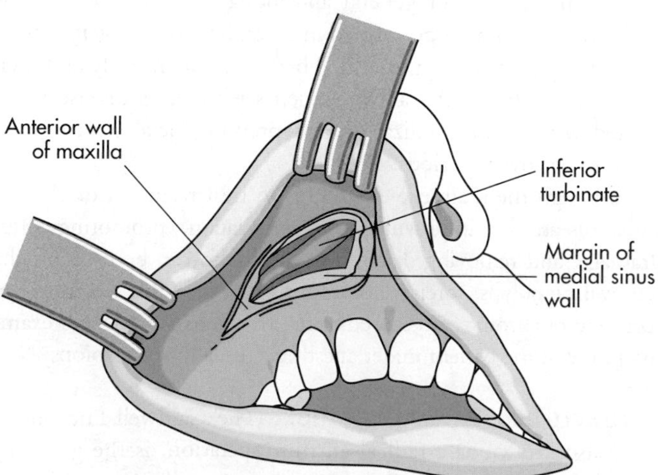

Figure 25-6 Caldwell-Luc operation. After removal of sinus mucosa or polypoid tissue, the surgeon makes a window into the nose along its floor, allowing dependent drainage from maxillary sinus. The incision is closed with absorbable sutures.

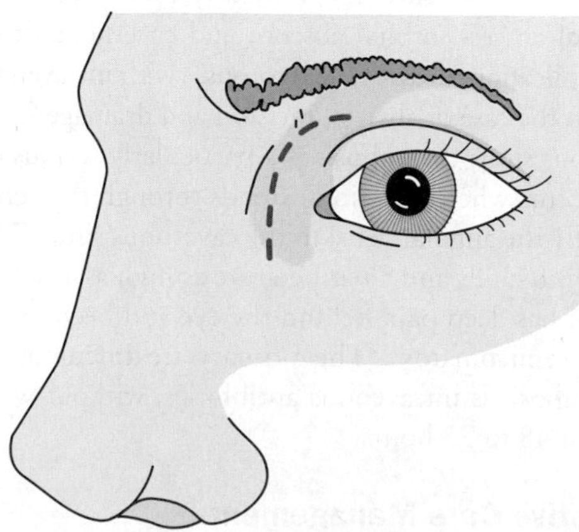

Figure 25-7 Medial canthal incision for external ethmoidectomy.

was common. The osteoplastic flap operation allows for complete removal of diseased mucosa of the frontal sinus and for obliteration of the sinus so that it is no longer functional or continuous with the inner nose.

The osteoplastic flap procedure is performed through a "gull-wing" or "crossbow" incision. In men the incision extends along the eyebrows and connects along the bridge of the nose. In women, for whom baldness usually is not a problem in later life, the incision connects both temporal areas a few centimeters posterior to the hairline. Both incisions give excellent postoperative cosmesis and are extended to the periosteum of the bone overlying the frontal sinus.

The skin overlying the sinus is reflected, and a radiograph of the frontal sinus (obtained before surgery) is used as a template for sawing the lateral and superior borders of the anterior frontal bone. The anterior bone is then reflected inferiorly, thus exposing the entire contents of the frontal sinus. The surgeon removes the mucosa under direct vision, using an operating microscope to ensure all fragments are removed. The surgeon then makes an incision in the left lower abdominal quadrant and obtains subcutaneous fat for adipose obliteration of the sinus. The bony flap and skin are then repositioned, and a pressure dressing applied to minimize postoperative swelling.

Pain in the frontal area is not significant after 24 hours after surgery. Pain in the abdominal area, however, often lasts several days, and serous drainage from this area is common after the drain is removed. Sutures are removed on about the fifth postoperative day. Because nasal packs are not used, special oral hygiene care is not needed. However, a dressing may be placed under the nose to catch drainage (Figure 25-8).

DIET. After FESS, patients may eat whatever they wish, although the nasal packing and postoperative swelling decrease appetite. After other types of sinus surgery, fluids are given freely for the first 24 hours, progressing to a soft diet. In all cases increasing protein intake aids in healing.

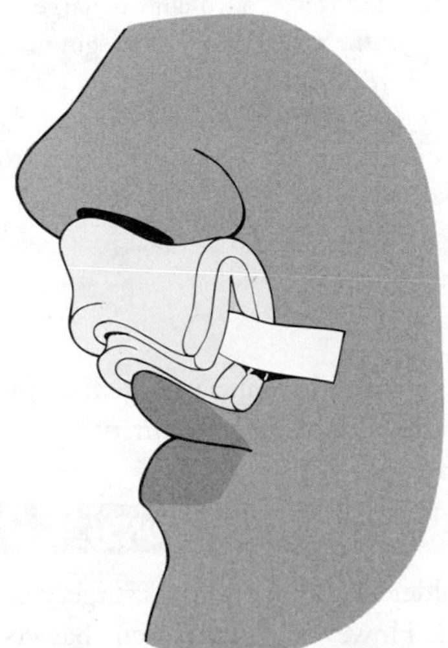

Figure 25-8 Sometimes called a mustache dressing or drip pad, a dressing is placed under nose to catch nasal drainage.

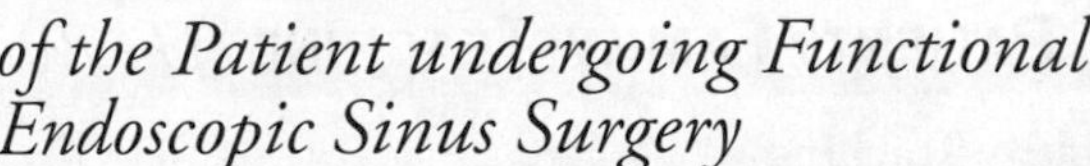

Nursing Management

of the Patient undergoing Functional Endoscopic Sinus Surgery

PREOPERATIVE CARE

Because FESS is an outpatient procedure, preadmission tests and preoperative teaching are scheduled a few days before surgery. The nurse reviews the postoperative routine at this time so the patient can determine in advance of surgery the preparations, if any, that will need to be made at home. The Patient/Family Teaching box covers all information that needs to be taught to the patient having sinus surgery.

POSTOPERATIVE CARE

If inflammation or infection is noted during the surgery, antibiotics are administered and continued for 10 to 14 days. Some surgeons also order a steroid nasal spray for a few days. To keep the mucosa moist, all patients begin normal saline sprays after packing is removed. Saline irrigations may be necessary for those with considerable nasal crusting.

The nurse reinforces self-care information before discharge and assesses the patient's progress via a telephone call within 24 hours.

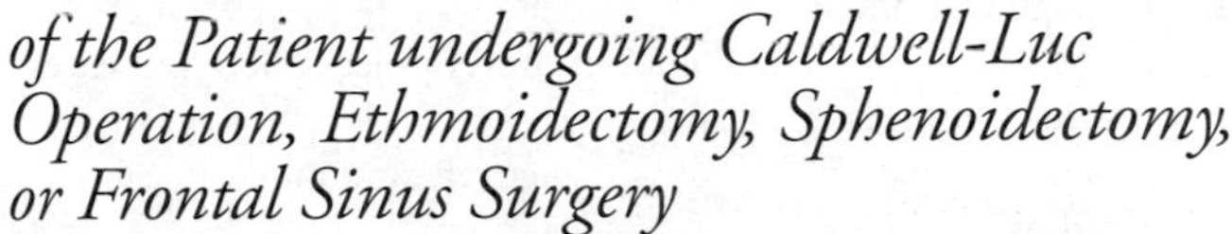

Nursing Management

of the Patient undergoing Caldwell-Luc Operation, Ethmoidectomy, Sphenoidectomy, or Frontal Sinus Surgery

PREOPERATIVE CARE

For the patient's convenience, preadmission tests and preoperative teaching should be scheduled for the same day, usually a few days before surgery. The patient is admitted to the hospital the morning of surgery. The Patient/Family Teaching box on p. 596 provides information for the patient having any sinus surgery.

POSTOPERATIVE CARE

Because general anesthesia is usual, the nurse positions the patient well on the side to facilitate removal of secretions and to maintain the airway. This position also prevents swelling of the surgical site and aspiration of bloody drainage. Cool mist is administered by face tent or collar to prevent drying of secretions and to keep mucous membranes moist.

When the patient recovers from anesthesia, the nurse elevates the head of the bed to a mid-Fowler's position to prevent edema and promote drainage. The nurse reminds the patient to sniff secretions to the back of the mouth, where they can be expectorated. Ice compresses are applied over the nose or over the maxillary or frontal sinuses for a few hours after surgery to help reduce swelling in the operative area, constrict blood vessels, reduce bleeding, and relieve pain.[4]

The nurse monitors the patient for:

- Excessive bleeding from the nose (Frequent swallowing is a clue.)
- Decreased visual acuity, especially diplopia, which indicates damage to the optic nerve or muscles of the globe of the eye

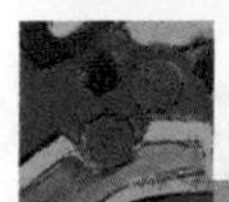

PATIENT/FAMILY TEACHING *The Patient Undergoing Sinus Surgery*

Preoperative Teaching

Determine patient's understanding of the surgical procedure. Clarify misconceptions and answer patient's and family's questions. Explain that patient will:

- Have nothing to eat or drink for 6 to 8 hours before surgery
- Receive a sedative before surgery
- Feel pressure, not pain, during surgery
- Have a nasal pack for 24 to 48 hours after surgery and may feel like he or she has a "head cold"
- Have a mustache dressing after surgery (see Figure 25-8)
- Have "black eyes" and swelling around the nose and eyes for 1 to 2 weeks after surgery
- Have a prescription for pain medication as needed

Postoperative Teaching

Precautions for the First Week

- Do not blow your nose until after your first office visit, usually 3 to 5 days after surgery. Blowing your nose puts too much pressure on the surgical site. After a Caldwell-Luc operation, do not blow the nose for 2 weeks.
- If you feel fluid or congestion in your nose, gently sniff back the fluid and spit it into a tissue.
- Try not to sneeze, since this will put too much pressure on the surgical site. If you must sneeze, keep your mouth open and sneeze through your mouth.
- Do not bend over, and do not lift heavy objects; both put excessive pressure on the surgical site.
- Avoid constipation (Valsalva's maneuver [straining] can cause bleeding).
- Additional precautions for patients with Caldwell-Luc operation include:
  —Do not chew on affected side until incision heals.
  —Use caution with oral hygiene to avoid injury to the incision.
  —Avoid wearing dentures for about 10 days.

Managing Pain

- The discomfort after surgery is more of an ache and pressure from the packing in the nose than actual pain.
- The pain may increase during the week after surgery because of swelling and secretions in the sinus.
- Most patients obtain relief by taking acetaminophen. If your physician expects you to have more pain, another medication will be prescribed.
- Never take aspirin or any product containing aspirin, since aspirin can cause bleeding.

Taking Care of Drainage

- Expect the drainage to increase after surgery.
- A small amount of bright red bleeding is normal and may continue for a week.
- Old blood that accumulated during the surgery is reddish brown, and it will drain for a week or more. It is of no concern.
- A small dressing (dry pad) will be placed beneath your nose to absorb any drainage.
- You may need to change the pad several times each day, depending on the amount of drainage. The drainage pad can be discontinued when the drainage stops.
- After initial bloody drainage stops, a thicker, yellowish green drainage may continue for several weeks.

Breathing Difficulties

- Your head may feel stuffy, and the mucous membranes of your nose may swell. This is normal.
- Stuffiness will increase during the first week after surgery and then decrease over the next couple of weeks, and breathing through your nose should improve.
- Keeping your head elevated and sleeping with an extra pillow will make you more comfortable, reduce swelling, and allow better drainage of nasal secretions.
- A cool mist humidifier at the bedside will help loosen secretions and prevent crusting of the nose. Be sure to follow the manufacturer's directions for cleaning the unit so that bacteria will not grow, be dispersed into the air, and infect you or others.
- At the postoperative visit, the physician will remove the packing and give you instructions for cleaning your nose.

Rest and Activity

- Since the body needs extra rest for at least a week to heal, take it easy the first week and then return to normal activities. The usual time to be off work or school is 5 to 7 days unless you work in a dusty or dirty environment.
- After a week, swimming, jogging, or other such exercises are usually permitted. If bright red bleeding occurs, stop activity until bleeding stops, and then gradually resume activity.

Self-Monitoring

- Report signs of infection (fever, purulent discharge) to surgeon.
- Expect ecchymoses of the nose and eyes to begin to change color over the next 1 to 2 weeks.
- Expect tarry stools from swallowed blood for a few days.
- Take prophylactic antibiotics as prescribed; do not stop until all medication is taken.

- Pain over the involved sinus, which may indicate an infection or inadequate drainage
- Elevated temperature (The temperature must be taken rectally or aurally; it cannot be taken orally because of packing in the nose, which causes mouth breathing.)

Because of increased dryness of the lips, the nurse provides frequent mouth care using a soft toothbrush and applies a lubricant. Mouthwash can be used to manage halitosis. If there is an oral incision, the nurse provides mouth care before meals to improve appetite and after meals to remove food debris, which could lead to infection. Liberal fluid intake is urged to prevent drying of secretions. Also, the patient may be thirsty because of dry mouth from mouth breathing.

GERONTOLOGIC CONSIDERATIONS

The care for an older adult having sinus surgery is the same as that already described. However, if the patient has coexisting disease, attention must be given to assessment of affected organs and functions. In addition, the patient may be hospitalized for a day or two to carefully monitor the status and prevent complications.

▶ ARE YOU READY?

In the postoperative client after frontal sinus surgery, which of the following findings would require immediate intervention?

1. Dry mucous membranes
2. Excessive swallowing
3. Headache
4. Edema

Infections of the Pharynx and Larynx

Acute Pharyngitis

Etiology and Epidemiology. Acute pharyngitis, or throat inflammation, is caused by hemolytic streptococci, staphylococci, other bacteria, filterable viruses, or fungi. Group A beta-hemolytic streptococci are the cause of up to 30% of the cases of acute pharyngitis. Viruses, however, account for about 70% of the cases. There is also increased evidence of gonococcal pharyngitis caused by the gram-negative diplococcus *Neisseria gonorrhoeae.* The disease is increasingly found in both men and women. When gonorrhea is suspected, a throat culture is indicated. A severe form of acute pharyngitis often is termed *strep throat* because of the frequency of streptococci as the causative organism.[5]

Pathophysiology. Dryness of the throat is a common complaint associated with pharyngitis. The throat appears red, and soreness may range from slight scratchiness to severe pain with difficulty in swallowing. A hacking cough may be present. Children often develop a very high fever, whereas adults may have only a mild elevation of temperature. Symptoms usually precede or occur simultaneously with the onset of acute rhinitis or acute sinusitis. Pharyngitis is also a common manifestation of infectious mononucleosis. The Clinical Manifestations box summarizes signs and symptoms of the different types of pharyngitis.

Collaborative Care Management. Acute pharyngitis usually is relieved by hot saline throat gargles and mild OTC analgesics. An ice collar also may provide comfort. For adults, the physician may prescribe acetylsalicylic acid administered orally as a gargle or in Aspergum. Lozenges containing a mild anesthetic may help relieve local soreness. Moist inhalations may help relieve throat dryness. A liquid diet usually is better tolerated than solid food, and fluids, at least 2.5 L/day, are encouraged. Oral hygiene may prevent drying and cracking of the lips and usually refreshes the mouth. The person should remain in bed if the temperature is elevated and should have extra rest if afebrile.

A throat culture is necessary to identify the infecting organism. If beta-hemolytic streptococci are identified, the drug of choice is penicillin. For the person allergic to penicillin, erythromycin or another antibiotic is prescribed. Persons with a history of bacterial endocarditis or rheumatic fever are usually given penicillin prophylactically if they are not allergic. The prescribed course of antibiotic therapy varies from 7 to 12 days, depending on the organism and the severity of infection. Patients must understand that they should continue therapy for the prescribed number of days even if they are symptom free.

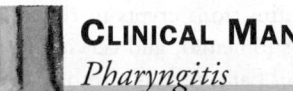

CLINICAL MANIFESTATIONS *Pharyngitis*

Group A Beta-Hemolytic Streptococcal

Sore throat
Slightly elevated temperature
Malaise

Gonococcal or Viral

Minimal discomfort
Fever
Diffuse sore throat

Infectious Mononucleosis (Epstein-Barr Virus)

Sore throat
Cervical lymphadenopathy
Fever

Fungal (Especially Candidiasis [Thrush])

Pus
Dysphagia
White plaques in mouth or on pharyngeal walls

The major role of the nurse is patient teaching (see the Patient/Family Teaching box). It is important to stress the need for strict hand washing, use of separate eating utensils, and covering one's mouth when coughing and sneezing to reduce the spread of infection.

Acute Follicular Tonsillitis

Etiology and Epidemiology. Acute follicular tonsillitis is an acute inflammation of the tonsils and their crypts. It is usually caused by streptococci, although staphylococci, pneumococci, gram-negative organisms, and viruses can also be causative agents. Acute tonsillitis is more likely to occur when the person's resistance is low, and it is common in children and young adults, especially mouth breathers or those with a history of asthma and chronic upper respiratory tract infections.

Pathophysiology. The onset is almost always sudden, and symptoms include sore throat, pain on swallowing, a feeling of fullness in the throat, fever, chills, general muscle ache, and malaise. These symptoms often last for 2 to 3 days. The pharynx and tonsils appear red, and the peritonsillar tissues are swollen.

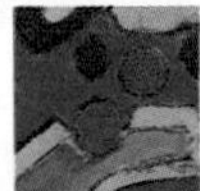

PATIENT/FAMILY TEACHING *The Patient With Pharyngitis or Tonsillitis*

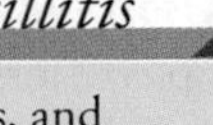

- Use warm saline gargles, ice collars, moist inhalations, and frequent mouth care for comfort.
- Drink at least 2 to 3 L of fluids daily.
- Observe for symptoms of recurrence requiring medical attention: fever, excessive pain, pus, dysphagia.
- To prevent reinfection, obtain prophylactic antibiotic therapy for pharyngitis if there is a history of rheumatic fever or infective endocarditis.

Sometimes a yellowish exudate drains from crypts in the tonsils. Occipital, tonsillar, submaxillary, submental, and cervical lymph nodes may be swollen and palpable. Earache may also be present.

Untreated or chronic tonsillitis can be the source of organisms that spread and adversely affect the heart and kidneys or lead to chorea and pneumonia. The incidence of these complications is decreasing with early diagnosis and the widespread use of penicillin.

A peritonsillar abscess is an uncommon local complication of acute follicular tonsillitis in which infection extends from the tonsil to form an abscess in the surrounding tissues. Pus behind the tonsil causes difficulty in talking, opening the mouth, and swallowing, often such that the person is unable to swallow. Pain is severe and may extend to the ear on the affected side.

Collaborative Care Management. Acute tonsillitis is treated with antibiotics to which the infecting organism is sensitive. The patient is encouraged to rest and drink generous amounts of fluids. Warm saline throat irrigations may be ordered, and antibiotics are given for streptococcal pharyngitis. Acetaminophen (Tylenol) and sometimes codeine sulfate may be ordered for pain and discomfort. An ice collar applied to the neck may relieve discomfort. Occasionally, in extreme cases, physicians may prescribe intramuscular or oral steroids to reduce inflammation.

Because the person with acute tonsillitis is usually cared for at home, the nurse should help in teaching the general public the care that is needed (see Patient/Family Teaching box, p. 597).

Peritonsillar abscess also is treated with antibiotics; if it is caused by anaerobic organisms, hydrogen peroxide (an oxidizing agent) in the form of a mouthwash may help relieve symptoms. In some cases of peritonsillar abscess, incision and drainage may be necessary. For this procedure, the patient's head usually is lowered, and suction is applied as soon as the incision is made to prevent the patient from aspirating the purulent drainage. Warm saline irrigations, an ice collar, or narcotics may relieve discomfort. If acute follicular tonsillitis is treated adequately, peritonsillar abscess is not likely to occur.[2]

Tonsillectomy (discussed later) may be done for recurrent attacks of acute tonsillitis, chronic infection, or repeated peritonsillar abscess. This procedure is usually performed 4 to 6 weeks after an acute attack has subsided.

Acute Laryngitis

Etiology and Epidemiology. Simple acute laryngitis is an inflammation of the mucous membrane lining the larynx, accompanied by edema of the vocal cords. It may be caused by a cold, sudden change in temperature, or irritating fumes.

Pathophysiology. Symptoms vary from a slight huskiness to complete loss of voice. The throat may be painful and feel scratchy, and a cough may be present.

Collaborative Care Management. Laryngitis in adults usually requires only symptomatic treatment. Individuals diagnosed with laryngitis are advised to remain indoors and to avoid using their voice for several days or weeks, depending on the severity of the inflammation. Steam inhalations may be soothing, and cough syrups or home remedies for coughs provide relief to some patients. Patients should avoid smoking or being near others who are smoking. Additional fluids by mouth help prevent dehydration and drying of the throat.

Chronic laryngitis occurs in people who use their voices excessively, who smoke a great deal, or who work continually around irritating fumes. Hoarseness usually is worse in the early morning and in the evening. The patient may have a dry, harsh cough and a persistent need to clear the throat. All persons with persistent hoarseness should be examined by laryngoscopy to rule out cancer of the larynx. Treatment of chronic laryngitis consists of removal of irritants, voice rest, correction of faulty voice habits, steam inhalations, and cough medications. Additional fluids by mouth are encouraged to prevent dehydration and drying of the throat.[5] The nursing role is mainly supportive and includes teaching the patient comfort and preventive measures, as mentioned above.

Chronic Enlargement of Tonsils and Adenoids

Etiology and Epidemiology. Tonsils and adenoids are lymphoid structures located in the oropharynx and nasopharynx. They reach full size in childhood and begin to atrophy during puberty. When they enlarge, it is usually a result of chronic infection, but sometimes the cause is not identifiable.

Pathophysiology. When adenoids enlarge, they cause nasal obstruction. The person breathes through the mouth, snores loudly, may have a dull facial expression, and may have reduced appetite because the blocked nasopharynx can interfere with swallowing. Hypertrophy of the tonsils does not usually block the oropharynx but may affect speech and swallowing and cause mouth breathing.

Collaborative Care Management. The tonsils and adenoids are removed when they become enlarged and cause symptoms of obstruction. No specific tests are used to determine whether surgery is indicated.

Before surgery, patients must be allowed nothing by mouth (remain NPO) after midnight, be infection free, and meet criteria for the specific form of anesthesia to be used. Tonsillectomy in adults may be performed with either general or local anesthesia. After removing the tonsils, the surgeon applies pressure to stop superficial bleeding. The surgeon ties off bleeding vessels with sutures or electrocoagulation. The nurse monitors the patient carefully for hemorrhage, especially when he or she is sleeping, since a large amount of blood may be lost without any external evidence of bleeding. The physician may be able to control minor postoperative bleeding by applying a sponge soaked in a solution of epinephrine to the site. The person who is bleeding excessively often returns to the operating room for surgical treatment to stop the hemorrhage. Use of sutures causes more pain and discomfort than electrocoagulation, and the patient may be unable to take solid foods for several days. Most otolaryngologists prescribe acetaminophen instead of aspirin for pain after a tonsillectomy because aspirin increases the tendency for bleeding.

The tough, yellow, fibrous membrane that forms over the operative site begins to break away between the fourth and eighth postoperative days, and hemorrhage may occur. The separation of the membrane accounts for the throat being more painful at this time. Pink granulation tissue soon becomes apparent, and by the end of the third postoperative week the area is covered with normal mucous membrane. The Guidelines for Safe Practice box outlines postoperative care. Postoperative assessments focus primarily on identification of complications of tonsillectomy, namely, hemorrhage and respiratory obstruction related to edema of local tissue.

Laryngeal Paralysis and Edema

Laryngeal Paralysis

Etiology and Epidemiology. Laryngeal paralysis may result from disease or injury of either the laryngeal nerves or the vagus nerve. Causes include aortic aneurysm, mitral stenosis, laryngeal cancer, subglottic or cervical esophageal tumors, bronchial carcinoma, neck injuries, severing or stretching of the recurrent laryngeal nerve during thyroidectomy, and prolonged intubation of patients in intensive care units.

Pathophysiology. One or both vocal cords may be paralyzed. If only one cord is involved, the airway is adequate and only the voice may be affected. Improvement of voice quality in persons with unilateral cord paralysis has been achieved by injecting a small quantity of Gelfoam or Teflon into the paralyzed cord. This swells the cord and pushes it toward the midline, where the other cord can approximate it better during phonation.

Bilateral paralysis impairs the airway and causes incapacitating dyspnea, stridor on exertion, and a weak voice. A sudden bilateral vocal cord paralysis is uncommon and usually results from a massive cerebrovascular accident or blunt trauma, both of which are usually incompatible with life. Treatment of bilateral cord paralysis is aimed at restoring the airway, not at improving the voice.

Collaborative Care Management. The primary diagnostic test is laryngoscopy. This and other tests used, along with their purposes, are listed in Table 25-4. If the patient is experiencing gastroesophageal reflux, the physician may order antacids, which neutralize gastric acid, or H_2 inhibitors, which reduce the amount of gastric acid produced. If the patient has signs and symptoms of an infection, appropriate antibiotics are prescribed. For patients with swelling of the vocal cords, systemic steroids are often ordered, and for those with spastic movements of the cords, botulinum may be injected.

TABLE 25-4 DIAGNOSTIC TESTS FOR LARYNGEAL PARALYSIS

Test	Purpose
Computed tomography scan	To visualize vocal cords to locate tumor or aneurysm
Electromyography	To check movement of vocal cords
Indirect laryngoscopy	To visualize interior of larynx for diagnostic purposes
Videostroboscopy (closed circuit television technique that records images of vocal cords while vibrating)	To observe vibrations and diagnose abnormalities

Treatment of cord paralysis may involve excision of nodules or polyps or a thyroplasty, in which a stent is inserted to reapproximate the vocal cords. A **tracheostomy** may be necessary to maintain the airway. Other possible procedures include an arytenoidectomy, in which a portion of one of the arytenoid cartilages is resected, thus increasing the diameter of the posterior portion of the glottis sufficiently to improve breathing.

Nursing care is directed at providing information specific to any of the treatments listed above and to prepare the patient for home care and any further follow-up care that may be needed.

Acute Laryngeal Edema

Etiology and Epidemiology. Acute **laryngeal edema** is a medical emergency, not to be confused with laryngeal paralysis. Laryngeal edema may be caused by anaphylaxis, urticaria, acute laryngitis, serious inflammatory disease of the throat, or edema after intubation.

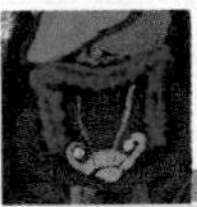

GUIDELINES FOR SAFE PRACTICE *Care of the Patient After Tonsillectomy*

- Position patient on side until fully awake after general anesthesia or in mid-Fowler's position when awake.
- Monitor for signs of hemorrhage: frequent swallowing (inspect throat), bright red vomitus, rapid pulse, restlessness.
- Promote comfort:
  —Give 30% cool mist via collar.
  —Apply ice collar to neck (will also reduce bleeding by vasoconstriction).
  —Use acetaminophen instead of aspirin.
- Give appropriate food and fluids.
  —Give ice-cold fluids and bland foods during initial period (e.g., ice chips, frozen juice bars, gelatin).
  —Milk is usually not given because it may increase mucus and cause patient to clear throat.
  —Advance to normal diet as soon as possible.
- Instruct patient to:
  —Avoid attempting to clear throat immediately after surgery (may initiate bleeding).
  —Avoid coughing, sneezing, vigorous nose blowing, and vigorous exercise for 1 to 2 weeks.
  —Drink lots of fluids (2 to 3 L/day) until mouth odor disappears.
  —Avoid hard, scratchy foods, such as pretzels, popcorn, or toast, until throat is healed.
  —Report signs of bleeding to physician immediately.
  —Expect more throat discomfort between the fourth and eighth postoperative days because of membrane separation.
  —Expect stool to be black or dark for a few days because of swallowed blood.
  —Resume normal activity immediately, as long as it is not stressful and does not require straining.

Pathophysiology. Acute laryngeal edema narrows or closes the airway, which must be immediately restored if life is to be maintained.

Collaborative Care Management. Treatment of acute laryngeal edema consists of administration of a corticosteroid or epinephrine and intubation or tracheostomy if necessary. Edema of the larynx caused by irradiation of the larynx or tumors of the neck may be chronic and may also require tracheostomy.

Nasal Deformities and Obstructions

Reconstruction of the Nose

Etiology and Epidemiology. The **nasal septum** is made up of cartilage and bone joined by a fibrous attachment. The septum separates the nose into two cavities, provides support, and acts as a shock absorber for the floor of the frontal fossa. Normally the septum of the nose is straight and thin. As a person ages, the septum tends to deviate to one side or the other, and an irregular projection may develop on it.

Deformities of the nose may be present from birth or develop as the result of trauma to the nose from sports injuries, automobile crashes, abnormal vasculature, nasal illicit drug use, and the like. Trauma can result in overgrowth of fibrous tissue that fills in the fracture and causes bowing of the septum. There can also be loss of nasal septal cartilage from trauma or infection, resulting in marked concavity, referred to as a saddle nose.

Although some deformities may seem minor to the casual observer, cosmetic appearance may be important to the person with an external nasal deformity. The patient's desire for a change in the size or shape of the nose may be unrelated to function and be for cosmetic reasons.

Pathophysiology. The primary effect of a deviated septum or nasal fracture is obstruction to breathing through the nose. A deviated septum may also alter the velocity with which air passes through the nose and hence can interfere with filtering, warming, and humidifying inspired air. As a result, the nasal mucosa becomes dry and crusty, nasal bleeding increases, and changes in the lining of the nose develop. Patients may also have trouble breathing through the nose or mouth, postnasal drip, nasal discharge, or loss of smell or taste.

Complications of nasal deformities are usually identified as physical or psychosocial. Physical complications prevent the normal exchange of air through the nasal pathway and can lead to chronic dryness and irritation of the nasal mucosa and decreased ability to breathe, especially at night when sleeping on the unaffected side. Psychosocial complications include alterations in body image, self-concept, and shyness, often to the point of social isolation, depending on the degree of deformity or the patient's perception of it.

Collaborative Care Management. The most common test used to confirm nasal fracture is x-ray examination. For cosmetic problems, high-tech tests, usually performed in the surgeon's office, allow the patient to examine several methods of repair and reconstruction and view what the repair might look like when completed.

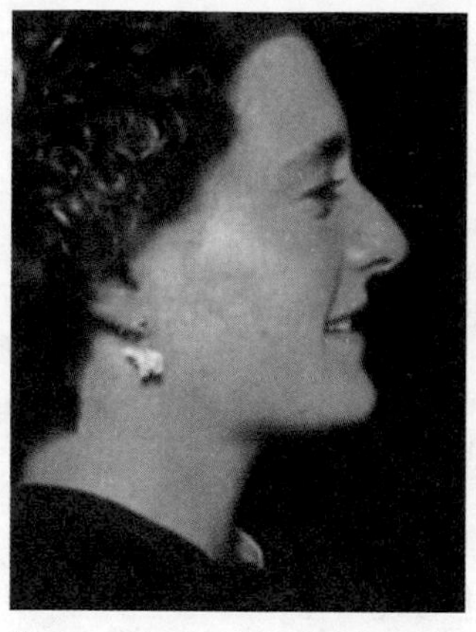

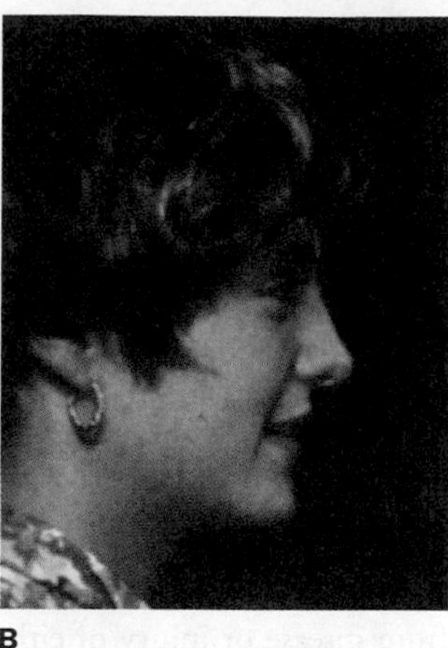

A B

Figure 25-9 Rhinoplasty. **A,** Preoperative lateral view. **B,** Postoperative lateral view.

Cosmetic surgery on the nose is referred to as rhinoplasty when the external nose is reconstructed and nasoseptoplasty when the septum is involved. Rhinoplasty and nasoseptoplasty are often combined, and most are done with the patient under local anesthesia. In a rhinoplasty, bone and cartilage may be removed from the nose if it is irregular, or they may be inserted if a defect such as a saddle nose is being corrected (Figure 25-9). The incision is usually made at the end of the nose inside the nostril so that it is not conspicuous.

To reconstruct the nasal septum, the surgeon makes an incision through the mucosa at the caudal end of the septal cartilage, elevates the septal mucous membranes, and separates the septal cartilage from its bony attachments and straightens it. The septal mucous membranes are then approximated to prevent bleeding.

The surgeon inserts nasal septal splints made of plastic or Silastic into the nose to prevent synechiae (a type of scar tissue) and to keep the septum in place. The nose may be packed for several days to prevent a hematoma from forming between the septal flaps and to support the septum. The patient is usually given antibiotics until the packing is removed. A surgeon removes the splints and nasal packing. Firm healing develops on about the tenth day. Ecchymosis and swelling are present around the eyes and nose for 10 to 14 days after surgery. It is several weeks before the final results of the surgery are evident.

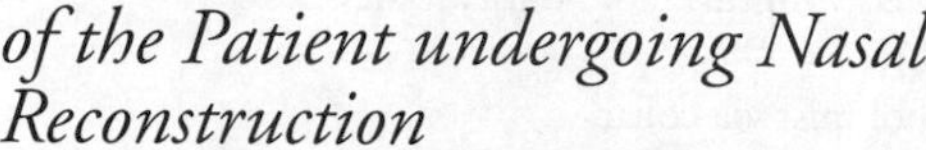

Nursing Management

of the Patient undergoing Nasal Reconstruction

PREOPERATIVE CARE

Preoperative care primarily focuses on facilitating open communication with the patient to ensure he or she understands the procedure and what it entails. It is important for the patient to be secure with the decision to have surgery and to possess a realistic expectation of the outcome. Depending on the extent of surgery needed, some surgeons prefer to revise the nose a little at a time to allow the patient to get used to the new look. Some changes are subtle and take a while to be noticed, but some changes are evident immediately. Subtle changes can sometimes turn to overt changes as a result of scar tissue or keloids in the nasal cavity. Sometimes patients return to the clinic for several steroid injections to minimize scarring.

POSTOPERATIVE CARE

After surgery the nurse places the patient in mid-Fowler's position to decrease local edema and administers a cool mist via a collar or face tent. Iced compresses are usually applied to the nose to reduce discoloration, bleeding, and discomfort and to hasten fluid resorption from the surgical site. Patients can usually apply their own iced compresses.

The nurse monitors the patient for signs of hemorrhage (see the Guidelines for Safe Practice box). Some oozing on the dressing below the nose is expected, and this dressing may be changed as necessary (see Figure 25-8). If bleeding becomes pronounced, the nurse notifies the surgeon and prepares equipment for repacking the nose. This equipment consists of a hemostat tray containing gauze packing, umbilical tape for posterior packing, a few small gauze sponges, a small catheter (for inserting a postnasal plug), packing forceps, tongue blades, and scissors. The surgeon may require a head mirror, good light, epinephrine 1:1000 or other vasoconstrictor, 4% topical lidocaine (Xylocaine) or 4% cocaine solution, applicators, a nasal speculum, and suction.

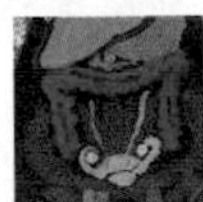

GUIDELINES FOR SAFE PRACTICE
Care of the Patient After Nasal Surgery

- Assess for signs of hemorrhage: excessive blood on nasal dressing, bright red vomitus, repeated swallowing (check back of throat with penlight for blood running down throat), rapid pulse, restlessness.
- Assess for signs of infection: fever, elevated white blood cell count.
- Take measures to relieve discomfort and promote effective breathing:
  —Place patient in mid-Fowler's position to decrease local edema.
  —Provide cool mist via collar or face tent.
  —Apply ice compresses over nose for 24 hours as needed.
  —Provide psychologic support and sedation as needed.
  —Use flashlight or penlight to examine back of throat to ensure packing has not slipped to back of throat, where it could gag patient.
  —Provide frequent oral care.
  —Change dressing under nose as needed (see Figure 25-8).
- Promote good nutrition:
  —Encourage food as tolerated.
  —Encourage increased fluid intake.
- Instruct patient to:
  —Avoid blowing nose for 48 hours after packing has been removed.
  —Avoid constipation and straining (Valsalva's maneuver) and vigorous coughing until healing occurs, since it can cause bleeding.
  —Expect stools to be tarry for several days.
  —Expect face to be discolored around eyes and nose for several days. (Cosmetic effect from nasal surgery cannot be judged for 6 to 12 months, when the tissue has returned to normal and scarring has resolved.)

Because packing blocks the passage of air through the nose, the patient creates a partial vacuum during swallowing and may complain of a sucking action when attempting to drink. Postnasal drainage, old blood in the mouth, dryness of the mouth from mouth breathing, and loss of the ability to smell often lead to anorexia. Frequent mouth care is important.

If the patient received intravenous anesthesia, clear liquids are recommended until nausea subsides. Progression to a regular diet can then be implemented. Activity is limited for a minimum of 7 to 10 days to prevent injury. Postoperative care, including patient/family teaching, is summarized in the Guidelines for Safe Practice box.

GERONTOLOGIC CONSIDERATIONS

Most nasal reconstructive procedures performed on older patients are required because of disease or trauma; few are simply cosmetic. This means that most older patients not only have age-related factors that increase the challenge of perioperative management but also have a significant recent problem that has precipitated the need for surgery.

Hypertrophied Turbinates

Etiology and Epidemiology. Longstanding allergic rhinitis and low-grade inflammation may cause permanent enlargement of the turbinates, especially the inferior turbinate.

Pathophysiology. The turbinates lose most of their normal ability to expand and shrink. This results in continuous nasal obstruction (Figure 25-10).

Collaborative Care Management. Hypertrophied turbinates may be medically treated with aerosols containing corticosteroids such as beclomethasone dipropionate (Beconase, Vancenase) or dexamethasone (Decadron, Turbinaire). These aerosols are used for their antiinflammatory effect.

Although not as common since the advent of corticosteroid aerosols, laser surgery may still be used to restore the airway by debulking (resection) of the hypertrophied mucosa of the turbinates. The care and teaching of the patient are the same as those for patients undergoing nasal surgery. The nurse explains the problem and potential treatment options to the patient and family. If surgery is necessary, the nurse instructs the patient before and after surgery about the procedure and care needs, as outlined in the Guidelines for Safe Practice box for nasal surgery.

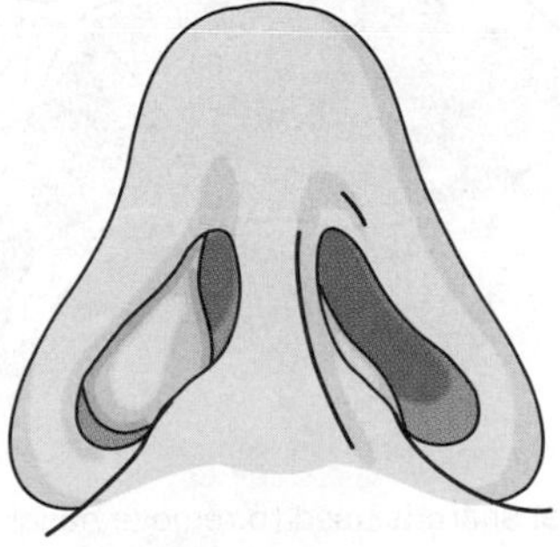

Figure 25-10 Hypertrophic turbinate.

Nasal Polyps

Etiology and Epidemiology. Nasal polyps are grapelike growths of the sinus mucosa that project into the cavities of the nose and paranasal sinuses. The exact cause of nasal polyposis is unknown, but some believe it is related to the inflammatory response. Supporting this theory is the fact that persons with chronic viral or bacterial infections have a higher incidence of nasal polyps. Nasal polyps are common and affect men twice as often as women. They are typically associated with allergies, cystic fibrosis, asthma, disorders of ciliary motility, chronic rhinitis, and chronic sinusitis.

Pathophysiology. Some patients with nasal polyps also have symptoms of asthma and intolerance to aspirin, indomethacin, and other nonsteroidal antiinflammatory drugs (NSAIDs). The cause of the triad of nasal polyps, asthma, and aspirin sensitivity is unknown, but the patient may have an acute asthmatic attack in response to infection, anesthesia, surgery, or the administration of aspirin, all of which could be considered stressors for the hyperresponsive airway of the person with asthma.

Collaborative Care Management. Nasal polyps can be treated with corticosteroid sprays or by local injection of a steroid into the polyp. Steroid sprays are used for long-term reduction of polyp size, for prevention of recurrence, and for reduction of the inflammatory response, thus reducing swelling. Antibiotics such as amoxicillin or erythromycin are prescribed when infection is present. Persistent polyps may require nasal polypectomy (Figure 25-11) or removal of polyps via a Caldwell-Luc operation, in which the maxillary sinus is entered. The nurse's major role is in patient teaching (see Patient/Family Teaching box).

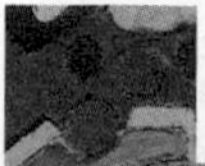

PATIENT/FAMILY TEACHING
The Patient With Nasal Polyps

- Elevate the head of the bed to decrease nasal edema and improve breathing through the nose.
- Increase humidity to thin secretions and reduce dryness of the nose. Use a central humidifier on the furnace or use a room humidifier. Increase fluid intake and use a saline nasal spray.
- Prevent respiratory infections by avoiding persons with upper respiratory tract infections and avoiding crowds. Notify the physician at the first sign of infection so that appropriate therapy can be started.
- Take medications as ordered. Be aware of side effects such as drowsiness if antihistamines are prescribed.
- Seek prompt medical attention if there are signs of recurrence of polyps.

Sleep Apnea

Etiology and Epidemiology. The Greek word *apnea* literally means "without breath." There are three types of **apnea**: obstructive, central, and mixed; of the three, obstructive is the most common. People with any type of untreated sleep apnea stop breathing repeatedly during their sleep, sometimes hundreds of times during the night and often for a minute or longer.

Sleep apnea is as common as adult diabetes, affecting more than 12 million Americans, according to the National Institutes of Health.[4] Risk factors include being male, overweight, and over the age of 40, but sleep apnea can strike anyone at any age, even children. Nonetheless, because of the lack of awareness by the public and health care professionals, the vast majority of cases remain undiagnosed and therefore untreated, despite the disorder's significant consequences.

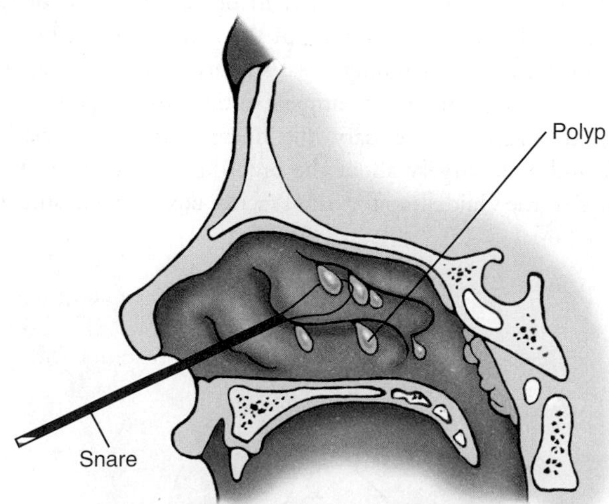

Figure 25-11 Nasal snare is used to remove nasal polyps. After nose is anesthetized, nasal snare is slipped around polyp, which is transected and removed with forceps.

Pathophysiology. Obstructive sleep apnea (OSA) is caused by a blockage of the airway, usually when the soft tissue in the rear of the throat collapses and closes during sleep. In central sleep apnea the airway is not blocked, but the brain fails to signal the muscles to breathe. Mixed apnea is a combination of the two. With each apnea event, the brain briefly arouses people so they can resume breathing; consequently sleep is extremely fragmented and of poor quality. Untreated, sleep apnea can cause high blood pressure and other cardiovascular disease, memory problems, weight gain, impotency, and headaches. Moreover, untreated sleep apnea may be responsible for job impairment and motor vehicle crashes.[3]

The most common signs of sleep apnea include (1) loud snoring, (2) choking or gasping during sleep, and (3) the need to fight sleepiness during the day, even while driving or at work.

Collaborative Care Management. Care begins with teaching patients the three basic steps that help many people with sleep apnea sleep better: (1) stop using alcohol or sleep medicines, since these relax the muscles in the back of the throat and make it harder to breathe; (2) if overweight, attempt to lose as much weight as possible; and (3) assume a lateral position for sleep instead of supine.

If the problem still persists, the patient care can wear a continuous positive airway pressure (CPAP) mask over the nose and mouth while sleeping. The mask keeps the airway open by adding pressure to the air being inhaled. The mask helps most people with sleep apnea, but sometimes surgery is necessary to remove tonsils or extra tissue from the throat. Patients should understand that if they lose weight or alter sleep habits, the sleep apnea may improve without additional medical or surgical management.

▶ ARE You READY?

Which of the following statements by the patient with sleep apnea indicates the need for further teaching?

1. "I try to lie on my side when I am sleeping."
2. "If I lose some weight, this disorder may get better."
3. "I have stopped taking sleeping pills at night."
4. "I drink 2 glasses of wine at night to help me to sleep."

Trauma to Upper Airway

Fractures of Nasal Bones and Septum

Fractures of the nasal bones and septum commonly occur from relatively minor injuries, such as falls, or from more severe injuries, such as automobile accidents or fights. If there is no displacement of the bone, no obstruction to the airway, and no cosmetic deformity, treatment is not needed. When airway obstruction or bone displacement occurs, a physician performs a simple reduction of the fracture. Most simple nasal fractures can be reduced by applying firm pressure on the convex side of the nose. Nasal fractures should be reduced within the first 24 hours if possible. Local anesthesia is often used. After 24 hours the reduction becomes more difficult and may require general anesthesia.

Fractures of Maxillary and Zygomatic Bones

Fractures of the maxillary and zygomatic bones are often seen after automobile accidents, fights, or severe falls in sporting events. These fractures are generally reduced with the patient under anesthesia. Patients may also require wiring of the teeth, with all the attendant problems of that procedure.

Epistaxis

Etiology and Epidemiology. **Epistaxis** (nosebleed) usually originates from the tiny blood vessels in the anterior part of the septum. Bleeding from the posterior part is more common in older adults and is more likely to be severe. Nosebleeds are more common in men than in women.

The most common cause of epistaxis is trauma to the nasal mucosa from damage by a foreign object. Other causes include picking the nose, local irritation of the mucous membrane from lack of humidity in the air, chronic infection, violent sneezing, or blowing the nose. Systemic causes include coagulation defects, such as hemophilia, leukemia, and purpura.

Pathophysiology. Although persons with hypertension do not have more nosebleeds than do normotensive persons, they tend to bleed more profusely when they do have a nosebleed. Nosebleed is usually unilateral, and some persons are more prone to nosebleed than are others. Persons with frequent nosebleeds should have a complete physical examination to determine the cause.

Collaborative Care Management. Most nosebleeds can be controlled with simple measures (see Guidelines for Safe Practice box). If these measures are ineffective, medical intervention is necessary. After identifying the site of the bleeding, the physician cauterizes the bleeding point with a silver nitrate stick or electrocautery. If the bleeding point cannot be seen, a postnasal pack may be inserted (Figure 25-12). Patients are admitted to the hospital because this procedure is extremely painful and may cause complications. For example, the pressure of the postnasal pack may stimulate the sinopulmonary reflex, causing the patient to stop breathing. In this situation the pack must be removed immediately. If no problems occur, the pack is left in place for 48 to 72 hours and then gently removed. Management includes adequate oxygenation, humidification, analgesia, bed rest, blood transfusions, intravenous fluids, systemic antibiotics, and sedation. If the posterior pack fails to control the bleeding, another pack may be placed and the patient taken to surgery for ligation of the internal maxillary artery or to the radiology department for embolization of the bleeding vessels.

Severe epistaxis causes apprehension because of the profuse bleeding from the nose and into the throat. The person is kept in mid-Fowler's position and is urged not to swallow blood, since doing so may cause nausea and vomiting. The nurse frequently checks the position of the postnasal pack by viewing the posterior oropharynx for bleeding or slippage. Nasal packs may slip out of place and cause airway obstruction. The nurse monitors the patient for complications (confusion, agitation, increased lethargy, and changes in vital signs, especially in respirations and pulse). Nasal packs also make eating and swallowing difficult; a liquid diet is usually better tolerated.

Patient education for epistaxis focuses on the proper treatment of nosebleeds and recognition of when medical care is needed. The proper method for stopping nosebleeds is presented in the Guidelines for Safe Practice box.

Malignancies of Upper Airway: Overview

Malignancies involving the upper airway can occur in several sites, including (1) the lip and oral cavity; (2) the pharynx: nasopharynx, oropharynx, and laryngopharynx; (3) the larynx;

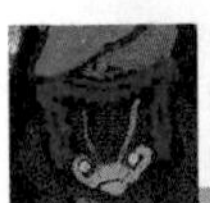

GUIDELINES FOR SAFE PRACTICE

Initial Care of the Patient With Epistaxis

- Have patient sit up, leaning forward with head tipped downward to prevent swallowing or aspiration of blood.
- Use fingers to compress soft tissues of nose against septum and maintain pressure for at least 5 minutes.
- Apply ice or cold compress to nose to constrict blood vessels.
- If bleeding does not stop with direct pressure, place a cotton ball soaked in a topical vasoconstrictor (e.g., phenylephrine [Neo-Synephrine]) into nose and apply pressure.
- Instruct patient not to blow nose for several hours after a nosebleed.
- Notify physician.

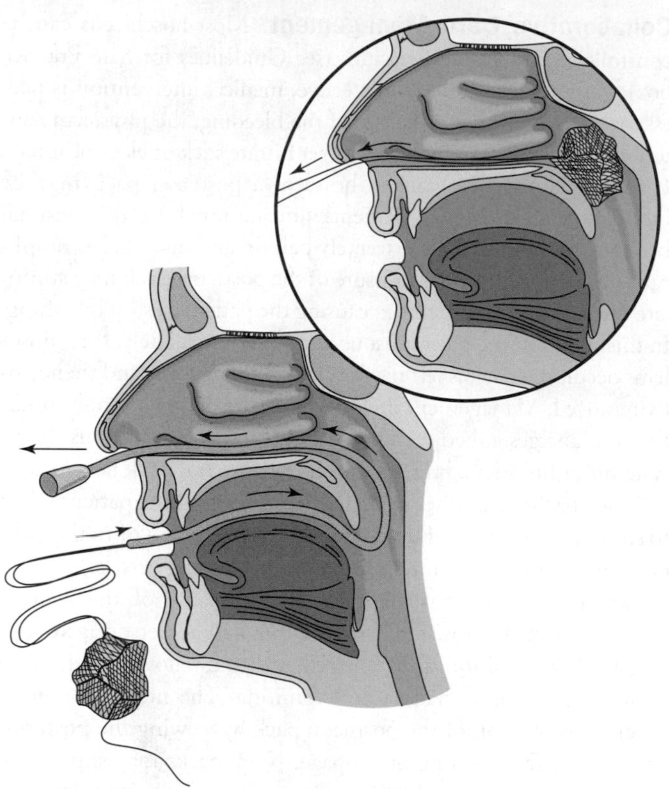

Figure 25-12 Postnasal packing. A pack is attached to catheter and then pulled through mouth to posterior aspect of nasopharynx.

(4) the paranasal sinuses; (5) the salivary gland; and (6) the thyroid gland.

Ninety percent of cancers of the head and neck are squamous cell carcinoma, which can metastasize to regional lymph nodes. Metastasis is most common in those areas with rich lymphatic supply, such as the floor of the mouth, tongue, pharyngeal wall, nasopharynx, and supraglottic larynx. There is little correlation between cervical lymph node metastases and the size of the primary lesion; even small lesions may have regional metastases. The lung is the most common site of distant metastasis. Metastases to the liver and skeleton are less common, and metastasis to the brain is rare.

The diagnosis is confirmed by biopsy, CT scan, and MRI. The CT scan is used to differentiate between benign and malignant lesions, determine tumor extension, and identify the presence of bony destruction. The MRI scan with gadolinium enhances tumor imaging in soft tissues and shows tumor extension and tumor secretions. The radiolucency of the tumor and its secretions are different, which is why both can be identified on MRI with gadolinium.

Treatment of squamous cell carcinomas of the head and neck depends on the size of the primary tumor and the presence of nodal metastasis. The usual system for staging head and neck cancer is the TNM (tumor, node, metastasis) system. This is an anatomic staging system that describes the extent of the primary tumor and the involvement of regional lymph nodes and/or distant metastasis (Box 25-2).

Persons with stage I or II cancer of the head and neck can be treated with either primary radiotherapy or surgical intervention with equal success. Radiotherapy is given either preoperatively or postoperatively, depending on the experience and wishes of the surgeon. Chemotherapy may also be used, but it is considered experimental at this time. A chemotherapeutic regimen used alone or as an adjuvant to radiotherapy and resection for squamous cell carcinoma of the head and neck has yet to be standardized.[1] Persons with stage III or IV disease are automatically placed in the advanced-stage category requiring a combination of radiotherapy, surgery, and chemotherapy.

Box 25-2 TNM System for Staging of Head and Neck Cancer

Stage I	T_1, N_0, M_0
Stage II	T_2, N_0, M_0
Stage III	T_3, N_0, M_0; T_1, T_2, or T_3, N_1, M_0
Stage IV	T_4, N_0 or N_1, M_0 Any T, N_2 or N_3, M_0 Any T, any N, M_1

T, Primary tumor extent or size; *N,* regional lymph node involvement (number, size, and location); *M,* presence or absence of distant metastases.

When cervical lymph node metastases are identified at the time of surgery, a neck dissection is performed. In the past a radical neck dissection involved removal of all affected nodes, lymphatic tissues with the submandibular gland, the sternocleidomastoid muscle, the internal jugular vein, and the spinal accessory nerve. Advances in surgical techniques have led to modified neck dissection, in which an attempt is made to preserve the sternocleidomastoid muscle, internal jugular vein, various chains or sections of lymph nodes, and spinal nerves by themselves or in combination. As previously stated, patients have radiation treatments before or after neck dissection, depending on surgeon preference, the condition of the patient, and the site of the tumor.

Persons at high risk for upper airway cancers are those who work in high-risk areas where toxic fumes are present, including secondhand smoke; those who consume alcohol; those with a family history of these cancers; and those 50 years of age and older. Referral to an ear, nose, and throat (ENT) specialist for further evaluation is necessary for anyone who meets high-risk criteria or questions the character of a noted lesion or node.

Carcinoma of Nasal Cavity and Paranasal Sinuses

Etiology and Epidemiology. Carcinoma of the nasal cavity has its highest incidence in men between 60 and 70 years of age. Exposure to certain substances has been implicated in some malignancies of the nasal cavity. These substances include wood dust and leather dust (inhaled by furniture workers), nickel compounds, chromate compounds, hydrocarbons, nitrosamines, and dioxane. The risk is higher among those who dip snuff, work in the shoe industry, or are textile and asbestos workers. However, the majority of persons have no history of exposure to high-risk substances.

Pathophysiology. Most patients with cancer of the nasal cavity or paranasal sinuses have signs and symptoms of a longstanding chronic sinusitis. Common complaints include a stuffy nose, sinus headache, and facial pain (see the Clinical Manifestations box).

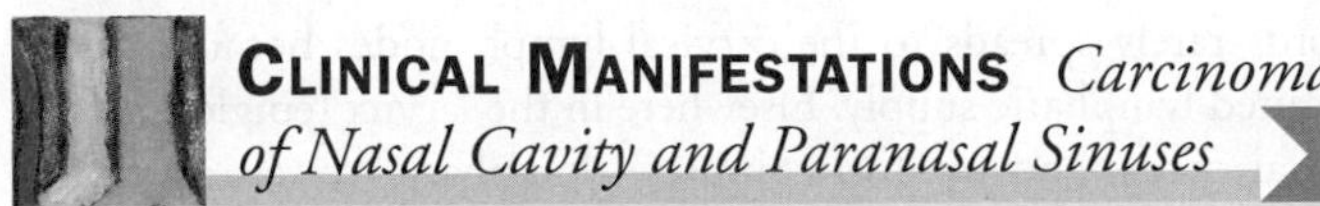

CLINICAL MANIFESTATIONS *Carcinoma of Nasal Cavity and Paranasal Sinuses*

Maxillary Sinus

The patient may have a bump on the hard palate. Nasal obstruction and bleeding occur as the tumor breaks into the nasal cavity. Swelling of the cheek occurs with pain. Swelling of the gums may cause toothache or result in ill-fitting dentures. If the tumor impinges on the infraorbital nerve, the patient may have numbness of the cheek, increased lacrimation, exophthalmos, and double vision (diplopia). More advanced tumors may result in displacement of the eye, extraocular muscle palsy, hyperesthesia of the cheek, and inability to open the mouth.

Frontal Sinus

Patients commonly have swelling and frontal pain that mimics a sinus headache. Pain occurs when the tumor invades bone and causes bony destruction. If the tumor invades the ethmoids and orbit, the eye on that side will be displaced, resulting in diplopia.

Sphenoid Sinus

A major complaint is steady, deep-seated temporoparietal headaches. Because of its close proximity to the cavernous sinus, a tumor extending into this area compresses the third, fourth, and sixth cranial nerves, causing diplopia.

Ethmoid Sinus

These tumors cause medial orbital swelling, puffiness of the face, decreased vision, excessive tearing (epiphora), and olfactory complaints. Death is caused by direct extension of the tumor into the vital areas of the skull.

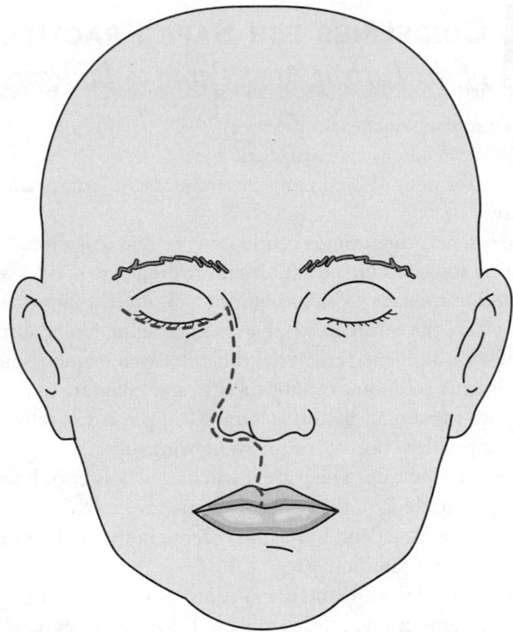

Figure 25-13 Weber-Fergusson incision for maxillectomy.

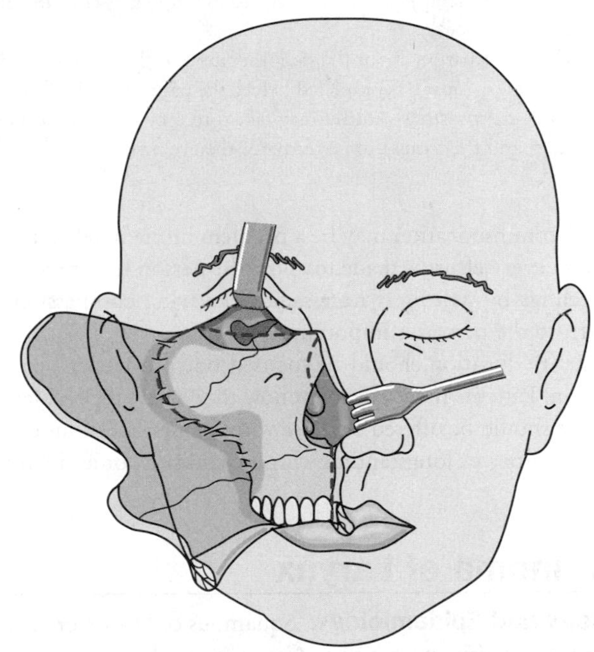

Figure 25-14 Demonstration of exposure and block removal of maxilla with eye preservation. If tumor extends through floor of orbit, the eye must be removed with the maxilla.

Collaborative Care Management. Treatment consists of radiotherapy followed by complete surgical excision of the maxilla. This combination eradicates the tumor more effectively than either radiation or surgery alone. Some surgeons prefer that radiation be given 8 to 10 weeks before surgery; other surgeons prefer surgery followed by radiotherapy. Chemotherapy used in conjunction with surgical intervention and radiation may improve long-term survival.

Surgery for maxillary sinus and palate tumors consists of removal of the entire jaw (maxillectomy), removal of the entire palate (hard and soft), and, when necessary, removal of one eye (orbital exenteration) (Figures 25-13 and 25-14). Split-thickness skin grafts are usually applied to the oral defect remaining after surgery. After healing, a dental prosthesis replaces the hard palate and floor of the nose. The patient then has nearly normal speech, swallowing, and appearance. Early diagnosis and treatment greatly affects the surgical outcome.

Radical surgery is required because of the danger of recurrence. Meningitis is a potential postoperative complication, and prophylactic antibiotics are usually prescribed. Maintenance of an airway postoperatively is critical for these patients, and sometimes a tracheostomy is performed. A nasogastric tube is inserted to ensure adequate liquid and caloric intake, since eating is difficult until the prosthesis is fitted. Several different prostheses are usually needed before a final one fits, since the cavity shrinks as healing progresses. Often they need to be readjusted and sized weekly.

The Guidelines for Safe Practice box summaries postoperative care. Persons who undergo radical surgery of this type have a number of emotional adjustments to make. With their physical appearance visibly altered, the person feels conspicuous and different. In addition to disfigurement, these patients have all the normal fears associated with surgery and cancer, including concerns about the future, the ability to live normally, and rejection. Anger and grief are common responses to the loss and the helplessness to control it.

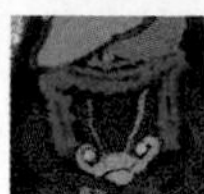

Guidelines for Safe Practice *Care of the Patient After Paranasal Surgery*

- Provide routine tracheostomy care.
- Administer feedings via nasogastric tube.
- Monitor for signs of meningitis: fever, headache, stiff neck, neck rigidity.
- Provide mouth care using a gentle spray or oral irrigation. Oral irrigating solutions include saline and hydrogen peroxide, weak sodium bicarbonate, or an antibiotic solution. It is important to know where the suture line is to avoid damaging it when irrigating the mouth. If the patient has difficulty swallowing, aspirate the irrigating solution from the mouth, and take care to prevent trauma to the sutures by the suction. Management of saliva may also be a problem because of the swallowing difficulty.
- Provide dressing care. The patient will have a bolster or bolus dressing or packing in the maxillary sinus cavity. Observe packing to ensure it is intact and not hanging loose in the back of the throat, where it can cause gagging.
- Assess the fit of the prosthesis and adjust as necessary. If the prosthesis creates pressure, it leads to pain. If eating causes nasal regurgitation, the prosthesis may need adjustment.
- Provide information on long-term follow-up care after discharge. A nurse sees the patient weekly for at least 6 weeks. If the patient receives radiotherapy postoperatively, follow-up visits continue for several more weeks.
- Provide information about the radiotherapy and the eye prosthesis. Radiotherapy must be completed before the patient can be fitted for an ocular prosthesis, and it may take 4 to 6 months for healing to occur and the patient to be ready for the eye prosthesis.

Oral communication may be a problem immediately after surgery, and every effort is made to allow the person to express needs and feelings by writing if necessary. Conveying compassion and concern to the person is important.[1]

Patient education should be focused on "prevention" or early detection. Patients must be taught how to identify the risk factors. Referrals should be offered to those with further questions or concerns, a history of longstanding chronic sinusitis, or an identified lesion.

Carcinoma of Larynx

Etiology and Epidemiology. Squamous cell carcinoma of the larynx is increasing in frequency. Cancer of the larynx is five times more common in men than in women, and it occurs most often in persons over 60 years of age. People who smoke or use other tobacco products are at risk of developing tumors of the larynx. Cancer of the larynx appears to be related to heavy smoking, heavy alcohol intake, chronic laryngitis, vocal abuse, and family predisposition to cancer. Because of the increase in the number of women who are heavy smokers, the incidence of carcinoma of the larynx among this group is increasing. Smoking and excessive alcohol use together constitutes a high risk for the development of laryngeal cancer.

Pathophysiology. Squamous cell carcinoma can arise from any part of the laryngeal mucous membrane. It is often preceded by leukoplakia. Cancer of the larynx limited to the true vocal cords rarely spreads to the cervical lymph nodes because of the limited lymphatic supply. Elsewhere in the larynx (epiglottis, false vocal cords, and pyriform sinuses), lymphatic vessels are abundant, and cancer of these tissues often spreads rapidly and metastasizes early to the deep lymph nodes of the neck. Tumors of the supraglottic and infraglottic portions of the larynx have a 35% to 40% incidence of metastasis to mid to low jugular nodes.[1]

The most common presenting symptom of laryngeal cancer is persistent hoarseness, often associated with otalgia and dysphagia. Anyone, but especially any smoker, who becomes progressively hoarse or is hoarse for longer than 2 weeks should be urged to seek medical attention at once. If treatment is given when hoarseness first appears (caused by the tumor's preventing the complete approximation of the vocal cord), a cure usually is possible. Signs of metastases of cancer to other parts of the larynx include a sensation of a lump in the throat, pain in the Adam's apple that radiates to the ear, dyspnea, dysphagia, enlarged cervical nodes, and cough.

Collaborative Care Management

Diagnostic Tests. Tests used in the diagnosis of laryngeal cancers are found in Table 25-5.

Medications. After laryngoscopy, only pain medications are usually prescribed. Preadmission medications such as digitalis preparations or diuretics are continued.

Diet. Tube feedings progressing to a soft diet are given postoperatively. Protein is encouraged for wound healing. Certain types of laryngeal surgery can cause specific dietary problems, so the specifics of dietary management for each surgery are discussed in the following pages.

Treatments. The primary therapy is surgical excision or radiotherapy. Patients with early-stage lesions (T_1 or T_2) that are localized to the glottis have an 85% to 90% cure rate when treated with either of these procedures. Surgery is either an endoscopic laser excision or partial **laryngectomy** (Table 25-6).

Table 25-5 Diagnostic Tests for Laryngeal Cancer

Test	Purpose
Barium swallow	To rule out metastasis to esophagus
Biopsy	For pathologic confirmation of diagnosis
Chest x-ray examination	To determine whether there is metastasis to lung, a second primary tumor, or chronic obstructive pulmonary disease
Computed tomography scan	To determine if there is metastasis to lymph nodes or adjacent structures
Direct and indirect fiberoptic laryngoscopy	To determine diagnosis; locate mass or ulceration

TABLE 25-6 LARYNGECTOMY SURGERY FOR CANCER

Type	Description	Voice Result	Swallowing Ability
Partial laryngectomy			
Hemilaryngectomy	Opening into larynx through thyroid cartilage with removal of diseased false cord, arytenoid, and one side thyroid cartilage	Hoarse voice	Initially need swallowing therapy to learn how to swallow without aspirating
Supraglottic partial laryngectomy	Horizontal incision passes above true cords (leaving cords intact) with removal of epiglottis and diseased tissue	Normal voice	Same as above
Total laryngectomy	Removal of epiglottis, thyroid cartilage, and 3-4 tracheal rings; closure of pharynx with trachea; permanent tracheostomy	No voice	No swallowing problem

Patients with more extensive tumors (T_3 or T_4) require a combined approach of surgical resection and preoperative or postoperative radiotherapy. Newer treatment regimens add chemotherapy with cisplatin and 5-fluorouracil along with radiotherapy in an attempt to preserve the larynx. Chemotherapy alone is never curative in these cancers.

If these therapies fail, if the tumor recurs, or the tumors are extensive with cartilaginous invasion, a total laryngectomy is required. Some patients also require a modified neck dissection. Complications related to the surgical wound include hematoma, wound dehiscence, tissue loss, pharyngocutaneous fistula, and carotid artery rupture. Complications of myocutaneous and free flaps include venous or arterial congestion, flap necrosis, and slough.

SURGICAL MANAGEMENT

HEMILARYNGECTOMY. In hemilaryngectomy, or vertical partial laryngectomy, half the larynx is removed (Figure 25-15). This procedure is usually well tolerated. The patient is not allowed to swallow for 7 to 10 days postoperatively, but difficulty in swallowing is not a long-term problem. The quality of the voice is adequate for communication.

Removal of more than half the larynx or a portion of the second vocal cord is called a *subtotal laryngectomy*. Removal of more of the second cord causes more difficulty in swallowing. Thin liquids are the most difficult to swallow, and thickened liquids and soft foods are recommended. Speech pathologists are often consulted to assist patients with swallowing technique.

SUPRAGLOTTIC LARYNGECTOMY. When cancer invades the supraglottis, a supraglottic laryngectomy (horizontal partial laryngectomy) is performed (Figure 25-16). Because the true vocal cords are preserved, the patient's voice quality is excellent. The major postoperative problem is the danger of aspiration because of difficulty swallowing. Aspiration may occur because the major reflex arc that causes closure of the larynx is initiated by sensory receptors in the supraglottic larynx, which has been removed. These patients need special swallowing training postoperatively. Patients take variable amounts of time to learn to swallow safely, and it may be 2 to 3 weeks or longer before oral feedings are started. When aspiration is suspected, the patient swallows a drink with methylene blue dye, grape juice, or food coloring added, and the nurse checks the color in tracheal secretions.

After a partial laryngectomy a temporary **tracheostomy tube** is inserted. It is removed when edema in the surrounding tissues subsides. The person is not on absolute voice rest but is advised not to use the voice until the surgeon gives specific approval (usually 3 days after surgery). In the past, whispering was allowed, but it is now believed that whispering can further damage the voice. The person usually adjusts readily to the relatively minor limitations of speech.[1]

TOTAL LARYNGECTOMY. When cancer of the larynx is advanced, a total laryngectomy may be performed. This includes removal of the epiglottis, thyroid cartilage (larynx), hyoid bone, cricoid cartilage, and three or four rings of the trachea. The pharyngeal opening to the trachea is closed, and the remainder of the trachea is brought out to the neck wound and sutured to the skin to form a permanent tracheostomy through which the patient breathes (Figure 25-17). The patient loses the sense of smell because breathing through the nose is impossible. Initially the person has a runny nose because sniffing in and out is not possible. The person has no voice because of loss of the larynx. Nursing care of the patient after a total laryngectomy is outlined in the Guidelines for Safe Practice box, p. 610.

RADICAL NECK DISSECTION. A radical neck dissection may be performed along with the laryngectomy when risk of metastasis to the neck is high (i.e., when the size and location of the primary tumor are known to result in metastasis or when palpable cervical lymph nodes are found during surgery). In a radical neck dissection the surgeon removes the submandibular salivary gland, sternocleidomastoid muscle, internal jugular vein, and spinal accessory nerves. This extensive surgery is done to ensure complete removal of node-bearing tissue or to prevent nodal spread. In some patients modifications of a radical neck dissection are performed. These are referred to as selective, modified, conservative, or functional neck dissections and are used when the nodal metastatic disease is not far advanced. Radical neck dissection causes atrophy of the trapezius muscle, and the shoulder droops on the side of surgery.

The physical therapist or nurse can assist patients with range-of-motion exercises, which will gradually replace the function of

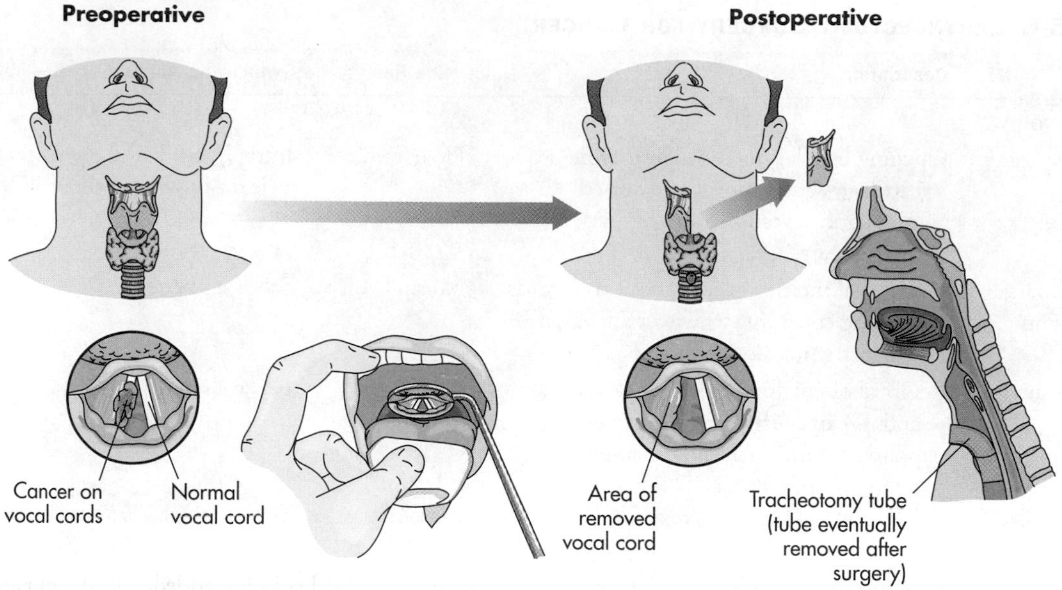

Figure 25-15 Technique of hemilaryngectomy (vertical partial laryngectomy).

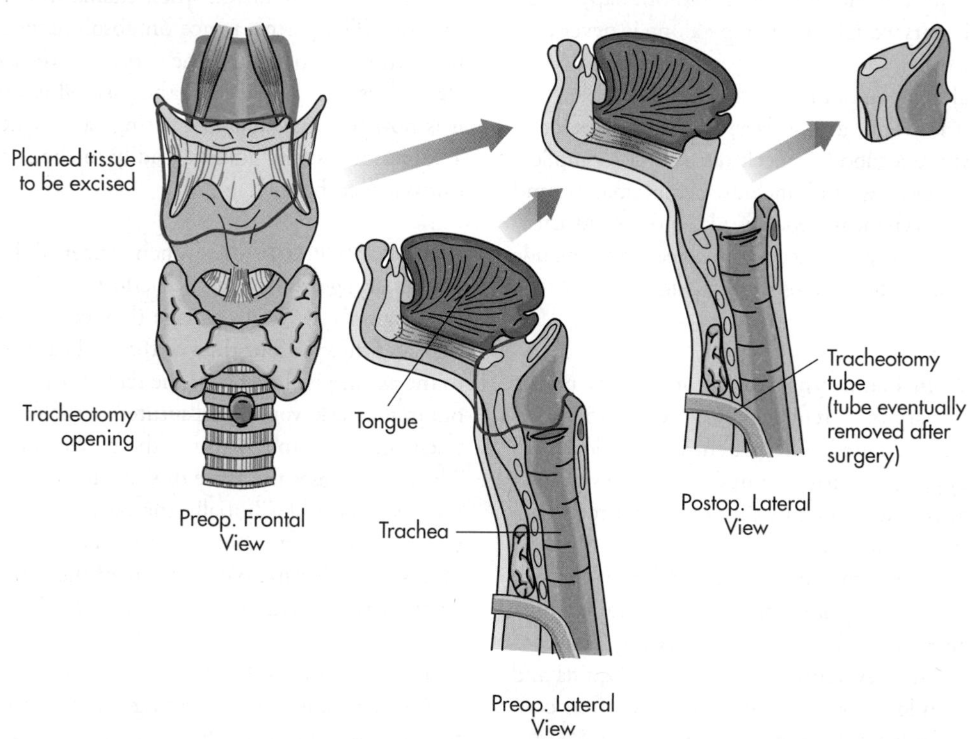

Figure 25-16 Technique of supraglottic laryngectomy (horizontal partial laryngectomy).

the lost muscles with that of other muscles. Initially the patient may have some difficulty lifting the head and must place the hands with fingers interlocked behind the head to lift it from the pillow.

The patient can breathe best in a mid-Fowler's position. This position helps reduce facial edema, improve circulation, and reduce or prevent headaches from lymphedema. Pressure dressings are not recommended in radical neck dissection, since they compromise the blood supply to the skin flaps protecting the vital neck structures.

Often a Hemovac (Figure 25-18) or another suction device is attached to drains placed in the incision in the operating room. Its purpose is to maintain constant drainage from the neck wound and prevent pressure on the skin flaps.

Radical neck dissection can be performed without laryngectomy for persons whose primary malignant lesion is in the oral cavity, oropharynx, or parasinuses. Often the procedure accompanies other procedures and is referred to as a composite resection. Composite resections may consist of radical neck dissection plus removal of the mandible; removal of the mandible with resection

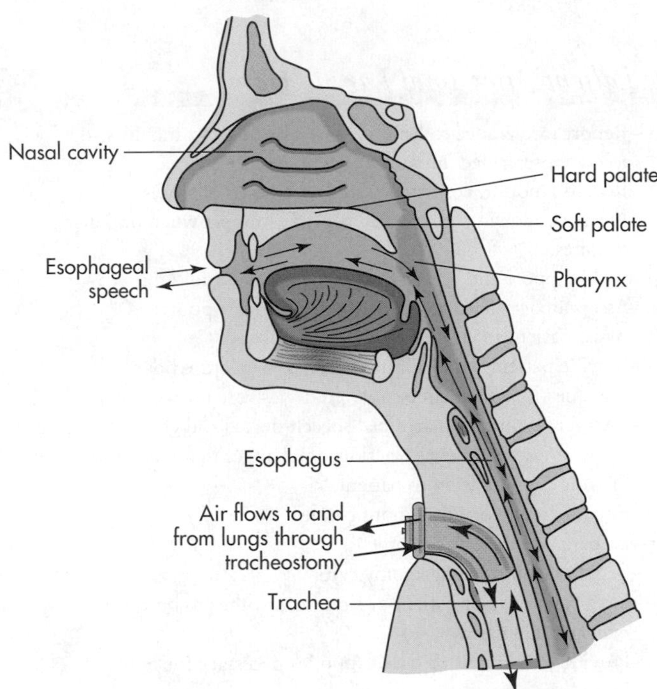

Figure 25-17 Permanent tracheostomy: no connections exist between trachea and esophagus.

of the floor of the mouth; or removal of the mandible, the floor of the mouth, and the tongue. Patients who undergo a composite resection usually have a tracheostomy.

Emotional reactions to this type of radical surgery may be profound, since disfigurement is readily visible. In addition to the usual fears of surgery and cancer, the patient having a composite resection may have fears of rejection and fears concerning the future. Nursing care for patients after a radical neck dissection is outlined in the Guidelines for Safe Practice box, p. 611.

RECONSTRUCTIVE SURGERY. Because of the extensive surgery required to treat malignancies of the head and neck, reconstructive surgery has become common practice. In the past, skin grafts and pedicle or rotation skin flaps were used for reconstruction. Today myocutaneous flaps and free flaps are most commonly used to reconstruct large deficits caused by extensive tumor resection and traumatic defects of the head and neck.

Myocutaneous Flaps. Myocutaneous flaps use the axial blood supply that supplies muscle mass, as well as cutaneous and subcutaneous tissue. The inclusion of muscle with its blood supply when transferring the skin allows for a much greater range of rotation of the flap. The pectoralis major, latissimus dorsi, trapezius, and sternocleidomastoid muscles can be used for myocutaneous flaps.

Free Flaps. Free flaps consist of harvested tissue separated from the donor site with the vein and artery. The vein and artery are anastomosed to recipient vessels close to the defect (microvascular anastomosis). It is also possible to harvest flaps containing soft tissue and bone to reconstruct the mandible after mandibulectomy.

To prevent clot formation in the recipient graft, the hematocrit is kept below 30% and sometimes as low as 25% before blood replacement is considered. Some surgeons order low-dose aspirin or even heparin to prevent clot formation. Persons with a below-normal hematocrit fatigue easily because of the blood's reduced oxygen-carrying capacity.[1]

Nursing Management

of the Patient undergoing Laryngeal Surgery

PREOPERATIVE CARE

Before surgery the physician tells the patient who is to undergo a total laryngectomy that breathing will occur through a permanent opening made in the neck and that normal speech will not be possible. This information is often depressing to the patient because it may threaten economic status, as well as quality of life. The patient meets with a speech pathologist before surgery to learn about options for postoperative rehabilitation and speech. In some instances a visit from another person who has undergone successful rehabilitation from total laryngectomy is helpful. In other instances the visit may depress the patient further. Careful assessment must be made to determine whether the patient will benefit from such a visit and whether the visit should be made preoperatively, immediately after surgery, or later in the recovery period. Even though the patient and significant other may be hesitant about the visit, they often indicate afterward that the visit was helpful and improved their outlook about the patient's future.

Many large cities have a Lost Chord Club or a New Voice Club, and the members are willing to visit hospitalized patients. Information regarding these clubs may be obtained by contacting the International Association of Laryngectomees (http://www.larynxlink.com/). Local speech rehabilitation centers may supply instructive films and other resources. The local chapters of the American Cancer Society and the local health department also have information. If possible, the family should also learn about the method of speech that the person will be learning.

POSTOPERATIVE CARE

Like all patients who have had head and neck surgery, patients who have undergone a laryngectomy require hemodynamic monitoring, airway monitoring, and wound and flap monitoring after surgery.

Maintaining a Patent Airway. Some degree of airway obstruction is common in patients after a partial laryngectomy, from either preoperative radiotherapy or swelling from surgery close to the airway. To prevent airway emergencies, the surgeon performs a tracheostomy at the time of surgery. A cuffed tracheostomy tube is generally inserted to (1) allow ventilation after surgery until the patient wakes from anesthesia, (2) prevent blood from the surgical site from entering the tracheobronchial tree, (3) prevent pharyngeal and gastric secretions from soiling the bronchial tree, and (4) maintain an adequate airway when edema from surgery or radiation is expected.

The tracheostomy cuff is kept inflated until the morning after surgery or until the patient can manage his or her secretions. The nurse suctions the patient every 2 to 4 hours to prevent the buildup of secretions in the tracheobronchial tree or in the tracheostomy

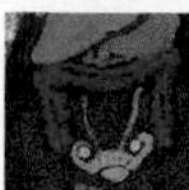

GUIDELINES FOR SAFE PRACTICE *Care of the Patient After Total Laryngectomy*

- Provide comfort care and airway management:
  —Elevate head of bed 45 degrees.
  —Encourage coughing and deep breathing every 4 hours.
  —Maintain oxygen to tracheostomy collar.
  —Assess airway patency every shift and as needed.
  —Assess vital signs, quality and rate of respiration, and skin color (pallor, cyanosis).
  —Auscultate lungs every shift and as needed.
- Provide care for suture line and stoma site as ordered by surgeon:
  —Assess suture line and stoma site every 4 hours.
  —Report erythema, purulent drainage, or hematoma.
  —Monitor drain function and output.
  —Maintain suction to drain at level ordered.
  —Milk tubing every 1 to 2 hours for 24 hours, and then every 4 hours and as needed.
  —Report changes in amount and color of drainage or air leak.
- Attend to fluid, food, and hygiene needs:
  —Monitor hydration and ensure adequate fluid intake to maintain healthy oral mucosa; provide mouth care at least three times daily.
  —Record intake and output every shift.
  —Weigh the patient daily at the same time and in the same amount of clothing.
  —Provide stoma and stoma vent care every shift and as needed.
  —Administer enteral feedings as ordered.
  —Assess patient's tolerance of feedings.
  —Assess bowel sounds every shift and as needed.
  —Report intolerance to feedings (nausea, fullness, inability to tolerate prescribed amount of feedings).
  —Record amount, consistency, and frequency of stools.
  —Assess swallowing ability, and provide support when oral diet resumes.
- Provide support and education for the patient and family:
  —Assess anxiety level and provide emotional support.
  —Assist patient in communicating.
  —Provide patient with writing materials or picture board.
  —Use questions that can be answered "yes" or "no."
  —Instruct about use of artificial speech device and encourage its use.
  —Be sensitive to patient's reactions to changes in appearance.
  —Provide time to listen to patient.
  —Encourage use of Lost Chord or New Voice Club.
  —Prepare patient for discharge.
  —Begin teaching laryngectomy care.
  —Monitor ability of patient or significant other to perform airway management care.
  —Provide patient with a list of supplies necessary for home care.
  —Provide information about soft diet.
  —Review written instructions in home-going booklet with patient and family.
  —Refer the patient to home nursing staff to assess patient's ability to perform self-care at home.
  —Refer the patient to a speech pathologist for voice and speech rehabilitation.

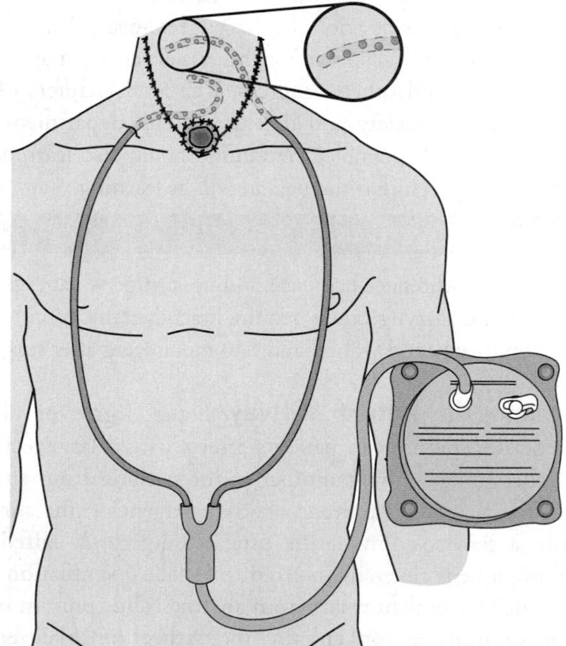

Figure 25-18 Hemovac apparatus for constant closed suction. In this system of wound drainage, suction is maintained by plastic container with spring inside that tries to force apart the lids and thereby produces suction that is transmitted through plastic tubing. Neck skin is pulled down tight, and no external dressing is required. The container serves as both suction source and receptacle for blood. It is emptied as required, and drainage tubes are left in neck for 3 days.

tube. The patient is suctioned orally before the cuff is deflated to prevent aspiration of secretions accumulated above the cuff. In some centers 3 to 5 ml of sterile saline may be instilled in the tube to soften and dislodge thickened secretions.

Patients receive cool mist therapy with a T tube. They also receive incentive spirometry and chest physiotherapy and, if necessary, aerosol and systemic bronchodilators.

When a cuffed tracheostomy tube is no longer necessary (not earlier than the third postoperative day), an uncuffed tube is inserted. Cuffless tubes are less harmful to the trachea, interfere less with swallowing, and minimize aspiration. Because there is no cuff, secretions cannot accumulate above the tube. Also, the cuffless tube allows the patient to occlude the tube with a finger and speak, which is a significant psychologic boost. Because the patient is able to expectorate secretions and has an adequate airway, the tracheostomy tube is plugged for increasing periods. The goal is to remove the tube and allow the opening to close by secondary intention. Some patients' tubes are removed 5 to 7 days after surgery; others remain in for up to 10 days.

Care for the person after a total laryngectomy is essentially the same as that described for tracheostomy later in the chapter, except these patients usually have a laryngectomy tube in place. It is shorter and wider in diameter than a tracheostomy tube. Some patients may not have a tube in the laryngeal stoma after the operation; instead, the stoma is a permanent one kept open initially by sutures because the surgeon believes there is less tissue reaction and a better laryngeal stoma if no tube is used. If a

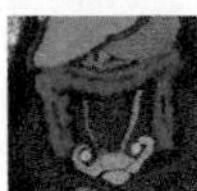

GUIDELINES FOR SAFE PRACTICE *Care of the Patient After Radical Neck Dissection*

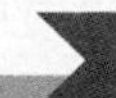

- Provide comfort care and airway management:
  - —Elevate head of bed 30 degrees.
  - —Maintain oxygen mist therapy if ordered.
  - —Encourage coughing, deep breathing, and use of incentive spirometer.
  - —Assess airway for signs and symptoms of increasing airway obstruction (stridor, dyspnea, increased pulse and respiratory rate).
  - —Monitor vital signs every 4 hours.
- Assess wound and provide care:
  - —Maintain venous access with large-bore needle.
  - —If hemorrhage occurs, page physician immediately, apply direct pressure, suction airway, and reassure patient.
  - —Care for suture line as ordered.
  - —Maintain drainage output, color, and consistency.
  - —Maintain suction to drain.
  - —Milk tubing every 1 to 2 hours for 24 hours, then every 4 hours and as needed.
  - —Check for air leak in drain.
  - —Assess patient for signs and symptoms of infection of suture line (erythema, pus, elevated temperature).
  - —Assess skin flap every shift for signs and symptoms of poor drain patency or infection (swelling, bleeding, oozing of suture line, or dehiscence).
  - —Monitor intake and output and record every shift.
- Prevent complications:
  - —Monitor shoulder droop secondary to loss of nerve supply to trapezius muscle and inability to raise hand over head.
  - —Reinforce need to do shoulder-strengthening exercise three times per day.
  - —Consult physical therapist with concerns about patient's exercises.
  - —Monitor for difficulty in swallowing related to postoperative swelling and xerostomia (dry mouth) from preoperative radiotherapy.
- Manage nutrition:
  - —Monitor patient's ability to ingest optimal caloric intake.
  - —Weigh daily at same time and with same amount of clothing.
  - —Consult with dietitian and physician if desired caloric intake can not be met.
  - —Explain about role of diet in wound healing.
- Provide patient and family support and education:
  - —Plan for specific time to provide emotional support.
  - —Monitor depression, which is not uncommon after disfiguring surgery.
  - —Identify members of patient support system, and involve them and patient in planning and giving care.
  - —Help patient verbalize feelings about having cancer, changes in body image, and changes in lifestyle.
  - —Refer patient to home care nursing staff to assess patient's ability to care for self at home.
  - —Provide optimal pain management.
  - —Encourage activity to prevent permanent disability.[5]
  - —Teach suture line care for home going (cleanse site with half-strength hydrogen peroxide followed by antibiotic ointment twice daily to keep incision line free of crusting).

laryngectomy tube is used, it remains until the wound is healed and a permanent fistula has formed—usually 3 to 6 months or longer.[1]

Maintaining Proper Positioning. To reduce venous and arterial pressure in the neck and decrease the risk of swelling and hemorrhage, the nurse elevates the head of the bed 30 to 45 degrees. The neck generally is maintained in a slightly flexed position to minimize tension on the suture lines. However, some patients require greater neck flexion or rotation to minimize tension or flexion of the flaps used for reconstruction. If the procedure is uncomplicated, the patient is usually up in a chair on the first postoperative day and is able to walk in the hall with assistance on the second day.

Managing the Wound. In head and neck surgery, complications are always a threat because of extensive undermining of subcutaneous tissues to elevate the skin flaps, contamination at the time of surgery when the upper aerodigestive tract is entered, and the poor quality of tissue in persons who receive preoperative radiotherapy.

The surgeon closes the surgical site with either interrupted or running sutures or staples and leaves the wound exposed (no dressing). Monitoring the wound site is critical to safe patient care, and the persons caring for the patient need to be familiar with the initial appearance of the wound so that any changes are readily apparent. Close postoperative monitoring of any type of skin flap is essential. Monitoring includes:

- Direct observation unless the wound is completely covered with a dressing. Some surgeons exteriorize (bring to the outside) a small segment of buried flaps for monitoring purposes.
- Use of Doppler to monitor patency of the anastomoses. The surgeon indicates the area where the Doppler is to be applied. Assessments are hourly for at least the first 24 hours.

The viability of skin flaps is indicated by their color, temperature, capillary refill, and induration. Slight erythema and induration of the skin flaps are normal in the early postoperative period. The incision should be kept free of crusting and exudates.

The nurse assesses the suture line for approximation, edema, color, and drainage. The nurse cleans the incision with half-strength hydrogen peroxide solution using clean technique; uses cotton swabs to remove crusts; and applies antibiotic ointment to the wound to seal the suture line. Drain exit sites and the tracheostomy incision receive the same care as the suture line. A minimal amount of bleeding from skin edges is normal in the immediate postoperative period. A more diffuse ooze of darker, red blood, along with swelling of the wound, indicates that a hematoma is developing, and the surgeon must be notified immediately. It is especially important to closely monitor the wounds of patients who received radiotherapy before surgery because they are more prone to wound dehiscence or the development of a pharyngocutaneous fistula.

Maintaining the Closed Drainage System. A closed drainage system with continuous suction is used to eliminate dead space and prevent accumulation of blood, serum, and other secretions under the skin flaps. Many drainage systems are available (e.g., Davol, Hemovac, Jackson-Pratt), and all provide a continuous negative pressure of 80 to 120 mm Hg. The nurse monitors them for function, air leaks, and the type and amount of drainage. If the drainage system is not functioning properly, a massive hematoma under tension can develop, which may require that the patient return to surgery for exploration, control of bleeding, and restoration of the drainage system.[1]

If air continuously seeps into the drainage system, negative pressure will not be maintained. Air leaks should be corrected immediately. If air leaks through the suture line, additional sutures may be added or a thick layer of antibiotic ointment applied to the incision line. In some situations a circular dressing is applied to the neck if no reconstruction flap is involved. If the air leak is minimal, the drain can be connected to wall suction. When a massive air leak occurs, the drain may need to be replaced and the leak obliterated. The nurse milks the tubing every 1 to 2 hours for the first 24 hours after surgery and then every 4 hours and as needed. As the nurse milks the tubing, he or she examines the wound to determine whether fluid is accumulating under the flaps.

The nurse records the type and amount of drainage every 8 hours. The amount of drainage in the first 16 hours can vary from less than 100 ml to 300 ml. Initially the drainage is sanguineous to serosanguineous. The nurse should report changes in the amount or color of drainage to the surgeon. The drains are removed when the drainage is less than 30 ml/day. Purulent or granular serous drainage mixed with air (with an odor to it) is considered abnormal and indicates a probable pharyngocutaneous fistula.

Nutrition. A nasogastric tube, inserted during the surgical procedure, is used for the instillation of food and fluids at regular intervals after both partial and total laryngectomy (Figure 25-19). The use of a nasogastric tube to give food is thought to minimize contamination of the pharyngeal and esophageal suture lines and to prevent fluid from leaking through the wound into the trachea before healing occurs. The nasogastric tube is removed as soon as the person can swallow safely. The person who has undergone a total laryngectomy requires careful attention during his or her first attempts to swallow, even though aspiration cannot occur because the trachea is no longer communicating with the esophagus. With a partial laryngectomy, especially a supraglottic laryngectomy, the patient has to relearn swallowing and is at significant risk for aspiration.

After tube feedings are discontinued, soft, formed foods, such as ice cream and mashed potatoes, are begun. The nurse instructs the patient to hold the breath, flex the head, and tilt it toward the unaffected side; place a small amount of food on the back of the tongue; swallow; and then cough to expel any food that entered the trachea. Other foods and fluids are added to the diet as the patient masters the swallowing technique.

After a total laryngectomy the patient does not receive normal olfactory sensations because breathing through the nose is impossible. Some patients report they are able to smell, and most have drainage from the nose for a time. See the Guidelines for Safe Practice boxes for a summary of postoperative care of the patient after a total laryngectomy (p. 610) and after neck dissection (p. 611).

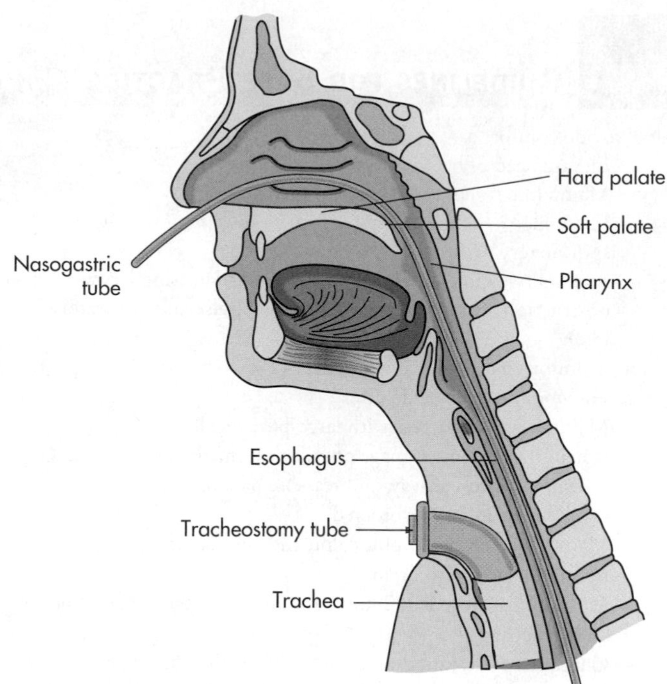

Figure 25-19 Position of tracheostomy tube and nasogastric tube after total laryngectomy.

Body Image. Some alteration of appearance is readily visible, which may cause the person to feel conspicuous. Anger, grief, or denial may be part of the normal response to the change in body image.

Speech Rehabilitation. Three types of speech are possible after a total laryngectomy: (1) tracheoesophageal speech; (2) esophageal speech; and (3) speech via an artificial larynx, or electrolarynx, which is learned immediately after surgery (Box 25-3).

For **tracheoesophageal speech**, a tracheoesophageal puncture (TEP) is made to create a tracheoesophageal fistula large enough for insertion of a valve prosthesis. Some surgeons create

Box 25-3 Speech Methods After Total Laryngectomy

- Tracheoesophageal prosthesis: Formation of a tracheoesophageal fistula with insertion of a silicone prosthesis that produces a sound in the esophagus (see Figure 25-20, *B*)
- Esophageal speech: Speech produced by expelling swallowed air (burping) across constricted tissue in the pharyngoesophageal segment
- External speech aids: Mechanical devices such as a vibrator or electronic artificial larynx used externally

the tracheoesophageal fistula after the larynx has been resected and a frozen section reveals that all the carcinoma has been removed. Other surgeons prefer to wait until the patient has completed postoperative radiotherapy, as long as 3 to 6 months after surgery, to allow time for edema of the incision to abate. Also, radiotherapy may shrink the skin around the incision. The tracheoesophageal fistula may require an overnight hospital stay, or the procedure may be performed in an outpatient setting. In this procedure the surgeon creates a small fistula from the superior wall of the tracheal stoma into the proximal wall of the esophagus. The surgeon pulls a red rubber catheter through the fistula into the esophagus at the 12 o'clock position of the laryngostoma and sutures it into place (Figure 25-20, *A*). The end of the catheter is occluded with a plug or an umbilical clamp, or a knot is tied in the catheter. The patient is discharged with the catheter in place. The prosthesis is inserted 5 to 7 days later by the speech pathologist or the surgeon (Figure 25-20, *B*). The speech pathologist teaches the patient how to speak with the TEP at this time.[1]

The prosthesis is a hollow silicone tube with a one-way valve that is open at the tracheal end and closed with a horizontal slit at the laryngopharyngeal end. When the patient talks, air pressure opens the closed end, permitting air to enter the laryngopharynx. When the patient stops talking, the laryngopharyngeal end closes, preventing saliva from draining into the trachea. Because air is diverted from the trachea into the esophagus, this form of speech is referred to as *tracheoesophageal speech.*

The stoma must be occluded during speech, either by placing a finger over the valve opening or by using a special tracheostomal valve inserted after the patient has learned to use the prosthesis. The patient or family must be taught to remove, clean, and reinsert the voice prosthesis rapidly so that the fistula does not stenose. Not all patients and families are comfortable with removing and cleaning the prosthesis, and considerable support by the speech pathologist may be necessary. The patient and family need to be taught how to place a rubber catheter into the fistula if the prosthesis comes out (see Figure 25-20, *A*). After placement, the catheter is knotted and taped to the chest. The patient should then see a physician.

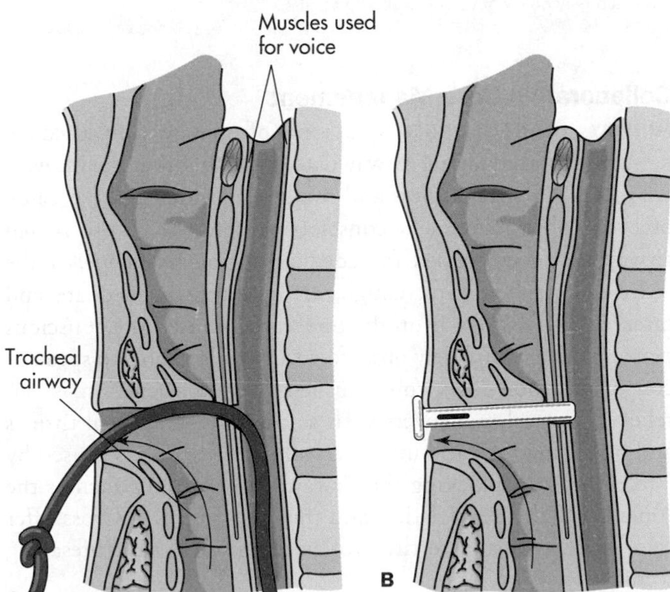

Figure 25-20 Tracheoesophageal puncture (TEP). **A,** Placement of red rubber catheter into TEP. Note knot in end of catheter to prevent passage of stomach contents. **B,** Placement of voice prosthesis into TEP.

Advantages of tracheoesophageal speech include more rapid restoration of voice; speech that is closer to normal in rate and phrasing; and speech that is more pleasing than with an electrolarynx. Disadvantages include reliance on a prosthesis and the possibility that the tracheoesophageal fistula may stenose. For these reasons, all three methods of speaking are still in use; in fact, some patients find it useful to use more than one method.

The speech pathologist teaches the patient to use **esophageal speech** after all therapy (including postoperative radiotherapy) is completed and swelling of the incision has abated. This may not occur until 3 to 6 months after surgery. To learn esophageal speech, the patient must first practice burping. This provides the moving column of air needed for sound, and folds of tissue at the opening of the esophagus act as the vibrating surface. The patient must learn to coordinate articulation with esophageal vocalization made possible by aspirating air into the esophagus. The new voice sounds are natural, although somewhat hoarse. The qualities of speech provided by the use of the nasopharynx are still present. The patient may have digestive difficulty while learning to speak; this is caused by swallowing air during practice, by unusual strain on abdominal muscles, and by nervous tension. Digestive difficulties usually abate with proficiency in speaking.

Most patients learn esophageal speech best at a specialized speech clinic; some individuals may need to go to a nearby city for this instruction. Motivation and persistent effort are essential in learning this kind of speech. Encouragement from the professional staff and from the patient's significant other is important to the patient's morale. Until recently, esophageal speech was the primary speech method used after laryngectomy. Although this method of speech was successful for many laryngectomees, others could never learn to use it. In addition, the use of radiotherapy after a total laryngectomy, which is increasing, causes fibrous tissue to form, making esophageal speech difficult to master. Information about esophageal speech can be obtained from the American Speech-Language-Hearing Association, the International Association of Laryngectomees, and the American Cancer Society.

The speech pathologist teaches use of an electronic artificial larynx 1 or 2 days after surgery. Various mechanical devices are available, and newer ones permit a natural type of speech, providing pitch inflection and volume control. The patient's speech pathologist, the local chapter of the American Cancer Society, or the local telephone company can provide information about purchasing these devices.[1]

GERONTOLOGIC CONSIDERATIONS

A total laryngectomy is traumatic for the patient in many ways. Because the older adult is even more susceptible to complications, anxiety, and poor wound healing, caring for an older patient who has undergone a laryngectomy is a challenge. The nurse should be knowledgeable about the patient's history and the presence of complicating, preexisting conditions that require monitoring during the

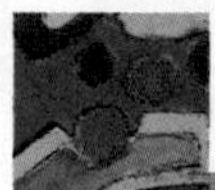

PATIENT/FAMILY TEACHING *Home Care of the Patient After Laryngectomy*

Home care of the patient after a laryngectomy can be difficult. It is frightening for both the patient and the family until they become familiar with the equipment and care needed. The nurse should help them feel comfortable with the new responsibilities by reinforcing instructions, providing detailed written instructions, allowing them to demonstrate techniques with nursing supervision, and planning time for questions and concerns.

Explain the following additional information to the patient and family:

- The nose normally filters and warms air that we breathe. This function is lost with a tracheostomy or stoma; therefore extra humidity is necessary to moisten the air. To increase humidity:
  —Use a cool mist in the room where you spend most of your time. Also use it in your bedroom at night.
  —Cover the stoma during the day with a dampened stoma cover, and moisten it when it dries.
  —Wash the stoma with a washcloth and warm water and soap daily to remove crusts of mucus that form inside and outside the stoma. Do not clean around the stoma with paper tissues, since they contain lint that can be inhaled into the stoma. Crusts that are difficult to remove can be softened with hydrogen peroxide or a few drops of saline solution.
  —Use a syringe or eyedropper to instill 3 to 5 ml of normal saline into your laryngectomy vent or stoma. This loosens mucous plugs before suctioning. Normal saline can be made by boiling 1 teaspoon of table salt in 1 quart of tap water for 20 minutes, cooling the solution, and placing it in a clean bottle with a lid. Make a new solution daily or at least every 2 days, because it does not contain a preservative.*
  —Keep the stoma covered when you go outside to prevent cold air, dust, or pollen from getting in the tube or stoma. Use a scarf, bib, crocheted cover, or shirt that buttons at the neck.
  —If the skin around the stoma becomes irritated, apply a thin coat of plain petroleum jelly or zinc oxide. Take care not to place it too close to the stoma to avoid inhaling it.
- You can bathe in a tub or take a shower, being careful to keep soap and water from entering the tube or stoma. A stoma shower guard or a handheld shower can be used.
- Keep shampoo and water out of the stoma. You may need someone to help you shampoo.
- Men can shave using an electric or a manual razor. Be sure to cover the stoma so that lather and particles do not fall into the opening.
- You may not swim because water would enter your lungs.
- Drink at least 8 to 10 glasses of fluid daily. More fluid is needed during hot weather or when home heating is in use.
- Avoid persons who have colds or the flu or are not feeling well.
- Call your physician immediately if you feel like you are getting a cold or other respiratory tract infection.
- You can use antihistamines or decongestants, but be aware that they dry secretions; drink extra fluids and increase humidity while taking them.
- Increasing your activity helps thin secretions and makes them easier to cough or suction up.
- Wear a medical identification bracelet or carry a card stating that you are a neck breather. Emergency cards stating, "I am a total neck breather" can be obtained from the local American Cancer Society.
- Persons who have undergone a total laryngectomy often have dry mouth and bad breath. Brush with fluoride toothpaste and floss your teeth at least after breakfast and at bedtime. Keep your mouth fresh and clean by using baking soda and salt gargle (1 teaspoon of salt, 1 teaspoon of baking soda, and 1 quart of water).
- Observe for complications, including hematoma, wound dehiscence, tissue loss, pharyngocutaneous fistula, and carotid artery rupture. If these are present, see a physician.

*This step may not be prescribed for all patients.

postoperative period. If the patient has preexisting communication difficulties, communication challenges are exacerbated in the postoperative phase. The patient may be referred for additional nursing care on discharge to the home. Home care of the patient after a laryngectomy is outlined in the Patient/Family Teaching box.

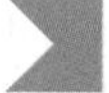

The Compromised Airway

Etiology and Epidemiology. The airway can be partially or completely obstructed by many conditions, several of which are discussed earlier in this chapter.

Pathophysiology. When the airway is completely obstructed, the conscious person has no breath sounds and displays signs of severe respiratory distress progressing to respiratory arrest. Airway obstruction is confirmed in the unconscious person when attempts to ventilate the person do not produce chest movement and no expiratory air passes from the individual's airway. With partial airway obstruction the individual displays respiratory distress and produces sounds such as gurgling, snoring, or stridorous ventilations.

Collaborative Care Management

AIRWAY MANAGEMENT. The type of intervention used to reestablish and maintain airway patency depends on the individual's level of consciousness and respiratory status and the cause of airway obstruction. The conscious person with an obstructed airway must be assessed for adequacy of air exchange. If the individual can talk and cough, air exchange is adequate and interventions can focus on the underlying cause. The conscious person with a completely obstructed airway is unable to speak or cough and soon loses consciousness if the obstruction is not relieved. Special maneuvers such as chest or abdominal thrusts and back blows are administered if the obstruction is caused by a foreign object blocking the airway. Organizations such as the American Heart Association and the American Red Cross offer training programs to certify proficiency in these basic lifesaving techniques.

In the unconscious individual the tongue falls back, covering the glottis. Lifting the chin moves the tongue forward, opening the airway. An alternative to keep the tongue from obstructing the unconscious person's glottis is to place the individual in a side-lying position.

When a person has a mechanical obstruction of the airway and is expected to be unconscious for some time, it may be necessary to use an **artificial airway.**

ARTIFICIAL AIRWAYS

ORAL AIRWAYS. The simplest type of artificial airway is an oropharyngeal airway, which keeps the tongue from falling back over the glottis. This type of airway is never used in a conscious individual, since it may cause vomiting or laryngospasm. An oropharyngeal airway must be inserted correctly to avoid pushing the tongue back against the glottis.

The esophageal gastric airway consists of a face mask with two ports. The lower port is for the esophageal tube, which is introduced into the esophagus to help prevent reflux of gastric contents. The upper port is for ventilation. The esophageal gastric tube airway is never inserted into a conscious person.

ENDOTRACHEAL TUBES AND TRACHEOSTOMY. When a person is no longer able to maintain his or her own airway, an endotracheal tube or a tracheostomy is necessary. In endotracheal intubation a tube is passed through either the nose or the mouth into the trachea (Figure 25-21, *A*), whereas in a tracheostomy an artificial opening is made in the trachea, into which a tracheostomy tube is inserted (Figure 25-21, *B*). An endotracheal tube is usually chosen initially as a means of providing the airway because most physicians consider it safer to do an emergency endotracheal intubation and then perform a tracheostomy as a nonemergency procedure in the operating room if prolonged support of the airway is needed. In this case the endotracheal tube is not removed until after the tracheostomy opening is made.[1] A tracheostomy is performed initially only if the use of an endotracheal tube is contraindicated as in severe trauma; burns; or laryngeal obstruction caused by tumor, infection, or vocal cord paralysis. In a choking emergency, a cricothyrotomy may be done to establish an airway. This is an incision into the larynx that is held open by means of a tube open at both ends to allow air exchange until a tracheostomy can be done.

Endotracheal tubes are made of rubber or plastic and usually have an inflatable cuff (Figure 25-22). The cuff is designed to prevent aspiration of gastric secretions, but is not 100% effective since "microaspiration" occurs in many patients. Cuffed tubes are always used for patients receiving mechanical ventilation because the cuff allows a closed system with the ventilator. Endotracheal tubes are inserted via the mouth or nose through the larynx into the trachea. If an oral endotracheal tube is used, a rubber airway or bite block is often necessary to prevent the patient from biting down on the tube and obstructing the airway.

Once the airway is secured, either by intubation or tracheostomy, the nurse aspirates secretions and provides well-humidified oxygen. If the patient is unable to sustain respiration, a mechanical ventilator is attached to either the endotracheal tube or the tracheostomy tube. Usually an endotracheal tube is not left in place longer than 10 to 14 days. If the patient is unable to maintain a patent airway after this time, a tracheostomy is performed.

Patients with endotracheal tubes can have two potentially fatal complications: accidental extubation and displacement of the endotracheal tube. Tips of endotracheal tubes have been shown to shift as much as 2 cm in the trachea when patients flex or extend their necks or laterally tip their heads. Usually the endotracheal tube is affixed to the patient's face with waterproof tape above and below the lips and around the tube to keep it in place. This method can cause facial skin breakdown and is of particular concern in patients with risk factors such as advanced age, low blood pressure, poor perfusion, and malnutrition. For this reason, commercially available endotracheal tube holders that use no tape are preferred (Figure 25-23).

Tracheostomy tubes are usually made of silicone, pliable plastic, or metal. Most adult-sized plastic tracheostomy tubes have a cuff that is inflated with air to fill the space between the outside of the tube and the trachea. The cuff, as on any cuffed tube, provides a sealed airway for positive-pressure mechanical ventilation and helps prevent aspiration of gastric secretions or tube feedings in the unconscious person. Low-pressure cuffs are least likely to damage the tracheal wall, although care is needed to ensure the

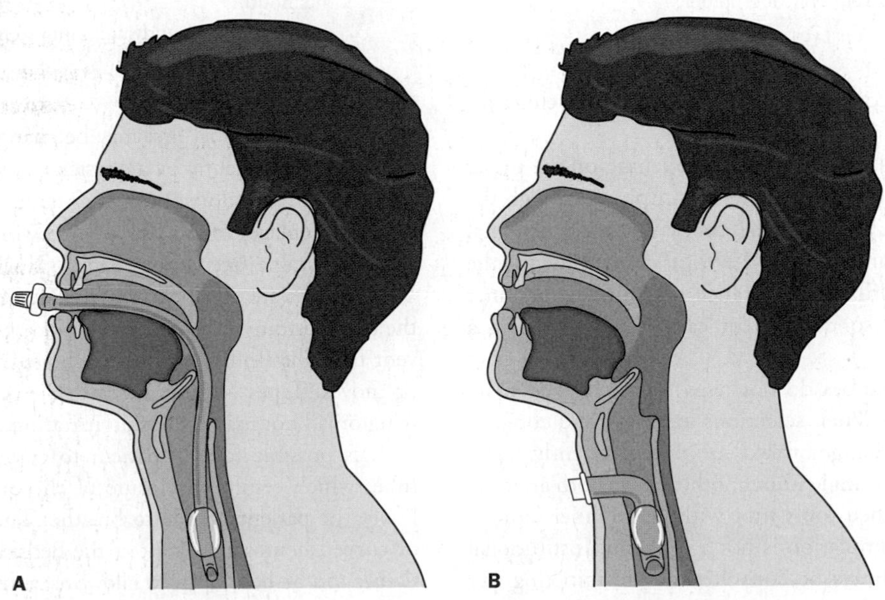

Figure 25-21 **A,** Position of endotracheal tube. **B,** Position of tracheostomy tube.

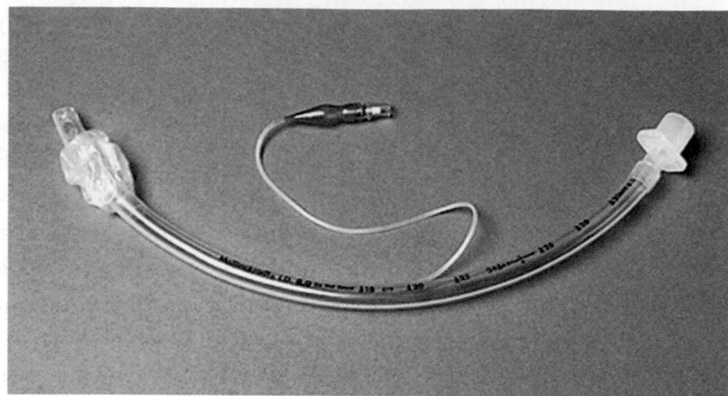

Figure 25-22 Endotracheal tube.

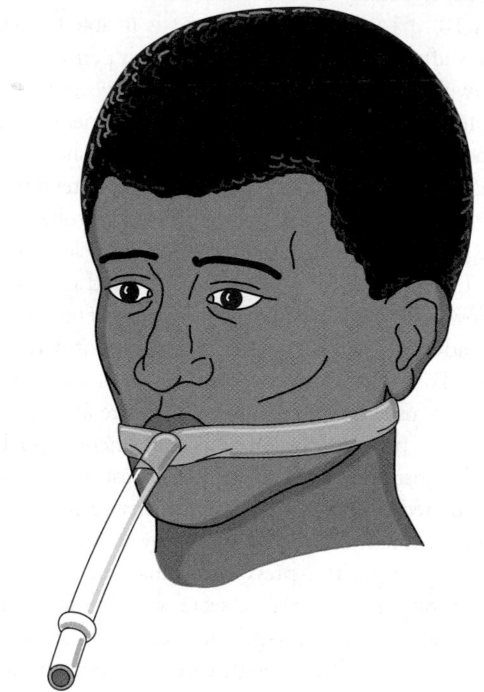

Figure 25-23 Comfit endotracheal tube holder.

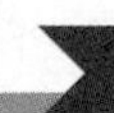

Guidelines for Safe Practice

Inflating and Deflating an Endotracheal or Tracheostomy Cuff

The cuff should be inflated to a volume that provides adequate occlusion around the tube without increasing the risk of tracheomalacia, tracheostenosis, tracheoesophageal fistula, or erosion through a major blood vessel. This means using only the minimum volume of air needed to seal the airway (no greater than 20 mm Hg or 25 cm H_2O). Alternatively, the clinician can determine pressure using the minimal leak technique for inflating the cuff as follows:

1. Using a 10 or 20 ml syringe, slowly inject air into the cuff.
2. As air is introduced, assess for air leak around the tube. This is determined by (a) the patient's ability to talk or make sounds and (b) the nurse's ability to feel air coming from the patient's nose or mouth.
3. When the airway is sealed and no passage of air around the tube can be detected, remove 0.5 ml of air. This creates a "minimal leak" and ensures that the lowest possible pressure is being exerted on the tracheal wall.
4. Auscultate over the trachea while ventilating the patient with either an Ambu bag or a mechanical ventilator. A small amount of air should be heard gurgling past the cuff.
5. If an adequate seal cannot be obtained with 25 ml of air, notify the physician.
6. The exact pressure in the cuff can be measured by connecting the pilot balloon to a handheld meter. To do this, inflate the balloon with a syringe, in the normal fashion, until a seal is obtained. Remove the syringe and attach the meter. Record the meter reading, in cm H_2O, and check the pressure in the cuff each shift to ensure consistency.

Although this technique limits pressure on tracheal tissue, it also creates the risk of secretions leaking around the cuff.

When deflating a cuff, proceed as follows:

1. Have patient cough up secretions if possible, then suction the tube and the mouth to decrease the risk of secretions being aspirated during deflation.
2. Deflate during exhalation so secretions are propelled toward the mouth.
3. Repeat coughing and suctioning to further clear secretions.

cuff is inflated with the correct amount of air (see Guidelines for Safe Practice box).

A fenestrated tracheostomy tube has an opening on the upper surface of the outer cannula that allows air inspired through the nose and mouth to pass through the tube. When the external opening is plugged, air can pass over the vocal cords, allowing the individual to talk. If ventilatory assistance is required, the inner cannula can be inserted so the patient can be connected to a mechanical ventilator.

Usually tracheostomy tubes do not need to be changed more than every 2 to 3 weeks. When secretions are thick and copious, the tube may have to be changed weekly or more frequently. Some tracheostomy tubes have a single lumen; others have both an inner and outer cannula. A tracheostomy tube without an inner cannula is used when mucus accumulation is not a problem. Institutional policies, which should always be consulted before initiating any interventions, determine who changes tracheostomy tubes and the procedures to be followed in maintaining the tube. In some agencies the outer cannula first may be changed only by an ENT surgeon and subsequently by a physician, specially prepared nurse, or a registered respiratory therapist. The nurse regularly removes and cleans or replaces the inner cannula, which may be either disposable or reusable (see Patient/Family Teaching box). Twill tapes or Velcro straps are attached to each side of the faceplate (flange) of the tracheostomy tube and secured on the side of the neck to prevent the tube from becoming dislodged when the patient coughs or moves. Tapes are not tied behind the patient's neck because lying on a knot may cause skin irritation and a pressure sore.

It is possible for the patient to cough out the tracheostomy tube, which results in closure of the opening for the tube and leaves the patient unable to breathe. Therefore a tracheal dilator or curved hemostat is kept at the bedside so that, if needed, the tissues can be held open to allow insertion of a new tracheostomy tube. A sterile replacement tracheostomy tube and one that is one size smaller also are kept at the bedside in case of accidental

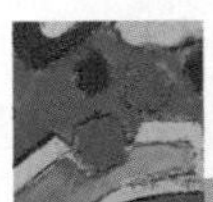

PATIENT/FAMILY TEACHING *Home Care of the Patient With a Permanent Tracheostomy Tube*

Increasing Environmental Humidity

Use a cool mist humidifier in the room where you spend most of your time.

Use it in your bedroom when you are napping or sleeping.

Suctioning the Tracheostomy Tube

1. Gather the supplies you need:
   - Suction machine
   - Suction catheter (No. 14 French whistle-tip)
   - Two nonsterile gloves
   - A clean basin or sink
   - Hydrogen peroxide
   - Clean 4 × 4 fine-mesh gauze pads
   - Jar of tapwater or normal saline (Use distilled water if you have well water.)
   - Clean cotton-tipped swabs
   - Clean pipe cleaners or small brush
   - Clean washcloth and towel
   - Tracheostomy tube ties
   - Clean scissors
   - Plastic or paper bag for disposal of soiled materials
2. Wash hands thoroughly with soap and water.
3. Sit or stand in front of the mirror (such as the mirror over the sink in the bathroom).
4. Put on gloves.
5. Suction the tracheostomy tube.
6. If your tube has an inner cannula, remove it. (If your tube does not have an inner cannula, go to step 12.)
7. Clean the inner cannula in the basin. Pour hydrogen peroxide over it until it is clean.
8. Clean the inner cannula with pipe cleaners or a small brush. Discard used pipe cleaners in a disposable bag.
9. Rinse the cannula thoroughly with normal saline, tapwater, or distilled water.
10. Dry inside and outside of the cannula with 4 × 4 fine-mesh gauze. Discard used gauze in a disposable bag.
11. Reinsert the inner cannula and lock it in place.
12. Remove the soiled gauze dressing from your neck and dispose of it in a disposable bag.
13. Inspect the skin around the stoma for any signs of irritation or infection, such as redness, hardness, tenderness, drainage, or a foul smell. If any of these are present, call your nurse or physician after you finish your tracheostomy tube care.
14. Soak cotton-tipped swabs in hydrogen peroxide. Use swabs to clean the exposed parts of the outer cannula and the skin around it. Discard in a disposable bag.
15. Wet the washcloth with tapwater, normal saline, or distilled water. Wipe away hydrogen peroxide and clean the skin around the stoma.
16. Dry the area around the stoma with the clean towel.
17. Change the ties using twill tape recommended to you.
18. Do not completely remove the old tie until you have a new one in place.
19. Cut twill tape as you have been taught.
20. Place fine-mesh gauze under the tracheostomy tie and neck plate by folding it or cutting a slit.
21. Remove your gloves and discard them in the same bag used for soiled gauze.
22. Wash your hands with soap and warm water.
23. Wash the basin and small brush with soap and warm water.
24. Put the washcloth and towel in the laundry.
25. Wash your hands again.

decannulation. Some surgeons prefer to place a retention suture on each side of the tracheostomy opening and tape the end of the suture to the skin. If the opening shows signs of closing, tension can be placed on the sutures to widen the opening.

Depending on the patient's condition, a tracheostomy can be either temporary or permanent; the person who has undergone a total laryngectomy has a permanent tracheostomy.

In addition to establishing and maintaining a patent airway, endotracheal intubation and tracheostomy help prevent aspiration by sealing off the trachea from the digestive tract in the unconscious or paralyzed person; permit removal of tracheobronchial secretions in the person who cannot cough adequately; and allow positive-pressure mechanical ventilation that cannot be given effectively by mask.

Nursing Management

of the Patient with an Endotracheal or a Tracheostomy Tube

The nurse must ensure adequate ventilation and oxygenation. The nurse assesses lung sounds regularly. Unless the individual's underlying pathologic condition alters lung ventilation, breath sounds should be heard bilaterally, and chest expansion should be symmetric. If an endotracheal tube is inserted too far, it will slip into one of the main-stem bronchi (usually the right) and occlude the opposite bronchus and lung, resulting in atelectasis on the obstructed side. Even if the endotracheal tube is still in the trachea, airway obstruction results if the end of the tube is located on the carina (the area at the lower end of the trachea at the point of bifurcation of the main-stem bronchi). Although these complications are more common with the use of an endotracheal tube, they can occur with a tracheostomy tube, especially in a small person with a short neck. In either situation the nurse pulls the tube back until it is positioned below the larynx and above the carina, and then fastens the tube securely in place.

For maximum ventilation and lung perfusion, the nurse turns and repositions the patient every 2 hours. The nurse assesses respiratory frequency, tidal volume, and vital capacity, and performs postural drainage, percussion, and vibration as appropriate.

Tube placement must be maintained. The tube is secured with tape or specially designed ties, and the nurse assesses placement at regular intervals. The endotracheal tube is marked to establish a landmark for position comparison and to measure and document the length of tube that extends beyond the patient's lips. A spare tube is always kept at the bedside. The nurse changes tapes or ties whenever soiled to decrease skin irritation.

Endotracheal and tracheostomy tubes irritate the trachea, resulting in increased mucus production, so the nurse must assess the patient regularly for excess secretions and suction him or her as often as necessary to maintain a patent airway (see Guidelines for Safe Practice box). Patients should not be suctioned routinely or when the airway can be cleared by coughing, since suctioning is mechanically irritating to the tissues and can cause bronchospasm. Indications that the patient needs to be suctioned include noisy respirations, adventitious breath sounds, moist cough that the patient is unable to clear, elevated pulse and respiratory rates, increase in peak inspiratory pressure on a mechanical ventilator, restlessness and agitation associated with a decrease in SpO_2 or PaO_2, or any other sign of respiratory distress. If mucus is blocking the inner cannula of a tracheostomy tube and cannot be removed by suction, the inner cannula is removed to open the airway. When the mucus is thick, the nurse should clean or replace the inner cannula at once because the outer tube may also become blocked. If, despite these measures, the patient becomes cyanotic, the nurse should summon the physician immediately. The amount of mucus subsides gradually, and the patient eventually may go for several hours without being suctioned. However, even when secretions are minimal, the patient can be apprehensive and need constant attendance.

Because endotracheal airways bypass the upper airway, which normally humidifies and warms inspired air, an external source of cool, humidified air must be provided to avoid mucosal irritation and thickening and crusting of bronchial secretions. Large-bore tubing is needed to provide mist, since water particles condense in small-bore tubing. The viscosity of secretions is noticeably different in patients who do not receive mist for even as short a period as 30 minutes.

Interventions to minimize the risk of infection are essential, since an endotracheal or tracheostomy tube provides a direct route for introduction of pathogens into the lower airway. All respiratory therapy equipment should be changed every 24 hours, and any equipment that touches the floor must be replaced. Water that condenses in equipment tubing must be removed but never poured back into the humidifier reservoir because it may contain pathogens.

The nurse must provide frequent mouth care for the patient with an endotracheal tube, which causes irritation and an increased volume of oropharyngeal secretions. The patient also has great difficulty swallowing (especially if an oral tube is used), and secretions tend to pool in the mouth and pharynx, particularly if the tube's cuff is inflated. This means that frequent oropharyngeal suctioning is needed. Mouth care is also important because an endotracheal tube or oral airway increases the risk of ulceration or abrasion of the lips and oropharynx. The nurse inspects the lips, tongue, and oral cavity regularly; cleans the oral cavity with swabs soaked in saline; and applies a moisturizing agent to cracked lips.

Adequate nutritional intake must be maintained. The person with an endotracheal tube is kept NPO, so nourishment is given by parenteral or enteral feedings. Enteral supplemental feedings are preferred because they maintain the function of the gut, provide more nutrition than intravenous feedings, pose less infection risk, and are more economical.

The patient with a tracheostomy tube is usually able to swallow and have a normal oral intake. Some experts prefer that the cuff on the tracheostomy tube be inflated while the patient is eating to prevent aspiration. Others believe the inflated cuff bulges into the esophagus and makes swallowing more difficult; therefore they prefer that the cuff be deflated (see Guidelines for Safe Practice box, p. 616). Nursing assessment determines which technique to use. The patient can swallow methylene blue dye before each feeding. If the dye does not appear in tracheal secretions, it is safe to proceed with the meal.

Patients with endotracheal tubes or tracheostomy tubes with the cuff inflated cannot talk. Therefore the call light should be kept within the patient's reach, the patient should be reoriented frequently, and an acceptable communication mode must be established. The nurse should ask questions so that the patient can indicate a simple "yes" or "no" response by nodding the head, using hand signals, or squeezing the nurse's hand. Some patients may be able to use an erasable board or notepad to communicate. The nurse needs to talk to the patient, explain all procedures, and reinforce that the ability to speak will return when the tube is removed. The nurse should encourage family and friends to talk to the patient and offer support.[1]

During the immediate extubation period, special precautions must be observed. The nurse monitors the patient for signs of upper airway obstruction secondary to laryngeal edema, including increased respiratory distress, increased restlessness, hoarseness, and laryngeal stridor. The nurse also assesses the adequacy of the cough and gag reflexes. Although nursing care of persons with either endotracheal or tracheostomy tubes is similar, patients with tracheostomies have additional nursing care needs. They are apprehensive and often fearful of choking. Thus, when feasible,

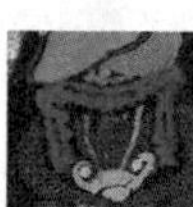

GUIDELINES FOR SAFE PRACTICE

Suctioning a Tracheostomy Tube

- Use gloves and goggles to protect yourself.
- Use a suction catheter with a diameter that does not exceed one half the diameter of the tracheostomy tube.
- Set suction pressure so that it is no more than 120 mm Hg when the tubing is occluded.
- Maintain sterility of all equipment that will come in contact with the patient's lower airway. This means wearing a sterile glove to handle the catheter, which must be sterile, and using sterile solution to rinse the catheter.
- Suction sterile water or saline through the catheter to test suction.
- Obtain baseline assessment of SpO_2, heart rate, and rhythm.
- Preoxygenate the patient with 100% oxygen for several breaths in preparation for suctioning.
- Instill sterile normal saline into the airway if secretions are thick and tenacious.
- Insert catheter until it meets resistance, then retract it 1 to 2 cm.
- Withdraw catheter while rotating it in a circle with suction being applied. Do not exceed 10 to 15 seconds for this step.
- Reoxygenate the patient for several breaths.
- Rinse catheter with sterile water.
- Repeat the above, including rinsing catheter, up to three times to clear airway.
- Suction oropharyngeal cavity on completion of tracheal suctioning.
- Dispose of equipment as per agency protocol.
- Repeat respiratory assessments.
- Document procedure, including patient's response.

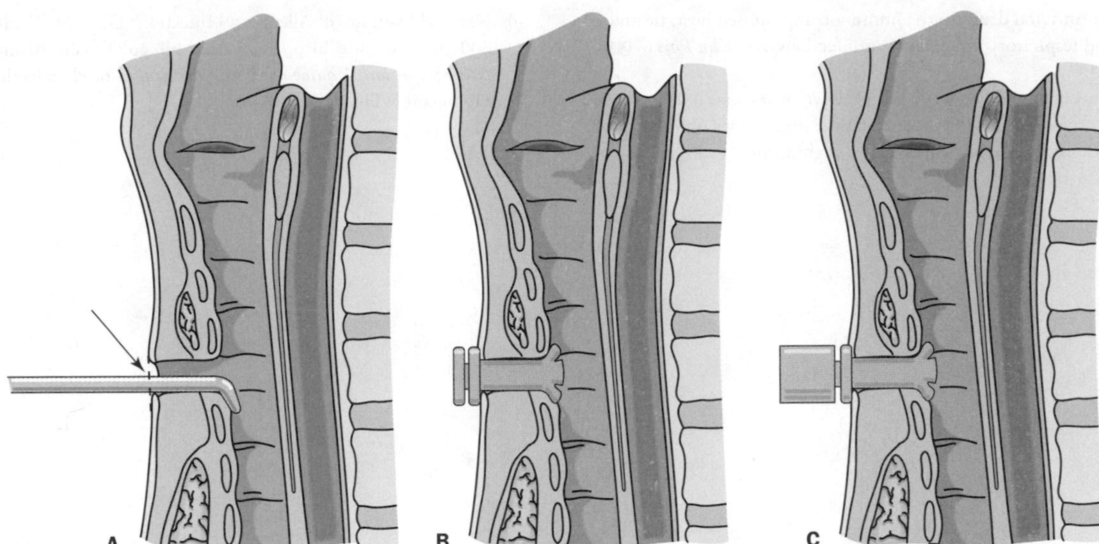

Figure 25-24 Tracheal button. **A,** Bent pipe cleaner is inserted into stoma to measure depth. Pipe cleaner is gently pulled back to hook on anterior tracheal wall. Distance from pipe cleaner bend to skin surface determines length of tracheostomy button. As an alternative, several different sizes of tracheal buttons are tried to determine which one is most comfortable. **B,** Solid plug inserted into tracheostomy button prevents button from being coughed out and allows patient to breathe through upper airway and vocalize. **C,** Hollow tube adaptor ("one-way" valve) replaces stoma plug to allow for suctioning and inspiration through button and expiration and vocalization through upper airway.

the surgeon or nurse thoroughly explains the procedure to the patient before surgery. Both the patient and the family need to understand that the patient will be unable to speak, that the nurses will use alternate methods to communicate with the patient, and that constant attendance will be provided until the patient can manage his or her own airway safely.

Analgesics and sedatives are given judiciously so as not to depress the respiratory center. Also, a small dressing may be placed under a tracheostomy tube. Although drainage should be minimal, during the immediate postoperative period the nurse inspects the wound frequently for bleeding and changes the dressings as they become soiled with mucous drainage.

Weaning From the Tracheostomy Tube. Patients who have had tracheostomies for a while may require progressive weaning before the tracheostomy tube can be safely removed (decannulation). The cuff is deflated to determine the patient's ability to handle secretions without aspiration. If no aspiration occurs, a smaller, uncuffed tube is inserted to determine the patient's ability to breathe around the tube and through the nose and mouth. Next, the opening of the tracheostomy tube is occluded for 24 hours to ensure the patient can breathe through the nose and mouth without difficulty. If the patient tolerates this procedure, the tracheostomy tube is removed and decannulation is accomplished. An occlusive dressing is applied to the stoma site to promote healing.

After removal of a tracheostomy tube, a temporary air leak occurs at the incision site. The nurse instructs the patient to occlude the opening with a finger in order to speak. The tracheal stoma is suctioned if needed. However, frequent use of the stoma for suctioning can delay closure and healing of the tracheostomy incision.

Some patients with a permanent tracheal stoma use a tracheal button, a hollow Teflon tube with a serrated distal end that is inserted into the tracheal stoma, where the end fits against the anterior tracheal wall (Figure 25-24). When the button is in place, a solid plug is inserted to spread the distal end flanges, which secures the tube in place. The button keeps the stoma tract open and allows the patient to breathe, vocalize, and clear secretions through the upper airway.

If the patient has difficulty breathing, the solid plug can be removed and the patient ventilated with an Ambu bag fitted with an adaptor. Routine suctioning through the tracheal button is discouraged, since the suction catheter tends to hit the posterior wall of the trachea, causing ulceration and bleeding. If the tracheostomy tube must be reinserted after several hours or days, it can be easily reinserted because the stoma has been kept open with the button. For patients with a permanent tracheostomy, care continues in the home as presented in the Patient/Family Teaching box, p. 617.

Critical Thinking

1. A 60-year-old patient who has been seen in the family practice clinic that you are working in as a registered nurse states that she was not given an antibiotic to treat her sinusitis. What possible responses would you make to the patient?
2. Should nurses recommend that patients use complementary and alternative therapies in managing their upper respiratory illnesses?

References

1. American Cancer Society: *All about laryngeal and hypopharyngeal cancer,* accessed June 2004 from website: http://americancancersociety.org/docroot/home/index.asp.

2. Colgan R et al: Antiviral drugs in the immunocompromised host: treatment of influenza and respiratory syncytial virus infections, *Am Fam Phys* 67(4): 763–766, 2003.
3. National Heart, Lung, and Blood Institute: *What are the signs and symptoms of sleep apnea?,* accessed June 2004 from website: http://www.nhlbi.nih.gov/health/dci/Diseases/SleepApnea/SleepApnea_Signs.html.
4. National Institutes of Allergy and Infectious Diseases: *Sinusitis,* accessed June 2004 from website: http://www.niaid.nih.gov/factsheets/sinusitis.htm.
5. *Nurse practitioner's quick reference to clinical facts,* Philadelphia, 2005, Lippincott Williams & Wilkins.

 Visit the Evolve website: http://evolve.elsevier.com/Monahan/medsurg

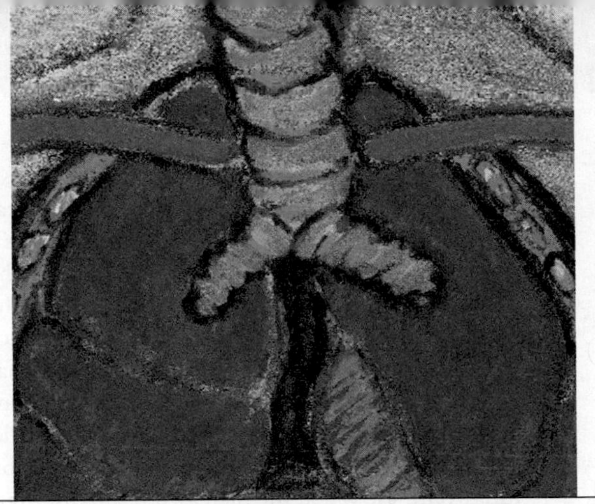

CHAPTER 26
Lower Airway Problems

by Pamela D. Dennison

OBJECTIVES

After studying this chapter, the learner should be able to:

1. Differentiate between restrictive and obstructive pulmonary disorders.
2. Compare community-acquired and hospital-acquired pneumonia.
3. Describe incidence, preventive measures, and current challenges in the diagnosis and treatment of tuberculosis.
4. Compare fungal infections of the respiratory tract.
5. Describe incidence, prevention, and therapy for lung cancer.
6. List five precautions to be observed in the care of chest tubes and a closed drainage system, and give the rationale for each.
7. Explain the pathophysiology of acute lung injury and acute respiratory distress syndrome.
8. Differentiate among a closed, an open, and a tension pneumothorax in terms of signs and symptoms, treatment, and nursing management.

KEY TERMS

Many diseases, both acute and chronic, affect the respiratory system. In recent decades the incidence of some pulmonary diseases such as lung abscess and bronchiectasis has decreased, whereas the incidence of other pulmonary diseases such as chronic bronchitis and emphysema has increased. In addition, the reduction in immunocompetence that occurs with cancer chemotherapy, immunosuppressant medications given after organ transplantation, or acquired immunodeficiency syndrome (AIDS) has resulted in an increase in opportunistic lung infections caused by microorganisms that were rarely pathogenic in the past.

Historically, acute respiratory infections were the major cause of morbidity and mortality from respiratory diseases. Since the 1960s, however, the most significant pulmonary diseases are chronic. Because most diseases of the respiratory tract are not reportable to the Centers for Disease Control and Prevention, the full extent of both acute and chronic illness is difficult to estimate. However, the Social Security Administration reports that disability payments to persons with chronic pulmonary problems are second only to payments to persons with heart problems, indicating chronic pulmonary diseases are a major health problem. Chronic lower respiratory disease is the fourth overall cause of death in the U.S. population.

Early symptoms of respiratory diseases are often ignored by the general population. The major factor preventing early diagnosis and treatment of pulmonary diseases (except for acute pulmonary disorders) is the insidious nature of their signs and symptoms. Medical attention is needed for cough, difficulty breathing, production of sputum, shortness of breath, and nose and throat irritations that do not subside within 2 weeks, since these symptoms suggest respiratory disease.

Classification of Pulmonary Disorders

One approach to the classification of lung diseases differentiates pulmonary disorders on the basis of etiology and how they affect ventilation. Usually lung diseases are divided into restrictive and obstructive ventilatory disorders. A third category, pulmonary vascular disorders, includes diseases that alter the lungs' ability to carry out respiration effectively.

Restrictive Disorders

In restrictive lung disease, expansion of the lungs is limited. Static lung volumes are diminished as a result of decreased lung or thoracic compliance. Restrictive pulmonary diseases are either intrinsic processes primarily affecting the lung parenchyma, or processes extrinsic to the lung such as obesity, kyphoscoliosis, chest trauma, and the muscular dystrophies. Intrinsic disorders result from chronic conditions (sarcoidosis, pulmonary fibrosis, and alveolar proteinosis) and are less common. Patients with a restrictive disorder may demonstrate respiratory alkalosis caused by a compensatory increase in respiratory rate to offset diminished lung volumes. When the increased respiratory rate no longer adequately compensates for the diminished lung volumes, hypoxemia occurs. Table 26-1 compares pulmonary function test results between restrictive and obstructive diseases. Individuals with restrictive disorders exhibit some degree of dyspnea, but they may become dyspneic only on exertion. As the restrictive disease progresses, however, they also become dyspneic at rest. In addition, individuals with restrictive disorders often have a dry, hacking cough. Table 26-2 lists major disorders that result in primarily restrictive ventilatory defects.

Pulmonary Vascular Disorders

Pulmonary vascular disorders include any process that results in the narrowing or occlusion of pulmonary blood vessels. In pulmonary vascular disease, efficiency of pulmonary respiration is compromised, usually resulting in hypoxemia. Clinically, patients have dyspnea, increased respiratory frequency, digital clubbing, atelectasis, and chest pain. Pulmonary vascular disease may result from primary pulmonary hypertension, circulatory problems, or lung disease. This chapter discusses pulmonary vascular disease related to pulmonary emboli and pulmonary infarction.

Obstructive Disorders

Obstructive lung disease includes any process that limits airflow on expiration. Both lung compliance (lung expansibility) and airway resistance are increased. These pathophysiologic changes alter the ability to move air out of the lungs, which results in characteristic changes in both static and dynamic lung volume measurement (see Table 26-1). Clinically, persons with obstructive lung disease may exhibit a prolonged expiration time, increased anteroposterior diameter of the thorax, and hyperresonance on percussion. Persons with pulmonary disorders characterized by the preceding description have been identified as having chronic obstructive pulmonary disease (COPD), which is discussed in Chapter 27.

TABLE 26-1 COMPARISON OF PULMONARY FUNCTION TEST RESULTS IN RESTRICTIVE AND OBSTRUCTIVE DISEASE

Test	Restrictive	Obstructive
FVC	Decreased	Decreased or normal
RV	Decreased	Increased
TLC	Decreased	Normal or increased
RV/TLC	Normal or increased	Significantly increased
FEV_1/ FVC	Normal or increased	Decreased
FEV_3/FVC	Normal or increased	Decreased

FVC, Forced vital capacity; *RV,* residual volume; *TLC,* total lung capacity; *FEV,* forced expiratory volume (in 1, 3 sec).

TABLE 26-2 RESTRICTIVE PULMONARY DISEASES

Type of Disorder	Disease Example
Parenchymal inflammation	Pneumonia, acute respiratory distress syndrome
Space-occupying lesion	Benign or malignant tumor
Diffuse pulmonary disease	Silicosis, fibrosis
Pleural disease	Pleural effusion
Lung collapse	Pneumothorax, atelectasis
Resectional surgery	Pneumonectomy
Neuromuscular disorder	Poliomyelitis, Guillain-Barré syndrome
Central nervous system depression	Narcotic overdose, cerebral edema

Restrictive Lung Disorders

Infectious Diseases

Acute Bronchitis

Etiology and Epidemiology. Bronchitis can be acute or chronic. (Chronic bronchitis is discussed in Chapter 27.) Acute inflammation of the conductive airways is common, especially among children and older adults. Acute bronchitis is an inflammation of the bronchi and usually the trachea; thus the more correct term for this illness is *tracheobronchitis.* Although acute bronchitis occurs most often in persons with chronic lung disease, it also occurs as an extension of an upper respiratory tract infection in persons without underlying lung disease and is therefore communicable. It may also be caused by physical or chemical agents such as dust, smoke, or volatile fumes. As air pollution increases, the incidence of acute bronchitis increases. It has a marked seasonal incidence that peaks in late winter or spring.[38] Acute bronchitis is typically viral, but bacterial pathogens such as *Streptococcus pneumoniae* and *Haemophilus influenzae* may also cause bronchitis either as a primary or a secondary infection (Box 26-1).

Pathophysiology. In the healthy person the defense mechanisms of the respiratory tract usually destroy or remove inhaled microbes. When defenses are weakened, however, the potentially pathogenic bacteria that normally reside in the nose and pharynx may colonize the mucosa of the trachea and bronchi. As part of the inflammatory process, blood flow to the affected area increases, causing an increase in pulmonary secretions. A painful cough with sputum production, low-grade fever, and malaise are common symptoms. The patient may have pain beneath the sternum caused by inflammation of the tracheal wall. Symptoms usually last 1 to 2 weeks but may continue for 3 to 4 weeks. Rhonchi and

Box 26-1 Infectious Causes of Acute Bronchitis

Viruses	Bacteria
Rhinovirus	*Streptococcus pneumoniae*
Adenovirus	*Haemophilus influenzae*
Influenza A and B	*Moraxella catarrhalis*
Parainfluenza virus	*Bordetella pertussis*
Respiratory syncytial virus	*Mycoplasma pneumoniae*
	Chlamydia pneumoniae (TWAR strain)

wheezes are heard on chest examination. If symptoms worsen and the patient has high fever, shortness of breath, pleuritic chest pain (pain on inspiration), rapid respirations, and rales (crackles) or signs of consolidation on physical examination of the chest, pneumonia is suspected.

Collaborative Care Management. Diagnosis is based on the history and symptoms. Most instances of acute bronchitis are caused by viruses and resolve spontaneously within 1 to 2 weeks; only a small proportion becomes complicated by bacterial superinfections. Bacterial cultures of sputum are of limited use, and viral cultures are unnecessary. Chest x-ray findings are usually normal.[38]

Acute bronchitis is often preceded by symptoms of an upper respiratory tract infection: coryza, malaise, chills, mild fever, back and muscle pain, and sore throat. Treatment of acute bronchitis is mainly symptomatic and supportive. It depends on the patient's age and the presence of other complicating illnesses. Frequently all that is needed is reassurance; increased fluid intake to 2 to 3 L/day to thin secretions; and mild analgesic-antipyretic therapy with aspirin, acetaminophen, or ibuprofen every 4 to 6 hours for comfort. If nocturnal cough prevents sleep, codeine or dextromethorphan may be prescribed. Over-the-counter cough and cold remedies are not recommended, since they may dehydrate bronchial secretions and make them more difficult to remove. For patients with wheezing or other respiratory discomfort, a bronchoactive medication such as an inhaled beta$_2$-agonist is often prescribed. Unless there is evidence of bacterial infection, antibiotics are avoided to reduce the development of antibiotic resistance, which is particularly problematic in older adults.[41] During known epidemics of influenza A virus, amantadine or rimantadine may be given early in the course of the disease to minimize symptoms.[19] All patients are urged to avoid environmental tobacco smoke, which is further irritating to the respiratory tract, and those who smoke are urged to quit.

Nursing care is supportive and is directed toward helping the patient with prescribed therapy and avoidance of future infection. Patient teaching is an important component of patient care (see Patient/Family Teaching box).

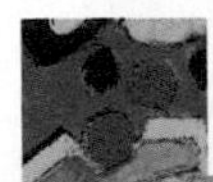

PATIENT/FAMILY TEACHING

The Patient With Tracheobronchitis

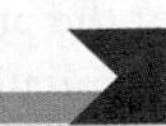

The nurse should teach the patient to cough effectively using the "huff cough" technique so airway mucus is expelled:

- Have the patient inspire deeply, hold the breath a few seconds, and cough two or three times with the mouth open and without taking another breath.
- Have the patient repeat this several times, then rest.

This type of controlled cough and forced expiration technique is believed to work because the cleansing action of cough in the large airways takes place primarily during the first one or two coughs of the cough sequence. The sequential nature of the coughing promotes the movement of mucus along the pulmonary tree from the lower airways to the mouth for expectoration.

The nurse should also explain the lack of benefit of antibiotic treatment and the risks of unnecessary antibiotic therapy. If a bronchoactive medication is ordered, the nurse teaches the patient how to use an inhaler with a spacer.

Pneumonia

Etiology and Epidemiology. Pneumonia is an acute inflammation of lung tissue. It can result from infectious agents being inhaled or transported to the lungs via the bloodstream. It can also be due to noxious fumes or radiation treatment. Pneumonia is the most common cause of death from infectious disease in the United States. The incidence of pneumonia is increasing with an aging population and with the relative underutilization of respiratory vaccines in the older adults.[10] Most types of pneumonia are communicable, with the mode of transmission depending on the infecting organism. There have been significant changes in pathogens causing bacterial pneumonia and dramatic shifts in antimicrobial resistance patterns. Pathogen resistance has led to the development of many new antimicrobial agents, including beta-lactamase inhibitors, fluoroquinolones, macrolides, and azalides.[22]

Pneumonia is classified as community-acquired pneumonia (CAP) or hospital-acquired pneumonia (HAP), depending on where the infection was acquired. With the rise in the elderly population, an increasingly important form of CAP is nursing home–acquired pneumonia (NHAP). HAP, also referred to as nosocomial pneumonia, includes the subset of ventilator-associated pneumonia (VAP).[42]

Pathophysiology. Pneumonia results in inflammation of lung tissue. Depending on the pathogen and the host's physical status, the inflammatory process may involve different anatomic areas of the lung parenchyma and the pleurae.

COMPLICATIONS. With the advent of antibiotics and better diagnostic measures such as x-ray procedures, complications during or after pneumonia are rare in otherwise healthy persons. Atelectasis, delayed resolution, lung abscess, **pleural effusion** (fluid in the pleural cavity), empyema, pericarditis, meningitis, and relapse were common complications in the past. The patient must understand the importance of strict adherence to the prescribed medical treatment. Careful and accurate observation and sufficient time for convalescence also help ensure that the average patient has a smooth recovery. Older adults and those with a chronic illness are likely to have a relatively long course of convalescence from pneumonia and are at higher risk for complications.

Community-Acquired Pneumonia. CAP is an acute infection of the pulmonary parenchyma that occurs in patients who are not hospitalized or residing in a long-term care facility for 14 days before the onset of illness; it is associated with symptoms of lower respiratory tract disease and accompanied by new infiltrates on x-ray or auscultatory findings consistent with pneumonia.[38]

CAP is a common problem and is associated with significant morbidity and mortality. It may affect healthy individuals, but more than 70% of cases occur in persons with preexisting disease (e.g., COPD, coronary artery disease, diabetes mellitus, malignancy, and alcohol abuse) or impaired defenses. The mortality rate for persons with CAP ranges from less than 1% among outpatients to 30% among those requiring hospitalization.[38] The incidence of specific pathogens varies among patient populations and is dictated by host and environmental factors. *S. pneumoniae* is the most common identifiable cause of pneumonia and the most frequent cause of fatal CAP[10]; *Mycoplasma pneumoniae* primarily affects adolescents and young adults, but it can cause severe pneumonia in older adults and debilitated persons. *H. influenzae* and aerobic gram-negative bacteria have increased as a cause and are responsible for 12% of cases of CAP. *Legionella pneumoniae* accounts for about 6% of cases of CAP but is associated with a disproportionately high rate of respiratory failure and death.[8]

CAP is heralded by the symptoms of fever, rigors, sweats, new cough with or without sputum, a change in the color of the sputum, chest discomfort, and the onset of dyspnea.

NHAP, a form of CAP, is a leading cause of morbidity, hospitalization, and death among older adults living in nursing homes. The annual Medicare expenditures for acute hospitalization exceed $3.5 billion, and as many as 28% of Medicare beneficiaries admitted with pneumonia come from skilled nursing facilities.[8] NHAP is defined as a new radiologic pulmonary infiltrate not solely attributable to heart failure, cancer, or pulmonary embolus, with at least one major criterion or two minor criteria. Major criteria are cough, sputum production, and fever; minor criteria are dyspnea, pleuritic chest pain, altered mental status, pulmonary consolidation, and increased white blood cell (WBC) counts.

Hospital-Acquired Pneumonia. HAP includes any case of pneumonia that starts 48 hours or more after hospital admission. It is the second most common nosocomial infection in the United States and the leading cause of death from nosocomial infections. Nearly 1% of patients admitted to the hospital develop pneumonia, and nearly one third of these die. Up to 60% of patients in intensive care units (ICUs) develop pneumonia.[7] The mortality rate is high because of coexisting diseases and the prevalence of gram-negative bacteria that are resistant to many antibiotics. The majority of HAP infections are caused by gram-negative aerobes; organisms commonly associated with HAP are *Pseudomonas aeruginosa, Enterobacter* species, *Klebsiella pneumoniae, Acinetobacter* species, and methicillin-resistant *Staphylococcus aureus.*[31] Risk factors for HAP are summarized in the Risk Factors box.

HAP occurs with aspiration of endogenous oropharyngeal bacteria into the lower respiratory tract. Oropharyngeal and tracheal colonization with gram-negative bacteria often occurs when patients have impaired defenses or serious underlying disease. Colonization of the stomach may lead to subsequent colonization of the airway and lower respiratory tract. Agents that increase gastric pH (e.g., antacids, H_2 antagonists) are associated with higher rates of nosocomial pneumonia in critically ill patients undergoing mechanical ventilation.

Intubation and mechanical ventilation greatly increase the risk of bacterial pneumonia. VAP is pneumonia in a patient treated with mechanical ventilation when pneumonia is neither present nor developing at the time of intubation. It is a serious problem that has an overall mortality rate of 54% to 71%, adds an additional 5 to 7 days to the hospital stay of surviving patients, and adds billions of dollars to the nation's health care costs.[31] Aspiration of bacteria from the oropharynx, leakage of contaminated secretions around the endotracheal tube, patient position, and cross-contamination from respiratory equipment and health care providers are important factors in the development of VAP.

Environmental factors implicated in the transmission of bacteria are contaminated ventilator tubing and inadequate hand washing by medical staff. Studies on hand washing repeatedly demonstrate lack of compliance with recommendations for prevention of infection. Nosocomial pneumonia can also be spread hematogenously to the lung from infections in wounds, soft tissue, or the urinary tract.

Risk Factors

Hospital-Acquired Pneumonia

- Treatment in an intensive care unit (ICU)
- Mechanical ventilation (Those requiring 48 hours or more of ventilation in an ICU have a 10% to 20% chance of developing pneumonia.)
- Endotracheal intubation or tracheostomy
- Recent surgery
- Debilitation or malnutrition
- Invasive devices
- Neuromuscular disease
- Depressed level of alertness
- Aspiration
- Antacid use
- Age 60 years or older
- Prolonged hospital stay
- Any serious underlying disease

Viral Pneumonia. Viruses cause approximately 8% of cases of pneumonia in hospitalized adults. The incidence of viral infection as a cause of pneumonia is underestimated because of the insensitivity of viral diagnostic methods. The importance of the different viruses as causes of pneumonia varies with the season and the age distribution of the population. Respiratory synctial virus is an increasingly recognized cause of pneumonia, but during outbreaks, influenza virus accounts for more than 50% of cases in adults. Some cases of viral pneumonia have a rapid, relentless, and fatal course with generalized alveolar and interstitial infiltrates, development of acute respiratory distress syndrome, and progressive respiratory failure.[40]

Collaborative Care Management. Approximately 80% of patients with CAP are treated as outpatients.[21] Usually individuals ages 55 years and younger who are in good health, without a serious preexisting condition such as COPD, diabetes, congestive heart failure, renal failure, liver disease, cerebrovascular accident, malignancy, or debilitation, can be treated on an outpatient basis as long as they respond well to oral therapy. Persons who develop systemic toxicity, debilitation, respiratory failure, or hypoxemia are usually hospitalized. Administration of parenteral antibiotics for 2 to 3 days often improves these patients' conditions sufficiently so that oral antibiotics can be substituted and treatment continued on an outpatient basis. Guidelines for the treatment of NHAP are being developed on the basis of initial studies. Initial indications are that a significant number of nursing home residents with pneumonia can be treated successfully with oral antibiotics in the nursing home.[21]

DIAGNOSTIC TESTS. Although the majority of patients with CAP are not hospitalized, the American Thoracic Society recommends that all patients with CAP be admitted to have several diagnostic tests (Table 26-3).

MEDICATIONS. The choice of initial therapy for CAP affects survival. The best approach is to give the right antibiotic at the right time—within 8 hours or less and within 4 hours if possible. Unless the clinical findings and Gram stain are classic for a specific organism, initial treatment of CAP is with a broad-spectrum antimicrobial. Therapy is modified when the results of culture and sensitivity are received.[11]

HAP (including VAP), with its high mortality rate, requires aggressive therapy. Therapy is often empiric and uses combinations of broad-spectrum antibiotics. Many experts recommend treatment with a third-generation cephalosporin or an anti-*Pseudomonas* penicillin-beta-lactamase inhibitor combined with an aminoglycoside. HAP caused by methicillin-resistant *S. aureus* is treated with vancomycin.[11]

Bronchoactive medications delivered as inhaled aerosols directly to the respiratory tract may be ordered to decrease respiratory symptoms of rhonchi and wheezing. The success of this therapy, which minimizes systemic drug exposure and side effects, depends on the effective use of aerosol delivery devices. The devices most commonly used to administer orally or nasally inhaled aerosols are the metered-dose inhaler (MDI) with or without a reservoir (holding chamber or spacer) device, the small-volume nebulizer, and the dry-powder inhaler (DPI).

With spontaneous breathing, the inhaled aerosol medication is distributed to both the lungs and the stomach because the medication is deposited in the oropharynx. The therapeutic effect is achieved by absorption in the airway; the systemic effects are caused by absorption in the airways and gastrointestinal tract. Studies have repeatedly demonstrated that only about 15% of the dose is delivered by MDI, DPI, or nebulizer. Patient technique may significantly decrease the amount of delivered dose. Nursing plays a major role in teaching and assessing the correct use of aerosol therapy devices (Figure 26-1).

A spacer is a molded plastic reservoir that can be fitted onto an inhaler to deliver medication more safely and effectively. This device makes it unnecessary to coordinate breathing as carefully as with the standard inhaler, and thus patients are medicated more effectively. With enhanced delivery of medication to the lungs, it may be possible to reduce the number and volume of puffs required, thereby reducing the cost of medication. Once the medication is in the spacer, the patient takes several breaths, inhaling each time from the spacer, to receive the entire dose. Inhalers with spacers can be used to deliver most bronchoactive medications.

TREATMENTS. Oxygen is given to maintain an adequate saturation level. Turning, coughing, and deep breathing to promote airway clearance and effective respiration are performed regularly.

DIET. A high-calorie, high-protein diet with frequent small feedings is usually prescribed.

HEALTH PROMOTION AND PREVENTION. Patients need to be instructed how to prevent recurrent episodes of pneumonia. Teaching the patient about the transmission of the disease and proper handling of secretions is important. Good hand washing is always a key element in the prevention process. High-risk adults and older adults should be informed about the vaccinations recommended.

▶ ARE YOU READY?

Which of the following poses the greatest risk for development of hospital-acquired pneumonia?

1. Endotracheal intubation
2. Enteral feeding
3. Oxygen therapy via nasal cannula
4. Use of oral thermometer

TABLE 26-3 PNEUMONIA: DIAGNOSTIC TESTS AND PURPOSES

Test	Purpose
Chest x-ray	Determine diagnosis; see extent of disease; demonstrate consolidation and distribution of lung involvement; document pleural effusion
Blood gases	Determine oxygenation status and respiratory support needs
Complete blood count	Determine diagnosis; check hemoglobin; observe for infection
Pulse oximetry	Determine oxygenation status
Cold agglutinins and complement fixation studies	Determine if cause is a virus
Thoracentesis	Obtain pleural fluid specimen for analysis if pleural effusion is present

NOTE: Routine sputum testing in not recommended because of low diagnostic yield and results that do not significantly contribute to patient management.

How To Use Your Metered-Dose Inhaler the Right Way

Using an inhaler seems simple, but most patients do not use it the right way. When you use your inhaler the wrong way, less medicine gets to your lungs. (Your doctor may give you other types of inhalers.)

For the next 2 weeks, read these steps aloud as you do them or ask someone to read them to you. Ask your doctor or nurse to check how well you are using your inhaler.

Use your inhaler in one of the three ways pictured below (**A** or **B** are best, but **C** can be used if you have trouble with **A** and **B**).

Steps for Using Your Inhaler

Getting ready
1. Take off the cap and shake the inhaler.
2. Breathe out all the way.
3. Hold your inhaler the way your doctor said (A, B, or C below).

Breathe in slowly
4. As you start breathing in **slowly** through your mouth, press down on the inhaler **one** time. (If you use a holding chamber, first press down on the inhaler. Within 5 sec, begin to breathe in slowly.)
5. Keep breathing in **slowly**, as deeply as you can.

Hold your breath
6. Hold your breath as you count to 10 slowly, if you can.
7. For inhaled quick-relief medicine (β_2-agonists), wait about 1 min between puffs. There is no need to wait between puffs for other medicines.

A. Hold inhaler 1 to 2 inches in front of your mouth (about the width of two fingers).

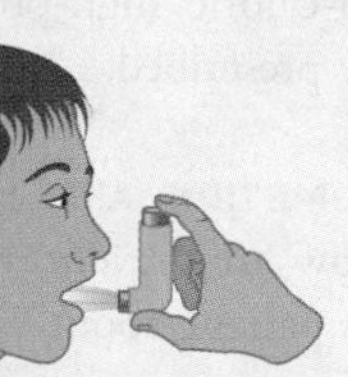

B. Use a spacer/holding chamber. These come in many shapes and can be useful to any patient.

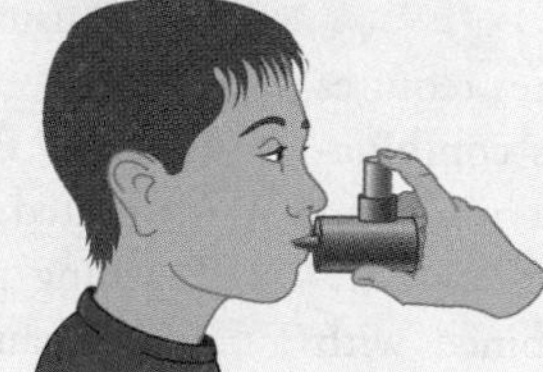

C. Put the inhaler in your mouth. Do not use for steroids.

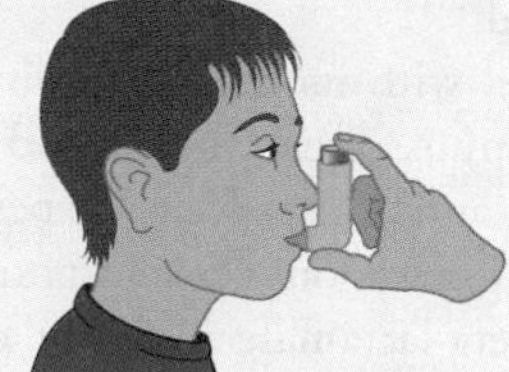

Clean Your Inhaler as Needed

Look at the hole where the medicine sprays out from your inhaler. If you see "powder" in or around the hole, clean the inhaler. Remove the metal canister from the L-shaped plastic mouthpiece. Rinse only the mouthpiece and cap in warm water. Let them dry overnight. In the morning, put the canister back inside. Put the cap on.

Know When to Replace Your Inhaler

For medicines you take each day (an example):
Say your new canister has 200 puffs (number of puffs is listed on canister) and you are told to take 8 puffs per day.

$$\text{8 puffs per day}\ \overline{)\ \text{200 puffs in canister}}\quad = \text{25 days}$$

So this canister will last 25 days. If you started using this inhaler on May 1, replace it on or before May 25.

You can write the date on your canister.

For quick-relief medicine take as needed and count each puff.

Do not put your canister in water to see if it is empty. This does not work.

Figure 26-1 How to use a metered-dose inhaler.

Nursing Management *of the Patient with Pneumonia*

Assessment

Health History. Assess for:

- History and character of onset and duration of cough, fever, chills, chest pain, sputum production (amount, color, consistency)
- Self-care modalities used to treat symptoms
- History of exposure to persons with upper respiratory tract infection or pulmonary irritants
- History of recent antibiotic use (Bacterial identification may be obscured by prior antibiotic use.)
- Patient's ability to maintain activities of daily living (ADLs)

Physical Examination. Assess for:

- Elevated temperature, either significant (102.2° to 104° F [39° to 40° C]) or low grade
- Tachycardia and tachypnea

- Accessory muscle retraction, central cyanosis, respiratory grunting on expiration, and restricted chest movement
- Decreased expansion on the affected side of the chest and increased tactile fremitus using palpation
- Dullness over areas of consolidation using percussion
- Bronchial breath sounds, inspiratory crackles (rales), decreased vocal fremitus caused by pleural effusion, and egophony caused by consolidation

NURSING DIAGNOSES, OUTCOMES, AND INTERVENTIONS

Nursing Diagnosis: Ineffective Airway Clearance

OUTCOMES. Common examples of expected outcomes for the patient with a diagnosis of *ineffective airway clearance* are:
Patient will:

- Demonstrate effective cough with expectoration (both cough and sputum production should decrease within 72 hours of treatment initiation).
- Return to prepneumonia status.

NURSING INTERVENTIONS. The nurse should ensure adequate fluid intake to thin secretions and enable the patient to expectorate them easily, since dehydration results in thick, tenacious secretions. If the patient does not have cardiovascular disease requiring fluid restriction, a fluid intake of 3 to 4 L/day should be provided. The best liquefying agent is water. The nurse should change the patient's position frequently to assist in mobilizing secretions. Also the nurse should assist with nebulizer therapy and support effective coughing by teaching the proper technique and splinting the chest if needed because of muscle soreness. The patient who is unable to clear his or her own airway should be suctioned using sterile technique.

The nurse should administer bronchoactive medications as ordered and monitor the patient for side effects and response to therapy.

RELATED NIC INTERVENTIONS. Airway Management, Cough Enhancement, Positioning, Respiratory Monitoring

Nursing Diagnosis: Impaired Gas Exchange

OUTCOMES. A common example of expected outcomes for the patient with a diagnosis of *impaired gas exchange* is:
Patient will:

- Demonstrate improved ventilation and adequate oxygenation of tissues, with return of arterial blood gas (ABG) results to baseline.

NURSING INTERVENTIONS. The nurse helps the patient breathe deeply and expand the chest to increase ventilation. The patient is placed in a position that facilitates breathing, typically upright or semiupright. A pillow placed lengthwise at the patient's back provides support and thrusts the thorax slightly forward, allowing freer use of the diaphragm. The patient who must be upright to breathe may find it restful to put the head and arms on a pillow placed on an overbed table or to sit up in a big armchair with a footrest to prevent dependent edema.

Oxygen by mask or cannula (Figures 26-2 and 26-3) is usually ordered when the partial pressure of oxygen (PaO_2) is less than 60 mm Hg. When supplemental oxygen is necessary, it may be administered by nasal prongs or by mask, depending on the patient's condition and the concentration of oxygen required. The nurse needs to be familiar with the various devices used to administer oxygen and must check the equipment frequently to ensure it is working properly. Table 26-4 compares oxygen delivery systems. Oxygen therapy is administered at the lowest concentration needed to achieve desired ABG values or pulse oximetry saturations.

The nurse should monitor the patient for signs of hypoxemia. The patient with hypoxemia may not be breathless or cyanotic because cyanosis does not occur until there is 5 g/dl or more of deoxygenated hemoglobin. In persons with anemia, all the available heme is completely saturated with oxygen, and thus these persons are never cyanotic, even though they may be hypoxemic. Thus an increase in the pulse rate or restlessness may be the first indication of hypoxemia. Patients receiving oxygen therapy should also be monitored with ABG studies and pulse oximetry.

RELATED NIC INTERVENTIONS. Airway Management, Oxygen Therapy, Respiratory Monitoring

Nursing Diagnosis: Activity Intolerance

OUTCOMES. A common example of expected outcomes for the patient with a diagnosis of *activity intolerance* is:
Patient will:

- Require minimal assistance with ADLs.

NURSING INTERVENTIONS. Activities need to be spaced to prevent fatigue and **respiratory distress**. The nurse should monitor

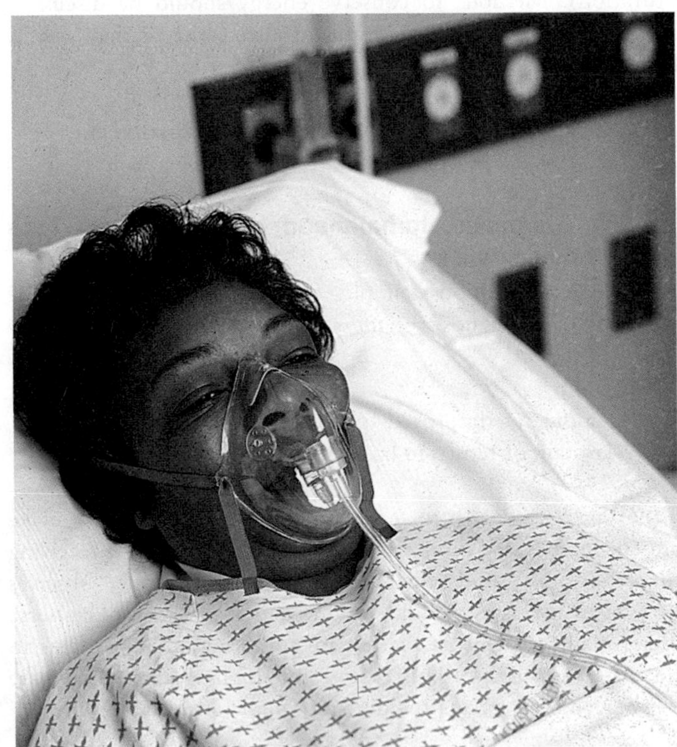

Figure 26-2 Simple oxygen mask.

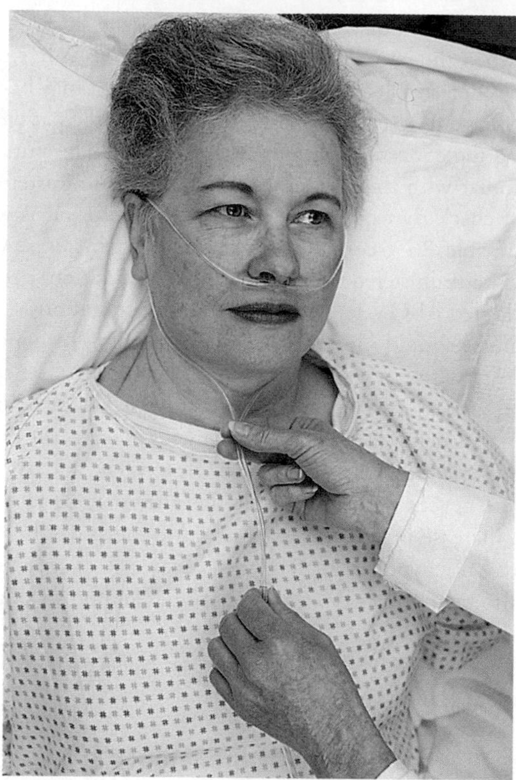

Figure 26-3 Nasal cannula.

response to physical activity and adjust activities to prevent overexertion. Activity levels are increased gradually on the basis of patient response. The nurse must carefully assess the need for supplemental oxygen with increased activity (based on oxygen saturation). Methods to conserve energy should be discussed. Other patient teaching points are listed the Patient/Family Teaching box.

Related NIC Interventions. Energy Management, Self-Care Assistance

Nursing Diagnosis: Imbalanced Nutrition: Less Than Body Requirements

Outcomes. Common examples of expected outcomes for the patient with a diagnosis of *imbalanced nutrition: less than body requirements* are:

Patient will:

- Demonstrate improved appetite.
- Maintain or return to baseline weight.

Nursing Interventions. The nurse monitors total daily intake and encourages oral fluids as permitted. If the patient is receiving intravenous (IV) fluids, the rate is monitored. The nurse observes the patient for signs of fluid volume deficit or excess. The nurse offers small, frequent meals that are appealing and appetizing to the patient. High-carbohydrate and high-protein foods are encouraged. The nurse provides oral care before and after meals.

Related NIC Interventions. Nutrition Management, Nutritional Counseling, Nutritional Monitoring

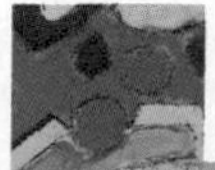

Patient/Family Teaching
The Patient With Pneumonia

The major teaching emphasis for patients with pneumonia is prevention of complications and recurring episodes. The nurse should:

- Assess the patient's understanding of pneumonia by asking questions such as, "How is pneumonia transmitted?" and "What are the risk factors?"
- Teach proper handling of secretions, including the importance of covering the nose and mouth with tissue when coughing or sneezing; discarding tissues in a paper or plastic bag for disposal; expectorating into an appropriate container; and washing the hands after coughing, sneezing, and expectorating.
- Explain the importance of follow-up care and the need for vaccinations to prevent respiratory infections.
- Explain that persons at risk for developing complications of influenza should receive an annual vaccine unless they are allergic to eggs or egg products or have had a previous reaction to vaccine.
- Tell the patient that the pneumonia polysaccharide vaccine is given only every 3 to 5 years. A booster vaccination is recommended 5 years after initial vaccination in all patients originally immunized before the age of 65.
- Teach the patient how to conserve energy and maintain good nutrition.

Evaluation

To evaluate the effectiveness of nursing interventions, compare patient behaviors with those stated in the expected patient outcomes.

Related NOC Outcomes. Activity Tolerance, Nutritional Status: Energy, Nutritional Status: Food & Fluid Intake, Respiratory Status: Gas Exchange, Respiratory Status: Ventilation, Vital Signs

Gerontologic Considerations

Respiratory tract infections, especially pneumonia, are important causes of disease and death in older adults. Risk factors for pneumonia in older adults include alcoholism, asthma, immunosuppressive therapy, chronic lung disease, heart disease, institutionalization, and age greater than 70 years. Nurses working with older persons need to be aware of their vulnerability to pneumonia, particularly because the atypical presentation in older patients may delay diagnosis and treatment. In these patients the usual symptoms and signs (cough, crackles, rhonchi, fever, chills, rigors, chest pain, and chest consolidation) may be absent. Instead they may have confusion; weakness; lethargy; failure to thrive; anorexia; abdominal pain; tachypnea; and episodes of falling, incontinence, delirium, or headache. Interventions are directed toward preventing pneumonia by teaching older adults to receive yearly vaccinations for influenza and pneumonia as indicated.

Older adults discharged from the hospital after being admitted with CAP who are otherwise in fairly good health still require 4 to 6 weeks before they feel completely well. Recuperation requires extra rest and gradual resumption of activities, including return to

TABLE 26-4 COMPARISON OF OXYGEN DELIVERY SYSTEMS

Delivery System	Indications	Concentration	Flow Rate	Considerations
LOW FLOW				
Nasal cannula	Patient with spontaneous respirations and oxygen requirements of less than 50%	32%-36%	2-6 L/min with no respiratory distress; 5-6 L/min with onset of respiratory distress	Oxygen concentration increases about 4% for each increase of 1 L/min. Efficacy is questionable in patients who are mouth breathing.
Simple face mask	Patient with spontaneous respirations	35%-60%	6-8 L/min	Flow should be *at least* 6 L/min to prevent accumulation and rebreathing of expired carbon dioxide. Claustrophobic patient may not tolerate this. Effective for patients who are mouth breathing.
Partial rebreather face mask	Patient with spontaneous respirations and oxygen requirements greater than 50%	65%-75%	6-10 L/min	Flow rates should be high enough to ensure reservoir bag remains inflated during inspiration *and* expiration.
Nonrebreather face mask	Spontaneously breathing patient with profound hypoxia or oxygen requirement	85%-95%	8-12 L/min	Flow rates should be high enough to ensure reservoir bag remains inflated during inspiration *and* expiration.
HIGH FLOW				
Venturi mask	Patient with spontaneous respirations	24%-50%	Varies (consult manufacturer's directions)	This works well for patients who require delivery of precise oxygen concentrations. This is prescribed by concentration, not flow rate.
POSITIVE PRESSURE				
One-way valve pocket mask	Patient requiring assistance or control of ventilation	50%-55% (with oxygen supplement)	10-15 L/min	Mask prevents direct contact between health care provider and patient. It is easier to use and obtain adequate tidal volumes than bag-valve mask. It should be used with oropharyngeal or nasopharyngeal airway in place to prevent gastric distention.
Bag-valve mask	Patient requiring assistance or control of ventilation	Approaching 100% with reservoir; 45%-50% without reservoir	10-15 L/min	Mask prevents direct contact between health care provider and patient. It should be used with oropharyngeal or nasopharyngeal airway in place to prevent gastric distention. It is difficult to use; inexperienced operators may not deliver adequate tidal volumes. This is short-term device of choice after endotracheal intubation.

From Somerson SJ et al: Mastering emergency airway management, *Am J Nurs* 96(5):25, 1996.

work. An adequate, balanced diet is essential, as are rest periods and adequate sleep at night.

Those with HAP have an even more protracted period of recovery because their pneumonia may be superimposed on a chronic condition such as COPD. Their activities are likely to be more restricted because of chronic shortness of breath and resultant fatigue.

Ideally older persons living alone should have someone in the home at least part of each day to assist with ADLs such as bathing, dressing, and meal preparation. The nurse or a social worker should make a referral to a home health agency before patients are discharged, unless they have a significant other to assist with these activities. These patients also need to be monitored closely by their health care provider and often need assistance in going to follow-up appointments.

Tuberculosis

In 1900 tuberculosis (TB) was the leading cause of death in the United States. It remained a major cause of death until the introduction of antituberculosis drug therapy in the late 1940s and early 1950s. Although TB is considered preventable and curable, it demands constant public health surveillance. In some states TB is still on the rise, particularly among specific populations such as those with AIDS, immigrants, and individuals of low-economic status.

Etiology and Epidemiology. TB is an infectious disease caused by the bacillus *Mycobacterium tuberculosis* or the tubercle bacillus, an acid-fast organism. The World Health Organization (WHO) estimates that approximately one third of the world's population is infected with *M. tuberculosis.*[48] This estimate has held steady for almost a decade while the number of diagnosed cases continues to increase. TB is responsible for more deaths of young and middle-aged adults than any other disease except AIDS. Each year there are approximately 8 million new TB cases and 3 million deaths attributed to TB.[26] The highest rates occur in sub-Saharan Africa and South Asia. The lowest rates are reported in Western Europe and North America. Targets for TB control established recently by the World Health Assembly include cure of 85% of the sputum smear–positive TB cases detected and detection of 70% of the estimated new sputum smear–positive TB cases.[49]

In the United States the epidemic of infection with the human immunodeficiency virus (HIV) has had a major impact on the incidence of TB. The United States experienced a resurgence of TB from 1986 to 1992 as a result of deteriorating public health services, increased incidence of HIV, increased international travel, and development of disease among immigrants who arrived with latent disease. In response, TB control programs enhanced efforts to promptly identify persons with active TB and initiate and complete appropriate therapy. In 2002 the incidence rate in the United States was 5.2 per 100,000, the ninth year with decreased incidence and the lowest rate since surveillance began in 1953. The decrease is true, however, only among individuals born in the United States. Foreign-born U.S. residents account for 51% of the cases of TB.[6]

TB continues to disproportionately affect poor, homeless, and HIV-infected persons. Cities with the highest number of persons positive for HIV, especially drug abusers, also have the highest number of TB cases. These cities more likely have a large number of immigrants, many of whom come from countries in which TB is endemic. A major concern is that many persons with HIV are infected with TB organisms resistant to most chemotherapeutic agents used to treat TB. These infected persons pass along their resistant organisms, complicating the treatment of newly infected persons. Because HIV infection is an important risk factor for developing TB among persons who have a positive tuberculin test, the Centers for Disease Control and Prevention (CDC) recommends that all HIV-infected persons be screened for active TB and, if infected, receive appropriate therapy. Also, persons with active TB and all tuberculin-positive persons should be evaluated for HIV infection. The CDC has set a goal of reducing the TB rate to less than 1 per 1 million people by 2010.[25]

Pathophysiology. When an individual with no previous exposure to TB (negative tuberculin reactor) inhales a sufficient number of tubercle bacilli into the alveoli, TB infection occurs. The body's reaction to the tubercle bacilli depends on the individual's susceptibility, the size of the dose, and the virulence of the organisms. Inflammation occurs within the alveoli (parenchyma) of the lungs, and natural body defenses attempt to counteract the infection.

Macrophages ingest the organisms and present the mycobacterial antigens to the T cells. CD4 cells secrete lymphokines that enhance the macrophages' capacity to ingest and kill bacteria. Lymph nodes in the hilar region of the lung become enlarged as they filter drainage from the infected site. The inflammatory process and cellular reaction produce a small, firm, white nodule called the *primary tubercle.* The center of the nodule contains tubercle bacilli. Cells gather around the center, and usually the outer portion becomes fibrosed. Thus blood vessels are compressed, nutrition of the tubercle is impaired, and necrosis occurs at the center. The area becomes walled off by fibrotic tissue, and the center gradually becomes soft and cheesy, a process known as caseation necrosis. This material may become calcified (calcium deposits), or it may liquefy (liquefaction necrosis). The liquefied material may be coughed up, leaving a cavity, or hole, in the parenchyma of the lung. The cavity or cavities are visible on chest x-ray films and result in the diagnosis of cavitary disease.

Most individuals who are exposed to TB and develop a TB infection (confirmed by a positive tuberculin test) do not develop an active case of TB. The only x-ray evidence of their TB infection is a calcified nodule known as a Ghon tubercle. The evidence on x-ray films of enlarged hilar lymph nodes and the Ghon tubercle is referred to as the *primary complex.*

Persons with the primary complex have become sensitized to the tubercle bacillus. This causes an antigen-antibody reaction when the person receives the antigen in the form of a purified protein derivative (PPD) or old tuberculin in a tuberculin test, and so the tuberculin test is said to be positive. This sensitization, once developed, usually remains throughout life unless something compromises the immune response. Evidence suggests that most persons who have a positive tuberculin reaction and take isoniazid (INH) prophylactically convert from a positive to a negative tuberculin test. This protection is believed to last for life. A positive tuberculin test does not mean that one has active TB, however, and nurses should explain this to persons undergoing the test.

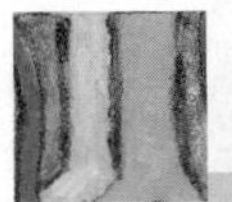

CLINICAL MANIFESTATIONS
Pulmonary Tuberculosis

Constitutional Symptoms	Pulmonary Symptoms
Low-grade fever	Cough productive of a scant amount of mucoid sputum
Pallor	Purulent, blood-stained sputum if cavitation has occurred
Chills	Dyspnea: late in the disease
Night sweats	Chest pain: late in the disease
Easy fatigability	
Anorexia	
Weight loss	

Data from O'Brien RJ, Nunn PP: The need for new drugs against tuberculosis, *Am J Respir Crit Care Med* 163(5):1055–1058, 2001.

TB is unlike other infections. Usually other infections disappear completely when overcome by the body's defenses, leaving no living organisms and generally no signs of infection. *However, persons who have been infected with tubercle bacilli harbor the organism for the remainder of their lives unless they receive prophylactic INH.* Tubercle bacilli remain in the lungs in a dormant, walled-off, or so-called resting, state. When a person is under physical or emotional stress, these bacilli may become active and begin to multiply. The symptoms of TB are presented in the Clinical Manifestations box.

The development of active TB is believed to be caused by defects in T-cell function, macrophage function, or both. However, it is generally accepted that only 1 out of 10 persons with a positive tuberculin test ever develops active TB, and the incidence is expected to be much lower among those who receive preventive therapy with INH. TB that occurs several years after the primary infection is known as *reactivation TB.*

TB is more likely to occur in persons with HIV infection because of progressive depletion and dysfunction of CD4 cells, along with defects in macrophage and monocyte function. Studies have estimated that patients who are coinfected with HIV and TB have higher rates of reactivation TB, higher rates of acute disease, higher rates of extrapulmonary disease, and malabsorption of anti-TB medications. Two mycobacterial organisms are found in persons with AIDS. In developed countries the *Mycobacterium avium-intracellulare* complex (MAC) is the organism found in middle-class AIDS patients who have no history of IV drug use, whereas pulmonary TB caused by *M. tuberculosis* is more common in AIDS patients from developing countries and in persons from inner-city minority populations who have a history of IV drug use.

The WHO has revised the international definitions used in TB control to establish consistent, clear, and relevant definitions of the basic terms used by everyone involved in these efforts[48] (Table 26-5).

Extrapulmonary TB has taken on increased importance because of its extremely high rate of occurrence, usually along with pulmonary TB, in persons with HIV infection. TB is spread to other parts of the body via blood (hematogenously) or lymph (lymphogenously).

Mycobacteria other than tubercle bacilli (MOTT), formerly referred to as atypical acid-fast bacilli, include *Mycobacterium kansasii,* MAC, *Mycobacterium xenopi, Mycobacterium marinum, Mycobacterium fortuitum,* and *Mycobacterium chelonae* (Table 26-6).

TABLE 26-5 CLASSIFICATIONS OF TUBERCULOSIS

Classification	Definition
Tuberculosis (TB) suspect	Any person with symptoms or signs suggestive of TB
Case of TB	Person in whom TB has been bacteriologically confirmed or diagnosed by clinician
Definite case of TB	Person with culture positive for *Mycobacterium tuberculosis* complex
Pulmonary TB, sputum smear positive	Two or more sputum smear examinations positive for TB, or one sputum smear examination positive for acid-fast bacilli (AFB) plus x-ray abnormalities consistent with active pulmonary TB; or one sputum smear positive for AFB plus sputum culture positive for *M. tuberculosis*
Pulmonary TB, sputum smear negative	At least three sputum specimens negative for AFB, x-ray abnormalities consistent with active TB, no response to course of broad-spectrum antibiotics, and decision by clinician to treat with full course of anti-TB chemotherapy
Extrapulmonary TB	TB of organs other than lungs (e.g., pleurae, lymph nodes, abdomen, genitourinary tract, skin, joints and bones, meninges); diagnosis based on 1 culture-positive specimen or histologic or strong clinical evidence consistent with active extrapulmonary TB, followed by decision by clinician to treat with full course of anti-TB chemotherapy
New patient	Person who has never had treatment for TB or who has taken anti-TB drugs for less than 1 month
Relapse	Patient previously treated for TB who has been declared cured or had treatment completed and is diagnosed with bacteriologically positive (smear or culture) TB
Failure	Patient who, while on treatment, is sputum smear positive at 5 months or later during course of treatment
Chronic	Patient who is sputum positive at the end of retreatment regimen

Adapted from World Health Organization: Revised international definitions in TB control, *Int J Tuberc Lung Dis* 5(11):1071-1072, 2001.

TABLE 26-6 MYCOBACTERIA OTHER THAN TUBERCLE BACILLI ASSOCIATED WITH HUMAN DISEASE

Organism	Sites Typically Involved	Suggested Therapy
M. avium-intracellulare complex (MAC)	Lung, disseminated (AIDS)	Amikacin; clofazimine (Lamprene); RIF, EMB, and clarithromycin
M. kansasii	Lung	INH, RIF, and EMB for 12-24 mo
M. xenopi	Lung	Amikacin, clofazimine, RIF, and EMB (perhaps clarithromycin and quinolone)
M. marinum	Skin, soft tissue	RIF, trimethoprim-sulfamethoxazole, or minocycline as single agents
M. fortuitum	Soft tissue, lung, disseminated	Amikacin (parenteral) and cefoxitin or imipenem for 4-6 wk
M. chelonae	Soft tissue	Often resistant to INH and PZA; may respond to 4 or more drugs; surgical excision of localized disease

AIDS, Acquired immunodeficiency syndrome; *EMB,* ethambutol; *INH,* isoniazid; *M., Mycobacterium; PZA,* pyrazinamide; *RIF,* rifampin.

These are strongly acid-fast organisms, but they differ from *M. tuberculosis* on culture. They are being isolated with increasing frequency from immunocompromised patients (persons with HIV infection or AIDS, transplant patients, and patients undergoing antineoplastic chemotherapy). MOTT have been found in soil and water and less commonly in food and are considered opportunistic organisms. MOTT identified in sputum specimens may mean that the person is colonized and does not have invasive disease. MOTT are often isolated from the sputum of patients with pneumoconiosis, chronic bronchitis, COPD, a history of TB, bronchiectasis, and chronic aspiration from esophageal disease.

MAC is the most common bacterial infection in patients with AIDS. It occurs in 30% to 50% of AIDS patients. Patients with MAC have fever, night sweats, weight loss, diarrhea, lymphadenopathy, and anemia. The diagnosis is usually made from isolator blood cultures, bone marrow, lymph node, or liver biopsy. It is also diagnosed by acid-fast smear of stool in patients with disseminated infection.

Multidrug-resistant (MDR) TB has become a major problem in the United States. The emergence of MDR TB means that increased efforts are required to find every TB patient and to ensure that he or she is initially treated with multidrug therapy to prevent further drug resistance. It is also important to protect other patients and health care workers from becoming infected by patients with MDR TB. The problem is especially great in institutions caring for large numbers of patients with HIV, many of whom also have MDR TB.

COMPLICATIONS. The complication of greatest concern is the development of a resistant strain of TB that may be extremely difficult to treat and will require hospitalization while effective drug therapy is sought. HIV may also develop, and it may not be possible to determine which of the two diseases occurred first. Rigorous treatment of both diseases is required, and hospitalization is often necessary.

Collaborative Care Management. The most critical issues in the management of TB involve the recognition of patients at risk and strategies to ensure completion of therapy. The increasing use of directly observed therapy (DOT) and directly observed therapy, short course (DOTS), has been key to controlling efforts in both developed and developing countries. The DOT and DOTS strategies for TB control are based on five[25]:

1. Government commitment to make TB a high-priority program and to provide resources for nationwide coverage
2. Use of sputum smear microscopy for case detection among persons with persistent cough
3. A regular and uninterrupted drug supply for treatment
4. Use of standardized courses of chemotherapy under proper case management conditions, including DOT ("supervised swallowing")
5. A recording and reporting system for monitoring treatment outcomes to reach targets of 85% cure, and training and supervision of health care workers and community volunteers

DIAGNOSTIC TESTS. Diagnostic testing for TB is slow and not ideally sensitive. Tests include the tuberculin skin test (or Mantoux test), sputum smear and culture, and chest x-ray examination. Skin testing is performed to evaluate the body's cell-mediated immune function and to determine the body's sensitivity to infectious agents or allergens. A positive reaction is manifested by induration (thickening or hardening) at the site of the injection within a specified time. Testing for *M. tuberculosis* with tuberculin-PPD is a common type of skin test. A positive reaction indicates that the individual has developed antibodies to the infectious agent, but it does not confirm active disease. A positive skin test reaction must be substantiated with other diagnostic evidence before active disease can be confirmed. Skin controls are sometimes administered to individuals along with the PPD skin test. If the reaction to the control is positive but the reaction to PPD is negative, it is unlikely that the individual has TB. If the reaction to the control is negative, the individual is *anergic* (i.e., has an altered cellular immunity system) and other tests must be performed to make the diagnosis of TB. The nurse should explain the purpose of the test and its procedure (see Guidelines for Safe Practice box).

Sputum smears and cultures are also used in the diagnosis of TB. If microscopic study of a slide prepared from the sputum of an individual reveals tubercle bacilli, the individual is said to have positive sputum, which confirms the diagnosis of TB. However, most persons with TB do not have positive sputum on smear, and a positive sputum culture is necessary to confirm the diagnosis.

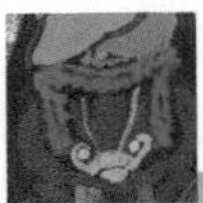

GUIDELINES FOR SAFE PRACTICE

Administering the Mantoux Test

1. Draw up 0.1 ml (or amount specified by manufacturer) of purified protein derivative (PPD), using a tuberculin syringe and ½-inch, 25- to 27-gauge needle.
2. Cleanse the site (ventral forearm) with alcohol and let dry.
3. Keeping skin slightly taut, insert the needle (bevel upward) just beneath the skin surface.
4. Inject the solution, creating a 6 to 10 mm bleb. Do not massage the area after withdrawing the needle.
5. Read the test site with a millimeter ruler 48 to 72 hours after injection. Lightly palpate the site to determine the presence or absence of induration. Measure the largest diameter of induration and record it in millimeters. Also note any erythema at the site. Erythema alone does not indicate a positive result.
6. Interpretation of induration:
   a. 10 mm or more: highly significant for past or present infection
   b. 5 through 9 mm: doubtful reaction; however, retesting may be required
   c. 0 through 4 mm: little or no sensitivity; however, if individual's history indicates exposure, repeat the test in 4 to 6 weeks, since it may take this long for a tuberculin test to convert from negative to positive

Results of chest x-ray films and sputum examinations either rule out the possibility or confirm a diagnosis of TB. Because it is impossible to differentiate between typical bacilli and MOTT by a sputum smear, cultures are obtained on all persons who test positive on the smear. Cultures are also used for antimicrobial susceptibility (sensitivity) studies. Despite the introduction of improved culture media, the tubercle bacillus grows slowly on artificial media, and culture reports are not available for 3 to 6 weeks. Newer approaches to culturing the bacillus are under development.

Blood-streaked sputum in the absence of pronounced coughing may be the first indication to the person that something is wrong. Pathologic changes may have occurred in the lungs, but sputum examination may not show tubercle bacilli. However, if the nodules produced in the parenchyma of the lung become soft in the center and then caseated and liquefied, the liquefied material may break through and empty into the bronchi and be raised as sputum. Cavities in the lung may appear on x-ray films and may be present in more than one lobe of the lung.

MEDICATIONS AND TREATMENTS. Current TB treatment regimens are effective yet problematic, but little research has addressed the development of new tools. When the ideal combination of available drugs is used, treatment requires a minimum of 6 months. Low-income countries aim for 8 months of therapy. Medical regimens for TB are associated with high levels of nonadherence.[39,49]

Accomplishing the goals of therapy requires individualization, often with creative innovations to foster patient compliance. Because of public health considerations related to TB, successful therapy needs to be viewed as the sole responsibility of those supervising patient care. To avoid the emergence of drug-resistant organisms, the Advisory Council for the Elimination of Tuberculosis recommends the following regimen for beginning therapy for TB.

SUSCEPTIBILITY TESTING. All persons from whom *M. tuberculosis* is isolated should have drug susceptibility testing performed on the first isolate. Drug susceptibility testing should also be performed on additional isolates from patients whose cultures fail to convert to negative within 3 months of beginning therapy.

INITIAL REGIMEN. Initial treatment involves four drugs (Table 26-7). During the first 2 months the patient receives INH, rifampin (RIF), pyrazinamide (PZA), and either ethambutol (EMB) or streptomycin (SM), with daily dosing for at least 2 weeks. Rifater combines INH, RIF, and PZA; and Rifamate is a combination of RIF and INH. These new combination medications enhance regimen adherence by decreasing the number of pills per day. When drug susceptibility results are available, the regimen should be altered as needed. Two models for dosing during the remaining period are:

1. The initial daily dosing followed by 6 weeks of twice-weekly dosing of the same four drugs followed by 4 months of twice-weekly dosing of INH and RIF
2. Daily dosing with INH, RIF, PZA, and EMB or SM until drug resistance is ruled out (8 weeks of dosing), followed by 4 months of INH and RIF

In 1998 the U.S. Food and Drug Administration approved the first new drug for pulmonary TB in 25 years. Rifapentine (Prifin) may be taken 2 times per week during the intensive phase and once a week during the continuation phase of treatment. Pyridoxine (vitamin B_6) is administered concurrently.

These first 2 months, when the bacterial burden is greatly reduced and patients become noninfectious, are called the *intensive* or *bactericidal* phase. The *continuation* or *sterilizing* phase of 4 to 6 months is required to eliminate persisting bacilli and minimize the risk of relapse. Sputum cultures should be monitored monthly for patients with positive cultures. Conversion to negative occurs in 85% of patients.[48]

Patients who are homeless or have limited incomes are referred to social services for assistance with food and shelter. To prevent infecting others, some patients should not return to their previous living conditions until their sputum cultures are negative for acid-fast bacilli. Environmental factors are of extreme importance in the transmission of the disease. A nutritionist should meet with the patient and significant others to review the basic food groups, the amount of each nutrient the patient requires, and ways to provide extra calories in small, frequent meals. A community health nurse should meet with the patient and significant other to develop a plan for follow-up care. Increased periods of rest are recommended to promote healing and prevent fatigue.

Health care and correctional facilities that are experiencing outbreaks of TB resistant to INH and RIF or that are resuming treatment of a patient who has been treated for TB in the past may need to begin patient treatment with five or six drugs as initial therapy. As global rates of MDR TB rise, patients are being treated with a combination of second-line drugs that are more expensive, more toxic, and less effective. The most common second-line

TABLE 26-7
COMMON MEDICATIONS *for Tuberculosis*

Drug	Action	Nursing Intervention
Isoniazid (INH)	Penetrates all body tissues and fluids, including cerebrospinal fluid; is bactericidal	Teach patient that alcohol interferes with metabolism of drug and increases risk of hepatic problems, and that antacids may interfere with absorption of drug.
Rifampin (RIF)	Penetrates all body tissues and fluids, including cerebrospinal fluid; is bactericidal	Tell patient that urine and sweat may appear orange temporarily; it may decrease effectiveness of oral contraceptives, anticoagulants, corticosteroids, and other drugs. Instruct patient to consult with health care providers prescribing other medications and alert them to this therapy.
Ethambutol (EMB)	Penetrates body tissues and fluids except cerebrospinal fluid; is bacteriostatic	Tell patient to take with food and have vision checked frequently. Assess lung sounds and character and amount of sputum periodically throughout therapy. Advise patient to report blurring of vision, constriction of visual fields, or changes in color perception immediately. Tell patient that renal and hepatic functions, CBC, and uric acid levels should be monitored routinely throughout therapy.
Pyrazinamide (PZA)	Prevents or reverses neuropathy associated with INH therapy; used in transport of amino acids, formation of neurotransmitters, and synthesis of heme	Instruct patient to take medication as directed. If a dose is missed, it may be omitted because an extended time is required to become deficient in vitamin B6. The best source of vitamins is a well-balanced diet with foods high in vitamin B_6 (bananas, whole-grain cereals, potatoes, lima beans, and meats). Tell patients taking vitamin supplements not to exceed the RDA.
Streptomycin (SM)	Inhibits protein synthesis in bacteria; has poor penetration of body tissues; is bactericidal	Monitor kidney function of patient monthly and check vestibular and general hearing monthly.

CBC, Complete blood count; *RDA,* recommended daily allowance.

drugs include *p*-aminosalicylic acid (PAS), cycloserine, clofazimine, thiacetazone, and quinolones.[39]

IMMUNOSUPPRESSED PATIENTS. HIV infection and other factors that compromise the immune system make patients more susceptible to resistant organisms. For this reason, patients with HIV and TB should be treated for a total of 9 months and for at least 6 months after their sputum converts to negative. If drug susceptibility results are not available, EMB or SM should be considered for the entire course of therapy because of the rapid progression of TB while the patient is receiving inadequate therapy. TB therapy poses additional risk for HIV patients because the medication regimen has the potential to interact with other medications, especially antiretroviral agents.

TREATMENT OF EXTRAPULMONARY TUBERCULOSIS. The regimen used for treating pulmonary disease is also used to treat extrapulmonary disease. Some experts believe that therapy should be for 9 months instead of 6 months for patients with disseminated TB, miliary disease, TB of bones and joints, and TB of the lymph glands.

TREATMENT OF TUBERCULOSIS DURING PREGNANCY. Therapy is essential for pregnant women who have TB. SM is not used because it may cause congenital deafness. Routine use of PZA is not recommended because the risk of birth defects in the fetus has not been determined. Nine months of therapy with INH, RIF, and EMB is recommended. Women may breastfeed while receiving TB therapy because the concentration of the drugs in breast milk is so low that drug toxicity does not develop in the newborn.

DIET. A well-balanced diet containing the essential food groups with a vitamin supplement is recommended. Persons who are homeless or have limited incomes may require food vouchers to obtain additional food. Those who are poorly nourished or underweight may benefit from six small feedings of high-calorie, high-protein foods daily rather than three large meals.

HEALTH PROMOTION AND PREVENTION. The major priority of TB prevention and control programs is that all persons with TB be promptly identified and treated with an adequate course of drug therapy.[47] A special effort must be made to identify TB among foreign-born U.S. residents from countries with high TB rates. These high rates reflect the global nature of TB as a public health problem. The *Healthy People 2010* document has set goals for reducing the incidence of TB and treating cases of diagnosed TB (see Healthy People 2010 box).[43]

Healthy People 2010

Objectives for Tuberculosis

- Reduce tuberculosis.
  Target: 1.0 new case per 100,000 population
- Increase the proportion of all tuberculosis patients who complete curative therapy within 12 months.
  Target: 90% of patients
- Increase the proportion of contacts and other high-risk persons with latent tuberculosis infection who complete a course of treatment.
  Target: 85%
- Reduce the average time for a laboratory to confirm and report tuberculosis cases.
  Target: 2 days for 75% of cases

From US Department of Health and Human Services: *Healthy people 2010: understanding and improving health,* Washington, DC, 2000, The Department.

PRIMARY AND SECONDARY PREVENTION. To eliminate TB, treatment is necessary to prevent the organism from being transmitted from one person to another. Persons with latent TB (positive PPD test, no clinical signs of disease) who are at risk for progression to active TB are treated with INH 300 mg/day for 6 to 12 months (Box 26-2). Preventive INH therapy is more than 90% effective in patients who adhere to a 52-week regimen.[19] It is a common misconception that INH therapy for latent infection is contraindicated in patients over age 35. If INH-associated hepatitis occurs, the symptoms are mild, nonspecific, and similar to those of any viral illness. Contraindications to the use of INH preventive therapy are (1) previous INH-associated liver disease; (2) severe adverse reactions to INH, such as fever, chills, rash, and arthritis; and (3) acute liver disease of any etiology.[19] Persons receiving INH preventive chemotherapy may receive pyridoxine concurrently to reduce the incidence of central nervous system (CNS) effects or peripheral neuropathies. A health care provider should see them monthly to reinforce the importance of adhering to the regimen and to monitor for any serious side effects. Because most patients with TB and HIV infection have a history of a positive tuberculin test, all persons with HIV infection should be considered for preventive therapy with INH.

Box 26-2 Priorities for Preventive Therapy With Isoniazid Among Tuberculosis-Infected Persons

1. Persons with human immunodeficiency virus (HIV) infection
2. Recent contacts of persons with infectious tuberculosis (TB)
3. Persons with recent skin test conversions
4. Persons with recent TB disease who have been inadequately treated
5. Persons with negative sputum cultures and stable fibrotic lesions on chest radiographs consistent with inactive TB
6. Persons with medical conditions that increase the risk of TB:
   - Leukemia or lymphoma
   - Silicosis
   - Diabetes mellitus
   - Gastrectomy
   - End-stage renal disease
   - Antibodies to HIV

VACCINATION. The search for a satisfactory TB vaccine continues. Currently bacille Calmette-Guérin (BCG) is used worldwide except in the United States and the Netherlands. Vaccination is compulsory in many developing countries and officially recommended in others. In the United States BCG is rarely used because the risk of TB is low. The vaccine contains attenuated tubercle bacilli that have lost their ability to produce disease. It produces a subclinical infection that results in sensitization of T lymphocytes and cross-immunity. In most instances it produces a positive PPD reaction, so it is administered only to persons who have a negative reaction to the tuberculin test. The vaccine should be given intradermally only by persons who have had careful instruction in the proper technique. A multiple-puncture disk is used to give the vaccine. BCG vaccine has important limitations: immunity decreases after 5 to 10 years, and the vaccine may cause adverse reactions in patients with compromised immune systems. The increased understanding of the *M. tuberculosis* genome has advanced the search for a more effective vaccine, but significant issues remain to be addressed before human subjects are identified for testing with new vaccines.[12]

PROTECTION OF HEALTH CARE WORKERS. Controlling the spread of TB to hospital employees is based on three tenets: tuberculin skin testing and chest x-ray studies for new employees, isolation of clinical cases, and a high level of suspicion for TB among new admissions. Concern about occupational transmission is heightened by the increasing incidence of TB (see Future Watch box). Recent transmissions to health care workers have resulted from failure to diagnose, delays in laboratory identification of TB, delays in recognition of drug resistance, and lapses in infection control practices. The prevention of nosocomial TB is supported by 1997 Occupational Safety and Health Administration (OSHA) standards that require (1) an active surveillance program using the tuberculin PPD test, (2) isolation of persons with suspected TB, (3) negative-pressure isolation rooms, and (4) the use of particulate respirators.[45]

To protect nurses and other health care providers caring for patients who have a positive TB smear or culture, the following measures are indicated:

- First and foremost, emphasis is on preventing the patient from expelling *M. tuberculosis* into room air. Patients are instructed to cover their noses and mouths with tissues when coughing and sneezing. Those who are too ill to do so or who are confused have a surgical mask put over their nose and mouth.

Future Watch

Isolation Precautions

The Centers for Disease Control and Prevention (CDC) is updating its Guideline for Isolation Precautions in Hospitals to address concerns about the transmission of infection to patients and health care workers. A draft of the new document is undergoing final revision before publication.

- The patient is placed in a private room, and the door to the hallway kept closed.
- If the patient must leave the room for tests or procedures, he or she wears a mask or particulate respirator with a one-way valve.
- The air pressure in the room is negative. This allows air to flow into the room when the door is open and prevents room air from moving out into the hallway.
- The air in the room is exchanged several times every hour, with two of the exchanges being with fresh air from the outside (the evidence is inconclusive as to the optimal number of air exchanges required). Air from the patient's room is directly vented to the outside and not recirculated within the hospital.
- High-energy particulate air (HEPA) filters are installed in ventilation ducts.
- Ultraviolet lights high on walls or ceilings in patient rooms are used to disinfect room air. They are placed so that they do not cause a risk to the patients or health care workers.
- Personnel caring for patients wear a disposable particulate respirator. The respirator fits snugly over the nose and mouth to prevent as much room air as possible from getting in around the edges. The particulate respirator filters out organisms as small as 1 μm; *M. tuberculosis* organisms are 3 to 5 μm. Compliance with the use of the particulate respirators has been a problem because of discomfort.
- All health care workers should know their tuberculin status. Workers who are tuberculin negative should be tested yearly with PPD. Those who have not had a recent test should receive a baseline tuberculin test on employment and then yearly. Workers who have inadvertently been exposed to a patient with TB (often before the diagnosis of TB is made) should have a tuberculin test 8 to 12 weeks after exposure. It takes this period for a test to convert from negative to positive. The CDC recommends that health care workers caring for patients who are receiving cough-inducing procedures, such as bronchoscopy and tracheal suctioning, be tested with tuberculin at least every 6 months.
- Health care workers who convert from a negative to a positive tuberculin test should have an examination to rule out active TB. Those refusing therapy should have a yearly chest x-ray examination.

Nursing Management *of the Patient with Tuberculosis*

ASSESSMENT

Health History. Assess for:

- Fever, chills, night sweats, anorexia, weight loss
- A history of a known exposure to a person with TB (Often the source of the infection is unknown and never determined. Close contacts of the patient need to be identified so that they may undergo examination to determine whether they are infected and have active disease or a positive tuberculin test.)

Physical Examination. Assess for:

- Productive cough
- Pallor
- Adventitious breath sounds
- Afternoon temperature elevation
- Tuberculin skin test reaction of 10 mm induration or more

NURSING DIAGNOSES, OUTCOMES, AND INTERVENTIONS

Nursing Diagnosis: Risk for Infection: Patient Reinfection and Prevention of Spread

OUTCOMES. Common examples of expected outcomes for the patient with a diagnosis of *risk for infection* (patient reinfection and control to prevent spread or environmental exposure) are:

Patient will:

- Explain measures such as compliance with chemotherapy regimen and measures to prevent spread of TB, such as covering the mouth and nose with tissues when coughing or sneezing and proper disposal of used tissues.
- State name, dose, actions, and side effects of prescribed medications.
- Explain the rationale for two, three, or four chemotherapy agents taken together.
- Explain the relationship between drug-resistant organisms and the need to take chemotherapy agents as directed.
- Explain why the health care provider should be notified immediately if for any reason chemotherapy agents cannot be taken (e.g., side effects).
- State where to receive a new supply of chemotherapy agents and the date they are to be obtained.
- State the need and plan for follow-up care.
- Describe signs and symptoms that indicate the need for immediate medical care (increased cough, hemoptysis, unexplained weight loss, fever, night sweats).
- State when and where the next sputum test or x-ray film is to be taken.

NURSING INTERVENTIONS. The most important factor in the transmission of TB is overcrowded living conditions. To prevent the transmission of TB from person to person, it is necessary to prevent contamination of the air with *M. tuberculosis.* This is accomplished by treating the patient with antituberculosis drugs and teaching the patient to cover the nose and mouth with a tissue when coughing, sneezing, and laughing so that droplet nuclei are not discharged into the air. Most persons who adhere to the antiinfective prescribed therapy and do not have mitigating factors such as immunosuppression convert their sputum from positive to negative in 2 to 3 weeks (see Patient/Family Teaching box).

RELATED NIC INTERVENTIONS. Infection Control, Infection Protection

Nursing Diagnosis: Ineffective Airway Clearance

OUTCOMES. Common examples of expected outcomes for the patient with a diagnosis of *ineffective airway clearance* are:

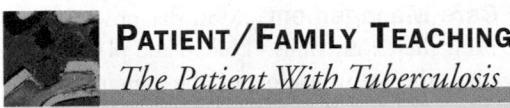

PATIENT/FAMILY TEACHING
The Patient With Tuberculosis

The nurse should teach the patient:

- The signs and symptoms that indicate need for referral such as increased cough, hemoptysis, unexplained weight loss, fever, night sweats
- How to prevent contamination of air with *Mycobacterium tuberculosis:*
  —Cover nose and mouth with disposable tissues when coughing, sneezing, or laughing.
  —Place used tissues in paper or plastic bag for disposal.
- The need for follow-up care
- The importance of the drug therapy:
  —Must be taken as prescribed
  —Should notify the health care provider if the chemotherapy cannot be taken for any reason
- Where to get new supplies of medications
- What the medication is and its side effects
- The rationale for the medications and dosing schedule

Patient will:

- Have clear breath sounds.
- Clear the airway by effective coughing.
- Have minimal sputum production.

NURSING INTERVENTIONS. To improve airway clearance, the nurse teaches the patient to sit upright in a chair or in bed. If the patient is confined to bed at home, he or she may find it helpful to sit on the side of the bed with the feet on a chair. The nurse teaches the patient to take two or three deep breaths, cover the mouth with tissues, and then cough. Using this method when coughing decreases fatigue because it requires less energy. Many patients can cough most effectively when the mouth is moist, and sips of water or a warm beverage can be encouraged before coughing. For patients with thick, tenacious sputum, the nurse encourages fluid intake to thin the secretions and make them easier to expectorate. Many experts consider water to be the most effective sputum-liquefying agent.

RELATED NIC INTERVENTIONS. Airway Management, Cough Enhancement, Positioning, Respiratory Monitoring

Nursing Diagnosis: Ineffective Therapeutic Regimen Management

OUTCOMES. A common example of expected outcomes for the patient with a diagnosis of *ineffective therapeutic regimen management* is:

Patient will:

- Demonstrate behaviors necessary to maintain the therapeutic regimen.

NURSING INTERVENTIONS. To encourage patient understanding of the complex therapeutic regimen and to promote adherence, nurses and other health care professionals should encourage open discussion and solicit questions and concerns from the patient and family. The nurse must be patient and may need to repeat the information often to promote understanding. To achieve continuity of teaching, care should be coordinated among acute care and home care personnel or public health clinicians. The nurse should answer all questions as completely as possible, supplying information appropriate to the patient's educational level and ability to comprehend what is being taught. Written materials with diagrams and drawings that reinforce the information are helpful. The nurse should review all written materials with the patient and, whenever possible, a family member before giving them to the patient. For patients who do not speak English, a translator and written materials in the patient's language are necessary. Concerns about interpersonal or financial problems indicate the need for a social services referral.

RELATED NIC INTERVENTIONS. Emotional Support, Mutual Goal Setting, Self-Modification Assistance

Nursing Diagnosis: Activity Intolerance

OUTCOMES. A common example of expected outcomes for the patient with a diagnosis of *activity intolerance* is:

Patient will:

- Be able to participate in ADLs.

NURSING INTERVENTIONS. During the acute phase of the illness, persons with TB experience fatigue and have difficulty completing ADLs. Increasing activity tolerance involves careful assessment of the physiologic response to activity and planning for progressive increases based on patient tolerance. In some settings activities may require measures to prevent exposure of susceptible individuals. Respiratory isolation may hinder patient interest in activity, especially when wearing a mask is required. The nurse needs to reinforce the need for isolation while also promoting a positive self-image and increasing activity.

RELATED NIC INTERVENTIONS. Energy Management, Self-Care Assistance

EVALUATION

To evaluate the effectiveness of nursing interventions, compare patient behaviors with those stated in the expected patient outcomes.

RELATED NOC OUTCOMES. Activity Tolerance, Aspiration Prevention, Compliance Behavior, Endurance, Respiratory Status: Ventilation, Self-Care: Activities of Daily Living (ADL), Symptom Control

GERONTOLOGIC CONSIDERATIONS

Many older persons were exposed to TB when they were children and have a positive tuberculin test. This indicates they have dormant tubercle bacilli walled off in their lungs. When subjected to physical or emotional stress, they may develop active TB. Also, with aging, the immune system may be less able to react to the tuberculin test or respond effectively to an infection. This increases the risk of undiagnosed infection, which can be transmitted to others. Thus it is recommended that older adults, including those in nursing homes, have a yearly chest x-ray examination. If an active case of TB is found in a nursing home resident, more frequent x-ray examinations of other residents are necessary.

Many older adults, especially those who are frail, have a poor appetite and need special attention to their nutritional needs. Other older persons with limited financial resources need help obtaining an adequate diet. Asking the person to keep a daily food diary can help determine whether the person's diet is sufficient to support healing of the TB.

Lung Abscess

Etiology and Epidemiology. A lung abscess is a pus-containing necrotic lesion of the lung parenchyma that often contains an air-fluid level. It may be associated with infections, pulmonary infarction, malignancy, and necrosis secondary to silicosis and coal miners' pneumoconiosis. Lung abscess secondary to aspiration is much less common since the introduction of antibiotic treatment, and the prognosis has improved, with a mortality rate of 15% to 20%. The prognosis is relatively poor, however, for elderly, debilitated, malnourished, and immunocompromised patients. Large abscesses and aerobic bacteria are associated with the worst outcomes.

Pathophysiology. Infected material lodges in the small bronchi and produces inflammation. Partial obstruction of the bronchus results in retention of secretions beyond the obstruction and the eventual necrosis of tissue. The necrotic lung tissue is coughed up, leaving an air-filled cavity in the lung. Aspirated food particles and perigingival debris, which contains both aerobic and anaerobic organisms, are the most common causes of lung abscess secondary to aspirated substances. Laboratory cultures of sputum or transtracheal aspirates are necessary to identify the causative organism. Lung abscess may follow bronchial obstruction caused by a tumor, foreign body, or stenosis of the bronchus. Metastatic spread of cancer cells to the lung parenchyma may also cause an abscess, and occasionally the infection appears to have been borne by the bloodstream. Bronchoscopy may be used to identify the infected segment and to obtain specimens for culture. Signs and symptoms of an acute lung abscess are presented in the Clinical Manifestations box.

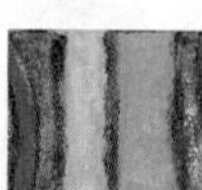

CLINICAL MANIFESTATIONS
Acute Lung Abscess

- High fever: 102° F (39° C)
- Chills and prostration
- Cough and sputum production common
- Night sweats, pleuritic chest pain, anemia, and occasionally hemoptysis
- Putrid sputum in about 50% of patients; foul odor evident in patient's room
- Weight loss in about 40% of patients (foul-smelling and foul-tasting sputum often causing anorexia)
- Mortality rate with primary abscess of 5%
- Up to one third of patients 45 years of age and older with a lung abscess also have carcinoma; consider diagnostic bronchoscopy for all high-risk patients, even if they respond well to therapy

Collaborative Care Management. Most diagnoses of lung abscess are made from chest x-ray films. If blood and pleural fluid cultures are negative, the identification of the causative agent requires an invasive procedure, such as bronchial lavage or percutaneous lung aspiration.

The course of lung abscess is influenced by the cause of the abscess and by the type of drainage that can be established. If the purulent material drains easily, the patient may respond well to segmental postural drainage, antibiotic therapy, and good general supportive care. Antibiotic therapy is based on the identified pathogen and may be continued for up to 8 weeks. Most cavities close within 6 weeks, but occasionally a cavity may persist for months. Foul-smelling sputum usually disappears within a few days, whereas cough and non–foul-smelling sputum may continue for a longer period. Usually the patient begins to feel better during the first week of therapy, but it may take up to 2 months for the temperature to return to normal. In some patients uninfected cavities or fibrosis may persist.

If the patient does not improve with the above therapy, bronchoscopy is performed to improve drainage and search for a possible obstruction to drainage, such as carcinoma or a foreign body. Rarely, surgical resection of the abscessed area is needed.

The individual with a lung abscess is very ill and requires hospitalization (see Guidelines for Safe Practice box). Of equal importance to caring for the patient with a lung abscess is the prevention of lung abscess in hospitalized patients. Nursing interventions that decrease the risk of lung abscess begin with monitoring patients who are at risk for aspiration (i.e., those with a reduced level of consciousness, depressed cough or gag reflexes, impaired swallowing, a tracheostomy, or an endotracheal tube). These patients should be elevated to the highest or best position for eating and drinking. Patients receiving enteral feedings should also be carefully positioned and closely monitored to ensure that the tube is in the stomach. The nurse provides frequent mouth care to persons with diminished levels of consciousness. Patients who are vomiting should be placed on their side in postanesthesia position to reduce the risk for aspiration. For patients unable to expectorate secretions from the mouth and oropharynx, oral suctioning may be necessary.

Empyema

Etiology and Epidemiology. Empyema is the presence of fluid containing pus within a body cavity, typically the pleural space. It usually occurs after pleural effusion secondary to other respira-

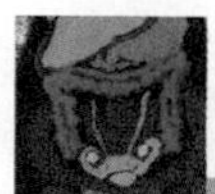

GUIDELINES FOR SAFE PRACTICE
The Patient With Lung Abscess

- Monitor vital signs at least every 4 hours because temperature may spike in afternoon and may persist for as long as 2 weeks.
- Place patient in comfortable position. If patient is conscious, he or she usually is more comfortable with head rest at 45 to 90 degrees.
- Help patient cough up sputum. This helps drain abscess.
- Collect sputum for culture and sensitivity tests to determine organism and antibiotic therapy. This monitors effectiveness of therapy and whether resistant organisms are developing.
- Do postural drainage. This facilitates drainage from the abscess.

tory diseases, such as pneumonia, lung abscess, TB, and fungal infections of the lung, and also after thoracic surgery or chest trauma. It is reported in 1% to 2% of patients hospitalized with CAP. Empyema can result from staphylococcal infection.

Pathophysiology. Empyema has three stages:

Stage I: Exudative phase—The empyema is in a fluid stage.

Stage II: Fibrinopurulent phase—The pleural effusion becomes infected with cellular debris.

Stage III: Organizing phase—The empyema is chronic and characterized by a thick, inelastic pleural peel that traps and compresses the lung.

The Clinical Manifestations box presents the signs and symptoms of empyema.

Collaborative Care Management. Treatment of empyema requires vigorous pleural drainage and antimicrobial therapy. Initial treatment is often serial **thoracentesis** with aspiration of the cavity and instillation of antibiotics into the pleural space. Oral or IV antibiotics may also be given. An alternative method of drainage is closed-chest drainage, in which a trocar is inserted between the ribs at the base of the cavity, a chest catheter is inserted through the trocar, the trocar is removed, and the tube is connected to water-seal drainage. Pus then drains from the cavity into the collection chamber. For closed drainage to be successful, the pus must be thin enough to drain out of the pleural space, and the lung must be able to reexpand to fill the pleural space. When the fluid is loculated, the chest tube may require ultrasound or computed tomography (CT)–guided placement. In some cases fibrinolytic agents may be instilled via the chest tube to promote drainage. The agents most commonly used include streptokinase and urokinase. Urokinase has the advantage of being less allergenic. Both work by activating plasminogen, which is converted to plasmin, which then degrades fibrin and clots, helping to liquefy the drainage. If none of these measures effectively drains the pleural space within a few days, or if the lung fails to reexpand to obliterate the space, surgery is necessary.

For second-stage empyema, a newer procedure of video-assisted thoracostomy has demonstrated good success. In instances of chronic empyema in which a fibrinous peel has formed on the visceral pleura, preventing the lung from reexpanding and filling the space left after drainage of the empyema cavity, decortication may be necessary. In decortication the surgeon removes the fibrinous peel from the visceral pleura by blunt dissection, freeing the lung so that it can reexpand and fill the pleural space. With both these procedures, two **chest tubes** are inserted into the pleural space and connected to water-seal drainage with additional suction. A repeat chest CT scan and assessment of the patient's clinical condition are important in evaluating response to therapy.

Nursing care depends on the type and effectiveness of the procedure and the patient's symptoms. Some patients require oxygen therapy. The nurse administers antibiotics and monitors the response. Activity is reduced initially, on the basis of patient tolerance, but progresses gradually to prevent debilitation. Coughing and deep breathing exercises may be indicated to improve ventilation. In some cases the patient goes through several treatments before the empyema space is closed. This can be frustrating, and the patient may become discouraged. A major nursing role is to support the patient and family and to keep them apprised of progress and any treatments during the various procedures.

CLINICAL MANIFESTATIONS
Empyema

- Fever
- Dyspnea
- Anorexia
- Pleuritic chest pain
- The following found on examination:
  —Unequal chest expansion
  —Weight loss with malaise
  —Pleural friction rub
  —Foul-smelling sputum
  —Decreased lung sounds in area of empyema

Fungal Infections

North America is home to three major endemic mycoses that give rise to major fungal infections of the lungs: histoplasmosis, coccidioidomycosis, and blastomycosis. The causative agents are found in soil. They are classified as deep mycoses because the parasite is involved in deeper tissues and internal organs. Most of the clinical presentations are mild and self-limiting, but each of these diseases can be problematic to certain populations and can become disseminated, requiring aggressive treatment. Table 26-8 summarizes the clinical manifestations and medical therapy for the three major fungal lung infections.

Histoplasmosis

ETIOLOGY AND EPIDEMIOLOGY. Inhalation of spores of *Histoplasma capsulatum* causes histoplasmosis. Spores are found in soil contaminated by the excrement of birds and bats, such as that around chicken coops, near bird roosts, and in caves. The excrement enhances the growth of the organism in soil by accelerating sporulation.[46] Activities that disturb contaminated soil sites are associated with exposure to the spores, and air currents may carry them for miles. Extensive skin testing suggests that as many as 50 million people in the United States have been infected by *H. capsulatum,* and up to 500,000 new infections occur yearly. Most healthy people who are infected remain asymptomatic.

PATHOPHYSIOLOGY. The inhaled spores are phagocytized by alveolar macrophages within which they germinate. The spores form yeast cells and multiply by budding. The patient has a primary infection with involvement of regional lymphatics and early dissemination to other organs via lymphatics and blood. Yeast cells spread to the liver, spleen, and bone marrow and are phagocytized by reticuloendothelial cells. The process in the lung involves necrosis and healing by fibrotic encapsulation, and eventually the original parenchymal foci and hilar lymph nodes show calcification.

The severity of illness after inhalation exposure to *H. capsulatum* depends on the intensity of exposure and the host's immune status. Some individuals are asymptomatic; others develop a flu-like pulmonary illness with cough, chest pain, dyspnea, headache, fever, arthralgia, anorexia, erythema nodosum, hepatomegaly, and splenomegaly. Patchy infiltrates may be seen on chest x-ray films.

TABLE 26-8 CLINICAL MANIFESTATIONS AND MEDICAL THERAPY FOR FUNGAL LUNG INFECTIONS

Type of Infection	Clinical Manifestations	Medical Therapy
Histoplasmosis	Severe infections; acute onset with fever, chest pain, dyspnea, prostration, weight loss, widespread pulmonary infiltrates, hepatomegaly, and splenomegaly; no symptoms in some persons, benign acute pneumonitis in others; without treatment, patient with disseminated disease dies	Drug(s) of choice: amphotericin B (Fungizone IV); cures 75% of patients Ketoconazole (Nizoral), 400 mg/day orally at bedtime or with meals
Coccidioidomycosis (Valley fever, San Joaquin Valley fever)	Asymptomatic upper respiratory tract infection in about 60% of those who inhaled spores; 40% have symptoms ranging from flulike illness to frank pneumonia; therapy required for only 10% of those with symptoms; remainder have spontaneous remission	Amphotericin B IV Ketoconazole orally
Blastomycosis	Skin lesions that appear as small papular or pustular lesions on exposed parts of body, such as hands and face Peripheral development of lesions; may become raised but do not itch	Amphotericin B IV; mandatory in immunocompromised patients Ketoconazole orally Miconazole (only for patients who cannot tolerate amphotericin or ketoconazole)

IV, Intravenously.

In most individuals T-cell immunity develops in 10 to 14 days, and the initial infection is self-limiting and does not require antifungal chemotherapy. However, some immunocompromised persons may develop a rapidly progressive primary infection that is fatal without antifungal therapy.

Chronic pulmonary histoplasmosis (CPH) develops almost exclusively in patients with underlying lung disease. They have recurrent episodes of necrotizing segmental or lobar granulomatous pneumonitis, which has a tendency toward cavity formation, contraction, fibrosis, and compensatory emphysema. Patients exhibit cough, dyspnea, fever, and weight loss.

Progressive disseminated histoplasmosis (PDH) occurs in 1 in 2000 exposed individuals with very low resistance to infection (infants, older adults, and immunocompromised persons). Disseminated histoplasmosis rarely occurs in people with no known immune disorder. Those who are infected have fever, weakness, weight loss, hepatosplenomegaly, leukopenia, and oropharyngeal ulceration. Adrenal insufficiency occurs in about 50% of cases.

COLLABORATIVE CARE MANAGEMENT. Skin testing for histoplasmosis is used only for screening purposes. In endemic areas, 90% to 95% of young adults have positive test results. The person should be tested with histoplasmin, tuberculin, blastomycin, and coccidioidin because of the likelihood of cross-reaction. The strongest skin reaction indicates the likely cause of the infection. Positive diagnosis of fungal disease may be based on direct demonstration of intracellular yeasts in smears of bone marrow; biopsy specimens of lymph nodes, liver, or spleen; or cultures of bone marrow, blood, or sputum. Agglutination, precipitation, and complement fixation tests may also be used to help establish the diagnosis of histoplasmosis. These serology tests become positive about 1 month after the primary infection. Titers of serial tests are used to determine activity of the infection. In histoplasmosis, chest x-ray films demonstrate a nodular infiltrate similar in appearance to TB. The WBC count is usually normal, although in acute cases it may increase to 13,000/mm^2. Leukopenia and anemia may be present in persons with disseminated disease.

In many cases the disease is self-limiting and no antifungal therapy is needed. When it is needed, treatment focuses on administering and monitoring the effects of medications. Antifungal therapy consists primarily of amphotericin B (Fungizone), itraconazole (Sporanox), or ketoconazole (Nizoral). The duration of therapy depends on the type of infection, the condition of the patient's immune system, and the agent used. Amphotericin B is given intravenously. The dose and length of therapy are determined by the difficulty in eradicating the infection and the likelihood of relapse. The therapy may last 2 to 3 weeks or 2 to 3 months. Amphotericin B has many toxic properties, including local phlebitis, systemic reactions, renal toxicity, hypokalemia, and anemia. In rare instances, anaphylaxis, bone marrow suppression, and cardiovascular and hepatic toxicity develop. Systemic toxicity (chills, fever, aching, nausea, and vomiting) can be lessened by premedication with acetaminophen along with 25 to 50 mg of diphenhydramine (Benadryl) orally. Heparin and hydrocortisone succinate (Solu-Cortef) are sometimes added to the infusions to minimize phlebitis. A bone scan should be performed before starting amphotericin B therapy.

A reversible azotemia occurs when amphotericin B is administered. The level of azotemia is monitored by biweekly blood urea nitrogen (BUN) or serum creatinine determinations. A BUN value of greater than 40 mg/dl or a creatinine level nearing 3 mg/dl indicates a need to reduce the drug or temporarily stop it. Therapy is not continued until the azotemia improves. Serum potassium levels are checked biweekly, and hypokalemia is treated with oral potassium. Anemia is common, and the hematocrit usually stabilizes at 25% to 35%.

Other antifungals that may be used are itraconazole and ketoconazole. Itraconazole is administered orally with food because food enhances its absorption. An initial loading dose is followed by lower maintenance doses. Treatment with itraconazole, 200 mg once or twice per day for 12 to 24 months, is indicated for all patients with CPH. Those patients requiring hospitalization for ventilatory insufficiency, general debilitation, or an inability to tolerate itraconazole are usually treated with amphotericin B.[46]

Itraconazole and amphotericin B are the treatment choices in PDH histoplasmosis. Persons with AIDS who develop PDH have a relapse rate of 80% after treatment. For this reason, the goal of therapy is lifelong suppression as opposed to cure. Amphotericin B, which is administered intravenously weekly or twice weekly, is highly effective but inconvenient and not well tolerated. Itraconazole, 200 mg once or twice daily, is the treatment of choice for those patients who have shown a positive response to a lengthy course of amphotericin B, usually for 12 weeks. Antigen levels may be monitored every 3 to 6 months to ensure that concentrations remain negative or low.[46]

Ketoconazole is also administered orally and is fairly well tolerated by patients. Toxicity appears to be minimal; pruritus, minor gastrointestinal intolerance, and liver function abnormalities have been reported. However, studies have shown that ketoconazole is less effective than itraconazole.[46]

Persons with mycotic diseases can be seriously ill and may require long-term therapy (2 to 3 months or more) with IV antifungal agents. Because the public does not understand these diseases, the patient and family need to feel comfortable in discussing concerns with the nurse. The nurse is responsible for providing information; clarifying misconceptions; and helping the patient and family understand the disease, its therapy, and the required follow-up care.

In the management of fungal disease, promoting comfort is also important. The nurse should position the patient to facilitate breathing. Measures such as the use of antipyretics and cool sponge baths can help reduce fever. Patients require close medical follow-up for 1 year to prevent relapse. The patient and family must understand the need to avoid infected areas or to wear a protective mask if they have to be in an infected area.

Coccidioidomycosis

Etiology and Epidemiology. Coccidioidomycosis is caused by inhalation of spores of *Coccidioides immitis,* which are found in desert soil and dispersed in dust in the spring. The disease is endemic in the desert areas of the Southwestern United States. Susceptibility to the infection is in part genetically determined. Coccidioidomycosis is 50 times more common in Filipino men and 10 times more common in African-American men than in Caucasian men. This increased susceptibility to progressive disease in these groups of men parallels their susceptibility to TB and is believed to be the result of a genetically determined impairment of their capacity to develop cellular immunity to infection.

Pathophysiology. The pathophysiologic process that occurs after inhalation of spores is believed to be similar to that described under Histoplasmosis. Disseminated disease is marked by hilar adenopathy, and fungi can be isolated from lymph nodes. A pneumonic disease with necrosis and cavitation may occur after development of delayed hypersensitivity. The disease process is controlled and resolved in most persons as a result of cellular immunity mechanisms. Approximately 60% of infected persons are asymptomatic, with the remainder having symptoms that range from flulike to frank pneumonia. Progressive disseminated coccidioidomycosis or progressive pulmonary disease is found only in persons whose ability to resist infection or develop immunity has been compromised in some way.[47]

X-ray films of the chest may show pneumonic infiltrate, hilar adenopathy, pleural effusion, or cavitary lesions 2 to 4 cm in size. These cavities usually close spontaneously within 2 years of detection. Approximately 5% of persons with primary pulmonary involvement have residual lung lesions such as cavities or nodules. Only about 0.5% of infected individuals go on to develop a severe, progressive mycosis.[47]

Extrapulmonary dissemination of coccidioidomycosis can occur. One of the sites of dissemination is the meningeal surface of the brain. If there is any indication of CNS involvement, a lumbar puncture is performed. A positive complement fixation titer in the spinal fluid is diagnostic of meningitis. Dissemination can also occur to skin, soft tissue, liver, and bones; the patient is monitored by physical examination of the skin, gallium scanning of soft tissue, and bone scans.

Collaborative Care Management. Coccidioidin, 1:10 or 1:100, is used to test for the disease. The test is read in 48 hours. It takes 3 to 6 weeks after exposure for the test to become positive. In severe disseminated disease the test may be negative, indicating that the patient's immune system is no longer able to respond.

As with histoplasmosis, agglutination, precipitation, and complement fixation tests may be used to help establish the diagnosis. These serology tests become positive about 1 month after the primary infection. Titers of serial tests are used to determine activity of the infection. Surgical intervention for lesions that are localized may involve either excision or drainage to facilitate healing. Management of coccidioidomycosis is otherwise similar to that of histoplasmosis.

Blastomycosis

Etiology and Epidemiology. Blastomycosis is caused by inhalation of *Blastomyces dermatitidis* spores, which are carried on air currents. The incidence of blastomycosis is difficult to report because it has no reliable skin test.

Pathophysiology. Although skin lesions that appear as small, nonitchy, papular or pustular lesions on exposed parts of the body, such as the hands and face, may be the first evidence of blastomycosis, the initial site of infection is the lung. Researchers assume that inhaled spores are phagocytized in the alveoli as part of the primary infection. Thus the pathogenesis of blastomycosis is similar to that of TB, histoplasmosis, and coccidioidomycosis. The infection spreads to other organs by lymph and blood. The skin, bones, and prostate are the most common sites of spread. Acute pulmonary blastomycosis in the form of a self-limiting pneumonia can occur. Otherwise, blastomycosis is a chronic progressive disease with a mortality rate of about 90% when untreated. For this reason, treatment is recommended for every person in whom the diagnosis is established.

Collaborative Care Management. Management of blastomycosis is similar to that for histoplasmosis. Nursing care should be adjusted to meet the patient's specific needs and other chronic problems, if present.

Occupational Lung Diseases

Etiology and Epidemiology. Many pulmonary diseases are believed to be caused by substances inhaled in the workplace. Occupational lung diseases are more common in blue-collar workers than in white-collar workers, in industrialized areas than in rural areas, and in small and medium-sized businesses than in larger industrial plants.

In some instances it is debatable whether a person's lung disease is clearly occupation specific. This is especially true in cases of bronchitis, asthma, emphysema, or cancer, since all these conditions can be caused or aggravated by several factors found in many different occupations and by nonoccupational factors such as smoking and air pollution.

Millions of Americans are believed to have job-related diseases. Because these diseases are not reportable, exact statistics do not exist. The U.S. Department of Health and Human Services has estimated that 400,000 persons develop job-related diseases each year and 100,000 people die from them. The National Heart, Lung, and Blood Institute reports that lung diseases cause more than half these deaths. More than $5 billion per year is paid out in workers' compensation for job-related illnesses and injuries.[5]

It is well documented that smokers develop occupational lung disease more often than nonsmokers and that smokers' lungs are more vulnerable to the effects of these diseases than are nonsmokers' lungs. The combined effects of cigarette smoke and industrial pollutants are great. The risk of developing chronic bronchitis, emphysema, lung cancer, and heart disease is much increased when the worker smokes. Some of these risks, such as lung cancer in persons who worked with asbestos and who also smoked, are becoming more widely known.

Occupational lung diseases are divided into several categories. The major ones are (1) the pneumoconioses, including silicosis and coal workers' pneumoconiosis (black lung disease); (2) asbestos-related lung disease; and (3) hypersensitivity diseases, including occupational asthma, allergic alveolitis (farmer's lung), and byssinosis (brown lung disease). Table 26-9 presents the etiology, epidemiology, pathophysiology, clinical manifestations, and prevention of the major occupational lung diseases.

Collaborative Care Management. Medical therapy depends on the patient's signs, symptoms, and complications. The nurse's major role is to be knowledgeable about the cause and prevention of occupational lung diseases so that he or she can present appropriate information and teaching to the public. The nurse may be key in determining that the patient's presenting symptoms are occupation related. A careful occupational history is essential. Questions such as, "Do you see dust or mist in the air?" "Do you blow dust from your nose or cough it up at the end of the day?" and "Are your symptoms different on the first day of the work week?" may provide significant clues to occupational exposure and risk.

Occupational lung diseases are preventable, but require concerted efforts by the public, government agencies, and industry. OSHA has initiated standards for preventing lung disease attributed to the workplace environment contamination. The American Association of Occupational Health Nurses is also promoting higher standards for protecting employees at the worksite. Measures recommended by the American Lung Association to reduce the incidence of occupation-related lung diseases include:

- Public education about the relationship between polluted air in the workplace and lung diseases
- General commitment to reduce, eliminate, or avoid air pollution in the workplace
- Elimination of the most prevalent and notorious lung hazard—cigarette smoke

Education of the public includes not only employers and employees but also engineers and planners who design operations; buyers and purchasers who select ingredients, cleaning agents, and equipment; and physicians and nurses who care for persons with occupation-related diseases. Many times, workers who are instructed about the hazards involved in certain occupations and workplaces help in determining preventive measures to combat or minimize the effects of hazards. The commitment to reduce, eliminate, or avoid pollution of workplace air requires full consideration of possible health effects whenever operations are planned and improvement of conditions whenever possible.

Sarcoidosis

Etiology and Epidemiology. Sarcoidosis is a multiorgan disease that affects the lungs more than 90% of the time.[9] The cause of sarcoidosis is unknown. However, a growing body of knowledge indicates it may result from exposure of a genetically susceptible host to specific environmental agents. It is worldwide in distribution and is most common in young and middle-aged adults. In the United States it is most common in African-American women.

Pathophysiology. Sarcoidosis may result from an antigen-antibody reaction manifested by a reticuloendothelial response in which both thymus-derived (T) cells and plasma (B) cells participate. It is believed that the antigen is airborne, since bilateral hilar lymphadenopathy is commonly present at the onset and bronchopulmonary macrophages are increased.

The central pathologic event involves the growth of noncaseating granulomas and proliferation of lymph tissue. The patient with sarcoidosis may initially complain of vague symptoms of malaise, fever, aching joints, or weakness. In addition to mediastinal lymph node enlargement, the patient may have ocular manifestations, such as uveitis and conjunctivitis, and dermatologic changes, such as erythema nodosum. Symptoms of pulmonary sarcoidosis are also nonspecific but may include a dry cough, dyspnea, chest pain, and in some cases bronchial hyperreactivity.[9]

Diagnosis of sarcoidosis is based on x-ray film findings, transbronchial lung biopsy, and organ biopsy showing noncaseating granulomas. Chest x-ray findings are abnormal in more than 90% of patients, typically showing bilateral hilar lymph node enlargement. Organ biopsy yields the most conclusive evidence of sarcoidosis and is most helpful in differentiating it from Hodgkin's lymphoma and TB.

Other tests useful in the diagnosis of pulmonary sarcoidosis include a gallium scan and bronchoalveolar lavage (BAL) with flexible fiberoptic bronchoscopy. The fluid obtained from BAL is examined to determine the degree of active inflammation in the lung and the need for therapy. Changes in pulmonary function tests (PFTs) are present in only 20% of patients with stage I sarcoidosis but are found in 40% to 70% of patients in the later stages. Gas exchange is preserved until late in the clinical course.[9]

Collaborative Care Management. In many patients sarcoidosis is a benign, self-limiting process that resolves within 2 years of diagnosis with no residual damage. Other patients have an acute or chronic form of the disease requiring corticosteroids or other therapy for more than 2 years.[9] The optimal treatment regimen for pulmonary sarcoidosis is still being determined. Corticosteroids have been the mainstay of treatment of symptomatic sarcoidosis for 40 years. However, toxicity from long-term usage has led to more widespread use of alternate therapy, including cytotoxic drugs such as methotrexate and immune modifiers such as hydroxychloroquine. New cytokine inhibitors, such a thalidomide and infliximab, have also increased the options for sarcoidosis therapy.

About 10% of patients develop chronic sarcoidosis. Among these patients, a subgroup develops refractory disease that fails to improve with the usual doses of corticosteroids. Patients with advanced pulmonary disease, including fibrosis, may die as a result of lung involvement. In severe cases, pulmonary hypertension and **cor pulmonale** (right ventricular decompensation) develop. Lung and other organ transplantations have been successfully performed in patients with end-stage sarcoidosis. However, after transplantation some patients develop recurrent sarcoid lesions, which are controlled by posttransplantation immunosuppression.

Nursing care needs vary with the severity of the patient's signs and symptoms and medical therapy. Care includes teaching the patient about the precautions and side effects of steroid therapy. Sarcoidosis can cause bone marrow suppression, with associated anemia and leukopenia. The cytotoxic agents directly affect the bone marrow; hence complete blood counts must be performed regularly, usually every 6 to 8 weeks. Sarcoidosis patients are often female and premenopausal. Thalidomide is associated with severe congenital malformations and cannot be prescribed to either a woman who may become pregnant or a man who may father a child.

Cancer of the Lung

Etiology and Epidemiology. Cancer of the lung may be either metastatic or primary. Metastatic tumors may follow malignancy anywhere in the body. Metastasis from the colon and kidney is common. Metastasis to the lung may be discovered before the primary lesion is known, and sometimes the location of the primary lesion is found only at autopsy.

Lung cancer is the leading cause of cancer death in both men and women in the United States. Increases in its incidence closely coincide with increases in cigarette smoking (Box 26-3). It is estimated that 87% of lung cancers are attributable to smoking.[1] The American Cancer Society estimated that in 2005 172,570 people would be diagnosed with lung cancer and 163,510 would die from the disease.[4] Lung cancer is the third most common type of cancer in the United States, after breast cancer and prostate cancer. Only 10% to 15% of people who develop lung cancer survive 5 years after diagnosis.[33]

The increase in death rates for both men and women is directly related to cigarette smoking. The cancer death rate for male cigarette smokers is more than double that for nonsmokers, and the death rate for female smokers is 67% higher than that for nonsmokers. The American Cancer Society projects that mortality from lung cancer among women will continue to rise until 2010.[4]

A history of smoking, especially for 20 years or more, is a prime risk factor. Other risk factors include exposure to certain industrial substances such as arsenic, specific organic chemicals, radon, and asbestos, particularly in those who smoke. Asbestos workers who smoke are estimated to have a 6 to 10 times greater incidence of lung cancer than the general population. Some evidence also suggests a genetic predisposition to lung cancer.

Because no effective treatment exists for lung cancer, emphasis is on prevention. The cure rate has not significantly improved since 1950 despite advances in surgery, chemotherapy, and radiation. Success with therapy is enhanced by early diagnosis and treatment. The American Cancer Society estimates that 72% of people have regional or distant metastases at diagnosis.[33]

LUNG CANCER SCREENING. Symptoms of lung cancer are not usually apparent until the disease is in the advanced stages. Some patients are diagnosed early in the disease progression when they are tested for another medical condition. Although numerous organizations recommend screening and early detection of breast, colorectal, and prostate cancers, currently no such recommendations exist for lung cancer. Because of the tremendous impact of lung cancer on individuals, families, and society, the interest in early detection and screening is growing. However, no lung cancer screening test has been shown to prevent the high mortality rates from the disease.[4,17] Newer studies show that when stage I cancer is resected, 5-year survival can be as high as 70%.[37]

Recent and current studies are examining the beneficial effect of a new x-ray technique called spiral or low-dose CT scanning in asymptomatic but at-risk populations. The populations identified as being at-risk and eligible for screening include smokers or former smokers who are (1) 60 years of age or older, (2) have at least a 10–pack-year smoking history, (3) have no known history of malignancy, and (4) are fit to undergo thoracic surgery. CT scanners are capable of detecting very small nodules and thus help diagnose lung cancer earlier.[3,4] Research is also attempting to identify biomarkers for lung cancer applied to sputum specimens.[17]

Pathophysiology. More than 90% of all lung cancers fall into four major histologic types: adenocarcinoma, large cell and squamous cell carcinoma, and small cell lung cancer (SCLC) (Figure 26-4). Small cell cancer grows the most rapidly and, in general, is the most responsive to cytotoxic chemotherapy.[19]

As with other types of cancer, lung cancer is staged. Staging for SCLC is a simple two-stage system, since more than 70% of SCLC cases are metastatic at the time of diagnosis and therefore inoperable for cure. The two stages are (1) limited (indicating a confined tumor) and (2) extensive (indicating metastasis). The TNM (tumor, node, metastasis) International Staging System for Lung Cancer is used for non–small cell lung cancer (NSCLC) (Box 26-4).

TABLE 26-9 MAJOR OCCUPATIONAL LUNG DISEASES

Type	Etiology and Epidemiology	Pathophysiology	Clinical Manifestations and Prevention
PNEUMOCONIOSES*			
Simple (chronic) silicosis	Inhaled silica dust; most common form seen in miners, foundry workers, and others who inhaled relatively low concentrations of dust for 10-20 yr	Dust accumulated in tissue causing tissue reaction with whorl-shaped nodules throughout lungs	Breathlessness with exercise; 20%-30% progress to complicated silicosis
Complicated silicosis (also called confluent silicosis)	Developed by 20%-30% of persons with chronic silicosis	Progressive massive fibrosis (PMF) throughout lungs causing decreased lung function and cor pulmonale	Breathlessness, weakness, chest pain, productive cough with sputum; death from cor pulmonale and respiratory failure
Acute silicoproteinosis	Rapidly progressive disease, leading to severe disability and death within 5 yr of diagnosis	Inflammatory reaction within alveoli, diffuse fibrosis Rapid progression to respiratory failure	Prevention: dust control and improved ventilation to reduce dust levels; use of special suits and breathing apparatus by sandblasters in enclosed spaces; some experts believe such protective measures still inadequate
Complicated progressive massive fibrosis (PMF)	Develops in 3% of persons with simple silicosis; occurs in miners with heavy deposits of coal dust in lungs; *may appear suddenly years after miner has left mines;* workers who smoke have 5-6 times more lung obstruction than nonsmoking workers; cigarette smoking causes chronic bronchitis and emphysema	Fibrosis developing in some of dust-laden areas; fibrosis spreading, and fibrotic areas coalescing; eventually most of lung stiffened and useless	Shortens life span; patients may die of respiratory failure, cor pulmonale, or superimposed infection. Most silicosis-associated deaths in persons over age 65 years National Institute for Occupational Safety and Health (NIOSH) concerned about number of young persons dying from silicosis; occupations include operators of machines used to crush, grind, mix, and blend materials; painters and paint spray operators; construction workers; and laborers More deaths in minorities; more women developing silicosis Prevention: dust control; abrasive blasting with silica sand, to prepare surfaces for painting, equals exposure to 200 times NIOSH recommendations; worker education about NIOSH recommendations for avoiding prolonged overexposure to silica dust

TABLE 26-9 MAJOR OCCUPATIONAL LUNG DISEASES—CONT'D

Type	Etiology and Epidemiology	Pathophysiology	Clinical Manifestations and Prevention
ASBESTOS-RELATED LUNG DISEASE			
	Asbestos causing lung cancer, malignant mesothelioma of pleura and periosteum, cancer of larynx, certain GI cancers, and asbestosis, a progressive fibrotic lung disease; risk increases with repeated exposure and length of time since first exposure; declared a human carcinogen by EPA and International Agency for Research on Cancer of WHO Total number of U.S. deaths eventually caused by exposure to asbestos estimated to exceed 200,000; 20%-25% of deaths from workers with heavy exposure are from lung cancer; cancer related to degree of exposure and to cigarette smoking, which enhances carcinogenic properties of asbestos; *asbestos workers who smoke are 90 times more likely to develop lung cancer than smokers with no exposure to asbestos* Four commercially important forms of asbestos: chrysotile, crocidolite, amosite, and anthophylline; chrysotile accounts for 95% of current world production; nearly all asbestos used in North America is mined in Quebec; crocidolite is 2-4 times more potent than chrysotile or amosite in causing mesothelioma; all forms equally potent as cause of lung cancer; new use of asbestos almost completely ended in United States and other developed nations as a result of government bans and market pressures; asbestos extensively and aggressively marketed by Canada and other exporting nations in developing world, where sales remain strong	Fibrosis caused by asbestos called asbestosis; asbestos fibers accumulate around terminal bronchioles; fibers surround iron-rich tissue, forming ferruginous bodies with characteristic picture on x-ray film; more asbestos bodies as more fibers are inhaled; after 20-30 yr of exposure, fibrosis begins in lungs; if heavy exposure, appears in 4-5 yr Occurs in persons exposed to crocidolite fibers of a certain size; needlelike shape of crocidolite fibers enables them to pass through lung tissue to pleura	After fibrosis begins, cough, sputum, weight loss, increasing breathlessness; most die within 1-5 yr of first symptoms Treatment with radical pleurectomy and pneumonectomy; survival only 1-2 yr Prevention: enforcement of regulations governing mining, milling, and use of asbestos; follow guiding principle of AHERA, that asbestos in a building poses no hazard to health unless fibers become airborne and can be inhaled; removal of asbestos required only when asbestos is visibly deteriorating or when renovation is imminent; protective masks necessary when working with asbestos

Continued

TABLE 26-9 MAJOR OCCUPATIONAL LUNG DISEASES—CONT'D

Type	Etiology and Epidemiology	Pathophysiology	Clinical Manifestations and Prevention
ASBESTOS-RELATED LUNG DISEASE—CONT'D			
	Asbestos Hazard Emergency Response Act (AHERA), passed in 1986, tightened controls on use of asbestos in United States; mesothelioma accounts for 7%-10% of deaths in asbestos workers; inoperable and always fatal; can occur after little exposure to crocidolite; has been reported in wives of asbestos workers and in persons living near asbestos plants; cigarette smoking not a contributing factor in these persons; inhalation of only a few fine, straight crocidolite factors are necessary; swallowing of asbestos-contaminated sputum responsible for cancer of larynx, esophagus, stomach, and intestines		
HYPERSENSITIVITY DISEASES			
	Fall into occupational category when antigen is found primarily in workplace; lung hypersensitivity can occur in bronchi, bronchioles, or alveoli; coarse dust causes bronchial reactions; fine dust provokes small airway and alveolar reactions		
Occupational asthma	More common in 10% of population who are atopic (genetic tendency to develop an allergy); nonatopic persons can also become sensitized; substances with antigenic properties include detergent enzymes, platinum salts, cereals and grains, certain wood dusts, isocyanate chemicals used in polyurethane paints and other	Hypersensitivity reaction mediated by histamine progressing to bronchoconstriction and increased mucus production; repeated attacks if cause unrecognized and asthma is untreated; may lead to permanent obstructive lung disease; asthmatic response that is well established can be	Wheezing a major symptom Prevention: total elimination of antigen; desensitization not successful

Lung cancer may metastasize to nearby structures, such as the prescalene lymph nodes, the esophageal walls, and the pericardium; or to distant areas, such as the brain, liver, kidneys, adrenal glands, or skeleton. The overall cure rate for all types of lung cancer is only about 10%.[4] Survival rates of patients with NSCLC depend on the size of the tumor, nodal status, and degree of metastasis.

A patient's signs and symptoms depend on several factors, including the location of the lesion. In approximately 10% of cases, patients are asymptomatic and the cancer is identified on a routine chest x-ray film. Of patients with cancer of the lung or bronchus who have symptoms, approximately 75% have a cough and approximately 50% have hemoptysis. Shortness of

TABLE 26-9 MAJOR OCCUPATIONAL LUNG DISEASES—CONT'D

Type	Etiology and Epidemiology	Pathophysiology	Clinical Manifestations and Prevention
HYPERSENSITIVITY DISEASES—CONT'D			
	products, agents used in printing, and some pesticides	provoked by other factors (house dust, cigarette smoke) and by fatigue, breathing cold air, and coughing	
Hypersensitivity pneumonitis (allergic alveolitis [farmer's lung])	Caused by fine organic dust inhaled into smallest airways; farmer's lung caused by moldy hay; allergic alveolitis caused by other dusts, including moldy sugar cane and barley, maple bark, cork, animal hair, bird feathers and droppings, mushroom compost, coffee beans, and paprika; often disease is named for cause (mushroom worker's lung, etc.); fungus spores growing in apparent antigen are thought in many cases to be real cause of disease	Alveoli are inflamed, inundated by WBCs, sometimes filled with fluid; if exposure infrequent or level of dust low, symptoms are mild, and treatment not sought; chronic form develops over time; eventually, fibrosis occurs, and may be so well established that it cannot be arrested	Symptoms begin hours after exposure to offending dust and include fatigue, shortness of breath, dry cough, fever, and chills; symptoms may be severe enough to require emergency treatment and hospitalization; acute attacks treated with steroids; recovery may take 6 wk, and patient may have residual lung damage; real cure is permanent separation of patient and antigen Prevention: properly dried and stored farm products (hay, straw, sugar cane); presumably fungi only grow in moist conditions
Byssinosis (brown lung)	Occupational disease occurring in textile workers; mainly cotton workers, but also afflicts workers in flax and hemp industries; cause is found in bales of raw cotton that contain not only cotton fibers but fragments of cotton plant; something in plant matter, rather than pure cotton, is cause	Chronic bronchitis and emphysema develop in time; constriction of bronchioles in response to something in crude cotton; symptoms of asthma and allergy persist as long as there is exposure to cotton antigen	Tightness in chest on returning to work after weekend away (Monday fever); strong relationship between amount of dust inhaled and symptoms; persistent, productive, tight chest with chronic bronchitis and emphysema; person leaves industry as respiratory cripple Prevention: dust control measures; pretreating bales of cotton by washing with steam and other agents may inactivate causative agent; try to detect persons who are likely to become sensitized to cotton dust and keep them out of high-risk areas

EPA, Environmental Protection Agency; *GI,* gastrointestinal; *NIOSH,* National Institute for Occupational Safety and Health; *WBC,* white blood cells; *WHO,* World Health Organization.
*Also known as "dust in the lungs."

breath and a unilateral wheeze are also common. Extrapulmonary intrathoracic signs and symptoms occur with peripheral pulmonary lesions that perforate into the pleural space. These include pain on inspiration, friction rub, pleural effusion, edema of the face and neck when the superior vena cava is involved, fatigue, and clubbing of the fingers. In the later stages of the disease, weight loss and debility usually indicate metastases, especially to the liver.

Collaborative Care Management

DIAGNOSTIC TESTS. Confirmed diagnosis of lung cancer requires histologic examination of the tumor. Specimens for examination

Box 26-3 Effects of Smoking on Lung Cancer Risk

- Smokers are 10 times more likely to develop lung cancer than those who never smoked.
- Heavy smokers are more likely to die of lung cancer than light smokers, suggesting a dose-response effect.
- Risk associated with smoking increases with the number of years a person smokes.
- Risk decreases steadily after a person stops smoking.
- Cigarette smokers have a higher death rate than pipe smokers.
- Nonsmoking wives of smokers have a significantly higher risk of lung cancer than nonsmoking wives of nonsmokers.

may be obtained by fiberoptic bronchoscopy, percutaneous transthoracic needle biopsy, endoscopic ultrasonography with fine-needle aspiration, sputum collection, or surgery (Table 26-10).

MEDICATIONS. Historically NSCLC has not been considered amenable to cytotoxic chemotherapy, but more recently developed regimens have improved response rates and survival. Combination therapy that includes cisplatin plus etoposide, vinorelbine, paclitaxel, docetaxel, or gemcitabine has demonstrated the best results. Patients who are most likely to benefit from chemotherapy include those with minimal weight loss, less extensive disease spread, and good functionality.[18] The Food and Drug Administration recently approved the drug erlotinib (Tarceva) in treatment of patients with advanced NSCLC. The medication is not used in combination with other chemotherapeutic agents. It has been shown to extend survival time for these patients.[20]

The most widely used chemotherapy regimens for SCLC, which is the most responsive type of lung cancer to cytotoxic agents, include cyclophosphamide, doxorubicin, and etoposide; cisplatin and etoposide; or ifosfamide, carboplatin, and etoposide.[17,18] Medications to control pain, hypertension, or other coexisting disease are also a part of the patient's treatment.

TREATMENTS. Radiotherapy given concurrently or alternating with chemotherapy appears to improve survival, but it may also increase the risks for myelosuppression and esophagitis.

SURGICAL MANAGEMENT. Assessment of surgical risk for pulmonary resection considers age, pulmonary reserve, presence of cardiovascular disease, and presence of disease so extensive it would require a pneumonectomy. Mortality and morbidity related to pulmonary resection increase significantly in persons older than 70 years of age. Some studies suggest higher mortality and morbidity in those 60 to 65 years of age. ABG studies and PFTs are used to measure pulmonary reserve.[17] A $Paco_2$ of greater than 45 mm Hg indicates inoperability, whereas a Pao_2 of less than 60 mm Hg suggests that pulmonary resection would be risky. An exception is when the low Pao_2 is caused by complete airway obstruction that results from desaturated blood entering the pulmonary veins from a perfused but nonventilated lung (ventilation-perfusion [V/Q] mismatch). The PFTs are used to evaluate the risk for pulmonary resection. A predicted postoperative forced expiratory volume in 1 second (FEV_1) of more than 800 ml is required in most adults. Most patients with an FEV_1 of less than 30% of predicted are unable to tolerate pneumonectomy.

Coronary artery disease is present in about 80 of every 1000 patients older than age 65. Previous myocardial infarction,

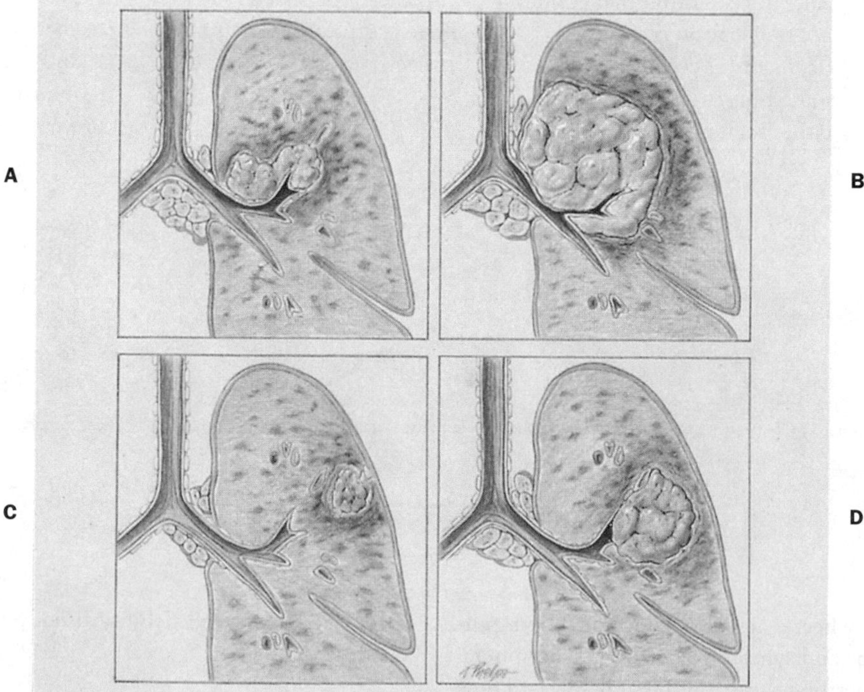

Figure 26-4 Cancer of the lung. **A,** Squamous (epidermoid) cell carcinoma. **B,** Small cell (oat cell) carcinoma. **C,** Adenocarcinoma. **D,** Large cell carcinoma.

BOX 26-4 International Staging System for Lung Cancer: TNM Descriptors for Non–Small Cell Lung Cancer

Primary Tumor (T)

Tx	Primary tumor cannot be assessed or tumor proven by the presence of malignant cells in sputum or bronchial washings and not visualized by imaging or bronchoscopy
T0	No evidence of primary tumor
Tis	Carcinoma in situ
T1	Tumor ≤3 cm in dimension; surrounded by lung or visceral pleura
T2	Tumor ≥3 cm in dimension; involves main bronchus; invades visceral pleura; associated with atelectasis
T3	Tumor of any size that directly invades the chest wall, diaphragm, mediastinal pleura, or parietal pericardium
T4	Tumor of any size that invades the heart, great vessels, trachea, esophagus, vertebral body, or carina; or tumor with pleural or pericardial effusion

Regional Lymph Nodes (N)

Nx	Regional lymph nodes cannot be assessed
N0	No regional lymph node metastasis
N1	Metastasis to ipsilateral hilar lymph nodes, intrapulmonary nodes
N2	Metastasis to ipsilateral mediastinal or subcarinal lymph nodes
N3	Metastasis to contralateral mediastinal, hilar, scalene, or supraclavicular lymph nodes

Distant Metastasis (M)

Mx	Presence of distant metastasis cannot be assessed
M0	No distant metastasis
M1	Distant metastasis present

Adapted from Hyer JD, Sivestri G: Diagnosis and staging of lung cancer, *Clin Chest Med* 21(1):95–106, 2000.

TABLE 26-10 LUNG CANCER: DIAGNOSTIC TESTS AND PURPOSES

Test	Purpose
Fiberoptic bronchoscopy	Used to obtain tissue for diagnosis from centrally located lesions. Tissue samples can be removed from visible tumors and peripheral lesions brushed and washed.
Transbronchial needle biopsy	Used when hilar or mediastinal lymph nodes are involved; done to obtain nodal tissue for examination.
Percutaneous transthoracic needle biopsy	Procedure of choice for diagnosing malignancy in peripheral lung nodules.
Endoscopic ultrasonography with fine-needle aspiration	Used for diagnosis and staging of lung cancer.
Cytologic analysis of sputum	Used to diagnose lung cancer. It is considered safest and least expensive test. In this approach, a sample of sputum is examined for bacteria and cancer cells. For best results, a 3-day pooled sample is used. Diagnostic yield also has been shown to increase with induction of sputum rather than spontaneous expectoration.
Video-assisted thoracoscopy or thoracotomy	Used to perform small diagnostic wedge excisions.
Lateral chest x-ray	Used in diagnosis and staging of lung cancer.
Contrast-enhanced computed tomography (CT) scan or magnetic resonance imaging (MRI)	Used to differentiate underlying mass from atelectasis, or inflammation or involvement of visceral pleura from involvement of parietal pleura, thus identifying chest wall invasion.
Positron emission tomography (PET)	Used in staging NSCLC; more sensitive than CT or MRI and aids in the diagnosis of both primary and metastatic sites.
Thoracentesis	Routinely performed if evidence of pleural effusion clinically or on CT scan.
Mediastinoscopy	Considered better than CT scan or MRI for assessing mediastinal metastases and effectiveness of preoperative radiotherapy or chemotherapy.

NSCLC, Nonsmall cell lung cancer.

especially within 6 months before surgery, increases the risk. Left ventricular dysfunction, including signs of heart failure, indicates high risk of death after pulmonary resection. Unstable angina or hypertension must be controlled before resection. Frequent premature ventricular contractions are signs of severe heart disease and are associated with increased perioperative complications and death. Pneumonectomy is associated with higher risk than lesser procedures, particularly for patients ages 70 and over, and especially with surgery of the right lung.

Endotracheal anesthesia is used for surgery involving the lung in which the pleural space is entered. Endotracheal anesthesia makes it possible to keep the uninvolved ("good") lung expanded and functioning when the chest is opened and atmospheric pressure enters the pleural space.

The pressure in the pleural space (the space between the visceral and parietal pleura) is subatmospheric (less than 760 mm Hg) and is referred to as negative. When the pleura is entered surgically or with trauma to the chest wall, atmospheric (positive) pressure enters the pleural space, and the lung on that side collapses. After resectional surgery of the lung (except pneumonectomy), the surgeon inserts one or two drainage tubes into the pleural space. Each tube is connected to a negative-pressure closed drainage system, which allows air and fluid to drain from the pleural space and prevents air or fluid from entering the pleural space. In all resectional surgery (except pneumonectomy) the remaining portions of the lung must overexpand and fill the space left by the resected portion. The removal of air and fluid from the pleural space aids in the expansion of the remaining portion of the lung and helps reestablish negative pressure in the pleural space.

Types of thoracic surgery along with indications are presented in Box 26-5. An exploratory thoracotomy confirms a suspected diagnosis of lung or chest disease. The usual approach is by a posterolateral parascapular incision through the fourth, fifth, sixth, or seventh intercostal space. Occasionally an anterior approach is used. The ribs are spread to give the best possible exposure of the lung and hemithorax. The pleura is entered and the lung examined, a biopsy usually taken, and the chest closed. This procedure may also be used to detect bleeding in the chest or other injury after trauma to the chest. Because the pleural space was entered, a chest tube and closed drainage system are necessary (Figure 26-5).

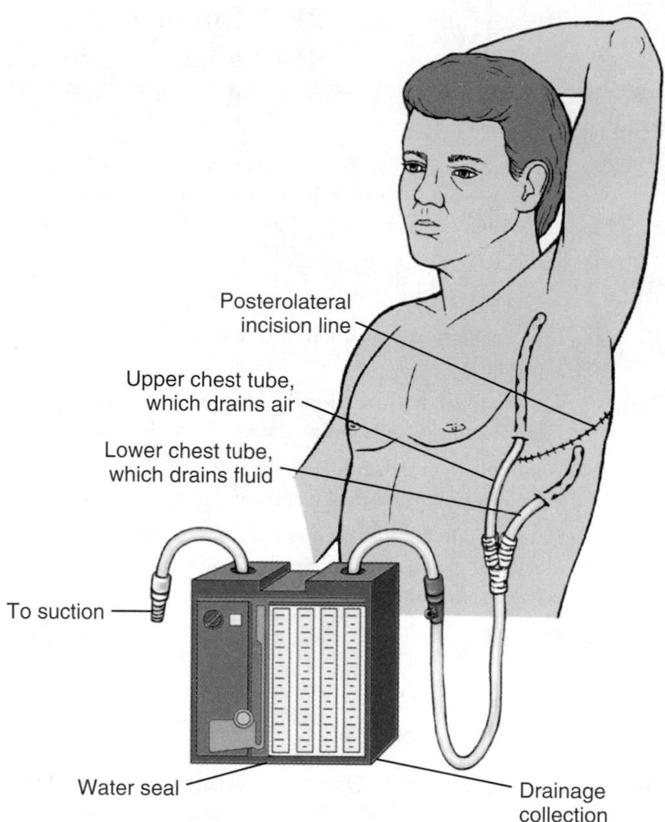

Figure 26-5 Closed chest drainage system.

A pneumonectomy (the removal of an entire lung) is most often performed to treat bronchogenic carcinoma (Figure 26-6). It may also be used to treat TB. However, a pneumonectomy is performed only in cases in which a **lobectomy** (removal of a lobe of the lung) or segmental resection (removal of a part of a lobe) will not remove all the diseased tissue. The surgeon makes a thoracotomy incision in either the posterior or anterior chest. Before removing the lung, the surgeon ligates, then cuts the pulmonary artery and vein. The main-stem bronchus leading to the lung is clamped, divided, and sutured or stapled. To ensure an airtight closure of the bronchus, the surgeon may place a pleural flap over it and suture it in place. This is not necessary if staples are used.

Box 26-5 Types of Thoracic Surgery and Indications for Use

- Exploratory thoracotomy: Confirmation of suspected diagnosis of lung or chest disease, especially carcinoma; to obtain a biopsy; being replaced by noninvasive procedures (thoracoscopy)
- Pneumonectomy: Removal of a lung; used for bronchogenic carcinoma when lobectomy will not remove all of lesion, or for tuberculosis when other surgery will not remove all of diseased lung
- Pneumonectomy: Lung reduction surgery to reduce lung volume and decrease tension on respiratory muscles in persons with emphysema
- Lobectomy: Removal of one lobe of lung; used for bronchogenic carcinoma confined to a lobe, bronchiectasis, emphysematous blebs or bullae, lung abscess, fungal infections, benign tumors, or tuberculosis
- Bilobectomy: Removal of two lobes from right lung; used for bronchogenic carcinoma when lobectomy will not remove all of disease
- Sleeve lobectomy: Resection of main bronchus or distal trachea with reanastomosis to a distal uninvolved bronchus; used for bronchogenic carcinoma to preserve functional parenchyma
- Segmental resection: Segmentectomy; removal of one or more lung segments; used for bronchiectasis, lung abscess or cyst, metastatic carcinoma, or tuberculosis
- Wedge resection: Removal of pie-shaped section from surface of lung; used for well-circumscribed benign tumors, metastatic tumors, or localized inflammatory disease, including TB
- Decortication: Removal of a fibrinous peel from visceral pleura; used for chronic empyema
- Thoracoplasty: Removal of ribs; used for residual air space after resectional surgery or chronic empyema space

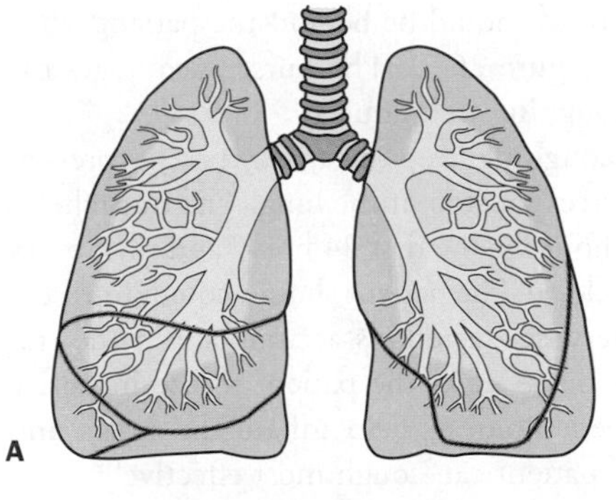

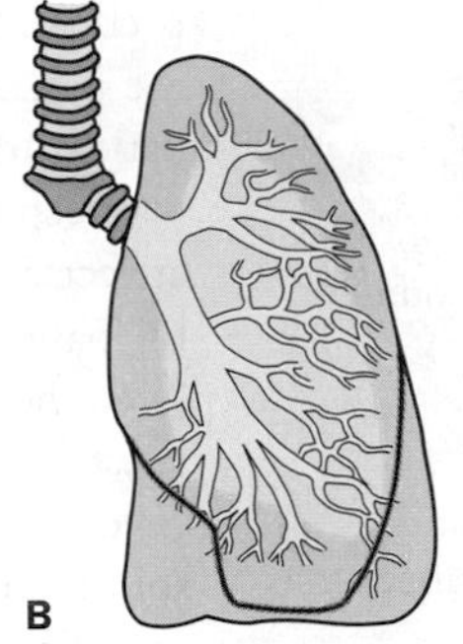

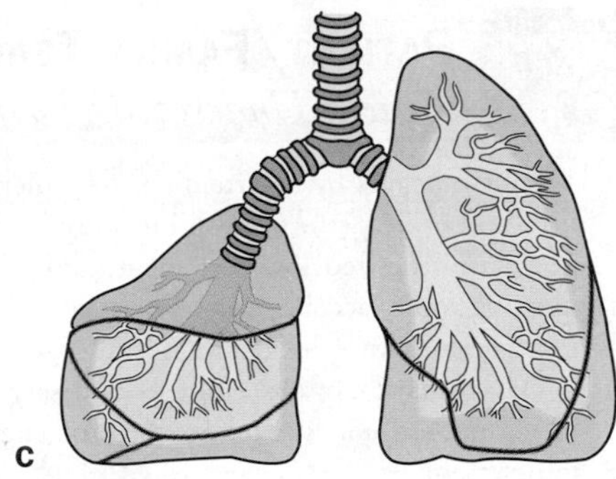

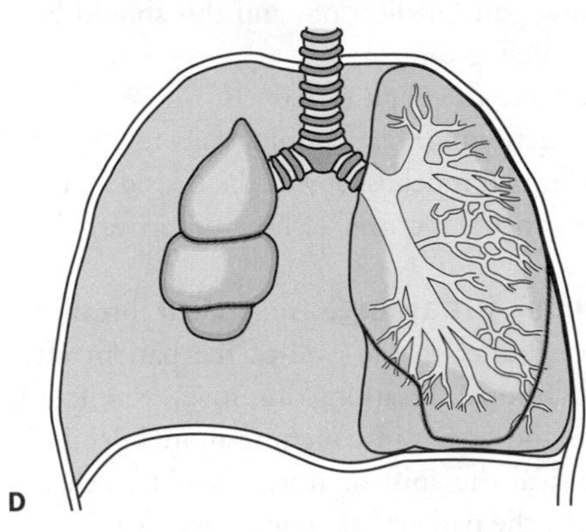

Figure 26-6 **A,** Normal lungs. **B,** Surgical absence of right lung after pneumonectomy. **C,** Surgical absence of right upper lobe after lobectomy. **D,** Complete collapse of right lung as a result of air in pleural cavity (pneumothorax).

The phrenic nerve on the operated side is crushed, causing the diaphragm on that side to rise and reduce the size of the remaining space. Because no lung is left to reexpand, drainage tubes are not usually used. Ideally, the pressure in the closed chest is slightly negative. The fluid left in the space consolidates in time, preventing the remaining lung and the heart from shifting toward the operated side (mediastinal shift).

In a lobectomy one lobe of the lung is removed (Figure 26-6, *C*). In addition to treating lung cancer, it is used to treat bronchiectasis, emphysematous blebs or bullae, lung abscesses, benign tumors, fungal infections, and TB. For a lobectomy to be successful, the disease must be confined to one lobe, and the remaining lung tissue must be capable of overexpanding to fill the space of the resected lobe. One or two chest tubes are connected to a closed drainage system for postoperative drainage.

In a segmental resection one or more segments of the lung are removed. This procedure is used in an attempt to preserve as much functioning lung tissue as possible. It is an extremely taxing procedure for the surgeon, since he or she must perform the dissection between segments carefully and slowly, and the identification of the segmental pulmonary artery and vein and bronchus is more difficult than when a lobe is involved. Because the right lung has 10 segments and the left lung 8, only a portion of a lobe or lobes may need to be removed. The most common indication for segmentectomy is bronchiectasis. Chest tube(s) and a closed drainage system are necessary after surgery. Because of air leaks from the segmental surface, the remaining lung tissue may take longer to reexpand.

In a wedge resection a well-circumscribed diseased portion is removed without regard to the segmental planes of the lung. The area to be removed is clamped, dissected, and sutured or stapled. Chest tube(s) and a closed drainage system are used after surgery. With decortication, a fibrinous peel is removed from the visceral pleura, allowing the encased lung to reexpand and obliterate the pleural space (see earlier discussion under Empyema). Chest tube(s) and chest suction facilitate the reexpansion of the lung. If the lung has been encased for a long time, it may be incapable of reexpanding after decortication. In this situation, thoracoplasty may be necessary.

DIET. The diet for a patient with lung cancer varies with the stage of the cancer and the therapy prescribed. However, good nutrition is always important for healing, so the patient is encouraged to eat well as tolerated throughout the course of the disease.

Nursing Management

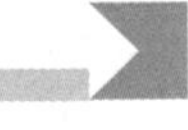

of the Patient undergoing Thoracic Surgery

PREOPERATIVE CARE

The nurse discusses the proposed surgery with both patient and family. The goal of teaching is to prepare the patient for what he or she is expected to do after surgery. Patients may be admitted to the hospital the day of surgery. To be effective, preoperative teaching is a responsibility shared by primary care clinicians and home care and acute care nurses. In some hospitals nurses from the operating room, recovery room, or ICU participate in the preoperative teaching. The goal is that the patient understands the impending surgery and has an opportunity to ask questions and express concerns. The Patient/Family Teaching box lists topics to address in the teaching plan. The nurse may refer patients to local cancer support groups and assistive agencies for information, support, and other services.

POSTOPERATIVE CARE

The care of the patient after thoracic surgery centers on promoting ventilation and reexpansion of the lung by maintaining a clear

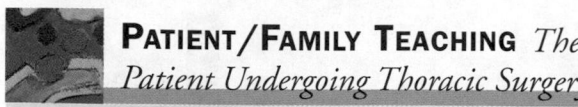

PATIENT/FAMILY TEACHING *The Patient Undergoing Thoracic Surgery*

The nurse begins by ascertaining the patient's understanding of the procedure to be performed and its purpose, as well as the amount of information desired by the patient, and adjusts teaching about the following topics accordingly:

- Patient's knowledge of procedure
- Explanation of procedure as necessary, including intubation for anesthesia, site of incision, and chest tube(s) and drainage system
- Oxygen
- Blood administration and intravenous infusions
- Pain medication, including patient-controlled analgesia if used
- What patient will be asked to do:
  —Coughing and deep breathing
  —Arm exercises
  —Ambulation
- Where patient will be taken after surgery:
  —To recovery—for how long
  —To intensive care unit—for how long
- Where family can wait during surgery

airway, maintaining the closed drainage system if one is used, promoting arm exercises to maintain full use on the operated side, promoting nutrition, and monitoring the incision for bleeding and subcutaneous emphysema. Care in the initial postoperative period takes place in an ICU. The patient remains in the ICU until successfully extubated and hemodynamically stable.

The patient is usually attached to a cardiac monitor. A Swan-Ganz catheter and central venous pressure line are used for hemodynamic monitoring. Oxygen is attached to the endotracheal tube in the immediate postoperative period. After extubation, humidified oxygen is given by cannula, usually at 6 L/min. An oxygen mask is not used because of the need to have the patient cough and raise secretions frequently. The nurse checks vital signs every 15 minutes until the patient is well recovered from anesthesia, every hour until the patient's condition has stabilized, and then every 2 to 4 hours. Blood pressure may fluctuate during the first 24 to 36 hours, and close monitoring of the patient is essential. Acute changes or disturbing trends (hypotension, hypertension) are reported to the surgeon.

Positioning the Patient in Bed. The patient is kept flat in bed or with the head elevated slightly (20 degrees) until blood pressure is stabilized to preoperative levels. Once blood pressure is stabilized, the patient can usually breathe best in semi-Fowler's position with a pillow under the head and neck but not under the shoulder and back because of the subscapular incision.

Initiating Coughing and Deep Breathing Exercises. The nurse helps the patient cough as soon as he or she is conscious and extubated. If the blood pressure is stable, the nurse helps the patient to a sitting position, using the hands to support the incision anteriorly and posteriorly. Firm, even pressure over the incision with the open palm of the hands or a surgical pillow is effective. The nurse's head should be behind the patient while the patient is coughing (Figure 26-7). The nurse encourages the patient to use the huff coughing technique.

Deep breathing and coughing keep the airway patent, prevent atelectasis, and facilitate reexpansion of the lung. The nurse helps the patient cough every hour for the first 24 hours and then every 2 to 4 hours around the clock. The patient should cough until the chest sounds clear. Otherwise, secretions accumulate in the tracheobronchial tree. The nurse urges the patient to use incentive spirometry 10 times every hour to help inflate the lungs and mobilize secretions. The patient can cough most effectively 20 to 30 minutes after receiving pain medication, and this should be a priority when planning nursing care.

When a patient is unable to cough effectively, the nurse performs tracheobronchial suctioning. If suctioning fails to clear the airway, the surgeon performs bronchoscopy at the bedside with a fiberoptic bronchoscope, since it is crucial to keep the airway clear.

Promoting Abdominal Breathing. Abdominal breathing exercises are a valuable adjunct to the care of the patient after chest surgery, since abdominal breathing improves ventilation without increasing pain and assists in coughing more effectively (Figure 26-8). The physical therapist or nurse should teach the exercises before surgery so the patient has time to practice them.

Promoting Comfort by Pain Relief. Medication for pain should be given as needed, as often as every 1 to 4 hours during the first 48 to 72 hours. The patient is often extremely uncomfortable and is reluctant to cough or turn unless pain is relieved. The tubes in the chest cause pain, and the patient may attempt rapid, shallow breathing to splint the lower chest and avoid

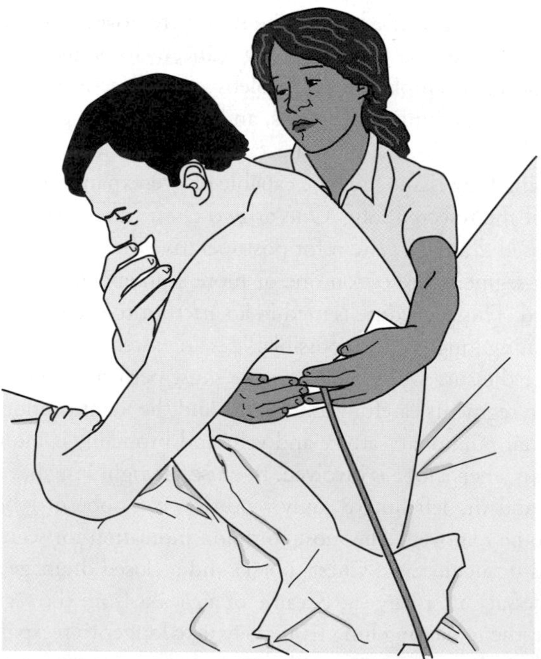

Figure 26-7 Nurse helps patient cough by splinting incision with firm support using her hands. This lessens muscle pull and pain as patient coughs. Note that nurse keeps her head behind patient while he coughs, and patient uses tissue to cover his mouth.

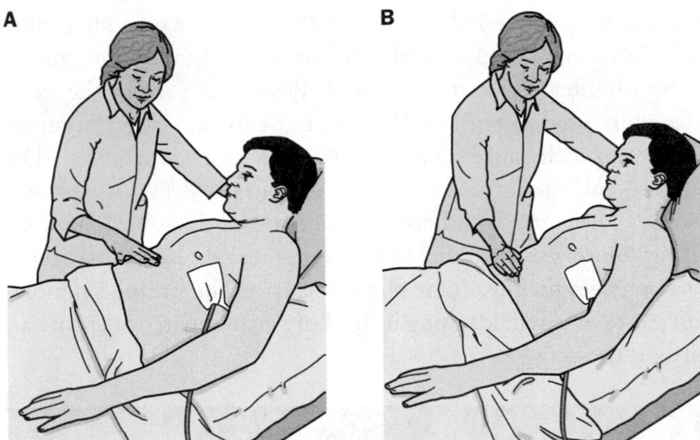

Figure 26-8 **A,** Physical therapist assists patient in learning augmented abdominal breathing. Patient is instructed to inhale through the nose, using abdominal muscles, and to concentrate on moving lower ribs under the therapist's hand. This exercise improves ventilation of base of lungs. **B,** Physical therapist places hand on upper abdomen while helping patient exhale fully.

motion of the catheters. This impairs ventilation, makes coughing ineffective, and causes secretions to be retained. It is a nursing responsibility to make the patient comfortable, since this facilitates deep breathing and coughing. Patient-controlled analgesia pumps and epidural catheters are widely used for pain medication management. Rarely an intercostal nerve block may be required.

Promoting Arm Exercises. The nurse usually begins passive range-of-motion (ROM) arm exercises the evening of surgery to prevent restriction of function. Most patients are reluctant to move the arm on the operated side, but with proper pain control, preoperative instruction, and postoperative follow-through, they do so readily. Both the patient and the nurse should understand that the longer the arm is unexercised, the stiffer it becomes. The patient should put both arms through active ROM two or three times a day within a few days. The recommended exercises are similar to those used after mastectomy. The exercises are best performed when the patient is upright or lying on the abdomen. Exercises such as elevating the scapula and clavicle, "hunching the shoulders," bringing the scapulae as close together as possible, and hyperextending the arm can be performed only in these positions. Because lying on the abdomen may not be possible at first, these exercises are performed with the patient sitting on the edge of the bed or standing.

Promoting Nutrition. The nurse encourages the patient to take fluids postoperatively and to progress to a general diet as soon as it is tolerated. Fluids help liquefy secretions and make them easier to expectorate. A diet adequate in protein and vitamins, especially vitamin C, facilitates wound healing.

Monitoring the Incision for Bleeding or Subcutaneous Emphysema. The nurse checks the dressing periodically for bleeding. Blood on the dressing is unusual and should be reported to the surgeon at once. The nurse records the time and amount of blood in the patient's record. The surgeon may reinforce the dressing. In the rare instance when bleeding persists, the patient may be taken back to surgery, the chest wall reopened, and the source of bleeding located and ligated.

Subcutaneous emphysema is not unusual after chest surgery. In subcutaneous emphysema, air leaks from the pleural space through the thoracotomy incision or around the chest tubes into the soft tissues. The presence of air under the skin is readily detected and has been described as feeling like "tissue paper" or "Rice Krispies" under the skin. Subcutaneous emphysema is most notable in the neck and chest; if considerable air is leaking, the patient's face and neck become swollen. Small amounts of air reabsorb over time and cause no problem. However, if subcutaneous emphysema worsens, the surgeon may remove the chest tube and insert one with a larger diameter, since air is leaking into the tissues faster than the tube is removing it. Additional suction may also be applied to the chest tube(s) in an attempt to remove air more rapidly. Rarely, a patient needs to return to surgery for closure of air leaks.

The patient with a pneumonectomy should have only a small amount (if any) of subcutaneous emphysema. Progressive subcutaneous emphysema after pneumonectomy is very serious and should be reported to the surgeon immediately because it could indicate a major leak in the bronchial stump. This is a rare occurrence, requiring immediate return to surgery for reclosure of the stump.

Maintaining Chest Tube and Drainage System. All patients who have resectional surgery of the lung, except those having a pneumonectomy, require drainage of the pleural space by one or two chest tubes connected to closed drainage. At the completion of the surgical resection, the surgeon inserts each tube into the pleural space through an incision in the chest wall and sutures the tubes in place (Figure 26-9). When two tubes are used, one catheter is inserted in the anterior chest wall above the resected area. This anterior or upper tube removes air from the pleural space. The second tube is inserted in the posterior chest, and this posterior or lower tube drains serosanguineous fluid that accumulates as a result of the surgery. The lower tube may be of a larger diameter than the upper tube to prevent it from becoming plugged with clots. When only one chest tube is used, it is usually placed anteriorly above the resected area of the lung.

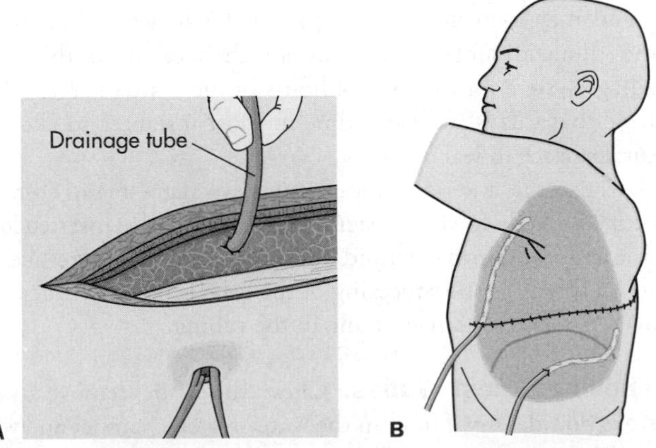

Figure 26-9 **A,** Drainage tube being inserted into pleural space. **B,** Note that both tubes are placed well into pleural space.

To initiate chest tube drainage, the chest tubes are connected to a closed-chest drainage system that allows for removal of fluid and air from the intrapleural space to promote lung reexpansion. (A commonly used system is the Pleur-Evac.) The water in a water-seal chest drainage system acts as a one-way valve, permitting the unidirectional flow of air or fluid out of the pleural space. As air and fluid drainage begins, the pressure in the pleural space becomes more negative. The more negative this pressure is, the more the lung expands. Lung expansion, in turn, forces more fluid and air out of the pleural space. This cycle continues until the lung is fully expanded and intrathoracic pressure returns to its normal (subatmospheric) level. A water-seal drainage system must be airtight between the pleural space and the water seal. Any air leak is an entry for atmospheric air into the pleural space, creating a positive pressure that collapses the lung. Suction may be applied to water-seal systems to encourage drainage. Suction must be maintained at the prescribed level for the patient. The water in the suction chamber of the drainage system bubbles when suction is present. A gentle, continuous level of bubbling is desired. If the water fails to bubble, the desired level of suction is not being attained, and the tubing should be checked for air leaks. If there are no leaks, the surgeon should be notified at once, because the air leak in the pleural surface may be so great that the amount of negative pressure is not sufficient to overcome it. (Chest tubes and closed drainage are shown in Figure 26-5.)

Dry suction chest drainage units have been developed that provide access to fluid samples, adjusting fluid levels and both negative and positive pressure relief. These devices also allow for adaptation to water seal.[16]

Maintaining Patency of Chest Tubes. In the past, chest tubes were "milked" or "stripped" to prevent the formation of clots that could plug the tubes. However, studies have shown that stripping the tube greatly increases the negative pressure exerted on the pleural space. Undesirable side effects of increased pressure include (1) lung entrapment in the chest tube eyelets and focal tissue infarction and (2) persistent pneumothorax. The **persistent pneumothorax** occurs when the lung's pleural surface, which normally has air leaks at the close of the procedure, does not seal off. Fibrin usually seals the air leaks; however, an increased amount of negative pressure may prevent the air leaks from sealing and may even increase the size of the air leaks. This is why some thoracic surgeons do not attach suction to the closed drainage system for the first 24 hours or more after surgery. They believe that this is sufficient time in most instances to allow the pleural surface to seal off.

Because the anterior (upper) tube evacuates mainly air, this tube is less likely to clot. Posterior tubes, which are inserted lower in the chest, drain more fluid and blood and are more likely to clot. However, gentle squeezing of the tube is usually sufficient to move the bloody drainage along in the tubing.

Removing Chest Tubes. Chest tubes are removed when there is no tidaling of fluid in the water-sealed chamber and when x-ray films confirm the full reexpansion of the lung. Most chest tubes are removed within 48 to 72 hours after surgery. If the patient has a persistent air space in the apex of the lung, the upper tube may be left in longer. Surgeons are concerned about leaving tubes in for long periods because of the risk of an ascending tube track infection. The patient should receive medication for pain 15 to 30 minutes before tube removal. Physicians vary in the exact procedure used to remove the tube, but generally a sterile suture set, 4 × 4 inch gauze squares, and 2-inch tape are required. The surgeon cuts the suture holding the tube in place, asks the patient to take a deep breath and hold it, and removes the tube. If a purse-string suture was used, the surgeon reties it and places a dry sterile dressing over the site. Some physicians cover the site with petroleum gauze or a Telfa dressing instead of gauze squares to ensure an airtight dressing.

▶ ARE YOU READY?

The nurse notes that there is no bubbling in suction chamber of the Pleur-Evac attached to the chest tube of a patient after a left lower lobectomy. Which of the following actions should the nurse take first?

1. Increase the suction setting
2. Check the tubing for air leaks
3. Clamp the chest tube
4. Place the patient supine

Providing Care After Pneumonectomy. The postoperative care discussed previously applies to all patients with resectional surgery except those undergoing pneumonectomy. Chest tubes are not necessary because there is no lung left to reexpand on the operated side.

The patient may lie on the back or operated side only. The patient is not allowed to lie with the operated side uppermost because of fear that the bronchial stump may leak, allowing fluid to drain into the unoperated side and drown the patient. In the operating room, after the chest is closed, a pneumothorax apparatus (which can instill or remove air) is used to check the pressure in the operative space, and air is removed or instilled as necessary to bring the pressure to slightly negative (slightly less than 760 mm Hg).

The surgeon palpates the patient's trachea at least daily to determine if it is in midline. Deviation of the trachea toward either the operated or unoperated side is a sign of mediastinal shift. If pressure builds up in the operated side, the trachea will deviate toward the unoperated side. The treatment is to remove air (positive pressure) with a pneumothorax apparatus. Mediastinal shift toward the "good" lung can seriously compromise ventilation and needs to be treated promptly. Deviation of the trachea toward the operated side indicates that more pressure (air) needs to be instilled into the empty space. The patient with a mediastinal shift resembles the patient in congestive heart failure. Neck veins are distended, the trachea is displaced to one side, pulse and respirations are increased, and dyspnea is present. Serous drainage collects in the operated space and over time congeals to the consistency of axle grease. This is often sufficient to keep the mediastinum from shifting toward the operated side. Persistent mediastinal shift toward the operated side may have to be treated with thoracoplasty (removal of ribs) to reduce the size of the remaining space and assist in maintaining the mediastinum in midline.

The remaining lung needs 2 to 4 days to adjust to the increase in blood flow. For this reason the nurse closely monitors the amount of fluids and blood given intravenously to prevent fluid overload. Central venous pressure monitoring is common. Crackles are often heard over the base of the remaining lung, and vascular markings will be more prominent on x-ray films. Any increase in crackles, in pulse or blood pressure, and in dyspnea may indicate circulatory overload and should be reported immediately. Treatment may include diuretics or digitalization along with discontinuing intravenous fluids.

In the immediate postoperative period (24 to 48 hours), hypotension, cardiac dysrhythmias, pulmonary edema, and subcutaneous emphysema may occur. Long-term complications include a residual air space, which results from failure of the remaining portions of the lung to reexpand and fill the space. If this space is small, no treatment is indicated. Later in the postoperative period empyema may occur, either alone or with a bronchopleural fistula. The signs, symptoms, and treatment of these two complications are outlined in Table 26-11.

If the pneumonectomy was performed because of the diagnosis of cancer, radiotherapy is usually ordered and may be started before the patient leaves the hospital. The Guidelines for Safe Practice box outlines additional special care required after a pneumonectomy while the patient is still hospitalized.

Patients with lung cancer treated with thoracic surgery are discharged from the hospital less than a week after surgery. Most require a family member or a home health aide to assist them until they regain strength and can care for themselves. Those who must leave their home to receive chemotherapy or radiotherapy need someone to drive them to treatments and to care for them after therapy. Both chemotherapy and radiotherapy can be extremely debilitating. Many patients become nauseated and require antiemetics to avoid dehydration.[44] Combination chemotherapy regimens are more toxic than a single agent but offer a better chance of survival. Patients with significant weight loss (10% or more) and decreased performance typically do not tolerate treatment well and have a poor response.[33]

Because of the poor prognosis for most patients with lung cancer, the nurse or hospital social worker should discuss available hospice services with the patient and family. If the patient and family opt to use this service, a hospice nurse is responsible for managing patient care, with the emphasis on keeping the patient as comfortable as possible. Some patients are able to remain at

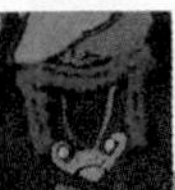

GUIDELINES FOR SAFE PRACTICE
The Patient After Pneumonectomy

- Encourage patient to do deep breathing and coughing (huff coughing technique) to prevent infection and maximize ventilation.
- Perform arm exercises (as described earlier in this chapter) to prevent restriction of motion.
- Talk with patient about resuming usual activities of daily living. Patients who have had a lung removed may have a lowered vital capacity, and exercise and activity should be limited to that which can be performed without dyspnea. Because the body must be given time to adjust to having only one lung, the patient's return to work may be delayed.
- Explain symptoms to be alert for and when to notify the physician. Tell the patient to observe for hoarseness, dyspnea, pain on swallowing, or localized chest pain and to call the physician, since these symptoms may be signs of complications.

TABLE 26-11 LONG-TERM COMPLICATIONS OF RESECTIONAL SURGERY

Complications	Signs and Symptoms	Treatment
EMPYEMA		
Pus in pleural space is a dreaded complication of thoracic surgery. Pus may drain from chest tube(s), or if chest tubes are already removed, pus can be obtained on thoracentesis (insertion of needle attached to syringe with 3-way stopcock used to remove fluid, blood, or pus from pleural space).	Unexplained elevation in temperature Evidence of pleural exudate on x-ray film	Dependent drainage by thoracentesis, intercostal chest tube, or open drainage with rib resection. Chest tube may be connected to closed drainage system or cut off and allowed to drain into chest dressings. Water seal not necessary if empyema space has thick wall and there is no danger of lung collapse. Over time, as empyema drains out tube, space becomes smaller and smaller and fills in with granulation tissue. If space persists, thoracoplasty is necessary.
BRONCHOPLEURAL FISTULA (BPF)		
Opening in sutured bronchus that permits communication between bronchus and pleural space. Space usually becomes infected, and empyema develops. Use of automatic stapling machine to close bronchus has reduced incidence of BPF.	Cough (usually nonproductive), fever, leukocytosis, anorexia, expectoration of purulent sputum, and evidence of pleural exudate on x-ray film	Chest tube connected to water-seal chamber because there is direct communication between bronchus (positive pressure being inspired) and pleural space. Persistent bronchopleural fistula is treated by thoracoplasty and muscle implant to seal off bronchus.

home with hospice services; others go to the hospital or a long-term care facility for management of ongoing problems and progressive debilitation.

Gerontologic Considerations

Many older individuals with lung cancer are not candidates for thoracic surgery, and some receive radiation as palliative therapy. For those who have surgery, adjunctive therapy with radiation or antineoplastic drugs, or both, may be necessary. The side effects of both radiation and chemotherapy may be more severe in older adults than in younger persons. Radiotherapy is usually given on an outpatient basis at the hospital, and chemotherapy may be administered in an outpatient clinic or at home. Special emphasis for the older adult is on fluid, dietary, exercise, and sleep requirements, all of which are affected by the therapy the patient receives.

Acute Lung Injury and Acute Respiratory Distress Syndrome

Etiology and Epidemiology. Acute lung injury (ALI) is a syndrome of severe, acute respiratory failure characterized by respiratory distress, severe impairment of oxygenation, and noncardiogenic pulmonary edema. ALI is defined as a syndrome of inflammation and increased permeability. Components include acute onset; bilateral infiltrates on chest x-ray films; a ratio of PaO_2 to fraction of inspired oxygen (FiO_2) of less than 300 mm Hg, regardless of positive end-expiratory pressure (PEEP); and pulmonary artery occlusion pressure of less than 18 mm Hg or no clinical evidence of left arterial hypertension.[13]

Acute respiratory distress syndrome (ARDS), also known as *adult respiratory distress syndrome,* has similar criteria but reflects more severe hypoxemia. In ARDS the PaO_2/FiO_2 ratio is less than 200 mm Hg. There has been much debate about the definitions, criteria, and names of these entities. The exact incidence of ALI and ARDS is not clear. The variability in diagnosis has made determination of incidence difficult.

Pathophysiology. Among the numerous risk factors for the development of ALI or ARDS are both direct and indirect causes of lung injury[45] (see the Risk Factors box). Four phases of ALI and ARDS have been recognized (Table 26-12).

Complications. Many complications are possible when a patient has ALI or ARDS, including dysrhythmias, pneumonia, gastrointestinal bleeding, disseminated intravascular coagulation, renal failure, and respiratory arrest.

Risk Factors

Clinical Disorders Associated With Acute Lung Injury or Acute Respiratory Distress Syndrome

Direct Lung Injury

Aspiration of gastric contents
Severe thoracic trauma
 –Pulmonary contusion
Diffuse pulmonary infection
 –Bacterial
 –Viral
 –Fungal: *Pneumocystis carinii*
Toxic gas (smoke) inhalation
Near drowning

Indirect Lung Injury

Severe sepsis
Shock
Acute pancreatitis
Severe nonthoracic trauma
Multiple long bone fractures
Hypovolemic shock
Drug overdose
Hypertransfusion (multiple transfusions)
Reperfusion injury
 –After lung transplant
 –After cardiopulmonary bypass

Adapted from Weinacker AB, Vaszar LT: Acute respiratory distress syndrome: physiology and new management strategies, *Ann Rev Med* 52:221-237, 2001.

Collaborative Care Management

Diagnostic Tests. No laboratory findings are specific for ALI or ARDS. Tests used to evaluate the patient and document the criteria for diagnosing the syndromes include PFTs, ABG studies, chest x-ray studies, lactic acid levels, and BAL. Results of PFTs indicative of ALI or ARDS are a V/Q-oxygen gradient increased to 300 to 500 mm Hg, which indicates an increased number of alveolocapillary units with a low (V/Q) ratio, a shunt factor greater than 15% to 20% (normal is 6%), below-normal compliance, and a low to normal pulmonary capillary wedge pressure. ABGs are markedly abnormal, with severe hypoxemia that may seem out of proportion to the chest x-ray film. Carbon dioxide levels initially are seen within normal or low-normal ranges. The blood pH is elevated at first in response to hyperventilation, but as ARDS worsens, the pH decreases. Lactic acid levels may increase with tissue hypoxia. Chest x-ray films show diffuse bilateral infiltrates with a normal cardiac silhouette. Infiltrates are generally focal and may be similar to those of severe cardiogenic pulmonary edema. CT scanning has demonstrated that alveolar consolidation and atelectasis occur most often in dependent lung zones.[27] Findings on BAL demonstrate a high neutrophil count and procollagen peptide III. The latter is a marker of pulmonary fibrosis and correlates with mortality.

Medications. No specific drug therapy exists for ALI and ARDS, but trials are looking at new therapies aimed at interfering with the toxic mediators thought to trigger the cascade of events. The medications being investigated include monoclonal or polyclonal antibodies to endotoxins, antiinflammatory agents, antioxidants, vasodilators, antiproteases, cytokine inhibitors, and surfactant.[19]

Treatments

Oxygen. Supplemental oxygen is the first choice of treatment in the management of impaired oxygen exchange. Although patients with ALI or ARDS may have some response in arterial oxygenation to supplemental oxygen administration, more oxygen is not necessarily better. Increasing the FiO_2 improves arterial

TABLE 26-12 PHASES OF ACUTE LUNG INJURY OR ACUTE RESPIRATORY DISTRESS SYNDROME

Phase	Description
Phase I: acute injury	Occurs within first 24 hr of injury Mild hypoxemia, dyspnea, tachypnea with or without evidence of pneumonia or pulmonary edema; clinically may see only respiratory alkalosis
Phase II: latent period	May last from several hours to 2 days Gradual development of patchy lung infiltrates (tend to be peripheral) Hypoxemia resistant to increases in supplemental oxygen administration Mechanical ventilation requiring higher concentrations of oxygen and positive end-expiratory pressure (PEEP) At tissue level, endothelial cell swelling, capillary congestion, microvascular destruction, and microatelectasis
Phase III: exudative phase	Occurs 2-10 days after injury Onset of acute respiratory failure Progressive dyspnea, tachypnea, hypoxemia, decreasing lung compliance Diffuse rales heard on examination Chest x-ray film showing patchy infiltrates that coalesce to become diffuse alveolar infiltrates Hemodynamic instability; may have signs of other organ involvement Signs of systemic inflammatory response syndrome At tissue level, edematous alveoli, edema accumulating in interstitial spaces, and alveolar consolidation secondary to accumulation of cellular debris and fibrin; hyaline membrane development; surfactant dysfunction impairing gas exchange; lungs showing microthrombus formation and occlusion
Phase IV: fibroproliferative phase	Occurs 10 days after lung injury Onset of severe physiologic abnormalities Intrapulmonary shunting leading to refractory hypoxemia and metabolic and respiratory acidosis Development of multiorgan involvement Fever, systemic inflammation, refractory hypoxia, loss of responsiveness to PEEP Results in remodeling of pulmonary microvascular system

Adapted from Van Soeren MH et al: Pathophysiology and implications for the treatment of ARDS, *AACN Clin Issues* 11(2):179-197, 2000.

oxygen saturation only when an intrapulmonary shunt is not responsible for oxygen desaturation. In ALI or ARDS, deoxygenated venous blood is shunted from the right side of the circulation to the left side. There is no alveolar contact; thus oxygen is not taken up in the shunted areas. Supplemental oxygen should be prescribed at the lowest concentration that will allow for adequate tissue oxygenation. The goal is to increase the hemoglobin saturation to 90% without risking oxygen toxicity.

MECHANICAL VENTILATION. Mechanical ventilation is the mainstay of supportive care in ALI or ARDS to provide adequate oxygenation and stabilize ventilation. Evidence continues to build that standard ventilation for patients with ALI or ARDS involves the use of small tidal volumes to protect the lungs and prevent ventilator-associated lung injury. The Acute Respiratory Distress Syndrome Network Study found a decrease in mortality and a decrease in ventilatory days by using a lower tidal volume of 6 ml/kg and a plateau pressure of less than or equal to 30 cm H_2O.[27] Permissive hypercapnia also limits ventilatory pressures by allowing $PaCO_2$ to rise, generally in the range of 60 to 100 mm Hg, with pH maintained at 7.25 or more without negative effects.

PEEP is a ventilator mode shown to increase the effectiveness of mechanical ventilation in certain patients. It involves the maintenance of positive pressure at the end of expiration, rather than allowing airway pressure to return to normal (atmospheric pressure), as usually occurs. With the maintenance of positive pressure, alveoli that would otherwise collapse on expiration are held open, thus increasing the opportunity for gas exchange across the alveolocapillary membrane. This is accomplished by the increase in functional residual capacity (FRC). The result is a decrease in physiologic shunting and the ability to achieve a higher level of PaO_2 with lower concentrations of delivered oxygen (FiO_2). PEEP can, however, decrease cardiac output, increase dead space, increase lung volumes, and stretch during inspirations. The lowest mean airway pressure that achieves an acceptable level of arterial oxygenation with a nontoxic FiO_2 should be used.[27]

Additional ventilation strategies have been devised to prevent further lung injury. They include high frequency, inverse-ratio ventilation, extracorporeal membrane oxygenation (ECMO), and prone positioning. Although they show promise, to date no method has been shown to be superior in minimizing lung injury and lengthening survival.

High frequency uses very small tidal volumes and allows higher end-expiratory lung volumes with less overdistention than conventional ventilation. The high respiratory rates allow the maintenance of normal or near-normal $PaCO_2$ levels. It limits lung overdistention and prevents cyclic lung collapse by maintaining end-expiratory lung volume.

Inverse-ratio ventilation increases the proportion of time spent in inspiration, which increases the mean airway pressure and the end-expiratory volume, creating auto-PEEP. Auto-PEEP increases applied PEEP and maintains alveolar inflation. The goal is to improve oxygenation, but it may take several hours to achieve maximal benefits. Hyperinflation and decreased cardiac output are risks of this technique, and it is often poorly tolerated by awake patients, thus requiring increased sedation and paralysis (see Nursing Care Plan).

ECMO is still experimental and may offer the most promise when combined with other strategies. Further research is being conducted on this modality.[27]

Prone positioning during mechanical ventilation improves oxygenation by opening consolidated, dependent lung regions. Ventral lung regions do not seem to be affected with atelectasis, as one might expect in the prone position, and ventilation is distributed more homogeneously with better ventilation of the dorsal lung areas. The prone position shifts the weight of the heart from the dorsal lung regions to the sternum and anterior rib cage and facilitates pulmonary drainage of dorsal segments. Most trials have shown best advantage early in the course of ALI or ARDS. Disadvantages include loss of the endotracheal tube, loss of vascular access, facial edema, and difficulties with cardiopulmonary resuscitation.

Additional information on mechanical ventilation and the requisite nursing care is included in Chapter 27.

Fluid Management. Fluid management has been controversial in the treatment of ALI or ARDS because the optimal left atrial filling pressure is unknown. It requires a balance between providing enough fluids to maintain adequate perfusion and creating more edema. Current recommendations suggest a conservative approach to fluid replacement therapy while maintaining adequate hemodynamics. In the exudative phase, red blood cells are recommended as volume expanders, since they also improve oxygen-carrying capacity. Later in the disease process, liberal amounts of fluid are needed to overcome increased pulmonary vascular resistance and alveolar pressures, to perfuse pulmonary capillaries, and to minimize dead space.

Other Modalities. Other modalities to improve ALI or ARDS outcomes include the use of nitric oxide. Nitric oxide plays numerous roles in the physiology and pathophysiology of the lung, including decreasing neutrophil adhesion, acting as a molecular reactant, and signaling vasoconstriction. Inhaled nitric oxide is a vasodilator that reduces pulmonary artery pressure and, in high doses, reverses hypoxic pulmonary vasoconstriction without causing systemic hypotension. Some studies have shown that inhaled nitric oxide improves oxygenation in patients with ARDS by reversing hypoxic pulmonary vasoconstriction in ventilated lung units. Larger studies have yet to show improvement in mortality for ALI or ARDS.[36]

The use of inhaled pulmonary surfactant in adults is being studied, based on success in neonates. Pulmonary surfactant reduces the alveolar surface tension and prevents alveolar collapse. The surfactant proteins are decreased in concentration and are of abnormal composition in patients with ALI or ARDS, rendering them dysfunctional. Some studies have demonstrated improvement in the PaO_2/FiO_2 ratio in patients given inhaled surfactant, but decreases in mortality have not been seen.[30]

Diet. The patient with ALI or ARDS is generally in a well-nourished but extremely hypermetabolic state.[40] The hypermetabolic stress response results in increased energy needs. Nutritional assessment and intervention are aimed at minimizing excessive protein losses, preserving lean body mass by providing adequate energy, and maintaining positive nitrogen balance. Nonintubated patients are able to maintain better spontaneous oral intake. Mechanically ventilated patients often require nutritional support administered systemically by total parenteral nutrition or by enteral nutrition. General nutrition prescriptions include 20% protein, 60% to 70% carbohydrate, and 20% to 30% fat.[40] Enteral nutrition should be the mode of choice unless the gastrointestinal tract is not functioning. The patient needs to be observed closely for nutrition-induced hypercapnia.

Health Promotion and Prevention. Prompt treatment of the underlying cause of ARDS is the major focus of preventive care. In addition, judicious use of the mechanical ventilator and oxygen therapy is required to avoid inducing ALI and ARDS as untoward complications of these treatment modalities.

Nursing Management

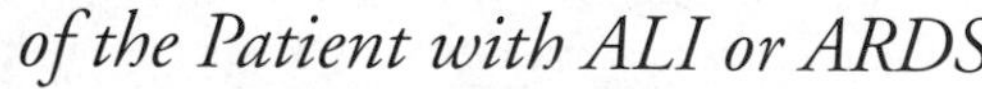

of the Patient with ALI or ARDS

Assessment

Health History. Assess for:

- Any pertinent background information and the history of the present illness (may need to be obtained from family members, since the patient is usually too ill to give details)

Physical Examination. Assess for:

- Dyspnea with tachypnea
- General respiratory distress
- Shallow inspiratory effort
- Mottled or cyanotic skin
- Rales or wheezes on auscultation (As ARDS progresses, lung sounds diminish.)

Nursing Diagnoses, Outcomes, and Interventions

Nursing Diagnosis: Impaired Gas Exchange

Outcomes. Common examples of expected outcomes for the patient with a diagnosis of *impaired gas exchange* are:

Patient will:

- Demonstrate improved ventilation and oxygenation.
- Maintain a PaO_2 of 50 to 60 mm Hg during acute phase of illness.
- Tolerate mechanical ventilatory assistance.
- Return to acceptable preillness levels of PaO_2, $PaCO_2$, and pH.

Nursing Interventions. The nurse provides oxygen therapy as ordered and monitors the patient for signs of hypoxemia and oxygen toxicity. A patent airway is maintained, and the nurse positions the patient for optimal oxygenation, usually with the head of the bed elevated 45 to 90 degrees. If an artificial airway is present, the necessary care is provided. An endotracheal tube must be secured to avoid movement either in or out of the established position. Because of the risk of an endotracheal tube slipping into the right main-stem bronchus, the nurse auscultates the lungs hourly to check the tube's placement. The tube is kept patent by suctioning if needed.

The nurse administers bronchoactive medications as ordered, checks ventilator settings frequently, and checks proper ventilator function to ensure delivery of adequate tidal volume and oxygen concentration. If the patient appears to be in respiratory distress even though the ventilator is functioning properly, the nurse assesses ABG levels.

RELATED NIC INTERVENTIONS. Airway Management, Oxygen Therapy, Respiratory Monitoring

Nursing Diagnosis: Ineffective Breathing Pattern

OUTCOMES. Common examples of expected outcomes for the patient with a diagnosis of *ineffective breathing pattern* are:
Patient will:

- Breathe effectively, maintaining adequate tissue perfusion.
- Demonstrate respiratory rate of 16 to 20 breaths/min.

NURSING INTERVENTIONS. The nurse positions the patient for maximal lung expansion, checks respirations regularly, auscultates lung sounds, and checks pulse oximetry and blood gas reports. The nurse also needs to observe and assess the patient for adequate tissue perfusion by checking color and blood flow distally. The patient requires frequent rest periods during care activities.

RELATED NIC INTERVENTIONS. Airway Management, Respiratory Monitoring

Nursing Diagnosis: Risk for Deficient Fluid Volume

OUTCOMES. Common examples of expected outcomes for the patient with a diagnosis of *risk for deficient fluid volume* are:
Patient will:

- Maintain fluid volume at functional level.
- Demonstrate pulmonary capillary wedge pressure (measure of pulmonary capillary pressure) of below 18 mm Hg.
- Exhibit stable vital signs.
- Maintain urinary output of at least 30 ml/hr.
- Have palpable peripheral pulses and extremities that are warm to touch.
- Demonstrate good skin turgor, moist mucous membranes.

NURSING INTERVENTIONS. The nurse monitors the pulmonary capillary wedge pressure and electrolytes and notifies the physician if the pressure is above or below the established range. If the pressure is below the established range, volume expanders or antihypotensive medications are administered as ordered. If the pressure is high, diuretics or vasodilators are administered as ordered. The nurse monitors urinary output, vital signs, and extremities every hour; checks skin turgor; and monitors fluid intake.

RELATED NIC INTERVENTIONS. Electrolyte Monitoring, Fluid Management, Hypovolemia Management

Nursing Diagnosis: Risk for Infection

OUTCOMES. Common examples of expected outcomes for the patient with a diagnosis of *risk for infection* are:
Patient will:

- Remain free from infection.
- Demonstrate vital signs within normal limits, with a temperature that is not elevated.
- Have negative cultures of pulmonary secretions and urine.

NURSING INTERVENTIONS. The nurse should always wash hands before any contact with the patient, use sterile procedures and equipment, and alert others to practice protective measures. The patient's airway is suctioned only when necessary to avoid trauma to tissue and introduction of bacteria. The nurse monitors vital signs frequently and may obtain cultures of urine and blood.

RELATED NIC INTERVENTIONS. Infection Control, Infection Protection

Nursing Diagnosis: Anxiety

OUTCOMES. Common examples of expected outcomes for the patient with a diagnosis of *anxiety* are:
Patient will:

- Display increased physiologic and psychologic comfort and decreased anxiety.
- Tolerate ventilator and artificial airway.
- Acknowledge and express fears.
- Communicate personal needs effectively with staff and family.
- Cooperate and assist with care.

NURSING INTERVENTIONS. The nurse identifies a method for the patient to communicate concerns and express feelings. It is difficult for patients to feel secure when unable to communicate vocally. The nurse provides simple explanations about procedures and orients the patient to the surroundings. The nurse also offers explanations about care routines and the environment to the family. The family is encouraged to approach, talk to, and touch the patient as they desire. The nurse keeps the patient and family informed about each aspect of treatment, with special attention to intubation and mechanical ventilation when necessary.

RELATED NIC INTERVENTIONS. Anxiety Reduction, Calming Technique

EVALUATION

To evaluate the effectiveness of nursing interventions, compare patient behaviors with those stated in the expected patient outcomes.

RELATED NOC OUTCOMES. Acceptance: Health Status, Anxiety Self-Control, Fluid Balance, Hydration, Knowledge: Infection Control, Respiratory Status: Ventilation, Risk Control, Vital Signs

Nursing Care Plan

Patient With Acute Respiratory Distress Syndrome on Mechanical Ventilation

Data A 28-year-old married man was admitted to the surgical intensive care unit after a motor vehicle accident. Injuries sustained include a ruptured spleen and liver laceration resulting in hypovolemic shock. The patient was taken to the operating room, where his spleen was removed and liver laceration repaired. His early postoperative course was unremarkable. On the third postoperative day, the patient began to experience respiratory difficulty with deterioration in his arterial blood gases (ABGs). Intubation and mechanical ventilation were necessary due to severe hypoxemia from acute respiratory distress syndrome (ARDS). His chest x-ray examination revealed diffuse interstitial and alveolar infiltrates.

The patient's wife visited daily and attempted to reassure and calm him when he became anxious and resisted the ventilator. Collaborative nursing actions included:

- Supporting oxygenation and ventilation to maintain Pao_2 over 60 mm Hg and maximize functional residual capacity
- Gradual weaning from Fio_2 and levels of positive end-expiratory pressure (PEEP) while monitoring ABGs
- Monitoring for signs of hypoxia

Nursing Diagnosis

Impaired gas exchange related to ARDS

Outcomes

- Patient will regain and maintain gas exchange within normal parameters as evidenced by normal ABGs, absence of hypoxemia, and regular rate and rhythm of respirations.

Related NOC Outcomes

- Comfort Level
- Respiratory Status: Airway Patency
- Respiratory Status: Gas Exchange
- Respiratory Status: Ventilation

Related NIC Interventions

- Airway Suctioning
- Artificial Airway Management
- Respiratory Monitoring

Nursing Interventions/Rationales

- Monitor respirations and assess breath sounds for adventitious findings hourly or more often as needed. *Respiratory rate increases initially as lung compliance decreases. Respiratory workload increases as compliance decreases.*
- Monitor ABGs as needed. *If the patient becomes fatigued and cannot initiate own respirations, carbon dioxide may be retained, adversely affecting ABGs.*
- Administer pulmonary toilet every 2 hours and as needed (turning, chest physiotherapy). *To maintain patent airway and prevent complications.*
- Monitor for signs of pulmonary complications and respiratory distress (asymmetrical chest excursion, sudden sharp chest pain, cyanosis, anxiety, subcutaneous emphysema). *When alveolar walls cannot withstand the positive pressure from PEEP, perforation can occur. As a result, air leaks into the pleural space, mediastinum, or its subcutaneous space. The result may be pneumothorax, pneumomediastinum, or subcutaneous emphysema, respectively.*
- Keep chest tube set up at bedside. *Emergency chest tube placement may be necessary if pneumothorax occurs.*
- Suction only when essential to prevent loss of PEEP secondary to disconnection from ventilator. *Suctioning may be needed to clear the airway, however, disconnecting the ventilator places the patient at risk for inadequate oxygenation.*
- Monitor required levels of PEEP and Fio_2. *To restore and maintain oxygenation.*
- Assess peripheral pulses, warmth and color of extremities. *To detect changes that indicate inadequate oxygenation and to determine effectiveness of ventilation.*
- Monitor mixed venous blood oxygen levels. *ARDS is an acute lung injury that affects capillary permeability, which permits proteins and fluids to leak out into alveoli and interstitial spaces, thus preventing normal gas exchange. Mixed venous blood oxygen levels reflect adequacy of oxygenation.*

Nursing Diagnosis

Decreased cardiac output related to decreased venous return

Outcomes

- Patient will have hemodynamic parameters within normal limits for adult man.

Related NOC Outcomes

- Cardiac Pump Effectiveness
- Circulation Status
- Tissue Perfusion: Abdominal Organs
- Tissue Perfusion: Cerebral
- Tissue Perfusion: Peripheral

Related NIC Interventions

- Acid-Base Management
- Acid-Base Monitoring
- Cardiac Care: Acute
- Electrolyte Management
- Fluid Management
- Hemodynamic Regulation

Nursing Interventions/Rationales

- Monitor temperature, blood pressure, and heart rate every hour or more frequently as needed. *To determine abnormalities so that corrective treatment can be initiated in a timely manner.*
- Monitor hemodynamic parameters (cardiac output, mean arterial pressure, central venous pressure). *To identify alterations in cardiac status and to help evaluate effectiveness of treatments. PEEP may cause*

decreased cardiac output by increasing intraalveolar pressures, thereby decreasing venous return to the heart.

- Assess and monitor ABGs to determine Pa_{O_2}. *Altered ABGs result from inadequate oxygenation. Early recognition allows for early correction of problems.*
- Monitor intake and output. *To identify adequacy of urinary function and fluid status. Normally, output approximates intake.*
- Assess peripheral circulation every 2 to 4 hours and as needed. *To identify adequacy of peripheral circulation.*
- Perform passive range-of-motion exercises every 4 to 6 hours. *To encourage venous blood return to the heart.*
- Administer prescribed adrenergic agents. *To improve cardiac output.*
- Notify physician of respiratory complications. *To facilitate the implementation of corrective treatments.*

Nursing Diagnosis

Risk for imbalanced nutrition: less than body requirements related to intubation

Outcomes

- Patient will remain within 5 pounds of preillness (or ideal) body weight.

Related NOC Outcomes

- Nutritional Status
- Nutritional Status: Food & Fluid Intake
- Nutritional Status: Nutrient Intake

Related NIC Interventions

- Nutrition Management
- Nutrition Therapy
- Nutritional Monitoring

Nursing Interventions/Rationales

- Administer hyperalimentation or enteral feedings as prescribed. *Acute illness increases metabolic demands on the body. Nutritional status must be maintained for healing to occur, strength to be maintained, and successful weaning of the patient from ventilation.*
- Monitor intake and output. *Decreased urinary output and concentrated urine are indications of inadequate fluid replacement.*
- Weigh daily. *To determine whether nutritional needs are being met and to evaluate the effectiveness of nutritional interventions.*
- Administer albumin and plasma expanders as prescribed. *Protein and volume expanders increase colloidal osmotic pressure, thus maintaining fluid within the intravascular compartment.*
- Monitor serum albumin levels. *Serum albumin levels reflect the adequacy of protein intake. Decreased levels are associated with peripheral edema caused by loss of osmotic pull from within the vascular space.*

Nursing Diagnosis

Anxiety related to ARDS and discomfort from intubation and mechanical ventilation

Outcomes

- Patient will remain free from anxiety related to intubation and mechanical ventilation.

Related NOC Outcomes

- Anxiety Self-Control
- Coping
- Psychosocial Adjustment: Life Change

Related NIC Interventions

- Anxiety Reduction
- Calming Technique
- Communication Enhancement: Speech Deficit
- Coping Enhancement
- Presence

Nursing Interventions/Rationales

- Assess for signs of anxiety. *Intensive care, mechanical ventilation, the inability to communicate, and fear of the unknown all contribute to feelings of fear and anxiety for the patient who is intubated and receiving mechanical ventilation. Restlessness, agitation, and resisting ventilation may be signs of fear or anxiety.*
- Explain the disease process to the family, including the benefits of mechanical ventilation and PEEP. *Knowledge often reduces fear and corresponding anxiety.*
- Allow patient and family to express their concerns and fears. *When patients and family members can communicate their fears, anxiety is often reduced. The patient's inability to communicate verbally does not mean that he or she cannot understand explanations regarding what is occurring or what to expect.*
- Explain procedures before performing them. *Patients have less fear and anxiety when they know what to expect.*
- Provide a means of communication between patient and spouse. *The ability to communicate allows some degree of control for the patient and allows him or her to communicate needs to health care providers and spouse.*
- Attempt to anticipate patient needs. *If patients' needs are met before they have to ask, their fears of the situation and not having needs met will be reduced. Conversely, if their needs are not met and they cannot communicate, their frustration will significantly increase their anxiety.*
- Administer prescribed light sedation and antianxiety medications if necessary. *Sedative and antianxiety medications produce relaxation, which reduces fighting or "bucking" of ventilator and promotes sleep. Positive-pressure exhalation is often uncomfortable for the patient, who may respond by resisting ventilation.*
- Provide distraction from ICU environment (soft music, television). *Distraction may minimize the perception of discomfort and reduce anxiety.*

Evaluation

Evaluation is based on comparing the patient's outcomes with desired outcomes.

GERONTOLOGIC CONSIDERATIONS

Mortality is significantly higher for patients with ALI or ARDS who are older than 55 years of age. The older adult may have a reduced ability to respond adaptively to environmental changes, and the processes of tissue repair are slowed or impaired. Older patients may also have chronic underlying health problems that contribute to the severity of the disease process and may influence the decision to withdraw life-sustaining therapy. Despite this, there is some evidence that ALI and ARDS are less severe in older patients, in whom lower levels of PEEP and FiO_2 are required to maintain PaO_2. The issue of age bias in treatment decisions deserves continued investigation, since studies have shown that older patients with underlying chronic illnesses survive more often than younger patients with chronic illnesses and many elderly ALI or ARDS survivors are not severely impaired after recovery.

Pulmonary Vascular Disorders

Pulmonary Embolism

Etiology and Epidemiology. Pulmonary embolism (PE) is not a disease per se; it is a complication of venous thrombosis. PE is caused by a clot or clots lodging in a pulmonary arterial vessel. Commonly the clot is from a deep venous thrombosis (DVT). Pulmonary emboli can cause massive occlusion of a major part of the pulmonary circulation and may be chronic or recurrent. Pulmonary infarction results when an embolus is large enough to interfere with the blood supply to a part of lung tissue, causing necrosis of lung parenchyma. **Embolism** without infarction does not cause permanent lung injury.

PE is a common cardiovascular and cardiopulmonary illness with an incidence in the United States of more than 1 per 100 and a mortality rate greater than 15% in the first 3 months after diagnosis.[23] The trend toward early discharge has been accompanied by an increased incidence of postdischarge venous thromboembolism. Thromboembolic risk does not end at discharge. About 50% of the deaths from PE occur within 2 hours of the event, and the embolism is often undetected. Emboli rarely occur without the presence of certain risk factors, although in some cases it may be difficult to identify the cause (see Risk Factors box). The most common reversible risk factor is obesity. Genetic predisposition to venous thrombosis is increasingly recognized as a significant contributing factor.[23]

Pathophysiology. Emboli travel from their site of origin through the right side of the heart and lodge in the pulmonary vasculature. The hemodynamic response to pulmonary embolism depends on the size of the embolus, coexistent cardiopulmonary disease, and neurohumoral effects. Acute PE increases pulmonary vascular resistance, often doubling it and, subsequently, pulmonary artery pressure. Increased right ventricular (RV) afterload can cause right ventricular dilation, hypokinesia, tricuspid regurgitation, and ultimately RV failure. As the RV wall stress increases, cardiac ischemia may develop because increased RV pressure compresses the right coronary artery, diminishes subendocardial perfusion, and limits myocardial oxygen supply. RV microinfarction leads to elevations of troponin, and RV overload causes elevations of pro-B-type natriuretic peptide and B-type natriuretic peptide (BNP).[14,34]

Risk Factors

Pulmonary Embolism

- Thrombophlebitis (deep venous thrombosis)
- Immobility
- Recent surgery (especially orthopedic or gynecologic)
- Obesity
- Congestive heart failure or myocardial infarction
- Recent fracture
- Estrogen therapy (oral contraceptives)
- Pregnancy

Acute PE impairs the efficient transfer of oxygen and carbon dioxide across the lung. Hypoxemia and an increase in the alveolar-arterial oxygen tension gradient are the most common gas exchange abnormalities. Total dead space increases. Ventilation and perfusion become mismatched, with blood flow from obstructed pulmonary arteries redirected to other gas exchange units. Shunting of venous blood into the systemic circulation may occur.

If the embolus blocks a larger vessel, the person may complain of sudden dyspnea, sharp upper abdominal or thoracic pain, and cough, and may have hemoptysis; shock may develop rapidly. If the area of infarction is smaller, the symptoms are much milder. The patient may have dyspnea, unexplained tachypnea, cough, pleuritic chest pain, slight hemoptysis, tachycardia, elevated temperature, and increased leukocyte count. An area of dullness or crackles may be detected when checking breath sounds. Table 26-13 presents the pathophysiology and clinical picture of a patient with PE.

COMPLICATIONS. Complications of PE include pulmonary infarction, pleural effusion, RV failure, gastrointestinal bleeding, and bleeding from other sites.

Collaborative Care Management

DIAGNOSTIC TESTS. To diagnose PE, one must think of it as a diagnostic possibility.[32] The diagnosis of PE is not easy to make with confidence. Clinical history, changes in blood chemistries, and plain chest x-ray films are often not definitive in establishing the diagnosis. Pulmonary angiography is the ultimate standard diagnostic test for PE; an abrupt cutoff of a vessel or a filling defect indicates the presence of an embolus. However, V/Q scanning is the recommended first test when PE is suspected because of the exclusionary value of a normal scan. High-probability scans have 87% specificity and sensitivity. Low- and intermediate-probability scan results indicate that more testing is needed. V/Q scanning is not a helpful diagnostic tool for patients with COPD.

D-dimer is frequently used in the diagnosis of PE because it is safe, noninvasive, rapid, and inexpensive. D-dimer is elevated in almost all patients with PE because of endogenous but ineffective fibrinolysis, which causes plasmin to digest some of the fibrin clot and release D-dimers into the systemic circulation. This normally occurs within 1 hour after thrombus formation. D-dimers have a half-life of 4 to 6 hours, but the continued fibrinolysis of a embolus increases the level for about 1 week.

Dead-space determination is another type of testing. A pulmonary embolus causes a decrease in blood flow to the alveoli, thus increasing alveolar dead space, which, in turn, decreases the carbon dioxide content of expired breath. Efforts are being direct-

TABLE 26-13 NORMAL FUNCTION, PRIMARY PATHOPHYSIOLOGY, AND CLINICAL MANIFESTATIONS OF PULMONARY EMBOLISM

Normal Function	Pathophysiology	Clinical Manifestations
PULMONARY VASCULATURE		
Carry venous blood received from right side of heart to alveolocapillary membrane in lung for oxygen–carbon dioxide exchange	Occlusion of pulmonary vessels because of increased vascular resistance, decreased cardiac output (usually occurs only in massive emboli), decreased lung perfusion	Elevated pulmonary artery pressure Dyspnea Hypotension Tachycardia High ventilation-perfusion (V/Q) ratio as shown on lung scan Hypocapnia and elevated arterial blood pH
AIRWAYS		
Carry oxygenated air to alveolocapillary membrane for exchange, and carry deoxygenated air out of lung	Airway constriction from lowered alveolar carbon dioxide levels	Underventilated lung areas as shown on lung scan Hypoxemia Tachypnea Cough
ALVEOLI		
Lung site where gas exchange takes place (alveolocapillary membrane)	Infarction of alveolar tissues caused by complete obstruction, resulting in extravasation of blood cells into alveoli (NOTE: Occurs only in more severe cases)	Hemoptysis Radiologic opacity
PLEURAE		
Maintain close approximation of lungs and chest wall Minimize friction during lung expansion and contraction	Transudate from damaged vascular structures (pleural effusion)	Pleural friction rub Chest pain during inhalation/exhalation

ed to improve the sensitivity of testing measures to dead-space increases to aid in the diagnosis of PE.[35]

Also of use in diagnosis are biomarkers such as troponin elevation, which indicates RV microinfarction, and elevations of pro-B-type natriuretic peptide and BNP, which indicate RV overload.[14]

Echocardiography is 90% specific and sensitive with PE of the pulmonary trunk and right and left pulmonary arteries. It shows an unexplained increase in RV volume or pressure. Spiral CT is under investigation for use in the diagnosis of PE. Because it can be completed in 20 to 30 seconds, if its sensitivity is strong, it will offer great advantage over traditional CT. Spiral CT is most helpful in diagnosing a centrally located embolus rather than one in the periphery of the lung field. It is not useful in patients with COPD who are suspected of having PE.

MEDICATIONS. A focus of medical treatment of PE is the prevention of venous thromboembolism. Anticoagulant therapy may either be prophylactic for persons at risk for DVT or curative for persons with an actual pathologic event. When the patient is not responsive to anticoagulant therapy or when it is contraindicated, surgical intervention may be necessary.

ANTICOAGULANT THERAPY. The goal of anticoagulant therapy is to limit the growth of the embolized thrombus and prevent reembolization by inhibiting coagulation and preventing deposition of new clots. Heparin is the mainstay of therapy for pulmonary emboli without hemodynamic compromise or bleeding. It substantially reduces morbidity and mortality by preventing further fibrin deposition on the thrombus. When there is strong suspicion of PE, heparin therapy should be started immediately while awaiting diagnostic confirmation. Short-acting intravenous unfractionated heparin is initiated with a bolus of 80 units/kg, followed by a continuous infusion of 18 units/kg/hr.[24] The patient is monitored by activated partial thromboplastin time (aPTT) every 4 to 6 hours. The goal is to achieve an aPTT of 1.5 to 2.5 times the control. Heparin may be given subcutaneously to patients with poor venous access. It is more difficult to achieve and maintain therapeutic values, however. For the patient with a major pulmonary embolus, the current recommendation is heparin therapy for at least 1 week.[24]

Low-molecular-weight heparins (LMWHs) are progressively replacing heparin in the treatment of DVT and being used with greater confidence to treat PE. LMWHs decrease the complexities involved in heparin administration and thromboplastin aPTT monitoring. They may be given subcutaneously once or twice per day. The specific agents used most often include aldeparin, dalteparin, and enoxaparin. Advantages of these medications include increased bioavailability, longer half-life, and simplified administration. Dosing adjustments are needed in patients with renal insufficiency because the drugs are renally excreted. Disadvantages include lack of a specific means to reverse the effect, difficulty monitoring their anticoagulant effect, and high cost.

Warfarin, 5 to 10 mg/day, is begun once the patient's condition is stable. Warfarin is monitored by prothrombin time (PT). The goal is to achieve a PT of 2 to 3 international normalized ratios (INR). Heparin and warfarin are continued until the PT is at the desired level. The length of anticoagulation treatment is 3 to 6 months. Lifelong anticoagulation is needed by a small population of patients, including those with irreversible acquired or genetic predisposition to venous thrombosis, major V/Q scan defects, and a history of recurrent thromboembolic events.

Inferior vena cava filters are recommended if anticoagulants are contraindicated or if the patient has a recurrent pulmonary embolus while receiving anticoagulant therapy. The filters may also be placed if the PE is severe (RV failure, hypotension). A filter may be placed percutaneously to protect the vascular bed from embolization. The filter does not lessen the occurrence or extension of venous thrombosis, nor is there evidence that filters have any advantages over anticoagulation. Complications associated with vena cava filters include perforation of the vessel wall, thrombosis at the access site, and leg edema.[24]

THROMBOLYTIC THERAPY. Thrombolytic therapy promotes immediate dissolution of the embolus and prompt return of pulmonary function in a patient who is hemodynamically unstable or severely hypoxic. It is not recommended for routine treatment of PE, and current evidence does not indicate a change in mortality rates. One of the thrombolytic agents (urokinase, streptokinase, or recombinant tissue plasminogen activator [rt-PA]) is used. Therapy can be delivered either systemically or directly into the pulmonary artery via selective catheterization, although systemic therapy appears to be superior. This therapy is often not applicable to many postsurgical patients because of the increased risk of bleeding complications at the surgical site.

TREATMENTS. A small group of patients with PE may be considered for a pulmonary embolectomy, the surgical removal of the thrombus from the pulmonary vasculature. This intervention is reserved for patients with hemodynamically massive PE who have contraindications to anticoagulant or thrombolytic therapy and who fail to respond to immediate aggressive medical support. This procedure is usually performed with the patient under general anesthesia, although it may be performed with a special IV suction catheter and the patient under local anesthesia.

DIET. Diet is as tolerated; the patient usually starts with fluids and progresses to soft foods.

HEALTH PROMOTION AND PREVENTION. Prevention is critical in reducing the death rate, morbidity, and cost of PE. Mechanical measures for hospitalized patients include graduated compression stockings and intermittent pneumatic compression devices, which stimulate endogenous fibrinolytic activity in addition to direct physical stimulation of increased venous blood flow. Perioperative prophylaxis is widely accepted, but because of abbreviated hospitalizations, most postoperative pulmonary emboli occur after hospital discharge.

Nursing Management 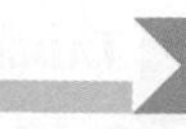

of the Patient with Pulmonary Embolism

ASSESSMENT

Health History. Assess for:

- Presence of risk factors (see Risk Factors box, p. 662)
- Recent onset of any of the following symptoms: dyspnea, substernal chest pain, hemoptysis, chest palpitations, pleuritic pain, cough, apprehension (sense of foreboding), or diaphoresis
- History of leg pain, especially in the calf or knee area; recent surgery; cigarette smoking; use of oral contraceptives; sedentary lifestyle; and recent travel with prolonged sitting and pressure on the back of the legs

Physical Examination. Assess for:

- Changes in skin color
- Complaint of dyspnea or chest pain
- Apprehensiveness, anxiety, nervousness
- Tachypnea, tachycardia
- Elevated temperature
- Pleural friction rub and localized, decreased breath sounds and crackles by auscultation
- Distended jugular veins, an accentuated pulmonic heart sound, and a tricuspid regurgitation murmur (signs of right-sided heart failure)

NURSING DIAGNOSES, OUTCOMES, AND INTERVENTIONS

Nursing Diagnosis: Ineffective Breathing Pattern

OUTCOMES. Common examples of expected outcomes for the patient with a diagnosis of *ineffective breathing pattern* are:
Patient will:

- Have respiratory rate of 16 to 20 breaths/min.
- Have clear breath sounds; no use of accessory muscles.

NURSING INTERVENTIONS. The nurse monitors the patient's respiratory rate, depth, and pattern, as well as breath sounds. The head of the bed is elevated to promote physiologic and psychologic ease of maximal inspiration. The nurse encourages use of controlled breathing techniques.

RELATED NIC INTERVENTIONS. Airway Management, Respiratory Monitoring

Nursing Diagnosis: Impaired Gas Exchange

OUTCOMES. A common example of expected outcomes for the patient with a diagnosis of *impaired gas exchange* is:
Patient will:

- Demonstrate improved gas exchange by PaO_2, $PaCO_2$, and pH within normal limits, or will return to baseline level with no cyanosis.

NURSING INTERVENTIONS. The nurse encourages the patient and helps him or her to deep breathe and cough every 4 hours and to use an incentive spirometer every hour. Oxygen therapy is administered as ordered and monitored with pulse oximetry. Prescribed activity is maintained; overexertion is avoided. The nurse may have to assist the patient with some activities and allow for rest time in between treatments.

RELATED NIC INTERVENTIONS. Airway Management, Oxygen Therapy, Respiratory Monitoring

Nursing Diagnosis: Ineffective Tissue Perfusion

OUTCOMES. Common examples of expected outcomes for the patient with a diagnosis of *ineffective tissue perfusion* are:
Patient will:
- Demonstrate adequate tissue perfusion with extremities warm and dry to touch and palpable peripheral pulses.
- Exhibit coagulation studies (PT, INR, PTT) within normal limits.

NURSING INTERVENTIONS. The nurse ensures that the patient's lower extremities are elevated and monitors for adequate pulses. Legs should not be not massaged, nor the bed gatched at the knees. Pneumatic compression devices are applied as ordered. The nurse measures the legs to determine if fluid is pooling in the lower extremities. The nurse administers anticoagulants as ordered; monitors PT, INR, and aPTT; and notifies the physician if PT or aPTT is below or above the desired therapeutic range. Opiates are used cautiously for pain if the patient is hypotensive.

RELATED NIC INTERVENTIONS. Circulatory Precautions, Pneumatic Tourniquet Precautions, Positioning

Nursing Diagnosis: Anxiety

OUTCOMES. Common examples of expected outcomes for the patient with a diagnosis of *anxiety* are:
Patient will:
- Report anxiety is at manageable level.
- Verbalize concerns and ask questions about prognosis and care plan.

NURSING INTERVENTIONS. The nurse offers support, makes the patient comfortable, teaches the patient relaxation strategies, and encourages the patient to verbalize fears and concerns. The nurse explains all treatments and procedures (see Patient/Family Teaching box).

RELATED NIC INTERVENTIONS. Anxiety Reduction, Calming Technique

EVALUATION

To evaluate the effectiveness of nursing interventions, compare patient behaviors with those stated in the expected patient outcomes.

RELATED NOC OUTCOMES. Anxiety Self-Control, Circulation Status, Coping, Respiratory Status: Ventilation, Tissue Perfusion: Peripheral, Vital Signs

GERONTOLOGIC CONSIDERATIONS

Older persons are at higher risk for developing PE because they are more likely to have surgery, such as knee and hip replacements, and they may be less active than younger persons. They are also more likely to have thrombophlebitis, which puts them at higher risk for PE. Diagnosis of PE in older adults is difficult because clinical and laboratory findings can be nonspecific and atypical. D-dimer studies may have a more limited role in the management of PE because values increase with age and many older patients suffer from multiple medical problems that influence D-dimer values.

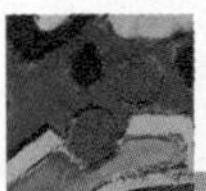

PATIENT/FAMILY TEACHING *The Patient With Pulmonary Embolism*

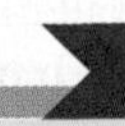

The nurse should teach the patient and family:
- About the prescribed anticoagulant therapy and prevention of future embolic events.
- The dose, side effects, and time of administration.
- About the need to wear a Medic-Alert bracelet or carry a card stating that he or she is taking an anticoagulant.
- To observe precautions to prevent bleeding while taking anticoagulant therapy. These precautions include using a soft toothbrush, not going barefoot, applying pressure to cuts to stop bleeding, and not taking any medication containing aspirin without conferring with a health care professional.
- To seek immediate medical attention if dyspnea, substernal chest pain, hemoptysis, chest palpitations, cough, diaphoresis, or feelings of unexplained apprehension occur.
- About risk factors associated with pulmonary embolism and how to avoid them: avoid wearing constrictive clothing such as rolled garters; avoid standing or sitting for prolonged periods; move about at least every 2 hours; and actively dorsiflex the feet while sitting. The importance of not smoking is also stressed, and referrals to smoking cessation resources are made if needed.

Chest Trauma

Chest wall trauma is most commonly seen after motor vehicle collisions and accounts for 8% of all trauma admissions.[28] It is both a marker of severe injury and a significant contributor to the morbidity and mortality of injured patients, with older patients and those with poor respiratory reserve being most vulnerable. A chest injury may affect the rib cage, pleurae and lungs, diaphragm, or mediastinal contents. Chest injuries are broadly classified into two groups: blunt and penetrating (Box 26-6). Blunt, or nonpenetrating, injuries damage the structures within the chest cavity without

Box 26-6 Penetrating and Nonpenetrating (Blunt) Chest Injuries

Penetrating	Blunt (Nonpenetrating)
Open pneumothorax (sucking chest wound)	Fractured ribs
Hemothorax	Flail chest
Tracheobronchial injury	Closed pneumothorax
Pulmonary contusion	Tension pneumothorax
Diaphragm rupture	Tracheobronchial injury
Mediastinal injury	Diaphragm rupture
	Mediastinal injury

disrupting chest wall integrity. Penetrating injuries disrupt chest wall integrity and alter intrathoracic pressures.

Trauma is the leading cause of death in those younger than 45 years of age and the fifth leading cause of death for those older than 65 years of age. Blunt chest trauma is second only to head and spinal cord trauma as the leading cause of death among trauma victims, and for almost 25% of all trauma patients who die, blunt chest trauma is reported as a predominant or contributing factor.[29] Penetrating wounds usually result from gunshot or stabbing injuries.

Older persons account for 12% of trauma admissions but consume 33% of each health care dollar spent on trauma patients.[2] Older adults are potentially more vulnerable to thoracic injury and have increased mortality rates. Aging frequently results in osteoporosis, exaggerated thoracic kyphosis, decreased muscle mass, thinning of intervertebral disks, shortening of vertebral bodies, and decreased chest wall compliance. Postmenopausal women are particularly susceptible to age- related loss of bone density. These factors can predispose the older adult to rib fractures in traumatic situations and increase the morbidity of such injuries. Age is a strong predictor of outcome with flail chest and is associated with increased mortality.[2]

Blunt Injuries

Blunt chest trauma is associated with three mechanisms of injury: rapid acceleration/deceleration, direct impact, and compression. An acceleration/deceleration injury is most commonly caused by a motor vehicle or motorcycle crash, a pedestrian injury, or a fall. These injuries create a shearing force that stretches tissue, organs, or blood vessels beyond their capacity, resulting in tear, leak, or rupture. Direct-impact injuries are caused by motor vehicle and motorcycle crashes and by a blunt object striking the chest. Direct-impact injuries can cause rib, sternal, or scapular fracture and injuries to the lung parenchyma, heart, or thoracic cage. Compression injuries result from the force of the rapid deceleration as the tissues strike a fixed object such as the sternum and ribs. Compression injuries can result in organ rupture, contusions, or bleeding.[29]

Rib Fractures

Etiology and Epidemiology. Rib fractures are the most common of all chest injuries and are identified in 10% of all patients after trauma. The overall incidence is probably higher because not all rib fractures are seen on chest x-ray examination or otherwise detected. Fractures of ribs 1 and 2 are called the "hallmark of severe trauma" because these ribs are short, thick, and well protected by the thoracic musculature. It requires tremendous force to fracture these bones. Ribs 4 through 9 are most often fractured, because they are less well protected by the chest muscles. Rib fractures are caused by blows, crushing injuries, or strain from severe coughing or sneezing spells.

Pathophysiology. If the rib is splintered or the fracture displaced, sharp fragments may penetrate the pleura and lung, resulting in a **hemothorax** (blood in the pleural space) or pneumothorax (air in the pleural space), which are penetrating injuries. Common signs and symptoms of rib fracture include pain at the site of injury that increases on inspiration, localized tenderness and crepitus on palpation, splinting of the chest, and shallow breathing.

Collaborative Care Management. Diagnosis of rib fractures can be difficult. Fractures are confirmed by chest x-ray findings but often are not visible. They may be diagnosed by clinical assessment alone with acute pain over a specific location along the rib. Uncomplicated rib fractures require no treatment except pain relief to ensure adequate ventilation.

Multiple fractured ribs cause severe pain, which may be more debilitating and harmful than the injury itself. Pain limits one's ability to cough and breathe deeply, resulting in sputum retention, atelectasis, and a reduction in functional residual capacity (FRC). These factors may result in decreased lung compliance, ventilation-perfusion mismatch, hypoxemia, and respiratory distress. Failure to control pain can have serious respiratory complications.

Close assessment of breathing and airway status is a priority. The nurse observes the patient for splinting of the chest and shallow breathing, which could lead to atelectasis. To improve breathing, the nurse places the patient in a position of comfort—usually Fowler's or semi-Fowler's position—and provides analgesia to relieve pain. The ideal pain management regimen would provide complete and prolonged analgesia, permit deep breathing and secretion clearance, and allow cooperation during chest physiotherapy. It would also improve respiratory dynamics, have minimal central nervous and systemic effects, and permit early ambulation. However, no single regimen meets all these criteria. The first-line management for relieving pain is commonly systemic opioids, either intermittent on-demand injections, continuous IV infusion, or patient-controlled analgesia. Nerve blocks for the intercostal nerve proximal to the fracture site are often used. Epidural anesthesia (EA) via the lumbar or the thoracic route using local anesthetic agents, opioids, or a combination has successfully managed pain in patients with multiple fractured ribs. The use of EA in patients with thoracic trauma who are older than 60 years of age is an independent predictor of both decreased mortality and decreased incidence of pulmonary complications.[28] Intrathecal opioids, interpleural analgesia, and thoracic paravertebral block are additional strategies to increase comfort. Oral analgesia drugs such as nonsteroidal antiinflammatory drugs and acetaminophen are useful for mild to moderate pain.

The nurse instructs the patient to use an incentive spirometer every hour, to rest and avoid strenuous activities for several days, and to take prescribed oral analgesics as needed for pain. The patient is also directed to contact the health care provider if pain relief is inadequate and to return to the emergency department immediately if shortness of breath, sudden sharp chest pain, or coughing up of blood occurs. If the patient is discharged with an epidural catheter for pain management, the nurse teaches specific care and arranges for a home health follow-up visit.

Flail Chest

Etiology and Epidemiology. **Flail chest** is a thoracic injury resulting in paradoxical motion of the chest wall segments. Flail chest is an indication of severe chest trauma, often as a result of a

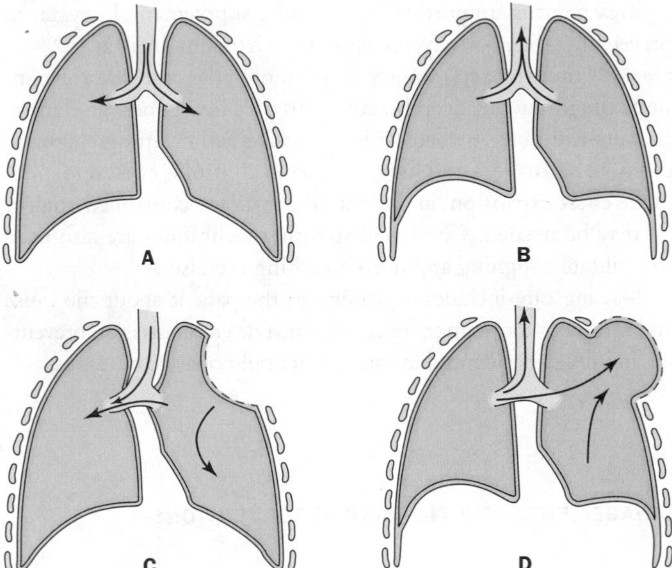

Figure 26-10 The effects of chest trauma. **A,** Inspiration. **B,** Expiration. **C** and **D,** Paradoxic motion. **C,** Area of lung underlying unstable chest wall sucks in on inspiration. **D,** Same area balloons out on expiration. Note movement of mediastinum toward opposite lung in inspiration.

direct-impact, high-speed mechanism of injury. This may occur in a motor vehicle accident or a severe fall.

Pathophysiology. Fracture of at least four consecutive ribs in two or more places is usually required to cause a flail chest, which is categorized by location as sternal, anterior, lateral, or posterior. With a flail, the chest wall no longer provides the rigid bony support necessary to maintain the bellows function required for normal ventilation. The result is paradoxical breathing, or paradoxical respiratory movement. During inspiration the dislocated segment is pulled inward by the subatmospheric **intrapleural pressure** (pressure in the pleural cavity) (Figure 26-10, *C*). During expiration the dislocated segment bulges outward as intrapleural pressure becomes less negative (Figure 26-10, *D*). Flail chest usually causes localized atelectasis secondary to decreased ventilation, resulting in hypoxemia. Because of the increased work of breathing, the individual may also develop hypercapnia and respiratory acidosis. Pulmonary contusion is another common occurrence. The signs and symptoms of flail chest are summarized in the Clinical Manifestations box, at right.

Collaborative Care Management. Chest x-ray studies are done to determine the extent of trauma, and ABGs are obtained to determine PaO_2 and $PaCO_2$. Oxygenation saturation is maintained at 90% or above with the use of supplemental oxygen if needed. In addition, management focuses on pain control and other measures to promote good ventilation, such as incentive spirometry and aggressive pulmonary physiotherapy, humidification of air, and early mobilization.

Treatment of patients in severe distress includes intubation and mechanical ventilation. Care focuses on the maintenance of proper gas exchange and observation for signs of hypovolemic shock that would require aggressive fluid resuscitation. Stabilization of the flail chest with surgical fixation has demonstrated improved long-term pulmonary function, fewer cases of pneumonia, and less ventilator time.[29] Complications of flail chest include pneumonia, tension pneumothorax, ARDS, and shock secondary to hemothorax.

Health history data to be collected include the nature of the injury and when it occurred. Often the patient is too badly injured to answer questions, and data are obtained from those accompanying the patient. Pain is severe and increases with each respiratory movement. Thus the flail segment should be splinted with the hands during coughing and deep breathing (see Figure 26-7). On physical examination the mediastinum is found to oscillate or flutter with each respiration, and breath sounds are decreased. If there is severe interference with cardiac function, neck veins will be distended. Pulse and respiratory rates are increased, and blood pressure falls if paradoxic motion is not relieved.

The nurse encourages the patient to request pain medication as needed to promote deep breathing and early mobilization. The nurse also instructs the patient to promptly report changes in respiratory status to the nurse or other health care professional.

CLINICAL MANIFESTATIONS
Flail Chest

- Severe chest pain
- Paradoxical breathing (asymmetric chest movement)
- Oscillation of mediastinum
- Increasing dyspnea
- Rapid, shallow respirations
- Accessory muscle breathing
- Restlessness
- Decreased breath sounds on auscultation
- Cyanosis
- Anxiety related to difficult breathing

Penetrating Injuries

Pulmonary Contusion

Etiology and Epidemiology. A pulmonary contusion is a serious injury to the lung parenchyma. It leads to interstitial hemorrhage with resulting alveolar collapse, atelectasis, and consolidation of the uninjured areas of the lung.

Pathophysiology. As edema forms around the area of initial injury, ventilation begins to decrease. The resulting hypoxia is due to shunting of blood through the unventilated lung (see Clinical Manifestations box, p. 668).

Collaborative Care Management. Chest x-ray films show patchy infiltrates or nonsegmental areas of opacification. This reflects the mechanical forces applied to the lung, resulting in the tearing of tissues.[29] These findings usually appear within 4 to 6 hours of injury and typically occur in areas that underlie rib, clavicular, or sternal fractures. Chest CT is the gold standard for diagnosis because it is more specific and sensitive than an x-ray film. A pulmonary contusion appears on a CT scan as an ill-defined area of consolidation.

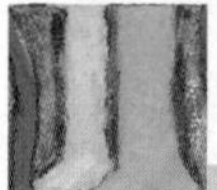

Clinical Manifestations
Pulmonary Contusion

Pulmonary contusion may vary from total absence of symptoms to the full spectrum of symptoms associated with noncardiogenic pulmonary edema. Signs and symptoms (some of which may be delayed) include:
- Increasing dyspnea
- Tachypnea
- Increasing restlessness
- Crackles noted on auscultation
- Hemoptysis

Treatment is supportive and includes supplemental oxygen to prevent hypoxemia (oxygen saturation is maintained at 90% or greater), incentive spirometry to promote adequate chest expansion, coughing and deep breathing to promote good ventilation, and repositioning in bed with aggressive activity progression to promote perfusion of all lung areas. Pain control is critical for adequate chest expansion, and epidural or patient-controlled analgesia may be needed. Chest wall splinting techniques are also used to facilitate coughing and deep breathing exercises.

Nursing care includes explaining to the patient about the cause and treatment for pulmonary contusion. The emphasis is on preventing injuries or accidents and thus further pulmonary contusions.

Table 26-14 Clinical Manifestations, Medical Management, and Nursing Interventions Related to Pneumothorax

Pneumothorax	Clinical Manifestations	Medical Management	Nursing Interventions
Closed (spontaneous)	Small or slowly developing pneumothorax may produce no symptoms. Larger or rapidly developing pneumothorax results in: Sharp pain on inspiration Increasing dyspnea Increasing restlessness Diaphoresis Hypotension Tachycardia Absence of chest movement on affected side Absence of breath sounds on affected side Hyperresonance on affected side	Observation on outpatient basis Supplemental oxygen Needle aspiration of air from pleural space, if present; insertion of chest catheter connected to flutter valve or closed drainage system If frequent recurrences, doxycycline or talc instilled into pleural space to cause adhesions between pleurae; if this procedure fails, lung portion with defect resected and parietal pleura abraded	Place patient in semi-Fowler's position. Administer oxygen. Obtain thoracentesis tray and closed drainage equipment. For outpatient or for patient after chest tube removal, instruct to: Report any increased dyspnea to physician. Avoid strenuous exercise or activity that increases rate and depth of breathing. Avoid holding breath. Follow physician's instructions about resuming normal activity.
Tension	Severe dyspnea Agitation Trachea deviated from midline toward unaffected lung (mediastinal shift) Jugular venous distention Absence of chest movement on affected side Hypotension, tachycardia Breath sounds absent on affected side Hyperresonance on affected side Diminished heart sounds Shock Subcutaneous emphysema Ineffective ventilation	True emergency Defect in chest wall covered with sterile dressing Insertion of chest tube connected to flutter valve or closed drainage system	This is a life-threatening event; carry out interventions immediately to relieve increased intrapleural pressure; interventions same as those listed for closed pneumothorax. Monitor vital signs frequently. Observe for cardiac dysrhythmias. Palpate for subcutaneous emphysema in upper chest and neck. Provide same discharge instruction as for closed pneumothorax.
Open	Sucking sounds at wound site with respiration Tracheal deviation (trachea moving toward unaffected side during inspiration and returns toward midline with expiration)	Occlusion of open wound Same as for closed pneumothorax	Occlude wound with nonporous covering. Perform same interventions as for closed pneumothorax. Provide same discharge instructions as for closed pneumothorax.

Pneumothorax

Etiology and Epidemiology. In pneumothorax, air is in the pleural space between the lung and the chest wall. A pneumothorax can occur spontaneously or as a result of penetrating or nonpenetrating chest injuries.

Pathophysiology. A closed pneumothorax is caused by fractured ribs that pierce the pleura. It can also occur when the rib cage is suddenly compressed. Air enters the pleural space, increasing intrapleural pressure and collapsing the lung (see Figure 26-6). A variant of closed pneumothorax is a spontaneous pneumothorax that results from the rupture of an emphysematous bleb on the lung surface. A spontaneous pneumothorax may also follow severe bouts of coughing in persons with a chronic pulmonary disease such as asthma. It commonly occurs as a single or recurrent episode in an otherwise healthy young man. If large enough and left untreated, a closed pneumothorax can become a tension pneumothorax.

A tension pneumothorax occurs when air enters the pleural space on inspiration but cannot leave it on expiration. Although usually a result of a closed pneumothorax, a tension pneumothorax can be caused by a penetrating chest injury. The accumulating air builds up positive pressure in the chest cavity, resulting in lung collapse on the affected side, mediastinal shift toward the unaffected side, and decreased venous return caused by compression of mediastinal contents (heart, great vessels).

An open pneumothorax occurs when a penetrating chest wound opens the intrapleural space to atmospheric pressure. Each time the person inspires, he or she sucks air into the intrapleural space, increasing intrapleural pressure. This is a life-threatening injury and can severely compromise breathing and lead to a tension pneumothorax. Blood also may leak into the pleural cavity, creating a hemothorax.

Collaborative Care Management. The clinical manifestations, medical management, and nursing interventions associated with the various types of pneumothorax are presented in Table 26-14. The nurse supports and informs the patient about the treatments and procedures for restoring lung function.

Critical Thinking

1. You are caring for a 67-year-old patient with lung cancer. His wife is always at his bedside. No other family members are available to assist with his care. He is not a candidate for surgical intervention, but he will have chemotherapy. What nursing interventions are important to institute with this patient? What are your responsibilities to his family? What referrals might be appropriate?
2. What can you do to help convince individuals who smoke to join a smoking cessation program? What are the benefits of such program? What strategies are used to help people quit smoking? Does age or gender make a difference in the strategies used?

References

1. Adjei AA: Primary lung cancer. In Rakel RE, Bope ET, editors: *Conn's current therapy 2001,* Philadelphia, 2001, Saunders.
2. Albaugh G et al: Age-adjusted outcomes in traumatic flail chest injuries in the elderly, *Am Surg* 66(10):978-981, 2000.
3. Altorki N, Kent M, Pasmantier M: Detection of early-stage lung cancer: computed tomographic scan or chest radiograph, *J Thorac Cardiovasc Surg* 121(6):1053-1057, 2001.
4. American Cancer Society: *Detailed guide: lung cancer,* accessed Sept 2005 from website: www.cancer.org.
5. American Lung Association: *Occupational lung diseases fact sheet,* 2003, accessed Jan 2005 from www.lungusa.org.
6. American Lung Association: *TB fact sheet,* 2004, accessed Jan 2005 from website: www.lungusa.org.
7. Amin A et al: Recommendations for management of community- and hospital-acquired pneumonia—the hospitalist perspective, *Curr Opin Pulm Med* 10(Suppl 1):S23-S27, 2004.
8. Andrews J et al: Community-acquired pneumonia, *Curr Opin Pulm Med* 9(3):175-180, 2003.
9. Baughman RP, Lower EE: New therapies for sarcoidosis, *Clin Pulm Med* 11(3):154-160, 2004.
10. Ben-David D, Rubinstein, E: Appropriate use of antibiotics for respiratory infections: review of recent statements and position papers, *Curr Opin Infect Dis* 15(2):151-156, 2002.
11. Blasi F et al: Newer antibiotics for the treatment of respiratory tract infections, *Curr Opin Pulm Med* 10(3):189-196, 2004.
12. Britton W, Palendera U: Improving vaccines against TB, *Immunol Cell Biol* 81(1):34-45, 2003.
13. Bryan CL, Homma A: Acute respiratory failure. In Rakel RE, Bope ET, editors: *Conn's current therapy 2001,* Philadelphia, 2001, Saunders.
14. Cardin T, Marinelli A: Pulmonary embolism, *Crit Care Nurs Q* 27(4): 310-322, 2004.
15. Critical/emergency care: products, *Nurs Manage* 34(12):22, 2003.
16. Dabbs AD et al: Striving for normalcy: symptoms and the threat of rejection after lung transplantation, *Soc Sci Med* 59(7):1473-1484, 2004.
17. Deslauriers J: Should screening for lung cancer be revisited? *J Thorac Cardiovasc Surg* 121(6):1031-1032, 2001.
18. Diasio RB: Adjuvant chemotherapy for adenocarcinoma of the lung—is the standard of care ready for change? *N Engl J Med* 350(17):1777-1779: 2004.
19. Dipiro JT: *Pharmacotherapy: a pathophysiologic approach,* Norwalk, Conn, 2002, Appleton & Lange.
20. Federal Drug Administration: *FDA news,* accessed Jan 2005 from website: www.fda.gov.
21. Fero TJ: Overview of national treatment guidelines for common respiratory tract infections, *Am J Ther* 11(Suppl 1):S9-S14, 2004.
22. File TM, Tan JS, Plouffe JF: Bacterial pneumonia: community-acquired and nosocomial in immunocompetent hosts. In Rakel RE, Bope ET, editors: *Conn's current therapy 2001,* Philadelphia, 2001, Saunders.
23. Goldhaber SZ, Elliott CG: Acute pulmonary embolism, part I, Epidemiology, pathophysiology and diagnosis, *Circulation* 108(22):2726-2729, 2003.
24. Goldhaber SZ, Elliott CG: Acute pulmonary embolism, part II, Risk stratification, treatment and prevention, *Circulation* 108(23):2834-2838, 2003.
25. Goldrick B: Once dismissed, still rampant: tuberculosis, the second deadliest infectious disease worldwide, *AJN* 104(9):68-70, 2004.
26. Jarahzadeh M, Sutjita M: Respiratory tract infections, *Top Emerg Med* 25(2):134-138, 2003.
27. Kane C, Galanes S: Adult respiratory distress syndrome, *Crit Care Nurs Q* 27(4):325-335, 2004.
28. Karmaker MK, Ho A: Acute pain management of patients with multiple fracture ribs, *J Trauma* 54(3):615-625, 2003.
29. Keough V, Pudelek B: Blunt chest trauma: review of selected pulmonary injuries focusing on pulmonary contusion, *AACN Clin Issues* 12(2):270-281, 2001.
30. Klein Y et al: Non-ventilatory-based strategies in the management of acute respiratory distress syndrome, *J Trauma* 57(4):915-924, 2004.
31. Kollef MH: Prevention of hospital-associated pneumonia and ventilator-associated pneumonia, *Crit Care Med* 32(6):1396-1405, 2004.
32. Koschel MJ: Pulmonary embolism: quick diagnosis can save a patient's life, *Am J Nurs* 104(6):46-50, 2004.
33. Kreamer KM: Getting the lowdown on lung cancer, *Nurs* 33(11):36-43, 2004.
34. Kruger S et al: Brain natriuretic peptide predicts right heart failure inpatients with acute pulmonary embolism, *Am Heart J* 147(1):60-65: 2004.

35. Kucher N, Goldhaber SZ: Cardiac biomarkers for risk stratification of patients with acute pulmonary embolism, *Circulation* 108(18): 2191-2194, 2003.
36. Marini JJ: Advances in the understanding of acute respiratory distress syndrome: summarizing a decade of progress, *Curr Opin Crit Care* 10(4): 265-271, 2004.
37. Morrissey BM, Albertson TE: To just say NO or I don't inhale? *Crit Care Med* 29(6):1284-1285, 2001.
38. Murray JF, Nadal JA, editors: *Textbook of respiratory medicine,* ed 3, Philadelphia, 2000, Saunders.
39. O'Brien RJ, Nunn PP: The need for new drugs against tuberculosis, *Am J Respir Crit Care Med* 163(5):1055-1058, 2001.
40. Pingleton SK: Nutrition in chronic critical illness, *Clin Chest Med* 22(1):149-163, 2001.
41. Steinman MA et al: Processes and outcomes of care in elderly patients with acute bronchitis, *J Gen Intern Med* 18(Suppl 1):296-297, 2003.
42. Thorne CD et al: Using the hierarchy of control technologies to improve healthcare facility infection control: lessons from severe acute respiratory syndrome, *J Occup Environ Med* 46(7):613-622, 2004.
43. US Department of Health and Human Services: *Healthy people 2010: understanding and improving health,* Washington, DC, 2000, The Department.
44. Walker WC, Glassman SJ, Rashbaum IG: Cardiopulmonary rehabilitation and cancer rehabilitation, *Arch Phys Med Rehabil* 82(3 Suppl 1):S56-S62, 2001.
45. Weinacker AB, Vaszar LT: Acute respiratory distress syndrome: physiology and new management strategies, *Ann Rev Med* 52:221-237, 2001.
46. Wheat J et al: Practice guidelines for the management of patients with histoplasmosis, *Clin Infect Dis* 30(4):688-695, 2000.
47. Williams PL: Coccidioidomycosis. In Rakel RE, Bope ET, editors: *Conn's current therapy 2001,* Philadelphia, 2001, Saunders.
48. World Health Organization: Revised international definitions in TB control, *Int J Tuberc Lung Dis* 5(3):213-215, 2001.
49. World Heath Organization: *Adherence to long term therapies: evidence for action*, 2003, accessed Jan 2005 from website: www.who.int/chronic-conditions.

Visit the Evolve website: http://evolve.elsevier.com/Monahan/medsurg

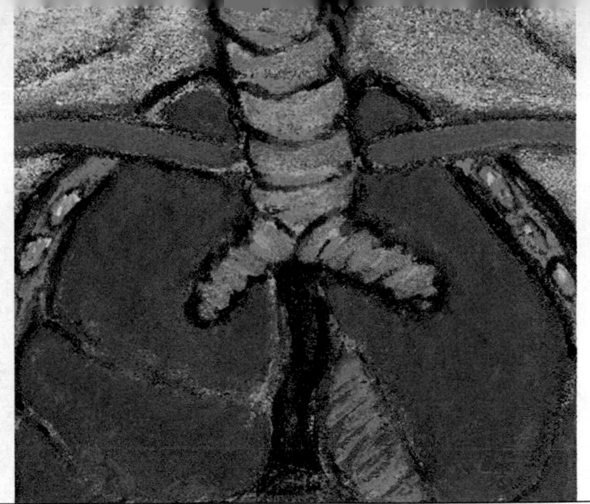

CHAPTER 27

Chronic Respiratory Problems

by Pamela D. Dennison

OBJECTIVES

After studying this chapter, the learner should be able to:

1. Explain the pathophysiology of and interventions for chronic bronchitis, pulmonary emphysema, and asthma.
2. Discuss the clinical manifestations and care management of adults with cystic fibrosis.
3. Describe interventions for managing patients with respiratory failure.
4. Discuss the care of the patient with an endotracheal tube and mechanical ventilation.
5. Discuss the indications for and advantages of noninvasive methods of providing mechanical ventilation.
6. Explain the clinical considerations in weaning patients from mechanical ventilation.
7. Describe the unique needs of the patient undergoing a lung transplant.

KEY TERMS

atelectasis, p. 675
bronchoconstrictor response, p. 685
bronchodilator, p. 675
intubation, p. 688
mucous plug, p. 685
postural drainage, p. 696
pursed-lip breathing, p. 674
spirometry, p. 675
status asthmaticus, p. 688
suctioning, p. 702
ventilator, p. 689
weaning, p. 703

The most significant pulmonary diseases are those that are chronic, and these have increased dramatically in recent years. The incidence can be expected to increase annually as the number of older adults in our society increases. Because most diseases of the respiratory tract are not reportable to the Centers for Disease Control and Prevention, the full extent of chronic illnesses such as asthma or chronic obstructive pulmonary disease (COPD) is difficult to estimate. However, known facts about disability from chronic pulmonary diseases indicate that these diseases are a major health problem and that they cause tremendous losses in productivity in the United States. The Social Security Administration reports that disability payments to persons with chronic pulmonary problems are second only to payments to persons with heart problems. COPD is the fourth leading cause of death in the United States; only heart disease, cancer, and stroke are responsible for more deaths.[1]

Early symptoms of respiratory diseases are probably those most often ignored by the general population. The major factor preventing early diagnosis and treatment of chronic pulmonary diseases is the insidious nature of their signs and symptoms. Medical attention is needed for cough, difficulty breathing, production of sputum, shortness of breath, and nose and throat irritations that do not subside within 2 weeks, since these symptoms suggest respiratory disease. Many individuals such as long-term smokers often ignore the symptoms of chronic pulmonary disease until disability results.

Chronic Obstructive Pulmonary Disease

Chronic obstructive pulmonary disease (COPD) is not a disease entity but a complex of conditions that contribute to airflow limitation. COPD is a chronic, slowly progressive disorder characterized by stable phases increasingly interrupted by worsening of symptoms, termed *acute exacerbations.* In 1995 the American Thoracic Society defined COPD as a disease state characterized by airflow obstruction resulting from chronic bronchitis or emphysema[2] (Figure 27-1). Asthma is discussed separately because of its unique characteristics of inflammation and degree of reversibility.

Most persons with COPD have one predominant disease entity, but often with manifestations of both. Why some individuals develop bronchitis and others develop emphysema is unknown. Hereditary or environmental factors or factors in the patient's history are believed to influence differences in susceptibility and the predominant type of disease.

Etiology and Epidemiology. Cigarette smoking is the primary causative factor of COPD in more than 90% of patients. Although the exact mechanism is unknown, cigarette smoking causes changes in the airways that limit airflow. However, only 15% to 20% of heavy smokers develop COPD.[53] This points to

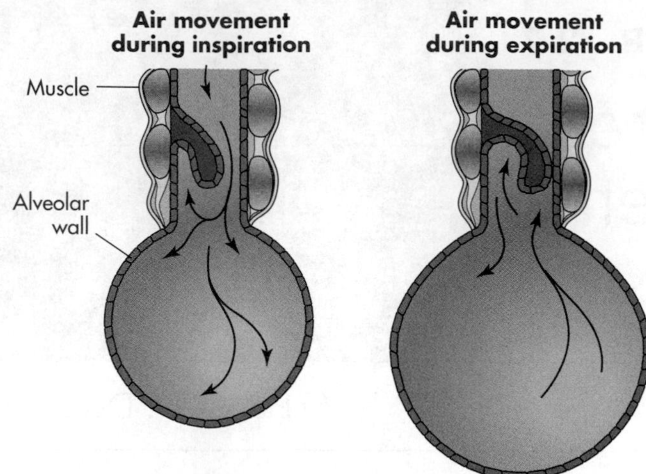

Figure 27-1 Mechanisms of air trapping in chronic obstructive pulmonary disease. Mucous plugs and narrowed airways cause air trapping and hyperinflation on expiration. During inspiration, airways enlarge, allowing gas to flow past obstruction. During expiration, airways narrow and prevent gas flow. This mechanism of air trapping, known as ball valving, occurs in asthma and chronic bronchitis.

environmental and genetic factors as additional causal agents. Imbalances in the amounts of proteases and antiproteases also play a role in the development of COPD, especially emphysema. Deficiencies in antiproteases can lead to enhanced lung parenchymal destruction. Alpha$_1$-antitrypsin (AAT) deficiency is the only known genetic abnormality that leads to COPD.[4] AAT is a serum protein produced by the liver and normally found in the lungs. Its main role is to protect the lungs from a breakdown product of white blood cells (WBCs) called neutrophil elastase. Severe AAT deficiency leads to premature emphysema. The majority of persons with AAT deficiency are misdiagnosed or undiagnosed. A high index of suspicion is needed when emphysema occurs in patients under age 60, even those with a significant smoking history.[7] Environmental tobacco smoke, also called secondhand smoke or passive smoking, is the exposure of nonsmokers to cigarette smoke and is a risk factor for COPD. High levels of air pollution, occupational exposure to toxins, and infections are also considered causative factors for a small percentage of patients with COPD.

COPD is a major health problem, the fourth leading cause of death in the United States, and the only one in the top five that continues to rise.[19] It is estimated that 11.2 million adults in the United States are diagnosed with COPD, but about 24 million Americans have evidence of impaired lung function, suggesting an underdiagnosis of COPD.[1] According to estimates by the National Heart, Lung, and Blood Institute, in 2004 the annual cost to the nation for COPD was $37.2 billion. This included $20.9 billion in direct health care expenditures, $7.4 billion in indirect morbidity costs, and $8.9 billion in indirect mortality costs.[37] Historically, COPD has had a greater prevalence and mortality rate among men compared with women. In 2002 studies revealed the incidence of COPD in women had surpassed the incidence in men (61,000 versus 59,000).[1] Significantly more women have chronic bronchitis (6.2 million women versus 2.9 million men).[1] The rates for emphysema remain higher for men, but the disparity has decreased.[56]

Pathophysiology. The pathophysiologic hallmarks of COPD are destruction of the lung parenchyma (characteristic of emphysema) and inflammation of the central airways (characteristic of chronic bronchitis) (Figure 27-2).[53] The functional consequence of these abnormalities is expiratory airflow limitation.

EMPHYSEMA. Emphysema is defined in terms of anatomic pathology as abnormal permanent enlargement of the air spaces distal to the terminal bronchioles, accompanied by destruction of their walls and without obvious fibrosis. However, recent data have shown that the destructive process is accompanied by an increase in the mass of collagen, suggesting alveolar wall fibrosis.[43] Still, the defining element of emphysema is the destructive process. Depending on how the acinus is destroyed, emphysema is classified as centriacinar or panacinar. In centriacinar emphysema the destruction is restricted to respiratory bronchioles and central portions of the acinus surrounded by areas of grossly normal lung parenchyma. In panacinar emphysema the whole acinus is uniformly involved; this type is less associated with smoking and more typically occurs in AAT-deficient persons.

As indicated above, evidence suggests that proteases released by polymorphonuclear leukocytes or alveolar macrophages are involved in destruction of the lung's connective tissue. Connective tissue in the lungs is primarily composed of elastin, collagen, and proteoglycan, which can be damaged and destroyed by enzymes such as proteases and elastase. Protease-antiprotease imbalances and cigarette smoke destroy connective tissue. Cigarette smoke directly blocks the inhibitory capacity of AAT and promotes an excess of neutrophils through the attractant effects of alveolar

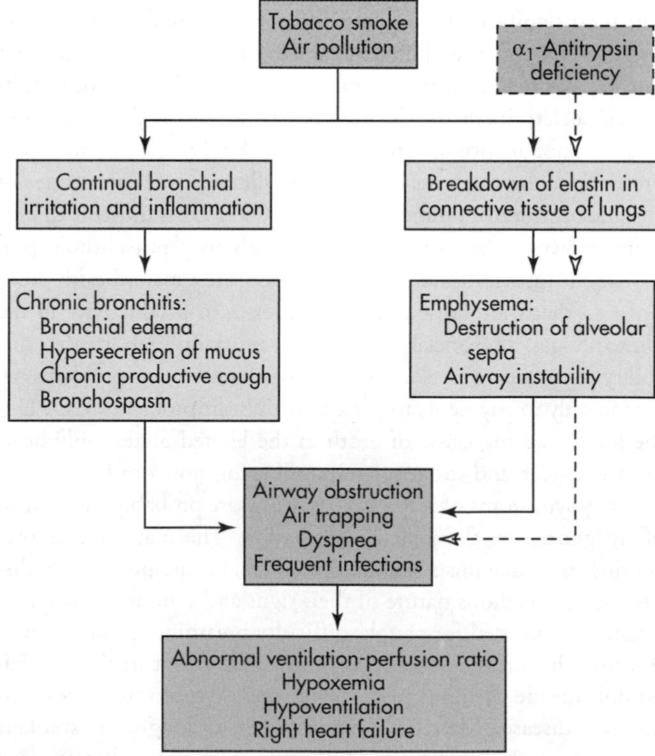

Figure 27-2 Pathogenesis of chronic bronchitis and emphysema. (*Dashed arrows* indicate role of alpha$_1$-antitrypsin deficiency, if present.)

macrophages. The neutrophils release elastases, which are capable of destroying the elastin structure of the lung. An established familial tendency to AAT deficiency indicates that relatives of persons with this type of emphysema should be screened and provided with counseling.

An estimated 1% of persons with COPD have AAT deficiency, but a recent study showed 116 million carriers worldwide among all racial groups.[17] The mean age for onset of dyspnea related to COPD is 40 to 45 years in persons with AAT deficiency. Their mean life expectancy is 50 to 65 years of age, with smokers dying about 10 years earlier than nonsmokers. Because AAT deficiency cannot be prevented, it is important that persons who have it do not smoke.

The clinical diagnosis of emphysema is inferred from the signs and symptoms of known pathophysiologic changes associated with the disease. Physiologic abnormalities characteristic of emphysema include:

- *Increased lung compliance:* Loss of elastic recoil resulting from destruction of elastin in lung parenchyma causes the lungs to become permanently overdistended (Figure 27-3). Thus, compared with normal lungs, emphysematous lungs have a larger increase in volume relative to the pressure change that occurs during inhalation.
- *Increased airway resistance:* Destruction of elastic lung tissue causes the small airways to either collapse or narrow, particularly during expiration (Figure 27-4). Thus air becomes trapped in the distal air spaces, contributing to the lungs' overdistended state. The overdistended lungs press down against the diaphragm, diminishing its ventilatory effectiveness. Use of accessory muscles for breathing, which is a

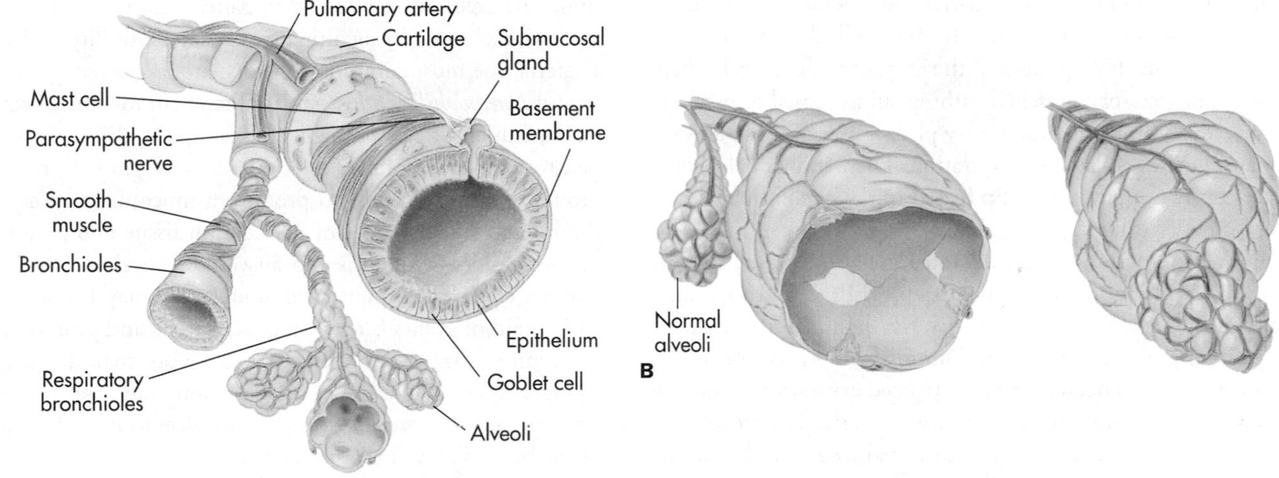

Figure 27-3 Airway obstruction caused by emphysema. **A,** Normal lung. **B,** Emphysema: enlargement and destruction of alveolar walls with loss of elasticity and trapping of air. *Left,* Panlobular emphysema showing abnormal weakening and enlargement of all air spaces distal to terminal bronchioles (normal alveoli shown for comparison only); *right,* centrilobular emphysema showing abnormal weakening and enlargement of respiratory bronchioles in proximal portion of acinus.

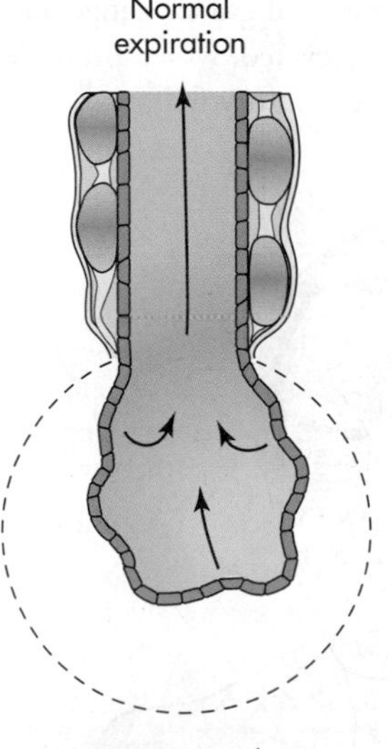

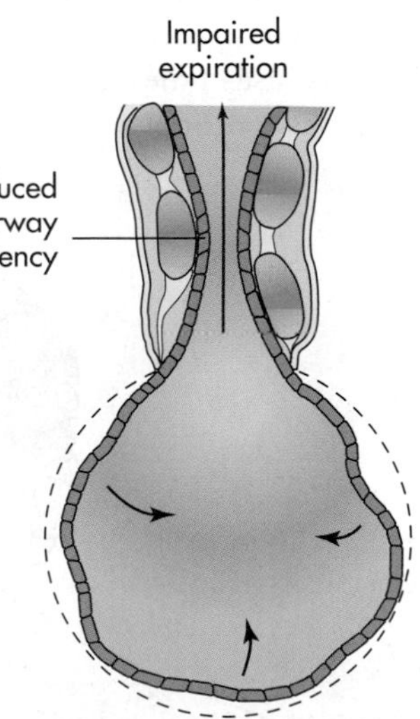

Figure 27-4 Mechanisms of air trapping in emphysema. Damaged or destroyed alveolar walls no longer support and hold airways open; alveoli lose their elastic recoil. Both these factors contribute to collapse of alveoli during expiration.

compensatory attempt to force the trapped air out of the lungs, causes an increase in intrapleural pressure, which further accentuates airway collapse.

- *Altered oxygen–carbon dioxide exchange:* Destruction of alveolar and respiratory bronchiole walls decreases alveolocapillary membrane surface area, which in turn may diminish diffusion of oxygen and carbon dioxide. Persons with emphysema are able to compensate for these destructive changes by increasing their respiratory rate. Thus arterial blood gases (ABGs) remain relatively normal, although mild hypoxemia may be present. Late in the course of the disease, extensive surface area loss and ventilation-perfusion (V/Q) inequalities usually cause respiratory acidosis and hypoxemia. The first sign of emphysema is an insidious onset of dyspnea, initially on exertion. With further disease progression, they have difficulty exhaling and constant dyspnea. There is minimal cough and sputum production. Persons with emphysema usually appear thin and manifest a "barrel chest" with an increased anteroposterior (AP) diameter from hyperinflation. The characteristic breathing pattern of the emphysematous individual includes accessory muscle breathing, an increased respiratory rate, and a prolonged expiratory phase resulting from airway narrowing or collapse on expiration. These individuals spontaneously exhibit **pursed-lip breathing**, which facilitates effective air exhalation (Figure 27-5).

Pulmonary function studies demonstrate an increased residual volume (RV), functional residual capacity (FRC), and total lung capacity (TLC). Diffusing capacity is significantly reduced because of lung tissue destruction. Diminished respiratory airflow is demonstrated by a decreased FEV_1 (forced expiratory volume in 1 second) and maximum midexpiratory flow rate. The vital capacity (VC) may be normal or only slightly reduced until late in the disease progression; thus the FEV_1/VC ratio is decreased.

ABGs are often near normal because of the individual's ability to compensate through an increased respiratory rate and tidal volume. Indeed, many people with emphysema overcompensate and develop a mild respiratory alkalosis from hyperventilation. Because resting hypoxemia is absent and ventilation is high, these individuals maintain a normal $Pa{CO_2}$ despite abnormal gas exchange. Late in the course of the disease, the $Pa{CO_2}$ is elevated, which promotes the development of cor pulmonale and respiratory failure.[51]

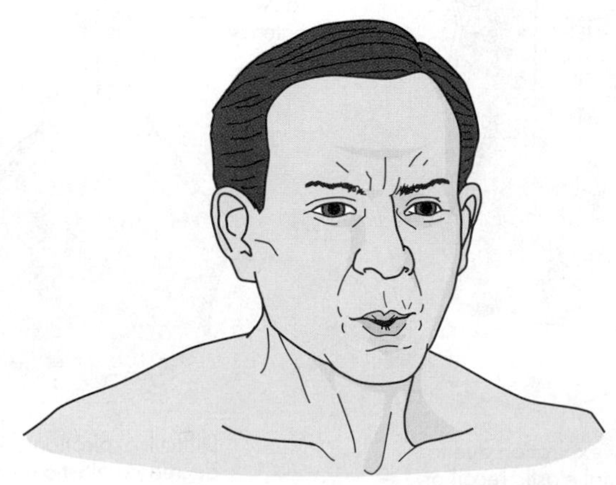

Figure 27-5 Pursed-lip breathing.

▶ ARE You READY?

The nurse recognizes which of the following clinical manifestations as the first sign of emphysema?

1. Thick, tenacious sputum
2. Increased respiratory rate
3. Dyspnea on exertion
4. Excessive cough

CHRONIC BRONCHITIS. Chronic bronchitis is defined in clinical terms as the presence of a chronic productive cough for 3 months in each of 2 successive years in a patient in whom other causes of chronic cough have been excluded.

The pathologic changes that typify chronic bronchitis are hypertrophy of mucus-secreting glands and chronic inflammatory changes in the small airways. Mucous gland hypertrophy and hyperplasia from chronic irritation cause excessive mucus production. The excessive mucus and impaired ciliary movement associated with chronic bronchitis increase susceptibility to infection. Bacteria, the most common of which are *Streptococcus pneumoniae* and *Haemophilus influenzae,* proliferate in the mucus secretions in the lumen of the bronchi. As bacteria multiply, they exert a neutrophilic chemotaxis, and pus cells migrate from between bronchial epithelial cells to produce a mucopurulent exudate in the lumen. The presence of granulation tissue and peribronchial fibrosis results in stenosis and airway obstruction. Small airways may be completely obliterated, and others may become dilated. This chain of events further traps secretions and promotes multiplication of bacteria. Some evidence exists that the pathologic changes occur initially in small airways and move to larger bronchi. The disease may progress to ulceration and destruction of the bronchial wall (Figure 27-6).

Persons with chronic bronchitis develop increased airway resistance as a result of bronchial wall tissue changes, mucosal edema, and excessive mucus production. Excess mucus in the airways not only obstructs airflow but also often causes bronchospasm, which further increases airway resistance.

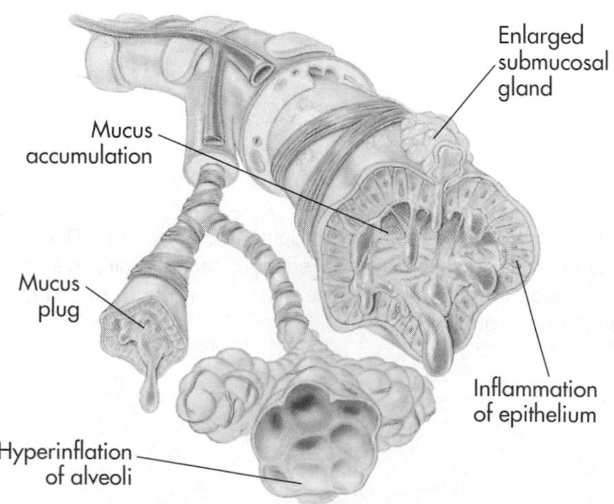

Figure 27-6 Airway obstruction caused by chronic bronchitis. Inflammation and thickening of mucous membrane with accumulation of mucus and pus, leading to obstruction; characterized by cough.

Oxygen–carbon dioxide exchange is altered. Airway obstruction results from all the pathophysiologic changes that increase airway resistance and cause V/Q mismatching at the alveolocapillary membrane by decreasing the amount of oxygenated air that reaches the alveoli. In addition, the obstructed airways may lead to **atelectasis** (lung collapse), which further diminishes the surface area available for respiration. The result of these pathophysiologic alterations is hypercapnia, hypoxemia, and respiratory acidosis.

Right ventricular decompensation (cor pulmonale) may develop. The hypercapnia and hypoxemia typically associated with chronic bronchitis cause pulmonary vascular vasoconstriction. The increased pulmonary vascular resistance results in pulmonary vessel hypertension that in turn increases vascular pressure in the right ventricle of the heart. The earliest symptom of chronic bronchitis is a productive cough, especially on awakening. This symptom is often ignored by cigarette smokers, who become so accustomed to an early-morning cough that they take it for granted; some of them even refer to it as their "cigarette cough."

Early in the course of chronic bronchitis, the symptoms tend to be episodic. As the disease progresses, the patient's symptoms are constantly present to some degree. The patient appears increasingly dyspneic, using accessory muscles to breathe. Chronic hypoxemia resulting in polycythemia causes the patient to appear cyanotic. Increased pulmonary vascular resistance caused by respiratory acidosis and hypoxemia increases pressure on the right side of the heart, ultimately resulting in right-sided heart failure (cor pulmonale). The person with late-stage chronic bronchitis and cor pulmonale appears stout or overweight from edema, and the skin appears dusky.

Patients with chronic bronchitis complicated by cor pulmonale often have chronic respiratory failure (gradual onset of Pao_2 of less than 50 mm Hg and a $Paco_2$ of more than 50 mm Hg). They are also prone to acute respiratory failure as a complication of a respiratory infection superimposed on their already diseased lung.

COMPLICATIONS. Infection and respiratory failure are the major complications.

CLINICAL MANIFESTATIONS. COPD progresses for about 30 years from inception to clinical manifestations. Decline in lung function develops insidiously and is almost always caused by decades of exposure to tobacco smoke. The normal decline in lung function as measured by FEV_1 is 25 to 30 ml/yr beginning at about age 35. The rate of decline of FEV_1 is steeper for smokers than for nonsmokers, and the heavier the smoking, the steeper the rate. Patients often do not complain of exertional dyspnea until their FEV_1 is between 40% and 50% of its expected value. Patients with COPD have usually smoked at least 20 cigarettes per day for 20 or more years before symptoms develop. They commonly are seen in the fifth decade with productive cough or an acute chest illness. Dyspnea on effort usually does not occur until the sixth or seventh decade.

Persons with COPD often unconsciously reduce their activities of daily living (ADLs) to accommodate their respiratory symptoms. They usually do not seek medical help until their symptoms are severely exacerbated, often by a respiratory infection, or until their respiratory symptoms interfere significantly with ADLs, resulting in diminished quality of life.[50]

Physical examination early in the disease may reveal only slowed expiration and wheezing on forced expiration. As obstruction progresses, hyperinflation becomes evident and the AP diameter of the chest increases. The diaphragm becomes limited in its motion. Breath sounds are decreased, expiration prolonged, and heart sounds often distant. Coarse crackles may be heard at the lung bases. Wheezes can often be elicited with forced expiration.

Collaborative Care Management

DIAGNOSTIC TESTS. Underdiagnosis of COPD is common. It may be undiagnosed in up to 50% of individuals who have the disease.[15]

PULMONARY FUNCTION AND SPIROMETRY TESTS. Pulmonary function and spirometry tests are used for diagnosis and to follow progression of disease. **Spirometry** testing can detect physiologic alterations that occur early in the disease. It measures airflow over time from fully inflated lungs. Although spirometry testing is sensitive in the identification of airflow obstruction, it does not identify the cause.[29]

FVC is the entire exhaled breath; FEV_1 is the amount of air exhaled in the first second. Normally the FEV_1/FVC ratio is 70%. In COPD both these measurements are reduced. Up to 30% of patients have an increase in FEV_1 after inhalation of a **bronchodilator**. Lung volumes (TLC, FRC, RV) are usually within normal limits until later in the course of the disease, when the lung volumes may be increased. Usually no loss of diffusing capacity occurs.

The Third National Health and Nutrition Examination Survey (NHANES III) indicated a high prevalence of undiagnosed COPD. As a result, the survey recommended the use of office spirometry to screen at-risk patients before symptoms appear and early intervention to preserve pulmonary function. Clinicians have not yet fully embraced this recommendation for screening as a part of primary care; only about 25% of health care providers have a spirometer in their offices.[15]

CHEST X-RAY FILMS. Chest x-ray films of patients with COPD typically demonstrate a low, flat diaphragm; increased AP diameter of the thorax; and overdistention of the lungs. Bullae may be present, and patients with chronic bronchitis may have increased bronchovascular markings.

ARTERIAL BLOOD GAS STUDIES. In the early stage of COPD, ABG studies show mild or moderate hypoxemia without hypercapnia. In the later stages patients have more severe hypoxemia and hypercapnia, and values may worsen during exacerbations, exercise, and sleep.

SPUTUM AND HEMATOLOGY STUDIES. Sputum studies are done for Gram stain, culture, and sensitivity. The most frequent pathogens cultured are *S. pneumoniae* and *H. influenzae.* Neutrophils and bronchial epithelial cells usually are found in chronic bronchitis. On complete blood count, erythrocytosis is frequently seen as Pao_2 levels fall below 55 mm Hg. AAT assay also may be done.

MEDICATIONS. The judicious use of appropriate medications in a stepwise approach is the recommended treatment strategy, with the goals of improving airflow and providing significant symptomatic relief.[24] Medications have yet to affect COPD mortality, so the focus is on improved morbidity outcomes.

BRONCHOACTIVE MEDICATIONS. COPD is not completely reversible, but most patients experience some improvement in dyspnea with the inhalation of bronchodilating and antiinflammatory medications.

ANTICHOLINERGIC AGENTS. Multiple cholinergic receptors in the lung stimulate muscle contraction and mucous gland secretion. Acute anticholinergic medication use in patients with COPD produces equal or greater bronchodilation than beta-agonists. Long-term anticholinergic use provides sustainable effects. Anticholinergic agents are considered first-line therapy for COPD.

Ipratropium (Atrovent) is currently the only anticholinergic available in the United States that is administered in a metered dose inhaler (MDI). The usual dose is 2 puffs four times daily, but the dose may be increased to 3 or more puffs four times per day. Ipratropium is well tolerated. Some patients have a cough and dry mouth as side effects of anticholinergic agents.

BETA-AGONISTS. Inhaled $beta_2$-agonists are the second choice of therapy for COPD management. Beta-agonists produce bronchodilation and improve hyperinflation, dyspnea, exercise capacity, and quality of life in patients with COPD. In addition to short-acting beta-agonists (albuterol, metaproterenol, pirbuterol), a long-acting agent, salmeterol, is now available in the United States. Beta-agonists may be delivered by inhaled, oral, subcutaneous, or intravenous (IV) routes. The preferred route is by inhalation to minimize side effects. Table 27-1 lists the commonly prescribed adrenergic agents that work at $beta_2$ sites in smooth muscles of the airways.

METHYLXANTHINES. Methylxanthines such as theophylline and caffeine have been used to treat patients with respiratory problems for decades. Theophyllines are known to increase respiratory muscle strength and prevent respiratory muscle fatigue. They are also mildly antiinflammatory and mitigate some lymphocyte responses. However, the role of theophylline in COPD management has been questioned, and use has fallen significantly. Theophylline has a narrow therapeutic range, interacts with numerous drugs, and is only a mild bronchodilator. Administering long-acting theophylline in the evening has been shown to reduce overnight decline in FEV_1 and morning respiratory symptoms. Current dosing recommendations include serum theophylline levels of 5 to 12 mg/L. Close monitoring for side effects and toxicity is required. Seizures and arrhythmias remain high-risk complications. The more common side effects include tremor and gastrointestinal (GI) distress.

COMBINATION THERAPY. Combinations of anticholinergics and beta-agonists are of added benefit in patients with stable COPD. Combination therapy may be achieved with the use of separate MDIs, a single MDI with the two medications combined, or nebulizer delivery of medications. The addition of theophylline to this regimen appears to increase symptomatic relief.

CORTICOSTEROIDS. The use of corticosteroids in COPD is controversial, although they are frequently prescribed for both acute and chronic regimens. During acute exacerbations corticosteroids can improve patient symptoms and reduce hospital stays. Steroids may also reduce the incidence of relapses after acute exacerbations in patients with a history of frequent exacerbations, and regular use of inhaled steroids may improve quality of life and decrease exacerbations in patients with severe disease. Thus some COPD patients benefit from chronic steroid use, but it may require 6 months of inhaled steroids to identify these patients. Therapy with inhaled corticosteroids is recommended by the National Heart, Lung, and Blood Institute; World Health Organization; and Global Initiative for Chronic Obstructive Lung Disease for (1) patients with symptomatic COPD who have a documented spirometric response to inhaled corticosteroids and (2) patients with moderate to severe COPD who have repeated exacerbations that require treatment with antibiotics or oral corticosteroids.[26] When corticosteroids are used, the dose should be maintained at the minimum level to achieve desired outcomes.

MUCOLYTICS. Mucus hypersecretion is a risk factor for more rapid disease progression. It increases the likelihood for hospitalization and symptomatic limitations. Unfortunately, little evidence is

TABLE 27-1 $BETA_2$-AGONISTS AND DOSAGES FOR METERED-DOSE INHALERS AND NEBULIZED SOLUTIONS

	MDI		
Drug	**Dose**	**mg/Puff**	**Nebulization**
Albuterol (Proventil, Ventolin)	2-3 puffs q4-6h	0.09	0.3-0.5 ml 0.5% solution in 3 ml saline q4-6h
Bitolterol (Tornalate)	2-3 puffs q6-8h	0.37	
Metaproterenol (Alupent, Metaprel)	2-3 puffs q4-6h	0.65	0.3 ml 5% solution in 2.5 ml saline q4-6h
Pirbuterol (Maxair)	2-3 puffs q4-6h	0.20	
Salmeterol (Serevent)	2 puffs q12h	0.50	
Terbutaline (Brethaire)	2-3 puffs q4-6h	0.20	

MDI, Metered-dose inhaler; *q,* every; *h,* hour.

currently available that mucokinetic agents reduce mucus production or enhance the elimination of mucus in patients with COPD.

ANTIBIOTICS. Chronic or prophylactic antibiotics are not routinely recommended for patients with COPD. Antibiotics can shorten the course of acute exacerbations that involve purulent sputum in association with increased sputum production or dyspnea. Lower-cost broad-spectrum antibiotics are preferred.

ALPHA$_1$-ANTITRYPSIN. Regular replacement of AAT in patients with deficiency may prevent the protease-antiprotease imbalance that damages the lungs. Although definitive proof of long-term benefits of AAT replacement therapy is still lacking, a growing body of evidence suggests that patients who are AAT deficient and receive replacement therapy have a slower rate of lung destruction as measured by spirometry and a chest computed tomographic scan. It may also reduce mortality.[2] IV infusion of AAT can be given on a weekly or biweekly basis but is most commonly administered monthly. Newer modes of delivery such as inhalation are under investigation.

ANTIDEPRESSANT AND ANTIANXIETY MEDICATIONS. Depression is frequently unrecognized in patients with COPD and may manifest as insomnia or anxiety. Multiple medications can successfully treat depressed patients with COPD; however, serotonin selective reuptake inhibitors (SSRIs) are the most commonly prescribed.

Anxiety is also common in COPD patients, with panic attacks occurring in a significant number. SSRI medications, which provide effective therapy and relative patient safety, are the primary medications used to treat anxiety in patients with COPD. Buspirone is an example of an anxiolytic that does not have respiratory depressant effects. However, it has only mild antianxiety effects and may not be adequate.

TREATMENTS

SMOKING CESSATION. No intervention other than smoking cessation has been shown to slow the rate of decline in lung function in patients with COPD. Approximately 60% of individuals who smoke say they want to quit. Helping individuals quit smoking is an important nursing consideration. The Lung Health Study showed that early intervention in individuals with mild to moderate airflow obstruction can decrease age-related decline in FEV_1.[15] A consideration for nurses teaching smoking cessation is role modeling. Statistics continue to show that nurses and nursing students smoke at a higher rate than the general population.[10]

Smoking cessation is a challenge at any age, but particularly for older patients who have been smoking for years. For each attempt to stop smoking, relapse rates approach 70% at 3 months and exceed 90% at 1 year.[31] The older adult may have tried many interventions, made multiple attempts to quit, and have high expectations for failure. On the other hand, older adults are more likely to value advice from physicians and health care providers and therefore more seriously contemplate smoking cessation. Some intervention studies have shown positive results from regular, brief calls and letters of encouragement from health care professionals. Counseling alone has been shown to result in a less than 5% sustained quit rate. When using nicotine replacement strategies, older patients need to be monitored closely for signs of nicotine excess (nausea, tachycardia, dizziness). A lower dose may be needed.[31]

OXYGEN THERAPY. Administration of supplemental oxygen is the only therapy proven to alter the course of advanced stages of COPD. Hypoxemia in patients with COPD adversely affects function and leads to death. Oxygen therapy is required for patients with COPD who are unable to maintain a PaO_2 greater than 55 mm Hg or oxygen saturation greater than 85% or more at rest and for those who cannot carry out ADLs (breathing, eating, dressing, toileting) without becoming short of breath. In these patients 1 to 2 L/min of oxygen is usually given via nasal prongs to relieve hypoxemia and decrease pulmonary hypertension, which in turn decreases the load on the right side of the heart. The goal of oxygen therapy is to provide oxygen to patients at rates sufficient to maintain oxygen saturations above 90% as close to 24 hours per day as possible.

Although supplemental oxygen improves alertness, endurance, and walking distance, not enough evidence is available to support continuous long-term oxygen therapy for patients who do not qualify based on resting oxygenation levels. Detailed oxygen assessment at rest and with activity is recommended for all patients with moderate to severe COPD. Patients with COPD with adequate resting daytime oxygen levels may have significant hypoxemia during activity or at night. Oxygen supplementation at these times can improve performance, quality of life, and sleep. It also may improve survival, especially if cor pulmonale or cardiac arrhythmias are present. Ambulatory oxygen is preferable to oxygen from stationary sources because it allows patients to exercise and improve cardiac output, thus improving tissue oxygenation.

A common misunderstanding expressed by patients requiring ongoing oxygen therapy is that they should use their oxygen only when they are symptomatic (i.e., short of breath) to avoid becoming habituated to the oxygen and thus requiring higher levels of oxygen. The nurse needs to clarify that habituation to oxygen will not occur. The nurse also stresses the importance of continual oxygen use to receive maximal benefits of the therapy.

Because many patients with COPD have chronic carbon dioxide retention, their stimulus to breathe is their low PaO_2 level. Patients must understand that high flow rates of oxygen (greater than 6 L/min) and high concentrations (greater than 40%) may elevate their PaO_2 to a level that removes the stimulus by which they breathe, resulting in respiratory failure. Long-term oxygen therapy has been shown to be of substantial benefit for patients with advanced COPD and chronic hypoxemia. Before discharge from the hospital, the nurse needs to determine ABG and oxygen saturation levels at rest, with exercise, and during sleep to evaluate the need for home use of oxygen. The Centers for Medicare and Medicaid Services (CMS), which fund Medicare, have established specific criteria for reimbursement of home oxygen and oxygen equipment under the durable medical equipment benefit.

CMS considers home oxygen therapy reasonable and necessary only for patients with significant hypoxemia who meet the criteria related to medical documentation, laboratory evidence, and specified health conditions. Required documentation includes a diagnosis of the disease requiring home use of oxygen; the oxygen flow rate; and an estimate of the frequency and duration of use (e.g., 2 L/min, 10 min/hr, 12 hr/day) and duration of need (e.g., 6 months, lifetime). The required laboratory evidence includes the results of a blood gas study ordered and evaluated by a physician within 2 days of discharge. Covered blood gas values include:

- PaO_2 of 55 mm Hg or less or oxygen saturation of 88% or less taken on room air at rest
- PaO_2 of 55 mm Hg or less or oxygen saturation of 88% or less during exercise
- PaO_2 between 56 and 59 mm Hg or oxygen saturation of 88% or less in the presence of heart failure, pulmonary hypertension, cor pulmonale, or hematocrit more than 56%

Covered health conditions include severe lung disease (COPD, interstitial lung disease, cystic fibrosis, lung cancer), hypoxia-related symptoms, or findings that might be expected to improve with oxygen therapy (pulmonary hypertension, heart failure caused by cor pulmonale, erythrocytosis, impairment of cognitive processes, nocturnal restlessness, morning headaches).

Medical supply companies bring the oxygen to the home, show the patient and caregivers how to use it, and check the equipment regularly. Oxygen for home use is available in three forms: liquid, tank, or oxygen concentrator. Either a mask or nasal cannula is used. Oxygen concentrators are the most widely used stationary oxygen delivery system. Concentrators are fairly quiet, efficient, and low maintenance. The cost of electricity to operate these units is not reimbursable, and oxygen concentrators are inoperable during an electrical power failure. Liquid oxygen is stored in large, insulated canisters of 60 to 120 pounds as a stationary source of oxygen delivery in the home. The reservoir units must be refilled frequently, so even though liquid oxygen is relatively inexpensive, its cost can be substantial, particularly in rural or remote areas.

Portable oxygen systems that weigh more than 10 pounds are mounted on wheels and allow for some mobility but are difficult to maneuver. Portable oxygen concentrators that can be operated from either a 12-volt battery or conventional AC electrical outlet are useful for travel. Ambulatory liquid oxygen systems that can be refilled in the home have vastly improved patient mobility and satisfaction. Technologic advances continue in development of lighter-weight and longer-lasting units.

Oxygen-conserving devices reduce the cost of home oxygen therapy by reducing the frequency of renewing the supply of liquid or gaseous oxygen. Oxygen-conserving devices use a mechanical reservoir or an anatomic reservoir that fills with 100% oxygen during exhalation and empties the oxygen into the lungs early in inspiration. Mechanical reservoirs include a nasal reservoir cannula and a pendant reservoir cannula. Both empty on inspiration and fill during exhalation. In both systems the effective bolus of 100% oxygen is about 20 ml. The cannula is more visible, but the pendant is less comfortable.

Another system for oxygen conservation is the pulsation of a bolus of oxygen during the first fourth to half of inspiration, when virtually all the oxygen delivered goes to the oxygen-exchanging areas of the lung with minimal distribution to anatomic dead space. These units have multiple manufacturers, and each functions differently. Most are battery powered. The quantity of oxygen in each pulse may be variable or fixed, and the pulse may occur with each breath or have a variable frequency based on the flow setting. Patient acceptance has been excellent. All oxygen-conserving devices provide 50% or more oxygen savings at rest, but the degree of conservation may vary substantially during exercise.

Another mode of oxygen delivery that may be used with COPD patients is transtracheal oxygen (TTO) delivery. TTO involves insertion of a catheter percutaneously between the second and third tracheal interspaces; this is held in place by a necklace and transparent film dressing. Oxygen enters the trachea via this catheter, thus significantly reducing oxygen delivery to airway dead space. Patients have been reported to use 37% to 58% less oxygen during TTO delivery, compared with continuous-flow nasal oxygen. In all patients receiving TTO, it is standard practice to titrate the dose of oxygen to ensure adequate oxyhemoglobin saturation, both at rest and during exercise. Not all patients are candidates for TTO. The ideal candidate has a strong desire to remain active, is willing to follow the care protocol, is not experiencing frequent exacerbations, has a caregiver willing to assist with problem solving and details of care, and has access to good medical follow-up. Relative contraindications to TTO include high-dose steroids and conditions that predispose the patient to delayed healing (e.g., diabetes, connective tissue disease, and severe obesity). Absolute contraindications include subglottic stenosis or vocal cord paralysis, herniation of the pleura into the insertion site, severe coagulopathy, uncompensated respiratory acidosis, and inability to practice self-care. Complications of TTO include catheter displacement, bacterial cellulitis, subcutaneous emphysema, hemoptysis, a severed catheter, and mucous balls that can result in acute respiratory distress and, in some cases, acute respiratory failure.

AEROSOL THERAPY. Aerosol therapy is one of the most effective ways to deliver bronchoactive medications with minimal side effects. Directions for teaching patients to use an inhaler with a spacer are described in the Patient/Family Teaching box.

VACCINATION. Pneumococcal and influenza vaccinations are recommended for all patients with COPD. Influenza vaccines usually become available by October, and the optimal time for vaccination is October through mid-November, before influenza become prevalent. Patients with COPD, their household contacts, and health

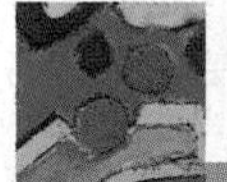

PATIENT/FAMILY TEACHING
Using an Inhaler With a Spacer

The nurse should teach the patient to:

- Exhale fully.
- Position nebulizer in mouth *without* sealing lips around it.
- Take a deep breath while releasing a puff of medication into spacer.
- Hold breath for 3 to 4 seconds at full inspiration.
- Exhale slowly through pursed lips.
- Take prescribed number of puffs—usually one or two.
- Take number of breaths necessary to receive the entire prescribed dose from the spacer.
- Rinse mouth after completing treatment.
- Wash inhaler and spacer with warm soapy water, rinse, and dry thoroughly after each use.

care workers who have contact with vulnerable patient populations are encouraged to receive vaccinations as soon as possible.[33]

ADDITIONAL THERAPY. Patients should be up and about as much as possible. Some use portable oxygen while walking or doing other tasks. To promote optimal daytime activity, nurses must assess adequacy of sleep and rest. Sleep disorders are pervasive in patients with COPD. Sleep is disturbed by symptoms, medications, gas exchange abnormalities, and sleep apnea.[30]

Pulmonary rehabilitation attempts to return patients to their highest possible functional capacity. The rehabilitative approach to the care of COPD patients has been shown to improve independence and quality of life, decrease hospital days, and improve exercise capacity (see Evidence-Based Practice box). Lung function is usually not improved.

Pulmonary health care teams consist of physicians, nurses, respiratory therapists, occupational therapists, physical therapists, dietitians, social workers, and psychologists or psychiatrists. The complex multidisciplinary rehabilitation team is ideal, but the nurse in a small community hospital or community health agency can provide effective rehabilitation activities for the person with COPD.[23]

Hospice is also considered for its palliative care. Since COPD is a progressive and ultimately fatal disease, palliative care should be the focus when physical or psychologic suffering becomes central. The provision of palliative care is not limited by the site of care (home, hospital, acute care, intensive care). The National Hospice Organization suggests that the following criteria be used for admission to a hospice program for patients with noncancerous conditions: disabling dyspnea at rest with progressive pulmonary disease, cor pulmonale, hypoxemia at rest (PaO_2 less than 55 mm Hg or oxygen saturation less than 88%) or hypercapnia ($PaCO_2$ greater than 50 mm Hg), unintentional progressive loss of 10% of body weight in 6 months, or resting tachycardia (more than 100 beats/min).[3]

Effective health care management programs for persons who have COPD require a multidisciplinary approach. Management programs should be designed to prevent premature morbidity and mortality from COPD, educate patients and families, minimize airflow limitation and retard its progression, correct secondary physiologic problems, and optimize functional capabilities.[50] A comprehensive management program benefits all patients, even those with severe disease.

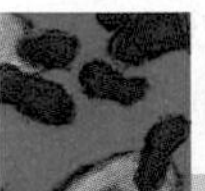
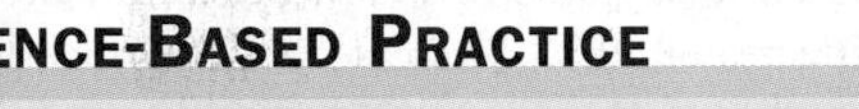

EVIDENCE-BASED PRACTICE

Topic Question: Is pulmonary rehabilitation beneficial for chronic obstructive pulmonary disease (COPD)?

Evidence Base: The review included reports of 23 randomized controlled trials that measured quality of life, exercise capacity, or both after pulmonary rehabilitation. The rehabilitation and treatment consisted of at lease 4 weeks of exercise training, psychoemotional support, and education. Controls groups did not receive the treatment.

Findings: There were statistically significant results in the quality of life and the exercise capacity of the participants.

Conclusions: Pulmonary rehabilitation programs are effective in relieving some of the symptoms of COPD such as dyspnea and fatigue. This improves the patient's quality of life.

Lacasse Y et al: *Pulmonary rehabilitation for chronic obstructive pulmonary disease (Cochrane Review).* In Cochrane Library, Issue 3, 2004, Chichester, UK, John Wiley & Sons, accessed July 2004 from website: www.cochrane.org.

SURGICAL MANAGEMENT

LUNG TRANSPLANTATION. COPD is the most frequent indication for lung transplantation.[47] The survival rate after transplantation for emphysema is the highest of any patient population with lung disease. Generally, it is considered an option for patients under age 65 with an FEV_1 below 30% of the predicted rate; without evidence of pulmonary hypertension; and with consideration given to the patient's functional status and quality of life, assessed after pulmonary rehabilitation. Long-term survival is generally better if emphysematous recipients undergo bilateral lung transplantation, rather than single lung. Single lung transplantation is generally performed when only one lung is available. Infection is the most significant complication. Lung transplantation is discussed more thoroughly later in the chapter.

LUNG VOLUME REDUCTION SURGERY. Lung volume reduction surgery (LVRS) is a surgical procedure for patients with severe emphysema. The hyperinflated portion of the lung or lungs is removed so that the patient's chest wall and diaphragm can return to normal positions, thereby easing breathing. Most often it is used as a bridge to transplantation that improves respiratory function for patients during the prolonged waiting time for donor organs.

Patient eligibility criteria for LVRS include:

- Severe limitation of pulmonary function, with FEV_1 less than 30% of that predicted, FVC less than 60%, and TLC greater than 8 L
- Impaired ADLs
- Maximally flattened diaphragm documented on chest x-ray examination
- No effective response to medical management
- Completion of 6 to 12 weeks of pulmonary rehabilitation
- Successful smoking cessation for at least 6 months

LVRS involves either mediastinoscopy or video-assisted thoracoscopic surgery. Regardless of the approach, the goal is to reduce lung volume by approximately 25%. The procedure involves deflating one lung by clamping one side of the bifurcated double-lumen endotracheal tube. Normal lung tissue turns gray, but the hyperinflated section of the lung remains pink from trapped air. The surgeon excises the hyperinflated area, then fills the patient's chest cavity with saline to inspect for air leaks. If none are detected, the surgeon repeats the procedure on the opposite lung. After surgery one or two chest tubes are placed and connected to a water-seal drainage system. No suction is used unless an air leak develops. Postoperative emphasis is on monitoring ABGs; early ambulation; and management of pain, usually with an epidural catheter.[49]

LVRS can improve both objective and subjective measures of lung performance in carefully selected COPD patients, with demonstrated positive effects of up to 5 years. The National Emphysema Treatment Trial showed most benefit for patients who had predominantly upper lobe emphysema and low exercise capacity.[50] Most studies demonstrate improvement in pulmonary function, decreased dyspnea, and enhanced exercise capacity. As of 2003, the CMS agreed to cover the costs of LVRS for patients who were not at high risk of death from the procedure, whose disease affected the upper lobes exclusively, and who had a combination of diffuse disease and low exercise capacity.[24] Pioneering work in bronchoscopic lung volume reduction may offer expanded options for nonsurgical candidates in the future.[52]

DIET. Improving nutrition is an important goal.[40] (See discussion under Nursing Interventions.)

HEALTH PROMOTION AND PREVENTION. Ideally, all types of COPD would be prevented if people quit smoking and respiratory irritants were removed from the environment. Although this is not likely to happen soon, continued efforts should be made to educate people about respiratory irritants and dangers. Public education must focus on the pulmonary health risks associated with inhaled irritants, regardless of their source. Increased public awareness of the vital role that clean air plays in pulmonary health is essential for the success of any legislative actions promoting air quality standards. Individuals must also understand the importance of personal responsibility to decrease their own health risk through smoking cessation. *Healthy People 2010* has set goals for reducing cases of chronic respiratory disease (see Healthy People 2010 box).[54]

Persons with a family history of emphysema should be screened for AAT deficiency. It is imperative that persons with this enzyme deficiency take active measures to prevent progressive lung damage from smoking, air pollution, and infection. Those at high risk for emphysema may require vocational counseling if their current work environment has inhaled irritants. These individuals should also be counseled to receive the influenza vaccine yearly and the pneumococcal vaccine every 3 to 5 years.

Nursing Management

of the Patient with Chronic Obstructive Pulmonary Disease

ASSESSMENT

Health History. Assess for:

- History, character, onset, and duration of symptoms
- Dyspnea, including its effects on ADLs and whether it is associated with any specific illness or event
- Cough
- Sputum production (amount, color, consistency)
- Pain in right upper quadrant (hepatomegaly)
- Smoking history
- Family history of COPD, respiratory illnesses
- Disease history, especially influenza, pneumonia
- History of respiratory tract infections, chronic sinusitis
- Past or present exposure to environmental irritants at home or at work
- Self-care modalities used to treat symptoms
- Current pattern of activity and rest, willingness to exercise
- Nutritional status—caffeine and alcohol use, history of eating disorders, weight history, food allergies, body mass index
- Medications taken and their effectiveness in relieving symptoms

Healthy People 2010

Selected Objectives for Reduction of Chronic Respiratory Diseases

- Reduce cigarette smoking by adolescents and adults.
- Reduce the proportion of nonsmokers exposed to environmental tobacco smoke.
- Reduce the proportion of persons exposed to air that does not meet the U.S. Environmental Protection Agency's health-based standards for ozone.

From US Department of Health and Human Services: *Healthy people 2010: understanding and improving health*, Washington, DC, 2000, The Department.

Physical Examination. Assess for:

- General appearance (Appearance and hygiene may be indicators of symptom interference with ADLs. Patient may appear underweight, overweight, or bloated, and skin color may be dusky or pale.)
- Increased AP diameter of chest ("barrel chest")
- Dependent edema and jugular venous distention
- Enlarged or tender liver
- Elevated temperature, tachycardia, tachypnea
- Use of accessory muscles of breathing, forward-leaning (tripod) posture, pursed-lip breathing, central cyanosis, clubbed fingers
- Sputum production: amount, color, consistency, time of day, change from baseline
- Signs of an altered sensorium (restlessness or lethargy), which may be the first indicator of hypoxia
- Auscultation of breath sounds, which may be distant as a result of increased AP diameter and decreased airflow; commonly reveal crackles (rales), especially in dependent lung fields; rhonchi (gurgles); and wheezes, especially on forced exhalation
- Relevant laboratory findings, including an elevated hemoglobin, hematocrit, and WBC count; alterations in ABGs; decreased FEV_1, decreased VC, normal diffusing capacity, and normal to increased lung volumes (TLC, FRC, RV)

NURSING DIAGNOSES, OUTCOMES, AND INTERVENTIONS

Nursing Diagnosis: Impaired Gas Exchange

OUTCOMES. Common examples of expected outcomes for the patient with a diagnosis of *impaired gas exchange* are:

Patient will:

- Demonstrate improved ventilation and oxygenation.
- Exhibit arterial blood $Pa{O_2}$, $Pa{CO_2}$, and pH levels at patient's baseline.
- Explain how and when to use oxygen therapy.

NURSING INTERVENTIONS. The nurse monitors ABGs for indications of hypoxemia, respiratory acidosis, and respiratory alkalosis. Hypoxemia and hypercapnia often occur simultaneously, and the signs and symptoms are similar. These include headache, irritability, confusion, increasing somnolence, asterixis (flapping tremors of extremities), cardiac dysrhythmias, and tachycardia. Morning headache is a frequent sign of hypercapnia. If hypocapnia is developing, tachypnea, vertigo, tingling of the extremities, muscular weakness, and spasm are often present. The presence of signs and symptoms associated with altered levels of PaO_2 and $PaCO_2$ depends more on the rate of change than on the degree. Rapidly changing signs usually indicate a rapid worsening of the patient's condition, whereas patients with longstanding hypoxemia and hypercapnia may be relatively asymptomatic because they have physiologically accommodated to increased $PaCO_2$ and decreased PaO_2.

The nurse is in a key role to assess the need for supplemental oxygen, to assess the response to therapy and acceptance of therapy, and to ensure that the patient meets Medicare criteria for home oxygen therapy. It is important for the nurse to educate the patient and family on the following points:

- Oxygen is to be delivered at the prescribed flow rate. Adjustments need to be discussed with the health care provider.
- Oxygen dries the nose membranes. Applying a water-soluble lubricant (K-Y Jelly) to the inside of the nose may reduce dryness and cracking. Petroleum jelly (Vaseline) should not be used because it may be inhaled.
- If humidification is used, the amount of water in the humidifier bottle must be checked every 6 to 8 hours and refilled as needed with sterile or distilled water.
- A new supply of oxygen must be ordered when the oxygen source reads one-fourth full.
- Safety precautions must always be observed. Oxygen is not flammable itself, but it supports combustion. No one should smoke in the room where oxygen is being used; patients using oxygen should stay away from gas stoves, gas space heaters, or kerosene heaters or lamps; the container should always be kept upright to prevent leakage; and an all-purpose fire extinguisher should be readily available in the home.
- The health care provider should be notified if breathing is more difficult or if restlessness, anxiety, tiredness, drowsiness, difficulty waking up, persistent headache, slurred speech, confusion, or cyanosis of the fingernails or lips occurs.

RELATED NIC INTERVENTIONS. Airway Management, Oxygen Therapy, Respiratory Monitoring

Nursing Diagnosis: Ineffective Airway Clearance

OUTCOMES. Common examples of expected outcomes for the patient with a diagnosis of *ineffective airway clearance* are:
Patient will:

- Demonstrate adequate airway clearance.
- Use effective methods of coughing.
- Use bronchoactive medications, including MDIs, dry powder inhalers (DPIs), nebulizers, and humidifiers appropriately.

NURSING INTERVENTIONS. Clearing of the airways is of utmost importance in meeting tissue demands for increased oxygen during periods of rest and increased activity. The nurse should teach the patient effective coughing maneuvers of sitting upright and using the huff coughing technique.

To thin secretions, a fluid intake of 3 to 4 L has traditionally been encouraged unless contraindicated. However, evidence suggests that this quantity of fluids may not be needed to keep secretions mobile. Although expectorants are sometimes prescribed, some experts believe they do more harm than good. Water is still considered the best expectorant, and the nurse should encourage adequate hydration without fluid overload.

Pulmonary physiotherapy techniques may be helpful to some patients with COPD, but many are not able to tolerate this intervention because of hypoxemia, age, debilitation, and other factors. The Global Initiative for Chronic Obstructive Lung Disease recommends manual or mechanical chest percussion and postural drainage in patients producing more than 25 ml of sputum each day as well, as in those with lobar atelectasis.[25] (These techniques are discussed under Cystic Fibrosis.)

RELATED NIC INTERVENTIONS. Airway Management, Cough Enhancement, Respiratory Monitoring

Nursing Diagnosis: Ineffective Breathing Pattern

OUTCOMES. Common examples of expected outcomes for the patient with a diagnosis of *ineffective breathing pattern* are:
Patient will:

- Demonstrate effective breathing pattern.
- Have inspiratory/expiratory ratio 5:10 seconds.
- Use forward-leaning postures, controlled breathing techniques (pursed-lip breathing), and diaphragmatic breathing (abdominal muscle breathing).
- Exhale with exertion.
- Demonstrate respiratory rate within near-normal limits, with moderate tidal volume.

NURSING INTERVENTIONS. The nurse encourages the patient to use controlled breathing techniques, including pursed-lip breathing, the forward-leaning position, and abdominal breathing, to control dyspnea and anxiety. The goal is a reduced respiratory rate and enhanced expiratory tidal volume, thus decreasing air trapping.

Pursed-lip breathing (see Figure 27-5) decreases dyspnea when it is used with activities that produce tachypnea, which leads to progressive air trapping. Pursed-lip breathing decreases the respiratory rate, increases tidal volume, decreases $PaCO_2$, and increases PaO_2 and SaO_2. Some patients use pursed-lip breathing intuitively, and others need to be taught. To teach it, the nurse asks the patient to (1) inhale through the nose for several seconds with the mouth closed and (2) exhale slowly (taking twice as long as inhalation) through pursed lips held in a narrow slit. One method of teaching this technique is by using a child's soap bubble wand and blowing one big soap bubble. This approach combines an enjoyable activity with a measurable means of visualizing a pursed-lip exhalation, provides immediate patient feedback, and promotes relaxation of the patient's upper body and decreased use of accessory breathing.

The nurse teaches the forward-leaning (tripod) position for exhalation. A forward-leaning position of 30 to 40 degrees with the head tilted at a 16- to 18-degree angle effectively improves exhalation (Figure 27-7). As mentioned previously, patients with

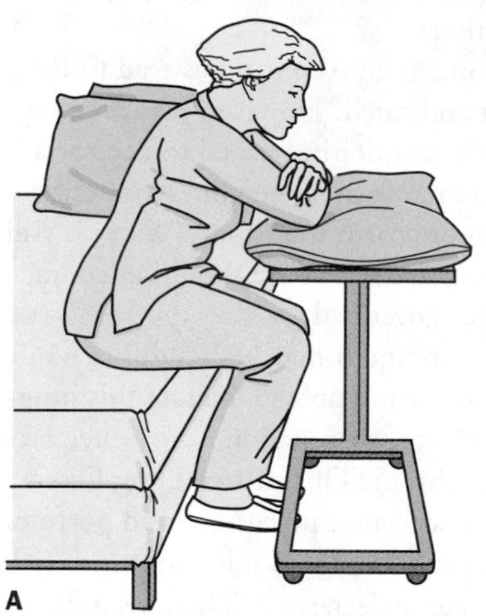

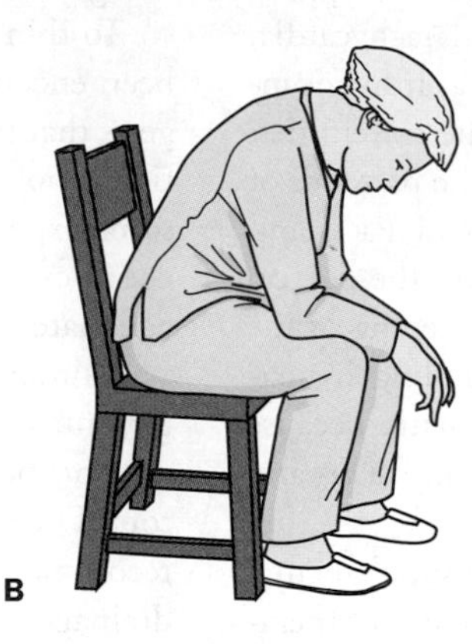

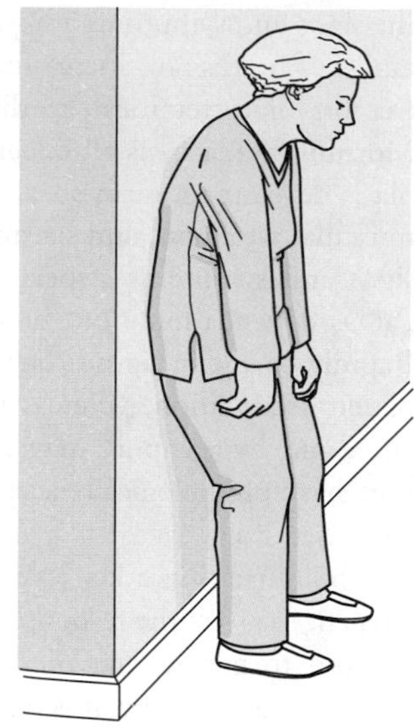

Figure 27-7 Forward-leaning position. **A,** Patient sits on edge of bed with arms folded on pillow placed on elevated bedside table. **B,** Patient in three-point position. Patient sits on chair with feet approximately 1 foot apart and leans forward with elbows on knees. **C,** Patient leans against wall with feet apart, allowing shoulders to sag forward with arms extended.

emphysema have increased TLC and RV with the diaphragm in a fixed, flattened position. Therefore the diaphragm cannot assist in exhalation as it does normally. Leaning forward allows removal of more air from the lungs on exhalation. The patient can achieve the forward-leaning position while sitting or standing. The patient sits on the edge of the bed or a chair and leans forward on two or three pillows placed on a table or overbed stand, or sits in a chair with the legs spread apart shoulder width (or wider, if the patient is obese) with the elbows on the knees and the arms and hands relaxed, or stands with the back and hips against the wall with the feet spread apart and about 12 inches (30 cm) from the wall. The patient then relaxes and leans forward. In these positions the patient cannot use the accessory muscles of respiration, and the upward action of the diaphragm is improved.

Abdominal breathing improves the breathing efficiency of persons with COPD because it assists in elevating the diaphragm. Abdominal breathing can be done in the sitting or lying position. The patient sits on the side of the bed or in a chair and holds a small pillow or a book against the abdomen. The patient exhales slowly while leaning forward and pressing the pillow or book against the abdomen. In the lying position, the patient places a hand on the abdomen and then "puffs out" the abdomen while inhaling and raises the hand as high as possible. The patient then exhales slowly through pursed lips while pulling in on the abdominal muscles. Manual pressure on the upper abdomen during expiration facilitates this maneuver (see Chapter 26). In addition to abdominal breathing, exercises to strengthen the abdominal muscles help patients use them more effectively in emptying their lungs. This controlled breathing pattern is used while performing various ADLs, from sitting, standing, walking, and climbing stairs to more complex activities. As this pattern becomes natural, the patient uses it automatically during periods of increased shortness of breath.

Environment plays a significant role in ease of breathing. Humidity of 30% to 50% is ideal and can be achieved with a humidifier. An air conditioner may reduce dyspnea by controlling the temperature and preventing entrance of pollutants from outside air. The cost of an air conditioner is a medically deductible expense for persons with COPD. Movement of cool air with a fan has also been shown to reduce dyspnea, perhaps from the stimulation of receptors on the face or decreased temperature of facial skin. Wearing a scarf over the nose and mouth in cold weather helps warm the air and prevent bronchospasm. Masks for this purpose are also available. Smoking cessation is essential, as is minimal exposure to air pollution and the avoidance of environmental tobacco smoke.

RELATED NIC INTERVENTIONS. Airway Management, Oxygen Therapy, Respiratory Management

Nursing Diagnosis: Activity Intolerance

OUTCOMES. Common examples of expected outcomes for the patient with a diagnosis of *activity intolerance* are:

Patient will:

- Maintain or work toward an optimal activity level.
- Pace activities.
- Plan for simplification of activities.
- Participate in planned muscle-conditioning program.
- Demonstrate how to carry out the exercise program to be followed at home, including specific exercises to be completed; frequency of each exercise; and criteria for monitoring physical response to exercises, such as heart rate increase or perceived fatigue.

NURSING INTERVENTIONS. To minimize the discomfort of dyspnea, individuals with COPD often avoid physical exertion. The result is gradual deconditioning and dyspnea at ever-lower levels of exertion. Fatigue and muscle wasting also result from deconditioning. Exercise training (aerobic exercise training, strength training, and inspiratory muscle training) improves aerobic capacity, endurance, strength, and functional performance in day-to-day life, and it reduces breathlessness and fatigue during exertion.[13] Patients should undertake both general exercises and specific muscle training.[33]

For general exercise conditioning, graded leg exercises performed by stationary cycling, stair climbing, and walking are safe and well tolerated. Oxygen during exercise is recommended for patients who have significant exercise desaturation and show improved exercise tolerance while using oxygen.

Leg-raising exercises, with each leg being raised alternately as the patient exhales, is one way to strengthen abdominal muscles. Another way is for the patient to raise the head and shoulders from the bed while he or she exhales. With practice and encouragement, the patient can do the exercises 10 times each morning and evening after clearing the lungs of secretions as completely as possible.

The term *muscle reconditioning* refers to a variety of muscle-toning exercises. For patients who are able to be out of bed, walking, using a treadmill, or riding a stationary bicycle is helpful. The exercise period starts slowly, with 10 minutes twice daily three times a week, increasing to 20 minutes twice daily three times a week. The patient needs to be assessed for his or her ability to carry out such an exercise program, and a staff member should be present during the exercise period.

Patients need to be encouraged not to rush (i.e., to allow ample time for activities). Supplemental oxygen may be needed before and during activities. Activities such as walking should be gradually increased. The nurse should provide positive feedback on progress and encourage new endeavors when the patient is ready. The nurse assists patients in balancing work, rest, and recreation to regulate energy expenditure.

New research suggests that the nurse should take a sleep history.[30] Physiologic changes during sleep can exacerbate COPD symptoms and disrupt sleep. Changes in sleep patterns may be early indicators of illness progression and changes in health status. Sleep affects breathing, even in healthy adults, by increasing airway resistance and decreasing ventilation, particularly during rapid-eye-movement sleep. Changes in airway caliber resulting from mild nocturnal bronchoconstriction and relaxation of upper respiratory muscles are common causes of increased airway resistance during sleep. Minute ventilation falls by about 0.5 to 1.5 L/min. In persons with COPD this increase in airway resistance and decline in minute ventilation during sleep can lead to hypoxemia and hypercapnia during sleep.[6] Hypoxemia is a common cause of arousal and sleep disruption as a result of the increased respiratory effort that occurs when the body corrects for increases in airway resistance or decreases in minute ventilation. Bronchospasm and coughing can prolong period of wakefulness.

Recurrent episodes of hypoxemia are seen in COPD patients during sleep. Effects of nocturnal hypoxemia include cardiac dysrhythmias, pulmonary hypertension, heart failure, and polycythemia. Hypoxemia during sleep may also adversely affect daytime cognition and function. Nurses need to routinely assess sleep and breathing patterns. For patients with COPD, therapies to promote rest should avoid benzodiazepines, since they can depress respiration. Trazodone is perhaps the most frequently prescribed hypnotic, since it reduces arousals and increases overall sleep quality. Melatonin has improved both duration and quality of sleep.[6]

RELATED NIC INTERVENTIONS. Energy Management, Exercise Promotion: Strength Training, Exercise Therapy: Ambulation, Sleep Enhancement

Nursing Diagnosis: Imbalanced Nutrition: Less Than Body Requirements

OUTCOMES. Common examples of expected outcomes for the patient with a diagnosis of *imbalanced nutrition* are:

Patient will:

- Explain dietary changes required after discharge.
- Maintain optimal weight for height, age, and gender.
- Describe food and fluid requirements and daily plan for achieving them.
- State specific foods to avoid.
- Discuss plan for frequent, small feedings that are easily chewable, increased time for eating, and use of supplemental oxygen as indicated.

NURSING INTERVENTIONS. Malnutrition plays a role in the deterioration of physical performance, the development of clinical complications, and overall prognosis. Loss of appetite affects many people with COPD, and evidence shows that hypoxia may be contributory. Hypoxia has an anorexic effect and is a key catabolic stimulus. In malnourished COPD patients hypoxia-induced cytokine release leads to anorexia and muscle wasting.[41] Other contributing factors are the feeling of satiety that occurs with small amounts of food because the flattened diaphragm compresses abdominal contents; dyspnea, which interferes with eating; and gastric irritation associated with the use of bronchodilators and steroids. Diminished total weight is correlated with a dramatic decrease in size and strength of respiratory muscle (especially the diaphragm). Physical reconditioning and endurance training combined with a balanced diet are essential to maintaining or improving energy metabolism and nutritional status.

To help the patient with COPD maintain adequate nutrition, the nurse explores the patient's and family's usual dietary habits and counsels the patient to select foods that provide a high-protein, high-calorie diet. It is important to counsel the patient to select foods that derive their calories from high fat rather than high carbohydrate levels. Persons with advanced chronic bronchitis or emphysema are unable to exhale the excess carbon dioxide that is a natural end product of carbohydrate metabolism. Therefore calories obtained from high-carbohydrate foods may elevate $Paco_2$ levels in persons with COPD. The nurse also advises the patient to take supplemental vitamins and prepackaged food supplements such as milk shakes or snack bars between meals because they are an excellent source of protein and calories. The patient is taught that smaller, more frequent meals are often tolerated better than three larger meals. Larger meals require more energy to digest and limit the downward movement of the diaphragm during inspiration. Patients are encouraged to select foods that are easy to chew and swallow to further conserve energy.[40]

RELATED NIC INTERVENTIONS. Nutrition Management, Nutritional Counseling

Nursing Diagnosis: Risk for Infection

OUTCOMES. Common examples of expected outcomes for the patient with a diagnosis of *risk for infection* are:
Patient will:
- Remain free from infection.
- Be afebrile.
- Exhibit sputum at baseline in color, amount, and consistency.
- Inform health care provider if signs of infection occur.

NURSING INTERVENTIONS. The most common complication of COPD, and the cause of most hospital readmissions, is respiratory infection that produces acute exacerbations (AECOPD). Bacteria, viruses, and atypical pathogens have been implicated as causes of AECOPD.[43] Pulmonary response to the infectious process includes increased respiratory rate, mucosal irritation, and increased mucus production. Because of these localized responses, patients may have bronchospasm and a change in their pattern of sputum production. If the infection remains untreated, the result is overall increased work of breathing with eventual respiratory failure. Patient teaching is an important component of infection prevention (see the Patient/Family Teaching box).

The nurse should also evaluate the person's knowledge of the care, cleansing, and use of inhalant and nebulizer equipment. Contaminated MDIs, DPIs, and nebulizer equipment are common sources of infection.

RELATED NIC INTERVENTIONS. Infection Control, Infection Protection

Nursing Diagnosis: Ineffective Coping (Individual and Family)

OUTCOMES. Common examples of expected outcomes for the patient with a diagnosis of *ineffective coping* are:
Patient will:
- Identify own coping mechanisms, both effective and ineffective.
- Identify stressors, threats to role.
- Use effective coping mechanisms (discussion with family, health care providers).
- Set realistic personal goals.
- Participate in ADLs and therapeutic regimens.
- State names and telephone numbers of appropriate community support services, such as home health provider, Visiting Nurses Association, home medical equipment supplier.

PATIENT/FAMILY TEACHING

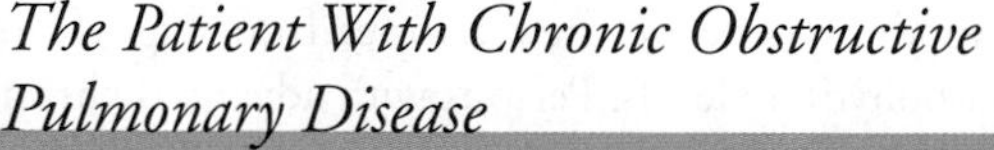

The Patient With Chronic Obstructive Pulmonary Disease

To decrease the risk of respiratory infections, the nurse should teach the patient to:
- Avoid large crowds, especially during known influenza seasons.
- Avoid contact with people who have an upper respiratory tract infection.
- Obtain influenza and pneumonia immunizations.
- Contact the health care provider if the following common signs and symptoms occur: change in sputum color, amount, and consistency; more frequent or productive cough; elevated temperature; change in behavior (e.g., more argumentative than usual), which indicates an increase in $PaCO_2$; increased fatigue; increased dyspnea; weight gain; or peripheral edema.

NURSING INTERVENTIONS. Persons who are short of breath are usually anxious and frightened. The nurse encourages the patient to talk about anxiety and fears with family members and health care professionals. The nurse should foster a realistic assessment of abilities and limitations, with a focus on those activities the patient is still able to do. Positive body responses should be stressed without negating the seriousness of the health issues involved. Vocational rehabilitation may be an option for some patients. Enrollment in pulmonary rehabilitation programs can also mitigate the sense of isolation and encourage ongoing involvement. The nurse encourages the patient to try new coping behaviors and gradually master them. Referral to professional counseling should be initiated if indicated.

Acute exacerbations in COPD are particularly stressful and affect quality of life. Patients may experience fear because of excessive breathlessness, which can trigger anxiety, depression, or panic. COPD patients are reported to perceive an acute exacerbation as a possible life threat. Nurses are in a unique position to determine needs for psychologic support that may enhance quality of life.[3] They should provide patients phone numbers for support services such as the home health nurse, medical equipment supplier, etc., and encourage them to call when needed.

COPD also affects the well-being of the family and caregivers. Spouses of COPD patients are more likely to report depressive symptoms compared with spouses of individuals without COPD. Nurses and other health care providers should be aware of the strain that COPD places on caregivers' mental health and consider methods of screening for depressive symptoms.[28,57]

RELATED NIC INTERVENTIONS. Coping Enhancement, Emotional Support, Support System Enhancement

EVALUATION

To evaluate the effectiveness of nursing interventions, compare patient behaviors with those stated in the expected patient outcomes.

RELATED NOC INTERVENTIONS. Acceptance: Health Status, Activity Tolerance, Appetite, Aspiration Prevention, Coping, Endurance, Knowledge: Infection Control, Knowledge: Health Resources, Nutritional Status: Food & Fluid Intake, Respiratory Status: Airway Patency, Respiratory Status: Gas Exchange, Risk Control, Vital Signs

GERONTOLOGIC CONSIDERATIONS

Many patients with COPD are older and may require additional time and support in learning how to take their medications, perform breathing exercises, and use oxygen properly. A multidisciplinary team, including social services, nutritional services, and physical therapy, may be necessary to assess the patient and assist the nurse with teaching. The patient's significant others need to be involved in each teaching activity so that they can assist the patient as necessary.[42]

In addition to the nursing care for COPD described in previous paragraphs, see the Nursing Care Plan.

Asthma

Asthma is a chronic inflammatory disorder of the airways that is characterized by an exaggerated **bronchoconstrictor response** (narrowing of the air passages) to a wide variety of stimuli. Airway hyperresponsiveness leads to clinical symptoms of wheezing and dyspnea after exposure to allergens, environmental irritants, viral infections, cold air, or exercise.

Etiology and Epidemiology. Asthma results from complex interactions among inflammatory cells, mediators, and other cells and tissues that reside in airways. An initial trigger may be the release of inflammatory mediators from bronchial mast cells, macrophages, T lymphocytes, and epithelial cells. These substances direct the migration and activation of other inflammatory cells to the airway, where they cause injury, abnormalities in autonomic neural control of airway tone, mucus hypersecretion, change in mucociliary function, and increased airway smooth muscle responsiveness. Box 27-1 lists common asthma triggers.

In sensitive individuals the inflammatory response causes recurrent episodes of wheezing, breathlessness, chest tightness, and cough, particularly at night and in the early morning. Early-phase reactions appear seconds after exposure and last about 1 hour. About half of all patients with asthma also experience a delayed, or late-phase, reaction. The symptoms are the same, but these reactions begin 4 to 8 hours after exposure and can last for hours or days. These episodes are usually associated with widespread but variable airflow obstruction that is often reversible either spontaneously or with treatment. Asthma begins most frequently in childhood and adolescence, but it can develop at any time in life.

Box 27-1 Common Factors Triggering Asthma Attack

- Environmental factors
  Change in temperature, especially cold air
  Change in humidity: dry air
- Atmospheric pollutants: cigarette and industrial smoke, ozone, sulfur dioxide, formaldehyde
- Strong odors: perfume
- Allergens: feathers, animal dander, dust mites, molds, allergens, foods treated with sulfites (beer, wine, fruit juices, snack foods, salads, potatoes, shellfish, fresh and dried fruits)
- Exercise
- Stress or emotional upset
- Medications: aspirin and nonsteroidal antiinflammatory drugs, beta-blockers (including eyedrops), cholinergic drugs (to promote bladder contraction and in eyedrops for glaucoma)
- Enzymes, including those in laundry detergents
- Chemicals: toluene and others used in solvents, paints, rubber, and plastics

Increases in the prevalence of asthma and in its mortality and morbidity rates have been seen in the past 2 decades. Asthma affects 17.3 million people in the United States with costs in excess of $6 billion.[9] Asthma accounts for approximately 500,000 hospital admissions annually, with an average length of stay of 5 days, and 2 million emergency visits. People with asthma experience 75% more sick days than controls.[48] Both hospitalizations for the treatment of asthma and deaths from it have increased. Most of the morbidity and all of the mortality involve acute exacerbations of asthma, and treatment of these events accounts for the majority of expenditures in money and health care resources. The reasons for the increase in morbidity and mortality are not well understood but may include lack of access to primary care, overuse and incorrect use of medications, or the inability to recognize the severity of symptoms.

Pathophysiology. Airflow limitation in asthma is recurrent and caused by a variety of changes in the airway (Figure 27-8). These changes include bronchoconstriction, edema, chronic **mucous plug** formation, and airway remodeling. Bronchoconstriction in the early asthmatic response is thought to be due to airway smooth muscle contraction, whereas bronchoconstriction in the late asthmatic response is due to airway inflammation.

ACUTE BRONCHOCONSTRICTION. Allergen-induced acute bronchoconstriction results from an immunoglobulin E–dependent release of mediators from mast cells. These mediators include histamine, tryptase, leukotrienes, and prostaglandins that directly contract airway smooth muscle. Aspirin and other nonsteroidal antiinflammatory drugs can also cause acute airflow obstruction in some patients, and this also involves mediator release from airway cells. Other stimuli, including exercise, cold air, and irritants, can cause acute airflow obstruction, but these mechanisms are less well defined.

AIRWAY EDEMA. Airway wall edema, even without smooth muscle contraction or bronchoconstriction, limits airflow in asthma. Increased microvascular permeability and leakage caused by

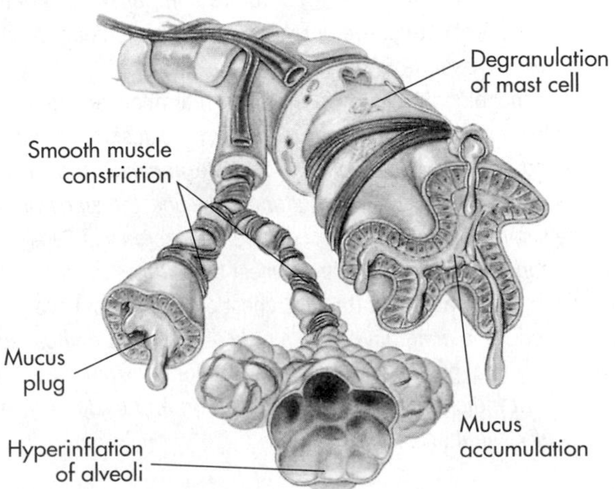

Figure 27-8 Bronchial asthma; thick mucus, mucosal edema, and smooth muscle spasm cause obstruction of small airways; breathing is labored and expiration difficult.

Nursing Care Plan

Patient With Chronic Obstructive Pulmonary Disease

Data A 68-year-old man was admitted to the hospital for severe shortness of breath and inability to care for himself at home. He was diagnosed with chronic obstructive pulmonary disease (COPD) about 9 years ago, most likely related to his 40-year history of cigarette smoking. He is widowed, lives alone, and ordinarily manages his care and disease without difficulty. The patient states that the cold, rainy weather has made his breathing much worse over the past couple of days. He complains of being severely fatigued and short of breath.

Physical examination reveals a thin appearing man who is diaphoretic, leaning forward in a sitting position, and in obvious respiratory distress. Vital signs are temperature, 100.8° F orally; heart rate, 104 beats/min; respiratory rate, 36 breaths/min and labored; and blood pressure, 146/92 mm Hg. He has wheezing and crackles throughout all lung fields. Humidified oxygen is initiated at 2 L/min via mask, 5% dextrose in water (D_5W) is started at 75 ml/hr, and 125 mg of methylprednisolone (Solu-Medrol) is administered intravenously. The respiratory care department is notified to provide the patient with an immediate breathing treatment as the nurse initiates an aminophylline drip.

Nursing Diagnosis

Impaired gas exchange related to chronic obstructive lung disease

Outcomes

- Patient will regain and maintain gas exchange within baseline.
- Patient will be free from changes in mental status.

Related NOC Outcomes

- Respiratory Status: Airway Patency
- Respiratory Status: Gas Exchange

Related NIC Interventions

- Cough Enhancement
- Oxygen Therapy
- Respiratory Monitoring

Nursing Interventions/Rationales

- Monitor respirations and assess breath sounds hourly and more often as needed. *To establish baseline for future comparisons to determine whether treatment is effective or different interventions are required to prevent further respiratory distress.*
- Monitor arterial blood gases (ABGs), oxygen saturation, and mentation. *To detect early signs of hypoxemia, respiratory acidosis, and respiratory alkalosis so corrective interventions may be implemented. Hypoxemia and hypercapnia often occur simultaneously, and the signs and symptoms are similar. Decreasing Pao_2 coupled with increasing $Paco_2$ is a sign of respiratory failure and may be manifest by changes in mentation.*
- Administer pulmonary toilet (turning, chest physiotherapy) every 2 hours and as needed. *To maintain patent airway and prevent complications.*
- Assess peripheral pulses and warmth and color of extremities. *To detect changes that indicate inadequate oxygenation and to determine effectiveness of ventilation.*
- Position for maximum ventilation. *A high Fowler's or sitting, forward-leaning position relieves pressure on the diaphragm and allows for improved lung expansion and ventilation. Improved ventilation prevents stasis of lung secretions. The forward-leaning position allows more air to be removed from the lungs on exhalation, prevents use of accessory muscles of respiration, and improves the upward action of the diaphragm.*
- Encourage slow, pursed-lip breathing. *Pursed-lip breathing decreases the respiratory rate, increases tidal volume, decreases $Paco_2$, and increases Pao_2, all of which help reduce dyspnea.*
- Encourage abdominal breathing and abdominal muscle exercises. *To improve breathing efficiency by elevating the diaphragm. Exercises strengthen the abdominal muscles and help patients empty their lungs more effectively.*
- Administer humidified oxygen therapy as prescribed. *Low-flow oxygen is generally prescribed because COPD patients chronically retain carbon dioxide and depend on their hypoxic drive to stimulate respirations. Apnea can occur if the oxygen delivery is too high.*

Nursing Diagnosis

Risk for infection related to inability to clear trapped secretions secondary to chronic lung disease

Outcomes

- Patient will remain free from infections.

Related NOC Outcomes

- Immune Status
- Risk Control

Related NIC Interventions

- Infection Protection
- Surveillance

Nursing Interventions/Rationales

- Assess white blood cell (WBC) count. *Patients with COPD are at high risk for lung infection because of trapping of secretions, which serve as media for bacterial growth. An elevated WBC count is associated with systemic infection and may indicate the presence of pneumonia.*
- Monitor for signs of systemic infection (chills, fever, diaphoresis). *Indicates the presence of actual or developing infection.*
- Obtain sputum culture and sensitivity as prescribed. *To identify causative organism of infection and to monitor effectiveness of therapy.*
- Maintain hydration. *To thin secretions, prevent stasis, and facilitate expectoration.*
- Administer antibiotics on time if prescribed. *To maintain steady blood levels to eradicate infectious organism.*
- Encourage patient to obtain influenza vaccine annually and the pneumococcal pneumonia vaccine as indicated by the Centers for Disease Control and Prevention. *Patients with COPD are at high risk for respiratory complications secondary to influenza or bacterial pneumonia. Vaccines reduce the risk for and duration of these illnesses.*

Nursing Diagnosis

Activity Intolerance related to dyspnea secondary to COPD

Outcomes

- Patient will report decreased fatigue.
- Patient will achieve heart rate, respirations, and blood pressure at baseline within 3 minutes after increased activity.

Related NOC Outcomes

- Activity Tolerance
- Endurance
- Energy Conservation

Related NIC Interventions

- Energy Management
- Progressive Muscle Relaxation
- Teaching: Prescribed Activity/Exercise

Nursing Interventions/Rationales

- Assess and monitor patient's response to activity (vital signs, dyspnea, signs of exertion). *To determine patient's response to self-care or other activities. Activity tolerance depends on the ability to physiologically adapt to changes in demand.*
- Assist the patient in sequencing activities to provide for rest periods. *Rest decreases myocardial oxygen consumption, allowing intervals of low energy demand. Decreased oxygen consumption allows more oxygen to be available for ventilation.*
- Provide an environment conducive to rest. *Environmental stimulation inhibits the patient's ability to enter a state of relaxation and subsequent rest.*
- Assist with activities of daily living as needed. *Patients are unable to perform self-care during periods of severe dyspnea. Activity increases metabolic demand and decreases available oxygen for breathing.*

Nursing Diagnosis

Risk for imbalanced nutrition: less than body requirements related to increased energy expenditure from difficulty breathing

Outcomes

- Patient will remain within 5 pounds of preillness (or ideal) body weight.
- Patient will gain weight as condition stabilizes and breathing effort decreases.

NOC Suggested Outcomes

- Nutritional Status
- Nutritional Status: Food & Fluid Intake
- Nutritional Status: Nutrient Intake

NIC Suggested Interventions

- Nutrition Management
- Nutrition Therapy
- Nutritional Monitoring

Nursing Interventions/Rationales

- Provide small, frequent meals and nutritional supplements. *Difficult breathing increases the metabolic demands on the body. Nutritional status must be maintained to meet the caloric needs of patients expending excessive calories on breathing and prevent weight loss, especially in patients who are below their ideal weight.*
- Monitor intake and output. *Decreased urinary output or concentrated urine is an indication of inadequate fluid replacement.*
- Weigh daily. *To determine whether nutritional needs are being met and to evaluate the effectiveness of nutritional interventions.*
- Administer albumin and plasma expanders as prescribed. *Protein and volume expanders increase colloidal osmotic pressure, thus maintaining fluid within the intravascular compartment.*
- Monitor serum albumin levels. *Serum albumin levels reflect the adequacy of protein intake. Decreased levels are associated with peripheral edema caused by loss of osmotic pull from within the vascular space.*

Nursing Diagnosis

Risk for ineffective therapeutic regimen management related to chronic disability secondary to COPD

Outcomes

- Patient will verbalize understanding of therapeutic regimen.
- Patient will report ability to adhere to therapeutic regimen.

Related NOC Outcomes

- Adherence Behavior
- Compliance Behavior
- Knowledge: Treatment Regimen

Related NIC Interventions

- Behavior Modification
- Referral
- Self-Modification Assistance

Nursing Interventions/Rationales

- Assess patient's understanding of the disease process. *To identify specific learning needs so teaching can be individualized. Patients with longstanding COPD may be familiar with how to control their disease, which will change the type and amount of teaching.*
- Provide verbal and written instructions as needed. *Teaching reinforces the need to comply with recommended management. Written material provides additional resources for home reference.*
- Teach the importance of maintaining prescribed medication dosages and schedules. *To maintain blood levels to control symptoms while also preventing underdosing or overdosing.*
- Stress the importance of compliance with follow-up care recommendations. *Follow-up care is essential for patients with COPD so complications can be identified early and corrective measures implemented.*

Evaluation

Evaluation is based on comparing the patient's outcomes with desired outcomes.

released mediators contribute to mucosal thickening and airway swelling. As a consequence, the airway becomes more rigid and interferes with airflow. In sudden-onset asthma, neutrophils predominate; eosinophils predominate in the slow-onset form of the disease.[48]

CHRONIC MUCOUS PLUG FORMATION. In severe, intractable asthma, airflow limitation is often persistent. This change may arise as a consequence of mucus secretion and the formation of mucous plugs.

AIRWAY REMODELING. In some patients with asthma, airflow limitation may be only partially reversible because of structural changes in the airway that accompany longstanding and severe airway inflammation. A histologic feature of asthma may be an alteration in the amount and composition of the extracellular matrix in the airway wall. The importance of airway remodeling and persistent airflow limitation suggest a rationale for early intervention with antiinflammatory therapy.

To prevent airway remodeling and to help standardize asthma management with the hope of improving outcomes, the National Asthma Education and Prevention Program (NAEPP) developed Guidelines for the Diagnosis and Management of Asthma. Under these guidelines asthma is classified into four categories:

1. *Mild intermittent*: Symptoms occur less than twice a week.
2. *Mild persistent*: Symptoms occur more than twice a week but less than daily.
3. *Moderate persistent*: Daily symptoms occur, including exacerbations more than twice a week.
4. *Severe persistent*: Symptoms occur continually, along with frequent exacerbations, limiting the patient's physical activity.

For each category a stepwise approach to symptom management has been outlined by the NAEPP for physicians to use in treating patients with asthma[19,35] (Table 27-2).

COMPLICATIONS. Complications of asthma include status asthmaticus and respiratory failure (see the Respiratory Failure section later in the chapter).

Persons who are severely affected by asthma and who have attacks that cannot be controlled with the usual medications have **status asthmaticus**. In status asthmaticus the symptoms of an acute attack continue despite measures to relieve them. Air trapping in the distal air spaces ultimately leads to respiratory muscle exhaustion and severe V/Q abnormalities with resultant respiratory failure and hypoxemia. Repeated attacks of status asthmaticus may cause irreversible emphysema, resulting in a permanent decrease in total breathing capacity.

Patients with status asthmaticus often demonstrate such severe respiratory distress that they are unable to talk. They may be moving minimal amounts of air into and out of the lungs; thus audible wheezing and adventitious lung sounds may not be present. During this phase of the attack, the patient appears cyanotic and may demonstrate both pulsus paradoxus and sensorium changes. This is a medical emergency, and the patient requires immediate therapy. Most patients arrive in the emergency department, where treatment is begun. Patients remain in the emergency department until their condition is stabilized. Most patients are then admitted to the hospital for ongoing therapy and observation.

Collaborative Care Management. The major focus in asthma treatment is education for an active partnership with the patient. It begins at the time of asthma diagnosis and is integrated into all aspects of care. Patients learn to treat inflammation and day-to-day symptoms themselves through a program of provider-guided comanagement or partnership that stresses collaboration. This self-management program is developed according to the needs of each patient, with sensitivity to cultural beliefs and practices. Desired outcomes include effective symptom management, improved quality of life, and the ability to engage in usual activities.

DIAGNOSTIC TESTS. Tests for asthma are described in Table 27-3.

MEDICATIONS. The objectives of medical management of asthma are to promote normal functioning and prevent recurrent symptoms, severe attacks, and side effects from medication. The chief aim of various medications is to afford the patient immediate, progressive, ongoing bronchial relaxation. Table 27-4 lists the drugs used to treat patients with asthma.

TREATMENTS. Patients, families, and health care professionals need an objective measure of airflow obstruction to guide them in managing asthma attacks promptly. Numerous clinical and experimental studies show that many patients with asthma cannot accurately evaluate the severity of airflow obstruction. Many patients manage their asthma with the aid of peak flow meters. Peak expiratory flow rate (PEFR) is the greatest airflow velocity that can be produced during a forced expiration that starts from fully inflated lungs. Peak flow monitoring is used to audit daily response to treatment, detect a buildup in airflow obstruction, assess the severity of an attack, evaluate response to therapy, and aid decisions about hospitalization. PEFR monitoring devices cost from $15 to $40 and are portable and easy to use. The normal range for peak flow is 500 to 700 L/min for men and 380 to 500 L/min for women. Peak flow rates vary with age, sex, race, height, smoking history, respiratory muscle strength, and effort. The NAEPP recommends that the peak flow value be at least 70% of the predicted value.[45]

Patients with moderate or severe persistent asthma are encouraged to measure PEFR daily and to keep a diary of their readings and symptoms. A system based on a traffic light has been developed: the green zone is equal to 80% or better, the yellow zone is 50% to 79%, and the red zone is less than 50%. Patients are taught that the yellow zone requires increasing bronchodilator use as needed and, if there is no improvement, adding either an antiinflammatory drug or beginning oral corticosteroids. The red zone indicates a need to contact the patient's health care provider.

Patients with status asthmaticus require emergent treatment. Humidified oxygen is given to achieve full saturation. Inhaled short-acting beta$_2$-agonists are given in large and frequent doses. Subcutaneous epinephrine may help patients who do not respond after several hours of inhaled beta$_2$-agonists. Treatment with bronchodilators is continuous until the desired clinical effect is achieved or until toxic side effects limit continued use. Noninvasive positive-pressure ventilation (NIV) is preferable to **intubation** and mechanical ventilation. If mechanical ventilation is required, MDIs and nebulizers may be used to deliver bronchodilators. MDIs require the use of a spacing device on the inspi-

TABLE 27-2 STEPWISE APPROACH TO ASTHMA MANAGEMENT

Long-Term Control	Quick Relief (Rescue)
STEP 1	
No daily medication needed	Short-acting bronchodilator: inhaled beta$_2$-agonist Use more than twice a week indicates need for long-term control therapy
STEP 2	
Daily antiinflammatory: either inhaled low-dose corticosteroid, or cromolyn or nedocromil; sustained-released theophylline is an alternative but not preferred; zafirlukast or zileuton may be considered	Inhaled beta$_2$-agonist, short acting Daily or increasing use indicates need for additional long-term therapy
STEP 3	
Daily antiinflammatory: either inhaled medium-dose corticosteroid or inhaled low- to medium-dose corticosteroid plus long-acting bronchodilator—either long-acting inhaled beta$_2$-agonist or oral agent If needed, inhaled medium- to high-dose corticosteroid and long-acting bronchodilator—either long-acting inhaled beta$_2$-agonist, sustained-release theophylline, or long-acting beta$_2$-agonist tablets	Inhaled beta$_2$-agonist, short acting Daily or increasing use indicates need for improved long-term control agent
STEP 4	
Daily antiinflammatory: inhaled high-dose corticosteroid and long-acting bronchodilator—either long-acting inhaled beta$_2$-agonist, sustained-release theophylline, or long-acting beta$_2$-agonist tablets and corticosteroid tablets long term (2 mg/kg/day)	Inhaled beta$_2$-agonist, short acting

Adapted from National Asthma Education and Prevention Program: *Guidelines for the diagnosis and management of asthma,* National Heart, Lung, and Blood Institute, USDHHS, NIH, accessed Sept 2005 from www.nhlbi.nih.gov.

TABLE 27-3 DIAGNOSTIC TESTS FOR ASTHMA

Test	Purpose
Pulmonary function/spirometry tests, which include forced expiratory volume in 1 sec (FEV$_1$) and peak expiratory flow (PEF)	Used for assessing degree of obstruction and its reversibility; also to establish baseline ventilatory function
Arterial blood gases	Obtained to identify presence of mild to severe hypoxemia and mild to severe respiratory acidosis
Induced sputum specimen examinations	Used to determine marked eosinophilia
Allergy testing	Done to identify allergen or other trigger responsible for onset of asthma symptoms
Exhaled breath testing	Being studied for use as noninvasive measure of airway inflammation; involves measurement of volatile mediator in exhaled breath, specifically, nitric oxide; other potential markers include ethane, pentane, and carbon monoxide[38]

ratory limb of the **ventilator** to optimize drug delivery. A minimum of 4 puffs and up to 10 to 20 puffs may be given. Patient-ventilator synchrony is essential, and an inspiratory pause may be useful. Nebulizers may increase barotrauma because they require added gas flow (8 L/min) when used with mechanical ventilation. This can be minimized by decreasing the minute ventilation, placing the nebulizer close to the ventilator, raising the tidal volume above 500 ml, and decreasing the inspiratory flow to 40 L/min.[36]

Corticosteroids are administered as soon as possible. The minimum dose is 40 mg of methylprednisolone every 6 hours. Evidence is accumulating that people with asthma are being managed with higher than needed doses of corticosteroids. Theophylline does not add to bronchodilation but may be helpful for its

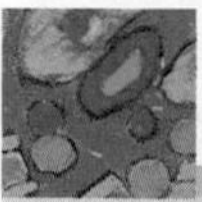

TABLE 27-4
COMMON MEDICATIONS *for Asthma*

Drug	Action	Nursing Intervention
Maintenance Medications		
Nonsteroidal Antiinflammatory Drugs		
Cromolyn (Intal) Nedocromil (Tilade)	Decrease airway inflammation and irritation	Teach patient: (1) use medication routinely, not more often than prescribed; (2) if a dose is missed, take as soon as possible and then continue other doses at regular intervals; (3) don't take a double dose; (4) don't discontinue taking without consulting physician or exacerbation of symptoms may occur; (5) don't discontinue concurrent glucocorticoid or bronchodilator therapy without consulting health care professional. Explain use of inhaler (Spinhaler or Halermatic devices) or how to use intranasally, depending on product.
Corticosteroids		
Beclomethasone (Vanceril, Beclovent, Beconase, Vancenase AQ) Budesonide (Pulmicort) Triamcinolone acetonide (Azmacort) Flunisolide (AeroBid) Fluticasone (Flovent)	Antiinflammatory	Teach patient: if using inhalation corticosteroids and bronchodilator, use bronchodilator first, wait 5 min before administering corticosteroid, unless otherwise directed by health care professional. Explain that inhalation corticosteroids should not be used to treat acute asthma episode. Systemic corticosteroids may be needed for acute attacks. Explain how to use regular peak flow monitoring to determine respiratory status and how to use inhaler or other device correctly. Explain need to avoid smoking, known allergens, and other respiratory irritants, and to notify physician if sore throat or sore mouth occurs.
Leukotriene Inhibitors/Receptor Antagonists		
Zafirlukast (Accolate) Zileuton (Zyflo) Montelukast sodium (Singulair)	Antiinflammatory	Teach patient: (1) take medication on empty stomach as directed, at evenly spaced times; (2) if dose is missed, take as soon as possible but do not double dose; (3) do not discontinue therapy without consulting physician; (4) do not discontinue or reduce other asthma medications unless instructed to do so. Explain the medication is not for acute asthma attacks but for maintenance. Explain side effects such as generalized flulike syndrome, fever, muscle aches and pain, weight loss, and worsening respiratory symptoms, and to report these to physician.
Theophylline		
Theophylline (Theo-Dur, Theo-Stat, Theobid, Theo-24, Uniphyl, T-Phyl)	Long-acting bronchodilator	Monitor vital signs and ABGs. Teach patient: (1) take medication exactly as prescribed; (2) take missed doses as soon as possible but do not double dose; (3) drink plenty of fluids (2000 ml/day minimum) to decrease viscosity of airway secretions; (4) try to avoid

antiinflammatory and diaphragmatic effects. The use of long-acting $beta_2$-adrenoceptor agonists (LABAs) is a relatively new development in therapy and is indicated for persons with persistent asthma who experience breakthrough symptoms despite using inhaled corticosteroids. LABAs are currently not recommended as sole therapy for asthma, since they do not inhibit allergen-induced increases in sputum eosinophils.[12]

HEALTH PROMOTION AND PREVENTION. In asthma, perhaps more than in any other disease, an effective partnership between the patient and the health care professional is essential. Knowing about the person's attitudes toward health and his or her lifestyle, such as type of work, leisure activities, social supports, learning style, and interest in self-care management, is an essential element in developing an effective management plan. The identification of asthma triggers requires involvement of both the patient and the health care professional. Avoidance of triggers can be an important component in preventing exacerbations. The *Healthy People 2010* document sets goals to reduce the problems and incidence of asthma (see Healthy People 2010 box).[54]

Healthy People 2010

Selected Objectives for Asthma Reduction

- Reduce deaths from asthma.
- Reduce hospital emergency room visits for asthma.
- Reduce asthma morbidity to no more than 25 hospitalizations per 10,000 for children younger than age 5, 7.7 per 10,000 for children/adults ages 5-64, and 11 per 10,000 for adults ages 65 and older.

From US Department of Health and Human Services: *Healthy people 2010: understanding and improving health,* Washington, DC, 2000, The Department.

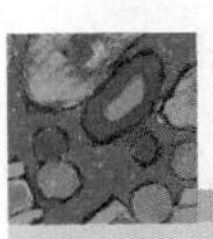

TABLE 27-4
COMMON MEDICATIONS *for Asthma—cont'd*

Drug	Action	Nursing Intervention
Maintenance Medications		
Theophylline—cont'd		
Theophylline ethylenediamine (aminophylline)		over-the-counter cough and cold medications; (5) refrain from smoking; (6) reduce intake of colas, coffee, chocolate. Advise patient to contact physician if usual dose of medication does not produce desired results, if symptoms worsen after treatment, or if toxic effects occur.
Anticholinergic		
Ipratropium (Atrovent)	Short-acting bronchodilator	Assess respiratory status and teach proper use of inhaler or nasal spray. Teach patient to notify physician if cough, fever, gastrointestinal distress, headache, or dizziness occurs.
Beta$_2$-Agonist		
Salmeterol (Serevent)	Long-acting bronchodilator	Assess respiratory status and teach proper use of metered-dose inhaler or powder inhalation. Seek consultation if any side effects are present. Teach patient: (1) medication is not used to treat acute asthma attacks; (2) missed doses should be taken as soon as possible, but do not double dose.
Rescue Medications		
Corticosteroids		
Prednisone Methylprednisolone (Medrol) Prednisolone (Orasone) Prednisolone sodium phosphate (Pediapred)	Antiinflammatory	Teach patient correct use of medication. Discuss side effects. Explain not to discontinue without consulting physician, to take as directed only.
Beta-Agonists		
Albuterol (Proventil, Ventolin) Metaproterenol (Alupent, Metaprel) Pirbuterol (Maxair) Epinephrine	Short-acting bronchodilators	Teach patient correct use of medication. Discuss side effects and when to notify physician of complications. Some of these medications should be taken with food.

Nursing Management

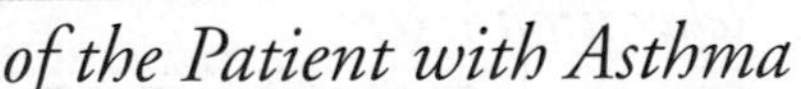

of the Patient with Asthma

ASSESSMENT

Health History. Assess for:

- History of asthma onset and duration
- Precipitating factors
- Any recent changes in medication regimen
- Medications used to relieve asthma symptoms
- Other medications
- Self-care methods used to relieve symptoms

Physical Examination. Assess for:

- General appearance
- Mental status; signs of altered sensorium or apprehension, which may indicate hypoxemia
- Tachycardia; pulsus paradoxus (diminished pulse with inspiration, confirmed by a 6 to 8 mm Hg drop in systolic blood pressure during inspiration); tachypnea; or other abnormality
- Dyspnea, use of accessory muscles for breathing, forward-leaning (tripod) posture, prolonged expiration, and cyanosis; palpation for decreased lateral expansion of the chest and decreased fremitus; percussion for hyperresonance and decreased diaphragmatic excursion; auscultation of breath sounds (may be absent or faint as the patient approaches exhaustion from the increased work of breathing; inspiratory and expiratory wheezing and rhonchi common)
- Relevant laboratory findings, including ABGs (during a short-term or moderate asthma attack, indicate respiratory alkalosis with mild hypoxemia; during a prolonged or severe attack, demonstrate respiratory acidosis with severe hypoxemia); PFTs (document a decreased FEV_1 and VC); and sputum examinations (show eosinophilia)

Nursing Diagnoses, Outcomes, and Interventions

Nursing Diagnosis: Ineffective Airway Clearance

Outcomes. Common examples of expected outcomes for the patient with a diagnosis of *ineffective airway clearance* are:

Patient will:

- Demonstrate effective airway clearance.
- Cough effectively.
- Have breath sounds that are clear or at baseline.

Nursing Interventions. During an asthma attack, secretions tend to become viscous and can plug airways, causing increased airway obstruction. Mobilizing secretions often prevents the need for intubation and artificial ventilation. To promote mobilization, the nurse should ensure adequate systemic fluid intake. Overhydration is not necessary, since research findings suggest it may not increase secretion clearance above levels obtained by normal hydration.[45] It is also important to provide extra humidity, teach effective cough maneuvers, provide adequate nutrition for energy, and medicate with short-acting rescue medications.

Related NIC Interventions. Airway Management, Asthma Management, Respiratory Management

Nursing Diagnosis: Ineffective Breathing Pattern

Outcomes. Common examples of expected outcomes for the patient with a diagnosis of *ineffective breathing pattern* are:

Patient will:

- Demonstrate effective breathing pattern.
- Have inspiratory/expiratory ratio of 5:10 seconds.
- Have respiratory rate within near-normal limits.

Nursing Interventions. The nursing role in improving breathing patterns and gas exchange is to help the patient assume a position of comfort, administer medication as ordered, and monitor for both therapeutic and adverse effects of medications. The nurse must also assess for possible medication overuse (see Table 27-4). The nurse encourages the patient to exercise and monitors the need for an inhaled beta$_2$-agonist 15 to 30 minutes before exercise.

Related NIC Interventions. Airway Management, Asthma Management, Vital Signs Monitoring

Nursing Diagnosis: Impaired Gas Exchange

Outcomes. Common examples of expected outcomes for the patient with a diagnosis of *impaired gas exchange* are:

Patient will:

- Demonstrate improved ventilation.
- Have arterial blood pH and $Paco_2$ at baseline levels.
- Maintain Pao_2 at optimal level for the patient.

Nursing Interventions. The nurse monitors blood gas results carefully. If respiratory alkalosis is present, the nurse encourages the patient to breathe more slowly. If respiratory acidosis and hypoxemia are present, oxygen is administered as prescribed. If oxygen and other therapeutic measures do not relieve the attack, intubation and ventilatory assistance may be required.

Related NIC Interventions. Airway Management, Oxygen Therapy, Respiratory Management

Nursing Diagnosis: Anxiety

Outcomes. Common examples of expected outcomes for the patient with a diagnosis of *anxiety* (mild, moderate, or severe) are:

Patient will:

- Demonstrate activities to control anxiety response to symptoms.
- Use progressive muscle relaxation.
- Use medications appropriately.

Nursing Interventions. The nurse should never leave the patient alone during an asthma attack. The nurse guides the patient in the use of relaxation techniques and respiratory maneuvers and encourages use of relaxation and other techniques to reduce anxiety (see Patient/Family Teaching box).

Related NIC Interventions. Anxiety Reduction, Simple Relaxation Therapy

Nursing Diagnosis: Ineffective Therapeutic Regimen Management

Outcomes. Common examples of expected outcomes for the patient with a diagnosis of *ineffective therapeutic regimen management* are:

Patient will:

- Describe the "stepped plan" and partnership approach to asthma management.
- Identify asthma triggers (e.g., allergens, infections, stress).
- Describe strategies for avoiding asthma triggers.
- State the importance of keeping a diary of symptoms and medications (time and dose).
- Explain home medication program.
- State name, dose, action, and side effects of each medication.
- Describe conditions under which medications might be increased (e.g., infection: start or increase antibiotics;

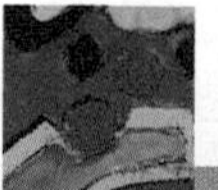

Patient/Family Teaching

Progressive Relaxation Exercises

The nurse should teach the patient to:

- Contract each muscle to a count of 10 and then relax it.
- Do exercises in quiet room while sitting or lying in a comfortable position.
- Do exercises to relaxing music, if desired.
- Have another person serve as a "coach" by giving the command to contract a specific muscle, count to 10, and relax the muscle.

Exercises that are helpful to some persons with chronic obstructive pulmonary disease include:

- Raise shoulders, shrug them, and relax for 5 seconds; then relax them completely.
- Make a fist of both hands, squeeze them tightly for 5 seconds, and then relax them completely.

increased stress or worsening of symptoms: increase corticosteroids).
- Demonstrate how to take inhaled medications, use of MDI, inhaler.
- Verbalize steps to take when an acute attack is beginning.
- Use peak flow meter to determine changes in medication regimen and when to call a health professional.
- Show card to be carried at all times giving data about the drug, dose of the drug, and name of the physician; or wear a Medic-Alert bracelet if receiving corticosteroid therapy.
- State plans for ongoing follow-up care, including plans for desensitization if appropriate.

NURSING INTERVENTIONS. The nurse assesses the patient's knowledge of asthma and teaches the information needed for the patient to become an effective partner in managing the disease (see Patient/Family Teaching box).

RELATED NIC INTERVENTIONS. Emotional Support, Patient Counseling, Teaching: Disease Process

EVALUATION

To evaluate the effectiveness of nursing interventions, compare patient behaviors with those stated in the expected patient outcomes.

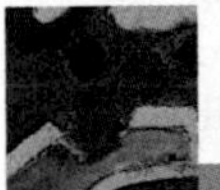

PATIENT/FAMILY TEACHING
The Patient With Asthma

Nursing interventions for the patient with asthma include teaching the patient:

- Signs and symptoms of an attack: tightness in chest, restlessness or vague feeling of uneasiness, dyspnea, increased wheezing, productive cough
- Importance of keeping a symptom diary to record timing of attacks, symptom patterns, possible precipitating factors, time and dose of self-administered medications, and their effectiveness
- Self-treatment of signs and symptoms:
  —Importance of taking bronchoactive medications as ordered
  —Conditions under which medication might be increased (e.g., change in peak flow readings, infection, increased stress, or worsening of symptoms)
  —Need to call someone in the event of an attack so as not to be alone
  —Importance of remaining calm, breathing slowly, and using relaxation techniques at the first sign of an attack
  —Need to call a physician or go to the nearest emergency facility if symptoms do not dissipate
  —Use of equipment such as a metered dose inhaler, inhaler with a spacer, and peak flow meter if one is prescribed (The patient should demonstrate use of the inhaler with each visit to the health care provider to reinforce correct technique.)
  —Importance of smoking cessation and avoidance of environmental tobacco smoke
  —Need to avoid large crowds during flu season
  —Importance of obtaining influenza and pneumococcal vaccines

RELATED NOC OUTCOMES. Anxiety Self-Control, Knowledge: Treatment Regimen, Respiratory Status: Airway Patency, Respiratory Status: Gas Exchange, Respiratory Status: Ventilation, Symptom Control, Vital Signs

GERONTOLOGIC CONSIDERATIONS

Although the goals of treatment of asthma are the same for persons of all ages, they may be more difficult to achieve in older adults. The Cardiovascular Health Study is one of the largest population-based examinations of heart and lung disease in older persons in the United States. This study explored the associations of asthma in older adults with quality of life, morbidity, and use of asthma medications. Results of the study indicated that asthma in older persons is associated with a lower quality of life. Participants who had asthma were much more likely to rate their general health as fair or poor and report their activity as less than the previous year. Results also indicated that asthma is underdiagnosed in older adults and is often associated with allergic triggers. Inhaled corticosteroids are underused.[22] This study provides considerable impetus for health care providers to prioritize the diagnosis and treatment of asthma in the older population.

Cystic Fibrosis

Cystic fibrosis (CF) is a multisystem disorder characterized by chronic airway obstruction and infection and by exocrine pancreatic insufficiency, with its effects on GI function, nutrition, growth, and maturation.

Etiology and Epidemiology. CF continues to be the most common fatal genetic disease among Caucasians. Numerous mutations of a single gene are responsible for CF. The gene encodes a membrane protein known as the CF transmembrane regulator (CFTR), and mutations of CFTR protein result in reduced secretion of chloride from epithelial cells. It is an autosomal recessive disease. When both parents are carriers (heterozygotes), there is a one-in-four chance with each pregnancy that the child will have CF (Figure 27-9).

In Caucasian populations 2% to 5% are carriers of a CF gene mutation. Approximately 25,000 individuals with CF live in the

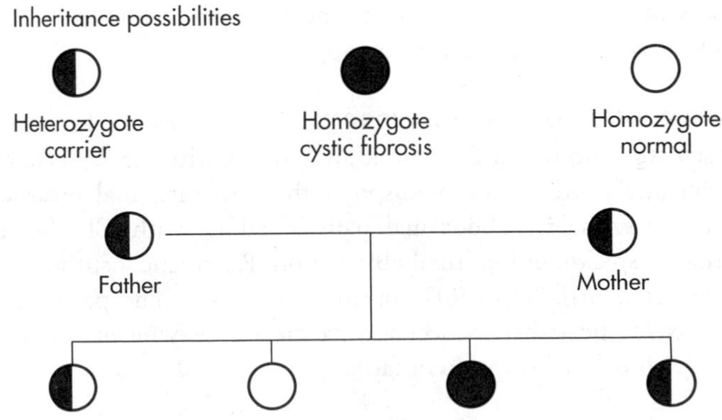

Figure 27-9 Inheritance of cystic fibrosis (CF) when both mother and father are carriers of CF gene.

United States. The number of adults with CF continues to increase steadily because of increased life expectancy and diagnostic advances. Two groups make up this adult CF population: (1) those diagnosed when infants or children and (2) those diagnosed as adolescents or adults. Statistics indicate that approximately 20% of the adult CF population is diagnosed after age 15.[21]

Reaching adulthood is now a realistic expectation for infants and children with CF. The average life expectancy in 1998 was 32.3 years.[21] The major contributing factors to this increased life expectancy include advancements in antibiotic therapies, new treatments, more aggressive management, and the availability of a network of about 115 comprehensive CF referral centers sponsored by the Cystic Fibrosis Foundation.

Pathophysiology. CF is an exocrine gland disease involving various systems (pulmonary, pancreatic/hepatic, GI, reproductive). Obstruction of the exocrine gland ducts or passageways occurs in nearly all adult patients with CF. Exocrine gland secretions are known to have decreased water content, altered electrolyte concentration, and abnormal organic constituents (especially mucous glycoproteins); however, the specific biochemical or physiologic defect that leads to obstruction is not known.

Pulmonary Involvement. Disease of the conducting airways in CF is acquired after birth. Either hypersecretion or failure to clear secretions at an early age accounts for mucus accumulation in bronchial regions. Failure to clear secretions from the airway probably initiates infection because mucous plaques and plugs serve as media for growth of bacteria.[36] Chronic airway infection is rarely eradicated. As lung disease progresses, bronchiolitis and bronchitis are evident, submucosal glands hypertrophy, and goblet cells increase. Bronchiectasis is a consequence of persistent obstruction-infection cycles. Bronchiectatic cysts occupy as much as 50% of the late-stage CF lung. *Pseudomonas aeruginosa* and *Staphylococcus aureus* are the organisms most frequently causing infection.[11] The earliest manifestation of lung involvement is generally cough, at first intermittent and then daily. It is often worse at night and on arising in the morning. Cough becomes productive, then paroxysmal, and is associated with gagging and emesis. Sputum is usually tenacious, purulent, and green. Recurrent pulmonary infections erode blood vessels such as the bronchial arteries, which branch from the aorta and the lung at high pressures and can lead to bleeding with hemoptysis.

Gastrointestinal and Pancreatic Involvement. Intestinal obstruction occurs in 20% of adult patients with CF. Generally, pancreatic insufficiency predisposes them to intestinal obstruction. Cramps and abdominal pain in adults with CF should arouse suspicion of intestinal obstruction. Pancreatic insufficiency is reported in 80% to 90% of adults with CF. The pathologic lesions in the pancreas decrease pancreatic enzyme production and lead to malabsorption of fat.

Other Involvement. In older children and young adults CF may be manifested by heat exhaustion after exercise or exposure to hot weather, or by dehydration after fever. In some young adults the only clinical manifestation of CF may be infertility. The varied signs and symptoms of CF are summarized in the Clinical Manifestations box.

Complications. Complications of CF include pneumothorax, hemoptysis, airway problems, GI problems, and respiratory failure. Patients with CF eventually succumb to progressive respiratory and cardiac failure. Because these patients have a fatal disease, they usually have do-not-resuscitate (DNR) orders and are not intubated or placed on mechanical ventilation. The patient and family have to be involved in the DNR decision, and nurses play an important role in supporting them in their decision.

Pneumothorax. A pneumothorax occurs secondary to rupture of a subpleural bleb. The incidence is 1% per year but increases with age. It occurs more frequently in the right side of the chest. It should be suspected any time a patient with CF experiences the acute onset of shortness of breath, chest pain, or hemoptysis. When a pneumothorax occurs, the surgeon makes a stab wound between the ribs and inserts a chest tube connected to a closed drainage system. After the lung is reexpanded, pleural sclerosis using doxycycline or talc may be induced. This procedure causes the visceral pleura to adhere to parietal pleura, obliterating the pleural space. If an air leak is persistent or pleural sclerosis fails, the surgeon may perform a partial pleurectomy, removing the portion of the pleura overlying the cysts that ruptured.

Hemoptysis. Hemoptysis occurs when a blood vessel is eroded as a result of chronic airway inflammation. It is more common in older CF patients and correlates with the presence of bronchiectasis. Patients with large-volume hemoptysis may describe a bubbling or gurgling sensation in one area of the chest. The patient may expectorate as much as 300 to 500 ml of blood in 24 hours. The patient is very anxious and should not be left alone.

During episodes of hemoptysis the nurse elevates the head of the bed 45 to 90 degrees and turns the patient's head to the left side to facilitate expectoration of blood. The nurse provides tis-

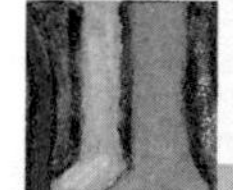

Clinical Manifestations
Cystic Fibrosis

Pulmonary

Chronic productive cough, recurrent bronchitis or pneumonia
Crackles and rhonchi, decreased pulmonary compliance, digital clubbing
Shortness of breath and dyspnea on exertion, wheezing, and weight loss; occur with respiratory complications and usually indicate need for vigorous therapy

Gastrointestinal

Frequent, bulky, greasy stools
Weight loss
Cramps and abdominal pain; should arouse suspicion of obstruction

Glucose Intolerance

Polyuria, polydipsia, polyphagia
Absence of ketoacidosis even with above signs

sues and an emesis basin and empties the basin frequently so the patient is not anxious over the amount of blood. The nurse measures the amount of hemoptysis and records the time and amount.

Hemoptysis usually subsides with conservative measures. Postural drainage and percussion are withheld during acute episodes of bleeding, usually for at least 24 hours. Vitamin K_1 (phytonadione [Mephyton]) may be given orally or subcutaneously. Bronchoscopy with endobronchial tamponade is another option and is most successful for patients with minimal bleeding. If hemoptysis becomes life threatening, surgical intervention, such as removal of the bronchiectactic lobe, may be necessary. Unfortunately, in most patients the pulmonary disease is too extensive to permit surgery.

AIRWAY PROBLEMS. Allergic bronchopulmonary aspergillosis is an allergic immune reaction to *Aspergillus* organisms that is characterized by airway inflammation and edema. This complication occurs in 1% to 10% of patients with CF. It should be considered when new lung infiltrates appear on x-ray films or increased cough, respiratory distress, wheezing, and the expectoration of rusty brown plugs of sputum occur. Treatment is with corticosteroids and oral antifungal agents for several months.

GASTROINTESTINAL PROBLEMS. GI problems are common, and treatment includes vitamin and pancreatic enzyme supplements. Supplemental fat-soluble vitamins aid digestion and improve weight. Most patients take multivitamins and vitamin E. Pancreatic enzyme supplement doses are individualized and titrated by patients to limit fatty stools to less than three per day. Approximately 90% of patients with CF require mealtime pancreatic enzyme supplements. The number and dose are prescribed on the basis of weight gain, the presence or absence of abdominal cramping, and the number of stools. When a patient can take nothing by mouth (is NPO), minimal doses of pancreatic enzyme supplements are necessary. If adequate intake cannot be maintained orally, IV feedings or gastrostomy may be necessary.

RESPIRATORY FAILURE. Respiratory failure leads to death in more than 90% of CF patients. Hypoxemia develops during exertion or sleep and progresses over years. Hypercapnia reflects severe airway obstruction. The principal mechanism underlying hypoxemia is a V/Q mismatch causing hypercapnia.

Collaborative Care Management. Management of CF often involves extensive and complicated treatment regimens that require many hours daily.

DIAGNOSTIC TESTS. The diagnosis of CF is confirmed by the presence of at least two of the following:

- A positive sweat test with a chloride level greater than 60 mEq/L
- Chronic sinopulmonary disease
- Chronic chest x-ray abnormalities: hyperinflation of the lung; mucoid impaction of bronchi, which is seen as branching, fingerlike shadows; or atelectasis of the right upper lobe
- Pancreatic exocrine insufficiency
- Obstructive azoospermia in men
- Laboratory evidence of CFTR dysfunction
- Positive family history of CF

MEDICATIONS. Lung infection is the major source of morbidity and mortality. By age 18, 80% of CF patients are chronically infected with *P. aeruginosa,* 40% with *S. aureus,* and 50% with *Burkholderia cepacia.*[18] Antibiotic therapy is a mainstay designed not to eradicate the bacteria from the airways but to reduce the number of bacteria and control progression of disease. Best results have been shown with early and vigorous use of antibiotics. Dosages need to be higher than in non–CF-related chest infections, and the choice is based on sputum culture and sensitivity. Combination therapy with two or three antibiotics for 10 to 14 days is recommended to prevent bacterial resistance. Shorter courses of antibiotic therapy are associated with exacerbation of symptoms. In both moderate and severe exacerbations, aerosolized (inhaled) antibiotics are used in conjunction with intravenous antibiotics. Organisms with multiple resistance profiles such as *B. cepacia* have emerged in the CF population. This reinforces the need for close monitoring of antibiotic susceptibility and strict adherence to isolation policies for infection control.

Dornase alfa (Pulmozyme) is a recombinant form of the naturally occurring human enzyme deoxyribonuclease I (DNase I), which is responsible for the breakdown of extracellular deoxyribonucleic acid (DNA). In patients with CF the viscosity of airway secretions is abnormally high because of an increased number of neutrophils and DNA in cellular breakdown products. Inhalation of dornase alfa may provide a modest improvement in lung function and decreased pulmonary exacerbation in patients with mild to moderate lung disease. The dosage is 2.5 mg aerosolized daily.

Bronchodilator use is controversial despite the fact that it is prescribed for more than 80% of CF patients. Most CF patients have some bronchodilation after aerosolized albuterol. This may serve to enhance secretion clearance. Some experts are concerned, however, that bronchodilators may be detrimental to cough clearance of secretions by decreasing airway tone, causing dynamic collapse of airways.[11]

TREATMENTS. Treatment goals include the control of infection, promotion of mucus clearance, and improved nutrition. The patient is encouraged to be as active and independent as possible.

Patients are often referred to pulmonary physiotherapy, respiratory therapy, social services, and genetic counseling. It is important to promote compliance with therapy. Approaches that promote a positive self-concept and foster the patient's ability to control the medical management have been successful. Care that provides continuity and fosters trust is essential to achieving expected patient outcomes.

As persons with CF move into adulthood, their medical care should transition from a pediatric to adult focus, and they need support in taking control of their health issues. One concern that often interferes with this transition to independence is the difficulty in acquiring adequate health insurance.[7] Health care professionals can be key in identifying useful resources.

PULMONARY PHYSIOTHERAPY (CHEST PHYSIOTHERAPY). Cough clears mucus from large airways, and chest vibration moves secretions from small airways to large ones. Daily pulmonary physiotherapy is one of the most important preventive and therapeutic aspects of care in patients with CF.

Pulmonary physiotherapy activities (segmental postural drainage, percussion, and vibration) may be performed by a physical therapist, nurse, or family member, or by the patient using new modalities. Pulmonary physiotherapy is physically demanding and time consuming but essential to care. The frequency and duration of treatment are individualized.

Segmental **postural drainage** with percussion and vibration combines the force of gravity with the natural ciliary activity of the small bronchial airways to move secretions upward toward the main bronchi and the trachea. From this point the patient can cough secretions up, or can be suctioned. All segments are usually drained by placing patients in various postural drainage positions (Table 27-5). Treatment may also be directed at draining specific areas of the lung. For example, if the right middle lobe of the lung is affected, drainage is accomplished best by way of the right middle bronchus. The patient lies supine with the body turned at approximately a 45-degree angle. The angle can be maintained by pillow supports placed under the right side from the shoulders to the hips. The foot of the bed is raised about 30 cm (12 inches). Most patients can maintain this position fairly comfortably for half an hour. If the lower posterior area of the lung is affected, the foot of the bed can be raised 45 to 50 cm (18 to 20 inches) with the patient assuming a prone position for drainage.

While the patient is in each position, the health care provider performs percussion with a cupped hand over the area being drained. This maneuver helps loosen secretions and stimulates coughing (Figure 27-10). After percussing the area for approximately 1 minute, the caregiver instructs the patient to breathe deeply. Vibration (pressure applied with a vibrating movement of the hand on the chest) is performed during the expiratory phase of the deep breath. This helps the patient exhale more fully. The procedure is repeated as necessary. When the patient cannot tolerate a head-down position, a modified position is used.

Positions that provide gravity drainage of the lungs can be achieved in several ways, depending on the person's age and general condition, as well as the lobe or lobes of the lungs where secretions have accumulated. Electric hospital beds can be tilted into a head-down position with little difficulty. If an electric bed is not available (e.g., in the home), blocks can be placed under the casters at the foot of the bed, or a hydraulic lift can be used.

Newer techniques such as positive expiratory pressure, a FLUTTER valve device, the Vest System and autogenic drainage, or active cycle breathing are alternatives to traditional and time-intensive chest physiotherapy. FLUTTER, a mucus-clearance device, is a small, handheld device in the shape of a pipe. Within the FLUTTER is a high-density stainless steel ball resting in a plastic cone. As the patient exhales, the ball rolls out of place and back many times, resulting in variance of endobronchial pressure and expiratory airflow. The oscillations loosen mucus from the airway walls, and the acceleration of airflow moves the mucus up the airways. The oscillations also decrease collapsibility of the airways. The Vest System is a portable, high-frequency chest compression system. It is an inflatable, tailored, fitted vest jacket

TABLE 27-5 POSITIONS FOR SEGMENTAL POSTURAL DRAINAGE, PERCUSSION, AND VIBRATION

Area of Lung	Position of Patient	Area to Be Percussed or Vibrated
UPPER LOBE		
Apical bronchus	Semi-Fowler's position, leaning to right, then left, then forward	Over area of shoulder blades with fingers extending over clavicles
Posterior bronchus	Upright at 45-degree angle, rolled forward against pillow at 45 degrees on left and then right side	Over shoulder blade on each side
Anterior bronchus	Supine with pillow under knees	Over anterior chest just below clavicles
MIDDLE LOBE		
Lateral and medial bronchus	Trendelenburg's position at 30-degree angle or with foot of bed elevated 35-40 cm (14-16 inches), turned slightly to left	Anterior and lateral right chest from axillary fold to midanterior chest
LINGULA		
Superior and inferior bronchus	Trendelenburg's position at 30-degree angle or with foot of bed elevated 35-40 cm (14-16 inches), turned slightly to right	Left axillary fold to midanterior chest
Apical bronchus	Prone with pillow under hips	Lower third of posterior rib cage on both sides
Medial bronchus	Trendelenburg's position at 45-degree angle or with foot of bed raised 45-50 cm (18-20 inches) on right side	Lower third of left posterior rib cage
Lateral bronchus	Trendelenburg's position at 45-degree angle or with foot of bed raised 45-50 cm (18-20 inches) on left side	Lower third of right posterior rib cage
Posterior bronchus	Prone Trendelenburg's position at 45-degree angle with pillow under hips	Lower third of posterior rib cage on both sides

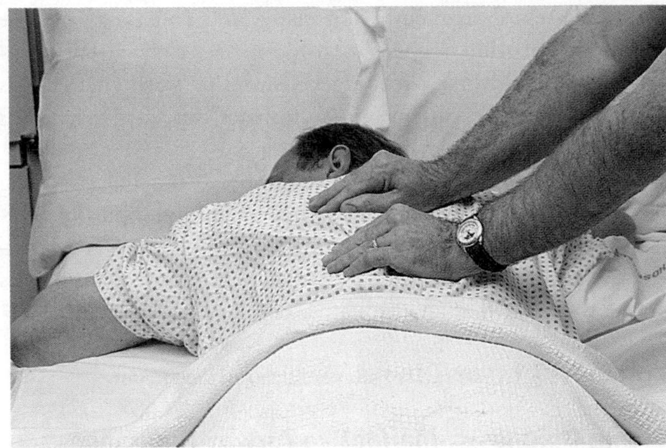

A

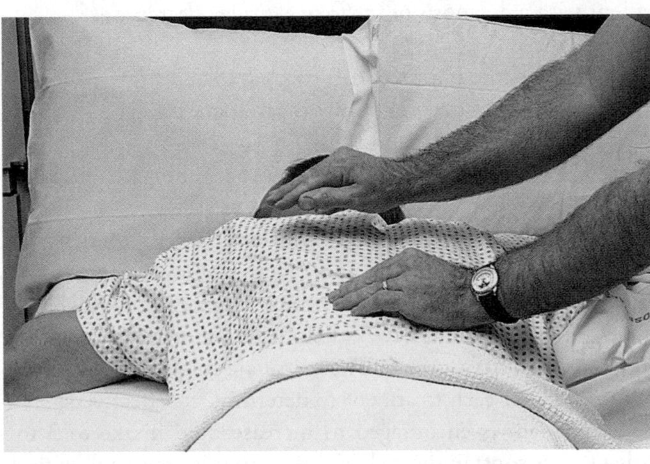

B

Figure 27-10 **A,** Hand position for chest wall percussion during physiotherapy. **B,** Chest wall percussion; alternating hand motion against patient's chest wall.

attached to a large pump that generates high-frequency oscillations. The resulting pressures cause the vest to inflate and deflate against the chest wall. In this passive technique, the vibrations cause transient increased airflow, resulting in improved mucus mobilization.[44]

Postural drainage and percussion should be planned to achieve maximal benefit. Some patients spend up to 8 hours per day involved with this treatment. The frequency of treatments depends on each person's needs, but care should be taken to avoid exhaustion, which results in shallow ventilation and negates the positive effects of the treatment. Because the patient may feel nauseated by the odor and taste of sputum, the procedure should be timed for at least 1 hour before meals. A short rest period after percussion while still in the postural drainage position often improves the effectiveness of treatment. Chest percussion is contraindicated in patients with pulmonary emboli, hemorrhage, exacerbation of bronchospasms, or severe pain and also over areas of resectable carcinoma.

LUNG TRANSPLANTATION. Lung transplantation has become accepted therapy for respiratory failure secondary to CF. Patients should be referred when their prognosis is about equal to the waiting time for donor lungs, currently about 2 years. The best indicator currently is an FEV_1 of less than 30% of predicted, although women and younger children may need a transplant before reaching this level. The transplanted lungs remain free of CF but are subject to secondary infection and acute or chronic rejection. Survival rates for lung transplant patients with CF is 73% at 1 year and 48% at 5 years.[20]

DIET. The diet may be as tolerated, but may need to be altered because of GI problems.

HEALTH PROMOTION AND PREVENTION. Because CF is a genetically inherited disease, identification of carriers who may pass on the defect and disease to offspring remains the most important preventive strategy. Early identification of carriers combined with genetic counseling minimizes the chance of offspring inheriting this lethal genetic disease. Family histories of possible incidences of CF should be followed up by genetic testing.

Patient teaching is an important component of patient care (see Patient/Family Teaching box).

Nursing Management

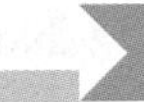

of the Patient with Cystic Fibrosis

ASSESSMENT

Health History. Assess for:

- Description of symptoms such as shortness of breath, dyspnea on exertion, fatigue, and wheezing
- Patient's understanding of CF pathophysiology and treatment regimens, including postural drainage and percussion; antibiotics; aerosol therapy with dornase alfa, bronchodilators, and antibiotics; and nutritional supplements such as pancreatic enzymes and vitamins
- Color, consistency, and frequency of stools
- Color, smell, and frequency of urination

PATIENT/FAMILY TEACHING
The Patient With Cystic Fibrosis

Because the adult patient with cystic fibrosis has had the disease for several years, teaching is more in the form of review and reinforcement. Information to review includes:

- Daily nutrition requirements, vitamins, and the need to check weight daily
- Daily pulmonary exercises and treatments, including postural drainage and percussion, as well as use of bronchoactive medication before postural drainage
- Usual dose, expected effects, and side effects of medications
- Clinical symptoms that indicate that the health care provider should be notified, such as signs of an acute respiratory tract infection (fever, increased fatigue, shortness of breath, increased production of sputum, or change in color of sputum); hemoptysis; and sudden, sharp chest pain
- Patient's knowledge and understanding of fertility, genetic testing, and contraceptive methods
- Patient's and family's knowledge of community and social resources for assistance with health care reimbursement programs, disability insurance, and support groups

- Description of appetite and ability to swallow food
- Daily eating pattern
- Medications taken at home and their effectiveness in decreasing stool frequency
- Onset, duration, intensity, and type of any abdominal discomfort
- Signs or symptoms of gastric reflux
- History of weight loss, including amount and time of onset
- Description of daily routine as it relates to work or school, pulmonary regimen, medications, and leisure activities
- Description of current coping strategies and support network
- Concerns about sexuality or fertility
- Method of financial support (job, family, other forms of assistance)
- Patient's and family's understanding of CF
- Symptoms and stage of grieving: anxiety, sleeplessness, hallucinations
- Patient and family strengths
- Patient support structure
- Normal adult developmental needs
- Need for genetic counseling, career counseling, or social services

Physical Examination. Assess for:

- Diminished breath sounds, wheezes, and adventitious breath sounds, which are most often heard in the upper lobes
- Chest pain on inspiration
- Cyanotic mucous membranes
- Digital clubbing
- Presence of a productive cough (observe color of sputum if possible)
- Presence of fever or tachypnea
- ABGs indicative of a falling PaO_2 or rising $PaCO_2$ and results of PFTs (decrease in tidal volume and FEV_1)
- Adverse effects of medications, such as renal toxicity from antibiotics and tachycardia from bronchodilators
- Nutritional and GI status; patient's weight; presence of bowel sounds on auscultation

NURSING DIAGNOSES, OUTCOMES, AND INTERVENTIONS

Nursing Diagnosis: Risk for Infection

OUTCOMES. Common examples of expected outcomes for the patient with a diagnosis of *risk for infection* are:
Patient will:

- Exhibit no signs of infection.
- Demonstrate decreased mucus in the airway.
- Maintain an environment free of pathogenic bacteria.
- Discuss ways of reducing risk of infection.
- Verbalize knowledge of when to take influenza and pneumococcal vaccines.

NURSING INTERVENTIONS. Because the adult with CF is extremely vulnerable to infection, the environment should be kept as free of pathogens as possible. The patient should wash his or her own hands frequently, especially after coughing, and the nurse should provide frequent mouth care, especially after postural drainage. The nurse encourages visitors to wash their hands before touching the patient and minimizes exposure to persons with upper respiratory tract infections.

The nurse monitors the patient's temperature regularly, along with the color, volume, and consistency of sputum. Sputum specimens must be collected correctly and sent for culture and sensitivity as indicated. Care must be taken to administer antibiotics on time to ensure that an adequate blood level is maintained.

RELATED NIC INTERVENTIONS. Infection Prevention

Nursing Diagnosis: Ineffective Airway Clearance

OUTCOMES. Common examples of expected outcomes for the patient with a diagnosis of *ineffective airway clearance* are:
Patient will:

- Demonstrate improved airway clearance.
- Demonstrate decreased mucus production.
- Have clear breath sounds.
- Report decreased fatigue and shortness of breath.

NURSING INTERVENTIONS. The nurse assists the patient with coughing, postural drainage, and percussion every 2 to 4 hours, depending on the severity of the infection. The newer FLUTTER valves and Vest System devices help promote independence with these needed interventions. The nurse auscultates breath sounds before and after each treatment to determine its effectiveness.

The patient is encouraged to increase fluid intake to 3 to 4 L/day unless contraindicated, and the room is kept cool, with the temperature below 70° F (21.1° C).

RELATED NIC INTERVENTIONS. Airway Management, Cough Enhancement, Respiratory Monitoring

Nursing Diagnosis: Imbalanced Nutrition: Less Than Body Requirements

OUTCOMES. Common examples of expected outcomes for the patient with a diagnosis of *imbalanced nutrition: less than body requirements* are:
Patient will:

- Demonstrate improved nutrition.
- Maintain weight within 20% of ideal weight.
- Maintain normal blood glucose level.
- Eat small, frequent meals.

NURSING INTERVENTIONS. Because the patient with CF often has difficulty maintaining nutrition, the nurse may need to be creative. The nurse performs baseline and periodic assessments of nutrition, including food history, recording of daily intake and output, and recording of daily weight. Blood glucose levels are monitored so that insulin can be given as prescribed according to blood glucose findings. The nurse works with the dietitian and the patient to provide small, frequent meals that are appealing to the patient. The nurse administers pancreatic enzymes and vitamins as ordered.

RELATED NIC INTERVENTIONS. Nutrition Management, Nutrition Therapy

Nursing Diagnosis: Anticipatory Grieving

OUTCOMES. Common examples of expected outcomes for the patient with a diagnosis of *anticipatory grieving* are:

Patient will:

- Manifest enhanced coping skills.
- Verbalize actual and potential losses.
- Identify own strengths and personal goals.
- Identify support person to assist with coping and achievement of goals.

NURSING INTERVENTIONS. The nurse can play a major role in helping the patient work through the grieving process by identifying the stage of grieving; allowing time for the patient to verbalize feelings, hopes, and fears; and supporting expressions of hope, while avoiding false reassurance. The nurse supports both patient and family through grief work and recommends CF support groups as indicated. The nurse may also refer the patient for genetic counseling, career counseling, or social services. The nurse intervenes for pathologic symptoms of grief, such as anxiety, sleeplessness, and hallucinations.

RELATED NIC INTERVENTIONS. Family Support, Grief Work Facilitation

EVALUATION

To evaluate the effectiveness of nursing interventions, compare patient behaviors with those stated in the expected patient outcomes.

RELATED NOC OUTCOMES. Coping, Family Coping, Immune Statue, Knowledge: Infection Control, Nutrition Status: Nutrient Intake, Respiratory Status: Airway Patency

GERONTOLOGIC CONSIDERATIONS

Only a few CF patients live into the sixth or seventh decade of life. However, 50% of patients can now expect to survive beyond age 30, so in a few years many more CF patients may be living at ages 55 and older. The Cystic Fibrosis Foundation is helpful to patients and families in terms of supplying names of health care resources and providing support to family caregivers.

▶ ARE You READY?

In planning care for the adult patient with cystic fibrosis, the nurse incorporates which of the following interventions?

1. Maintain room temperature above 75° F
2. Encourage fluid intake to 3-4 L/day
3. Administer cough suppressants
4. Decrease protein in diet

Respiratory Failure

Etiology and Epidemiology. Respiratory failure is impairment of the lung's ability to maintain adequate oxygen and carbon dioxide homeostasis. Analysis of ABGs and pulse oximetry are required for diagnosis. Respiratory failure is classified as acute (ARF), chronic (CRF), or acute-on-chronic (AOCF). ARF is any rapid change in respiration resulting in hypoxemia, hypercarbia, or both. It occurs over hours to days, and the term *acute respiratory failure* connotes a sense of urgency. CRF develops over months to years, allowing compensatory mechanisms to improve oxygen transport and buffer respiratory acidemia. AOCF is ARF superimposed on CRF, as in a patient with COPD who experiences an acute exacerbation.

Respiratory failure may also be classified according to the underlying pathophysiology as hypoxemic respiratory failure or hypoxemic-hypercapnic respiratory failure. Patients often demonstrate characteristics of both during the course of the illness. Hypoxemic respiratory failure is characterized by a low PaO_2 (less than 55 mm Hg) and a normal or low $PaCO_2$. The result of V/Q mismatch is best demonstrated by acute respiratory distress syndrome (ARDS). Hypoxemic-hypercapnic respiratory failure is characterized by a low PaO_2 (less than 55 mm Hg) and an elevated $PaCO_2$ (greater than 50 mm Hg). An elevated $PaCO_2$ normally increases ventilatory drive, so this form of respiratory failure indicates the patient is not able to sense the elevated $PaCO_2$ (COPD) or the lungs and chest are not able to respond (parenchymal or muscular inefficiency).[5]

Many disorders can lead to or are associated with respiratory failure (Box 27-2).

Pathophysiology. The respiratory system is made up of two basic parts: the gas exchange organ (the lungs) and the pump (the respiratory muscles and the respiratory control mechanisms). Any alteration in the function of the gas exchange unit or the pump can result in respiratory insufficiency or failure. Regardless of the underlying condition, the resultant events or processes that occur in respiratory failure are the same. With inadequate ventilation, the arterial oxygen falls and tissue cells become hypoxic. Carbon dioxide accumulates, leading to a fall in pH and respiratory acidosis.

BOX 27-2 Disorders Associated With Respiratory Failure

Pulmonary Disorders

Severe infection
Pulmonary edema
Pulmonary embolism
Chronic obstructive pulmonary disease
Cystic fibrosis
Acute respiratory distress syndrome
Cancer
Chest trauma (flail chest)
Severe atelectasis
Airway compromise secondary to trauma, infection, or surgery

Nonpulmonary Disorders

Central nervous system disturbance secondary to drug overdose, anesthesia, head injury
Neuromuscular disorders (e.g., Guillain-Barré syndrome, myasthenia gravis, multiple sclerosis, poliomyelitis, muscular dystrophy, spinal cord injury)
Postoperative reduction in ventilation after thoracic and abdominal surgery
Prolonged mechanical ventilation

ARF is defined by predetermined physiologic criteria. These criteria are sudden onset of:

- PaO_2 of 50 mm Hg or less (measured on room air)
- $PaCO_2$ of 50 mm Hg or more
- pH of 7.35 or less

Hypercapnia and hypoxemia are present in CRF. In CRF the pH usually stays within the range of 7.35 to 7.40 because of compensation. Patients with CRF develop AOCF as a result of a secondary insult to their compromised pulmonary system, usually in the form of a respiratory infection. The individual can no longer compensate for the altered lung function, and a dramatic decrease in pH (below 7.35), accompanied by severe hypoxemia, occurs. Because carbon dioxide retention (hypercapnia) preexists in patients with AOCF, the $PaCO_2$ is less relevant than pH and PaO_2 in determining respiratory status. In fact, these patients often display few clinical signs or symptoms, even though they may have major blood gas derangements.

Underlying blood gas alterations are the basis for the clinical signs and symptoms associated with respiratory failure (see Clinical Manifestations box). The signs and symptoms of hypoxemia, hypercapnia, and respiratory acidosis are presented together because the blood gas derangements causing them usually occur simultaneously. It is important for the nurse to recognize that the signs and symptoms associated with hypoxemia and hypercapnia depend more on the rate of change in value than on absolute value. The patient with COPD may show few signs until severe ARF occurs.

COMPLICATIONS. Complications of respiratory failure and mechanical ventilation include impaired gas exchange from a plugged tube, kinked tube, or cuff herniation; fluid volume excess; electrolyte imbalance; stress ulcer and GI bleeding; infection; increased intracranial pressure secondary to altered cerebral perfusion; tissue hypoxia; and cardiopulmonary arrest.

One-year survival after respiratory failure is 28% to 72%. The prognosis is best for those with kyphoscoliosis or neuromuscular disease and worst for those with pneumoconiosis and pulmonary fibrosis. Men with COPD who require mechanical ventilation have a survival rate of about 50% at 1 year.[45]

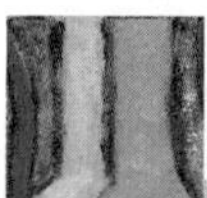

CLINICAL MANIFESTATIONS
Respiratory Failure

Secondary to Hypercapnia, Hypoxemia, and Respiratory Acidosis

Headache
Irritability
Confusion
Increasing somnolence, coma
Asterixis (flapping tremor)
Cardiac dysrhythmia
Tachycardia
Hypotension
Cyanosis

Secondary to Increased Work of Breathing

Dyspnea
Exhaustion

Secondary to Pressure on Right Side of Heart

Peripheral edema
Neck vein distention
Hepatomegaly

ARE You READY?

In the patient with respiratory failure, the nurse monitors for adult respiratory distress syndrome characterized by which of the following arterial blood gas results?

1. PaO_2 50 and $PaCO_2$ 32
2. PaO_2 60 and $PaCO_2$ 40
3. PaO_2 65 and $PaCO_2$ 48
4. PaO_2 80 and $PaCO_2$ 55

Collaborative Care Management

DIAGNOSTIC TESTS. Usual diagnostic tests are ABGs, chest x-ray studies, pulmonary spirometry, and sputum for culture and sensitivity. All these are done to determine the severity of the disease and the treatment needs. Additional tests are based on other needs the patient may develop.

MEDICATIONS. The medications prescribed depend on the patient's symptoms and the underlying cause.

TREATMENTS. Therapy is based on the severity of the failure, ventilation needs, and the underlying cause. Oxygen therapy and support ventilation are usually prescribed. Other complications the patient experiences are treated as needed.

MECHANICAL VENTILATION. When respiratory failure progresses despite medical therapy, mechanical ventilation often becomes necessary. The goals of mechanical ventilation are to correct potentially life-threatening blood gas and acid-base abnormalities; provide support during bronchoactive pharmacologic therapy; and rest the muscles of respiration, allowing them to recover from fatigue. In respiratory failure, adjustments are made to the ventilator to promote respiratory muscle rest. Respiratory muscles require 48 to 72 hours to achieve full recovery. Rest can be achieved in any mode of ventilation that minimizes patient effort. Mechanical ventilation can be provided noninvasively by face or nasal mask or by intubation.

Noninvasive Modes. Noninvasive mechanical ventilation (NIV) is the delivery of mechanical ventilation without the use of an invasive airway. It is becoming the treatment of choice for respiratory failure, although the specific indications are still somewhat controversial. At least two of the following criteria should be present before initiation: moderate to severe shortness of breath with accessory muscle use and evidence of respiratory muscle fatigue, acidosis, hypercapnia, or a respiratory rate of greater than 25 breaths/min.[25] NIV has been shown to improve ABGs and reduce intubation and mortality rate in patients suffering from exacerbation of COPD complicated by acute hypercapnic respiratory failure.[8] NIV may also be an option to support patients with respiratory failure who refuse intubation. The American Thoracic Society believes it justifiable to use NIV in do-not-intubate patients with a reversible cause of ARF.[8]

The methods include negative-pressure ventilation and nasal and face mask intermittent positive-pressure ventilation (IPPV). Most centers use a face or nasal mask and pressure support ventilation (PSV), also called noninvasive positive-pressure ventilation (NPPV). Ventilation is delivered via a volume- or pressure-cycled ventilator or a continuous positive airway pressure (CPAP) or bilevel positive airway pressure (BiPAP) ventilation device.

A tight-fitting mask allows ventilatory assistance and provides for brief periods off the ventilator, during which the patient can speak, inhale nebulized medications, expectorate, and swallow liquids. NIV methods may be used for up to 1 week. They have been effective in relieving symptoms, decreasing respiratory rate, increasing tidal volume, improving gas exchange, decreasing the length of the hospital stay, and decreasing in-house mortality.[27] Complications are few compared with other methods of ventilatory support and include local skin breakdown and aspiration; also, some patients cannot tolerate the mask.

With NIV the positive pressure is applied during the patient's inspiration via IPPV or PSV or throughout the respiratory cycle at a constant pressure (CPAP). The NPPV may also be set to different levels during inspiration and expiration through the use of BiPAP. These positive-pressure modes reduce the work of breathing, decrease respiratory muscle fatigue, and increase minute ventilation. NIV requires an alert, cooperative, hemodynamically stable patient. Relative contraindications include copious secretions, aspiration risk, and impaired mental status. This approach to ventilatory support requires careful attention to a properly fitting mask and time from the clinicians to stay with the patient to explain the device, titrate pressures, troubleshoot problems, and provide support and close, ongoing assessment.[5]

Intubation. If the patient with respiratory failure is not a candidate for NIV or if NIV is not maintaining adequate ventilation, intubation is required for mechanical ventilation.

Ventilator Modes. Ventilator modes determine whether the machine controls the breaths and, if so, how many, or whether, to some degree, the patient controls the breaths with assistance from the machine. The most common modes are assist/control (A/C), synchronized intermittent mandatory ventilation (SIMV), and CPAP (Table 27-6).

In the A/C mode the ventilator senses each time the patient begins to inspire and delivers a breath. If the patient is unable to trigger the machine, the ventilator delivers the preset number of breaths at the set tidal volume. The A/C mode, also called continuous mechanical ventilation, gives the patient complete ventilatory support. This mode is the most frequently used in respiratory failure to ensure respiratory muscle rest. Tidal volumes of 5 to 7 ml/kg are used with respiratory rates of 20 to 24 breaths/min.

TABLE 27-6 VENTILATOR MODES

Type	Description
Assist/control (A/C)	Each breath ventilator assisted. If patient unable to trigger machine, ventilator continues to deliver preset number of breaths at set tidal volume.
Bilevel positive airway pressure (BiPAP)	Positive pressure applied to spontaneous breathing, allowing independent settings for inspiratory positive pressure and expiratory positive pressure.
Continuous positive airway pressure (CPAP)	Positive pressure applied during respiration and maintained throughout entire respiratory cycle. Decreases intrapulmonary shunting.
Controlled mandatory ventilation (CMV)	Delivers preset volume at fixed rate regardless of patient's effort to breathe.
Independent lung ventilation (ILV)	Each lung ventilated separately. Used in unilateral lung disease. Requires intubation with double-lumen tube.
Intermittent mandatory ventilation (IMV)	Delivers preset number of breaths. Patient may take unassisted breaths.
Positive end-expiratory pressure (PEEP)	Applies positive pressure at end of expiration. Decreases intrapulmonic shunting.
Pressure support ventilation (PSV)	Selected amount of positive pressure applied to airway during patient's spontaneous respiratory efforts. Amount of pressure gradually reduced until patient receives no assistance.
Synchronized intermittent mandatory ventilation (SIMV)	Intermittent ventilator breaths synchronized with patient's spontaneous breaths. Reduces competition between patient and ventilator.
High-frequency ventilator	Special positive-pressure ventilator used in some patients.
High-frequency positive-pressure ventilation (HFPPV)	Extremely short inspiratory times with total volume equivalent to dead space. Rate 60-100 cycles/min.
High-frequency jet ventilation (HFJV)	Small volumes less than anatomic dead space pulsed through jet injector catheter at 100-600 cycles/min.
High-frequency oscillation ventilation (HFO)	Small volume of gas continuously vibrated in airways at rates up to 4000 cycles/min.

Adapted from Stillwell S: *Mosby's critical care nursing reference*, ed 3, St Louis, 2002, Mosby.

SIMV allows the patient to take additional breaths over the set rate of the ventilator. The volume of extra breaths is determined by the patient's ability and effort to breathe spontaneously. In SIMV the number of ventilator breaths can be gradually reduced until the patient is breathing on his or her own.

In the CPAP mode the machine delivers a set airway pressure throughout inspiration and exhalation, and the patient determines respiratory rate, tidal volume, inspiratory flow, and inspiratory time. Additional pressure can be added to assist the inspiratory muscles.

Different kinds of ventilators are available to deliver these modes (Table 27-7; Figures 27-11 and 27-12). In adults there are two basic types: pressure-cycled and volume-cycled ventilators. Volume-cycled ventilators, the ones used most frequently, deliver a constant volume of air with each breath. The volume is preset and delivered to the patient at whatever pressure is necessary to attain that volume. A volume-cycled machine should have a pressure cutoff valve that allows a pressure limit to be set. If the pressure required to deliver the set volume exceeds the pressure limit, the machine will turn off before the entire volume is delivered. The pressure limit on a volume-cycled machine usually has an audible alarm. The nurse can set the limit slightly above the pressure required to ventilate the patient (approximately 5 cm H_2O). The alarm will then go off if the patient coughs, accumulates secretions, or starts to resist the machine. Box 27-3 describes the functionality of the volume-cycled ventilator.

Pressure-cycled ventilators deliver a volume of gas to the airway using positive pressure during inspiration. The positive pressure is delivered until the preselected pressure has been reached; the machine then cycles off. Exhalation occurs passively. The disadvantage of pressure-cycled ventilators is that a varying tidal volume may be delivered as a result of changes in airway resistance or compliance.

Suctioning the Patient. When the patient on a ventilator needs **suctioning,** a closed system is preferred. In closed-system endotracheal suctioning, the nurse inserts an adaptor at the endotracheal tube–ventilatory circuitry interface (Figure 27-13). This allows patients to be suctioned without disconnecting them from the ventilator. The benefits of this form of suctioning are (1) continuation of the oxygen supply, (2) the stability of PEEP, and (3) a reduced

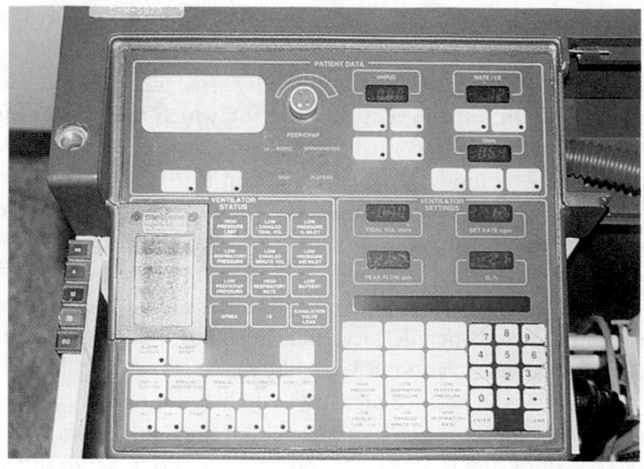

Figure 27-11 Front display panel of ventilator for monitoring airway pressures and volumes.

incidence of ventilator-assisted pneumonia. Refer to the Guidelines for Safe Practice box for the steps in closed-system suctioning.

General Care of the Patient on a Ventilator. When care is planned for the patient on a mechanical ventilator, knowing the patient's ability to breathe spontaneously in the event of accidental disconnection from the ventilator is imperative. In most facilities respiratory therapists regularly monitor ventilator function and settings, but the nurse is also responsible for maintaining the ventilator settings. Usually a checklist is used to verify the settings on an hourly basis.

The nurse assesses the patient regularly and any time a ventilator alarm sounds. The cause of an alarm sounding can be a dysfunction anywhere from the person's lungs to the machine. Troubleshooting is carried out in a systematic manner, starting with the patient and moving toward the machine (Box 27-4). If the alarm continues to sound and the cause cannot be determined or the patient is in respiratory distress, the nurse disconnects the patient from the machine and manually ventilates with an Ambu bag (or anesthesia bag) with oxygenated air until the problem can be resolved.

Patients who have a prolonged course of mechanical ventilation need to be evaluated for tracheostomy. If a course of mechanical

Table 27-7 Types of Mechanical Ventilators

Types	Basic Function Mode
Positive-pressure ventilator (requires intubation)	Types of positive-pressure ventilators are based on how inspiratory phase is ended.
Pressure-cycled ventilator (requires intubation)	Inspiration ends at a preset pressure limit; time and volume are variable.
Time-cycled ventilator (requires intubation)	Inspiration is preset for given time interval; volume and pressure are variable.
Volume-cycled ventilator (requires intubation)	Preset volume of air is delivered. Time and pressure are variable. However, volume-cycled ventilators often have pressure- and time-cycled capacities.
Negative-pressure ventilator (intubation not required)	Thorax, at least, is encapsulated. When ventilator expands, it creates negative pressure by pulling thorax outward. Air rushes into airways because of pressure gradient created.
High-frequency ventilation (requires intubation)	Several variants are available. All use high respiratory rates to deliver small tidal volumes at low pressures.

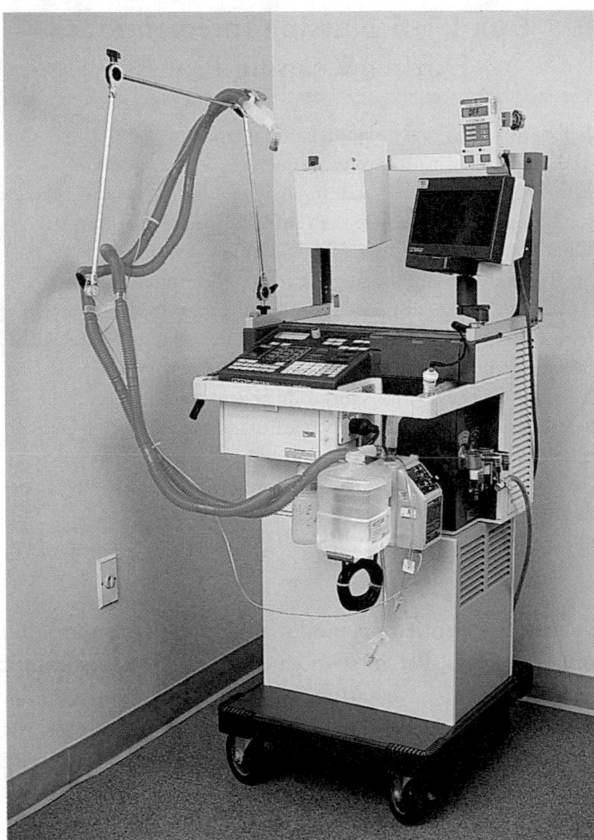

Figure 27-12 Mechanical ventilator.

Box 27-3 Adjustable Functions With Volume-Cycled Ventilators

- Tidal volume: volume of air in a normal breath
- FiO_2: oxygenation concentration delivered through the ventilator
- Alarm systems: vary from machine to machine; basic alarms usually present
  - —High-pressure alarm: increased resistance somewhere in system from lungs to machine
  - —Low-pressure alarm: system not reaching minimal pressure required for ventilation
  - —Low-volume alarm: volume of ventilation does not equal the amount set
- Control modes: degree of ventilation that is controlled by the ventilator; can vary from complete ventilator control to almost total patient control

ventilation is projected to go beyond 2 weeks, a tracheostomy is usually placed for patient comfort and communication and to avoid the complications associated with prolonged endotracheal tube placement.

Weaning From the Ventilator. Prolonged mechanical ventilation is dangerous and expensive. The incidence of pneumonia increases with each day on mechanical ventilation. Most patients can be extubated once the precipitating cause of ARF resolves and the patients are medically stable. The decision to wean a person from the ventilator is based on clinical evidence of improved physical

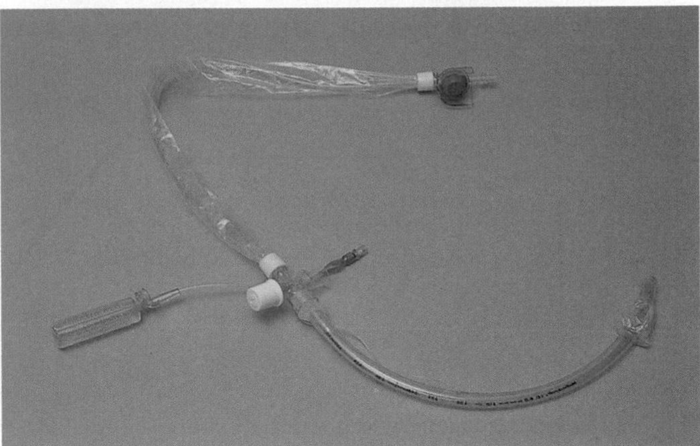

Figure 27-13 Closed-system suctioning tube.

status. **Weaning** is most successful when the health care team plans it in partnership with the patient. Weaning protocols are used in a number of settings and are overseen by highly skilled clinicians.

Some nurse experts divide the weaning process into three phases: preweaning, weaning, and extubation. During the preweaning stage, the nurse ensures the patient has normal electrolytes, including phosphate, calcium, and magnesium. Malnutrition is avoided, but the patient should not be overfed. Overfeeding with carbohydrates and extra calories may result in increased carbon dioxide production and increased ventilatory demand. The recommended 24-hour caloric intake is 1500 to 2500, which should ensure adequate calories for energy expenditure. Protein intake is important, and 1 to 1.5 mg/kg has been suggested. Tube feedings containing these requirements are given to prepare the patient for weaning.

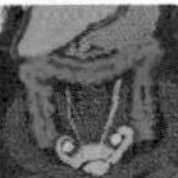

GUIDELINES FOR SAFE PRACTICE
Closed-System Suctioning

- Wash hands for 10 seconds, as recommended by the Centers for Disease Control and Prevention, and put on gloves.
- Select a catheter that is half the diameter of the artificial airway. The catheter has a suction valve at one end, has a patient connector at the other end, and is enclosed in a plastic sheath.
- Attach suction valve to suction source. Select suction pressure between 80 and 120 mm Hg. Set maximum pressure by pinching suction tubing closed.
- Attach patient connector to ventilator tubing and the endotracheal tube (ET). Use the ventilator to hyperoxygenate and hyperinflate the patient's lungs before suctioning.
- Open access valve and advance catheter through the connector into the ET and trachea.
- Using the suction valve, apply suction for not more than 10 seconds as the catheter is withdrawn. Repeat as necessary.
- Provide 100% oxygen and have patient take deep breaths while suctioning.
- Withdraw catheter and close access valve.
- Clean suction tip by attaching a normal saline unit–dose vial or syringe containing normal saline to irrigation port. Squirt the saline on the catheter tip and apply suction until the catheter is clean and saline is sucked out of the catheter.
- Remove gloves and wash hands for 10 seconds.

Box 27-4 Patient and Ventilator Assessment

Patient Assessment

Inspection

Does the person appear to be in respiratory distress?
Is the person's chest moving with machine-cycled inspiration?
Is the chest moving bilaterally?

Auscultation

Are breath sounds present?
Are adventitious sounds present?
Are breath sounds coordinated with ventilator inspiration?

Assessment of Tubing to Machine

Is there an air leak around the endotracheal cuff?
Is there excess condensation in the tubing? (Always remove water from the tubing system. Do not empty back into the humidifier reservoir.) NOTE: Not all ventilators have humidifiers.

Assessment of Machine

Are all ventilator settings and readouts correct?

Weaning is initiated when the patient meets certain physiologic criteria:

- Acceptable ABGs
- Tidal volume greater than 10 ml/kg
- VC greater than 15 ml/kg
- Fraction of inspired oxygen (FiO_2) less than 0.5
- Maximum inspiratory pressure greater than 220 cm H_2O (usually 230 to 240 cm H_2O preferred)
- Normal hematocrit (Most patients on long-term ventilator support have hematocrits below 30%. They are usually not transfused until their hematocrit falls to about 25%. There is general agreement that weaning is most successful when the patient's hematocrit is 30% or higher.)

Nursing interventions during the weaning process are listed in Box 27-5. The weaning process is individualized to meet the patient's needs. The three most common methods of weaning are T-piece weaning, SIMV weaning, and PSV weaning.

For T-piece weaning, the nurse places the patient in an upright position, disconnects the ventilator, and connects a T-piece to the endotracheal tube cuff to provide oxygenated humidified air. The nurse observes the patient for signs of respiratory distress and reconnects the ventilator when he or she indicates fatigue. Some patients may be able to breathe for only a few minutes on their own; others may do well for 30 minutes. Time off the ventilator is gradually increased. With SIMV weaning, the patient remains connected to the ventilator. The number of synchronized mandatory breaths delivered by the machine is gradually reduced, allowing the patient to take an increasing number of breaths independently. The patient is disconnected from the ventilator when predetermined physiologic criteria are maintained. With PSV weaning, the patient also remains connected to the ventilator, and the level of preset positive pressure during inspiration is gradually reduced until the patient is receiving no assistance. This mode eases breathing by reducing airflow resistance of artificial airways.

Box 27-5 Nursing Interventions During Weaning Process

- Before initiating weaning, prepare the patient.
- Teach effective breathing techniques.
- Inform the patient that weaning may require several attempts, each for a longer period, before the ventilator can be disconnected.
- Obtain baseline vital signs, tidal volume, and vital capacity.
- Stay with the patient during the initial weaning process.
- Coach the patient as needed to breathe more slowly and deeply, with emphasis on increasing the time of exhalation.
- Suction as needed.
- Monitor for the clinical signs of hypoxemia and hypercapnia (increased respiratory rate, tachycardia, dysrhythmias, increased blood pressure, agitation, diaphoresis, or increased somnolence).
- Reconnect the ventilator if the patient cannot breathe on his or her own.

Noninvasive ventilation modes are being used more often in weaning protocols. Patients who are able to breathe comfortably after weaning and have satisfactory ABGs are extubated. Some patients may receive supplemental oxygen by face mask for 24 hours. The nurse observes the patient closely for signs of respiratory distress and increased efforts to breathe (e.g., respirations less than 8 breaths/min or more than 30 breaths/min; increase in respiratory rate of 10 breaths/min or more from starting rate; increase or decrease in heart rate by 20 beats/min; increase or decrease in blood pressure by 20 mm Hg; decrease in PaO_2 or increase in $PaCO_2$; or pH less than 7.35). If a patient develops respiratory distress, reintubation may be necessary.

Patients who have a projected course of mechanical ventilation beyond 2 weeks usually have a tracheostomy done to make them more comfortable, facilitate communication, and avoid complications from the endotracheal tube. Patients with a prolonged course may be transferred to a transitional ventilator unit for specialized but less intensive care.

Failure to wean successfully. Some patients cannot be weaned from a ventilator. Reasons include underlying obstructive lung disease, severe chest wall deformities, neuromuscular disease, and prolonged hospitalizations secondary to multisystem organ failure. Additional factors that contribute to weaning failure include malnutrition, recurrent aspiration, electrolyte abnormalities, occult infection, and steroid myopathy.[38]

Because of the number of patients who require long-term ventilatory support and thus may be difficult to wean, the North American Nursing Diagnosis Association has approved two nursing diagnoses: Dysfunctional Ventilatory Weaning Response (mild, moderate, or severe) and Impaired Spontaneous Ventilation (major or minor). With either diagnosis, related factors are noted. For Dysfunctional Ventilatory Weaning Response, the related factors are pathophysiologic, such as muscle weakness; situational, such as fear of separation from the ventilator; and treatment errors, such as rushing the weaning process. Related factors for Impaired Spontaneous Ventilation include physiologic, such as respiratory muscle fatigue; and psychosocial, such as depression.

Care of the patient who cannot be weaned. Patients who require prolonged mechanical ventilation may be cared for in a specialized respiratory unit of a hospital or long-term care facility or at home. Chronic ventilator units have a larger nurse/patient ratio than critical care units. Thus the patient's acute care needs must be resolved before transfer. These units usually continue weaning efforts, often using a slower, more individualized approach. Few patients find it possible to go home on a ventilator, because of the lack of suitable space and a significant other who can assume responsibility for the ventilator 24 hours a day, 7 days a week. If the patient and significant others decide that the patient will be discharged home, careful planning is required to ensure that the home can accommodate the patient and the necessary equipment. The home assessment is best made by a nurse from the health care agency that will be monitoring home care.

Patients and families also may choose to be taken off the ventilator. Once the patient indicates that this is his or her choice, the care team meets to discuss how the patient's wishes can best be accommodated. To ease the patient's anxiety, sedation, usually a morphine infusion, is started before the ventilator is disconnected. A comfort measures–only approach to care is then adopted. Hospice involvement is encouraged.

DIET. Diet is as tolerated. However, the patient may be NPO, depending on the acuity and severity of the respiratory failure.

HEALTH PROMOTION AND PREVENTION. Prevention of respiratory failure focuses on early identification of persons at high risk for developing ARF. In the inpatient setting every person with an increased risk of developing respiratory failure should have a preventive care plan, including:

- Keeping the airway clear by instituting regular deep breathing and coughing maneuvers and using nasotracheal suctioning if necessary
- Maintaining an optimal activity level
- Using sedatives or analgesics judiciously
- Assessing regularly for signs and symptoms indicating deterioration of respiratory status

Nursing Management *of the Patient with Respiratory Failure*

ASSESSMENT

Health History. Assess for:

- History of past or present associated disorders, recent change in respiratory status, change in sputum (color, viscosity, odor), increased dyspnea, change in mental status, complaints of chest tightness or pain
- Current medications and any recent changes in medication regimen
- Self-care modalities used
- A family member or friend who may be able to provide objective information about changes in the patient

Physical Examination. Assess for:

- Abnormalities of general appearance, such as wasting appearance, breathing difficulty, postural changes
- Variations in mental status, which may range from agitation to somnolence
- Changes in vital signs to identify tachycardia, tachypnea, bradypnea, or apnea (Respiratory rates of less than 8 breaths/min result in alveolar hypoventilation; rates over 35 breaths/min cannot be sustained.); hypotension; or other abnormality
- Respiratory status abnormalities, the extent of which depends on what the patient can tolerate and the underlying cause of respiratory failure
- Relevant laboratory studies, including ABGs for blood gas derangements associated with ARF, sputum culture and sensitivity, and bedside spirometry (which typically shows a VC less than 15 ml/kg ideal body weight)

NURSING DIAGNOSES, OUTCOMES, AND INTERVENTIONS

Nursing Diagnosis: Impaired Gas Exchange

OUTCOMES. Common examples of expected outcomes for the patient with a diagnosis of *impaired gas exchange* are:

Patient will:

- Demonstrate improved ventilation and oxygenation.
- Have PaO_2, $PaCO_2$, and pH within acceptable baseline limits.
- Demonstrate mental status at prerespiratory failure level.
- Exhibit respiratory rate within or near normal levels, with moderate tidal volume.
- Have no dyspnea or preacute illness level of dyspnea.

NURSING INTERVENTIONS. Severe hypoxemia is incompatible with life. Thus it is imperative for the nurse to initiate oxygen therapy rapidly if severe hypoxemia is present. The effectiveness of oxygen therapy is evaluated with ABG measurements and pulse oximetry. Supplemental oxygen should be provided to maintain a PaO_2 of 60 to 90 mm Hg. Persons without underlying pulmonary disease can receive oxygen by either high-flow or low-flow systems. However, hazards are associated with prolonged exposure to high concentrations of oxygen. *Oxygen toxicity* is the term used to describe the damage to lung tissue that results from prolonged exposure to high oxygen concentrations. Although the exact effects of oxygen in any one individual may depend on the person's underlying pathologic condition, exposure to greater than 60% oxygen for more than 36 hours or exposure to 90% oxygen for more than 6 hours may result in atelectasis and alveolar collapse. Breathing very high concentrations of oxygen (80% to 100%) for prolonged periods (24 hours or more) is often associated with the development of ARDS. Thus a firm principle is to use the lowest amount of oxygen necessary to achieve an acceptable PaO_2.

Special precautions must be taken when administering oxygen to patients with COPD who are carbon dioxide retainers to avoid further elevation of their $PaCO_2$ levels, resulting in carbon dioxide narcosis or coma. These patients must receive supplemental oxygen via a controlled oxygen therapy system. The preferred mode is a nasal cannula or Venturi mask. A nasal cannula has the advantage of allowing the patient to talk, eat, and drink. However, the actual concentration of oxygen delivered to the lungs by cannula depends on the patient's ventilatory pattern. The Venturi mask

(Figure 27-14) provides oxygen at controlled ranges of 24% to 40% but may be poorly tolerated. Regardless of the oxygen delivery system used, the patient's response to oxygen therapy can be accurately assessed only by ABG measurements or pulse oximetry. The goal is to achieve a PaO_2 of 60 mm Hg, which allows an arterial saturation of 90% or greater.

Adequate oxygenation is essential for life. Therefore if adequate oxygenation cannot be maintained without a concurrent rise in $PaCO_2$ (hypercapnia), oxygen therapy must be provided by alternative delivery modes. (See previous section on Mechanical Ventilation.) Although carbon dioxide narcosis might be precipitated if a chronically hypoxemic person receives high concentrations of oxygen, treatment of the hypoxemia is the first priority in the patient's care.

Nursing interventions for patients with ARF must be implemented in a firm but empathetic manner. The patient may be agitated or nearly exhausted from hypoxemia, hypercapnia, and the increased work of breathing. It is imperative that the patient be gently guided in respiratory maneuvers to improve breathing. The nurse must be alert for signs and symptoms indicating that the patient's condition has changed from acutely ill but adequately ventilating to critically ill with insufficient ventilation to maintain body functions. Nursing interventions include:

- Frequent assessment of respiratory status, vital signs, level of consciousness, tolerance of ventilatory support, ventilator settings
- Facilitation of use of controlled breathing techniques
- Review of pertinent laboratory data, especially electrolytes, hematocrit
- Judicious administration of analgesia, especially opiates

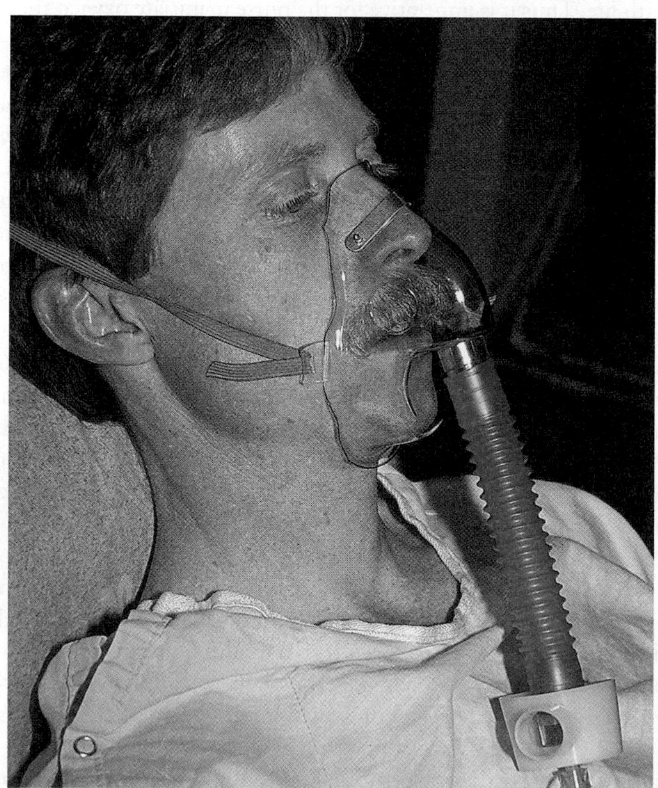

Figure 27-14 Venturi mask.

RELATED NIC INTERVENTIONS. Airway Management, Oxygen Therapy, Ventilation Assistance, Vital Signs Monitoring

Nursing Diagnosis: Ineffective Airway Clearance

OUTCOMES. Common examples of expected outcomes for the patient with a diagnosis of *ineffective airway clearance* are:
Patient will:

- Demonstrate effective airway clearance.
- Use effective coughing maneuvers.
- Have breath sounds clear or at baseline level.
- Use nebulizers, MDIs, and humidifiers appropriately.

NURSING INTERVENTIONS. Airways clogged with excess mucus are one of the most reversible precipitating components of ARF. Causes of mucus clogging are many, and positive-pressure ventilation itself may contribute to increased mucus production. Monitoring is basic to effective intervention; and patients' breath sounds need to be auscultated at least every 1 to 2 hours in the acute phase of respiratory failure.

The nurse helps patients cough effectively using the huff technique; changes the patient's position every 2 hours; elevates the patient's head and chest; guides the patient in performing frequent deep breathing exercises or using the sigh mechanism on the ventilator; encourages the patient to be out of bed as tolerated; and promotes sufficient fluid intake to mobilize secretions (3 to 4 L, unless contraindicated, has traditionally been encouraged, but some evidence suggests that this quantity may not be needed). In addition, humidification of the airway is maintained to further liquefy secretions, and nasotracheal suctioning is done if the patient is unable to cough effectively.

RELATED NIC INTERVENTIONS. Airway Management, Mechanical Ventilation, Respiratory Monitoring

Nursing Diagnosis: Decreased Cardiac Output

OUTCOMES. Common examples of expected outcomes for the patient with a diagnosis of *decreased cardiac output* are:
Patient will:

- Maintain adequate cardiac output.
- Have blood pressure within acceptable limits.
- Demonstrate heart rate and rhythm within acceptable limits.
- Have palpable and equal peripheral pulses.
- Maintain urinary output of greater than 30 ml/hr.

NURSING INTERVENTIONS. Decreased cardiac output may be a complication of ARF or may be a precipitating factor related to underlying cor pulmonale. Diminished cardiac output causes tissue hypoxia, which creates a metabolic acidosis in addition to the respiratory acidosis caused by the respiratory failure. Thus the nurse must assess vital signs and hemodynamic parameters (arterial, central venous, pulmonary, and left atrial pressures) at least every hour during ARF. In addition, the nurse must monitor the patient for signs of inadequate tissue perfusion (urinary output of less than 30 ml/hr, cool extremities with decreased peripheral pulses) and for cardiac arrhythmias.

RELATED NIC INTERVENTIONS. Cardiac Care, Circulatory Care: Mechanical Assist Device, Oxygen Therapy, Vital Signs Monitoring

Nursing Diagnosis: Imbalanced Nutrition: Less Than Body Requirements

OUTCOMES. Common examples of expected outcomes for the patient with a diagnosis of *imbalanced nutrition: less than body requirements* are:

Patient will:

- Maintain nutritional intake adequate to balance metabolic needs.
- Maintain weight at preacute illness weight or make progress toward an established goal weight.

NURSING INTERVENTIONS. Individuals with ARF are at increased risk for nutritional deficits because of the increased work of breathing. The overall focus of nutritional interventions is to prevent or correct malnutrition. Nutritional intake affects ventilatory drive, respiratory muscle function, and the amount of oxygen consumed and carbon dioxide produced from metabolic processes. Nutritional status can have a major impact on the individual's ability to be successfully weaned from the ventilator. The nurse focuses on providing appropriate nutrition to meet the patient's specific metabolic needs while on the ventilator and during and after weaning from it. Nutritional support by either enteral supplementation or parenteral hyperalimentation may be necessary. Whenever feasible, the enteral route should be used because it poses fewer risks and is more economical. It is advisable to supply at least 50% of total calories in the form of lipids to minimize high levels of carbon dioxide production.

RELATED NIC INTERVENTIONS. Nutrition Management, Nutrition Therapy

EVALUATION

To evaluate the effectiveness of nursing interventions, compare patient behaviors with those stated in the expected patient outcomes.

RELATED NOC OUTCOMES. Circulation Status, Mechanical Ventilation Response: Adult, Nutritional Status: Nutrient Intake, Respiratory Status: Ventilation, Tissue Perfusion: Pulmonary, Vital Signs

GERONTOLOGIC CONSIDERATIONS

Care for older adults with respiratory failure is similar to that for older adults with COPD. Some evidence does exist that those older than 70 years are especially susceptible to long-term ventilator dependence. Elderly patients with COPD and subsequent respiratory failure have poor outcomes, which are more a product of the disease process than age.[42]

Lung Transplantation

Etiology and Epidemiology. Successful transplantation of the lungs became a reality in the 1980s. The first lung transplant was performed in the United States in 1983 on a patient with pulmonary fibrosis. (A heart-lung transplant was performed in 1981.) Lung transplants may involve a single lung, two lungs, or a lobe of a lung. Many of the patients who need lung transplants have a history of primary pulmonary hypertension. Other diseases that cause problems severe enough to require a lung transplant include emphysema, CF, sarcoidosis, and pulmonary fibrosis. It is a last-resort treatment for lung failure.[46,55]

The procedure is usually limited to patients less than 60 years old who are not active smokers and who suffer from advanced lung disease. Single lung transplantation is used for restrictive lung disease, since the decreased compliance and increased pulmonary resistance of the recipient's remaining lung result in preferential ventilation and perfusion of the transplanted lung. Double lung transplants are typically used in persons with emphysema or CF. Most lobe transplants are for CF patients.[46]

COMPLICATIONS. This is an extreme measure for preserving life in a patient who has damaged and diseased lungs. The survival rate ranges as high as 80% at 1 year after transplant and 60% at 4 years after transplant, but this is not without some long-term problems for the patient. The major one is the ongoing immunosuppression process from antirejection drugs. Complications include lymphoproliferative disorders, pulmonary edema, infections, phrenic nerve injury, atrial fibrillation, and deep venous thrombosis.[39,46,55]

Posttransplant lymphoproliferative disorders (PTLD) are a heterogeneous group of diseases that occur often after lung transplant. Lung transplant recipients are at a higher risk for PTLD than other solid organ transplant recipients. The intensive posttransplant immunosuppressive regimens coupled with a greater degree of pulmonary transplant lymphoid tissues likely contribute. PTLD can occur anytime after transplantation, with highest incidence in the first year. Manifestations vary from asymptomatic pulmonary nodules to marked constitutional symptoms, including fever, lethargy, and weight loss. A biopsy of lung tissue is required for diagnosis. PTLD is often confined to the transplanted lung, but in single lung transplant patients it is occasionally seen in both the transplanted and the native lung.

Risk factors for PTLD include pediatric age, age over 55 years, cytomegalovirus infection, specific immunosuppressive regimens, and Epstein-Barr virus seroconversion. Treatment in patients with less aggressive disease begins with a decrease in immunosuppression. This therapy may, in fact, be curative in early lesions. Other treatment options include antivirals (acyclovir, ganciclovir), but this approach has been minimally effective. Chemotherapy may be used in disseminated disease, but patients have difficulty tolerating this treatment and the side effects. Radiotherapy with surgical resection for PTLD may have a role in specific situations. The use of anti-B-cell monoclonal antibodies has shown promise.[46]

Infection is a risk for any transplant recipient but is of particular concern for lung transplant recipients. Obliterative bronchiolitis causes severe deterioration of lung function in as many as 50% of lung transplant recipients after the first year. It is mostly irreversible, and the only viable treatment option is retransplantation. The cause of this condition has not been determined. Possibilities include chronic rejection, viral infection, cyclosporine toxicity, long-term denervation of the lung, the lack of lymphatics, and the loss of bronchial blood supply. Patients experience a cough and progressive dyspnea. Obliterative bronchiolitis is diagnosed with fiberoptic bronchoscopy and transbronchial lung biopsy.[14,16]

Collaborative Care Management. Single lung transplants are performed through an anterolateral thoracotomy (Figure 27-15).

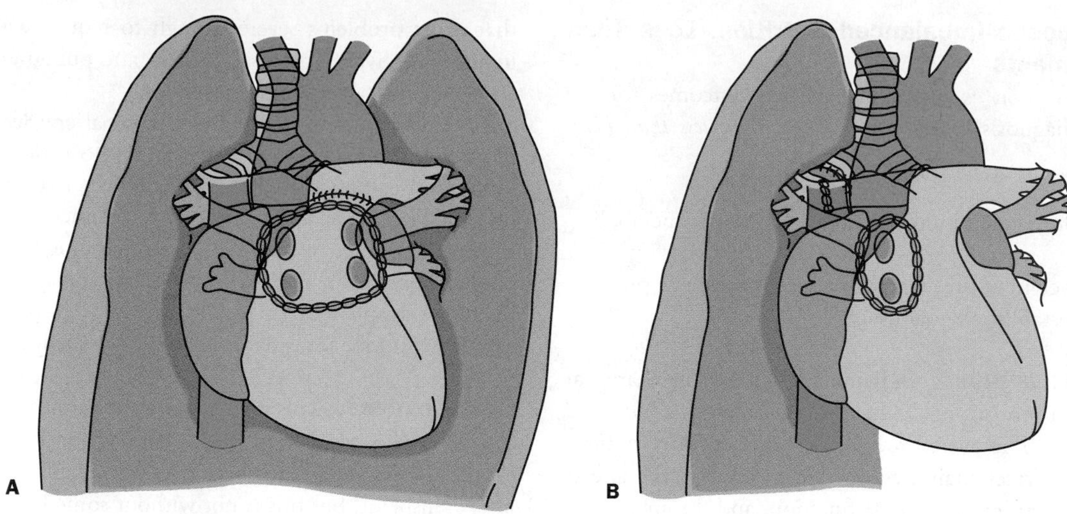

Figure 27-15 Anastomoses for **A,** double lung, and **B,** single lung transplantation.

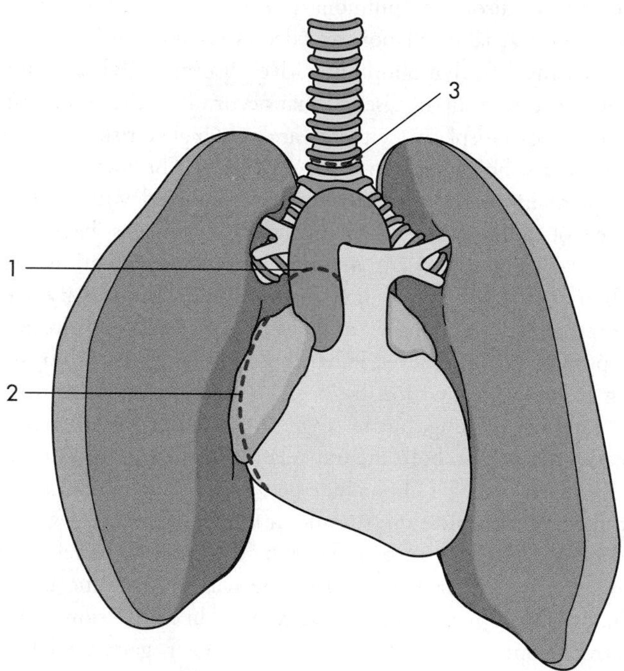

Figure 27-16 Anastomotic sites in heart-lung transplant. *1,* Aorta; *2,* right atria; *3,* trachea.

Some patients, especially those with primary pulmonary hypertension, require cardiopulmonary bypass. The double lung transplant procedure has been modified to a bilateral single lung transplant procedure with individual bronchial anastomoses (Figure 27-16). Cardiopulmonary bypass is required in the double lung procedure.

When heart-lung procedures are performed with the use of cardiopulmonary bypass, the recipient's heart is first removed and the phrenic nerves isolated. Enough left atrium is removed to allow the donor's right lung to fit into the right pleural space. The lungs are then removed individually and the donor's heart-lung bloc is placed into the recipient's chest. Tracheal anastomosis completes the surgical process.

The patient is cared for in an intensive care setting after surgery. The most important aspects of care are promoting adequate airway clearance and gas exchange and preventing major complications associated with lung transplant. Poor gas exchange is a common complication and may be caused by reperfusion edema of the lung, impaired cough, infection, or rejection. Appropriate immunosuppressive therapy is initiated, and the patient is monitored closely for signs of rejection.

It is common for the patient undergoing lung transplantation to experience two or three episodes of acute rejection during the first 6 weeks after transplantation (see Clinical Manifestations box).[14] As with other solid organ transplants, treatment of rejection involves enhancement of immunosuppression, but corticosteroids are not used for the first 7 to 14 days after the lung transplant procedure, since they jeopardize healing of the tracheal and bronchial anastomoses. Once healing has occurred, immunosuppressive therapy using drugs such as cyclosporine begins, but these drugs also reduce the body's ability to fight infections. Research is being conducted to enhance the delivery of the drugs to improve their effectiveness in the rejection process (see Future Watch box).

Aggressive respiratory care is critical. It is difficult for the patient to clear the airway because the transplanted lung (or lungs) is denervated below the level of the trachea and mucociliary clearance is decreased. Care includes frequent position changes and deep breathing, along with postural drainage and coughing. Supplemental oxygen is necessary. Patients with lung transplants are prone to cardiovascular complications from hypervolemia or hypovolemia, myocardial irritability, or decreased contractility. Hemodynamic status is carefully managed to maintain adequate cardiac output without fluid overload that can lead to pulmonary edema and elevated pulmonary vascular resistance.

CLINICAL MANIFESTATIONS
Lung Transplant Rejection

- Fever
- Dyspnea
- Nonproductive cough
- Malaise
- Decreased oxygen saturations
- Abnormal pulmonary function tests

Future Watch

An Inhaled Antirejection Drug?

A transplanted lung is highly susceptible to rejection, more so than any other transplanted organ. Patients who have had a lung transplant are being tested with an experimental version of inhaled cyclosporine that may significantly increase their chances of survival. It is delivered directly to the lungs and helps prevent immune cells from attacking the transplanted organ. In a recent study over 2 to 5 years, patients using the inhaled antirejection medication were four times more likely to survive than those taking a placebo. Also, patients using the inhaled cyclosporine had a significantly lower rate of rejection. Researchers will seek U.S. Food and Drug Administration approval for the new therapy.

Lung transplants: inhaled antirejection drug shows promise, *Nursing* 34(7):26, 2004.

Patients are at risk for dysrhythmias because of the use of cardiopulmonary bypass.[39]

The use of anticoagulants with cardiopulmonary bypass or excessive replacement of blood products puts patients at risk for bleeding from coagulopathy. Careful monitoring of coagulation studies and blood loss from mediastinal tubes is imperative. Administration of platelets or fresh frozen plasma may be necessary. Additional care needs include nutritional support, comfort measures, and promotion of adequate sleep.

Preparation for discharge involves teaching the importance of adherence to the regimen and regular follow-up monitoring. Postrecovery patients are cautioned about daily activities and exercising. Although they might experience an increased ability to participate in exercises, research has found limitations to exercise for up to 2 years.[34] Quality of life before and after transplantation is still controversial. Although the surgery is often a last-hope-for-survival procedure, its impact on the patient's quality of life is still being evaluated[32] (see Research box).

Research

Lanuza DM et al: Prospective study of functional status and quality of life before and after lung transplantation, *Chest* 118(1):115-122, 2000.

This study looked at the impact of lung transplants on patients' ability to function and their quality of life (QOL). The researchers monitored 10 participants before their transplants through 3 months after surgery. Researchers looked at the patients' perceived status, moods, respiratory functioning, and satisfaction with their QOL and health status. The study used a QOL instrument, respiratory function tests, and mood and satisfaction with health status scales.

The results showed the participants' overall lung function was significantly improved after the surgery, as was their health status and QOL perception. However, the researchers cautioned that this study only reported satisfaction and QOL up to 3 months after surgery. Other studies have found questionable results about the patient's limitations and QOL after lung transplant surgery. They recommended further studies be done following patients for longer periods after surgery to evaluate their perspective on health status and QOL.

Preparing for Practice

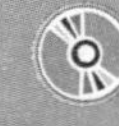

CD-ROM Activity Select Exercise Three: Chronic Obstructive Pulmonary Disease on the Companion CD.

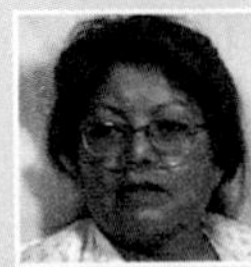

Patient: *Sally Begay,* **Room 304**

Sally Begay, a 58-year-old Navajo woman, was admitted with a rule out diagnosis of Hantavirus that was subsequently determined to be pneumonia. Ms. Begay has a history of hypertension, coronary disease, and myocardial infarction.

Assessment

View the patient's **Report**.

Review the patient's **Medical Record.** Read the entire History & Physical; Physicians' Orders; and Diagnostics sections.

Conduct a **Patient Interview**. As you conduct your interview, focus primarily on data that will be helpful in planning care for this patient. Record the data you collect.

Nursing Diagnoses, Outcomes, and Interventions

1. It is essential to take a current health history to properly evaluate a respiratory disorder. For each of the following complaints, write two questions that could be used to further evaluate each symptom. *Hint*: Use information in the Nursing Management section for each disease state if needed.
   Dyspnea
      Cough
   Sputum production
      Hemoptysis
      Wheezing
      Chest pain
      Upper respiratory symptoms
      Pain in right upper quadrant (hepatomegaly—enlarged liver)
2. How long has Sally Begay had bronchitis?
3. In addition to the respiratory diagnoses of pneumonia, what other medical diagnoses does Sally Begay have?
4. Read the sections in this chapter describing COPD, emphysema, and chronic bronchitis (see pp. 671 to 675). Define each.
5. Name four risk factors in the etiology of COPD.
6. Review the results of the chest x-ray that was ordered for Sally Begay in the Diagnostics section of the **Medical Record**. Focus on the radiologic report by Dr. Kawasaka. What findings listed in the chest x-ray report are consistent with COPD? *Hint*: The general discussion of chest x-ray studies in Chapter 24 of the textbook may be helpful in understanding the results.
7. You have determined that a nursing diagnosis of *ineffective breathing pattern* is appropriate for Ms. Begay. What nursing interventions would you implement to address this problem?
8. How should the effectiveness of the interventions be evaluated?

Critical Thinking

1. A patient has just been admitted to your unit with a history of COPD. She is developing respiratory complications. What nursing interventions are appropriate? What laboratory tests do you want to review?
2. Consider the trend of increasing the life expectancy for patients with CF. What ethical issues arise from this trend? What is the nurse's responsibility when discussing these issues?
3. A patient with asthma is on your unit. This patient has had many episodes of status asthmaticus in the past. What preparations should you make in case she has another episode while hospitalized? What nursing assessments are important?

References

1. American Lung Association: *COPD fact sheet*, accessed Jan 2005 from website: www.lungusa.org.
2. American Thoracic Society: COPD: definitions, epidemiology, pathophysiology, diagnosis and staging, *Am J Respir Crit Care Med* 152(5, Pt 1): 1713–1735, 1995.
3. Andenaes R, Kalfoss M, Wahl A: Psychological distress and quality of life in hospitalized patients with chronic obstructive pulmonary disease, *J Adv Nurs* 46(5):523–530, 2004.
4. Banasik J: Diagnosing alpha$_1$-antitrypsin deficiency, *Nurse Pract* 26(1): 58–62, 2001.
5. Bryan CL, Homma A: Acute respiratory failure. In Rakel RE, Bope ET, editors: *Conn's current therapy 2001,* Philadelphia, 2001, Saunders.
6. Carlson BW, Mascarella JJ: Changes in sleep patterns in COPD: a new vital sign in the management of people with chronic obstructive pulmonary disease, *Am J Nurs* 103(12):71–74, 2003.
7. Carson AR, Hieber KV: Adult pediatric patients, *Am J Nurse* 101(3):46–55, 2001.
8. Chu CM et al: Noninvasive ventilation in patients with acute hypercapnic exacerbation of chronic obstructive pulmonary disease who refused endotracheal intubation, *Crit Care Med* 32(2):372–377, 2004.
9. Cicutto LC, Downew GP: Biological markers in diagnosing, monitoring and treating asthma: a focus on noninvasive measurements, *AACN Clin Issues Adv Pract Acute Crit Care* 15(1):97-111, 2004.
10. Clark E et al: Cognitive dissonance and undergraduate nursing students' knowledge of and attitudes about smoking, *J Adv Nurs* 46(6):586–594, 2004.
11. Colombo JL: Long-acting bronchodilators in cystic fibrosis, *Curr Opin Pulm Med* 9(6):504–508, 2003.
12. Corbridge SJ, Corbridge TC: Severe exacerbations of asthma, *Crit Care Nurs Q* 27(3):207–228, 2004.
13. Covey MK, Larson JL: Exercise and COPD: aerobic and strengthening exercises are crucial in patients with chronic obstructive pulmonary disease, *Am J Nurs* 104(5):40–43, 2004.
14. Dabbs AD et al: Striving for normalcy: symptoms and the threat of rejection after lung transplantation, *Soc Sci & Med* 59(7):1473–1484, 2004.
15. De Jong SR, Veltman RH: The effectiveness of a CNS-led community-based COPD screening and intervention program, *Clin Nurse Spec* 18(2):72–79, 2004.
16. De Perrot M et al: Twenty-year experience of lung transplantation at a single center: influence of recipient diagnosis on long-term survival, *J Thorac Cardiovasc Surg* 127(5):1493–1501, 2004.
17. De Serres FJ: Worldwide racial and ethnic distribution of 1-antitrypsin deficiency: summary of an analysis of published genetic epidemiologic surveys, *Chest* 122:1818–1829, 2002.
18. Dipiro JT et al: *Pharmacotherapy,* Norwalk, Conn, 1999, Appleton & Lange.
19. Doherty DE: Identification and assessment of chronic obstructive pulmonary disease in the elderly, *J Am Med Dir Assoc* 4(5):S116–S120, 2003.
20. Donaldson SH, Boucher RC: Update on pathogenesis of cystic fibrosis lung disease, *Curr Opin Pulm Med* 9(6):486–491, 2003.
21. Elpern EH, Cheatham J: Inpatient care of the adult with an exacerbation of cystic fibrosis, *AACN Clin Issues* 12(2):293–304, 2001.
22. Enright PL et al: Underdiagnosis and undertreatment of asthma in the elderly, *Chest* 116(3):603–613, 1999.
23. Ferrari M et al: Minimally supervised home rehabilitation improves exercise capacity and health status in patients with COPD, *Am J Phys Med Rehabil* 83(5):337–343, 2004.
24. Gillick MR: Medicare coverage for technological innovations—time for new criteria? *N Engl J Med* 350(21):2199–2203, 2004.
25. Gronkiewicz C, Borkgren-Okonek M: Acute exacerbation of COPD: nursing application of evidence-based guidelines, part 2, *Crit Care Nurs Q Adv Respir Manage* 27(4):336–352, 2004.
26. Highland KB: Inhaled corticosteroids in chronic obstructive pulmonary disease: is there a long-term benefit? *Curr Opin Pulm Med* 10(2):113–119, 2004.
27. Hill N: Non-invasive mechanical ventilation for post-acute care, *Clin Chest Med* 22(1):35–54, 2001.
28. Kanervisto M, Paavilainen E, Astedt-Kurki P: Impact of chronic obstructive pulmonary disease on family functioning, *Heart Lung* 32(6):360–367, 2003.
29. Kanner RE: Chronic obstructive pulmonary disease. In Rakel RE, Bope ET, editors: *Conn's current therapy 2001,* Philadelphia, 2001, Saunders.
30. Kutty K: Sleep and chronic obstructive pulmonary disease, *Curr Opin Pulm Med* 10(2):104–112, 2004.
31. Lantz MS, Gianbuco V: Smoking cessation: the key to treating older smokers? Don't quit helping, *Geriatrics* 56(5):58–59, 2001.
32. Lanuza DM et al: Prospective study of functional status and quality of life before and after lung transplantation, *Chest* 118(1):115–122, 2000.
33. Larson JL, Covey MK, Corbridge S: Inspiratory muscle strength in chronic obstructive pulmonary disease, *AACN Clin Issues Adv Pract Acute Crit Care* 13(2):320–332, 2002.
34. Mathur S, Reid DW, Levy R: Exercise limitation in recipients of lung transplants, *Phys Ther* 84(12):1178–1187, 2004.
35. Murphy KR et al: Asthma: helping patients breathe easier, *Nurs Pract* 29(10):38–55, 2004.
36. Murray JF, Nadal JA, editors: *Textbook of respiratory medicine,* ed 3, Philadelphia, 2000, Saunders.
37. National Heart, Lung, and Blood Institute: *Morbidity and mortality chartbook,* 2004, USDHHS.
38. Nevins ML, Epstein SK: Weaning from prolonged mechanical ventilation, *Clin Chest Med* 22(1):13–33, 2001.
39. Nielsen TD et al: Atrial fibrillation after pulmonary transplant, *Chest* 126(2):496–501, 2004.
40. Pingleton SK: Nutrition in chronic critical illness, *Clin Chest Med* 22(1):149–163, 2001.
41. Raguso C et al: Chronic hypoxia: common traits between chronic obstructive pulmonary disease and altitude, *Curr Opin Clin Nutr Metab Care* 7(4):411–417, 2004.
42. Rosenthal RA, Kavic SM: Assessment and management of the geriatric patient, *Crit Care Med* 32(4):S92–S105, 2004.
43. Sethi S: New developments in the pathogenesis of acute exacerbations of chronic obstructive pulmonary disease, *Curr Opin Infect Dis* 17(2):113–119, 2004.
44. Silverman E et al: Current management of bronchiectasis: review and 3 case studies, *Heart Lung* 32(1):59–64, 2003.
45. Snow V, Lascher S, Mottur-Pilson C: The evidence base for management of acute exacerbations of COPD: clinical practice guidelines, part 1, *Chest* 119(4):1185–1189, 2001.
46. Snyder LD, Palmer SM: Posttransplant lymphoproliferative disorders in lung transplant, *Curr Opin Organ Transpl* 9(3):325–331, 2004.
47. Starnes VA et al: A decade of living lobar lung transplantation: recipient outcomes, *J Thorac Cardiovasc Surg* 127(1):114–122, 2004.
48. Tamul PC, Peruzzi WT: Assessment and management of patients with pulmonary disease, *Crit Care Med* 32(4):S137–S145, 2004.
49. Theander K, Unosson M: Fatigue in patients with chronic obstructive pulmonary disease, *J Adv Nurs* 45(2):172–177, 2004.
50. Tomas LHS, Varkey B: Improving health-related quality of life in chronic obstructive pulmonary disease, *Curr Opin Pulm Med* 10(2):120–127, 2004.

51. Troosters T, Gosselink R, Decramer M: Chronic obstructive pulmonary disease and chronic heart failure: two muscle diseases? *J Cardiopulm Rehabil* 24(3):137–145, 2004.
52. Trow TK: Lung-volume reduction surgery for severe emphysema: appraisal of its current status, *Curr Opin Pulm Med* 10(2):128–132, 2004.
53. Turato G, Zuin R, Saetta M: Pathogenesis and pathology of COPD, *Respiration* 68(2):117–128, 2001.
54. US Department of Health and Human Services: *Healthy people 2010: understanding and improving health,* Washington, DC, 2000, The Department.
55. US National Library of Medicine and National Institutes of Health Medline Plus: *Lung transplant,* accessed Nov 2005 from website: www.nlm.nih.medlineplus/ency/article.
56. Varkey AB: Chronic obstructive pulmonary disease in women: exploring gender differences, *Curr Opin Pulm Med* 10(2):98–103, 2004.
57. Witt WP et al: The mental health impact of living with a spouse with chronic obstructive pulmonary disease, *J Gen Intern Med* 19(Suppl 1): 222–223, 2004.

evolve Visit the Evolve website: http://evolve.elsevier.com/Monahan/medsurg

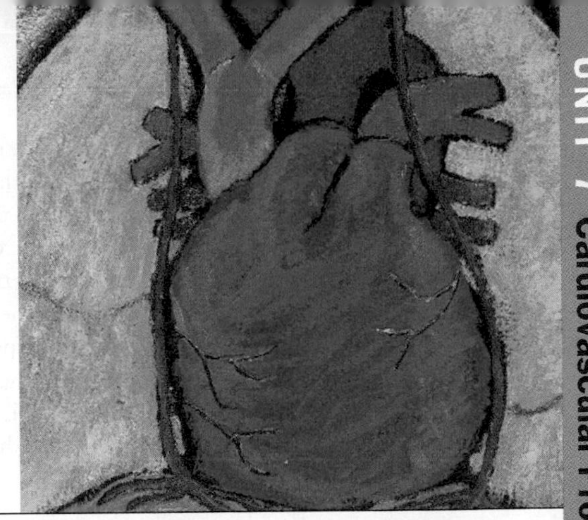

CHAPTER 28

Assessment of the Cardiovascular System

by Shelley Yerger Huffstutler

OBJECTIVES

After studying this chapter, the learner should be able to:

1. Describe the health history and physical examination data relevant to a cardiovascular examination.
2. Discuss the basic structure and function of the heart and peripheral vasculature.
3. Explain the conduction system of the heart in relation to the cardiac cycle.
4. Analyze factors that affect cardiac output.
5. Discuss physiologic changes that occur in the cardiovascular system with aging.
6. Differentiate common manifestations of altered cardiac functioning.
7. Explain the significance of various diagnostic tests used to assess cardiac functioning.
8. Compare nursing care of patients undergoing various cardiovascular diagnostic testing procedures.

KEY TERMS

action potential, p. 717
afterload, p. 722
automaticity, p. 716
cardiac cycle, p. 719
cardiac output, p. 720
conductivity, p. 716
contractility, p. 716
depolarization, p. 718
diastole, p. 714
excitability, p. 716
murmurs, p. 730
palpitation, p. 727
preload, p. 721
refractory period, p. 719
repolarization, p. 718
resting membrane potential, p. 717
stroke volume, p. 720
syncope, p. 727
systole, p. 714

Cardiovascular disease (CVD) in the United States represents a continuing crisis of epidemic proportions, with nearly 960,000 individuals dying from heart disease and stroke each year. CVD has been the leading cause of death in this country every year since 1900, with the exception of 1918, the year of the great influenza epidemic. According to the most recent statistics, if all forms of major CVD were eliminated, life expectancy would rise almost 7 years. Furthermore, although it is often perceived as a disease of older age, approximately 50% of CVD diagnoses and 15% of CVD deaths are in patients under 65 years of age.[1]

The cardiovascular system consists of the heart and great vessels, as well as the arteries and veins of the peripheral vascular system. The primary purpose of the cardiovascular system is to pump the blood and distribute it to all areas of the body. This chapter reviews the anatomy and physiology of the cardiovascular system, discusses the components of a cardiovascular health history and physical examination, and describes various cardiovascular diagnostic tests and their associated nursing care.

Anatomy and Physiology of the Heart

The heart is a relatively small organ that weighs 300 g and is approximately the size of a fist. It is located in the middle of the mediastinum, and the lungs partially overlap it. This pulsatile four-chambered pump beats approximately 72 times per minute, pumping more than 5 L of blood each minute, or about 2000 gal/day. It continuously propels oxygenated blood into the arterial system and receives poorly oxygenated blood from the venous system. The heart muscle rests on the diaphragm and is tilted forward and to the left so that the apex of the heart is rotated anteriorly.

The heart is enclosed by the pericardium, which consists of two layers: the inner layer (visceral pericardium) and the outer layer (parietal pericardium). The two pericardial surfaces are separated by a pericardial space that normally contains approximately 10 to 20 ml of thin, clear pericardial fluid. This lubricating fluid moistens the contact surfaces of the pericardial layers and reduces the friction produced by the pumping action of the heart. The visceral pericardium encases the heart and extends several centimeters onto each of the great vessels. The parietal pericardium is attached anteriorly to the manubrium and xiphoid process of the sternum, posteriorly to the vertebral column, and inferiorly to the diaphragm.

The three layers of the heart are the (1) epicardium, the outer layer of the heart, which is the same structure as the visceral pericardium; (2) myocardium, the middle layer of the heart, which is composed of striated muscle fibers and is responsible for the heart's contractile force; and (3) endocardium, the innermost layer of the heart, which consists of endothelial tissue. The endocardium lines the inside of the chambers of the heart and covers the heart valves.

Chambers

The heart is divided in half by a muscular wall (septum) (Figure 28-1). Each half has an upper collecting chamber (atrium) and a lower pumping chamber (ventricle). Oxygen-poor venous blood enters the right atrium, flows from the right atrium to the right ventricle (mainly by gravity) when the tricuspid valve is opened, and is pumped into the pulmonary artery to the lungs. Oxygen-rich blood returns from the lungs to the left atrium, enters the left ventricle when the mitral valve is opened, and is ejected into the aorta for distribution to the peripheral tissues.

The right atrium is a thin-walled structure that serves as a reservoir for venous blood returning to the heart. Venous blood returns to the heart via the superior and inferior vena cavae and the coronary sinus, which drains venous blood from the heart muscle. Blood is temporarily stored in the right atrium during right ventricular **systole** (contraction). During ventricular **diastole** (filling), approximately 80% of the stored blood from the right atrium flows by gravity into the ventricle through the tricuspid valve. The remaining 20% of the venous return is delivered to the ventricles during atrial systole. This additional 15% to 20% of the venous return, which is actively propelled into the ventricles, is called the *atrial kick*.

The right ventricle is normally the most anterior structure of the heart and is situated immediately beneath the sternum. The right ventricle receives venous blood from the right atrium during ventricular diastole. During ventricular diastole this blood is propelled through the pulmonic valve into the pulmonary artery and then to the lungs. Because the pulmonary system is a low-pressure system, the overall workload of the right ventricle is much lighter than that of the left ventricle. The right ventricle has a crescent-shaped chamber and a thin outer wall that is 4 to 5 mm thick. This thin structure is suitable for right ventricular systole because the right ventricle contracts against low resistance.

The thin-walled left atrium receives oxygenated blood from the four pulmonary veins and serves as a reservoir during left ventricular systole. Blood flows by gravity from the left atrium into the left ventricle through the opened mitral valve during ventricular diastole. Left atrial contraction then propels the remaining 20% of the blood stored in the atrium to the left ventricle. This atrial kick stretches the ventricle and prepares it for ventricular ejection. Blood is then ejected through the aortic valve into the systemic arterial circulation during ventricular systole. The left ventricle must contract against the high-pressure systemic circulation to deliver blood flow to the peripheral tissues. Therefore the left ventricular chamber is surrounded by 8 to 15 mm of thick muscle, approximately two to three times the thickness of the right ventricle. The thick muscle and ellipsoidal-sphere shape contribute to the powerful expulsive ability of the left ventricle.

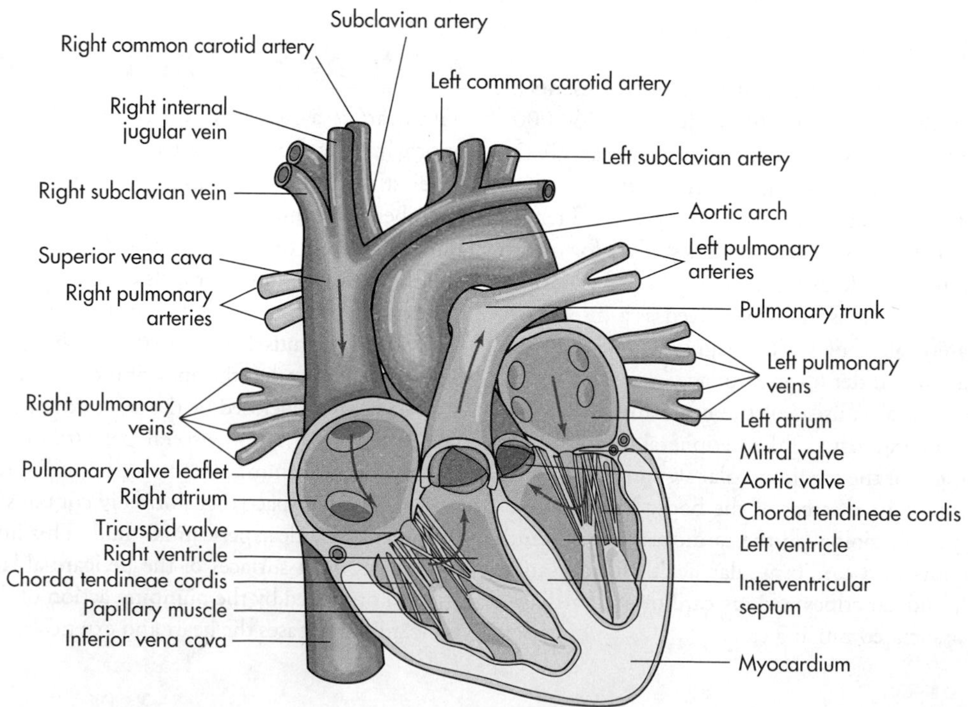

Figure 28-1 Heart in frontal section; course of blood through chambers.

Valves

The four cardiac valves are flaplike structures that maintain unidirectional (forward) blood flow through the heart chambers. These valves open and close in response to pressure and volume changes within the cardiac chambers. The cardiac valves are classified into two types: the atrioventricular (AV) valves, which separate the atria from the ventricles, and the semilunar valves, which separate the pulmonary artery and the aorta from their respective ventricles.

Atrioventricular Valves. The AV valves are the tricuspid valve, located between the right atrium and the right ventricle, and the bicuspid (or mitral) valve, located between the left atrium and left ventricle. The tricuspid valve contains three leaflets held in place by fibrous cords called the chordae tendineae cordis, which in turn are anchored to the ventricular wall by the papillary muscles. The mitral valve on the left side of the heart is a bicuspid valve with two valve cusps or leaflets. It also is attached to chordae tendineae cordis, which extend to the papillary muscles (Figure 28-2). The chordae tendineae cordis are extremely important because they support the AV valves during ventricular systole to prevent valvular prolapse into the atrium. Some leaflet overlapping occurs during closure of the AV valves, which helps prevent the backward flow of blood. Damage to the chordae tendineae cordis or to the papillary muscles allows for the regurgitation of blood back into the atrium during ventricular systole, resulting in increased pressure and volume. During diastole the AV valves serve as a type of funnel, facilitating blood flow from the atria to the ventricles.

Semilunar Valves. The semilunar valves are the pulmonic and aortic valves. The pulmonic valve lies between the right ventricle and the pulmonary artery. The aortic valve lies between the left ventricle and the aorta. The structural design of the semilunar valves is different and simpler than that of the AV valves; each consists of three cuplike cusps (see Figure 28-2). These valves are open during ventricular systole (contraction) to permit blood flow into the aorta and the pulmonary artery. They are closed during diastole (relaxation) to prevent retrograde flow from the aorta and the pulmonary artery back into the ventricles.

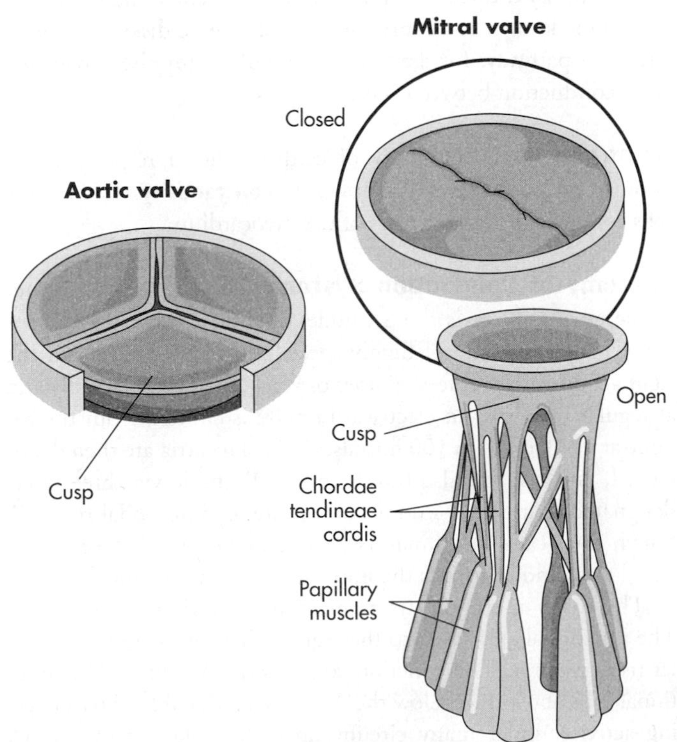

Figure 28-2 Aortic and mitral (bicuspid) valves.

Coronary Arteries

The coronary arteries arise from the aorta (just behind the cusps of the aortic valve) in an area known as Valsalva's sinus. The function of the coronary artery system is to provide an adequate blood supply to the myocardium.

There are two main coronary arteries, the left and the right (Figure 28-3). The left coronary artery (LCA) divides into two branches: the left anterior descending (LAD) artery and the circumflex coronary artery (CCA). The LAD branch supplies the left ventricular myocardium, septum, anterior papillary muscle, and parts of the right ventricle. In addition, the LAD artery usually supplies the anterior apex and some part of the posterior apex. The CCA typically emerges at a sharp 90-degree angle from the LCA and is then directed toward the lateral left ventricle and apex. The CCA and its branches supply most of the left atrium, the lateral wall of the left ventricle, and part of the posterior wall of the left ventricle. Diagonal branches arise between the LAD artery and the CCA and are distributed along the free wall of the left ventricle.

Two important external landmarks—sulci, or grooves—are used in tracing the coronary circulation. The first is the AV groove, which encircles the heart between the atria and the ventricles. The second is the interventricular groove, which divides the right and left ventricles. The meeting of the two anatomic grooves on the posterior side of the heart is known as the crux of the heart. The location of the crux is significant because this is where the AV node is located. The terms *dominant left circulation* and *dominant right circulation* refer to whether the left or the right coronary artery turns at the crux of the heart and supplies the posterior interventricular groove. If the CCA extends as far as the posterior interventricular groove, the circulation is considered to be dominant left. This condition occurs in only 10% to 15% of the population.

The right main coronary artery (RCA) arises from the right Valsalva's sinus off the aorta and courses around the right AV groove. Its branches supply the right ventricle; a portion of the septum; and, in more than 50% of all persons, the sinoatrial (SA) node. In approximately 67% of all persons, the RCA turns at the crux of the heart and descends in the posterior interventricular groove. These hearts are classified as dominant right. The posterior descending branch of the RCA then supplies the posterior aspect of the septum and the posterior left papillary muscle before terminating in several branches to the left ventricular wall.

Great variation exists in the branching pattern of the coronary arteries. In approximately 18% of the population, the CCA reaches the crux of the heart with the RCA; this is the "balanced" coronary artery pattern. In the remaining persons, no true posterior interventricular branch exists; rather, many branches from either main coronary artery supply the posterior septum.

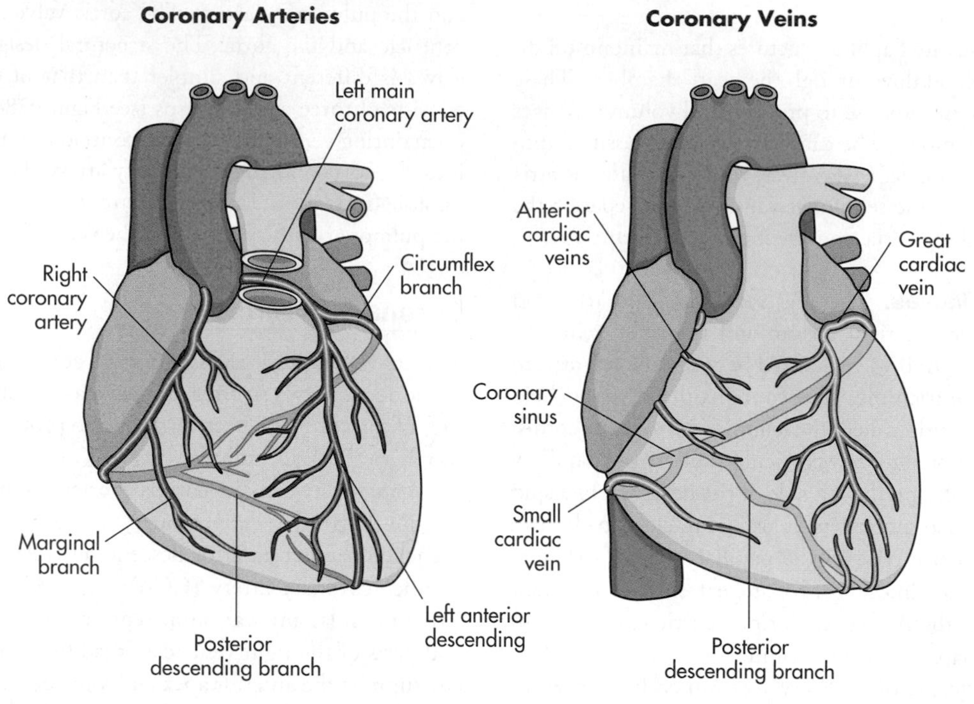

Figure 28-3 Coronary blood vessels.

Blood flow to the myocardium occurs almost exclusively during diastole, when coronary vascular resistance is diminished. During systole, coronary vascular resistance is increased because of the increased ventricular wall tension produced by ventricular contraction. During diastole, blood enters the coronary arteries at the pressure that exists at that moment in the aortic arch. This is termed *aortic diastolic pressure.*

Coronary venous drainage is accomplished via three subdivisions of the heart's venous system: (1) the thebesian veins drain a portion of the right atrial and right ventricular myocardium, (2) the anterior cardiac veins drain a large portion of the right ventricle, and (3) the coronary sinus and its branches drain the left ventricle and receive most myocardial venous return.

Conduction System

Properties of Cardiac Muscle. The mechanical contraction of the heart is the product of a stimulus-response process. The four properties of automaticity, excitability, conductivity, and contractility are integral components of the electromechanical events in the heart.

AUTOMATICITY. The heart's ability to initiate impulses regularly and spontaneously is known as **automaticity**, or rhythmicity. Although most cardiac cells have this ability, it is the prominent property of the SA node, making this cluster of cells the dominant pacemaker in the normal heart. Pacemaker cells are known to have lower resting membrane potentials than other myocardial cells and exhibit spontaneous depolarization.

EXCITABILITY. The ability of cardiac cells to respond to a stimulus by initiating a cardiac impulse is known as **excitability**. Excitatory cells differ from pacemaker cells in that pacemaker cells do not require a stimulus to initiate an impulse.

CONDUCTIVITY. The ability of cardiac cells to respond to a cardiac impulse by transmitting the impulse along cell membranes is referred to as **conductivity**. Cells that specialize in this function are found in the conduction system. Adjacent cells are connected end to end by a thickened portion of the sarcolemma or surface membrane known as an intercalated disk. These disks act as low-resistance pathways for the transmission of an impulse and ensure rapid conduction between cells.

CONTRACTILITY. The ability of cardiac cells to respond to an impulse by contracting is known as **contractility**. Contractile cells compose the largest mass of the myocardium.

Anatomy of Conduction System. The pacemaking center of the normal heart is the SA node, or sinus (Figure 28-4). It is composed of a group of highly specialized tissues located in the right atrium adjacent to the superior vena cava. Automatically and at regular intervals, an electrical impulse is emitted from the SA node at a rate of 60 to 100 impulses/min. The atria are then depolarized, and the impulse travels to the AV node via three tracts designated as anterior, middle, and posterior internodal tracts. A fourth tract called Bachmann's bundle branches off the anterior nodal tract and transmits the impulse to the left atrium.

The three internodal tracts meet at the atrionodal junction. The junctional area refers to the region where atrial and ventricular tissues merge. This junction contains the AV node. The junctional cells above and below the AV node are capable of pacemaking activity under many circumstances (e.g., failure of the SA node to fire). The AV node itself is located on the right side of the

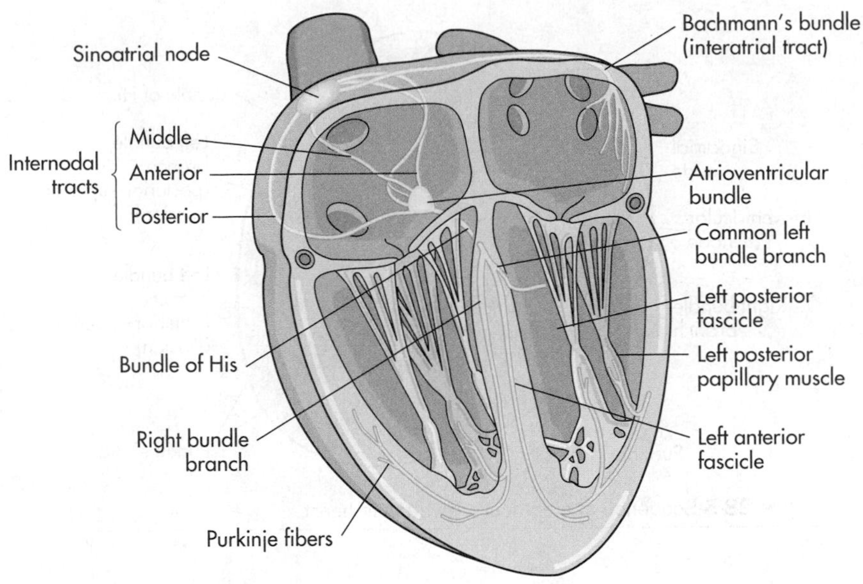

Figure 28-4 Heart's conduction system.

interatrial septum. These cells lack the ability to initiate electrical impulses (i.e., automaticity), but they are uniquely responsible for a brief physiologic delay in the conduction of the impulse to the ventricles.

The bundle of His begins anatomically at the "tail" of the AV node. It is a short, thick cable of fibers separated by collagen septa that bifurcates into the right bundle branch (RBB) and the left bundle branch (LBB). The RBB extends down the right side of the interventricular septum and is covered by a connective tissue sheath. It extends to the anterior papillary muscle of the right ventricle, where it merges with the Purkinje system. It lies close to the septal surface for much of its length, and therefore its functional ability is vulnerable to right ventricular pressure changes.

The LBB bifurcates into anterior and posterior fascicles. The anterior fascicle extends anteriorly down the left side of the interventricular septum to the anterior papillary muscle. The posterior fascicle is shorter and thicker and extends to the posterior papillary muscle of the left ventricle. Both fascicles connect with the Purkinje system and share equally in the spread of the impulse to the left ventricle.

Purkinje fibers lie as a network on the endocardial surface and penetrate the myocardium of both ventricles. They are responsible for transmitting the impulse to both ventricular free walls. Purkinje cells are elongated and contain intercalated disks, which contribute to the superior conductivity of myocardial tissue.

Sequence of Cardiac Activation. Depolarization (activation of the cardiac muscle) is initiated by an impulse from the SA node. The impulse first spreads through the right atrium and then activates the left atrium. Atrial activation normally is accomplished in 0.11 second or less. Shortly after the impulse reaches the left atrium, it also activates the junctional region and subsequently the AV node. The AV node delays the impulse about 0.1 second before the impulse enters the bundle of His and is transmitted along the bundle branches. Within the ventricles, the first structure to be activated is the ventricular septum. The septum is activated by the impulse traveling from the left side to the right side (Figure 28-5).

The impulse then continues down the remaining length of the bundle branches and into the Purkinje network, activating the ventricular walls almost simultaneously. Activation of the ventricular muscle then proceeds from the apex back toward the base of the heart to complete the process.

Depolarization of the cardiac musculature proceeds from endocardium to epicardium. Repolarization in the atria follows this same pathway. In contrast, repolarization of the ventricular musculature proceeds from epicardium to endocardium. Knowledge of the sequence of activation is fundamental to analysis of the electrocardiogram (ECG).

ACTION POTENTIAL. The resting myocardial cell has a membrane potential (i.e., an electrical charge) as a result of the relative distribution of sodium and potassium ions extracellularly. Whenever the cell is stimulated, the membrane potential changes. A graphic record of this change forms the basis for an ECG. The change in electrical potential in response to a stimulus is known as the **action potential**. The two components of the action potential are depolarization and repolarization.

RESTING MEMBRANE POTENTIAL. In the resting state the inside of the cell is negative with respect to the outside (Figure 28-6). Initiation and conduction of cardiac impulses depend on the cell's ability to maintain an electrical potential gradient when the cell is at rest. The main factor that contributes to the 290 mV **resting membrane potential** is the cell's permeability to potassium and not to sodium. The sodium-potassium exchange pump is responsible for actively transporting sodium out of the cell and potassium into the cell. The hydrolysis of adenosine triphosphate provides the energy for the functioning of this pump. Because more sodium is pumped out of the cell than potassium is moved in, a net outward current of positive ions further enhances the cell's negativity during the resting phase.

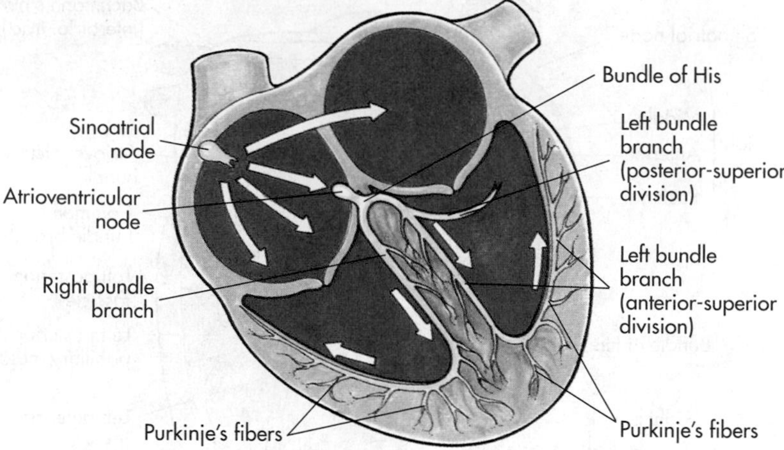

Figure 28-5 Sequence of electrical activation in heart.

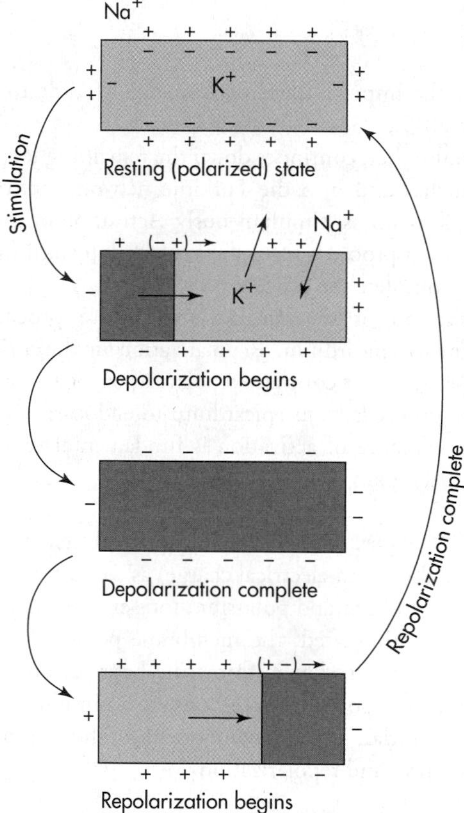

Figure 28-6 Process of depolarization and repolarization. *Na^+*, Sodium; *K^+*, potassium.

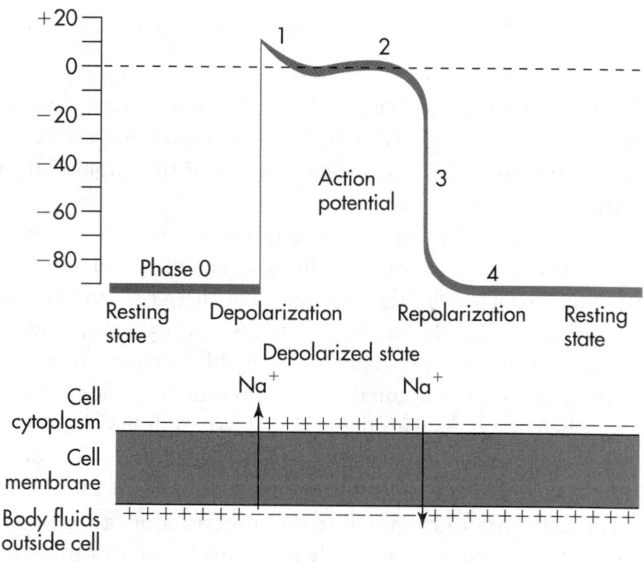

Figure 28-7 Phases of action potential of cardiac muscle. *Na^+*, Sodium.

DEPOLARIZATION. The initiation of a cardiac impulse begins with the process of **depolarization**. Depolarization indicates the rapid reversal of the resting membrane potential, which results from the following sequence of events: (1) the cell membrane permeability to sodium increases either spontaneously, in pacemaking cells, or in response to a stimulus; (2) a rapid influx of sodium occurs; and (3) potassium moves out of the cell. This movement of ions across the membrane creates an electrical current. When the amount of sodium entering the cell reaches a critical level, an electrical impulse is generated. The impulse may spread as a wave of depolarization to adjacent cells.

REPOLARIZATION. Repolarization is the process by which the cell is returned to the resting state. The cell membrane permeability to sodium decreases, and sodium leaves the cell. Potassium returns through an active ion transport system.

PHASES OF ACTION POTENTIAL

PHASE 0. Phase 0 is the tall upstroke of the action potential that occurs when the cell is stimulated, causing the cell membrane to become permeable to sodium ions. Fast sodium channels open to allow sodium to rush into the cell, creating a positive intracellular membrane potential of 0 to 120 mV (Figure 28-7).

PHASE 1. Phase 1 represents a brief period of rapid repolarization secondary to an outward positive current carried mainly by potassium ions. Sodium influx is abruptly terminated as soon as

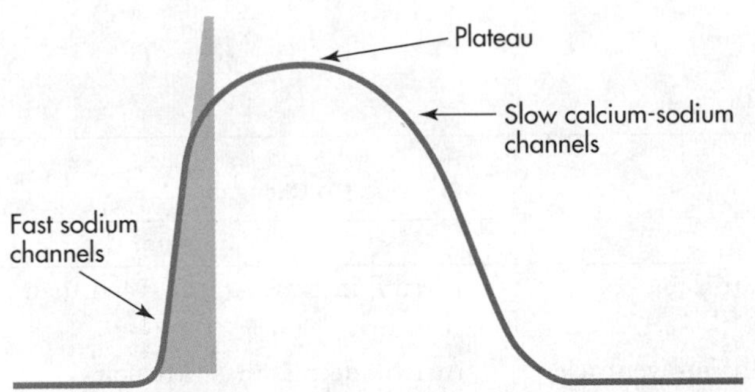

Figure 28-8 Differing effects of fast sodium channels and slow calcium-sodium channels on action potential. Flow of sodium throughout fast sodium channels initiates action potential, and then these channels close *(shaded area)*. Flow of current through slow calcium channels is responsible for plateau and duration of action potential.

the cell depolarizes. These two factors cause a slight decline in intracellular positivity.

PHASE 2. Phase 2 of the action potential is often referred to as the plateau phase. It is sustained by an influx of positive ions, primarily calcium, through the slow calcium channels into the cell (Figure 28-8). This supplies the cell with the calcium needed for contraction. This inward current results in a prolonged **refractory period** by maintaining the cell in a depolarized state, allowing time for completion of muscular contraction.

PHASE 3. During phase 3 the sodium pump, along with the increased loss of intracellular potassium, causes a rapid restoration of negativity to the cell.

PHASE 4. Phase 4 is the return of the cell to the resting membrane potential.

REFRACTORINESS. The inability of cardiac cells to respond to successive stimuli is known as refractoriness. During the absolute refractory period, no stimulus will produce a response. This period begins with depolarization and extends through a portion of the repolarization period until the sodium ion carrier sites are again free to transport the sodium ions necessary for depolarization (Figure 28-9).

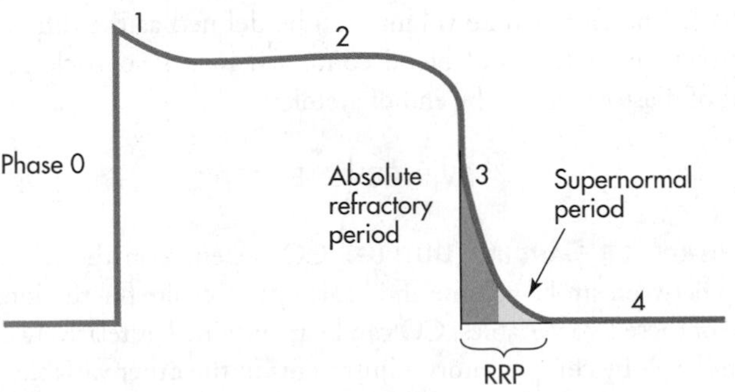

Figure 28-9 Schematic of action potential showing absolute and relative refractory period *(RRP)*. Strong stimulus will produce response in first part of RRP, and mild stimulus will do so in later part of RRP (supernormal period).

Refractoriness progressively diminishes in the relative refractory period, which occurs in the final stage of repolarization. During this interval a stimulus of sufficient strength will produce a response. When the resting state is attained, the cell is no longer refractory and a mild stimulus will initiate a cardiac impulse. This is known as the supernormal period.

Cardiac Cycle. The action potential itself does not cause the myofibrils to contract. The electrical stimulation initiates muscular contraction by stimulating the release of calcium ions in the sarcoplasmic reticulum of the muscle. Calcium ions then catalyze the chemical reaction that promotes the interdigitating and sliding of the actin and myosin filaments along each other, producing muscular contraction (see Chapter 51).

The **cardiac cycle** has two phases, diastole and systole. Relaxation and filling of both atria and then both ventricles take place during diastole. Contraction and emptying of both atria and then both ventricles occur during systole.

DIASTOLE. The diastolic phase of the cardiac cycle is subdivided into (1) isovolumetric ventricular relaxation, (2) rapid ventricular filling, (3) slow ventricular filling, and (4) atrial systole (Table 28-1 and Figure 28-10, *A*). Isovolumetric relaxation begins as soon as the aortic and pulmonic valves close. During this time the myocardial muscle relaxes, and ventricular pressure falls. However, the falling ventricular pressure is still higher than atrial pressure; therefore the AV valves remain closed and, as a result, blood collects in the atria. As ventricular pressure begins to drop more rapidly to its low diastolic level, the higher pressure in the atria pushes the AV valves open and allows blood to flow rapidly into the ventricular cavity. This second phase of diastole, rapid ventricular filling, lasts for approximately the first third of diastole and causes intraventricular pressure to rise. As ventricular pressure increases, it impedes further rapid filling, and the resultant slowing of ventricular filling marks the third phase of diastole. This phase of slow ventricular filling is referred to as diastasis. Both the atrial and the ventricular chambers are relaxed, and blood entering the atria flows passively into the ventricles. During the phase of atrial systole, electrical depolarization spreads through the atria and pauses at the AV node for 0.10 second. The atrial musculature then contracts, propelling an additional 20% to 30% of blood into the ventricle before ventricular contraction.

SYSTOLE. The ventricular systolic phase of the cardiac cycle is subdivided into phases of (1) isovolumetric ventricular contraction, (2) maximal ventricular ejection, and (3) reduced ventricular ejection (see Table 28-1 and Figure 28-10, *B*). During the isovolumetric ventricular contraction phase, myocardial tension and intraventricular pressure increase, while no change occurs in blood volume or muscle fiber length. At this time the aortic valve is closed because pressure in the aortic root exceeds left ventricular pressure. The higher pressure in the aortic root is the result of a previous systole that has just ejected blood into the aorta. As this aortic blood is distributed to the periphery, aortic pressure falls slowly. At the same time, intraventricular pressure and tension are increasing. When intraventricular pressure exceeds aortic root pressure, the aortic valve opens and maximal ventricular ejection begins. Blood from the ventricles is pumped into the pulmonary

TABLE 28-1 EVENTS DURING THE CARDIAC CYCLE

Phase	Valves: Pulmonic and Aortic	Valves: Mitral and Tricuspid	Actions	Pressure (P) Changes
DIASTOLE				
Isovolumetric relaxation	Closed	Closed	Blood collects in atria.	Atrial P increases until greater than ventricular P.
Rapid ventricular filling	Closed	Open	Blood flows rapidly into ventricles from pressure differential.	Atrial P decreases; ventricular P increases.
Slow ventricular filling	Closed	Open	Blood flows passively into ventricles.	Same as for rapid filling
Atrial systole	Closed	Open, then closed	Atrial contraction pushes additional blood into ventricles.	Ventricular P becomes greater than atrial P.
SYSTOLE				
Isovolumetric contraction	Closed	Closed	Myocardial tension increases.	Ventricular P increases; aortic P decreases until ventricular P is greater than aortic P.
Maximal ventricular ejection	Open	Closed	Blood is pumped from ventricles into pulmonary artery and aorta.	Ventricular P decreases.
Reduced ventricular ejection	Open, then closed	Closed	Some blood is ejected.	Ventricular P decreases rapidly when ventricles relax.

and systemic circulations. As the ejection rate starts to slow, the phase of reduced ventricular ejection, or protodiastole, begins. The ventricles remain contracted, but little blood is ejected from the ventricle into the aorta. Ventricular pressure actually falls slightly below aortic root pressure, but some blood is still ejected simply because of the momentum built up by the contraction. At the end of systole, ventricular relaxation begins suddenly, and intraventricular pressure rapidly falls. The higher pressure in the large arteries and in the aortic root immediately pushes blood back toward the ventricles, thus snapping shut the semilunar valves.

Cardiac Output. The amount of blood ejected from the left ventricle into the aorta per minute is called the **cardiac output** (CO). Although the right ventricle ejects an equivalent amount of blood into the pulmonary artery, it is not included in the measurement of total CO. Rather, CO is equivalent to stroke volume (SV) (volume of blood ejected from the left ventricle with each contraction) times heart rate (HR) (number of heartbeats per minute):

$$CO = SV \times HR$$

The average CO ranges from 4 to 8 L/min in the adult man. However, during periods of strenuous exercise, the CO may reach 20 to 25 L/min. Because cardiac requirements vary according to individual body size, a more accurate means of assessing tissue perfusion is to compute the cardiac index. The cardiac index is obtained by dividing the CO by the person's total body surface area:

$$\text{Cardiac index} = \text{CO (L/min)}/\text{Body surface area (m}^2\text{)}$$

Therefore the cardiac index represents the CO in terms of liters per minute per square meter of body surface. This corrects an individual's CO to match body size. The normal range for the cardiac index is 2.4 to 4.0 L/min. For example, the average 70 kg man has an approximate cardiac index of 3 L/min.

STROKE VOLUME. **Stroke volume** is the amount of blood ejected by the left ventricle into the aorta per beat. At the completion of each filling phase, or diastole, the ventricle contains approximately 120 ml of blood (end-diastolic volume [EDV]) (Figure 28-11). Under normal circumstances the heart ejects approximately two thirds of the EDV. The blood that is ejected is called the ejection fraction. The volume of residual blood in the ventricle at the end of systole is known as the end-systolic volume (ESV). Therefore stroke volume can be defined as the difference between the volumes of blood contained in the ventricle at the end of diastole and at the end of systole:

$$SV = EDV - ESV$$

CONTROL OF CARDIAC OUTPUT. CO depends on the relationship between stroke volume and heart rate. Despite fluctuations in one of these two variables, CO can be maintained at relatively constant levels by compensatory adjustments in the other variable. For example, if the heart rate slows, the time for ventricular filling (diastole) is lengthened. This lengthened period allows for an increase in preload and a subsequent increase in stroke volume. Conversely, if the stroke volume falls, the heart rate can increase to compensate temporarily and maintain CO. Therefore the actual

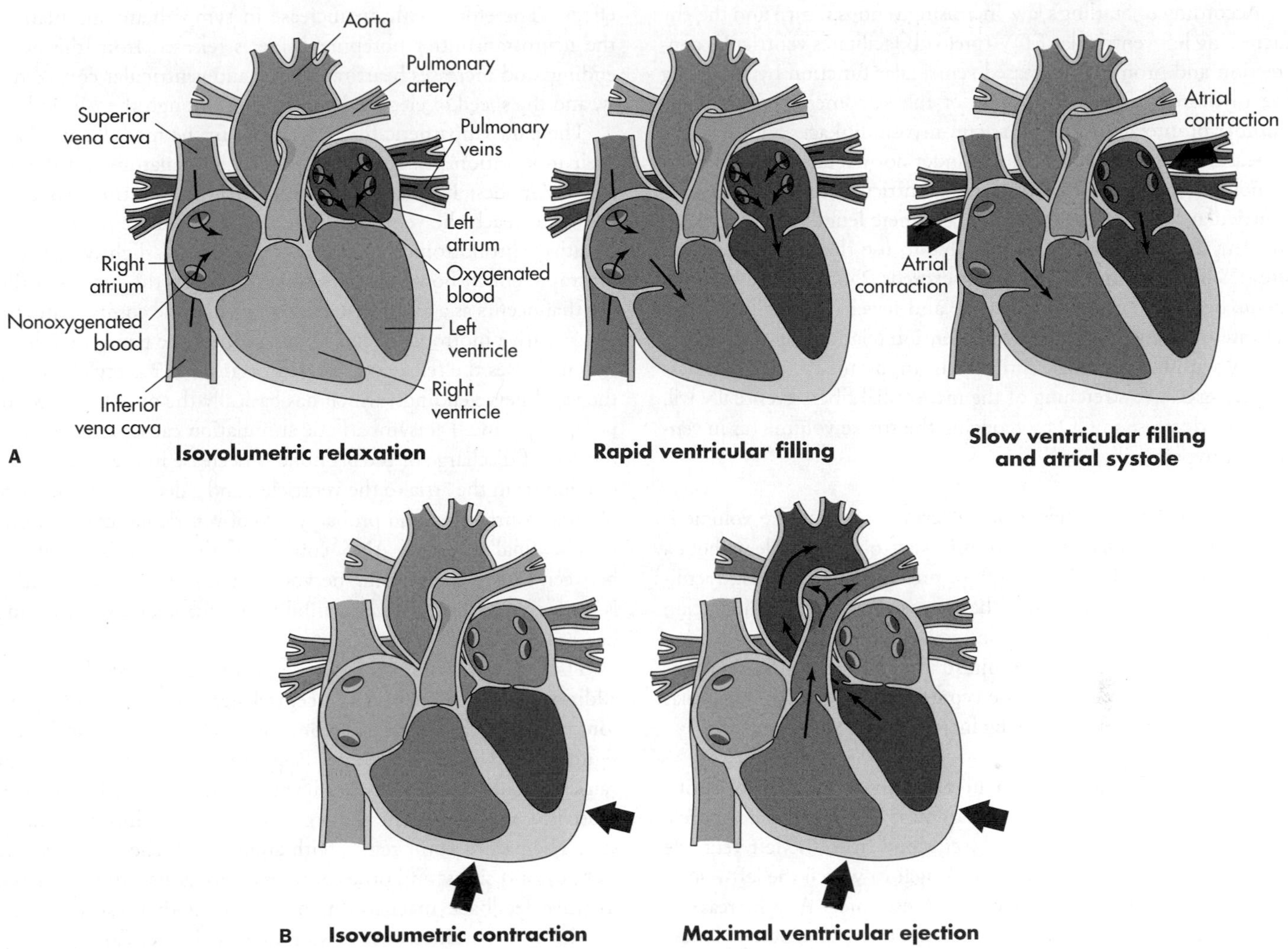

Figure 28-10 Events during cardiac cycle. **A,** Diastole. **B,** Systole.

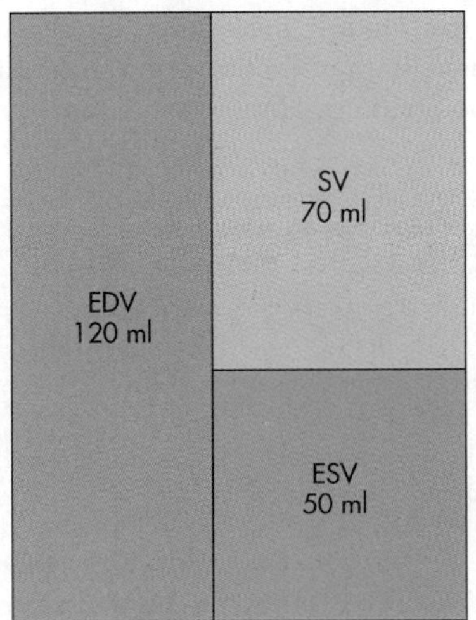

Figure 28-11 Representation of normal ventricular function, illustrating relationship between end-diastolic volume *(EDV)*, stroke volume *(SV)*, and end-systolic volume *(ESV)*.

determinants of CO are the mechanisms regulating stroke volume and heart rate.

CONTROL OF STROKE VOLUME. Stroke volume, and ultimately CO, is determined by three factors: preload, contractility, and afterload.

PRELOAD. Starling's law of the heart states that myocardial fibers respond with a more forceful contraction when they are stretched. An example of this phenomenon is increasing the stretch of a rubber band to obtain a more forceful recoil when the rubber band is released. Myocardial fibers can be stretched by increasing the volume of blood delivered to the ventricles during diastole. The degree of myocardial stretch before contraction is expressed in terms of preload.

Preload is defined as the volume of blood distending the ventricles at the end of diastole. Preload is based on the amount of venous return and the ejection fraction, which determines the amount of blood left in the ventricle at the end of systole.

According to Starling's law, increasing venous return and thereby increasing left ventricular EDV (preload) facilitates ventricular contraction and promotes increased ventricular function by stretching the myocardial fibers. Stretching of the sarcomeres increases the number of interaction sites for actin-myosin linkages and therefore increases ventricular contraction. Under normal conditions the sarcomere is stretched to 2 mm during ventricular diastole. Maximal ventricular force is developed at a sarcomere length of 2.2 mm. At this length, actin and myosin are able to use the most interaction sites. When myocardial stretching exceeds 2.4 mm, the myofilaments become partially disengaged, and fewer contractile sites are activated. Because Starling's length-tension relationship is functional only within physiologic limits, it is important to note that prolonged, excessive stretching of the myocardial fibers eventually will lead to a decrease in CO by reducing the stroke volume (as in ventricular hypertrophy).

CONTRACTILITY. Another major determinant of stroke volume is contractility, a change in the inotropic state of the muscle without a change in myocardial fiber length or preload. Increased contractility (inotropism) is a function of the increased intensity of interaction at the actin-myosin linkages. Contractility can be increased by sympathetic stimulation or by administration of medications such as calcium or epinephrine. Increased contractility improves ventricular emptying during systole, thereby increasing the stroke volume.

AFTERLOAD. The third factor involved in the control of stroke volume is **afterload,** which is the amount of tension the ventricle develops during contraction to eject blood from the left ventricle into the aorta. The major impedance against which the left ventricle must pump is peripheral vascular resistance. Any increase in pressure resulting from hypertension or vasoconstriction produces increased resistance to pumping and requires an increase in ventricular tension to eject blood. The afterload on the heart is affected not only by the amount of aortic pressure but also by the size of the heart. This relationship between ventricular tension, arterial pressure, and ventricular size is known as Laplace's law:

$$\text{Ventricular tension} = \text{Arterial pressure} \times \text{Ventricular radius}$$

Both hypertension and dilation of the ventricular chamber increase ventricular tension (increase afterload). Therefore, if arterial pressure increases, the ventricle must pump against higher resistance to empty adequately. Also, if ventricular radius increases, ventricular volume will increase. Thus at the same level of aortic pressure, the afterload against which an enlarged or dilated left ventricle must work is greater than that encountered by a normal-sized ventricle. This would result in an impaired ventricular emptying, thereby reducing stroke volume and CO.

CONTROL OF HEART RATE. The autonomic nervous system (ANS) regulates the heart rate through the sympathetic and the parasympathetic nervous systems. The sympathetic fibers arise from the thoracic spinal cord and reach the entire atria and ventricles, as well as the SA and AV nodes. Control of the heart by the ANS is mediated by neurotransmitters. The sympathetic neurotransmitter is norepinephrine. The sympathetic fibers have both positive chronotropic (increase rate) and inotropic (increase force) effects. Therefore, with an increase in sympathetic stimulation, the neurotransmitter norepinephrine is released from the nerve endings and increases heart rate, atrial and ventricular contractility, and the speed of electrical conduction through the AV node.

The parasympathetic fibers originate in the medulla and have their innervation primarily in the atrial musculature and the SA and AV nodes; however, parasympathetic stimulation has been shown to reach the ventricles. The parasympathetic fibers have a negative chronotropic effect and may exert a slightly negative inotropic effect; however, in the healthy heart, the increased filling that occurs as a result of a lengthened diastole compensates for this negative inotropic effect. Stimulation of the parasympathetic system causes the release of the neurotransmitter acetylcholine at the vagal nerve endings, which has basically the opposite effect of norepinephrine. Parasympathetic stimulation causes a decrease in the rate of discharge of the SA node, a decrease in the rate of conduction from the atria to the ventricles, and a decrease in the force of atrial contraction and probably also of ventricular contraction.

The final effect of ANS control of the heart is a balance between these two opposing nervous systems. Normally, the heart is under the control of vagal inhibition and maintains a resting heart rate of 60 to 90 beats/min.

The effects of the ANS can be greatly influenced by several additional factors, such as the central nervous system and pressoreceptor reflexes. Impulses from the cerebral cortex can have a significant effect on heart rate. Pain, fear, anger, and excitement can cause substantial increases in heart rate. Also, reflex changes caused by stimulation of the pressoreceptors can influence heart rate. The baroreceptor reflex, with afferent branches in the aortic arch, carotid sinus, and other pressoreceptor zones, functions as a negative feedback mechanism to regulate both pressure in the arteries and resistance of vessels in the vasculature. Consequently, an episode of hypotension would cause a sudden drop of blood pressure in the aorta or carotid sinus and would stimulate the pressoreceptors less intensely. Subsequently, stimulation of the cardiac inhibitory center would decrease in frequency, resulting in a reflex increase in heart rate.

Other important factors involved in the control of heart rate include body temperature, medication, catecholamines, arterial blood gas tensions, hormones other than epinephrine, and plasma electrolyte concentrations. However, these are beyond the scope of this chapter.

▶ ARE You READY?

Blockage of which artery correlates to decreased perfusion of the left ventricular myocardium?

1. Left anterior descending artery
2. Left circumflex artery
3. Anterior coronary artery
4. Circumflex coronary artery

Anatomy and Physiology of Peripheral Vascular System

The vascular system is a closed circuit consisting of the systemic and pulmonary circulations. Blood circulates from the left side of the heart to the tissues and back to the right side of the heart. It then flows through the lungs and back to the left side of the heart. The main components of the vascular system are the arteries, capillaries, and veins.

Arteries

Arteries are thick-walled vessels that transport oxygen and blood via the aorta from the heart to the tissues. Figure 28-12 shows the principal arteries. As the arteries approach the tissues, they branch into smaller vessels called arterioles.

Arteries are composed of three tissue layers:

1. Inner layer of endothelium (intima)
2. Middle layer of connective tissue, smooth muscle, or elastic fibers (media)
3. Outer layer of connective tissue (adventitia)

The media forms the major portion of the vessel wall and in larger arteries is composed primarily of elastic and connective tissue. This enables the artery to respond to alterations in blood volume while maintaining a constant flow. The smaller arteries and arterioles have much less elastic fiber; the smooth muscle contracts and relaxes in response to nervous, chemical, and hormonal factors.

Capillaries

Capillaries, composed of a single layer of cells, are minute, thin-walled vessels located in the tissues. The capillaries connect the arterioles to the smallest veins and venules, allowing for the exchange of essential cellular products. Nutrients, oxygen, and regulatory substances move into the cells; waste products, carbon dioxide, and cellular secretions move from the cells into the blood.

Veins

Veins are thin-walled vessels that transport deoxygenated blood from the capillaries back to the right side of the heart. Veins are composed of the same three layers as arteries (intima, media, and adventitia), but in contrast to arterial walls, venous walls have little smooth muscle or connective tissue. This makes the veins distensible, enabling them to accumulate large volumes of blood. The sympathetic nervous system innervates the veins, causing venoconstriction, decreased venous volume, and increased circulating blood volume. Major veins, particularly those in the lower extremities, have one-way valves that promote blood flow against gravity and thereby prevent retrograde flow. Additionally, the squeezing action of skeletal muscle contraction creates an opposing force against gravity. Figure 28-13 shows the major veins in the body.

Principles of Blood Flow

Blood flow is brought about by a pressure difference between the various parts of the circulatory system. Blood flow is influenced by multiple factors, including vessel length, vessel radius, blood viscosity, pressure difference between the two ends of the vessel, cross-sectional area of the vessel, and wall tension. The rate of flow is directly related to pressure differences between the two ends of the vessel and inversely related to vessel length, vessel radius, and blood viscosity. The cross-sectional area of a vessel influences the velocity of flow; therefore, as the cross-sectional area decreases, the velocity increases, and vice versa. The relationship between wall tension, pressure, and radius is described by Laplace's law, which states that wall tension becomes greater as the radius increases. Wall tension is also inversely related to wall thickness; therefore the thicker the wall of the vessel, the lower the tension; and the thinner the wall of the vessel, the greater the tension.

Physiologic Changes With Aging

The number one cause of death in people 65 years of age and older is cardiovascular disease. Age-related changes in the chemical composition, cells, and tissues of the heart and blood vessels influence many aspects of cardiovascular function. Despite the physiologic changes of aging, however, the heart is able to meet day-to-day demands and function adequately. Only under unusual circumstances or increased stress is the changing function of the heart apparent. Coronary atherosclerosis is more prevalent in older adults, but it commonly manifests as an occult or silent condition.

Heart

Progressive left ventricular hypertrophy occurs with aging because of thickening of the ventricular septa and increasing circumference of all four cardiac chambers. This is accompanied by a concomitant rise in systolic blood pressure. Heart weight increases in women but not in men. By age 40 years, the circumference of the aortic valve generally surpasses that of the pulmonic valve. In both genders the leaflet thickness and calcification of the mitral and aortic valves increase progressively and significantly with advancing age. These rigid valves can lead to audible systolic murmurs, usually of an ejection nature.

An increase in average myocyte (muscle cell) size explains the increase in heart mass; however, the simultaneous change in the amount and functional properties of myocardial collagen plays a key role in the development of age-related cardiovascular abnormalities. The increased connective tissue contributes to myocardial stiffness and decreased cardiac compliance. The amount of subendocardial fat increases, and the endocardium undergoes fibrosis, thickening, and sclerosis.[6]

Peak-systolic left ventricular wall stress decreases with aging. Increasing left ventricular wall thickness and increasing body surface area with age are presumed to be contributing factors. The isovolumetric relaxation period also is prolonged, resulting in incomplete relaxation during early diastolic filling. However, enhanced ventricular filling occurs later in diastole as a result of a compensatory, augmented atrial contribution to ventricular filling.

Arteries

The degenerative changes that occur in the walls of the blood vessels as part of normal aging cause problems in the transport of blood and nutrients to the tissues. Increased thickness in the intimal wall results from fibrosis and is further affected by the accumulation of collagen and calcium. The elastic fibers of the media become thin and calcified, greatly decreasing the elasticity and flexibility of the vessels and increasing peripheral vascular resistance.

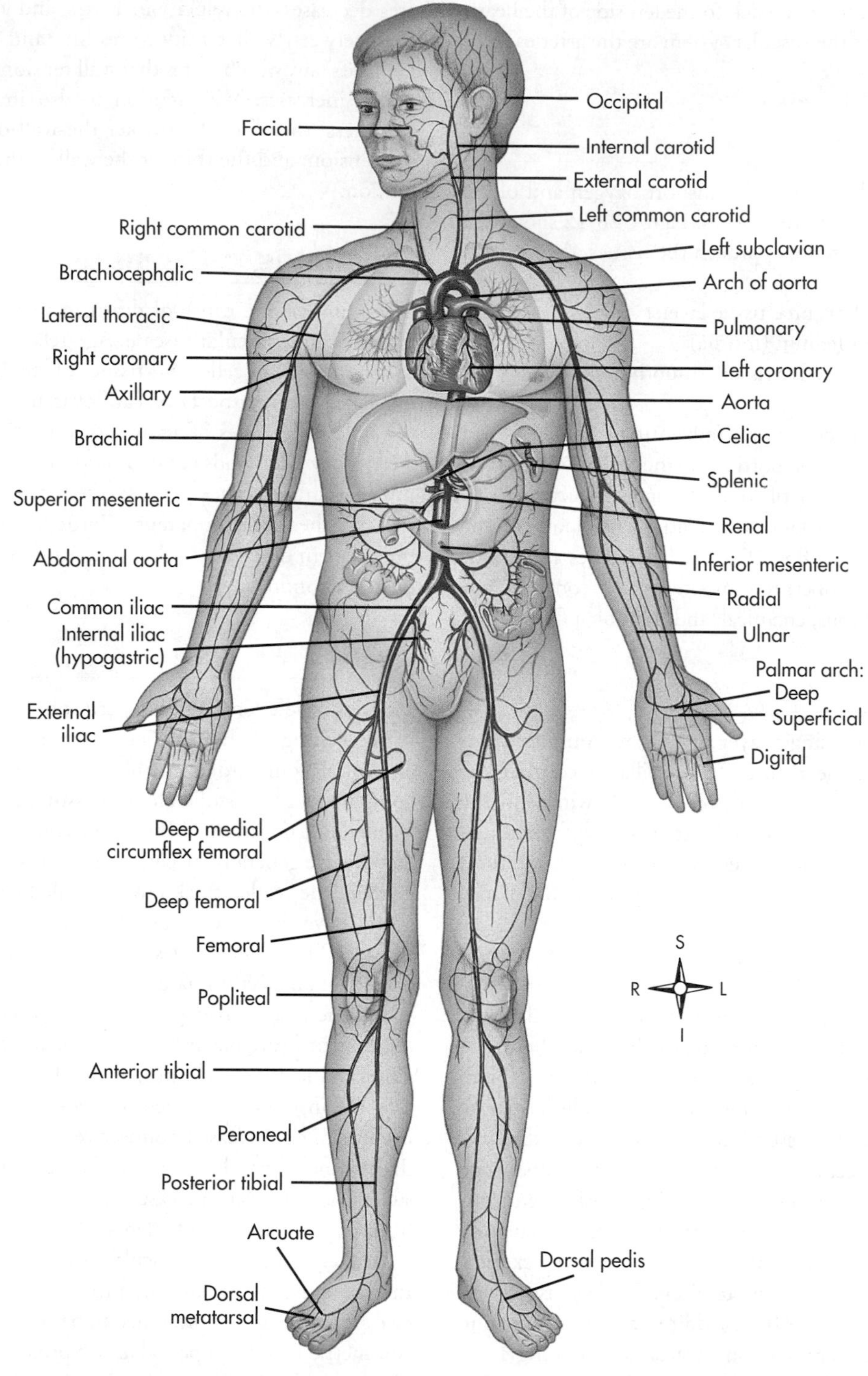

Figure 28-12 Principal arteries of body.

The result is a rise in blood pressure and decreased flow through the vessels. This results in a decreased supply of oxygen and nutrients to the tissues coupled with an accumulation of cellular secretions, waste products, and carbon dioxide.

Both the aorta and its branches and the large pulmonary arteries and their branches undergo progressive dilation and elongation with age. Because the enlargement is both transverse and longitudinal, the aorta tends to become tortuous. However, the large pulmonary arteries do not dilate longitudinally because the vessels are anatomically shorter and maintain a considerably lower pressure. The generalized loss of elasticity in the arterial system can also lead to a sluggish baroreceptor response. The baroreceptors are then less able to modulate blood pressure, particularly during rapid postural change.

Conduction System

Prolonged AV conduction with disturbances in cardiac rate and rhythm occurs in healthy aging persons as a result of fibrosis and fatty infiltration. Fibrotic changes occur predominantly in the

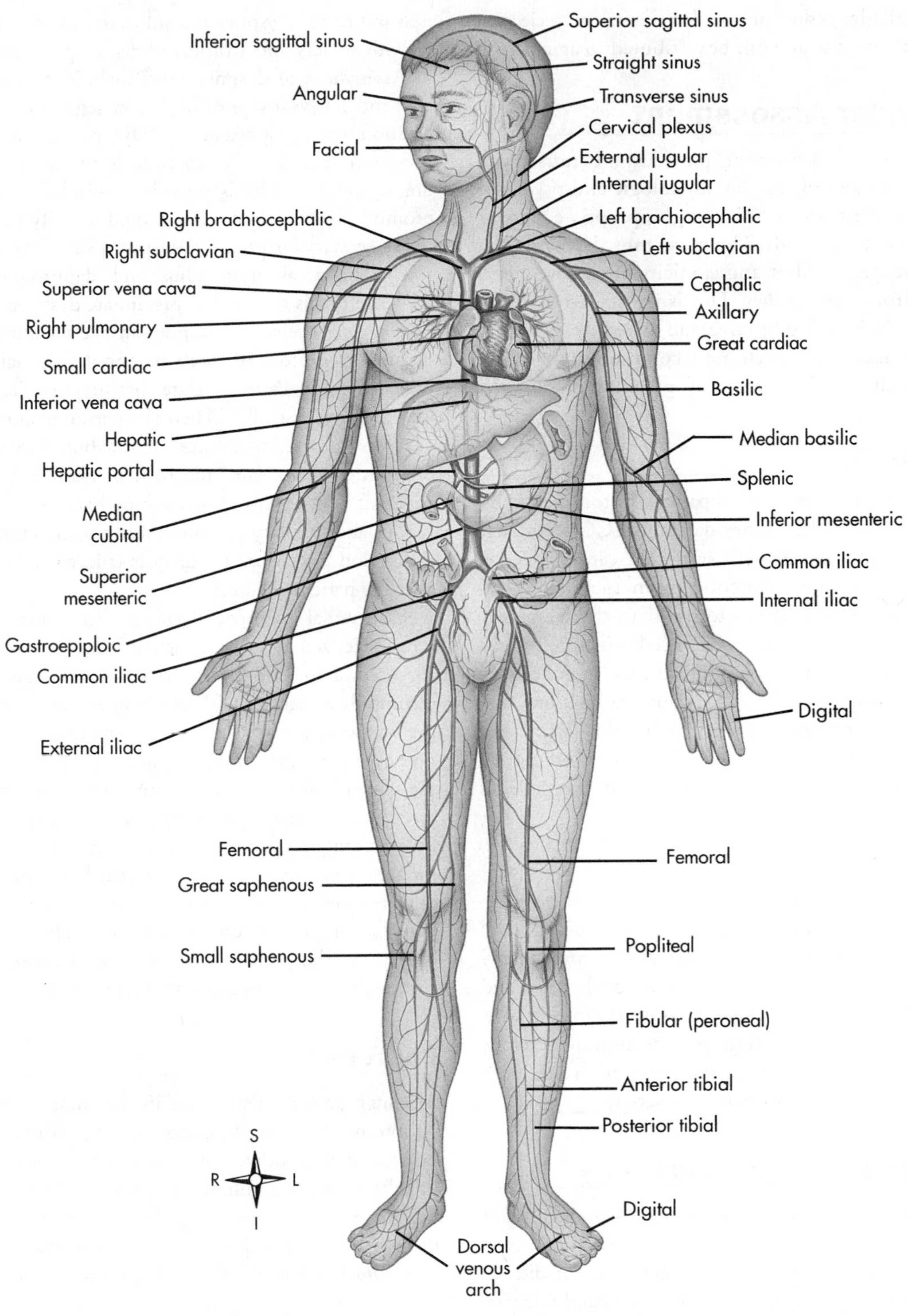

Figure 28-13 Principal veins of body.

ventricular system, whereas fatty deposits tend to occur in the SA and AV nodes, as well as in the atria.

Exercise and Cardiovascular Response

Age-related changes in the cardiovascular system are significantly more pronounced in response to exercise. The overall increase in heart rate during vigorous exercise is less in older persons. Older persons without significant coronary artery disease may demonstrate greater stroke volume increases compared with younger adults to compensate for the lesser increases in heart rate. Persons of all ages exhibit comparable increases in left ventricular EDV during upright exercise at low workloads. At higher workloads, in older persons whose heart rate increase is less, increases in left ventricular volume and stroke volume may continue throughout physical exercise.

Left ventricular ejection fraction has been shown to decrease, or fail to increase, with more exercise in persons with coronary artery disease. Similarly, reductions in left ventricular ejection fraction from rest to exercise also can be attributed to aging.

Cardiovascular Assessment

Systematic cardiovascular assessment provides the nurse with baseline data useful in identifying the physiologic and psychosocial needs of the patient and in planning appropriate nursing interventions to meet these needs. The nurse must be aware that patients of different ages, genders, and ethnicity often have different presentations from one another. This is particularly true for gender differences. "Classic" subjective and objective signs and symptoms of heart disease are much more common in men than women, who more often have an "atypical" presentation.

Health History

Data obtained by means of a detailed patient history can be as diagnostically significant as laboratory data and ECG recordings in the assessment of the patient with suspected cardiac disease. Accurate assessment attempts to identify both modifiable and nonmodifiable cardiovascular risk factors and to determine the psychodynamic family relationships that need to be addressed during treatment. Classic symptoms of heart disease include dyspnea, chest pain or discomfort, edema, syncope, palpitations, and fatigue. Cardiovascular function, which may be adequate at rest, may be insufficient during exercise or exertion. Therefore careful attention is directed to the effects of activity on the patient's symptoms.

Personal Habits

The collection of data regarding nutrition, smoking, alcohol intake, exercise, and medications is essential. It is particularly important to assess the diet in terms of calorie, cholesterol, and sodium content; smoking and alcohol consumption history, including the frequency and duration of consumption; exercise participation, both type and amount; and medication use, both prescription and over the counter (including herbals).[5]

Cardiovascular History: Self and Family

The nurse should determine whether the patient has any significant cardiovascular history, including hypertension, hyperlipidemia, coronary artery disease, heart failure, peripheral vascular disease, murmurs, aneurysms, deep venous thromboses, Raynaud's disease, and arterial or venous ulcers. A personal history of other related diseases such as diabetes mellitus, renal disease, or blood dyscrasias should also be explored. If any family members have a significant cardiovascular history, it is important to obtain a detailed account of their experience and treatment if possible.

Dyspnea

Dyspnea, one of the most common and distressing symptoms of cardiopulmonary disease, is described as an abnormally uncomfortable awareness of breathing. The patient complains of shortness of breath. Dyspnea is a subjective experience and is associated with anxiety and a variety of disease processes.

Assessment of dyspnea must include the factors that precipitate and relieve dyspnea and data regarding the patient's body position when dyspnea occurs. Dyspnea on exertion is a common symptom of cardiac dysfunction. In the early stages of heart failure, dyspnea usually is provoked only by effort and is relieved promptly by rest. The nurse should identify the amount of exertion necessary to produce dyspnea, since the lower the cardiac reserve (heart's ability to adjust and adapt to increased demands), the less effort is required to precipitate dyspnea.

Orthopnea refers to dyspnea in the recumbent position. It is usually a symptom of more advanced heart failure than is exertional dyspnea. Patients relate that they require two or more pillows to sleep restfully. When the person assumes the recumbent position, gravitational forces redistribute blood from the lower extremities and splanchnic bed, increasing venous return. The augmentation of intrathoracic blood volume elevates pulmonary venous and capillary pressures, resulting in a transient pulmonary congestion. Orthopnea usually is relieved in less than 5 minutes after the patient sits upright.

Paroxysmal nocturnal dyspnea, also known as cardiac asthma, is characterized by severe attacks of shortness of breath that generally occur 2 to 5 hours after the onset of sleep. This condition is commonly associated with sweating and wheezing. Classically, the person awakens from sleep, arises, and quickly opens a window to get some fresh air. These frightening attacks are precipitated by the same physiologic mechanisms that cause orthopnea. The diseased heart is unable to compensate for increased blood volume by pumping extra fluid into the circulatory system, and pulmonary congestion results. Paroxysmal nocturnal dyspnea is typically relieved by the patient changing from a supine to sitting position or getting out of the bed. However, unlike simple orthopnea, the patient with paroxysmal nocturnal dyspnea may require 20 minutes or more to obtain relief.

Chest Pain

Although pain or discomfort in the chest is one of the cardinal symptoms of cardiac disorders, chest pain can also be precipitated by various noncardiac conditions such as anxiety, acute musculoskeletal injuries, pulmonary disorders (e.g., pleurisy and pulmonary embolism), esophageal spasm or reflux, and peptic ulcer disease. To evaluate chest pain accurately, the nurse should assess:

- *Onset*: When was the chest pain first noticed (e.g., date, time)?
- *Manner of onset*: Did the pain or discomfort start suddenly or gradually (e.g., quick, slow, vacillation)?
- *Duration*: How long did the pain last (e.g., seconds, minutes, hours)?
- *Precipitating factors*: What factors were associated with the onset of pain (e.g., exertion, food, anxiety, emotions)?
- *Location*: Where did the pain originate? Did it radiate? To what area (e.g., shoulder, jaw, neck, arms)?
- *Quality*: What did the pain feel like? Can the patient describe it (e.g., sharp, dull, ache, pressure)?
- *Intensity*: How severe was the pain (based on 1 to 10 scale)?

- *Chronology and frequency*: Has this pain occurred in the past? If so, how often (e.g., establish timeline)?
- *Associated symptoms*: Did any other signs or symptoms occur at the same time (e.g., nausea, sweating, dizziness, shortness of breath)?
- *Aggravating factors*: What made the pain worse (e.g., activity, positioning, stress)?
- *Relaxing factors*: What made the symptoms less intense (e.g., rest, nitroglycerin, oxygen use)?

The same list of factors can also be used to evaluate leg pain. The responses can assist the examiner in establishing a diagnosis of peripheral vascular disease. Furthermore, the analysis can help differentiate arterial from venous disease.

Syncope

Syncope is defined as a generalized muscle weakness with an inability to stand upright, accompanied by loss of consciousness. The most common cause of syncope is decreased perfusion to the brain. Any condition that results in a sudden reduction of CO and thus reduced cerebral blood flow could potentially cause a syncopal episode. In patients with cardiovascular disorders, conditions such as orthostatic hypotension, hypovolemia, or a variety of dysrhythmias (e.g., heart block and severe ventricular dysrhythmias) may precipitate syncope.

Palpitations

Palpitation is a common subjective phenomenon defined as an unpleasant awareness of the heartbeat. It may be precipitated by a change in cardiac rate or rhythm or by an increase in myocardial contractility. Patients may describe their heartbeat as "pounding," "racing," or "skipping." Palpitations that occur either during or after strenuous activity are considered physiologic. Palpitations that occur during mild exertion may suggest the presence of heart failure, anemia, or thyrotoxicosis. Other noncardiac factors that may precipitate palpitations include nervousness; heavy meals; lack of sleep; and a large intake of caffeine-containing beverages, alcohol, or tobacco.

Fatigue

Fatigue and lassitude have many causes and therefore are not diagnostic of cardiovascular disorders. However, fatigue may be a direct consequence of heart failure. The exact physiologic mechanism is not known, but it is probably a consequence of an inadequate CO. Fatigue can occur during effort or at rest and generally worsens as the day progresses. Fatigue that occurs after mild exertion may indicate a low cardiac reserve, with the heart unable to meet even small increases in metabolic demands.

Physical Examination

Physical examination of the cardiovascular system includes the standard assessment techniques of inspection, palpation, percussion, and auscultation. Before beginning the cardiovascular examination, the examiner should obtain vital signs. Respiration, pulse, temperature, and blood pressure provide initial information about the patient's baseline physiologic status.

Inspection

Skin Color. The examiner notes the color of the patient's skin and mucous membranes. A person's "normal" color depends on race, ethnic background, and lifestyle and is an indication of adequate CO and circulation. Pallor may indicate anemia, hypoxia, or peripheral vasoconstriction. Cyanosis, a bluish discoloration of the skin, is most easily observed by examining the earlobes, oral mucosa at the base of the tongue, lips, and nail beds. (Refer to Chapter 64 for more details on assessment of skin color.)

There are two types of cyanosis: central and peripheral. In central cyanosis the tongue is characteristically cyanotic. This form of cyanosis is caused by low arterial oxygen saturation and generally is seen in patients who have congenital heart defects or pulmonary diseases that interfere with ventilation or diffusion. Peripheral cyanosis results from low CO and generally is accompanied by decreased skin temperature and mottling. In contrast to central cyanosis, no cyanosis of the tongue is present.

The examiner also assesses skin color of the extremities. It is important to note any erythema or pigmentation changes, as well as shiny or dry, scaly skin, which may indicate a vascular disorder. Hair distribution, venous pattern, and size of the extremities should be assessed.

Neck Vein Distention. A general estimate of venous pressure can be obtained by observation of the neck veins (Figure 28-14). Normally, when a person is supine, the neck veins are distended. However, when the head of the bed is elevated to a 45-degree angle, the neck veins are collapsed. If jugular distention is present, jugular venous pressure can be assessed by measuring from the highest point of visible distention to the sternal angle. Measurements above 3 cm are considered elevated.

The jugular veins reflect venous tone, blood volume, and right atrial pressure. Therefore distended neck veins suggest increased

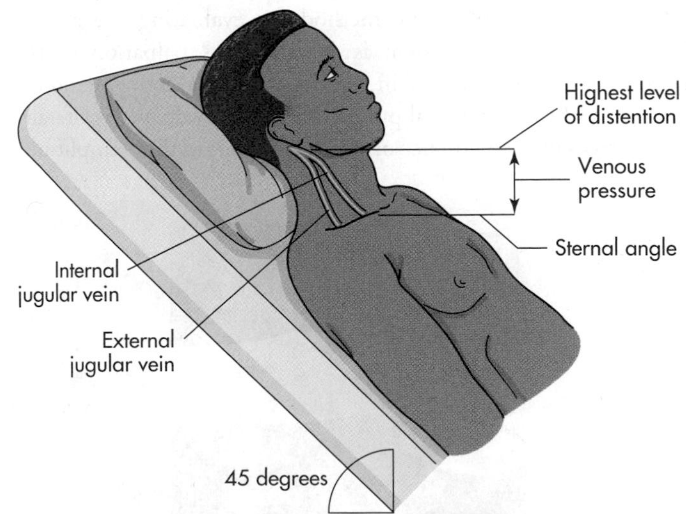

Figure 28-14 Position of internal and external jugular veins used in measuring venous pressure.

venous pressure, which may be caused by right-sided heart failure, circulatory volume overload, superior vena caval obstruction, or tricuspid valve regurgitation.

Respirations. The rate and character of the patient's respirations are important to assess. Normally an adult breathes comfortably at a rate of 12 to 20 breaths/min. Particular attention is paid to the ease or difficulty in breathing and the patient's general demeanor.

Pulsations. Inspection of the anterior chest is best accomplished with the patient lying supine, either flat or with the head slightly elevated. The examiner observes the precordium for the apical impulse, which is a pulsation of the chest wall caused by the forward thrusting of the left ventricle during systole. When visible, the apical impulse occupies the fourth or fifth intercostal space, at or inside the midclavicular line. The apical impulse was formerly known as the *point of maximal impulse.* The apical impulse is not always visible, but it is palpable in about half of adults.

Clubbing and Capillary Refill. The examiner assesses the nails for clubbing and capillary refill. The exact cause of clubbing is not known; however, clubbing of the fingers is common in congenital heart defects and pulmonary AV fistulas with right-to-left shunting (Figure 28-15). Capillary filling, or blanching, is an indicator of peripheral circulation to the fingers and toes and can be tested in all nail beds. The examiner presses a thumbnail against the edge of a patient's fingernail or toenail and then quickly releases it. The normal response is whitening (blanching) of the area when pressure is applied and brisk return of color when pressure is released. Lack of the blanching response may indicate lack of circulation to the finger or toe because of arterial insufficiency secondary to atherosclerosis or spasm; however, severe vasoconstriction may be the causative factor.

Palpation

Peripheral Pulses. One method for evaluating the arterial flow of the vascular system is simultaneous palpation of the extremities to determine skin temperature. A second method is palpation of the peripheral pulses, which are evaluated bilaterally on the basis of their absence or presence, rate, rhythm, amplitude, quality, and equality. Each pulse, except the carotids, is palpated on the left and right side simultaneously to evaluate contralateral symmetry (Figure 28-16). Pulses are rated on a scale of 0 to 4 as follows:

0	Absent
+	Palpable, but diminished
++	Normal, or average
+++	Full and brisk
++++	Full and bounding, often visible

Several abnormalities may be detected during palpation of pulses. A hypokinetic (weak) pulse signifies a narrowed pulse pressure, a decreased difference between the systolic and diastolic pressures. It usually is produced by a low CO and is associated with increased peripheral vascular resistance. This type of pulse is often detected in such conditions as severe left ventricular failure, hypovolemia, or mitral and aortic valve stenosis. A hyperkinetic (bounding) pulse represents a widened pulse pressure. It usually is associated with increased left ventricular stroke volume and decreased peripheral vascular resistance. This type of pulse is often found in hyperkinetic circulatory states caused by exercise, fever, anemia, or hyperthyroidism.

Pulsus alternans is a condition in which the heart beats regularly, but the pulses vary in amplitude. It is caused by an alternating left ventricular contractile force and usually indicates severe depression of myocardial function. Pulsus alternans may be detected by palpation but is more accurately assessed by auscultation of the blood pressure.

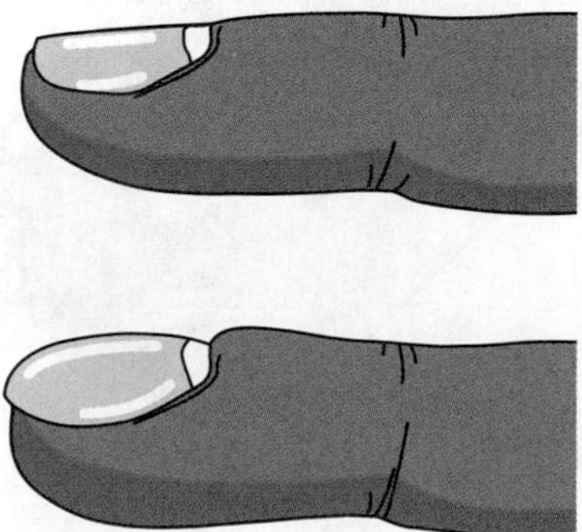

Figure 28-15 Comparison of normal nail *(top)* and digital clubbing *(bottom)*.

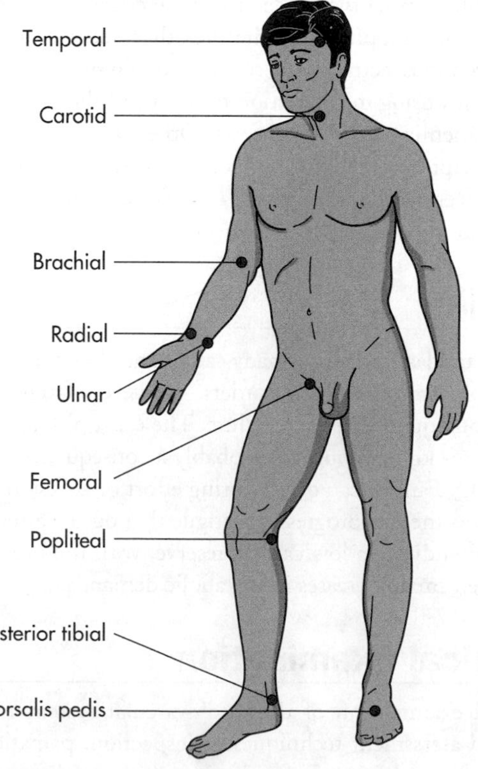

Figure 28-16 Body sites at which peripheral pulses are most easily palpated.

Pulsus paradoxus signifies a reduction in the amplitude of the arterial pulse during inspiration. Variations in pulse strength can be palpated, but a paradoxical pulse is most readily detected by sphygmomanometry. Pulsus paradoxus is an accentuation of the normal decrease in systolic arterial pressure with inspiration. This is a result of decreased left ventricular stroke volume and the transmission of negative intrathoracic pressure to the aorta. Pulsus paradoxus may occur in conditions such as cardiac tamponade and constrictive pericarditis, but it also may occur in patients with chronic obstructive pulmonary disease who have wide swings of intrapleural pressure during respiration.

Normally the apical impulse is felt as a single, light tap. The presence of anything other than a single, light tap may suggest a myocardial pathologic condition and should be reported to the physician. A thrill, or palpable murmur, indicates the presence of significant turbulent blood flow across an intracardiac shunt or a severely stenotic valve. A thrill is often described as a vibration similar to that of a cat's purr and is more readily palpated after the patient exhales forcefully. Having the patient in a left lateral position or leaning forward may accentuate the vibration.

Edema. Edema is an accumulation of fluid in the interstitial spaces. It may be localized to one particular body part, organ, or tissue; or it may have a generalized distribution. Retention of considerable amounts of extracellular fluid may occur without associated edema. In fact, weight gains of up to 7 kg of water can occur before the abnormality is detected. Because early manifestations of edema may be subtle, careful comparison of daily weights is required to determine weight gains resulting from fluid retention. Normally, basal body weight varies little from day to day; therefore subtle weight gains resulting from fluid retention are readily detectable.

Nonpitting peripheral edema is caused by gravity flow or by interruption of the venous return to the heart as a result of constricting clothing or pressure on the veins of the lower extremities. The presence or absence of peripheral edema, especially in the feet, ankles, legs, and sacrum, is an important indicator of cardiovascular function. This edema often disappears on elevation of the body part. In contrast, pitting edema does not disappear with elevation of the extremity or body part, and it may indicate fluid overload or a pathologic condition (e.g., heart failure). Pitting edema is described as an indentation left in the skin after a thumb or finger has applied gentle pressure. Table 28-2 depicts a scale commonly used to assess pitting edema.

Percussion

The use of percussion in cardiac assessment is extremely limited, since the chest x-ray study is much more accurate. Usually only the left border of cardiac dullness can be determined, since this is located near the apical impulse, or within the midclavicular line. Cardiac dullness to percussion is characteristic of cardiac hypertrophy. Unfortunately, mild to moderate degrees of cardiac hypertrophy are not usually detectable by percussion.

Auscultation of Heart Sounds

The first heart sound (S_1), called *lub*, is thought to be produced by the almost simultaneous closures of the mitral and tricuspid

TABLE 28-2 PITTING EDEMA SCALE

Scale	Description	Measurement
1+	Barely perceptible pit	2 mm (3/32 in)
2+	Deeper pit; rebounds in a few seconds	4 mm (5/32 in)
3+	Deep pit; rebounds in 10-20 sec	6 mm (1/4 in)
4+	Deeper pit; rebounds in >30 sec	8 mm (5/16 in)

+1 2 mm · +2 4 mm · +3 6 mm · +4 8 mm

From Wilson S, Giddens J: *Health assessment for nursing practice,* ed 2, St Louis, 2001, Mosby.

valves. S_1 lasts approximately 0.10 second and signals the onset of ventricular systole. S_1 is generally loudest at the apex but can be heard over the entire precordium. S_1 is longer and lower pitched than the second heart sound (S_2), called dub (the first and second heart sounds together are referred to as lub-dub), and S_1 corresponds to the beat of the carotid pulse. S_2 is caused by the closure of the semilunar valves (aortic and pulmonic) and is loudest at the base of the heart. It is described as shorter, higher pitched, and "snappier" than S_1 (Figure 28-17).

The diaphragm chest piece of the stethoscope is most useful for listening to high-pitched sounds and murmurs. These include S_1, S_2, ejection sounds, and clicks. The examiner places the diaphragm firmly on the chest wall so that an indentation is present on the patient's skin when the diaphragm is removed. The bell chest piece is most useful for detecting low-pitched sounds and murmurs. These include the third heart sound (S_3), the fourth heart sound (S_4), and mitral and tricuspid diastolic rumbles. The bell is placed lightly on the chest wall, barely creating an airtight seal. If the bell is placed firmly on the skin, it acts as a diaphragm.

Splitting of S_1 and S_2. The two main components of S_1 (closure of the mitral and tricuspid valves) are asynchronous, since left ventricular systole usually occurs slightly ahead of right ventricular systole. The S_1 may be split in persons who have RBB block,

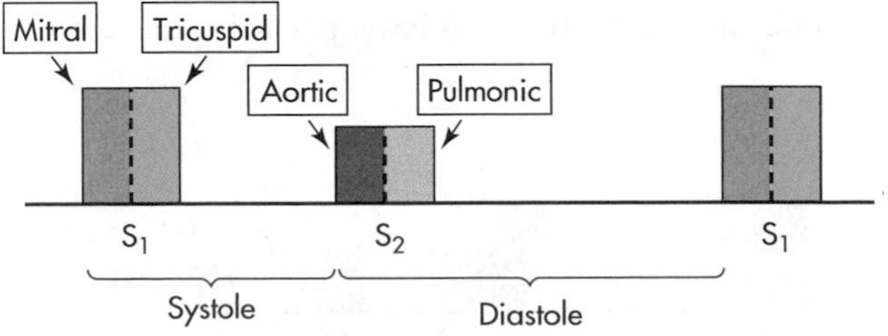

Figure 28-17 Heart sound S_1 is closure of mitral and tricuspid valves: S_2 is closure of aortic and pulmonic valves. Systole is interval between S_1 and start of S_2; diastole is S_2 to start of S_1. Diastole is longer than systole.

left-sided mechanical defects (e.g., mitral stenosis) or tricuspid valve dysfunction associated with pulmonary hypertension.

Because left ventricular contraction slightly precedes right ventricular contraction, the aortic valve also normally closes slightly before the pulmonic valve. On inspiration, intrathoracic pressure decreases and facilitates an increase in venous blood return to the right side of the heart. This increased blood return delays the closure of the pulmonic valve and results in a normal physiologic split S_2. On expiration, closure of the aortic and pulmonic valves occurs almost simultaneously and therefore is heard as a single sound. In conditions of increased blood flow or increased right ventricular pressure, there may be a "fixed" split of S_2; that is, both components of S_2 are heard on both inspiration and expiration. A fixed split is considered abnormal and may occur in RBB block, pulmonary hypertension, and right ventricular failure related to atrial or ventricular septal defects.

Extra Heart Sounds. Extra heart sounds include ejection sounds (systolic clicks), opening snaps, S_3, and S_4. The two most common extra heart sounds are S_3 and S_4, or ventricular gallop and atrial gallop, respectively (Figure 28-18).

Ventricular diastolic gallop, or S_3, is a faint, low-pitched sound produced by rapid ventricular filling in early diastole. It occurs when the volume of early filling is increased or ventricular compliance is decreased. Ventricular "gallop" recalls the gallop of a horse, which is mimicked at heart rates greater than 100 beats/min. When this sound is present in healthy children and young adults, it is almost always a normal condition and is referred to as a physiologic S_3. An S_3 heard in an older person usually is a pathologic sign, commonly one of the first signs of serious heart disease or cardiac decompensation. S_3 is typically present in such conditions as left-to-right shunts, mitral regurgitation, heart failure, and constrictive pericarditis.

Atrial diastolic gallop, or S_4, is a low-frequency sound that occurs under circumstances of altered ventricular compliance, either left or right. S_4 occurs late in diastole when atrial systole ejects blood into a noncompliant ventricle. Because the presence of an audible S_4 is related to a decrease in left ventricular compliance and an increase in left ventricular end-diastolic pressure, it is often heard in patients with hypertensive cardiovascular disease and idiopathic hypertrophic subaortic stenosis. An S_4 commonly is identified in patients with acute myocardial infarction or coronary artery disease, especially during an attack of angina pectoris. In addition, an S_4 may be present when CO and stroke volume are increased, such as in severe anemia, thyrotoxicosis, and large AV fistulas. Although the S_4 sound occurs close to S_1, it can be easily differentiated because S_4 is lower pitched than S_1.

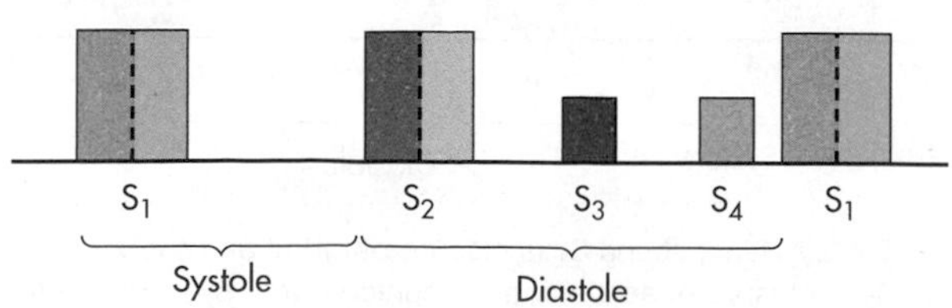

Figure 28-18 Location of extra heart sounds during cardiac cycle.

Murmurs. **Murmurs** are audible vibrations of the heart and great vessels that occur because of turbulent blood flow. They may be produced by hemodynamic events or by structural alterations in the heart or in the walls of the great vessels. In general, murmurs are heard most distinctly over the area of the valve or altered cardiac structure responsible for the vibrations. The major factors involved in the production of cardiac murmurs include (1) increased velocity of blood flow through normal or abnormal valves; (2) forward flow through a stenotic or irregular valve orifice; (3) backward (regurgitant) blood flow through an incompetent valve, septal defect, or patent ductus arteriosus; and (4) turbulent blood flow produced in a dilated chamber, such as in a ventricular or aortic aneurysm.[6]

Murmurs generally are characterized according to timing (position in the cardiac cycle), intensity, quality, pattern, posture, pitch, location, and direction of radiation. These characteristics provide data concerning the location and nature of the cardiac abnormality.

Pericardial Friction Rub. A pericardial friction rub is an extra heart sound originating from the pericardial sac as the heart moves. It is often a sign of inflammation, infection, or infiltration. The sound is high pitched and scratchy, like pieces of sandpaper being rubbed together. The sound is best heard with the diaphragm of the stethoscope while the patient is in an upright position and leaning forward.

Assessment measures and variations in normal findings relevant to the care of older adults are presented in the Gerontologic Assessment box, which also identifies common disorders that may be responsible for abnormal assessment findings.

Diagnostic Tests

Cardiovascular diseases usually are diagnosed by integrating diagnostic test results with findings from the patient interview and physical examination. The diagnostic tests ordered most commonly in patients with heart disease include blood tests, urinalysis, electrocardiography, invasive hemodynamic monitoring, sonic studies, dynamic studies, radiography, scintigraphic studies, and angiography.

The nurse may be directly or indirectly involved in these tests and procedures. It is essential that the nurse understand the various tests or procedures and the importance of the data to an accurate diagnosis. This information enables the nurse to prepare the patient adequately before any diagnostic procedure and to document relevant signs and symptoms while caring for the patient.

Laboratory Tests

A complete blood cell count is ordered for all patients with documented or suspected heart disease. Data concerning red blood cells (RBCs) and white blood cells are helpful in diagnosing infectious heart disease and myocardial infarction (Table 28-3). The RBC count may be elevated as a physiologic response to inadequate tissue oxygenation. The erythrocyte sedimentation rate is a measurement of the rate at which RBCs "settle out" of anticoagulated blood in 1 hour. The rate of settling is increased if the proportion of globulin to albumin increases or if fibrinogen levels are exces-

Gerontologic Assessment

- Count the pulse for a full minute at rest and after exertion.
  –The pulse is often slower and may be irregular because older adults are more prone to decreased cardiac output and dysrhythmias.
- Monitor changes in blood pressure.
  –Systolic blood pressure in older adults may normally be as high as 160 mm Hg (compared with 140 mm Hg in younger adults). A widened pulse pressure also may be observed.
  –Check blood pressure with patient in a lying, sitting, and standing position to detect postural hypotension, since vasomotor control is decreased in older adults.
- Auscultate carefully.
  –Murmurs are common from thickening and calcification of the valves. Also, extra heart sounds may be present on auscultation. S_4 often occurs in older people with no known cardiac disease. However, an S_3 is associated with congestive heart failure and is always abnormal over age 35. When assessing the heart, note that the apical impulse may be harder to locate.
- Monitor for signs of mental confusion, lethargy, indigestion, and weakness.
  –These may be early signs of cardiac disease. Angina is common with ischemic heart disease.
- Always use caution when palpating and auscultating the carotid artery because pressure in the carotid sinus area can cause a reflex slowing of the heart rate.
  –Creating pressure on this area is a particular risk with older adults because circulation may already be compromised by atherosclerosis.

Common Disorders in Older Adults

Atherosclerosis
Congestive heart failure
Angina pectoris
Myocardial infarction
Dysrhythmias
Valvular disorders
Left ventricular hypertrophy
Hypertension
Peripheral vascular disease

sively increased. Nonspecific increases in globulin and fibrinogen levels occur when the body responds to injury or inflammation, as seen with infectious heart disorders and myocardial infarction.

Blood coagulation tests, including prothrombin time, international normalized ratio, and activated partial thromboplastin time, measure the rapidity of blood clotting. These tests are useful during anticoagulation therapy (see Table 28-3). A blood urea nitrogen (BUN) determination is a useful indicator of renal function. Decreased CO leading to a low renal blood supply and reduction in glomerular filtration rate will elevate the BUN.

Blood Lipids. The blood (plasma) lipids are composed mainly of cholesterol, triglycerides, phospholipids, and free fatty acids, all of which are insoluble in water and require a "carrier" for transport. The carriers for plasma lipids are the proteins to which they are bound, hence the name *lipoproteins*. Lipoproteins have four major classes: chylomicrons, very low–density lipoproteins (VLDLs), low-density lipoproteins (LDLs), and high-density lipoproteins (HDLs), all of which contain varying levels of cholesterol, triglycerides, and phospholipids.

Chylomicrons are composed mainly of triglycerides and originate in the intestine after the absorption of dietary fat. Chylomicrons should not be found in the plasma after 12 to 14 hours of fasting. Elevated chylomicron levels do not appear to be associated with heart disease.

VLDLs are composed primarily of triglycerides and are synthesized in the liver. Sustained elevations of VLDLs are associated with both atherosclerosis and coronary artery disease.

LDLs are composed of approximately 50% cholesterol and are thought to have the greatest correlation with coronary artery disease. The LDLs are believed to enter the arterial intima and produce arterial endothelial injury. This process can result in progressive atherosclerotic plaque formation and eventually ischemic heart disease. Lipoprotein (a), or Lp(a), is a protein associated with LDL. High plasma levels of Lp(a) have been correlated with an increased risk for atherothrombotic cardiovascular disease. Structurally Lp(a) is similar to plasminogen, which explains its ability to interfere with the processes involved in plasmin generation and clot lysis.

HDLs are composed of mostly protein with a modest amount of cholesterol and a considerable amount of phospholipids. This lipoprotein appears to have the lowest atherogenic potential. In fact, studies have demonstrated that HDLs are inversely associated with coronary heart disease. The HDLs are believed to carry cholesterol away from tissues, including atheromatous plaques, and provide some protection against coronary heart disease.

The National Cholesterol Education Program Expert Panel on Detection, Evaluation, and Treatment of High Blood Cholesterol established and updates criteria for cholesterol and lipid assessment that include total cholesterol, LDL, HDL, and triglyceride levels (Table 28-4). Adjustments in target levels are made for individuals with coronary artery disease risk factors such as hypertension, diabetes mellitus, or family history of premature coronary disease.

Evaluation of individual blood lipid components is important, but the most significant predictor of coronary artery disease is the ratio of total cholesterol to HDL. This ratio is calculated by dividing the HDL level into the total cholesterol level (e.g., 50 HDL to 200 total cholesterol = 4:1). The acceptable ratio is 5:1 with the optimal ratio being 3.5:1.

Before blood lipid tests are performed, the patient must fast for 12 hours and may not take any alcoholic beverages or lipid-influencing drugs (e.g., estrogens, oral contraceptives, steroids, salicylates). Because lipid levels may fluctuate greatly from day to day, repeated blood samples are obtained before a definitive diagnosis of hyperlipidemia is made.

Amino Acids. Homocysteine is an amino acid, produced in the human body, that may irritate blood vessels and lead to atherosclerosis. High homocysteine levels in the blood can also cause cholesterol to change to LDL, which is more damaging to the arteries.[4] In addition, high homocysteine levels can make blood clot more easily, increasing the risk of thrombi that might cause a

TABLE 28-3 SELECTED LABORATORY TESTS FOR CARDIOVASCULAR DISORDERS

Test	Normal Values	Significance in Heart Disorders
Serum red blood cell count	Men: 4,600,000-6,200,000/mm^3 Women: 4,200,000-5,400,000/mm^3	Decreased in subacute endocarditis Increased with inadequate tissue oxygenation
Serum white blood cell count	4500-11,000/mm^3	Decreased in some congenital heart disease with right-to-left shunt Increased in acute and chronic heart inflammations and in acute myocardial infarction
Erythrocyte sedimentation rate	Men: up to 15 mm/hr Women: up to 20 mm/hr	Increased in acute myocardial infarction and infectious heart disease
Prothrombin time	12-14 sec 100% compared to control	Indicates rapidity of blood clotting; used to monitor anticoagulant therapy with warfarin (Coumadin)
International normalized ratio	2-3	Ratio of patient's prothrombin time to normal standard prothrombin time of testing laboratory; used to monitor anticoagulant therapy with warfarin
Activated partial thromboplastin time	20-35 sec	More sensitive than prothrombin time; used to monitor heparin therapy
Blood urea nitrogen	11-23 mg/dl	Increased with decreased cardiac output
Serum proteins	6-8 g/dl	Level below 5 g/dl seen with edema
Homocysteine	<12 μmol/L	Increases risk of atherosclerosis
C-reactive protein	<6 mg/L	Increases indicate inflammatory process

TABLE 28-4 INITIAL CLASSIFICATION OF TOTAL, LOW-DENSITY LIPOPROTEIN, AND HIGH-DENSITY LIPOPROTEIN CHOLESTEROL AND TRIGLYCERIDES

Classification	Total Cholesterol (mg/dl)	Low-Density Lipoprotein Cholesterol (mg/dl)	High-Density Lipoprotein Cholesterol (mg/dl)	Triglycerides (mg/dl)
Optimal	<200	<100	>60	—
Normal or near optimal	200	100-129	>40	<150
Borderline high	200-239	130-159	—	150-199
High	≥240	160-189	—	200-499
Very high		≥190	—	>500

From the Third report of the National Cholesterol Education Program (NCEP) Expert Panel on Detection, Evaluation, and Treatment of High Blood Cholesterol in Adults (Adult Treatment Panel III), Executive Summary, NIH Publication 01-3670, May 2001, National Institutes of Health, National Heart, Lung, and Blood Institute.

myocardial infarction or stroke. Up to 20% of people with heart disease are found to have high homocysteine levels. Homocysteine levels can be measured at any time of day using a simple blood test and do not require any special preparation. An optimal homocysteine level is less than 12 μmol/L. Although no studies have yet proven that lowering homocysteine levels ultimately helps reduce the risk of strokes, heart attacks, and other cardiovascular events, research is ongoing, and the amino acid is now classified as a risk factor for heart disease.[3]

Highly sensitive C-reactive protein (HS-CRP) is considered an acute phase reactant, a substance that is increased during an inflammatory process. It is not known whether HS-CRP is directly involved in the development of atherosclerosis, but since atherosclerotic heart disease is believed to be an inflammatory process, elevated HS-CRP is considered to be a marker of risk.[7] When HS-CRP is elevated, the risk of developing atherosclerosis is increased three to six times.[9] Levels of HS-CRP are measured using a specific assay, but only in the absence of evidence of acute inflammation. The routine assay has no ability to predict the risk of an actual atherosclerotic event.

Enzyme Studies. Enzymes, which are located in all tissues, catalyze the body's biochemical reactions. When cell membranes are damaged, as in myocardial infarction, enzymes leak out of the damaged myocardial cell and escape into the serum. The different enzymes are released into the blood at varying times after a myocardial infarction, and it is crucial to evaluate the enzyme level in relation to the time of onset of the chest pain or other symptoms. Refer to Chapter 29 for a more detailed description of the time course of cardiac enzymes after a myocardial infarction.

The serum enzyme measurements that are used to detect myocardial necrosis are serum aspartate aminotransferase (AST), creatine kinase (CK), troponin I, lactate dehydrogenase (LDH), and hydroxybutyrate dehydrogenase (HBD). Because these enzymes are located in various body tissues, numerous conditions other than myocardial damage may produce enzyme elevations; for example, the brain, pancreas, and liver are all rich sources of AST. If a person developed chest pain concurrently with pancreatic or liver disease, an elevated AST level may be mistaken for myocardial necrosis. Fortunately, three of the enzymes, CK, troponin I, and LDH, have isoenzymes that are thought to be present almost exclusively in myocardial muscle.[2]

The CK molecule has two subunits, which have been identified as M, associated with muscle; and B, associated with brain. The brain and gastrointestinal tract contain modest amounts of the BB dimer, and skeletal muscle contains large amounts of the MM form. Heart muscle contains huge quantities of MM, but it also contains the MB hybrid form of CK. Because CK-MB is not found in any other tissue, its presence in the serum is a sensitive indicator of myocardial damage.

Cardiac troponin I is normally present in minuscule amounts and is also specific to heart muscle. It is immediately released from damaged myocardial cells and is present in the blood for about 1 week after release.[8] Of the five LDH isoenzymes, LDH1 has been found to be the most sensitive indicator of myocardial damage; however, the use of LDH isoenzymes has largely been replaced by troponin and CK-MB.[10]

Serologic Tests. Syphilis can play an important role in the development of aortic disorders. The patient may have aortic insufficiency, aortic aneurysms, or disease of the orifices of the coronary arteries. Because of the relationship between syphilis and heart disease, a routine VDRL (Venereal Disease Research Laboratory) test is performed on all cardiac patients.

Urinalysis. A routine urinalysis is performed to determine the effects of cardiovascular disease on renal function. Detection of myoglobin in the urine plays a role in the diagnosis of myocardial infarction. Although clinical experience with this test remains limited, it may prove to be a sensitive indicator of myocardial damage. Destruction of striated muscle by infarction liberates myoglobin, which is small and can filter through the glomerulus and be excreted in the urine.

▶ ARE You READY?

Which of the following laboratory values is most closely correlated with coronary artery disease?

1. High-density lipoproteins
2. Low-density lipoproteins
3. Very low density lipoproteins
4. Chylomicrons

Radiologic Tests

Chest Radiography. An x-ray film of the chest may be taken to determine the overall size and configuration of the heart, as well as the size of the individual cardiac chambers. Most abnormalities of heart size and calcification in the heart muscle, valves, and great vessels can be detected with standard posteroanterior and lateral views of the chest.

Cardiac Fluoroscopy. Cardiac fluoroscopy facilitates observation of the heart from varying views while the heart is beating. Fluoroscopy can be used to detect ventricular aneurysms, monitor prosthetic valve movement, or assess the position of cardiac calcifications during the cardiac cycle. Because of the radiation risk associated with fluoroscopy, many institutions no longer use this diagnostic technique.

Special Tests

Electrocardiogram. The ECG is a graphic representation of the electrical forces produced within the heart. The ECG is an essential tool for cardiac evaluation that is used for a wide variety of diagnostic purposes (Box 28-1), but it must be combined with other data sources for accurate diagnosis. A resting ECG may be normal, even in the presence of heart disease. Conversely, abnormal variances may be seen in the ECG of a normal heart.

Standard 12-Lead Electrocardiogram. The ECG tracing represents the net electrical activity or electrical potential variations of the atria and ventricles as each depolarizes and repolarizes. The electrical currents passing through the heart can be detected by electrodes and measured when they reach the surface.

The conventional 12-lead ECG machine uses electrodes to measure the electrical potential differences between a series of locations on the body surface. Each pair of electrodes, consisting of a positive and a negative terminal, constitutes an ECG lead. Representative tracings obtained from the 12 leads are shown in Figure 28-19. The standard lead sites are right arm, left arm, right leg, and left leg. The chest (or precordial) electrodes are placed across the chest wall in six different locations. These 10 sites are combined in pairs through a switching network in the ECG machine. Effective contact between the skin and electrode is established by the use of electrode jelly, which contains electrolytes and an abrasive capable of penetrating the waterproof layer of the skin.

LIMB LEADS. The standard bipolar limb leads, designated by Roman numerals I, II, and III, are created by electrodes applied to the right arm (RA), left arm (LA), and left leg (LL) (Figure 28-20). The right leg (RL) electrode acts as a grounding electrode. Lead I records the difference between the RA and LA potentials. Lead II records the difference between the RA and LL potentials. Lead III records the difference between the LA and LL potentials. The augmented unipolar limb leads are designated by the abbreviated

Box 28-1 Diagnostic Uses for Electrocardiogram

The electrocardiogram may be used to evaluate:

- Tachycardia, bradycardia, or dysrhythmias
- Sudden onset of dyspnea
- Pain in the upper part of the trunk and in the extremities
- Syncopal episodes
- Shock state or coma
- Preoperative status
- Postoperative hypotension
- Hypertension, murmurs, or cardiomegaly
- Artificial pacemaker function

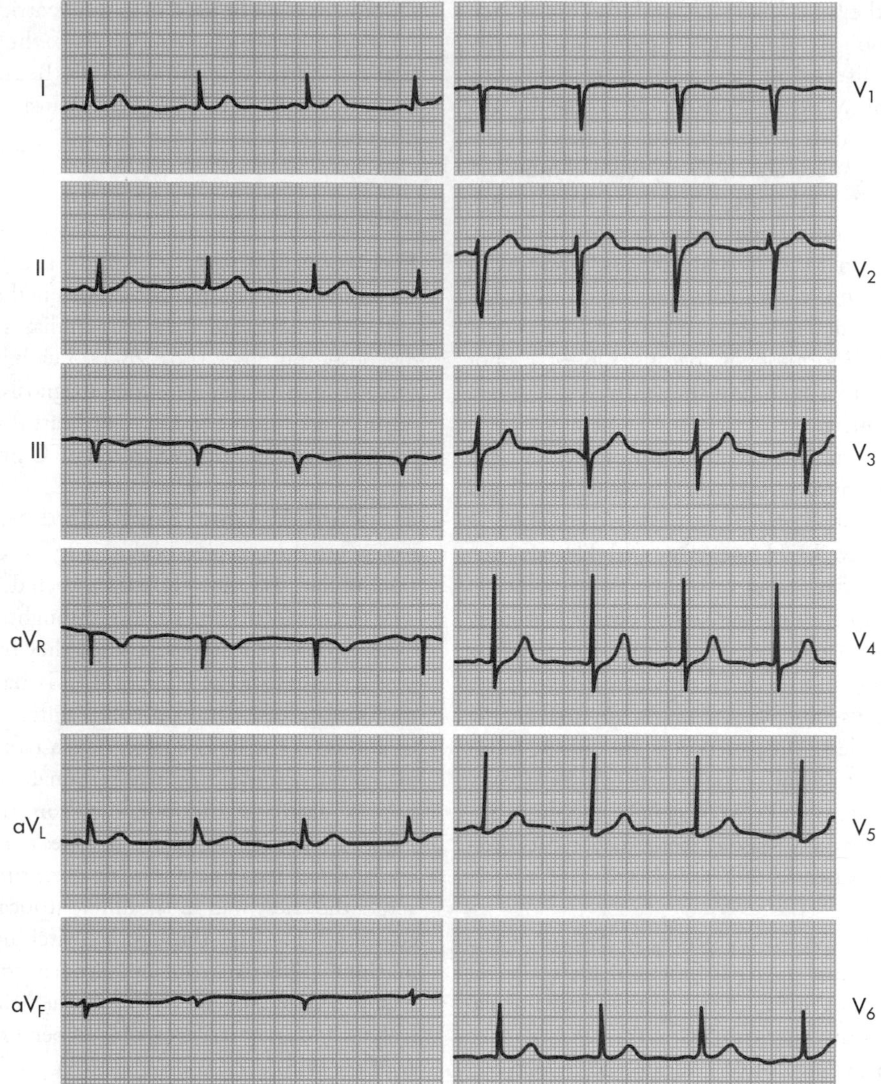

Figure 28-19 Twelve-lead electrocardiogram showing normal sinus rhythm.

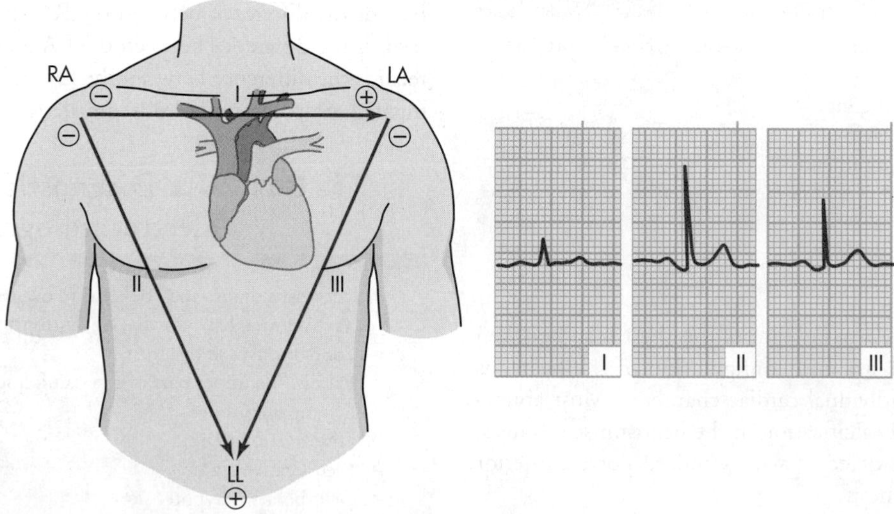

Figure 28-20 Schematic representation of standard limb lead system. *RA*, Right arm; *LA*, left arm; *LL*, left leg.

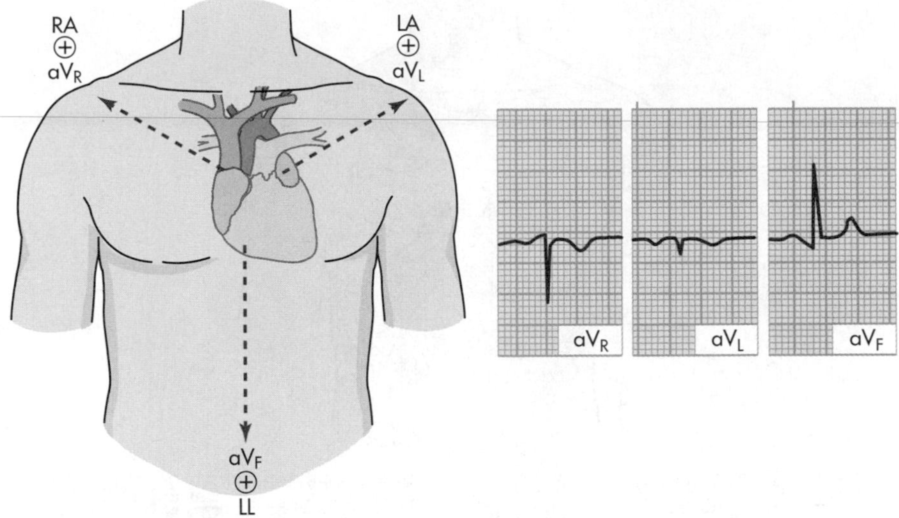

Figure 28-21 Schematic representation of augmented unipolar limb lead system. *RA,* Right arm; *LA,* left arm; *LL,* left leg.

forms aV_R, aV_L, and aV_F. For these leads the right arm (R), left arm (L), and left leg (F) become the respective positive electrodes (Figure 28-21). For clinical purposes the amplitude of the recordings from these electrodes is augmented by approximately 50% to produce a tracing that is easier to interpret. Together, the augmented and standard limb leads provide the six frontal plane leads.[11]

PRECORDIAL LEADS. The six precordial or chest leads are designated by the symbols V_1 through V_6. These leads register the electrical variations of the heart in the horizontal plane (Figure 28-22). The positive electrode is placed on six different sites across the chest (Figure 28-23).

Monitoring. To perform continuous cardiac monitoring, the conventional ECG leads have been modified to eliminate cumbersome wiring. The most popular leads for continuous cardiac monitoring are lead II and lead V_1. The patient wears two, three, or five electrodes, which are attached by small lead wires to a cable connected to a wall-mounted monitor with an oscilloscope screen.

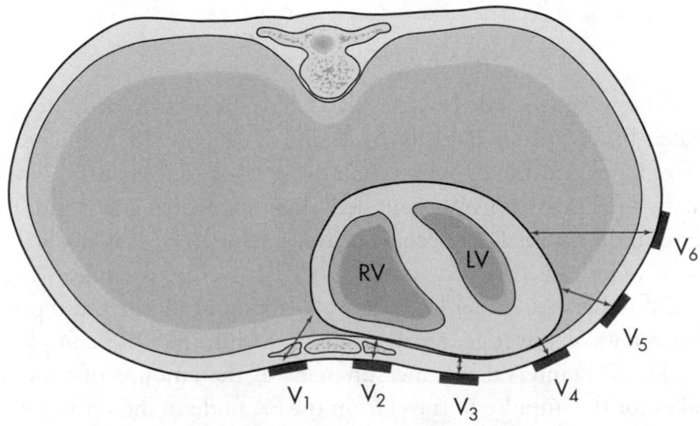

Figure 28-22 Cross-section of heart showing precordial leads V_1 through V_6 in a horizontal plane. *RV,* Right ventricle; *LV,* left ventricle.

Lead II is produced by placing the negative electrode on the right arm (modified and placed near the right shoulder below the clavicle) and the positive electrode on the left leg (modified and placed on the lower left rib cage eighth intercostal space).

Lead V_1 is produced by placing the negative electrode on the left arm (modified and placed near the left shoulder below the clavicle) and the positive electrode at the fourth intercostal space to the right of the sternum. With these modifications, V_1 is known as MCL_1. The MCL_1 lead is the most helpful lead for determining the origin of premature beats and determining the presence of bundle branch blocks.

An alternative type of continuous monitoring is known as telemetry. The telemetry system requires no cables that would restrict patient mobility. The electrical impulses are transmitted through an antenna to an oscilloscope at another location.

Electrocardiogram Tracing. The ECG tracing is recorded on graph paper that is divided into millimeter squares. The millimeter squares are grouped and divided into larger squares by thick lines that occur every fifth square (Figure 28-24). Horizontally each millimeter square represents 0.04 second of elapsed time. Each thick line denotes the passage of 0.20 second. Fifteen hundred small, or 300 large, squares represent 1 minute. With this information, the examiner can determine the duration of any complex or interval on the ECG by counting the number of small squares and multiplying by 0.04. Heart rate may be measured or estimated by various methods (Box 28-2).

Vertically, each small square is 1 mm in height and represents 0.1 mV of voltage. Thus each large square is 5 mm and represents 0.5 mV. The voltage or amplitude of a wave or complex in a given lead indirectly indicates the electrical activity of the muscle below the positive electrode. Hypertrophied myocardium produces abnormally high voltage in some leads, whereas infarcted myocardium may produce no voltage or only low-voltage waves.

The baseline of the ECG tracing is known as the isoelectric line. Waves are deflections, either above (positive) or below (negative) the isoelectric line. The direction of deflection is determined

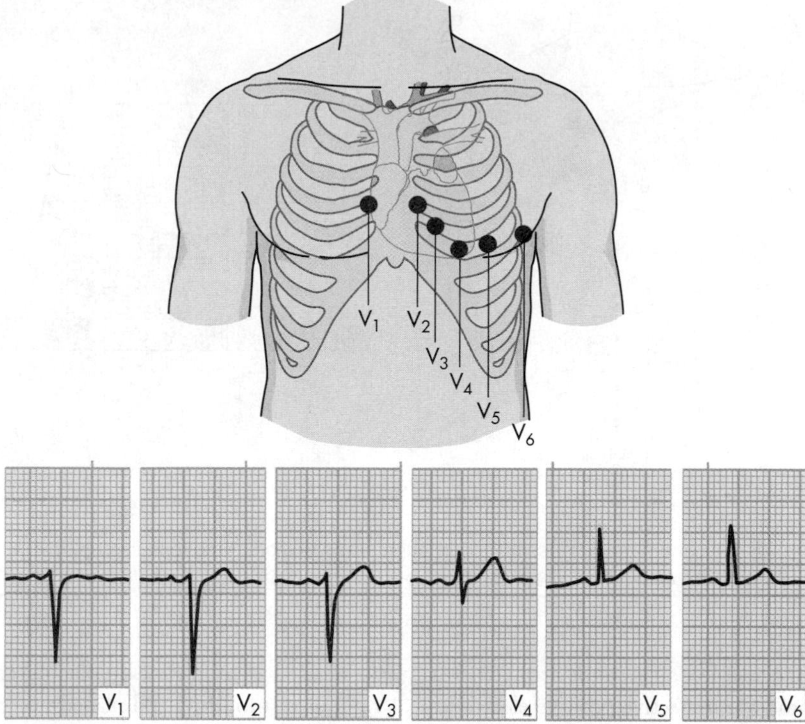

Figure 28-23 Anatomic placement of precordial leads.

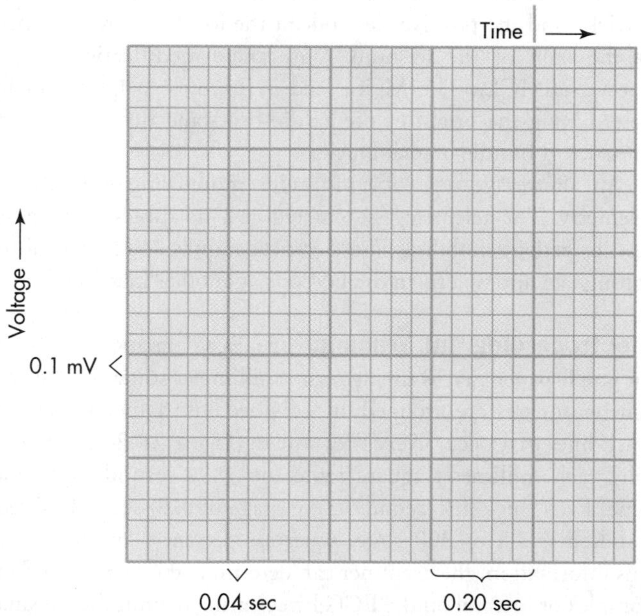

Figure 28-24 Components of electrocardiograph paper.

by (1) the direction in which the electrical impulse flows, (2) the distance between the source of the impulse and the positive electrode, and (3) the site of the electrode. As a rule, when the flow of electrical current is directed toward the positive electrode, the deflection will be positive, and when the flow of current is directed away from the positive electrode, the deflection will be negative (Figure 28-25).

Box 28-2 Three Methods for Estimating Heart Rate From Electrocardiogram Tracing

1. Measure the interval between consecutive QRS complexes, determine the number of small squares, and divide 1500 by that number. This method is used only when the heart rhythm is regular.
2. Measure the interval between consecutive QRS complexes, determine the number of large squares, and divide 300 by that number. This method is used only when the heart rhythm is regular.
3. Determine the number of R-R intervals within 6 seconds and multiply by 10. The electrocardiograph paper is conveniently marked at the top with slashes that represent 3-second intervals. This method can be used when the rhythm is irregular. If the rhythm is extremely irregular, an interval of 30 to 60 seconds should be used.

The waves recorded by the ECG have been arbitrarily designated by the letters P, Q, R, S, T, and U (Figure 28-26). The P wave represents the depolarization of the atria (Table 28-5). Normally the P wave is gently rounded, does not exceed 2 to 3 mm in amplitude, and is 0.11 second or less in duration. It is normally positive in leads I, II, aV_F, and V_4 to V_6. It is negative in lead aV_R and variable in all other leads. Repolarization of the atria also produces a wave, but it generally is hidden within the QRS complex.

The P-R interval is a measurement of the amount of time it takes for the impulse to travel from the SA node to the ventricular musculature. It includes the normal physiologic delay of impulse conduction by the AV node. This interval is measured from the

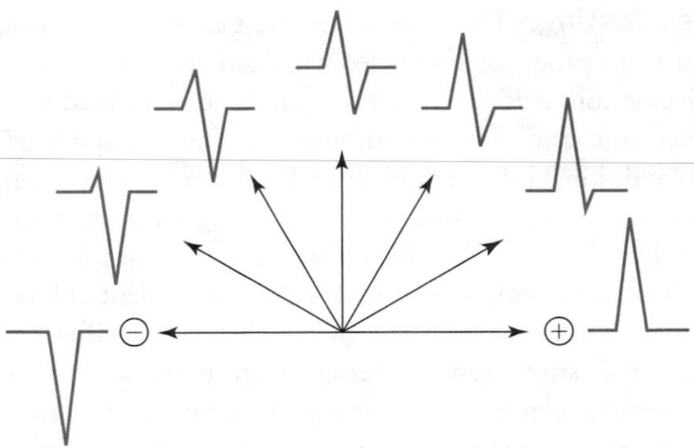

Figure 28-25 Several vectors and their resultant electrocardiographic complex. NOTE: (1) Current perpendicular to axis produces equiphasic deflection, and (2) current parallel to axis results in tallest or deepest complex possible.

TABLE 28-5 ELECTRICAL ACTIVITY OF HEART AND RESULTANT ELECTROCARDIOGRAM FINDINGS

Electrical Activity of Heart	Electrocardiogram Events
Sinoatrial node fires	Not recorded
Wave of depolarization spreads through atria	P wave
Slight pause at atrioventricular node	Isoelectric baseline between P wave and QRS complex
Atrial repolarization	Not recorded; overpowered by electrical activity of ventricles
Ventricular depolarization	QRS complex
Ventricular repolarization	T wave

beginning of the P wave to the beginning of the QRS complex. Normally the P-R interval measures 0.12 to 0.20 second.

The QRS complex represents depolarization of the ventricles and is often the most significant portion of the ECG. The Q wave is a negative initial deflection from the isoelectric line and may not always be present. A small Q wave of less than 0.04-second duration is a normal finding in leads I, II, III, aV_L, aV_F, and V_4 to V_6. The first positive deflection from the isoelectric line is an R wave. The negative deflection following an R wave is an S wave. The full duration of the QRS complex is measured from the first deflection from the isoelectric line (whether it is a Q or an R wave) to the point where the QRS complex ends and the ST segment begins. The normal QRS complex is 0.05 to 0.10 second.

The ST segment represents the plateau (phase 2) of the action potential. It is normally isoelectric because all cells are at zero potential and no current flows. Slight elevation no greater than 1 mm or a subtle depression no greater than 0.5 mm is considered normal. Abnormal elevations or depressions of the ST segment

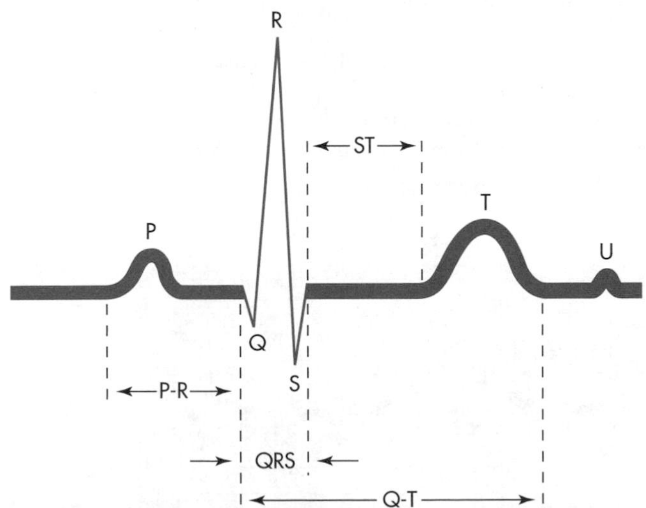

Figure 28-26 Schematic drawing of electrocardiographic waves produced by cardiac cycle.

can occur as a result of myocardial muscle injury, conduction disturbances, hypertrophy, and the effect of digitalis.

The T wave represents phase 3 of the action potential, when the ventricles are being rapidly repolarized. It is normally rounded, slightly asymmetric, and of the same polarity as the QRS complex. The height of the T wave should not exceed 5 mm in a limb lead or 10 mm in a precordial lead. It is normally a positive wave in leads I, II, and V_3 to V_6. The T wave is a negative deflection in lead aV_R and variable in all other leads.

The effective refractory period is present during the beginning of the T wave. At the peak of the T wave, more of the fast sodium channels have recovered and therefore a stronger-than-normal stimulus can produce a successful action potential. However, some fibers are still unresponsive, and electrical chaos and subsequent ventricular fibrillation may occur. The approximate location of this vulnerable period is illustrated in Figure 28-27.

The Q-T interval is measured from the beginning of the QRS complex to the end of the T wave. It represents the entire duration of ventricular depolarization and repolarization. The normal Q-T value varies with age, gender, and heart rate but generally should be less than half the preceding R-R interval. The termination of the T wave is sometimes difficult to determine, and measuring the Q-T interval accurately is not always easy.

The U wave is a small wave sometimes seen after the T wave. It usually deflects in the same direction as the T wave and is best

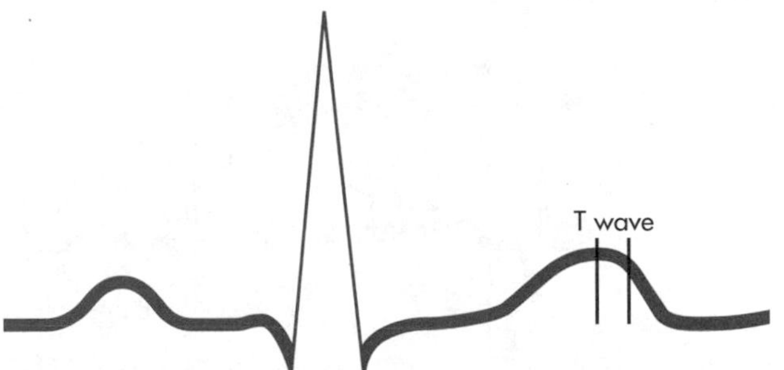

Figure 28-27 Approximate location of vulnerable period of ventricular repolarization.

seen in lead V_3. It has been suggested that the U wave represents late repolarization of papillary muscle.

Normal Sinus Rhythm. The term *normal sinus rhythm* implies that cardiac electrical activity is within normal limits. This means that the following criteria are met (Figure 28-28):

- P waves are present and regular.
- The atrial rate (P waves) is between 60 and 100 beats/min.
- Each P wave is followed by a QRS complex.
- The P-R interval and QRS duration are within established norms.

Electrocardiogram Signal Averaging. ECG signal averaging involves amplification of electrical signals from the heart that have a voltage too small to be recorded by a standard ECG. It is used to detect low-amplitude, high-frequency signals in the terminal portion of the QRS complex to identify patients at risk for ventricular tachycardia. Approximately 200 identical QRS complexes are grouped and averaged, resulting in a waveform that appears smooth and continuous. Signal averaging minimizes the noise that contaminates the ECG signal and thereby exposes signals of a microvolt level normally hidden within the noise. The rate of postinfarction sudden death precipitated by ventricular tachycardia that degenerates into ventricular fibrillation is approximately 10% to 15%.[12] Thus early identification of this life-threatening complication is essential.

Dynamic Studies

Holter Monitor. Resting ECGs supply valuable information about a person's cardiovascular status. However, for patients who experience chest pain or palpitations only during exertion, a more dynamic method for studying the ECG may be necessary. The Holter monitor is used to obtain a continuous graphic tracing of a patient's ECG during daily activities. It is helpful in documenting episodic dysrhythmias. The Holter monitor is a small, portable ECG monitor about the size of a large transistor radio that can be carried with a shoulder strap. The patient is attached to the Holter monitor for approximately 24 hours. During this time the patient keeps a log or diary of daily activities. The log includes activities, medications taken, and unusual sensations the person experiences while attached to the monitor. At the end of the monitoring period, the physician compares the ECG with the patient's log to determine whether any correlations exist between the ECG and the patient's activities.

Stress Testing. The exercise stress test evaluates cardiovascular response to a progressively graded workload. The stress test may be invasive or noninvasive. Stress testing may be performed for a variety of reasons and is often combined with an echocardiogram to obtain additional information about heart function (Box 28-3).

The exercise test can be performed using a treadmill or a stationary bicycle with adjustable resistance to pedaling. Various protocols are used during the procedure, but the patient's blood pressure and ECG are monitored closely during and after the test. Because the stress test is designed to progressively increase myocardial oxygen demand, some patients may experience untoward effects (e.g., ventricular tachycardia, a significant change in peak systolic blood pressure, premature ventricular contractions, or chest pain), and the test may need to be terminated.

Adequate preparation for stress testing is important. Although the procedure is not painful, it can be fatiguing; patients may be anxious because they will be exercising at a level that might produce symptoms such as dyspnea, palpitations, and chest pain. The nurse reviews the purpose and method of stress testing and encourages the patient to[7]:

- Avoid coffee, tea, and alcohol the day of the test.
- Avoid smoking and taking nitroglycerin 2 hours before the test.
- Wear comfortable, loose-fitting clothes. (Women are advised to wear a brassiere for support.)
- Wear sturdy, comfortable walking shoes.
- Consult with the physician about taking any medications before the test.

Box 28-3 Indications for Performing Stress Test

- Evaluation of the patient with symptoms suggestive of coronary artery disease
- Determination of the patient's physical work capacity and aerobic capacity
- Determination of the patient's functional capacity after a myocardial infarction and as an aid in planning an exercise rehabilitation program
- Evaluation of exercise-induced dysrhythmias
- Evaluation of the symptom-free person more than 40 years old who is at risk for coronary artery disease
- Evaluation of pharmacologic interventions for dysrhythmias, angina, or ischemia

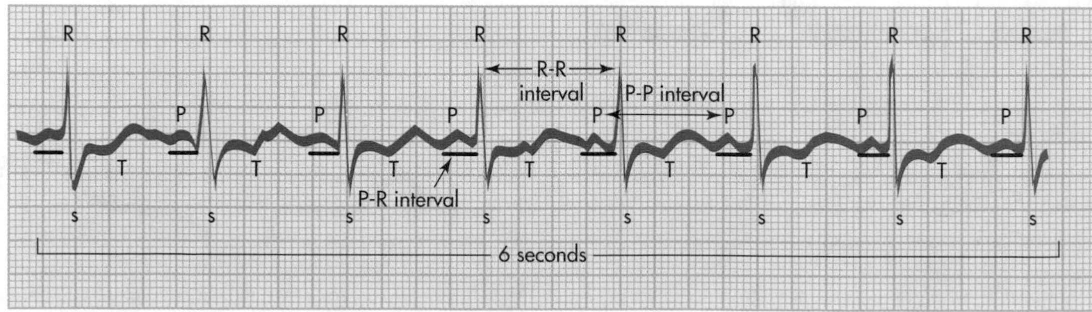

Figure 28-28 Normal sinus rhythm showing R-R, P-P, and P-R intervals.

Scintigraphic Studies

Various types of myocardial imaging can be used to identify myocardial infarctions, evaluate myocardial perfusion, and assess left ventricular function. Myocardial imaging studies are relatively safe and noninvasive techniques for evaluating myocardial function. Myocardial imaging is occasionally combined with stress testing to improve the depth and accuracy of information about myocardial function.

Stannous Pyrophosphate Scan. The pyrophosphate scan, referred to as "hot spot" imaging, typically uses technetium 99m stannous pyrophosphate. A minute dose of the radioisotope is injected into an antecubital vein, and the heart is visualized after about 2 hours. The healthy myocardium shows a homogeneous distribution of the radioisotope, whereas a damaged heart shows an increased uptake of the radioactive material. A gamma scintillation camera is used to identify the area of increased uptake (hot spot). The test is best performed 1 to 3 days after the infarction.

Thallium Imaging. Thallium imaging is referred to as "cold spot" imaging because the uptake of the isotope is greater in healthy myocardial tissue than in the infarction area; thus this area remains a cold spot. A gamma scintillation camera is used to detect the distribution of the radioisotope. Thallium imaging, which most often is combined with exercise testing, can provide valuable information about the extent and severity of myocardial infarction.

Thallium scanning can be helpful in quantifying the amount of myocardium at risk during acute infarction by use of two resting scans to localize the affected area. The resting scan is obtained very early in the infarction, and a redistribution scan is obtained 3 to 4 hours later. The total area of ischemia and infarction is visible on the initial scan. A smaller cold spot is visible during the redistribution scan if the ischemic tissue has successfully extracted the isotope. This technique is useful in evaluating the efficacy of therapeutic interventions such as thrombolytic therapy, as well as providing direction for further treatment based on the degree of myocardium still in jeopardy. Risk is minimal because the amount of thallium injected is small.

Pharmacologic Myocardial Perfusion Imaging. Dipyridamole is a potent coronary vasodilator. By blocking cellular reuptake of adenosine, dipyridamole acts to increase blood and tissue concentrations of adenosine, which in turn promotes optimal coronary vasodilation. In normal coronary arteries, dipyridamole increases blood flow three to four times that of baseline values. In stenosed arteries the increase in flow is less, and with severe stenosis a flow increase may not occur.

Adenosine perfusion imaging may be used as an alternative to dipyridamole because of its significantly shorter half-life (2 to 10 seconds for adenosine versus several minutes for dipyridamole). Adenosine also elicits more consistent maximal coronary vasodilation over a shorter period than does dipyridamole. Side effects are common, however, and include headache, dyspnea, chest pain, and facial flushing. Side effects generally disappear within 1 to 2 minutes and rarely require the administration of aminophylline as an antagonist.

Technetium 99m Sestamibi Myocardial Perfusion (SPECT) Imaging. Technetium 99m sestamibi (Cardiolite) is a nonredistributing radionuclide agent used to evaluate outcomes of thrombolytic and other interventional therapy for acute myocardial infarction. Typically technetium 99m sestamibi is administered in the emergency department, followed by thrombolytic or interventional therapy. Once hemodynamic stability has been established, perfusion imaging is performed. Because minimal redistribution occurs with this agent, delayed images still delineate the initially nonperfused myocardial region. Improvements noted in repeat scintigraphy provide accurate assessment of salvaged myocardium.

Multiple Gated Acquisition Scanning. Multiple gated acquisition (MUGA) scanning has the ability to demonstrate cardiac wall motion to enable assessment of injury and residual cardiac function. The technique lends itself well to the portable imaging techniques required to scan acutely ill patients.

Gated blood pool imaging is a noninvasive radionuclide technique. ECG leads are applied, and the ECG is synchronized to a computer and a gamma scintillation camera. A small amount of technetium 99m is injected intravenously. After the radioactivity reaches a state of equilibrium (approximately 3 to 5 minutes), the patient is placed supine with the gamma scintillation camera positioned over the precordium. The computer then constructs an average cardiac cycle that represents the summation of several hundred heartbeats. Enough data are generated so that an outline of the left side of the heart in all phases of the cardiac cycle can be seen.

Gated blood pool imaging offers several advantages. Because all RBCs are tagged, their counts reflect blood volume. Thus, if the heart can be positioned to isolate the left ventricle on the scan, the left ventricular ejection fraction can be determined. The ejection fraction may provide an early indicator of deteriorating cardiovascular functioning. This information is extremely useful in patients with heart failure or low CO. Right ventricular ejection fraction also can be determined but is less accurate. The effects of pharmacotherapeutics (e.g., nitroglycerin, vasodilators) on ventricular function can also be evaluated. Stress-testing ventriculography can be performed to evaluate the ejection fraction during exercise. Some patients with coronary artery disease demonstrate a normal ejection value at rest but experience a decline under the stress of exercise.

Positron Emission Tomography. Positron emission tomography (PET) is a radionuclide-based imaging technique that uses short-lived radionuclides as tracers to evaluate both perfusion and metabolic events. The tracers are administered by intravenous injection or inhalation. Myocardial uptake is proportional to the quantity of tracer delivered by the blood flow. The tracer elements readily pass through the tissues and are detected by counters placed on opposite sides of the body.

Under normal circumstances the well-perfused, aerobically metabolizing myocardium prefers free fatty acids for energy production. When ischemia is present, more glucose and less fatty acid tend to be used. PET is particularly useful in demonstrating this process because the radioisotopes are incorporated into biochemically relevant components. It also provides the basis for medical management of asymptomatic coronary atherosclerosis and is useful in evaluating the effectiveness of interventions such as thrombolysis and percutaneous transluminal coronary angioplasty.

Sonic Studies

Echocardiography. Echocardiography uses ultrasound to assess cardiac structure and mobility noninvasively. It is useful in the diagnosis of a variety of cardiac conditions (Box 28-4). A small transducer is placed on the patient's chest at the level of the third or fourth intercostal space near the left lower sternal border. The transducer transmits high-frequency sound waves and then receives these waves back from the patient as they are reflected from different structures. The ultrasonic beam that is reflected back from the patient's heart produces "echoes" that are viewed as lines and spaces on an oscilloscope. These lines and spaces represent bone, cardiac chambers and valves, the septum, and muscle. A copy of the echocardiogram is recorded on paper.

Because echocardiography is a noninvasive procedure, it is safer than cardiac catheterization and is usually performed first. There are virtually no contraindications to the echocardiogram, and it can be performed at the bedside of critically ill patients. No special preparation is necessary for the test, and the patient can eat and take medications without interruption. Patient teaching regarding the echocardiogram should include the purpose of the test and the facts that it is painless and takes approximately 30 to 60 minutes. The patient lies quietly in a supine position during the test with the head elevated 15 to 20 degrees. The patient may resume normal activities as soon as the test is completed.

Transesophageal Echocardiography. Transesophageal echocardiography (TEE) allows high-resolution ultrasonic imaging of the cardiac structures and great vessels via the esophagus. It permits echocardiography to be used effectively with patients who have chronic pulmonary disease or are mechanically ventilated and poor candidates for ultrasound testing. This technique uses a transducer affixed to the tip of a modified, flexible endoscope that is advanced into the esophagus and manipulated to produce clear posterior images of the heart. The left atrium, left atrial appendage, and aortic and mitral valves are easily visualized. It is, however, unable to visualize the aortic arch and arch vessels. Box 28-5 summarizes indications for TEE.

Box 28-4 Conditions Detected or Evaluated by Echocardiography

- Abnormal pericardial fluid
- Valvular disorders, including prosthetic valves
- Ventricular aneurysms
- Cardiac tumors, such as atrial myxomas
- Some forms of congenital heart disease, such as atrial septal defects
- Cardiac chamber size
- Stroke volume and cardiac output
- Some myocardial abnormalities, such as idiopathic hypertrophic subaortic stenosis
- Wall motion abnormalities

Box 28-5 Clinical Indications for Transesophageal Echocardiography

- Aortic dissection or aneurysm
- Mitral valve prosthetic dysfunction
- Mitral valve regurgitation
- Infective endocarditis
- Congenital heart disease
- Intracardiac thrombi (especially left atrium and left atrial appendage)
- Cardiac tumor
- Intraoperative assessment: left ventricular function, adequacy of valve repair or replacement

The procedure can be performed at the bedside without contrast dye and with the patient under conscious sedation. The patient receives nothing by mouth for at least 4 to 6 hours before the test. Preprocedure assessment includes any history of esophageal dysfunction or surgery. Initially the patient assumes a chin-to-chest position to facilitate passage of the endoscope through the oropharynx. The scope is advanced 30 to 35 cm to allow posterior visualization of the left atrium by the transducer. To view the left ventricle, the scope is advanced into the stomach and flexed upward for an inferior view. The procedure usually takes about 5 to 20 minutes. The patient is carefully monitored throughout the test and resuscitation equipment is kept readily available. Cardiac rhythm, vital signs, and oxygen saturation (SaO_2) are monitored throughout the procedure. The patient is given a topical anesthetic by spray or gargle to reduce coughing or gagging during probe insertion. Conscious sedation is initiated and maintained with diazepam (Valium) or midazolam (Versed).

The priority for posttest monitoring is the prevention of aspiration. The patient is given nothing by mouth until the gag reflex fully returns. The patient is kept in an upright or side-lying position to support ventilation. Throat lozenges and saline rinses can help alleviate throat discomfort. Other potential complications include esophageal perforation, pharyngeal bleeding, dysrhythmias, and transient hypoxemia.

Phonocardiography

Phonocardiography involves recording electrically amplified cardiac sounds. Special microphones attached to the patient's chest pick up cardiac sounds produced by pressure changes in the heart and great vessels. The sounds are graphically recorded on special phonograph paper. Phonocardiography can be helpful in determining the exact timing and characteristics of murmurs and extra heart sounds. Phonocardiograms may be used in conjunction with echocardiograms so that a comparison can be made between sound (phono) and motion (echo). Patient preparation is similar to that described for the echocardiogram.

Cardiac Catheterization

Cardiac catheterization is an extremely valuable diagnostic tool for obtaining detailed information about the structure and function of the cardiac chambers, valves, and coronary arteries. Cardiac catheterization may include studies of the right side of the heart, the left side of the heart, and the coronary arteries. Indications for cardiac catheterization are summarized in Box 28-6.

Right-Sided Heart Catheterization. Right-sided heart catheterization is performed to evaluate congenital heart disease and valvular disorders. Blood samples and pressure readings are taken, and cineradiographs of the right chambers of the heart and the pulmonary arterial circulation are made. A cardiac biopsy may be obtained in a heart transplant patient to assist in determining whether the body is rejecting the new heart.

To perform a catheterization of the right side of the heart, the physician inserts a catheter via cutdown or percutaneously into a large vein (e.g., the medial cubital, brachial, or internal jugular). The catheter is then threaded with the use of fluoroscopy into the superior vena cava, the right atrium, the right ventricle, the pulmonary artery, and arterioles. As the catheter passes through the various chambers and vessels, blood samples are taken to determine the oxygen content and saturation. Blood pressure measurements also are recorded (Figure 28-29). The pressure is highest in the right ventricle because of the stronger ventricular contractions. Normally the pulmonary artery pressure is approximately 25/10 mm Hg, or approximately one fifth the systemic blood pressure. Elevations in chamber pressures such as an elevated right atrial pressure can indicate valvular problems or possibly right ventricular failure.

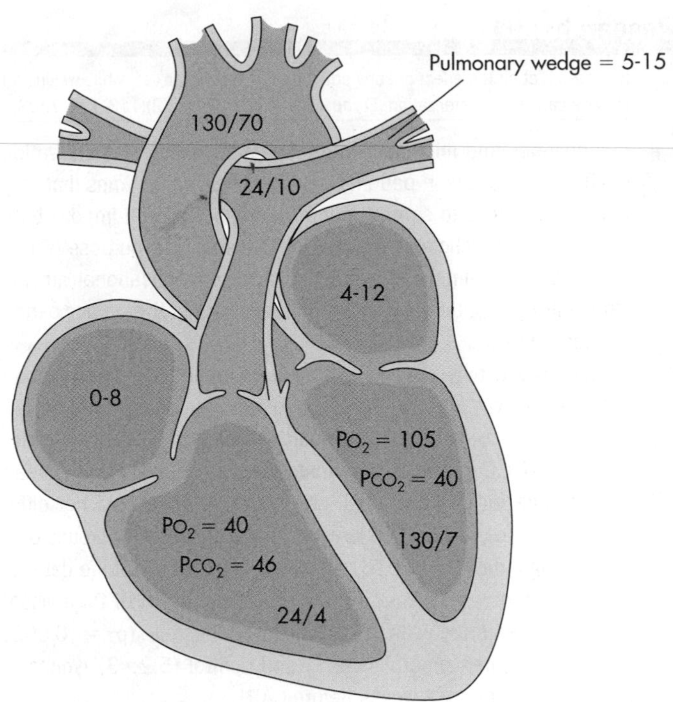

Figure 28-29 Pressure readings and blood gases in millimeters of mercury (mm Hg) in chambers of heart and major blood vessels.

Left-Sided Heart Catheterization. Left-sided heart catheterization is performed to evaluate pressures on the left side of the heart, valvular competency, and left ventricular function. A catheter is passed into the aorta from either the brachial or the femoral artery with the use of fluoroscopy. After reaching the aorta, the catheter is manipulated around the aortic arch, down the ascending aorta, and through the aortic valve into the left ventricle. Pressure-gradient measurements are obtained to detect pressure changes across the valves.

Ventricular angiography may be performed during left-sided heart catheterization. This involves the injection of contrast material into the ventricle while radiographs are taken. Information about contractility, aneurysm formation, valvular disorders, and ejection fraction can be obtained.

Selective coronary arteriography also may be performed during left-sided heart catheterization. The catheter is threaded to the aortic root, and the tip of the catheter is then advanced into the right and left coronary arteries. Contrast medium is injected into each coronary artery, which outlines the entire coronary circulation, and cineangiographic films are taken to monitor the progression of the dye. This outlines the number and severity of stenotic segments and the presence of collateral vessels.

Introduction of the dye may temporarily displace blood flow in the coronary arteries and may produce transient ischemia and chest pain. Sublingual nitroglycerin may be administered to relieve the discomfort. In addition, medications such as isosorbide (Isordil) may be given to dilate the vessels and achieve greater visualization. Occasionally, injection of contrast material into the right coronary artery may suppress the SA node, producing bradydysrhythmias, and administration of intravenous atropine may be required.

Box 28-6 Indications for Cardiac Catheterization

- Confirmation of suspected heart disease, including congenital heart disease, valvular disease, and myocardial disease
- Determination of the location and severity of the disease process
- Preoperative assessment to determine whether cardiac surgery is indicated
- Evaluation of ventricular function after surgical revascularization
- Evaluation of the effect of medical treatment modalities on cardiovascular function
- Performance of specialized cardiac interventions such as internal pacemaker placement

Preparing for Catheterization. Preparation for cardiac catheterization is extremely important. The nurse should provide information about the procedure, care after the test, common sensations that may be experienced during the catheterization, and a brief description of the room environment during the test. Even after careful preparation most patients remain apprehensive about both the procedure and the possible results (see Research box). It is important to include the family in all pretest teaching if possible. The nurse asks the patient concerning any history of allergy, especially to iodine, shellfish, and contrast media. The meal before the procedure is usually withheld. If the procedure is scheduled for later in the day, the patient may be permitted a clear liquid breakfast. A mild sedative may be given before the procedure, and an antibiotic may be ordered as a prophylactic measure. The nurse assesses the presence and quality of peripheral pulses and marks them before the test.

Research

Harkness K et al: The effect of early education on patient anxiety while waiting for elective cardiac catheterization, *Europ J Cardiovasc Nurs* 2(2):113-121, 2003.

A supply-demand mismatch with respect to cardiac catheterization (CATH) often results in patients experiencing waiting times that vary from a few weeks to several months. Long delays can impose both physical and psychologic distress on patients. The purpose of this study was to examine the effect of a psychoeducational nursing intervention on patient anxiety at the beginning of the waiting period for elective CATH.

This was a two-group randomized controlled trial. Intervention patients received a nurse-delivered, detailed information and education session within 2 weeks of being placed on the waiting list for elective CATH. Control group patients received usual care. The mean waiting time for CATH was 13.4±7.2 weeks, which did not differ between groups ($p = 0.509$). Anxiety increased in both groups over the waiting time ($p = 0.028$). Health-related quality of life deteriorated over the waiting time in both groups ($p < 0.05$). On a visual analog scale, there was a significant difference ($p = 0.002$) between the intervention (4±2.7) and control (5.2±3) groups in self-reported anxiety 2 weeks before CATH.

The waiting period before elective CATH has a negative impact on patients' perceived anxiety and quality of life, and a simple intervention, provided at the beginning of the waiting period, may positively affect the experience of waiting.

Relatively little discomfort is involved in a right-sided heart catheterization, although the patient may feel pressure in the femoral or antecubital area. During a left-sided heart catheterization, the patient may experience a warm, flushing sensation for approximately 30 seconds as the contrast medium is injected. The patient also may experience nausea and "fluttering" sensations produced by catheter manipulation or catheter advancement through the heart.

The body's physiologic responses to cardiac catheterization are numerous and vary with each person. Therefore it is essential that the patient understand the importance of reporting any unusual sensations that occur during and after the catheterization.

Nursing Care After Catheterization. The postprocedure nursing care after both types of heart catheterization is similar. These procedures generally last from 1 to 3 hours and can be tiring for the patient. Many patients prefer to rest or sleep after the examination. The nurse monitors the patient's pulse and blood pressure every 15 minutes for 1 hour and then every 30 minutes for 3 hours. It is essential to check the pulses distal to the catheter insertion site to determine the patency of the cannulated artery. The amplitude of the pulse may be slightly diminished for approximately 24 hours because of arterial spasm or edema at the site. At times thrombus formation may totally obliterate the distal pulse, and surgery may be necessary to restore circulation.

If a femoral approach was used, the patient is initially placed on bed rest and monitored for signs of bleeding, inflammation, tenderness, or edema at the insertion site. Various modalities are currently being used to prevent bleeding at the puncture site. Historically, sandbags or weights were used; however, these have been replaced by hemostatic plugs and vascular closure devices that provide external compression. Frequent puncture site observation is a priority in any postprocedure monitoring protocol.[2] The patient should not have the head of the bed elevated more than 30 degrees and should keep the affected leg extended.

If the brachial site is used, the arm is kept straight for several hours, usually with an arm board, but the patient can be up in the room as soon as vital signs are stable. If any bleeding occurs from the cutdown site, the nurse applies firm pressure directly over the site and notifies the physician.

Intake and output are monitored in all patients regardless of the approach used to ensure an adequate intake to flush the dye from the circulation and to monitor the patient's renal status. Hypotension may develop as a result of the diuretic effect of the contrast material used during angiography.

Complications of cardiac catheterization are not common; however, cardiac dysrhythmias such as ventricular fibrillation can occur. The development of tachycardia or any dysrhythmia is reported to the physician immediately.

Contrast Angiography and Venography

Contrast angiography, or arteriography, is a standard in vascular diagnostic imaging. It is the most invasive test used in the evaluation of peripheral vascular disease and has the greatest risk for the patient. Angiography assists in the diagnosis of arterial emboli, arterial trauma, aneurysm, Buerger's disease, and reevaluation of the patency of arteries after grafting. The procedure involves inserting a radiopaque catheter into the vessel with the patient under local anesthesia, followed by injection of a contrast medium. X-ray films are obtained that visualize the arterial system.

Venography is performed in a similar manner except that the venous system is examined. It is the definitive test in the diagnosis of deep venous thrombosis; another common use of this test is with patients suspected of having incompetent vein valves. The test takes about an hour and is uncomfortable for the patient.

The procedure and nursing interventions are similar to those for a cardiac catheterization. The nurse assesses the patient for allergies to contrast media before the procedure, obtains informed consent, and explains that it is common to experience a flushing or burning sensation after injection of the contrast medium.

A pressure dressing may or may not be placed at the insertion site after the procedure. The extremity is kept straight while the site is closely monitored for hemorrhage, hematoma, and inflammation. Potential complications include an allergic reaction to the contrast medium, thrombi, perforation of the vessel, emboli, renal failure, and pseudoaneurysms. Creatinine levels are monitored to evaluate renal function.

Digital Subtraction Angiography

Digital subtraction angiography, or digital vascular imaging, is a computerized fluoroscopic procedure that visualizes the vascular system. It is less expensive and quicker than angiography.

Contrast medium is injected through a catheter, and x-ray films are taken with the patient under local anesthesia. A state-of-the-art video system displays the vessels on a television monitor while a computer subtracts images that are not necessary. Separate injections are required for different views of the limb. Pretest and posttest nursing care is similar to that provided for arteriography.

Electrophysiologic Study

The electrophysiologic (EP) study systematically assesses the heart's electrical stability. This procedure requires electrode placement within the heart to record intracardiac electrical activity. The degree of invasiveness depends on the area of the heart to be studied. More detailed information about the heart's electrical activity can be obtained with the EP study than with the surface ECG because of the proximity of the catheters to the cardiac conduction system. The test demonstrates the exact sequence of atrial and ventricular activation, localizes areas of conduction disturbances (such as accessory pathways, areas of ischemia and infarction, and dysrhythmia foci), and evaluates the effectiveness of antidysrhythmic management. Although EP studies are used more often than in the past, they are not routinely ordered. Their use is currently reserved for persons not responding to standard treatment.

An EP study is performed using fluoroscopy to guide the pacing electrodes into position. The electrodes are typically inserted through the femoral, brachial, or basilic veins. Arterial cannulation is performed only when left ventricular stimulation is necessary. Before the test antidysrhythmic drugs usually are discontinued for approximately five half-lives to prevent pharmacologic interference with the study. Three to six intracardiac pacing catheters are inserted and connected to a multichanneled electrogram. A surface ECG is recorded simultaneously for comparison and evaluation. When indicated, dysrhythmias may be initiated by applying a series of programmed extra stimuli to areas of the heart, and the effects of various antidysrhythmic drugs are evaluated. Pacing also may be used to terminate a tachycardia by inhibiting impulse transmission in conduction pathways.

The EP study usually lasts 2 to 4 hours. At completion of the test, catheters are removed and pressure applied at the insertion site, followed by application of a pressure dressing. Patients may be closely monitored in a telemetry or intensive care unit after the test. Complications of EP studies are similar to those of cardiac catheterization. Patients are closely monitored for hemorrhage, perforation, hematoma, pulmonary emboli, deep venous thrombus, infection, cerebrovascular accident, angina, and dysrhythmia.

The nurse plays a key role in preparing patients for an EP study. Reinforcing teaching about the indications for the test, the procedure itself, and its risks may allay anxiety for the patient and family. A description of the equipment used and the room's appearance is also helpful. It is important that patients know they will be awake throughout the procedure.

Postprocedural monitoring includes vital signs; peripheral pulses; insertion site; and color, warmth, and sensation of extremities. Initially these observations are performed every 15 minutes and then gradually reduced to every 4 hours. The affected extremity is immobilized, and the patient is placed on bed rest for 4 to 6 hours. Documentation of any changes in rhythm and frequency of ectopy is essential.

Invasive Hemodynamic Monitoring

Invasive hemodynamic monitoring (also see Chapter 10) is not a typical diagnostic test, but it is used to evaluate the hemodynamic status of the critically ill patient and has greatly increased the data base for health professionals planning and evaluating therapeutic modalities. Numerous devices are used in hemodynamic monitoring.

Central Venous Pressure. Central venous pressure (CVP) measurements reflect the pressures in the right atrium and provide information regarding changes in right ventricular pressure. The CVP is used to monitor blood volume and the adequacy of venous return to the heart. Because the CVP reflects the pressure in the great veins as blood returns to the right side of the heart, a low (or falling) reading may indicate an inadequate blood volume (hypovolemia). A high (or rising) CVP usually is secondary to left-sided heart failure. Unfortunately, the patient's hemodynamic status may be severely compromised before representative changes in the CVP are evident. Normal values for CVP vary with different equipment; however, a range of 5 to 15 cm H_2O is considered acceptable. It is important to note that a change or a trend in the CVP is more important than the actual numerical value.

Intraarterial Blood Pressure Measurement. In the critically ill patient the CO may be decreased to such an extent that standard blood pressure readings may be inaccurate. As the stroke volume falls, Korotkoff sounds become increasingly more difficult to auscultate. Invasive arterial blood pressure monitoring will more accurately reflect actual blood pressure.

Arterial catheters are most commonly placed in the radial, brachial, and axillary arteries, although other vessels may be used. The patient with an arterial line requires frequent observation. It is essential that the extremity with the arterial line be kept uncovered so the insertion site can be monitored for bleeding. The pulse, color, sensation, and temperature of the extremity distal to the catheter are assessed every 2 hours.

Pulmonary Artery and Pulmonary Capillary Wedge Pressures. A balloon-tipped catheter (Swan-Ganz catheter) may be introduced into the pulmonary artery to obtain essential information regarding left ventricular function. The pulmonary artery catheter permits the measurement of the pulmonary artery end-diastolic pressure (PAEDP) and the pulmonary capillary wedge pressure (PCWP) (Table 28-6). The best indicator of left ventricular function is the left ventricular end-diastolic pressure (LVEDP). Elevations in LVEDP result from impaired left ventricular contractility that does not permit adequate emptying of the ventricles. The PAEDP and the PCWP are similar in a healthy person. However, in the presence of increased peripheral vascular resistance such as that found in pulmonary embolism, the PAEDP will rise while the PCWP remains normal. Therefore, to evaluate the true LVEDP, the health care provider must monitor PCWP.

Insertion of the pulmonary artery catheter is accomplished using several different approaches. These include a small incision (cutdown) in an antecubital vein or percutaneously through the internal jugular or subclavian veins. The catheter is threaded

TABLE 28-6 PULMONARY ARTERY AND CAPILLARY WEDGE PRESSURES

Type	Common Abbreviation	Normal Values (mm Hg)
Left ventricular end-diastolic pressure	LVEDP	12-15 (Elevations result from inadequate emptying of ventricles.)
Pulmonary artery end-diastolic pressure	PAEDP	4-12 (Elevations result from increased peripheral vascular resistance.)
Pulmonary capillary wedge pressure	PCWP	4-12 (Levels >25 mm Hg indicate imminent pulmonary edema.)

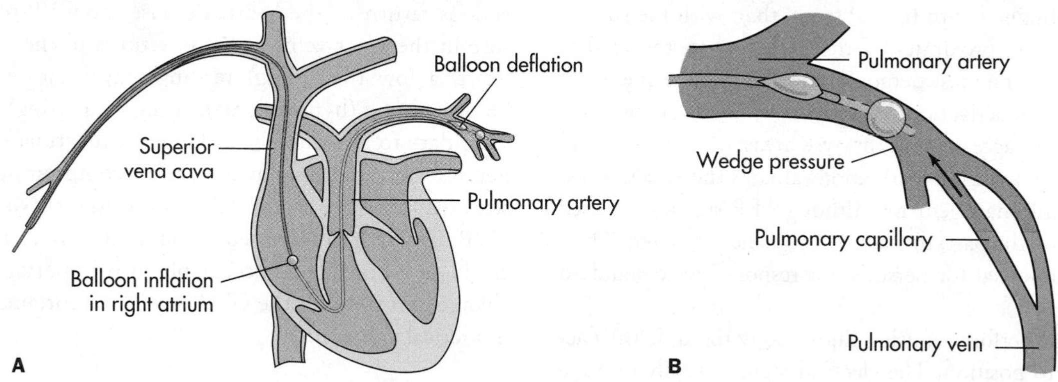

Figure 28-30 A, Flow-directed, balloon-tipped catheter showing inflation of balloon in right atrium and consequent "floating" of catheter through right ventricle and out to distal pulmonary artery branch. Balloon is deflated, advanced slightly, and reinflated slightly to obtain pulmonary capillary wedge pressure (PCWP). **B,** During initial positioning of balloon-tipped catheter in pulmonary artery, balloon is deflated. Catheter is then advanced and balloon is reinflated just long enough to obtain PCWP.

through the superior vena cava, through the tricuspid valve, and into the pulmonary artery. The balloon is then inflated, which causes the catheter to wedge in a distal branch of the pulmonary artery (Figure 28-30). Measurement of PAEDP is continuous. The PCWP is measured when the balloon is inflated, usually every 2 to 4 hours. It reflects pressures in the pulmonary capillary bed and left-sided heart function.

Three- and four-lumen catheters are also available that allow measurement of additional hemodynamic parameters. Some catheters have a third lumen that contains a thermistor used to determine CO by the thermodilution technique. A fourth lumen that ends at the level of the right atrium can be used to monitor CVP and to obtain blood samples. A four-lumen thermodilution catheter is illustrated in Figure 28-31.

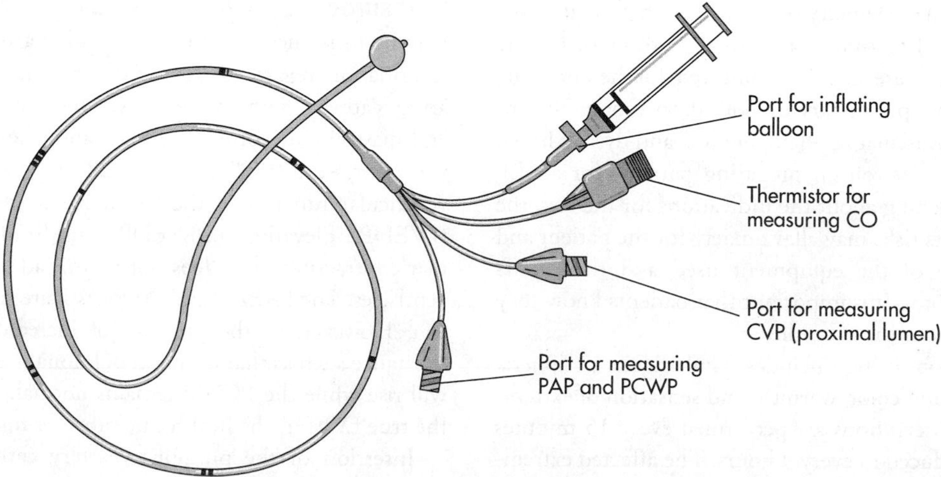

Figure 28-31 Four-lumen thermodilution pulmonary artery catheter for measuring cardiac output *(CO)*, central venous pressure *(CVP)*, pulmonary artery pressure *(PAP)*, and pulmonary capillary wedge pressure *(PCWP)*.

Noninvasive Vascular Tests

Doppler Ultrasound. Doppler ultrasound, or ultrasound imaging, aids in the diagnosis of carotid artery disease, peripheral artery disease, venous occlusive disease, valvular insufficiency, and deep venous thrombosis. Ultrasonic waves directed at an artery or vein reflect off RBCs, producing a waveform or audible sound. Arterial waveforms should be pronounced, with peaks and valleys reflective of the systolic and diastolic pressures; a flattened waveform indicates obstruction. Venous waveforms are in phase with respirations and are of continuous amplitude.

Ankle-Brachial Index. The ankle-brachial index is the most commonly used parameter for overall evaluation of arterial status in the lower extremity. Blood pressure measurements are obtained over both the dorsalis pedis and posterior tibial arteries using a regular blood pressure cuff. A Doppler probe is then placed over the pulse, and the cuff is inflated to above systolic pressure. The point at which the pulse returns as the cuff deflates is recorded as the systolic endpoint number. Typically the higher of the two pressures is used as the indication of vascular status. This number is divided into the higher of two brachial artery pressures (e.g., an ankle pressure of 70 mm Hg with a brachial pressure of 140 mm Hg gives an index of 0.5). Normal foot arteries have an index of 1.0 to 1.2. Indexes below 1.0 indicate arterial obstruction.

Impedance Plethysmography. Venous outflow in the lower extremities is measured by inflation and deflation of pneumatic cuffs around the thighs. The assumption is that because blood is a good conductor of electricity, the electrical resistance will change as blood volume is altered. Electrodes are attached to obtain measurements and determine quality of blood flow. Sharp rises in venous volume suggest venous occlusion, such as blood clots. If a deep venous thrombosis is present in a major vessel, the increase in blood volume during the test is less than expected because the veins are already full.[6] During the procedure the patient is kept supine with the leg elevated and knee flexed.

Exercise Testing. The treadmill test is used to obtain an objective measurement of the severity of intermittent claudication. This test is similar to the test used to evaluate the heart, except the walking speed is usually 1.5 to 2 miles/hr with a grade elevation of 10% to 20% and a time limit of 5 minutes. A walking tolerance of 5 minutes suggests mild disease, and 1 minute indicates severe disease. Patients are instructed to wear loose-fitting clothing and good walking shoes. The exercise is stopped at the maximal level of exertion or when symptoms become disabling.

Magnetic Resonance Imaging. Magnetic resonance imaging (MRI) creates a three-dimensional image of the blood vessels for evaluation of the vascular network, measurement of blood flow velocities, and assessment of stages of vascular disease. MRI does not require ionizing radiation or any contrast media and may be preferred to arteriography. However, MRI is expensive and time consuming, which makes it a less likely choice for routine screening. The patient is informed that the noise level during the test may be high and require the use of earplugs. Confinement in a relatively small space is sometimes problematic for patients who have a tendency toward claustrophobia.

References

1. American Heart Association: *Heart disease and stroke statistics,* accessed July 2004 from website: http://www.americanheart.org/presenter.jhtml?identifer=1200000.
2. Best DG, Grainger P: Cardiac biomarkers: new kids on the block, *Can J Cardiovasc Nurs* 12(3):10–16, 2002.
3. Braunwald E et al, editors: *Harrison's principles of internal medicine: disorders of the cardiovascular system,* accessed July 2004 from website: http://harrisons.accessmedicine.com/server-java/Arknoid/amed/harrisons/co_chapters/ch225/ch225_p01.html.
4. Cesari M et al: Inflammatory markers and cardiovascular disease, *Am J Cardiol* 92(5):522–528, 2003.
5. Clare SA, Sandys NP: A nurse-led approach to secondary prevention of CHD in primary care, *Professional Nurse* 18(1):38–41, 2002.
6. Docherty B: Adult/elderly care nursing: cardiorespiratory physical assessment for the acutely ill, *Brit J Nurs* 11(11):750–752, 754–758, 2002.
7. George EL, Tasota FJ: Predicting heart disease with C-reactive protein, *Nursing* 33(5):70–71, 2003.
8. Lai CS et al: Prevalence of troponin-I elevation during out of hospital cardiac arrest, *Am J Cardiol* 93(6):754–756, 2004.
9. MacKenzie JR: Predicting CAD events: C-reactive protein, a marker for atherosclerotic risk, *Nurse Practitioner* 29(6):14–15, 19, 22–24, 2004.
10. Mandadi VR et al: Predictors of troponin elevation after percutaneous coronary intervention, *Am J Cardiol* 93(6):747–750, 2004.
11. Robinson SL: Is it an MI? What the leads tell you, *RN* 67(5):48–54, 2004.
12. Somers MP et al: Additional electrocardiographic leads in the ED chest pain patient: right ventricular and posterior leads, *Am J Emerg Med* 21(7):563–573, 2003.

Visit the Evolve website: http://evolve.elsevier.com/Monahan/medsurg

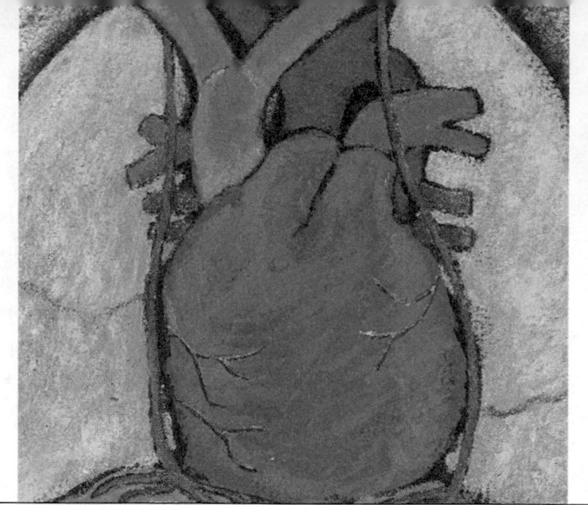

CHAPTER 29

Coronary Artery Disease and Dysrhythmias

by Kathy Henley Haugh

OBJECTIVES

After studying this chapter, the learner should be able to:

1. Discuss the role of risk factors in the pathogenesis of coronary artery disease.
2. Recognize the signs and symptoms of coronary artery disease.
3. Explain the collaborative management of stable angina pectoris and acute coronary syndromes.
4. Discuss the nursing role in the care of the patient with coronary artery disease.
5. Recognize common dysrhythmias associated with the cardiac conduction system.
6. Discuss the collaborative care management of patients with cardiac dysrhythmias.
7. Describe the basic components of cardiopulmonary resuscitation.

KEY TERMS

angina, p. 746
angioplasty, p. 761
antiplatelet agent, p. 757
atrioventricular block, p. 787
automaticity, p. 773
biomarkers, p. 755
bradycardia, p. 776
cardioversion, p. 789
defibrillation, p. 789
dyslipidemia, p. 748
dysrhythmia, p. 753
pacemakers, p. 790
Q wave infarctions, p. 752
reentry, p. 775
remodeling, p. 761
telemetry, p. 789
tachycardia, p. 776
thrombolytics, p. 757

Patients with coronary artery disease (CAD) often seek health care after experiencing angina or myocardial infarction (MI). CAD is directly implicated in other cardiovascular diagnoses such as dysrhythmias, heart failure, and cardiomyopathy. All nurses need to be familiar with the collaborative care management of CAD because of its high prevalence in the industrialized world. This chapter discusses the origins and management of CAD. It also discusses the recognition and management of common dysrhythmias.

Coronary Artery Disease

Etiology and Epidemiology. Coronary heart disease (CHD), which encompasses acute MI, angina pectoris, atherosclerotic cardiovascular disease, and all other forms of acute and chronic ischemic heart disease, is the leading cause of death in the industrialized Western world, accounting for one of every five deaths in 2001. It is estimated that 13,200,000 Americans have CHD; 7,800,000 have experienced MI; and 6,800,000 have angina. Approximately 865,000 Americans experienced a new or recurrent MI in 2001, with 184,757 deaths. CHD remains the number one health problem in the United States and the leading cause of premature, permanent disability.[4]

CAD is a generic designation for many different conditions that involve obstructed blood flow through the coronary arteries. The most prevalent etiologies of CAD are atherosclerosis, coronary vasospasm, and microvascular angina. Microvascular **angina** results from poor function of the smaller blood vessels that supply the heart. Atherosclerosis is by far the most common cause of CAD and is the focus of this chapter.

Both individual risk factors and the presence of concurrent disease states influence the incidence of CAD. Some populations have an increased occurrence of CAD because of definable characteristics or risks. Risk factors are classically categorized as nonmodifiable and modifiable. Nonmodifiable risk factors include age, gender, race, family history, and genetics. Modifiable risk factors include diabetes, hypertension, tobacco use, sedentary lifestyle, obesity, and stress (see Risk Factors box). The American Heart Association (AHA) has not firmly established hyperhomocysteinemia as an independent risk factor; however, it has established guidelines for monitoring homocysteine levels in high-risk individuals.[19] C-reactive protein, another measure of inflammation, is also considered a marker for an increased risk of cardiovascular disease and of adverse outcomes in patients with acute coronary syndrome (ACS). People in a high-risk group have about a

Risk Factors

Coronary Artery Disease

Established Risk Factors

- Age and gender
- Family history and genetics
- Diabetes
- Hypertension
- Tobacco use
- Sedentary lifestyle
- Dyslipidemia
- Obesity

Risk Factors Requiring More Research

- Stress
- Race
- Hyperhomocysteinemia

twofold increase in relative risk for cardiovascular disease compared with those in a low-risk group. Current guidelines suggest that highly sensitive C-reactive protein can be used as an independent marker of risk, but should not yet be used for mass screening or to guide therapy.[20] Table 29-1 links the major risk factors for CAD with their specific physiologic effects.

AGE AND GENDER. Clinical evidence of CAD is rarely apparent before the second and third decades of life, but CAD is already a leading cause of mortality in men 35 to 45 years old. Overall, CHD makes up more than half of all cardiovascular events for persons less than 75 years of age. The average age of a person having a first heart attack is 65.8 for men and 70.4 for women. Eighty-four percent of individuals who die of CHD are 65 years of age or older. However, about 80% of CHD deaths in people under age 65 occur during the first attack.[4] The incidence of CAD in women significantly increases after menopause, and one in three women over age 61 has some form of CAD. The theoretical cardioprotective benefits of estrogen stimulated a wide variety of research regarding the effects of hormone replacement therapy (HRT). Unfortunately, researchers through large-scale studies instead found an increase in cardiovascular events in women taking HRT. Therefore HRT is no longer recommended for preventing heart disease in women. With increasing longevity in the Western world, the incidence of CAD among both male and female octogenarians and nonagenarians also will increase.

RACE. CAD is nondiscriminatory, affecting all races, but the independent role of race in the development of CAD is unclear. Other risk factors such as hypertension, obesity, lifestyle (including cultural practices), ethnic traditions, access to health care, and individual choices may play a more significant role in the development of CAD than race alone.

FAMILY HISTORY AND GENETICS. The likelihood that an offspring will have CAD increases if the biologic parent manifests CAD before the age of 55, but it is difficult to determine the

TABLE 29-1 ROLE OF RISK FACTORS IN CORONARY ARTERY DISEASE

Risk Factor	Physiologic Effect
Age and gender	Decrease in elasticity of arteries with age Estrogen in females lowers serum cholesterol, decreases systemic vascular resistance, and improves endothelium-dependent vasodilation
Heredity: family history of coronary artery disease	Undetermined—genetic research pending
Diabetes	Damage to intima Modified lipid metabolism from insulin
Hypertension	Decreased elasticity of blood vessels Tearing effect on arteries Increased resistance to ejection of ventricular volume
Tobacco use (nicotine)	Decreased high-density lipoproteins Displacement of oxygen from hemoglobin Increased catecholamines in response to nicotine, increasing heart rate, and increasing blood pressure Increased platelet adhesiveness Accelerated atheroma formation Coronary spasm
Sedentary lifestyle	Altered lipid metabolism Altered insulin sensitivity
Hypercholesterolemia, familial hyperlipidemia	More substrate provided for lesion formation Increased levels of low-density lipoproteins, increasing atherogenesis

independent role of genetics in the pathogenesis of CAD. Confounding variables include environmental factors and individual lifestyle choices that significantly influence the development of CAD. Genetics may directly affect the incidence of CAD through the differential coding of genes responsible for lipid metabolism (apolipoprotein E), homocysteine metabolism, angiotensin-converting enzyme (ACE) levels, and coagulation.

DIABETES. Heart disease is the leading cause of diabetes-related deaths. Adults with diabetes have heart disease death rates about two to four times higher than adults without diabetes.[8] Hyperinsulinemia, a consequence of peripheral insulin resistance, can occur up to a decade before hyperglycemia is even diagnosed. Elevated levels of circulating insulin may begin the process of atheroma formation by initiating damage to the arterial intima. Impaired insulin regulation is associated with a variety of atheromatous processes, including elevated triglycerides, decreased high-density lipoprotein (HDL) levels, elevated very-low-density lipoprotein (VLDL) levels, coagulation disorders, increased vascular resistance, obesity, and hypertension.

HYPERTENSION. Hypertension, defined as a measured elevation in blood pressure above 140/90 mm Hg on at least three occasions, increases the incidence of CAD twofold to threefold. National Heart, Lung, and Blood Institute guidelines define blood pressures of 120 to 139 mm Hg systolic and 80 to 89 mm Hg diastolic as prehypertension.[28] Hypertension affects the ability of the blood vessel to constrict and dilate. Shearing forces on the intimal lining caused by hypertension predispose the artery to atherosclerosis. In addition, the heart must work harder to pump against an increased resistance to blood flow. Adequate control of hypertension with medication and lifestyle modifications may decrease the incidence of CAD in the hypertensive population.

TOBACCO. The risk of death from CAD is significantly higher in smokers than in nonsmokers, and the risk is proportional to the amount of tobacco used. In addition, approximately 35,000 nonsmokers die from CHD yearly secondary to environmental smoke.[7] Cigarette smokers have the highest incidence of CAD; however, pipe and cigar smokers, as well as tobacco chewers, also have an increased risk of developing CAD compared with nonusers.

SEDENTARY LIFESTYLE. In 1996 the surgeon general released a seminal report on physical activity and health. This report noted that the incidence of CAD is higher in individuals who do not participate in regular physical activity compared with those who exercise. Exercise is associated with a decrease in total cholesterol, low-density lipoprotein (LDL) cholesterol, and triglycerides. Up to 60% of U.S. adults reported no pattern of regular exercise during the study period in the early 1990s.[25] The Centers for Disease Control and Prevention (CDC) data collected during 2000 and 2001 showed that these numbers had not yet improved, with 54.6% of Americans ages 18 and older considered not active enough to meet physical activity recommendations.[9]

DYSLIPIDEMIA. Research findings consistently report an association between abnormal blood cholesterol levels **(dyslipidemia)** and CAD. In 2001, 50.7% of the U.S. population had total cholesterol levels greater than 200 mg/dl, 45.8% had LDL cholesterol levels greater then 130 mg/dl, and 26.4% had HDL cholesterol levels less than 40 mg/dl.[4] LDLs are the most atherogenic of the lipid compounds, transporting 60% to 70% of the body's cholesterol. An increased triglyceride level, in combination with a high LDL level, is also a strong predictor of heart disease and MI. Research also indicates that elevated plasma lipoprotein (a) levels are predictive of premature CAD in men. Hyperlipidemia may be either primary (familial) or secondary to some other process, such as concomitant disease states (e.g., diabetes) or lifestyle factors, such as diet, sedentary activity levels, and smoking. Excess lipids in the circulation result in endothelial injury and increase the available substrate for foam cell production, an early step in the development of atherosclerotic lesions.

OBESITY. Obesity is also associated with an increased risk of cardiovascular disease. Sixty-four percent of the U.S. adult population was defined as overweight in 2001, and 15.3% of children ages 6 to 11 were defined as overweight.[4] Although obesity is commonly cited as a significant coronary risk factor, the extent to which it has an independent effect in predisposing a person to CAD is controversial. But obese persons are more prone to glucose intolerance, hypertension, elevated triglycerides, and low levels of HDL. In addition, obese individuals often demonstrate other behaviors, such as sedentary lifestyles, that are known risk factors for CAD.

STRESS. Much discussion has taken place over the years about the relationship between stress and CAD. Catecholamines, released during the stress response, increase platelet aggregation and may also precipitate vasospasm. A complete understanding of the effects of stress on circulation, lipid metabolism, and coagulability still requires additional research.

HOMOCYSTEINE. Homocysteine is an amino acid synthesized during protein catabolism by the conversion of methionine to cysteine. Homocysteine is believed to contribute to vascular disease by altering coagulation, activating the inflammatory response, and contributing to endothelial dysfunction. The metabolism of homocysteine depends on vitamin B_6, folate, and vitamin B_{12}. Levels of homocysteine greater than 15 μmol/L are predictive of increased mortality and morbidity. The AHA recommends screening for total homocysteine in patients with a personal or family history of premature cardiovascular disease.[18]

Pathophysiology. CAD refers to the development and progression of plaque accumulation in the coronary arteries. Figure 29-1 illustrates the dynamic nature of CAD. Stages along the continuum are stable angina and ACS; the most severe presentation is MI. A patient with CAD may seek treatment at any point along this continuum and may move back and forth along the continuum over time.

STABLE ANGINA. The coronary arteries are small arteries that provide oxygen to the beating heart, a surface that is constantly moving (see Chapter 28). The arteries lie on the epicardial surface

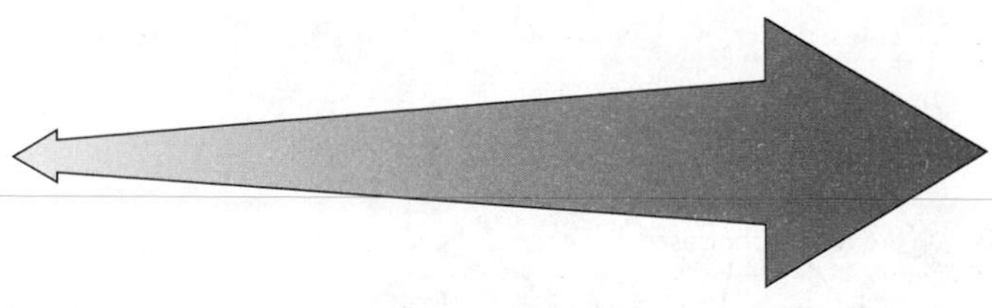

Figure 29-1 Continuum of coronary artery disease. Arrow depicts increased severity of continuum to the right.

and branch frequently. The small size of the arteries, constant tension, and turbulence at the bifurcations all contribute to the development of atherosclerotic lesions.

Normally the endothelium of the coronary artery allows for unrestricted blood flow to the myocardium. Any kind of trauma or irritant, including high cholesterol, hypertension, and smoking, can disrupt this protective endothelium. Infectious pathogens such as *Chlamydia pneumoniae*, hepatitis A virus, *Helicobacter pylori*, and cytomegalovirus have also been implicated in endothelial injury. The body's response to the injury involves a complex interplay of chemical mediators designed to protect the area.

Platelets adhere to the collagen and release adenosine diphosphate (ADP). Circulating platelets with ADP-specific surface receptors become activated and bind to the released ADP. Endothelial injury also triggers the release of thromboxane A_2, which causes local vasoconstriction to minimize the extent of injury and further stimulates platelet aggregation (Figure 29-2). Endogenous nitric oxide acts to protect the artery through vascular relaxation.

The intima also releases prostacyclin in response to the effects of thromboxane A_2. Prostacyclin works to restore equilibrium by local vasodilation and opposing platelet aggregation. With repeated injury, however, the deteriorating intima cannot produce sufficient prostacyclin to balance the process, and platelet aggregation forces predominate. Activation of the various platelet factors also causes the glycoprotein (GP) IIb/IIIa receptor sites to change shape and build fibrinogen bridges with adjacent platelets. Platelets and accumulating monocytes also release powerful growth factors into the arterial wall that stimulate the proliferation and migration of medial smooth muscle cells into the intima. This increases the permeability of the vessel wall to cholesterol. The accumulation of cholesterol produces a fatty streak that protrudes into the lumen of the artery. Endothelial injury also causes the release of leukocyte-soluble adhesion molecules and chemotactic factors. These factors mediate the attachment of monocytes to endothelial cells and encourage monocyte migration into the subintima.[20] Smooth muscle cells and fibrous tissue then form a fibrous cap over the fatty streak.

The fatty streak continues to grow, accumulating macrophages, mast cells, and activated T cells and invading both the intima and media. Involvement of the media affects the vessel wall's ability to vasodilate and vasoconstrict. The artery continues to supply oxygen and nutrients to the myocardium as long as the blockage is less than 70% of the arterial lumen. Stable plaques may even occlude the coronary artery by more than 70% and still not cause symptoms.

The presence of risk factors appears to accelerate the atherogenesis, decreasing the oxygen supply. The presence of risk factors can also increase the myocardium's demand for oxygen (see Table 29-1). Concomitant conditions such as anemia, smoking (carbon monoxide displaces oxygen in the bloodstream), and hypovolemia further compromise delivery of oxygen to the myocardium. The demand for oxygen can be met only by an adequate blood supply. As long as supply is greater than or equal to demand, aerobic metabolism occurs. When demand is greater than supply, the myocardium must switch to anaerobic metabolism for nourishment. Anaerobic metabolism produces lactic acid, which is believed to be responsible for ischemic anginal pain. This pain is the most common initial symptom of CAD, but it does not have to be present for the diagnosis of CAD to be made. Myocardial oxygen demand increases with any condition causing an increase in heart rate, resistance to ejecting blood volume, or myocardial size. With stable angina the patient usually experiences a known threshold beyond which myocardial oxygen demand exceeds supply.

ACUTE CORONARY SYNDROME. Atherosclerosis may remain stable if the blockage in the coronary artery does not progress beyond 70%; if collateral (alternate) vessels develop to supply the myocardium; and, most important, if the fibrous cap remains intact. Inflammation plays a critical role in plaque destabilization. Lipoprotein-associated phospholipase A_2 (Lp-PLA_2) hydrolyzes oxidized LDL, generating proinflammatory mediators that increase adhesion molecules, cytokine production, and the migration of monocytes into the intima. Monocytes differentiate into macrophages that engulf oxidized LDLs to become foam cells. Pressure within the lesion (plaque) can increase to the point of plaque rupture. Activated macrophages also cause the secretion of connective tissue enzymes that break down collagen, weakening the fibrous cap.[20] Smaller, soft, lipid-rich lesions appear to be the most likely to rupture. Rupture of the fibrous cap exposes the inner plaque to the circulating blood, activating clotting factors and causing both collagen accumulation and smooth muscle cell proliferation (Figure 29-3). The process of platelet activation is once again initiated to seal the rupture.

The presence of certain risk factors also contributes to this destructive pathophysiologic process. Nicotine from tobacco use increases platelet adhesion and increases the potential for clotting at the site of disruption. Catecholamines released during the stress response also increase platelet aggregation.

Plaque rupture has several possible outcomes (Figure 29-4, *A* and *B*). The area can heal over with the platelet plug absorbed into the plaque under a new cap, in which case the larger plaque further narrows the vessel lumen and may precipitate symptoms. The second outcome leaves a residual fibrous clot extending into the lumen, partially obstructing the artery. A third possible outcome is complete obstruction of the coronary artery with the fibrous clot. This is termed *coronary thrombosis* or *coronary occlusion* and is the first stage of MI (Figure 29-4, *C*). Acute coronary occlusion triggers a rapid series of physiologic events. Myocardial ischemia distal to the occlusion occurs immediately. Ischemia alters the integrity and permeability of the myocardial cell membrane to vital electrolytes. This instability depresses myocardial contractility and predisposes the patient to sudden

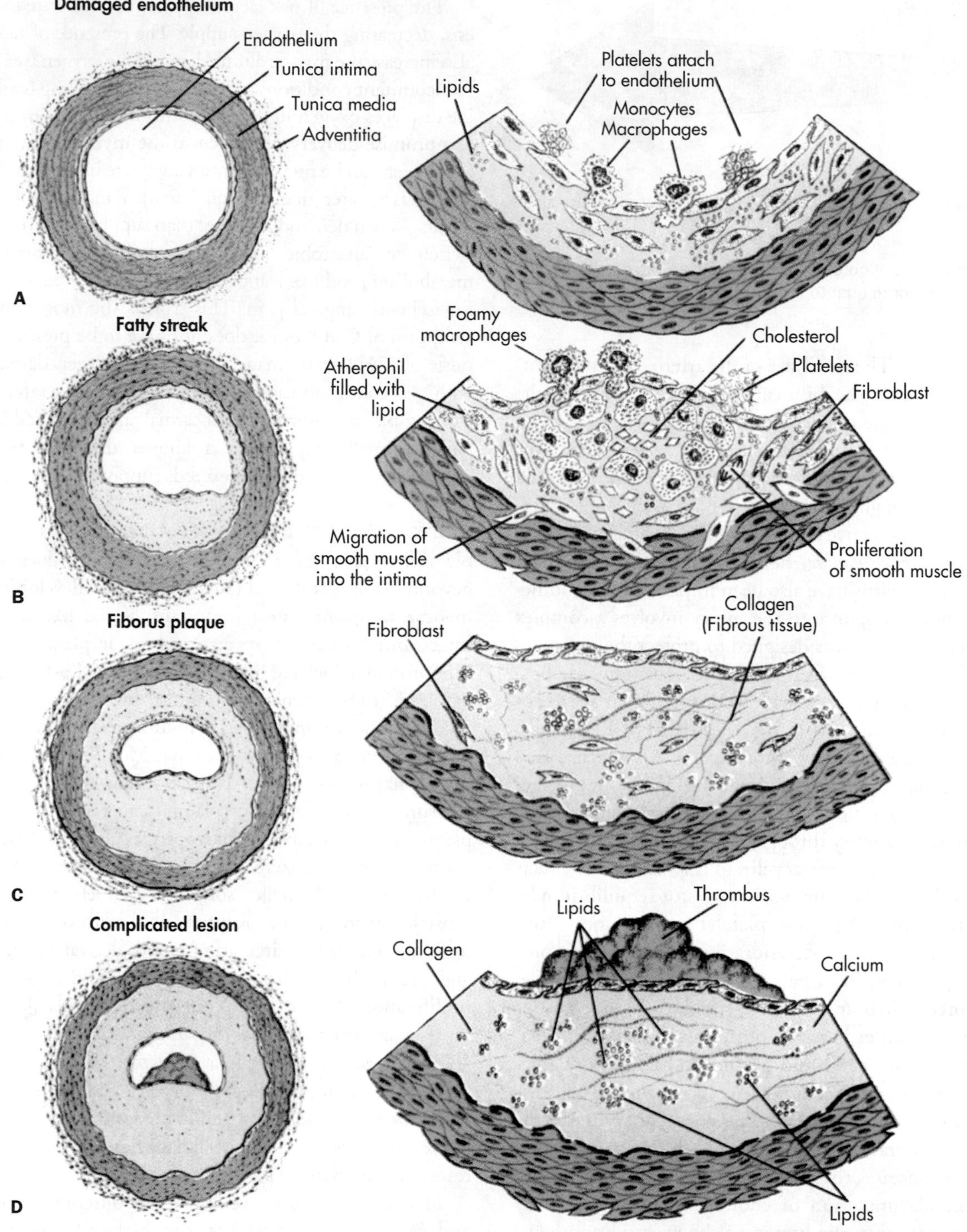

Figure 29-2 Progression of atherosclerosis. **A,** Thromboxane stimulates platelet aggregation. Inflammatory response initiates monocyte activity. **B,** Medial smooth muscle migrates into intima, increasing permeability of the wall to cholesterol. **C,** Fibrous cap seals plaque. **D,** Macrophages secrete enzymes that weaken fibrous cap. Rupture of plaque stimulates thrombus formation and acute coronary syndrome.

death from dysrhythmias. Figure 29-5 illustrates the spiraling series of events that occurs in the cardiovascular system from myocardial ischemia.

The body activates the process of fibrinolysis to lyse the clot and restore blood flow. However, if clot lysis does not immediately restore blood flow, ischemia continues in the area of myocardium distal to the obstruction. Time is a critical factor in this scenario. Ongoing myocardial ischemia for 20 minutes or longer can result in tissue death. This is termed *acute myocardial infarction* (AMI). A zone of ischemia, made up of potentially viable tissue, surrounds the infarcted area of myocardium. The final size of an infarct depends on whether this marginal area in the ischemic zone succumbs to the effects of prolonged ischemia (Figure 29-6). The entire thickness of the myocardium may not become

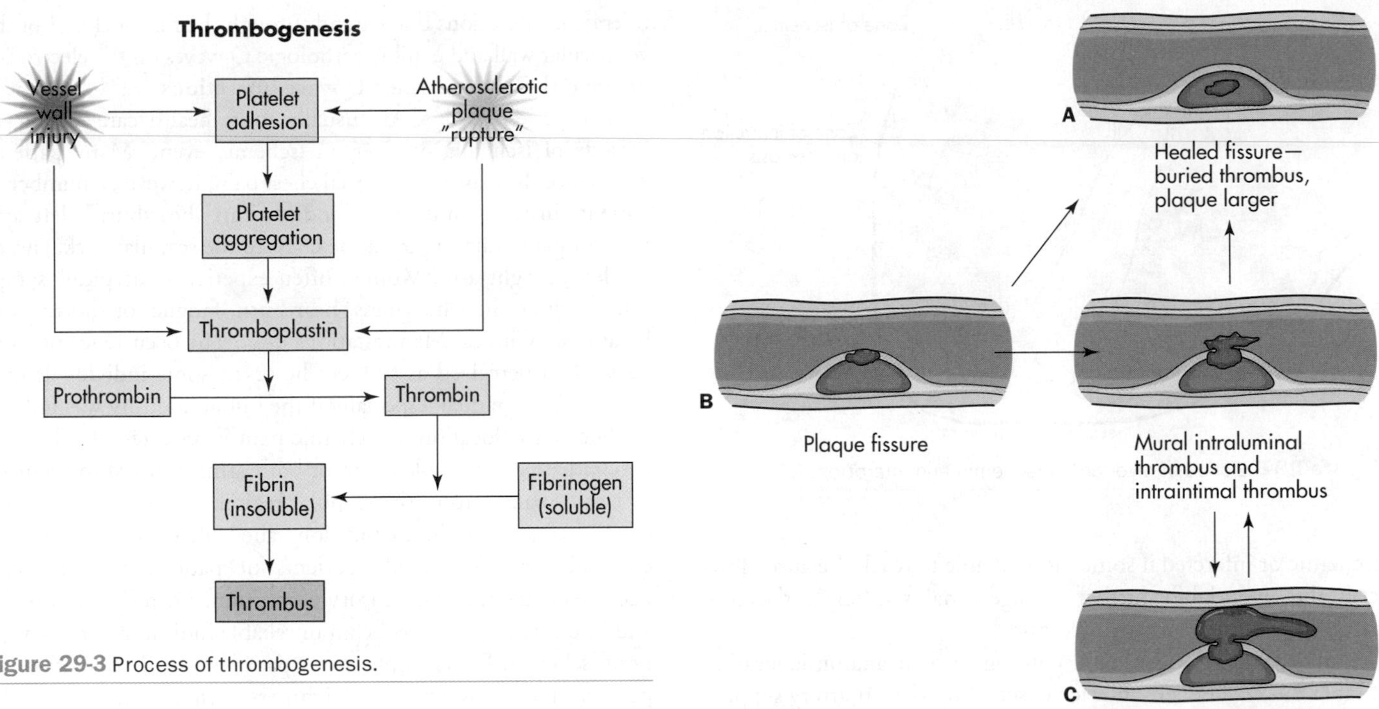

Figure 29-3 Process of thrombogenesis.

Figure 29-4 Possible pathophysiologic scenarios after plaque fissure. **A,** Clot is resorbed into plaque, healing over area of fissure, but with smaller lumen resulting. **B,** Clot remains at site of fissure, decreasing lumen diameter. **C,** Clot extends into lumen, completely obstructing lumen (myocardial infarction).

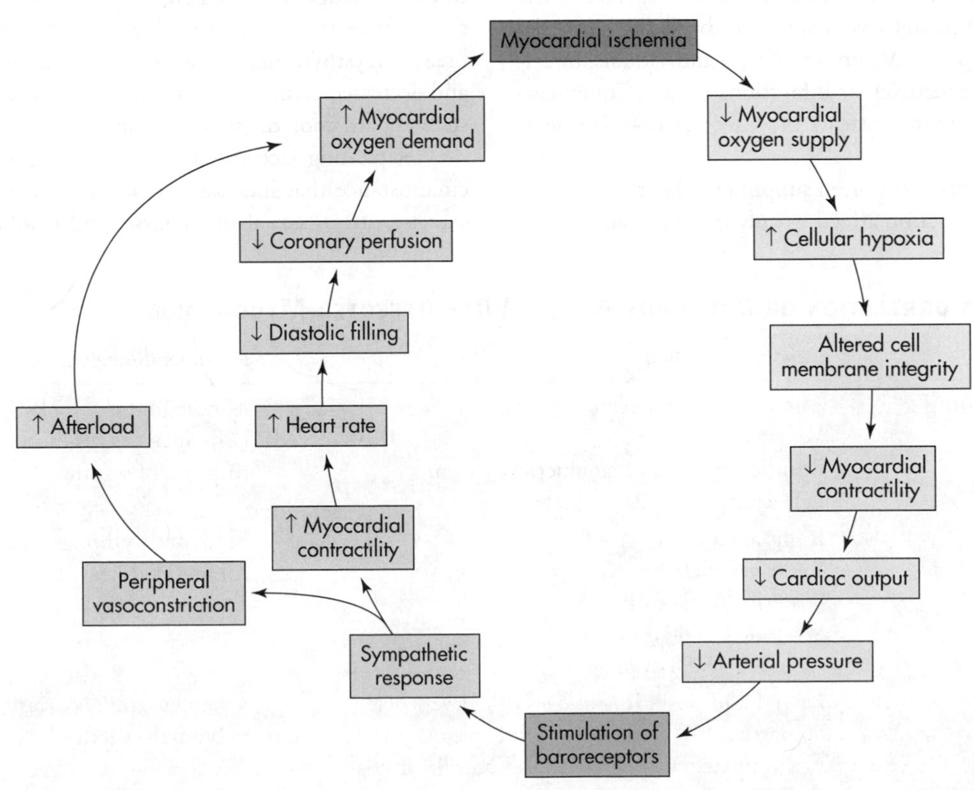

Figure 29-5 Effects of prolonged myocardial ischemia.

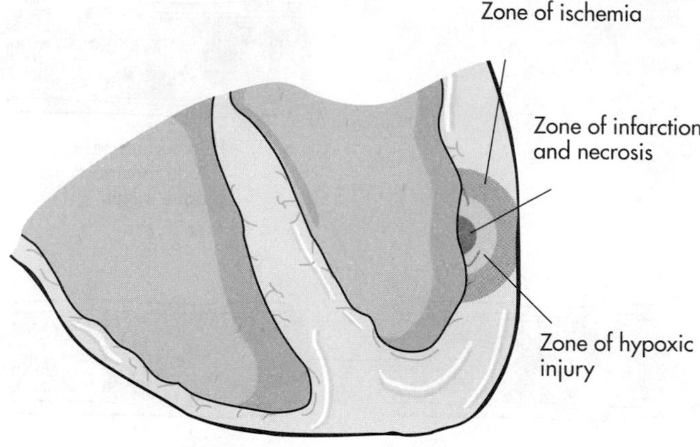

Figure 29-6 Zones of myocardial ischemia and infarction.

ischemic or infarcted if some blood is able to reach the area. However, the potential for further damage remains as long as the coronary artery lumen is atherosclerotic.

Infarctions are classified according to their anatomic location (Table 29-2). The left anterior descending (LAD) artery supplies the anterior surface of the left ventricle and the bundle branches of the conduction system. This area of the heart is responsible for most of the contractility necessary to eject blood into the aorta. This portion of the heart requires a substantial source of oxygen to generate the force needed to pump against the aorta's high-pressure system. Lesions in the LAD artery that lead to anterior infarctions are often associated with a decrease in contractility and cardiac output that results in heart failure. Sudden death secondary to ventricular dysrhythmias may also occur.

The right coronary artery supplies the inferior surface of the left ventricle, the entire right ventricle, and both the sinoatrial (SA) and atrioventricular (AV) nodes in most individuals. Inferior infarctions or right ventricular infarctions may be complicated by transient or permanent heart blocks or right-sided heart failure.

The circumflex artery most often supplies the lateral surface of the left ventricle. Obstruction affecting only this area is often well tolerated. Infarctions that extend through the full thickness of the ventricular wall and exhibit pathologic Q waves on the electrocardiogram (ECG) are termed **Q wave infarctions.**

The patient with CAD usually seeks health care during an episode of ischemia or after an ischemic event. Many patients experience the classic midsternal chest pain; however, a number of patients instead complain of indigestion; "heartburn"; left arm pain; or pain radiating from the chest to the scapula, neck, jaw, or the left or right arm. Women often experience "atypical" symptoms such as chest heaviness, heartburn, fatigue, or shortness of breath (see Clinical Manifestations box). The occurrence of angina is often perceived as sudden; however, some individuals may perceive it as gradual, especially if the initial intensity was mild.

The classic location of ischemic pain is retrosternal. The pain may radiate down the left arm or both arms, upward to the neck or jaw, or backward to the scapular region. Some patients do not experience pain at all, a condition called silent ischemia. This is especially true for elderly patients or patients with diabetes because of alterations in sensory perception. Therefore the quality and intensity of pain may be an unreliable indicator of the severity of ischemia. For example, some patients with MI describe the pain as "mild indigestion" or "tightness," whereas others describe the pain as excruciating and viselike.

Symptoms of stable angina are often of short duration, ending when the demand for oxygen is decreased. Symptoms of unstable angina are of longer duration and usually require intervention. Symptoms of MI continue until blood flow is restored or the myocardium dies.

In addition to chest pain, patients may complain of dizziness, dyspnea, nausea, vomiting, or anxiety. Patients experiencing an AMI often report a feeling of doom or as though they are "going to die." Changes in vital signs may include tachycardia or bradycardia, increased or decreased blood pressure, and shortness of breath. Dysrhythmias may develop from myocardial ischemia, and decreased cardiac output can result in classic shock symptoms such as pale, cool, diaphoretic skin.

Precipitating factors for stable angina symptoms include any circumstance that increases myocardial oxygen demand, such as exercise, stress, sexual intercourse, and smoking. ACS may have

TABLE 29-2 CORRELATION OF CORONARY ARTERY WITH AFFECTED MYOCARDIUM

Coronary Artery	Structure Supplied	Potential Complications
Left anterior descending	Anterior surface of left ventricle Ventricular septum Bundle branches of conduction system Left atrium	Bundle branch blocks Left-sided heart failure Rupture of septum
Right coronary	Right atrium Right ventricle Posterior surface of left ventricle SA node (55% of people) AV node (90% of people)	Bradydysrhythmias and heart blocks Right-sided heart failure
Circumflex	Lateral and posterior surfaces of left ventricle Sinoatrial (SA) node (45% of people) Atrioventricular (AV) node and bundle of His (10% of people)	When circumflex artery supplies SA node, bradydysrhythmias a possibility

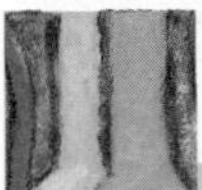

CLINICAL MANIFESTATIONS *Coronary Artery Disease*

Subjective

Pain: midsternal, jaw, or left arm
Pain radiation to the scapula, neck, jaw, or arm
Indigestion, heartburn
Dizziness
Dyspnea
Nausea
Anxiety
Feeling of doom

Objective

Clutching, rubbing, or stroking chest
Vomiting
Tachycardia, bradycardia
Shortness of breath
Elevated blood pressure (or hypotension in some patients)
Dysrhythmias
Altered neurologic status, if decreased cardiac output
Crackles, if decreased contractility creates left ventricular failure
Presence of S_3 or S_4 gallop
Diminished pulses
Pallor

Diagnostic Indicators

Electrocardiogram: ST elevation or depression, Q waves, T wave abnormalities
Laboratory: elevated CK-MB, troponin I, glucose, white blood cells, erythrocyte sedimentation rate

Alternative Presentations

Women: chest heaviness, heartburn, fatigue, shortness of breath
Older or diabetic patients: shortness of breath, syncope, fatigue, confusion

similar precipitating factors or no identifiable precipitating event. The onset of ACS can occur at rest or on awakening if platelets are stimulated.

COMPLICATIONS. The most common complications of CAD are heart failure, dysrhythmias, and pericarditis. The likelihood of complications increases with severe multivessel CAD and with AMI. Additional complications include cardiogenic shock, ventricular septal defect, free wall rupture, ventricular aneurysms, and ischemic cardiomyopathy. Nursing research has investigated the association between the meaning patients attach to having an MI and the occurrence of complications (see Research box).

HEART FAILURE. Heart failure in CAD occurs in response to decreased contractility secondary to an ischemic myocardium. A hypokinetic or akinetic myocardium does not generate the inotropic action needed to sustain adequate cardiac output. The amount of ischemic or infarcted myocardium determines the onset and severity of heart failure. Heart failure is most often seen in patients having large MIs, particularly MIs involving the anterior surface of the myocardium. The use of ACE inhibitors in the acute setting to reduce afterload may limit postinfarction remodeling, reducing the risk of heart failure. Heart failure is discussed in Chapter 30.

DYSRHYTHMIAS. Dysrhythmias often occur secondary to the ischemic processes of CAD. Ischemia alters the stability of the myocardial cell membrane, and ischemia of the specialized conduction pathways (SA node, AV node, and bundle branches) can result in heart blocks. Individuals with right coronary artery blockages and inferior MIs may experience heart block and bradycardia, since the right coronary artery most often supplies the SA and AV nodes. Patients with LAD artery blockages may have complete or incomplete bundle branch blocks and ventricular dysrhythmias, since the LAD artery supplies the bundle branch system and a disproportionately large surface of the anterior myocardium. Direct damage to the myocardial cell creates electrolyte imbalances that alter the cells' action potential. Dysrhythmias are not usually treated unless they are considered hemodynamically significant. Management of common dysrhythmias is presented later in the chapter.

Research

Cherrington CC et al: Illness representation after acute myocardial infarction: impact on in-hospital recovery, *Am J Crit Care* 13(2):136, 2004.

Forty-nine patients with myocardial infarction treated with percutaneous transluminal coronary angioplasty and beta-blockers were studied to determine the relationship between illness representation at the time of myocardial infarction and the occurrence of in-hospital complications. The researchers also studied the role of anxiety and depression in mediating this relationship. Patients were interviewed 24 to 48 hours after admission using three tools: the Illness Perception Questionnaire (IPQ), which measures five concepts of illness representation; Spielberger State Anxiety Inventory (SSAI); and the second edition of the Beck Depression Inventory (BDI). The researchers reviewed medical records at discharge for the occurrence of complications, including dysrhythmias, myocardial ischemia, heart failure, cardiac arrest, reinfarction, and cardiac death. The sample included equal numbers of men and women, the mean age was 60.8 years, and the majority of subjects had some education beyond high school. Because of the geographic location, all subjects in the sample were white.

The researchers found that as illness representation became more negative, the odds of experiencing a complication increased by 1.051. Patients found to have a negative representation of having a myocardial infarction were also more likely to be depressed or anxious compared with patients with a positive representation. Nurses must be alert to the significance and meaning patients attach to having a myocardial infarction, since a negative representation may be associated with a higher risk of complications.

PERICARDITIS. After an AMI the heart's pericardial lining can become inflamed, and fluid may accumulate between the parietal and visceral layers. The patient complains of severe precordial chest pain that closely resembles that of the original infarction. The presence of a characteristic pericardial friction rub is helpful in making the differential diagnosis. Pericarditis is usually treated with nonsteroidal antiinflammatory drugs or occasionally corticosteroids. Pericarditis is presented in greater detail in Chapter 30.

Collaborative Care Management

DIAGNOSTIC TESTS. When a patient has signs or symptoms of CAD, a variety of diagnostic tests are used to confirm the diagnosis of MI and to guide therapeutic options (Box 29-1).

ELECTROCARDIOGRAPHY. The ECG remains a critical tool in diagnosing CAD and is most useful while the patient is symptomatic. Because the ECG represents only one point in time, serial 12-lead ECGs, continuous monitoring, or both are the standard of care for the evaluation of chest pain. ST segment elevation is the hallmark of acute myocardial ischemia that is progressing toward infarction[21] (STEMI) (Figure 29-7). ST elevation resolves when blood flow is restored or the MI is complete. If the full thickness of the myocardium becomes necrotic, significant Q waves evolve over the next week. Future ECGs continue to show the Q wave, indicating that the patient suffered an MI in the past. When only the subendocardial surface infarcts (non–Q wave MI), Q waves do not develop. T wave abnormalities such as T wave inversion may also occur at the time of acute infarction. Non–ST segment elevation MI (NSTEMI) refers to an ACS that does not cause ST elevation but does produce elevated serum troponin levels. Normal or nonspecific findings on ECG do not always exclude the possibility of MI.

Gender and ethnicity affect ECG interpretation in subtle ways. Women with an MI may not exhibit the dramatic ST elevation of acute injury, perhaps because of less cardiac muscle mass, estrogens, and dampening of the ECG signal by breast tissue. Early repolarization patterns and ST segment elevation at the J point (the point where the QRS complex ends and the ST segment begins) are more prevalent in African-Americans. Comparison with the patient's prior ECG, when possible, helps with the differential diagnosis. Acute pericarditis, digitalis effects, electrolyte imbalances, hypothermia, subarachnoid hemorrhages, and ventricular hypertrophy may all affect the ST segment and should be considered with the patient's presentation. The presence of a left bundle branch block creates additional challenges to ECG interpretation.[1]

The 12-lead ECG represents 12 different anatomic views of the myocardium (see Chapter 28). ST changes occur in leads that are specific to the area of myocardium involved. Table 29-3 shows the relationship of specific leads to the affected area of myocardium. Additional leads are necessary to reveal damage to the right ventricle or posterior wall of the left ventricle. These 15- and 18-lead ECGs use the right chest wall and posterior thorax sites for localizing damage to the myocardium.

ST segment monitoring is an important part of patient monitoring to detect ischemia in patients who are seen with ACS and

Box 29-1 Diagnostic Tests for Coronary Artery Disease

12-Lead Electrocardiogram

Serial tests or continuous monitoring

ST segment elevation is a critical marker for myocardial ischemia progressing to infarction.

Elevation of greater than 1 mm in 2 contiguous leads plus the presence of new Q waves indicate a high probability of myocardial infarction (MI).

ST depression reflects ischemia that may resolve with improved perfusion.

Normal or nonspecific findings do not rule out the possibility of MI.

Serum Biomarkers

Serum Troponin

Composed of three proteins: troponin C, troponin I, and troponin T

Levels are normally undetectable.

Myocardial damage causes levels of troponin I to rise within 3 hours.

Levels remain elevated for up to 7 days (see Table 29-4).

Creatine Kinase

Confirms the presence of myocardial damage

Levels rise within 3 to 9 hours and return to normal in 1 to 3 days.

Levels decrease at 12 hours and help determine the endpoint of myocardial damage and the presence of reinfarction.

Myoglobin

Levels increase within 1 hour and return to normal within 24 to 36 hours.

Blood Chemistry and Complete Blood Count

Elevated glucose levels may occur in response to stress.

White blood cell count may elevate to 12,000 to 15,000/mm^3 in response to injured cardiac tissue. Elevation may last 3 to 7 days.

Erythrocyte sedimentation rate may remain elevated for several weeks.

C-Reactive Protein

Elevations are believed to be associated with an increased risk of adverse outcomes in persons with acute coronary syndrome.

Stress Testing

With or without nuclear imaging

Pharmacologic agents may be used to simulate the exercise response in patients who cannot exercise.

Cardiac Catheterization

Left-sided catheterization may include both angiography and ventriculography.

Other Options

Resting cardiac magnetic resonance imaging
Positron emission tomography
Multiple gated acquisition (MUGA) scanning
Technetium 99m SPECT scans
Multislice computed tomography (CT)
Electron bean CT
Radionuclide angiography scans

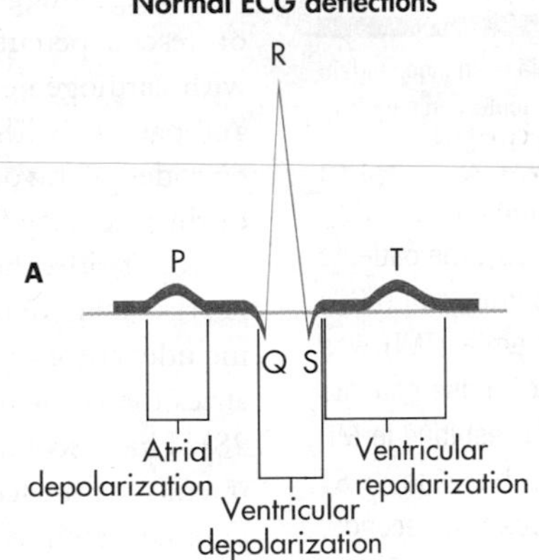

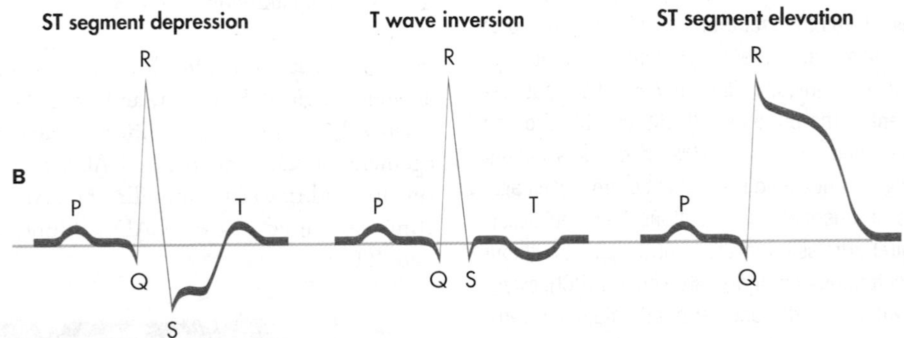

Figure 29-7 Electrocardiogram (ECG) and coronary artery disease. **A,** Normal ECG. **B,** ECG alterations associated with ischemia and injury.

TABLE 29-3 CORRELATION OF ELECTROCARDIOGRAPHIC FINDINGS WITH CARDIAC ANATOMY

Acute Changes In Leads	Anatomic Location of Infarct
II, III, aV_F	Inferior
I, aV_L, V_4-V_6	Lateral
V_1-V_3	Anteroseptal
V_1-V_6	Anterolateral
R:S ratio > 1 in V_1 and V_2	Posterior
Upright T waves in V_1, V_8, V_9, RV_4, RV_5 (right precordial lead placement)	Right ventricular

those who receive thrombolytic therapy or coronary interventions. ST segment monitoring is also useful in detecting silent ischemia. Research supports the value of ST segment monitoring in ACS (see Research box, p. 756).

BLOOD TESTS. Biomarkers provide definitive information about the presence and severity of myocardial damage and are drawn immediately in patients experiencing unrelenting chest pain. Biomarkers are especially valuable in evaluating patients who are seen for possible thrombolytic therapy. The most specific biomarker for MI is serum troponin, which is composed of troponin C, troponin I, and troponin T. Any elevation of serum troponin indicates myocardial cell damage. Cardiac troponin I that is already elevated on admission is associated with an increase in both complications and mortality (Table 29-4). However, elevated troponin levels may also reflect minor myocardial injury from causes other than ACS.

Injured myocardial cells release another biomarker, the enzyme creatine kinase (CK), during AMI. CK elevation confirms the presence of myocardial damage. Brain tissue and skeletal muscle also release CK with injury, but the isoenzyme CK-MB is specific to the myocardium. Myoglobin, an oxygen-binding protein found in cardiac and skeletal muscle, is another early biomarker for MI.

Blood chemistry tests and a complete blood count (CBC) are performed to determine concurrent disease states and help with differential diagnosis. C-reactive protein, another measure of inflammation, is also considered a marker for an increased risk of cardiovascular disease. The AHA and CDC have established risk guidelines for C-reactive protein as follows: concentrations of less than 1.0 mg/L are considered low risk, 1.0 to 3.0 mg/L are average risk, and higher than 3.0 mg/L are high risk. People in the high-risk group have about a twofold increase in relative risk for cardiovascular disease compared with those in the low-risk group.[20]

STRESS TESTING AND ECHOCARDIOGRAPHY. Stress testing is a noninvasive test that highlights areas of the myocardium that do not receive adequate perfusion at peak exercise and relates the significance of coronary artery blockages to the patient's functional status. The ECG tracings recorded during the exercise component of the test can also indicate which coronary arteries might be involved. Echocardiography is another noninvasive test that may be used (see Chapter 28).

Research

Pelter MM, Adams MG, Drew BJ: Transient myocardial ischemia is an independent predictor of adverse in-hospital outcomes in patients with acute coronary syndromes treated in the telemetry unit, *Heart and Lung* 32(2):71, 2003.

This study investigated the value of ST segment monitoring in 237 patients admitted with acute coronary syndrome (ACS). The patients were monitored using continuous 12-lead electrocardiogram (ECG) ST segment monitoring. Transient myocardial ischemia (TMI) was detected in 17% of patients (n = 39). Thirty-five of these patients had TMI, and four patients had sustained ischemia resulting in MI. TMI was defined as a change from the patient's baseline in ST amplitude of 1 mV in at least 1 ECG lead for at least 60 seconds. The occurrence of ischemic events ranged from 1 to 8 in the TMI group with an average duration of 43 minutes (range, 2 to 90 minutes). Of particular interest was the fact that only 10 patients (26%) had chest pain or an anginal equivalent symptom during at least one episode of TMI; TMI was clinically silent in 74% of the patients with TMI. Forty-six percent of the patients with TMI by ECG also had in-hospital complications compared with 10% of patients without TMI ($p < 0.001$). This significance held even after controlling for age, gender, and prognosis. In-hospital complications included occurrence of MI after hospital admission in those ACS patients without MI who underwent percutaneous coronary intervention (PCI), extension of MI if admitted with MI, cardiovascular death, major dysrhythmia necessitating intervention, hemodynamic compromise necessitating intervention, and unplanned transfer from the telemetry unit to the CCU because of acute complications. A significantly higher proportion of patients with ischemia had hypotension, acute MI, and abrupt closure after PCI, compared with those patients without ischemia. In addition, patients with ischemia were more likely to sustain an MI or die compared with patients without TMI. Patients with ischemia had a longer duration of hospitalization. The presence of TMI was the only independent predictor of adverse outcome.

Table 29-4 Cardiac Biomarker Levels in Acute Myocardial Infarction

Cardiac Enzyme	Elevation (hr)	Peak Elevation (hr)	Duration (hr)
Creatine kinase MB	3-9	12-18	1-3
Troponin T	3-5	10-24	10-14
Troponin I	3-6	10-24	7
Myoglobin	1	4-6	1-2

Additional Noninvasive Studies. Radionuclide myocardial perfusion imaging has been helpful in diagnosing AMI in the emergency room. Normal resting perfusion imaging studies have been used to exclude MI and avoid unnecessary hospitalizations. Options for scanning are listed in Box 29-1.

Cardiac Catheterization. Cardiac catheterization is indicated for patients who have recurrent symptoms despite intensive medical management, and for patients with one or more recurrent, severe, or prolonged (longer than 20 minutes) ischemic episodes. The AHA recommends diagnostic catheterization in the following emergent or urgent situations: candidates for primary or rescue percutaneous coronary interventions (PCI), patients with cardiogenic shock who are candidates for revascularization, and patients with spontaneous episodes of myocardial ischemia or episodes of myocardial ischemia provoked by minimal exertion during recovery from STEMI.[5]

Right-sided heart catheterization provides information on the heart's hemodynamic status. Left-sided heart catheterization includes coronary angiography and left ventriculography, and visualizes the coronary arteries, as shown in Figure 29-8 (see Chapter 28). Fluoroscopic imaging allows direct visualization of the contractility of the left ventricle. Ventriculography can identify areas of poor contractility (hypokinesis), overcompensation (hyperkinesis), nonmovement (akinesis), and asynergy (dyskinesis). An infarcted area is usually akinetic.

Medications. Box 29-2 lists the basic principles of CAD management in an A-E format, and drug therapy plays a major role. Figures 29-9 and 29-10 outline treatment algorithms for the management of stable angina and ACS that incorporate both drug therapy and risk factor modification. An overview of medications commonly used to treat CAD is found in Table 29-5, pp. 759 and 760.

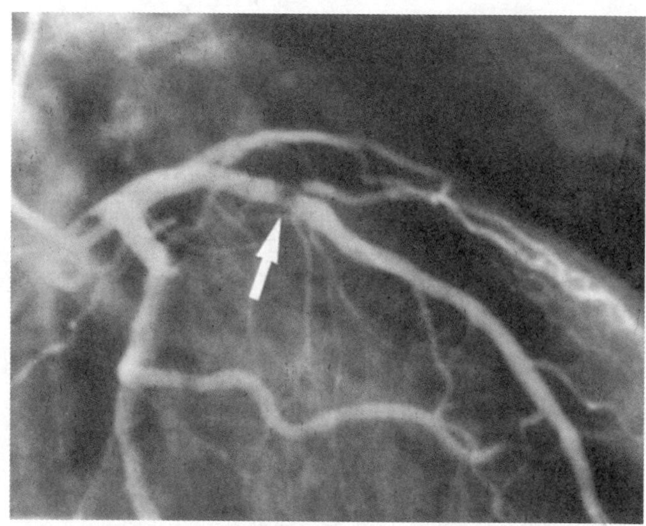

Figure 29-8 Coronary arteriogram showing coronary artery thrombus (*arrow*) in patient with unstable angina.

Box 29-2 Guidelines for Management of Stable Angina

- **A**spirin and antianginals
- **B**eta-blocker and blood pressure
- **C**holesterol and cigarettes
- **D**iet and diabetes
- **E**ducation and exercise

From Gibbons RJ et al: ACC/AHA 2002 guideline update for the management of patients with chronic stable angina: summary article: a report of the American College of Cardiology/American Heart Association Task Force on Practice Guidelines (Committee on the Management of Patients With Chronic Stable Angina), *Circulation* 107(1):149–158, 2003.

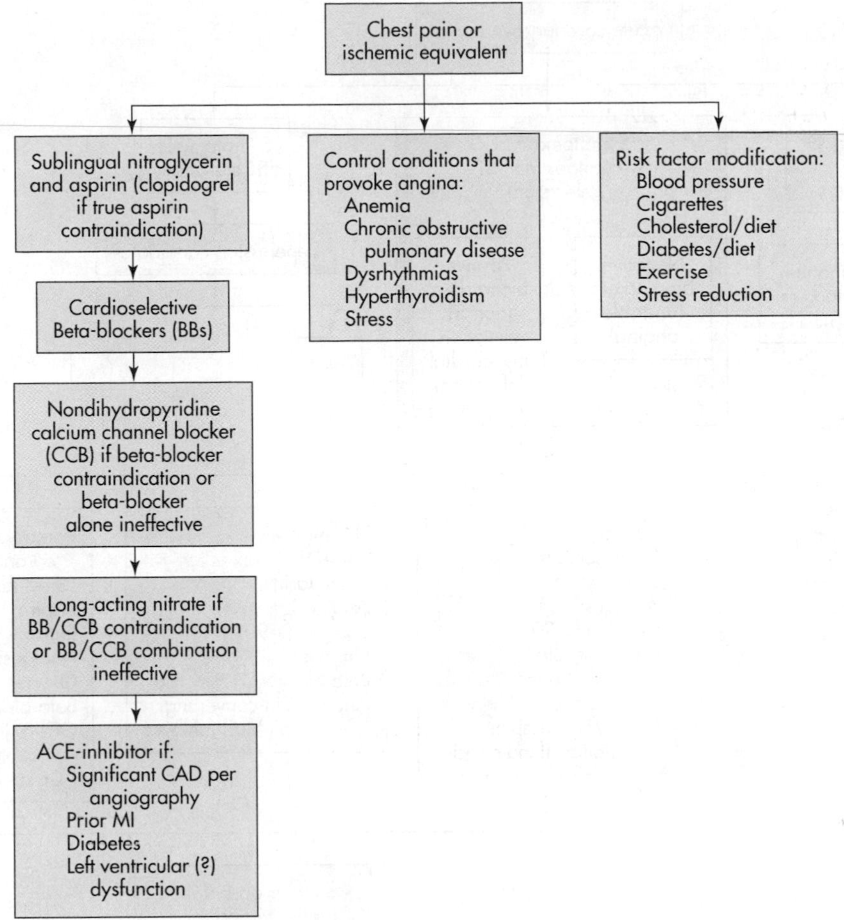

Figure 29-9 Algorithm for management of chronic stable angina. *ACE,* Angiotensin-converting enzyme; *CAD,* coronary artery disease; *MI,* myocardial infarction.

ANTIPLATELET AGENTS. Aspirin is the primary **antiplatelet agent** used in the prevention and treatment of CAD. Aspirin is given in the emergency department (or in the prehospital setting) to any patient suspected of having an MI. Aspirin blocks the formation of thromboxane A_2, inhibiting platelet aggregation; research has demonstrated that a single daily dose of 81 mg (one baby aspirin) can effectively sustain the desired antiplatelet effect. Enteric-coated forms can be prescribed for individuals who cannot tolerate pure aspirin.

Thienopyridines have an irreversible effect on the platelets that is sustained for the life of the platelet but takes several days to become manifest. Clopidogrel (Plavix) prevents platelet activation by blocking ADP-induced platelet binding. It is used for individuals who cannot tolerate aspirin and for patients undergoing PCIs. Ticlopidine (Ticlid) is rarely used because of the associated risk of neutropenia.

THROMBOLYTICS. Patients seen with a STEMI at a facility without the capability of performing primary PCIs within 90 minutes receive thrombolytic therapy unless contraindicated. **Thrombolytics** activate thrombolytic processes to lyse the clot that is occluding the lumen of the coronary artery. Therapy should be initiated within 30 minutes of arrival at the facility. Symptom onset should be within the prior 12 hours, and ST elevation should be greater than 0.1 mV in at least two contiguous leads.[5] Prehospital administration of thrombolytics may be initiated by rescue personnel trained and supported by expert practitioners; however, prehospital thrombolysis is not generally accepted practice at this time, although protocols continue to be established and evaluated.

Thrombolytics are administered intravenously when the ECG confirms the diagnosis of AMI. Commonly used thrombolytics include tissue plasminogen activators such as reteplase (Retavase), alteplase (Activase), tenecteplase (TNK-tPA), and streptokinase (Streptase). Streptokinase activates the conversion of plasminogen to plasmin, which degrades fibrin and fibrinogen into fragments. Tissue plasminogen activators also activate plasmin, but preferentially at the site of occlusion. Depending on the chosen agent, heparin may or may not be given concurrently. The risk of bleeding associated with the use of thrombolytic agents necessitates thorough screening of all patients for bleeding risks (see Guidelines for Safe Practice box, p. 762). When contraindications to thrombolytic therapy exist, primary PCI is initiated without delay. The reperfusion of previously ischemic myocardium results in numerous biochemical and cellular events, which can include myocyte necrosis, dysrhythmias, and depressed myocardial contractility.

GLYCOPROTEIN IIB/IIIA RECEPTOR INHIBITORS. GP IIb/IIIa antagonists have been used successfully to affect the final pathway in platelet-thrombus formation in both ACSs and in conjunction

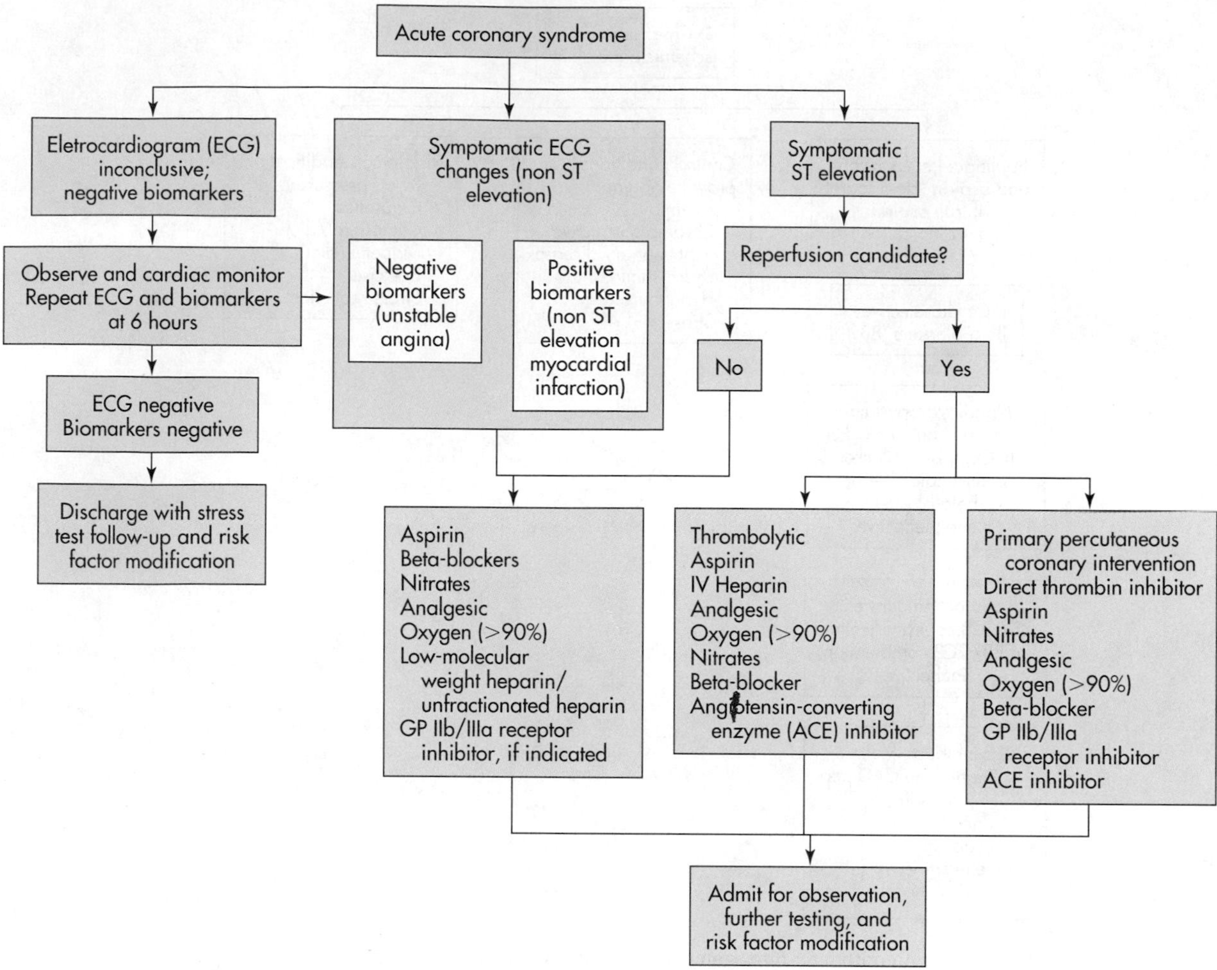

Figure 29-10 Algorithm for management of acute coronary syndrome. *GP*, Glycoprotein; *IV*, intravenous.

with PCI. By binding to the GP IIb/IIIa receptor site, these drugs block the binding of fibrinogen to the platelet, thereby preventing platelet aggregation and clot formation. Approved agents currently include tirofiban (Aggrastat), eptifibatide (Integrilin), and abciximab (ReoPro). Inhibition of platelet aggregation persists for up to 48 hours after abciximab is discontinued; effects of eptifibatide and tirofiban are reversed when the infusion is discontinued.

ANTICOAGULANTS. Anticoagulants are often prescribed for the patient with ACS. Intravenous unfractionated heparin binds to antithrombin III, inactivating coagulation factors Xa, IXa, and thrombin, thereby blocking the conversion of fibrinogen to fibrin. Weight-adjusted doses are administered to achieve activated partial thromboplastin (aPTT) levels of 50 to 70 seconds. Low-molecular-weight heparins (LMWH) have a more predictable dose-response curve and an increased plasma half-life compared with unfractionated heparin. Enoxaparin (Lovenox) is the only LMWH approved for use in ACS.[6]

DIRECT THROMBIN INHIBITORS. Bivalirudin (Angiomax) is used for anticoagulation in ACS patients undergoing coronary interventions. It is a synthetic analog of recombinant hirudin that binds to thrombin to inhibit the final step in the coagulation pathway. It is more predictable than conventional heparin and is active against clot-bound thrombin with continued efficacy after plasma clearance.

NITRATES. Nitrates are effective in the treatment of both stable angina and ACS. Nitrates cause vasodilation, reducing the amount of blood returning to the heart from the venous system, thus decreasing preload. This decreases both the workload of the heart and the myocardial oxygen demand. Nitrates also dilate the peripheral arteries, decreasing the resistance against which the left ventricle must pump, decreasing afterload, and reducing myocardial oxygen demand. In addition, nitrates act specifically to dilate coronary arteries that are not atherosclerotic, increasing collateral flow to the ischemic parts of the myocardium.

Many nitrate preparations are available for use. Sublingual nitroglycerin is used most commonly for acute episodes of angina. The tablets, absorbed within minutes from beneath the tongue, are highly effective in relieving the acute symptoms of angina. Intravenous nitroglycerin may be used for patients experiencing prolonged chest pain. Nitrates are also available as topical preparations, ointments, and patches that provide a sustained therapeutic effect. Shorter-acting ointment preparations are used during the hospitalization as medications are initiated and adjusted, since

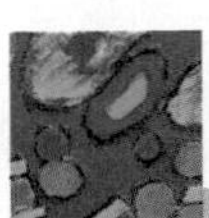

TABLE 29-5
COMMON MEDICATIONS *for Coronary Artery Disease*

Drug	Action	Nursing Intervention
Antiplatelet Agents		
Aspirin Clopidogrel	Aspirin: inhibits thromboxane-induced platelet aggregation Clopidogrel: prevents platelet activation by blocking ADP-induced platelet binding	Aspirin should be prescribed unless true hypersensitivity reaction is present or patient has severe risk of bleeding.
Glycoprotein IIb/IIIa Receptor Inhibitors		
Tirofiban (Aggrastat) Eptifibatide (Integrilin) Abciximab (ReoPro)	Interrupt final pathway in platelet thrombus formation by binding to GP IIb/IIIa receptor site	Observe patients for bleeding complications. Ensure correct weight-based dose. Monitor platelet counts.
Thrombolytics		
Alteplase (recombinant t-PA) (Activase) Reteplase (r-PA) (Retavase)	Activate thrombolytic processes to lyse clot associated with plaque rupture and vessel occlusion of MI Streptokinase: activates conversion of plasminogen to plasmin, which degrades fibrin and fibrinogen into fragments	Carefully screen patients before administration of thrombolytic agents. Monitor for reperfusion, reocclusion, and bleeding complications with thrombolytic administration.
Tenecteplase (TNK-tPA) Streptokinase (Streptase)	Tissue plasminogen activators (tPA) also activate plasmin, but preferentially at site of occlusion	Direct interventions toward preventing bleeding complications.
Anticoagulants		
Unfractionated heparin Low-molecular-weight heparin (LMWH) (Enoxaparin [Lovenox])	Prevent growth of established thrombus by rapidly inhibiting thrombin LMWH: affects predominantly factor Xa, with less effect on thrombin	With unfractionated heparin, measure heparin partial thromboplastin times (aPTTs) 6 hr after any change in dose. Dose is weight based. Maintain therapeutic levels between 50 and 70 sec. LMWH does not require heparin aPTTs. Monitor hemoglobin, hematocrit, and platelets for downward trends. Observe platelets for heparin-induced thrombocytopenia. Recurrent ischemia, active bleeding, and hypotension may signify subtherapeutic or supratherapeutic dosages and should be evaluated immediately.
Direct Thrombin Inhibitors		
Bivalirudin (Angiomax)	Binds to thrombin, preventing further platelet aggregation and clot formation	Used with percutaneous coronary interventions. Monitor for bleeding, back pain, pain, nausea, headache, hypotension.
Nitrates		
Isosorbide dinitrate (Isordil) Isosorbide mononitrate (Imdur) Nitroglycerin	Decrease myocardial oxygen demand: Venodilate (decrease preload) Peripherally vasodilate (decrease afterload) Increase myocardial oxygen supply Coronary vasodilate	Administer sublingual nitrates with patients lying or sitting. Titrate intravenous nitroglycerin to relieve symptoms or limit side effects such as headache or systolic BP <90 mm Hg. Replace intravenous preparations with oral or topical preparation when patient has been symptom free for 24 hr. Use caution in patients with known aortic stenosis. Anticipate headache, and administer analgesics as appropriate. Tolerance to nitrates can develop within 24 hr. A nitrate-free interval of 6-8 hr may improve responsiveness to therapy. Clean topical nitrates from skin surface before applying new dose. Appropriate areas of application include any hair-free area, preferably in noticeable areas when initial dose is being determined. Rotate application areas. Wear gloves when applying topical preparations.

Continued

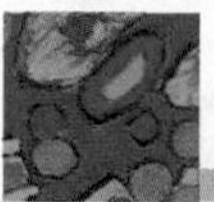

TABLE 29-5
COMMON MEDICATIONS *for Coronary Artery Disease—cont'd*

Drug	Action	Nursing Intervention
Beta-Blockers		
Atenolol (Tenormin) Metoprolol (Lopressor) Esmolol (Brevibloc)	Decrease myocardial oxygen demand: Decrease contractility Slow impulse conduction Decrease BP (through renin interaction) Slow heart rate, thereby increasing diastolic filling time and coronary perfusion Decrease morbidity and mortality after acute MI	Give intravenous metoprolol in 5 mg increments over 1-2 min. Atenolol may be prescribed intravenously instead of metoprolol. Intravenous preparations are followed by oral preparations after patient is stabilized. Monitor ECG and BP. Monitor for atrioventricular block (including measuring P-R interval), symptomatic bradycardia, hypotension, left ventricular failure (rales, decreased cardiac output), and bronchospasm. Target heart rate for beta-blockade at discharge is 50-60 beats/min.
Calcium Channel Blockers		
Diltiazem (Cardizem) Verapamil (Calan)	Decrease afterload and preload, thereby decreasing workload of heart and decreasing remodeling of left ventricle Long-term consequences of remodeling: increased oxygen demand and heart failure	These are prescribed when vasospasm is considered part of pathologic condition or significant hypertension exists. Monitor for symptomatic bradycardia, prolonged P-R intervals, advanced heart blocks, hypotension, heart failure.
Angiotensin-Converting Enzyme Inhibitors		
Captopril (Capoten) Enalapril (Vasotec) Benazepril (Lotensin) Lisinopril (Prinivil) Fosinopril (Monopril)	Decrease myocardial oxygen demand Venodilate (decrease preload)	Monitor for adverse effects: angioneurotic edema, cough, hypotension, hyperkalemia, pruritic rash, renal failure. With first doses, take BP before and 30 min after administration.
Analgesics		
Morphine sulfate	Blunts deleterious consequences of sympathetic stimulation with pain Vasodilates, decreasing preload	Establish baseline vital signs, level of consciousness, and orientation. Monitor for hypotension, respiratory depression, changes in level of consciousness. Doses are usually given in increments of 2-5 mg.
Anxiolytics		
Alprazolam (Xanax)	Binds receptors at several sites within CNS, including limbic system and reticular formation	Monitor for lessening anxiety, which may allow for reduction of doses of analgesics.
Oxygen		
	Increased arterial oxygen saturation	Monitor for adequate arterial oxygenation with finger pulse oximetry. Maintain saturation levels above 90%.
Cholesterol-Lowering Agents		
Atorvastatin (Lipitor) Lovastatin (Mevacor) Pravastatin (Pravachol) Rosuvastatin (Crestor) Simvastatin (Zocor) Ezetemibe (Zetia) Gemfibrozil (Lopid) Niacin (nicotinic acid)	Reduce substrate for lipid deposition in coronary artery	Side effects vary with drug class. Intolerance to side effects may limit usefulness of certain medications. Obtain lipid levels at regular intervals to monitor for success in effecting changes. Teach patients that cholesterol-lowering agents do not substitute for dietary modifications (see Table 29-7).

ADP, Adenosine diphosphate; *BP,* blood pressure; *CNS,* central nervous system; *ECG,* electrocardiogram; *GP,* glycoprotein; *MI,* myocardial infarction.

they can be quickly removed from the skin surface if hypotension occurs.

BETA-BLOCKERS. Most beta-blockers used to treat stable angina and ACS are cardioselective, blocking predominantly the beta-1 receptor and causing a decrease in the force of contraction, a slowing of heart rate, and a slowing of impulse conduction. These three mechanisms of action combine to decrease myocardial oxygen demand. In addition, by slowing the heart rate, beta-blockers indirectly increase the blood supply to the myocardium by increasing diastole, thus increasing the time available for coronary artery perfusion. Beta-blockers also decrease blood pressure through their effect on the renin-angiotensin system.

The use of beta-blockers is associated with a decreased incidence of morbidity and mortality when they are administered within 48 hours of MI and continued for 2 to 3 years after AMI. Beta-blockers may be administered intravenously in the emergency department and then orally once the patient is stabilized.

CALCIUM CHANNEL BLOCKERS. The role of calcium channel blockers in the management of CAD is limited. Nondihydropyridine calcium channel blockers (diltiazem [Cardizem] or verapamil [Calan]) may be used when beta-blockers are contraindicated. These agents inhibit the influx of calcium through the slow calcium channels. They slow the heart rate and decrease myocardial oxygen demand. They also indirectly increase myocardial oxygen supply by increasing the time for coronary perfusion during diastole. These agents also block the calcium used for myocardial contractility, decreasing the force of contraction (and hence oxygen demand).

ANGIOTENSIN-CONVERTING ENZYME INHIBITORS. ACE inhibitors may be used in the management of CAD to decrease preload and afterload and the overall workload of the heart. ACE inhibitors are recommended for patients with chronic stable angina who have significant CAD documented by angiography, who have diabetes, or who have left ventricular systolic dysfunction.[16] Decreasing workload prevents **remodeling** of the left ventricle, which involves the development of hypertrophy in the unaffected left ventricle that attempts to compensate for the loss of function in the infarcted area. The long-term consequence of remodeling can be a steady increase in myocardial oxygen demand for the enlarged muscle and the onset of heart failure.[5]

ANALGESICS. Despite the use of thrombolytics, acetylsalicylic acid, and heparin to open the coronary arteries and decrease chest pain, severe chest pain often persists. Pain activates the sympathetic nervous system, increasing heart rate and producing vasoconstriction. These changes decrease myocardial oxygen supply and increase myocardial oxygen demand. The immediate administration of intravenous opioid analgesics interrupts these deleterious effects of pain. The drug of choice is morphine sulfate, which not only blunts the sensation of pain, but also promotes vasodilation, thereby decreasing preload.

ANXIOLYTICS. Alprazolam (Xanax) and other anxiolytics may be administered to patients who experience significant anxiety.

OXYGEN. Oxygen is administered to the patient with ACS to maintain arterial oxygen saturation levels above 90%. This simple but effective intervention is key to increasing myocardial oxygen supply. Oxygen may be administered by nasal cannula or mask.

CHOLESTEROL-LOWERING AGENTS. Because considerable evidence links hypercholesterolemia to atherosclerosis, drugs that can reduce plasma lipids and lipoproteins are often prescribed in the treatment of patients with CAD. Drug classes include hydroxymethylglutaryl–coenzyme A (HMG-CoA) reductase inhibitors, niacin, absorption inhibitors (bile acid resins, ezetamibe), and fibrates. The statin group of drugs (HMG-CoA reductase inhibitors) increases receptor activity that removes LDL from the blood, and blocks the production of LDLs. These lipid-lowering agents are especially useful as adjuncts to dietary management for patients with familial hypercholesterolemia (Table 29-6). In high-risk persons the recommended LDL cholesterol goal is 100 mg/dl. Latest clinical trial evidence recommends an LDL cholesterol goal of 70 mg/dl, especially for patients at very high risk. Combination therapy is instituted to obtain desirable LDL, HDL, and triglyceride levels.[17]

TREATMENTS. Patients with AMI may experience alterations in tissue perfusion to the skin, brain, kidneys, and other organs in addition to alterations in myocardial perfusion. Meticulous monitoring is an essential aspect of care. These alterations occur from a decrease in cardiac output that results from impaired myocardial contractility. Nurses, because of their ongoing presence at the bedside, assume most of the responsibility for monitoring for altered perfusion. Frequent measurement of vital signs is essential. The nurse performs head-to-toe assessments that include level of consciousness and orientation, breath sounds, heart sounds, pulse amplitude, rhythm strips, bowel sounds, urinary output, and skin turgor and hydration. Abnormal findings require immediate collaboration with the physician to prevent further complications.

INTRAAORTIC BALLOON PUMP. Patients who experience hemodynamic instability after an MI may benefit from placement of an intraaortic balloon pump (IABP). The IABP, inserted into the descending thoracic aorta, inflates during diastole, augmenting early diastolic pressure and coronary artery perfusion. The balloon deflates rapidly at the end of diastole, decreasing afterload and increasing cardiac output. A more complete description of the IABP is found in Chapter 30.

PERCUTANEOUS CORONARY INTERVENTIONS. An estimated 1,051,000 coronary interventional procedures were performed in the United States in 2001.[4] These procedures can be performed in conjunction with diagnostic cardiac catheterization or as a separate procedure.

Percutaneous Transluminal Coronary Angioplasty. With balloon **angioplasty** the physician first inserts a guidewire across and beyond the lesion in the blocked artery, then advances a catheter with a cylindric balloon over the guidewire, and positions the balloon centrally in the blockage. The balloon, filled with radiopaque dye and saline, is inflated at pressures great enough to

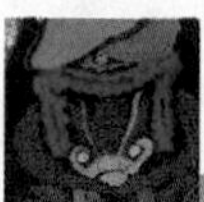

GUIDELINES FOR SAFE PRACTICE *The Patient Receiving Thrombolytic Therapy*

Patient Eligibility

Within 6 to 12 hours of symptom onset
Symptom duration of at least 30 minutes
Electrocardiogram (ECG) pattern strongly suggestive of acute myocardial infarction (ST elevation or new left bundle branch block)

Patient Screening

Screen for bleeding risks: history of cerebral hemorrhage at any time, ischemic stroke within 3 months (except acute ischemic stroke within 3 hours), intracranial neoplasm, active bleeding, suspected aortic dissection, severe hypertension, known bleeding disorders, current anticoagulation therapy, traumatic or prolonged cardiopulmonary resuscitation (over 10 minutes), major surgery within 3 weeks, significant closed head or facial trauma within 3 months, arteriovenous malformation.
Establish baseline vital signs and physical examination for overt or covert bleeding, such as unexplained hypotension or tachycardia, rigid abdomen, subtle neurologic changes.

Monitor for Successful Reperfusion

Resolution of chest pain
Resolution of ECG ST changes
Presence of reperfusion dysrhythmias, such as accelerated idioventricular rhythm
Early peak of cardiac biomarkers

Minimize Risk of Bleeding

Continue assessment for bleeding, including intracranial, internal, retroperitoneal, and puncture sites.
Monitor for frank and occult blood (heme, guaiac).
Monitor for any change in neurologic status in first 24 hours.
Monitor laboratory values for therapeutic ranges.
Use caution with patient transfers.
Limit and coordinate venipunctures; avoid establishing noncompressible intravenous access sites.
Apply pressure to all venous and arterial access sites.
Avoid arterial punctures after fibrinolysis.
Maintain a safe, clean environment.

Monitor for Reocclusion

Recurrence of chest pain
Return of ST abnormalities
Evidence of hemodynamic compromise

Support Patient and Family During Crisis

Approach in a calm, quiet manner.
Provide simple explanations of procedures and care.
Offer realistic reassurance.
Encourage family presence when interventions permit.

TABLE 29-6 DRUGS USED TO LOWER BLOOD LIPIDS

Drug Class	Lipid and Lipoprotein Effects	Side Effects
Hydroxymethylglutaryl– coenzyme A reductase inhibitors: Atorvastatin, fluvastatin, lovastatin, pravastatin, simvastatin, rosuvastatin	↓ LDL 18%-60% ↑ HDL 5%-15% ↓ TG 7%-30%	Myopathy Increased liver enzymes
Bile acid sequestrants: Cholestyramine, colesevelam, colestipol	↓ LDL 15%-30% ↑ HDL 3%-5% TG: no change or ↑	Bloating Constipation Decreased absorption of other drugs
Ezetemibe	↓ LDL 18%-25% when used alone or added to a statin	Angioedema Diarrhea, abdominal pain Arthralgia, back pain Fatigue
Niacin (nicotinic acid): Immediate release, extended release, sustained release	↓ LDL 15%-30% ↑ HDL 15%-35% ↓ TG 20%-50%	Flushing Hyperglycemia Hyperuricemia Upper gastrointestinal distress Hepatotoxicity
Fibric acids: Clofibrate, fenofibrate, gemfibrozil	↓ LDL 5%-20% (may increase if high TG) ↑ HDL 10%-20% ↓ TG 20%-50%	Dyspepsia Gallstones Myopathy

From US Department of Health and Human Services: *National Cholesterol Education Program: third report of the Expert Panel on Detection, Evaluation, and Treatment of High Blood Cholesterol in Adults (Adult Treatment Panel III)*, NIH Pub No 01-3305, Washington, DC, 2001, National Institutes of Health, National Heart, Lung, and Blood Institute.

HDL, High-density lipoprotein; *LDL*, low-density lipoprotein; *TG*, triglyceride.

reconfigure the blockage. This reconfiguration includes both controlled dissection (splitting) of the intima and to a lesser extent vessel dilation (Figure 29-11). The controlled dissection creates a wider passage for arterial blood flow. At times, the dissection may create enough turbulence to stimulate clot formation and obstruct the coronary lumen. In these situations, GP IIb/IIIa receptor inhibitors or additional interventional measures (such as intracoronary stenting) may be necessary.

The major limitation of percutaneous transluminal coronary angioplasty (PTCA) is the strong chance of lesion recurrence or restenosis, usually within 6 months. Restenosis occurs in response to the controlled injury caused by balloon inflation. In approximately 30% of procedures, the arterial wall continues to heal with smooth muscle proliferation into the arterial lumen. Although this is not the same lipid accumulation that caused the original blockage, it nevertheless compromises myocardial blood flow and results in myocardial ischemia. Arterial constriction can also occur with intimal hyperplasia.

Stents. Intracoronary stents help maintain the patency of the treated coronary arteries and decrease the incidence of restenosis (see Figure 29-11). Bare-metal stents remain in the coronary artery as a scaffold and endothelialize over 3 weeks, gradually decreasing the risk of thrombus formation on the foreign material. Stent thrombosis most frequently occurs in the first days to weeks after stent implantation. Patients usually are seen with severe chest pain and often exhibit ST segment elevation. The incidence of stent thrombosis is decreased with the administration of aspirin and loading doses of platelet ADP-receptor inhibitor therapy before the procedure, and treatment with aspirin and other platelet inhibitors after the procedure. Drug-eluting stents have been studied as one avenue of decreasing stent thrombosis. The use of sirolimus, an immunosuppressive that blocks growth factors or cytokines that stimulate smooth muscle cell proliferation, was approved in 2002. The stent is coated in sirolimus, which is slowly released over 30 days. Paclitaxel (Taxol), a drug approved for the treatment of various cancers, is being evaluated as another stent-coating agent. Because of concern that endothelialization may simply be delayed and not prevented, and late stent thrombosis may still develop in patients who are treated with drug-eluting stents, clopidogrel and aspirin therapy are administered for 6 months after the PCI. Most coronary stents in current use are stainless steel; some are weakly ferromagnetic. Therefore magnetic resonance imaging (MRI) procedures are considered safe when clinically indicated.

Other PCIs. Less commonly used PCI procedures include directional coronary atherectomy, laser therapy, transluminal extraction catheterization, and rotablation. These procedures are especially beneficial for specific types of lesions. The effect of hypothermia during PCI for MI is being evaluated in a prospective, international study[23] (see Future Watch box).

Procedural complications associated with PCI include allergic dye reactions, contrast nephropathy, and access site complications. Patients with known allergic reactions to contrast dye should be pretreated with steroids and a histamine$_1$ blocker. Patients at greatest risk for contrast nephropathy include those

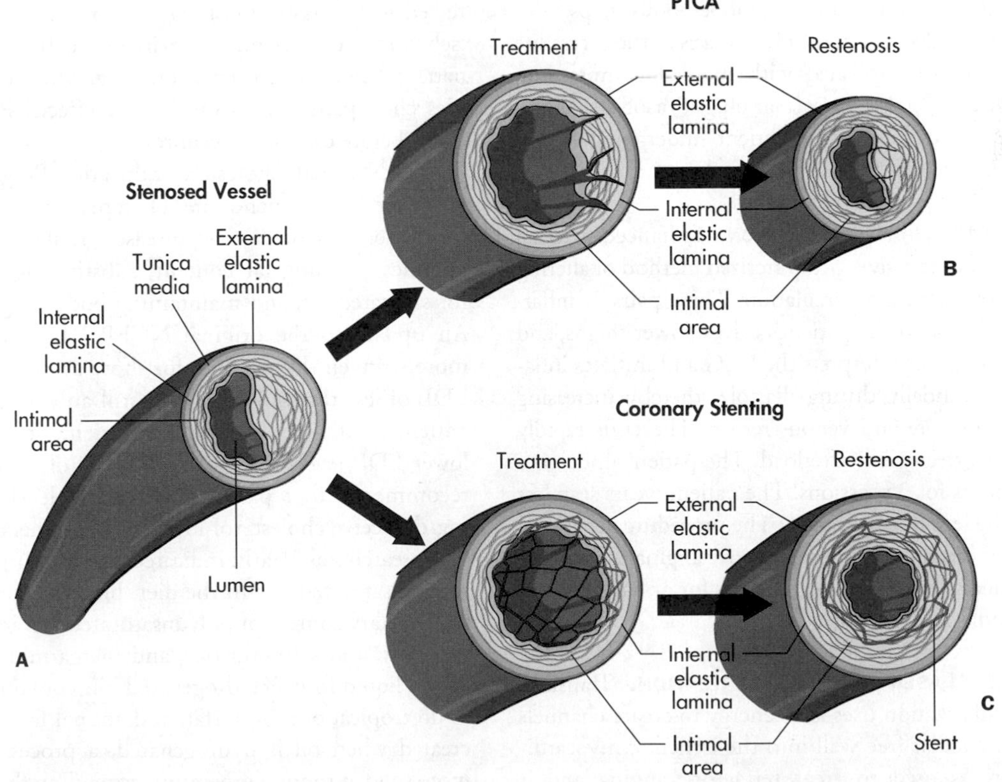

Figure 29-11 Possible mechanisms of restenosis after percutaneous transluminal coronary angioplasty (PTCA) and coronary stenting. **A,** Atherosclerosis. **B,** PTCA to left and restenosis following PTCA on right. **C,** Coronary stenting to left and restenosis of stent to right.

Future Watch

Hypothermia, Myocardial Infarction, and Percutaneous Coronary Intervention

An international, multicenter, prospective, randomized trial is currently in progress to investigate the effects of cooling on patients with myocardial infarction (COOL MI). The patient's body temperature is cooled as blood contacts a catheter filled with circulating cool saline that is placed into the inferior vena cava via the femoral vein during percutaneous coronary intervention. The patient's temperature is reduced to 91° F (33° C) over 1 hour. The patient's core temperature is maintained at this temperature for 24 hours and then gradually rewarmed using precision catheter properties. The patient is sedated but conscious throughout the period. In preliminary data from 42 patients, mean infarct size was 58.5% smaller and the median infarct size was 77.8% smaller in the treatment group. Four hundred patients are to be studied before conclusions can be drawn. A second study, COOL AID, is being conducted to evaluate cooling effects in acute ischemic brain damage.

Radiant Medical Clinical Trials: *COOLing for myocardial infarction (COOL MI)*, accessed Dec 2004 from website: http://radiantmedical.com/clinical/clinical_trials.htm.

with diabetes, preexisting renal insufficiency, or volume depletion. A rise in creatinine concentration 24 to 48 hours after the procedure is considered diagnostic. Adequate hydration both before and after the procedure is an important preventive measure.[24]

Postprocedure protocols are carefully implemented to prevent or promptly identify complications. The patient undergoing interventional procedures requires close monitoring for vessel occlusion, bleeding and hematoma formation, thromboembolism, pseudoaneurysms, and contrast dye reactions. Hemostasis at the access site after the procedure is accomplished with manual compression, suture-mediated devices (Perclose), vascular plugs (VasoSeal, Angio-Seal), and procoagulants. Care of the patient undergoing PCI is summarized in the Guidelines for Safe Practice box.

Enhanced External Counterpulsation. Enhanced external counterpulsation is a noninvasive, computerized method of altering blood flow to improve coronary circulation. Three pairs of inflatable cuffs are secured around the patient's calves, lower thighs, and upper thighs. The computer interprets the ECG and initiates inflation of the cuffs sequentially during diastole, thereby increasing coronary perfusion pressure and venous return. The cuffs rapidly deflate during systole, decreasing afterload. The patient undergoes 1- to 2-hour treatments for 35 sessions. The patient wears seamless "tights" to protect the legs from abrasion. The procedure is believed to stimulate angiogenesis over time and improve angina. It is generally used for individuals who are not candidates for or have not had success with traditional PCI or surgery.

Transmyocardial Laser Revascularization. Transmyocardial laser revascularization uses laser energy to create channels through the left ventricular free wall into the ischemic myocardium. The procedure is used to treat refractory angina and is believed to increase blood flow to the myocardium through the channels and stimulate angiogenesis to increase collateral blood flow. It can be performed percutaneously, similar to other PCIs, or surgically, through a median sternotomy or left thoracotomy approach. Depending on the type of laser used, myocardial channels are created from thermal ablation or breaking of molecular bands within the myocardial cells. Complications may include cardiac tamponade and heart failure.

Surgical Management. Coronary artery bypass graft (CABG) surgery bypasses the obstruction in a coronary artery by grafting an artery or vein to the coronary artery beyond the blockage, reestablishing blood flow (Figure 29-12). The decision to operate depends on the location of the coronary lesion and the surgical risks and benefits. CABG is indicated for patients with significant left main CAD; for patients with three-vessel disease and a left ventricular ejection fraction (LVEF) of less than 0.50; and for patients with two-vessel disease with significant proximal LAD CAD and either an LVEF of less than 0.50 or evidence of significant ischemia with stress testing. The increased use of antiplatelet therapy for ACS increases the risk of bleeding complications with CABG. The use of eptifibatide, if discontinued at least 2 hours before surgery, appears to cause less bleeding than other GP IIb/IIIa inhibitors. It is recommended that, when possible, clopidogrel be held for 5 days before surgery.[12]

Although CABG surgery is not curative because the grafts can occlude, it improves the quality of life for many patients. Heart transplants may be used in selected patients whose hearts are so badly damaged that conventional therapy is of no benefit. Chapter 30 presents more information on CABG and transplant surgery.

Diet. The patient being evaluated for acute chest pain is given nothing by mouth (NPO) until the diagnosis of MI can be ruled out. Keeping the patient NPO prevents blood from being redirected to the gastrointestinal system at a time when the heart is ischemic and demanding an increased blood flow. Keeping the patient NPO also prevents vomiting, which commonly accompanies chest pain due to vagal nerve effects. Patients may also be NPO before cardiac procedures.

The National Cholesterol Education Program III (NCEP III) guidelines recommend the Therapeutic Lifestyle Changes diet for patients with cardiac disease (Table 29-7). Diet teaching includes reducing fat content, substituting polyunsaturated fat for saturated fat, and maintaining body weight at normal levels. An update to the original NCEP III guidelines recommends more stringent lipid values for those at high risk for CAD.[27] An LDL of less than 100 mg/dl is still an overall goal for high-risk patients, but for very high-risk patients it may be preferable to lower LDL levels to less than 70 mg/dl. The 2004 update also recommends that patients with LDL levels from 100 to 129 mg/dl receive cholesterol-lowering drug therapy.[17]

Research has clearly indicated that when polyunsaturated fats replace saturated fats in the diet, blood cholesterol levels tend to fall. Dietary sources of polyunsaturated fats include corn, cottonseed, soy, and safflower oils; and margarines incorporating these oils in liquid form. Hydrogenated oils contain more saturated fat, as do tropical oils, butterfat, and animal fats. Transfatty acids are created when oil is hydrogenated, a process that makes an oil more solid at room temperature, extending the product's shelf life. When an unsaturated fat converts to a transfatty acid, it then acts in the body in much the same way as a saturated fat. Transfatty acids increase LDLs and total cholesterol and may even decrease

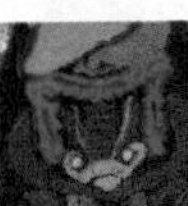

GUIDELINES FOR SAFE PRACTICE *The Patient Undergoing Percutaneous Coronary Intervention*

General Concepts to Reinforce

Indications for the procedure
Rationale for percutaneous coronary intervention (PCI) versus other interventions
PCI not a surgical intervention: no incisions, no general anesthesia
Risk factors associated with procedure, including a less than 1% chance of emergency surgery in uncomplicated PCIs

Preprocedure Preparation

Tests performed before procedure: electrocardiogram (ECG), complete blood count (CBC), platelets, basic chemistry, prothrombin time, partial thromboplastin time, international normalized ratio
Anxiolytics for anxiety
Intravenous access started to give medications and fluids; if radial access, contralateral arm used
Nothing by mouth (NPO) after midnight, except medications, clear liquid breakfast if late procedure
If groin access, groin shaved and scrubbed
Pedal pulses marked (femoral access); Allen's test documented as normal/abnormal (radial access)
Cardiac monitor placed
Premedicate for contrast allergy and contrast-induced nephropathy (CIN)
Hold oral anticoagulants and low-molecular weight heparin
Clopidogrel, 600 mg PO, and aspirin, 325 mg PO
Hold metformin and other hypoglycemics per protocol

Intraprocedure Expectations

Catheter laboratory environment—cool, sterilely draped, staff with masks and gowns, camera close to body
Anxiolytics for anxiety
Cardiac monitor at all times
Local anesthetic to access site; arm support if radial access
Back or arm discomfort possible from positioning—notify staff (morphine, fentanyl)
Chest pain or anginal equivalent possible with intervention
Fluoroscopy used to visualize all interventions
Need to cough to clear dye and deep breathe to provide a better picture of anatomy
Duration of procedure from 30 minutes to 2 hours

Postprocedure Expectations

Groin: need to keep affected leg still until after sheath removed; clear dressing over access site; while femoral sheath is in, head of bed (HOB) elevated less than 30 degrees; flexible sheaths allow HOB elevation up to 60 degrees; sheath pulled when activated clotting time is less than 180; after sheath is removed, HOB needs to be flat with patient on bed rest for 1 to 4 hours depending on hemostasis method; vital signs and neurovascular assessments every 15 minutes for first hour, every 30 minutes ×2, then every hour until stable; perform orthostatic checks after bed rest.
Radial: sheath removed immediately and dressing applied; may receive medication to decrease arterial spasm for sheath removal; wristband applied to obtain hemostasis and arm board positioned to minimize mobility. Vital signs and neurovascular assessments every 15 minutes while wristband on. Wristband removed after 1 to 2 hours and pressure dressing applied (for 24 hours). Wrist immobilized for 2 to 4 hours after wristband removed. Keep arm at heart level for 24 hours. Can walk after sheath removal with care taken to evaluate for effects of sedation and fluid shifts before ambulation.
Back pain (most often occurs with femoral approach); may logroll with assistance; back rubs, pain medication available
ECG: routine ECG after procedure; discontinue monitor after 6 hours
Notify staff if access site feels warm or wet; any pain (anginal, back, leg); inability to void with abdominal fullness
NPO until sheath pulled; fluids encouraged, unless contraindicated, to flush dye from system
Hold metformin for 48 hours
Continue CIN protocols
Monitor CBC and platelets if glycoprotein IIb/IIIa inhibitor used

Discharge Expectations

Provide all teaching relevant to angina or myocardial infarction patient (see Nursing Management) plus the following:

- Femoral site: groin restrictions—no heavy lifting, no tub baths for 2 days
- Radial site: don't drive, avoid wrist movement, do not lift more than 1 pound for 2 days; avoid strenuous arm movement for 5 days; no tub baths for 3 days
- Carry stent card and apply for MedicAlert jewelry.
- Take aspirin daily; if stent, take clopidogrel per stent protocol (bare metal versus drug eluting).
- Reinforce signs and symptoms of restenosis and use of nitroglycerin per protocol.

HDLs. Patients should avoid transfatty acid products such as stick margarines, shortenings, and foods prepared with these products. Fatty acids from fish oil decrease triglyceride levels, platelet aggregation, and blood pressure.

The nurse and dietitian work collaboratively with the patient and family to plan realistic changes in the diet. Dietary complementary and alternative therapies continue to be a focus of research and may prove beneficial in reducing the risks of coronary events[14] (see Complementary & Alternative Therapies box).

For patients with hyperhomocysteinemia, interventions focus on ways to lower total homocysteine levels. Effective measures include increasing the consumption of vitamin-enriched or fortified ready-to-eat cereal that contains 100% of the recommended daily allowance of folic acid (folate), pyridoxine hydrochloride (vitamin B_6), and cyanocobalamin (vitamin B_{12}). Additional sources of folate, vitamin B_6, and vitamin B_{12} include fish, fortified grains and cereals, fruits, legumes, meats, and vegetables. Supplemental vitamins may also be given.

HEALTH PROMOTION AND PREVENTION. Every patient with CAD needs a comprehensive educational plan aimed at promoting health that is based on the individual's unique risk factors. The Patient/Family Teaching box presents an overview of health promotion guidelines for patients with CAD.

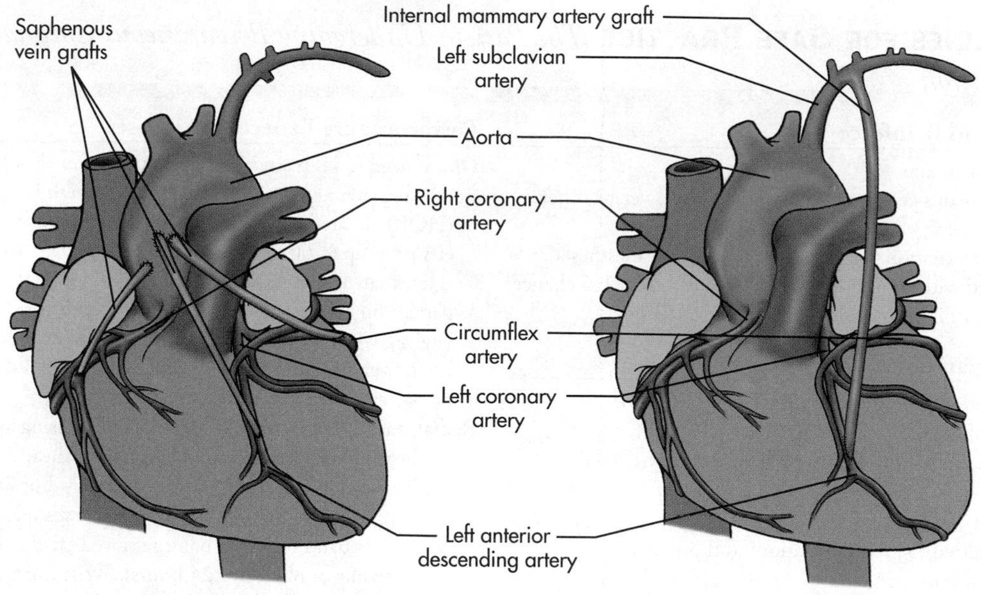

Figure 29-12 Coronary artery bypass graft surgery. Common grafts: saphenous vein and internal mammary artery.

TABLE 29-7 The Therapeutic Lifestyle Changes Diet

Nutrient	Recommended Intake
Saturated fat	Less than 7% of total calories
Polyunsaturated fat	Up to 10% of total calories
Monounsaturated fat	Up to 20% of total calories
Total fat	25%-35% of total calories
Carbohydrate	50%-60% of total calories
Fiber	20-30 g/day
Protein	Approximately 15% of total calories
Cholesterol	Less than 200 mg/day
Total calories (energy)	Balance energy intake and expenditure to maintain desirable body weight, prevent weight gain

From US Department of Health and Human Services: *National Cholesterol Education Program: third report of the Expert Panel on Detection, Evaluation, and Treatment of High Blood Cholesterol in Adults (Adult Treatment Panel III)*, NIH Pub No 01-3305, Washington, DC, 2001, The Department.

Complementary & Alternative Therapies

Drinking hot tea has been advocated throughout the years as a remedy for numerous ailments. This complementary therapy reduced the risk of myocardial infarction (MI) in 4807 men and women monitored for more than 5 years. Individuals who drank more than three cups of black tea reduced their risk of MI by 43% compared with those who did not. The threat of a fatal coronary event was reduced by 70%. Women had more favorable results than men. The researchers postulate that flavonoids within the tea mediate an estrogenic effect, creating the cardioprotective effects.

Geleijnse JM et al: Inverse association of tea and flavonoid intakes with incident myocardial infarction: the Rotterdam Study, *Am J Clin Nutr* 75(5):880-886, 2002.

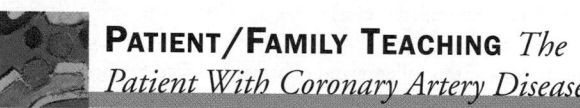

Patient/Family Teaching *The Patient With Coronary Artery Disease*

Risk Factor Modification

- Provide specific verbal and written instructions on smoking cessation, stress management, and diet modification.
- Consider referral to a smoking cessation program or outpatient cardiac rehabilitation program.
- Encourage adherence to a diet low in calories, saturated fats, and cholesterol.
- Discuss the benefits of stress management techniques in decreasing negative effect on oxygen demand. Refer to individual or group counseling as needed.

Resumption of Activity

- Discuss the benefits of exercise and encourage a regular exercise program.
- Provide specific instructions on activities that are permissible and those to avoid.
- Discuss resumption of driving and return to work.
- Discuss guidelines for resuming sexual relations.

Medications

- Ensure understanding of the role of aspirin.
- Instruct patient that recurrent symptoms lasting more than 1 to 2 minutes should prompt the patient to stop all activities, sit down, and take a sublingual nitroglycerin (NTG) tablet. This may be repeated at 5-minute intervals for two additional tablets if needed. If symptoms persist, patient should call emergency medical services (911). (High-risk patients may be taught to call after the first NTG.)
- Teach correct use and storage of nitroglycerin (see Patient/Family Teaching box, p. 768).
- Instruct patient on the purpose, dose, and major side effects of each medication prescribed.

Before the patient's hospital discharge, the nurse thoroughly reviews with the patient and family all medications, their purpose, dose, and possible side effects and establishes a medication schedule suited to the patient's lifestyle. This collaborative effort promotes adherence to the medical regimen. The nurse reminds the patient to discuss drug side effects with his or her health care provider and not to discontinue any medications without consultation.

The importance of exercise in preventing disease progression cannot be overstated. A regular exercise regimen can decrease LDLs, increase collateral circulation, decrease resting heart rate, and decrease blood pressure. Despite these benefits, patients with known cardiac disease must take precautions to prevent overtaxing the already compromised balance of myocardial oxygen supply and demand. Activity guidelines promote conditioning and simultaneously prevent overexertion that could further increase myocardial oxygen demand. The family is included, if possible, in all discussions of activity progression after MI. Disagreements over acceptable activity are a major source of conflict between spouses and patients, adding to the stress of this crisis situation. The nurse also facilitates discussion regarding the stress of this illness on children of all ages, who commonly exhibit behavior changes, sleep disturbances, and somatic complaints in response to the stress of an MI involving a parent.

Many of the *Healthy People 2010* goals target the primary prevention of CAD (see Healthy People 2010 box).[26] The ability to meet these goals depends on the development of new and creative approaches that minimize accessibility barriers related to culture, ethnicity, race, and socioeconomic status.[11]

Healthy People 2010

Objectives Related to Heart Disease

- Reduce coronary heart disease deaths to no more than 166 per 100,000 people.
- Increase the proportion of adults ages 20 years and older who are aware of the early warning symptoms and signs of a heart attack and the importance of accessing rapid emergency care by calling 911.
- Increase the proportion of eligible patients with heart attacks who receive artery-opening therapy within an hour of symptom onset.
- Increase the proportion of adults ages 20 years and older who call 911 and administer cardiopulmonary resuscitation when they witness an out-of-hospital cardiac arrest.
- Increase the proportion of eligible persons who had an out-of-hospital cardiac arrest with witnesses who receive their first therapeutic electrical shock within 6 minutes after collapse recognition.
- Reduce the mean total blood cholesterol levels among adults to 199 mg/dl.
- Reduce the proportion of adults with high total blood cholesterol levels to no more than 17%.
- Increase to at least 80% the proportion of adults who have had their blood cholesterol checked within the preceding 5 years.
- Increase the proportion of persons with coronary heart disease who have their low-density lipoprotein–cholesterol level treated to reach a goal of less than or equal to 100 mg/dl.

From US Department of Health and Human Services: *Healthy people 2010: understanding and improving health,* Washington, DC, 2000, The Department.

▶ ARE You READY?

Which of the following is the most specific biomarker for myocardial infarction?

1. CK-MB
2. Myoglobin
3. Serum troponin
4. C-reactive protein

Nursing Management

of the Patient with Coronary Artery Disease

ASSESSMENT

Health History. Assess for:

- Chest pain: location, severity, intensity, quality, duration, time of onset (Patient may be asymptomatic; classic pattern is retrosternal pain that may radiate down the left arm or both arms, upward to neck or jaw, or backward to scapular region; MI pain may be described as crushing or worst pain ever experienced.)
- Precipitating factors (e.g., exercise, stress, smoking)
- Measures attempted to control pain (e.g., nitroglycerin, lying down, eating or drinking, using antacids); effectiveness
- Other symptoms (e.g., indigestion, heartburn, nausea, abdominal pain, malaise, dizziness, dyspnea, anxiety or feeling of doom)
- Risk factors for CAD (e.g., positive family history, lipid profile, tobacco use, history, stress levels, exercise pattern)
- Other illnesses (e.g., diabetes, hypertension, bleeding disorders, recent trauma or surgery); current management regimens and allergies
- Medications in use—prescription, over the counter, herbal products, nutritional supplements
- Support systems, insurance coverage, financial resources for rehabilitation
- Current employment, activity level

Physical Examination. Assess for:

- Posture indicating presence of chest pain (e.g., clutching or rubbing chest, leaning forward)
- Changes in vital signs: tachycardia or bradycardia, hypertension or hypotension
- Dyspnea or shortness of breath, rales (crackles)
- Presence of S_3 or S_4
- Dysrhythmias
- Altered level of consciousness, syncope
- Vomiting
- Declining urinary output
- Pale, cool, diaphoretic skin

Nursing Diagnoses, Outcomes, and Interventions

Nursing Diagnosis: Acute Pain

Outcomes. Common examples of expected outcomes for the patient with a diagnosis of *acute pain* are:

Patient will:

- Be free from chest pain or anginal equivalent.
- Be able to effectively control angina through the use of medications.

Nursing Interventions. Because ischemic cardiac pain results from an imbalance between myocardial oxygen supply and demand, treatment of pain attempts to increase myocardial oxygen supply while reducing myocardial oxygen demand (see Guidelines for Safe Practice box). Immediate nursing interventions include administering prescribed oxygen, opioids, and nitrates; and assisting with measures to open an occluded artery (reperfusion therapy). Before medication administration, the nurse validates the absence of allergies and bleeding risks and establishes baseline vital signs, level of consciousness, and orientation. The nurse observes the patient for any deviations from this baseline after the administration of nitrates, thrombolytics, and opioids. It is helpful to have the patient rate the chest pain on a scale of 0 to 10, where 0 is no pain and 10 is the worst pain ever. The patient's pain ratings over time provide a baseline from which to evaluate the effectiveness of the immediate interventions. Morphine and fentanyl are the preferred analgesics for cardiac pain.

Because of the vasodilatory effects of nitrates, the nurse instructs the patient to lie down before administration. An ECG may also be obtained before the first dose of nitroglycerin is given. When the patient has documented CAD and the treatment strategy has already been determined, nitroglycerin administration can be initiated before a diagnostic ECG. This prevents additional delays in treatment. Because of the vasodilator effects of nitroglycerin on cerebral arteries, many patients receiving nitroglycerin complain of headache that may be severe enough to require analgesic administration. The Patient/Family Teaching box provides detailed information about the safe and effective use of sublingual nitroglycerin.

Topical nitrates, supplied as ointments, creams, and pastes, may also be used. The nurse administering the medication must handle these preparations carefully and use clean gloves when applying the medication. The nurse places the topical nitrate on the chest or upper arm, avoiding areas with excess hair, and rotates the site of application with each dose. Topical nitrates can be easily removed if untoward effects develop, and this advantage proves useful during dose adjustments in the early phases of treatment.

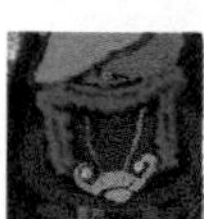

Guidelines for Safe Practice
The Patient Experiencing Angina

- Stay with patient. Ask for assistance in obtaining needed equipment (e.g., 12-lead electrocardiogram [ECG] and oxygen setup).
- Assess for presence of chest pain (or anginal equivalent). Document baseline intensity.
- Obtain baseline vital signs. Continue to monitor vital signs every 5 minutes during interventions.
- Apply oxygen when available. Monitor changes in oxygen saturation.
- Ensure intravenous access (two sites).
- Obtain an ECG as soon as possible. For diagnostic purposes an ECG should be performed before administration of nitroglycerin. If patient has known coronary artery disease, nitroglycerin may be administered before ECG. Set up continuous ST segment monitoring. Obtain serial ECGs as indicated.
- Ensure that patient has received aspirin.
- Administer nitroglycerin and morphine per orders until pain resolves. If pain is not responsive to sublingual nitroglycerin and morphine, anticipate additional interventions such as intravenous nitroglycerin.
- Treat alterations in vital signs with appropriate medications. If ECG indicates acute myocardial infarction, anticipate and prepare for thrombolytic therapy or primary percutaneous coronary intervention.
- Obtain laboratory specimens as indicated. Specimens may include complete blood count, chemistry, coagulation studies, and cardiac biomarkers (troponin and creatine kinase MB).
- Assess patient's level of anxiety and offer realistic reassurance. Explain all interventions. Approach patient and family in a calm, confident manner. Minimize environmental stimulation.

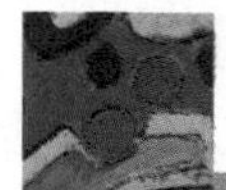

Patient/Family Teaching
Use and Storage of Nitroglycerin

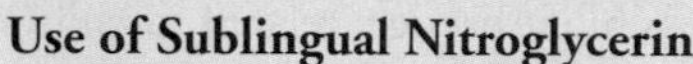

Use of Sublingual Nitroglycerin

Sit or lie down at onset of angina or chest pain.

Place tablet under the tongue and allow tablet to dissolve; do not chew.

If pain is not relieved within 5 minutes, take a second tablet. A third tablet can be used after an additional 5 minutes if pain persists. Continuing pain after three tablets and 15 minutes indicates a need to receive immediate medical evaluation. (High-risk patients may be taught to call 911 after the first nitroglygerin.)

Tablet will cause a tingling sensation under the tongue.

Rest for 15 to 20 minutes after taking nitroglycerin to avoid faintness.

A tablet may, with the physician's permission, be taken 10 minutes before an activity known to trigger an anginal attack.

Anticipate the occurrence of hypotension, tachycardia, and headache in response to the medication.

Headache may persist for 15 to 20 minutes after administration.

Keep a record of the number of anginal attacks experienced, the number of tablets needed to obtain pain relief, and the precipitating factors if known.

Note: Sublingual spray is administered following the same guidelines as above.

Storage of Nitroglycerin

Carry tablets for immediate use if necessary. Do not pack in luggage when traveling.

Keep tablets in tightly closed, original container. Protect tablets from exposure to light and moisture.

Store tablets in a cool, dry place.

Check expiration date on prescription. Discard tablets after 6 months once the bottle has been opened. Plan for replacement of supply.

Oral nitrates typically replace topical nitrates for long-term therapy. Nitrate tolerance develops rapidly with ongoing use, and it is important to provide a nitrate-free interval, usually at night, to minimize its development.

Intravenous nitroglycerin may be used in the treatment of ACS. During the administration of intravenous nitroglycerin, the nurse frequently monitors the patient's blood pressure. Intravenous nitroglycerin is typically titrated to keep the patient pain free while maintaining a systolic blood pressure above 90 mm Hg.

Thrombolytics are used emergently to open the blocked coronary artery, increase the blood supply to the myocardium, and relieve pain. Before thrombolytic administration, all members of the health care team participate in screening the patient for bleeding risks (see Guidelines for Safe Practice box, p. 762). No question can be asked too often in this situation. Thrombolytic therapy must be administered without delay, preferably within 4 to 6 hours of symptom onset, although benefits are still possible up to 12 hours later. The nurse assisting in the administration of thrombolytics must be knowledgeable about all current treatment protocols to minimize the preparation time. The nurse obtains baseline vital signs and completes a physical examination for signs and symptoms of overt or covert bleeding. During the administration of thrombolytics, the nurse monitors the patient's pain status and assesses the ECG for resolution of ST segment elevation. Should increasing pain or further signs of myocardial injury develop, the nurse anticipates the possibility of emergency interventional cardiac procedures (PCI or bypass surgery) and helps mobilize the cardiac team. PCI is the preferred method for revascularization when it can be done quickly and safely (see Guidelines for Safe Practice box, p. 765).

Treatment efforts also address the need to decrease the patient's myocardial oxygen demand. MI patients are often started on intravenous beta-blockers in the emergency room, and the nurse further decreases myocardial oxygen demand by modifying the patient's environment in subtle ways such as adjusting the room temperature and restricting visitors who increase the patient's anxiety or prevent the patient from resting. In addition, the nurse attempts to decrease the patient's anxiety level by approaching the patient in a calm, quiet manner (often the opposite occurs in the hectic setting of the emergency department or coronary care unit) and carefully explaining all care and procedures. Anxiolytics may also be administered to decrease the sympathetic effects of the stress response.

RELATED NIC INTERVENTIONS. Analgesic Administration, Anxiety Reduction, Cardiac Precautions, Medication Management, Pain Management

Nursing Diagnosis: Anxiety

OUTCOMES. A common example of an expected outcome for the patient with a diagnosis of *anxiety* is:

Patient will:

- Experience only manageable levels of anxiety, permitting patient to seek and process information.

NURSING INTERVENTIONS. Nursing interventions to relieve anxiety are best directed at its cause. For the MI patient, the threat of death is real and is a common source of severe anxiety. Psychologic support, realistic reassurance, brief explanations about care (to the extent desired by the patient), and family visiting should be priorities for a patient with an MI.[10] All interventions aimed at reducing anxiety should also include the family, who are also likely to experience high levels of anxiety and may even make the patient's level of anxiety worse.

Anxiolytics may be prescribed to decrease patient anxiety, especially during the acute phase of MI. Severe anxiety is common and increases the patient's myocardial oxygen demand at a time of decreased oxygen supply. Persistent anxiety may be managed with stress reduction techniques alone or in combination with anxiolytics. Stress reduction techniques include relaxation therapy, guided imagery, music therapy, and exercise. Supportive listening is a simple but effective intervention, especially when combined with realistic reassurance and appropriate sharing of information. All these interventions are beneficial, but research indicates that a structured exercise program eventually offers the best overall outcomes for the patient with CAD.

RELATED NIC INTERVENTIONS. Anxiety Reduction, Presence, Simple Relaxation Therapy

Nursing Diagnosis: Activity Intolerance

OUTCOMES. Common examples of expected outcomes for the patient with a diagnosis of *activity intolerance* are:

Patient will:

- Tolerate gradually increasing levels of activity.
- Verbalize the guidelines for resuming sexual activity.

NURSING INTERVENTIONS. Initially the patient experiencing chest pain is restricted to bed rest. This activity restriction decreases myocardial oxygen demand until biomarkers peak and a definitive diagnosis of MI can be made or ruled out. After the patient is hemodynamically stable and free of chest pain, activity can be increased gradually (see Guidelines for Safe Practice box). Assessment for activity tolerance includes monitoring for changes in blood pressure in response to position changes, dysrhythmias, appropriate changes in blood pressure and heart rate in response to activity, and symptoms such as dyspnea or chest pain. The presence of symptoms or hemodynamic changes necessitates cessation of activity until the patient stabilizes and the potential for cardiac ischemia decreases.

Before discharge or soon thereafter, postinfarction patients may undergo stress testing to determine a safe individual exercise level. Patients ideally enroll in outpatient cardiac rehabilitation programs. These programs supervise the progression of activity and offer variety in modes of exercise (bicycle, steps, weights), although outpatient programs vary in their effectiveness in creating and sustaining lifestyle changes[2] (see Research box). Unfortunately, not all insurance companies recognize the benefit of structured rehabilitation programs, and financial constraints may prevent patients from enrolling. In these situations standardized home exercise programs are recommended (see Patient/Family Teaching box). Activity prescriptions consider the location and extent of myocardial damage, results of stress testing when available, and specific patient needs. The activity pyramid (Figure 29-13) may help patients and families appreciate the progressive nature of building activity into their daily lives. The base of the pyramid emphasizes the importance of at

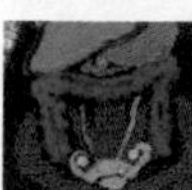

GUIDELINES FOR SAFE PRACTICE
Advancing Activity Levels

Activity Progression—Admission

0 to 12 hours: bed rest with bedside commode
12 to 24 hours: orthostatic check; out of bed to chair with meals, ad lib in room

Activity Progression—Day 2 to Discharge

Duration: first session, walk 1 to 2 minutes; increase duration 1 to 2 minutes per session if patient tolerates (see Criteria)
Frequency: initially one to four times per day for less than 10 minutes
Intensity: maintain heart rate no greater than 20 beats/min over baseline; patient should be able to converse on ambulation without shortness of breath

Criteria for Progressing Activity

Heart rate* within 20 beats/min of standing baseline heart rate
Systolic blood pressure* within 20 mm Hg of standing baseline blood pressure
Absence of chest pain, pressure, or anginal equivalent; shortness of breath; dysrhythmia; fatigue; lightheadedness; diaphoresis

*Blood pressures and heart rate checks are taken with patient in a standing position preambulation and immediately postambulation. Postambulation heart rate should be measured by taking pulse for 10 seconds and multiplying by 6.

least 30 minutes of moderately intense exercise on most, if not all, days of the week. More structured and varied activity options are built on this base. The ultimate goal is to decrease the amount of time spent in the sedentary activities found at the peak of the pyramid.[13]

The nurse includes information about returning to work and sexual activity as part of the overall activity guidelines. Return to work is individualized to the patient's occupation. A patient with a desk job and low stress levels receives different guidelines than the patient with high occupational stress or heavy labor demands.

Medications often improve a patient's tolerance of activity. Nitroglycerin taken before an activity that is known to cause angina may allow the patient to complete the activity without experiencing chest pain. Beta-blockers decrease the sympathetic response to exercise, allowing patients to exercise at an increased intensity but with a safer heart rate. Both myocardial oxygen demand and efficiency improve with the use of beta-blockers.

Fatigue commonly limits the patient's exercise tolerance and can be related to medications, particularly beta-blockers. The nurse informs the patient about potential fatigue and what to do if it occurs. The patient taking beta-blockers is cautioned not to discontinue the medication abruptly, since this can result in rebound angina and hypertension. The nurse encourages the patient to discuss concerns with a primary care provider. Interventions for medication-induced fatigue include altering the dose; prescribing another type or class of medication; and offering counseling or referral, particularly if the fatigue is associated with depression.

The patient with ACS requires additional guidance about resuming sexual activity safely. For the patient with unstable angina, nitroglycerin may be taken before intercourse if intercourse causes angina. For the post-MI patient, guidelines for sexual activity are based on successful progression through a home walking or structured outpatient exercise program. Traditional parameters for resuming intercourse include being able to climb two flights of stairs or walk at a pace of 3 to 4 miles/hr without dyspnea or chest pain. The patient's spouse or partner, who may also have fears about the effects of sexual activity on the patient's heart, should be included in all counseling and educational sessions (see the Patient/Family Teaching box, p. 773).

Beta-blockers cause impotence in some men. The nurse is honest in communicating the side effects of these drugs, since the patient who is aware of the possibility of impotence may be better able to cope with the problem should it occur. Herbal supplements, marijuana, and cocaine are additional drugs that may alter sexual function and place the myocardium at risk. Patients should consult with their primary care provider before using sildenafil (Viagra) or any other drug for erectile dysfunction because of their vasodilatory effects.

Research

Aldana SG et al: Cardiovascular risk reductions associated with aggressive lifestyle modification and cardiac rehabilitation, *Heart and Lung* 32(6):374, 2003.

Researchers compared the impact of three cardiac rehabilitation approaches on cardiovascular risk factors in 84 patients who had undergone bypass surgery or percutaneous coronary intervention. The traditional program studied included the first three of a standard four-phase approach: phase 1, in-hospital walking and bed exercises; phase 2, supervised outpatient aerobic exercise for 1 to 3 months; phase 3, supervised exercise in a community setting for 6 to 12 months; and phase 4 (not studied), lifelong fitness and exercise programs. The Ornish approach includes a low-fat vegetarian diet; stress management techniques, moderate aerobic exercise, and group support meetings. The third group was a control group who chose not to participate in these two options, and returned home without additional structured rehabilitation.

Data were collected at baseline, 3 months, and 6 months and included blood lipids, glucose concentrations, diet (3-day diet diary), weight, body mass index (BMI), waist-to-hip ratio, blood pressure, exercise participation, anginal pain frequency, and adherence. Ornish program participants had significantly greater reductions in anginal frequency, body weight, BMI, systolic blood pressure, total cholesterol, low-density lipoprotein cholesterol, glucose, and dietary fat and increases in complex carbohydrates. The traditional rehabilitation group had significant reductions in anginal pain severity and waist-to-hip ratio and increased high-density lipoprotein cholesterol, but they also demonstrated significantly increased body weight, BMI, and systolic blood pressure. The control group experienced the greatest reduction in anginal pain severity, but also had significantly higher systolic blood pressure, total cholesterol, and low-density lipoprotein cholesterol.

A major limitation of this study was self-selection into the three groups. The groups were matched for income and demographic measures; however, motivation and education may have confounded the findings. Nevertheless, the study reinforced the value of cardiac rehabilitation, since both the Ornish program and the traditional rehabilitation program (to a less extent) helped participants deal positively with cardiovascular risk factors.

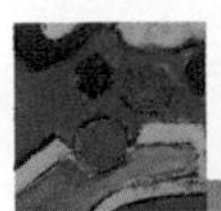

PATIENT/FAMILY TEACHING
Home Walking Program

- *Count pulse:* Take your pulse before, during, and immediately after your walk. Stop and rest if your heart rate is higher than 20 beats/min over resting heart rate, and then continue at a slower pace.
- *Safety:* Carry your nitroglycerin with you and use as directed if symptoms occur.
- *Warm-up*: Start with 1 minute of arm and chest exercises followed by 4 or 5 minutes of stationary walking. This gradually increases blood flow to the muscles, preventing injury.
- *Duration:* Walk at moderate intensity for 5 to 10 minutes. Increase your time by 1 to 2 minutes each time you walk with a goal of a 30- to 45-minute walk.
- *Intensity:* Stay within a heart rate not higher than 20 beats/min above your resting heart rate and less than 120 beats/min initially. If you are taking beta-blockers, stay within 20 beats/min of your baseline.
- *Cool down:* Cool down with 5 to 10 minutes of low-intensity walking followed by stretching. The purpose is to gradually decrease effort and prevent a drop in blood pressure, causing dizziness.
- *General tips:*
  —Preferably walk on a level surface. If you must walk uphill, go more slowly.
  —Walk at least three times per week.
  —In the summer do not walk if the temperature is higher than 85° F or if the humidity is higher than 75%.
  —Wear loose clothing. Drink plenty of water to prevent dehydration.
  —In the winter do not walk outside if the temperature is lower than 40° F. Wear a hat and a face scarf.
  —Avoid exercise for 1 to 2 hours after eating. Patients with diabetes should have a light snack before walking.
  —Do not use tobacco for 1 hour before exercise.

Patients with CAD frequently have numerous concerns related to sexuality. They may be concerned about the occurrence of chest pain during sexual intercourse or their ability to perform sexually. If the patient and the nurse have established a therapeutic relationship, the nurse is usually able to address these concerns with the patient. The nurse reassures the patient that concerns about sexuality after MI or with the diagnosis of CAD are normal and that it is particularly important to discuss them openly with his or her partner.

RELATED NIC INTERVENTIONS. Cardiac Care: Rehabilitative, Energy Management, Exercise Promotion, Teaching: Prescribed Activity/Exercise

Nursing Diagnosis: Risk for Injury

OUTCOMES. A common example of an expected outcome for the patient with a diagnosis of *risk for injury* (bleeding) is:
Patient will:

- Not experience bleeding, or bleeding will be effectively controlled and treated if it occurs.

NURSING INTERVENTIONS. The patient who receives thrombolytic therapy has an increased risk of bleeding, and the nurse has primary responsibility for frequently assessing the patient for any indications of bleeding. Relevant findings include the onset of bleeding from the nose or gums, excessive bruising, frank blood in the urine or guaiac-positive stool, unexplained hypotension or tachycardia, and a rigid abdomen. Subtle symptoms such as headache and visual disturbances may be indicative of cerebral hemorrhage and require evaluation with cerebral imaging. CBC and blood coagulation studies are performed at prescribed intervals and monitored for trends indicative of bleeding.

In addition to monitoring for bleeding complications, the nurse acts to prevent patient injury. The nurse assists in all transfers to ensure minimum abrasion to skin surfaces. The nurse limits the number of venipunctures and applies direct manual pressure to the puncture site until complete hemostasis is obtained. Arterial punctures are avoided once thrombolytic therapy is begun, especially at sites that cannot easily be compressed to control bleeding.

Anticoagulation therapy is often used in the treatment of ACS. Anticoagulation prevents future clot formation but does not lyse existing clots. Nursing interventions for the patient receiving anticoagulants (e.g., heparin) are the same as those for the patient receiving thrombolytics. During the administration of intravenous unfractionated heparin, the nurse monitors the patient's partial thromboplastin time (aPTT) to evaluate the therapy's effectiveness. The nurse follows established algorithms and adjusts the dosage of heparin to keep the aPTT in the therapeutic range of 50 to 70 seconds. If patients are receiving warfarin (Coumadin) for other health problems, it is important to ensure that their INR (international normalized ratio) is less than 1.6 before they undergo any invasive procedure.

Antiplatelet therapy, both aspirin and other drugs, is often used for ACS and PCIs. The purpose of antiplatelet therapy is to minimize clot formation, especially in the area of unstable plaque or at the site of coronary intervention. Nursing interventions include physical assessment for bleeding, prevention of physical injury, and maintenance of hemostasis at puncture sites. The nurse reminds patients to read over-the-counter product labels carefully to avoid using any other aspirin-containing product.

RELATED NIC INTERVENTIONS. Bleeding Precautions, Environmental Management, Medication Management, Risk Identification

Patient/Family Teaching. Patient and family teaching is one of the most important aspects of the nursing care provided to patients who are experiencing CAD. Teaching is a priority during the diagnostic, emergency room, coronary care unit, hospital, and rehabilitative phases of care. The nurse needs to be extremely knowledgeable about the disease and its pharmacologic and interventional management to help patients and families become full partners in disease management. Relevant aspects of teaching are discussed under each nursing diagnosis and highlighted in the Patient/Family Teaching boxes.

After the patient's condition stabilizes, the nurse makes appropriate referrals for inpatient cardiac rehabilitation and initiates discharge planning. The experienced staff nurse recognizes when she or he is able to meet the patient's needs and when it is more appropriate to refer the patient to someone with greater expertise, ability, or time for either immediate crisis intervention or long-term follow-up care.

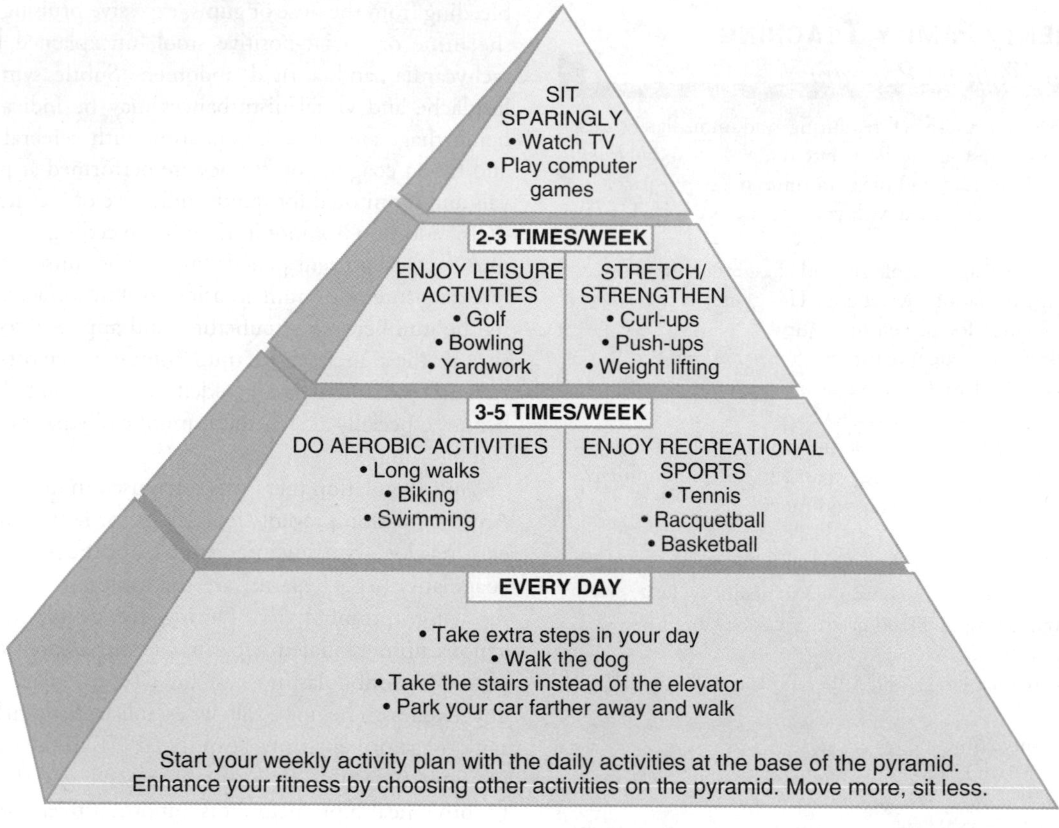

Figure 29-13 Activity pyramid.

Evaluation

To evaluate the effectiveness of nursing interventions, compare patient behaviors with those stated in the expected patient outcomes.

Related NOC Outcomes. Activity Tolerance, Anxiety Level, Blood Coagulation, Cardiac Disease Self-Management, Comfort Level, Knowledge: Medication, Pain Control, Risk Control, Stress Level

Gerontologic Considerations

The prevalence of CAD increases with age. In assessing chest pain in the older adult, the nurse is aware that older adults may experience atypical signs and symptoms and often delay seeking care. Older patients often experience "silent MIs" and come to the emergency department with shortness of breath, heart failure, or pulmonary edema, but without chest pain. Absence of chest pain as a classic symptom often impedes recognition of the older person's heart attack. Older adults may therefore delay seeking medical care for the evaluation of their "heart condition," especially when they have a long history of angina. Older adults also may delay seeking care because they are reluctant to go to the hospital, do not want to bother anyone, or are lonely and depressed. Diminished cardiac reserve and altered response to inotropic medications place the older patient at risk for heart failure or cardiogenic shock.

Older adults may also be especially sensitive to certain medications. The nurse carefully observes for side effects and drug interactions and anticipates that the older patient may require higher doses of vasoactive agents to achieve desired effects. However, secondary prevention interventions appear to be just as effective in older adults as in younger patients, and nurses should encourage older adults to get involved in secondary prevention programs to fully realize their rehabilitation potential.[31]

> **▶ ARE You READY?**
>
> In assessing a patient for eligibility to receive thrombolytic therapy, the nurse recognizes which of the following as the greatest bleeding risk?
>
> 1. Severe chest pain that started 8 hours ago
> 2. History of cerebral hemorrhage 3 years ago
> 3. Facial trauma 8 months ago
> 4. Elevated troponin levels

Cardiac Dysrhythmias

Etiology and Epidemiology. Normal sinus rhythm (NSR) begins with the spontaneous depolarization of the SA node. The impulse passes through the atria to the AV node and then through the bundle of His and bundle branches to the Purkinje fibers (see Figure 28-4). A rhythm is classified as "normal" when it meets the following criteria: presence of one upright and consistent-appearing P wave before each QRS complex, all P-R intervals between 0.12 and 0.20 second, a consistent-appearing QRS complex of less than 0.12 second, a consistent R-R interval, and a heart rate between 60 and 100 beats/min (Figure 29-14). All rhythm strips displayed are from lead II.

Cardiac dysrhythmias occur as the result of alterations in impulse formation or propagation. The anatomic site of the dys-

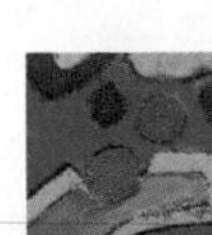

PATIENT/FAMILY TEACHING *Guidelines for Sexual Activity After Myocardial Infarction*

Stages of Sexual Response

Arousal: flushed; breathing and heart rate increase; blood pressure goes up slightly
Plateau: increase in respirations, blood pressure, and heart rate
Orgasm (15 to 20 seconds): further increases in pulse and blood pressure
Resolution: return to resting state within seconds; angina or palpitations most likely to occur during resolution

General Guidelines

Sexual foreplay at a relaxed pace allows your heart rate and blood pressure to increase more slowly.
Hugging, stroking, and touching are safe ways to get back in touch with your partner.
Talk with your partner. Express your feelings.
Extramarital affairs or sex with new partners may produce more stress.
Avoid positions for sex that you find uncomfortable.
Have sex in a pleasant, comfortable environment.
Do not take very hot or cold baths or showers before or after sex.
Be rested before sex.
Do not have sex after a heavy meal or drinking alcohol.
If you have any questions about side effects of any drug, do not stop taking the drug, but talk to your health care provider.
Masturbation and manual or oral stimulation are not harmful to your heart. Anal intercourse may lead to an irregular heartbeat. Avoid this choice unless you clear it with your health care professional.

function helps classify the dysrhythmia, but the underlying etiology varies with each specific dysrhythmia. Common causes include underlying cardiac disease, sympathetic stimulation, vagal stimulation, electrolyte imbalances, and hypoxia.

Benign dysrhythmias such as sinus bradycardia and occasional premature beats are common in the general population, but dysrhythmias are more prevalent in patients with cardiac disease. In patients with CAD a benign rhythm may have negative consequences because the myocardium is already compromised. Common dysrhythmias and their management are presented in the Collaborative Care Management section.

Pathophysiology. An understanding of normal cardiac electrophysiology, presented in Chapter 28, is necessary to grasp the pathophysiology of dysrhythmias. Alterations in impulse formation and propagation arise from one of three main pathophysiologic processes: altered automaticity, altered conduction resulting in delays or blocks, and reentry mechanisms.

ALTERATIONS IN AUTOMATICITY. **Automaticity,** the ability to depolarize spontaneously without external stimulation, is a property normally confined to the cells of the SA node. Depolarization, however, is not unique to the SA node and occurs all along the electrical impulse pathway (Figure 29-15). These nonpacemaker cells may be responsible for dysrhythmias. The SA node usually depolarizes at a faster rate than other potential pacemaker cells because of the steep slope of phase 4, allowing sinus cells to reach threshold at a faster rate (Figure 29-16). A variety of conditions can alter the automaticity of the SA node and produce faster or slower than usual heart rates. Vagal stimulation decreases this slope, resulting in a slower heart rate (Figure 29-17). Sympathetic stimulation and hypoxia steepen phase 4, resulting in a faster heart rate (Figure 29-18).

If the rate of phase 4 depolarization found in the AV node or ventricular conduction system increases, enhanced automaticity is said to exist. The result may be premature beats or tachycardias. Some causes of enhanced automaticity are hypoxia, catecholamines, atropine, hypokalemia, hypocalcemia, heat, trauma, and digitalis toxicity.

Even cells that do not normally have automaticity may develop abnormal automaticity if the resting membrane potential or threshold potential is altered. Making the threshold potential less negative slows the heart rate, since more time is needed to reach threshold (Figure 29-19). If the resting membrane potential is made less negative, automaticity increases because it is easier to reach threshold (Figure 29-20). Abnormal automaticity is not easily suppressed by the activity of the usual pacemakers.

One variation of automaticity often associated with ventricular dysrhythmias is afterdepolarization. Afterdepolarizations arise from fluctuations in the cellular membrane potential occurring after phase 0 has been initiated. If the fluctuation reaches threshold amplitude, an early action potential, an "afterdepolarization," occurs. Afterdepolarizations can occur soon after phase 0 is initiated or later, after repolarization is complete. Delayed afterdepolarizations are often associated with increased intracellular calcium, catecholamines, and digoxin toxicity.

ALTERATIONS IN CONDUCTION. When the rate or amplitude of depolarization decreases, conduction also decreases. Any condition that decreases the amplitude of the action potential, such as ischemia, hypercalcemia, or calcification of the conducting fibers,

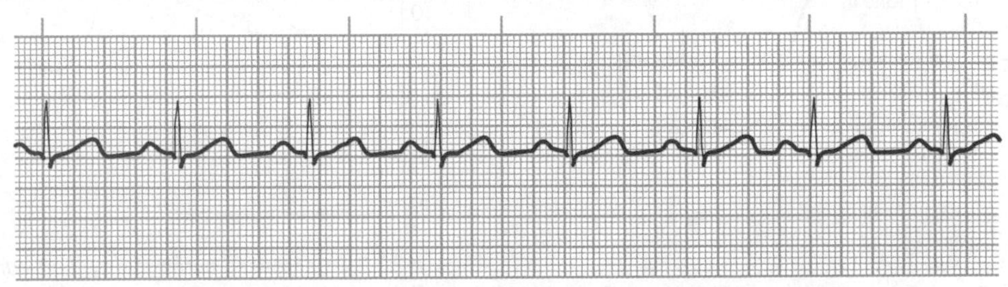

Figure 29-14 Normal sinus rhythm; heart rate, 80 beats/min.

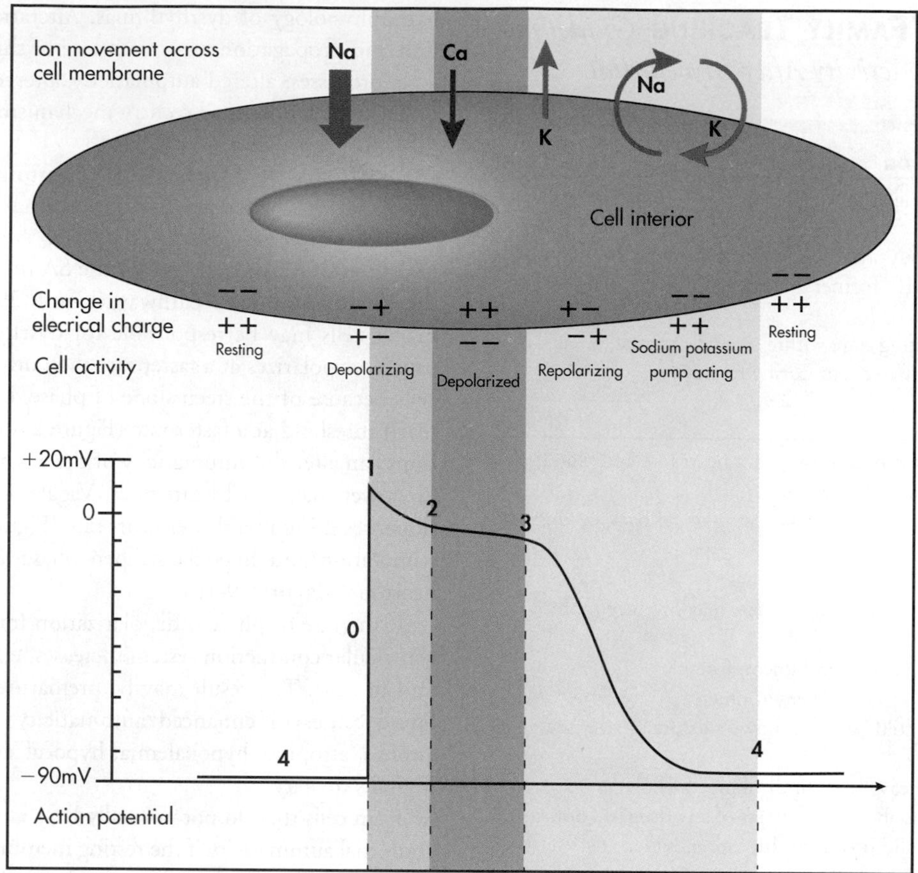

Figure 29-15 Phases of action potential of a cardiac cell. In resting phase *(4)*, cell membrane is polarized. Cell's interior has net negative charge, and membrane is more permeable to potassium ions *(K)* than to sodium *(Na)*. When cell is stimulated and begins to depolarize *(0)*, sodium ions enter cell, potassium leaves cell, calcium *(Ca)* channels open, and sodium channels close. In its depolarized phase *(1)*, cell's interior has net positive charge. In plateau phase *(2)*, calcium and other positive ions enter cell and potassium permeability declines, lengthening action potential. Then *(3)*, calcium channels close and sodium is pulled from cell by sodium-potassium pump. Cell's interior then returns to its polarized, negatively charged state *(4)*.

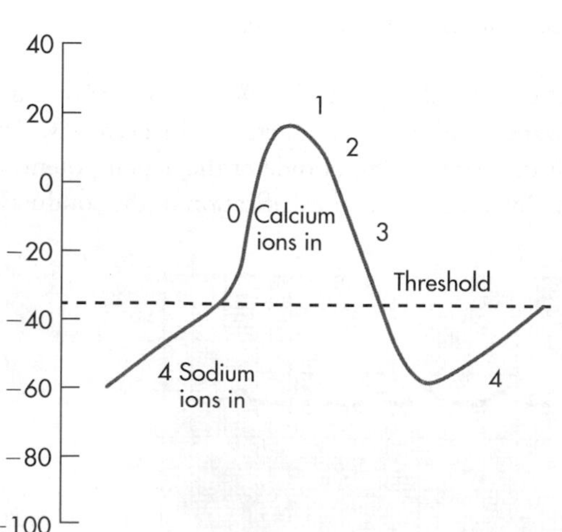

Figure 29-16 Action potential recorded from pacemaker cell.

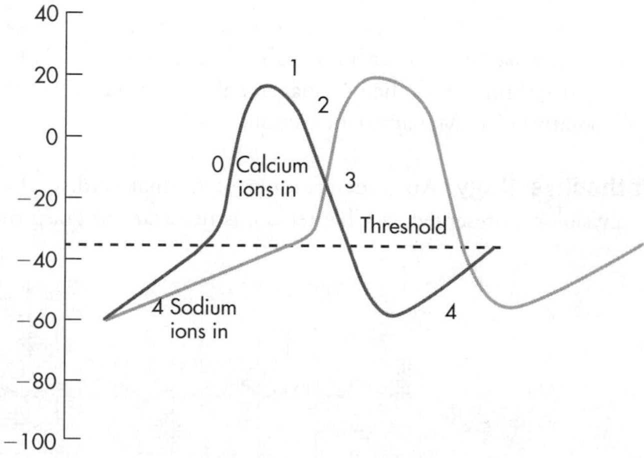

Figure 29-17 Decreased automaticity. *Left curve*: Normal action potential recorded from pacemaker cell. *Right curve*: Vagal stimulation decreases rate of phase 4 depolarization, decreasing heart rate.

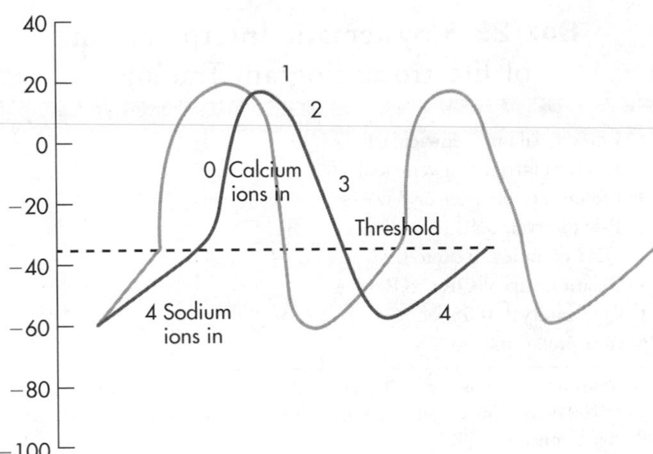

Figure 29-18 Increased automaticity. *Left curve*: Sympathetic stimulation and hypoxia steepen phase 4 depolarization, increasing heart rate. *Right curve*: Normal action potential recorded from pacemaker cell.

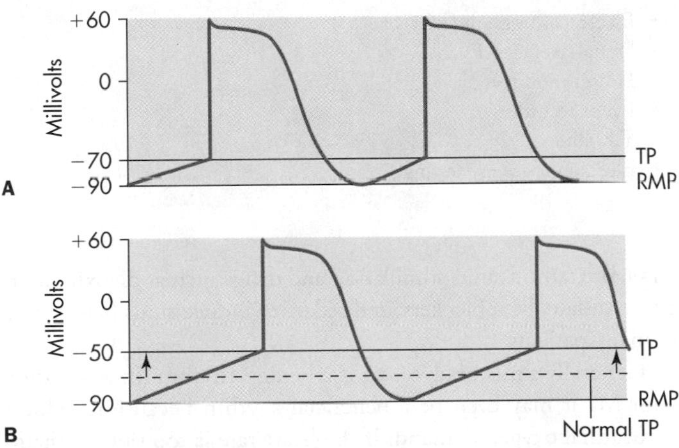

Figure 29-19 Decreased automaticity. **A,** Normal action potential recorded from nonpacemaker cell. **B,** Making threshold potential *(TP)* less negative increases time needed to reach threshold, decreasing heart rate. *RMP,* Resting membrane potential.

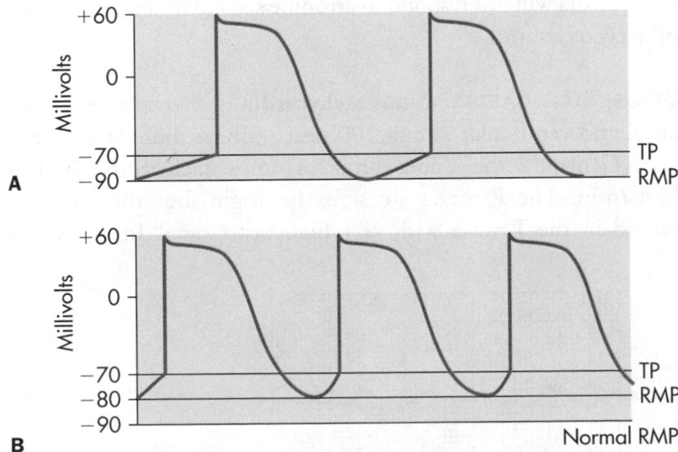

Figure 29-20 Increased automaticity. **A,** Normal action potential recorded from nonpacemaker cell. **B,** Making resting membrane potential *(RMP)* less negative makes it easier to reach threshold, increasing heart rate. *TP,* Threshold potential.

can cause cardiac conduction disturbances. Abnormalities in conduction can occur anywhere in the conduction system, including the SA node, AV node, and bundle branches. The severity of the impaired conduction ranges from a slight delay to complete cessation or block of impulse transmission.

REENTRY. **Reentry** involves impulse transmission around a unidirectional block. Reentry occurs when an impulse is delayed within a pathway of slow conduction long enough that the impulse is still viable when the remaining myocardium repolarizes. The impulse then reenters surrounding tissue and produces another impulse. This typically occurs when two different pathways share an initial and final segment. The first impulse travels down the faster pathway, leaving behind its refractory tail. Should a second, early impulse follow, it is blocked because that path is refractory. The second impulse then enters the slow pathway and can return retrogradely through the fast path, initiating a circuitous pattern (Figure 29-21).

CLINICAL MANIFESTATIONS. Many patients with dysrhythmias are asymptomatic as long as cardiac output meets the body's metabolic demands. The clinical manifestations associated with most dysrhythmias relate to decreases in cardiac output from slow or fast heart rates (see Clinical Manifestations box). Significant changes in heart rate may not allow adequate time for the ventricles to fill and empty. In addition, patients may complain of palpitations (e.g., a "racing heart" or "skipping beats") related to changes in heart rate and stroke volume. These symptoms often create acute anxiety.

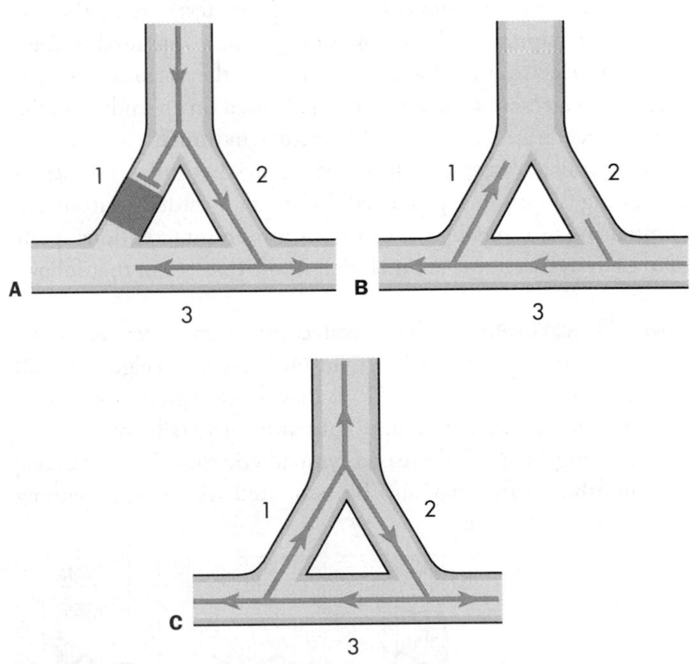

Figure 29-21 Reentry. **A,** Shaded area shows refractory area after first impulse passes down path 1. Premature impulse is then blocked from entering path 1 but can travel down path 2. **B,** Path 1 is no longer refractory to stimulation; therefore premature impulse can travel backward up path 1. **C,** Reentry down path 2 establishes circuitous pathway.

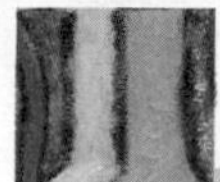

CLINICAL MANIFESTATIONS
Cardiac Dysrhythmias

General

Palpitations (racing heart, skipped beats)
Anxiety
Fatigue

Altered Cardiac Output

Pallor or cyanosis
Cool, clammy skin
Shortness of breath
Rales
Decreased blood pressure
Confusion
Dizziness
Weakness
Presyncope
Syncope with loss of consciousness
Chest pain
Atrial thrombi (may dislodge to cause systemic emboli)

Collaborative Care Management. The diagnosis of dysrhythmias begins with the 12-lead ECG. Each dysrhythmia exhibits characteristic changes in the ECG tracing. A systematic approach to analyzing the ECG rhythm helps distinguish the different dysrhythmias (Box 29-3). Table 29-8 outlines the rhythm criteria that define each common dysrhythmia and their common associated causes. Some rhythms, especially fast rhythms, seem to defy interpretation using the ECG alone. Additional diagnostic tests (Box 29-4) are often needed to determine the dysrhythmia itself and, most important, its cause. These tests are further discussed in Chapter 28. Electrophysiology studies are used to determine the electrophysiologic properties of the various dysrhythmias. Management is then determined based on an understanding of the mechanism responsible for the dysrhythmia.

The collaborative management of dysrhythmias focuses on alleviating symptoms produced by altered cardiac output and eliminating or reversing the cause. Common interventions specific to each dysrhythmia are included in the discussion that follows.

SINUS BRADYCARDIA. Sinus **bradycardia** is characterized by atrial and ventricular rates of less than 60 beats/min (Figure 29-22), but in all other respects is a NSR. It may develop gradually or occur suddenly for a brief period. Bradycardia generally results from increased vagal tone or decreased sympathetic tone. It is commonly seen in athletes and may also be associated with sleep, vomiting, and MI. Carotid sinus stimulation and drugs such as digoxin, morphine sulfate, beta blockers, and sedatives induce sinus bradycardia in many patients.

Generally sinus bradycardia is a benign rhythm. In association with MI it may even be a beneficial rhythm because it reduces myocardial oxygen demand. If the heart rate is too slow to maintain adequate cardiac output, however, the patient may be predisposed to syncope and heart failure. Administration of atropine is usually effective in increasing the heart rate. Secondary interventions include transcutaneous pacing, dopamine, epinephrine, and isoproterenol. Postcardiac transplant patients with unstable bradycardia will not respond to atropine secondary to denervation of nervous control.

SINUS TACHYCARDIA. Sinus **tachycardia** is characterized by an atrial and ventricular rate of 100 beats/min or more (Figure 29-23). Generally the upper limit of sinus tachycardia is 160 beats/min. The P waves are sinus in origin, but they may be buried in the T wave with very high heart rates. Intervals and

Box 29-3 Systematic Interpretation of Electrocardiogram Tracing

- Rate (atrial and ventricular)
- Rhythm (atrial and ventricular)
- Presence or absence of P waves
- P-R interval, 0.12 to 0.20 second
- QRS complex, 0.06 to 0.12 second
- Relationship of QRS to P wave
- Q-T interval, 0.55 sec
- Interpretation

NOTE: A normal sinus rhythm has an atrial (P) and ventricular (QRS) rate of 60 to 100 beats/min, a regular rhythm (constant P-P and R-R intervals), and a P wave before every QRS.

Box 29-4 Diagnostic Tests for Cardiac Dysrhythmias

- Electrocardiogram (ECG)
- Signal-averaged ECG
- Holter monitor
- Event recorder
- Tilt table
- Electrophysiology testing

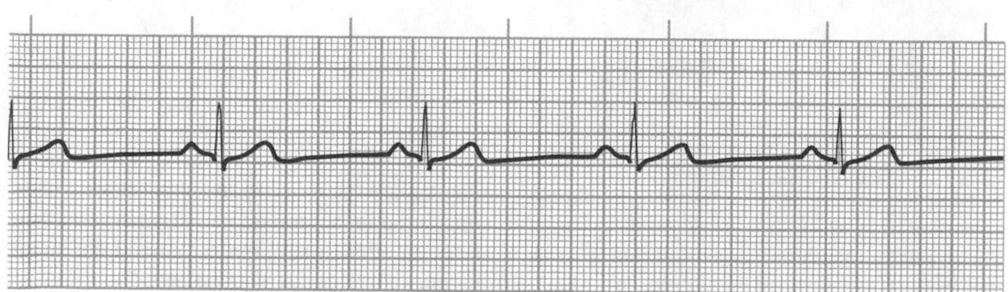

Figure 29-22 Sinus bradycardia; heart rate, 40 beats/min.

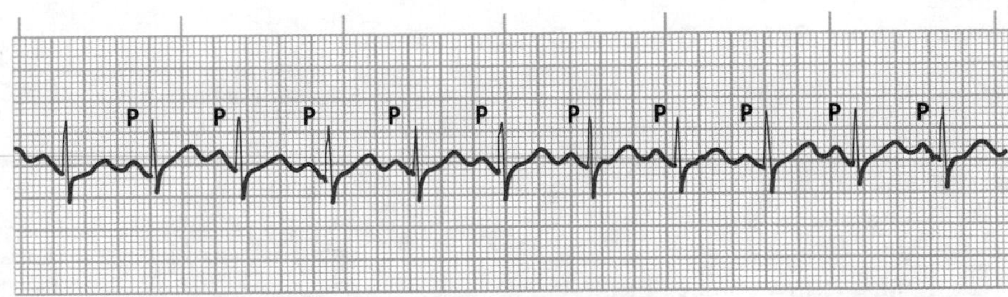

Figure 29-23 Sinus tachycardia; heart rate, 110 beats/min.

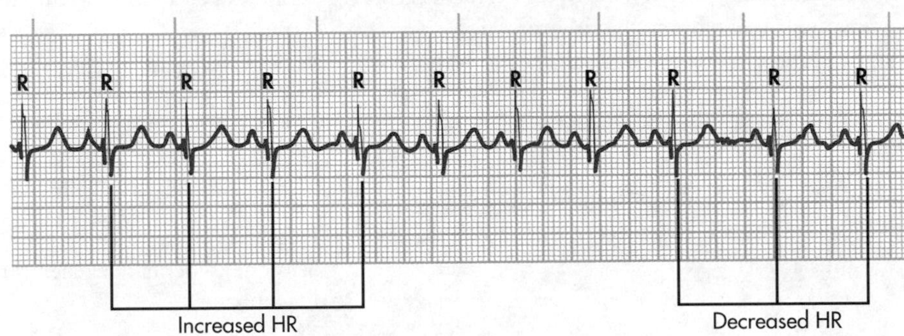

Figure 29-24 Sinus dysrhythmia. Heart rate increases with inspiration and decreases with expiration; overall heart rate *(HR)*, 100 beats/min.

complexes are within normal limits. The onset of sinus tachycardia usually is gradual, as the sinus node rate increases in response to higher metabolic needs.

Sinus tachycardia is associated with the ingestion of alcohol, caffeine, and tobacco and is a normal physiologic response to exertion, fever, fear, excitement, acute pain, or any condition that requires a higher basal metabolism. Clinically, sinus tachycardia can be a short-term compensatory response to heart failure, anemia, hypovolemia, and hypotension. Sinus tachycardia is also seen with hyperthyroidism and may be produced by drugs such as atropine and amphetamines.

Generally, sinus tachycardia is a benign rhythm that slows with resolution of the cause. The patient may complain of palpitations or have no symptoms. In the patient with a compromised myocardium the tachycardia increases myocardial oxygen demand and may cause a decrease in cardiac output with resultant lightheadedness, chest pain, and heart failure. Sinus tachycardia can usually be slowed with digoxin, beta-blockers, or diltiazem if necessary.

SINUS DYSRHYTHMIA. Sinus dysrhythmia is typically found in young adults and older persons. Sinus dysrhythmia is an irregular rhythm in which P-P intervals vary by more than 0.16 second. The P waves have a consistent shape, and the P-R interval and QRS duration are within normal limits. Changes in P-P intervals are accompanied by changes in R-R intervals (Figure 29-24). The cyclic pattern of changing P-P or R-R intervals often correlates with the patterns of inspiration and expiration. During inspiration the intervals shorten as the heart rate increases. Conversely, the intervals lengthen during expiration.

Sinus dysrhythmia is not treated unless the bradycardic phase is severe, causing symptoms. With slower heart rates, some patients may experience palpitations or dizziness if the P-P intervals are unusually long. Atropine may be effective in treating symptomatic bradycardia.

SICK SINUS SYNDROME. Tachycardia-bradycardia syndromes are characterized by the presence of bradycardia with intermittent episodes of tachydysrhythmias. The episode of tachydysrhythmia often is followed by a long pause before returning to bradycardia. Sick sinus syndrome (SSS) is one type of tachycardia-bradycardia syndrome. In SSS the bradycardia and tachycardia are both sinus in origin. Complications of this inefficient rhythm include heart failure and stroke resulting from thromboembolism. In addition, cerebral blood flow may be decreased, producing confusion in the elderly. SSS is associated with ischemia or degeneration of the SA node.

Some patients may remain free of symptoms or complain only of palpitations. For the patient with severe symptoms, the heart rhythm is stabilized with a permanent implantable pacemaker for the slow phase and the administration of digoxin or beta-blockers to control the ventricular rate of the tachycardic phase.

SINUS EXIT BLOCK AND SINUS ARREST. Sinus exit block occurs when an impulse originates in the SA node but is immediately blocked (Figure 29-25). No P wave or QRS complex is generated, resulting in a long pause. The next impulse occurs in a time interval representing the normal P-P interval. The term *sinus arrest* implies that the SA node never fired; therefore there is no P or QRS complex. The next impulse is asynchronous to the normal P-P interval.

Sinus exit block and sinus arrest may occur as a result of medications such as digoxin, hypoxia, myocardial ischemia, and injury to the SA node. The patient becomes symptomatic from a decrease in cardiac output when the pauses are long or frequent.

TABLE 29-8 COMPARISON OF SELECT CARDIAC DYSRHYTHMIAS

Dysrhythmia	ECG Diagnostic Criteria	Etiologic Factors
DYSRHYTHMIAS OF SINUS NODE		
Sinus bradycardia	P waves present followed by QRS Rhythm regular Heart rate <60 beats/min	Athletes Vagal stimulation Digitalis, beta-blockers, sedatives
Sinus tachycardia	P waves present followed by QRS Rhythm regular Heart rate 100-160 beats/min	Increased metabolic demands Compensatory mechanism for heart failure, shock, hemorrhage, anemia
Sinus dysrhythmia	Phasic shortening of P-P and R-R intervals with inspiration, lengthening with expiration	Respiratory variation in impulse initiation by SA node
Sick sinus syndrome	Sinus bradycardia alternating with sinus tachycardia	SA node ischemia, degeneration Hypertension Ischemia Digoxin
Sinus exit block and sinus arrest	Isoelectric line (pause) without P or QRS; P wave returns in synchrony (exit block) or asynchrony (sinus arrest)	Hypoxia Ischemia SA node ischemia, degeneration Digoxin
ATRIAL DYSRHYTHMIAS		
Premature atrial beats	Early P wave QRS may or may not be normal Pause follows QRS	Stress Ischemia Atrial enlargement Caffeine, nicotine
Wandering atrial pacemaker	P waves of different appearances or buried in QRS; varying P-R intervals	Cardiac disease Drug toxicity
Atrial tachycardia	P wave present (may be hidden in previous T wave), QRS usually normal, heart rate usually 150-250 beats/min	Sympathetic stimulation, caffeine, nicotine, drug toxicity Pulmonary disease Heart disease
Atrial flutter	Atrial rate 240-400 beats/min; F waves usually in a ratio to QRS complexes such as 2:1, 3:1; QRS complexes normal	Pulmonary disease Valve disease Cardiac surgery
Atrial fibrillation	Rapid, indiscernible P waves (>350 beats/min) Ventricular rhythm irregularly irregular Ventricular rate varies	Rheumatic heart disease Atrial ischemia Coronary atherosclerotic disease Hypertension Thyrotoxicosis Cardiac surgery Alcohol
JUNCTIONAL DYSRHYTHMIAS		
Premature junctional beat	Early beat P before, during, or after QRS P inverted or retrograde P-R interval <0.12 sec if P before QRS QRS normal	Increased metabolism Nicotine, caffeine Ischemia Electrolyte imbalance

TABLE 29-8 COMPARISON OF SELECT CARDIAC DYSRHYTHMIAS—CONT'D

Dysrhythmia	ECG Diagnostic Criteria	Etiologic Factors
Junctional rhythm	P before, during, or after QRS P inverted or retrograde P-R interval <0.12 sec if P before QRS QRS normal Rate 40-60 beats/min: junctional rhythm Rate 60-100 beats/min: accelerated junctional rhythm Rate > 100 beats/min: junctional tachycardia	Accelerated: Heart disease Caffeine Pain Digoxin
VENTRICULAR DYSRHYTHMIAS		
Premature ventricular beats	Early, wide, bizarre QRS, not associated with P wave Rhythm irregular	Stress, acidosis, ventricular enlargement Electrolyte imbalance Myocardial infarction Digitalis toxicity Hypoxemia, hypercapnia
Accelerated idioventricular rhythm (AIVR), ventricular tachycardia (VT)	P not associated with QRS, QRS wide and bizarre VT: ventricular rate >100, usually 140-240 beats/min AIVR: rate 40-100 beats/min	VT: hypoxemia, drug toxicity, electrolyte imbalance, bradycardia, coronary artery disease AIVR: reperfusion of ischemic myocardium
Torsades de pointes	No associated P waves Wide, bizarre QRSs twist along isoelectric line Heart rate >100 beats/min	Medications Electrolyte imbalance Congenital long Q-T interval
Ventricular fibrillation	No recognizable complexes Wavy line of varying amplitude	Myocardial infarction Electrocution Drowning
Ventricular asystole	No complexes "Straight line"	Myocardial infarction Chronic diseases of conducting system
IMPULSE CONDUCTION DEFICITS		
First-degree AV block	P-R interval prolonged, >0.20 sec	Rheumatic fever Myocardial infarction Cardiac medications
Second-degree AV blocks		
Mobitz I	P waves usually occurring regularly at rates consistent with SA node initiation P-R interval lengthened before nonconducted P wave; QRS may be widened	Acute myocardial infarction Increased vagal tone Electrolyte imbalance Infection
Mobitz II	Constant P-R intervals Nonconducted P waves at random or patterned intervals	Coronary artery disease Myocardial infarction Rheumatic heart disease Digoxin
Complete third-degree AV block	Atria and ventricles beat independently P waves have no relation to QRS Ventricular rate as low as 20-40 beats/min if ventricular; 40-60 beats/min if junctional	Digitalis toxicity Coronary artery disease Myocardial infarction
Bundle branch block	Same as normal sinus rhythm except QRS duration >0.12 sec	Hypoxia Acute myocardial infarction Heart failure Coronary atherosclerosis Hypertension

AV, Atrioventricular; *ECG,* Electrocardiogram; *SA,* sinoatrial.

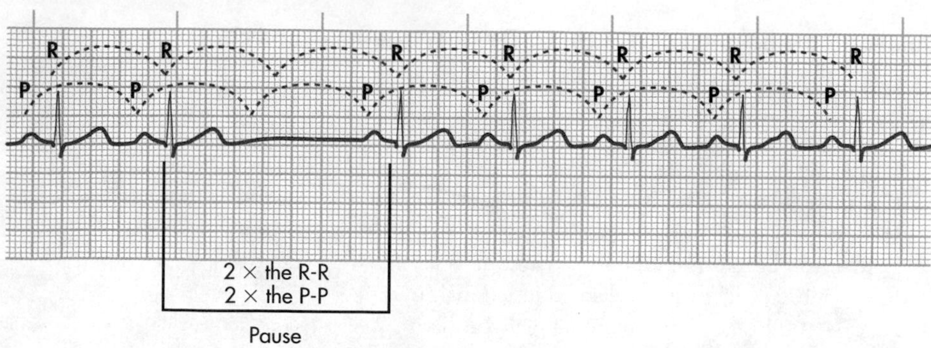

Figure 29-25 Sinus exit block. Pause equal to two complete cardiac cycles; overall heart rate, 70 beats/min.

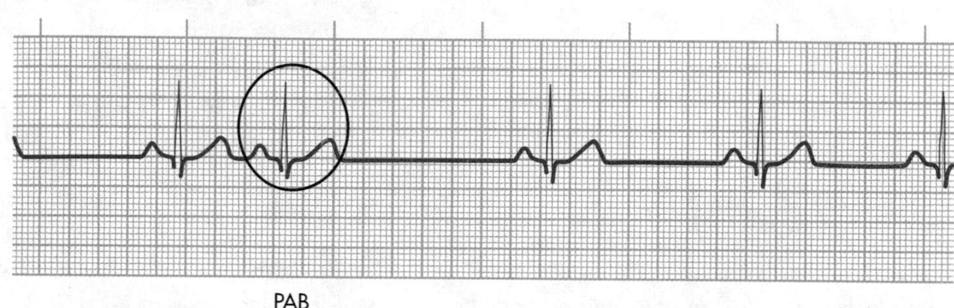

Figure 29-26 Premature atrial beat *(PAB)* in a sinus bradycardic rhythm; heart rate, 40 beats/min.

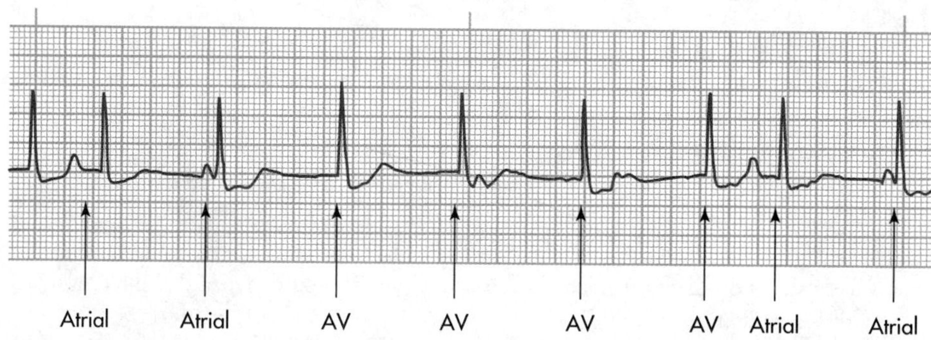

Figure 29-27 Wandering atrial pacemaker; ≠ indicater sites of origin; heart rate, 90 beats/min. *AV,* Atrioventricular node.

The patient may feel palpitations from the increased stroke volume that accompanies the next beat after the pause. When the patient is symptomatic, atropine may be administered to increase the heart rate and cardiac output. Definitive therapy includes insertion of a permanent pacemaker.

Premature Atrial Beat. A premature atrial beat (PAB) is initiated by an ectopic focus in the atria (Figure 29-26) and is characterized by a premature P wave with a contour different from that of a sinus P wave. The location of the ectopic focus within the atria determines its shape. The QRS complex may or may not be normal. The PAB is often followed by a pause. The atrial impulse may be nonconducted (blocked) because of refractoriness of the AV node at the time the impulse arrives. The nonconducted atrial beat (blocked PAB) is a common cause of irregularity in the heart rhythm.

The PAB may be associated with stress or the use of caffeine or tobacco products. It also is seen in the clinical setting with hypoxia, atrial enlargement, infection, inflammation, and myocardial ischemia. Frequent PABs may warn of impending atrial fibrillation (AF) or tachycardia. In the absence of organic disease, no treatment is required. Often the elimination of caffeine and tobacco will suppress the atrial focus. Premature atrial beats may produce palpitations, but cardiac output is generally not affected unless PABs or blocked beats are frequent.

Wandering Atrial Pacemaker. Wandering atrial pacemaker occurs when at least three ectopic sites create impulses for the cardiac rhythm (Figure 29-27). The ECG shows P waves of different shapes and P-R intervals of different lengths. The impulse can originate from the area around the AV node, which creates inverted P waves from retrograde conduction. Impulses from this lower area may also stimulate the atria at the same time as or after the ventricle. The P waves then appear to be buried in the QRS or even occur inverted after the QRS.

Wandering atrial pacemakers usually signify underlying heart disease or drug toxicity. The patient is usually asymptomatic unless the heart rate increases or decreases enough to affect cardiac output. The nurse monitors for changes in the rhythm and in the patient's symptoms.

ATRIAL TACHYCARDIA. In atrial tachycardia the atrial rate is approximately 150 to 250 beats/min. P waves are present but may be hidden in the T waves of the preceding beats when the ventricular rate is high. When the P waves vary in appearance, the rhythm is called multifocal atrial tachycardia. The QRS complex generally is normal, and the ventricular rhythm is regular (Figure 29-28). Transient episodes of atrial tachycardia occur in young adults in the absence of heart disease. The dysrhythmia is associated with rheumatic heart disease, pulmonary disorders, stress, hypoxia, caffeine, marijuana, and sympathomimetics.

The patient may complain of palpitations, lightheadedness, and anxiety during a tachycardic episode. Short, infrequent episodes require no treatment. Generally, hemodynamic changes are not severe unless the episode is prolonged, the rate is greater than 200 beats/min, or underlying disease exists. Lengthy episodes may respond to carotid sinus pressure or vagal stimulation. Some patients can be taught to perform Valsalva's maneuvers to slow the rate. Adenosine may be used in the acute situation. Depending on the electrophysiology associated with the atrial tachycardia, one of the following interventions is generally selected: AV nodal blockade with beta-blockers, calcium channel blockers, or digoxin; cardioversion; or antidysrhythmics (procainamide [Pronestyl], amiodarone [Cordarone], or sotalol [Betapace]). For long-term management, symptomatic atrial tachycardia arising from reentry is treated with beta-blockers or calcium channel blockers. If these agents do not control the dysrhythmia, ablation of the ectopic focus with or without pacemaker insertion may be recommended instead of additional antidysrhythmic drugs.

Atrial tachycardia with block is characterized by the same rapid atrial rate, but some impulses are not conducted into the ventricles (i.e., they are blocked). The AV nodal conduction ratio is usually 2:1, producing a ventricular rate of 75 to 125 beats/min. This dysrhythmia is associated with organic heart disease, and both digitalis toxicity and potassium deficit can cause it. Treatment depends on the clinical picture and often is aimed at correcting the underlying cause. Digitalis antibody may be indicated for hemodynamic compromise secondary to digitalis toxicity.

ATRIAL FLUTTER. In atrial flutter the atria depolarize at a rate of 240 to 400 beats/min. The atrial depolarizations produce flutter (F) waves that give the baseline a sawtooth appearance (Figure 29-29). The QRS configurations are normal. There is no measurable P-R interval because it is difficult to determine electrocardiographically which atrial impulse actually is conducted to the ventricles. With rapid atrial rates, the AV node physiologically prevents conduction of each atrial impulse. The ventricles often respond to the impulses at a regular rate. The number of flutter waves to QRS complexes is expressed as a ratio (e.g., atrial flutter, 3:1 block).

Reentry is the primary pathophysiologic process. Atrial flutter usually indicates underlying disease. It is associated most commonly

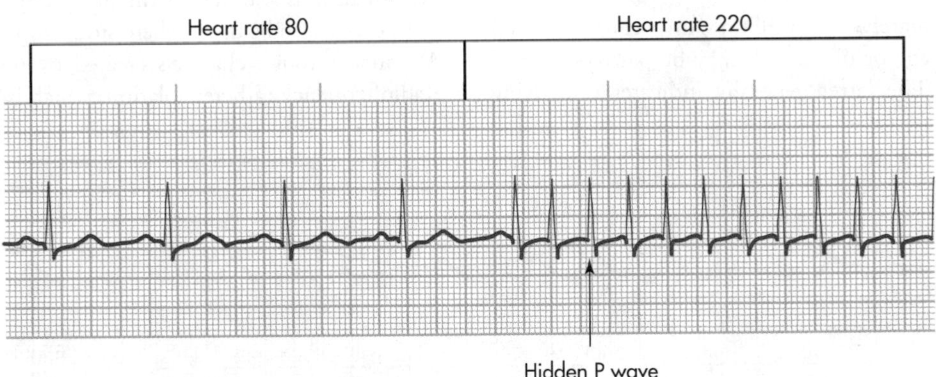

Figure 29-28 Normal sinus rhythm; heart rate, 80 beats/min, progressing to atrial tachycardia; heart rate, 220 beats/min.

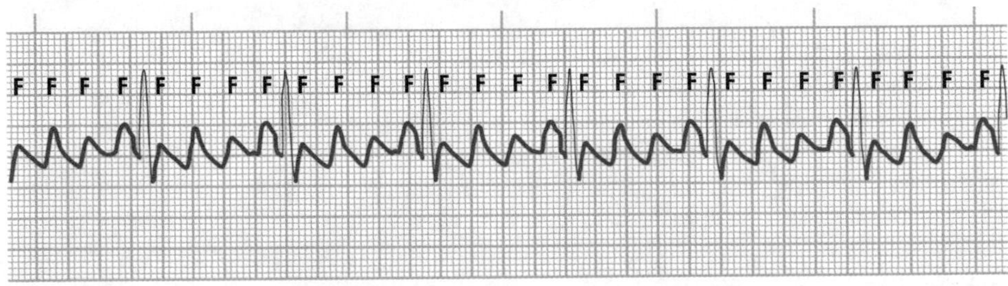

Figure 29-29 Atrial flutter, 4:1 block. Atrial heart rate, 260 beats/min; ventricular heart rate, 60 beats/min.

with CAD, pulmonary embolism, mitral valve disease, thoracic surgical procedures, and chronic obstructive pulmonary disease.

The potentially rapid or slow ventricular rate of atrial flutter may result in decreased cardiac output. The major goal of treatment is control of the ventricular rate. Diltiazem, digoxin, or beta-blockers usually succeed in slowing the ventricular rate. If these drugs do not slow the heart rate, amiodarone may be tried. Atropine may be used to augment the heart rate when the ventricular response is slow. Drugs used to terminate the rhythm include procainamide, disopyramide (Norpace), propafenone (Rythmol), sotalol, flecainide (Tambocor), amiodarone, dofetilide (Tikosyn), and ibutilide (Corvert). Azimilide, currently under investigation, is a promising treatment for supraventricular dysrhythmias.

Cardioversion is highly successful in converting atrial flutter to sinus rhythm. It may be the initial treatment if the patient is unstable. Care must be taken to prevent cardioembolic events (see Atrial Fibrillation). Pacing may be used when pharmacologic intervention and external cardioversion have been unsuccessful. For long-term management, radiofrequency ablation is often used to interrupt the reentry circuit. This procedure is successful in the majority of cases.

Atrial Fibrillation. AF is the most rapid atrial dysrhythmia (Figures 29-30 and 29-31). The atria depolarize chaotically at rates of 350 to 600 beats/min. AF is generated and perpetuated by one or more rapidly firing ectopic foci, with reentry being the pathophysiologic process in many cases. Paroxysmal AF in young adults has been associated with distinct electrically active foci within the pulmonary veins. The baseline in AF is composed of irregular undulations without definable P waves. The QRS complex usually is normal, but the ventricular rhythm is "irregularly irregular."

AF affects approximately 2.2 million Americans, most of whom are 65 years of age or older.[3] AF may be paroxysmal and transient, or chronic. The latter generally indicates underlying heart disease. AF is typically associated with pericarditis, thyrotoxicosis, cardiomyopathy, CAD, hypertension, rheumatic mitral valve disease, cardiac surgery, heart failure, pulmonary disease, and excessive alcohol intake ("holiday heart"). The underlying cause should be corrected whenever possible.

AF causes irregularity in the ventricular rhythm and impairs the ventricular filling that normally occurs with synchronous atrial contractions (atrial kick), thus decreasing cardiac output. Symptoms include fatigue, dyspnea, and dizziness. Thrombi may form in the stagnant blood in the atria and cause emboli, which can lodge in the pulmonary or peripheral blood vessels. The goal of therapy is to prevent complications through control of the ventricular rate and the restoration of NSR. The severity of the patient's symptoms, hemodynamic instability, and risk of embolization guide treatment decisions.

Drugs used to control fast ventricular rates include diltiazem, verapamil, digoxin, and beta-blockers. Digoxin is not as effective in controlling the heart rate variations that occur with exercise. In AF with a slow ventricular response, atropine may be necessary to increase the heart rate and cardiac output. When medications are ineffective in controlling the rate and the patient is symptomatic from an ineffective cardiac output, cardioversion may be necessary to restore NSR and a more normal heart rate.

Several antidysrhythmics may be successful in converting AF to NSR. The same drugs may be used to maintain patients in NSR once successful cardioversion occurs. Suggested AHA guidelines for the indication of these drugs are summarized in Box 29-5.[3] These drugs can have a prodysrhythmic effect. Therefore patients require careful monitoring, often within the hospital.

External cardioversion (see p. 789) is the most commonly used nonpharmacologic approach for restoring NSR. Internal atrial defibrillation is another treatment option. The surgical maze procedure may also be used, where sinus impulses are rerouted to the AV node through channels created by multiple atrial incisions. Radiofrequency catheter ablation, which isolates and treats specif-

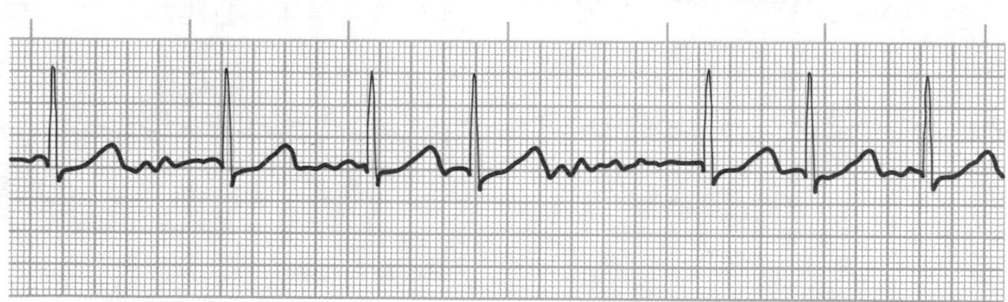

Figure 29-30 Rate-controlled atrial fibrillation; ventricular heart rate, 70 beats/min.

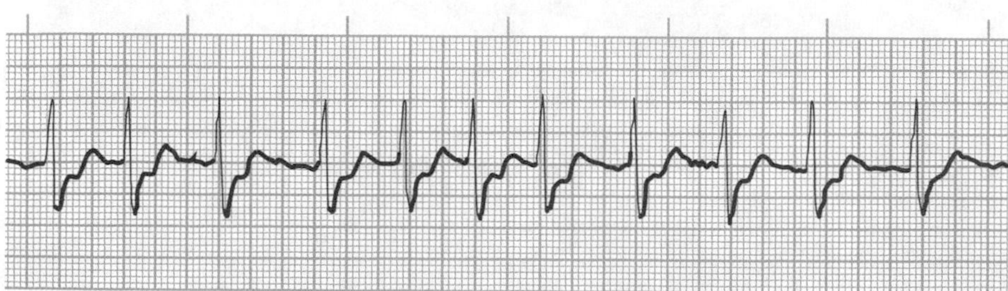

Figure 29-31 Atrial fibrillation with rapid ventricular response. No distinguishable P waves; ventricular heart rate, 110 beats/min.

Box 29-5 Antidysrhythmic Selection in Atrial Fibrillation

Pharmacologic Cardioversion

Atrial Fibrillation Less Than or Equal To 7 Days' Duration

Dofetilide
Flecainide
Ibutilide
Propafenone

Atrial Fibrillation Longer Than 7 Days' Duration

Dofetilide

Maintenance of Sinus Rhythm

Patients Without Coronary Artery Disease

First line: flecainide, propafenone, sotalol
Second line: amiodarone, dofetilide
Third line: disopyramide, procainamide, quinidine

Patients With Heart Failure

Amiodarone
Dofetilide

Patients With Coronary Artery Disease

First line: sotalol
Second line: amiodarone, dofetilide
Third line: disopyramide, procainamide, quinidine

Patients With Hypertension and Left Ventricular Hypertrophy

Amiodarone

Patients With Hypertension and Minimal Left Ventricular Hypertrophy

First line: flecainide, propafenone
Second line: amiodarone, dofetilide, sotalol
Third line: disopyramide, procainamide, quinidine

Clinical Trials

Azimilide
Dronedarone
Tedisamil

Data from ACC/AHA/ESC guidelines for the management of patients with atrial fibrillation: executive summary: a report of the American College of Cardiology/American Heart Association Task Force on Practice Guidelines and the European Society of Cardiology Committee for Practice Guidelines and Policy Conferences (Committee to Develop Guidelines for the Management of Patients With Atrial Fibrillation), *Circulation* 104(17):2118–2150, 2001.

ic areas of atrial activity, is successful in selected situations. Ablation of the AV node with subsequent placement of a permanent pacemaker may be used in individuals with permanent symptomatic AF. This procedure does not, however, abolish the fibrillatory activity of the atria. Other treatment options include single and dual site atrial pacing and newer implantable atrial defibrillators.

The risk of systemic emboli is high with persistent AF. Patients ideally are stabilized on warfarin therapy for 4 weeks with an INR goal of 2 to 3 before an elective pharmacologic or electrical cardioversion attempt. If the patient is hemodynamically unstable or has refractory symptoms, however, the need to electrically cardiovert may take priority. Transesophageal echocardiography may be helpful in determining the presence of atrial thrombi. If no thrombi are found, the patient may be electrically cardioverted. After successful conversion to NSR, thrombi may still form until the atria contract effectively and in synchrony. Therefore anticoagulation therapy is continued for at least 4 weeks after conversion to NSR. If conversion to NSR is unsuccessful, the patient is maintained indefinitely on warfarin therapy. If the patient cannot tolerate warfarin, aspirin therapy, with a daily dose of 325 mg, is recommended. Ximelagatran, an oral thrombin inhibitor, is currently under investigation as an alternative to warfarin therapy.

PREMATURE JUNCTIONAL BEATS. Premature junctional beats (PJBs) arise from an ectopic focus either (1) at the junction of the atria and the AV node or (2) at the junction of the AV node and the bundle of His. If the PJBs arise from the first junction, the P wave will be inverted and premature and will precede the QRS complex. In the second case, the P wave is either hidden in the QRS or is inverted and follows the QRS (Figure 29-32). The abnormal timing and inversion of the P wave are caused by depolarization of the atria in a retrograde fashion. The QRS is normal, but the P-R interval is less than 0.12 second.

PJBs may occur in the normal heart. They also may result from digitalis toxicity, ischemia, hypoxia, pain, fever, anxiety, nicotine, caffeine, or electrolyte imbalance. Treatment, when needed, is directed toward correcting the underlying cause.

JUNCTIONAL RHYTHMS. When the SA node fires at a rate less than 40 to 60 beats/min, the automatic cells in the AV junction

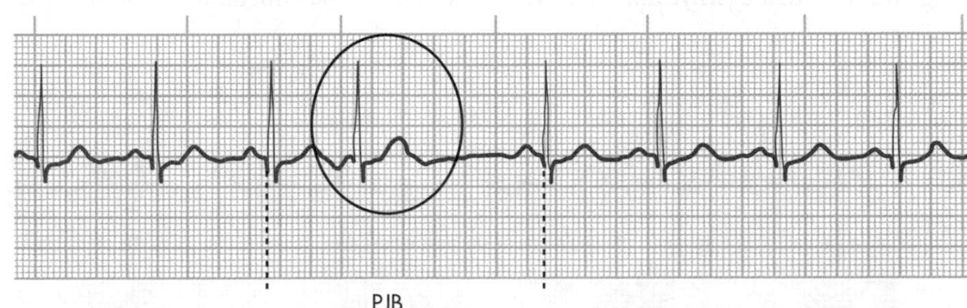

Figure 29-32 Sinus rhythm with premature junctional beat; heart rate, 80 beats/min.

may initiate impulses (escape beats) to stabilize the rhythm. A succession of beats from the junction is a junctional escape rhythm. The P waves may occur before, during, or after the QRS. The QRS is normal, and the ventricular rhythm is regular. A junctional escape rhythm occasionally is found in the well-trained athlete or as a complication of an acute inferior wall MI. Junctional escape rhythm generally is not treated unless the loss of atrial kick produces symptoms of low cardiac output. These patients may require artificial pacing.

When the automaticity of a junctional pacemaker increases to a rate greater than 60 beats/min, it may usurp the SA node as the pacemaker of the heart. A rate of 60 to 100 beats/min is called an accelerated junctional rhythm (Figure 29-33). An accelerated junctional rhythm may be due to heart disease, pain, anemia, caffeine, or amphetamines.

A junctional tachycardia exists when the rate exceeds 100 beats/min. Junctional tachycardia is associated with digitalis toxicity, acute rheumatic fever, and heart disease; treatment is aimed at the underlying cause. If the rate is interfering with cardiac output, vagal maneuvers may be attempted followed by digoxin, beta-blockers, or diltiazem administration.

Both junctional tachycardia and AT may be collectively referred to as supraventricular tachycardia (SVT), indicating that the rhythm originates above the ventricles. Symptomatic SVT from reentry may be treated with beta-blockers or calcium channel blockers. If these agents do not control the dysrhythmia, ablation of the irritable focus with or without pacemaker insertion may be recommended instead of antidysrhythmics.

Premature Ventricular Beats. A premature ventricular beat (PVB) is an early beat arising from an ectopic focus in the ventricles. The characteristic wide, bizarre QRS (usually greater than 0.12 second) makes the PVB readily identifiable on the ECG tracing. There is no associated P wave, and the T wave records in the opposite direction from the main QRS deflection. Most PVBs are followed by a pause until the next normal impulse originates in the SA node.

If PVBs are of different configurations on the ECG tracing, they are said to be multifocal. This indicates the presence of more than one ectopic focus in the ventricles, or one ectopic focus with multiple reentry pathways, each producing complexes of differing forms. Premature ventricular beats also may exhibit varying degrees of prematurity. The relationship of the PVB to the Q, R, S, and T waves of the preceding beat is important. An electrical impulse of any kind that stimulates the heart near the peak of the T wave (thereby preventing full repolarization of the ventricles) may precipitate a more dangerous or lethal dysrhythmia. The frequency and morphology of PVBs determine their importance. When every other beat is a PVB, the term *bigeminy* is used; every third beat, *trigeminy*, and so forth (Figure 29-34). Two PVBs together are termed a *couplet*.

PVBs occur in the absence of heart disease and increase in number with age. However, the incidence and frequency of occurrence are higher in the population with heart disease. Clinically, PVBs are associated with AMI, heart failure, digitalis toxicity, hypoxia, stimulants, catecholamines, and electrolyte imbalances. In the latter cases treatment of the underlying cause may abolish the dysrhythmia.

Ventricular Rhythms and Tachycardia. If the SA node and AV junction fail to initiate impulses, a ventricular pacemaker cell automatically begins to initiate impulses at a rate of 20 to 40 beats/min. This is known as an idioventricular rhythm (Figure 29-35). P waves, when seen, are not associated with the ventricular rhythm, and the QRS complex is greater than 0.12 second, wide, and bizarre.

If the rate of the ventricular-initiated rhythm increases to 40 to 100 beats/min, it is known as an accelerated idioventricular rhythm (AIVR). An AIVR may be seen in hypoxia, in digitalis toxicity, as a complication of an AMI, and as a reperfusion dysrhythmia after thrombolytic therapy. Suppression of the heart's dominant and perhaps only rhythm could be hazardous. Therefore idioventricular rhythms are not treated except to correct underlying abnormalities.

If the cardiac output is low and symptoms of heart failure, syncope, or hypotension develop, the patient may require a temporary or permanent pacemaker. Atropine may be helpful in stimulating the return of SA node activity.

By definition, three or more successive PVBs constitute ventricular tachycardia (VT) (Figure 29-36). The ventricular rate is regular or slightly irregular, and is greater than 100 beats/min, usually 140 to 240 beats/min. P waves may be present but are not associated with the QRS complexes. VT may complicate any form of heart disease and may be a direct result of a PVB striking during the heart's action potential vulnerable period. Conditions that favor its occurrence include hypoxemia, drug toxicity, electrolyte imbalance, and bradycardia. Abnormal automaticity can occur in the postinfarction period from the loss of fast depolarizing sodium channels, contributing to the development of VT. VT can also be attributable to ischemia, nonischemic heart disease, and drugs, and can even be found in the structurally normal heart (e.g., long QT syndrome). Reentry is often involved. Treatment is based on the underlying electrophysiology of the dysrhythmia, which may be difficult to establish.

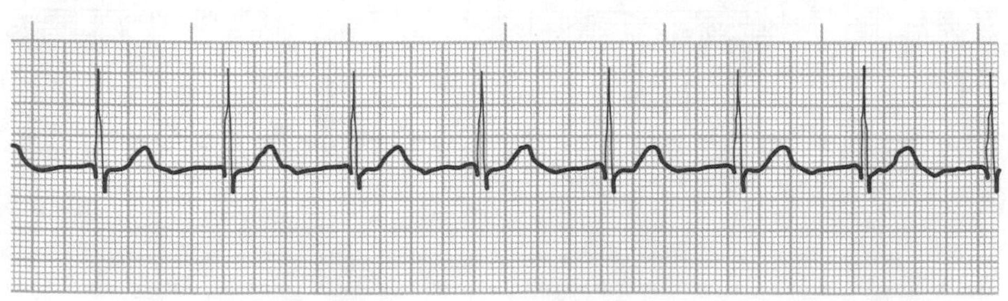

Figure 29-33 Accelerated junctional rhythm with hidden P waves; heart rate, 70 beats/min.

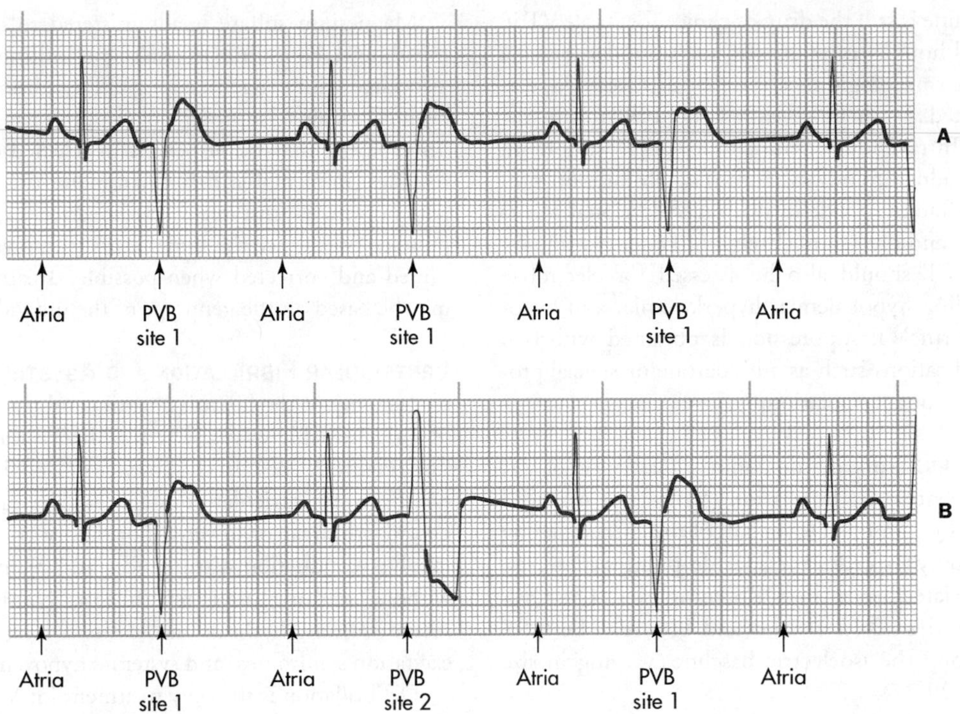

Figure 29-34 Bigeminy. **A,** Sinus rhythm with unifocal bigeminy premature ventricular beats (PVBs); heart rate, 70 beats/min. **B,** Sinus rhythm with multifocal bigeminy PVBs; heart rate, 70 beats/min.

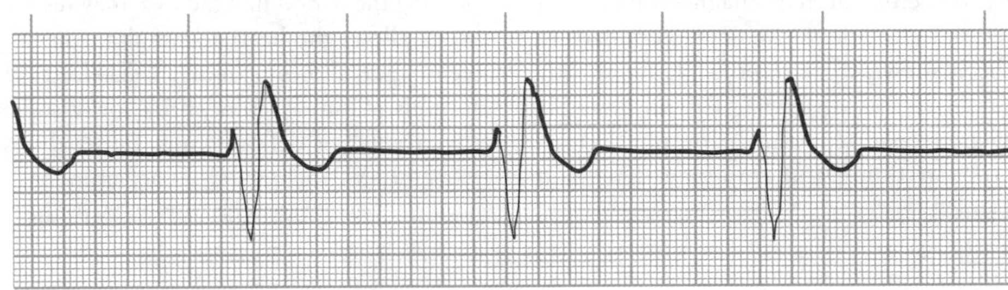

Figure 29-35 Idioventricular rhythm; ventricular heart rate, 30 beats/min.

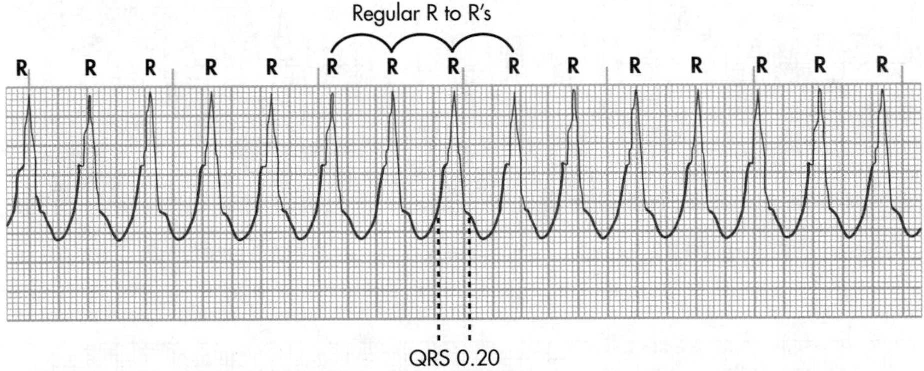

Figure 29-36 Ventricular tachycardia with regular R-R intervals and QRS greater than 0.12 second; heart rate, 150 beats/min.

VT is classified as sustained (lasting more than 30 seconds) or nonsustained. Nonsustained VT may occur in patients with or without cardiac disease and is associated with palpitations or recurrent syncope. In the presence of severe ventricular dysfunction, nonsustained VT may be a precursor to sustained VT and sudden death. As the heart rate increases, cardiac output decreases, since the ventricles do not have sufficient time to fill and empty. Symptoms vary depending on the length of the VT and the rate.

Intravenous lidocaine administration was standard therapy for VT for many years, but more efficacious antidysrhythmics are now available. Lidocaine is still the drug of choice for stable VT in many institutions, although some centers use amiodarone as a first-line agent. If pharmacologic measures are unsuccessful, cardioversion is attempted. With pulseless VT, defibrillation is the standard of care. Intravenous amiodarone and vasopressin (Pitressin) have been added to advanced cardiac life support protocols to treat VT refractory to defibrillation. Additional agents include procainamide and bretylium (Bretylol). Patients with persistent or recurrent VT should also be assessed for electrolyte abnormalities, including hypokalemia, hyperkalemia, and hypomagnesemia. Long-term VT suppression is obtained with oral antidysrhythmic medications such as amiodarone or special procedures such as radiofrequency ablation.

Torsades de Pointes. Torsades de pointes, a variation of VT, can also progress to ventricular fibrillation (VF) if not managed appropriately. A long Q-T interval (over half of the corresponding R-R interval) commonly precedes torsades de pointes. P waves, when seen, are dissociated from the QRS complexes. The QRS complexes are longer than 0.12 second and bizarre. The QRS complexes "twist" along the isoelectric baseline, varying in size and direction (Figure 29-37).

The initiating electrophysiologic mechanism may be triggered activity or reentry. The rhythm may result from prolonged repolarization, represented on the ECG as a prolonged Q-T interval. Prolongation may occur secondary to various medications or electrolyte abnormalities (hypokalemia or hypomagnesemia), or it may be congenital. Alterations in ion movement secondary to genetic mutations have been shown to be responsible for slightly more than 50% of researched cases of long QT syndrome. Six genetic variants currently are recognized. Cardiac output decreases from inadequate ventricular filling and emptying that result from the increased heart rate.

Magnesium sulfate is administered to stabilize the electrical membrane. Potassium may also be indicated. When torsades is associated with congenital long QT syndrome, beta-blockers have been efficacious. Isoproterenol (Isuprel) has also been used. Overdrive pacing may be of benefit in selected cases. With recurrent torsades, implantable defibrillators are used as prophylaxis. The patient who is unstable is cardioverted or defibrillated as with pulseless VT. Once the initial crisis is resolved, the cause is determined and corrected when possible. Treatment modalities soon may be based on the genotype of the individual.

Ventricular Fibrillation and Asystole. In VF the ventricular activity of the heart is chaotic, and the ECG tracing consists of unidentifiable waves. The fibrillatory waves may be coarse or fine (Figure 29-38). In the absence of depolarization there can be no effective ventricular contraction. The most common cause is CAD with areas of lowered fibrillatory thresholds. It frequently involves conduction disturbances and reentry. It can also occur without warning after reperfusion. Nonischemic causes may include antidysrhythmic medications, long QT syndromes, preexcitation syndromes, and systemic hypoxemia.

Defibrillation is the only treatment for VF, and it must be performed as soon as possible. Automated external defibrillators (AEDs) eliminate the need for rhythm recognition and can be manipulated quickly to allow for rapid defibrillation. While awaiting an AED, bystander cardiopulmonary resuscitation (CPR) may prolong the period in which VF may respond to defibrillation. The shock allows the heart to simultaneously depolarize, stopping all reentry and allowing an organized electrical rhythm to return. The administration of epinephrine or vasopressin may increase the effectiveness of defibrillation. Other drugs that may be used for refractory VF include lidocaine, amiodarone, bretylium, and magnesium. For those who survive VF, the long-term use of beta-

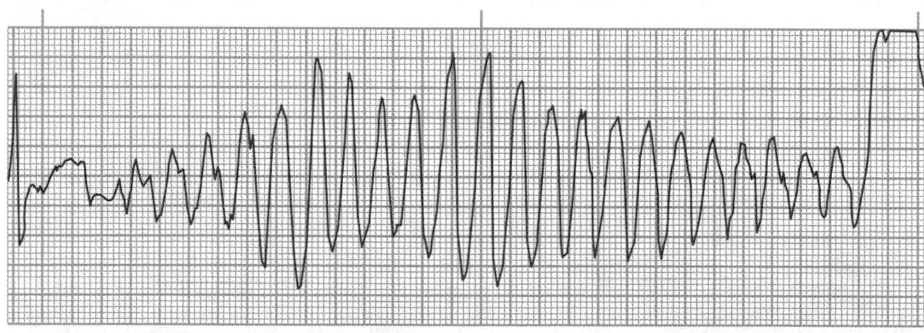

Figure 29-37 Torsades de pointes; heart rate, 240-250 beats/min.

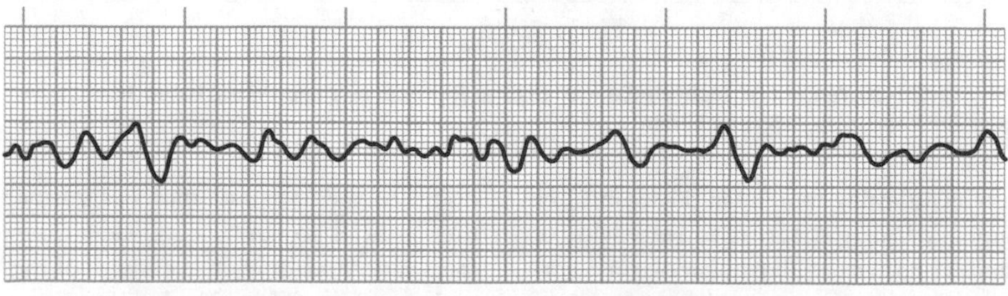

Figure 29-38 Coarse ventricular fibrillation; heart rate, not measurable.

blockers may decrease the recurrence rate. An implantable defibrillator is the treatment of choice for survivors.

In asystole the ECG tracing is a flat line and no electrical activity is noted; all pacemaker cells have failed. The patient has no blood pressure, pulse, or audible heartbeat; respirations quickly cease. CPR must be instituted immediately. Epinephrine, atropine, and external pacing are all used in the effort to restore cardiac excitability.

Pulseless electrical activity is the term used to describe the presence of electrical activity in the absence of a heartbeat. CPR is instituted immediately along with measures to restore contraction. These may include pericardiocentesis, if tamponade is inhibiting contraction, or the administration of calcium to stimulate contractile force. Medications may include epinephrine and atropine.

ATRIOVENTRICULAR BLOCK. A block to impulse conduction can occur at any point along the conduction pathways. One common area is the AV junction. The severity of the **atrioventricular block** is identified by degrees, that is, first-, second-, or third-degree AV block. First-degree AV block is present when the P-R interval is longer than 0.20 second, indicating a conduction delay in the AV node (Figure 29-39). It usually is found in association with rheumatic fever, digoxin, beta-blockers, acute inferior MI, and increased vagal tone. When a first-degree AV block occurs in isolation, the patient is usually asymptomatic and no treatment is necessary.

Second-degree AV block may be subdivided into two categories. Type I (Wenckebach, or Mobitz type I) is characterized by a P-R interval that progressively lengthens until a P wave is not followed by a QRS complex (Figure 29-40). The nonconducted impulse arrives at the AV node during the refractory period. The ratio of P waves to QRS complexes may be 5:4, 4:3, 3:2, or 2:1 and creates a clustered appearance. The pathologic condition is usually within the AV node and produces QRS complexes of less than 0.12 second.

Any drug that slows AV conduction may cause a type I block, but such blocks are most often seen in the patient with an acute inferior wall MI, digitalis toxicity, increased vagal tone, electrolyte imbalance, or acute myocarditis or after cardiac surgery. Type I blocks often are transient and reversible, and treatment is not required unless the patient becomes symptomatic. Atropine may be effective in increasing cardiac output.

Type II (Mobitz type II) second-degree AV block is less common but more serious. A type II block is characterized by nonconducted sinus impulses despite constant P-R intervals for the conducted P waves. The nonconducted P waves may occur at random or in patterned ratios (e.g., 2:1, 3:1) (Figure 29-41). The QRS complexes are widened unless the block is within the bundle of His.

Type II blocks may occur in patients with CAD, MI, rheumatic heart disease, cardiomyopathy, and chronic fibrotic disease of the conduction system. If cardiac output is decreased, a temporary pacemaker usually is inserted prophylactically until the conduction stabilizes. If the block is persistent, the patient benefits from a permanent pacemaker. Atropine may be used to reduce vagal tone and improve conduction through the AV node. However, this is effective only if the site of block is the AV node. If the block is below the AV node, atropine is not effective.

In third-degree AV block (complete heart block) all the sinus or atrial impulses are blocked, and the atria and ventricles beat independently. Either a junctional or a ventricular pacemaker cell

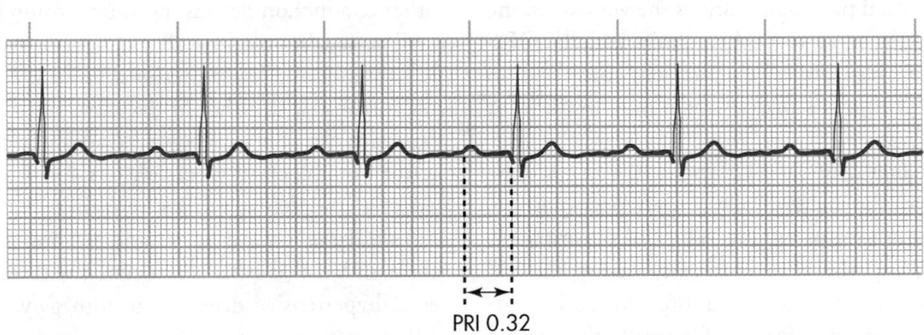

Figure 29-39 First-degree heart block. P-R interval *(PRI)* greater than 0.20 second.

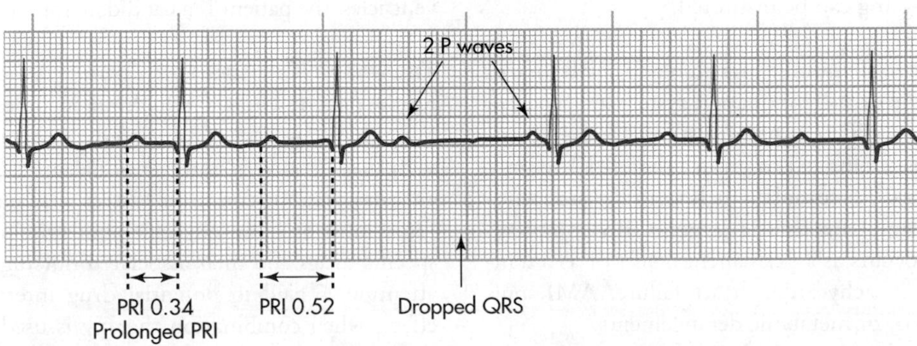

Figure 29-40 Mobitz I heart block; atrial heart rate, 60 beats/min; ventricular heart rate, 50 beats/min. *PRI*, P-R interval.

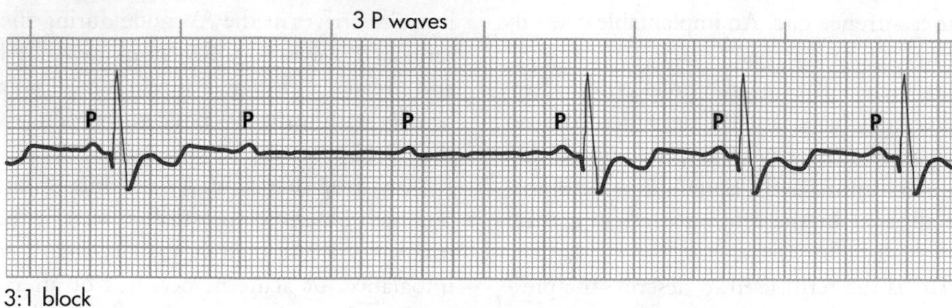

Figure 29-41 Mobitz II with a 3:1 heart block.

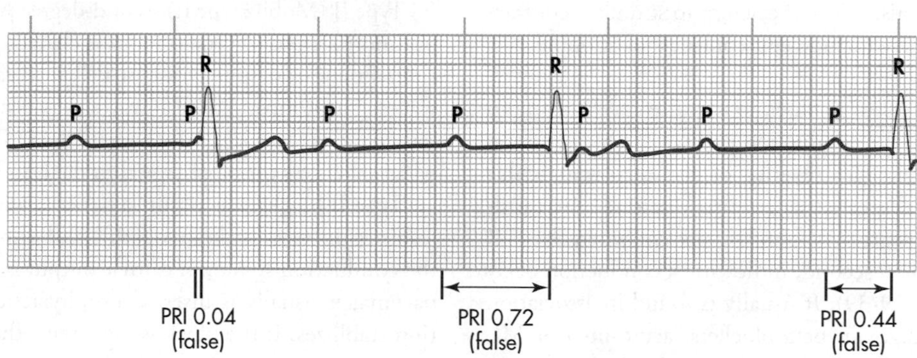

Figure 29-42 Separate P waves and QRS complexes of third-degree heart block; atrial heart rate, 70 beats/min; ventricular heart rate, 30 beats/min. *PRI*, P-R interval.

drives the ventricles. The lesion is usually in the bundle of His or the bundle branches but may also be at the AV junction. The rate and dependability of the ventricular rhythm are related to the level of the lesion. If a junctional pacemaker drives the ventricles, the ventricular rate will be at least 40 to 60 beats/min and the QRS complexes are narrow. This block may be a transient complication of inferior posterior MI or digitalis toxicity, or it may result from severe heart disease.

If a ventricular pacemaker drives the ventricles, the rate will be 20 to 40 beats/min, and the patient may experience syncope, heart failure, altered mentation, or angina. The QRS complex is abnormally wide, indicating that the block lies below the AV junction (Figure 29-42). The prognosis is more serious if complete heart block accompanies anterior MI. Generally the patient requires a permanent pacemaker. Epinephrine or isoproterenol administered intravenously may increase the ventricular rate temporarily until artificial pacing can be instituted.

Bundle Branch Block. In bundle branch block (BBB) one or both bundle branch paths of the conduction system are blocked. The impulse must travel a different path to stimulate the ventricle; therefore the QRS is prolonged to greater than 0.12 second. Instead of a synchronous QRS complex, each ventricle independently depolarizes, creating characteristic jagged QRS complexes (Figure 29-43). A BBB occurs as a permanent defect or as a transient block secondary to tachycardia, heart failure, AMI, pulmonary embolus, hypoxia, or metabolic derangements.

The right bundle branch is the more delicate of the two bundles and has a longer refractory period in some persons. In the younger patient right BBB often results from right ventricular hypertrophy, whereas CAD usually is the cause in the older patient. One classic ECG pattern is an M-shaped QRS in V_1 and V_2. In the absence of other conduction defects, no intervention is necessary.

The left bundle branch has a main trunk that bifurcates into left anterior and left posterior divisions. A block may occur in the main trunk or in either of the divisions. (Blocks of the anterior or posterior division are known as left anterior hemiblock or left posterior hemiblock, respectively.) A block in the main trunk produces a complete left BBB, resulting in a QRS greater than 0.12 second; large R waves in V_5 and V_6; and deep, wide S waves in V_1 through V_3. Left BBB is associated with severe CAD, valvular disease, hypertensive disease, cardiomegaly, and acute anterior wall MI. It also may occur as a result of degenerative changes in the conduction system. Whenever sufficient blockage is present to leave the heart dependent on just one fascicle for conduction to the ventricles, the patient is a candidate for a permanent pacemaker.

Treatment Options for Dysrhythmias. Collaborative care for the patient with a dysrhythmia includes diagnosing the specific dysrhythmia and its associated cause and treating the disorder with medications or interventional procedures. Table 29-9 presents medications commonly used to manage dysrhythmias. The nurse must be knowledgeable about the mechanism of action of specific drugs and their associated nursing interventions. Careful attention is paid to potential drug interactions and synergistic effects when combination therapy is used. The metabolism and excretion of medications may be impaired in older adults and in patients with decreased perfusion to the kidneys and liver. The

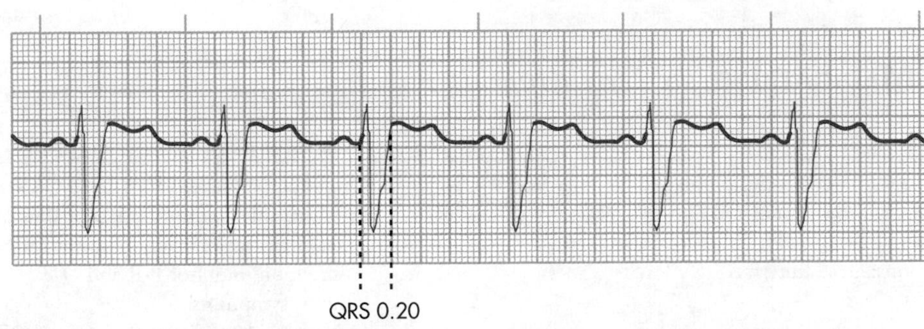

Figure 29-43 Sinus rhythm with bundle branch block; heart rate, 60 beats/min.

nurse must be aware of new agents approved for the management of cardiac dysrhythmias and how to monitor their safe use.

Nursing management of the patient experiencing dysrhythmias focuses on interventions to decrease oxygen demand. The nurse spaces activities and encourages frequent rest periods. While medication therapy is being adjusted, patients are on continuous ECG monitoring (**telemetry**). Rhythms are documented every 4 to 8 hours and as needed. The nurse provides skin care to minimize the irritation of the monitoring electrodes.

The nurse must be alert to changes in the patient's rhythm. Assessments for changes in cardiac output are documented. Emergency drugs should be available, and intravenous access is ensured. Ancillary equipment such as defibrillators, oxygen, suction, and temporary pacemakers are kept available and in good working condition.

Interventions such as cardioversion, defibrillation, coronary ablation, pacemaker therapy, automatic implantable cardioverter-defibrillators, and CPR are also part of the collaborative care strategies used for patients with dysrhythmias.

CARDIOVERSION AND DEFIBRILLATION. Cardioversion and defibrillation use electrical energy to convert a cardiac dysrhythmia to a rhythm that is hemodynamically stable, preferably a sinus rhythm. Electrophysiologically, the electrical countershock produces a simultaneous depolarization of a critical mass of cardiac fibers, thus halting the asynchronous chaos of a fibrillation or the rapid firing of a tachycardia. In some cases, especially in elective cardioversion, the shock is delivered more than once until the required level of voltage is reached. Once the heart is fully depolarized, the SA node is better able to resume control.

Defibrillation applies an unsynchronized electrical countershock during a VF emergency or pulseless VT. The paddles from the defibrillator are placed at the third intercostal space to the right of the sternum and the fifth intercostal space on the left midaxillary line. Conducting gel or saline pads are applied between the paddles and the skin to ensure conductance and to minimize skin burning. The button on each paddle is depressed simultaneously to release 200 to 360 watt-seconds (joules, or J) to the patient. Defibrillation must be performed quickly for VF and most cases of VT.

Cardioversion differs from defibrillation in that the electrical discharge is synchronized with the R wave to avoid triggering VF from accidental discharge during the vulnerable period of repolarization. Indications for cardioversion include hemodynamically unstable atrial flutter, AF, and atrial tachycardia. Body size and patient stability are used to guide the amount of energy selected, usually 100 to 360 J. Biphasic defibrillators require less energy and have proven more effective in converting AF to NSR. Appropriate levels of anticoagulation should be established for patients with atrial flutter or fibrillation rhythms before treatment with cardioversion. Patches may be placed in either the right anterior and left posterior or right anterior and left lateral positions. Occasionally the simultaneous use of two sets of patches and two defibrillators is needed for large patients or resistant rhythms. Patients should be NPO before the procedure. The nurse prepares patients psychologically for what to expect during cardioversion and reassures them that they will be sedated with intravenous diazepam (Valium), midazolam (Versed), or fentanyl. An anesthesiologist is nearby. Elective cardioversion should be performed in a special laboratory and not the patient's room. The defibrillator is synchronized so that the impulse is not initiated until the next R wave occurs. This eliminates the danger of entering the vulnerable period. For most elective procedures, the amount of watt-seconds or joules required for conversion is lower than that required for defibrillation. The nurse monitors the patient after cardioversion until vital signs are stable. Although the procedure itself is often successful, the rate of recurrence is high.

Internal atrial cardioversion may be an alternative when external cardioversion fails. Two small electrode catheters are placed in the right atrium and coronary sinus to accomplish the cardioversion. A bipolar catheter is placed in the right ventricle to precisely time the cardioversion. Energy levels are typically 1 to 100 J. The patient is under conscious sedation during the procedure.

RADIOFREQUENCY CATHETER ABLATION. Radiofrequency catheter ablation (RFCA) involves the insertion of a catheter, usually through the patient's femoral or jugular vein, which delivers programmed electrical stimulation to recreate the patient's dysrhythmia and localize the area for ablation. The site of origin for the dysrhythmia, or the pathway necessary for its propagation, is then destroyed using radiofrequency energy, a form of high-frequency electromagnetic waves. The thermal energy causes coagulation necrosis in the area selected for ablation. Cryoablation, the use of freezing temperatures, may also be used to destroy the site of origin. The amount of damage caused by the catheter is relatively small because the energy used can be precisely regulated and focused. The patient remains in the electrophysiology laboratory for a short interval after the procedure for observation.

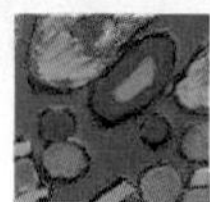

TABLE 29-9
COMMON MEDICATIONS *for Dysrhythmias*

Drug	Action	Nursing Intervention
Quinidine Procainamide Disopyramide*	Inhibit sodium influx during phase 0 depolarization Prolong action potential and effective refractory period in atrium, bundle of His, and ventricle Indications: atrial flutter, AF, SVT, VT	Quinidine: monitor Q-Tc, P-R, QRS; may cause tinnitus. Procainamide: administer PO or slow IV push followed by maintenance infusion; monitor for hypotension with IV initiation; monitor P-R and Q-Tc; may cause systemic lupus symptoms. Disopyramide: monitor P-R, Q-Tc, QRS; may cause anticholinergic effects.
Lidocaine Mexiletine Tocainide Moricizine†	Moderately inhibit sodium influx during phase 0 depolarization, decreasing automaticity; increase electrical stimulation threshold of ventricle, His-Purkinje system; shorten repolarization and action potential Indications: VT	Lidocaine: administer by IV push followed by maintenance infusion; toxic effects include confusion, psychosis, decreased hearing, seizures.
Flecainide Propafenone‡	Decrease sodium influx during phase 0 depolarization; reduce membrane responsiveness; inhibit automaticity; increase effective refractory period with little effect on action potential duration Indications: life-threatening dysrhythmias—not first-line drugs	Propafenone: significantly decreases inotropic activity; use with caution in LV dysfunction.
Propranolol Acebutalol Esmolol Metoprolol	Inhibit beta-adrenergic receptors and slow ventricular rate through action on slow calcium channels of AV node that are coupled with beta-1 receptors Indications: dysrhythmias of abnormal automaticity, triggered activity, or reentry	Administer PO or slow IV push. Monitor P-R and blood pressure. Teach patient not to discontinue abruptly. Monitor for heart failure in susceptible patients.
Amiodarone§ Sotalol§	Block outward potassium channels or facilitate slow inward sodium current; lengthen refractory period Depress SA node automaticity and conduction in AV node Indications: VF and VT, atrial flutter and AF (but not FDA approved for atrial dysrhythmias)	Amiodarone: increases warfarin effect; may cause thyroid dysfunction, pulmonary toxicity, blue-gray skin discoloration. Half-life: 15-100 days with PO onset 1-3 wk Monitor P-R and Q-Tc. Sotalol: normalize potassium and magnesium before therapy. Monitor P-R and Q-Tc.
Ibutilide Dofetilide	Block outward potassium channels or facilitate slow inward sodium current; lengthen repolarization by prolonging action potential Indications: atrial flutter and AF	Ibutilide: for IV cardioversion of AF in critical care unit. Q-Tc should be less than 0.44 sec before infusion. Dofetilide: adjust dose to creatinine clearance and Q-Tc.
Diltiazem Verapamil	Increase effective refractory period in AV node; inhibit calcium ion influx across cell membrane during cardiac depolarization; slow SA and AV node conduction times	Administer PO or slow IV push. Avoid in patients with accessory pathways or wide-complex tachycardia.

Attempts are then made to reinitiate the dysrhythmia, using electrical or pharmacologic stimulation. If the dysrhythmia recurs, additional ablation bursts are administered until the site is destroyed.

Indications for catheter ablation include AV node reentry tachycardias, accessory pathways (such as Wolff-Parkinson-White syndrome), focal atrial tachycardia, atrial flutter, and bundle branch reentry. Ectopic areas in and near the pulmonary vein are also target sites for catheter ablation in AF. Ablation is also an alternative in select cases of VT. Complications related to RFCA are rare but may include problems at the access site, catheter-induced thrombi, and myocardial perforation. The most common complication of AV node–associated dysrhythmias is heart block.

Patients are given anticoagulants up to 4 to 6 hours before the procedure, and anticoagulation is reinitiated after transseptal access is obtained. Intracardiac echo may be used to help guide the placement of the catheter.[30]

Patient teaching is a major focus of nursing intervention for RFCA because preprocedure anxiety is often high (see Patient/Family Teaching box, p. 792). Electrophysiology procedures, both diagnostic and therapeutic, are increasing in number and scope, and nursing research is evolving in this area, with a focus on developing best practice approaches[15] (see Research box).

PACEMAKERS. Pacemakers are typically inserted when patients experience symptomatic chronic or recurrent dysrhythmias that are unresponsive to pharmacologic therapy. Pacemakers may be placed internally for permanent pacing or used externally to address a temporary need. Permanent pacemakers use a pulse generator, powered by a sealed lithium battery, as the "control center" for the pacemaker's functions (Figure 29-44). The generator attaches to one or two leads that are positioned in the right ventricle or right atrium (Figure 29-45). These leads

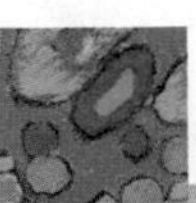

TABLE 29-9
COMMON MEDICATIONS *for Dysrhythmias—cont'd*

Drug	Action	Nursing Intervention
Verapamil—cont'd	Indications: atrial flutter, AF, SVT	May cause hypotension. Direct depressant effect on contractility; use with caution in LV dysfunction.
Adenosine	Depresses SA node and slows conduction through AV node; can interrupt reentry pathways through AV node Indications: SVT	Administer rapid IV push followed by 20 ml flush. Half-life: 10 sec Transient side effects include flushing, labored breathing, chest pain. Effects blocked by methylxanthines and caffeine.
Atropine	Increases heart rate by antagonizing acetylcholine receptors, blocking vagal stimulation, increasing automaticity of SA node and conduction in AV node Indications: symptomatic bradydysrhythmia	Administer intravenously or endotracheally. Increases oxygen demand with increased heart rate.
Calcium chloride	Cation needed for cardiac contractility Indications: asystole	Give slow IV push: extravasation will result in necrosis.
Digoxin	Direct suppression of AV node Indications: AF, atrial flutter, SVT	Check apical pulse for 1 min; if less than 50 beats/min, notify primary care provider. Hypokalemia increases risk of digoxin toxicity. Monitor for therapeutic drug levels. Administer PO or slow IV push. Will increase contractility.
Epinephrine	$Beta_1$ and $beta_2$ agonist increasing automaticity Indications: asystole, refractory VT/VF	Give intravenously or endotracheally. Increases oxygen demand.
Isoproterenol	Causes increased contractility and heart rate by acting on $beta_1$ and $beta_2$ receptors in heart Indications: symptomatic bradydysrhythmias	Give intravenously.
Magnesium sulfate	Reduces SA node impulse formation, prolongs conduction time in myocardium Indications: documented hypomagnesemia with dysrhythmias, torsades de pointes	Monitor magnesium levels.

AF, Atrial flutter; *AV,* atrioventricular; *FDA,* Food and Drug Administration; *IV,* intravenous; *LV,* left ventricular; *PO,* by mouth; *SA,* sinoatrial; *SVT,* supraventricular tachycardia; *VF,* ventricular flutter; *VT,* ventricular tachycardia.

*Use of quinidine, procainamide, and disopyramide is decreasing due to newer, safer, and more efficacious drugs.

†Use of these drugs, including lidocaine (historically a first-line choice for VT), is gradually decreasing in favor of safer, more efficacious antidysrhythmics.

‡These drugs are not recommended for use in patients with coronary artery disease because of increased incidence of mortality and nonfatal cardiac arrest in patients after myocardial infarction.

§Among the most widely used antidysrhythmics.

are flexible, insulated wires with electrodes for sensing the heart's rhythm and delivering electrical impulses when necessary. The leads are introduced into the myocardium transvenously under fluoroscopic visualization through the subclavian or jugular vein with the aid of a guidewire to facilitate correct placement of the leads against the atrial or ventricular endocardium. A subcutaneous pocket is created surgically to enclose the generator, most often infraclavicularly.

The pacemakers in use today have multiple capabilities that can be identified through a five-letter pacemaker code (Table 29-10). The last two letters of the code describe the pacemaker's specific features such as antitachycardic pacing and rate-responsive pacing. When an antitachycardic pacemaker senses a heart rate above its programmed limit, it paces at a heart rate just above the patient's tachycardia to take control of the heart. The pacemaker then slows the rhythm to an acceptable rate. Rate-responsive pacemakers allow pacing at accelerated heart rates when the pacemaker senses programmed indicators of increased activity such as changes in oxygen saturation, cardiac output, or blood temperature.

Pacemaker insertion can be performed with the patient under local anesthesia. Before insertion of a permanent pacemaker, the nurse thoroughly educates the patient about the indications for the pacemaker, the procedure itself, pacemaker care, and potential complications (see the Patient/Family Teaching box, p. 794). Complications of pacemaker therapy include pacemaker malfunction, cardiac perforation and tamponade, pneumothorax and hemothorax, and infection. Nursing responsibilities before and after permanent pacemaker implantation are summarized in the Guidelines for Safe Practice box, p. 794.

Figure 29-46 shows the ECG appearance of pacemaker-stimulated heartbeats. Paced beats are readily identifiable by the sharp spike that precedes the ECG complex. The paced QRS

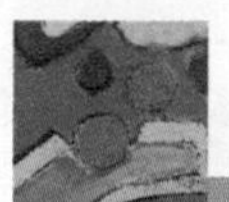

PATIENT/FAMILY TEACHING *The Patient Undergoing Radiofrequency Catheter Ablation*

Preprocedure

Teach patient about:
- Indication for procedure
- Potential complications
- Withholding of antidysrhythmics per physician orders
- Avoiding caffeine and alcohol 24 hours before procedure
- Taking nothing by mouth for 8 hours before the procedure
- Intravenous access for fluids, sedation, and cardiac medications
- Preparation of femoral site and right side of the neck
- Potential for indwelling urinary catheter insertion
- Preprocedure tests: clotting studies, chest x-ray study, baseline electrocardiogram

Intraprocedure

Teach patient to expect:
- Sedation throughout procedure
- Possible discomfort in groin and neck—local anesthetic used
- Cardiac monitor at all times
- Sterile drapes to prevent infection at access sites
- Medications readily available to test effectiveness of procedure or to treat dysrhythmias should they occur

Postprocedure

Teach patient about expected care routines:
- Access sheath pulled immediately after procedure
- Vital signs, access site, and neurovascular checks every 15 minutes for 1 hour, then every 30 minutes until patient is stabilized
- Baseline 12-lead electrocardiogram obtained
- Bed rest—duration dependent on hemostasis and sheaths used; analgesic and backrubs for back pain
- Need to report any pleuritic or chest pain

Discharge Instructions

Teach patient about:
- Likelihood of discharge on same day
- Use of daily aspirin
- Avoiding prolonged sitting for first day
- Avoiding strenuous activity for 72 hours
- Avoiding driving for 24 hours
- Signs and symptoms of infection or complications at access site
- Signs and symptoms of dysrhythmia recurrence

Research

Gianakos S et al: Time in bed after electrophysiologic procedures (TIBS IV): a pilot study, *Am J Crit Care* 13(1):56, 2004.

Nurse researchers challenged the common practice of keeping patients in bed for 4 hours after electrophysiology procedures that used a femoral venous approach. Sixty-eight patients were randomized to 2 hours (n = 31) or 4 hours (n = 37) of bed rest. Patients were similar with regard to age, gender, number of sheaths used, and procedural heparin use. Medications given during the electrophysiology procedure included midazolam and fentanyl for conscious sedation. Postprocedure femoral access site care included a gauze dressing over the catheter insertion site, extension of the affected leg, and elevation of the head of bed 30 to 45 degrees. Sandbags and pressure dressings were not used. Medications for pain management included acetaminophen, 650 mg; or one to two tablets of oxycodone, 5 mg, plus acetaminophen, 325 mg.

The groups had no significant differences with regard to bleeding incidence, hematomas, use of analgesics, or patient satisfaction. This study supported the nurses' belief that bed rest after electrophysiologic studies via a femoral vein approach could safely be reduced to 2 hours. Nurses should continue to challenge existing protocols through research. Time-in-bed studies should increasingly explore patient safety as new devices for closure of arterial and venous punctures are employed.

complex is wide because initiation of the impulse occurs in the ventricle (as with a PVB).

If a pacemaker should malfunction, the patient usually experiences a recurrence of symptoms. However, the nurse must also be able to diagnose the following ECG indicators of pacemaker malfunction: loss of sensing, loss of capture, and failure to pace. Table 29-11, p. 795, describes common pacemaker problems and interventions to troubleshoot them. A Nursing Care Plan for a patient undergoing pacemaker insertion in on pp. 796 and 797.

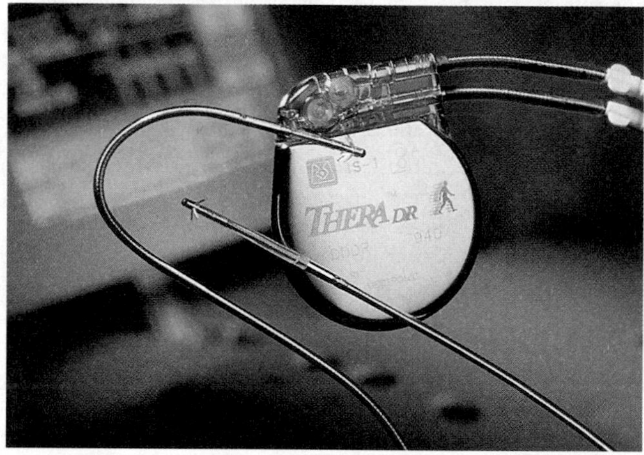

Figure 29-44 Permanent pacemaker (pulse generator) that can be implanted in subcutaneous tissue below patient's clavicle or in abdomen. Pacing wires are then threaded to patient's heart.

Temporary pacemakers are indicated for the short-term management of dysrhythmias until the patient's rhythm stabilizes or a permanent pacemaker can be inserted. The pacer wire is advanced transvenously to the right ventricle, and the leads are attached to an external pulse generator box (Figure 29-47, p. 798). Transvenous pacemakers can include devices that combine pulmonary artery catheters with the pacemaker. The environment must be kept free from electrical hazards that could trigger dysrhythmias. Temporary epicardial pacing is used after cardiac surgery. The epicardial wires are lightly sutured to the right atrium and right ventricle during the surgical procedure, and are brought out through the chest wall and sutured to the skin. When both atrial and

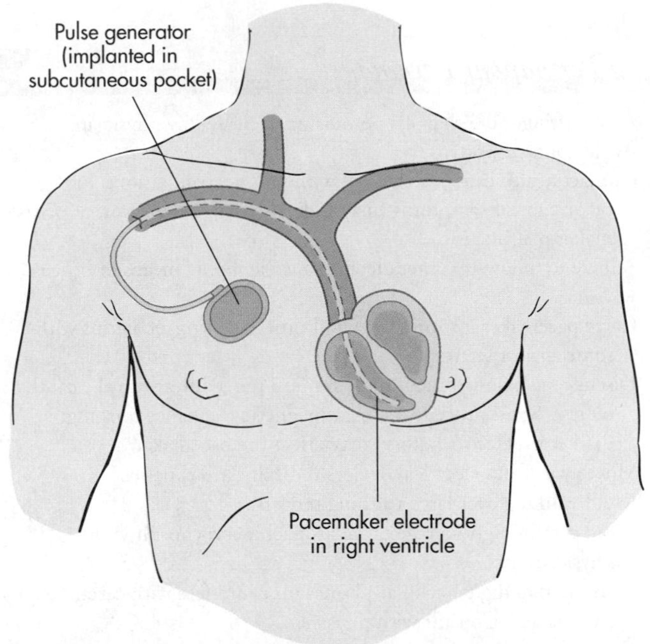

Figure 29-45 Permanent pacemaker placement.

ventricular wires are used, atrial wires exit to the right of the sternum and ventricular wires exit to the left. Care of the patient with a temporary pacemaker is summarized in the Guidelines for Safe Practice box, p. 798.

External cardiac pacemakers are primarily used for patients with unstable rhythms in emergency situations and require the application of two electrodes to the chest wall, one over the cardiac apex and the other on the back beneath the left scapula (Figure 29-48, p. 799). An electrical current flows between the electrodes and is controlled by the device operator. Most external pacing devices function in the demand mode. An oscilloscope allows monitoring of the pacemaker activity. External pacing is uncomfortable for the patient, and the nurse plans for pain management and offers encouragement and support.

Transthoracic pacing uses a transthoracic needle to place electrodes into the ventricle, which are then attached to, and controlled by, an external generator. This procedure is used only in emergency situations where other measures have failed. Transesophageal pacing utilizes a pacing electrode inserted into the lower esophagus via a nasal catheter electrode or gelatin pill electrode. Transesophageal pacing is beneficial for overdrive atrial pacing, that is, pacing the atria at a faster rate to take control and slow the rate. It has been less successful as a route for ventricular pacing.

IMPLANTABLE CARDIOVERTER DEFIBRILLATORS. More than half the deaths from CAD in the United States each year are sudden deaths occurring within 24 hours of the onset of symptoms, commonly before the patient reaches the hospital. The pathophysiology of sudden cardiac death remains obscure, since only 20% of sudden deaths are directly associated with MI. Researchers theorize that the cause of sudden cardiac death is not occlusive thrombosis or myocardial damage but a derangement in the heart's electrical stability, most often deteriorating into VF.[4] The incidence of sudden death is greater in patients with cardiomyopathy, prolonged Q-T intervals, myocarditis, prodysrhythmic medications, and electrolyte imbalance.

The implantable cardioverter-defibrillator (ICD) is indicated for the treatment of clinically significant and hemodynamically important dysrhythmias that do not respond to antidysrhythmic therapy. The ICD consists of a pulse generator and two or three lead systems that continuously monitor heart activity and automatically deliver a

TABLE 29-10 INTERSOCIETY COMMISSION FOR HEART DISEASE CODES FOR PACEMAKERS

Chamber(s) Paced	Chamber(s) Sensed	Modes of Responses (sensing function)	Programmable Functions	Special Tachydysrhythmia Functions
V: ventricle	V: ventricle	T: triggered	P: programmable	B: bursts
A: atrium	A: atrium	I: inhibited (demand)	M: multiprogrammable	N: normal rate competition (dual demand)
D: double (dual)	D: double (dual)	D: double (dual function: T and I)	O: none (permanent pacemakers only)	S: scanning E: external
	O: none	O: none (continuous)		
		R: reverse		

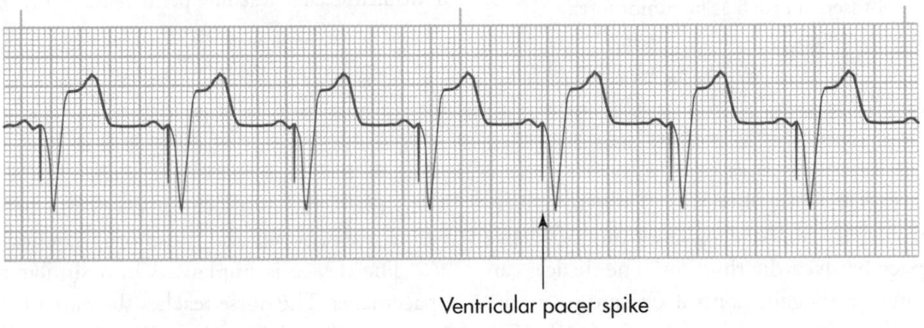

Figure 29-46 Ventricular pacemaker rhythm with pacer spikes.

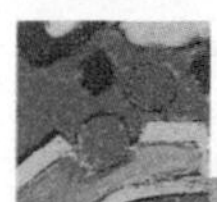

PATIENT/FAMILY TEACHING *The Patient With a Permanent Pacemaker*

Procedural

Teach patient about:
- Indication for pacemaker
- Potential complications
- Nothing by mouth for 8 hours before the procedure
- Pretests, including baseline 12-lead electrocardiogram and bleeding function studies
- Cardiac monitor at all times during the procedure
- Intravenous access for fluids, cardiac medications, and sedation
- Prep and shave of area where generator will be implanted
- Anesthesia of access sites
- Analgesics offered postprocedure
- Restricted movement of affected arm for 24 hours
- Routine chest x-ray to check placement

Discharge Instructions

Teach patient to:
- Monitor site for infection and bleeding the first week.
- Avoid immersion of site in water for 3 days (tub bath OK).
- Leave Steri-Strips in place for about 1 week.
- Limit range of motion of affected arm and wear loose covering over incision for 1 week.
- Avoid lifting more than 10 pounds until cleared by physician.
- Avoid contact sports.
- Contact health care professional with fatigue, palpitations, or recurrence of symptoms (may indicate battery depletion or pacemaker malfunction).
- Adhere to follow-up schedule via transtelephonic means or office visits.
- Carry pacemaker information at all times; can trigger alarms with some airport security.
- Discuss any planned medical or surgical procedures with the cardiologist. Some procedures (e.g., magnetic resonance imaging, diathermy, electrocautery) may affect the pacemaker.
- Move away from electrical devices if dizziness is experienced.
- Avoid working over large running motors.
- Avoid certain high-voltage or radar machinery; consult with physician first.
- Be aware that digital cellular phones may interfere with certain pacemakers. Consult with physician.
- Take radial pulse; notify health care professional for rates outside those programmed (may indicate pacemaker malfunction or battery depletion).

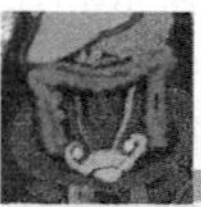

GUIDELINES FOR SAFE PRACTICE *The Patient Undergoing Permanent Pacemaker Insertion*

Preprocedure

- Establish assessment baselines: vital signs, 12-lead electrocardiogram (ECG), peripheral pulses, heart and lung sounds, mental status.
- Teach patient per patient/family education guidelines.
- Maintain nothing-by-mouth status for 8 hours.
- Establish intravenous (IV) access for administration of fluids, sedation, and emergency drugs.
- Assess anxiety level and intervene appropriately with active listening, reassurance, education, and sedation as needed.

Intraprocedure

- Shave and scrub access site.
- Maintain sterile field.
- Cardiac monitor at all times.
- Assess patient's anxiety level and intervene appropriately with reassurance and sedation as needed.

Postprocedure

- Monitor for complications of insertion such as pneumothorax, hemothorax, perforation, tamponade.
- Be alert to lead dislodgement, manifested by ECG changes or hiccups if diaphragm is being paced.
- Control pain: provide analgesics and nonpharmacologic interventions (positioning, distraction) as needed.
- Obtain baseline ECG and monitor for loss of sensing, loss of capture, or failure to pace.
- Assess insertion site for bleeding and infection.
- Ensure bed rest for 12 hours.
- Restrict range of motion of affected arm for 12 to 24 hours.
- Apply ice pack to minimize pain and swelling for first 6 hours.
- Do not administer aspirin or heparin for 48 hours.
- If defibrillation is necessary, anteroposterior placement is preferable; avoid area surrounding generator site.
- If patient is symptomatic from pacer malfunction, enforce bed rest, follow safety precautions for syncope potential, monitor vital signs frequently, and obtain a 12-lead ECG to diagnose malfunction.
    - —Monitor by continuous telemetry, obtain IV access (with atropine at bedside), provide oxygen if needed, perform chest x-ray study to check lead position, and use pacemaker magnet to convert pacemaker to fixed mode if indicated.
- Provide discharge teaching per patient/family teaching guidelines.

countershock to correct a perceived dysrhythmia. The pacemaker-cardioverter-defibrillator models can pace patients out of tachycardic rhythms and can pace bradycardic rhythms. The devices can override the heart's pacemaker to gain control or cardiovert the heart at different energy outputs if overpacing is ineffective. Records of the dysrhythmic event can be retrieved to evaluate the sequence of events and the appropriateness of ICD therapy.

The device is implanted in a similar manner to a permanent pacemaker. The nurse teaches the patient about situations that may cause malfunction of the ICD, such as MRI or diathermy. Special

TABLE 29-11 TROUBLESHOOTING PACEMAKER MALFUNCTION

Problem	Definition	ECG Finding	Physiologic Effect	Nursing Action
Loss of sensing—oversensing	Pacemaker senses extraneous signal as impulse and therefore does not pace.	Pause	Decreased cardiac output	Decrease sensitivity of pacemaker. Check for electromagnetic interference and proper grounding of equipment (temporary pacemaker).
Loss of sensing—undersensing	Pacemaker does not sense heart's own impulse and therefore thinks it has to pace the heart.	Inappropriate pacing (extra beats)	Danger of pacing in vulnerable period, causing ventricular tachycardia	Increase sensitivity to heart's rhythm.
Loss of capture	Pacemaker fires but does not depolarize ventricle.	Spike present but without QRS complex	Decrease in cardiac output	Increase milliamperes (energy delivered); turn to left side (bring lead in better contact with endocardium). Check all connections (temporary pacemaker). Determine cause of ventricle not responding and correct electrolyte abnormality, ischemia, lead dislodgement.
Failure to pace	Electrical impulse never initiated.	Pause without spikes	Decrease in cardiac output	Keep external or temporary pacemaker at bedside. Assess response and treat symptoms until cause determined and corrected (dislodged lead, battery depletion, malfunctioning pulse generator).

ECG, Electrocardiogram.

precautions are also necessary during procedures such as lithotripsy and radiotherapy. Electrical interference may occur with stereo systems, high-powered motors, and arc welders. Emotional support is critical because patients and family members commonly respond to the ICD with anxiety, depression, fear, and anger. The strongest predictor of a poor quality-of-life outcome may be linked with ICD shocks.[22] Phantom shocks, also reported in the literature, can contribute to anxiety and depression after the procedure. Teaching guidelines are included in the Patient/Family Teaching box, p. 799.

PATIENT/FAMILY TEACHING. Patient and family teaching is an integral part of the nursing care for patients experiencing dysrhythmias. Lifestyle modifications may include the elimination of caffeine, alcohol, or other substances believed to contribute to the disorder. Stress reduction measures are often encouraged. The nurse directly addresses the patient's and family's fears and concerns, recognizing the challenges of living with a potentially life-threatening dysrhythmia. The nurse teaches the patient about the specific dysrhythmia, the treatment plan, and the importance of seeking medical attention promptly if symptoms recur. Patients should also know how to take the pulse and the types of pulse changes that need to be reported. The nurse reviews the common side effects of the antidysrhythmic agents with the patient and encourages the patient to discuss the incidence and severity of side effects with a health care professional. Patients are cautioned not to adjust the dose or discontinue the use of any prescribed medication. Follow-up is essential in monitoring medication therapy and response.

Nursing Care Plan

Patient Receiving Permanent Pacemaker

Data A 65-year-old woman is admitted to the cardiac care unit for unstable angina and suspected acute myocardial infarction. Her presenting symptoms are unusual fatigue and indigestion. Her medical history includes type 2 diabetes mellitus of 20 years' duration and hypertension, which has been controlled with medication for the past 7 years. Before a diagnostic cardiac catheterization can be performed, the patient develops symptomatic bradycardia ranging between 40 and 50 beats/min. Electrocardiogram reveals a Mobitz type II second-degree atrioventricular block. Atropine is administered and temporary pacing initiated. Further diagnostic tests indicate that the patient has suffered an acute myocardial infarction. Because of the patient's increased risk for heart failure as a result of bradycardia and the ischemic blood supply to her conduction system, the decision is made to proceed with permanent pacemaker placement. A DDD pacemaker is placed 3 days after her admission to the hospital. Her postoperative course is uncomplicated, and plans are made for her discharge to home. The patient's daughter, who will be caring for her at home, voices concern about what to do should the pacemaker fail.

Nursing Diagnosis

Risk for infection related to surgical implantation of foreign device

Outcomes

- Patient will remain free from signs of wound and systemic infection.
- Patient will accurately demonstrate sterile technique in caring for surgical incision.
- Patient will accurately list symptoms associated with infection.

Related NOC Outcomes

- Immune Status
- Knowledge: Infection Control
- Risk Control

Related NIC Interventions

- Infection Control
- Infection Protection
- Surveillance
- Wound Care

Nursing Interventions/Rationales

- Assess insertion site for signs of localized wound infection (redness, swelling, tenderness, warmth). *To recognize the presence of wound infection so treatment can be initiated and systemic infection prevented.*
- Assess for signs of systemic infection (fever, fatigue, elevated white blood cell count). *To recognize the presence of systemic infection so prompt treatment can be initiated.*
- Teach patient how to maintain sterile technique when changing dressing or cleaning incisional site. *Microorganisms can readily penetrate through nonintact skin such as a surgical incision. Sterile technique reduces the risk of contamination and subsequent wound infection.*
- Teach patient the signs and symptoms of localized and systemic infection. *So the client will recognize impending infection and seek assistance quickly.*
- Encourage patient to avoid handling of or unnecessary contact with surgical site. *To decrease the risk of wound contamination and subsequent wound infection.*
- Encourage a high-protein, high-calorie diet. *Proteins and calories are necessary for wound healing.*

Nursing Diagnosis

Impaired physical mobility related to incisional site pain, activity restrictions, and fear of lead displacement

Outcomes

- Patient will verbalize prescribed restrictions.
- Patient will describe resources to assist with activities of daily living (ADLs) until physical mobility improves.

Related NOC Outcomes

- Adherence Behavior
- Knowledge: Prescribed Activity
- Mobility

Related NIC Interventions

- Pain Management
- Positioning
- Self-Care Assistance
- Teaching: Prescribed Activity/Exercise

▶ ARE You READY?

In emergent treatment for a patient in ventricular fibrillation, the nurse's first action is to:

1. Administer intravenous magnesium sulfate
2. Set-up for placement of transcutaneous pacemaker
3. Prepare the patient for cardioversion
4. Defibrillate the client

Cardiopulmonary Resuscitation

The AHA estimates that 400,000 to 460,000 individuals die of heart disease each year in the emergency room or before they even reach the hospital, often from VF.[4] Sudden death from ischemic heart disease is one of the most serious medical emergencies, and it seems reasonable to assume that many of these deaths might be prevented by prompt and appropriate intervention. Lay rescuers are increasingly being trained to use AEDs, since the time from collapse to defibrillation is the single greatest determinant of survival. Access to AEDs is increasing at sites with concentrated populations (e.g., sporting events, airlines, and shopping malls). AEDs are used only when the patient is unresponsive, has no effective breathing, and has no signs of circulation (cardiopulmonary arrest).

Cardiopulmonary arrest is characterized by the cessation of breathing and circulation and signifies a state of clinical death. It is characterized by unresponsiveness, cessation of respiration, pallor and cyanosis, absence of heart sounds and blood pressure, loss of palpable pulse, and dilation of the pupils. Immediate and definitive action must be instituted within 4 to 6 minutes after the arrest, or biologic death occurs.

Basic life support is an emergency procedure that consists of recognizing an arrest and initiating proper CPR techniques to maintain life until the victim either recovers or is transported to a medical facility where advanced life-support measures are available. The "ABCD" mnemonic of CPR stands for airway, breathing, circulation, and defibrillation or definitive treatment (Table

Nursing Interventions/Rationales

- Provide analgesics before activity while hospitalized. Encourage the patient to self-administer analgesics at home before activities requiring arm movement. *Appropriate timing of pain medication allows the patient to perform ADLs with less pain and more independence. Controlling pain decreases the risk for complications caused by immobility.*
- Explore with the patient activities requiring assistance and community resources to help during times of physical immobility (family, friends, church, neighbors, home health aides). *Encouraging the patient to list activities requiring assistance (meals, shopping, bathing) helps the patient identify the most appropriate community or family resources for her needs.*
- Reinforce the need to limit activities that stress the incision site for 4 weeks (lifting more than 25 pounds or activities that require placing the arms over the head). *Limiting activities that overuse the affected arm will help stabilize the pacemaker until fibrotic tissues forms around the pacemaker and electrodes, decreasing the risk for electrode displacement.*

Nursing Diagnosis

Fear related to lack of knowledge deficit of pacemaker function and care

Outcomes

- Patient and family will report feelings of comfort with functioning of pacemaker.
- Patient will verbalize understanding of symptoms that indicate pacemaker malfunction that need to be reported immediately.
- Patient will accurately demonstrate pulse checks, transtelephonic recording.

Related NOC Outcomes

- Anxiety Self-Control
- Comfort Level
- Coping
- Fear Self-Control

Related NIC Interventions

- Anxiety Reduction
- Coping Enhancement
- Emotional Support
- Teaching: Procedure/Treatment

Nursing Interventions/Rationales

- Provide teaching and information regarding pacemaker function and reliability. *To prevent distortions and correct misconceptions. Misinterpretation can increase fear and anxiety.*
- Teach skills to enhance control: instruct patient how to self-monitor for symptoms of pacemaker malfunction (daily pulse checks, transtelephonic recordings). *Understanding home care (including monitoring for pacemaker malfunction) increases the patient's confidence in her ability to comply with treatment recommendations. Knowing when to worry versus appropriate expectations helps the patient identify areas requiring medical attention or follow-up care.*
- Provide written materials that reinforce teaching. *Written information provides a later resource for information that may have been forgotten or misunderstood.*
- Obtain referral for home health nurse visit at least once before the patient's first follow-up visit with cardiologist to monitor the surgical site, assess knowledge retention, and answer patient questions. *The availability of follow-up care provides positive reinforcement of the patient's actions for self-care and decreases the patient's fears and anxiety.*
- Arrange for the patient to meet with another patient who successfully lives at home independently with a permanent pacemaker. *Learning from the successes of others helps the patient identify misconceptions and areas where assistance may be needed and builds self-confidence in own ability to care for self at home.*

Evaluation

Evaluation is based on comparing the patient's outcomes with desired outcomes.

29-12). Safe implementation of CPR by health care professionals for adult victims involves five steps. The procedure is under continuous review and evaluation and has been updated to simplify CPR training and improve its effectiveness.[4a]

Step 1: Assess Level of Consciousness

Persons who appear to be unconscious may be asleep, deaf, or intoxicated. Unconsciousness is confirmed by shaking the victim's shoulders and shouting, "Are you OK?" If the person does not respond, the emergency response system (911) is activated immediately, an AED is obtained if possible, and the victim is cautiously placed in the supine position on a firm surface, remembering the potential for head injury. The AED is used as soon as it is available for witnessed arrests and in-hospital deaths. If the arrest is the result of asphyxia (e.g., drowning, drug overdose) or if the response time for an out-of-hospital arrest is greater than 5 minutes, CPR is initiated immediately and the AED is used after the first 2-minute cycle.[4a] The emergency response system is also activated at this time.

Step 2: Open the Airway

The tongue is the most common cause of airway obstruction in the unconscious person. The head tilt–chin lift and the jaw thrust are the two recommended methods for opening and maintaining the airway (Figures 29-49 and 29-50). Jaw thrust (without head tilt) is the safest approach to use for a victim with a suspected neck injury but the head tilt–chin lift maneuver is substituted immediately if a jaw thrust does not successfully open the airway. The rescuer must carefully support the head to avoid turning or tilting it backward. While maintaining an open airway, the rescuer takes 3 to 5 seconds to look, listen, and feel for spontaneous breathing. The rescuer places an ear over the victim's nose and mouth while looking at the victim's chest to see if it moves with respiration, listens for air escaping during exhalation, and feels for air movement against the face.

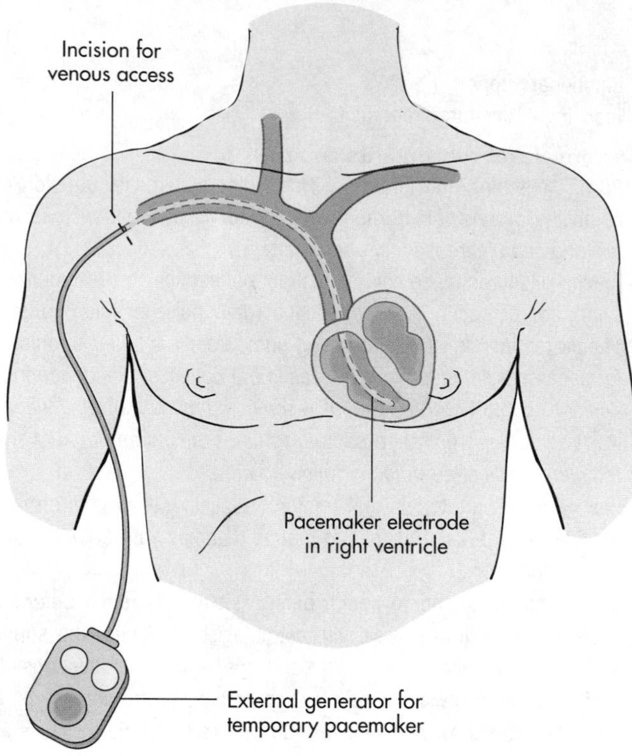

Figure 29-47 Transvenous temporary pacemaker placement.

Step 3: Initiate Artificial Ventilation

Mouth-to-Mouth Ventilation. To initiate artificial ventilation, the rescuer gives two breaths lasting 1 second each, and observes for a visible rise in the chest. Healthcare providers may need to try a couple of times to adequately open the airway and deliver effective breaths. Abdominal thrusts are implemented if a foreign body is obstructing the airway. If the patient does not resume breathing, the rescuer continues mouth-to-mouth ventilation. One breath is delivered every 5 seconds (10–12 breaths per minute) when rescue breathing is performed without chest compressions.

1. Maintain victim in head tilt–chin lift or jaw thrust position.
2. Pinch nostrils.
3. Take a normal breath and place mouth around outside of victim's mouth, forming a tight seal. Use a rescue airway if available.
4. Blow into victim's mouth.
5. Adequate ventilation is demonstrated by:
    a. Rise and fall of chest
    b. Hearing and feeling air escape as victim passively exhales
    c. Feeling the resistance of the victim's lungs expanding

Mouth-to-Nose Ventilation. Mouth-to-nose ventilation is indicated when the mouth is seriously injured or a tight seal cannot be established around the mouth. The rescuer places one hand on the forehead to tilt the head back and uses the other hand to lift the lower jaw and close the mouth. After taking a normal breath, the rescuer seals the mouth around the victim's nose and begins blowing until the lungs expand. Occasionally, when mouth-to-nose ventilation is used, it may become necessary to open the victim's mouth or lips to allow air to escape on exhalation because the soft palate may produce nasopharyngeal obstruction.

Mouth-to-Stoma Ventilation. Direct mouth-to-stoma artificial ventilation is performed for the laryngectomy patient. For the patient with a temporary tracheostomy tube, mouth-to-tube ventilation should be initiated after the cuff is inflated.

Mouth-to-Barrier Ventilation. An alternative to direct mouth-to-mouth ventilation is use of a barrier device such as a face shield and mask device. Most mask devices have a one-way valve so that exhaled air does not enter the rescuer's mouth; many face shields

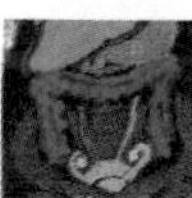

GUIDELINES FOR SAFE PRACTICE *The Patient With a Temporary Pacemaker*

Assess Patient's Tolerance of Heart Rhythm

Perform patient assessment: mental status, blood pressure and rhythm, urinary output, skin color and warmth, pulses, heart sounds, and lung sounds.
Perform continuous electrocardiographic (ECG) monitoring.

Check System for Proper Functioning

Check pacing threshold (the minimum amount of milliamperes needed to pace the heart) every 12 hours; set milliampere level two to three times the threshold as a safety margin; adjust as needed and notify physician.
Replace battery in generator or connecting cable for failure to pace as necessary.
Adjust sensitivity for undersensing or oversensing; notify physician.
Secure all connections; secure generator box to patient (preferably) or bed.

Maintain Electrical Safety

Wires must be connected and secured to the correct connector ports (atrial/ventricular, positive/negative).
Maintain insulation cover over uninsulated ends.
Wear rubber gloves when handling exposed terminals.
Do not touch the patient and electrical equipment at the same time.
Prevent liquids from coming in contact with the generator, cables, or insertion site.
Keep ungrounded electrical equipment from contact with the patient.

Monitor for Complications at Insertion Site

Inspect site daily for infection.
Change dressing every 48 hours using central line dressing sterile technique.

Assess Patient Safety and Comfort

Explain the purpose of the pacemaker to decrease anxiety.
Position patient comfortably, avoiding accidental tension on external wires and generator.
When mobility is limited, help the patient find diversional activities.

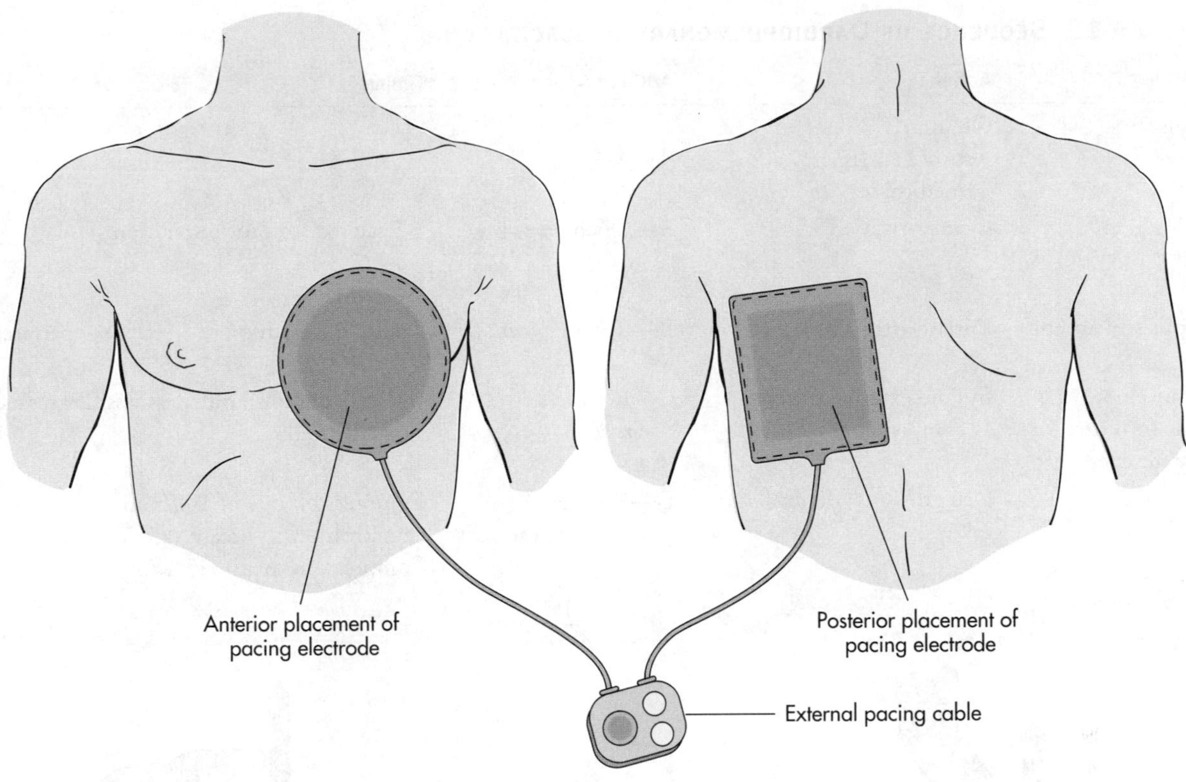

Figure 29-48 Transcutaneous external pacing.

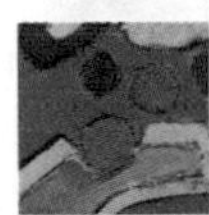

PATIENT/FAMILY TEACHING *The Patient With an Implantable Cardioverter-Defibrillator*

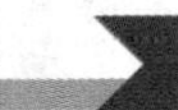

Procedural

Teach patient about:

- Indication for implantable cardioverter-defibrillator (ICD)
- Potential complications
- Nothing by mouth for 8 hours before the procedure
- Pretests, including baseline 12-lead electrocardiogram and bleeding function studies
- Cardiac monitor at all times during the procedure
- Intravenous access for fluids, cardiac medications, and sedation
- Prep and shave of area where generator will be implanted
- Anesthesia of access sites
- Sterile field during procedure
- Analgesics available after procedure
- Restricted arm movement for 24 hours if implant site is infraclavicular
- Routine chest x-ray to check placement

Discharge Instructions

Insertion Site

Teach patient to:

- Monitor site for infection and bleeding the first week.
- Avoid immersion of site in water for 3 days.
- Remove Steri-Strips in about 1 week.
- Wear loose covering over incision for 1 week.

Activity

Teach patient to:

- Avoid contact sports and ham radios.
- Increase activity gradually after implantation of device (should be at full preimplant activity level once incision has healed).
- Follow driving restrictions and dicuss concerns with cardiologist.
- Seek guidance from cardiologist about: flying, excessive heights, industrial facilities, welding
- Avoid swimming or boating alone.

Health Care Follow-up

Teach patient to:

- Adhere to schedule for important follow-up care.
- Sit or lie down if signs or symptoms of decreasing cardiac output with dysrhythmia occur.
- Notify health care professional for:
  - —Signs or symptoms of dysrhythmia similar to those before ICD
  - —Rapid, irregular heart rate
  - —Chest pain or shortness of breath

Safety

Teach patient to:

- Carry ICD information at all times—will alarm some airport security.
- Consult with cardiologist before undergoing diagnostic or surgical interventions.
- Move away from devices if dizziness experienced.
- Avoid working over large, running motors.
- Learn how to take radial pulse; notify health care professional for rates outside those programmed.

NOTE: Patient and others in physical contact with patient will experience a mild sensation with shock delivery.

TABLE 29-12 SEQUENCE OF CARDIOPULMONARY RESUSCITATION

Findings	Action	ABCs of Action	Timing
No response	Obtain AED Activate emergency medical services		
Absence of respirations; cyanosis, dilated pupils	Open airway	A—Open *airway*	3-5 sec to assess for respiration
Respirations still absent	Initiate artificial ventilation	B—Restore *breathing*	Deliver 1 breath every 5 sec, 2 sec per breath (12/min)
Carotid pulse not palpable (omitted with lay rescuers)	Initiate external cardiac compressions	C—Restore *circulation*	10 sec to establish pulselessness (lay rescuers omit)
ECG: ventricular fibrillation	Drug therapy; defibrillation	D—Provide *definitive* treatment	Compression rate of 100/min Compression-to-breath ratio of 30:2 Compression depth 1.5-2 in

ECG, Electrocardiogram.

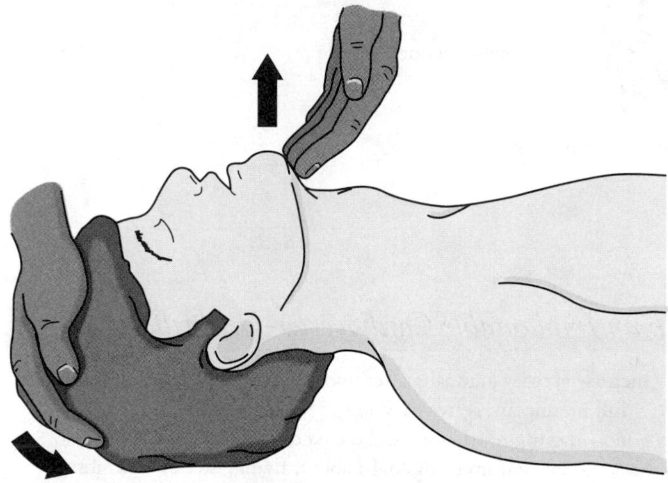

Figure 29-49 Head tilt–chin lift maneuver for opening airway. Place one hand on forehead and place tips of fingers of other hand under lower jaw near chin. Bring chin forward while pressing forehead down.

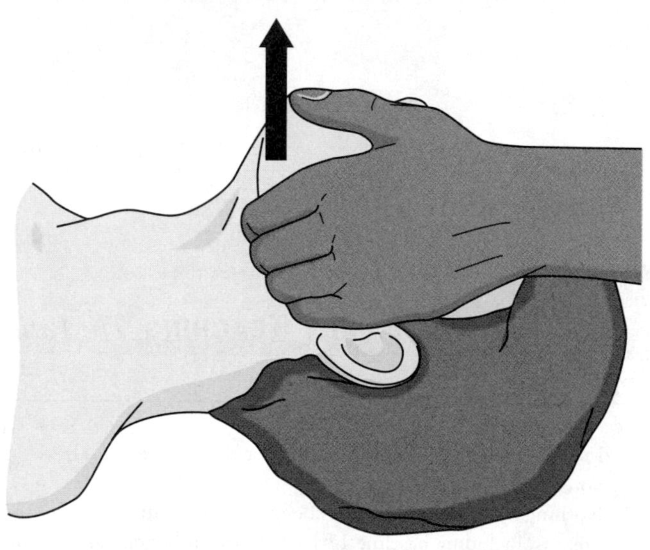

Figure 29-50 Jaw thrust maneuver for opening airway.

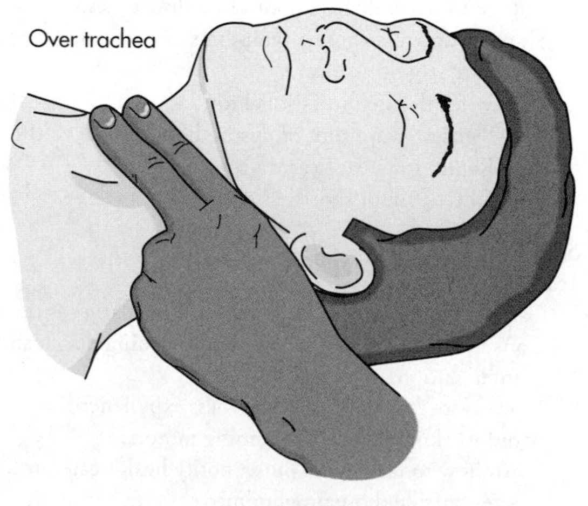

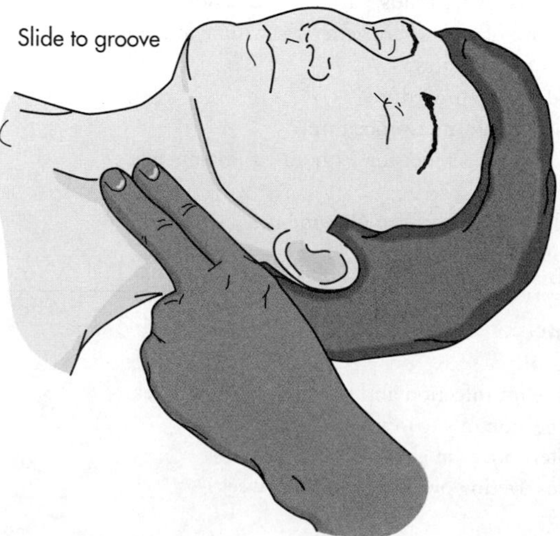

Figure 29-51 Locating carotid artery.

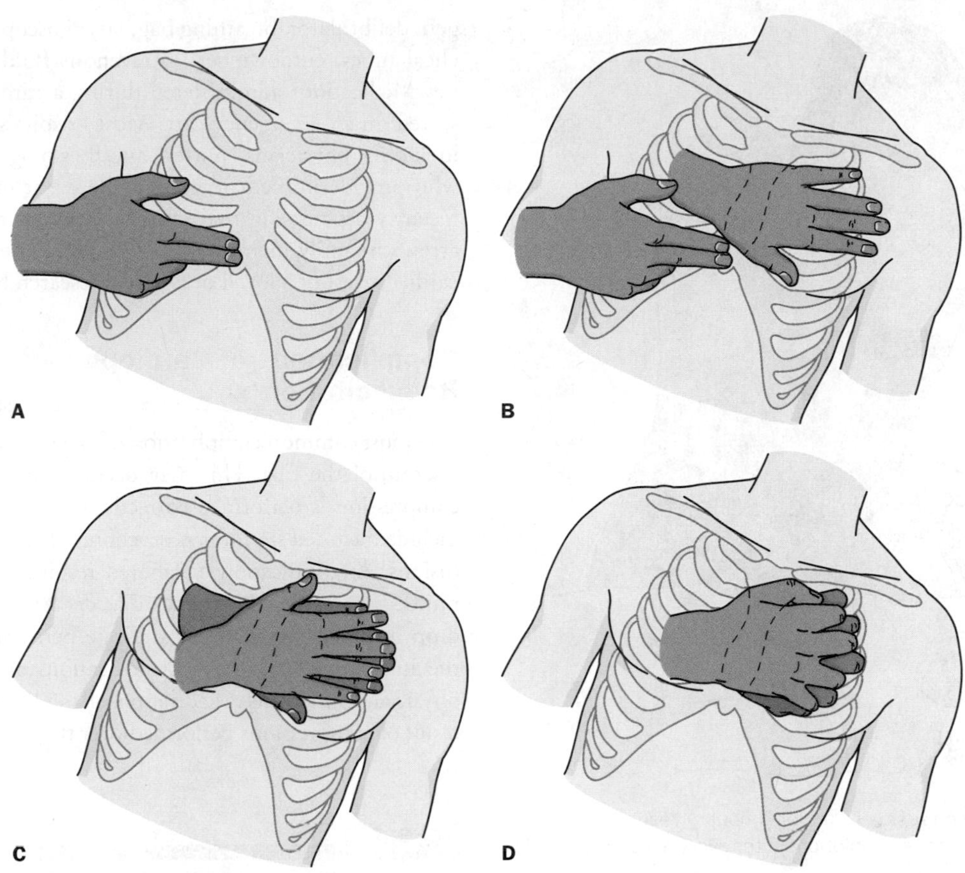

Figure 29-52 Positioning of hands on sternum in external cardiac compression. **A,** Middle finger locates xiphoid process; index finger is positioned next to middle finger. **B,** Heel of opposite hand is placed on sternum next to index finger. **C,** First hand is removed from landmark position and placed on top of other hand so that heels of both hands are parallel and fingers point away. **D,** Fingers may be interlocked to avoid pressure on ribs.

have no exhalation valves, which cause air leakage around the shield. The barrier device (face mask or face shield) is positioned over the victim's mouth and nose, ensuring an adequate air seal.

Step 4: Assess Circulation

The rescuer palpates the carotid pulse to determine whether cardiac compression is needed. The carotid pulse is located by finding the larynx and sliding the fingers laterally into the groove between the trachea and the sternocleidomastoid muscle (Figure 29-51). Other signs of circulation might include movement or coughing. If the carotid pulse is not palpable in approximately 10 seconds, the rescuer initiates cardiac compressions. The carotid pulse is palpated because it is accessible and the carotid arteries are central. Sometimes these pulses persist when more peripheral pulses are no longer palpable. If the pulse is absent, cardiac arrest is confirmed and external chest compression is initiated. Lay rescuers are no longer being taught to check for a pulse because their accuracy in pulse assessment is only about 65%.

Step 5: Initiate External Cardiac Compression

External cardiac compression (sometimes called external cardiac massage) is the rhythmic compression of the heart between the lower half of the sternum and the thoracic vertebra. This intermittent pressure compresses the heart, raises intrathoracic pressure, and produces an artificial pulsatile circulation. Correctly performed cardiac compressions can produce a peak systolic blood pressure of more than 100 mm Hg. The diastolic pressure is close to 0 mm Hg, however, and the mean blood pressure in the carotid arteries is approximately 40 mm Hg, or about one-fourth normal. The technique for performing external cardiac compression is as follows:

1. Take a position close to the victim's side. Using the middle finger of one hand, locate the xiphoid process (Figure 29-52, *A*). Place the index finger of the same hand on the sternum directly next to the middle finger. Using the index finger as a landmark, place the heel of the opposite hand on the sternum in the center of the chest between the nipples next to the index finger (Figure 29-52, *B*). Then place the first hand on top of the hand on the sternum (Figure 29-52, *C*). Fingers may be interlocked to avoid pressure on the patient's ribs (Figure 29-52, *D*). Positioning near the victim's shoulders facilitates smooth transitions from chest compressions to rescue breathing.
2. To perform effective external cardiac compression, take a position directly over the victim's shoulders, keeping the elbows locked in a straight position, and depress the lower sternum $1\frac{1}{2}$ to 2 inches pushing hard and fast. The compressions are regular, smooth, and uninterrupted. After each compression, release the pressure completely to allow the

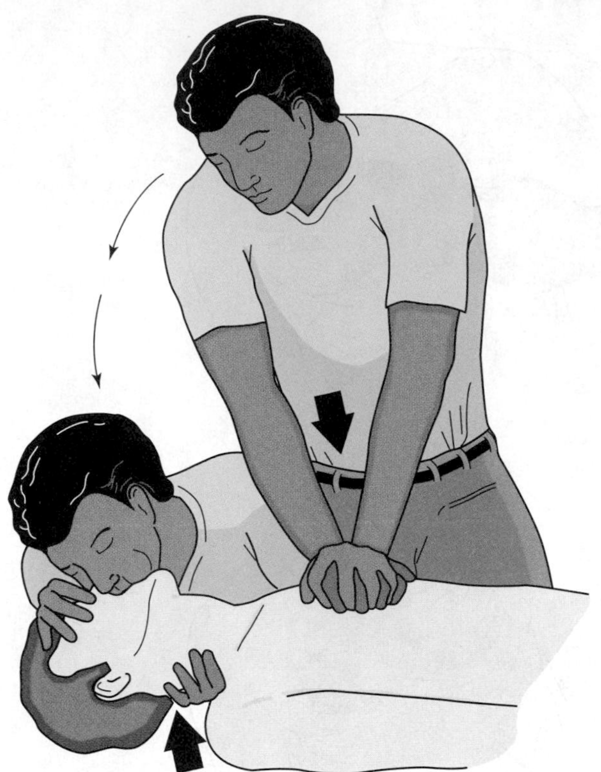

Figure 29-53 One-person rescuer cardiopulmonary resuscitation. Rescuer delivers two effective ventilations after every 15 compressions.

heart to refill. Establish a compression rate of 100/min with a ratio of compressions to breaths of 30:2. Deliver two full breaths after every 30 compressions (Figure 29-53).

3. When two rescuers are available to administer CPR, one rescuer is positioned at the victim's side and performs external cardiac compression while the second rescuer remains at the victim's head to perform artificial ventilation. The cardiac compression rate of 100 per minute and the compression to ventilation rate of 30:2 remains the same. Compressions are paused to allow for a full breath to be delivered. Rescuers should rotate the compressor role approximately every 2 minutes.
4. After the first minute of CPR, again palpate the carotid pulse to assess the effectiveness of CPR and to check for the return of spontaneous circulation. If two rescuers are performing CPR, the person ventilating the victim also assesses pulses and monitors for the return of spontaneous breathing. Continue to perform CPR until one of the following takes place:
   a. Spontaneous circulation and ventilation return.
   b. Another rescuer takes over basic life support.
   c. The victim is transported to an emergency facility.
   d. The victim is pronounced dead by a physician.
   e. The rescuer is exhausted and unable to continue.

Advanced Cardiac Life Support

The AHA regularly reviews and updates algorithms for advanced life support. The AHA website (www.americanheart.org) provides the most current practice guidelines and information about training sessions for beginning and advanced cardiac life support. Equipment needs include an ECG machine, suction device, oxygen, defibrillator, breathing bag, laryngoscope, variety of endotracheal tubes, cutdown set, intravenous fluids, and tracheostomy set. Medications administered during a cardiac arrest are usually stored on an emergency cart. Most hospitals have trained teams, including physicians, nurses, anesthesiologists, and technicians, who provide immediate care in the event of a cardiac arrest. In recent years nursing research has explored the effects of cardiac arrest on family members, including the effects of witnessing the cardiac arrest of a loved one[29] (see Research box).

Complications of Cardiopulmonary Resuscitation

The most common complication of external cardiac compression is fracture of the ribs. This may occur even when external cardiac compression is performed correctly. Other possible complications include fractured sternum, costochondral separation, and lung contusions. Any indication of labored respiration, paradoxical pulse, muffled heart sounds, tachycardia, decreased breath sounds, or a drop in blood pressure may indicate pericardial tamponade from the injection of intracardiac medications and is reported to the physician immediately. Laceration of the liver also may occur as a result of compressions performed over the xiphoid process.

Research

Wagner JM: Lived experience of critically ill patients' family members during cardiopulmonary resuscitation, *Am J Crit Care* 13(5):416, 2004.

The presence of family members during cardiopulmonary resuscitation (CPR) is now a focus of nursing research. Using a qualitative design, Wagner interviewed six family members who were present at the onset of CPR in the coronary care unit at one 700-bed urban community hospital. Interviews were conducted within 24 hours of the event. Open-ended questions addressed where the family was at the time of the event, feelings and emotions experienced, support during the event, and communication with the health care team during the event. The overall theme from the research was: "Should we go or should we stay?" In the throes of CPR, two subthemes emerged: "What is going on?" and "You do your job." At this point, family members negotiated to stay in the room or acquiesced to the request that they leave. Family members wanted information and expected answers, yet trusted the health care team to do their job. After the crisis, family members moved into a phase Wagner calls "breaking the rules." During this time family members increased their vigilance regarding their loved ones. Formal and informal permission of the health care workers allowed a renegotiation of visiting hours and family presence, but only after the patient's condition was fully stabilized.

Wagner concluded that the health care team takes control during CPR simply by determining whether family members are allowed to stay during CPR. This health care team control leads to the sense of a loss of autonomy by families who seek to be with their critically ill family member. Control by the health care team denies the family the opportunity to be vigilant, a need expressed by families after observing CPR. A lack of communication during resuscitation intensifies this loss of autonomy. Wagner suggests that further study of family members' perceptions during CPR needs to occur, including the study of a liaison role between family members and the health care team during CPR.

Preparing for Practice

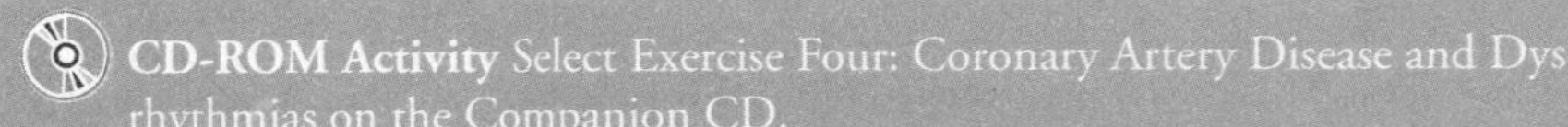

CD-ROM Activity Select Exercise Four: Coronary Artery Disease and Dysrhythmias on the Companion CD.

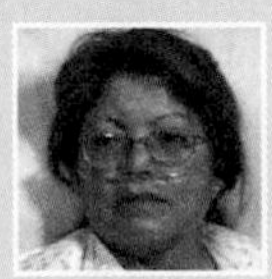

Patient: *Sally Begay,* **Room 304**

Sally Begay, a 58-year-old Navajo woman, was admitted with a rule out diagnosis of Hantavirus that was subsequently determined to be pneumonia. Ms. Begay has a history of hypertension, coronary disease, and myocardial infarction (MI).

Assessment

View the patient's **Report.**
Review the patient's **Medical Record;** examine the History & Physical report in detail.
Conduct a **Patient Interview**. As you conduct your interview, focus primarily on data that will be helpful in planning care for this patient. Record the data you collect.

Nursing Diagnoses, Outcomes, and Interventions

1. When obtaining a health history to determine cardiac disease, identify and describe six important clinical manifestations to inquire about. *Hint:* Use information on p. 752 if needed.
2. Sally Begay is a woman of the Navajo Indian tribe. What role does race play in the development of coronary artery disease?
3. The medical record indicates that Ms. Begay is experiencing chest pain. How might you differentiate chest pain of cardiac origin from the chest pain she is experiencing because of pneumonia?
4. Sally Begay's significant medical history lists "MI five years ago, mild CHF, and stable angina" in the section on heart disease in the History & Physical. What is angina?
5. Describe what occurs during an episode of angina. *Hint:* Refer to pp. 748 and 749.
6. According to Sally Begay's history, where is her pain localized, and what causes her to experience most of her chest pain?
7. Formulate a plan of care that reflects your knowledge of the factors that could provoke Ms. Begay's angina during this admission. Identify nursing interventions that address those factors. *Hint:* Refer to p. 749 for a discussion of increased myocardial oxygen demands.
8. Sally Begay had an MI 5 years ago. What is an MI, and what happens during the process?

Critical Thinking

1. A 49-year-old man is admitted to the emergency department to rule out MI. His chest pain began at an intensity of 3 out of 10 at 7:45 AM on his drive to work. He reported that he had to make a presentation for which he did not feel prepared and had gotten little rest the night before. At work, he drank some coffee and took ibuprofen for the pain. He tried to give the ibuprofen time to work, but the unrelenting pain finally caused him to confide in a co-worker around 9 AM. He asked his co-worker if he thought Maalox or "something else" might get rid of the pain. It took an additional 30 minutes before he decided to go to the emergency department. He tried to "tough it out" with pain rated at 8 out of 10. On arrival in the ED at 10:30 AM, his pain had reached 10/10, radiated to his left arm and up into his jaw. It was described as "gnawing and unrelenting."
   a. What diagnostic tests will be done in the emergency department to rule out MI? What is being looked for on these diagnostic tests to confirm or rule out MI?
   b. What collaborative interventions are indicated for patients experiencing MI and being screened for reperfusion therapy? Consider the eligibility requirements for both thrombolytic therapy and primary PCIs.
   c. The patient receives a stent of the right coronary artery. How will you explain the procedure to his wife? What will you teach her regarding his postprocedure care?
   d. The patient is to be discharged today after successful stenting. He lives with his wife of 22 years, a 17-year-old son, and a 13-year-old daughter. He works in middle management at a local company that has been downsizing. His wife is a physical therapist at a long-term nursing facility. Their home is two stories and has all modern conveniences. He and his family attend church weekly and are involved in various activities. A cholesterol screen done on admission showed a total cholesterol of 202. He does not routinely take any medications. He smokes one half to one pack of cigarettes a day, but only at the office. He smoked a pack and a half a day until 5 years ago. He does not use alcohol. As the nurse responsible for his discharge *today,* develop a comprehensive teaching plan based on what you would *expect* the medical orders to be for this patient. Consider diet, medications, activity, and risk factor modification.
2. The rhythm strip illustrates which of the following rhythms?
   a. Sinus tachycardia
   b. Atrial tachycardia
   c. Ventricular tachycardia

Discuss possible causes of this rhythm and its treatment.

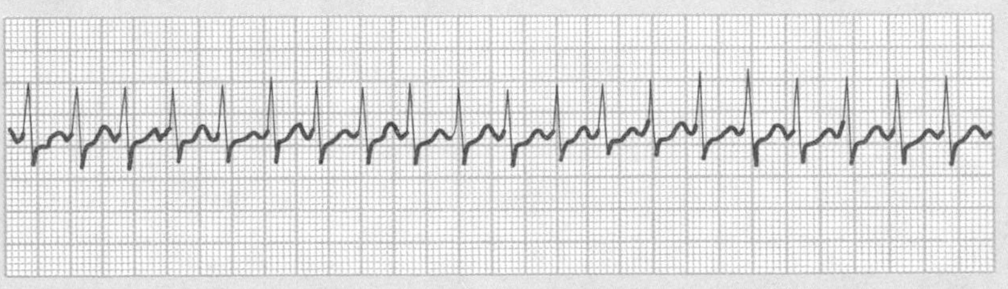

References

1. Adams-Hamoda MG et al: Factors to consider when analyzing 12-lead electrocardiograms for evidence of acute myocardial ischemia, *AJCC* 12(1): 9-16, 2003.
2. Aldana SG et al: Cardiovascular risk reductions associated with aggressive lifestyle modification and cardiac rehabilitation, *Heart and Lung* 32(6): 374-382, 2003.
3. American College of Cardiology, American Heart Association: ACC/AHA/ESC guidelines for the management of patients with atrial fibrillation: executive summary: a report of the American College of Cardiology/American Heart Association Task Force on Practice Guidelines and the European Society of Cardiology Committee for Practice Guidelines and Policy Conferences (Committee to Develop Guidelines for the Management of Patients With Atrial Fibrillation), *Circulation* 104(17):2118-2150, 2001.
4. American Heart Association: *Heart disease and stroke statistics—2004 update,* Dallas, 2003, The Association.

4a. American Heart Association: 2005 American Heart Association guidelines for cardiopulmonary resuscitation and emergency cardiovascular care. *Circulation* 112(suppl I):iv-1-iv-5, 2005.

5. Antman EM et al: ACC/AHA guidelines for the management of patients with ST-elevation myocardial infarction: executive summary: a report of the American College of Cardiology/American Heart Association Task Force on Practice Guidelines (Committee to Revise the 1999 Guidelines on the Management of Patients With Acute Myocardial Infarction), *J Am College Cardiol* 44(3):671-719, 2004.
6. Braunwald E et al: ACC/AHA 2002 guideline update for the management of patients with unstable angina and non–ST-segment elevation myocardial infarction: summary article: a report of the American College of Cardiology/American Heart Association Task Force on Practice Guidelines (Committee on the Management of Patients With Unstable Angina), *Circulation* 106(14):1893-1900, 2002.
7. Centers for Disease Control and Prevention: Annual smoking-attributable mortality, years of potential life lost, and economic costs—United States, 1995-1999, *Morbid Mortal Weekly Rep* 51(14):300-303, 2002.
8. Centers for Disease Control and Prevention: *National diabetes fact sheet: general information and national estimates on diabetes in the United States, 2002,* Atlanta, 2003, US Department of Health and Human Services.
9. Centers for Disease Control and Prevention: Prevalence of physical activity, including lifestyle activities among adults—United States, 2000-2001, *Morbid Mortal Weekly Rep* 52(32):764-769, 2003.
10. Cherrington CC et al: Illness representation after acute myocardial infarction: impact on in-hospital recovery, *Am J Crit Care* 13(2):136-145, 2004.
11. Chyun DA et al: Coronary heart disease prevention and lifestyle interventions: cultural influences, *J Cardiovasc Nurs* 18(4):302-318, 2003.
12. Eagle KA et al: ACC/AHA 2004 guideline update for coronary artery bypass graft surgery: summary article: a report of the American College of Cardiology/American Heart Association Task Force on Practice Guidelines (Committee to Update the 1999 Guidelines on Coronary Artery Bypass Graft Surgery), *J Am College Cardiol* 44(5):1146-1154, e213-310, 2004.
13. Franklin BA, Swain DP, Shephard RJ: New insights in the prescription of exercise for coronary patients, *J Cardiovasc Nurs* 18(2):116-123, 2003.
14. Geleijnse JM et al: Inverse association of tea and flavonoid intakes with incident myocardial infarction: the Rotterdam Study, *Am J Clin Nutr* 75(5): 880-886, 2002.
15. Gianakos S et al: Time in bed after electrophysiologic procedures (TIBS IV): a pilot study, *Am J Crit Care* 13(1):56-58, 2004.
16. Gibbons RJ et al: ACC/AHA 2002 guideline update for the management of patients with chronic stable angina: summary article: a report of the American College of Cardiology/American Heart Association Task Force on Practice Guidelines (Committee on the Management of Patients With Chronic Stable Angina), *Circulation* 107(1):149–158, 2003.
17. Grundy SM et al: Implications of recent clinical trials for the National Cholesterol Education Program Adult Treatment Panel III Guidelines, *J Am College Cardiol* 44(3):720-732, 2004.
18. Malinow MR, Bostom AG, Krauss RM: Homocyst(e)ine, diet, and cardiovascular diseases: a statement for healthcare professionals from the Nutrition Committee, American Heart Association, *Circulation* 99(1):178-182, 1999.
19. Pearson TA et al: AHA guidelines for primary prevention of cardiovascular disease and stroke: 2002 update: consensus panel guide to comprehensive risk reduction for adult patients without coronary or other atherosclerotic vascular diseases, *Circulation* 106(3):388–391, 2002.
20. Pearson TA et al: Markers of inflammation and cardiovascular disease: application to clinical and public health practice: a statement for healthcare professionals from association, *Circulation* 107(3):499-511, 2003.
21. Pelter MM, Adams MG, Drew BJ: Transient myocardial ischemia is an independent predictor of adverse in-hospital outcomes in patients with acute coronary syndromes treated in the telemetry unit, *Heart and Lung* 32(2): 71-78, 2003.
22. Prudente LA: Phantom shock in a patient with an implantable cardioverter defibrillator: case report, *Am J Crit Care* 12(2):144-146, 2003.
23. Radiant Medical Clinical Trials: *COOLing for myocardial infarction (COOL MI),* accessed Dec 2004 from website: http://radiantmedical.com/clinical/clinical_trials.htm.
24. Thompson EJ, King SL: Acetylcysteine and fenoldapam: promising new approaches for preventing effects of contrast nephrotoxicity, *Crit Care Nurse* 23(3):39-46, 2003.
25. US Department of Health and Human Services: *Physical activity and health: a report of the surgeon general,* Washington, DC, 1996, The Department.
26. US Department of Health and Human Services: *Healthy people 2010: understanding and improving health,* Washington, DC, 2000, The Department.
27. US Department of Health and Human Services: *National cholesterol education program: third report of the Expert Panel on Detection, Evaluation, and Treatment of High Blood Cholesterol in Adults (Adult Treatment Panel III),* NIH Pub No 01-3305, Washington, DC, 2001, The Department.
28. US Department of Health and Human Services: *The seventh report of the Joint National Committee on Prevention, Detection, Evaluation, and Treatment of High Blood Pressure,* NIH Pub No 04-5230, Washington, DC, 2004, The Department.
29. Wagner JM: Lived experience of critically ill patients' family members during cardiopulmonary resuscitation, *Am J Crit Care* 13(5):416-420, 2004.
30. Weiss EM, Buescher T: Atrial fibrillation: treatment options and caveats, *AACN Clinical Issues* 15(3):362-376, 2004.
31. Williams MA et al: Secondary prevention of coronary heart disease in the elderly (with emphasis on patients ≥75 years of age): an American Heart Association scientific statement from the Council on Clinical Cardiology Subcommittee on Exercise, Cardiac Rehabilitation, and Prevention, *Circulation* 105(14):1735-1743, 2002.

Visit the Evolve website: http://evolve.elsevier.com/Monahan/medsurg

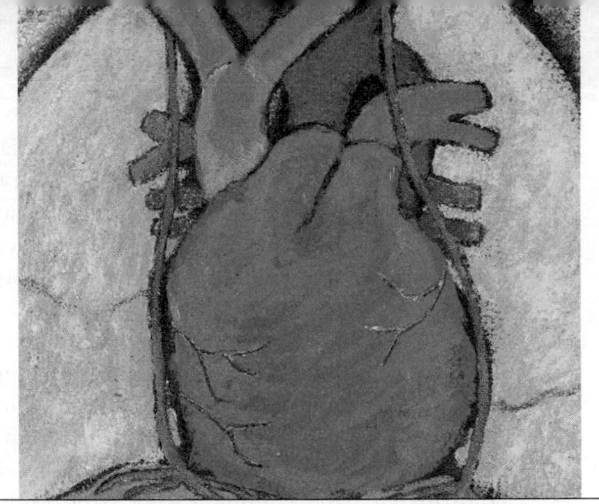

CHAPTER 30

Heart Failure, Valvular Problems, and Inflammatory Problems of the Heart

by Kathy Henley Haugh, Kathryn B. Reid

OBJECTIVES

After studying this chapter, the learner should be able to:

1. Discuss the collaborative management of patients with heart failure, pericarditis, endocarditis, and myocarditis.
2. Explain the pathophysiology that produces the clinical manifestations associated with heart failure.
3. Develop a care plan for the patient with progressive heart failure.
4. Differentiate between the various forms of cardiac valve problems in terms of etiology, impact on the heart's function, clinical manifestations, and treatment.
5. Identify at least three important aspects of patient and family education for patients with cardiac valve disorders.
6. Describe six indications for cardiac surgery.
7. Discuss the nursing management of patients after heart surgery.

KEY TERMS

annuloplasty, p. 842
cardiac tamponade, p. 806
cardiomyopathy, p. 829
cold cardioplegia, p. 841
commissurotomy, p. 842
contractility, p. 809
heart failure, p. 809
infective endocarditis, p. 806
intraaortic balloon pump, p. 822
mediastinitis, p. 846
mitral valve prolapse, p. 836
orthopnea, p. 814
paroxysmal nocturnal dyspnea, p. 814
pericarditis, p. 805
regurgitation, p. 831
remodeling, p. 810
stenosis, p. 831
valvuloplasty, p. 842
ventricular assist device, p. 822

Heart disease can be divided into two general types: congenital and acquired. Congenital heart disease is caused by some error in the embryologic development of the heart's structures. Acquired heart disease results from inflammation, infection, chemical agents, or a diminished blood supply, and its onset may be sudden or gradual. Heart disease can also be classified according to its specific etiologic agent (e.g., rheumatic fever, infective endocarditis, valvular scarring). Any of these problems can eventually lead to cardiac failure.

Inflammatory Heart Disease

Pericarditis

Etiology and Epidemiology. **Pericarditis** is an inflammatory process of the visceral or parietal pericardium. It can be acute or chronic and can spread from or to the myocardium. Pericarditis can develop as a bacterial, viral, or fungal infection. It may also occur as a complication of systemic disease processes such as rheumatoid arthritis, systemic lupus erythematosus, malignancy, uremia, or as a complication of myocardial infarction (Dressler's syndrome). Pericarditis also occurs secondary to trauma or interventions such as cardiac surgery (postpericardiotomy syndrome), radiation, or chemotherapy. Myopericarditis has been reported after smallpox vaccination in some individuals.

Pathophysiology. In acute pericarditis the membranes surrounding the heart become inflamed and rub against each other, producing the classic pericardial friction rub. The friction rub sounds scratchy and harsh on auscultation and persists throughout both systole and diastole. It is best heard at the end of expiration with the patient leaning forward. The patient complains of severe precordial chest pain, which may closely resemble that of acute myocardial infarction. The pain intensifies when the person is lying supine and decreases in a sitting position. The pain also may intensify when the patient breathes deeply. The pain of pericarditis often radiates to the trapezius muscle.

Fever typically occurs, accompanied by leukocytosis and a rise in the erythrocyte sedimentation rate (ESR). Malaise, myalgias, and tachycardia are common. The onset of bacterial pericarditis is associated with high fevers, shaking chills, and night sweats. The electrocardiogram (ECG) shows P-R depression and upward concave

ST elevation. These changes reflect pericardial inflammation over the entire surface of the heart. When ST elevation is present, plasma troponin I also may be elevated. Computed tomography (CT), magnetic resonance imaging (MRI), and echocardiography (transthoracic or transesophageal) are useful tools for diagnosing complications, such as effusion and constriction. Thickening and calcification of the pericardium, which can be seen on echocardiography, occur more commonly with bacterial or fungal pericarditis.

The acute inflammation causes an accumulation of fluid within the pericardial sac called a pericardial effusion. The fluid may be serous, purulent, or hemorrhagic. Serous effusions usually accompany viral and immunoreactive pericarditis; purulent effusions indicate bacterial disorders. Hemorrhagic effusions usually occur from tuberculosis, trauma, and malignancies.[43] An echocardiogram provides the most definitive diagnosis of the effusion. The ECG may exhibit low-voltage QRS complexes. When fluid accumulation is gradual, the patient may not develop symptoms until as much as 1 L of clear or serosanguinous fluid is present. Excessive fluid in the pericardial sac can cause compression of the heart **(cardiac tamponade)**, which decreases venous return to the heart, resulting in decreased ventricular filling and ultimately decreased stroke volume. These events can rapidly lead to cardiac failure, shock, and death. The three classic symptoms of tamponade, referred to as Beck's triad, are hypotension, jugular venous distention, and muffled heart sounds. Additional signs include tachycardia, pulsus paradoxus, and a narrowed pulse pressure.

Chronic pericarditis can also occur. Adhesive pericarditis occurs when the pericardial layers adhere to each other, restricting movement of the heart. Chronic constrictive pericarditis results from fibrosis of the pericardial sac that can develop secondary to surgery, uremia, or radiation. The thick, fibrous pericardium tightens around the heart, decreasing cardiac filling and output. Patients exhibit symptoms of heart failure from the heart's diminished ability to pump.

Collaborative Care Management. Treatment is specific to the underlying cause of the pericarditis. It is critical to differentiate the pain of pericarditis from that of myocardial infarction, since thrombolytic administration in the presence of pericardial effusion may result in hemorrhage. In uncomplicated cases, therapy is primarily supportive and includes administration of nonsteroidal antiinflammatory drugs (NSAIDs), including ibuprofen or indomethacin. Colchicine or corticosteroids may be prescribed if the inflammation is refractory to nonsteroidal agents. The pericarditis can recur after the antiinflammatory drug therapy is completed; colchicine is the drug of choice for recurrent pericarditis.

A pericardiocentesis (pericardial tap) may be performed to remove excess fluid from large effusions and to obtain fluid for diagnostic evaluation. Recurrent effusions may be treated with percutaneous alternatives, such as balloon pericardial windows or instillation of sclerosing agents. Surgery may also be used to treat recurrent effusions, to provide for continuous drainage of pericardial fluid when necessary, and to obtain a biopsy. Procedures may include a subxiphoid approach or subdiaphragmatic laparoscopic, video-assisted thoracoscopic, and flexible pericardioscopic techniques.[43] Complications include atelectasis and infection. The nurse monitors the amount and quality of the drainage and reports increases or changes to the physician.

Chronic constrictive pericarditis, defined as chronic fibrous thickening of the pericardial sac, is most often associated with tuberculosis, cardiac surgery, and radiation. The rigid pericardium interferes with normal diastolic filling, and the patient manifests signs and symptoms of right-sided heart failure (see p. 814). Pericardial thickening and myocardial tethering can be seen on echocardiography. Doppler echocardiography, CT, and MRI studies provide additional details. Diuretics may be tried initially to draw fluids from around the pericardium; however, removal of the pericardium (pericardiectomy) is the definitive treatment to restore cardiac function. Postoperative care is similar to that for other open cardiac surgeries (see p. 848). Treatment may also include medications to restore the heart's pumping efficiency.

With both acute and chronic pericarditis, the nurse monitors the patient's vital signs and heart sounds for changes that might indicate cardiac tamponade. Analgesics are used as needed to control pain and facilitate lung expansion. Antiinflammatory medications and comfort measures are used to treat fever and general malaise. Nursing interventions include encouraging adequate fluid intake, spacing activities to allow rest periods, and using distraction or other nonpharmacologic methods to manage discomfort.

PATIENT/FAMILY TEACHING. The nurse teaches the patient and family about the nature of the disease and the purpose and correct use of all medications, including the management of side effects. The nurse teaches the patient measures to decrease fatigue and provides information on how to minimize the risks of complications. The nurse emphasizes that any return of symptoms could indicate recurrence of the pericarditis and needs to be promptly reported to the primary care provider.

Infective Endocarditis

Etiology and Epidemiology. **Infective endocarditis** (IE) involves the endocardium, most often of the heart valves. Acute IE develops rapidly, often on otherwise normal heart valves, and if untreated can result in death within days to weeks. Subacute IE develops gradually, usually on previously damaged heart valves, and responds well to treatment. IE is classified by the causative organism, including hemolytic streptococci, *Staphylococcus aureus, Staphylococcus epidermidis,* and enterococci.

Individuals at high risk for IE are those with underlying pathologic cardiac conditions, including rheumatic valve disease, congenital heart disease, and degenerative heart disease. Mitral valve prolapse is a leading risk factor. Endocarditis develops in 1% to 4% of persons who have prosthetic heart valve implants. In some cases IE occurs after invasive procedures such as oral surgery, gynecologic procedures, implantation of internal cardiac devices, and insertion of indwelling urinary catheters or renal shunts. Intravenous (IV) drug users are also at high risk because of the possibility of bacteremia from contaminated needles and syringes. Human immunodeficiency virus (HIV) infection is also a risk factor for IE. Box 30-1 identifies categories of IE and specific patient populations at risk.

Pathophysiology. A damaged cardiac valve or a ventricular septal defect produces turbulent blood flow that allows bacteria to settle on the low-pressure side of the valve or defect. IE from IV

Box 30-1 Categories of Infective Endocarditis With Patient Populations at Risk

- Native-valve infective endocarditis (IE)
  - —Congenital heart disease: bicuspid aortic valve, ventricular septal defects, patent ductus arteriosus, and tetralogy of Fallot
  - —Chronic rheumatic heart disease
  - —Mitral valve prolapse with valve regurgitation
  - —Degenerative valve lesions: calcific aortic stenosis
  - —Hypertrophic cardiomyopathy
- Prosthetic-valve IE: mechanical and bioprosthetic
- Intravenous drug users IE
- Intravascular devices and procedures
  - —Infections of implantable pacemakers and cardioverter-defibrillators
  - —Intravascular lines
  - —Surgically constructed systemic pulmonary shunts or conduits
- Residual valvular damage resulting from a previous attack of endocarditis

drug abuse most commonly affects the tricuspid valve. The hallmark of IE is a platelet-fibrin-bacteria mass on the valve, called a *vegetation* (Figure 30-1). The organisms surround the heart valve, become embedded in the valve matrix, and cause vegetative growths that may scar and perforate the leaflets. Emboli occur if the vegetative growths break free of the valves and enter the bloodstream. If the emboli become trapped in organs such as the spleen or kidney, abscesses may form.

In acute IE the onset is swift, with septicemia and fever above 100° F (38° C). The patient with subacute IE has a more insidious onset, with vague complaints of malaise and general achiness. Low-grade fever is usually present, although a high fever may occur with *S. aureus* infection. Other commonly reported symptoms include headache, arthralgia, arthritis, low back pain, myalgias, anorexia, weight loss, chest pain, night sweats, and occasional hemoptysis. Physical examination may reveal splenomegaly; clubbing of the fingers; Osler's nodes (small, raised, tender, bluish areas) on the fingers or toe pads; and small capillary hemorrhages (petechiae) in the conjunctiva, in the mouth, and on the extremities. Janeway lesions (nontender lesions on the palms or soles) and Roth's spots (retinal lesions) are additional findings unique to IE. Auscultation reveals murmurs over the affected cardiac valves.

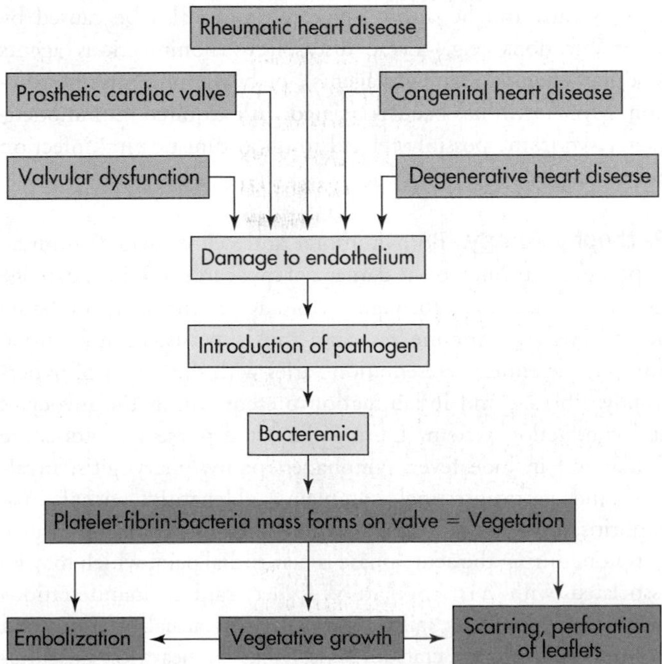

Figure 30-1 Infective endocarditis. Relationship of endothelial damage, bacteria introduction, and subsequent vegetative growth.

Diagnostic tests include blood cultures to guide antibiotic therapy, echocardiography (preferably transesophageal in the high-risk patient) to demonstrate valvular vegetations and function, and occasionally cardiac catheterization to evaluate ventricular and valvular function. The Duke criteria have been used as an objective mode of diagnosis,[12] although modifications to these defining criteria were recommended in 2000 (Box 30-2).[25] Laboratory tests usually reveal an increased white blood count and ESR. A normocytic normochromic anemia may also be present.

Collaborative Care Management. The major aim of therapy is to eliminate all microorganisms from the vegetative growths and prevent complications. Cellular and humoral host defenses

Box 30-2 Modified Duke Criteria for Diagnosis of Infective Endocarditis

Major Criteria

Blood cultures positive for infective endocarditis (IE)
Evidence of endocardial involvement (intracardiac mass, abscess, new partial dehiscence of a valvular prosthesis, new valvular regurgitation)

Minor Criteria

Predisposing heart disease or injection drug use
Temperature of more than 100° F (38° C)
Vascular phenomenon
Immunologic phenomenon
Microbiologic evidence

Definite Endocarditis

Histologic or microbiologic evidence of infection at surgery or autopsy
Two major criteria
One major criterion and three minor criteria
Five minor criteria

Possible Endocarditis

One major criterion and one minor criterion
Three minor criteria

No Endocarditis

Negative findings at surgery or autopsy for a patient who received antibiotic therapy for 4 days or less
Firm alternative diagnosis
Resolution of illness with antibiotic therapy for 4 days or less
Failure to meet criteria for possible endocarditis

From Li IS et al: Proposed modifications to the Duke criteria for the diagnosis of infective endocarditis, *Clin Infect Dis* 30(4):633-638, 2000.

are impaired over the affected areas because the colonized bacteria are embedded in the valve matrix, preventing host defenses from reaching the bacteria. If IE goes untreated for weeks or months, the incidence of embolic complications and progressive involvement of the heart valves greatly increases. Therefore antibiotic therapy is initiated as soon as three blood cultures have been obtained to identify the infecting organism. Blood cultures should be repeated 3 to 4 days into therapy. Antibiotic therapy continues even after symptoms abate, usually for 4 to 6 weeks. Outpatient IV antibiotic administration may be considered when barriers to adherence are low, therapeutic regimens are uncomplicated, and support systems are in place. Outpatient management is contraindicated for IV drug abusers and those with prosthetic heart valves. Peak and trough drug levels are evaluated to ensure the desired therapeutic outcomes of antibiotic administration and avoid adverse patient outcomes. The nephrotoxic effects of many antibiotics necessitate ongoing assessment of renal function throughout treatment. Deteriorated heart valves may be surgically repaired or replaced with prosthetic valves when IE is refractory to medical therapy or the patient's cardiac and hemodynamic status is compromised. When pacemakers or implantable defibrillators are implicated in causing the infection, complete removal may be required for cure.

The nurse monitors the patient for new murmurs or changes in preexisting murmurs. With impaired valve function, the patient is at risk for developing heart failure. Changes in breath sounds and fluid status can alert the staff to early signs of heart failure. The nurse continuously assesses the patient for signs and symptoms of embolic events and dysrhythmias. Decreased tissue perfusion also affects the peripheral vasculature and alters the person's activity tolerance. When bed rest is necessary, active or passive range-of-motion exercises are performed regularly.

PATIENT/FAMILY TEACHING. The nurse teaches the patient to avoid excessive fatigue and to stop activity immediately if chest pain, dyspnea, lightheadedness, or faintness occurs. The nurse encourages 30 to 60 minutes of rest between all activities, teaches patients to avoid infection, and initiates referrals for outpatient IV management. The nurse teaches the patient to monitor for complications, including signs and symptoms of heart failure and embolic events. The nurse instructs the patient to inform all primary care providers, including physicians and dentists, about the history of IE so that antibiotic therapy, if clinically indicated, can be administered before intrusive procedures. Prophylactic antibiotics are recommended for those at high and moderate risk. Those at high risk include patients with prosthetic heart valves, previous bacterial endocarditis, complex cyanotic congenital heart disease, and surgically constructed pulmonary shunts. Those at moderate risk include patients with most other congenital cardiac disorders, acquired valve disease, hypertrophic cardiomyopathy, and significant mitral valve prolapse. Current American Heart Association (AHA) recommendations for the use of prophylactic antibiotics are presented in Box 30-3. The patient is instructed to use a soft-bristled toothbrush and floss regularly to protect the gums from infection and prevent dental caries. Good dental hygiene is of utmost importance in decreasing the risk of recurrent IE in susceptible patient populations (see Nursing Care Plan).

Box 30-3 American Heart Association Recommendations for Antibiotic Prophylaxis of Infective Endocarditis

Dental, Oral, Respiratory Tract, or Esophageal Procedures

Pathogen: *Streptococcus viridans*
Antibiotic of choice: amoxicillin, 2 g, 1 hour before procedure
Alternatives if unable to take oral preparation or if allergic to penicillin:
—Ampicillin, intravenous (IV)
—Clindamycin, oral or IV
—First-generation cephalosporins (e.g., cefazolin IV)
—Azithromycin or clarithromycin

Genitourinary and Nonesophageal Gastrointestinal Procedures

Pathogen: *Enterococcus faecalis*
Antibiotic of choice: parenteral ampicillin or oral amoxicillin

Myocarditis

Etiology and Epidemiology. Myocarditis is an inflammatory disease of the myocardium that causes an infiltrate in the myocardial interstitium and injury to adjacent myocardial cells. Myocarditis may be a primary disease with an unknown origin or occur secondary to an identifiable cause such as drug hypersensitivity or toxicity, connective tissue disease, sarcoidosis, or infection. The inflammatory process often develops secondary to endocarditis or pericarditis. Myocarditis may be classified as acute or chronic.

Viral infection, typically with a strain of picornaviruses, is the most common cause of myocarditis. The subset of coxsackievirus B accounts for nearly 50% of the cases, and coxsackievirus A, echovirus, and poliovirus account for most of the remainder.[46] Other viruses include influenza A and B, rubella, mumps, rabies, Epstein-Barr, and hepatitis. Myocarditis can also be caused by other infections (e.g., Lyme disease), by noninfectious agents (cocaine, chemotherapeutic agents), or by an autoimmune reaction. Myocarditis has been associated with acquired immunodeficiency syndrome possibly related to opportunistic viral infection or HIV itself.[19]

Pathophysiology. Both humoral and cell-mediated immune responses contribute to the damage of myocarditis. Direct damage to the myocardium through cytotoxic mechanisms probably occurs. An autoimmune response causes persistent myocardial disease. The clinical presentation varies with the extent of hypertrophy, fibrosis, and inflammation present within the myocytes and conduction system. During the acute phase symptoms are flulike and include fever, lymphadenopathy, pharyngitis, myalgias, and gastrointestinal complaints. Hepatitis, encephalitis, nephritis, and orchitis also can occur. The most common cardiac symptom during the acute phase is pericardial pain, which may be associated with a friction rub. Other cardiac manifestations include signs of heart failure, syncope, pericardial effusion, and ischemia. Pulmonary crackles (rales) may be heard on auscultation. ECG changes include ST segment elevation, T wave flattening or inversion, appearance of Q waves, and prolonged Q-T interval. These abnormalities may disappear after recovery or persist for several years. Ventricular ectopy can include multiple forms of premature ventricular beats and ventricular tachycardia.

Preliminary laboratory findings are nonspecific and include elevation of the ESR, viral titers, and levels of various enzymes (such as lactate dehydrogenase, creatine kinase, and the transaminases). Mild to moderate leukocytosis with atypical lymphocytes may be seen. Chest radiographs may show the heart size to be normal or enlarged. Echocardiography shows dilated chambers, depressed systolic function, and mild or no pericardial effusion. Although the diagnosis of myocarditis may be suspected clinically, it must be confirmed histologically by endomyocardial biopsy while lymphocytic infiltration and myocyte damage are present (within 6 weeks of the acute illness). Autoimmune myocarditis is diagnosed through additional testing for autoimmune serum markers or the presence of intercellular adhesion molecules on cardiac myocytes.

Collaborative Care Management. Postbiopsy monitoring focuses on the potential for hematoma or bleeding at the cannulation site, cardiac tamponade, or pneumothorax. The site is inspected for bleeding, ecchymosis, or swelling. The nurse reports shortness of breath, changes in breath sounds, dyspnea, and alterations in respiratory rate and pattern of breathing. The nurse monitors vital signs closely to assess for continued hemodynamic stability.

Medical therapy includes antibiotics, treatment of heart failure, and management of dysrhythmias. Monitoring for heart failure is an important nursing responsibility. Immunosuppressive therapy may be used to prevent irreversible myocardial damage in persons with autoimmune myocarditis. Anticoagulation therapy is often prescribed to prevent intraventricular thrombi and embolic events. Pacemakers or defibrillators may be indicated for dysrhythmias. The prognosis is variable, depending on the cause and the patient. Ventricular assist devices may be indicated for patients progressing to dilated cardiomyopathy.

The cornerstone of management is supportive care, including bed rest to decrease metabolic demand. Measures to decrease cardiac workload include frequent rest periods, a quiet environment, and the use of semi-Fowler's position. Patients are commonly anxious about the sudden onset of heart disease and its implications for the future. The nurse provides emotional support and encourages patients to verbalize their concerns.

PATIENT/FAMILY TEACHING. The nurse emphasizes the importance of an extended period of energy conservation. The risk of myocardial damage increases with exercise. The nurse teaches the need for slow progression in activity, with frequent rest periods. The use of NSAIDs in viral myocarditis appears to increase the myocardial damage, and the nurse emphasizes the need to avoid these drugs. The patient is instructed about a heart-healthy diet and the early symptoms of heart failure that need to be reported promptly.

Heart Failure

Etiology and Epidemiology. **Heart failure** occurs when the myocardium cannot maintain a sufficient cardiac output to meet the body's metabolic needs. Failure can result from either systolic or diastolic dysfunction. Systolic dysfunction causes inadequate pumping of blood from the ventricle and decreases cardiac output. Any process that alters myocardial **contractility** can produce systolic dysfunction. Many disease processes are implicated, but ischemic heart disease and hypertension are the most prevalent causes (Box 30-4).

Diastolic dysfunction (stiff heart syndrome) occurs when the ventricle does not fill adequately during diastole. Inadequate filling decreases the amount of blood available in the ventricle for cardiac output. Systolic function is often normal. Hypertension and coronary artery disease (CAD) are again the primary causes of diastolic dysfunction, but it also occurs secondary to aging, infiltrative diseases (such as myocarditis), and constrictive pericarditis (see Box 30-4).[22]

The causes for both systolic and diastolic dysfunction are similar, but they affect the ventricles in different ways. Systolic dysfunction is the more common form of heart failure, although the percentage of patients with chronic heart failure and intact left ventricular systolic function is increasing. Nearly all patients with systolic dysfunction develop some degree of diastolic dysfunction over time.

Approximately 5 million Americans have heart failure, and 550,000 new cases are diagnosed each year. It is the most common diagnosis in hospitalized patients over the age of 65 years.[1] Over the past 20 years, hospital discharges for heart failure increased from 377,000 to 999,000, a 165% increase. Fifty percent of patients die within 5 years of diagnosis. Heart failure is the only major cardiovascular disorder that is increasing in incidence, prevalence, and mortality rate.[4]

CAD is the precipitating cause of heart failure in two thirds of patients.[20] An increase in the number of survivors of myocardial infarction is in part responsible for the increase in the number of patients with heart failure.[38] Hypertension is present as a risk factor in 75% of patients with heart failure.[17] Additional contributors include diabetes, cigarette smoking, obesity, an elevated total cholesterol–to–high-density lipoprotein cholesterol ratio, an abnormally high or low hematocrit level, and proteinuria (see Risk Factors box, p. 812).[32]

Morbidity from heart failure has made this diagnosis the number one reason for hospital admission. Management of heart failure is also extremely expensive. Direct costs for 2004—including inpatient care, professional care, medications, medical equipment,

BOX 30-4 Common Causes of Heart Failure

Systolic	Diastolic
Coronary artery disease	Coronary artery disease
Hypertension	Hypertrophy
Metabolic disorders	Fibrosis of advanced age
Myocarditis	Constrictive pericarditis
Alcohol	Myocarditis
Cocaine	Hypertension
Cardiac valve disease	Aortic stenosis
Dilated cardiomyopathy	Ventricular remodeling
	Collagen diseases
	Cardiomyopathy

Nursing Care Plan

Patient With Infective Endocarditis

Data A 68-year-old patient underwent a routine colonoscopy and polyp removal 6 six weeks ago. His significant history includes aortic regurgitation, which was diagnosed 4 years ago. In the weeks following the colonoscopy, the patient's wife noticed a decrease in his normal activity level, increased complaints about muscle aches, and his need to rest more frequently while performing simple yard work. Two days ago the patient developed night sweats. When he visited his health care provider, the provider noted that the patient had a low-grade fever of 100° F (37.7° C); small, raised, tender, bluish areas on his fingers; multiple petechiae over his extremities; and an increase in intensity from his baseline aortic murmur. On questioning, the patient recalled that he had been instructed about antibiotic prophylaxis before invasive procedures but forgot to mention his valve problem when consulting the gastrointestinal specialist. The patient was admitted and a transesophageal echocardiogram was performed, which confirmed the presence of vegetation on the aortic valve. A diagnosis of infective endocarditis was confirmed. Blood cultures were quickly obtained and antibiotic therapy initiated. The patient responded well to treatment and will be discharged next week with plans for ongoing administration of intravenous ampicillin at home.

Nursing Diagnosis

Acute pain related to inflammation and infection of endocardial tissues (valves)

Outcomes

- Patient will report control of pain by rating pain less than 3 on a scale of 0 to 10.

Related NOC Outcomes

- Comfort Level
- Pain Control
- Pain Level

Related NIC Interventions

- Analgesic Administration
- Coping Enhancement
- Pain Management
- Medication Management

Nursing Interventions/Rationales

- Administer analgesics routinely and before pain is severe. *Analgesics control pain more effectively when they are given routinely during the early stages of infection. Mild to moderate pain is more easily controlled than severe pain. Analgesics lower pain to tolerable levels, working synergistically with nonpharmacologic strategies.*
- Teach patient regarding self-administration of prescribed pain medications, including correct dosage, intervals between dosing, and potential side effects. *Allows patient to be in control and decreases the risk for overdosing or underdosing.*
- Assess and document patient response to analgesic medications. *The effectiveness of medications needs to be evaluated to minimize risk of side effects and tolerance. Ineffective strategies need to be replaced with more effective alternatives. Patients who require pain medications more frequently than prescribed may need a higher dosage of medication or a different analgesic.*
- Encourage adequate rest. *Sleep deprivation lowers pain threshold.*

Nursing Diagnosis

Risk for decreased cardiac output related to infective cardiac process

Outcomes

- Patient will maintain cardiac output within normal limits as evidenced by blood pressure within normal range for patient; warm, dry skin; absence of cardiac dysrhythmias; strong and equal peripheral pulses; and clear lung sounds.

Related NOC Outcomes

- Circulation Status
- Hemodynamic Regulation
- Knowledge: Treatment Program

Related NIC Interventions

- Cardiac Care
- Cardiac Pump Effectiveness
- Medication Management

Nursing Interventions/Rationales

- Monitor for signs of cardiac compromise. *To determine if cardiac function is being compromised. Signs of cardiac compensation resulting from sympathetic stimulation from low cardiac output include tachycardia; decreased blood pressure; cold, clammy skin; restlessness; weak peripheral pulses; decreased urinary output; and dyspnea.*
- Monitor for signs of decreased tissue perfusion secondary to embolization. *Patients with endocarditis are at increased risk for embolism. A complete physical assessment is performed to establish a baseline and at least every 8 hours thereafter to detect significant changes. Early detection of abnormalities enables prompt intervention to minimize serious complications.*

and home health care—were estimated to be in excess of $23.7 billion.[1] The prevalence of heart failure and its associated morbidity create multiple socioeconomic dilemmas for the health care system, especially as older adults increase in number.

Pathophysiology

Systolic and Diastolic Dysfunction. Systolic and diastolic heart failure both occur secondary to myocardial injury. The progression of heart failure depends in large part on the degree of ventricular **remodeling** that occurs after myocardial injury (Figure 30-2). Remodeling involves an increase in the intraventricular dimension, an increase in collagen formation leading to fibrosis, and myocyte changes that adversely affect contractility. Remodeling increases myocardial oxygen demands, decreases myocardial perfusion, and increases the potential for dysrhythmias.

The ventricle changes shape and dimensions, decreasing its effectiveness as a pump. Increases in diastolic pressure may further change the shape of the left ventricle (LV), resulting in papillary muscle rearrangement and mitral insufficiency. Accelerated programmed cell death (apoptosis, or cell "suicide") decreases the number of myocytes available for pumping and occurs for as yet undetermined reasons.[22]

- Teach patient the importance of maintaining antibiotic schedules. *Treating the underlying cause will prevent further destruction of heart valves and reduce the pain associated with the disease.*
- Encourage physical and emotional rest. *To decrease metabolic demands and hence decrease excessive oxygen consumption.*

Nursing Diagnosis

Activity intolerance related to decreased cardiac output secondary to infective endocarditis

Outcomes

- Patient reports decreased fatigue.
- Pulse, respiration, and blood pressure return to normal for patient within 3 minutes after increased activity.

Related NOC Outcomes

- Activity Tolerance
- Endurance
- Energy Conservation

Related NIC Interventions

- Energy Management
- Teaching: Prescribed Activity/Exercise
- Progressive Muscle Relaxation

Nursing Interventions/Rationales

- Assess and monitor patient's response to exercise (vital signs before and after exercise, dyspnea, signs of exertion). *Activity intolerance depends on the ability to physiologically adapt to changes in demand. Heart rate and blood pressure should increase with increasing demand but decrease to near baseline within 3 minutes after activity ceases.*
- Teach the patient to report dyspnea, chest pain, palpitations, and fatigue during activity. *Abnormal subjective responses indicate intolerance of activity.*
- Teach the patient to perform activities more slowly. *Energy conservation minimizes the risk of exceeding the heart's oxygen requirements.*
- Assist the patient in sequencing activities to provide for rest periods. *Rest decreases myocardial oxygen consumption, allowing intervals of low energy demand.*
- Provide an environment conducive to rest. *Environmental stimulation inhibits the patient's ability to enter a state of relaxation and subsequent rest.*

Nursing Diagnosis

Risk for ineffective therapeutic regimen management (individual and family) related to complexity of therapeutic regimen, knowledge deficits

Outcomes

- Patient will verbalize understanding of therapeutic regimen.
- Patient will report adherence to therapeutic regimen.

Related NOC Outcomes

- Adherence Behavior
- Compliance Behavior
- Knowledge: Treatment Regimen

Related NIC Interventions

- Behavior Modification
- Family Support
- Referral
- Self-Modification Assistance

Nursing Interventions/Rationales

- Provide verbal and written instructions for pathophysiology of endocarditis, treatment plan, medications, and signs and symptoms of endocarditis that need to be reported. *Teaching reinforces the need to comply with recommended management. Written material provides additional resource for home reference.*
- Teach the importance of appropriate antibiotic prophylaxis. *Adhering to antibiotic recommendations helps decrease the risk of disease recurrence.*
- Emphasize the importance of good oral care, avoidance of trauma to the gums, and regular dental checkups. *Proper oral hygiene decreases the risk of pathogen entry via the oral mucosa. Trauma provides a pathway in the oral mucosa for pathogenic entry.*
- Teach the importance of wearing an identification bracelet or necklace to inform health care providers of heart condition. *Proper identification can decrease the risk of inadvertent exposure to pathogens without appropriate prophylaxis.*
- Stress the importance of compliance with follow-up care recommendations. *Repetitive explanations may help improve adherence behaviors. Follow-up care is essential to prevent further cardiac compromise.*

Evaluation

Evaluation is based on comparing the patient's outcomes with desired outcomes.

In most cases heart failure begins with left ventricular systolic dysfunction. Common causes of decreased left ventricular contractility include CAD, systemic hypertension, and aortic stenosis. CAD decreases contractility by diminishing the oxygen supply to the myofibrils. Hypertension causes the LV to contract more forcefully to eject blood into the aorta. Over time, the muscle fibers thicken (hypertrophy) and increase the myocardial oxygen consumption. Failure occurs when the heart's need for oxygen can no longer be met. In aortic stenosis the LV must also increase its pumping force to deliver blood through the tight valve.

The diminished pumping power of the LV results in ejection fractions (EFs) of less than 40%. Blood remains in the LV at the end of systole. Left atrial pressure must increase to empty the blood volume from the left atrium (LA) into the LV. When the LA cannot completely empty its volume, blood backs up into the pulmonary circulation and increases the pressure within the fragile pulmonary capillaries. The increased pressure drives fluid out of the smaller pulmonary capillaries into the interstitium and alveoli. High pulmonary pressures then impede the flow of blood from the right ventricle (RV) to the lungs. The RV must generate more force to move blood into the pulmonary system.

Risk Factors

Heart Failure

- Coronary artery disease (precipitating cause in two thirds of patients)
- Hypertension (present in 75% of patients)
- Advanced age
- Diabetes
- Cigarette smoking
- Obesity
- Elevated total cholesterol-to-high-density lipoprotein cholesterol ratio
- Abnormally high or low hematocrit
- Proteinuria

The remaining blood backs up into the RA and ultimately the peripheral venous circulation.

RV dysfunction most often results from LV dysfunction. Primary pulmonary hypertension and chronic obstructive pulmonary disease are other possible causes. The high pulmonary pressures impede the RV's ability to pump blood to the pulmonary vessels, and the RV must generate higher pressures to overcome the resistance.

With LV diastolic dysfunction, the LV is abnormally "stiff" (noncompliant) during diastole and does not fill at the normal lower pressures. Myocardial fibrosis and ventricular hypertrophy are possible causes of ventricular noncompliance. Fibrotic changes that prevent the ventricle from expanding occur with aging, myocardial infarction, and constrictive pericarditis. Hypertrophy results from hypertension, cardiac valve disease, and the remodeling that follows myocardial infarction. The increased muscle mass is often thick, stiff, and noncompliant. Elevated calcium concentrations also inhibit diastolic relaxation. Calcium concentrations rise when the sarcoplasmic reticulum is unable to remove calcium from the myofibril, as occurs with ischemia, hypertrophy, and advanced age.[11]

A stiff LV is not able to expand effectively to receive additional blood volume. With higher preloads, congestion may develop within the heart as atrial pressures increase to overcome the higher ventricular pressures. With low preload, the net result is a decrease in stroke volume (the actual volume pumped per beat), although the EF in diastolic heart failure may be normal.

Altered myocardial contractility and filling result in hemodynamic instability, and the body responds to these changes through complex neurohormonal and endocrine responses, principally through the sympathetic nervous system (SNS) and the renin-angiotensin-aldosterone system (Figure 30-3).

Sympathetic Nervous System. Baroreceptors in the carotid sinus and aortic arch sense the drop in cardiac output and activate the SNS to release more catecholamines. Beta-receptor stimulation increases both heart rate and contractility and also causes the

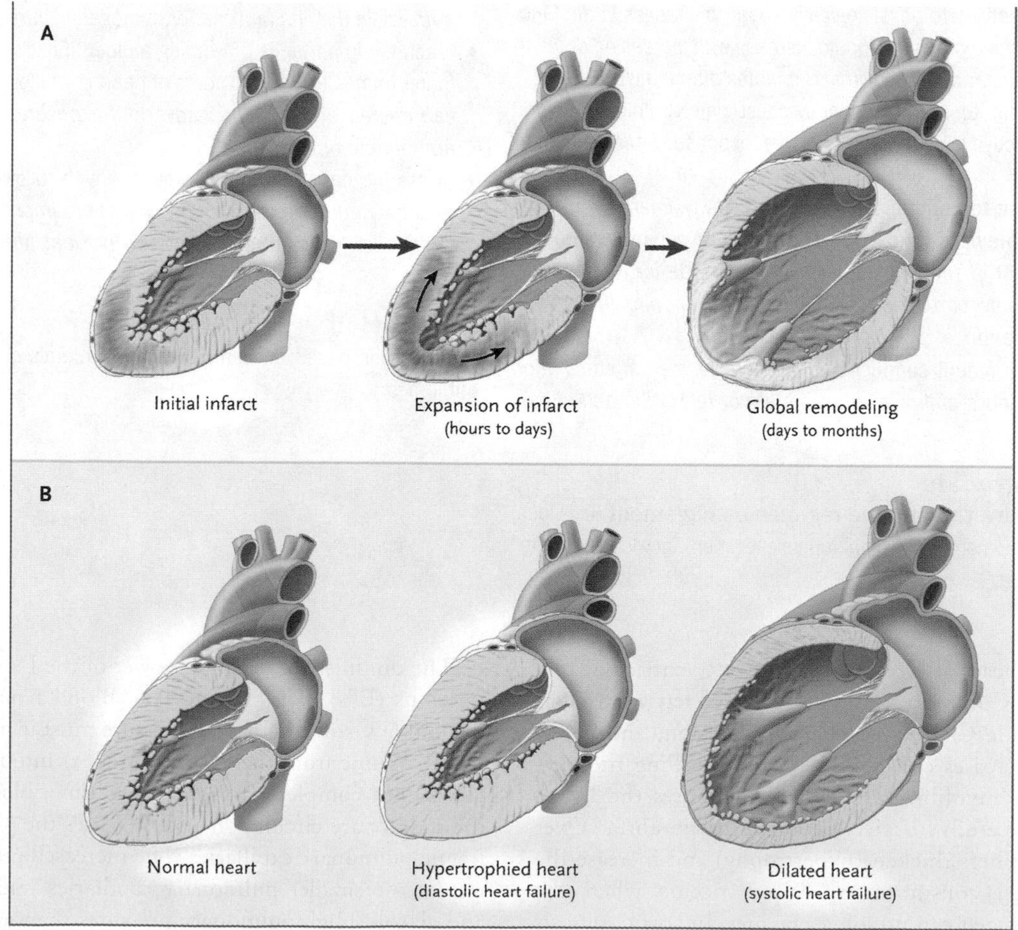

Figure 30-2 Ventricular remodeling after infarction **(A)** and in diastolic and systolic heart failure **(B)**.

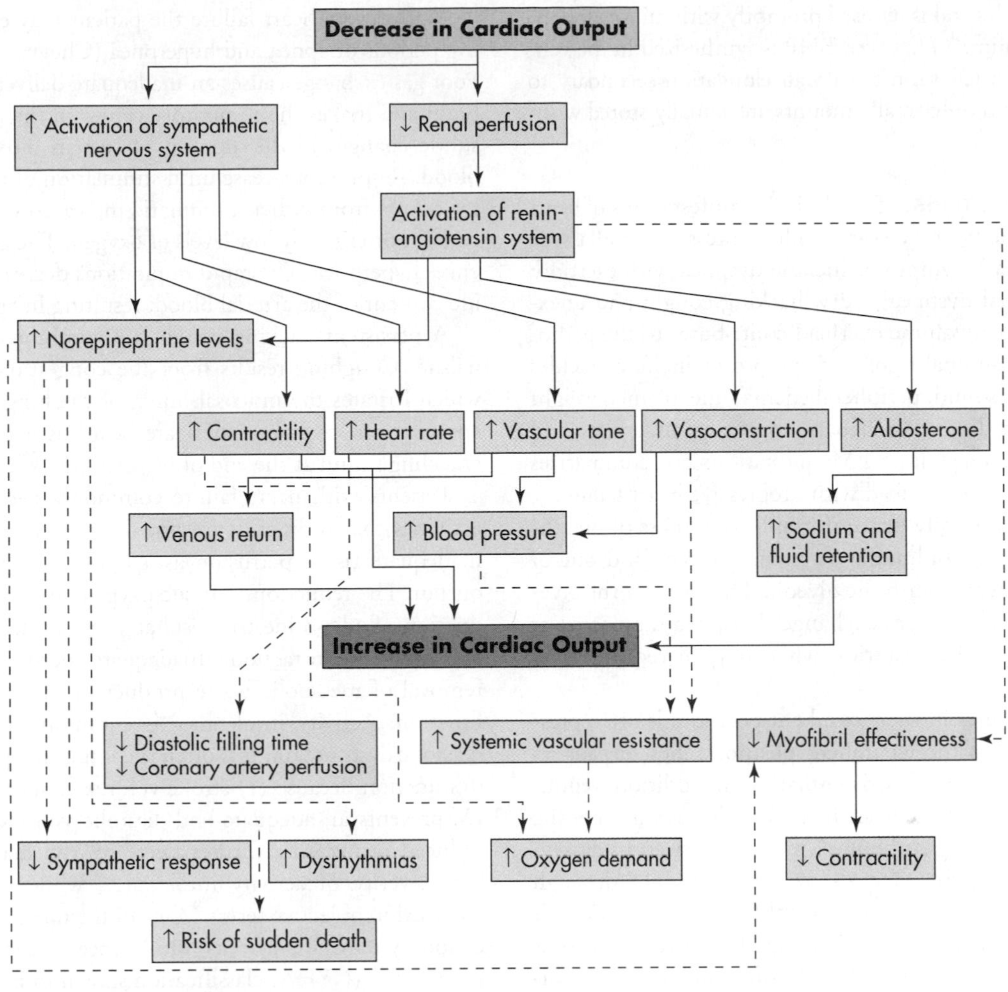

Figure 30-3 Effects of neurohormonal activation on the heart.

release of renin from the kidneys, increasing vascular tone. Alpha-receptor stimulation increases systemic arteriolar tone, causing a rise in blood pressure. The concomitant rise in venous tone increases the amount of blood returning to the right side of the heart. The increases in heart rate, contractility, and venous return initially all work to increase cardiac output.

Unfortunately these mechanisms lose their effectiveness over time. With increasing heart rates, the time for diastole shortens and less time is available for ventricular filling. Coronary blood flow (and oxygen delivery) decreases because the coronary arteries are perfused only during diastole. An increase in contractility requires more oxygen, and an increase in blood pressure raises the systemic vascular resistance (SVR). The SVR is the pressure the LV must overcome to eject its blood volume. The additional work required of the LV again increases myocardial oxygen demand. High levels of norepinephrine eventually decrease the heart's ability to respond to sympathetic stimulation and may cause cardiac dysrhythmias and sudden death. As heart failure progresses, the ratio of alpha- and beta-receptor sites is altered. Excessive levels of catecholamines can become directly cardiotoxic, increasing myocyte hypertrophy, fibrosis, and remodeling and worsening the failure.

Renin-Angiotensin-Aldosterone System. Insufficient cardiac output decreases renal perfusion and activates the renin-angiotensin system, triggering vasoconstriction to correct a perceived hypovolemia. Aldosterone secretion is also increased, resulting in sodium and fluid retention. The increases in fluid volume and blood pressure increase cardiac output but quickly outlive their usefulness. In systolic dysfunction, any additional fluid volume increases the amount of fluid the failing ventricle must pump. Vasoconstriction increases SVR, which requires the ventricle to increase its pressure to eject its volume.

Other Factors. Progressive heart failure also activates the release of endothelin, produced by vascular endothelial cells, and arginine vasopressin, released by the posterior pituitary gland. These neurohormones cause additional vasoconstriction and increases in preload. The deleterious effects of cytokines, such as tumor necrosis factor-alpha and interleukin-6, have also been implicated in the pathophysiology of progressive heart failure.

Natriuretic Peptides. Stretching of myocardial tissue from the combined effects of all of these factors promotes the release of two endogenous natriuretic peptides: atrial natriuretic peptide (ANP) and B-type natriuretic peptide (BNP).[10] These peptides lower the levels of angiotensin II, aldosterone, and endothelin, thereby promoting the desired effects of arterial and venous vasodilation, diuresis, and inhibition of sodium reabsorption. ANP is stored within the atria and ventricles and is released promptly with minor stretching of the myocardium.[16] However, BNP is synthesized in the ventricles in response to left ventricular wall elongation secondary to myocardial stress, and only small amounts are actually stored within the ventricles.[27]

CLINICAL MANIFESTATIONS. The clinical manifestations of heart failure occur secondary to elevated filling pressures and tissue hypoperfusion. Classic symptoms include dyspnea with exertion; orthopnea, nocturnal dyspnea; a dry, hacking cough; and unexplained fatigue. When volume overload contributes to the pathologic condition, additional signs and symptoms include crackles (rales), a third heart sound, peripheral edema, unexplained weight gain, jugular venous distention, hepatic engorgement, ascites, and worsening dyspnea. The Clinical Manifestations box summarizes common symptoms encountered with progressive heart failure.

Dyspnea, an abnormally uncomfortable awareness of breathing, occurs when high pulmonary pressures force fluid out of the pulmonary capillaries into the alveoli. The fluid in the alveoli interferes with effective gas exchange. Dyspnea may occur at rest or only with physical exertion when oxygen requirements increase.

Orthopnea, dyspnea in the recumbent position, is often present in heart failure. In the recumbent position, chest expansion diminishes, resulting in decreased ventilation. In addition, venous return to the right side of the heart increases with elevation of the legs. Patients experiencing orthopnea often must sleep using several pillows or sitting in a semi-Fowler's position. Although orthopnea may occur immediately after the patient lies down, it typically does not occur for 2 to 5 hours. The patient awakens suddenly with severe shortness of breath, often in panic, a condition called **paroxysmal nocturnal dyspnea**. The severe dyspnea resolves after being upright for 10 to 30 minutes.

With severe heart failure the patient may experience alternating periods of apnea and hyperpnea (Cheyne-Stokes respiration). Poor gas exchange causes an inadequate delivery of oxygen to the brain and makes the respiratory center in the brain insensitive to subtle changes in the amount of carbon dioxide in the arterial blood. Respirations cease until stimulation of the respiratory center occurs from either a dramatic increase in the carbon dioxide content or critically low levels of oxygen. The patient then experiences hyperpnea. The rapid respirations decrease the carbon dioxide content of the arterial blood, resulting in apnea.

A persistent hacking cough is a common symptom of heart failure. Coughing results from the congestion of trapped fluid, which irritates the mucosal lining of the lungs and bronchi. On auscultation, crackles (rales) are heard as a moist popping and crackling sound at the end of inspiration.

Patients with heart failure commonly become fatigued after activities that ordinarily are not tiring. The fatigue results from inadequate tissue perfusion as a result of the decreased cardiac output. The reduction in tissue oxygen decreases the aerobic production of adenosine triphosphate, the immediate energy source for muscle contraction. Inadequate perfusion also decreases removal of metabolic waste products, further decreasing muscle function. Activity intolerance is common in both systolic and diastolic dysfunction. It is often the initial symptom with diastolic dysfunction because (1) stroke volume cannot increase when the LV prevents an adequate end-diastolic volume and (2) exercise-induced tachycardia further decreases the diastolic filling time. The severity of activity intolerance, while subjective, is often recorded in objective terms.[9] One of the most widely used classification systems for activity intolerance is the New York Heart Association (NYHA) classification shown in Box 30-5.

Angina can occur from decreased blood flow to the myocardium. The balance of myocardial oxygen supply and demand is precarious

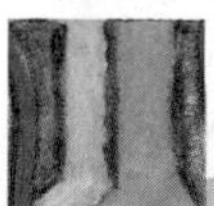

CLINICAL MANIFESTATIONS *Heart Failure*

Respiratory

Dyspnea
Orthopnea
Paroxysmal nocturnal dyspnea
Persistent hacking cough
Alternating periods of apnea and hyperpnea
Crackles (rales)

Cardiovascular

Angina
Jugular venous distention
Tachycardia
Decrease in systolic blood pressure with increase in diastolic blood pressure
S_3 or S_4 heart sounds

Gastrointestinal

Enlargement and tenderness in the right upper quadrant of the abdomen
Ascites
Nausea
Vomiting
Bloating
Anorexia
Epigastric pain

Cerebral

Altered mental status (confusion, restlessness)

Generalized

Fatigue
Decrease in activity tolerance
Postural dizziness
Edema (peripheral, pitting)
Cool extremities
Weight gain

Psychosocial

Anxiety

Box 30-5 New York Heart Association Classification of Heart Failure

- Class I: No symptoms, tolerates ordinary physical activity
- Class II: Comfortable at rest; ordinary physical activity results in symptoms
- Class III: Comfortable at rest; less than ordinary physical activity results in symptoms
- Class IV: Symptoms may be present at rest; symptoms with any physical activity

in even the most stable patient with heart failure. Angina is most likely to occur in patients with preexisting CAD.

Engorgement of the low-pressure peripheral venous system results from pressure increases in the right side of the heart. Distention of the internal jugular vein (jugular venous distention) is often observed with the patient in a semi-Fowler's position. With sharply elevated venous pressure, pulsations of the earlobes may occur when the patient sits upright.

High venous pressures force fluid into the extravascular tissue. The patient often notices this as pitting, nontender edema in dependent areas, usually the lower extremities. As the edema becomes more pronounced, it progresses up the legs into the thighs, external genitalia, and lower portion of the trunk. If the tissue becomes extremely engorged, the skin may crack and fluid may "weep" from the tissues. Increasing fluid volume is most often responsible for the unexplained weight gain experienced by patients in heart failure. Fluid volume increases as urinary output diminishes from poor renal perfusion.

The liver also becomes engorged with intravascular fluid, resulting in enlargement and tenderness in the right upper quadrant of the abdomen. Altered hepatic blood flow adversely affects liver function. Among its many functions, the liver metabolizes aldosterone and antidiuretic hormone and many of the medications used to treat heart failure. Pressure increases within the portal system can force fluid through the blood vessels into the abdominal cavity. The resulting ascites can create nausea, vomiting, bloating, and epigastric pain and put pressure on the diaphragm, resulting in respiratory distress.

Tachycardia is often present as the SNS attempts to compensate for the low cardiac output. The skin becomes cool and clammy as the SNS triggers vasoconstriction and stimulates the sweat glands. Additional physical assessment findings include a decrease in systolic blood pressure with an increase in diastolic blood pressure. S_3 and S_4 heart sounds, reflecting resistance to ventricular filling, are often heard over the mitral or right ventricular area. Confusion and restlessness can occur if cerebral blood flow diminishes.

A patient with heart failure may be stabilized on medications, but become symptomatic when new insults or stresses to the heart occur (Box 30-6). Triggers include infections; active ischemia from CAD; tachydysrhythmias such as atrial fibrillation; surgery; and ineffective control of chronic conditions such as hypertension, pulmonary disease, or diabetes. These triggers increase the metabolic demand of the myocardium or interfere with its ability to contract or fill and can undo the fragile balance temporarily achieved through therapeutic modalities. For example, the likelihood of angina with heart failure increases when additional stress occurs.

Box 30-6 Precipitating Events in Heart Failure

Factors Increasing Myocardial Demand

Increases in Ventricular Volume to Be Pumped

Hypervolemia from high-output states (e.g., pregnancy, anemia, hyperthyroidism, infection)
Aortic regurgitation
Mitral regurgitation
Excessive sodium intake
Excessive administration of fluids
Renal failure

Increase in Ventricular Force Needed to Eject Blood

Poorly controlled systemic hypertension
Pulmonary hypertension
Significant aortic stenosis
Significant pulmonic stenosis

Factors Interfering With Heart's Ability to Contract or Fill

Myocardial ischemia
Myocardial infarction
Cardiomyopathy
Myocarditis
Ventricular aneurysm
Excessive alcohol intake
Mitral stenosis
Cardiac tamponade
Constrictive pericarditis
Dysrhythmias

Exacerbations of heart failure frequently require stabilization within the hospital setting and a reevaluation of management.

COMPLICATIONS

ACUTE PULMONARY EDEMA. Acute pulmonary edema is a medical emergency that may develop as a result of severe ventricular failure. Any of the events presented in Box 30-6 can cause decompensation in chronic heart failure, resulting in pulmonary edema.

Pulmonary edema arises from left ventricular overload. The volume overload increases left atrial pressure, resulting in increased pulmonary vein and pulmonary capillary pressures. Pulmonary capillary hydrostatic pressure quickly exceeds the intravascular oncotic pressure and forces fluid and sodium into the interstitium. The high interstitial pressure then forces fluid into the alveoli. The surfactant that keeps the alveoli expanded loses its effectiveness. The fluid-filled alveoli collapse, preventing the exchange of oxygen and carbon dioxide, and unoxygenated blood returns to the left side of the heart. Red blood cells also enter the alveoli, producing the characteristic blood-tinged sputum. The fluid then rapidly moves into the bronchioles and bronchi, creating the acute life-threatening symptoms that characterize this medical emergency: profound dyspnea, pallor, audible wheezing, and cyanosis.[44] Restlessness, anxiety, and tachycardia also develop from the acutely impaired gas exchange.

The air hunger of pulmonary edema triggers acute anxiety and causes catecholamine release that results in increased oxygen demand and can confound treatment. Morphine sulfate is administered because it blunts the sympathetic response and increases venous capacitance, thereby lowering left atrial pressure. It is not administered in heart failure for its analgesic effect. Nursing interventions include raising the head of the bed, positioning the patient to maximize chest expansion, and approaching the patient in a calm and reassuring manner.

Arterial blood gas or pulse oximetry results determine the need for supplemental oxygen. Oxygen may be administered at 40% to 70% by face mask to quickly achieve oxygen saturations above 90%. Humidification aids in the removal of secretions. Intubation becomes necessary for patients who do not respond to conventional measures, and ensures the delivery of adequate tidal volumes and oxygen concentrations to decrease the work of breathing. Intubation also facilitates the removal of secretions by suctioning. Aminophylline may be administered to dilate the bronchi, increase urinary output, and increase cardiac output. Other prescribed medications may include inotropic agents, diuretics, afterload reducers, and adjunct medications such as dopamine hydrochloride to increase renal perfusion. The significant diuresis that typically occurs with treatment requires careful monitoring to prevent electrolyte imbalance.

DYSRHYTHMIAS. Atrial fibrillation is a common complication of heart failure. The backup of blood into the atria causes atrial enlargement and ischemia. The ischemia alters the electrical stability necessary for impulse initiation and conduction and increases both the automaticity and irritability of the atrial tissue. Atrial fibrillation can provoke heart failure or trigger an exacerbation.

Ischemia and irritability in the ventricles can also result in premature ventricular beats. As the disease progresses, premature beats may lead to more lethal dysrhythmias that are difficult to manage because of altered cardiac metabolism, but the prophylactic use of antidysrhythmic agents is not supported through clinical research. Amiodarone may be used for symptomatic ventricular dysrhythmias. Implantable cardiac defibrillators may be beneficial for symptomatic ventricular dysrhythmias in select patients with heart failure. The management of dysrhythmias is discussed in Chapter 29.

MULTISYSTEM FAILURE. Heart failure affects every organ system, and multiple organ system failure can occur. Clinical manifestations and treatment are specific to the organ that is underperfused. Renal failure is a common problem.

▶ ARE YOU READY?

Which of the following findings associated with aortic stenosis?

1. Left atrial dilation
2. Left vertricular dilation
3. Left atrial hypertrophy
4. Left ventricular hypertrophy

Collaborative Care Management. In 2001 the American College of Cardiology and the AHA reconceptualized the approach to the management of heart failure in the adult. They implemented staging as a tool to emphasize preventive efforts in heart failure (Table 30-1), before an indication for diagnostic testing.

DIAGNOSTIC TESTS. A variety of diagnostic tests may be used in the diagnosis and management of heart failure (Box 30-7 and Tables 30-2 and 30-3).

MEDICATIONS. Pharmacologic agents play a central role in the management of heart failure. Prescribed agents include diuretics, angiotensin-converting enzyme (ACE) inhibitors, and inotropes (Table 30-4). These medications decrease the pressure generated by the volume of blood that the heart must pump (preload), decrease the resistance the heart must overcome to eject its volume (afterload), and increase the force of myocardial contraction (positive inotropic action). Beta-blockers blunt many of the neurohormonal mechanisms responsible for the downward spiraling nature of heart failure. Most protocols for the treatment of heart failure evolved from research about systolic heart failure. Diastolic heart failure is managed using many of the same medications, but the approach to managing pulmonary congestion is individualized to the patient's preload. Box 30-8 outlines the pharmacologic management of heart failure endorsed by the Quality of Care and Outcomes Working Group on Heart Failure.[24] Figure 30-4 is an algorithm for the pharmacologic management of systolic heart failure.

ANGIOTENSIN-CONVERTING ENZYME INHIBITORS. ACE inhibitors block the enzyme that converts angiotensin I to angiotensin II, thereby blocking both vasoconstriction and aldosterone production. The resulting decrease in SVR reduces afterload. The resulting mild hypotension is usually well tolerated because of the accompanying increase in cardiac output. The decrease in aldosterone production reduces sodium and water retention, resulting in a decrease in preload. Renal blood flow increases, promoting natriuresis. ACE inhibitors also block the catabolism of bradykinins, promoting further vasodilation, and they inhibit cardiac remodeling by decreasing hypertrophy and collagen formation. Because of their combined effects on afterload, preload, and remodeling, ACE inhibitors are considered the drugs of choice for all patients with heart failure. ACE inhibitor therapy is the only therapy that has been conclusively shown to reduce mortality and morbidity in heart failure.

ACE inhibitors are prescribed for patients who are asymptomatic but are known to have low EFs, and for patients who require long-term therapy after experiencing an acute episode of heart failure. Research indicates that ACE inhibitors remain underprescribed and underdosed despite their proven effectiveness.[17] Side effects such as hypotension, cough, and renal impairment may deter clinicians from maximizing their use of these important drugs.

Angiotensin II blockers are direct antagonists of the angiotensin II receptor. By blocking the binding of angiotensin II to its receptor site, the drugs interrupt the vasoconstrictor and aldosterone-producing effects of angiotensin II. Preload and afterload are decreased. Angiotensin II blockers do not block the catabolism of bradykinin and do not cause the angioedema or cough associated with the bradykinin-mediated effects of ACE inhibitors. However, the beneficial effects of bradykinin on vasodilation and remodeling are also absent. ACE inhibitors remain the drugs of choice for all heart failure patients.

DIURETICS. Diuretics are administered when clinical signs of volume overload exist. Commonly administered diuretics include

TABLE 30-1 STAGES OF HEART FAILURE AND MANAGEMENT RECOMMENDATIONS

Stage	Definition	Patient Examples	Therapeutic Recommendations
A	High risk for developing heart failure but without structural abnormalities or symptoms	Patients with hypertension, CAD, diabetes mellitus Patients using cardiotoxic agents Patients with family history of cardiomyopathy	Control systolic and diastolic hypertension. Counsel patient to avoid behaviors that increase risk of heart failure (alcohol, illicit drug use, smoking, inactivity). Treat lipid disorders. Control rate for tachydysrhythmias. Treat thyroid disease. Administer ACE inhibitors in patients with CAD, diabetes mellitus, or hypertension with associated cardiovascular risk factors.
B	Structural heart disease but has never developed symptoms of heart failure (asymptomatic left ventricular systolic dysfunction)	Patients with previous myocardial infarction, left ventricular systolic dysfunction, asymptomatic valvular disease	Follow stage A recommendations *plus* administer ACE inhibitors to patients with history of myocardial infarction or decreased EF. Administer beta-blockers to all patients with recent MI or decreased EF. Repair valve if indicated. Provide consistent follow-up care.
C	Past or current symptoms of heart failure associated with structural heart disease	Patients with known structural heart disease, dyspnea and fatigue, decreased exercise tolerance	Follow stage A and B recommendations *plus* administer diuretics if patient has fluid retention. Give ACE inhibitors and beta-blockers to all patients. Give digitalis to treat symptoms. Withdrawal of drugs adversely affects myocardium (NSAIDs, antidysrhythmics, calcium channel blockers).
D	End-stage disease with refractory heart failure requiring specialized interventions	Patients with marked symptoms at rest despite maximum medical therapy	Follow stage A, B, and C recommendations *plus* provide aggressive control of fluid retention. Perform heart transplantation when eligible. Refer patient to heart failure program for continuous inotropic infusions for palliation, ventricular assist device, or cardiac resynchronization therapy. Provide hospice care when indicated.

From Hunt SA et al: ACC/AHA guidelines for the evaluation and management of chronic heart failure in the adult: executive summary: a report of the American College of Cardiology/American Heart Association Task Force on Practice Guidelines (Committee to Revise the 1995 Guidelines for the Evaluation and Management of Heart Failure), *Circulation* 104:2996-3007, 2001.

ACE, Angiotensin-converting enzyme; *CAD*, coronary artery disease; *EF*, ejection fraction; *MI*, myocardial infarction; *NSAIDs*, nonsteroidal antiinflammatory drugs.

loop diuretics, thiazides, and potassium-sparing diuretics. Diuretics increase urinary output, causing a decrease in blood volume, preload, and ultimately cardiac workload. Diuretics can be administered intravenously to treat acute heart failure and orally for long-term management of fluid overload. Patients with chronic heart failure are likely to benefit from combination diuretic therapy. Electrolyte imbalance is a serious concern with both loop and thiazide diuretics, and can predispose the patient to dysrhythmias. Potassium-sparing diuretics such as spironolactone (Aldactone) block the remodeling and fibrotic effects of aldosterone on the myocardium, and are considered cardioprotective for NYHA class III and IV heart failure patients when used as an adjunct to conventional therapy. Hyperkalemia is a concern that must be monitored for closely.[47]

Box 30-7 Diagnostic Tests for Heart Failure

Chest Radiograph

Vascular congestion causes dense whitened areas.
Cardiomegaly is present in chronic heart failure from hypertrophy or dilation.
The presence of Kerley's B lines reflects lymphatic drainage of the overloaded pulmonary vessels.
The presence of liver congestion suggests right-sided heart failure.

Laboratory Tests

B-type natriuretic peptide:
—Concentrations of 80 pg/ml accurately diagnose heart failure.
—Elevated levels are associated with poorer outcomes.
Other common laboratory test findings are summarized in Table 30-2.

Electrocardiogram

This may be normal or reflect underlying cardiac pathologic condition.

Echocardiography

Echocardiography is the most useful test for evaluating heart failure.
Severity of heart failure is reflected in left ventricular ejection fraction (EF) and size:
—EF below 40% confirms left ventricular dysfunction.

Cardiac Catheterization

Diastolic dysfunction shows as an elevated end-diastolic pressure with normal and decreased ventricular volume
See Table 30-3 for a summary of hemodynamic findings in heart failure.

Other

Exercise stress testing can rule out coronary artery disease as a contributing factor in heart failure.
Multiple gated acquisition (MUGA) scanning accurately determines EF and assesses right ventricle.

Table 30-2 Common Laboratory Value Abnormalities With Heart Failure

Laboratory Value	Alteration	Rationale
Sodium	Decreased	Increased total body water dilutes body fluid
Chloride	Decreased	Associated with sodium loss
Potassium	Increased	Depressed effective renal blood flow and low glomerular filtration rate
Blood urea nitrogen	Increased	Decreased renal perfusion
Creatinine	Increased	Impaired renal function
Red blood cell count	Decreased	Decreased production of erythropoietin with renal involvement
Liver function tests	Increased	Hepatic congestion
PaO_2	Decreased	Fluid in alveoli limiting oxygen exchange
$PaCO_2$	Decreased	Compensatory increase in respiratory rate decreases carbon dioxide

Table 30-3 Altered Hemodynamic Findings in Heart Failure

Hemodynamic Variable	Finding in Heart Failure	Rationale
Cardiac output/index	Decreased	Systolic or diastolic dysfunction
Systemic vascular resistance	Increased	Compensate for decreased cardiac output
Pulmonary artery wedge pressure	Increased when left side of heart affected	End-diastolic pressure or volume in left ventricle increased because of inadequate emptying or inability to relax during diastole
Central venous pressure	Increased when right side of heart affected	Reflects increased pressure and volume within right side of heart

Beta-Blockers. Beta-blockers interrupt the negative effect of the SNS on the failing heart. They decrease the heart rate and allow more complete emptying of the LA, thereby improving left ventricular volume. Myocardial oxygen demand decreases along with the decrease in heart rate and contractility. Beta-blockers blunt neurohormonal mechanisms, decrease remodeling, improve overall myocardial function, and decrease dysrhythmias. Beta-blocker therapy is usually initiated once the patient is stabilized with ACE inhibitors and diuretic therapy.

Inotropes. Digitalis preparations remain the most widely prescribed inotropic agents. Digoxin, the most common form of digitalis, inhibits the sodium-potassium pump, increasing intracellular sodium levels. The excess sodium is forced out of the cell in exchange for calcium, increasing the force of contraction, increasing cardiac output, and decreasing end-diastolic pressure. Digoxin also blocks the slow calcium channels of the atrioventricular nodes, slowing the heart rate and increasing time for ventricular filling. In addition, digoxin blunts the neurohormonal

Box 30-8 Quality Indicators Endorsed by American Heart Association/American College of Cardiology for Management of Heart Failure

Medication Measures

Patients with heart failure, left ventricular systolic dysfunction, and no contraindications to angiotensin-converting enzyme (ACE) inhibitors should be prescribed ACE inhibitors. Angiotensin-receptor blockers or a hydralazine-nitrate combination should not be substituted for ACE inhibitors in patients who tolerate ACE inhibitors.

Patients hospitalized with heart failure and left ventricular systolic dysfunction should be treated with digoxin.

Patients with New York Hospital Association class II and III heart failure, left ventricular systolic dysfunction, and no contraindication to beta-blockers should be prescribed beta-blockers.

General Medical Interventions

Vaccinations against influenza and pneumonia

Anticoagulation to prevent emboli associated with atrial fibrillation

Evaluation of ischemia

Treatment of hyperlipidemia for coronary artery disease

From Krumholz HM et al: American Heart Association/American College of Cardiology First Scientific Forum on Assessment of Healthcare Quality in Cardiovascular Disease and Stroke: measuring and improving quality of care: a report of the Quality of Care and Outcomes Research Working Group on Heart Failure, *Circulation* 101(12):1483, 2000.

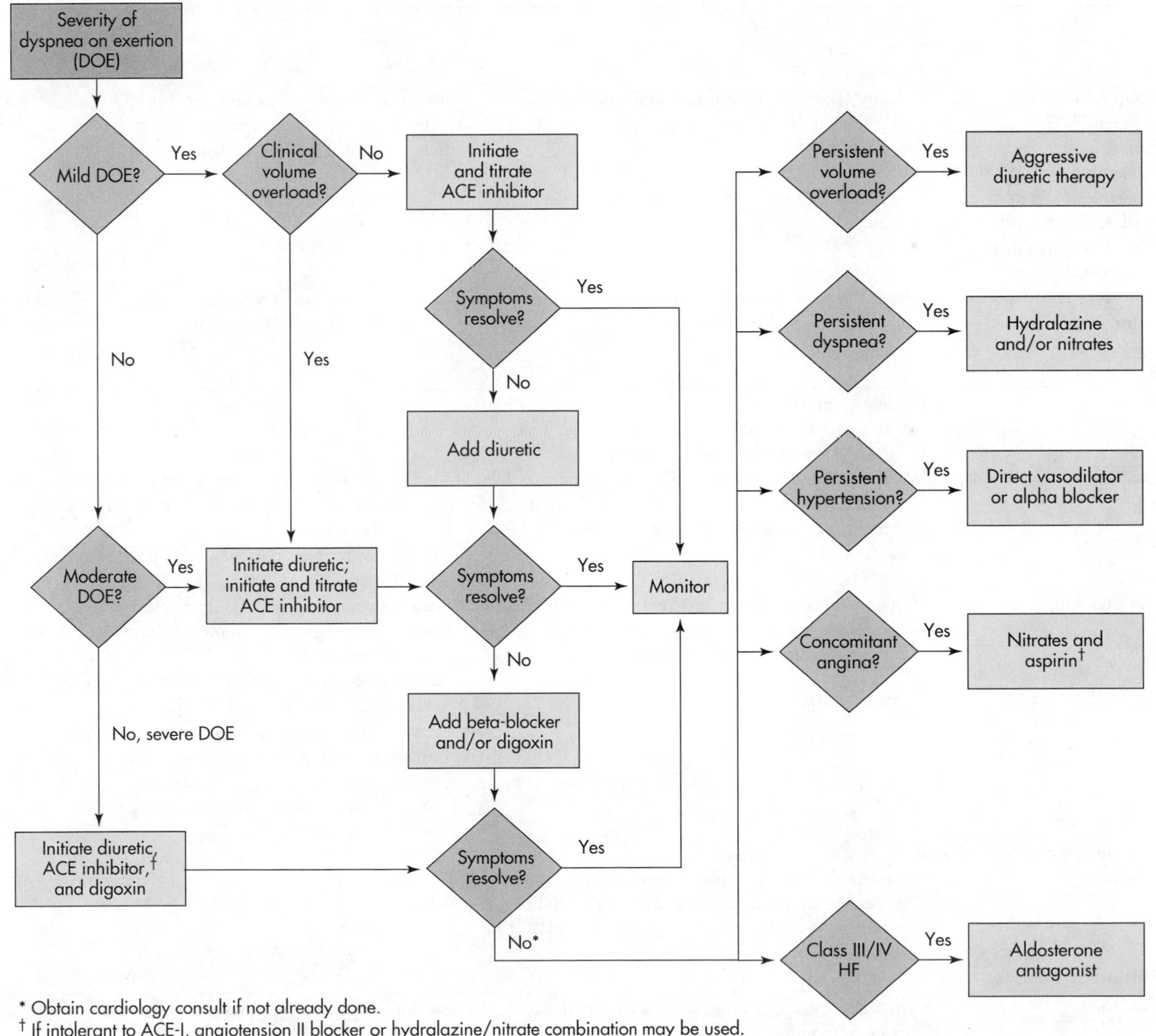

Figure 30-4 Algorithm for management of systolic heart failure *(HF)*. Class III/IV patients may require the addition of nesiritide to conventional therapy. *ACE*, Angiotensin-converting enzyme.

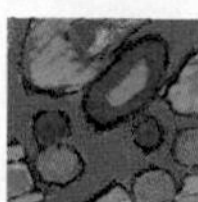

TABLE 30-4
COMMON MEDICATIONS *for Heart Failure*

Drug	Action	Nursing Intervention
Angiotensin-Converting Enzyme Inhibitors		
Captopril* Enalapril* Fosinopril* Lisinopril* Quinapril* Ramipril* Perindopril Benazepril* Trandolapril Moexipril	Block vasoconstriction and aldosterone, decreasing systemic vascular resistance, afterload, and preload	Be alert for presence of volume depletion from diuretics before initiating ACE inhibitor therapy (may need to correct hypovolemia before ACE inhibitor therapy). Closely monitor for hypotension at initiation of therapy; maintain patient on bed rest for 3 hr after initial dose. Monitor laboratory values for hyperkalemia, renal insufficiency (increasing blood urea nitrogen and creatinine), and neutropenia (decreasing white blood cell count). Be alert to side effects limiting compliance: cough, rash, and angioedema.
Diuretics		
	Decrease volume overload Increase urinary output Decrease preload	
Loop Diuretics Furosemide Bumetanide Torsemide	Enhance excretion of sodium, chloride, potassium, calcium, and magnesium	Monitor laboratory values for hypokalemia, hyperglycemia, hyperuricemia. Observe patient for postural hypotension and rashes.
Thiazides Hydrochlorothiazide Thiazide-related drug: metolazone	Block reabsorption of sodium, chloride, water in distal tubule	Same as for loop diuretics
Aldosterone Antagonists Spironolactone Eplerenone	Inhibit action of aldosterone, interfere with sodium reabsorption in distal tubule	Monitor for increasing potassium levels, especially when administered with ACE inhibitors.
Inotropes		
	Increase contractility Increase cardiac output Decrease left ventricular end-diastolic pressure	
Digoxin	Inhibits sodium-potassium pump, increasing intracellular calcium; slows heart rate by slowing conduction through atrioventricular node; blunts neurohormonal mechanisms	Be alert for cardiac dysrhythmias and clinical manifestations of toxicity (confusion, nausea, anorexia, visual disturbance). Monitor for hypokalemia, which can increase potential for toxicity.
Dobutamine	Stimulates beta$_1$-receptors, increases intracellular calcium and contractility; increases myocardial oxygen demand; decreases afterload; increases cardiac output	Record accurate weight for correct dose. Communicate signs and symptoms of hypovolemia when therapy initiated. Be alert to dysrhythmias that may require decrease in dose or discontinuation of therapy. Be aware of safe intravenous administration, including onset of action within 1 to 2 min, titrating dose to blood pressure and heart rate, tapering drip when discontinuing therapy, and monitoring site for infiltration.
Phosphodiesterase Inhibitors		
Milrinone	Vasodilates by relaxing vascular smooth muscle, decreasing afterload and preload; increases cardiac output by increasing cyclic adenosine monophosphate levels	Observe for chest pain, hypotension, dysrhythmias. Administer loading dose over 10 min. Note onset within 5 to 15 min.
Natriuretic Peptides		
Nesiritide	Vasodilates, causing reduced preload and afterload; promotes sodium-rich diuresis	Do not shake vial or infusion bag while mixing. Administer via infusion pump. Use caution if patient's systolic blood pressure is <90 mm Hg.

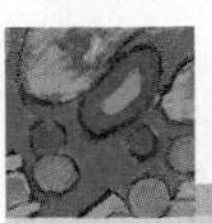

TABLE 30-4 COMMON MEDICATIONS *for Heart Failure—cont'd*

Drug	Action	Nursing Intervention
Beta-Blockers		
Metoprolol Carvedilol Bisoprolol	Blunt neurohormonal mechanisms Decrease oxygen demand Vasodilate by alpha$_1$-blockade	Initiate only after patients have been stabilized with conventional therapy (ACE inhibitors, diuretics, digoxin). Monitor for bradycardia, heart block, hypotension. Anticipate initial worsening of heart failure on initiation of therapy. Provide patient education, including support through initiation period and warnings not to stop medication abruptly.
Angiotensin II Receptor Blockers		
Losartan* Candesartan* Irbesartan Olmesartan Valsartan* Telmisartan Eprosartan	Produce direct antagonism of angiotensin II receptors	Monitor for adverse effects: dizziness, upper respiratory tract infection, hyperkalemia.
Vasodilators		
	Decrease cardiac workload Improve stroke volume and cardiac output	
Nitrates: isosorbide dinitrate	Venodilates, reducing preload	Monitor for headache and hypotension.
Hydralazine	Directly dilates arterioles, decreasing afterload	Monitor for headache, nausea, tachycardia, lupuslike syndrome.
Nitroprusside	Dilates arteries and veins; decreases left ventricular filling pressure	Monitor for severe hypotension, increased cyanide levels if prolonged.
Prazosin	Dilates arteries and veins	Monitor for dizziness, headache, hypotension.
Dopamine Agonist		
Dopamine	At low doses, stimulates dopaminergic receptors in renal vessels, increasing renal blood flow, increasing diuresis; increases myocardial contractility; vasodilates peripheral arterioles	Note onset of action within 10 min; monitor site for infiltration. If extravasation occurs, prepare phentolamine (Regitine) to infiltrate site. Titrate drip to blood pressure and urinary output. Taper dose when discontinuing. Use lowest dose possible to avoid increasing afterload.
Analgesics		
Morphine sulfate	Decreases anxiety Promotes venous pooling, decreasing preload and workload	Monitor vital signs before and after administration, with special attention to respiration depression. Evaluate effect on anxiety.
Anticoagulants		
Warfarin	Blocks synthesis of vitamin K–dependent clotting factors	Patients with history of systemic or pulmonary embolism or recent atrial fibrillation should be anticoagulated to an INR of 2-3. Communicate bleeding precautions and safety measures to all caregivers. Teach importance of follow-up coagulation studies, minimizing changes in intake of vitamin K, and safety to prevent bleeding.
Aspirin	Inhibits platelet aggregation	Avoid other medications that contain aspirin. Observe and report any signs of bleeding.

ACE, Angiotensin-converting enzyme; *INR,* international normalized ratio.
*Most often used.

mechanisms of heart failure, an action that is now believed to be the key to its effectiveness, as opposed to its ability to increase contractile force. Digoxin does not benefit all patients and can even be deleterious in diastolic dysfunction. It has not been shown to influence mortality rates.

Dobutamine (Dobutrex), a sympathomimetic agent, acts primarily on beta$_1$-receptors, stimulating cyclic adenosine monophosphate (cAMP), which increases intracellular calcium and results in a greater contractile force. The increase in cardiac output causes the body's sympathetic stimulation to decrease, slightly decreasing afterload. Milrinone (Primacor) blocks the activity of phosphodiesterase, which breaks down cAMP, resulting in an increase in contractility that improves stroke volume and cardiac output. Milrinone also increases vasodilator activity and relaxes smooth muscle, thereby decreasing both afterload and preload.

Natriuretic Peptides. Nesiritide (BNP) is the newest medication approved for patients with class III or IV heart failure. Nesiritide is a potent vasodilator that promotes diuresis and natriuresis, decreasing preload and vascular resistance. It also decreases plasma norepinephrine and aldosterone levels.[48]

Vasodilators. Nitrates dilate both arteries and veins when given intravenously, reducing cardiac workload. Nonparenteral nitrates predominantly affect the systemic veins, reducing preload. Hydralazine (Apresoline) is a direct arteriolar vasodilator that reduces afterload and therefore cardiac workload. Nitroprusside (Nipride) and prazosin (Minipress) also dilate both arteries and veins and can be given to stabilize patients with acute heart failure.

Adjunctive Pharmacologic Agents. Dopamine hydrochloride (Intropin) in low dosages (2 to 5 mcg/kg/min) may be used in combination with inotropes, vasodilators, or diuretics to treat heart failure. Low-dose dopamine stimulates dopaminergic receptors in the renal vessels, resulting in an increased renal blood flow and a more effective diuresis. The net result is an increase in cardiac output. Dosages between 5 and 10 mcg/kg/min may be used to increase myocardial contractility. Dosages above 10 mg/kg/min stimulate alpha-receptors, cause profound vasoconstriction, and are not used.

Morphine sulfate decreases anxiety and sympathetic stimulation and is used in acute episodes of heart failure. Morphine also promotes venodilation, reducing both preload and cardiac workload.

Supplemental oxygen is appropriate when inadequate gas exchange occurs, as evidenced by oxygen saturation levels below 90%. Mechanical ventilation may occasionally be necessary to reduce the work of breathing.

Heart failure can increase the risk of blood clots from stagnant blood flow. Anticoagulation is currently recommended for heart failure patients with a history of systemic or pulmonary embolism, recent onset of atrial fibrillation, or existing left ventricular thrombi. Low-dose aspirin therapy may be indicated for its antiplatelet activity.

Treatments. The goal of treatment for heart failure is to improve cardiac performance without increasing cardiac workload. Medications are the mainstay of treatment; however, adjunctive therapies are effective in specific patient populations.

Ventricular Assist Devices. In chronic heart failure beta-receptor responsiveness diminishes (downregulation), causing the heart's mechanisms to fail and medications to become ineffective. It then becomes necessary to decrease cardiac workload through nonpharmacologic devices such as the **intraaortic balloon pump** (IABP) and **ventricular assist device** (VAD). The IABP decreases afterload, thus decreasing the workload of the heart. It also increases coronary perfusion during diastole when the balloon inflates. The IABP is discussed in more detail later in this chapter.

Patients in low-output states or with a structural abnormality may require stabilization with a VAD. The VAD withdraws blood from the ventricle or atrium and infuses it directly into either the pulmonary or systemic circulation, thus resting the failing ventricle (Figure 30-5). In 2002 VADs were approved as "destination therapy" for patients with class IV heart failure; that is, they may be used in refractory heart failure without the patient having to be listed concomitantly for a heart transplant.[41] Before that time, VADs were only used as a bridge to transplantation. In addition to decreasing preload, reducing workload, and improving perfusion, VADs have also been shown to reverse remodeling in some individuals, leading to safe removal of the VAD. The device is surgically implanted in the left upper abdomen; sepsis, thromboembolism, and device failure are the most serious complications (see the Guidelines for Safe Practice box).

Cardiac Resynchronization Therapy. Abnormalities of the heart's conduction system are common in patients with heart failure. The most common abnormality is a left bundle branch block, which causes the RV to contract earlier than the LV. This asynchronous contraction is often severe enough to reduce the EF and worsen heart failure symptoms. Biventricular pacemakers pace both ventricles to contract simultaneously so as to resynchronize ventricular contractions, optimize LV filling, and improve cardiac output.[15] The delay in electrical conduction is decreased, resulting in a narrower, more normal QRS complex on the ECG tracing. Biventricular pacing is known as cardiac resynchronization therapy (CRT). CRT pacemakers have at least three leads: right atrial, right ventricular, and a third lead most often placed transvenously into the coronary sinus to pace the left side of the heart (Figure 30-6). The CRT device may also include an implantable cardioverter-defibrillator for patients who are at high risk for sudden death from ventricular tachycardia or ventricular fibrillation. Patient teaching related to CRT is included in the Patient/Family Teaching box.

Ultrafiltration. Patients with both heart failure and renal failure may benefit from ultrafiltration (hemofiltration) or hemodialysis to reduce blood volume.[39] The two primary methods of ultrafiltration are continuous arteriovenous hemofiltration (CAVH) and continuous arteriovenous hemofiltration and dialysis (CAVHD). Patients who are hypotensive and are receiving maximal inotrope support can seldom tolerate removal of large fluid volumes through hemodialysis. For these patients, CAVH or CAVHD may be appropriate alternatives.

Continuous Positive Airway Pressure. Continuous positive airway pressure (CPAP) is beneficial in patients with obstructive sleep apnea, a condition common in patients with heart failure. CPAP may also have cardiovascular benefits, including

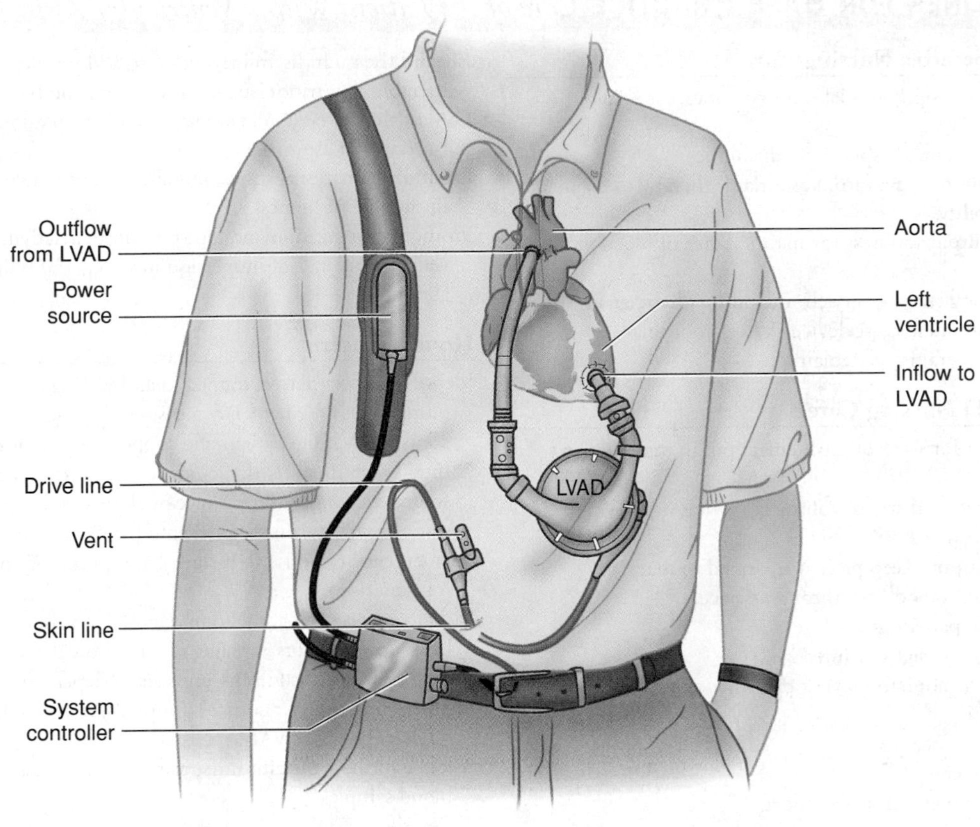

Figure 30-5 Patient with a left ventricular assist device *(LVAD)*.

reduction of preload, afterload, and blood pressure and improvement in cardiac output. CPAP may also help slow ventricular remodeling, although the mechanism of action is not understood.[5]

SURGICAL MANAGEMENT. Surgical interventions can reverse the course of heart failure arising from some causes. Corrective surgeries include pericardiectomy, valve replacements or valvuloplasty, surgical repair of septal defects, and ventricular aneurysmectomies. Revascularization through coronary artery bypass graft (CABG) surgery may also benefit patients who have severe angina, although the surgery is accompanied by significant morbidity and mortality.

In progressive heart failure, transplantation may be the only option. Ischemic heart disease and dilated cardiomyopathies account for the majority of cardiac transplant procedures. Survival rates are good and remain steady at 70% at 5 years (see p. 853). Criteria for heart transplantation continue to change as surgical experience improves. The primary limiting factor is the availability of donor hearts. Because of this shortage, new treatment strategies such as stem cell infusions are being researched (see Future Watch box). Surgical strategies under investigation include endoventricular circular patch plasty (Dor procedure), which replaces nonfunctional myocardium with a patch; myosplints, passive synthetic restraints with epicardial pacing; and an acorn cardiac support device that reshapes the heart to promote the reversal of remodeling. Surgeries that have met with limited success include partial left ventriculectomy (reduction ventriculoplasty) and dynamic cardiomyoplasty, which involves wrapping the myocardium with the latissimus dorsi muscle.

DIET. A "no–added salt" diet is recommended for patients with mild heart failure. This diet eliminates salt in food preparation and avoids obviously salted foods. Diets restricted to 2 g of sodium daily decrease extracellular water and blood volume. Sodium restrictions of less than 2 g/day are rarely ordered because the diet is unpalatable, resulting in poor patient adherence. The use of salt substitutes requires careful attention to potassium content if patients are taking potassium-sparing diuretics. Teaching emphasizes foods that are permitted on the sodium-restricted diet. A printed list of foods permitted and foods to avoid goes home with the patient and family.

Fluid restrictions may also be necessary for patients with acute or chronic heart failure. Such restrictions consider the patient's weight fluctuations, intake and output ratios, and electrolyte status. When teaching about fluid restrictions, the nurse educates the patient about what counts as fluid intake, including Jell-O, ice cream, pudding, and sauces. Fluid restrictions are often unnecessary. For patients with diuretic-induced thirst, an upper limit of 64 oz (2 L) daily is an appropriate guideline. The nurse teaches the

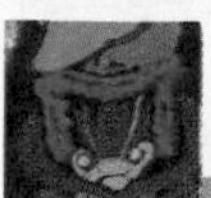

GUIDELINES FOR SAFE PRACTICE *Care of the Patient With a Ventricular Assist Device*

Immediate Postoperative Nursing Care

Frequently monitor vital signs and laboratory values, especially coagulation status.
Administer prophylactic broad-spectrum antibiotics.
Provide intravenous inotropes and/or vasodilator therapy to maintain hemodynamic stability.
Monitor input and output to assess for maintenance of blood volume and regular voiding.
Take a multidisciplinary team approach, including physicians, transplant and ventricular assist device (VAD) coordinator, nurses, respiratory therapists, chaplain.

Ongoing Post-VAD Nursing Care

Continuously monitor for signs of mechanical pump malfunction or failure.
Record pump rate, flow, and stroke volume and vital signs every 12 hours.
Monitor input and output. Keep patient hydrated to maintain adequate volume and blood flow through device.
Keep hand pump with patient at all times.
Continuously monitor for signs of infection.
Use sterile dressing technique to prevent driveline or power source infection.
Stabilize driveline entry site.
Maintain personal hygiene.
Provide psychosocial and emotional support.
Expand the multidisciplinary team to add physical or occupational therapists, nutritionists, social workers, and home health workers.
Prevent thromboembolic events via anticoagulation specific to device (warfarin or aspirin).
Optimize nutritional status; initially patient may need tube feeding until sense of fullness abates.
Promote mobilization and return to normal activities. Encourage daily walks, avoidance of immersion in water, and blunt trauma to abdomen.

Home Concerns

Identify support person trained in and willing to provide hand pumping as an emergency measure. This person must pass a training course. Teach the patient and support person how to change the vent filter (keep the filter dry, clean, and unobstructed), battery to power source exchanges, significance of alarms, safety precautions (water, static electricity, no magnetic resonance imaging), dressing care, and emergency response to include hand pumping (no cardiopulmonary resuscitation).
Visually inspect the home for electrical hazards, electrical support, back-up generators, labeling of circuit breakers.
Notify local electrical utility of patient's dependence on VAD.
Identify community resources (hospitals, first responders) with knowledge of the VAD.
Arrange for home health nurse as needed to assess VAD site, obtain blood samples.

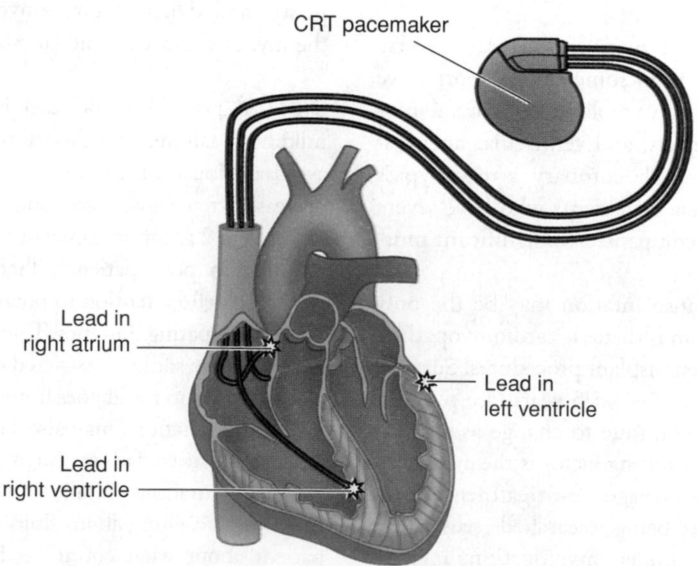

Figure 30-6 Cardiac resynchronization therapy *(CRT)*.

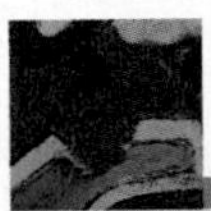

PATIENT/FAMILY TEACHING *The Patient Undergoing Cardiac Resynchronization Therapy*

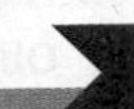

Preprocedure

Teach difference in purpose between a standard pacemaker and cardiac resynchronization therapy (CRT). Goal is to decrease heart failure symptoms and increase activity tolerance.

If implantable defibrillator is planned, explain purpose of device and what a shock would feel like (see Chapter 29).

Explain purpose of contrast agent when used for transvenous placement and prophylactic measures such as acetylcysteine for high creatinine levels and steroids and diphenhydramine for possible allergic reactions if known contrast allergy.

Advise patients that they will be given medication to relax them and control pain during the procedure.

Postprocedure

Remind patient to ask for analgesia as needed.

Explain purpose of prophylactic antibiotics.

Keep incision dry for 10 days. Teach patient signs and symptoms of infection.

Instruct patient to avoid arm movement above shoulder for 2 weeks and to avoid lifting more than 10 pounds for 1 month.

Remind patient of need to resume anticoagulation therapy as prescribed after 48 hours.

Discharge Instructions

Teach patient to:

- Keep scheduled clinic appointments.
- Call health care provider for tachycardia, near syncope, shocks.
- Use cell phones on opposite side from implant.
- Carry identification card.
- Avoid security wand screening at airports.
- Contact cardiologist before invasive procedures, such as electrocautery.
- Avoid magnetic fields, including magnetic resonance imaging.
- Refrain from driving until cleared by physician (may be up to 6 months).
- Avoid sports with vigorous arm extension.
- Avoid high altitudes.

patient alternatives to satisfy thirst, such as sugarless hard candy, Popsicles, and ice chips.

Supervised weight loss programs are indicated for obese patients with heart failure. Other patients may need nutritional supplementation because of cachexia-related weight loss. Albumin levels may decrease as a result of nutritional deficiencies and fluid overload. Serum albumin levels below 3 g/dl indicate malnutrition and require further assessment and intervention. Alcohol is restricted to one drink per day, defined as one glass of beer or wine or a mixed drink containing no more than 1 oz of alcohol. Minimizing caffeine intake is advisable for patients with tachycardic heart rhythms.

HEALTH PROMOTION AND PREVENTION. One of the 16 *Healthy People 2010* objectives related to heart disease and stroke is specifically targeted at reducing hospitalizations related to heart failure (see Healthy People 2010 box). Effective disease management and the prevention of disease progression and complications are the keys to achieving this goal. Patient and family education is a critical strategy and begins at the time of diagnosis. A multidisciplinary approach demands the effective use of appropriate specialists and careful coordination of their services. Patients and families are taught about the disease itself; recommended diet and activity modifications; safe and appropriate use of all medications; and other general strategies such as effective control of concurrent illnesses (e.g., hypertension, CAD, and diabetes), stress management, and preventive measures such as smoking cessation and the annual flu vaccine. Patient education is discussed further under Nursing Management.

The complexity of heart failure requires a team approach to care. Multidisciplinary health care professionals collaborate with the patient and family to improve quality of life. Advanced practice nurses can make substantial contributions to the effective management of patients with heart failure. All health care professionals emphasize the importance of follow-up and regimen adherence. Patients must be able to recognize risks for decompensation and the early associated signs and symptoms. Adherence directly affects mortality, and lack of adherence is a major cause of

Future Watch

Stem Cells and Heart Failure

Stem cells are cells at an early stage of maturation that are capable of becoming any specific type of cell. Researchers at the Texas Heart Institute and two hospitals in Rio de Janeiro successfully performed stem cell transplants on 14 Brazilian patients with end-stage ischemic heart disease. Bone marrow mononuclear cells were harvested from each of these patients' bone marrow and then transplanted into the myocardium after 4 hours. The stem cells were introduced by a femoral catheter directly into the left ventricle. The weakest areas of the heart were identified and directly injected with the cells. Each patient received an average of 15 injections, with approximately 2 million stem cells per injection. There were no procedural complications, and the patients were discharged after 3 days.

In comparison with a group of seven control patients, those patients injected with the stem cells had a significantly lower incidence of heart failure and angina after 2 months. Noninvasive studies showed less ischemia with improvement in global left ventricular function. Invasive studies at 4 months showed an improved ejection fraction and a reduction in end-systolic volume. Serum creatinine and B-type natriuretic peptide levels were relatively higher in the control patients. Researchers cannot explain the exact mechanism responsible for the improvement, but believe that the stem cells either become new blood vessels and heart muscle cells or stimulate the heart to develop new blood vessels and myocardial cells.

Perin EC et al: Transendocardial, autologous bone marrow cell transplantation for severe, chronic ischemic heart failure, *Circulation* 107(18):2294-2302, 2003.

Healthy People 2010

Objectives for Heart Failure

Reduce hospitalizations of older adults with congestive heart failure as the principal diagnosis.

- *Adults Ages 65-74 Years:* Reduce hospitalizations from the 1997 rate of 13.2 per 1000 population to a 2010 target of 6.5 per 1000 population.
- *Adults Ages 75-84 Years:* Reduce hospitalizations from the 1997 rate of 26.7 per 1000 population to a 2010 target of 13.5 per 1000 population.
- *Adults Ages 85 Years and Older:* Reduce hospitalizations from the 1997 rate of 52.7 per 1000 population to a 2010 target of 26.5 per 1000 population.

From US Department of Health and Human Services: *Healthy people 2010: understanding and improving health,* Washington, DC, 2000, The Department.

hospitalization. The nurse discusses the importance of adherence and assists the patient in removing barriers such as knowledge deficits, self-confidence, cost, side effects, and complexity of protocols. Family and social support is critical in helping the patient sustain a commitment to heart failure management. Caregivers need special attention and should never be made to feel like outsiders. Telehealth is increasingly used to provide the needed follow-up and support to patients with heart failure.

Nursing Management *of the Patient with Heart Failure*

ASSESSMENT

Health History. Assess for:

- History of current episode (onset, duration)
- Paroxysmal nocturnal dyspnea (frequency, severity, duration)
- Orthopnea (frequency, severity, self-treatment)
- New-onset dyspnea on exertion (related activities, severity)
- Fatigue (severity, duration, self-treatment)
- Lower extremity edema
- Persistent cough
- Recent weight gain (documented or perceived, appetite changes)
- Presence of comorbid health conditions, treatment
- Medications in use (prescription, over the counter, natural products)
- Diet and activity history
- Concerns and anxieties of the patient and significant others and the effectiveness of support systems

Physical Examination. Assess for:

- Presence of third heart sound
- Respiratory distress, including increased effort and respiratory rate
- Pulmonary crackles
- Elevated jugular venous pressure
- Peripheral edema (severity)
- Increase in daily weight without increased intake
- Abdominal distention
- Cool extremities and decreased pulses
- Alterations in level of consciousness
- Decreased urinary output

NURSING DIAGNOSES, OUTCOMES, AND INTERVENTIONS

Nursing Diagnosis: Impaired Gas Exchange

OUTCOMES. Common examples of expected outcomes for the patient with a diagnosis of *impaired gas exchange* are:

Patient will:

- Have a resting pulse oximetry above 90% or have values that are consistent with baseline.
- Be eupneic, without respiratory distress.
- Have lungs clear to auscultation, or at baseline.
- Have pink skin and mucous membranes.

NURSING INTERVENTIONS. The less effective oxygenation of the blood as it passes through the congested lungs greatly reduces the oxygen content of the blood. The patient may be more comfortable and better able to rest while receiving oxygen because it helps reduce dyspnea and fatigue. Oxygen is usually administered by nasal cannula at 2 to 6 L/min.

The nurse positions the patient in a semi-Fowler's position; encourages the use of the incentive spirometer; and teaches relaxed, controlled breathing to improve gas exchange. The nurse also monitors the patient's respiratory rate, depth, and ease; breath sounds; skin color; and pulse oximetry to evaluate improvement or deterioration in gas exchange.

Mechanical ventilation is necessary when the work of breathing significantly increases cardiopulmonary demands. However, because of the complications associated with mechanical ventilation in patients with heart failure, alternatives such as noninvasive positive pressure ventilation may be considered as a first-line attempt.

RELATED NIC INTERVENTIONS. Airway Management, Oxygen Therapy, Respiratory Monitoring

Nursing Diagnosis: Ineffective Tissue Perfusion

OUTCOMES. Common examples of expected outcomes for the patient with a diagnosis of *ineffective tissue perfusion* are:

Patient will:

- Have improved hemodynamic parameters (cardiac output, central venous pressure, pulmonary artery wedge pressure, blood pressure, and heart rate), or parameters that remain at baseline.
- Have improved peripheral pulses, capillary refill time, and skin temperature, or parameters that remain at baseline.
- Be free of signs of systemic circulatory insufficiency (hepatomegaly, nausea, dependent edema), or signs consistent with baseline.

NURSING INTERVENTIONS. The nurse actively works to improve existing alterations in cardiac output by reducing cardiac workload, promoting venous return, and minimizing myocardial oxygen requirements. Interventions include placing the patient in a semi-Fowler's position or position of comfort; avoiding Valsalva's maneuver, which triggers abrupt changes in venous return to the heart; and promoting a calm, quiet, comfortable environment.

Maintaining safe and effective IV access is important in the management of patients with heart failure who require cardioactive IV medications and frequent blood work analysis. Ongoing assessments focus on identifying changes in cardiac output and include vital signs, hemodynamic parameters, telemetry monitoring, heart sounds, level of consciousness, presence and severity of edema, peripheral temperature, capillary refill, urinary output, and laboratory values. With acute heart failure, assessments occur hourly or even more frequently while medications are being adjusted. When the patient stabilizes, the frequency of assessments becomes a nursing judgment.

Anorexia may occur when venous engorgement affects the gastrointestinal system. The nurse helps the patient select a diet that meets baseline nutrient needs so that catabolism does not occur. Smaller, more frequent meals reduce stress on the gastrointestinal tract. The nurse also uses this opportunity to discuss the no-added salt diet, enlisting the assistance of a nutritionist if appropriate. It is important to involve the family in all discussions related to recommended changes in diet. The use of stool softeners minimizes the risk of Valsalva's maneuvers. Increasing fiber in the diet as a measure to avoid constipation may not be well tolerated by some patients with heart failure because of intestinal edema and bloating.

RELATED NIC INTERVENTIONS. Fluid Monitoring, Nutrition Management, Vital Signs Monitoring

Nursing Diagnosis: Excess Fluid Volume

OUTCOMES. Common examples of expected outcomes for the patient with a diagnosis of *excess fluid volume* are:
Patient will:

- Have urinary output greater than 30 ml/hr (exception: renal failure).
- Have a balanced intake and output (or as prescribed).
- Have a stable weight.
- Adhere to sodium and fluid restrictions.

NURSING INTERVENTIONS. The nurse works with the patient to determine how to best manage fluid and sodium restrictions. The physician orders the total amount of fluid permitted, and the nurse and patient develop a schedule that divides the fluid allowance throughout the day according to patient preferences. The nurse ensures that all IV medications are administered in the minimal acceptable volume to prevent unnecessary fluid intake.

Assessment of fluid balance is ongoing. Parameters include peripheral edema; intake and output; laboratory values for sodium, potassium, blood urea nitrogen (BUN), and creatinine; and diuretic response to administered medications. The nurse records the patient's weight daily with the patient in similar clothing, using the same scale, with an empty bladder, and before eating. Weight gain indicates fluid retention: 1 kg of weight gain represents 1 L of retained fluid. The frequency of assessment can decrease as the patient's condition stabilizes.

Patients with pitting edema may be at risk for skin breakdown caused by poor nourishment of the skin and cracks in the skin surfaces. The nurse appropriately positions the patient to minimize pressure points and shearing. Positioning is especially important for the patient confined to bed and at risk for the development of sacral edema. Skin care includes gentle cleansing and the application of lotion to decrease disruptions in skin integrity. The use of 4-inch foam and other pressure-relieving mattresses is a standard preventive intervention.

RELATED NIC INTERVENTIONS. Fluid Monitoring, Electrolyte Monitoring, Hypervolemia Management, Skin Surveillance

Nursing Diagnosis: Activity Intolerance

OUTCOMES. Common examples of expected outcomes for the patient with a diagnosis of *activity intolerance* are:
Patient will:

- Tolerate a progressive increase in activity and accomplish activities of daily living (ADLs) with decreased dyspnea.
- Demonstrate appropriate heart rate and blood pressure responses to exercise.

NURSING INTERVENTIONS. Patients with heart failure often experience severe fatigue and have little ability to perform even basic ADLs. Dyspnea often limits the amount of activity the patient tolerates. Bed rest reduces myocardial oxygen demand during acute episodes of heart failure while medications are being adjusted and until the severity of symptoms resolves. The nurse organizes the environment to limit myocardial oxygen demand by providing a bedside commode, placing toiletry and other items within easy reach, and assisting with ADLs as needed.

As the acute stage resolves, the patient gradually progresses to sitting, walking in the room, and finally walking in the hall. The nurse helps the patient space activities and avoids the hour after meals when gastrointestinal perfusion needs are greatest. The nurse monitors the patient's ability to tolerate activity by evaluating pulse and blood pressure response to activity and the absence of symptoms. Fatigue and dizziness may occur in some patients receiving aggressive diuretic therapy.

The patient's ability to tolerate activity while hospitalized guides the discharge activity prescription. An explanation of the importance of exercise can encourage patients to gradually return to daily activities. Patients with EFs as low as 13% can safely exercise without experiencing exercise-related complications or adversely affecting cardiac output or wall motion.[2] Heart failure patients without ischemia receive detailed exercise prescriptions that include activity frequency, intensity, type, and duration. Patients with heart failure need to recognize their individual tolerance levels for physical activity and limit activity until their symptoms resolve. Cardiac rehabilitation programs are especially beneficial for patients who are anxious about exercising on their own. Walking on level surfaces at least four times a week is a reasonable alternative to a structured outpatient exercise program. The nurse teaches the patient to discontinue walking if the heart rate increases by more than 20 beats/min or if chest discomfort, excessive fatigue, severe shortness of breath, or syncope occur. Pacing activities to decrease myocardial oxygen demand is the guiding principle. Patients with heart failure and ongoing ischemia may need to undergo revascularization before beginning a conditioning program.

At times, successful home management after discharge can be achieved through the use of support systems such as services to deliver nutritional meals or supplemental education about the proper use of mobility aids (e.g., bedside commodes, shower seats) to decrease cardiac workload. The nurse explores the patient's home support network and initiates referrals to community agencies as appropriate.

Nursing interventions that promote restful sleep help ensure that the patient can meet the challenges of increasing activity. These interventions include offering back rubs, providing comfortable bedding, closing doors, turning off televisions and phones, decreasing alarm volumes, minimizing bright lights, and promoting quiet conversations. Sedatives may be beneficial in the acute care setting (see Research box).

Alterations in sexual activity may occur as a result of the patient's activity intolerance and the limitations of the disease process (hypoperfusion, fatigue), medications, depression, fear, or altered body image. The nurse supports partner communication and provides honest information about drug side effects, counseling the patient concerning energy conservation measures, positioning, and the atmosphere for sexual intercourse.

RELATED NIC INTERVENTIONS. Energy Management, Exercise Promotion, Self-Care Assistance, Sleep Enhancement

Research

Erickson VS et al: Sleep disturbance symptoms in patients with heart failure, *AACN Clin Issues: Adv Practice Acute Crit Care* 14(4):477-487, 2003.

Researchers surveyed 84 heart failure (HF) patients to determine the presence of sleep disturbances in this population. Each patient completed a sleep survey during a regularly scheduled clinic visit. Patients were asked to indicate the presence of 16 common sleep disturbances, such as unable to sleep flat, stop breathing, wake with anxiety, and wake with choking feeling. Six additional items addressed specific hours of sleep, naps, and the use of medications. Seventy percent of the patients were men with a mean age of 54 years and a mean left ventricular ejection fraction of 22%. Ischemia was the cause of HF in 45% of patients; obesity was present in 39%; 8.3% were self-identified smokers; and 13.3% were taking beta-blockers. (The authors noted that the sample was obtained before the increased emphasis on beta-blockers in the management of HF.)

Fifty-six percent of the patients reported trouble sleeping. The authors noted this percentage is similar to that with other chronic disease states, such as hypertension, diabetes, arthritis, and depression. The most frequently reported problems were inability to sleep flat (51%), restless sleep (44%), trouble falling asleep (40%), awakening early (39%), restless legs (38%), trouble returning to sleep (32%), being a light sleeper (32%), and needing to use sleeping pills (32%). Of those reporting the use of medication, benzodiazepines, zolpidem (Ambien), and antidepressants were the medications used most often. Severity of HF, age, gender, etiology, obesity, smoking, and the use of beta-blockers were tested as predictors of sleep disturbance. No variables were found to be significant predictors. The authors suggest that without significant predictors of sleep disturbance in this population, nurses must be vigilant in assessing patients for sleep disturbances to identify concerns and intervene appropriately.

Nursing Diagnosis: Hopelessness

OUTCOMES. Common examples of expected outcomes for the patient with a diagnosis of *hopelessness* are:

Patient will:

- Demonstrate initiative and self-direction in decision making.
- Express confidence in the future.

NURSING INTERVENTIONS. Heart failure is a chronic illness with a poor prognosis. Patients need counseling regarding the effects of heart failure on self-concept and role performance. Approximately one in five people with heart failure suffers clinical depression (see Research box). Quality of life remains a priority, and the nurse encourages patients to be active, using energy conservation guidelines to promote optimal functioning. The patient with heart failure needs support in learning to accept uncertainty in life.[34] Patient teaching includes techniques for stress management, relaxation strategies, and support groups.

The nurse involves the patient and family in the management plan and discussion of prognosis. Patients with heart failure are encouraged to complete advance directives concerning their health care preferences. All individuals involved in the patient's care need updates on these preferences.

Research

Havranek EP et al: Predictors of the onset of depressive symptoms in patients with heart failure, *J Am College Cardiol* 44(12):2333-2338, 2004.

Researchers at 14 outpatient clinics studied 245 patients prospectively for the development of depression. All patients had ejection fractions less then 40%, were older than 30 years of age, had been diagnosed with heart failure (HF), and were without depressive symptoms at baseline. Patients completed two questionnaires (the Medical Outcomes Study-Depression [MOS-D] questionnaire and a Kansas City Cardiomyopathy Questionnaire [KCCQ]) and received a full clinical evaluation, including an assessment of social and economic status. The MOS-D does not assess somatic symptoms that are common in HF; therefore this tool was chosen as a screening tool for depression with this population. The KCCQ is specific to patients with HF and measures symptoms, physical function, social function, self-efficacy, and quality of life.

At 1-year follow-up, 21.2% of the 245 patients without depressive symptoms at baseline had developed significant depressive symptoms. Patients who developed depressive symptoms were nearly twice as likely to live alone. Other independent predictors of depressive symptoms included alcohol abuse, perception of medical care as an economic burden, and KCCQ scores indicative of poor function. Patients without any of these four factors had a 7.9% incidence of new depression. When one factor was present, the 1-year incidence was 15.5%, when two were present the incidence was 36.2%, and when three were present the incidence was 69.2%. No patient had all four factors. The authors noted that living alone as a predictor of depression was unique to this HF population when compared with other populations where predictors of depression have been studied (postmyocardial infarction, general population). The authors suggest all patients with HF should be screened for depression, and sequential screening should be initiated for those with any of the four predictors identified in this study.

RELATED NIC INTERVENTIONS. Emotional Support, Hope Instillation, Presence, Support Group

Patient/Family Teaching. The Guidelines for Safe Practice box summarizes the major components of the care plan for a patient with heart failure, which serves as the foundation for teaching (see the Patient/Family Teaching box, p. 832). The nurse must provide a large amount of information and uses a variety of educational strategies to help the patient and family learn. An explanation of heart failure and its probable cause is the foundation for teaching. The nurse teaches the patient signs and symptoms, what to do if symptoms worsen, and the importance of self-monitoring for symptoms (including daily weights).

The nurse carefully reviews the safe use of all medications, including purpose and side effects. The nurse works with the physician and patient to schedule medications to minimize the disruption of daily routines. Administering diuretics in the morning minimizes sleep disturbances but may not be compatible with employment demands. Using individualized algorithms, many patients can be taught to adjust their diuretic dose (and electrolyte supplementation) to weight fluctuations. The patient on ACE-inhibitor or spironolactone therapy should avoid potassium-containing salt substitutes. The nurse teaches the patient taking digoxin about the signs and symptoms of toxicity. Because of the potential for heart failure to initially worsen with the initiation of beta-blocker therapy, the nurse provides the patient with established parameters for when to seek care. The nurse cautions patients to avoid all over-the-counter and prescription medications, especially NSAIDs and alternative medications such as herbal products, without first consulting their primary care provider.[14]

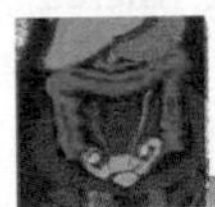

GUIDELINES FOR SAFE PRACTICE
The Patient With Heart Failure

- Support oxygenation:
  —Administer oxygen by nasal cannula at 2 to 6 L/min for oxygen saturation greater than 90%.
  —Give oxygen as needed for dyspnea.
  —Patient should be well supported in a semi-Fowler's position.
  —Encourage use of incentive spirometry every 4 hours.
- Balance rest and activity:
  —Reinforce importance of energy conservation and planning for activities to avoid fatigue.
  —Encourage activity within prescribed restrictions; monitor for intolerance to activity (dyspnea, fatigue, increased pulse rate that does not stabilize).
  —Assist with activities of daily living as necessary; encourage independence within patient's limitations.
  —Provide diversional activities that assist in conservation of energy.
  —Provide a calm, quiet environment.
- Perform head-to-toe assessment each shift, including laboratory values, daily weights, and intake and output.
- Provide skin care, particularly over edematous areas; use prophylactic measures to prevent skin breakdown.
- Assist in maintaining an adequate nutritional intake while observing prescribed dietary modifications (offer smaller meals with supplements).
- Monitor for constipation; give prescribed stool softeners.
- Give prescribed medications and monitor for adverse effects.
- Provide patient and family opportunities to discuss their concerns and time to learn about the diagnosis and care plan.

EVALUATION

To evaluate the effectiveness of nursing interventions, compare patient behaviors with those stated in the expected patient outcomes.

RELATED NOC OUTCOMES. Acceptance: Health Status, Activity Tolerance, Appetite, Cardiac Pump Effectiveness, Fluid Balance, Fluid Overload Severity, Hope, Respiratory Status: Gas Exchange, Self-Care Status, Urinary Elimination

GERONTOLOGIC CONSIDERATIONS

Alarmingly, heart failure is now the most common Medicare diagnosis-related group, and more Medicare spending is devoted to heart failure management than to any other diagnostic group.[20] Heart failure is the most common cause of hospitalization in patients over 65 years of age. Older patients with heart failure may not exhibit the common clinical manifestations of dyspnea, crackles (rales), and edema. Confusion, fatigue, and failure to thrive may be the only clinical manifestations.[26]

Primary health care providers make adjustments in medications to account for the physiologic changes seen in older patients. Nurses caution older patients to make position changes slowly while taking diuretics, since they may not be able to adapt quickly to venous pooling. Older patients are also especially sensitive to the first-dose hypotensive effect of ACE inhibitors. When even mild renal impairment is present, older adults may develop acute renal insufficiency. The nurse monitors BUN, creatinine, and potassium routinely when older patients are taking ACE inhibitors and diuretics. The routine use of NSAIDs by the older population decreases the effectiveness of ACE inhibitors. All older patients taking digoxin must be carefully monitored for signs and symptoms of toxicity because of their increased risk for toxicity from decreased renal function and lean body mass. In addition, simple tasks such as daily weights can be more challenging to older persons. They may need special scales for standing and large numbers for reading.

Older individuals may not adhere to their medication regimen for a multitude of reasons, including cognition, sensory perception, lack of social support, inadequate financial resources, and lack of motivation. A multidisciplinary approach for follow-up care after discharge can reduce the rate of readmission for this population. Older patients with heart failure who follow up with nurse practitioner clinics and home health care nurses have significantly fewer exacerbations than patients not managed by these professionals. All health care providers must consider the impact of physiologic changes associated with aging, including sensory and motor deficits and comorbid processes, on the willingness and capacity of older patients to adhere to the heart failure regimen.

Cardiomyopathy

Etiology and Epidemiology. The term **cardiomyopathy** (CMP) refers to a group of heart muscle disorders that impair the structural or functional abilities of the myocardium. CMP may occur as a primary disorder or secondary to another disease process. CMP is most commonly caused by irreversible damage from ischemic heart disease, but may also result from genetic factors, viral infections, or toxins (such as alcohol).[7] CMP causes specific progressive structural changes within the myocardium. There are three major categories of CMP: dilated CMP, hypertrophic CMP, and restrictive CMP (Figure 30-7).

In dilated CMP the LV dilates but does not experience a proportional increase in contractility. Possible causes for dilated CMP include ischemia, damage from inflammatory processes, toxins such as ethanol and chemotherapy, or heredity. Longstanding hypertension and valve disorders also contribute to the development of dilated CMP.

Hypertrophic CMP refers to a dilated, hypertrophied, and hypercontractile ventricle. Hypertrophic CMP may represent a defect of muscle development and therefore may have a hereditary component.[13] *Hypertrophic obstructive cardiomyopathy* (HOCM) is the term used when the septum hypertrophies asymmetrically, obstructing left ventricular ejection.

Restrictive CMP occurs when the LV is of normal or small size and the muscle mass is normal or increased (Table 30-5). Infiltrative and proliferative disorders such as amyloidosis and sarcoidosis are common causes for restrictive CMP. CMP is classified as idiopathic when a specific etiology cannot be identified.

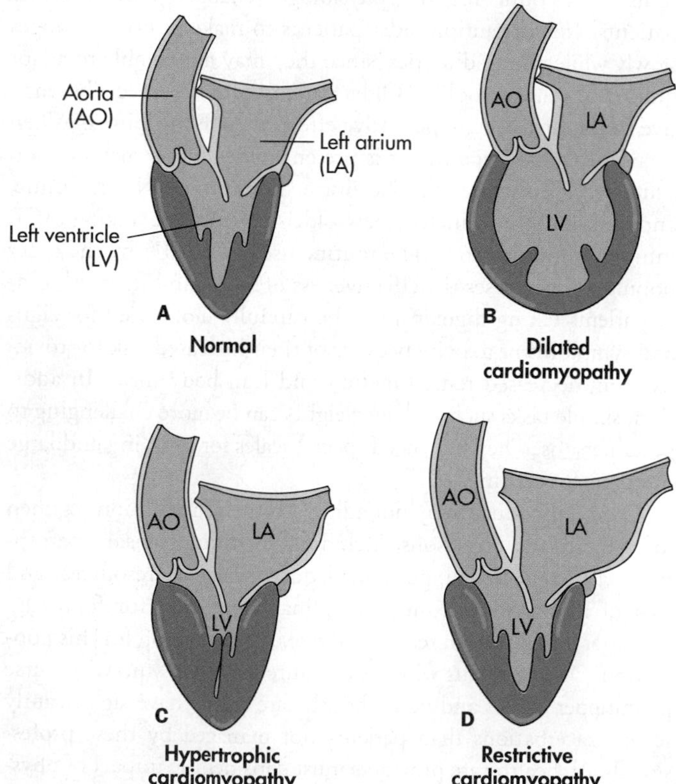

Figure 30-7 Major distinguishing pathophysiologic features of three types of cardiomyopathy. **A,** Normal heart. **B,** In dilated cardiomyopathy, heart has a globular shape and the largest circumference of the left ventricle is not at its base but midway between apex and base. **C,** In hypertrophic type, wall of left ventricle is greatly thickened; left ventricular cavity is small, but left atrium may be dilated because of poor diastolic relaxation of ventricle. **D,** In restrictive (constrictive) type, left ventricular cavity is of normal size but, again, left atrium is dilated because of reduced diastolic compliance of ventricle.

Pathophysiology. In dilated CMP the ventricular chamber dilates in response to constant stress. Dilation of the LV increases its volume capacity (increased compliance). The stretching of the myocardial fibers, however, displaces the sarcomeres beyond the limits of the Starling curve. As a result, optimal cross-linkages for contractility do not occur, decreasing contractility. Fibrosis can also inhibit the ability to contract. Therefore in dilated CMP the patient has a larger capacity for ventricular volume but a decrease in contractility. These changes result in decreased cardiac output, stroke volume, and EF. The decrease in cardiac output is reflected in the major signs and symptoms, including fatigue, weakness, and overt manifestations of left-sided heart failure.

In hypertrophic CMP muscle mass increases but without an increase in LV chamber size. Fibrotic infiltrates of the myocardium increase the stiffness of the ventricle, creating additional hypertrophy. Compliance to left ventricular filling decreases, and the LA dilates in an attempt to increase volume. When the hypertrophied ventricle contracts, the ventricle easily ejects the small available volume of blood, but cannot increase cardiac output to meet increases in demand, as would occur with exercise. This results in syncope, serious dysrhythmias, or sudden death. Heart failure is the eventual outcome as the disease progresses. Metabolic needs increase, create an imbalance between the high oxygen demand and the reduced cardiac output, and may precipitate angina. Clinical manifestations include those of dilated CMP plus an increased cardiac impulse, a high EF in the early stages, and a decreased EF when heart failure ensues.

In restrictive CMP the LV is fibrotic and thickened secondary to infiltrates. The ventricle loses its ability to stretch, thereby decreasing compliance; the heart cannot adequately fill, thereby decreasing cardiac output. Heart failure ensues. As in hypertrophic CMP, the LA often dilates. The patient may have symptoms of infection and amyloid infiltration.

Collaborative Care Management. Diagnostic tests for CMP include chest x-ray studies, echocardiogram, 12-lead ECG, and physical examination. The nurse monitors for subtle changes in systemic perfusion (e.g., mental status, heart rhythm, vital signs, peripheral perfusion, oxygenation, fluid status). The nursing assessment also seeks to determine how the illness has affected the patient's quality of life. The nurse considers the patient holistically, including the planned medical management and special needs, such as those related to the disbelief and shock that follow the sudden onset of viral CMP.

Management focuses on decreasing the workload of the heart, improving contractile efficiency, managing symptoms, and preventing complications. Medications include all those used in heart failure. Pacing of activities decreases workload, and restriction of activities with high metabolic equivalents may be beneficial. Even everyday conversation may create extreme dyspnea, and the nurse cautions the patient to pace this activity to minimize cardiac workload. Proper positioning and supplemental oxygen facilitate breathing. Assessment for orthostatic blood pressure changes and the initiation of appropriate safety measures decrease the risk of injury. Complications include altered renal function and electrolyte imbalance from diuretic therapy, as well as thromboemboli from stagnant blood flow within the myocardium. Anticoagulation may be prescribed (see Chapter 31

TABLE 30-5 PATHOPHYSIOLOGIC EFFECTS OF CARDIOMYOPATHIES

Pathophysiology	Type of Cardiomyopathy: Dilated	Hypertrophic	Restrictive
Major symptoms	Fatigue, weakness, palpitations	Dyspnea, angina pectoris, fatigue, dizziness (syncope), palpitations	Dyspnea, fatigue
Chamber size	Increased	Normal or decreased	Decreased or normal
Hypertrophy	Left ventricular myocardium	Left ventricular myocardium and interventricular septum	Left ventricular myocardium
Alterations of chamber volume	Volume increased	Volume decreased, particularly in left ventricle	Volume normal to decreased
Alterations of chamber compliance	Compliance increased	Compliance decreased, particularly in left ventricle	Compliance decreased, particularly in left ventricle
Ventricular filling pressure	Increased	Normal or increased	Increased
Alterations of systolic function (myocardial contractility)	Contractility decreased in left ventricle	Contractility increased or vigorous	None
Cardiac output	Decreased	Normal	Normal or decreased
Associated conditions	Alcoholism, pregnancy, infection, nutritional deficiency, exposure to toxins	Possible inherited defect of muscle growth and development	Infiltrative disease
Eventual cardiovascular event	Left-sided heart failure	Left-sided heart failure	Heart failure

Adapted from Huether SE, McCance KL: *Understanding pathophysiology*, ed 3, St Louis, 2004, Mosby.

for related nursing interventions). Dysrhythmias can occur if ischemia creates enhanced automaticity, reentry, or conduction defects. Ventricular dysrhythmias are the leading cause of death in hypertrophic CMP, and implantable defibrillators are often recommended after one or more documented episodes of ventricular tachycardia or ventricular fibrillation.

The value of pacemaker therapy continues to be investigated with regard to improving cardiac output in dilated CMP and high-output HOCM. In hypertrophic CMP removal of the septum (septal myotomy-myomectomy) or reduction of the left ventricular mass through a partial ventriculectomy (the Batista procedure) has been used with success in select patients. Cardiac transplantation may be an appropriate intervention for the patient refractory to conventional management

PATIENT/FAMILY TEACHING. The nurse provides appropriate explanations of all treatments and interventions to facilitate adherence to the recommended regimen and restore the patient's sense of confidence. Many of the teaching guidelines appropriate to patients with heart failure are also appropriate for patients with CMP. Patients with CMP are at an increased risk of sudden death because of dysrhythmias, and the nurse refers interested family members to an appropriate agency for instruction in cardiopulmonary resuscitation. Treatment options may seem limited to the patient and family, but the nurse emphasizes the importance of follow-up care.

Valvular Heart Disease

The cardiac valves are responsible for ensuring unidirectional blood flow through the heart. The term **stenosis** of the valve refers to narrowing of the valve lumen, which interferes with the forward flow of blood through the valve. The term *valvular insufficiency* refers to incomplete closing of the valve, causing **regurgitation,** or backward leaking of blood through the valve (Figure 30-8). Both stenosis and regurgitation negatively affect the overall function of the heart by increasing the size of the affected cardiac chamber and causing hypertrophy of the affected heart muscle. See Chapter 28 for a review of valve structure and function.

When a cardiac valve is mildly stenotic or regurgitant, the heart initially compensates and maintains function despite gradual chamber dilation and myocardial hypertrophy. However, over time the myocardium's compensatory ability begins to fail. Excessive myocardial hypertrophy and chamber dilation result in decreased contractility, reduced EF, and ultimately ventricular failure. Medical therapy supports cardiac function with the use of inotropes, diuretics, and dietary sodium restriction, but if symptoms continue to worsen, surgical valve repair or replacement may become necessary.

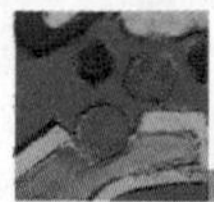

PATIENT/FAMILY TEACHING *Heart Failure*

- Monitor for signs and symptoms of recurrent heart failure, and report these signs and symptoms to the primary care provider:
  —Weight gain of 1 to 1.5 kg (2 to 3 lb)
  —Loss of appetite
  —Shortness of breath
  —Orthopnea
  —Swelling of ankles, feet, or abdomen
  —Persistent cough
  —Frequent nighttime urination
- Avoid fatigue and plan activity to allow for rest periods. Incorporate activities of daily living, occupational activity, and sexual activity into daily routine by pacing activities.
- Plan and eat meals within prescribed sodium restrictions:
  —Avoid salty foods.
  —Avoid drugs with high sodium content (e.g., some laxatives and antacids, Alka-Seltzer); read all labels.
  —Eat several small meals rather than three large meals per day.
- Take prescribed medications:
  —If several medications are prescribed, develop a method to facilitate accurate administration.
  —If taking digoxin, check own pulse rate daily; report a rate of less than 50 beats/min to primary care provider.
  —If taking diuretics:
    —Weigh self daily at same time of day.
    —Eat foods high in potassium and low in sodium (such as oranges, bananas) if on potassium-depleting diuretics.
  —If taking vasodilators:
    —Report signs of hypotension (lightheadedness, rapid pulse, syncope) to physician.
    —Avoid alcohol.
- Adopt healthy lifestyle choices: establish a daily routine, develop support groups, stop smoking, limit alcohol intake to no more than one drink per day, minimize risk of infections.
- Comply with follow-up appointments.

The symptoms produced by valvular heart disease and the complications that develop are primarily related to decreased cardiac input, and the general management follows the guidelines presented for patients with heart failure. Table 30-6 presents an overview of the specific valvular disorders and the diagnostic findings associated with each. Table 30-7 compares the common clinical manifestations associated with each disorder.

Mitral Stenosis

Etiology and Epidemiology. Mitral stenosis impedes the blood flow from the LA to the LV during ventricular diastole (ventricular filling). Mitral stenosis is usually caused by thickening or fibrotic changes in the mitral valve, and is the most common disorder of the mitral valve. The primary cause is rheumatic fever, which leads to an inflammatory process on the mitral valve's chordae tendineae cordis or commissures (leaflets). Less common causes of mitral stenosis include bacterial vegetation, thrombus formation, calcification of the mitral annulus, and atrial myxoma (tumor).

Forty percent of persons with rheumatic heart disease develop mitral stenosis, and two thirds of all persons with rheumatic mitral stenosis are women. With the decreasing incidence of rheumatic fever in industrialized countries, the incidence of rheumatic mitral stenosis has substantially declined, although it remains a common disorder in developing countries.

Pathophysiology. In mitral stenosis the mitral valve leaflets become thickened and fibrotic from calcification and scar tissue formation. As the valve leaflets become stiff and fused, the valve lumen progressively narrows and becomes immobile. The chordae tendineae may also shorten and thicken, and the mitral valve orifice may decrease from its normal size of 4 to 6 cm^2 to less than 1 cm^2 (Box 30-9).

Progressive mitral stenosis causes the left atrial pressure to elevate as a result of incomplete emptying of the LA. This causes the myocardium to compensate with left atrial dilation and hypertrophy. In addition, high pressures in the LA lead to elevated pulmonary venous, capillary, and arterial pressures. Eventually, sustained elevation of left atrial pressure can cause pulmonary hypertension and subsequent right ventricular hypertrophy. Increased pressure in the pulmonary vasculature causes fluid leakage across the pulmonary capillary membrane into the lung interstitium and can lead to pulmonary edema (Figure 30-9).

Persons with mitral stenosis experience a reduction in cardiac output that is directly related to the degree of stenosis. Persons with mild to moderate stenosis can generally maintain a normal cardiac output at rest but may be unable to tolerate exercise.

Mitral stenosis also increases the risk for cardiac dysrhythmias. Atrial fibrillation develops in 50% of persons with mitral stenosis, causing a further decrease in cardiac output. In addition, atrial fibrillation may allow blood to pool in the LA, resulting in thrombus formation and possible embolization to vital organs.

Many persons with mitral stenosis remain symptom free for as long as 20 years after the initial attack of rheumatic carditis. Symptoms may develop gradually or abruptly depending on the severity of the stenosis (see Table 30-7). When acute symptoms develop, the disease progresses rapidly and death occurs within 5 to 10 years unless surgical correction takes place.

The primary symptom of mitral stenosis is dyspnea, largely a result of reduced lung compliance. Dyspnea on exertion, paroxysmal nocturnal dyspnea, and orthopnea occur as a result of pulmonary hypertension. The symptoms may be precipitated by emotional stress, respiratory infection, sexual intercourse, or atrial fibrillation. Some persons experience a dry cough, dysphagia, or bronchitis because of bronchial irritation from the enlarged LA. Pressure exerted on the laryngeal nerve by an engorged pulmonary artery can cause hoarseness. Fatigue and weakness occur as a result of decreased cardiac output. Hemoptysis, usually a late sign, occurs from the rupture of a bronchial vein. Eventually right-sided heart failure leads to jugular venous distention, pitting edema, and hepatomegaly.

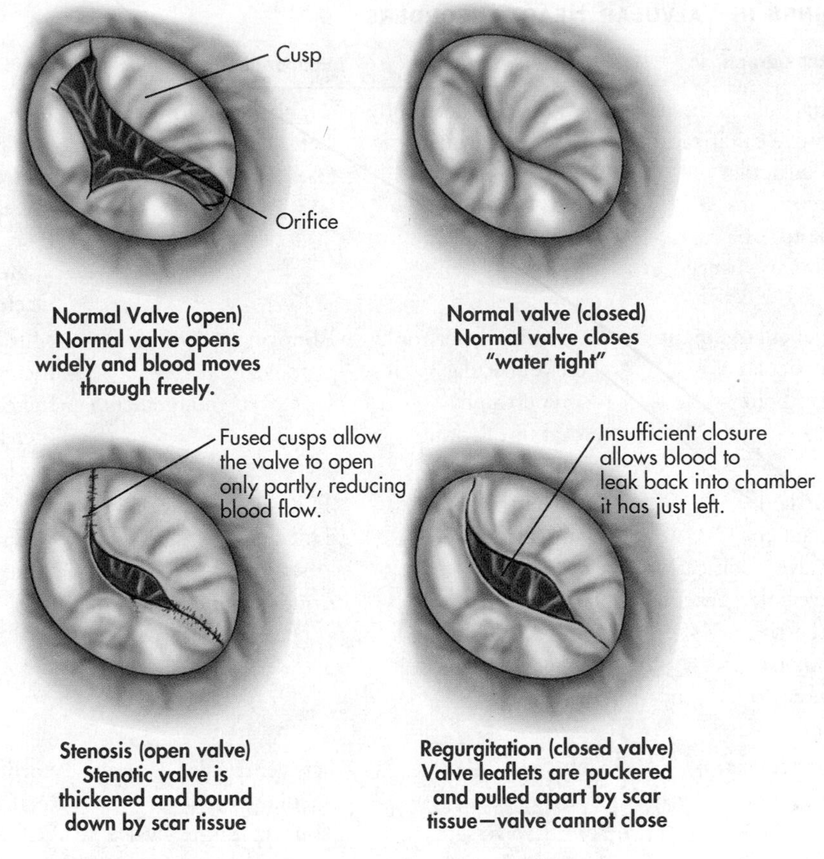
Cusp
Orifice
Normal Valve (open)
Normal valve opens widely and blood moves through freely.
Normal valve (closed)
Normal valve closes "water tight"
Fused cusps allow the valve to open only partly, reducing blood flow.
Insufficient closure allows blood to leak back into chamber it has just left.
Stenosis (open valve)
Stenotic valve is thickened and bound down by scar tissue
Regurgitation (closed valve)
Valve leaflets are puckered and pulled apart by scar tissue—valve cannot close

Figure 30-8 Valvular diseases.

Collaborative Care Management. The diagnosis of mitral stenosis is established by the clinical symptoms, such as an opening snap on auscultation, created by the forceful opening of mitral valve, followed by a diastolic rumbling or murmur that results from the increased velocity of blood flow. The diastolic murmur is absent when the valve is severely calcified. ECG changes indicate right ventricular hypertrophy, and chest x-ray films show left atrial enlargement. The most sensitive and noninvasive diagnostic test is the echocardiogram, which shows an impedance of blood flow, fusion of valve leaflets, and poor leaflet separation during diastole. Mitral stenosis also can be diagnosed with cardiac catheterization (see Table 30-6).

Mildly symptomatic patients with mitral stenosis are treated with diuretics; digitalis is used to control heart rate in the event of atrial fibrillation. Anticoagulation therapy with warfarin (Coumadin) may be used to prevent thrombus formation in patients with moderate to severe mitral stenosis or a history of thromboembolism. Medical therapy also includes antibiotic prophylaxis before dental or surgical procedures to reduce the risk of bacterial endocarditis.

More definitive intervention is indicated when the disease causes either loss of exercise tolerance or pulmonary hypertension. Percutaneous valvuloplasty using balloon dilation provides a nonsurgical alternative to reopen the valve. Surgical commissurotomy can also be performed while the valve leaflets remain mobile. Both commissurotomy and valvuloplasty allow patients to retain their natural valve and reduce the need for long-term anticoagulant therapy. Mitral valve replacement using open heart surgery and cardiopulmonary bypass is performed when the valve is severely fibrotic or calcified. In general, patients undergoing mitral valve replacement require permanent anticoagulation therapy.

PATIENT/FAMILY TEACHING. Patients with symptomatic disease are prescribed a sodium-restricted diet to help prevent fluid retention and progressive heart failure. The nurse teaches the patient about the dietary restriction and helps the patient adjust activity to his or her level of tolerance. Family involvement in both diet and activity teaching is encouraged to support adherence. Patients with moderate to severe stenosis are advised to avoid activities that require sudden increases in cardiac output. Patients receiving anticoagulant therapy receive instruction about the safe use of the drug and measures to follow to prevent bleeding (see Chapter 31).

Mitral Regurgitation

Etiology and Epidemiology. Mitral regurgitation (mitral insufficiency) occurs when the mitral valve fails to completely close during ventricular systole, allowing blood to flow backward into the LA. Mitral regurgitation can be either an acute or chronic condition.

Mitral regurgitation can be caused by rheumatic heart disease and is often present in conjunction with mitral stenosis. Mitral regurgitation occurs more commonly in men than in women and is the most prevalent lesion in patients who experience heart failure with active rheumatic carditis. With the exception of congenitally malformed mitral valves and connective tissue disorders,

TABLE 30-6 FINDINGS IN VALVULAR HEART DISORDERS

Disorder	Chest Radiograph	Electrocardiogram	Echocardiogram	Cardiac Catheterization
Mitral stenosis	Left atrial enlargement Mitral valve calcification Right ventricular enlargement Prominence of pulmonary artery	Left atrial hypertrophy Right ventricular hypertrophy Atrial fibrillation	Thickened mitral valve Left atrial enlargement	Increased pressure gradient across valve Increased left atrial pressure Increased PCWP Increased right-sided heart pressure Decreased CO
Mitral regurgitation	Left atrial enlargement Left ventricular enlargement	Left atrial hypertrophy Left ventricular hypertrophy Atrial fibrillation Sinus tachycardia	Abnormal mitral valve movement Left atrial enlargement	Mitral regurgitation Increased atrial pressure Increased LVEDP Increased PCWP Decreased CO
Aortic stenosis	Left ventricular enlargement Aortic valve calcification May have enlargement of left atrium, pulmonary artery, right ventricle, right atrium	Left ventricular hypertrophy	Thickened aortic valve Thickened ventricular wall Abnormal movement of aortic leaflets	Increased pressure gradient across valve Increased LVEDP
Aortic regurgitation	Left ventricular enlargement	Left ventricular hypertrophy Tall R waves Sinus tachycardia	Left ventricular enlargement Abnormal mitral valve movement Increased movement of ventricular wall	Aortic regurgitation Increased LVEDP Decreased arterial diastolic pressure
Tricuspid stenosis	Right atrial enlargement Prominence of superior vena cava	Right atrial hypertrophy Tall, peaked P waves Atrial fibrillation	Abnormal valvular leaflets Right atrial enlargement	Increased pressure gradient across valve Increased right atrial pressure Decreased CO
Tricuspid regurgitation	Right atrial enlargement Right ventricular enlargement	Right ventricular hypertrophy Atrial fibrillation	Prolapse of tricuspid valve Right atrial enlargement	Increased atrial pressure Tricuspid regurgitation Decreased CO

PCWP, Pulmonary capillary wedge pressure; *CO,* cardiac output; *LVEDP,* left ventricular end-diastolic pressure.

mitral regurgitation is primarily a disease of middle-aged and older persons. Other causes of mitral regurgitation include endocarditis; coronary heart disease; dilated CMP; a leaky prosthetic mitral valve; mitral valve prolapse; congenital malformation of the mitral valve; and connective tissue disorders such as Marfan syndrome, amyloidosis, and ankylosing spondylitis.

Weakness, rupture, or fibrosis of a papillary muscle secondary to ischemic heart disease, ventricular aneurysm, or acute myocardial infarction can also cause acute mitral regurgitation. Papillary muscle dysfunction allows the valve leaflets to flop in the direction of the LA during systole, and the blood flows backward. In addition, rupture of the chordae tendineae cordis or perforation of a mitral valve cusp can cause acute mitral regurgitation.

Pathophysiology. In chronic mitral insufficiency or regurgitation a variable amount of blood from the LV is shunted back through the mitral valve to the LA. This backflow of blood causes both the LA and LV to dilate and hypertrophy. Increasing preload and left atrial pressure also raise the pulmonary venous and arteriolar pressures and eventually cause right-sided heart failure (Figure 30-10). As the ventricle hypertrophies, it becomes dysfunctional and cardiac output decreases. Concurrently, the LA is often fibrillating, diminishing the cardiac output even further.

Fatigue and weakness are the primary symptoms of mitral regurgitation. Right-sided heart failure causes hepatic congestion, edema, ascites, and distended neck veins in severe cases. Some persons experience palpitations or paroxysmal nocturnal dyspnea.

Progressive dyspnea on exertion and pulmonary edema from an elevated left atrial pressure are the primary symptoms of acute regurgitation. The increased atrial pressure is transmitted immediately to the pulmonary veins, causing the congestive symptoms. Because the ventricle has not yet hypertrophied, the cardiac output remains sufficient and fatigue is not a problem. Although persons with mitral regurgitation commonly develop atrial fibrillation, thrombus formation in the atria is less common than with

TABLE 30-7 CLINICAL MANIFESTATIONS OF VALVULAR STENOSIS AND REGURGITATION

Manifestation	Aortic Stenosis	Mitral Stenosis	Aortic Regurgitation	Mitral Regurgitation	Tricuspid Regurgitation
Cardiovascular outcome*	Left ventricular failure	Right ventricular failure	Left-sided heart failure	Left-sided heart failure	Right-sided heart failure
General symptoms	Fatigue	Fatigue, weakness	Fatigue, weakness	Fatigue, weakness	Peripheral edema (with heart failure)
Respiratory effects	Dyspnea on exertion	Dyspnea on exertion, orthopnea, paroxysmal nocturnal dyspnea; predisposition to respiratory infections; hemoptysis; pulmonary hypertension; edema	Dyspnea with effort	Dyspnea; occasional hemoptysis	Dyspnea
Central nervous system effects	Syncope, especially on exertion	Neural deficits only associated with emboli (e.g., hemiparesis)	Syncope	None	None
Gastrointestinal effects	None	Ascites; hepatic angina with hepatomegaly	None	None	Ascites; hepatomegaly (with heart failure)
Pain	Angina pectoris	Chest pain	Chest pain (anginal)	None	Palpitations
Heart rate, rhythm	Bradycardia, dysrhythmias (with heart failure)	Palpitations (atrial fibrillation)	Palpitations, water-hammer pulse	Palpitations	Atrial fibrillations
Heart sounds	Systolic murmur	Diastolic murmur; accentuated first heart sound; opening snap	Diastolic and systolic murmurs	Murmur throughout systole	Murmur throughout systole
Most common causes	Congenital; rheumatic fever	Rheumatic fever	Bacterial endocarditis; aortic root disease	Floppy valve; coronary artery disease	Congenital

Data from Braunwald E, editor: *Heart disease: a textbook of cardiovascular medicine,* ed 7, Philadelphia, 2005, Elsevier; Hancock EW: Valvular heart disease, *Sci Am Med* 1(I-XI):1, 1992.
*If disease not treated.

mitral stenosis because backflow and the resulting turbulence of the blood limit pooling.

Collaborative Care Management. The diagnosis of mitral regurgitation is made from the clinical symptoms and from auscultation of a blowing, high-pitched systolic murmur and third heart sound. The first heart sound (S_1) may not be heard, depending on the severity of regurgitation. A chest x-ray examination reveals left atrial enlargement and occasional left ventricular dilation. The ECG shows left ventricular hypertrophy and, less commonly, right ventricular hypertrophy (see Table 30-6). An echocardiogram may identify mitral valve cusp prolapse, ruptured chordae tendineae cordis, and enlargement of the LA and LV. Definitive diagnosis is

Box 30-9 Relationship of Mitral Orifice Size to Emergence of Symptoms

>2.6 cm^2	No symptoms with exertion
2.1-2.5 cm^2	Symptoms with extreme exertion
1.6-2.0 cm^2	Symptoms with moderate exertion
<1.5 cm^2	Symptoms with minimal exertion

From Fuster V et al: *Hurst's the heart,* ed 7, New York, 2004, McGraw-Hill.

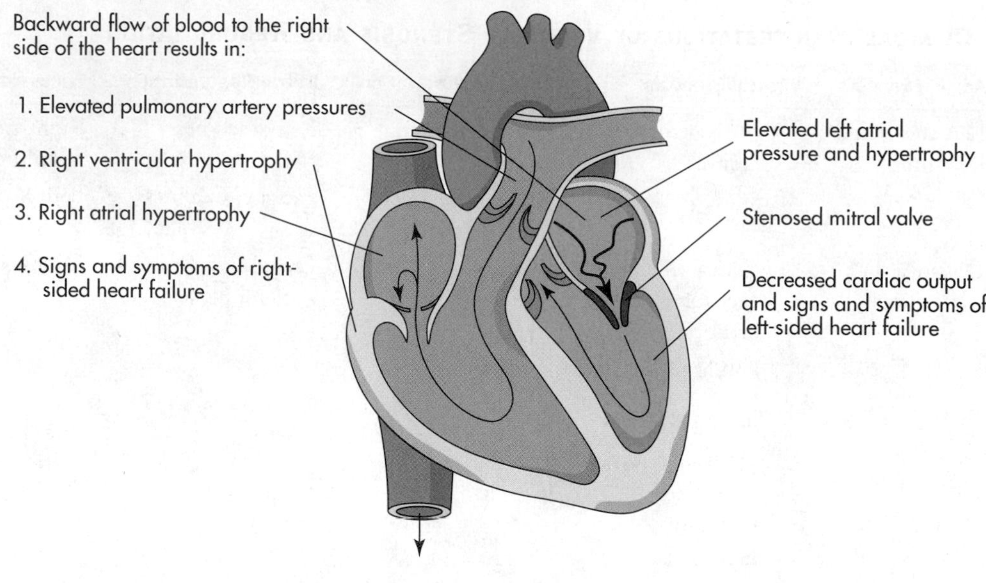

Backward flow of blood to the right side of the heart results in:
1. Elevated pulmonary artery pressures
2. Right ventricular hypertrophy
3. Right atrial hypertrophy
4. Signs and symptoms of right-sided heart failure
Elevated left atrial pressure and hypertrophy
Stenosed mitral valve
Decreased cardiac output and signs and symptoms of left-sided heart failure

Figure 30-9 Effects of mitral stenosis.

made through cardiac catheterization, which assesses left ventricular function and the degree of regurgitation.

Patients with mild mitral regurgitation who develop new-onset atrial fibrillation may need to undergo controlled cardioversion to restore normal sinus rhythm and maximize cardiac output. Patients with longstanding atrial fibrillation or a history of thromboembolism receive long-term anticoagulation.

Mitral regurgitation that progresses despite medical therapy necessitates valve repair or prosthetic replacement. Individuals with intact left ventricular function and without other severe noncardiac disease may be candidates for open heart surgery and valve replacement.

PATIENT/FAMILY TEACHING. Patient teaching is directed primarily at symptom management and is similar in most respects to the education provided to patients with mitral stenosis.

Mitral Valve Prolapse

Etiology and Epidemiology. **Mitral valve prolapse** occurs when abnormalities in the mitral valve leaflets, chordae tendineae cordis, or papillary muscles allow prolapse of the mitral valve leaflets backward into the LA during ventricular systole. Mitral valve prolapse is also known as Barlow's syndrome and as a "floppy" or "billowing" mitral valve. Mitral valve prolapse is the most common valvular disorder in the United States. It occurs in approximately 4% to 7% of adults, most commonly young women. In many patients, mitral valve prolapse is a benign, asymptomatic disorder and may remain undiagnosed.

Mitral valve prolapse may be caused by a variety of factors. Its incidence is possibly linked to an autosomal dominant inherited trait, and it is also associated with other inherited connective tissue disorders such as Marfan syndrome, Ehlers-Danlos syndrome, and osteogenesis imperfecta. Other causes of mitral valve prolapse

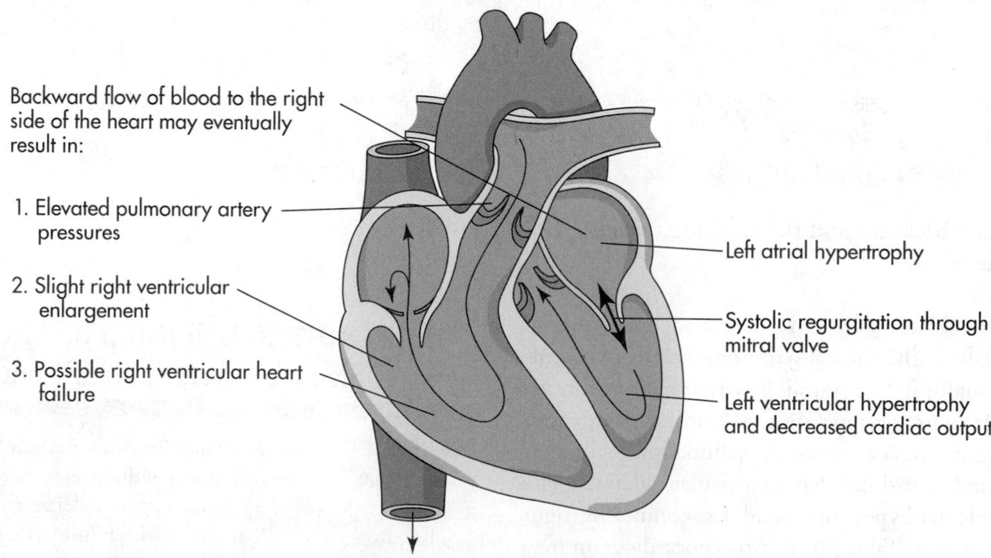

Backward flow of blood to the right side of the heart may eventually result in:
1. Elevated pulmonary artery pressures
2. Slight right ventricular enlargement
3. Possible right ventricular heart failure
Left atrial hypertrophy
Systolic regurgitation through mitral valve
Left ventricular hypertrophy and decreased cardiac output

Figure 30-10 Effects of mitral regurgitation.

include endocarditis, CAD, myocarditis, CMP, cardiac trauma, and hyperthyroidism.

Pathophysiology. In mitral valve prolapse the leaflets of the mitral valve become enlarged or thickened, and the chordae tendineae cordis may become elongated. These changes permit the valve leaflets to billow upward into the LA during ventricular systole. Depending on the degree of prolapse and the integrity of the valve leaflets, mitral regurgitation may occur. The subsequent pathophysiology parallels that of mitral regurgitation. In addition, research suggests that individuals with mitral valve prolapse may experience some autonomic nervous system dysfunction causing excessive catecholamine release, leading to a wide array of subjective complaints.

Many cases of mitral valve prolapse are asymptomatic. Individuals who are symptomatic report palpitations, which are secondary to dysrhythmias and tachycardia. Other symptoms include lightheadedness, syncope, fatigue, lethargy, weakness, dyspnea, and chest tightness. In addition, hyperventilation, anxiety, depression, panic attacks, and atypical chest pain may occur. Many of the symptoms of mitral valve prolapse are vague and are not necessarily related to the degree of prolapse.

Although mitral valve prolapse is generally benign, as many as 15% of individuals develop mitral regurgitation and subsequent left ventricular failure. In addition, individuals with mitral valve prolapse are at increased risk for embolic stroke. On physical examination most individuals have a midsystolic click and, if mitral regurgitation is present, a late-systolic murmur. In the absence of auscultatory findings, mitral valve prolapse may be detected on echocardiography.

Collaborative Care Management. ECGs of individuals with mitral valve prolapse are normal unless the person is symptomatic from dysrhythmias. The most common rhythm disturbances include premature ventricular contractions, supraventricular tachycardia, and atrial tachydysrhythmias. Mitral valve prolapse is diagnosed principally by echocardiography, although cardiac angiography may be used to confirm the diagnosis. Individuals who experience palpitations require 24-hour ambulatory ECG monitoring to determine the severity of the dysrhythmia.

Asymptomatic individuals with mitral valve prolapse usually do not require treatment. Symptomatic individuals may require medications to control dysrhythmias (see Chapter 29). Beta-blockers are the treatment of choice for managing palpitations and chest pain.

All persons with mitral valve prolapse need regular follow-up care and should have an echocardiogram every few years to monitor disease progression. The severity of mitral regurgitation associated with the valve prolapse determines the necessity for surgical intervention. Antibiotic prophylaxis against endocarditis is indicated before dental and surgical procedures for individuals who have a systolic murmur or echocardiographic evidence of mitral valve leaflet thickening. Asymptomatic individuals do not usually require antibiotic prophylaxis.

PATIENT/FAMILY TEACHING. The nurse encourages patients to avoid caffeine, which may exacerbate the incidence of tachycardia and atrial dysrhythmias. These episodes can be frightening for the patient and family, who need to thoroughly understand the problem and how to control or respond to it. No additional dietary restrictions are needed. Activity is also unrestricted, although symptomatic patients may need to adjust their activities in response to the nature and severity of their symptoms.

Aortic Stenosis

Etiology and Epidemiology. Aortic stenosis occurs when the aortic valve leaflets become stiff, fused, or calcified and impede blood flow from the LV into the aorta during ventricular systole. Aortic stenosis is caused by congenital malformations of the aortic valve, inflammatory heart disease (endocarditis), or degenerative disease (calcification). Aortic stenosis generally impedes the outflow of blood from the LV at the level of the aortic valve, although obstruction to flow can also occur above and below the valve itself. Conditions such as hypertrophic CMP may lead to subvalvular aortic stenosis. Coarctation of the aorta is a supravalvular lesion that may mimic aortic stenosis.

The causes of aortic stenosis vary with the patient's age. In patients less than 30 years old, aortic stenosis is typically caused by a congenitally stenotic aortic valve. Between the ages of 30 and 65 years, aortic stenosis is more commonly caused by progressive stenosis of a congenital bicuspid aortic valve, and less commonly by rheumatic heart disease. Although less than 2% of the general population have a congenital bicuspid aortic valve, 50% of these individuals develop aortic calcification and stenosis by the age of 50.[29] In persons over 65 years old, aortic stenosis is caused by degeneration and sclerosis of the valve, and the incidence is equally distributed between men and women. Except in older persons, men are three or four times more likely to develop isolated aortic stenosis.

Pathophysiology. Aortic stenosis occurs when the aortic valve narrows and obstructs the flow of blood into the aorta during systole (Figure 30-11). Resistance to blood flow from the LV causes an increase in left ventricular systolic pressure. This pressure increase and the LV's compensatory efforts to increase cardiac output lead to left ventricular hypertrophy. Even though the LV pumps harder to meet the body's needs, the stenotic valve effectively blocks any increase in blood flow from the heart. Hence, in advanced aortic stenosis, cardiac output becomes fixed despite the LV's attempts to increase blood flow.

Worsening left ventricular hypertrophy leads to a constellation of problems late in the course of the disease, including pulmonary congestion, syncope, and myocardial ischemia. Pulmonary congestion occurs when the stenosis significantly interferes with the forward movement of blood. Syncope and myocardial ischemia occur because of the fixed-flow condition and the inability of the LV to meet the body's changing needs. The severity of aortic stenosis is determined by the pressure gradient between the LV and the aorta.

Aortic stenosis develops gradually, and symptoms do not appear until late in the course of the disease. Life expectancy without medical or surgical intervention is generally less than 4 years after the onset of symptoms. Early symptoms of aortic stenosis include fatigue and dyspnea. The combination of dyspnea, exertional angina, and syncope or near-syncopal episodes indicates

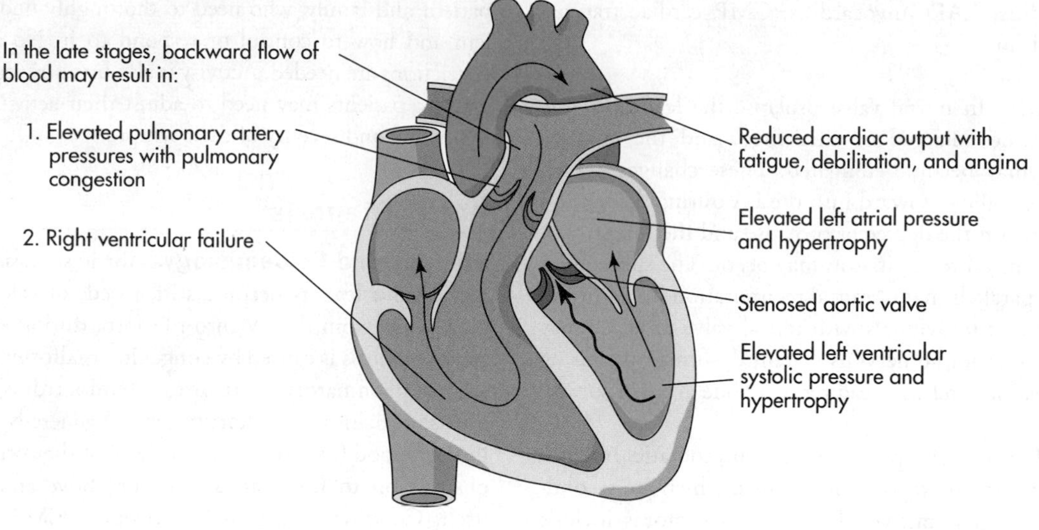
In the late stages, backward flow of blood may result in:
1. Elevated pulmonary artery pressures with pulmonary congestion
2. Right ventricular failure
Reduced cardiac output with fatigue, debilitation, and angina
Elevated left atrial pressure and hypertrophy
Stenosed aortic valve
Elevated left ventricular systolic pressure and hypertrophy

Figure 30-11 Effects of aortic stenosis.

severe aortic stenosis. Individuals who develop symptomatic heart failure survive less than 2 years, whereas patients with either syncope or angina survive 5 years and 3 years, respectively. In addition, 15% of those with symptomatic aortic stenosis and 5% of asymptomatic patients suffer sudden cardiac death.

In addition to dyspnea, fatigue, heart failure, angina, and syncope, an array of physical findings is present in individuals with aortic stenosis. The hallmark clinical findings include a grade III/VI or IV/VI systolic ejection murmur over the aortic area radiating upward into the carotid arteries and a pulse pattern that demonstrates a delayed systolic upstroke (Table 30-8). Other clinical findings depend on the degree of heart failure and pulmonary edema.

Collaborative Care Management. A diagnosis of aortic stenosis is made from the clinical symptoms and diagnostic tests (see Table 30-6), including an ECG, chest x-ray studies, echocardiogram, and cardiac catheterization.

The ECG is normal early in the course of aortic stenosis. Late changes include left ventricular hypertrophy, nonspecific ST depression, and T wave inversion that indicates subendocardial ischemia. The chest x-ray film may reveal aortic calcification. The echocardiogram reveals valve leaflet defects and increased ventricular wall thickness. Cardiac catheterization definitively diagnoses aortic stenosis and quantifies the severity of the disease. Cardiac catheterization may be used to evaluate left ventricular function, coronary vessel patency, and the degree of associated aortic and mitral regurgitation before cardiac surgery.

Percutaneous balloon valvuloplasty may be used to alleviate aortic stenosis. The technique involves cardiac catheterization and the introduction of a balloon catheter into the aortic valve orifice. The balloon is repeatedly inflated until the valve lumen is further opened, thus relieving some of the stenosis. Patients receive the same care provided to individuals undergoing cardiac catheterization but may also be monitored in an intensive care unit for 24 to 48 hours after the procedure. Although balloon valvuloplasty improves symptoms for some individuals, the procedure carries a high morbidity and mortality rate and is currently used primarily for patients who are poor candidates for cardiac surgery and cardiopulmonary bypass.

The definitive therapy for patients with aortic stenosis is valve replacement with a prosthetic aortic valve. Although the surgery carries significant risks, most individuals experience substantial improvement in their general health and exercise tolerance.

TABLE 30-8 AUSCULTATORY DIFFERENCES IN VALVULAR HEART DISEASE

Valvular Disorder	General Findings	Murmurs
Mitral stenosis	S_1 snapping, louder Palpable thrill at apex	Soft, low pitched, rumbling Diastolic
Mitral regurgitation	S_1 soft or absent S_3 present Palpable thrill at apex	High pitched, blowing Pansystolic
Aortic stenosis	S_2 soft Left-sided S_4 Systolic thrill at heart base	Low pitched, harsh, rasping Midsystolic
Aortic regurgitation	S_3 present Systolic thrill over aortic area	High pitched, blowing Diastolic
Tricuspid regurgitation	Systolic thrill at lower left sternal border	High pitched, blowing Pansystolic

PATIENT/FAMILY TEACHING. Patients with aortic stenosis have an unrestricted diet unless heart failure is present, in which case the nurse instructs patients to restrict their daily intake of sodium and fluid. Activity levels are carefully monitored because patients are at risk for sudden cardiac death. The nurse cautions patients against undue physical exertion or stress, which may precipitate acute heart failure or dysrhythmia. Patients and families need ongoing teaching and support to effectively manage the disease in their daily lives. The nurse also reminds patients of the importance of seeking prophylactic antibiotic treatment against endocarditis before any invasive dental procedure or surgery.

Aortic Regurgitation

Etiology and Epidemiology. Aortic regurgitation occurs when an incompetent aortic valve allows blood to flow backward from the aorta into the LV during diastole. An incompetent aortic valve may result from disease of the valve cusps or the aortic root. Common causes of aortic regurgitation include inflammatory diseases (rheumatic heart disease, bacterial endocarditis), a congenital bicuspid aortic valve, or idiopathic dilation of the aortic root (CMP). Less common causes include traumatic rupture of an aortic valve cusp, rheumatoid arthritis, ankylosing spondylitis, Reiter's syndrome, connective tissue disorders (Marfan syndrome, Ehlers-Danlos syndrome, osteogenesis imperfecta), and syphilitic aortitis. The incidence of aortic regurgitation related to rheumatic heart disease has decreased significantly during the past 20 years. Except in cases of rheumatic heart disease, aortic regurgitation is more common in men than in women.

Acute aortic regurgitation occurs with sudden dilation of the aortic root and is most commonly associated with an ascending dissecting aortic aneurysm (see Chapter 31). The most common risk factor for acute aortic dissection is systemic hypertension. Selected connective tissue disorders, especially Marfan syndrome, also pose a risk for acute aortic dissection.

Pathophysiology. In chronic aortic regurgitation the backward flow of blood through the incompetent, leaky aortic valve increases the volume of blood in the LV (Figure 30-12). This increased blood volume and subsequent increase in left ventricular end-diastolic pressure increase stroke volume and sustain cardiac output. Over time, however, left ventricular dilation and hypertrophy occur. Ultimately, the LV loses its ability to compensate for the increased pressure and volume, leading to decreased stroke volume and cardiac output and finally left ventricular failure. Progressive aortic regurgitation can also lead to increased left atrial pressures, left atrial chamber dilation, pulmonary congestion, pulmonary hypertension, and possibly right-sided heart failure.

In acute aortic regurgitation the LV cannot compensate for the sudden dramatic increase in workload, and patients develop fulminant pulmonary edema. Left ventricular decompensation and failure occur rapidly, and these patients require emergent lifesaving care.

Individuals with chronic aortic regurgitation may remain asymptomatic for 20 years or report only mild dyspnea on exertion. With disease progression and gradual left ventricular decompensation, symptoms of heart failure and pulmonary edema develop, including progressively severe dyspnea, orthopnea, paroxysmal nocturnal dyspnea, and angina. The development and progression of these symptoms reflect advanced disease. Other symptoms vary depending on the cause.

The hallmark physical finding in individuals with aortic regurgitation is a diastolic murmur that is loudest over the aortic area (see Table 30-8). The duration of the murmur reflects the severity of the regurgitation. Other classic physical findings of chronic aortic regurgitation include decreased diastolic pressure, widened pulse pressure, and subsequent water-hammer pulse. Water-hammer pulse sounds can be auscultated over the femoral arteries, and some persons demonstrate a head bobbing with each heartbeat. Individuals with acute aortic regurgitation do not demonstrate the changes in pulse pressure because of the sudden onset of the disease.

Collaborative Care Management. The diagnosis of aortic regurgitation is made based on the diastolic murmur and widened pulse pressure (see Tables 30-5 and 30-7). Persons with chronic aortic regurgitation exhibit evidence of left ventricular hypertrophy on the ECG and cardiomegaly on the chest x-ray film. Patients with acute aortic regurgitation may exhibit only nonspecific ST or T wave changes with a normal heart size. Echocardiography is useful in assessing left ventricular function, hypertrophy, and aortic root dilation.

Persons with asymptomatic aortic regurgitation do not require treatment beyond yearly follow-up with a chest x-ray examination and ECG. Persons with symptomatic aortic regurgitation are managed medically until a decision can be made concerning valve surgery. Digitalis and diuretic therapy are indicated for individuals who demonstrate heart failure. Afterload-reducing agents may also be used.

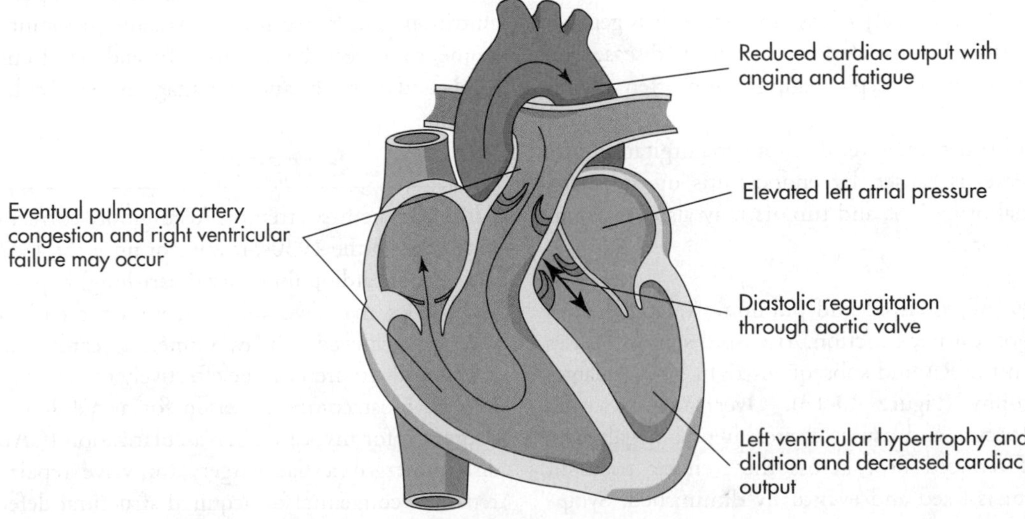

Figure 30-12 Effects of aortic regurgitation.

Because of the high mortality rate associated with symptomatic aortic regurgitation, all symptomatic individuals are evaluated for aortic valve replacement surgery. Operative mortality is significantly reduced when the surgery is performed before the development of left ventricular dysfunction. Early intervention is also associated with an improved quality of life.

PATIENT/FAMILY TEACHING. Patients with aortic regurgitation must understand the nature and potential seriousness of their disease and commit to regular medical follow-up care and evaluation. Asymptomatic patients do not need to restrict their diet or activity in any way. The nurse instructs symptomatic patients to reduce their intake of sodium to help control the symptoms of heart failure and to adapt their activity as needed to changes in their symptoms. Patients need to be knowledgeable about the safe use of any prescribed medications. The nurse reminds patients that it is important to request prophylactic antibiotic therapy against endocarditis before undergoing any dental or surgical procedure.

Tricuspid and Pulmonic Valve Disorders

Etiology and Epidemiology. Tricuspid stenosis is a restriction of the tricuspid valve orifice that impedes blood flow from the RA to the RV during right ventricular diastole (filling). Conversely, tricuspid regurgitation involves an incompetent tricuspid valve that allows blood to flow backward from the RV to the RA during ventricular systole. Pulmonic stenosis is a restriction of the pulmonic valve orifice impeding blood flow out of the RV into the pulmonary vasculature during systole. Pulmonic regurgitation involves an incompetent pulmonic valve that allows blood to flow backward into the RV during diastole.

Disorders of the tricuspid and pulmonic valves are significantly less common than disorders of the valves on the left side of the heart. The right side of the heart is a low-pressure system, with less potential for inflammatory changes and calcification. Mitral and aortic valve diseases often also involve the tricuspid or pulmonic valves.

Disorders of the tricuspid valves are primarily caused by rheumatic fever. Less common causes include endocarditis or congenital malformations of the valve cusps. Tricuspid stenosis is generally seen in women with a history of rheumatic heart disease who suffer from mitral stenosis. Tricuspid regurgitation often accompanies tricuspid stenosis.

Pulmonic valve disorders are rare. Pulmonic regurgitation, like tricuspid valve disease, is caused by endocarditis or rheumatic fever. Congenital malformations and tumors may also cause pulmonic valve dysfunction.

Pathophysiology. All tricuspid and pulmonic valve disorders have similar effects on cardiac function. Tricuspid stenosis causes increased pressure in the RA and subsequent right atrial enlargement and hypertrophy (Figure 30-13). Over time, systemic venous congestion occurs and causes ascites, hepatomegaly, and edema. Because of reduced flow across the stenotic tricuspid valve, cardiac output is fixed and eventually diminished. Symptoms of tricuspid stenosis are generally overshadowed by those associated with mitral or aortic valve dysfunction. Fatigue is present because of decreased cardiac output. Tricuspid regurgitation involves the same pathologic consequences as tricuspid stenosis, except that the backward flow of blood into the RA during systole serves to increase the workload of the RV. Therefore right ventricular dilation, hypertrophy, and failure are present in tricuspid regurgitation but not in tricuspid stenosis. The pathophysiologic mechanisms affecting cardiac function in pulmonic stenosis and pulmonic regurgitation are identical to those described for tricuspid disorders.

Disorders of the tricuspid and pulmonic valves ultimately lead to symptoms of right-sided heart failure and decreased cardiac output. The ECG shows tall, peaked P waves (atrial hypertrophy) in both tricuspid stenosis and tricuspid regurgitation. Right ventricular hypertrophy is evident on ECG with tricuspid regurgitation, pulmonic stenosis, and pulmonic regurgitation. Atrial fibrillation may also be present. In tricuspid stenosis a high-pitched diastolic murmur can be auscultated along the left sternal border. In the other disorders of the tricuspid and pulmonic valves, the murmur is harsh and can be heard throughout systole. The chest x-ray film shows right atrial enlargement, right ventricular enlargement (except in tricuspid stenosis), and a prominent shadow of the superior vena cava. Echocardiogram is used to determine the degree of valve dysfunction.

Collaborative Care Management. Care for patients with tricuspid and pulmonic valve disorders focuses on the management of right-sided heart failure and decreased cardiac output. The care is similar to that previously outlined for mitral and aortic valve disorders. One exception is that patients do not experience dyspnea and pulmonary complications with tricuspid or pulmonic valve disease, unless these disorders occur concurrently with aortic and mitral valve disease.

PATIENT/FAMILY TEACHING. Patient and family teaching for patients with tricuspid and pulmonic valve disorders is targeted toward symptom management, which may vary substantially from patient to patient. The nurse encourages patients to modify activities to match their tolerance level and to plan for chronic fatigue. Congestion within the gastrointestinal tract may lead to chronic anorexia, and the nurse emphasizes the importance of adequate nutrition. The nurse teaches patients to monitor their edema at home, to protect the skin from breakdown, to use all medications safely and correctly, and to manage expected side effects.

Cardiac Surgery

Although the first attempts to surgically correct cardiac problems date back to the 1930s, it was not until the 1950s and the development of cardiopulmonary (heart-lung) bypass and new surgical techniques that favorable outcomes for patients could be predictably achieved. Today, numerous cardiac disorders in both adults and children can be effectively treated with surgery.

The most common reason for an adult to undergo cardiac surgery is for myocardial revascularization (CABG), but patients also undergo cardiac surgery for valve repair or replacement, repair of congenital or acquired structural defects, implantation of devices, and cardiac transplantation (Table 30-9). Cardiac surgery is classified as either open heart or closed heart, depending

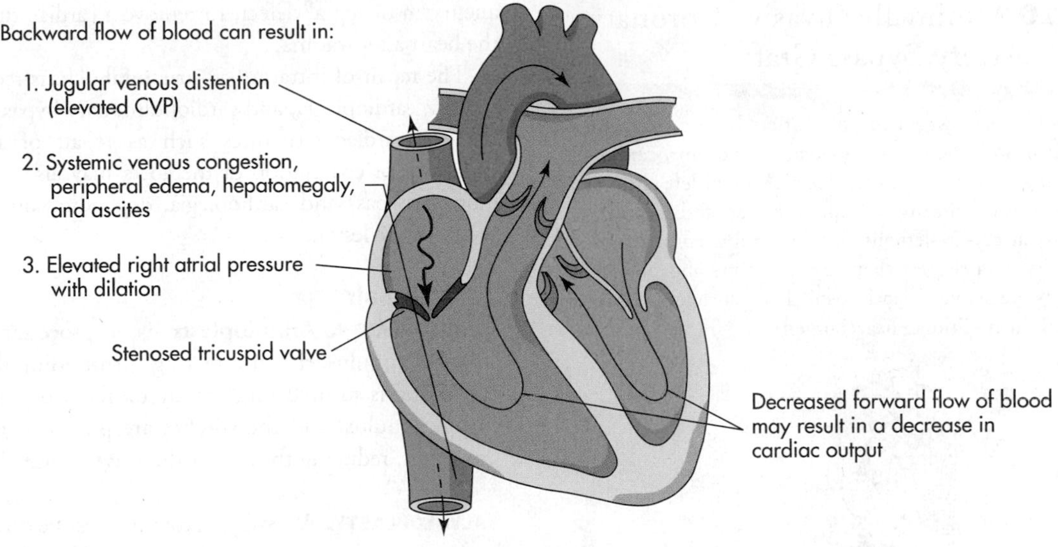
Backward flow of blood can result in:
1. Jugular venous distention (elevated CVP)
2. Systemic venous congestion, peripheral edema, hepatomegaly, and ascites
3. Elevated right atrial pressure with dilation
Stenosed tricuspid valve
Decreased forward flow of blood may result in a decrease in cardiac output

Figure 30-13 Effects of tricuspid stenosis.

TABLE 30-9 INDICATIONS FOR CARDIAC SURGERY AND ASSOCIATED PROCEDURES

Indication	Procedure
Ischemic heart disease	Coronary artery bypass graft
Structural abnormalities	Valve repair Valve replacement Atrial septal defect repair Ventricular septal defect repair Ventricular aneurysm resection Atrial tumor resection Aortic aneurysm (thoracic) repair
Implantation of devices	Automatic implantable cardioverter-defibrillator Ventricular assist device Artificial heart chamber
Transplantation	Replacement of diseased heart with healthy heart

on whether the heart is "opened" during the course of the surgery. Cardiac surgery involving the repair of internal structural defects is open heart, whereas myocardial revascularization is a closed heart procedure.

Coronary Artery Bypass Graft

CABG is a common choice for treating coronary artery obstruction. The graft allows blood to bypass the obstructed portion of the coronary artery and provides improved blood flow and increased oxygen to the myocardial tissue distal to the lesion. Although CABG does not cure the underlying heart disease, it does reduce the incidence of angina and prevents myocardial ischemia and infarction.

Patients can undergo a single bypass or simultaneously receive multiple bypass grafts, depending on the nature and severity of their coronary disease. The surgical procedure has traditionally involved closed heart surgery with access obtained via a median sternotomy, **cold cardioplegia** in which heart activity is stopped, and extracorporeal circulation initiated via a cardiopulmonary bypass machine. More recent advances in cardiac surgery led to the development of the minimally invasive direct coronary artery bypass for individuals with only one diseased coronary artery. In this surgery, the surgeon achieves access to the heart via a smaller incision at the left sternal border of the anterior thorax instead of the larger median sternotomy, and neither cardioplegia nor cardiopulmonary bypass is used (Box 30-10).[40] Multiple CABGs are also now being performed via median sternotomy, but without the use cardioplegia and cardiopulmonary bypass. These advances, referred to as "off-pump" or "beating heart" procedures, have reduced the incidence of complications after surgery and facilitate a speedier recovery. The average length of hospital stay is 4 or 5 days for patients undergoing traditional CABG surgery, but as little as 2 or 3 days for the less invasive off-pump procedures.[42]

The graft used to bypass the affected coronary artery must be either a vein or artery. Although vein grafts have been the mainstay of bypass procedures in the past, arterial grafts improve both long-term patency and perfusion of the myocardium and now are increasingly used. The most common donor vein is a long portion of the saphenous vein, although occasionally a cephalic vein from the forearm is used. After vein harvesting, the graft is anastomosed to the coronary artery distal to the obstructive lesion, and the proximal end is anastomosed to the ascending aorta. The donor graft is reversed before insertion because of the presence of directional valves in the vein segment (see Figure 29-12). Preoperative Doppler studies of venous flow help pinpoint optimal segments of veins for use as grafts. This enables the surgeon to use minimally invasive vein harvesting to remove only the necessary segments, rather than the entire length of the vein.

The artery most commonly used for CABG is an internal mammary artery (right or left). Only the distal end of the artery is dissected away from the tissues and anastomosed to the coronary

Box 30-10 Minimally Invasive Coronary Artery Bypass Graft

This surgical technique allows for coronary artery bypass graft surgery to be performed without the use of a median sternotomy, cardiopulmonary (heart-lung) bypass, or cardioplegia. A small left chest incision allows the surgeon to directly visualize the heart and complete an internal mammary artery–to–left anterior descending coronary artery bypass. Preliminary data suggest that operative time and postoperative complications are reduced, and hospital stay averages 2 days as opposed to 5 days for traditional heart surgery.

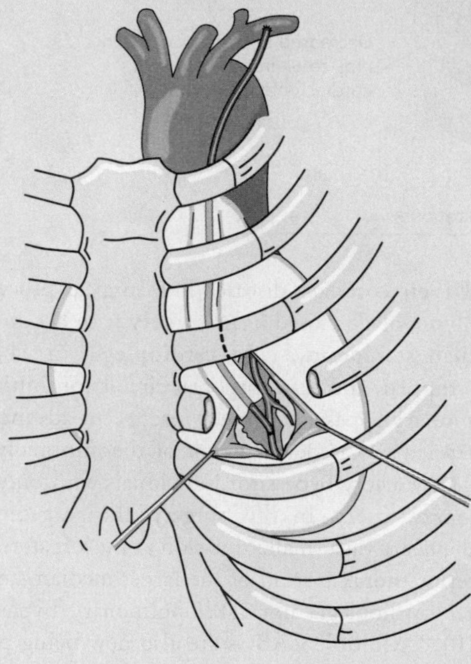

Through a pericardial window, anastomosis of the left internal mammary artery to the left anterior descending coronary artery is performed under direct vision.

artery distal to the obstructive lesion. The proximal segment is left in place. The surgeon may also use the radial artery from the forearm or occasionally the gastroepiploic artery.

Long-term patency rates for internal mammary artery grafts exceed those for saphenous vein grafts. Studies have shown that 40% to 50% of saphenous vein grafts close within 2 years, whereas 90% of internal mammary artery grafts remain patent 10 years after surgery. However, internal mammary artery grafts are contraindicated for patients with diabetes mellitus because of the impact of reduced arterial circulation to the chest wall, as well as in obese or large-breasted individuals.

Correction of Structural Defects

Cardiac surgery may also be used to repair structural problems such as valve dysfunction. Surgical options include either valve repair (annuloplasty, valvuloplasty, or commissurotomy) or replacement with a valve prosthesis (Box 30-11). Less commonly, adults undergo cardiac surgery to repair structural defects such as a ventricular aneurysm or septal defect, to remove a cardiac tumor, or to repair the heart after trauma.

The repair of intracardiac structural defects requires open heart surgery, cardioplegia, and cardiopulmonary bypass. Surgery involving extracardiac structures such as repair of a thoracic aortic aneurysm or coarctation of the aorta may also include cardiopulmonary bypass and cardioplegia, depending on the location and extent of the lesion.

Valve Repair

ANNULOPLASTY. **Annuloplasty** is a procedure to reduce an enlarged annulus, the fibrous ring surrounding the valve. A prosthetic ring is sutured into the circumference of the mitral or tricuspid annulus, and the stitches are pulled together toward the prosthesis, reducing the size of the valve orifice (Figure 30-14).

VALVULOPLASTY. **Valvuloplasty** involves the direct repair of torn leaflets or clefts by open heart surgery. The advantages of operative valve repair over valve replacement include (1) higher survival rates; (2) fewer cardiac complications, particularly thromboembolism; (3) lower operative morbidity and mortality rates; (4) potential improvement in left ventricular function; (5) reduced need for anticoagulation; and (6) lower cost. Mitral valvuloplasty has gained increasing acceptance as the surgery of choice for mitral regurgitation, including cases of rheumatic origin.

COMMISSUROTOMY. Mitral **commissurotomy** involves the separation or incision of the stenosed valve leaflets at their borders, or commissures. Either an open or a closed technique may be used, although open commissurotomy is currently the procedure of choice. An open commissurotomy usually is performed through a median sternotomy or a right anterolateral thoracotomy incision to allow for proper visualization of the mitral valve. Cardiopulmonary bypass is initiated, the LA is opened, and the commissures are incised with a scalpel. The newly mobilized valve leaflets are attached to the chordae tendineae cordis. The disadvantages of this approach include those associated with open heart surgery in general. Advantages include fewer thrombotic and embolic complications and fewer atrial tears with resultant hemorrhage. If the valve disease appears to be too advanced to repair, valve replacement can be performed immediately.

A closed commissurotomy (without bypass) is performed through a left posterolateral thoracotomy. The fifth rib is removed and the atrium palpated to detect the presence of any thrombi. If a thrombus is present, the procedure is converted to an open procedure to allow for clot removal. Otherwise, the surgeon inserts a finger through a small incision, dividing the papillary muscle lon-

Box 30-11 Types of Valve Repair

- Annuloplasty: Repair of ring or annulus of incompetent or diseased valve
- Valvuloplasty: Repair of valve, suturing of torn leaflets
- Commissurotomy: Dilation of valve; repair of a leaflet, commissure, fibrous band, or ring

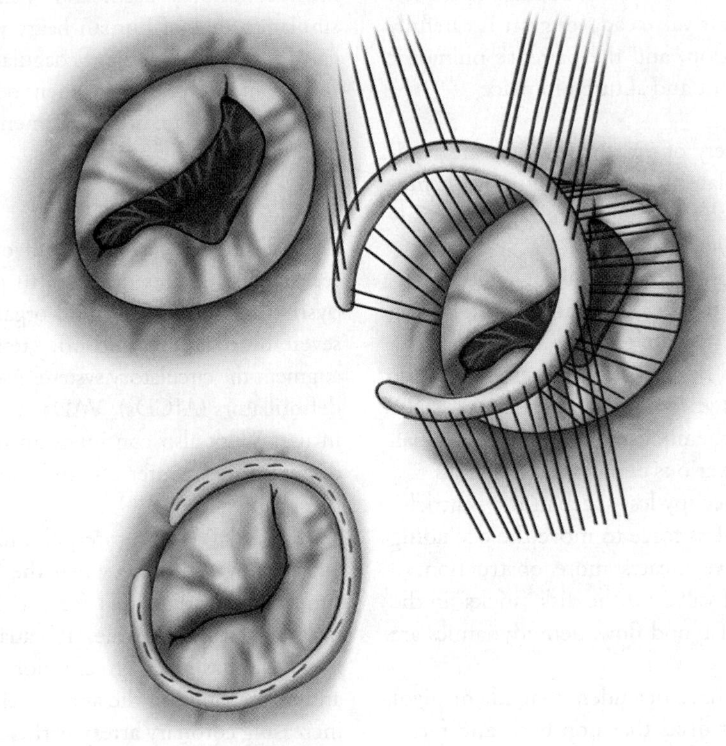

Figure 30-14 Annuloplasty.

gitudinally from the apex toward the base (Figure 30-15). The surgeon digitally examines the atrium for thrombi and examines the valve for calcium particles. Some surgeons digitally open the fused commissures and use a dilator to open the valve and relieve the stenosis. The advantages of the closed approach include a shorter operating time, a simpler procedure, and less blood replacement. Systemic emboli, atrial wall tears, inadequate alleviation of the stenosis, and mitral regurgitation are all risks associated with this approach.

Valve Replacement. Valve replacement is considered when the valve is so stenosed and calcified that repair would not achieve long-term relief. The decision carefully considers the patient's general health status and level of myocardial functioning, since valve replacement carries a significant operative mortality.

The heart usually is approached by a median sternotomy, and cardiopulmonary bypass is initiated. The diseased valve leaflets are excised at the annulus, and the remaining annuli are sized with an obturator. The loose chordae tendineae are excised to prevent their becoming tangled in the new valve, and the prosthetic valve is sutured into the new annulus. The operative mortality rate for aortic valve replacement is less than 5% but increases to 10% for mitral valve replacement. Risk factors include physiologic and chronologic age, chronicity, type of valvular lesion, and left ventricular dysfunction. Mortality rates for valvular replacement surgery increase in persons older than 70 years.

The Ross procedure is an alternative method of aortic valve replacement using the patient's own pulmonic valve, which has all the characteristics of the patient's aortic valve. This procedure is specifically indicated for young patients with a long life expectancy. Primary indications include isolated aortic valve disease, severe aortic stenosis, and severe aortic regurgitation with or without dilation of the aortic root. A routine midline sternotomy is performed and cardiopulmonary bypass is initiated. Extreme care is

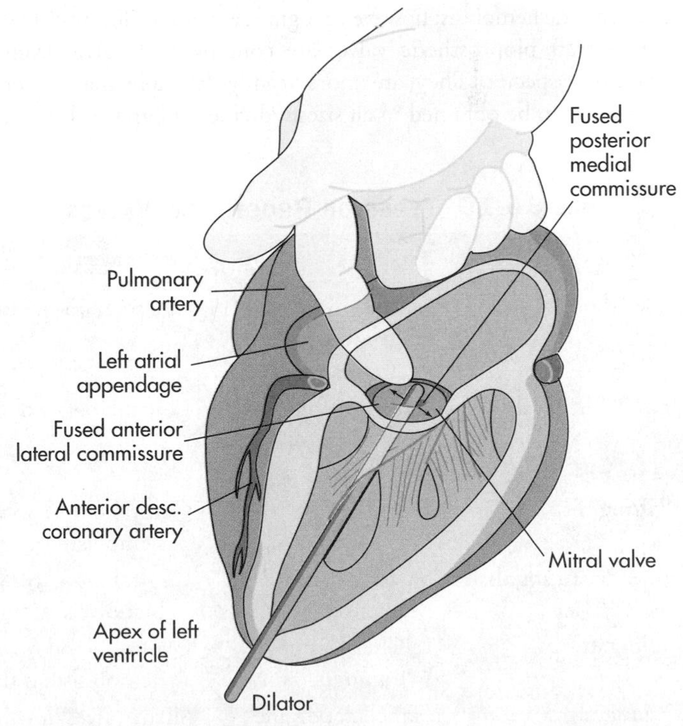

Figure 30-15 Technique of closed mitral commissurotomy using mitral dilating instrument.

taken in removing the pulmonic valve to avoid damage to the left main coronary artery. A homograft valve cadaver graft is carefully inserted into the pulmonic position, and the patient's pulmonic valve is inserted into the aortic root and sutured in place.

TYPES OF VALVES. A wide variety of prosthetic valves are available (Table 30-10). The ideal replacement valve is durable, hemodynamically accurate, nonhemolytic, nonthrombogenic, easily inserted, and anatomically suitable.

Caged-ball prosthetic valves consist of a metal cage with a synthetic, freely moving ball inside; the cage is attached to a sewing ring (Figure 30-16). The ring and struts of the cage are covered by a synthetic cloth. The cloth-covered ring is sutured carefully into the existing valve annulus. Within 2 to 3 months, tissue covers the cloth and the incidence of thromboembolism decreases. Caged-ball valves come in different sizes and various designs and materials.

Caged disk prosthetic valves occupy less space in the ventricles than do other valves and require less force to move the occluding disk. However, this type of valve creates more obstruction to blood flow than do other types of valves. If the disk "sticks" in the cage, causing total obstruction of blood flow, hemodynamics are seriously compromised.

Tilting disk prosthetic valves have occluders that tilt or pivot within a ring rather than balls or disks that pop back and forth. Several varieties are available. This type of valve produces nearly central blood flow through its orifice, which more closely approximates flow through a normal valve; however, the areas under the pivoting points are more susceptible to thrombus formation as a result of blood stasis.

Stenting allografts are human heart valves that are supported or "stented" by an underlying frame. Allografts provide relatively normal hemodynamic characteristics with central flow, no thromboemboli, and little hemolysis; however, allografts are not readily available.

Xenograft bioprosthetic valves are composed of valves from nonhuman species. They are more readily available than other valves and can be obtained in all sizes. Porcine xenograft valves are most commonly used, and their hemodynamic performance is similar to that of human heart valves. Patients with this type of valve may not require anticoagulants. Porcine valves remain patent for about 10 years but then begin to experience calcification. Therefore they are not recommended for use in young people.

Implanted Devices

Cardiac surgery may also involve the implantation of a variety of technologic devices designed to prevent sudden death from fatal dysrhythmias, prevent end-organ damage in individuals with severe heart failure, and offer temporary support to the heart to augment the circulatory system. Automatic implantable cardioverter-defibrillators (AICDs), VADs, and artificial heart chambers are all in use. Work also continues on the artificial heart. The AICD is discussed in Chapter 29, and the left VAD is discussed earlier in this chapter.

The IABP is a counterpulsation device that augments the circulation by pumping when the heart is in diastole. Box 30-12 summarizes indications for use of an IABP. When the balloon inflates during diastole, it causes an intraaortic pressure rise known as diastolic augmentation. This raises the diastolic pressure and forces blood in the aortic arch to flow in a retrograde fashion, increasing coronary artery perfusion. When the balloon deflates at the end of diastole, it reduces pressure in the aorta, and blood from the aortic arch moves into the space that was occupied by the balloon. This reduces the resistance the ventricle must overcome during systole. The LV empties more effectively, leaving more space for ventricular filling, which also reduces preload.

The intraaortic balloon is inserted percutaneously or by cutdown into the right or left femoral artery and advanced into the thoracic aorta. An axillary approach may also be used. It is sutured into place after the balloon tip has been correctly positioned just distal to the left subclavian artery. The balloon catheter is attached to a pump that inflates and deflates it with helium. The timing of the inflation-deflation sequence is extremely important in obtain-

TABLE 30-10 TYPES OF PROSTHETIC VALVES

Type	Examples	Advantages	Disadvantages
Caged ball	Starr-Edwards Braunwald-Cutter McGovern-Cromie	Durable, low incidence of endocarditis	Large size that may obstruct blood flow
Single tilting disk	Hufnagel Cross-Jones Kay-Shiley	Low incidence of thromboemboli	Disk may stick, causing severe obstruction of blood flow
Tilting disk	Björk-Shiley Wada-Cutter	Central blood flow, low incidence of hemolysis	Higher incidence of thrombus
Bileaflet tilting disk	St. Jude Medical Medtronic-Hall	Central blood flow, low incidence of hemolysis	Higher incidence of thrombus
Allograft	Lillehei-Kaster homograft valve	Central blood flow, low incidence of hemolysis, no thromboemboli	High incidence of calcification
Xenograft	Hancock porcine Carpentier-Edwards porcine	Silent valves, low incidence of thromboembolism or hemolysis	High incidence of calcification over time

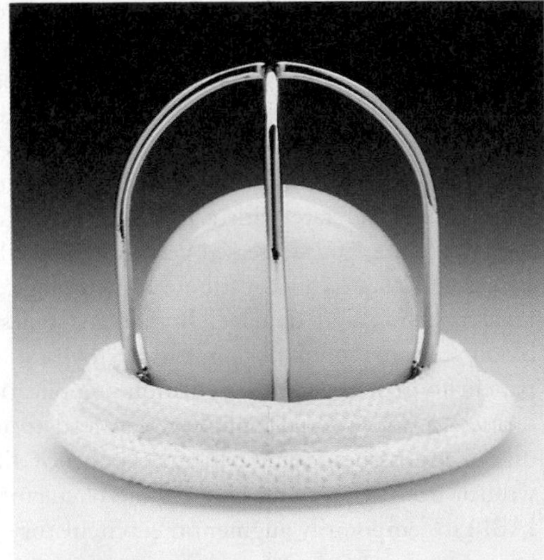

A

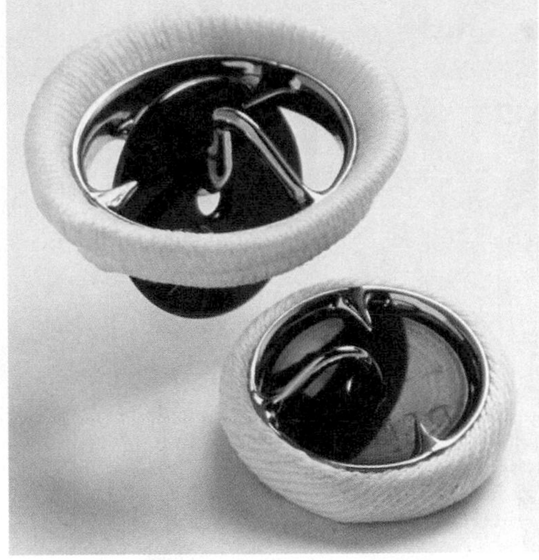

B

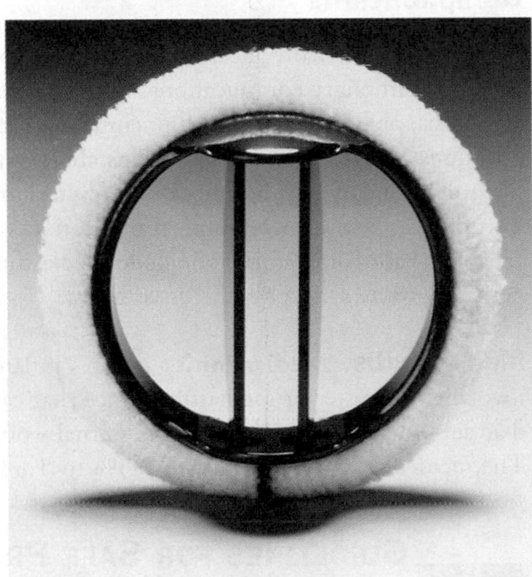

C

Figure 30-16 **A,** Starr-Edwards caged-ball prosthetic valve. **B,** Medtronic-Hall caged-disk prosthetic valve. **C,** St. Jude Medical tilting-disk heart valve.

Box 30-12 Intraaortic Balloon Counterpulsation: Indications for Use

- Cardiogenic shock secondary to acute myocardial infarction
- Other low cardiac output states
- During emergency diagnostic procedures on unstable cardiac patients
- In unstable cardiac patients before and during open heart surgery
- Assistance in removing patients from cardiopulmonary bypass after surgery
- Drug-resistant, life-threatening dysrhythmias
- Unstable angina pectoris
- Severe acute myocardial infarction

ing maximal counterpulsation effect. The ECG is used to trigger the balloon, which inflates just at the beginning of ventricular diastole, immediately after closure of the aortic valve. The balloon remains inflated during diastole and then deflates immediately before the next ventricular systole, just before the aortic valve reopens (Figure 30-17).

The IABP is used to provide temporary assistance to the patient's circulation until the underlying condition can be corrected. It is not indicated for persons whose underlying disease is so severe that eventual weaning from the IABP is considered impossible. Although patients have been maintained on the pump from several hours to several months, the usual time interval is 2 or 3 days. The patient undergoing intraaortic balloon counterpulsation requires intensive nursing observation and care (see the Guidelines for Safe Practice box).

Cardiopulmonary Bypass

Many heart surgery procedures require either partial or total cardiopulmonary bypass. In partial, or left heart, bypass, blood is drained from the LA and LV and passed through a pulsatile or roller pump, which returns the blood to the common femoral artery or the descending aorta. This type of bypass does not interrupt the pulmonary circulation.

In total cardiopulmonary bypass the heart-lung bypass machine provides artificial oxygenation and circulation of the blood throughout the surgical procedure. Venous blood is removed from

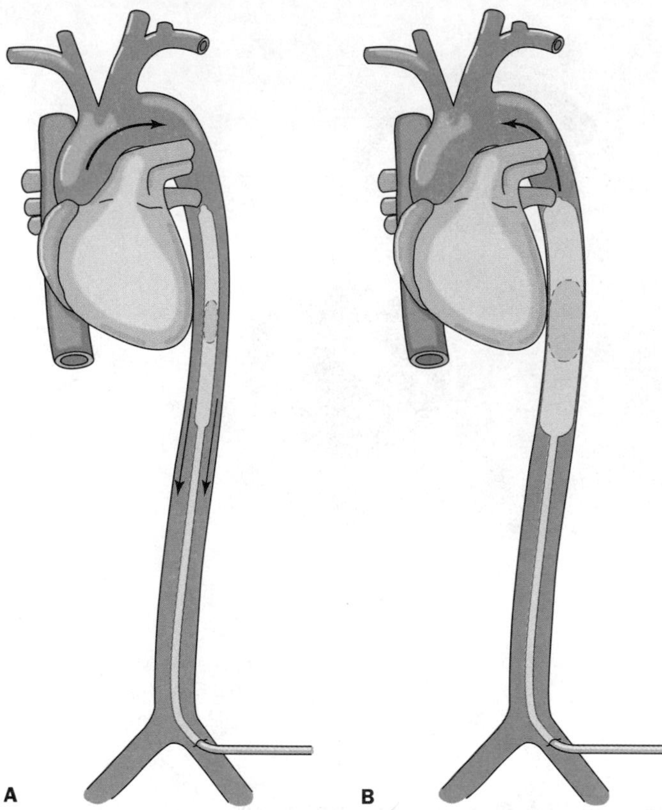

Figure 30-17 Representation of intraaortic balloon positioned just distal to left subclavian artery. **A,** Balloon is deflated, allowing forward blood flow during systole. **B,** Balloon is inflated to increase coronary perfusion during diastole.

the body through large cannulas placed in either the RA or the inferior or superior vena cava (Figure 30-18). The blood passes through an oxygenating mechanism and is then pumped back into the arterial circulation through large cannulas placed in either the ascending aorta or the femoral artery. In addition to providing artificial oxygenation and circulation, the cardiopulmonary bypass machine also provides a way to administer medications and control body temperature during the procedure. The bypass machine can induce systemic hypothermia by cooling the perfusion solution mildly (86° to 95° F [30° to 35° C]) or profoundly (59° F [15° C]) to lower the metabolic needs and oxygen consumption of the body's vital organs and tissues.

Cardioplegia involves the intentional stoppage of the heart during bypass surgery. The aorta is clamped and a cold cardioplegic solution is infused into the heart and coronary arteries, causing the heart to stop beating. This induced cardiac arrest provides the surgical team with a quiet heart on which to operate. The chilled solution also reduces myocardial oxygen demand and contains an alkaline solution that helps preserve the myocardial tissue.

Once the surgical repair is complete, the blood in the bypass machine is rewarmed, slowly bringing the patient's core body temperature back to near normal. The heart is restarted, the lungs are reexpanded, and weaning from cardiopulmonary bypass begins. The autologous blood from the bypass machine is collected and returned to the patient. Systemic anticoagulation is required during the surgery to prevent thrombus formation within the bypass machine. Anticoagulation also prevents the patient from developing a thrombus during periods of reduced blood flow and cardiac output. Anticoagulation is reversed with protamine sulfate at the end of cardiopulmonary bypass.

Cardiopulmonary bypass has allowed for dramatic advancements in heart surgery, but its use is accompanied by a number of potentially serious complications. Cardiopulmonary bypass creates a shocklike state with a low hematocrit, decreased systolic blood pressure, and decreased perfusion of the body's organs and tissues. This state can contribute to neurologic, myocardial, and renal ischemia and damage. Both platelet destruction and red blood cell hemolysis occur during bypass, predisposing the patient to postoperative coagulation complications.[31] Thrombus formation and arterial embolism can lead to infarction of vital organs and tissues. Some patients experience difficulties in being weaned from bypass and may require circulatory assistance (e.g., IABP) to temporarily augment their circulatory system.

Complications

Many factors can complicate the patient's recovery after cardiac surgery. Pulmonary complications are most common and include atelectasis, pleural effusion, and pneumonia. Cardiovascular complications include hemodynamic instability and dysrhythmias. Neurologic changes, fluid imbalance, fever, immobility, and sleep disturbances are all common complications that can impede recovery. Late complications include mediastinitis and the postpericardiotomy syndrome discussed below.

Mediastinitis. Mediastinitis is an inflammatory process involving the anterior mediastinal space that can occur after cardiac surgery from separation of the sternal wound and infection. The incidence of mediastinitis is 0.5% to 5% of cardiac surgery

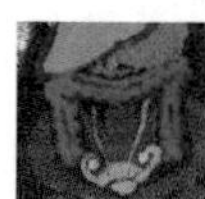

Guidelines for Safe Practice
The Patient With an Intraaortic Balloon Pump

- Monitor vital signs and cardiac indices per protocol.
- Titrate vasopressor and antidysrhythmic agents to keep patient values within established parameters.
- Monitor peripheral pulses and circulation hourly until balloon is removed.
- Position patient to keep affected leg extended, avoiding hip flexion.
  —Keep head of bed elevated to no more than 30 degrees to prevent balloon migration.
- Tilt patient to alternate sides every 2 hours to prevent skin breakdown.
  —Ensure that appropriate pressure-relieving devices are in place on the bed.
- Monitor the insertion site regularly.
  —Keep dressing clean and dry.
  —Change dressing every 24 to 72 hours per protocol using sterile technique.
- Provide teaching to patient and family about the purpose and function of the intraaortic balloon pump (IABP).
  —Provide reassurance and support as needed.
  —Reinforce that the IABP is assisting the patient's heart function, not replacing it.

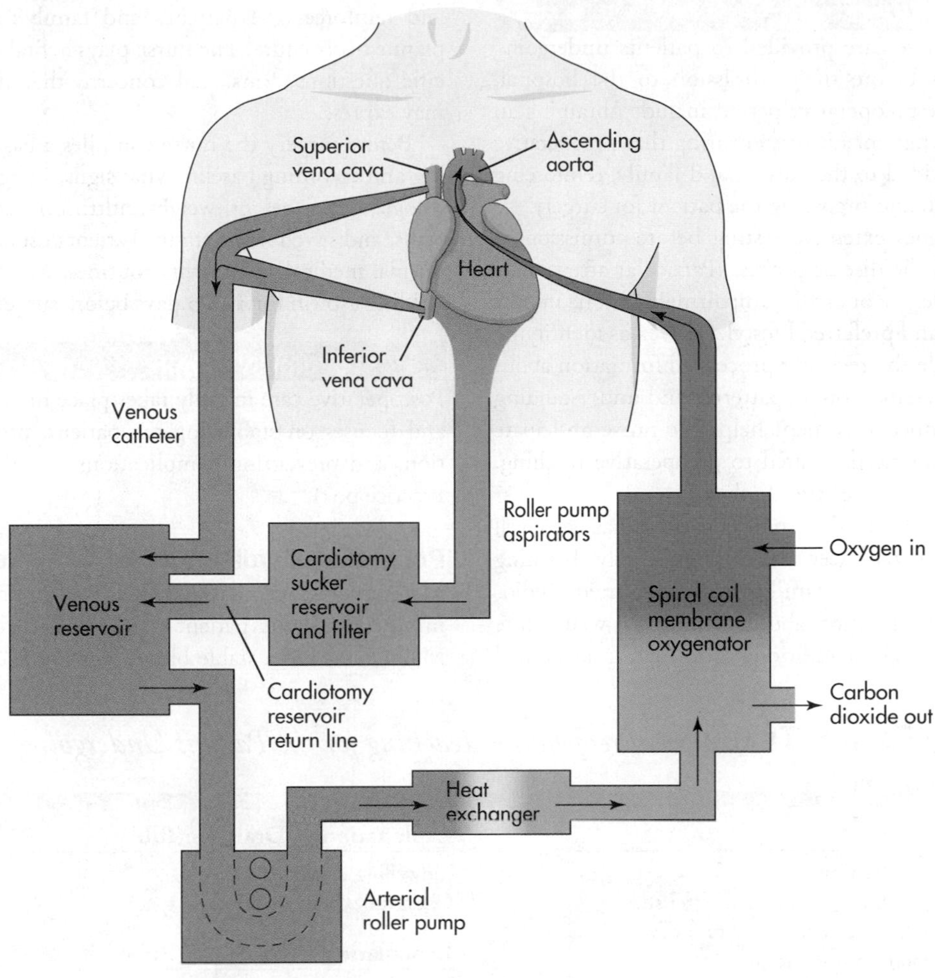

Figure 30-18 Setup for cardiopulmonary bypass.

patients, and it typically occurs 4 to 30 days after surgery.[35] Signs and symptoms include pain, erythema, and tenderness of the incisional area; serous or purulent wound drainage; grating of the sternum with coughing; fever; elevated white blood cell count; and positive wound cultures.[18] The most common infecting organisms are normal skin flora such as *S. epidermidis; S. aureus; Candida albicans;* and *Pseudomonas, Klebsiella, Enterobacter,* and *Aspergillus* organisms. Risk factors for development of mediastinitis include nutritional deficiency, diabetes, obesity, smoking, and the use of the internal mammary artery for bypass grafting.[28] Stress to the sternal wound may also predispose the patient to mediastinitis. Potential stressors include vomiting, coughing, external cardiac massage, and heavy lifting.

Treatment of mediastinitis depends on the invasiveness of the infection and includes parenteral antibiotic therapy, surgical debridement, mediastinal irrigation, and dressing changes. Severe cases of mediastinitis may require muscle or omental flaps to revascularize and support the affected area. Mediastinitis is best prevented through careful hand washing, meticulous aseptic technique, and antibiotic prophylaxis during the perioperative period. Prevention is clearly the most effective intervention.

Postpericardiotomy Syndrome. Postpericardiotomy syndrome is a form of a postcardiac injury syndrome that affects between 10% and 40% of patients undergoing cardiac surgery. Symptoms may appear 1 week to several months after surgery and include fever, malaise, and pleuropericardial pain. An important physical finding is the presence of a pericardial friction rub on auscultation. Diagnostic studies may reveal nonspecific ST-T wave changes on ECG, bilateral pleural effusions on chest x-ray studies, and pericardial effusion on echocardiogram. Associated laboratory values include an increased eosinophil count, increased white blood cell count, and anemia.

Although the cause of postpericardiotomy syndrome is not completely clear, the most accepted explanation is that it is an autoimmune reaction to cardiac injury that leads to the production of anticardiac antibodies. The autoimmune reaction produces the inflammatory changes seen in the typical patient. Treatment is directed toward reducing the fever and pain and consists of administering aspirin, NSAIDs, or corticosteroids. Postpericardiotomy syndrome generally resolves spontaneously within several days to several weeks.

Nursing Management
of the Patient undergoing Cardiac Surgery

Care of the person undergoing cardiac surgery involves a multidisciplinary team approach. Careful attention to discharge planning is essential because the patient's hospital stay is usually only 4 or 5 days.

PREOPERATIVE CARE

Much of the preoperative care provided to patients undergoing cardiac surgery occurs before their admission to the hospital. Important goals for the preoperative period include obtaining an accurate and complete patient history, ensuring that preoperative teaching has been provided to the patient and family, reinforcing that teaching as needed, and preparing the patient for surgery.

The patient undergoes extensive testing before admission to evaluate the severity of the disease process. Particular attention is given to assessing the degree of cardiac impairment and its impact on the patient's ADLs and preferred lifestyle, as well as identifying factors that may impede the recovery process. Information about the patient's support systems, coping patterns, and understanding of the disease and planned treatment helps the nurse anticipate the patient's and family's needs related to preoperative teaching, postoperative recovery, and care after discharge.

Preoperative teaching for cardiac surgery patients has been well researched and standardized[3] (see the Patient/Family Teaching box). Ideally patients and their families receive printed, audiotaped, or videotaped information about the surgery well before admission. The nurse provides additional information as needed and reinforces the patient's and family's understanding of the planned procedure. The nurse plays a vital role in addressing specific questions, fears, and concerns that the patient and family may express.

Before surgery the nurse compiles a baseline data base, assessing and recording baseline vital signs, integrity of all pulses, neurologic status, height, weight, nutritional status, elimination patterns, and psychologic status. Patients usually continue with their normal medical and activity routines, with the exception of withholding aspirin for 1 to 3 days before surgery.

POSTOPERATIVE CARE

Postoperative care initially takes place in an intensive care setting and focuses on stabilizing the patient, promoting cardiac function, and preventing complications (see the Guidelines for Safe Practice box).

Promoting Cardiac Output and Perfusion. The nurse monitors and records vital signs and arterial pressures every 15 minutes until the patient is stable, and then hourly thereafter. Maintenance of a stable blood pressure is critical to the patient's

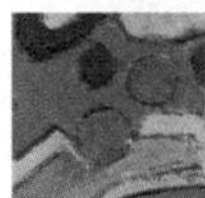

PATIENT/FAMILY TEACHING *Preoperative Teaching for the Patient Undergoing Cardiac Surgery*

General Information

Places of care during hospitalization
—Coronary care unit or intensive care unit after surgery
—Return to general patient care unit in 2 or 3 days
Visiting hours and location of waiting rooms

Description of Surgery

Simple explanation of anatomy of heart and effect of the patient's cardiovascular disorder (e.g., incompetent valve, obstructed coronary artery)
Explanation of surgical procedure, including planned incision
Definition of any unfamiliar terms (e.g., bypass, extracorporeal)
Length of time in surgery: 2 to 4 hours
Length of time until able to see family (usually 1½ to 2 hours after surgery)

Preparation for Surgery

Shower or bath night before surgery with special antimicrobial soap
Surgical shave: shaving of entire chest and abdomen, neck to groin and left midaxillary line to right
Legs shaved if saphenous vein grafts will be used
Preoperative medication

Explanation of Monitors

Round patches on chest connected to a cardiac monitor that records patient's heartbeats
Monitor makes beeping sound all the time

Explanation of Lines

Intravenous routes for fluid and medications
Central venous line in neck or chest to monitor fluid status
Pulmonary artery catheter in chest or neck to measure pulmonary pressures and monitor fluid status
Plastic connector line to obtain blood samples without a needlestick

Explanation of Drainage Tubes

Indwelling urinary catheter
Chest tube: bloody drainage expected

Explanation of Breathing Tube

Tube in windpipe connected to machine called ventilator
Unable to speak with tube in place but can mouth words and communicate in writing
Tube removed when patient is fully awake and stable
Secretions in lungs or tube removed by nurse using a suction catheter
Food and oral fluids not permitted until breathing tube is removed

Explanation and Demonstration of Activities and Exercises

Purpose of activity: to promote circulation, keep lungs clear, and prevent infection
Activity includes:
—Turning from side to side in bed
—Sitting on edge of bed
—Sitting in chair the night of or morning after surgery
Range-of-motion exercises
Deep breathing using sustained maximal inspiration
Movement somewhat restricted by tubes and lines, but nurse will assist patient

Relief of Pain

Some pain, but not excruciating (different pain from original angina if this was present)
Frequent pain medication to relieve the pain, but patient should always tell nurse when pain is present

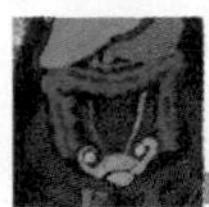

GUIDELINES FOR SAFE PRACTICE *The Patient Who Has Undergone Cardiac Surgery*

I. Monitoring
 A. Cardiovascular
  1. Blood pressure and pulse (rate, pulse deficit)
  2. Pulmonary artery pressure (PAP), pulmonary capillary wedge pressure (PCWP), cardiac output (CO), central venous pressure (CVP), left atrial pressure (LAP)
  3. Electrocardiogram for signs of dysrhythmias
  4. Body temperature
  5. Skin color, temperature, capillary filling
  6. Signs of hypovolemic shock (decreased CVP, decreased LAP, decreased PCWP, decreased CO)
  7. Signs of cardiac tamponade (cessation of chest drainage, restlessness, decreased blood pressure, increased CVP, increased PAP, increased LAP)
 B. Respiratory
  1. Respirations: rate, depth, quality
  2. Breath sounds
  3. Chest tubes for patency and drainage
  4. Autotransfuse chest tube drainage
 C. Neurologic
  1. Level of consciousness
  2. Pupillary size and reaction
  3. Orientation
  4. Movement and sensation of extremities
 D. Gastrointestinal
  1. Nausea
  2. Anorexia
 E. Urinary
  1. Output (amount)
  2. Color
  3. pH and specific gravity
 F. Fluid and electrolyte balance
  1. Intake/output balance
  2. Daily weights
  3. Serum potassium and calcium levels
  4. Flow rates of parenteral fluids
 G. Presence of discomfort: pain, fatigue
 H. Ability to sleep
 I. Behavior: depression, fear, disorientation, hallucinations

II. Promoting oxygen–carbon dioxide exchange
 A. Provide preoxygenation and suction during intubation; suction as necessary after extubation.
 B. Position with head only slightly elevated; turn side to side.
 C. Encourage breathing exercise; incentive spirometry.
 D. Give analgesics before breathing and coughing exercises.
 E. Encourage range-of-motion exercises and progressive activity.

III. Promoting comfort
 A. Give opioid analgesics every 3 hours during the first 24 hours, then as needed.
 B. Give frequent mouth care.
 C. Control environment for comfort.
 D. Change bed linens when diaphoresis is present (assure patient that this is common).
 E. Plan activities to permit periods of sleep.
 F. Provide back rubs for backache.
 G. Splint incision during coughing.
 H. Encourage patient to share feelings and experiences.
 I. Support family visiting.

IV. Promoting activity
 A. Provide for passive then active range-of-motion exercises.
 B. Encourage ambulation when permitted.
 C. Initiate sternal precautions if median sternotomy approach is used.

V. Teaching
 A. Promote progressive return to physical activity as recommended by the physician.
 B. Initiate rehabilitation exercise program.
 C. Sexual activity is usually permitted in 3 to 4 weeks.
 D. Signs of overexertion include fatigue, dyspnea, pain.
 E. Encourage patient to eat a balanced diet with any prescribed modifications (such as no added salt or low cholesterol).
 F. Medications
  1. Name, dosage, schedule, action, and side effects of prescribed medications
  2. Use of prescribed medications as needed
 G. Signs that may persist include dyspnea, pain, night sweats.
 H. Signs requiring medical attention include fever, increasing dyspnea, or chest pain with minimal exertion.
 I. Importance of ongoing medical care.

recovery, and pharmacologic agents are used aggressively to keep the patient's blood pressure within the desired range. Postoperative hypertension can lead to excessive postsurgical bleeding, cardiac tamponade, and excessive oxygen demand in the weakened myocardium. Postoperative hypertension can also result from the patient awakening from anesthesia and experiencing anxiety and acute pain. Appropriate pain management and patient reassurance assist in the management of postoperative hypertension. An unstable low blood pressure must also be aggressively treated. Causes include hypovolemia and cardiogenic shock.

The nurse measures central venous pressure, pulmonary artery pressure, pulmonary capillary wedge pressure, and cardiac output as indicated by the patient's condition. The nurse monitors peripheral pulses for bilateral strength and symmetry, and compares apical and radial pulses for evidence of a pulse deficit. Skin color, temperature, and capillary refill are assessed for evidence of adequate tissue perfusion. Urinary output, a reliable indicator of cardiac output, is assessed hourly.

The patient's ECG is monitored continuously and compared with the preoperative baseline. Cardiac dysrhythmias are common and may be triggered by operative trauma, anesthesia, extracorporeal circulation, alterations in potassium levels, hypotension, hypovolemia, and hypoxia. Supraventricular tachycardia commonly occurs after cardiac surgery because of edema or inflammation in the atrial tissue. Atrial flutter, atrial fibrillation, or other supraventricular tachycardias produce decreased left ventricular diastolic filling and a subsequent deterioration in cardiac output.[23] Postoperative dysrhythmias are aggressively managed with antidysrhythmic agents (see Chapter 29) or temporary cardiac pacing.

Temporary epicardial pacing may be used to manage cardiac dysrhythmias and low cardiac output. Atrial pacing can effectively restore a normal sinus rhythm. Bradydysrhythmias after cardiac surgery are transient and may be associated with low cardiac output. Temporary pacing may be required to increase the heart rate and augment cardiac output. Temporary pacing wires are a potential source of lethal ventricular dysrhythmias if they come in contact with a ground current, and the electrodes must be insulated with either a rubber cap or glove when not in use.[21]

Patients with mechanical or bioprosthetic heart valves are at high risk for developing systemic emboli. Anticoagulation is necessary to prevent thrombus formation on the valve surface. Warfarin, the most commonly used anticoagulant, is used long term. The maintenance dose of warfarin is based on the INR (international normalized ratio), which allows for greater standardization in anticoagulant monitoring than the use of the traditional prothrombin time. See Chapter 31 for a discussion of the patient teaching associated with anticoagulant use.

Maintaining Blood Volume and Chest Drainage. Mediastinal and possibly pleural chest tubes are placed during surgery to drain the surgical area. Refer to Chapter 26 for further information about the care of a patient with a chest tube. The nurse assesses and records chest tube drainage hourly to monitor for postsurgical bleeding. Drainage should not exceed 100 ml/hr during the first 2 postoperative hours and should not exceed approximately 500 ml during the first 24 hours. A sudden increase or cessation in drainage from the chest tubes may signify a postoperative bleeding problem, and the surgeon is notified immediately. Sudden cessation can also indicate clotting in the tubes.

Clotting predisposes the patient to cardiac tamponade, as the drainage builds up around the heart. Cardiac tamponade requires immediate emergent intervention, and the nurse needs to be familiar with its classic clinical manifestations (see Clinical Manifestations box).

Excessive blood loss through the chest tubes can lead to hypovolemic shock unless the patient's blood volume is maintained. Treatment of postoperative hypotension includes fluid resuscitation and gentle rewarming of the patient's core body temperature. Ideally the chest drainage system allows for the collection of bloody chest drainage for later autotransfusion in the event of a bleeding complication. This avoids the risks of transfusion reaction and disease transmission. Postoperative bleeding may require correction of clotting abnormalities or surgical reexploration of the chest. Refer to Chapter 19 for further discussion of hypovolemic and cardiogenic shock management.

Persistent cardiogenic shock that is unresponsive to these standard interventions may be treated with a temporary mechanical assist device. Intraaortic balloon counterpulsation can be used at any point during the preoperative, perioperative, or postoperative period. The use of a VAD may also provide circulatory assistance if the myocardial performance is insufficient to meet the body's needs. Administration of inotropic agents also helps stimulate myocardial performance.

Although patients are rewarmed before cardiopulmonary bypass is terminated, body temperature frequently remains unstable, leading to postoperative hypothermia. Persistent hypothermia causes shivering, increases myocardial workload and oxygen demand, and increases carbon dioxide and lactic acid production. Measures to gently rewarm the patient include the use of heat lamps, thermal blankets, and perfusion blankets and the infusion of vasodilating agents. Once the patient's body temperature has rewarmed, cool or diaphoretic skin can be an important indicator of shock.

Promoting a Patent Airway and Effective Gas Exchange. Intubation and mechanical ventilation are maintained until the patient is stable and fully recovered from anesthesia. The nurse monitors and records the rate, depth, and quality of respirations and assesses the patient's breath sounds. The effectiveness of coughing efforts and sputum production are monitored. Arterial blood gas and oxygen saturation monitoring provide evidence of effective gas exchange. A postoperative chest x-ray examination verifies proper lung reexpansion and chest tube placement after the surgical procedure. In general, patients are awake and extubated within 4 to 18 hours after cardiac surgery.

The lack of alveolar expansion and ventilation during cardiopulmonary bypass contributes to decreased surfactant production and alveolar collapse in the postoperative period. Therefore the nurse promotes aggressive pulmonary hygiene every 1 to 2 hours while the patient is awake. Administration of adequate pain medication helps the patient cough, breathe deeply, and use an incentive spirometer more effectively. Splinting the surgical incision with a small pillow or folded blanket provides extra support during coughing. Patients who are unable to clear excessive pulmonary secretions may require nasotracheal suctioning. Frequent position changes while in bed and early ambulation are also critical interventions to prevent pulmonary complications after cardiac surgery.

Monitoring Fluid Balance. Accurate recording of intake and output is essential for the first few postoperative days. Careful observation of hourly urinary output, as well as urine color, pH, and specific gravity, provides essential information about renal function. Urinary output should be at least 30 ml/hr. Red blood cells may be present in the urine initially as a result of cardiopulmonary bypass. Fluids are limited at first to reduce the chance of fluid overload and to decrease cardiac workload. Daily weights are obtained, and diuretics are administered if fluid retention occurs.

Renal insufficiency after heart surgery can be caused by complications of cardiopulmonary bypass. The destruction of red blood cells can cause obstruction in the kidneys. If low-perfusion states occurred during the surgical procedure, the kidneys themselves may have been damaged, resulting in acute tubular necrosis. If acute renal failure is severe and prolonged, temporary hemodialysis is initiated. Up to 25% of cardiac surgery patients may experience some form of renal failure after bypass.

The nurse checks serum electrolyte levels, particularly serum potassium, magnesium, and phosphorus, several times during the

CLINICAL MANIFESTATIONS
Cardiac Tamponade

- Diminished or absent point of maximal impulse
- Diminished heart sounds
- Tachycardia
- Paradoxical pulse
- Narrowed pulse pressure
- Distended neck veins (increased central venous pressure)

first 24 hours and at least daily thereafter. Supplemental electrolytes may be needed in the immediate postoperative period, particularly if diuretics are in use. The serum glucose may be initially elevated from the stress of surgery and cardiopulmonary bypass, but this is temporary and usually does not require intervention.

The nurse obtains hemoglobin and hematocrit values and prothrombin times daily to assess the extent of blood loss and the effect of replacement therapy. Plasma and plasma expanders are given to avoid hypovolemia and to maintain a normal osmotic gradient in the blood. Crystalloid solutions are administered to ensure adequate circulating volume.

Monitoring Neurologic Status. Patients usually awaken within 1 to 2 hours after surgery. Failure to awaken may be the result of unusually deep anesthesia or embolization of air, calcium, fat, or thrombotic particles to the brain. A sluggish return of consciousness may be caused by poor cerebral perfusion or microembolization during cardiopulmonary bypass.

In the immediate postoperative period the nurse frequently checks pupil size, equality, and reaction to light. Pupil dilation may be caused by excessive carbon dioxide in the blood or by cardiac medications such as atropine. Constricted pupils may be caused by opioids or dopamine. Disorientation and restlessness may be signs of hypoxia or embolization in addition to being symptoms of pain, fatigue, fear, or sensory overload.[36]

Pain management is critical in the postoperative period, and patients are kept as comfortable as possible. In addition to patient comfort, pain management reduces stress on the heart, decreases the need for oxygen, and promotes healing. Other comfort measures include positioning, controlling environmental temperature, providing frequent oral hygiene, and encouraging visits from concerned family or friends.

Promoting Activity. After cardiac surgery the patient is weak and tires easily. Activity periods are organized so that rest periods can be frequent and uninterrupted. If a median sternotomy was performed, the nurse takes precautions to protect the healing sternum from injury. Sternal precautions include reducing pressure on the arms and upper body while moving in bed, out of bed, or out of a chair.[30] In addition, patients are instructed to lift no more than 10 pounds for up to 6 weeks, and not to be behind a steering wheel for at least 4 weeks.

Passive arm exercises are started shortly after surgery, followed by active exercises as the patient gains strength. The nature and extent of activity depend on the patient's situation, but most patients are assisted out of bed the first day after surgery. Activity progresses steadily from dangling at the bedside to sitting in a chair. Ambulation begins in the room and, if tolerated, progresses to walking in the halls. Close supervision is necessary during ambulation; if the activity causes excessive fatigue, dyspnea, or an increased pulse or respiratory rate, it is discontinued, the patient is returned to bed, and the physician is consulted before further activity is attempted. Many patients experience a prompt and satisfying improvement in their activity tolerance after corrective cardiac surgery.

Supporting Nutrition. Gastrointestinal symptoms, such as anorexia and nausea, may occur after cardiac surgery from preexisting gastrointestinal disease, drug therapy, perioperative hypoperfusion or hypotension, systemic hypothermia, stress, and anxiety. Although anorexia occurs more commonly than nausea, the latter is more distressing. The nurse institutes comfort measures to decrease nausea and administers antiemetics if needed. Small amounts of food may be more palatable than a large meal.

Promoting Psychologic Adaptation. The psychologic ramifications of heart surgery, sleep deprivation, and sensory overload can be overwhelming. Some patients experience a period of depression or disorientation after surgery, and others may become unreasonably fearful or hallucinatory. The disorientation can even progress to panic. The nurse is alert to subtle behavioral changes and reassures the patient and family that these reactions are common and do not mean the patient is "losing his or her mind." Physiologic causes of the behavior must be ruled out.

It is helpful to the patient and family if the nursing staff members attempt to personalize the patient's experience as much as possible. It is easy to lose sight of the person behind the monitoring equipment in an intensive care unit.[8] Calling the patient by his or her preferred name, using frequent physical contact, orienting the patient to time and place, and including the patient in any discussions that are held at the bedside are all simple strategies that can help decrease the sense of isolation.

Patient/Family Teaching. In preparation for discharge after cardiac surgery, the nurse and care team explore the safety and appropriateness of the patient's normal daily activities. The patient generally is allowed to do anything that does not cause fatigue or pain but is advised against attempting too much too soon. Patients are instructed to resume activities slowly and progress gradually to more energy-consuming tasks.[6] Sexual intercourse usually is permitted within 3 to 4 weeks after surgery. The physician will want the patient to return for frequent medical follow-up visits, at which time advice will be given regarding the resumption of additional activities. The nurse provides definitive instructions about climbing stairs; attempt only two or three steps the first time, climb slowly, and plan to rest two or three times while climbing one flight of stairs.

The family is also instructed about the patient's activity guidelines. If the patient was an invalid before surgery, the family may be fearful about any increase in activity, which can create tension between the patient and family. Referral to a structured cardiac rehabilitation program can be an effective strategy for achieving ongoing support and supervision.

The nurse cautions the patient and family that no major improvement may be noticed immediately after the operation. It can take as much as 3 to 6 months before the full results of the surgery can be evaluated. Many patients are able to return to work, but the physician needs to provide them with specific directions regarding timing and intensity. Patients are informed that some dyspnea and pain may still be present after discharge. Discharge instructions for cardiac surgery patients and a list of symptoms to report are presented in the Patient/Family Teaching box.

GERONTOLOGIC CONSIDERATIONS

As the population ages, the number of very old patients (between 80 and 100 years old) undergoing cardiac surgery continues to increase. Advanced age alone is not a contraindication to cardiac

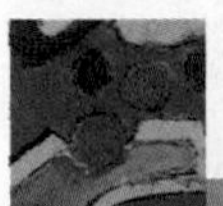

PATIENT/FAMILY TEACHING *Discharge Instructions After Cardiac Surgery*

Incision Care

Cleaning twice a day
Care of sterile strips, staples, sutures
Incision massage with cocoa butter after 10 days

Showering

Washing with soap that is unscented, gentle, bactericidal
No tub baths until incisions completely healed

Activity

No lifting greater than 10 pounds
No driving for 6 weeks
No prolonged sitting
Activity as tolerated; cardiac rehabilitation if ordered
May resume sexual activity when comfort level allows, usually 3 weeks

Nutrition

Low-sodium, low-fat, heart-healthy diet
Increased protein intake for 4 to 6 weeks

Medications

Pain medications: do not drive or operate machinery if taking opioids

Symptoms to Report

Incision red (like a sunburn)
Area around incision feels warm
Incision swollen
Incision with increased or different drainage (pus)
Fever above 100.5° F (38° C)
Unusual pain
Return of presurgical symptoms:
If angina occurs, rest and take nitroglycerin; seek medical attention for angina unrelieved by three nitroglycerin tablets or for frequent occurrence of angina.
Shortness of breath
Palpitations (skipping of heartbeat)
Heart beating too fast or too slow
Severe bruising or bleeding
Worsening fatigue
Flu symptoms (aches, chills, fever, loss of appetite)

Miscellaneous

Women wear a bra to help support chest
TED stockings
Daily weights—notify physician for gain of 6 pounds in 2 days
Incentive spirometer three times a day
Prevent constipation with fiber, fluids, and stool softeners

surgery, but consideration of the special needs of the older patient is essential to a successful postoperative recovery.

Cardiovascular age-related changes include decreased cardiac output, decreased vasomotor responsiveness, decreased cardiac conduction tissue, and increased aortic calcification. These changes can predispose the very old patient to decreased tolerance for sudden fluctuations in fluid volume status, orthostasis, or heart rhythms. Age-related changes in renal and hepatic function can alter the pharmacokinetics of drugs; endocrine and immune system dysfunction can contribute to impaired skin integrity and wound healing. Changes in mobility, functional status, and neuropsychologic status can impair postoperative progress and delay recovery. In addition, very old patients often have significant coexisting medical problems that can complicate recovery from surgery. Discharge planning is particularly important for this population, who are likely to experience a longer period of convalescence and may have limited social supports in the community.

ARE YOU READY?

Following Coronary artery bypass graft surgery, the nurse would expect how much chest tube drainage in the first 24 hours?

1. Less than 150 ml
2. 150–250 ml
3. 300–500 ml
4. 600–800 ml

Heart Transplantation

Etiology and Epidemiology. Since the first heart transplant was performed in 1967, the procedure has steadily evolved into a mainstream treatment for end-stage cardiac disease. The medical management of heart failure (see pp. 816 to 826) has also improved dramatically, and both the morbidity and mortality associated with the condition have decreased significantly. However, heart transplant is still considered an important option of last resort when medical therapy is no longer effective. Transplant is primarily used with patients experiencing rapidly decompensating new-onset heart failure and those with chronic failure who no longer respond satisfactorily to comprehensive medical therapy. Primary cardiomyopathy (see p. 829) is a common precipitating cause.

An imbalance between supply and demand exists for heart transplants, just as it does for all major organs, and the waiting time to receive a heart may be prolonged. As the patient's condition deteriorates, extended hospitalization may be required. These patients are typically physiologically unstable and require continuous complex care, including multiple drugs and supportive technologies such as an IABP or VAD. About 25% of those awaiting a transplant die before a suitable organ can be found.

About 3800 patients are on the heart transplant waiting list, and just over 2000 transplants are performed each year.[33] The number of transplants performed has remained fairly stable and even declined in recent years as transplant teams have become increasingly skilled in selecting viable donor hearts. This number is also somewhat constrained by the fact that living donors are, of course, not an option with heart transplants. In the United States approximately 75% of heart transplants are performed in men and a similar percentage are performed in Caucasians. The Organ Procurement and Transplantation Network reported in 2003 that 85.3% of heart transplant patients survived for 1 year and 70.6% survived for 5 years.[33] Although most potential transplant candidates are both free from major organ system diseases and less than 60 years of age, heart transplant is following the trend of other major organ transplants in seeing a significant increase in the percentage of potential recipients who are over 65.

Collaborative Care Management. Donor matching includes ABO blood group compatibility and negative lymphocyte cross matching. HLA screening has not proven to be of significant benefit and is not usually performed. Organ viability issues make time

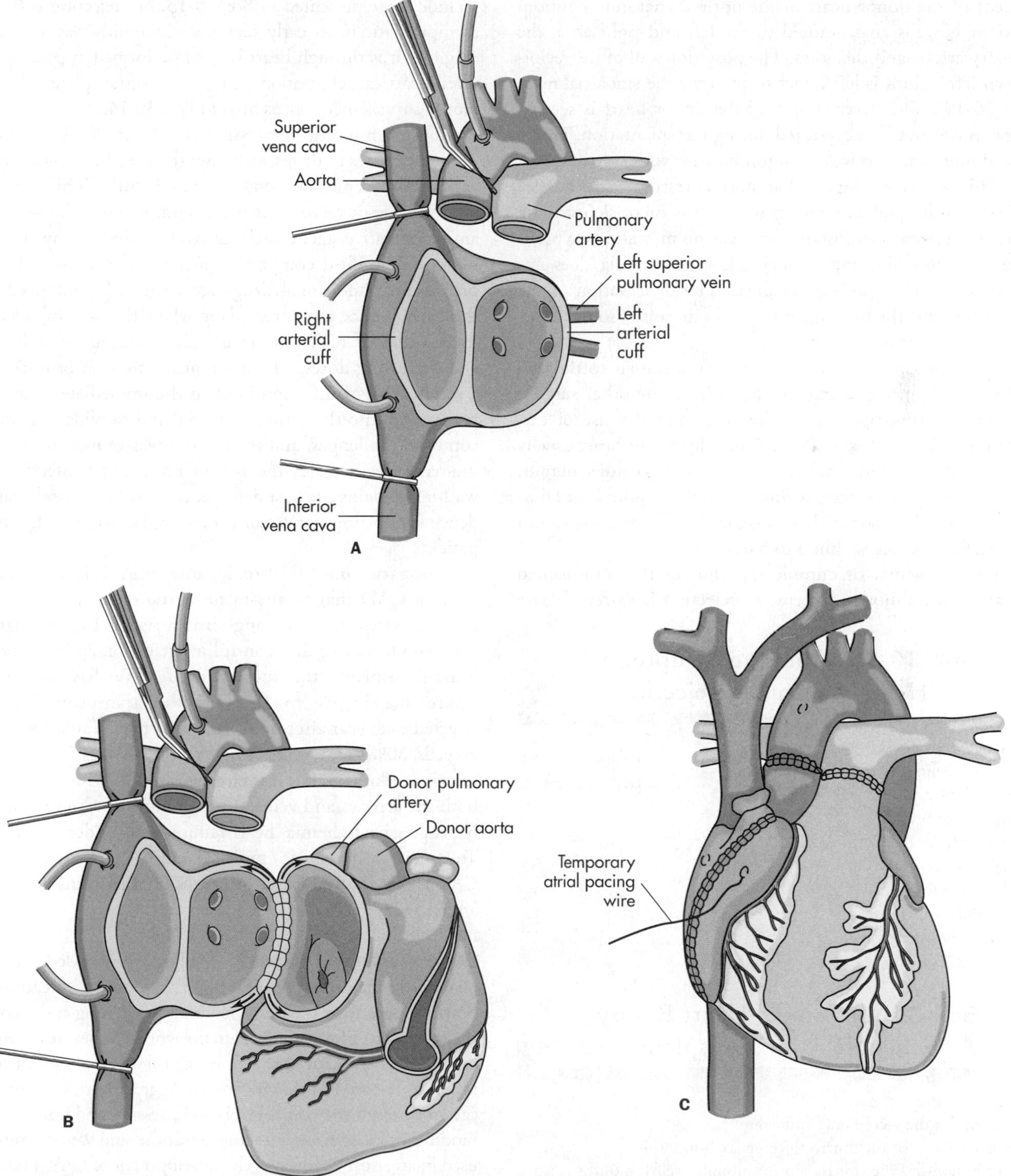

Figure 30-19 **A,** Recipient arterial cuffs and great vessels after cardiectomy. **B,** Beginning of left atrial suture line. *Arrows* indicate direction of suture line. **C,** Completed cardiac transplant.

constraints extremely important in heart transplantation. Although all heart transplant organs are obtained from cadaver sources, transplant surgeons have steadily decreased their use of hearts from persons who experienced sudden cardiac death because of the low long-term viability of these organs.

The surgical procedure developed by Lower and Shumway has been the gold standard for heart transplant for more than 30 years. It involves the excision of the recipient's damaged heart and placement of the donor heart in the normal anatomic position. The donor heart is anastomosed to the left and right atria, the pulmonary artery, and the aorta. The posterior wall of the recipient's own left atrium is left intact to preserve the sinoatrial node (Figure 30-19). The nerve supply of the donor heart is severed during removal and is not restored during transplantation. Therefore the donor heart receives no autonomic nervous system innervation. This results in a higher than normal resting heart rate (90 to 110 beats/min) and an inability to abruptly increase heart rate in response to stress. Orthostatic hypotension may also be a problem because normal compensatory reflex tachycardia does not occur in response to position changes. The denervation of the heart also prevents the transmission of pain impulses, so the recipient will not experience angina.

Postoperative care after heart transplant is similar to the care provided after bypass grafting (see p. 848) or any other surgical procedure requiring opening of the chest and the use of cardiopulmonary bypass (see p. 845). A healthy donor heart usually functions well and rapidly stabilizes the recipient's cardiac output. Intensive hemodynamic monitoring is initially required, and dysrhythmias are a common early problem. Transfer to a step-down unit is usually possible within 3 to 5 days.

Hyperacute, acute, or chronic rejection of the transplanted heart can occur, although hyperacute rejection is extremely rare with appropriate ABO matching and an aggressive immunosuppression protocol. Acute rejection occurs when surface antigens on the transplanted heart are recognized as foreign. It commonly occurs in the first few weeks after transplant but can appear anytime thereafter. Up to 50% of heart transplant recipients have at least one rejection episode in the first year, and a complex regimen of antirejection medications must be taken for life. Most episodes can be successfully reversed. Common symptoms of rejection include those presented in Box 30-13, but rejection is frequently asymptomatic in its early stages, and the only way to accurately diagnose it is through heart biopsy, performed as part of a right-sided heart catheterization. A typical posttransplant schedule for biopsy surveillance is presented in Box 30-14.

Routine immunosuppression usually involves at least three different classes of drugs, although the specific selection of drugs varies from center to center. A calcineurin inhibitor such as cyclosporine or tacrolimus is one component. The second is an antiproliferative agent such as azathioprine or mycophenolate mofetil. The third component includes corticosteroids such as prednisone. Additional drugs are frequently employed during the early weeks after transplant when the risk of rejection is high. Cases of rejection are usually managed by adding drugs and increasing doses. The immunosuppression protocol creates a serious risk of infection both in the immediate postoperative period and into the future. Bacterial and candidal infections are common challenges, and the use of invasive monitoring devices dramatically increases the risk of nosocomial infection. Hand washing remains the best defense; there is no research-based evidence supporting the use of protective isolation with transplant patients.[45]

Coronary allograft vasculopathy (CAV) is an accelerated form of CAD that occurs in heart transplant patients and is a major obstacle to their long-term survival. Despite significant gains in preventing and controlling rejection and infection after heart transplant, the incidence of CAV has not declined. Approximately 5% to 10% of heart transplant patients are affected each year after transplant, and the cumulative incidence exceeds 50% by 5 years. The exact pathology of the disorder remains unknown, but it is clearly immune mediated and affects both the arteries and veins of the donor heart, producing rapidly progressive ischemia, heart failure, and sudden cardiac death. Treatment at present is empirical and not particularly effective. CAV is the leading cause of death in heart transplant patients after 1 year.[37]

PATIENT/FAMILY TEACHING. Medication knowledge and compliance are major focuses of patient and family education after a heart transplant, as is education about preventing and recognizing the early signs of infection. Patients who were severely debilitated before the transplant may require a prolonged period of rehabilitation to restore health and fitness. Aggressive risk factor modification through the control of blood pressure and lipid levels, diet modification, exercise, smoking cessation, and weight control, are used in an effort to forestall the development of CAV. Heart transplant recipients need to make a commitment to regular follow-up care, including the intensive screening protocol of biopsies that are designed to monitor for rejection.

Box 30-13 Common Symptoms of Heart Transplant Rejection

- Fatigue or weakness
- "Just not feeling right"
- Fever of 100.5° F (38° C) or higher
- Shortness of breath
- Tachycardia or dysrhythmia
- Swelling of the hands or feet
- Sudden weight gain
- Hypotension
- Flulike aches and pains

Box 30-14 Sample Heart Biopsy Schedule After Transplant

- Weekly for the first month
- Biweekly for the second and third months
- Once a month for the fourth through sixth months
- Every 3 months twice for the ninth through twelfth months
- Once a year for the second through fifth years
- Every other year thereafter

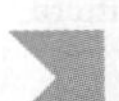

Preparing for Practice

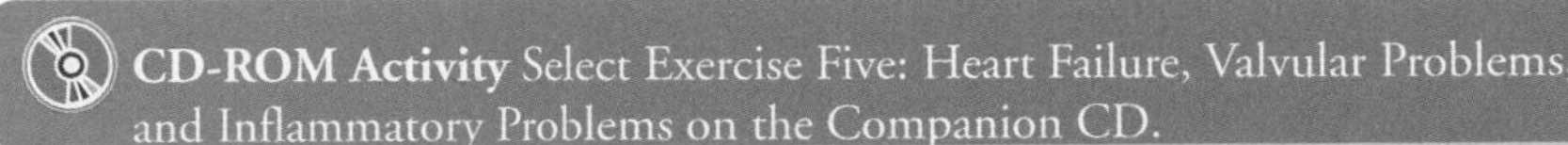

CD-ROM Activity Select Exercise Five: Heart Failure, Valvular Problems, and Inflammatory Problems on the Companion CD.

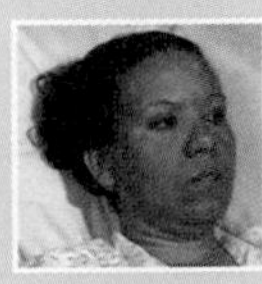

Patient: *Carmen Gonzales,* **Room 302**

Carmen Gonzales, an older Hispanic female, presents with an infected leg that has become gangrenous. She has Type 2 diabetes mellitus, as well as complications of congestive heart failure and osteomyelitis.

Assessment

View the patient's **Report**.

Open the patient's **Medical Record** and familiarize yourself with her care. Specifically search for any information that addresses heart failure or risk for heart failure.

Conduct a **Patient Interview**. As you conduct your interview, focus primarily on data that will be helpful in planning care for this patient. Record the data you collect.

Nursing Diagnoses, Outcomes, and Interventions

1. What information did you find in the History & Physical that addresses Carmen Gonzales' status in relation to heart failure?
2. If you had conducted the initial assessment in the emergency department, would you have gathered any additional assessment data (history or physical examination) related to heart failure? *Hint:* Refer to pp. 814 and 815 if needed.
3. Several events can affect the development of heart failure in a patient. Review Box 30-4 and list the factors that are likely to be the etiology of heart failure for Carmen Gonzales.
4. Based on what you have learned thus far about Carmen Gonzales, identify two specific triggers that are likely to have precipitated temporary decompensation of her status with regard to heart failure.
5. What information in Carmen Gonzales' profile gives you additional clues about the presence of symptoms of heart failure?
6. Use your assessment findings and responses to questions 1 through 5 to formulate an appropriate nursing diagnosis for Ms. Gonzales. Identify three priority nursing interventions and the expected outcome of care.

? Critical Thinking

1. A 59-year-old woman was discharged 2 weeks ago with the diagnosis of heart failure after her second myocardial infarction in 18 months. She now comes to the emergency department with acute shortness of breath, chest pain, a positive S_3, and significant bilateral crackles. Her ECG shows new-onset atrial fibrillation at 150 beats/min and evidence of her prior anterolateral myocardial infarction. Her serum electrolytes are normal, except for a potassium level of 3.2 mEq/L. Her hemoglobin and hematocrit are 7.3 g/dl and 25%, respectively; on discharge, they were 11.2 g/dl and 30.3%. Discuss the likely precipitating events for her heart failure exacerbation, including the pathophysiology.
2. A 72-year-old man has undergone a triple CABG operation without complications and is preparing for discharge tomorrow. What factors do you need to assess about his home situation to appropriately plan for his discharge? What factors would either impair or facilitate his recovery after discharge?

References

1. American Heart Association: *Heart disease and stroke statistics—2004 update,* Dallas, 2003, American Heart Association.
2. Appleton B: The role of exercise training in patients with chronic heart failure, *Brit J Nurs* 13(8):452-456, 2004.
3. Asilioglu K, Celik SS: The effect of preoperative education on anxiety of open cardiac surgery patients, *Patient Educ Counsel* 53(1):65-70, 2004.
4. Bertoni AG et al: Heart failure prevalence, incidence, and mortality in the elderly with diabetes, *Diabetes Care* 27(3):699-703, 2004.
5. Bosen DM: New strategies for treating patients with heart failure, *Nursing* 33(12):44-47, 2003.
6. Brooks D et al: The 2 minute walk test as a measure of functional capacity in cardiac surgery patients, *Arch Phys Med Rehabil* 85(9):1525-1530, 2004.
7. Bush NJ, Griffen-Sobel JP: Chemotherapy-induced cardiomyopathy, *Oncol Nurs Forum* 31(2):185-187, 2004.
8. Contrada RJ et al: Psychosocial factors in outcomes of heart surgery: the impact of religious involvement and depressive symptoms, *Health Psychol* 23(3):227-238, 2004.
9. Costello J, Boblin S: What is the experience of men and women with congestive heart failure? *Can J Cardiovasc Nurs* 14(3):9-20, 2004.
10. Dao Q et al: Utility of B-type natriuretic peptide in the diagnosis of congestive heart failure in an urgent-care setting, *J Am College Cardiol* 37(2):379-385, 2001.
11. Deaton C, Grady KL: State of the science for cardiovascular nursing outcomes: heart failure, *J Cardiovasc Nurs* 19(5):329-338, 2004.
12. Durack DT et al: New criteria for diagnosis of infective endocarditis: utilization of specific echocardiographic findings, *Am J Med* 96:200, 1994.
13. Elliott P, McKenna WJ: Hypertrophic cardiomyopathy, *Lancet* 363(9424):1881-1891, 2004.
14. Feldman PH et al: A randomized intervention to improve heart failure outcomes in community based home health care, *Home Health Care Services Q* 23(1):1-23, 2004.
15. Gura MT, Foreman L: Cardiac resynchronization therapy for heart failure management, *AACN Clin Issues* 15(3):326-339, 492-494, 2004.
16. Harrison A et al: B-type natriuretic peptide predicts future cardiac events in patients presenting to the emergency department with dyspnea, *Ann Emerg Med* 39(2):131-138, 2002.
17. Heart Failure Society of America: HFSA guidelines for management of patients with heart failure caused by left ventricular systolic dysfunction—pharmacological approaches, *J Cardiac Failure* 5(4):357-382, 1999.
18. Holcomb SS: Managing a sternal wound infection after cardiac surgery, *Nursing* 34(9):68-69, 2004.
19. Holcomb SS: Recognizing and managing myocarditis, *Nursing* 34(4):32cc1-2, 32cc4, 2004.
20. Hunt SA et al: ACC/AHA guidelines for the evaluation and management of chronic heart failure in the adult: executive summary: a report of the American College of Cardiology/American Heart Association Task Force on Practice Guidelines (Committee to Revise the 1995 Guidelines for the Evaluation and Management of Heart Failure), *Circulation* 104:2996-3007, 2001.

21. Hyett JM: Caring for a patient after CABG surgery, *Nursing* 34(7):48-49, 2004.
22. Jessup M, Brozena S: Heart failure, *N Engl J Med* 348:2007-2018, 2003.
23. Kern LS: Postoperative atrial fibrillation: new directions in prevention and treatment, *J Cardiovasc Nurs* 19(2):103-107, 2004.
24. Krumholz HM et al: American Heart Association/American College of Cardiology First Scientific Forum on Assessment of Healthcare Quality in Cardiovascular Disease and Stroke: conference proceedings, measuring and improving quality of care: a report of the Quality of Care and Outcomes Research Working Group on Heart Failure, *Circulation* 101(12):1483, 2000.
25. Li IS et al: Proposed modifications to the Duke criteria for the diagnosis of infective endocarditis, *Clin Infect Dis* 30(4):633-638, 2000.
26. Luggen AS: Early management of heart failure, *Geriatr Nurs* 25(4):251-253, 2004.
27. Maisel AS et al: Rapid measurement of B-type natriuretic peptide in the emergency diagnosis of heart failure, *N Engl J Med* 347(3):161-167, 2002.
28. Matorell C et al: Surgical site infections in cardiac surgery: an 11 year perspective, *Am J Infect Control* 32(2):63-68, 2004.
29. McCann GP, Hillis WS: Surgery in asymptomatic aortic stenosis, *BMJ* 328(7431):63-64, 2004.
30. Milgrom LB et al: Pain levels experienced with activities after cardiac surgery, *Am J Crit Care* 13(2):116-125, 2004.
31. Murphy GJ, Angeline GD: Side effects of cardiopulmonary bypass: what is the reality? *J Cardiac Surg* 19(6):481-488, 2004.
32. Nichols GA et al: The incidence of congestive heart failure in type 2 diabetes: an update, *Diabetes Care* 27(8):1879-1884, 2004.
33. OPTN/SRTR: Transplant statistics—2003 annual report, accessed from website: www.ustransplant.org.
34. Paul S, Sneed NV: Strategies for behavior change in patients with heart failure, *Am J Crit Care* 13(4):305-313, 2004.
35. Rao N et al: Prevention of postoperative mediastinitis, *J Healthcare Qual* 26(1):22-28, 60, 2004.
36. Redeker NS, Ruggiero J, Hedges C: Patterns and predictors of sleep pattern disturbance after cardiac surgery, *Res Nurs Health* 27(4):217-224, 2004.
37. Rhodes LR: Cardiac allograft vasculopathy, *Crit Care Nurs Q* 27(1):10-16, 2004.
38. Roger VL et al: Trends in heart failure incidence and survival in a community based population, *JAMA* 292(3):344-350, 2004.
39. Rosenthal K: Using ultrafiltration to treat heart failure, *Nursing* 34(4):17, 2004.
40. Shirai K et al: Minimally invasive coronary artery bypass grafting versus stenting for patients with proximal left anterior descending coronary artery disease, *Am J Cardiol* 93(8):959-962, 2004.
41. Stahovich M, Chillcott S, Ferber L: Management of adult patients with a left ventricular assist device, *Rehabil Nurs* 29(3):100-103, 2004.
42. Thanikachalam M et al: The history and development of direct coronary surgery without cardiopulmonary bypass, *J Cardiac Surg* 19(6):516-519, 2004.
43. Troughton RW, Asher CR, Klein AL: Pericarditis, *Lancet* 363(9410): 717-727, 2004.
44. Trupp RJ: Patient identification and management in congestive heart failure, *CE-Today for Nurse Practitioners* 3(8):5, 2004.
45. Wade CR et al: Postoperative nursing care of the cardiac transplant recipient, *Crit Care Nurs Q* 27(1):17-30, 2004.
46. Wisniewski A: Muscle up your knowledge of myocarditis, *Nursing* 34(10):17, 2004.
47. Wrenger E et al: Interaction of spironolactone with ACE inhibitors or angiotensin receptor blockers: analysis of 44 cases, *Brit Med J* 327(7407):147-149, 2003.
48. Yancy CW et al: Safety and feasibility of using serial infusions of nesiritide for heart failure in an outpatient setting (from the FUSION I trial), *Am J Cardiol* 94(5):595-601, 2004.

Visit the Evolve website: http://evolve.elsevier.com/Monahan/medsurg

CHAPTER 31

Vascular Problems

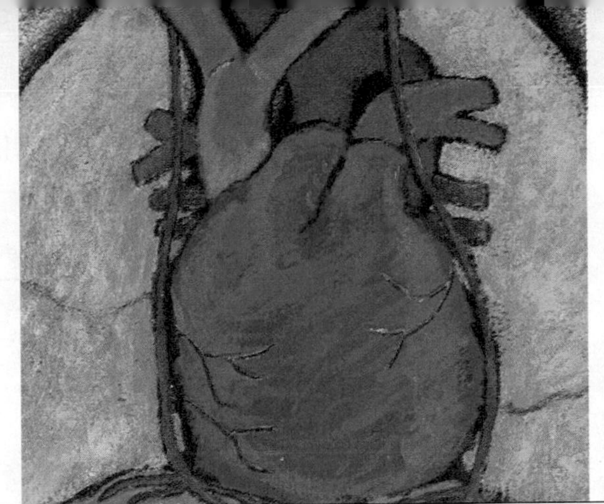

by Carol Lynn Maxwell-Thompson, Kathryn B. Reid

OBJECTIVES

After studying this chapter, the learner should be able to:

1. Discuss the pathophysiology of arterial and venous disease.
2. Prepare a teaching plan for a person with primary hypertension.
3. Discuss the use of pharmacologic agents in the management of vascular diseases.
4. Identify the risk factors associated with the development of vascular disease.
5. Compare the collaborative management of arterial and venous disease.
6. Describe the preoperative and postoperative nursing care for patients undergoing vascular surgery.
7. Develop a care plan for a patient undergoing amputation related to the complications of vascular disease.

KEY TERMS

aneurysm, p. 883
ankle-brachial index, p. 869
deep venous thrombosis, p. 885
embolectomy, p. 881
hypertension, p. 857
intermittent claudication, p. 869
phantom limb pain, p. 876
Raynaud's phenomenon, p. 875
thrombolytics, p. 880
Unna's boot, p. 893

Hypertension

Etiology and Epidemiology. **Hypertension** is defined as a consistent elevation of the systolic blood pressure above 140 mm Hg, a diastolic blood pressure above 90 mm Hg, or a report of taking antihypertensive medication.[10] Early diagnosis and effective management of hypertension are essential because it is a major modifiable risk factor for cerebrovascular, cardiac, vascular, and renal diseases. The higher the blood pressure, the greater the risk for heart attack, heart failure, stroke, and kidney disease. It is estimated that more than 60 million people in the United States have hypertension, but barely half of these individuals are actually diagnosed with the condition. According to the Joint National Committee on the Prevention, Detection, Evaluation, and Treatment of High Blood Pressure (JNC), more than half of individuals from 60 to 69 years of age and three fourths of those 70 and older are affected by hypertension.[10] It is often called "the silent killer," since the condition may proceed undetected and uncontrolled, leading to irreparable end-organ damage. The importance of hypertension as a health problem in the United States is reflected in several specific *Healthy People 2010* goals (see the Healthy People 2010 box).[41]

The two major types of hypertension are essential (primary) and secondary. Primary hypertension accounts for more than 90% of all cases and has no known cause, although it is theorized that genetic factors, hormonal changes, and alterations in sympathetic tone all may play a role in its development. Secondary hypertension develops as a consequence of an underlying disease or condition (Box 31-1). Treatment for secondary hypertension focuses on correcting or controlling the underlying disease process, although only 1% to 2% of cases are curable.

Healthy People 2010

Objectives Related to Hypertension

- Reduce the proportion of adults with high blood pressure to less than 28%.
- Increase the proportion of adults with high blood pressure whose blood pressure is under control to more than 18%.
- Increase the proportion of adults with high blood pressure who are taking action (e.g., losing weight, increasing physical activity, or reducing sodium intake) to help control their blood pressure to more than 82%.
- Increase the proportion of adults who had their blood pressure measured within the preceding 2 years and can state whether or not their blood pressure was normal or high to more than 90%.

From US Department of Health and Human Services: *Healthy people 2010: understanding and improving health,* Washington, DC, 2000, The Department.

Box 31-1 Causes of Secondary Hypertension

Renal Causes

Chronic kidney disease
—Chronic glomerular nephritis or pyelonephritis
—Polycystic kidney disease
—Collagen disease of the kidney
—Obstructive uropathy
Renovascular disease
—Renal artery stenosis

Adrenal and Endocrine Causes

Cushing's syndrome
Chronic steroid therapy
Primary aldosteronism
Pheochromocytoma
Thyroid or parathyroid disease

Other Associated Factors

Excessive alcohol intake
Oral contraceptives
Cocaine, other drugs
Head trauma or cranial tumor
Pregnancy-induced hypertension
Coarctation of the aorta

The prevention and treatment of hypertension is a major public health issue in the United States. When blood pressure is controlled, cardiovascular and renal disease and stroke may be prevented. The prevalence of risk factors in the American population is high. According to the JNC, 122 million people in America are overweight or obese, consume large amounts of dietary sodium and alcohol, and do not eat adequate amounts of fruits and vegetables; less than 20% exercise regularly.[10]

Both modifiable and nonmodifiable factors play a role in the development of hypertension (see the Risk Factors box). In general, the risk of hypertension increases with age, except for the rare condition called hypertensive crisis, which typically occurs in patients 40 to 50 years old. Hypertension is more common among men than women until after menopause, when the incidence in women increases. The incidence of hypertension also varies significantly among different races and cultural groups and is of particular concern among African-Americans of both genders. Hypertension is twice as prevalent among African-Americans as among Caucasians and is also usually more severe.

Factors that may contribute to hypertension in African-Americans include obesity, elevated blood glucose levels, diet, and other lifestyle variables. For reasons that are not fully understood, the incidence and severity of hypertension are particularly high among African-Americans living in the southeastern United States compared with those in other areas.[25]

The seventh report of the JNC has refined and streamlined blood pressure guidelines. The aim of the new guidelines is to prevent and slow the progression of high blood pressure and the arterial stiffness and renal damage that occur with the disease. Because of the risk of cardiovascular complications associated with hypertension, a new classification termed *prehypertension* has been introduced for individuals with blood pressures ranging from 120 to 139 mm Hg systolic (SBP) or 80 to 89 mm Hg diastolic (DBP) (Table 31-1). The purpose of this more stringent classification is to identify at-risk individuals and to promote lifestyle changes to decrease blood pressure. SBP continues to rise with age and is the source of the most common form of hypertension. DBP rises until about 50 years of age and then typically stabilizes.[5] Many health care providers have been taught that an elevated DBP is more important to treat than an elevated SBP; however, according to the JNC, although an elevated DBP presents a more serious cardiovascular risk before the age of 50, an elevated SBP becomes more important as a person ages.[10]

Risk Factors

Hypertension

- Age (older than 55 for men, 65 for women)
- Cigarette smoking
- Obesity (body mass index of greater than 30 kg/m^2)
- Physical inactivity
- Dyslipidemia
- Diabetes mellitus
- Family history of hypertension or premature cardiovascular disease
- Microalbuminuria or glomerular filtration rate of less than 60 ml/min
- African-American race

Pathophysiology. Blood pressure is controlled by a complex set of interrelated mechanisms that involve the control of vascular tone and sodium and water balance. The sympathetic nervous system and the renal renin-angiotensin system provide overall control, and cardiac output and peripheral vascular resistance are the primary regulating factors. Baroreceptors within the carotid sinus and the aortic arch along with chemoreceptors in the medulla oblongata sense changes in the blood pressure and cause the vasomotor center to respond to those changes through the sympathetic and parasympathetic nervous systems. The renin-angiotensin system contributes to the control of blood pressure through release of angiotensin II (a potent vasoconstricting agent) and the production of aldosterone, which leads to sodium and water retention (Figure 31-1). Despite a detailed understanding of the mechanics and regulation of blood pressure, the exact cause of hypertension remains unknown.[43]

Hypertension usually occurs without any symptoms, yet can be profoundly damaging to the blood vessels of major organ systems, including the brain, heart, and kidneys. In the early phases of hypertension, few pathologic changes can be found in the structure of the blood vessels. Over time, however, chronically elevated blood pressure causes widespread pathologic changes that interfere with effective blood flow, especially to the body's vital organs. Most important, shearing forces from the elevated blood pressure damage the intimal layers of the blood vessels, leading to increased fibrin accumulation and vessel edema. Both the large and small arteries in the body may become atherosclerotic, tortuous, and weak. These changes result in narrowing of the vessel lumen, thereby decreasing blood flow to the organ or tissue supplied. As the damage progresses, the vessel can become occluded

TABLE 31-1 CLASSIFICATION AND MANAGEMENT OF BLOOD PRESSURE FOR ADULTS*

BP Classification	SBP* (mm Hg)	DBP* (mm Hg)	Lifestyle Modification	Initial Drug Therapy: Without Compelling Indication	Initial Drug Therapy: With Compelling Indications
Normal	<120	and <80	Encourage	No antihypertensive drugs indicated.	Drug(s) for compelling indications.†
Prehypertension	120-139	or 80-89	Yes		
Stage 1 hypertension	140-159	or 90-99	Yes	Thiazide-type diuretics for most. May consider ACE inhibitor, ARB, BB, CCB, or combination.	Drug(s) for compelling indications.† Other antihypertensive drugs (diuretics, ACE inhibitor, ARB, BB, CCB) as needed.
Stage 2 hypertension	≥160	or ≥100	Yes	Two-drug combination for most‡ (usually thiazide-type diuretic and ACE inhibitor, ARB, BB, or CCB).	Same as for Stage 1

From Chobanian A et al: The seventh report of the Joint National Committee on Prevention, Detection, Evaluation, and Treatment of High Blood Pressure, *JAMA* 289(DOI 10.1001), 2003.
ACE, Angiotensin-converting enzyme; *ARB*, angiotensin receptor blocker; *BB*, beta-blocker; *BP*, blood pressure; *CCB*, calcium channel blocker; *DBP*, diastolic blood pressure; *SBP*, systolic blood pressure.
*Treatment determined by highest BP category.
†Treat patients with chronic kidney disease or diabetes to BP goal of <130/80 mmHg.
‡Initial combined therapy should be used cautiously in those at risk for orthostatic hypotension.

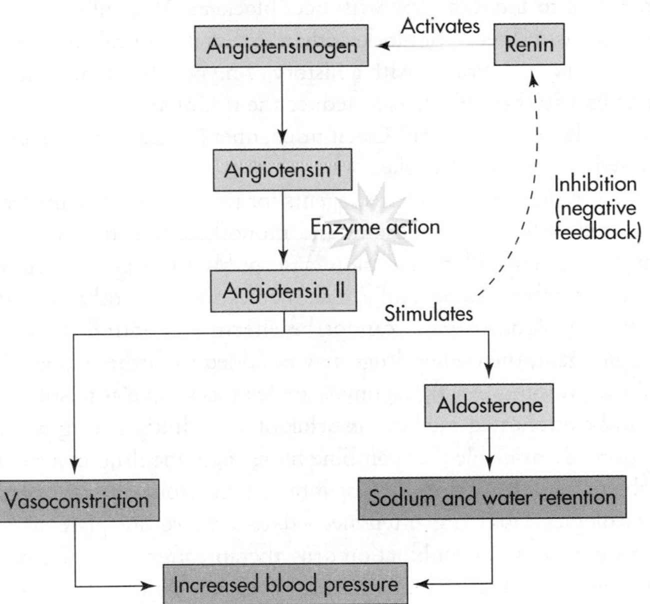

Figure 31-1 Effects of the renin-angiotensin system on blood pressure.

or even rupture, causing an abrupt cessation of blood flow to the area. Finally, these pathophysiologic changes decrease local autoregulatory controls of blood flow, as the vessels are less able to constrict and dilate in response to tissue needs. Over time these changes greatly increase the person's risk for coronary artery disease, cerebrovascular disease, renal artery and parenchymal disease, and peripheral vascular disease.

Although hypertension in itself is largely asymptomatic, symptoms of end-organ damage become evident as the disease progresses. Symptoms of coronary artery disease and cerebrovascular disease may not be evident until the affected blood vessel is more than 80% occluded or an acute occlusion or vessel rupture occurs. Clinical manifestations of advanced, untreated hypertension are presented in the Clinical Manifestations box.

COMPLICATIONS. Progressive damage to major body organs is the most common complication of essential hypertension. It primarily occurs when control is ineffective or erratic because of regimen adherence problems. End-organ damage can eventually lead to encephalopathy, renal failure, left ventricular failure, and retinal hemorrhage. Hypertensive crisis produces significant and immediate risks of acute complications such as myocardial infarction and cerebrovascular accident. Untreated hypertensive crisis results in significant morbidity and mortality, as high as 90% within 2 years. When hypertensive crisis is treated successfully, however, the survival rate approaches 94% at 1 year. Appropriate ongoing follow-up monitoring appears to be the key variable and is clearly linked to the effectiveness of patient education.

Collaborative Care Management

DIAGNOSTIC TESTS. The initial diagnosis of hypertension is made on the basis of two or more elevated blood pressure readings,

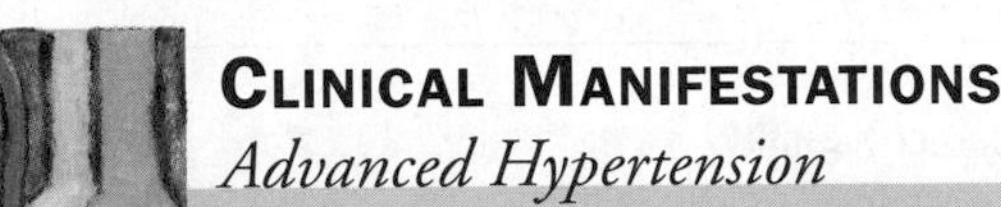

CLINICAL MANIFESTATIONS
Advanced Hypertension

- Headache, especially early-morning headache
- Blurred vision
- Spontaneous nosebleed
- Depression

NOTE: Hypertension is usually asymptomatic in its early stages.

supine and sitting, obtained on at least two separate occasions. At the time of diagnosis the hypertension is classified based on the degree of blood pressure elevation (see Table 31-1). If the systolic and diastolic blood pressures fall into different categories, the higher category is used to classify the person's disease.[9]

In taking blood pressures, the nurse must ensure that the equipment, whether it is aneroid, mercury, or electronic, is in good working order and its accuracy is validated. The patient should sit quietly for at least 5 minutes in a chair with feet on the floor and arm supported at heart level. An appropriate size cuff that encircles at least 80% of the arm should be used. Caffeine, smoking, and exercise should be avoided for 30 minutes before the reading is taken. Two different readings should be taken and the average recorded.

Once the initial diagnosis of hypertension is made, additional specific diagnostic tests may be ordered to (1) rule out an underlying cause, (2) evaluate the presence and extent of organ damage and cardiovascular disease, and (3) identify other risk factors or disorders that could affect the person's treatment.[9] Some of the available tests are presented in Box 31-2.

Medications. Lifestyle modification is the first-line intervention for all patients with hypertension, but pharmacologic therapy is the cornerstone of disease treatment. The goals of medication therapy are to reduce the blood pressure and prevent cardiovascular and renal morbidity and mortality. Management guidelines for hypertension recommended by the JNC are summarized in Table 31-1 and presented as a treatment algorithm in Figure 31-2.

Drug selection is made on an individual basis with consideration of the patient's age, gender, cultural background, and lifestyle. In general, treatment is started with a low dose of a drug from one drug category that ideally can be administered once a day to support patient adherence. Either the frequency of administration or the dose may be increased later based on the patient's therapeutic response. Adjustments are made based on a series of blood pressure readings obtained over several weeks. Other classes of drugs may be added or a new drug substituted if the previous medication is unsuccessful in controlling the patient's hypertension after approximately 2 to 3 months of treatment. Figure 31-3 illustrates the sites of blood pressure regulation and the action of major categories of antihypertensive drugs. The vast array of drug categories and combinations used in the treatment of hypertension are presented in Tables 31-2 and 31-3.

The JNC report recommends diuretics and beta-blockers as first-line therapy in uncomplicated stage 1 and 2 hypertension. Angiotensin-converting enzyme (ACE) inhibitors, calcium antagonists, alpha$_1$-blockers, alpha$_2$-agonists, and direct vasodilators are used as first-line therapy only when diuretics and beta-blockers are contraindicated.[10] Age and cultural differences in response to certain classes of blood pressure medications are important considerations in treatment decisions. ACE inhibitors are most effective in the Caucasian young adult population, who tend to have higher levels of renin than African-Americans and older patients. ACE inhibitors have also proven effective with diabetic patients experiencing proteinuria and patients with a history of heart failure. On the other hand, diuretics are highly effective in the African-American and older populations because these groups tend to have higher levels of intracellular sodium. Studies have shown that African Americans have a poorer blood pressure response to monotherapy with beta-blockers, ACE inhibitors, or angiotensin II receptor blockers than to diuretics or calcium channel blockers.[25] Patients with a history of myocardial infarction are treated with beta-blockers to reduce the risk of another infarction or sudden cardiac death. Calcium channel blockers may be used to reduce the risk of stroke.

Diuretics are the preferred agents for treating older adults with isolated systolic hypertension, and monotherapy is the preferred approach. The elderly are more susceptible to drug interactions and are often taking additional medications for other disease states. If blood pressure cannot be effectively controlled with a single agent, then other drugs may be added to further reduce the blood pressure. Dosing regimens are kept as simple as possible to avoid complicated medication schedules.[11] Multiple drug preparations are available that combine more than one drug in a single tablet (see Table 31-3). Two or more agents from different pharmacologic classes are often needed to achieve adequate blood pressure control. Combination drug therapy often allows for convenient once-daily dosing that improves adherence.[11] Combination antihypertensive agents include nonpotassium-sparing diuretics and potassium-sparing diuretics, beta-blockers and diuretics, ACE inhibitors and diuretics, angiotensin II antagonists and diuretics, and calcium channel blockers and ACE inhibitors. One recently approved combination agent, Caduet, is used for the treatment of high blood pressure and high cholesterol. Caduet combines a long-acting calcium channel blocker, amlodipine, with the lipid-lowering statin, atorvastatin. This is the first medication to treat two different conditions in one tablet.[42]

Drug interactions are important considerations in the treatment of hypertension. Studies have shown that nonsteroidal antiinflammatory drugs (NSAIDs) can elevate blood pressure in the normotensive population. The effect of antihypertensive agents that act

Text continued on p. 864.

Box 31-2 Diagnostic Tests for Hypertension

Routine Tests

Complete blood count
Sodium, potassium, and fasting blood glucose
Blood urea nitrogen, creatinine, uric acid
Lipid profile
—High- and low-density lipoprotein cholesterol
—Fasting serum triglycerides
Urinalysis
Electrocardiogram

Other Tests

Echocardiogram
Carotid and femoral ultrasound
Serum C-reactive protein
Microalbuminuria or albumin/creatinine ratio*
Additional tests targeted at identifying causes of secondary hypertension

*Albuminuria is associated with an increased risk of cardiovascular complications.

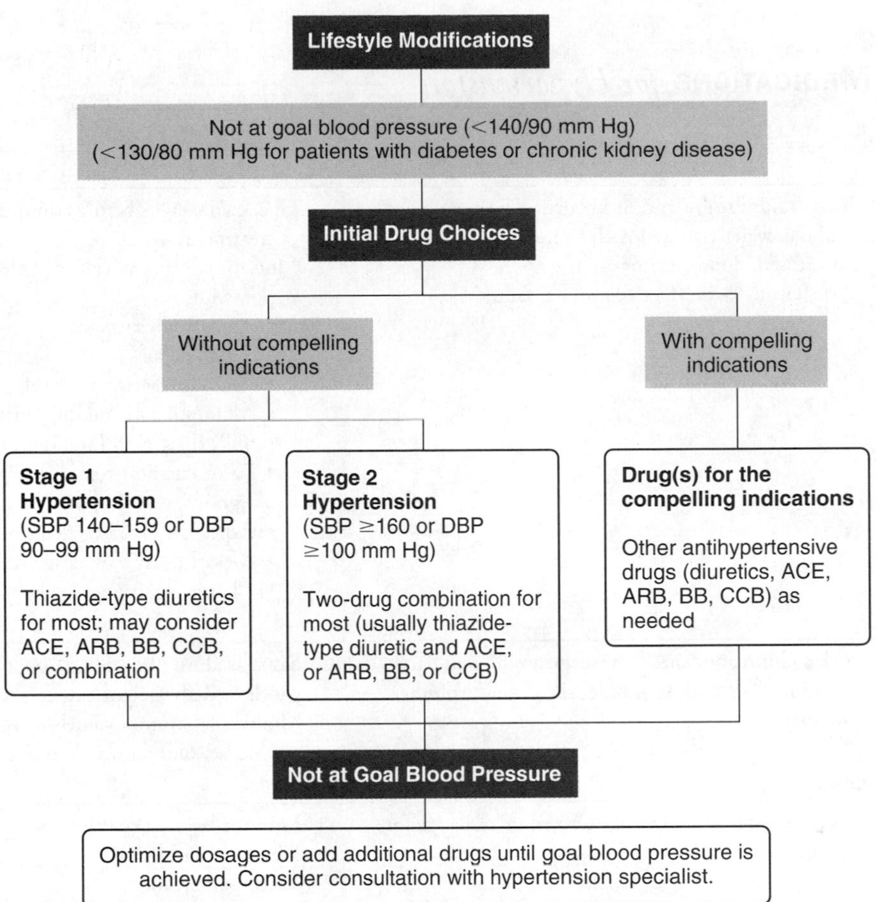

Figure 31-2 Algorithm for treatment of hypertension. *ACE*, Angiotensin-converting enzyme; *ARB*, angiotensin receptor blocker; *BB*, beta-blocker; *CCB*, calcium channel blocker; *DBP*, diastolic blood pressure; *SBP*, systolic blood pressure.

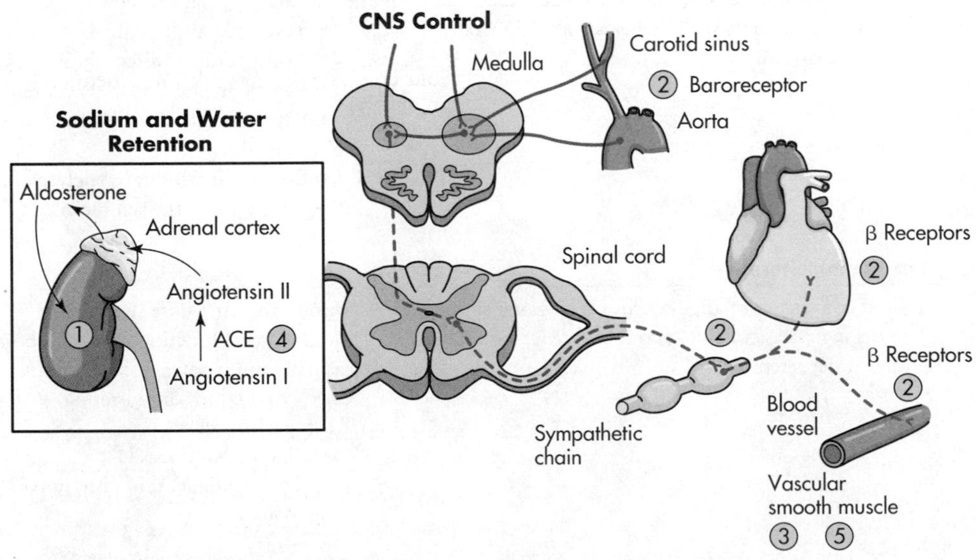

Figure 31-3 Sites of blood pressure regulation and action of antihypertensive drugs. *1*, Diuretics. *2*, Adrenergic inhibitors. *3*, Vasodilators. *4*, Angiotensin-converting enzyme *(ACE)* inhibitors. *5*, Calcium antagonist. *CNS*, Central nervous system.

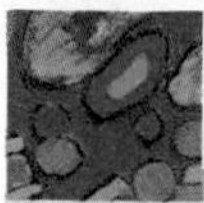

TABLE 31-2
COMMON MEDICATIONS *for Hypertension*

Drug	Action	Nursing Intervention
Thiazide Diuretics		
Chlorothiazide (Diuril) Chlorthalidone Hydrochlorothiazide (Microzide, HydroDIURIL) Polythiazide (Renese) Indapamide (Lozol) Metolazone (Mykrox, Zaroxolyn)	Block sodium reabsorption in cortical part of ascending tubule; water excreted with sodium, producing decreased blood volume NOTE: Thiazides ineffective in renal failure	Check vital signs before administering in early days of treatment. Monitor laboratory values of electrolytes, particularly potassium. Monitor patient's weight. Teach patient to: • Take drugs early in the day. • Maintain a liberal fluid intake. • Take drug with food if GI upset occurs. • Eat potassium-rich diet (e.g., fruits, legumes, whole grains, cereals, potatoes). • Expect an increased frequency and volume of urination. • Report muscle weakness, cramping, fatigue, nausea. • Change positions slowly.
Loop Diuretics		
Bumetanide (Bumex) Furosemide (Lasix) Torsemide (Demadex)	Block sodium and water reabsorption in medullary portion of ascending tubule; cause rapid volume depletion	Same as above, but potassium loss can be severe. Monitor daily weight to assess response to treatment. Monitor laboratory values for increases in uric acid, glucose, blood urea nitrogen.
Potassium-Sparing Diuretics		
Amiloride (Midamor) Triamterene (Dyrenium) Eplerenone (Inspra) Spironolactone (Aldactone)	Inhibit aldosterone; sodium excreted in exchange for potassium	Monitor laboratory values for potassium excess. Weigh patient daily. Teach patient to: • Expect increased volume of urine. • Avoid potassium-rich foods. • Report drowsiness or GI side effects.
Beta-Blockers		
Acebutolol (Sectral) Atenolol (Tenormin) Betaxolol (Kerlone) Bisoprolol (Zebeta) Carvedilol (Coreg) Labetalol (Normodyne, Trandate) Metoprolol (Lopressor) Nadolol (Corgard) Penbutolol (Levatol) Pindolol Propanolol (Inderal) Timolol (Blocadren)	Block beta-adrenergic receptors of sympathetic nervous system, decreasing heart rate and BP NOTE: Beta-blockers should not be used in patients with asthma, chronic obstructive pulmonary disease, congestive heart failure, and heart block; use with caution in patients with diabetes and peripheral vascular disease.	Establish baseline vital signs and laboratory values before treatment. Check BP and pulse before administration. Teach patients to: • Change positions slowly. • Take drug as prescribed. • Avoid abruptly discontinuing use. • Report any decline in sexual responsiveness. • Report incidence of fatigue, drowsiness, difficulty breathing. • Be alert to signs of hypoglycemia if diabetic because drugs mask the symptoms.
Angiotensin-Converting Enzyme Inhibitors		
Benazepril (Lotensin) Captopril (Capoten) Enalapril (Vasotec) Fosinopril (Monopril) Lisinopril (Prinivil, Zestril) Moexipril (Univasc) Perindopril (Aceon) Quinapril (Accupril) Ramipril (Altace) Trandolapril (Mavik)	Inhibit conversion of angiotensin I to angiotensin II, thus blocking release of aldosterone and reducing sodium and water retention	Monitor for first-dose syncope. Monitor renal function through laboratory work, potassium levels. Check BP before administering. Teach patient to: • Change positions slowly. • Report fatigue, skin rash, impaired taste, chronic cough.

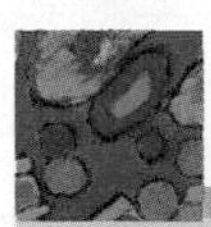

TABLE 31-2
COMMON MEDICATIONS *for Hypertension—cont'd*

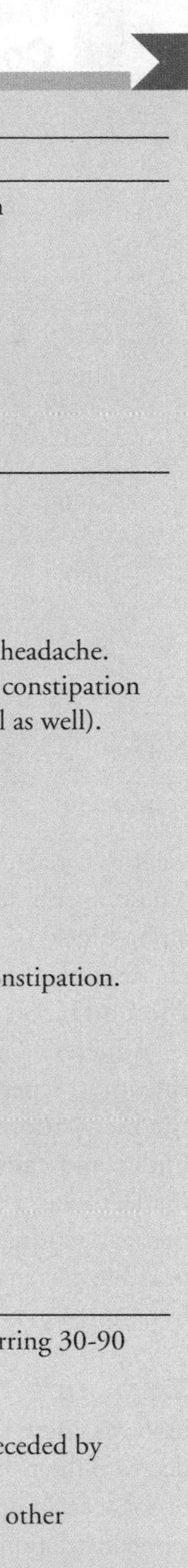

Drug	Action	Nursing Intervention
Angiotensin II Antagonists		
Candesartan (Atacand) Eprosartan (Teveten) Irbesartan (Avapro) Losartan (Cozaar) Olmesartan (Benicar) Telmisartan (Micardis) Valsartan (Diovan)	Selectively block binding of angiotensin I to angiotensin II receptors found in many tissues and vascular smooth muscle, which blocks its vasoconstrictive and aldosterone-secreting effects	Monitor for first-dose syncope, especially in volume-depleted patients. Check BP before administering. Teach patient per ACE inhibitor teaching. Check vital signs before administering (bradycardia is common).
Calcium Channel Blockers		
Nondihydropyridines Diltiazem extended release (Cardizem CD, Cardizem LA, Dilacor XR, Tiazac) Verapamil sustained release (Calan, Isoptin SR) Verapamil extended release (Covera-HS, Verelan PM, Calan SR)	Inhibit influx of calcium into muscle cells; act on vascular smooth muscles to reduce spasms and promote vasodilation; also inhibit calcium movement in heart muscle	Monitor renal and liver function tests. Teach patient to: • Take drugs before meals. • Change positions slowly. • Report peripheral edema, fatigue, and headache. • Adjust diet and fluid intake to control constipation (drugs inhibit smooth muscle in bowel as well).
Dihydropyridines Amlodipine (Norvasc) Felodipine (Plendil) Isradipine (DynaCirc) Nicardipine sustained release (Cardene SR) Nifedipine long-acting (Adalat CC, Procardia XL) Nisoldipine (Sular)	As above; primarily affect vascular smooth muscle	As above. Drugs do not cause significant constipation.
Alpha$_1$-Blockers		
Doxazosin (Cardura) Prazosin (Minipress) Terazosin (Hytrin)	Block synaptic receptors that regulate vasomotor tone; reduce peripheral resistance by dilating arterioles and venules	Monitor closely for first-dose syncope occurring 30-90 min after first administration. Give first dose at bedtime. Monitor BP and pulse. Syncope may be preceded by tachycardia. Perform other intervention as described for other adrenergic blockers.
Central Alpha$_2$-Agonists and Other Centrally Acting Drugs		
Clonidine (Catapres) Clonidine patch (Catapres-TTS) Methyldopa (Aldomet) Reserpine Guanfacine (Tenex)	Activate central receptors that suppress vasomotor and cardiac centers, causing a decrease in peripheral resistance NOTE: Rebound hypertension may occur with abrupt discontinuation of drug (except with methyldopa).	Check vital signs before administration. Teach patient to: • Change positions slowly. • Avoid hot baths, steam rooms, saunas. • Use gum or hard candies to counteract dry mouth. • Be cautious driving or operating machinery if drowsiness or sedation occurs. • Report any decline in sexual responsiveness.
Direct Vasodilators		
Hydralazine (Apresoline)	Dilate peripheral blood vessels by directly relaxing vascular smooth muscle	Check BP and pulse before each dose. Palpitations and tachycardia are common during first week of therapy.

Continued

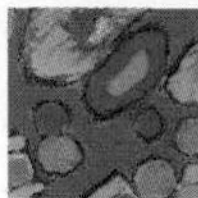

TABLE 31-2
COMMON MEDICATIONS *for Hypertension—cont'd*

Drug	Action	Nursing Intervention
Direct Vasodilators—cont'd		
Minoxidil (Loniten)	NOTE: Usually used in combination with other antihypertensives, since they increase sodium and fluid retention and can cause reflex cardiac stimulation	Teach patient to: • Change positions slowly because dizziness is common. • Avoid hot baths, steam rooms, saunas. • Take drug with meals. • Be prepared for nasal congestion and excess lacrimation. • Report constipation or peripheral edema.
Peripheral-Acting Adrenergic Antagonists		
Guanadrel (Hylorel) Guanethidine (Ismelin) *Rauwolfia serpentina* (Raudixin) Reserpine (Serpasil, Serpalan)	Deplete catecholamines in peripheral sympathetic postganglionic fibers Block norepinephrine release from adrenergic nerve endings	Check vital signs before administration. Teach patient to: • Change positions slowly (dizziness is common). • Avoid hot baths, steam rooms, saunas. • Use stool softeners as needed to prevent constipation. • Report edema in hands or feet. • Use gum or hard candy to relieve dry mouth. • Report any decline in sexual responsiveness.

BP, Blood pressure; *GI,* gastrointestinal.

via the renal prostaglandin pathway is reduced by NSAID use. These agents include the thiazides, loop diuretics, beta-blockers, alpha-blockers, and ACE inhibitors. The combination of calcium channel blockers and NSAIDs appear to have little or no adverse effect on blood pressure.

Adherence is the primary concern with hypertension drug therapy. Hypertension is usually completely asymptomatic, and the medications prescribed often represent a substantial financial outlay and cause predictable side effects. Therefore every effort is made to keep the regimen as simple as possible and to adjust dosages gradually to minimize adverse effects. It is occasionally possible to reduce drug dosages slightly after a year of successful hypertension control.

TREATMENTS. The primary treatment for all stages of hypertension involves lifestyle modification to both lower blood pressure and decrease the risk of cardiovascular disease (Table 31-4).[10] Avoidance of tobacco in any form is essential. Cigarette smoking causes direct vasoconstriction of blood vessels and significant increases in blood pressure, thereby counteracting the benefit of antihypertensive therapy and increasing the risk of cardiovascular disease. The role of stress is less clear, but the use of relaxation and stress management strategies is often helpful in blood pressure control.

SURGICAL MANAGEMENT. Surgery does not play a role in the treatment of primary hypertension. It can, however, be used to treat secondary causes of hypertension such as the adrenal tumor pheochromocytoma, which secretes excessive amounts of catecholamines, or to correct selected renal problems.

DIET. Diet plays an important role in hypertension management. Excess body weight is closely correlated with high blood pressure, and weight loss of as little as 10 pounds can reduce blood pressure in many overweight persons.[6] Weight reduction also reduces other cardiovascular risk factors. Therefore all patients with hypertension who are above their ideal body weight should be assisted in developing a daily regimen that includes caloric restriction and increased physical activity.

Because dyslipidemia is a major independent risk factor for cardiovascular disease, dietary management of dyslipidemia is an important adjunct to antihypertensive therapy. In general, fat intake does not increase blood pressure, and large of amounts of omega-3 fatty acids may actually play a role in lowering blood pressure. Studies have indicated that the use of olive oil contributes to a significant reduction in total and saturated fatty acid levels and decreases both blood pressure and the amount of antihypertensive drug required for effective disease management.[6]

High levels of sodium intake lead to higher blood pressure, although the increase is widely variable. Therefore moderate sodium limitation of 2 to 4 g/day is recommended for all persons with high blood pressure. Because most dietary sodium is contained in processed foods, effective dietary counseling includes teaching patients and families to read food labels and select lower sodium choices.

Evidence exists of an inverse relationship between serum levels of potassium, calcium, and magnesium and blood pressure. Although evidence is insufficient to support the use of supplements, enriched dietary intake of these three important electrolytes may help lower blood pressure and protect against hypertension. Dietary counseling, therefore, focuses on helping patients identify foods rich in potassium, calcium, and magnesium. Potassium-rich food sources are also an essential component of patient teaching for patients taking potassium-wasting diuretics.

Alcohol consumption is a risk factor for both hypertension and stroke, and all persons with hypertension are advised to limit alcohol intake to no more than one beverage equivalent per day.

HEALTH PROMOTION AND PREVENTION. Multiple factors interact to result in hypertension, which is self-managed in the community and home setting. Thus the average adult has numerous

TABLE 31-3 COMBINATION DRUGS FOR HYPERTENSION

Combination Type	Fixed-Dose Combination	Trade Name
ACE inhibitors and CCBs	Amlodipine-benazepril	Lotrel
	Enalapril-felodipine	Lexxel
	Trandolapril-verapamil	Tarka
ACE inhibitors and diuretics	Benazepril-hydrochlorothiazide	Lotensin HCT
	Captopril-hydrochlorothiazide	Capozide
	Enalapril-hydrochlorothiazide	Vaseretic
	Fosinopril-hydrochlorothiazide	Monopril HCT
	Lisinopril-hydrochlorothiazide	Prinzide, Zestoretic
	Moexipril-hydrochlorothiazide	Uniretic
	Quinapril-hydrochlorothiazide	Accuretic
ARBs and diuretics	Candesartan-hydrochlorothiazide	Atacand HCT
	Eprosartan-hydrochlorothiazide	Teveten HCT
	Irbesartan-hydrochlorothiazide	Avalide
	Losartan-hydrochlorothiazide	Hyzaar
	Olmesartan-hydrochlorothiazide	Benicar HCT
	Telmisartan-hydrochlorothiazide	Micardis HCT
	Valsartan-hydrochlorothiazide	Diovan HCT
BBs and diuretics	Atenolol-chlorthalidone	Tenoretic
	Bisoprolol-hydrochlorothiazide	Ziac
	Metoprolol-hydrochlorothiazide	Lopressor HCT
	Nadolol-bendroflumethiazide	Corzide
	Propranolol hydrochlorothiazide	Inderide LA
	Timolol-hydrochlorothiazide	Timolide
Centrally acting drug and diuretic	Methyldopa-hydrochlorothiazide	Aldoril
	Reserpine-chlorthalidone	Demi-Regroton, Regroton
	Reserpine-chlorothiazide	Diupres
	Reserpine-hydrochlorothiazide	Hydropres
Diuretic and diuretic	Amiloride-hydrochlorothiazide	Moduretic
	Sprionolactone-hydrochlorothiazide	Aldactazide
	Triamterene-hydrochlorothiazide	Dyazide, Maxzide

From Chobonian A et al: Seventh report of Joint National Committee on Prevention, Detection, Evaluation, and Treatment of High Blood Pressure, *JAMA* 289:(DOI 10.1001), 2003.
ACE, Angiotensin-converting enzyme; *CCB*, calcium channel blocker; *ARB*, angiotensin receptor blocker; *BB*, beta-blocker.

opportunities to change his or her daily lifestyle to reduce the risk or affect the course of the disease. Dietary guidelines and weight management strategies are important for patients with the disease but also can reduce the risk of hypertension in normotensive individuals. The same applies to activity. Patients with hypertension are encouraged to develop a pattern of regular aerobic exercise, which may help control their hypertension, but also contributes to weight loss and reduces cardiac risk factors.

Moderate regular aerobic exercise has been shown to result in continuous and long-term decreases in both systolic and diastolic blood pressure at rest and during exercise. Some experts believe that regular exercise can be as beneficial as drug therapy in the treatment of hypertension.[21] Patients are cautioned to avoid strenuous exercise, particularly activities such as weight lifting that involve heavy lifting or Valsalva's maneuver. Sustained moderate exertion is preferable to bursts of effort. Current activity guidelines recommend that the person with hypertension engage in moderately intense physical activity, such as 30 to 45 minutes of brisk walking, at least 4 days a week.

Numerous herbal products are believed to have effects on blood pressure and are used by many patients. The Complementary & Alternative Therapies box reports the results of one study exploring the effects of tea consumption on blood pressure.

Nursing Management 

of the Patient with Hypertension

ASSESSMENT

Health History. Assess for:

- Family history of heart disease, hypertension, stroke, diabetes, hyperlipidemia
- History of hypertension: treatment prescribed; adherence and follow-up care
- History or symptoms of cardiovascular, cerebrovascular, or renal disease; diabetes; hyperlipidemia
- Smoking history, alcohol use
- Usual diet, history of weight gain or loss

TABLE 31-4 LIFESTYLE MODIFICATIONS TO MANAGE HYPERTENSION*†

Modification	Recommendation	Approximate SBP Reduction (Range)
Weight reduction	Maintain normal body weight (body mass index 18.5-24.9 kg/m^2).	5-20 mm Hg/10 kg weight loss
DASH eating plan	Consume diet rich in fruits, vegetables, and low-fat dairy products with reduced content of saturated and total fat.	8-14 mm Hg
Dietary sodium reduction	Reduce dietary sodium intake to no more than 100 mmole/day (2.4 g sodium or 6 g sodium chloride).	2-8 mm Hg
Physical activity	Engage in regular aerobic physical activity such as brisk walking (at least 30 min/day, most days of the week).	4-9 mm Hg
Moderation of alcohol consumption	Limit consumption to no more than 2 drinks (1 oz or 30 ml ethanol; e.g., 24 oz beer, 10 oz wine, or 3 oz 80-proof whiskey) per day in most men and to no more than 1 drink per day in women and lighter weight persons.	2-4 mm Hg

From Chobonian A et al: Seventh report of Joint National Committee on Prevention, Detection, Evaluation, and Treatment of High Blood Pressure, *JAMA* 289:(DOI 10.1001), 2003.
SBP, Systolic blood pressure; *DASH,* Dietary Approaches to Stop Hypertension.
*For overall cardiovascular risk reduction, stop smoking.
†The effects of implementing these modifications are dose and time dependent, and could be greater for some individuals.

- Activity and exercise pattern
- Occupation, stress level, and stress management
- Patient's knowledge of hypertension and its treatment
- Social and environmental factors that may influence understanding of and compliance with treatment

Physical Examination. Assess for:
- Blood pressure elevations on two or more occasions with reading taken in both arms at different times
- Abnormalities in height and weight
- Presence of arteriolar narrowing or hemorrhage on funduscopic eye examination
- Carotid bruits, distended neck veins, or enlarged thyroid gland
- Heart murmurs, S_3, S_4, increased rate, or evidence of left ventricular hypertrophy
- Abdominal bruits, aortic pulsations, masses, or organomegaly
- Extremities: warmth, color, edema; quality of peripheral pulses; femoral artery bruits

Complementary & Alternative Therapies

Tea and Hypertension

The researchers in this study looked at the relationship between blood pressure and tea consumption in a population of 1500 Chinese adults without a history of hypertension. Forty percent of the study population were self-reported habitual tea drinkers, consuming at least 4 to 20 oz of mostly green or oolong tea daily for at least a year. This group was found to be 45% less likely to develop hypertension than nonhabitual tea drinkers in the study population. Participants who drank more than 20 oz of tea daily were 65% less likely to develop hypertension despite the presence of significant risk factors such as obesity, smoking, and alcohol consumption.

Yang YC et al: The protective effect of habitual tea consumption on hypertension, *Arch Intern Med* 164(14):1534, 2004.

- Laboratory test results (complete blood count, chemistries, lipids, blood urea nitrogen [BUN], creatinine), electrocardiogram, urinalysis

NURSING DIAGNOSES, OUTCOMES, AND INTERVENTIONS

Nursing Diagnosis: Ineffective Health Maintenance

OUTCOMES. Common examples of expected outcomes for the patient with a diagnosis of *ineffective health maintenance* are: Patient will:
- Verbalize knowledge about the disease process and its effective management.
- Make lifestyle modifications to reduce risk factors.
- Accurately describe action of prescribed medications and expected side effects.

NURSING INTERVENTIONS. The effective treatment of hypertension requires a lifelong commitment to therapy and lifestyle modifications. Nursing interventions focus on teaching the patient and family about the disease, its associated risk factors, and the importance of adherence to the medical regimen. Although drug therapy plays a central role in hypertension management, effective treatment also relies on lifestyle modification to reduce major risk factors. The nurse focuses patient teaching on smoking cessation, diet modification, weight control, exercise, and stress management.

Cigarette smoking is a major risk factor for cardiovascular disease and an important target of any health promotion effort. Nicotine constricts the blood vessels, which increases peripheral vascular resistance and contributes to a chronic elevation in blood pressure. The nurse explores the issue of smoking cessation directly and openly with the patient and ensures that the patient and family have information about options to support quitting and community resources available to assist them with this difficult challenge.

The primary diet modifications recommended for patients with hypertension mirror those recommended for heart-healthy living in general. The nurse encourages the patient to reduce the intake of dietary fats and use only moderate amounts of sodium. Dramatic changes are not necessary. Excess sodium elevates blood pressure because it contributes to fluid retention. Saturated fats have no direct effect on blood pressure and are targeted primarily because of their etiologic role in cardiac disease. A patient with both hypertension and hyperlipidemia has an increased risk of major adverse cardiovascular events such as heart attack and stroke. Reduction of saturated fat intake also makes it easier for the patient to lose weight and maintain a stable body weight. Blood pressure typically but not always drops as the patient loses weight, and less medication may be required. The nurse also discusses alcohol use as part of the overall plan. Alcohol has little direct effect on hypertension, and the patient can continue moderate alcohol intake, but alcohol potentiates the effects of certain antihypertensive medications and can increase the risk of adverse reaction. The negative effects of alcohol on major target organs such as the liver and heart are well documented.

Regular aerobic exercise helps reduce resting blood pressure, improves the heart's response to exercise and physical exertion, and assists the patient in effective weight control. The nurse encourages the patient to begin an exercise plan gradually and slowly work up to a regular program of 30 to 45 minutes of aerobic exercise at least three or four times a week. The nurse cautions the patient to avoid weight lifting and other forms of exercise that involve bursts of activity or Valsalva's maneuver.

The nurse also explores the role of stress in the patient's life and the patient's willingness to use stress reduction strategies. Patients may need help identifying their sources of life stress and recognizing their own unique responses to stress. Simple measures such as relaxation techniques and improved coping mechanisms can be suggested to any patient. Patients who are interested in self-management strategies may be encouraged to explore the use of biofeedback as part of their hypertension treatment plan.

Lifestyle modifications are a critical component of management, but the vast majority of patients also depend on drugs to control their hypertension, and they need to know how to use these medications safely. Once initiated, drug therapy is usually required for life.[43] Patients need to know the name, dosage, action, and side effects of each blood pressure medication prescribed; the nurse provides the patient and family with this information in writing for home reference. The nurse encourages the patient to keep an updated list of all medications with his or her health insurance information for easy reference in case of emergency. Family members, especially the spouse or partner, are included in the medication education process if possible. Significant others play an essential role in adherence, particularly for older persons. Many antihypertensive medications cause a variety of side effects, and the nurse encourages the patient to discuss any severe adverse effects with the health care provider. Numerous options are available in the antihypertensive drug arsenal, and patients can be switched to a different drug if the prescribed agent is unacceptable.

Common side effects of antihypertensive medications include potassium depletion and orthostatic hypotension. Potassium depletion occurs primarily with the use of diuretics and can usually be managed by eating foods high in potassium or taking a potassium supplement. Many drugs can lead to orthostatic hypotension. It is often worse in the morning when blood pressure is normally lower, after alcohol use, and after active exercise.[3] The nurse instructs the patient to change positions slowly and sit down immediately if feeling faint. The nurse advises the patient to avoid standing in one position for long periods because this promotes venous pooling. Hot showers and baths, hot tubs, saunas, and steam baths all promote vasodilation and should be used with caution.

RELATED NIC INTERVENTIONS. Exercise Promotion, Health Education, Medication Management, Risk Identification, Smoking Cessation Assistance, Teaching: Disease Process, Weight Management

Nursing Diagnosis: Risk for Ineffective Therapeutic Regimen Management

OUTCOMES. Common examples of expected outcomes for the patient with a diagnosis of *risk for ineffective therapeutic regimen management* are:

Patient will:

- Maintain weight within recommended range.
- Consume a heart-healthy diet with moderate alcohol intake and increased potassium, calcium, and magnesium intake.
- Exercise moderately for 30 to 45 minutes 4 days per week.
- Stop using all tobacco products.
- Take antihypertensive medication as prescribed.

NURSING INTERVENTIONS. Adherence is a major multidimensional concern that is neither easily understood nor accomplished. The absence of symptoms associated with hypertension makes adherence a greater challenge, especially in the face of financial constraints and troublesome drug side effects. The nurse encourages patients to be involved in the care plan and in all decisions about disease management. The nurse also encourages patients to have their blood pressure checked regularly at community sites such as health fairs, grocery stores, and walk-in clinics. A log of blood pressure readings can be kept and brought to the health care provider's office on each visit. These records give the provider more information about the status of the patient's blood pressure control than can be obtained in a single office measurement. The nurse also stresses the importance of keeping regular follow-up visits for ongoing disease management.

RELATED NIC INTERVENTIONS. Family Support, Referral, Self-Modification Assistance, Support Group

Patient/Family Teaching. The diagnosis of hypertension is usually unexpected and not accompanied by any noticeable symptoms. Yet, once the diagnosis is made, the patient is asked to modify meal patterns and food choices; adopt daily exercise routines; and adhere to the use of new medications with a variety of side effects. Effective adherence is a huge challenge, and individualized teaching is the nurse's best tool for addressing it. All the material discussed under Collaborative Care Management and Nursing Management is part of the nurse's patient teaching content. The key variable is establishing an effective working partnership with the patient and motivating him or her to take responsibility for the regimen.

Evaluation

To evaluate the effectiveness of nursing interventions, compare patient behaviors with those stated in the expected patient outcomes.

Related NOC Outcomes. Adherence Behavior, Knowledge: Diet, Knowledge: Disease Process, Knowledge: Health Behavior, Knowledge: Treatment Regimen, Risk Detection

Gerontologic Considerations

Hypertension can occur at any point in the adult life span, but becomes increasingly prevalent with aging. Therefore the entire overview of hypertension and its management is relevant to older adults. Lifestyle changes can be particularly difficult for this age-group, and the nurse needs to be sensitive to these challenges. Economic issues are frequently important for older adults, as medication costs chip away at fixed incomes. Polypharmacy issues are also common, and the nurse reviews all medications in use and explores the use of generic alternatives or combinations where possible.

Older adults are also more vulnerable to the side effects of hypertension medication, and the development of orthostatic hypertension can pose a significant risk for falls. Failing memory may also interfere with medication compliance, and patients may benefit from the use of weekly medication boxes that can be filled by family, friends, or visiting nurses.[40] Hypertension is a community-managed problem, and the nurse who manages care for the elderly must plan holistically to meet the patient's needs for safe medication, side effect management, and follow-up care.

▶ Are You Ready?

Which statement from the patient with stage 1 hypertension indicates the need for further teaching?

1. "I am glad that my blood pressure can be controlled without medication."
2. "I will need to take diuretics to help lower my blood pressure."
3. "I will have to stop smoking."
4. "It is important that I get enough exercise."

Arterial Disorders

Arterial disease can affect any artery of the body and can manifest as either an acute or chronic condition. Disruption of the arterial blood flow can result from narrowing or complete obstruction of the wall of the vessel from a variety of causes (Box 31-3). The symptoms of arterial disease are directly related to the severity of interruption in blood flow, which impedes the delivery of oxygen and nutrients to the tissues and causes accumulation of waste products and carbon dioxide. If the tissue needs for oxygen and nutrients exceed the supply, ischemia and necrosis can result.

Box 31-3 Causes of Decreased Arterial Blood Flow

- Atherosclerotic plaque
- Arterial spasm
- Embolus or thrombus
- Changes in blood pressure
- Increased blood viscosity or hypercoagulability
- Arteriovenous fistula
- Trauma
- Heart failure
- Compartment syndrome

Chronic Arterial Occlusive Disease

Etiology and Epidemiology. Chronic arterial occlusive disease (also referred to as *peripheral vascular disease,* or PVD) results from the progressive narrowing, degeneration, and eventual obstruction of the arteries of the extremities. The lower extremities are most frequently involved, and arteriosclerosis obliterans is the most common form. The process of atherosclerosis combines with the process of diffuse arteriosclerosis or calcification to produce widespread, slowly progressive narrowing of the arteries. The superficial femoral, iliac, and popliteal arteries are the most common sites of involvement. Plaque typically develops at points of arterial branching or bifurcation (Figure 31-4).

Risk factors known to predispose individuals to chronic arterial occlusive disease are the same as those identified for other forms of cardiovascular disease (see the Risk Factors box). Modifiable risk factors include smoking, obesity, stress, and a sedentary lifestyle. The presence of a positive family history and other relat-

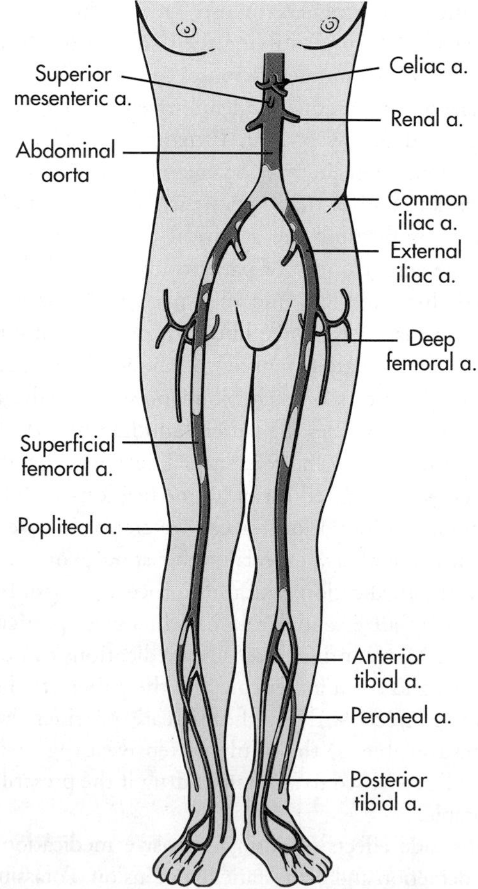

Figure 31-4 Common sites of atherosclerosis.

Risk Factors

Chronic Arterial Occlusive Disease

- Male gender
- Increasing age
- Smoking
- Hypertension
- Atherosclerosis
- Obesity
- Diabetes mellitus
- Stress
- Family history of peripheral vascular disease or atherosclerosis
- Sedentary lifestyle
- Hyperlipidemia

ed diseases, including hypertension, atherosclerosis, diabetes, and hyperlipidemia, also increases the risk for arterial occlusive disease. Chronic occlusive disease is more prevalent in men than in women. It is strongly associated with aging, and symptoms usually develop between the ages of 50 and 70 years. Approximately 10% of adults over the age of 70 are believed to experience symptoms of arterial occlusive disease.[26]

Pathophysiology. The atherosclerotic plaque formation that occurs with arteriosclerosis obliterans causes thickening of the intima and media of the artery, resulting in partial or complete obstruction of the vessel lumen. The calcification of arteriosclerosis further weakens the arterial wall and increases the chance for both thrombus and aneurysm formation. The disease usually occurs segmentally, with lengths of normal vessel interspersed with diseased portions. As blood flow to the affected tissues decreases, the body attempts to compensate by vasodilating the arteries to improve blood flow to the area, as well as by developing additional blood vessels in the affected areas and enhancing other sources of blood supply, a process known as collateral circulation.[38] In slowly progressive disease this collateral circulation may successfully reduce the overt symptoms.

Symptoms develop as the disease progresses and the compensatory mechanisms become inadequate. The affected vessel is frequently more than 70% occluded before the onset of symptoms.[30] **Intermittent claudication**, an aching pain or cramping sensation that occurs in the muscle with activity, is the classic symptom. The pain is usually distal to the site of obstruction and disappears within 1 to 2 minutes after cessation of exercise.[38] Calf muscles are commonly involved when disease affects the femoral artery. Muscles of the lower back, buttocks, thigh, and foot are also commonly affected. Symptoms initially occur when the individual has walked one half to two blocks and appear even more rapidly when the person walks uphill.

Exercise tolerance decreases as the disease worsens. Sedentary patients may not develop claudication if they do not walk enough to cause ischemia. Pain that occurs at rest, termed *rest ischemia,* indicates severe disease. Rest pain typically occurs at night and is accompanied by coldness, numbness, and tingling of the extremity.[27] Any factor that decreases cardiac output and peripheral arterial blood flow such as elevating the extremities can trigger the pain. The patient may be awakened at night and need to sit up or walk around. Gravity improves perfusion of the tissues and relieves or lessens the pain. In advanced arteriosclerosis obliterans, rest ischemia may lead to necrosis, ulceration, and gangrene, particularly in the toes and distal foot.

Other symptoms of chronic occlusive disease include hair loss on the affected extremity; thick, brittle, and slow-growing nails; and impaired motor function. The skin typically appears shiny and taut and is fragile, dry, and scaly. It also feels cooler than normal to the touch. The extremity becomes extremely pale when elevated above the level of the heart for 5 minutes and then exhibits reactive hyperemia, or redness, when lowered, which persists for more than 15 seconds.[20] Reddish discoloration, or rubor, may be present whenever the extremity is in a dependent position. Bruit, a blowing sound, may be auscultated over the obstructed vessel where the blood flow is turbulent. A Doppler ultrasound may be necessary to hear either pulses or bruit in obstructed vessels. The signs and symptoms of chronic arterial occlusive disease are summarized in the Clinical Manifestations box.

COMPLICATIONS. The major complications of chronic arterial occlusive disease include injury, infection, gangrene, and acute occlusion. Many of these problems, if not identified and treated promptly, can result in the loss of the limb through amputation. Insufficient arterial blood flow causes ischemia, necrosis, and possibly arterial ulcers. Arterial ulcers are found at the distal point of arterial perfusion such as the tips of the toes and are typically located on or between the toes or on the upper surface of the foot over the metatarsal heads (Figure 31-5). Arterial ulcers are extremely painful and have a pale, dry base with surrounding shiny skin. The ulcer base may have a yellow film. Arterial ulcers are often described as punched out in appearance.

Collaborative Care Management

DIAGNOSTIC TESTS. Chronic arterial occlusive disease is initially diagnosed through a careful history and physical examination, and may be confirmed by measuring the **ankle-brachial index** (ABI). The ABI measures the difference in blood pressure and blood flow in the upper and lower extremities and is an objective measurement of the degree of stenosis present in a vessel.[22] The test is described in more detail in Chapter 28. In a healthy person the pressure in the leg should be the same as or slightly higher

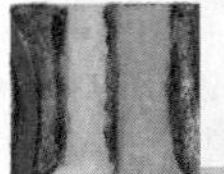

CLINICAL MANIFESTATIONS

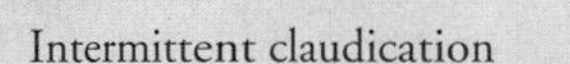

Chronic Arterial Occlusive Disease

- Intermittent claudication
- Rest pain in advanced disease
- Diminished hair growth on affected extremities
- Thick, brittle, slow-growing nails
- Shiny, thin, fragile, taut skin
- Dry and scaly skin
- Cool skin temperature
- Diminished or absent pulses
- Pale, blanched appearance with extremity elevation
- Reddish discoloration (rubor) with extremity in dependent position
- Reactive hyperemia
- Decreased motor function
- Ulcer formation with advanced disease
- Ankle-brachial index of 0.5 to 0.95

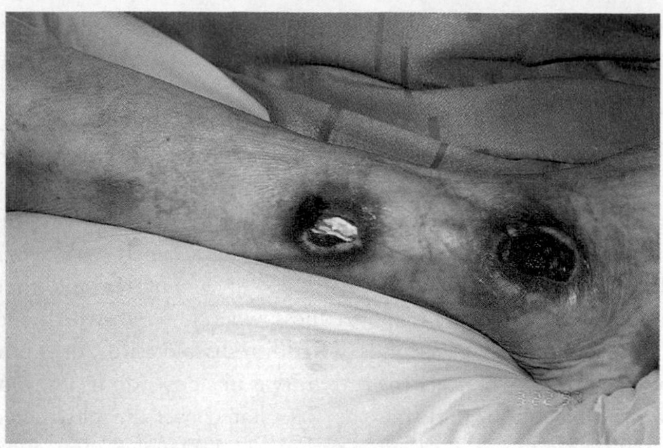

Figure 31-5 Arterial ulcers of lateral malleolus and distal lateral portion of leg. Note round, smooth shape.

than the pressure in the arm, yielding an ABI of about 1. Patients with arterial insufficiency have an ABI of 0.5 to 0.95. Patients experiencing ischemic rest pain typically exhibit an ABI of 0.5 or less, and in the presence of severe tissue damage and ischemia the ABI can be 0.25 or lower. Other noninvasive tests include ultrasonography, segmental limb pressure, pulse volume recordings, and exercise testing.[1] Arteriography is used to localize the site and severity of the disease process and is an essential part of any plan for surgical intervention.

MEDICATIONS. Therapy for chronic arterial occlusive disease follows the general outline of cardiovascular disease management and includes both lifestyle modification and pharmacologic therapy. Pharmacologic therapy is used in PVD management to improve blood flow and prevent thrombus formation in affected extremities. Although they are commonly prescribed, vasodilators have no proven effectiveness in treating chronic arterial occlusive disease, since the dilating capabilities of the affected vessels are already maximized by the time symptoms appear.

Pharmacologic agents that are helpful in treating patients with chronic arterial occlusive disease include pentoxifylline (Trental) and thromboxane A_2 inhibitors such as aspirin and clopidogrel (Plavix). Pentoxifylline increases erythrocyte flexibility and reduces blood viscosity, directly improving the supply of oxygenated blood to the ischemic tissue.[32] Antiplatelet agents inhibit the formation of arterial thrombi that are composed primarily of platelets. Aspirin is the classic antiplatelet drug, but dipyridamole (Persantine) and ticlopidine (Ticlid) are also commonly prescribed. Clopidogrel interferes with platelet aggregation by interfering with the adenosine diphosphate binding receptors. The effectiveness of antiplatelet agents in improving circulation through diseased arteries has not been proven and continues to be studied. Antiplatelet and anticoagulant medications are also used after surgical bypass interventions to prevent reocclusion. Drugs commonly used to treat chronic arterial occlusive disease are presented in Table 31-5.

TREATMENTS. A variety of interventional radiologic procedures may be used in the management of PVD, including percutaneous transluminal angioplasty (PTA), laser surgery, atherectomy, and intravascular stent placement. These procedures are used when the disease has become incapacitating.[12] None of the described interventions is without risk. Rethrombosis, embolism, vasospasm, and

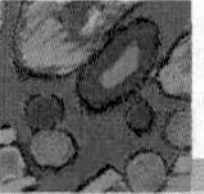

TABLE 31-5
COMMON MEDICATIONS *for Arterial Occlusive Disease*

Drug	Action	Nursing Intervention
Antiplatelet Medications		
Aspirin Ticlopidine (Ticlid) Dipyridamole (Persantine) Clopidogrel (Plavix)	Inhibit platelet aggregation, prolong bleeding time	Administer with food to reduce GI distress. Monitor coagulation times. Assess for signs of bleeding.
Xanthine Derivatives		
Pentoxifylline (Trental)	Increases flexibility of RBCs, thereby facilitating passage through microcirculation; decreases RBC aggregation; increases fibrinolytic activity	Monitor for side effects—GI upset, tremor. Monitor for effect on claudication and exercise tolerance. Therapeutic effect may take 2-4 wk.
Dihydropyridines		
Nifedipine (Adalat, Procardia) Isradipine (DynaCirc) Felodipine (Plendil) Nimodipine (Nimotop) Amlodipine besylate (Norvasc)	Selectively block influx of calcium ions across cell membrane of vascular smooth muscle; decrease peripheral resistance, increasing blood flow; primarily indicated for Raynaud's phenomenon	Monitor blood pressure. Teach patient to change position slowly and report edema, fatigue, or headache.
Vasodilators		
Hydralazine (Apresoline) Minoxidil (Loniten, Minodyl)	Cause vasodilation and decrease peripheral vascular resistance; useful in peripheral vascular disease only if small vessels can dilate in response to stimulation	Monitor blood pressure and pulse. Teach patient to change positions slowly, take drug with meals, and report constipation or peripheral edema.

GI, Gastrointestinal; *RBC,* red blood cell.

both local and systemic bleeding are all possible complications, especially when patients are also receiving anticoagulants.

PERCUTANEOUS TRANSLUMINAL ANGIOPLASTY. PTA is an adaptation of the well-known coronary balloon angioplasty procedure (see Chapter 29). It can be used for both diagnostic and treatment purposes. PTA can be used to dilate any artery of the body except for the carotids. Angioplasty has been used to successfully treat stenosis in the coronary, aortic, iliac, femoral, popliteal, tibial, mesenteric, and renal arteries; but calcified and fibrous lesions cannot be treated in this manner. A catheter is inserted into a major artery and advanced under fluoroscopic guidance to the site of obstruction. If a red thrombus (deep venous thrombus or embolus) is found, it can be treated with either thrombolytic therapy or thrombectomy. If a white or yellow-white atherosclerotic plaque is seen, the vessel is either dilated with the balloon to increase blood flow, or treated with a surgical bypass or recanalization procedure.[15] Patients are typically placed on anticoagulants after the procedure to reduce the risk of immediate restenosis and then placed on long-term antiplatelet therapy.

LASER-ASSISTED BALLOON ANGIOPLASTY. Laser energy is used to vaporize the obstructive plaque and open the occluded artery so that balloon angioplasty can be effectively performed. The use of the laser is designed to reshape the artery and reduce the incidence of restenosis.

INTRAVASCULAR STENTS. Restenosis is a persistent problem after any revascularization procedure. Stents have been developed that can be inserted into the affected artery to provide structure and support vessel patency.

INTRAVASCULAR ULTRASOUND. This procedure is used as a diagnostic adjunct with other more definitive treatment strategies. Ultrasound accurately measures the stenotic area to allow for the safe removal of the atheroma without vessel injury. It can also assist in placing stents or evaluating their placement.

PERIPHERAL ATHERECTOMY. This percutaneous procedure directly removes the obstructing atheroma or plaque from the diseased artery.

TREATMENT OF ARTERIAL ULCERS. Treatment for arterial ulcers focuses on protecting and restoring skin integrity, preventing infection, and maximizing circulation to the affected area. Treatment options include wound debridement; medications such as platelet inhibitors, antilipids, and ACE inhibitors; and surgical revascularization. Before healing can occur, necrotic tissue must be removed through mechanical debridement, chemical debridement with an enzymatic agent such as streptokinase-streptodornase (Varidase), or autolytic debridement with hydrocolloid and film dressings. Nonrestrictive bandages are used to support circulation and healing. If these treatments do not heal the ulcer, the patient may need to undergo amputation of the affected area. The diabetic patient is particularly vulnerable to the development of ulcers, which may become chronic. Treatment is difficult, and outcomes unpredictable. Prevention is the highest priority.

SURGICAL MANAGEMENT. Surgical procedures are typically used in the management of arterial disease that is disabling, does not respond to more conservative treatment, or threatens the patient with loss of the limb. Surgery may be the treatment option of choice for severe occlusion, or it may be used when more conservative interventions fail to reverse the severe ischemia. The open form of arterial bypass or the bypass graft reestablishes blood flow. Bypass grafting is the most commonly used and successful surgical option (Box 31-4). An autologous graft of the patient's own saphenous vein is preferred because of the reduced risk of restenosis and graft failure. Synthetic grafts such as polytetrafluoroethylene, commonly known as Gore-Tex grafts, and grafts from human umbilical cord veins have also been successfully used.[24]

The aorta and the renal, iliac, femoral, popliteal, and anterior and posterior tibial arteries are common sites of severe obstruction. The surgeon determines the optimal graft placement to reestablish arterial flow. Grafting from the femoral to the popliteal artery is common (Figure 31-6). Patients with occlusion of the distal aorta may undergo aortoiliac bypass. A femoral-femoral bypass shifts blood from one femoral artery to the other and may be a procedure of last resort for patients who have had prior aortic surgery and are not candidates for further surgery on the aorta. Angioplasty and percutaneous procedures may be combined with open surgeries to improve the success. Lytic agents may also be used for recanalization of a recently occluded vessel.

DIET. A heart-healthy, low-fat, low-cholesterol diet is recommended to slow progression of the disease. Additional dietary needs are based on the presence of other comorbid conditions, such as obesity, diabetes, dyslipidemia, and hypertension.

HEALTH PROMOTION AND PREVENTION. Arterial occlusive disease is frequently well established before symptoms develop and a firm diagnosis is made. Therefore specific preventive efforts for this chronic condition are rarely applicable. However, patients can profit from the general prevention guidelines that apply to all cardiovascular diseases and are discussed in the various Collaborative Care Management sections throughout the chapter. Individuals are specifically encouraged to avoid smoking; control body weight; and effectively control hypertension, diabetes, and blood lipid levels.

Daily activity can help maintain a normal body weight, and increasing daily activity in a carefully planned way can decrease

BOX 31-4 Options for Surgical Repair of Acute Arterial Occlusion

- Endarterectomy: A direct opening made into the artery to remove the obstruction
- Embolectomy: Removal of an embolus from an artery
- Femoral-femoral bypass: A graft from one femoral artery to the other
- Axillofemoral bypass: A graft from the axillary artery to the femoral artery; created subcutaneously on the side of the chest
- Femoral-popliteal bypass: A graft from the femoral artery to the popliteal artery
- Aortoiliac bypass: A graft from the aorta to the iliac arteries; incision made from the xiphoid process to the pubis

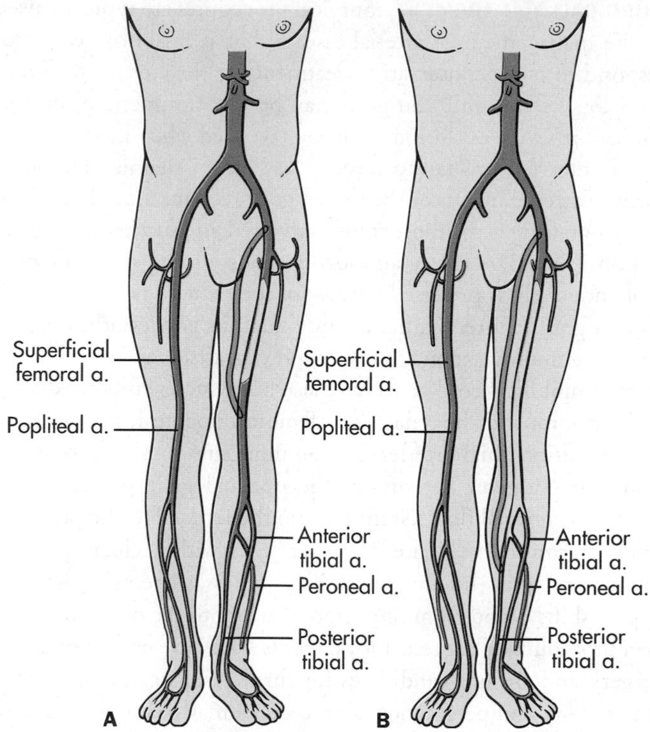

Figure 31-6 **A,** Femoral-popliteal bypass graft around occluded superficial femoral artery. **B,** Femoral–posterior tibial bypass graft around occluded superficial femoral, popliteal, and proximal tibial arteries.

blood lipids, help control hypertension, and improve arterial blood flow by stimulating the development of collateral circulation in the occluded regions. A daily walking program is suggested for all patients with arterial occlusive disease. Participation in a structured, holistic rehabilitation program is recommended, if possible, because the patient can receive the professional support and monitoring that can ensure safety.

▶ ARE YOU READY?

Which clinical manifestation is the classic symptom of chronic arterial occlusive disease?

1. Hair loss on the affected extremity
2. Impaired motor function
3. Intermittent claudication
4. Thick, brittle, slow-growing nails

Nursing Management

of the Patient with Arterial Occlusive Disease

ASSESSMENT

Health History. Assess for:

- Presence, severity, and location of intermittent claudication; presence of rest pain, if any
- Exercise or walking tolerance
- History of hypertension, diabetes, coronary artery disease; treatment used, adherence to regimen
- Smoking history; attempts to quit, if any
- Dietary patterns
- Daily activities and usual exercise routine, if any
- Impact of disease on activities of daily living (ADLs)
- Home living situation and effect on mobility
- Effect of disease on family, work, social activities
- Effects of disease on sexuality (impotence)

Physical Examination. Assess for:

- Quality of peripheral pulses, by palpation (1 to 4) or Doppler
- Shiny skin, thick nails, and diminished hair on extremities
- Signs of skin breakdown
- Postural color changes; reactive hyperemia, presence and severity
- Muscle wasting, presence and severity
- Cool skin temperature
- Numbness or tingling in extremity; presence, location, and severity
- ABI of less than 1
- Elevated cholesterol and triglyceride levels

NURSING DIAGNOSES, OUTCOMES, AND INTERVENTIONS

Nursing Diagnosis: Ineffective Peripheral Tissue Perfusion

OUTCOMES. A common example of an expected outcome for the patient with a diagnosis of *ineffective peripheral tissue perfusion* is: Patient will:

- Promote effective tissue perfusion through daily exercise, temperature control, clothing modifications, positioning, and smoking cessation.

NURSING INTERVENTIONS. The nurse encourages patients to incorporate lifestyle modifications into their daily activities to improve oxygen delivery to the tissues. Maintaining an environmental temperature of about 70° F (21° C) is recommended. Avoiding exposure to the cold is critical because cold triggers vasoconstriction and is likely to induce ischemia and pain. Socks, layered clothing, and blankets are used for warmth, but the nurse cautions patients about the dangers associated with heating pads and hot water bottles. The nurse encourages the patient to avoid constrictive or restrictive clothing such as girdles, rolled garters, tight shoes or shoelaces, tight waistbands, and socks with tight banding that could impede circulation.

Positioning is also an important intervention to support perfusion. The patient maintains the legs in a position of slight dependency, so that gravity enhances tissue perfusion. If the patient experiences rest pain at night, the head of the bed is elevated 4 to 6 inches. The legs are not elevated above the level of the heart, since this would impede arterial flow. The patient is encouraged to avoid crossing the legs at the knees, which places pressure on the arteries of the leg, and to avoid sitting in a slumped or slouched posture that could cause acute constriction of the arteries in the pelvis. Both pressure on and massage of the extremities should be avoided. The skin is fragile and breaks down easily, and massage can promote embolus formation.

Eliminating smoking can also improve perfusion. Nicotine causes vasoconstriction and promotes vasospasm, and inhaled carbon dioxide reduces the oxygen-carrying capacity of the blood. The importance of smoking cessation in PVD cannot be overstated. The nurse explores the patient's understanding of the effects of smoking, prior efforts to quit, interest in quitting, and knowledge of options available to support quitting. Referral for community support is an important strategy.

RELATED NIC INTERVENTIONS. Circulatory Care: Arterial Insufficiency, Exercise Therapy: Ambulation, Lower Extremity Monitoring, Skin Surveillance

Nursing Diagnosis: Risk for Impaired Skin Integrity

OUTCOMES. Common examples of expected outcomes for the patient with a diagnosis of *risk for impaired skin integrity* are:
Patient will:

- Maintain skin integrity.
- Avoid injury and infection.

NURSING INTERVENTIONS. The skin of the extremities is at high risk for breakdown because of decreased tissue oxygenation. The nurse teaches the patient to carefully inspect the skin daily for dryness, redness, and injury. A mirror can be used to inspect areas that are difficult to see such as the heels and the plantar surfaces of the toes. If the patient is hospitalized, the nurse performs a complete skin assessment at least once each day and equips the bed with antipressure devices to prevent skin breakdown. The feet are cleaned daily using a mild soap. The skin is gently dried, and a moisturizing lotion such as lanolin is applied as necessary to counteract dryness. Cotton, nonconstricting socks are recommended and should be changed daily to prevent moisture buildup and irritation. Properly fitted shoes are extremely important, and the nurse recommends the use of soft leather shoes that allow the feet to breathe.

Sensation may be decreased in the feet, particularly in diabetic patients, and this increases the chance for injury. It is important for the patient to learn how to protect the feet from abrasion and irritation as much as possible. The use of direct heat is contraindicated. Toenails are trimmed straight across using nail clippers. Corns, calluses, and other minor foot problems should be evaluated by a podiatrist and not self-treated. The patient is encouraged to contact the health care provider immediately if ulceration, infection, or skin breakdown is detected.

RELATED NIC INTERVENTIONS. Circulatory Precautions, Foot Care, Nail Care, Teaching: Foot Care

Nursing Diagnosis: Risk for Activity Intolerance

OUTCOMES. Common examples of expected outcomes for the patient with a diagnosis of *risk for activity intolerance* are:
Patient will:

- Increase walking tolerance.
- Be free of claudication pain.

NURSING INTERVENTIONS. Activity improves circulation through rhythmic muscle contraction and stimulates the formation of collateral circulation that can increase blood flow to the ischemic area. The nurse encourages the patient to exercise or walk frequently to the point of pain to decrease the incidence and severity of claudication. The exercise should be slow and progressive. Walking is the preferred exercise, but swimming and use of a stationary bicycle can also be incorporated into the plan. The patient is instructed to avoid bed rest as much as possible. The goal is an exercise tolerance of 30 to 45 minutes of steady walking twice a day. Exercise is halted immediately when pain occurs. The patient rests and resumes walking when the pain has completely subsided. If initial walking tolerance is poor, the nurse encourages the patient to walk and rest repeatedly as needed until the cumulative 30 to 45 minutes of activity is achieved.

Buerger-Allen exercises can also be beneficial for patients with advanced disease who have minimal exercise tolerance. The patient lies flat with the legs elevated above the heart for 2 to 3 minutes and then relaxes with the legs in a slightly dependent position for an additional 2 to 3 minutes. The patient then proceeds to exercise the feet (flexion, extension, inversion, eversion), ankles (rotations and pumps), and knees (flexion, extension) for 30 seconds in each position. The exercises are repeated several times a day.

Alternative and complementary therapies have also demonstrated some possible effectiveness in managing the pain associated with intermittent claudication (see the Complementary & Alternative Therapies box).

RELATED NIC INTERVENTIONS. Activity Therapy, Energy Management, Exercise Therapy: Ambulation, Teaching: Prescribed Activity/Exercise

Patient/Family Teaching. Most of the nursing interventions presented for patients with chronic arterial occlusive disease fall into the category of patient and family education. The disease is chronic and progressive and is best managed by lifestyle modifications that support peripheral perfusion and prevent injury. The patient needs to incorporate these measures into her or his daily lifestyle in a way that is comfortable and acceptable (see the Patient/Family Teaching box).

Complementary & Alternative Therapies

Vascular Disease

Complementary and alternative therapies have a long history in the management of vascular disease. Vitamin E has long been known to be useful in improving the pain of intermittent claudication. Studies have confirmed its effectiveness and clarified that positive outcomes are associated with daily doses of 400 to 800 mg. About 3 months of treatment are required before positive outcomes are seen. Other approaches have less clear outcomes. Gingko biloba appears to have a minimally positive effect on the discomfort of intermittent claudication. Garlic has also shown promise, but the doses required are too high to be palatable for most individuals. Horse chestnut seed extract appears to have a positive effect on chronic venous insufficiency, and early studies have shown it to be as effective as the use of compression stockings. The extract is already being widely used in Europe with acceptable side effects.

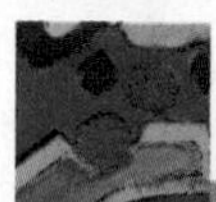

PATIENT/FAMILY TEACHING *The Patient With Peripheral Vascular Disease*

- Avoid trauma to the feet.
  - —Wear properly fitted shoes; avoid going barefoot; wear socks, preferably cotton, with your shoes.
  - —Avoid the use of heating pads and hot water bottles; use layered clothing for warmth.
  - —Do not self-treat any calluses, corns, or ingrown toenails; see a podiatrist or nurse specialist for care.
- Avoid use of all medications on the feet unless prescribed by the health care provider.
- Care for the feet daily.
  - —Wash with mild soap and dry well.
  - —Inspect the feet daily for injury or abrasion, using a mirror to visualize hard to access places.
- Exercise regularly; 30-45 minutes of daily walking is recommended.
- Prevent vasoconstriction.
  - —Avoid the use of any tobacco products.
  - —Avoid wearing tight or constrictive clothing.
  - —Avoid crossing the legs.
- Maintain control of other related chronic conditions.
  - —Control blood pressure.
  - —Keep diabetes under control.
  - —Follow a low-fat diet.
  - —Monitor blood lipids with health care provider.

EVALUATION

To evaluate the effectiveness of nursing interventions, compare patient behaviors with those stated in the expected patient outcomes.

RELATED NOC OUTCOMES. Activity Tolerance, Circulation Status, Endurance, Energy Conservation, Risk Control, Symptom Severity, Tissue Integrity: Skin & Mucous Membranes, Tissue Perfusion: Peripheral

GERONTOLOGIC CONSIDERATIONS

Chronic arterial occlusive disease is primarily a disease of later life and almost exclusively affects older adults. All the interventions previously discussed also apply to this population. Several factors make interventions with this population more challenging. Lifestyle patterns and habits are usually deeply entrenched, and change is difficult to achieve. The presence of arthritis and other chronic diseases can make it difficult for older adults to increase their activity, and diabetes frequently complicates disease management. None of the measures are curative and a great deal of damage has already occurred before diagnosis. The presence of adequate social support can often determine the success or failure of the interventions presented. The nurse carefully assesses patients for vision or hearing losses that may make it more difficult for them to learn the self-care regimen. Potential obstacles in the home environment also need to be considered and modified if possible.

Buerger's Disease (Thromboangiitis Obliterans)

Etiology and Epidemiology. Buerger's disease is an obstructive vascular disorder caused by segmental inflammation in the arteries and veins; it was first described by Leo Buerger, an American surgeon, in 1908. It typically occurs in men between 20 and 40 years old and is rare in women. Although Buerger's disease occurs worldwide, its incidence is much higher in the Middle East and Asia and in persons of Jewish heritage. The incidence of Buerger's disease is directly related to cigarette smoking—the disease does not occur in nonsmokers. The increased incidence in women since the 1980s is attributed to the increased prevalence of smoking. The underlying cause of the disease remains unknown. It primarily affects the vessels of the lower extremities, particularly the tibial arteries and vessels of the foot. Usually more than one limb is involved. Only 30% of patients with Buerger's disease have upper extremity involvement, primarily in the vessels of the forearm and hand. In rare cases the disease can affect the aorta and cerebral, coronary, pulmonary, iliac, or renal arteries.

Pathophysiology. Buerger's disease is characterized by an inflammatory response in the arteries, veins, and nerves. It is theorized that the inflammation is an autoimmune response that is triggered by nicotine in genetically susceptible persons. The affected area is infiltrated by white cells and becomes fibrotic as healing occurs. The presence of inflammatory thrombi causes occlusion of the veins and arteries. The pathologic process differs from that of atherosclerotic disease because small and medium-sized arteries *and* veins are involved. Arteriogram findings reveal a classic tapering or abrupt occlusion of peripheral vessels with collateral vessels exhibiting a corkscrew appearance.

Symptoms of Buerger's disease include slowly developing claudication, cyanosis, and coldness in the affected extremity. Rest pain is common. Recurrent superficial thrombophlebitis occurs in both the upper and lower extremities, and necrotic lesions form at the tips of the finger and toes. The risk of gangrene increases in the presence of collagen disease or atherosclerosis and in response to stress or cold weather.

Collaborative Care Management. The goals of treatment are to halt disease progression and avoid amputation. Buerger's disease is difficult to treat, and management focuses on helping the patient quit smoking. Smokeless tobacco such as snuff or chewing tobacco, nicotine replacement gums and patches, and exposure to large amounts of secondary passive smoke can all aggravate the disease process. Anticoagulants, vasodilators, and antiplatelet agents have no proven effectiveness, but calcium channel blockers can be beneficial in reducing the severity of the vasospastic episodes. Daily intravenous (IV) infusions of iloprost, a prostacyclin analog, have achieved some success in Europe, and intraarterial thrombolytic therapy with low-dose streptokinase has also achieved modest success. Surgical revascularization is seldom effective because of the diffuse nature of the disease and the involvement of distal vessels. Gene therapy has been successful in stimulating the development of collateral circulation in controlled research studies.

Spinal cord stimulators have been used in select cases to control chronic ischemic pain. Sympathectomy may be needed to eliminate vasospasm and improve healing of superficial ischemic ulcerations, but to be effective it must be performed early in the disease process. Amputation of the involved extremity may become necessary if other treatments fail.

PATIENT/FAMILY TEACHING. It is crucial for the nurse to help the patient with Buerger's disease and his or her family understand the direct relationship between cigarette smoking and the disease process. Complete abstinence from smoking is essential if the disease is to be successfully controlled. Most patients improve when they stop smoking. In addition to supporting the patient's smoking cessation efforts, the nurse teaches the patient to avoid exposure to the cold and to protect the extremities from injury and trauma.

Raynaud's Disease

Etiology and Epidemiology. Raynaud's disease is an episodic vasospastic disorder of the small cutaneous arteries, usually involving the fingers and toes. It affects an estimated 5% to 10% of the population, 93% of whom are women.[14] When Raynaud's disease occurs in isolation, it is called Raynaud's syndrome. When it occurs in conjunction with another disease process, such as systemic sclerosis, systemic lupus erythematosus, rheumatoid arthritis, hematologic disorders, trauma, and arterial obstruction, it is termed **Raynaud's phenomenon**. The disease is characterized by bilateral, intermittent vasospasm of the small arteries in the digits. The symptoms are commonly precipitated by exposure to the cold, emotional upset, caffeine ingestion, and tobacco use and occur more frequently in winter and in damp, cool climates. Other contributing factors include occupation-related trauma and pressure to the fingertips such as that experienced by typists, pianists, and workers who use handheld vibrating equipment.

Pathophysiology. Vasoconstriction occurs as the result of activation of the $alpha_1$-receptors in the blood vessels by norepinephrine. Persons with Raynaud's disease may have an increased number of $alpha_1$-receptors or a decreased number of beta-receptors and calcitonin, which are responsible for vasodilation. The pathologic sequence of Raynaud's disease or phenomenon is not completely understood.

Symptoms of Raynaud's disease are symmetric and occur bilaterally in two distinct phases. In the ischemic phase the fingers are cold, pale, and numb. This is followed by a hyperemic phase in which redness, swelling, and throbbing pain in the fingers develop from rebound vessel dilation. The vasospasm is confined to the digits and does not usually include the thumb. Only the tip of the finger distal to the metacarpophalangeal joint is typically affected. Toes may also be affected in the same pattern. The classic triphasic color changes of pallor, cyanosis, and rubor of one or more digits of both hands is considered to be diagnostic for Raynaud's disease (Figure 31-7), although the cyanotic phase is not always present.[14] Normal radial and ulnar pulses are usually preserved. Episodes typically last just minutes, but in severe cases they can persist for hours. Lesions and gangrenous ulcers on the fingertips can develop from persistent ischemia. A positive antinuclear antibody is present in 25% of patients.

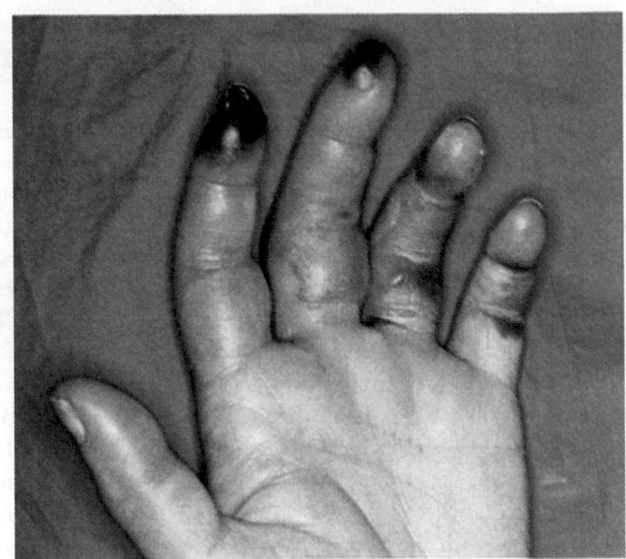

Figure 31-7 Raynaud's phenomenon.

Collaborative Care Management. Raynaud's disease has no known cure and in mild cases does not require treatment because the episodes are self-limiting, but it is important to rule out any underlying treatable conditions. Treatment for primary Raynaud's disease focuses on preventing vasospasm and includes keeping the extremity warm and advising the patient to avoid tobacco, since both cold and nicotine are frequent vasospasm triggers. Drug therapy includes the use of calcium channel blockers, vascular smooth muscle relaxants, and vasodilators, although their effectiveness is highly variable. A prostacyclin analog, iloprost, has been successfully used to improve circulation and decrease pain in research subjects.[34] Biofeedback techniques to increase skin temperature and prevent spasm have been used successfully with selected patients. Sympathectomy may be necessary in severe cases. Persistent, uncontrolled spasms can cause gangrene and necessitate amputation.

PATIENT/FAMILY TEACHING. Education for patients with Raynaud's disease focuses on reassuring them that episodes of vasospasm can be effectively managed in most cases. The nurse explores ways to help the patient minimize exposure to the cold through the use of layered clothing, including socks and mittens, which do not constrict the fingers and allow the fingers to touch and warm each other. The nurse cautions the patient to avoid direct contact with ice and frozen food and to use gloves when handling cold products. Stress management and relaxation techniques can often be effective in decreasing the frequency of vasospastic episodes and preventing the need for surgical intervention. Interventions and support for smoking cessation efforts are critical, and the patient is referred to appropriate community support services.

Nursing Management
of the Patient undergoing Amputation

Amputation is a surgical intervention commonly used in the treatment of advanced PVD. Amputation is usually considered to be a last-resort treatment that is only used when other medical and surgical interventions have failed to preserve the limb. Amputation, although radical and traumatic for the patient, can sometimes provide dramatic relief from chronic pain, offer the potential to walk again with the use of a prosthesis, and improve the patient's quality of life.[13]

More than 110,000 amputations are performed each year in the United States, and 91.7% of them are lower extremity amputations.[19] Diabetes is the underlying pathologic condition that results in severe PVD in more than 50% of all cases. Amputation occurs in patients with diabetes 15 times more frequently than in other patients with chronic arterial occlusive disease. Birth defects, trauma, and malignancy are other possible causes of amputation.

Chronic tissue ischemia that results in necrosis and then gangrene is the most common pathologic sequence that results in amputation. Peripheral pulses become decreased or absent as the ischemia worsens and the patient experiences progressive pain. Gangrene in diabetic patients is typically the dry type. The tissues dry, become cold and black, and actually begin to separate from the body. The toes are usually affected first, and then the gangrene moves steadily upward toward the knee. Moist gangrene is more common after limb trauma when the area is filled with blood and infectious material.

The goal of amputation is to preserve as much of the functional length of the extremity as possible while removing all infected or ischemic tissue. Lower extremity amputations are roughly classified as below-knee (B-K) or above-knee (A-K) amputations (Box 31-5). Before the 1960s most leg amputations were performed above the knee to increase the chance for successful wound healing. As diagnostic testing improved, clinicians were able to more accurately assess the adequacy of perfusion to the extremity and perform B-K amputations more frequently and with greater success. B-K amputations preserve the knee joint, which allows the patient an increased range of motion and improves the likelihood of successful prosthesis fitting after surgery. A B-K amputation is usually made at the lower third of the leg, leaving a 12 to 18 cm stump. An A-K amputation can be made at any level, although a longer stump makes it easier to fit a prosthesis.

The two major techniques for amputation are closed and open. With the closed method the surgeon cuts the bone approximately 2 inches shorter than the skin flap, creating a stump that is suitable for weight bearing with a prosthesis. The incision is closed with the sutures placed in a posterior position to avoid the weight-bearing area, reducing the chance of irritation from the prosthesis. Drains are inserted to prevent excessive swelling and to allow for removal of old blood, fluid, and infectious matter. The open amputation is used most commonly when the limb is infected. The bone and muscle are cut at the same level, and the wound is left open to allow drainage. Wound closure is usually achieved at a future point through a second surgical procedure.

Box 31-5 Types of Amputations

- Below-knee (B-K) amputation
- Above-knee (A-K) amputation
- Amputation of the foot and ankle (Syme's)
- Amputation of the foot between metatarsus and tarsus (Hey's or Lisfranc's)
- Hip disarticulation: removal of the limb from the hip joint
- Hemicorporectomy: removal of half of the body from the pelvis and lumbar areas

Preoperative Care

The preoperative period focuses on the careful evaluation and preparation of the patient for surgery. The medical goal is to ensure that the patient is in the best possible physical state to undergo extensive surgery. Diagnostic testing is completed using Doppler ultrasound, thermography, radioisotope clearance, and arteriogram to accurately assess the limb's circulation and determine the likelihood of successful healing after surgery. Control of diabetes is critical but may be difficult if infection is present in the affected limb. A physical therapy consultation is initiated to plan an effective exercise program that can begin to strengthen the muscles needed for crutch walking and postoperative rehabilitation. The nurse initiates teaching about transfer techniques and the safe use of crutches and walkers before surgery, when pain is not as distracting. An over-bed trapeze increases the patient's independence in self-care activities.

The nurse focuses on teaching and patient support in the preoperative period. Amputation can have tremendous psychologic implications for the patient. This radical change in body image can evoke feelings of loss, anger, fear, shock, and denial. A period of anger and depression is expected, and the nurse validates the appropriateness of these emotions and encourages the patient to express the feelings. The nurse assesses the patient's coping resources and the support systems available. The patient's family should be involved in this process to the degree that it is comfortable for the patient. A thorough home assessment is an important step in discharge planning.

Preoperative teaching focuses on the care that will be delivered in the postoperative period, pain management strategies, plans for prosthesis fitting, and a basic introduction to stump care routines. The patient is told to anticipate the occurrence of phantom limb sensation, which is an aching, tingling, itching, or simple "awareness" of the amputated part. Phantom limb sensation is an expected but still disconcerting aspect of amputation. Sensations typically decrease over time but initially can be quite strong. If chronic pain has been present in the extremity, the patient is also taught about the possibility of **phantom limb pain**. Phantom limb pain is similar to the ischemic pain experienced before surgery and represents a complex management problem. Phantom sensation occurs in most patients, but fortunately phantom pain is much less common.

Postoperative Care

Maintaining Physiologic Stability. Monitoring for complications is an important aspect of initial postoperative nursing care. The nurse closely monitors vital signs and pulse oximetry values until the patient stabilizes. The nurse assesses the wound dressing and drainage systems at least every 2 hours to monitor for excessive bleeding, since hemorrhage is the primary immediate complication of amputation. A surgical tourniquet is kept available at the bedside in case of acute bleeding. Some serosanguinous drainage is expected, but the appearance of bright red blood should be reported immediately. Tachycardia and hypotension are classic indicators of bleeding and early shock. The stump dressing is not usually disturbed for the first 2 to 3 days, but the nurse assesses the operative site as thoroughly as possible. The nurse maintains intake and output records and accurate flow rates for all IV lines. Respiratory care and assessment are also critical. The nurse encourages the patient to begin deep breathing, position changes, and coughing as needed to clear the airway, as soon as he or she is alert. Effective pain management is a critical intervention because severe pain can adversely affect vital signs, decrease the ability to breathe deeply and clear the airway, and compromise the ability to participate in self-care.

Maintaining Appropriate Stump Positioning. The stump is elevated on pillows to reduce postoperative pain and swelling for the first 24 hours. Stump positioning and exercise become critical interventions after this initial period. The stump is supported but not elevated because of the risk of flexion contractures. The flexor muscles in the extremities are stronger than the opposing extensors, and the patient needs to effectively counteract the flexion pull to prevent hip and knee contractures. Position changes are made at least every 2 hours, and the patient is encouraged to lie prone for at least 20 to 30 minutes twice a day to stretch the hip flexor muscles. Positioning is also used to prevent both the abducted and adducted position. Any change in normal hip alignment makes it difficult for the patient to achieve an acceptable prosthesis fit and normal gait. The patient continues to work with the physical therapist to strengthen the muscles needed for ambulation and is encouraged to be out of bed for increasing intervals each day.

Conditioning the Stump. Stump care is a critical nursing intervention in the early postoperative period, and it remains a major management concern throughout the healing and rehabilitation period. Some surgeons apply an immediate temporary prosthesis after amputation. These devices are composed of a rigid plastic bandage that is applied around the closed stump and attached to a prosthetic pylon with an ankle and foot assembly. The device is applied in the operating room while the patient is still anesthetized. Its main advantages are the potential for early weight bearing and reduction of edema. The major disadvantage is the inability to directly assess wound healing in the stump. If delayed prosthesis fitting is planned, the stump is initially wrapped snugly in dressings and Ace wraps to provide compression and minimize edema. Examples of standard prostheses are illustrated in Figure 31-8.

Proper stump bandaging helps shape the stump for eventual prosthesis fitting and weight bearing. A compression bandage is worn at all times, except for needed skin care, and must be correctly reapplied whenever it becomes loose or wrinkled. The shrinker bandage typically is reapplied at least daily, and the nurse teaches the patient how to correctly apply the bandage as soon as possible. The bandages need to be washed and changed regularly, and the nurse instructs the patient in the importance of keeping these wrappings clean. Figure 31-9 illustrates the correct method of applying compression or shrinker bandages to A-K and B-K amputations.

Daily stump care is also part of the conditioning process. The nurse closely monitors incision healing and instructs the patient to carefully assess the stump each day for signs of redness or irritation. The stump is washed daily after healing is complete and thoroughly air dried before rewrapping. No lotion, oil, or powder should be applied to the stump surface without specific orders from the surgeon or rehabilitation specialist. The goal is to achieve a well-healed and appropriately shaped stump whose surface skin is tough enough to absorb the pressures of weight bearing with a prosthesis. Guidelines for care of a patient after an amputation are summarized in the Guidelines for Safe Practice box.

Supporting Independence in Self-Care. The physical therapist continues to work with the patient on range of motion, ambulation with an assistive device, and general conditioning. Building upper body strength, particularly triceps strength, is emphasized because these muscles are critical to crutch walking. The therapist teaches the patient the principles of safe transferring, and the patient practices this skill on the unit under the nurse's supervision. The loss of the weight and mass of the amputated limb can significantly alter the patient's center of gravity, and the nurse is alert to the patient's need for support while relearning upright balance. A fall can have serious adverse consequences on wound healing.

Patient/Family Teaching. Hospitalizations for all conditions are being steadily shortened, and planning for discharge must begin before surgery. The nurse creates a teaching plan that includes time for the patient to learn stump care, transfer techniques, safe ambulation, prevention of complications and contractures, and the importance of follow-up care from the multidisciplinary care team. Referral to a prosthetist may not occur until after discharge, and achieving a good prosthetic fit can take as long as 2 years because the healing stump continues to shrink and change shape. The process is slow and often frustrating, and the nurse needs to help the patient and family anticipate the long-term nature of the rehabilitation period (see the Nursing Care Plan).

GERONTOLOGIC CONSIDERATIONS

Lower limb amputations are commonly performed on older patients. The patient's previous ability to walk and perform self-care profoundly affects the transition to independence after amputation. Use of a prosthesis for ambulation requires strength and energy. If the older adult is already weakened from other debilitating health problems, it may not be possible to fit a prosthesis, even if the stump heals adequately. Wheelchair mobility may be a more realistic option. Most older adults also require at least short-term admission to a rehabilitation facility after discharge to continue with needed therapy.

Acute Arterial Occlusive Disease

Etiology and Epidemiology. Acute arterial occlusion can occur in both healthy and diseased arteries. The occlusion can result from an arterial thrombus that forms in an atherosclerotic artery, an

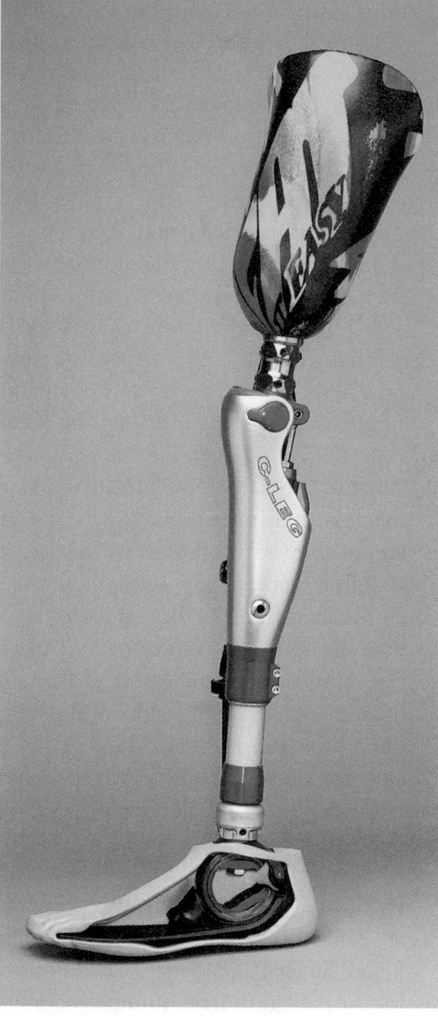

A

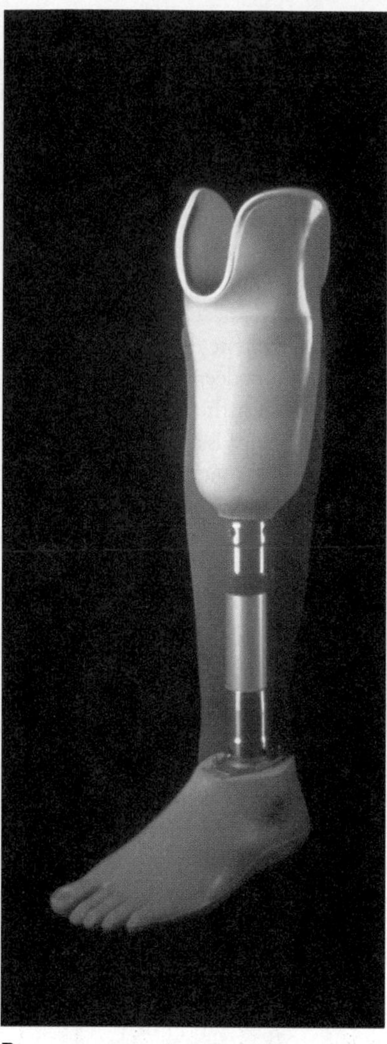

B

Figure 31-8 Permanent lower-extremity prostheses. **A,** Above-knee prosthesis. **B,** Below-knee prosthesis.

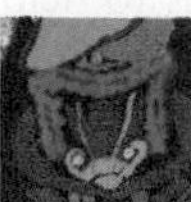

GUIDELINES FOR SAFE PRACTICE *Care of the Patient After an Amputation*

- Assess stump and monitor drainage for color and amount; report signs of increased drainage.
- Position patient with no flexion at hip or knee to avoid contractures; encourage prone position.
- Maintain patient in low Fowler's or flat position after above-knee amputation.
- Support stump with pillow for first 24 hours (according to physician preference and avoiding flexion); place rolled bath blanket along outer aspect of leg to prevent external rotation.
- Encourage exercises to prevent thromboembolism:
  —Active range of motion of unaffected leg, ankle rotations and pumps
  —Use of overhead trapeze when moving in bed
  —Push-ups from sitting position in bed
  —Quadriceps sets
  —Lifting stump and buttocks off bed while lying flat on back to strengthen abdominal muscles
- Teach care of stump:
  —Inspect for redness, blister, and abrasions.
  —Wash stump with mild soap, rinse with water, and pat dry.
  —Avoid use of alcohol, oils, and creams.
  —Remove stump bandage or stump sock and reapply as needed; use firm smooth figure-of-eight Ace wrapping (see Figure 31-9) to reduce swelling and shape stump (if rigid dressing not used).
- Encourage patient to walk using correct crutch-walking technique:
  —Keep elbows extended; limit elbow flexion to 30 degrees or less.
  —Avoid pressure on axilla.
  —Bear weight on palms of hands, not on axilla.
  —Maintain upright posture (head up, chest up, abdomen in, pelvis in, foot straight).
- Monitor patient's ability to use a prosthesis.

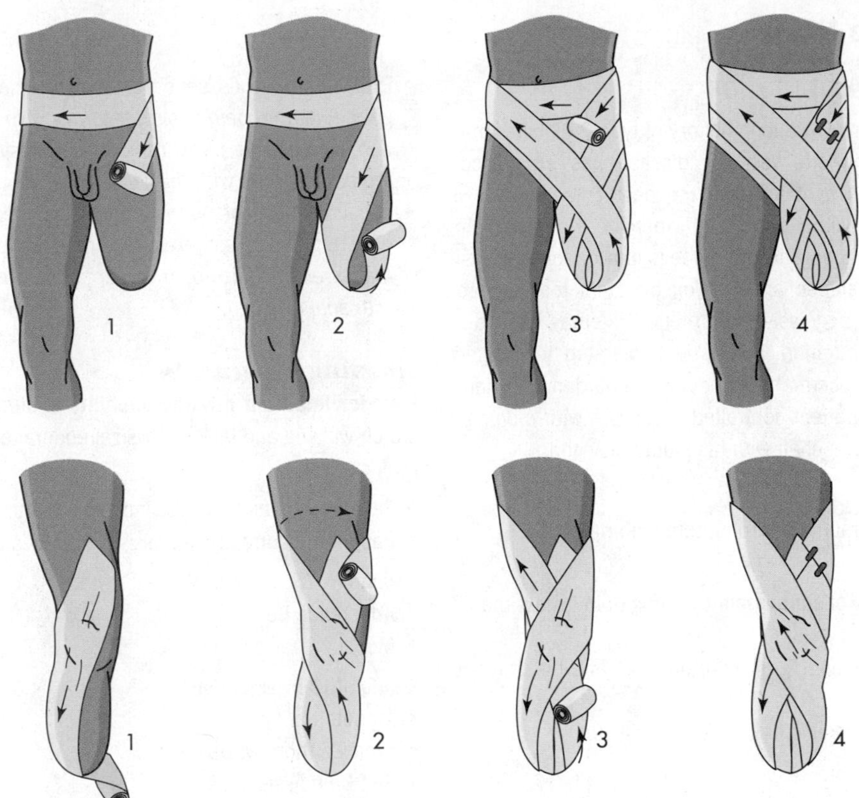

Figure 31-9 *Top,* Correct method for bandaging midthigh amputation stump. Note that bandage must be anchored around patient's waist. *Bottom,* Correct method for bandaging midcalf amputation stump.

embolism in a healthy artery, or trauma. The occlusion typically occurs suddenly and without warning. An embolus that forms in the heart or an atherosclerotic aneurysm is the most common cause. The embolus dislodges and travels to the lungs if it originates in the right side of the heart or to anywhere in the systemic circulation if it originates in the left side of the heart. The occlusion typically occurs at sites of vessel bifurcation or narrowing.

Acute arterial occlusion can occur in any patient in the presence of appropriate risk factors. Patients with rheumatic heart disease, artificial heart valves, myocardial infarction, and atrial fibrillation are at particular risk because of a high incidence of thrombus formation with these conditions. Postoperative vascular surgery patients, patients who have undergone invasive arterial procedures, and trauma patients with lacerated or compressed arteries are also at risk.

Pathophysiology. When an acute arterial occlusion occurs, the blood supply distal to the obstruction is abruptly interrupted. The extent and severity of the resulting symptoms depend on the location and size of the obstruction and the patency of the surrounding vessels. When PVD is already present in the extremity, symptoms are likely to be much more severe. Acute embolic occlusion usually occurs suddenly, and the pain is severe and unrelenting. Neither rest nor activity relieves it. The primary symptoms of acute occlusion can be clearly described through the "six Ps" of neurovascular assessment: the limb exhibits pain, pallor, pulselessness, paresthesia, paralysis, and poikilothermia (coolness to the touch) (see the Clinical Manifestations box). Development of paralysis in the affected limb is considered a late and ominous sign that usually reflects the ischemic death of nerve cells supplying the extremity. Patients are often unable either to rest or sleep because of the severity of the pain.

COMPLICATIONS. Severe ischemia rapidly progresses to necrosis and gangrene and requires limb amputation if prompt intervention

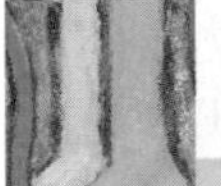

CLINICAL MANIFESTATIONS
Acute Arterial Occlusion

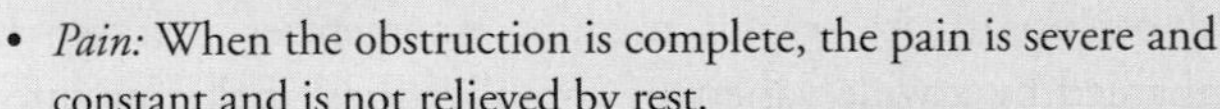

- *Pain:* When the obstruction is complete, the pain is severe and constant and is not relieved by rest.
- *Pallor:* The limb typically appears pale or mottled.
- *Pulselessness:* The peripheral pulses are either diminished or completely absent over the path of the affected vessel.
- *Paresthesia:* Numbness, tingling, and burning in the extremity are common when ischemia is severe.
- *Poikilothermia:* The limb is typically cool, if not frankly cold, to the touch.
- *Paralysis:* Mobility of the part is limited. Development of frank paralysis is an ominous sign because it may indicate the ischemic death of nerves in the extremity.

NOTE: Symptoms typically occur suddenly and are severe. If perfusion is not rapidly restored, the limb will develop signs of necrosis and gangrene, often in a matter of hours.

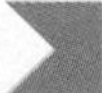

Nursing Care Plan

Patient Undergoing Amputation

Data A 70-year-old patient with a long history of type 2 diabetes mellitus, hypertension, and peripheral vascular disease has experienced increasing claudication in his right leg over the past 6 months. He is unable to walk across a room without pain and experiences pain at night, which forces him to get out of bed and put his legs in a dependent position. One month ago he developed an ulcer on his great toe that progressed to gangrene despite aggressive treatment. Yesterday, he underwent a right below-knee amputation. The patient tolerated the surgery well, although he expresses concern about becoming a burden to his family. Currently he is receiving patient-controlled analgesia with morphine and may be helped to sit up in a chair with his stump elevated.

Nursing Diagnosis

Acute pain related to tissue trauma and phantom limb pain

Outcomes

- Patient will verbalize control of stump pain by rating pain as less than 3 on scale of 0 to 10.
- Patient will verbalize understanding of phantom pain and measures to control discomfort.
- Patient will use nonpharmacologic pain relief strategies.

Related NOC Outcomes

- Comfort Level
- Pain Control
- Pain Level

Related NIC Interventions

- Analgesic Administration
- Coping Enhancement
- Pain Management

Nursing Interventions/Rationales

- Assess character, intensity, and location of pain. *To establish baseline for later comparisons.*
- Administer prescribed analgesics. *Analgesics decrease the transmission and perception of pain stimulus. Adequate pain control is essential for optimal physical therapy and rehabilitation.*
- Explain the causes, sensations, and methods of treatment for phantom pain. *Phantom pain is similar to pain experienced before the amputation. Warning the patient about the possibility of phantom pain helps the patient cope with the sensations.*
- Encourage use of nonpharmacologic measures to control or reduce pain (e.g., relaxation exercises or distraction). *Many nonpharmacologic measures minimize pain perception and work in a synergistic manner with analgesics.*

Nursing Diagnosis

Risk for impaired physical mobility related to lack of experience with crutch-walking and lack of physical endurance

Outcomes

- Patient will maintain baseline range of motion (ROM).
- Patient will correctly use assistive devices for ambulation.

Related NOC Outcomes

- Adherence Behavior
- Mobility

Related NIC Interventions

- Amputation Care
- Exercise Therapy: Balance
- Self-Care Assistance

Nursing Interventions/Rationales

- Assess upper extremity strength, cardiopulmonary status, and endurance. *Upper body strength and optimal conditioning are essential to achieve mobility and perform bed-to-chair transfers and crutch walking.*
- Teach ROM and strengthening exercises. *To build endurance, strength, and flexibility.*
- Teach positioning and exercises to prevent flexion and abduction contractures. *Contractures will prevent proper fitting of prosthesis and thus limit rehabilitation progress.*
- Dangle or assist patient in sitting up in chair 12 to 24 hours after surgery. *To prevent loss of muscle strength from disuse or bed rest.*
- Teach the purpose and benefits of exercise and interventions. *Understanding why exercise is necessary and beneficial fosters exercise compliance.*

does not successfully restore perfusion. The window of opportunity for successful treatment can be mere hours in severe cases. Acute arterial occlusions are serious medical emergencies that can be accompanied by a wide variety of complications, including infection; reocclusion; and a range of other respiratory, circulatory, and renal complications.

Collaborative Care Management

Diagnostic Tests. The diagnosis of acute occlusion is primarily established through physical assessment of the affected limb. Noninvasive tests such as Doppler ultrasonography and ABI measurements are commonly used. Magnetic resonance imaging or angiography may be used to map the location and severity of the obstruction before surgical intervention.

Medications. Drug therapy may be used as a primary treatment modality or as a follow-up to interventions such as embolectomy. The goal of drug therapy is to dissolve the clot and prevent further clot formation. Anticoagulant therapy with continuous IV heparin is usually initiated immediately to prevent further enlargement of the thrombus. However, heparin does not dissolve existing clots. Emboli may be treated with thrombolytic agents when the risks associated with ischemia outweigh the risk of bleeding. **Thrombolytics** can also prevent complications associated with the more invasive procedures. Urokinase is the most commonly used drug. Its effectiveness depends on the severity and location of the obstruction. A percutaneous arterial catheter is inserted into the femoral artery and advanced to the site of obstruction. This allows the drug to be directly administered to the thrombus. The thrombus is dissolved over 24 to 48 hours. The risk of bleeding complications is high; therefore patients need to be carefully selected and screened.

Arterial thrombi and emboli can also trigger severe vessel spasm. Spasmolytic agents such as papaverine (Pavabid), tolazoline (Priscoline), and calcium channel blockers may be administered to relieve or prevent arterial spasm. Blood pressure control is also important for any patient with an acute arterial condition,

Nursing Diagnosis

Risk for impaired skin integrity related to incision and effects of diabetes on wound healing

Outcomes

- Patient's wound will show evidence of progressive healing.
- Patient will accurately demonstrate stump care and prosthesis care.
- Patient will maintain blood glucose within normal limits.

Related NOC Outcomes

- Tissue Integrity: Skin & Mucous Membranes
- Wound Healing: Primary Intention

Related NIC Interventions

- Incision Site Care
- Skin Surveillance

Nursing Interventions/Rationales

- Assess stump for drainage or bleeding, edema, proximal pulses, and tissue perfusion. *Drainage or bleeding may indicate lack of healing or complications such as infection. Edema, absent proximal pulses, and decreased tissue perfusion indicate compromised circulation, which predisposes the patient to skin breakdown.*
- Maintain dressing without wrinkles or constriction. *To prevent compromised circulation and resultant skin breakdown.*
- Teach patient how to care for stump and prosthesis. *Meticulous skin care helps prevent infection and loss of skin integrity. Care of the prosthesis prevents contamination of stump wound.*
- Teach signs and symptoms of decreased stump perfusion that need to be reported. *Cool skin or loss of sensation may indicate tissue compromise. Tissue compromise must be quickly recognized and reported so that immediate corrective treatments can be implemented to prevent further tissue damage.*
- Monitor blood glucose levels before each meal and at bedtime. *Stress of surgery and infection can result in hyperglycemia and decreased healing, which predispose the patient to skin breakdown.*

Nursing Diagnosis

Anticipatory grieving related to loss of limb

Outcomes

- Patient will verbally express feelings of loss and grief.
- Patient will verbalize plan for resocialization.
- Patient will participate in stump care.

Related NOC Outcomes

- Coping
- Family Coping
- Grief Resolution

Related NIC Interventions

- Emotional Support
- Grief Work Facilitation
- Support System Enhancement

Nursing Interventions/Rationales

- Assess significance of loss to patient and family. *The significance of the loss varies. Plans to facilitate grief depend on the patient's reaction to the loss.*
- Encourage patient and family to verbalize feelings. *Allows the opportunity for patient and family to ventilate feelings of anger and grief in a safe environment. Recognizing and verbalizing feelings is an essential step in working through grief.*
- Allow privacy for the expression of grief. *Grief is a personal experience that many individuals chose to deal with privately, at least initially. The patient may be reluctant to cry or demonstrate other expressions of grief unless privacy is provided.*
- Refer to support group or counseling as appropriate. *Effective support and resolution of grief are necessary for the patient to successfully cope with needed lifestyle adjustments and changes.*

Evaluation

Evaluation is based on comparing the patient's outcomes with desired outcomes.

especially if surgical intervention is planned. Drug therapy is used as needed to manage the patient's blood pressure. A pain service may be consulted in the preoperative period to help manage the patient's severe ischemic pain. Both patient-controlled analgesia and epidural administration are used successfully.

Anticoagulant therapy may also be initiated after successful treatment of the thrombus. Any patient considered to be at risk for future embolization is usually prescribed long-term anticoagulant therapy with an oral agent such as warfarin (Coumadin) to prevent future episodes.

TREATMENTS. Treatment of an acute arterial occlusion may involve the use of an endovascular procedure that allows for treatment within the artery itself to remove blockages. Possible procedures are adaptations of procedures in use for the treatment of coronary artery disease and include balloon angioplasty or PTA, intraluminal ultrasound, laser angioplasty, mechanical atherectomy, and stent placement (see the descriptions in Chapter 29).

Patients are kept on bed rest after interventional procedures until the invasive arterial lines and thrombolytic agents can be discontinued. Protocols vary based on the nature and extent of the intervention, but bed rest is commonly maintained for 6 to 24 hours.

SURGICAL MANAGEMENT. Surgery is indicated in the event of life- or limb-threatening arterial occlusion when other measures have failed to restore blood flow. An open **embolectomy** or thrombectomy may be performed to remove the obstructive clot from the vessel lumen. Bypass graft procedures may also be performed.

DIET. Diet does not play a major or direct role in the treatment of acute arterial occlusion. Patients usually receive nothing by mouth (NPO) while the workup is completed and treatment decisions are made. An empty stomach minimizes aspiration risks associated with both interventional and surgical procedures. The NPO status is extremely important when general anesthesia is used, particularly with abdominal procedures. Patients are gradually advanced to a normal diet after surgery. Ileus is common after surgery on the aorta, and meticulous abdominal assessment is important. Once a normal oral diet is resumed, attention is again directed toward encouraging the patient to adhere to a heart-healthy diet of low-fat, low-cholesterol foods. Diet is particularly important when diabetes complicates the management of vascular problems.

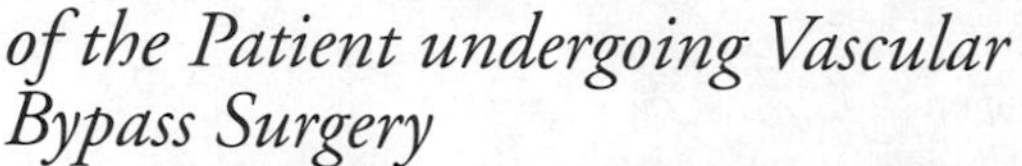

Nursing Management *of the Patient undergoing Vascular Bypass Surgery*

PREOPERATIVE CARE

Preoperative care focuses on the physical, emotional, and psychosocial preparation of a severely stressed patient. The patient may be undergoing a variety of emergency tests and procedures and is likely to have extensive needs for teaching and support. Pain, medication effects, anxiety, and uncertainty all influence the ability of the patient and family to absorb the information being presented. The nurse performs frequent vital sign and neurovascular assessments to monitor for changes in patient status. The nurse is an important liaison between the patient and the rest of the treatment team and attempts to keep the channels of communication open. General care and monitoring before surgery are summarized in the Guidelines for Safe Practice box.

POSTOPERATIVE CARE

The patient receives meticulous general surgical care, since the complications of vascular surgery can affect virtually any organ system. The more invasive the procedure, the greater the risk of complications. Surgery involving the aorta creates the greatest risk. Potential complications include bleeding, infection at the graft site, heart failure, myocardial infarction, dysrhythmias, stroke, renal failure, and injury to adjacent organs and tissues (e.g., ureters, bowel, nerves). The nurse is responsible for meticulous postoperative monitoring of all major body systems.

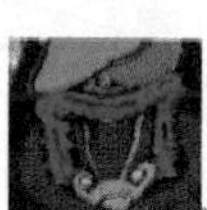

GUIDELINES FOR SAFE PRACTICE
The Patient With an Acute Arterial Occlusion

- Monitor the affected limb for any change in circulatory status. Monitor temperature, color, sensation, and pain. A change in these parameters may indicate worsening occlusion.
- Monitor peripheral pulses bilaterally for presence, strength, quality, and symmetry.
- Keep the extremity warm, but do not apply direct heat or heat lamps.
- Avoid chilling.
- Maintain bed rest unless activity is specifically ordered.
- Keep the extremity flat or in a slightly dependent position to promote perfusion.
- Use an overbed cradle to protect a painful extremity from the pressure of linens.
- Use a sheepskin and 4-inch foam mattress beneath the extremity.
- Do not elevate the bed at the knee; instruct the patient not to cross the legs at the knee or ankle.
- Do not apply any restraint to the affected limb.
- Keep the head of the bed low to support circulation to the lower extremities.
- Monitor the effects of anticoagulant and thrombolytic therapy. Monitor international normalized ratio, partial thromboplastin time, platelets, and other coagulation studies.

Supporting Circulation and Perfusion. Patients with vascular disease also frequently have problems with coronary artery disease or hypertension. The nurse integrates data from vital sign measurements, cardiac monitoring, pulse oximetry, arterial blood gases, cardiac enzymes, electrolytes, and Swan-Ganz catheter measurements to accurately assess the impact of the surgery on the patient's heart and to anticipate and identify the onset of any complications.

Graft patency is a priority concern in the postoperative period because of the significant risk of reocclusion from thrombosis, restenosis, or debris. The nurse monitors the patient's peripheral pulses and limb temperature, as well as the degree of pain, pallor, sensation, and movement.

The initiation of anticoagulant therapy increases the risk of bleeding from the suture line and graft anastomoses. The nurse closely monitors appropriate laboratory values such as hemoglobin, hematocrit, and coagulation studies, which can alert the clinician to potential bleeding. Body excretions, particularly nasogastric secretions, are tested for blood. The nurse also monitors all incision and arteriogram sites for signs of bleeding. Measuring the patient's abdominal girth and limb circumferences provides an objective means to detect distention from either internal bleeding or edema.

Preventing Respiratory Complications. Atelectasis is the most common cause of fever in the first 24 hours after surgery. Atelectasis can progress rapidly to pulmonary infection if aggressive pulmonary toilet measures are not instituted. The nurse encourages the patient to breathe deeply and cough to clear the airway as needed and to use an incentive spirometer frequently. Early ambulation is important after vascular surgery and helps prevent the complications of immobility. The nurse helps patients out of bed the first day after surgery as long as they are hemodynamically stable. Activity is then steadily progressed. Patients with abdominal and chest incisions need lots of encouragement plus effective pain management to assist them in complying with essential respiratory and ambulation protocols. Chest percussion and postural drainage are initiated if needed.

Supporting Fluid Balance. The kidneys are at particular risk after bypass surgery because many of the procedures involve the aorta or femoral arteries. Hypotension, hypovolemia, and trauma to the kidneys or ureters during surgery can all lead to acute postoperative renal failure. The nurse carefully measures and records the patient's intake, output, and daily weight; monitors laboratory values of BUN, creatinine, and serum electrolytes; and assesses the urine for signs of myoglobinuria, which is indicative of tissue damage.

Promoting Wound Healing. Wound healing problems and infection are common after vascular surgery, particularly in diabetic and malnourished patients. The nurse cleans the incision with saline solution at least twice daily and teaches this technique to the patient or a family member. With the surgeon's approval, the patient may shower a few days after surgery. An antibacterial soap without lotions or perfume is suggested. Tub baths are not recommended because of the risk of contamination from standing water. The nurse teaches the patient and family the signs and symptoms of wound infection, complications to monitor for after discharge, and the importance of promptly reporting any complications to the surgeon. Infection in the graft is an extremely serious complication with a high mortality rate. Graft infection is usually accompanied by high fever, prolonged ileus, and a rapidly rising white blood cell count.

Patient/Family Teaching. Hospitalization for patients undergoing vascular surgery is brief, and the patient and family need to receive adequate education for self-care at home. If the nurse or family questions the patient's and family's ability to provide adequate care, a home health referral is promptly initiated. Patients receive standard discharge teaching concerning diet, activity, wound care, and resumption of normal activities. A daily walking program is usually recommended. If possible, the patient is referred to a structured vascular rehabilitation program. Exercise helps support blood flow, improves overall function, and increases the patient's general sense of well-being. Heavy lifting is restricted for at least 6 weeks after surgery. Sexual activity may be resumed as soon as the patient's comfort level permits. The nurse also provides the patient with information on decreasing the risk of vascular problems and future complications. A summary of discharge instructions for the patient after vascular surgery is presented in the Patient/Family Teaching box.

PATIENT/FAMILY TEACHING
Discharge Teaching After Bypass Graft Surgery

- Shower daily, cleaning the incision gently with a mild antibacterial soap without lotion or perfume added. Pat dry. Use a shower chair or stool to prevent falling if any instability is present. Avoid tub baths until healing is complete.
- Monitor the incision daily for signs of infection—redness, swelling, increased pain, discharge, or suture or staple separation. Promptly report any of these symptoms to the surgeon.
- Advance activity gradually as tolerated. Initiate a daily walking regimen. Expect to feel fatigued, and plan for rest periods throughout the day. Avoid lifting anything heavier than 10 pounds until approved by surgeon.
- Resume a low-fat, low-cholesterol diet as tolerated. Use supplements as needed to ensure adequate calories, protein, and vitamin C during the healing period. Four to six small meals a day are often better tolerated than three large ones.
- Avoid constipation and straining at stool. Eat a high-fiber diet with plenty of fluids to avoid constipation. Remain active. Take a stool softener daily plus a bulk-forming laxative if constipation cannot be managed through diet and fluids alone.
- Use prescribed pain medications as needed to ensure adequate rest and activity. Take oral medication with food to prevent gastric irritation.

GERONTOLOGIC CONSIDERATIONS

Most individuals with vascular disease are older and have multiple health care needs. The presence of diabetes, coronary artery disease, poor nutrition, and other chronic illnesses and conditions may complicate surgical recovery. An acute arterial occlusion is an abrupt emergency situation that disrupts the patient's and family's normal patterns of support and interaction. The older person's sudden need for significant support and physical assistance can have a tremendous impact on all concerned. The nurse uses the multidisciplinary care team to coordinate the patient's care and effectively plan for needed care and support after discharge. Discharge planning needs to be proactive, especially when the need for home care can be anticipated.

Aneurysms

Etiology and Epidemiology. An **aneurysm** is a point of weakness, dilation, or outpouching of arteries to at least 1.5 times their normal size with a tendency for enlargement and possible rupture. The word *aneurysm* comes from the Greek word *aneurysma* meaning widening. Aneurysms occur most commonly in the aorta, but they can occur in any artery of the body. Other common sites include the femoral and popliteal arteries. Aneurysm disease is the thirteenth leading cause of death in the United States.[2] Over 33,000 elective aneurysm repairs are performed each year to prevent rupture. Most abdominal aneurysms never rupture, and elective repair is performed only when the risk of rupture is high.

Aneurysms are three times more common in men than women and typically develop between the ages of 50 and 70 years. The prevalence of aneurysms in men with an aortic diameter of 3 cm or larger increases by about 6% each decade. Aneurysms of at least 4 cm in diameter occur in about 1% of men 55 to 64 years of age. They are rare in women younger than 55 years of age. Aneurysms are caused by atherosclerotic disease, trauma, syphilis, and congenital abnormalities of the vessel; infection and connective tissue disorders that weaken the vessel wall are also contributory. Cigarette smoking, hypertension, diabetes, PVD, hypercholesterolemia, and a genetic predisposition are all linked to the development of aneurysms. Smoking is the strongest risk factor, and more than 90% of patients with aneurysms have a smoking history.[2] Abdominal aortic aneurysms (AAAs) show evidence of familial or genetic patterns, and individuals with conditions such as Marfan syndrome or Ehlers-Danlos syndrome type IV experience an increased risk of AAA.[35] The steady aging of the population and improved diagnostic tools have increased the frequency with which aneurysms are diagnosed.

Pathophysiology. The abdominal aorta supplies blood to the abdomen and lower extremities and is the most common site for aneurysm formation. Aneurysms may occur at other sites in the aorta or in other arteries, but the most common site is in the infrarenal abdominal aorta. More than 90% of infrarenal AAAs are related to degenerative diseases such as atherosclerosis and the destruction of elastin and collagen fibers.[31] Inflammatory mechanisms or trauma can also contribute to their formation. Factors that weaken the vessel wall act in combination with the forceful turbulent blood flow in this region to gradually dilate the vessel.

Box 31-6 lists terms used to describe various types of aneurysms. A fusiform aneurysm involves a circumferential dilation of the vessel wall and is relatively uniform in shape. A saccular aneurysm is a localized outpouching that occurs on just one side of the artery. A narrow neck connects the aneurysm sac to the vessel wall. Saccular aneurysms are more likely to rupture. A dissecting aneurysm develops from a tear in the arterial intima that causes an accumulation of blood in the newly formed cavity between the intima and the media. Dissecting aneurysms are further classified by the type of tear and the degree of hematoma or bleeding. Dissecting aneurysms are strongly associated with arterial hypertension and hemodynamic instability and most often develop in the thoracic aorta.

Aneurysms can even affect the aortic valve. The growth rate of aneurysms is unpredictable, but in general the larger the aneurysm, the greater the risk of rupture. An estimated 50% of all aneurysms larger than 6 cm in diameter rupture within 1 year. Repair is recommended if the aneurysm is 4 cm in diameter or greater and the patient does not have any medical contraindications for surgery. Aneurysms also have the potential for thrombosis or embolization, causing an abrupt decrease in blood flow below the aneurysm.[18]

At the time of presentation, patients with AAA may be symptomatic or asymptomatic or may have a rupture, but most patients are asymptomatic. Abdominal aneurysms may be felt as a palpable mass on abdominal examination, and a systolic bruit may be heard. The patient may complain of abdominal or back pain. If the aneurysm leaks or ruptures, the patient develops severe pain, signs of shock, decreased red blood cell count, and increased white blood cell count. Symptoms of thoracic aneurysms vary and depend on the size and location of the aneurysm and its effect on surrounding tissues. Most patients are again asymptomatic. Patients may experience anterior chest wall, back, flank, or abdominal pain or may develop signs of shock if the aneurysm leaks. Symptoms such as dyspnea, cough, and wheezing may develop if the aneurysm puts pressure on the trachea or bronchus.

Collaborative Care Management. Most aneurysms are discovered on a routine physical examination or as an unexpected finding from the use of x-ray studies or ultrasound performed for an unrelated health issue. Figure 31-10 depicts an AAA between the renal and iliac arteries. Once the diagnosis is established, the primary therapeutic goal is to prevent aneurysm rupture through control of blood pressure and smoking cessation. Patients who are symptom free and have small aneurysms of less than 4 cm may be treated conservatively with careful monitoring through ultrasonography or computed tomography to assess for changes in the aneurysm size. The risk of rupture with aneurysms greater than 6 cm outweighs the risks of intervention. Regardless of whether interventions are planned, maintenance of blood pressure in an optimal range is a high priority of care.

Surgical repair has been standard for aneurysms requiring intervention, but surgery on the abdominal or thoracic aorta is complex and dangerous, potentially affecting all body systems.[18] In 1991 the surgeon Juan Parodi first repaired an AAA with a less invasive endovascular stent grafting procedure. This endovascular procedure requires fewer hospital days, has a shorter recovery time, and is less expensive. The procedure can be performed with the patient under monitored sedation or spinal or general anesthesia. An individual is considered a candidate for the endovascular procedure if life expectancy is greater than 1 year, the aneurysm is infrarenal and larger than 4.5 cm, and the iliac arteries are larger than 10 mm and can accommodate passage of the graft.[31] The complications are the same as for the open surgical procedures, plus an added risk of leakage or migration of the stent graft and an increased incidence of thrombolic complications caused by atheromatous plaques that are disrupted during the procedure. Figure 31-11 shows an endograft successfully placed within the vessel. Patients undergoing an endovascular procedure must also be compliant with a lifelong imaging surveillance program to monitor for graft leakage, increased growth of the aneurysm, and the graft's durability and placement.

Box 31-6 Types of Vessel Aneurysms

- Fusiform: These aneurysms involve an entire circumferential segment of the vessel, which results in a diffuse dilated lesion.
- Saccular: These aneurysms involve only a portion of the circumference of the vessel, and the vessel appears to have an outpouching.
- Mycotic: These rare, infectious aneurysms of the aorta are caused by:
  —Staphylococci
  —Streptococci
  —Salmonellae
- Pseudoaneurysms: The adventitia is dilated, although the media and intimal layers are unaffected. There may be a clot with a false lumen that acts like a pseudoaneurysm.

Adapted from Dzau VJ, Creager MA: Diseases of the aorta. In Braunwald et al, editors: *Harrison's principles of internal medicine,* ed 15, New York, 2001, McGraw-Hill.

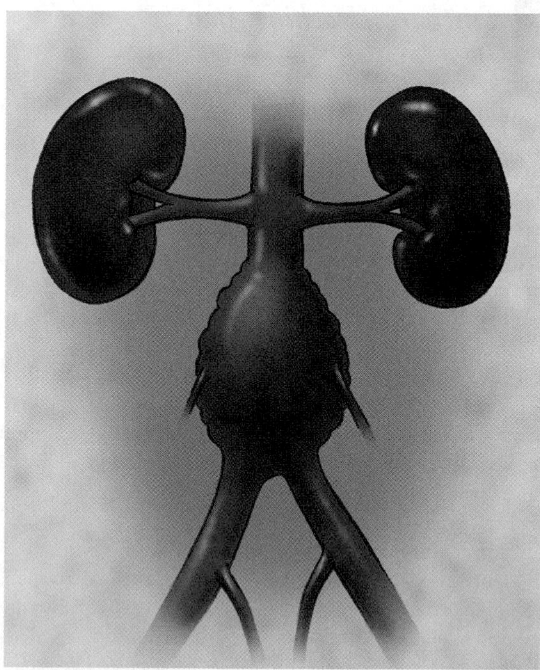

Figure 31-10 Abdominal aortic aneurysm situated between renal arteries and iliac arteries.

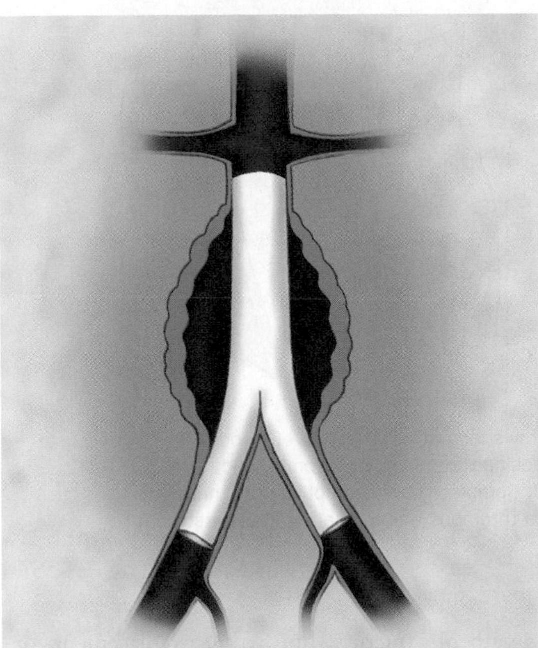

Figure 31-11 Endograft successfully placed in abdominal aorta.

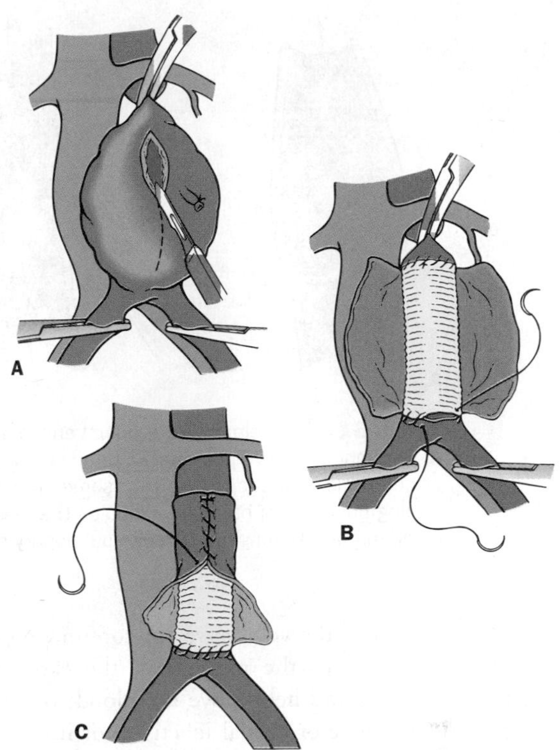

Figure 31-12 Surgical repair of an abdominal aortic aneurysm. **A,** Incising the aneurysmal sac. **B,** Insertion of synthetic graft. **C,** Suturing native aortic wall over synthetic graft.

Endovascular repair of AAAs is a rapidly evolving technology. The decision to repair an AAA with an endovascular stent graft or by open surgery is made collaboratively with the patient and family after a careful workup and discussion of all risks and benefits. The open surgical repair also involves the use of a synthetic graft to support the weakened area (Figure 31-12). Care of the patient undergoing aneurysm repair surgery is similar to that provided to patients undergoing vascular bypass surgery.

The patient's length of hospital stay depends on the procedure selected, type of anesthesia used, patient's general condition, and complications after the procedure. The patient is carefully assessed for incisional bleeding, pain, and lower extremity neurovascular status. The nurse monitors vital signs and pulse oximetry along with lower extremity pulses, sensation, movement, and temperature. Urinary output is monitored closely because of the close proximity of the renal arteries. Creatinine is measured to assess the patient's renal status for toxic effects from the procedure or the contrast dye used with intraoperative fluoroscopy. Antibiotics are given to prevent wound and graft infections. If no complications develop, the patient who undergoes an endovascular procedure could be discharged as early as the first postoperative day, but the usual hospital stay is 2 or 3 days.

PATIENT/FAMILY TEACHING. The decision regarding whether to undergo surgical repair or endovascular repair of an aneurysm is difficult. The nurse can play an essential role in helping the patient and family sort through the available data and make an informed choice. The nurse helps ensure that the patient's decision is respected and supported. The nurse reinforces the importance of blood pressure control and regular medical follow-up care, especially if surgery is not planned. Discharge education for patients undergoing aneurysm repair is similar to that provided to patients after vascular bypass surgery.

▶ ARE You READY?

The nurse assesses for which of the following in the patient with a ruptured or leaking abdominal aortic aneurysm?

1. Decreased pulse rate
2. Elevated blood pressure
3. Decreased serum sodium
4. Increased white blood cell count

Venous Disorders

The most common venous disorders result from incompetent valves in the veins and obstruction of venous return to the heart, usually as a result of a thrombus.

Deep Venous Thrombosis

Etiology and Epidemiology. A variety of different terms are used to describe the disorder that results from the process of clot formation within a vein (Figure 31-13). The term *phlebothrombosis* refers to the actual presence of a clot in a vein. Thrombus formation is commonly accompanied by some degree of vein wall inflammation, and the terms *phlebitis* and *thrombophlebitis* reflect this inflammation. Thrombus formation occurs in either the superficial or deep veins of the body. Superficial thrombophlebitis occurs in the majority of patients receiving IV therapy. **Deep venous thrombosis** (DVT) is more serious and carries the risk of potentially fatal embolization.

Venous thrombosis typically results from at least one element of Virchow's triad: venous stasis, damage to the endothelial lining of the vein, and hypercoagulopathy. Venous return to the heart is

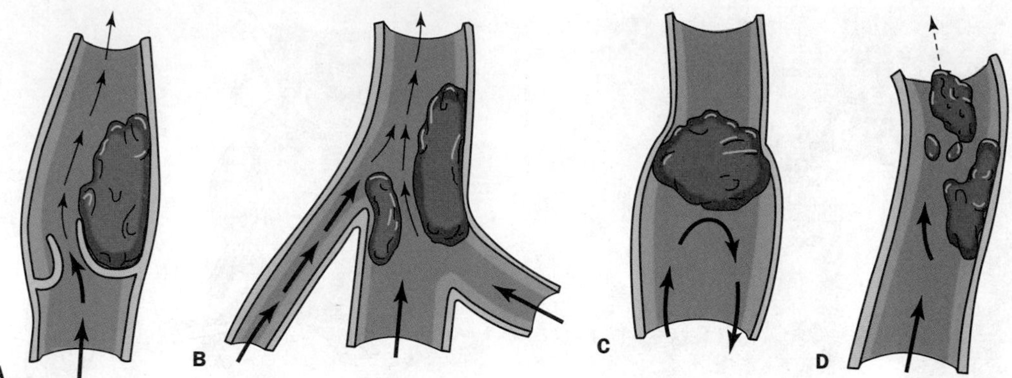

Figure 31-13 Development of deep venous thrombosis with arrows indicating direction of blood flow. **A,** Thrombus in valve pocket of a deep vein with blood flowing beside thrombus. **B,** Thrombi tend to form at bifurcations of deep veins with some slowing of blood flow. **C,** Complete occlusion of vein by thrombus forcing backflow of blood. **D,** Embolus that has broken off from a thrombus and is floating in bloodstream could migrate to lungs and cause pulmonary embolus.

supported by the action of the vein valves in conjunction with the rhythmic contractions of the muscles in the extremities, which compress the veins and help move the blood toward the heart. Any period of relative or partial inactivity or immobility, such as prolonged sitting, surgery, or bed rest, impairs venous return. A decrease in muscle tone and activity in the legs causes pooling and venous distention. The distention causes minor damage to the endothelial lining of the veins and valves, and platelets are attracted to the site.[4] This can result in the development of a thrombus. The presence of IV catheters, central lines, and pacemaker wires and the irritation of drugs and IV solutions contribute to endothelial damage. Any increase in viscosity or hypercoagulability of the blood increases the likelihood of thrombus formation. Dehydration, pregnancy, clotting disorders, sickle cell anemia, malignancy, polycythemia, systemic lupus erythematosus, and oral contraceptive use all can contribute to the subtle alteration in coagulability that results in thrombus formation. The presence of atherosclerosis and varicosities also increases the risk. Travel, especially air travel and journeys longer than 4 hours, has been theorized to contribute to the development of DVT and pulmonary emboli.[7]

Most thrombi form in the veins of the pelvis and lower extremities, but they can also form in the vessels of the upper extremities and those leading directly to the heart. Upper extremity DVT is typically associated with venous compression or deep venous instrumentation from central venous catheters used for total parenteral nutrition, dialysis access, and hemodynamic monitoring. Venous thrombi can dislodge and become emboli. An embolus can travel from the site where it formed through the larger veins and into the right side of the heart, where it may be ejected into the pulmonary arteries.

Approximately 2.5 million Americans are diagnosed with DVT each year, and as many as 50% of these persons develop pulmonary emboli.[16] Approximately 50,000 to 200,000 deaths are associated with pulmonary embolism each year. DVT occurs more commonly in women and persons over 40 years old. No racial variances have been identified. At increased risk are patients undergoing various types of surgery: general, orthopedic, gynecologic-obstetric, urologic, and neurosurgical procedures. Patients with hip fracture, hip or knee replacement, or reconstruction are particularly at risk.[17] The multiple risk factors for DVT are presented in the Risk Factors box.

It is estimated that 90% of pulmonary emboli begin as thrombi in the lower extremities, usually in the popliteal, femoral, and pelvic veins. Calf thromboses rarely embolize, although the reason for this is unknown. DVT is a relatively common occurrence in both hospital and community settings, and it is the third most common form of cardiovascular disease.

Pathophysiology. Thrombi develop from platelets, fibrin, and both red and white blood cells. They form in areas where the blood flow is slow or turbulent. Three primary factors, called Virchow's triad, trigger the formation of DVT: vessel wall damage, venous stasis, and hypercoagulability. Once formed, a clot can enlarge and extend. The venous valves may be damaged by the associated inflammatory response, causing postphlebitic syndrome. Muscle spasm and changes in intravascular pressure can cause the developing thrombus to dislodge and move toward the heart and lungs. The lungs are rich in heparin and plasmin activators and can effectively dissolve some thrombi; however, if the thrombus is not successfully dissolved, it can lodge in an artery and obstruct perfusion to the lung segment. The development of a pulmonary embolus is an extremely dangerous condition that carries a significant mortality risk. The pulmonary arteries become partially or totally obstructed depending on the size of the embolus, and the circulation to a lung segment or the entire lung may be affected. If the area of obstruction is large, the lung may undergo severe infarction with massive tissue destruction.[16] Pulmonary embolism is clearly the most serious outcome of DVT and is the major reason that treatment is immediate and aggressive. The development of a major pulmonary embolism can be rapidly fatal.

Clinical manifestations of DVT vary substantially according to the size and location of the thrombus and the adequacy of the collateral circulation (see the Clinical Manifestations box). Approximately 80% of all patients with DVT are completely asymptomatic.[17] Possible symptoms include pain or tenderness in the affected area, unilateral edema or swelling of the affected extremity,

Risk Factors

Deep Venous Thrombosis

Venous Stasis

Heart disease
Dehydration
Immobility (bed rest for more than 72 hours, prolonged sitting [automobile or air travel for longer than 4 hours])
Paralysis
Incompetent vein valves
Obesity (more than 20% over ideal body weight)
Pregnancy
Surgery lasting more than 45 minutes
Age over 40 years
Female gender (occurs more often in women)

Vessel Wall Injury

Trauma
–Fracture, especially involving the pelvis and long bones
–Extensive burns
Infection
Venipuncture
Intravenous infusion of irritant solutions
Central and peripheral intravenous catheters, pacemaker wires
History of deep venous thrombosis, varicose veins
Previous major surgery

Hypercoagulability

Alterations in hemostatic mechanisms
–Hemolytic anemias
–Increased viscosity (polycythemia vera)
–Inherited coagulation disorders
Trauma or surgery
Malignancy
Oral contraceptive use
Dehydration

and redness or warmth if the phlebitis is extensive (Figure 31-14). Superficial thrombophlebitis produces a palpable, firm, cordlike vein; and the area surrounding the affected vessel is usually tender, reddened, and warm. Fewer than 20% of all patients exhibit the classic Homans' sign (calf tenderness with dorsiflexion of the foot).

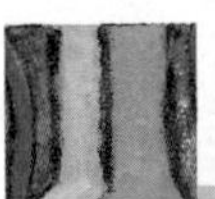

CLINICAL MANIFESTATIONS
Deep Venous Thrombosis

- Local pain or tenderness
- Unilateral edema or swelling
- May be bilateral if deep venous thrombosis (DVT) is located in the vena cava
- Local warmth, redness
- Mild fever
- Tender, palpable venous cord in the popliteal fossa
- Positive Homans' sign in fewer than 20% of all patients with DVT
- No symptoms in approximately 50% of all patients

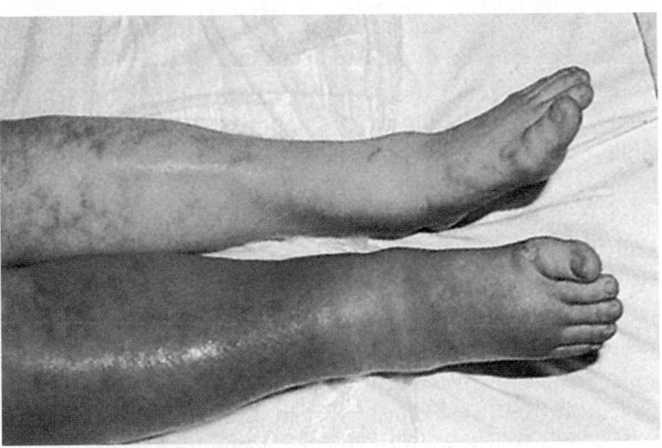

Figure 31-14 Deep venous thrombosis with phlebitis.

COMPLICATIONS. Recurrence of DVT and the development of pulmonary embolus are the two most significant complications of the disorder. It is not always possible to prevent these complications, but the measures outlined below are the best available strategies for prevention.

Collaborative Care Management

DIAGNOSTIC TESTS. Noninvasive testing with impedance plethysmography and ultrasonography is being used increasingly to determine the presence of a DVT. Plethysmography measures changes in electrical resistance to blood flow, and ultrasonography evaluates the sound of blood flowing through the veins. Duplex scanning combines traditional Doppler scanning with B-mode ultrasonography and is an accurate bedside, noninvasive, initial screening test. Positive tests may need to be confirmed by contrast venography. Although the venogram is the gold standard for diagnosing a DVT, it may mistakenly identify filling defects in the vein as a DVT. A venogram is more accurate in diagnosing peripheral thrombi, but is less effective in diagnosing pelvic, renal, or vena caval thrombi. The venogram is irritating to the veins and can itself trigger phlebitis and thrombus formation. The dye injection is uncomfortable for the patient and also creates a risk for allergic reaction to the contrast dye. Other tests that aid in the evaluation of the DVT include radiolabeled fibrinogen scans and D-dimer testing. The fibrinogen becomes visible at the site of thrombosis, but it takes 24 to 36 hours for sufficient fibrinogen to reach the site and make it visible. D-dimer testing is an agglutination assay blood test that uses venous blood to assess the degree of agglutination occurring.

MEDICATIONS. The treatment goals for pharmacologic therapy of DVT include decreasing the risk for pulmonary embolism, stopping further thrombosis, dissolving the existing thrombi, and preventing postphlebitic syndrome. Anticoagulant therapy is the first line of treatment in both preventing and treating DVT. Anticoagulant therapy to prevent a DVT involves administering either standard (unfractionated) heparin or low-molecular-weight heparin (LMWH) intermittently by subcutaneous injection.

Unfractionated heparin is extracted from animal tissues such as porcine intestine mucosa and bovine lung tissue, and binds to plasma antithrombin III to inactivate thrombin and other clotting factors, thereby interrupting coagulation. Unfractionated heparin is administered by IV or subcutaneous injection, and its effectiveness is monitored by the activated partial thromboplastin time (aPTT). Newer LMWHs are also approved for DVT prophylaxis (Table 31-6). Like unfractionated heparin, the LMWHs are administered subcutaneously once or twice a day, but the dose is determined by the patient's weight, and no blood testing is required.[29] Enoxaparin (Lovenox) is approved for DVT prophylaxis in nonsurgical patients and in patients recovering from hip, knee, and abdominal surgery.

Anticoagulant therapy used to treat a diagnosed DVT is more aggressive and involves the administration of heparin either subcutaneously or intravenously (or an LMWH subcutaneously), along with warfarin sodium, an oral agent. The goal of heparin therapy is to prevent new clots from forming and the existing thrombus from extending or growing. Heparin cannot dissolve existing thrombi, but it does block the conversion of fibrinogen to fibrin and prevents further extension of the thrombus.

IV heparin administration requires hospitalization and frequent aPTT monitoring, and so LMWH has quickly become the option of choice for treating an existing DVT.[29] Blood levels are quickly established and easily maintained without constant laboratory monitoring, and earlier discharge is possible as long as the patient is able to successfully administer the drug at home. Studies indicate that LMWH can be used safely as a long-term preventive measure, but most patients are still gradually converted to oral warfarin for long-term treatment. Oral anticoagulation with warfarin is initiated along with the LMWH or IV heparin therapy to prevent recurrence of thrombi. Warfarin takes several days to reach a therapeutic concentration, and most authorities recommend starting it immediately. Others advocate beginning warfarin administration after 3 to 5 days of heparin therapy.[28] A standard beginning dose of 5 to 10 mg is administered and is then gradually adjusted until a therapeutic international normalized ratio (INR) of 2.0 to 3.0 is achieved. Warfarin therapy is usually continued for at least 6 months after an initial episode of thrombosis.

Thrombolytic therapy with streptokinase, urokinase, or tissue plasminogen activator may also be used to treat DVT and pulmonary embolus. These agents activate the conversion of plasminogen to plasmin and actively dissolve existing thrombi, but thrombi in the veins of the lower extremities are usually older and larger than those which cause acute arterial occlusions and often do not respond as well to thrombolytics. Bleeding is the major adverse consequence of anticoagulant therapy, although heparin-induced thrombocytopenia, or white clot syndrome, can also occur. This serious complication occurs in 5% to 10% of patients receiving heparin therapy and can be life threatening.

TABLE 31-6 LOW-MOLECULAR-WEIGHT HEPARINS AND THEIR APPROVED INDICATIONS

Low-Molecular-Weight Heparin	Indications
Enoxaparin (Lovenox)	Total hip arthroplasty Hip fracture Total knee arthroplasty
Danaparoid (Orgaran)	Total hip arthroplasty
Dalteparin (Fragmin)	Total hip arthroplasty
Ardeparin (Normiflo)	Total knee arthroplasty

TREATMENTS. Patients with DVTs have traditionally been restricted to bed rest for 5 to 7 days while therapeutic blood levels of unfractionated heparin were being established. Activity restriction is generally not ordered for patients receiving LMWH. These patients are usually permitted to walk as tolerated and may be allowed to continue employment while receiving LMWH therapy.[28] Some physicians, however, still prefer to order bed rest for the initial treatment of DVT. If severe edema or pain is present in the extremity, the patient remains on bed rest with the leg elevated. Local moist heat and mild analgesics may be used to decrease the pain and inflammation. Heat and elevation improve venous return, decrease venous congestion, and decrease pain. After the acute episode resolves, graduated compression stockings (GCSs) are used to improve venous return and decrease swelling.

SURGICAL MANAGEMENT. Surgery does not play a major role in the management of DVT, although the thrombus may be removed via thrombectomy if the circulation in the extremity is compromised. Surgical intervention may also be used for patients who do not respond well to anticoagulant therapy or who experience recurrent DVT and pulmonary emboli. The primary surgical option is a transvenous filtration device placed in the vena cava to trap emboli before they reach the heart and pulmonary vessels. Two devices in current use are the Greenfield filter and the bird's nest filter. The Greenfield filter (Figure 31-15) is inserted either surgically or by interventional radiology through an incision in the jugular or femoral vein and is then advanced to the superior vena cava. The bird's nest filter is a web of stainless steel wires that is inserted percutaneously through the femoral vein or occasionally through the subclavian or jugular veins. Both filters intercept and trap emboli and are permanently implanted. They rarely become dislodged or occluded. Indications for use of a vena caval filter are summarized in Box 31-7, and the guidelines for care of a patient with a filter are presented in the Guidelines for Safe Practice box.

DIET. Patients with DVT have no dietary restrictions. Patients receiving warfarin may need to restrict their intake of foods high in vitamin K because the vitamin acts as an antidote to the action

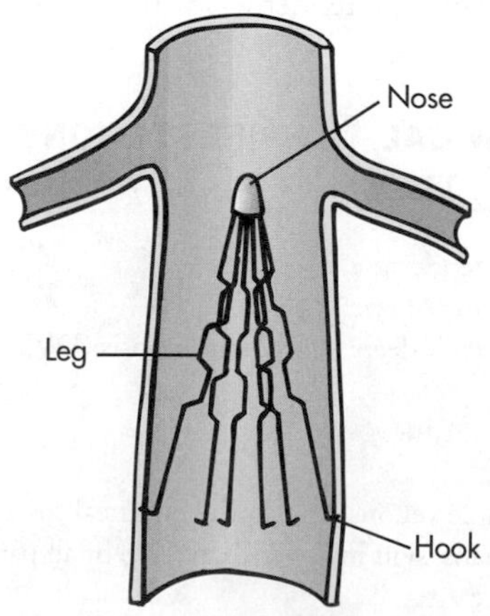

Figure 31-15 Greenfield filter placed in the vena cava.

BOX 31-7 Indications for Vena Caval Filter Placement

- Recurrent thromboembolism despite anticoagulation
- Confirmed deep venous thrombosis or thromboembolism with a contraindication to anticoagulation therapy
- Complication of anticoagulation requiring discontinuation of therapy
- Recurrent pulmonary embolism with associated pulmonary hypertension and cor pulmonale
- Free-floating thrombus
- Postpulmonary embolectomy
- Prophylaxis in high-risk patients

Adapted from Aquila A: Deep vein thrombosis, *J Cardiovas Nurs* 15(4):25-44, 2001.

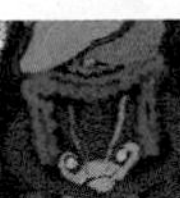

GUIDELINES FOR SAFE PRACTICE
The Patient With a Vena Caval Filter

- Assess venipuncture site for signs of bleeding or infection. Maintain an adhesive covering over the insertion site.
- Immobilize the extremity after the procedure per institution protocol or physician's order.
- Assess peripheral pulses, temperature, color, and sensation in affected extremity per protocol. Assess for pain and presence of positive Homans' sign.
- Assess respiratory status and monitor pulse oximetry or blood gases as indicated. Position in partial or high Fowler's position.
- Implement bleeding precautions and associated safety measures if systemic anticoagulation is to be continued. Monitor appropriate laboratory test results (e.g., activated partial thromboplastin time, platelets, hemoglobin, hematocrit, international normalized ratio).
- Teach the patient:
  —To monitor for:
    —Signs of infection at insertion site
    —Signs of systemic bleeding (e.g., blood in urine, stool, gums; nosebleeds; easy bruising)
  —Bleeding precautions for home use if anticoagulation is to be continued (e.g., use of soft toothbrush, electric razor, stool softeners)
  —To monitor for symptoms of complications:
    —Bleeding and infection
    —Deep venous thrombosis
    —Swelling and warmth in extremity
    —Sudden chest pain, dyspnea, tachypnea, restlessness
    —Filter occlusion: localized pain, venous stasis or swelling, unusual symptoms

of warfarin and can disrupt its therapeutic blood level. Obese patients may also be advised to attempt to achieve a more optimal body weight.

HEALTH PROMOTION AND PREVENTION. DVTs are common complications of routine hospital admissions, and preventing their incidence is a major nursing concern. DVTs are usually attributed to the effects of immobility. Early ambulation remains the single best preventive measure available; and the nurse carefully explains the importance of this intervention and other preventive interventions in common use, including the use of antiembolic stockings, graduated compression stockings (GCSs), external pneumatic compression (EPC) sleeves, and the administration of low-dose heparin.[36] Each of these devices is designed to increase the venous return from the lower extremities and prevent venous stasis. Frequent leg and ankle exercises also help prevent DVT.

Antiembolic stockings provide moderate consistent compression to the legs from the toes to either the knees or thighs. GCSs apply different degrees of compression to different parts of the legs. The pressure is recorded as 100% at the ankle and then decreases to 70% compression at midcalf and 40% at midthigh. Pneumatic compression devices consist of soft plastic sleeves that are applied to the legs and attached to an air pump, which regulates the flow of air into the sleeves. This provides gentle intermittent compression by inflating and deflating the sleeves at regular intervals to stimulate venous return (Figure 31-16). Both GCS and EPC devices are contraindicated in patients with arterial disease, severe edema, phlebitis, leg fractures, or skin breakdown.

All patients need instruction about the risks associated with prolonged sitting and the importance of taking breaks for walking every 1 to 2 hours during long car trips. Exercising on airplanes is more difficult but equally important. Patients are also instructed to maintain a high fluid intake to avoid dehydration when traveling, to avoid sitting with the ankles or knees crossed, to consider using compression stockings when traveling, and to perform ankle and leg exercises every hour if possible. Young women are informed about the risks of DVT associated with the use of estrogen-containing oral contraceptives, particularly if they also smoke cigarettes. Not all episodes of DVT can be prevented, but the risks can be decreased through some of these basic measures (Box 31-8).

Nursing Management
of the Patient with Deep Venous Thrombosis

ASSESSMENT

Health History. Assess for:
- History of DVT, treatment
- Significant risk factors (e.g., female, advancing age, prolonged sitting or immobility, recent extensive air travel)
- Oral contraceptive use, duration

Physical Examination. Assess for:
- Pain or tenderness in calf or thigh muscle at rest or with exercise
- Tenderness over affected area with palpation
- Abrupt pain on attempted dorsiflexion of the foot (Homans' sign)
- Warmth or redness over affected area
- Engorgement of collateral veins in affected area
- Unilateral or bilateral extremity edema; increase in leg circumference over the affected area
- Sudden onset of chest pain, dyspnea, or tachypnea, which may indicate pulmonary embolus
- Positive results from Doppler ultrasonography, venography, or plethysmography

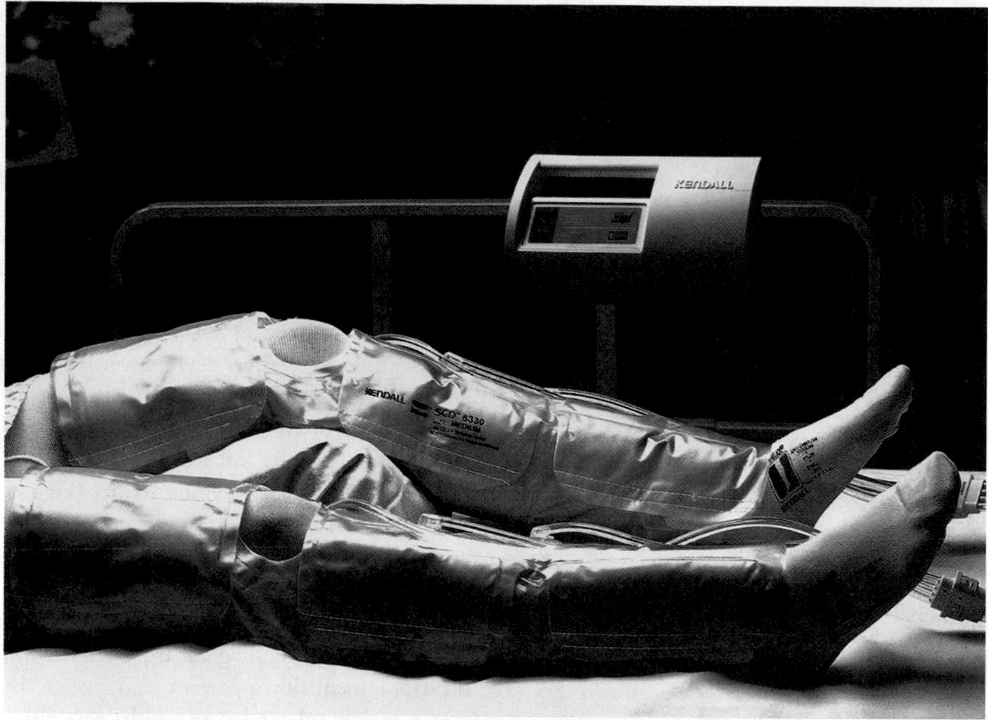

Figure 31-16 Pneumatic compression devices, such as the Kendall sequential compression device, are commonly used to prevent deep venous thrombosis in high-risk patients.

Box 31-8 Nursing Interventions to Prevent Deep Venous Thrombosis

- Identify risk factors that predispose the patient to deep venous thrombosis; reevaluate patient status frequently.
- Implement ordered prophylactic regimen.
  —Nonpharmacologic (mechanical)
    —Graduated compression stockings
    —Intermittent (external) pneumatic compression
    —Venous foot pump
  —Pharmacologic
    —Subcutaneous low-dose unfractionated heparin
    —Subcutaneous low-molecular-weight heparin
    —Oral anticoagulants
- Document patient tolerance to ordered prophylactic regimen.
- Assess all extremities on a regular basis for:
  —Pain and tenderness
  —Unilateral edema
  —Erythema
  —Warmth
- Encourage early ambulation and the performance of active leg exercises every hour while patient is awake.
- Perform passive range-of-motion exercises every shift if patient is immobile.
- Monitor for low-grade fever to detect thrombophlebitis.
- Encourage fluid intake to avoid dehydration; maintain accurate intake and output records.
- Use stool softeners to avoid straining, which increases venous pressure.
- Avoid use of knee gatch on bed.
- Provide patient education:
  —What deep venous thrombosis is and why it develops
  —Risk factor awareness
  —Signs and symptoms
  —Methods to prevent deep venous thrombosis
    —Engage in regular activity such as walking, cycling, and swimming to promote venous return.
    —Avoid prolonged sitting and standing.
    —Elevate legs with prolonged sitting.
    —Avoid constrictive garments: garters, girdles, tight-fitting stockings.

Adapted from Aquila A: Deep vein thrombosis, *J Cardiovasc Nurs* 15(4):25-44, 2001.

Nursing Diagnoses, Outcomes, and Interventions

Nursing Diagnosis: Ineffective Peripheral Tissue Perfusion

Outcomes. A common example of an expected outcome for the patient with a diagnosis of *ineffective peripheral tissue perfusion* is:

Patient will:

- Maintain adequate circulation to lower extremities as evidenced by palpable distal pulses and warm, pink extremities.

Nursing Interventions. The nurse monitors the adequacy of the perfusion to the affected extremity through regular neurovascular assessment, including all pulses distal to the site of the obstruction, the degree of pain and paresthesia if any, temperature changes, and degree of swelling. Calf and thigh circumferences are recorded each shift. When monitoring leg circumference, the nurse marks the site to be used for measurement directly on the skin to ensure the tape measure is consistently placed on the same site for each measurement.

The presence and severity of the pain, edema, and redness of the involved extremity determine the patient's activity level. If the extremity is red, edematous, and painful, bed rest with the leg elevated is usually prescribed. Patients receiving an LMWH may have no activity restrictions, although some physicians are hesitant to allow patients to walk because of the perceived risk of pulmonary embolus. Patients receiving traditional heparin therapy may be kept in bed for 5 to 7 days. Once out of bed, the patient is encouraged to walk frequently, avoid prolonged standing and sitting, and avoid crossing the legs at the knee or ankle. Compression stockings are applied to both legs unless contraindicated.

The nurse also carefully monitors the patient for signs of complications related to anticoagulant therapy or pulmonary embolus. The nurse monitors all laboratory results and implements bleeding precautions to protect the patient. These include assessing the patient for signs of bleeding, holding all venipuncture sites for at least 5 minutes, avoiding the use of intramuscular medications, and checking all body excretions (urine, stool, any emesis) for blood. The patient's records should be clearly marked to indicate the anticoagulated state to anyone performing venipuncture.

RELATED NIC INTERVENTIONS. Circulatory Care: Venous Insufficiency, Embolus Care: Peripheral, Embolus Precautions, Lower Extremity Monitoring

Nursing Diagnosis: Acute Pain

OUTCOMES. Common examples of expected outcomes for the patient with a diagnosis of *acute pain* are:

Patient will:

- State that pain is absent.
- Experience decreased leg edema.

NURSING INTERVENTIONS. Patients with DVT experience both physical and psychologic discomfort. Leg pain is managed with mild analgesics as needed, elevation of the affected leg, and restriction of activity. The nurse assesses the patient's comfort level frequently. Warm soaks may be applied to the affected leg for comfort if active phlebitis is present. NSAIDs are frequently used for both their pain-relieving and antiinflammatory effects. The patient is likely to be extremely anxious during the early days of treatment because the risk of pulmonary embolus is very real. The nurse encourages the patient to participate in all care decisions and keeps the patient and family informed about laboratory results and test findings. The nurse encourages the patient to express fears and concerns and offers realistic comfort and reassurance when possible.

RELATED NIC INTERVENTIONS. Analgesic Administration, Anxiety Reduction, Heat/Cold Application, Pain Management, Simple Relaxation Therapy

Patient/Family Teaching. Patients who experience DVT need extensive education because they are likely to require long-term anticoagulation at home. Patients need to know how to monitor their anticoagulant therapy and prevent complications. The nurse instructs the patient about the major action and side effects of the anticoagulants, the rationale for long-term management, and the planned schedule for laboratory monitoring of coagulation levels (see the Patient/Family Teaching box). The nurse instructs the patient to assess for and report any excessive bruising or bleeding.

The patient may also be instructed to wear compression stockings after discharge, and the nurse provides instruction about their safe and appropriate use. The patient needs more than one pair of the stockings so that they can be washed regularly. The correct fit is ensured by careful ankle, calf, and thigh circumference measurement before purchase. The stockings should be smoothly applied before getting out of bed in the morning and worn throughout the day. The skin is carefully inspected for bruising and signs of irritation or breakdown whenever the stockings are removed. The legs and feet are cleansed routinely.

PATIENT/FAMILY TEACHING

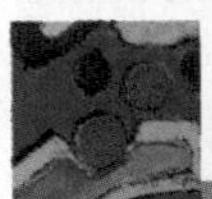

The Patient Receiving Oral Anticoagulant Therapy

Patient teaching should include information about the action, dosage, and side effects of medication, as well as the following instructions:

- Consult with pharmacist about the concurrent use of any other medications, since warfarin causes multiple adverse drug reactions.
- Avoid taking any aspirin-containing over-the-counter (OTC) medications, since aspirin increases the effect of anticoagulants.
- Read all OTC medication labels carefully.
- Take the drug at the same time each day.
- Never discontinue the drug without specific instruction from the health care provider.
- Monitor for signs of bleeding and report them to the health care provider:
  —Bleeding gums
  —Nosebleeds
  —Blood in the urine or stool
  —Cuts that do not stop bleeding despite application of direct pressure
- Keep scheduled follow-up appointments for blood tests to monitor anticoagulant levels.
- Maintain a log of dosage taken and relevant laboratory values.
- Eat dark green and yellow leafy vegetables in moderation. These are rich sources of vitamin K, which can counteract the effect of warfarin.
- Avoid the use of multivitamins with high vitamin K content.
- Use a soft toothbrush for oral care and avoid the use of straight razors for shaving.
- Use alcohol only in moderation, since it increases the anticoagulant effect.
- Wear a MedicAlert tag or bracelet that identifies the use of anticoagulants.

EVALUATION

To evaluate the effectiveness of nursing interventions, compare patient behaviors with those stated in the expected patient outcomes.

RELATED NOC OUTCOMES. Anxiety Level, Circulation Status, Comfort Level, Pain Control, Tissue Perfusion: Peripheral

GERONTOLOGIC CONSIDERATIONS

DVT is common in older adults, and preventive measures are particularly important for this age-group. Early ambulation and avoidance of prolonged bed rest are important measures during any hospitalization, particularly after surgery. Compression stockings and the administration of subcutaneous heparin are essential preventive measures. Older adults are also more likely to need home care assistance after discharge for teaching, follow up, and support.

Varicose Veins

Etiology and Epidemiology. Varicose veins are prominent, abnormally dilated veins that develop most often in the lower extremities because of the effects of gravity on venous pressure. In 1891 Trendelenburg first concluded that varicose veins were caused by vein valve incompetence combined with abnormally high hydrostatic pressure in the lower extremities. Few individuals younger than 25 develop varicose veins, except for young women who have had multiple pregnancies. By 40 years of age, 25% of men and more than 50% of women have some varicosities. The incidence rate increases to 50% of men and more than 64% of women by age 50.[23] A hereditary component is theorized to play a role in the development of varicose veins, but obesity, prolonged standing, and the effects of chronic diseases such as cirrhosis and heart failure are also well documented.

Pathophysiology. Venous blood flow in the legs begins in the capillaries and moves through the superficial veins that lie next to the skin. The blood then moves into the penetrating or communicating veins to the deep veins, which return the blood to the heart. Venous blood flow from the lower extremities is constantly working against gravity and is assisted by the unidirectional intraluminal valves in the veins that help move the blood toward the heart. Activity causes intermittent compression of the veins by the leg muscles and also supports venous blood flow. Over time, the accumulated pressure on the vein valves can cause them to become incompetent. Risk factors such as obesity, prolonged standing, pregnancy, and chronically elevated intraabdominal pressure can significantly contribute to elevated pressure within the veins. As the valves fail, the veins appear progressively swollen and enlarged and may become hard and tortuous (Figure 31-17). The patient may be asymptomatic or may develop swelling and a feeling of heaviness, pressure, or chronic fatigue in the legs, particularly after standing for any length of time.

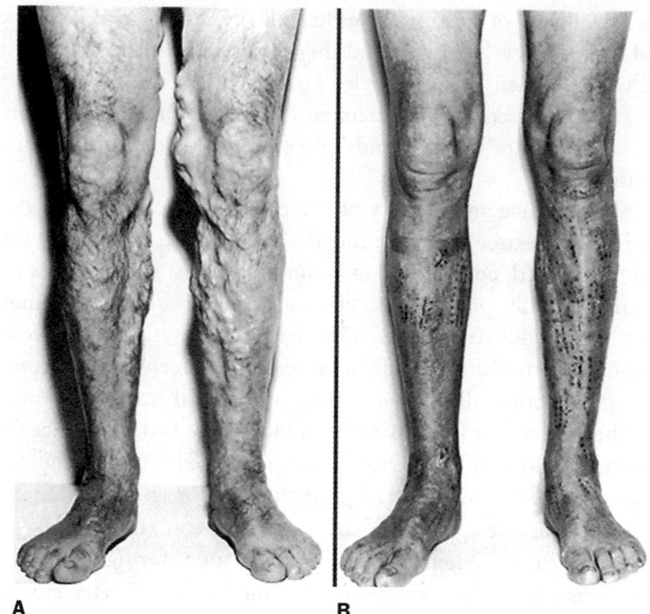

Figure 31-17 Extensive varicosities (incompetence of greater saphenous systems). **A,** Appearance before surgery. **B,** Appearance 2 weeks after surgery.

Collaborative Care Management. Varicose veins are a common problem in primary care. Noninvasive vascular testing is done to distinguish varicose veins from more serious venous disease. Trendelenburg's test is commonly used to evaluate valve competence. The patient lies supine and elevates the leg. A tourniquet is then applied to the upper thigh and the patient is helped to a standing position. If the veins fill immediately, varicosities are present.

Treatment depends on the severity of the disease. Primary interventions include teaching the patient about the importance of regular exercise, leg elevation, and avoidance of prolonged standing. Elastic stockings or another form of external support are usually recommended. Custom-fitted stockings are prescribed to be worn whenever the legs cannot be elevated. The appearance and weight of these stockings have improved over time, but they still may be unacceptable to many women. They are also somewhat difficult to put on, which makes them challenging for older patients and those with arthritis.

Sclerotherapy is an option for patients with small, localized varicosities. A sclerosing agent, usually 1% to 3% sodium tetradecyl, is injected into the vein.[37] Ligation, stripping, and excision of veins are traditional surgical options for more severe disease and can usually be performed as outpatient surgery if no untoward complications develop. Outpatient laser treatment has also proven effective in eradicating smaller, localized varicose veins.[8]

PATIENT/FAMILY TEACHING. The patient with varicose veins needs to understand the relationship between gravity and varicose filling. The nurse assists the patient to find ways to minimize prolonged sitting or standing during daily activities, and ways to elevate the legs above the level of the heart at intervals throughout the day. The nurse also encourages the patient to maintain an optimal body weight and explore whether symptoms can be improved by weight loss. The nurse also encourages the patient to wear compression stockings. The patient may need to experiment with different types and brands until a style and weight can be found that provide the needed support and are acceptable to the patient for daily use. The nurse reinforces the importance of applying compression stockings before getting out of bed in the morning. Discharge teaching after vein surgery includes monitoring wound healing, assessing for signs of infection, resting with the legs elevated at intervals throughout the day, walking regularly, and avoiding prolonged sitting and standing.

Venous Ulcers

Etiology and Epidemiology. Venous ulcers are called venous stasis ulcers. Leg ulcers can be caused by many conditions, including venous hypertension, infection, diabetes mellitus, malignancy, connective tissue disorders, rheumatoid arthritis, and damage from DVT or venous stasis. External insults such as trauma, pressure, and insect bites are other possible causes. Venous ulcers account for more than 85% of all vascular ulcers. One in four Americans over the age of 65 (more than 1.5 million people) annually develop extremity ulcers, the vast majority of which are the result of chronic venous disease.[39] Treatment is prolonged and is estimated to cost from $750 million to $1 billion each year. Most ulcers result from a coexisting disease process or trauma, but risk factors include a positive family history, pregnancy, obesity, and an occupation that requires prolonged standing.

Pathophysiology. Venous ulcers typically develop from a pattern of increased venous tension and valve incompetence that leads to venous stasis, poor venous return, edema, and ultimately ulceration. The pattern is similar in most ways to the pathology of other venous disorders. It is theorized that fibrin cuffs may develop around the dermal capillaries in response to prolonged venous hypertension. These cuffs prevent sufficient oxygen and nutrients from reaching the tissue. The decreased circulation results in ulceration. An alternative theory suggests that capillaries are damaged from prolonged venous stasis and cellular permeability increases owing to the release of inflammatory substances from the white cells.

Chronic venous hypertension causes varicosities, stasis dermatitis, and lipodermatosclerosis. The varicosities are the direct result of the incompetent valves, but only 3% of patients with varicosities develop ulcers. Stasis dermatitis occurs from edema and blistering. Stasis dermatitis is often the first sign of ulcers. Lipodermatosclerosis occurs when fibrotic tissue develops in response to longstanding extremity edema. The fibrotic tissue replaces the normal tissue and fat in the legs. The leg becomes larger at the calf and smaller at the ankle, and the skin is tough and thick. Venous ulcers are often located over the medial or lateral malleolus but can develop on other parts of the leg.

The ulcers typically exhibit irregular, ill-defined margins; vary in size; and range in appearance from red granulation tissue to fibrinous or necrotic tissue (Figure 31-18). Venous ulcers usually produce copious serous exudate. The surrounding skin is brown or brawny in appearance because of the accumulation of waste products from hemolyzed red blood cells. Edema and distention of the veins on the medial aspect of the foot are also common.

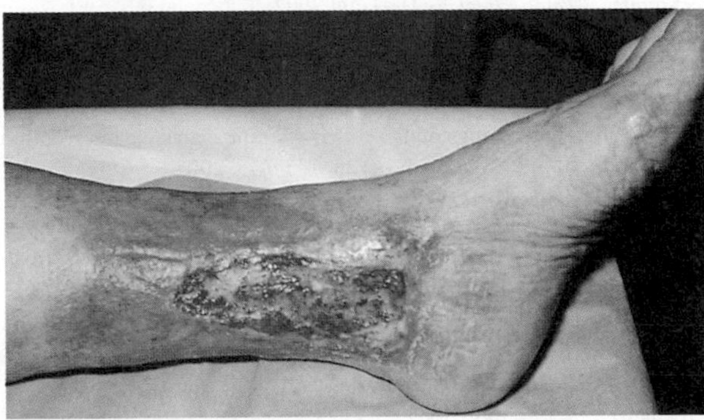

Figure 31-18 Classic venous ulceration in malleolar region.

Collaborative Care Management. Venous ulcers heal slowly and often recur. The diagnosis is made by clinical examination, but diagnostic tests are usually performed to evaluate both the arterial and venous systems. Doppler ultrasound, color duplex scanners, photoplethysmographs, or air plethysmographs are used to evaluate the venous system. Patients must understand that treatment will be a lifelong process. Venous ulcers are treated with a combination of compression, elevation, and topical wound care. Compression is directed at improving blood flow and venous return to the heart. It also decreases edema and assists in the healing process. Several bandaging techniques are in common use, including Unna's boot, the Setopress, and four-layer compression devices such as Profore.[33] The Research box below presents the findings of a study that compared the effectiveness of four-layer compression with the use of **Unna's boot**. Elastic stockings may also be used as part of treatment and to prevent recurrence of the ulcer. Compliance with high-pressure stockings is poor, however, as reported in the Research box on p. 894. As in other conditions, compression hose are applied before getting out of bed and removed before going to bed. Intermittent compression devices can also be beneficial to patients with venous ulcers.

Unna's boot was developed by Paul Unna in the late 1800s and is the model for other compressive devices used to treat venous ulcers. It is composed of a continuous compression bandage that contains glycerol and zinc oxide with the option to include diphenhydramine lotion. The extremity is covered by an elastic compression dressing that is wet when applied and requires up to 12 hours to dry. Unna's boot disintegrates in water, so bathing is prohibited during treatment. Skin and circulatory assessments are

Research

Polignano R et al: A randomized controlled study of four layer compression versus Unna's boot for venous ulcers, *J Wound Care* 13(1):21-24, 2004.

This study compared healing rates, handling properties, and patient comfort associated with the use of a four-layer bandage system (Profore) versus the traditional Unna's boot for the treatment of venous ulcers. Sixty-eight patients were drawn from various vascular clinic settings and randomized to receive treatment with either Unna's boot or the four-layer bandage system. Healing was recorded for 24 weeks. Staff evaluated ease of application, and patients rated comfort with the treatment.

At the end of the study period, complete healing had been obtained for 74% of the four-layer bandage system group and 66% of the Unna's boot group. The time to closure was not significantly different between the groups. Staff rated the quality of application more favorably for the four-layer bandage system, and it was rated as significantly easier to apply. The initial appearance of the two systems was comparable, but the appearance of the layer bandage deteriorated more than that of the Unna's boot over the study period. No significant differences were found in patient comfort, and the researchers concluded that the four-layer bandage is a viable and effective alternative to Unna's boot for the treatment of venous leg ulcers.

Research

Jull AB et al: Factors influencing adherence with compression stockings after venous leg ulcer healing, *J Wound Care* 13(3):90-92, 2004.

This study investigated the factors influencing patient adherence to the use of compression stockings after the healing of a venous leg ulcer. A sample of 129 patients was drawn from the practice of a leg ulcer specialty service. The participants were questioned about their use of compression stockings in the first 6 months after treatment for a leg ulcer. Fifty-two percent reported daily wearing of the ordered stockings, 16% reported that they wore them most days, 5% reported that they wore them occasionally, and 22% had not worn them at all after discharge. The remainder did not provide data.

The most important variables in the decision to wear the stockings or not were the beliefs that the stockings were worthwhile and that they were uncomfortable to wear. Other commonly cited factors such as cosmetic appearance and cost, difficulty putting them on, age, and gender did not significantly influence the decision for this population.

essential components of care. Excessive boot pressure can cause arterial compression, and both peripheral pulses and capillary perfusion are carefully monitored after the boot is applied.

Patients with stasis dermatitis may be treated with a topical steroid cream. A hydrocolloid dressing such as DuoDERM may be applied over the cream. Any open wound needs to be kept clean, and normal saline is an appropriate choice for cleaning noninfected wounds. Infected ulcers may require topical or systemic antibiotics and daily wound care. Alginates, hydrocolloids, hydrogels, foams, and transparent films may all be used on the infected ulcer. Ideally, a nurse wound care specialist develops the overall plan for wound care to be implemented by the patient and family at home. A compression wrap is usually applied over the base dressing.

Surgical intervention is of limited value but may be necessary to prevent the recurrence of venous ulcers and promote healing. Thrombosed veins may be surgically removed. Split-thickness skin grafting may be necessary to cover the wound after excision of the ulcer. Skin grafts and tissue transfer for topical treatment are used to manage ulcers. The subfascial endoscopic perforator surgery is used to identify incompetent perforator veins and ligate them, which theoretically contributes to ulcer healing after the procedure.[39]

PATIENT/FAMILY TEACHING. Patient/family teaching is an important part of nursing care for patients with venous ulcers, which are difficult and time consuming to heal. From 70% to 80% of them recur, so their management becomes a lifelong process. Patients may be admitted to an acute care institution for portions of their care, but most of the wound management takes place in the home. The wound cleansing and dressing routines can be complex and time consuming. Home health assistance may be indicated initially, but most patients are expected to manage their ongoing wound care with the family's help. The nurse plays an essential role in teaching the patient and family about wound care techniques and the rationale for all interventions. The patient and family also need to know where to find wound care supplies in their community and how to effectively compare the wide range of products available. Compression, elevation, and optimal skin care are the essential components for healing. The nurse also discusses supportive measures such as weight loss or control, rest, optimal nutrition, and avoidance of prolonged standing.

? Critical Thinking

1. A 62-year-old woman is recovering from a recent myocardial infarction. She is in atrial fibrillation. She suddenly complains of a severe pain in her left leg. The nurse notes that pulses are absent, and the leg is cool to the touch. On further questioning the woman states that her leg feels somewhat numb. What is the likely cause of her symptoms? What are the appropriate next steps in her care?
2. You are addressing a community group of young pregnant women. One of them raises the issue of varicose veins and asks you if it is true that they are inevitable. What information would you provide these women about varicose veins and their prevention?

References

1. Abou-Zamzam AM: Detection and treatment of peripheral arterial occlusive disease, *J Clin Outcomes Manage* 11(5):308-320, 2004.
2. Anderson L: Abdominal aortic aneurysm, *J Cardiovasc Nurs* 15(4):1-14, 2001.
3. Andrade SE et al: Hypertension management: the care gap between the clinical guidelines and clinical practice, *Am J Managed Care* 10(7 part 2): 481-486, 2004.
4. Aquila A: Deep vein thrombosis, *J Cardiovasc Nurs* 15(4):25-44, 2001.
5. Asmar R: Benefits of blood pressure reduction in elderly patients, *J Hypertension* 21(6 suppl):25-30, 2003.
6. Bacon SL et al: Effects of exercise, diet and weight loss on high blood pressure, *Sports Med* 34(5):307-316, 2004.
7. Ball K: Deep vein thrombosis and airline travel—the deadly duo, *AORN* 77(2):345, 348-349, 351-352, 357-359, 2003.
8. Bender M: Vanishing veins: a new laser treatment can leave your legs blemish free for good, *Health* 18(3):23-24, 2004.
9. Berg AO et al: Screening for high blood pressure: recommendations and rationale, *Am J Nurs* 104(11):82-85, 2004.
10. Chobanian A et al: The seventh report of the Joint National Committee on Prevention, Detection, Evaluation, and Treatment of High Blood Pressure, *JAMA* 289(DOI 10.1001), 2003.
11. Clifford-Middel M: Simplifying dosing regimens appears to improve treatment adherence in patients with high blood pressure in ambulatory settings, *Evidence-Based Nurs* 7(4):11, 2004.
12. Cynamon J, Rosado M: Angiography and catheter directed interventional techniques, *J Vasc Technol* 26(1):41-44, 2002.
13. DeGodoy JMP et al: Quality of life after amputation, *Psychol Health Med* 7(4):397-400, 2002.
14. Desai R, Korn JH: Diagnosis and management of Raynaud phenomenon: presence of an underlying condition may warrant aggressive intervention, *J Musculoskel Med* 20(3):124, 126-128, 133-135, 2003.
15. Dugdill S: Peripheral arterial disease: strategies for treatment, *Practice Nurse* 28(4):50, 52, 54, 2004.
16. Goldhaber S, Morrison R: Pulmonary embolism and deep vein thrombosis, *Circulation* 106(12):1436-1438, 2002.
17. Gorski L: Clinical update: deep vein thrombosis, *Home Healthcare Nurse* 19(5):307-310, 2001.
18. Hall S: Endovascular repair of abdominal aortic aneurysms, *AORN* 77(3):630-642, 645-648, 2003.
19. Hazelgrove JF, Rogers PD: Phantom limb pain—a complication of lower extremity wound management, *International J Lower Extremity Wounds* 1(2):112-124, 2004.

20. Holman JR: Peripheral arterial disease: tips on diagnosis and management, *Consultant* 44(1):101-103, 107-108, 2004.
21. Ketelhut R et al: Regular exercise as an effective approach in antihypertensive therapy, *Med Sci Sports Exercise* 36(1):4-8, 2004.
22. Kupinski AM: Segmental pressure measurement and plethysmography, *J Vasc Technol* 26(1):32-38, 2002.
23. Leach MJ: Making sense of the venous leg ulcer debate: a literature review, *J Wound Care* 13(2):52-56, 2004.
24. Lipsitz EC, Veith FJ: Surgical therapy for the patient with lower extremity ischemia, *J Vasc Technol* 26(1):45-51, 65-66, 2002.
25. Luggen A: Research review: hypertension management in African Americans, *Geriatr Nurs* 25(1):60-61, 2004.
26. Michael A, Reisner C: Intermittent claudication in older people, *Geriatr Med* 34(6):61-62, 64, 2004.
27. Mohler ER: Peripheral arterial disease: identification and implications, *Arch Intern Med* 163(19):2306-2314, 2003.
28. Morris BA et al: Venous thromboembolism: prevention and treatment, *RN* 65(10):24hf3-24hf9, 2002.
29. Nadeau C, Varrone J: Treat DVT with low molecular weight heparin, *Nurse Practitioner* 28(10):22-29, 2003.
30. Olson KWP, Treat-Jacobson D: Symptoms of peripheral arterial disease: a critical review, *J Vasc Nurs* 22(3):72-77, 2004.
31. Palec D: Endovascular repair of abdominal aortic aneurysm: new technology is helping to save lives, *Am J Nurs* 101(4):24AA, 24CC, 24EE, 24GG-24II, 2001.
32. Patel MD, Thompson PD: Drug treatment of claudication, *ACC Current J Rev* 13(3):16-20, 2004.
33. Polignano R et al: A randomized controlled study of four layer compression versus Unna's boot for venous ulcers, *J Wound Care* 13(1):21-24, 2004.
34. Pope J et al: Iloprost and cisaprost for Raynaud's phenomenon in progressive systemic sclerosis, *Cochrane Library,* ID No. CD000953, 2005.
35. Powell JT, Greenhalgh RM: Small abdominal aortic aneurysms, *N Engl J Med* 348(19):1895-1901, 2003.
36. Rice K, Walsh E: Minimizing venous thromboembolic complications in the orthopaedic patient, *Orthop Nurs* 20(6):21-27, 2001.
37. Rigby KA et al: Surgery versus sclerotherapy for the treatment of varicose veins, *Cochrane Library,* ID No. CD004980, 2005.
38. Sieggreen M, Kline R: Arterial insufficiency and ulceration: diagnosis and treatment options, *Adv Skin Wound Care* 17(5):242-251, 2004.
39. Sieggreen M, Kline R: Recognizing and managing venous leg ulcers, *Adv Skin Wound Care* 17(6):302-322, 2004.
40. Tzourio C: Vascular factors and cognition: toward a prevention of dementia? *J Hypertension* (Suppl) 21(5):15-19, 2003.
41. US Department of Health and Human Services: *Healthy people 2010: understanding and improving health,* Washington, DC, 2000, The Department.
42. Wimett L, Laustsen G: Caduet treats two cardiovascular conditions at once, *Nurse Practitioner* 29(6):56-57, 2004.
43. Woods A: Loosening the grip of hypertension, *Nursing* 34(12):36-43, 2004.

evolve Visit the Evolve website: http://evolve.elsevier.com/Monahan/medsurg

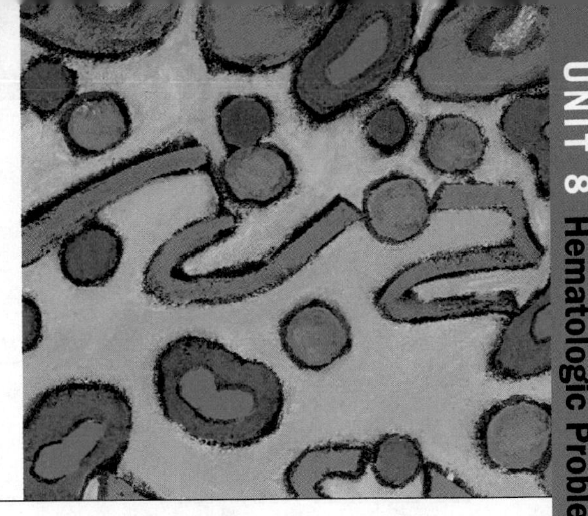

CHAPTER 32

Assessment of the Hematologic System

by Peggy Ellis

OBJECTIVES

After studying this chapter, the learner should be able to:

1. Recall the structure and function of the organs, tissues, and cells of the hematologic system.
2. Discuss changes that occur within the hematologic system as a result of normal aging.
3. Identify essential data to be collected as part of the assessment of the hematologic system.
4. Describe common diagnostic tests used in the assessment of the hematologic system.
5. Explain the nursing implications of hematology-related diagnostic tests.

KEY TERMS

activated partial thromboplastin time, p. 905
bone marrow, p. 897
erythrocytes, p. 897
hematocrit, p. 904
hematopoiesis, p. 897
hemoglobin, p. 897
international normalized ratio, p. 905
leukocytes, p. 897
lymphangiography, p. 905
lymphatic system, p. 899
mononuclear phagocyte system, p. 897
prothrombin time, p. 905
thrombocytes, p. 897

Anatomy and Physiology

Diseases associated with the hematologic system are diverse in their underlying pathologic manifestations, disease course, and response to treatment. Most often the accompanying symptoms result from altered **hematopoiesis** (blood cell production) or interference with the normal development and function of the blood components: **erythrocytes** (red blood cells [RBCs]), **thrombocytes** (platelets), and **leukocytes** (white blood cells [WBCs]). Normally a balance is maintained between the rate of production of normal blood cells and the rate of destruction. Disorders of the blood occur when this balance is lost. Disturbances in the coagulation mechanism also result in blood disorders.

Components of the Hematologic System

The hematologic system includes blood and its components; **bone marrow;** and the **mononuclear phagocyte system** (MPS) (previously known as the reticuloendothelial system), which is located throughout the body. The MPS function is phagocytizing foreign materials and lysing (breaking down) RBCs.

Blood. Blood is an aqueous solution (plasma) that contains water, proteins, electrolytes, and inorganic and organic constituents. Cells make up 7% to 9% of the blood. The cell components of blood include erythrocytes, leukocytes, thrombocytes, and plasma cells. All normal cells are derived from a single stem cell that can divide into lymphoid and myeloid stem cells. These stem cells can, in turn, become progenitor cells that divide along a specific single pathway (Figure 32-1). This process, known as hematopoiesis, takes place in the bone marrow of the flat bones in adults. Activity is highest in the iliac crests, sternum, ribs, and proximal epiphysis of long bones. Production may occur in all the long bones during periods of increased demand, such as during hemorrhage or cell destruction (hemolysis).

ERYTHROCYTES. An erythrocyte (RBC) is a nonnucleated biconcave disk that is soft and pliable. These characteristics enable the RBC to change its shape during passage through the microcirculation and to function efficiently as a gas carrier (oxygen and carbon dioxide). The major component of the RBC is **hemoglobin** (Hgb), a protein that transports oxygen and carbon dioxide and maintains normal pH through a series of intracellular buffers. The Hgb molecule contains globin (two pairs of polypeptide chains) and four heme groups, each containing an atom of ferrous iron. Thus each Hgb molecule can unite with four oxygen molecules to form oxyhemoglobin (a reversible reaction). Carbon dioxide is carried by the globin portion of the

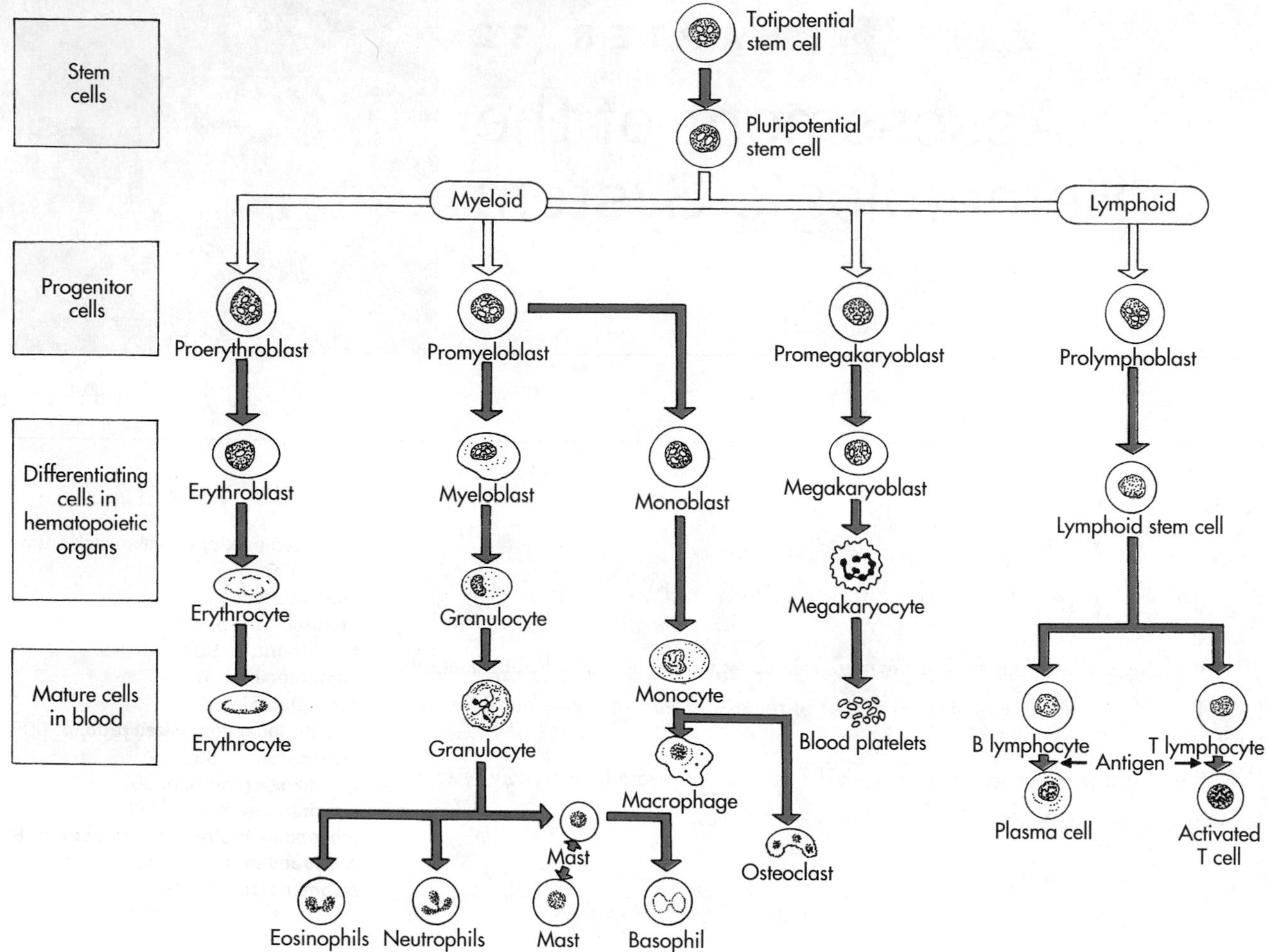

Figure 32-1 Scheme of stem cell differentiation.

Hgb molecule. In a normal person 99% of the hemoglobin molecules are saturated with oxygen.

Immature RBCs are called reticulocytes. They are released in the bloodstream where they circulate until they mature. Reticulocytes normally make up approximately 1% of the RBCs. Production of RBCs in the bone marrow requires adequate amounts and use of vitamin B_{12}, folic acid, proteins, enzymes, and minerals (iron, copper). Erythropoiesis (RBC formation) can be greatly stimulated by the secretion of the hormone erythropoietin from the kidneys; this occurs when the numbers of RBCs falls below normal (such as with severe blood loss) or when demand for oxygen increases (tissue hypoxia).

The RBCs circulate for 120 days and are then destroyed by the macrophages of the MPS. Most of the iron is removed from the heme and can be used to form new heme groups. Small amounts of iron lost daily in urine and feces and through menstrual flow must be replaced by iron ingestion. The remainder of the heme is broken down to form bilirubin and is secreted into the bile. Energy in the form of adenosine triphosphate is required to maintain cell membrane integrity and the relatively low sodium and high potassium content of the RBCs. When breakdown of RBCs is accelerated, there is an increase in bilirubin in the blood and urobilinogen in the urine.

LEUKOCYTES. Leukocytes make up the body's mobile defense system against foreign invaders. These cells are formed both in the bone marrow (granulocytes, monocytes, and some lymphocytes) and in the lymphatic tissue (lymphocytes). These cells are classified into two groups: polymorphonuclear granulocytes (neutrophils, basophils, and eosinophils) and nongranular leukocytes (monocytes and lymphocytes). The average life span of a leukocyte is 4 or 5 days, but once activated it lives only 6 to 8 hours in circulation. Monocytes that lodge in tissue become macrophages and can live months to years until they are destroyed in the process of phagocytosis.

Neutrophils, also referred to as segmented neutrophils (or "segs"), make up 50% to 70% of circulating leukocytes. Immature forms are called bands or stabs. In response to inflammation or infection, transient increases in neutrophils occur (neutrophilia). Neutrophils provide defense in two ways. First, they release the contents of their granules, which contain enzymes to kill and digest bacteria. Second, they are capable of direct phagocytosis of foreign organisms (see Figure 20-5).

Eosinophils constitute about 4% of circulating leukocytes. Although not significant in bacterial infections, eosinophils are active in parasitic infections by attaching to the organism and releasing chemicals to aid in destruction of the invader. Eosinophils also participate in the allergic response by preventing local inflammation from spreading throughout the body.

Basophils are less than 1% of circulating leukocytes. The granules of the basophil contain heparin, histamine, and small quantities of bradykinin and serotonin. These substances are released during the process of inflammation. In the allergic response the immunoglobulin E (IgE) antibody attaches to the basophil, causing the release of chemicals and resulting in the localized tissue reaction commonly seen with the allergic response.

Circulating monocytes make up 2% to 8% of the total number of leukocytes. These cells are larger than granulocytes and have a kidney-shaped nucleus. The majority of monocytes are tissue based and become macrophages as they leave the circulation. The tissue macrophage is the first line of defense against infection. These tissue macrophages participate in phagocytosis of dead and injured cells, cell fragments, and microorganisms.

Lymphocytes make up the remaining 20% to 40% of leukocytes. These cells have a round to oval nucleus. The majority of lymphocytes originate in lymphoid tissue, but some are made in the bone marrow. The two types of lymphocytes are circulating T lymphocytes originating from the thymus and noncirculating B lymphocytes. Refer to Chapter 20 for further information on the role of leukocytes in inflammation and the immune response.

THROMBOCYTES. Thrombocytes (platelets) are not cells but granular, disk-shaped, nonnucleated cell fragments. Their production is regulated by thrombopoietin, which is produced in the liver and kidneys. They are important in the blood clotting process and also play a role in inflammation (see Research box). Approximately two thirds of all platelets are within the circulatory system, and the remaining one third is present in the spleen as a reserve pool. The life span of a platelet is approximately 6 to 10 days. Platelets originate from the stem cells that process megakaryocytes, which are precursors to platelets and are essential to hemostasis and coagulation (see Figure 32-1).

Research

Cambien B et al: Antithrombotic activity of TNF-alpha, *J Clin Invest* 112(10): 1589, 2003.

Some researchers have suggested that thrombosis and inflammation are closely related. Tumor necrosis factor–alpha (TNF-alpha) is a cytokine that is active in inflammation and the immune response. In this study, researchers gave mice TNF-alpha in the same dose as would be found in sepsis. Then they tested bleeding times of the mice and examined the fibrinogen binding and platelet aggregation. The results demonstrated that mice who received TNF-alpha had a significantly increased bleeding time. This indicates the TNF-alpha has a strong antithrombotic activity. After treatment with TNF-alpha the platelets showed a decrease in fibrinogen binding and reduced platelet aggregation. These results indicate that TNF-alpha decreases platelet activation and inhibits thrombi formation during inflammation. This effect is not due to the action of TNF-alpha on platelets but to its effects on other chemicals related to vessel injury.

The coagulation process occurs in stages and usually takes about 5 to10 minutes. An individual with a shorter clotting time than this may be prone to develop intravascular thrombi, and an individual with a longer clotting time may have a tendency to bleed more than normal. In the first stage, platelets and plasma proteins agglutinate at the injury site and adhere to the injured vessel walls (Figure 32-2). Platelets are attracted to the site by exposure of collagen-containing subendothelial tissue. In the presence of calcium, platelets become spiny-shaped spheres that release strong biochemical mediators and form thromboplastin. Adhesion to the site of injury is enhanced by the binding of the platelet to fibrinogen and is also promoted by von Willebrand's factor. In the second stage the thromboplastin activates the conversion of prothrombin to thrombin in the presence of calcium. Thrombin leads to the development of the fibrin mesh and platelet aggregation. In the third stage, thrombin and fibrinogen form fibrin. In the presence of calcium a fibrin clot forms. In the fourth stage the clot breaks into fibrin split products and is removed, a process called fibrinolysis.

The coagulation process is often described as a cascade made up of two independent pathways that join to form a common pathway. This cascade is a series of enzymatic reactions with each step leading to the next. The intrinsic pathway is slower. It involves the circulating coagulation factors of high-molecular-weight kininogen, factor XII, prekallikrein, factor XI, factor IX, factor VIII, factor X, factor V, and prothrombin. It is measured by the activated partial thromboplastin time. The extrinsic pathway involves tissue factor, factor VII, factor X, factor V, and factor II. It is measured by prothrombin time. These two pathways join together to form the common pathway, which proceeds to clot formation.

Mononuclear Phagocyte System. The MPS includes circulating monocytes and their precursor cells in the bone marrow. Also included are more or less fixed mononuclear phagocytic cells (also called macrophages) found in blood channels in the spleen and liver (Kupffer's cells), in the lymphatic system, in serosal cavities of the body, in the lungs, in general connective tissue, and in the bone marrow.

The MPS is primarily responsible for phagocytosis, the process of engulfing and removing "wasted" white blood cells. In addition to phagocytosis, the MPS processes the Hgb of RBCs that have reached the end of their life span, splitting Hgb into an iron-containing substance and bilirubin.

Lymphatic System. The **lymphatic system** is an alternative pathway by which fluid can flow between the interstitial spaces and the blood. Its chief function is to remove proteins from the tissue spaces. All tissues of the body contain lymph channels with the exception of the central nervous system, bone, and the superficial skin layers. Lymph fluid circulates throughout the body at a rate of 120 ml/hr. The lymphatic system also plays an important role in the regulation of tissue volume and interstitial fluid pressure.

The normal lymph node consists of connective tissue encapsulating a fine mesh of reticular cells. The reticuloendothelial cells function chiefly in the phagocytosis of cellular debris. The primary

Sequence of Events		Substances Involved
Stage 1 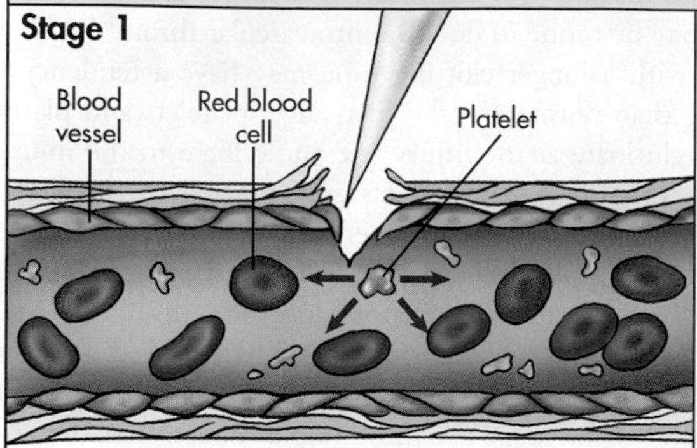 Blood vessel Red blood cell Platelet	• Injury occurs to vessel (intrinsic pathway) or tissue (extrinsic pathway) • Vessel constricts • Platelets release platelet factors	*Intrinsic:* Factor XII: Hageman factor, contact factor High–molecular weight kininogen (HMWK) Prekallikrein Kallikrein Factor XI: Plasma thromboplastin antecedent (PTA) Factor IV (Ca^{++}): Calcium Factor IX: Plasma thromboplastin component (PTC), Christmas factor Factor VII: Serum prothrombin conversion accelerator (SPCA) Factor VIII: Antihemophilic globulin (AHG), antihemophilic factor (AHF) Phospholipid *Extrinsic:* Factor III: Thromboplastin, tissue thromboplastin Factor VII: SPCA Tissue factor Ca^{++}
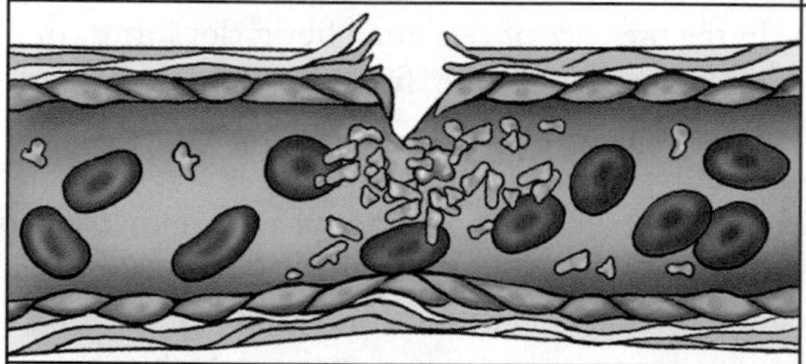	• Platelet factors attract more platelets • Platelets aggregate around wound • Prothrombin activator formed	Factor III: Thromboplastin, tissue thromboplastin Factor X: Stuart-Prower factor Factor V: Proaccelerin, labile factor Phospholipid Factor IV (Ca^{++}): Calcium Factor II: Prothrombin
Stage 2 Thromboplastin **Prothrombin** → **Thrombin**	• Thromboplastin converts prothrombin to thrombin	Factor II: Prothrombin Factor IV (Ca^{++}): Calcium
Stage 3 Thrombin **Fibrinogen** → **Fibrin**	• Thrombin converts fibrinogen to fibrin threads	Factor I: Fibrinogen
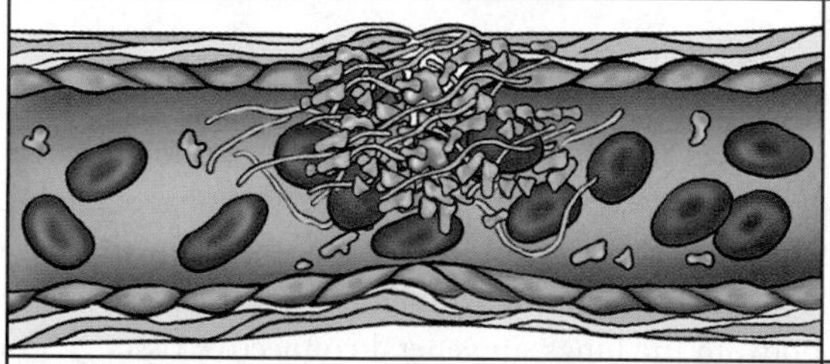	• Fibrin threads tangle with platelets and trap red blood cells, forming a clot • Factor XIII stabilizes clot and it begins to retract and harden	Factor XIII: Fibrin-stabilizing factor, fibrinase Factor IV (Ca^{++}): Calcium
Stage 4 **Plasminogen** → **Plasmin**	• Plasminogen converts to plasmin	
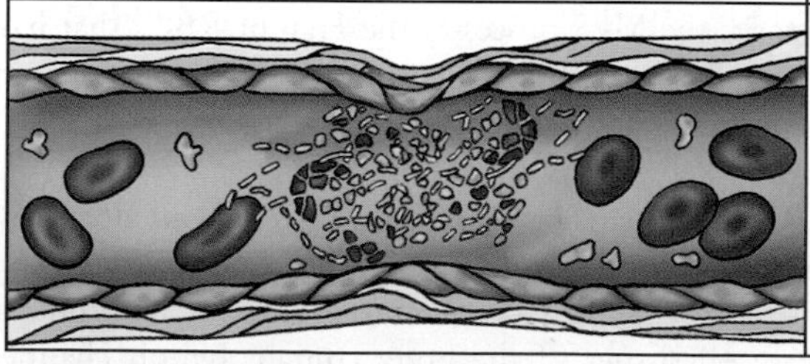	• Plasmin breaks the clot into fibrin split products, dissolving it	

Figure 32-2 Formation of a blood clot.

function of lymphocytes, which are the main cells constituting the lymph nodes, is to provide an immune response to antigens presented to the node from the structure being drained by the node.

Lymph node enlargement, or lymphadenopathy, results from an increase in the number and size of lymphoid follicles with proliferation of lymphocytes and reticuloendothelial cells. Lymphadenopathy also may occur when the node is invaded by cells normally not present (leukemic cells, cancer cells) or when lymph channels and nodes are surgically removed. In lymphomas the actual nodal structure is destroyed by the malignant cells.

Normally lymph nodes are not palpable. With disease and the consequent increase in size, the nodes become palpable.

Physiologic Changes With Aging

The effect of aging on hematopoiesis is under study, but to date there have been no clear, clinically significant findings. There is some indication that the cellularity of human marrow decreases with age, perhaps as a result of an increase in fat from osteoporosis. In addition, some research demonstrates a decrease in bone marrow production of cells.

In human beings the total number of leukocytes and differential counts show no variation through middle age and no gross changes in old age. In general, however, the leukocyte count does not rise as high in response to infection in older persons; that may be because they have a diminished marrow granulocyte reserve.

The Hgb level decreases after middle age, although the decrease in women seems to be relatively less than that in men. Unexplained anemia in older adults has been noted, but iron absorption is not impaired. This anemia does not appear to be solely a function of age and may be related to reduced ingestion of iron because of the side effect of constipation. Serum iron and iron-binding capacity decrease in older people, and low serum vitamin B_{12} and folic acid levels occur in a significant number of older persons—but without anemia. Obvious signs and symptoms of hematologic disorders in a younger individual may be mistaken for normal aging in an older person. Fatigue, activity intolerance, and pallor may be attributed to advanced age. It is important when assessing an older patient to be aware of the normal physiologic changes and to distinguish those from pathologic changes related to hematologic dysfunction (see Gerontologic Assessment box). Older people are also more likely to have a chronic illness and a higher risk for malignancy. Both these situations may cause an anemia of otherwise unexplained origin.

No age-related changes in platelets have been reported. Some of the plasma coagulation factors have been reported to increase with age (factors I, V, VII, and IX). Partial thromboplastin time may be shortened. The RBC sedimentation rate increases significantly, but this rate is of limited value in detecting disease in older adults.

Gerontologic Assessment

- Obtain a thorough history of chronic illness such as diabetes, heart disease, and renal failure. These diseases can cause hematologic abnormalities.
- Gather detailed information about diet and nutritional status. Older adults are at risk for malnutrition and vitamin deficiency that can cause hematologic problems.
- Question the patient about changes in usual activity tolerance and ability to perform activities of daily living; muscular and skeletal pain, which is often attributed to arthritis; and changes in taste, smell, and vision. These diverse, nonspecific symptoms can all reflect hematologic disorders.
- Obtain orthostatic vital signs. Changes in vital signs are systemic manifestations of hematologic disorders.
- Inspect the skin for lesions and note color. Platelet dysfunction can cause petechiae, ecchymoses, and purpura. Jaundice can be indicative of hemolytic disease or pernicious anemia. Contrary to popular belief, pallor is not a reliable indicator of anemia.

Common Disorders in Older Adults

Mental status (dehydration and hypoxia may be attributed to dementia)
Iron deficiency anemia
Anemia of chronic disease
Folic acid and pernicious anemia
Chronic leukemia
Lymphoma

▶ ARE You READY?

In reviewing laboratory values, which result is indicative of inflammation?

1. Elevated neutrophils
2. Elevated thrombocytes
3. Decreased eosinophils
4. Decreased basophils

Health History

A thorough health history is essential in the assessment of hematologic status. A variety of primary hematologic disorders exist, and many of their symptoms are nonspecific and common to many diseases. This diverse array of symptoms includes shortness of breath, fatigue, bruising, tarry stools, constipation, lymphadenopathy, flulike illness, pallor, and musculoskeletal pain. Further complicating the assessment is the fact that secondary effects from a disease of another body system may manifest in abnormal hematologic findings. For example, the anemia associated with renal insufficiency is the consequence of disease outside the hematopoietic system.

A thorough history includes detailed information about the person's symptoms and a detailed review of systems. Other key areas are family history, drug history, exposure to chemicals, and general nonspecific complaints offered by the patient. Since the history assists not only in assessing the patient's health status but also in identifying needs for health information and instruction, assessing for good health practices relating to hematologic system function is essential (see Patient/Family Teaching box). A thorough history of lifestyle activities such as exercise and diet is important. Exercise has been shown to promote coagulation and fibrinolysis. Long-term exercise lowers plasma levels of fibrinogen and fibrinolytic activity. Obesity as measured by body mass index

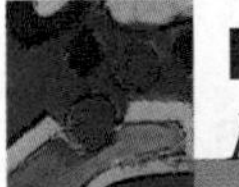

PATIENT/FAMILY TEACHING
Hematologic Health

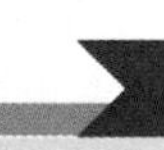

To maintain the hematologic system health, adults should:

- Eat a well-balanced diet, including four to six small meals per day, following the guidelines of MyPyramid.
- Seek early treatment when symptoms of infection are present.
- Report continued weakness, dyspnea, or extreme fatigue unrelated to excessive work, stress, or sleeplessness.
- Report excessive bruising or bleeding.
- Report excessive joint and bone pain.
- Maintain good hygiene, especially oral hygiene.
- Wash hands frequently.
- Avoid contact with individuals who have diagnosed infections.

(BMI) and waist-to-hip ratio is associated with increased hemostasis but decreased fibrinolytic activity. A relationship may also exist between saturated fatty acids in the diet and clotting. Alcohol is often associated with a delay in coagulation, but heavy alcohol consumption has been shown to increase coagulation and lower fibrinolytic activity in some people. Habitual smokers seem to have increased clotting and decreased fibrinolysis.[1]

Family History

The possibility of inherited hematologic disorders such as sickle cell disease and malignant tumors necessitates a detailed family history. Questions regarding disease or presence of symptoms among relatives should include reference to parents and siblings (a genogram is an excellent tool to visualize the family's history). Specific disorders such as hemophilia may involve questions related to grandfathers, uncles, and nephews. Female relatives need to be considered for other disorders. Questions should explore instances of severe or prolonged bleeding after minor trauma, dental extractions, or surgery and the occurrence of jaundice or anemia in relatives.

Drugs and Chemicals

Drugs may induce or potentiate hematologic disease (Box 32-1). Most notable are the hematologic effects of the cytotoxic drugs used in cancer chemotherapy and the neutropenia associated with chloramphenicol.[2] A thorough history of drugs ingested by a person is a crucial part of assessment. Many individuals regularly take a sleeping aid, a relaxing agent, or an over-the-counter pain medication. Analgesics, tranquilizers, laxatives, and sedatives often are overlooked by persons when asked about drugs. Specific, often rephrased questioning is necessary to obtain a complete drug history. Obtaining information about over-the-counter medication is important because drugs such as aspirin and ibuprofen, as well as alcohol, delay coagulation. Long-term use of these drugs can cause easy bruising and bleeding.[2] It is also important to ask about the use of herbs and natural supplements. Supplements such as agrimony or alfalfa may affect clotting times. Other herbs such as lysine and motherwort can affect the actions of anticoagulants.

Certain chemicals may also exert a potentially harmful effect on the hematopoietic system. To elicit information about exposure to chemicals, an occupational history is useful.

Fever

Fever is a common manifestation of many hematologic disorders and an important symptom to explore during the history. Fever typically occurs in lymphoma, primarily Hodgkin's disease and leukemia. Severe chills may accompany hemolytic disorders. Night sweats commonly are associated with both lymphoma and leukemia.

Fatigue and Malaise

Fatigue and malaise are difficult symptoms to evaluate because they accompany many physical and emotional disorders. The history should include questions about these symptoms. When combined with physical and laboratory findings, they are of some diagnostic value. In addition, the person's subjective description of such symptoms lends some insight into perception of the illness, the extent to which the illness is affecting daily living, and the patient's ability to adapt to changes in homeostasis.

Physical Examination

The nurse performs a thorough physical examination in the assessment of a person with a hematologic disorder. Particular

Box 32-1 Selected Drugs Implicated in Hematopoietic Suppression*

- Acetophenetidin (1, 3)
- Acetyl sulfisoxazole (3)
- Acetylsalicylic acid (aspirin) (1, 2, 3)
- *p*-Aminosalicylic acid (3, 4)
- Ammonium thioglycolate (3)
- Amodiaquine hydrochloride (3)
- Arsenicals (1, 2, 3, 4)
- Arsphenamine (1, 2)
- Benzene (1, 2, 3, 4)
- γ-Benzene hexachloride (1, 3)
- Beta-naphthoxyacetic acid (2)
- Bishydroxycoumarin (3, 4)
- Carbamazepine
- Carbamide (urea) (2)
- Carbon tetrachloride (1)
- Chloramphenicol (1, 2, 3, 4)
- Chlordane (1)
- Chlordiazepoxide (Librium) (3)
- Chlorophenothane (DDT) (1, 2)
- Chlorothiazide (3)
- Chlorpheniramine maleate (3)
- Chlorpromazine (Thorazine) (3)
- Chlorpropamide (2)
- Chlortetracycline (1, 3)
- Cinophen (3)
- Coldricine (2, 3)
- Cycloheximide (3)
- Dextromethorphan hydrobromide (2)
- Diethylstilbestrol (2)
- Dipyrone (3)
- Ethinamate (2)
- Fumagillin (3)
- Hair lacquer (3)
- Imipramine hydrochloride (3)
- Iproniazid (1)
- Isoniazid (1, 3, 4)
- Lead (1)
- Lithium carbonate (1)
- Mephenytoin (Mesantoin) (1, 2)
- Meprobamate (1, 2, 3)
- Methapyrilene hydrochloride (4)
- Methylpromazine (3)
- Mezapine (2)
- Nitrofurantoin (4)
- Novobiocin (4)
- Nystatin (2)
- Oxyphenbutazone (2)
- Penicillin (1, 2, 3, 4)
- Phenobarbital (1, 2, 3, 4)
- Phenylbutazone (Butazolidin) (1, 2, 3)
- Phenytoin (Dilantin) (4)
- Pipamazine (1)
- Primidone (1)
- Prochlorperazine (Compazine) (2, 3)
- Pyrimethamine (Daraprim) (1, 2, 3)
- Quinacrine hydrochloride (Atabrine) (1, 2)
- Quinidine (2)
- Quinine (2, 3)
- Reserpine (2)
- Stibophen (2)
- Streptomycin (1, 2, 3)
- Sulfamethoxypyridazine (Kynex) (2, 3, 4)
- Tetracycline (3)
- Thioridazine hydrochloride (3)
- Tolazoline hydrochloride (1, 2)
- Tolbutamide (Orinase) (2)
- Trifluoperazine (Stelazine) (3)
- Trimethadione (Tridione) (1, 2)

*These drugs have produced dyscrasias when given alone. *1*, Pancytopenia; *2*, thrombocytopenia; *3*, leukopenia; *4*, anemia.

attention is given to target organs and alterations known to reflect hematologic disease.

Skin

Skin manifestations of hematologic disease are often readily visible. Petechiae, ecchymoses, and purpura are associated with decreased platelets (thrombocytopenia) and other bleeding disorders. Jaundice may be associated with pernicious anemia, hemolytic disease, or primary liver dysfunction. The layperson typically associates pallor with disorders of the blood, but this may be deceptive because many healthy persons have pale complexions, whereas some severely anemic patients may have ruddy complexions. Pallor is also often difficult to determine in dark-skinned persons. It is more noticeable in the sclera, conjunctiva, tongue, buccal mucosa, lips, and nail beds; thus it is extremely important to check these sites on all patients. Other skin changes that appear pathologic may be normal for a particular patient. Therefore it is essential to establish individual norms.

The nurse may also observe changes in skin texture. Except in severe cases, the patient most likely will not be aware of such changes. With iron deficiency anemia, dry skin, dry hair, and brittle nails occur. Severe itching, especially on the palms, often is associated with Hodgkin's disease and also may occur with polycythemia vera, especially after bathing. In persons with leukemia and lymphoma, infiltrative lesions of the skin may occur on any part of the body.

Head and Neck

The nurse examines the sclerae of the eyes for jaundice and the conjunctivae for pallor. Retinal hemorrhages may occur in persons with severe anemia and thrombocytopenia. Questions also may elicit a history of visual disturbances.

The nurse observes the oral mucosa for pallor, bleeding tendency, and ulceration. The tongue may be very smooth in association with both pernicious anemia and nutritional deficiencies. The neck is observed primarily for lymph nodes. Nodes may be so large they are visible, but palpation is always used in their assessment. A "lump" on the neck often is the reason for seeking medical attention. Enlarged tumors may obstruct breathing or cause coughing or difficulty in swallowing.

Chest

The nurse exerts firm pressure with the fingertips along the sternum and ribs to elicit any tenderness that may be present. Such tenderness may reflect a leukemic process or multiple myeloma. Lung sounds are assessed for signs of pneumonia, another common occurrence with leukemia or multiple myeloma.

Abdomen

The nurse uses percussion and palpation over the abdomen, with special attention to the liver and spleen. Both organs are prone to enlargement in association with hematologic disease. Ascites may be a late manifestation of liver failure that can be associated with a hematologic disease process.

Back and Extremities

The nurse evaluates the skeletal system primarily for pain, joint deformity, and arthritis. Bone pain may be associated with malignant conditions of hematologic origin. Persons with hemolytic processes or some hematologic malignancies have an increased uric acid production and a corresponding increase in the incidence of gout. Joint deformities are associated with bleeding disorders, and pathologic fractures may be a late sign of a hematologic disorder.

Lymph Nodes

Lymph nodes are widely distributed in the body and are routinely examined by palpation. In the healthy adult the only palpable nodes are in the inguinal region and occasionally in the axilla. In disease, cervical, supraclavicular, or other nodes may become palpable. Any enlarged lymph node may reflect a disease process and must be evaluated thoroughly. The nurse evaluates the size, consistency, and mobility of an enlarged node. Enlarged lymph nodes may be painful if they impinge on other organs. Further evaluation of lymph nodes requires x-ray examination, lymphangiography, or biopsy.

Nervous System

Many neurologic abnormalities may develop in persons with hematologic disorders. These catastrophic complications are caused by bleeding or infection within the central nervous system. Infiltration of malignant leukemic or lymphomatous cells may produce signs and symptoms of a cerebral tumor or stroke. In addition, some of the lymphomas, especially Hodgkin's disease, may produce dementia as a remote effect. Therefore initial physical examination should include assessment of mental status, cranial nerve function, sensory function (pain, touch, position, vibratory sensation), and motor function (strength, reflexes, plantar response). It is important to know an individual's baseline assessment status. The nurse should note deviations from the baseline.

Diagnostic Tests

Laboratory Tests

Extensive blood examinations are part of the diagnostic workup of a person suspected of having a hematologic disorder. A list of these tests according to the blood cell under study along with reference intervals for adults is found in Table 32-1. The most common laboratory tests are Hgb and hematocrit (Hct) levels; RBC indices; reticulocyte count; and peripheral smear, which includes a WBC count and differential WBC count. The information obtained from such studies provides important clues to the pathology of the disorder. In addition to their diagnostic value, blood studies are used to monitor a patient's progress and response to treatment. The confirmation of a hematologic disease often depends on an examination of a peripheral blood smear and results of the bone

TABLE 32-1 LABORATORY TESTS OF BLOOD CELL STRUCTURE AND FUNCTION

Laboratory Tests	Reference Intervals
ERYTHROCYTE TESTS	
RBC count	Male: 4,600,000-6,100,000/mm^3 Female: 4,000,000-5,400,000/mm^3
Hemoglobin	Male: 13-18 g/dl Female: 12-16 g/dl
Hematocrit	Male: 45%-52% Female: 37%-48%
Reticulocyte count	1%-2% of the total RBC count
Mean corpuscular hemoglobin concentration	32%-36%
Mean corpuscular volume	80-95/mm^3
Red cell fragility	Morphologic description in stained smear
THROMBOCYTE (PLATELET) TESTS	
Platelet aggregation	60%-100%
Platelet count	150,000-400,000/mm^3
Bleeding time (Ivy method)	1-9 min
LEUKOCYTE TESTS	
White blood cell count with differential	5000-10,000/mm^3 Granulocytes: Neutrophils (PMN, segs) 55%-70% Eosinophils 1%-4% Basophils up to 1% Monocytes 2%-6% Lymphocytes 25%-40%

RBC, Red blood cells; *PMN,* polymorphonuclear; *segs,* segmented neutrophils.

marrow examination. Culture and sensitivity results are important to rule out other sources of fever, malaise, or abnormal complete blood count results.

Hemoglobin and Hematocrit. The Hgb test measures the amount of Hgb in the peripheral blood by weight. The packed RBC volume, or **hematocrit** (Hct), is the ratio of RBC volume to the whole blood volume. The two measurements are usually taken together and commonly parallel each other. The Hct level is usually three times that of the Hgb.

Red Blood Cell Indices. The RBC indices consist of the mean corpuscular volume (MCV), mean corpuscular hemoglobin (MCH), and mean corpuscular hemoglobin concentration (MCHC). The MCV estimates the average size of the RBC. Both the MCH and MCHC measure the content of Hgb in RBCs. The MCHC is considered more accurate than the MCH because it measures the entire blood volume of Hgb rather than just that from a single cell. The RBC indices provide a differential diagnosis of the type of anemia.

Hemoglobin Electrophoresis. Normal and abnormal Hgb can be assessed through electrophoresis. This test is performed when a disease associated with an abnormal Hgb type is suspected (hemoglobinopathy). There are many types of Hgb, but the most common in the adult erythrocytes are A_1, A_2, and F, with type A making up 95% to 98% of the total Hgb (Box 32-2). In infants Hgb F makes up 50% to 80% of the total Hgb and is referred to as fetal Hgb. The test is used to diagnose sickle cell anemia, aplastic anemia, Hgb C disease, some thalassemias, and other rare hemoglobinopathies.

Reticulocyte Count. The number of reticulocytes (immature RBCs) circulating in the blood provides useful information about the erythropoietic activity of the bone marrow. In anemia the bone marrow should respond with an increase in activity that would lead to an increased reticulocyte count.

Peripheral Blood Smear. Each blood cell possesses microscopic features that identify and set the cell apart from other cell types. Examination of the peripheral blood smear provides information concerning the cause of a blood disorder. The nurse observes the color, size, shape, and contents of the RBCs (Box 32-3). Color indicates the amount of Hgb contained in the RBC and is described as *normochromic* for normal or *hypochromic* for decreased. When RBCs in a smear vary in size, the condition is referred to as *anisocytosis.* The size of individual RBCs is described as *macrocytic* (large), *normocytic* (normal), or *microcytic* (small). When RBCs vary in shape, the condition is referred to as *poikilocytosis.* Variations in cell shape are the basis for descriptive names of cell types such as *leptocytes* (flat and elongated), seen in thalassemias; and *spherocyte* (round), seen in acquired hemolytic anemia.

A differential WBC count can provide useful information about what might be causing alterations in the WBCs. A decreased platelet count may indicate a tendency for bleeding.

Box 32-2 Normal and Abnormal Hemoglobins

Normal Values

In adults the total hgb is composed of the following types and percentages:

- Hgb A_1: 95%-98%
- Hglb A_2: 2% to 3%
- Hgb F: 0.8% to 2%

NOTE: In infants and children the types and percentages for normal values are different.

Abnormal Values

- Hgb A_2: any variant significantly less or greater than 2% to 3% of the total
- Hgb F: >2% of the total
- Hgb C: any amount
- Hgb S: any amount

Hgb, Hemoglobin.

BOX 32-3 Descriptive Cell Characteristics in Anemia

Size	Hemoglobin
Macrocytic (large)	Normochromic
Normocytic (normal)	Hypochromic (decreased)
Microcytic (small)	

Often results of a peripheral blood smear, when combined with data from the history, physical examination, and other laboratory tests, determine the medical diagnosis.

Iron Studies. Serum iron measures the concentration of iron that is bound to transferrin, which is normally 50 to 150 mg/dl. The total iron-binding capacity (TIBC) measures the amount of iron that could still bind to the receptor sites on the transferrin. The serum iron and TIBC should vary conversely and are both used to evaluate microcytic anemia. Serum vitamin B_{12} and serum folate, as well as bilirubin, are also useful in identifying causes and types of anemia (Table 32-2).

Coagulation Studies

ACTIVATED PARTIAL THROMBOPLASTIN TIME. **Activated partial thromboplastin time** (aPTT) (normally 25 to 35 seconds) measures the number of seconds in which a clot forms. It evaluates the intrinsic pathway but not the extrinsic pathway. It is used to evaluate and identify congenital and acquired deficiencies in the coagulation system and to monitor the effectiveness of heparin therapy.

PROTHROMBIN TIME AND INTERNATIONAL NORMALIZED RATIO. The **prothrombin time** (PT), normally 10 to 13 seconds or 60% to 140% of normal clotting activity, also measures the time needed to form a clot, but specifically measures factors I, II, V, VII, and X in the coagulation cascade and the extrinsic pathway. The PT is used to monitor warfarin (Coumadin) therapy and to screen for vitamin K deficiency and disseminated intravascular coagulation (DIC).

The PT may be reported as time in seconds, as a percentage of normal clotting activity, or as an **international normalized ratio** (INR). The INR reflects the relationship of the patient's PT to a normal control. This measurement is more accurate than the PT reported as time in seconds for anticoagulation control. The normal INR range for warfarin therapy is 2.5 for low-dose therapy and 2.5 to 3.5 for high-dose therapy. This may vary from patient to patient, depending on the reason for the anticoagulant therapy and specific treatment goals. The INR increases or decreases in response to the same conditions that affect the PT.

BOX 32-4 Coagulation Factor Deficiencies

- Vitamin K deficiency: decreased VII, IX, X
- Liver disease: decreased II, V, VII, IX, X
- Hemophilia A: decreased VIII
- Hemophilia B: decreased IX
- Disseminated intravascular coagulation: decreased V, VI

FIBRIN SPLIT PRODUCTS. During the process of fibrinolysis, or clot breakdown, fibrinogen is broken down into fragments called fibrin split products or fibrin degradation products. These products interfere with normal clotting. The normal fibrin split products test (protamine sulfate test) is negative. Increased levels of these products occur in DIC, deep venous thrombosis, pulmonary embolism, and infarcts. They are also a measure of rejection in patients with organ transplants.

COAGULATION FACTOR ASSAY. To diagnose specific disorders of the coagulation pathway, it is necessary to isolate specific factor level abnormalities. The coagulation factor assay measures factors of the intrinsic and extrinsic pathway separately (Box 32-4).

ARE You READY?

In the patient with increased reticulocyte count, the nurse assesses for clinical manifestations of which of the following?

1. Thrombocytopenia
2. Hemophilia
3. Leukocytopenia
4. Anemia

Radiologic Tests

Lymphangiography. **Lymphangiography** is a radiologic technique used for visualization of the lymphatic system flow and nodes to detect the presence or stage of disease or to guide therapy. This procedure is especially valuable when used with computed tomography (CT) in the assessment of para-aortic nodes that are anatomically too deep in the abdomen to allow for evaluation by palpation. For this procedure the radiologist makes a small

TABLE 32-2 LABORATORY VALUES IN ANEMIA

	Anemia of Chronic Disease	Iron Deficiency	Vitamin B_{12} Deficiency	Folate Deficiency	Thalassemia
Mean corpuscular hemoglobin	Normal	Decreased	Increased	Normal	Decreased
Iron	Normal	Slightly decreased	Elevated	Elevated	Elevated
Total iron-binding capacity	Slightly decreased	Elevated	Normal	Normal	Normal
Bilirubin	Normal	Normal	Elevated	Elevated	Elevated
Vitamin B_{12}	Normal	Normal	Decreased	Normal	Normal
Folate	Slightly decreased	Normal	Normal	Decreased	Slightly decreased

incision between the toes or fingers and instills dye. After approximately 30 minutes, the lymphatic system is outlined. An iodine-based dye is then injected; radiographs are taken then and again 24 and 48 hours after the instillation of the dye. In addition, because the dye remains in the lymph nodes for as long as 6 months after the initial study, disease status and response to therapy can be periodically evaluated with routine abdominal roentgenograms.

Patient preparation includes information regarding the type and length of procedure, associated sensations, and aftercare. The patient is usually allowed to have food and fluids before the procedure. A consent form is necessary. Local anesthesia is used before the needle insertion. The patient may experience discomfort associated with needle puncture and lying still for the procedure, which may last up to 3 hours. The patient may experience a sensation of warmth and flushing as the iodine-based dye is injected. The examiner may ask the patient to walk to enhance visualization. An assessment of the patient's allergy status, particularly to iodine, is necessary because of the contrast media used.

After the procedure the affected limb is elevated for 24 hours. The nurse assesses the patient for signs of bleeding or adverse reactions to the dye. The dissection site may require a few sutures, and mild analgesia (acetaminophen or nonsteroidal antiinflammatory drugs) may be indicated.

The nurse carefully assesses the affected extremity for any changes in sensorimotor function, which suggest possible nerve damage. The nurse should inform the patient that the first dye injected may lead to a blue discoloration of the skin, stool, and urine. Complications include infection and, rarely, pneumonia if the dye migrates to the lung through the thoracic duct. The nurse instructs the patient and family to report any respiratory problems to the physician.

Computed Tomography. CT is used to assess abdominal lymph nodes. The CT scan is used as a monitoring tool to evaluate the patient's disease process, remission during chemotherapy, and response after treatment. Assessment by periodic CT scans (every 6 to 12 months) helps evaluate the remission or detect a relapse. Lymph nodes may also be evaluated by biopsy or endoscopy (mediastinoscopy, laparoscopy).

Special Tests

Bone Marrow Examination. The bone marrow examination is an adjunct to the peripheral blood smear. Generally the bone marrow is examined when the diagnosis is not clearly established from the peripheral blood smear or when further information is needed. The examiner obtains a bone marrow specimen by bone marrow aspiration or biopsy. Cells contained in the bone marrow include erythrocytes, granulocytes in all stages of maturation, megakaryocytes (from which platelets develop), lymphocytes, and plasma cells. Bone marrow examination is used to evaluate abnormal blood cells, monitor the effects of bone marrow depressants, monitor the patient's response to treatment, and help diagnose disorders associated with abnormal hematopoiesis.

Bone Marrow Aspiration. Aspiration is the most common procedure for obtaining a bone marrow sample. The procedure is possible because normal bone marrow is soft and semifluid and can be removed by needle aspiration. Bone marrow aspiration is most often performed in persons with severe anemia, neutropenia (decreased number of WBCs), acute leukemia, and thrombocytopenia (decreased number of platelets).

Legal Alert

Informed consent

Patients have the right to refuse to give consent for treatment or testing. This right continues up to the time the test is begun even if prior consent has been given. This is based on the common law right of freedom from bodily invasion. In some circumstances the patient's right of refusal can be denied by the court. They include:

1. Preservation of life if the patient does not have an incurable or terminal illness
2. Protection of minor dependents
3. Prevention of irrational self-destruction
4. Protection of the public's health

Education, preparation, and emotional support of the patient before bone marrow aspiration can reduce anxiety. Emotional support of the patient and family is necessary because of the potential life-threatening diagnoses that may result from the examination (see Legal Alert).

Procedure. The most common site for bone marrow aspiration is the posterior iliac crest (Figure 32-3). Other sites include the sternum and the anterior and posterior iliac spines. The examiner shaves the skin surrounding the puncture site (if necessary) and cleanses it with an antiseptic such as providone-iodine (Betadine). Sterile towels are placed around the site. The skin and periosteum are anesthetized to decrease pain. The physician first infiltrates the most superficial layer of the skin with procaine, then after a few seconds advances the needle until it meets bone. He or she then injects procaine to anesthetize the periosteum.

The examiner inserts the marrow aspiration needle. After entering the marrow cavity, the examiner removes the marrow stylet from the needle and attaches a sterile syringe. The examiner draws back the syringe plunger until marrow appears in the syringe. As the plunger is drawn back and suction is exerted, the patient experiences a brief, sharp pain, sometimes described as a burning sensation. At this point, the nurse's hands placed gently on the patient's shoulder and a calm reminder to lie still might prevent a sudden jerk or movement.

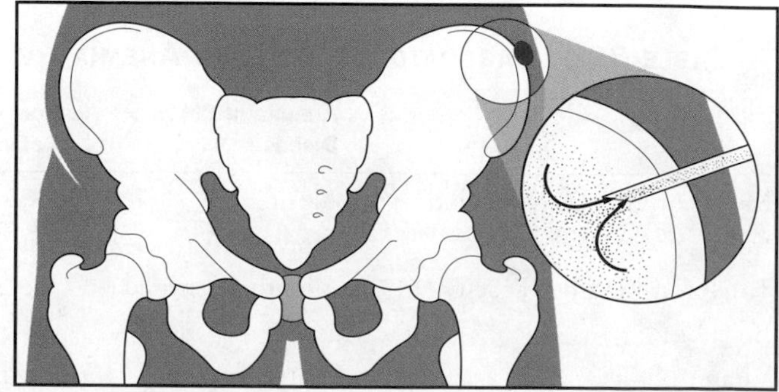

Figure 32-3 Most common site for bone marrow aspiration.

After removal of the needle, the nurse applies a pressure dressing over the aspiration site to stop the minimal bleeding that occurs. The patient should lie on the biopsied side to maintain pressure on the site for 10 to 15 minutes. If the patient has thrombocytopenia, pressure is applied for 15 minutes. The nurse monitors the site every 15 minutes for 1 hour after the procedure. An ice bag may be applied to the site to alleviate discomfort and prevent bleeding.

Some individuals may complain of tenderness at the aspiration site for a few days. Most often, no pain or discomfort is experienced after the procedure.

Bone Marrow Biopsy. A bone marrow biopsy is indicated when a large sample of bone marrow is needed. Persons most likely to undergo a bone marrow biopsy are those with pancytopenia (a decrease in more than one cell type), myelofibrosis, metastatic tumor, lymphoma, and multiple myeloma. The most common site for bone marrow biopsy is the posterosuperior iliac spine. The sternum and proximal tibia may also be used. The initial steps in the biopsy procedure are similar to those outlined for bone marrow aspiration. The use of a Jamshidi needle allows for a core of marrow to be collected (Figure 32-4).

From microscopic examination of the bone marrow, the examiner can determine iron stores and the morphology of the progenitor cell. Large immature cell changes may be observed; infiltration with leukemic cells and absence of cells, as in aplastic anemia, can be determined.

As with bone marrow aspiration, emotional support before, during, and after the procedure is indicated. Both the patient and family may be stressed and anxious while awaiting results.

Other diagnostic tests are discussed throughout the text along with the specific disorders to which they pertain.

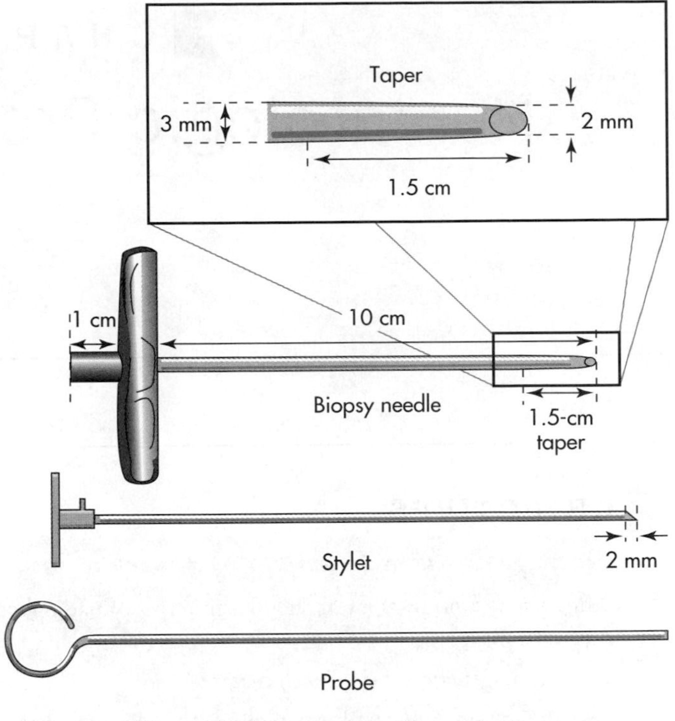

Figure 32-4 Bone marrow biopsy needle.

References

1. Lee KW, Lip GYH: Effects of lifesyle on hemostasis, fibrinolysis, and platelet reactivity: a systematic review, *Arch Intern Med* 163:2368, 2003.
2. Spratto GR, Woods AL: *PDR nurse's drug handbook*, Clifton Park, NJ, 2004, Thomson Delmar Learning.

evolve Visit the Evolve website: http://evolve.elsevier.com/Monahan/medsurg

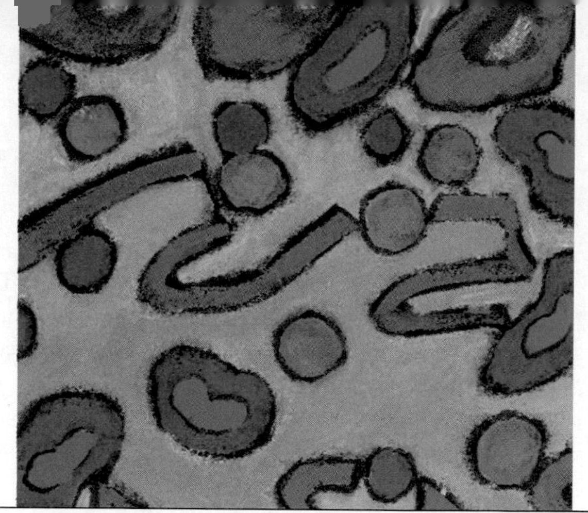

CHAPTER 33

Hematologic Problems

by Ann L. Garrigues

OBJECTIVES

After studying this chapter, the learner should be able to:

1. Differentiate among types of anemias in terms of pathophysiology, assessment, and interventions.
2. Explain the genetics of sickle cell disease.
3. Describe the nursing care for patients with sickle cell disease.
4. Differentiate among disorders of hemostasis, platelets, and coagulation (thrombocytopenia, thrombocytosis, hemophilia, vitamin K deficiency, and disseminated intravascular coagulation) in terms of pathophysiology, treatment, and nursing interventions.
5. Describe the nursing interventions and therapeutic modalities for the four major types of leukemia.
6. Identify gerontologic considerations important to the assessment and treatment of hematologic disorders in older adults.
7. Explain the differences between Hodgkin's disease and non-Hodgkin's lymphoma and the management of each.

KEY TERMS

anemia, p. 908
coagulation factors, p. 923
erythrocytes, p. 908
lymphocytes, p. 928
platelets, p. 910
primary hemostasis, p. 923
secondary hemostasis, p. 923
stem cells, p. 911
transfusion reactions, p. 910
vitamin K, p. 927

Management of persons with problems of the hematologic system is challenging to the nurse because of the diversity and vagueness of the presenting symptoms. Disease processes are as diverse as the components that make up the hematologic system. For this reason, a thorough assessment is necessary to determine the cause of the patient's health concerns. Interventions focus on supporting the patient's return to optimal function and resolution of the hematologic alteration. Treatment options vary, depending on the patient's age, health status, and history of illness.

Disorders Associated With Erythrocytes

Common disorders of **erythrocytes** (mature red blood cells) include underproduction (anemias), overproduction (erythrocytosis), and impaired hemoglobin (Hgb) synthesis (hemoglobinopathies). **Anemia** refers to a deficiency in the number of circulating red blood cells (RBCs) available for oxygen transport. This condition is determined by an overall decrease in the number of RBCs, the concentration of RBCs (hematocrit [Hct]), and the Hgb concentration of the RBCs. Anemias can be further subdivided by RBC size (macrocytic or microcytic) or by the concentration of Hgb (hyperchromic or hypochromic). Anemias can also be classified by their causative factors (Table 33-1). Some causative factors include blood loss, bone marrow dysfunction, nutritional deficits, hemolysis, Hgb defects, and chronic disease.

Anemia Caused by Blood Loss

Etiology, Epidemiology, and Pathophysiology

Acute Blood Loss. The anemia associated with acute blood loss is the direct result of a decrease in circulating RBCs. The adult of average build has a total blood volume of approximately 6000 ml. Usually an adult can lose 500 ml of blood without serious or lasting effects because of the spleen's ability to release stored red cells. If the loss reaches 1000 ml or more, serious acute consequences may result.

TABLE 33-1 TYPES OF ANEMIA AND CLINICAL MANIFESTATIONS

Type	Causes	Clinical Manifestations
SECONDARY TO BLOOD LOSS		
Acute	Hemorrhage	Early: weakness, cool moist skin, tachycardia, hypotension Late: decreased Hgb and Hct
Chronic	Gastrointestinal or other malignancy, bleeding ulcers, bleeding hemorrhoids, hypermenorrhea	Decreased RBCs, Hgb, Hct, MCV, and MCHC; fatigue
SECONDARY TO IMPAIRED PRODUCTION OF RED BLOOD CELLS		
Aplastic anemia	Drugs, chemicals, radiation, chemotherapy, virus, congenital, autoimmune mechanism	Pancytopenia, pallor of skin and mucous membranes, fatigue, palpitations, exertional dyspnea, bleeding tendency, infection
Anemia of chronic disease	Chronic illness, renal disease, diabetes	Decreased serum iron concentration; fatigue
HEMOLYTIC ANEMIAS		
Hereditary spherocytosis	Genetic: inherited as autosomal dominant trait	Spherocytes and increased reticulocytes on peripheral blood smear; fatigue, exertional dyspnea
Thalassemia	Genetic: decreased synthesis of 1 globin chain of Hgb	Microcytosis, hypochromic RBCs, decreased growth at pubescence, eventual cardiac failure
Sickle cell disease	Genetic hemoglobinopathy	Sickled cells on peripheral blood smears; painful episodes, vasoocclusive crises, chronic leg ulcers, chronic renal and ocular problems
Enzyme deficiency anemia	Genetic: deficiency of glucose-6-phosphate dehydrogenase (G6PD)	Decreased levels of G6PD; hemolytic episodes
Hemolytic anemia	Drug-induced or autoimmune response	Splenomegaly, jaundice (may or may not be present depending on cause), pallor
NUTRITIONAL ANEMIAS		
Iron deficiency anemia	Chronic blood loss, inadequate intake	Microcytosis, low serum iron concentration; fatigue, exertional dyspnea
Megaloblastic anemia	Deficiency in vitamin B_{12} or folic acid	Macrocytosis; glossitis, and neurologic abnormalities with vitamin B_{12} deficiency

Hgb, Hemoglobin; *Hct,* hematocrit; *RBCs,* red blood cells; *MCV,* mean corpuscular volume; *MCHC,* mean corpuscular hemoglobin concentration.

Signs and symptoms of acute blood loss include those associated with hypovolemia and hypoxemia (see Table 33-1). Weakness; stupor; irritability; and cool, moist skin may be observed. Vital signs indicate hypotension and tachycardia. Decreased Hgb and Hct levels may not be evident until several hours after the blood loss has occurred. The severity of the patient's symptoms correlates with the severity of the blood loss. Acute blood loss is associated with trauma, surgery, platelet dysfunction, and coagulation disorders.

CHRONIC BLOOD LOSS. The body has remarkable adaptive powers and can adjust fairly well to a severe reduction in RBCs and Hgb, provided the condition develops gradually. A person may remain asymptomatic even though the total RBC count drops to almost half its normal amount. For example, patients with chronic kidney failure tolerate Hgb levels of less than 8.0 g/dl without difficulty. With chronic anemia, determinations of RBC counts, Hgb and Hct levels, mean corpuscular volume (MCV), mean corpuscular Hgb concentration (MCHC), and reticulocyte counts are important diagnostic tests. All indices usually are below normal (see Table 32-1 for normal values).

Chronic blood loss is the most common cause of iron deficiency anemia. When blood loss is continuous and moderate, the bone marrow compensates by increasing the production of RBCs. However, if the cause of chronic blood loss is not corrected, the patient becomes iron deficient and develops symptoms of anemia (see Table 33-1).

Collaborative Care Management. Successful treatment of anemia caused by blood loss requires immediate identification of the source of the loss and institution of appropriate treatment. In addition, transfusion therapy or iron supplements may be needed.

Blood transfusions are not indicated for the asymptomatic patient with chronic anemia because of the increased risks associated with them. Transfusions are used only in cases of severe symptoms (Table 33-2). Transfusion of whole blood is rarely indicated even in situations of surgical hemorrhage. Instead, packed red blood cells are used because they reduce the incidence of pulmonary edema and circulatory overload. If colloids and clotting factors are needed, plasma, **platelets** (thrombocytes), and cryoprecipitate may be transfused as separate products.

Patients need to be educated about the risks and benefits of transfusion therapy. The nurse may need to address concerns regarding acquired immunodeficiency syndrome (AIDS) and hepatitis. The nurse also needs to explore the patient's belief system regarding the use of blood products. Certain cultural and religious belief systems (e.g., Jehovah's Witness) prohibit the receipt of blood products. The health care team needs to respect these beliefs, despite any ethical dilemmas they create.

If transfusion therapy is indicated, the nurse must carefully monitor the patient during the process. **Transfusion reactions** can occur even though laboratory testing was done to verify compatibility of the product. Because transfusion reactions generally occur within the first 15 to 20 minutes after the infusion is started, the nurse must observe hospital protocols for administering blood products and monitor the patient carefully for adverse reactions. The nurse should also teach the patient reportable signs and symptoms.

In addition to transfusion therapy, iron supplementation is used to replace depleted iron stores from increased blood cell production (see Iron Deficiency Anemia). Patients experiencing chronic blood loss are encouraged to eat a well-rounded diet that includes foods rich in iron and vitamins.

Patients with low Hgb levels may exhibit chronic fatigue and activity intolerance as a result of tissue hypoxia. The nurse should space activities and allowing frequent rest periods, thus optimizing the patient's limited energy reserves.

Occupational health nurses may do routine screening for anemia in high-risk populations. Fecal occult blood screening is recommended for persons over the age of 50. Most screening takes place during routine physical examinations and includes blood tests. Nurses in all settings teach about dietary needs for iron and vitamins. They can teach persons with low incomes to identify inexpensive food sources of the vitamins and minerals necessary for hematologic health. Nurses can also become politically active to ensure adequate government funding for low-cost nutritional programs for persons with marginal incomes.

Women who have long-term blood loss because of heavy menstrual bleeding are at risk for anemia, as are other persons with long-term, slow blood loss. These women need to be informed of the risks and of the need for continued monitoring of RBC indices. The nurse should also teach them energy conservation techniques to decrease fatigue.

Aplastic Anemia

Etiology and Epidemiology. Aplastic anemia (anemia resulting from impaired erythrocyte production) affects all age-groups and both genders. In approximately half of patients with aplastic anemia in the United States, no etiologic agent is identifiable. Identified causes of aplastic anemia include antineoplastic drugs and exposure to certain drugs, including chloramphenicol, sulfonamides, and anticonvulsant agents such as phenytoin (Dilantin). Insecticides such as chlorophenothane (DDT) and chemicals, particularly benzene, also are thought to cause aplastic anemia. Infections associated with the pathogenesis of aplastic anemia include hepatitis (types B and C), Epstein-Barr virus infection, cytomegalovirus infection, and miliary tuberculosis. The defect leading to aplastic anemia is most likely injury or destruction of a common stem cell that affects all subsequent cell populations. Aplastic anemia may also be congenital (Fanconi's anemia).[13]

Pathophysiology. Aplastic anemia usually is characterized by depression or cessation of activity of all blood-producing elements. The person has a decrease in the number of white blood cells (WBCs) (leukopenia); a decrease in the number of platelets (thrombocytopenia); and a decrease in the formation of RBCs, which leads to anemia (Table 33-3). The process may be chronic or acute, depending on the causative factor.

Symptoms of aplastic anemia usually develop gradually over weeks or months but in some cases can have an abrupt onset. Pallor of the skin and mucous membranes is characteristic but not always a good indicator since pallor may be difficult to determine (see Chapter 32). In addition, fatigue, palpitations, and exertional dyspnea are usually present. Infections of the skin and mucous membranes occur with severe granulocytopenia; hemorrhagic symptoms (bleeding into the skin and mucous membranes and spontaneous bleeding from the nose, gums, vagina, and rectum) occur with severe thrombocytopenia. Findings on physical examination are often unremarkable. The complete blood count characteristically reveals a pancytopenia (a marked decrease in the numbers of all cell types) with a low reticulocyte count. Definitive diagnosis of aplastic anemia is made by bone marrow examination. Attempts at bone marrow aspiration may yield a "dry tap" because of hypocellularity and a decrease in active marrow, so a bone marrow biopsy is often necessary.

TABLE 33-2 TRANSFUSION GUIDELINES FOR SYMPTOMATIC PATIENT WITH ANEMIA

Component	Indications	Patient Symptoms
Red blood cells	Hemoglobin <8 g/dl	Shortness of breath, fatigue
Platelets	$<20,000/mm^3$	Bleeding, petechiae, bruising
Granulocytes	$<500/mm^3$	Sepsis, failure of antibiotic therapy
Fresh frozen plasma	Deficiency of coagulation factors	Hemorrhage
Cryoprecipitate	Deficiency of factors VII and XIII	Diagnosis of hemophilia; uncontrolled hemorrhage

TABLE 33-3 NORMAL BLOOD CELL FUNCTION CORRELATED WITH PATHOPHYSIOLOGY AND CLINICAL MANIFESTATIONS OF APLASTIC ANEMIA

Normal Function	Pathophysiology	Clinical Manifestations
RED BLOOD CELLS		
Major component is Hgb, which transports oxygen to cells and carbon dioxide from cells to lungs	Reduction or depletion of hematopoietic stem cells, with decreased production of erythrocytes, platelets, and leukocytes Decreased tissue oxygenation	Pallor of skin and mucous membranes; fatigue and exertional dyspnea Low Hgb and Hct levels
PLATELETS		
Adhesion and aggregation capabilities to plug small breaks in small blood vessels Release of thromboplastin, which, in presence of calcium ions, converts prothrombin into thrombin in initial step of coagulation process	Fewer platelets available for blood coagulation	Bleeding tendency, as evidenced by ecchymosis, purpura, and petechiae Bleeding from nose, mouth, vagina, and rectum Low platelet count
WHITE BLOOD CELLS		
Neutrophils as primary defense against bacterial infection through phagocytosis Monocytes for removal of dead and injured cells, cell fragments, and microorganisms Lymphocytes participate in cellular immune response (T cell) and humoral immune response (B cell)	Fewer WBCs increasing susceptibility to infection as a result of decreased phagocytosis and decreased immune response	Repeated infections; frequent sick days

Hct, Hematocrit; *Hgb,* hemoglobin; *WBCs,* white blood cells.

Fanconi's anemia is an autosomal recessive inherited disorder that is characterized by pancytopenia, or deficiency of all bone marrow elements. Heart, kidney, and skeletal abnormalities may also be present. It is usually lethal by age 20, but new treatment modalities using bone marrow transplantation (BMT) and **stem cells** (hemocytoblasts) to repopulate the patient's body with RBCs, lymphocytes, and platelets are being researched in such places as St. Jude's Hospital in Memphis, Tennessee.[13,15]

Collaborative Care Management. The immediate treatment for aplastic anemia is removal of the causative agent, if known. In the past, treatment for aplastic anemia was aimed primarily at stimulating hematopoiesis through the administration of steroids and androgen therapy. Because these agents have proved to be of limited value and can produce toxic side effects, BMT from a donor with identical human leukocyte antigen (HLA) has emerged as the treatment of choice for persons with severe aplastic anemia who are younger than age 40 years. Other individuals are treated with immunosuppressive therapy. BMT centers are reporting survival rates of 80% in young people, and 40% to 70% in older people.[12]

The prognosis for persons with aplastic anemia depends primarily on the severity of the anemia, the method of treatment, and general supportive care. Also, a higher treatment success rate occurs in patients who receive BMT early and have not received blood products, especially from the potential bone marrow donor. Patients who have undergone transfusion have a higher mortality rate from graft-versus-host disease. If transfusions are essential, leukocyte-poor RBCs and platelets should be given. Patients who are not successfully treated often die of complications associated with repeated hemorrhage and infection.

Nursing care is based on careful assessment and management of the complications of pancytopenia and is primarily focused on preventing infection and monitoring for signs of bleeding. To prevent infection in the hospitalized patient who is immunosuppressed, the care plan should include:

- Provision of a private room
- Use of protective isolation
- Provision of and instruction of the patient on meticulous hygiene
- Assessment and maintenance of protective oral care regimens
- Monitoring of invasive lines for signs of infection
- Avoidance of bladder catheterization
- Instruction for family and visitors on careful hand washing

Nursing interventions aimed at the prevention of bleeding episodes include:

- Monitoring invasive line sites
- Testing urine and stool for blood
- Minimizing venipuncture and injections
- Avoiding rectal temperatures, medications, and enemas
- Instructing the patient on the use of soft sponges for oral care

Decreased oxygen-carrying capacity of the blood decreases oxygen supply to the tissues, leading to fatigue with activity. Measures to prevent fatigue include providing frequent rest periods, avoiding fatigue-producing activities, and monitoring the patient for signs of excessive fatigue or shortness of breath with activities. Education is important in the prevention of infection and the avoidance of bleeding episodes in the bone marrow–suppressed patient (see Patient/Family Teaching box). Patients are often hospitalized for several weeks, depending on the type of treatment received. The nurse needs to assist the patient in developing coping strategies, such as music and art therapies, to deal with the anxiety and isolation of prolonged hospitalization.

Hemolytic Anemias

Hemolytic anemia is defined as the premature destruction of erythrocytes occurring at such a rate that the bone marrow is unable to compensate for the loss. Hemolysis can occur either extravascularly or intravascularly. In the case of extravascular hemolysis the spleen removes erythrocytes from the circulation at an accelerated rate, usually because of some perceived problem with the erythrocytes. Examples of this type of hemolytic anemia are the autoimmune anemias and hereditary spherocytosis (HS).

Intravascular hemolysis, in which erythrocytes lyse and spill cell contents into the plasma, occurs as a result of an enzyme deficiency in the erythrocyte membrane or mechanical factors such as dialysis or a prosthetic heart valve, which can prematurely weaken the erythrocyte. Hemolytic anemias can also develop as a result of abnormal Hgb synthesis, as in thalassemia and sickle cell disease.

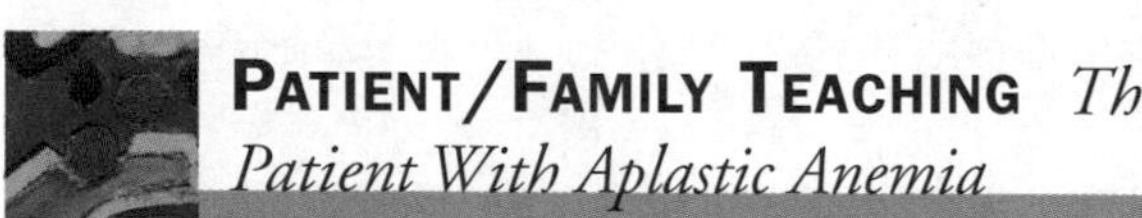

PATIENT/FAMILY TEACHING *The Patient With Aplastic Anemia*

- Prevent infection.
  - —Use good hand-washing technique.
  - —Avoid contact with those who have infections.
  - —Avoid sharing eating utensils and bath linens.
  - —Take a bath every day (or every other day if skin is dry); keep perineal area clean.
  - —Use good oral hygiene.
  - —Eliminate intake of raw meats, fruits, or vegetables.
  - —Report signs of infection immediately to health care provider.
- Prevent hemorrhage.
  - —Observe for signs such as bloody urine, stool, and petechiae, and report these to physician.
  - —Use a soft toothbrush or swab for mouth care; avoid use of dental floss.
  - —Keep mouth clean and free of debris.
  - —Avoid enemas or other rectal insertions.
  - —Avoid picking or blowing the nose forcefully.
  - —Avoid trauma, falls, bumps, and cuts; avoid contact sports.
  - —Avoid use of aspirin or aspirin preparations (anticoagulant effect).
  - —Use an electric razor.
  - —Use adequate lubrication and be gentle during sexual intercourse.
- Prevent fatigue.
  - —Take frequent rest periods between activities of daily living and other activities.
  - —Avoid excessive workload or heavy lifting, and ask for assistance with strenuous activity.
  - —Increase time necessary for routine care.
  - —Decrease activity if shortness of breath, dizziness, or sensation of heaviness in extremities occurs.

In these cases the spleen identifies the RBC as being "abnormal" and destroys it.

Autoimmune Hemolytic Anemia

Etiology and Epidemiology. Autoimmune hemolytic anemias are classified as warm-reacting, cold-reacting, and drug-induced forms. Warm-reacting forms are usually idiopathic and are more commonly seen in women. Associated disease entities are systemic lupus erythematosus, rheumatoid arthritis, chronic lymphocytic leukemia, and myeloma. Immunoglobulin A has also been identified as an etiologic factor in warm-reacting hemolytic disease.

Cold-reacting disease is less common and affects mostly older adults, with an increased incidence in older women. An example of cold-reacting disease is Raynaud's phenomenon. Cold-reacting disease is also associated with mononucleosis, *Mycoplasma pneumoniae,* Epstein-Barr virus, mumps, and legionnaires' disease.

A reaction to drugs causes approximately one fifth of the autoimmune hemolytic anemias. Drugs causing this type of autoimmune reaction are methyldopa, penicillin, quinine, and quinidine.

Pathophysiology. In warm-reacting anemias, antibodies (immunoglobulin G [IgG]) develop against an individual's own erythrocytes. These antibodies combine more readily at body temperature. Antibody-coated RBCs are destroyed by the mononuclear phagocyte system, particularly the spleen. In episodes of severe hemolysis, dyspnea, palpitations, and congestive heart failure can occur. Jaundice, pallor, and splenomegaly are common.

In cold-reacting disease, immunoglobulin M antibodies react with antigens on the erythrocyte, optimally in cold temperatures (below 88° F [31° C]). Ischemia occurs when red cells clump in the capillary beds, causing cyanosis, pain, and paresthesias. Hemoglobinuria also occurs.

Methyldopa (Aldomet) is associated with production of an autoantibody and a positive Coombs' test result in approximately 20% of patients, and with a hemolytic anemia that is indistinguishable from an idiopathic autoimmune hemolytic anemia in 1% of patients. Infrequently, high-dose penicillin produces hemolysis through production of an antibody that requires the presence of penicillin on the RBC membrane for its effects to occur.

Collaborative Care Management. Diagnosis is confirmed by demonstrating the presence of the antibody or complement on the RBCs (direct Coombs' test) or in the serum (indirect Coombs' test). Additional laboratory findings show a decreased Hct, increased reticulocyte count, and increased bilirubin level. The treatment depends on the cause of the hemolysis.

Mild cases require no treatment. When treatment is indicated, 70% of persons respond to the administration of corticosteroids or danazol (Cyclomen), a gonadotropin inhibitor. Splenectomy is performed for those patients not sufficiently responsive to steroids or danazol and often is successful in controlling or ameliorating the disease. Transfusions may be given cautiously for life-threatening anemia, but this therapy may be difficult and dangerous because of the autoantibody reacting not only with the patient's RBCs but also with all donor cells. Plasmapheresis may be indicated for critically ill patients. Nursing management consists of teaching the patient about the drug therapy, preparing the patient for surgery if indicated, and helping the patient and family cope with the illness. Teaching includes preventive measures such as avoiding exposure to cold for persons with cold-reacting anemias.

Hereditary Spherocytosis

Etiology and Epidemiology. HS is the most common problem of alteration in erythrocyte shape. This anomaly occurs in approximately 1 of every 5000 persons. It affects all races and both genders fairly equally. HS, inherited as an autosomal dominant trait, is characterized by a membrane abnormality that leads to osmotic swelling of the RBC and susceptibility to destruction by the spleen. It usually is detected in childhood but may appear initially in adulthood.

Pathophysiology. In HS a defect is present in the proteins that form the structure of the erythrocyte, giving the cells a thick, spherical appearance. The abnormal cell becomes increasingly permeable to sodium, leading to increased energy demands by the cell. The circulating spherocytes become trapped in the spleen because of the cell's inability to traverse the spleen's microcirculation. Hemolysis occurs in the spleen.

Collaborative Care Management. Diagnosis depends on observation of spherocytes on the peripheral blood smear and laboratory demonstration of increased osmotic fragility of the RBCs. The reticulocyte count usually is elevated, as is the serum bilirubin level. Bilirubin is derived from the breakdown of the Hgb released by the destroyed RBCs. Occasionally, red cell survival time needs to be determined. This is accomplished by labeling the cells with radioactive chromium and measuring the rate of decrease of radioactivity for 1 to 2 weeks (chromium survival). Symptoms of spherocytosis include those typically associated with anemia (pallor, fatigue, exertional dyspnea), jaundice from the increased serum bilirubin level, and an enlarged spleen from the increased RBC destruction.

The treatment for HS is splenectomy. This corrects the hemolysis, but the underlying spherocytosis persists. The gallbladder is often also removed because of the increased incidence of gallstones (50%) in patients with HS. Patients should be given pneumococcal and *Haemophilus influenzae* vaccines before splenectomy. Subtotal splenectomy has some beneficial effects for the management of HS, since the spleen's phagocytic function remains intact as opposed to the loss associated with total splenectomy.[1]

Routine postoperative care is indicated for persons who have undergone splenectomy or cholecystectomy. Nursing management includes careful monitoring for infection, continuing monitoring for signs of anemia, and wound management if splenectomy was performed. Genetic counseling is indicated for couples considering childbirth (see Ethical Alert). Energy conservation techniques should be included in the teaching plan.

Enzyme Deficiency Anemia

Etiology and Epidemiology. Deficiency of enzymes in the pathways that metabolize glucose and generate adenosine triphosphate (Embden-Meyerhof and pentose phosphate shunt pathways) commonly leads to premature RBC destruction, known as enzyme deficiency anemia. The most common clinically significant enzyme abnormality is that of glucose-6-phosphate dehydrogenase (G6PD). This defect is autosomal recessive and occurs in a mild form among African-Americans. A more severe form can occur in certain population groups from the Mediterranean area and may cause chronic hemolytic anemia.

Ethical Alert

Genetic Counseling

Ethical dilemmas can arise when genetic counseling is offered to families when a child has a genetic disorder or one or more parents has a genetic disorder or is a carrier of a genetic disorder. It is often the nurse's responsibility to talk to the parents about seeking genetic counseling and to refer them to a center or person who can assist them. Some individuals believe it is not appropriate to take the risk of having children when there is a chance they will have a genetic disease. On the other hand, some individuals believe it is not appropriate to interfere with "nature" in this matter. The nurse should be aware that this can be a sensitive and traumatic topic for families. (See Chapter 5 for more information about genetics and disease.)

Pathophysiology. The enzyme G6PD is responsible for the antioxidant reactions in the RBCs. The lack of this enzyme renders the cell susceptible to oxidizing agents. Exposure to these agents results in damage to the Hgb on the RBC membrane and the subsequent release of Hgb into the circulation.

Hemolytic episodes in G6PD deficiency can be caused by viral and bacterial infection or oxidant drugs (antimalarials, antipyretics, sulfonamides, quinidine, and vitamin K derivatives). Diagnosis is established by laboratory confirmation of the lack of the G6PD enzyme. Hemolytic episodes persist for 7 to 10 days after exposure to oxidizing agents. Symptoms include back pain, jaundice, and hemoglobinuria.

Collaborative Care Management. Treatment is based on recognition of the disorder and cessation of the offending drugs. During a hemolytic episode, hydration and blood transfusions may be necessary. Prompt treatment of infections is also important in managing these patients. Nursing care centers on the education of patients and their families on avoiding precipitating drugs.

Sickle Cell Disease

Etiology and Epidemiology. Normal Hgb is composed of heme (related to iron) and globin (protein component). The globin part is composed of two pairs of polypeptide chains, alpha and beta. Each of the polypeptide chains has a specific amino acid sequence and number, any deviation of which results in abnormal Hgb synthesis. Disorders of Hgb synthesis are categorized as hemoglobinopathies.

Sickle cell disease is an umbrella term for a group of inherited hemoglobinopathies in which abnormal sickle hemoglobin (Hb S) partially or completely replaces normal adult hemoglobin (Hb A). Two of the most common forms of sickle cell disease in the United

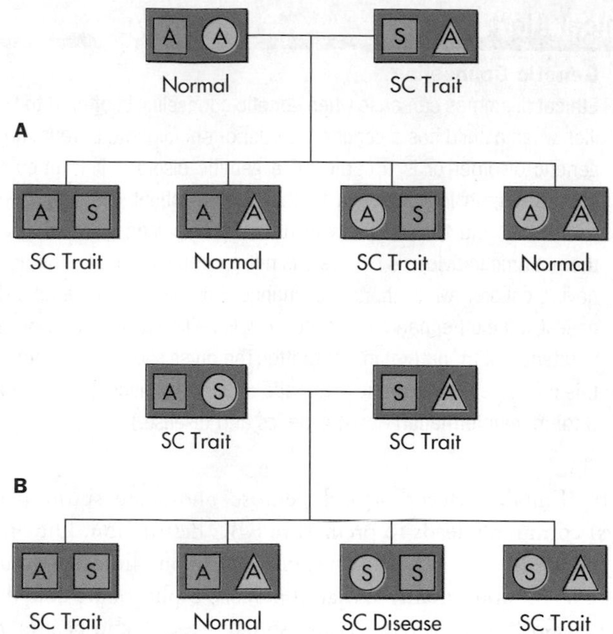

Figure 33-1 **A,** When one parent has sickle cell *(SC)* trait (Hb SA), a 50% probability (2/4) exists that a child will have sickle cell trait. **B,** When both parents have sickle cell trait, there is a 25% probability (1/4) that a child will have sickle cell disease and a 50% probability of sickle cell trait.

States are sickle cell trait (SCT) and sickle cell anemia. SCT is the heterozygous form of the disease in which the affected individual has both normal (Hb A) and sickle (Hb S) hemoglobin. Sickle cell anemia, also known as hemoglobin SS disease, is the homozygous form in which the affected individual has predominantly sickle hemoglobin (Hb SS) (Figure 33-1). In addition to the classic disease of sickle cell anemia, a group of sickling syndromes is also associated with Hb S (Table 33-4).

Sickle cell anemia is the most common genetic disorder in the United States. It is a chronic hemolytic anemia, which occurs predominantly in the African-American population. An estimated 70,000 African-Americans in the United States have sickle cell anemia, and 10% of African-Americans have sickle cell trait. To a lesser extent, sickle cell disease also occurs in persons from Asia Minor, India, the Mediterranean area, and the Caribbean area.

Table 33-4 Types of Sickle Cell Disorders

Term	Characteristic	Hemoglobin Molecule
Sickle cell trait	Carrier of Hb S Asymptomatic carriers	Hb SA
Sickle cell disease	Presence of sickling with associated symptoms	Hb SS
Sickle cell syndromes	Diseases associated with Hb S	Hb SC (sickle cell Hb C) Hb SD (sickle cell Hb D) Hb S-beta (sickle cell–thalassemia disease)

Pathophysiology. The basic abnormality lies within the globin fraction of the Hgb, where a single amino acid (valine) is substituted for another (glutamic acid) in the sixth position of the beta chain. This single amino acid substitution profoundly alters the properties of the Hgb molecule, and Hb S is formed instead of normal Hb A. Hb S has normal oxygen-carrying capacity. However, when the oxygen tension of RBCs decreases, Hb S polymerizes, causing the Hgb to distort and realign the RBC into a sickle shape (Figure 33-2). The sickle cell in circulation leads to increased blood viscosity, which prolongs circulation time. This slower circulation time causes an increase in the hypoxic time of the cell, promoting further sickling. The development of sickle cells leads to plugging of the small circulation, further decreasing cellular pH and oxygen tension (Figure 33-3). Anaerobic metabolism occurs, with resulting tissue ischemia in any organ. This cycle leads to further hypoxia, infarction of organs, and a painful

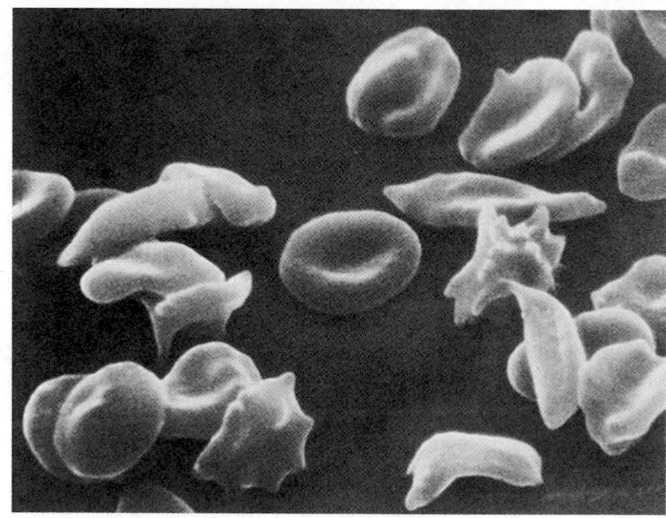

Figure 33-2 Sickled red blood cells.

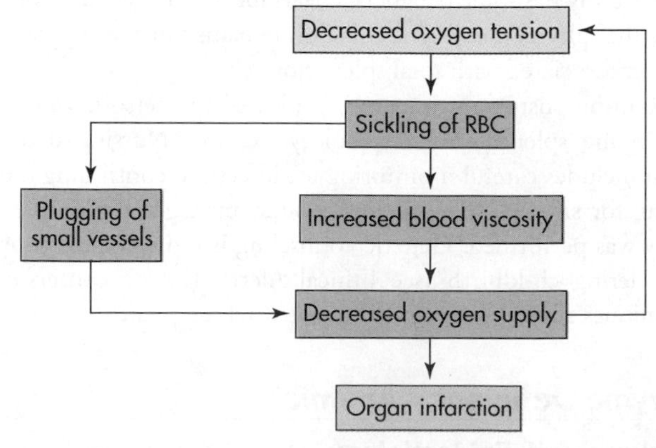

Figure 33-3 Physiologic effects of red blood cell (*RBC*) sickling.

crisis. The affected cells have a shortened life span. They survive in the circulation only 7 to 20 days, compared with the normal 105 to 120 days, because they are identified as abnormal and destroyed by the spleen.

Sickle cell disease is often diagnosed in early childhood and may be fatal by middle age.[14] The course of the disease is characterized by gradations of sickling and symptoms, which vary both in occurrence and intensity. Periods of exacerbation when symptoms are at their worst are called *crises*. These crises can be of various types: vasoocclusive (referred to as a painful episode), sequestration, aplastic or megaloblastic, or hyperhemolytic crisis (see Clinical Manifestations box).

The painful vasoocclusive episode is the most common event in sickle cell disease. The pain is a manifestation of localized bone marrow necrosis affecting the periarticular areas of the long bones, spine, pelvis, ribs, and sternum. The frequency of these episodes varies greatly. Some patients experience one or two episodes per month, whereas others have only one or two per year. The duration of the episode also varies and may last from 1 to 10 days. Physical and probably emotional factors (such as stress) precipitate painful episodes. Physical factors include events that cause dehydration or change the oxygen tension in the body, such as infection, fever, anesthesia, overexertion, exposure to cold or high altitudes, high Hgb levels, ingestion of alcohol, and smoking (see Nursing Care Plan).

Aplastic crises are transient periods during which erythropoiesis ceases and anemia worsens rapidly as a result of the shortened life span of the RBCs. Aplastic crises can be due to infection or bone marrow necrosis. Diagnosis of aplastic crisis can be made by bone marrow examination. Megaloblastic crisis can also occur in some cases as a result of the depletion of bone marrow stores of folic acid. These crises may be treated or prevented by administration of folic acid. Another cause of exacerbation of anemia is acute splenic sequestration. This occurs when the spleen suddenly increases in size, blood pools in it, and hypovolemia with signs of shock develops. In hyperhemolytic crises RBC destruction is accelerated and anemia, jaundice, and reticulocytosis occur.

Complications of sickle cell anemia relate to the major effects of the sickling process on many body systems. Thrombosis and infarction resulting from anoxia may occur in the brain, kidneys, bone marrow, and spleen. Increased intracranial pressure may occur. In younger patients death may result from cerebral hemorrhage or shock, although the incidence of first and subsequent strokes in children younger than 18 years of age has been significantly reduced through regular monthly transfusion therapy (chronic transfusion therapy).

Bacterial infection, another complication, is a major cause of morbidity and mortality in patients with sickle cell anemia. These persons are particularly susceptible, primarily because most experience functional asplenia (no spleen function). Persons with other hemoglobinopathies, such as Hb SC (sickle-hemoglobin C disease) and Hb AS (sickle cell trait), seem to be at lower risk for infection. Infection usually occurs in tissues damaged by lack of blood flow caused by sickling in the vessels, especially the lungs, urinary tract, and bones. Meningitis; sepsis; and urinary tract infections, which may be a chronic problem, are common. Alterations in skin integrity, such as leg ulcers, which occur on the malleoli and tend to heal poorly, are common skin manifestations.

Bony complications involve the growth plates, resulting in uneven bone growth. Avascular necrosis, especially in the shoulders and hips, can lead to arthritis and eventually necessitate total joint replacement. The vertebrae are also susceptible to bony collapse.

Pulmonary complications include pneumonia, infiltrates, and pulmonary infarction. Fat embolism (arising from the bone marrow) may also occur. Long-term pulmonary complications include pulmonary hypertension and cor pulmonale. Multiorgan failure, including pulmonary, renal, neurologic, and hepatic involvement, may occur in the person with sickle cell disease.

Cardiovascular complications may result from an increased cardiac workload. The patient should be assessed for dysrhythmias and murmurs.

Priapism (prolonged, painful erection) can result from a sickle cell crisis. There is no effective therapy. The best treatment is avoidance of prolonged sexual activity, alcohol, and dehydration.

Although many patients may die during childhood from cerebral hemorrhage or shock, the mortality rate is decreasing and life expectancy is slowly increasing. In older patients, death usually results from progressive renal damage and uremia.

Clinical Manifestations
Sickle Cell Disease

Acute Episodes

Pain: usually in the back, chest, or extremities; may be localized, migratory, or generalized
Fever: low grade, 1 to 2 days after onset of pain
Vasoocclusive crises: occlusion of blood vessels by the sickled cells; may occur in areas such as the brain (cerebrovascular accident), chest, liver, or penis (priapism)
Jaundice: caused by increased red blood cell destruction and the release of bilirubin

Chronic Problems

Leg ulcers: usually of the medial malleolus
Renal problems: renal insufficiency from repeated infarctions
Ocular problems: microinfarctions of the peripheral retina leading to retinal detachment and blindness
Musculoskeletal: necrosis of the femoral head

Collaborative Care Management

Diagnostic Tests. A metabisulfate test, or sickling test, is used to screen for both sickle cell anemia and SCT. The diagnosis of sickle cell anemia can be confirmed with Hgb electrophoresis.

Medications. Hydroxyurea is a part of current therapy because it has been shown to decrease the number and severity of pain episodes, the need for transfusions, and episodes of acute chest syndrome and hospitalization.[4] Erythropoietin, supplemental iron, folic acid, and vitamin B_{12} are given to promote RBC production. Antibiotics are given early in the course of infection to

Nursing Care Plan

Patient With Sickle Cell Crisis

Data A 24-year-old African-American man with a 14-year history of sickle cell disease is admitted to the hospital in sickle cell crisis and congestive heart failure. He has severe joint pain in his upper and lower extremities, moderate fever (101° F [38.3 C]), and shortness of breath. Physical examination reveals crackles in both lower lung lobes; cyanosis of the lips and nail beds; dry, scaly skin on both legs; and 2+ pitting edema with a small (2 cm) reddened area over each medial malleolus. His hemoglobin is 9 g/dl.

Physician orders include 4 L/min of oxygen by nasal cannula, bed rest with bathroom privileges, and morphine sulfate given intravenously (IV) via patient-controlled analgesia. He is to receive 2 units of packed red blood cells followed by IV fluids.

The patient expresses concern about the outcome of his disease, including his ability to breathe, support his family, care for his son, engage in sexual relations with his wife, and participate in athletic events. The patient states that he had his son before understanding the genetic nature of his disease. He fears having more children because he does not want to pass on the sickle cell trait.

Nursing Diagnosis

Anxiety related to threat to self-esteem, health status, and role functioning

Outcomes

- Patient will report reduction in anxiety after use of coping strategies.

Related NOC Outcomes

- Acceptance: Health Status
- Anxiety Self-Control
- Coping

Related NIC Interventions

- Anxiety Reduction
- Calming Technique
- Coping Enhancement

Nursing Interventions/Rationales

- Provide opportunities for patient to explore concerns about the effects of his disease. *Making the unknown known and correcting any misconceptions that may exist reduce anxiety.*
- Assess patient's knowledge of sickle cell anemia and crisis and correct any misunderstandings. *Misinformation or misunderstandings often lead to fear and anxiety that can be relieved by providing accurate information.*
- Teach relaxation measures and encourage their use when feeling anxious. *Relaxation decreases the psychomotor responses to anxiety.*
- Teach patient to avoid situations that cause crises (see text). *Crises can often be avoided if patients understand factors that promote crisis and can learn to avoid them. Understanding how to avoid crises reduces fear, which in turn reduces anxiety.*

Nursing Diagnosis

Risk for infection related to spleen dysfunction and altered primary and secondary defense mechanisms

Outcomes

- Patient will remain free from infection.

Related NOC Outcomes

- Immune Status
- Nutritional Status
- Risk Control

Related NIC Interventions

- Infection Control
- Infection Protection
- Skin Surveillance

Nursing Interventions/Rationales

- Monitor for signs of localized infection (redness, warmth, tenderness, swelling) and systemic infection (elevated white blood cell count, fever, lethargy). *Treatment for infection can be instituted more quickly when signs of infection are recognized early.*
- Use good hand-washing techniques and maintain medical asepsis. *Aseptic technique decreases the patient's contact with pathogenic organisms. Infection is predicated on the type and number of organisms to which a person is exposed, as well as the patient's resistance to infection.*
- Restrict persons (staff members, visitors) with active infections. *Restricting persons with infections decreases the patient's exposure to infectious agents.*

Nursing Diagnosis

Acute pain in joints related to disease process

Outcomes

- Patient will report adequate control of pain as evidence by rating pain less than 2 on a scale of 0 to 10.

Related NOC Outcomes

- Comfort Level
- Pain Control
- Pain Level

Related NIC Interventions

- Analgesic Management
- Coping Enhancement
- Pain Management

Nursing Interventions/Rationales

- Assess effectiveness of analgesics at least every 4 hours. Consult physician if analgesia is not effective in reducing or controlling pain. *The pain from sickle cell crisis can be excruciating, and large doses of medication may be necessary. Alternative medications need to be considered when currently prescribed medications do not control pain.*

avoid precipitating a crisis. Medications to manage both acute and chronic pain are individualized to the patient's current needs, so frequent reassessment is just as important as initial assessment. Opioids are titrated to give the best pain control for the individual; they are not given by a routine protocol. Drugs used in addition to the opioids include antihistamines, nonsteroidal antiinflammatory drugs, and ketorolac.

TREATMENTS. Hydration and pain management are still essential treatments. Helping the patient find appropriate

- Identify pain relief measures the patient has found useful for relieving pain in the past. *Often pain control methods that are effective for one kind of pain will be effective for other types of pain.*
- Support joints gently when assisting patient with range-of-motion exercises. *Improper support or lack of support increases stress on joints and exacerbates pain.*
- Use moist heat or massage, if helpful. *Heat dilates blood vessels and increases circulation to the area, which may increase comfort.*
- Use nonpharmacologic pain relief measures (relaxation, distraction, biofeedback, music, self-hypnosis). *Nonpharmacologic measures may decrease physiologic responses to pain and potentiate the effect of analgesics.*
- Teach patient the importance of drinking 4 to 6 L of fluid daily. *Dehydration is a primary cause of red blood cell sickling. If the patient understands this, compliance is more likely.*

Nursing Diagnosis

Risk for situational low self-esteem related to change in disease status, pain, and fear of future disability

Outcomes

* Patient will verbalize satisfaction with life, self, and control of disease.

Related NOC Outcomes

- Acceptance: Health Status
- Psychosocial Adjustment: Life Change
- Self-Esteem

Related NIC Interventions

- Coping Enhancement
- Emotional Support
- Self-Esteem Enhancement

Nursing Interventions/Rationales

- Assess patient's knowledge regarding his disease. *The extent of the patient's knowledge about his disease should be acknowledged. It is necessary to determine what the patient does and does not know before teaching can be planned.*
- Provide opportunities for patient to discuss his feelings about the inability to fulfill his expected role at this time. *Verbalization of concerns decreases their impact and assists in problem solving.*
- Assist patient in identifying personal strengths. *Focusing on strengths and positive aspects of life provides a basis for personal growth.*
- Assist patient in exploring alternative ways to meet role expectations. *Concern over losses may immobilize patient. Providing assistance in exploring alternatives helps the patient refocus and seek new methods of reaching desired goals.*
- Refer patient to a support group or for counseling. *To minimize dependent behaviors. Research shows that increased social support from family and groups increases recovery from disease and disability and facilitate rehabilitation.*
- Provide resources for family planning and genetic counseling. *Persons and groups with in-depth knowledge of family planning methods help patients identify family planning methods that conform to their cultural and religious values.*

Nursing Diagnosis

Sexual dysfunction related to fatigue, pain, and fear of pregnancy

Outcomes

- Patient will verbalize satisfaction with sexual functioning and relationship.

Related NOC Outcomes

- Endurance
- Sexual Functioning

Related NIC Interventions

- Energy Management
- Sexual Counseling

Nursing Interventions/Rationales

- Discuss coital positions that require less energy for the patient. *Coitus requires energy and involves neuromuscular activity; side-lying or male-inferior position is less demanding for male patients.*
- Suggest coitus at times of day when patient is less fatigued (morning, afternoon). *Fatigue increases with continued daily activities and demand on cardiovascular system.*
- Discuss the need for genetic counseling and contraception. *Knowledge and use of reliable contraception methods to prevent pregnancy reduces fear that contributes to sexual dysfunction.*

Evaluation

Evaluation is based on comparing the patient's outcomes with desired outcomes.

pain relief with and in addition to medications can be a challenge (see Research box). Oxygen therapy should be administered during an acute crisis to prevent hypoxemia. Frequent blood transfusions (every 3 to 4 weeks) in children younger than 18 years of age have been shown to prevent both initial strokes and second or third strokes. Exchange transfusions have been done with varying degrees of success during vaso-occlusive crises.

Patients with sickle cell anemia can be considered for BMT. A problem is the lack of HLA-identical donors because of the genetic

Research

Elander J et al: Pain management and symptoms of substance dependence among patients with sickle cell disease, *Soc Sci Med* 57(9):1683, 2003.

The study looked at substance dependence in patients with sickle cell disease, a common problem since these patients use a variety of medications to control pain. The researchers interviewed sickle cell disease patients who were taking analgesics for pain management. The study found that 31% of the sample met the DSM-IV criteria for substance dependence. The researchers recommended that health care providers seek a better pain management regimen for patients with sickle cell disease. Those who prescribe medications should become more aware of how the patients are coping with pain and find additional ways to assist them.

component of the disease. Research is continuing for the use of unrelated cord blood stem cell transplantation.

Genetic counseling is important in the prevention of sickle cell disease and is recommended for persons considering childbirth (refer to the Ethical Alert box, p. 913). Parents who both have SCT should be informed that the risk of giving birth to an infant with sickle cell disease is one out of four births. Diagnosis of sickle cell disease can be done early in the first trimester of pregnancy.

DIET. A diet rich in protein, calcium, vitamins, and adequate fluids should be encouraged. Iced liquids should be avoided because they may precipitate a crisis.

Nursing Management *of the Patient with Sickle Cell Anemia*

ASSESSMENT

Health History. Assess for:

- Present and prior symptoms
- History of chronic fatigue, chest pain, dyspnea, joint pain, and swelling

Physical Examination. Assess for:

- Changes in vital signs: fever, palpitations, shortness of breath
- Delayed capillary refill
- Signs of pain: abdominal, back, chest or joint pain; headache
- Decreased urinary output
- Enlarged spleen, liver, or lymph nodes

NURSING DIAGNOSES, OUTCOMES, AND INTERVENTIONS

Nursing Diagnosis: Ineffective Tissue Perfusion (Peripheral)

OUTCOMES. A common example of expected outcomes for the patient with a diagnosis of *ineffective tissue perfusion (peripheral)* is:

Patient will:

- Identify factors that promote vasodilation and improve peripheral circulation.

NURSING INTERVENTIONS. The nurse monitors the patient for signs of pain that indicate blood vessel occlusion. Changes in pain or mental status are reported to the physician. Constrictive clothing should be avoided. To prevent vasoconstriction, the nurse encourages the patient not to smoke.

The vasoocclusive nature of painful episodes requires adequate hydration to decrease blood viscosity. The nurse advises patients who are supposedly in a steady state of their disease to drink 4 to 6 quarts of water daily; this requirement increases to 6 to 8 quarts of water daily during a painful episode. If intravenous hydration is necessary, careful attention must be given to venous access, with avoidance of multiple punctures and infiltration.

Oxygen is given for dyspnea or excessive fatigue with exertion. Reducing activity strain lessens the demand for oxygen. Promoting frequent rest periods while assisting the patient with difficult activities also reduces the demand.

RELATED NIC INTERVENTIONS. Neurologic Monitoring, Peripheral Sensation Management, Positioning

Nursing Diagnosis: Pain

OUTCOMES. Common examples of expected outcomes for the patient with a diagnosis of *pain* are:

Patient will:

- Verbalize that pain is reduced.
- Rate pain as 4 or less on a scale of 0 (no pain) to 10 (maximum pain).
- Experience less fatigue or dyspnea on exertion.

NURSING INTERVENTIONS. The nurse helps the patient who experiences weakness and fatigue from the anemia in planning daily activities to include rest periods. Pain medication is given before activities that may increase discomfort. Nursing care for painful episodes involves all the principles of pain management. The goal is to relieve the pain but not overmedicate. This usually involves the use of both narcotic and nonnarcotic analgesics. Astute evaluation of the effectiveness of pain medication is most important. Managing pain in a sickle cell crisis may include the use of patient-controlled analgesia.

RELATED NIC INTERVENTIONS. Medication Management, Pain Management

Nursing Diagnosis: Ineffective Family Therapeutic Regimen Management

OUTCOMES. A common example of expected outcomes for the patient with a diagnosis of *ineffective family therapeutic regimen management* is:

Family and patient will:

- Encourage each other and maintain a normal life.

NURSING INTERVENTIONS. Patients with sickle cell disease are sometimes labeled as difficult or malingerers because of their behavior patterns, which are influenced by anxiety about their chronic illness. The nurse should encourage counseling, use of support groups, and verbalization of fears and anxieties. The nurse should support the patient and family while they are implementing behavior and lifestyle changes necessary to cope with a chronic illness.

Many patients with genetic disorders such as sickle cell disease are now deciding when or whether they want to have children. Some forms of birth control, such as the intrauterine device (IUD), are not as highly recommended as other forms, such as the diaphragm or spermicides, for persons with sickle cell disorders. An IUD has a higher incidence of infection than the diaphragm or spermicides. Tubal ligation, vasectomy, and oral contraceptives are other possible choices for birth control, but they are associated with significant risk. To make a wise decision about contraception, couples require accurate information about options, side effects, and risks. Such family counseling must be performed by knowledgeable persons.

RELATED NIC INTERVENTIONS. Coping Enhancement, Counseling, Mutual Goal Setting, Support Group

Patient/Family Teaching. Patient teaching is an important component of patient care (see Patient/Family Teaching box).

EVALUATION

To evaluate effectiveness of nursing interventions, compare patient behaviors with those stated in the expected patient outcomes.

RELATED NOC OUTCOMES. Circulation Status, Comfort Level, Knowledge: Illness Care, Knowledge: Treatment Regimen, Pain Control, Tissue Perfusion: Peripheral

Thalassemia

Etiology and Epidemiology. Thalassemia is one of the most common inherited single-gene disorders in the world. This inherited disorder of Hgb synthesis primarily affects persons of Mediterranean descent, but it also occurs in those of Southeast Asian, Chinese, and African descent.

Pathophysiology. Thalassemia is characterized by a decreased synthesis of one of the globin chains of Hgb. The beta chain is most often affected (beta-thalassemia). As a result, Hgb synthesis declines and the alpha globin chain accumulates in the erythrocyte. These alterations result in decreased RBC production and a chronic hemolytic anemia.

Thalassemia has two presentations (Table 33-5). The heterozygous state, thalassemia minor, is associated with a mild anemia (usually asymptomatic). No therapy is required. The homozygous condition, thalassemia major (also called Cooley's anemia), is characterized by a severe anemia. The RBCs are characteristically hypochromic (low MCHC) and microcytic (low MCV). Diagnosis is by Hgb electrophoresis. Growth failure usually begins between ages 10 and 12 years. Death usually occurs during the young adult years, between ages 17 and 30.

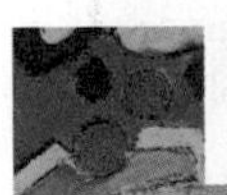

PATIENT/FAMILY TEACHING

The Patient With Sickle Cell Disease

The nurse should include the following information when teaching an individual with sickle cell disease:

- Information about the disease
- Avoidance of situations that cause crises (infection, high altitudes, overexertion, emotional stress, alcohol, cigarette smoking); avoidance of trauma
- Importance of adequate fluid intake
- Availability of psychologic support services and social resources
- Importance of medical follow-up care

TABLE 33-5 TYPES OF THALASSEMIA

Type	State	Symptoms	Therapy
Thalassemia minor	Heterozygous	Mild anemia; usually asymptomatic	None required
Thalassemia major	Homozygous	Severe anemia Low MCHC Low MCV	Transfusion

MCHC, Mean corpuscular hemoglobin concentration; *MCV,* mean corpuscular volume.

Collaborative Care Management. The common treatment for thalassemia is transfusion therapy. BMT is usually considered in children with thalassemia major who are less than 5 years of age. Transfusions may be administered either to alleviate severe symptoms or to maintain the Hgb at a near-normal level to allow for a more normal lifestyle. The latter approach incurs the risk of producing iron overload from frequent transfusions, a problem that can be ameliorated by the use of an iron-chelating agent such as deferoxamine. Splenectomy may help decrease transfusion requirements in some patients. Allogenic BMT has been successful in a small number of patients.

The nurse must be familiar with transfusion therapy and sensitive to the emotional needs of patients receiving frequent transfusions. Because the average age at which death occurs is 17 to 30 years, the nurse should be aware of the hopelessness and depression that may occur in this population. Patients and their families need education about the disease process and rationales for treatment. Couples should be referred for genetic counseling.

Iron Deficiency Anemia

Etiology and Epidemiology. Iron is a fundamental part of the Hgb molecule, and its deficiency leads to production of RBCs with a decreased amount of Hgb and ultimately to fewer RBCs. The average adult body contains approximately 4 g of iron, 3 g of which are in Hgb, 500 mg to 1 g in iron stores in the liver and bone marrow, and the rest in certain tissues and enzyme systems. The body loses approximately 1.5 mg of iron daily; this loss is usually compensated for with daily dietary intake. Iron deficiency anemia is common in young women who have poor nutrition, older adults, and those in lower socioeconomic areas.

Pathophysiology. The tenuous balance between intake and losses of iron may be compromised by chronic blood loss, either physiologic (such as menstruation) or pathologic (from gastrointestinal [GI] or other bleeding), as well as by poor nutrition,

Box 33-1 Identifying and Preventing Iron Deficiency Anemia in Older Adults

Since older adults may be prone to develop iron deficiency anemia, the nurse should include the following steps in the care plan:

- Assess for dyspnea, bleeding, paleness, and clubbing.
- Observe the patient's laboratory studies for hemoglobin and iron levels.
- Listen carefully to the patient's comments about nutritional habits and general health status.
- Check whether the patient is taking an iron supplement or vitamin with iron.
- Check the patient's nutritional patterns.
- Assess the dietary iron intake.
- Offer strategies on how to increase iron intake in the diet.
- Talk to the patient about the importance of preventing iron deficiency anemia.

especially in older adults (Box 33-1). This compromise results in an iron deficiency anemia.

Gradual development of iron deficiency anemia may permit adaptation with few clinical signs. Some persons may develop fatigue and exertional dyspnea. Severe iron deficiency anemia causes the nails to become brittle and spoon shaped (concave) and to develop longitudinal ridges (see Clinical Manifestations box). The papillae of the tongue atrophy, and the tongue has a smooth, shiny, bright red appearance. The corners of the mouth may be cracked, reddened, and painful (cheilosis). The RBCs are characteristically hypochromic and microcytic, and the anemia is evident in a peripheral blood smear and blood cell indices. Diagnosis is confirmed by a low serum iron level and elevated serum iron-binding capacity or by a low serum ferritin level or absent iron stores in the bone marrow.

Collaborative Care Management. The first step in medical therapy is to determine and correct the cause of the iron deficiency. Iron is then administered to replace iron stores in the body. Oral iron supplementation usually is given in the form of ferrous sulfate.

Patient teaching is one of the major nursing interventions, especially with a patient newly diagnosed with iron deficiency anemia. Because ferrous sulfate may irritate the GI tract, the patient is instructed to take it after meals and with orange juice or vitamin C to increase absorption. The nurse tells the patient that the stools will be black or tarry and that symptoms of diarrhea or nausea should be reported to the health care provider. Constipation is a major side effect of iron supplementation, and a stool softener may be needed. When the patient cannot tolerate oral iron preparations or is unable to absorb iron properly, parenteral iron is administered intravenously and, rarely, with Z-track intramuscular injection.

Poor diet is rarely the sole cause of iron deficiency anemia but is usually a contributing factor. The nurse assesses the person's dietary habits and knowledge of principles of nutrition. Persons with insufficient financial means for food, medication, or medical attention may be referred to community resources, including a dietitian, social worker, or Meals-on-Wheels.

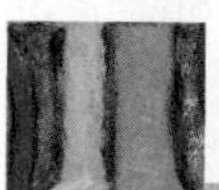

CLINICAL MANIFESTATIONS
Iron Deficiency Anemia

Mild

Fatigue and exertional dyspnea

Severe

Brittle, spoon-shaped nails with longitudinal ridges
Smooth, shiny tongue
Cheilosis

ARE You READY?

Which clinical manifestation is associated with iron deficiency anemia?

1. Peripheral neuropathy
2. Smooth, shiny, bright red tongue
3. Thickened nails
4. Decreased bleeding time

Megaloblastic or Macrocytic Anemia

Megaloblastic anemia refers to anemia with characteristic morphologic changes caused by defective deoxyribonucleic acid (DNA) synthesis and abnormal RBC maturation. On the peripheral blood smear, macrocytic RBCs and hypersegmented neutrophils (increased number of nuclei) are present. In the bone marrow, erythroid precursors can be found that are two to three times larger than normal, with nuclei that are immature relative to their cytoplasmic development.

Most megaloblastic anemias are caused by deficiency of either vitamin B_{12} (cobalamin) or folic acid (Table 33-6). Deficiency of vitamin B_{12} can result from dietary deficiency, surgery, malabsorption, or pernicious anemia. Pernicious anemia is the most common cause of vitamin B_{12} deficiency. Vegetarians can develop vitamin B_{12} deficiency as a result of dietary habits. Both vitamin B_{12} and folic acid are essential in the synthesis of DNA, and their deficiency leads to impaired nuclear development in cells throughout the body. Deficiency of either leads to anemia and often leukopenia and thrombocytopenia. Administration of medication that interferes with DNA metabolism, such as chemotherapeutic agents and anticonvulsants, can also cause megaloblastic anemia. It is essential that the cause of the anemia be identified before medications are started. Failure to recognize a combined vitamin B_{12} and folate deficiency, plus treatment of the folate deficiency only, can result in worsening of neurologic problems. A subacute neurologic syndrome can occur and may progress.

Vitamin B_{12} Deficiency

Etiology and Epidemiology. Vitamin B_{12}, obtained from dietary sources, combines with intrinsic factor in the stomach and is carried to the ileum, where it is absorbed and transported by a carrier protein to the body tissues. Patients who have had a total gastrectomy or ileal resection need parenteral vitamin B_{12} injections for life. Anemia is caused by a lack of intrinsic factor, which allows absorption of vitamin B_{12}.

TABLE 33-6 ETIOLOGY AND PATHOPHYSIOLOGY OF MEGALOBLASTIC OR MACROCYTIC ANEMIAS

Anemia	Etiology	Pathophysiology
Vitamin B_{12} (or cobalamin) deficiency	Poor dietary intake Malabsorption syndrome Pernicious anemia	Deficiency results in impaired synthesis of DNA, resulting in morphologic changes in blood and marrow.
Folic acid deficiency	Poor dietary intake Chronic alcoholism Malnutrition Pregnancy	Folic acid is an essential element required for DNA synthesis and RBC maturation; deficiencies result in morphologic changes in blood and marrow.
Pernicious anemia	Autoimmune reaction Loss of parietal cells Overgrowth of intestinal organisms Gastrectomy Ileal resection Tapeworms Inflammatory bowel disease Celiac disease	Intrinsic factor produced by stomach is absent or deficient, resulting in malabsorption of vitamin B_{12}.

DNA, Deoxyribonucleic acid; *RBC*, red blood cell.

Pathophysiology. Diagnosis of vitamin B_{12} deficiency is made by demonstration of a low serum vitamin B_{12} level in a patient with macrocytic anemia and megaloblastic bone marrow. In addition to the general symptoms associated with anemia, patients with vitamin B_{12} deficiency may manifest neurologic abnormalities, particularly a peripheral neuropathy and a loss of balance resulting from an abnormality of the posterior and lateral columns of the spinal cord (subacute combined degeneration).

Loss of proprioception and diminished vibratory sense have been reported in up to 40% of persons with vitamin B_{12} deficiency. Other neurologic manifestations, including mental status changes, impaired memory, dementia, and depression, are often overlooked or mistaken for Alzheimer's disease in older adults. Diagnosis of pernicious anemia is confirmed by an abnormal Schilling test result, which demonstrates the inability to absorb vitamin B_{12} unless intrinsic factor also is administered.

Collaborative Care Management. Treatment of vitamin B_{12} deficiency consists of parenteral administration of vitamin B_{12}, usually once a month by a nurse in an outpatient setting, for patients who have any condition that interferes with absorption from the small bowel or who are not producing intrinsic factor. Oral administration is used only in cases of nutritional deficiency. Vitamin B_{12} is available in oral, intramuscular, subcutaneous, and intranasal forms. The most common cause of relapse in persons with pernicious anemia is their reluctance to continue therapy for life. The nurse must help the patient understand the nature of the illness and the absolute necessity for continued treatment.

Folic Acid Deficiency

Etiology and Epidemiology. Folic acid deficiency anemia may be caused by dietary deficiency, often in association with chronic alcoholism, overcooking of vegetables, malabsorption syndromes, and medications that inhibit the enzyme involved in normal folate absorption through the intestinal wall. Pregnancy causes an increase in the need for and use of folic acid. Deficiencies during pregnancy may result in neural tube defects.

Pathophysiology. The pathophysiology depends on the underlying cause of the disease. Signs and symptoms are also associated with the underlying disease and anemia in general. Laboratory findings include macrocytic anemia, megaloblastic changes in the bone marrow, and a low serum folate level.

Collaborative Care Management. Most persons respond promptly to oral folic acid and a well-balanced diet. Daily requirements for folic acid are 100 to 200 mg. The body is able to store approximately a 4-month supply of folic acid. Persons with anemia caused by dietary deficiency can be treated with 1 mg of folic acid per day for a 3-month period. Return visits to nursing clinics and community health nurse home visits help the person incorporate dietary modifications into daily life. Patients who drink alcohol excessively may be referred to Alcoholics Anonymous. Patients with financial limitations are referred to appropriate community resources. The nurse provides patients with information about food sources of folic acid and instructions about proper preparation. Foods rich in folic acid include organ meats, eggs, cabbage, broccoli, citrus fruits, and Brussels sprouts. Boiling, steaming, and canning of folic acid–rich foods reduce the amount of available vitamin. Persons who consume large amounts of fast foods are susceptible to folic acid deficiency.

Anemia of Chronic Disease

Etiology and Epidemiology. Anemia of chronic disease (ACD) is one of the most common types of anemia, second only to iron deficiency anemia. It is a normochromic, normocytic, hypoproliferative type of anemia. This anemia commonly accompanies such diseases as chronic inflammatory disorders, some infections, malignancy, AIDS, Crohn's disease, and other systemic disorders.

Pathophysiology. The pathophysiology of ACD is not fully understood but is thought to be related to the failure of erythropoietin (EPO) to stimulate RBC production. Immune activation contributes to the inability of EPO to stimulate the bone marrow. Also contributing to ACD are certain treatments such as chemotherapy, which suppress the marrow's ability to produce RBCs. Symptoms include fatigue, weakness, dyspnea, and anorexia, as well as symptoms of the underlying disease.

Collaborative Care Management. Diagnosis is based on findings of low serum iron, decreased total iron-binding capacity, and increased serum ferritin. Treatment is supportive and related to appropriate management of the underlying disease process. The anemia is usually mild, but transfusions may be given in more severe cases. EPO therapy has also been shown to improve the anemia associated with chronic disease. The nurse should give the patient information about the relationship of the anemia to the underlying disease process. Patients need to maximize periods of high energy and to allow frequent rest periods to avoid fatigue. The nurse should inform patients about risks and benefits of transfusion therapy. Instructions about the self-administration of EPO may also be required.

Erythrocytosis

Erythrocytosis refers to an abnormal increase in erythrocytes. The increase may be a primary disorder (polycythemia vera) or occur secondary to hypoxia (from high altitudes or from pulmonary and cardiac disease) or certain EPO-producing tumors. With hypoxia, RBCs increase as a compensatory mechanism to carry additional oxygen. Principal laboratory tests used to determine the nature of erythrocytosis include arterial oxygen concentration, RBC volume, and plasma volume.

Polycythemia Vera

Etiology and Epidemiology. Polycythemia vera is a myeloproliferative disorder of the pluripotent stem cell. The etiology is unknown. The incidence is about 5 persons per 1 million.[6] Polycythemia vera affects both men and women of all ages, with a median age of 60 years. Without treatment, 50% of symptomatic patients die within 18 months. The median survival time (MST) with treatment is 7 to 15 years. The disease is found mainly among Jewish men of European descent.

Pathophysiology. Polycythemia vera (primary polycythemia) is a bone marrow disorder characterized by erythrocytosis, usually with a simultaneous leukocytosis and thrombocytosis. Hypervolemia (increased blood viscosity from the increased RBC mass) and platelet dysfunction occur.

Symptoms usually are absent in the early stages. As hypervolemia develops, headaches, vertigo, tinnitus, and blurred vision occur. Thromboses with embolization may result from the increased blood viscosity, and the skin may develop a more reddened appearance. Platelet dysfunction may lead to nosebleeds, ecchymoses, and GI bleeding (see Clinical Manifestations box).

Thromboembolic events occur in over one third of persons with polycythemia vera and include deep venous thrombosis, cerebral infarction, myocardial infarction, pulmonary embolism, arterial embolism, and splenic infarction. On physical examination splenomegaly typically is found in persons with polycythemia vera, but it is not common in other types of erythrocytosis. Laboratory tests demonstrate an increased total RBC volume and a plasma volume that is either increased or normal. The Hct at sea level is greater than 53%. Arterial oxygen concentration is usually normal.

Complications of polycythemia vera include thrombosis, hemorrhage, hyperuricemia, aquagenic pruritus, acid-peptic disease, splenomegaly, hepatomegaly, myelofibrosis, and acute leukemia. Only about 2% of patients develop leukemia unless the treatment includes leukemogenic therapies, in which case the incidence increases. The major causes of death are thrombosis (40%), hemorrhage (9%), and leukemia-myelofibrosis (10%).

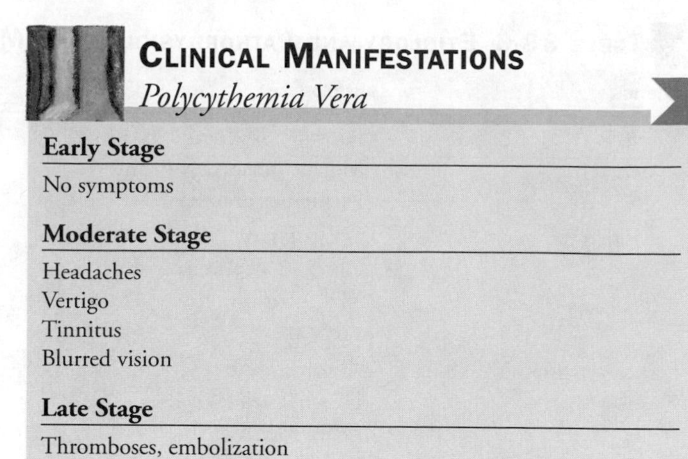
CLINICAL MANIFESTATIONS
Polycythemia Vera

Early Stage
No symptoms

Moderate Stage
Headaches
Vertigo
Tinnitus
Blurred vision

Late Stage
Thromboses, embolization
Nosebleeds, ecchymoses, gastrointestinal bleeding

Collaborative Care Management. The goal of therapy is to decrease the red cell mass. Treatment options are phlebotomy, use of alkylating agents, radioactive phosphorus, or interferon. Leukemia transformation may be a significant risk in younger persons treated with myelosuppressive therapy. Usual treatment is periodic phlebotomy aimed at maintaining the Hct and Hgb at a normal level. For patients with secondary erythrocythemia, the underlying cause is treated.

Patient teaching is an important component of patient care (see Patient/Family Teaching box).

PATIENT/FAMILY TEACHING
The Patient With Polycythemia Vera

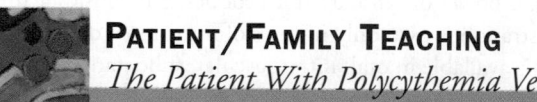

The nurse should teach the patient with polycythemia vera the following:

- Nature of the disorder
- Importance of continued medical care, blood tests, and phlebotomy
- Name, dosage, frequency, desired action, and side effects of prescribed medications
- Signs of thromboembolic events that require immediate medical attention
- Need to maintain hydration to decrease blood viscosity
- Importance of quitting or avoiding smoking

Platelet and Coagulation Disorders

Normal hemostatic function requires vascular integrity, normal numbers and function of platelets, and normal clotting factors. Although each of the essential components arises separately and is independently regulated, their balanced interplay is necessary to protect the body from excessive bleeding or excessive thrombi formation.

Primary hemostasis involves the formation of a platelet plug over a damaged area of endothelial cells lining a blood vessel. Primary hemostasis is completed with the formation of the platelet plug. **Secondary hemostasis** is the formation of a fibrin clot overlying the platelet plug. This process requires sequential activation in the cascade of clotting factors (see Chapter 32). The major steps are the formation of thrombin from prothrombin, leading to the formation of fibrin from fibrinogen.

A fibrinolytic mechanism that leads to clot lysis balances clot formation. Two enzymes are involved in clot lysis: plasminogen and plasmin. Plasminogen is the inactive form that circulates in the blood. It is converted to plasmin by active Hageman factor in addition to other factors. Plasmin then degrades and dissolves the clot. Streptokinase is a fibrinolytic enzyme.

Anticoagulants also help balance clot formation. A naturally occurring anticoagulant is heparin, which interferes with activation of several **coagulation factors**, including thrombin. Coumarin derivatives interfere with synthesis of coagulation factors II, VII, IX, and X in the liver by interfering with vitamin K. Heparin interferes with the intrinsic mechanism, whereas warfarin interferes with the extrinsic mechanism.

Platelet Disorders

Disorders of platelet function include both increased and decreased numbers of platelets (Box 33-2). The term *thrombocytosis* is defined as the presence of an abnormally high number of circulating platelets (Box 33-3). Mild bleeding syndromes may be caused by quantitatively normal but functionally defective platelets. The most common cause of such platelet abnormalities is drugs, particularly aspirin. Aspirin inhibits the release of intrinsic platelet adenosine diphosphate and produces a defect in platelet aggregation, which remains for the platelet's life span. A variety of familial and nonfamilial platelet disorders also has been described. Defective platelet function typically occurs in persons with uremia. The abnormality may be detected by a test of bleeding time or, more sensitively, by platelet aggregation tests. Patients with disorders of platelet function have clinical manifestations and patient care needs similar to those of persons with thrombocytopenia, although the bleeding abnormality usually is mild.

Thrombocytopenia

Etiology and Epidemiology. Thrombocytopenia is defined as a lower than normal number of circulating platelets. Laboratory values for a normal adult platelet count range from 150,000 to 400,000/mm^3. The many types of thrombocytopenia may result from (1) decreased platelet production, (2) decreased platelet survival, (3) increased platelet destruction (most common form), (4) sequestration of blood in the spleen, (5) consumption of platelets, or (6) loss from hemorrhage.

The most common cause of increased platelet destruction is idiopathic thrombocytopenic purpura (ITP). ITP can be divided into acute and chronic forms. Acute ITP is self-limiting, lasts less than 6 months, and generally follows a viral illness (usually in children). Chronic ITP, also termed *autoimmune thrombocytopenic purpura*, occurs most often in the second and third decades of life, affects women two or three times more often than men, and is caused by production of an autoantibody (IgG) directed against a platelet antigen.[11]

Box 33-2 Disorders Associated With Platelets and Coagulation

Platelets

Thrombocytopenia—decreased number of platelets
Thrombocytosis—increased number of platelets
Bleeding syndromes—disorders of platelet function

Coagulation

Congenital
Hemophilia A—deficiency of factor VIII
Hemophilia B—deficiency of factor IX
Von Willebrand's disease—decrease of factor VIII and defective platelet function

Acquired
Vitamin K deficiency—decrease of factors II, VII, IX, and X
Disseminated intravascular coagulation—stimulates first the clotting process, then the fibrinolytic process

Box 33-3 Thrombocytosis

Thrombocytosis can be categorized as reactive (hyperactive bone marrow) or essential (myeloproliferative syndrome).

Associated Conditions

Polycythemia vera
Myelofibrosis
Splenectomy
Iron deficiency anemia
Chronic inflammatory diseases
Hemorrhagic thrombocythemia (thrombocytosis)
Advanced carcinomas

Clinical Manifestations

Thrombosis
Increased bleeding tendencies
Platelet counts of greater than 1,000,000/mm^3

Collaborative Care

Control of underlying cause
Myelosuppressive drug therapy
Plasmapheresis to reduce circulating number of platelets

Box 33-4 Selected Drugs Typically Causing Thrombocytopenia

- Alcohol
- Aspirin
- Chemotherapeutic agents
- Chloroquine
- Digitoxin
- Estrogens
- Gold salts
- Heparin
- Methyldopa
- Nonsteroidal anti-inflammatory agents
- Oral hypoglycemic agents
- Penicillin
- Phenobarbital
- Quinidine
- Quinine
- Rifampin
- Sulfonamides
- Thiazides

Platelet destruction may also be drug induced. Approximately 70 drugs (some of which are listed in Box 33-4) have been shown to induce thrombocytopenia. Platelet counts generally return to normal within 1 to 2 weeks after the drug is withdrawn; some drugs such as gold salts may require several months.

Secondary thrombocytopenia may result from aplastic anemia, acute leukemia, and conditions causing splenomegaly (such as cirrhosis or lymphomas, which lead to sequestration of blood in the spleen). Sequestration of blood in the spleen results in splenomegaly. Consumption of platelets is seen in conditions such as disseminated intravascular coagulation (DIC), where the platelet supply is simply used up. Hemorrhage from any cause also results in loss of large numbers of platelets.

Pathophysiology. The major signs of thrombocytopenia observable by physical examination are petechiae, ecchymoses, and purpura. Petechiae occur only in platelet disorders. The person may give a history of hypermenorrhea, epistaxis, and gingival bleeding. The patient is questioned about recent viral infections, which may produce a transient thrombocytopenia; drugs in current use; and the extent of alcohol ingestion.

Collaborative Care Management. The most commonly used tests for assessment of platelets are platelet count, peripheral blood smear, and bleeding time (Table 33-7). In addition, a bone marrow examination is performed to determine the presence of megakaryocytes (precursors of platelets in the bone marrow). Examination of the bone marrow also reveals the presence or absence of primary bone marrow abnormalities, such as neoplastic invasion, aplastic anemia, or fibrosis.

The most common treatments for ITP are corticosteroid and immunoglobulin therapy and splenectomy. Steroids appear to decrease both antibody production and phagocytosis of the antibody-coated platelets. Splenectomy removes the principal organ involved in destruction of the antibody-coated platelets. Other therapeutic modalities include danazol or immunosuppressive drugs, but these have the potential for severe side effects and are usually reserved for severe cases that have not responded to other therapies. Plasma exchange may have some efficacy in acute ITP.

Transfusion with platelet concentrates may be used in persons with thrombocytopenic bleeding. It is not usually helpful for ITP because the transfused platelets have a short survival time and are rapidly destroyed by the same mechanism as the person's own platelets. When platelet production is impaired, the platelet concentrates increase the platelet count for approximately 1 to 3 days.

Platelets may be obtained from random or HLA-compatible donors. Random donors are easier to obtain and often provide effective platelets for considerable periods, but use of these platelets may eventually lead to decreased efficacy. Because platelets are not always matched for ABO antigens and the infused platelets usually are contaminated with some erythrocytes, antibodies to these antigens may develop, impairing platelet transfusion effectiveness. An attempt should be made, then, to obtain platelets from an HLA-compatible donor. The effectiveness of platelet transfusions may be monitored by performing a platelet count before and 1 hour after transfusion. No increase in the platelet count indicates that the transfusion was ineffective. Platelets must be transfused within several days of collection, or they lose their viability. Their survival in a recipient ranges from 48 to 72 hours, compared with a normal

TABLE 33-7 Common Bleeding/Coagulation Blood Tests

Test	Description	Normal Value
Bleeding time	Evaluation of vascular and platelet factors—the time it takes for small stab wound to stop bleeding	1-9 min
Clotting time	Time required for solid clot to form (less sensitive test than PTT)	5-10 min
Prothrombin time (Pro-time) (PT)	Indicates rapidity of blood clotting (indicative of adequacy of extrinsic coagulation pathway; factors I, II, V, VII, X)	11-12.5 sec; 85%-100%, compared with control levels
Partial thromboplastin time (PTT)	More sensitive test than PT to evaluate adequacy of intrinsic coagulation pathway (fibrin clot formation)	60-70 sec
Activated partial thromboplastin time (aPTT)	Modified PTT; more sensitive; quicker to perform; commonly used to monitor heparin therapy and hemophilia	30-40 sec
International normalized ratio (INR)	Mathematic calculation that standardizes PT by correcting for variability in sensitivities of thromboplastin reagents used in testing	Therapeutic range: 2.0-3.5 in most instances

platelet life span of 10 days. Transfusions often must be administered twice weekly.

A primary concern in the nursing care of persons with decreased numbers of platelets is the concomitant bleeding tendency. Bleeding associated with trauma is likely with a platelet count less than 60,000/mm^3. Spontaneous hemorrhage may be a life-threatening possibility when the platelet count is below 20,000/mm^3. Ongoing nursing assessment of the patient is essential and includes alertness for an increase in ecchymoses or petechiae, bleeding from other sites, and any change in mental status. The need for avoiding trauma is obvious. Persons with platelet counts below 20,000/mm^3 should have bleeding precautions instituted, including:

- Test all urine and stools for blood (guaiac).
- Do not take temperatures rectally.
- Do not administer intramuscular injections.
- Apply pressure to all venipuncture sites for 5 minutes and to all arterial puncture sites for 10 minutes.

Patient teaching is an important component of patient care (see Patient/Family Teaching box).

Thrombotic Thrombocytopenic Purpura

Etiology and Epidemiology. Thrombotic thrombocytopenic purpura (TTP) is a rare disorder of young adults, occurring more commonly in women than in men. In the majority of cases the etiology is unknown. The increased incidence within families suggests a genetic component. There is also an increased incidence in persons with an immune system disorder (rheumatoid arthritis, systemic lupus erythematosus, or sarcoidosis). TTP has also been associated with lymphoma; pregnancy; bacterial endocarditis; and certain drugs, including iodine, sulfonamides, penicillin, oral contraceptives, and cyclosporine.

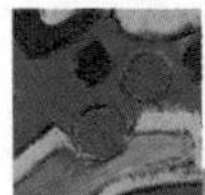

PATIENT/FAMILY TEACHING

The Patient With Thrombocytopenia

Patient teaching should include information about:

- The nature of thrombocytopenia
- Signs of decreased platelet count (petechiae, ecchymoses, gingival bleeding, hematuria, hypermenorrhea)
- The name, dosage, frequency, and side effects of prescribed medications and the importance of not stopping corticosteroid medications abruptly
- Guidelines for preventing injury, such as:
  - —Use a soft toothbrush or swab for mouth care.
  - —Do not use dental floss.
  - —Keep mouth clean and free of debris.
  - —Avoid intrusions into rectum (e.g., rectal medications, enemas).
  - —Use an electric shaver.
  - —Apply direct pressure for 5 to 10 minutes if any bleeding occurs.
  - —Avoid contact sports, elective surgery, and tooth extraction.
  - —Avoid blood-thinning drugs, such as aspirin, which decrease sticking ability of platelets.
  - —Increase knowledge of contents of over-the-counter medications and effects on platelet function.
- The need for follow-up medical care

Pathophysiology. The underlying problem in TTP relates to the depletion of circulating platelets as a result of abnormal clotting processes. The cause of the abnormality in the clotting process is unknown but is thought to be related to vascular injury and hypercoagulability of circulating platelets. The resulting platelet aggregation results in thrombus formation; the thrombus then lodges in the microvasculature of susceptible organs, such as the heart, brain, kidneys, pancreas, and adrenal glands. Symptoms of the disease include fever (with no infection noted), anemia, nausea, anorexia, weakness, petechiae, and hematuria. Additional symptoms are related to the organ involved and include kidney failure and neurologic changes.

Collaborative Care Management. Diagnosis of TTP is made by peripheral blood smear. Findings include low platelet counts and red cell fragmentation. Other laboratory features are anemia, reticulocytosis, increased serum lactate dehydrogenase (LDH), normal or increased blood urea nitrogen, and increased fibrin degradation products (FDPs).

Plasma exchange using fresh frozen plasma is the treatment of choice for TTP. Survival rates are about 85%.[11] Treatment is most effective if it is initiated as soon as TTP is suspected. Exchanges should be continued until platelet counts and serum LDH levels are near normal. Other therapies include vincristine, cyclosporine, azathioprine, immunoglobulin, and splenectomy. Monitoring the patient's mental status is important because coma associated with TTP is not uncommon. Monitoring renal and cardiac function is necessary for early treatment of complications. Renal dysfunction occurs in 50% to 75% of patients with TTP.

Patients may require prolonged treatment with plasma exchanges and may require placement of central venous access devices. Patients and families need to be taught correct management of these devices. Other points to be included in the teaching are listed in the Patient/Family Teaching box at left.

Coagulation Disorders

Hemophilia

Etiology and Epidemiology. Hemophilia is a hereditary coagulation disorder. Hemophilia A (factor VIII deficiency), hemophilia B (factor IX deficiency), and hemophilia C (factor XI deficiency) are inherited as sex-linked recessive disorders and are therefore almost exclusively limited to males (Figure 33-4). The incidence of hemophilia A is 1:10,000 of the male population, and for hemophilia B, 1:100,000. Hemophilia C is rare, with an incidence of 2% to 3% of all hemophilias. The most common "other" form of hemophilia is von Willebrand's disease (vWD), which affects 1% to 3% of the U.S. population but is often overlooked or undertreated in women. In vWD there is a lack of von Willebrand's factor or the factor does not function as it should in platelet adhesion or as a carrier of factor VIII.

Pathophysiology. The diagnosis of hemophilia usually is made in infancy or early childhood. The clinical history is one of lifelong bleeding tendency. A history of excessive bleeding after circumcision or dental extractions commonly is obtained. Persons with hemophilia may give a history of bleeding into any part of

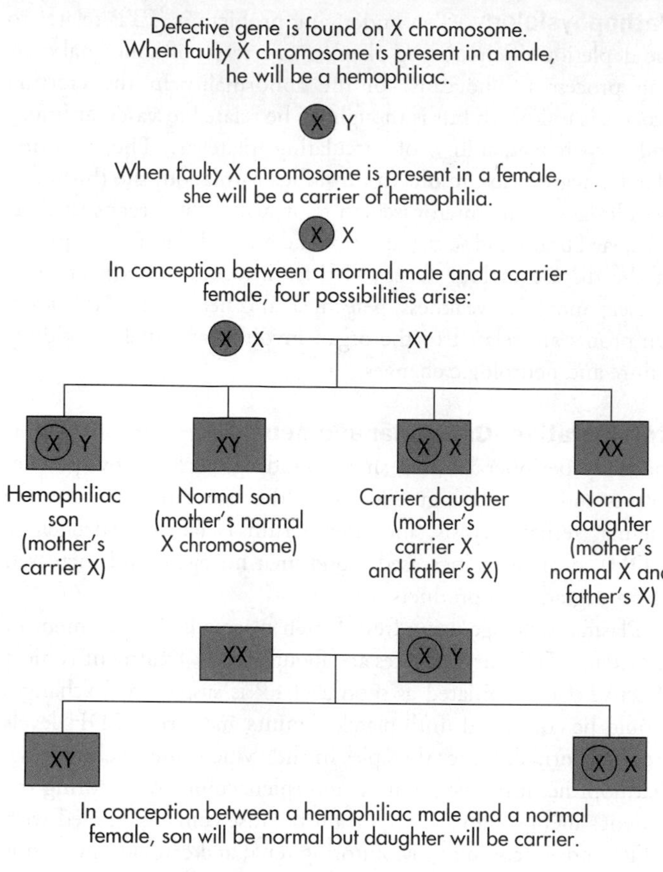
Defective gene is found on X chromosome.
When faulty X chromosome is present in a male, he will be a hemophiliac.
X Y
When faulty X chromosome is present in a female, she will be a carrier of hemophilia.
X X
In conception between a normal male and a carrier female, four possibilities arise:
X X
XY
X Y
XY
X X
XX
Hemophiliac son (mother's carrier X)
Normal son (mother's normal X chromosome)
Carrier daughter (mother's carrier X and father's X)
Normal daughter (mother's normal X and father's X)
XX
X Y
XY
X X
In conception between a hemophiliac male and a normal female, son will be normal but daughter will be carrier.

Figure 33-4 Pattern of inheritance of hemophilia.

the body—spontaneously or after trauma (see Clinical Manifestations box). Women with vWD often have a history of easy bruisability, heavy menstrual flow, or postpartum hemorrhage.

A diagnosis of hemophilia is made by specific assays for factors VIII, IX, and XI. The partial thromboplastin time (PTT), which reflects the intrinsic pathway of coagulation, is prolonged in hemophilia A, hemophilia B, and hemophilia C. The platelet count and prothrombin time (PT) are normal.

Complications associated with hemophilia are the direct result of the bleeding tendency. Commonly the person experiences repeated episodes of spontaneous bleeding into the joints, resulting in joint deformities. Life-threatening bleeding involves retroperitoneal, intracranial, and peritracheal soft tissue hemorrhages.

Collaborative Care Management. Treatment is replacement of the deficient coagulation factor when bleeding episodes do not respond to local treatment (ice bags, manual pressure or dressings, immobilization, elevation, or topical coagulants such as

CLINICAL MANIFESTATIONS
Hemophilia

- History of lifelong bleeding tendency
- Repeated episodes of spontaneous bleeding into joints
- Excessive bleeding after dental extractions
- Life-threatening hemorrhages: retroperitoneal, intracranial, peritracheal

fibrin foam and thrombin). Because the deficient factors are contained in plasma, the treatment used for many years was fresh plasma and blood or fresh frozen plasma. In major hemorrhages adequate blood levels were difficult to maintain without overloading the person's circulation with large volumes of blood and plasma. The discovery of cryoprecipitate in 1964 led the way to the development of commercially prepared concentrated preparations such as fibrinogen, factor VIII, and a concentrate containing the four vitamin K–dependent factors (factors II, VII, IX, and X). Concentrates avoid the problem of circulatory overload and produce fewer adverse effects (e.g., urticarial or febrile reactions) in some patients.

In the 1980s the possibility of contamination with a hepatitis virus or human immunodeficiency virus (HIV) was a drawback to the use of some pooled blood concentrates. A number of persons with hemophilia A developed AIDS from transfusions of factor VIII concentrate. This problem has been corrected with the testing of blood donors for evidence of HIV and with heat treatment of the factor VIII concentrates, which kills HIV. The ability to test for the hepatitis C virus has decreased the per-unit risk for developing the disease to 0.001%.

In classic hemophilia the treatment of choice for an acute bleeding episode is infusion of concentrates of the antihemophilic factor (AHF) (factor VIII). One such concentrate is cryoprecipitate, with a concentration of AHF 15 to 40 times that of normal plasma. Two new recombinant products made from clones of factor VIII are now on the market (Recombinate and Kogenate). In 1997 a recombinant factor IX was approved for use. The use of these recombinant factors has eliminated most, if not all, danger of transmission of HIV or hepatitis (viral) C to patients.

DDAVP (D-amino-8-D-arginine vasopressin) has been demonstrated to increase the factor VIII level in persons with vWD and mild hemophilia A. It is given nasally for mild cases and intravenously for moderate or severe cases. DDAVP does not carry the risk of transmitting hepatitis, AIDS, or other disorders.

The outlook for the person with hemophilia has been greatly improved by the availability of transfusion and recombinant therapy. In the past many persons with factor VIII deficiency died in infancy or in the first 5 years of life. Surgical procedures can now be performed to prevent joint deformity, thus increasing quality of life. Today many persons with moderate or mild hemophilia live normal, productive lives.

Adults with hemophilia generally are knowledgeable about their disease. They should be aware of the possibility of hemorrhage after dental extraction, injury, or surgery. They should carry a card or wear a Medic-Alert tag that includes their name, blood type, physician's name, and disorder to avoid delay in medical treatment if they accidentally sustain injury and lose consciousness.

Pain control and the threat of spontaneous bleeding episodes are ongoing stressors the person must confront. Those persons who are able to meet the demands of their illness and adapt their lifestyles accordingly are able to live productive lives. Genetic counseling, aimed at explaining the pattern of inheritance of hemophilia, can help potential parents realistically evaluate their ability to raise a child afflicted with hemophilia and to anticipate ways to meet the demands placed on both them and the child.

The National Hemophilia Foundation (www.hemophilia.org) is an organization dedicated to hemophilia research and other functions, including the establishment of standards for chapters, publication of literature, production of films, and promotion of federal health care legislation. Local chapter services include special camps for children with hemophilia; parent, child, and adult counseling; group therapy sessions for parents; and a newsletter that reports advances in hemophilic care. A chapter may function as a liaison between hospitals and families with insurmountable bills.

Vitamin K Deficiency

Etiology and Epidemiology. **Vitamin K**, a fat-soluble vitamin, is a cofactor in the synthesis of clotting factors II, VII, IX, and X. Approximately 50% of required vitamin K is obtained from a normal diet, and 50% is produced by intestinal bacteria. Vitamin K deficiencies can be anticipated in persons who have a decreased intake and who are given broad-spectrum antibiotics (such as neomycin sulfate) that decrease the growth of intestinal bacteria. Interference with vitamin K absorption occurs with primary intestinal disease (e.g., ulcerative colitis, Crohn's disease), biliary disease, and malabsorption syndromes. Drugs such as coumarin derivatives and large doses of salicylates, quinine, and barbiturates interfere with vitamin K function.

Pathophysiology. Symptoms of vitamin K deficiency are those of hypoprothrombinemia superimposed on the underlying disease. Bleeding is similar to that of other coagulation disorders (i.e., bleeding of the mucous membranes and into the tissues). Postoperative hemorrhage may be observed. In severe cases GI bleeding may be massive.

Collaborative Care Management. A prolonged PT and PTT are diagnostic features of vitamin K deficiency. The levels of vitamin K–dependent clotting factors are also decreased. Treatment consists of therapy for the underlying disorder and cessation of causative drugs. For mild disorders a water-soluble vitamin K preparation (menadione) is given orally or parenterally. In severe disorders a fat-soluble vitamin K preparation (phytonadione) may be given. Fresh frozen plasma will partially correct the disorder immediately, whereas vitamin K therapy, which does not have the complications of fresh frozen plasma, takes 6 to 24 hours to be effective.

Nursing management includes monitoring vital signs and patient teaching regarding safety precautions to prevent bruising or bleeding episodes. The nurse instructs the patient to avoid trauma, use a soft-bristled toothbrush, avoid intramuscular injections, and apply direct pressure immediately on any bleeding sites.

Disseminated Intravascular Coagulation

DIC is a response of the body's hemostatic mechanisms to a variety of diseases or injuries. DIC is a complicated and potentially fatal process characterized first by clotting and secondarily by hemorrhage. It always occurs in response to another disease or condition.[3]

Etiology and Epidemiology. DIC is essentially an imbalance between the processes of coagulation and anticoagulation. Many disease states alter the normal balance of clotting and fibrinolytic factors, which under normal conditions prevents bleeding while maintaining the fluidity of the blood. DIC may be directly or indirectly initiated by conditions that trigger at least one of three mechanisms: factor XII formation, activation of factors II and X, or tissue thromboplastin release. A stimulus such as sepsis, anoxia, or a burn most likely causes activation of the intrinsic clotting system by the release of factor XII after endothelial cell wall damage and platelet aggregation. DIC may be caused by factor VII activation from massive trauma or the release of tissue thromboplastin from an amniotic fluid embolus entering the maternal circulation. Proteolytic enzymes in snake venom can cause direct activation of factors II and X (Box 33-5). Mortality rates vary because of the multiple precipitating factors associated with DIC. Death usually results from uncontrolled bleeding or multiple organ failure.

Pathophysiology. The primary disease initiates the clotting process. This response is generalized and occurs throughout the vascular system, creating a state of hypercoagulability. The fibrinolytic processes, which normally operate to limit clot extension and dissolve clots, are then stimulated (Figure 33-5). As clotting factors are depleted and fibrinolysis continues, a state of hypocoagulability develops.

The most common sequela of DIC is hemorrhage. This paradox is caused by (1) decreased platelets; (2) depletion of clotting factors II, V, VIII, and fibrinogen in the clotting process; and (3) the production of FDPs through fibrinolysis. The FDPs act as anticoagulants and increase the hemorrhagic tendency.

As the disorder progresses, clinical manifestations may include bleeding of the mucous membranes and tissues, manifested as petechiae and ecchymoses; oral, GI, genitourinary, and rectal bleeding; and bleeding after injections and venipunctures. Hypoxia, tachypnea, hemoptysis, hypotension, acidosis, and fever may also be present (see Clinical Manifestations box).

Box 33-5 Common Precipitating Factors Associated With Disseminated Intravascular Coagulation

Infections
- Hepatitis
- Sepsis
- Gram-negative infections
- Glomerulonephritis

Neoplastic
- Adenocarcinoma
- Acute leukemias
- Pheochromocytoma

Other Factors
- Snakebites
- Blood transfusion reaction
- Surgery
- Anaphylaxis
- Polycythemia vera
- Shock

Obstetric
- Retained dead fetus
- Abruptio placentae
- Amniotic fluid embolus
- Toxemia
- Septic abortion

Vascular
- Aortic aneurysm
- Fat embolus
- Vasculitis

Trauma
- Crush injury
- Brain injury
- Burns
- Ischemia

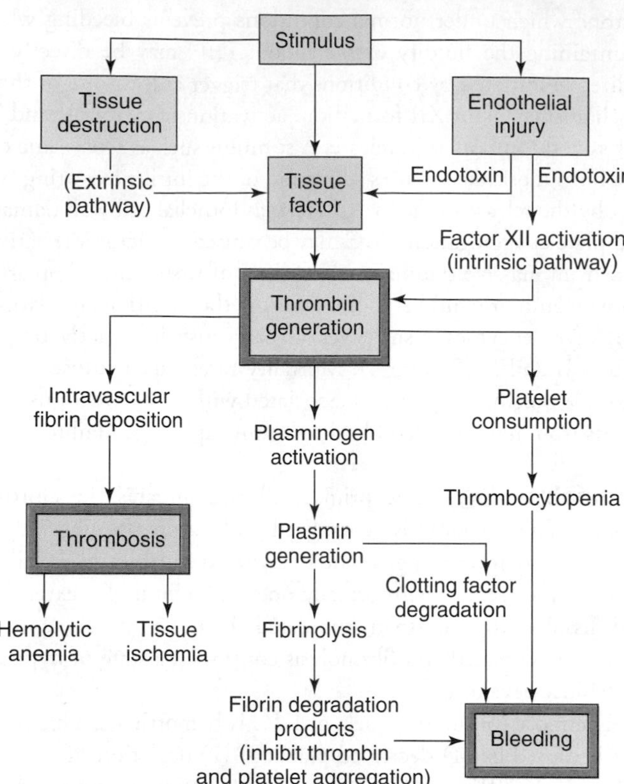

Figure 33-5 Pathophysiology of disseminated intravascular coagulation.

Collaborative Care Management. Clinical suspicion of DIC is confirmed by laboratory findings (Table 33-8). Abnormal RBCs may be found on a peripheral smear; fibrinolysis may be reflected in increased FDPs, increased D-dimers, and a prolonged thrombin time. The management of DIC always begins with treatment of the primary disease. Once this has been initiated, the goal is to control the bleeding and restore normal levels of clotting factors. Blood products such as fresh frozen plasma, platelet packs, cryoprecipitate, and fresh whole blood may be administered to replace the depleted factors. Heparin has been used to inhibit the underlying thrombotic process; however, it too often promotes rather than decreases bleeding, and its use is controversial.

Nursing management is extremely challenging for the patient with DIC, who is critically ill and commonly has numerous sites of bleeding. The nurse should note and record the amount and nature of drainage from chest and nasogastric tubes, oozing from surgical incisions, and progressive discoloration of the skin. Continual observation for new bleeding sites and for an increase or decrease in bleeding is an integral part of the nursing plan, especially if heparin therapy is being used. These persons' susceptibility to bleeding presents special problems; medications should be given orally or intravenously if at all possible, and small-gauge needles should be used when other injections are necessary. The precautions previously described for patients with thrombocytopenia are applicable to patients with DIC (see the Patient/Family Teaching box on p. 925.

Maintaining fluid balance assumes great importance. Persons with DIC usually lose large quantities of blood and receive frequent transfusions and other fluid replacement. In addition to monitoring blood infusion rates carefully, the nurse must be alert for signs of fluid overload, such as a slow, bounding pulse and increasing central venous pressure. The nurse records hourly urinary output not only as another indication of cardiac function but also because of the possibility of renal thrombi formation and subsequent kidney failure.

Commonly the patient is comatose, and the presence of purpura, numerous intravenous lines, and drainage tubes makes the patient's appearance especially upsetting to the family. Most of the primary conditions associated with DIC are sudden, and the family requires preparation and help in understanding this catastrophic occurrence. Emotional support of the family is paramount because of the sudden onset of DIC. Depending on the cause and severity of DIC, the family may need support and referrals during the grieving process.

Disorders Associated With White Blood Cells

The WBC (leukocyte) system is composed of neutrophils, lymphocytes, monocytes, basophils, and eosinophils. All but the lymphocytes derive from a common stem cell. The primary function of WBCs is to provide for humoral and cellular response to infection. Neutrophils are primarily responsible for phagocytosis and the destruction of bacteria and other infectious organisms. **Lymphocytes** are the principal cells involved in immunity, which is responsible for the development of delayed hypersensitivity and the production of antibodies. Any compromise in the integrity of the WBC system renders a person susceptible to infection.

Neutropenia

Etiology and Epidemiology. Neutropenia is defined as a neutrophil count of less than $2000/mm^3$. Neutropenia may occur as a primary hematologic disorder, but more often it is associated with other disorders, including malignant diseases of the bone marrow, aplastic anemia, megaloblastic anemia, use of chemotherapeutic agents, and hypersplenism.

Pathophysiology. Severe neutropenia, sometimes referred to as agranulocytosis, occurs as a reaction to a variety of drugs and chemicals, including sulfonamides, propylthiouracil, and chloramphenicol. The degree of susceptibility to infection is in direct proportion to the degree of neutropenia. Persons with severe neutropenia are at risk of contracting a life-threatening infection.

Collaborative Care Management. Specific treatment consists of removing the offending agent. Granulocyte transfusion may be used for the patient with severe, life-threatening neutropenia. Neutropenic precautions are instituted to protect the patient from infection.

A person with a compromised WBC system is highly susceptible to life-threatening infections. Teaching focuses on avoiding potential sources of infection and recognizing the earliest signs of infection. If infection is suspected, the patient should report to the primary health care provider. Meticulous hand washing by hospital personnel and visitors is mandatory. The environment should be kept scrupulously clean and dustless, and persons with

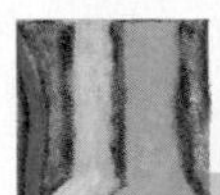

CLINICAL MANIFESTATIONS *Disseminated Intravascular Coagulation*

Neurologic

Confusion
Irritability
Headache
Dizziness
Seizures
Fevers
Increased intracranial pressure
Vertigo
Decreased level of consciousness

Sensory

Blurred vision, intraocular hemorrhage
Inner ear bleeding
Conjunctival hemorrhage
Epistaxis

Cardiovascular

Tachycardia
Chest pain
Hypotension
Absence of peripheral pulses
Abnormal or increased bleeding from venipuncture or intravenous insertion sites

Respiratory

Hemoptysis
Diffuse infiltrates on x-ray study
Hypoxia
Dyspnea
Tachypnea
Pulmonary embolus
Pulmonary edema

Genitourinary

Progressive oliguria
Hematuria
Kidney failure
Bleeding around indwelling Foley catheters
Severe bleeding during menstruation
Vaginal bleeding
Proteinuria

Gastrointestinal

Melena
High-pitched bowel sounds
Nausea
Vomiting
Abdominal distention
Hematemesis

Integumentary

Cool, moist skin
Cyanosis
Petechiae
Mottling
Ecchymoses
Purpura

General

Acidosis
Acral cyanosis

TABLE 33-8 LABORATORY PROFILE OF DISSEMINATED INTRAVASCULAR COAGULATION

Diagnostic Test	Normal Value	Expected Value in DIC
Bleeding time (Ivy method)	1-9 min	Prolonged
Platelet count	150,000-400,000/mm^3	Decreased
Prothrombin time	11-12.5 sec	Prolonged
Partial thromboplastin time (PTT)	PTT: 60-70 sec aPTT: 30-40 sec	Prolonged
Factor assay (I, II, V, VII, VIII, IX, X, XI, XII, XIII)		Decreased levels of factors I, II, V, VIII, X, and XIII
Fibrinogen level	200-400 mg/dl	Decreased
Fibrinogin/fibrin degradation products	<10 mg/ml	Increased
RBC smear		Damaged RBC
Euglobulin lysis time	>2 hr	Normal or prolonged
D-Dimer	Qualitative—Negative Quantitative—<250 ng/ml	Increased
Thrombin time	10-12 sec	Usually prolonged

Data from Pagana KD, Pagana TJ: *Mosby's manual of diagnostic and laboratory tests*, ed 2, St Louis, 2002, Mosby.
aPTT, Activated partial thromboplastin time; *DIC,* Disseminated intravascular coagulation; *RBC,* red blood cell.

any type of infection should not be allowed contact with the patient. Family members and hospital personnel need frequent reminders of this. Mild colds and respiratory tract infections, taken for granted in daily life, are serious threats to patients with decreased numbers of WBCs.

Patients should be in private rooms with posted neutropenic precautions. When this is not possible, cautious screening of roommates for a potential source of infection is mandatory. The patient should be instructed to wear a mask whenever leaving his or her room. To decrease the risk of exposure to bacteria, fresh fruits, vegetables, and flowers are not permitted.

Neutrophilia

Neutrophilia is defined as a neutrophil count greater than 10,000/mm^3. Such an increase is a normal response to infections, primarily bacterial infections. Prolonged elevation of the neutrophil count, especially in the absence of an apparent cause, demands a diligent search for the underlying cause. Persistent elevated neutrophil counts are associated with leukemia, polycythemia vera, myeloid metaplasia, and various systemic and inflammatory disorders.

Leukemias

An estimated 34,810 new cases of leukemia were diagnosed in the United States during 2005. The survival rate for leukemia patients 50 years ago was 0%. A study from 1960 through 1963 showed leukemia patients had a 14% chance of living 5 years. Forty years later the 5-year survival rates have more than tripled.[7] Leukemia is most common in Caucasian males.

Leukemia is a malignant disorder of the hematopoietic system involving the bone marrow and lymph nodes; it is characterized by uncontrolled proliferation of leukocytes, myelocytes, and their precursors. With rare exceptions the bone marrow is involved at the onset, with infrequent manifestations in other hematopoietic organs that lead to organ enlargement (splenomegaly, hepatomegaly). The proliferation of one type of cell often interferes with the normal production of other hematopoietic cells, resulting in the development of immature cells, thrombocytopenia, and anemia. The immaturity of the WBCs leads to decreased immunocompetence and increased susceptibility to infections.

The cause of leukemia is unknown, but some predisposing relationships have been discovered. Persons with specific chromosomal aberrations, such as occur with Down syndrome, von Recklinghausen's neurofibromatosis, and Fanconi's anemia, have an increased incidence of acute leukemia.[13] Chronic exposure to chemicals such as benzene, drugs that cause aplastic anemia, and radiation has been associated with an increased incidence of the disease. An increased risk for development of acute leukemia also has been noted after cytotoxic therapy for Hodgkin's disease; non-Hodgkin's lymphoma; multiple myeloma; polycythemia vera; and breast, lung, and testicular cancers.

Leukemia is a broad term with a complex disease classification system. However, the disease can be grouped into four primary categories according to the dominant type of WBC involvement and the rate of cell growth. Basically the four kinds of leukemia are lymphoblastic (also known as lymphocytic), myelogenous, acute, and chronic. The four major types or categories are acute lymphoblastic leukemia (ALL), acute myelogenous leukemia (AML), chronic lymphoblastic leukemia (CLL), and chronic myelogenous leukemia (CML).

Cancerous changes in lymphocytes develop into the lymphoblastic leukemias. When granulocytes and monocytes are the predominant type of cell undergoing malignant transformation, the leukemia is classified as myelogenous. Leukemia is either acute or chronic according to the progression of cell differentiation. Acute leukemia, which affects immature cells, has a rapid onset and progression. In chronic leukemia more mature cells are affected and cell growth progresses slowly. These mature cells, although abnormal, can still carry on some normal cell functions. Thus the chronic form of leukemia may progress over many years.

Acute leukemias have a rapid onset and a short course ending in death if untreated. The paucity of normal WBCs leads to numerous infections such as pneumonia and septicemia. Early symptoms include fever and bruising from low WBC and platelet counts; lymphadenopathy; and pallor, malaise, and fatigue from anemia. The WBC count may be normal, decreased, or increased. Other symptoms include bone pain, increased abdominal girth from oliguria, hepatosplenomegaly, dehydration, DIC, central nervous system symptoms of nausea and vomiting, headache, and blurred vision.

Chronic leukemias have a more insidious onset. The MST is 3 to 4 years for patients with CML and 2 to 10 years for those with CLL, depending on the stage at diagnosis. Nonspecific flulike symptoms are the usual presentation of chronic leukemia. Early signs include fatigue, weakness, anorexia, and weight loss characteristic of a chronic hypermetabolic state. An enlarged spleen and liver usually can be palpated. The WBC count usually is considerably elevated. See Table 33-9 for a synopsis of the four types of leukemia, symptoms, cell type, and commonly used chemotherapeutics.

Acute Lymphoblastic Leukemia

Etiology and Epidemiology. As mentioned earlier, the etiology of ALL is unknown. Eighty percent of persons affected by ALL are between 2 and 4 years of age. An estimated 3970 cases occur annually.[2] The incidence of the disease declines past the age of 10 years.

Pathophysiology. ALL is a malignant disorder arising from a single lymphoid stem cell with impaired maturation and accumulation of the malignant cells in the bone marrow. Diagnosis is confirmed by bone marrow aspiration or biopsy, which typically shows different stages of lymphoid development, from very immature to almost normal cells. The degree of immaturity is a guide to the prognosis: the greater the number of immature cells (increased percentage of lymphocytes and presence of blast cells on a peripheral smear and bone marrow aspiration), the poorer the prognosis.

Signs and symptoms of ALL include anemia, bleeding, lymphadenopathy, and a predisposition to infection. A blood smear may show immature lymphoblasts. The platelet count and Hct level are reduced in most patients.

Collaborative Care Management. Perhaps more dramatically than in any other malignant disorder, chemotherapy has improved the prognosis of children with ALL. Untreated patients

TABLE 33-9 CLINICAL MANIFESTATIONS AND COMMON CHEMOTHERAPEUTIC AGENTS USED IN DIFFERENT LEUKEMIAS

Leukemia	Peak Age (yr)	Characteristic Symptoms	WBC Level	Bone Marrow Cell Predominance	Common Chemotherapeutic Agents
Acute lymphoblastic leukemia (ALL)	2-4	Fever, infections of respiratory tract, anemia, bleeding of mucous membranes, ecchymoses, lymphadenopathy	Decreased, normal, or increased	Lymphoblasts	Regimens with vincristine and prednisone, 6-mercaptopurine, methotrexate
Acute myelogenous leukemia (AML)	12-20, after 55	Same as ALL except less lymphadenopathy	Increased, normal, or decreased	Myeloblasts	Cytarabine, 6-thioguanine, doxorubicin (Adriamycin), daunomycin
Chronic lymphoblastic leukemia (CLL)	50-70	Weakness, fatigue, lymphadenopathy, pruritic vesicular skin lesions, thrombocytopenia, anemia, splenomegaly	Increased (20,000-100,000/mm^3)	Lymphocytes	Alkylating agents (e.g., chlorambucil), glucocorticoids
Chronic myelogenous leukemia (CML)	30-50	Weakness, fatigue, anorexia, weight loss, splenomegaly	Increased (15,000-500,000/mm^3)	Granulocytes	Hydroxyurea (Droxia) and imatinib (Gleevec); busulfan (Busulflex) (rarely used now)

WBC, White blood cell.

have a MST of 4 to 6 months. With current chemotherapy regimens, the MST is close to 5 years, approximately 50% of children with ALL can be cured, and complete remissions are obtained in more than 90% of patients.[2]

Chemotherapeutic protocols for ALL involve three phases: (1) induction, often using vincristine and prednisone; (2) consolidation, using a modified course of intensive therapy to eradicate any remaining disease; and (3) maintenance, usually a combination of drugs, usually including the antimetabolites 6-mercaptopurine and methotrexate. In most chemotherapeutic regimens, vincristine and prednisone are administered intermittently during the maintenance program. Appropriate duration of therapy in patients who remain disease free remains unsettled, but in most centers it is approximately 3 years. The use of "prophylactic" treatment of the central nervous system (e.g., intrathecal administration of methotrexate with or without craniospinal radiation) has greatly diminished recurrences. Because the blood-brain barrier does not allow parenterally infused chemotherapy to reach the leukemic cells, the central nervous system acts as a sanctuary for the leukemia. Intrathecal administration of chemotherapy, craniospinal radiation, or both eradicate the leukemic cells.[9]

Patient teaching is an important component of patient care (see Patient/Family Teaching box).

▶ ARE YOU READY?

In evaluating a patient's laboratory results, the nurse associates which of the following findings with acute lymphoblastic leukemia? (Choose all that apply.)

1. Anemia
2. Thrombocytosis
3. Decreased bleeding time
4. Decreased hematocrit
5. Leukocytosis
6. Immature lymphoblasts

Acute Myelogenous Leukemia

Etiology and Epidemiology. AML is a disease of the pluripotent myeloid stem cell. The cause of the malignant transformation is unknown. AML can occur at any age but occurs most often at adolescence and after age 55. An estimated 11,960 cases occur

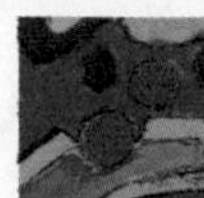

PATIENT/FAMILY TEACHING
The Patient With Leukemia

Patient teaching should include information about:
- The nature of the disease process and the effects of therapy
- How to prevent infection and bleeding
- Symptoms requiring immediate medical attention (fever, bleeding)
- Medications: name, side effects, etc.
- Importance of good nutrition and adequate fluid intake
- How to do meticulous oral care to prevent stomatitis
- Regimen of chemotherapy administration and periodic blood counts
- Available community resources (American Cancer Society, Leukemia and Lymphoma Society)
- The need for regular medical follow-up care

annually.[2] Other terms for AML include *acute nonlymphocytic, acute granulocytic*, and *acute myelocytic leukemia*.

Pathophysiology. AML arises from a single myeloid stem cell and is characterized by the development of immature myeloblasts in the bone marrow. Clinical manifestations are the same as for ALL (see Table 33-9). The WBC count may be low, normal, or high. Bone marrow aspiration reveals a significant increase in myeloblasts.

Collaborative Care Management. Therapy includes the use of cytarabine, and doxorubicin or daunorubicin (see Future Watch box, below). Elderly patients who cannot tolerate the severity of the therapy may elect to take hydroxyurea (which has a lower cure rate, but results in few early deaths and a better quality of life). Complete remission occurs in 50% to 75% of treated patients, and the MST is approximately 2 to 3 years. Approximately 20% of patients are in complete remission at 5 years and are capable of prolonged disease-free periods (remission). Although patients in remission clearly have an improved quality of life, induction of therapy is arduous, often requiring weeks in the hospital with intensive supportive care (blood component replacement and antibiotic therapy).

BMT with the use of HLA-identical allogeneic bone marrow is being used with increasing frequency. Transplanting the patient's own (autologous) bone marrow obtained after a remission with chemotherapy or radiotherapy is another option. Several studies have shown the advantages of BMT with the benefits of colony-stimulating factor, as compared with salvage chemotherapy. Autologous peripheral stem cell transplantation is a method of retrieving stem cells from the patient's blood. The blood undergoes centrifuge to remove cancerous clones and is then stored for reinfusion after the patient's bone marrow has been destroyed. In the untreated patient or the patient who is unresponsive to therapy, the MST is approximately 2 to 3 months.[10]

Patient teaching is an important component of patient care (see Patient/Family Teaching box for patients with leukemia, at left).

Future Watch

Garlic Remedy

Garlic has been used since early Egyptian times as a remedy for tumors. Several types of garlic compounds have been shown to inhibit tumor growth through apoptosis in a variety of types of cancers. Ajoene, a garlic-derived compound, demonstrated some effect in clinical trials using the compound topically for skin cancer. Now trials are testing its use in leukemia. It has been shown to inhibit proliferation and induce apoptosis in the myeloblasts in patients with chronic myeloid leukemia. It also enhanced the effect of other antineoplastic drugs such as cytarabine and fludarabine. Researchers continue to test the drug's effectiveness in clinical trials in acute myeloid leukemia (AML). They predict it could be the new antileukemia agent for AML in the future.

Hassan HTA: Ajoene (natural garlic compound): a new anti-leukemia agent for AML therapy, *Leukemia Res* 28(7):667, 2004.

Chronic Lymphoblastic Leukemia

Etiology and Epidemiology. As with other types of leukemia, the etiology of CLL is unknown. An estimated 8190 new cases occur annually.[3] The incidence of CLL increases with age; it is rare under age 45. Approximately 95% of CLL patients are older than 50 years.[2] CLL is more common in men than in women.

Pathophysiology. CLL is characterized by a proliferation of small, abnormal, mature B lymphocytes, often leading to decreased synthesis of immunoglobulins and depressed antibody response. The accumulation of abnormal lymphocytes begins in the lymph nodes, then spreads to other lymphatic tissues and the spleen. The number of mature lymphocytes in the peripheral blood smear and bone marrow is greatly increased.

The onset is insidious, with weakness, fatigue, and lymphadenopathy. Symptoms include pruritic vesicular skin lesions, anemia, thrombocytopenia, and an enlarged spleen (see Table 33-9). The WBC count is elevated to between 20,000 and 100,000/mm^3; this increases blood viscosity, and a clotting episode may be the first manifestation of disease. Bone marrow biopsy shows infiltration of lymphocytes.

Collaborative Care Management. The MST of persons with CLL is 4.5 to 5.5 years. As a rule, persons are treated only when symptoms appear, particularly anemia, thrombocytopenia, or enlarged lymph nodes and spleen. Chemotherapeutic agents used in the treatment of CLL are most often one of the alkylating agents, such as chlorambucil, or one of the glucocorticoids (see Future Watch box, p. 933). Although no treatment is curative, remissions may be induced by chemotherapeutics or radiation of the thymus, spleen, or entire body.

Patient teaching is an important component of patient care (see Patient/Family Teaching box for patients with leukemia, at left). Education is necessary regarding the course of the disease and benefits and possible side effects of treatment. This is especially important because of the age of the affected population and the advantages of conservative therapy. Some persons do well without treatment, especially if they are asymptomatic.

Future Watch

Pivanex for Leukemia

Pivaloyloxymethyl butyrate (Pivanex), an anticancer agent, inhibits histone delacetylases (HDAC) in the cells. HDAC is a group of enzymes that augment cell growth. By slowing HDAC proliferation, Pivanex retards tumor growth, causing destruction of cancer cells. Thus far, Pivanex has demonstrated some positive results in this process. This clinical trial will study the effectiveness of Pivanex versus docetaxel alone and Pivanex plus docetaxel in the treatment of chronic lymphoblastic leukemia (CLL) and malignant melanoma. Preliminary research has shown Pivanex to be effective in treating CLL. Since CLL is the most common form of leukemia in the United States, researchers are hoping the clinical trials will prove the drug is an effective new treatment for this disease.

Phase II clinical studies to study Pivanex in leukemia and melanoma, *Cancer Weekly* June 22, 2004, p. 22.

Chronic Myelogenous Leukemia

Etiology and Epidemiology. Research has found that CML results from an acquired injury to the DNA of a stem cell in the bone marrow. Scientists do not understand what produces this change, but they do know that this injury is not inherited and is not present at birth. The Philadelphia chromosome, a translocation of chromosomes 22 and 9, distinguishes CML from other types of leukemia.[7]

CML accounts for approximately 14% of all cases of leukemia. The incidence is about 4600 cases per year. The frequency of CML increases with age from about 1/1,000,000 children in the first decade of life, to 1/100,000 at age 50, and 1/10,000 at 80 years of age or older.[3,7]

Pathophysiology. The primary defect in CML is an abnormal stem cell leading to uncontrolled proliferation of the granulocytic cells. As a result of this proliferation, the number of circulating granulocytes increases sharply.

CML is characterized by the classic symptoms of chronic types of leukemia, including fatigue, weakness, anorexia, weight loss, and splenomegaly (Table 33-10). The WBC ranges from 15,000 to 500,000/mm^3, depending on the stage of the disease. The peripheral blood smear demonstrates granulocytes in varying degrees of maturity, from blast cells to mature neutrophils, and granulocytic hyperplasia in the bone marrow.

CML commonly changes from a chronic indolent phase into an accelerated phase that progresses rapidly into a fulminant neoplastic process sometimes indistinguishable from an acute leukemia. The accelerated phase of the disease (blastic phase) is characterized by increasing numbers of granulocytes in the peripheral blood, often with a corresponding anemia and thrombocytopenia. Fever and adenopathy also may develop. Of patients with CML, 50% to 60% progress to the blastic phase. Once the CML enters the blastic phase, the chemotherapeutic regimen is similar to that of AML.

The overall survival rate for CML is poor. Only 30% of patients survive 5 years after diagnosis. After the onset of a blast crisis, the life expectancy decreases to 2 to 4 months. Imatinib (Gleevec) was approved by the Food and Drug Administration under its "accelerated approval" regulations in May 2001. Imatinib is approved for the treatment of three stages of CML: CML myeloid blast crisis, CML accelerated phase, and CML in the chronic phase after failure of treatment with interferon. Imatinib inhibits the translocation-created enzyme and blocks the rapid growth of WBCs. The long-term efficacy of the drug has not yet been tested, but individuals in the three stages of CML for which the drug is intended are often rapidly approaching terminal disease if standard treatments do not induce remission. Clinical trials have indicated that many patients will improve.[3]

Complications of CML include those associated with treatment options. Hemorrhage, infection, and mucositis can occur as a result of chemotherapy or the disease process. During the blast phase, lytic bone lesions, soft tissue infiltrates, and epidural tumors causing cord compression may complicate the course of the disease. Prognosis in this phase is grave. Widespread organ damage may occur, caused by large numbers of leukemic cells occluding the vasculature.

Collaborative Care Management

DIAGNOSTIC TESTS. Table 33-11 describes diagnostic tests for CML.

MEDICATIONS. The goal of treatment for CML is to control the proliferation of WBCs. Two commonly used medications used are hydroxyurea and busulfan. Of these two, hydroxyurea is most commonly used because of the high incidence of toxic side effects associated with busulfan. The major side effect of hydroxyurea is reversible myelosuppression. Busulfan toxicity includes potentially fatal myelosuppression, organ fibrosis (lung, heart, and bone marrow), and a wasting syndrome similar to Addison's disease. Patients taking hydroxyurea must be instructed about compliance with daily medications and have their blood counts monitored at frequent intervals.

Once CML has converted to the blast phase of the disease, aggressive therapy becomes necessary. Anthracyclines and cytosine arabinoside have been used, but with less than a 20% remission rate. Some success has been seen with the use of the biologic response modifier interferon-alpha, and current studies are further evaluating the long-term effects of this medication. Toxicity

TABLE 33-10 SYMPTOMOLOGY OF PHASES OF CHRONIC MYELOGENOUS LEUKEMIA

Symptomology	Stable	Accelerated	Blast Crisis
Presence of symptoms	None to minimal	Moderate	Pronounced
Splenomegaly	Mild	Increased	Marked
WBC count	Slight elevation	Erratic	Very high
Differential	<1% blasts	Increase in immature cells	>25% blasts

WBC, White blood cell.

TABLE 33-11 DIAGNOSTIC TESTS FOR CHRONIC MYELOGENOUS LEUKEMIA

Test	Purpose
WBC	Most distinguishing characteristic of CML: WBC count, which may be >100,000/mm^3 at time of diagnosis, with elevated eosinophil and basophil counts
Differential count	To observe for shift to left, which is seen in CML
Leukocyte alkaline stain	To differentiate CML from other types of leukocytosis
Genetic karyotyping	To verify presence of Philadelphia chromosome, which is indicative of CML

CML, Chronic myelogenous leukemia; *WBC,* white blood cell.

associated with the use of interferon-alpha manifests as fever, chills, malaise, arthralgia, fatigue, and headache. These symptoms usually resolve after 2 weeks of therapy. Late signs of toxicity include hepatitis, proteinuria, hypothyroidism, depression, and psychosis. Imatinib is given orally once daily and continued for as long as the patient benefits from it. Like the other drugs used to treat CML, imatinib has side effects and adverse reactions that require careful monitoring. These include fluid retention and edema, GI irritation, hematologic toxicity, hepatotoxicity, and toxicities from long-term use (liver, kidney, immunosuppression seen in animal studies for the drug). In 2% to 8% of adult patients taking imatinib, fluid retention is sudden and severe, with ascites, effusions in the lung and pericardium, and pulmonary edema.

TREATMENTS. The only potential curative therapy for CML is BMT. Transplants with HLA-matched sibling donors are the most successful if they are done early in the course of the disease in patients who are younger than 50 years of age and who are in good underlying health. Transplant-related complications include graft-versus-host disease, sepsis, and uncontrolled bleeding. These present significant risk to the patient.

DIET. Diet is generally unrestricted. Patients who are considered neutropenic (absolute neutrophil count less than 500/mm^3) should be placed on a low-pathogen diet, which excludes fresh, uncooked fruits and vegetables.

Nursing Management

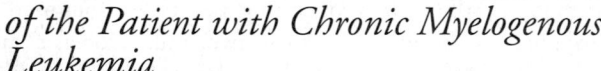

of the Patient with Chronic Myelogenous Leukemia

ASSESSMENT

Health History. Assess for:
- Fatigue, weakness
- History of arthralgia, malaise
- Decreased exercise tolerance
- Tenderness in the left upper quadrant
- Sensation of abdominal fullness
- Anorexia, weight loss
- Abnormal bruising or bleeding

Physical Examination. Assess for:
- Altered vital signs, including elevated temperature
- Pallor
- Shortness of breath
- Bruising
- Abdominal tenderness
- Splenomegaly
- Lymphadenopathy

NURSING DIAGNOSES, OUTCOMES, AND INTERVENTIONS

Nursing Diagnosis: Risk for Infection

OUTCOMES. Common examples of expected outcomes for the patient with a diagnosis of *risk for infection* are:
Patient will:
- Maintain normal body temperature.
- List precautions needed to remain free from signs of infection.

NURSING INTERVENTIONS. Patients who are neutropenic from either chemotherapy or leukemia are at an increased risk for infection and sepsis. Interventions aimed at reducing patient risk begin with careful hand washing before patient contact. The nurse must also instruct visitors and patients about the necessity of good hand washing. Proper perineal care after urination and bowel movements also decreases the risk of infection.

Patients should have private rooms and be placed in protective isolation. A low-pathogen diet eliminating raw fruits and vegetables is appropriate. Foods from outside sources (carry-out, fast foods) and fresh plants and flowers should be discouraged. The nurse carefully monitors the skin, oral cavity, phlebotomy sites, and invasive line sites for signs of infection; maintains all invasive lines aseptically; and monitors the patient's temperature.

RELATED NIC INTERVENTIONS. Environmental Management, Infection Control, Infection Protection

Nursing Diagnosis: Risk for Injury

OUTCOMES. Common examples of expected outcomes for the patient with a diagnosis of *risk for injury* are:
Patient will:
- Demonstrate appropriate measures to prevent bleeding episodes.
- Identify injury-prevention measures.

NURSING INTERVENTIONS. Bleeding is a constant risk for the patient with CML. The nurse monitors platelet counts daily during hospitalizations. Platelet transfusions may be indicated for patients whose platelet counts are below 20,000/mm^3 and who exhibit signs of bleeding.

The nurse assesses the skin daily for petechiae and ecchymosis, assesses intravenous lines and all invasive sites for bleeding, and monitors stool and urine for blood. Any changes in mental status, severe headache, changes in visual and pupillary response, restlessness, or widening pulse pressure should be reported immediately. All invasive procedures should be avoided. The patient should use electric razors to avoid potential trauma, soft-bristled toothbrushes for oral care, and stool softeners to prevent constipation. The nurse instructs the patient to avoid straining with bowel movements or blowing the nose forcefully.

RELATED NIC INTERVENTIONS. Bleeding Precautions, Environmental Management, Health Education

Nursing Diagnosis: Ineffective Coping

OUTCOMES. Common examples of expected outcomes for the patient with a diagnosis of *ineffective coping* are:

Patient will:

- Identify effective coping strategies to deal with chronic illness.
- Participate in support groups.

NURSING INTERVENTIONS. The nurse informs patients about the disease progression, complications, and treatment options available. The nurse provides information so that the patient can understand the terminology and make informed decisions about the care and treatment delivered.

CML is a chronic disease with a poor prognosis. Patients and family members must cope with actual and potential losses, as well as with the fear of future treatments and possible side effects. Actively listening as patients and families verbalize their concerns while creating a nonjudgmental atmosphere facilitates coping. Helping the patient establish personal goals helps promote feelings of self-worth despite chronic illness.

Additional strategies to facilitate coping include relaxation, guided imagery, and music therapy. The nurse should also encourage patients to seek out support groups. Many organizations provide assistance to persons with cancer, and patients may need assistance locating available help. Sources of assistance include:

- American Cancer Society (www.cancer.org)
- American Red Cross (www.redcross.org)
- Leukemia and Lymphoma Society (www.leukemia.org)
- National Coalition for Cancer Survivorship (www.canceradvocacy.org)

The nurse's establishment of a therapeutic relationship with the patient and family allows the patient to vent feelings and fears regarding living with the diagnosis of CML. Teaching sessions should include sufficient time for questions. The family should be included whenever possible (see Patient/Family Teaching box for the patient with leukemia, p. 932).

RELATED NIC INTERVENTIONS. Coping Enhancement, Counseling, Emotional Support, Support Group

EVALUATION

To evaluate effectiveness of nursing interventions, compare patient behaviors with those stated in the expected patient outcomes.

RELATED NOC OUTCOMES. Acceptance: Health Status, Blood Loss Severity, Coping, Knowledge: Infection Control, Personal Safety Behavior, Risk Control, Risk Detection

GERONTOLOGIC CONSIDERATIONS

CML is a disease that primarily affects older adults. The typical symptoms of CML may be confused with characteristic changes of aging (Table 33-12). Some persons may be asymptomatic; others may report vague symptoms such as malaise, fatigue, headache, and weight loss.

Disorders Associated With the Lymph System

Lymphedema

Etiology and Epidemiology. Lymphedema is an abnormal accumulation of lymph within the tissues that is caused by an obstruction in flow. Lymphedema can be classified as primary or secondary. Primary lymphedema results from hypoplastic, aplastic, or hyperplastic development of the lymphatic vessels. Symptoms may manifest at birth, during puberty, or in middle age. Secondary or acquired lymphedema most often develops from trauma to the lymph nodes. Common causes include surgical removal of lymph nodes, radiation-induced fibrosis, inflammation, lymphomas, and parasitic infections.

Primary lymphedema affects women more commonly than men. Filarial infections, prevalent in tropical climates, are the most common worldwide cause of secondary lymphedema.

Pathophysiology. The lymphatic vessels carry lymph from the tissues back into the venous circulation. This system is made up of small, thin vessels that are found throughout the body in close proximity to the veins. The lymphatics begin as capillaries that drain the tissues of lymph (a fluid similar to plasma) and tissue fluid that contains cells, cellular debris, and proteins. The lymph flows through the lymph nodes, which remove noxious agents such as bacteria and toxins. The flow then drains into the thoracic duct and

TABLE 33-12 CHRONIC MYELOGENOUS LEUKEMIA IN OLDER ADULTS

Assessment Findings in CML	Changes Associated With Aging
Skin changes: petechiae, ecchymoses	Increased fragility and decreased skin turgor
Oral cavity: swollen, gums	Ill-fitting dentures
Neurologic: headache, confusion, decreased nerve response	Alzheimer's disease, dementia
Musculoskeletal: joint pain, inflammation, bone pain	Degenerative joint disease
Genitourinary: hematuria, urinary tract infection	Benign prostatic hypertrophy

CML, Chronic myelogenous leukemia.

the right lymphatic duct, which empty into the bloodstream at the junction of the internal jugular vein and subclavian vein (Figure 33-6).

Pathophysiologic changes may include (1) roughening of the surface of the lymphatic vessel, (2) dilation of some lymph channels with thickening and edema of the lymphatic tissue, and (3) fibrosis and separation of elastic fibers that may be present in inflammatory states. Recurrent episodes of lymphedema may cause fibrosis and hyperplasia of lymph vessels, leading to a severe enlargement of the extremity, called elephantiasis.

Lymphedema of the lower extremities begins with mild swelling at the ankle, which gradually extends to the entire limb. Initially the edema is soft and pitting, but it then progresses to firm, rubbery, nonpitting edema. Left leg swelling is more common than right leg swelling. This condition is aggravated by prolonged standing, pregnancy, obesity, warm weather, and menstruation.

Complications of lymphedema include infection and deformity. These complications are infrequent and can usually be avoided with adherence to the treatment regimen.

Collaborative Care Management

Diagnostic Tests. Diagnostic tests include the use of lymphangiography. Radioisotope lymphography involves injection of the isotope into the foot, with subsequent scanning. A CT scan may show a honeycomb pattern in the subcutaneous compartment.

Medications. Diuretics can be prescribed to temporarily decrease the size of the limb. Long-term antibiotic therapy may be indicated to control recurrent cellulitis and infection.

Treatments. Treatment consists of elevating the foot of the bed on blocks at least 8 inches high, wearing compression support stockings, and using an intermittent pneumatic compression device. Monitoring the circumference of the extremities can help in determining the effectiveness of treatments.

Surgical Management. Surgery is restricted to severe cases of lymphedema that are unsuccessfully treated by medical management. In general, surgery is directed toward restoring lymphatic function or improving the patient's symptoms. The most common reason is to reduce the size and bulk of the limb. Surgery also may be used to decrease the incidence of recurrent infections and to improve the cosmetic appearance of the involved limb. The surgical approaches are varied. Microsurgery involving vein grafting to small lymph vessels has been successful.

Diet. No special diet is required to treat lymphedema; however, patients receiving diuretic therapy require adequate potassium and should avoid salty and spicy foods that predispose them to fluid retention and edema.

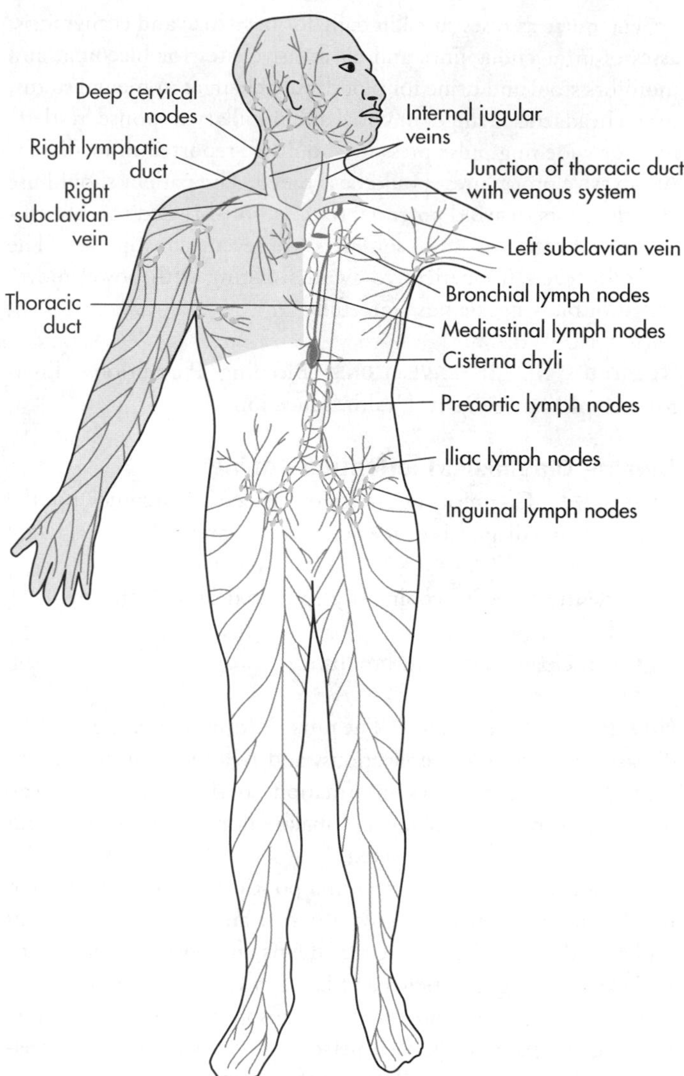

Figure 33-6 Lymph pathways of lower limb drain into subclavian vein.

Nursing Management

of the Patient with Lymphedema

Assessment

Health History. Assess for:

- Onset of swelling in affected limb
- Functional limitation secondary to swelling
- History of surgical removal of lymph nodes, radiotherapy, recurrent inflammation, parasitic infection
- Swelling associated with prolonged standing, pregnancy, obesity, warm weather, or menstruation

Physical Examination. Assess for:

- Presence of edema (pitting or nonpitting)
- Location of edema (more common in left leg)
- Comparable size of extremities
- Texture of skin (firm, rubbery)

Nursing Diagnoses, Outcomes, and Interventions

Nursing Diagnosis: Risk for Infection

Outcomes. A common example of an expected outcome for the patient with a diagnosis of *risk for infection* is:

Patient will:

- Remain free from signs and symptoms of infection.

Nursing Interventions. The nurse monitors the skin daily for intactness, swelling, redness, and lesions. It is important to provide meticulous care to the skin, especially the feet. The nurse reminds the patient to complete the entire course of prescribed antibiotics and to avoid application of nonprescribed topical ointments and creams.

RELATED NIC INTERVENTIONS. Infection Control, Infection Protection

Nursing Diagnosis: Disturbed Body Image

OUTCOMES. A common example of an expected outcome for the patient with a diagnosis of *disturbed body image* is:
Patient will:

- Express acceptance of appearance.

NURSING INTERVENTIONS. The nurse encourages the patient to express concerns regarding swelling of the affected limb. The nurse presents strategies for altering clothing and shoes to accommodate the swelling. The nurse also teaches about the importance of adherence to measures that decrease edema.

RELATED NIC INTERVENTIONS. Body Image Enhancement, Counseling, Coping Enhancement

Patient/Family Teaching. Patient and family teaching are an important aspect of care for the patient with lymphedema (see Patient/Family Teaching box).

EVALUATION

To evaluate the effectiveness of nursing interventions, compare patient behaviors with those stated in the expected patient outcomes.

RELATED NOC OUTCOMES. Body Image, Risk Control, Risk Detection, Self-Esteem

GERONTOLOGIC CONSIDERATIONS

Older adult patients with lymphedema may be at increased risk for nonadherence to the prescribed regimen. If the patient has other chronic diseases, restricted mobility, lack of support systems, or difficulty with self-care activities, the nurse should refer the patient to a home care agency for additional assistance after discharge. Meeting with family members or other patient caregivers is important for continuity of care. Teaching sessions may need to be extended to the home environment after discharge.

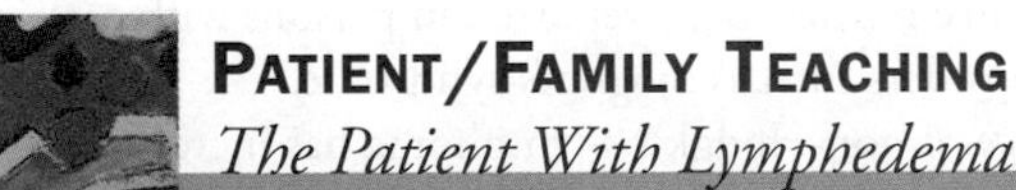

PATIENT/FAMILY TEACHING
The Patient With Lymphedema

The nurse instructs the patient to:

- Perform passive and active exercises of involved limb.
- Exercise on a regular basis.
- Avoid standing still for long periods.
- Elevate affected extremity.
- Elevate foot of bed on 8-inch blocks.
- Use pneumatic external compression pump if ordered.
- Wear compression support stockings.
- Avoid constrictive clothing.
- Take medications as prescribed.
- Adhere to any dietary restrictions that are indicated.

Hodgkin's Disease

Etiology and Epidemiology. Hodgkin's disease is a malignant disorder of lymph nodes first described by Thomas Hodgkin in 1832. The etiology is unknown, but the disease may have a genetic component. An increased incidence among siblings has been reported. An infectious etiology is under debate. The Epstein-Barr virus has been associated with the development of Hodgkin's disease and is noted in the history of up to 40% of patients who develop Hodgkin's disease. The peak incidence of disease occurs in the third decade of life, with a second peak after age 60. Men are more frequently affected than women. An estimated 8000 persons are diagnosed with Hodgkin's disease in the United States annually.[5]

Pathophysiology. The presence of the Reed-Sternberg cell is the pathologic hallmark of the disorder, but four histologic subtypes of Hodgkin's disease have been recognized: lymphocyte predominance, nodular sclerosis, mixed cellularity, and lymphocyte depletion. The lymphocyte predominance and nodular sclerosis types have the best prognosis, and lymphocyte depletion the worst. Nodular sclerosis is the most common type, accounting for 40% to 70% of cases. Nodular sclerosis typically manifests in the supraclavicular and cervical nodes. The origin of the Reed-Sternberg cell is unclear, but it may originate from the B lymphocyte or macrophage. The most important prognostic indicator is the stage of the disease at the time of diagnosis. Accurate staging is crucial to the subsequent treatment regimen. The diagnostic workup is often arduous and difficult, and explanation of the many facets of the complex diagnostic procedures helps provide the emotional support so often needed during this time.

Systemic symptoms associated with Hodgkin's disease include fatigue, weakness, anorexia, unexplained fever, night sweats, and generalized pruritus. Physical examination may show painless enlargement of the lymph nodes, liver, and spleen. Lymphadenopathy is most common in the cervical, axillary, and inguinal nodes. A chest roentgenogram may identify a mediastinal mass. A bone marrow biopsy is performed to determine whether the marrow is involved. The disease may spread via the lymph system to the liver, spleen, vertebrae, uterus, and bronchi. The liver and spleen are evaluated by radionuclide scanning or by a CT scan. Lymphangiography, which requires an experienced operator for accurate results, is performed to evaluate the intraabdominal nodes. A staging laparotomy is performed in some circumstances to obtain a biopsy specimen of retroperitoneal lymph nodes and both lobes of the liver and to remove the spleen.

Classification of the disease into stages (Box 33-6) allows for comparison of persons with similar disease involvement and their response to a given treatment regimen. Over time such comparisons have identified the treatment course most appropriate for a described disease.

Collaborative Care Management. Radiotherapy (Figure 33-7) is used for stages IA, IB, IIA, and IIB. This treatment yields a cure rate of approximately 80% in stages I and II. Combination

Box 33-6 Ann Arbor Clinical Staging Classification of Hodgkin's Disease

- Stage I: Presentation in a single lymph node region or in a single extralymphatic site
- Stage II: Involvement of two or more lymph node regions on the same side of the diaphragm; or localized involvement of an extralymphatic site and one or more lymph node regions on the same side of the diaphragm
- Stage III: Presentation in lymph node regions on both sides of the diaphragm, which may also be accompanied by involvement of the spleen, or by localized involvement of an extralymphatic site, or by both
- Stage IV: Disseminated (multifocal) involvement of one or more extralymphatic organs (e.g., bone marrow, lung, or liver tissue), with or without associated lymph node involvement

NOTE: The presence or absence of fever, night sweats, or significant weight loss is denoted by the suffix letters *B*, presence, or *A*, absence.

Research

Wettergren L et al: Determinants of health-related quality of life in long-term survivors of Hodgkin's lymphoma, *Qual Life Res* 13(8):1369, 2004.

The study looked at the health-related quality of life (HRQL) in long-term survivors of Hodgkin's lymphoma. The purpose of the study was to get a better understanding of these patients' quality of life to improve care and rehabilitation. Participants completed a quality-of-life scale, Hospital Anxiety and Depression scale, Short Form-12 health survey questionnaire (SF-12), and Sense of Coherence scale. No significant differences existed between the mean scores for the survivors of Hodgkin's lymphoma and the control group except on the SF-12. The survivors perceived themselves as being in a poorer state of health than the control group. However, the perception of HRQL between the two groups was similar. Perhaps the survivors viewed their lives as still good just because they had survived Hodgkin's disease for approximately 14 years or more. The study indicated a need for further research in this area.

chemotherapy is the treatment of choice for stages IIIB and IV. Therapy of stage IIIA is controversial and involves chemotherapy, radiotherapy, or a combination. The most commonly used chemotherapy combination is the MOPP regimen, which consists of mechlorethamine (nitrogen mustard), vincristine (Oncovin), prednisone, and procarbazine (Table 33-13). This regimen is administered in a 2-week course each month, with prednisone added during the first and fourth courses. The drugs are administered for at least 6 months or for two or three courses after the attainment of complete remission. Complete remissions are achieved in approximately 80% of these patients; long-term, disease-free remissions and probable cures occur in half this group. With treatment, the patient with Hodgkin's disease can continue to live a long and productive life (see Research box).

Continuing chemotherapy beyond the attainment of complete remission has not been shown to improve survival. Combinations such as ABVD (doxorubicin [Adriamycin], bleomycin, vinblastine [Velban], and dacarbazine; see Table 33-13) are likely to be added to the treatment regimen if relapse occurs, and complete remission can again be attained. Use of alternating courses of MOPP and ABVD has not significantly increased the complete remission rates, but at 8 years, freedom from progression increased from 36% with MOPP alone to 65% with the alternating therapy. Unfortunately, the toxicity from the treatment was greater than from either therapy used alone. Omitting dacarbazine from the therapy greatly reduces the toxicity, and the death rate from stage IV Hodgkin's disease has been significantly reduced with this protocol.

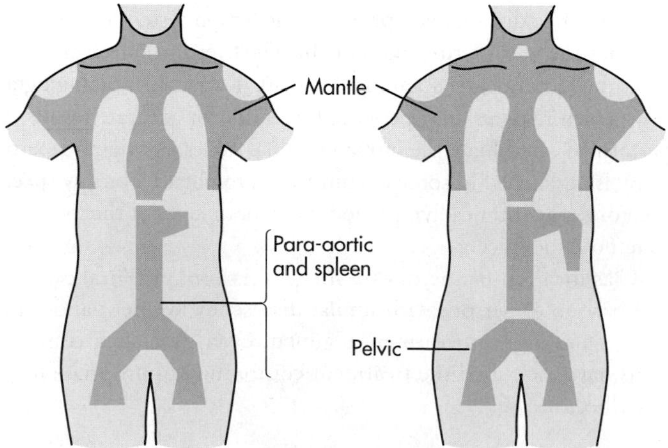

Figure 33-7 Diagram of mantle and inverted Y–fields used in total lymphoid radiotherapy of Hodgkin's disease.

Decreasing the patient's risk for infection and skin damage is important in Hodgkin's disease. The patient and family should be knowledgeable regarding the treatment regimen and potential side effects. As with other hematologic disorders, the patient should avoid all types of potential injury.

Non-Hodgkin's Lymphoma

Etiology and Epidemiology. The non-Hodgkin's lymphomas include a broad spectrum of lymphoid malignant diseases with different histopathologies, disease courses, and responses to therapy. The cause is unknown, although viruses have been implicated. An association between the development of non-Hodgkin's lymphoma and immunosuppressed status, particularly in persons with AIDS and organ transplant recipients, has been reported. An increased incidence has also been reported in persons with certain autoimmune disorders such as Sjögren's syndrome.

The incidence of non-Hodgkin's lymphoma has increased over the past 20 years. In 2005 approximately 56,390 new cases were diagnosed in the United States, with 20,610 deaths estimated for that year.[8] Men are more commonly affected than women, with the greatest incidence occurring in those over 60 years of age. Burkitt's lymphoma, a high-grade tumor, is most common in children and persons with AIDS.

Pathophysiology. Accurate identification of the pathologic histology is crucial to the determination of the treatment plan. One classification separates the non-Hodgkin's lymphomas into lymphocytic, histiocytic, and mixed-cell types, each of which may appear as nodular or diffuse on microscopic examination. These

TABLE 33-13 CHEMOTHERAPEUTIC REGIMENS FOR TREATMENT OF HODGKIN'S DISEASE

Drugs	Dose	Method	Schedule	Cycle
MOPP				
Mechlorethamine (nitrogen mustard)	6 mg/m^2	IV	Days 1 and 8	2 wk with 2-wk rest period
Vincristine (Oncovin)	1.4 mg/m^2	IV	Days 1 and 8	
Prednisone	40 mg/m^2	PO	Days 1-14	
Procarbazine	100 mg/m^2	PO	Days 1-14	
ABVD				
Doxorubicin (Adriamycin)	25 mg/m^2	IV	Days 1 and 15	2 wk with 2-wk rest period
Bleomycin	10 mg/m^2	IV	Days 1 and 15	
Vinblastine (Velban)	6 mg/m^2	IV	Days 1 and 15	
Dacarbazine (DTIC-Dome)*	375 mg/m^2	IV	Days 1 and 15	

IV, Intravenous, *PO,* oral.
*NOTE: Dacarbazine may be omitted (MOPP/ABV).

have been subdivided into "favorable" and "unfavorable" histology (Box 33-7). In general, a nodular pattern of cell structures conveys a more favorable prognosis than a diffuse pattern. A lymphocytic cytology is more favorable than a histiocytic one, and a mixed cellularity–histiocytic type is intermediate in its prognosis.

Patients most often have nontender peripheral lymphadenopathy that may appear bulky. The liver and spleen may be moderately enlarged. Other symptoms include unexplained fever, night sweats, and weight loss.

Collaborative Care Management. The diagnosis of non-Hodgkin's lymphoma is made by examination of pathologic lymph node tissue. Accurate histologic classification is important, and often slides are sent to major cancer centers for consultation. Once the diagnosis is made, the extent of the disease (staging) must be determined. As with Hodgkin's disease, accurate staging is a crucial factor in determining the treatment regimen. The staging workup is similar to that for Hodgkin's disease, except that staging laparotomies are less often needed. Explanations of the extensive workup and its importance in determining the treatment plan are an important focus of patient teaching during the diagnostic period.

The complexity of the disease and the array of treatment regimens used require nurse-physician discussion of the treatment plan. It is especially important that the goals of therapy be shared, whether the goals are for cure or only local or systemic palliation.

In general, radiotherapy is the initial treatment when the disease is localized. Local field radiation is used. Total nodal radiation is reserved for patients whose disease is more widespread. Chemotherapy is the mainstay of treatment of non-Hodgkin's lymphomas that are not localized (Table 33-14).

Nodular, poorly differentiated lymphocytic lymphoma is the most commonly occurring non-Hodgkin's lymphoma. In some patients, observation is reasonable until the disease shows signs of progression. Treatment with a single alkylating agent, most often chlorambucil, is effective in that it produces a response rate that extends survival. Combination chemotherapy produces higher response rates, including complete remissions, but is not yet shown to be curative. The MST is 7 to 10 years.

In diffuse histiocytic lymphoma, which includes most of the cases previously designated as reticulum cell sarcoma, combination chemotherapy has been superior to single-agent therapy. Survival is significantly prolonged in those who demonstrate a complete response, and a significant minority of this group is cured. Chemotherapy regimens produce complete responses in 40% to 60% or more of patients whose MST is well over 3 years.

In nodular histiocytic and nodular mixed histiolymphocytic types, complete responses have been achieved with single agents, and 50% to 70% of those treated with COP, COPP, MOPP, and other combinations have shown an MST of 55 months for those who attained a complete response and 13 months for those who attain only a partial response (see Tables 33-13 and 33-14).

Hodgkin's disease most often affects young adults; therefore special attention needs to be given to minimizing the impact of the illness and its treatment on their lives, not only during the treatment period, but later as well. Before the initiation of treatment, therapy-induced sterility should be discussed. For young women receiving radiotherapy alone, the ovaries can be surgically relocated outside the field of radiation. Sterility commonly occurs in association with chemotherapy. For women, the ability to conceive and bear normal children may return after therapy is completed. For men, sterility is more commonly permanent. For this

BOX 33-7 Non-Hodgkin's Lymphomas

"Favorable" Histology

Nodular, poorly differentiated lymphocytic lymphoma
Nodular, mixed lymphocytic and histiocytic lymphoma
Well-differentiated lymphocytic lymphomas of the nodular or diffuse type

"Unfavorable" Histology

Nodular histiocytic lymphoma
Diffuse poorly differentiated lymphocytic
Diffuse histiocytic lymphoma
Diffuse mixed lymphoma
Diffuse undifferentiated lymphoma

TABLE 33-14 CHEMOTHERAPEUTIC REGIMENS FOR TREATMENT OF NON-HODGKIN'S LYMPHOMAS

Drugs	Dose	Method	Schedule	Cycle
COP				
Cyclophosphamide (Cytoxan)	800-1000 mg/m^2	IV	Day 1	3 wk
Vincristine (Oncovin)	2 mg	IV	Day 1	
Prednisone	60 mg/m^2	PO	Days 1-5	
CHOP				
Cyclophosphamide	750 mg/m^2	IV	Day 1	3 wk
Hydroxydaunomycin (doxorubicin)	50 mg/m^2	IV	Day 1	
Vincristine	1.4 mg/m^2	IV	Day 1	
Prednisone	100 mg/m^2	PO	Days 1-5	
CHOP-BLEO				
Cyclophosphamide	750 mg/m^2	IV	Day 1	3 wk or 4 wk
Hydroxydaunomycin (doxorubicin)	50 mg/m^2	IV	Day 1	
Vincristine	2 mg	IV	Days 1 and 5	4 wk
Prednisone	100 mg	PO	Days 1-5	
Bleomycin	15 unit/m^2	IV	Days 1 and 5	
COPP				
Cyclophosphamide	400-650 mg/m^2	IV	Days 1 and 8	4 wk
Vincristine	1.4 mg/m^2 (max, 2 mg)	IV	Days 1 and 8	
Procarbazine	100 mg/m^2	PO	Days 1-10	
Prednisone	40 mg/m^2	PO	Days 1-14	
BACOP				
Vleomycin	5 unit/m^2	IV	Days 15 and 22	4 wk
Doxorubicin, cyclophosphamide	25 mg/m^2 10-15 mg/kg	IV	Days 1 and 8	
Vincristine	650 mg/m^2	IV	Days 1 and 8	
Procarbazine	1.4 mg/m^2 (max, 2 mg)	IV	Days 1 and 8	
Prednisone	60 mg/m^2	PO	Days 15-28	
PRO-MACE				
Prednisone	60 mg/m^2	IV	Days 1 to 14	Follow with MOPP regimen (see Table 33-13); then restart Pro-MACE

reason the option of sperm banking should be discussed before beginning either radiotherapy or chemotherapy.

To allow for work and career development, every effort should be made to schedule treatment at times that least interfere with work and other important events in the person's life. The nurse has a crucial role in helping patients develop a realistic approach to the illness and successfully meet the demands and limitations imposed by the illness and its treatment.

Persons with lymphomas have periods of remission and recurrence. Such peaks and valleys are stressful and disruptive. Many patients describe subsequent courses of treatment after a recurrence as more stressful than the initial treatment. Comments include, "Is it worth it? I don't have the same faith." Other patients, realistically encouraged by the initial response to treatment, are more optimistic: "It worked the first time. It will work again." Because of the stress involved in therapy, the patient needs strong support systems. The health care team can provide some of the needed support and guidance as the person learns to incorporate the illness into daily life.

Patient teaching is an important component of patient care (see Patient/Family Teaching box, p. 942).

Infectious Mononucleosis

Etiology and Epidemiology. Infectious mononucleosis is an acute disease caused by a herpeslike virus, the Epstein-Barr virus.

TABLE 33-14 CHEMOTHERAPEUTIC REGIMENS FOR TREATMENT OF NON-HODGKIN'S LYMPHOMAS—CONT'D

Drugs	Dose	Method	Schedule	Cycle
PRO-MACE—CONT'D				
Methotrexate	1.5 g/m^2	IV	One time	Follow with MOPP regimen (see Table 33-13); then restart Pro-MACE
Doxorubicin	25 mg/m^2	IV	Days 1 and 8	
Cyclophosphamide	650 mg/m^2	IV	Days 1 and 8	
Etoposide (VP-16)	120 mg/m^2	IV	Days 1 and 8	
Leucovorin	50 mg/m^2	IV	q6h for 5 days	
M-BACOD				
Methotrexate	200 mg/m^2	IV	Days 8 and 15	Repeat cycles every 3 wk
Bleomycin	4 unit/m^2	IV	Days 1 and 21	
Doxorubicin	45 mg/m^2	IV	Days 1 and 21	
Cyclophosphamide	600 mg/m^2	IV	Days 1 and 21	
Vincristine	1 mg/m^2	IV	Days 1 and 21	
Dexamethasone	6 mg/m^2	PO	Days 1-5 and 21-25	
Leucovorin rescue	10 mg/m^2	PO	q6h for 8 doses, beginning 24 hr after each methotrexate dose	
MACOP-B				
Methotrexate	100 mg/m^2, then 300 mg/m^2	IV	Wk 2, 6, 10	Cycles may be repeated
Leucovorin rescue	15 mg	PO	q6h for 6 doses beginning 24 hr after each methotrexate dose	
Doxorubicin	50 mg/m^2	IV	Wk 1, 3, 5, 7, 9, 11	
Cyclophosphamide	350 mg/m^2	IV	Wk 1, 3, 5, 7, 9, 11	
Vincristine	1.4 mg/m^2	IV	Wk 2, 4, 8, 10, 12	
Prednisone	75 mg	PO	Daily doses tapered over last 15 days	
Bleomycin	10 unit/m^2	IV	Wk 4, 8, 12	
NOTE: CNS prophylaxis is also given to patients with bone marrow involvement after bone marrow remission.				
Methotrexate	12 mg	IT	Wk 6-8	Cycles may be repeated
Cytarabine	30 mg/m^2	IT	Wk 6-8	

CNS, Central nervous system; *IT*, intrathecal; *IV*, intravenous; *PO*, oral; *q6h*, every 6 hr.

It occurs more often in young persons, with the highest incidence occurring between 15 and 30 years of age.

Pathophysiology. Signs and symptoms of infectious mononucleosis are varied (see Clinical Manifestations box). It is a benign disease with a favorable prognosis. The onset may be subtle, appearing almost as flulike symptoms. Malaise is a common early complaint, and it is often accompanied by fever, lymphadenopathy, sore throat, headache, generalized aches and pains resembling those of influenza, and moderate enlargement of the liver and spleen. Pruritus, palatal petechiae, jaundice, and rash may be present. The mode of transmission is via intimate contact, with the spread of the virus through the saliva. Rupture of the spleen and encephalitis are rare complications.

Collaborative Care Management. Diagnosis is established by the heterophil agglutination or monospot blood test. This test is based on the presence of a substance in the blood of a person with infectious mononucleosis that causes clumping, or agglutination, of the washed erythrocytes (antigen) of another animal. The test result is almost always positive after 10 to 14 days of the illness. Other laboratory findings are a great increase in the number of mononuclear leukocytes (hence the name of the disease) and an increase in atypical lymphocytes. At the height of the disease, the WBC count may range between 10,000 and 20,000 cells/mm^3.

Infectious mononucleosis is self-limiting; with rest, affected persons usually recover spontaneously within 2 to 3 weeks. Effectiveness of antiviral therapy has not been established. The use of

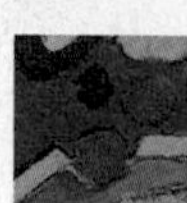

PATIENT/FAMILY TEACHING
The Patient With Non-Hodgkin's Lymphoma

Patient teaching includes information about:
- The disorder, its treatment, and prognosis
- Name, dosage, frequency, and side effects of medications
- Arrangements for chemotherapy or radiation treatments and for periodic blood cell counts
- Symptoms requiring immediate medical attention (fever, bleeding, bone pain)
- Need for continued medical follow-up care
- Resources available in the community: financial assistance and local support groups (American Cancer Society)

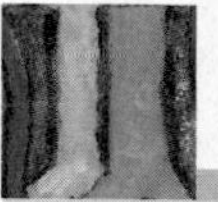

CLINICAL MANIFESTATIONS
Infectious Mononucleosis

Mild

Fever
Malaise
Fatigue

Moderate

Enlarged lymph nodes
Sore throat
Headache
Generalized aches
Moderate enlargement of liver and spleen

Severe (Rare)

Rupture of spleen
Encephalitis

corticosteroids may be indicated in severe cases with tonsillar enlargement and potential airway obstruction. Acetaminophen is effective in relieving fever, sore throat, and myalgias. Most persons can return to activities that do not require heavy exertion in 1 to 2 weeks and to normal activities in 4 to 6 weeks. Some persons have persistent fatigue for several months. Nursing management is supportive and focuses on the relief of symptoms and promotion of rest.

The patient should avoid heavy lifting or contact sports for at least 1 month or until the splenomegaly is resolved. An enlarged spleen is susceptible to rupture. Fluids should be increased as tolerated. Appropriate hand washing is always important in disease-spread prevention. Young adults should be told about the mode of transmission and incubation period of mononucleosis. Persons with mononucleosis should be cautioned against donating blood for at least 6 months after the onset of illness. Reassurance should be given that isolation is not necessary, but that the oral secretions of a person with acute mononucleosis should be considered infectious.

? Critical Thinking

1. A 63-year-old man recently diagnosed with CML is extremely anxious about his diagnosis. He is still actively employed and also enjoys a variety of recreational activities. He has heard many horror stories about chemotherapy. What would you explain to him regarding the initial therapy for CML? What nursing interventions might help him cope with his anxiety? How does this treatment differ from treatment for acute types of leukemia? Are there community resources available to aid the patient and his family?
2. Identify differences in nursing interventions for a patient with non-Hodgkin's lymphoma versus Hodgkin's disease.

References

1. Bader-Meunier B et al: Long-term evaluation of the beneficial effect of subtotal splenectomy for management of hereditary spherocytosis, *Blood* 97(2):399-403, 2001.
2. Cancer Group Institute: *Acute leukemia*, accessed Sept 2005 from website: www.cancergroup.com.
3. Cancer Group Institute: *Chronic leukemia*, accessed Sept 2005 from website: www.cancergroup.com.
4. Dressler D: Coping with a coagulation crisis, *Nursing 2004* 34(5):58-62, 2004.
5. Hematology and oncology: anemias. In Beers MH, Berkow R, editors: *The Merck manual*, ed 17, Section 11, Chapter 127, accessed July 2004 from website: www.merck.com.
6. Hematology and oncology: myeloproliferative disorders. In Beers MH, Berkow R, editors: *The Merck manual*, ed 17, Section 11, Chapter 130, accessed July 2004 from website: www.merck.com.
7. Hematology and oncology: platelet disorders. In Beers MH, Berkow, R, editors: *The Merck manual*, ed 17, Chapter 133, accessed Sept 2005 from website: www.merck.com.
8. Leukemia and Lymphoma Society: *Leukemia*, accessed October 2005 from website: www.leukemia-lymphoma.org.
9. National Cancer Institute: *Adult acute lymphoblastic leukemia (PDQ): treatment*, accessed Aug 2004 from website: www.cancer.gov/cancertopics.
10. National Cancer Institute: *Adult acute myeloid leukemia (PDQ): treatment*, accessed Aug 2004 from website: www.cancer.gov/cancertopics.
11. National Heart, Lung, and Blood Institute: *Idiopathic thrombocytopenic purpura*, accessed July 2004 from website: www.nhlbi.nih.gov/health/dci.
12. National Library of Medicine and National Institutes of Health: *Idiopathic aplastic anemia*, accessed Aug 2004 from website: www.nlm.nih.gov/medlineplus.
13. National Organization for Rare Disorders: *Anemia, Fanconi's*, accessed July 2004 from website: www.rarediseases.org.
14. Rucknagel DL: Progress and prospects for the acute chest syndrome of sickle cell anemia, *J Pediatr* 138(2):160-162, 2001.
15. *Stem cell/bone marrow transplant*, accessed July 2004 from website: www.stjude.org/clinicalscience.

evolve Visit the Evolve website: http://evolve.elsevier.com/Monahan/medsurg

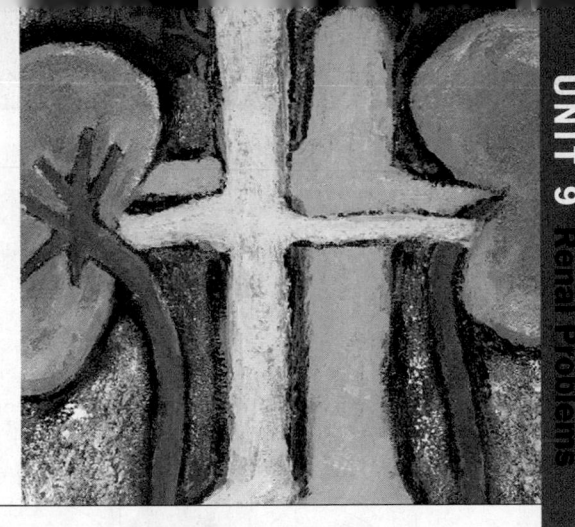

CHAPTER 34

Assessment of the Renal System

by Kelly A. Weigel, Cynthia K. Potter

OBJECTIVES

After studying this chapter, the learner should be able to:

1. List the major functions of the kidney.
2. Describe the anatomy of the kidney.
3. Identify subjective and objective data essential to the assessment of renal function.
4. Correlate significant urinary tract symptoms with common etiologies.
5. Describe common diagnostic tests used to identify renal alterations.
6. Explain guidelines for caring for patients after select urologic diagnostic procedures.

KEY TERMS

Anatomy and Physiology

The major organs of the renal system are the kidneys, which are retroperitoneal organs that maintain the body's homeostasis. The kidneys produce and secrete hormones and enzymes that help regulate red blood cell production, blood pressure, and calcium and phosphate metabolism. By excreting metabolic end products and varying the excretion of water and solutes, the kidneys regulate body fluid volume, acidity, and electrolytes, thus maintaining normal body blood composition (Box 34-1).

Anatomy

Upper Urinary Tract. The kidneys are two limabean–shaped organs that lie outside the peritoneal cavity against the posterior abdominal wall (Figure 34-1). Each kidney is about 11 cm long, 5 cm wide, and 3 cm thick.[3] The kidneys lie on either side of the abdominal aorta, inferior vena cava, and lumbar spine between the twelfth thoracic and third lumbar vertebrae. The right kidney is slightly lower than the left because of the space occupied by the liver.

The kidneys are encased in a fibrous coat known as the renal capsule. Each kidney and capsule is embedded in a fatty layer that protects against injury. An adrenal gland lies above each kidney within the fatty layer. Renal fascia, a layer of connective tissue, and surrounding organs help hold the kidneys in place and protect them from trauma. On the medial aspect of each kidney is a concave notch known as the hilum. The renal arteries and nerves enter the kidney, and the renal veins, lymphatics, and ureters exit, at the hilum.

When the kidney is cut longitudinally and opened, three distinct areas can be seen: the cortex, medulla, and renal sinus (Figure 34-2). The renal cortex, the outermost 1 cm, is pale and has a granular appearance. Most parts of the **nephron**, the functional unit of the kidney, lie in this area.

The inner 5-cm portion of the kidney is the renal medulla, which contains 8 to 10 triangular wedges or pyramids. The bases of the pyramids face the cortex, and their apices, or renal papillae, face the center of the kidney. The pyramids have a striated appearance because of the segments of the nephrons and collecting ducts located here.[3]

The third section of the kidney is the renal sinus. This is a cavity that contains blood vessels, the calyces, the renal pelvis, and

Box 34-1 Functions of the Kidney

- Regulation of body fluid volume and osmolality
- Regulation of electrolyte balance
- Regulation of acid-base balance
- Excretion of metabolic waste products, toxins, and foreign substances
- Production and secretion of hormones

NOTE: Additional related functions such as blood pressure regulation and red blood cell production occur as a result of the above.

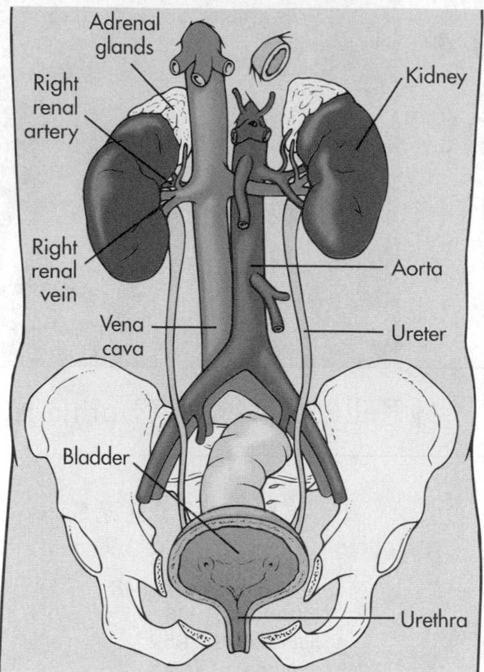

Figure 34-1 Organs and structure of urinary system.

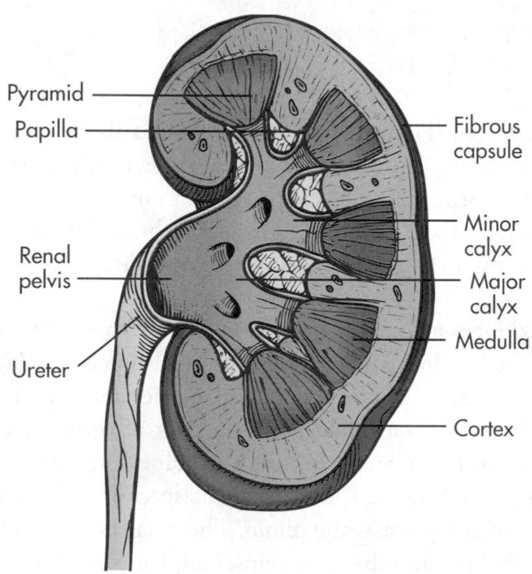

Figure 34-2 Frontal section of the kidney.

structures formed by the expanded upper end of the ureter. Before entering the kidney, the ureter dilates to form the renal pelvis. The renal pelvis branches into two or three calyces. Each major calyx branches into several minor calyces. The minor calyces collect the urine that drains from the collecting ducts.

The nephron is the functional unit of the kidney. Each kidney contains approximately 1 million nephrons.[3] The two types of nephrons, cortical and juxtamedullary, are named according to their location within the renal parenchyma (the essential and distinctive tissue of an organ). The cortical nephrons account for 85% of the total nephrons and perform excretory and regulatory functions. The juxtamedullary nephrons make up the remaining 15% and play an important role in the concentration and dilution of urine by generating a steep osmotic gradient. The structures of the nephron involved in the process of urine formation include the renal corpuscle, the renal tubules, and the collecting duct (Figure 34-3). The renal corpuscle consists of the glomerulus and Bowman's capsule and is responsible for the formation of ultrafiltrate from the blood. The renal tubules consist of the proximal convoluted tubule, the loop of Henle, and the distal convoluted tubule and are responsible for the resorption and secretion that alter the volume and composition of the ultrafiltrate to form the final urine product. The collecting duct receives tubular fluid from many nephrons and transports the fluid from the cortex to the minor calyx.

The kidneys are highly vascular organs, receiving about 20% of the cardiac output in the resting state, or about 1200 ml/min. Arterial blood is supplied by the renal arteries, which branch directly off the abdominal aorta (see Figure 34-1). Although 70% of human beings have one renal artery supplying each kidney, about 30% have one or more accessory renal arteries that also branch off the aorta and supply a part of the kidney.

The renal artery branches into approximately five segmental arteries, dividing the kidney into vascular segments. The segmental arteries branch to form the lobar arteries that supply each pyramid. The lobar arteries then branch several more times so blood can move efficiently through each nephron. Each nephron has its own blood supply; blood enters the glomerulus through the afferent arteriole and exits through the efferent arteriole. Blood then flows through the peritubular capillaries that surround the nephron's tubules. Ultimately the peritubular capillaries empty into venules that return the filtered blood to the general circulation via the renal venous system.[2]

The ureters (see Figure 34-2), approximately 30 cm long, arise as extensions of the renal pelvis and empty into the bladder in an area known as the trigone (Figure 34-4). The trigone is a fold of

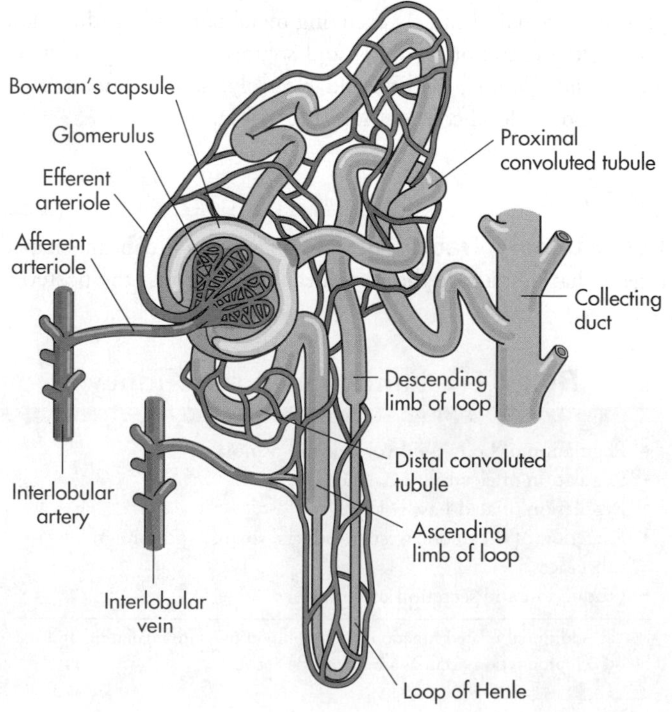

Figure 34-3 Nephron.

mucous membrane that serves as a valve preventing the backflow, or reflux, of urine into the ureters when the bladder contracts. The ureters are composed of smooth muscle and are innervated by the sympathetic and parasympathetic nerves.[2] The function of the ureters is to propel urine from the renal pelvis to the bladder.

Lower Urinary Tract. The bladder, located behind the symphysis pubis (see Figure 34-1), serves as a collecting bag for urine. The mucous membrane lining the bladder is arranged in folds called rugae. These rugae, together with the elasticity of the muscular walls, enable the bladder to distend to hold large amounts of urine. Two sphincter muscles control excretion of urine from the urinary bladder via the urethra. A layer of smooth muscle encircles the base of the bladder at the junction of the urethra, forming the internal urethral sphincter, which is under involuntary control. A second sphincter, the external urethral sphincter, is located below the bladder. It is composed of skeletal muscle and is under voluntary control. If both of these sphincters relax, urination occurs. If the external sphincter does not relax, the internal sphincter does not open, and urination is prevented.

The urethra serves as the outlet for urine from the bladder. The male urethra is about 20 cm long, whereas the female urethra is about 4 cm long. The urinary meatus is the opening through which urine exits the body.

The walnut-sized prostate gland is a male reproductive gland that encircles the upper part of the male urethra (see Figure 34-4). The gland is doughnut shaped, with the urethra passing through the "hole." When the prostate is enlarged, it squeezes the urethra, obstructing the flow of urine. Numerous prostatic ducts empty into the urethra. Bacteria from urinary tract infections may travel up these ducts, causing inflammation and infection of the prostate.

Physiology

A clear understanding of the physiology of the kidneys is needed to understand the many physiologic and chemical changes that occur with kidney failure.

Ultrafiltration. **Ultrafiltration** is the process by which the fluid part of urine is formed. As blood passes through the capillary bed of the glomerulus, the pressure of plasma forces fluid across the semipermeable membrane of the glomerulus into Bowman's capsule (Figure 34-5). The volume of this glomerular filtrate approximates 180 L/day. Of the total volume, 99% is resorbed by the kidneys. Because of the kidneys' tremendous capacity for resorption, the average urinary output of an adult is only 1 to 2 L/day.

Ultrafiltration is measured as the glomerular filtration rate (GFR). Clinically GFR is defined as the amount of glomerular filtrate formed in 1 minute. The larger the body surface area, the greater the GFR. The GFR in an average-sized adult is approximately 125 ml/min (7.5 L/hr). At this rate, a volume of approximately 60 times the plasma volume is filtered each day. The average GFR of a woman is about 10% less than that of a man. Glomerular filtrate is formed by the same forces that affect fluid transport between vascular and interstitial spaces in other tissues of the body. These forces include hydrostatic pressure and oncotic pressure.

The rate of renal perfusion exceeds the metabolic and oxygen needs of the kidneys but facilitates efficient clearance of metabolic

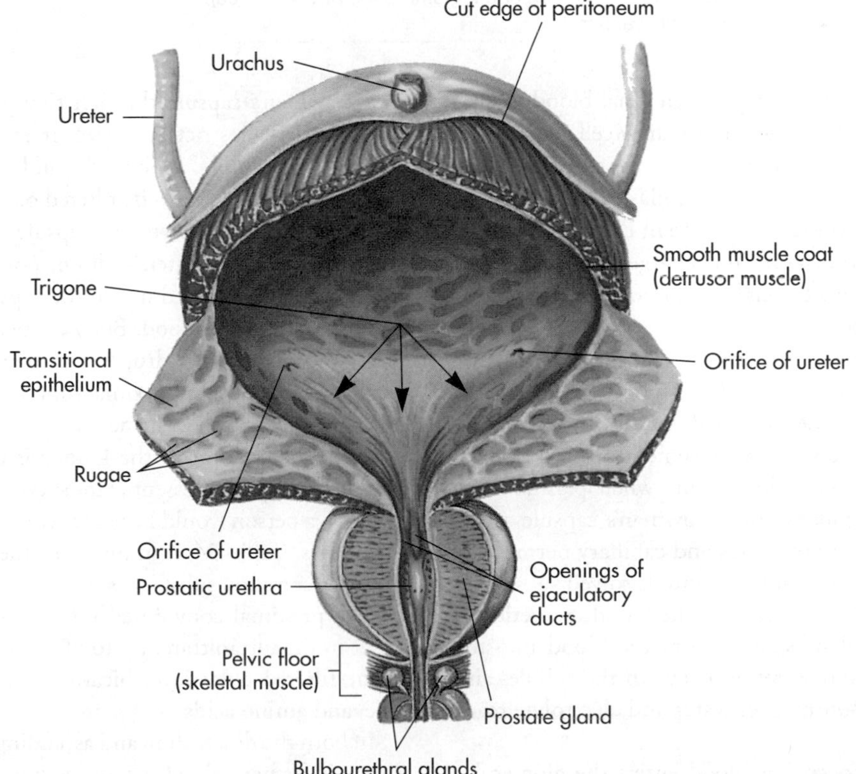

Figure 34-4 Interior of urinary bladder and associated structure in the male.

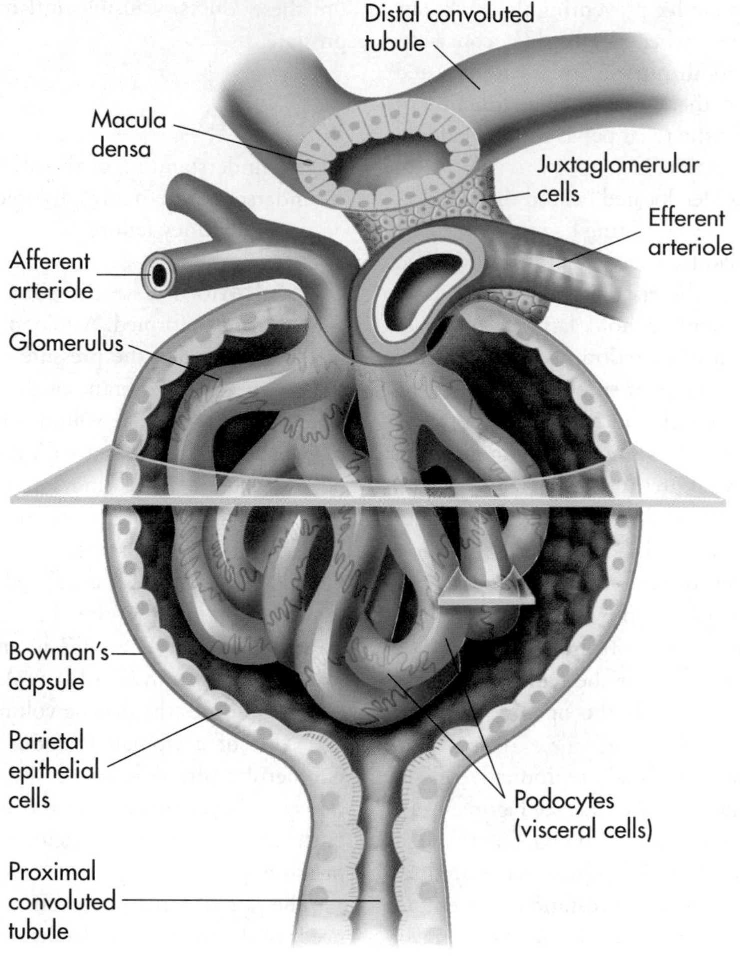

Figure 34-5 Cross section of the glomerulus, Bowman's capsule, and juxtaglomerular apparatus.

wastes. A severe or prolonged interruption in renal blood flow or cardiac output affects urine formation and kidney cell viability.

Urine formation begins when blood enters the afferent arteriole of the nephron. The filtrate, which is similar to plasma minus proteins, begins to be transformed into urine in Bowman's capsule and tubules. Molecular size, shape, and charge are the primary determinants of what can pass through the glomerular membrane and become part of the filtrate.

The kidneys maintain a stable internal environment by balancing the fluid and solute composition of the blood within narrow ranges. Three intricate processes are used: filtration, resorption, and secretion. **Filtration** refers to the movement of fluid across a semipermeable membrane. Filtration occurs when plasma flows through the glomerular capillaries into Bowman's capsule as the result of osmotic and capillary pressures and capillary permeability. **Resorption** is the movement of water and dissolved substances from the tubular fluid (filtrate) back into the blood. **Secretion** is the movement of fluid and substances from the blood into the tubular fluid. Resorption and secretion occur in the tubules and collecting duct. Box 34-2 summarizes water and electrolyte regulation by the nephron.

Effective ultrafiltration occurs as blood enters the glomerular capillaries, and water and small molecules begin to be filtered out into Bowman's capsule through tiny pores in the capillary wall. The pore size restricts the size of molecule that can leave the blood. For example, blood cells and proteins are too large, but urea is the correct size to be filtered out of the blood. The ultrafiltrate moves from Bowman's capsule into the proximal tubule where most of the water, sodium, potassium, calcium, chloride, and bicarbonate filtered out in the capsule originally are resorbed and returned to the blood. Body waste products such as hydrogen ions, phosphate, and drugs and their metabolites are secreted from the blood in the proximal tubules.[2,3] Table 34-1 presents the normal composition of urine.

A major function of the kidney is conservation of water and electrolytes, which is essential for survival. If conservation were not possible, a person would be volume and electrolyte depleted in 3 to 4 minutes. Table 34-2 summarizes the filtration and resorption values of common substances.

The proximal convoluted tubule resorbs 85% to 90% of the water in the ultrafiltrate; up to 80% of filtered sodium; and most of the filtered potassium, bicarbonate, chloride, phosphate, glucose, and amino acids.

In both the descending and ascending loops of Henle, the ultrafiltrate is further refined as more sodium and water is resorbed and magnesium is reclaimed from the tubules. Final adjustment in

Box 34-2 Water and Electrolyte Regulation of Nephron

Bowman's Capsule

Ultrafiltrate from plasma enters Bowman's capsule and flows into the proximal convoluted tubule

Proximal Convoluted Tubule

Passive resorption of 65% of glomerular filtrate with sodium, potassium, chloride, bicarbonate, magnesium, phosphate, glucose, amino acids, and urea

Secretion of hydrogen ions and some drugs and toxins

Loop of Henle

Resorption: 25% of the glomerular filtrate with sodium, calcium, potassium, magnesium, chloride, and urea

Distal Convoluted Tubule

Resorption: 9% of the glomerular filtrate with sodium, chloride, bicarbonate, water, and urea

Secretion of hydrogen, potassium, and ammonia

Collecting Duct

Resorption of water dependent on presence of antidiuretic hormone

Sodium resorbed and potassium secreted if aldosterone present

Calcium resorbed if parathyroid hormone present

Acid-base balance regulation continuing

TABLE 34-1 NORMAL URINE VALUES

Laboratory Test	Normal Adult Values
Calcium (24 hr)	100-250 mg/day (diet dependent; based on average calcium intake of 600-800 mg/24 hr)
Chloride	110-250 mEq/day
Creatinine	Men: 1-2 g/24 hr Women: 0.8-1.8 g/24 hr
Glucose	Negative
Osmolality	250-900 mOsm/kg
Protein	30-150 mg/24 hr (method dependent)
pH	4.5-8.0
Phosphorus	0.9-1.3 g/day (diet dependent)
Potassium	25-123 mEq/24 hr (markedly intake dependent)
Sodium	27-287 mEq/24 hr (diet dependent; output lower at night)
Specific gravity	1.007-1.030 (range in SI units)
Urea nitrogen	6-17 g/day
Uric acid	250-750 mg/day
Volume	Men: 800-2000 ml/day Women: 800-1600 ml/day
Color	Pale to darker yellow
Clarity	Clear
Ketones	None
Red blood count	0-5/high-power field
White blood count	0-5/high-power field
Bacteria	None; occasional in voided specimen
Casts	0-4 hyaline casts/low-power field
Crystals	Interpreted by physician
Culture	Negative

Data from Chernecky CC, Berger BJ: *Laboratory tests and diagnostic procedures,* ed 4, St Louis, 2004, Saunders.

TABLE 34-2 AVERAGE FILTRATION AND RESORPTION VALUES FOR SEVERAL COMMON SUBSTANCES

Substance	Amount Filtered (per day)	Amount Excreted (per day)	Percent Resorbed
Water (L)	180	1.8	99.0
Sodium (g)	630	3.2	99.5
Glucose (g)	180	0.0	100.0
Urea (g)	54	30.0	44.0
Potassium (g)	35	2.0	94.0
Calcium (g)	5	0.2	96.0
Amino acids (g)	10	0.3	97.0

urine composition is made in the distal convoluted tubule and the collecting ducts. The primary solutes affected in this area are potassium, bicarbonate, hydrogen ions, and, again, sodium and chloride. This final refinement of the urine is accomplished primarily by feedback mechanisms regulated by the hormones aldosterone and antidiuretic hormone (ADH, or vasopressin).

ADH exerts hormonal regulation of salt and water balance. ADH is produced by the hypothalamus and stored and released by the pituitary gland in response to changes in plasma osmolarity. Plasma osmolarity refers to the concentration of ions in the blood. If water intake is low or if water loss is high, ADH is released, causing the kidneys to retain water. ADH acts on the collecting ducts, increasing their permeability to water. As a result, more water is resorbed into the bloodstream.[1,4] Aldosterone is a steroid secreted by the adrenal cortex. It acts on the distal tubule to increase resorption of sodium. It is not, however, the only means of sodium control.

As the filtrate moves from the proximal to the distal tubule and finally into the collecting ducts, it becomes increasingly concentrated and acidic. The final pH of the urine is usually between 5 and 6, and the total amount of urine leaving the body is reduced to between 1 and 2 L/day. Considering the total blood volume filtered, an incredible amount of filtrate concentration occurs between the glomerulus and the ureter.[2] The nephron's intricate work successfully maintains the extracellular pH within a narrow range and finely tunes the fluid and electrolyte composition to sustain the complex, delicate processes of the body. Figure 34-6 illustrates the mechanism of urine formation.

Electrolyte Balance. A constant ebb and flow of electrolytes (electrically charged particles) occurs along the anatomic path of the ultrafiltrate. Electrolytes are filtered out in Bowman's capsule only to be mostly resorbed in the proximal tubules. Ultimately their concentration is adjusted in the distal nephron under the influence of hormones (primarily aldosterone and ADH). The specific mechanisms for moving electrolytes across the tubular membranes are both passive and active. Passive movement of electrolytes occurs when there is a concentration difference of molecules across the semipermeable membrane; molecules move from an area of greater concentration to one of lesser concentration. Active movement of electrolytes or active transport requires the expenditure of energy and enables the movement of molecules regardless of concentration gradients. Active and passive movement allows the kidney to maintain optimal electrolyte balance. See Chapter 17 for a discussion of fluid and electrolyte regulation.

Maintenance of Acid-Base Balance. For normal cell function, plasma pH for arterial blood must be maintained in a narrow range, between 7.35 and 7.45. This balance is achieved by maintaining a blood bicarbonate/carbon dioxide ratio of 20:1. The respiratory system and kidneys work together to maintain

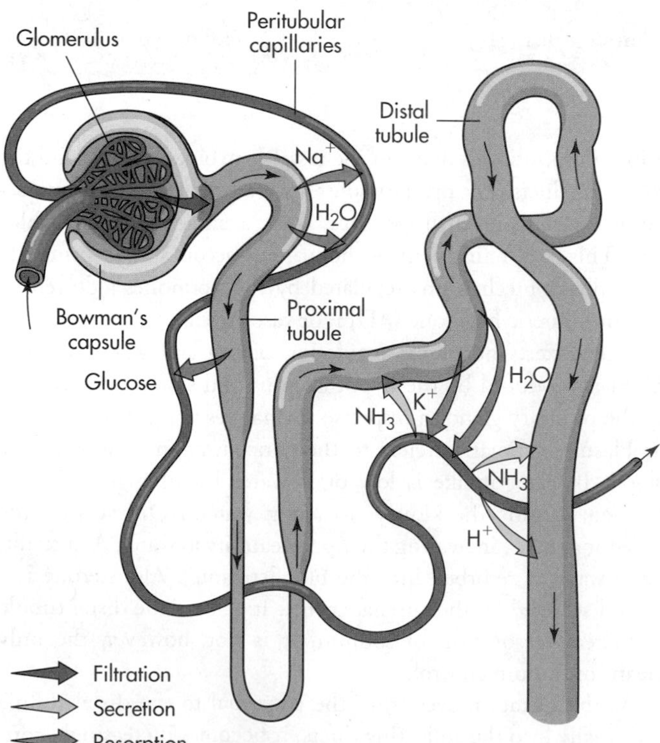

Figure 34-6 Mechanisms of urine formation—filtration, resorption, and secretion—and where they occur in the nephron. *Na^+*, Sodium; *H_2O*, water; *NH_3*, ammonia; *K^+*, potassium; *H^+*, hydrogen.

this ratio. The lungs vary the carbon dioxide content of the blood, and the kidneys principally secrete or retain bicarbonate and hydrogen ions in response to the pH of the blood. These two substances must move in or out of the blood at precisely the right time for the pH to remain stable. The exchange is accomplished in both the proximal tubules and the collecting ducts of the nephron. See Chapter 18 for a discussion of acid-base balance.

Erythropoiesis. The kidneys play a crucial role in red blood cell production via the process of **erythropoiesis**. Decreased tissue oxygenation stimulates special cells in the kidneys (thought to be the epithelial cells of the peritubular capillaries) to produce about 90% of the body's erythropoietin (EPO).[3] EPO stimulates the bone marrow to produce proerythroblasts, which develop into erythrocytes. Hypoxia and anemia generally trigger an increase in production of erythropoietin. Treatment with genetically engineered erythropoietin (epoetin alfa [Epogen, Procrit]) can improve the hematocrit and reduce the need for blood transfusions in patients with anemia secondary to chronic kidney failure, anemias associated with malignancies, and other disorders. With a synthetic form of erythropoietin, patients achieve a near-normal production of erythrocytes.

Calcium and Phosphorus Regulation. Serum calcium and phosphorus regulation is one of the kidney's most important functions. Calcium is crucial for bone formation, cell division and growth, blood coagulation, hormone response, and cellular electrical activity. Phosphate is a component of all intermediates of glucose metabolism, a part of the structure of all high-energy transfer compounds such as adenosine triphosphate, and an integral part of the crystalline structure of bones.

The kidneys influence the reciprocal calcium and phosphorus balance by converting the inactive form of vitamin D absorbed from the gut, to its active form, 1,25-dihydroxycholecalciferol. Parathyroid gland secretion of parathyroid hormone (PTH) is regulated by this form of vitamin D and calcium concentration. Under the influence of PTH, calcium resorption is increased and phosphate resorption is decreased.[1]

Blood Pressure Regulation. The kidneys play an active role in the regulation of blood pressure, primarily by regulating plasma volume and vascular tone. Blood pressure is manipulated through the kidneys' response to several mechanisms that alter the total volume of blood in the circulatory system. These mechanisms include ADH response, the renin-angiotensin system, and aldosterone response. As previously discussed, ADH release by the pituitary causes the kidneys to resorb water, which increases blood pressure.

The renin-angiotensin system and aldosterone response also influence the regulation of blood pressure. Renin is a hormone released by the juxtaglomerular apparatus of the nephron in response to sodium and potassium depletion, a drop in renal artery blood pressure, or sympathetic stimulation. Renin stimulates the conversion of angiotensinogen (a substance produced by the liver) to angiotensin I. Conversion of angiotensin I to angiotensin II by angiotensin-converting enzymes from the lung produces a powerful vasoconstriction and release of aldosterone, resulting in increased blood pressure. Aldosterone is released from the adrenal glands and acts on the kidneys to resorb sodium and water, increasing circulating blood volume and pressure (Figure 34-7).

Prostaglandin and bradykinin, hormones produced by the kidney and other tissues, help elevate blood pressure and increase renal blood flow as well. They are released in response to renal ischemia, the presence of ADH and angiotensin II, and sympathetic stimulation.[4] Acting locally and rapidly inactivated, they provide an immediate mechanism for improving renal blood flow.[4]

Excretion of Metabolic Wastes and Toxins. Metabolic wastes are excreted into the glomerular filtrate. Creatinine contained in the glomerular filtrate is excreted unchanged into the urine. Other wastes, such as urea, are excreted unchanged in the glomerular filtrate but are resorbed in part during passage through the nephron. Thus the amount of waste material excreted in urine is only a portion of that which was originally contained in the glomerular filtrate.

Most drugs are either excreted directly by the kidneys or first metabolized by the liver to inactive forms and then excreted by the kidneys. Because of the role of the kidneys in drug excretion, some drugs are contraindicated and the doses of others adjusted when renal function is impaired. Examples include many antibiotics, salicylates, and long-acting barbiturates.

Micturition. Micturition (urination) is a complex sensorimotor process. Urine flows from the renal pelvis and is propelled through the ureters by peristaltic action. About 200 to 300 ml of urine can collect in the bladder before the urge to void is felt. As

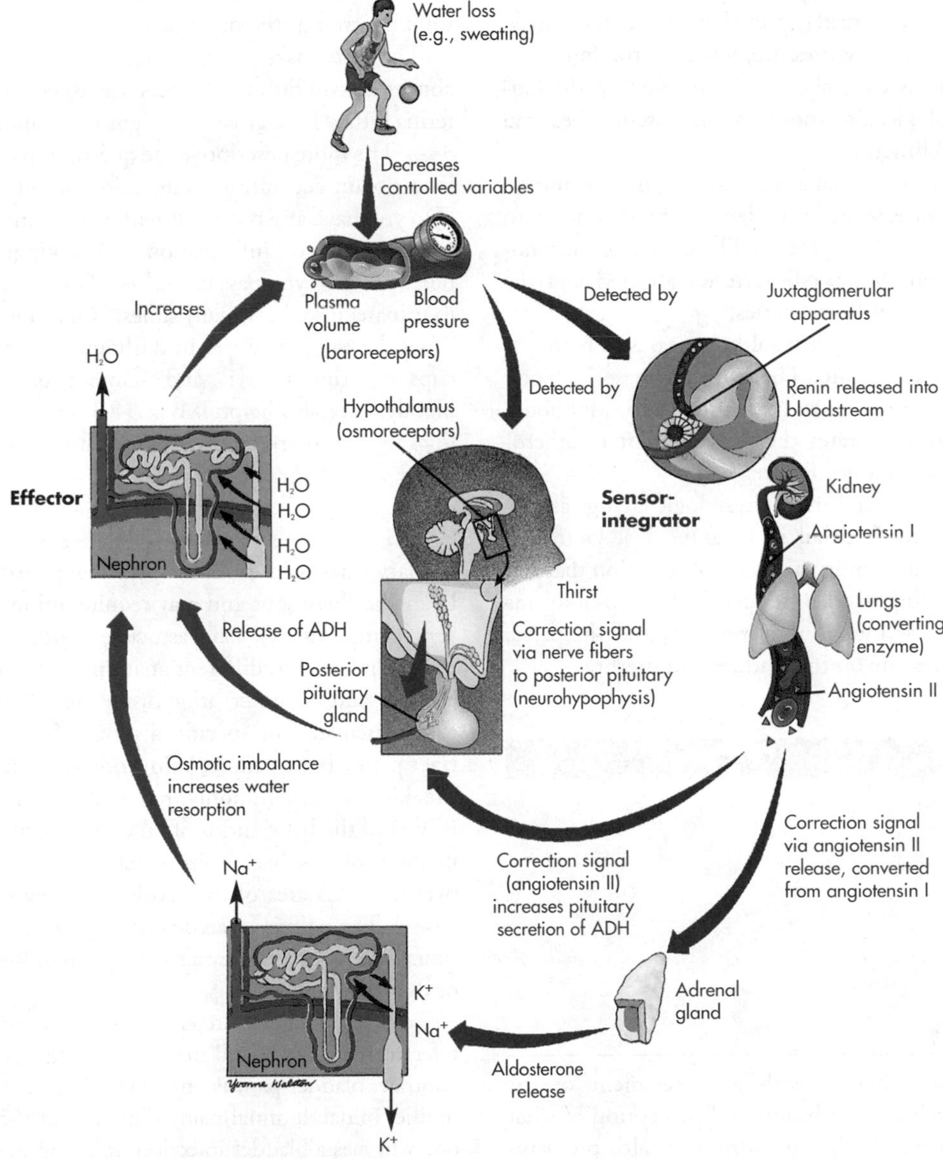

Figure 34-7 Renin-angiotensin system. Decreased blood pressure triggers hypothalamus to rapidly release antidiuretic hormone *(ADH)* from posterior pituitary gland. ADH increases water resorption by kidneys. Decreased blood pressure is also sensed by each nephron's juxtaglomerular apparatus, which responds by secreting renin. Renin triggers formation of angiotensin II, which stimulates release of aldosterone from adrenal cortex. Aldosterone boosts water *(H_2O)* resorption by increasing sodium *(Na^+)* resorption. These mechanisms work together to increase blood pressure. *K^+*, Potassium.

the bladder wall is stretched, baroreceptors cause reflex stimulation of parasympathetic nerves to the bladder, resulting in bladder contractions. When the motor nerves to the external urinary sphincter are inhibited, the muscle relaxes, opening the sphincter and permitting urine to be expelled.

When the motor nerves to the external urinary sphincter are activated, the sphincter remains contracted. This allows for voluntary control of urination even if the bladder muscles are also contracting. The end products of ultrafiltration are finally eliminated in this last step, and homeostasis is maintained.

Physiologic Changes With Aging

A variety of changes occur in the kidney and urinary tract in response to aging. A direct relationship exists between blood supply to the kidneys and renal function. The rate of blood flow to the kidneys is 5 to 10 times greater than that to the heart, liver, and brain. Glomerular capillary pressure, which is the force that promotes ultrafiltration, is controlled by blood flow to the kidneys. Therefore physiologic alterations in the vascular bed can lead to changes in renal function.

Arteriosclerotic changes in renal arteries are the most common form of renal vascular disease. Arteriosclerotic changes occur to some extent in the normal aging process. The degree of morphologic change depends on the specific arteries affected and the extent of involvement within those arteries.

Aging is also known to cause predictable increases in both systolic and diastolic blood pressure. This slow increase in blood pressure begins early in life and continues through adulthood. Untreated hypertension accelerates the development of atherosclerosis, which can lead to kidney failure.

Prostatic hypertrophy is a common physiologic change associated with aging (discussed in detail in Chapter 57). Untreated prostatic hypertrophy results in urinary tract obstruction that can lead to kidney failure. Aging women frequently develop problems with stress incontinence as muscle tone weakens and the pelvic organs put increasing pressure on the bladder and urethra.

▶ ARE You READY?

Which of the following causes sodium retention by the kidneys?

1. Angiotensin
2. Antidiuretic hormone
3. Aldosterone
4. Angiotensinogen

Health History

Baseline renal assessment begins with an assessment of the patient's subjective overall state of health and perception of what constitutes good health, rather than a listing of health problems and comorbidities. The interview then explores any patient concerns or health problems, especially any urinary tract symptoms. Table 34-3 defines terms used to describe common urologic symptoms and their clinical significance. When a kidney problem is suspected, the nurse asks the patient directly about each of these symptoms.

Urination

Obtaining baseline data concerning the person's usual voiding patterns, such as frequency and amount of urine with each void, is helpful when changes are anticipated. Persons who are admitted to a hospital or nursing facility are questioned about their ability to carry out toileting independently. All persons should be questioned about any changes noted in voiding patterns. If changes have occurred, the nurse must obtain more detailed information pertaining to onset, duration, and measures the person has taken to deal with problems.

When asking questions about urination, the nurse must be aware that some patients are reluctant to answer, either because of embarrassment or misunderstanding. A calm, matter-of-fact approach helps put the person at ease. Many persons are not familiar with terms such as *voiding* or *urination*, and the nurse may need to use more colloquial words and confirm that the person understands the questions.

The nurse asks specific questions to elicit information about abnormal conditions. Patients are asked directly in nonmedical terms if they have any of the signs or symptoms outlined in Table 34-3. The more descriptive the question, the more likely the nurse is to obtain accurate relevant information. For example, asking, "Do you have any problems with urination?" is less likely to elicit useful diagnostic information than asking, "Do you experience burning when you pass urine?" or "Do you have to get up at night to urinate; if so, how many times?" Questions such as "How many times do you pass water in 24 hours?" "Do you pass less than 2 cups of urine a day?" and "Does your urine look cloudy or bloody?" are also helpful. Box 34-3 reviews health history guidelines related to upper urinary tract disorders.

Pain

Urinary tract pain deserves special emphasis, since the cause can be medically serious and may require immediate attention to prevent complications. Pain associated with urinary tract disorders may be referred to different anatomic locations depending on the etiology and the innervation of the area affected. (See Chapter 35 for a discussion of specific disease processes that cause urinary tract pain.) For example, pain from inflammation or infection of the kidney is commonly referred to the costovertebral angle (CVA) of the back and is often called "flank pain." Patients complaining of low back pain of renal origin experience tenderness over the CVA area of the involved kidney when that area is percussed. The pain is often described as severe. If the cause is infectious, these patients may also complain of lower urinary tract pain or dysuria.

Pain involving the ureter or upper urinary tract is also generally referred to the back and manifests as vague, chronic back pain. In contrast, bladder pain is often experienced as lower, crampy, spasmodic, midabdominal pain. This type of pain is typical of someone who has a bladder infection. It is important to remember that pain intensity varies from person to person. For example, patients with peripheral neuropathy commonly seen in advanced diabetes or patients with paresthesias from spinal cord lesions may experience remote, decreased, or even no pain from renal or urinary tract disease. The nursing implication of this deviation is that pain cannot be relied on as a warning sign of disease in these populations.

TABLE 34-3 CLINICAL SIGNIFICANCE OF COMMON URINARY TRACT SYMPTOMS

Symptom	Definition	Clinical Significance
Dysuria	Pain, burning with voiding	Urinary tract infection
Frequency	Voiding multiple times during the day in either large or small amounts	Urinary tract infection, retention, hyperglycemia with increased fluid intake, prostatic hypertrophy
Urgency	Need to void immediately	Urinary tract infection, bladder irritation, trauma, tumor
Nocturia	Awakening to void; abnormal when it occurs multiple times during sleep cycle	Diuretics, prostatic hypertrophy, kidney failure or insufficiency, increased fluid intake, congestive heart failure
Hesitancy	Difficulty initiating voiding	Partial urethral obstruction, neurogenic bladder
Incontinence	Loss of voluntary control of urination	Urinary tract infection, urethral obstruction, posturinary catheter removal, central nervous system or spinal cord disease, postprostatectomy, laxity of perineal muscles in older women
Frothing	Excessive foaming of urine	Presence of protein in urine
Foul odor	Foul smell associated with urine	Urinary tract infection
Polyuria	Urinary output >3000 ml/24 hr	Diabetes mellitus, hormonal abnormality, diabetes insipidus, high-output kidney failure
Oliguria	Urinary output <400 ml/24 hr	Kidney failure, urinary retention or obstruction
Anuria	Urinary output <100 ml/24 hr	Kidney failure, total obstruction (trauma, mass)
Myoglobinuria	Red-brown, at times black, pigment in urine	Muscle tissue breakdown after extreme physical exertion or massive trauma (myoglobin is muscle hemoglobin); can result in kidney failure
Hematuria	Red blood cells in urine; may be gross (visible to eye) or microscopic (detectable with urine screen and microscope)	Renal calculi, urinary tract infection, inflammation of kidney or bladder, trauma to kidney or urinary tract, posturinary catheter removal, menses

Box 34-3 Health History Related to Upper Urinary Tract Disorders

Change in Usual Voiding Pattern

Dysuria: pain or burning on urination
Frequency of urination: frequent voiding
Nocturia: need to void at night
Polyuria: excretion of unusually large amounts of urine
Oliguria: decreased capacity to form and pass urine
Anuria: inability to urinate, cessation of urine production
Questions: onset and duration, pattern, severity, associated symptoms, efforts to treat and their outcome
Pain
—Location: kidney (flank, costovertebral angle); ureter (along course of ureter to groin)
—Questions: character, intensity, onset and duration, precipitating factors, relieving factors, accompanying symptoms

Change in Appearance of Urine

Hematuria: bright red bleeding, rusty brown, cola colored; at beginning, end, or throughout voiding
Proteinuria: deep yellow, foamy
Color changes caused by food or drugs
Passage of stone
May be a single stone or gravel-like material; may be associated with hematuria, fever, and pain

Patient's Perception of Problem

Degree of concern about the symptom and the patient's opinion as to its cause

Patient History Relating to Upper Urinary Tract Disorders

Concurrent disorders
Medical history
—Infancy, childhood
Previous disorders (urinary tract infection, kidney stones, other kidney disease)
Serious injuries
Hospitalizations, surgery
Gynecologic history
Medication history: current and recent prescription and non-prescription drugs taken
Family history: polycystic kidney disease, renal calculi, renal tubular acidosis, hypertension, diabetes mellitus, renal or bladder cancer
Diet and nutritional state
Sociocultural history
Psychosocial history

From Brundage D: *Renal disorders,* St Louis, 1992, Mosby.

Physical Examination

Moderate or severe renal disease can cause significant observable pathologic changes. For example, the quantity of urine excreted in 24 hours offers critical diagnostic data. Polyuria, oliguria, and anuria (see Table 34-3) are all clinically significant and require further evaluation.

Obtaining an accurate assessment of urinary output is often difficult in a hospital setting. Urine may be inadvertently discarded, or the patient may void into the toilet. The nurse must explain the importance of accurate urine collection and verify that the patient understands. All staff members need to be aware if a patient's output is being measured. In some cases, such as patients in shock or acute kidney failure, an indwelling catheter must be inserted to ensure accurate assessment of urinary output. However, the risks and benefits of inserting an indwelling urinary catheter must always be assessed before placement occurs.

The actual appearance of the urine is clinically important as well. The nurse inspects the urine for gross variations from normal. Normal urine varies from pale to deep yellow, depending on specific gravity. A very dark color suggests that urine may be concentrated (high specific gravity) or may have an increased excretion of bilirubin. Certain medications and foods also can change the color of urine. Cloudy urine may result from precipitation of phosphate salts in alkaline urine or from bacterial growth. Vaginal discharge also may give the urine a cloudy appearance.

Hematuria (blood in the urine) may be detected overtly or microscopically. In gross hematuria the urine may be pink tinged to cherry red. If blood is observed in the urine of a woman having her menstrual period, the vaginal orifice can be blocked with cotton balls and another specimen obtained to ascertain the source of the blood. Hematuria with pain may be the result of calculi, a clot from renal bleeding, or bladder infection.

The physical appearance of the patient with kidney failure can change noticeably. For example, kidney failure commonly causes edema of the eyelids, hands, feet, and ankles (or even the sacrum in immobile bed-bound patients). To assess changes in edema and fluid balance, the nurse must weigh the patient daily, at the same time of day and using the same scale for consistency. The skin may be pale or even have a frosted appearance *(uremic frost)* when the kidneys stop functioning completely. The breath may have an ammonia-like odor as waste products accumulate in the body. Kidney failure is presented in detail in Chapter 36.

Assessment measures and variations in normal findings relevant to the care of older adults are presented in the Gerontologic Assessment box. Also identified are disorders common in older adults, which may be responsible for abnormal assessment findings.

Gerontologic Assessment

Urinary Problems

- Determine pattern of urination and any related personal habits.
- Problems with urinary control are not unusual in older adults, and individuals establish personal methods of coping such as use of incontinence products and timing of fluid intake.
- Assess for contributing factors if functional (environmental) incontinence is a problem.
- Mobility problems, diuretic use, or mental changes may be contributing factors.
- Assess for signs of urinary tract infection that are commonly manifested in older persons. Usual signs of fever and pain or burning with urination may be minimal or absent; confusion and anorexia may be the only symptoms.
- Monitor kidney function during diagnostic testing.
- When older adults undergo extensive testing that may lead to dehydration, marginal kidney function can be compromised.

Common Disorders in Older Adults

- Urinary incontinence
- Urinary tract infections
- Benign prostatic hyperplasia
- Cancer of kidney, bladder, or prostate
- Kidney failure
- Dysuria

Diagnostic Tests

Special examinations of the urinary system are performed to identify the location and nature of existing disease. The accuracy of the test findings often depends on the patient's cooperation in restricting or augmenting fluids and collecting specimens at designated times. The nurse should give the patient clear, precise directions; written instructions are a valuable supplement to verbal directions for patients who can see and read.

Many of the diagnostic tests used to assess renal function can be performed in an ambulatory setting. Therefore it is important to make certain that the patient understands all instructions in preparation for the test. Some examinations must be performed with patients under sedation; if so, the nurse instructs patients to arrange for someone to take them home after the procedure.

Laboratory Tests

Blood Tests. Several serum tests can be performed to evaluate kidney function. The two most common are tests for blood urea nitrogen (BUN) and creatinine levels, by-products of protein breakdown and muscle metabolism, respectively. The kidneys, as long as they function normally, maintain serum levels of BUN and creatinine within a narrow, predictable range. Of the two, BUN varies the most because it can be influenced by a high-protein diet or events such as gastrointestinal bleeding. Creatinine remains relatively constant. With severe renal disease and the loss of nephrons and corresponding function (acute or chronic kidney failure or end-stage renal disease), the complete blood count, iron studies, and blood chemistry analyses become altered as homeostasis is lost. Table 34-4 summarizes blood tests used in the evaluation of renal function.

Urine Tests

URINALYSIS. A urinalysis is performed in two parts. The first part (the urine screen) consists of dipping a reagent strip into a clean-catch urine specimen and noting the color changes in each section of the strip, which tests for substances such as glucose and albumin. This may be followed by a microscopic examination, which is performed whenever the results from the urine screen are abnormal or abnormalities are suspected. The examination focuses on analysis of urine sediment, the solid matter found in

TABLE 34-4 SELECTED RENAL FUNCTION TESTS

Test	Normal Results	Purpose or Significance	Pretest Preparation and Posttest Care
BLOOD TESTS			
Serum creatinine	Men: 0.85-1.5 mg/dl Women: 0.7-1.25 mg/dl	Test indicates ability of kidneys to excrete creatinine. Serum creatinine gives rough estimate of glomerular filtration rate.	No specific preparation is needed for test. Diet and metabolic rate have little effect on serum creatinine value.
Blood urea nitrogen	5-20 mg/dl	Test indicates ability of kidneys to excrete nitrogenous wastes.	Blood urea nitrogen can be affected by high-protein diet, blood in gastrointestinal tract, hepatic disease, medications, hydration status, and catabolic state (injury, infection, fever, poor nutrition).
URINE TESTS			
Urine specific gravity	1.003-1.029	Test measures ability of kidneys to concentrate urine.	First morning void usually is in high normal range in healthy person. False high is caused by presence of radiographic dyes.
Urine osmolality	250-900 mOsm/L	Test is excellent indication of renal function. Osmolality is total concentration of particles in solution.	No special preparation is needed.
Fishberg concentration test	Urine volume: 300/ml/12 hr Specific gravity: 1.024 or greater Urine osmolality: 850 mOsm/kg or greater	Test is used to determine ability of kidney to conserve fluid and to establish differential diagnosis for diabetes insipidus and psychogenic polydipsia.	No fluid can be taken during test period. Test period is 8-12 hr, usually during night. First morning void ensures maximal concentration. Three hourly urine specimens are collected for volume, specific gravity, and osmolality after test period. Patient should be observed for signs of vascular collapse.
Urine chemistry	Sodium: 110-250 mEq/24 hr Potassium: 25-123 mg/24 hr Calcium: 100-250 mg/24 hr	Urine electrolytes reflect ability of kidney to excrete and resorb electrolytes.	Abnormal results may be caused by disease processes other than renal disorders (e.g., elevated urine calcium in hyperparathyroidism or prolonged immobilization).
Creatinine clearance	Men: 90-140 ml/min Women: 85-125 ml/min	Results provide rate at which kidneys remove creatinine from plasma. Because diet and metabolic state have little influence on it, creatinine clearance provides rough estimate of glomerular filtration rate.	See Guidelines for Safe Practice box on p. 955 for collecting a timed urine specimen.

the urine after centrifuging. Normal urine contains almost no sediment. Interpretation of abnormal sediment is difficult, and the findings are carefully correlated with data from the patient's history and physical examination. Table 34-5 summarizes normal and abnormal urinalysis findings.

Clean-Catch Urine Specimens. Ideally all urinalysis specimens should be clean-catch specimens (see Guidelines for Safe Practice box at left), but this is particularly important if a urinary tract infection is suspected. Specimens should be transported to the laboratory within 30 minutes or promptly refrigerated. Clean-catch specimens are also obtained for toxicologic analysis (drugs or chemicals), cytology (abnormal cells), and pregnancy testing. A catheterized specimen may be indicated if midstream urine cannot be collected. However, catheterization should only be used if absolutely necessary. The risk of bacterial contamination is significant any time a catheter is introduced into the bladder.

Timed Urine Collection. A timed urine collection involves pooling all the urine a patient excretes over a specific period. This test is often required for urologic diagnosis. The duration of urine collections may vary from 2 to 24 hours, with 24-hour collections being the most common. The pooled urine specimen is examined for sugar, protein, sediment (blood cells and casts), 17-ketosteroids, electrolytes, catecholamines, and breakdown products of protein metabolism. These tests provide information on (1) the ability of the kidneys to excrete and conserve various solutes, (2) the production of various hormones that are excreted in the urine, (3) changes in the body's regulation of glucose metabolism, (4) identification of organisms difficult to recognize through routine urine cultures, and (5) the presence of abnormal cells and debris in the urine.

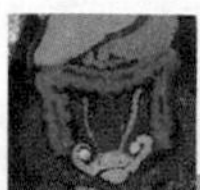

Guidelines for Safe Practice
Collecting a Midstream Urine Specimen

Equipment Needed

Sterile container for the urine
Three sponges (cotton or gauze) saturated with cleansing solution

General Directions

Touch only the outside of collecting container.
Collect urine in container well after urinary stream is started.

Special Directions

Female

Cleanse meatus with one front-to-back motion with each of three cleansing sponges.
Keep labia separated throughout procedure.

Male

Cleanse glans with each of three cleansing sponges.
Retract foreskin if penis is uncircumcised.

The accuracy of findings in a timed urine collection depends on proper collection of the specimen. Whether the specimen is obtained in the hospital or the home, the nurse needs to tell the person exactly how to collect it and verify his or her understanding (see Guidelines for Safe Practice box, p. 955).

Timed urine tests also may involve collecting urine from more than one source. The person may pass urine from the urethra and also drain urine from a nephrostomy tube. In addition, urine may drain from ureteral catheters, with urine being collected separately from each kidney. Depending on the test's purpose, the urine col-

Table 34-5 Urinalysis Findings

Test	Normal	Abnormal
Color	Pale to darker yellow	Red indicates hematuria (possibly urinary obstruction, renal calculi, tumor, kidney failure, cystitis).
Clarity	Clear	Cloudy urine may indicate debris or bacterial sediment (UTI).
pH	4.5 -8.0 (average 6.0)	pH is alkaline on standing or with UTI. Acidity is increased with renal tubular acidosis.
Specific gravity	1.007-1.030	Specific gravity usually reflects fluid intake; the less the fluid intake, the higher the specific gravity. If specific gravity remains low (1.010-1.014), renal disease or pituitary disease (deficit of ADH) is suspected.
Protein	0-8 mg/dl	Proteinuria may occur with high-protein diet and exercise (particularly prolonged). It is also seen in renal disease.
Glucose	None	Glycosuria occurs after high intake of sugar or with diabetes mellitus.
Ketones	None	Ketonuria occurs with starvation and diabetic ketoacidosis.
Red blood cells	0-5 cells/high-power field	Red blood cells indicate injury to kidney tissue (see Color, above).
White blood cells	0-5 cells/high-power field	White blood cells indicate UTI.
Casts	0-4 hyaline casts/low-power field	Casts are seen with UTI, renal disease.

ADH, Antidiuretic hormone; *UTI*, urinary tract infection.

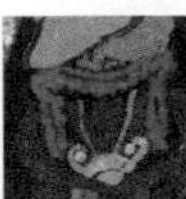

GUIDELINES FOR SAFE PRACTICE
Collecting a Timed Urine Specimen

- Instruct the patient to empty the bladder and discard the urine at the appointed time to start the test.
- Save the urine from all subsequent voidings.
- Provide specific directions for storing the urine. Some specimens need to be kept cold during the collection period, some need preservatives, and some need no special care.
- Instruct the patient to void into a separate receptacle before defecating to avoid contaminating the specimen.
- Instruct the patient to empty the bladder and add the urine to the collection at the appointed time to end the test.
- Send the designated amount (properly labeled) to the laboratory.
- If an aliquot (5 to 10 ml sample of the total specimen) is the designated amount, measure the total amount collected and record, and mix the specimen well before removing the aliquot.

lected from each source may be collected in separate containers or combined.

CLEARANCE TESTS. When renal disease is suspected, the amount of damage that has occurred, if any, must be assessed. Clearance tests are the most practical and efficient way to identify losses in renal function. These tests measure the amount of blood that a person's kidneys can "clear," or filter out of a substance, in a given amount of time. When the results are compared with normal values, changes in renal function become apparent. Clearance tests also are used to monitor the direction of change and the rate of change in renal function over time.

The *creatinine clearance test* is the most practical and widely used of all clearance tests. **Creatinine** is a substance that results from the breakdown of muscle tissue. Produced at a relatively fixed and uniform rate throughout the day, creatinine can be measured readily in the blood and is not influenced by dietary intake. Creatinine is excreted through the kidneys, filtered at the glomerulus, and passed practically unchanged through the renal tubules. Creatinine is an ideal, naturally occurring substance that, when blood and urine values are compared, allows an estimation of changes in GFR and overall kidney function. A person's creatinine clearance value is expressed in terms of milliliters per minute and is determined according to the following formula:

$$\text{Creatinine clearance (ml/min)} = \text{Urine volume (ml/min)} \times \frac{\text{Urine creatinine concentration (mg/ml)}}{\text{Plasma creatinine concentration (mg/ml)}}$$

A morning-to-morning 24-hour urine collection is obtained. Immediately after the final urine specimen is collected, a blood specimen is drawn to determine the serum creatinine level. Both blood and urine specimens are sent together for analysis. Analysis of the total urine volume for the test period is essential to accurately determine renal function. If one void is accidentally discarded, the test must be repeated. Accurate collection of all urine in the prescribed time is essential for the validity of the test. A shorter period when obtaining an accurate 24-hour urine collection is not possible.

The *Cockroft and Gault equation* (CGE) may also be used to assess and estimate kidney function. No urine collection is necessary for the CGE. The equation is:

$$\text{Creatinine clearance (ml/min)} = \frac{(140 - \text{Age}) \times (\text{IBW}) \times 0.85 \text{ if female}}{72 \times \text{SCR}}$$

where IBW is ideal body weight (kg) (men = 50 kg ++ 2.3 kg/in over 5 ft; women = 45.5 kg + 2.3 kg/in over 5 ft) and SCR is serum creatinine.

The *sodium excretion test* measures tubular function. Specifically this test provides information about the kidneys' ability to appropriately excrete or conserve sodium; in chronic kidney failure either inappropriate retention or excretion of sodium can occur. Knowledge of urinary excretion of this electrolyte is helpful in calculating the patient's sodium intake requirements. Current and past sodium excretion studies are compared to determine changes in tubular function. The sodium excretion test is performed by analyzing the sodium content of a 24-hour urine collection.

Radiologic Tests

A number of radiologic examinations are used to visualize the urinary tract. Because the kidneys lie retroperitoneally, any accumulation of flatus or feces in the intestine can obstruct the view on the x-ray film. To ensure adequate visualization, bowel cleansing is necessary before the x-ray films are taken.

X-ray films of the urinary tract may be ordered in conjunction with other abdominal studies. Visualizing the urinary tract may be difficult if the patient has recently undergone barium studies. Performing urinary tract examinations before barium contrast studies of the gastrointestinal tract can prevent this problem. Table 34-6 summarizes the common radiologic tests used to assess kidney function.

Special Tests

Measurement of Residual Urine. Normally the bladder contains little or no urine after voiding; however, certain disease states prevent the bladder from emptying completely. Some common conditions associated with incomplete emptying of the bladder are benign prostatic hypertrophy, urethral strictures, and interruptions in bladder innervation (neurogenic bladder). Urine remaining in the bladder after voiding is called **residual urine**.

One way to determine the amount of residual urine is to catheterize the person immediately after voiding. This may be performed on a one-time basis or repeated with each void. If the residual volume is large, an indwelling catheter may be left in place. Residual urine volumes of 50 ml or less indicate near-normal or returning bladder function.

A second way to determine the amount of residual urine is the use of a portable ultrasound instrument at the patient's bedside. This noninvasive study is accurate in measuring bladder volumes greater than 200 ml.

To avoid inserting a catheter, the examiner may take an x-ray film of retained urine. A radiopaque substance is injected intravenously. As the dye is excreted in the urine, it passes into the

TABLE 34-6 COMMON RADIOLOGIC AND SPECIAL TESTS FOR URINARY TRACT

Purpose	Procedure	Pretest Preparation and Posttest Care
RETROGRADE PYELOGRAPHY		
Visualization of urinary tract	1. Ureteral catheterization required 2. Radiopaque material (Hypaque, Renografin) gently injected 3. X-ray films taken of renal collecting structures	Patient may experience discomfort in region of kidneys as dye is injected. Pain may be experienced if too large a volume of dye is injected and renal pelvis becomes distended.
INTRAVENOUS PYELOGRAPHY (IVP)		
Determination of size and location of kidneys, degree of obstruction Demonstration of cysts, renal stones, or tumors Outline of filling of renal pelvis Outline of ureters and bladder	1. X-ray film of abdomen (KUB) taken to identify size and position of kidneys 2. Radiopaque dye given intravenously 3. X-ray films of kidneys taken at 3-, 5-, 10-, and 20-min intervals	Bowel cleansing is required. Inform patient that feeling of warmth, flushing of face, and salty taste in mouth may occur as dye is injected. Inform patient that numerous x-ray films are taken during procedure; this does not indicate a problem. Assess patient before test for any history of allergy to iodine, shellfish, or dyes, and carefully monitor for signs and symptoms of reaction to dye, including respiratory distress, diaphoresis, urticaria, instability of vital signs, or unusual sensations. Emergency equipment should be available. Force fluids after test to help excrete contrast material and prevent kidney failure.
KIDNEY, URETER, AND BLADDER (KUB) X-RAY FILMS		
Gross visualization of KUB Location of calcifications and stones possible	X-ray plain film of abdominal region obtained	Bowel cleansing sometimes is ordered.
COMPUTED TOMOGRAPHY (CT) SCAN		
Visualization of kidneys and renal circulation using an x-ray beam rotated around body Gold standard for diagnosis of renal stones Stages and evaluates renal cell carcinoma and renal venous thrombosis	Whole body CT scanner segments kidneys Can be performed with intravenous contrast dye	If dye is used, the same implications apply as listed for IVP.

urinary bladder. A sufficient amount of urine containing the radiopaque material is allowed to accumulate in the bladder, and the person is then instructed to void. An x-ray film is taken, revealing any urine retained in the bladder. This means of determining residual urine is used in conjunction with other studies to visualize the urinary tract.

Cystometrography. Cystometric examination is performed to evaluate bladder tone. The examination is indicated for patients with incontinence or evidence of neurologic bladder dysfunction. An indwelling urinary catheter is inserted before the examination. With the person in a supine position, a liter bag of normal saline or sterile distilled water and a cystometer are connected to the catheter. Fluid is instilled at a constant and specified rate; measurements of the pressure that the bladder musculature exerts on the fluid are recorded after the instillation of every 50 ml of fluid. The person is asked to report feelings of fullness, the need to void, and any urgency or discomfort. Fluid is instilled until urgency occurs or sensation is determined to be absent. During cystometric examination a cholinergic drug (bethanechol chloride [Urecholine]) may be administered to determine its effect on enhancing the tone of a flaccid bladder, or anticholinergic medication may be given to assess relaxation in a hyperactive bladder. No specific care is required after cystometric examination.

Other urodynamic tests may be used to evaluate the neuromuscular function of the urinary sphincter. Electromyography

TABLE 34-6 COMMON RADIOLOGIC AND SPECIAL TESTS FOR URINARY TRACT—CONT'D

Purpose	Procedure	Pretest Preparation and Posttest Care
MAGNETIC RESONANCE IMAGING (MRI)		
Gold standard for diagnosis of renal venous thrombosis	Uses electromagnetic energy to provide visualization of structures No dye needed No radiation	Contraindicated with cardiac pacemakers, implanted metallic clips, some heart valves, and life support devices. Patient may need sedation. Patient must lie still in confined space for 30-90 min. Prepare patient for sounds from pulsing of magnetic field during scanning.
RENAL ANGIOGRAPHY		
Visualization of renal circulation Particularly useful in evaluating renal artery stenosis and polyarteritis nodosa	Similar to IVP; however, contrast dye often injected directly into femoral artery by passing catheter through artery to level of renal arteries	Nursing implications are same as for IVP. Observe patient for dye-induced acute kidney failure and bleeding at arterial puncture site, especially within first 4 hr. Check pressure dressing for fresh bleeding. Check puncture site for tenderness or swelling. Assess vital signs and distal pulses frequently (every 15 min for 3-4 hr). Maintain bed rest for 8 hr after procedure.
ISOTOPE GLOMERULAR FILTRATION RATE		
Uses isotope that is eliminated by kidney to accurately measure glomerular filtration rate	Radioisotope injected and blood samples collected for 4-6 hr to track clearance of isotope	Reassure patient that only trace doses of isotope are used, and there is no risk related to radioactivity.
ULTRASOUND		
Uses sound waves to determine size and texture of kidneys Test of choice to exclude urinary tract obstruction Can grossly differentiate cystic and solid masses	Sound waves reflecting off kidneys; computer interpreting different tissue densities	Procedure is painless and noninvasive. A full bladder is required to delineate abdominal structures.

aids in the assessment of functional or psychologic voiding disturbances. Electromyography may also be used to evaluate sphincter tone and determine whether nerve pathways are intact.

Ultrasonography. Sound waves may be used to detect renal or urinary problems such as tumors, congenital defects, obstruction, abnormalities in size or shape of the kidneys or bladder, or abnormal fluid accumulations. Ultrasonography is a harmless, noninvasive procedure. A transducer placed over the kidney or bladder emits high-frequency sound waves that bounce back to a sensor. Electronic conversion of the sound waves produces an image of the underlying structure. The only preparation for an ultrasonography test is fluid intake to ensure a full urinary bladder, which is required for the test. Ultrasonography is often the first screening test used when renal or bladder dysfunction is suspected.

Kidney Biopsy. Kidney (or renal) biopsy is the most accurate diagnostic tool for determining the type and stage of a pathologic condition involving the kidneys. This test aids in differentiating diagnoses, following the progression of disease processes, selecting therapy, and determining prognosis of the illness. The biopsy can be performed either through a skin puncture (percutaneous) or through an incision (open renal biopsy) over the kidney.

Because the kidney is such a vascular organ, hemorrhage after a biopsy is a potential threat. Throughout the procedure, care is taken to prevent and detect early blood loss. Before performing a biopsy, the health care provider completes a thorough medical evaluation with particular attention to any abnormality in bleeding or coagulation time. Medications that alter clotting function are withheld. These include aspirin, nonsteroidal antiinflammatory drugs, platelet inhibitors, and warfarin. The patient's blood usually is typed and cross-matched for 2 units of blood. The risk of bleeding is greatest in the first 12 hours after biopsy.[5,6]

Preparation before either type of biopsy includes discussing the procedure with the patient and answering any questions. Informed consent is required, since renal biopsy is an invasive procedure. The biopsy may be performed in the operating room or radiology department.

The procedure for percutaneous (closed) renal biopsy is as follows. Before the biopsy, the patient is taken to the radiology department for localization of the kidney. This is accomplished with a plain x-ray, a dye contrast x-ray, or fluoroscopic location. The lower pole of the kidney is located and marked on the skin in ink. The lower pole is the site for obtaining the biopsy specimen because it contains the fewest blood vessels. The patient is then transported to the area where the biopsy will be performed. The percutaneous biopsy is performed with ultrasound or computed tomography to guide the placement of the biopsy needle.

Sedation is not generally required unless the patient is restless or unable to relax sufficiently to follow instructions during the procedure. The patient is placed in a prone position over a sandbag or firm pillow. The physician identifies the location for biopsy, and a local anesthetic agent is injected. As the biopsy needle is inserted, the patient is instructed to take a breath and hold it, since the kidneys move up and down with respiration. The patient may feel pressure or pain in the kidney region as the needle punctures the tough renal capsule. The needle is withdrawn immediately, and direct pressure is applied to the site for 20 minutes. A pressure dressing is then applied, and the patient is turned supine and kept flat for at least 4 hours. A small sandbag may be placed over the biopsy site to help prevent bleeding. The nursing care associated with renal biopsy is summarized in the Guidelines for Safe Practice box.

An open biopsy carries less risk of hemorrhage and provides better visualization of the kidney. However, it is a more invasive procedure with associated risks of anesthesia, wound infection, and longer recovery time. The procedure for an open biopsy is similar to that used for kidney surgery. Nursing care for this type of surgery is discussed in Chapter 35. Most biopsies are performed by the percutaneous method.

▶ ARE You READY?

Which of the following statements by the patient scheduled for renal biopsy indicates that teaching was effective?

1. "I should take my Coumadin with a sip of water."
2. "I will be put to sleep for this procedure."
3. "I will have to stay flat on my back for four hours after the test."
4. "I will have a catheter during the procedure."

Endoscopy. Technologic advances make it possible to visualize the urinary tract directly and indirectly. Endoscopy allows for assessment of both structure and function of the organs and tissues of the urinary tract. Visualization of the urinary tract is used not only for diagnosis but also for evaluation of the patient's response to therapy over time.

GUIDELINES FOR SAFE PRACTICE
Care of the Patient After Percutaneous Renal Biopsy

- Maintain the patient motionless in a supine position for 4 hours after the biopsy.
- Instruct the patient to avoid coughing for first 4 hours after the biopsy because it increases abdominal venous pressure.
- Take blood pressure and pulse on the following schedule:
  —Every 15 minutes for the first hour
  —Every 30 minutes for the second hour
  —Every hour for the next 2 hours or until stable
- Notify the physician of increases in pulse of more than 10 to 20 beats/min above the baseline or decreases in blood pressure of more than 10 mm Hg, unless instructed otherwise.
- Maintain bed rest for 24 hours.
- Observe urine for hematuria for first 24 hours after the biopsy.
- Instruct patient to:
  —Avoid heavy lifting and strenuous activities for 10 to 14 days after the biopsy.
  —Increase fluid intake unless contraindicated.
  —Report any signs of renal bleeding or infection.

CYSTOSCOPY. Cystoscopy is the direct examination of the bladder with an instrument called a cystoscope (Figure 34-8). The cystoscope relies on a flexible optic fiber to illuminate the urinary tract. The instrument is attached to the light source and then slowly passed through the urinary tract, enabling direct visualization of the urethra, ureteral orifices, and bladder. Since the procedure is invasive, informed consent is required. The patient is asked to drink 2 to 3 L of fluid 2 hours before the procedure to ensure a continuous flow of urine in the event specimens need to be collected. Patients undergoing general anesthesia for the procedure receive fluids intravenously. If x-ray films are to be taken during the procedure, bowel preparation is necessary.

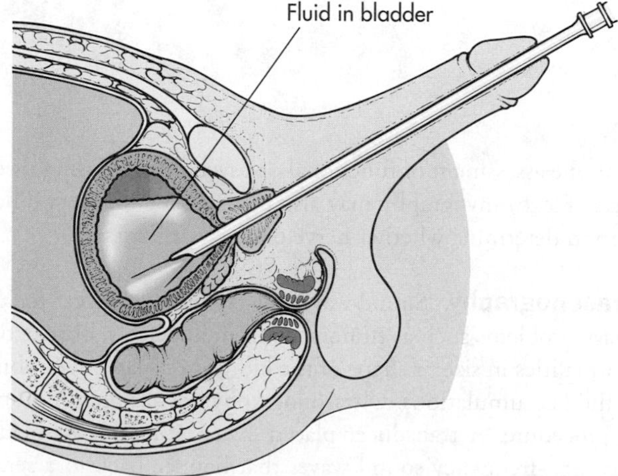

Figure 34-8 Cystoscope inserted for examination of bladder.

The cystoscopic examination may be performed with or without anesthesia. General anesthesia is rarely required for cystoscopy, unless the person is unable to cooperate and the procedure is absolutely necessary. The need for painful manipulation during the procedure may also necessitate general anesthesia. In these cases anesthesia reduces the possibility of urethral trauma or bladder perforation caused by the patient's sudden vigorous movement during the examination.

Much of the discomfort felt during this procedure is the result of contraction or spasm of the bladder sphincters, which can be decreased through deep-breathing exercises and general relaxation. A sedative such as diazepam (Valium) or midazolam (Versed) and an opioid such as morphine or meperidine hydrochloride (Demerol) are usually given an hour before the examination.

If the patient is relatively comfortable, the cystoscope may be passed with little pain, provided there is no obstruction in the urethra. A local anesthetic such as procaine (usually 4%) may be instilled into the urethra before insertion of the cystoscope.

When the patient is awake, he or she will feel a strong desire to void immediately after the instrument is passed into the urethra. This feeling is due to the pressure exerted by the instrument against the internal sphincter. During the examination the bladder is distended with normal saline for visualization. As the bladder becomes increasingly distended, the urge to void increases.

A number of additional tests may be performed during cystoscopic examination. *Cystography* involves the injection of a radiopaque dye such as methiodal (Skiodan) or air as a contrast medium to visualize the bladder and determine its size, shape, and presence of irregularities. Bladder capacity can be measured through instillation of distilled water. A voiding *cystourethrogram* can reveal reflux of urine into the ureters on voiding, a bladder malfunction that can lead to pyelonephritis.

Ureteral catheterization (with a nylon, radiopaque, size 4 to 6 F catheter) can be performed through the cystoscope. The catheter is inserted into the ureteral opening in the bladder, then carefully advanced up the ureter and into the renal pelvis (Figure 34-9). This procedure may involve one or both ureters. Ureteral catheterization is performed (1) when culture and analysis of urine from individual kidneys is required, (2) when tests of renal function are to be performed on the kidneys separately, and (3) when visualization of the urinary tract is desired, and intravenous pyelogram visualization has been inadequate, obstruction is present, or sensitivity to intravenous radiopaque material is noted.

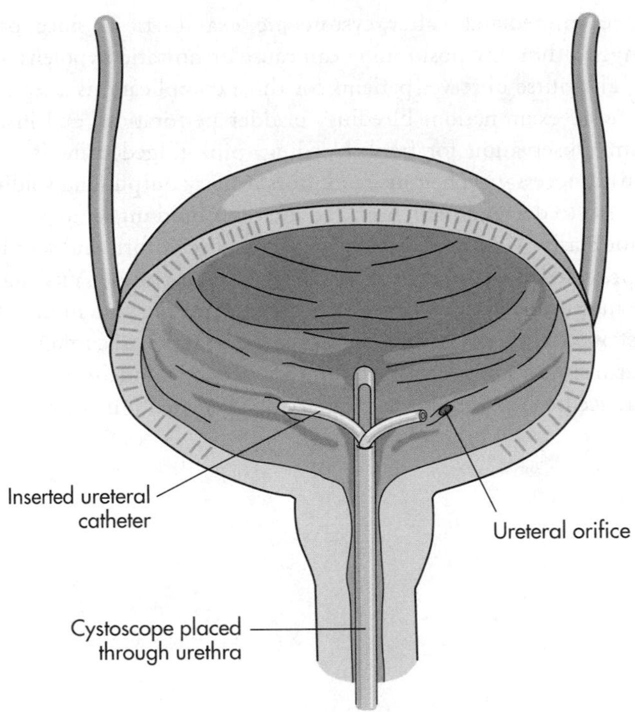

Figure 34-9 Ureteral catheterization through cystoscope. Note ureteral catheter inserted into left orifice. Right ureteral catheter is ready to be inserted.

The nurse verifies the patient's understanding of the procedure as part of preprocedural teaching. If local anesthesia is to be used, the nurse must describe what the patient can expect to feel during the procedure. The patient should not stand or walk

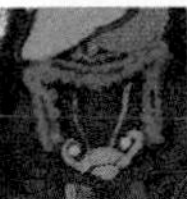

GUIDELINES FOR SAFE PRACTICE *Care of the Patient After Cystoscopy*

- Ensure that vital signs are stable and that the patient has a patent airway immediately postprocedure if the procedure was done using general anesthesia or if a medication such as midazolam (Versed) has been used for relaxation and sedation. This is the first priority.
- Ensure a comfortable transition to the recovery area. If patient does not have an indwelling catheter, ask if he or she needs to void. If the patient does not void, check the bladder for distention and discomfort. If a catheter is in place and no urine is flowing, check the bladder for distention and the catheter and tubing for clots or kinking.
- Follow physician's order for catheterization if the patient has a full bladder. If the catheter is obstructed, follow standard guidelines and orders for irrigation or catheter change.
- Check for signs of frank bleeding from the bladder once urine is flowing. If the urine is grossly bloody, recheck pulse and blood pressure (and hematocrit if possible) and have the urologist evaluate whether this is expected bleeding or excessive bleeding. NOTE: Some bleeding is normal, but excessive, continuous bleeding indicates serious trauma to the bladder wall, perhaps even bladder perforation, and should be recognized and treated promptly. This complication is rare but possible.
- Medicate for pain as ordered if vital signs permit. Pain should not be severe but might be mild to moderate once sedation wears off.
- Explain to the patient and family that any time an instrument is passed into the bladder, it is possible for an infection to develop. Tell them to report any signs of infection or bleeding. Describe these to the patient.
- Monitor urinary output and make sure that it is consistent with intake.
- Discharge the patient when bleeding is minimal and he or she is awake, is voiding normally, and has stable vital signs. The patient may have mild pain with urination for a short time after the procedure.
- Ensure that the patient has either a follow-up appointment or a number to call to reach the clinic or physician.

alone immediately after cystoscopic examination, since prolonged lithotomy positioning can cause orthostatic hypotension.

The nurse observes patients for three complications after cystoscopic examination: bleeding, bladder perforation, and infection. Observation for frank bleeding (pink-tinged urine is normal) is necessary. The nurse monitors urinary output and voiding pattern to detect obstruction, and increases fluid intake to prevent urine stasis. Mild analgesics are given for discomfort, and warmth is provided if the patient complains of being chilled. Vital signs are monitored as necessary. The nurse informs the patient that the first void after cystoscopic examination may be uncomfortable. Warm sitz baths may provide comfort. See the Guidelines for Safe Practice box, p. 959, for a summary of associated nursing care.

References

1. Brenner BM, Rector FC: *Brenner and Rector's the kidney,* ed 7, Philadelphia, 2004, Saunders.
2. Guyton AC, Hall JE: *Textbook of medical physiology,* ed 10, Philadelphia, 2000, Saunders.
3. Lancaster LE: *Core curriculum for nephrology nursing,* ed 4, Pittman, NJ, 2001, Jannetti.
4. McCance KL, Huether SE: *Pathophysiology: the biologic basis for disease in adults and children,* ed 4, St Louis, 2002, Mosby.
5. Post TW, Rose BD: *Approach to the patient with renal disease including acute renal failure,* 2001, accessed from website: http://www.uptodate.com.
6. Rose BD: *Indications for and complications of renal biopsy,* 2001, accessed from website: http://www.uptodate.com.

Visit the Evolve website: http://evolve.elsevier.com/Monahan/medsurg

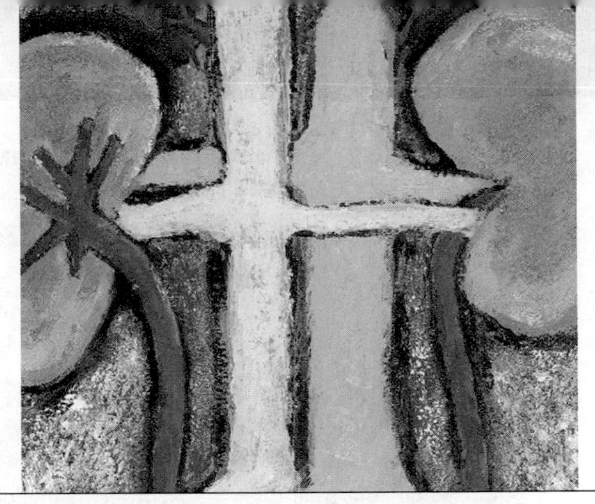

CHAPTER 35

Kidney and Urinary Tract Problems

by Cynthia K. Potter, Kelly A. Weigel, Carol J. Green

OBJECTIVES

After studying this chapter, the learner should be able to:

1. Describe the etiology, pathophysiology, and management of lower urinary tract infections and pyelonephritis, including the importance of public awareness and patient teaching.
2. Compare glomerulonephritis and the nephrotic syndrome in terms of pathophysiology, clinical manifestations, and management.
3. Discuss the common vascular and obstructive problems of the kidney.
4. Discuss the common cancers of the urinary tract.
5. Implement management strategies for persons requiring urinary catheterization.
6. Explain the causes and treatments of renal calculi.
7. Differentiate types of urinary incontinence and their management.
8. Develop a care plan for patients undergoing urinary diversion surgery.
9. Contrast the common types of urinary diversion procedures and management of urinary stomas.
10. Discuss the pathophysiology and management of polycystic kidney disease.

KEY TERMS

bacteriuria, p. 961
extracorporeal shock wave lithotripsy, p. 979
glomerulonephritis, p. 968
hydronephrosis, p. 975
nephrectomy, p. 974
nephrolithiasis, p. 977
nephrosis, p. 970
pyelonephritis, p. 966
stenosis, p. 974
urinary diversion, p. 985
urolithiasis, p. 977
urosepsis, p. 967

Urinary system diseases are a significant cause of morbidity and mortality in the United States. Renal function is threatened when disease involves the kidneys. Disease within the urinary drainage system produces damage at the site of the disease process; spreads upward and produces damage in the kidney; or obstructs the flow of urine, which also produces kidney damage. The primary objective for treatment of disease in any part of the urinary tract is early detection and adequate therapy focused on preserving or improving renal function. This chapter describes common disorders of the urinary system. Diseases of the prostate are discussed in Chapter 57.

Inflammatory Disorders

The kidneys are susceptible to inflammation caused by bacterial infection, altered immune response, drugs and other chemicals, toxins, and radiation. Inflammation may be acute or chronic.

Urinary Tract Infections

Urinary tract infections (UTIs) are among the most common infections affecting humans throughout their life span. Lower UTIs affect the urinary bladder (cystitis), prostate (prostatitis), or urethra (urethritis). Upper UTIs affect the renal parenchyma and renal pelvis (pyelonephritis). UTIs may manifest as bacteria in the urine (**bacteriuria**), bacteria in the blood originating from the genitourinary tract (bacteremia), or sepsis resulting from a UTI (urosepsis). Uncomplicated UTIs occur in persons without structural or functional abnormalities of their voiding mechanisms and in those who respond readily to antibiotics. Complicated UTIs are seen in persons with anatomic or functional abnormalities of their voiding mechanisms, persons who have undergone genitourinary procedures, or in those with indwelling urinary catheters or pathogens that are resistant to commonly used antibiotics. Table 35-1 summarizes genitourinary abnormalities associated with increased incidence of UTIs.

TABLE 35-1 GENITOURINARY ABNORMALITIES ASSOCIATED WITH INCREASED INCIDENCE OF URINARY TRACT INFECTIONS

Abnormality, Lesion, or Problem	Examples
Obstruction	Stricture, congenital abnormality, tumor, prostatic hypertrophy, renal stone, renal cyst, diverticulum
Urinary instrumentation	Cystoscopy, prostatectomy
Foreign body	Indwelling catheter, ureteric stent, nephrostomy tube
Metabolic disease or illness	Diabetes mellitus, postrenal transplantation
Urinary diversion	Ileal conduit
Functional abnormality	Neurogenic bladder, vesicoureteral reflux

Adapted from Cohen J, Powderly G, editors: *Infectious diseases,* ed 2, St Louis, 2004, Mosby.

Etiology and Epidemiology. UTIs account for more than 5 million office visits in the United States annually.[14] UTIs are taken seriously because, if left untreated, they can cause more serious problems. UTIs occur more frequently in women than men until after 50 years of age, when the incidence is similar. School-aged girls account for approximately 1% of infections. This rate increases by approximately 1% per decade, up to almost 10% in older adult women.[14] The incidence increases to 30% for persons older than 80 years regardless of whether they live at home or in a chronic care facility. The increased incidence of UTIs in men after the age of 50 may be due to age-related decreases in prostatic fluid, which provides protection from UTIs.[28] Infection in the lower urinary tract is associated with increased incidence of acute kidney infection (pyelonephritis) as a result of ascending microorganisms.

UTIs are caused by inflammation of some portion of the urinary tract from the invasion of pathogenic bacteria (Box 35-1). About 80% of UTIs are caused by the gram-negative rod *Escherichia coli,* which is normally found in the intestine. *Klebsiella* organisms are associated with about 5% of cases. Other causative pathogens are *Proteus, Enterobacter,* and gram-positive cocci such as *Staphylococcus* and *Streptococcus* organisms.[31]

Many factors place an individual at risk for a UTI (see Risk Factors box). Contrary to the beliefs of many, the risk of developing a UTI is not associated with dietary practices; personal hygiene practices, including wiping; and the use of tampons or tight clothing. Rather, the development of UTI depends on a series of complex interactions that allow bacterial colonization of the periurethral area, bacterial ascent into the urinary bladder, multiplication of bacteria in the urine, tissue invasion, and a resultant immune reaction.[5]

A major factor contributing to the development of UTI in women is a short urethra, which facilitates the entry of organisms from the vagina and rectal area into the bladder. Some women

Box 35-1 Bacteria Associated With Urinary Tract Infections

Gram-Negative Organisms

Escherichia coli
Klebsiella pneumoniae
Citrobacter organisms
Enterobacter organisms
Proteus mirabilis
Pseudomonas aeruginosa

Gram-Positive Organisms

Enterococci
Coagulase-negative staphylococci
Staphylococcus aureus
Group B streptococci

Adapted from Cohen J, Powderly G, editors: *Infectious diseases,* ed 2, St Louis, 2004, Mosby.

Risk Factors

Urinary Tract Infection

Women

Sexual intercourse
Pregnancy
Diaphragm use
Spermicides
Diabetes mellitus
History of urinary tract infection
Delayed postcoital voiding

Men

Lack of circumcision
Prostatic hypertrophy
Acquired immunodeficiency syndrome
Homosexual activity

Both

Obstruction of urinary flow
  –Congenital abnormalities
  –Renal calculi
  –Ureteral occlusion
Vesicoureteral reflux
Residual urine in the bladder
  –Neurogenic bladder
  –Urethral stricture
Instrumentation of the urinary tract
  –Indwelling urinary catheter
  –Intermittent catheterization
  –Urethral dilation
  –Cystoscopy

develop routine postcoital UTIs. In men the presence of zinc in the prostatic fluid acts as an antibacterial agent that helps prevent UTIs. Men who are not circumcised have a greater incidence of UTIs than men who are circumcised.

Bladder catheterization is responsible for a large number of hospital-acquired UTIs. Even when performed without a break in aseptic technique, catheterization results in a significant rate of bladder infection (see Guidelines for Safe Practice box). Drug-resistant strains of *Staphylococcus* and *Pseudomonas* organisms, along with various other organisms typically found in hospitals, are frequently associated with nosocomial UTIs. Prevention and control of all UTIs can be most significantly influenced by lowering of the rate of nosocomial infection. New technologies such as antiinfective lubricants are currently being tested to decrease the incidence of these infections[19] (see Research and Legal Alert boxes).

Legal Alert

Indwelling Urinary Catheters

Urinary catheters are a significant source of nosocomial infections, yet it is estimated that less than half the patients who have indwelling catheters actually need them. In many cases the patient has no physician order or documented reason for the catheter placement. To prevent possible litigation, the nurse needs to:

- Obtain an order for catheter placement from the physician.
- Document the reason for which an indwelling urinary catheter is needed.
- Document assessment of the patient's urinary status while the catheter is in place.
- Consult with the attending physician on a regular basis so that the catheter can be removed as soon as possible.

Pathophysiology. The mode of entry of bacteria into the genitourinary tract cannot always be traced with certainty; however, four major pathways exist:

1. *Ascending infection from the urethra:* This is the most common cause of genitourinary tract infection in adults. Because the female urethra is short and rectal bacteria tend to colonize the perineum and vaginal vestibule, women are especially susceptible to ascending UTIs.
2. *Hematogenous spread:* This occurs infrequently, except in the case of tuberculosis, renal abscesses, and perinephric abscesses. Bacteremia is more likely to complicate a UTI when structural and functional abnormalities exist than when the urinary tract is normal.
3. *Lymphatogenous spread:* Rarely, bacterial pathogens are thought to travel through lymphatics to the bladder, prostate, and female genitourinary tract.
4. *Direct extension from another organ:* This occurs from intraperitoneal abscesses, especially those associated with inflammatory bowel disease, fulminant pelvic inflammatory disease in women, paravesical abscesses, and genitourinary tract fistulas.

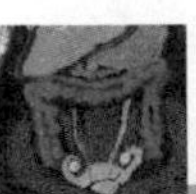

GUIDELINES FOR SAFE PRACTICE
Care of Indwelling Urinary Catheters

- Insert using proper sterile technique.
- Cleanse meatal catheter junction one or two times per day with an antimicrobial soap.
- Use a sterile closed drainage system, and empty every 8 hours.
- Use sterile technique if the collecting system is opened for irrigations; however, do not irrigate regularly.
- Keep urine collection bags below the level of the bladder.
- Follow the institutional policy for routine catheter change.

Research

Use of Indwelling Catheters in Hospitalized Patients

The researchers conducted a random review of 285 charts of hospitalized patients ages 65 years and older who had indwelling urinary catheters. They found that only 46% of patients had appropriate indications for urinary catheterization; 33% of patients had no written order for the use of the indwelling catheterizations; and only 13% had explicitly documented reasons for catheter placement. The investigators concluded that, based on findings from similar studies in other hospitals, interventions are needed to decrease the inappropriate use of indwelling urinary catheters.

Gokula RR, Hickner JA, Smith MA: Inappropriate use of urinary catheters in elderly patients at a Midwestern community teaching hospital, *Am J Infect Control* 32(4):196-199, 2004.

Structural and functional abnormalities of the urinary tract, obstruction of urine flow, and impaired bladder innervation increase the risk for developing a UTI. A protective layer within the bladder interferes with bacterial adherence, and efficient emptying of the bladder decreases the number of bacteria within the bladder. Whenever urinary stasis occurs, such as with incomplete emptying of the bladder, renal calculi, or genitourinary obstructions, bacteria have a greater opportunity to grow. Urinary stasis also causes more alkaline urine, which facilitates bacterial growth. During micturition, urine may flow back up the ureters (vesicoureteral reflux) and carry bacteria from the bladder up through the ureters to the kidney pelvis, leading to pyelonephritis.

To colonize the urinary tract, bacteria attach or adhere to the urothelium via rodlike structures called pili. In addition, bacteria may secrete toxins that promote their survival. Women who have recurrent UTIs may have receptors on the mucosal surface of their genitourinary tract; these receptors act as binding sites for bacteria and other pathogens.[26]

The clinical manifestations that prompt a patient to seek medical attention for a UTI typically include urinary frequency, urgency, dysuria (burning on urination), cloudy or foul-smelling urine, suprapubic discomfort, and hematuria. In asymptomatic persons, UTIs are identified only on routine examination of the urine.

COMPLICATIONS. UTIs alone do not lead to deterioration of renal function. However, complicated UTIs and recurring UTIs can lead to serious problems such as pyelonephritis, sepsis, or kidney failure. Complicated UTIs occur after urologic surgery or invasive urinary procedures. Complicated UTIs are more difficult to treat and place the patient at increased risk for spread of the infection to the blood (bacteremia), which can result in permanent kidney damage (see Chapter 36). Recurring UTIs increase the risk for kidney failure because of scar tissue, which causes strictures and distention. Pyelonephritis is discussed later in the chapter.

Collaborative Care Management

DIAGNOSTIC TESTS. Although a urine culture confirms the presence of infection, a urinalysis is useful for screening for a possible UTI in persons with symptoms (dysuria, urgency, and frequency). The presence of nitrites and leukocyte esterase indicates the presence of bacteria and white blood cells, respectively. In the past a positive urine culture with colony counts in excess of 10^5 organisms/ml of urine in a properly obtained and stored midstream specimen (see Chapter 34) was considered the diagnostic standard for women with an uncomplicated UTI. However, 30% to 50% of women with an uncomplicated UTI have lower colony counts despite the presence of white blood cells (pyuria) on urinalysis.[28]

Urine cultures are not routinely indicated in women with isolated episodes of frequency and dysuria. However, a urine culture should be obtained for a first infection or for recurrent infection before drug therapy is initiated to confirm the organism's sensitivity to antimicrobials and protect against the development of drug-resistant organisms. Because 24 to 48 hours are required to obtain results of urine cultures, an antibiotic that is effective against the suspected causative organism may be prescribed until results are available. In most situations reculturing the urine is not necessary when the symptoms resolve after antibiotic therapy.

A more extensive urologic workup is usually recommended for men with a first UTI episode, all patients with complicated infection or bacteremia, and those with suspected obstruction or renal stones. The rationale for the recommended workup in men is to assess for possible underlying anatomic problems because UTIs are not as common in men as they are in women. Ultrasound studies of the kidneys and pelvis are used during the initial diagnostic workup if obstruction or other structural abnormalities are suspected. In the past the intravenous pyelogram was part of the urologic workup; however, computed tomography (CT) with contrast has become the procedure of choice.

MEDICATIONS. Although many UTIs clear spontaneously, symptoms can last for months. The goal of therapy is, therefore, to eliminate the infection to prevent future occurrences and potential complications. Antibiotics are not indicated for most patients with asymptomatic bacteriuria (a condition in which large numbers of bacteria are present, but symptoms are not) or for those with indwelling catheters unless symptoms are present.[17] If a patient with a chronic indwelling catheter must be treated, the catheter should be replaced before antibiotics are started.

For patients who are symptomatic (dysuria, frequency, urgency, low-grade fever), antibiotics are usually given as a single dose or for 3 days when the UTI is uncomplicated. Persons who are pregnant, are elderly, have diabetes, or have recurrent UTIs are usually treated for 7 days. Trimethoprim-sulfamethoxazole (Bactrim) and nitrofurantoin (Macrodantin) are considered first-line agents, since they are usually effective against most pathogens that cause UTIs. These drugs are the most widely used antibiotics for the treatment of patients with uncomplicated UTIs in the outpatient setting.

Other agents may also be used to treat UTIs. The cephalosporins are usually reserved for culture-documented infections. Ampicillin and amoxicillin have fallen out of favor because they are now ineffective against approximately 30% of common urinary pathogens. The fluoroquinolones (e.g., ciprofloxacin) are expensive and powerful antibiotics and are reserved for the treatment of complicated UTIs and resistant organisms.[12]

TREATMENTS. Increasing fluid intake to 3 to 4 L/day may improve patient comfort. Fluids help dilute the urine; reduce irritation and burning; and provide a continual flow of urine, which minimizes stasis and multiplication of bacteria in the urinary tract. Increasing fluid intake does not, however, eradicate or kill bacteria.

DIET. In addition to increasing fluid intake, limiting or avoiding the intake of caffeine, alcohol, spicy foods, and tomatoes may enhance comfort, since they are known bladder irritants. Urine acidification may be helpful and can be accomplished by taking vitamin C or drinking cranberry juice. Acidification is thought to prevent the attachment of bacteria to the bladder wall, thereby increasing their elimination from the bladder. None of these measures, however, influences bacterial death.

HEALTH PROMOTION AND PREVENTION. The most important defenses against UTI are large urine volume, free urine flow, and complete emptying of the bladder to prevent urinary stasis. Patients are advised to avoid prolonged periods with a full bladder. Women are instructed to void after intercourse. Estrogen replacement therapy (especially vaginal estrogen) may decrease the incidence of a UTI in postmenopausal women. Urinary catheterization should be performed only when absolutely necessary, and the catheter should be removed as soon as possible. Education of the public (Figure 35-1) and efforts by health care providers can assist in decreasing the incidence of UTIs and their complications. The Complementary & Alternative Therapies box lists foods, vitamins, and minerals that support urinary health.

▶ ARE You READY?

The most common cause of genitourinary tract infection in adults is spread of infection via:

1. Another organ
2. The blood stream
3. The lymph system
4. The urethra

Nursing Management

of the Patient with Urinary Tract Infection

ASSESSMENT

Health History. Assess for:

- Presence and length of time since onset of frequency, urgency, dysuria, chills, and fever
- Predisposing factors such as diaphragms, spermicidals, and sexual intercourse
- History of previous UTIs

Physical Examination. Assess for:

- Elevated temperature
- Urine analysis and culture, presence of blood in urine, abnormal urinalysis results, positive urine culture
- Abdominal and costovertebral tenderness

JAMA PATIENT PAGE

Urinary Tract Infections

Water is the most vital substance your body requires. Water is very important for the basic chemical reactions that keep the body functioning. Many of the unusable by-products of these chemical reactions are then processed through the kidneys and eliminated from the body through the urinary tract as **urine**.

The normal function of the urinary system can be disrupted by structural abnormalities or disease. For example, infection can cause inflammation that can interrupt the normal operation of the urinary system. If you suspect you have a urinary tract infection or a problem with your urinary system, consult with your doctor, so that you can be tested and given proper treatment. Left untreated, an infection has the potential to cause more serious, even life-threatening, difficulties and permanent damage to your urinary tract.

An article in the March 22/29, 2000, issue of *JAMA* looks at the effectiveness of 2 different medications to treat a specific type of urinary tract infection, **pyelonephritis**, which is inflammation of the upper urinary tract and kidney. The article stresses the importance of testing and of receiving the correct medication.

TYPES OF URINARY TRACT INFECTIONS:

The most common types of urinary tract infections are:

- **Urethritis** – Inflammation of the **urethra** (the tube-like structure that allows urine to pass from the bladder to be eliminated outside the body)
- **Cystitis** – Inflammation of the **bladder** (the balloon-like structure that stores urine before elimination through the urethra)
- **Pyelonephritis** – A more serious condition that is characterized by inflammation of the upper urinary tract, which includes the kidneys and the **ureters** (the 2 tube-like structures that connect each kidney to the bladder)

If you are prescribed an antibiotic for an infection, it is important that you finish all of the pills even if the symptoms have gone away and you are feeling better.

COMMON SYMPTOMS:

- More frequent urge to urinate, even though only a small amount is eliminated
- Pain or burning sensation during urination
- Greenish-yellow or white discharge from, or itching in, your penis or vagina

If you have any of these symptoms see your doctor; you may have a urinary tract infection or a sexually transmitted disease. If you are diagnosed with a sexually transmitted disease you need to let your sex partner(s) know so that they can also be treated.

- Pain in the back that is just above the waist
- Pain in your side or groin area
- Fever, chills, nausea, and vomiting
- Pus or blood in the urine

If you have any of the above symptoms see your doctor immediately; you may have pyelonephritis or another serious problem

PREVENTING URINARY TRACT INFECTIONS:

- Drink plenty of fluids—at least 8 to 10 cups (64 to 80 ounces) of water a day. You need to increase your fluid intake beyond this if you are physically active or when you are in a warm environment.
- Urinate frequently
- Wash your genitals daily, especially before and after sexual relations
- Urinate after sexual relations
- Practice safer sex (e.g., wearing a condom during sexual relations)
- Women should always wipe from front to back after having a bowel movement
- Women should not use feminine hygiene products that contain deodorants

URINARY TRACT INFECTIONS IN CHILDREN:

Urinary tract infections can cause life-threatening and permanent damage to a child's urinary system. Therefore, it is important to receive treatment as soon as possible. Though the signs are similar for children and adults, they may not be as easy to observe in children. The child may have a fever and chills, experience nausea and vomiting, complain of pain in the abdomen, back, or pelvis, and complain about pain during urination. The child may also be irritable or not want to eat. For children with repeated urinary tract infections the child's doctor may suggest tests to determine if there are any abnormalities in the child's urinary system.

FOR MORE INFORMATION:

- National Kidney and Urologic Diseases Information Clearinghouse
  3 Information Way
  Bethesda, MD 20892-3580
  301/654-4415
  or www.niddk.nih.gov
- American Foundation for Urologic Disease
  Answers to Your Questions About Urinary Tract Infections
  (800) 242-2383
  or www.afud.org

INFORM YOURSELF:

To find this and previous *JAMA* Patient Pages, check out the AMA's Web site at www.ama-assn.org/consumer.htm.

URINARY TRACT INFECTIONS

From JAMA, March 22/29, 2000—Vol 283, No. 12

Figure 35-1 Sample patient education page for urinary tract infections.

NURSING DIAGNOSES, OUTCOMES, AND INTERVENTIONS

Nursing Diagnoses: Impaired Urinary Elimination

OUTCOMES. Common examples of expected outcomes for the patient with a diagnosis of *impaired urinary elimination* are: Patient will:

- Report completing all of prescribed antimicrobials.
- Report resolution of symptoms.
- Verbalize the need for follow-up care.

NURSING INTERVENTIONS. The nurse stresses to patients how important it is that they complete the full course of antibiotic therapy even after symptoms resolve to prevent recurrence of the infection and development of antibiotic resistance. Female patients are advised that spermicidal jellies, diaphragms, antibiotics, and estrogen deficiency favor the colonization of enteric

Complementary & Alternative Therapies

Foods, Vitamins, and Minerals That Promote Urinary Health

- Cranberries and blueberries—inhibit binding of bacteria to bladder walls
- Vitamin C, 250 to 500 mg twice a day—acidifies urine
- Beta carotene, 25,000 to 50,000 unit/day—supports immune function
- Zinc, 30-50 mg/day—supports immune function
- Garlic—has antibacterial activity
- Celery seed—contains apiol, which has antibacterial activity
- Parsley—has urinary antiseptic activities
- Asparagus—promotes urinary tract health

Data from University of Maryland Medical Center, 2005 website: http://umm.edu/altmed

organisms in the region between the urethra and rectum. Voiding after coitus and preventing urinary stasis by completely emptying the bladder may reduce recurrence of infection. Postmenopausal women who experience vaginal dryness may benefit from vaginal estrogen, which increases circulation to the urogenital area.[5]

Treatment success for UTI depends directly on patient understanding and compliance with prescribed regimens. A visit to the practitioner 7 to 14 days after the initial infection provides an opportunity to obtain urine cultures and discuss the need for further treatment. Patient education about the specific problem, drug requirements, and need for follow-up care may increase compliance with drug regimens and preventive measures.

RELATED NIC INTERVENTIONS. Fluid Management, Infection Protection, Medication Management, Urinary Elimination Management

Nursing Diagnosis: Acute Pain

OUTCOMES. Common examples of expected outcomes for the patient with a diagnosis of *acute pain* are:

Patient will:

- Report control of pain by rating pain as less than 3 on a scale of 1 to 10.
- Report loss of sense of urgency and frequency in voiding.

NURSING INTERVENTIONS. The nurse encourages patients to increase fluid intake to 3 L/day unless contraindicated (see discussion above). Fluid flushes the urinary bladder and decreases bacterial count when urination occurs. Acidifying the urine with cranberry juice or ascorbic acid makes it difficult for some microbes to live and grow. Emptying the bladder completely every 2 to 3 hours helps eliminate bacteria from the bladder and reduces urinary stasis, which may protect against reinfection. Alcohol and caffeine should be avoided, since they irritate the urinary bladder.

Over-the-counter pain medication such as acetaminophen or ibuprofen may provide adequate pain relief for some patients. For others, prescribed medications such as phenazopyridine (Pyridium) or a combination of phenazopyridine and antibiotic (e.g., Azo-Gantrisin) may be necessary. Nonpharmacologic pain relievers include warm sitz baths or a heating pad applied to the lower abdomen, both of which relieve spasms caused by UTIs. Increasing fluid intake relieves pain by flushing bacteria from the bladder.

RELATED NIC INTERVENTIONS. Analgesic Administration, Fluid Management, Pain Management

EVALUATION

To evaluate the effectiveness of nursing interventions, compare patient behaviors with those stated in the expected patient outcomes.

RELATED NOC OUTCOMES. Comfort Level, Hydration, Knowledge: Treatment Regimen, Symptom Control, Urinary Elimination

GERONTOLOGIC CONSIDERATIONS

An estimated 10% to 20% of persons 65 years and older have bacteria in their urine (bacteriuria). UTIs are the most common cause of bacterial sepsis in older adults. Structural changes of the urinary system associated with aging add to susceptibility. Bladder muscles in older adult women may atrophy and weaken, and men may develop prostatic hypertrophy, both of which lead to incomplete bladder emptying and retention. Decreased prostatic secretions in men and decreased estrogen in women, which favors vaginal bacterial colonization, also increase UTI susceptibility. UTIs are prevalent among persons who live in long-term care facilities perhaps in part because of the many comorbid illnesses that predispose them to UTIs. Most infections in older adults are asymptomatic. Antibiotic treatment has no benefit for asymptomatic persons.

Pyelonephritis

Etiology and Epidemiology. Acute **pyelonephritis** is an infection of the upper urinary tract that involves both the parenchyma and kidney pelvis (Figure 35-2). It is one of the leading causes of infections in the blood (bacteremia) and accounts for more than 100,000 hospital admissions per year.[7] Pregnant women with bacteriuria are at significant risk for developing pyelonephritis. Other risk factors that increase susceptibility to pyelonephritis include instrumentation of the urinary tract, diabetes, and female gender.

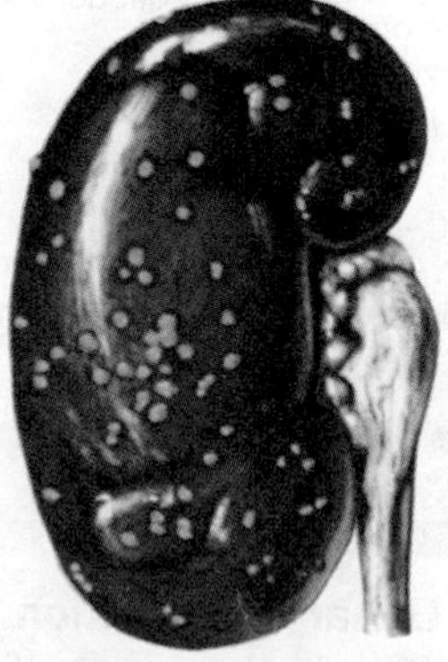

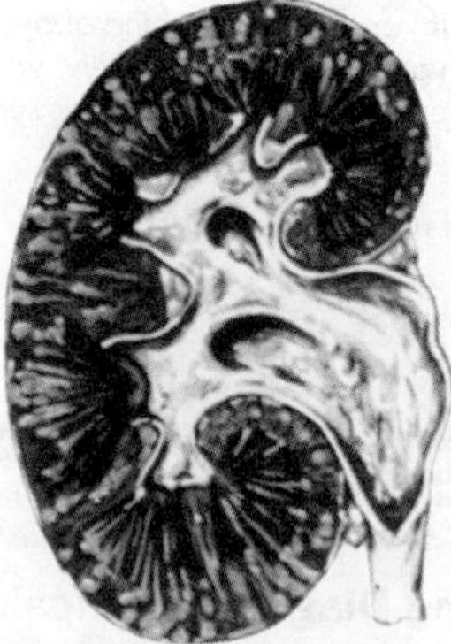

Figure 35-2 Appearance of kidney in acute pyelonephritis. **A,** Kidney is swollen with multiple abscesses on the surface. **B,** Abscesses appear as yellowish gray streaks on cross section.

Pathophysiology. As discussed previously, pyelonephritis usually begins in the lower urinary tract and ascends into the kidneys. Lower UTIs may be asymptomatic, and kidney involvement may be the first indication of lower urinary tract disease. As in lower UTI, *E. coli* is the most common organism identified in pyelonephritis. Other causes are gram-negative bacilli and enterococci. The diagnostic workup of a person with pyelonephritis often reveals previously unknown urinary tract obstruction or another chronic kidney disease.

Pyelonephritis may be acute or chronic. *Acute pyelonephritis* may temporarily affect renal function, but rarely progresses to kidney failure. *Chronic pyelonephritis* permanently destroys renal tissue through repeated inflammation and scarring. The process of developing chronic kidney failure from repeated kidney infections occurs over a number of years or after several extensive and fulminant infections. Pyelonephritis is the original diagnosis in an estimated 13% of all persons with end-stage renal disease.[16]

Clinical manifestations of acute pyelonephritis may include those of lower UTIs in addition to the following typical signs of inflammation: chills and fever, malaise, flank pain, costovertebral angle tenderness, and leukocytosis. Urinalysis demonstrates the presence of white blood cells, casts, and bacteria. In chronic pyelonephritis the only symptom may be persistent bacteriuria until extensive scarring and atrophy result in renal insufficiency, as manifested by hypertension, increased blood urea nitrogen (BUN), and decreased creatinine clearance.

Collaborative Care Management. Optimal treatment of pyelonephritis includes early detection of the bacterial infection through urine culture, antibacterial therapy based on identified sensitivities, and detection and treatment of any underlying systemic disease or urinary tract abnormality. The course of antibiotic therapy usually lasts 10 to 14 days. Opioids or anti-inflammatory drugs may be given for pain, which is primarily felt in the flank area. Pain eases as the inflammation resolves. In chronic pyelonephritis, an evaluation is indicated to determine the cause of recurrent infections, such as obstruction caused by kidney stones. If structural abnormalities are found, surgery may be indicated. Antibiotic therapy is usually consistent with the goal of reducing and controlling the bacterial population of the urinary tract to prevent renal damage.

Nursing interventions and patient outcomes are the same as those for UTIs. The nurse encourages patients to take measures to prevent recurrent urinary infections and report signs of infection, including increased flank pain, fever, chills, frequency, or urgency. The nurse stresses the importance of follow-up care. Urine cultures are completed periodically until the infection is cleared. The most significant efforts to prevent pyelonephritis are through early detection and adequate treatment of lower UTIs (see Patient/Family Teaching box).

PATIENT/FAMILY TEACHING
Pyelonephritis

Patients with pyelonephritis will most likely be cared for at home; therefore the nurse teaches them to:

- Continue the course of antibiotic therapy even after symptoms resolve to ensure that bacteria have been eliminated, and to prevent recurrence of infection and antibiotic resistance.
- Drink 3 L of fluids per day unless contraindicated.
- Monitor urinary output and report if urine volume is less than fluid intake.
- Monitor daily weight and report sudden increases.

Urosepsis

Etiology and Epidemiology. UTIs may remain localized or spread to the bloodstream, producing bacteremia and sepsis, known as **urosepsis**. Urosepsis can occur in anyone, but the risk is greatest in immunocompromised individuals; older women; and patients with diabetes mellitus, severe UTIs, indwelling urinary catheters, or kidney stones. Mortality from urosepsis ranges between 20% and 60% depending on how quickly it is recognized and treated.[25]

Pathophysiology. The pathophysiology of urosepsis is complex. Gram-negative organisms, such as *E. coli*, are most commonly responsible for urosepsis, although gram-positive and other organisms have also been implicated. Bacteria migrate to the bloodstream from the genitourinary tract, where they release endotoxins that damage cells. Damaged cells release proinflammatory cytokines and set the complement cascade into motion (see Chapter 20). Widespread inflammation alters metabolism and results in a cascade of multiorgan failure secondary to severe sepsis and septic shock. Altered mental status and fever or hypothermia are the most common early signs of urosepsis. Other manifestations include tachycardia, tachypnea, hypotension, oliguria, and leukopenia.

Collaborative Care Management. Diagnosis of urosepsis is based on culture results, laboratory data, clinical manifestations, and presence of risk factors. Treatment begins with prevention. Patients who are infected with multiresistant organisms should be isolated to prevent cross-infection with patients who are immunocompromised or have indwelling urinary catheters. Indwelling catheters should be removed as early as the patient's condition allows, since they provide a portal of entry into the urinary bladder. When indwelling catheters must be used, drainage systems should be closed and minimal system integrity breaks should occur. Good hand washing and Standard Precautions can significantly reduce the risk of transferring microbes from one patient to another.[25]

Diagnosed urosepsis is treated with aggressive antibiotic therapy, appropriate adjunctive therapies, and adequate life-support measures. Broad-spectrum antibiotics such as the cephalosporins or aminoglycosides are started as soon as cultures are obtained and continued until sensitivity results are known. Antimicrobial selections are then altered based on culture and sensitivity results and the predominant bacteria found in the hospital environment. Adjunctive and life-support therapies may include corticosteroids to reduce inflammation associated with gram-negative infections, sympathomimetic agents (isoproterenol, dopamine, dobutamine) to maintain blood pressure, and fluid and electrolyte management to support circulation during shock. Naloxone, an opiate antagonist, may reverse the course of endotoxic shock.[25]

Patients with urosepsis are acutely ill and are treated in the critical care environment. The nurse teaches families about the disease process and treatment measures. As the patient recovers, the focus of teaching changes to prevention of future urinary tract or kidney infections, the need to maintain prescribed treatment regimens even when the patient begins to feel better, and the need for close follow-up care for several months after the initial infection.

Acute Glomerulonephritis

Etiology and Epidemiology. Acute glomerulonephritis is a disease that affects the glomerular capillaries. Etiologic factors are many and varied; they include immunologic reactions (systemic lupus erythematosus, streptococcal infection), vascular injury (hypertension), metabolic disease (diabetes mellitus), and disseminated intravascular coagulation. **Glomerulonephritis** exists in acute, latent, and chronic forms. The most common form of acute glomerulonephritis occurs 1 to 3 weeks after a group A beta-hemolytic streptococcal infection. Common sites of the primary infection include the pharynx or tonsils and the skin (impetigo).

Preschool-age and grade school–age children (2 to 6 years old) are most likely to develop acute glomerulonephritis. Spontaneous recovery usually occurs after this acute illness. The severity of the acute illness does not relate to the prognosis. Persons with mild illness may develop chronic disease, and those with severe illness may completely recover over a period of months and have no recurrence.[31]

Pathophysiology. Acute poststreptococcal glomerulonephritis is the result of an antigen-antibody reaction where insoluble immune complexes develop and become entrapped in glomerular tissue, producing swelling and death of capillary cells. Renal function is impaired by scarring and obstruction of circulating blood through the glomerulus.

Clinical manifestations reflect damage to the glomeruli, with leaking of protein and red blood cells into the urine; varying degrees of decreased glomerular filtration; and retention of metabolic waste products, sodium, and water (see Clinical Manifestations box). The patient typically reports shortness of breath, mild headache, weakness, anorexia, and flank pain. The classic signs associated with acute glomerulonephritis are proteinuria, hematuria, and azotemia.

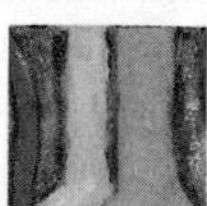

CLINICAL MANIFESTATIONS
Acute Glomerulonephritis

Early	Late
Hematuria	Circulatory congestion
Proteinuria	Hypertension
Azotemia	Edema
Increased urine specific gravity	Kidney failure
Elevated erythrocyte sedimentation rate	
Oliguria	
Elevated antistreptolysin O titer	

COMPLICATIONS. Besides the obvious complications such as sepsis from infection and kidney failure from extensive kidney damage, other complications may arise as a result of fluid overload. These fluid-related complications include congestive heart failure, pulmonary edema, and, rarely, increased intracranial pressure. Each must be treated aggressively, and the patient may require critical care management. Cardiac glycosides may be prescribed to prevent congestive heart failure.

Collaborative Care Management

DIAGNOSTIC TESTS. Urinalysis provides important data, such as the presence of proteinuria, hematuria, and cell debris (red cells and casts). Hematuria and proteinuria can take several months to resolve. Serum BUN and urine creatinine clearance tests indicate renal function status. Tests to determine infection include white blood cell count, erythrocyte sedimentation rate, and antistreptolysin O titer.

MEDICATIONS. Patients with poststreptococcal glomerulonephritis may be given a course of prophylactic antibiotics, with penicillin being the drug of choice. Prophylactic therapy may be continued for months after the acute phase of illness to prevent recurrence of the streptococcal infection. Immunosuppressants and steroids may be indicated to reduce inflammation. Symptomatic salt and water retention is treated by diuretics and angiotensin II receptor blocking agents.[8] Hyperkalemia may need to be treated with potassium-binding resins, such as sodium polystyrene sulfate (Kayexalate). Spontaneous diuresis usually occurs in 7 to 10 days. Diuretic therapy is implemented when severe fluid overload develops. Elevated blood pressure is controlled by antihypertensive drugs only after fluid control has failed.

TREATMENTS. No specific treatment exists for acute glomerulonephritis. General management focuses on prevention.

DIET. Fluid retention is often a problem and is managed by dietary sodium restriction. Dietary protein is also restricted, usually to 1 to 1.2 g/kg body weight/day when BUN and creatinine levels are elevated. It is important that the diet contain sufficient carbohydrates to prevent protein from being used for energy,

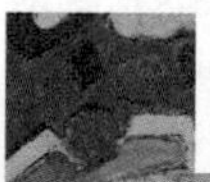

PATIENT/FAMILY TEACHING
Acute Glomerulonephritis

Patient and caregiver teaching regarding acute glomerulonephritis includes:

- Nature of the illness
- Effect of diet and fluids on fluid balance and sodium retention
- Need for avoiding infections, which can exacerbate illness
- Medication regimen
- Expectations and information about recovery:
  - —Recovery period may be as long as 2 years; therefore close follow-up care is essential.
  - —Proteinuria, hematuria, and cellular debris may exist microscopically, even when other symptoms subside.
  - —Fatigue may be present, although the patient usually feels well. Exercise should be balanced with rest to avoid fatigue.

which will result in muscle wasting and nitrogen imbalance. Caloric requirements are 25 to 35 kcal/day. The nurse monitors the patient for weight loss, since loss of protein stores may occur. Potassium intake should be restricted if the glomerular filtration rate is less than 10 ml/min (see Patient/Family Teaching box).

HEALTH PROMOTION AND PREVENTION. Prevention of acute poststreptococcal glomerulonephritis involves prompt medical treatment of sore throats and upper respiratory tract infections. Cultures should be obtained and antibiotics prescribed when indicated.

> **ARE YOU READY?**
>
> Which of the following clinical manifestations is commonly associated with acute poststreptococcal glomerulonephritis?
> 1. Painful urination
> 2. Hematuria
> 3. Polyuria
> 4. Lower abdominal pain

Nursing Management

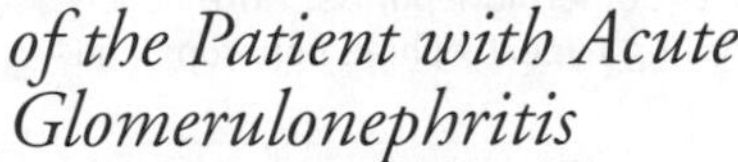

of the Patient with Acute Glomerulonephritis

ASSESSMENT

Health History. Assess for:

- Recent infection or symptoms of infection
- Change in pattern of urination, either in frequency, color, or volume
- Shortness of breath, headaches, weakness, nausea, vomiting, or loss of appetite
- Recent weight gain or swelling

Physical Examination. Assess for:

- Adequate intake and output
- Elevated temperature or weight changes
- Hypertension or edema
- Signs or symptoms of infection

NURSING DIAGNOSES, OUTCOMES, AND INTERVENTIONS

Nursing Diagnosis: Excess Fluid Volume

OUTCOMES. Common examples of expected outcomes for the patient with a diagnosis of *excess fluid volume* are:

Patient will:

- Maintain preillness weight.
- Remain free from edema.
- Achieve blood pressure within his or her normal limits.

NURSING INTERVENTIONS. Edema and fluid overload are anticipated and treated initially with dietary sodium and fluid restrictions. Sodium intake is usually restricted to 2 to 4 g/day, but the amount varies with the severity of fluid retention. Sodium restriction is maintained until dependent edema and circulatory overload are no longer present. Strict recording of fluid intake and output is necessary to determine the extent of fluid retention.

The nurse weighs the patient daily using correct procedure (see Chapter 17). The nurse monitors vital signs every shift and assesses the apical heart rate for dysrhythmias. The patient is monitored for jugular vein distention, which is indicative of fluid overload and congestive heart failure, and for periorbital, pretibial, pedal, and sacral edema. The lungs are auscultated for adventitious sounds. Because antihypertensive and diuretic therapy is usually prescribed, serum potassium levels are also monitored closely.

RELATED NIC INTERVENTIONS. Electrolyte Monitoring, Fluid/Electrolyte Management, Fluid Management, Vital Signs Monitoring

Nursing Diagnosis: Risk for Infection

OUTCOMES. Common examples of expected outcomes for the patient with a diagnosis of *risk for infection* are:

Patient will:

- Be free from signs and symptoms of infection (e.g., fever, leukocytosis).
- Verbalize need to avoid persons with infections.

NURSING INTERVENTIONS. Mild infections may reactivate glomerulonephritis; therefore the patient must be protected from exposure to infection, particularly from persons with upper respiratory tract infections. If the patient is suspected of having an upper respiratory tract infection, cultures are obtained and, when indicated, antibiotics are prescribed. When possible, any procedure such as urinary catheterization that may lead to nosocomial infection is avoided.

RELATED NIC INTERVENTIONS. Infection Protection, Surveillance

Nursing Diagnosis: Readiness for Enhanced Coping

OUTCOMES. Common examples of expected outcomes for the patient with a diagnosis of *readiness for enhanced coping* (individual and family) are:

Patient will:

- Verbalize concerns and feelings about restricted activity.
- Implement prescribed care plan.
- Participate in diversional activities to prevent boredom while on prolonged bed rest.

NURSING INTERVENTIONS. Bed rest is prescribed during the acute phase of the illness. Ambulation is allowed when blood sedimentation rates and blood pressure return to normal and edema abates. If ambulation causes an increase in proteinuria or hematuria, bed rest is reinstituted. Because the period of bed rest may be extensive, the nurse may need to reinforce the importance of bed rest as the patient starts to feel better. The importance of diversional activities should not be ignored. When bed rest is resumed after a period of ambulation, the person may become depressed as a result of the perceived setback in recovery. Helping the patient express concerns can serve as the impetus for making realistic plans about the illness and its sequelae.

RELATED NIC INTERVENTIONS. Coping Enhancement, Decision-Making Support, Emotional Support, Teaching: Individual

EVALUATION

To evaluate the effectiveness of nursing interventions, compare patient behaviors with those stated in the expected patient outcomes.

RELATED NOC OUTCOMES. Family Coping, Fluid Balance, Electrolyte & Acid/Base Balance, Knowledge: Disease Process, Knowledge: Treatment Regimen, Vital Signs

GERONTOLOGIC CONSIDERATIONS

Because of preexisting structural and age-related changes in the kidney, the older adult patient is more likely to develop chronic glomerulonephritis and has an increased risk for complications. Treatment remains the same, regardless of age.

Chronic Glomerulonephritis

Etiology and Epidemiology. Although chronic glomerulonephritis (CGN) may follow the acute form of the disease, most persons have no history or source of predisposing infection, and evidence suggests the disease results from immunologic mechanisms.[6] The course of CGN is extremely variable. Some persons with minimal impairment in renal function continue to feel well and show little progression of disease. In others, renal deterioration progresses either insidiously or rapidly and results in end-stage renal disease.

Pathophysiology. CGN is an autoimmune disease caused by loss of tolerance to self-antigens. It is characterized by progressive destruction of glomeruli and gradual loss of renal function. The glomeruli have varying degrees of hypercellularity and become sclerosed (hardened). The kidney decreases in size. Eventually tubular atrophy, chronic interstitial inflammation, and arteriosclerosis occur (Figure 35-3).

Various symptoms of renal dysfunction may lead the person to seek health care. These include headache, especially in the morning; dyspnea on exertion; blurred vision; lassitude; and weakness or fatigue. Other signs of CGN include edema, nocturia, and weight loss.

Early in the disease process urinalysis may reveal albumin, casts, and blood, despite normal renal function tests. The kidneys' ability to regulate the internal environment begins to decrease as more glomeruli become scarred, resulting in fewer functional nephrons. When few nephrons remain intact, hematuria and proteinuria decrease, the specific gravity of the urine becomes fixed at 1.010 (equal to plasma), and the urea nitrogen level in the blood increases.

Collaborative Care Management. No specific therapy exists to arrest or reverse CGN. Treatment of kidney failure begins when the illness progresses to end-stage renal disease (see Chapter 36). With any exacerbation of hematuria, hypertension, and edema, the patient is returned to bed rest, and treatment similar to that for acute glomerulonephritis is instituted. Signs of pulmonary edema and congestive heart failure are closely monitored.

Women with CGN who become pregnant appear to be susceptible to toxemia and spontaneous abortion. The woman who has had nephritis of any nature should be urged to see a physician if she plans to become pregnant. When pregnancy does occur, the woman should be monitored closely by an obstetrician who specializes in high-risk pregnancies.

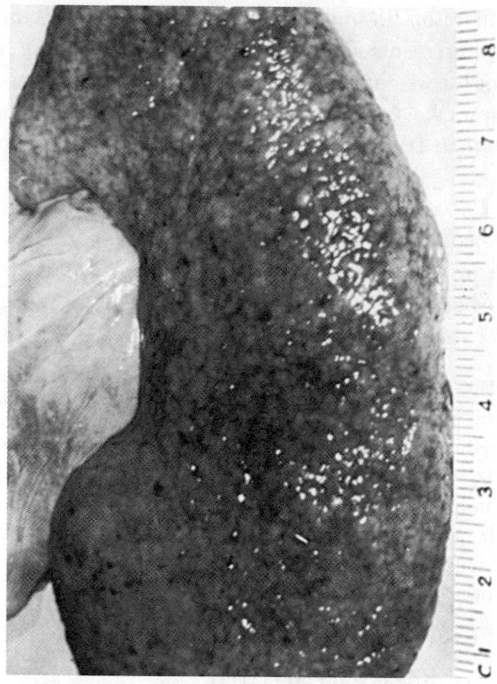

Figure 35-3 End-stage chronic glomerulonephritis. Note pebbly surface corresponding to surviving hypertrophied nephrons and atrophy.

Nursing care involves teaching the patient to maintain a healthy lifestyle, avoid infections, eat a balanced diet within prescribed limits, take prescribed medications, maintain follow-up health care, and report any exacerbation in signs or symptoms to the health care provider. If complications occur, specific treatment is symptomatic and supportive.

HEALTH PROMOTION AND PREVENTION. No preventive measures exist for CGN because predisposing factors have not yet been identified. Infections should be treated promptly, as discussed under Acute Glomerulonephritis, to reduce the possibility of the acute disease progressing to CGN. The nurse encourages patients to receive ongoing treatment for symptoms to slow the progression of disease.

Nephrotic Syndrome

Nephrotic syndrome **(nephrosis)** is not a single disease entity but a constellation of symptoms, including albuminuria, hypoalbuminemia, edema, hyperlipidemia, and lipuria. Nephrotic syndrome damages the glomeruli with resultant severe proteinuria, with losses of up to 3.5 g of protein per day.

Etiology and Epidemiology. Nephrotic syndrome has been associated with allergic reactions (insect bites, pollen, acute glomerulonephritis), infections (herpes zoster), systemic disease (diabetes mellitus, lupus erythematosus, amyloidosis, Goodpasture's syndrome, sickle cell disease), circulatory problems (severe congestive heart failure, chronic constrictive pericarditis), cancers (Hodgkin's disease; lung, colon, and breast cancer), renal transplantation, and pregnancy. Many persons with chronic kidney failure develop nephrotic syndrome. Known glomerular disease is the most common precipitating event in adults. Some individuals have periods of remission and exacerbation. The etiology of nephrotic syndrome in children is usually idiopathic (unknown).

Nephrotic syndrome is seen most often in children with minimal change nephropathy, which results in loss of negative charges in the basement membrane, thus allowing negatively charged proteins to pass through and be wasted in the urine. The prevalence is about 15 cases per 100,000 in the pediatric population, with 2 to 7 new cases per year. In adults the most common cause of nephrotic syndrome is membranous glomerulopathy.

Pathophysiology. The initial physiologic change in nephrotic syndrome is damage to cells in the glomerular basement membrane from immune complex deposition, nephrotoxic antibodies, or other nonimmune mechanisms. These changes result in increased membrane porosity and permeability with significant proteinuria. As protein continues to be excreted, serum albumin is decreased (hypoalbuminemia), thus decreasing the serum osmotic pressure (Box 35-2). The capillary hydrostatic fluid pressure in all body tissues becomes greater than the capillary osmotic pressure, and generalized edema results (Figure 35-4). As fluid is lost into the tissues, the plasma volume decreases, stimulating secretion of aldosterone to retain more sodium and water. This additional fluid also passes out of the capillaries into the tissue, leading to even greater edema.

Clinical manifestations of nephrotic syndrome include severe generalized edema *(anasarca)*, significant proteinuria, hypoalbuminemia, and hyperlipidemia. Hyperlipidemia develops from increased hepatic production of lipids or perhaps from interference of lipid utilization. Urine volume and renal function may be either normal or greatly altered. Altered renal function and symptoms of kidney failure occur as a result of progressing glomerulonephritis. Loss of appetite and fatigue are common.

COMPLICATIONS. Like glomerulonephritis, nephrotic syndrome can lead to kidney failure and complications involving fluid overload in the periphery resulting from protein shifts. At the vascular level, the patient may become hypovolemic because of changes in osmotic pressure.

Box 35-2 Nephrotic Syndrome

- Normal function:
  - —Glomerular capillaries are impermeable to serum proteins.
  - —Plasma proteins create colloid osmotic pressure to retain intravascular fluid.
- Pathophysiology:
  - —Glomerular capillaries become permeable to serum proteins, resulting in proteinuria and decreased serum osmotic pressure.
  - —Glomerular filtration rate decreases.
- Clinical manifestations:
  - —Patient may develop severe generalized edema, pronounced proteinuria, hypoalbuminemia, and hyperlipidemia.

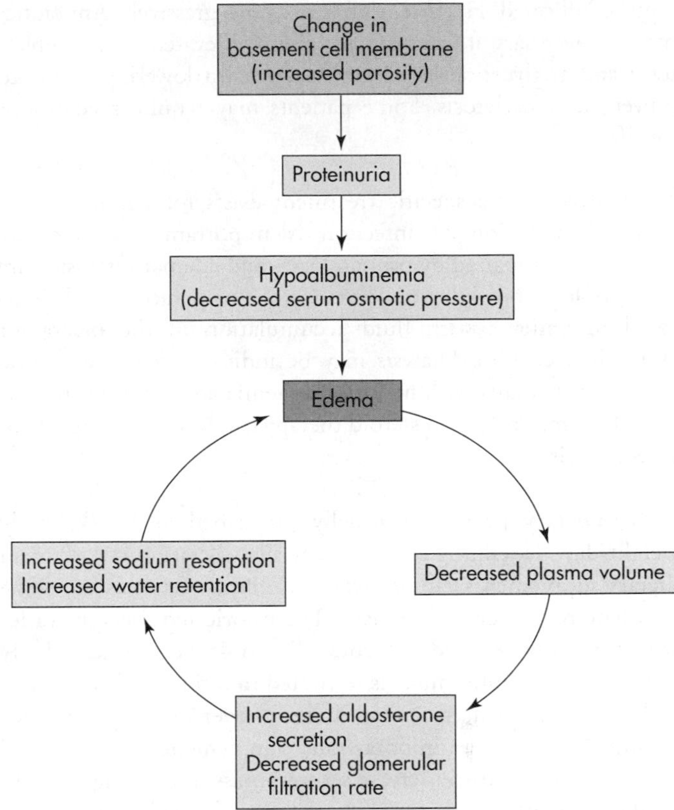

Figure 35-4 Pathophysiologic changes in nephrotic syndrome.

Collaborative Care Management. Treatment of nephrotic syndrome focuses on relieving symptoms and preventing complications to prevent progressive renal damage. Immunosuppressive agents, corticosteroids, diuretics, and antihypertensives are often used to control symptoms.

DIAGNOSTIC TESTS. Laboratory tests include urinalysis for protein, casts, and erythrocytes and serum tests for protein and lipid analysis. Dipstick urine protein may be as high as +3 or +4. Hyperlipidemia and elevated serum cholesterol, elevated triglycerides, and elevated low-density and very low–density lipid levels are common findings. Serum albumin can fall below 2 g/dl. Periodic determinations of proteinuria and measures of renal function are performed to monitor response to treatment and level of kidney function. Renal biopsy is sometimes used to obtain a definitive diagnosis or determine the extent of kidney damage. Biopsy may reveal minimal to extensive changes, including hypercellularity, changes in the epithelium, fatty deposits in the tubules, sclerosing of the glomeruli, and deposition of immunoglobulins along the capillary walls. Persons with extensive damage generally do not respond to treatment and develop end-stage renal disease.

MEDICATIONS. Corticosteroids may be useful in controlling the illness, but responses vary. Even patients responsive to steroids may experience relapses for several years.[27] Prednisone is the drug of choice. Cyclophosphamide or azathioprine is used for patients unresponsive to steroids. Immunosuppressants and angiotensin-converting enzyme inhibitors significantly reduce protein loss in the urine. Slow resolution of edema with diuretics and albumin may be indicated. Hypertension is treated aggressively. Antibiotics may be necessary if infection is present. Elevated serum cholesterol and triglyceride levels are treated with lowering agents to prevent atherosclerosis. Some patients may require medications for life.[1]

TREATMENTS. No specific treatment exists for nephrotic syndrome. Prevention of infection is important because body defenses are impaired by protein losses and edematous tissues are susceptible to breakdown. Thoracentesis or paracentesis is indicated in patients with fluid accumulation in the pleural or abdominal cavities. Dialysis may be indicated for severe cases. Nephrotic patients with hypoalbuminemia are at risk for thromboembolism. Prolonged steroid therapy can lead to osteopenia or osteoporosis.

DIET. Dietary protein is usually prescribed at 1 g/kg body weight/day, depending on the glomerular filtration rate. Protein dietary supplements can be given with meals. Calories should be adequate to prevent catabolism. The caloric requirement varies with the individual; adults require 35 to 45 kcal/kg ideal body weight/day. Sodium intake is restricted to 0.5 to 1 g/day to control edema. Patients receiving diuretics over prolonged periods should eat foods high in potassium. Supplements are prescribed only after attempts to increase serum potassium through dietary intake have failed. Limiting dietary fat is of little benefit in controlling cholesterol or triglyceride levels, since they are caused by liver overproduction rather than dietary intake (see Patient/Family Teaching box).

HEALTH PROMOTION AND PREVENTION. Nephrosis is often progressive; therefore the nurse teaches patients and caregivers measures that may slow the disease's progress, such as control of the underlying condition. The nurse informs them about the effects of nephrotic syndrome on the kidneys and the possible need for dialysis or renal transplant in the future.

PATIENT/FAMILY TEACHING
Nephrotic Syndrome

Nephrotic syndrome is often progressive; therefore teaching includes:

- Effects of nephrotic syndrome on the kidneys and the possible need for dialysis or renal transplant in the future
- Medication regimen: name, dose, actions, side effects, and the need to finish antibiotic prescription (as appropriate)
- Information about nutritional needs and restrictions:
  —The need for increased calories and adequate protein to meet nutritional needs
  —The need for limiting the intake of dietary sodium
- How to self-assess fluid status, including signs and symptoms of hypovolemia and hypervolemia
- Signs and symptoms requiring medical attention: increased edema, dyspnea, fatigue, headache, or infection
- Importance of health habits to prevent infection, including exercise, adequate rest and sleep, and avoidance of sources of infection
- Need for follow-up care to monitor renal function

Nursing Management
of the Patient with Nephrotic Syndrome

ASSESSMENT

Health History. Assess for:

- Predisposing factors
- Length of time since onset of symptoms
- History of weight changes, loss of appetite, fatigue

Physical Examination. Assess for:

- Degree of edema
- Change in daily weights
- Intake and output (liquids and solids)
- Abdominal girth
- Skin condition

NURSING DIAGNOSES, OUTCOMES, AND INTERVENTIONS

Nursing Diagnosis: Imbalanced Nutrition: Less Than Body Requirements

OUTCOMES. Common examples of expected outcomes for the patient with a diagnosis of *imbalanced nutrition: less than body requirements* are:
Patient will:

- Consume a diet high in protein and calories, but low in sodium.
- Maintain stable weight.

NURSING INTERVENTIONS. A sodium-restricted diet is usually prescribed. The protein prescription varies according to the amount of protein lost in the urine over 24 hours. Appetite is diminished as a result of fluid retention and decreased food palatability. Small frequent feedings may be better tolerated. Vitamin supplements with iron may be prescribed. After assessing the patient's food preferences, the nurse should work with the dietitian to develop a diet plan. Whenever possible, the protein should be of high biologic value (lean meat, fish, poultry, and dairy products). The nurse teaches patients how to assess their own fluid status, including signs and symptoms of hypovolemia and hypervolemia.

The nurse offers oral hygiene at regular intervals. Mouth care can help reduce the unpleasant metallic taste and breath odor that are partially responsible for the anorexia of renal failure. The nurse monitors laboratory data, including serum protein, lipids, and calcium, to assess protein stores. The patient is weighed daily and interventions implemented for excessive weight loss or gain.

RELATED NIC INTERVENTIONS. Diet Staging, Nutrition Management, Nutritional Counseling, Nutritional Monitoring

Nursing Diagnosis: Risk for Infection

OUTCOMES. Common examples of expected outcomes for the patient with a diagnosis of *risk for infection* are:
Patient will:

- Be free from signs and symptoms of infection.
- Maintain intact skin.

NURSING INTERVENTIONS. Persons with nephrosis are at increased risk for infections because urinary protein losses impair body defenses. They should, therefore, be protected from potential sources of infection. It is also important to remember that corticosteroid use may mask signs of infection. Nonetheless, the nurse teaches patients the signs and symptoms of infection and when to report them. When infection is suspected, it is important to address the problem immediately. The nurse obtains specimens for culture and sensitivity testing; administers antibiotics at prescribed times to maintain therapeutic blood levels; and stresses the importance of completing the prescribed course of medication to the patient and caregiver. Invasive procedures should be avoided or performed under strict aseptic technique.

Edematous tissue is particularly susceptible to skin breakdown and infection. Careful positioning and frequent position changes may increase comfort while also protecting the skin. Air or water mattresses may increase comfort and relieve skin pressure. Men may develop scrotal edema; if so, a scrotal support provides comfort and aids in reducing swelling.

RELATED NIC INTERVENTIONS. Fluid/Electrolyte Management, Infection Protection, Skin Surveillance, Surveillance

EVALUATION

To evaluate the effectiveness of nursing interventions, compare patient behaviors with those stated in the expected outcomes.

RELATED NOC OUTCOMES. Immune Status, Nutritional Status: Food & Fluid Intake, Nutritional Status: Nutrient Intake, Risk Control, Tissue Integrity: Skin & Mucous Membranes

GERONTOLOGIC CONSIDERATIONS

With age, interest in eating may decline because of changes in the sensory organs, which alter the taste of food. A major component of the treatment for nephrotic syndrome is maintaining a high-protein, low-sodium diet. Older adults may lack the resources to comply with the prescribed diet. In addition, they are more likely to have complications related to steroid therapy because of excess levels of circulating free glucocorticoids.

Chemical-Induced Nephritis

Etiology and Epidemiology. Chemical-induced nephritis, also known as acute or chronic interstitial nephritis, is an idiosyncratic reaction that results in renal damage associated with interstitial edema and infiltration with inflammatory cells, T lymphocytes, and monocytes. Chronic lesions cause interstitial fibrosis. This disease process was first noted in patients sensitive to the sulfonamides. Many other substances are now associated with chemical-induced nephritis, including those listed in Box 35-3.

Pathophysiology. Chemical-induced nephritis usually begins within days or weeks of exposure to the chemical. The inflammatory process disrupts the ability of the glomeruli to filter. Furthermore, the capillary membrane becomes permeable to plasma proteins and red blood cells, which results in mild to moderate proteinuria and hematuria. Eosinophils in the urine signify an allergic interstitial nephritis.

Box 35-3 Substances Associated With Nephritis

Antibiotics

Sulfonamides
Methicillin, penicillin
Cephalosporins
Sulfamethoxazole-trimethoprim (Bactrim)
Rifampin
Gentamicin
Amphotericin B

Other Medications

Cimetidine
Phenytoin
Allopurinol
Nonsteroidal antiinflammatory drugs (e.g., fenoprofen)
Diuretics

Infections

Streptococci
Legionella

Solvents

Carbon tetrachloride
Methanol
Ethylene glycol

Heavy Metals

Lead
Arsenic
Mercury

Other Substances

Pesticides
Poisonous mushrooms

Clinical manifestations of nephritis include fever, eosinophilia, hematuria, mild proteinuria, and rash. A precipitous decrease in renal function results in an acute rise in serum creatinine. Oliguria, or urine output of 400 ml or less in a 24-hour period, may occur from interstitial inflammation severe enough to obstruct and impede urine flow. Kidney size is normal or slightly enlarged. Urinalysis is used to demonstrate protein, red cell, or white cell casts in the urine. Lumbar pain is possible because of distention of the renal capsule from diffuse kidney swelling. Serum toxicology screening may identify the source of the nephritis.

Collaborative Care Management. Medical management includes immediate withdrawal of the suspected chemical. Hemodialysis or charcoal kidney dialysis may be required to remove the nephrotoxins from the blood. Plasmapheresis may be indicated for treatment of some cases of idiopathic nephritis. Steroids are often administered because of their antiinflammatory effect. If renal function is severely compromised, dietary sodium and protein restrictions may be instituted.

The nurse assesses the patient for signs of fluid and electrolyte imbalance, including edema, blood pressure changes, and adventitious breath sounds. The person needs to understand the rationale for maintaining fluid balance and any sodium restrictions. Care is similar to that for the patient with acute kidney failure (see Chapter 36).

HEALTH PREVENTION AND PROMOTION. Identifying causative agents and removing them from the environment is the best method of preventing chemical-induced interstitial nephritis. Solvents should be kept in well-ventilated areas, and all household chemicals should be clearly labeled.

Frequently people are exposed to nephrotoxic chemical agents as a result of their medical regimen. Health care professionals must be aware of these agents and the signs and symptoms of chemical-induced interstitial nephritis. The prognosis may be improved with early detection and removal of the causative agent.

Industrial exposure to chemicals is a major risk factor for nephritis. Occupational health professionals should be aware of potential risks and should educate employees regarding appropriate preventive measures.

Vascular Disorders

Vascular renal disease results from one of two processes: (1) disease of the main renal arteries, or renal artery stenosis; and (2) sclerosis of renal arterioles, or nephrosclerosis.

Renal Artery Stenosis

Etiology and Epidemiology. Renal artery **stenosis** is a narrowing of one or both renal arteries and their branches. It is the cause of approximately 2% to 5% of all cases of hypertension. Stenosis of the renal artery is caused by atherosclerosis in 90% of cases and fibromuscular dysplasia in about 10% of cases.[33] In both instances the end result is a narrowing of the lumen of the arteries supplying the kidneys (Figure 35-5). Patients at risk include those with severe hypertension, bruits, other vascular disease, and a history of smoking.

Pathophysiology. Renal artery stenosis results in a major reduction of blood flow to the kidneys. The decrease in renal perfusion stimulates the secretion of renin and activation of the renin-angiotensin-aldosterone system.[33] The end result is acceleration of hypertension, which, if untreated, leads to further pathologic changes in the kidneys. See the Clinical Manifestations box for common clinical findings in persons with renal artery stenosis.

Collaborative Care Management. Diagnostic testing depends on the patient's clinical picture. Renal artery stenosis is usually diagnosed with renal arteriography, duplex Doppler ultrasound, and/or magnetic resonance imaging (MRI).[39]

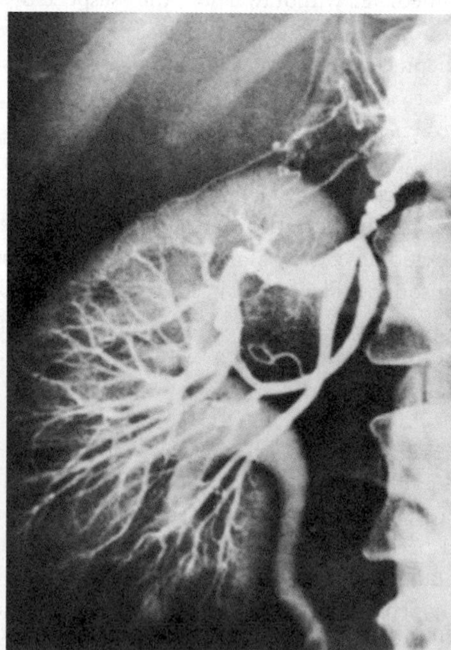

Figure 35-5 Renal arteriogram showing stenosis of right renal artery.

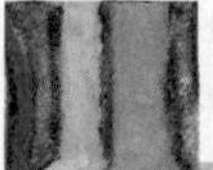

CLINICAL MANIFESTATIONS
Renal Artery Stenosis

- Hypertension (usually abrupt onset)
- Abdominal bruits
- Disparity in kidney size
- Unexplained azotemia

Medical treatment for patients with renal artery stenosis secondary to atherosclerotic disease includes antihypertensive therapy to control blood pressure, aspirin to decrease platelet aggregation, cholesterol-lowering drugs, and smoking cessation. When significant stenosis exists in the renal artery, percutaneous angioplasty with or without stenting or surgical bypass of the stenotic area may be performed to improve circulation.[37]

Complications after an angioplasty include hematoma at the puncture site, azotemia from the dye, and emboli. **Nephrectomy** may be indicated for persons unresponsive to medication and those with restenosis after percutaneous angioplasty (see Patient/Family Teaching box).

Nephrosclerosis

Etiology and Epidemiology. Whereas renal artery stenosis results in hypertension, hypertension can cause nephrosclerosis or damage to the renal arteries, arterioles, and glomeruli. Hypertension is the second major cause of end-stage renal disease.[23] An estimated 10% of individuals with essential hypertension develop severe renal damage, and approximately 1% develop end-stage renal disease and die unless supportive care is provided. Some researchers believe that one's susceptibility to nephrosclerosis may be genetically based. Nephrosclerosis is more common in African-Americans. Other risk factors include a history of hypertension and factors that increase the risk for hypertension (e.g., obesity, diabetes mellitus, positive family history, smoking history, and lack of exercise).

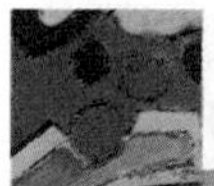

PATIENT/FAMILY TEACHING
Renal Artery Stenosis

Teaching for the patient with renal artery stenosis and his or her caregiver includes:

- Importance of follow-up care for regular blood pressure checks and measurement of renal function:
  —How to monitor the patient's blood pressure at home and the need to apprise the health care provider of patient's status
  —How to recognize the signs of decreasing renal function and the need to report those symptoms promptly
- Need for periodic noninvasive studies such as ultrasound to screen for restenosis
- Behaviors that lower cholesterol:
  —Maintaining a diet low in animal fat
  —Increasing aerobic exercise

Pathophysiology. Nephrosclerosis affects the renal vasculature. Renal arterial vessels show thickening and narrowing of their lumens, and some glomerular capillaries are sclerosed and collapsed. Renal blood flow can be reduced as a result of these vascular changes, causing kidney ischemia. The renal tubules can also be affected, resulting in tubular atrophy. Proteinuria results from glomerular damage. Nocturia may occur from moderate loss of tubular concentrating ability. Urinary casts may be present from tubular injury.

Patients with nephrosclerosis resulting from hypertension often have target organ damage elsewhere such as left ventricular hypertrophy or retinopathy. Signs and symptoms of nephrosclerosis are the same as those for chronic kidney failure (see Chapter 36). By the time clinical manifestations of disease develop, the disease has progressed to an extreme point. Deterioration in renal function progresses gradually.

Collaborative Care Management. Although seldom done, renal biopsy can confirm the diagnosis of hypertensive nephrosclerosis. Treatment goals for patients with nephrosclerosis focus on early detection and treatment of hypertension. Causative factors are sought, and treatment to lower blood pressure is initiated (see Chapter 31). When significant renal damage exists, stabilizing the person's current level of function or slowing deterioration of the kidney tissue is the goal while control of hypertension continues.

Nursing management of patients with nephrosclerosis is the same as that outlined for chronic kidney failure (see Chapter 36). The goals for nursing care center on providing comfort and maintaining self-care in daily living. During drug therapy, the nurse teaches the patient to monitor closely for tachycardia, hypotension, and marked sodium and water retention (see Patient/Family Teaching box).

Obstructive Disorders

Structural or functional changes in the urinary tract can impede the normal flow of urine. Obstruction can occur in any portion of the urinary tract from the meatus to the renal tubules (Figure 35-6).

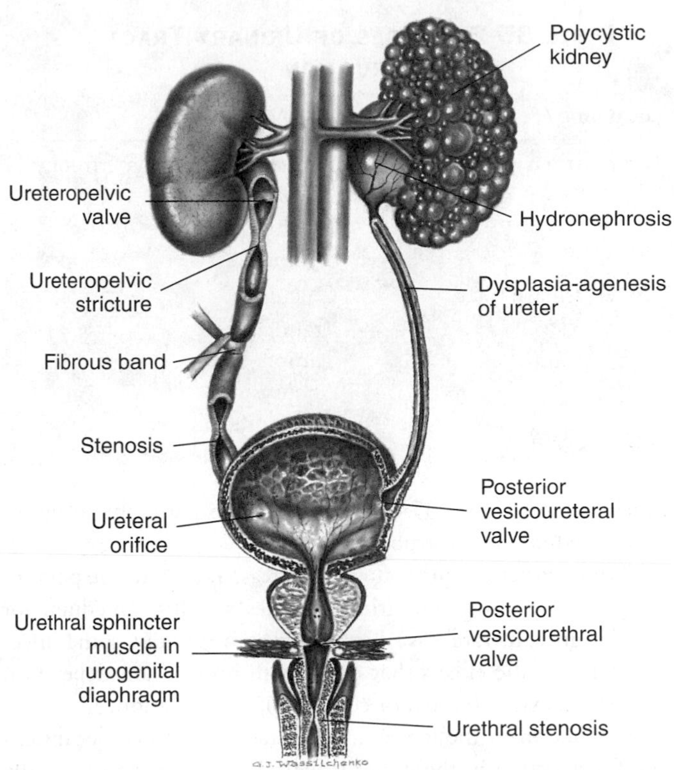

Figure 35-6 Major sites of urinary tract obstruction.

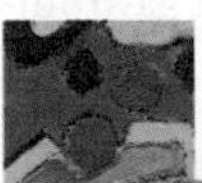

PATIENT/FAMILY TEACHING
Nephrosclerosis

Teaching for the patient with nephrosclerosis and his or her caregiver includes:

- Need for follow-up care
- Self-monitoring techniques to determine adequacy of blood pressure control:
  - —Assessing vital signs
  - —Measuring fluid intake and output
  - —Recording daily weights
- Lifestyle modifications to prevent hypertension:
  - —Dietary modifications
  - —Exercise
- Medication actions, dosages, schedules, and potential side effects
- Explanation about the possible need for dialysis or transplant in the future if end-stage renal disease develops

Patients with obstructions usually have characteristic clinical manifestations, depending on the location and extent of the obstruction. Less than 5% of cases of acute kidney failure are due to urinary tract obstruction. This section describes major concepts related to obstruction of the urinary system and the care of patients with obstructive disorders. Subsequent sections discuss specific obstructive disorders (renal calculi, urinary strictures, and tumors). Benign prostatic hypertrophy is discussed in Chapter 57.

Hydronephrosis

Etiology and Epidemiology. **Hydronephrosis** is the dilation of the renal calyces and pelvis proximal to the obstruction. Hydronephrosis may occur either unilaterally or bilaterally, depending on the site of the obstruction. Hydronephrosis is more common in men after age 60 years because of prostate enlargement. It is more common in women between the ages of 20 and 60 years as a result of pregnancy and uterine cancer. Table 35-2 summarizes causes of urinary tract obstructions.

Pathophysiology. Obstruction of any part of the urinary system from the urethra to the kidney generates backflow of urine and pressure on the renal tubules, causing tubular dysfunction. Partial obstruction may produce slow dilation of structures above the obstruction without functional impairment. As the obstruction increases, pressure builds up in the tubular system behind the obstruction, causing a backflow of urine and dilation of the ureter *(hydroureter)*. The urine backup eventually reaches the kidney, causing dilation of the kidney pelvis *(hydronephrosis)*, which may range in size from mild to severe (Figure 35-7). Pressure buildup in the renal pelvis leads to destruction of kidney tissue and eventually

TABLE 35-2 CAUSES OF URINARY TRACT OBSTRUCTION

Location	Major Causes
Lower urinary tract	Benign prostatic hypertrophy Calculi Urethral strictures Tumors
Upper urinary tract	Calculi Trauma Tumor Aneurysms Congenital anomaly

kidney failure. Figure 35-8 summarizes the pathophysiology of uncorrected urinary obstruction.

With obstruction, urine flow is decreased, even to the point of stagnation. The stagnant urine provides a culture medium for bacterial growth; rarely is obstruction seen without some infection. The specific effects that occur with obstruction depend on its location, extent (partial or complete), and duration.

Obstruction in the lower urinary tract causes bladder distention. Obstruction in the upper urinary tract can progress rapidly to hydronephrosis because of the small size of the ureters and kidney pelvis. The increased pressure in the ureters extends into the kidney pelvis and increases the pressure in the tubules; this along with progressive vasoconstriction in the kidney leads to decreased glomerular filtration rate. Urinary stasis in the dilated pelvis leads to infection and calculi, which add to the renal damage. The unaffected kidney must increase its workload to maintain elimination of waste products. With prolonged obstruction, the unaffected kidney hypertrophies and may function almost as effectively alone (80%) as both kidneys did before the obstruction; however, bilateral obstruction leads to kidney failure.

Symptoms of hydronephrosis depend on the onset and duration of the obstruction. Persons with a slowly developing obstruction may be asymptomatic. Pain radiating to the groin is common in persons with rapidly progressing obstruction (see Clinical Manifestations box). The pain is caused by stretching of the tissues and by hyperperistalsis. An acute upper urinary tract obstruction causes pain, nausea, vomiting, local tenderness, spasm of the abdominal muscles, and a mass in the kidney region. Because the amount of pain is proportional to the rate of stretching, a slowly

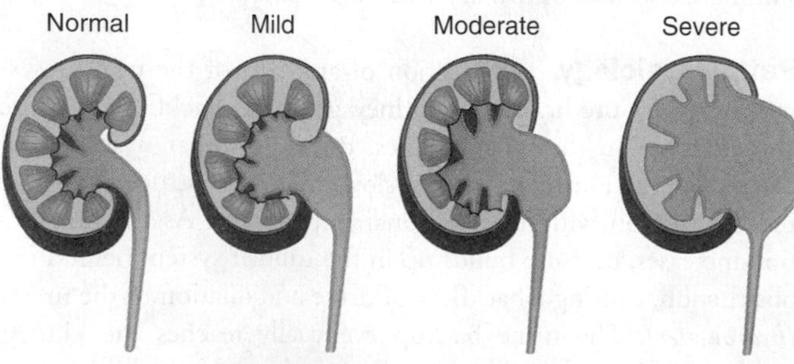

Figure 35-7 Hydronephrosis. Progressive enlargement of renal pelvis and calyces caused by obstruction of upper urinary tract.

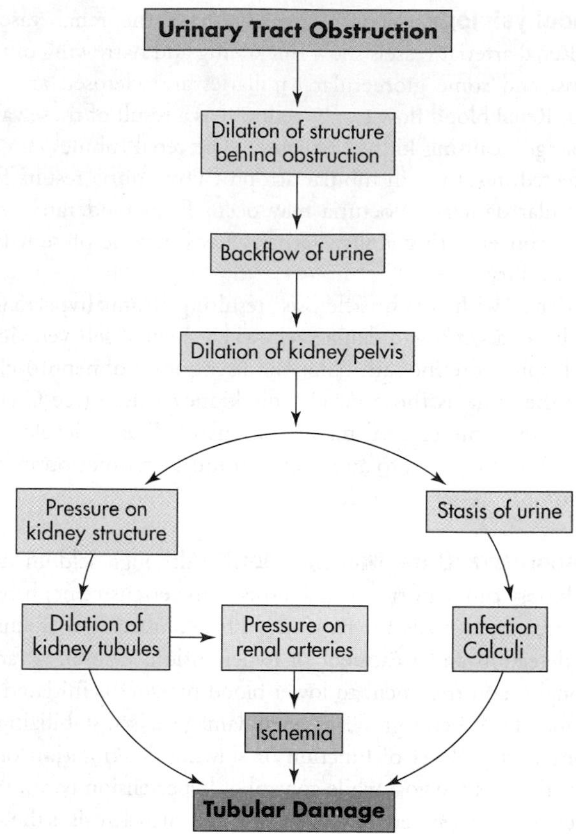

Figure 35-8 Pathophysiology of uncorrected urinary obstruction.

developing hydronephrosis may cause only dull flank pain, whereas a sudden blockage of the ureter (e.g., from a stone) causes a severe, stabbing (colicky) pain in the flank or abdomen. The pain may radiate to the genitalia and thigh and is caused by the increased peristaltic action of the smooth muscles of the ureter in an effort to dislodge the obstruction and force urine past the blockage.

The nausea and vomiting frequently associated with acute obstruction are caused by a reflex reaction to the pain and usually abate as soon as the pain is relieved. An extremely dilated kidney, however, may press on the stomach, causing continued gastroin-

CLINICAL MANIFESTATIONS
Urinary Tract Obstruction

Chronic Hydronephrosis

No symptoms
Intermittent pain
Elevated blood urea nitrogen and creatinine

Acute Hydronephrosis

Renal colic
Changes in urinary output
Hematuria
Palpable bladder
Hypertension
Hesitancy, urgency, incontinence, postvoid dribbling, decreased force of stream

testinal symptoms. If renal function has been seriously impaired, nausea and vomiting may indicate uremia. (See Chapter 36 for discussion of uremia.)

When the bladder is distended from lower urinary tract obstruction, the patient experiences lower abdominal discomfort and feels the need to void, although voiding may not be possible. The bladder may be palpated above the symphysis pubis. With partial obstruction, as seen in benign prostatic hypertrophy, the patient first complains of increasing urinary frequency because the bladder fails to empty completely with each void and therefore refills more quickly to the amount that causes the urge to void (usually 250 to 500 ml). Nocturia, hematuria, and pyuria may also be present.

Collaborative Care Management. Early recognition and management are essential, since declines in renal function are related to the duration and extent of the obstruction. Bladder outlet obstruction can be determined by placing an indwelling urinary catheter or by using an ultrasonic bladder scanner. If the cause is not determined by either of these two methods, an ultrasound or CT scan is used. Further diagnostic studies vary depending on whether an upper or lower tract obstruction is suspected. Urinalysis may lend important clues to the etiology, and serum renal function studies help determine impairment in renal function.

Medical management is specific to the cause of the urinary obstruction. Treatment centers on preserving or restoring renal function. When an obstruction is relieved early, defects in function usually disappear completely. Complete obstruction warrants immediate action. If the obstruction is below the level of the bladder, an attempt should be made to insert an indwelling catheter. Often relief of an obstruction is achieved by balloon dilation of the stenosis, placement of nephrostomy tubes, or stenting. Surgical relief of the obstruction is most often reserved for patients with fibrosis involving both ureters. Dialysis may be necessary before surgical interventions in patients with acute kidney failure.

Clinical manifestations depend on the location (upper or lower), degree of obstruction (partial or complete), and duration and cause of the obstruction. For example, patients with an obstruction resulting from a kidney stone may be seen with severe pain (see next section). In contrast, patients with chronic or partial obstructions may be asymptomatic or have intermittent pain. Patients with acute, sudden obstruction are frequently acutely ill and may have severe colic. Opioids, such as morphine and meperidine, in combination with antispasmodic drugs, such as propantheline bromide (Pro-Banthine), and belladonna preparations, are usually necessary to relieve severe, colicky pain.

When patients are relieved of a bilateral obstruction, initial urinary output may be 200 ml/hr or greater, depending on their hydration status before the obstruction. This phenomenon is called *postobstructive diuresis.* During this diuresis, the nurse should monitor intake and output, body weight, and basic serum electrolytes and provide fluid replacement as indicated. Fluid is usually replaced with 0.45% normal saline with or without dextrose. Fluid replacement may be delayed in patients who are edematous or hypertensive at the beginning of diuresis.[35]

Nursing interventions for the person with urinary obstruction are specific for the underlying cause and are described in the following sections on calculi, tumors, and urinary strictures. Important focuses of care for the person with a urinary obstruction include pain management, fluid balance assessment, prevention of urinary complications, and patient teaching. In addition, the patient should be monitored for signs and symptoms of infection and electrolyte imbalances (see Patient/Family Teaching box).

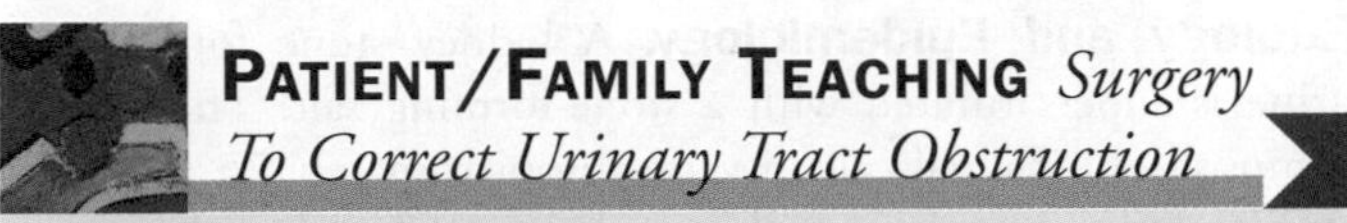

PATIENT/FAMILY TEACHING *Surgery To Correct Urinary Tract Obstruction*

Teaching for the patient and caregiver after surgery to correct urinary tract obstruction includes:
- Postoperative care of incisions
- Care and management of indwelling catheters (if applicable)
- Medication regimen, including expected effects, schedule, dosage, and side effects
- Signs and symptoms of infection and recurrent obstruction that need to be reported

Renal Calculi

Urinary stones **(urolithiasis)** may develop at any level in the urinary system but are most frequently found within the kidney **(nephrolithiasis)**. Nephrolithiases are commonly referred to as renal calculi or kidney stones. Figure 35-9 illustrates the most common locations of calculi formation.

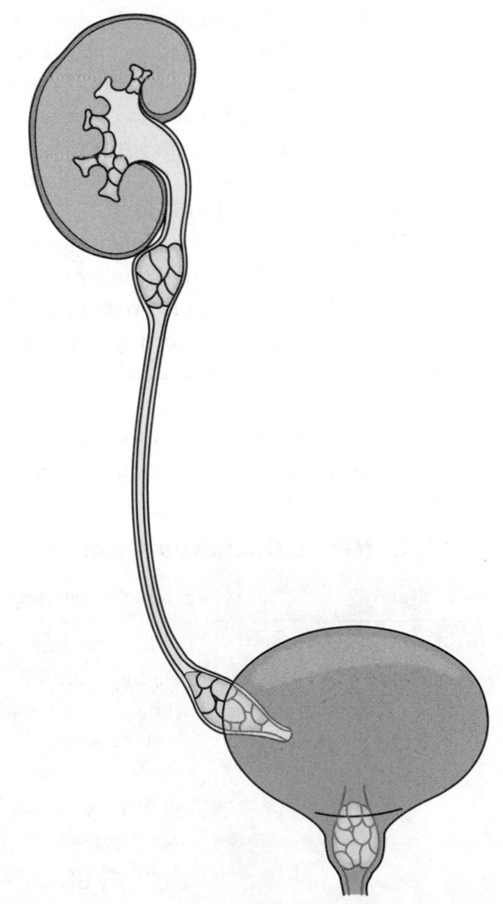

Figure 35-9 Most common locations of renal calculi formation.

Etiology and Epidemiology. A kidney stone forms when urine is supersaturated with a stone-forming salt. The mineral composition of renal calculi varies. Approximately 75% of renal stones consist of calcium salts (oxalates or phosphates), and the remaining stones are composed of struvite, uric acid, or cystine.

Risk factors can be identified in 90% of persons with kidney stones. In addition to inadequate hydration, risk factors for the development of calcium stones include hypercalciuria and high protein and sodium intake. UTIs increase the risk of developing struvite stones. Excess intake of dietary purine found in red meat, fish, and poultry and a disorder in purine metabolism (i.e., gout) are primary risk factors for formation of uric acid stones. Although rare, an autosomal recessive inheritance of homocystinuria can cause development of cystine stones.

Estimates indicate that kidney stones affect about 720,000 people in the United States each year[15] and account for 7 to 10 of every 1000 hospital admissions.[29] Renal calculi are 2.5 times more common in men than women and in persons between the ages of 20 and 50 years old. Approximately 50% of persons who develop renal calculi have a recurrence within 5 years.[15] Fortunately most stones pass without medical intervention.

Pathophysiology. Kidney stones are primarily made of a crystalline component, which requires three major steps for formation: nucleation, growth, and aggregation. Nucleation starts or seeds the stone process and may be initiated by a variety of materials such as protein, foreign bodies, or crystals. The initial crystal serves as the core for further growth and aggregation. Table 35-3 lists the common contributing factors for each type of stone. It is now believed that persons who form stones may lack inhibitor substances in the urine that naturally slow or inhibit stone formation. Although it was once thought that a calcium-restricted diet would reduce the risk of recurrent calcium stone formation, studies have shown that in some patients a low-calcium diet may increase the risk for recurrent stone formation.[23]

Pain associated with the passage of a kidney stone (renal calculi) is referred to as *renal colic.* Pain is the primary symptom in an acute episode of renal calculi. The classic presentation is sudden onset of severe flank pain usually combined with tenderness over the costovertebral angle. Radiation of the pain may indicate the location of the stone in the urinary tract. For example, if the stone is in the kidney pelvis, the pain is caused by hydronephrosis and is more dull and constant in character, occurring primarily in the costovertebral angle. As the stone moves down the ureter, excruciating and intermittent pain is caused by spasm of the ureter and anoxia of the ureter wall from the pressure of the stone. The pain follows the anterior course of the ureter down to the suprapubic area and radiates to the external genitalia.

As the stone moves down the ureter closer to the bladder, the person has an urge to urinate or a burning sensation during urination. Pain can vary widely depending on the location of the stone, degree and acuity of obstruction, and variations in individual anatomy. Often a stone is "silent," causing no symptoms for years. This is especially true of very large stones that develop over a long period and remain lodged in the renal pelvis. Extremely small, smooth stones may be passed asymptomatically. Hematuria is present in about 95% of persons. Many patients experience nausea and vomiting, but only a few have abdominal pain.

Complications. Complications occur as a result of untreated obstruction. If urine flow is not reestablished, severe pain and hydronephrosis with resultant kidney failure may occur. In addition, stasis of urine increases the risk of infection.

Collaborative Care Management

Diagnostic Tests. An x-ray film called a flat plate of the abdomen or KUB (kidneys, ureters, and bladder) is often one of the first diagnostic studies obtained. It can reveal radiopaque stones larger than 2 mm. During the past decade the spiral CT has become the standard radiographic diagnostic test when available. An intravenous pyelogram (IVP) is a radiographic study used to evaluate potential structural and anatomic abnormalities of the urinary tract. An ultrasound may be considered in patients allergic to contrast dye. Serum electrolytes (BUN and creatinine), a complete blood count, urinalysis, and urine culture should be obtained from patients who have acute renal colic.

Because recurrence of renal calculi is common, stone composition is usually analyzed to help direct preventive therapy. Additional studies are carried out after the acute episode has subsided. Successive determinations of serum calcium, phosphorus, protein, electrolytes, and uric acid levels may be performed to identify the underlying disease that influenced stone formation. The urine pH may be measured with a dipstick each time the patient voids to determine the urine acidity or alkalinity. A pH of less than 6 is seen with calcium and uric acid stones; a pH of greater than 7.2 is seen with struvite stones. A nitroprusside urine test may be per-

Table 35-3 Renal Calculus Composition and Contributing Factors

Composition of Stone	Factors Contributing to Stone Formation
Calcium (oxalate and phosphate)	Low urine volume, hypercalciuria (resulting from primary hyperparathyroidism, renal tubular acidosis, immobilization, hyperthyroidism), hypocitruria (resulting from chronic diarrhea, renal tubular acidosis, increased dietary protein loads), hyperuricuria (resulting from inflammatory bowel disease, small bowel resection, dietary excess [e.g., spinach, Swiss chard, rhubarb]), medullary sponge disease
Uric acid	Low urine volume, high purine diet, gout
Struvite	Urinary tract infection
Cystine	Hereditary disorder of amino acid metabolism

formed to check for cystine. An accurate 24-hour urine specimen is collected to measure calcium, oxalate, phosphorus, and uric acid levels. A 24-hour urine specimen may be collected with the patient eating a normal diet or after a 3-day low-calcium, low-phosphorus diet.

MEDICATIONS. Treatments are aimed at relieving pain, preserving renal function, preventing infection, and restoring fluid and electrolyte balance. The majority of stones less than 5 mm pass spontaneously. Patients who are unable to tolerate oral fluids or who have pain despite oral analgesics should be given intravenous (IV) fluid and IV medications for pain. IV opioids or nonsteroidals (ketorolac [Toradol]) are good choices for analgesia. IV fluids may be necessary to restore fluid volume in patients who are dehydrated. Lastly, antiemetics may be indicated for patients with nausea and vomiting.[15]

Although management of kidney stones varies depending on the type of stone, certain recommendations hold for all patients with stones (Box 35-4). In general, fluid intake should be increased to 3 L/day, and dietary oxalate and sodium should be limited (see Evidence-Based Practice box). For calcium stones, a chelating agent such as cellulose phosphate is administered with meals if the problem is thought to be due to increased absorption of calcium in the bowel. The chelating agent binds to calcium and impedes absorption in the small bowel. Thiazide diuretics, particularly hydrochlorothiazide, decrease the calcium content in the urine by increasing resorption of calcium in the renal tubules. Because hyperparathyroidism is the second most common cause of calcium stones, a serum parathyroid level should be obtained. Those with hyperparathyroidism require surgical resection of the parathyroid adenoma (see Chapter 38).

Prophylaxis for uric acid stones consists of alkalinizing the urine by administering sodium bicarbonate or citrate solution. Also, allopurinol (Zyloprim) is usually prescribed to inhibit synthesis of uric acid. The gold standard treatment for struvite stones is complete surgical removal and treatment of the infection with antibiotics. Cystine stones can be treated with penicillamine, which acts by combining with cystine to form a soluble compound.

TREATMENTS. Although 75% to 80% of urinary calculi are passed spontaneously,[27] some stones may fail to pass and cause

BOX 35-4 Stone Clinic Recommendations for Conservative Therapy for Renal Calculi

- High fluid intake: Drink 10 10-oz glasses of fluid (3 L) per day.
- Low-oxalate diet: Limit dark greens, nuts, chocolate, vitamin C.
- Low-sodium diet: Limit sodium to 2 g/day.
- Low purine: Limit meat to 2 moderate servings per day.
- Citrus fruit juice intake: Drink at least 10 oz per day; lemonade encouraged (2 L/day).
- Calcium restriction in the presence of hypercalcemia: Limit dairy products to 2 servings per day.

From Rakel RE, Bope ET: *Conn's current therapy,* Philadelphia, 2001, Saunders.

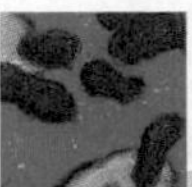

EVIDENCE-BASED PRACTICE

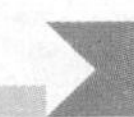

Topic Question: Is increased water intake effective for the primary and secondary prevention of urinary calculi?

Evidence Base: One trial with 199 patients studied the impact of increased water intake on the recurrence of urinary calculi.

Findings: The recurrence rate of urinary calculi was lower (12%) in subjects with increased water intake compared with subjects (27%) who received no intervention.

Conclusions: Increased water intake reduces the risk of recurrence of urinary calculi and prolongs the average interval between recurrences. However, further research is needed.

Qiang W, Ke Z: Water for preventing urinary calculi (Cochrane Review). In *Cochrane Library,* Issue 3, Chichester, UK, 2004, John Wiley & Sons.

obstruction. In these instances, ureteral stent(s) may be passed through a cystoscope up the ureter. This procedure relieves the obstruction in more than 85% of patients.

In general, four modalities are available for interventional treatment: **extracorporeal shock wave lithotripsy** (ESWL), percutaneous nephrostolithotomy, rigid and flexible ureteroscopy, and open surgery.[18] ESWL has become the most commonly used treatment modality. Open surgical procedures are used in less than 1% of patients, having been replaced by less invasive techniques that fragment stones.

EXTRACORPOREAL SHOCK WAVE LITHOTRIPSY. Although there are several categories of lithotripsy, the most common is ESWL. The overall success rate for ESWL is 90%. ESWL is performed by generating external shock waves that are transmitted through the skin and soft tissues and directed on the stone. In the past the patient was submerged in water to transmit the shock; however, newer machines require only a cushion of water to transmit the shock (Figure 35-10). The energy delivered with the shock causes the stone to fragment into small pieces that are often passed spontaneously or can be removed with an endoscope. An electrocardiogram (ECG) should be obtained on all patients before the procedure to determine abnormal rhythms, since shock wave delivery is controlled by the patient's ECG. Patients with pacemakers may need reprogramming. Patients should be instructed to discontinue anticoagulants (warfarin, aspirin, and nonsteroidal anti-inflammatory drugs) before the procedure to decrease the risk of bleeding.[18]

Redness or bruising on the skin at the lithotripsy site, pain, and hematuria are the most commonly reported symptoms following the procedure. Patients are discharged after the procedure if there are no complications; they are informed that small particles may pass in the urine for several days after lithotripsy. Pain may occur from passing fragments of the pulverized stone through the lower urinary tract and persist for up to 3 days. Opioids may be prescribed for pain management. If large fragments of the stone are formed, a percutaneous nephrostomy may be needed to allow passage of the fragments. Nursing care includes pain management and

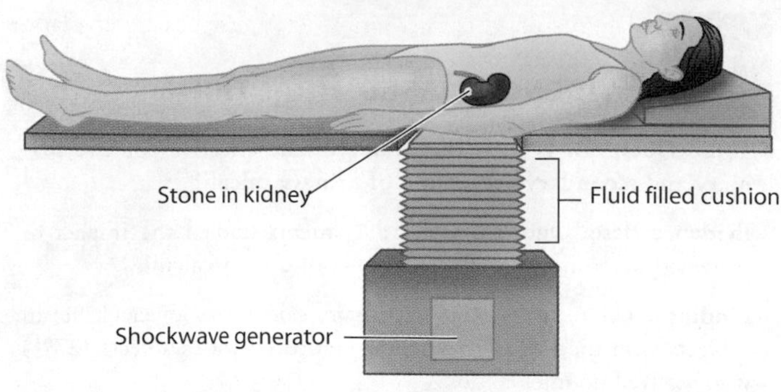

Figure 35-10 Extracorporeal shockwave lithotripsy.

monitoring for complications, including flank pain, bleeding, decreased urinary output, symptoms of obstruction, and fever.

SURGICAL MANAGEMENT

PERCUTANEOUS NEPHROLITHOTOMY. This procedure is carried out with the patient under general anesthesia. A fine needle with a guidewire is inserted into the renal pelvis under ultrasound guidance. A series of dilators are passed over the guidewire. When the surgeon visualizes the stone, he or she breaks it up with ultrasound, electrohydraulic, laser, or pneumatic lithotripsy and evacuates the fragments. A nephrostomy tube is then inserted and sutured to the skin. Complications are few and the risk of hemorrhage low.

URETEROSCOPY. This procedure is used most frequently to remove stones less than 2 cm in the distal and middle ureter. A ureteroscope is inserted directly to the level of the stone. Stones are removed with a basket or graspers, and a stent is placed.

DIET. Specific dietary instructions depend on the stone's composition. Box 35-4 lists conservative measures recommended for all persons with kidney stones. Because of potential adverse effects on the bones and the overall incidence of stones, calcium and protein restrictions are not always (or consistently) recommended.

HEALTH PROMOTION AND PREVENTION. Measures can be taken to decrease the potential for renal stones in persons at high risk. Adequate hydration (intake of 3 L/day or more unless contraindicated) helps prevent urinary stasis that can lead not only to stone formation but also to a UTI. Persons with indwelling catheters need scrupulous aseptic technique in catheter care to prevent infection and require adequate hydration and patent catheter drainage to flush away deposits at the catheter tip.

Nursing Management *of the Patient with Renal Calculi*

ASSESSMENT

Health History. Assess for:

- Location, intensity, radiation of pain
- Dietary and medication history
- Previous abdominal surgery
- Genitourinary abnormalities
- Voiding history

Physical Examination. Assess for:

- Flank and costovertebral tenderness
- Intake and output
- Strain urine for stones

NURSING DIAGNOSES, OUTCOMES, AND INTERVENTIONS

Nursing Diagnosis: Acute Pain

OUTCOMES. Common examples of expected outcomes for the patient with a diagnosis of *acute pain* are:

Patient will:

- Report satisfactory control of pain by rating it as 3 or less on a scale of 1 to 10.
- Report use of relaxation and distraction as a method of pain control.

NURSING INTERVENTIONS. Renal colic is an excruciating type of pain. Morphine, other opiates, or antispasmodics are given to control pain. If the patient can tolerate oral fluids during the acute pain phase, they should be forced. Fluids increase urinary output and dilate the ureters, which relieves pressure on the ureter and may decrease pain. Dilating the ureters also facilitates passage of the calculi. If the patient cannot tolerate oral fluids or is nauseated or vomiting, antiemetics may be administered. Relaxation techniques such as music therapy and guided imagery are also useful.

RELATED NIC INTERVENTIONS. Analgesic Administration, Anxiety Reduction, Pain Management

Nursing Diagnosis: Risk for Infection

OUTCOMES. A common example of expected outcomes for the patient with a diagnosis of *risk for infection* is:

Patient will:

- Remain free from infection.

NURSING INTERVENTIONS. The presence of renal calculi can lead to an increased incidence of infection in susceptible patients. The nurse monitors the patient for any signs of a UTI and encourages the patient to increase fluid intake to at least 3.5 to 4 L/day. Liquids should be caffeine free, since caffeine acts as a diuretic. Prophylactic antibiotics are frequently indicated and should be administered as directed.

RELATED NIC INTERVENTIONS. Fluid Management, Infection Protection, Surveillance

Nursing Diagnosis: Impaired Urinary Elimination

OUTCOMES. Common examples of expected outcomes for the patient with a diagnosis of *impaired urinary elimination* are:

Patient will:

- Remain free from UTI.
- Maintain fluid output equal to fluid intake.

NURSING INTERVENTIONS. The nurse carefully monitors input and output. Deficits in urinary output may indicate inadequate fluid intake or urinary obstruction from the stone. Urinary output is normal in the presence of unilateral obstruction. Urinary diversion devices (nephrostomy or ureterostomy) should be assessed frequently for correct placement and patency. The tubing should be kept free of kinks to prevent reflux of urine.

The urine of all persons with relatively small stones is strained by placing two opened gauze sponges over a funnel. Stones vary in size and may be no larger than the head of a pin. The stones are saved for inspection by the physician and sent to the laboratory for analysis.

Refer to the Patient/Family Teaching box for guidelines related to urinary calculi.

RELATED NIC INTERVENTIONS. Fluid Management, Fluid Monitoring, Urinary Elimination Management

EVALUATION

To evaluate effectiveness of nursing interventions, compare patient behaviors with those stated in the expected patient outcomes.

RELATED NOC OUTCOMES. Comfort Level, Infection Severity, Knowledge: Infection Control, Pain Control, Pain: Disruptive Effects, Pain Level, Urinary Elimination

GERONTOLOGIC CONSIDERATIONS

Renal stones commonly occur between the ages of 20 and 50 years; however, older adults remain at risk, especially when a history of recurrent stone formation is present. Risk factors, treatments, and medications are the same for older adults as for younger adults. Also see the Nursing Care Plan.

Urethral Strictures

Etiology and Epidemiology. A urethral stricture is a narrowing or constriction of the lumen of the urethra. Urethral strictures can be congenital or acquired. Congenital urethral strictures can occur in isolation or in combination with other urinary tract anomalies. The majority of acquired urethral strictures result from trauma secondary to accidents or instrumentation (traumatic catheter placement or removal or a chronic indwelling urinary catheter), inflammation or pressure from the outside by adjacent structures, or growing tumors. Urethral strictures occur more often in men than in women, primarily because of the length of the urethra.

Pathophysiology. Strictures are scars in the urethral epithelium. When the urethra is completely severed and anastomosed, strictures frequently occur at the surgical site. As the scar tissue contracts, the length of the urethra may shorten and the lumen narrow. Inflammation is another cause of urethral stricture, since it produces hyperplasia of the urethral lining. *Balanitis xerotica obliterans,* a chronic skin disease of the penis, is the major cause of inflammatory strictures.[3] Other causes include gonorrhea, chlamydia, and tumors that exert pressure on the exterior of the urethra.

The first symptoms of urethral stricture are usually a decrease in the urinary stream and difficulty initiating the stream. Other symptoms are those of a UTI and urinary retention. Severe urethral strictures result in complete urinary obstruction, leading to hydronephrosis.

Collaborative Care Management. Special imaging studies (retrograde urethrography and voiding cystourethrography) are used to diagnose the length, location, and diameter of the stricture. Urethral strictures can be repaired with urethroplasty, dilation, or stent placement.[41] Dilation is accomplished by inserting splinting catheters of increasing size into the urethra past the area of the stricture.

Nursing care involves teaching patients the early signs and symptoms of urethral stricture, such as decreased urine stream and retention, so that early treatment can be initiated. If dilation is used as treatment, patients can be taught to perform this procedure at home.

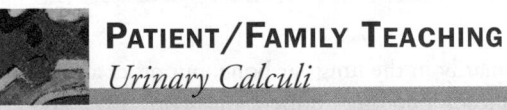

PATIENT/FAMILY TEACHING
Urinary Calculi

Teaching for the patient with urinary calculi and his or her caregiver includes:

- Need for intake of at least 3 L of fluids per day
- Importance of emptying the bladder at regular intervals
- The name, dosage, and side effects of medications prescribed to acidify or alkalinize the urine
- Signs and symptoms that need to be reported to the health care provider:
  —Signs of calculi recurrence (costovertebral pain or pain radiating to external genitalia)
  —Signs of urinary tract infection (burning on urination, frequency, urgency, or fever)

Tumors of the Kidney

Etiology and Epidemiology. Although the exact causes of renal cell carcinoma have not been identified, certain risk factors have been linked to the disease. The strongest risk factor is tobacco use (cigarette, pipe, or cigar). Obesity; exposure to analgesics; autosomal dominant polycystic kidney disease; and occupational exposure to cadmium, asbestos, leather tanning, and certain petroleum products have been implicated in the development of renal cell carcinoma.[32] The majority of renal cell carcinomas start in the proximal convoluted tubule.

In the United States in 2004 there were approximately 35,710 new cases of renal cell cancer and about 12,480 deaths from the disease.[2] Renal cell carcinomas account for approximately 3% of adult cancers and occur twice as often in men as in women. This type of cancer is most commonly seen in persons 40 to 70 years old, with onset rarely occurring before the age of 30 years. At the time of diagnosis, about one third of persons have metastatic disease.[32] The most common sites of metastasis are the lung, lymph nodes, liver, and bone.

Pathophysiology. Renal carcinomas usually develop unilaterally but may occur bilaterally (Figure 35-11). There are five distinct cell

Nursing Care Plan

Patient With Renal Calculi Undergoing Nephrostomy Tube Placement for Obstruction

Data A 55-year-old male reported to the emergency department with sudden onset of severe right flank pain. Diagnostic evaluation demonstrated the presence of right-sided renal calculi with obstruction. A right nephrostomy tube was placed and connected to gravity drainage. Urinary output is blood-tinged with some small clots. A small amount of crusted drainage is at the insertion site, which is without erythema. The patient's blood pressure is 160/94 mm Hg; heart rate is 100 beats/min; and temperature is 98.2° F (37° C) orally. He guards his right flank during examination. Small pinpoint granules can be seen in his strained urine. The patient is anxious about caring for his nephrostomy and voices concern about pain management.

Nursing Diagnosis

Acute pain related to renal calculi and placement of nephrostomy tube

Outcomes

- Patient will return to pain-free status.

Related NOC Outcomes

- Pain Control
- Pain Level

Related NIC Interventions

- Analgesic Administration
- Pain Management

Nursing Interventions/Rationales

- Assess location, severity, frequency, duration, and quality of pain. Use pain scale to rate patient's perception of pain. *Provides baseline data to assess effectiveness of pain control interventions. Rating pain helps the nurse estimate the degree of pain and plan for appropriate interventions.*
- Apply warm compresses to flank area. *Warmth decreases inflammation and promotes relaxation.*
- Administer prescribed analgesics. *Provides pain relief by altering the perception of pain and blocking pain pathways to the brain.*
- Encourage use of relaxation techniques such as focused breathing, music, and guided imagery if acceptable to patient. *Promotes comfort and decreases the need for narcotic analgesics by altering the perception of pain.*
- Allow patient to assume position of comfort. Side lying may enhance comfort. *There are no contraindications to the patient assuming the most comfortable position during acute pain.*
- Increase fluid intake. *Fluids increase urinary output, which helps dilate the ureter and may decrease pain as the stone progresses toward the bladder.*

Nursing Diagnosis

Risk for infection related to urinary stasis and break in skin integrity (insertion and presence of nephrostomy tube)

Outcomes

- Patient will remain free from infection.

Related NOC Outcomes

- Immune Status
- Risk Control

Related NIC Interventions

- Infection Protection
- Surveillance
- Wound Care

Nursing Interventions/Rationales

- Assess temperature, nephrostomy site, urinary frequency and urgency, and abdomen for tenderness. *Establishes a baseline for later comparisons. Changes from baseline data may indicate the presence of infection.*
- Maintain strict asepsis when changing nephrostomy dressing. *To decrease the potential for bacterial contamination of surgical site. The surgical incision allows a portal of entry for microorganisms.*
- Assess nephrostomy site for erythema, drainage, tenderness, induration, or swelling. *Indicates actual or developing localized infection.*
- Monitor for signs of systemic infection (chills, fever, diaphoresis). *Indicates actual or developing systemic infection.*
- Obtain (tissue or fluid) sample for culture and sensitivity if indicated. *To identify causative organism of infection and to monitor effectiveness of therapy.*
- Maintain hydration and voiding schedule. *To prevent bladder distention and urinary stasis, which contributes to the multiplication of pathogens.*
- Administer prophylactic antibiotics as prescribed. *To maintain steady blood levels to decrease the risk of infection.*

types: clear cell, papillary, chromophobe, collecting duct, and "unclassified." Clear cell type is the most common type. Renal cell carcinoma is staged using the TMN system or the Robson system. The TMN system provides information about the tumor (T), distant metastases (M), and regional lymph node involvement (N).

The Robson system, which is more widely used in the United States, categorizes tumors in stages. In stage I disease the tumor margins are well defined (encapsulated) and compress the kidney parenchyma during growth, rather than infiltrating the tissue. The upper pole of the kidney is usually involved, and the tumor is usually large at the time of diagnosis. In stage II the tumor invades the fat surrounding the kidney. Stage III consists of local metastasis either through direct extension or through the renal vein or lymphatics (lymph node involvement). Distant metastases during stage IV are primarily in the lungs or bone, but other areas, such as the liver, spleen, opposite kidney, or brain, may also be involved. Prognosis is based on the stage and advancement of the disease at diagnosis. Factors influencing the prognosis include the patient's overall health and nutritional status.

Painless hematuria is the most frequent sign of renal cell carcinoma. Unfortunately, the hematuria is often intermittent, lessening the person's concern, which may cause a delay in seeking treatment. Any person with hematuria should have a complete urologic examination, since immediate investigation of the first signs of hematuria positively affects the prognosis. Other signs and symptoms include dull flank pain, palpable mass, unexplained weight loss, fever, and polycythemia. Some persons may be totally asymptomatic and are diagnosed by a radiologic abnor-

Nursing Diagnosis

Impaired urinary elimination related to presence of renal calculi and nephrostomy tube

Outcomes

- The patient will achieve preillness urinary elimination pattern.

Related NOC Outcomes

- Urinary Elimination

Related NIC Interventions

- Tube Care: Urinary
- Urinary Elimination Management

Nursing Interventions/Rationales

- Assess intake. *To determine the adequacy of fluid intake. Increased intake facilitates the passage of stones and prevents stasis, which can contribute to infection.*
- Assess urinary output and presence of clots in nephrostomy collection bag. *Deviations from normal indicate potential mechanical blockage.*
- Strain all urine for calculi and send for analysis. *Data help determine treatment strategies for specific stone types.*
- Encourage high fluid intake (3 L/day). *Promotes passage of stones, and prevents urinary stasis.*
- Assess for dysuria, urgency, frequency, or incontinence. *Indications of infection or altered renal function.*
- Maintain patency and position of nephrostomy tube, avoiding kinks in tubing and keeping urinary drainage bag in dependent position. *Prevents reflux of urine into kidney and dislodgement of tube; allows for gravity drainage of urine.*

Nursing Diagnosis

Anxiety related to home management of nephrostomy tube

Outcomes

- Patient will perform self-care for nephrostomy tube without anxiety.

Related NOC Outcomes

- Anxiety Self-Control
- Coping
- Knowledge: Treatment Procedure(s)

Related NIC Interventions

- Anxiety Reduction
- Coping Enhancement
- Teaching: Psychomotor Skill

Nursing Interventions/Rationales

- Assess level of anxiety. *Provides a baseline for planning interventions.*
- Encourage patient and family to express fears and concerns. *Provides opportunity to validate patient's and family's feelings. Identifies concerns and fears so that appropriate interventions can be planned and implemented.*
- Assist patient in identifying primary support systems. *Adequate support mechanisms help reduce the patient's anxiety.*
- Teach (demonstrate and provide written instructions) patient and wife, partner, or caregiver regarding care of nephrostomy tube. *Knowledge decreases anxiety. Written instructions provide resource for later referral if needed.*
- Observe patient and wife performing nephrostomy care. *To correct procedure and to provide reinforcement of learning. Reinforcement builds self-confidence and decreases anxiety.*
- Provide emergency numbers for home support. *Knowledge of ready resources or support helps reduce anxiety.*

Evaluation

Evaluation is based on comparing the patient's outcomes with desired outcomes.

mality detected on ultrasound or by abdominal CT scan. Hypertension may also be present as a result of stimulation of the renin-angiotensin system.

Collaborative Care Management

DIAGNOSTIC TESTS. Most renal tumors are detected incidentally when an ultrasound or abdominal CT has been obtained for some other abdominal complaint. An IVP is usually done in the diagnostic workup of hematuria. If a mass is identified, further diagnostic imaging is usually indicated (ultrasound, CT scan, or MRI). Biopsy confirms the diagnosis.

TREATMENT. Unless the person is a poor surgical risk or has extensive metastases, the diseased kidney is removed (radical nephrectomy) through a transabdominal, flank, or extraperitoneal approach. Radical nephrectomy, performed to prevent metastases, includes the removal of the kidney, adrenal gland, proximal ureter, renal artery and vein, and surrounding fat and renal fascia.

Laparoscopic nephrectomy is a safe and minimally invasive alternative to a radical nephrectomy. The laparoscopic technique offers a smaller incision (Figure 35-12), shorter length of stay, and shorter recovery period.[20] Nephron-sparing surgery is indicated in those who have only one kidney or a small tumor and allows persons with only one kidney to maintain life without dialysis.

Neither standard chemotherapy nor radiation used before or after nephrectomy has been shown to be effective. Other therapies include the use of hormones, immunotherapy, alpha-interferon, and interleukin-2 therapy. The use of chemotherapeutic agents in

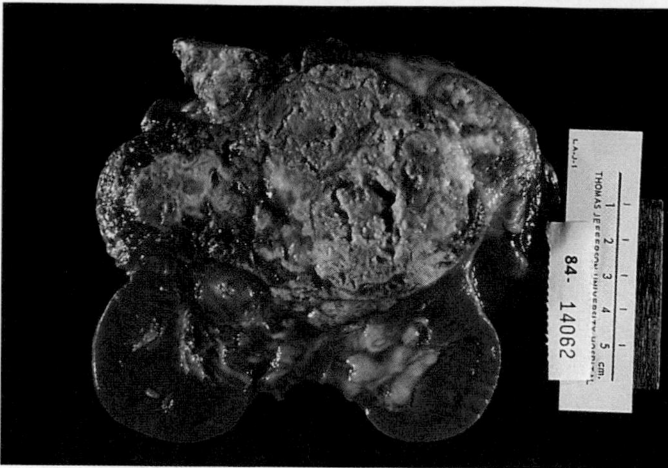

Figure 35-11 Renal cell carcinoma.

combination with immunomodulation agents has shown some benefit. Interleukin-2 has shown some promise for the treatment of renal cell carcinoma with partial to complete regression of tumor in clinical trials. Five-year survival rates after treatment of stage I, II, and IIIA tumors are 70%.[2]

Management of the patient after nephrectomy is similar to that for persons undergoing major abdominal surgery (see Chapter 43) and urinary diversion (discussed later in the chapter). Many nonsurgical therapies for renal cell carcinoma are experimental. It is imperative that patients fully understand the expected outcomes and risks and benefits of each option. The diagnosis of cancer is frightening for patients and their families. Information on support groups such as "I Can Cope" through the American Cancer Society may be helpful to persons facing cancer.

Tumors of the Bladder

Etiology and Epidemiology. The bladder is the most common site of cancer in the urinary tract. An estimated 60,240 persons in the United States were diagnosed with cancer of the bladder in 2004.[2] Cancer of the bladder occurs three times more often in males than in females and is the fourth most common tumor in men. Most cases occur in men between 60 and 80 years old. Although environmental exposure to aromatic amines found in many industries (rubber, electric, paint, and textiles) is a major risk factor in the development of bladder cancer, tobacco exposure is now the greatest risk factor. Other risk factors include exposure to certain chemotherapeutic agents, pelvic irradiation, and chronic infections.

There are three types of bladder tumors: transitional cell carcinoma accounts for 90% of cases, followed by squamous cell carcinoma (8%) and adenocarcinoma (1% to 2%). One of the earliest developments in transitional cell carcinoma is the loss of genetic material on the long arm of chromosome 9.

Pathophysiology. Most neoplasms are of the transitional cell type because the urinary tract is covered with transitional epithelium. The majority of persons diagnosed with bladder cancer initially have superficial disease. Superficial bladder tumors develop via the papillary or invasive pathways. The majority of bladder tumors begin as papillomas. Although most papillomas are noninvasive, some infiltrate to deeper tissues; therefore all papillomas of the bladder are considered premalignant and are usually removed when identified. As the name implies, tumors that develop via the invasive pathway usually infiltrate deeper tissues and have a high risk of metastasis.

Carcinomas of the bladder are graded and staged according to the definitions in Table 35-4. Grading is done by the TMN classi-

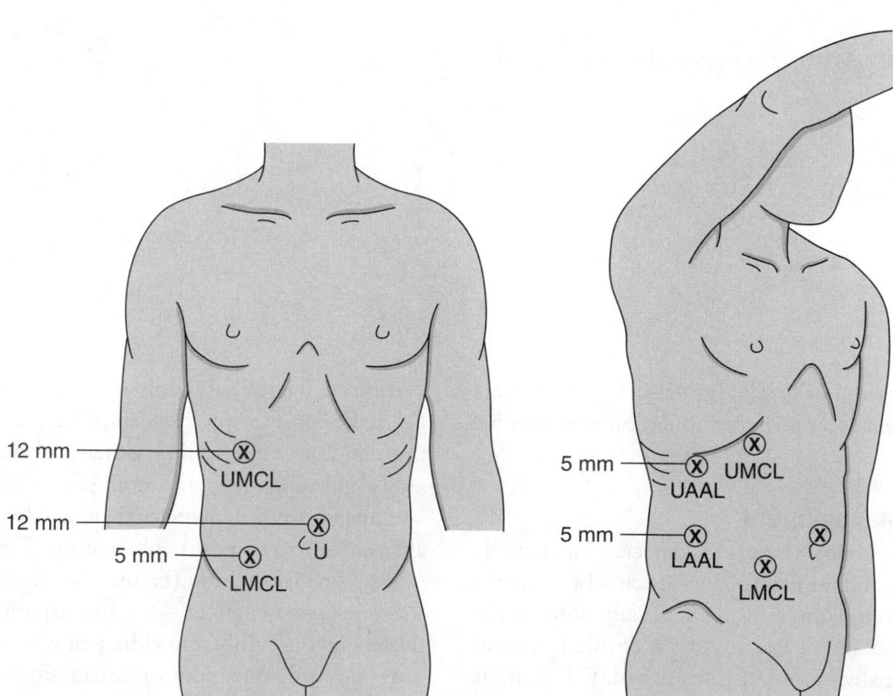

Figure 35-12 Port placement for laparoscopic nephrectomy. *LAAL*, Lower anterior-axillary line; *LMCL*, lower midclavicular line; *U*, umbilicus; *UAAL*, upper anterior-axillary line; *UMCL*, upper midclavicular line.

TABLE 35-4 GRADING AND STAGING CARCINOMAS OF THE BLADDER

GRADES	DIFFERENTIATION
I	Well differentiated
II	Medially differentiated
III	Poorly differentiated
IV	Anaplastic
STAGES	**TISSUE INVOLVEMENT**
0	Mucosa
A	Submucosa
B	Muscle
C	Perivesical fat
D	Lymph nodes

fication system. Grade I and II bladder tumors are usually superficial, whereas grade III and IV tumors are usually invasive.

Painless hematuria is the first sign of a bladder tumor in most patients, The intermittent nature of the hematuria may cause delay in seeking treatment. Hematuria may be accompanied by urgency and dysuria. Some patients are asymptomatic until obstruction of the bladder outlet or ureters occurs. Painless hematuria may also be seen in nonmalignant urinary tract disease and in cancer of the kidney; however, any hematuria should be investigated. Cystitis may also be an early sign of disease, since the tumor acts as a foreign body in the bladder, causing inflammation. Pain in the pelvic region may indicate regional or distant involvement.

Collaborative Care Management

DIAGNOSTIC TESTS. Urinalysis that reveals blood with no apparent cause warrants further investigation. An IVP reveals filling defects in the bladder and upper tracts. A cystoscopy permits visual inspection and facilitates biopsy of suspicious lesions. Cytologic analysis on a total voided urine sample may reveal malignant cells before the lesion can be visualized by cystoscopy. Urine can also be tested for tumor markers. A chest x-ray study and bone scan may be ordered to rule out metastases. A CT scan and MRI may be indicated to evaluate surrounding tissues and organs.

When a tumor is detected by cystoscopy, initial staging and treatment are done by transurethral resection of the bladder tumor. Clinical determination of the invasiveness of the tumor is important in establishing a therapeutic regimen and predicting the prognosis.

TREATMENTS. Treatment options include intravesical chemotherapy, surgery, and radiotherapy. Intravesical chemotherapy or immunotherapy involves instilling the agent directly into the bladder via a catheter. This technique is used in patients with superficial disease or to reduce recurrence in patients whose tumors have been surgically removed. Because of limited absorption of the drugs from the bladder, the main side effect is irritation with voiding. Mitomycin, thiotepa, doxorubicin, and bacillus Calmette-Guérin are the most common agents used.[13]

SURGICAL MANAGEMENT. The most common surgical options include transurethral resection or laser photocoagulation and partial or radical cystectomy. Transurethral resection is used to grade and stage tumors and to remove superficial tumors. Laser photocoagulation is reserved for superficial bladder cancer. Cystectomy provides the best control of local disease. If the entire bladder is removed (radical cystectomy), diversion of the urinary tract is necessary. A long, vertical abdominal incision is present, along with one or more pelvic drains. A nasogastric tube is inserted in the operating room, and the patient is given nothing by mouth until gastrointestinal function returns. Radiotherapy or radiation directed at the bladder and standard chemotherapy are treatment options often used along with the surgery.

Partial removal of the bladder (segmental resection) is usually performed for tumors of the bladder dome. During the immediate postoperative period, bladder capacity is usually less than 60 ml. However, the elastic tissue of the bladder regenerates, increasing bladder capacity to 200 to 400 ml within several months.

Urinary diversion procedures are required for persons undergoing radical cystectomy. Other indications for diversion procedures include birth defects, neurogenic bladder, chronic progressive pyelonephritis, and irreparable trauma to the urinary tract. A urinary diversion establishes an uninterrupted flow of urine, most often via a stoma where the urine is collected in an appliance attached to the skin's surface. The flow of urine may be diverted at any level of the urinary system. The most common urinary diversion procedure in the United States is the ileal conduit, followed by the colon conduit.[22]

With the *ileal conduit,* the ureters are excised from the bladder and transplanted into one end of a 15 to 20 cm segment of ileum resected from the intestinal tract. The remaining intestinal segments are anastomosed, and gastrointestinal function is expected to return to its normal preoperative state after healing. The end of the resected ileum into which the ureters are connected is sutured closed, and the other end is brought through the abdominal wall to the skin surface to create a stoma (Figure 35-13). The urinary bladder may be removed or left intact, depending on the reason for the diversion. The ileal segment functions as a passageway for urine, rather than as a reservoir.

The *colon conduit* (colonic loop) is performed similarly to an ileal conduit except that a segment of colon (ascending, descending, transverse, or sigmoid) acts as the conduit for the urine. The colon conduit has reduced the incidence of urinary reflux for some persons. Preoperative and postoperative nursing care and ongoing management are the same as those for ileal conduit surgery.

The *continent urostomy* has an internal reservoir made from intestine that holds urine. The stoma must be catheterized at regular intervals to drain the reservoir. The *Kock continent ileal reservoir* (Figure 35-14) is formed from loops of the small intestine. The *ileocecal (or Indiana) pouch* consists of portions of large intestine and ileum (Figure 35-15).

Cutaneous ureterostomy is performed when the patient's physical condition prohibits more extensive surgical procedures and is rarely used as a permanent form of diversion. One or both ureters are excised from the bladder and brought out through the skin, either on the flank or the anterior abdominal wall, to create a small stoma. When both ureters are involved, each may be brought out to the skin surface separately, resulting in two stomas, or the ureters

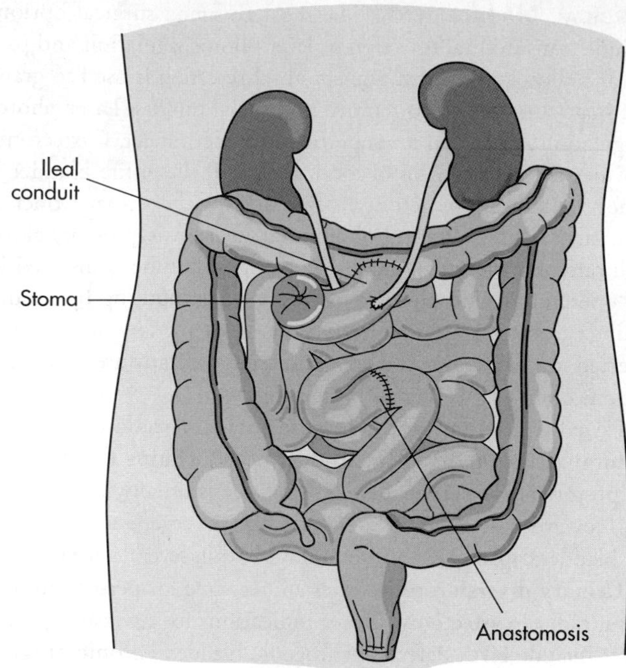

Figure 35-13 Ileal conduit or ileal loop.

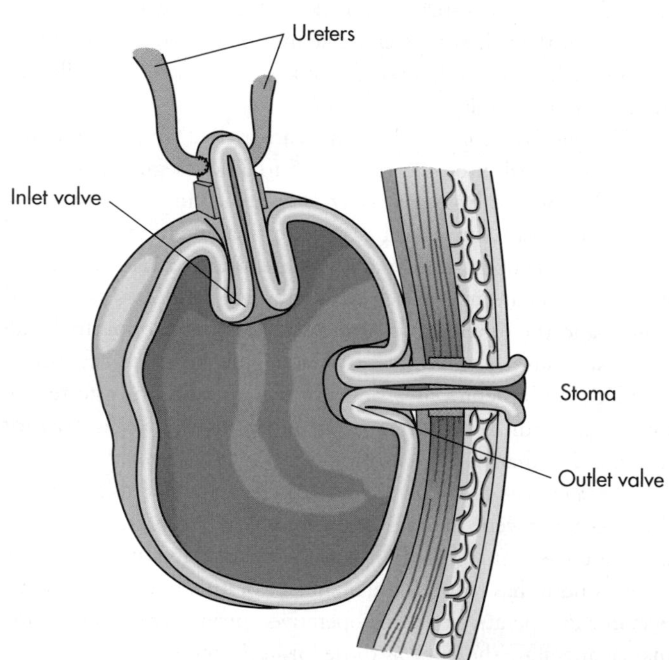

Figure 35-14 Kock continent ileal urinary reservoir.

may be joined and brought out through the abdominal wall to form only one stoma.

For the Kock pouch procedure, the ureters are connected to the pouch above a valve. This valve prevents reflux of urine to the kidney. A second valve placed in the intestinal segment leading to the stoma prevents the leakage of urine, thus maintaining continence. For the ileocecal pouch, which utilizes a segment of ileum and large bowel, the ureters are anastomosed to the colon portion of the reservoir in a manner to prevent reflux. The ileocecal valve is used to provide continence, and the section of ileum that

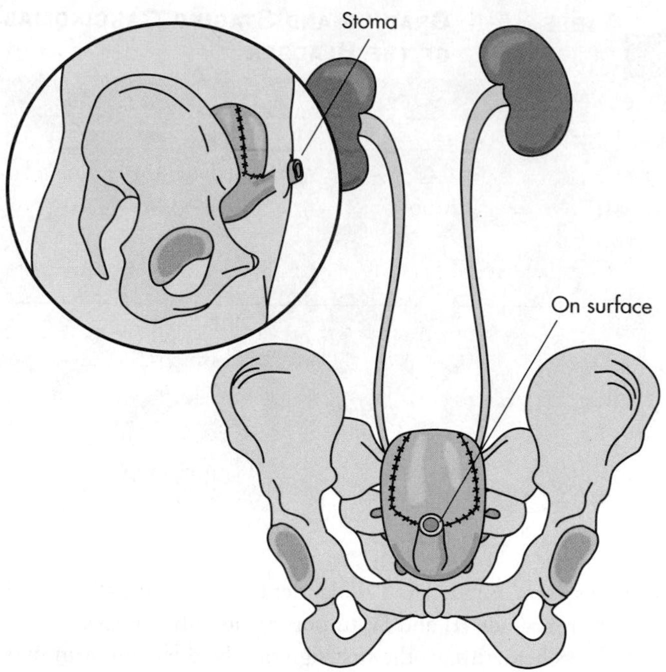

Figure 35-15 Ileocecal continent urinary reservoir (Indiana pouch).

extends from the intestinal reservoir to the skin is narrowed (plicated) to prevent urine leakage. The end of the intestinal segment is brought out onto the skin to form the stoma. The stoma for the continent urostomy is usually flush to the skin and placed lower on the abdomen than the ileal conduit stoma.

Stoma assessment is an important postoperative consideration. The ileal conduit, colon conduit, and continent urostomy stomas should be edematous and beefy red after surgery. Pallor or a gray color may indicate ischemia. Early complications after surgery include breakdown of the anastomosis in the gastrointestinal tract, leakage from the ureteroileal or ureterosigmoid anastomosis, paralytic ileus, obstruction of the ureters, wound infection, mucocutaneous separation, and stomal necrosis. Complications that may occur after hospitalization include stomal problems (retraction, stenosis, or hernia) and UTIs.

The *orthotopic neobladder* is an alternative to urinary diversion for patients who have a competent sphincter without cancer in the urethra, trigone, or bladder neck. A reservoir is constructed, and the patient's urethra is attached to the reservoir. This procedure produces good results, preserves the patient's ability to void, and eliminates the need for a stoma.[40]

Medications. Epidural and parenteral opioids are given for the first 4 to 5 days after surgery to control surgical pain. Opioids may be administered via patient-controlled analgesia. After the patient begins oral intake, oral analgesia can be used.

Postsurgical Complications. The person with a urinary diversion is at greater risk for a UTI because of the shorter distance from the urinary diversion to the kidneys. The nurse teaches the patient the signs and symptoms of a UTI (cloudy urine, blood in urine, strong odor to urine, flank pain, fever, and malaise). Urine cultures are obtained by catheter from the ileal or colon conduit stoma. A specimen taken from the pouch is likely to be contaminated. A pouch with an antireflux valve is recommended to reduce infection from bacteria found in the pouch.

Bowel segments used in continent reservoirs are subject to bacterial colonization leading to pouchitis and pyelonephritis. In addition, mucus, which can cause obstruction and be a source of infection, may be produced for about 1 year after surgery. Daily pouch irrigation with normal saline should be incorporated into care routines.

Problems with the peristomal skin include erythema and irritation from contact with urine, candidal infections, allergic dermatitis, and pseudoverrucous (wartlike) lesions. Problems with the stoma include bleeding, stenosis, or hernia. A small amount of bleeding from the stomal mucosa may occur when the stoma is cleansed. Bleeding generally stops within a few seconds. If bleeding persists or is unusually severe, the physician is notified. Blood that originates from the urinary tract rather than the stoma may be related to complications such as infection or calculi.

Interaction of urine with the bowel epithelium causes altered transport of electrolytes. When the ileum or colon is used, the conduit mucosa resorbs chloride from the urine, and the patient may develop a metabolic hyperchloremic acidosis. A person with optimal renal function has no difficulty excreting the resorbed chloride. When renal function is compromised, the patient is more likely to develop electrolyte problems. This resorption can also occur in those with internal reservoirs because the urine is retained within the internal pouch until the stoma is catheterized and the urine drained. Follow-up urologic care visits and electrolyte studies are imperative. Early in the postoperative period, as the suture lines heal, urine may leak into the peritoneal cavity, causing peritonitis. Patients usually are seen with painful, rigid abdomen; fever; and absent bowel sounds.

DIET. No specific dietary modifications are necessary for the patient with bladder cancer. Anorexia and nausea are problems that need to be addressed. High-caloric supplements are encouraged to prevent weight loss or wasting. Fluid intake of at least 2 L/day is recommended to avoid dehydration. The patient should avoid substances that irritate the bladder, including alcohol, tea, spices, and smoking.

Nursing Management

of the Patient with Urinary Diversion Surgery

ASSESSMENT

Health History. Assess for:

- Acceptance of diagnosis
- Urinary history, including frequency, hematuria, infections

Physical Examination. Assess for:

- Elevated temperature
- Level of pain and degree of relief from medications
- Signs of infection at surgical site
- Patency of urinary drainage system
- Intake and output

NURSING DIAGNOSES, OUTCOMES, AND INTERVENTIONS

Nursing Diagnosis: Risk for Impaired Urinary Elimination

OUTCOMES. Common examples of expected outcomes for the patient with a diagnosis of *risk for impaired urinary elimination* are:

Patient will:

- Maintain patent urinary drainage system.
- Maintain urinary output of at least 30 ml/hr.

NURSING INTERVENTIONS. The basic needs of patients requiring urologic surgery are the same as those of any other surgical patient (see Chapter 15). Special emphasis must be placed on promotion of ventilation and adequate urinary output, prevention of distention and hemorrhage, and attention to drainage tubes and dressings (see Guidelines for Safe Practice box).

Before urinary diversion surgery a complete cleansing of the bowel is required. Bowel preparation reduces the possibility of fecal contamination when the bowel is resected and used to form the conduit or internal reservoir. The cleansing routine consists of a low-residue diet for 2 days followed by a clear liquid diet for 24 hours before surgery and nothing by mouth after midnight the night before surgery. Large-volume oral bowel cleansing solutions (GoLYTELY or Colyte) or a special laxative and fluid program may be prescribed the day before surgery. Cleansing enemas may be ordered to supplement the clean-out procedure. Intestinal antibiotics such as erythromycin or neomycin may also be administered orally.

During the postoperative period, the decreased bladder size is of major importance for patients who have had segmental resections. The patient returns from surgery with catheters draining the bladder both from a cystostomy and from the urethra to avoid obstruction of drainage. The bladder becomes distended rapidly if obstruction occurs, resulting in disruption of the bladder suture line.

As soon as the urethral catheter is removed, the patient becomes acutely aware of the small bladder capacity. Most patients need to void at least every 20 minutes; consequently the nurse needs to reassure them that bladder capacity will gradually increase. Total fluid intake should be 3 L throughout the day unless contraindicated by another medical condition. Large quantities of fluid

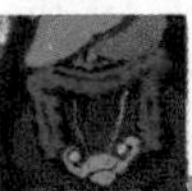

GUIDELINES FOR SAFE PRACTICE
The Patient After Urologic Surgery

- Promote ventilation.
  —Encourage breathing exercises.
  —Encourage frequent self-turning in bed.
  —Encourage ambulation.
- Monitor patency and output of urinary catheters.
- Prevent complications.
  —Change wet dressings to protect skin.
  —Restrict food and oral fluids if bowel sounds are absent.
  —Encourage fluids to 3 L/day when permitted.
  —Monitor for bright red blood on dressings or in urine.
- Administer analgesics to control pain.

should not be ingested at one time, however, and fluids should be limited for several hours before going out.

After an ileal or colon conduit procedure, stents are usually in place in the stoma for 1 week to 10 days to promote urinary drainage. The patient with a continent urostomy generally has a catheter, stents, or both in the stoma sutured in place to allow drainage from the reservoir. A drain tube is placed into the pelvic area for drainage of blood and surgical fluids. All tubes are placed below the level of the kidney so they can drain by gravity. The newly created internal reservoir must be protected from distention to prevent leakage at the anastomosis.

A nasogastric tube with suction is in place until effective intestinal peristalsis has returned. The nasogastric tube is maintained to prevent pressure on the intestinal anastomosis. The patient may have nothing by mouth until peristalsis returns. IV fluids are given until adequate intake of oral liquids is tolerated. Once peristalsis resumes, clear liquids are started and the diet is advanced gradually.

After any type of urinary diversion, the nurse initially monitors urinary output every hour and reports output less than 30 ml/hr. Edema of the stoma or of the ureteral anastomosis site may prevent urine drainage, leading to hydronephrosis or a break in the anastomosis. Decreased urinary output may be associated with other complications such as dehydration, obstruction of the ureters, or compromised renal function. Symptoms of peritonitis (fever, abdominal distention, and pain) coupled with decreased urinary output indicate intraperitoneal leakage of urine at either the intestinal or the ureterointestinal anastomosis. If this occurs, emergency surgery is required to repair the leak.

Urine is initially pink but should change to clear by the third postoperative day. Bright red blood or clots are reported immediately, since they may indicate infection at the site of anastomosis. Mucus, a normal discharge from the intestinal segment, is usually secreted from an ileal or colon conduit or continent urostomy.

Postoperative instruction is started as soon as the patient feels able to participate in urostomy care. During the active phases of teaching, the nurse removes the pouch more often than is recommended after discharge. The nurse teaches the patient (or caregiver) how to manage the assembly, apply, and empty the selected pouch.

RELATED NIC INTERVENTIONS. Fluid Management, Fluid Monitoring, Urinary Elimination Management

Nursing Diagnosis: Risk for Impaired Skin Integrity

OUTCOMES. Common examples of expected outcomes for the patient with a diagnosis of *risk for impaired skin integrity* are:

Patient will:

- Maintain bright pink or red stoma with surrounding healed skin.
- Demonstrate correct application and maintenance of appliance.

NURSING INTERVENTIONS. Skin care is an important consideration after urinary diversion surgery. Leakage of urine on surrounding skin can cause skin breakdown. For urinary diversions that exit to the skin's surface, care must be taken to prevent urine leakage onto the surrounding skin and abdominal incision. For the ileal or colon conduit, a transparent pouch is placed around the stoma in the operating room. The pouch allows visualization of the stoma, catheter or stents, and stoma sutures.

The stoma should be bright pink or red. Any evidence of gray or black discoloration is reported to the surgeon, since this may indicate decreased circulation, which leads to necrosis of the stoma. Careful assessment of the stoma that is in contact with a catheter is imperative because improper positioning of a catheter may exert pressure on the stoma mucosa, leading to necrosis. The nurse changes the pouch within 24 to 48 hours after surgery to allow for better visualization and assessment of the stoma and the peristomal skin. The nurse observes the abdominal incision at least daily for healing of the suture line.

In the early postoperative period the pouch is positioned so that it drains to the side of the bed to facilitate drainage and emptying. The urostomy pouch is emptied through a valve at the bottom. Drainage tubing and a collection bag can be attached to the valve of the pouch to allow continuous drainage during the postoperative period (Figure 35-16). The procedure for changing the pouch is outlined in the Guidelines for Safe Practice box.

Stoma edema begins to subside within 7 days after surgery, but the stoma continues to decrease gradually in size for the next 6 to 8 weeks. Therefore before discharge the nurse teaches the patient how to measure the stoma and adjust the pouch size to accommodate the smaller stoma. Too large an opening can lead to skin problems for persons with an ileal or colon conduit. Too small an opening may restrict circulation or cause trauma to the stoma. The opening should be no more than 2 to 3 mm larger than the stoma.

Several types of pouches are available (Figures 35-17 and 35-18). All have two characteristics in common: a pouch to collect the urine

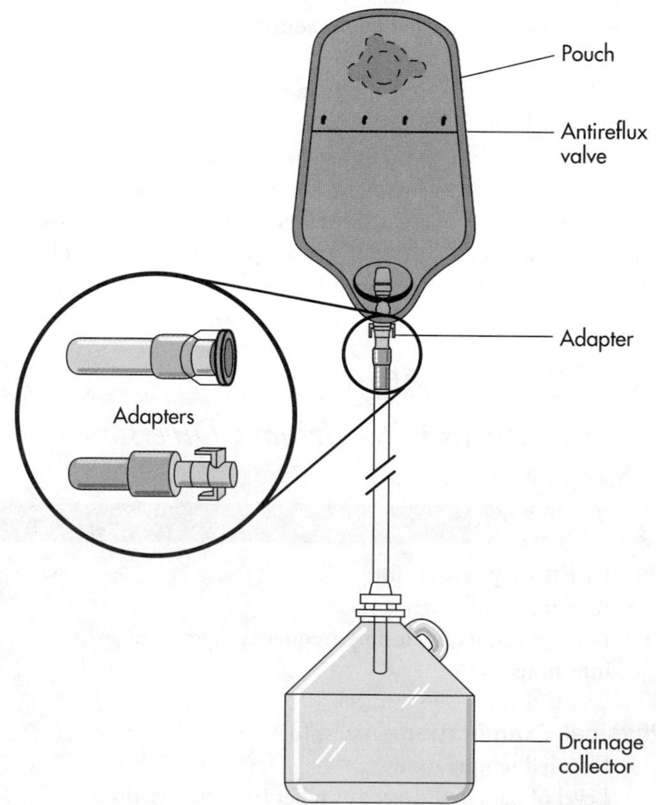

Figure 35-16 Urostomy pouch connected to continuous drainage.

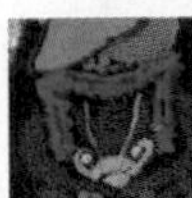

GUIDELINES FOR SAFE PRACTICE
Changing a Urinary Pouch

1. Explain procedure to patient, being sure to include sensory information.
2. Assemble all supplies.
3. Empty the pouch and gently remove it from the skin.
4. Cleanse the peristomal skin with mild soap and water. Rinse and pat dry. Gently wash mucous secretions off the stoma.
5. Place a rolled piece of gauze or cotton balls over the stomal opening to absorb draining urine while caring for the skin.
6. Measure the diameter of the stoma and cut a corresponding opening in the skin barrier and the pouch or select the corresponding size of precut pouch.
7. Apply skin sealant around the stoma if desired. Allow the area to dry completely.
8. Attach the pouch to the skin barrier. The pouch and skin barrier may be applied to the skin separately or together. In the early postoperative period it is easier to attach the pouch to the skin barrier and then apply the system in once piece to the skin.
9. Apply the pouch and skin barrier around the stoma, keeping the adhesive area free of wrinkles or creases. Press gently but firmly into place. The valve at the bottom of the pouch must be closed or attached to the drain tubing and a collection bag.

and an outlet or valve at the bottom for easy emptying every 3 to 4 hours. The basic types of pouches are (1) semidisposable pouches that fit onto a permanent disk or faceplate and (2) one- or two-piece disposable pouches. The pouches adhere to the body with a skin barrier to form a watertight seal. The type of pouch selected depends on the patient's preference, body build, and special needs, such as physical or visual impairment. The enterostomal therapy nurse can assist the patient in selecting the appropriate pouch. Although many pouches can be worn for 5 to 7 days, they are generally changed more frequently to reduce the risk of infection.

Before discharge the nurse must be certain that the patient can manage the urinary drainage system and can detect any deviations from normal. A return visit or an opportunity for telephone consultation with the primary nurse involved in the teaching or the enterostomal therapy nurse is extremely helpful. The majority of patients with bladder cancer who undergo urinary diversion require home nursing care for stoma and pouch maintenance. Patients with a continent diversion should be informed that they will need a follow-up cystogram to assess the anatomic integrity of the reservoir.

RELATED NIC INTERVENTIONS. Incision Site Care, Ostomy Care, Skin Surveillance

Nursing Diagnosis: Risk for Disturbed Body Image

OUTCOMES. Common examples of expected outcomes for the patient with a diagnosis of *risk for disturbed body image* are:
Patient will:

- Participate in care of urinary diversion.
- Verbalize feelings regarding change in body appearance and function.

NURSING INTERVENTIONS. Any procedure for diversion of urine that results in an external stoma leads to a significant change in body image. Reactions may vary depending on the reason for the procedure, but virtually every person requires time and much support while adapting to the altered means of urine elimination.

The enterostomal therapy nurse specializes in the care of and instruction to persons who have or will have an ostomy. If possible, the enterostomal therapy nurse should have a preoperative meeting with the patient. If time permits, a meeting with the patient and a representative from the United Ostomy Association can be arranged. The United Ostomy Association has experienced volunteers who have coped well with an ostomy and are willing to visit patients and provide support, reassurance, and personal experiences. A postoperative or home visit can also be arranged

Before surgery the nurse may give the patient booklets designed for the person having a urinary diversion. A simple drawing supplements and clarifies explanations of the surgical procedure. The booklet defines terms such as stoma, urostomy, and pouch. Some persons need this additional information to assist them in accepting the surgery. Others may be unable to review written materials until after surgery. The patient with an ileal or colon conduit is informed of the need to wear the pouch, the frequency of changing and emptying the pouch, and the function of the urinary stoma.

The nurse informs patients undergoing continent urostomy procedures of the need to catheterize the stoma at regular intervals and to irrigate the internal reservoir to remove mucus. The nurse assures patients that he or she will provide stoma care immediately after surgery and help the patients to master self-care before

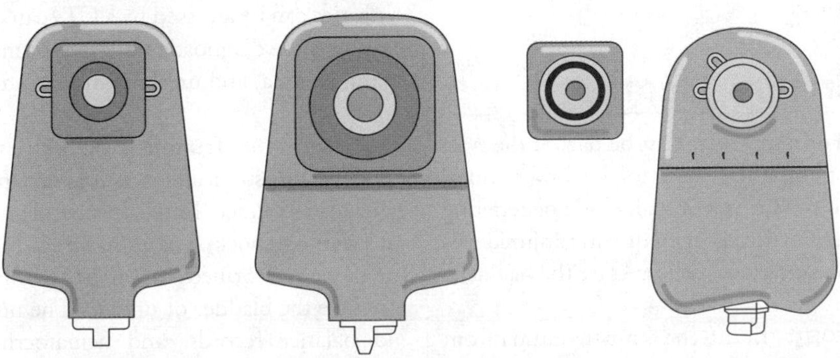

Figure 35-17 Disposable one- and two-piece pouches.

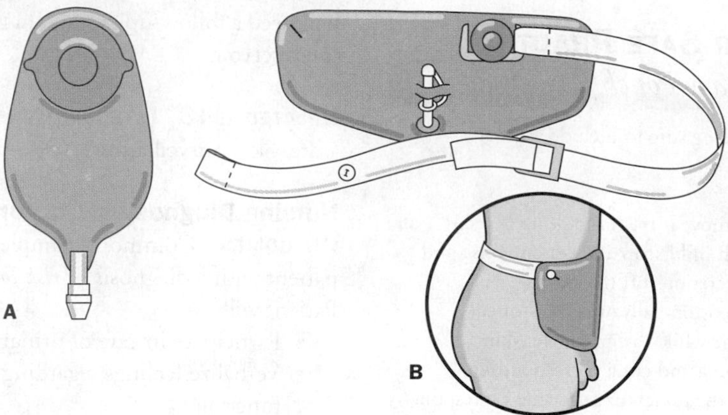

Figure 35-18 Reusable pouches. **A,** One-piece pouch. **B,** One-piece nonadhesive pouch.

discharge. Patients who have an orthoptic neobladder must be taught that urination will require increased pressure by abdominal straining and pelvic floor muscle relaxation. Because of the risk of inefficient voiding, patients should be taught to void when the bladder feels full or every 3 to 4 hours.

RELATED NIC INTERVENTIONS. Active Listening, Anxiety Reduction, Body Image Enhancement, Coping Enhancement, Counseling, Emotional Support

EVALUATION

To evaluate the effectiveness of nursing interventions, compare patient behaviors with those stated in the expected outcomes.

RELATED NOC OUTCOMES. Body Image, Coping, Ostomy Self-Care, Self-Esteem, Tissue Integrity: Skin & Mucous Membranes, Urinary Elimination

GERONTOLOGIC CONSIDERATIONS

The older adult is at increased risk for developing cancer of the bladder. The disease is most common in the 60- to 90-year-old age-group. Older adults may not tolerate radiation and chemotherapy well. Modifications in stoma care and appliances may be necessary for older patients with decreased dexterity because of arthritis or sensory deficits. Home nursing care may be necessary to manage ostomy care. Because of age-related skin changes, fitting the pouch may be difficult, and preventing skin breakdown may be a challenge.

Trauma to the Urinary Tract

Assessing the integrity of the urinary tract must be part of the evaluation of any person with traumatic injury to the lower trunk. Injuries particularly related to the urinary tract include penetrating and blunt trauma. The kidney is the most frequently injured urinary tract structure in trauma situations, followed by the bladder.

Etiology and Epidemiology. Blunt abdominal trauma from motor vehicle accidents, falls, and assaults accounts for the majority of renal and bladder trauma. Pelvic fractures can cause bladder perforation and urethral tearing. A sharp blow to the body, particularly to the lower back, may result in contusion, tearing, or rupture of a kidney. The mobility and anatomic location of the ureters make injuries from blunt trauma rare; most external ureteral injuries occur from gunshot wounds.

Pathophysiology. Renal injuries are classified into one of five grades based on radiographic and clinical history, ranging from contusion or hematoma to a shattered kidney[21] (Figure 35-19). Urinary output may be scant or absent after trauma to the urinary tract. Although hematuria is present when trauma occurs to the kidney, bladder, and urethra, hematuria is absent in approximately 40% of persons with renal vascular injuries.[4] The amount of hematuria does not necessarily correlate to the degree of kidney trauma. The initial symptoms of trauma to the kidney are usually hematuria and pain or tenderness of the upper abdominal quadrant and flank on the involved side. Persons with bladder injury may report abdominal pain and distention. The inability to urinate is common is persons with bladder and urethral trauma. Signs of shock may be present if hemorrhage is extensive.

Collaborative Care Management.

DIAGNOSTIC TESTS. Urine is evaluated for hematuria. A complete blood count and chemistry profile is also obtained. Urethral catheterization should never be attempted in persons with blood at the urinary meatus. A urology consult must be initiated.

A CT scan or MRI is used to assess renal injuries. A cystography is the imaging test appropriate for bladder injuries. Ureteral injuries can be assessed by a CT scan or IVP. Retrograde urethrography is the diagnostic test used for males suspected of having urethral trauma, and urethroscopy is indicated for females.

TREATMENTS. Treatment of injuries focuses on stabilizing the patient and surgically repairing any perforations or lacerations of the urinary tract. Initial treatment includes controlling bleeding, preventing shock, and promoting urinary drainage. A cystotomy may be performed to provide urinary drainage when injuries involve the bladder or urethra. The nurse monitors vital signs, fluid balance records, and hematocrit levels to assess bleeding. Reports of pain may indicate ureteral colic, signifying obstruction of the ureter by a clot. Surgery is required to control severe hemorrhage; otherwise the kidney is allowed to heal spontaneously. Bed

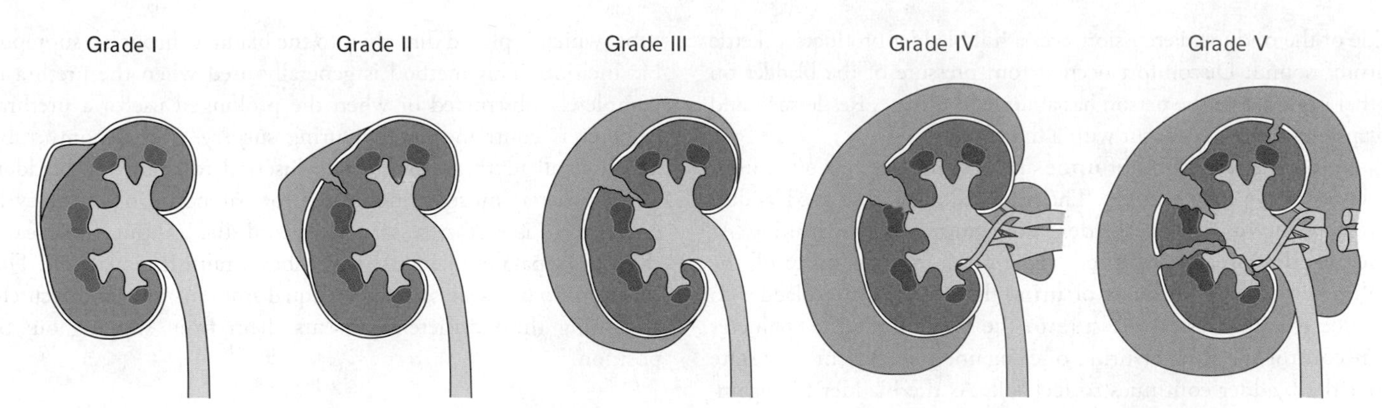

Grade I
- Renal contusion (cortical)
- Perirenal hematuria

Grade II
- Renal laceration (limited to cortex)
- Perirenal hematuria

Grade III
- Deep laceration (involving medulla), or
- Segmental arterial thrombosis without parenchymal laceration

Grade IV
- Deep laceration (involving collecting system)

Grade V
- Renal arery thrombosis
- Avulsion of renal pedicle, or
- Shattered kidney

Figure 35-19 Severity of renal injury.

rest is maintained until gross hematuria resolves; thereafter, activity progresses according to tolerance and absence of hematuria.

When urethral injuries are suspected, great care must be taken when inserting urinary catheters to prevent further urethral injury. A urologist may need to insert the catheter during a retrograde ureterogram or cystogram (see Chapter 34).

Nephrectomy may be indicated depending on the severity of the trauma. Adequate waste removal can be maintained by the remaining kidney or by less than half of one functioning kidney. Care of the person after nephrectomy is similar to that for persons with abdominal or urinary diversion procedures. Much of the patient's concern depends on the type of surgery and cause of the trauma. Because the surgery temporarily or permanently alters urinary elimination, patients are concerned about the degree of change that will occur. Refer to the Patient/Family Teaching box.

Urinary Retention

Urinary retention is the inability to empty the urinary bladder. The kidneys are producing sufficient urine, but the person is unable to expel urine from the bladder.

PATIENT/FAMILY TEACHING
Blunt Kidney Trauma

Common causes of blunt kidney trauma are motor vehicle accidents, contact sports, and falls; therefore health promotion teaching is an important nursing intervention. Teaching includes preventive strategies such as:

- Wearing a seat belt when in an automobile
- Following safety rules when riding a bicycle or walking
- Wearing protective equipment when participating in contact sports

Persons with one kidney should be cautioned about participation in contact sports.

Etiology and Epidemiology. Causes of urinary retention are either mechanical or functional (Box 35-5). Anatomic causes may be congenital or acquired and include anatomic blockage of urine flow in the lower urinary tract. Functional causes include impairment of urine flow in the absence of mechanical obstruction.

The incidence of urinary retention increases with age, particularly in men.[24] Because of the multifactorial etiology of urinary retention, it is difficult to predict the frequency of occurrence. Urinary retention can be acute or chronic. Acute urinary retention, if unrelieved, may lead to acute kidney failure or bladder rupture. Chronic retention (greater than 300 ml) is associated with a recurrent UTI, kidney stones, and hydronephrosis, which were discussed previously.

Pathophysiology. Urinary retention may be related to bladder outlet obstruction, deficient detrusor muscle strength, or both. Acute urinary retention is often associated with a large volume of fluid intake and delayed urination, which causes distention of the detrusor muscle and impaired contractility. The end result and primary feature of urinary retention is the inability to void. The bladder becomes distended with urine and is sometimes displaced to either

Box 35-5 Causes of Urinary Retention

Mechanical Causes	Functional Causes
Congenital or Anatomic	Neurogenic bladder dysfunction
Urethral stricture	Ureterovesical reflux
Urinary tract malformation	Decreased peristaltic activity of the ureter
Spinal cord malformation	Detrusor muscle atrophy
Acquired	Atrophy (e.g., fear of pain after surgery)
Renal calculi	Medications (i.e., anesthetics, opioids, sedatives, and antihistamines)
Urinary tract infection	
Trauma	
Tumor	
Pregnancy	

side of the midline. Percussion over a full bladder produces a "kettle drum" sound. Discomfort occurs from pressure of the bladder on other organs, and the person has an urge to urinate. Restlessness and diaphoresis also may occur with a full bladder.

Voiding 25 to 50 ml of urine at frequent intervals often indicates *retention with overflow.* The intravesical (within the bladder) pressure increases as the bladder continues to fill with urine. As the bladder overfills, it taxes the restraining capability of the sphincter. A small amount of urine flows out of the bladder to reduce the intravesical pressure to the level where the sphincter can control the flow of urine once again. The patient may state that the bladder continues to feel full. As the bladder fills again, the cycle is repeated. The urine specific gravity is normal or high in the presence of retention with overflow because the kidney's ability to produce urine is not impaired.

COMPLICATIONS. Complications from treatment of urinary retention are related to catheterization. It is normal to note some dribbling of urine for a few hours after a urethral catheter has been removed because of dilation of the sphincter muscles by the catheter. Dribbling of urine that persists longer than a few hours may indicate damage to the sphincters.

Another problem that may arise after removal of a catheter is inability to void. The nurse encourages the patient to drink fluids and then attempt to void. Efforts are made to provide comfortable positioning and privacy to facilitate voiding. A patient with adequate fluid intake should void within 8 hours. Patients with edema of the bladder neck may require temporary catheter reinsertion to facilitate urinary drainage. Cystitis (inflammation of the bladder) may develop after catheter removal because of incomplete emptying of the bladder as muscle tone is being reestablished.

Collaborative Care Management. Urinary retention is a urologic emergency and, if untreated, can lead to kidney damage. Interventions for urinary retention are aimed at reestablishing urine flow.

DIAGNOSTIC TESTS. The diagnosis of urinary retention is based on determining the amount of residual urine after voiding attempts. Urine yield of 250 to 300 ml on catheterization after voiding is indicative of retention. Postvoid residual should be less than 25% the person's total bladder capacity. If an attempt to pass an average-sized catheter (14 to 16 F) fails, a urologist needs to be consulted. Cystoscopy may be indicated.

MEDICATIONS. Medication use in urinary retention depends on the cause. Retention caused by sensory or neurologic problems may be treated with cholinergic medications. This group of medications stimulates bladder contraction and should not be used if obstruction is suspected. Bethanechol chloride (Urecholine) may be prescribed to initiate voiding by stimulating the detrusor muscle of the bladder. Urinary retention from prostate enlargement is discussed in Chapter 57.

TREATMENTS. When obstruction occurs below the bladder, continuous drainage must be provided to prevent damage to the kidney. One means of providing drainage is the use of a *cystostomy* tube, which is placed directly into the bladder through a suprapubic incision. This method is generally used when the urethra is completely obstructed or when the prolonged use of a urethral catheter is contraindicated. During surgery, a cystostomy tube and a small urethral catheter are inserted to drain the bladder. Both catheters must be monitored for patency. Once patency is ensured, it is not necessary to record the output from each catheter separately, since both tubes drain the bladder. The catheters do not necessarily drain equal amounts of urine. Securely anchoring these catheters prevents them from slipping out of position.

SURGICAL MANAGEMENT. If a ureter becomes obstructed, a catheter must be placed directly into the renal pelvis. This prevents kidney damage from pressure within the kidney because of continued urine formation. For a complete obstruction, a *nephrostomy* or *pyelostomy* tube may be inserted (surgically or under radiologic guidance) into the renal pelvis. The surgical incision is located laterally and posteriorly in the kidney region. An alternate form of drainage for a ureteral obstruction is the surgical placement of an *ureterostomy* tube passed through an incision in the upper outer quadrant of the abdomen into the ureter above the obstruction. The catheter is then passed through the ureter to the renal pelvis. If the ureter is unobstructed or partially obstructed, the renal pelvis may be drained by a ureteral catheter, which is passed up the ureter to the renal pelvis through a cystoscope.

All catheters must be firmly anchored to prevent trauma to tissues and accidental dislodgement. When a catheter is inserted during surgery, it is usually sutured in place and affixed to the skin. When not sutured in place, the tube is anchored to the skin at two points using adhesive, with some slack in the tubing between the anchor points. Care must be taken to prevent kinking of the tubes while the patient is in the side-lying position in bed.

Unobstructed drainage of catheters leading to the renal pelvis is of the utmost importance. The normal renal pelvis has only a 5- to 8-ml capacity; if the catheter is obstructed for even a few minutes, the resulting pressure can damage renal structures. In some patients, nephrostomy tubes may be left in place for several months, serving as a form of urinary diversion for long-term use. The person at home with a catheter draining the kidney pelvis must know how to obtain medical assistance quickly if the catheter becomes obstructed or dislodged.

DIET. No dietary modifications are necessary. Fluid intake should be encouraged. Optimally, 2 to 3 L of fluids per day provide prophylaxis for UTIs.

▶ ARE YOU READY?

A patient with an 800-ml total bladder capacity is being evaluated for urinary retention. In completing a postvoid residual approximately how many milliliters of urine should the nurse expect?

1. 50
2. 100
3. 200
4. 400

Nursing Management
of the Patient with Urinary Retention

ASSESSMENT

Health History. Assess for:

- Voiding pattern, including frequency and volume
- Pain or burning on urination (dysuria)
- Sensation of need to void or bladder fullness immediately after voiding
- Fluid intake and output

Physical Examination. Assess for:

- Urine color, clarity, and odor
- Bladder displacement above the symphysis pubis after voiding

NURSING DIAGNOSES, OUTCOMES, AND INTERVENTIONS

Nursing Diagnosis: Urinary Retention

OUTCOMES. Common examples of expected outcomes for the patient with a diagnosis of *urinary retention* are:
Patient will:

- Void several times a day in adequate amounts.
- State bladder feels empty.
- Remain free from palpable bladder after voiding.
- Maintain unobstructed drainage of urine.

NURSING INTERVENTIONS. Reestablishing urine flow is an immediate treatment goal for obstruction. However, before catheterization is considered, noninvasive measures are attempted to stimulate voiding of urine. These measures may include: having the patient assume a position that facilitates voiding (positional stimuli: male standing upright; female sitting upright), running water (auditory stimuli), or pouring water over the perineum or placing the patient's hands in water (tactile stimuli). Sitting in lukewarm water may help relax the urinary sphincters. Providing privacy and encouraging use of the bathroom whenever possible also help promote voiding. The nurse can teach the patient to "double void" to promote complete bladder emptying. After voiding, the patient attempts a second void 5 minutes later to completely empty the bladder.

If noninvasive measures are not effective, periodic complete emptying of the bladder is necessary to eliminate residual urine (an excellent culture medium for bacteria) and maintain a good blood supply to the bladder wall by avoiding high pressures within the bladder. A urologist evaluates patients for the appropriateness of this form of management. The urologist assesses the potential for success, using input from the nurse, psychologist, social worker, and other health care professionals; however, teaching is generally a nursing responsibility. An individual catheterization regimen is planned using either clean or sterile technique as appropriate. The patient needs to know the expectations of the treatment plan to promote cooperation.

The type of catheter used to provide drainage in the presence of obstruction depends on location of the blockage (Table 35-5). A size 14 F catheter is generally used for an adult. A special silicone catheter without a balloon is used for intermittent catheterization. The nurse records the volume of urine obtained with each catheterization so that the catheterization schedule can be adjusted as needed. The adult bladder should not be permitted to hold more than 300 to 500 ml at any time, since greater amounts lead to overdistention and increased susceptibility to infection. The frequency of catheterization is determined by the amount of residual urine.

If intermittent self-catheterization is required, the patient needs to understand the rationale for the procedure and the importance of emptying the bladder on a regular basis (see Patient/Family Teaching box, p. 994). The goals of intermittent catheterization are generally to prevent urinary retention and its sequelae (UTI and kidney damage) and to achieve continence. The patient's fears of causing damage by incorrect placement of the catheter can be alleviated by illustrating the basic anatomy of the genitalia and urinary tract.

Most patients require much support initially when performing self-catheterization but usually become comfortable over time. Initially, the nurse encourages women to self-catheterize while sitting on the commode, using palpation to locate the urethral meatus or a mirror to visualize the meatus. Men may sit or stand for self-catheterization. It is important that men use generous amounts of lubricant to avoid urethral irritation; women generally do not require as much lubrication because of the shorter urethra. Family members may be taught catheterization if the patient is unable to perform self-catheterization. Clean technique has been shown to be effective in home use.

The patient may wear a leg bag drainage system during the day, but disconnect the tubing and change to a regular drainage bag at night. The drainage bag should hold at least 2000 ml for

TABLE 35-5 TYPES OF CATHETERS

Type of Catheter	Description	Use
Whistle-tip	Open slant end	Hematuria or blood clots in urine
Robinson	Closed end, multiple lumen	Intermittent catheterization
Foley	Balloon (5 or 30 ml) to secure catheter in bladder	Constant drainage
Coudé	Tapered curved end	Suspected prostatic hypertrophy
Ureteral	4 to 6 F size (urethral catheters usually 14 to 16 F)	Drain ureters
Malecot	Batwing-shaped tip	Drain renal pelvis, nephrostomy drainage
De Pezzer	Mushroom-shaped tip	Drain renal pelvis, nephrostomy drainage

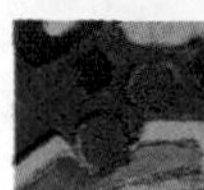

PATIENT/FAMILY TEACHING
Intermittent Catheterization

Teaching about intermittent catheterization is designed to enable the patient and family to:

- Explain the need for adequate fluid intake (approximately 30 ml/kg body weight per day)
- Explain the reason for the intermittent catheter drainage
- State the need for regular, periodic, complete emptying of the bladder
- Demonstrate self-catheterization using clean technique (unless sterile technique is prescribed)
- Describe how to adapt the catheterization routine to the individual lifestyle
- State how to obtain needed supplies
- Describe symptoms of urinary tract infection requiring medical care
- State plans for ongoing urologic care

overnight collection. To lessen contamination, the caregiver is taught to wash the hands and then wipe the catheter and tubing with 70% alcohol before disconnection and reconnection. The disconnected ends of the drainage bags are protected with sterile gauze secured in place with a rubber band or protected with a connector cap. The drainage system should be kept as clean as possible by daily washing with soap and water, and kept at a level lower than the urinary bladder to prevent urine reflux.

Persons requiring catheter drainage at home on a temporary or permanent basis must be able to safely maintain the urinary drainage system. The nurse instructs a family member in care of the catheter and drainage system in case the patient is unable to perform care. A written list of needed supplies and where they can be obtained is helpful to avoid confusion.

The person needs to be well informed about adaptations that can be made with the urinary drainage system to allow a return to an optimal level of activity. A shower or tub bath with a catheter in place is generally permitted unless a surgical incision is unhealed. The adhesive tape holding the catheter in place needs to be replaced after bathing. Leg bags are available in a variety of sizes and are concealed by clothing. Indwelling catheters do not need to be removed before intercourse. The man can fold the indwelling catheter over the penis to facilitate insertion during intercourse. This information needs to be included in all teaching because patients may hesitate to ask.

The person with a urinary catheter of any type needs follow-up medical care and needs to contact the health care provider for back pain, fever, or other urinary tract symptoms. When bladder drainage is discontinued, the nurse educates the patient about signs and symptoms of urinary retention, changes in the color and clarity of the urine, incontinence, and dysuria. Often the first indicators of dysfunction are subjective comments from the patient. This information enhances detection of early recurrence of urinary drainage problems.

If the hospital or outpatient teaching time is short, follow-up care may be required by a home health care nurse to help the person adapt the catheterization routine to life routines and to assist with any difficulties. Ongoing urologic care, including periodic urine cultures, is essential.

RELATED NIC INTERVENTIONS. Tube Care: Urinary, Urinary Catheterization, Urinary Catheterization: Intermittent, Urinary Retention Care

Nursing Diagnosis: Risk for Infection

OUTCOMES. Common examples of expected outcomes for the patient with a diagnosis of *risk for infection* are:

Patient will:

- Remain free from UTI.
- Demonstrate correct technique when performing self-catheterization.

NURSING INTERVENTIONS. Urethral catheterization with an indwelling catheter is the most common means of draining the bladder. Because catheterization is the major cause of UTIs, strict asepsis must be practiced when inserting and assembling the drainage equipment. The nurse must carefully evaluate the need for urethral catheterization. If resistance is met or the catheter is difficult to insert, the nurse discontinues the procedure and notifies the health care provider. Traumatic catheterization predisposes the patient to a UTI, formation of urethral strictures, and bleeding. In patients with urethral disorders, resistance may be encountered with a standard catheter; special equipment, such as catheter dilators or filiform-tipped catheters, may be needed. Catheterization after urologic surgery and the use of special catheter equipment are not nursing procedures.

The urethral catheter is changed when it is in danger of becoming obstructed by sediment within its lumen. Before discharge, the person going home with an indwelling urethral catheter needs to learn to change the catheter or have a family member demonstrate the ability to insert a catheter.

Clean (not sterile) catheterization technique is usually prescribed for home use. Hand washing is required before each catheterization, and the meatal area is cleansed with soap and water. In intermittent catheterization, after the catheter is inserted and the bladder is drained, the catheter is removed, washed with soap and water, and dried on a clean surface. Once dry, the catheter is stored in a closed container for the next use. The catheter is reused until it becomes either too soft or too hard to be directed properly.

Even though the clean technique is suitable for home use, sterile technique is necessary during hospitalization to decrease the possibility of nosocomial infection. When hospitalized, the patient who customarily performs self-catheterization may continue to use clean technique, but preferably a sterile catheter will be used each time. Specimens for culture must be obtained by the usual sterile catheterization technique to avoid contamination of the specimen. The nurse informs the patient about why sterile technique is necessary in the hospital setting.

RELATED NIC INTERVENTIONS. Infection Protection, Perineal Care, Surveillance, Tube Care: Urinary, Urinary Catheterization

EVALUATION

To evaluate the effectiveness of nursing interventions, compare patient behaviors with those stated in the expected patient outcomes.

RELATED NOC OUTCOMES. Risk Control, Urinary Elimination

GERONTOLOGIC CONSIDERATIONS

Older patients are at increased risk for urinary retention because of decreased bladder tone and increased incidence of chronic disease. Changes in bladder muscle tone and prostatic enlargement in men play a key role. Although treatment options remain the same, the older patient must be fully evaluated regarding the ability to take part in treatment plans. Because of decreases in dexterity and sensory function, such as vision, catheterization and catheter care may be difficult.

Urinary Incontinence

Etiology and Epidemiology. Urinary incontinence is the involuntary, unpredictable expulsion of urine from the bladder and is encountered in several temporary and permanent conditions. There are several major types of incontinence: urge (the inability to suppress a sudden need to urinate), stress (intermittent leakage of urine resulting from a sudden strain, such as a cough or sneeze), overflow (characterized by dribbling, urgency, or frequency), and functional (inability to reach a toilet).

Approximately 12 million to 15 million Americans have urinary incontinence. The prevalence of incontinence is 1.5% to 5% in men and 10% to 25% in adult women under the age of 65 years. Urinary incontinence affects about 33% of women and 20% of men over age 60 who are noninstitutionalized.[30] For persons who are institutionalized, the incidence increases to 50%. It is estimated that more than $15 billion per year are spent managing patients with incontinence. Because of missed diagnoses and underreporting, the problem may be even more widespread. Risk factors related to urinary incontinence are found in the Risk Factors box.

Pathophysiology. Most cases of incontinence are related to bladder or urethral dysfunction. As the bladder fills, the pressure within the bladder gradually increases. In the person with normal bladder function the detrusor muscle within the bladder wall responds by relaxing to accommodate the greater volume. When the bladder has filled to capacity, usually between 400 and 500 ml of urine, the parasympathetic stretch receptors located within the bladder wall are stimulated. The stimuli are transmitted through afferent fibers of the reflex arc for micturition. Impulses are then carried through the efferent fibers of the reflex arc to the bladder, causing contraction of the detrusor muscle. Completion of this reflex arc can be interrupted and voiding postponed through release of inhibitory impulses from the cortical center, which results in voluntary contraction of the external sphincter. If any part of this complex control system is interrupted, urinary incontinence results.

Urge incontinence is the involuntary loss of urine associated with an abrupt and strong desire to void (urgency). When active detrusor contractions overcome urethral resistance, urine leakage occurs. This type of incontinence has many potential causes, including UTIs, obstruction, and neurologic diseases (multiple sclerosis or stroke). Urge incontinence can also be brought on by hearing running water, standing up after lying down, and rapid changes in temperature. Urge incontinence is more prevalent in older adults. The amount of urine lost can range from a few drops to the entire bladder contents.

Stress incontinence occurs as a result of dysfunction in the closure capabilities of the urethra or defective support structures.[9] The patient experiences a loss of 50 ml or less of urine as a result of increased abdominal pressure. Any activity leading to an increase in intraabdominal pressure on the bladder can result in urinary incontinence. These activities include lifting, exercising, coughing, sneezing, or laughing. Stress incontinence occurs primarily in women.

Increased distention of the bladder causes detrusor storage pressure to exceed urethral pressure, which results in *overflow incontinence.* Presenting symptoms include frequent or constant dribbling. Overflow incontinence can result from spinal cord injury, stroke, diabetic neuropathy, or radical pelvic surgery.

In *functional incontinence,* the urinary tract is normal but other factors contribute to either the inability to reach toileting facilities or the inability to perceive a full bladder. Lack of awareness of a full bladder is seen in those who are confused, demented, acutely ill, or sedated.

Finally, incontinence may be caused by a disturbance of the urethrobladder reflex resulting from spinal cord lesions or damage to peripheral nerves of the bladder. Disturbances in the urethrobladder reflex may be seen in persons with spinal cord malformations, injuries, or tumors and in those with compression of the spinal cord caused by fractures of the vertebrae, herniated disk, metastatic tumor, or postoperative edema of the spinal cord. The neurologic dysfunction results in detrusor inadequacy or *neurogenic bladder.* Three types exist: reflex, spastic, and flaccid. The person with a neurogenic bladder has no control over bladder function.

COMPLICATIONS. The incontinent patient is at a high risk for developing skin breakdown because of exposure of skin to urine. Any break in the integrity of the skin can greatly increase the risk of serious infection. Another complication of incontinence is depression related to social isolation.

Risk Factors

Urinary Incontinence

Type	Example
Stress/urge	Loss of urethrovesical junction in women
	Urethral irritation from infection or radiation after prostatectomy
	Obesity
	Sphincter incompetence
	Pelvic relaxation
	Multiple sclerosis
	Urinary tract infections
	Stroke
	Medications: hypnotics, tranquilizers, sedatives, diuretics
Overflow	Retention with bladder distention
	Fecal impaction
	Benign prostatic hyperplasia
Functional	Altered mental status
	Physical disabilities
	Physical barriers

Collaborative Care Management

DIAGNOSTIC TESTS. Evaluation of the patient begins with a voiding diary that includes voiding patterns and circumstances surrounding the episodes of incontinence. A urinalysis is performed to rule out a possible UTI as the cause of incontinence. Postvoid residual is assessed, since elevations may indicate an abnormality in bladder contraction or outlet resistance. Further diagnostic tests may be indicated if the cause of incontinence cannot be determined from these initial steps. A cystometrogram is a useful test, especially for urge incontinence; it assesses the relationship between pressure and volume in the bladder primarily during the filling phase. Many other urodynamic studies can be used to determine the cause of incontinence (uroflowmetry, electromyography, pressure flow studies). An ultrasound of the bladder, cystoscopy, and IVP may also be done to assess the structures and function of the urinary tract.

MEDICATIONS. Medication management for the treatment of incontinence is based on the identified cause (Table 35-6). These medications need to be used cautiously in older adults who may be taking multiple medications for other conditions. Bladder outlet obstruction should be ruled out before use of medications.

TREATMENTS. The U.S. Department of Health and Human Services has established treatment protocols and algorithms for the management of the incontinent adult. Treatments can be categorized as behavioral, pharmacologic, and surgical. A combination of therapies is often used. The type of therapy is guided by the type of incontinence (Table 35-7).

Behavioral therapy includes education about lifestyle changes and dietary modifications such as fluid restriction and avoidance of caffeine and other irritants. Behavioral techniques include bladder retraining, timed voiding, prompted voiding, and pelvic muscle exercises. Bladder retraining encompasses timed voiding (e.g., every 2 to 3 hours) in which the interval is gradually increased.

Pelvic floor physiotherapy, often referred to as Kegel exercises, helps the patient suppress unwanted bladder contractions. These exercises involve the voluntary contraction and relaxation of the muscles that support the bladder and urethra. The goal of pelvic floor physiotherapy is to strengthen the pelvic muscles, thus preventing the downward rotation of the urethra and involuntary loss of urine. Because it is difficult for some women to isolate these muscles, a variety of methods have been used, including vaginal weights, vaginal electrical stimulation, and biofeedback. Vaginal weights, called vaginal cones, are inserted into the vagina and require contraction of the pelvic muscles to maintain their position. Biofeedback uses electromyography or vaginal pressure measurements that provide visual and/or auditory signals to an individual with respect to performance with pelvic floor muscle contraction.

The person with a brain tumor, meningitis, or traumatic injury to the brain that prevents adequate voluntary control of bladder function may benefit from a bladder retraining program. If the person's condition or response prohibits such a program, an internal or external drainage device should be used.

Persons with spinal cord injuries experience a transitory period of *spinal shock* in which urinary retention occurs (see Chapter 50). An indwelling catheter is placed to facilitate urinary drainage and prevent bladder distention. After the acute stage, management depends on the exact nature of any residual neurogenic bladder dysfunction. Persons with a lesion above the sacral segments and with an intact urethrobladder reflex may initiate voiding by pinching or stroking trigger areas of the thighs or suprapubic area. In persons with a lower motor neuron lesion,

TABLE 35-6
COMMON MEDICATIONS *for Urinary Incontinence*

Drug	Action	Nursing Intervention
Stress Incontinence		
OTC antihistamines Pseudoephedrine (Sudafed)	Antihistamine Alpha-adrenergic substance that causes vasoconstriction of mucous membranes	Do not use in patients with CV disease, hypertension, hyperthyroidism, increased intraocular pressure. Do not exceed recommended dosage.
Estrogen Estradiol vaginal ring (Estring) Vaginal estrogen cream	Female sex hormone Increases circulation to perineal area	Monitor for vaginal irritation and potentially serious side effects. Be certain to correctly apply or insert.
Overactive Bladder (Urge)		
Antispasmodics/anticholinergics Oxybutynin (Ditropan, Ditropan XL)	Relaxes urinary tract smooth muscles by inhibiting acetylcholine at postganglionic sites	Do not use in patients with hypersensitivity, obstructive GI disorders, glaucoma, or myasthenia gravis.
Tolterodine (Detrol) Dicyclomine (Bentyl) Hyoscyamine (Cystospaz)	Antimuscarinic agents Prevent bladder contractions by blocking effects of acetylcholine at muscarinic receptors sites	Do not use in patients with glaucoma, hypersensitivity, renal or hepatic dysfunction. Ensure adequate fluid intake to prevent constipation.
Tricyclic antidepressants Imipramine (Tofranil) Doxepin (Sinequan)	Inhibit presynaptic uptake of norepinephrine and serotonin	Do not use in patients with hypersensitivity, concomitant MOA inhibitors, CV disorders, impaired renal or hepatic function.

OTC, Over-the-counter; *CV*, cerebrovascular; *GI*, gastrointestinal; *MOA*, monoamine oxidase.

TABLE 35-7 INCONTINENCE: TYPES, CAUSES, AND TREATMENTS

Type	Common Causes	Treatments
Stress	Pelvic floor muscular weakness; hypermobility of urethra	Behavioral therapy Kegel exercises Surgery: bladder neck suspension or sling Alpha-adrenergic agonists
Urge	Detrusor overactivity related to urinary tract problems: urinary tract infection, kidney stones Central nervous system problems: stroke, spinal cord injury	Behavioral therapy Bladder relaxants
Overflow	Obstruction: (1) stricture, enlarged prostate; (2) neurogenic bladder (e.g., multiple sclerosis, certain spinal cord lesions)	1. Surgery 2. Catheterization (intermittent or chronic)
Functional	Dementia, immobility	Behavioral therapy Absorbent padding

the use of *Credé's* method, which consists of exerting manual pressure over the bladder, may provide more complete bladder emptying. The physician must determine the appropriateness of this technique, based on the person's complete urologic status. Many individuals with neurogenic bladder dysfunction are taught intermittent self-catheterization using clean technique to prevent infection and to manage incontinence. Maintenance of a regular schedule for catheterization is stressed, and the frequency is determined on an individual basis.

SURGICAL MANAGEMENT. Many surgical procedures are used to treat incontinence. The classic treatment has been surgical bladder neck suspension to return the bladder neck and urethra to their proper position. Treatment for a nonfunctioning sphincter includes a sling procedure, artificial urinary sphincter, or intraurethral bulking agents. Periurethral bulking is a relatively simple procedure performed with the patient under local anesthesia or sedation. This treatment involves injecting material around the urethra to increase urethral resistance.

Other interventions include occlusive and supportive devices. Supportive devices improve continence by supporting the bladder neck. Tampons, traditional pessaries, contraceptive diaphragms, and intravaginal devices have been used for this purpose. Occlusive devices can occlude the urethra or bladder neck externally or internally via the urethra. For men, a clamp-type device is placed across the penile urethra. For women, occlusive devices may be inserted through the vagina or the urethra. An external occlusive device is a type of foam pad placed over the urethral meatus.[38]

Finally, neuromodulation, modification of sensory or motor function through electrical stimulation, can be tried when other conservative methods have failed. Although the precise mode of action is unclear, this method has been successful in inhibiting bladder activity.

DIET. Nutritional alterations for the patient with urinary incontinence involve scheduling fluid intake and avoiding bladder stimulants such as alcohol, chocolate, and coffee. Fluid intake after dinner should be reduced or avoided.

Nursing Management

of the Patient with Urinary Incontinence

ASSESSMENT

Health History. Assess for:
- Frequency of incontinence
- Precipitating events (stress, fear, coughing, sneezing, laughing, exercise)
- Pain or burning with incontinence
- Urge to void before incontinent episodes

Physical Examination. Assess for:
- Volume of urine
- Characteristics of urine
- Ability to follow directions, functional status, and ability to perform ADLs
- Physiologic reason for incontinence (e.g., spinal cord injury)

NURSING DIAGNOSES, OUTCOMES, AND INTERVENTIONS

Nursing Diagnosis: Urinary Incontinence

OUTCOMES. Common examples of expected outcomes for the patient with a diagnosis of *urinary incontinence* (stress, urge, total, functional, reflex) are:

Patient will:
- Achieve optimal urinary control.
- Demonstrate perineal exercises (if appropriate).
- Describe actions to control voiding (as appropriate), measures to maintain skin integrity, and plans for follow-up care.

NURSING INTERVENTIONS. When incontinence is caused by confusion or acute illness, control can usually be established through use of a persistent bladder retraining schedule. The nurse develops a voiding schedule and the patient strictly adheres to it until he or she gradually relearns to recognize and react appropriately to the urge to void. A successful program (Box 35-6), leading to complete rehabilitation or continence, requires the patient to be mentally competent. Otherwise, someone else must always remind the person to follow the schedule.

People ordinarily void on awakening, before retiring, and before or after meals. Consuming caffeinated beverages such as coffee creates a diuretic effect, and the urge to void occurs in about 30 minutes. Using this knowledge, the nurse can set up a schedule for placing the person on a bedpan or taking the person to the toilet. A record of involuntary voiding is kept for a few days to determine the normal voiding pattern. If the schedule based on the pattern of incontinence is not successful, toileting every 1 to 2 hours is carried out on a 24-hour basis, with intervals progressively increased. See the Evidence-Based Practice box.

When possible, toileting should be carried out in surroundings that remind the person of the voiding function, that is, the bathroom. If this is not possible, a bedside commode can be an adequate substitute. Many men can void into a urinal more easily if allowed to stand at the bedside. The use of a bedpan is unfamiliar and distasteful to most persons, but for women who must remain in bed, voiding into a bedpan can be facilitated by elevating the head of the bed as much as possible. This position is more consistent with the position normally assumed for voiding and facilitates complete bladder emptying. Few persons can void adequately in the supine position.

Providing adequate amounts of fluids, a minimum of 3 L/day, is necessary to ensure that adequate amounts of urine are produced and present in the bladder to stimulate the voiding reflex at the proper times. Fluids may be given at scheduled times, the largest portion being given during the day before 4 PM to decrease the frequency of voiding through the night. Persons with restricted fluid intake because of medical problems should receive the prescribed amount of fluid.

Occasionally the use of an indwelling catheter for the incontinent patient is justified. Reasons include the need to protect a surgical incision or to permit healing of a pressure ulcer in the area. Indwelling catheterization, however, presents many potential dangers, such as development of a UTI, urethritis, epididymitis, and urethral fistulas. All other means to manage the incontinence should be exhausted before resorting to catheterization.

For men, external drainage can be accomplished with a condom catheter (Figure 35-20). Several commercial products are available. Before applying the condom, the nurse cleans and dries the penis thoroughly and checks for edema, skin breaks, or discoloration. The nurse then inverts the condom and rolls it onto the penis. There should be no roll at the top that could cause constriction. At least 2.5 cm (1 inch) of the condom should remain between the meatus and drainage tube to allow for penile erection, without allowing twisting and interference with drainage.

The nurse removes the external catheter daily and washes and inspects the skin. Frequent assessment is necessary to determine whether edema or irritation is present and to ensure proper

Box 35-6 Bladder Retraining

- Establish patient's usual voiding patterns.
- Plan toileting based on the patient's usual pattern; assist patient as necessary.
- If no voiding pattern can be determined, plan toileting for every 1 to 2 hours.
- Encourage patient to use normal toilet position.
- Encourage patient to empty bladder completely.
- Provide for a fluid intake of 3 L/day for adequate urine volume.
- Schedule majority of fluid intake before 4 PM.

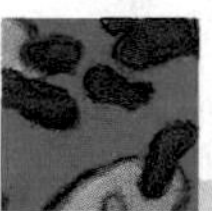

Evidence-Based Practice

Topic Question: Is bladder retraining an effective treatment for urinary incontinence?

Evidence Base: Five trials involved 149 female subjects. Three hypotheses were tested: bladder retraining is better than no bladder retraining; bladder retraining is better than other treatments; and combining bladder retraining with another treatment is better than the other treatment alone.

Findings: Limited evidence suggested that bladder retraining may be more effective than no bladder retraining, but the other two hypotheses could not be supported because of the trials' variable quality and small size.

Conclusions: Bladder retraining may be more effective than no bladder training. The evidence was insufficient to determine if bladder retraining is more effective than other treatments. More research is needed.

Wallace SA et al: Bladder training for urinary incontinence in adults (Cochrane Review). In *Cochrane Library,* Issue 3, Chichester, UK, 2004, John Wiley & Sons.

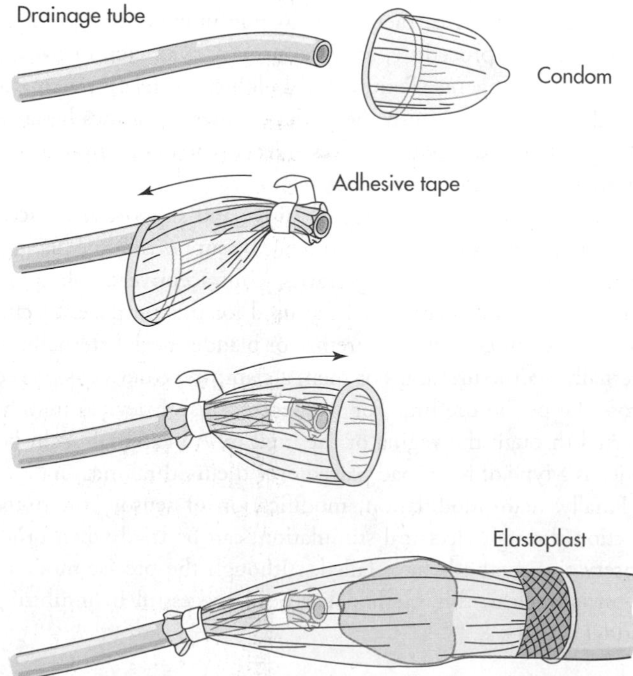

Figure 35-20 One method of making an external drainage apparatus.

drainage. This is especially important in men with loss of sensation. The external device can be attached to either a leg bag or to straight drainage.

For persons who need external urinary drainage indefinitely, a rubber appliance (sometimes called an incontinence urinal) may be used (Figure 35-21). Two appliances are recommended to allow for cleaning and drying of one device while the other is in use. They should be washed with mild soap and water, turned inside out, and thoroughly dried before application to prevent skin irritation.

Most persons prefer to manage their own incontinence if they can. The nurse should support and encourage self-care, offering assistance as necessary and instruction in basic principles of skin care, equipment selection, and maintenance (see Patient/Family Teaching box). The choice of management method should take into account the person's ability to manage as independently as possible.

RELATED NIC INTERVENTIONS. Prompted Voiding, Self-Care Assistance: Toileting, Urinary Catheterization, Urinary Catheterization: Intermittent, Urinary Habit Training, Urinary Incontinence Care

Nursing Diagnosis: Risk for Situational Low Self-Esteem

OUTCOMES. Common examples of expected outcomes for the patient at with a diagnosis of *risk for situational low self-esteem* are: Patient will:

- Verbalize feelings and concerns without self-deprecating statements.
- Socialize with others.

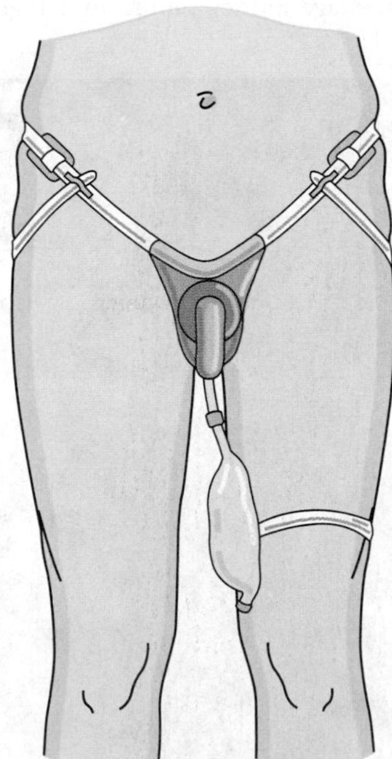

Figure 35-21 Rubber urinary appliance. Bag is emptied by drain valve at bottom of bag.

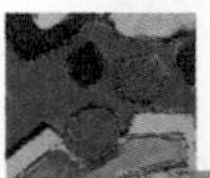

PATIENT/FAMILY TEACHING
Urinary Incontinence

Teaching for the incontinent patient includes:

- Explanation of the rationale for activities, such as the toileting schedule, mobility, and fluid requirements in order to increase the probability that the person will follow through with treatment plans.
- Use of perineal exercises (Kegel exercises) to help control incontinence or strengthen muscles after catheter removal. Stress incontinence can be prevented if perineal exercises are taught before and after childbirth.
- Explanation regarding care of any drainage system, measures to maintain skin integrity, signs and symptoms of urinary tract infection (frequency or dysuria) that need to be reported.
- Information about how to obtain and maintain any needed supplies and equipment (commode, protective padding, and drainage systems).

NURSING INTERVENTIONS. Persons who are incontinent may feel isolated from their families and familiar surroundings, which may lead to decreased self-esteem. These patients frequently respond well to bladder retraining programs. When nurses believe it is easier to change bed linen than to establish an appropriate bladder retraining program, they do a disservice to the individual and create more work for themselves. The person may have an increased risk of developing a UTI and skin breakdown, and feelings of worthlessness are increased. Urinary incontinence should not be considered inevitable in older adults or institutionalized person.

RELATED NIC INTERVENTIONS. Emotional Support, Self-Esteem Enhancement

EVALUATION

To evaluate the effectiveness of nursing interventions, compare patient behaviors with those stated in the expected outcomes.

RELATED NOC OUTCOMES. Self-Care: Toileting, Self-Esteem, Symptom Control

GERONTOLOGIC CONSIDERATIONS

Changes that occur with aging lead to decreased sensation and bladder muscle control, which may result in urinary incontinence. Because persons are often embarrassed about the loss of bladder control, they do not seek assistance and often become socially isolated.

Older patients, especially those with decreased ambulatory abilities, may not be able to reach the toilet in time to void. Confusion, disorientation, and medications such as diuretics may also hamper the patient's ability to reach the toilet in time. Portable commodes, urinals, and appropriate timing of medications help manage functional incontinence. It is important to set realistic goals for the older patient to restore maximal efficiency of incontinence management. Prompted voiding and individualized toileting schedules may be effective ways of decreasing incontinence in older memory-impaired adults.

Congenital Disorders

Approximately one third of all congenital abnormalities affect the genitourinary tract.[10] These deviations range in severity from minor anomalies that do not require correction to those which are incompatible with life. Box 35-7 lists some of the more common congenital malformations of the lower urinary tract. Details about the management of congenital disorders are covered in most pediatric nursing texts. However, renal cystic disorders and congenital conditions of the upper urinary tract contribute to adult morbidity and are discussed in this chapter.

Polycystic Kidney Disease

Etiology and Epidemiology. Renal cystic disorders encompass a relatively large group of diseases characterized by the formation of one or more fluid-filled cavities that arise in any part of the kidney. Cysts may develop in utero or after birth and may be inherited or acquired. They range in size from slightly larger than a single nephron in their formative stage, to large cysts that replace the majority of kidney mass. Renal cysts may be benign, producing little or no damage, or severe enough to compromise function, resulting in kidney failure. They may be a primary renal disorder or may appear as a result of nonrenal disorders.

The major cystic diseases of the kidney are cystic, medullary, and polycystic. Cystic kidney disease includes simple cysts, which are commonly seen in patients over 50 years of age, and acquired cystic kidney disease seen in patients with either kidney disease (e.g., glomerulonephritis) or other disease that affects the kidney (e.g., diabetes). Medullary cystic kidney disease is a rare, inherited disorder. Polycystic kidney disease is a genetic disorder in which numerous fluid-filled cysts grow within the kidney. Only polycystic kidney disease is discussed in detail here.

Polycystic kidney disease has two inherited forms (autosomal dominant and autosomal recessive) and one noninherited form (acquired cystic kidney disease). Autosomal dominant polycystic kidney disease (ADPKD) is the most common form. The majority of cases are associated with a PKD1 gene located on chromosome 16. ADPKD is one of the five leading causes of kidney failure (see Chapter 36). It affects between 1 in 500 and 1 in 1000 live births in all racial groups, regardless of gender, worldwide. In the United States about 500,000 people have ADPKD.[11] There is some variability in gene expression, which accounts for some individuals developing symptomatic disease by age 20 and others dying of unrelated problems later in life.

Pathophysiology. ADPKD affects both kidneys in the majority of patients. Cysts are diffusely scattered through the renal parenchyma, with islands of normal tissue between them (Figure 35-23). The cysts arise from all segments of the nephron and collecting system. Cysts can range in size from a few millimeters to several centimeters. The kidneys may reach five times their normal size and be studded with cysts of various sizes. One of the most devastating features is that ADPKD undergoes relentless progression to end-stage kidney failure in a high percentage of

Box 35-7 Congenital Malformation of Lower Urinary Tract

- Duplication of ureters: Partial or complete
- Hydroureters: Dilation of ureters
- Exstrophy of urinary bladder: Eversion of bladder on outer abdominal wall
- Hypospadias: Opening of urethra on underside of penis (Figure 35-22, *A*)
- Epispadias: Opening of urethra on dorsum of penis (Figure 35-22, *B*)

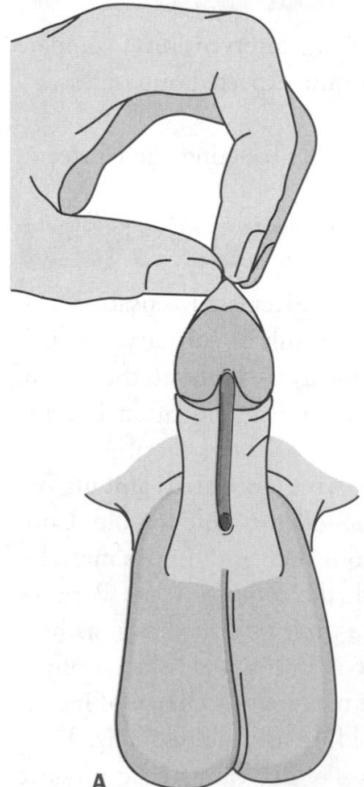

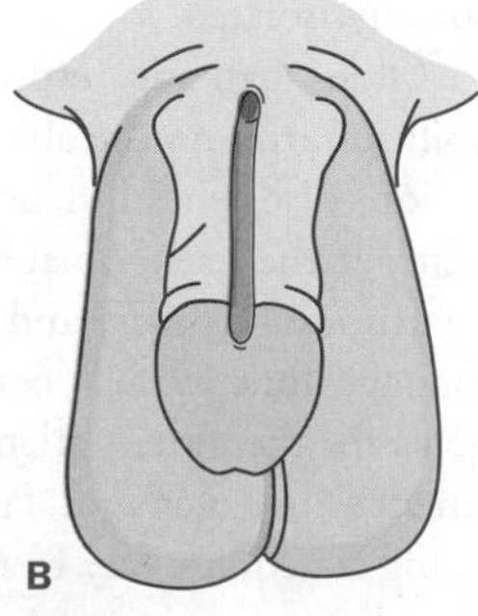

Figure 35-22 **A,** Hypospadias. **B,** Epispadias.

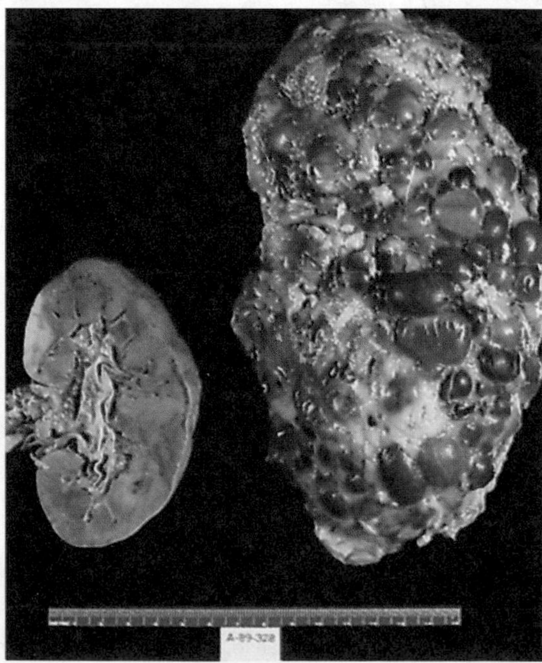

Figure 35-23 Normal kidney *(left)*; polycystic kidney *(right)*.

patients, usually in the fourth or fifth decade of life. Loss of renal function occurs as the cysts enlarge and compress adjacent parenchyma, causing ischemia of surrounding tissue. The process of cyst formation begins with increased division of epithelial cells within a few renal tubule cells. This causes enlargement of the tubule and formation of "cysts." Cystic enlargement also causes occlusion of the normal tubules.

In addition to renal cysts, persons with ADPKD may develop cysts in the liver, pancreas, and spleen. As many as 10% to 20% of patients have cerebral and abdominal aneurysms.[12] Abdominal and inguinal hernias are relatively common in patients with ADPKD.

Abdominal or flank pain and hematuria are the most common early symptoms in patients with ADPKD. The pain is often caused by bleeding into the cyst. It may be dull and aching, a vague sense of heaviness, or knifelike and stabbing. Hematuria occurs when a cyst ruptures in the renal pelvis. Patients with polycystic disease are prone to cyst infections and serious infections of the kidney parenchyma, which are manifested by pain, fever, leukocytosis, pyuria, and positive blood and urine cultures. Hypertension develops in approximately 50% of patients at some time in the course of the disease, often several years before measurable functional renal impairment. If hypertension is uncontrolled, renal destruction is accelerated. Later in the disease process, some patients notice increased abdominal girth, and in many cases the kidneys can be palpated.

Collaborative Care Management

DIAGNOSTIC TESTS. An ultrasound that shows five or more total cysts distributed through both kidneys confirms the diagnosis of polycystic disease in patients with a consistent family history. CT or MRI can be used when the results of the ultrasound are unclear.

TREATMENTS. Because there is no therapy directed at the disease process, the goals of management are to alleviate symptoms and slow the onset of renal dysfunction. Hypertension should be controlled, since it has been shown to accelerate the decline in renal function. Limiting dietary sodium and protein intake and avoiding nephrotoxic drugs appears to lengthen the functional duration of the kidneys.[8] Infections are treated vigorously with antibiotics, since scarring may lead to further disease progression. Antibiotics are usually taken until renal pain resolves and the urine clears of pus, which may take several months. Infections that are difficult to eradicate with oral antibiotics are treated with parenteral antibiotics. When patients are admitted to the hospital, intake and output must be closely monitored.

Analgesics may be used to help control flank pain. Surgical aspiration or laparoscopic decompression of cysts has been found to improve discomfort, but not slow the progression of the disease. When urinary bleeding from ruptured cysts becomes severe and gross hematuria is present, bed rest and increased hydration are often instituted. Refer to the Patient/Family Teaching box.

HEALTH PROMOTION AND PREVENTION. Prevention is the key to decreasing the incidence of ADPKD. Prevention occurs only by prospectively identifying those with the disorder so that they have an opportunity to determine whether or not to bear children. Because it is an autosomal dominant disorder, patients with the gene may expect that each child will have a 50/50 chance of inheriting the disease. Family history is a crucial part of the counseling process. Family members may be unwilling to reveal or may not know whether other family members had this disease. Often persons do not learn they have the ADPKD gene until they are beyond the childbearing period.

Challenges exist in helping the person deal with an illness on an individual basis when relatives have died of the same disease and children have not yet developed symptoms. Counseling may be required about family health care and the individual's role in passing on a potentially fatal disease to children.

PATIENT/FAMILY TEACHING
Polycystic Disease

Teaching for the patient with polycystic disease and his or her family is important because patients are at increased risk for chronic renal failure. Therefore teaching includes:

- Signs and symptoms of infection and bleeding that need to be reported
- How to monitor urinary output and the need for reporting changes
- Information regarding the long-term complications and typical disease progression of autosomal dominant polycystic kidney disease, which cannot be prevented but may be slowed through measures such as the control of hypertension

Critical Thinking

1. You are caring for a 68-year-old patient who underwent urinary diversion surgery 3 days ago as treatment for urinary obstruction. You note blood clots in the tubing and urinary drainage bag. What conclusions can you draw about this patient's situation, and how should you respond?
2. What procedure should you follow when you insert an indwelling urinary catheter and do not obtain urine?

References

1. Agha IA: *Nephrotic syndrome*, American Accreditation HealthCare Commission, accessed Oct 2003 from website: http://www.nlm.nih.gov/medlineplus/ency/article/000490.htm#Treatment.
2. American Cancer Society: accessed from website: http://www.cancer.org.
3. Brandes SB: Urethral stricture disease. In Hanno PM, Malkowicz SB, Wein AJ, editors: *Clinical manual of urology*, ed 3, New York, 2001, McGraw-Hill.
4. Brandes SB, Yu M: Urologic trauma. In Hanno PM, Malkowicz SB, Wein AJ, editors: *Clinical manual of urology*, ed 3, New York, 2001, McGraw-Hill.
5. Cohen J, Powderly G, editors: *Infectious diseases*, ed 2, St Louis, 2004, Mosby.
6. Couser WG: Pathogenesis of damage in glomerulonephritis, *Nephrol Dialysis Transplant* 13(suppl):10-15, 1998.
7. Dolan JG: Pyelonephritis. In Rakel RE, Bope ET, editors: *Conn's current therapy*, Philadelphia, 2001, Saunders.
8. Falk RJ, Jennette JC, Nachman PH: Primary glomerular disease. In Brenner BM, Rector FC, editors: *Brenner and Rector's the kidney*, ed 7, Philadelphia, 2004, Saunders.
9. Foster HE: Female urology and incontinence. In Weiss RM, George NJR, O'Reilly PH, editors: *Comprehensive urology*, London, 2001, Mosby.
10. Gearhart JP, Baker LA: Congenital diseases of the lower urinary tract. In Weiss RM, George NJR, O'Reilly PH, editors: *Comprehensive urology*, London, 2001, Mosby.

11. Grantham JJ: Cystic diseases of the kidney. In Goldman L, Ausilleo D, editors: *Cecil textbook of medicine,* Philadelphia, 2004, Saunders.
12. Grantham JJ, Nair V, Winklhofer F: Cystic diseases of the kidney. In Brenner BM, Rector FC, editors: *Brenner and Rector's the kidney,* ed 7, Philadelphia, 2004, Saunders.
13. Grossfeld GD, Carroll PR: Urothelial carcinoma: cancers of the bladder, ureter and renal pelvis. In Tanagho EA, McAninch JW, editors: *Smith's general urology,* ed 16, New York, 2003, McGraw-Hill.
14. Hanno PM: Lower urinary tract infections in women. In Hanno PM, Malkowicz SB, Wein AJ, editors: *Clinical manual of urology,* ed 3, New York, 2001, McGraw-Hill.
15. Irby PB: Renal calculi. In Rakel RE, Bope ET, editors. *Conn's current therapy,* Philadelphia, 2001, Saunders.
16. Kohn IJ, Weiss JP: Pyelonephritis. In Hanno PM, Malkowicz SB, Wein AJ, editors: *Clinical manual of urology,* ed 3, New York, 2001, McGraw-Hill.
17. Kunin CM: Urinary tract infections and pyelonephritis. In Goldman L, Ausilleo D, editors: *Cecil textbook of medicine,* Philadelphia, 2004, Saunders.
18. Lingerman JE, Lifshitz DA, Evan AP: Surgical management of urinary lithiasis. In Walsh PC et al, editors: *Campbells' urology,* ed 8, Philadelphia, 2002, Saunders.
19. Maki DG, Tambyah PA: Engineering out the risk for infections with urinary catheters, *Emerg Infect Dis* 7(2):342, 2001.
20. Malkowicz SB, Sanchez-Ortiz RF, Wein AJ: Adult genitourinary cancer. In Hanno PM, Malkowicz SB, Wein AJ, editors: *Clinical manual of urology,* ed 3, New York, 2001, McGraw-Hill.
21. McAninch JW, Safir MH: Genitourinary trauma. In Weiss RM, George NJR, O'Reilly PH, editors: *Comprehensive urology,* London, 2001, Mosby.
22. McDougal WS: Use of intestinal segments and urinary diversion. In Walsh PC et al, editors: *Campbells' urology,* ed 8, Philadelphia, 2002, Saunders.
23. Menon M, Resnick MI: Urinary lithiasis: etiology, diagnosis and medical management. In Walsh PC et al, editors: *Campbells' urology,* ed 8, Philadelphia, 2002, Saunders.
24. Mikel G: Urinary retention: management in the acute care setting, *AJN* 100:40, 2001.
25. Naber KG et al: EAU guidelines for the management of urinary and male genital tract infections, *Eur Urol* 40(5):576-588, 2001.
26. Nguyen HT: Bacterial infections of the genitourinary tract. In Tanagho EA, McAninch JW, editors: *Smith's general urology,* ed 16, New York, 2003, McGraw-Hill.
27. Niaudet P: *Treatment of idiopathic nephrotic syndrome in children,* 2001, accessed from website: http://uptodate.
28. Nicolle LE: Bacterial urinary tract infections in women. In Rakel RE, Bope ET, editors: *Conn's current therapy,* Philadelphia, 2001, Saunders.
29. Pahira JJ, Razack AA: Nephrolithiasis. In Hanno PM, Malkowicz SB, Wein AJ, editors: *Clinical manual of urology,* ed 3, New York, 2001, McGraw-Hill.
30. Peggs J: Urinary incontinence. In Rakel RE, Bope ET, editors: *Conn's current therapy,* Philadelphia, 2001, Saunders.
31. Rose BR: *Course of poststreptococcal glomerulonephritis,* 2001, accessed from website: http://uptodate.
32. Sachdiva KS et al: *Renal cell carcinoma,* 2004, accessed from website: http://emedicine.com/med/topic2002.htm.
33. Safian RD, Textor SC: Renal-artery stenosis, *N Engl J Med* 344:431, 2001.
34. Reference deleted in proofs.
35. Shinghal R, Payne CK: Emergency room urology. In Hanno PM, Malkowicz SB, Wein AJ, editors: *Clinical manual of urology,* ed 3, New York, 2001, McGraw-Hill.
36. Reference deleted in proofs.
37. Textor SC, Wilcox CS: Renal artery stenosis: a common, treatable cause of renal failure? *Ann Rev Med* 52:421, 2001.
38. Wein AJ, Rovner ES: Voiding function and dysfunction. In Hanno PM, Malkowicz SB, Wein AJ, editors: *Clinical manual of urology,* ed 3, New York, 2001, McGraw-Hill.
39. Wilcox CS: Renovascular hypertension. In Massry SG, Glassock RJ: *Massry and Glassock's textbook of nephrology,* ed 4, Philadelphia, 2001, Lippincott Williams & Wilkins.
40. Wood DP et al: Incidence and significance of positive urine cultures in patients with an orthotopic neobladder, *J Urol* 169(6):2196-2199, 2003.
41. Zinman L: Urethral stricture disease. In Weiss RM, George NJR, O'Reilly PH, editors: *Comprehensive urology,* London, 2001, Mosby.

Visit the Evolve website: http://evolve.elsevier.com/Monahan/medsurg

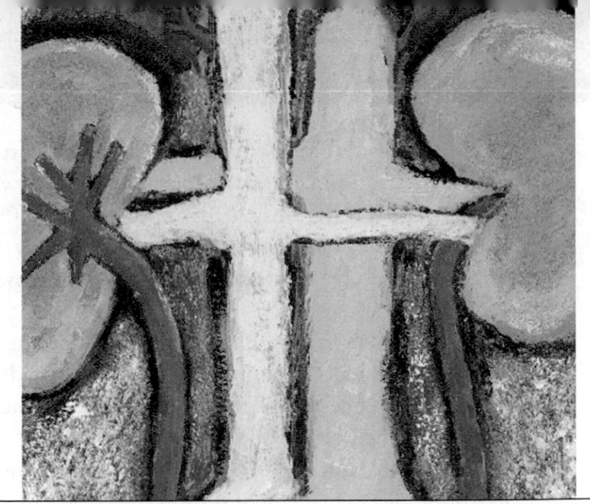

CHAPTER 36
Kidney Failure

by Kelly A. Weigel, Cynthia K. Potter, Carol J. Green

OBJECTIVES

After studying this chapter, the learner should be able to:

1. Explain the pathophysiologic changes and clinical manifestations of acute and chronic kidney failure.
2. Differentiate between the medical and nursing management of patients during the oliguric and diuretic phases of acute kidney failure.
3. Explain the benefits of continuous renal replacement therapy for patients with kidney failure.
4. Identify treatment goals for patients with chronic kidney failure.
5. Describe the physiologic principles of dialysis.
6. Compare the nursing assessment and management of patients undergoing hemodialysis, peritoneal dialysis, and kidney transplantation.
7. Identify factors that affect organ donation and candidate selection for transplantation.
8. Describe the preoperative and postoperative nursing care of organ donors and recipients.
9. Describe the major complications associated with organ transplantation.
10. Discuss immunosuppression in the transplant recipient.

KEY TERMS

arteriovenous fistula, p. 1020
diuresis, p. 1006
erythropoiesis, p. 1018
hemodialysis, p. 1020
intrarenal, p. 1003
nephrotoxicity, p. 1004
oliguric, p. 1004
peritoneal dialysis, p. 1022
postrenal, p. 1004
prerenal, p. 1003
ultrafiltration, p. 1007

Kidney failure is one of the most significant causes of death and disability throughout the world. More than 8 million people in the United States alone have moderate to severe kidney dysfunction.[3,24] Because of the complexity of renal function, organ failure affects all body systems and compromises the ability to independently sustain life.

Kidney failure, also known as renal failure, may occur in several forms. Acute kidney failure develops within hours to days, whereas chronic kidney failure develops slowly and progressively over several years. *Renal insufficiency* exists when the loss of kidney function is significant, but not so much that the internal environment becomes inconsistent with life. *Uremia*, also known as *uremic syndrome*, is a syndrome of kidney failure characterized by elevated blood urea nitrogen (BUN) and creatinine levels. *Azotemia* refers to elevated levels of serum urea and creatinine. *Azotemia* and *uremia* are sometimes inappropriately interchanged; both terms refer to the buildup of nitrogenous waste products in the blood, but the person with azotemia does not manifest sign and symptoms, whereas the person with uremia does.

Acute Kidney Failure

Etiology and Epidemiology. Acute kidney failure (AKF) is an abrupt decline in kidney function manifested by increases in BUN and plasma creatinine levels. Urinary output is generally less than 40 ml/hr (oliguria) but may be normal or even increased. Depending on cause, AKF is classified as prerenal, intrarenal (intrinsic), or postrenal (Box 36-1). About 55% to 70% of cases of AKF are due to **prerenal** factors such as intravascular volume depletion, decreased cardiac output, and vascular failure secondary to vasodilation or obstruction. **Intrarenal** causes account for 25% to 40% of cases of AKF. Intrarenal failure is caused by damage to the kidney tissues and structures and includes tubular necrosis, nephrotoxicity, and alterations in renal blood flow. Acute tubular necrosis (ATN) is responsible for approximately 90% of all cases of intrarenal AKF. **Postrenal** failure (approximately 5% of cases) is generally caused by obstruction of urine flow between the kidney and the urethral meatus.

AKF is a common problem. It affects approximately 5% of all hospitalized patients and up to 30% of patients admitted to intensive care areas. The mortality rate for AKF approaches 50%, making it one of the leading causes of inpatient death.[17] Recovery from an episode of AKF depends on the underlying illness, the patient's condition, and management during the period of renal shutdown. The major cause of AKF is infection.[17] For those in whom AKF has been caused by an acute event or a superimposed injury with preexisting glomerular disease, return of kidney function is determined by the extent of scarring and obliteration of functional nephrons that occurred during the acute episode of kidney failure.[17] Research indicates that the prognosis for these patients may not be as favorable as for those with AKF resulting from toxic or ischemic injury. AKF is also known as acute renal failure (ARF).

Pathophysiology. The kidneys receive approximately one fourth of the cardiac output; therefore they are sensitive to alterations in perfusion. An ischemic episode can rapidly result in nephron damage. Because a urinary output of at least 400 ml/day is necessary for adequate excretion of wastes, the resulting decrease in glomerular filtration rate (GFR) that occurs in AKF is responsible for the increased BUN and serum creatinine levels.

The kidneys' response to hypoperfusion is the release of renin, an adaptive response to maintain perfusion to the glomerular bed. AKF develops when this adaptive response is ineffective in maintaining normal kidney function. The pathophysiology of AKF is not completely understood. Nephrotoxic factors and ischemia may be the cause.

Although a variety of conditions contribute to the development of AKF, ATN is the most common. ATN is classified as *postischemic* or *nephrotoxic.* Ischemic events causing ATN occur most commonly after surgery. Ischemia results in inflammation and causes cell swelling, injury, and necrosis along any part of the nephron. Necrosis associated with **nephrotoxicity** is generally limited to the proximal tubules. Three theories explain the oliguria associated with ATN (Table 36-1 and Figure 36-1). Oliguria probably occurs as a result of a combination of all three mechanisms.

Phases. AKF can be divided into four phases: onset, oliguric, diuretic, and recovery (Table 36-2). The onset is the initial phase of injury to the kidney. Reversal or prevention of kidney dysfunction is possible at this stage by early intervention. The **oliguric** phase follows within 1 day of onset. Major problems during the oliguric phase include inability to excrete fluid loads, regulate electrolytes, and excrete metabolic waste products. During the diuretic phase, large amounts of fluid (4 to 5 L/day) and elec-

Box 36-1 Causes of Acute Kidney Failure

Prerenal

Hypovolemia
Hemorrhage
Dehydration
Vomiting
Diabetes insipidus
Cirrhosis
Diarrhea
Inappropriate use of diuretics
Diaphoresis
Burns
Peritonitis
Pancreatitis

Decreased Cardiac Output
Congestive heart failure
Myocardial infarction
Tamponade
Dysrhythmias

Systemic Vasodilation
Sepsis
Acidosis
Vasodilating medications
Anaphylaxis

Hypotension or Hypoperfusion
Cardiac failure
Shock

Intrarenal (Intrinsic)

Tubule or Nephron Damage
Acute tubular necrosis (most common cause)
Glomerulonephritis
Rhabdomyolosis

Vascular Changes
Coagulopathies
Malignant hypertension
Abdominal aortic aneurysm
Sclerosis
Renovascular disease

Nephrotoxins
Antibiotics (gentamicin, tobramycin, amphotericin B, polymyxin B, neomycin, kanamycin, vancomycin)
Chemicals (carbon tetrachloride, lead, ethylene glycol [antifreeze])
Heavy metals (arsenic, mercury)
Iodinated radiographic contrast media (intravenous pyelogram dye)
Drug-induced interstitial nephritis (nonsteroidal antiinflammatory agents, tetracyclines, furosemide, thiazides, phenytoin, penicillins, cyclosporine, tacrolimus, sulfonamides, cephalosporins)

Postrenal

Ureteral and Bladder Neck Obstruction
Calculi
Neurogenic bladder
Neoplasms
Prostatic hyperplasia

TABLE 36-1 PATHOPHYSIOLOGIC THEORIES OF OLIGURIA OF ACUTE TUBULAR NECROSIS

Theory	Pathophysiology
Tubular obstruction	Tubular necrosis causes cell sloughing or ischemic edema, which results in tubular obstruction. Glomerular filtration rate (GFR) is decreased as result of obstruction.
Back leak	GFR remains normal while tubular resorption of filtrate is increased. Ischemia is underlying cause.
Decreased blood flow	Exact mechanism is unknown. Ischemic blood flow may be responsible for changes in glomerular permeability and decrease in GFR. Arteriolar constriction may be associated with release of angiotensin II.

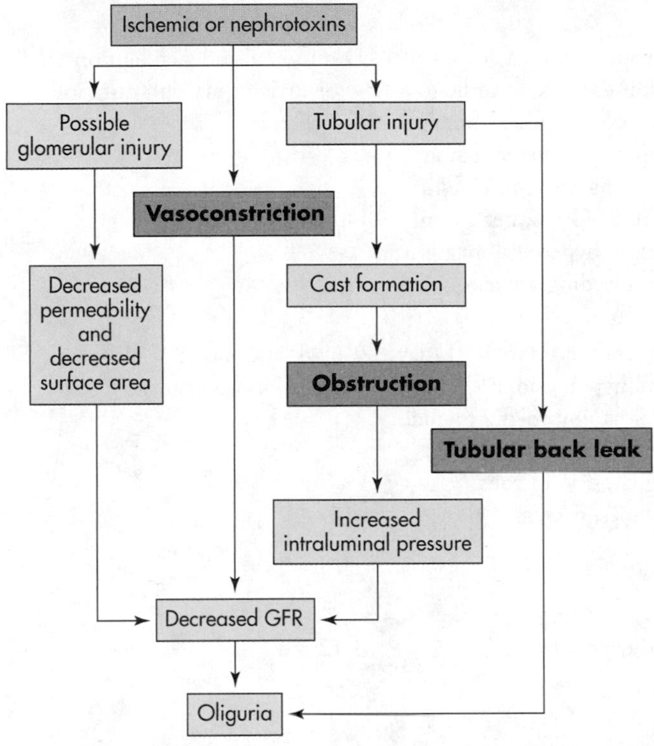

Figure 36-1 Pathogenesis of acute kidney failure. *GFR,* Glomerular filtration rate.

trolytes are lost. The recovery phase may last up to 12 months. Most patients are left with some residual renal dysfunction.

With decreased kidney function, fluids are retained in the body, resulting in fluid overload and edema (see Chapter 17). When fluid overload is excessive, congestive heart failure and pulmonary edema may occur. Hypertension may accompany AKF when the person is hypervolemic.

Inability to excrete fluid leads to decreased urinary output. Either oliguria or anuria (urinary output less than 100 ml/day) may be present, although oliguria is more common. Classically the patient in AKF shows a decrease in urinary output to between 50 and 400 ml/day within 1 to 2 days. The urine specific gravity is low (<1.010), and the osmolality of the urine approaches that of the person's serum (280 to 320 mOsm). These fixed ranges are due to the kidney's inability to resorb sodium and water, which results in the elimination of very dilute urine.[9]

ELECTROLYTE AND ACID-BASE IMBALANCE. Fluid and electrolyte imbalance occurs in the patient with AKF. The three major electrolyte problems are hyperkalemia, sodium imbalance, and metabolic acidosis.

HYPERKALEMIA. In the normal individual the potassium ion is exchanged in the distal convoluted tubule of the nephron for either a sodium or a hydrogen ion; healthy persons cannot conserve the potassium ion. However, in AKF, with many tubular cells not functioning, no mechanism exists to remove potassium from the body. *Hyperkalemia* (the most sudden hazard in oliguric AKF) is said to exist when the serum concentration of this ion reaches a level of 5.5 mEq/L or higher. Serum concentrations of 7 to 10 mEq/L can be quickly reached in AKF and are incompatible with normal cardiac function and life.

The most reliable indicators of potassium toxicity are changes on the electrocardiogram (ECG), such as widened QRS complexes and peaked T waves, and laboratory determinations of serum potassium. Occasionally neuromuscular symptoms such as paresthesias and paralysis (distal to proximal) are seen.[8] Changes in the patient's pulse are not indicators of the amount of potassium excess.

SODIUM IMBALANCE. *Hyponatremia* in AKF most often develops with overhydration. The oliguric patient cannot excrete large volumes of urine; as the administration of sodium-free or low-sodium intravenous or oral fluids continues, the serum is diluted, and the serum concentration of sodium falls.

Hyponatremia is usually accompanied or caused by hypervolemia. The situation typically occurs when an acutely ill patient receives numerous drugs and fluids in an attempt to treat coexisting life-threatening problems. When the volume of drugs and fluids cannot be reduced to a safe level, dialysis is required to remove the excess fluid and restore sodium balance.

Signs and symptoms of hyponatremia include warm, moist, flushed skin; cerebral edema; and mental status changes such as confusion, delirium, coma, and convulsions. Serum sodium concentrations are less than 130 mEq/L. The hematocrit and hemoglobin values fall suddenly in the absence of bleeding because of hemodilution.

Increases in the total body content of sodium also can occur in AKF when the patient is receiving medications high in sodium content and excess sodium in the diet. Edema and increasing blood pressure indicate retention of sodium and water, even though the serum sodium concentration is normal or below normal.

METABOLIC ACIDOSIS. Acidosis develops when hydrogen ion secretion and bicarbonate ion production diminish in the tubules. The pH of the blood decreases, the plasma bicarbonate content

TABLE 36-2 PHASES OF ACUTE KIDNEY FAILURE

Phase	Physiologic Effect	Symptoms	Duration
Onset	Initial phase of injury; hypotension, ischemia, hypovolemia	Subtle	Hours to days
Oliguric			
Urinary output: <400 ml/24 hr	Inability to excrete metabolic wastes: increased serum urea nitrogen and creatinine; BUN may increase 20 mg/dl/day	Nausea, vomiting; drowsiness, confusion; coma; gastrointestinal bleeding; asterixis; pericarditis	1-3 wk; may extend to several weeks in older patients
or			
Urinary output: <30 ml/24 hr	Inability to regulate electrolytes: hyperkalemia, hyponatremia, acidosis, hypocalcemia, hyperphosphatemia Inability to excrete fluid loads: fluid overload, hypervolemia Hematologic dysfunction: anemia, platelet dysfunction, leukopenia May still require dialysis	Nausea, vomiting; cardiac dysrhythmias, electrocardiogram changes; Kussmaul's respiration; drowsiness, confusion; coma; edema; congestive heart failure; pulmonary edema; neck vein distention; hypertension; fatigue; bleeding; infection	Duration also dependent on type of toxic injury and duration of ischemia
Diuretic (urinary output: >1000 ml/24 hr)	Increased production of urine (deficit in concentrating ability of tubules and osmotic diuretic effect of high BUN); slowly increasing excretion of metabolic wastes; hypovolemia; loss of sodium; loss of potassium; high BUN initially, gradually returns to baseline	Urinary output of up to 4-5 L/day; postural hypotension; tachycardia; improving mental alertness and activity; weight loss; thirst; dry mucous membranes; decreased skin turgor	2-6 wk after onset of oliguria; duration varies
Recovery	Kidneys returning to normal functioning; some residual renal insufficiency; 30% of patients do not attain full recovery of GFR	Decreased energy levels	3-12 mo

BUN, Blood urea nitrogen; *GFR,* glomerular filtration rate.

decreases, and central nervous system symptoms of drowsiness progressing to stupor and coma may appear (see Chapter 18). Although the lungs cannot totally compensate for the increasing acid load, they help determine the rate at which acidosis develops and the frequency of or need for dialysis. In compensating for increased metabolic acid loads, the lungs attempt to excrete more carbon dioxide by taking rapid breaths.

INABILITY TO EXCRETE METABOLIC WASTES. Decreased kidney function alters the body's ability to eliminate metabolic waste products, producing the typical signs and symptoms of uremia. BUN and serum creatinine values rise sharply. In the person who has already sustained illness and trauma, BUN values may increase at a rate of 30 mg/dl/day. Signs and symptoms include neurologic manifestations such as confusion, convulsions, coma, and asterixis (hand flapping tremor).

Other pathologic changes also occur as a result of uremia. Bruising and bleeding may result from changes in platelet function. Gastrointestinal (GI) bleeding may result from a lesion such as an angiodysplasia (vascular dilation), which is associated with uremia and decreased platelet function.[25] Decreased cellular immunity causes an increased risk of infection. Pericarditis is thought to develop as a result of pericardial irritation from accumulated metabolic wastes. A pericardial friction rub may be present on auscultation.

The increased output associated with the diuretic phase indicates that the damaged nephrons are healing and are able to begin excreting urine. Daily urine volume increases slowly, although within 1 to 2 days **diuresis** up to or exceeding 4 to 5 L/day may occur. Although fluid can be excreted, the kidneys are not yet healed. Often the person is unable to excrete proportional amounts of waste products, and the BUN and creatinine may rise or remain elevated as urinary volume increases. At times, excessive excretion of sodium and potassium occurs during diuresis. Complete recovery of renal function requires weeks to months. Renal function is normal or near normal when the kidney can both concentrate and dilute urine, control serum electrolytes, and excrete nitrogenous wastes.

COMPLICATIONS. The leading complication of AKF is the development of chronic kidney failure (CKF). Approximately 50% of patients have some residual impairment of glomerular filtration. About 5% never regain kidney function and require long-term hemodialysis or kidney transplantation.[24]

Collaborative Care Management

DIAGNOSTIC TESTS. When altered kidney function is suspected, BUN, creatinine, and electrolyte levels are obtained. Urinalysis is done to determine specific gravity, osmolality, and urine sodium content. Additional studies include a complete blood count (CBC), arterial blood gases, and urine protein. Table 36-3 lists laboratory values in AKF.

Radiographic examinations of the kidney and surrounding structures are used to help determine the cause of AKF, particularly in postrenal failure. Ultrasonography, computed tomography (CT), intravenous pyelography, and magnetic resonance imaging can be done to rule out obstructive causes of kidney failure. These procedures also determine the size and thickness of the kidneys. Enlarged kidneys may represent hydronephrosis. To visualize stones, a plain x-ray film of the abdomen or KUB (kidneys, ureters, and bladder) may be obtained. Cystoscopy may be performed to visualize obstructions. If the etiology of AKF is unknown, a renal biopsy may be done.

MEDICATIONS. The use of medications in the treatment of AKF depends on the underlying cause and the presenting symptoms. Hypovolemia is treated with hypotonic solutions such as 0.45% saline. If hypovolemia is due to blood or plasma loss, packed red blood cells (RBCs) and isotonic saline are administered. Volume replacement rates must match volume losses on a 1:1 basis. Loop diuretics are used to manage altered electrolyte and fluid levels. Doses of up to 320 mg/day of furosemide may be required to produce adequate diuresis.

Kidney failure from nephrotoxins or ischemia is treated with agents that increase renal blood flow. These include mannitol and loop diuretics. Low-dose dopamine is still used extensively in the management of hospital-acquired AKF, despite a lack of significant supporting data.[18] Inflammatory states as in acute glomerulonephritis are treated with glucocorticosteroids.

Patients with impaired renal function may have altered responses to therapeutic doses of many medications. Uremia alters the protein-binding sites, absorption, distribution, and metabolism of many drugs.[6] Nonsteroidal antiinflammatory drugs (NSAIDs) and angiotensin-converting enzyme (ACE) inhibitors are contraindicated in patients with AKF.

TREATMENTS. When conservative management is not effective, dialysis is required. Dialysis, the process by which waste products in the blood are filtered through a semipermeable membrane, is indicated when the patient with AKF is fluid overloaded or has rapidly progressive azotemia, hyperkalemia, and metabolic acidosis. Three methods of dialysis are used: hemodialysis, peritoneal dialysis (discussed later in the chapter), and continuous renal replacement therapy (CRRT).

CONTINUOUS RENAL REPLACEMENT THERAPY. CRRT provides continuous (8 to 24 hours or more) **ultrafiltration** of extracellular fluid and clearance of uremic toxins. It must be administered in a critical care setting. This therapy may or may not necessitate the use of a hemodialysis machine and both arterial and venous access. CRRT that does not require a hemodialysis machine relies on the patient's own blood pressure to power the system and requires both arterial and venous vascular access, usually via catheters placed in the femoral vessels. In most patients a mean arterial blood pressure of 60 mm Hg is required to maintain adequate blood flow through this system. Whether or not a hemodialysis machine is used, success of CRRT depends on the maintenance of blood flow through the hemofilter, which is made up of a collection of hollow fibers. Blood flows through the inside of these hollow fibers, each of which serves as a

TABLE 36-3 LABORATORY VALUES IN ACUTE KIDNEY FAILURE

Finding	Prerenal	Intrarenal	Postrenal
BLOOD VALUES			
Blood urea nitrogen (BUN)	Increased	Increased	Increased
Creatinine	Normal	Increased	Increased
BUN/creatinine ratio	20:1 or greater (increased)	10:1 or less (not increased because both values elevated)	Normal to slightly increased
URINE VALUES			
Urea	Decreased	Decreased	Decreased
Creatinine	About normal	Decreased	Decreased
Specific gravity	1.020 or more (increased)	Fixed and may be high	Variable
Volume	Oliguria	Nonoliguria or oliguria	Oliguria or polyuria Anuria
Osmolality	400 mOsm or more (increased)	250-350 mOsm (low and fixed; similar to plasma osmolality)	Variable: increased or similar to plasma osmolality

semipermeable membrane. The ultrafiltration system is composed of outflow and return tubing, the hemofilter, and an ultrafiltration collection receptacle (Figure 36-2).

During CRRT, water, electrolytes, and other solutes are removed as the patient's blood passes through the hollow fibers of the hemofilter. The resulting ultrafiltrate is a protein-free fluid with solute and electrolyte concentrations similar to those of plasma. The plasma proteins and cellular components of the blood remain in the hemofilter circuit and return to the venous circulation. The ultrafiltrate is collected in a receptacle and discarded. The mass transfer of water and solutes across a semipermeable membrane is a result of *convection* and *diffusion.* The convection forces applied through the fibers of the hemofilter depend primarily on the blood pressure. The higher the blood pressure, the greater the hydrostatic pressure within the hemofilter. Diffusion is the process by which solutes are passively transported across a semipermeable membrane. Diffusion depends on the presence of a concentration gradient across the membrane. In CRRT a concentration gradient is established by infusing dialysate into the nonblood side of the hemofilter.

Removal of plasma water and electrolytes by CRRT is a gradual process that closely resembles the kidney's normal function. Because the process is gradual, rapid fluctuations in fluid and electrolyte status do not occur. Therefore CRRT is recommended for patients with AKF who are too hemodynamically unstable to tolerate hemodialysis or peritoneal dialysis, such as patients with advanced cardiac disease, metabolic acidosis, abdominal wounds, cerebral edema, or sepsis.

Five variations of CRRT are in use: continuous venovenous hemofiltration, continuous arteriovenous hemofiltration, continuous venovenous hemodialysis, continuous arteriovenous hemodialysis, and slow continuous ultrafiltration. Each of these is designed to meet the renal replacement needs of a specific group of patients.

Continuous venovenous hemofiltration (CVVH) is favored by most clinicians.[9] Access to the patient's blood is obtained with a double-lumen catheter generally placed in a large central vessel. A significant benefit to this type of CRRT is that it does not require arterial access. Blood is pumped through a hemofilter by a specialized dialysis machine. This action of pumping generates hydraulic pressure for ultrafiltration. Fluid volume and electrolyte balance are controlled through pumped exchange of replacement fluids. Hourly ultrafiltrate loss is replaced by prescribed amounts of a sterile intravenous electrolyte solution. Systemic heparinization is usually instituted to prevent clotting; however, heparin requirements may be relatively low in patients with coagulopathy or thrombocytopenia.

Continuous arteriovenous hemofiltration (CAVH) removes large amounts of plasma, water, and solutes at rates of 400 to 800 ml/hr. Patients with AKF, mild to moderate azotemia, and electrolyte disturbances can have CAVH as the primary method of dialysis while in the intensive care unit. This type of CRRT is less desirable because it requires the patient's own blood pressure to move the blood through the hemofilter and affords less reliable blood flow rates. This system also has the disadvantage of requiring arterial access. Because of heparinization required to prevent system thrombosis and the patient's hemodynamic instability, cannulation of the arterial vessel puts the patient at increased risk for bleeding. In addition, cannulation of the artery incurs a risk of distal atheroembolic or artery-occlusive complications.

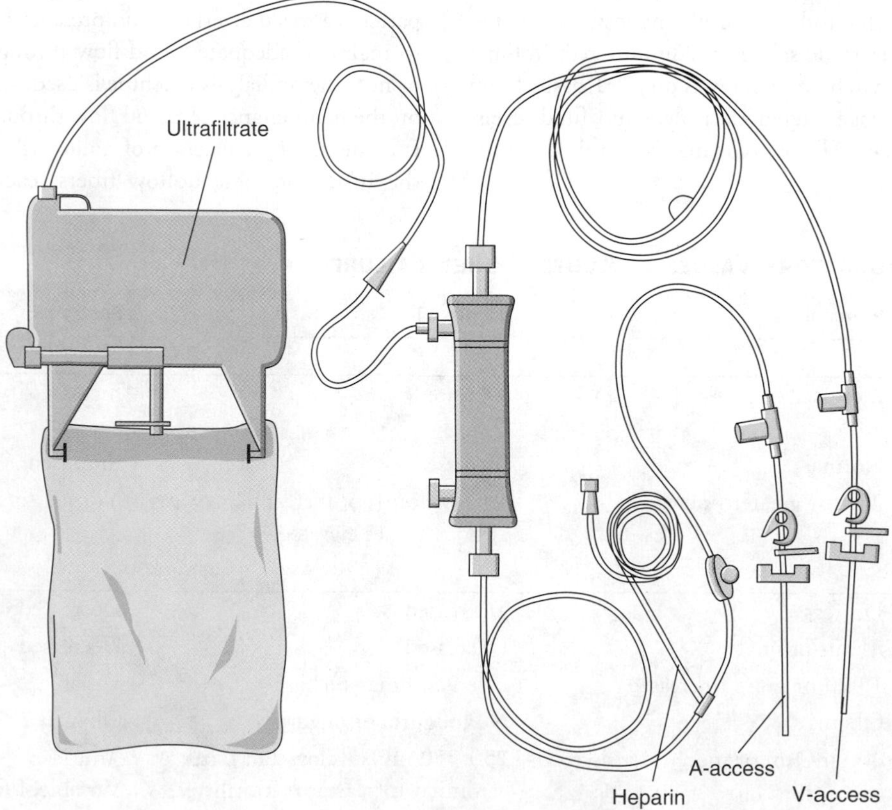

Figure 36-2 The ultrafiltration circuit. *A,* Arterial; *V,* venous.

Continuous venovenous hemodialysis (CVVHD) is the most recently developed mode of CRRT. Like CVVH, the benefit of this mode is that it does not require arterial access. Sterile dialysate fluid is pumped into the ultrafiltration compartment of the hemofilter. The dialysate flows countercurrent to the blood flow, which increases diffusion of solutes from the blood to the ultrafiltration compartment.

Continuous arteriovenous hemodialysis (CAVHD) combines the convective transport of CAVH with diffusion dialysis. Like CAVH, this mode requires both arterial and venous blood access. Solute removal is much greater than in CAVH because, as in CVVHD, sterile dialysate solution is pumped countercurrent to the blood flow, which increases the diffusion of solutes from the blood into the ultrafiltration compartment of the hemofilter. CAVHD can be used as primary dialysis therapy in a wide variety of critically ill patients, including patients with AKF who have severe azotemia, electrolyte imbalances, and acid-base disturbances.

Slow continuous ultrafiltration (SCUF), which is used to control fluid balance, slowly removes small amounts of plasma water and solutes at a rate of 150 to 300 ml/hr. SCUF is highly effective in patients with severe congestive heart failure (see Chapter 30) who do not respond to diuretic therapy. Fluid removal by ultrafiltration can greatly reduce preload in these patients. This method is unsuitable for patients with AKF who have azotemia or significant electrolyte abnormalities, since only small amounts of solutes are removed.

During the diuretic phase, medical management centers on maintaining adequate fluid balance and regulating electrolytes. Even though the patient may be excreting large volumes of urine, dialysis may still be necessary to control electrolyte balance. Protein restrictions are continued until BUN and serum creatinine levels decline.

DIET. Dietary management is important for patients with all types of kidney failure. Close collaboration between nurses, dietitians, and physicians is necessary to institute a diet that provides enough calories to avoid catabolism while preventing a surplus of nitrogen. Catabolism leads to an increased BUN level because of the breakdown of muscle for protein. For the patient with CKF, recommended daily allowance of protein is 0.75g/kg body weight/day or 20% of caloric intake.[7] For the patient with AKF, protein intake recommendations depend on the patient's estimated degree of catabolism.[7] Carbohydrate intake should be maintained at around 100 g/day. Sodium and potassium are restricted, as is free water in patients for whom hyponatremia is an issue. Dietary supplements are usually prescribed. Patients who are unable to take in sufficient nutrients may be candidates for total parenteral nutrition and administration of fat emulsions, which provide a nonprotein source of calories.

HEALTH PROMOTION AND PEVENTION

PRIMARY PREVENTION. The incidence of AKF can be reduced by the identification and control of environmental risk factors. A significant factor in preventive care is the control of nephrotoxic drugs, which is primarily a function of the Food and Drug Administration (FDA). Identification of nephrotoxic drugs and chemicals, enforced labeling of these substances, and drug dispensing only by prescription are examples of the FDA's attempts to promote public health. Proper labeling and storage of potentially toxic drugs and chemicals in the home can further reduce the number of accidental ingestions of nephrotoxic substances. Cleaners and solvents should be used in well-ventilated areas.

SECONDARY PREVENTION. Prevention of AKF includes increased medical supervision of persons with sore throats and upper respiratory tract infections and detection and treatment of individuals with bacteriuria and obstructive disease of the urinary system to monitor and prevent glomerulonephritis associated with bacterial infections. The greatest incidence of AKF occurs in persons with major trauma, extensive burns, surgery of the heart or large blood vessels, massive blood loss, and severe myocardial infarction. Frequent monitoring of urinary output and detection of excessive losses of body fluid in these patients can help identify inadequate renal perfusion before kidney failure develops.

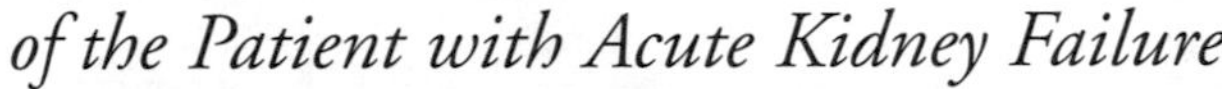

Which of the following is a risk factor for prerenal acute kidney failure?

1. Acute tubular necrosis
2. Intravascular volume depletion
3. Nephrotoxic agents
4. Renal calculi

Nursing Management
of the Patient with Acute Kidney Failure

ASSESSMENT

Health History. Assess for:

- Recent changes in voiding patterns
- Weight gain (fluid retention)
- Nausea or vomiting
- Flank pain
- Muscle weakness
- Changes in concentration, thinking ability
- Patient and family history of renal disease or trauma
- Medication use (prescription and over the counter)
- Recent surgery, anesthesia, or trauma
- History of hypertension
- Exposure to nephrotoxins
- Fatigue or lethargy
- Changes in bowel habits

Physical Examination. Assess for:

- Amount of urine excreted in 24 hours
- Increases or decreases in blood pressure, particularly with postural changes
- Fluid status: peripheral, periorbital, or sacral edema; lung sounds; skin turgor; daily weight
- Halitosis
- Mental status changes
- Tachycardia, tachypnea
- Weight (compared with ideal body weight)
- Ecchymosis
- Pallor

Nursing Diagnoses, Outcomes, and Interventions

Nursing Diagnosis: Deficient Fluid Volume/Excess Fluid Volume

Outcomes. Common examples of expected outcomes for the patient with a diagnosis of *deficient fluid volume* or *excess fluid volume* are:

Patient will:

- Be free from pulmonary edema.
- Demonstrate absence or control of peripheral edema.
- Achieve blood pressure readings between 135/80 and 100/60 mm Hg.
- Achieve balanced electrolytes: sodium 125 to 145 mEq/L, potassium 3.0 to 5.5 mEq/L, and bicarbonate greater than 14 mEq/L.

Nursing interventions. During the acute stage of illness, most patients are cared for in the intensive care unit because of the need for constant monitoring of blood pressure, ECG, pulmonary, and mental status. Many patients require mechanical ventilation and hemodynamic monitoring via a Swan-Ganz catheter to monitor intravascular fluid volume. Patients who cannot tolerate hemodialysis because of hemodynamic instability may be treated with CRRT. The goals of nursing management for patients undergoing CRRT are optimization of the patient's fluid volume and hemodynamic status, maintenance of ultrafiltration system patency, prevention of blood loss from line disconnection, and prevention of infection. These patients require one-to-one nursing care to continuously monitor blood pressure, administer and titrate medications, and maintain the system's patency. Emotional support is important for all patients and their families while in a critical care setting.

Control of fluids is essential during the oliguric phase of AKF because of the kidneys' deceased ability to excrete urine. The nurse needs to record all observations about the patient's state of hydration so that hour-to-hour and day-to-day comparisons can be made. Any finding indicating fluid retention is reported to the health care provider. Edema can first be noted in dependent areas such as the feet and legs, in the presacral area, and around the eyes (periorbital). It is important to remember, however, that edema may not be detected until the person has gained 5 to 10 pounds (2 to 5 kg) in fluid. Accuracy in measurement of daily weight is essential. The nurse observes carefully for signs of pulmonary edema and congestive heart failure (see Guidelines for Safe Practice box and Chapter 30).

Central venous or arterial monitoring lines help provide data for short-term comparisons in managing the fluid balance of the critically ill person. All fluid (parenteral and oral) input must total only slightly more than daily output to avoid severe overhydration. Devices that allow precise control of intravenous fluids help avoid fluid overload when giving parenteral fluids to anuric or oliguric patients. Accuracy in fluid balance records is essential.

Related NIC interventions. Electrolyte Management, Electrolyte Monitoring, Fluid Management, Fluid Monitoring

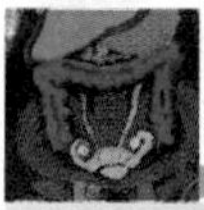

Guidelines for Safe Practice *The Patient With Acute Kidney Failure*

- Maintain fluid and electrolyte balance.
  —Maintain fluid restrictions.
  —Monitor intravenous fluids carefully.
  —Keep accurate records of intake and output.
  —Weigh patient daily.
  —Monitor vital signs frequently, including postural signs.
  —Assess fluid status of patient frequently.
  —Administer phosphate-binding medications as prescribed.
  —Monitor serum electrolytes.
  —During diuretic phase:
    —Assess for changes in mental status indicative of altered serum electrolyte levels.
    —Assess for presence of irregular apical pulse indicative of hypokalemia.
- Maintain nutrition.
  —Provide fluid in small amounts during oliguric phase; ginger ale and other effervescent soft drinks may be tolerated better than other fluids.
  —Provide a diet:
    —Restricted in protein, as prescribed.
    —High in carbohydrates and fat during protein restriction.
    —Low in potassium during hyperkalemia and high in potassium during hypokalemia.
  —Take measures to relieve nausea (antiemetics and comfort measures).
- Prevent injury.
  —Assess orientation; reorient confused patient.
  —When the patient is ambulatory, assess motor skills and monitor ambulation; assist patient as necessary.
  —Assess patient for signs of bleeding.
  —Perform guaiac tests on stool, emesis, and nasogastric returns.
  —Protect patient from bleeding (e.g., instruct patient to use soft toothbrush).
- Prevent infection.
  —Avoid sources of infection.
  —Assess for signs and symptoms of infection.
  —Maintain asepsis for indwelling lines or catheters.
  —Perform pulmonary hygiene.
  —Turn weak or immobile patients every 2 hours and as needed.
  —Provide meticulous skin care.
  —Bathe patient with superfatted soap.
  —Administer prescribed antipruritic agents.
- Facilitate coping.
  —Encourage development of nurse-patient relationship to assist patient in expressing feelings as desired.
  —Promote patient independence.
  —Assist patient in exploring alternative ways of coping.

Nursing Diagnosis: Imbalanced Nutrition: Less Than Body Requirements

OUTCOMES. Common examples of expected outcomes for the patient with a diagnosis of *imbalanced nutrition: less than body requirements* are:
Patient will:

- Assist with control of protein catabolism: BUN less than 100 mg/dl, creatinine less than 12 mg/dl, and absence of skin breakdown.
- Verbalize the need to maintain a diet high in calories and fat and restrict protein and potassium.

NURSING INTERVENTIONS. Most patients with AKF are too ill to tolerate oral feedings. Oral intake can exacerbate nausea as a result of the altered biochemical environment and accompanying GI tract irritation. If the patient is able to tolerate oral feedings, dietary protein and potassium are restricted to modest amounts. The aim is to increase protein available for tissue building and the palatability of the diet without leading to metabolic waste buildup or hyperkalemia.

A high-carbohydrate, high-fat diet is encouraged. Calories in the form of carbohydrates and fats provide energy and spare body protein stores, thus decreasing nonprotein nitrogen production. The body recycles urea to synthesize amino acids for protein building so that some regeneration of tissues can occur despite curtailed protein intake. A nutrition consultation may be beneficial in helping patients determine their caloric needs.

RELATED NIC INTERVENTIONS. Fluid/Electrolyte Management, Nutrition Management, Nutritional Counseling, Nutritional Monitoring, Weight Management

Nursing Diagnosis: Risk for Infection

OUTCOMES. Common examples of expected outcomes for the patient with a diagnosis of *risk for infection* are:
Patient will:

- Remain free from infection.
- Verbalize methods to decrease risks for infection.

NURSING INTERVENTIONS. Preventing infection is an important nursing intervention. Infection leads to tissue breakdown with production of metabolic wastes, which are difficult to eliminate for the patient with AKF. The nurse maintains aseptic technique during all treatments, especially with invasive lines and catheters. Pruritus frequently occurs and may lead to skin lesions from scratching. Measures to relieve pruritus include bathing the patient with a superfatted soap and administering prescribed antipruritic medications as necessary.

To compensate for increased metabolic acid loads, the lungs attempt to excrete more carbon dioxide. The nurse carries out pulmonary hygiene measures to maximize this pathway for acid excretion, to maintain maximal lung expansion, and to prevent atelectasis.

RELATED NIC INTERVENTIONS. Environmental Management, Infection Protection, Nutrition Management, Surveillance

Nursing Diagnosis: Risk for Injury

OUTCOMES. A common example of expected outcomes for the patient with a diagnosis of *risk for injury* is:
Patient will:

- Remain free from injury.

NURSING INTERVENTIONS. The patient with AKF is weak, may be confused, and may experience postural hypotension; thus the risk of falls is increased. The nurse continually assesses the amount of supervision required during daily care and takes appropriate actions to prevent injury. The confused, agitated, or restless patient must be protected from injury; side rails may need to be elevated and padded.

The nurse determines positioning and activity daily based on the person's energy level and respiratory function. The patient with AKF experiences fatigue and activity intolerance. Anemia may also contribute to fatigue. As the patient's energy level increases, the nurse encourages walking as an aerobic exercise.

The nurse provides meticulous skin care to prevent skin breakdown from edema. Bleeding also may occur from changes in platelet and endothelial function. Nursing interventions include measures to prevent and detect bleeding. (Further information on protection from bleeding is found in Chapter 33.)

RELATED NIC INTERVENTIONS. Environmental Management: Safety, Fall Prevention, Risk Identification

Patient/Family Teaching. Patient and family teaching is an important part of nursing care for a patient with acute kidney failure (see Patient/Family Teaching box).

EVALUATION

To evaluate the effectiveness of nursing interventions, compare patient behaviors with those stated in the expected patient outcomes.

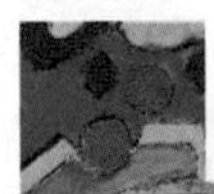

PATIENT/FAMILY TEACHING *The Patient With Acute Kidney Failure*

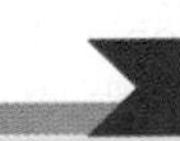

Teaching for the patient with acute kidney failure and his or her family includes information about:

- Cause of kidney failure and problems with recurrent failures
- Identification of preventable environmental or health factors contributing to the illness, such as hypertension and nephrotoxic drugs
- Prescribed medication regimen, including name of medication, dosage, reason for taking, desired and adverse effects
- Prescribed dietary regimen
- The risk of hypokalemia and reportable symptoms (muscle weakness, anorexia, nausea and vomiting, lethargy)
- Signs and symptoms of returning kidney failure (decreased urinary output without decreased fluid intake, signs of fluid retention, increased weight)
- Signs and symptoms of infection; methods to avoid infection
- Need for ongoing follow-up care
- Options for future; explanation of transplantation and dialysis if these are a possibility

RELATED NOC OUTCOMES. Activity Tolerance, Electrolyte & Acid/Base Balance, Fluid Balance, Knowledge: Disease Process, Nutritional Status

GERONTOLOGIC CONSIDERATIONS

Mortality in AKF is greatest in the older population partially because of the prevalence of heart disease, hypertension, and diabetes in this population. Chronic illness and polypharmacy in the aging population can tax the kidneys. Early signs of AKF are vague and may be attributed to other causes. In the older person, signs of acute infection may be absent or diminished. Changes in mental status related to electrolyte imbalances may be attributed to early signs of dementia. In older men, decreased urinary output, a sign of kidney failure, may be mistakenly attributed to benign prostatic hypertrophy.

Although the treatment for AKF remains the same regardless of the patient's age, older adults do not easily tolerate treatment strategies. Intravascular volume overload is particularly difficult to treat because of the increased risk of congestive heart failure. Older patients are much more likely to succumb to the severity of AKF because of an increased risk of complications such as pneumonia and sepsis.

Chronic Kidney Failure

Etiology and Epidemiology. CKF exists when the kidneys are no longer capable of maintaining an internal environment that is consistent with life and damage to the kidneys is irreversible. For most individuals the transition from health to a state of chronic or permanent illness is a slow process that occurs over a number of years. Recurrent infections and exacerbations of nephritis, obstruction of the urinary tract, systemic disease, and destruction of blood vessels from diabetes and longstanding hypertension can all lead to scarring in the kidney and progressive loss of function (Box 36-2). Some individuals, however, develop total irreversible loss of kidney function acutely. Such loss of function usually develops in a few hours or days and follows direct traumatic kidney insult. When only 10% of kidney function remains, the person is considered to have end-stage renal disease (ESRD). The causes of ESRD, in order of prevalence, are (1) diabetes mellitus 44%, (2) hypertension 28%, (3) glomerulonephritis 8%, and (4) other.[24]

Chronic kidney disease remains a significant health problem in the United States. More than 300,000 people have ESRD, and the number increases annually by 7%. The disease can affect persons of all ages, but the peak incidence is between 20 and 64 years old.

Box 36-2 Causes of Chronic Kidney Failure

Glomerular Dysfunction
- Glomerulonephritis
- Diabetic nephropathy
- Hypertensive nephrosclerosis

Systemic Disease
- Sickle cell anemia
- Scleroderma
- Polyarteritis nodosa
- Systemic lupus erythematosus
- Human immunodeficiency virus–associated nephropathy
- Vasculitis

Urinary Tract Obstruction
- Prostatic and bladder tumors
- Lymphadenopathy
- Ureteral obstruction
- Calculi

Other
- Chronic pyelonephritis
- Nephrotic syndrome
- Polycystic kidney disease
- Kidney infarction
- Cyclosporine nephrotoxicity
- Multiple myeloma

Pathophysiology. CKF differs from AKF in that the damage to the kidneys is progressive and irreversible. CKF progresses through four stages: decreased kidney reserve, kidney insufficiency, kidney failure, and ESRD (Box 36-3). In practice, however, these stages are not sharply differentiated. Severe symptoms occur at the kidney failure stage. As many as 50% of nephrons are destroyed before renal deficits are apparent.

The specific pathophysiologic mechanisms depend on the underlying disease causing kidney destruction. The following general pathophysiologic mechanism summarizes these changes. During CKF some of the nephrons, including the glomeruli and tubules, are thought to remain intact, whereas others are destroyed *(intact nephron hypothesis)*. The intact nephrons hypertrophy and produce an increased volume of filtrate with increased tubular resorption despite a decreased GFR. This adaptation permits the kidney to function until about three fourths of the nephrons are destroyed. The solute load then becomes greater than can be resorbed, producing an osmotic diuresis with polyuria and thirst. Eventually more nephrons are damaged, resulting in retention of waste products and oliguria.

Although the clinical course of CKF varies, some common features exist. Signs and symptoms result from disordered fluid and electrolyte balance, alterations in regulatory functions of the body, and retention of solutes. Anemia results from impaired RBC production because of decreased secretion of erythropoietin by the kidney. Patients may report lethargy, dizziness, and fatigue. In addition, the life span of RBCs is shortened as a result of uremia and superimposed nutritional anemia resulting from dietary restrictions and poor GI absorption of iron. Azotemia and acidosis are present, and potassium and hydrogen ion excretion is impaired. Fluid and sodium balance is abnormal and may involve either abnormal retention or secretion of sodium and water; therefore urine volume can be increased, normal, or decreased.

Hyperuricemia is a common finding in ESRD, although the varied serum levels of uric acid do not seem to have a definite relationship with the level of kidney function. Increased levels of serum phosphate are characteristic, and calcium levels may be low or normal. These findings result from decreased kidney excretion of phosphate and a simultaneous reduction in ionized serum calcium. Through increased production of parathyroid hormone (PTH), the body may reestablish a normal serum calcium level, at the expense of the bone matrix.

Hypertension may or may not be present. As ESRD develops, blood pressure is elevated because of increased total body water, release of a vasopresser by the kidney, and inadequately secreted vasodepressors. Glucose intolerance may be seen, although usually not of sufficient severity to warrant treatment. The rising blood glucose level appears to be the result of an altered biochemical environment produced by the failing kidneys and does not signify the development of diabetes mellitus. As kidney failure progresses, the patient develops increased pigmentation of the skin,

Box 36-3 Stages of Chronic Kidney Failure

Decreased Kidney Reserve (Kidney Impairment)

40% to 75% loss of nephron function
GFR: 40% to 50% of normal
BUN and serum creatinine levels normal
Patient asymptomatic

Kidney Insufficiency

75% to 80% loss of nephron function
GFR: 20% to 40% of normal
BUN and serum creatinine levels begin to rise
Mild anemia; mild azotemia, which worsens with physiologic stress
Nocturia, polyuria

Kidney Failure

GFR: 10% to 20% of normal
BUN and serum creatinine levels increase
Anemia, azotemia, metabolic acidosis
Urine specific gravity low
Polyuria, nocturia
Symptoms of kidney failure present

End-Stage Renal Disease

85% loss of nephron function
GFR: 10% of normal
BUN and serum creatinine at high levels
Anemia, azotemia, metabolic acidosis
Urine specific gravity fixed at 1.010
Oliguria
Symptoms of kidney failure present

BUN, Blood urea nitrogen; *GFR,* glomerular filtration rate.

which becomes sallow or brownish. Uremic frost, though a rare occurrence, is a pale deposit of crystals on the skin caused by kidney failure and uremia. Metabolic waste products, unable to be excreted by the kidney, are instead excreted through the small capillaries of the skin. With more advanced and insufficiently treated kidney failure, the patient may develop muscular twitching, numbness in the feet and legs, pericarditis, and pleuritis. These signs usually resolve when the patient is treated with medication and/or dialysis.

The symptoms of uremia usually develop so slowly that the patient and family often cannot identify the time of onset. These symptoms include lethargy, headaches, physical and mental fatigue, weight loss, irritability, and depression. Anorexia, persistent nausea and vomiting, shortness of breath, and pitting edema are symptomatic of severe loss of kidney function. Pruritus may be present. CKF affects all body systems (Table 36-4).

As ESRD develops, most women note changes in their menstrual cycle. Bleeding may occur at more widely spaced intervals, may be heavier or lighter than normal, or may cease altogether. This obvious change in the reproductive cycle is usually accompanied by changes in fertility. Ovulation may occur normally or may occur only a few times a year. Pregnancy in uremic women is of much lower incidence than in the normal population. However, ESRD cannot be used as an effective method of birth control. In men erectile dysfunction may occur as CKF progresses toward ESRD. Dialysis may be indicated to return or maximize reproductive function. It should be stressed that the sexual activity of some persons with CKF may remain normal despite changes in reproductive ability.

The point at which the patient becomes obviously symptomatic and displays signs typical of kidney failure occurs when approximately 80% to 90% of renal function has been lost (Figure 36-3). At this level of kidney function, creatinine clearance values fall to 10 ml/min or less.

Hypertriglyceridemia occurs in approximately 30% to 70% of persons with CKF. Atherosclerosis may develop as a result of an elevated ratio of high-density lipoproteins (HDL) to low-density lipoproteins. The production of HDL decreases because of decreased lipolytic activity caused by uremia.

Catabolism and proteinuria contribute to the negative nitrogen balance common in CKF. Muscle mass diminishes.

COMPLICATIONS. Many of the complications of ESRD and its treatments have been discussed. Fluid and electrolyte imbalances, shock, sepsis, and bleeding are described earlier. Other complications include anemia, hypertension, hyperkalemia, congestive heart failure, pulmonary edema, pericarditis, atherosclerosis, peptic ulcer disease, osteodystrophy, peripheral neuropathy, and metabolic encephalopathy.

Treatment options for CKF place the patient at risk for other complications. Those treated with hemodialysis often require multiple hospital admissions for problems with vascular access devices. Infection, clotting, and displacement create a need for additional surgical intervention, making proper care of these devices crucial. Complications can arise from improper technique, manipulation of the catheter, and exit-site care of the dialysis catheter. Research does not support the effectiveness of a particular care protocol over others.

Peritonitis is an ever-present threat during peritoneal dialysis. Aseptic technique must be strictly maintained during insertion of the catheter and throughout the procedure. The nurse should be knowledgeable about each patient's medication regimen and set appropriate medication schedules for the dialysis patient.

Collaborative Care Management

DIAGNOSTIC TESTS. Because of the multisystemic effects of CKF, many serious abnormalities in laboratory values are characteristic of persons with CKF. Serum creatinine levels are essential in the evaluation of kidney function. Increased levels of creatinine are seen only when a significant number of nephrons are destroyed, resulting in impaired creatinine excretion. A 12- or 24-hour urinary creatinine clearance test is used to evaluate kidney function and determine the degree of dysfunction. This test is the most specific indicator of kidney function. The creatinine clearance rate is equal to the GFR. Measurements of serum and urinary creatinine levels and urinary volume are necessary to complete the test. A creatinine clearance of less than 10 ml/min is indicative of severe kidney impairment. Creatinine clearance is

TABLE 36-4 BODY SYSTEM MANIFESTATIONS IN CHRONIC KIDNEY FAILURE

Causes	Signs and Symptoms	Assessment Parameters
HEMATOPOIETIC SYSTEM		
Decreased erythropoietin production	Anemia	Hematocrit
Decreased survival time of RBCs	Fatigue	Hemoglobin
Bleeding	Defects in platelet function	Bleeding time
Blood loss during dialysis	Decreased hematocrit	Observe for bruising, hematemesis, or melena
Decreased activity of platelets and endothelin	Ecchymosis	
	Bleeding	
CARDIOVASCULAR SYSTEM		
Fluid overload	Hypervolemia	Vital signs, body weight
Renin-angiotensin mechanism	Hypertension	Body weight, vital signs
Fluid overload, anemia	Tachycardia	Electrocardiogram
Chronic hypertension	Dysrhythmias	Heart sounds
Calcification of soft tissues	Congestive heart failure	Monitor electrolytes
Uremic toxins in pericardial fluid	Pericarditis	Assess for pain, pericardial friction rub
Fibrin formation on epicardium		
RESPIRATORY SYSTEM		
Compensatory mechanisms for metabolic acidosis	Tachypnea	Respiratory assessment
Uremic toxins	Kussmaul's respirations	Arterial blood gas results
Fluid overload	Uremic fetor (or uremic halitosis)	Inspection of oral mucosa
		Vital signs
	Tenacious sputum	Pulse oximetry
	Pain with coughing	
	Elevated temperature	
	Hilar pneumonitis	
	Pleural friction rub	
	Pulmonary edema, frothy sputum	
GASTROINTESTINAL SYSTEM		
Change in platelet activity	Anorexia	Monitor intake and output
Serum uremic toxins	Abdominal distention	Hematocrit
Electrolyte imbalances	Gastrointestinal bleeding	Hemoglobin
Urea converted to ammonia by saliva	Nausea and vomiting	Guaiac test for all stools
	Diarrhea	Assess quality of stools
	Constipation	Assess for abdominal pain

calculated based on 24-hour urine results (including serum and urinary levels) and data on body weight and height. The BUN/creatinine ratio is also useful in evaluating kidney function. The creatinine level changes only in response to kidney dysfunction, whereas the BUN level changes in response to dehydration or protein breakdown.

Blood chemistry analysis, CBC, and urinalysis are performed to evaluate the degree of impairment in patients with CKF (Table 36-5). Because urinary output declines with the progression of kidney failure, urinalysis may not provide as much information as other laboratory tests.

Radiographic examinations are of little use in the evaluation of the patient with ESRD. A KUB film can evaluate kidney size, shape, and position. The patient with ESRD often has atrophic kidneys. Ultrasound or CT may be ordered to evaluate possible obstruction. In patients with AKF or chronic kidney insufficiency, CT is preferably performed without contrast because of the nephrotoxicity potential of the contrast agent.

TABLE 36-4 BODY SYSTEM MANIFESTATIONS IN CHRONIC KIDNEY FAILURE—CONT'D

Causes	Signs and Symptoms	Assessment Parameters
NEUROLOGIC SYSTEM		
Uremic toxins	Lethargy, confusion	Level of orientation
Electrolyte imbalances	Convulsions	Level of consciousness
Cerebral swelling resulting from fluid shifting	Stupor, coma Sleep disturbances	Reflexes Electroencephalogram
	Unusual behavior	Electrolyte levels
	Asterixis	Assess for asterixis
	Muscle irritability	
SKELETAL SYSTEM		
Decreased calcium absorption	Renal osteodystrophy	Serum phosphorus Serum calcium
Decreased phosphate excretion	Joint pain Retarded growth	Assess for joint pain Parathyroid hormone level
INTEGUMENTARY SYSTEM		
Anemia	Pallor	Observe for bruising
Pigment retained	Pigmentation	Assess color of skin
Decreased size of sweat glands	Pruritus	Assess integrity of skin
Decreased activity of oil glands	Ecchymosis	Observe for scratching
Dry skin; phosphate deposits	Excoriation	
Excretion of metabolic waste products through skin	Uremic frost	
GENITOURINARY SYSTEM		
Damaged nephrons	Decreased urinary output Decreased urine specific gravity Proteinuria Casts and cells in urine Decreased urine sodium	Monitor intake and output Serum creatinine BUN Serum electrolytes Urine specific gravity Urine electrolytes
REPRODUCTIVE SYSTEM		
Hormonal abnormalities	Infertility	Monitor intake and output
Anemia	Decreased libido	Monitor vital signs
Hypertension	Erectile dysfunction	Hematocrit
Malnutrition	Amenorrhea	Hemoglobin
Medications	Delayed puberty	

RBCs, Red blood cells; *BUN,* blood urea nitrogen.

▶ ARE You READY?

Which of the following diagnostic studies is the most specific indicator of kidney function in a patient with renal disease?

1. Serum BUN
2. Serum creatinine
3. BUN/creatinine ration
4. 12- or 24-hour urinary creatinine clearance

MEDICATIONS. Patients with either AKF or CKF typically receive multiple drugs to manage the associated complications. Currently, the drug-approval process in the United States requires drug-dosing recommendations for patient with kidney failure as a part of the product labeling. In kidney failure a number of factors can affect drug absorption: uremic gastroparesis, changes in gastric pH, gut wall edema, and alterations in first-pass metabolism.[19] As a result, many common doses for drug therapy must be adjusted for the patient with kidney failure. Clearance of drugs that are

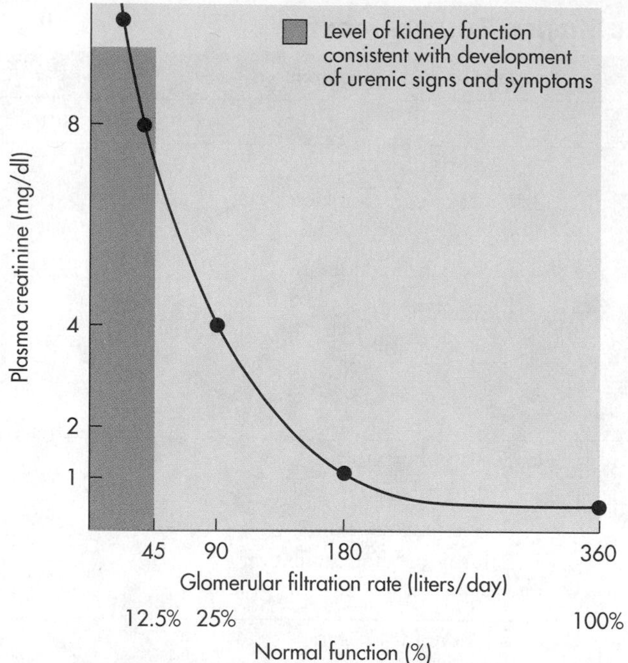

Figure 36-3 Glomerular filtration and plasma creatinine levels.

metabolized by the kidneys, such as insulin, meperidine, and numerous antibiotics, is greatly reduced in kidney failure. Patients must be closely monitored for adverse reactions associated with drug overdose (Boxes 36-4 and 36-5).

Initial management of patients with CKF focuses on controlling symptoms, preventing complications, and delaying the progression of kidney failure. Medications are used to control blood pressure, regulate electrolytes, and control intravascular fluid volume.

Hypertension is controlled by the use of a variety of antihypertensive agents, including ACE inhibitors, angiotensin II receptor antagonists, calcium channel antagonists, diuretics, and beta-blockers. If blood pressure cannot be controlled with a single agent, combination therapy may be instituted. Immunosuppressive therapy may be instituted in patients with glomerulonephritis. Intravascular fluid volume is also regulated by the use of diuretics.

Electrolyte imbalances are corrected by the use of sodium bicarbonate for metabolic acidosis. Hyperkalemia is treated with diuretic therapy or sodium polystyrene sulfate (Kayexalate). In severe hyperkalemia insulin may be administered intravenously with dextrose to temporarily decrease the serum potassium level. Calcium and phosphorus levels are maintained by the use of phosphate-binding agents, calcimimetic agents, calcium supplements, and vitamin D analogs.

TREATMENTS. Treatment goals include stabilization of the internal environment by controlling fluid and electrolyte balance, preventing infection, controlling existing diseases, correcting anemia, and preventing complications (Box 36-6).

FLUID CONTROL. Changes in the ability to regulate sodium and water excretion are often the first clinical signs of kidney failure. The ability to excrete sodium and water can vary considerably from one patient with CKF to the next. Although volume problems for most patients involve hypervolemia resulting from a marked inability to excrete sodium and water, some patients are unable to conserve these substances, and hypovolemia results. With significant inability to either excrete or conserve body fluid, the patient can develop severe fluid imbalances in a relatively short time. The health care team needs to identify fluid imbalances and prescribe an intake of sodium and water equivalent to the amount of these substances excreted in a 24-hour period. The desired effect is to maintain the person in a normotensive, normovolemic state.

ELECTROLYTE CONTROL

Hyperkalemia. Hyperkalemia is defined as a serum potassium level greater than 5.5 mEq/L, although the level at which hyperkalemic complications occur may vary, depending on the steady-state value for a given patient. Potassium retention occurs in CKF because of a direct reduction in nephron excretory ability. Hyperkalemia can be controlled by decreasing dietary intake of foods high in potassium, such as citrus fruits, green leafy vegetables, and salt substitutes. Exchange resins, such as sodium polystyrene sulfonate, are also effective in removing potassium$^+$ from the body. The resin exchanges sodium ions for potassium$^+$ and calcium in the GI tract. Sodium polystyrene sulfonate can be given either as an oral preparation or by retention enema. It is usually given with sorbitol to enhance potassium$^+$ excretion via the bowel. The use of a retention enema requires that the solution be retained in the colon for 30 to 60 minutes or longer.[8] In severe situations hemodialysis may be instituted.

Metabolic acidosis. Metabolic acidosis occurs because the damaged kidneys are unable to excrete the normal load of acids generated by metabolism. When the GFR drops 30% to 40%, metabolic acidosis begins to develop primarily because of a reduced capacity of the distal tubules to produce ammonia and an impaired resorption of bicarbonate. Although hydrogen ion retention and bicarbonate loss continue, the plasma pH is maintained at a level compatible with life by other buffering mechanisms, particularly the bone salts.

Hypocalcemia and hyperphosphatemia. When the kidneys fail, the ability to excrete phosphorus decreases, and a cycle of hypocalcemia-hyperphosphatemia results in significant bone demineralization. Several factors are responsible for these imbalances. A state of acidosis results in dissolution of the alkaline salts of bone that serve as buffers, since the kidney is no longer able to maintain acid-base balance. As a result, calcium and phosphorus are released into the bloodstream. Reduced glomerular filtration and excretion of inorganic phosphate lead to an elevation of plasma phosphate with a concomitant decrease in serum calcium. Decreased serum calcium concentrations stimulate the secretion of PTH, which results in resorption of calcium from the bones. Normally PTH also inhibits tubular resorption of phosphates, increasing their excretion, but the failing kidney is unable to excrete phosphorus so the level rises. The kidneys are also unable to complete the synthesis of vitamin D to its active form, 1,25-dihydroxycholecalciferol, which is necessary for absorption of calcium from the GI tract and deposition of calcium in the bones. This acquired resistance to vitamin D decreases calcium absorp-

TABLE 36-5 LABORATORY FINDINGS IN CHRONIC KIDNEY FAILURE

Test	Normal Values	Findings in Chronic Kidney Failure
SERUM CREATININE		
Male	0.6-1.5 mg/dl	Elevated
Female	0.5-1.1 mg/dl	Findings >4 mg/dl indicates significant kidney impairment
Elderly	Decreased (because of decreased muscle mass)	May rise to 30 mg/dl before symptoms appear
BUN		
Adults	7-20 mg/dl	Values >100 mg/dl indicate severe kidney impairment*
Elderly	8-21 mg/dl	
BLOOD CHEMISTRY		
Sodium	135-145 mEq/L	Decreased or increased
Potassium	3.5-5 mEq/L	Increased
Calcium		Decreased
Total	8.5-10.5 mg/dl	
Ionized	4.5-5.6 mg/dl	
Phosphorus	2.7-4.5 mg/dl	Increased
Magnesium	1.2-1.9 mEq/L	Increased
Serum pH	7.35-7.45	Decreased (metabolic acidosis) or normal
Serum bicarbonate	22-26 mEq/L	Decreased
COMPLETE BLOOD COUNT		
Hemoglobin		Decreased
Male	10-17 g/dl	
Female	11.5-15.5 g/dl	
Elderly	Decreased	
Hematocrit		Decreased (may rise to near normal with epoetin therapy)
Male	39%-49%	
Female	33%-43%	
Elderly	Decreased	
CREATININE CLEARANCE		
Male	70-150 ml/min	Decreased
Female	85-130 ml/min	Findings <50 ml/min indicative of kidney impairment
Elderly	Decreased up to 30% in absence of renal disease	Decrease reflects decreases in GFR
URIC ACID (SERUM)		
Male	2.1-8.5 mg/dl	Increased
Female	2.0-6.8 mg/dl	Findings >12 mg/dl indicate serious kidney impairment
Elderly	3.5-8.5 mg/dl	

BUN, Blood urea nitrogen; *GFR,* glomerular filtration rate.
*Increased levels dependent on protein intake, liver disease, and hydration status.

tion, permits further retention of phosphorus, and contributes to secondary hyperparathyroidism. The result of these complex disturbances is growth arrest or retardation in children and bone pain and deformities known as *renal osteodystrophy* in adults.

Elevated plasma phosphate, calcium-phosphate product, PTH, and excess calcium from long-term ingestion of calcium-containing phosphate binders also contribute to the increased incidence of cardiovascular calcification, cardiovascular disease and increased mortality in patients with chronic kidney disease.[2]

The aim of treatment is to decrease serum phosphorus levels. This is accomplished by restricting the intake of dietary phosphorus (eliminating dairy products and restricting protein) and of phosphate binders. The reduction of serum phosphorus toward normal is often associated with a small increase in serum calcium, a decline in serum PTH, and a reduced incidence of overt secondary hyperparathyroidism.

In dialysis patients predialysis serum phosphorus levels are ideally maintained between 4.5 and 6 mg/dl. To bind the phosphorus,

Box 36-4 Drugs That Are Prescribed Differently for Dialysis Patients

- Vancomycin: Large molecule is poorly cleared by all forms of dialysis (but may be cleared to a greater degree by continuous hemofiltration techniques); dose of 1 g once weekly usually results in consistently therapeutic drug levels (usual dose: 1 g twice daily).
- Aminoglycosides (e.g., netilmicin): These are cleared to a variable degree by both hemodialysis and peritoneal dialysis; dose likely to be greatly reduced (e.g., one third of usual daily dose every 2 days), and monitoring of plasma levels required; note that even if nephrotoxicity is no longer an issue, ototoxicity is still a serious complication of therapy.
- Morphine: Smaller doses are likely to be effective; accumulation of metabolites normally cleared by the kidney such as morphine-6-glucuronide can cause profound narcosis and respiratory depression; morphine-6-glucuronide is not cleared by dialysis, and clearance will take days to weeks in the anephric patient.
- Meperidine: Accumulation of normeperidine (a metabolite) can cause seizures; great care needed with use for longer than 24 hours.
- Digoxin: Clearance of digoxin is reduced; transient profound hypokalemia is common with hemodialysis, increasing the risk of arrhythmia.

From Frasser D, Vinning M: Urologic nephrology. In Weiss RM, George N, O'Reilly PH, editors: *Comprehensive urology,* London, 2001, Mosby.

Box 36-5 Drugs Requiring Caution in Patients With Kidney Impairment

- Angiotensin-converting enzyme (ACE) inhibitors: Avoid in those with renal artery stenosis. Renal blood flow depends on efferent arteriolar tone, and reduction of this by ACE inhibition may seriously damage renal function, sometimes irreversibly; these drugs pose risk of profound hypotension in patients with heart failure or volume depletion; these hazards are shared by angiotensin-receptor antagonists.
- Aminoglycosides: These have a narrow therapeutic range and, with prolonged treatment, are toxic within it; have predominantly renal excretion; pose a high risk of ototoxicity and nephrotoxicity in those with renal impairment; toxicity mainly relates to trough plasma concentration, so once-daily (or less frequent) dosing may be safer if their use is essential; netilmicin is probably the least nephrotoxic.
- Nonsteroidal antiinflammatory drugs: Risk of nephrotoxicity arises partly from effect on prostaglandin-mediated renal vasoregulation; damage caused by other insults to the kidney (e.g., hypoxia, hypotension, or sepsis) is likely to be enhanced; they increase the risk of peptic ulceration in uremic patients.
- Tetracyclines: These have an antianabolic effect, increasing blood urea, and should be avoided in those with renal impairment.
- X-ray contrast medium: Toxicity is enhanced by kidney failure, particularly with diabetes mellitus, myeloma, dehydration, and low cardiac output states; even nonionized contrast can cause acute kidney failure; intravenous urogram relies on the excretion of the contrast by the kidney and so will not be helpful in the presence of advanced kidney failure.

From Frasser D, Vinning M: Urologic nephrology. In Weiss RM, George N, O'Reilly PH, editors: *Comprehensive urology,* London, 2001, Mosby.

phosphate binders must be taken with meals and with snacks. The available agents for intestinal phosphate binding include calcium carbonate and calcium acetate. Another substance used for phosphate binding is sevelamer (Renagel), a nonabsorbed, phosphate-binding polymer. Sevelamer binds phosphate ions through a combination of ion exchange and hydrogen bonding without elevating serum calcium levels. Like other phosphate binders, it must be ingested during the meal. Historically phosphate binders containing aluminum were the mainstay of therapy. Because the kidney is the major route of aluminum excretion, prolonged ingestion of aluminum-containing phosphorus binders results in the accumulation of aluminum in kidney failure. Consequences of aluminum overload include dementia, myopathy, osteomalacia, and anemia.[21] Risks of calcium-containing phosphate binders include hypercalcemia and diarrhea. If calcium carbonate is given with meals, less calcium is absorbed and the risk of hypercalcemia is reduced. It is critical that nurses adjust the medication times to coincide with meal delivery to enhance phosphate binding and to minimize calcium absorption.

Some patients may benefit from the administration of the active form of vitamin D (calcitriol, 0.25 mcg/day). Indications for use include inadequate control of serum phosphorus, hypocalcemia, bone pain, myopathy, and rising serum PTH concentrations.[5]

TREATMENT OF CONCURRENT DISORDERS

Anemia. Anemia universally accompanies chronic kidney disease. Hematocrit values of 16% to 22% were not uncommon in the days before erythropoietin (EPO). When untreated, the anemia of chronic kidney disease is associated with a number of physiologic abnormalities, including decreased tissue oxygen delivery and use, increased cardiac output, cardiac enlargement, ventricular hypertrophy, angina, congestive heart failure, and decreased cognition and mental acuity.[11] The primary cause of anemia in these patients is insufficient production of erythropoietin by the diseased kidneys. The introduction and subsequent clinical success of EPO, the recombinant form of human erythropoietin, have confirmed this hormone's primary role in regulating the erythropoietic cascade. Patients treated with this agent have an increased hematocrit, a decreased need for blood transfusions, and improved energy levels. This increase in hematocrit enables the patient with CKF to carry out normal daily activities.

EPO is administered subcutaneously or intravenously, three times a week, in a calculated dose of 50 unit/kg body weight. It is usually administered during a scheduled dialysis treatment. Darbepoetin alfa, a long-acting form of the drug, may be administered weekly. Patients who are in a predialysis state, receiving peritoneal dialysis, or receiving other home dialysis regimens learn to self-administer one of these agents.

Iron is a necessary component of **erythropoiesis**, and therapy with EPO is hindered if patients do not have adequate iron stores. Iron stores should be evaluated before and during therapy. Iron deficiency may occur with EPO as a result of an internal shift of iron from stores to RBCs during the acute correction of anemia. Iron deficiency is a major factor in the pathogenesis of anemia in patients with chronic kidney disease. A number of factors may

BOX 36-6 Treatment Goals for Patient With Chronic Kidney Failure

- Stabilization of the internal environment as demonstrated by:
  —Mental alertness, attention span, and appropriate interactions
  —Absence or control of peripheral and pulmonary edema
  —Control of electrolyte balance within the following limits:
    —Sodium: 125 to 145 mEq/L
    —Potassium: 3-5.5 mEq/L
    —Bicarbonate: >15 mEq/L
    —Calcium: 9-11 mg/dl
    —Phosphate: 3-5 mg/dl
    —Serum albumin: 2 g/dl
  —Control of protein catabolism and protein metabolic wastes as indicated by the following parameters:
    —Urea nitrogen: <100 mg/dl
    —Creatinine: <10 mg/dl
  —Absence of joint inflammation and pain
  —Control of anemia
    —Hematocrit: ≥33%
    —Hemoglobin: 11-12 g/dl
    —Ferritin: >50-100 ng/ml
    —Iron saturation: >20%
- Absence of infection
- Absence of bleeding
- Blood pressure controlled at 135/80 mm Hg sitting, <10 mm Hg postural change on standing
- Control of coexisting disease, including:
  —Heart failure
  —Anemia
  —Dehydration
- Absence of toxicity from inadequately excreted medications
- Nutrient intake sufficient to maintain positive nitrogen balance
- Anorexia and nausea controlled
- Pruritus controlled

contribute to the iron deficiency, including decreased dietary intake and GI absorption of iron, chronic GI bleeding, and chronic inflammatory responses associated with infection or autoimmune disease. In these conditions, iron stores may be adequate, but the availability of usable iron for the production of hemoglobin is reduced because iron is not released from the stores. Because iron is necessary for continued RBC production, virtually all patients receiving EPO eventually require supplemental iron.

Folate and vitamin B_{12} are important cofactors in the production of RBCs and play a role in the formation and development of deoxyribonucleic acid (DNA). Shortages of these vitamins hinder the formation of DNA and thus RBCs. Folate can be taken orally at a dose of 1 mg/day, and vitamin B_{12} can be replaced with a monthly intramuscular injection of 100 to 1000 mcg based on the vitamin B_{12} blood level.

Blood pressure may rise during EPO therapy, especially during the early stage of treatment when the hematocrit is rising. About 25% of patients experience this rise in blood pressure. Regulating a dialysis patient's blood pressure involves reevaluating dietary sodium intake, the dialysis prescription, and antihypertensive medications.

Gastrointestinal disturbances. In patients with uremia, disturbances in fluid, electrolyte, and waste composition of body fluids produce changes in osmotic gradients in all cells. When these changes occur in the cells of the GI tract, anorexia, nausea, and vomiting result. Persons with uremia are subject to bleeding of the GI tract associated with lesions such as an angiodysplasia and decreased platelet function. Urea is broken down to ammonia by the action of intestinal bacteria. Because ammonia is a mucosal irritant, ulceration and bleeding can occur. Persons with chronic kidney disease also have decreased salivary flow. The smell and taste of ammonia resulting from urea breakdown increase anorexia. Treatment includes vinegar mouthwashes to neutralize ammonia and antacids every 2 to 4 hours to decrease GI irritation. Dietary control of uremia helps control disturbances in fluid, electrolyte, and water composition of body fluids and thus helps control nausea and vomiting.

DIALYSIS. Long-term intermittent hemodialysis was first used for the treatment of CKF in 1960. Before that, hemodialysis was reserved for the treatment of AKF. Once kidney failure was determined to be irreversible, hemodialysis was withdrawn. Many industrialized countries throughout the world continue to withdraw dialysis after irreversible kidney failure is confirmed.

In 1972 the U.S. Congress enacted legislation that provides some payment of health care costs for all U.S. citizens with ESRD. Under this legislation, any person with CKF is provided benefits under Medicare. This legislation enables many persons to live longer by undergoing chronic hemodialysis.

Many technologic advances have been made in the treatment of persons with ESRD. Drastic changes in dialyzers (artificial kidneys) allow for more efficient and comfortable hemodialysis treatments. The dialysis machines, which control blood flow through the dialyzer, have also undergone significant improvement, and some allow patients to dialyze at home. Developments in peritoneal dialysis permit patients to treat themselves with continuous and intermittent peritoneal dialysis. Home dialysis affords persons more control in meeting their own health care needs (see Future Watch box).

Dialysis involves the movement of fluid and particles across a semipermeable membrane. It can help restore fluid and electrolyte balance, control acid-base balance, and remove waste and toxic material from the body. This treatment can sustain life successfully in both acute and chronic situations that require substitution for or augmentation of normal kidney function. Specifically, dialysis is used to remove excessive amounts of drugs and toxins, correct serious electrolyte and acid-base imbalances, maintain kidney function when shutdown occurs as a result of

Future Watch

Kidney Dialysis Goes Home

Home Dialysis Plus, a Portland company, is working with Oregon State University (OSU) to develop a portable kidney dialysis machine that will enable renal failure patients to perform hemodialysis at home. Developers announced that the technology will allow them to reduce the artificial kidney to the size of about four sugar cubes. The new smaller kidney will provide better surface area and increase dialysis efficiency from 28% to 90%. The dialysis machine will be reduced from the size of a refrigerator to the size of a piece of carry-on luggage. Developers are hopeful that OSU's new microtechnology will lead the way to development of a wearable or implantable dialysis device in the future.

Portable kidney dialysis machine developed, accessed Feb 2004 from Oregon State University website: http://www.eurekalert.org/pub_releases/2004-02/osu-pkd020204.php.

transfusion reactions, replace kidney function temporarily in persons with AKF, and permanently substitute for the loss of kidney function in persons with ESRD.

Physiologic principles of dialysis. Dialysis is based on three principles: diffusion, osmosis, and ultrafiltration (Figure 36-4). Diffusion involves the movement of particles from an area of greater to an area of lesser concentration. In the body this usually occurs across a semipermeable membrane. Diffusion is involved in the clearance of solute from the patient's body in both hemodialysis and peritoneal dialysis. Diffusion results in the movement of urea, creatinine, and uric acid from the patient's blood into the dialysate. This solution contains fewer particles of substances to be removed from the bloodstream and high concentrations of particles of substances to be added to the blood (Figure 36-5). Because the dialysate contains no protein waste products, concentration of these substances in the blood decreases because of random movement of the particles across the semipermeable membrane into the dialysate. The same principle applies to the movement of potassium ions. Although blood has a high concentration of RBCs and protein, these molecules are large and do not diffuse through the membrane pores; thus they are not lost from the blood.

Osmosis involves the movement of water across a semipermeable membrane from an area of lesser to an area of greater concentration (osmolality) of particles. Osmosis is responsible for movement of extra fluid from the patient, particularly in peritoneal dialysis. Figure 36-5 shows that glucose has been added to the dialysate to make its particle concentration greater than that of the patient's blood. Fluid then moves through the pores of the membrane from the patient's blood to the dialysate.

Ultrafiltration involves the movement of fluid across a semipermeable membrane as a result of an artificially created pressure gradient. Ultrafiltration is more efficient than osmosis for removal of fluid and is used in hemodialysis for this purpose. During dialysis osmosis and diffusion or ultrafiltration and diffusion occur simultaneously.

Hemodialysis. Hemodialysis involves moving the patient's blood from the body, through a dialyzer (Figure 36-6) in which diffusion and ultrafiltration occur, and then back into the patient's circulation (Figure 36-7). Figure 36-8 shows an example of a hemodialysis machine. Hemodialysis requires access to the patient's bloodstream and a mechanism to transport the blood from the patient to the dialyzer (area in which the exchange of fluid, electrolytes, and waste products occurs) and then return the blood to the patient.[12] Currently the means of gaining access to the patient's bloodstream include the arteriovenous fistula; the arteriovenous graft; and catheterization of the femoral, interjugular, or subclavian veins (Table 36-6).

The access of choice for the hemodialysis patient is the **arteriovenous fistula** (AVF). This peripheral access is created in the operating room using the patient's native vessels. The artery and vein are anastomosed, allowing the arterial blood to be diverted into the vein. The increased blood flow through the vein stimulates intimal hyperplasia of the vein with a thickening of the vein wall (Figure 36-9). The vein "matures" over 6 to 12 weeks and is then able to be cannulated by the dialysis needles. A well-matured AVF is able to provide the high blood flow required for the dialysis procedure. If the fistula is cannulated before proper maturation, infil-

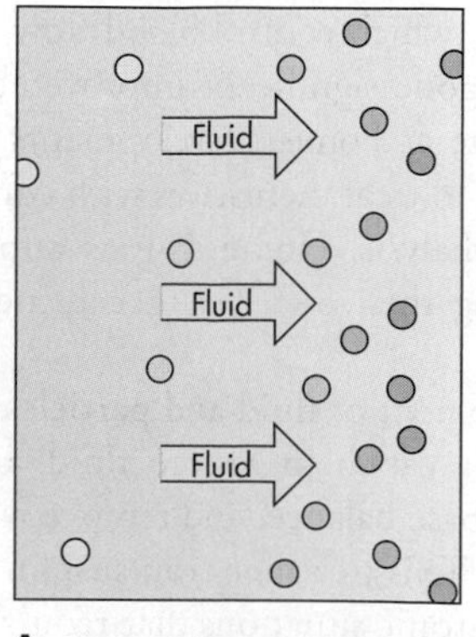

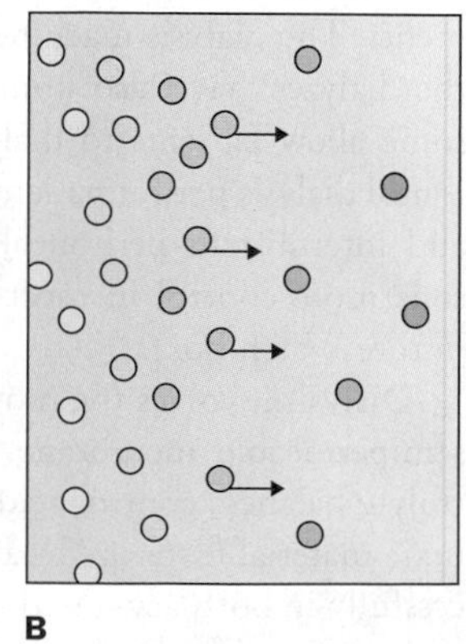

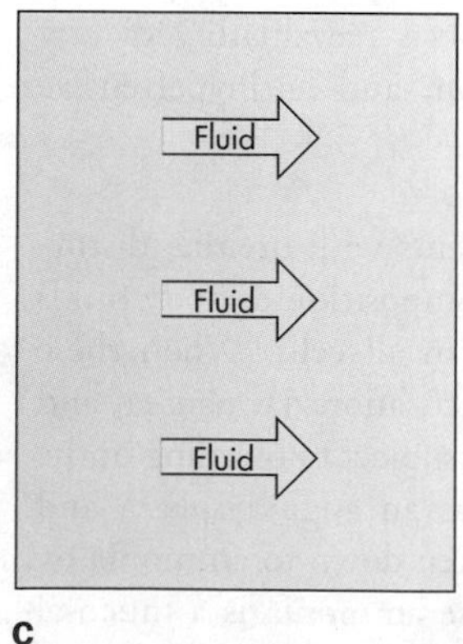

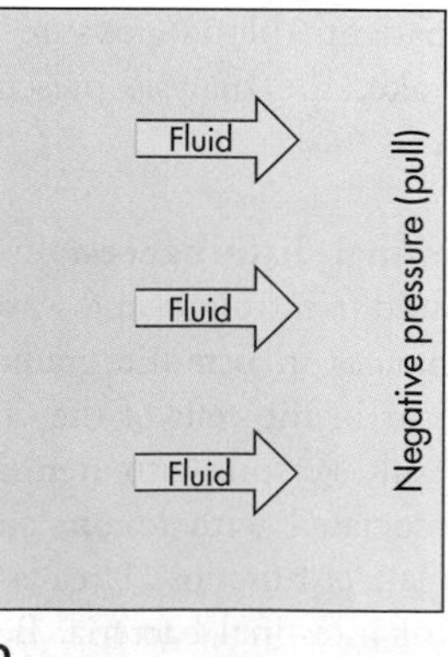

Figure 36-4 Semipermeable membrane. Dialysis is based on principles of osmosis **(A)**, diffusion **(B)**, and ultrafiltration. Ultrafiltration occurs when either positive pressure **(C)** or negative pressure **(D)** is placed on the system. Ultrafiltration can be maximized by simultaneously exerting both positive and negative pressure on the system.

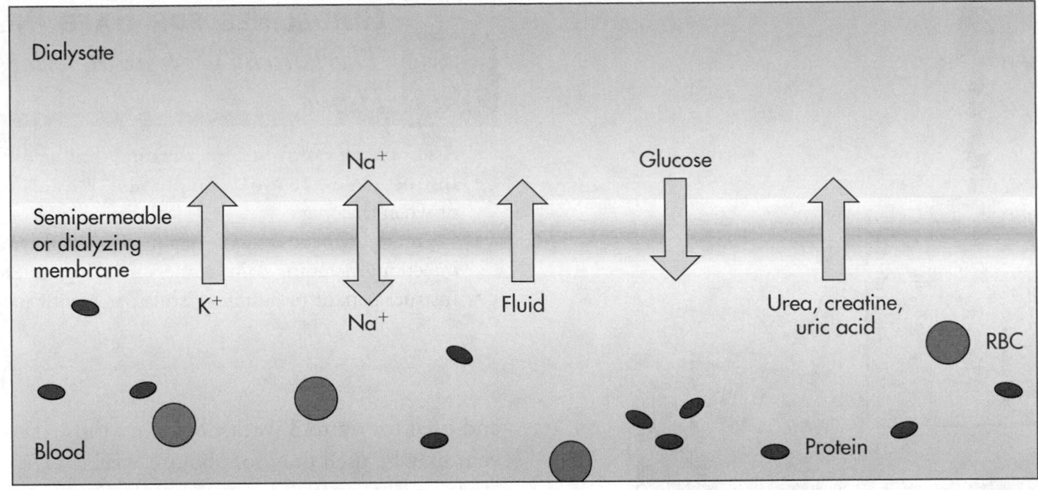

Figure 36-5 Osmosis and diffusion in dialysis. Net movement of major particles and fluid is illustrated. *K^+*, Potassium; *Na^+*, sodium; *RBC*, red blood cell.

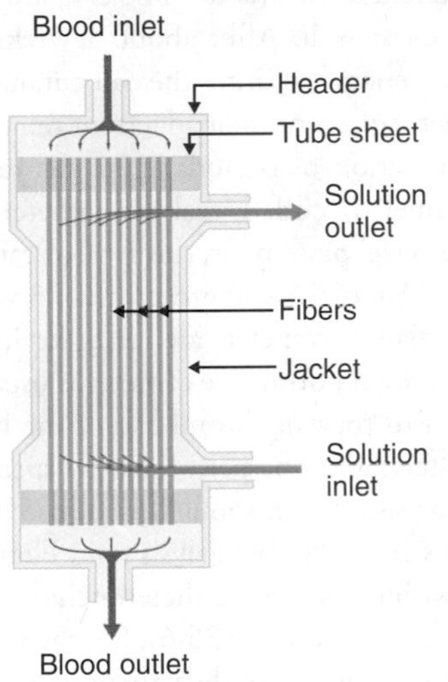

Figure 36-6 Hollow fiber dialyzer.

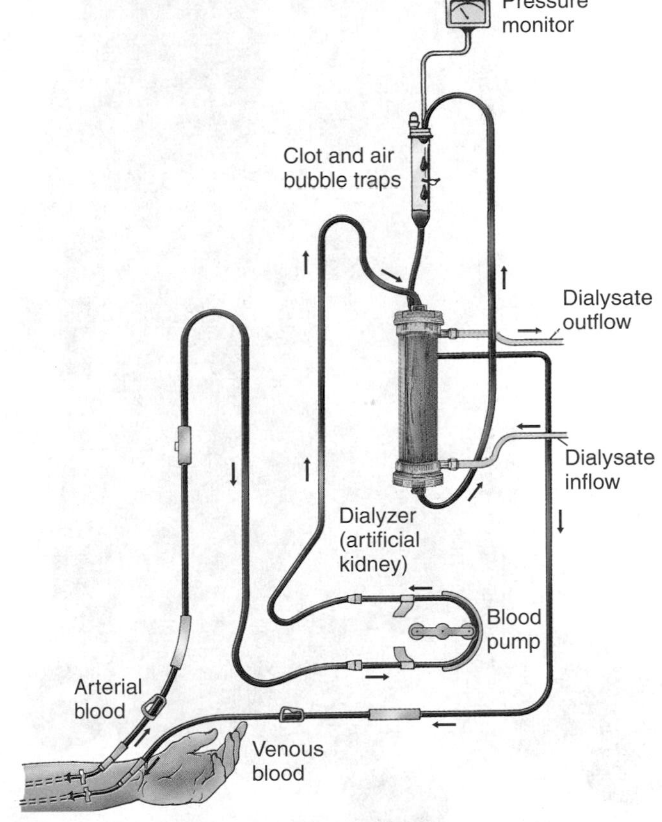

Figure 36-7 A hemodialysis circuit.

tration of the dialysis needle may occur. The patient may experience pain, edema, and hematoma[14] (see Guidelines for Safe Practice box).

Many patients do not have blood vessels that will support the development of an adequate AVF. Those patients with comorbid conditions such as vascular disease, diabetes, long-term hypertension, or advanced age may not be candidates for a fistula. These patients are candidates for placement of the arteriovenous graft (AVG). The AVG is placed in the operating room by anastomosing a piece of tubular, synthetic material to an artery; tunneling the material through the soft tissue; and finally anastomosing the graft to the vein. As with the AVF, blood flow is diverted into the graft material with outflow through the vein. After about 3 weeks the AVG becomes engrafted into the subcutaneous tissue and is ready for cannulation with dialysis needles. Over time, because of the increased blood flow, the venous outflow tract may become thickened, predisposing the AVG to thrombosis. Nursing implications for the patient with the AVG are the same as those for the patient with an AVF (Figure 36-10).

Dialysis catheters may also be used for hemodialysis access. These catheters may be placed in the femoral, internal jugular, or subclavian veins. In rare instances the catheters may be placed in other large vessels such as the inferior vena cava. The vessel of choice for the dialysis catheter is the internal jugular vein.

Temporary dialysis catheters are devices put in place at the patient's bedside or in a radiology suite for short-term dialysis use. These catheters are usually made of a firm plastic substance. This type of catheter is usually indicated for the patient with AKF or

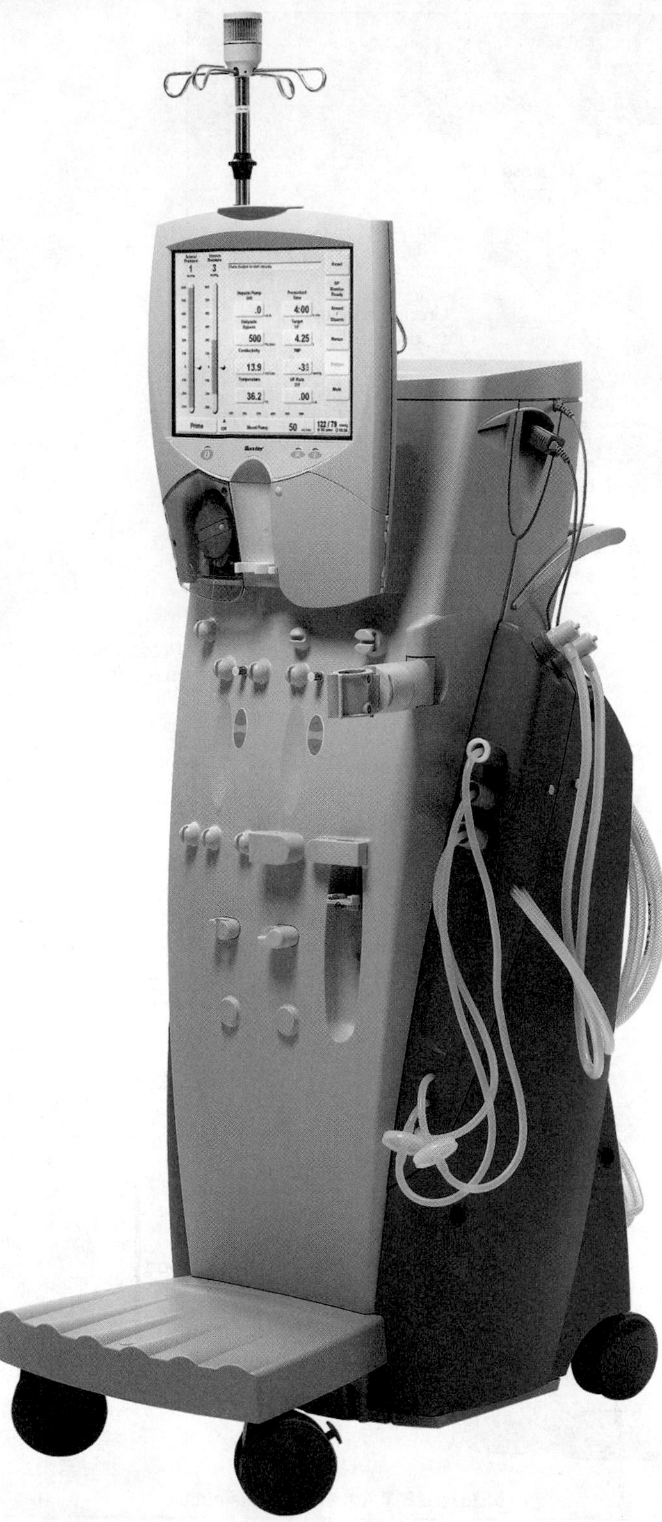

Figure 36-8 Baxter 1550 Hemodialysis Instrument.

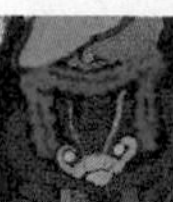

GUIDELINES FOR SAFE PRACTICE

The Patient With an Arteriovenous Fistula

- Assess patency of fistula by palpating thrill or auscultating bruit.
- Instruct patient to avoid compression of fistula by tight clothing or when sleeping.
- Instruct patient to assess fistula for signs and symptoms of infection, including pain, redness, swelling, or excessive warmth.
- Instruct patient to monitor fistula patency by palpating the thrill daily.

during the 3-week postoperative period after placement of an AVF or AVG (Figure 36-11). The procedure for placing these catheters is the same as that for placing any central venous catheter. The temporary dialysis catheter is large, usually about 12 F. Two lumina are present, one for outflow to the dialysis machine and one for return of blood to the patient. Temporary dialysis catheters placed in the internal jugular vein may be left in place and used for up to 3 weeks; however, those placed in the femoral vein may be used only for about 1 week.

Tunneled, cuffed hemodialysis catheters may be placed for long-term dialysis use. These catheters are made of a soft, silicone-like substance and are placed in the operating room or radiology suite. If the catheter is placed in the internal jugular vein, a tunnel is made in the subcutaneous tissue. The exit site of the catheter is on the anterior chest wall. After about 4 weeks the cuff of the catheter becomes engrafted into the subcutaneous tissue. This anchors the catheter, preventing inadvertent removal, and acts as a barrier to the migration of bacteria. Like the temporary dialysis catheter, the tunneled, cuffed dialysis catheter has two ports. Regardless of the vessel placement, this type of catheter may be left in place for long-term dialysis of greater than 3 weeks' duration.

Once placed, dialysis catheters are ready for immediate use. At the end of dialysis, each port of the catheter is usually instilled with high-dose heparin to prevent thrombosis of the lumina. Access of the dialysis catheter should be performed by specially trained persons only. The dialysis catheter should not be used for routine intravenous procedures except in the dialysis unit. Functional complications associated with the dialysis catheter include thrombosis of the catheter and infections (see Table 36-6). See the Guidelines for Safe Practice box, p. 1024, for care of the patient with a dialysis catheter.

Immediately before dialysis the nurse weighs the patient, takes vital signs, and assesses the patient's physical status. A sample of blood may be drawn to determine the level of serum electrolytes and waste products. Many patients expect to leave the dialysis treatment with a feeling of well-being. Few persons feel this way; most experience some minor discomfort that diminishes within several hours after dialysis. The greatest feeling of well-being seems to occur the day after dialysis.

Peritoneal dialysis. Peritoneal dialysis is used to treat AKF and CKF in the hospital or at home. Peritoneal dialysis involves instilling dialyzing fluid into the peritoneal cavity. The peritoneum serves as the dialyzing membrane (Figure 36-12). Peritoneal dialysis can be continuous for up to 36 hours or done intermittently in the hospital setting. The procedure, once instituted, becomes largely a nursing responsibility. Many patients find peritoneal dialysis to be advantageous because it allows them greater control (Box 36-7).

Procedure. Access to the peritoneum is gained through the introduction of a catheter into the peritoneal space. For patients who

TABLE 36-6 DIALYSIS ACCESS

Type	Usable	Comments
HEMODIALYSIS		
Central venous catheter (femoral, jugular, subclavian; avoid subclavian where possible)	Immediately	Usual maximum life of 2 wk. Complications include venous stenosis, which may prevent subsequent fistula or graft from being successful (particularly with subclavian catheters).
Tunneled central venous catheter	Immediately	May last 1 yr or more. Main complications are sepsis and catheter blockage.
Arteriovenous fistula	2-6 wk	May last indefinitely. Requires adequate artery and vein: Doppler studies can help assess patients with diabetes mellitus and peripheral vascular disease. Avoid cannulation of veins of forearm and wrist in patients likely to require fistula formation.
Arteriovenous graft	1-2 wk	More prone to thrombosis and infection than a fistula. Alternative for those whose vessels are inadequate for fistula formation.
PERITONEAL DIALYSIS ACCESS		
Hard cannula	Immediately	Usable for 1 wk.
Tenckhoff catheter	2 wk	Can be placed by minilaparotomy, laparoscopy, or percutaneous technique. Risk of fluid leaks increased by using the catheter sooner than 2 wk.

From Frasser D, Vinning M: Urologic nephrology. In Weiss RM, George N, O'Reilly PH, editors: *Comprehensive urology,* London, 2001, Mosby.

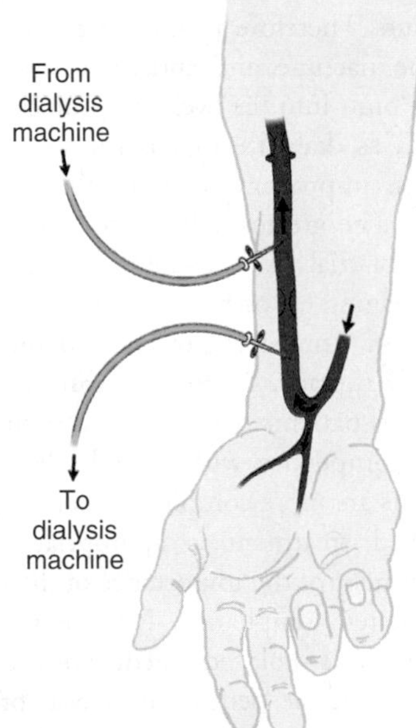

Figure 36-9 Arteriovenous fistula.

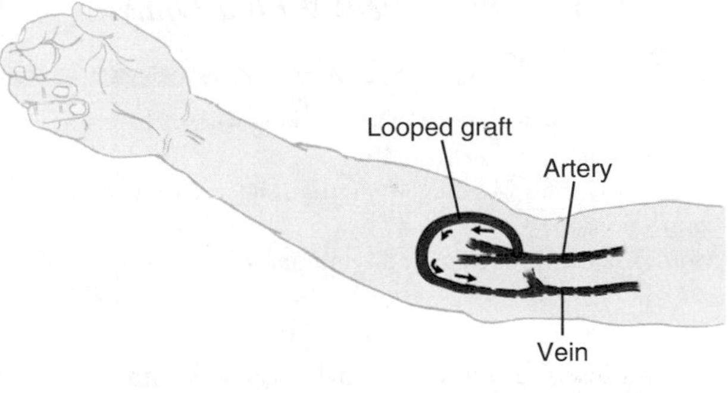

Figure 36-10 Arteriovenous graft.

require sporadic dialysis, a sterile catheter is inserted for each dialysis procedure. For the chronically ill person treated on a routine basis, a Tenckhoff peritoneal catheter can be placed into the peritoneal space; the catheter remains in place until it malfunctions or until another treatment option, such as transplantation, is selected. Because these catheters present a continuous portal of entry for organisms into the peritoneum, each patient must be thoroughly instructed in the care of the catheter and the signs and symptoms of local or peritoneal infection, which must be reported to the physician.

For all patients, the nurse records weight, blood pressure, and pulse before the procedure is initiated. These values serve as baseline information against which to assess changes during treatment. For persons undergoing insertion of a peritoneal catheter before dialysis, the nurse assesses their knowledge of the procedure and their anxiety level. A mild sedative may help the severely anxious person to better tolerate the insertion of the catheter. It is important that patients void before catheter insertion to decompress the bladder and prevent accidental puncture during catheter placement.

To insert a peritoneal catheter, the physician cleanses the abdomen and anesthetizes a small area in the midline of the abdomen about 5 cm (2 inches) below the umbilicus. The physician makes a small

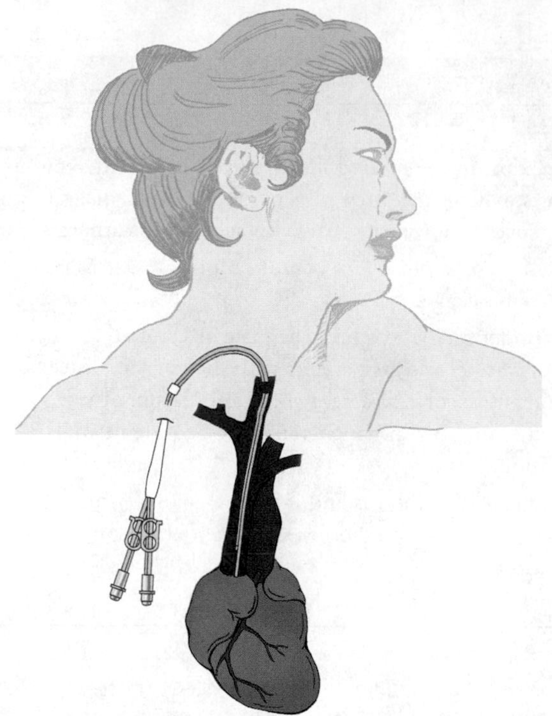

Figure 36-11 Venous catheter for temporary hemodialysis access.

GUIDELINES FOR SAFE PRACTICE
Care of the Patient With a Dialysis Catheter

- Maintain sterile technique when working with catheters or catheter exit site.
- Assess patient for bleeding at insertion site and tubing connections.
- Monitor patient for signs and symptoms of infection.

incision and inserts a multilumen nylon catheter into the peritoneal cavity. A dressing is placed around the protruding catheter.

Approximately 2 L of warm, sterile dialysate is attached by tubing to the catheter and allowed to run into the peritoneal cavity as rapidly as possible. This usually takes about 10 minutes. The tubing is then clamped. The maximal osmosis of fluid and diffusion of particles into the dialysate occurs in 20 to 30 minutes. At the end of the dwell time (amount of time the dialysate is left in the peritoneal cavity), the tubing is unclamped and the fluid is allowed to flow by gravity from the abdomen. Fluid should drain in a steady stream. Drainage time should average about 10 to 15 minutes. The first drainage may be pink-tinged as a result of the trauma of catheter insertion; however, drainage should clear with the second or third cycle. At no time should fluid draining from the abdomen be grossly bloody. After fluid has drained from the abdomen, another cycle is started immediately. Dialysis is initiated for the person with a permanent catheter by carefully cleansing the catheter and surrounding skin with a bactericidal agent before the catheter is connected to the dialysate line. After the infusion of dialysate has been completed, the permanent catheter is again cleansed and a sterile cap is applied to the tip.

If the procedure is temporary, the catheter is removed, and the incision is covered with a dry, sterile dressing. The small abdominal wound from the catheter should heal completely in 1 to 2 days[13] (see Guidelines for Safe Practice box).

Other approaches to peritoneal dialysis. Several advances in the management of patients with ESRD have led to two variations of peritoneal dialysis. Continuous ambulatory peritoneal dialysis (CAPD) and continuous cyclic peritoneal dialysis (CCPD) are primarily for home and self-dialysis use.

CAPD is a method of self-dialysis that is practical, relatively inexpensive compared with hemodialysis, and conducive to independence. CAPD involves continuous contact of dialysate with the peritoneal membrane. Approximately 2 L of dialysate is maintained in the peritoneal cavity and exchanged by the patient through a permanent peritoneal catheter four or five times each day. No special equipment is required for the exchanges, but patient education is imperative. CAPD allows the patient to lead a fairly normal life. Exchanges can take place at home or at work by connecting an empty bag to the catheter and opening a clamp to allow drainage. A full dialysate bag is then instilled, and the patient has completed an exchange.

CCPD differs from CAPD in that a machine known as a cycler is used to instill and drain dialysate from the patient (Figure 36-13). The machine has a series of time-controlled clamps. The timers open and close the clamps in sequence to allow for instillation and drainage of dialysate from the patient. The cycle times for patients with CKF generally allow for the patient to be dialyzed in 6 to 8 hours. Therefore a patient can connect to the cycler at bedtime, set the machine, and undergo dialysis while sleeping. Several alarms are built into the cycler to protect the patient from malfunctions such as dialysate that is too hot or cold, long or short dwell times, improper return of fluid, and changes in catheter pressures. The greatest advantage of CAPD and CCPD over other forms of dialysis is the unprecedented freedom the patient has in managing his or her own care.

Compliance is of utmost importance to the success of any CAPD and CCPD therapy. Conditions causing noncompliance in peritoneal dialysis patients have not been adequately analyzed. From studies on compliance with chronic drug regimens, it is known that patients are more compliant when they are convinced that the prescribed treatment is appropriate and beneficial. Frequent reinforcement of the importance of the treatment also is associated with better compliance. For the CAPD or CCPD patient, special emphasis is placed on education about the importance and technique of the peritoneal dialysis prescription. The nurse should repeat the instructions at least every 6 months and monitor patients for changes in compliance.[14]

Evaluating Dialysis Effectiveness. Numerous outcome studies have demonstrated a correlation between the delivered dose of hemodialysis and patient mortality and morbidity.[14] Clinical signs and symptoms alone are not reliable indicators of hemodialysis adequacy. To ensure that ESRD patients treated with chronic hemodialysis receive a sufficient amount, the delivered dose should be measured and monitored routinely.[19] *Kinetic modeling,* or prescription dialysis, is a tool developed by dialysis practitioners in the past decade to compute how much dialysis an individual needs.

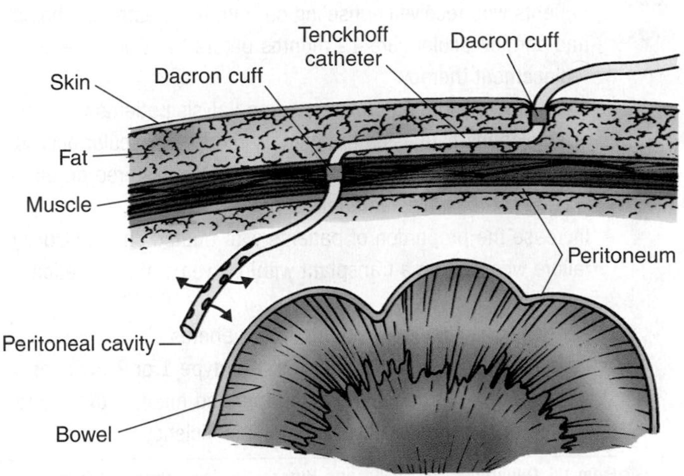

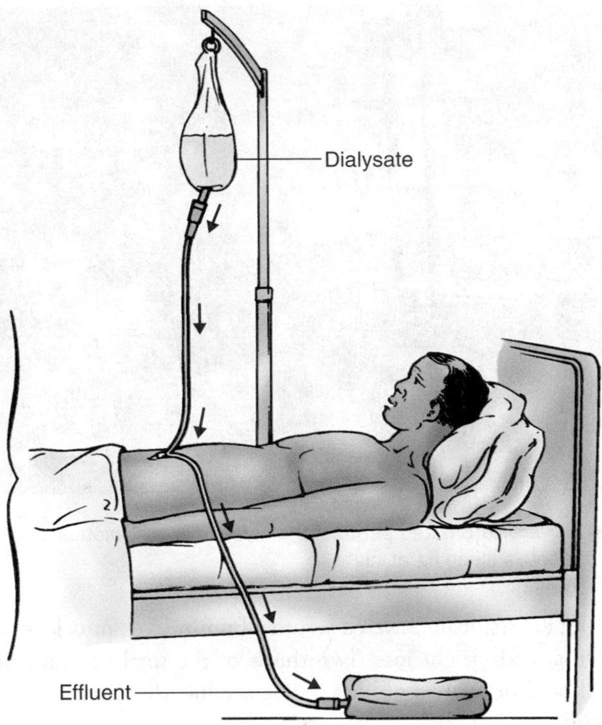

Figure 36-12 Manual peritoneal dialysis via an implanted Tenckhoff catheter.

Box 36-7 Advantages of Peritoneal Dialysis

- Provides a steady state of blood chemistry values
- Is a process that is easily taught to patients
- Allows patients to dialyze alone in any location without the need for machinery
- Requires few dietary restrictions; because of loss of protein in dialysate, usual diet is high protein
- Provides patients with more control over daily life
- Can be used for patients who are hemodynamically unstable

Kinetic modeling monitors the effectiveness of the delivered prescription. Nephrology practitioners usually prescribe hemodialysis based on the mathematic formula Kt/V, where K represents individual patient parameters of dialyzer clearance, t equals of dialysis, and V is the volume of urea distribution. In addition, care providers must determine and periodically reassess the patient's normalized protein catabolic rate. Using serum urea levels as the kinetic factor, practitioners are able to determine an expected outcome of treatment. If the patient's Kt/V is calculated to be inadequate, the patient's dialysis time or blood flow may be increased. A peritoneal dialysis patient may need to increase the number of dialysis exchanges.[13] See Nursing Care Plan, pp. 1028 and 1029.

SURGICAL MANAGEMENT. Kidney transplantation (discussed later) reverses many of the pathophysiologic changes associated with kidney failure. It also eliminates the dependence on dialysis and the need for dietary restrictions, provides the opportunity to return to normal life activities, and is more cost-effective than dialysis after the first year.

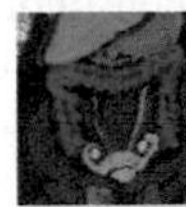

GUIDELINES FOR SAFE PRACTICE
Peritoneal Dialysis

- Regulate fluid volume and drainage.
  —Assess vital signs.
  —Monitor mental status.
  —Record fluid balance after each cycle.
  —Turn patient side to side to facilitate drainage.
  —Elevate head of bed.
- Promote comfort.
  —Administer analgesics as ordered.
  —Provide diversional activities.
  —Encourage side-to-side movement.
  —Assist with oral care and feeding.
- Prevent complications.
  —Assess respiratory effort.
  —Encourage frequent small meals.
  —Use aseptic technique.
  —Culture dialysate as directed.
  —Monitor temperature.
  —Observe for nausea, vomiting, abdominal tenderness, and cloudy outflow.

DIET. The goals of diet therapy are to (1) reduce the quantity of metabolic waste that requires excretion by the kidney, (2) provide sufficient calories and protein for growth and repair while limiting excretory demands on the kidney, (3) minimize metabolic bone disease, and (4) minimize fluid and electrolyte disturbances. The dietary protein restriction is calculated at 1 to 1.5 g/kg ideal body weight. Adequate protein intake is reflected by a BUN/creatinine ratio of 10:1. Excessive intake of protein results in nausea and vomiting, apathy, weakness, and neurologic symptoms. Insufficient

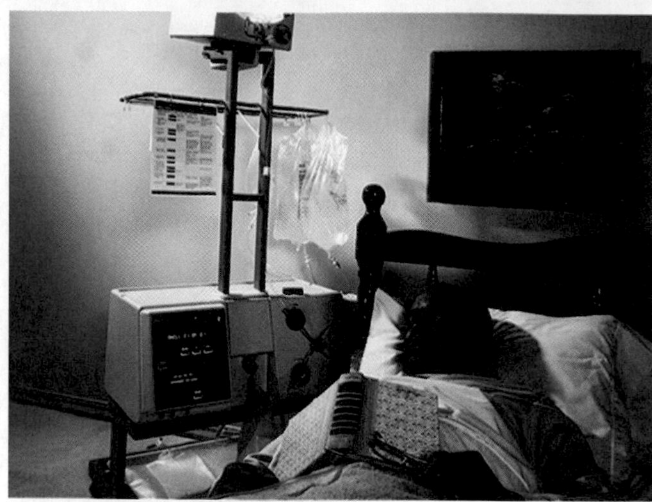

Figure 36-13 Automated peritoneal dialysis cycler, which is used while patient is sleeping at night.

protein intake results in lowered serum albumin level, muscle wasting, edema, and weight loss. Two thirds of the total protein consumed should be protein of high biologic value, that is, containing the essential amino acids.

Ample calories are obtained from carbohydrates and fats because they do not require renal excretion of their metabolic byproducts. This spares protein for growth and repair. Catabolism of existing protein stores liberates nitrogenous wastes. For this reason, sources of potential infection such as indwelling catheters are avoided. When infection is noted, it is immediately treated.

Health Promotion and Prevention

Primary prevention. Obstruction and infection of the urinary tract and hypertensive disease are common and often asymptomatic causes of kidney damage and failure. A significant reduction in the incidence of CKF can be achieved through increasing attention to general health promotion. Yearly physical examinations in which blood pressure is measured, urinalysis is performed, and the person is questioned about dysuria or urinary tract pain assist in early detection of diseases that may lead to CKF. Meticulous blood glucose control in diabetic persons is critical in reducing kidney failure.

Secondary prevention. General health maintenance can reduce the number of individuals who progress from kidney insufficiency to frank kidney failure. The aim of care is to adequately treat medical problems and closely supervise the person's health status in times of stress (e.g., infection or pregnancy).

Healthy People 2010. *Healthy People 2010* has targeted chronic kidney disease as a focus area for specific improvement. The objectives developed include reduction of the rates of new cases of ESRD, deaths from cardiovascular disease in persons with CKF, and kidney failure resulting from diabetes (see Healthy People 2010 box).[23]

Kidney disease outcomes quality initiative. Despite significant improvements in dialysis technology, many opportunities for further improvement remain. The publication of the National Kidney Foundation–Dialysis Outcomes Quality Initiative (DOQI) Clinical Practice Guidelines in 1997 represented the first comprehensive effort to give evidence-based guidance to clinical care teams. The initial four areas covered by the guidelines included hemodialysis adequacy, peritoneal dialysis adequacy, management of vascular access, and management of anemia. Each recommendation in the guidelines is accompanied by a rationale, enabling dialysis caregivers to make informed decisions about the proper care plan for each patient.[10a]

In 2000 the National Kidney Foundation revised these guidelines, expanding the DOQI to encompass the spectrum of chronic kidney disease well before the need for dialysis. Prevention and early intervention can delay or prevent the need for dialysis and improve outcomes for patients with ESRD. More recently, guidelines related to nutrition, bone metabolism and disease, hypertension, and management of dyslipidemias have been added. To reflect this expansion, the initiative is now known as the Kidney Disease Outcomes Quality Initiative.

Healthy People 2010

Objectives Related to Chronic Renal Disease

- Reduce the rate of new cases of end-stage renal disease.
- Reduce deaths from cardiovascular disease in persons with chronic kidney failure.
- Increase the proportion of treated chronic kidney failure patients who receive counseling on nutrition, treatment choices, and cardiovascular care 12 months before the start of renal replacement therapy.
- Increase the proportion of new hemodialysis patients who use arteriovenous fistulas as the primary mode of vascular access.
- Increase the proportion of dialysis patients registered on the waiting list for transplantation.
- Increase the proportion of patients with treated chronic kidney failure who receive a transplant within 3 years of registration on the waiting list.
- Reduce kidney failure resulting from diabetes.
- Increase the proportion of persons with type 1 or 2 diabetes and proteinuria who receive recommended medical therapy to reduce progression to chronic renal insufficiency.

From US Department of Health and Human Services: *Healthy people 2010: understanding and improving health*, Washington, DC, 2000, The Department.

▶ ARE YOU READY?

Which of the following is an appropriate dietary intake of protein for a patient with chronic kidney failure with an ideal body weight of 165 pounds?

1. 50 g
2. 85 g
3. 125 g
4. 165 g

Nursing Management

of the Patient with Chronic Kidney Failure

ASSESSMENT

Health History. Assess for:

- Current medications
- Recent changes in patterns of elimination (abrupt or gradual decrease in urinary output)
- Fatigue, lethargy
- Nausea, vomiting
- Pruritus
- Chronic diseases or conditions
- Muscle weakness
- Difficulty with concentration, confusion
- History of hypertension
- Exposure to nephrotoxins

Physical Examination. Assess for:

- Amount of urine excreted in 24 hours
- Increased or decreased blood pressure, particularly with postural changes
- Fluid status: presence of peripheral, periorbital, or sacral edema; lung sounds; skin turgor; daily weight
- Halitosis (ammonia smell to breath)
- Disorientation, confusion
- Tachycardia, dysrhythmias
- Weight (compared to ideal body weight)
- Ecchymosis
- Pallor
- Increased pigmentation

NURSING DIAGNOSES, OUTCOMES, AND INTERVENTIONS

Nursing Diagnosis: Excess Fluid Volume

OUTCOMES. A common example of expected outcomes for the patient with a diagnosis of *excess fluid volume* is:

Patient will:

- Be free from respiratory distress, peripheral edema, hypertension, or other signs and symptoms indicating fluid and electrolyte imbalance.

NURSING INTERVENTIONS. The person with CKF must learn to identify signs of imbalances, take fluids in the prescribed amounts, and eat within the prescribed limits. This requires careful monitoring of intake and output. Controlling sodium intake can be an extremely challenging for both the nurse and patient. Any sudden increase in weight indicates accumulating fluid, and the nurse must discuss the source of this fluid with the patient. When the patient is not acutely ill and is responsible for diet restrictions, the problem can often be traced to excess sodium ingestion, which produces thirst. To avoid this cycle of sodium-driven thirst leading to increased fluid ingestion and overhydration, the nurse teaches the patient about the amount of sodium and fluid allowed in the diet and restrictions to observe when purchasing prepared foods. The patient should check the words *sodium* and *salt* on all food labels and avoid salt substitutes, since these substitutes contain large amounts of potassium (see Guidelines for Safe Practice box, p. 1030).

Sometimes patients are unable to explain their increasing thirst and sodium ingestion. At this point the question of self-medication is raised. The person may be taking over-the-counter antacids that are high in sodium. If the nurse cannot identify the cause of the hypervolemia, he or she asks the patient to list all foods and fluids ingested over the previous 3 days. This list can be used to uncover dietary indiscretions and can serve as a teaching tool to reinforce the prescribed diet.

Nursing care of the patient during hemodialysis centers around (1) monitoring physical status before and during dialysis for evidence of physiologic imbalance and change, (2) providing comfort and safety, and (3) helping the patient understand and adjust to the care and changes in lifestyle. This latter objective involves educating the person on the specifics of the treatment program (especially diet and medications) and how these relate to altered kidney function. The nurse encourages the patient to express concerns and feelings and tries to help the individual work through these feelings. If dialysis is performed at home, the patient and dialysis partner must be able to institute all the care described. Hemodialysis treatments last 3 to 5 hours (see Box 36-7).

RELATED NIC INTERVENTIONS. Fluid Management, Fluid Monitoring, Electrolyte Management, Electrolyte Monitoring, Nutrition Management

Nursing Diagnosis: Imbalanced Nutrition: Less Than Body Requirements

OUTCOMES. Common examples of expected outcomes for the patient with a diagnosis of *imbalanced nutrition: less than body requirements* are:

Patient will:

- Accurately explain dietary plan, including fluid, protein, potassium, and sodium restrictions.
- Maintain estimated ideal body weight and lean body mass.

NURSING INTERVENTIONS. Persons usually need help planning diets within the prescribed sodium, potassium, phosphorus, and protein limits. Modifying the diet to the individual's preferences can help maintain appropriate intake of food. Dietary teaching and meal planning can be approached using an exchange system similar to that used for persons with diabetes. The nurse should refer patients for counseling by a registered dietitian specializing in kidney disease.

The nurse can promote compliance with a modified diet by attempting to decrease emotional tension at the dinner table. Food that is attractively arranged and flavorful is also likely to promote appetite. Herbs and other flavorings can add variety to foods that are prepared without sodium. When the GI tract is ulcerated, bland foods may be tried in an attempt to increase ingestion.

The nurse instructs patients that the adverse effects of iron on the GI tract (nausea and constipation) can be avoided or minimized by taking iron on a full stomach and by adding a stool softener or laxative to the medication regimen. Furthermore, patients should avoid simultaneous ingestion of iron and phosphate binders, since

Nursing Care Plan

The Patient With Kidney Failure Undergoing Dialysis

Data A 52-year-old man has a long history of diabetes mellitus and hypertension. He worked full time until 3 months ago, at which time his kidney function had decreased to the point of requiring hemodialysis. The patient is married and has three adolescent children. Because of financial hardship, his wife had to take a full-time job. The patient finds his present situation depressing and confides that he seems to be losing control over his life.

Nursing assessment reveals that the patient is scheduled for hemodialysis three times weekly. His treatments take about 4 hours each. He had a functioning arteriovenous fistula in his left arm. His blood pressure ranged from 180/100 to 190/110 mm Hg before dialysis and 120/70 to 100/64 mm Hg after dialysis. He often complains of a headache during dialysis.

Nursing Diagnosis

Excess fluid volume related to fluid accumulation secondary to kidney failure

Outcomes

- Patient will maintain fluid volume status within established parameters.

Related NOC Outcomes

- Electrolyte and Acid/Base Balance
- Fluid Balance

Related NIC Interventions

- Acid-Base Management
- Fluid/Electrolyte Management
- Hemodialysis Therapy
- Hypervolemia Management

Nursing Interventions/Rationales

- Assess weight, lung sounds, and extremities for presence of edema. *To determine fluid volume so that treatment parameters can be identified.*
- Monitor intake and output. *Some patients continue to urinate small amounts, but it is inadequate to clear all waste products. Intake is limited and must be monitored to prevent fluid volume overload.*
- Monitor laboratory data: blood urea nitrogen (BUN); serum creatinine, sodium, potassium, calcium, magnesium, and phosphorus levels; hemoglobin and hematocrit. *Nitrogenous waste and electrolytes accumulate between treatments. Anemia and blood losses associated with hemodialysis are complications associated with kidney failure.*
- Teach patient the need for maintaining treatment fluid restrictions. *To prevent excess intake, which can lead to hypervolemia.*
- Teach patient the need for restricting sodium intake. *Sodium intake stimulates thirst, which can lead to excessive fluid intake and subsequent hypervolemia.*

Nursing Diagnosis

Risk for infection related to frequent invasive procedure

Outcomes

- Patient will remain free from infections.

Related NOC Outcomes

- Immune Status
- Risk Control

Related NIC Interventions

- Hemodialysis Therapy
- Infection Protection
- Surveillance

Nursing Interventions/Rationales

- Maintain Standard Precautions for exposure to blood and body fluids. *To protect both patient and nurse.*
- Maintain sterile technique when performing access site puncture and discontinuing hemodialysis. *To prevent site contamination with microorganisms.*
- Assess site for signs of localized infection (warmth, redness, swelling, tenderness). *To detect infection so that treatment can be initiated.*
- Monitor temperature and white blood cell count. *To detect systemic infection so that treatment can be initiated.*
- Follow routine testing policies for hepatitis B and C and human immunodeficiency virus antibodies. *To identify change in patient status. Patients are monitored monthly and staff is monitored yearly.*

Nursing Diagnosis

Risk for ineffective therapeutic regimen management related to change in life status and dependency on dialysis

Outcomes

- Patient will verbalize (and demonstrate) adherence to therapeutic regimen as prescribed.

Related NOC Outcomes

- Family Normalization
- Health Beliefs: Perceived Control
- Health Beliefs: Perceived Resources

phosphate binders impede the absorption of oral iron. The risk of constipation is also high in persons with CKF because of the fluid restrictions and required medication therapy. Stool softeners or laxatives may be needed.

Related NIC Interventions. Fluid/Electrolyte Management, Nutrition Management, Nutritional Counseling, Nutritional Monitoring, Weight Management

Nursing Diagnosis: Risk for Infection

Outcomes. Common examples of expected outcomes for the patient with a diagnosis of *risk for infection* are:

Patient will:

- Remain free from infection.
- Maintain intact skin and mucous membranes.

Nursing Interventions. Tissue breakdown leads to infection. Edematous skin poses a high risk for skin breakdown; therefore daily skin care is important. The nurse should provide meticulous care of the dialysis access. Patients with CKF should avoid others with infections and seek medical attention when symptoms of infections, GI bleeding, or other problems first appear.

For patients undergoing peritoneal dialysis, care must be taken to avoid contaminating the solution or the tubing. The

- Knowledge: Treatment Regimen

Related NIC Interventions
- Family Support
- Financial Resource Assistance
- Mutual Goal Setting
- Role Enhancement
- Self-Modification Assistance

Nursing Interventions/Rationales
- Monitor for indications of noncompliance with treatment plan (abnormal laboratory data, missed appointments, excess fluid weight gain, verbalizations of noncompliance). *To determine whether patient is adhering to the prescribed treatment plan.*
- Determine factors that may interfere with patient's ability to adhere to treatment plan. *To assist patient with treatment plan adherence.*
- Encourage patient to participate in decision making about his own care. *Allows patient some control over his situation and increases the likelihood of adherence to treatment plan.*
- Prepare patient and family for community dialysis center by reviewing location of center and introducing them to a center representative who can review policies and procedures with them. *Preparing the patient and family will give them time to work through their fears about the unknown, reduce anxiety, and increase the likelihood of compliance.*
- Acknowledge the impact that chronic renal failure and hemodialysis has on the family. *The family is subjected to disruption, expenses, and considerable alterations in family routines to accommodate a patient with end-stage renal failure on dialysis.*
- Explore with patient and family their perception of the demands that the illness has made on them. *The family's perceptions and ability to cope affect patient outcomes both positively and negatively.*
- Support patient and family coping skills. *Previously successful coping skills can strengthen the family in new situations.*
- Refer to support group as appropriate. *Group members often provide mutual support and share beneficial information with one another.*

Nursing Diagnosis
Situational low self-esteem related to chronic kidney failure requiring machine dependency and loss of family status

Outcomes
- Patient will verbalize feelings and concerns.
- Patient will demonstrate behaviors that indicate positive self-esteem.

Related NOC Outcomes
- Acceptance: Health Status
- Body Image
- Grief Resolution
- Self-Esteem

Related NIC Interventions
- Body Image Enhancement
- Mutual Goal Setting
- Self-Esteem Enhancement
- Support Group

Nursing Interventions/Rationales
- Monitor patient's response to illness and treatments. *To determine the effect of health status changes so that appropriate interventions can be planned.*
- Allow patient to grieve over his losses. *Grieving is a necessary part of recovery.*
- Acknowledge patient's grief about being dependent on a machine. *Demonstrates empathy and validates patient's feelings.*
- Support strengths, self-confidence, determination, and motivation to live. *Dialysis patients are not disabled in all aspects of life. Many patients live near-normal lives while maintaining treatment schedules.*
- Help patient develop or continue interests beyond dialysis and return to as near a normal life as possible. *Patient may tend to withdraw from social activities because of new schedule and feelings of loss. Focusing on other interests will help the patient place less focus on his dependency.*
- Monitor for excessive expressed concerns about losses, depression, self-neglect, and noncompliance. *These may be indications of suicidal ideation, which needs to be identified and treated quickly.*
- Explore patient's feelings about changes in sexual functioning. *Renal failure characteristically produces infertility and decreased libido and can interfere with the patient's marital and sexual life.*

Evaluation
Evaluation is based on comparing the patient's outcomes with desired outcomes.

nurse performs cultures of the dialysate fluid routinely to rule out infection, assesses the patient for signs of peritonitis, and teaches the patient to recognize the symptoms at home. Signs of peritonitis include an elevated temperature, chills, abdominal pain or tenderness, nausea and vomiting, and cloudy outflow of solution. If these signs develop, the patient should contact the health care provider immediately (see Patient/Family Teaching box).

RELATED NIC INTERVENTIONS. Environmental Management, Infection Protection, Nutrition Management, Surveillance

Nursing Diagnosis: Risk for Injury. Possible etiologic factors associated with the risk for injury include sensorimotor deficits, lack of awareness of environmental hazards, fatigue, and decreased level of consciousness.

OUTCOMES. A common example of expected outcomes for the patient with a diagnosis of *risk for injury* is:

Patient will:
- Remain free from injury.

NURSING INTERVENTIONS. Extensive tissue damage must be avoided, since it can liberate a lethal amount of potassium (largely an intracellular cation) into the system of the person with CKF.

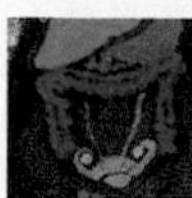

GUIDELINES FOR SAFE PRACTICE *The Patient With Chronic Kidney Failure*

- Maintain fluid and electrolyte balance.
  —Monitor for fluid and electrolyte excess.
    —Assess intake and output every 8 hours.
    —Weigh patient every day.
    —Assess presence and extent of edema.
    —Auscultate breath sounds.
    —Monitor pulse and blood pressure every 8 hours.
    —Assess level of consciousness every 8 hours.
  —Encourage patient to remain within prescribed fluid restrictions.
  —Provide small quantities of fluid spaced over the day to stay within fluid restrictions.
  —Encourage a diet high in carbohydrates and within the prescribed sodium, potassium, phosphorus, and protein limits.
  —Administer phosphate-binding agents with meals as prescribed.
- Prevent infection and injury.
  —Promote meticulous skin care.
  —Encourage activity within prescribed limits while avoiding fatigue.
  —Protect confused person from injury.
  —Protect person from exposure to infectious agents.
  —Maintain good medical-surgical asepsis during treatments and procedures.
  —Avoid aspirin products.
  —Encourage use of soft toothbrush.
- Promote comfort.
  —Medicate patient as needed for pain.
  —Medicate with prescribed antipruritics, use emollient baths, keep skin moist, and control environmental temperature to modify pruritus.
  —Encourage use of damp cloth to keep lips moist; give good oral hygiene.
  —Encourage rest for fatigue; however, encourage self-care as tolerated.
  —Provide calm, supportive atmosphere.
- Assist with coping in lifestyle and self-concept.
  —Promote hope.
  —Provide opportunity for patient to express feelings about self.
  —Identify available community resources.

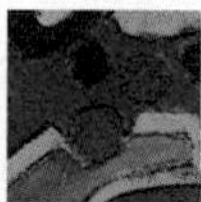

PATIENT/FAMILY TEACHING *Dialysis*

Teaching for person undergoing dialysis includes information about:
- The process of dialysis and its relationship to body needs
- Common side effects of treatment, means of controlling mild symptoms, and means of obtaining medical attention for severe or persistent complications
- Changes in medication schedule required before and after dialysis
- Work and activity schedules as physical capabilities permit

Specific information for persons undergoing hemodialysis includes:
- Appropriate care of the permanent peritoneal catheter
- How to care for the vascular access site, including the prevention of infection and clotting

Specific information for persons undergoing peritoneal dialysis includes:
- Appropriate care of the peritoneal dialysis access site
- Signs and symptoms of infection of the peritoneal cavity or catheter site, and where to obtain care if these occur

Other important nursing activities include helping the patient control blood loss. The nurse advises the patient to use a soft toothbrush for oral care; to observe for melena and report this without delay to the physician; to avoid aspirin, since it is normally excreted by the kidneys and may rapidly build to toxic levels and prolong bleeding time; and to avoid regular use of NSAIDs because of increased risk of GI bleeding and prolonged bleeding time.

The buildup of osmotically active particles and fluid in the body that occurs with kidney failure produces changes in brain cells that may lead to confusion and impaired decision-making ability. Fluid accumulation and hypertension can produce visual changes. The nurse assesses the person's environment for potential for injury. At times the person may need help in limiting activities to a level commensurate with mental processes and level of awareness. For example, blurred vision and delayed reaction time contraindicate driving a motor vehicle.

RELATED NIC INTERVENTIONS. Environmental Management: Safety, Fall Prevention, Risk Identification

Nursing Diagnosis: Ineffective Coping

OUTCOMES. Common examples of expected outcomes for the patient with a diagnosis of *ineffective coping* are:

Patient will:
- Describe methods of effective coping.
- Exhibit ability to perform activities of daily living (ADLs) and desired activities independently.

NURSING INTERVENTIONS. The goals of therapy for patients with ESRD include not only preservation of life, but also restoration of optimal quality of life, which is related to their function in the physical-medical, ADL, psychologic, and social-occupational dimensions.[10]

Optimal psychosocial care of patients with CKF requires careful and sophisticated psychosocial patient assessment. The physician, nurse, and social worker accomplish this assessment as a collaborative effort. Common psychologic problems include dysphoric moods (anxiety, depression, frustration, and anger), impaired body image (with a perceived loss of physical attractiveness), impaired self-esteem, and suicidal crises.

Noncompliance with the treatment regimen is a common behavioral problem; this may encompass treatment participation, diet and fluid restriction, and medications, as well as noncompliance with other medical diagnostic and therapeutic procedures. Several factors contribute to noncompliance: the intrusive and demanding aspects of chronic dialysis regimen, feelings of frustration and depression, a desire to maintain control over one's life and deny the unpleasant reality of chronic illness, a need to indirectly express anger toward staff members, and attempts to balance health concerns with a short-term need for pleasure.

Interventions that may effectively reverse significant patient noncompliance include (1) providing further information about the rationale for treatment procedures or restrictions, (2) helping the patient regain as much constructive control as possible over life's activities, (3) communicating with staff members to gather information and to design and implement a program to reward increased patient compliance, and (4) working with family members to educate them and enlist their support.

Social problems for patients with ESRD include strains in intimate relationships, loss of vocational function, and restriction of social and leisure activities. The introduction of a serious life-threatening illness such as ESRD is an added stress dimension to the already enormous demands placed on the contemporary family system. Role changes are common in families; spouses often take on the role responsibilities of the sick partner while maintaining their own roles. This leads to reduced rest and leisure for the spouse and lowers physical reserves. Families and patients must make major adjustments in thinking and living, while trying to maintain and nurture relationships. Nursing staff must be aware that professional caregivers may need to provide additional social support for patients, especially when family members take little responsibility for either physical or emotional support. These staff members may be viewed as important "significant others" for the patient with ESRD (see Research box).

Vocational dysfunction is a result of decreased physical capacities, the time-intensive requirements of dialysis, depression and cognitive impairment, governmental policies about reimbursement for dialysis medical care, and the reluctance of employers to hire individuals with kidney disease. The problems of vocational function are complex, particularly for patients with limited skills whose previous work involved manual labor. Implications for nursing and social work consist of identifying patients beginning dialysis and providing vocational counseling.

Each year more than 10,000 deaths in the United States are preceded by decisions to withdraw dialysis.[4] Because patient autonomy in the United States is the overriding legal imperative to accepting treatment, patient wishes must be honored. If the patient believes that the burdens of a life with impaired quality are so great that continuation of therapy offers no benefit but only prolongs a miserable existence, then discontinuing dialysis is reasonable. This is not considered suicide by the major religious groups (Protestant, Catholic, Jewish, Muslim, and Buddhist). Patients are apprehensive about the process of dying; they fear pain and discomfort. Nurses can assure patients and families that death associated with complications of kidney failure, usually hyperkalemia, is generally quiet, peaceful, and without pain or discomfort. Hospice care is helpful for patients who wish to remain at home (see Chapter 8 for a discussion of end-of-life care).

RELATED NIC INTERVENTIONS. Anxiety Reduction, Coping Enhancement, Decision-Making Support, Emotional Support, Teaching: Individual

Patient/Family Teaching. Patient and family teaching is an important part of nursing care for a patient with CKF (see Patient/Family Teaching box).

Research

Schneider RA: Chronic renal failure: assessing the Fatigue Severity Scale for use among caregivers, *J Clin Nurs* 13(2):219-225, 2004.

Quality of life for caregivers of persons with end-stage renal disease has not been well addressed, yet the physical and psychologic status of this group can be important in the patients' recovery or adaptation. The purpose of the study was to test the Fatigue Severity Scale for potential usefulness in assessing fatigue among a nonmedical population of caregivers of end-stage renal disease patients.

Subjects completed a short battery of measures at either a dialysis center or at home. The results suggest that physical fatigue may be more prominent than mental fatigue as a feature of caregiver quality of life. Results of the study suggest that intervention may need to focus more on rest and respite as opposed to psychosocial support or counseling.

The Fatigue Severity Scale, which has been used for multiple sclerosis patients, may prove to be useful as a short assessment of fatigue among the nonmedical population of end-stage renal disease caregivers. Physicians, nurses and allied health professionals will be called on more frequently to assess and intervene with fatigued and overburdened caregivers, in addition to patients themselves. A more thorough understanding of the nature of caregiver fatigue may drive changes or innovations with caregivers who are too often overlooked in the current era of scarce resources.

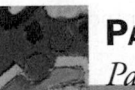

PATIENT/FAMILY TEACHING *The Patient With Chronic Kidney Failure*

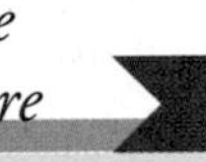

Teaching for person with chronic kidney failure and his or her family includes information about:

- Relationships between symptoms and their causes
- Relationships among diet, fluid restriction, medication, and blood chemistry values
- Preventive health care measures: oral hygiene, prevention of infection, avoidance of bleeding
- Dietary regimen, including fluid restrictions
  —Prescribed sodium, potassium, phosphorus, and protein restrictions
  —Label reading and identification of nutritional content of foods
  —Use of small, frequent feedings to maintain nutrient intake when anorexic or nauseated
  —Fluid prescription and sources of fluid in diet
  —Avoidance of salt substitutes containing potassium
- Monitoring for fluid excess
  —Accurate measurement and recording of intake and output
  —Monitoring for weight gain and edema
- Medications
  —Actions, doses, purpose, and side effects of prescribed medications
  —Avoidance of over-the-counter drugs, especially aspirin, cold medications, and nonsteroidal antiinflammatory drugs
- Measures to control pruritus
- Planning for follow-up health care
  —Symptoms requiring immediate medical attention: changes in urinary output, edema, weight gain, dyspnea, infection, increased symptoms of uremia
  —Need for continual medical follow-up

EVALUATION

To evaluate the effectiveness of nursing interventions, compare patient behaviors with those stated in the expected patient outcomes.

RELATED NOC OUTCOMES. Acceptance: Health Status, Adaptation to Physical Disability, Coping, Electrolyte & Acid/Base Balance, Fluid Balance, Knowledge: Disease Process, Nutritional Status

GERONTOLOGIC CONSIDERATIONS

The older patient with ESRD is more likely to develop complications as a result of age-related stressors placed on the kidneys. The GFR decreases 10% every 10 years after the age of 50 years. The older patient is more likely to experience kidney insufficiency, predominantly related to atherosclerosis. Older adults often have multiple risk factors such as diabetes and hypertension, which increase the risk of kidney failure. Once faced with ESRD, all persons, particularly older adults, need to consider their overall health when choosing a treatment option.

The nurse evaluates the patient's home environment and resources to determine the best treatment options. Obstacles for older patients may include lack of transportation to a dialysis center. Lack of motor skills or a chronic illness such as osteoarthritis may prohibit elderly patients from performing home dialysis. Options for the older patient include home health care or extended-care facilities. Agencies such as Help on Wheels offer free transportation to and from dialysis treatments.

Kidney Transplantation

Etiology and Epidemiology. Kidney transplantation is the oldest and most common type of transplant procedure, with the first kidney transplant dating back to the early 1950s. The procedure is now well established as a viable and desirable treatment for ESRD. Although transplant procedures are expensive, the current success rates have made transplantation a cost-effective treatment option, since it is less expensive than dialysis after the first year. A patient undergoing chronic hemodialysis costs the federal government, through Medicare, about $50,000 per year. The cost of a kidney transplant is approximately $75,000 for the first year and $12,500 per year for follow-up care.[24] If the transplanted kidney functions for 5 years (the actual rate approaches 75%), the cost is $125,000, as opposed to $250,000 for 5-year chronic hemodialysis. Other financial factors that increase the cost-effectiveness of transplantation are the potential earning power of the transplant recipient and the discontinuation of disability benefits previously required. In short, transplantation can restore dignity and quality to the lives of patients and families dealing with ESRD and provide the potential for patients to become productive members of society again.

In spite of the successes, kidney transplantation is not available to all who need it. Since 1988, 188,193 kidney transplants have taken place in the United States. However, more than 58,000 people are currently registered candidates for kidney transplantation.[15] In addition, many other patients who are approaching ESRD are in need of transplants before they require dialysis. This approach is particularly advantageous for children, whose physical and mental development is significantly impaired by kidney failure, and for patients with diabetes, who have a much higher mortality rate on dialysis than nondiabetics. However, because of the serious shortage of organ availability, many organ candidates will die before organs become available.

Pathophysiology. Kidney transplantation is primarily used to treat patients experiencing ESRD resulting from glomerular diseases, diabetes mellitus, polycystic kidney disease, and hypertension. The advantages of kidney transplantation include the reversal of many of the pathophysiologic changes associated with kidney failure as kidney function is restored.

ORGAN PROCUREMENT. Organ procurement organizations located in major cities are responsible for organ recovery in the United States and provide services on a local, state, and regional basis. They provide 24-hour assistance to evaluate potential donors, discuss donation with the next of kin, and assist with physical assessment and hemodynamic monitoring to maintain organ function until surgical removal. Additionally, they provide for organ recovery and placement through the United Network for Organ Sharing (UNOS), follow-up bereavement support to donor families and information regarding the outcome of the donation, and feedback to the donor hospital regarding transplant outcomes.[22]

ORGAN DONORS. UNOS estimates that a new patient is added to the national patient waiting list for organ transplantation every 20 minutes and that seven people die every day while waiting for organ transplants. The shortage of organs reflects both organ accessibility and availability. Only an estimated 40% of organs from people who die meeting donor eligibility criteria are actually donated each year.[15] Despite extensive public awareness campaigns and laws mandating that all families be given the opportunity to donate the organs of a loved one who dies, the ratio of potential to actual donors has been little affected. The three primary sources of organs are from living donors, non–heart beating donors, and deceased donors (see Guidelines for Safe Practice box).

LIVING DONORS. Living donors have been used in kidney transplantation since 1954. In the past, donors were restricted to blood relatives (i.e., parents, children, siblings). More recently, the donor pool has expanded to include unrelated donors, who are not blood relatives but have an emotional relationship with the potential recipient (e.g., spouse, stepparent, stepchild, friend). The advantages of a living donor include (1) improved patient and graft survival rates, (2) immediate availability of an organ, (3) the ability to schedule the surgery when the recipient is in the best possible medical condition, and (4) immediate functioning of the organ because there is minimal preservation time. More than 62,400 live donor kidney transplants have been performed in the United States, accounting for about 33% of the total[15] (see Ethical Alert).

NON–HEART BEATING DONORS. Patients who have been declared dead by traditional cardiopulmonary criteria rather than brain death criteria are another source of transplantable organs. Organ procurement takes place after the heart has stopped beat-

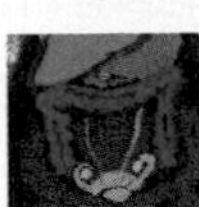

GUIDELINES FOR SAFE PRACTICE
Talking With Families About Organ and Tissue Donation

- Nurse, physician, and health care team identify potential donor.
- Death is declared and discussed with family. Make certain the family understands that brain death is irreversible.
- Allow time for family to assimilate information.
- Notify local organ procurement organization to determine suitability for organ and tissue donation.
- Attempt to determine the beliefs of the potential donor (donor card or driver's license signed).
- Identify legal next of kin and other family members who need to be included in the discussion.
- Provide a comfortable, private place for discussions between health care providers, procurement coordinator, and family.
- Respect cultural beliefs and differences.
- Acknowledge the family's pain; speak slowly and with compassion.
- Provide adequate, accurate information on the options available for discontinuing life support.
- Provide adequate, accurate information about organ and tissue donation, including informed consent and required evaluations.
- Ensure that the family understands that there is no cost to the donor family, and that donation will not interfere with the timing of the funeral service or open casket service.
- Provide time for the family to discuss the request and make their decision.
- Request written consent only after the family has had time to make their decision and has given an affirmative response.
- Respect the family's decision. Avoid being judgmental or condescending if the family chooses not to donate.

Ethical Alert

Live Organ Donations

Ethical concerns arise when people donate organs or portions of organs. These include the risk of surgical complications for the healthy donor, loss of income if the donor is a primary wage earner, uncertain outcomes for the recipient, and the donor's guilt if the recipient dies. The donor's concerns must be weighed against the recipient's risk of dying while awaiting a deceased donor of the right match. Respect for autonomy supports the donor's right to assume these risks if the donor's decision is informed, free from coercion, and truly autonomous.

ing. Before the institution of brain death criteria, these donors were the major source of transplantable kidneys, but problems with extended ischemia and resultant cellular and tissue damage limited their usefulness. Now, organs are procured from non–heart beating donors by in situ organ preservation immediately after cardiopulmonary arrest, and from patients who die after choosing to forgo life-sustaining treatment.[20]

DECEASED DONORS. The criteria for deceased donors have been liberalized to include increasing age (up to 72 years), diabetes, hypertension, some infections, high-risk social history but negative human immunodeficiency virus (HIV) test, some hemodynamic instability, some chemical imbalances, and increased organ preservation time. These expanded criteria increase the deceased donor supply by about 25%.[15] A careful evaluation, including histologic assessment of the recovered organs, is made before transplantation, and careful long-term follow-up is provided to ensure that patient and graft survival rates are comparable to those obtained with traditional deceased donors.

ORGAN RECIPIENTS. Appropriate recipient selection is important for both a successful outcome and the best use of this scarce resource. Candidacy is determined by a wide variety of medical and psychosocial criteria that vary among transplant centers. These factors include disease status, therapeutic benefits of transplantation, age, functional ability, and presence of family support. A careful evaluation is completed before transplant to identify and minimize potential complications after transplant. Contraindications for transplantation include disseminated malignancies, chronic infections (except hepatitis B and C), and ongoing psychosocial problems such as noncompliance with medical regimens and chemical dependency.[22]

COMPLICATIONS. The primary complications associated with kidney transplantation are transplant failure (rejection), hypertension, infection, and malignancies.

TRANSPLANT FAILURE. The major reason for transplant failure is rejection. The three types of rejection are hyperacute, acute, and chronic. A special type of rejection that occurs in recipients of allogeneic bone marrow transplants is graft-versus-host disease, which is discussed in Chapter 21 (see Clinical Manifestations box).

Hyperacute rejection. Hyperacute rejection occurs at the time of transplantation or within 48 hours after the transplant. It is mediated by the humoral immune system. Preformed circulating cytotoxic antibodies to incompatible ABO blood group antigens, antigens on the vascular endothelium, or histocompatibility antigens are responsible for the hyperacute rejection. The combination of the preformed antibody with the antigen causes activation of complement, entrapment of formed blood elements and clotting factors, massive intravascular coagulation, and necrosis of the graft from decreased perfusion. The degranulation of phagocytic cells causes the release of hydrolytic enzymes that also cause tissue destruction.

Hyperacute rejections are rare because of careful cross-matching and tend to be isolated to kidney transplants. A special type of hyperacute rejection is accelerated rejection, which occurs over 3 to 5 days and may be reversed if detected early.

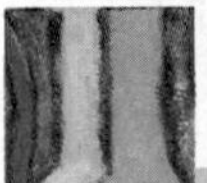

CLINICAL MANIFESTATIONS
Renal Transplant Rejection

- Fever greater than 100° F (37.7° C); may be masked by steroid therapy
- Pain or tenderness over grafted kidney
- Sudden weight gain (2 to 3 pounds in 24 hours)
- Edema
- Hypertension
- General malaise
- Elevated serum creatinine and blood urea nitrogen
- Decreased creatinine clearance
- Ultrasound or biopsy evidence of rejection

Acute rejection. Acute rejection usually occurs from 1 week to 3 months after the transplant and may recur at any time after the first incident. Acute rejection is mediated by both humoral and cellular immunity. In acute rejection, transplanted antigens are trapped by macrophages. This macrophage-antigen interaction stimulates differentiation and maturation of various B cell and T cell subsets, which cause destruction of the transplanted tissue directly or indirectly through activation of other immune cells. Acute rejection is treated by pharmacologic interventions consisting of increased doses of steroids, monoclonal antibodies (e.g., muromonab-CD3 [Orthoclone OKT3]), or polyclonal antibodies such as antithymocyte globulin or antilymphocyte globulin.

Chronic rejection. Chronic rejection occurs 3 months or longer after transplantation. It is mediated by both the cellular and humoral immunity and results in slow, progressive loss of graft function. Chronic rejection remains the major unresolved problem in transplantation, since it is less responsive to immunosuppressive therapies.

HYPERTENSION. Hypertension is a well-known complication of kidney failure that is rarely cured by kidney transplant. In fact, hypertension occurs in approximately 70% of kidney transplant recipients and up to 90% of patients transplanted with other solid organs such as hearts, livers, lungs, and pancreata. Hypertension has been associated with several antirejection drugs such as prednisone, cyclosporine, and tacrolimus.

INFECTION. Infection remains a major cause of morbidity and mortality after transplantation because of suppression of the body's normal defense mechanisms. Advancing age plus the presence of other illnesses such as diabetes mellitus, lupus erythematosus, and malnutrition further impairs the immune response. The signs and symptoms of infection can be subtle, and prompt diagnosis and treatment are essential.

The most common infections observed in the first month after transplantation are similar to those acquired by any postoperative patient, including wound and intravenous line infections, pneumonia, and urinary tract infections. Viral infections, especially cytomegalovirus (CMV), Epstein-Barr virus, herpes simplex virus, and varicella zoster virus, may occur as primary or reactivated infections. Reactivation of dormant viruses can occur from pharmacologic immunosuppression. Primary infections that occur after transplantation often can be traced to an exogenous source such as the donated organ or blood transfusion. Common organisms responsible for infection in transplant recipients are presented in Box 36-8.

MALIGNANCIES. The incidence of malignancies is significantly higher in transplant recipients than in the general population. Transplant recipients, compared with the general public, develop colon, lung, prostate, stomach, esophagus, pancreas, ovary, and breast cancer twice as often; melanoma, leukemia, and cervical and vulvovaginal cancers five times as often; testicular and bladder cancers three times as often; and kidney cancer 15 times as often.[1] The increased incidence is related to an altered immune system caused by chronic immunosuppressive therapy.

Box 36-8 Organisms Responsible for Infections in Transplant Recipients

Bacterial Infections

Gram-negative organisms, including *Pseudomonas aeruginosa, Serratia marcescens, Providencia rettgeri, Enterobacter cloacae, Legionella pneumophila*, and various *Nocardia* species

Viral Infections

Herpesviruses, including herpes simplex viruses 1 and 2; varicella-zoster virus; cytomegalovirus; and Epstein-Barr virus

Fungal Infections

Candidal species (most often *Candida albicans*) and other fungi, including *Aspergillus fumigatus, Cryptococcus neoformans, Coccidioides immitis*, and *Histoplasma capsulatum*

Parasitic Infections

Including *Pneumocystis carinii* and *Toxoplasma gondii*

Collaborative Care Management

DIAGNOSTIC TESTS. Kidney transplantations involve maximal histocompatibility testing, especially in situations involving a live donor. ABO compatibility, human leukocyte antigen matching, white blood cell cross-match, and mixed lymphocyte cross-match are all performed. Other routine laboratory tests include CBC, renal panel, liver panel, partial thomboplastin time, prothrombin time, viral titers, and creatinine clearance. Potential recipients are also screened for HIV, CMV, and Epstein-Barr virus, which are contraindications to renal transplantation.

MEDICATIONS. In the absence of immunosuppression, transplanted organs are rejected within about 2 weeks. Therefore patients undergoing kidney transplant are started on the full regimen of immunosuppressive therapy, which is maintained for life. The goal of drug therapy is to adequately suppress the immune response to prevent rejection of the transplanted kidney while maintaining sufficient immunity to prevent overwhelming infection. By using a combination of medications that affect differing phases of the immune response, effective immunosuppression can be achieved with lower doses of each drug while minimizing side effects (Figure 36-14). Immunosuppressive protocols are highly variable among transplant centers, with different combinations of medications used. Table 36-7 presents an overview of agents used for renal transplantation immunosuppression.

DIET. Before surgery the patient with ESRD continues on the kidney failure diet that has been prescribed. One of the major benefits of successful kidney transplantation is the ability to eat without the extensive restrictions of protein, fluid, sodium, and potassium that are characteristic of the management of ESRD. However, the patient needs to continue to control sodium and calorie content after transplantation to manage the side effects of high-dose steroid administration that is required for immunosuppression.

TREATMENTS. Patients awaiting kidney transplant continue on their regular schedule of dialysis right up to the time of transplant.

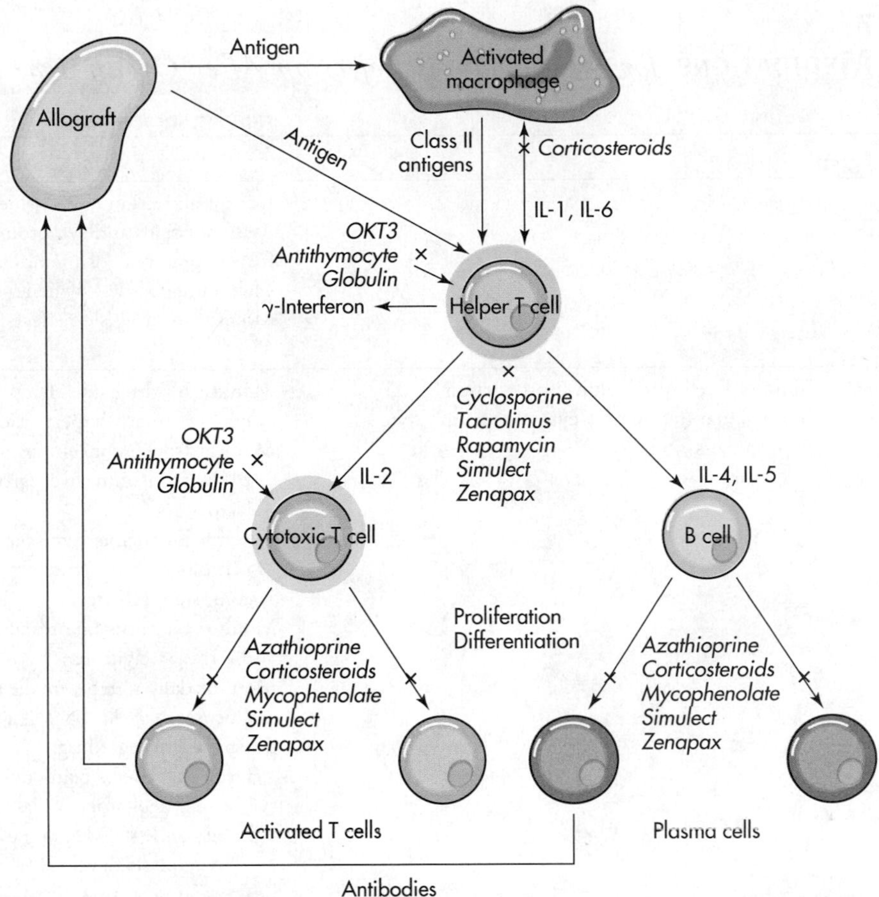

Figure 36-14 Sites of action for immunosuppressive agents. *IL*, Interleukin.

Dialysis is conducted as close to the time of surgery as possible to ensure that the patient is in the best possible metabolic condition to withstand the rigors of surgery. Living donor kidneys usually begin to function immediately after surgery. Deceased donor kidneys may experience a delay in functioning, and the patient might need to have dialysis resumed for a short time after surgery to maintain physiologic homeostasis.

SURGICAL MANAGEMENT. The donor kidney is carefully dissected free with its renal artery and vein intact. The ureter is also dissected with great care to preserve the periureteral vascular supply. The kidney is removed; flushed with a chilled, sterile electrolyte solution; and prepared for transplant into the recipient. The procedure takes about 2 hours.

The transplanted kidney is placed extraperitoneally, in the iliac fossa (Figure 36-15). Generally, the peritoneal cavity is not entered. The patient's own kidneys are not removed, unless they are infected or are causing significant hypertension, in order to maintain erythropoietin production, blood pressure control, and prostaglandin synthesis and metabolism. Efficient revascularization is critical to prevent ischemic injury to the kidney.

The donor ureter is used to the extent possible. If long enough, the donor ureter is tunneled through the bladder submucosa and sutured in place. This allows the bladder to clamp down on the ureter as it contracts for micturition, thereby preventing reflux of urine up the ureter into the transplanted kidney. The entire transplant surgery takes about 3 hours.

Nursing Management

of the Patient undergoing Kidney Transplant Surgery

PREOPERATIVE CARE

Nursing care in the preoperative phase includes emotional and physical preparation for surgery. The nurse informs the patient that there is a 20% chance the kidney will not function immediately and dialysis may be required for the first few weeks. In addition, the nurse stresses the rationale for immunosuppressive therapy and the importance of preventing infection after surgery.

To ensure that the patient is in optimal physical condition for surgery, an ECG, chest x-ray examination, and laboratory studies are performed. Dialysis is often required to achieve optimal fluid, electrolyte, and acid-base balance, as well as to remove excess nitrogenous wastes. Because dialysis may be required after transplant, the patency of the vascular access must be maintained. The nurse wraps the extremity containing the vascular access in Kerlix and labels it "dialysis access." This identification reminds all caregivers to avoid using the affected extremity for blood pressure measurement, phlebotomy, or intravenous infusions.

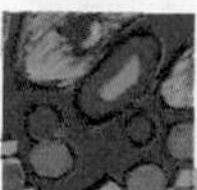

TABLE 36-7
COMMON MEDICATIONS *for Prevention of Rejection After Organ Transplantation*

Drug	Action	Nursing Intervention
All Immunosuppressive Agents		
		Institute infection control measures. Assess for signs and symptoms of infection. Inspect oral mucous membranes. Maintain good oral hygiene, including flossing. Monitor for drug side effects.
Calcineurin Inhibitors		
Cyclosporine (Sandimmune, Neoral)	Inhibits T-cell interleukin-2 production Inhibits maturation of T-cytotoxic lymphocyte precursors	Monitor for drug side effects: acute and chronic nephrotoxicity, hypertension, dyslipidemia. Monitor trough concentrations, serum creatinine, BUN, potassium, liver enzymes, and coagulation factors. Monitor for edema, hypertension, jaundice, and neurologic status (tremors, paresthesias, headache, confusion, seizures). Monitor GI status (anorexia, nausea, vomiting, diarrhea, weight loss). Monitor daily weight, intake and output, blood glucose. Teach patient regarding: Drug side effects being dose related Use of a depilatory if hirsutism develops Need for dental cleaning every 6 mo if gingival hyperplasia develops Decrease dose as prescribed. Administer diuretics and hypertensive agents as prescribed.
Tacrolimus (Prograf)	Prevents production and release of interleukin-2 Inhibits maturation of T-cytotoxic lymphocyte precursors	Tacrolimus: Monitor blood glucose levels and administer prescribed insulin or oral hypoglycemic agent.
Sirolimus (rapamycin, Rapamune)	Suppresses lymphocyte proliferation Inhibits B cells from synthesizing antibody	Sirolimus: Administer via central line over 4-6 hr.
Antiproliferative Agents		
Azathioprine (Imuran)	Suppress proliferation of rapidly dividing cells, including sensitized B and T cells Alkylating agent that interferes with DNA, RNA, and protein synthesis	Monitor hematocrit, white blood cell count, platelet count, liver enzymes, coagulation factors. Monitor for infection, bleeding, jaundice, nausea, vomiting, abdominal pain, hematuria, and hair loss. Administer prescribed oral antifungal agent.
Cyclophosphamide (Cytoxan)		Reduce dose as prescribed. Encourage increased fluid intake, especially water.

POSTOPERATIVE CARE

Care of the Donor. The postoperative care of a living donor is similar to that provided after a nephrectomy (see Chapter 35). The donor can easily be forgotten in the transplant process because of the attention focused on the recipient. The pain of a nephrectomy is significant, and adequate analgesia is essential to ensure comfort, promote ambulation, and prevent atelectasis and pulmonary complications. Most donors are discharged within 3 to 5 days and can usually return to work in 1 month. The majority of kidney donors feel good about the donation because of the improved health of their family member or significant other.

Care of the Recipient. The first priority of care for the recipient is maintenance of fluid and electrolyte balance. Rapid diuresis may take place soon after the blood supply to the kidney is reestablished, especially in living donor transplants. This diuresis is related to the kidney's ability to filter BUN, which acts as an osmotic diuretic; the abundance of fluids administered intravenously during the operation; and renal tubular dysfunction, which inhibits the kidney from concentrating urine normally. Urinary output during this phase may be as high as 1 L/hr, but decreases when BUN and serum creatinine levels return to normal. The nurse measures the patient's urinary out-

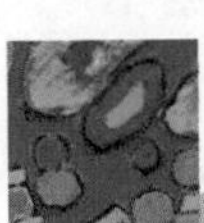

TABLE 36-7
COMMON MEDICATIONS *for Prevention of Rejection After Organ Transplantation—cont'd*

Drug	Action	Nursing Intervention
Corticosteroids		
Prednisone	Suppresses inflammatory response; prevents proliferation of T-cytotoxic lymphocytes	Monitor daily weight, blood glucose, wound healing. Monitor for blood in stool or emesis, complaints of acid indigestion, esophageal or gastric burning, changes in muscle strength. Encourage low-sodium intake; low-fat, low-cholesterol diet (especially in presence of high serum cholesterol levels). Administer antacids, H_2 receptor blockers as prescribed. Administer with food to decrease gastric irritation. Administer oral antifungal agent if prescribed. Teach patient regarding: Need for controlling intake to maintain ideal weight Need for consistent exercise to counteract muscle weakness Hyperglycemic effect of corticosteroids Avoid skin trauma and use of adhesive tape.
Monoclonal Antibodies		
Muromonab-CD3 (Orthoclone OKT3)	Monoclonal antibody that removes circulating T lymphocytes	Administer prescribed acetaminophen, diphenhydramine, and hydrocortisone at time of IV infusion.
Chimeric anti-IL-2 receptor antibody (basiliximab [Simulect])	Monoclonal antibody against IL-2 receptor Blocks T-cell activation and proliferation	Monitor daily weight, lung sounds, GI status (nausea, vomiting, diarrhea), intake and output, temperature.
Daclizumab (humanized anti-Tac, Zenapax)	Polyclonal antibody directed against lymphocytes	Monitor for peripheral edema, headache, photophobia.
Antilymphocyte globulin	Reduces circulating lymphocytes	Monitor platelet count and report if below $100,000/mm^3$. Administer prescribed diuretics.
Antithymocyte globulin	Decreases lymphocyte proliferation	Arrange for outpatient infusion to complete course of therapy after discharge.
Purine Synthesis Inhibitor		
Mycophenolate mofetil (CellCept)	Inhibits purine synthesis Suppresses T-cytotoxic lymphocyte proliferation	Monitor daily weight, GI status (nausea, vomiting, diarrhea, abdominal cramping, dyspepsia), intake and output, white blood cell count. Administer antiemetics and antidiarrheals as ordered.

BUN, Blood urea nitrogen; *GI,* gastrointestinal; *DNA,* deoxyribonucleic acid; *RNA,* ribonucleic acid; *IV,* intravenous; *IL-2,* interleukin-2.

put hourly and replaces it with intravenous fluids for the first 12 to 24 hours. Dehydration is avoided to prevent renal hypoperfusion and possible tubular damage. The nurse closely monitors the patient's electrolyte levels to detect hypokalemia, which is often associated with rapid diuresis or the kidney tubules' inability to concentrate.

Delayed graft function occurs in 20% of patients receiving deceased donor kidneys that have been preserved for longer than 24 hours. The ischemic damage from prolonged preservation results in ATN, which can last from several days to weeks, followed by gradually improving kidney function. Dialysis may be necessary initially, but is discontinued when the patient's urinary output increases and serum creatinine and BUN levels normalize.

A sudden decrease in urinary output in the early postoperative period may be caused by dehydration, rejection, vascular thrombosis, or an obstruction that impedes urine flow. Any decrease in output is thoroughly investigated. A blood clot in the Foley catheter is a common cause of early obstruction. Because the catheter remains in the bladder for 3 to 5 days after surgery to allow the bladder anastomosis to heal, its patency must be ensured. The physician may order careful, sterile catheter irrigation to dislodge the occluding clots.

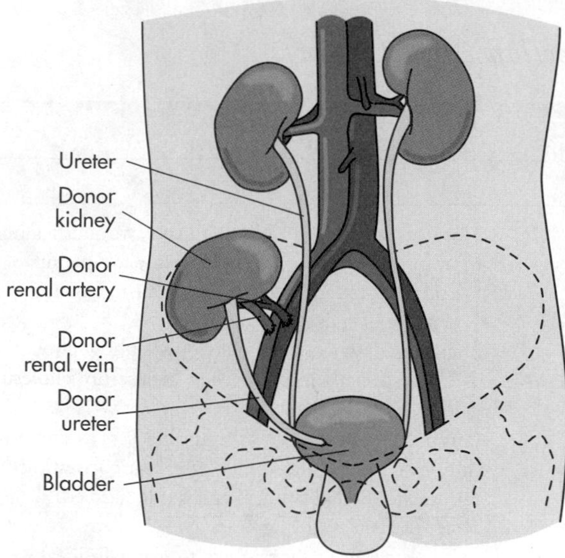

Figure 36-15 Location of a transplanted kidney showing anastomosis of renal artery, renal vein, and ureter.

Most patients undergo ultrasonography within 24 hours of transplantation to assess the kidney's vascular supply and look for any fluid collections, such as hematoma, lymphocele, or urine leak. The presence of hydronephrosis, with or without a dilated ureter, may indicate obstruction.

Patient/Family Teaching. Patient and family education is an integral part of a smooth transition from hospital to home. The first priority for discharge preparation is medication teaching. Patients and their families must be able to explain the action, dosage, and potential adverse effects of all medications. The nurse supplies a written list of discharge medications with the administration schedule for the patient to use as a home resource. Other key discharge instructions are found in the Patient/Family Teaching box.

Critical Thinking

1. A 65-year-old man is seen at your clinic with complaints of voiding in small amounts and constant feelings of urgency despite having voided. He also complains of bouts of incontinence. His postvoid residual volume is 300 ml. Both BUN and creatinine levels are elevated. What are some risk factors that may contribute to this patient's problem? What diagnostic examinations might be ordered? He is admitted for kidney failure to a general medical unit. His blood pressure is stable. What nursing interventions are appropriate? What are treatment options?
2. A 50-year-old woman receiving CAPD enters the emergency room with complaints of severe abdominal pain and cramping. She is nauseated and febrile. Her CAPD catheter site is red and swollen. Her white blood cell count is elevated. What do you suspect her diagnosis to be? Will she receive her dialysis while she has these symptoms? If so, how will dialysis be accomplished?

References

1. Bertram L et al: Cancer after kidney transplantation in the United States, *Am J Transplant* 4(6):905-913, 2004.
2. Bro S: How abnormal calcium, phosphate, and parathyroid hormone relate to cardiovascular disease, *Nephrol Nurs J* 30(3):275-281, 2003.
3. Cohen LM, Germain MJ, Poppel DM: Practical consideration in dialysis withdrawal, *JAMA* 289(16):2113-2119, 2003.
4. Coresh J et al: Prevalence of chronic kidney disease and decreased kidney function in the adult US population: Third National Health and Nutrition Examination Survey, *Am J Kidney Dis* 41(1):1-12, 2003.
5. Eknoyan G, Levin A, Levin NW: Bone metabolism and disease in chronic kidney disease, *Am J Kidney Dis* 42 (4)(suppl 3):S1-201, 2003.
6. Frasser D, Vinning M: Urologic nephrology. In Weiss RM, George N, O'Reilly PH, editors: *Comprehensive urology*, London, 2001, Mosby.
7. Greene JH, Hoffart N: Nutrition in renal failure, dialysis and transplantation. In Lancaster LE, editor: *Core curriculum for nephrology nursing*, Pittman, NJ, 2001, Janetti.

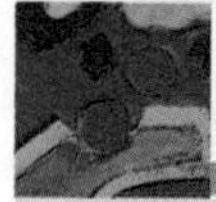

PATIENT/FAMILY TEACHING *Kidney Transplantation*

- Teach patient and family to monitor for signs and symptoms of rejection or infection and report them to the primary care provider:
  —Flank pain
  —Fever
  —Changes in urinary pattern
  —Sudden weight gain
  —Difficulty breathing
  —Edema
- Encourage patient to maintain activity limitations until directed otherwise:
  —Heavy lifting (more than 20 pounds) is avoided for the first 6 weeks until the incision heals completely.
  —Regular exercise is encouraged to counteract the proximal muscle weakness associated with steroid administration.
  —Most patients can return to work in 6 to 12 weeks.
  —Sexual intercourse may be resumed after 4 to 6 weeks.
- Instruct patient to follow written list of discharge medications and the administration schedule. Patient should be able to explain the action, dosage, and potential adverse effects of all medications on discharge.
- Monitor weight and cholesterol:
  —Steroids commonly stimulate appetite, and both steroids and cyclosporine increase the risk for hyperlipidemia. A dietitian may need to be consulted regarding dietary changes to minimize weight gain and control cholesterol levels.
  —Instruct patient to avoid foods and fluids that have hidden sources of sodium (fast food and convenience foods) to minimize salt- and water-retaining effects of steroids.
- Encourage women of childbearing age to postpone pregnancy for at least 1 year after transplant to ensure stable renal function and allow for lower doses of immunosuppressive drugs.

8. Kamel K, Halperin M: Treatment of hypokalemia and hyperkalemia. In Brady HR, Wilcox CS, editors: *Therapy in nephrology and hypertension: a companion to Brenner and Rector's the kidney,* Philadelphia, 1999, Saunders.
9. Kasiske BL, Keane WF: Laboratory assessment of renal disease: clearance, urinalysis and renal biopsy. In Brenner BM, editor: *Brenner and Rector's the kidney,* ed 7, Philadelphia, 2003, Saunders.
10. Kutner NG, Zhang R, McClellan WM: Patient-reported quality of life early in dialysis treatment: effects associated with usual exercise activity, *Nephrol Nurs J* 27(4):357-367, 2000.

10a. Levey MD et al: National Kidney Foundation practice guidelines for chronic kidney disease: evaluation, classification, and stratification, *Ann Intern Med* 139:137-147, 2003.

11. National Kidney Foundation: K/DOQI clinical practice guidelines for anemia of chronic kidney disease, 2000, *Am J Kidney Dis* 37(suppl 1): S182-S238, 2001.
12. National Kidney Foundation: K/DOQI clinical practice guidelines for hemodialysis adequacy, 2000, *Am J Kidney Dis* 37(suppl 1):S5-S64, 2001.
13. National Kidney Foundation: K/DOQI clinical practice guidelines for peritoneal dialysis adequacy, 2000, *Am J Kidney Dis* 37(suppl 1):S65-S136, 2001.
14. National Kidney Foundation: K/DOQI clinical practice guidelines for vascular access, 2000, *Am J Kidney Dis* 37(suppl 1):S137-S181, 2001.
15. Organ Procurement and Transplant Network: National data, accessed from website: http://www.unos.org/data/about/viewDataReports.asp, 2004.
16. Reference deleted in proofs.
17. Pichette V, Leblond FA: Drug metabolism in chronic renal failure, *Current Drug Metab* 4(2), 2003.
18. Redden D, Szczech LA, Owen WF: Acute renal failure. In Rakel RE et al, editors: *Conn's current therapy,* Philadelphia, 2001, Saunders.
19. Richard CJ: Renal disorders. In Lancaster LE, editor: *Core curriculum for nephrology nursing,* Pittman, NJ, 2001, Jannetti.
20. Rudich SM et al: Renal transplantations performed using non-heart-bearing organ donors: going back to the future? *Transplantation* 74(12):1715-1720, 2002.
21. Salusky IB, Goodman WG: Adynamic renal osteodystrophy: is there a problem? *J Am Soc Nephrol* 12:1978-1985, 2001.
22. United Network for Organ Sharing: *United Network for Organ Sharing annual report 2003,* accessed from website: http://www.unos.org/ContentDocuments/UNOS_Annual_Report_2003.pdf
23. US Department of Health and Human Services: *Healthy people 2010: understanding and improving health,* Washington, DC, 2000, The Department.
24. US Renal Data System: *USRDS 2003 annual report: atlas of end-stage renal disease in the United States, National Institutes of Health, National Institute of Diabetes and Digestive and Kidney Diseases,* Bethesda, Md, 2003, The System.
25. Wish JB, Weigel KA: Management of anemia in chronic kidney disease (predialysis) patients: nephrology nursing implications, *Nephrol Nurs J* 28(suppl)(3):341-345, 2001.

Visit the Evolve website: http://evolve.elsevier.com/Monahan/medsurg

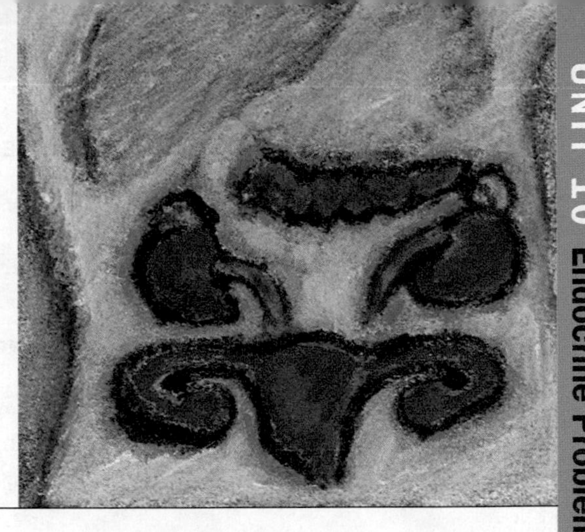

CHAPTER 37

Assessment of the Endocrine System

by Margaret M. Ulchaker

OBJECTIVES

After studying this chapter, the learner should be able to:

1. Describe the locations of endocrine glands and the mechanisms that control hormone synthesis and release from them.
2. Explain the functions of the hormones secreted by the pituitary, thyroid, parathyroid, adrenal cortex, adrenal medulla, and pancreas.
3. Compare the biologic effects of deficit and excess of each major hormone.
4. Describe the physiologic changes that occur within the endocrine system with aging.
5. Outline data essential to the assessment of patients with actual or potential health problems of the endocrine system.
6. Discuss the common diagnostic tests used to identify endocrine dysfunction, and explain the meaning of the results.

KEY TERMS

circadian rhythms, p. 1042
diurnal, p. 1041
endogenous, p. 1059
exogenous, p. 1059
hormone, p. 1041

The endocrine system is a cellular communication system involving hormones. A **hormone** is a molecule secreted from one organ that travels in the systemic circulation and affects a distant organ or organs. The endocrine system consists of the anterior and posterior pituitary, thyroid, parathyroid, adrenal cortex, adrenal medulla, pancreas, gonads, pineal body, and thymus glands. Specialized endocrine cells are also located along the gastrointestinal (GI) tract. The hormones from these endocrine glands are vital to the life transactions of the organism, including differentiation, reproduction, growth and development, metabolism, adaptation, and aging. The neuroendocrine response to stressors, which involves the nervous system, the adrenal medulla, and other endocrine glands, is briefly discussed in Chapter 14; the GI hormones are discussed in Chapter 40; and the gonads are discussed in Chapter 55. The thymus, which is critical to development of immunocompetent T lymphocytes, is discussed in Chapter 20.

Anatomy and Physiology

General Endocrine Processes

A hormone may:

- Stimulate another endocrine gland to produce another hormone with specific tissue effects (e.g., thyroid-stimulating hormone [TSH] stimulates the thyroid gland to secrete thyroxine [T_4] and triiodothyronine [T_3])
- Inhibit another endocrine gland's production of a hormone (e.g., somatostatin inhibits growth hormone [GH])
- Have a direct effect on specific tissues (e.g., insulin promotes glucose transport into insulin-sensitive cells)

A hormone's effects on the end organ tissue are mediated via several mechanisms, depending on the hormone's structure (Table 37-1). Peptide hormones (e.g., insulin) bind to cell surface receptors and trigger a secondary cascade of intracellular signals, resulting in the final event: the transportation of glucose into the cell. Steroid hormones bind to the nucleus of the target cell and result in altered protein synthesis.

Mechanisms of Hormone Action

The secretion and release of hormones do not occur at a uniform rate. Many hormones are secreted in a pulsatile fashion and may have **diurnal** (occurring during the day) variations. Physiologic levels of hormones are determined by the amount of hormone produced, an intact transport system, adequate receptors, feedback systems, and metabolic degradation of the hormone.

TABLE 37-1 STRUCTURAL CATEGORIES OF HORMONES

Structural Category	Examples
Peptide hormones	Growth hormone Parathyroid hormone Follicle-stimulating hormone Luteinizing hormone Thyroid-stimulating hormone Thyrotropin-releasing hormone Oxytocin Prolactin Calcitonin Glucagon Adrenocorticotropic hormone Endorphins Melanocyte-stimulating hormone Hypothalamic hormones or factors (e.g., corticotropin-releasing hormone) Somatostatin
Amino acid derivatives	Epinephrine Norepinephrine
Steroid hormones	Estrogens Progestins Thyroxine (T_4) Triiodothyronine (T_3)

From McCance KL, Huether SE: *Pathophysiology: the biologic basis for disease in adults and children,* ed 4, St Louis, 2002, Mosby.

Hormone Release. Hormone release is influenced by negative feedback systems, intrinsic rhythmicity, the nervous system, excretion, and metabolism. Understanding these mechanisms helps clarify the rationale for the various types of diagnostic testing used to assess pathologic conditions of the endocrine system.

ENDOCRINE AXIS AND FEEDBACK LOOPS. Understanding hormonal feedback loops is important not only for diagnosis, but also for therapeutic monitoring. In a negative feedback system a gland responds to a low hormone level by releasing an additional hormone. As the level of this second hormone returns to normal, its further release is inhibited. Thyroid hormone regulation is an example of a negative feedback system (Figure 37-1). In the example of the thyroid, it is important to recognize that (1) the earliest marker of excess thyroid hormone in the circulation is a suppressed TSH and (2) the earliest marker of deficiency of thyroid hormone is an elevated TSH. Changes in TSH normally occur before circulating thyroid hormone levels are out of the normal range and really reflect the pituitary's assessment of ambient thyroid levels. TSH levels return to normal very slowly (6 to 8 weeks) after correction of ambient thyroid hormone levels. Therefore measuring TSH at time intervals shorter than this will not yield meaningful information.

Although negative feedback control is a distinguishing feature of the endocrine system, it does not control all hormones. Examples of hormones with other mechanisms of control include estrogen in males, testosterone in females, placental hormones, and hormones produced by ectopic tumors.

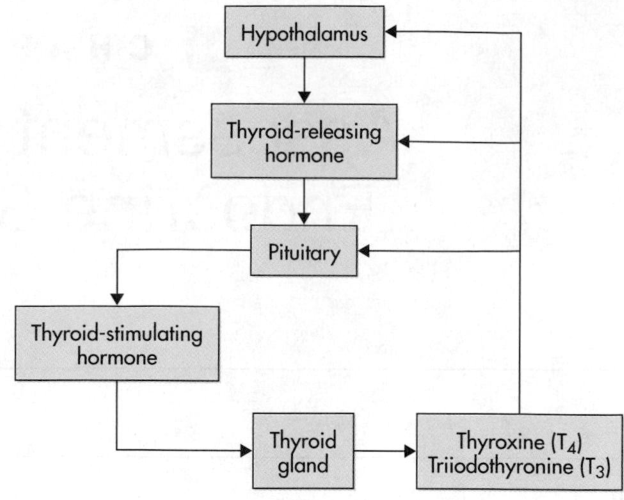

Figure 37-1 Endocrine axis feedback loop.

INTRINSIC RHYTHMICITY. A second factor regulating hormone levels is intrinsic rhythmicity. The intrinsic rhythms can vary over minutes, days, or weeks. For example, prolactin (PRL), cortisol, and GH demonstrate daily **circadian rhythms** (Figure 37-2). In

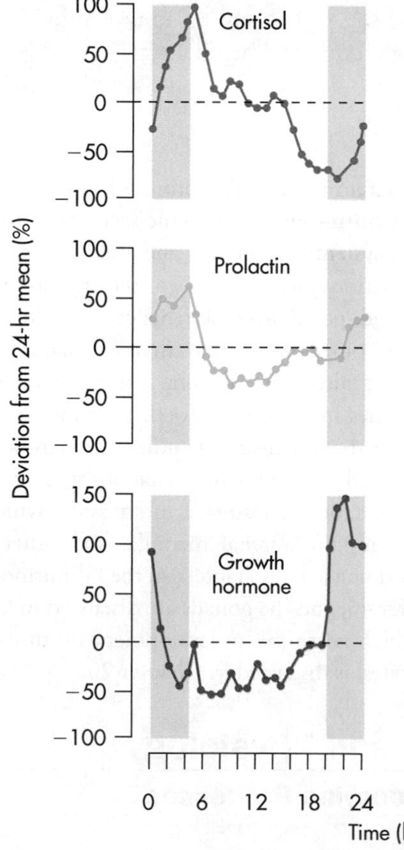

Figure 37-2 Intrinsic rhythms of cortisol, prolactin, and growth hormone.

addition to circadian rhythms, hormone secretion may demonstrate pulsatile or cyclic patterns.

These intrinsic rhythms are controlled by various factors. The environmental factor of sleep-wake patterns influences the circadian rhythms of GH, adrenocorticotropic hormone (ACTH), and cortisol. Age, growth, and development influence the intrinsic rhythmicity of gonadotropins and gonadal steroids. Neurogenic factors influence the intrinsic rhythm of other hormones such as PRL. Extrinsic factors such as pain, trauma, infection, or other stressors also influence levels of selected hormones. These extrinsic factors can override the normal feedback mechanisms or intrinsic rhythmicity and increase secretion of hormones to above normal levels.

NERVOUS SYSTEM. The central nervous system influences hormone release. The hypothalamus contains neurons and neurosecretory cells. Nerve tracts connect the hypothalamus with the posterior lobe of the pituitary. This neuroregulatory system is discussed in the section on endocrine structures and hormonal function.

The autonomic nervous system is also involved in hormone release. As the autonomic nervous system responds to a stressor, the adrenal medulla is stimulated to release epinephrine.

EXCRETION AND METABOLISM. The level of hormones is affected by excretion or metabolic inactivation. The liver and kidneys are primarily responsible for hormonal inactivation and excretion, and diseases of these organs can result in increased hormone levels.

Hormone Transport. Hormones may be transported through the circulatory system either in a free state or bound to plasma proteins. Hormones transported in the free state are biologically active. The concentration of free hormones is balanced by the concentration of bound hormones. As the level of free hormones falls, plasma proteins release enough of the bound hormone to reach equilibrium.

Hormone Action. Hormones stimulate responses by binding either with cell surface receptors or intracellular receptors. Steroid hormones such as adrenal steroids; gonadal steroids; and active derivatives of vitamin D, T_4, and T_3, which are lipid soluble, act through intracellular receptors. These hormones freely cross the cell membrane and combine with their specific intracellular receptor. The steroid-receptor complex is changed in size and conformation and is translocated to the nucleus, where it combines with acceptor sites located in the nucleus near the deoxyribonucleic acid (DNA) sequences. The binding of the hormone-receptor complex initiates transcription of DNA, translation of ribonucleic acid, and synthesis of protein (Figure 37-3).

Water-soluble hormones (hypothalamic releasing hormones, anterior and posterior pituitary hormones, parathyroid hormone [PTH], calcitonin, insulin, glucagon, and biogenic amines) bind to cell surface receptors. The hormone, acting as a first messenger, combines with its specific receptor on the cell membrane, and this hormone-receptor combination activates a second messenger located inside the cell. The second messenger then initiates a sequence of events in the cytoplasm that results in altered cell function. Cyclic adenosine monophosphate (cAMP) has been identified as the second messenger for several hormones. It is hypothesized that the combination of the hormone with the receptor activates adenylate cyclase, which causes the formation of 39,59-cAMP from adenosine triphosphate. The cAMP activates protein kinases, which phosphorylate specific proteins in the stimulated cell and result in altered cell function.

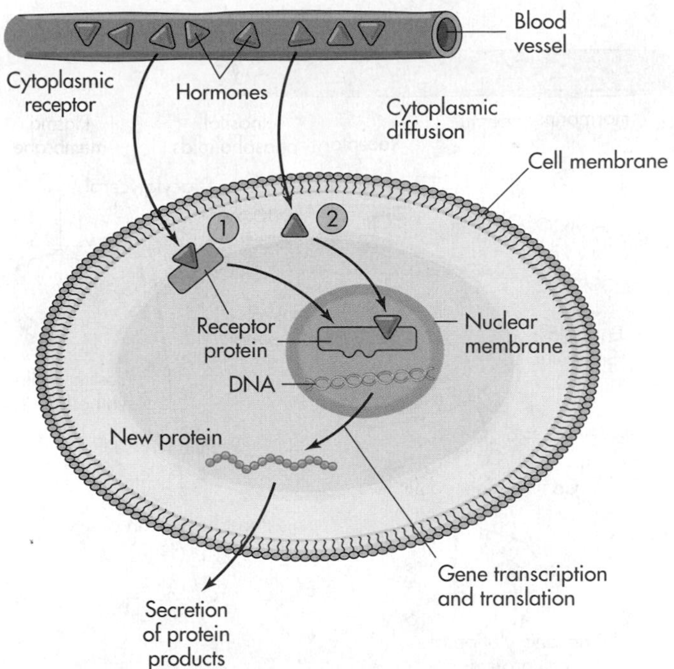

Figure 37-3 Lipid-soluble hormones receptor activity. *DNA*, Deoxyribonucleic acid.

Although cAMP has been identified as a second messenger for several hormones, other compounds serve as second messengers (Figures 37-4 and 37-5). GH is mediated by insulin-like growth factor-I (IGF-I), its second messenger. Calcium ions, calmodulin, adenosine, and prostaglandins are some of the other potential second messengers.

Endocrine Structures and Hormonal Function

The endocrine structures are located throughout the body. In addition to the glands depicted in Figure 37-6, endocrine cells occur throughout various parts of the GI tract.

Hypothalamus and Pituitary Gland. The hypothalamus, a part of the diencephalon, consists of numerous poorly defined nuclei. On its inferior surface the hypothalamus is continuous with the pituitary stalk. Although a small area of the brain, the hypothalamus receives input directly or indirectly from almost every other part of the brain and is a major controller of the anterior and posterior pituitary gland.

The pituitary gland, which is approximately 1 cm in size, lies in the sella turcica of the sphenoid bone. This gland is composed of two functionally distinguishable components: the adenohypophysis (anterior pituitary) and the neurohypophysis (posterior pituitary). The posterior pituitary is a continuation of the pituitary

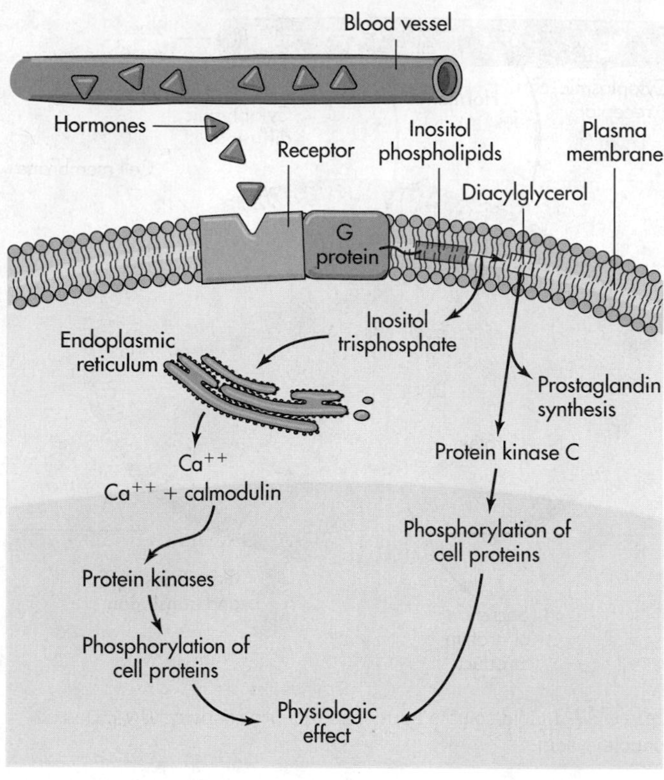

Figure 37-4 Calcium (*Ca^{++}*) as a second messenger.

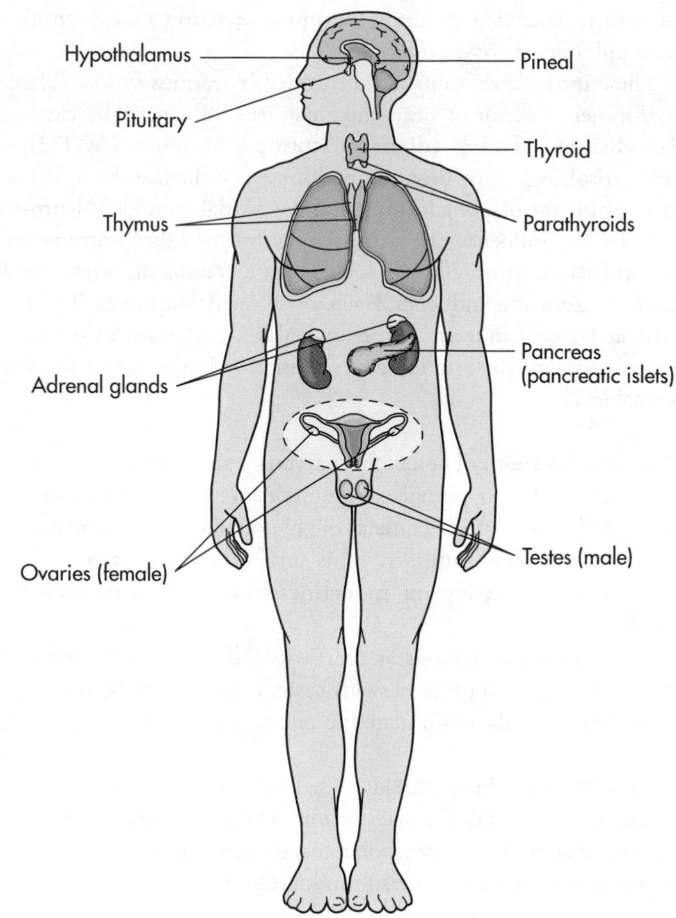

Figure 37-6 The endocrine system.

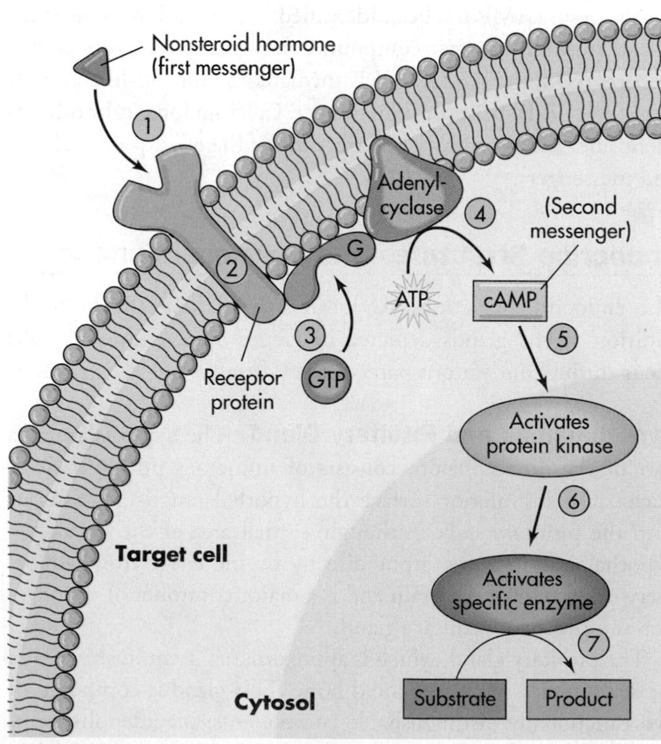

Figure 37-5 Cyclic adenosine monophosphate (*cAMP*) as a second messenger. *ATP*, Adenosine triphosphate; *GTP*, guanosine triphosphate.

stalk. The anterior pituitary, which makes up 75% of the total gland, arises embryonically from an outpouching of ectoderm and fuses with the posterior pituitary.

Hypothalamic-Pituitary Relationship. The hypothalamus serves as a critical link between the rest of the nervous system and the endocrine system, controlling both the posterior and anterior pituitary glands (Figure 37-7). By its control of the anterior pituitary gland, the hypothalamus exerts global control over the entire endocrine system. The hypothalamus is connected to the posterior pituitary gland by nerve tracts that originate in the paraventricular and supraoptic nuclei of the hypothalamus. Posterior pituitary hormones are actually synthesized in the hypothalamus and transported along nerve axons to the posterior pituitary gland, where they are stored.

The hypothalamus and anterior pituitary glands are connected by the hypothalamic-hypophyseal portal blood supply. Blood entering the anterior pituitary gland has first passed through the hypothalamus. The hypothalamus regulates anterior pituitary function by the synthesis of releasing or inhibiting hormones and their secretion into the hypothalamic-hypophyseal portal blood supply. These hormones are released in the anterior pituitary gland and stimulate or inhibit release of appropriate hormones.

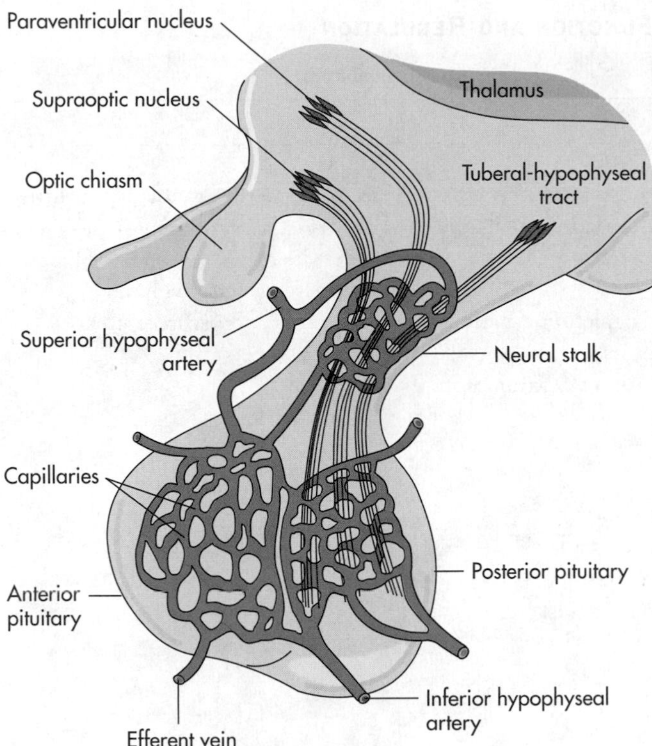

Figure 37-7 Hypothalamic-pituitary connections. Hypothalamus connects to posterior pituitary gland by nerve tracts. Connection between hypothalamus and anterior pituitary gland is vascular.

PITUITARY HORMONES. Most trophic hormones from the pituitary are stimulated by hypothalamic factors. PRL is an exception and is under tonic inhibition via an inhibiting factor, dopamine. Therefore interference with inhibition via pituitary stalk sections or compression or certain medications can raise PRL levels. Very high levels of thyrotropin-releasing hormone (TRH), such as in severe hypothyroidism, can also stimulate PRL release and raise circulating blood levels.

The known releasing and inhibiting hormones and factors include growth hormone–releasing hormone and growth hormone release–inhibiting hormone (or somatostatin) for GH; TRH for TSH; corticotropin-releasing hormone for ACTH; gonadotropin-releasing hormone for follicle-stimulating hormone (FSH) and luteinizing hormone (LH); and prolactin-inhibiting hormone and prolactin-releasing hormone for PRL.

The posterior pituitary gland stores and releases two hormones: antidiuretic hormone (ADH) (vasopressin) and oxytocin. Both these hormones are synthesized in the paraventricular and supraoptic nuclei of the hypothalamus. The blood levels of these two hormones are controlled by multiple factors that act either as stimulators or inhibitors. Table 37-2 defines the regulation and function of ADH and oxytocin.

Six hormones are produced in specific cells located throughout the anterior pituitary gland. Table 37-3 lists the hormones and their regulation and functions.

Thyroid Gland. The thyroid gland, consisting of two lobes connected by an isthmus, is located below the thyroid cartilage on the superior portion of the trachea (Figure 37-8). The gland weighs approximately 20 g and is composed of two distinct cell types: follicular cells and parafollicular cells. The thyroid is highly vascular and receives adrenergic and cholinergic innervation.

Iodine is necessary for the synthesis of thyroid hormone. The thyroid gland has the ability to trap and concentrate iodide. Thyroid hormone is produced in response to one of the following stimuli: TSH, TRH, low serum iodide levels, and factors affecting the binding capacity of thyronine-binding globulin (TBG).

The follicular cell is the functional unit of the thyroid, responsible for T_4 and T_3 production. The follicle consists of a ring of epithelial cells that surround a colloid-filled center. Thyroglobulin is produced by the follicular cells and stored in the colloid. When thyroid hormone is needed, the follicle converts thyroglobulin to T_4 and T_3, which are secreted into the blood. T_3 is the more potent of the two hormones and is generated largely by peripheral conversion of T_4 to T_3.

Thyroid hormone is transported via binding proteins; TBG is the protein with the greatest affinity for T_4 and T_3. Less than 1% of thyroid hormone is free and therefore active. The bound hormone acts as a reservoir to protect the cells against sudden large increases or shortages of thyroid hormone.

The parafollicular cells synthesize and secrete the hormone calcitonin, which is involved in calcium metabolism. Serum calcium levels influence the release of calcitonin. As the serum calcium level rises, calcitonin acts to maintain a normal level by opposing the action of PTH. Its physiologic significance in adults is unknown, as evidenced by the fact that no apparent adverse effects have been noted from the lack of calcitonin in patients who have had thyroidectomies. Table 37-4, p. 1050, lists the thyroid hormones, their regulation, and their function.

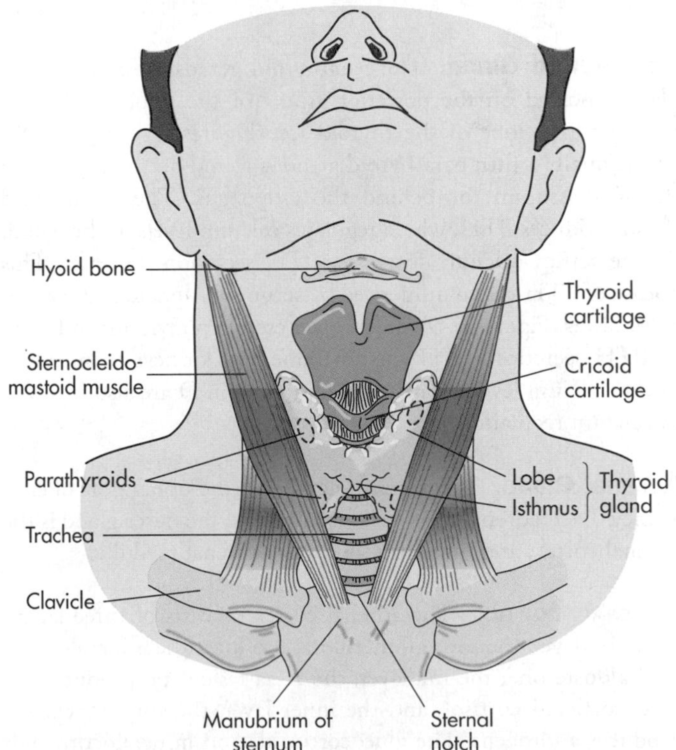

Figure 37-8 Midline neck structures; note thyroid gland in anterior aspect of neck.

TABLE 37-2 POSTERIOR PITUITARY HORMONES: THEIR FUNCTION AND REGULATION

Target Organ	Function	Stimulators	Inhibitors
ANTIDIURETIC HORMONE (ADH, VASOPRESSIN)			
Kidneys	Major regulator of osmolality and body water volume Increases permeability to water of collecting ducts in kidney, resulting in increased water resorption May stimulate water intake by stimulating perception of thirst	**Primary** Increased serum osmolality (as little as 1% increase) via hypothalamic osmoreceptors **Others** Modest volume depletion via atrial volume receptors Modest hypotension via baroreceptors Stressors Psychologic Pain Nausea and vomiting Chemicals Cholinergic agonist Beta-adrenergic agonist Barbiturates Morphine Nicotine	**Primary** Decreased serum osmolality (as little as 1%) via osmoreceptors Modest increased volume and blood pressure via atrial volume receptors and baroreceptors Chemicals Alcohol Alpha-adrenergic agonist
OXYTOCIN			
Breast tissue and uterus	Results in milk let-down in lactating breast Causes increased uterine contraction after labor has begun; role in initiating labor unclear	**Primary** Suckling via neurogenic reflex conducted from afferent fibers in nipple to hypothalamus **Others** Uterine contraction via neurogenic reflex from afferent fibers in uterus	Stressors Psychologic Physical Alpha-adrenergic stimulation

Parathyroid Gland. The parathyroid glands are four minute glands located on the posterior aspect of the upper and lower poles of each lobe of the thyroid (see Figures 37-6 and 37-8). Occasionally a fifth parathyroid gland is found on the thyroid, in the mediastinum, or behind the esophagus. The parathyroid gland produces PTH, which regulates calcium levels in the blood. As the serum calcium decreases, PTH secretion increases. This release of PTH is also influenced by serum phosphate and magnesium levels (Figure 37-9). Hypomagnesemia may result in failure of PTH secretion. PTH acts on bone and kidneys to maintain serum calcium levels. Calcitonin and vitamin D are also involved in calcium regulation.

Adrenal Gland. The adrenal glands cap the upper pole of each kidney. Each adrenal consists of two glands: the outer gland is the adrenal cortex, and the inner core is the adrenal medulla.

ADRENAL CORTEX. The adrenal cortex consists of three layers: the outer layer, the zona glomerulosa, produces the mineralocorticoid aldosterone; the midlayer, the zona fasiculata, produces the glucocorticoid cortisol; and the inner layer, the zona reticularis, produces androgens. The glucocorticoids and mineralocorticoids are not only secreted and used daily, but are secreted as part of the physiologic response to stress. The glucocorticoids and mineralocorticoids are critical to maintain life. Lack of an adrenal cortex is synonymous with death if the missing hormones are not replaced. Figure 37-10 illustrates the feedback control of glucocorticoids, and Table 37-5, p. 1051, outlines the regulation and functions of the adrenal cortex hormones.

ADRENAL MEDULLA. The adrenal medulla makes up approximately 10% of the total gland and produces two catecholamines: epinephrine and norepinephrine. The adrenal medulla arises embryonically from the neural crest and is really a modified sympathetic ganglion innervated by preganglionic splanchnic nerves. As the sympathetic nervous system stimulates the adrenal medulla, epinephrine and norepinephrine are released. They travel via the blood to various organs and bind to receptors on target cells. Norepinephrine is also released from the terminal postganglionic sympathetic fibers. Approximately 85% of the secretions of the adrenal medulla is epinephrine; the remaining 15% is norepinephrine. Norepinephrine is a potent stimulant of alpha-adrenergic receptors, whereas epinephrine stimulates both alpha- and beta-adrenergic receptors (Table 37-6, p. 1052).

In the presence of major stressors (i.e., physiologic, psychologic, or pathologic) increased amounts of epinephrine and norepinephrine are released as an adaptive mechanism. In contrast to the life-threatening consequences of an absent or nonfunctioning adrenal cortex, the absence of an adrenal medulla is compatible with life.

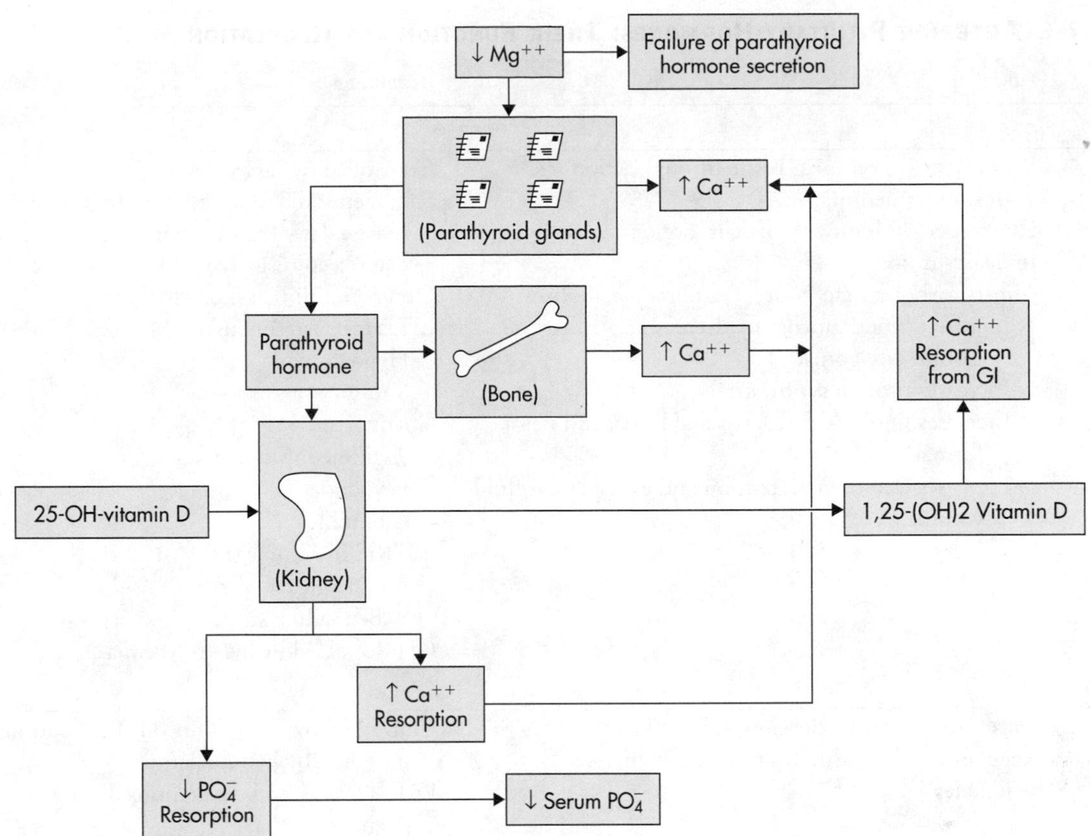

Figure 37-9 Regulation and function of parathyroid hormone. *Ca*$^{++}$, Calcium; *Mg*$^{++}$, magnesium; *PO*$_4^-$, phosphate; *1,25-(OH)2 Vitamin D*, 1,25-dihydroxycholecalciferol; *25-OH-vitamin D*, 25-hydroxy vitamin D.

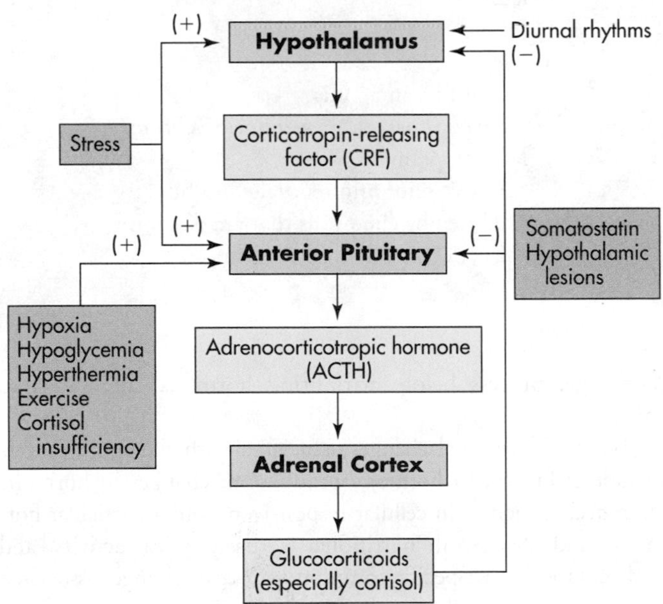

Figure 37-10 Feedback control of glucocorticoid synthesis and secretion.

Pancreas. The pancreas is both an exocrine and an endocrine gland. It lies retroperitoneally behind the stomach, with its head and neck in the curve of the duodenum, its body extending horizontally across the posterior abdominal wall, and its tail touching the spleen. Endocrine function resides in the cells in the islets of Langerhans. More than 1 million islet cells are spread throughout the pancreas, comprising 1% to 2% of the pancreatic mass. The islets of Langerhans consist of four cell types: (1) *alpha* cells, which secrete glucagon; (2) *beta* cells, which make up 70% of the cells and secrete insulin; (3) *delta* cells, which secrete somatostatin; and (4) cells that secrete pancreatic polypeptide. Somatostatin inhibits gastric motility and emptying; gallbladder contraction; intestinal absorption of fats, amino acids, glucose, and other nutrients; and insulin and glucagon secretion. Pancreatic polypeptide inhibits pancreatic exocrine secretion and contraction of the gallbladder.

INSULIN. Insulin, a peptide hormone, is secreted as a prohormone; an enzymatic reaction occurs to produce the active hormone, insulin. Insulin is an anabolic hormone and the only hormone that lowers blood glucose levels to maintain glucose homeostasis. (See Chapter 39 for detailed information on diabetes mellitus.)

GLUCAGON. The primary target of glucagon is the liver, where it stimulates glycogenolysis (breakdown of glycogen to glucose). When glycogenolysis fails to provide enough glucose, glucagon promotes amino acid transport from the muscle and stimulates gluconeogenesis (formation of glycogen from fatty acids and proteins, rather than carbohydrates). As a result of autoimmune pancreatic destruction, individuals with type 1 diabetes mellitus lose glucagon secretion early in the course of the disease. In response to hypoglycemia, the individual with type 1 diabetes must rely on the effects of the adrenergic response and the secretion of catecholamines.

TABLE 37-3 ANTERIOR PITUITARY HORMONES: THEIR FUNCTION AND REGULATION

Target Organ	Function	Regulation
GROWTH HORMONE (GH)		
Whole body	Possibly works on most tissue through action of somatomedin(s) Concerned with growth of cells, bones, and soft tissues Increases mitosis Affects carbohydrate, protein, and fat metabolism: Increases blood glucose by decreasing glucose use; insulin antagonist Increases protein synthesis Increases lipolysis, free fatty acid levels, and ketone formation Increases electrolyte retention and extracellular fluid volume	Controlled by GHRH/GHIH Shows episodic secretion with increases after eating (particularly high-protein diet) and after onset of deep sleep (usually within 1-2 hr after falling asleep) Other stimuli that increase GH: Exercise (strenuous) Hypoglycemia Stressors Chemicals: Arginine infusion Levodopa Clonidine TRH in acromegaly Adrenergic agonists Beta-adrenergic antagonists GH decreased by hyperglycemia
PROLACTIN (PRL)		
Breast, gonads	Necessary for breast development and lactation Regulator of reproductive function in males and females	Controlled by PRH and PIH; PRL chronically inhibited by hypothalamus PRL shows episodic secretions during later hours of sleep Other stimulants: Stressors Suckling Chemicals: Estrogen TRH Dopamine antagonist Conventional and newer antipsychotics Metoclopramide Selective serotonin reuptake inhibitors PRL inhibited by chemicals that are dopamine agonists (levodopa, bromocriptine)

SOMATOSTATIN. Somatostatin is a natural inhibitor of glucagon and helps maintain glucose homeostasis in the nondiabetic person. Synthetic somatostatin analogs are used to successfully treat acromegaly, to reduce pancreatic polypeptide levels and prevent recurrent pancreatitis in patients with pseudocysts, and to treat gastrin-producing tumors and vasoactive intestinal polypeptide–producing tumors. When administered to an individual with type 1 diabetes, a somatostatin analog can increase the risk of hypoglycemia.

Physiologic Changes With Aging

Changes in the endocrine system occur with normal aging. Signs and symptoms of endocrine dysfunction may be subtle, progress slowly, and often mimic normal changes associated with aging. In general, health care practitioners must search for and rule out a pathologic process before attributing hormonal alterations to aging.

Types of hormonal changes associated with the aging process include reduction in hormone production; changes in hormone clearance; reduction in cellular responsiveness to a particular hormone; and changes in nutritional status, physical activity, and body composition. Specific common endocrine changes associated with aging are the following:

- Menopause with loss of ovarian function is a naturally occurring event. The earliest hormonal signs of menopause are rising levels of gonadotropins (FSH and LH), which are trying to stimulate the failing ovaries.
- Androgen production in males declines with age but only within the normal reference range. Libido and sexual performance do not correlate well with absolute testosterone levels within the normal range. Sperm production may

TABLE 37-3 ANTERIOR PITUITARY HORMONES: THEIR FUNCTION AND REGULATION—CONT'D

Target Organ	Function	Regulation
THYROID-STIMULATING HORMONE (TSH)		
Thyroid gland	Necessary for growth and function of thyroid; controls all functions of thyroid	Controlled by TRH and negative feedback from plasma T_4 and T_3 levels Increased $T_4 \rightarrow$ decreased TSH Decreased $T_4 \rightarrow$ increased TSH
ADRENOCORTICOTROPIN HORMONE (ACTH)		
Adrenal cortex gland	Necessary for growth and maintenance of size of adrenal cortex Controls release of glucocorticoids (cortisol) and adrenal androgens Minor role in release of mineralocorticoids (aldosterone)	Controlled by CRH and negative feedback by cortisol levels Shows episodic secretion with rhythm that peaks between 6 and 8 AM Circadian pattern (24-hr pattern) related to sleep-wake pattern and caused by increased CRH Physiologic and psychologic stressors (e.g., hypoglycemia, infections, pain, anxiety) increase ACTH caused by increased CRH (override negative feedback); changes in cortisol influence ACTH Increased cortisol $\rightarrow$ decreased ACTH Decreased cortisol $\rightarrow$ increased ACTH
GONADOTROPINS: FOLLICLE-STIMULATING HORMONE (FSH), LUTEINIZING HORMONE (LH)*		
Gonads	Stimulate gametogenesis and sex steroid production in males and females	Secretion controlled by GnRH Amount of FSH secreted decreased by inhibin in males Amount of LH secreted decreased by testosterone in males Sex steroids in females exert positive feedback on FSH and LH at certain times in normal menstrual cycle and negative feedback at other times

CRH, Corticotropin-releasing hormone; *GHIH,* growth hormone–inhibiting hormone; *GHRH,* growth hormone–releasing hormone; *GnRH,* gonadotropin-releasing hormone; *PIH,* prolactin-inhibiting hormone; *PRH,* prolactin-releasing hormone; *TRH,* thyrotropin-releasing hormone.
*Previously called interstitial cell–stimulating hormone (ICSH) in males.

decrease somewhat with aging; however, fertility is well preserved in many octogenarians.

- Changes in PTH levels are not uncommon in older adults. In response to decreased intake of calcium (dietary and supplements) and vitamin D intake or production via decreased exposure to sunlight, many older patients have mild elevations in PTH levels and a negative calcium balance. This has a negative impact on bone density and increases fracture risk.
- Reduced insulin sensitivity rather than reduced insulin secretion is responsible for the high prevalence of impaired glucose tolerance and type 2 diabetes mellitus in older adults. This is related to factors that worsen insulin resistance, including (1) physical inactivity, (2) altered body composition with increased fat mass and decreased lean muscle mass, (3) obesity, and (4) the use of certain medications such as thiazide diuretics and beta-blockers.

▶ ARE YOU READY?

Based on the endocrine system's negative feedback system, which of the following is the earliest marker of excess thyroid hormone?

1. Elevated TSH
2. Elevated thyroxine
3. Decreased TSH
4. Decreased thyroxine

Health History

The health history must be comprehensive, with special attention given to growth patterns in children and altered reproductive function in adults (menstrual disturbances, infertility, impotence). Specific questions should be targeted to the suspected endocrine dysfunction. The health history should include the

TABLE 37-4 THYROID GLAND HORMONES: THEIR FUNCTION AND REGULATION

Function	Regulation
THYROXINE (T_4) AND TRIIODOTHYRONINE (T_3)	
Regulates protein, fat, and carbohydrates catabolism in all cells Regulates metabolic rate of all cells Regulates body heat production Acts as insulin antagonist Maintains GH secretion, skeletal maturation Affects central nervous system development Necessary for muscle tone and vigor Maintains cardiac rate, force, and output Maintains secretions of GI tract Affects respiratory rate and oxygen utilization Maintains calcium mobilization Affects red blood cell production Stimulates lipid turnover, free fatty acid release, and cholesterol synthesis Regulates sympathetic nervous system activity	T_4 and T_3 levels controlled by TSH Hormones show diurnal variation with peak during late evening Influences on amount secreted: Gender Pregnancy Gonadal steroid and adrenal corticosteroids; increased steroids → increased levels of T_4 and T_3 Exposure to extreme cold increases levels Nutritional state Chemicals: Somatostatin (GHIH) = ↓ levels Dopamine = ↓ _levels Catecholamines = ↑ levels
CALCITONIN	
Lowers serum calcium by opposing bone-resorbing effects of PTH, prostaglandins, and calciferols by inhibiting osteoclastic activity Also lowers serum phosphate levels May also decrease calcium and phosphorus absorption in GI tract	Elevated serum calcium—major stimulant for calcitonin Other stimulants: Gastrin Calcium-rich foods (regardless of serum Ca^{++} levels) Pregnancy Lowered serum calcium—suppresses calcitonin release

CA^{++}, Calcium; *GH*, Growth hormone; *GHIH*, growth hormone–inhibiting hormone; *GI*, gastrointestinal; *PTH*, parathyroid hormone; *TSH*, thyroid-stimulating hormone.

reason for seeking care, history of present illness, a review of systems, social history, and family history. Areas requiring particular focus are discussed below.

Cognitive Function

Abnormalities in endocrine function can result in cognitive impairment. Difficulties in concentration can be seen in a variety of endocrinopathies such as hyperthyroidism, hypothyroidism, pheochromocytoma, and Addison's disease (primary adrenal insufficiency). Depression can be another manifestation of endocrinopathies; however, the incidence of depression is high with chronic medical conditions in general.

Intake: Food, Fluids, and Electrolytes

Endocrine dysfunction can result in an alteration of the patient's fluid, electrolyte, and nutritional status. A thorough assessment of food and fluid intake via an accurate 24-hour dietary recall is helpful. Changes in appetite can accompany endocrine dysfunction (e.g., hyperthyroidism can cause a voracious appetite). Part of the treatment plan for endocrine dysfunction may include specific dietary recommendations for intake of food and fluids (e.g., carbohydrate consistency in diabetes mellitus, fluid restriction in syndrome of inappropriate antidiuretic hormone [SIADH]), in addition to vitamin and mineral supplementation (1,25-dihydroxycholecalciferol in secondary hyperparathyroidism).

Elimination Pattern

The endocrine system regulates water and electrolyte homeostasis. The nurse assesses urine frequency, volume, and characteristics (color, turbidity, odor, specific gravity). Urine volume is excessive in diabetes insipidus and may be excessive in diabetes mellitus; it is subnormal in SIADH. The presence or absence of nocturia or dysuria should be noted. In conjunction with assessment of urinary output, the nurse assesses the volume and type of oral fluid intake (patients with diabetes insipidus crave cold liquids).

Bowel habits also may be affected by endocrine dysfunction. The color, characteristics, and frequency of bowel movements are all important to assess. Constipation can be a manifestation of hypothyroidism or dehydration secondary to diabetes insipidus.

Energy Level

Many factors, including endocrine function and dysfunction, affect energy levels. A confounding variable is the presence of depression or dysphoria, a common comorbid condition in individuals with chronic medical conditions. A number of hormones such as T_4, T_3, testosterone, and GH can affect energy levels. Assessment of sleep patterns is also critical. Sleep patterns can be worsened by hyperthyroidism. However, poor sleep patterns unrelated to endocrine dysfunction also reduce energy levels.

TABLE 37-5 ADRENAL CORTEX HORMONES: THEIR FUNCTION AND REGULATION

Function	Regulation
GLUCOCORTICOIDS (CORTISOL)	
Overall effect: maintain blood glucose level by increasing gluconeogenesis and decreasing rate of glucose use by cells Increases protein catabolism Promotes lipolysis Antiinflammatory Degrades collagen Decreases T-lymphocyte participation in cell-mediated immunity by decreasing circulating level of T lymphocytes Increases neutrophils by increasing release and decreasing destruction Decreases new antibody release Decreases eosinophils, basophils, and monocytes Decreases scar tissue formation Increases red blood cell formation and possibly increases platelet formation Increases gastric acid and pepsin production Promotes sodium and water retention Maintains emotional stability	Level of cortisol is controlled by CRH and ACTH. Cortisol shows episodic secretion with circadian rhythm that peaks between 6 and 8 AM; this circadian pattern follows circadian pattern of CRH and ACTH. Physiologic and psychologic stressors (e.g., hypoglycemia, hypoxia, pain, infection, trauma, anxiety) result in increased cortisol via increased CRH and ACTH. This stress response overrides negative feedback cortisol normally exerts on ACTH.
MINERALOCORTICOIDS (ALDOSTERONE)	
Maintains sodium and volume status Increases sodium resorption in distal tubules Increases potassium and hydrogen excretion in distal tubules	Major regulator is renin-angiotensin system. When vascular volume or sodium is decreased, renin-angiotensin system is activated (see Chapters 17 and 34), and angiotensin II stimulates release of mineralocorticoids. Increased serum potassium directly stimulates adrenal cortex to release mineralocorticoids. CRH-ACTH system is a weak regulator.
ADRENAL ANDROGENS	
Responsible for some secondary sex characteristics in females; in males, acts as gonadal steroids	Major regulator is CRH-ACTH system.

ACTH, Adrenocorticotropin hormone; *CRH,* corticotropin-releasing hormone.

Perceptions of Body Characteristics

Body image is a critical component of the ego. Endocrine dysfunction can be marked by numerous physical signs and symptoms such as hirsutism (polycystic ovary syndrome [PCOS], Cushing's syndrome), hair loss (thyroid disease), hoarse voice (hypothyroidism), proptosis and ophthalmopathy (Graves' disease), darkening skin pigmentation (Addison's disease), excessive sweating (hyperthyroidism, acromegaly), and changes in soft tissues and bony structures (acromegaly). Reviewing family photographs can reveal gradual changes in appearance, which can help define a rough date of onset of an endocrine disorder such as Cushing's syndrome or acromegaly.

Reproductive and Sexual Function

Endocrine dysfunction can both directly and indirectly affect reproductive and sexual function. Both are intimately integrated with body image and self-image. The reproductive history should include assessment data on menarche, menses patterns, and pregnancies in women; or onset of puberty, erectile function, and testicular size and volume in men. The sexual history should encompass partner issues, frequency and type of sexual contact, arousal capabilities, ability to achieve orgasm, and sexually transmitted diseases. Fertility potential is negatively affected by many endocrine disorders (mild hypothyroidism, hyperprolactinemia, PCOS). On the other hand, individuals may not desire conception and may have specific concerns about contraception.

Physical Examination

A comprehensive physical examination should focus on pigmentation, skin texture, growth patterns, and visual fields. Special attention should be directed to endocrine glands suspected of being diseased.

Objective assessment begins during the professional nurse's initial encounter with the patient.

- Observation of the patient's facies. Does the patient have:
  - Facial plethora as seen in Cushing's syndrome?
  - Facial hirsutism as seen in PCOS, Cushing's syndrome, and adrenal disorders?
  - Graves' ophthalmopathy?

TABLE 37-6 EFFECTS OF ADRENAL-MEDULLARY-SYMPATHETIC STIMULATION ON BODY ORGANS

Organ	Effect*
Heart	Increased conduction velocity, automaticity, contractility, rate, and stroke volume caused by $beta_1$-stimulation
Blood vessels	
Coronary vessels, brain, lungs	Dilation caused by $beta_2$ stimulation and autoregulatory phenomena
Skin, mucosa, abdominal viscera, renal and salivary gland vessels	Constriction caused by $alpha_1$-receptor stimulation; renal vessels also have dopaminergic receptors
Veins	Constriction caused by $alpha_1$ stimulation
Bronchial muscles	Relaxation caused by $beta_2$ stimulation
Gastrointestinal tract	Inhibition of production of gastrointestinal secretions; decreased motility and contraction of sphincters
Gallbladder	Relaxation
Kidney	Increased renin secretion caused by $beta_2$ stimulation
Urinary bladder	Relaxation of detrusor muscle and contraction of sphincter
Skin	Pilomotor muscle contraction and localized sweating
Liver	Glycogenolysis and gluconeogenesis caused by $beta_2$ stimulation
Pancreas	Decreased secretion of exocrine cells; $beta_2$ stimulation causes increased secretion of islet beta cells, but alpha stimulation causes decreased secretion of islet cells; alpha effect predominates
Fat cells	Lipolysis
Brain	Increased alertness, restlessness
Eyes	Dilation of pupils and relaxation of ciliary bodies

*These total effects would be seen in physiologic responses to stressors.

- The handshake. Are the patient's hands:
  - Large and "doughy" as in acromegaly?
  - Sweaty and clammy as in hypoglycemia, hyperthyroidism, or pheochromocytoma?
- Observation of the patient's demeanor. Is the patient:
  - Anxious as in hyperthyroidism or pheochromocytoma?
  - Lethargic as in hypothyroidism or hypopituitarism?

A thorough multisystem physical examination by a skilled clinician assists in narrowing the differential diagnosis (Table 37-7).

Assessment measures and variations in normal findings relevant to the care of older adults are presented in the Gerontologic Assessment box, which also lists disorders common in older adults that may be responsible for abnormal assessment findings.

Diagnostic Tests

Selection of laboratory tests to assess endocrine function of the suspect gland is based on the history and physical examination. Laboratory tests should be ordered to confirm or refute a clinical suspicion. Routine screening for endocrine conditions is limited to a few situations such as congenital hypothyroidism and phenylketonuria. For any diagnostic testing, appropriate patient preparation is critical if accurate results are to be obtained (see Guidelines for Safe Practice box).

Principles of Laboratory Evaluation

Some basic principles guide the measurement and interpretation of hormone levels in the body. Basal hormone output is generally assessed by measuring serum values. Serum values of protein-bound hormones (e.g., T_4) may be elevated by high levels of binding proteins as seen in pregnancy. In such situations, measurement of the active free or unbound hormone better reflects basal hormone production.

Timing of the hormone measurement may be important in hormones with circadian rhythms such as cortisol. Many hormones, such as gonadotropins, are secreted in a pulsatile fashion, such that measuring the peak (highest) versus the trough (lowest) levels may yield widely divergent values. The relationship to food ingestion is also important when feeding may stimulate or suppress hormone production (e.g., eating carbohydrates stimulates insulin production but suppresses GH production).

Measuring a trophic hormone (one that stimulates organ growth) is another marker of mild hyperfunctioning or hypofunctioning of an endocrine gland. An example is the measurement of TSH in the evaluation of the thyroid gland.

Dynamic Testing

In many instances of endocrine dysfunction, the extreme ends of the normal range and the pathologic range overlap, and dynamic testing is necessary. In suspected cases of hyperfunction, the clini-

Gerontologic Assessment

Neurologic

Hoarseness, progressive deafness, unsteady gait, and muscle weakness may be caused by hypothyroidism.
Confusion, lethargy, and memory problems may result from hypothyroidism, hyperthyroidism, hyponatremia, hypernatremia, or hypoglycemia.
Neurologic symptoms such as paresthesias, blurred vision, headache, and inability to sense temperature may be attributed to complications from diabetes.

Cardiovascular

Count the pulse for 1 full minute. Check for signs and symptoms of angina and congestive heart failure. Both may occur with hyperthyroidism.
Check for orthostatic hypotension, which may occur in hypernatremia.

Eyes

Ophthalmopathy is rarely found in older patients who are newly diagnosed with hyperthyroidism.
Visual problems may be a result of complications of diabetes.

Skin and Hair

Assess for dry skin, poor skin turgor, and thin or fine hair. Some of these may occur with thyroid dysfunction.
Persons with frequent yeast or fungal infections may have diabetes mellitus.

Musculoskeletal

Assess ability to perform activities of daily living and other activities.
Lack of energy, muscle weakness, and apathy occur with hypernatremia and thyroid and pancreatic dysfunction.
Arthralgias may occur with adrenal insufficiency.
Fractures and loss of height may occur from osteoporosis secondary to decreased estrogen.

Gastrointestinal

Assess for changes in bowel habits.
Constipation may occur with hypothyroidism.
Diarrhea may occur with hyperthyroidism.
Weight loss, nausea, and abdominal pain may occur with adrenal insufficiency.
Anorexia and weight loss may occur with hypothyroidism or hyperthyroidism.

Psychosocial

Apathy is often the most apparent symptom of hyperthyroidism in an older adult.
Depression and withdrawal are often found in persons with hypothyroidism. The cause of these psychologic symptoms is unclear.

Common Disorders in Older Adults

Hypothyroidism
Type 2 diabetes mellitus

GUIDELINES FOR SAFE PRACTICE
Preparing the Patient for Diagnostic Tests

- Explain the purpose of the test.
- Explain what to expect before, during, and after the test.
- Ensure patient is prepared as ordered. For example, fasting hormone assays are generally performed after an overnight fast with blood drawn at 8 AM because of circadian hormonal rhythms.
- Dietary preparation for certain tests is critical. Iodide-containing foods such as cabbage and iodine supplements must be eliminated from the diet of a patient scheduled to undergo a radioiodine uptake scan.

cian attempts to suppress the gland. For example, the dexamethasone suppression test is an attempt to suppress production of cortisol; a glucose-loading test is an attempt to suppress secretion of GH. Failure to normally suppress the elevated hormone indicates a significant pathologic state. On the other hand, in suspected cases of hypofunction, the clinician attempts to stimulate the gland. For example, a cosyntropin (a synthetic subunit of ACTH) stimulation test attempts to stimulate the adrenal glands to produce cortisol. Failure to normally stimulate the gland indicates a pathologic state.

Urine Assessment of Hormonal Status

A 24-hour urine collection of either the hormone itself or its metabolites can yield an integrated marker of hormone production. This is frequently used in suspected adrenal cortisol disorders (Cushing's syndrome) and adrenal medullary disorders (pheochromocytoma). In addition to measurement of the desired hormone or metabolite, it is common to measure the 24-hour urine creatinine as a marker of the completeness of the collection.

Imaging Studies in Endocrinology

A variety of imaging techniques are used for the assessment of endocrine glands:

- Ultrasound (thyroid, parathyroid)
- Nuclear medicine scans (thyroid, parathyroid)
- Computed tomography (CT) and magnetic resonance imaging (MRI)
- Functional imaging studies—nuclear medicine studies based on physiologic and pathophysiologic processes such as cellular metabolism, tissue perfusion and local synthesis, uptake, or storage of hormones and their receptors (e.g., metaidobenzylguanidine scintigraphy, fludeoxyglucose F 18 positron emission tomography scan [PET], Octreoscan)

Plain-film x-ray studies have generally been replaced by the technologies in the preceding list.

TABLE 37-7 PHYSICAL ASSESSMENT CUES IN ENDOCRINE DYSFUNCTION

Physical Assessment	Potential Endocrine Dysfunction
DERMATOLOGIC SYSTEM	
Erythema, facial plethora, purplish striae, thin skin, moon facies, supraclavicular fat pads, thin hair or hair loss	Cushing's syndrome
Hyperpigmentation, poor skin turgor, dry mucous membranes	Adrenal insufficiency
Pallor, decreased perspiration, cool and dry skin, coarse skin texture, periorbital edema, nonpitting edema, thin hair or hair loss	Hypothyroidism Hypopituitarism
Smooth warm skin, increased perspiration, flushing, onycholysis	Hyperthyroidism
NEUROLOGIC SYSTEM	
Confusion	Hypoglycemia Cushing's syndrome Myxedema (severe hypothyroidism) Hyperglycemia with incipient diabetic ketoacidosis
Decreased mentation	Hypoglycemia Myxedema Cushing's syndrome Hyperglycemia with incipient diabetic ketoacidosis
Decreased neurologic tone, decreased deep tendon reflexes	Hypothyroidism
Spasms, positive Trousseau's sign, positive Chvostek's sign	Hypoparathyroidism
Seizures	Hypoglycemia Hypoparathyroidism Adrenal insufficiency
Hoarseness, speech changes	Hypothyroidism
Blurred vision	Hypoglycemia Hyperglycemia
Exophthalmos, proptosis	Graves' disease
CARDIOVASCULAR SYSTEM	
Bradycardia	Hypothyroidism
Tachycardia, palpitations, increased blood pressure, angina	Hyperthyroidism
RESPIRATORY SYSTEM	
Dyspnea	Hyperthyroidism
Kussmaul's respirations, acetone breath	Diabetic ketoacidosis
GASTROINTESTINAL SYSTEM	
Constipation, weight gain	Hypothyroidism

Imaging studies are ordered after a thorough history, physical examination, and chemical examination and hormonal evaluation of the patient. Incidental lesions (incidentalomas) are frequently encountered in otherwise normal people when scans are carried out for unrelated reasons such as trauma or vague pain in the region. Autopsy studies show that 20% of individuals may have incidentalomas—benign, nonfunctioning lesions in the pituitary or adrenal glands. An obvious diagnostic pitfall then arises in attributing clinical significance to incidentalomas and subjecting patients to unnecessary and perhaps major surgery. The opinion of the skilled, experienced endocrinologist is of paramount importance in these diagnostic dilemmas.[12,20,21,28]

Assessing Function of Individual Endocrine Glands

Endocrine dysfunction is broadly categorized into hyposecretory and hypersecretory disorders. These may be further categorized into primary, secondary, or tertiary dysfunctions. Diagnostic tests confirm clinical suspicions: if underactivity is suspected, a stimulation test is indicated; if overactivity is suspected, a suppression test is indicated.

Using the thyroid gland as an example, categories of dysfunction are:

1. Primary dysfunction: hypothyroidism resulting from intrinsic disease of the gland

TABLE 37-7 PHYSICAL ASSESSMENT CUES IN ENDOCRINE DYSFUNCTION—CONT'D

Physical Assessment	Potential Endocrine Dysfunction
GENITOURINARY SYSTEM	
Diarrhea, weight loss	Hyperthyroidism
Polyphagia	Hyperglycemia Hyperthyroidism
Polyuria, polydipsia	Diabetes mellitus Diabetes insipidus
Salt craving, weight loss	Adrenal insufficiency
Decreased urinary output	Adrenal insufficiency Syndrome of inappropriate antidiuretic hormone
Increased urinary output	Uncontrolled diabetes mellitus Diabetes insipidus
MUSCULOSKELETAL SYSTEM	
Weakness, fatigue	Hypoglycemia Hyperglycemia Hypothyroidism Hyperthyroidism Hypopituitarism Acromegaly
Muscle cramps	Hypoparathyroidism Adrenal insufficiency
Muscle wasting	Cushing's syndrome
Fractures, low bone mass	Cushing's syndrome Hyperparathyroidism Vitamin D deficiency Hyperthyroidism
PSYCHOSOCIAL SIGNS	
Depression	Hypothyroidism Diabetes mellitus Adrenal insufficiency
Emotional lability	Cushing's syndrome Hyperthyroidism
Anxiety	Hyperthyroidism
NONSPECIFIC	
Cold intolerance, decreased body temperature	Hypothyroidism
Heat intolerance, increased body temperature	Hyperthyroidism

2. Secondary dysfunction: secondary hypothyroidism caused by pituitary disease and deficiency of biologically active TSH
3. Tertiary dysfunction: hypothyroidism caused by hypothalamic dysfunction, resulting in deficiency of biologically active TRH with resultant deficiency of TSH and ultimately reduced T_4 and T_3 levels

The disease process at each of these levels (the individual endocrine gland, the pituitary gland, or the hypothalamus) may be due to either an intrinsic destruction of that organ (autoimmune thyroid disease damaging the thyroid gland and causing primary hypothyroidism, autoimmune adrenal gland disease damaging the adrenal glands and causing primary adrenal insufficiency, or hypophysitis damaging the pituitary gland and causing secondary hypothyroidism) or a secondary process such as metastatic disease (breast cancer metastasizing to the hypothalamic area and causing tertiary hypothyroidism, lung cancer metastasizing to the adrenal glands and causing primary adrenal insufficiency, or chronic kidney failure causing failure of activation of vitamin D and secondary hyperparathyroidism). Uncommonly, hyperfunctioning of an endocrine gland can result from ectopic hormone production (e.g., ACTH production from carcinoma of the lung, GH production from a pancreatic tumor).

Endocrine dysfunction can also be the result of iatrogenic or factitious disease. Iatrogenic disease usually is caused by overdosing or underdosing of hormone replacement therapy (e.g., levothyroxine), although occasionally it may be related to a side effect of a concurrently administered medication (lithium-induced hypothyroidism; amiodarone-induced hypothyroidism or hyperthyroidism). Factitious disease can involve a patient intentionally overdosing, such as taking levothyroxine in an attempt to lose weight.

Pituitary Gland

Pituitary Function Testing

PROLACTIN. The assessment of basal PRL levels generally suffices for evaluating PRL excess. Before further evaluation, it is critical to rule out hypothyroidism, renal disease, pregnancy, and adverse effects of medications (cimetadine, metoclopramide, etc.). Absolute PRL levels may be of value in distinguishing a tumor from other causes of hyperprolactinemia. A value in excess of 150 mcg/L nearly always is diagnostic for a tumor. However, PRL levels lower than 150 mcg/L may be associated with either a tumor or other causes. PRL deficiency is generally seen as a part of panhypopituitarism. A clinical clue to underlying pituitary destruction is postpartum failure of lactation.[5,22-24,31]

GROWTH HORMONE. Basal levels of GH alone are not sufficient to diagnose excessive (acromegaly) or deficient states. IGF-I and its principal binding protein, insulin-like growth factor binding protein 3 (IGF-BP3), are frequently measured to assess both deficiency and excess of growth hormone. Patients with high GH levels usually have characteristic clinical features. Basal GH levels in the fasting state in the morning with concurrent IGF-I levels are usually the initial step in evaluation of a patient. In an individual with elevated basal GH levels, the next step in the evaluation process is a glucose suppression test, whereby a baseline GH level is measured, a glucose load is administered, and then a postglucose load GH level is measured. Failure to suppress GH levels with a glucose load confirms autonomous secretion of GH and is consistent with the presence of a tumor.[5,14,22,33]

Isolated GH deficiency in a prepubertal patient is associated with growth retardation. In the adult, GH deficiency is generally associated with panhypopituitarism, such that other hormonal deficiencies are also present. Stimulation of GH secretion may be performed via (1) insulin tolerance, (2) arginine stimulation, (3) GH-releasing hormone stimulation, and (4) levodopa stimulation. Because no single stimulation test is 100% reliable, two tests are generally performed.

Although the insulin tolerance test (ITT) is the gold standard for diagnosing GH deficiency in adults, it has numerous disadvantages. The test is contraindicated for patients with seizure disorders or ischemic heart disease. And, because an ITT induces hypoglycemia, patients experience the related unpleasant symptoms. The sensitivity and specificity of the arginine/GH-releasing hormone stimulation test are comparable to those of the ITT, but side effects are fewer, with vasodilation and flushing being the most common. Thus the arginine/GH-releasing hormone stimulation test is a suitable diagnostic alternative to the ITT.[5,14,22,33]

ADRENOCORTICOTROPIC HORMONE. ACTH measurements are typically performed with the patient in the fasting and basal state in conjunction with cortisol determinations (see Table 37-5).

GONADOTROPINS: FOLLICLE-STIMULATING HORMONE AND LUTEINIZING HORMONE. FSH and LH can be measured in the basal and stimulated state, the stimulation being measured via administration of gonadotropin-releasing hormone (see Chapter 55 for discussion of ovarian function). In situations of progressive pituitary dysfunction, the first hormones lost are generally FSH and LH. Hence measurement of FSH and LH is commonly part of the anterior pituitary workup in situations of suspected hypopituitarism.[1,22]

ANTIDIURETIC HORMONE. ADH may be inappropriately produced to excess, as in SIADH, or may be deficient, related to posterior pituitary dysfunction. ADH deficiency results in DI, in which the patient is unable to concentrate the urine with resultant polyuria and increased thirst. Patients generally crave liquids, especially ice cold liquids, and report sleep disturbances owing to nocturia and thirst. An overnight water deprivation test is the test of choice to diagnose DI. During such tests, it is critical that the nurse closely monitor the patient for dehydration, hypotension, and vascular collapse. If the patient tolerates the test, the nurse measures fasting serum and urine osmolality, plasma ADH, and electrolytes. A positive water deprivation test will reveal a serum osmolality in excess of 300 mOsm/L in the context of inappropriately dilute urine as reflected by a low urine osmolality. The serum sodium may be elevated. To determine whether the DI is central (posterior pituitary dysfunction) or related to unresponsiveness of the kidneys to ADH (nephrogenic diabetes insipidus), a baseline urine osmolality and serum osmolality is taken. Then 5 units of aqueous vasopressin are given subcutaneously. In central DI, in response to administration of vasopressin, the urine osmolality rises and serum osmolality falls. In nephrogenic DI neither urine nor serum osmolality changes.[15,19,25,30,34]

Pituitary Imaging. Imaging of the anterior and posterior pituitary consists of contrast-enhanced CT or MRI, with MRI being the preferred approach. Plain-film x-ray studies are generally not useful, but may be done in some cases to identify pituitary macroadenomas (e.g., acromegaly).

Petrosal Sinus Sampling. Inferior petrosal sinus sampling may be indicated to localize an adenoma not clearly visualized on MRI or CT scanning. Levels of ACTH in the petrosal sinuses are measured and compared with ACTH levels in a vein in the forearm. A central-to-peripheral ACTH ratio of more than 3 after corticotropin-releasing hormone administration almost always indicates a pituitary source.

Thyroid Gland

Thyroid Function Testing. The mainstay of screening for thyroid disease is the third-generation TSH assay, which can distinguish low-normal TSH levels from truly suppressed TSH levels as in hyperthyroidism. Measurement of a free T_4 level in turn complements the TSH. The American Thyroid Association recommends measurement of a third-generation TSH level and a free T_4 level as the initial tests to be performed in an individual with suspected thyroid disease. Either a total T_3 or free T_3 level may be measured in suspected cases of T_3 toxicosis. As a result of the great improvement in reliable free T_4 assays, clinicians have stopped ordering total T_4 levels. Measurement of free T_4 levels eliminates confusion in situations involving increased TBG proteins with resultant elevation in the total T_4 levels. Increased binding proteins in response, for example, to estrogen therapy or pregnancy yield an elevated total T_4 value but a normal free T_4 value. TRH stimulation tests used to be carried out in the setting of equivocal hyperthyroidism. These tests are no longer needed in the context of the third-generation TSH assays and the modern free T_4 and free T_3 assays.[2,8,18] Thyroid autoantibodies are useful to define underlying autoimmune thyroid disease but cannot be used to predict hypothyroidism, euthyroidism, or hyperthyroidism.

Thyroid Imaging

ULTRASOUND. Ultrasound of the thyroid can accurately define the thyroid anatomy, including volume, echogenicity, and presence and size of nodules and cysts. Thyroid ultrasound may also be used for guidance with fine-needle aspirations of suspicious thyroid nodules. An endocrinologist experienced in ultrasonography should ideally perform thyroid ultrasound.[3,8]

RADIOACTIVE IODINE UPTAKE TEST. The thyroid has tremendous affinity for iodine; the normal 24-hour uptake of a tracer dose of ^{123}I is in the range of 5% to 35%. The radioactive iodine uptake test (RAIU) is generally ordered in hyperthyroid patients to enable calculation of a therapeutic ^{131}I dose. A low RAIU may be seen in thyroiditis, hypothyroidism, previous thyroid ablation, recent excess iodine uptake (diet, medication, iodinated contrast media), factitious hyperthyroidism, or malabsorption of the ^{123}I tracer dose secondary to illness.[8]

NUCLEAR THYROID SCAN. After a dose of labeled pertechnetate or radioactive iodine is given, a scintillation scan is carried out. The distribution of the radioactivity yields an image of the thyroid anatomy; however, the anatomic detail is not nearly as good as the ultrasound image. The nuclear medicine scan can yield information about the functioning of thyroid nodules. A "cold" nodule is one that fails to pick up the radioactive material and thus raises the issue of malignancy. A "hot" nodule, on the other hand, concentrates the radioactivity within the nodule with little or no uptake throughout the rest of the gland. This is indicative of a hyperfunctioning benign nodule.[8]

Patient isolation may not be necessary for RAIU or nuclear thyroid scans. Such isolation is necessary only for large ablative doses of ^{131}I such as those used in the treatment of thyroid cancer, although many centers now give larger ablative doses to individuals on an outpatient basis. Each hospital's nuclear medicine department has written policies and procedures for the care of patients receiving radioactive materials.

Parathyroid Glands

Parathyroid Function Testing. PTH may be produced in excess (hyperparathyroidism) or be deficient (hypoparathyroidism). The clinical history and physical examination, as well as the baseline serum calcium and phosphorus levels, yield important clinical information. The availability of sensitive intact PTH molecule assays has greatly increased the ease of diagnosis. In individuals with normal renal function, PTH excess results in increased mobilization of calcium from bone, decreased renal calcium excretion, and increased phosphorus excretion. Primary hyperparathyroidism is generally the result of a solitary parathyroid adenoma, although occasionally it is related to hyperplasia of all four parathyroid glands. Either of these situations results in an elevated serum calcium level, normal to subnormal serum phosphorus level, and elevated intact PTH level (see Figure 37-9). The serum alkaline phosphatase levels may be elevated to varying degrees.[6,7,32]

Secondary hyperparathyroidism occurs in response to a disorder that tends to cause hypocalcemia, such as (1) intestinal malabsorption (e.g., after gastric bypass surgery), (2) failure of vitamin D hydroxylation associated with liver disease or kidney failure, or (3) excessive catabolism of vitamin D as a side effect of certain medications. In secondary hyperparathyroidism, the intact PTH level is elevated and serum calcium is low normal or mildly subnormal. The phosphorus level varies depending on the primary cause of the disordered calcium balance; the alkaline phosphatase level is generally elevated to varying degrees.[32]

Tertiary hyperparathyroidism occurs with chronic, sustained secondary hyperparathyroidism (most commonly chronic kidney failure) where an adenoma forms in one of the parathyroid glands. Intact PTH levels are generally very high, along with hypercalcemia, in a patient with known prior secondary hyperparathyroidism.[32]

Hypoparathyroidism generally occurs after surgery in the parathyroid or thyroid area or after radiotherapy to the region. Intact PTH levels are inappropriately low normal to subnormal with low serum calcium levels.

Parathyroid Imaging. Attempts to identify hyperfunctioning adenomas are improving. The most common imaging techniques are ultrasound or a sestamibi scan; however, even with these, the ability to obtain a diagnostic image meets with variable success. Reduced bone mineral density (osteopenia and osteoporosis), particularly involving cortical bone (assessed best in the forearm), may be an important parameter to consider when surgery is being contemplated for an otherwise asymptomatic patient. When surgery is performed, intraoperative intact PTH measurements with a rapid assay can confirm successful removal of the adenoma.

Adrenal Gland

Adrenal Cortex

ADRENOCORTICAL FUNCTION TESTS. The principal parameters of cortisol metabolism that are used in diagnosis are ACTH level, serum cortisol level, and 24-hour urinary free cortisol level (Table 37-8). The principal parameters of mineralocorticoid metabolism are plasma aldosterone and plasma renin. Concurrent measurement of electrolytes and glucose are also generally carried out.

CORTISOL

Suspected Pathologic Cortisol Excess. Initially a 24-hour urine free cortisol level is measured as a marker of integrated cortisol production. When results are elevated, an overnight dexamethasone suppression test is conducted. The patient takes an oral dose

TABLE 37-8 DIURNAL PATTERN OF SERUM CORTISOL AND ADRENOCORTICOTROPIC HORMONE LEVELS

Analyte	Time	Serum Level
Cortisol	8 AM	4.3-2.4 mcg/dl
	4 PM	3.1-16.7 mcg/dl
Adrenocorticotropin hormone	7-10 AM	9-52 pg/ml

of 1 mg dexamethasone at 11 PM before sleep. The next morning at 8 AM a fasting serum cortisol is measured. Normally cortisol is suppressed to less than 5 mcg/dl.

If this low-dose dexamethasone suppression test is abnormal (the cortisol is not suppressed), additional testing is needed to clarify the primary mechanism involved in the cortisol excess. Possible causes include ACTH-dependent pituitary Cushing's disease, ectopic ACTH-dependent tumor, adrenal adenoma, and adrenal carcinoma.

The next stage in the workup is the high-dose dexamethasone suppression test. ACTH and cortisol values (serum and 24-hour urine) are measured after a patient takes dexamethasone, 0.5 mg, four times a day for 48 hours. Patients with pituitary Cushing's disease show some suppression of the 24-hour urine free cortisol level to less than 50% reduction from baseline, as well as some suppression of the ACTH level, indicating some responsiveness of the feedback loop.[4,11,26] Patients with either ectopic ACTH-dependent Cushing's or primary adrenal Cushing's syndrome show no change in their 24-hour urine free cortisol levels after these doses of dexamethasone. In primary adrenal Cushing's syndrome the ACTH levels are low throughout the testing period, whereas in ectopic ACTH-dependent Cushing's syndrome, the ACTH levels are high. Occasionally 24-hour urine collections are ordered for 17-hydroxyketosteroids and 17-ketosteroids as markers of cortisol metabolism. A corticotropin-releasing hormone stimulation test may be useful in distinguishing pituitary from ectopic ACTH production.[26,29]

Occasional patients with Cushing's syndrome have a normal low-dose dexamethasone suppression test. When the clinical suspicion is high for Cushing's syndrome despite a normal low-dose dexamethasone suppression test, further testing is warranted.[13]

Suspected Hypocortisolism. Declining cortisol reserve is readily assessed by the cosyntropin stimulation test, generally done in the fasting state. A baseline serum cortisol level is drawn and then 250 mcg of cosyntropin is injected either intravenously (IV) or intramuscularly (IM). A follow-up serum cortisol is drawn 30 minutes after IV administration or 60 minutes after IM administration of cosyntropin. The normal response is a peak stimulated cortisol level in excess of 20 mcg/dl.[16]

ALDOSTERONE EXCESS. Clinically the principal issue is the presence of hyperaldosteronism in a patient with (1) hypertension and (2) hypokalemia or borderline low potassium levels, unrelated to diuretic use. Aldosterone can be measured in the basal state as a plasma aldosterone level; it can also be assessed via a 24-hour urine. If salt loading with resultant volume expansion fails to suppress aldosterone levels, there is high likelihood of autonomous secretion of aldosterone from an adenoma or tumor. Plasma renin levels are low in patients with autonomous aldosterone secretion; in patients with secondary hyperaldosteronism, renin levels are elevated.[10,27,28,35,36]

ADRENOCORTICAL IMAGING. A CT scan with contrast is the most common imaging technique.[21] Occasionally, right and left adrenal vein catheterization and sampling of the adrenal veins is needed to define the source of the hormonal excess when a neoplasm is not clearly imaged.

Adrenal Medulla

ADRENOMEDULLARY FUNCTION TESTS. These tests are performed to diagnose a pheochromocytoma, a tumor (benign or malignant) producing excess catecholamines in a patient with hypertension (intermittent or persistent). Caffeine; alcohol; smoking; use of nicotine patches, gum, or spray; aspirin; bananas; and riboflavin in large doses should be discontinued during all assessments for catecholamine excess. The individual should stop taking all medications if possible. The initial screening test is a 24-hour urine determination for catecholamine metabolites: vanillylmandelic acid and metanephrines. In individuals with a true pheochromocytoma, the 24-hour urine results are generally elevated considerably outside of the reference range and not just "borderline high" (Table 37-9).[9,17]

In equivocal situations plasma catecholamines may be assessed. Fasting before the test is required. The patient is positioned comfortably in the supine position for at least 30 minutes in a dark, quiet room. Blood is drawn from an indwelling heparinized catheter to assess plasma catecholamines. The combination of the 24-hour urine catecholamines and plasma catecholamines usually confirms or refutes the diagnosis of pheochromocytoma. Rarely a clonidine suppression test may be required.[9,17]

ADRENOMEDULLARY IMAGING. To detect a pheochromocytoma, most endocrinologists prefer MRI over CT scanning. In addition, specialized imaging may be necessary when the aforementioned adrenomedullary function testing is nondiagnostic or the neoplasm is thought to be extraadrenal.[9]

Endocrine Pancreas

Assessment of insulin secretory capacity is accomplished via a C peptide (connecting peptide) test. When insulin is secreted by the

TABLE 37-9 URINARY ADRENOMEDULLARY SECRETIONS IN ADULTS: 24-HOUR URINE

Analyte	Normal Values
Epinephrine	2-24 mcg/24 hr
Norepinephrine	15-10 mcg/24 hr
Total metanephrines	Males: 110-480 mcg/g creatinine Females: 150-510 mcg/g creatinine
Dopamine	52-480 mcg/24 hr
Vanillylmandelic acid	<6.0 mg/24 hr

beta cells in the islets of Langerhans, it is actually secreted as proinsulin. An enzymatic reaction occurs and cleaves each proinsulin molecule, resulting in the production of one molecule of insulin and one molecule of C peptide. Measurement of C peptide provides an indirect marker of insulin secretory capacity. If insulin levels were measured in an insulin user, both **endogenous** (produced within the body) and **exogenous** (originating outside the body) insulin would be measured. In contrast, C peptide measures only endogenous insulin production, since C peptide is purified out of exogenous insulin. Glucagon levels are measured in cases of suspected glucagonomas.

Clinical measurement of somatostatin levels is rare. Diagnostic criteria for diabetes mellitus are discussed in detail in Chapter 39.

▶ ARE You READY?

Tertiary dysfunction of an endocrine gland with dysfunction is related to:

1. Intrinsic disease of the gland
2. Pituitary gland disease
3. Dysfunction of the hypothalamus
4. Disorders of the brainstem

References

1. American Association of Clinical Endocrinologists, AACE Hypogonadism Task Force: American Association of Clinical Endocrinologists medical guidelines for clinical practice for the evaluation and treatment of hypogonadism in adult male patients—2002 update, *Endocrine Practice* 8(6): 439-456, 2002.
2. American Association of Clinical Endocrinologists, AACE Thyroid Task Force: American Association of Clinical Endocrinologists medical guidelines for the evaluation and treatment of hyperthyroidism and hypothyroidism, *Endocrine Practice* 8(6):457-469, 2002.
3. American Association of Clinical Endocrinologists, American Association of Endocrine Surgeons, Thyroid Carcinoma Task Force: AACE/AAES medical/surgical guidelines for clinical practice: thyroid carcinoma, *Endocrine Practice* 7(3):202-220, 2001.
4. Arnaldi G et al: Diagnosis and complications of Cushing's syndrome: a consensus statement, *J Clin Endocrinol Metab* 88(12):5593-5602, 2003.
5. Becker KL: *Principles and practice of endocrinology*, ed 3, Philadelphia, 2001, Lippincott, Williams & Wilkins.
6. Bilezikian JP, Silverberg SJ: Asymptomatic primary hyperparathyroidism, *N Engl J Med* 350(17):1746-1751, 2004.
7. Bilezikian JKP et al: Clinical presentation of primary hyperparathyroidism. In Bilezikian JP, editor: *The parathyroids*, ed 3, New York, 2001, Raven.
8. Braverman LE, Utiger RD: *Werner and Ingbar's the thyroid*, ed 9, Philadelphia, 2004, Lippincott, Williams & Wilkins.
9. Bravo EL, Tagle R: Pheochromocytoma: state-of-the-art and future prospects, *Endocrinol Rev* 24(4):539-553, 2003.
10. Conn JW: Presidential address, part I, Painting background; part II, Primary aldosteronism, a new clinical syndrome, *J Clin Lab Med* 45(1):3-17, 1955.
11. Cushing H: The basophil adenomas of the pituitary body and their clinical manifestation, *Bull Johns Hopkins Hospital* 50:137, 1932.
12. Dunnick NR, Korobkin M: Imaging of adrenal incidentalomas: current status, *Am J Roentgenol* 179:559-568, 2002.
13. Findling JW, Raff H, Aron DC: The low-dose dexamethasone suppression test: a reevaluation in patients with Cushing's syndrome, *J Clin Endocrinol Metab* 89(3):1222-1226, 2004.
14. Freda PU: Pitfalls in the biochemical assessment of acromegaly, *Pituitary* 6(3):135-140, 2003.
15. Janicic N, Verbalis JG: Evaluation and management of hypo-osmolality in hospitalized patients, *Endocrinol Metab Clin North Am* 32(2):459-482, June 2003.
16. Kenward D, White KG, Addison's Disease Self-Help Group: Adrenal insufficiency, *Lancet* 362(9383):1881-1893, 2003.
17. Kudva YC, Sawka AM, Young WF: Clinical review 164: the laboratory diagnosis of adrenal pheochromocytoma: the Mayo Clinic experience, *J Clin Endocrinol Metab* 88(10):4533-4539, 2003.
18. Ladenson PW et al: American Thyroid Association guidelines for detection of thyroid dysfunction, *Arch Intern Med* 160(11):1573-1575, 2000.
19. Maghnie M: Diabetes insipidus, *Hormone Res* 59(Suppl 1):42-54, 2003.
20. Mansmann G et al: The clinically inapparent adrenal mass: update in diagnosis and management, *Endocrinol Rev* 25(2):309-340, 2002.
21. Mayo-Smith WW et al: State-of-the-art adrenal imaging, *Radiographics* 21:995-1012, 2001.
22. Melmed S: *The pituitary*, ed 2, Malden, Mass, 2001, Blackwell.
23. Molitch ME: Disorders of prolactin secretion, *Endocrinol Metab Clin North Am* 30(3):585-610, 2001.
24. Molitch ME: Medical management of prolactin-secreting pituitary adenomas, *Pituitary* 5(2):55-65, 2002.
25. Morello JP, Bichet DG: Nephrogenic diabetes insipidus, *Ann Rev Physiol* 63:607-630, 2001.
26. Morris DG, Grossman AB: Dynamic tests in the diagnosis and differential diagnosis of Cushing's syndrome, *J Endocrinol Invest* 26(7 Suppl):64-73, 2003.
27. Mulatero P et al: Extensive personal experience: increased diagnosis of primary aldosteronism, including surgically correctable forms, in centers from five continents, *J Clin Endocrinol Metab* 89:1045-1050, 2004.
28. National Institutes of Health: NIH State-of-the-science statement on management of the clinically inapparent adrenal mass ("incidentaloma"). *NIH Consens State Sci Statements* 19(2):1-25, Feb 4-5, 2002.
29. Reimondo G et al: The corticotrophin-releasing hormone test is the most reliable noninvasive method to differentiate pituitary from ectopic ACTH secretion in Cushing's syndrome, *Clin Endocrinol* (Oxf) 58(6):718-724, 2003.
30. Robertson GL: Antidiuretic hormone: normal and disordered function, *Endocrinol Metab Clin North Am* 30(3):671-694, 2001.
31. Schlechte JA: Prolactinoma, *N Engl J Med* 349(21):2035-2041, 2003.
32. Silverberg SJ, Fitzpatrick LA, Bilezikian JP: Hyperparathyroidism. In Becker KL, editor: *Principles and practice of endocrinology and metabolism*, ed 3, Philadelphia, 2001, Lippincott.
33. Vance ML: Perioperative management of patients undergoing pituitary surgery, *Endocrinol Metab Clin North Am* 32(2):355-366, 2003.
34. Verbalis JG: Management of disorders of water metabolism in patients with pituitary tumors, *Pituitary* 5(2):119-132, 2002.
35. Williams JS, Williams GH: Fiftieth anniversary of aldosterone, *J Clin Endocrinol Metab* 88(6):2364-2372, 2003.
36. Young WF: Minireview: primary aldosteronism—changing concepts in diagnosis and treatment, *Endocrinology* 144(6):2208-2213, 2003.

evolve Visit the Evolve website: http://evolve.elsevier.com/Monahan/medsurg

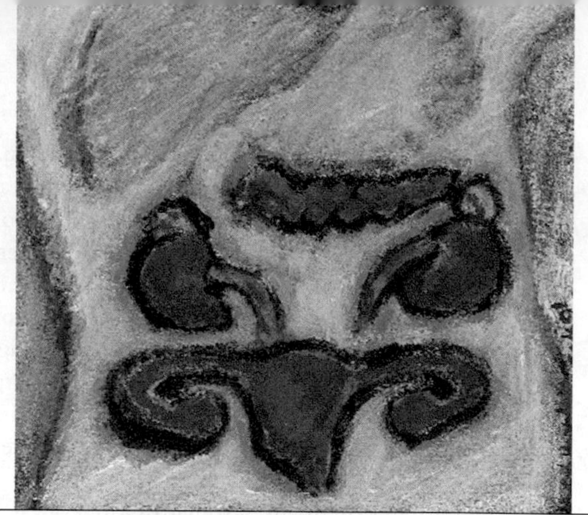

CHAPTER 38

Pituitary, Thyroid, Parathyroid, and Adrenal Gland Problems

by Margaret M. Ulchaker

OBJECTIVES

After studying this chapter, the learner should be able to:

1. Differentiate between the pathophysiology of hypersecretion and hyposecretion of the anterior and posterior pituitary, thyroid, parathyroid, and adrenal glands.
2. Correlate the clinical manifestations, including history, physical examination, and diagnostic test findings, with hypersecretion and hyposecretion of the anterior and posterior pituitary, thyroid, parathyroid, and adrenal glands.
3. Develop a nursing care plan for a patient with hypersecretion or hyposecretion of the anterior or posterior pituitary, thyroid, parathyroid, or adrenal gland.
4. Explain reasons for surgery of the pituitary, thyroid, parathyroid, or adrenal gland.
5. Formulate a nursing care plan for an individual having surgery on the pituitary, thyroid, parathyroid, or adrenal gland.
6. Describe self-care skills needed by a patient receiving long-term hormonal replacement therapy for pituitary, thyroid, parathyroid, or adrenocortical insufficiency.
7. Develop a teaching plan for a patient receiving long-term hormonal replacement therapy for pituitary, thyroid, parathyroid, or adrenocortical insufficiency.

KEY TERMS

dopaminergic, p. 1063
euthyroid, p. 1075
exophthalmos, p. 1074
galactorrhea, p. 1062
hyperplasia, p. 1060
hypersecretion, p. 1060
hypogonadism, p. 1064
hyposecretion, p. 1060
iatrogenic, p. 1060
myxedema, p. 1074
natriuresis, p. 1070
polydipsia, p. 1072
polyuria, p. 1072
proptosis, p. 1074

Endocrine dysfunction of the pituitary, parathyroid, thyroid, and adrenal glands generally results in **hyposecretion** or **hypersecretion** of the particular gland. Although the primary dysfunction may be localized in a particular gland, the effects are usually systemic. Clinical manifestations vary from mild symptoms, treated on an outpatient basis, to medical emergencies requiring surgical intervention or treatment in an intensive care unit. Types of pathologic processes involved in decreased hormone production include:

- Congenital (e.g., a biosynthetic defect such as in congenital adrenal hyperplasia)
- Inflammatory (e.g., autoimmune thyroid disease, infection)
- Ischemic (e.g., hemorrhagic infarction of the adrenals or pituitary, ischemic injury to the parathyroid glands during surgery)
- Destructive (surgical removal, radiation, or trauma of glands)
- Neoplastic (benign or malignant)
- **Iatrogenic** (caused by treatment; e.g., medication-related side effects)

The pathologic processes involved in excess hormone production include:

- **Hyperplasia** or hypertrophy of endocrine glands
- Inflammation (e.g., acute or subacute thyroiditis resulting in acute discharge of preformed thyroid hormone from the gland, causing transient thyrotoxicosis)
- Stimulation of receptors on the gland with resultant hormone release (e.g., production of thyroid-stimulating immunoglobulin in Graves' disease; stimulation of thyrotropin-stimulating hormone [TSH] receptors by a TSH-producing pituitary neoplasm; stimulation of adrenocorticotropic hormone [ACTH] receptors from ACTH ectopically produced by a carcinoma of the lung)
- Neoplasia (benign or malignant)
- Stimulation of hormone production secondary to administration of medications for cardiovascular, psychiatric, neurologic, and gastrointestinal disorders
- Exogenous administration of hormones

Disorders of the endocrine glands controlled by the hypothalamus and pituitary gland (thyroid and adrenocortical glands and gonads) that result in hyposecretion or hypersecretion are classified as intrinsic (primary), secondary, or tertiary. Disease of the thyroid and adrenal glands and gonads are classified as intrinsic or primary dysfunction. Secondary dysfunction occurs when the problem results from anterior pituitary dysfunction, and tertiary problems arise from hypothalamic dysfunction.

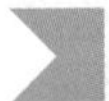

Pituitary Disorders

Pituitary dysfunction may manifest as hypersecretion, hyposecretion, or nonfunctioning tumors. Function, as defined in endocrinology, refers to whether the gland or tumor is producing hormones.

Anterior Pituitary Gland

Hyperfunction

Etiology and Epidemiology. Hyperfunction of the anterior pituitary gland may involve one or more hormones. Tumors and hyperplasia are common causes of anterior pituitary hyperfunction. Pituitary hypersecretion can result from a discrete functioning tumor producing one hormone to excess with relative hyposecretion of the remaining gland secondary to compression of the normal pituitary gland by the tumor. Hypersecretion is occasionally related to idiopathic hyperplasia of cells producing one trophic hormone. The cause of pituitary tumors is generally unknown.

Pathophysiology

PITUITARY TUMORS. Pituitary tumors (adenomas) are classified by size as macroadenomas (more than 10 mm in diameter) or microadenomas (10 mm or less in diameter). Pituitary tumors may also be classified according to hormone production as prolactin (PRL) secreting (about 60%, the most common), growth hormone (GH) secreting (about 20%), ACTH secreting (about 10%), and other (about 10%).

Functioning pituitary tumors resulting in pituitary hypersecretion are usually benign. The clinical picture varies, depending on which hormone is secreted (see Clinical Manifestations box). Clinical manifestations may include neurologic symptoms as the tumor enlarges, compressing adjacent structures and blood vessels.

In addition to the manifestations of hormone excess or deficiency, patients may complain of headaches or visual disturbances

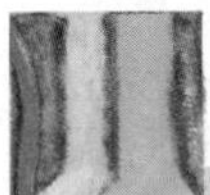

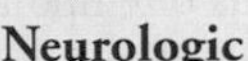

CLINICAL MANIFESTATIONS *Pituitary Hormone–Secreting Tumors*

Neurologic

Visual defects often first seen as losses in superior temporal quadrants with progression to hemianopia or scotomas and finally to total blindness
Headache
Somnolence
Rarely, signs of increased intracranial pressure (hydrocephalus, papilledema)
With very large tumors, disturbance in appetite, sleep, temperature regulation, and emotional balance because of hypothalamic involvement
Behavioral changes and seizures with expansion causing compression of the temporal or frontal lobe (very rare)

Endocrine

Prolactin Hypersecretion

Decreased testosterone (men); decreased estradiol (women)

Females

Menstrual disturbances, such as irregular menses, anovulatory periods, oligomenorrhea, or amenorrhea
Infertility
Galactorrhea
Manifestations of ovarian steroid deficit (vaginal mucosal atrophy and decreased vaginal lubrication leading to dyspareunia)

Males

Loss of libido and erectile function
Reduced sperm count and infertility
Gynecomastia
Galactorrhea (rare)

Growth Hormone Hypersecretion (Acromegaly)

Macroadenomas with resultant headache and visual changes
Changes in facial features (coarsening of features; increased size of nose, lips, and skin folds; prominence of supraorbital ridges; growth of mandible resulting in prognathism and widely spaced teeth; soft tissue growth resulting in facial puffiness)
Increased size of hands and feet, weight gain
Deepening of voice from thickening of vocal cords
Increases in vertebral bodies resulting in kyphosis
Enlarged tongue, salivary glands, spleen, liver, heart, kidney, and other organs; cardiomegaly resulting in increased blood pressure and signs and symptoms of congestive heart failure
Elevated blood pressure
Snoring, sleep apnea, and respiratory failure
Dermatologic changes: acne, malodorous diaphoresis, oiliness, skin tags
Hypertrophy progressing to atrophy of skeletal muscles
Backache, arthralgia, or arthritis from joint damage and bony overgrowth
Nerve entrapment syndromes such as carpal tunnel syndrome from bony overgrowth and changes in nerve size
Impaired glucose tolerance progressing to diabetes mellitus
Changes in fat metabolism resulting in hyperlipidemia
General changes in mobility: lethargy and fatigue
Radiographic findings indicative of bony proliferation in hands, feet, skull, ribs, and vertebrae
Electrolyte changes: increased urinary excretion of calcium; elevated serum phosphorus level

when the neoplasm extends out of the sella turcica and impinges on the optic chiasm. Sudden expansion of the tumor can result from hemorrhage into the tumor *(pituitary apoplexy)*, causing a severe headache and other neurologic symptoms. The abrupt loss of pituitary function is a medical emergency with resultant hypotension and vascular collapse from loss of ACTH secretion. Pituitary apoplexy may occur years after surgery or radiotherapy for the original tumor.

PROLACTIN HYPERSECRETION. PRL inhibits gonadotropin-releasing hormone (Gn-RH) and is necessary for lactation. PRL secretion by the pituitary is controlled primarily by the inhibitory factors of the hypothalamus, chiefly dopamine.[10] Normal levels are usually less than 20 ng/ml. As mentioned previously, PRL-secreting adenomas are a major cause of PRL excess. Other pathophysiologic mechanisms responsible for PRL excess include dopamine antagonists, chronic kidney failure (decreased clearance), neurogenic secretion triggered by chest irritation (rib fracture, thoracotomy, herpes zoster), hypothyroidism, and medications (Box 38-1).[45]

The clinical manifestations of PRL excess are the same, regardless of the cause. Classic manifestations are **galactorrhea** (milk secretion not associated with childbirth or nursing) and amenorrhea in women and decreased libido or erectile dysfunction in men.

GROWTH HORMONE HYPERSECRETION (ACROMEGALY). In most instances hypersecretion of somatotropin, or GH, is related to a pituitary tumor, generally a macroadenoma. In rare instances there may be an ectopic GH-producing tumor (e.g., in the pancreas) and also GH-releasing hormone–producing tumors. The clinical features of acromegaly usually evolve slowly over time, and a review of old family photographs can often show changes evolving for more than 10 years before diagnosis (Figure 38-1). Men and women are equally affected.

Excess of GH affects all growing cells; if it occurs before the epiphyses close, *gigantism* results with excess growth of the skeleton and soft tissues. *Acromegaly,* which occurs after the epiphyses close, is characterized by an increase in connective tissue, soft tissue, and cartilage, giving the characteristic growth and thickening of the hands, face, and feet (see Clinical Manifestations box, p. 1061). The soft tissue features may regress slowly after the cessation of the high GH levels; however, the bony changes are permanent.

In addition to the local effects of the tumor (mass effect), which impinges on other brain and skull structures, and other effects of GH excess, especially diabetes mellitus, untreated acromegaly results in hypertension, cardiomegaly, and premature cardiovascular death. GH excess is also associated with an increased risk of colon cancer.[21]

Most of the adverse effects of chronic GH hypersecretion are caused by stimulation of excessive amounts of insulin-like growth factor-I (IGF-I), which is secreted by the liver. The growth-promoting effects of IGF-I lead to the characteristic proliferation of bone, cartilage, and soft tissue and increase in the size of other organs. The insulin resistance and carbohydrate intolerance seen in acromegaly appear to be direct effects of GH, not IGF-I excess.

PITUITARY ADRENOCORTICOTROPIC HORMONE HYPERSECRETION. A pituitary adenoma producing ACTH is the most common noniatrogenic cause of Cushing's syndrome (discussed later in this chapter). In general, these tumors are microadenomas and the remaining pituitary function is normal. Larger tumors may compress the normal pituitary gland and cause hypofunction, loss of several trophic hormones, varying degrees of hypopituitarism, or other mass effect such as optic chiasm impingement with homonymous bitemporal hemianopia. Occasionally, the microadenoma is not visualized with the usual imaging modalities, and inferior petrosal sinus sampling is needed to assess for the ACTH excess. This is of immense value for the neurosurgeon undertaking transsphenoidal surgery.

Collaborative Care Management

DIAGNOSTIC TESTS

PITUITARY ADENOMA. Diagnosis of a pituitary tumor is made based on the history and physical examination, radiologic studies,

Box 38-1 Stimulants of Prolactin Secretion

Physiologic

Sleep
Stress (physical and psychologic)
Pregnancy, lactation

Pathologic

Prolactinoma
Primary hypothyroidism
Chronic kidney failure
Polycystic ovary syndrome
Cushing's disease
Hypothyroidism
Acromegaly
Chest wall trauma
Spinal cord injury
Idiopathic

Pharmacologic

Psychotropic agents
Antidepressants
—Tricyclics
—Selective serotonin reuptake inhibitors
—Monoamine oxidase inhibitors
Anxiolytics
—Benzodiazepines
Antiemetics
—Metoclopramide
Opiates
—Methadone
—Morphine
H_2 blockers
—Ranitidine
—Cimetadine
—Famotidine
Antihypertensive agents
—Reserpine
—Methyldopa
Calcium channel blockers
—Verapamil
Hormones
—Estrogens
—Thyrotropin-releasing hormone

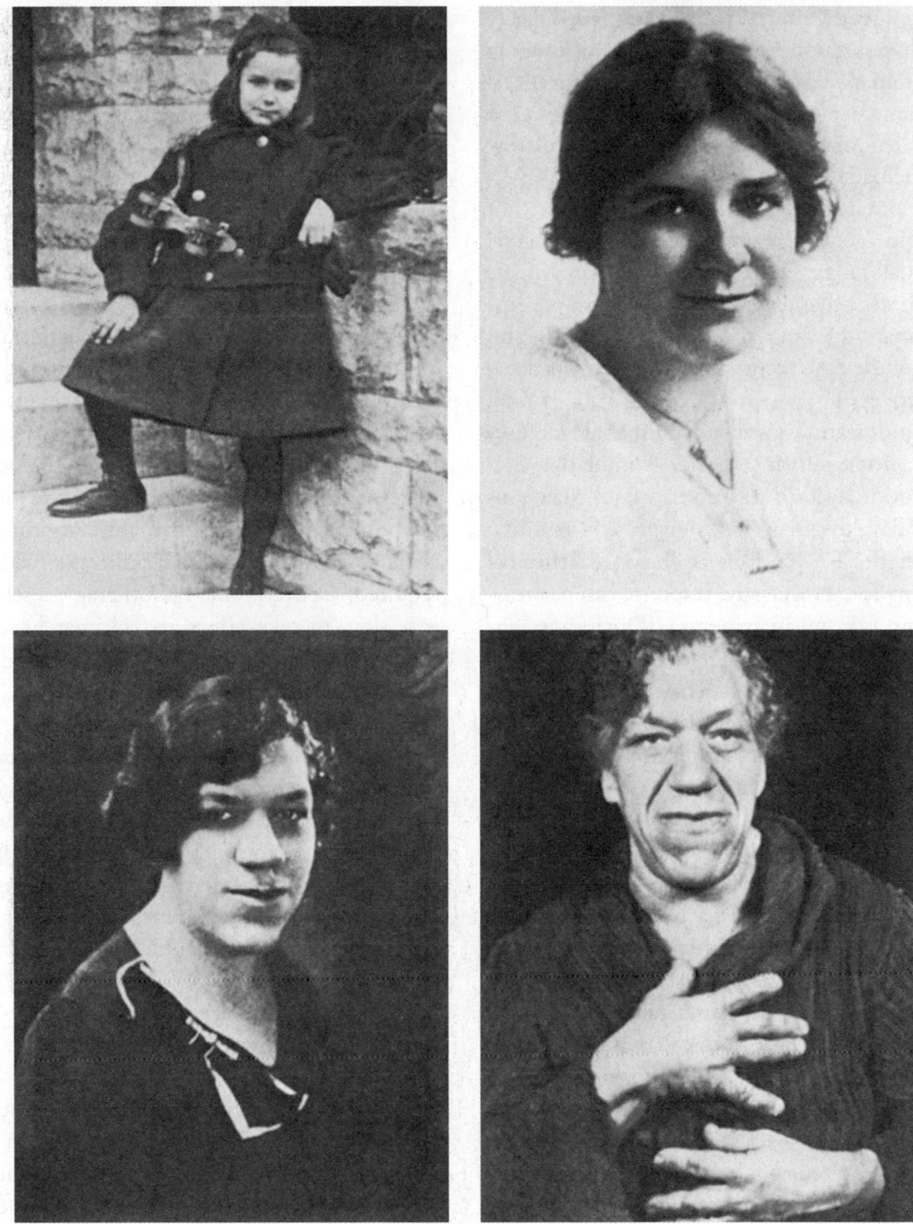

Figure 38-1 Progression of acromegaly in a woman from ages 9 to 52 years.

and laboratory determination of hormone levels. Imaging studies, including magnetic resonance imaging (MRI) with contrast of the sella turcica, can detect pituitary tumors. Presence of a functioning tumor is indicated by elevated pituitary hormone levels.

PROLACTIN HYPERSECRETION. Evaluation of patients with galactorrhea or unexplained gonadal dysfunction with normal or low plasma gonadotropin levels should include a thorough history relating to menstrual status, pregnancy, fertility, sexual function, and symptoms of hypothyroidism or hypopituitarism. An accurate medication history is critical to accurate diagnosis. PRL levels less than 150 ng/ml are more likely caused by medication than by tumor. Although PRL levels greater than 150 ng/ml are considered diagnostic for adenoma, levels may exceed 3000 ng/ml. The clinician should evaluate basal PRL levels; gonadotropins; and thyroid, liver, and renal function tests. Serum testosterone levels in men and pregnancy tests in women with amenorrhea should also be performed.

GROWTH HORMONE HYPERSECRETION. Diagnosis of acromegaly is usually clinically obvious and can be confirmed by assessment of GH secretion. Other tests to confirm the diagnosis include suppression with oral glucose and IGF-I measurement.[28] Because of the effects of GH or IGF-I, persons with GH excess may also have elevated postprandial plasma glucose, elevated serum phosphorus, and hypercalciuria. Radiographs show enlargement of the frontal and maxillary sinuses and thickening of the soft tissues.

MEDICATIONS. Prolactinomas are usually managed medically with **dopaminergic** (having a dopamine-like effect) medications such as bromocriptine (Parlodel), cabergoline (Dostinex), or pergolide (Permax). Cabergoline typically has fewer side effects than bromocriptine, which frequently causes nausea and occasionally vomiting, dizziness, and hypotension. In addition to acute lowering of PRL levels, these dopaminergic agents can have long-term effects on neoplasm size, with some neoplasm shrinkage and fibrosis. The natural history of microadenomas appears to be benign, and most remain stable in size. Macroadenomas, on the other hand, have a problematic potential for progressive growth when patients are not treated with dopaminergic agents. Treatment with dopamingeric agents and transsphenoidal surgery is recommended for patients with large neoplasms and extrasellar extension. Surgery is not commonly used as the primary treatment of microadenomas and macroadenomas because of the high recurrence rates; many patients are placed on medical therapy.[46,62]

Octreotide acetate (Sandostatin), a somatostatin analog, is useful for the treatment of acromegaly and thyroid-stimulating adenomas. Originally octreotide acetate was given as subcutaneous injections three times a day; it can now be given as a monthly depot injection (Sandostatin LAR). This is the most effective adjunctive medical therapy for acromegaly; response can be measured with serial IGF-I and GH measurements.[27] Dopamine agonists paradoxically lower GH levels in some acromegalic patients; however, their efficacy and tolerability are inferior to those of octreotide acetate. The GH receptor antagonist pegvisomant may be the drug of choice in patients who are either nonresponders or only partial responders to somatostatin analogs.[18,54,67]

TREATMENTS. Patients with pituitary hypersecretion may exhibit high anxiety levels in response to the body changes induced by neurologic or endocrine alterations and uncertainty about diagnosis, treatment method, and effects of treatment. Particular stressors may include visual loss, infertility, sexual dysfunction, or immobility. Although some patients in whom neurologic symptoms are diagnosed require immediate surgical treatment, most patients have a diagnostic workup in the outpatient setting and time to learn about their illness and its implications.

PITUITARY ADENOMAS. Treatment goals for patients with pituitary adenomas are to correct hypersecretion of the anterior pituitary hormones, preserve normal secretion of other anterior pituitary hormones, and remove or suppress the adenoma. Treatments include surgery, radiation, or medications. Patients with macroadenomas usually require a combination of therapies to achieve these goals.

Pituitary radiation is usually reserved for patients who have had incomplete resection of large pituitary adenomas. Conventional radiation using high-energy sources is most commonly used. Response to radiotherapy is usually slow. Hypopituitarism is a common complication after radiotherapy. Heavy-particle radiation with alpha particles or protons is also used. Advantages of this type are the ability to precisely focus the radiation beam, limiting exposure of surrounding tissues and achieving a more rapid response to therapy than with conventional radiation. Use of this type of radiation is usually limited to smaller tumors and those without extrasellar extension. Hypopituitarism also may occur after this treatment.

PROLACTIN HYPERSECRETION. Goals of treatment for patients with PRL hypersecretion are control of PRL levels, cessation of galactorrhea, and return to normal gonadal function. All patients with PRL-secreting adenomas should be treated either medically or surgically to avoid the risk of further tumor expansion, hypopituitarism, and visual impairment. Treatment of patients with microadenomas is also recommended to prevent osteoporosis secondary to persistent **hypogonadism** (decreased secretion of sex hormones by the ovaries or testes) and to restore fertility.

GROWTH HORMONE HYPERSECRETION. Treatment goals for patients with acromegaly are to halt progression of the disorder and to prevent complications and death. The objectives of therapy are removal or destruction of the tumor, reversal of GH hypersecretion, and maintenance of normal anterior and posterior pituitary function. Many patients are seen with advanced manifestations of acromegaly (Figure 38-2). The soft tissue features may regress slowly after normalization of the high GH levels; however, the bony changes are permanent. Surgical intervention is less successful with larger tumors; adjuvant medical treatment may be required. Conventional radiotherapy is seldom used now because it is slow to take effect and ultimately results in panhypopituitarism. Other radiologic therapies include particle beam radiation and Gamma Knife radiosurgery.

SURGICAL MANAGEMENT. Some physicians consider transsphenoidal resection of a pituitary adenoma to be the primary form of treatment. Surgical success is related to tumor size and the amount of invasion into the sella turcica. Although the microsurgical approach is preferred, subfrontal approach via craniotomy (see Chapter 48) is sometimes required for patients with suprasellar tumor extension. If residual tumor is present, radiation or dopamine agonists such as bromocriptine may be indicated. The surgical outcome for patients with PRL-secreting adenomas is related to tumor size and basal PRL level. Surgery is indicated if severe visual field defects are present.

In the transsphenoidal procedure the surgical approach to the pituitary is from the nasal cavity through the sphenoid sinus or from the mouth through a gingival incision (Figure 38-3). Under microscopic visualization, the surgeon incises the inferior sellar

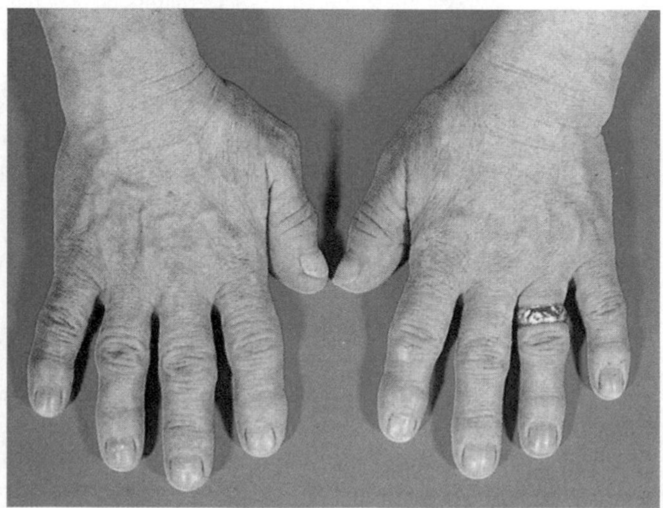

Figure 38-2 Hands of patient with acromegaly may appear broad and spadelike.

floor and dura and removes the adenoma. Normal pituitary tissue is preserved when possible. Complications, more common in persons with large or invasive tumors, include postoperative hemorrhage, cerebrospinal fluid (CSF) leak, and visual impairment (Box 38-2). The most common complication is transient diabetes insipidus (DI) lasting from days to weeks; permanent DI is rare.[70] Additional complications include syndrome of inappropriate antidiuretic hormone (SIADH) with symptomatic hyponatremia, surgical hypopituitarism, pituitary apoplexy or other types of pituitary hemorrhage (see Hyposecretion: Hypopituitarism), infection, and meningitis.[68]

Postoperative routines include management of incisional discomfort and headache and prevention of complications. After surgery, because of the caution against coughing and the nasal packing necessitating mouth breathing, patients are at risk for ineffective gas exchange. The nurse instructs patients about mouth breathing and deep breathing exercises before surgery, provides an opportunity for practice and a return demonstration, and then monitors for compliance with deep breathing exercises at least every 2 hours for the first 1 to 3 postoperative days. Assessment of vital signs and breath sounds every 4 to 8 hours helps identify any impairment of air exchange. Maintenance of adequate fluid intake helps prevent drying of mucus secretions and the formation of mucous plugs.

Persistent headaches may indicate meningitis and should be reported to the physician immediately. A firm mattress, range-of-motion exercises, back massage, frequent ambulation, and heat may be used to ameliorate back and joint discomfort in persons with GH-secreting tumors. Early ambulation helps prevent deterioration in mobility and joint movement. The nurse monitors the patient's postoperative vision and visual fields for changes. Rearranging the room to place necessary articles in line with intact vision may be necessary. Although additional visual compromise after transsphenoidal resection is rare, the visual pathway can be damaged during surgery or as a result of hemorrhage.

Box 38-2 Complications of Pituitary Tumors

Neurologic

Compression of optic chiasm or other brain tissue; visual loss
After surgery: cerebrospinal fluid leak, meningitis, increased intracranial pressure, neurologic deficit, visual impairment
Pituitary apoplexy

Endocrine

Syndromes of excess hormone: acromegaly, Cushing's syndrome; suppression of gonadotropic hormones; infertility or sexual dysfunction
Iatrogenic syndromes of hormonal deficit: diabetes insipidus, adrenal insufficiency, hypopituitarism (deficit in one or more anterior pituitary hormones: adrenocorticotropic hormone, growth hormone, thyroid-stimulating hormone, or gonadotropin)
Recurrence of pituitary tumor

DIET. Dietary changes may be necessary for patients with acromegaly or Cushing's syndrome. Carbohydrate intolerance or frank diabetes mellitus may be associated with both these disorders (see Chapter 39 for dietary management of patients with diabetes). Congestive heart failure may occur in patients with acromegaly, and sodium and fluid restrictions may be indicated.

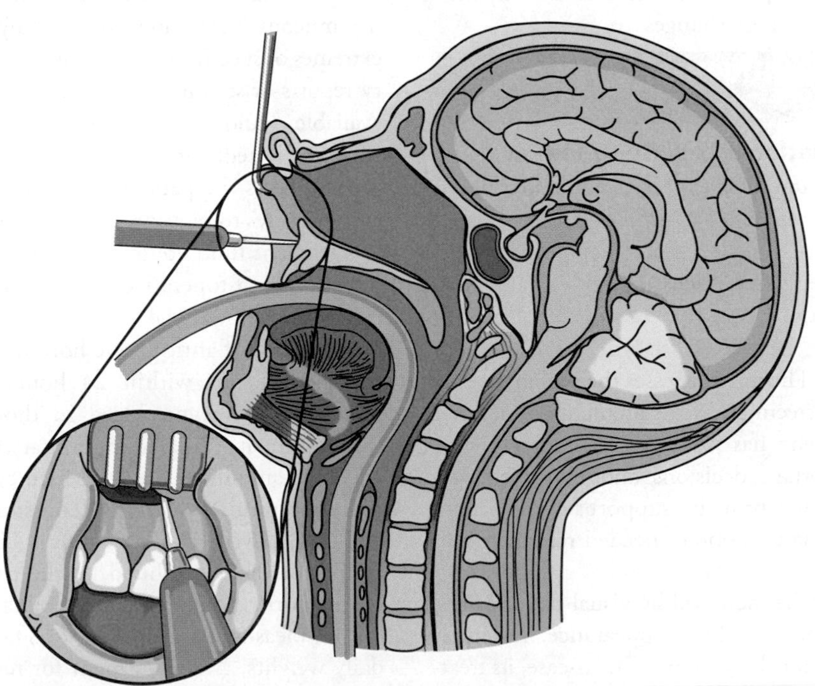

Figure 38-3 Transsphenoidal approach in anterior pituitary surgery with incision in the gingival mucosa.

Nursing Management
of the Patient with a Pituitary Tumor

ASSESSMENT

Health History. Assess for:

- Sensory alterations, particularly vision and visual fields, and other peripheral sensory changes
- Temporal or frontal headache of moderate intensity, arthralgias, backache
- Coarsening of facial features; increase in ring, glove, or shoe size; increase in sweating or oiliness of skin
- Changes in energy level (lethargy or fatigue) or decrease in mobility
- Psychosocial concerns: behavioral changes such as anxiety, irritability, concerns about self-image
- History of menstrual changes in females, erectile dysfunction in males, changes in libido; fertility concerns
- Use of oral contraceptives or psychotropic drugs
- Knowledge level related to disorder, treatment, and potential outcome of treatment

Physical Examination. Assess for:

- Functioning of cranial nerves II, III, IV, and VI (see Chapter 47)
- Retinal changes indicative of papilledema or elevated blood pressure
- Alertness and emotional status
- Peripheral nerve functioning (see Chapter 47)
- Body appearance and description
- Mobility and joint functioning (see Chapter 51)
- Blood pressure, pulse, respirations, and temperature
- Body weight and height
- Presence of organomegaly, particularly cardiac and hepatic, and signs associated with these changes

NURSING DIAGNOSES, OUTCOMES, AND INTERVENTIONS

Nursing Diagnosis: Situational Low Self-Esteem

OUTCOMES. A common example of expected outcomes for the patient with a diagnosis of *situational low self-esteem* is:
Patient will:

- Talk positively about self when discussing body characteristics, changes, and functions.

NURSING INTERVENTIONS. The nurse assesses the patient for factors posing a threat to self-esteem and for statements of negative self-appraisal. The patient who has just been diagnosed with a pituitary tumor faces important decisions and may feel overwhelmed or helpless. The nurse provides support for the patient to ask questions, seek information, obtain needed resources, and make decisions about care.

Threats to self-esteem can be increased by visual disturbances, infertility, immobility, or changes in body appearance. The nurse needs to assess the patient's knowledge about the disease, its treatment, and anticipated effects on body appearance and functions; the patient and significant others need to know that although changes in body characteristics and vision are not always reversible, progressive changes can be stopped. Sexual dysfunction associated with PRL excess is usually reversible. The nurse can help the patient and family cope with irreversible changes. Participation of the patient and family or significant others in a support group can enable them to learn how others have coped. It is also important to reassure the patient and family about the normalcy of individual responses to stressors. Enabling the patient to maintain an optimal level of independence in activities of daily living (ADLs) and personal control of his or her situation to the extent possible significantly supports self-esteem.

RELATED NIC INTERVENTIONS. Body Image Enhancement, Coping Enhancement, Self-Esteem Enhancement

Nursing Diagnosis: Deficient Fluid Volume

OUTCOMES. Common examples of expected outcomes for the patient with a diagnosis of *deficient fluid volume* are:
The patient will:

- Exhibit physical signs of fluid balance.
- Return to baseline weight.
- Have elastic skin turgor and moist mucous membranes.
- Have blood pressure and pulse within normal range.
- Have serum electrolytes and hematocrit within normal limits.
- Have urine specific gravity of 1.010 to 1.025.
- Have a fluid intake of at least 2 L/day, orally or parenterally (unless restrictions are prescribed).
- Explain measures to prevent fluid deficit.

NURSING INTERVENTIONS. The nurse regularly assesses risk factors for deficient fluid volume. The nurse weighs the patient daily before breakfast with the patient wearing the same clothing, with an empty bladder, and on the same scale. The patient is assessed every 8 hours for signs of deficient fluid: decreased skin turgor, dry mucous membranes, postural hypotension, tachycardia, and extremes of specific gravity of urine. The nurse monitors laboratory reports of serum osmolality, sodium levels, and hematocrit as available. Fluid intake of at least 2 L/day is encouraged unless contraindicated; parenteral therapy is maintained as ordered. The nurse teaches the patient and family about diet and fluid needs and measures to prevent insufficient intake as appropriate.

Deficient fluid volume is a potential problem in any patient during the postoperative period. However, the patient who has had a transsphenoidal surgery is at higher risk because inadequate release of antidiuretic hormone (ADH) may cause DI. DI usually develops within 24 hours and is usually temporary because ADH is produced in the hypothalamus and travels through the hypothalamic-pituitary portal circulation; therefore adequate amounts can be released even if damage occurs to the posterior pituitary gland. Remissions may occur for up to 2 weeks, followed by a recurrence. The signs and symptoms are similar to those exhibited by the patient with DI (see Antidiuretic Hormone Hyposecretion: Diabetes Insipidus). Intake and output measurements every 4 to 8 hours, specific gravity checks, daily weights, and assessment for reports of thirst help identify the presence of DI. If a deficit in ADH does occur, treatment depends on the severity. Increasing intake of oral fluids sufficiently to satisfy thirst may treat mild deficits. In patients with severe ADH deficits or those unable to tolerate oral fluids, desmopressin (synthetic vasopressin) is administered.

Before pituitary surgery, intravenous cortisol administration is initiated. Postoperative ACTH deficiency can result in severe deficient fluid volume (see Adrenal Cortex Hyposecretion: Adrenal Insufficiency). Cortisol replacement is necessary after surgery to prevent life-threatening adrenal crisis. All patients should be monitored for potential glucocorticoid deficiency and early signs and symptoms of adrenal insufficiency. Monitoring includes the adequacy of ADH; vital signs every 4 hours; and observation of energy level, alertness, appetite, and stated feelings of well-being. If these data reveal abnormalities, serum sodium, potassium, and glucose levels may be obtained. Increased urinary output, hypotension while lying down, orthostatic hypotension, persistent nausea, vomiting, fatigue and tiredness, hyponatremia, hyperkalemia, hypoglycemia, and acidosis indicate inadequate ACTH and glucocorticoid secretion. Hydrocortisone or the equivalent and fluid replacement are provided. If the ACTH deficit is permanent, the patient requires treatment as discussed later for persons with chronic adrenal insufficiency.

RELATED NIC INTERVENTIONS. Electrolyte Monitoring, Fluid/Electrolyte Management, Fluid Monitoring, Shock Prevention

Nursing Diagnosis: Risk for Infection

OUTCOMES. Common examples of expected outcomes for the patient with a diagnosis of *risk for infection* are:

The patient will:

- Remain free from infection, as evidenced by absence of persistent headache, CSF leak, and nuchal rigidity.
- Have adequate knowledge, as evidenced by patient's and family's ability to describe disease process, effects on bodily function, and goals of treatment.
- Explain nature of the disorder, medications, treatment regimen, surgical intervention, expected outcomes of treatment, and plan for follow-up care.
- Understand and participate in perioperative routines and care.

NURSING INTERVENTIONS. Nursing priorities after transsphenoidal surgery are preventing infection and maintaining the integrity of the surgical incision between the upper gum and lip. The nurse assesses the patient every shift for signs of infection, including fever, rhinorrhea, nuchal rigidity, and persistent headache. It is also important to teach the patient the importance and methods of mouth care. Oral incisional care consists of rinsing the mouth with saline or mouthwash and cleansing the teeth with a swab. Brushing the teeth and using dental floss are forbidden until the suture line heals.

Clear liquids are given as soon as the patient is alert and no longer nauseated from the anesthetic. The diet is advanced as tolerated. Foods that could irritate the mucous membranes and disrupt the suture line are avoided because of the mouth incision.

Increased intracranial pressure (ICP) can disrupt the incision in the sella turcica and dura. After the tumor is resected, the sella turcica is packed with muscle or fat from the abdomen or thigh. (NOTE: It is important that the patient be prepared for this additional incision.) The floor of the sella turcica is reconstructed with bone or cartilage. This patching, although strong, can be disrupted by increased ICP, which causes pressure on the incision. Activities such as bending over, straining, coughing, sneezing, and nose blowing are forbidden. To reduce cerebral edema, the head of the bed is elevated at least 30 degrees. In most cases these interventions prevent disruption of the patch and incision.

After surgery the patient's nose is packed for 24 to 48 hours, and a gauze sling is worn under the nose to absorb drainage. CSF leakage occurs if the patching and incision in the sella turcica are disrupted. The nurse monitors the patient for signs of CSF leakage: complaints of postnasal drip, even with the packing in place; increased swallowing (observation or patient's report); or the appearance of a halo ring on the gauze sling (CSF is clear and, when mixed with serous fluid on gauze, forms a halo surrounding the serous drainage).

Nasal drainage can be differentiated from CSF based on glucose content. Although the nurse can assess the glucose content of nasal drainage with a dipstick for glucose, fluid should be sent to a laboratory for confirmation. If a CSF leak occurs or is suspected, bed rest with the patient's head elevated is indicated until the leakage is ruled out or stops. Occasionally, patients must return to surgery for repair of the leakage site in the sella turcica.

If a documented CSF leak occurs, the patient is at high risk for infection, including meningitis. Besides restricting the patient's activities to prevent or control a CSF leak, the nurse monitors the patient for signs of an infection. Antibiotics are administered as prescribed.

RELATED NIC INTERVENTIONS. Environmental Management, Infection Control, Infection Protection

Patient/Family Teaching. Patient and family teaching is an important part of nursing care for patients undergoing surgery for a pituitary tumor (see Patient/Family Teaching box).

EVALUATION

To evaluate the effectiveness of nursing interventions, compare patient behaviors with those stated in the expected patient outcomes.

RELATED NOC OUTCOMES. Electrolyte & Acid/Base Balance, Fluid Balance, Hydration, Infection Severity, Nutritional Status: Food & Fluid Intake, Self-Esteem

Hyposecretion: Hypopituitarism

Etiology and Epidemiology. Hypopituitarism, or hyposecretion of the pituitary gland, may be congenital or related to tumor, infarction, autoimmune dysfunction, infection (bacterial or viral), or trauma (surgery or radiation) (Box 38-3). The spectrum can extend from missing all of the trophic hormones *(panhypopituitarism)* to isolated hormone deficiency. In some instances the hypopituitarism may be reversible, as when a macroadenoma that had been compressing the normal pituitary is removed. Acute loss of anterior pituitary function is generally vascular with acute infarction of a pituitary tumor and ischemic damage to the surrounding normal pituitary gland (pituitary apoplexy) or simply an ischemic infarction of the pituitary as seen in Sheehan's syndrome (postpartum pituitary necrosis).

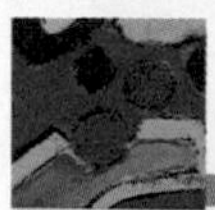

PATIENT/FAMILY TEACHING *The Patient Undergoing Pituitary Surgery*

Preoperative

The relationship of the patient's symptoms to a pituitary tumor and hormone excess. The use of a model of a brain during the educational process helps the patient better understand the pathology and treatment of his or her illness.

Definition of a *tumor*. Many individuals assume that tumor means cancer. These tumors are usually not malignant.

Planned diagnostic tests, including computed tomography or magnetic resonance imaging.

Available treatment for the tumor. On the basis of signs and symptoms, the physician has a high index of suspicion for the type of tumor and potential treatment. This information is initially provided by the physician and later reinforced by the professional nurse.

Basic preoperative and postoperative teaching, similar to that for any surgical patient (see Chapters 13 and 15).

Dietary instruction about prescribed changes as needed, and ways to meet dietary requirements.

Medication therapy: hormonal agents that may be used as replacement therapy.

Step-by-step instructions on performing a subcutaneous injection if prescribed. The nurse provides teaching and multiple opportunities for practice and return demonstration.

Expected outcomes from the treatment, including reversibility or irreversibility of signs and symptoms.

The importance of and plans for follow-up care.

Perioperative and Postoperative

Treatment regimen for any hormonal deficiencies that have occurred. If antidiuretic hormone (ADH), adrenocorticotropic hormone (ACTH), or glucocorticoid deficiency occurred after surgery, diagnostic tests are done before the patient leaves the hospital to determine whether the deficiencies are permanent. If so, the patient needs the same education required by any patient with diabetes insipidus (for ADH deficiency) or adrenocortical insufficiency (for ACTH deficiency) (see discussions in this chapter). Follow-up diagnostic tests to evaluate hormonal status are performed 4 to 6 weeks after surgery if no hormonal deficiencies develop.

Care needs related to irreversible changes in body appearance, joint and back pain, and visual problems. Information shared may include ways to minimize body changes with makeup and clothes, frequent showers to help control increased sweating and oily skin, pain management techniques, modification of activities to decrease stress and strain on the joints and back, and referral to a society to aid the visually impaired.

Discharge planning, including self-care and responsibility for follow-up care. The patient should know when to return to see the endocrinologist (initially in 1 to 4 weeks, depending on postoperative hormone deficits, and then every 3 to 6 months pending hormonal stability) and neurosurgeon (initially in 1 to 2 weeks and then in 6 weeks).

Sequelae of hypopituitarism related to individual hormonal deficiencies are outlined in Figure 38-4. The incidence of hypopituitarism is unknown.[44]

Pathophysiology. Symptoms of hypopituitarism vary widely, depending on the cause and the endocrine dysfunction present (see Clinical Manifestations box). If a tumor is present, the patient may exhibit some of the symptoms previously described. If the tumor arises from regions surrounding the pituitary, such as the third ventricle or hypothalamus, the neurologic signs and symptoms are more severe and include manifestations of increased ICP (see Chapter 48).

Endocrine dysfunction may be a result of hypothalamic damage or primary pituitary disease. The most frequent pathophysiologic change involves lack of synthesis and secretion of gonadotropins.[44]

Box 38-3 Causes of Hypopituitarism

- Tumors: craniopharyngioma, primary central nervous system tumors, nonsecreting pituitary tumors
- Ischemic changes: Sheehan's syndrome (ischemic changes after postpartum hemorrhage or infection resulting in shock)
- Developmental abnormalities
- Infections: viral encephalitis, bacteremia, tuberculosis
- Autoimmune disorders
- Radiation damage, particularly after treatment of secreting adenomas of pituitary gland
- Trauma, including surgery

Collaborative Care Management. Medical management focuses on identifying patients with deficiency syndromes, treating the underlying problem, and supplying the appropriate hormonal replacement. Failure to replace hormones results in increased mortality.[66] The target gland hormone (thyroid, cortisol, or gonadal steroids) is replaced as necessary. If a woman of childbearing age desires fertility, gonadotropins must be replaced. However, PRL does not need to be replaced.

GROWTH HORMONE DEFICIENCY. Isolated GH deficiency is generally seen only in childhood and responds to GH therapy; GH deficiency in adults is usually part of panhypopituitarism.

Replacing GH in adults requires daily subcutaneous injections starting at a dose of 0.006 mg/kg actual body weight/day and titrating upward to yield an IGF-I level in the upper half of the normal range. Anticipated patient outcomes include increased well-being, physical endurance, and improvement in body composition and bone mineral density.[1,2,20] The use of GH outside of these scenarios is experimental. The high cost of GH therapy may be prohibitive for some, although most manufacturers do have compassionate need programs.

THYROID-STIMULATING HORMONE DEFICIENCY Isolated TSH deficiency is uncommon; TSH deficiency is generally part of panhypopituitarism. Therefore concurrent cortisol deficiency is to be anticipated and its replacement mandatory. TSH itself is not

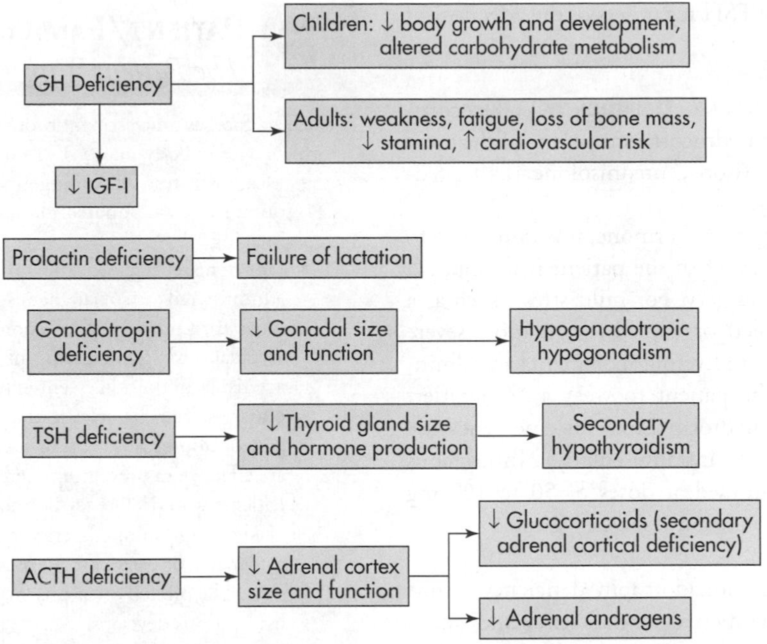

Figure 38-4 Sequelae of individual anterior pituitary hormone deficiency. *ACTH,* Adrenocorticotropic hormone; *GH,* growth hormone; *IGF,* insulin-like growth factor; *TSH,* thyroid-stimulating hormone.

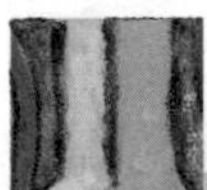

CLINICAL MANIFESTATIONS *Hypopituitarism*

- Manifestations based on cause, such as bacteremia, viral hepatitis, autoimmune disorders, and trauma
- Manifestations such as vision changes, papilledema, or hydrocephalus if cause is tumor
- Manifestations of gonadotropin deficiency:
  —Decreased serum levels of follicle-stimulating hormone, luteinizing hormone, and gonadal steroids
  Children: delayed puberty
  —Adults
    —Women: oligomenorrhea or amenorrhea, uterine and vaginal atrophy, potential atrophy of breast tissue, loss of libido, decreased body hair
    —Men: loss of libido, decreased sperm count, erectile dysfunction, decreased testicular size, decreased total body hair
- Manifestations of growth hormone (GH) deficiency
  —Children
    —Stunted growth (below third percentile) with normal body proportions, excessive subcutaneous fat, poor muscle development
    —Immature facial features, immature voice
    —Slow growth of nails and thin hair
    —Delayed puberty but eventual normal sexual development
    —Decreased levels of GH
  —Adults
    —Onset of hypopituitarism before puberty resulting in short stature
    —Appearance older than chronologic age
    —Moderate obesity
    —Decreased muscle mass and weakness
    —Lassitude
    —Emotional lability
    —Decreased basal levels of GH or decreased response to provocative testing
    —In some persons, normal GH levels with low level of somatomedins (insulin-like growth factor I)
- Manifestations of prolactin deficiency
  —Failure to lactate by postpartum woman
  —Decreased serum levels of prolactin
- Manifestations of thyroid-stimulating hormone (TSH) deficiency
  —Signs and symptoms of secondary hypothyroidism
  —Decreased serum level of TSH and thyroid hormone
- Manifestations of adrenocorticotropic hormone (ACTH) deficiency
  —Signs and symptoms of secondary ACTH insufficiency; *no hyperpigmentation*
  —Decreased serum levels of ACTH, glucocorticoids, and adrenal androgens (aldosterone levels may be normal)

available for replacement therapy; a thyroid hormone preparation is used. Replacement with levothyroxine is similar to that for the primary hypothyroid patient. Thyroid hormone replacement accelerates the metabolism of glucocorticoids such that failure to replace glucocorticoids concurrently can precipitate an acute adrenal crisis. Monitoring of thyroxine (T_4) levels, generally with the free T_4 blood test, is done on a regular basis as an evaluation of therapy. Because T_4 is converted to triiodothyronine (T_3) in the periphery, circulating T_3 levels may also be monitored. Monitoring of TSH levels is obviously of no value, since the patient with

TSH deficiency will have a low TSH regardless of the adequacy of their replacement.[44]

Adrenocorticotropic Hormone Deficiency. Glucocorticoid deficiency is replaced with hydrocortisone or one of the more potent synthetic analogs. Cortisone, prednisolone, and prednisone are also used for therapy.

Because cortisol is a primary stress hormone, it is imperative to augment these physiologic doses when the patient is ill, injured, or undergoing anesthesia and surgery. For mild stress, such as a viral illness, the dose is doubled or tripled. With more severe stress, such as surgery, threefold to fivefold increments are administered. The nurse instructs the patient to wear a Medic-Alert bracelet that states a need for hydrocortisone for emergency use (50 to 100 mg intravenously or intramuscularly). Intravenous hydrocortisone should be continued at doses of 50 to 100 mg every 6 hours until the acute condition resolves.

Gonadotropin Deficiency. Gonadotropin deficiency results in secondary hypogonadism, with estrogen deficiency and amenorrhea in women and erectile dysfunction and infertility in men. Testosterone and estrogen replacement is similar to that used in primary gonadal failure. Testosterone deficiency in men can lead to osteoporosis, loss of muscle mass and decrease in physical endurance; therefore treatment of testosterone deficiency should be considered in older men even if sexual function is not a priority for them.[3]

In the absence of pituitary destruction, the majority of patients with gonadotropin deficiency have hypothalamic GnRH deficiency. Replacement of GnRH in a pulsatile fashion with a subcutaneous infusion pump can restore fertility as well as estrogen or androgen production.

Prolactin Deficiency. Failure of lactation in the postpartum woman is a useful clinical clue to PRL deficiency. No PRL replacement preparation is available for clinical use, and chronic PRL deficiency does not appear to have any long-term adverse sequelae apart from the lactation issue.

Patient/Family Teaching. Patient and family teaching for the patient with hypopituitarism is presented in the Patient/Family Teaching box.

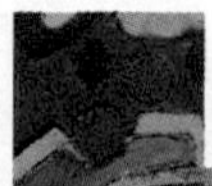

Patient/Family Teaching
The Patient With Hypopituitarism

Teaching focuses on treatment protocols and helping the patient cope with changes in body image. The nurse provides information about:

- Diagnostic tests, including blood tests and radiologic procedures such as computed tomography or magnetic resonance imaging.
- Hormone replacement therapy. Growth hormone therapy is administered via subcutaneous injections; therefore the patient must learn proper self-injection technique. Treatment with gonadal (sex) steroids helps initiate development of sexual characteristics in the adolescent entering puberty and restores secondary sexual characteristics in adults. Treatment with gonadotropins restores fertility. Additionally, gonadal steroids are effective in preventing premature decrease in bone mass. Patients who decline sex hormone therapy, particularly women, need to be monitored periodically for the development of osteopenia or osteoporosis, must take adequate calcium, and should be offered other pharmacotherapy if osteopenia or osteoporosis develops.

Box 38-4 Etiologic Factors Associated With Syndrome of Inappropriate Antidiuretic Hormone

- Pulmonary disorders: malignant neoplasms (e.g., small cell adenocarcinoma of lung), tuberculosis, ventilator patients receiving positive pressure, lung abscesses
- Other malignancies: duodenum, pancreas, prostate, lymphoma, sarcoma, leukemia, Hodgkin's lymphoma, non-Hodgkin's lymphoma
- Central nervous system disorders: tumors, infection, trauma, cerebrovascular accident, surgery
- Drugs such as clofibrate, chlorpropamide, thiazides, vincristine, cyclophosphamide, general anesthetic agents, opioids, tricyclic antidepressants, carbamazepine
- Stressors: fear, acute infections, pain, anxiety, trauma, surgery

Posterior Pituitary Dysfunction

Diseases of the posterior pituitary may result in excess secretion as in SIADH or undersecretion with resultant central DI.

Antidiuretic Hormone Hypersecretion: Syndrome of Inappropriate Antidiuretic Hormone

Etiology and Epidemiology. The most common causes of SIADH are small cell carcinoma of the lung (80% of cases) and medications: vincristine, selective serotonin reuptake inhibitors, and especially the sulfonylurea drug chlorpropamide (Box 38-4).

Pathophysiology. Inappropriate free water retention in relation to the patient's volume status results in a hypoosmolar state with a dilutional hyponatremia. Despite the expansion in intracellular volume, edema is not present; this volume expansion enhances glomerular filtration and decreases proximal tubular sodium resorption, resulting in **natriuresis** (urinary sodium excretion). These features contrast with the volume overload of congestive heart failure and cirrhosis and the hyponatremia seen in Addison's disease. The hypoosmolality of the plasma creates an osmotic gradient across the cell membranes (including the blood-brain barrier) with resultant flow of water into all cells.[59]

Severity of the clinical symptoms depends on the absolute serum sodium level and the rapidity of its fall (see Clinical Manifestations box). A rapid fall in serum sodium levels can result in rapid-onset cerebral edema and death, whereas a gradual fall over several weeks may result only in lethargy. In general, patient symptoms may be coordinated with the following serum sodium levels: 121 to 125 mEq/L, nausea and malaise; 115 to 120 mEq/L, headache, lethargy, obtundation; and 110 to 114 mEq/L, seizures and coma.

CLINICAL MANIFESTATIONS *Syndrome of Inappropriate Antidiuretic Hormone*

Early Signs and Symptoms

Anorexia
Nausea
Vomiting
Weight gain
Muscle weakness
Irritability
Mild disorientation
Malaise
Anger
Anxiety
Uncooperativeness

Late Signs and Symptoms

Lethargy
Headache
Decreased deep tendon reflexes
Coma
Seizures

Fluid and Electrolyte Changes

Decreased plasma sodium and plasma osmolality
Increased urinary sodium and urine osmolality
Decreased urinary volume
Absence of edema
Low normal to subnormal uric acid levels (a dilutional effect)

Collaborative Care Management. Medical management of acute SIADH focuses on treating the etiologic factor (e.g., carcinoma or infection) and correcting, or at least restoring toward normal, the plasma sodium level and plasma osmolality. Water restriction is the first priority of management. Water may be restricted to as little as 500 ml/day. Oral salt intake is increased if the patient is able to take oral nutrients.

Chronic SIADH and hyponatremia are first treated with water restriction. If water restriction alone cannot prevent hypoosmolality, pharmacologic treatment is added. Demeclocycline, a tetracycline derivative, blocks the action of ADH on the renal tubule and collecting duct cells and decreases urine osmolality. Lithium carbonate and phenytoin have also been used to treat SIADH.

If the patient's plasma sodium level is less than 120 mEq/L and the patient is exhibiting central nervous system manifestations such as nausea, vomiting, lethargy, and headaches, more rapid correction of the low plasma sodium level is necessary. This severe hyponatremia is treated with hypertonic saline (3% sodium chloride) and a loop diuretic such as furosemide (Lasix) or ethacrynic acid. The goal of this therapy is not to return the plasma sodium level to normal but to increase it to 125 to 130 mEq/L, or to administer enough sodium chloride to relieve symptoms or increase the plasma sodium by 25 mEq/L.

This correction needs to be made cautiously to avoid potential complications from either too rapid or too slow correction. Too rapid an increase in the plasma sodium level can produce a hypertonic plasma solution and a fluid shift from the intracellular to the extracellular compartment. A rapid fluid shift can result in central pontine myelinolysis, which is demyelination of the pons. This demyelination results in dysfunction of the nerve tracts that travel through or originate in the pons, causing bulbar palsies, quadriplegia, coma, and death. During treatment with hypertonic saline or loop diuretics, plasma osmolality and serum sodium are monitored every 2 to 4 hours. Note that 3% sodium chloride is used for sodium replacement, not for volume replacement.

Nursing care includes identifying persons at risk of SIADH and monitoring neurologic and fluid volume status. For high-risk patients, the nurse monitors daily weights, intake and output, daily serum and urinary sodium levels and osmolality, vital signs, and neurologic status. Any decrease below normal in serum sodium, any signs of fluid retention (increased weight or decreased output), and any neurologic changes (headaches, nausea, or decreased level of consciousness) must be reported. If the serum sodium level is below 125 mEq/L, laboratory results need to be reported immediately.

For patients with diagnosed SIADH being treated aggressively with hypertonic sodium or loop diuretics, the frequency of monitoring is increased to every 1 to 2 hours. Any deterioration in neurologic status is reported immediately.

For patients with chronic SIADH, weights are monitored daily to weekly and any increases not attributed to dietary changes or any reports of nausea, headache, or lethargy reported. Monitoring by the nurse in the outpatient department is the same as that described for high-risk patients.

The nurse should explain the rationale for fluid restrictions and methods to relieve discomfort from thirst. Fluid intake should be spaced throughout the 24-hour period. Ice chips should be encouraged to allow more frequent relief of thirst with less fluid intake. Mouth care is provided frequently.

PATIENT/FAMILY TEACHING. Patient and family teaching is presented in the Patient/Family Teaching box.

Antidiuretic Hormone Hyposecretion: Diabetes Insipidus

Etiology and Epidemiology. The etiology of DI may be either central (loss of production of ADH) or nephrogenic (lack of a renal response to ADH). This discussion focuses on central DI, the endocrine cause of DI. Central DI may be transient (as

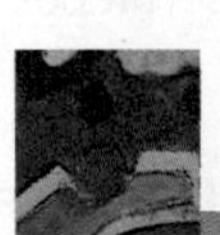

PATIENT/FAMILY TEACHING *The Patient With Syndrome of Inappropriate Antidiuretic Hormone*

Teaching focuses on the purpose and management of fluid restriction. The nurse stresses the need for self-monitoring on a long-term basis. Additional information includes:

- Methods to accurately measure body weight and intake and output.
- Medication therapy. Diuretics may be used long term; some patients use salt tablets with diuretics to replace urinary sodium losses and prevent volume depletion.
- Diet. Some patients may be prescribed a high-sodium diet.

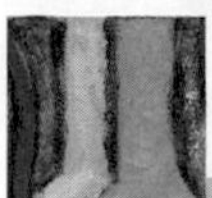

Clinical Manifestations
Diabetes Insipidus

- Polyuria: as much as 20 L of urine/day excreted; urine dilute, with a specific gravity of 1.005 or less or an osmolality of 200 or less
- Polydipsia secondary to increased thirst
- Only slightly elevated serum osmolality because water intake is usually maintained
- Abnormal results of tests for urine concentration
  —Water deprivation test (see Chapter 37): no increase in urine concentration with either pituitary or nephrogenic diabetes insipidus (DI)
  —Antidiuretic hormone replacement: increase in urine osmolality with pituitary DI but no response with nephrogenic DI
- Sleep disturbance from polyuria
- Inadequate water replacement results in:
  —Hyperosmolality: irritability, mental dullness, coma, hyperthermia
  —Hypovolemia: hypotension, tachycardia, dry mucous membranes, poor skin turgor

after transsphenoidal surgery for anterior pituitary adenomas) or permanent. The permanent causes of central DI include sarcoidosis, posterior hypophysectomy, pituitary tumors, head trauma, encephalitis, and meningitis. In many instances no underlying cause is found, and the case is labeled idiopathic.[38]

Pathophysiology. The lack of adequate ADH results in inadequate water resorption in the kidneys. The resulting loss of excessive water from the body **(polyuria)** produces dehydration and an increase in serum osmolality that stimulates thirst and **polydipsia** (see Clinical Manifestations box). Patients characteristically crave cold liquids and drink copious amounts of liquids during the day and night to maintain some semblance of fluid balance. The amount needed varies depending on the severity of the ADH deficiency. When inadequate water replacement occurs, central nervous system and vascular changes from hyperosmolality and volume depletion can result.

Collaborative Care Management. The person with pituitary DI is treated with a vasopressin synthetic analog (desmopressin [DDAVP]) rather than vasopressin itself (Table 38-1). Both DDAVP and vasopressin bind to the V2 receptors in the renal tubule. However, vasopressin also binds to the V1 receptors in smooth muscle of arterioles and other tissues and causes pressor side effects of exogenous ADH (abdominal cramping, hypertension, and angina). In addition, DDAVP has a more potent antidiuretic effect and longer duration of action. For persons who have some residual anterior pituitary function (partial DI), chlorpropamide and clofibrate, which stimulate release of endogenous ADH, may occasionally be prescribed.

Temporary DI associated with head trauma or surgery is treated with parenteral DDAVP. After transsphenoidal surgery, nasal packing and edematous nasal mucosa preclude using the nasal route for medications. The most common treatment for persons with nephrogenic DI is a low-sodium, low-protein diet and thiazide diuretics. The low-sodium diet and thiazide diuretics induce mild volume depletion. This volume depletion enhances sodium chloride and water resorption in the proximal part of the kidney tubule, resulting in less water being delivered to the collecting tubules where ADH should be; therefore less water is excreted. The diuretic also increases the osmolality of the medullary interstitial space and thus promotes more water resorption in collecting tubules that are less permeable because of inadequate ADH. Protein restriction helps control water loss by decreasing solute excretion. Nephrogenic DI can also be treated by administering nonsteroidal antiinflammatory agents, which impair prostaglandin production in the kidney and increase urinary concentrating ability.[47]

For patients with clinical evidence of hypernatremia such as mental status changes and hyperthermia, water replacement must be instituted. Fluid replacement is calculated by estimating the patient's water deficit and adding the insensible water loss and urinary loss. Fluid replacement must be done carefully and gradually over 48 hours to avoid cerebral edema, seizures, or even death. Too rapid correction of hypernatremia by fluid administration may create an osmotic gradient, with plasma osmolality being less than intracellular osmolality and the entry of water into the brain. The exact fluid administered depends on the patient's needs.[38]

Nursing interventions for the person with DI focus on maintaining fluid and electrolyte balance. Intake and output, daily weights, urine specific gravity, vital signs (orthostatic), skin turgor, and neurologic status are monitored every 1 to 2 hours during the acute phase, then every 4 to 8 hours until discharge, and again on return to the physician's office or outpatient clinic. The nurse provides the patient with adequate fluid and adequate rest periods during the day, since nocturia may disrupt sleep cycles.

Patient/Family Teaching. Patient and family teaching for the patient with hyposecretion of antidiuretic hormone is presented in the Patient/Family Teaching box.

Table 38-1 Common Preparations of Desmopressin Used for Treatment of Diabetes Insipidus

Medication	Dosage	Route of Administration
Desmopressin nasal spray	10-40 mcg/day administered in 1-3 doses	Intranasal
Desmopressin acetate rhinal tube	10-40 mcg/day administered in 1-3 doses	Intranasal
Desmopressin tablets	Initial dose: 0.05 mg bid Optimal dose: 0.05-0.6 mg bid	Oral
Desmopressin parenteral solution	1-2 mcg bid	Subcutaneous

bid, Twice a day.

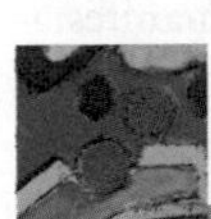

PATIENT/FAMILY TEACHING *The Patient With Hyposecretion of Antidiuretic Hormone (Diabetes Insipidus)*

The nurse instructs the patient and family about:

- Diagnostic tests, including their purposes, procedures, and required monitoring (see Chapter 37).
- The dosage, route, and frequency of prescribed medications. The patient is taught that if nasal congestion occurs, drug effectiveness may decrease, and polyuria and thirst will result.
- The need to observe for signs of volume excess (weight gain, edema).

ARE You READY?

Which nursing diagnosis is appropriate for a patient with diabetes insipidus?

1. Excess fluid volume related to sodium retention
2. Excess fluid volume related to water resorption
3. Deficient fluid volume related to sodium excretion
4. Deficient fluid volume related to water excretion

Thyroid Disorders

Thyroid disease is relatively common, with a gender predisposition to females. Diseases of the thyroid may result in hypersecretion, hyposecretion, or thyroid enlargement (goiter). A goiter refers to any enlargement of the thyroid and does not indicate any particular pathologic process or dysfunction.

Hypersecretion: Hyperthyroidism

Hyperthyroidism refers to elevated serum thyroid hormone levels and may be due to several causes. *Thyrotoxicosis* refers to the toxic effects or manifestations of excess thyroid hormone. The mildest form of hyperthyroidism is subclinical hyperthyroidism, which is generally devoid of symptoms and is characterized by normal free T_4 and free T_3 levels with suppressed TSH.[65] In addition to being a precursor of overt hyperthyroidism, thyrotoxicosis has been associated with a fivefold increased risk of atrial fibrillation in older persons[8] (see Research box).

Research

Auer J et al: Subclinical hyperthyroidism as a risk factor for atrial fibrillation, *Am Heart J* 142:838-842, 2001.

Atrial fibrillation is a well-known clinical manifestation of hyperthyroidism. The objective of this study was to determine whether subclinical hyperthyroidism increases the risk of atrial fibrillation. The authors studied 23,638 individuals and classified them according to their thyroid-stimulating hormone concentration. Rates of atrial fibrillation were group 1 (euthyroidism), 2.3%; group 2 (hyperthyroidism), 13.8%; and group 3 (subclinical hyperthyroidism), 12.7%. The relative risk of atrial fibrillation in group 3 (subclinical hyperthyroidism) versus group 1 (euthyroidism) was 5.2; that is, having subclinical hyperthyroidism increased the relative risk of atrial fibrillation by more than fivefold. No significant difference was found between the rates of atrial fibrillation in the hyperthyroid versus subclinical hyperthyroid groups. Implications include the importance of treating patients with subclinical hyperthyroidism to decrease the risk of atrial fibrillation with its inherent risks of cerebrovascular and pulmonary embolic events.

Etiology and Epidemiology. The causes of hyperthyroidism are summarized in Table 38-2. Drug-induced hyperthyroidism is now more common, especially with the wider use of the antiarrhythmic agent amiodarone.[15,41]

Graves' disease is the most common cause of hyperthyroidism, accounting for more than 60% of all cases. In addition to the symptoms and signs of hyperthyroidism, Graves' disease is characterized by a smooth diffuse goiter, variable degrees of ophthalmopathy, and occasionally an infiltrative dermopathy. Graves' disease has an autoimmune basis and is seen more commonly in patients with other autoimmune diseases such as type 1 diabetes mellitus, systemic lupus erythematosus, rheumatoid arthritis, pernicious anemia, or Addison's disease.

TABLE 38-2 CHARACTERISTICS OF HYPERTHYROIDISM

Classification	Characteristics
Graves' disease	Autoimmune; genetic component
Toxic multinodular goiter	Autonomous function of thyroid; multiple nodules
Toxic solitary adenoma	Single adenoma of follicular cells that secretes and functions independent of thyroid-secreting hormone (TSH) May selectively hypersecrete T_3, resulting in T_3 toxicosis
Hyperthyroidism caused by metastatic thyroid cancer	Rare; thyroid cancer cells do not usually concentrate iodine efficiently; may occur with large follicular carcinomas
TSH-secreting pituitary adenoma	A rare form of pituitary adenoma; treatment involves surgical removal
Chorionic hyperthyroidism	Chorionic gonadotropin has weak thyrotropin activity. Tumors such as choriocarcioma, embryonal cell carcinoma, and hydatidiform mole have high concentrations of chorionic gonadotropins that can stimulate T_4 and T_3 secretion; hyperthyroidism resolves with treatment of tumor.
Struma ovarii	Ovarian dermoid tumor made up partly of thyroid tissue that secretes thyroid hormone

Toxic multinodular goiter, or Plummer's disease, does not have an autoimmune basis and is generally seen in patients over 50 years old who have had longstanding, progressively enlarging goiters. Solitary toxic nodules, or hot nodules, can also cause hyperthyroidism and may have selective overproduction of T_3. Solitary toxic nodules are essentially always benign.

The incidence of hyperthyroidism in adults is estimated at 0.02% to 0.06%. Graves' disease, like other autoimmune diseases, is more common in women. There is some familial predisposition to autoimmune thyroid disease.

Pathophysiology

HYPERMETABOLISM. Hyperthyroidism results from autonomous production of thyroid hormone, independent of TSH from the pituitary gland. The first hormonal sign of emerging hyperthyroidism is therefore a suppressed TSH. The hyperthyroidism of Graves' disease results from an immunoglobulin that stimulates the TSH receptor on the thyroid gland, resulting in hypertrophy of the gland and overproduction of thyroid hormone. This immunoglobulin, thyroid-stimulating immunoglobulin, can be measured in the patient's serum as a marker of Graves' disease activity.

Toxic solitary nodules and multinodular goiters are benign tumors autonomously overproducing thyroid hormone. The underlying cause of these entities is unknown.

Excess thyroid hormone in the circulation increases metabolic rate, increases activity of the sympathetic nervous system, and affects fat and carbohydrate metabolism (Box 38-5). The degree of excess thyroid hormone correlates fairly well with the clinical picture. Severely toxic patients can have high-output congestive heart failure; cardiac arrhythmias; and even thyroid storm, which is life-threatening. Patients generally exhibit multiple manifestations of hyperthyroidism rather than a solitary sign or symptom. An exception would be atrial fibrillation in older adults as the sole manifestation of hyperthyroidism.[16]

GRAVES' OPHTHALMOPATHY. Ophthalmopathy may have an infiltrative or noninfiltrative cause. Both types of ophthalmopathy may be present in a given patient (Box 38-6). In *infiltrative ophthalmopathy* the retrobulbar connective tissue and extraocular muscle volume are expanded because of fluid retention resulting from the accumulation of glycosaminoglycans. The increase in tissue mass forces the eye forward **(proptosis)** up to the limits of the restraining action of the extraocular muscles **(exophthalmos)** (Figure 38-5). The pressure in the retrobulbar space increases because of the increased tissue and limited forward movement, causing periorbital and lid edema and pressure on the optic nerve. The stretched, enlarged extraocular muscles do not function well and commonly result in diplopia.

Noninfiltrative changes occur as a result of the thyrotoxicosis and usually resolve when the hyperthyroidism is treated. These changes, including lid retraction and lid lag, are due to sympathetic nervous system overstimulation resulting in contraction of the eyelid levator muscle.

Glycosaminoglycans and fluid accumulation also occur in the connective tissue in other parts of the body. This accumulation is particularly seen in the pretibial area—a condition called pretibial **myxedema**.

The risk of ophthalmopathy may be increased in cigarette smokers.[29] Significant preexisting ophthalmopathy in patients with Graves' disease may be exacerbated by radioiodine (RAI) therapy.

Box 38-5 Hyperthyroidism: Pathophysiologic Alterations and Clinical Manifestations

Common Signs and Symptoms

Increased metabolic rate, heat production, and oxygen consumption caused by the overall increase in metabolism, characterized by:

- Heat intolerance
- Increased body temperature
- Warm, moist skin
- Increased appetite
- Weight loss
- Muscle fatigue

Protein, Fat, and Carbohydrate Metabolism

The entire cycle of synthesis, degradation, and clearance is accelerated. Because of the increased lipolysis and increased lipid metabolism, especially lipid degradation, serum cholesterol and triglyceride levels may decline. The patient with preexisting diabetes mellitus may experience rising blood glucose levels because of increased glycogenolysis, increased intestinal glucose absorption, and increased insulin degradation.

Cardiovascular Function

The hypermetabolic state coupled with increased sensitivity to catecholamines increases myocardial oxygen consumption, shortens the systolic interval, and increases cardiac output. Signs and symptoms include tachycardia, palpitations, elevated blood pressure with a widened pulse pressure, atrial fibrillation, angina, dyspnea, and high-output congestive heart failure.

Central Nervous System Function

Thyroid hormone synergizes with other centrally acting hormones and neurotransmitters, and this is accelerated in hyperthyroidism. Signs and symptoms include nervousness; anxiety; restlessness; decreased attention span; insomnia; emotional lability; and fine rhythmic tremors of the hands, tongue, and eyelids.

Reproductive Function

Secretion and metabolism of gonadotropins and gonadal steroids are altered. Signs and symptoms include delayed sexual development in the prepubertal patient and increased libido, decreased fertility, and altered menses in the postpubertal patient.

Calcium and Phosphorus Balance

Thyroid hormone excess increases the mobilization of calcium from bone and the urinary excretion of calcium and phosphorus. Bone mass may decline, and proximal muscle weakness may occur.

Gastrointestinal Function

Increased motility of the gastrointestinal tract may lead to increased frequency of bowel movements.

Box 38-6 Graves' Ophthalmopathy

Signs

Bright-eyed stare, resulting from retraction of upper eyelid
Lid lag: on downward gaze, upper lid lagging behind globe movement, and sclera seen between lid and limbus
Lid movement: jerky and spasmodic
Lid closure problematic when significant proptosis exists
Periorbital edema

Symptoms

Sense of irritation and excessive tearing
Feeling of pressure behind eyes
Complaints of blurred vision or diplopia; eyes easily tired

Complications

Corneal ulceration from exposure and excess drying
Optic nerve involvement (optic neuropathy)
Myopathy of extraocular muscles

For this reason some endocrinologists prefer to treat such patients with antithyroid drug therapy rather than RAI.

THYROID STORM. Thyroid storm is a medical emergency in which patients develop severe manifestations of the signs and symptoms of hyperthyroidism. These include an elevated temperature; increased tachycardia or onset of dysrhythmias; blood pressure and respiratory rate increased above baseline; worsening tremors and restlessness; worsening mental status, including a delirious or psychotic state or coma; and sometimes abdominal pain.

Thyroid storm is a rare, severe manifestation of hyperthyroidism, usually seen in an individual with Graves' disease. Symptoms result from a severe increase in metabolism and are usually precipitated by a major stressor such as infection, trauma, or surgery. The use of medications to suppress thyroid activity before surgery decreases the risk of thyroid storm, since less hormone is available to be released into the circulation with manipulation of the gland. Thyroid crisis also may occur in a person who has been inadequately treated or who stops taking prescribed therapy.

Collaborative Care Management. The choice of therapy is based on the patient's age, gender, and reproductive status and the cause and severity of hyperthyroidism. The most toxic patients are treated with antithyroid drugs initially and thereafter with RAI therapy or ongoing antithyroid drug therapy. The potential for permanent remission with antithyroid drugs exists only for patients with Graves' disease.

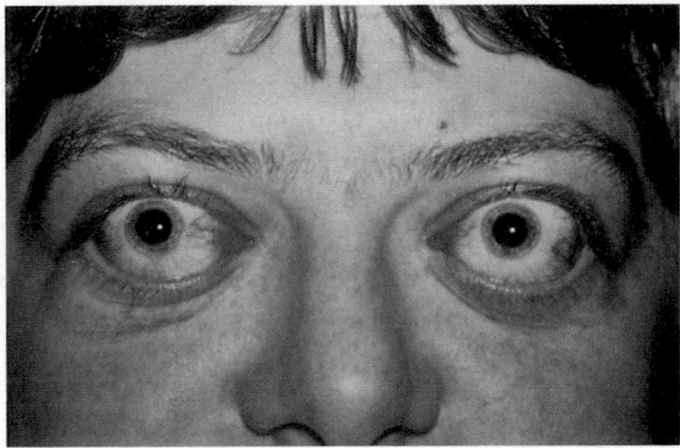

Figure 38-5 Classic Graves' ophthalmopathy.

DIAGNOSTIC TESTS. After a comprehensive history and physical examination, a TSH level should be the initial test ordered; TSH will be suppressed in all cases of hyperthyroidism. A free T_4 level confirms the magnitude of the hyperthyroidism. T_3 levels may be ordered if T_3 toxicosis is suspected (solitary nodules). The free T_4 in T_3 toxicosis may be normal or mildly elevated.

Ultrasound is also used to define the size of the gland, pathologic condition, or presence of nodules. An endocrinologist experienced in ultrasound is best able to interpret findings in the context of the clinical picture. A 24-hour radioactive iodine uptake (RAIU) test is elevated in almost all cases of hyperthyroidism. A near-zero RAIU is found in subacute thyroiditis, painless thyroiditis, and factitious disease. RAIU findings are inaccurate if the patient has received iodine in the weeks preceding the test. Other tests, such as the thyroid-binding globulin, can be used to calculate the free T_4 index if the patient has recently received iodine.

MEDICATIONS. The two commonly used antithyroid drugs (thionamides) are propylthiouracil (PTU) and methimazole (Tapazole). These drugs block the synthesis of thyroid hormone within the gland and may have some immunomodulatory properties. PTU also may block the peripheral conversion of T_4 to T_3, which is of additional value in severely toxic patients. Until the preformed thyroid hormone still stored in the thyroid gland is released and the excessive amounts of thyroid hormone in the circulation are metabolized, no significant clinical effects of the antithyroid drugs are seen. Given that the half-life of T_4 is 7 days, several weeks must elapse before seeing significant improvement. PTU is generally taken three times a day with a total daily dose of 300 to 450 mg. Methimazole is generally taken twice a day or in daily doses of 10 to 60 mg. The dosage of antithyroid drug is gradually tapered as the patient becomes **euthyroid**, and treatment is generally maintained for 12 to18 months.[23]

Twelve to 18 months after cessation of antithyroid drug therapy, approximately 50% of patients with Graves' disease are in remission. One study found that maintaining total thyroid suppression with antithyroid drug therapy and treating the drug-induced hypothyroidism with concurrent thyroid hormone will increase the remission rate to more than 90%. However, this study was carried out in a Japanese population but was unable to be reproduced in other populations, suggesting that genetics may play a role in the response to this approach.[65a] In the event of patient relapse, options include a further course of antithyroid drug therapy, RAI therapy, or surgery. In general, the best remission rates with antithyroid drug therapy in Graves' disease are seen in women with smaller goiters.

Side effects of antithyroid drugs include agranulocytosis; hence baseline and subsequent periodic monitoring of the white blood cell count is recommended. It is important to note baseline values, since many patients with Graves' disease have borderline-low white blood cells. The nurse instructs patients to look for signs and symptoms of leukopenia (e.g., sore throat, fever, sepsis) and other side effects (e.g., jaundice) and notify the health care provider if these occur.

Beta-adrenergic blockers such as propranolol are used to treat the tachycardia, arrhythmias, tremors, and agitation associated with the sympathetic nervous system stimulation. The doses required are generally high and give prompt symptomatic relief. The dose is titrated down as the hyperthyroidism is controlled. These drugs should be prescribed cautiously to patients with asthma or congestive heart failure, since exacerbation of symptoms can occur in response to the negative inotropic side effects of the beta-adrenergic blockers. If beta-adrenergic blockers are contraindicated or not tolerated, calcium channel blockers may be used.

TREATMENTS. Patients with thyroid storm are critically ill and are managed in a critical care unit. The immediate focus of care is to lower the metabolic rate as fast as possible, treat the precipitating cause, and support physiologic functioning (see Guidelines for Safe Practice box). The doses of medications used to treat thyroid storm are higher than those used in less critically ill patients because of accelerated metabolism of the drugs. Doses are adjusted according to patient response. Patients may require continual monitoring during rapid treatment.[23]

High-priority interventions focus on managing the patient's cardiovascular status and hyperthermia. Rapid atrial fibrillation is often the first cardiac alteration noted; other dysrhythmias are possible. Angina and high-output congestive heart failure may occur in hyperthyroid patients, often in those with underlying heart disease. Interventions for these patients are designed to normalize cardiac output. The nurse monitors cardiovascular status every hour and reports to the physician any changes, such as increased tachycardia, dysrhythmias, or signs of congestive heart failure (see Chapter 30). Cardiac workload is decreased by decreasing physical and emotional stressors. The nurse also monitors temperature every hour and reports any elevations. Room temperature is maintained in the cool range and external cooling devices used as ordered.

As the acute crisis subsides, the nurse continues to try to normalize cardiac output and temperature.

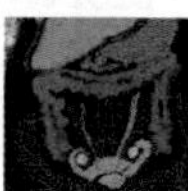

GUIDELINES FOR SAFE PRACTICE
The Patient With Thyroid Storm

- Monitor the patient's temperature, intake and output, neurologic status, and cardiovascular status every hour.
- Initiate an intravenous (IV) line for medications and fluids.
- Administer increasing doses of oral propylthiouracil (PTU) as ordered (200 to 300 mg every 6 hours may be given) after a loading dose of 800 to 1200 mg orally. PTU is the preferred antithyroid drug in this situation because it also inhibits the peripheral conversion of T_4 to T_3.
- Administer iodide preparations as ordered: sodium iodide given IV twice daily or an oral preparation.
- Administer dexamethasone, 2 mg IV every 6 hours. Glucocorticoids help inhibit the release of thyroid hormone.
- Administer beta-adrenergic blockers IV, as ordered. Noncardioselective beta-adrenergic blockers can worsen asthma or congestive heart failure because they constrict bronchial smooth muscles and reduce cardiac output.
- Initiate measures to lower body temperature, including external cooling devices, cold baths, and acetaminophen. Salicylates are contraindicated because they inhibit thyroid hormone binding to protein carriers and thus increase free thyroid hormone levels.
- Initiate other supportive therapy as ordered, including oxygen, cardiac glycosides, and treatment measures for the precipitating event.
- Maintain a quiet, calm, cool, private environment until the crisis is over.
- Maintain continuity of care.
- Decrease stressors by use of patient education, comfort measures, or family support.

RADIOIODINE THERAPY. Therapeutic RAI therapy with ^{131}I is a more definitive therapy for hyperthyroidism resulting from Graves' disease and is the only long-term therapy, other than surgery, for toxic multinodular goiter or solitary toxic nodules. RAI therapy is contraindicated in pregnancy. The dose is individualized based on the thyroid size and 24-hour ^{123}I uptake. Hypothyroidism is to be anticipated, since it is impossible to titrate the dose of ^{131}I to achieve a euthyroid state without a high failure rate and the need for retreatment. Pending TSH and free T_4 levels, replacement therapy with levothyroxine is initiated and maintained.[5,23]

The radiation dose for ^{131}I therapy for hyperthyroidism is usually 6000 to 7000 rad, equivalent to the radiation exposure for an intravenous pyelogram. Depending on the severity of the hyperthyroidism and the dose administered, a euthyroid state generally results sometime between 6 weeks and 6 months after therapy. Repeat treatment may be needed in 10% to 20% of patients.

The RAI is gradually eliminated from the body over a few days, primarily via the urine. Therefore appropriate hygienic measures should be used. Small amounts of RAI appear in the saliva; patients should be instructed to not share food, drink, or utensils with others and should avoid kissing for several days after receiving RAI therapy. Close contact with children should be minimized. A woman who has received ^{131}I therapy should defer pregnancy for 6 months and not breastfeed for 6 months.

SURGICAL MANAGEMENT. Hyperthyroidism is rarely managed surgically. Surgery is indicated for (1) failure of antithyroid drug therapy, (2) failure of or contraindication to RAI therapy, (3) large goiters with compressive symptoms, or (4) concurrent thyroid cancer.

Subtotal thyroidectomy, removal of approximately 80% of the thyroid gland, is generally the procedure of choice; total thyroidectomy is reserved for thyroid cancer. The rate of hypothyroidism is less with subtotal thyroidectomy than with RAI therapy; however, the relapse rate may be higher over time. Before surgery, patients are given antithyroid medication to achieve a euthyroid state. The risks of thyroidectomy include damage to the recurrent laryngeal nerve, hypoparathyroidism, tracheal and esophageal injury, and the usual postoperative complications.

DIET. Increased food intake and weight loss are characteristic of untreated hyperthyroidism. Increased nutrient and calorie intake are necessary to meet the increased metabolic requirements. Cessation of weight loss with treatment can signal the return of the euthyroid state in older patients. While hyperthyroidism is present, caloric intake needs to be increased, with attention to appropriate distribution of calories from macronutrients. Supplemental vitamins and trace minerals may be prescribed.

> **▶ ARE YOU READY?**
>
> Which of the following are clinical manifestations of hyperthyroidism?
> 1. Fatigue, weight gain, cold intolerance
> 2. Decreased pulse rate, slurred speech
> 3. Abdominal pain, constipation, heat intolerance
> 4. Nervousness, weight loss, tachycardia

Nursing Management *of the Patient with Hyperthyroidism*

ASSESSMENT

Health History. Assess for:

- Emotional and mental status changes
- Palpitations or chest pain
- Dyspnea, with or without exercise
- Changes in hair, skin, nails, or amount of sweating
- Visual disturbances and irritations; eye fatigue
- Appetite and history of nutritional intake and weight changes
- Sleep patterns (e.g., insomnia)
- Muscle tremors
- Increased stool frequency and stool bulk
- Heat intolerance
- Weakness, fatigue, and decreased ability to complete ADLs
- Changes in menses or libido
- Knowledge: disease, treatment, care needs

Physical Examination. Assess for:

- Shortened attention span, emotional lability, hyperkinesia, tremors
- Increased systolic blood pressure, decreased diastolic pressure, widened pulse pressure, tachycardia at rest, dysrhythmias, murmurs
- Warm, flushed, sweaty skin; dermopathy; fine, thinning hair
- Eyelid lag, proptosis, exophthalmos, diplopia, injected conjunctiva, decreased acuity
- Decreased weight, increased appetite and intake, decreased serum triglycerides and cholesterol levels
- Proximal muscle weakness, decreased muscle tone, difficulty rising from sitting position
- Decreased serum levels of TSH measured by a third-generation assay; elevated free T_4 or free T_3 levels

NURSING DIAGNOSES, OUTCOMES, AND INTERVENTIONS

Nursing Diagnosis: Risk for Activity Intolerance

OUTCOMES. Common examples of expected outcomes for the patient with a diagnosis of *risk for activity intolerance* are:

Patient will:

- Demonstrate no further decrease in activity tolerance and show a gradual increase in activity over 2 to 3 months.
- Show evidence of adequate tissue perfusion and cardiac output: no change in mental status, breath sounds clear, no edema formation, heart rate within 20 beats/min of baseline, and gradual decrease in resting heart rate.

NURSING INTERVENTIONS. The nurse promotes a balance of activity and rest. The first step is to document baseline vital signs and vital signs in response to activity and to monitor the patient's response to and ability to tolerate activity. Activity may be self-limited because of fatigue. A relaxing environment allows the patient rest periods during the day; however, sympathetic nervous system activation may make trying to rest frustrating, especially if the patient is unable to sleep at night. Work requiring concentration for long periods may be difficult. The patient may need assistance in coping with activity restrictions that interfere with occupational and financial demands. Usually activity restrictions are not imposed unless the patient has symptoms of tachycardia, atrial fibrillation, or other cardiovascular problems. Thyroid storm mandates complete bed rest and admission to an intensive care unit.

RELATED NIC INTERVENTIONS. Energy Management, Self-Care Assistance, Sleep Enhancement

Nursing Diagnosis: Anxiety

OUTCOMES. Common examples of expected outcomes for the patient with a diagnosis of *anxiety* are:

Patient will:

- Show signs of decreased anxiety and effective coping.
- Rate self as less anxious or less stressed on a scale of 0 to 10, with 0 meaning no stress and 10 meaning the worst stress.
- List three ways to cope with feelings regarding body changes.
- Identify home maintenance difficulties and methods to deal with difficulties until health stabilizes.

NURSING INTERVENTIONS. The nurse provides information regarding the physiologic reasons for changes in appearance, fatigue, activity intolerance, heat intolerance, and sleep disturbances. Providing symptomatic relief can decrease anxiety and feelings of frustration and powerlessness. The nurse helps the patient identify coping strategies to deal with feelings. Previously effective coping methods may be successful again. The environment should be supportive and allow the patient to participate in his or her care to the fullest extent possible. The nurse helps the patient explore relaxation techniques to decrease anxiety.

A Nursing Care Plan for the patient with hyperthyroidism is found on p. 1078.

RELATED NIC INTERVENTIONS. Anxiety Reduction, Calming Technique

Patient/Family Teaching. Patient and family teaching for the patient with hyperthyroidism is presented in the Patient/Family Teaching box, p. 1080.

Nursing Care Plan

Patient With Hyperthyroidism

Data The patient is a 28-year-old woman who states she feels overwhelmed, cries frequently, and fears losing control. She has lost 15 pounds during the past 2 months. She is persistently hungry even though she eats large quantities of food. She is heat and noise intolerant and feels clumsy.

Physical examination reveals temperature, 98.8° F (37° C) orally; blood pressure, 140/60 mm Hg; heart rate, 132 beats/min; and respirations, 24 breaths/min. Electrocardiogram confirms sinus tachycardia at 98 beats/min. She has a staring gaze with proptosis (equal bilaterally), lid lag, and globe lag. Her right eye is slightly reddened. Her skin is warm, and she is sweating. She complains of lower extremity weakness and has a fine tremor of both hands. She startles to sudden noises. Her thyroid is visibly enlarged.

Thyroid studies confirm the presence of hyperthyroidism (Graves' disease). The patient is placed on methimazole (Tapazole) and Lugol's solution in preparation for a thyroidectomy, which will take place in 2 weeks.

Nursing Diagnosis

Imbalanced nutrition: less than body requirements related to increased metabolic needs

Outcomes

- Patient will regain weight to within 5 pounds of ideal for height.

Related NOC Outcomes

- Nutritional Status
- Nutritional Status: Food & Fluid Intake
- Nutritional Status: Nutrient Intake

Related NIC Interventions

- Nutrition Management
- Nutrition Therapy
- Nutritional Monitoring

Nursing Interventions/Rationales

- Monitor weight at least weekly and more often if needed. *To determine whether nutritional needs are being met or further intervention is required.*
- Monitor serum albumin, hemoglobin, and lymphocyte levels. *To determine whether nutrition is adequate to meet metabolic and bodily needs or further intervention is needed.*
- Encourage a high-calorie, high-protein, high-carbohydrate diet with selections from all food groups. *Increased nutrient intake is needed to meet increased metabolic demands and prevent further weight loss.*
- Encourage the intake of six meals per day as tolerated. *To provide adequate nutrients consistently throughout the day to meet metabolic demands.*

Nursing Diagnosis

Risk for disturbed sensory perception (visual) secondary to Graves' disease

Outcomes

- Patient will remain free from visual loss.

Related NOC Outcomes

- Risk Control: Visual Impairment
- Vision Compensation Behavior

Related NIC Interventions

- Emotional Support
- Environmental Management
- Eye Care

Nursing Interventions/Rationales

- Assess for photophobia, visual acuity, and ability to close eyes. *To determine the extent of injury (if any) that has occurred and to prevent any further damage.*
- Protect the eyes from irritants through (1) patches or glasses, (2) artificial tears, and (3) elevating head of bed at night. *Protective measures can prevent corneal injury and minimize risk for loss of vision.*
- Teach patient to avoid lying prone at night and to wear eye shields if eyes do not close completely. *To protect the eyes from injury while sleeping and to prevent drying of cornea.*

Nursing Diagnosis

Activity intolerance related to generalized muscular weakness and increased metabolic rate secondary to Graves' disease

Outcomes

- Patient will report ability to perform daily (or desired) activities without experiencing fatigue.

Related NOC Outcomes

- Activity Tolerance
- Energy Conservation
- Nutritional Status: Energy

Related NIC Interventions

- Energy Management
- Nutrition Management
- Sleep Enhancement

Nursing Interventions/Rationales

- Assess severity of fatigue and patient's understanding of the physiologic cause. *A baseline assessment of the patient's fatigue is essential for later comparisons to determine effectiveness of interventions.*
- Encourage patient to prioritize daily activities and let go of unessential tasks. *Fatigue compromises one's ability to participate in daily activities. It is important that the patient's available energy be used to complete high-priority activities.*
- Explore strategies to (1) modify existing activities, conserving energy when possible; (2) seek assistance or delegate activities; and (3) pace activities throughout the day to allow a balance between activity and rest. *Many daily activities can be modified to consume less energy, but this requires the patient to think about routine activities in a different way. Accepting the reality of fatigue may allow the patient to consider seeking assistance or delegating activities.*
- Encourage patient to obtain at least 8 hours of uninterrupted sleep at night. *Effective nighttime sleep patterns may decrease daytime fatigue. The patient should avoid stimulants and exercise before bedtime, since either may interfere with the ability to fall asleep.*

Nursing Diagnosis

Deficient knowledge related to lack of prior experience or access to information about disease

Outcomes

- Patient will accurately describe disease process and treatments.

Related NOC Outcomes
- Knowledge: Diet
- Knowledge: Disease Process
- Knowledge: Energy Conservation
- Knowledge: Health Resources

Related NIC Interventions
- Teaching: Disease Process
- Teaching: Prescribed Activity/Exercise
- Teaching: Prescribed Diet
- Teaching: Prescribed Medication

Nursing Interventions/Rationales
- Teach patient how and when to take prescribed medications. *Knowledge and understanding increase the likelihood of compliance with medication routine to achieve euthyroid state.*
- Teach patient about side effects of medications that need to be reported. *To prevent injury from drug side effects that may further complicate existing condition.*
- Teach patient about signs and symptoms that need to be reported immediately (increased tachycardia, lightheadedness, etc.). *To detect complications early so that corrective action can be taken.*
- Teach patient about required care needs (diet, activities, rest). *To maintain maximal health and prevent complications while becoming regulated on medications and awaiting surgery.*
- Repeat teaching frequently. *Stress interferes with learning. There is too much information to learn at one time; therefore repetitive teaching enhances learning.*
- Provide written materials to enforce verbal teaching. *Patients who are ill or stressed do not always remember information taught. Written materials allow the patient to review important information and to proceed at their own pace.*
- Provide information about community resources that may be useful to patient and family. *The patient may not be aware of available community resources.*

Nursing Diagnosis
Ineffective coping related to personal vulnerability and environmental stimuli

Outcomes
- Patient will identify and use coping mechanisms effectively.

Related NOC Outcomes
- Coping
- Decision-Making

Related NIC Interventions
- Calming Technique
- Coping Enhancement
- Decision-Making Support

Nursing Interventions/Rationales
- Discuss reasons for emotional lability. *If the patient understands that her emotional lability is part of the disease process, she may be better able to cope.*
- Maintain a calm, relaxed environment. *Excessive external stimuli produce anxiety, which interferes with the patient's ability to cope.*
- Provide privacy (e.g., a private room). *To reduce external stimuli and stress.*
- Explain all procedures and interventions. *Knowledge reduces fear and anxiety, allowing the patient to better cope with the stressful situation.*
- Encourage avoidance of all stimulants (coffee, tea, caffeinated sodas). *To reduce physiologic stressors that can accelerate metabolic rate and prevent sleep or rest.*
- Encourage patient to identify previous coping mechanisms or explore new ones. *Mechanisms that have been beneficial in the past may help in her current situation.*
- Encourage patient to use relaxation techniques. *Relaxation promotes rest. A well-rested person is better able to use coping strategies than one who is fatigued.*

Nursing Diagnosis
Decreased cardiac output related to increased sympathetic stimulation

Outcomes
- Patient will have cardiac output within normal limits.
- Patient will remain free from cardiac dysrhythmias.

Related NOC Outcomes
- Cardiac Pump Effectiveness
- Circulation Status
- Vital Signs

Related NIC Interventions
- Cardiac Care
- Cardiac Care: Acute
- Vital Signs Monitoring

Nursing Interventions/Rationales
- Assess vital signs, especially heart rate and rhythm, at least every 4 hours or more often as indicated. *To detect changes from baseline that indicate cardiac compromise.*
- Teach patient to report palpitations, chest pain, or dizziness. *These symptoms are indicative of cardiac compromise and need to be evaluated.*
- Assess daily weight; intake and output; and signs of edema, jugular vein distention, and lung crackles. *To detect fluid volume changes that may be related to cardiac compromise secondary to tachycardia.*
- Decrease known stressors, explain all interventions, and listen to the patient. *Decreasing external stress decreases anxiety and the workload on the heart.*
- Balance periods of activity with periods of rest. *Activity is better tolerated when the patient is well rested. Frequent rest periods decrease the workload of the heart.*
- Administer prescribed medications and monitor for drug effectiveness. *To control symptoms, prevent excessive cardiac workload, and determine whether the selected medications are serving their intended purpose.*
- Report any changes in cardiac status to the physician. *Early detection of atrial fibrillation or thyroid storm allows for prompt treatment and prevents cardiac crisis.*

Evaluation
Evaluation is based on comparing the patient's outcomes with desired outcomes.

PATIENT/FAMILY TEACHING
The Patient With Hyperthyroidism

The nurse helps the patient learn to incorporate the therapeutic regimen into activities of daily living. In addition, the patient needs to plan how to achieve rest, adequate nutrition, and energy conservation at home and at work. The nurse can reinforce and clarify information about risks, benefits, consequences of the treatment, and the requirements for follow-up care. Patients may express concern about the effects of environmental radiation if radioiodine (RAI) therapy is an option.

The teaching plan should include information about:

- The disease process
- Treatment options
- Expected outcomes, the need for drug therapy for extended periods, and the potential complications of therapy
- Prescribed medications
- Precautions to be observed if treated with RAI
- Signs and symptoms of complications

EVALUATION

To evaluate the effectiveness of nursing interventions, compare patient behaviors with those stated in the expected patient outcomes.

RELATED NOC OUTCOMES. Activity Tolerance, Anxiety Level, Anxiety Self-Control, Energy Conservation, Self-Care: Activities of Daily Living (ADL)

GERONTOLOGIC CONSIDERATIONS

Older adult patients have less clear-cut clinical findings of hyperthyroidism. They may have weight loss, fatigue, and irritability; but goiter, tachycardia, eye changes, or tremor may be absent. In fact, subclinical hyperthyroidism, or "apathetic" or "masked" hyperthyroidism, is typical in older persons and needs to be treated.[55] RAI therapy is the treatment of choice in older patients.

When caring for an older adult with hyperthyroidism, the nurse must remember that hyperthyroidism can cause new-onset atrial fibrillation and an increased metabolism of drugs such as digoxin, theophylline, and warfarin, which are frequently taken in this age-group. Research has also shown that older Caucasian women with low serum TSH concentrations have increased risk of vertebral and hip fractures (see Research box).[9]

Nonthyroid disease may or may not raise the serum T_3 or T_4 in older persons and may suppress serum TSH. This is an important consideration because older persons typically have more than one chronic illness.

Research

Bauer DC et al, for Study of Osteoporotic Fractures Research Group: Risk for fracture in women with low levels of thyroid-stimulating hormone, *Ann Intern Med* 134:561, 2001.

From 1986 to 1988, 9704 Caucasian women over the age of 65 were enrolled in a prospective study of risk factors for fracture. The researchers took baseline serum samples, spine radiographs, and measurements of bone mass of the calcaneus by single-photon absorptiometry. Approximately 80% of these women had bone mineral density measurements of the proximal femur performed 2 years later and spine x-ray studies performed 3.7 years later. These women were then grouped by subsequent fracture into four groups: those with hip fractures, those with vertebral fractures, those with nonspine fractures, and those without fracture. After the observation period baseline values for thyroid-stimulating hormone (TSH) levels were measured, the mean TSH was similar in all groups. The women in each of the fracture groups had lower baseline calcaneal and femoral neck bone mineral density values. Results indicated that women with a low serum TSH (0.1 lmU/ml) had a 3.6-fold increased risk of hip fracture and a 4.5-fold increased risk of vertebral fracture. Limitations of the study include that not all women had TSH levels assayed and serum thyroxine levels were not measured.

Hyposecretion: Hypothyroidism

Etiology and Epidemiology. Hypothyroidism refers to low levels of thyroid hormone and encompasses:

- Congenital hypothyroidism (cretinism), which is detected through routine screening at birth
- Primary thyroid failure (e.g., Hashimoto's disease, other types of thyroiditis)
- Secondary thyroid failure (pituitary disease causing TSH deficiency)
- Tertiary thyroid failure resulting from thyrotropin-releasing hormone (TRH) deficiency with resultant TSH deficiency
- External thyroid gland destruction (i.e., after surgery, after ^{131}I therapy, from antithyroid drugs, or from medication side effects such as those from amiodarone or lithium)
- Miscellaneous (i.e., environmental iodine deficiency and peripheral resistance to thyroid hormone, both of which are rare)

In primary autoimmune thyroid failure, declining T_4 production causes increased TSH production with resultant hypertrophy of the remaining functioning thyroid tissue. Progressive thyroid enlargement over time can ensue with resulting clinical goiter. A goiter is any enlargement of the thyroid gland (Figure 38-6). If this enlargement is not associated with hyperthyroidism or hypothyroidism, cancer, or inflammation, it is referred to as a *simple goiter. Endemic goiters* refer to those which occur in a particular geographic region and from a common cause, such as iodine deficiency. *Sporadic goiter* describes those which occur sporadically in regions that are not the locus of endemic goiters. Box 38-7 lists goitrogenic factors. In many instances mild iodine deficiency is responsible for thyroid enlargement in pregnancy.

The most common cause of primary hypothyroidism in the United States is Hashimoto's disease. Patients are generally euthyroid or hypothyroid at presentation. Some may be asymptomatic with mild elevations in TSH, a condition called mild thyroid failure. Goiter formation in Hashimoto's disease is common in younger patients, and the goiter tends to enlarge over time if the patient is not receiving suppression therapy with exogenous thyroid hormone. Older individuals frequently have an autoimmune form of the disorder with thyroid atrophy (atrophic thyroiditis).[58]

Hypothyroidism affects an estimated 1% of the general population. In older persons the prevalence rates may exceed 10%. Hypothyroidism has a gender predisposition to females. Congen-

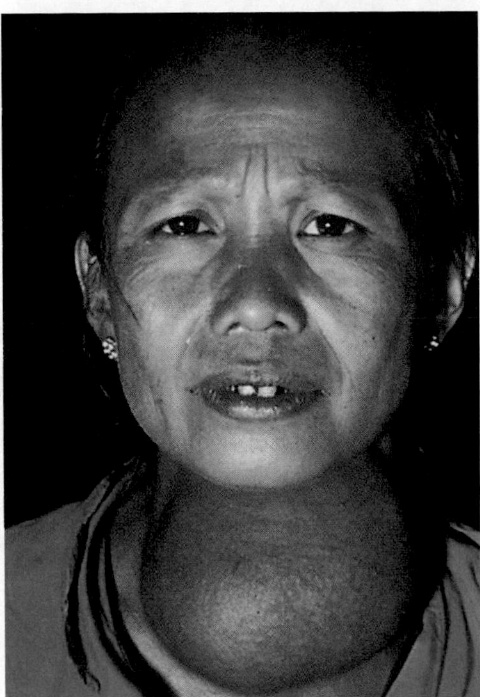

Figure 38-6 Simple goiter.

Box 38-7 Goitrogenic Factors

- Iodine deficiency
- Foods with goitrogenic properties (cabbage, turnips, soybeans)
- Lithium
- Intrinsic abnormality in thyroid hormone synthesis

ital hypothyroidism is detected in 1 of every 4000 to 5000 newborns (see Risk Factors box).

Risk Factors

Hypothyroidism

- History of thyroid disease
- History of radiation to neck
- Presence of other autoimmune disorders
  - –Type 1 diabetes mellitus
  - –Pernicious anemia (vitamin B_{12} deficiency)
  - –Vitiligo
  - –Addison's disease
- Family history of thyroid disease
- Family history of other autoimmune disorders
- Amiodarone treatment
- Lithium treatment

Pathophysiology

THYROIDITIS. Thyroiditis may be classified as acute, subacute, or chronic (Table 38-3). Hashimoto's disease is the most common form of chronic thyroiditis; most patients have thyroid enlargement owing in part to the trophic effects of the compensatory increase in TSH. Secondary and tertiary hypothyroidism is associated with low levels of TSH such that thyroid growth is not stimulated. The characteristic histologic picture includes infiltration with lymphocytes and varying degrees of fibrosis. Progressive glandular destruction results in an initial decline in T_4 levels and subsequent elevation in TSH.[56]

T_3 levels fall into the subnormal range after T_4 levels. Thyroid autoantibodies (antimicrosomal [thyroid peroxidase] and antithyroglobulin) are present in more than 90% of patients with Hashimoto's disease.

HYPOMETABOLISM. Regardless of the cause, a lack of thyroid hormone results in a general depression of the basal metabolic rate and slows the development or functioning of almost every system of the body, including the integumentary, cardiovascular, nervous, musculoskeletal, alimentary, and reproductive systems. Manifestations of hypothyroidism in infants are not usually seen until several months after birth, when signs such as retardation of mental and physical development occur and are usually irreversible.

In adults early signs and symptoms are vague, cover a wide range of body systems, and present a challenge for diagnosis. Symptoms include hypermenorrhea, infertility, menstrual cycle irregularity, hoarseness, carpal tunnel syndrome, constipation, hair loss, xeroderma, bradycardia, depression, and macrocytic anemia. Patients may complain of tiredness, lethargy, and weakness resulting in the inability to carry out a normal day's activities. Intolerance to cold and constipation may develop. Both men and women may note loss of libido. The majority of patients have multiple symptoms and signs, depending on the severity of the hypothyroidism (Box 38-8).

As the disease progresses, mental dysfunction occurs, appetite decreases, and changes in physical characteristics are noted. One major physical change is an accumulation of hyaluronic acids and alteration of ground substances, producing mucinous edema (myxedema) and third-space fluid effusions. Figure 38-7 illustrates the puffiness characteristic of myxedema facies. In the periphery the edematous tissues feel thickened or "doughy." The patient may report muscle and joint discomforts and chest pain. Severe hypothyroidism with markedly elevated TSH levels, secondary in part to the elevated TRH, results in concurrent elevation in PRL and potentially galactorrhea and amenorrhea.[58]

Occasionally patients with undiagnosed severe hypothyroidism are seen for coronary artery bypass graft (CABG) with advanced coronary artery disease. The dilemma then arises as to what to treat first—the hypothyroidism or the coronary artery disease. Clinical studies have documented the safety and efficacy of CABG in known hypothyroid patients, with thyroid hormone replacement therapy being deferred until after surgery. If hypothyroidism is not treated, myxedema coma develops.

MYXEDEMA COMA. Myxedema coma represents the most severe form of hypothyroidism and ultimately can occur in any patient with untreated, prolonged hypothyroidism. Precipitating factors include sedatives, opioids, exposure to cold, surgery, infections, and trauma. The patient has all the classic symptoms of hypothyroidism and also is comatose and has severe hypothermia. Therapy focuses on treating the underlying cause or precipitating event.

TABLE 38-3 THYROIDITIS: TYPES AND CHARACTERISTICS

Type	Characteristics
Acute thyroiditis	Bacterial infection of the thyroid. Causative agents include pyogenic bacteria, miliary tuberculosis, fungi, and *Pneumocystis carinii.* Symptoms include fever and a tender thyroid mass. This form of thyroiditis is rare in developed countries.
Subacute thyroiditis	A form of thyroiditis of increasing frequency. Etiology unknown, but possible autoimmune factor. Symptoms include self-limiting form of hyperthyroidism and nontender, enlarged thyroid gland, which may be followed by hypothyroidism. Symptomatic treatment during hyperthyroid phase consists of beta-adrenergic blockers, but not antithyroid medications. Patient monitored annually for hypothyroidism.
Postpartum thyroiditis	Occurs within a few months after delivery in 1% to 5% of pregnancies. Clinical course is similar to that of painless thyroiditis with transient toxic and hypothyroid phases that may be so mild as to go unnoticed in some patients. Permanent hypothyroidism may occur more frequently after postpartum thyroiditis than after painless thyroiditis.
Silent (painless) thyroiditis	Nontender thyroiditis associated with the presence of thyroid antoantibodies. The erythrocyte sedimentation rate is not elevated; goiter may or may not be present. Often considered a form of chronic thyroiditis; permanent hypothyroidism may result.
Chronic thyroiditis Hashimoto's thyroiditis	Autoimmune process characterized by lymphocytic infiltration of the thyroid, inflammation, and fibrosis. May present with large goiter.

Box 38-8 Hypothyroidism: Pathophysiologic Alterations and Clinical Manifestations

Common Signs and Symptoms

Decreased metabolic rate, heat production, and oxygen consumption leading to:

- Cold intolerance and perhaps decreased body temperature
- Cool, dry skin
- Decreased appetite
- Weight gain
- Myxedema facies with facial and periorbital edema, enlarged tongue, deepened or hoarse voice
- Fatigue
- Anemia

Protein, Fat, and Carbohydrate Metabolism

The entire cycle of synthesis, degradation, and clearance is slowed. Because of decreased lipolysis and decreased lipid metabolism, especially lipid degradation, serum cholesterol and triglyceride levels may increase. The patient with preexisting diabetes mellitus may experience decreased blood glucose levels because of decreased glycogenolysis, decreased intestinal glucose absorption, and decreased insulin degradation.

Cardiovascular Function

The hypometabolic state, coupled with decreased sensitivity to catecholamines, reduces the inotropic and chronotropic effects on the heart, resulting in decreased cardiac output. Additionally, polysaccharide infiltration can occur in the myocardium. Signs and symptoms include bradycardia, cardiomegaly, pericardial and pleural effusions, hyponatremia, decreased free water excretion, hypotension, and low-output congestive heart failure.

Central Nervous System Function

Thyroid hormone is synergized with other centrally acting hormones and neurotransmitters; this is decreased in hypothyroidism. Signs and symptoms include apathy; lethargy; depression; slowed, slurred speech; somnolence; paresthesias; hypoactive deep tendon reflexes; and coma.

Reproductive Function

Secretion and metabolism of gonadotropins and gonadal steroids is altered. Signs and symptoms include decreased libido, decreased fertility, altered menstrual patterns with or without anovulation, erectile dysfunction, and oligospermia.

Gastrointestinal Function

Decreased motility of the gastrointestinal tract may lead to constipation.

Collaborative Care Management

DIAGNOSTIC TESTS. Studies of thyroid function to diagnose hypothyroidism include the free T_4 index and serum TSH assay. Decreased levels of free T_4 and T_3 and an elevated TSH level confirm the diagnosis of a patient who has primary hyposecretion and no other disease.

Acute illness and presence of nonthyroid disease may alter levels of T_3, T_4, and TSH. Free T_4 and TSH levels may fall significantly in severe illness, a condition called *euthyroid sick syndrome.* As the illness resolves, the TSH may rise slightly as homeostasis is established. The professional nurse must be aware of these adaptive changes to illness and not be confused by the fluctuations in TSH, T_4, and T_3.

Thyroid antibody tests and fine-needle aspiration biopsy may be done to confirm the presence of chronic thyroiditis, Hashimoto's disease, or other pathologic conditions.[30] If a goiter in a hypothyroid patient shows progressive growth while the patient is receiving optimal replacement therapy, then concurrent thyroid

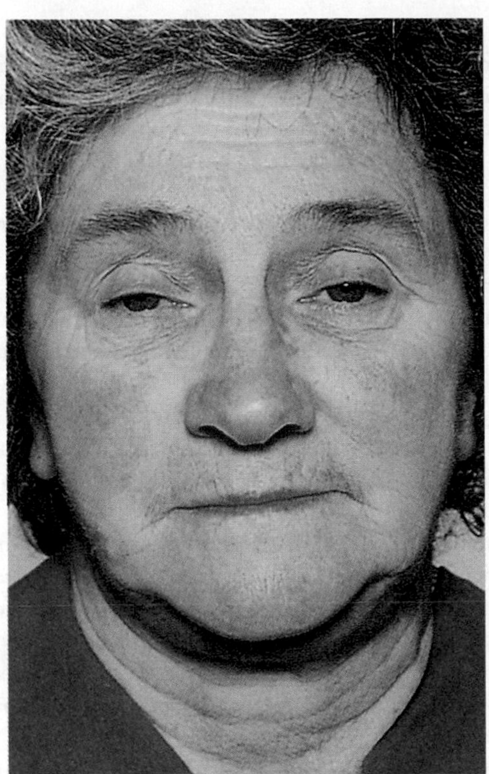

Figure 38-7 Adult with hypothyroidism.

cancer needs to be ruled out. The best way to assess change in thyroid size over time is with serial ultrasound studies.[35]

MEDICATIONS

GOITER SUPPRESSION. Apart from the unusual situations of iodine deficiency and goitrogenic drugs, most goiters are of unknown etiology, manifesting as euthyroid Hashimoto's disease, colloid nodules, or euthyroid multinodular goiters. The principle of suppression therapy is to exogenously supply thyroid hormone, thus rendering the thyroid redundant, with a decrease in TSH to the lower end of normal. This facilitates shrinkage of the goiter or at least cessation of growth. Goiter shrinkage tends to occur most readily in Hashimoto's disease. In some instances, because of the autonomous nature of the thyroid disorder, exogenous thyroid supplementation results in elevated free T_4 levels and a suppressed TSH, rendering suppression therapy impossible.

REPLACEMENT THERAPY. Standard replacement therapy for hypothyroidism is daily oral levothyroxine; the replacement dose is generally 1.6 to 1.8 mcg/kg body weight. The dosage should be titrated slowly, particularly in older individuals and those with coronary artery disease, until a normal metabolic rate is attained. The optimal dose is determined based on clinical parameters and a normal TSH and free T_4. It is important to note that the free T_4 is normalized long before the TSH, which may take more than 8 weeks.

Patient teaching should emphasize taking levothyroxine on an empty stomach to ensure consistent bioavailability. Failure to follow this guideline may be the reason for a patient suddenly requiring progressively larger doses of levothyroxine. The compounds interfering with absorption of levothyroxine include fiber, calcium, iron, and soy products.[51] Concurrent use of T_3 in conjunction with levothyroxine was thought to have some benefit based on one study. However, several subsequent studies failed to confirm a benefit of concurrent T_3 with levothyroxine even in depressed patients.[19,61,64,71] (see Research box).

Symptoms of hypothyroidism generally start to improve within a few days of replacement therapy. Complete resolution of all symptoms may take a couple of months in some patients, depending on the severity of the hypothyroidism and the rapidity of replacement to euthyroid hormone levels. The patient with hypothyroidism who remains hypothyroid either from lack of treatment or undertreatment with levothyroxine is at increased risk for dyslipidemia and cardiovascular disease.

The major side effects of therapy relate to either underreplacement or overreplacement, with resultant symptoms of either

Research

Walsh JP et al: Combined thyroxine/liothyronine treatment does not improve well-being, quality of life, or cognitive function compared to thyroxine alone: a randomized controlled trial in patients with primary hypothyroidism, *J Clin Endocrinol Metab* 88(10):4543-4550, 2003.

In the management of patients with hypothyroidism, the use of combined T_4/T_3 treatment is controversial. A few studies have reported that combination treatment improved well-being and cognitive function to a greater degree than did the traditional treatment of T_4 alone.

This double-blind study used a cohort of 110 subjects (101 women, 9 men; mean age 48 years) with primary hypothyroidism (mean duration 8 years). Subjects had been treated with a constant dose of levothyroxine (T_4) (mean daily dose 136 mcg) for at least 2 months. Subjects were randomized to a 10-week treatment period with (1) their usual dose of T_4 or (2) a T_4 dose 50 mcg lower than their usual dose in combination with 10 mcg of T_3. After this initial 10-week period, all subjects entered a treatment period during which they received their prior dose of T_4 alone. Subsequently, patients crossed over to the opposite treatment for an additional 10 weeks.

At baseline and at the end of each 10-week treatment period, subjects were examined and laboratory samples collected for TSH, free T_4, and free T_3. Additionally, patients completed three questionnaires: the Short Form 36 (assessing physical functioning, general health, vitality, social functioning, and mental health), the General Health Questionnaire-28 (measuring psychologic dysfunction), and the Thyroid Symptom Questionnaire (assessing symptoms commonly present in patients taking T_4). Subjects also completed 10 visual analog scales (VASs) regarding well-being, anxiety, and related symptoms.

Subjects in both groups achieved a euthyroid state. Combination treatment with T_4/T_3 showed no statistical improvement over T_4 treatment alone regarding (1) quality of life scores ($p<0.05$), (2) 8 out of 10 VAS assessing symptoms ($p<0.05$), (3) Thyroid Symptom Questionnaire scores ($p<0.05$), and (4) subjective satisfaction with treatments scores ($p<0.05$). However, subjects in the combined T_4/T_3 group scored worse on the General Health Questionnaire-28 and the VAS measuring anxiety and nausea ($p<0.05$) than did subjects treated with T_4 alone.

The authors concluded that combined treatment of T_4/T_3 at the doses used in this study did not result in any improvement in cognitive function, quality of life, or well-being.

hypothyroidism or hyperthyroidism. Inappropriately rapid dose titration can precipitate angina, myocardial infarction, and tachyarrhythmias (e.g., atrial fibrillation) in predisposed individuals. These sequelae can also occur with chronic overdosing of levothyroxine, leading to accelerated bone loss with reduced bone mineral density and fracture predisposition.

TREATMENTS. The patient with myxedema coma is frequently in both respiratory and cardiac failure and requires close monitoring in an intensive care unit. Manifestations are those of severe hypothyroidism with an emphasis on (1) hypothermia; (2) respiratory dysfunction related to respiratory muscle weakness (myopathy), sleep apnea, and decreased ventilatory drive in response to hypoxia and hypercapnia; (3) reduced cardiac output caused by bradycardia and decreased stroke volume (or overt congestive cardiac failure in patients with underlying cardiac disease); (4) slowed drug metabolism and clearance resulting in potential drug toxicity (e.g., digoxin toxicity); and (5) concurrent adrenal insufficiency, which may require stress doses of glucocorticoids.

Therapy for the patient with myxedema coma includes supportive care (cardiovascular, respiratory, and fluid balance support) and administration of thyroid hormone. Intubation and mechanical ventilation may be necessary for patients in respiratory failure. The hypothermic patient needs to be gradually rewarmed and additional heat loss prevented; however, rapid rewarming can cause vascular collapse. Treatment protocols vary; options for thyroid hormone therapy include T_4 and T_3. Some patients with myxedema coma may also have adrenal insufficiency; intravenous hydrocortisone in stress doses should be maintained until the serum cortisol value is greater than 20 mcg/dl or the cosyntropin test is within normal limits without exogenous glucocorticoids.

Nursing interventions include care of the comatose patient; surveillance of respiratory, cardiovascular, and fluid status; care of the patient with respiratory insufficiency; preventive care for problems of immobility; and assistance with the medical regimen.

SURGICAL MANAGEMENT. Pharmacologic therapy is the treatment of choice for patients with hypothyroidism. Surgery is indicated for large goiters producing persistent compression symptoms despite being euthyroid with the patient receiving replacement therapy. The degree of shrinkage of large goiters is generally limited with optimal thyroid hormone replacement. Patients should be informed that surgical intervention might be needed to relieve symptoms.

Subtotal thyroidectomy is indicated for (1) compression symptoms and (2) concerns about the possibility of concurrent thyroid cancer. Compression symptoms may manifest as choking sensations, dysphagia, or inspiratory stridor related to compression or deviation of the esophagus and trachea. These compression symptoms may be accentuated by asking the patient to raise his or her arms above the head. This is known as Pemberton's sign.

DIET. Adequate nutrition in the form of well-balanced meals is advocated for patients with hypothyroidism. Patients may be advised to follow a weight-reduction diet. If iodine deficiency or excessive intake of goitrogenic foods (such as cabbage) is a problem, the nurse provides pertinent dietary instructions. In severe hypothyroidism, apathy, anorexia, and self-care deficit may combine to limit food intake, and steps must be taken to achieve adequate intake. Fluid restriction and occasionally sodium modifications are necessary in severe hyponatremia.

HEALTH PROMOTION AND PREVENTION. Primary prevention of hypothyroidism focuses on the identification and treatment of dietary iodine deficiency. Dietary iodine deficiency results from living in an area with low iodine levels in the water and soil. In the United States the Great Lakes region was an area of dietary iodine deficiency, but the use of iodized salt has essentially eliminated the problem. Elsewhere in the world, however, dietary iodine deficiency is still problematic, and the World Health Organization estimates that 200 million people have goiters related to iodine deficiency.[16]

Secondary prevention of hypothyroidism focuses mainly on routine newborn screening and prompt treatment to prevent the irreversible brain damage, growth retardation, and other sequelae of hypothyroidism. The case for routinely screening older adults for hypothyroidism has significant merit. Screening of patients, especially women, with risk factors for hypothyroidism is reasonable.

Tertiary prevention of hypothyroidism focuses on ongoing iodine replacement in the iodine-deficient patient, as well as encouraging compliance with thyroid hormone replacement therapy.

Nursing Management *of the Patient with Hypothyroidism*

ASSESSMENT

Health History. Assess for:

- Changes in physical energy level and activity or mental and neurologic status
- Changes in skin, hair (head or body), nails
- Chest pain; syncope
- Changes in appetite and weight with typical nutritional intake
- Changes in bowel elimination
- Headache, muscle, or joint pain; intolerance to cold
- Changes in sexual function:
  - Women: changes in menses or libido, infertility
  - Men: changes in libido

Physical Examination. Assess for:

- Intellectual functioning; memory; speech pattern; somnolence, lethargy, or confusion
- Body weight and temperature
- Skin pigmentation, temperature, nonpitting edema
- Quality and quantity of head and body hair, thyroid examination
- Pulse rate and blood pressure
- Respiratory rate, breath sounds
- Bowel sounds
- Muscle strength, tone, and mass; range of motion; deep tendon reflexes; joint movement

NURSING DIAGNOSES, OUTCOMES, AND INTERVENTIONS

Nursing Diagnosis: Activity Intolerance

OUTCOMES. A common example of an expected outcome for the patient with a diagnosis of *activity intolerance* is:
Patient will:

- Show a gradual increase in activity tolerance over 2 to 3 months.

NURSING INTERVENTIONS. Nursing interventions for the patient with hypothyroidism vary greatly, depending on the severity of disease. The hypothyroid state is reversed slowly, requiring 2 to 3 months for the patient to return to his or her baseline health status. Increasing activities gradually promotes activity to the level of patient tolerance. The nurse monitors cardiovascular response to new activities. If the patient complains of chest pain or develops an unacceptable heart rate, the activity is stopped and then resumed at a slower rate. Blood pressure, pulse, and respirations should be monitored before, during, and after each new activity.

RELATED NIC INTERVENTION. Energy Management

Nursing Diagnosis: Disturbed Body Image

OUTCOMES. Common examples of expected outcomes for the patient with a diagnosis of *disturbed body image* are:
Patient will:

- Relate body image changes to hypothyroidism and will verbalize that most changes are reversible.
- Understand that sexual function will increase as thyroid status returns to normal.

NURSING INTERVENTIONS. The nurse provides information that helps the patient and significant others understand the relationship of body changes to hypothyroidism. This includes information about reversible body changes and the relationship between the sexual problems and hypothyroidism.

RELATED NIC INTERVENTIONS. Body Image Enhancement, Self-Esteem Enhancement

Nursing Diagnosis: Constipation

OUTCOMES. A common example of expected outcomes for the patient with a diagnosis of *constipation* is:
Patient will:

- Attain and maintain a bowel pattern that was typical before onset of illness.

NURSING INTERVENTIONS. The nurse determines the patient's normal pattern of bowel function and monitors current bowel elimination. The nurse encourages adequate fluid intake and a diet high in fiber, along with ambulation and adequate exercise to promote peristalsis and bowel motility. Stool softeners may be prescribed as needed.

RELATED NIC INTERVENTIONS. Constipation/Impaction Management, Fluid Monitoring, Nutrition Management

Nursing Diagnosis: Risk for Impaired Skin Integrity

OUTCOMES. A common example of expected outcomes for the patient with a diagnosis of *risk for impaired skin integrity* is:
Patient will:

- Have intact skin.

NURSING INTERVENTIONS. The nurse assesses the skin at least daily for areas of redness and pressure. Emollients are applied daily and after bathing. The number of baths is limited to avoid overdrying the skin. Tepid water is used because hot water depletes skin of moisture, especially in older patients. Superfatted soaps are used and the skin patted dry to avoid friction.

Preventive care measures such as use of sheepskin pads, soft sheets, and padding of bony prominences should be instituted as indicated. If the patient is unable to turn, the nurse helps him or her turn every 2 hours. Ambulation is encouraged when possible. Fluid intake is increased unless contraindicated by cardiac or renal disease to increase moisture in the skin. Use of a humidifier in the home increases moisture in the air and thus in the skin. A diet with adequate protein, carbohydrates, and vitamins is essential to promote optimal nutritional status.

RELATED NIC INTERVENTIONS. Pressure Management, Pressure Ulcer Prevention, Skin Surveillance

Patient/Family Teaching. Patient and family teaching is an important part of nursing care for the patient with hypothyroidism (see Patient/Family Teaching box).

EVALUATION

To evaluate the effectiveness of nursing interventions, compare patient behaviors with those stated in the expected patient outcomes.

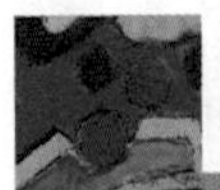

PATIENT/FAMILY TEACHING
The Patient With Hypothyroidism

The nurse teaches the patient and family or significant others how to continue the care plan, with an emphasis on compliance with medications and follow-up care. The teaching plan includes:

- Nature of the disorder, diagnostic tests, and treatment; need for lifelong thyroid hormone replacement therapy
- Medications: dosage, method of administration (on an empty stomach; taking substances that may inhibit levothyroxine absorption at a different time), and side effects of hypothyroidism and hyperthyroidism
- Self-monitoring of vital signs, weight, skin integrity, and bowel function
- Measures to prevent skin breakdown and constipation
- Need for periods of rest alternating with activity
- Need for continued follow-up care

The patient with a large goiter may need help with altered body image related to disfigurement. The goiter may be concealed by the use of scarves and high-collared shirts. An open and trusting relationship is necessary so the patient can share feelings and concerns.

RELATED NOC OUTCOMES. Body Image, Bowel Elimination, Energy Conservation, Hydration, Nutritional Status: Food & Fluid Intake, Risk Control, Tissue Integrity: Skin & Mucous Membranes

GERONTOLOGIC CONSIDERATIONS

The nurse assesses older adult patients for decreased alertness, decreased mobility, or increased susceptibility to cold, which are signs and symptoms more typically found with hypothyroidism in older persons. The nurse also assesses for signs of myxedema, as seen with untreated hypothyroidism, and for signs of drug toxicity because of decreased metabolic activity.

The nurse needs to help older patients plan a way to remember to take replacement therapy appropriately—first thing in the morning and on an empty stomach. The nurse teaches them to monitor for drug side effects and to report signs of angina or congestive heart failure, which may be provoked by initial doses of thyroid hormone replacement. Measures to prevent constipation, which often occurs with hypothyroidism and especially in older persons, also need to be promoted.

Thyroid Cancer

Etiology and Epidemiology. Thyroid cancer is less prevalent than other forms of cancer and generally has a much better prognosis. Papillary thyroid cancer is the most common type and is linked to prior radiation exposure to the head and neck. Some cancers may be familial (e.g., medullary thyroid cancer) and are associated with other endocrine neoplasms (multiple endocrine neoplasia [MEN]). Most thyroid cancers arise in a solitary nodule; the risk of a solitary nodule being malignant is greater in younger patients and in men.

Pathophysiology. Five types of primary thyroid cancer can occur, the majority arising from thyroid follicular epithelium (Table 38-4).[16] Papillary thyroid cancer is generally diagnosed on the basis of a fine-needle aspiration biopsy where characteristic papillary structures can be seen. A follicular neoplasm, on the other hand, may be hard to classify as benign or malignant on the basis of fine-needle aspiration alone, and further histologic analysis is needed for definitive diagnosis. Follicular cancers may spread via the bloodstream to the bone, lung, or liver. Malignant follicular and papillary lesions may produce some thyroid hormone, but generally not enough to cause hyperthyroidism. Medullary cancer of the thyroid arises in the parafollicular (or C) cells and may spread early to cervical nodes and metastasize to the liver, lungs, or bone. Anaplastic thyroid cancer and thyroid lymphomas are uncommon.

Collaborative Care Management

DIAGNOSTIC TESTS. Thyroid nodules may be discovered by the patient or on routine examination. Additionally, nodules may be discovered during diagnostic imaging for other diseases (e.g., MRI of the cervical spine for cervical disc disease or trauma). A thorough history should be carried out, focusing on any radiation exposure to the head or neck, compression symptoms (e.g., dysphagia), or symptoms of hypothyroidism or hyperthyroidism. Physical examination should document the size of the nodule, whether any additional nodules are palpable, and any lymphadenopathy.

Thyroid function is assessed via a TSH assay to confirm a euthyroid state. A suppressed TSH suggests a benign hyperfunctioning nodule. A thyroid ultrasound is done to identify anatomy and any lesions. If a solitary nodule is hyperfunctioning, the contralateral lobe shows suppression and shrinkage. Ultrasonography cannot definitively classify nodules as being benign or malignant; fine-needle aspiration is required. Ultrasound may be helpful for needle guidance to ensure accurate needle placement in fine-needle aspiration of smaller thyroid nodules. Ultrasonography may readily differentiate a solid from a cystic lesion; after aspiration of a cystic lesion ultrasonography can assist with needle guidance for fine-needle aspiration of the cyst wall. Cystic lesions containing clear fluid on aspiration are generally benign; those with a bloody aspirate may be malignant.

Radionuclide of malignant thyroid nodules shows absence of uptake of the RAI isotope—the so-called cold nodule; however, only approximately 20% of cold nodules are malignant. A hyperfunctioning, or hot, nodule on radionuclide scanning demonstrates uptake of the RAI in the nodule with suppression of the uptake in the rest of the gland. Hot nodules are always benign. Fine-needle aspiration of the thyroid consists of insertion of a 22-gauge needle, with or without ultrasound guidance, into the nodule. The patient is generally placed in the supine position with the neck extended. Usually several needle insertions into the nodule are made to ensure that a representative and adequate sample is obtained and submitted to the pathologist for cytologic evaluation. Most patients describe the discomfort as comparable to that of a routine phlebotomy, and the nurse should reassure the patient.

Lesions are classified as (1) diagnostic or highly suspicious for malignancy, (2) indeterminate, or (3) benign. Lesions that are diagnostic or highly suspicious for malignancy must be removed. Indeterminate lesions are generally removed.[52,63] Occasionally physicians elect to monitor indeterminate lesions while treating them with exogenous thyroid hormone suppression therapy. A thyroid nodule that shrinks on serial ultrasound examinations is usually benign. A thyroid nodule that expands while the patient is taking suppression therapy is highly suspicious of malignancy. Repeat fine-needle aspiration may be carried out to confirm the diagnosis. Sudden expansion of a benign thyroid nodule can occur as a result of hemorrhage into the nodule. Most benign nodules are simple colloid nodules and do not need to be removed unless causing compressive symptoms.

TREATMENTS. The lowest risk of recurrence of thyroid cancer (papillary and follicular) results from total thyroidectomy with ^{131}I ablation of any thyroid remnants. The dosage of ^{131}I is much higher than that used to treat hyperthyroidism. After such ablation therapy, the patient must be placed in isolation in the hospital, usually in a corner room. All urine and feces must be collected and disposed of in a radiation sewage disposal system. The patient must use disposable plates, cups, and utensils. The patient is not allowed visitors, and contact with health care professionals is strictly minimized. The isolation must continue until the total-body ^{131}I burden falls to less than 30 mCi as measured by a Geiger counter. In the patient with normal renal function, this ordinarily is achieved within 3 days. For the next several days the patient needs to follow the radiation safety instructions for the patient with hyperthyroidism undergoing ^{131}I therapy.[43] However, outpatient treatment with large doses of ^{131}I is done at some centers.

Thyroid hormone replacement with levothyroxine is started the day after the ^{131}I treatment. The treatment goal is a TSH level slightly below the lower limits of the reference range. This will take several weeks to achieve. T_4 and TSH levels are monitored 6 to 12 weeks after surgery. Serum thyroglobulin is measured and monitored as a marker of residual autonomously functioning thyroid tissue. A measurable serum thyroglobulin may indicate neoplastic tissue either in the thyroid bed or elsewhere. For further evaluation, an RAI body scan is done in one of two ways. The conventional way calls for withdrawal of thyroid hormone replacement and a low iodine diet for several weeks until the TSH becomes frankly elevated. An elevated TSH is needed to obtain RAI uptake into any remnant of neoplastic thyroid tissue. Patients naturally complain of severe symptoms of hypothyroidism throughout this whole process. The alternative approach is to use recombinant TSH injections (Thyrogen) to stimulate thyroglobulin levels and/or uptake of RAI. This approach is much more comfortable for the patient; however, the RAI scan yield may be somewhat less than with the conventional approach.

If the RAI scans prove positive, repeat ablative doses of ^{131}I may be administered, or if the recurrence is localized to the neck, repeat surgical removal may be performed. Generally, after the patient has had two consecutive negative scans, most physicians monitor either basal or thyrogen-stimulated thyroglobulin levels. Monitoring basal serum thyroglobulin levels may be inadequate, since patients who have undetectable basal serum thyroglobulin levels on suppression therapy may have local tumor recurrence or distant metastases.[5,43,53]

Patients with lymphoma of the thyroid are rarely treated with surgery. Radiotherapy is the treatment of choice; compressive symptoms usually respond rapidly to treatment.

SURGICAL MANAGEMENT. Total thyroidectomy is the treatment of choice for patients with bilateral disease, large unilateral tumors, papillary tumors, or a history of neck radiation. Advantages of total thyroidectomy include the ability to treat recurrences or metastases outside the thyroid with RAI. Performing a lobectomy alone may result in a 5% to 10% rate of recurrence in the opposite thyroid lobe, a high recurrence rate, and a high incidence of subsequent pulmonary metastases.[43] Serum thyroglobulin is used to monitor therapy after surgery. Neck dissection is indicated for patients with palpable metastases in cervical nodes. Radioablation with ^{131}I of the remaining thyroid tissue is performed 1 month after surgery while the patient is hypothyroid.

Treatment for the patient with medullary cancer of the thyroid is total thyroidectomy with removal of the lymph nodes in the center of the neck. The prognosis for anaplastic thyroid cancer is extremely poor. Invasion of local structures may make curative surgical resection impossible; radiation or chemotherapy may be offered as palliation.

Lifelong suppression therapy with levothyroxine follows surgery for any thyroid cancer. Dosages should be high enough to suppress serum TSH levels. Monitoring of T_4 and TSH levels should be done 6 to 12 weeks after surgery.

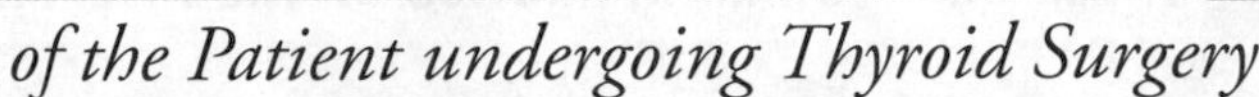

Nursing Management

of the Patient undergoing Thyroid Surgery

Care of the patient with a thyroid nodule first focuses on helping the patient through the diagnostic process. Thyroid nodules occur frequently, and most are not malignant. No single diagnostic test is completely reliable. Depending on patient characteristics and physician philosophy, various tests may be performed. The nurse prepares the patient for each test, focusing particularly on education.

PREOPERATIVE CARE

The patient having thyroid surgery needs care focused on producing and maintaining a euthyroid state. The patient with a diagnosis of cancer may have difficulty coping. The nurse provides patient teaching regarding general perioperative care (see Unit 3) on an outpatient basis. The nurse also teaches the patient to avoid straining the suture line by placing both hands behind the neck for support when coughing or moving the head and neck.

POSTOPERATIVE CARE

Immediate postoperative interventions are listed in the Guidelines for Safe Practice box, p. 1090. In addition to routine monitoring, the nurse checks the patient for major complications that can occur after thyroid surgery: recurrent laryngeal nerve injury, hemorrhage, transient hypocalcemia, and respiratory obstruction. Signs of these complications are reported immediately to the health care team.

Sore throat or hoarseness after surgery may be related to intubation during surgery; such hoarseness should clear gradually. If hoarseness persists or worsens, it is reported to the surgeon. Hoarseness may be a first sign of laryngeal nerve damage, which can result in vocal cord spasm and respiratory distress. Unilateral nerve injury usually causes hoarseness; bilateral injury may result in airway obstruction. An emergency tracheostomy may be necessary, and equipment for this should be available at the patient's bedside.

The nurse monitors the patient for hemorrhage for the first 12 to 24 hours after surgery. Hemorrhage can result in incisional bleeding or in compression of the trachea or surrounding tissue. If hemorrhage causes compression, the patient exhibits signs of respiratory distress. In such cases, the nurse loosens the dressing. If this does not relieve the respiratory distress, the surgeon may need to remove surgical clips or sutures. The patient may have to be taken back to surgery for ligation of the leaking blood vessels and wound closure.

Although the risk is minimal, the parathyroid glands can be injured during surgery, such that ischemia or inflammation blocks the normal release of parathyroid hormone (PTH). If the level of PTH drops, symptoms of hypocalcemia can occur. If not treated promptly, hypocalcemia can result in tetany with contraction of the glottis and respiratory obstruction, leading to death. Tetany typically appears 24 to 48 hours after surgery. Treatment for hypocalcemia is calcium carbonate or calcium gluconate given intravenously. Oral calcium is then necessary until normal parathyroid function returns. Permanent hypoparathyroidism is uncommon after total thyroidectomy.

The nurse must know that respiratory obstruction can occur from (1) recurrent laryngeal nerve damage causing vocal cord spasms that close off the larynx, (2) tracheal compression from hemorrhage, (3) tissue swelling or (4) tetany. The nurse should be prepared to assist in the management of all these problems.

TABLE 38-4 CHARACTERISTICS OF THE FIVE TYPES OF THYROID CANCER

	Cancers of Follicular Epithelium				Cancer of Parafollicular Tissue
Characteristics	**Papillary**	**Follicular**	**Anaplastic**	**Thyroid Lymphoma**	**Medullary**
Incidence of all thyroid cancers	65%	20%	5%	5%	5%
Age	Young persons	After 40 yr	After 60 yr	After 40 yr	After 50 yr
Female/male ratio	2-3:1	2-3:1	F > M	F > M	F = M
Metastasis	By intraglandular lymphatics and regional lymphadenopathy; slow-growing tumor	By blood vessels to distant sites (bone, lung, liver); occurs early	By direct invasion to adjacent structures; highly malignant	By lymphatic system; gland fixed to other structures	By intraglandular lymphatics and blood vessels
Prognosis	Good; rarely causes death in young persons if occult or intrathyroidal	Good if minimally invasive lesion	Prognosis varies with cell type; for giant cell, very poor (< 6 mo from diagnosis); for small cell, better (5-yr survival rate of 20%-50%)	Good	Moderate; 10-yr survival estimated at 60%; worst prognosis in multiple endocrine neoplasia (MEN), type III
Symptoms	Asymptomatic	Nodule (may have been present for years)	Hoarseness, inspiratory stridor, pain, dysphagia (signs of invasion of adjacent areas)	May have long history of previous goiter; rapid enlargement of goiter, hoarseness, dysphagia, pressure sensation, dyspnea, some pain	Tumors potentially producing adrenocorticotropic hormone resulting in Cushing's syndrome; serotonin, prostaglandins, and other hormones possibly produced, resulting in flushing and diarrhea
Tumor	Occult (< 1.5 cm in diameter), intrathyroidal (> 1.5 cm in diameter but does not extend	Well differentiated to poorly differentiated; cyst formation and calcification possible	Two cell forms: giant cell and small cell	Usually of nodular histiocytic form	Tumors varied from 1-2 mm in diameter to masses several centimeters in diameter

TABLE 38-4 CHARACTERISTICS OF THE FIVE TYPES OF THYROID CANCER—CONT'D

	Cancers of Follicular Epithelium				Cancer of Parafollicular Tissue
Characteristics	**Papillary**	**Follicular**	**Anaplastic**	**Thyroid Lymphoma**	**Medullary**
Tumor—cont'd	through thyroid capsule), and extrathyroidal (extends through thyroid capsule); well differentiated; psammoma body found in 40% of tumors and virtually diagnostic of malignant nature; tumors appearing as "cold" spots on nuclear thyroid scan				
Other	Growth partially dependent on thyroid-stimulating hormone; thyroid hormone can cause regression of metastatic lesions; ^{131}I sometimes used for nonresectable lesions; may have history of prior radiation therapy to head and neck for other diseases	Suppressive thyroid therapy possibly causing regression of metastatic lesions; radiation therapy with ^{131}I sometimes used when vascular invasion or metastasis present	External beam radiation sometimes used	Strong association with Hashimoto's thyroiditis; may have lymphoma at other sites	80% of cases sporadic Occurs as a familial form as part of MEN type II or III; in MEN II, medullary thyroid carcinoma, pheochromocytomas, and hyperparathyroidism found; in MEN III, medullary thyroid carcinoma, pheochromocytomas, mucosal neuromas, and marfanoid habitus found; skeletal abnormalities; also occurs as a non-MEN familial form

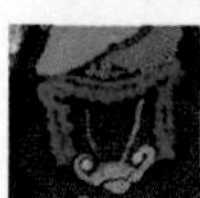

GUIDELINES FOR SAFE PRACTICE *Care of the Patient After Thyroid Surgery*

- Monitor for and report signs of complications:
  —Laryngeal nerve damage; hoarseness, weak voice
  —Hemorrhage or tissue swelling
    —Bleeding on dressing: check back of dressing by slipping hand gently under neck and shoulders
    —Choking sensation
    —Difficulty in coughing or swallowing
    —Sensation of dressing being too tight even after it is loosened
  —Hypocalcemia (tetany)
    —Early signs: tingling around mouth or of toes and fingers, decreasing serum calcium levels
    —Later signs: positive Chvostek's and Trousseau's signs (see Chapter 17), grand mal seizures
  —Respiratory distress associated with any of signs just listed
- Provide emergency care:
  —Keep emergency supplies readily available:
    —Tracheostomy set (for laryngeal nerve damage), oxygen and suction equipment, suture removal set (for respiratory obstruction from hemorrhage)
    —Intravenous calcium gluconate or calcium chloride (for tetany)
  —For acute respiratory distress:
    —Call for immediate medical help.
    —Raise head of bed.
    —Loosen dressing over incision.
    —Give calcium as ordered, if signs and symptoms of tetany are present.
    —If loosening the dressing does not relieve symptoms of respiratory distress and if medical help is not readily available, remove clips or sutures as instructed.
- Provide comfort:
  —Avoid tension on suture lines; encourage patient to support head when turning by placing both hands behind neck.
  —Give prescribed analgesics as necessary.
- Maintain nutritional status:
  —Start soft foods as soon as tolerated (only fluids may be tolerated initially).
  —Encourage a high-carbohydrate, high-protein diet.
- Teach patient:
  —Range-of-motion exercises for neck when suture line is healed to prevent permanent limitations
  —Need for lifelong thyroid hormone replacement therapy after a total thyroidectomy
  —Any special care measures related to the underlying disease
  —Need for follow-up care

The patient who has undergone a total thyroidectomy must immediately initiate l-thyroxine replacement therapy. Dosage should be calculated as per the guidelines for the patient with hypothyroidism based on actual body weight (see Hyposecretion: Hypothyroidism).

GERONTOLOGIC CONSIDERATIONS

Thyroid nodules have been identified in 5% of persons older than age 60 years, and 90% of these nodules are found to be benign. The older person needs special consideration when undergoing surgical intervention (see Unit 3).

Parathyroid Gland Disorders

Hypersecretion: Hyperparathyroidism

Hyperparathyroidism refers to elevated PTH levels caused by excessive release of PTH from the parathyroid glands. Primary hyperparathyroidism and hypercalcemia of malignancy are the most common causes of elevated serum calcium, accounting for approximately 90% of cases. Secondary hyperparathyroidism results from malabsorption syndrome or a defect in mineral homeostasis, such as renal failure, with a resultant increase in PTH secretion from the parathyroid glands. The serum calcium level is not elevated in secondary hyperparathyroidism.

Primary Hyperparathyroidism

Etiology and Epidemiology. The most frequent cause of primary hyperparathyroidism is a solitary adenoma (85%) involving one of the four parathyroid glands. The remaining 15% of patients usually have hyperparathyroidism of all four glands or, in rare instances, primary parathyroid cancer.

It is postulated that the "set point" for negative feedback on PTH secretion by ambient ionized calcium levels is elevated. In essence, this means that PTH secretion is not "switched off" in the adenoma or hyperplastic cells when serum calcium levels are at the upper limit of normal. Parathyroid adenomas are thought to represent clonal expression of mutant cells, in turn related to loss of function of tumor suppressor genes.[11]

Primary hyperparathyroidism may also be part of a MEN syndrome. The type I syndrome, or MEN I, consists of pituitary adenoma, pancreatic islet cell tumor, and primary hyperparathyroidism. The type II syndrome, or MEN IIA, consists of pheochromocytoma, medullary thyroid cancer, and primary hyperparathyroidism. An appropriate workup for these entities is prompted by family history, relevant symptomatology, and physical findings.

The incidence of primary hyperparathyroidism is approximately 1 in 500 to 1000 individuals, with women being affected more often than men by 3:1. The majority of patients are postmenopausal, in the sixth decade of life, and asymptomatic. They are frequently incidentally diagnosed via a routine serum chemistry panel that includes measurement of calcium levels. Some patients may be diagnosed after a workup for suspected secondary causes of osteoporosis or osteopenia.[12-14]

Pathophysiology. Elevation in PTH levels raises serum calcium via several mechanisms: (1) increased bone resorption; (2) enhanced activation of vitamin D to 1,25-hydroxycholecalciferol, with resultant enhanced calcium resorption from the gastrointestinal tract; and (3) enhanced renal tubular resorption of calcium from the glomerular filtrate.

Box 38-9 Hypersecretion of Parathyroid Hormone: Pathophysiologic Alterations and Clinical Manifestations

- Increase in calcium resorption from bone resulting in hypercalcemia, decreased bone mass, bone cysts, and fractures that can be characterized by bone pain and arthralgias
- Alteration in urinary calcium excretion during course of the disease
- Early: hypocalciuria
- Later: hypercalciuria with polyuria, polydipsia, nephrolithiasis, and kidney failure
- Decreased renal bicarbonate and phosphate resorption
- Hyperchloremic acidosis
- Increased gastrin secretion causing peptic ulcer disease
- Increased renal activation of vitamin D producing calcitriol (1,25-dihydroxycholecalciferol), increasing gastrointestinal calcium absorption, thereby adding to the hypercalcemia
- Depression of nerve and muscle activity from hypercalcemia
- Cardiac muscle signs and symptoms, including hypertension and electrocardiographic changes such as shortened Q-T intervals and dysrhythmias
- Neuromuscular signs and symptoms, including impaired mentation, apathy, lethargy, somnolence, hypoactive deep tendon reflexes, fasciculation of the tongue, muscle weakness, and myalgias (lower limbs more than upper limbs)
- Gastrointestinal signs and symptoms, including anorexia, nausea, vomiting, and constipation
- Hypercalcemia causing pancreatitis

In addition, PTH enhances the renal excretion of phosphate with resultant decrease in the serum phosphate level. Primary hyperparathyroidism is characterized by hypercalcemia with low to subnormal serum phosphate. Excess bone resorption results in declining bone mass, especially in cortical bone. This is best assessed with bone density measurements in the forearm. Although rare, cysts may form in the bone in severe cases of hyperparathyroidism, giving rise to osteitis fibrosa cystica.

Most patients with mild hyperparathyroidism are asymptomatic. In contrast, patients with more advanced disease are seen with renal calculi; bone pain; and vague, generalized arthralgias (Box 38-9).

Collaborative Care Management

DIAGNOSTIC TESTS. The initial diagnostic tests for primary hyperparathyroidism are serum calcium, phosphorus, and PTH levels. Various PTH assays are available, including C-terminal, N-terminal, midmolecule, and intact PTH. The most reliable and clinically useful assay is the intact PTH assay. The combination of an elevated serum calcium, low normal to subnormal serum phosphate, and elevated intact PTH level generally confirms the diagnosis (see Chapter 37).

Results of tests indicative of primary hyperparathyroidism include elevated serum calcium, decreased serum phosphate, and elevated PTH levels; elevated 24-hour urinary calcium excretion; and reduced bone mineral density and renal calculi on radiographic examination.

When the results do not meet these criteria, an alternative explanation for hypercalcemia must be sought (Box 38-10). Malignancy is the most common alternative explanation for hypercalcemia when primary hyperparathyroidism is not present. In general, patients with hypercalcemia of malignancy usually have obvious features of malignancy such as cachexia and weight loss; many have a previously diagnosed malignancy. Malignant cells can produce a PTH-like compound, parathyroid hormone–related protein, which can bind to and stimulate PTH receptors with resultant hypercalcemia. This so-called humoral hypercalcemia of malignancy is usually seen in patients with a large tumor burden, and patients generally have a poor prognosis related to the underlying malignancy.

MEDICATIONS AND TREATMENTS. Acute medical intervention to lower serum calcium is reserved for patients who are symptomatic from the hypercalcemia (anorexia, nausea, vomiting) and generally have serum calcium levels greater than 13 mg/dl. Long-term medical management is rarely undertaken except when patients are poor surgical candidates.

The immediate treatment is to correct any dehydration and promote fluid intake of at least 2 L/day unless contraindicated. Activity is encouraged to promote resorption of calcium by the bone. Thiazide diuretics promote renal calcium retention and are contraindicated in this setting. Loop diuretics such as furosemide reduce renal calcium resorption, but should be used cautiously because of the long-term risk of worsening bone disease. If given to a patient with dehydration, furosemide may exacerbate prerenal kidney failure.

Diuresis results in significant lowering of serum calcium and symptomatic patient improvement. Effects are temporary and cease when treatment is discontinued. Bisphosphonates (intravenous pamidronate or oral alendronate) have been used to control the hypercalcemia of primary hyperparathyroidism. Effects are also transient. Oral and intravenous phosphate is seldom used because of concerns about ectopic calcifications in soft tissues. Phosphate can interfere with the absorption of calcium, renal hydroxylation of vitamin D, and bone resorption.

Patients who are not surgical candidates are checked regularly to monitor disease progress. The nurse evaluates the patient's serum calcium and electrolytes, albumin, creatinine, and alkaline

Box 38-10 Causes of Hypercalcemia (Other Than Hyperparathyroidism)

- Malignancy
- Leukemia, lymphoma, multiple myeloma
- Vitamin D intoxication
- Granulomatous diseases (sarcoidosis)
- Other endocrine disorders: thyrotoxicosis, adrenal insufficiency
- Milk-alkali syndrome
- Immobilization
- Medications (thiazides, lithium, aminophylline, gonadal steroids)

phosphatase levels at regular intervals. Bone densitometry and renal ultrasound are done every 1 to 2 years.[14]

DIET. Dietary calcium intake for the patient with hyperparathyroidism should be moderate, with high intake being clearly undesirable. Low calcium intake may also be undesirable, since this could further stimulate PTH secretion and exacerbate bone disease.

The patient with significant hypercalcemia that is being managed medically needs careful monitoring to ensure adequate hydration, normal electrolytes, normal blood urea nitrogen and serum creatinine, and normal serum phosphorus with optimal control of the serum calcium. Patients need a fluid intake of at least 2 L/day, assuming the absence of limiting cardiac or renal processes, and must further increase their fluid intake when outside temperatures are high because of increased insensible fluid losses via sweat.

SURGICAL MANAGEMENT. Surgery is the definitive therapy for primary hyperparathyroidism and is usually curative. Surgical intervention prevents progression of preexisting complications of the disease (renal calculi, overt bone disease, fracture, life-threatening hypercalcemia) and prevents development of complications in high-risk patients. High risk is defined as[14]:

- Serum calcium more than 1 mg/dl above the upper limit of normal
- Age greater than 50 years
- Marked hypercalciuria (more than 400 mg/24 hr)
- Creatinine clearance reduced by more than 30% compared with age-matched individuals
- Bone mineral density at the distal radius more than 2.5 standard deviations below peak bone mass (a T-score of less than −2.5)
- Patients in whom medical surveillance is not desirable or possible

In most cases the procedure is removal of a solitary adenoma. In the case of four-gland hyperplasia, the approach is to remove three and a half glands, leaving the half-gland remnant in the neck or autotransplanting it in the nondominant forearm. The half-gland is left to prevent permanent hypoparathyroidism. Operative success can be readily confirmed by intraoperative PTH assay; results are available within 15 minutes. This intraoperative assay has assisted in reducing the need for repeat surgery for hyperparathyroidism.[60]

In some centers parathyroidectomy is performed as an ambulatory procedure with local anesthesia, and results are comparable to those with the patient under general anesthesia. Minimally invasive surgery with or without perioperative radioisotope localization of abnormal parathyroid tissue is being carried out in several centers. Persons with parathyroid hyperplasia, multiglandular disease, and abnormal neck anatomy are generally not suited for the minimally invasive approach.

PREOPERATIVE LOCALIZATION TESTING. In the patient with no prior neck surgery, an experienced parathyroid surgeon finds the abnormal parathyroid gland(s) in more than 90% of instances without any prior localization procedure. In the patient who has had prior neck surgery with resultant distortion of anatomic landmarks, however, most physicians support the use of preoperative localization to reduce the length of surgery and increase operative success. Several preoperative localization tests have been used, including ultrasonography, CT, MRI, and radioisotope (technetium-sestamibi) scintigraphy. This latter dual-isotopic method is currently the preferred method in clinical practice. It is not uncommon for studies to be falsely positive, and two different studies are frequently ordered to increase confidence in the localization.

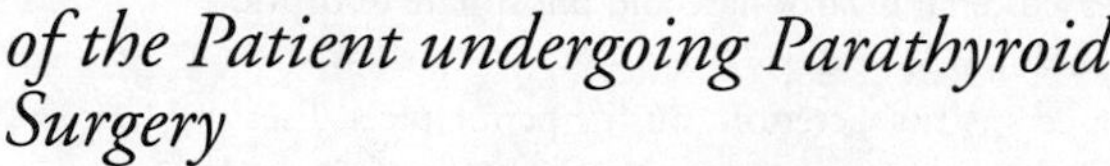

Nursing Management

of the Patient undergoing Parathyroid Surgery

PREOPERATIVE CARE

Routine preoperative assessment and teaching are discussed in Chapter 13. The patient having parathyroid surgery requires explanations regarding the pathophysiology of hyperparathyroidism and hypercalcemia. If renal damage has occurred, some changes may not be reversible. The family should be involved, if possible, particularly if mental status changes are present. The nurse should assess the home environment and availability of caregivers after surgery.

Patients with primary hyperparathyroidism have an increased risk of fall injuries as a result of musculoskeletal weakness or altered mental status. The patient with altered mental status should be placed in an environment where he or she can be observed closely; nursing interventions to promote safety and increase orientation are important. Patients with weakness need assistance for changing positions and walking and should wear nonskid slippers. The room should be free of unnecessary equipment. A gradual increase in activity and the incorporation of isometric exercise may improve endurance.

Hypercalcemia associated with primary hyperparathyroidism presents a risk for decreased cardiac functioning. The nurse monitors the patient's vital signs every 2 to 4 hours and instructs the patient to report any palpitations or vertigo. If cardiac dysfunction occurs, the patient may need continuous cardiac monitoring. The patient treated with digitalis therapy must be monitored closely for digitalis toxicity because the myocardium is unusually sensitive to digitalis in the presence of hypercalcemia; the dosage of digitalis may need to be decreased.

If the patient is hospitalized before surgery, increasing fluid intake before imposing "nothing by mouth" restrictions is important. Increasing the fluid intake decreases the urinary mineral concentration and helps prevent formation of renal calculi. A fluid intake of at least 2 L/day should be the goal unless contraindicated. The nurse monitors continually for renal calculi, straining the urine through a gauze mesh to collect any small calculi that pass (see Chapter 35). Intake and output are measured and the patient is observed for flank pain, hematuria, and nausea and vomiting. The patient is advised to avoid foods high in calcium (Box 38-11) to limit hypercalcemia.

POSTOPERATIVE CARE

Postoperative care requirements specific to parathyroid surgery are detailed in the Guidelines for Safe Practice box, p. 1094. Potential physiologic complications include hemorrhage, hypocalcemia, and

Box 38-11 Foods High in Calcium

Almonds	332 mg/1 cup
Blackstrap molasses	137 mg/1 tbsp
Brazil nuts	260 mg/1 cup
Broccoli spears	132 mg/1 cup
Cabbage (cooked)	220 mg/1 cup
Canned mackerel	221 mg/3 oz
Cheese (blue cheese, cheddar, American)	About 100-150 mg/1 oz
Collard greens (cooked)	289 mg/1 cup
Custard	280 mg/1 cup
Dandelion greens (cooked)	252 mg/1 cup
Egg	27 mg/1 egg
Green beans	80 mg/1 cup
Ice cream	175 mg/1 cup
Ice milk	292 mg/1 cup
Kale (cooked)	147 mg/1 cup
Lima beans	75 mg/1 cup
Macaroni (enriched) and cheese, baked	398 mg/1 cup
Milk (whole, 2%, skim, buttermilk)	290 mg/1 cup
Mustard greens (cooked)	193 mg/1 cup
Oranges	50 mg/1 orange
Oysters	226 mg/1 cup
Peanut halves	107 mg/1 cup
Pizza (cheese)	107 mg/1 slice
Raisins	124 mg/1 cup
Rhubarb (cooked)	212 mg/1 cup
Salmon, canned	167 mg/3 oz
Sardines	372 mg/3 oz
Spinach (drained solids)	212 mg/1 cup
Turnip greens (cooked)	250 mg/1 cup
White sauce, medium	305 mg/1 cup
Yogurt	295 mg/1 cup

airway obstruction. The nurse routinely monitors the patient's respiratory, cardiovascular, neurologic, and fluid volume status. A tracheostomy set should be at the patient's bedside for emergency use. The serum calcium level decreases within 24 hours, and the patient is monitored for tetany. Parathyroid function usually returns to normal within 5 to 7 days after a partial parathyroidectomy because the remaining tissue resumes normal functioning.

If mild hypocalcemia occurs, oral calcium is given. Severe hypocalcemia can occur if there has been extensive decrease in bone mass. As the PTH level declines, the calcium-deficient bones extract larger-than-normal quantities of calcium from the extracellular fluids—the "hungry bone syndrome." For patients with severe hypocalcemia, calcium chloride or calcium gluconate is given intravenously. These calcium preparations should be readily available for immediate administration if necessary. If permanent hypoparathyroidism results because the remaining tissue does not resume normal secretion or because a total parathyroidectomy is done, the patient will need continued treatment.

Indications for critical care management for the patient with hyperparathyroidism are similar to those for the patient recovering from thyroid surgery. Intensive care monitoring and nursing are needed if complications develop, such as hemorrhage, respiratory distress, or significant electrolyte imbalance.

Although rare, complications of parathyroid resection include vocal cord spasm, hemorrhage, tracheal obstruction, and laryngeal stridor. Chronic complications include hoarseness from recurrent laryngeal nerve damage and permanent hypoparathyroidism.

After surgery the patient usually has adequate parathyroid tissue to maintain calcium and phosphorus metabolism. The nurse monitors the patient for development of hypocalcemia. If the remaining parathyroid gland or glands are too small or nonfunctioning, some of the tissue removed can be implanted into the forearm. The excised gland must be cryopreserved at the time of surgery to allow reimplantation.

Secondary and Tertiary Hyperparathyroidism

Etiology and Pathophysiology. Failure to absorb adequate amounts of calcium and vitamin D from the gastrointestinal tract, failure to activate vitamin D in the liver or the kidney, and excessive catabolism of vitamin D result in downward drift in serum calcium. To maintain normal serum calcium, a compensatory increase in PTH secretion *(secondary hyperparathyroidism)* occurs. Secondary hyperparathyroidism is therefore a situation of hyperplasia in response to compromised calcium balance most commonly caused by gastrointestinal or renal disease. Chronic secondary hyperparathyroidism can occasionally result in *tertiary hyperparathyroidism* where a PTH-producing adenoma is formed and is unresponsive to the normal feedback loop. Exceptionally high PTH levels ensue with resultant hypercalcemia. In both secondary and tertiary hyperparathyroidism, a marked decrease in bone mass is to be expected.[11]

Collaborative Care Management. Treatment of secondary hyperparathyroidism revolves around treating the underlying disease responsible for the derangement of calcium balance. If the disease is progressive and irreversible (e.g., chronic renal failure), augmentation of calcium intake and supplementation with 1,25-hydroxycholecalciferol, in addition to normalizing the serum phosphate elevation, minimizes the secondary hyperparathyroidism.

In the case of tertiary hyperparathyroidism, surgical therapy is needed to remove the autonomously functioning adenoma. This will ultimately return the patient to a state of secondary hyperparathyroidism, previously discussed. Postoperative nursing measures are the same as for the patient with primary hyperparathyroidism who has undergone surgical excision.

PATIENT/FAMILY TEACHING. Care of patients with secondary hyperparathyroidism primarily involves teaching about the pathophysiology of the disease and the prescribed medication regimen. Teaching needs of patients with tertiary hyperparathyroidism who have undergone surgical excision of an adenoma are the same as those of the patient with primary hyperparathyroidism. After surgery the patient exhibits secondary hyperparathyroidism and needs medication instruction.

Hyposecretion: Hypoparathyroidism

Etiology and Epidemiology. Hypoparathyroidism is an uncommon endocrine disorder in which hypocalcemia occurs as a result of inadequate PTH secretion or impaired PTH action in target tissues.

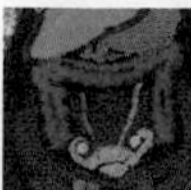

GUIDELINES FOR SAFE PRACTICE *Care of the Patient After Parathyroidectomy*

Care for the patient after parathyroidectomy is similar to that after thyroid surgery. Priorities of care are lowering serum calcium levels and preventing renal complications. In most patients serum calcium levels return to normal within 24 hours. However, mild hypocalcemia may occur after a rapid decrease in serum calcium levels. This transient decrease is usually treated with intravenous calcium infusion.

Patients with significant parathyroid bone disease have an increased risk of postoperative hypocalcemia. Treatment is usually intravenous calcium infusion and frequent monitoring of serum calcium levels. These patients may require supplemental calcium and an active vitamin D metabolite for weeks or months after surgery.

In addition, the nurse should:

- Monitor respiratory status and vital signs every 2 to 4 hours to detect changes in neurologic status and neuromuscular and cardiac function; provide explanations for frequent vital signs and neurologic assessments.
- Have tracheostomy tray and intravenous calcium preparations readily available.
- Report any signs of respiratory obstruction, laryngeal stridor, recurrent laryngeal nerve damage, or hemorrhage.
- Assess patient for quality of voice, dyspnea, choking sensation; tracheal obstruction may occur with vocal cord spasm or hemorrhage.
- Assess mental status and motor strength; implement safety interventions if signs of decreased mental status or weakness are present.
- Keep head of bed elevated 30 degrees to facilitate respirations. Encourage deep breathing, coughing, and turning.
- Monitor serum calcium, magnesium, and electrolytes; assess for presence of tetany and paresthesias.
- Encourage fluids, at least 2 L/day unless contraindicated, to maintain fluid balance and promote calcium excretion; avoid dehydration.
- Monitor and record input and output; weigh patient daily; assess for signs of fluid volume imbalance.
- Strain urine for renal calculi; teach patient signs of renal colic (see Chapter 35).
- Encourage early ambulation to promote bone resorption, decrease muscle atrophy, and decrease complications associated with immobility; inactivity will decrease the rate of calcium deposition in the bone.
- Teach the patient and family to recognize signs of hypercalcemia (anorexia, nausea, vomiting, constipation, weakness, apathy, somnolence, coma), hypocalcemia (paresthesias, muscle cramps, irritability, convulsions), and infection and to notify physician if these signs occur.
- Avoid medications that may cause increase serum calcium levels, including thiazides, vitamin D preparations.
- Provide information regarding calcium in the diet: recommendations for dietary intake of calcium depend on serum levels; hypercalcemia is to be prevented, but intake must allow for sufficient serum levels to promote bone remodeling.
- Provide information for follow-up care; stress importance of periodic assessment of serum calcium levels and potential for recurrence of hyperparathyroidism.

Transient hypoparathyroidism is often a complication of neck surgery. The risk of transient hypoparathyroidism after parathyroid or thyroid surgery is approximately 1% to 10%. Recovery often occurs within days to weeks after surgery. Permanent hypoparathyroidism can be the result of congenital absence of the parathyroids as in DiGeorge syndrome or destruction of the glands. Gland destruction can occur secondary to surgery, particularly radical head or neck surgery; infarction; infiltrative disorders such as hemochromatosis and Wilson's disease; or autoimmune disease. Hypoparathyroidism can also result from impaired secretion as in hypomagnesemia, or from impaired action as with pseudohypoparathyroidism.

Pathophysiology. Most cases of hypoparathyroidism are diagnosed when hypocalcemia occurs after neck surgery. Symptoms vary, depending on the onset, duration, and extent of hypocalcemia (see Clinical Manifestations box). Mild cases may be relatively asymptomatic. The biochemical hallmark of pseudohyperparathyroidism is PTH resistance. Patients who have pseudohypoparathyroidism have additional skeletal and developmental abnormalities. Short stature, stocky body, short neck, and mental retardation are commonly present. In contrast to other hypoparathyroid entities, the biochemical hallmark of pseudohypoparathyroidism is PTH resistance with elevated PTH levels in addition to hypocalcemia and hyperphosphatemia.[11]

Collaborative Care Management. PTH replacement therapy for PTH-deficient patients is not a clinically viable option. Currently, PTH therapy with teriparatide, the synthetic form of PTH, is only approved for the treatment of osteoporosis. Dietary measures to increase calcium intake and decrease phosphate intake have a negligible therapeutic effect and are not recommended. Thus the generally used treatment is calcium supplementation (either as calcium carbonate or calcium citrate) coupled with vitamin D supplementation, generally in the form of calcitriol (1,25-dihydroxycholecalciferol), for ease of adjustment and titration. Because the loss of PTH action at the level of the kidney results in renal calcium wasting or hypercalciuria, augmenting calcium and vitamin D to achieve a midnormal serum calcium level causes significant hypercalciuria and risk of renal calculi. Hence the goal of therapy is to maintain low-normal levels of serum calcium to control symptoms and minimize the risk of hypercalciuria and renal stone formation. Fluid intake should be increased to decrease the urinary mineral concentration and formation of renal calculi. A fluid intake of at least 2 L/day is recommended unless contraindicated. Fluid intake must be increased in hot weather because of an increase in insensible fluid losses.

Patients need an eye examination every 1 to 2 years to screen for cataracts, as well as careful clinical follow-up monitoring to ensure adherence to and success of their therapeutic regimen. Nonadherence can have serious sequelae, including tetany, seizures, and mental status changes. Presence of a positive Chvostek's sign or Trousseau's sign during a patient follow-up examination is indicative of a subtherapeutic regimen.

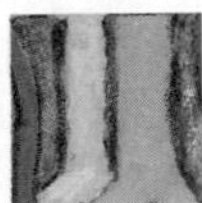

CLINICAL MANIFESTATIONS
True Hypoparathyroidism

- Changes in nerve activity affecting peripheral motor and sensory nerves
  —Paresthesias around mouth, tips of fingers, and sometimes in the feet
  —Tetany with positive Chvostek's and Trousseau's signs (see Chapter 17); spasms of wrists, fingers, forearms, feet, and back
  —Seizures that may consist of syncopal spells, tonic spasms of the total body, or the more typical tonic-clonic activity
  —Hyperventilation, laryngospasm, bronchospasm, respiratory alkalosis
  —Other neurologic signs: headache; papilledema; elevated cerebrospinal fluid pressure; local signs that mimic a cerebral tumor; extrapyramidal neurologic signs and symptoms, including gait changes, tremors, rigidity, and spasms; symptoms seen almost exclusively in patients with calcification of the basal ganglia
- Irritability, depression, anxiety, emotional lability, impairment of memory and cognitive function, confusion, frank psychosis
- Cardiovascular manifestations (effect of hypocalcemia)
  —Prolonged Q-T and ST intervals and occasional dysrhythmias
  —Resistance to effects of digitalis preparations
  —Decreased cardiac output secondary to congestive heart failure
- Cataract formation
- Dental manifestations (depending on age of onset)
  —Enamel defects seen on the tooth crown
  —Delayed or absent tooth eruption
  —Defective dental root formation
- Fragile nails; thin, patchy hair; dry, scaly skin; mucocutaneous candidiasis; impetigo herpetiformis
- Gastrointestinal malabsorption

PATIENT/FAMILY TEACHING. Patient and family teaching is presented in the Patient/Family Teaching box.

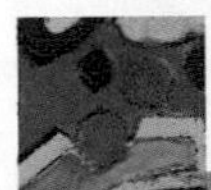

PATIENT/FAMILY TEACHING
The Patient With Hypoparathyroidism

Teaching content includes:
- Basic pathophysiology of the disease
- Medication administration:
  —Calcium is administered in divided doses.
  —Carbonate formulation taken with food as hydrochloric acid is needed for absorption.
  —Citrate formulation can be taken irrespective of food intake.
  —Vitamin D and phosphate binders are taken.
- The need for ongoing medical follow-up care every 3 to 6 months
- Self-monitoring for signs of:
  —Hypocalcemia (muscle spasms, tetany, declining mental status)
  —Hypercalcemia (thirst, polyuria, decreased muscle tone, constipation)
- Complications (renal calculi manifesting as renal colic, i.e., flank pain with or without radiation to the groin)
- Importance of diet: foods high in calcium but low in phosphorus (processed cheese, yogurt, milk)
- Importance of wearing a Medic-Alert bracelet

Adrenal Gland Disorders

Disorders of the adrenal gland may be classified as disorders of the cortex or medulla. Hyperfunction gives rise to distinct clinical syndromes: Cushing's syndrome, hyperaldosteronism, and pheochromocytoma, with symptoms occurring as a result of excess hormone production. Hypofunction of the adrenal cortex in terms of cortisol production is fatal if untreated. In contrast, lack of the adrenal medulla, which occurs after bilateral adrenalectomy, is compatible with normal bodily function.[69]

Adrenal Cortex

Cortisol Hypersecretion: Cushing's Syndrome

Etiology and Epidemiology. Excess circulating glucocorticoids can occur as a result of disorders at different levels of the hypothalamic-pituitary-adrenal axis (Figure 38-8). Clinical manifestations of glucocorticoid excess (Figure 38-9) are readily identified on a careful clinical examination. Milder degrees of glucocorticoid excess pose a diagnostic challenge, as does the pseudo–Cushing's syndrome seen in some patients with depression or obesity. In addition, diagnostic dilemmas occur in the patient with an incidentally discovered adrenal nodule on abdominal CT scanning for other reasons (adrenal incidentaloma).[25,40,42]

The most common cause of noniatrogenic Cushing's is a pituitary adenoma (approximately 60% of cases) in which excess ACTH production results in excess glucocorticoid production.[24] Second to pituitary adenoma is primary adrenal neoplasm or hyperplasia (approximately 25% of cases), with ectopic ACTH or corticotropin-releasing hormone (CRH) accounting for the remaining 15%. The most common ectopic source is an ACTH-producing pulmonary neoplasm such as a bronchial carcinoid or lung cancer. Cushing's syndrome, whether of pituitary or primary adrenal origin, is more common in women than in men. The incidence of pituitary Cushing's (Cushing's disease, in which a tumor produces excess ACTH) is estimated at 5 to 25 cases per 1 million persons per year. The incidence of iatrogenic Cushing's syndrome

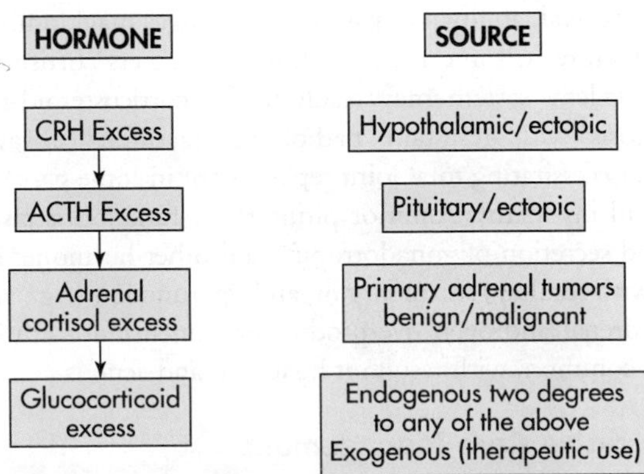

Figure 38-8 Hypothalamic-pituitary-adrenal axis and Cushing's syndrome: possible pathways to cortisol excess. *ACTH,* Adrenocorticotropic hormone; *CRH,* corticotropin-releasing hormone.

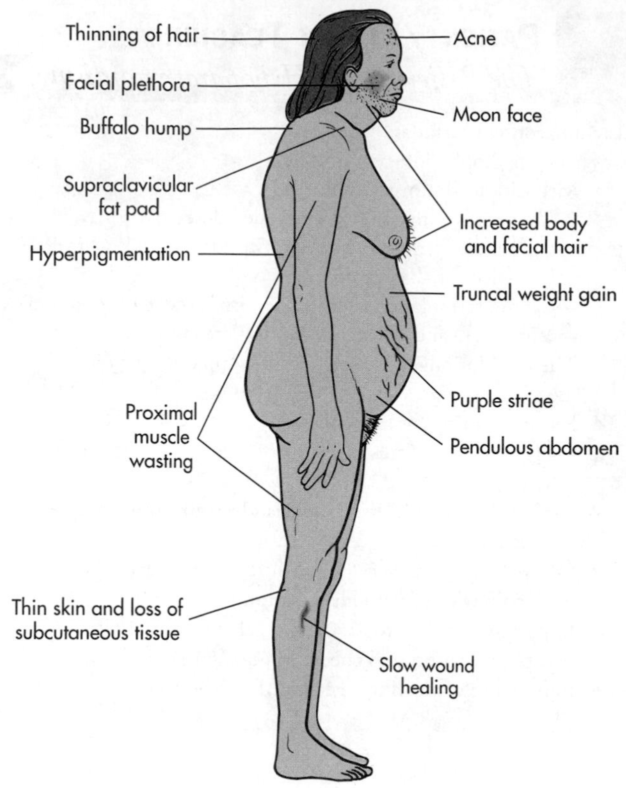

Figure 38-9 Common characteristics of Cushing's syndrome.

is unknown, but because more than 10 million patients in the United States are receiving chronic glucocorticoid therapy, the incidence is thought to be high.

Pathophysiology. Regardless of the etiology of noniatrogenic Cushing's syndrome, the first discernible abnormality is the loss of diurnal variation in cortisol secretion. The morning serum cortisol levels may be at the high end of the normal range, but the evening level may not show the normal decline. Therefore a single fasting serum cortisol is not a reliable marker of cortisol excess.

The pathophysiologic sequelae of cortisol excess involve multiple systems (Box 38-12). In many instances patients may be treated for the secondary metabolic dysfunction such as diabetes mellitus or hypertension before a diagnosis of Cushing's syndrome is considered. Emotional lability and psychiatric changes may dominate the clinical picture in some patients. Effects of excess cortisol on the musculoskeletal system may result in (1) corticosteroid-induced osteoporosis with resultant pathologic fractures; (2) avascular necrosis, necessitating total joint replacement in some patients; and (3) steroid myopathy. Anterior pituitary dysfunction is also common, and secretion of gonadotropins and other hormones may be altered with resultant secondary organ hypofunction (e.g., amenorrhea). Adrenal androgen overproduction concurrent with cortisol excess is common, with resultant hirsutism and acne.

Collaborative Care Management

Diagnostic Tests. The most important initial diagnostic test in the patient with suspected Cushing's syndrome is confirmation of excess glucocorticoid production. The 24-hour urine free cortisol is probably the single best test for diagnosing Cushing's syndrome. The false-positive rate is less than 4% and the false-negative rate less than 6%. The 1-mg overnight dexamethasone suppression test is also a useful screening test; it has a false-negative rate of less than 2%, but a high false-positive rate (see Chapter 37).

Once glucocorticoid excess has been documented, it must be determined whether it is ACTH dependent (pituitary, ectopic) or ACTH independent (adrenal neoplasm). In ACTH-independent Cushing's syndrome the ACTH is appropriately low to subnormal secondary to pituitary suppression, whereas in the ACTH-dependent Cushing's syndrome the ACTH is high normal to frankly elevated.

Pituitary Cushing's syndrome can be evaluated by an 8-mg overnight dexamethasone suppression test (see Chapter 37) in which 8 mg of dexamethasone is taken at 11 PM and the fasting serum cortisol is measured at 8 AM the next day. The patient with pituitary Cushing's syndrome exhibits a more than 50% reduction in the morning serum cortisol measurement. This test carries a sensitivity of 89% and a specificity of 100% and has clear advantages over some of the other diagnostic tests.[7,26]

If ACTH levels are borderline, a CRH stimulation test is of value. CRH is administered as an intravenous bolus, and serum values for cortisol and ACTH are drawn at 15-, 30-, 60-, 90-, and 120-minute intervals. Pituitary Cushing's syndrome will result in a rise in ACTH levels; in ectopic and adrenal Cushing's syndrome, no significant change occurs in the ACTH level.[48,57] False-positive tests for cortisol excess can occur (Box 38-13). Imaging studies are indicated if cortisol excess is clearly documented and dynamic tests indicate the source (i.e., pituitary versus adrenal versus ectopic) (Table 38-5). If the lesion is not visible by imaging techniques, bilateral inferior petrosal sinus sampling for ACTH levels is of value in lateralizing the tumor for the transsphenoidal surgeon.

Medications. Medical therapy for Cushing's syndrome is reserved for when patients fail surgical therapy, surgical therapy is not feasible, or the effects of radiotherapy are still pending. All these therapies revolve around inhibition of cortisol production in the adrenal glands. Medications used include ketoconazole, metyrapone, aminoglutethemide, and mitotane.

Treatments. Pituitary irradiation for failed transsphenoidal surgery for pituitary Cushing's syndrome has the serious disadvantages of delayed effectiveness, perhaps for several years; the risk of panhypopituitarism; and potential neurologic damage. Conventional irradiation induces remission in 20% to 50% of adults. Stereotactic irradiation such as the Gamma Knife radiosurgery is an alternative in patients with adenomas smaller than 30 mm and located at least 3 to 5 mm from the optic chiasm.[31,39] If pituitary irradiation is used, pituitary dysfunction or panhypopituitarism may result.

Surgical Management. Definitive management of noniatrogenic Cushing's syndrome revolves around identifying the cause; surgical cure is possible. In the case of pituitary Cushing's, transsphenoidal surgery should cure 80% to 90% of patients. Morbidity is low and mortality is less than 1%. Complications include permanent DI and panhypopituitarism.[68]

Box 38-12 Hypercortisolism: Pathophysiologic Alterations and Clinical Manifestations

Protein, Fat, and Carbohydrate Metabolism

Altered Protein Metabolism

Excessive catabolism of proteins results in loss of muscle mass, causing:

- Proximal muscle wasting and weakness, which may be characterized by difficulty getting up from low chairs, difficulty climbing stairs, or generalized weakness and fatigue
- Depletion of protein matrix of bone, resulting in osteoporosis, compression fractures of spine, backache, bone pain, and pathologic fractures
- Loss of collagen support of skin, resulting in thin, fragile skin that bruises easily, ecchymosis at trauma sites, and purple striae
- Poor wound healing

Altered Fat Metabolism

Changes in fat metabolism involve abnormal deposition of fat in the face, producing moon face (see Figure 38-9); in the interscapular area, producing a "buffalo hump"; and in the mesenteric bed, producing truncal obesity. Redistribution of fat with these characteristic features may be seen in patients without overt obesity. Body weight usually is increased.

Altered Carbohydrate Metabolism

Increased hepatic gluconeogenesis and impaired insulin utilization result in postprandial hyperglycemia and occasionally frank diabetes mellitus with all its signs and symptoms (see Chapter 39). Patients with concurrent diabetes mellitus may experience worsening hyperglycemia.

Inflammatory and Immune Response

Cortisol excess results in decreased lymphocytes, particularly T lymphocytes; decreased cell-mediated immunity; increased neutrophils; and altered antibody activity. These changes increase vulnerability to viral and fungal infections such as *Pneumocystis carinii* or other fungal infections. Early signs of infection, such as fever, may not be seen. Poor wound healing may also be related to infections.[17]

Water and Mineral Metabolism

Cortisol itself possesses mineralocorticoid activity; therefore cortisol excess results in characteristic signs and symptoms of increased mineralocorticoid activity even though the level of aldosterone is normal. These include:

- Sodium and water retention, which may accentuate body weight increase, may cause edema, and may expand blood volume; serum sodium usually normal
- Hypertension, which is found in almost every patient with excessive cortisol and may be caused by increased volume or increased sensitivity of arterioles to circulating catecholamines
- Hypochloremia and metabolic alkalosis (with severe cortisol excess) because of increased excretion of potassium and chloride (most often seen with ectopic Cushing's syndrome); hypokalemia unusual except with ectopic adrenocorticotropic hormone (ACTH)
- Increased calcium resorption from the bones and renal calculi from hypercalciuria, resulting in renal colic

Emotional Stability

Various emotional changes may occur, from irritability and anxiety, mild depression and poor concentration and memory, to severe depression and psychosis. Euphoria and sleep disorders are frequently noted. These may be the presenting signs and symptoms.

Hematologic Alterations

The patient may have a normal to high red blood cell count, hemoglobin, and hematocrit (may account in part for facial plethora). Leukocytosis, lymphopenia, and eosinopenia may be noted, as are increases in various clotting factors and platelets, resulting in thromboembolic phenomena.

Excessive Androgen Activity

If excessive androgens are present, female patients exhibit virilization, including:

- Hirsutism, manifested initially as fine, downy coat of hair on face and body
- Male pattern hair loss
- Acne
- Changes in menstrual cycle, varying from irregularities to oligomenorrhea to amenorrhea
- Changes in libido

Other Findings

Hyperpigmentation on the skin and mucous membranes may be present and indicates elevation of ACTH, which may be from an ectopic site or the pituitary. ACTH (which has melanotropic activity) levels are higher, and therefore hyperpigmentation is more common and significant from ectopic sources than from the pituitary.

In the case of adrenal tumors, adrenalectomy is the treatment of choice; adrenalectomy is done laparoscopically in select patients. Bilateral adrenalectomy is the second line of management for patients who have failed transsphenoidal surgery for pituitary Cushing's syndrome. The mortality rate from adrenalectomy is 4% to 10% with a 1% risk of recurrent Cushing's syndrome as a result of growth of an adrenal remnant. In the case of bilateral adrenalectomy for failed transsphenoidal surgery, there is a 10% to 20% risk of Nelson's syndrome. Nelson's syndrome involves progressive enlargement of an ACTH-secreting pituitary tumor and associated hyperpigmentation and mass effects, including visual field compromise and headache. Definitive therapy for ectopic tumors producing ACTH involves resection of the primary neoplasm (generally the lung), if feasible.[69]

After surgery, patients with unilateral solitary adrenal tumors, ACTH-producing pituitary tumors, or ectopic ACTH-producing tumors have suppression of the normal ACTH-adrenal axis and require temporary physiologic cortisol replacement. Recovery of the normal ACTH-adrenal axis may take 6 to 24 months with gradual tapering of the cortisol replacement dose. Bilateral adrenalectomy patients require lifelong glucocorticoid and mineralocorticoid replacement (see section on Addison's disease for discussion of glucocorticoids and mineralocorticoids).

After adrenal surgery the patient is usually managed in the intensive care unit because of the high risk for adrenal crisis and the need for invasive monitoring to maintain fluid and electrolyte balance (see Guidelines for Safe Practice box, p. 1099). Hemodynamic monitoring (central venous pressure, blood pressure, pulse, and at times

Box 38-13 Causes of a False-Positive Elevation of Cortisol

- *Acute or chronic illnesses:* Acute stressors may result in high cortisol levels and abnormal dexamethasone tests; these tests must be repeated after patient's condition is stable.
- *Obesity:* This results in high levels of urinary 17-hydroxycorticosteroids and 17-ketogenic steroids and abnormal screening suppression tests, but urine free cortisol, serum cortisol, and response to standard suppression test are normal.
- *Pregnancy, estrogen therapy, and oral contraceptives:* Elevated estrogen associated with these factors can increase serum cortisol and give abnormal results on a screening cortisol suppression test, but urine free cortisol and response to standard suppression test are normal.
- *Alcoholism:* Alcoholics may have both clinical and diagnostic characteristics of Cushing's syndrome, but abstinence from alcohol reverses signs, symptoms, and abnormal test results.
- *Depression:* Endogenous depression results in increased cortisol levels, loss of diurnal rhythm, increased urine free cortisol, increased urine 17-hydroxycorticosteroids and 17-ketogenic steroids, and abnormal screening suppression tests; however, patients with depression have increased cortisol in response to insulin-induced hypoglycemia, whereas patients with true Cushing's syndrome do not.

pulmonary capillary wedge pressure) is continuous. In addition, the nurse monitors daily serum electrolyte concentrations, blood glucose levels every 4 hours, daily weights, and hourly intake and output.

Intravenous cortisol replacement is continued for 24 to 48 hours after surgery. Fluids are given based on the clinical data and usually include saline-dextrose solutions. On the second postoperative day, mineralocorticoids may be started. By the third postoperative day the patient is usually able to tolerate oral glucocorticoids and a normal diet. If unusual weakness or anorexia, nausea, or vomiting occurs, glucocorticoids are increased. If unusual hypotension occurs, mineralocorticoids and fluids are adjusted appropriately.

A major complication of surgery is poor wound healing and infection related to the excess cortisol. Strict aseptic technique is used with wound care. Other postoperative needs are similar to those described for the patient with adrenal insufficiency. Replacement therapy is necessary throughout life.

For the patient who has had a unilateral adrenalectomy, monitoring, hormonal support, fluid therapy, and other care needs are the same during the immediate postoperative period as for the patient with a bilateral adrenalectomy. After the patient's condition has stabilized and physiologic and psychologic crises have been successfully avoided, the glucocorticoid support is slowly withdrawn; eventually a single gland can secrete enough hormone for both daily living and additional stressors. While glucocorticoids are being withdrawn, the nurse continues monitoring for signs and symptoms of adrenal insufficiency and crisis, since the remaining gland may have atrophied. If signs and symptoms occur, glucocorticoids are restarted and then again slowly withdrawn.

Persons with Cushing's syndrome caused by pituitary adenoma and treated by transsphenoidal resection may experience the complications described for hyperpituitarism. Persons treated with bilateral adrenalectomy require lifelong glucocorticoid and mineralocorticoid replacement therapy. Adrenal crisis is a potential complication.

DIET. Diet modifications are prescribed according to individual patient needs. Calories, sodium, lipids, and cholesterol are commonly restricted. If the patient becomes hyperglycemic or develops diabetes mellitus, dietary management of blood glucose levels is indicated.

HEALTH PROMOTION AND PREVENTION. Most causes of excessive cortisol production are not preventable. One exception is the ectopic secretion of ACTH from bronchogenic carcinoma, whose incidence could be decreased through elimination of smoking. No screening tests are available for secondary prevention. Evaluation of adrenal function depends on the primary health care provider's clinical suspicion. Tertiary preventive activities should be a major focus of nursing care. Nurses help patients deal with their chronic health problems, carry out self-monitoring practices to identify exacerbations early, and maintain their therapeutic regimens. These practices help prevent progression of problems. Patients receiving long-term glucocorticoid therapy are an important group for nurses to target for teaching.

Nursing Management *of the Patient with Cushing's Syndrome*

ASSESSMENT

Health History. Assess for:

- Changes in body proportions, weight, hair distribution, pigmentation, bruising, delayed wound healing
- Discomfort, particularly back pain

TABLE 38-5 DIAGNOSTIC IMAGING FOR CORTISOL EXCESS

Suspected Source	Diagnostic Imaging	Disadvantage
Pituitary	Magnetic resonance imaging	Pituitary lesion that is source of adrenocorticotropic hormone (ACTH) excess is not seen in 50% of patients because of lesion's small size. Pituitary lesion that is noted may be incidentaloma and not the source of ACTH excess.
Adrenal	Adrenal computed tomography (CT)	Adrenal lesion noted may be incidentaloma and not the cause of cortisol excess.
Ectopic ACTH	Chest CT Abdominal CT	CT scan may miss a lesion that is present.

- Frequent infections: skin, respiratory, yeast infections
- Changes noted in behavior, concentration, memory
- Nutritional data
- Usual 24-hour food and fluid intake
- Increase in thirst
- Complaints of weakness, fatigue, or difficulty doing normal activities
- Changes in urinary output
- Changes in menstrual history, secondary sexual characteristics, libido, or feelings about self
- Knowledge level: condition, treatment, diagnostic tests

Physical Examination. Assess for:

- General body appearance (presence of moon facies, buffalo hump, truncal obesity, proximal muscle wasting, hyperpigmentation, purple striae, ecchymoses, thin skin, facial plethora, acne, unhealed wounds)
- Affect and its appropriateness to situation, short-term memory, concentration
- Blood pressure, pulse, edema, jugular vein distention
- Intake and output, weight
- Muscle mass and tone, strength, ability to stand up from a sitting position; unexplained osteopenia
- Urinary output, glycosuria
- Sexuality in the female: secondary sexual characteristics, body and scalp hair distribution, acne
- Abnormal glucose tolerance, hypokalemia

NURSING DIAGNOSES, OUTCOMES, AND INTERVENTIONS

Nursing Diagnosis: Disturbed Body Image

OUTCOMES. Common examples of expected outcomes for the patient with a diagnosis of *disturbed body image* are:

Patient will:

- Have improved body image, as evidenced by speaking about self in positive terms.
- Participate in ADLs and leisure activities as tolerated.

NURSING INTERVENTIONS. A major focus of care is helping the patient deal with changes in body image, sexuality, and self-concept. Patients should know that some body changes are reversible with treatment. To help increase self-concept, the nurse assists patients in setting realistic goals. Clear explanations about changes in sexual characteristics and changes that will occur with treatment help patients cope. Including the patient's significant other can help alleviate anxiety regarding roles and relationships.

Resuming usual activities can help the patient restore a positive body image. This may require assistance with some activities that expend energy such as bathing. In addition, the nurse should space the patient's activities and provide rest periods. When electrolyte and fluid balance and glucose metabolism have stabilized, the patient's energy level and hence activity level will increase. The patient can then assume a more active role in self-care. The nurse should reassure the patient that symptoms should subside with treatment.

RELATED NIC INTERVENTIONS. Body Image Enhancement, Coping Enhancement, Self-Esteem Enhancement

Nursing Diagnosis: Risk for Infection

OUTCOMES. Common examples of expected outcomes for the patient with a diagnosis of *risk for infection* are:

Patient will:

- Detect early signs and symptoms of infection.
- Verbalize measures to prevent infection.

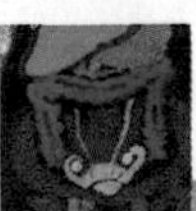

GUIDELINES FOR SAFE PRACTICE *The Patient undergoing Adrenal Surgery*

Preoperative

Provide supportive care.
Assist patient with usual preoperative care.
Maintain nutritional status with a high-protein, prescribed-calorie diet with adequate minerals and vitamins.
Assist with correction of fluid and electrolyte imbalance.
Assist with hormonal therapy as prescribed.
Assist with measures to prevent or treat crisis of adrenal hormonal excess or deficit.
Administer prescribed intravenous fluids and glucocorticoids before surgery.

Postoperative

Establish monitoring schedule to detect complications of surgery and:
—Adrenal crisis
—Blood pressure alterations
—Blood glucose alterations
—Fluid and electrolyte imbalances
Because the patient may have unusual activity intolerance, pace postoperative activities with alternate periods of rest and a gradual increase in self-care.
Provide measures to minimize effects of postural hypotension:
—Supply Ace bandages or elastic stockings.
—Assess effects of posture on blood pressure.
—Assist or accompany the patient during ambulation while blood pressure remains labile.
Provide measures to decrease risk of infection in the immunosuppressed patient (e.g., strict surgical asepsis, deep breathing, and avoiding contact with persons with infections).
Administer cortisol replacement as typically prescribed:
—Intravenous route for the first 24 to 48 hours
—Oral route when patient is able to tolerate food by mouth
Administer mineralocorticosteroid (fludrocortisone) replacement, if prescribed, typically when cortisol replacement is less than 40 to 50 mg/24 hours in the patient with bilateral adrenalectomy.
Assist patient and family in learning about required hormonal replacement:
—Bilateral adrenalectomy: maintenance dose of cortisol and mineralocorticoids
—Unilateral adrenalectomy: doses of cortisol dependent on degree of suppression of hypothalamic-pituitary-adrenal axis

NURSING INTERVENTIONS. The nurse takes the patient's temperature every 4 hours and monitors the white blood cell count. The nurse checks the mouth, lungs, and skin every shift for early signs of infection and reports them immediately, if present. The nurse also teaches the patient to self-assess the skin daily for signs of pressure or injury. Protective pads and an alternating air pressure mattress can help prevent skin breakdown, a source of potential infection. It is important to remember that the usual signs of inflammation may be masked by excess cortisol production.

The patient's exposure to possible pathogens must be minimized. The nurse teaches the patient and family proper handwashing techniques. Staff and visitors with signs and symptoms of upper respiratory tract infections are limited, as is visitation by young children. Invasive procedures are avoided when possible, and aseptic technique is used when they must be done.

Routine turning, coughing, and deep breathing are instituted every 2 hours; oral hygiene is given before breakfast, after meals, and at bedtime.

RELATED NIC INTERVENTIONS. Infection Control, Infection Protection, Skin Surveillance

Nursing Diagnosis: Risk for Injury

OUTCOMES. Common examples of expected outcomes for the patient with a diagnosis of *risk for injury* are:

Patient will:

- Avoid falling or injuring self.
- Verbalize measures to decrease risk of injury.

NURSING INTERVENTIONS. The patient with excess cortisol production is at risk for injury because of decreased bone mass. The nurse assists the patient in identifying potential sources of trauma and ways to minimize the risk of injury, such as wearing shoes with nonskid soles. The nurse encourages the patient to do exercises that increase muscle tone and strength and to walk and perform isometric leg exercises to decrease the risk of thromboembolic events. Avoidance of injury is important because of the risk of increased bleeding. The nurse inspects the skin for areas of ecchymosis.

RELATED NIC INTERVENTIONS. Environmental Management, Exercise Therapy: Muscle Control, Fall Prevention

Patient/Family Teaching. Patient and family teaching for the patient with Cushing's syndrome is presented in the Patient/Family Teaching box.

EVALUATION

To evaluate the effectiveness of nursing interventions, compare patient behaviors with those stated in the expected patient outcomes.

RELATED NOC OUTCOMES. Body Image, Fall Prevention Behavior, Infection Severity, Risk Control, Self-Esteem

Aldosterone Hypersecretion: Primary Aldosteronism

Etiology and Epidemiology. Primary aldosterone excess is characterized by high levels of aldosterone with suppressed renin levels, hypertension, and hypokalemia.[22] Recent studies show that hypokalemia may be absent in a significant number of patients.[49,74] Primary aldosterone excess must be distinguished from secondary aldosterone excess, which results from a variety of conditions (Box 38-14) causing hypoperfusion of the juxtaglomerular apparatus cells and therefore elevated renin levels. The most common cause of secondary aldosteronism is congestive heart failure.

Primary aldosteronism affects up to 12% of the hypertensive population and is twice as common in women as men, for unknown reasons. It is now the most common cause of secondary hypertension. Findings suggestive of primary aldosteronism include hypertension with hypokalemia, hypertension that is difficult to control, and hypertension with an adrenal incidentaloma.

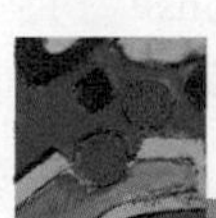

PATIENT/FAMILY TEACHING *The Patient With Hypersecretion of Cortisol (Cushing's Syndrome)*

Education of patients and significant others is ongoing. Information includes:

- Treatment goals and rationales.
- Diet: low sodium, foods rich in vitamin K, and limited carbohydrates. A weight-reduction diet may be indicated. The nurse teaches the patient to monitor body weight and to look for signs of fluid retention.
- Infection prevention.
- Complications.
- Signs and symptoms of adrenal insufficiency and excess.
- Medications, including the name, dosage, side effects, desired effects, interactions, and any necessary precautions. Persons with bilateral adrenalectomy require lifelong hormone replacement.
- Importance of wearing a Medic-Alert bracelet outlining diagnosis and treatment.
- Relationship between stress and hormone levels. Consulting with the health care provider during times of great emotional or physical stress is beneficial; adjustment in medication dosages may be necessary. Assisting the patient in developing effective coping and relaxation methods to manage stress is an important intervention.
- Need for perioperative stress doses of steroids for persons with chronic adrenal insufficiency who needs surgery for an unrelated adrenal problem. This information should be included in discharge instructions.

Box 38-14 Exogenous Causes of Secondary Aldosteronism

- Cardiac failure
- Liver disease
- Hypovolemic states
- Pregnancy
- Idiopathic cyclic edema
- Renal artery stenosis
- Bartter's syndrome (hypertrophy and hyperplasia of the juxtaglomerular cells)

Pathophysiology. Primary aldosteronism is due to bilateral angiotensin-responsive adrenal hyperplasia (also known as idiopathic aldosteronism) in 70% of patients and unilateral aldosterone-producing adrenal cortical adenoma in 25% of patients. The remaining patients have rare causes: unilateral zona glomerulosa hyperplasia, glucocorticoid-suppressible aldosteronism, and aldosterone-producing adrenocortical carcinoma.

The excess aldosterone produced stimulates the resorption of sodium in the renal tubules in exchange for potassium. The resultant volume expansion raises blood pressure without creating edema. Serum sodium levels tend to be at the upper end of the normal range or slightly elevated. Most persons have hypokalemia, except those with rare familial forms of primary aldosteronism. Most patients are asymptomatic; however, occasional neuromuscular complaints related to hypokalemia are reported. Excessive urinary loss of hydrogen ions results in mild alkalosis.[73]

Collaborative Care Management. In the patient suspected of having primary aldosteronism (hypertension and hypokalemia), diagnostic testing should be done after withholding hypertensive medication for 2 to 4 weeks. Many antihypertensive agents, especially spironolactone and angiotensin-converting enzyme (ACE) inhibitors, affect the renin-angiotensin system. Peripheral alpha$_1$-adrenergic blockers have the least potential to interfere with diagnostic testing for primary aldosteronism. Fasting early morning plasma aldosterone concentration (PAC) and plasma renin activity (PRA) levels are generally the first approach to document excess PAC with suppressed PRA. A PAC/PRA ratio of greater than 20 ng/ml/hr is deemed suspicious.[50,74]

After primary aldosteronism has been confirmed, adrenal CT or MRI is performed. The scan may show unilateral adrenal adenoma, show bilateral hyperplasia, or be near normal. When unilateral hyperplasia is suspected, bilateral adrenal vein sampling for aldosterone levels may be carried out to show which adrenal gland is overproducing aldosterone.

Definitive therapy for primary aldosteronism is surgical removal of a unilateral adenoma, unilateral hyperplastic adrenal gland, or adrenal cancer. Aldosterone-producing adenomas can be removed laparoscopically.[33] Patients may have residual hypertension on the basis of underlying essential hypertension even after successful removal of an adrenal tumor.

Pharmacologic therapy is used for all other etiologies. Spironolactone is the mainstay of drug therapy; when it is not tolerated, amiloride may be used. Eplerenone, a selective aldosterone-receptor antagonist, is approved by the Food and Drug Administration for treatment of uncomplicated essential hypertension and post–myocardial infarction congestive heart failure. Studies are ongoing to determine whether it is as effective as spironolactone for treatment of mineralocorticoid hypertension. Alternatives for patients intolerant to spironolactone also include a diuretic with the addition of a calcium channel blocker, beta-blocker, or ACE inhibitor.[37,74]

Dietary sodium restriction (less than 100 mEq/day), alcohol avoidance, regular aerobic exercise, and weight control are important in successful patient management. Evaluation and consultation with a registered dietitian are helpful. Spironolactone and/or amiloride corrects the hypokalemia, and long-term potassium supplementation is frequently not needed.

PATIENT/FAMILY TEACHING. Patient and family teaching for the patient with hypersecretion of aldosterone is presented in the Patient/Family Teaching box.

Adrenal Cortex Hyposecretion: Adrenal Insufficiency

Etiology and Epidemiology. Adrenal insufficiency or cortisol deficiency results from alteration in any step in the hypothalamic-pituitary-adrenal axis (CRH deficiency, ACTH deficiency, or primary adrenal disease). Dysfunction may be temporary (transient ACTH deficiency after removal of an ACTH-producing pituitary adenoma) or permanent (adrenal suppression resulting from chronic glucocorticoid therapy).

Permanent primary adrenal insufficiency is most commonly (70% of cases) a result of acute autoimmune destruction (Addison's disease) of the adrenal glands. Patients with autoimmune adrenal failure may also have other autoimmune disease with endocrine gland failure. Tuberculosis of the adrenal gland accounts for 20% of cases of primary adrenal failure. The remaining 10% of cases are due to metastatic cancer, adrenal hemorrhage, surgical removal, acquired immunodeficiency syndrome, fungal infections, congenital adrenal hypoplasia, and other rare disorders.[6]

Pathophysiology. The major distinguishing feature between primary and secondary adrenal insufficiency lies with the degree of skin pigmentation and mineralocorticoid deficiency. Patients with primary adrenal failure have a large compensatory increase in ACTH and concurrent increase in melanocyte-stimulating hormone with resultant increase in skin pigmentation. In contrast, pallor is present in secondary adrenal failure where ACTH secretion is low. Patients with primary adrenal insufficiency are mineralocorticoid deficient; in contrast, patients with secondary adrenal insufficiency are not mineralocorticoid deficient and therefore do not exhibit electrolyte disturbances or hypotension.

Because of increased ADH secretion, slight hemodilution may be seen in secondary adrenal deficiency caused by water retention; the patient may have a mild decrease in serum sodium. In the patient with primary adrenal failure, loss of mineralocorticoid action results in enhanced sodium excretion with characteristic

PATIENT/FAMILY TEACHING
The Patient With Hypersecretion of Aldosterone

Nursing care, including teaching needs, for the care of the patient after adrenal surgery is discussed in the text. For patients who have had unilateral adrenalectomy, lifelong steroid replacement is not necessary.

Patients treated nonsurgically need instructions regarding:

- Medications, including dosage, side effects, therapeutic effects, drug interactions, and any special precautions necessary
- Dietary needs; a consult with a dietitian provide instructions for a low-sodium, high-potassium diet
- Signs and symptoms to report to the health care provider, including signs of hypokalemia, weight gain, edema, weakness, palpitations, headache, or dyspnea

hyponatremia, hyperkalemia, dehydration, and hypotension. Progressive dehydration can lead to adrenal crisis *(addisonian crisis)* with shock, renal failure, and death.[6]

The pathophysiologic changes and clinical manifestations of adrenal insufficiency are outlined in Box 38-15. The clinical presentation depends on the severity of the adrenal insufficiency and the rate of decline of adrenal function. In the majority of patients with primary autoimmune adrenal insufficiency, the rate of decline in adrenal function is gradual and the early symptoms, such as fatigue, may be vague and nonspecific. The clinical manifestations outlined in Box 38-15 represent advanced adrenal insufficiency.

Collaborative Care Management

DIAGNOSTIC TESTS. A random serum cortisol level does not definitively diagnose adrenal insufficiency, since it may be in the low normal range and does not reflect physiologic reserves to combat stress. Serum cortisol levels may be inappropriately normal during the stress of acute illness; normally levels should be elevated above 20 mcg/dl.

In suspected acute adrenal insufficiency with advancing shock, serum cortisol levels should be drawn, then stress doses of intravenous hydrocortisone given until the crisis is over or the diagnosis is excluded. In persons with chronic adrenal insufficiency, the rapid cosyntropin (synthetic ACTH) stimulation test is most useful (see Chapter 37). However, this test does not distinguish between primary and secondary adrenal insufficiency, since it may take weeks or months after loss of ACTH secretion for the adrenal glands to atrophy. A 24-hour urinary free cortisol determination is not useful in the diagnosis of adrenal insufficiency, since approximately 20% of patients have normal results and the test gives no indication of the physiologic reserve in response to stress.

MEDICATIONS

CHRONIC ADRENAL INSUFFICIENCY. No universal agreement exists on appropriate doses or timing of replacement. Based on recent data showing that the daily cortisol production rate in normal adults is lower than previously thought, the traditional daily dose of 25 to 30 mg of hydrocortisone is excessive. Because the normal diurnal secretion of cortisol peaks in the early morning, approximately three fourths of the total daily dose is generally given in the morning and one third at night (e.g., hydrocortisone 15 mg at 8 AM and 5 mg at 5 PM). However, three-times-daily dosing of hydrocortisone (10 mg at 8 AM, 5 mg at noon, and 5 mg at 5 PM) more closely mimics normal cortisol secretion. Side effects of excess replacement are similar to those seen in Cushing's syndrome.[6]

Because of the negligible mineralocorticoid activity of these glucocorticoids, concurrent use of the mineralocorticoid fludrocortisone is needed in primary adrenal insufficiency. Doses are adjusted to maintain the patient symptom free with normal electrolytes. No reliable laboratory tests are available to assess optimal replacement therapy.

STRESS STEROID DOSING. The body's increased demand for glucocorticoids during periods of stress must be met with increased glucocorticoid administration. It is difficult to precisely define stress; however, most would agree on a fever above 100° F (38° C), vomiting and diarrhea secondary to gastroenteritis, major trauma, and surgical procedures. Doubling of the glucocorticoid dose is generally advocated during minor stress such as low-grade fever and vomiting or diarrhea. If oral replacement is not feasible, parenteral administration is necessary. Patients may be taught intramuscular glucocorticoid administration when they live in remote areas or have no access to an emergency room. For major stress such as major trauma and major surgical procedures, parenteral hydrocortisone at a dosage of 200 mg/day is generally given in divided doses. This, in turn, is rapidly tapered to the maintenance dose as the patient recovers.

DIET. The nurse encourages fluids and continually monitors the patient's hydration status. Nursing interventions include measures to decrease nausea, vomiting, and diarrhea in an effort to main-

BOX 38-15 Hypocortisolism: Pathophysiologic Alterations and Clinical Manifestations

Metabolism of Protein, Carbohydrate, and Fats

As a result of decreased glucocorticoids, carbohydrate metabolism is particularly affected by decreased gluconeogenesis and glycogenesis. Signs and symptoms include hypoglycemia, inability to tolerate prolonged fasts, weakness, lightheadedness, and fatigue.

Hypothalamic-Pituitary-Adrenal Axis

Adrenocorticotropic hormone (ACTH) levels increase as a result of a diminished negative feedback on secretion of ACTH. ACTH stimulates melanocyte-stimulating hormone. As a result, a generalized hyperpigmentation occurs. An increase in pigmentation in skin fold creases and the buccal mucosa may be early clues.

Catecholamine Activity

As glucocorticoids potentiate the catecholamine response, diminished catecholamine activity yields a poor response to endogenous and exogenous stressors. Hypovolemic shock as characterized by hypovolemia, hypotension, and tachycardia may occur.

Emotional Stability

Glucocorticoids in normal amounts assist in maintaining emotional stability. Glucocorticoid deficiency may lead to dysphoria, apathy, or depression.

Water and Mineral Metabolism

Aldosterone is the primary adrenal mineralocorticoid, and deficiency results in loss of both water and sodium. Potassium is abnormally conserved. Signs and symptoms include dehydration and hypovolemia (decreased weight, increased blood urea nitrogen, increased hematocrit, decreased skin turgor), hyponatremia, hyperkalemia, decreased bicarbonate with acidosis, muscle weakness, fatigue, postural hypotension, and hypovolemic shock. Glucocorticoid deficiency has similar, but milder, effects on water and mineral metabolism.

tain fluid and electrolyte and nutritional balance. The patient should be weighed daily. A high-sodium, low-potassium diet is indicated.

TREATMENTS. The major complication of adrenal insufficiency is acute adrenal crisis—a potentially life-threatening critical care issue for both the undiagnosed and the previously diagnosed patient. Patients who come into the health care facility with unexplained weakness or confusion and a history of chronic disease that may be managed with corticosteroids should be assessed for the possibility of adrenal crisis. The patient may be unable to give an accurate medical history that would alert the health care team to the possibility of adrenal insufficiency.

Frequent monitoring is necessary to detect changes, to evaluate effectiveness of therapy, to detect side effects of therapy (e.g., fluid overload), and to prevent or detect complications. Of particular concern are changes in mental status and respiratory depression. Monitoring for fluid status may include taking vital signs as often as every 15 minutes, intake and output hourly, and weights daily. Hemodynamic monitoring may help determine the exact amount of fluids needed. The fluid deficit is usually corrected in 4 to 6 hours. Stress doses of intravenous hydrocortisone are mandatory, as is aggressive treatment of any precipitating illness.

Until the patient's condition stabilizes, the nurse monitors serum electrolytes daily or more frequently as necessary. During the early phase of illness, the nurse conducts a neurologic assessment at least every 4 hours for signs of hyponatremia (dizziness, confusion, or neuromuscular irritability); this assessment can be done while the nurse is taking vital signs. If serum potassium levels are elevated, cardiac monitoring is instituted to assess for changes in T wave or QRS complexes or for changes in rhythm. The hyperkalemia usually resolves quickly with glucocorticoid and mineralocorticoid therapy, and the patient may actually need potassium after the acute period. Until the serum potassium level returns to normal, the nurse ensures that the patient does not inadvertently receive potassium in intravenous fluids or medications. Measures to prevent infections and trauma, which can increase cell death and the release of potassium into the extracellular space, are incorporated into the nursing care plan.

Monitoring for signs and symptoms of hypoglycemia and monitoring blood glucose levels are done on a routine basis, such as every 4 hours. Glucose is given in intravenous fluids as prescribed; when food is allowed, snacks may be incorporated between meals to avoid long periods of fasting. If symptoms of hypoglycemia occur, the blood glucose is checked, if possible, and treatment is initiated (see Chapter 39).

A focus of care is avoiding additional stressors. These patients should do nothing for themselves and should be protected from all stimuli and from exposure to infection. To decrease stressors, the same nurse should provide care for the first several hours while the patient's condition stabilizes. One-on-one care may be necessary. To prevent aspiration, the patient is given nothing by mouth until nausea and vomiting subside and mental status returns to baseline. After several hours, oral liquids may be given, and oral glucocorticoids may be started within 48 hours. The patient may experience a severe headache; comfort measures should be provided.

After the patient's condition has stabilized, attention focuses on achieving an improved state of well-being and preparing for discharge; the care plan is modified as the patient recovers from crisis to a state of chronic adrenal insufficiency.

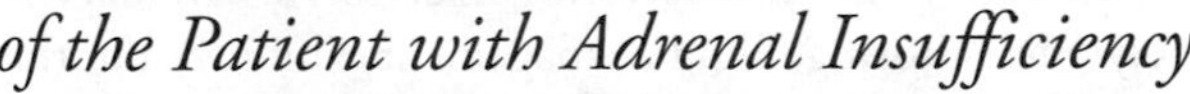

In reviewing laboratory results for a patient diagnosed with suspected adrenal insufficiency, the nurse correlates which finding to this disorder?

1. Hypernatremia
2. Hyperkalemia
3. Hyperglycemia
4. Hypercalcemia

Nursing Management *of the Patient with Adrenal Insufficiency*

ASSESSMENT

Health History. Assess for:

- Weakness, fatigue, muscle pain, dizziness, changes in behavior, lethargy, depression, changes in attention or ability to do work and activities, symptoms of hypoglycemia
- Changes in skin pigmentation
- Anorexia, nausea, vomiting, salt craving, weight loss, and abdominal pain; usual 24-hour food and fluid intake
- Changes in bowel habits; urinary output
- Sexual, females: menstrual history, changes in body and axillary hair
- Knowledge of disease, treatment, expectations

Physical Examination. Assess for:

- Affect, attention, activity level
- Hyperpigmentation, axillary or body hair distribution, skin turgor
- Blood pressure and pulse, especially with postural changes; heart rhythm
- Weight, 24-hour intake and output, abdominal tenderness
- Muscle strength, muscle wasting, ability to do ADLs

NURSING DIAGNOSES, OUTCOMES, AND INTERVENTIONS

Nursing Diagnosis: Deficient Fluid Volume

OUTCOMES. A common example of an outcome for the patient with a diagnosis of *deficient fluid volume* is:

Patient will:

- Maintain fluid balance.

NURSING INTERVENTIONS. Nursing interventions include monitoring the patient for signs of hypovolemia, including weakness, muscle cramps, and changes in vital signs. The nurse closely monitors daily weights and hourly and daily intake and output. Minimum hourly urinary output should be greater than 30 ml. If the patient has had vomiting or diarrhea, monitoring for electrolyte imbalance is important. Vital signs indicating fluid volume deficit are hypotension, tachycardia, decreased pulse volume, and temperature increase or decrease. The nurse also monitors the patient for postural hypotension. Other findings suggestive of fluid volume deficit include dry mucous membranes, thirst, decreased urinary output, decreased skin turgor, sunken eyeballs, weakness, and confusion. Laboratory data are evaluated for hemoconcentration, and fluid replacement is administered as ordered. Fluid intake of at least 2 L/day should be encouraged, unless contraindicated. A diet with normal sodium content (approximately 3 g/day) should be encouraged. Discharge instructions include measures to prevent excessive fluid losses during strenuous exercise, hot temperatures, and vomiting or diarrhea. Sodium intake should be increased when excessive diaphoresis is expected; potassium intake (depending on baseline values) may need to be increased to compensate for gastrointestinal losses.

A Nursing Care Plan for the patient with adrenal insufficiency is found on p.1106.

RELATED NIC INTERVENTIONS. Electrolyte Management, Electrolyte Monitoring, Fluid Management, Fluid Monitoring

Patient/Family Teaching. Patient and family teaching for the patient with adrenal insufficiency is presented in the Patient/Family Teaching boxes below and on p. 1105.

EVALUATION

To evaluate the effectiveness of nursing interventions, compare patient behaviors with those stated in the expected patient outcomes.

RELATED NOC OUTCOMES. Electrolyte & Acid/Base Balance, Fluid Balance, HydrationHyH

GERONTOLOGIC CONSIDERATIONS

Feedback mechanisms involved in maintaining glucocorticoid levels are not affected by age. Additionally, basal plasma levels of glucocorticoids tend to not change with age. The production rate of cortisol declines, but is matched by a corresponding decrease in the metabolic clearance rate of cortisol. Diurnal rhythmicity of cortisol secretion essentially remains intact with age. The amount of fibrous tissue in the gland increases and the gland shrinks somewhat after age 50.

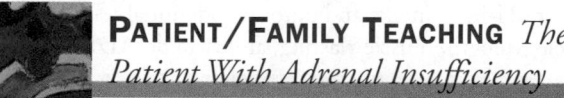

PATIENT/FAMILY TEACHING *The Patient With Adrenal Insufficiency*

The initial teaching during the acute phase relates to proposed diagnostic tests and immediate interventions. After the patient's condition is stable, the nurse provides information about the disease and long-term needs. Instructions about replacement therapy are similar to those given to patients taking therapeutic doses of glucocorticoids, but some important differences exist (see Patient/Family Teaching box, p. 1105). Additional teaching should include the effect of stressors on the disease and methods to reduce or eliminate stress. The patient and significant others should be able to describe:

- Discharge medication regimen, the need for continued treatment, and situations that require an increase in medication dosage
- Medical follow-up plan
- Symptoms indicating adrenal crisis and the need for medical attention
- Need for continual medical follow-up care
- Need to wear a Medic-Alert bracelet
- Need to carry identification card with information concerning physician and current medication

Adrenal Medulla Hypersecretion: Pheochromocytoma

Etiology and Epidemiology. Pheochromocytoma is a catecholamine-producing tumor arising from cells of the adrenal medulla and sympathetic ganglia: 90% of tumors occur within the adrenal gland and 10% are extraadrenal; 10% of the adrenal tumors are bilateral; 10% of all tumors are malignant. Pheochromocytomas may be part of the MEN type II (hyperparathyroidism, medullary thyroid cancer) or MEN type III (medullary thyroid cancer, multiple mucosal neuromas, marfanoid habitus). Pheochromocytomas may occur in up to 0.3% of the hypertensive population. Familial tumors account for approximately 10% of pheochromocytomas.[72]

Both men and women are affected equally; the usual age at diagnosis is 40 to 60 years. Pheochromocytomas are usually benign and curable but, if unrecognized or untreated, can be fatal.

Pathophysiology. Pheochromocytomas release excessive amounts of catecholamines, mainly norepinephrine; associated symptoms include the five Ps:

1. Pressure: paroxysmal increases in blood pressure
2. Palpitations
3. Pallor
4. Perspiration: profuse and generalized
5. Pain: paroxysmal pulsatile headaches, chest and abdominal pain

Most patients come in for health care in a hypertensive crises; the hypertension may be resistant to standard treatment for essential hypertension. In tumors secreting mainly epinephrine, paroxysmal hypotension, shock, tremors, anxiety, epigastric pain, diaphoresis, and chest pain are common manifestations. Labile hypertension is characteristic. Episodes may be spontaneous or precipitated by maneuvers that increase intraabdominal pressure such as lifting, straining, or bending. Episodes may also be precipitated by anesthesia and diagnostic tests. Tumor manipulation and induction of anesthesia can cause hypertensive crisis, arrhythmias, or stroke as a result of extensive catecholamine release. The clinical signs of pheochromocytoma include hypertension (paroxysmal in 50% of cases, or treatment resistant), orthostatic hypotension, weight loss (obesity is uncommon), constipation, tremors, pallor, hypertensive retinopathy, hyperglycemia, and hypercalcemia.

Collaborative Care Management. The most useful screening test measures 24-hour urine total metanephrines. Twenty-four hour vanillylmandelic acid test has a false-positive rate greater than 15% and is the least specific test. The 24-hour urine collection should be started at the onset of a hypertensive episode. Plasma catecholamine determinations are not as sensitive or specific as the 24-hour measurements. Radiologic imaging is best achieved with MRI or CT of the adrenals and abdomen. If MRI and CT

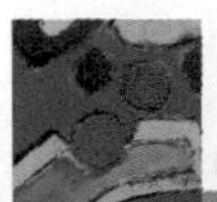

PATIENT/FAMILY TEACHING *The Patient Taking Replacement Doses of Glucocorticoids and Mineralocorticoids*

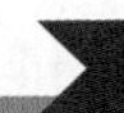

- Follow medication regimen.
  - —Take drugs with meals or snacks.
  - —Take glucocorticoids as directed.
  - —Take mineralocorticoids in the morning.
  - —Do not omit a drug dose.
  - —Keep sufficient medication on hand (on person and at home).
  - —If unable to retain oral form of drug, take parenteral form as instructed.
  - —Carry drugs on person or in carry-on luggage when traveling; do not ship drugs with luggage; make sure traveling companion knows how to give the injectable form of glucocorticoid.
  - —Carry extra doses in case of delays or illness.
- Wear a Medic-Alert bracelet or necklace that lists condition, drugs and dosage, and name and phone number of physician.
- Monitor self for increased stressors (fever, infections, dental work, accidents, or family or personal crises), and increase dose of glucocorticoids as instructed.
- Monitor self daily for signs and symptoms of insufficient drug therapy (anorexia, nausea, vomiting, weakness, depression, dizziness, polyuria, and weight loss) and report immediately (larger drug dose may be necessary).
- Monitor self daily for signs and symptoms of excessive drug therapy (rapid weight gain, round face, edema, or hypertension) and report immediately (smaller drug dose may be necessary).
- Eat a well-balanced diet, choosing foods from all food groups.
- Maintain a regular schedule with adequate sleep, regular meals, and regular exercise (irregular health habits increase glucocorticoid needs).
- See physician as instructed; consult as necessary if questions arise concerning therapy.

are negative, ^{123}I metaiodobenzylguanidine scintigraphy would be the next step.[17,34]

Laparoscopic removal of both adrenal and extraadrenal pheochromocytomas is the treatment of choice. Laparoscopic partial adrenalectomy has been successful in preserving adrenal cortical function in persons with hereditary forms of pheochromocytoma.[17,32,34]

Surgery without catecholamine blockade is associated with a 24% to 50% mortality rate. Catecholamine blockade is best accomplished with the administration of the alpha-adrenergic blocker phenoxybenzamine, followed by beta-adrenergic blockers. Phenoxybenzamine is started 2 weeks before surgery. The most common side effect is nasal congestion. Metyrosine (Demser), recently added to preoperative protocols, decreases catecholamine tumor content by 50% to 80%, thus reducing intraoperative blood loss and the amount of vasoactive medication needed to control blood pressure. Calcium channel blockers are used as an alternative in some centers. Correcting volume depletion with a liberal salt diet and, if necessary, intravenous normal saline is critical to prevent postoperative hypotension.

Before surgery, the nurse institutes measures to help stabilize the patient's hemodynamic status, monitors the clinical state, prepares the patient for tests and surgery, and prevents episodes of hypertension. Patients experiencing hypertensive crises should be in an intensive care unit, since frequent cardiac, blood pressure, and neurologic monitoring is required. If phentolamine infusion is necessary, the nurse checks the blood pressure every 15 minutes and gives the drug by controlled infusion at a rate to keep the blood pressure at a prescribed level. During this time the nurse informs the patient about planned diagnostic tests and treatments and prepares the patient for surgery. Activities that precipitate paroxysms, such as bending, Valsalva's maneuver, palpating the abdomen, and lifting, should be limited. Hypertension can also occur with inadequately treated postoperative pain.

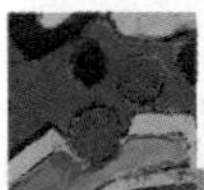

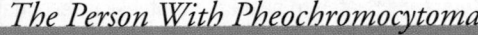

PATIENT/FAMILY TEACHING *The Person With Pheochromocytoma*

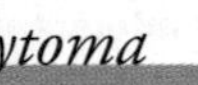

For patients treated medically or surgical patients without remission of symptoms, nursing care focuses on helping them attain the skills necessary for self-care. Teaching includes:

- Information about the disease and its relationship to the signs and symptoms
- Medication regimen: purpose, dosage, expected effects, and side effects
- Blood pressure self-measurement
- Measures to prevent paroxysms: preventing constipation, avoiding Valsalva's maneuver, and avoiding bending or flexing the body
- Importance of follow-up care
- Need to wear Medic-Alert bracelet and carry wallet card

After surgery the nurse closely monitors blood pressure, pulse, cardiac rhythm, neurologic status, and the effectiveness of treatment. Blood glucose levels are monitored until homeostasis returns, as elevated catecholamine levels lead to increased insulin production. After the hypertensive period, hypotension may occur; thus nursing care focuses on continual monitoring and administration of fluids or plasma expanders as prescribed.

Catecholamine levels should return to baseline approximately 6 weeks after surgery. Surgery results in complete remission of symptoms in most patients; therefore discharge teaching for most patients involves helping them plan for resumption of normal activities, maintain an adequate diet, and follow-up with the physician.

PATIENT/FAMILY TEACHING. Patient and family teaching for the patient with pheochromocytoma is presented in the Patient/Family Teaching box above.

Nursing Care Plan

Patient With Adrenal Insufficiency

Data A 47-year-old man is admitted from the emergency department with complaints of feeling so tired that he is unable to get out of bed. For the past 2 months he has experienced loss of appetite, nausea, vomiting, and diarrhea with increasing fatigue. He thought he was having relapses of the flu, which was prevalent during the winter months. He is an accountant and voices concern that his job may be interfering with his ability to fully recover.

Physical examination reveals a tan-appearing Caucasian man who looks ill. He has cool, sweaty skin; poor skin turgor; and dry oral mucous membranes. His respiratory rate is 20 beats/min, and lungs are clear bilaterally. His temperature is 98° F (36.5° C) orally; heart rate, 110 beats/min; blood pressure, sitting 40/50 mm Hg, lying 90/60 mm Hg; and weight, 70 kg (with a 3 kg weight loss during past month). He complains of lightheadedness when the head of the bed is elevated.

Laboratory findings include white blood cell count, 16,000/mm^3; blood glucose, 60 mg/dl; serum sodium, 130 mEq/L; chloride, 86 mEq/L; hemoglobin, 15 g/dl; hematocrit, 46%; blood urea nitrogen, 39 mg/dl; serum creatinine, 0.8 mg/dl; and serum potassium, 5.4 mEq/L.

Physical and laboratory findings confirm the presence of adrenal insufficiency.

Nursing Diagnosis

Activity intolerance related to postural hypotension secondary to adrenal insufficiency

Outcomes

- Patient will be able to perform desired activities of daily living without experiencing fatigue.

Related NOC Outcomes

- Activity Tolerance
- Energy Conservation
- Nutritional Status: Energy

Related NIC Interventions

- Energy Management
- Nutrition Management
- Sleep Enhancement

Nursing Interventions and Rationales

- Provide bed rest for first 24 hours. *To conserve energy and reduce metabolic demands until corticosteroid levels are normalized.*
- Avoid any unnecessary activities such as bathing for first 12 hours. *To conserve energy and reduce metabolic demands until corticosteroid levels are normalized.*
- Offer patient support by explaining that energy will return when hormone levels return to normal. *To reduce anxiety and fear, which increase metabolic demand and contribute to fatigue.*
- Gradually increase activities after hormone levels are returned to normal. *Patient has been ill for several months and may be much weaker than anticipated. Activities should be gradually increased until endurance improves.*

Nursing Diagnosis

Ineffective coping related to inability to respond to stressors secondary to adrenal insufficiency

Outcomes

- Patient will demonstrate adequate coping as evidenced by absence of signs of stress (tachycardia, restlessness, lack of attention, increased blood pressure).

Related NOC Outcomes

- Coping
- Decision-Making
- Role Performance
- Social Support

Related NIC Interventions

- Coping Enhancement
- Decision-Making Support
- Role Enhancement
- Support System Enhancement

Nursing Interventions/Rationales

- Decrease environmental stressors (noise, lights, temperature changes). *Patient has reduced ability to respond to any stressors. External stressors need to be controlled or eliminated until patient is able to cope in his usual manner.*
- Explain all procedures and interventions. *Understanding reduces fear and anxiety, both of which contribute to stress.*
- Maintain consistency of care providers for first 24 hours. *Consistency of personnel increases the patient's trust and reduces stress.*
- Provide care in a calm, unhurried manner. *Stress can be readily transferred from nurse to patient. If the nurse is calm, the patient is more likely to be calm.*
- Encourage family members to remain with patient, if they are comforting to him. *The presence of family members often increases comfort and security and reduces stress. If the patient does not find family members comforting, their presence will increase stress.*

Nursing Diagnosis

Deficient fluid volume related to inability to conserve fluid secondary to glucocorticoid deficiency

Outcomes

- Patient will have normal fluid status as evidenced by blood pressure within normal parameters and absence of hemoconcentration.

Related NOC Outcomes
- Electrolyte & Acid/Base Balance
- Fluid Balance
- Hydration

Related NIC Interventions
- Electrolyte Management
- Electrolyte Monitoring
- Fluid Management
- Fluid Monitoring

Nursing Intervetions/Rationales
- Monitor intake and output hourly. *Loss of fluid volume predisposes the patient to renal compromise and possible acute renal failure. Intake should approximate output.*
- Monitor blood pressure and heart rate hourly until normal. *To compare with baseline and detect increasing physical instability or determine the effectiveness of interventions.*
- Weigh daily. *To determine fluid and nutritional needs. Fluid deficit results in weight loss. Fluid restoration results in weight gain.*
- Administer intravenous fluids as prescribed (usually 5% dextrose in normal saline) and monitor fluid status. *Surveillance allows for early identification of problems with replacement therapy so that solutions or infusion rates can be adjusted or changed. Fluid volume deficiency results from excessive loss of sodium and water from glucocorticoid deficiency.*
- Monitor hematocrit, hemoglobin, blood urea nitrogen, and serum creatinine daily. *To determine the presence of hemodilution or hemoconcentration, and to monitor renal function.*
- Administer cortisol as prescribed. *Replacement cortisol is the primary treatment for cortisol deficiency.*

Nursing Diagnosis
Risk of injury related to weakness and hypoglycemia

Outcomes
- Patient will remain free from falls.

Related NOC Outcomes
- Fall Prevention Behavior
- Risk Control
- Symptom Control

Related NIC Interventions
- Environmental Management: Safety
- Fall Prevention
- Surveillance: Safety

Nursing Interventions and Rationales
- Keep bed in lowest position. *To increase ease with which patient can get into bed and decrease the possibility of falling.*
- Keep side rails up at all times unless patient refuses. *Side rails provide protection from falling out of bed when sleeping. If patient refuses side rails, they must be left down because they are considered restraints.*
- Monitor blood glucose levels every 4 hours. *Hypoglycemia and weakness can lead to injury.*
- Instruct patient to call for assistance when getting into or out of bed. *Patient is weak and fatigued. The assistance of another person is needed to decrease the risk for falls and injury.*

Nursing Diagnosis
Deficient knowledge (disease and treatment) related to lack of previous experience with current illness

Outcomes
- Patient will verbalize understanding of disease and its treatment.

Related NOC Outcomes
- Knowledge: Disease Process
- Knowledge: Treatment Regimen

Relatted NIC Interventions
- Teaching: Disease Process
- Teaching: Individual
- Teaching: Prescribed Medication

Nursing Interventions/Rationales
- Explain all care to patient and family so that no unexpected events occur. *To decrease stress so patient is capable of hearing and understanding information provided.*
- Focus on immediate care rather than home care at this time. *Patient is only capable of handling information about what is happening now. He will not likely retain information regarding home care until he is stable and less fatigued.*
- Repeat teaching frequently. *Stress interferes with learning. There is too much information to learn at one time, and the patient is very fatigued; therefore repetitive teaching enhances learning.*
- Provide written materials to enforce verbal teaching. *Patients who are ill or stressed do not always remember information taught. Written materials allow the patient to review important information and proceed at their own pace.*
- Provide information about community resources that may be useful to patient and family. *The patient may not be aware of available community resources.*

Evaluation
Evaluation is based on comparing the patient's outcomes with desired outcomes.

Critical Thinking

1. A 52-year-old Caucasian man is seen with hypertension with a blood pressure of 190/102 mm Hg, tachycardia, and diaphoresis. What endocrine abnormalities could be responsible for his hypertension? What questions would you ask him? What diagnostic tests might his physician order?
2. Endocrine disorders may cause a number of physical changes that can adversely affect body image and self-esteem. As you consider several endocrine disorders and their physical sequelae, formulate a plan to help the patient cope with changes in body image and self-esteem.

References

1. Ahmad AM et al: Body composition and quality of life in adults with growth hormone deficiency: effects of low-dose growth hormone replacement, *Clin Endocrinol* (Oxf) 54(6):709-717, 2001.
2. American Association of Clinical Endocrinologists: AACE medical guidelines for clinical practice for growth hormone use in adults and children—2003 update, *Endocrine Pract* 9(11):64-76, 2003.
3. American Association of Clinical Endocrinologists, AACE Hypogonadism Task Force: American Association of Clinical Endocrinologists medical guidelines for clinical practice for the evaluation and treatment of hypogonadism in adult male patients—2002 update, *Endocrine Pract* 8(6): 439-456, 2002.
4. American Association of Clinical Endocrinologists, AACE Thyroid Task Force: American Association of Clinical Endocrinologists medical guidelines for the evaluation and treatment of hyperthyroidism and hypothyroidism, *Endocrine Pract* 8(6):457-469, 2002.
5. American Association of Clinical Endocrinologists/American Association of Endocrine Surgeons Thyroid Carcinoma Task Force: AACE/AAES medical/surgical guidelines for clinical practice: management of thyroid cancer, *Endocrine Pract* 7(3):202-220, 2001.
6. Arle W, Allolio B: Adrenal insufficiency, *Lancet* 361(9372):1881-1893, 2003.
7. Arnaldi G et al: Diagnosis and complications of Cushing's syndrome: a consensus statement, *J Clin Endocrinol Metab* 88(12):5593-5602, 2003.
8. Auer J et al: Subclinical hyperthyroidism as a risk factor for atrial fibrillation, *Am Heart J* 142(5):838-842, 2001.
9. Bauer DC et al, for Study of Osteoporotic Fractures Research Group: Risk for fracture in women with low levels of thyroid-stimulating hormone, *Ann Intern Med* 134(7):561-568, 2001.
10. Ben-Jonathan N, Hnasko R: Dopamine as a prolactin inhibitor, *Endocrine Rev* 22(6):724-763, 2001.
11. Bilezikian JP, Marcus R, Levine MA, editors: *The parathyroids,* ed 2, San Diego, 2001, Academic Press.
12. Bilezikian JP, Silverberg SJ: Asymptomatic primary hyperparathyroidism, *N Engl J Med* 350(17):1746-1751, 2004.
13. Bilezikian JP et al: Clinical presentation of primary hyperparathyroidism. In Bilezikian JP, editor: *The parathyroids,* ed 3, New York, 2001, Raven.
14. Bilezekian JP et al: Summary statement for a workshop on asymptomatic primary hyperparathyroidism: a perspective for the 21st century, *J Clin Endocrinol Metab* 87(12):5353-5362, 2002.
15. Bogazzi F et al: The various effects of amiodarone on thyroid function, *Thyroid* 11(5):511-519, 2001.
16. Braverman LE, Utiger RD: *Werner and Ingbar's the thyroid,* ed 9, Philadelphia, 2004, Lippincott, Williams & Wilkins.
17. Bravo EL, Tagle R: Pheochromocytoma: state-of-the-art and future prospects, *Endocrine Rev* 24(4):539-553, 2003.
18. Clemmons DR et al: Optimizing control of acromegaly: integrating a growth hormone receptor antagonist into the treatment algorithm, *J Clin Endocrinal Metab* 88(10):4759-4767, 2003.
19. Clyde PW et al: Combined levothyroxine plus liothyronine compared alone in primary hypothyroidism: a randomized controlled trial, *JAMA* 290(22):2952-2958, 2003.
20. Colao A et al: Improved cardiovascular risk factors and cardiac performance after 12 months of growth hormone (GH) replacement in young adult patients with GH deficiency, *J Clin Endocrinol Metab* 86(5):1874-1881, 2001.
21. Colao A et al: Systemic complications of acromegaly: epidemiology, pathogenesis, and management, *Endocrine Rev* 25(1):102-152, 2004.
22. Conn JW: Presidential address: part I, Painting background; part II, Primary aldosteronism, a new clinical syndrome, *J Clin Lab Med* 45(1):3-17, 1955.
23. Cooper DS: Hyperthyroidism, *Lancet* 362(9382):459-468, 2003.
24. Cushing H: The basophil adenomas of the pituitary body and their clinical manifestation, *Bull Johns Hopkins Hospital* 50:137, 1932.
25. Dunnick NR, Korobkin M: Imaging of adrenal incidentalomas: current status, *Am J Roentgenol* 179:559-568, 2002.
26. Findling JW, Raff H, Aron DC: The low-dose dexamethasone suppression test: a reevaluation in patients with Cushing's syndrome, *J Clin Endocrinol Metab* 89(3):1222-1226, 2004.
27. Freda PU: Clinical review 150: somatostatin analogs in acromegaly, *J Clin Endocrinol Metab* 87(7):3013-3018, 2002.
28. Freda PU: Pitfalls in the biochemical assessment of acromegaly, *Pituitary* 6(3):135-140, 2003.
29. Hegedius L, Brix TH, Vestergaard P: Relationship between cigarette smoking and Graves' ophthalmopathy, *J Endocrinol Invest* 27(3):265-271, 2004.
30. Hollowell JG et al: Serum TSH, T_4 and thyroid antibodies in the United States population (1988-1994): National Health Nutrition Examination Survey (NHANES III), *J Clin Endocrinol Metab* 87(2):489-499, 2002.
31. Hoybye C et al: Adrenocorticotrophic hormone–producing pituitary tumors: 12- to 22-year follow-up after treatment with stereotactic radiosurgery, *Neurosurgery* 49(2):284-291, 292, 2001.
32. Jaroszewski DE et al: Laparoscopic adrenalectomy for pheochromocytoma, *Mayo Clin Proc* 78(12):1501-1504, 2003.
33. Kim AW et al: Outcome of laparoscopic adrenalectomy for pheochromocytomas vs. aldosteronomas, *Arch Surg* 139(5):526-529, 529-531, 2004.
34. Kudva YC, Sawka AM, Young WF: Clinical review 164: the laboratory diagnosis of adrenal pheochromocytoma: the Mayo Clinic experience, *J Clin Endocrinol Metab* 88(10):4533-4539, 2003.
35. Ladenson PW et al: American Thyroid Association guidelines for detection of thyroid dysfunction, *Arch Intern Med* 160(11):1573-1575, 2000.
36. Lamberts SWH, de Herder WW, van der Lely AJ: Seminar: pituitary insufficiency, *Lancet* 352(9122):127-134, 1998.
37. Lim PO, Young WF, MacDonald TM: A review of the medical treatment of primary aldosteronism, *J Hypertens* 19(3):353-361, 2001.
38. Maghnie M: Diabetes insipidus, *Hormone Res* 59(Suppl 1):42-54, 2003.
39. Mahmoud-Ahmed AS, Suh JH: Radiation therapy for Cushing's disease: a review, *Pituitary* 5(3):175-180, 2002.
40. Mansmann G et al: The clinically inapparent adrenal mass: update in diagnosis and management, *Endocrine Rev* 25(2):309-340, 2002.
41. Martino E et al: The effects of amiodarone on the thyroid, *Endocrine Rev* 22(2):240-254, 2001.
42. Mayo-Smith WW et al: State-of-the-art adrenal imaging, *Radiographics* 21:995-1012, 2001.
43. Mazzaferri EL, Kloos RT: Clinical review 128: current approaches to primary therapy for papillary and follicular thyroid cancer, *J Clin Endocrinol Metab* 86(4):1447-1463, 2001.
44. Melmed S: *The pituitary*, ed 2, Malden, Mass, 2001, Blackwell.
45. Molitch ME: Disorders of prolactin secretion, *Endocrinol Metab Clin North Am* 30(3):585-610, 2001.
46. Molitch ME: Medical management of prolactin-secreting pituitary adenomas, *Pituitary* 5(2):55-65, 2002.
47. Morello JP, Bichet DG: Nephrogenic diabetes insipidus, *Ann Rev Physiol* 63:607-630, 2001.
48. Morris DG, Grossman AB: Dynamic tests in the diagnosis and differential diagnosis of Cushing's syndrome, *J Endocrinol Invest* 26(7 Suppl):64-73, 2003.
49. Mulatero P et al: Extensive personal experience: increased diagnosis of primary aldosteronism, including surgically correctable forms, in centers from five continents, *J Clin Endocrinol Metab* 89:1045-1050, 2004.
50. National Institutes of Health: State-of-the-science statement on management of the clinically inapparent adrenal mass ("incidentaloma"), *NIH Consens Sci Statements* 19(2):1-25, Feb 4-5, 2002.

51. Neafsey PJ: Levothyroxine and calcium interaction: timing is everything, *Home Health Nurse* 22(5):338-343, 2004
52. Oertel YC: Extensive personal experience: a pathologist trying to help endocrinologists to interpret cytopathology reports from thyroid aspirates, *J Clin Endocrinol Metab* 87(4):1459-1461, 2002.
53. Pacini F et al: Prediction of disease status by recombinant human TSH-stimulated serum Tg in the postsurgical follow-up of differentiated thyroid carcinoma, *J Clin Endocrinol Metab* 86(12):5686-5690, 2001.
54. Paisley AN, Trainer PJ, Drake WM: The place of pegvisomant in the acromegaly treatment algorithm, *Growth Horm IGF Res* 12(Suppl A): S101-106, 2004.
55. Parle JV: Prediction of all-cause and cardiovascular mortality in elderly people from one low serum thyrotropin result: a 10-year cohort study, *Lancet* 358(9285):861-865, 2001.
56. Pearse EN, Farwell AP, Braverman LE: Thyroiditis, *N Engl J Med* 348(26):2646-2655, 2003.
57. Reimondo G et al: The corticotrophin-releasing hormone test is the most reliable noninvasive method to differentiate pituitary from ectopic ACTH secretion in Cushing's syndrome, *Clin Endocrinol* (Oxf) 58(6):718-724, 2003.
58. Roberts CGP, Ladenson PW: Hypothyroidism, *Lancet* 363(941):793-803, 2004.
59. Robertson GL: Antidiuretic hormone: normal and disordered function, *Endocrinol Metab Clin North Am* 30(3):671-694, 2001.
60. Rolighed L et al: Primary hyperparathyroidism: intraoperative PTH-measurements, *Scand J Surg* 93(1):43-47, 2004.
61. Sawka AM et al: Does a combination regimen of thyroxine (T_4) and 3,5,3' triiodothyronine improve depressive symptoms better than T_4 alone in patients with hypothyroidism? Results of a double-blind, randomized, controlled trial, *J Clin Endocrinol Metab* 88(10):4551-4555, 2003.
62. Schlechte JA: Prolactinoma, *N Engl J Med* 349(21):2035-2041, 2003.
63. Sclabas GM et al: Fine-needle aspiration of the thyroid and correlation with histopathology in a contemporary series of 240 patients, *Am J Surg* 186(6):702-709, 709-710, 2003.
64. Siegmund W et al: Replacement therapy with levothyroxine plus triiodothyronine (bioavailable molar ration 14:1) is not superior to thyroxine alone to improve well-being and cognitive performance in hypothyroidism, *Clin Endocrinol* (Oxf) 60(6):750-757, 2004.
65. Toft AD: Clinical practice: subclinical hyperthyroidism, *N Engl J Med* 345(7):512-516, 2001
65a. Toft AD: Thyroxine suppression therapy in Graves' disease, *Baillere's Clin Endocrinol Metabol* 11(3):537-548, 1997.
66. Tomlinson J et al: Association between premature mortality and hypopituitarism, *Lancet* 357:425, 2001.
67. van der Lely AJ et al: Long-term treatment of acromegaly with pegvisomant, a growth hormone receptor antagonist, *Lancet* 358(9295):1754, 2001.
68. Vance ML: Perioperative management of patients undergoing pituitary surgery, *Endocrinol Metab Clin North Am* 32(2):355-366, 2003.
69. Vaughan ED: Diseases of the adrenal gland, *Med Clin North Am* 88(2):443-466, 2004.
70. Verbalis JG: Management of disorders of water metabolism in patients with pituitary tumors, *Pituitary* 5(2):119-132, 2002.
71. Walsh JP et al: Thyroxine and triiodothyronine are not more effective than thyroxine alone in unselected patients with hypothyroidism, *J Clin Endocrinol Metab* 88(10):4543-4550, 2003.
72. Walther MM: Pheochromocytoma. In Rakel RE, Bope ET, editors: *Conn's current therapy,* Philadelphia, 2002, Saunders.
73. Williams JS, Williams GH: Fiftieth anniversary of aldosterone, *J Clin Endocrinol Metab* 88(6):2364-2372, 2003.
74. Young WF: Minireview: primary aldosteronism—changing concepts in diagnosis and treatment, *Endocrinology* 144(6):2208-2213, 2003.

Visit the Evolve website: http://evolve.elsevier.com/Monahan/medsurg

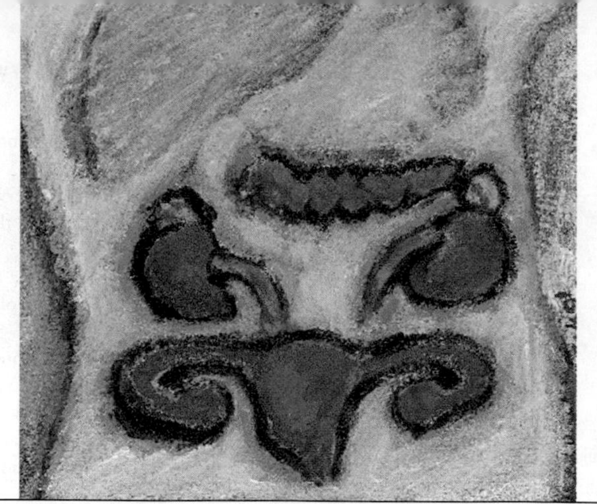

CHAPTER 39

Diabetes Mellitus and Hypoglycemia

by Margaret M. Ulchaker

OBJECTIVES

After studying this chapter, the learner should be able to:

1. Differentiate among type 1, type 2, and gestational diabetes mellitus (DM).
2. Contrast the epidemiologic and etiologic factors of type 1 and type 2 DM.
3. Differentiate the pathophysiologic bases for type 1 and type 2 DM.
4. Describe the common manifestations of uncontrolled type 1 and type 2 DM.
5. Differentiate the pathophysiology, clinical manifestations, and management of persons with diabetic ketoacidosis from those of persons with hyperglycemic hyperosmolar nonketotic coma.
6. Describe the chronic complications of DM, the relationship between metabolic control and the chronic complications, and the management of the complications.
7. Compare the comprehensive care of patients with type 1 and type 2 DM, including the roles of dietary management, education, and exercise.
8. Describe physiologic insulin regimens in type 1 DM.
9. Analyze the oral agents used in the treatment of type 2 DM in terms of mechanism of action, dosage ranges, metabolic effects, side effects, and contraindications.
10. Discuss hypoglycemia as a consequence of diabetes management, including causes, signs and symptoms, treatment, and prevention.
11. Develop a nursing care plan for an individual with stable DM.
12. Describe the surgical considerations for the individual with DM.
13. Discuss sick-day management guidelines for the individual with DM.
14. Differentiate fasting and reactive hypoglycemia on the basis of causes, clinical manifestations, and management.

KEY TERMS

albuminuria, p. 1121
counterregulatory hormones, p. 1113
euglycemia, p. 1116
gluconeogenesis, p. 1118
glucotoxicity, p. 1111
glycogenolysis, p. 1118
glycosuria, p. 1114
hypertriglyceridemia, p. 1114
insulin resistance, p. 1111
ketone bodies, p. 1118
lipolysis, p. 1114
macrovascular, p. 1116
microalbuminuria, p. 1120
microvascular, p. 1116
nephropathy, p. 1120
neuropathy, p. 1121
polyphagia, p. 1114
retinopathy, p. 1118

Diabetes Mellitus

"Diabetes mellitus is a group of metabolic diseases characterized by hyperglycemia resulting from defects in insulin secretion, insulin action, or both."[6,9] The basis of the abnormalities in carbohydrate, protein, and fat metabolism in diabetes is the deficient action of insulin on the target tissues of skeletal muscle, adipose tissue, and the liver. Uncontrolled diabetes mellitus (DM) may result in long-term damage, dysfunction, and failure of various organs. Diabetes cannot be cured, but it can be controlled.

By nature, DM can be significantly influenced by daily self-care. No other disease demands so much of the patient's self-knowledge and skills. Thus the professional nurse has the challenge and responsibility of helping patients gain the knowledge, skills, and attitudes necessary for self-care.

Standards of care for DM, both national (American Diabetes Association [ADA][6]) and international (World Health Organization, St. Vincent Declaration), have been in existence for some years. These standards of care encompass diabetes evaluation, management, and education. Despite their publication and dissemination to the health care community and patients alike, these protocols have yet to become standard practice. Fewer than 10% of patients with diabetes in the United States go to endocrinologists for diabetes care, as the standards recommend; with the declining number of endocrinologists, this percentage can only worsen. Thus primary care physicians provide the bulk of diabetes care. One way for patients to identify providers of excellent care is at the National Committee for Quality Assurance (NCQA) website, which lists physician recipients of the NCQA/ADA Provider Recognition award (www.ncqa.org/dprp). Numerous studies demonstrate a large gap between current recommendations for diabetes care and actual practice patterns of primary care physicians[42,72,82] (for one such study, see Research box below). Additionally, nurses' knowledge of diabetes is far from optimal (see Research box at right).[29] Diabetes care delivered by a dedicated specialty team has been demonstrated to confer a survival advantage of up to 15 years.[60,107]

Classification

The current diagnostic and classification system for diabetes was first published by the ADA's Expert Committee on the Diagnosis and Classification of Diabetes Mellitus in July 1997[9] (Table 39-1). This system reflects the etiology and pathophysiology of diabetes, with the two major categories being type 1 DM (previously termed *insulin-dependent diabetes mellitus* or *juvenile-onset diabetes mellitus*) and type 2 DM (previously termed *non-insulin-dependent diabetes mellitus* or *maturity-onset diabetes mellitus*).

This chapter focuses on type 1 and type 2 DM, which are the two most common types. Table 39-2 compares the characteristics of type 1 and type 2 DM. Both the categories and their characteristics are important for understanding this chapter.

Research

Putzer GJ et al: Prevalence of patients with type 2 diabetes mellitus reaching the American Diabetes Association's target guidelines in a university primary care setting, *Southern Med J* 97(2):145-148, 2004.

The researchers randomly selected charts of 218 patients with type 2 diabetes mellitus who received their diabetes care at a particular university primary care medical practice. Data were abstracted to assess the primary care physicians' abilities to attain six American Diabetes Association (ADA) treatment goals and four ADA-recommended health services. The mean number of items attained was 4.9 out of 10. The majority of patients attained goals for low-density lipoprotein cholesterol, hemoglobin A_{1c}, diastolic blood pressure, and triglyceride levels; most had received some ADA-recommended diabetes education. However, the majority of patients (1) had not had an annual microalbumin screen, (2) had not had an annual ophthalmologic evaluation, (3) had not met treatment goals for high-density lipoprotein cholesterol, (4) had not met treatment goals for systolic blood pressure, and (5) were not taking aspirin daily. Only one patient had met all 10 goals.

Further studies are needed to determine why ADA goals are not met in primary care settings. The results of this study have tremendous implications not only for day-to-day glycemic control, but also ultimately for morbidity and mortality from diabetes mellitus.

Research

El-Deirawi KM, Zuvaikat N: Registered nurses' actual and perceived knowledge of diabetes mellitus, *J Nurses Staff Dev* 17(1):5-11, 2001.

The researchers assessed the perceived versus actual knowledge of diabetes mellitus in a group of registered nurses employed at a home health agency and a community hospital. Two tools were used to assess knowledge: the Diabetes Basic Knowledge Test (DBKT) and the Diabetes Self-Report Tool. The nurses' actual and perceived diabetes knowledge was positively correlated ($r = 0.402$; $p < .0001$). However, the mean score on the DBKT was low, at 72.2%. The results of this study raise concerns about the competency of nurses who care for patients with diabetes mellitus. They also underscore the importance of nurses attaining initial knowledge of diabetes mellitus and then updating their knowledge through ongoing continuing education. Given that diabetes mellitus is a chronic disease that (1) affects a high percentage of the U.S. population, (2) carries with it such enormous morbidity and mortality, and (3) is a major public health problem in the United States, it is critical that nurses possess accurate and current knowledge of the disease.

Etiology and Epidemiology

Table 39-3 summarizes the known etiologic factors of type 1 and type 2 DM; however, our understanding of the etiology of each type of DM is still unfolding. In relation to type 1 DM, genetics seems to have a permissive role that allows environmental factors, perhaps viruses, to trigger the onset of diabetes by stimulating an autoimmune response. In regard to type 2 DM, individuals with a family history of diabetes are at high risk. Other risk factors for type 2 DM are a history of impaired glucose tolerance (IGT) or gestational DM, particularly in obese individuals. The conversion rate from IGT to type 2 DM is approximately 7% per year and varies with ethnic background. Seventy percent of individuals with prior gestational DM develop type 2 DM later in life. **Glucotoxicity**, the toxic effects of hyperglycemia on the pancreatic islets, may be another causal factor in type 2 DM. **Insulin resistance**, or the inability of the insulin-sensitive tissues (skeletal muscle, liver, and adipose tissue) to respond normally to insulin-stimulated glucose uptake, has a role in the pathogenesis of type 2 DM.

In the United States an estimated 18.2 million people (6.3% of the population) have diabetes; one third of these are undiagnosed. DM is the seventh leading cause of death by disease in the United States. The prevalence of diabetes varies with race and ethnicity, is slightly greater in women, and increases significantly with age (Table 39-4). Each year approximately 1.3 million new cases are diagnosed, 95% of which are type 2 DM. However, studies have shown that 8% to 45% of children with newly diagnosed diabetes are actually diagnosed with type 2 DM, not type 1.[17]

Figure 39-1 depicts the risks of major complications when persons with diabetes are compared with nondiabetic persons. In addition, as many as 50% of men with diabetes and 35% of

TABLE 39-1 CLASSIFICATION OF DIABETES MELLITUS AND OTHER DISORDERS OF GLUCOSE TOLERANCE

Type	Defining Characteristics
TYPE 1 DIABETES MELLITUS (DM)	
Immune mediated	Insulinopenic (insulin deficient) and dependent on exogenous insulin to sustain life Onset generally before age 30 yr, but may occur at any age, including geriatric years Generally lean, rarely obese Variable rate of beta-cell destruction Clinical presentation usually rapid In 85%-90%, one or more of following autoantibodies are present when fasting hyperglycemia is initially detected: Glutamic acid decarboxylase autoantibodies Tyrosine phosphatase IA-2 or IA-2-beta autoantibodies (specific islet cell autoantibodies) Strong human leukocyte antigen (HLA) associations Major susceptibility locus within HLA complex on chromosome 6; provides 40%-50% of the inheritable risk (HLA DR/DQ)
Idiopathic diabetes	No immunologic evidence for beta-cell destruction No HLA association Strongly inherited Most individuals affected of African or Asian origin Episodic ketoacidosis with varying degrees of insulin deficiency between episodes
TYPE 2 DM	
	Episodic absolute requirement for exogenous insulin No requirement for exogenous insulin to sustain life at least initially Ranges from a picture of predominantly insulin resistance with mild relative insulin deficiency to more severe insulin secretory defects with insulin resistance Usually obese; those not obese by traditional criteria usually have abdominal adiposity Onset usually after age 40 yr, but may occur at any age, including in obese, inactive children No autoimmune or HLA association
OTHER	
Genetic defects of beta-cell function	Previously termed *maturity-onset diabetes of youth*—impaired insulin secretion without defects in insulin action Autosomal dominant inheritance Abnormalities in three genetic loci determined to date

women with diabetes have sexual problems from neuropathy and other factors.

Diabetes is a disease that kills women more readily than men. A woman with diabetes has four times the risk of cardiovascular disease compared with her nondiabetic counterpart. A man with diabetes has only twice the risk of cardiovascular disease compared with his nondiabetic counterpart. This risk is even greater in certain minority populations. Diabetes was the sixth leading cause of death listed on death certificates in 2000. Diabetes may be underrepresented as a cause of death; reportedly, only 35% to 40% of individuals with DM have it listed in any location on the death certificate.[17]

Diabetes is a costly disease in terms of morbidity and mortality, and also in dollars and cents. In 2002 the annual total costs for diabetes in the United States were $132 billion: $92 billion in direct costs and $40 billion in indirect costs. One out of every 10 health care dollars in the United States was attributed to DM. In 2002 alone, DM was responsible for almost 88 million disability days; additionally, diabetes caused 176,000 cases of permanent disability at a cost of $7.5 billion. In the United States in 2002, the annual cost of providing health care to an individual without DM was $2560 compared with a staggering $13,243 for an individual with DM. When adjusted for age, sex, race, and ethnicity, the individual with DM had 2.4-fold higher medical expenditures than the individual without DM.[5,17]

Pathophysiology

The hallmark of diabetes is insulin deficiency, either absolute or relative. In *absolute* insulin deficiency the pancreas produces either no insulin or very little insulin, as in type 1 DM. In *relative* insulin deficiency the pancreas produces either normal or excessive amounts of insulin, but the body is unable to use it effectively and glucose levels remain elevated. This latter defect, known as insulin resistance, is seen in type 2 DM (Figure 39-2). Fundamentally, failure of the pancreas to produce enough insulin to overcome this insulin resistance precipitates clinical type 2 DM in predisposed individuals.

TABLE 39-1 CLASSIFICATION OF DIABETES MELLITUS AND OTHER DISORDERS OF GLUCOSE TOLERANCE—CONT'D

Type	Defining Characteristics
OTHER—CONT'D	
Genetic defects in insulin action	No distinguishing characteristics
Diseases of exocrine pancreas	Pancreatitis, trauma, infection, pancreatectomy, pancreatic carcinoma, cystic fibrosis, hemochromatosis
Endocrinopathies	Acromegaly, Cushing's syndrome, glucagonoma, pheochromocytoma
Drug induced	Permanent destruction of beta cells (Vacor [rat poison], intravenous pentamidine) Impairment of insulin action (nicotinic acid, glucocorticoids, thiazide diuretics) Impairment of insulin secretion, thereby precipitating DM in individual with insulin resistance (e.g., drug-induced hypokalemia)
Infections	Congenital rubella, cytomegalovirus
Uncommon forms: immune mediated	Stiff-man syndrome, antiinsulin receptor antibodies
Genetic syndromes associated with DM	Turner's syndrome, Down syndrome, Klinefelter's syndrome
Gestational DM	Pregnancy related
Prediabetes	Affects an estimated 41 million people in United States (NOTE: Some have both IGT and IFG.)
Impaired glucose tolerance (IGT)	Glucose levels higher than normal but do not meet diagnostic criteria for DM Affects an estimated 16 million people in United States ages 40-74 Generally obese Approximately 7% per year progression to overt type 2 DM; higher in some ethnic populations Insulin resistant and at increased cardiovascular risk
Impaired fasting glucose (IFG)	Fasting glucose levels higher than normal but lower than those in IGT or DM Affects an estimated 35 million people in United States ages 40-74

Adapted from American Diabetes Association: Clinical practice recommendations 2004, *Diabetes Care* 27(Suppl1):S1-S150, 2004; Centers for Disease Control and Prevention: *National diabetes fact sheet: general information and national estimates on diabetes in the United States 2002,* Atlanta, 2003, US Department of Health and Human Services, Centers for Disease Control and Prevention; Pugliese A: Genetics of type 1 diabetes, *Endocrinol Metab Clin North Am* 33(1):1-16, 2004.

This absolute or relative insulin deficiency results in significant abnormalities in the metabolism of body fuels. The body needs fuel for all its functions, including growth and repair of tissues. The fuel comes from ingested food, which is composed of carbohydrates, proteins, and fats. It is important to emphasize to patients that diabetes is not a disease of glucose alone, although diagnostic criteria use the plasma glucose level as the marker for diagnosis and control of the disease. Because the most common word used in the diabetes vocabulary is *sugar,* some patients with longstanding or new diabetes believe that eliminating sugar from the diet means the battle is won. Nurses must help patients understand that diabetes is a disease that affects how the body utilizes all foods (carbohydrates, fats, and proteins).

Hormones. The hormones involved in glucose metabolism include those from the pancreas (insulin and glucagon) (Table 39-5), pituitary gland (growth hormone and adrenocorticotropic hormone), adrenal cortex (cortisol), autonomic nervous system (norepinephrine), and adrenal medulla (epinephrine) (Table 39-6). Insulin is the only hormone that lowers blood glucose levels. The other hormones, called **counterregulatory hormones**, elevate blood glucose levels. Insulin is synthesized by the beta cells in the islets of Langerhans within the pancreas. Insulin ensures that the body is able to use glucose for energy. Insulin binds to insulin receptors on the surface of the insulin-sensitive tissues (skeletal muscle, liver, and adipose tissue). In response, a cascade of events (postreceptor events) allows glucose to move from the bloodstream into the cell. Adiponectin is the only adipocytokine that enhances insulin sensitivity. Low levels of adiponectin have been shown to be predictive of the development of type 2 DM and coronary artery disease.

Consequences of Insulin Deficiency: Absolute or Relative. The insulin-requiring organs are the liver, skeletal muscle, and adipose tissue. Of these, the liver is the most insulin sensitive. The consequences of either absolute or relative insulin deficiency at the level of these organs are (1) liver—hyperglycemia, hypertriglyceridemia, and ketone production; (2) skeletal muscle—failure of glucose uptake and amino acid uptake; and (3) adipose

TABLE 39-2 CHARACTERISTICS OF TYPE 1 AND TYPE 2 DIABETES MELLITUS

Characteristic	Type 1 Diabetes Mellitus	Type 2 Diabetes Mellitus
Insulin status	Insulin secretion increased	Insulin secretion increased, decreased, or normal
Age	Usually under 30 yr but may occur at any age	Usually over 40 yr but may occur at any age
Clinical presentation	Rapid	Slow
Body build	Lean or normal usually	80%-90% overweight
Family history	Weak	Strong
Autoantibodies to glutamic acid decarboxylase and tyrosine phosphatase IA-2 or IA-2-beta	Sensitivity 96.7 % for development of type 1 DM	Absent
Human leukocyte antigen association	Positive (DR/DQ)	Negative
Incidence	10% of total	90% of total
Symptoms	Polyuria, polydipsia, polyphagia, weight loss	No symptoms or may have same symptoms as type 1 May have symptomatic complications when diagnosed
Ketones	Prone	Resistant except during infection or with stressors
Complications	Related to degree and duration of hyperglycemia Not present at time of diagnosis	Related to degree and duration of hyperglycemia May be present at diagnosis in 20% or more of cases because of delay in diagnosis
Treatment	Insulin, diet, exercise	Diet, exercise, oral agents, insulin
Racial distribution	More common in Caucasians	More common in African-Americans and Hispanics Highest in Native Americans

Adapted from American Diabetes Association: Clinical practice recommendations 2004, *Diabetes Care* 27(Suppl):S1-S150, 2004; Pugliese A: Genetics of type 1 diabetes, *Endocrinol Metab Clin North Am* 33(1):1-16, 2004; Redondo MJ et al: Heterogeneity of type 1 diabetes: analysis of monozygotic twins in Great Britain and the United States, *Diabetalogia* 44(3):354-362, 2001; Verge CF et al: Late progression to diabetes and evidence for chronic beta-cell autoimmunity in identical twins of patients with type 1 diabetes, *Diabetes* 44(10):1176-1179, 1995.

tissue—uncontrolled **lipolysis** resulting in elevated free fatty acid levels in the circulation (Figure 39-3). This situation is worsened by the consumption of dietary carbohydrate, which is metabolized into glucose and fails to be used by the liver and skeletal muscle, with resultant progressive hyperglycemia (elevated blood glucose levels) and **glycosuria** (abnormal amounts of glucose in the urine).

When the blood glucose level reaches the renal threshold (approximately 180 mg/dl) in normal kidneys, the kidneys cannot keep up with resorbing the glucose from the glomerular filtrate, and glycosuria results. Glucose attracts water, and an osmotic diuresis occurs, resulting in *polyuria* (increased urination). This polyuria results in the loss of water and electrolytes, particularly sodium, chloride, potassium, and phosphate. The loss of water and sodium results in thirst and increases fluid intake *(polydipsia)*. Losses of electrolytes such as potassium, magnesium, and phosphorus occur with the osmotic diuretic effect of glycosuria. Extreme hunger and increased food intake **(polyphagia)** are triggered as the cells become starved of their fuel. In type 1 DM this cycle of glucose loss in the urine and the inability to use glucose for energy results in rapid weight loss. Patients with type 2 DM generally do not have sufficient insulin deficiency to result in pathologic ketosis and major weight loss. In both types of DM, dehydration and electrolyte disturbance lead to fatigue and listlessness.

Serum lipids (triglycerides, very-low-density lipoproteins, and sometimes cholesterol) may be elevated. Serum ketones may also be elevated. Total body levels of electrolytes (sodium, potassium, chloride, phosphate) can be depleted, even though the serum levels may be elevated (e.g., hyperkalemia). This results from transcellular shifts secondary to acidosis (from ketones). The severity of this altered metabolism depends on the severity of the absolute or relative insulin deficiency. Early recognition of symptoms and diagnosis (before dehydration, weight loss, and ketogenesis) is best achieved by increased awareness of diabetes among both the public and health care professionals.

In mildly insulin-deficient conditions, altered glucose metabolism with hyperglycemia and glycosuria may occur only after meals. Glucose levels and protein metabolism may be normal in the fasting state. As the deficiency increases in severity, hyperglycemia, glycosuria, and protein catabolism are present all the time. Altered lipid metabolism resulting in elevated levels of triglycerides (**hypertriglyceridemia**) occurs even in mildly insulin-deficient states. Abnormally high production of ketones may be seen only in markedly insulin-deficient states, usually in persons with type 1 DM.

If the alterations just described are not corrected or adequately controlled, acute and chronic complications can occur. Acutely,

TABLE 39-3 ETIOLOGIC FACTORS IN TYPE 1 AND TYPE 2 DIABETES MELLITUS

Factor	Type 1 Diabetes Mellitus	Type 2 Diabetes Mellitus
Genetic	Human leukocyte antigen (HLA) association (particularly DR/DQ genes)	Not associated with HLA antigens
Heredity	Unknown Familial aggregates rare Less than 50% concordance in monozygotic twins Greater risk for child to develop type 1 if father has type 1 (6%) than if mother has type 1 (3%)	Unknown except for class of genetic defects of beta-cell destruction, which is inherited dominantly
Autoimmune basis	Strong autoimmune basis as seen by: Insulitis (inflammation of islets of Langerhans with lymphocytic infiltration) Presence of autoantibodies to tyrosine phosphatase IA-2 or IA-2-beta (specific islet cell autoantibodies), insulin, or glutamic acid decarboxylase	None
Environmental basis	Viral infections possible environmental trigger; as counterregulatory hormones increase in response to stress of illness, islets unable to respond with needed increased insulin secretion to maintain euglycemia	Modern lifestyle of poor eating and nutritional habits and inactivity resulting in obesity, providing stimuli for those who are predisposed

Adapted from American Diabetes Association: Clinical practice recommendations 2004, *Diabetes Care* 27(Suppl1):S1-S150, 2004; Pugliese A: Genetics of type 1 diabetes, *Endocrinol Metab Clin North Am* 33(1):1-16, 2004; Redondo MJ et al: Heterogeneity of type 1 diabetes: analysis of monozygotic twins in Great Britain and the United States, *Diabetalogia* 44(3):354-362, 2001; Verge CF et al: Late progression to diabetes and evidence for chronic beta-cell autoimmunity in identical twins of patients with type 1 diabetes, *Diabetes* 44(10):1176-1179, 1995.

TABLE 39-4 PREVALENCE OF DIABETES BY RACE AND ETHNICITY

Race and Ethnicity	Diagnosed
Non-Hispanic Caucasian Americans	8.4% of all ≥ 20 yr of age
Non-Hispanic African-Americans	11.4% of all ≥ 20 yr of age 25% of those 65-74 yr of age
Latinos	8.2% of all ≥ 20 yr of age
Mexican Americans	24% of those 45-74 yr of age
Puerto Ricans	26% of those 45-74 yr of age
Cuban Americans	16% of those 45-74 yr of age
Native Americans	
Overall population receiving health care from Indian Health Service	14.5%
Alaskan Natives	6.8%
Native Americans in Southeast United States	27%
Pima Indians of Arizona	50% of those 30-64 yr of age; highest rate of diabetes mellitus in world
Japanese and Filipino residents of Hawaii	2 times more likely than non-Hispanic Caucasians of similar age living in Hawaii
Other Pacific Islanders/Asian Americans	Limited data available, but some subgroups have high risk

Adapted from American Diabetes Association: *Diabetes statistics*, accessed July 2004 from website: www.diabetes.org/statistics; Centers for Disease Control and Prevention: *National diabetes fact sheet: general information and national estimates on diabetes in the United States 2002*, Atlanta, 2003, US Department of Health and Human Services, Centers for Disease Control and Prevention.

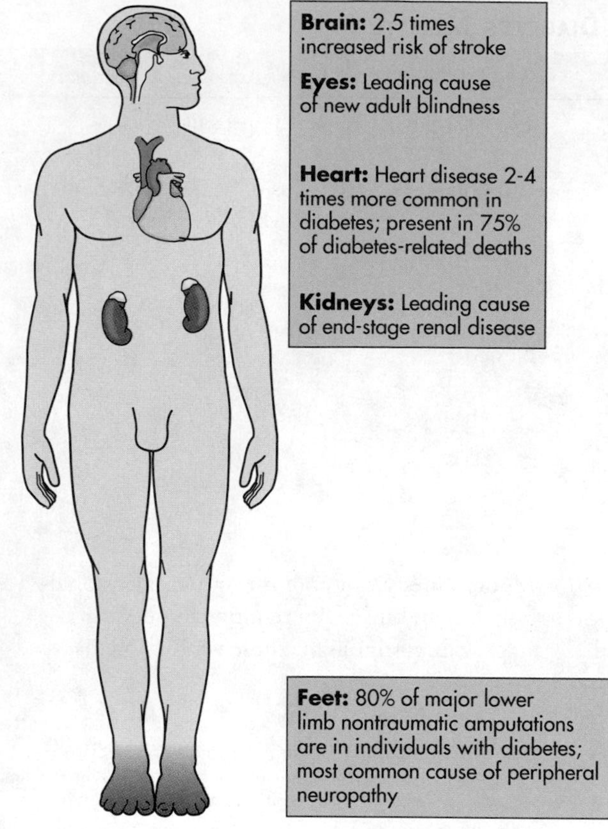

Figure 39-1 Diabetes complications.

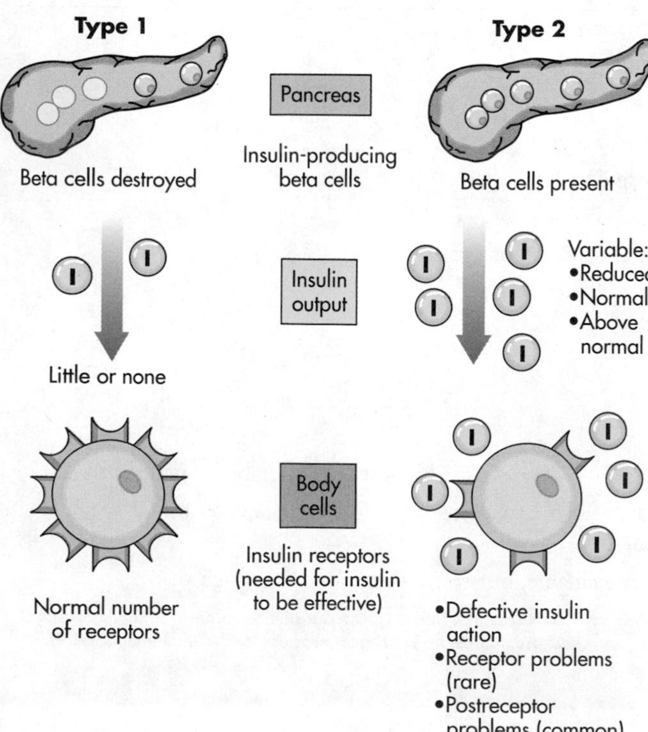

Figure 39-2 Insulin defects in type 1 and type 2 diabetes mellitus.

the patient can develop nausea, vomiting, and other alterations; fluid and electrolyte problems worsen; and the patient's condition can advance to hyperglycemic hyperosmolar nonketotic coma (HHNC) or diabetic ketoacidosis (DKA). The mortality rate in DKA approaches 10%, and the mortality rate in HHNC reaches 70%. Chronically, the patient can develop **microvascular** (small blood vessel) and **macrovascular** (large blood vessel) complications or neuropathy.

The classic symptoms of diabetes are polyuria, polydipsia, and polyphagia. These "polys" are nearly always present in individuals with newly diagnosed type 1 DM and can be present in individuals with newly diagnosed type 2 DM (see Clinical Manifestations box). However, many persons with type 2 DM have subtle symptoms of acute metabolic changes or chronic complications.

When differentiating between type 1 and type 2 DM, clinicians can readily classify most individuals on the basis of age, body weight, and family history. Some elements of a patient's history may make diagnosis difficult (e.g., age 30 to 40 years, unavailable family history [adopted], and weight loss to less than 120% of ideal body weight). However, an understanding of the basic pathophysiology readily clarifies the situation. Glutamic acid decarboxylase antibodies and/or pancreatic islet cell antibodies are positive in 85% to 90% of type 1 DM patients, and insulin levels are low or subnormal (see Tables 39-1 to 39-3). In a patient already being treated with insulin (before a definitive diagnostic classification), a C-peptide level can provide clarification of endogenous insulin production. A molecule of C peptide is generated when the insulin precursor molecule proinsulin, produced in the islet cells, is converted to insulin. Hence for every molecule of insulin secreted by the pancreatic islets, a molecule of C peptide is produced.

An important clue to the correct classification of type 2 DM patients is the presence of other components of the dysmetabolic syndrome—a syndrome encompassing varying degrees of glucose intolerance, hypertension, hypertriglyceridemia, low levels of high-density lipoprotein (HDL) cholesterol, abdominal obesity, hyperuricemia, and elevated levels of plasminogen activator inhibitor type 1. All these factors are mediated and modulated by the control of insulin resistance.[74-76] Insulin resistance essentially blocks the normal uptake of glucose into insulin-sensitive tissues. The earliest abnormality in glucose metabolism occurs in skeletal muscle as insulin-mediated glucose uptake decreases. A compensatory hyperinsulinemia develops as the pancreatic islets increase production and secretion of insulin in an effort to maintain **euglycemia** (normal blood glucose levels). Eventually, pancreatic

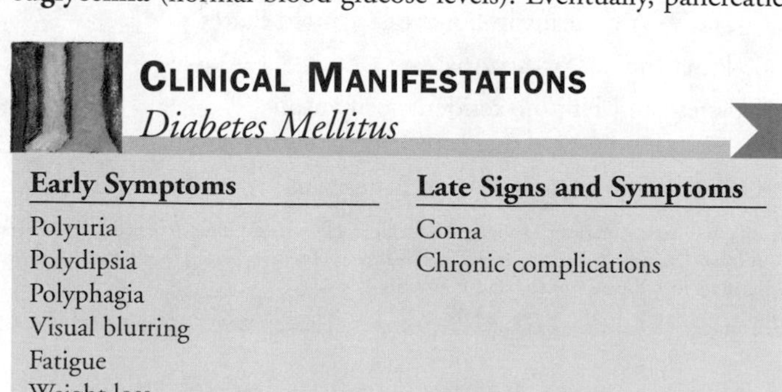

CLINICAL MANIFESTATIONS
Diabetes Mellitus

Early Symptoms	Late Signs and Symptoms
Polyuria	Coma
Polydipsia	Chronic complications
Polyphagia	
Visual blurring	
Fatigue	
Weight loss	

TABLE 39-5 EFFECTS OF PANCREATIC HORMONES

Insulin Promotes, Glucagon Inhibits	Insulin Inhibits, Glucagon Promotes
Glucose uptake into skeletal muscle and liver	Hyperglycemia
Glycogenesis (glycogen synthesis)	Gluconeogenesis (conversion of amino acids into glucose) Glycogenolysis (glycogen breakdown)
Protein anabolism (protein synthesis)	Protein catabolism (protein breakdown)
Lipogenesis (fat synthesis and deposition)	Lipolysis (fat breakdown)

NOTE: Insulin is the only hormone that lowers blood glucose levels.

TABLE 39-6 EFFECTS OF EXTRAPANCREATIC GLUCOSE-ELEVATING HORMONES

Cortisol	Catecholamines	Growth Hormone
Gluconeogenesis	Gluconeogenesis	Gluconeogenesis
Lipolysis	Lipolysis	Lipolysis
Secretion controlled by pituitary adrenocorticotropic hormone; deficiency or excess affects glucose control	Inhibits insulin release	Decreases glucose uptake into skeletal muscle

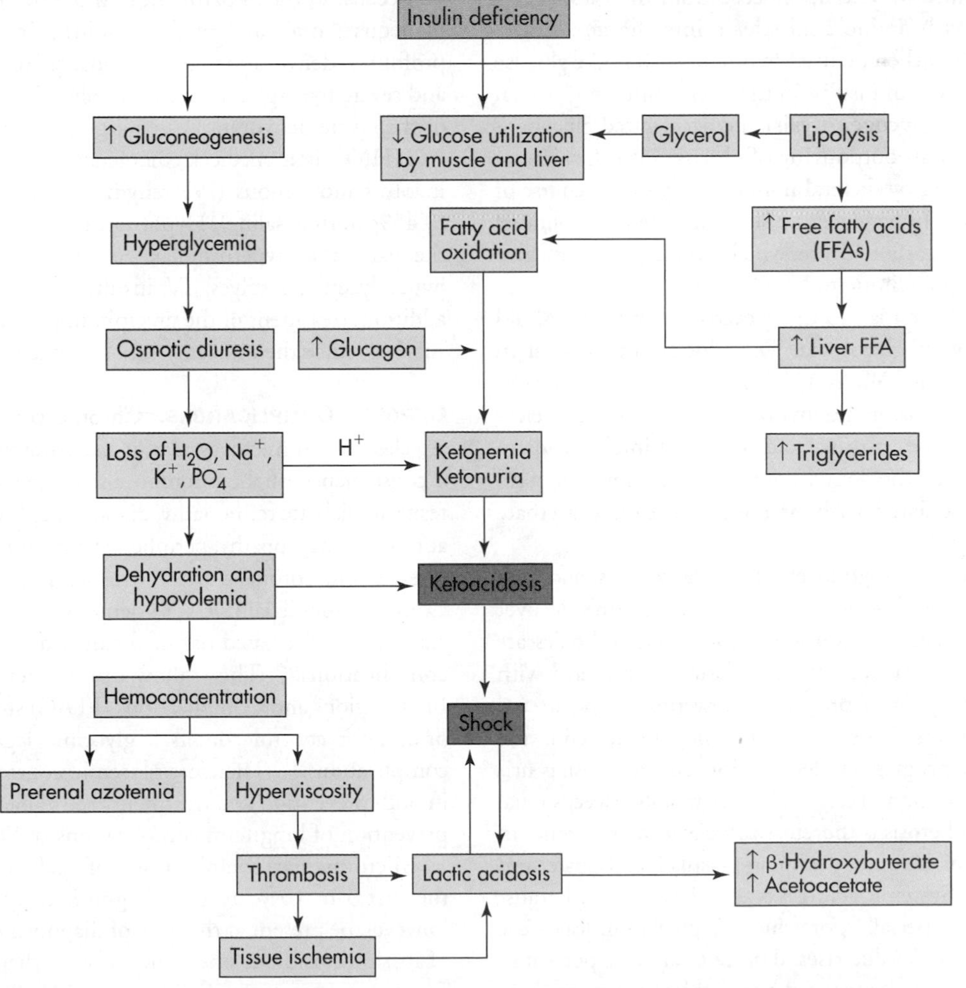

Figure 39-3 Pathophysiology of insulin deficiency. *H_2O*, Water; *Na^{++}*, sodium; *K^+*, potassium, *PO_4^-*, phosphate; H^+, hydrogen.

exhaustion occurs, and the necessary insulin production falls off. Once the pancreas is no longer able to secrete enough insulin to overcome the insulin resistance, type 2 DM occurs. Progressive loss of beta cell (the insulin-producing cells in the pancreatic islets of Langerhans) mass and function is typical of type 2 DM.

Complications. The complications of diabetes are classified as acute or chronic. Acute complications include hypoglycemia, DKA, and HHNC. Information on hypoglycemia in individuals with diabetes is presented later in the chapter. Cigarette smoking increases the risk of the development and progression of every known complication of DM. Aggressive attempts at smoking cessation are critical.

Acute Complications

Diabetic Ketoacidosis. DKA is the extreme consequence of severe insulin deficiency at the insulin-sensitive tissues: adipose tissue, skeletal muscle, and liver (see Figure 39-3). DKA can be precipitated by illness or omission of insulin. Lack of insulin in adipocytes results in failure to suppress lipolysis, with resultant release of free fatty acids into the circulation and weight loss. The free fatty acids in turn serve as a substrate for the liver to synthesize triglyceride and ketone bodies. Lack of insulin in skeletal muscle results in failure to take up glucose from the plasma and protein catabolism with amino acid release into the circulation. These amino acids may then be used by the liver to make glucose **(gluconeogenesis)**. Lack of insulin in the liver results in glycogen breakdown to glucose **(glycogenolysis)** and accelerated gluconeogenesis. This results in an outpouring of glucose into the circulation that cannot be used by skeletal muscle. Early in the course of insulin deficiency, this hyperglycemic state may be compounded by ingestion of dietary carbohydrate, which gets digested into glucose and is unable to be eliminated.

Progressive hyperglycemia rapidly exceeds the renal threshold for glucose, resulting in glycosuria. The blood glucose level in hyperglycemia may be as high as 1500 mg/dl. Glycosuria acts as an osmotic diuretic, resulting in dehydration, with water and electrolyte losses. An increase in thirst and oral fluid intake tends to minimize the severity of the dehydration early on; however, nausea and vomiting associated with progressive ketosis exacerbate the dehydration.

With insulin deficiency, high levels of free fatty acids, and high levels of counterregulatory hormones (especially glucagon), the liver produces excessive amounts of **ketone bodies**. Ketone bodies are acidic and must be cleared from the circulation or buffered with alkali (bicarbonate) to prevent progressive lowering of the arterial pH and systemic acidosis. Early on, the ketones are cleared in the urine; however, with progressive dehydration and decreasing urinary output, the production of ketone bodies rapidly exceeds renal clearance. Progressive ketosis is therefore associated with ketones in the urine, rising plasma ketones, declining plasma bicarbonate, and declining arterial pH. Systemic acidosis is also associated with transcellular shifts of ions, especially potassium, as potassium leaves the cells and serum potassium value rises, despite total body potassium depletion. Potassium depletion caused by renal losses may be compounded by gastrointestinal losses (vomiting and diarrhea).

Failure to recognize emerging and worsening DKA results in progressive dehydration, ketosis, acidosis, circulatory collapse, tissue hypoxia, and shock. The advent of tissue hypoxia results in lactate accumulation and lactic acidosis, which dramatically increase the mortality rate.

Treatment of DKA involves rehydration, insulin administration, and electrolyte repletion (see Guidelines for Safe Practice box). Each medical institution has its own protocol for DKA management.

Hyperglycemic Hyperosmolar Nonketotic Coma. HHNC is the acute complication of type 2 DM. The pathophysiology and clinical issues are similar to those of DKA, with the following exceptions. In HHNC:

- Dehydration is profound, with fluid deficit as high as 8 to 9 L.
- The degree of hyperglycemia is greater, with serum glucose levels in the range of 600 to 2000 mg/dl.
- The serum osmolarity is 350 mOsm/L or higher.
- Sufficient ketosis is absent because individuals with type 2 DM have insulin secretion to prevent ketosis.
- An underlying central nervous system problem (e.g., cerebrovascular disease) is usually present, which impairs the patient's thirst perception.
- A concurrent illness is usually present.

Because of the impairment in thirst perception, the patient has inadequate oral fluid intake, resulting in the primary defect of profound dehydration. As a consequence, hemoconcentration and severe hyperglycemia occur. Polyuria disappears early because of the severe dehydration. Lethargy and somnolence may result.

HHNC is a medical emergency. The primary management involves intravenous (IV) rehydration with hypotonic solutions (0.45% normal saline). Hypotonic solutions are indicated because the patient is hyperosmolar. As the patient is rehydrated, the hyperglycemia resolves. IV insulin is generally not needed. In addition, treatment of the precipitating illness is critical to patient survival, since the mortality rate approaches 70%.

Chronic Complications. Chronic complications of diabetes are classified as microvascular or macrovascular. These changes are a consequence of the duration and degree of hyperglycemia and result in diabetic retinopathy, diabetic nephropathy, peripheral and autonomic neuropathy, peripheral vascular disease, cerebrovascular disease, and coronary artery disease. The Diabetes Control and Complications Trial (DCCT) demonstrated that intensive therapy resulted in a decreased risk of the development and progression of complications.[24] The follow-up Epidemiology of Diabetes Interventions and Complications (EDIC) study demonstrated that prior poor control confers a glycemic legacy for microvascular complications.[114] Therefore glycemic control should be a priority in both prevention and treatment. See Table 39-7 for discussion of prevention of long-term complications of DM.

Microvascular complications of diabetes rarely occur within the first 5 to 10 years after diagnosis of type 1 DM. They may, however, be present at the time of diagnosis of type 2 DM because of its slow, insidious onset and delay in diagnosis.

Microvascular Complications

Diabetic Retinopathy. Diabetic **retinopathy** is the leading cause of new blindness among adults 20 to 74 years of age in the United

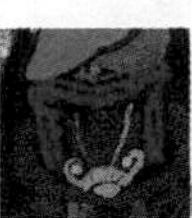

GUIDELINES FOR SAFE PRACTICE *Diabetic Ketoacidosis (DKA): Management Principles and Priorities*

Monitoring

Fingerstick blood glucose determinations every hour
Serum potassium initially and then every hour
Bicarbonate initially and then every 2 hours
Arterial blood gas studies initially and then every 2 to 4 hours
Electrocardiogram initially and then as needed
Additional monitoring depending on patient status: continuous cardiac tracing, central venous pressure, Swan-Ganz catheter, nasogastric intubation, and indwelling urinary catheter
Intake and output monitoring

Intravenous Rehydration

Fluid deficit possibly in excess of 6 L
Normal saline at 500 ml/hr for the first hour, then 250 ml/hr
Avoidance of hypotonic solutions (0.45% normal saline) because they may increase the risk of cerebral edema

Intravenous (IV) Regular Insulin

IV regular insulin is given to control gluconeogenesis, lipolysis, and ketogenesis and to promote skeletal muscle glucose uptake.
It should be given as constant infusion, starting at rate of 0.1 unit/kg body weight. If IV volume is not a concern (i.e., congestive heart failure), a more dilute solution is easier to titrate. Dilute as 50 ml regular insulin in 500 ml normal saline; then 1 unit = 10 ml. Titrate drip hourly by 0.1-unit (1-ml) increments until glucose reaches goal of 70 to 150 mg/dl.
IV bolus of regular insulin has a half-life of 5 minutes and is of no value.
When the patient begins to take oral fluids with carbohydrates, additional insulin must be given subcutaneously to match the carbohydrate load.
When the patient is recovering and ready to eat, resume routine insulin program. Do not discontinue IV insulin infusion until 2 hours after subcutaneous insulin dosage to prevent loss of control of hepatic glucose output and disposal.

Electrolyte Repletion

Give IV potassium once renal output is established.
—If serum potassium is 3 mEq/L or less, give 40 to 60 mEq/hr.
—If serum potassium is 3 to 4 mEq/L, give 30 mEq/hr.
—If serum potassium is 4 to 5 mEq/L, give 20 mEq/hr.
—If serum potassium is 6 mEq/L or more, withhold potassium replacement until serum potassium is less than 6 mEq/L.
If necessary, give half as potassium chloride and half as potassium phosphate to also replace phosphate losses.
Patient may need magnesium replacement depending on serum values.
IV bicarbonate is indicated only if arterial pH is 7.0 or less and patient has complicating medical problems such as hypotension, shock, or dysrhythmia. If given, it should be by slow IV infusion. Goal is an arterial pH 7.0 or more. Concern with bicarbonate is association with the potentially fatal complication of cerebral edema.

White Blood Count With Differential

Leukocytosis may be present. Determine whether leukocytosis is indicative of underlying sepsis or is the leukocytosis with left shift that is commonly seen in DKA.

Treatment of Underlying Cause (Sepsis, Myocardial Infarction)

In a patient with diabetes who acutely loses glycemic control, silent myocardial infarction must be ruled out.

Patient Education

Prevention and early intervention
Mortality risk of DKA

States. Between 12,000 and 24,000 new cases of blindness from diabetic retinopathy occur each year.[17] A diagnosis of diabetic retinopathy results in an elevenfold increased risk of blindness compared with the risk in the general population. The DCCT[24] demonstrated that intensive therapy resulted in a statistically significant decreased risk of development and progression of retinopathy. Good visual acuity does not exclude significant retinopathy.

The earliest lesion is the microaneurysm in the retinal vessels. Having one dot-blot hemorrhage results in a twentyfold increased risk of blindness compared with the general population. Soft exudates ("cotton-wool spots") are areas of ischemia in the retina resulting from reduced retinal blood flow. Hard exudates are deposits of lipid on the retina, resulting from leaking retinal blood vessels. Early retinal changes (background retinopathy) may progress to a more serious state, proliferative retinopathy.[31,88]

Proliferative retinopathy, or neovascular disease, results when the ischemic retina responds with the formation of new, fragile blood vessels on the retina. These fragile vessels bleed, causing vitreous hemorrhage (hemorrhage into the vitreous fluid of the eye) and sometimes retinal detachment. This hemorrhage can be repetitive and lead to permanent visual loss. Early laser photocoagulation to seal off the leaking retinal vessels to preserve vision is now the standard treatment, based on the results of the Diabetic Retinopathy Study (DRS).[25] The DRS demonstrated a 60% reduction in severe visual loss with the use of argon laser treatment. However, laser photocoagulation does destroy some normal retina in the process; peripheral vision and night vision are most affected. Without laser photocoagulation, progressive hemorrhage and subsequent blindness are inevitable. Laser photocoagulation is an outpatient surgical procedure performed in the ophthalmologist's office.

In severe cases the extent of vitreous hemorrhage necessitates a vitrectomy, where surgical instruments are placed into the eyeball and the hemorrhagic fluid removed by suction and replaced with fluid. This inpatient surgical procedure is also vision preserving.[31,88] (See Chapter 61 for further discussion of vitrectomy.)

Macular edema can occur in nonproliferative or proliferative disease. The macula is the part of the retina responsible for central vision. Macular edema and loss of vision result from the leaking of fluid and lipid into the macula of the eye. The Early

TABLE 39-7 PREVENTION OF LONG-TERM COMPLICATIONS OF DIABETES MELLITUS

Complication	Early Detection	Early Intervention
Retinopathy	Annual dilated funduscopic examination	Care by an ophthalmologist or retinal specialist Control of hyperglycemia Control of hypertension
Nephropathy	Annual examination of urine for albumin or protein excretion Measurement of serum creatinine and creatinine clearance	Control of hyperglycemia Control of hypertension and other cardiovascular risk factors Limiting protein intake Avoiding nephrotoxic agents
Atherosclerosis	History of risk factors and symptoms Examination: electrocardiogram and serum lipid measurements, peripheral pulses, ankle-brachial indices, assessment for carotid bruits	Control of hyperglycemia Control of hypertension Weight control Exercise Control of lipids
Neuropathy	History of symptoms of pain, numbness, paresthesias, etc. Examination: orthostatic blood pressures, muscle strength, reflexes, sensory function	Control of hyperglycemia Avoidance of neurotoxic agents Education about importance of routine evaluation, foot care, and specific treatment of neuropathy
Foot problems	History of symptoms of numbness, infection, and peripheral vascular insufficiency Complete foot examination Ankle-brachial indices	Control of hyperglycemia Control of atherogenic risk Education about importance and methods of foot care Referral to podiatrist Referral for orthotics or custom shoes

Treatment Diabetic Retinopathy Study established the benefit of laser photocoagulation in macular edema with a 50% reduction in severe visual loss.[27]

The ADA recommends an annual ophthalmic examination for early detection, diagnosis, and treatment of retinopathy.[6] One goal of *Healthy People 2010* is to increase the proportion of adults with diabetes who have an annual dilated eye examination to 75%.[101,108] The DCCT demonstrated that intensive therapy resulted in a significant decrease in the risk of development and progression of diabetic retinopathy.[24] In addition, blood pressure control is critical, since hypertension accelerates the development and progression of retinopathy.

Diabetic Nephropathy. Diabetic **nephropathy** is the leading cause of end-stage renal disease in the United States, accounting for approximately 43% of new cases. Twenty percent of all persons with diabetes have nephropathy. In 2000 alone, 41,046 individuals with DM began treatment for end-stage renal disease. Unless aggressively treated, nephropathy rapidly progresses and may result in end-stage renal disease, requiring dialysis, transplantation, or both. In 2000, 129,183 persons with diabetes underwent dialysis or transplantation treatment.[17]

The characteristic renal lesion is nodular glomerulosclerosis, or Kimmelstiel-Wilson syndrome. This syndrome involves nodular masses of laminated hyaline material that occur randomly throughout the kidney and is associated with proteinuria, edema, and hypertension. Kimmelstiel-Wilson lesions are seen only in DM and occur in 10% to 35% of individuals with DM.[61]

Laboratory abnormalities of renal disease generally do not occur until 10 years or more after the onset of type 1 DM,[43] but they may be present at diagnosis in persons with type 2 DM. The natural history of diabetic nephropathy begins with early glomerular hypertrophy and hyperfiltration with an elevated glomerular filtration rate. Microscopic amounts of albumin in the urine, or **microalbuminuria**, is the earliest laboratory abnormality and is asymptomatic. Microalbuminuria can be assessed via a radioimmunoassay on either

Healthy People 2010

Objectives Related to Diabetes Mellitus

- Prevent diabetes: reduce new cases to 2.5 per 1000 people per year (age-adjusted baseline: 3.5 new cases per 1000 people in 1994 to 1996) and reduce the overall rate of diabetes that is clinically diagnosed to 25 overall cases per 1000 people (age-adjusted baseline: 40 overall cases, including new and existing cases, of diabetes per 100,000 people).
- Reduce complications among people with diabetes: end-stage renal disease, blindness, and lower extremity amputation.
- Reduce deaths from cardiovascular disease in persons with diabetes to 309 deaths per 100,000 persons with diabetes (age-adjusted baseline: 343 per 100,000 persons with diabetes).
- Reduce the diabetes death rate to no more than 45 deaths per 100,000 people (age-adjusted baseline: 75 per 100,000 in 1997) and the diabetes-related death rate to 7.8 per 1000 persons with diabetes (age-adjusted baseline: 8.8 per 1000 persons with diabetes listed anywhere on the death certificate in 1997).

From US Department of Health and Human Services: *Healthy people 2010: understanding and improving health*, Washington, DC, 2000, The Department.

a spot or a timed urine collection. Microalbuminuria is present if the urinary albumin level is greater than or equal to 30 mcg/mg creatinine on a random urine specimen or if the excretion rate is 20 mcg/min (30 mg/24 hr) on a timed specimen.[23] Dipstick results are much less accurate. The development and progression of microalbuminuria can be reduced through meticulous glucose control[24] and blood pressure control, especially with angiotensin-converting enzyme (ACE) inhibitors.

Microalbuminuria has additional significance, since it increases the risk for retinopathy and autonomic neuropathy. Microalbuminuria has poor prognostic implications in regard to both cardiovascular disease and mortality in both type 1 and type 2 DM patients.[2]

Microalbuminuria may progress to **albuminuria** or clinical proteinuria (300 mg albumin/24 hr, which is equivalent to 500 mg total protein/24 hr) and end-stage renal disease. Proteinuria also has poor prognostic implications in terms of cardiovascular disease and the mortality rate in both type 1 and type 2 DM patients.[45] Renal disease, even at this point, can remain asymptomatic, detectable only by objective measures. Glycemic control still plays a role in reducing risks of progression. The ADA recommends an annual laboratory examination for urinary albumin and protein.[6]

Hypertension is the factor that most often accelerates diabetic nephropathy. Aggressive blood pressure control decreases the rate of deterioration and improves survival.[11] Studies demonstrate that in a person with diabetes, the lower the blood pressure within the normal range, the lesser the albuminuria.[61]

ACE inhibitors also have an important role in clinical proteinuria. The U.S. Food and Drug Administration (FDA) approved the ACE inhibitor captopril for use in patients with clinical proteinuria to slow progression to end-stage renal disease, even in the absence of hypertension.[59] The use of ACE inhibitors in microalbuminuria is well studied with promising results, and FDA approval is pending. The angiotensin receptor blockers irbesartan and losartan have been shown to retard the progression of nephropathy in patients with type 2 DM.[22,55]

Reduction in dietary protein intake may be of additional benefit, although clinical trials have not been conclusive. In patients with renal disease, a restriction of protein to 0.8 mg/kg actual body weight is recommended.[33]

The ADA recommends annual screening for albuminuria, beginning at the time of diagnosis in individuals with type 2 DM and after 5 years' DM duration in individuals with type 1. One of three methods may be used for screening: measurement of the albumin-to-creatinine ratio on a random spot urine collection, a timed overnight urine albumin and creatinine collection, or a 24-hour urine test for albumin, creatinine, and creatinine clearance.

Diabetic Neuropathy. Diabetic **neuropathy** affects 60% to 70% of individuals with diabetes.[17] The most common forms of neuropathy are peripheral and autonomic (Table 39-8).

Symmetric sensory peripheral polyneuropathy. In symmetric sensory peripheral polyneuropathy, sensory changes and subsequent sensory loss occur symmetrically in a glove-and-stocking distribution. The lower extremities are generally affected first because they contain the longest nerves in the body; upper extremity involvement may follow. Comprehensive assessment of neuropathy is critical because most patients with mild to moderate neuropathy are asymptomatic; even the patient with severe damage can remain asymptomatic.

The health care provider should perform a thorough neurologic examination assessing sensation, vibration, and deep tendon reflexes. Routine assessment with a monofilament is widely performed during follow-up examinations. However, monofilament testing assesses only a patient's risk of foot ulceration. Once a patient has an abnormal monofilament examination, extensive nerve damage has already occurred. When patients do get symptoms of neuropathy, they can experience abnormal sensations such as paresthesias, numbness, and pain. Pain can range from minimal in the toes to sharp, stabbing, lancinating pain in a glove-and-stocking distribution. Abnormal sensations tend to worsen in the evening and may make it difficult for the patient to fall asleep. Even the light pressure of the bed sheet may be uncomfortable. Commonly patients are unaware of sensory loss, so proper foot care is critical. In addition to sensory involvement, motor neurons may also be affected. The impairments occur slowly and are progressive.[16]

Painful peripheral neuropathy. The glove-and-stocking distribution of pain is common in persons with painful peripheral neuropathy (PPN). Patients may exhibit loss of vibratory sense, increased or decreased temperature sensation, loss of fine motor skills, and gait changes resulting from dorsiflexion weakness. Pain management of PPN involves antidepressants, anticonvulsants, and topical agents such as capsaicin cream. Other medications used include clonidine and mexiletine. Gabapentin is perhaps the most commonly used agent, although its use is not FDA approved. Opioids are not generally recommended because of their suboptimal effect in treating chronic pain and concerns about the potential for addiction. Nonpharmacologic therapies include heat and cold, massage, relaxation, biofeedback, physical therapy, and psychotherapy. See Chapter 50 for further discussion of PPN.

Autonomic neuropathy. Damage to the autonomic nervous system may also occur, resulting in alterations in many body systems (see Table 39-7). An easy and quick assessment of autonomic function is the R-R trend analysis in response to deep breathing and Valsalva's maneuver using a special electrocardiograph machine. A patient with intact autonomic function has great variability in the heart rate with deep breathing and Valsalva's maneuver. Patients with autonomic neuropathy lose that heart rate variability. A patient may experience none, some, or all of the dysfunctions. Commonly the only symptom is fatigue with exercise resulting from an inability to increase the heart rate to increase cardiac output. Another common symptom is dizziness on postural change.[109]

Autonomic neuropathy carries a poor prognosis, with up to a 50% 5-year mortality rate, generally because of silent ischemia resulting in silent myocardial infarctions or cardiac dysrhythmias.[46,58,111,113] Improvement in glycemic control can improve autonomic function.[35]

Other neuropathies. Cranial nerve palsies (of cranial nerves III, IV, VI, and VII) occur more commonly in persons with diabetes than in those without. The onset is acute, and the course

TABLE 39-8 CLASSIFICATION OF DIABETIC NEUROPATHY

Type	Signs and Symptoms
Peripheral sensory polyneuropathy	Classic symmetric glove-and-stocking distribution Paresthesia Hyperesthesia Pain (characteristics vary; may be sharp, stabbing, lancinating, aching, etc.) with nocturnal intensification Loss of sensation to pinprick, vibration, temperature Loss of deep tendon reflexes Muscle wasting and weakness
Autonomic	Orthostatic hypotension Cardiac denervation Anhidrosis Gustatory sweating Gastroparesis, with delayed gastric emptying, nausea, emesis Diarrhea Bladder atony Erectile dysfunction
Mononeuropathy	Cranial nerve palsy (III, IV, VI, and VII) Ulnar nerve palsy Carpal tunnel syndrome
Amyotrophy	Acute anterior thigh pain or numbness Weakness to hip flexion on examination Quadriceps wasting
Radiculopathy	Follows dermatomal distribution on trunk Paresthesia Hyperesthesia Pain Numbness

is self-limiting. Ulnar nerve palsies may be a result from a mononeuritis of acute onset or from nerve entrapment. Carpal tunnel syndrome is twice as common in individuals with diabetes as in nondiabetic individuals (see Chapter 53 for further discussion). Diabetic amyotrophy (muscle wasting and weakness) is an acute event involving anterior thigh numbness or pain, which can be excruciating. Quadriceps muscle wasting and resultant weakness on hip flexion may occur within a few days. No specific diagnostic tests are indicated. Supportive therapy with analgesics and maintenance of walking are critical. Amyotrophy generally resolves spontaneously in 6 to 8 weeks, although severe cases may persist up to 6 to 12 months.

MACROVASCULAR COMPLICATIONS. Statistics of macrovascular disease comparing diabetic with nondiabetic individuals are stunning. Cardiovascular disease is two to four times more prevalent in persons with diabetes and is responsible for approximately 75% of diabetes-related deaths. Middle-aged persons with diabetes have coronary disease death rates two to four times higher than those of their nondiabetic peers. The stroke risk in persons with diabetes is two to four times higher.[17]

Individuals with diabetes develop the same macrovascular changes as those without diabetes. However, in persons with diabetes, these changes occur at an earlier age, are more severe, and are more extensive in the vascular tree. Patients with type 2 DM have a higher rate of macrovascular changes than those with type 1 DM.[83] Risk factors that must be aggressively addressed include dyslipidemia and hypertension.[6,37]

A unifying hypothesis in microalbuminuria, albuminuria, proteinuria, and cardiovascular disease and mortality is the Steno hypothesis. The Steno hypothesis is based on the common cause, which appears to be endothelial dysfunction in a multitude of vascular beds in the body, with the resultant end-stage disease depending on the vascular bed involved.[23] A large family study of type 2 DM in Finland and Sweden showed that of all of the individual components of the metabolic syndrome, microalbuminuria confers the strongest risk of cardiovascular death.[45]

Dyslipidemia. Dyslipidemia affects an estimated 50% of people with diabetes. Elevated low-density lipoprotein (LDL) cholesterol, elevated triglycerides, and low HDL cholesterol are risk factors for atherosclerosis. Because of insulin resistance, the lipid profile in the patient with type 2 DM is commonly characterized by hypertriglyceridemia and low HDL cholesterol level with varying degrees of hypercholesterolemia.[6] The LDL is characteristically of the small, dense variety, which is more prone to oxidation and has enhanced atherogenic potential. In type 1 DM, lipid disorders are generally seen only if the patient has a familial dyslipidemia or renal disease. Evidence-based medical data from clinical trials support aggressive screening, diagnosis, and treatment of dyslipidemia and the use of statins in individuals with DM to reduce cardiovascular events and mortality rates.[41,73, 81,84,87]

Hypertension. Hypertension affects approximately 70% of adults with diabetes. Hypertension in the patient with type 1 DM implies renal disease, microalbuminuria, or proteinuria, until proven otherwise. In contrast, hypertension in the patient with type 2 DM can either be a result of coexistent renal disease or be essential hypertension. Regardless of the etiology, blood pressure must be aggressively monitored and hypertension diagnosed early because it exacerbates retinopathy, nephropathy, and macrovascular disease. In the individual with DM, hypertension is diagnosed at a blood pressure of 130/85 mm Hg. The goal blood pressure is less than 130/80 mm Hg, or lower in patients with nephropathy.[64]

Lifestyle modification (weight loss, sodium restriction, exercise) should be the primary modality of treatment. When this fails, the pharmacologic agent chosen should be metabolically neutral (i.e., not worsen insulin resistance or dyslipidemia or cause electrolyte disturbance). ACE inhibitors are the antihypertensives of choice, unless contraindicated. The Heart Outcomes Prevention Evaluation (HOPE) trial demonstrated a reduced risk of microvascular and macrovascular events in individuals with DM treated with the ACE inhibitor ramipril.[39,40] In patients intolerant of ACE inhibitors because of cough, angiotensin receptor blockers are good alternatives in light of data showing they decrease proteinuria. Beta-blockers have an important role in the post–myocardial infarction/angina patient and in the patient with heart failure. Calcium channel blockers are effective in lowering blood pressure and specifically reduce the risk of stroke.[48] The benefits of beta-blockade in these patients outweigh the theoretic problems of masking hypoglycemia, delaying recovery from hypoglycemia, and worsening insulin resistance. The majority of patients with diabetes require multiple antihypertensives to meet blood pressure goals.[6]

The Diabetic Foot. Three major factors play a role in the diabetic foot: neuropathy, ischemia, and sepsis. Diabetes is responsible for more than 60% of major lower limb nontraumatic amputations in the United States. From 2000 to 2001, approximately 82,000 nontraumatic amputations were performed in individuals with DM in the United States.[17]

Sensory impairment leads to painless trauma and the potential for ulceration. Motor impairment contributes to wasting of intrinsic muscles in the feet, resulting in foot deformity. Foot deformities alter the normal gait and pressure distribution. Friction and resultant callosities may develop and cause pressure necrosis and ulceration. Complete foot off-loading is critical to fully heal neuropathic ulcers.[13,14] Painless trauma can result in fractures in the ankle or forefoot and ultimately in significant deformity known as Charcot's (or neuropathic) arthropathy. Anhidrosis (decreased or absent sweat secretion) as a manifestation of autonomic neuropathy can result in excessive dryness and cracking of the skin, which also contributes to infection. Macrovascular and microvascular alterations produce tissue ischemia and may lead to sepsis. This triad of neuropathy, ischemia, and sepsis can result in gangrene and ultimately amputation.[13,14,16] Aggressive glycemic control and hospitalization for IV antibiotics to limit the spread of infection are necessary. Amputation of affected toes is often necessary. The area must be kept dry to prevent wet gangrene. Wet gangrene is gangrene coupled with inflammation; septicemia and shock may occur.

Podiatric care is critical to attaining and maintaining foot health. Proper toenail trimming and the use of orthotic, extra-depth, extra-width, or custom-molded shoes can prevent ongoing trauma and ultimately amputation associated with the diabetic foot.[15]

Collaborative Care Management

In the past, patients with diabetes were often hospitalized to initiate management. Hospitalization now occurs only if the patient experiences acute metabolic decompensation. Patients need to establish goals with their health care team members for management of their diabetes. Collaborative care focuses on:

- Using diagnostic tests to determine the presence of DM or complications (microvascular or macrovascular)
- Establishing goals related to the level of daily control
- Using medications, treatments, diet, and activities to manage diabetes on a day-to-day basis
- Using medications, treatments, and diet to manage acute and chronic complications of diabetes
- Working as a multidisciplinary team

Achievement and maintenance of metabolic control requires the judicious use of medications, diet, activity, monitoring, and education.

Diagnostic Tests. Diagnostic criteria for diabetes are found in Box 39-1. Frequent monitoring of diagnostic tests (blood glucose, lipids) is a method of assessing glycemic control.

The definition of *control* has changed dramatically over the years. Before the discovery of insulin in 1921, control was defined as the avoidance of early death or coma. The current definition is normalcy—normalization not only of glucose levels but also of other metabolic parameters, such as lipids and blood pressure (Table 39-9).

The relationship between glycemic control and microvascular complications of diabetes was debated for years, despite evidence of a definite relationship.[55,56,70] The control and complications issue, however, was proved beyond doubt in 1993 when results of the 10-year, nationwide, DCCT were published.[24] The DCCT, a clinical trial of over 1400 persons with type 1 diabetes, compared conventional therapy with intensive therapy consisting of three or more insulin injections daily or insulin pump therapy, random home blood glucose monitoring (HBGM) before meals and at bedtime, and a more precise carbohydrate-consistent meal plan. The intensive therapy group had a statistically significant reduction in both development and progression of microvascular complications (Table 39-10). The DCCT found that the lower the hemoglobin A_{1c} (HbA_{1c}) (a marker of diabetes control), the lower the risk of complications. As a result of this landmark study, the ADA recommends intensive therapy for all individuals with type 1 DM, with few exceptions, such as advanced age and end-stage complications.[6]

The EDIC study, a continuation of the DCCT, highlighted the surprising finding that 4 years after switching patients from conventional therapy to intensive therapy, better glycemic control did not reverse the damaging metabolic cascade initiated by prior poor glycemic control. The EDIC study concluded that intensive

Box 39-1 Diagnostic Criteria for Diabetes Mellitus, Impaired Glucose Tolerance, Impaired Fasting Glucose, and Gestational Diabetes Mellitus

Nonpregnant Adults

Diabetes Mellitus

Diagnosis of diabetes mellitus in nonpregnant adults should be restricted to those who have one of the following:

- Fasting plasma glucose level of 126 mg/dl. *Fasting* is defined as no caloric intake for at least 8 hours.
- Symptoms of diabetes mellitus (such as polyuria, polydipsia, unexplained weight loss) coupled with a casual plasma glucose level of 200 mg/dl. *Casual* is defined as any time of day, without regard to the time interval since the last meal.
- Two-hour postprandial plasma glucose level of 200 mg/dl during an oral glucose tolerance test. The test should be performed according to World Health Organization criteria, using a glucose load containing the equivalent of 75 g of anhydrous glucose dissolved in water.

In the absence of unequivocal hyperglycemia with acute metabolic decompensation, these criteria should be confirmed by repeat testing on a second occasion. The oral glucose tolerance test is not recommended for routine clinical use. A normal hemoglobin A_{1c} (HbA_{1c}) does not rule out the presence of diabetes, since the earliest defect is in postprandial control. Hence the HbA_{1c} is not part of the diagnostic package.

Impaired Glucose Tolerance

Diagnosis is made with a 2-hour postprandial plasma glucose level of 140 mg/dl to 200 mg/dl during an oral glucose tolerance test. The test should be performed according to World Health Organization criteria, using a glucose load containing the equivalent of 75 g of anhydrous glucose dissolved in water.

Impaired Fasting Glucose

This diagnosis requires a fasting plasma glucose level between 100 and 126 mg/dl.

Gestational Diabetes

After an oral glucose load of 100 g, gestational diabetes is diagnosed if two plasma glucose values equal or exceed:

- Fasting: 95 mg/dl
- 1 hour: 180 mg/dl
- 2 hour: 155 mg/dl
- 3 hour: 140 mg/dl

Adapted from American Diabetes Association: Clinical practice recommendations 2004, *Diabetes Care* 27(Suppl 1):S1-S150, 2004.

Table 39-9 Goals for Control: Normalization of Metabolic Parameters

Time	Levels
TARGET BLOOD GLUCOSE LEVELS IN NONPREGNANT STATE: EUGLYCEMIA	
Fasting	70-100 mg/dl
1 hour postprandially	< 120 mg/dl
2-4 AM	70-100 mg/dl
TARGET LIPID LEVELS (ADULTS)*	
Total cholesterol	< 200 mg/dl
High-density lipoprotein cholesterol	> 50 mg/dl in women, > 40 mg/dl in men
Triglycerides	< 150 mg/dl
Low-density lipoprotein cholesterol	< 70 mg/dl
TARGET BLOOD PRESSURE (ADULTS)†	< 130/80 mm Hg

*Grundy SM et al, for Coordinating Committee of the National Cholesterol Education Program: Implications of recent clinical trials for the National Cholesterol Education Program Adult Treatment Panel III Guidelines, *Circulation* 110(2):227-239, 2004. NOTE: These guidelines are the result of expert panel and do not reflect data from randomized clinical trials and evidence-based medicine.

†National High Blood Pressure Education Program Working Group: National High Blood Pressure Education Program Working Group report on hypertension in diabetes, *Hypertension* 23(2):145-158, 159, 1994.

therapy should be initiated as soon as is safely possible after the onset of type 1 DM.[114]

The control and complications issue in type 2 DM was answered by two clinical trials. Intensive therapy for type 2 DM, however, involves different regimens, aimed at both reducing insulin resistance and augmenting insulin secretion or replacing insulin. The Kumamoto study of intensive insulin therapy in type 2 DM patients demonstrated a statistically significant relationship between control and complications.[65] The United Kingdom Prospective Diabetes Study (UKPDS), a 20-year prospective study in type 2 DM, demonstrated that both intensive glycemic control and intensive blood pressure control reduced the risk of microvascular and macrovascular complications of DM (see Research boxes).[93-98] Despite the weight of all of this evidence, glucose control for the majority of patients remains suboptimal and is indeed worsening.[18]

Blood Parameters

Short-Term Control. HBGM is a critical component of the treatment regimen for patients with either type 1 or type 2 DM. Glucose levels are "vital signs" to persons with diabetes. HBGM is the only accurate method of monitoring glucose control on a

TABLE 39-10 REDUCTION IN COMPLICATION RISK WITH INTENSIVE THERAPY

Complication	Risk Reduction (%)
Clinically significant retinopathy	76
Severe retinopathy, laser surgery	45
Microalbuminuria	35
Albuminuria	56
Clinically significant neuropathy	60

Data from Diabetes Control and Complications Trial Research Group: The effect of intensive treatment of diabetes on the long-term complications in insulin-dependent diabetes mellitus, *N Engl J Med* 329:977, 1993.

Research

UK Prospective Diabetes Study Group: Association of glycaemia with macrovascular and microvascular complications of type 2 diabetes (UKPDS 35): prospective observational study, *BMJ* 321:405, 2000.

The United Kingdom Prospective Diabetes Study (UKPDS), conducted at 23 centers in England, Scotland, and Northern Ireland, was a prospective clinical trial of the intensive control of blood glucose and blood pressure in patients with newly diagnosed type 2 diabetes. A total of 4585 Caucasian, Asian Indian, and African-Caribbean subjects participated in the trial. In the glucose control part of the study, subjects were randomized to groups treated with conventional therapy (diet and exercise) versus intensive therapy (sulfonylureas, metformin, or insulin treatment). The UKPDS concluded that intensive glucose therapy resulted in a reduced risk of development of diabetic complications. In addition, complete data were obtained on 3642 subjects to enable analysis in the epidemiologic portion of the trial, which analyzed the effect of lowering hemoglobin A_{1c} on the risk of developing complications.

daily basis and allows the person with diabetes to make any necessary changes in the diabetes regimen. Results should be recorded in a logbook. Minimally, nonpregnant individuals with type 1 DM should perform HBGM before meals and at bedtime. Patients using an insulin pump perform HBGM up to 12 or more times per day. The frequency of HBGM in type 2 DM patients is determined by the treatment regimen and varies from once to several times per day. Postprandial HBGM is critical even in the diabetic patient with a normal HbA_{1c}. Approximately 50% of persons with diabetes who have a normal HbA_{1c} have a 2-hour postprandial glucose level in excess of 200 mg/dl. The higher the HbA_{1c}, the more likely it is that a patient will have an elevated postprandial glucose level. Unfortunately, according to *Healthy People 2010*, only 42% of persons with diabetes 18 years of age or older perform HBGM at least once daily.[101,108] A recent study demonstrated that the provision of free glucose monitoring supplies by a health maintenance organization to enrollees with DM improved the frequency of HBGM, medication compliance, and glycemic control.[90]

HBGM uses capillary whole blood obtained by a fingerstick and correlates well with laboratory values when accurate techniques are used. Plasma glucose values are approximately 10% higher than whole blood values (see Guidelines for Safe Practice box). The

Research

UK Prospective Diabetes Study Group: Association of systolic blood pressure with macrovascular and microvascular complications of type 2 diabetes (UKPDS 36): prospective observational study, *BMJ* 321:412, 2000.

Of the 4585 subjects in the glucose control study, 4801 Caucasian, Asian Indian, and African-Caribbean subjects were eligible for the blood pressure control study. Of these, complete data were obtained on 3642 subjects to enable analysis in the epidemiologic part of the study. A total of 1148 patients with hypertension were randomized to groups with tight blood pressure control (less than 150/85 mm Hg) versus less tight blood pressure control (less than 180/105 mm Hg) using a beta-blocker or an angiotensin-converting enzyme (ACE) inhibitor. Additional agents were prescribed as necessary to meet the blood pressure goals.

The intensively treated group had a significant decrease in risk of events compared with the conventionally treated group. However, regardless of whether a subject was in the intensive treatment or the conventional treatment group, for every 10 mm Hg decrease in systolic blood pressure, the following risk reductions were noted:

Complication	Risk Reduction (%)	p-Value
Any diabetes endpoint	12	<0.0001
Diabetes-related death	17	<0.0001
All-cause mortality	12	<0.0001
Myocardial infarction	12	<0.0001
Cerebrovascular accidents	19	<0.0001
Peripheral vascular disease	16	<0.0001
Microvascular complications	13	<0.0001
Congestive heart failure	15	<0.0001

There was no threshold at which a lower blood pressure did not reduce complications; the lower the systolic blood pressure, the lower the risk of complications. The trial also noted that beta-blockers and ACE inhibitors may have additional benefits in reducing complications over and above those related to lowering blood pressure.

For every 1% reduction in the mean hemoglobin A_{1c} (HbA_{1c}), the following risk reductions were noted:

Complication	Risk Reduction (%)	p-Value
Any diabetes endpoint	21	<0.0001
Deaths related to diabetes	21	<0.0001
Myocardial infarction	14	<0.0001
Microvascular complications	37	<0.0001

There was no threshold of diabetes control for risk reduction: no level below which a lower HbA_{1c} did not result in a lower risk of complications, nor a level above which a higher HbA_{1c} did not result in a higher risk of complications. In other words, the lower the HbA_{1c}, the lower the risk of complications.

majority of available glucose meters use a "no blot" technique—the user does not blot or wipe the blood off the test strip. The user inserts a test strip into the meter and applies a drop of capillary blood to the strip, which is impregnated with either glucose oxidase or another chemical. A chemical reaction occurs, and the meter displays the result. Test time varies among manufacturers, ranging from 5 to 45 seconds. All marketed glucose meters must be approved by the FDA and yield accurate results when proper technique is used. Meters must be calibrated to each test strip lot according to manufacturers' specifications. The most common source of errors in HBGM results is user technique, followed by problems with the test strips. Because a chemical is embedded in the test strip, any factors that can affect the chemical (light, heat, cold, humidity) will alter the result. Use of control solution is the only way to test the accuracy of the strips. Control solution, produced by the meter's manufacturer, is glucose solution in a known concentration that yields a standard result. Unfortunately, control solution is often not readily available in pharmacies and is an additional cost to the individual, the insurance company, or both.

Alternate site testing (the use of anatomic sites other than the fingertips) is FDA approved for certain blood glucose meters. Blood glucose results from alternate site testing do *not* correlate with fingerstick blood glucose results when blood glucose levels are rapidly changing, such as postprandially and when the patient is hypoglycemic. Therefore patients should always monitor blood glucose via a fingerstick postprandially or if they suspect hypoglycemia. Alternate site testing can be accurately used in the fasting and premeal states.[30,54,57] Many patients have difficulty obtaining an adequately sized sample from alternate sites, most commonly the forearm. Additionally, because a larger aperture in the lancing device is needed to obtain an alternate site sample, and pressure is placed on the anatomic site, areas of skin puncture and erythema can develop, which can be cosmetically displeasing.

A continuous glucose monitoring system, the Medtronic CGMS System Gold, measures interstitial glucose every 5 minutes for 72 hours. The system consists of a sensor that is inserted subcutaneously in the abdomen and a reading device that is worn at the waist. Fingerstick blood glucose levels are used to calibrate the device before use and then at least four times daily to provide reference points for comparison. To obtain the most valuable data analysis, the patient should also enter into the system meal times, exercise, etc. The system does not provide a real-time display of blood glucose levels; data are downloaded to a computer and then retrospectively analyzed. The CGMS System Gold is currently not available for purchase and daily use by individuals with diabetes. Another system, the GlucoWatch G2 Biographer, monitors interstitial blood glucose levels. The watchlike device uses alkaline batteries to create a low electrical current that wicks interstitial fluid into sensors on the underside of the device. Skipped readings are common because of glitches such as the device being bumped, excessive perspiration, or rapid temperature changes. The displayed readings are approximately 17 minutes behind capillary readings because of the delay in compartmentalization of glucose. Mild to moderate skin irritation occurs as a result of the wicking process. The GlucoWatch G2 Biographer is FDA approved for trend detection in glucose levels, not to replace HBGM. Fingerstick blood glucose readings must be done every 12 hours to calibrate a new sensor, and should be done anytime medication is taken or hypoglycemia is suspected, since the GlucoWatch is not FDA approved for adjusting doses. The GlucoWatch G2 biographer retails for approximately $875, with the disposable autosensors costing about $150 for 16 autosensors.

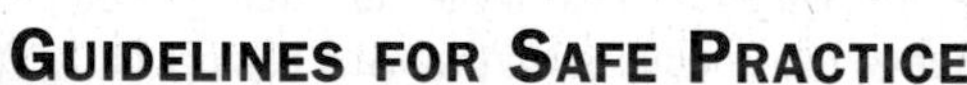

GUIDELINES FOR SAFE PRACTICE

Procedure for Capillary Blood Glucose Monitoring

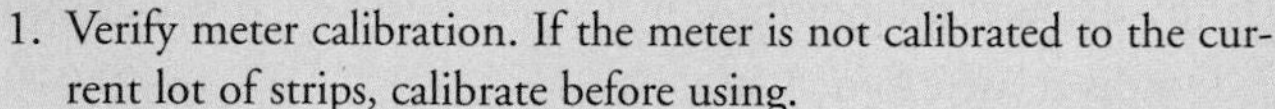

1. Verify meter calibration. If the meter is not calibrated to the current lot of strips, calibrate before using.
2. Use control solution when opening a new box or bottle of test strips or any time the glucose result does not make sense in the context of the clinical setting.
3. Cleanse finger with either soap and water or alcohol. If alcohol is used, wait for the finger to dry.
4. Place lancet in a fingerstick device.
5. Prick finger.
6. Gently squeeze finger to obtain an adequate sample of blood. NOTE: If alcohol was used to cleanse the finger, discard the first drop of blood.
7. Follow manufacturer's instructions to perform the test.
8. Discard lancet, cap of lancing device, and any other part of the equipment that may have been contaminated by blood in a hazardous waste receptacle.
9. Record glucose result, noting date, time, result, and action taken.

LONG-TERM CONTROL. Long-term glycemic control is achieved by monitoring HbA_1C, which reflects the average blood glucose level over a period. Glucose in the blood readily attaches to hemoglobin. Once attached, it remains so throughout the life span of the erythrocyte (90 to 120 days). The HbA_{1c} provides an objective measure of control and is not influenced by age, sex, duration of diabetes, or recent blood glucose levels. The HbA_{1c} reflects glycemic control over the past 3 months but can be affected by hemoglobin variants, such as hemoglobin S found in sickle cell anemia. High-performance liquid chromatography reveals patients with variants. The HbA_{1c} should be used in conjunction with HBGM results to assess glycemic control. Unfortunately, in the United States the majority of individuals with diabetes fall far short of having the ADA-recommended quarterly HbA_{1c} measurements; only 24% of individuals with diabetes have an HbA_{1c} measurement done at least once per year.[101,108]

URINE PARAMETERS

GLUCOSE MONITORING. Urine glucose monitoring should not be used to assess glycemic control. Glucose spills into the urine when serum glucose reaches the renal threshold (approximately 180 mg/dl). A urine glucose result always gives retrospective data, never current blood glucose levels. It only reflects blood glucose levels hours before, when the renal threshold is exceeded.

KETONE MONITORING. Individuals with type 1 DM should perform ketone monitoring when ill and when HBGM results exceed 300 mg/dl. Ketone monitoring is performed by using test strips impregnated with acetoacetate, which are dipped into the urine. Test time varies, depending on the manufacturer. Negative results are indicated by a beige color on the test strip. Urine ketones are positive at the trace level; as ketone levels rise, the color turns to deeper shades of purple. The Precision Xtra is a combination blood glucose and blood ketone meter. Blood ketone monitoring is useful for children and persons with insulin pumps, who can become rapidly ketotic at lower than typical glucose levels. Patients who are color blind cannot accurately read urine ketone strips. In persons with type 1 DM, the presence of ketones in the blood or urine is a dangerous sign and requires prompt attention to insulin, diet, and fluid intake to avoid DKA. Individuals with type 2 DM should monitor ketones during periods of illness. Ketones can be present in a type 2 DM patient with significant hyperglycemia, hypertriglyceridemia, dehydration, or electrolyte depletion. As with type 1 DM, positive ketones require prompt attention.

ANKLE-BRACHIAL INDICES. Ankle-brachial indices (ABIs) are part of clinical recommendations for assessment of vascular disease and risk.[67] The nurse places a sphygmomanometer cuff of appropriate size on the upper arm and, using a handheld Doppler, auscultates the systolic pressure at the radial artery. This procedure is repeated for the opposite arm. Then, with a cuff of appropriate size placed on the lower leg proximal to the ankle, the nurse auscultates systolic pressure at both the dorsalis pedis and the posterior tibial pulses.[8] The nurse repeats the procedure on the opposite leg and calculates an index for each pedal site (ankle pressure divided by brachial artery pressure).

An index greater than 1.2 indicates calcific disease. Calcification of blood vessels is a common consequence of longstanding diabetes, which may be complicated by hypertension and dyslipidemia. An index below 0.9 signifies diminished blood flow and implies arterial disease. Abnormal results require a complete noninvasive lower extremity evaluation consisting of segmental pressures, pneumoplethysmography, and photoplethysmography. The clinical importance of an ABI extends beyond the peripheral arterial tree; a reduced ABI is a marker of systemic cardiovascular risk. An isolated reduced posterior tibial index carries a threefold higher risk of all-cause mortality and a fourfold higher risk of coronary heart disease mortality.[20]

Medications and Treatments.

Type 1 DM and type 2 DM are two separate and distinct pathophysiologic entities, and their pharmacologic treatment regimens differ significantly.

TYPE 1 DIABETES MELLITUS: INSULIN. Treatment of type 1 DM involves a triad: insulin, diet, and exercise. Because type 1 DM is characterized by insulinopenia, physiologic insulin replacement is the first management component. The discovery of insulin, an "extract of pancreatic origin," by Banting and Best in 1921 and treatment of the first patient that same year occupy a major place in medical history. Insulin products over the years have become increasingly pure and plentiful.[12,85]

PROPERTIES OF INSULIN. Three properties of insulin preparation are identified in the prescription: source, strength, and type or kinetics. Animal-source insulins, extracts from pancreata of pigs or cows, have been discontinued from the U.S. market. Human insulin is derived by recombinant deoxyribonucleic acid (DNA) technology (Humulin from *Escherichia coli;* Novolin from *Saccharomyces cerevisiae* [bakers' yeast]). The strength of insulin in the United States is U-100: 100 units of insulin per milliliter of volume. A rare patient requiring very large doses of insulin may need U-500 insulin, which must be specially ordered. Insulins used to treat diabetes are detailed in Table 39-11.[69]

Insulins differ in their speed of onset, peak, and duration of action and are classified as rapid acting, intermediate acting, or long acting. Dietary carbohydrate and activity must be coordinated with insulin action so that (1) insulin is available for optimal metabolism when the food that was eaten is absorbed, and (2) food is available while insulin is acting to prevent hypoglycemic reactions. Regular insulin and intermediate-acting insulins (NPH and Lente) require that the patient eat a supplemental snack of 15 g of carbohydrate to match the peak action of the insulin (e.g., a 10 AM snack after a 7 AM injection of regular insulin). When the insulin prescription is changed, careful patient monitoring is necessary to identify the clinical effect.

▶ ARE You READY?

The nurse administers 10 units of regular insulin and 12 units of NPH insulin at 7 AM. At what time is the patient most susceptible to hypoglycemia related to the NPH insulin?

1. 8 AM
2. 4 PM
3. 8 PM
4. 11 PM

PHYSIOLOGIC REPLACEMENT OF INSULIN

Normal Glucose Metabolism. In a person without diabetes, insulin is secreted by the pancreas in two fashions: basal and prandial (Figure 39-4). Insulin is secreted in a basal fashion in the fasting state and between meals to control hepatic glucose output and disposal. In persons without diabetes who live a "day life" (awake during the day and asleep at night), counterregulatory hormones are at their nadir between midnight and 2 AM; therefore blood glucose levels are at their lowest point. After 3 to 4 AM the counterregulatory hormones rise, causing an increase in hepatic glucose output, which can continue until 10 or 11 AM. In a nondiabetic person, to maintain euglycemia, the pancreas responds by increasing secretion of insulin by approximately 50%. This is the concept of "the happy liver"—the liver needs to "see" insulin continuously to control glucose output and production in the fasting state. Prandial insulin is secreted by the nondiabetic pancreas in response to the ingestion of dietary carbohydrate. Native prandial insulin is secreted biphasically, with the first phase or peak occurring in 1 minute and the second phase or peak occurring in 60 minutes. First-phase insulin secretion serves to shut off hepatic glucose output in the context of an anticipated glucose load from a meal. The pancreas tailors the amount of insulin to the amount of carbohydrate ingested.

Intensive Insulin Therapy Regimens. The challenge in the treatment of type 1 DM is physiologic insulin replacement: one must "think like a pancreas." Joslin aptly described the challenge: "Everyone knows it requires brains to live long with diabetes, but to use insulin successfully requires more brains."[47]

Intensive therapy using multiple daily insulin injections has become the gold standard since the publication of the DCCT. Conventional therapies, which use once- and twice-daily insulin

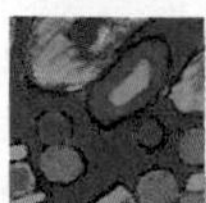

TABLE 39-11 COMMON INSULINS *for Diabetes Mellitus*

Type	Onset (hr)	Peak (hr)	Duration (hr)	Retarding Agent	Appearance
Rapid Acting					
Analogs					
Aspart	0-0.2	0.75-1.5	3-4	None	Clear
Lispro	0-0.2	1	3	None	Clear
Insulin					
Regular	0.5	2.5-3.5	6-8	None	Clear
Intermediate Acting					
Insulin					
Humulin or Novolin NPH	1.5	4-12	22	Protamine sulfate	Cloudy suspension
Humulin Lente	2.5	7-15	22	Zinc	Turbid solution
Long Acting					
Analog					
Glargine	1-2	None	24+	None	Clear
Insulin					
Humulin Ultralente	4	None	28	Zinc	Turbid solution
Combinations					
Insulins					
Humulin 50/50 (50% NPH, 50% regular)	0.5	2-5	22	Protamine sulfate	Cloudy suspension
Humulin or Novolin 70/30 (70% NPH, 30% regular)	0.5	1.5-16	22	Protamine sulfate	Cloudy suspension
Analogs, Insulins					
Humalog Mix 75/25 (75% NPH, 25% Lispro)	0-0.2	1-6.5	22	Protamine sulfate	Cloudy suspension
Novolog Mix 70/30 (70% NPH, 30% Aspart)	0-0.2	1-4	22	Protamine sulfate	Cloudy suspension

From *Physician's desk reference*, ed 58, Montvale, NJ, 2001, Medical Economics.

injection programs, were shown to be less effective in the management and control of diabetes. The "split-mix" insulin regimen, using either premixed or self-mixed insulin, is one conventional therapy regimen. Premixed insulin combines two types of insulin in a preset proportion. For example, 1 unit of Humulin or Novolin 70/30 provides 0.7 units of NPH insulin and 0.3 units of regular insulin. A disadvantage of premixed insulins is that they do not allow fine tuning of the insulin regimen. Thus if one strives for fasting blood glucose levels consistently within the euglycemic range of 70 to 100 mg/dl with a split-mix regimen, an unacceptable incidence of nocturnal hypoglycemia occurs because the predinner intermediate-acting insulin has its peak effect during the counterregulatory nadir (approximately 12 midnight to 2 AM) (Figure 39-5).

Three injections per day: regular or rapid-acting analog and intermediate-acting insulin. An example of this regimen with a prescribed daily insulin dose of 60 units follows. Approximately two thirds of the total daily insulin dose (40 units) is given in the morning before breakfast, with one third of that dose (13 units) being given as regular or rapid-acting analog (RAA) insulin; the remaining two thirds of the prebreakfast dose (27 units) is given as NPH or Lente. In the evening the remaining one third of the total daily dose (20 units) is delivered: 50% (10 units) as regular or RAA insulin before dinner and 50% (10 units) as NPH or Lente at bedtime. Moving the predinner NPH/Lente to bedtime (10 PM to 1 AM) moves the insulin peak to dawn and can reduce nocturnal hypoglycemia as much as fivefold. Therefore the dose is 13 units of RAA and 27 units of NPH/Lente before breakfast, 10 units of RAA before dinner, and 10 units of NPH/Lente at bedtime. The drawback of this insulin regimen is the lack of flexibility with regard to the timing of lunch because of the emerging peak effect from the prebreakfast dose of NPH/Lente insulin (see Figure 39-5).

Three injections per day: Ultralente basal with premeal regular or rapid-acting analog insulin. In this regimen approximately 50% of the total daily insulin dose is given as Ultralente, divided into two injections given before breakfast and before dinner. The Ultralente insulin acts as basal insulin to control hepatic glucose output and disposal in the fasting state, and it is given regardless of whether dietary carbohydrate is consumed. Then regular or RAA insulin is given before each meal (before snacks also if using RAA insulin), with the dosage titrated to the amount of carbohydrate planned. This regimen provides more flexibility in meal timing, and patients may compensate for addition or deletion of carbohydrate at each meal with the adjustment of the premeal insulin dose. Because of these advantages, this regimen is com-

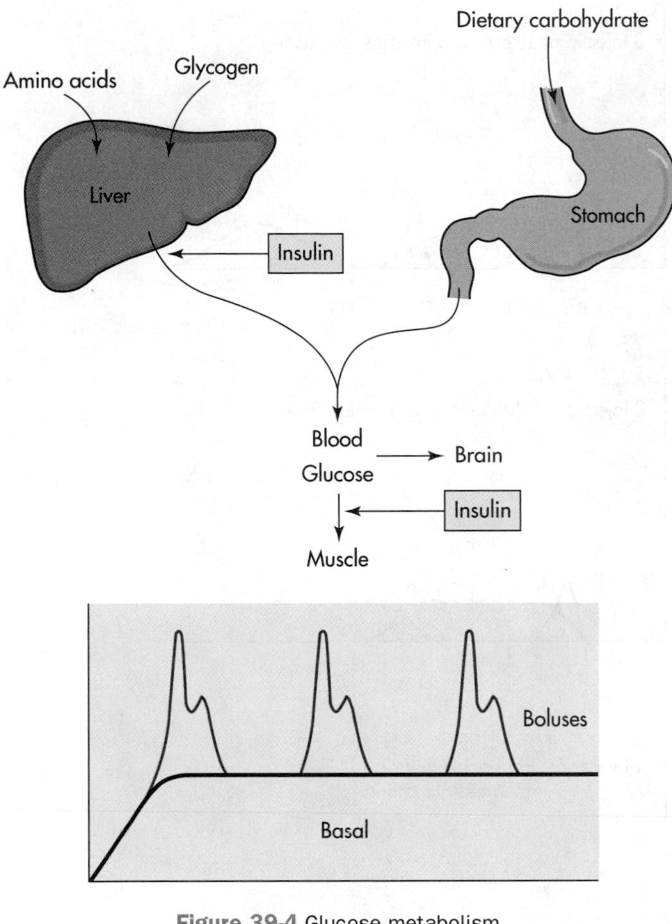

Figure 39-4 Glucose metabolism.

monly known as "the poor man's pump." It is not useful for treating individuals with a pronounced dawn hormonal surge (adolescents and pregnant women) or individuals with longstanding diabetes, in whom insulin kinetics may be erratic (see Figure 39-5).

Four injections per day: premeal rapid-acting analog and bedtime insulin glargine. Insulin glargine is a true basal insulin analog with no peak effect and more than 24 hours' duration of action. Insulin glargine injected once daily at bedtime controls hepatic glucose output and production in the fasting state.[85] Premeal RAA insulin is taken before consuming carbohydrates, with the dosage titrated to the amount of carbohydrate planned. Approximately 40% to 60% of the total daily dose is insulin glargine, with the remaining being RAA. This regimen is another example of "the poor man's pump." Because insulin glargine has a low pH, it can never be mixed in an insulin syringe with any other insulin or precipitation will occur (see Figure 39-5).

Four injections per day: premeal regular and overnight NPH/Lente insulin. With this regimen, typically, about 20% of the total daily dose is given as NPH/Lente at bedtime (10 PM to 1 AM), with the remaining 80% given as regular insulin and distributed proportionately between the carbohydrate loads at each of the three meals. It must be remembered that the overnight NPH/Lente insulin dose does not cover the full 24-hour basal requirements. Therefore a portion of the premeal regular insulin dose is covering the basal requirements. If persons have longer than 6 hours between injections of regular insulin, they generally experience "insulin run-out hyperglycemia," because if the liver does not "see" insulin, it uncontrollably releases more glucose (see Figure 39-5).

Four injections per day: prebreakfast Ultralente and rapid-acting analog, prelunch and predinner rapid-acting analog, and overnight NPH/Lente insulin. This regimen is ideal for persons who use RAA insulin, require flexibility, and have a significant dawn hormonal surge. The substitution of RAA for regular insulin in the previously described regimen would result in significant insulin run-out hyperglycemia because of the short duration of action of RAA. The insulin run-out issue with RAA can be managed by the addition of a small dose of Ultralente insulin before breakfast to control hepatic glucose output and disposal during the day, with the bedtime NPH/Lente insulin providing coverage during the night (see Figure 39-5). This regimen allows flexibility in doses and the interval between injections and mealtimes to best control postprandial glucose levels.

In modern clinical practice, most intensive therapy insulin injection regimens revolve around insulin glargine and RAA because of the superior kinetics and predictability with reduced risk of hypoglycemia. When cost constraints prevail, older insulin formulations may be used.

Continuous subcutaneous insulin infusion or insulin pump therapy. Insulin pump therapy using a portable external insulin infusion pump offers the most physiologic insulin delivery. The pump holds only quick-acting insulin, usually RAA. The pump is preprogrammed to deliver varying hourly basal rates. For example, the pump can be programmed to deliver less insulin during the midnight to 2 AM counterregulatory nadir and then to increase insulin delivery in the dawn hours, thus matching the individual's needs. In addition to being the most physiologic insulin delivery system, an insulin pump is also the most flexible (see Figure 39-5).

Current insulin pumps are no larger than a pager (Figure 39-6). The ideal candidate for the pump is a person who has failed to control diabetes on one of the aforementioned insulin regimens, someone who is pregnant or contemplating pregnancy, or someone who desires increased daily flexibility. Disadvantages include the initial capital outlay of approximately $5000 and the cost of maintenance supplies, although most insurance companies cover 70% to 100%; the continuous presence of a needle or Teflon-like cannula placed subcutaneously in the abdomen; and the potential risk of sepsis. Attention to sterile technique and changing the infusion site every 24 to 48 hours minimize the risk of sepsis. Insulin pump therapy should be initiated only in an educated, motivated patient under the care of a diabetes team educated and skilled in pump therapy and offering 24-hour support for the patient.[1,6,44, 112]

The greatest risk is the potential for rapid-onset DKA if insulin delivery is interrupted by partial occlusion of the tubing, needle, or cannula or accidental removal of the needle or cannula. A good safety net is to have patients with pumps change the infusion site if the capillary blood glucose level is greater than 300 mg/dl and the elevation is not a result of excess carbohydrate intake.

Pumps deliver insulin in two fashions: (1) basals, automatic delivery of small amounts of insulin every few minutes to cover

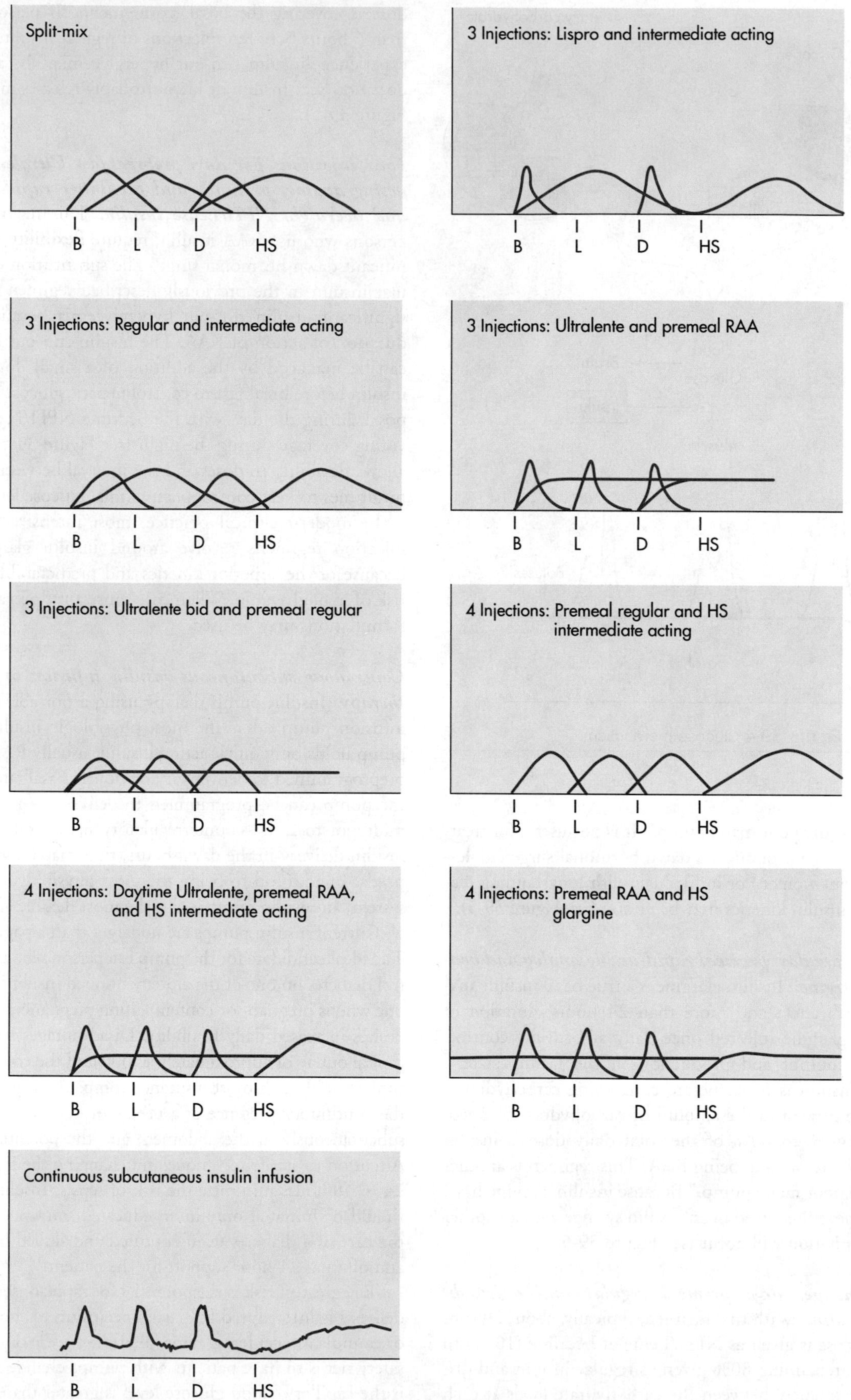

Figure 39-5 Insulin delivery programs. *RAA*, Rapid-acting analog; *B*, breakfast; *L*, lunch; *D*, dinner; *HS*, at bedtime; *bid*, twice a day.

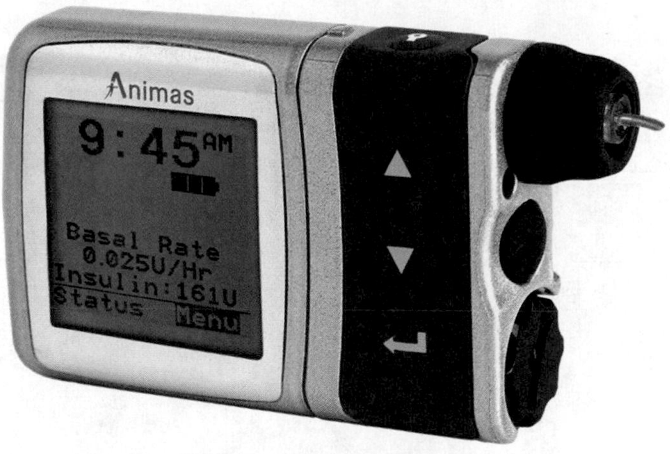

Figure 39-6 Insulin infusion pump.

hepatic glucose output and disposal; and (2) boluses, "spikes" of insulin that the patient programs to be delivered when he or she is ready to eat. Exercise with a pump is facilitated by the ability to program a temporary basal reduction for planned physical activity, thus eliminating the need for individuals to consume additional carbohydrates before exercise. "Smart pumps" allow patients to preprogram the pump with insulin-to-carbohydrate ratios. At meals or snack time, the patient programs the number of grams of carbohydrate he or she plans on consuming, and the pump calculates the insulin dose needed based on the preprogrammed insulin-to-carbohydrate ratios.

Insulin Algorithms as a Component of Intensive Therapy. An insulin algorithm is a plan for additional insulin to be administered for episodes of hyperglycemia; each patient should have an individualized plan. Via an algorithm, additional insulin is given over and above the baseline or usual insulin dose on the basis of fingerstick blood glucose levels. For example, for a patient taking 0.5 to 0.8 units/kg body weight, an additional unit of RAA or regular insulin would be expected to lower blood glucose levels by approximately 50 mg/dl (Box 39-2). In smart pumps, a patient can program (1) an insulin sensitivity factor (ISF)—the amount (in mg/dl) that an additional unit of insulin would lower the blood glucose; (2) a target glucose level (in mg/dl); and (3) the estimated duration of a bolus of RAA. When the patient has elevated blood glucose and needs additional insulin to lower the blood glucose level, he or she enters the current blood glucose level into the pump. The pump calculates the number of units of insulin needed to lower the blood glucose to the target level, taking into account the ISF and the duration and action of insulin from prior boluses the patient may have taken to correct for hyperglycemia. This reduces the risk of overcompensating with insulin by forgetting about the effects of insulin previously administered.

Insulin algorithms must be differentiated from "sliding scales." In a sliding scale no baseline insulin is administered to control either hepatic glucose output and disposal or prandial needs; insulin is administered on a contingency basis every 4 to 6 hours on the basis of the prevailing fingerstick blood glucose level (Box 39-3). In other words, with a sliding scale, quick-acting insulin is given only after hyperglycemia has already occurred. Sliding-scale insulin dosing makes no physiologic sense and results in an "unhappy liver" manifested by hyperglycemia and perhaps ketosis. A health care team can readily precipitate nosocomial DKA by using sliding-scale insulin dosages.[99]

Inhaled rapid-acting insulin is under clinical investigation, and early results have been promising in terms of glycemic control. In the trials, inhaled quick-acting insulin is administered to cover prandial requirements; intermediate- or long-acting insulin is injected to cover basal requirements.[19,68] Concerns about inhaled insulin center on the vasodilatory properties of insulin and the theoretic potential for pulmonary hypotension and pulmonary edema, especially in patients with cardiac dysfunction. Additionally, the inhaled dose of insulin is approximately tenfold greater than the subcutaneous dose.

Box 39-2 Sample Algorithm for Hyperglycemia

Premeal, for every 50 mg/dl elevation in blood glucose above 120 mg/dl, add 1 unit of RAA or regular insulin to the baseline dose:

Blood Glucose (mg/dl)	Add RAA or Regular Insulin (units, SC)
≥170	1
≥220	2
≥270	3

At bedtime, for every 50 mg/dl elevation in blood glucose above 150 mg/dl, add 1 unit of RAA or regular insulin to the baseline dose:

Blood Glucose (mg/dl)	Add RAA or Regular Insulin (units, SC)
≥200	1
≥250	2
≥300	3

RAA, Rapid-acting analog; *SC*, subcutaneously.

Box 39-3 Sample Sliding Scale

Give no baseline insulin. Give RAA or regular insulin every 4 hours based on fingerstick blood glucose values as follows:

Blood Glucose (mg/dl)	Give RAA or Regular Insulin (units, SC)
≥200	2
≥250	6
≥300	10

RAA, Rapid-acting analog; *SC*, subcutaneously.

TYPE 2 DIABETES MELLITUS: MEDICATIONS. Pharmacotherapy for type 2 DM can be directed at (1) decreasing insulin resistance and increasing insulin sensitization (metformin hydrochloride and the thiazolidinediones), (2) interfering with the digestion and absorption of dietary carbohydrate (alpha-glucosidase inhibitors), (3) augmenting insulin secretion and action (secretagogues: sulfonylureas, repaglinide, and nateglinide), or (4) providing exogenous insulin (Table 39-12).

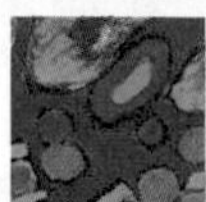

TABLE 39-12 COMMON MEDICATIONS *for Type 2 Diabetes Mellitus*

Parameter	Metformin	Pioglitazone	Rosiglitazone	Sulfonylureas
Mode of action	↓ Hepatic glucose ↑ Skeletal muscle glucose use	↑ Skeletal muscle glucose use ↓ Hepatic glucose	↑ Skeletal muscle glucose use ↓ Hepatic glucose	↑ Insulin secretion ↓ Hepatic glucose production
Glucose effects	Fasting and postprandial	Fasting and postprandial	Fasting and postprandial	Fasting and postprandial
Hypoglycemia as monotherapy	No	No	No	Yes
Weight gain	No	Possible	Possible	Possible
Insulin levels	↓	↓	↓	↑
Side effects	GI (self-limiting symptoms of nausea, diarrhea, anorexia)	Edema	Edema	Potential allergic reaction if sulfa allergy Potential drug interactions (first-generation agents) SIADH
Lipid effects	↓	↑ HDL, ↓ triglycerides LDL concentration unaltered Possible change in particle composition	Increase in total cholesterol, LDL, and HDL concentration Possible change in particle composition	↑ or ↓
Usual starting dose for a 70-kg man	500 mg bid with meals or extended release (XR), 500 mg with evening meal	15 mg once daily	4 mg daily either single or divided dose Better results with divided dose	Varies with each agent Glyburide, 2.5 mg once daily Glipizide extended release (Glucotrol XL), 5 mg once daily Glyburide (Glynase), 3 mg once daily Glimeperide (Amaryl), 2 mg once daily
Maximum dose	850 mg tid with meals or extended release, 2000 mg with evening meal	45 mg once daily	8 mg daily as either single or divided dose Better results with divided dose	Varies with each agent: Glyburide, 10 mg bid Glucotrol XL, 20 mg once daily Glynase, 6 mg bid Amaryl, 8 mg once daily
Contraindications	Type 1 diabetes Renal or hepatic dysfunction History of ETOH abuse Chronic conditions associated with hypoxia (asthma, COPD, CHF) Acute conditions associated with potential for hypoxia (CHF, acute MI, surgery) Situations associated with potential renal dysfunction (e.g., IV contrast)	Type 1 diabetes	Type 1 diabetes	Type 1 diabetes

DECREASING INSULIN RESISTANCE OR INCREASING INSULIN SENSITIVITY. Metformin (Glucophage) and the thiazolidinediones work via different mechanisms. Metformin primarily inhibits uncontrolled hepatic glucose production, whereas the thiazolidinediones enhance skeletal muscle glucose uptake—the earliest defect in evolving type 2 DM.

Metformin, a true insulin sensitizer, decreases hepatic glucose production and enhances peripheral glucose use. Because it is an antihyperglycemic agent and does not stimulate insulin secretion, it cannot induce hypoglycemia when used as monotherapy. Ideal candidates for treatment with metformin are overweight or obese patients with type 2 DM. The potentially fatal side effect of lac-

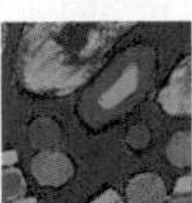

TABLE 39-12
COMMON MEDICATIONS *for Type 2 Diabetes Mellitus—cont'd*

Parameter	Repaglinide	Nateglinide	Acarbose	Miglitol
Mode of action	↑ Insulin secretion	↑ Insulin secretion	Alpha-glucosidase inhibition ↓ Carbohydrate digestion and absorption from GI tract	Alpha-glucosidase inhibition ↓ Carbohydrate digestion and absorption from GI tract
Glucose effects	Postprandial and fasting	Postprandial	Postprandial	Postprandial
Hypoglycemia as monotherapy	Yes; less than that seen with sulfonylureas	No	No	No
Weight gain	No	No	No	No
Insulin levels	↑	↑	↓ or no change	↓ or no change
Side effects	Rare hypoglycemia	Very rare hypoglycemia, since effects are glucose dependent	GI (flatulence, abdominal distention, diarrhea)	GI (flatulence, abdominal distention, diarrhea)
Lipid effects	No change	No change	↓ or no change	↓ or no change
Usual starting dose for a 70-kg man	0.5 mg before meals	120 mg tid	25 mg tid with first bite of each meal	25 mg tid with first bite of each meal
Maximum dose	16 mg daily in divided doses at meals and snacks	120 mg tid	100 mg tid with first bite of each meal	100 mg tid with first bite of each meal
Contraindications	Type 1 diabetes	Type 1 diabetes	Type 1 diabetes Inflammatory bowel disease Bowel obstruction Cirrhosis Chronic conditions with maldigestion or malabsorption	Type 1 diabetes Inflammatory bowel disease Bowel obstruction Cirrhosis Chronic conditions with maldigestion or malabsorption

GI, Gastrointestinal; *SIADH,* syndrome of inappropriate antidiuretic hormone; *HDL,* high-density lipoprotein; *LDL,* low-density lipoprotein; *bid,* twice a day; *XR,* extended release; *qid,* four times daily; *tid,* three times daily; *ETOH,* ethanol; *COPD,* chronic obstructive pulmonary disease; *CHF,* congestive heart failure; *MI,* myocardial infarction; *IV,* intravenous.

tic acidosis generally occurs only when metformin is used in patients for whom it is contraindicated—those with renal insufficiency, liver disease, alcohol excess, or underlying hypoxic states (congestive heart failure, chronic obstructive pulmonary disease, significant asthma, acute myocardial infarction). Metformin should be discontinued on the morning of an elective surgical procedure that may require general anesthesia because of the risk of hypoxia, which can cause lactic acidosis. Metformin should also be discontinued on the morning of any elective procedures using contrast materials (e.g., IV pyelogram, cardiac catheterization), since contrast materials can directly cause renal shutdown and drug accumulation. In both these situations, metformin should not be restarted for 48 hours after the surgery or procedure, pending documentation of a normal serum creatinine level. Adjustments in the individual's diabetes regimen have to be made for this period to maintain glycemic control. In the UKPDS, despite similar levels of glycemic control, the subset of obese type 2 DM patients treated with metformin had a statistically significantly lower cardiovascular event and death rate than the other groups.[95] Thus metformin must be modulating other aspects of the metabolic syndrome.

Thiazolidinediones, better known as the glitazones (pioglitazone [Actos] and rosiglitazone [Avandia]), are antihyperglycemic insulin-sensitizing agents that bind to the peroxisome proliferator-activated receptor-gamma (PPARG), a nuclear receptor, and amplify the insulin signal. Glitazones stimulate skeletal muscle glucose uptake directly; in addition, and perhaps more important, they may do so indirectly via effects on adipose tissue with reduction in circulating free fatty acids. Free fatty acids induce insulin resistance. In addition to glucose-lowering properties, glitazones have purported beneficial effects on other components of the metabolic syndrome. These agents may also assist in preservation of beta cell function via reduction in lipid deposition within the islets of Langerhans—a concept known as lipotoxicity that is documented in animals. These agents can be safely used in patients with renal insufficiency without the need for dosage adjustment. A contraindication to their use is liver disease or elevations in hepatic transaminases. Hepatic transaminases should be monitored at baseline before treatment and then periodically thereafter at the clinical judgment of the health care provider. At any point during treatment, if hepatic transaminases are more than three times the upper limit of normal, the glitazone should be discontinued. It is suspected that an alternative explanation will ultimately be found for the hepatic transaminase elevation. These agents are contraindicated in patients with New York grade III or grade IV congestive heart failure. The most common adverse effect is edema. Clinically, glucose lowering is very gradual with these agents, with maximum effect of a given dose being seen at 8 to 12 weeks.[69]

Interfering With Carbohydrate Digestion and Absorption. Alpha-glucosidase inhibition by acarbose (Precose) and miglitol (Glyset) has a primary mode of action of decreasing postprandial blood glucose levels via direct interference with the digestion and absorption of dietary carbohydrate. These agents are most commonly used as adjunctive therapy rather than as monotherapy. Both these agents need to be taken with the first bite of the meal. Increased intestinal gas formation, the most common side effect, is minimized with slow dose titration and does improve with continued administration.

Augmenting Insulin Secretion: Secretagogues. Sulfonylureas enhance insulin secretion and action. First-generation sulfonylureas (chlorpropamide, tolazamide, tolbutamide), although efficacious, have a higher risk of side effects, such as sustained hypoglycemia, the chlorpropamide flush (an Antabuse-like reaction), protein-binding interference with certain medications, and the syndrome of inappropriate diuretic hormone (SIADH). The second- and third-generation sulfonylureas are preferred because of their increased milligram potency, shorter duration of action, and better side effect profile.

Prior concerns about possible cardiotoxicity of sulfonylureas have generally disappeared, given the emergence of data to support the safety of these agents from the cardiovascular prospective in the UKPDS.[93] Glimepiride, a third-generation sulfonylurea, has benefits in terms of a reduced risk of hypoglycemia, potentially lower risk of adverse cardiovascular effects, and perhaps reduced potential for secondary failure.

One of the meglitinides, repaglinide (Prandin), is taken before meals to lower blood glucose levels by stimulating the release of insulin from the islet cells. Because of the risk of hyperglycemia, the patient must be monitored carefully.

Nateglinide (Starlix), a phenylalanine derivative, is given before meals to produce an abrupt spurt of insulin. Hypoglycemia is rare. Switching from a sulfonylurea to nateglinide can result in a slight rise in fasting glucose levels; however, the HbA_{1c} may be maintained or lowered, since postprandial glucose levels are significantly improved and they contribute more to the HbA_{1c} than fasting or premeal glucose levels do. Both repaglinide and nateglinide are useful in patients with sulfa allergy and patients experiencing hypoglycemia with sulfonylureas.

To achieve the ADA goal HbA_{1c}, the vast majority of type 2 DM patients require combination therapy. Beginning pharmacotherapy with an insulin-sensitizing agent appears physiologically logical and ideally will help delay or prevent sulfonylurea failure, which is frequently seen after 5 to 6 years of sulfonylurea monotherapy. In addition, it is hoped that insulin sensitization will decrease many of the other components of the metabolic syndrome and reduce macrovascular disease. This hypothesis is currently being tested in several clinical trials.

Providing Insulin Therapy in Type 2 Diabetes Mellitus. Insulin therapy in patients with type 2 DM is frequently needed because of progressive decline in beta cell function, especially after 10 to 15 years of the disease. Insulin therapy is indicated when patients are in a state of acute metabolic decompensation and are more insulin resistant because of the stress of illness. In these patients short-term insulin therapy can reestablish glycemic control and metabolic stability. Reevaluation of insulin secretory capacity via a C-peptide test is important so that patients do not remain on a regimen of insulin unnecessarily.

In a person with type 2 DM and a low-normal C-peptide level or a lean person with a normal C-peptide level, insulin therapy will probably be needed, along with maintenance of diet, exercise, and oral agents. The use of a single daily dose of insulin glargine or intermediate-acting insulin at bedtime may be sufficient. The theory is that this bedtime dose will maximally control both the dawn hepatic glucose output and disposal and the peak insulin resistance. The bedtime insulin dose assists in achieving the best possible fasting blood glucose level and minimizes glucotoxicity. Minimizing glucotoxicity maximizes the daytime pancreatic insulin secretory capability and minimizes the daytime insulin dose. In addition, the appetite-stimulating effect of insulin is minimized, which assists in weight control. Occasionally patients with type 2 DM may require multiple injections, just like patients with true type 1 DM. The exact needs of each patient are determined on the basis of the premeal and bedtime blood glucose levels.

In contrast, insulin therapy in the C peptide–positive overweight patient with type 2 DM should be avoided if possible. Insulin is lipogenic, and the weight gain may further exacerbate the insulin-resistant state. Diet, exercise, and appropriate oral agents should be aggressively used before insulin therapy is contemplated. A bedtime dose of intermediate-acting insulin or insulin glargine is the ideal starting point, along with the continuation of oral agent therapy. Combination therapy with oral agents usually helps maintain glycemic control with a lower insulin dosage. Insulin therapy must not be viewed as a substitute for diet and exercise, but as an adjunct. Commonly, insulin therapy in the obese C peptide–positive patient not only fails to improve glycemic control on a sustained basis but also increases appetite, resulting in weight gain, increased hyperglycemia, and increased hyperinsulinemia, thus perpetuating the insulin-resistant state and the components of the metabolic syndrome.[75-77]

Insulin therapy is necessary for the type 2 DM patient who becomes C-peptide negative. Such individuals are usually lean and look phenotypically more like an individual with type 1 DM. In these individuals, just as in type 1 DM patients, intensive insulin therapy with carbohydrate gram counting is needed. An insulin pump may be an option for selected individuals. It is also important to note that in the geriatric years, 10% of newly diagnosed individuals will have bona fide type 1 DM, again requiring intensive therapy and carbohydrate gram counting.

COMPLICATIONS OF MEDICATIONS

INSULIN HYPERSENSITIVITY. Hypersensitivity to insulin itself is uncommon. Rarely a patient with a sulfa allergy cross-reacts with NPH insulin, which contains protamine sulfate. A rare patient who is allergic to zinc may react to the Lente insulins. Patients may react to preservatives within insulin. A switch in insulin manufacturer may eliminate the latter problem. Insulin hypersensitivity reactions are generally local reactions, consisting of wheals at injection sites. However, systemic symptoms and anaphylaxis can occur. When systemic reactions occur, local reactions may also be present. Formal desensitization is an option for patients with true insulin allergy.

HYPOGLYCEMIA. Hypoglycemia, or a blood glucose level of less than 60 mg/dl, is a potential complication of therapy with insulin or oral hypoglycemic agents. Hypoglycemia is caused by a disturbance in the balance between insulin or secretagogues, carbohydrates, and activity (Box 39-4).

Signs and Symptoms. The common signs and symptoms of hypoglycemia may be adrenergic (caused by activation of the sympathetic nervous system) or neuroglycopenic (caused by depression of central nervous system activity as the brain receives an insufficient supply of glucose) (Box 39-5). Adrenergic symptoms generally precede neuroglycopenic symptoms. The particular signs and symptoms in a given individual may vary with the absolute blood glucose level, the rapidity of the decrease in blood glucose level, and the duration of hypoglycemia. In addition, signs and symptoms commonly vary throughout a person's life.

A rapid drop in plasma glucose results primarily in manifestations from increased sympathetic nervous system activity. In slow-developing hypoglycemia, as might be seen with long-acting insulin or with oral hypoglycemic agents, the central nervous system signs and symptoms predominate. If a rapid drop occurs and is allowed to persist, all signs and symptoms usually occur.

Hypoglycemia may occur during sleep. The only symptoms may be nightmares, sweating, restless sleep, headache on awakening, elevated fasting blood glucose value, or feelings of total exhaustion on awakening. Nighttime hypoglycemia may be part of the Somogyi phenomenon (see p. 1152).

Patients with long-standing diabetes may become less sensitive to hypoglycemia and may have very low blood glucose levels before some, if any, symptoms occur. Sustained recurrent hypoglycemia results in an increase in glucose transporter numbers at the blood-brain barrier to maintain the cerebrospinal fluid glucose level as close to normal as possible. This is why patients with recurrent hypoglycemia can maintain consciousness at lower blood glucose levels without experiencing significant adrenergic symptoms compared with individuals without diabetes. Euglycemia with elimination of hypoglycemia results in a reduction of the glucose transporter number at the blood-brain barrier to a normal level. Consequently, when glucose levels fall slightly into the hypoglycemic range, the patient experiences adrenergic symptoms.[89]

Patients with DM who are treated with beta-adrenergic antagonists (beta-blockers) may be at special risk for hypoglycemia. These beta-adrenergic antagonists block or inhibit the appearance of early signs and symptoms of hypoglycemia by blocking the sympathetic nervous system. In addition, these drugs prevent or block gluconeogenesis and glycogenolysis, thus inhibiting the normal endogenous response to hypoglycemia, making it more difficult to reverse the problem.

Signs and symptoms similar to those of hypoglycemia may occur when the blood glucose level is elevated and drops rapidly

Box 39-5 Signs and Symptoms of Hypoglycemia

Adrenergic Symptoms	Neuroglycopenic Symptoms
Pallor	Headache
Diaphoresis	Mental confusion
Tachycardia	Circumoral paresthesia
Piloerection	Fatigue
Palpitations	Incoherent speech
Nervousness	Coma
Irritability	Diplopia
Sensation of coldness	Emotional lability
Weakness	Convulsions
Trembling	
Hunger	

Box 39-4 Causes of Hypoglycemia During Treatment With Exogenous Insulin or Secretagogues

- Unphysiologic insulin regimen
- Overdosage of insulin or sulfonylureas
- Inconsistent carbohydrate intake
- Omission of meal
- Omission of planned snack
- Uncompensated exercise
- End-stage renal disease
- End-stage liver disease
- Alcohol consumption

to a level that is still in an elevated range. The sudden rapid drop in blood glucose stimulates the physiologic neuroendocrine response to stressors. Thus a patient whose glucose level drops rapidly from 500 to 300 mg/dl may demonstrate the same signs and symptoms as a patient whose glucose drops to 40 mg/dl. Patients with uncontrolled diabetes may complain of feeling hypoglycemic, even though their plasma glucose levels are high. The nurse should discuss this phenomenon with patients with uncontrolled diabetes and reassure them that this "relative hypoglycemia" associated with improved glycemic control generally lasts only a few weeks.

Most hypoglycemia is mild and easily self-treated. The majority of cases of severe hypoglycemia result from patient error: inadequate carbohydrate intake at meals, missed snacks, uncompensated activity, or incorrect insulin dosing (insulin type or quantity).

Diagnosis and Treatment. A fingerstick blood glucose value should be obtained to verify hypoglycemia (blood glucose level of 60 mg/dl or lower). In a conscious patient, treatment consists of 15 g of quick-acting carbohydrate (e.g., three or four glucose tablets, 4 ounces of juice [no added sugar], or three hard candies). The fingerstick blood glucose value should be rechecked in 15 minutes. If the blood glucose level remains at 60 mg/dl or lower, the patient should self-treat again. If a glucose meter is not readily available, treatment should be taken regardless. In an unconscious patient, oral administration of glucose should never be attempted. In the hospital setting one ampule of 50% dextrose is given by IV push. Recovery is usually within 1 minute. In the outpatient setting a friend or family member should inject 1 mg of glucagon subcutaneously; this causes the liver to release its glycogen store. The unconscious patient given subcutaneous glucagon generally regains consciousness in 10 to 20 minutes. After recovery the patient should be given a snack of 45 g of carbohydrate to aid in replacing glycogen stores. Patients commonly are nauseated after receiving glucagon and may vomit. Seizures can occur when hypoglycemia is severe.[21]

Side Effects of Oral Agents. Oral agents may cause hypoglycemia. Potential adverse effects of the oral agents are noted in Table 39-12.

Surgical Management. Pancreas transplantation has been proven effective in improving the quality of life in persons with diabetes by eliminating the need for exogenous insulin, frequent blood glucose monitoring, and dietary restrictions. Currently a pancreas transplant is indicated for persons with end-stage renal disease who are planning to or have had a kidney transplant. A pancreas transplant may be done at the time of the kidney transplant or after the kidney transplant. Studies comparing simultaneous pancreas-kidney transplantation, living related donor kidney transplantation, and cadaveric kidney transplantation conflict in terms of survival advantage; some studies show advantage to simultaneous pancreas-kidney transplantation, whereas others show advantage to living related donor kidney transplantation.[52,66]

A group of investigators in Edmonton, Alberta, Canada, have treated 17 patients with type 1 DM with islet cell transplantation via the Edmonton Protocol. After transplant, these patients received triple immunosuppressive therapy. A significant percentage ultimately still required insulin therapy. Eleven of the 17 still have DM, based on ADA diagnostic criteria. Risks of immunosuppression persist. Further research is needed to explore the relationship between immunosuppressants and glucose metabolism, and safer immunosuppressive agents need to be developed.[80]

Diet. Nutritional management is the cornerstone of therapy in all types of DM.[6] Patients need to be referred early to a registered dietitian, preferably one who is also a certified diabetes educator, for nutritional education and the development of meal plans that are flexible and fit their lifestyles. Food issues are never simple for patients, and an initial understanding can often determine the success of their management. If no dietitian is available, the professional nurse should provide basic nutritional information until the patient can be formally counseled by a dietitian.

The current nutritional management for diabetes is to maintain a reasonable weight and control blood glucose and lipid levels without compromising health. Current nutritional recommendations for people with diabetes are similar to those for healthy individuals without diabetes, as developed by the National Research Council, the American Heart Association, and the American Cancer Society (Box 39-6).

Most persons need 25 kcal/kg desired body weight to maintain their weight and meet basic metabolic needs. With this as the basis, calories are added or subtracted based on the patient's activity level, age, and need to lose or gain weight (Table 39-13).

Another dietary component that is manipulated is fiber. A high-fiber, moderate-carbohydrate (40% to 50% of daily calories) diet decreases insulin requirements, cholesterol, and both fasting and postprandial glucose serum levels. Fiber can increase satiety, which might help with weight reduction. Fiber delays gastric emptying and decreases peak blood glucose, so when fiber is introduced into the diet, blood glucose should be monitored, and insulin or any oral agents may need to be adjusted. Adding fiber gradually helps minimize abdominal discomfort and flatulence. Increasing water intake also helps.

Principles of Dietary Management. Recommendations need to be made with the awareness that eating habits are difficult if not impossible to change overnight. Changes should be instituted gradually as the professional nurse helps the patient adopt a diet that is as close to ideal as possible.

To increase success, dietary planning should consider:

- Religious, cultural, and personal preferences of the patient
- Lifestyle components: family eating patterns, finances, and work schedule
- Amount, timing, and level of exercise; work; and sleep
- Actions of prescribed medications: onset, duration, and peak
- Self-perception of desired body weight

Carbohydrates must be distributed on a consistent basis so that the blood level of nutrients matches the blood level of insulin or any oral hypoglycemic agent. Relative consistency in timing of meals is also important for the person who needs to lose weight. Distribution of carbohydrates helps prevent large increases in postprandial blood glucose and allows the blood glucose to return to the preprandial level before the next meal regardless of whether the patient is receiving insulin or oral agents.

BOX 39-6 Target Nutritional Goals for Patients With Diabetes Mellitus

Calories

Sufficient to achieve and maintain weight as close to desirable body weight as possible

Carbohydrate

Varies in relation to assessment and protein and fat intake; usually 40% to 60% of total calories

Liberalized, individualized emphasis on total carbohydrate intake versus eliminating simple sugars only

Carbohydrate consistency at meals

Modest amounts of sucrose and other refined sugars acceptable contingent on metabolic control and body weight

Protein

Usual dietary intake of protein double the amount needed

Exact ideal percentage of total calories debatable; usually 12% to 20% of total calories

Recommended dietary allowance (RDA): 0.8 g/kg body weight for adults; RDA modified for children, pregnant and lactating women, older adults, and those with special medical conditions

Avoidance of excess dietary protein intake in renal disease

Fat

Usually 30% or less of total calories, but may be as high as 40%

Polyunsaturated fats, 6% to 8%

Saturated fats, less than 10%

Monounsaturated fats, remaining percentage

Cholesterol, less than 300 mg/day

May need to be further modified, depending on lipid profile

Fiber

Up to 40 g/day

25 g/1000 kcal for low-calorie intakes

Alternative Sweeteners

Use of various nutritive and nonnutritive sweeteners

Sodium

3000 mg/day or less

Modified for special medical conditions (e.g., hypertension, edema)

Alcohol

Two or less equivalents per day (1 equivalent = 1.5 ounces distilled liquor, 4-ounce glass of wine, or 12-ounce glass of beer)

Vitamins and Minerals

Despite a lack of scientific evidence that individuals with diabetes mellitus (DM) who eat a well-balanced diet require vitamin or mineral supplementation, the RDAs were developed based on a healthy population. Also, given that many vitamins and minerals are excreted in excess in the urine of individuals with DM, supplementation with a general multivitamin is prudent and rarely harmful.

TABLE 39-13 GUIDELINES FOR ESTIMATING CALORIE REQUIREMENTS

Level	Activities	Calorie Requirements
Light, more than 55 years old, obese, or inactive	Less than for "light" below	10 cal/lb (22 kcal/kg) of desired body weight (DBW)
Light	Ambulating in hospital, washing clothes, walking 2.5-3 miles/hr, carpentry, electrical work, golfing, sailing	10-12 cal/lb (22-26 kcal/kg) DBW
Moderate	Weeding and hoeing, bicycling, dancing, tennis, walking 3.5-4 miles/hr, scrubbing floors, work involving loading and stocking	12-14 cal/lb (26-32 kcal/kg) DBW
Heavy	Climbing, walking uphill with full load, basketball, football, swimming	14-16 cal/lb (31-35 kcal/kg) DBW
Weight reduction		Subtract 500 cal from total daily calories for 1 lb weight loss per week

SYSTEMS FOR LEARNING AND MAINTAINING DIETARY PLANS. Once the goals of nutritional therapy are established, patients are taught one of several methods for manipulating calories and food.

EXCHANGE SYSTEM. Historically the exchange system was the most widely used method. The American Dietetic Association and the ADA divided foods into six groups with exchange lists (or choices), based on the amount of carbohydrate, protein, and fat contained in foods. There are six exchange lists: starch/bread, meat and meat substitutes, vegetables, fruit, milk, and fat. Each exchange list contains foods in specific serving sizes that contain approximately equal amounts of carbohydrates, proteins, fats, and calories. Because of this, these foods can be substituted or exchanged for one another. For example, in the fruit list, one 4-ounce apple equals 12 cherries equals 4 ounces of orange juice. Using the suggested serving size is an important point. The patient should weigh and measure foods. The exchange system offers a wide variety and combinations of foods that can be eaten. Implementation of the system requires knowing the caloric, carbohydrate, protein, and fat content of different foods. Labels on food products and convenience foods and recipe books list carbohydrate, protein, and fat content. The total number of exchanges for each day is determined by the total calorie, carbohydrate, fat, and protein prescription.

Once the dietary prescription has been made and the caloric amount decided, a meal plan such as the one shown in Figure 39-7 can be developed. Resources other than the one depicted in the figure are available from the ADA. Some are simple and have pictures of foods and a place to write in the number of exchanges from each group to be used.

It is important to maintain consistency with the distribution of exchanges and not "borrow from lunch and add to dinner." Box 39-7 shows an example of the nutritional information found on cereal boxes. In terms of carbohydrate, protein, and fat content, one serving of cereal is equal to about 1⅓ bread exchanges.

TOTAL GRAM COUNTING OF CARBOHYDRATE. Total gram counting of carbohydrate is now the most popular meal-planning system for persons with both type 1 and type 2 DM. With this system the patient counts the total amount of carbohydrate available in the meal or snack. Only carbohydrates are initially tracked. Insulin is then matched to the carbohydrate planned. Carbohydrate gram counting helps people understand the relationship between food ingested and blood glucose levels. One disadvantage of this method is that patients may minimize carbohydrate intake and increase their intake of fat and protein, which is clearly undesirable. Successful focus on carbohydrate gram counting occurs in the context of an overall healthy meal plan.[6,32]

MYPYRAMID. Another system that can be used to help patients with meal plans is the MyPyramid food guidance system developed by the U.S. Department of Agriculture (see Chapter 3).[100] This guide recommends less meat and poultry than does the exchange list.

POINT SYSTEM. With the point-counting system, foods are assigned points for the number of calories and carbohydrate, protein, and fat content. The total daily food allowance is written as the number of calorie and carbohydrate points, and the person is instructed to select foods according to a point distribution. This system is similar to the exchange list but is less well known.

BOX 39-7 Nutrition Information Per Serving of Cereal

- Serving size: 1 ounce (1¼ cup)
- Serving per package: 20 (1-ounce servings)
- Calories: 110
- Protein: 4 g
- Carbohydrate: 20 g
- Sodium: 320 mg
- Percentage of vitamins and minerals
- Ingredients: whole-oat flour, wheat starch, salt, sugar, calcium carbonate, etc.

DIETETIC FOODS, SWEETENERS, AND ALCOHOL. The diabetic diet does not require the use of special or dietetic foods. If used, these foods must be counted into the meal plan; the substitutions made in these products do not necessarily mean that they are low in calories or useful for people with diabetes. Foods that are labeled "sugar free" are only "sucrose free"—not carbohydrate free. These foods frequently are sweetened with alternative sweeteners such as fructose or maltose, or one of the sugar alcohols such as sorbitol, mannitol, or xylitol. Sugar alcohols are not absorbed or digested as well as other carbohydrates and therefore contribute only 2 kcal/g compared with the 4 kcal/g of other carbohydrates. Intake of large amounts of foods containing sugar alcohols can produce osmotic diarrhea.

Various sweeteners other than sugar are available in the United States, including saccharine, aspartame (Equal), acesulfame-K (Sunette), and sucralose (the first sugar substitute made from sugar). All these products are called low- or no-calorie sweeteners. Patients commonly ask how much of the sweeteners can be consumed safely. The accepted daily intake (ADI) is generous and is usually reported as an amount per kilogram of body weight (2.2 pound = 1 kg). For example, 50 mg/kg is the ADI for aspartame. For a 110-pound person this represents twelve 12-ounce cans of 100% aspartame-sweetened soda pop or 71 packets of Equal per day for a lifetime.

The term *net carbs*, *net carb effect*, and *impact carb* have not been defined or approved by the FDA. Food manufacturers created these terms to market their products. The concept is to subtract the grams of fiber and sugar alcohols from the total carbohydrate. Most nutritionists disagree with the use of the "net carb" concept. Some organizations suggest counting half the grams of sugar alcohol as carbohydrates, since half the sugar alcohol on average is digested. Fiber is not digested; some organizations suggest subtracting the grams of fiber from the total carbohydrate content only if the serving of food contains more than 5 g of fiber. Patients utilizing a "net carb" calculation can underestimate the total carbohydrates that are ultimately digestible to glucose, then underdose their insulin, with resultant hyperglycemia.

Alcohol does not furnish carbohydrate, protein, or fat, but it yields 7 kcal/g when metabolized and must be included in caloric calculations if weight loss is necessary. Some alcohol may be permitted, but the patient must be instructed about the caloric value of pure alcohol; the high carbohydrate content of beer, cordials, wine, and mixed drinks; the inhibiting effect of alcohol on gluconeogenesis with the possible precipitation of hypoglycemia; and the alcohol-induced increase in triglyceride levels.

The general rule is to allow a maximum of two drinks per day (1 drink = 1½ ounces of liquor, 5 ounces of wine, or 12 ounces of beer) and to consume alcohol with food. Lower-carbohydrate alcohol (e.g., light beer, rum with diet cola) is preferable. Alcohol should never be calculated as part of the carbohydrate load of a meal. Hypoglycemia is especially common if alcohol is consumed without food, since the liver's priority is to metabolize alcohol and liver glucose output is then reduced.[6,102]

NCIDE MEAL PLAN	Patient: JANE SMITH		Date: 08/22/05
Calories: 1200	Fat: 40 g		Carbohydrate: 150 g
MEAL	**FOOD**	**SERVINGS**	**SAMPLE MENUS**
BREAKFAST	FRUIT	0	
	STARCH	1	1 1/4 cup puffed rice cereal
	MILK	1	8-oz vanilla soy milk
	MEAT	0	
	FAT	0	
	OTHER	0	
Snack	STARCH	1	1 pack reduced calorie peanut butter crackers
LUNCH	FRUIT	1	4-oz apple
	STARCH	3	3-oz bagel
	VEGETABLE	2	1/2 cup raw cauliflower, 5 oz raw bell pepper
	MILK	0	
	MEAT	1	1 slice light cheese
	FAT	1	2 Tb light mayonnaise
	OTHER	0	
Snack	MILK	1	Reduced-calorie yogurt
DINNER	FRUIT	0	
	STARCH	4	1 1/2 cup macaroni and cheese, 1/2 cup peas
	VEGETABLE	3	Tossed salad (2 cups lettuce, one bell pepper ring, 2-oz tomato, 1/4 cup broccoli [cooked])
	MILK	0	
	MEAT	4	1 slice light cheese, 3-oz tuna in spring water
	FAT	1	2 Tb vinegarette dressing
	OTHER	0	
Snack	OTHER	1	Sugar Free gelatin

Figure 39-7 Sample meal plan.

▶ ARE YOU READY?

Which of the following is included in the dietary teaching for a patient with diabetes mellitus?

1. 40% to 60% of calories should be carbohydrates.
2. Fat intake should be less than 10% of total calories.
3. Alternative sweeteners are contraindicated.
4. Sodium should be less than 2000 mg per day.

Health Promotion and Prevention

PRIMARY PREVENTION

PRIMARY PREVENTION OF TYPE 1 DIABETES MELLITUS. Primary prevention of type 1 DM is under active research in both basic science studies and clinical research trials.[28,105] All type 1 DM prevention programs are experimental and focus on arresting the autoimmune process (see Future Watch box).[7] If an individual has a family member (aside from an identical twin) with type 1 DM, the risks of developing the disease are low (Table 39-14).

PRIMARY PREVENTION OF TYPE 2 DIABETES MELLITUS. Primary prevention of type 2 DM takes on a different focus. Abdominal obesity and a high waist-hip ratio (more than 0.85 for women; more than 0.90 for men) are significant risk factors for type 2 DM. Individuals with abdominal obesity are hyperinsulinemic and are at increased risk not only for type 2 DM, but for all components of the metabolic syndrome, as previously described.[75-77]

Primary prevention of type 2 DM involves identification and modification of risk factors (see Risk Factors box). Primary prevention should be directed toward lifestyle changes that include exercise, weight loss or control, and knowledge of risk factors. It is important that persons with type 2 DM be made aware of the familial tendencies and risks for siblings of the individual with either type of diabetes (see Table 39-14).[101,108]

Prevention of type 2 DM is an area of intense study. For example, the Diabetes Prevention Program studied 3200 subjects with type 2 DM in individuals with IGT. The study group that practices intensive lifestyle changes (including diet and exercise) had a 58% risk reduction in the development of type 2 DM; in individuals ages 60 and older, the risk reduction was a dramatic 71%. Another group treated with metformin group experienced a 31% risk reduction.[53]

Thiazolidinediones have been shown in clinical trials to reduce the risk of development of type 2 DM in the high-risk group of individuals with prior gestational DM.[10] A Finnish lifestyle modification study demonstrated a 58% risk reduction in the development of type 2 DM in patients with IGT who were randomized to a program of intensive diet and exercise.[92]

In the HOPE trial in the cohort of nondiabetic patients at high risk for developing cardiovascular disease, individuals who were treated with ramipril, 10 mg/day, had a 34% risk reduction

Future Watch

Preserving Beta Cell Function

The Type 1 Diabetes TrialNet Study Group comprises investigators from the United States, Canada, Australia, New Zealand, and Europe. It is funded by the National Institutes of Health, the Juvenile Diabetes Research Foundation, and the American Diabetes Association. The two major goals of TrialNet are to identify relatives of persons with type 1 diabetes mellitus (DM) who may be at risk for DM and to enroll them in clinical research trials in an attempt to preserve beta cell function. The first clinical research study to be conducted is an observational study of relatives of individuals with type 1 DM who have positive autoantibodies indicating ongoing autoimmune destruction of their pancreatic islets.

Participants in this observational study may be eligible to ultimately enroll in one of several intervention trials being planned. The first trial will test two immunosuppressive agents, mycophenolate mofetil alone or in combination with daclizumab, both of which are currently approved by the U.S. Food and Drug Administration for use in individuals who have received organ transplants. One obvious issue is the short- and long-term sequelae of the use of immunosuppressive agents in healthy individuals.

American Diabetes Association: TrialNet Study: further research to prevent and treat type 1 diabetes, *Diabetes Today*, accessed Aug 2004 from website: www.diabetes.org.

TABLE 39-14 ESTIMATED RISK OF DEVELOPING DIABETES MELLITUS

Relationship to Person With Diabetes	Approximate Rate of Developing Diabetes
No diabetes in family	Type 1: 0.3%
Identical twin with type 1	Type 1: 36%
One parent with type 1	Type 1: 3%
Sibling with type 1	Type 1: 3%
No diabetes in family	Type 2: 14%
Identical twin with type 2	Type 2: almost 100%
One parent with type 2	Type 2: 20%-30%
Both parents with type 2	Type 2: 35%-55%

Adapted from American Diabetes Association, Expert Committee on the Diagnosis and Classification of Diabetes Mellitus: Report of the Expert Committee on the Diagnosis and Classification of Diabetes Mellitus, *Diabetes Care* 24(Suppl 1):S5, 2001; Redondo MJ et al: Heterogeneity of type 1 diabetes: analysis of monozygotic twins in Great Britain and the United States, *Diabetalogia* 44(3):354-362, 2001.

Risk Factors

Type 2 Diabetes Mellitus

- Family history of diabetes
- Overweight (body mass index of 25 or more kg/m^2)
- Race (Native American, Hispanic-American, African-American, Asian-American, Pacific Islander)
- Age of 45 years or older
- Previously identified impaired glucose tolerance or impaired fasting glucose
- Hypertension (more than 140/90 mm Hg in adults)
- History of gestational diabetes mellitus or delivery of babies over 9 pounds
- High-density lipoprotein cholesterol of 35 mg/dl or less, and/or triglyceride level of 250 mg/dl or more
- Polycystic ovary syndrome
- History of vascular disease

in the development of type 2 DM.[39,40] In the West of Scotland trial the use of pravastatin reduced the risk of developing type 2 DM by 30%.[34] Other trials have shown reduction in the risk of developing type 2 DM in hypertensive patients treated with angiotensin-receptor blockers.[22,48]

HEALTHY PEOPLE 2010. The surgeon general's report *Healthy People 2010* established several goals that give the previously discussed primary prevention recommendations more momentum (see Healthy People 2010 box, p. 1120).[62,101,108] One goal is to reduce overweight prevalence to not more than 15% among people ages 20 or older (baseline: 23% for people ages 20 through 74 in 1988 to 1994). Another goal directed toward prevention of type 2 DM is to increase to at least 30% the proportion of adults ages 18 years and older who engage regularly, preferably daily, in moderate physical activity for at least 30 minutes (baseline: 15% of people ages 18 and older were active for at least 30 minutes five or more times per week in 1992). The need for patient education is outlined in the *Healthy People 2010* goal to increase to at least 60% the proportion of people with chronic and disabling conditions who receive formal patient education, including information about community and self-help resources, as an integral part of the management of their condition (age-adjusted baseline: 45% of persons with diabetes in 1998).

SECONDARY PREVENTION. From 85% to 90% of individuals with type 1 DM have autoantibodies at the time of initial fasting hyperglycemia. Therefore the ADA does not recommend screening for type 1 DM in either the general population or in higher-risk individuals (siblings of type 1 DM individuals) until clinical trials demonstrate the efficacy and safety of treatments to prevent or delay type 1 DM.[6] Observational and interventional treatment trials are being planned (see Future Watch box, p. 1140).

On the other hand, the prevalence of undiagnosed type 2 DM is high, with as many as 8 million people in the United States undiagnosed. Individuals with components of the metabolic syndrome are in the high-risk group. Box 39-8 outlines the ADA recommendations for screening for undiagnosed type 2 DM.[6]

TERTIARY PREVENTION. Tertiary prevention is the major focus of diabetes management. Both chronic and acute complications occur often, and nurses who work with patients who have diabetes must be involved in tertiary prevention to reduce severe complications of diabetes (see Table 39-8). Cardiovascular disease is the leading cause of death among people with diabetes, accounting for more than half of all deaths. Health behaviors aimed at reducing cardiovascular disease risk factors could have a major effect on morbidity and mortality from DM. The Medical Research Council Heart Protection Study has demonstrated a major benefit in reducing cardiovascular events in patients with DM treated with 3-hydroxy-3-methylglutaryl coenzyme A (HMGCo-A) reductase inhibitors (statins).[41] The major emphasis of tertiary preventive education is on the early detection and interventions listed in Table 39-8.

Complementary and Alternative Therapies. Chromium and vanadium are two trace elements that positively affect glucose tolerance. Chromium picolinate has been studied in humans. Trials with vanadium have been limited to animals at this time (see Complementary & Alternative Therapies box below). Cinnamon has also been shown to positively affect glucose tolerance (see Complementary & Alternative Therapies box, p. 1142).[51]

Complementary & Alternative Therapies

Chromium Picolinate

Chromium increases (1) insulin binding to the insulin receptor, (2) insulin receptor numbers, and (3) phosphorylation of the insulin receptor. Studies have demonstrated that supplementation with chromium picolinate improves blood glucose and hemoglobin A_{1c} levels in persons with type 2 diabetes mellitus. The safe, effective dosage appears to be in the 200 to 800 mcg/day range.

Box 39-8 Screening for Type 2 Diabetes Mellitus in Asymptomatic Individuals

- Screening for type 2 diabetes mellitus (DM) may be done with an oral glucose tolerance test or with a fasting plasma glucose (FPG) test. In clinical settings, the FPG is preferred because of the ease of testing, patient acceptance, convenience, and lower cost.
- Screening for type 2 DM should be considered at 3-year intervals, beginning at age 45, especially in individuals with a body mass index (BMI) (weight [kg]/height [m^2]) of 25 kg/m^2 or more.
- Screening should be considered at a younger age or more frequently in individuals who are overweight and who have one or more of the risk factors listed in the Risk Factors box.
- Screening should be performed in children and adolescents who are overweight and have 2 or more additional risk factors.
- Overweight in children and adolescents is defined as one of the following:
  —BMI over than the 85th percentile for age and sex
  —Weight for height over 85th percentile
  —Weight 120% of ideal body weight or more, with ideal body weight defined as the 50th percentile for height
- Additional risk factors to be considered in children and adolescents are:
  —Family history of type 2 DM in first-degree (parents, siblings) or second-degree (grandparents, aunts, uncles) relatives
  —Belonging to a specific racial or ethnic group (Native Americans, Hispanic Americans, African Americans, South Pacific Islanders)
  —Having signs of insulin resistance (acanthosis nigricans, hypertension, dyslipidemia)

From American Diabetes Association: Clinical practice recommendations 2004, *Diabetes Care* 27(Suppl 1):S1-S150, 2004.

Complementary & Alternative Therapies

Cinnamon

Studies have shown that extracts from cinnamon enhance the activity of insulin in vitro. These polyphenolic polymers may function as antioxidants and potentiate insulin action. One study of the use of cinnamon in individuals with type 2 diabetes mellitus demonstrated an improvement in fasting serum glucose and fasting total cholesterol, low-density lipoprotein cholesterol, and triglyceride levels compared with placebo.[51] Because of the paucity of data, however, no formal recommendations have been made on the use of cinnamon as an adjunct to the treatment of type 2 diabetes mellitus.

Nursing Management *of the Patient with Diabetes Mellitus*

A Nursing Care Plan for a patient with type 2 DM is found on p. 1144.

Assessment

Establishing a therapeutic relationship with the patient with diabetes is challenging as the professional nurse interacts with the patient at some time and place in the "diabetes life span." Many persons with type 2 DM have diabetes of 10 or more years' duration at the time of diagnosis as a result of the insidious onset of the disease. However, having diabetes for 30 years does not imply 30 years of optimal management. People can be "experienced" at doing the wrong thing. Many patients and health care professionals alike believe myths about diabetes (Box 39-9). The professional nurse is in an ideal position to educate patients and peers and dispel the myths of diabetes; it is imperative that the professional nurse be knowledgeable regarding current diabetes management.

Economic issues are a key concern to persons with diabetes. Many persons with diabetes do not have adequate insurance coverage, since the cost of private insurance may be prohibitive, some companies will not insure people with diabetes, and group plan benefits may be limited. A referral to a social worker may be indicated to help the patient obtain information regarding available insurance plans. Most pharmaceutical companies have compassionate need programs to provide prescription medications at either no cost or a reduced cost to individuals meeting specific income criteria.

Depression commonly occurs with any chronic illness; prevalence rates in individuals with diabetes may be as high as 32%. A referral to a behavioral psychologist or psychiatric clinical nurse specialist may be indicated.

Box 39-9 Myths of Diabetes Mellitus

- Diabetes is just a touch of sugar.
- You have borderline diabetes mellitus if you don't take insulin.
- My diabetes will always control me.
- *Symptom free* means complication free.
- Complications are inevitable.
- If you have diabetes, you are doomed to illness and early death.

Health History. Assess for:

- Psychosocial-emotional status: perception of the meaning of the diagnosis and how it affects the patient's life, future plans, day-to-day activities (e.g., work, social activities, family role, meals); identification of life stressors; current coping strategies; support systems; level of education, literacy
- Knowledge level: concept of diabetes, effect of uncontrolled metabolic state, potential treatment
- Family history of food buying, cooking, diabetes
- Cardiovascular drugs, history of blood pressure problems, chest pain or leg pain with exercise
- Smoking history, environmental hazards
- Changes in vision or speech, dizziness, confusion, headache, symptoms of neuropathy (tingling, numbness, pain at rest that disappears with activity)
- Weight changes, history of gastrointestinal problems (indigestion, diarrhea, constipation)
- Urinary frequency or incontinence
- Women—menstrual history, history of changes noted with intercourse (if sexually active); men—problems with erectile dysfunction or amount of ejaculate (if sexually active)
- Blurred vision, decreased acuity, most recent eye examination
- Financial security, insurance

Physical Examination. Assess for:

- Weight and height
- Emotional state, responsiveness, attention, alertness, comprehension, appropriateness of response
- Neuromuscular: visual acuity (with and without glasses); range of motion, muscle strength (both upper and lower extremities); touch, temperature, pain, vibratory sense (especially lower extremities), position sense, deep tendon reflexes
- Blood pressure (both lying and standing), peripheral pulses, ankle-brachial indices
- Bowel sounds, gastrointestinal masses
- Urinary output and fluid intake
- Vaginal discharge, irritation
- Skin intactness, temperature, lesions, moisture, hair distribution, texture (especially in lower extremities), turgor
- Results of diagnostic tests:
  - Blood/plasma glucose levels in the fasting or postprandial state may be normal (euglycemia), high (hyperglycemia), or low (hypoglycemia).
  - HbA_{1c} may be normal or elevated.
  - Serum lipids may be normal or abnormal.
  - Urine and blood ketones may be negative or positive.
  - Urine microalbumin-creatinine ratio and serum creatinine, as markers of renal function, may be normal or abnormal.

Nursing Diagnoses, Outcomes, and Interventions

Nursing Diagnosis: Risk for Deficient Fluid Volume

Outcomes. Common examples of expected outcomes for the patient with a diagnosis of *risk for deficient fluid volume* are:

Patient will:

- Exhibit physical signs of fluid balance.
- Return to baseline weight.
- Have elastic skin turgor and moist mucous membranes.
- Have blood pressure, pulse, serum electrolytes, and hematocrit within normal range.
- Have urine specific gravity of 1.010 to 1.025.
- Have a fluid intake of 2.5 to 3 L/day, orally or parenterally (unless restrictions are prescribed).
- Explain measures to prevent fluid deficit.

NURSING INTERVENTIONS. To improve fluid status, the patient needs to improve his or her metabolic status and to ingest an adequate amount of fluid. The nurse explores possible causes of fluid loss (dehydration) with the patient, and reinforces the relationship between fluid loss and high blood glucose levels. For example, the nurse may state, "Glucose attracts water, and when blood glucose is high, glucose goes out in the urine, pulling water with it, thus increasing urination." The nurse stresses that increased thirst is nature's way of telling the person to drink more fluids; if the person is not drinking, fluid losses will not be controlled. This illustration can help the patient visualize how to manage the diabetes using tools such as HBGM and testing for urine and blood ketones. In addition to teaching about these tests, the nurse educates patients about diet and medications and provides emergency telephone numbers of the physician and diabetes team.

RELATED NIC INTERVENTIONS. Fluid/Electrolyte Management, Fluid Management, Fluid Monitoring, Teaching: Disease Process

Nursing Diagnosis: Ineffective Therapeutic Regimen Management

OUTCOMES. Common examples of expected outcomes for the patient with a diagnosis of *ineffective therapeutic regimen management* are:

Patient will:

- Describe the rationale for following prescribed treatment regimen.
- Describe and follow prescribed health regimen, including medications and exercise plan.
- Perform self-monitoring.

NURSING INTERVENTIONS

EXERCISE. In all persons with diabetes, exercise is an important part of the medical management and deserves careful and thorough explanation before implementation. Physical activity has important physiologic and psychologic implications. Exercise is also a wonderful insulin sensitizer, enhancing glucose uptake into skeletal muscle. The exact mechanism is unknown, but it occurs in both type 1 and type 2 DM. For example, children who go away to summer camp can decrease their insulin dosage by 25% or more as a consequence of the insulin sensitization resulting from exercise.

Many persons with type 2 DM have insulin resistance and excess weight. Any type of therapy that decreases resistance and promotes weight loss has potential benefit. Both clinical experience and various studies have shown exercise to be of value in both insulin resistance and weight loss. For maximal benefit, the exercise program should be done on a regular basis. Even then, the effect on glucose may be short lived.

Exercise plans for persons with diabetes cannot be discussed without exploring the risks and benefits of such programs (Boxes 39-10 and 39-11). Exercise is contraindicated during periods of hyperglycemia (fingerstick blood glucose value of 250 mg/dl or higher) and ketosis. The combination of hyperglycemia, ketosis, and exercise exerts a physiologic stress on the body, resulting in progressive hyperglycemia.

The exercise prescription may look something like Figure 39-8 and consists of type of exercise, intensity, duration, and frequency. Before entering into any type of exercise program, all patients should have a complete history and physical examination, with particular attention to the cardiovascular system and any long-term complications. An exercise stress test is recommended for patients with DM who are considered to be at high risk for cardiovascular disease. High-risk factors include:

Box 39-10 Benefits of Exercise for the Patient With Diabetes Mellitus

- Improves insulin sensitivity
- Lowers blood glucose during and after exercise
- Improves lipid profile
- May improve hypertension
- Increases energy expenditure
- Assists with weight loss
- Preserves lean body mass
- Promotes cardiovascular fitness
- Increases strength and flexibility
- Improves sense of well-being
- Improves survival

Data from American Diabetes Association: Clinical practice recommendations 2004, *Diabetes Care* 27(Suppl 1):S1-S150, 2004; Gulati M, Pandey DK, Arnsdorf MF: Exercise capacity and the risk of death in women: the St. James Women Take Heart Project, *Circulation* 108(13):1554-1559, 2003; Myers J et al: Exercise capacity and mortality among men referred for exercise testing, *N Engl J Med* 346(11):793-801, 2002.

Box 39-11 Risks of Exercise for the Patient With Diabetes Mellitus

- Precipitation or exacerbation of cardiovascular disease, angina, or dysrhythmias, followed by sudden death
- Hypoglycemia, if taking insulin or oral agents
- Exercise-related hypoglycemia
- Late-onset postexercise hypoglycemia
- Hyperglycemia after very strenuous exercise
- Worsening of long-term complications:
  —Proliferative retinopathy
  —Peripheral neuropathy
  —Autonomic neuropathy
- Traumatic foot ulcerations

Data from American Diabetes Association: Clinical practice recommendations 2004, *Diabetes Care* 27(Suppl 1):S1-S150, 2004.

Nursing Care Plan

Nursing Care Plan
Patient With Diabetes Mellitus

Data The patient is an obese, 62-year-old married woman with an 8-year history of type 2 diabetes mellitus controlled by oral hypoglycemic agents. She has been referred to a short-term ambulatory diabetes education program for instruction on insulin administration to achieve better blood glucose control. The patient states that she has an inconsistent sleep-activity schedule and does not exercise regularly. She has accurate knowledge of dietary modifications and has successfully lost weight; however, within a few months she gains the weight back. She performs regular foot checks, wears well-fitted shoes, and has no skin breakdown, but complains of loss of sensation in both feet. Although she performed self-glucose monitoring in the past, she does not currently have a working blood glucose monitor at home. Her fasting blood glucose is 220 mg/dl. Physical assessment reveals 1+ peripheral pulses; extremities warm and dry, with color consistent with the rest of her body; patellar and Achilles tendon reflexes 3+ (on scale of 1 to 4); decreased perception to touch in lower extremities; and decreased vibration and pinprick sensation to great toes bilaterally. She weighs 200 pounds and is 5 foot, 4 inches tall. Her blood pressure is 134/84 mm Hg; heart rate, 92 beats/min; and respirations, 24 breaths/min. Her urine is negative for microalbuminuria. Her vision is 20/40 on the Snellen chart.

Nursing Diagnosis
Risk for deficient fluid volume related to hyperglycemia

Outcomes
- Patient will maintain serum glucose level within normal parameters.
- Patient will remain free of fluid imbalance.

Related NOC Outcomes
- Blood Glucose Level
- Fluid Balance
- Hydration

Related NIC Interventions
- Fluid Management
- Fluid Monitoring
- Hypoglycemia Management

Nursing Interventions/Rationales
- Monitor blood glucose levels. *Increased blood glucose levels increase the osmolarity of the serum, which results in fluid being pulled from the tissues into the vascular space and elimination by the kidneys via osmotic diuresis.*
- Assess and monitor for fluid volume deficiency. *Diabetic patients are at increased risk for hypovolemia caused by osmotic diuresis secondary to hyperglycemia. The earlier fluid volume deficiencies are identified, the quicker fluid balance can be restored.*
- Encourage the intake of 2 to 3 L of fluid per day. *To replace fluid losses and prevent hypervolemia and cellular dehydration.*
- Teach patient the relationship between high blood glucose levels and fluid loss. *To help the patient understand the need for blood glucose control and to increase the likelihood of compliance with therapeutic regimen.*
- Teach patient signs and symptoms of fluid volume depletion and the need to report such manifestations quickly. *To facilitate early recognition and treatment.*

Nursing Diagnosis
Imbalanced nutrition: more than body requirements

Outcomes
- Patient will achieve weight loss to within 20 pounds of ideal weight.
- Patient will select correct dietary choices within prescribed diet.

Related NOC Outcomes
- Nutritional Status
- Nutritional Status: Food & Fluid Intake
- Nutritional Status: Nutrient Intake

Related NIC Interventions
- Eating Disorders Management
- Nutrition Management
- Weight Management
- Weight Reduction Assistance

Nursing Interventions/Rationales
- Obtain a thorough diet history. *To assess the patient's current dietary intake so that dietary alterations to maintain blood glucose control can be planned.*
- Encourage patient to become involved in setting goals for dietary changes, documenting food intake, and planning meals. *Changes are more likely to be made when the patient is involved in planning those changes. Patients know their own likes and dislikes, financial resources, and ability to make dietary changes. Participation allows the patient greater control over the situation.*
- Set realistic weight control goals. *Setting goals that are unrealistic and unachievable produces frustration and hopelessness, which may discourage the patient from trying to control her weight.*
- Help the patient identify an acceptable weight loss schedule. *Permanent weight loss is generally gradual and based on sound dietary principles. Fad diets should be avoided. The patient's agreement with the weight loss plan increases the probability of compliance.*
- Teach or reinforce earlier teaching about the selected system of dietary management. *Knowledge increases the likelihood of compliance.*
- Teach the patient how to handle sick days and unplanned social events. *To prepare the patient to deal appropriately with unusual dietary events or inability to intake food.*
- Teach the patient the need for maintaining food intake distribution throughout the day. *To maintain consistency of blood glucose levels after the administration of insulin.*

Nursing Diagnosis
Risk for infection related to altered tissue perfusion secondary to chronic hyperglycemia

Outcomes
- Patient will remain free from infection.
- Patient will accurately verbalize the relationship between poor blood glucose control and risk for infection.
- Patient will accurately list signs and symptoms of infection.

Related NOC Outcomes

- Immune Status
- Knowledge: Infection Control
- Tissue Integrity: Skin & Mucous Membranes

Related NIC Interventions

- Skin Surveillance
- Surveillance
- Teaching: Disease Process

Nursing Interventions/Rationales

- Teach the patient the relationship between infection and metabolic control. *If the patient understands that good metabolic control decreases the risk for infection, she is more likely to comply with prescribed treatments. Metabolic control reduces the extent of neuropathy that occurs from chronic hyperglycemia.*
- Monitor for signs of localized infections (heat, redness, warmth, pain) and systemic infections (elevated white blood cell count, fever, lethargy). *Early detection of infection results in treatment being implemented more quickly.*
- Teach the patient the signs of localized and systemic infections. *The patient is usually the first to identify early infections.*
- Teach patient to inspect feet daily for signs of infection. *Diabetic neuropathy (sensory loss) increases the patient's risk for foot infections. The need for foot care cannot be overemphasized.*

Nursing Diagnosis

Deficient knowledge (self-administration of insulin, care of equipment, home monitoring of blood glucose) related to lack of previous exposure to information or skill

Outcomes

- Patient will accurately verbalize disease process; need for blood glucose control; and signs of infection, hyperglycemia, and hypoglycemia.
- Patient will accurately demonstrate self-administration of insulin.

Related NOC Outcomes

- Knowledge: Medication
- Knowledge: Treatment Regimen

Related NIC Interventions

- Teaching: Prescribed Medication
- Teaching: Psychomotor Skill

Nursing Interventions/Rationales

- Support and encourage patient as necessary to self-inject insulin. *At first patients may be afraid to self-inject. Adults who perform self-injections have minimal discomfort and come to realize they are capable of performing this skill.*
- Demonstrate and have patient return demonstrate home blood glucose monitoring (HGBM), correcting technique as needed. *The patient needs to be taught the skill before performing it. Evaluation of patient skill is necessary to ensure accuracy.*
- Teach the patient about the effect of activity, dietary intake, and insulin on blood glucose. Instruct patient on timing of blood glucose monitoring. *To help the patient understand that all aspects of care are interrelated. HBGM provides immediate feedback about previous behaviors and reinforces the value of therapeutic measures.*
- Teach the signs and symptoms and treatment measures for hyperglycemia and hypoglycemia. *This knowledge decreases the fear of reactions and allows for quick intervention if hyperglycemia or hypoglycemia does occur.*
- Teach about the care of insulin and supplies. *To ensure that insulin remains stable and equipment is sterile.*
- Refer to dietitian for further teaching regarding any dietary modifications that need to be made now that the patient is receiving insulin. *The dietitian enforces previous teaching, assesses for new dietary needs, and teaches new information.*

Nursing Diagnosis

Ineffective health maintenance related to ineffective coping skills

Outcomes

- Patient will independently maintain blood glucose control via diet, monitoring, and self-administration of insulin.
- Patient will state at least one change that will help her improve her blood glucose control.

Related NOC Outcomes

- Health Promoting Behavior
- Knowledge: Health Resources
- Knowledge: Treatment Regimen
- Participation in Health Care Decisions

Related NIC Interventions

- Coping Enhancement
- Health System Guidance
- Self-Modification Assistance
- Teaching: Disease Process

Nursing Interventions/Rationales

- Counsel patient regarding effects of lack of exercise and diet on blood glucose levels. *Change in behavior is more likely to occur if the patient understands the relationships between lifestyle, activity, diet, and glucose control.*
- Explore willingness and ability to change behaviors: sleep-activity, diet, and exercise. *Goals are more likely to be achieved if the patient agrees that the changes will be beneficial.*
- Engage patient in mutual problem solving as opposed to prescribing. *Increasing patients' sense of control can help with self-esteem and enhance attitudes toward change.*
- Explore sources for long-term support in learning more effective ways of coping (i.e., weight loss, exercise, diabetes management). *Changing lifestyle, eating behaviors, and coping skills is difficult; support over long periods is usually required.*

Evaluation

Evaluation is based on comparing the patient's outcomes with desired outcomes.

- Age over 35 years
- Age less than 25 years with (1) type 1 DM of less than 15 years' duration or (2) type 2 DM of more than 10 years' duration
- Presence of any risk factor for cardiovascular disease
- Presence of microvascular complications of DM
- Presence of peripheral vascular disease
- Presence of autonomic neuropathy

The Detection of Silent Myocardial Ischemia in Asymptomatic Diabetic Subjects study, which used adenosine technetium-99m sestamibi single-photon emission computed tomography (SPECT) myocardial perfusion imaging, demonstrated that autonomic neuropathy was the strongest predictor of myocardial ischemia.[111]

Once the patient with DM has been cleared for an exercise program, special precautions may be indicated (see Guidelines for Safe Practice box). Studies have repeatedly shown that physical fitness or exercise capacity is a major predictor of survival in individuals with and without diabetes.[38,63] The professional nurse should use this fact to motivate patients to engage in routine aerobic exercise.

INSULIN SELF-ADMINISTRATION. Patients taking insulin should be able to name the prescribed type of insulin, doses and peak effects, and how the exercise regimen and diet are coordinated with the insulin. They should know insulin measurement (units) and the need for similarly calibrated syringes and insulin pens. In addition, they must know how to handle insulin needs on sick days.

For safe insulin administration, patients must know how to draw insulin into the syringe, use the insulin pen device (if pertinent), mix two insulins (if pertinent), select and prepare the injection site, use consistent injection sites, rotate within those sites, and inject insulin (Box 39-12). Most patients have some fears related to self-injection and should start practicing as soon as insulin treatment is deemed necessary.

Preparing the Insulin Dose. The nurse teaches the patient to rotate or roll the vial or pen of cloudy insulin to return any precipitated particles to solution and to draw the required dose of insulin into the syringe using correct technique. Current insulin syringes have little or no dead space, thus eliminating a potential

Name: ______________________ Date: __________

Mode: (type of exercise)*

( ) Cycling ( ) Jumping rope
( ) Walking
( ) Swimming ( ) Other __________
* Can change/rotate

Intensity: (how hard)

Perceived exertion scale
6
7 Very, very light
8
9 Very light
10
11 Fairly light
12
13 Somewhat hard
14
15 Hard
16
17 Very hard
18
19 Very, very hard
20

Duration: (how long)*

Slow (stretch-warm up) __________
Faster (training) __________
Slow (cooling down) __________
* Start slow and build up

Frequency: (how often) Type of exercise How often

Aerobic: __________ __________
Other: __________ __________

Physician: __________

Figure 39-8 Sample exercise prescription.

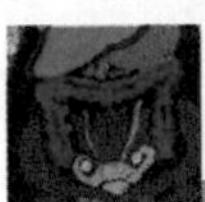

GUIDELINES FOR SAFE PRACTICE *Exercise Program for Patient With Diabetes Mellitus*

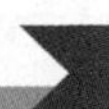

Exercise Type

Aerobic (low impact for type 2 diabetes mellitus)
Starting with light level

Exercise Session

Each session should eventually include:
—Warm-up stretching and limbering exercises, 5 to 10 minutes
—Aerobic exercise with heart rate in target zone (as defined by physician) or perceived exertion rating, 20 to 30 minutes
—Light exercise and stretching to cool down, 15 to 20 minutes

Exercise Frequency

Three to 5 times per week

Special Precautions

Consider insulin or oral agent regimen (may need to decrease insulin).
Consider the plan for food intake. Discuss with health care provider. May need to take extra carbohydrate before exercise.
Check blood glucose before, during, and afterward (for baseline).
If glucose level is higher than 250 mg/dl, check ketones. If negative or normal, okay to exercise. If positive, take insulin; do not exercise until ketones are negative or normal.
Exercise should not cause shortness of breath and should be stopped with any onset of chest pain or dyspnea.
Carry diabetes identification card and bracelet.
Carry a source of easily absorbed carbohydrate (three glucose tablets or hard candies).
Do not exercise in extreme heat or cold. In temperature extremes, try to exercise indoors (recreation center, walking in mall).
Inspect feet daily and after exercise.

Precautions for Selected Persons

Persons with insensitive feet should choose good shoes for walking and avoid running and jogging. Swimming and cycling may be included in the exercise program.
Persons with proliferative retinopathy should avoid exercises associated with Valsalva's maneuver, those which jar and jolt the head, and exercises with the head in a low position.
Persons with hypertension should avoid exercises associated with Valsalva's maneuver and intense exercises involving the torso and arms. (Exercises involving the lower extremities are preferred.)

source of error. The patient can practice the procedure using saline solution and a syringe.

If the patient is using an insulin pen, when a new cartridge is started, the patient must do an "air shot" of 8 to 10 units to prime the cartridge. Then, for subsequent injections, the patient must do an "air shot" of 2 units before each injection. The patient should anchor the pen securely after inserting the needle and before injecting the insulin, thus reducing the risk of bruising. The needle should be kept in the subcutaneous tissue for a count of 10 before removing it.

Patient fear of pain is greatly reduced if the nurse self-injects sterile saline (rather than the traditional orange or sponge), thus demonstrating no discomfort with injection. Given the superior insulin absorption from the abdomen, patients can be taught to give their first injection in the upper abdomen. For the first injection, the nurse may elect to delay teaching about the preparation and focus first on self-injection. Adults may be better able to focus on preparing the syringe after experiencing self-injection.

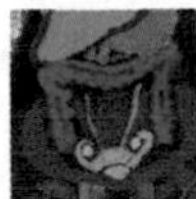

GUIDELINES FOR SAFE PRACTICE *Mixing Two Insulins in One Syringe*

1. Gather equipment.
2. Wash hands.
3. Roll vial of longer-acting insulin. *Never mix insulin glargine in a syringe with any other insulin.*
4. Cleanse tops of vials with alcohol.
5. Draw up air equivalent to the dose of the longer-acting insulin, and inject the air into that vial. (Do not draw up this insulin.) Remove needle from vial.
6. Draw up air equivalent to the dose of the rapid-acting analog (RAA) or regular insulin, inject the air into the bottle, and withdraw the RAA or regular insulin to the correct dose. Remove all air, and readjust to the correct dose. Remove needle.
7. Insert needle into the vial of the longer-acting insulin, and draw up the correct dose.
8. If an error is made, discard the insulin in the syringe and start over.

Mixing Two Insulins. If the patient is using two insulins, they may be mixed in one syringe so that only one injection is necessary (see Guidelines for Safe Practice box). As mentioned earlier, insulin glargine can never be mixed in a syringe with any other insulin, since its lower pH will result in precipitation. A relative contraindication is mixing a crystalline zinc insulin (Lente or Ultralente) with other types of insulins. Most practitioners permit patients to mix other insulins with Lente or Ultralente and inject immediately. The mix-and-inject immediately routine is recommended, regardless of which insulins are being mixed together.

Mixing two insulins in the same syringe is one of the more complex psychomotor skills the patient has to learn; therefore it needs to be started early. A major risk of mixing two insulins in one syringe is contamination of the two vials of insulin. Cross-contamination can be avoided by always withdrawing from the lispro or regular insulin vial first, since injecting minute amounts of RAA or regular insulin into a vial of longer-acting insulin is less problematic than the RAA or regular insulin being contaminated by the longer-acting insulin.

If the patient has difficulty mastering the skill of mixing two insulins, he or she may take two separate injections each time or

Box 39-12 Professional Prompter Worksheet for Diabetes Education

Teaching Survival/Initial Skills

Concentrate on survival. These are the skills every patient must know before discharge. The patient cannot go further without this foundation.

Assess patient's knowledge via a pretest.

Type 1 Diabetes Mellitus Survival/Initial Skills (S1)

Address psychologic and family factors.

Ensure patient can give insulin correctly (i.e., see the increments, inject correctly, use proper sites, reuse syringe, know time and action of insulin).

Monitor blood glucose and urine ketones.

Recognize and treat hypoglycemia.

Type 2 Diabetes Mellitus Survival/Initial Skills (S2)

Address psychologic and family factors.

Explain what diabetes is (insulin resistance versus insulin deficiency).

Treat with diet, oral agent, and insulin if necessary, or combination therapy.

Monitor blood glucose and urine ketones.

Recognize and treat hypoglycemia if patient is taking sulfonylureas or insulin.

Tools to Use for Survival/Initial Teaching

Barrier check

Initial assessment

Take-home instruction sheet

American Diabetes Association curriculum guidelines

Referral to specialty practice or center

Referral to group class in local hospital

Assessment (S1 and S2)

Perform complete assessment, including diabetes knowledge.

Barriers (S1 and S2)

Define Barrier

Fatigue

Pain

High anxiety

Blindness

Teaching Tools

Give instructions a second time.

Identify source of anxiety and address it before proceeding.

Use audio material and devices.

Refer patient to specialty center.

Overview of Diabetes (S2)

Determine whether patient can:

- Verbalize that diabetes is a disease in which the body is unable to use carbohydrate foods properly because of lack of insulin or inability to use insulin
- Define high blood sugar in terms of blood glucose (normal versus diabetes); list symptoms
- Define which type of diabetes he or she has
- Describe essential parts of diabetes management: knowledge, self-care, meal planning, exercise, and medication; can state the effect each of these has on the blood glucose level
- Explain the effect of activity on blood glucose
- Explain the effect of illness or stress on blood glucose

Stress and Psychologic Adjustment (S1 and S2)

Determine whether patient:

- Has adapted to having diabetes
- Expresses feelings about having diabetes
- Acknowledges losses—grief process (fear, anxiety, denial, anger, bargaining, depression, acceptance)

Family Involvement and Social Support (S1 and S2)

Determine whether patient and family:

- Can identify one feeling a person with diabetes may experience
- Can state ways diabetes has affected the family
- Have an adequate support person or network

Nutrition (S1 and S2)

Determine whether patient:

- Has an individualized meal plan
- Can state reasons for maintaining consistency (if appropriate) of meal spacing, proper mealtimes, and snacks to avoid hypoglycemia or hyperglycemia
- Can describe the relationship of insulin or oral agent, activity, and caloric intake to glycemic control
- Can explain diet changes for sick-day management, exercise, use of alcohol, change in meal schedule, and restaurant dining
- Knows the importance of attaining and maintaining ideal body weight
- Can state the effects of dietary fiber

Exercise and Activity

Determine whether patient:

- Can state how exercise affects diabetes control
- Can describe the cautions and risks of exercise
- Knows when one should not exercise
- Has a personal exercise program

Medications (S1 and S2)

Determine whether patient can verbalize or demonstrate the following.

Insulin

The function of insulin (rapid, quick, intermediate, or long acting)

Differentiation of insulin types

Medication schedule—amounts and times taken

Correct technique for insulin preparation:

—Inject insulin at room temperature.
—Rotate bottle to mix (cloudy insulin).
—Inject air.
—Withdraw proper amount of insulin.
—Rid syringe of air bubbles.

Correct technique for drawing up insulin, two types:

—Rotate bottle to mix (cloudy) insulin.
—Inject air into both bottles.
—Withdraw clear (regular) insulin first.
—Add proper amount of second insulin.

Correct technique for insulin administration:

—Clean site with alcohol.
—Gather skin and insert needle all the way.

Box 39-12 Professional Prompter Worksheet for Diabetes Education—cont'd

—Inject insulin, holding needle steady (needle should go in at 90-degree angle unless person is thin).
—Use consistent sites; rotate within those sites (abdomen, arm, leg, buttocks).

Correct technique for use of an insulin pen device:
—Use 8- to 10-unit "air shot" for first prime of a new pen or pen cartridge.
—Use subsequent 2-unit "air shot" before each injection to prime air out of cartridge.

Storage of insulin:
—Store insulin in the refrigerator.
—For travel, insulin can be stored at room temperature (57° to 85° F) up to 1 month.

Disposal of syringes in sealable can or special disposal unit
Fact that insulin can cause hypoglycemia

Oral Agents

Action of oral agent
Medication schedule—amount and time to be taken
Need to eat three carbohydrate-consistent meals a day
Can cause hypoglycemia

Relationships Among Nutrition, Exercise, Medication, and Blood Glucose Levels (S1 and S2)

Determine whether patient can verbalize or demonstrate:

- Effect of food on blood glucose
- Effect of insulin oral agents on blood glucose
- Effect of oral agents on insulin resistance
- Effect of physical activity on blood glucose
- Effect of illness on blood glucose

Monitoring and Use of Results (S1 and S2)

Determine whether patient can verbalize or demonstrate:

- Need for monitoring glucose
- Normal range of blood glucose and acceptable targets
- Capillary blood glucose monitoring:
  —Loads and operates lancing device
  —Holds arm down to the side to get better drop of blood
  —Obtains large hanging drop of blood
  —Places blood on strip properly
  —Waits appropriate amount of time according to directions
  —Reads meter and records results
  —Uses meter (knows name of meter, strips to use; how to calibrate and use control solutions; how to clean, insert battery; and understands readout)
- Whether alternate site blood glucose monitoring can be performed with his or her meter and, if so, appropriate or inappropriate time to do so to enable accurate results
- Checking ketones:
  —Knows how to do it
  —Knows when to do it
- When and whom to call for help

Acute Complications: Hyperglycemia

Determine whether patient can verbalize or demonstrate:

- Definition and cause of hyperglycemia
- Symptoms of hyperglycemia
- Illness and sick-day rules:
  —What to do about insulin or oral agents when ill
  —How often to check glucose and ketones
  —When to call physician
  —Sick-day eating

Acute Complications: Hypoglycemia (S1 and S2)

Determine whether patient can verbalize or demonstrate:

- Definition and cause of hypoglycemia
- Symptoms of hypoglycemia
- Treatment of hypoglycemia (wears diabetes identification)
- When to call physician, nurse practitioner

Chronic Complications

Determine whether patient can verbalize or demonstrate:

- Possible long-term complications.
- Importance of prevention; primary role of glycemic control.
- The organs and body systems at risk in diabetes:
  —Eyes
  —Blood vessels
  —Blood pressure
  —Feet
  —Kidneys
  —Neurologic
  —Reproductive
- Reasons for good foot care, including daily cleansing and inspection/appropriate footwear
- Reason for yearly dilated funduscopic examination (and last date)
- Need for blood pressure control; blood pressure goal

Foot, Skin, and Dental Care

Determine whether patient can verbalize or demonstrate the importance of good health habits:

- Dental
- Skin
- Feet
- Signs of infection
- Effect of smoking, alcohol, and drug abuse

Behavior Change Strategies, Goal Setting, and Problem Solving

Determine whether patient can verbalize or demonstrate:

- The need for a planned system of medical care, including follow-up and education
- The benefits and responsibilities of goal setting for self-help care
- The importance of being well informed, equal partner to make choices

Use of Health Care System and Community Resources

Determine whether patient is aware of resources that can help:

- American Diabetes Association
- Self-management classes
- Services for the blind
- Juvenile Diabetes Research Foundation
- Local diabetes associations

Continued

Box 39-12 Professional Prompter Worksheet for Diabetes Education—cont'd

Necessary Take-Home (S1 and S2)

Determine whether patient:

- Feels comfortable doing all skills under survival
- Knows the skills and is able to simulate them in a normal day (i.e., take you through a day and list all diabetes-related activities as patient would do them)
- Knows whom to call, the telephone number, and when to call
- Has a return appointment card with health care provider's name and phone number listed
- Has instructions written on:
  - —Take Home Instruction form
  - —Choice to Better Daily Living form
- Has a schedule of the diabetes classes if patient chooses to attend them
- Has a meal plan and has consulted with a dietitian (If dietitian is unavailable and you must instruct on meal plan, refer to section on nutrition.)

Adapted from Eaks GA: *Professional prompter worksheet,* Kansas City, Kan, 1993, University of Kansas Medical Center, Cray Diabetes Education Center.

have a family member, significant other, or friend prefill the syringes. A 7- to 10-day supply of insulin (including mixed insulin) can be predrawn.

Injection Sites. Two principles govern injection sites: consistency and rotation. Consistent use of sites is critical because insulin absorption varies dramatically depending on the anatomic site. The upper abdomen provides the quickest absorption, followed by the arms, legs, and lower buttocks. The abdominal site is also not affected by exercise. Consistent use of a specified injection site for a specified injection time helps eliminate some variability in glucose levels. For example, the patient could use the abdomen for the prebreakfast injection, the arm for the predinner injection, and the buttocks for the bedtime injection. The rotation of injections among the designated anatomic sites helps prevent lipodystrophy. Ideally, injections should be given 1 inch apart while trying not to reuse an injection site within a 2- to 4-week period. The injection site should be cleansed with 70% isopropyl alcohol before use.

Lipodystrophy can occur with repeated injections, causing poor absorption of medication (Figure 39-9). Two forms of lipodystrophy can occur: hypertrophy and atrophy. Hypertrophy is thickening of an injection site from the development of fibrous scar tissue as a result of repeated injections. A hypertrophic area is usually devoid of nerve endings, and the patient likes to reuse it because injections are painless, but absorption is erratic. Atrophy is loss of subcutaneous fat from unknown causes; however, an immunologic process has been implicated.[79] Lipodystrophies may be partially caused by impurities in insulin; the development of purified insulins has decreased this problem, but rotation of sites is still important. Recommended sites for subcutaneous injection are illustrated in Figure 39-10.

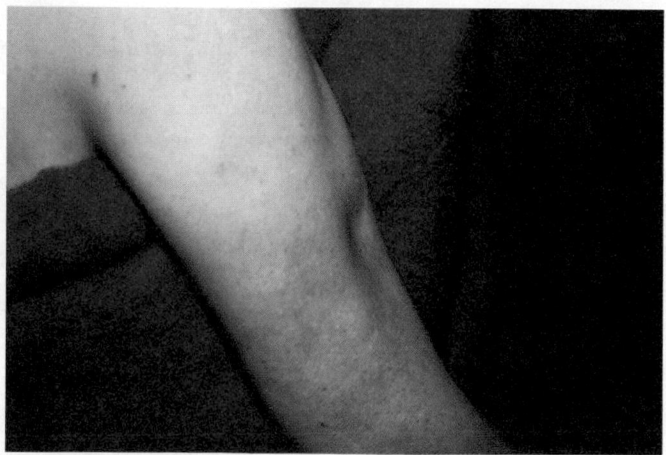

Figure 39-9 Lipodystrophy of the arm.

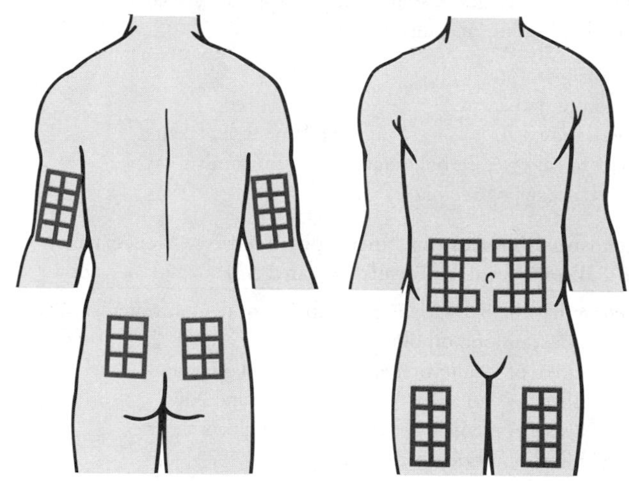

Figure 39-10 Insulin injection sites.

Injection of Insulin. Insulin should be administered subcutaneously. In the past the subcutaneous tissue was pinched up before injection. With the current insulin syringes, with needles from 0.25 to 0.5 inch long, the patient does not need to pinch up the subcutaneous tissue unless he or she is very thin or cachectic. Rather, the subcutaneous tissue is gently gathered or, if the patient is obese, stretched tautly. With these shorter-needle syringes, the needle is inserted at a 90-degree angle. There is no need for routine aspiration. Injections should produce little, if any, discomfort. Use of the techniques described in the Patient/Family Teaching box can minimize painful injections.

Although disposable syringes are designed for single use, many patients with DM reuse their own insulin syringes until the needle dulls. Insulin has bacteriostatic additives that inhibit bacterial growth. With reuse of the syringe, however, the light coating of

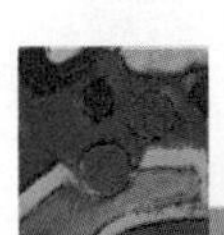

PATIENT/FAMILY TEACHING
Steps To Eliminate Painful Insulin Injections

- Inject insulin that has been at room temperature for 15 minutes. Do not inject cold insulin.
- Wait until the topical alcohol has dried before injecting insulin.
- Keep muscles in the area of injection relaxed, not tensed.
- Penetrate the skin quickly. Use the hingelike action of the wrist to "dart" the needle in.
- Do not change the direction of the needle on insertion or withdrawal.
- Do not use dull needles.
- Use the shortest possible needles, depending on adiposity.
- Use the finest gauge needles.

lubrication on the needle is lost and injections may be more uncomfortable. Some studies also demonstrate physical damage to the bevel of the needle after even a single use, thereby creating the potential for inaccurate drawing up of insulin and perhaps incomplete insulin delivery when syringes are reused. In patients who practice good hygiene and good injection technique, however, the reuse of syringes is safe and practical.

Safe disposal of syringes and lancets used at home is critical. Sharps disposal containers are available for purchase at drugstores, or needles and syringes can be placed in a hard-sided receptacle, such as a detergent or bleach bottle. Patients should call their local government office for information on disposal.

Storage of Insulin and Other Supplies and Care of Syringes. Patients need to develop a home storage system for insulin and equipment. Insulin is stable for 30 days at room temperature; however, it is a good idea to refrigerate extra insulin. Insulin can be prefilled in syringes for 7 to 10 days. After drawing up the insulin into the syringe, the patient may draw approximately 5 units of air into the syringe, which provides some buffer if the plunger is accidentally pushed. Prefilled syringes should be stored in the refrigerator with the needles facing downward. All equipment should be stored out of the reach of children.

Patients should always have an extra vial of each type of insulin they use. Insulin has an expiration date, which should be checked at purchase; patients should purchase only the amount that can be used before the expiration date. When traveling on an airplane, patients should hand carry insulin and supplies to prevent loss. It is also recommended that they bring twice as many supplies as they anticipate using.

For persons unwilling or unable to use syringes, a variety of injection aids are available (Figure 39-11). Pen devices for insulin delivery facilitate taking injections away from home. The Autoject by Owen Mumford not only injects the needle but also injects the insulin; it gives a virtually pain-free injection and retails for approximately $40. Jet-spray injectors are also available but are expensive, retailing for approximately $400 to $600. Although jet-spray injectors are designed to reduce discomfort and enhance insulin absorption, some patients actually find them more uncomfortable and report inconsistencies with insulin delivery as a result of the variable pressure settings needed in different anatomic sites.

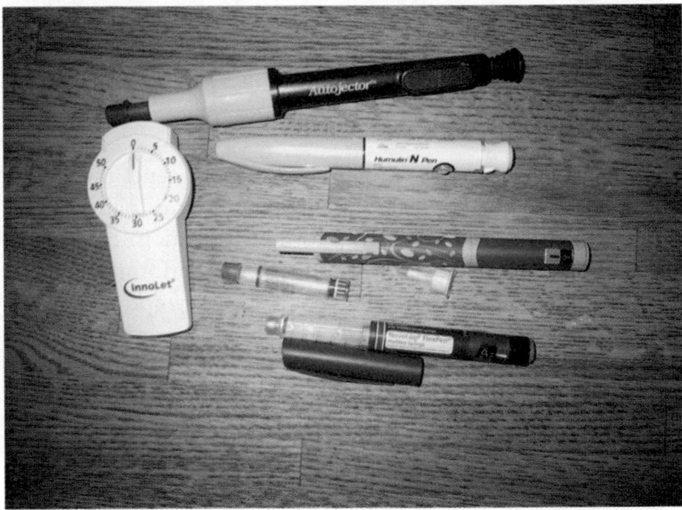

Figure 39-11 Insulin injection aids.

Measures to Assist the Sensory-Impaired Individual. Adaptation of equipment may be necessary for the sensory-impaired person. A number of aids for the visually handicapped are advertised in diabetes publications or are available from the American Foundation for the Blind or local agencies for the visually impaired. Special syringes with plunger locks, attachable devices for locking the plunger, and attachable needle and insulin bottle guides to facilitate entry of the needle into the bottle can be purchased. Persons who have failing vision may also use a small magnifying adapter that can be clipped to a syringe.

Persons with poor vision may draw air instead of insulin into the syringe and should be cautioned to invert the vial completely and insert the needle only a short distance. Visually impaired persons are often advised to use only about two thirds of a vial of insulin. Some persons have a family member or a friend draw the last doses from the vial. Another option is to know how long to use a vial before the level gets so low that the needle is not covered (e.g., if the vial holds 1000 units and the person is taking 40 units/day, he or she should stop using the vial on the twenty-second day unless assisted by a sighted person).

MANAGING ORAL AGENTS. Patients taking oral agents must be equally prepared to handle their medication. Each patient must know the name of the medication, dose, peak effects, and how the diet and exercise regimens are coordinated with medication therapy. If taking secretagogues, patients must be educated about hypoglycemia symptoms and treatment. Patients must know how to handle illness. Oral agents should be kept out of the reach of children, at room temperature, and out of direct sunlight. The medication should be hand carried when traveling to decrease the risk of loss.

SELF-MONITORING OF METABOLIC STATUS. All persons with diabetes should perform HBGM if possible. Meters are affordable (less than $80), and most manufacturers provide discount coupons or no-cost meters with the purchase of test strips. Home blood glucose meters correlate well with venous samples when correct technique is used (see Guidelines for Safe Practice box, p. 1126).

Although health care professionals recommend the use of physiologic parameters to monitor glucose status, patients continue to use symptoms as guides for self-regulation. Health care providers must emphasize the importance of performing a home blood glucose test to correlate a subjective symptom with an objective measure. All patients should use a diary or log to record the date, time, and monitoring results. Other diary notations may include medications, food intake, activity level, and illnesses so that the person can begin to see the relationship between blood glucose or urine ketone levels and the treatment regimen. Although many meters have large memories for results and may be downloaded to a computer by patients or providers, no meter manufacturer provides printing capability in a log book format, linking date, time and glucose result. Therefore the traditional paper log frequently provides both patients and health care providers with more comprehensive data on which to base changes in a patient's treatment regimen.

As patients gain expertise, they may manipulate insulin, diet, and exercise independently on the basis of monitoring results. Patients gain increasing independence on the basis of ability, interest, and encouragement by caregivers.

MANAGING HYPOGLYCEMIA. Patients receiving insulin or sulfonylureas must be educated about hypoglycemia (plasma blood glucose level of 60 mg/dl or lower). Patients must know:

- Causes of hypoglycemia (see Box 39-4)
- Signs and symptoms of hypoglycemia (see Box 39-5)
- Appropriate treatment of hypoglycemia
- How to obtain an identification card, Medic-Alert bracelet, or necklace and the importance of carrying or wearing it at all times
- The importance of carrying a quickly absorbed glucose source
- Methods to prevent further episodes of hypoglycemia

Because hypoglycemia can occur suddenly, family members and friends also should learn the symptoms and how to handle a reaction. Most hypoglycemia is mild and easily treated. If a patient is awake but groggy, another person can put corn syrup, honey, or cake icing in the patient's mouth between the gum and cheek. This will be absorbed through the oral mucosa, and the patient will usually be aroused sufficiently to take a glass of juice, milk, or sugar-sweetened coffee or tea (Box 39-13).

Glucagon should be prescribed for all individuals with type 1 DM. Significant others should be educated in its proper use. All patients should strive for prevention of hypoglycemia. Information about hypoglycemia should be included as part of the survival skills during the initial management phase. A good time to teach about hypoglycemia is after teaching about insulin injection and self-monitoring. It is helpful to illustrate survival teaching using simulation and going through a typical day with patients, letting them take the lead in relating all the diabetes-related activities in sequence. At this time, information about insulin reaction can be taught in relationship to time and action of insulin.

Box 39-13 Carbohydrates for Relief of Hypoglycemia*

- 4 ounces apple or orange juice
- 6 ounces carbonated soda drink (regular, not diet)
- ½ cup regular gelatin dessert (not diet)
- 4 cubes or 2 packets of sugar
- 3 pieces of hard candy
- 3 to 4 glucose tablets or equivalent to yield 15 g of carbohydrate

*Items listed provide 12 to 15 g of carbohydrate.

Somogyi Phenomenon. The Somogyi phenomenon is characterized by hyperglycemia after hypoglycemia. As is true in healthy persons without diabetes, the hypoglycemia in persons with diabetes stimulates the production of counterregulatory hormones (glucocorticoids, growth hormone, epinephrine). These hormones promote glycogenolysis and gluconeogenesis. In individuals without diabetes the blood glucose level remains in the normal range because with minimal elevations, insulin secretion is stimulated. In individuals with diabetes the blood glucose rises to abnormally high levels because insulin secretion is absent or altered. In some instances the signs and symptoms of hypoglycemia are subtle and may not be recognized. Or hyperglycemia following the hypoglycemia may be recognized in the early morning and mistaken for the dawn phenomenon. The assumption is made that the patient needs higher doses of insulin, but this treatment worsens the problem (Figure 39-12).

The signs and symptoms of the Somogyi phenomenon can be any of those normally associated with hypoglycemia but commonly consist only of night sweats, nightmares, restless sleep, and a headache on arising. With both the Somogyi phenomenon and the dawn phenomenon, the patient has glycosuria, relatively normal blood glucose levels with positive ketones (remember that counterregulatory hormones stimulate lipolysis and beta-oxidation of fats), and wide fluctuations in blood glucose unrelated to meals.

To differentiate the Somogyi from the dawn phenomenon, the patient should perform overnight HBGM at 2 AM and 4 AM. In the Somogyi phenomenon hypoglycemia will occur, followed by hyperglycemia. In the dawn phenomenon no overnight hypo-

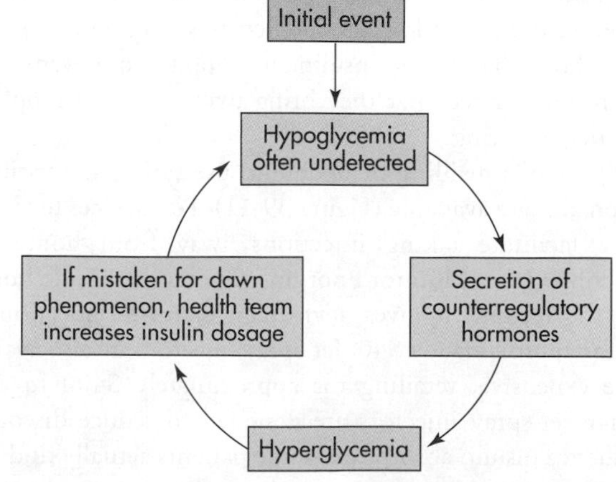

Figure 39-12 Sequence of events in Somogyi phenomenon.

glycemia will occur; rather, blood glucose levels will rise consistently overnight. Decreasing the dose of insulin precipitating the hypoglycemia treats the Somogyi phenomenon. Treatment of the dawn phenomenon consists of increasing the dose of the insulin, which is affecting nocturnal glucose levels.

A primary nursing role is to document reports of hypoglycemia, glucose intake, and laboratory results and to assess for the presence of night sweats, nightmares, and early-morning headaches. The nurse should also correlate these complaints and laboratory results with mealtimes. Such data help identify the phenomenon.

RELATED NIC INTERVENTIONS. Health Education, Risk Identification, Teaching: Procedure/Treatment

Nursing Diagnosis: Risk for Infection

OUTCOMES. Common examples of expected outcomes for the patient with a diagnosis of *risk for infection* are:

Patient will:

- List signs and symptoms of infection.
- State methods to decrease the risk for infection.
- Verbalize the need to do HBGM, at the frequency prescribed by the health care team.
- Identify factors that increase blood glucose.

NURSING INTERVENTIONS. Persons with uncontrolled diabetes are at increased risk of infection. The effectiveness of the skin as a first line of defense can be diminished. Uncontrolled diabetes leads to loss of fat deposits under the skin, loss of glycogen, and catabolism of body proteins. Hyperglycemia can hamper the inflammatory response and wound healing and impair leukocyte function, migration of leukocytes to the site of infection, phagocytosis, and bacterial killing, all of which are involved in combating infection. Circulatory impairments can also delay healing. The skin must be kept supple and as free of pathogenic organisms as possible. This is especially true in warm, moist areas that encourage growth of organisms (between the toes, under the breasts, and in the axillae and groin). It is extremely important that persons with diabetes carry out hygienic measures for prevention of infection daily, with special emphasis on foot care. They should seek medical attention immediately if an infection occurs.

Foot problems in diabetes involve the interaction of three major factors: neuropathy, ischemia, and sepsis. The need for foot care cannot be overemphasized. The patient's feet should be thoroughly assessed at every follow-up visit to identify patients at risk.[115] Peripheral neuropathy must be assessed objectively by measuring reaction to pinprick, vibration, and temperature and by assessing deep tendon reflexes (Box 39-14). Subjective sensations of paresthesias, pain, and numbness appear only after years of damage. The decreased ability to perceive a standard nylon filament pressure on the foot is a sign of advanced neuropathy with predisposition to foot ulceration. Once protective sensory loss is determined, the risk of the patient's foot being injured can be categorized[36] (Table 39-15).

Box 39-14 Assessment of the Feet of the Patient With Diabetes Mellitus

- *Color:* Compare one foot with the other.
- *Temperature:* Compare both feet with upper legs; assess for lines of demarcation.
- *Sensory function:* Test for pinprick and vibratory sense.
- *Reflexes:* Test Achilles and quadriceps tendon reflexes.
- *Pulses:* Check dorsalis pedis and posterior tibial pulses (ankle-brachial indices should be performed by diabetes team).
- *Lesions:* Examine for calluses, cuts, bruises, cracks, or infection.
- *Hair growth:* Assess if there is hair growth on toes or if it stops proximal to the toes.
- *Self-care:* Discuss self-care regimen being used.

Each person with diabetes is responsible for practicing preventive care on a daily basis through a thorough foot examination (see Patient/Family Teaching box, p. 1154, top). Podiatric consultation may be necessary for orthotics to relieve pressure areas and to treat calluses and corns. Extra-depth and custom-made shoes can be purchased in specialty stores. Medicare reimburses patients who meet certain foot problem criteria for a percentage of the cost of the shoes.

Improvement in metabolic control is the primary way to prevent infections. The patient and significant others must understand the relationship of poor blood glucose control to infection. They must also understand that infection can worsen glycemic control. Awareness of the signs and symptoms of infections and management of sick days is critical (see Patient/Family Teaching box, p. 1154, bottom). All illnesses influence the status of diabetes control; in most instances the person with diabetes needs increased insulin. A patient taking oral agents may need an increased dosage or even temporary insulin therapy during a concurrent illness.

TABLE 39-15 Risk Categories and Associated Footwear Guidelines

Category	Clinical Findings	Footwear Changes
0	Has protective sensation	Education on proper footwear
1	Has lost protective sensation	Add soft insole to shoe of proper contour and fit
2	Has lost protective sensation and has foot deformity	Depth footwear or custom shoe for severe deformity, molded insoles
3	Has lost protective sensation and has history of foot ulcer	Inspect type and condition of footwear and insoles at every visit

From Gillis W. Long Hansen's Disease Center, Bureau of Primary Health Care: *Comprehensive lower extremity amputation prevention programs: risk management categories for the foot*, accessed Aug 2004 from website: www.bphc.hrsa/gov/htm.

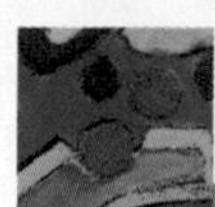

PATIENT/FAMILY TEACHING *Foot Care for the Patient With Diabetes Mellitus*

- Never soak feet.
- Wash feet daily and dry them well, paying attention to the area between the toes.
- Inspect feet daily. Look for:
  —Color changes
  —Swelling
  —Cuts
  —Cracks in the skin
  —Redness
  —Blisters
  —Temperature changes
- Never walk barefoot. Always wear shoes or slippers.
- Wear well-fitting shoes and clean socks.
- After bathing, when toenails are soft, cut nails straight across. Do not cut into the corners. File edges smooth with an emery board. If you have visual problems, have someone else cut your toenails for you.
- If feet are dry, apply lotion or cream; do not put lotion between the toes.
- Do not perform "bathroom surgery." Do not self-treat corns, calluses, warts, or ingrown toenails. Consult a podiatrist.
- Bathwater should be no warmer than 90° F. Test water temperature on your inner forearm, just as you would a baby's bottle, before immersing hands or feet.
- Do not use heating pads or hot water bottles.
- Enhance your circulation by:
  —Not smoking
  —Avoiding crossing legs when sitting
  —Protecting your hands and feet when exposed to cold
  —Avoiding tight elastic on socks
  —Exercising regularly
  —Using sunscreen
- *Any foot problem is a medical emergency.* Consult your primary care provider, podiatrist, or diabetes team immediately if any foot problem arises. Delay in seeking care can cost you your feet.

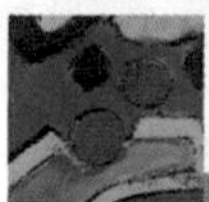

PATIENT/FAMILY TEACHING *Sick-Day Guidelines*

To determine when to call your physician or nurse about being sick or "out of sorts," go through the checklist and check what you have:

_____ Unable to keep down fluids or food
_____ Unable to eat regular foods for more than 1 day
_____ Signs of infection: redness, warmth, swelling, pus, tenderness any place
_____ Symptoms of dehydration: dry mouth, fever, thirst, dry flushed skin, vomiting, abdominal pain, severe nausea, diarrhea, rapid breathing
_____ Vomiting more than three times or diarrhea lasting longer than 3 hours
_____ Increased urination and increased thirst
_____ Coughing and bringing up yellow or green material
_____ Any symptoms getting worse
_____ Home blood glucose monitoring consistently showing elevated blood glucose beyond specified levels
_____ Fever present
_____ Ketones present
_____ Any questions about how to take care of yourself and control your diabetes
_____ Questions about adjusting insulin or oral agents

Information to have ready for physician or nurse when you call:

_____ Length of time you have been sick
_____ Your temperature
_____ What's bothering you (a list of symptoms)
_____ Test results: urine ketones and blood glucose
_____ Diabetes medication: type, time you take, and amount, as well as amount taken today
_____ Other medications you take; medication allergies; type, amount, time of medications recently taken
_____ Pharmacy phone number

Remember:

- Always take your insulin or oral agent.
- Drink plenty of fluids, including broth.
- Test urine ketones and blood glucose every 4 hours; record results.
- Eat carbohydrates according to your meal plan; replace with liquids if necessary.
- Know all your caregivers' phone numbers and names.

When you get better, return to your normal eating plan and medication dosage. This information applies to short-term illness (1 to 2 days). If you are unable to eat or have vomiting or diarrhea, call immediately.

RELATED NIC INTERVENTIONS. Infection Control, Infection Protection, Skin Surveillance

Nursing Diagnosis: Imbalanced Nutrition

OUTCOMES. Common examples of expected outcomes for the patient with a diagnosis of *imbalanced nutrition* (more than or less than body requirements) are:

Patient will:

- Exhibit signs of nutritional adequacy.
- Maintain weight, or lose or gain weight as appropriate.
- Have blood glucose, HbA_{1c}, and lipid measurements that are moving toward normal.
- Distribute food intake throughout the day.
- Verbalize dietary plan and ways to achieve dietary modifications.

NURSING INTERVENTIONS. Both the nurse and the dietitian are involved in nutritional education for the patient and family. A dietary history should be part of the professional nurse's initial assessment. Information about cultural or social food habits that are identified in the dietary history needs to be incorporated into the dietary plan. For example, it may be necessary to make accommodations for a vegetarian diet or for limited quantities of fast foods.

Because of the difficulty in changing food habits, the patient should be involved in setting goals for dietary changes. Compromises that may be necessary include:

- Identifying an acceptable weight loss schedule for the obese person
- Incorporating an alcoholic beverage into the daily plan, if desired
- Distributing food in a different pattern (e.g., a large noon meal and a small evening meal)
- Adding desserts to some meals

The patient and dietitian should identify the system for maintaining the dietary plan. The nurse documents the selected system in the nursing care plan so that everyone involved uses the same terminology and food groupings. The mutually established goals, including compromises and sociocultural practices, are also documented so that the patient is not given conflicting information. Significant others are included in the teaching.

After dietary goals are established, the nurse helps the patient apply dietary knowledge. This can be done through simulations in which the person chooses foods from restaurant menus, food models, or other learning tools; through patient participation in documenting food intake, blood and urine results, activity, and medications; and through discussions on how these factors interrelate.

The nurse evaluates patient and family satisfaction with the plan. After the initial management phase the patient should (1) be able to manage the diet for 1 week, (2) know whom to contact if unusual events requiring adjustments occur, and (3) know how to handle sick days. Ultimately patients should be able to:

- Manage dietary needs on a daily basis, making adjustments for normal life changes
- Select appropriate foods from restaurant menus or at social occasions
- Manage dietary needs while traveling or during shift work
- Manage dietary needs at unplanned social events (e.g., "happy hour" after work, unexpected business dinner)
- Evaluate success in dietary management through evaluating weight changes and HbA_{1c} or through HBGM
- Eliminate excess salt, decrease saturated fat intake, decrease caffeine intake, and make a conscious effort to include adequate vitamins and minerals
- Keep up-to-date on new findings about dietary management and consult health team members about the new recommendations
- Manipulate diet, exercise, and medications together to cover a variety of daily situations
- Work with others in the household to help them incorporate principles of healthy eating into the diet

RELATED NIC INTERVENTIONS. Nutrition Management, Nutrition Therapy, Nutritional Counseling, Nutritional Monitoring

Patient/Family Teaching. Joslin summarized the critical importance of patient education: "There is no disease in which an understanding by the patient of the methods of treatment avails as much."[47] Ideally patient education is integrated with traditional medical care of patients with diabetes. The ADA and the American Association of Diabetes Educators (AADE) have worked closely over the past decade to improve the quality of diabetes education and management. The AADE and the National Certification Board for Diabetes Educators are responsible for the certification of health care professionals as certified diabetes educators. Local chapters of the AADE are present in many major U.S. cities. To locate the nearest chapter, go to the AADE website: www.aadenet.org. The American Nurses Credentialing Center and the AADE have developed an advanced certification: Board Certified—Advanced Diabetes Management (BC-ADM). Eligible health care providers consist of nurse practitioners, clinical nurse specialists, and dietitians or pharmacists who hold a minimum of a master's degree in their discipline. The ADA has two accreditation programs. The ADA Provider Recognition Program recognizes physicians who have documented the delivery of exemplary diabetes care to patients on both a clinical and an educational basis (see a listing at www.ncqa.org/dprp). The ADA also has a Diabetes Education Recognition Program that recognizes programs that deliver comprehensive diabetes education. Some states also have state-specific accreditation programs.[6] The content areas of patient education programs accredited by the ADA are outlined in Box 39-15.

Adjustment to a chronic illness such as diabetes is ongoing. The degree to which patients with DM adjust, as evidenced by taking control of the disease management, often depends on how well they adapt emotionally to their diagnosis. Helping the person begin to cope with chronic illness may be one of the first nursing care priorities. Patients must have a chance to work through their feelings of loss, shock, disbelief, identity change, or anger in response to the crisis. They need to feel accepted, regardless of their behavior.

A major responsibility of the professional nurse is helping patients gain self-management skills for any chronic health problem through teaching and counseling. Self-management skills are probably the major determinant of how well the health problem is controlled and the quality of life maintained, particularly for persons with diabetes. Research confirms that patient education has a positive effect on patient outcomes. Teaching and management are instituted in a manner to avoid overwhelming the patient. Despite the compelling evidence linking glycemic, blood pressure, and lipid control with decreased long-term complications of diabetes, fewer than 18% of individuals reach targets for control. The nurse is in a unique position to educate and motivate patients with DM to optimize well-being and minimize long-term diabetic complications.

The major problem confronting the professional nurse when dealing with a knowledge deficit in the person with DM is, "How much do I teach?" A pretest is ideal for assessing what the patient knows, or does not know, about diabetes. The bottom line is that patients have to survive in the real world. Hence the patient's ability to perform day-to-day survival skills should always be validated.

The ADA suggests that diabetes education be continuous and take place in three stages: (1) survival/initial stage, (2) in-depth stage, and (3) continuous stage. Stages 2 and 3 emphasize knowledge and skills needed to be completely self-sufficient in daily

Box 39-15 Fifteen Content Areas of Diabetes Education

1. **Overview of Diabetes Mellitus**
   Definition of diabetes mellitus
   Effects of alterations in metabolism of carbohydrates, proteins, and fats
   Classification of diabetes (e.g., type 1, type 2, gestational)
2. **Stress and Psychologic Adjustment**
   Grieving and adaptation to living with a chronic disease
   Expressing feelings openly
   Unrealistic expectations
   Effect of stress on metabolic control
   Recognizing the need for professional help
   Stress management
3. **Family Involvement and Social Support**
   Diabetes as a family challenge
   Learning to recognize and work with adverse family dynamics
   Need for support
4. **Nutrition**
   Individualized meal plan to control weight, glucose, and lipids
   Composition of the diet
   Achieving and maintaining desired body weight and glucose control
   Advice on alcohol use
   Eating on special occasions
   Reading and interpreting nutrition labels
5. **Exercise and Activity**
   Benefits and risks
   Effects of exercise on therapeutic plan
   Preparing for exercise (food and medication; companion)
   Heart rate monitoring
   Monitoring necessary before starting exercise
   Monitoring necessary when establishing an exercise program
6. **Medications**
   Goals of treatment
   Oral agents
   —Action on blood glucose
   —Side effects
   —Drug interactions
   Insulin
   —Action on blood glucose
   —Cautions (especially Somogyi phenomenon)
   —Strengths, purities
   —Injection techniques
   —Complications of treatment: hypoglycemia, lipodystrophy
   Glucagon
   —How to buy, store, and use
7. **Monitoring and Use of Results**
   Goals
   Types of blood glucose monitoring equipment available
   Quality control of monitors
   How to use blood glucose monitoring to achieve and maintain good glucose control: performing tests accurately, interpreting test results, frequency of testing, taking action appropriate to test results
   Ketone testing
   Hemoglobin A_{1c} test: how to relate to average blood glucose level
8. **Relationships Among Nutrition, Exercise, Medication, and Blood Glucose Levels**
   Balancing nutrition, exercise, and medications
   Adjusting each factor in relation to the others
   Adjusting times of monitoring
   Identifying times for snacks
   Effects of exercise on blood glucose
9. **Acute Complications: Hyperglycemia and Hypoglycemia**
   Definitions of hyperglycemia and hypoglycemia
   Prevention of each
   Early recognition, treatment, and record keeping
   Hypoglycemia unawareness
   Dawn phenomenon and Somogyi phenomenon
   What to do for diabetic ketoacidosis and hyperosmolar coma
   Effects of illness on diabetes
   Monitoring glucose and ketones
   Sick-day guidelines (including diet)
10. **Chronic Complications: Prevention, Detection, and Treatment**
    Kinds of complications: microvascular and macrovascular, neuropathy
    Examples of each kind of complication (especially those likely to occur in your population)
    Possible causes of complication
    Self-care for prevention or delay of complications
    Coping strategies (support groups, counseling, stress management)
11. **Foot, Skin, and Dental Care**
    Daily self-care measures
    Relationship of problems to diabetes care
    The need for regular evaluation of feet and teeth
12. **Behavioral Change Strategies, Goal Setting, Risk Factor Reduction, and Problem Solving**
    Changing behaviors through goal setting
    Rights of patient
    Responsibility of patient
    Patient-professional partnership in planning care
    Taking care of self when sick
13. **Benefits, Risks, and Management Options for Improving Glucose Control**
    Study results (Diabetes Control and Complications Trial, Epidemiology of Diabetes Interventions and Complications, UK Prospective Diabetes Study Group)
    Therapeutic care plans—maps to good health and quality of life
    —Blood glucose control
    —Blood pressure control
    —Lipid control
    —Aspirin use
    Use of angiotensin converting enzyme inhibitors in normotensive patients
14. **Preconception Care, Pregnancy, and Gestational Diabetes**
15. **Use of Health Care Systems and Community Resources**
    Planned follow-up
    Patient's responsibility
    Names and telephone numbers of health care team members
    Emergency care
    Community resources
    Planning for travel
    Educational resources and need for continuing education
    Insurance and employment regulations and reimbursement

Adapted from American Diabetes Association: Clinical practice recommendations 2004, *Diabetes Care* 27(Suppl 1):S1-S150, 2004.

management and to gain flexibility in management, insight, and self-determination. Professional tools can facilitate learning (see Box 39-12). The person with type 1 or 2 DM first must master survival or initial knowledge; other areas, such as dealing with complications and in-depth information about hyperglycemia and ketoacidosis, are left for stages 2 and 3 teaching.

Other teaching tools are available from pharmaceutical companies, the ADA, and health care institutions with diabetes centers. It is important to assess the patient's education and reading level before giving out educational materials.

EVALUATION

To evaluate the effectiveness of nursing interventions, compare patient behaviors with those stated in the expected patient outcomes.

RELATED NOC OUTCOMES. Activity Tolerance, Adherence Behavior, Energy Conservation, Fluid Balance, Knowledge: Diet, Knowledge: Treatment Regimen, Nutritional Status: Food & Fluid Intake, Nutritional Status: Nutrient Intake, Risk Control, Symptom Control, Tissue Integrity: Skin & Mucous Membranes, Weight Control

GERONTOLOGIC CONSIDERATIONS

The prevalence of DM increases with age along with insulin resistance. In the age-group 60 years and older, 20.9% of individuals (10.3 million) have DM.[6,7,7a] DM prevalence estimates in individuals over 80 years of age are as high as 40%. An estimated 42% of individuals with type 2 DM are 65 years of age or older, rendering diabetes a major clinical problem. In addition, when persons with IGT are included, the prevalence of abnormal glucose tolerance (IGT and DM) rises to 40% of the geriatric population.

Accurate diagnosis of diabetes is a problem. Because of the insidious onset of type 2 DM, the initial diabetes presentation in an older adult is often painful diabetic neuropathy or other diabetic complications without prior documentation of hyperglycemia.

The etiology of geriatric insulin resistance is complex and may include genetic factors, obesity (increase in the ratio of fat body mass to lean body mass), physical inactivity, renal insufficiency, infections or illness, medications (corticosteroids, thiazide diuretics), and perhaps nutritional factors (increase in carbohydrate intake).[77,110] Insulin resistance at the cellular level may be due to decreased receptor numbers, receptor binding, and postreceptor defects. The prevalence of the metabolic syndrome rises dramatically with age, with its attendant risk of developing type 2 DM.

Worsening insulin resistance is not an inevitable consequence of aging and may be prevented by physical fitness, control of obesity, good nutritional habits, and avoidance of medications that exacerbate insulin resistance (thiazide diuretics, beta-blockers, corticosteroids). Clearly, lifestyle changes need to be made before the geriatric years as the primary preventive strategy. However, improvements are clearly attainable in later life, even in individuals who have developed overt diabetes. The evidence to date supports glycemic control in older adults to reduce the risk of chronic complications of diabetes.

Special considerations and therapeutic principles must be used when approaching the older patient (Boxes 39-16 and 39-17).

MANAGEMENT OF THE PATIENT WITH DIABETES MELLITUS WHO IS UNDERGOING SURGERY

Most nurses working in acute care settings care for individuals with diabetes who are undergoing surgery. Understanding patient concerns and the metabolic consequences of surgery will facilitate patient recovery. In many instances the patient's greatest concern is not the admitting medical problem; rather, it concerns diabetes management and loss of glycemic control.

Box 39-16 Special Considerations for Older Patients With Diabetes Mellitus

- Accuracy of diagnosis (may be missed if relying on fasting plasma glucose alone)
- Accuracy of classification of diabetes; C-peptide level needed
- Mental status: depression or dementia
- Visual acuity
- Fine motor skills
- Social support systems
- Diabetes knowledge and education potential
- Blood glucose monitoring: patient, family, friend
- Diet and meal planning: poor or variable intake or compulsive overeating
- Activity level: inactivity leading to weight gain and decreased insulin sensitivity
- Increasing ratio of fat to lean body mass
- Diabetic complications
- Concurrent illnesses
- Concurrent pharmacotherapy
- Increased risk of adverse drug reaction

Box 39-17 Therapeutic Principles in Older Patients With Diabetes Mellitus

- Set realistic goals for glycemic control in the context of age, general condition, diabetic complications, and life expectancy.
- Treat patients with true type 1 diabetes mellitus with intensive therapy (i.e., multiple daily insulin injections and carbohydrate-consistent meal plan).
- Avoid unnecessary insulin therapy.
- Review potential for diet therapy with patient and family. A 5% to 10% weight reduction may be significant.
- Increase physical activity safely whenever possible.
- Use antihyperglycemic agents such as metformin, thiazolidinediones, or acarbose if not contraindicated.
- Consider nateglinide, with its negligible risk of hypoglycemia. If using a sulfonylurea, consider glimepiride, since its reduced risk of hypoglycemia may be safer. Use sulfonylureas at low doses.
- Combination therapy with oral agents and insulin may be of value for selected patients.
- Physiologic intensive insulin therapy with multiple daily insulin injections is the safest option for severely insulinopenic patients. Modify glycemic control goals, if necessary.

The perioperative management of the patient with diabetes may be complicated by poor control of blood glucose levels and other conditions such as hypertension, diabetic nephropathy, autonomic neuropathy, coronary artery disease, and systemic atherosclerosis. Counterregulatory hormones increase during anesthesia, surgery, and recovery and result in hyperglycemia.

Poor control of blood glucose levels can negatively affect the patient's recovery. Hyperglycemia may precipitate DKA, retards wound healing, and promotes thrombosis as a result of hypercoagulability. Tight glycemic control can have a dramatic effect on reducing wound infections, morbidity, and mortality.[103,104]

Effects of Surgery on Metabolic Control of Diabetes Mellitus. The person with DM faces the risk of developing hypoglycemia or hyperglycemia during the perioperative period. During this period, persons are not usually given anything by mouth and are given IV fluids. This decreases total carbohydrate intake and also decreases insulin needs; however, the effects of surgery on counterregulatory hormones usually increase the need for insulin. The stressors of surgery cause the release of glucocorticoids and catecholamines, which elevate blood glucose levels.

Management of Glucose Control in Patients Treated With Insulin. Various protocols may be used to maintain glucose control in the person receiving insulin. Neither hyperglycemia nor hypoglycemia should be allowed to occur. A commonly used perioperative protocol is beginning an IV infusion of dextrose the morning of surgery and giving half the usual insulin dose subcutaneously as intermediate-acting insulin. This insulin covers hepatic glucose production during the intraoperative period and prevents hyperglycemia. If the patient is taking insulin glargine, the full dose should be given, since insulin glargine is used to control hepatic glucose output and disposal in the fasting state, not to cover carbohydrates consumed. If the surgery is lengthy, blood glucose levels are checked intraoperatively, and insulin or extra glucose is given as needed.

During the postoperative period the person is maintained by IV glucose infusion until food can be taken. Insulin is given either by dividing the normal daily dose equally over a 24-hour period and giving it subcutaneously or by separate IV infusion. If a standard dose of insulin is being given, extra insulin may be given via an algorithm based on fingerstick blood glucose checks every 4 to 6 hours.

Management of Glucose Control in Individuals Not Receiving Insulin. Persons with diabetes who are not normally managed with insulin receive an IV infusion of dextrose on the morning of surgery, after fasting during the night. Such patients may be able to meet their usual insulin needs with their endogenous insulin supply, but in times of stress they may require exogenous insulin. As mentioned previously, patients with type 2 DM who are treated with metformin should discontinue the drug the morning of elective surgery that may require general anesthesia and should remain off metformin until resuming oral intake. After surgery the nurse checks blood glucose and urine ketone levels every 4 to 6 hours; if hyperglycemia is present, exogenous insulin may be needed.

Resumption of Diet. All persons with diabetes, whether or not they are treated with insulin, should receive 125 to 250 g of carbohydrate per day until their normal diet is resumed. Fewer grams of carbohydrate than this may result in starvation ketosis. The patient resumes the normal diabetes regimen as soon as possible. The nurse monitors blood glucose and urine ketone levels frequently, even after the patient's usual diet and medication are resumed. The increase in catabolism because of the surgery remains for some time, and additional insulin may continue to be needed. By the time patients are discharged, they should be back on their normal regimens along with an appropriate algorithm for correction of hyperglycemia.

Hypoglycemia Without Diabetes Mellitus

Hypoglycemia in the nondiabetic person is characterized by subnormal plasma glucose levels, generally less than 50 mg/dl. It may be asymptomatic; may cause adrenergic symptoms (anxiety, irritability, palpitations, diaphoresis, pallor); or, if severe, may cause neuroglycopenic symptoms. Neuroglycopenic symptoms include mental confusion, seizures, and coma and may result in severe trauma (e.g., motor vehicle accidents). A firm diagnosis rests with the documentation of Whipple's triad: (1) appropriate signs and symptoms, (2) subnormal blood glucose level, and (3) response to normalization of blood glucose with carbohydrate ingestion.[49,91]

Box 39-18 Etiology of Fasting Hypoglycemia

Insulin Excess

Surreptitious exogenous insulin
Sulfonylurea ingestion (accidental in individual without diabetes mellitus, surreptitious use, pharmacy dispensation error)
Insulin-producing islet cell tumor (insulinoma)—benign or malignant
Islet hyperplasia

Decreased Hepatic Glucose Production

Advanced renal disease
Advanced liver disease
Ethanol use, especially with poor nutrition
Severe sepsis
Severe malnutrition

Counterregulatory Hormone Deficiencies

Hypopituitarism
Adrenocorticotropic hormone deficiency
Growth hormone deficiency
Primary adrenal failure (Addison's disease)

Hypothyroidism

Rare

Non–Islet Cell Tumors

Mesenchymal tumors, generally clinically obvious, with limited life expectancy

Autoimmune Disease

Antibodies that stimulate the insulin receptor (rare)

Classification

Hypoglycemia may be broadly classified as either fasting or nonfasting (reactive) hypoglycemia. Fasting hypoglycemia generally results in neuroglycopenic symptoms, whereas reactive hypoglycemia is usually associated with more adrenergic symptoms.

Etiology

The etiology of fasting hypoglycemia is presented in Box 39-18. Reactive hypoglycemia generally occurs 3 to 5 hours after meals, in relation to either a primary delay in insulin secretion (idiopathic) or a rapidly rising postprandial glucose value as a result of rapid gastric emptying (postgastric surgery). Failure of the pancreas to keep pace with this rapidly rising postprandial glucose level results in later insulin hypersecretion and hypoglycemia. Individuals with true idiopathic reactive hypoglycemia, reflecting an insulin secretory defect, are at increased risk for developing type 2 DM.

Collaborative Care Management

Diagnosis of fasting hypoglycemia is performed in the hospital via a 72-hour fast to document a subnormal glucose level with simultaneous increased insulin and C-peptide levels. Insulinomas (insulin-secreting tumors of the pancreas) are the most common

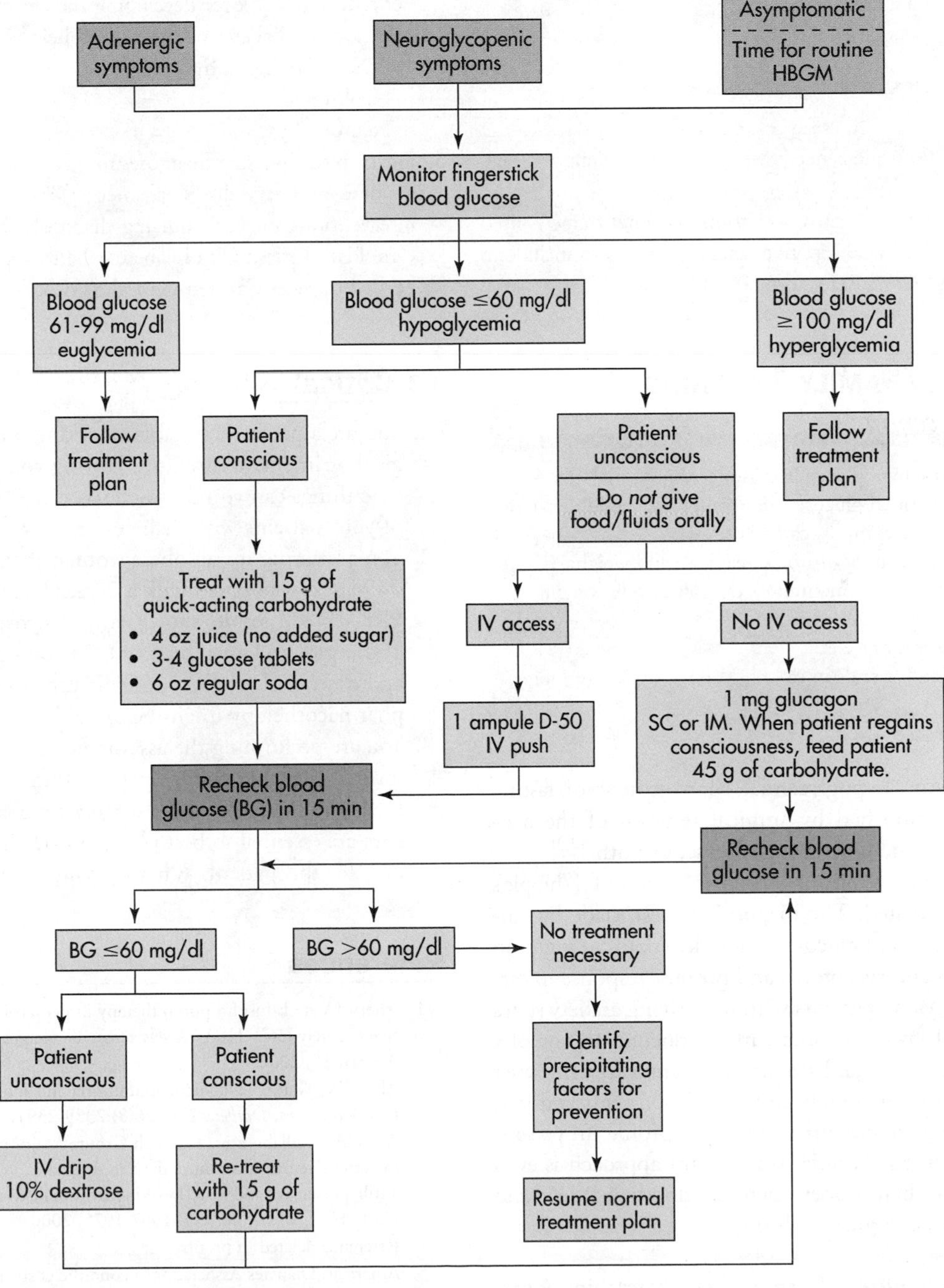

Figure 39-13 Algorithm for treating hypoglycemia. *HBGM*, Home blood glucose monitoring; *IV*, intravenous; *D-50*, 50% dextrose; *SC*, subcutaneous; *IM*, intramuscular.

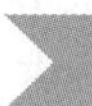

Preparing for Practice

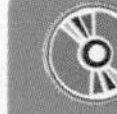

CD-ROM Activity Select Exercise Six: Diabetes Mellitus and Hypoglycemia on the Companion CD.

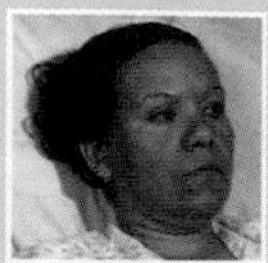

Patient: *Carmen Gonzales,* **Room 302**

Carmen Gonzales, an older Hispanic female, presents with an infected leg that has become gangrenous. She has type 2 diabetes mellitus, as well as complications of congestive heart failure and osteomyelitis.

Assessment

View the patient's **Report**.

Open the patient's **Medical Record** to familiarize yourself with her care. Specifically, click on the following areas as part of your review: Physicians' Orders, Nurses' Notes, and Expired MAR.

Conduct a **Patient Interview**. As you conduct your interview, focus primarily on data that will be helpful in planning care for this patient. Record the data you collect.

Nursing Diagnoses, Outcomes, and Interventions

1. What are Carmen Gonzales's needs with respect to dietary management?
2. Carmen Gonzales needs to learn how to manage her diabetes mellitus during times of illness. List five teaching points to include in sick-day guidelines. *Hint*: Refer to p. 1154.
3. To help Carmen Gonzales reduce her risk for developing foot infection because of diabetes mellitus, create a list of actions she should take, using the following categories:
   Inspection
   Foot care
   Foot wear
   Measures to avoid injury
   Measures to increase general circulation
   What to do if you develop a foot problem (*Hint*: Use the Patient/Family Teaching box on p. 1154 if needed.)
4. What information should you provide to Carmen Gonzales to help her reduce her risk for developing the chronic microvascular complications of diabetes mellitus listed below?
   Diabetic retinopathy
   Nephropathy
   Neuropathy
5. Develop two nursing diagnoses for Carmen Gonzales that relate to diabetes and its self-management. Write outcomes and sample interventions for each nursing diagnosis. *Hint*: Use the Nursing Care Plan: Patient with Diabetes Mellitus (p. 1144) and adapt it as needed to meet Carmen Gonzales's needs.

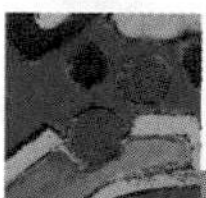

PATIENT/FAMILY TEACHING
Hypoglycemia

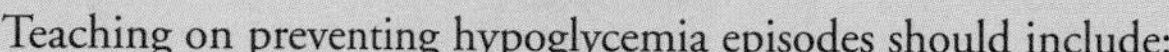

Teaching on preventing hypoglycemia episodes should include:
- Delay the postprandial glucose rise through increased dietary fiber and the use of complex carbohydrates.
- Enhance insulin sensitivity through exercise and weight restrictions to achieve or maintain a desirable body weight.
- Carry simple carbohydrates with you.
- Wear a Medic-Alert bracelet.
- Include family and friends in teaching about signs, symptoms, and treatment.

organic cause of fasting hypoglycemia. Management of fasting hypoglycemia is accomplished by surgical removal of the neoplasm, management of the underlying disease, or both.[49,91]

Reactive hypoglycemia is overdiagnosed as a result of Whipple's triad not being documented. The diagnosis is best made by randomly documenting a blood glucose level of less than 50 mg/dl in association with signs and symptoms and prompt response to carbohydrate ingestion. Many patients with underlying anxiety states are misdiagnosed with hypoglycemia with no documentation of a truly low blood glucose level and are placed on unnecessarily strict diets, usually low in carbohydrates and high in proteins and fats, with resultant weight gain and an adverse lipid profile. In persons with true idiopathic hypoglycemia, this dietary approach is even more deleterious given their propensity to develop type 2 DM and the metabolic syndrome (Figure 39-13).

Patient/Family Teaching. Patient and family teaching as part of nursing care for the patient with hypoglycemia is presented in the Patient/Family Teaching box.

Critical Thinking

1. You are a professional nurse working on a busy medical-surgical or intensive care unit. During your work day, what specific things can you do to enhance the "diabetes knowledge" of your patients with diabetes?
2. You are caring for an obese woman (height, 5 feet 3 inches; weight, 210 pounds) with a 2-year history of type 2 DM. Her HBGM results show fasting glucose levels of 130 to 160 mg/dl and an HbA_{1c} of 8.2% on her regimen of diet and exercise. Develop a care plan for this patient. What pharmacotherapy might be prescribed for her treatment?
3. You are performing the assessment and preoperative teaching for a 55-year-old woman patient with a long history of type 1 DM. She is scheduled for surgery for a laminectomy. What data are essential to best plan her care? Develop a teaching plan for this patient. What are some perioperative concerns?

References

1. Ahern JA et al: Insulin pump therapy in pediatrics: a therapeutic alternative to safely lower HbA_{1c} levels across all age groups, *Pediatr Diabetes* 3(1):10-15, 2002.
2. Allen KV, Walker JD: Microalbuminuria and mortality in long-duration type 1 diabetes, *Diabetes Care* 26(8):2389-2391, 2003.
3. ALLHAT Collaborative Research Group: Major cardiovascular events in hypertensive patients randomized to doxazosin vs. chlorthalidone: the antihypertensive and lipid-lowering treatment to prevent heart attack trial (ALLHAT), *JAMA* 283(15):1967-1975, 2000.
4. Reference deleted in proofs.
5. American Diabetes Association: Economic costs of diabetes in the U.S. in 2002, *Diabetes Care* 26(3):917-929, 2003.
6. American Diabetes Association: Clinical practice recommendations 2004, *Diabetes Care* 27(Suppl 1):S1-S150, 2004.

7. American Diabetes Association: *Diabetes statistics*, accessed July 2004 from website: www.diabetes.org/statistics.

7a. American Diabetes Association: Total prevalence of diabetes and prediabetes, accessed 2005 from website: www.diabetes.org/diabetes_statistics/prevalence.jsp.

8. American Diabetes Association: TrialNet study: further research to prevent and treat type 1 diabetes, *Diabetes Today*, accessed Aug 2004 from website: www.diabetes.org.

9. American Diabetes Association, Expert Committee on the Diagnosis and Classification of Diabetes Mellitus: Report of the Expert Committee on the Diagnosis and Classification of Diabetes Mellitus, *Diabetes Care* 24(Suppl 1):S55, 2001.

10. Azen SP et al: TRIPOD (Troglitazone in the Prevention of Diabetes): a randomized, placebo-controlled trial of troglitazone in women with prior gestational diabetes mellitus, *Control Clin Trials* 19(2):217-231, 1998.

11. Bakris GL: Hypertension and nephropathy, *Am J Med* 115(Suppl 8A): 49S-54S, 2003.

12. Bliss M: *The discovery of insulin,* Chicago, 1982, University of Chicago Press.

13. Boulton AJ, Armstrong DG: Trials in neuropathic diabetic foot ulceration: time for a paradigm shift? *Diabetes Care* 26(9):2689-2690, 2003.

14. Boulton AJ, Armstrong DG: Off-loading in trials of neuropathic foot ulceration: further evidence of the need for a paradigm shift, *Diabetes Care* 27(2):636-637, 2004.

15. Boulton AJ, Jude EB: Therapeutic footwear in diabetes: the good, the bad, and the ugly? *Diabetes Care* 27(7):1832-1833, 2004.

16. Boulton AJ et al: Diabetic somatic neuropathies, *Diabetes Care* 27(6):1458-1486, 2004.

17. Centers for Disease Control and Prevention: *National diabetes fact sheet: general information and national estimates on diabetes in the United States,* Atlanta, 2003, US Department of Health and Human Services, Centers for Disease Control and Prevention.

18. Centers for Disease Control and Prevention: Preventive-care practices among persons with diabetes—United States, 1995 and 2001, *JAMA* 288(22):2814-2818, 2002.

19. Chan NH et al: Inhaled insulin in type 1 diabetes, *Lancet* 357:2001.

20. Criqui MH et al: The sensitivity, specificity, and predictive value of traditional clinical evaluation of peripheral arterial disease: results from noninvasive testing in a defined population, *Pathophysiol Nat History Periph Vascular Dis* 71:516, 1985.

21. Cryer PE, Davis SN, Shamoon H: Hypoglycemia in diabetes, *Diabetes Care* 26(6):1902-1912, 2003.

22. Dahlöf B et al, for LIFE study group: Cardiovascular morbidity and mortality in the Losartan Intervention for Endpoint Reduction in Hypertension study (LIFE): a randomized trial against atenolol, *Lancet* 359(9311):1004-1110, 2002.

23. Deckert T et al: Albuminuria reflects widespread vascular damage: the Steno hypothesis, *Diabetalogia* 32:219, 1989.

24. Diabetes Control and Complications Trial Research Group: The effect of intensive treatment of diabetes on the long-term complications in insulin-dependent diabetes mellitus, *N Engl J Med* 329:977, 1993.

25. Diabetic Retinopathy Study Research Group: Photocoagulation treatment of proliferative diabetic retinopathy: clinical application of Diabetic Retinopathy Study (DRS) findings, DRS Report No 8, *Ophthalmology* 88(7):583-600, 1981.

26. Eaks GA: *Professional prompter worksheet,* Kansas City, Kan, 1993, University of Kansas Medical Center, Cray Diabetes Education Center.

27. Early Treatment Diabetic Retinopathy Study Research Group: Photocoagulation for diabetic macular edema: Early Treatment Diabetic Retinopathy Study report number 1, *Arch Ophthalmol* 103(12):1796-1806, 1985.

28. Eisenbarth GS, Jasinski JM: Disease prevention with islet autoantigens, *Endocrinol Clin Metab Clin North Am* 33(1):59-74, 2004.

29. El-Deirawi KM, Zuraikat N: Registered nurses' actual and perceived knowledge of diabetes mellitus, *J Nurses Staff Dev* 17(1):5-11, 2001.

30. Ellison JM, Stegmann JM, Colner SL: Rapid changes in postprandial blood glucose produce concentration differences at finger, forearm, and thigh sampling sites, *Diabetes Care* 25(6):961-964, 2002.

31. Frank RN: Diabetic retinopathy, *N Engl J Med* 359(1):48-58, 2004.

32. Franz MJ: Prioritizing diabetes nutrition recommendations based on evidence, *Minerva Med* 95(2):115-123, 2004.

33. Franz MJ, Wheeler ML: Nutrition therapy for diabetic nephropathy, *Curr Diab Rep* 3(5):412-417, 2003.

34. Freeman DJ et al: Pravastatin and the development of diabetes mellitus: evidence for a protective treatment effect in the West of Scotland Coronary Prevention Study, *Circulation* 103(3):357-362, 2001.

35. Gaede P et al: Multifactorial intervention and cardiovascular disease in patients with type 2 diabetes, *N Engl J Med* 348(5):383-393, 2003.

36. Gillis W. Long Hansen's Disease Center, Bureau of Primary Health Care: *Comprehensive diabetes lower extremity amputation prevention programs: risk and management categories for the foot,* accessed Aug 2004 from website: www.bphc.hrsa/gov/htm.

37. Grundy SM et al, for Coordinating Committee of the National Cholesterol Education Program: Implications of recent clinical trials for the National Cholesterol Education Program Adult Treatment Panel III Guidelines, *Circulation* 110(2):227-239, 2004.

38. Gulati M, Pandey DK, Arnsdorf MF: Exercise capacity and the risk of death in women: the St James Women Take Heart Project, *Circulation* 108(13):1554-1559, 2003.

39. Heart Outcomes Prevention Evaluation (HOPE) Study Investigators: Effects of ramipril on cardiovascular and microvascular outcomes in people with diabetes mellitus: results of the HOPE study and MICRO-HOPE sub-study, *Lancet* 355(9200):253-259, 2000.

40. Heart Outcomes Prevention Evaluation (HOPE) Study Investigators: Effects of an angiotensin-converting enzyme inhibitor, ramipril, on cardiovascular events in high risk patients, *Lancet* 342(3):145-153, 2002.

41. Heart Protection Study Collaborative Group: MRC/BHF Heart Protection Study of cholesterol lowering with simvastatin in 20,536 high risk individuals: a randomized placebo-controlled trial, *Lancet* 360(9326):7-22, 2002.

42. Heisler M et al: How well do patients' assessments of their diabetes self-management correlate with actual glycemic control and receipt of recommended diabetes services? *Diabetes Care* 26(3):738-743, 2003.

43. Hovind P et al: Predictors for the development of microalbuminuria and macroalbuminuria in patients with type 1 diabetes: inception cohort study, *BMJ,* April 19, 2004, doi:10.1136/bmj.38070.450891.FE.

44. Hunger-Dathe W et al: Insulin pump therapy in patients with type 1 diabetes mellitus: results of the Nationwide Quality Circle in Germany (ASD) 1999-2000, *Exp Clin Endocrinol Diabetes* 111(7):428-434, 2003.

45. Isomaa B et al: Cardiovascular morbidity and mortality associated with the metabolic syndrome, *Diabetes Care* 24(4):683-689, 2001.

46. Jermendy G: Clinical consequences of cardiovascular autonomic neuropathy in diabetic patients, *Acta Diabetol* 40(Suppl 2):S370-S374, 2003.

47. Joslin EP: *Diabetic manual,* ed 10, Philadelphia, 1959, Lea & Febiger.

48. Julius S, Kjeldsen SE, Weber M: Outcomes in hypertensive patients at high cardiovascular risk treated with regimens based on valsartan or amlodipine: the VALUE randomized trial, *Lancet* 363(9426):2022-2031, 2004.

49. Kaltsas GA, Besser GM, Grossman AB: The diagnosis and medical management of advanced neuroendocrine tumors, *Endocrinol Rev* 25(3):458-511, 2004.

50. Reference deleted in proofs.

51. Khan A et al: Cinnamon improves glucose and lipids of people with type 2 diabetes, *Diabetes Care* 26(12):3215-3218, 2003.

52. Knoll GA, Nichol G: Dialysis, kidney transplantation, or pancreas transplantation for patients with diabetes mellitus and renal failure: a decision analysis of treatment options, *J Am Soc Nephrol* 14(2):500-515, 2003.

53. Knowler WC et al, for Diabetes Prevention Program Research Group: Reduction in the incidence of type 2 diabetes with lifestyle intervention or metformin, *N Engl J Med* 346(6):393-403, 2002.

54. Koschinsky T, Jungheim K, Heinemann L: Glucose sensors and the alternate site testing–like phenomenon: relationship between rapid glucose changes and glucose sensor signals, *Diabetes Technol Ther* 5(5):829-842, 2003.

55. KROC Collaborative Study Group: Blood glucose control and the evolution of diabetic retinopathy and albuminuria, *N Engl J Med* 311:364, 1984.

56. Lauritzen T et al: Continuous subcutaneous insulin (2-year Steno study data), *Lancet* 1(8339):1445-1446, 1983.
57. Lee DM, Weinert SE, Miller EE: A study of forearm versus finger stick glucose monitoring, *Diabetes Technol Ther* 4(1):13-23, 2002.
58. Lee KH et al: Prognostic value of cardiac autonomic neuropathy independent and incremental to perfusion defects in patients with diabetes and suspected coronary artery disease, *Am J Cardiol* 92(12):1458-1461, 2003.
59. Lewis EJ et al, for Collaborative Study Group: The effect of angiotensin-converting enzyme inhibition on diabetic nephropathy, *N Engl J Med* 329(20):1456-1462, 1993.
60. Mandrup-Poulson T: *Personal communication*, Gentofte, Denmark, 1992, Steno Diabetes Center.
61. Mogensen CE, Cooper ME: Diabetic renal disease: from recent studies to improved clinical practice, *Diabet Med* 21(4):4-17, 2004.
62. Murphy D and staff of Division of Diabetes Translation, National Center for Chronic Disease Prevention and Health Promotion, Centers for Disease Control and Prevention: *Diabetes prevention and control: a public health imperative,* accessed Aug 2004 from website: www.cdc.gov/nccdphp/promising_practices/diabetes/progress_to_date.htm.
63. Myers J et al: Exercise capacity and mortality among men referred for exercise testing, *N Engl J Med* 346(11):793-801, 2002.
64. National High Blood Pressure Education Program Working Group: National High Blood Pressure Education Program Working Group report on hypertension in diabetes, *Hypertension* 23(2):145-158, 159, 1994.
65. Ohkubo Y et al: Intensive insulin therapy prevents the progression of diabetic microvascular complications in Japanese patients with non-insulin-dependent diabetes mellitus: a randomized prospective 6-year study, *Diabetes Res Clin Pract* 28(2):103-117, 1995.
66. Ojo AO et al: The impact of simultaneous pancreas-kidney transplantation on long-term patient survival, *Transplantation* 71(1):82-90, 2001.
67. Orchard TJ, Strandness DE: *Assessment of peripheral vascular disease in diabetes: report and recommendations of an international workshop sponsored by the American Heart Association and the American Diabetes Association,* New Orleans, Sept 18-20, 1992, *Diabetes Care* 16(8):1199, 1995.
68. Owens DR, Zinman B, Bolli G: Alternative routes of insulin delivery, *Diabet Med* 20(11):886-898, 2003.
69. *Physicians' desk reference,* ed 58, Montvale, NJ, 2001, Medical Economics.
70. Pirart J: Diabetes mellitus and its degenerative complications: a prospective study of 4400 patients observed between 1947 and 1973, parts 1 and 2, *Diabetes Care* 1:168-188, 252-263, 1978.
71. Pugliese A: Genetics of type 1 diabetes, *Endocrinol Metab Clin North Am* 33(1):1-16, 2004.
72. Putzer GJ et al: Prevalence of patients with type 2 diabetes mellitus reaching the American Diabetes Association's target guidelines in a university primary care setting, *Southern Med J* 97(2):145-148, 2004.
73. Pyorala K et al, Scandinavian Simvastatin Survival Study (4S): Cholesterol lowering with simvastatin improves prognosis of diabetic patients with coronary heart disease: a subgroup analysis of the Scandinavian Simvastatin Survival Study (4S), *Diabetes Care* 20(4):614-620, 1997.
74. Reaven GM: Role of insulin resistance in human disease, Banting lecture 1988, *Diabetes* 37(12):1595, 1988.
75. Reaven GM: Role of insulin resistance in human disease (syndrome X): an expanded definition, *Ann Rev Med* 44:121-131, 1993.
76. Reaven GM: Syndrome X, *Clin Diabetes* 3-4:32-52, 1994.
77. Reaven G: Age and glucose intolerance: effect of fitness and fatness, *Diabetes Care* 26(2):539-540, 2003.
78. Redondo MJ et al: Heterogeneity of type 1 diabetes: analysis of monozygotic twins in Great Britain and the United States, *Diabetalogia* 44(3):354-362, 2001.
79. Richardson T, Kerr D: Skin-related complications of insulin therapy: epidemiology and emerging management strategies, *Am J Clin Dermatol* 4(10):661-667, 2003.
80. Ryan EA et al: Successful islet transplantation: continued insulin reserve provides long-term glycemic control, *Diabetes* 51(7):2148-2157, 2002.
81. Sacks FM et al, for Cholesterol and Recurrent Events Trial Investigators: The effect of pravastatin on coronary events after myocardial infarction in patients with average cholesterol levels, *N Engl J Med* 335(14):1001-1009, 1996.
82. Saddine JB, Engelau MM, Beckles GL: A diabetes report card for the United States: quality of care in the 1990s, *Ann Intern Med* 136(8):565-574, 2002.
83. Saydah SH, Fradkin J, Cowie CC: Poor control of risk factors for vascular disease among adults with previously diagnosed diabetes, *JAMA* 291(3):335-342, 2004.
84. Scandinavian Simvastatin Survival Study Group: Randomised trial of cholesterol lowering in 4444 patients with coronary heart disease: the Scandinavian Simvastatin Survival Study (4S), *Lancet* 344(8934):1383-1389, 1994.
85. Sheehan JP: The gift of insulin, *J Lab Clin Med* 115(2):267-268, 1990.
86. Reference deleted in proofs.
87. Shepherd J et al, for West of Scotland Coronary Prevention Study Group: Prevention of coronary heart disease with pravastatin in men with hypercholesterolemia, *N Engl J Med* 333(2):1301-1307, 1995.
88. Sjolie AK, Moller F: Medical management of diabetic retinopathy, *Diabet Med* 21(7):666-672, 2004.
89. Smith D, Amiel SA: Hypoglycemia unawareness and the brain, *Diabetalogia* 45(7):949-958, 2002.
90. Soumerai SB et al: Effects of health maintenance organization coverage of self-monitoring devices on diabetes self-care and glycemic control, *Arch Intern Med* 164(6):645-652, 2004.
91. Thompson GB: Diagnosis and management of insulinomas, *Endocrine Pract* 8(5):385-386, 1992.
92. Tuomilehto J et al: Prevention of type 2 diabetes mellitus by changes in lifestyle among subjects with impaired glucose tolerance, *N Engl J Med* 344(18):1343-1360, 2001.
93. UK Prospective Diabetes Study Group: UK prospective diabetes study XI: biochemical risk factors in type 2 diabetic patients at diagnosis compared with age-matched normal subjects, *Diabet Med* 11(6):533-544, 1994.
94. UK Prospective Diabetes Study Group: UK prospective diabetes study XVI: overview of 6 years' therapy of type 2 diabetes: a progressive disease, *Diabetes* 44(11):1249-1258, 1995.
95. UK Prospective Diabetes Study Group: Effect of intensive blood-glucose control with metformin on complications in overweight patients with type 2 diabetes (UKPDS 34), *Lancet* 352(9131):854-865, 1998.
96. UK Prospective Diabetes Study Group: Intensive blood-glucose control with sulphonylureas or insulin compared with conventional treatment and risk of complications in patients with type 2 diabetes (UKPDS 33), *Lancet* 352(9131):837-853, 1998.
97. UK Prospective Diabetes Study Group: Association of glycaemia with macrovascular and microvascular complications of type 2 diabetes (UKPDS 35): prospective observational study, *BMJ* 321(7258):405-412, 2000.
98. UK Prospective Diabetes Study Group: Association of systolic blood pressure with macrovascular and microvascular complications of type 2 diabetes (UKPDS 36): prospective observational study, *BMJ* 321(7258):412-419, 2000.
99. Ulchaker MM, Sheehan JP: Iatrogenic brittle diabetes: the hold-the-insulin decision, *Diabetes Educ* 17:111, 1991.
100. US Department of Agriculture, Human Nutrition Information Service: *Dietary guidelines for Americans,* Washington, DC, 2005, The Department, website: www.mypyramed.gov.
101. US Department of Health and Human Services: *Healthy people 2010: understanding and improving health,* Washington, DC, 2000, The Department.
102. Van De Wiel A: Diabetes mellitus and alcohol, *Diabetes Metab Res Rev* 20(4):263-267, 2004.
103. Van den Bergh GH: Role of intravenous insulin therapy in critically ill patients, *Endocrine Pract* 10(Suppl 2):17-20, 2004.
104. Van den Bergh G et al: Intensive insulin therapy in the critically ill patients, *N Engl J Med* 345(19):1359-1367, 2001.
105. Vendrame F, Gottlieb PA: Prediabetes: prediction and prevention trials, *Endocrinol Clin Metab Clin North Am* 33(1):75-92, 2004.
106. Verge CF et al: Late progression to diabetes and evidence for chronic beta-cell autoimmunity in identical twins of patients with type I diabetes, *Diabetes* 44(10):1176-1179, 1995.

107. Verlato G et al: Attending the diabetes center is associated with increased 5-year survival probability of diabetic patients: the Verona Diabetes Study, *Diabetes Care* 19(3):211-213, 1996.
108. Vinicor F et al: Healthy people 2010: diabetes, *Diabetes Care* 23(6): 853-855, 2000.
109. Vinik AI et al: Diabetic autonomic neuropathy, *Diabetes Care* 26(5): 1553-1579, 2003.
110. Volpi E, Nazemi R, Fujita S: Muscle tissue changes with aging, *Curr Opin Clin Nutr Metab Care* 7(4):405-410, 2004.
111. Wackers FJ et al: Detection of silent myocardial ischemia in asymptomatic diabetic subjects: the DIAD study, *Diabetes Care* 27(8):1954-1960, 2004.
112. Weissberg-Benchell J, Antisdel-Lomaglio J, Seshadri R: Insulin pump therapy: a meta-analysis, *Diabetes Care* 26(4):1079-1087, 2003.
113. Whang W, Bigger JT: Comparison of the prognostic value of RR-interval variability after acute myocardial infarction in patients with versus those without diabetes mellitus, *Am J Cardiol* 92(3):247-251, 2003.
114. Writing Team for the Diabetes Control and Complications Trial/Epidemiology of Diabetes Interventions and Complications Research Group: Retinopathy and nephropathy in patients with type 1 diabetes 4 years after a trial of intensive therapy, *N Engl J Med* 342(6):381-389, 2000.
115. Yetzer EA: Incorporating foot care education into diabetic foot screening, *Rehabil Nurs* 29(3):80-84, 2004.

Visit the Evolve website: http://evolve.elsevier.com/Monahan/medsurg

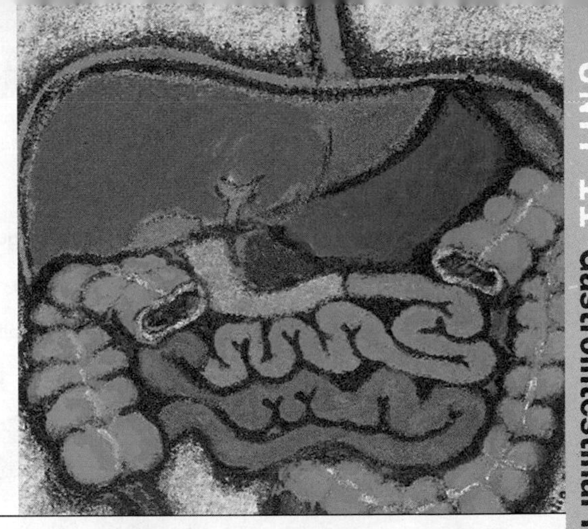

CHAPTER 40

Assessment of the Gastrointestinal, Biliary, and Exocrine Pancreatic Systems

by Shelley Yerger Huffstutler

OBJECTIVES

After studying this chapter, the learner should be able to:

1. Describe the anatomy and physiology of the gastrointestinal system and its accessory organs.
2. Discuss age-related physiologic changes that occur in the gastrointestinal system.
3. Identify health history and physical examination data essential to the nursing assessment of the gastrointestinal system.
4. Explain the significance of findings from diagnostic tests for various problems of the gastrointestinal tract.
5. Analyze the rationale for nursing interventions associated with various diagnostic tests of the gastrointestinal, biliary, and exocrine pancreatic systems.

KEY TERMS

acini, p. 1167
ascites, p. 1173
Blumberg's sign, p. 1175
borborygmi, p. 1174
chyme, p. 1169
dysphagia, p. 1172
endoscopic retrograde cholangiopancreatography, p. 1181
esophagogastroduodenoscopy, p. 1181
melena, p. 1172
rugae, p. 1166
peristalsis, p. 1166
steatorrhea, p. 1172
stomatitis, p. 1173

The gastrointestinal (GI) system, also termed the *digestive system* and *alimentary canal,* consists of the GI tract and its accessory organs. Its primary function is to convert ingested nutrients and fluids into a form that can be used by the cells of the body. This goal is accomplished through the processes of ingestion, digestion, and absorption. The second major function of the GI system is the storage and final excretion of the solid waste products of digestion. Proper function of the GI system is essential to the maintenance of proper nutrition and health.

Anatomy and Physiology

The upper portion of the GI tract consists of structures that aid in the ingestion and digestion of food, including the mouth, esophagus, stomach, and duodenum, plus the related organs of the biliary system and exocrine pancreas. The lower GI tract consists of the small and large intestines, the rectum, and the anus. The GI system is primarily composed of a hollow, muscular tube approximately 9 m (30 feet) long that stretches from the mouth to the anus (Figure 40-1).

Although this muscular tube is located within the body, it is actually an extension of the external environment. The walls of the GI tract successfully prevent most harmful agents from entering the body and essential body fluids and materials from leaving the body. The composition of the walls is predominantly smooth muscle; however, the mouth and upper esophagus, along with a portion of the rectum and anus, consist of voluntary muscle.

Mouth

The mouth is made up of the lips, cheeks, tongue, hard and soft palates, teeth, and salivary glands (Figure 40-2). These structures begin the digestive process by mechanically breaking down and lubricating the food. Because digestive enzymes can function only on the exposed surfaces of food particles, the teeth must begin the breakdown of food. No other portion of the GI system can perform the function of the teeth in their absence.

The lubrication of food is accomplished by the action of the watery and mucous secretions of the salivary, parotid, sublingual, and submandibular glands of the mouth. Approximately 1 L of saliva is produced each day. Saliva contains ptyalin (amylase), which hydrolyzes starch to maltose. After chewing and moistening are completed, the muscular tongue pushes the food bolus back to the pharynx to initiate swallowing (deglutition). Small amounts of saliva, which contain immunoglobulin A (IgA) antibodies to many normal environmental microorganisms, are produced continually to keep the tissues of the mouth moist and clean.

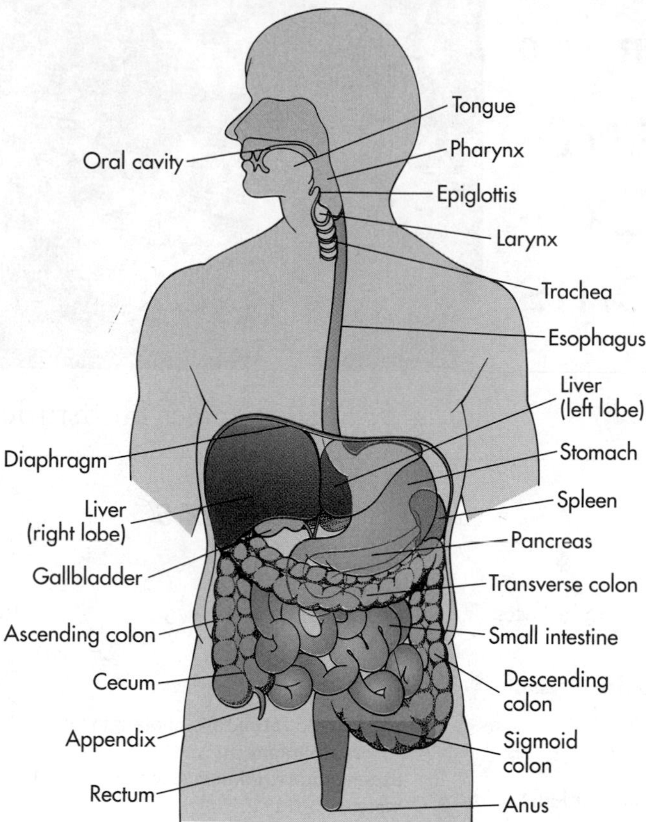

Figure 40-1 Organs of the gastrointestinal system and related structures.

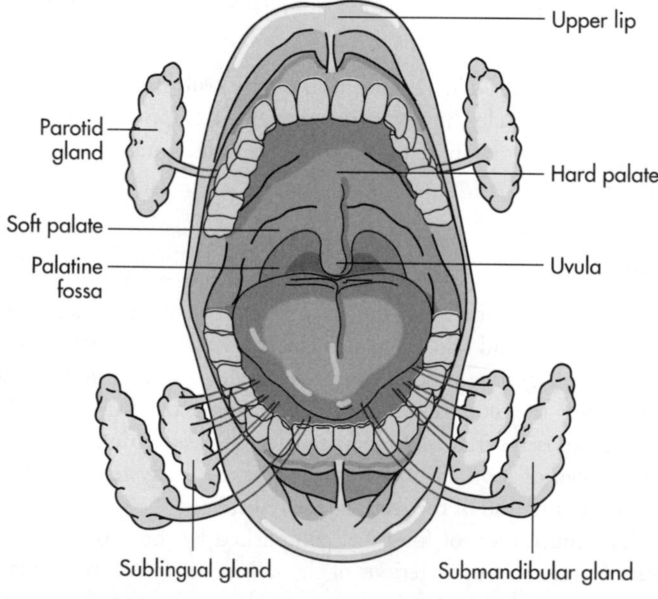

Figure 40-2 Structures of the mouth.

Esophagus

The esophagus begins at the lower end of the pharynx. It is a hollow, muscular tube 25 cm (10 in) in length that lies behind the trachea, passes through the thorax, and connects the mouth and stomach. The upper third is composed of skeletal muscle, and the lower two thirds are smooth muscle. Sphincters that help prevent the reflux of gastric contents are located at both ends of the esophagus. These sphincters are normally closed, except during the act of swallowing.

The primary function of the esophagus is to move the food bolus by **peristalsis** from the pharynx to the stomach. The esophagus does not secrete enzymes, and only mechanical digestion takes place. The secretion of mucus assists in the movement of the food bolus and protects the walls of the esophagus from abrasion by partially digested food.

Swallowing is a complex physiologic mechanism that must be accomplished without compromising respiration. It consists of three phases: (1) the voluntary phase, in which the tongue forces the bolus of food into the pharynx; (2) the involuntary pharyngeal phase, in which the food moves into the upper esophagus; and (3) the esophageal phase, in which food moves down into the stomach. The esophageal muscles are activated by the glossopharyngeal and vagal nerves, which create rhythmic peristaltic waves that propel the food toward the stomach. Food is prevented from passing into the trachea by the closing of the epiglottis and the opening of the esophagus.

Stomach

The stomach is roughly J shaped and lies in the upper abdomen to the left of midline. It is positioned to the left of the liver, to the right of the spleen, and posterior to both organs. It is a muscular pouch whose shape changes with its contents. Its three major regions are the fundus, body, and antrum (Figure 40-3). The cardiac sphincter protects the opening from the esophagus, and the pyloric sphincter protects the exit to the duodenum. The **rugae**, or longitudinal folds, of the stomach enable it to quadruple in size and increase from a resting volume of 50 ml to a capacity of approximately 1500 ml for food digestion, without major changes in pressure. The stomach has an outer serous layer, three layers of smooth muscle, and an inner mucosal layer. The outermost layer of smooth muscle is longitudinal, the middle layer is circular, and the inner layer is oblique. The rugae are found on the inner mucosal layer.

The stomach primarily serves as a reservoir but also has digestive and secretory functions. Food is stored in the stomach until partially digested. The fundus contains chief cells, which secrete digestive enzymes, and parietal cells, which secrete water, hydrochloric acid (HCl), and the intrinsic factor that is essential for the absorption of vitamin B_{12}. The HCl is responsible for the highly acidic medium of the stomach (pH of 0.9 to 1.5), which is needed to activate the enzymes that initiate protein digestion. This highly acidic pH also serves a protective function, destroying most ingested microorganisms. Gastric acid secretion is under the control of parasympathetic stimulation via the vagus nerve, as is the secretion of gastrin and histamine. Gastrin is a hormone secreted from endocrine cells in the gastric glands of the stomach in response to vagal stimulation and mechanical distention of the stomach. The secretion of histamine$_2$ (H_2) also increases gastric acid secretion. Approximately 2 to 2.5 L of gastric secretions are produced each day. The gastric mucosa is covered by a thick mucous gel layer produced by the densely packed epithelial cells of the mucosa. The mucous layer is almost completely impermeable to hydrogen ions. The mucosal epithelial cells also secrete bicarbonate, which acts as

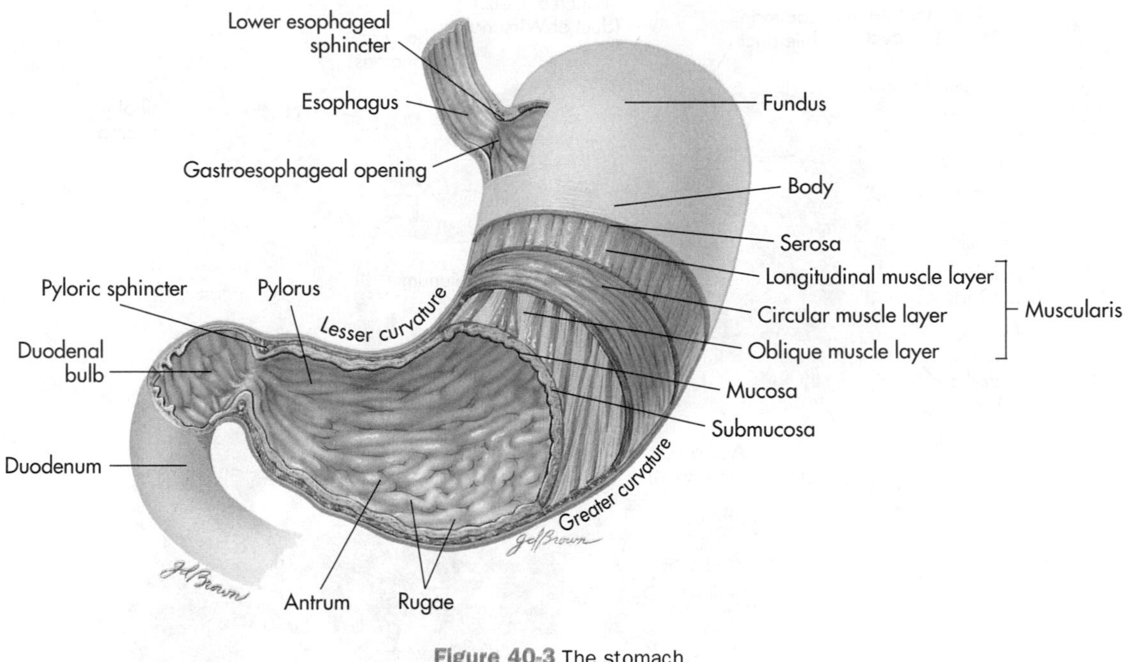

Figure 40-3 The stomach.

a buffer and helps neutralize the acidic secretions. The combined actions of these two mechanisms are so effective that, although the gastric secretions have a pH of less than 2.0, the intraluminal pH of the mucosa is maintained at about 7.0.

Gastric emptying is controlled by both hormonal and autonomic nervous system activity. Parasympathetic stimulation by the vagus nerve increases both peristalsis and secretion. Sympathetic stimulation inhibits them. The peristaltic contractions of the stomach, which propel the chyme toward the antrum, occur at a frequency of about 3 to 5 contractions per minute. The pylorus closes during antral contraction, and larger food particles are propelled back toward the body of the stomach for further mixing. Gastric contents are emptied into the duodenum between peristaltic contractions. Although the pylorus is not a true anatomic sphincter, it does help prevent the backflow of duodenal contents and bile salts into the stomach.

Gallbladder and Biliary Ductal System

The gallbladder is a pear-shaped organ that lies on the inferior surface of the liver. It is composed of serous, muscular, and mucous layers and has a usual capacity of 50 ml, although it can increase in size under normal conditions. Innervation of the gallbladder is from the parasympathetic and sympathetic nervous system. The cystic duct connects the gallbladder with the remaining structures of the ductal system—the hepatic ducts and common bile duct.

The gallbladder's major function is to store and concentrate bile. Bile, which is formed in the liver, is excreted into the hepatic ducts, which unite to form the common bile duct. The common bile duct passes behind the pancreas, is joined by the pancreatic duct, and empties into the duodenum. The sphincter of Oddi regulates the flow of bile into the duodenum. A second sphincter is located above the junction with the pancreatic duct and controls the flow of bile in the common bile duct. When this sphincter is closed, bile moves back into the gallbladder, where it is concentrated fivefold to tenfold. Because bile can be released directly into the duodenum from the liver, the gallbladder is not essential to life. Bile salts emulsify fats for action by intestinal lipases and facilitate the absorption of fats, fat-soluble vitamins, and cholesterol.

Approximately 600 to 800 ml of bile is produced daily. The release of bile from the gallbladder or liver is controlled by cholecystokinin (CCK), which is released from the walls of the duodenal intestinal mucosa when lipids, amino acids, and hydrogen ions enter the duodenum from the stomach. CCK travels via the blood to the gallbladder and causes contraction of the gallbladder's smooth muscle and relaxation of the sphincter at the end of the common bile duct (the sphincter of Oddi), so that bile can be emptied into the duodenum.

Most of the bile salts are reabsorbed from the intestine into the enterohepatic circulation and returned to the liver, where they can be recirculated. The system is so efficient that only 15% to 25% of the bile salt pool needs to be replaced by the liver each day.

Pancreas

The pancreas is an elongated, flattened organ located in the posterior abdomen, with its head lying within the curve of the duodenum and its tail resting against the spleen. The pancreas has both exocrine and endocrine functions. The exocrine functions are carried out by the acinar cells and duct system, and the endocrine functions are carried out by islets of Langerhans cells (Figure 40-4). Exocrine functions are discussed in this chapter. The endocrine functions are discussed in Chapter 37.

The pancreas is divided into three parts: head, body, and tail. Each of these parts, which are composed of lobules, is formed from groups of secretory cells termed **acini**. The acini drain into a ductal system that ultimately reaches the main pancreatic duct (or

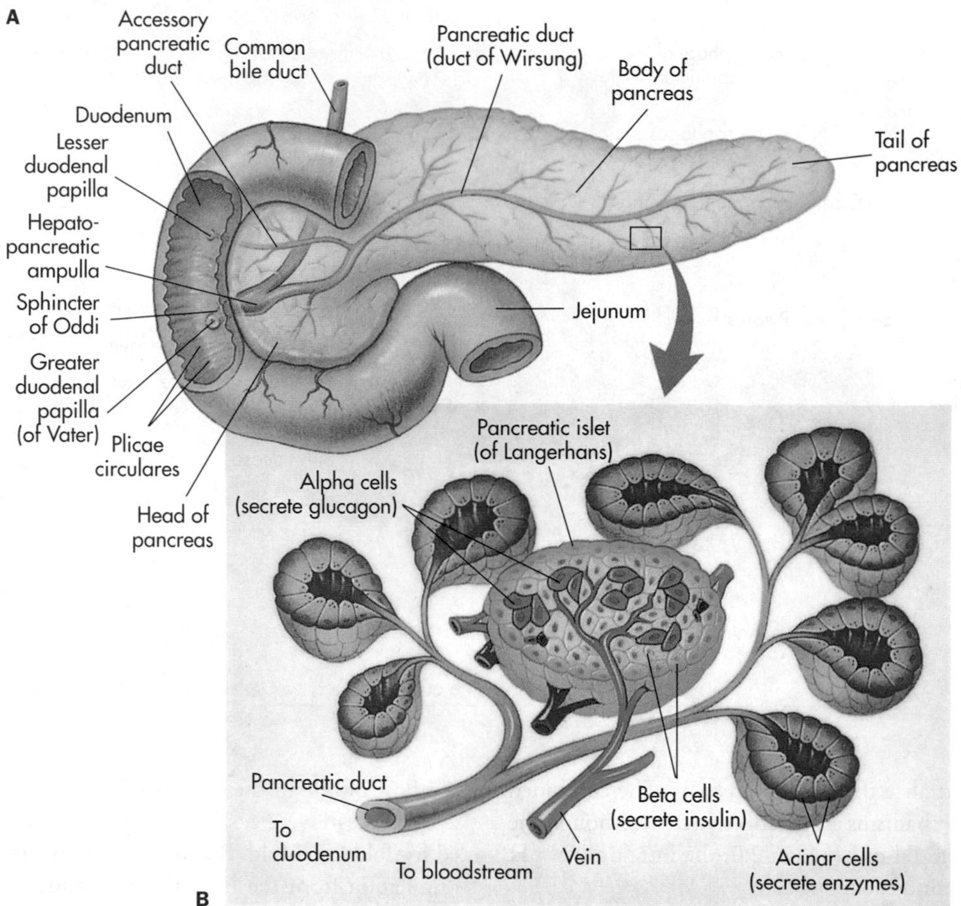

Figure 40-4 **A,** Pancreatic ductal system. **B,** Note both endocrine and exocrine glandular cells of pancreas.

duct of Wirsung). This major duct extends the entire length of the gland. At the head of the pancreas the ductal secretions enter the duodenum through the ampulla of Vater. The sphincter of Oddi controls its opening.

Approximately 2 L of pancreatic secretions are produced daily. The ductal epithelium produces a balanced electrolyte secretion, and the acini secrete digestive enzymes in an inactive precursor state. The pancreatic secretions contain trypsin, which breaks down protein; pancreatic amylase, which breaks down starch; and lipase, which hydrolyzes fat into glycerol and fatty acids. The pancreatic acini also produce an enzyme inhibitor that prevents the activation of the secretions before they reach the duodenum. The production of the pancreatic secretions is controlled by the action of the parasympathetic nervous system, gastrin, and hormones released from the duodenum during digestion.

Intestines

The small intestine is about 2.5 cm (1 inch) wide and 6 m (20 feet) long and fills most of the abdomen (see Figure 40-1). It consists of three parts: (1) the duodenum, which connects to the stomach; (2) the jejunum, or middle portion; and (3) the ileum, which connects to the large intestine.

The large intestine is about 6 cm (2.5 inches) wide and 1.5 m (5 feet) long. It also consists of three parts: (1) the cecum, which connects to the small intestine; (2) the colon; and (3) the rectum. The ileocecal valve prevents backward flow of fecal contents from the large intestine to the small intestine. The vermiform appendix, which has no known function, is an appendage close to the ileocecal valve. The colon is subdivided into four sections: the ascending, transverse, descending, and sigmoid colons. The points at which the colon changes direction are named for adjacent organs: the hepatic flexure (liver) and the splenic flexure (spleen). The rectum is 17 to 20 cm (7 to 8 inches) long, ending in the 2- to 3-cm anal canal. The opening of the anus is controlled by a smooth muscle internal sphincter and a striated muscle external sphincter.

Table 40-1 summarizes the major digestive enzymes. The actions and stimuli for secretion of the major GI hormones are presented in Table 40-2.

Small Intestine. The primary functions of the small intestine are the digestion of food and the absorption of nutrients. This process occurs primarily in the jejunum and ileum. The duodenum contains the opening for the bile and pancreatic ducts, which allow bile and pancreatic secretions to enter the intestine. Mucus-producing glands are concentrated where gastric contents are emptied and digestive secretions enter the duodenum. The mucus helps protect the duodenum from the acids in the gastric chyme and the actions of the digestive enzymes.

TABLE 40-1 DIGESTIVE ENZYMES

Source	Action
MOUTH	
Ptyalin (salivary amylase)	Breaks starch into maltose (polysaccharides to disaccharides)
STOMACH	
Gastric pepsin	Breaks protein into polypeptides
Gastric lipase	Digests butterfat
PANCREAS	
Pancreatic amylase	Breaks starch into maltose (polysaccharides to disaccharides)
Trypsin	Splits polypeptide chains
Pancreatic lipase	Splits emulsified fat into monoglycerides
SMALL INTESTINE	
Maltase	Breaks maltose into glucose
Dextrinase	Breaks alpha-limit dextrin to glucose
Lactase	Breaks lactose into galactose and glucose
Sucrase	Breaks sucrose into glucose and fructose
Enteropeptidase	Activates trypsin
Peptidases	Splits polypeptides into amino acids
Intestinal lipase	Splits neutral fats into glycerol and fatty acids

Digestion begins in the mouth and stomach, but it takes place primarily in the small intestine. The intestinal mucosa is impermeable to most large molecules, so proteins, fats, and complex carbohydrates must be broken down into small particles before they can be absorbed. The intestinal mucosa also secretes surface enzymes that aid in digestion and about 2 L/day of serous fluid that acts as a diluting agent to facilitate absorption. Carbohydrate digestion, which begins in the mouth, is completed in the small intestine as disaccharides are broken down into monosaccharides (glucose, fructose, and galactose) by the action of intestinal enzymes and pancreatic amylase. Protein digestion, which begins in the stomach, is completed as polypeptides are broken down into peptides and amino acids by the action of pancreatic trypsin. Fat digestion is accomplished by emulsification into small droplets by the action of bile and pancreatic lipase. The droplets are then further broken down into glycerol and fatty acids. The release of digestive secretions is stimulated by the hormones secretin and CCK (also called pancreozymin) and by the action of the parasympathetic nervous system.

The inner mucosal surface of the small intestine is covered with millions of villi, which are the functional units for absorption. Each villus is equipped with a blind-end lymph vessel (lacteal) in its center, which is surrounded by capillaries, venules, and arterioles (Figure 40-5). These structures bring blood to the surface of the intestine and provide a network for absorption into the portal blood or lymphatic system. Ninety percent of absorption occurs within the small intestine by either active transport or diffusion. Active transport requires metabolic energy expenditure and is used to absorb amino acids, monosaccharides, sodium, and calcium. Fatty acids and water diffuse passively, primarily into the lymphatics.

The contents of the small intestine **(chyme)** are propelled toward the anus by regular peristaltic movements. Both segmental and propulsive movements occur. The segmental movements primarily involve the circular muscles of the intestine. Slow contractions move the chyme back and forth in small segments of the intestine (1 to 4 cm). This movement mixes the chyme and facilitates digestion and absorption. Segmental peristaltic movements increase after meals. The propulsive peristaltic movements involve intestinal segments 10 to 20 cm long. Contraction occurs in the proximal segment, with relaxation in the distal segment. Chyme advances slowly and normally takes 3 to 10 hours to move from the stomach to the colon. Parasympathetic stimulation, primarily through branches of the vagus nerve, increases peristaltic activity. Sympathetic stimulation is primarily inhibitory.

Large Intestine. Minimal chemical digestion takes place in the large intestine. It functions primarily to absorb water and electrolytes from the chyme and store the food waste (feces) until defecation. Reabsorption occurs predominantly in the right or ascending colon. The colon can absorb six to eight times more

TABLE 40-2 MAJOR GASTROINTESTINAL HORMONES

Hormone	Action	Stimulus for Secretion
Gastrin	Stimulates secretion of gastric acid and pepsinogen; increases gastric blood flow; stimulates gastric smooth muscle contraction and motility	Secreted from antrum of stomach and duodenum in response to vagal stimulation, epinephrine, solutions of calcium salts, and alcohol; inhibited by an antral stomach pH of less than 2.5
Secretin	Stimulates secretion of bicarbonate-containing solution by pancreas and liver; inhibits gastric acid secretion and motility	Secreted by duodenum in response to low pH chyme (less than 3.0) entering duodenum
Cholecystokinin	Stimulates contraction of gallbladder and secretion of pancreatic enzymes; slows gastric emptying	Secreted in duodenum and jejunum in response to presence of fatty and amino acids
Enterogastrone	Inhibits gastric secretion and motility; relaxes sphincter of Oddi	Secreted in duodenum in response to presence of partially digested proteins and fats

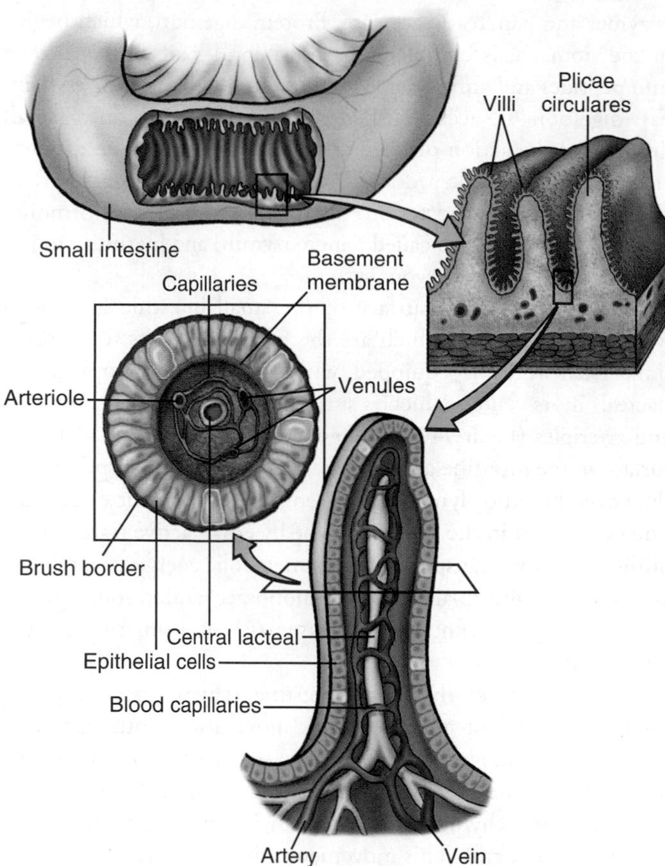

Figure 40-5 Adaptations in wall of small intestine assist digestion and absorption of foods. Note plicae circulares covered with villi, the capillary bed and central lacteal in each villus, and brush border of microvilli.

fluid than is delivered to it daily, and only approximately 100 ml of fluid is left in the colon to be mixed with the fecal residue.

The large number of microorganisms found in the large intestine further break down the residual proteins that were not digested or absorbed in the small intestine. The breakdown of amino acids produces ammonia, which is converted to urea by the liver. These intestinal bacteria also play a vital role in the synthesis of vitamin K and some of the B vitamins. The only significant secretion of the colon is mucus, which protects the intestinal walls and helps the fecal matter adhere into a mass.

Approximately 450 ml of chyme reach the cecum each day. The transit time in the large bowel is slow, taking about 12 hours to reach the rectum. The fecal contents in the colon are pushed forward by mass movements that occur only a few times each day. These mass movements are stimulated by gastrocolic reflexes initiated when food enters the duodenum from the stomach, especially after the first meal of the day.

The rectum is well innervated with sensory fibers. Parasympathetic fibers are responsible for the contraction of the rectum and relaxation of the internal anal sphincter. The defecation reflex occurs when feces enter the rectum. Afferent impulses are transmitted to the sacral segments of the spinal cord; subsequently, reflex impulses are transmitted back to the sigmoid and rectum, initiating relaxation of the internal anal sphincter.

Physiologic Changes With Aging

GI complaints are extremely common in older persons. Distinct changes occur in the GI system with aging, although these changes are incompletely understood. Most aging-related changes do not interfere with normal function, but it is important for nurses to be cognizant of the changes and incorporate appropriate modifications when planning care for older patients. In addition, the GI effects of other chronic illnesses such as diabetes require careful consideration because they are usually more important than the effects of aging itself.

In the mouth, teeth darken and may loosen or fracture and the gums recede. Salivary gland output decreases, which causes mouth dryness and increased susceptibility to infection and tissue breakdown. Taste bud sensitivity decreases, which can negatively affect both appetite and nutrition. Aging causes decreased motility and strength of peristalsis in the esophagus, but these changes appear to have minimal significance in healthy persons. Some deterioration in the lower esophageal sphincter (LES) may increase the frequency of esophageal reflux.

Gastric motility and emptying diminish slightly but progressively with age, and gastric acid secretion also decreases steadily after age 50. Achlorhydria (absence of free HCl) is relatively common. These changes can produce minor problems in digestion but are usually asymptomatic. Chronic gastritis is common in older persons, but the condition is usually the result of bacterial colonization by *Helicobacter pylori,* not aging.

No significant structural changes in the biliary system are associated with aging. However, the composition of the bile becomes increasingly lithogenic (likely to produce calculi), possibly because of an increase in biliary cholesterol. The incidence of gallstones increases with each decade.[2]

The pancreas exhibits ductal hyperplasia and fibrosis with aging, but these changes are not necessarily associated with altered function. The output of pancreatic secretions steadily declines after age 40, but related problems with absorption have not been substantiated.

Age-related changes in small intestinal function are important and can lead to poor nutrition, even with adequate intake. Nutrient absorption, particularly the absorption of carbohydrates, is impaired. Absorption of water-soluble vitamins remains intact, but the absorption of vitamin D is defective in many older persons, and the active transport of calcium is also impaired. Decreased production of secretory IgA can lead to an increase in the frequency and severity of infections.

Chronic constipation is one of the most common complaints in older persons, yet the segmental mass movements and contractions of the large intestine have been found to be unchanged as long as the individual remains physically active. The incidence of both diverticula and polyps in the colon increases with age. The rectum has decreased elasticity and a steady decrease in volume, which can

▶ ARE YOU READY?

Which of the following disorders is associated with the patient with decreased trypsin secretion?

1. Altered protein breakdown
2. Altered starch breakdown
3. Altered vitamin absorption
4. Altered fat absorption

result in sphincter failure. However, the sensation of rectal fullness remains intact, and most problems with bowel incontinence in older persons are not attributable to them effects of aging.

Health History

A thorough health history is necessary to adequately assess the health status of persons with potential dysfunction of the GI system.[6]

Patient/Family History

The nurse asks the patient about previous GI problems; hospitalizations; surgeries; and past and current medication use, both over-the-counter and prescribed. The use of antacids and laxatives is particularly important. The nurse inquires about the presence of GI problems in the nuclear or extended family, including cancer and disorders such as inflammatory bowel disease, which have a documented hereditary link.

Diet and Nutrition

The adequacy of the diet, in terms of both quality and quantity, can be quickly estimated through comparison of the daily intake with standard recommendations. Nutritional assessment has particular significance in GI disorders, since it may reveal changes in eating patterns that are characteristic of specific illnesses or disorders. The nutritional assessment includes an exploration of usual eating patterns and any changes that may be the result of illness or specific symptoms. The assessment explores changes in appetite, food preferences and intolerances, food allergies, planned and unplanned changes in weight, adherence to special or therapeutic diets, and use of dietary or vitamin supplements. A 24-hour dietary recall may be a useful tool to approximate caloric and specific nutrient intake and analyze the overall adequacy of the diet. Symptoms related to food intake should also be carefully assessed. Changes in appetite and symptoms such as dysphagia, nausea, and discomfort are carefully explored.

Lifestyle, economic, and cultural factors affecting nutrition are also assessed. Food has multiple social and emotional values for individuals that are distinct from its role in nutrition. Financial resources, access to food preparation and storage facilities, and religious or social beliefs may all influence both the quality and quantity of the diet. Lifestyle factors can have a direct or indirect effect on GI function. GI symptoms commonly develop or worsen in response to life stressors. Open-ended questions are most effective for exploring beliefs and feelings about food.

A complete nutritional assessment includes an evaluation of the patient's use of sugar and salt substitutes, coffee, alcohol, and tobacco (both chewing and smoking). The presence of dentures is an essential consideration because dentures may significantly influence food selection and chewing.

Abdominal Pain

Although pain is not an early or common manifestation of GI disease, it is frequently the reason individuals seek medical attention. The nurse assesses its onset; duration; character; location; and relationship to meals, stressful events, activity, or medications. The patient is asked to identify the site of pain in the abdomen. Pain may be experienced anywhere along the length of the GI tract in a specific localized pattern or a general, nonspecific pattern, or it may be referred to another somatic or skeletal region that shares the same nerve innervation (Figure 40-6). Abdominal pain may be continuous, episodic, or associated with eating. The pain sensation is thought to arise from the distention or sudden contraction of a hollow viscus; therefore local stretching or traction on pain-sensitive

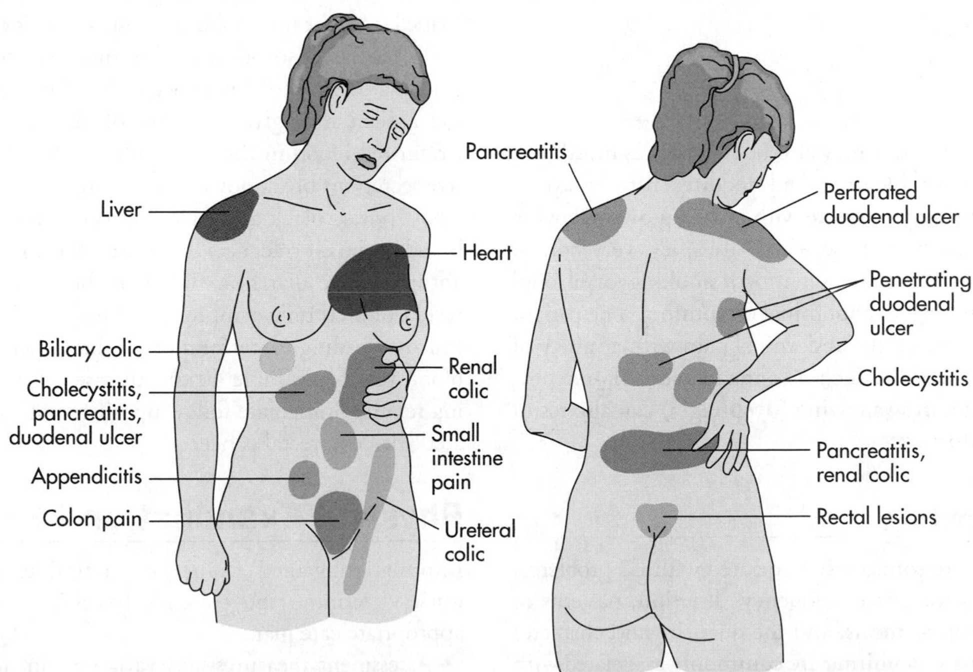

Figure 40-6 Common sites of referred pain. Note that location of the pain may not be directly over or even near the site of the organ.

Research

Pagel JM et al: Retrospective analysis of a guideline for evaluating nontraumatic abdominal pain in older patients presenting to the emergency department, *J Clin Outcomes Manage* 10(11):589-595, 2003.

This study examined the potential impact of a guideline for evaluating nontraumatic abdominal pain in the emergency department (ED) in patients ages 50 years or older. A retrospective chart review was used with patients who came to an academic medical center ED over a 3-month period with a primary complaint of abdominal pain discovered at triage, abdominal pain noted in the history, and/or abdominal tenderness noted on physical examination. The guideline included indications for surgical consultations and radiologic and laboratory studies and recommended that analgesic medications be given early in the evaluation. The researchers measured the number of patients who received imaging studies, surgical consultation, and parenteral opioids, and calculated point estimates and 95% confidence intervals to compare care received with care recommended by the guideline.

One hundred eighteen of 143 charts of eligible patients were available for analysis. The average age was 66.8 years, 56% of the patients were women, and 29% were admitted to the hospital. Thirty-four patients received a surgical consultation, whereas 100 met guideline criteria for consultation. Twenty-four of the 42 abdominal radiographs ordered were not indicated, and 41 patients received pain medications.

The researchers concluded that this guideline would increase the number of surgical consultations and the number of patients who receive analgesia during their ED stay and decrease the number of abdominal radiographs. A prospective review of the guideline is needed to assess its impact on outcomes.

structures will elicit the pain response. The painful area may exhibit local muscle guarding, which serves as a protective mechanism. The pain associated with pancreatic or biliary dysfunction is usually severe (see Research box).[9]

Food Intolerance

Abdominal pain or discomfort may also be reported as heartburn, indigestion, belching, or bloating and requires further exploration. The discomfort may interfere with chewing or swallowing food. Specific foods, such as those which are spicy, very hot, or very cold, may precipitate the discomfort; smoking or alcohol consumption may also trigger abdominal discomfort. The patient may have already self-treated the abdominal pain with a variety of over-the-counter preparations such as antacids and H_2-receptor antagonists. Difficulties in swallowing **(dysphagia)** can also result in abdominal discomfort.

Nausea and Vomiting

Nausea and vomiting are commonly associated with GI problems, and the nurse assesses for onset, frequency, duration, patterns of occurrence, relationship to meals, and the quantity and character of the emesis. Nausea and vomiting are commonly associated with medication administration. Red blood in emesis is indicative of recent bleeding. "Coffee-ground" emesis may indicate old bleeding in the stomach. The presence of bile produces a green color and a bitter taste; brown vomitus may contain fecal matter.

Fatigue and Weakness

Persons with GI system problems often complain of fatigue or weakness. Inadequate nutrient intake, abnormal fluid and electrolyte status, and increased metabolic demands may all contribute to the problem. It is important for the nurse to carefully consider other problems that may contribute to the symptoms, including cardiac, respiratory, renal, and other metabolic disorders.[3] These complaints may be present in a wide variety of situations, but their careful assessment is essential for planning an overall approach to care. Resolution of these problems usually takes time. Fatigue and weakness may also contribute to weight loss, particularly when associated with persistent anorexia, nausea, vomiting, or abdominal pain.

Elimination Patterns

Patterns of bowel elimination vary significantly among healthy individuals, and these patterns are commonly altered by GI system disorders. The nurse assesses the individual's usual elimination pattern; explores any changes that have occurred; and assesses the use of laxatives, suppositories, or other products to support bowel elimination.

Changes in the normal pattern of bowel elimination may represent a physiologic alteration, a pathologic condition, or simply a change in normal diet and activity patterns. Constipation is a classic example. Constipation may be a temporary response to a change in diet or activity, or it may be a sign of bowel obstruction. Constipation may also result from the administration of opioids that slow peristalsis. Diarrhea may indicate enteritis or invasion by a parasite. Obstruction in the descending colon may produce small, ribbon-shaped stools or no stool if the obstruction is complete.

When fat absorption is abnormal, **steatorrhea** (bulky, foul-smelling, fatty stools) may occur. If biliary obstruction is present, the patient may give a history of clay-colored (grayish) stools. Bright red blood in the stool indicates lower GI bleeding. Digestive secretions break down blood from the upper GI tract, and the stool appears black and sticky (tarry). Sometimes the presence of blood in the GI tract acts as a powerful cathartic and may produce abrupt, severe diarrhea. Blood in the stool **(melena)** may be a recent or a chronic symptom and may result from erosion of the mucosa, leading to perforation of the muscle wall or rupture of a blood vessel (see Table 40-6). All cases of melena or rectal bleeding require immediate follow up, since both are symptoms associated with colorectal cancer.

Physical Examination

Information gained from the physical examination helps the nurse determine the patient's baseline status and develop an appropriate care plan.

Assessment measures and variations in normal findings relevant to the care of older adults are presented in the Gerontologic Assessment box. Also identified are disorders common in older

Gerontologic Assessment

- *Inspect abdomen.* Peristalsis may be more easily observed in older patients because the abdominal musculature is thinner and has less tone. These patients usually have increased deposits of subcutaneous fat on the abdomen because the ratio of fat to water increases with aging.
- *Palpate abdomen gently.* Abdominal palpation is often easier because the abdominal wall is softer and thinner. The liver and kidneys are usually palpable if the patient is not obese.
- *Assess thoroughly for pain.* Older adults often verbalize less pain than younger adults when experiencing an acute abdomen.
- *Obtain a week-long diary of dietary intake.* Food patterns may vary during the course of the month based on monthly income.

Common Disorders in Older Adults

Gastroesophageal reflux disease
Gastritis
Gallstones

adults, which may be responsible for the abnormal assessment findings.

Mouth

Assessment of the mouth provides data about the patient's ability to salivate, masticate, and swallow. The nurse observes the lips for symmetry, color, moisture, swelling, cracks, or lesions. If asymmetry is noted, the nurse assesses the ability to masticate and swallow. A tongue blade and penlight are needed to improve visualization, and gloves should be worn for all examinations of the mouth. In certain situations, a mask and eye shield may also be appropriate.

The lips are normally reddish and are good indicators of pallor or cyanosis. Dryness may indicate dehydration, and cracks or fissures can occur with excessive dryness, exposure to cold, poorly fitting dentures, or a riboflavin deficiency. When cracks occur in the corners of the mouth they are referred to as angular **stomatitis**. Swelling of the lips is usually the result of an inflammatory response. Lesions on the lips may be benign or malignant. A commonly encountered benign lesion is herpes simplex (cold sore, fever blister), which is caused by a virus and can create enough discomfort to limit mastication.

The enamel surface of the teeth should be white but will darken with surface stains (tea, coffee, tobacco). Common abnormalities of the teeth include caries, loose or broken teeth, and absence of some or all teeth. The gums, or gingivae, are normally pink, attach to the teeth, and fill the interdental surfaces. Recession of the gum line is common in older individuals. If the person is partially or completely edentulous (without teeth), the nurse examines the gingivae for areas of redness caused by improperly fitting dentures, partial plates, or implants. The person is then asked to insert the dentures so their correct fit and comfort for chewing can be assessed.

The buccal mucosa is light pink, although patchy pigmentation may be seen in dark-skinned patients. The nurse examines the mucosa for moisture, white spots or patches, debris, areas of bleeding, or ulcers resulting from ill-fitting dentures or braces. Dryness and debris may indicate dehydration. White, curdy patches, which are removable with some effort, may be caused by candidiasis (thrush). White, nonremovable patches (leukoplakia); white plaques within red patches; or red, granular patches (erythroplakia) may be premalignant lesions and should be reported to the physician. A round or oval white ulcer surrounded by an area of redness is indicative of an aphthous ulcer (canker sore) (see Chapter 41).

While the tongue is depressed with a tongue blade and the person says "Ah," the nurse observes the soft palate for symmetry and the effective functioning of cranial nerve X, the vagus, which is necessary for effective swallowing. The uvula, soft palate, tonsils, and posterior pharynx are observed for signs of inflammation. Tongue mobility and function are essential to mastication, taste, and swallowing. Normally movement is not limited in any direction, but the tongue deviates toward the paralyzed side with paralysis of the twelfth cranial nerve (hypoglossal). A thin, white coating and large papillae on the dorsum of the tongue are normal findings. A thick coating indicates poor oral hygiene, and a smooth, red surface suggests a nutritional deficiency. The nurse examines the ventral surface for leukoplakia, ulceration, or nodules, any of which may indicate malignancy.

Any distinctive odor of the breath is noted. A foul odor may occur after the ingestion of certain foods; with poor hygiene or oral infections; and with some metabolic dysfunctions such as diabetic ketoacidosis, liver disease, and bowel obstruction. Normally the mandible slides forward and down without difficulty, and a "cracking" sound is audible when the mouth is opened widely. With a gloved finger, the nurse carefully checks the interior of the mouth for areas of tenderness, ulcers, and lumps.

Abdomen

Examination of the abdomen determines the presence of (1) tenderness, (2) organ enlargement, (3) masses, (4) spasm or rigidity of the abdominal muscles, and (5) fluid or air in the abdominal cavity. Physical examination of the abdomen is performed in the following order: inspection, auscultation, percussion, and palpation. Auscultation is performed before percussion and palpation because the latter two may alter the frequency and intensity of bowel sounds.

The surface of the abdomen can be divided anatomically into either four quadrants or nine regions (Figure 40-7). For examination, the patient is placed in a supine position and kept as relaxed as possible. Good lighting should be available.

Inspection. The nurse inspects the skin of the abdomen for color, texture, scars, rashes, lesions, symmetry, contour, and visible peristalsis. The abdomen is normally flat but will be rounded in an obese person and may appear scaphoid in a thin or emaciated person. The integrity and turgor of the skin are reliable indicators of total body hydration. Abdominal distention may be caused by air or fluid in the GI tract or fluid in the peritoneal space (**ascites**). Air may collect from swallowing or from gas produced by bacterial action in the bowel. Decreased peristalsis prevents the accumulated air from moving through the GI tract. Fluid may also accumulate from decreased peristalsis and be a symptom of

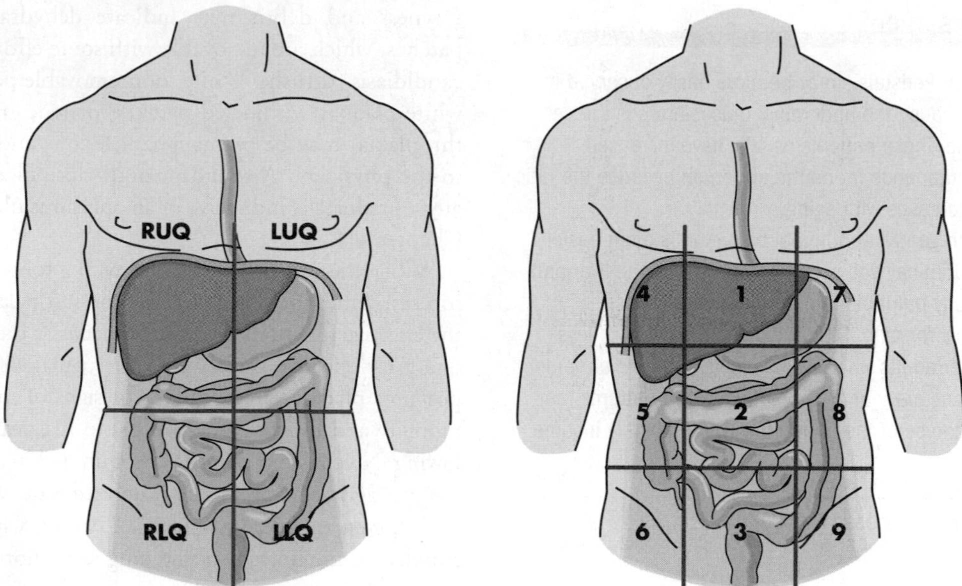

Figure 40-7 Anatomic divisions of abdomen. **Left,** Abdomen divided into four quadrants. **Right,** Abdomen divided into nine topographic regions: *1,* Epigastrium; *2,* umbilical; *3,* suprapubic; *4,* right hypochondrium; *5,* right lumbar or flank; *6,* right inguinal or iliac; *7,* left hypochondrium; *8,* left lumbar or flank; *9,* left inguinal or iliac.

partial or complete bowel obstruction. Ascites usually results from increased portal hypertension secondary to liver or heart disease.[7]

Measurement of abdominal girth provides a baseline for the evaluation of any increase or decrease in size related to distention. The nurse places a measuring tape around the abdomen at the level of or 2.5 cm below the umbilicus. It is important to lightly mark the measurement site on the patient's skin with a waterproof pen so that all subsequent measurements are taken at the same level.

Inspection includes assessment for jaundice, which is a common symptom in biliary tract or liver disease. A slight aortic pulsation may be present in the epigastric area, but peristalsis is not normally visible. Table 40-3 summarizes common findings from abdominal inspection.

Auscultation. Auscultation is used primarily to assess peristalsis. In the normal abdomen, bowel sounds caused by fluid and air movement can always be heard. Their intensity and frequency depend mainly on the phase of digestion. Most intestinal sounds occur at a rate of 5 to 34 per minute (although some may not be audible for up to 5 minutes) and are high pitched and gurgling. A normal peristaltic wave produces audible sounds of air and fluid movement through the intestine. The sounds are the loudest to the right of and below the umbilicus. Abnormalities may include either extreme. A virtual absence of normal sounds occurs when bowel motility is inhibited by inflammation or paralytic ileus. Exaggerated peristalsis produces waves of loud, gurgling sounds called **borborygmi**, which may result from infection or obstruction.

Bowel sounds are auscultated by placing the diaphragm of the stethoscope lightly against the abdomen and listening to all quadrants systematically. The stethoscope is warmed in the hands before placement on the abdomen. It may take 5 full minutes to determine that bowel sounds are completely absent, but the absence of any bowel sounds in 2 minutes clearly indicates a problem. Sounds that occur at a rate of about 1 per minute are hypoactive. The bell of the stethoscope may be used to auscultate for vascular sounds, such as bruits over the aorta and renal and iliac arteries. These sounds are not considered to be normal assessment findings. Box 40-1 outlines the location of the organs within the quadrants of the abdomen. A summary of common findings from auscultation is found in Table 40-4. Optimal areas for auscultation of vascular sounds are illustrated in Figure 40-8.

Percussion. Percussion of the abdomen is used primarily to confirm the size of various organs and to determine the presence of excessive amounts of fluid or air. Normally, percussion over the abdomen is tympanic because of the small amount of swallowed air within the GI tract. A dull or flat percussion note is found over a solid structure. Dull sounds normally occur over the liver and spleen or a bladder filled with urine. Abnormal percussion findings occur because of ascites or abnormal masses. Ascites classically produces a shifting dullness, which is caused by fluid movement to dependent areas. Interpreting the sounds of abdominal percussion may be difficult in obese individuals.

The examiner percusses the four quadrants beginning with the thoracic and moving downward systematically. The degree of tympany, from soft to pronounced, is recorded. Tympanic sounds should be heard beginning at the ninth interspace in the left upper quadrant of the abdomen.

Palpation. Palpation is of value in determining the outlines of abdominal organs; the presence and characteristics of any abdominal masses; and the presence of direct tenderness, guarding, rebound tenderness, and muscular rigidity. Bending the patient's knees slightly, placing a small pillow under the head, and positioning the patient's arms flat on the bed can help relax the abdominal muscles and make palpation easier. In the presence of

TABLE 40-3 COMMON FINDINGS FROM ABDOMINAL INSPECTION

Finding	Interpretation
Scars or striae	May be result of pregnancy, obesity, ascites, tumors, edema, surgical procedures, or healed burned areas
Engorged veins	May be caused by obstruction of vena cava or portal vein and circulation from abdomen
Skin color variation	May be caused by jaundice (yellow), inflammation (red), or intraabdominal hemorrhage (blue)
Visible peristalsis	May be caused by pyloric or intestinal obstruction; normally peristalsis not visible except for slow waves in thin persons
Visible pulsations	Normally slight pulsation of aorta, visible in epigastric region
Visible masses and altered contour	Observe for hernias, distention of ascites, and obesity; instructing patient to cough may bring out hernia "bulge" or elicit pain or discomfort in abdomen; marked concavity possibly caused by malnutrition
Spider angioma	Appear on upper part of body and blanch with pressure; commonly result from liver disease

Box 40-1 Anatomic Locations of Organs Within Each Abdominal Quadrant

Right Upper Quadrant (RUQ)	Left Upper Quadrant (LUQ)
Liver	Stomach
Gallbladder	Spleen
Duodenum	Left kidney
Right kidney	Pancreas
Hepatic flexure of colon	Splenic flexure of colon

Right Lower Quadrant (RLQ)	Left Lower Quadrant (LLQ)
Cecum	Sigmoid colon
Appendix	Right ovary and tube
Left ovary and tube	

gallbladder disease, normal palpation of the liver elicits sharp pain and a positive inspiratory arrest (Murphy's sign). The acute onset of pain causes the patient to stop inspiration abruptly, midway through the breath. Abnormal findings from palpation may include (1) direct tenderness over an organ capsule, (2) rebound tenderness, (3) muscular rigidity, or (4) masses that are large enough or close enough to the surface to be felt. Distinction should be made between a distended abdomen that is firm to the touch and one that is soft to the touch.

Light palpation is used to elicit tenderness and cutaneous hypersensitivity. The nurse uses the pads of the fingertips, with the fingers together, and presses gently, depressing the abdominal wall about 1 cm. All quadrants are palpated using smooth movements.

Deep palpation is used to delineate organs and masses and should be performed only by properly trained persons, since improper technique can result in injury. The nurse again uses the palmar surface of the fingers but presses more deeply using a single- or two-handed technique. Known tender or painful areas should be assessed last. Rebound tenderness is tested by pressing slowly but firmly over the painful site. The fingers are then quickly withdrawn. Acute pain on withdrawal reflects peritoneal inflammation (positive **Blumberg's sign**). This maneuver (Figure 40-9) can be extremely painful and should never be performed unnecessarily.[4]

Rectum

The normal perineal and perianal skin resembles the skin on the rest of the body with no breaks in integrity. Abnormal findings may include pruritus ani, coccygeal or pilonidal sinus tract openings, fistulas, fissures, external hemorrhoids, or rectal prolapse. Internal hemorrhoids may appear when the patient bears down.

▶ ARE YOU READY?

An abdominal assessment should be performed in what order?

(1) Auscultation	1. 2, 3, 4, 1
(2) Inspection	2. 2, 4, 1, 3
(3) Palpation	3. 2, 1, 4, 3
(4) Percussion	4. 2, 3, 1, 4

TABLE 40-4 COMMON FINDINGS FROM ABDOMINAL AUSCULTATION

Finding	Interpretation
Absence of bowel sounds in 5 min	Peritonitis, paralytic ileus, and hypokalemia
Repeated, high-pitched bowel sounds occurring at frequent intervals	Increased peristalsis caused by gastroenteritis, early pyloric obstruction, early intestinal obstruction, or diarrhea
Bruit	Abnormal sound caused by turbulence of blood flow through partially occluded or diseased aorta or renal artery
Hum and friction rub	Heard over liver and splenic areas, indicating increased venous blood flow, possibly related to peritoneal inflammation

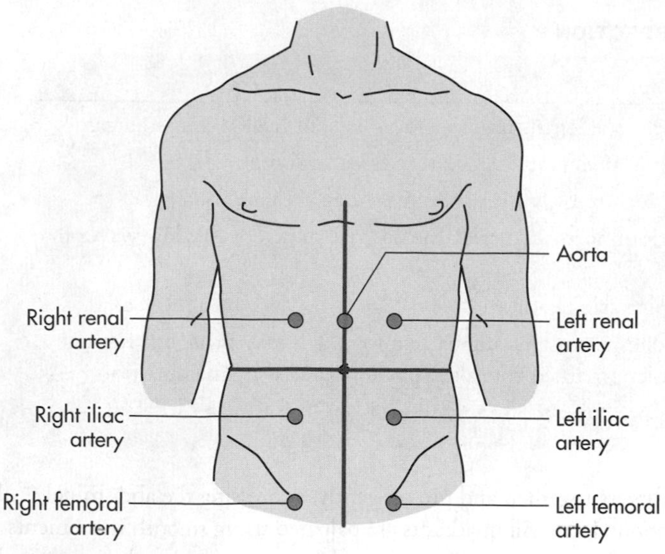

Figure 40-8 Sites for auscultation of vascular sounds in abdomen.

Diagnostic Tests

Many of the examinations and tests for diagnosing problems of the GI system are both time consuming and unpleasant. Several of the tests are intrusive, uncomfortable, and embarrassing, which adds to the patient's stress. Representatives from the radiology department or laboratory may assume responsibility for instructing patients about diagnostic tests, since the tests are usually performed on an outpatient basis. Most institutions also have printed educational material for the patient and family. It remains the nurse's responsibility to meet the patient's educational and psychologic needs by answering, in a caring manner, questions concerning the test procedure, rationale for its use, and specific test preparation. Diagnostic tests are sequenced to make the most effective use of time and equipment. The nurse ensures the patient is prepared physically and mentally to avoid the preventable repetition of time-consuming and expensive tests.

Laboratory Tests

Numerous tests may be used as part of the evaluation of GI, biliary, and exocrine pancreatic function.[2] Table 40-5 summarizes major blood and urine tests that may be ordered.

Stool Examination. Stool specimens are collected for culture; determination of fat content; and examination for the presence of ova, parasites, and fresh or occult blood. Special collection procedures may be necessary to enhance the identification of bacteria (salmonellae, shigellae, and *Staphylococcus aureus*), ova, and parasites. A fresh, warm stool specimen is optimal for laboratory analysis.

Fecal urobilinogen is responsible for the brown color of the stool. These specimens are sent promptly to the laboratory because urobilinogen breaks down rapidly. Biliary obstruction may cause decreased amounts to be present and turns the stool light or clay colored. Stool color also may vary in response to food intake and artificial colors in foods. For example, beets may cause red stool, whereas greenish black stool may be due to ingestion of licorice. Other fecal color changes are identified in Table 40-6.

Detection of occult or hidden blood in the stool is useful in identifying bleeding in the GI tract. Fecal occult blood testing (FOBT) may use either the traditional guiaic smear test (Hemoccult, Coloscreen) or the newer flushable reagent pad (EZ Detectt, ColoCARE), which is available over the counter for home use. Both tests are nonspecific and are vulnerable to both false positives and false negatives. Meat, poultry, or fish eaten within 3 days before testing can cause a false-positive test, as can ingestion of aspirin or antiinflammatory drugs within 7 days. Vitamin C in quantities greater than 500 mg/day may cause a false-negative test if consumed 3 days before testing. Determination of fecal fat may be done as part of a workup for malabsorption. Elevations in fecal fat are present with biliary or pancreatic obstructions and many intestinal malabsorption disorders.

Radiologic Tests

Visualization of the GI tract may be performed by barium swallow, upper GI series, or barium enema. Barium is a radiopaque sub-

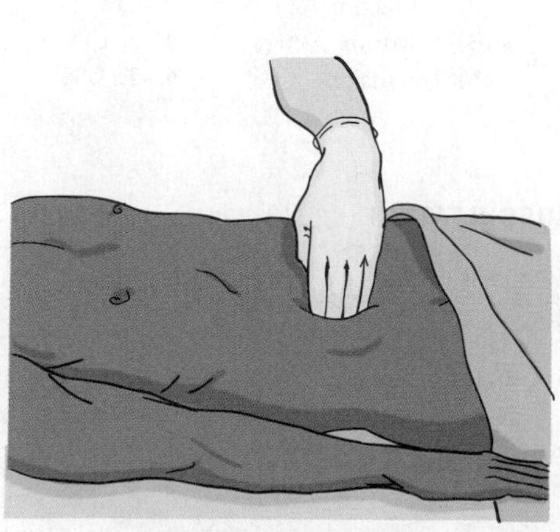
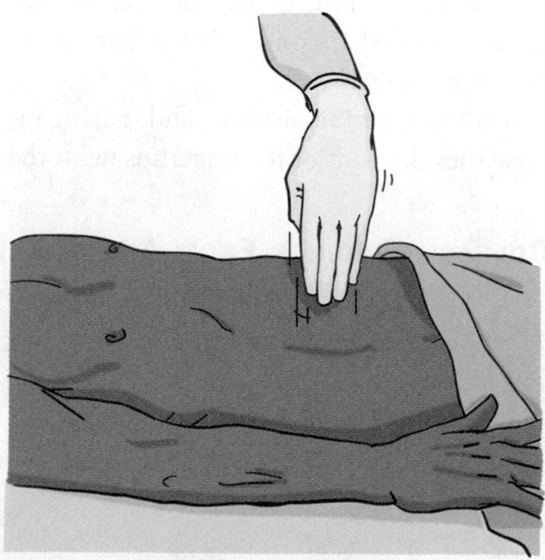

Figure 40-9 Palpating for rebound tenderness.

TABLE 40-5 MAJOR GASTROINTESTINAL, BILIARY, AND EXOCRINE PANCREAS BLOOD AND URINE TESTS

Blood Test	Reference Interval	Description and Purpose
STOMACH		
Stomach gastrin (fasting serum)	0-100 pg/ml (0-1 mg/L)	Gastrin is a gastric hormone that is a powerful stimulus for gastric acid secretion. Elevated levels are found in those with pernicious anemia and Zollinger-Ellison syndrome.
Helicobacter pylori	None	*H. pylori* detected in serum is a highly sensitive but less specific indicator of active infection; *H. pylori* infection predisposes person to peptic ulcer disease.
BILIARY SYSTEM		
Total bilirubin Conjugated (direct)	0.3-1 mg/dl 0.1-0.4 mg/dl	Bilirubin is excreted in bile. Obstruction in biliary tract contributes primarily to rise in conjugated (direct) values.
Alkaline phosphatase	35-150 unit/L	Alkaline phosphatase is found in many tissues, with high concentrations in bone, liver, and biliary tract epithelium. Obstructive biliary tract disease and carcinoma may cause significant elevations.
PANCREAS		
Amylase	25-125 unit/L	Amylase is secreted normally by acinar cells of pancreas. Damage to these cells or obstruction of pancreatic duct causes enzyme to be absorbed into blood in significant quantities. It is a sensitive yet nonspecific test for pancreatic disease.
Lipase	10-140 unit/L	Lipase is a pancreatic enzyme normally secreted into duodenum. It appears in blood when damage occurs to acinar cells. It is a specific test for pancreatic disease.
Calcium	8.4-10.6 mg/dl	Calcium levels may be low in cases of severe pancreatitis or steatorrhea, since calcium soaps are formed from sequestration of calcium by fat necrosis.
INTESTINE		
Total protein (albumin, globulin)	Total protein: 6-8 g/dl Albumin: 3.5-5.5 g/dl Globulin: Alpha_1 0.2-0.4 g/dl Alpha_2 0.5-0.9 g/dl Beta 0.6-1.1 g/dl Gamma 0.7-1.7 g/dl	Although primarily a reflection of liver function, serum protein level is also a measure of nutrition. Malnourished patients have greatly decreased levels of serum protein.
D-Xylose absorption test	Blood levels of 25-40 mg/dl 2 hr after ingestion	D-Xylose is a monosaccharide that is easily absorbed by normal intestine but not metabolized by body. It does not require biliary or pancreatic function. D-Xylose is administered orally and assists in diagnosis of malabsorption.
Lactose tolerance test	Rise in blood glucose level of >20 mg/dl	Oral dose of lactose is administered. In absence of intestinal lactase, lactose is neither broken down nor absorbed and plasma glucose levels do not rise. Test assists in diagnosis of lactose intolerance.
Carcinoembryonic antigen (CEA)		CEA is protein normally present in fetal gut tissue. It is typically elevated in persons with colorectal tumors. Although not useful as screening tool, it is useful in determining prognosis and response to therapy.
URINE		
5-Hydroxyindoleacetic acid (5-HIAA) Quantitative Qualitative	<5 ng/ml 2-6 mg/24 hr Negative	Carcinoid tumors are serotonin secreting and are derived from neuroectoderm tissue. This neurohormone is metabolized to 5-HIAA by the liver and excreted in urine.
Urine bilirubin	Negative	Bilirubin is not normally excreted in urine. Biliary stricture, inflammation, or stones may cause its presence.
Urobilinogen	0.5-4 mg/24 hr	This is a sensitive test for hepatic or biliary disease. Decreased levels are seen in those with biliary obstruction and pancreatic cancer.
Urine amylase	<17 unit/hr	Rise in level usually mimics rise in serum amylase. However, level remains elevated for 7-10 days, which allows for retrospective diagnosis.

TABLE 40-6 INTERPRETATION OF FECES COLOR

Color/Appearance	Interpretation
White	Barium
Gray, tan (clay)	Lack of bile, biliary obstruction
Red	Lower gastrointestinal (GI) bleeding
Black	
Tarry	Rapid peristalsis with bile present
Dry	Upper GI bleeding
Green	Rapid peristalsis with bile present

stance that, when ingested or given by enema, outlines the passageways of the GI tract for viewing by fluoroscopy or x-ray films.

Nursing responsibilities related to these tests commonly involve supervision of the cleansing of the GI tract with enemas and laxatives. It is important for the nurse to monitor the patient's fluid and electrolyte status because extensive bowel cleansing may cause significant fluid losses, particularly in older persons. The nurse provides psychologic support to the patient because the procedures can be intrusive and uncomfortable. The nurse also addresses the patient's educational needs, explaining the procedure, the rationale for use, and procedural steps.

Upper Gastrointestinal Series. An upper GI series involves visualization of the esophagus, stomach, duodenum, and upper jejunum through the use of a contrast medium. It is a fluoroscopic x-ray test that permits the examination of the structure, position, peristaltic activity, and motility of the organs. It can assist in the detection of tumors, ulceration, inflammation, abnormal anatomy, or malposition.

An upper GI series involves swallowing the contrast medium (usually barium), which is prepared in a flavored milkshake form. The barium is unpleasant tasting and may cause vomiting. It is administered cold to increase its palatability. The barium outlines the structures as it flows by gravity through the esophagus and stomach into the intestinal loops. Films are taken at intervals during the test, which takes about 45 minutes. The procedure is termed a *barium swallow* if only the function of the esophagus is to be evaluated; this takes about 15 minutes. If the small bowel is the primary focus, it may be termed a *small bowel series*.

The only preparation for an upper GI series is nothing-by-mouth (NPO) status for at least 6 hours before the test. After an upper GI series, the patient is prescribed a laxative to hasten elimination of the barium; barium that remains in the colon may harden and be difficult to expel, leading to fecal impaction. The stool should return to its normal color (barium is white) after the barium is expelled.

The upper GI series used to be the foundation of a diagnostic workup for many GI disorders, but with the ready availability of endoscopy, the test is now seldom used.

Barium Enema. A barium enema clearly outlines most of the large intestine through the use of a contrast medium. It is used to detect colon polyps, tumors, and chronic inflammatory bowel disease. If both an upper GI series and a barium enema are to be performed, the barium enema is done first to prevent barium from the upper GI series from entering the colon. The procedure involves the instillation of barium through a rectal tube with an inflatable balloon to hold the barium in the colon. The patient is then placed in various positions while the radiologist observes on a monitor as the barium flows through the colon. The procedure takes about 30 minutes. The instillation and retention of the barium can cause the patient considerable embarrassment and discomfort.

Preparation for a barium enema involves thorough cleansing of the bowel by laxatives, enemas, or both. Thorough preparation is essential because retained fecal material obscures the normal bowel anatomy. The patient may be asked to restrict dairy products, follow a liquid diet for 24 hours before the test, and remain NPO for at least 8 hours before the test. Laxatives may also be administered after the test to facilitate removal of the barium. The stools may be white tinged for several days. Inpatients are closely monitored for complications after the test, such as perforation of the bowel. Outpatients are instructed to report abdominal pain and to monitor carefully for constipation.

Ultrasonography. Ultrasonography involves the use of high-frequency sound waves that are transmitted into the abdomen and create echoes that vary with tissue density. The echoes bounce back to a transducer and are electronically converted into pictorial images of the organs. This reveals organ size, shape, and position and is useful in diagnosing cysts, tumors, and stones. Ultrasonography has become the procedure of choice for diagnosing gallbladder disease because it does not expose the patient to radiation. The procedure is both painless and safe.

Patient preparation is straightforward. The patient remains NPO for 8 to 12 hours before the test, since gas in the bowel may interfere with the results. If the gallbladder is the focus of the test, the patient is instructed to eat a low-fat meal the evening before the test so that bile will accumulate in the gallbladder, thereby enhancing visualization. The patient resumes a normal diet and activity after the test.

Computed Tomography. Computed tomography (CT) can also be used to assess patients with gallbladder, biliary ductal system, or pancreatic problems. It is helpful in identifying problems similar to those described for ultrasonography. In a CT scan, multiple x-rays are passed through the abdomen, and a computer reconstructs the data into two-dimensional images on a television screen. Still photographs can also be taken of the images. Contrast media can be used with the CT scan to better visualize the biliary tract or to accentuate differences in tissue density in the pancreas. The test is comparable to ultrasonography in effectiveness. It is used less often because of its significantly higher cost and moderate radiation exposure for the patient. It is extremely useful with obese individuals, however, because increased tissue density limits the effectiveness of ultrasound transmission.

The patient should remain NPO for 8 to 12 hours before the test. If contrast medium is to be used, the patient should be assessed for allergies to iodine, seafood, or contrast medium. Barium studies, if necessary, should be done at least 4 days before the CT scan or after the scan, since the barium can interfere with test results. There are no special after-care considerations. The patient may resume pretest diet and activity.

Radionuclide Imaging. GI scintigraphy is used to pinpoint the site of GI bleeding, particularly at sites in the lower GI tract that are not possible to visualize with endoscopy. For GI scintigraphy, an intravenous injection of technetium 99m sulfur colloid is administered. This radionuclide then pools at the bleeding site. No pretest preparation is required, and no discomfort is experienced. Patients in unstable condition may not be candidates for this test if they are unable to travel safely to the nuclear medicine department for the 30 minutes required for the test.

Cholecystography. Oral cholecystography involves the radiographic examination of the gallbladder after the administration of a contrast medium. A normal liver will remove radiopaque drugs, such as iodoalphionic acid (Priodax), iopanoic acid (Telepaque), and iodipamide methylglucamine (Cholografin Meglumine), from the bloodstream and store and concentrate them in the gallbladder. The dye-filled gallbladder shows on x-ray examination as a dense shadow. Lack of a shadow indicates a nonfunctioning gallbladder. Stones, which are not radiopaque, show as dark patches on the film. Ultrasonography has largely replaced this once commonly used test in the diagnosis of gallbladder disease. Cholecystography is primarily used today when the ultrasound picture is inconclusive.

Cholangiography. Cholangiography involves x-ray examination of the bile ducts to confirm the presence of stones, strictures, or tumors. The radiopaque substance may be administered intravenously or injected directly into the common bile duct with a needle or catheter during surgery or endoscopy. After surgery on the common bile duct, a radiopaque drug such as iodipamide methylglucamine is instilled through a drainage tube to determine the patency of the duct. The dye also may be injected through the skin and abdominal wall directly into a bile duct (percutaneous transhepatic cholangiography). The technique is useful in visualizing the location and extent of a pathologic process such as obstructive jaundice, and permits decompression of the liver. Complications from the test are rare, but include bile leakage leading to peritonitis or bleeding caused by accidental rupture of a blood vessel.

The patient remains NPO for about 8 hours before the test. The injection of the contrast medium may cause temporary pain or a feeling of pressure or epigastric fullness. The nurse carefully monitors the patient's vital signs and looks for bleeding or adverse reactions to the dye. The patient typically rests in bed for about 6 hours after the test, lying on the right side as much as possible. The nurse monitors the needle insertion site for signs of bleeding or infection.

Special Tests

Esophageal Function Tests. Several diagnostic tests may be used to evaluate the function of the esophagus and aid in the diagnosis of esophageal reflux or motility problems. These tests can be performed by having the patient swallow two or three tiny tubes that are attached to an external transducer. Once the tubes are in the stomach, they are slowly pulled back into the distal esophagus at varying levels. Lower esophageal sphincter pressure, swallowing activity, pH, and effectiveness of clearance can all be measured in about 30 to 45 minutes. However, 24-hour pH monitoring is still considered to be the gold standard for the accurate diagnosis of esophageal reflux.

In preparation for these tests, the nurse instructs the patient to (1) remain NPO for 8 hours before the procedure(s); (2) avoid alcohol and smoking the day before; and (3) avoid medications such as antacids, H_2-receptor antagonists, proton pump inhibitors, and anticholinergics before the test(s).[8] Sedation is not required but may be used if the patient experiences persistent choking or gagging during the procedure. After removal of the tubes, a mild sore throat is common. Esophageal tests may include any or all of the tests described below.

MANOMETRY. This test measures the pressure in the lower esophageal sphincter and records the duration and sequence of peristaltic movements within the esophagus. Readings are taken at various levels in the esophagus with the patient at rest and during swallowing. Baseline sphincter pressure is normally about 20 mm Hg. The test is used primarily to diagnose esophageal reflux, but the graphic record of muscular activity during swallowing may also help document the presence of achalasia or esophageal spasm.

pH MONITORING. This test evaluates the competency of the LES by obtaining a single measurement of the esophageal pH. An electrode attached to a manometry catheter is placed above the LES. Normally, the esophagus maintains a pH greater than 6.0. Serial measurements may be obtained by maintaining the electrode in place for 24 hours. The probe must be inserted transnasally and connected to a recording box similar to a Holter monitor that is worn about the waist. The patient can then be monitored at home while eating a normal diet; 24-hour pH monitoring is the most sensitive and specific diagnostic test for abnormal acid reflux.

ESOPHAGEAL CLEARANCE TEST. In conjunction with the previous two tests, esophageal clearance tests evaluate the function of both the upper and lower esophageal sphincters, along with the body of the esophagus, in response to swallowing. Normally, esophageal function allows for the complete clearance of acid material from the esophagus in less than 10 swallows. Readings are recorded from the catheter tip to determine the rate and efficiency of acid clearance.

ACID PERFUSION TEST (BERNSTEIN TEST). Confusion surrounding the origin of heartburn symptoms is often resolved with the Bernstein test, which attempts to reproduce the pain. Small quantities of HCl are instilled into the distal esophagus by nasogastric tube. The test is positive if the acid produces pain. Saline is instilled to rinse out the acid, and an antacid may be administered to relieve the discomfort.

Gastric Function Tests

GASTRIC ANALYSIS (BASAL GASTRIC SECRETION AND GASTRIC ACID STIMULATION TESTS). Examination of the fasting contents of the stomach can be helpful in establishing a diagnosis of gastric disease. The purpose of the test is to quantify gastric acidity in the fasting and stimulated states. Abnormal secretion may be related to ulcers, malignancy, pernicious anemia, or Zollinger-Ellison syndrome. A nasogastric tube is inserted, and gastric contents are aspirated. Gastric contents may then be aspirated every 15 minutes for 90 minutes.

The nurse instructs the patient to restrict food, fluid, and smoking for 8 to 12 hours before the test. The flow of gastric acid is then stimulated by betazole hydrochloride, histamine phosphate, or pentagastrin administered subcutaneously. The person may experience side effects from the medication, including flushing, a feeling of warmth, slight headache, or itching. Epinephrine is given to counteract the effects of histamine if sensitivity occurs.

TUBELESS GASTRIC ANALYSIS (DIAGNEX BLUE TEST). Tubeless gastric analysis may be used for detection of gastric achlorhydria. The test indicates the presence of free HCl but cannot be used to determine the amount of free HCl that is present. A gastric stimulant such as caffeine is given, and then a cation exchange resin containing azure A is given orally an hour later. If free HCl is present in the stomach, introduction of the resin causes a substance to be released in the stomach that will be absorbed from the small intestine and excreted by the kidneys as blue dye within 2 hours. Absence of detectable amounts of blue dye in the urine indicates that free HCl probably was not secreted.

SCHILLING TEST. The Schilling test evaluates vitamin B_{12} absorption. In the normal GI tract, vitamin B_{12} combines with the intrinsic factor that is produced by the parietal cells in the gastric mucosa and is absorbed in the distal portion of the ileum. Pernicious anemia develops if intrinsic factor is lacking or malabsorption exists. This is a concern in patients who have had the terminal ileum removed for disorders such as Crohn's disease.

The patient is kept NPO for 8 to 12 hours before the test and then administered an oral preparation of radioactive vitamin B_{12}, followed by an intramuscular injection of nonradioactive vitamin B_{12} to saturate the tissue-binding sites. Urinary B_{12} levels are measured after urine is collected for 24 to 48 hours. With normal absorption of vitamin B_{12}, the ileum absorbs more vitamin B_{12} than the body needs and excretes the excess into the urine. With impaired absorption of vitamin B_{12}, little or no vitamin B_{12} is excreted into the urine. Intrinsic factor preparations may also be administered to differentiate intestinal problems from pernicious anemia.

UREA BREATH TEST. Testing for *H. pylori* is both technically difficult and expensive.[3] The urea breath test (UBT) is based on the principle that the *H. pylori* organism is able to produce large amounts of urease, a surface enzyme that catalyzes the breakdown of urea in gastric secretions into bicarbonate and ammonia. Patients are administered an oral solution of carbon isotope–labeled urea in water. If *H. pylori* is present in the stomach, the urea is metabolized. The labeled bicarbonate is excreted in the form of labeled carbon dioxide, which can be collected and measured. The patient exhales into a balloon or other receptacle, and the carbon dioxide is measured with a scintillation counter. The sample can be collected 20 minutes after the solution is ingested. The test has minimal risks associated with radioactivity and is estimated to be 97% sensitive and 100% specific for *H. pylori*.

Biopsy

UPPER GASTROINTESTINAL BIOPSY. A biopsy of the oral cavity or tongue may be done on any lesion or ulcerated area that requires a differential diagnosis. This procedure is usually performed with a local anesthetic. After the biopsy, the biopsy site is assessed for bleeding. Biopsy of the stomach is typically performed during fiberoptic endoscopy.

INTESTINAL BIOPSY. Biopsy of the small or large bowel may also be performed during the course of endoscopic examination to allow tissue analysis of lesions, polyps, or masses. A knife blade or snare is typically used to obtain the tissue sample. The procedure is usually not painful, although the patient may feel pressure. Bleeding from the site of the biopsy is uncommon. If bleeding does occur, the patient is instructed to report this to the physician and to curtail physical activity until examined by a physician.

Endoscopy

Endoscopy allows for direct visualization of portions of the GI tract by means of a long, flexible, fiberoptic scope (Figure 40-10). Images are seen through an eyepiece or projected onto a video screen. The remote control tip moves in multiple directions. Endoscopy may be used for direct inspection, biopsy, and removal of polyps and stones. In addition, GI bleeding may be controlled endoscopically through laser, photocoagulation, or the injection of sclerosing agents. The upper GI tract may be visualized as far as the duodenum by insertion of a fiberscope through the mouth. A fiberscope is inserted through the rectum for visualization of the rectum (proctoscopy), sigmoid colon (sigmoidoscopy), or entire colon (colonoscopy).

Today most endoscopic procedures are performed on an ambulatory basis, even with older adults. Oral fiberscope insertion is uncomfortable and may precipitate gagging or choking despite the use of topical anesthetic sprays or gargles. Premedication with an intravenous sedative such as midazolam (Versed) or diazepam (Valium) or an analgesic such as meperidine (Demerol) is used. Thus the patient is conscious but sedated; amnesia is often experienced when high doses of these drugs are used.

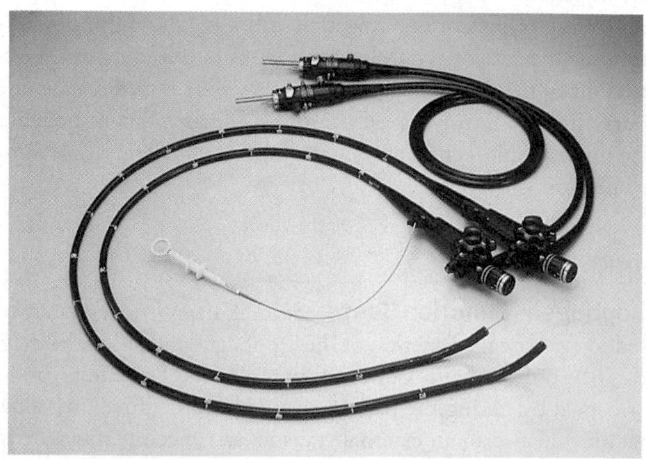

Figure 40-10 Flexible colon fiberscopes.

Esophagogastroduodenoscopy. Upper GI endoscopy may be limited to the esophagus (esophagoscopy), stomach (gastroscopy), or duodenum (duodenoscopy); or it may involve examination of the entire region (**esophagogastroduodenoscopy** [EGD]) (Figure 40-11). This is particularly useful for identifying the source of upper GI bleeding and for differentiating gastric malignancies from benign ulcers, and gastric ulcers from duodenal ulcers. Other uses include visualization of esophageal strictures, varices, tumors, achalasia, and hiatal hernias, and the surgical removal of gastric polyps.[4]

Preparation for an EGD involves instructing the patient to remain NPO for 8 hours before the test. Because air is typically introduced as the endoscope is advanced to improve visibility, the nurse tells the patient that he or she will likely experience a feeling of pressure or fullness. The entire test lasts about 15 to 30 minutes unless additional treatments are planned.

After the procedure the nurse monitors the patient carefully for signs of dyspnea, pain, bleeding, or acute dysphagia. Vital signs are taken every 30 minutes for 3 to 4 hours, and no oral food or fluids are administered until the nurse determines that the gag reflex is fully intact. Throat lozenges or saline gargles may be used to relieve sore throat after the test. Complications are rare but include aspiration, perforation, and bleeding.

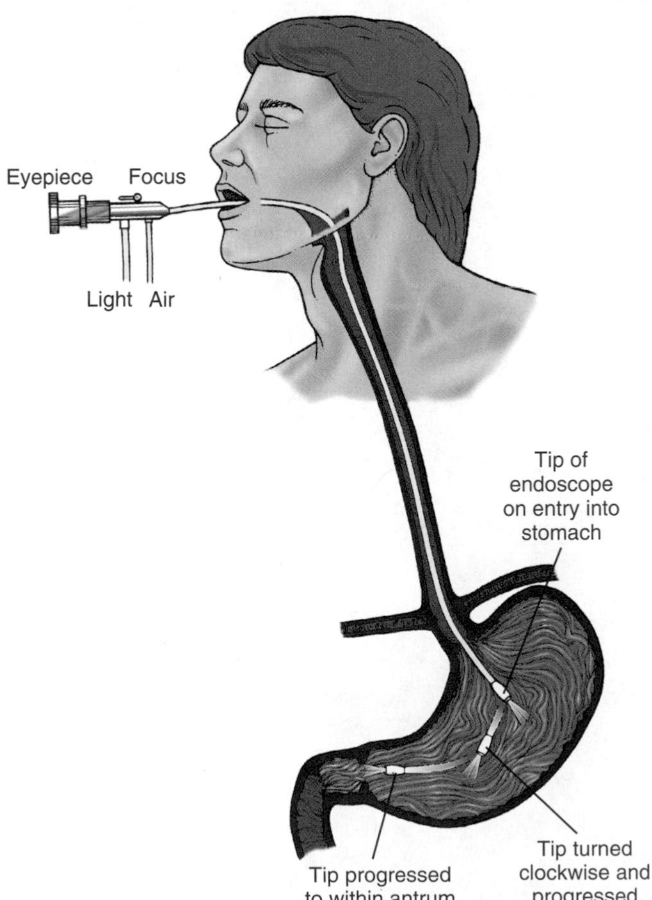

Figure 40-11 Flexible endoscope shown passing through mouth and esophagus to stomach. *Dotted lines* show how endoscope is moved to allow visualization of all areas of stomach.

Endoscopic Retrograde Cholangiopancreatography. **Endoscopic retrograde cholangiopancreatography** (ERCP) also involves the oral insertion of an endoscope, but this device has a side-viewing tip and a cannula that can be maneuvered into the papilla of Vater (Figure 40-12). Dye may be injected to outline the pancreatic and biliary ducts. The procedure may be combined with papillotomy to enlarge the sphincter and release gallstones. Glucagon may be administered to minimize spasm in the duodenum and sphincter.

Care after the procedure is similar to that for an EGD. The nurse monitors the patient carefully for signs of abdominal pain, nausea, and vomiting, which might indicate pancreatitis.

Colonoscopy. Fiberoptic colonoscopy allows the examination of the entire colon in most patients. It is used to evaluate benign and malignant growths, remove polyps, take biopsy specimens, and localize sites of bleeding. A colonoscopy is the current gold standard for diagnosing colorectal cancers.

Thorough bowel preparation is essential before the test, which is especially difficult for older persons. A 1-day preparation with an oral osmotic solution is now standard because it reduces overall fluid and electrolyte loss. A gallon of polyethylene glycol (Colyte) solution is administered rapidly (8 ounces every 15 minutes) and induces a profuse watery diarrhea within 30 to 60 minutes, which lasts about 4 hours. In some cases the patient may receive a 2- to 3-day preparation consisting of a clear liquid diet, strong laxatives, and an enema the day of the test. All patients are NPO for about 8 hours before the test.[1]

Patients are sedated before the colonoscopy. The fiberoptic colonoscope, which is 105 to 185 cm (42 to 72 inches) long, visualizes the mucosa of the colon as it is advanced along its length. Air is introduced as the colonoscope is advanced to

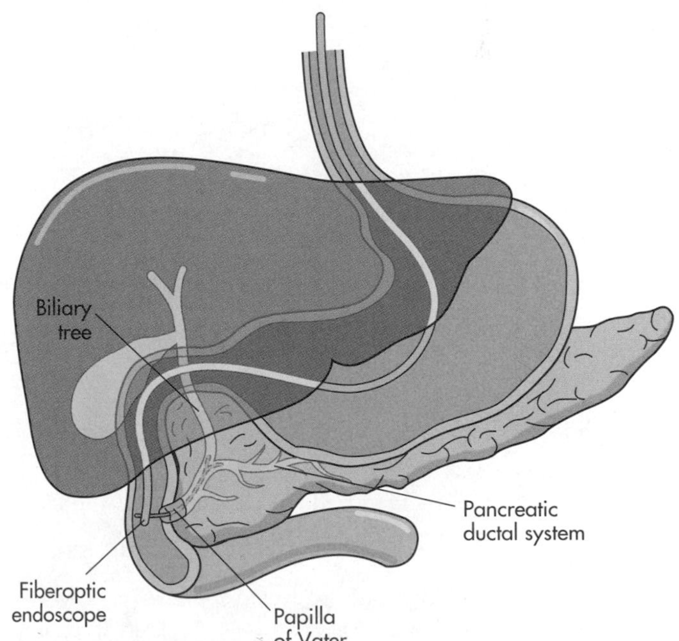

Figure 40-12 Endoscopic retrograde cholangiopancreatography (ERCP).

increase visualization and may cause abdominal cramping. The procedure lasts from 20 to 60 minutes.

Afterward the nurse assumes responsibility for carefully monitoring the patient and ensuring full recovery from sedation. Any changes in vital signs or development of severe abdominal pain, rectal bleeding, or fever is immediately reported to the physician. Arrangements for transportation home are important because the patient should not drive.

Sigmoidoscopy may be performed rather than colonoscopy. The cost of a sigmoidoscopy is considerably less than a colonoscopy but the procedure only allows for visualization of the anus, rectum, and distal sigmoid colon.[5] However, approximately 75% of all polyps and tumors of the large intestine can be visualized with a flexible sigmoidoscope.[6] Pretest preparation instructions vary widely. The patient may be instructed to prepare with a 2-day clear liquid diet and pretest fasting. Fleet enemas may be ordered, or a cleansing enema may be preferred. The knee-chest position and a strong urge to defecate that is produced by the larger-diameter sigmoidoscope make this an uncomfortable and unpopular procedure for patients. Sedation is not usually used. Aftercare involves monitoring for distention, increased tenderness, and bleeding. The patient may initially pass large amounts of flatus from the instillation of air during the procedure. Slight rectal bleeding may occur if biopsies have been taken.

References

1. Ayers DMN: Using a colonoscopy to survey intestinal health, *Nursing* 33(3):65, 2003.
2. Bartz S: Gastrointestinal disorders in the elderly, *Ann Long Term Care* 11(7):33-39, 2003.
3. DiBaise JK: Risk factors for *H pylori* resistance, *Am J Gastroenterol* 97(4):792, 2002.
4. LeBlond R, DeGowin R, Brown D: *DeGowin's diagnostic examination*, ed 8, New York, 2004, McGraw-Hill.
5. Li CZ: Viewing the small intestine via capsule endoscopy, *Nursing* 34(4):70-71, 2004.
6. Lynch HT: Cancer family history and genetic testing: are malpractice adjudications waiting to happen? *Am J Gastroenterol* 97(3):518-520, 2002.
7. Mehta M: Assessing the abdomen, *Nursing* 33(5):54-55, 2003.
8. Nightengale J, Hogg P: The gastrointestinal advanced practitioner: an emerging role, *Radiography* 9(2):151-160, 2003.
9. Pagel JM et al: Retrospective analysis of a guideline for evaluating nontraumatic abdominal pain in older patient presenting to the emergency department, *J Clin Outcomes Manage* 10(11):589-595, 2003.

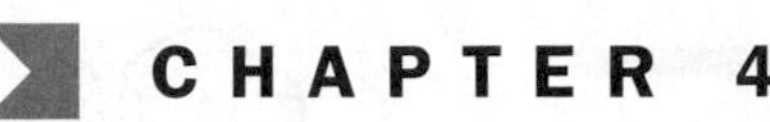 Visit the Evolve website: http://evolve.elsevier.com/Monahan/medsurg

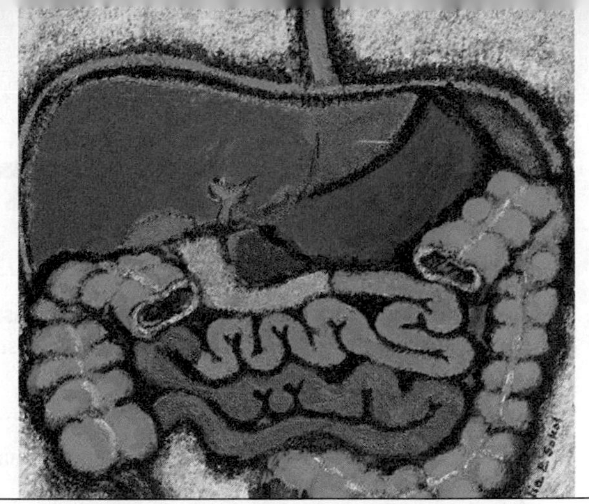

CHAPTER 41

Mouth and Esophagus Problems

by Judith K. Sands

OBJECTIVES

After studying this chapter, the learner should be able to:

1. Describe lifestyle modifications for the prevention of common oral and esophageal disorders.
2. Discuss the pathophysiology underlying common problems of the mouth and esophagus.
3. List the major clinical manifestations of common oral and esophageal disorders.
4. Discuss the collaborative care management of common problems of the mouth and esophagus.
5. Use the nursing process to describe nursing care of patients with major esophageal disorders.

KEY TERMS

achalasia, p. 1195
aphthous stomatitis, p. 1184
Barrett's epithelium, p. 1188
fundoplication, p. 1190
gastroesophageal reflux disease, p. 1187
gingivitis, p. 1183
hiatal hernia, p. 1193
leukoplakia, p. 1186
odynophagia, p. 1189
plaque, p. 1183
pyrosis, p. 1188
water brash, p. 1189
xerostomia, p. 1187

Problems involving the mouth and esophagus include a number of common disorders that affect millions of adults. The majority of the disorders are managed by the individual in the home and rarely involve admission to the acute care setting. The nurse's role includes patient and family education directed toward prevention and health promotion, as well as self-care management.

Problems of the Mouth

Tooth and Gum Disease

Progressive tooth loss used to be considered a virtually inevitable consequence of aging. Advances in our understanding of dental health and new approaches to tooth maintenance have changed these perspectives substantially, and the preservation of natural teeth is now a primary goal. This heavy emphasis on prevention is clearly reflected in the *Healthy People 2010* goals for oral health (see Healthy People 2010 box).

Etiology and Epidemiology. Tooth decay is by far the most common problem affecting the teeth. Plaque formation is the most important factor in tooth decay, but familial tendency, poor oral hygiene, poor health, and perhaps a diet high in simple or refined sugars also play a role.

The periodontium is the tissue that surrounds and supports the teeth. Disease of the periodontium is the most common cause of tooth loss in adults after age 50. At any time, an estimated 25% to 75% of the adult population with natural teeth have some evidence of the disease. Bacterial plaque is again the most important contributor to the problem; other factors are dental malocclusion, caries, dietary deficiencies, and systemic diseases such as diabetes.

Pathophysiology. Dental **plaque** is a soft, colorless mass composed of proliferating bacteria that adheres to the teeth. Acids produced by these bacteria slowly destroy the enamel and dentin of the teeth, creating cavities, which are the visible evidence of decay. Food, particularly carbohydrates, stimulates bacterial acid production. Simple sugars have the greatest effect. Plaque begins to collect on the teeth within 2 hours of eating, and the more frequently carbohydrates are ingested, the longer it takes for the pH of the mouth to return to normal.

Gingivitis, the earliest form of periodontal disease, is characterized by reddened gums, swelling, and easy bleeding. Inflammation causes the gingivae to separate from the tooth surface, forming pockets that can collect bacteria, food particles, and pus. Progressive gingivitis can result in receding gums, resorption of alveolar bone, and loosening of the teeth (Figure 41-1). Bleeding

Healthy People 2010

Goal and Objectives Related to Oral Health

Goal

Prevent and control oral and craniofacial diseases, conditions, and injuries and improve access to related services.

Objectives

Reduce the proportion of children, adolescents, and adults with untreated dental decay.
Increase the proportion of adults who have never had a permanent tooth extracted because of dental caries or periodontal disease.
Reduce the proportion of older adults who have had all their natural teeth extracted.
Reduce periodontal disease.
Increase the proportion of the U.S. population served by community water systems with optimally fluoridated water.
Increase the proportion of adults and long-term care residents who use the oral health system each year.
Increase the proportion of local health departments and community-based centers, including community migrant and homeless health centers, that have an oral health component.
Increase the number of states (and the District of Columbia) that have an oral and craniofacial health surveillance system.
Increase the number of tribal, state (including the District of Columbia), and local health agencies serving jurisdictions of 250,000 or more persons that have in place an effective public dental health program directed by a dental professional with public health training.

From US Department of Health and Human Services: *Healthy people 2010: understanding and improving health,* Washington, DC, 2000, The Department.

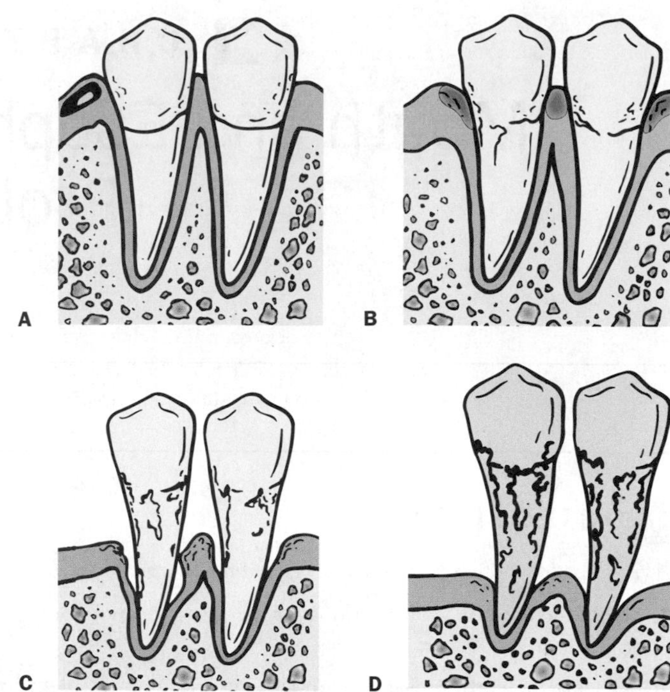

Figure 41-1 Progression of periodontal disease. **A,** Calculus (calcification of dental plaque) deposited on teeth at gum line. **B,** Gingivae become swollen and tender. **C,** Inflammation spreads, pockets develop between gums and gingivae, and gums recede. **D,** Alveolar bone is destroyed and teeth loosen.

of the gums with normal tooth brushing is a common early sign. There is usually no pain.

Collaborative Care Management. Prevention is the most appropriate management strategy for both dental decay and periodontal disease. It should start in childhood and continue throughout life. Widespread fluoridation of water supplies has decreased the incidence of tooth decay significantly. Fluoride makes tooth enamel more resistant to acids and is widely available in toothpastes, dental rinses, and mouthwashes. Fluoride may also be applied in concentrated forms by a dentist. Sealants and bonding preparations can be applied in childhood to increase tooth resistance to decay.

Treatment of periodontal disease includes the removal of decayed tooth structures and their replacement with restorative barriers. Progressive gingivitis may require aggressive measures such as scaling or root planing to control or correct the problem. If control is not possible, the individual may face the need for tooth extraction and the fitting of dentures.

PATIENT/FAMILY TEACHING. Good oral hygiene with frequent brushing and regular flossing is the mainstay of prevention for tooth and gum disease. Health care providers take every opportunity to reinforce this principle and instruct individuals in correct techniques. Regular checkups and professional cleaning facilitate early identification and intervention. Restricting the amount of simple sugar in the diet is a standard recommendation, and adequate or supplemental vitamin C is believed to reduce plaque. It is increasingly recognized that access to affordable dental care is a significant obstacle to the achievement of public health goals related to oral health.

▶ ARE You READY?

The nurse is preparing an educational offering about disorders of the mouth for a group of senior adults. Which of the following statements about gingivitis should be included in this presentation?

1. Pain is usually intense.
2. Bleeding of the gums is an early sign.
3. Tooth loss occurs despite treatment.
4. Systemic blood infections are common if left untreated.

Mouth Infections

Etiology and Epidemiology. A wide variety of primary oral infections can be triggered by various bacteria and viruses. Any of the structures of the mouth may develop infection, which can seriously affect the individual's ability to eat and drink. Oral infections may also occur secondary to vitamin deficiencies, other systemic diseases or treatments, or local trauma or stress. Common examples include the following.

Aphthous stomatitis produces well-circumscribed, shallow ulcers (canker sores) that are often covered with a grayish white or yellow exudates on the soft tissues of the mouth, including the lips, tongue, insides of the cheeks, pharynx, and soft palate (Figure 41-2). The lesions are acutely painful but noncontagious and are of uncertain, although perhaps autoimmune, origin. Aphthous ulcers are a chronic problem. They affect up to 25% of the population at some time[15] and usually first appear in the teenage years. Healing usually occurs in 1 to 3 weeks.

Herpes simplex is a viral infection that produces characteristic blisters referred to as cold sores or fever blisters. The virus is usually acquired in early childhood; an estimated 80% to 90% of the adult population may be infected.[15] The virus is harbored in a dormant state by cells in the sensory nerve ganglia. Reactivation of the virus can occur with emotional stress, fever, or exposure to cold or ultraviolet light. The lesions typically appear on the mucocutaneous border junction of the lips in the form of small vesicles, which then erupt and form painful, shallow ulcers.

Acute necrotizing ulcerative gingivitis, also called trench mouth, is an acute inflammatory gum disease caused by a tremendous proliferation of normal mouth flora, such as spirochetes and fusiform bacilli. It is commonly triggered by poor oral hygiene, nutritional deficiencies, alcoholism, infection, or an immunocompromised condition. The disease is not infectious.

Candidiasis (thrush) is caused by an increase in the number of *Candida albicans,* a yeastlike fungus normally found in the gastrointestinal (GI) tract, vagina, and oral cavity and on the skin. Overgrowth of the organism may result from antibiotic depletion of normal flora or immunosuppression from steroid therapy, chemotherapy, or human immunodeficiency virus infection. The condition is painful and, if widespread, can interfere with oral nutrition.

Glossitis, inflammation of the tongue, can accompany a wide variety of local and systemic infections, nutritional deficiencies, and chemical irritation. Patients experience pain or burning sensations, and the tongue exhibits mild or patchy erythema or a completely erythematous surface.

Parotitis is an inflammation of the salivary or parotid glands. The viral infection known as mumps, which affects the parotid glands, occurs primarily in the pediatric population, although it can occur in unimmunized adults. Acute bacterial parotitis typically occurs in debilitated or older patients in whom poor oral hygiene, dehydration, minimal oral intake, or medications have resulted in chronic dry mouth. As the natural secretions diminish, bacteria invade the gland. The causative organism is often *Staphylococcus,* and the infection may be serious. Sudden-onset pain and acute swelling occur, and the infection can become chronic and

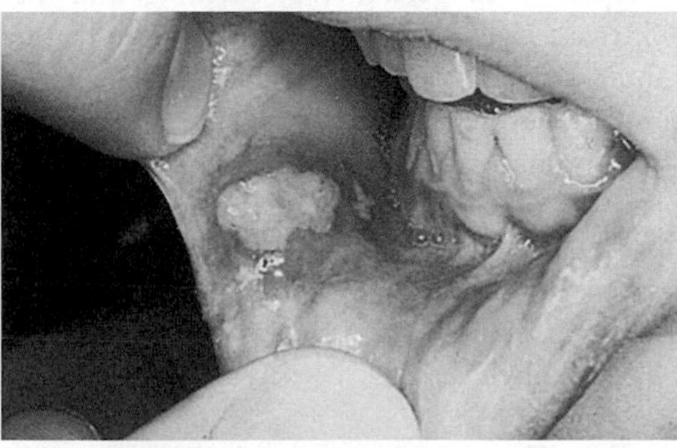

Figure 41-2 Major aphthous ulcer.

recurrent. An acute form of the inflammation, known as surgical mumps, can also occur in postoperative patients.

Pathophysiology. Most infectious diseases of the mouth have similar signs and symptoms. The mucosa throughout the mouth is thin, and evolving vesicles and bullae break open rapidly forming ulcers. These ulcers may be further traumatized by the teeth and can readily become infected by the abundant oral flora. Many of the causative organisms are the same as those which cause common skin infections. Table 41-1 summarizes the clinical manifestations of common disorders.

Collaborative Care Management. Most oral infections are self-limiting and heal spontaneously without the need for direct intervention. Supportive or palliative care includes brushing and flossing, rinsing with mouthwashes, and diet modification to reduce irritation.

PATIENT/FAMILY TEACHING. Patient and family teaching is directed at self-care management, since virtually all mouth infections are treated at home. The nurse discusses the proper use of antibiotics, rinses, and anesthetic ointments, as well as the importance of maintaining regular oral hygiene despite discomfort. Herpesvirus lesions can be spread by direct contact to other areas of the body and to others, so the nurse stresses the importance of good hand washing. The nurse also provides specific information about symptoms that indicate complications requiring medical intervention.

Cancer of the Mouth

Etiology and Epidemiology. Cancer may develop on the lips, tongue, palate, floor of the mouth, or other portions of the oral cavity. With the exception of cancer of the tongue, oral cancer is clearly linked to a history of smoking and alcohol consumption, and the risk increases with heavy use.[32] It has proven difficult to separate the unique effects of smoking and alcohol use, but their combined effects are theorized to cause a breakdown in the body's defense mechanisms as evidenced by a decrease in immunoglobulin A levels. The role of viruses, particularly the herpesviruses, is also being thoroughly researched. The precise etiology of oral cancer remains unknown, and the etiologic factors discussed are theorized to act as cocarcinogens with as yet unidentified primary factors.

Oral cancers account for approximately 3% of cancers in men and 2% of cancers in women; the incidence is higher among African-Americans.[16] Most oral cancer occurs in persons over 45 years old, and the incidence increases with age, but recent years have shown an increase in oral malignancies in younger adults.[16] Many oral cancers are believed to be preventable through lifestyle changes (e.g., alcohol and cigarette smoking reduction). The importance of prevention is reflected in the *Healthy People 2010* objectives (see Healthy People 2010 box, p. 1186).

Pathophysiology. More than 90% of oral cancers arise from the squamous cells that line the surface oral epithelium; epidermoid, basal cell, and other carcinomas also may occur.[32] The majority of tumors appear on the lateral or ventral surfaces of the tongue. They are often asymptomatic and frequently go unnoticed by the patient. A single lesion is typical.

TABLE 41-1 MOUTH INFECTIONS

Infection	Clinical Manifestations	Collaborative Management
Aphthous stomatitis (canker sore)	Painful, small mucosal ulcerations occurring anywhere in oral cavity	Palliative: mouthwashes, hydrocortisone-antibiotic ointment (e.g., fluocinonide [Lidex] ointment in benzocaine [Orabase]); heals in 1-3 wk
Herpes simplex stomatitis (cold sore, fever blister)	Painful vesicles and ulcerations of mouth, lips, or edge of nose; may have prodromal itching or burning; fever, malaise, lymphadenopathy may occur	Palliative: mouthwashes, fluids, soft diet; topical or systemic acyclovir (Zovirax) in severe cases
Acute necrotizing ulcerative gingivitis (trench mouth)	Painful hemorrhagic gums with ulceration, foul mouth odor, fever, lymphadenopathy	Oral antibiotics, analgesics, topical hydrogen peroxide, good oral hygiene, referral to dentist for removal of plaque or tartar
Candidiasis (thrush)	Creamy white, curdlike patches closely adherent to mucosa; mucosa bleeds and ulcerates when patches scraped off; condition is painful	Oral or topical nystatin, ketoconazole, clotrimazole; amphotericin B for immunocompromised patients
Parotitis	Fever, swelling, and pain in glands with abrupt onset	Local heat and cold, frequent oral hygiene, adequate hydration; broad-spectrum antibiotics occasionally needed Salivary secretion stimulated with lozenges, hard candies, and lemon slices

Healthy People 2010

Objectives Related to Oral Cancer

- Reduce the oropharyngeal cancer death rate from a baseline of 3 per 100,000 to 2.7 per 100,000.
- Increase the proportion of oral and pharyngeal cancers detected at the earliest stage.
- Increase the proportion of adults who, in the past 12 months, report having had an examination to detect oral and pharyngeal cancers.

From US Department of Health and Human Services: *Healthy people 2010: understanding and improving health*, Washington, DC, 2000, The Department.

The tongue has an abundant supply of blood vessels and lymphatic drainage channels, so spread of the cancer to adjacent structures can be rapid. Despite the ease of examination of the oral cavity, most cancers are not diagnosed in early stages, and the 5-year survival rate remains poor. Metastasis has already occurred in 60% of patients at the time of diagnosis.[16] The cure rate for cancer involving the lips, which is similar to skin cancer, is high, partly because the lesion is so readily apparent. Tumors of the parotid gland are usually benign, whereas those arising in the submaxillary glands have a high rate of malignancy and tend to grow rapidly. Clinical manifestations of parotid and submaxillary gland tumors may include palpable masses, enlarged lymph nodes, dysphagia, chronic ear pain, and visible lesions.

Oral cancer usually is first seen as a painless lesion resembling a nonhealing ulcer. Both red and white mouth lesions are frequently found in smokers. The vast majority of these lesions are asymptomatic, and the primary concern is their cancer-causing potential. The term **leukoplakia** refers to white lesions that occur on the mucosa of the cheeks, lips, gingivae, and palate (Figure 41-3). They are more common in men and in those over 60 years old.

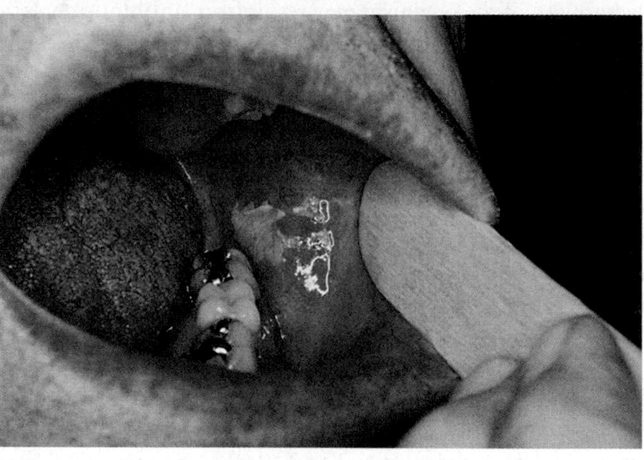

Figure 41-3 Leukoplakia.

One classic variety, stomatitis nicotina (also called smokers' patch), is clearly linked to heavy smoking, especially pipe smoking. These grayish white lesions appear on the palate and are theorized to be related to high heat exposure from the smoke. The lesions disappear if the person stops smoking, and they do not appear to increase the cancer risk unless found on the floor of the mouth. Snuff dippers' lesion is another classic form of leukoplakia. Similar lesions may develop from chronic cheek or lip biting and from friction trauma associated with ill-fitting dentures. Erythroplasia or erythroplakia are lesions similar to leukoplakia in many respects but are bright red and velvety in appearance. They are also associated with a significantly higher risk of cancer, and biopsy is strongly recommended for any persistent red lesion that does not have an obvious cause.[32]

Collaborative Care Management. Biopsy is the primary diagnostic test used in cases of suspected oral cancer. It may be used to evaluate lymph nodes, leukoplakia or erythroplakia lesions, ulcers, or neck masses that do not resolve spontaneously within 1 to 2 weeks. Ultrasonography is an excellent adjunct for evaluating masses that are close to the surface. Computed tomography scans may be used to evaluate deeper, less defined masses and delineate bone involvement.

Treatment of oral cancer depends on the location and stage of the tumor. Early-stage cancer is usually treated by either radiation or surgery, depending on the size and accessibility of the tumor. More invasive cancers may require both modalities, and advanced oral cancers are treated palliatively. Early lesions are highly curable with radiation if they are confined to the mucosa. Radiation, which has the advantage of preventing widespread tissue destruction, may be delivered by external beam or through the insertion of needles or seeds. If both radiation and surgery are planned, the radiotherapy is usually administered after the surgery, since irradiated tissue is more susceptible to infection and breakdown. Care of the patient being treated with radioactive needle implants is summarized in the Guidelines for Safe Practice box.

Several surgical options exist for the treatment of oral cancers. Confined local excision is possible in some situations, but many of the procedures are radical and involve extensive resection. Examples include partial mandibulectomy, partial (hemiglossectomy) or total (glossectomy) removal of the tongue, and resections of the floor of the mouth or buccal mucosa. Because many oral cancers metastasize early to the cervical lymph nodes, the surgery usually also includes functional or radical neck dissection, with removal of the regional and deep cervical lymph nodes and their channels.[33] In advanced cases the surgical procedure may also include removal of the sternocleidomastoid muscle or other neck muscles, internal jugular vein, thyroid gland, submaxillary gland, and spinal accessory nerve. A more complete discussion of radical neck dissection can be found in Chapter 25 in the discussion of laryngeal cancer.

The extent of excision can create significant aesthetic and functional problems for the patient, including problems with speech, chewing, swallowing, and airway management. High-dose radiotherapy commonly causes stomatitis; xerostomia; dental decay; and changes in taste, which may be long term. The **xerostomia** (severe dry mouth) begins 1 to 2 weeks after treatment is started and may persist throughout life. Dental decay, especially at the gingival margins, results from decreased salivary secretion and altered pH of the saliva. Tissue reconstruction may require repeated follow-up surgery, and a multidisciplinary approach to patient care is essential.

PATIENT/FAMILY TEACHING. Depending on the aggressiveness of the treatment, the patient may need to acquire significant new self-care skills. Good mouth care is essential to minimize tooth decay and infection and to promote healing. Patient and family teaching, as presented in the Patient/Family Teaching box, p. 1188, is an important part of nursing care for the patient recovering from oral cancer surgery.

Patients may need to adapt to significant changes in body image and function after treatment for oral cancer. Patients need honest information about the changes to expect and their degree of permanence. Family members are included in all teaching, and the nurse encourages them to help the patient avoid social isolation. Referrals are made as necessary for speech therapy and ongoing dental care.

Problems of the Esophagus

Gastroesophageal Reflux Disease

Etiology and Epidemiology. **Gastroesophageal reflux disease** (GERD) is a relapsing and often chronic disease process that results from esophageal reflux. Most cases in adults are attributed to the inappropriate relaxation of the lower esophageal sphincter (LES) in response to an unknown stimulus; slowed or delayed gastric emptying and ineffective clearing of the esophagus may also play a role.[10] Reflux allows gastric and duodenal contents to move back into the distal esophagus. The presence of a hiatal hernia, which displaces the LES into the thorax, was formerly believed to be the primary cause of GERD. However, hiatal hernia has now been found to be a common condition in the adult population and, although most persons with hiatal hernias do experience reflux, the reverse has not been found to be true. The reason for the relaxation of the LES remains unclear, although a number of environmental and physical factors appear to influence its tone and contractility.

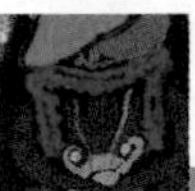

GUIDELINES FOR SAFE PRACTICE *The Patient With Radioactive Needle Implants in Oral Tissue*

Implant Care

- Check needle patency several times each day.
- Do not pull on the strings. Any movement could alter the placement or direction of the radiation or loosen the needles.
- Monitor linens, bed areas, and emesis basin for needles that may dislodge.
- Ensure that a protective container is present in the room to contain any needles that might dislodge.

Patient Care

- Assist with gentle oral hygiene every 2 hours while patient is awake.
- Encourage the patient to avoid hot and cold foods and beverages, as well as smoking.
- If the patient has dentures, encourage their removal at night for comfort. Assess gums for irritation and bleeding whenever dentures are removed.
- Provide viscous lidocaine (Xylocaine) solutions or lozenges as needed when oral discomfort interferes with nutrition.
- Provide the patient with an alternate means of communication; talking around implanted needles is usually difficult or impossible.
- Assist the patient in implementing the mouth care regimen prescribed by the physician.

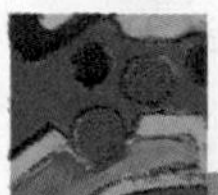

PATIENT/FAMILY TEACHING *Self-Care Strategies for the Patient Recovering from Surgery for Oral Cancer*

Mouth Care

Good mouth care is essential to promote healing and minimize tooth decay and infections.

Follow the prescribed mouth care regimen (e.g., irrigation, soft toothbrush, fluoride treatment).

—Use sterile water, dilute peroxide and saline, or bicarbonate solution as prescribed by the physician.

—Avoid commercial mouthwashes until healing is complete.

Diet and Eating

Provide for privacy while mastering adapted feeding techniques.

Modify the consistency of the diet as indicated to minimize discomfort and promote swallowing.

Eat slowly.

Avoid the use of forks or any utensil that could traumatize healing tissues.

Avoid both very hot and very cold foods to support comfort and healing.

Use liquid supplements as needed to supplement nutrition and maintain weight.

Rinse the mouth carefully with water or prescribed solution after eating.

A decrease in LES tone is associated with the ingestion of a wide variety of foods and drugs. These include fatty foods; caffeine-containing substances such as chocolate, cola, coffee, and tea; nicotine; and drugs such as calcium channel blockers, theophylline, and possibly nonsteroidal antiinflammatory drugs. Elevated levels of estrogen and progesterone and conditions that elevate intraabdominal pressure, such as obesity, pregnancy, or heavy lifting, have also been implicated, but a causal link has not been proven.[21] Population studies of the link between lifestyle factors and reflux continue to provide conflicting results.[10] Genetic factors may also be important. Reflux is much more common after a meal, and more than 60% of reflux sufferers have delayed gastric emptying.

GERD is a common disorder in all age-groups. Occasional heartburn is estimated to affect more than 60 million Americans, with 15% of the population experiencing heartburn at least weekly and up to 45% of adults experiencing heartburn at least once a month.[26] The actual incidence of mild disease may be even higher, since many individuals simply accept reflux as an occasional mild problem that can be tolerated or effectively self-treated. Fewer than 25% of all reflux sufferers ever consult a health care provider about their symptoms, and the advent of over-the-counter proton pump inhibitor (PPI) drugs further decreases the likelihood that mild to moderate reflux sufferers will seek medical help. Treatment costs exceed $1 billion annually. No documented gender or cultural patterns are associated with reflux, but older adults experience decreased esophageal peristalsis and a higher incidence of hiatal hernia, which together increase the likelihood of reflux in this population.

Pathophysiology. Two zones of high pressure, termed the upper and lower esophageal sphincters, normally prevent the reflux of gastric contents. The zones maintain a constant pressure and relax only during swallowing. Esophageal reflux occurs when either gastric volume or intraabdominal pressure is elevated or when LES sphincter tone is decreased. Periodic reflux occurs in most persons and is usually asymptomatic.

The normal physiologic response to occasional reflux is immediate swallowing. One or more rapid swallows induce peristaltic contractions to clear the reflux and neutralize the acid with the bicarbonate-rich saliva. However, the esophagus has only a limited ability to withstand the damaging effects of acid reflux, and GERD develops when the mucosal barrier breaks down and an inflammatory response is initiated.[18]

The degree of esophageal inflammation is related to the number, duration, and acidity or alkalinity of the reflux episodes. The effectiveness and efficiency of esophageal clearance also are important, particularly at night, when the swallowing rate and salivation decrease by two thirds and a recumbent position interferes with clearance. An inflamed esophagus gradually loses its ability to clear refluxed material quickly and efficiently, and the duration of each episode gradually lengthens. Despite the central role of *Helicobacter pylori* infection in peptic ulcer disease, there is currently no evidence that it contributes to the development of GERD.[2]

Chronic reflux causes hyperemia and inflammation. Minor capillary bleeding is common, although frank bleeding is rare. Repeated episodes of inflammation and healing can gradually produce a change in the epithelial tissue that makes it more resistant to acid. However, the presence of this new tissue, termed **Barrett's epithelium**, is also associated with a higher risk of adenocarcinoma.[25] Over time, fibrotic tissue changes can also occur and produce esophageal stricture.

The clinical manifestations of GERD are consistent in nature, but vary substantially in severity (see Clinical Manifestations box). The irritation of chronic acid reflux produces the primary symptom of heartburn **(pyrosis)**. The pain is described as a substernal or retrosternal burning sensation that tends to radiate upward and may involve the neck, jaw, or back. The pain typically occurs 20 minutes

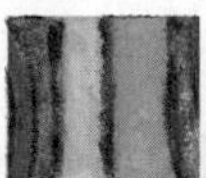

CLINICAL MANIFESTATIONS *Gastroesophageal Reflux Disease*

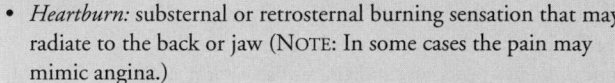

- *Heartburn:* substernal or retrosternal burning sensation that may radiate to the back or jaw (NOTE: In some cases the pain may mimic angina.)
- *Regurgitation* (not associated with nausea or belching): a sour or bitter taste perceived in the pharynx
- *Water brash:* reflex hypersecretion of the salivary glands that does not have a bitter taste
- *Frequent belching, flatulence*
- *Dysphagia or odynophagia* (difficult or painful swallowing): usually occurs only in severe cases
- *Nocturnal cough, wheezing, hoarseness*

to 2 hours after eating. An atypical pain pattern that closely mimics angina may also occur and needs to be carefully differentiated from true cardiac disease. Although heartburn is the classic symptom of reflux, most episodes of acid reflux do not trigger the sensation of heartburn.[27] By some estimates, as few as 20% of reflux episodes cause heartburn. It is theorized that prolonged contraction of the longitudinal muscle of the lower esophagus in response to reflux may also contribute to the sensation of heartburn.

The second major symptom of GERD is regurgitation, which is not associated with either belching or nausea. The person experiences a feeling of warm fluid moving up the throat. If the fluid reaches the pharynx, a sour or bitter taste is perceived.[29] **Water brash**, a reflex salivary hypersecretion that does not have a bitter taste, occurs less commonly.

In severe cases GERD can produce dysphagia or **odynophagia** (painful swallowing). Belching and a feeling of flatulence are other common complaints. Nocturnal cough, wheezing, or hoarseness all may occur with reflux, and it is estimated that more than 80% of adult asthmatics may experience reflux.[10] The frequency and severity of reflux episodes usually determine the severity of the symptoms.

COMPLICATIONS. If GERD is not successfully controlled, it can progress to serious and even life-threatening problems. Esophageal ulceration and hemorrhage may result from severe erosion, and chronic nighttime reflux is accompanied by a significant risk of aspiration. Adenocarcinoma can develop from the premalignant tissue called Barrett's epithelium. Gradual or repeated scarring can permanently damage esophageal tissue and produce stricture.

Collaborative Care Management

DIAGNOSTIC TESTS. Mild cases of GERD are diagnosed from the classic symptoms, and treatment is initiated without further diagnostic workup. Millions of people self-diagnose and treat occasional heartburn without consulting a primary care provider. More severe and persistent cases may require other screening tools. A variety of esophageal motility and pH tests may be performed, but 24-hour pH monitoring is considered the gold standard for diagnosis.[23] Esophageal tests are described in more detail in Chapter 40. Tests for GERD are summarized in Box 41-1.

MEDICATIONS. Drug therapy, the cornerstone of GERD management, usually begins with the occasional use of over-the-counter agents to treat heartburn. Antacids were the mainstay of GERD treatment until the 1980s and are still effective in dealing with occasional heartburn, usually producing prompt relief of symptoms. The choice of antacid is usually based on palatability and patient preference. Alginates may be used as an alternative. Alginates (such as aluminum hydroxide–magnesium carbonate [Gaviscon]) combine alginic acid with an antacid, which forms viscous foam that floats on top of the gastric contents. This theoretically creates a mechanical barrier to reflux and limits acid contact with the mucosa when reflux occurs.

Since their release for over-the-counter purchase, histamine$_2$ (H_2)-receptor antagonists have been heavily marketed as first-line agents for occasional heartburn. Ease of use and absence of side effects have ensured their popularity. The American Gastroenterological Association issued a consensus statement in 2002 declaring that over-the-counter H_2-receptor antagonists and antacids remain first-line treatment for patients with mild GERD symptoms.[31] These drugs also support tissue healing, although complete resolution of esophageal inflammation is exceedingly difficult to achieve and sustain. GERD is a chronic disease, and relapse is a constant concern. Healing rates with H_2-receptor antagonists range from 50% to 70% at 8 weeks.[31] However, when taken at night, they also have the advantage of improved nocturnal gastric acid control.

Severe GERD is now routinely treated with PPIs, which are superior to H_2-receptor antagonists in treating erosive esophagitis and its complications.[20] A single daily dose, taken 15 to 30 minutes before a meal, decreases acid secretion by 90% to 95% and supports healing within 4 to 6 weeks. Symptom relief is achieved in about 78% of patients.[31] All first-generation PPIs appear to have equivalent effectiveness, but individual variation in response is common. Second-generation esomeprazole (Nexium) appears to be slightly more effective for patients with severe reflux (see Research box).[2] Ongoing use of PPIs appears to be necessary to sustain healing in severe cases.[5]

The research effort is ongoing to find agents that can prevent reflux rather than simply suppress acid secretion. Bethanecol (Urecholine) and metoclopramide (Reglan) are motility drugs that increase the rate of gastric emptying, and they have always

Box 41-1 Diagnostic Tests for Gastroesophageal Reflux Disease

Esophageal pH Monitoring

pH probe is inserted nasally and positioned 5 cm above the lower esophageal sphincter.

Monitoring is conducted for 18 to 24 hours while the patient eats normally and engages in usual activities.

A pH drop below 4 is considered to be a reflux episode.

Tubeless pH Monitoring

A small device is attached to the wall of the esophagus endoscopically and monitors reflux episodes over a 10- to 14-day period.

Endoscopy

Endoscopy accurately documents the type and extent of mucosal injury, but it cannot diagnose the nature or severity of reflux.

Biopsy

A biopsy may be combined with endoscopy to confirm or rule out the presence of Barrett's epithelium or cancer.

Manometry

Manometry provides information on the functional ability of the sphincters and muscles.

Other Tests

Barium swallow documents the presence of hiatal hernia.

Acid perfusion (Bernstein) test links acid levels and heartburn symptoms.

Research

Miner P et al: Gastric acid control with esomeprazole, lansoprazole, omeprazole, pantoprazole and rabeprazole: a five way crossover study, *Am J Gastroenterol* 98(12):2616-2620, 2003.

This study compared intragastric pH values in 34 patients after 5 days of treatment with standard doses of the five currently approved proton pump inhibitors (PPIs). The patients were between 18 and 60 years of age, and all reported symptoms of gastroesophageal reflux disease. All participants were negative for *Helicobacter pylori* infection and exhibited no evidence or history of esophageal erosions or ulcers. The participants were also screened for use of nicotine, alcohol, and nonsteroidal antiinflammatory drugs. They were randomly assigned to treatment with one of the five PPIs and received the standard dose once daily before their usual breakfast. Antacid use was permitted for treating breakthrough heartburn. Twenty-four hours of intragastric pH monitoring was performed after 5 consecutive days of treatment.

All five PPIs successfully suppressed gastric acid (as measured by a pH greater than 4) for at least 10 hours in the 24-hour measuring cycle. Esomeprazole maintained the pH above 4 for a significantly longer period than any of the other four PPIs. No other differences were noted among the drugs.

seemed to have a logical role in GERD therapy, but their use has been limited by frequent undesirable side effects. New prokinetic agents are currently in development. The use of baclofen (Lioresal), a gamma-aminobutyric acid agonist that may inhibit relaxation of the LES, is being studied. Drug therapy for GERD is summarized in Table 41-2.

TREATMENTS. Endoscopic treatments have recently been developed that show some promise in treating complex GERD not accompanied by significant hiatal hernia, but these approaches are still experimental.[7] Radiofrequency ablation of the LES (Stretta procedure) (Figure 41-4) is undertaken with a balloon tipped four-needle catheter that delivers the energy to the tissue and may generate scarring that decreases the amount of reflux.[8]

A second new treatment involves the endoscopic placement of sutures below the gastroesophageal junction (EndoCinch) to reinforce the sphincther.[17] Another approach involves the endoscopic injection of an inert vinyl polymer (Enteryx). Theoretically the material expands into a spongy mass, thickening the LES.[8] A great deal of additional study is needed to confirm the long-term safety and efficacy of these approaches.

SURGICAL MANAGEMENT. Antireflux surgery is usually performed in patients with severe GERD who do not respond to aggressive medical management. The need for and high cost of long-term pharmacologic management and the development of laparoscopic surgical techniques have stimulated a new look at surgical interventions.[6] The surgical procedures involve **fundoplication**, the wrapping and suturing of the gastric fundus around the esophagus to reinforce the LES and anchor it below the diaphragm. These procedures are also used to correct hiatal hernia (p. 1193).

Evidence continues to accumulate, however, that antireflux surgery is no more effective at preventing Barrett's epithelium and the subsequent risk of esophageal cancer than standard medical intervention.[12] Surgical success is difficult to sustain over time, and many patients still require the use of PPIs to control heartburn symptoms.[8]

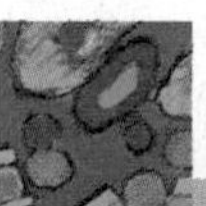

TABLE 41-2
COMMON MEDICATIONS *for Gastroesophageal Reflux Disease*

Drug	Action	Nursing Intervention
Antacids		
Aluminum- or magnesium-based product	Neutralize gastric acids	Evaluate effectiveness. Monitor frequency of use. Monitor for constipation or diarrhea, and help patient adjust product use as needed.
Antacid Plus Alginic Acid		
Aluminum hydroxide–magnesium carbonate (Gaviscon)	Neutralizes gastric acid; forms viscous foam that prevents reflux or buffers its effects	Same as for antacids
Histamine$_2$-Receptor Antagonists		
Cimetidine (Tagamet) Ranitidine (Zantac) Famotidine (Pepcid) Nizatadine (Axid)	Reduce gastric acid secretion and support tissue healing	Instruct patient to take drugs at intervals with meals (if ordered). Monitor for common side effects: fatigue, headache, diarrhea.
Proton Pump Inhibitors		
Omeprazole (Prilosec) Lansoprazole (Prevacid) Pantoprazole (Protonix) Rabeprazole (Aciphex) Esomeprazole (Nexium)	Inhibit enzyme system of gastric parietal cells and suppress gastric acid production by more than 90%	Instruct patient to take drugs before a meal, usually at breakfast. Monitor for side effects (rare): abdominal cramping, headache, diarrhea.

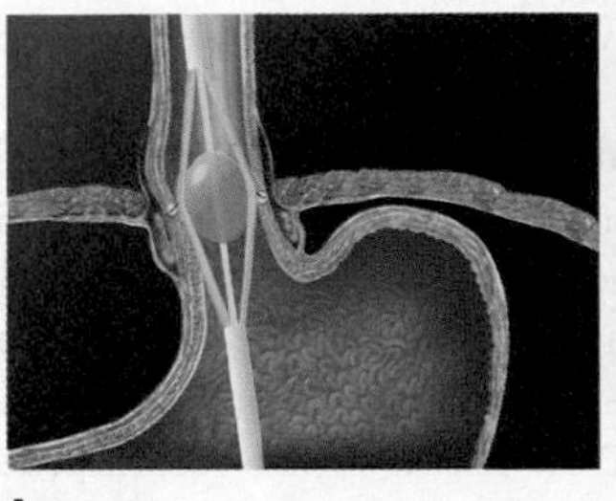

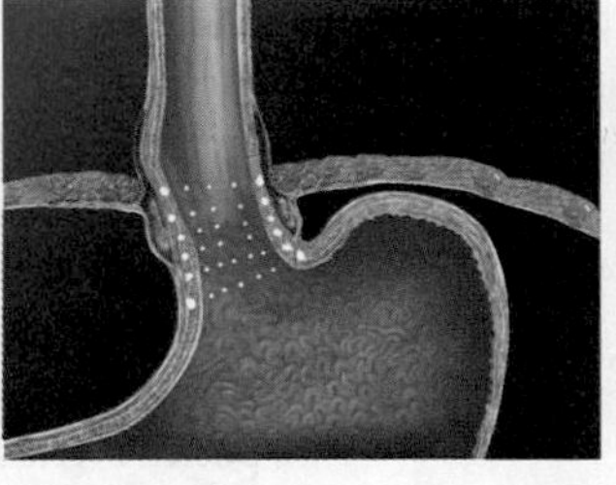

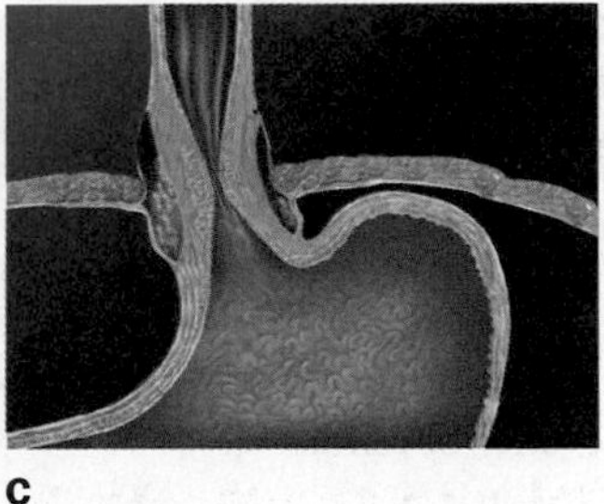

Figure 41-4 Stretta procedure. **A,** Endoscopic placement of Stretta catheter. **B,** Radiofrequency delivery to gastroesophageal junction. **C,** Heat-induced collagen contraction, reduction in reflux episodes, and improvement in gastroesophageal reflux disease symptoms.

DIET. Modification of diet and eating patterns may relieve symptoms in mild GERD. Certain foods have been shown to affect LES pressure, although no studies have proven their role in reflux disease. Fatty foods, chocolate, and alcohol all appear to decrease LES pressure, and patients are usually encouraged to avoid them. Adequate dietary protein stimulates the release of gastrin and cholecystokinin, which increase LES pressure. Other foods such as tomato-based products, coffee, and cola provoke heartburn by direct esophageal irritation.[22] Patients are encouraged to modify their diet by limiting the intake of foods that predictably increase the incidence of heartburn. Weight loss and avoidance of overeating may also reduce the frequency of reflux episodes. A smaller evening meal and fasting for several hours before bedtime can be particularly effective in reducing nocturnal reflux.

HEALTH PROMOTION AND PREVENTION. Primary prevention does not play a major role in GERD because the condition does not have readily identifiable, preventable etiologic factors. Standard preventive measures might include maintaining an optimal body weight and avoiding overeating, particularly at night. Prevention also includes avoiding activities that increase intraabdominal pressure and the likelihood of reflux such as heavy lifting, wearing constrictive clothing, and working in a stooped or bent-over position.

The most significant issue in secondary prevention is the need for health care professionals to directly inquire about a patient's experience with heartburn. Patients rarely report heartburn to their health care provider unless directly asked or until the symptoms become severe. If identified and recognized early, the disease may be more responsive to treatment. It is also important for health care professionals to carefully explore the patient's use of over-the-counter medications to self-treat heartburn.

Nursing Management

of the Patient with Gastroesophageal Reflux Disease

ASSESSMENT

Health History. Assess for onset; frequency; duration; severity; and precipitating, aggravating, and alleviating factors for classic symptoms:

- Heartburn
- Regurgitation or water brash
- Dysphagia or odynophagia
- Belching or flatulence
- Nocturnal cough
- Hoarseness or wheezing—day or night
- Diet and meal pattern
- Relationship of symptoms to food intake, meal pattern, and activity
- Use of over-the-counter medications, particularly antacids, H_2-receptor antagonists, and proton pump inhibitors

Physical Examination. Assess for:

- Body weight
- Evidence of reflux aspiration on auscultation

NURSING DIAGNOSES, OUTCOMES, AND INTERVENTIONS

Nursing Diagnosis: Acute Pain

OUTCOMES. A common example of an expected outcome for the patient with a diagnosis of *acute pain* is:

Patient will:

- Report few or no episodes of heartburn.

NURSING INTERVENTIONS. The nurse discusses the medication regimen with the patient and provides written information about the safe use and expected side effects of all medications. PPIs are taken once a day before breakfast and rarely induce mild GI side effects. Patients need to be aware of the cost of these drugs, which may be prohibitive without insurance coverage. Adherence to the daily drug regimen is essential to achieve and sustain healing. Antacids and over the counter H_2-receptor antagonists may also be used on an as-needed basis until the heartburn is controlled.

The nurse also explores the patient's use of other medications. Anticholinergics, calcium channel blockers, xanthine derivatives, and diazepam all appear to lower the LES pressure and may need to be avoided. The nurse discusses their use with the primary care provider.

Symptom relapse is a common problem after GERD treatment. The nurse reinforces the importance of seeking prompt medical evaluation if a return of heartburn or other GERD-related symptoms occurs.

RELATED NIC INTERVENTIONS. Medication Administration: Oral, Medication Management, Pain Management

Nursing Diagnosis: Ineffective Health Maintenance

OUTCOMES. Common examples of expected outcomes for the patient with a diagnosis of *ineffective health maintenance* are:
Patient will:

- Incorporate lifestyle changes into daily activities to reduce reflux.
- Identify changes in the daily diet that can help control the incidence and severity of reflux.

NURSING INTERVENTIONS. Lifestyle changes have always been an important aspect of GERD treatment. However, few of these recommendations have proven efficacy through research, and it is easy to minimize their value given the development of newer, more potent pharmacologic agents. However, significant anecdotal evidence indicates that lifestyle modifications can be effective in controlling the incidence and severity of heartburn.

The nurse ensures the patient is informed about daily living choices that can help prevent reflux and prevent relapse once healing is accomplished. The nurse encourages the patient to reduce consumption of foods that are associated with lowering LES sphincter pressure. A low-fat diet with limited use of caffeine-containing beverages, alcohol, and chocolate is ideal. Adequate protein intake is encouraged for its LES-enhancing ability. Individual responses to food vary substantially, and patients are encouraged to limit intake of specific foods that consistently induce heartburn. Use of an H_2-receptor antagonist with meals containing potentially irritating foods can also safely reduce the incidence of heartburn.

Modifying meal size and timing are the two most important strategies the nurse offers. Eating four to six small meals a day is recommended. Large meals increase gastric pressure and volume and delay gastric emptying. These factors increase the frequency and severity of reflux episodes. Simple strategies such as eating slowly and chewing thoroughly facilitate digestion and reduce belching. Eating a light evening meal and avoiding nighttime snacking are particularly important. The patient should not eat for at least 3 hours before bedtime. Nighttime reflux is troublesome because the combination of inactivity and a recumbent position dramatically decreases the effectiveness of esophageal clearance. Evening snacking exacerbates the problem. It may also be helpful for the patient to elevate the head of the bed for sleep, using a foam wedge, to limit the effects of recumbency on reflux incidence.

Weight reduction helps lower intraabdominal pressure and may reduce the severity of reflux in obese patients. Most patients notice a reduction in symptom severity with even a relatively modest weight loss and should be encouraged to attempt the change. Achieving an "ideal weight" is not necessary to have a positive effect on reflux. Other recommended lifestyle changes include avoiding increases in intraabdominal pressure caused by constrictive clothing, straining, weight lifting, or working in a bent-over or stooped position. Smoking cessation is recommended because smoking causes a rapid and significant drop in LES pressure. Evening smoking, particularly while resting in bed, is of greatest concern, especially when combined with snacking. The nurse works with the patient to identify strategies that most effectively reduce the incidence and severity of symptoms.

RELATED NIC INTERVENTIONS. Health Education, Risk Identification, Teaching: Disease Process, Teaching: Prescribed Diet

Patient/Family Teaching. Patient and family teaching is an important part of nursing care for the patient with GERD (see Patient/Family Teaching box).

EVALUATION

To evaluate the effectiveness of nursing interventions, compare patient behaviors with those stated in the expected patient outcomes.

RELATED NOC OUTCOMES. Client Satisfaction: Symptom Control, Comfort Level, Knowledge: Diet, Knowledge: Disease Process, Symptom Control

GERONTOLOGIC CONSIDERATIONS

Esophageal function remains effective into advanced age, although some decline in esophageal peristalsis is expected, and a decrease in saliva production impairs the efficiency of esophageal clearance. Even routine reflux becomes protracted and increases the risk of irritation. Older patients need to be assessed for heartburn, since they typically underreport their symptoms. They also appear to be particularly vulnerable to alkaline reflux from the

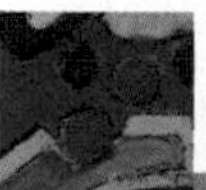

PATIENT/FAMILY TEACHING *Diet and Lifestyle Modifications to Manage Gastroesophageal Reflux Disease*

Diet

Eat four to six small meals daily.
Follow a low-fat, adequate-protein diet.
Reduce intake of chocolate, tea, and all foods and beverages that contain caffeine.
Limit or eliminate alcohol intake.
Eat slowly, and chew food thoroughly.
Do not eat for 2 to 3 hours before bedtime.
Remain upright for 1 to 2 hours after meals when possible; never eat in bed.
Avoid any food that directly produces heartburn.
Reduce body weight if indicated.

Lifestyle

Eliminate or reduce smoking.
Avoid evening smoking; never smoke in bed.
Avoid constrictive clothing over the abdomen.
Avoid activities that involve straining, heavy lifting, or working in a bent-over position.
Elevate the head of the bed at least 6 to 8 inches for sleep.
Never sleep flat in bed.

duodenum. Acid combined with bile and pancreatic juice is believed to be more damaging to the mucosa than acid alone. Alkaline reflux typically occurs at night and causes respiratory symptoms such as choking, paroxysmal coughing, and wheezing. Patients with frequent nighttime awakenings from coughing should be evaluated for GERD. The risk of aspiration is high. Treatment approaches are the same as those outlined for other forms of GERD.

Hiatal Hernia

Etiology and Epidemiology. The opening in the diaphragm that allows the esophagus to pass from the thorax to the abdomen is called the esophageal hiatus. A **hiatal hernia** develops when the distal esophagus, and possibly a portion of the stomach, moves into the thorax through the hiatus. There are four main types of hiatal hernia. Type I, also known as a sliding hernia, is by far the most common.[28] In type I the gastroesophageal junction and a portion of the stomach are displaced upward into the thorax (Figure 41-5, *A*). The hernia is usually freely movable and slides back and forth into the thorax in response to changes in position and abdominal pressure. Type II and III hernias may represent more advanced stages of type I. They are usually referred to as paraesophageal hernias.[28] In type II the gastroesophageal junction is normally positioned in the hiatus but a portion or all of the fundus of the stomach lies in the thorax above the hiatus (Figure 41-5, *B*). Type III is a combination of types I and II where both the gastroesophageal junction *and* the stomach lie above the hiatus in the thorax. Type IV refers to the herniation of other abdominal viscera into the thorax as well and is extremely rare in adults.

All types of hiatal hernias develop from an enlarged hiatal opening and laxness of the ligaments that support the hiatus. Since intraabdominal pressure is positive and thoracic pressure is negative, the more mobile greater curvature of the stomach rolls up into the posterior mediastinum. The exact cause of the anatomic enlargement of the hiatal opening is unknown. It may represent a congenital anatomic defect, but aging, trauma, surgery, and prolonged increases in intraabdominal pressure may all play a role.

Hiatal hernias are believed to be common in the adult population, although their true incidence can only be estimated. Their incidence is roughly estimated at 25% to 30% in the general population and as high as 60% in the over-60 age-group. Hiatal hernias affect women more commonly than men, although their incidence increases in both sexes with aging.

Pathophysiology. Most adults with hiatal hernias are completely asymptomatic. Development of symptoms is rare before middle age. Hiatal hernias are usually small, but their relative size is not necessarily related to the presence or severity of symptoms.

Sliding hernias cause no functional problems. When symptoms are produced, they are directly related to chronic reflux. Reflux occurs from the exposure of the LES to the low-pressure environment of the thorax where sphincter function is significantly impaired. The clinical manifestations mimic GERD (see Clinical Manifestations box, p. 1188).

Most type II and III paraesophageal hernias are also asymptomatic; reflux is not a common problem, but heartburn and chest pain may be reported. Symptoms result from mechanical problems such as distention and obstruction. Occult bleeding is fairly common because venous engorgement in the herniated portion of the stomach causes the mucosal surfaces to rub against each other and ooze. Occult bleeding leads to iron deficiency anemia, but frank hemorrhage is rare. Ulceration of the fundus from mechanical trauma in the hiatus is also fairly common and can contribute to the severity of the bleeding.

COMPLICATIONS. The risk of anatomic complications is fairly high with all forms of paraesophageal hernias; these complications can be life threatening. Obstruction, strangulation, and acute volvulus are all possible complications necessitating emergent surgery. The risk of these serious complications has fueled a great deal of debate over the need for elective repair of all diagnosed type II and higher hiatal hernias, rather than adopting a wait-and-see policy.

Collaborative Care Management

DIAGNOSTIC TESTS. Unless acute complications develop, most hiatal hernias are diagnosed as part of a workup for GERD, and

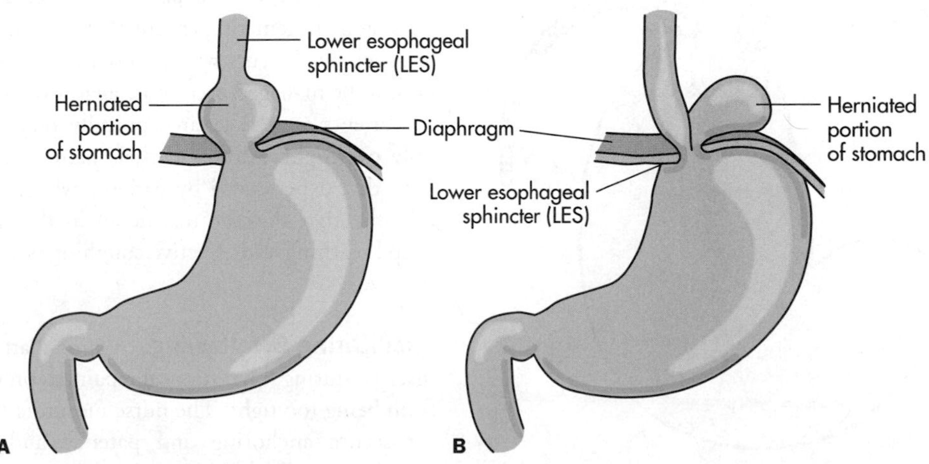

Figure 41-5 Hiatal hernia. **A,** Sliding hernia (type I). **B,** Paraesophageal hernia (type II).

the diagnostic tests are similar (see Box 41-1). The barium swallow with fluoroscopy is the most useful test. Paraesophageal hernias are usually clearly visible, and sliding hernias can be easily demonstrated when the patient is moved into positions that increase intraabdominal pressure. Additional findings in individuals with paraesophageal hernias may include low hemoglobin and hematocrit levels from chronic low-grade bleeding, which will be evident on routine blood tests.

MEDICATIONS. Antacids, H_2-receptor antagonists, and PPIs are used as needed to manage reflux-related heartburn if it accompanies the hernia (see Table 41-2).

DIET. The recommended diet modifications for hiatal hernia follow the general guidelines outlined in the section on antireflux therapy. The diet also focuses on reducing obesity if possible. Obesity can significantly increase intraabdominal pressure and worsen the severity of both the hernia and the symptoms of reflux.

TREATMENTS. No specific treatments are used in the management of hiatal hernia.

SURGICAL MANAGEMENT. Surgery is the only effective treatment for paraesophageal hernias. Regardless of the type of hernia, the surgical repair involves reduction of the hernia and its sac and partial closure of the widened hiatus. A fundoplication antireflux procedure may also be performed, wrapping the stomach fundus around the LES to stabilize it. The Nissen fundoplication is the most commonly used antireflux procedure (Figure 41-6). The fundus of the stomach is wrapped a full 360 degrees around the lower esophagus to reinforce the LES.

These surgeries may be performed transthoracically, transabdominally, or laparoscopically.[28] Although open procedures have some advantages in terms of access and completeness of repair, the laparoscopic approach has become the surgery of choice for patients because of its low degree of invasiveness and shortened recovery time. The surgery is technically difficult and requires a skilled and experienced surgeon. Follow-up studies have demonstrated that laparoscopic repairs are associated with a relatively high incidence of reherniation, up to 40%, but most of the recurrent hernias are small and asymptomatic.[28]

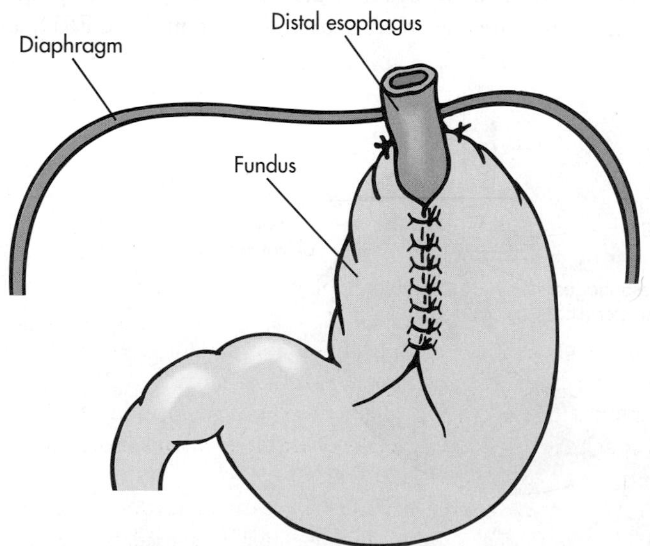

Figure 41-6 Nissen fundoplication for repair of hiatal hernia.

A variety of other surgical approaches are in use that involve various degrees of fundoplication, posterior instead of anterior wrapping, and fixation to the diaphragm instead of the abdominal wall for stability. Physician preference plays a major role in the decision.

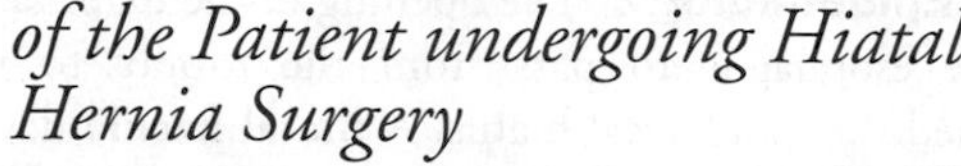

Nursing Management
of the Patient undergoing Hiatal Hernia Surgery

PREOPERATIVE CARE

Preoperative teaching focuses on instructing the patient in deep breathing, the correct use of an incentive spirometer, and splinting the incision effectively for coughing. All surgical approaches involve the diaphragm, and pulmonary hygiene is essential in preventing respiratory complications. The high, long incisions of open procedures make pulmonary hygiene painful, and it is essential to discuss the pain management plan with the patient. If a thoracic approach is used, teaching also includes management of chest tubes. The small incisions, decreased pain, and brief hospital stay associated with laparoscopic fundoplication explain its popularity with patients.

Patients who are overweight are encouraged to lose weight if possible before surgery, and smokers are encouraged to significantly reduce or eliminate their use of tobacco. The nurse also teaches about the nasogastric (NG) tube that is inserted during surgery and the planned time frame for resuming oral feedings.

POSTOPERATIVE CARE

Facilitating Airway Clearance. Prevention of respiratory complications is the primary postoperative consideration. The head of the bed is elevated 30 degrees to facilitate lung expansion. The nurse assists the patient out of bed as soon as possible and supports the incision for coughing. Regular lung auscultation, incentive spirometry, and chest physical therapy are routinely used. Adequate analgesia is essential to the success of the respiratory protocol. It should be provided via patient-controlled analgesia or aggressive nursing management, particularly before ambulation or chest physical therapy. Patients with a smoking or pulmonary disease history need to be managed even more aggressively.

Patients treated laparoscopically may remain in the hospital only overnight. Although their pain is usually significantly less than that experienced by patients with major incisions, it is still essential that they be instructed in the importance of frequent deep breathing and effective coughing (see the Nursing Care Plan, p. 1196).

Facilitating Swallowing. A large-diameter NG tube is usually inserted during open surgical repairs to prevent the fundoplication from being too tight. The nurse monitors the tube postoperatively for secure anchoring and patency and regularly assesses the drainage, which should consist of normal yellowish green gastric secretions within the first 8 hours after surgery. It should not contain fresh blood. It is essential that the stomach remain decompressed to prevent vomiting, which could disrupt the fundoplication sutures.

The NG tube is carefully placed by the surgeon and is usually neither moved nor repositioned. The nurse carefully follows orders concerning irrigation. Sterile solutions are generally preferred for irrigation in the early postoperative period. Frequent oral and nasal hygiene are important for comfort because the large tube is irritating. An NG tube may not be used with the laparoscopic procedures.

The patient is offered oral fluids after peristalsis has been reestablished. Some surgeons prefer to use gastrostomy feedings to avoid stress on the surgical repair and facilitate healing, but most patients progress to a near-normal diet within 6 weeks. Temporary dysphagia is almost universal because of the tight wrap around the LES. The food storage area of the stomach is also decreased. The nurse encourages the patient to eat multiple small meals throughout the day, gradually exploring tolerance to different foods and consistencies. Few foods need to be completely restricted. An upright position is also helpful. Support and encouragement during early feeding attempts are essential. Relatively few dietary restrictions are in place by discharge.

Many patients also experience temporary or persistent gas bloat after surgery from a decreased ability to belch. The nurse teaches the patient to avoid carbonated beverages and gas-producing foods. Patients who swallow a lot of air during meals need to eat and drink slowly and chew food thoroughly. Excess air in the stomach that cannot be relieved by belching produces significant abdominal discomfort. Frequent position changes and ambulation are often effective strategies for clearing air from the GI tract. Even with successful repair, reflux may continue to be a problem, and the antireflux diet, medications, and lifestyle modifications discussed for GERD management may need to be continued. This can be discouraging for patients who anticipate a complete cure with surgery.

GERONTOLOGIC CONSIDERATIONS

Muscle weakness develops in the esophageal hiatus with aging. It is estimated that 60% of the over-60 age-group is affected by hiatal hernia. Reflux symptoms in older patients should be investigated and the possibility of hiatal hernia determined. The management, as outlined in the preceding discussion, is applicable to the older as well as the younger adult population, and the refinement of laparoscopic fundoplication techniques reduces the risk of surgery in this population. Open procedures are associated with an increased risk of surgical complications, particularly respiratory complications, and meticulous nursing management is essential.

Achalasia

Etiology and Epidemiology. Motility disorders of the esophagus are conditions in which the normal motor function of the esophagus is disturbed. The disorder may be a primary esophageal problem or secondary to another systemic disease. **Achalasia** is a primary motility disorder in which the lower esophageal muscles and sphincter fail to relax appropriately and in synchrony in response to swallowing. This can result in mechanical or functional obstruction to food passage. Failure of the LES to close adequately after swallowing can also occur, resulting in chronic reflux or regurgitation. Achalasia is characterized clinically by slowly progressive dysphagia and regurgitation of swallowed food. Esophageal spasm is a common component of motility disorders, and the spasm is often intense enough to mimic angina.[34]

The cause of the disorder is unknown, although a familial link is possible. Achalasia usually develops between 20 and 40 years of age, but it also occurs in children and older adults.[11] Both sexes are affected about equally, and there appear to be no cultural differences in incidence.

Pathophysiology. Achalasia is theorized to result from a neuromuscular defect in the inner circular muscle layer of the esophagus. Resting pressure in the LES is elevated, and the sphincter fails to relax with swallowing. Degeneration and loss of ganglion cells cause a defect in the innervation of the esophagus with resultant aperistalsis. There is also a significant reduction in the synthesis of important mediators of esophageal relaxation such as nitric oxide.[34] Considerable functional obstruction results, and, as the disease progresses, the portion of the esophagus surrounding the constriction becomes dilated and the muscle walls hypertrophy. Although the severity of achalasia varies widely, the obstruction may be so severe that little or no food can enter the stomach. In extreme cases the esophagus may hold 1 L or more of food and fluid above the constricted area. Slowly progressive dysphagia and regurgitation are the classic symptoms. Symptoms may progress over as much as 2 years before the person seeks help.

Spasm may be provoked by cold or hot liquids or foods and is often worsened by stress or overeating. Dysphagia is present with both liquids and solid foods. Many patients report heartburn, which may prompt an initial diagnosis of GERD. The heartburn may be caused by fermentation of undigested food in the esophagus, which also creates a foul mouth odor. Chest pain, variable weight loss, and aspiration of retained food may all occur.

Barium studies clearly illustrate the classic "rat tail" narrowing of achalasia. The proximal esophageal dilation may be mild or massive (Figure 41-7). Esophageal manometry, which reveals an elevated resting LES pressure, failure to relax in response to swallowing, and diminished or absent peristaltic waves in the esophagus, is the gold standard for diagnosis. Endoscopic ultrasonography has added a new diagnostic capability and facilitates the estimation of the length and thickness of the LES muscle.[1]

Collaborative Care Management. Achalasia treatment is aimed at controlling the symptoms. It does not correct the underlying pathologic condition. Drugs that relax smooth muscles such as nitrates and calcium channel blockers have been used, but their effectiveness is usually limited and of short duration.[11] The injection of botulinum toxin type A (Botox) into the LES through an endoscope showed initial promise, but its positive effects are not sustained and symptoms recur within 6 months.[34] Repeat treatment is possible but not as effective, and the fibrotic changes brought on by the drug make other interventions more difficult. Analgesics may be needed for severe pain.

Esophageal dilation has been a mainstay of treatment for achalasia for centuries.[11] Various techniques have been used, but pneumatic balloon dilation is currently believed to be the most effective. The procedure involves passing polyurethane balloons on a catheter

Nursing Care Plan

Patient Undergoing Hiatal Hernia Repair

Data The patient is a 56-year-old man who is 40 pounds overweight, is a moderately heavy cigarette smoker, and has a 5-year history of progressively worsening heartburn. Esophageal studies and barium swallow under fluoroscopy revealed severe reflux and a large sliding hiatal hernia that shifted into the thorax with minimal position change. His esophagus was inflamed and minimally ulcerated with no signs of cancer. His surgeon recommended surgical repair because of the size of the hernia and the rapid progression of his symptoms, to which the patient agreed.

It is now late afternoon and the patient has returned to his room after successful and uneventful surgical repair of the hiatal hernia via Nissen fundoplication. He has a nasogastric (NG) tube in place connected to low suction. He is receiving intravenous fluids, cimetidine, and antibiotics. His incision is intact, with a Jackson Pratt drain in place. The planned abdominal approach was successful, and no chest tubes are in place. He is groggy but alert when addressed by name. He complains of incisional pain. His wife is present and concerned, but emotionally supportive.

Nursing Diagnosis

Acute pain related to surgical incision

Outcomes

- Patient will report pain as less than 3 on a scale of 0 to 10 following pain control measures.
- Patient will splint his incision to reduce pain when coughing and deep breathing.
- Patient will report satisfaction with pain control methods.

Related NOC Outcomes

- Comfort Level
- Pain Control
- Pain Level

Related NIC Interventions

- Analgesic Administration
- Coping Enhancement
- Pain Management

Nursing Interventions/Rationales

- Ask patient to rate pain using a scale of 0 to 10. *Allows nurse to determine extent of patient's pain and evaluate the effectiveness of interventions. If current interventions do not control the patient's pain, other methods of control are necessary, such as a change in analgesic medication.*
- Administer prescribed analgesics to prevent pain from becoming severe. *Analgesics decrease the transmission and perception of pain stimuli. Severe pain is more difficult to control than moderate pain; therefore pain should be treated before it becomes severe.*
- Encourage patient to report pain before it is severe. *Administering pain control medications during the early stages of pain prevents the pain from becoming severe. Only the patient can determine the degree of his pain.*
- Encourage patient to use patient-controlled analgesia if prescribed. *Allows patient control over the pain process.*
- Encourage nonpharmacologic measures to reduce pain. *Relaxation, music, and other nonpharmacologic measures minimize pain perception.*

Nursing Diagnosis

Risk for ineffective airway clearance related to incisional pain, temporarily limited mobility, and history of cigarette smoking

Outcomes

- Patient will remain free from airway compromise.
- Patient will maintain clear breath sounds.

Related NOC Outcomes

- Aspiration Prevention
- Respiratory Status: Airway Patency
- Respiratory Status: Gas Exchange

Related NIC Interventions

- Aspiration Precautions
- Cough Enhancement
- Positioning
- Respiratory Monitoring

Nursing Interventions/Rationales

- Maintain bed in semi-Fowler's position (at least 30 degrees). *Positions diaphragm and lungs in most effective position to facilitate breathing, and allows for maximal lung expansion.*
- Perform pulmonary assessment every 2 to 4 hours or more often as needed. *To detect retained secretions or atelectasis so treatment can be implemented early.*
- Provide adequate opioid analgesia for incisional pain (or monitor patient-controlled analgesia use if prescribed). *Adequate pain control facilitates pulmonary hygiene and mobility. Patients who are in severe pain are reluctant to move or breathe deeply.*
- Supervise pulmonary hygiene (incentive spirometry, chest percussion and vibration) at least every 4 hours. *Prevents atelectasis and facilitates expulsion of secretions.*
- Reposition and encourage deep breathing exercises at least every 2 hours. *Movement and position changes facilitate expulsion of secretions and prevent atelectasis.*
- Splint incision for deep breathing exercises, coughing, and position changes. *Splinting of incision controls pain. Pain control facilitates the ability to breathe deeply, cough, and move.*
- Medicate patient half an hour before ambulation. *Patient will be able to walk better if pain is first controlled by analgesia.*

across the lower esophagus and then inflating the balloon to a predetermined volume. The procedure is repeated as needed. Esophageal tearing is the primary concern, and the risk of perforation is small but serious. The success rate is 60% to 90%, and many patients obtain long-term relief. Dilation is an outpatient procedure that can be repeated in 2 to 3 months if needed. Dilation can also be successfully used to treat other causes of esophageal spasm and stricture.

Severe unrelieved achalasia may require surgical intervention with esophagomyotomy, which releases the stricture through longitudinal incisions. A success rate of 90% is reported with the sur-

Nursing Diagnosis

Impaired swallowing related to functional changes in fundoplication surgery

Outcomes

- Patient will remain free from choking and subsequent aspiration.

Related NOC Outcomes

- Aspiration Prevention
- Swallowing Status
- Swallowing Status: Esophageal Phase

Related NIC Interventions

- Aspiration Precautions
- Positioning
- Surveillance

Nursing Interventions/Rationales

- Maintain initial nothing-by-mouth status and monitor for patency of NG tube. *NG tube must remain patent to prevent fluid accumulation in the stomach and vomiting.*
- Do not irrigate or reposition the NG tube. *Stomach must remain decompressed to prevent vomiting.*
- Report fresh blood occurring in drainage after the first 8-hour postoperative period. *Tube movement or vomiting can disrupt sutures and cause fresh bleeding.*
- Offer frequent oral and nasal hygiene. *To increase comfort while the NG tube is in place.*
- Initiate feedings with 30 ml of clear liquids after peristalsis is reestablished. *The capacity of the stomach is significantly reduced; therefore initial feedings must be smaller.*
- Evaluate presence and severity of dysphagia. *Fundoplication and reduced stomach capacity make swallowing difficult initially.*
- Advance feedings to multiple small feedings and from liquids to solids as tolerated. *The ability to swallow will improve slowly but steadily.*
- Encourage techniques to prevent gas bloating (chewing thoroughly; eating slowly; sitting up to eat; and avoiding air swallowing, using straws, carbonated beverages, gas-producing foods, and excessive talking while eating). *Fundoplicaton may make belching difficult if not impossible. Retained air and gas can produce significant abdominal discomfort.*
- Encourage patient to walk after meals. *To stimulate peristalsis and movement of food and fluids into the intestines.*

Nursing Diagnosis

Deficient knowledge (reflux management) related to lack of previous exposure or access to resources

Outcomes

- Patient will accurately describe dietary and lifestyle measures to prevent reflux.
- Patient will verbalize participation in self-care measures to prevent reflux.

Related NOC Outcomes

- Knowledge: Diet
- Knowledge: Disease Process
- Knowledge: Health Behavior
- Knowledge: Health Resources

Related NIC Interventions

- Teaching: Disease Process
- Teaching: Individual
- Teaching: Prescribed Diet

Nursing Interventions/Rationales

- Teach patient about necessary dietary modifications (eat a low-fat diet; avoid tea, coffee, chocolate, caffeine-containing foods; strictly limit or eliminate alcohol intake; eat four to six small meals daily; eat slowly and chew thoroughly; remain in upright position 1 to 2 hours after eating; avoid eating in bed, nighttime snacking, foods that induce heartburn; reduce overall body weight). *Fundoplication reduces the severity of reflux but does not eliminate it. Foods that lower the lower esophageal sphincter (LES) pressure need to be avoided. Overloading the stomach increases the occurrence of reflux. Reflux is worse at night, so the stomach needs to be empty before retiring for the night.*
- Discuss lifestyle habits that promote reflux (smoking, straining, lifting, stooping, constrictive clothing) and modifications that can help reduce those habits. *Smoking decreases LES pressure significantly and can induce reflux. Heavy lifting and straining increase intraabdominal pressure and reflux. Reflux is more common and severe at night when the patient is recumbent and has a full stomach.*
- Encourage use of antacids for occasional heartburn. *Antacids neutralize exisiting acid and may decrease pain associated with reflux.*
- Encourage patient to report frequent or severe reflux episodes. *Surgical repair rarely completely eliminates acid reflux; therefore alternative treatments may be necessary.*
- Repeat teaching frequently and provide written information about home care. *Stress such as surgery interferes with learning. Repetitive teaching enhances learning. Written materials provide a resource for later review as needed.*

Evaluation

Evaluation is based on comparing the patient's outcomes with desired outcomes.

gery, which may involve thoracic, abdominal, and more recently minimally invasive thoracoscopic or laparoscopic approaches.[11] The evolution of minimally invasive techniques has significantly increased the appeal of more definitive surgical correction for achalasia. Antireflux fundoplication may be included, based on surgeon preference. Surgery is usually recommended after two or three dilations have failed to provide lasting relief.

PATIENT/FAMILY TEACHING. Dysphagia is the primary challenge of motility disorders, and the nurse works with the patient

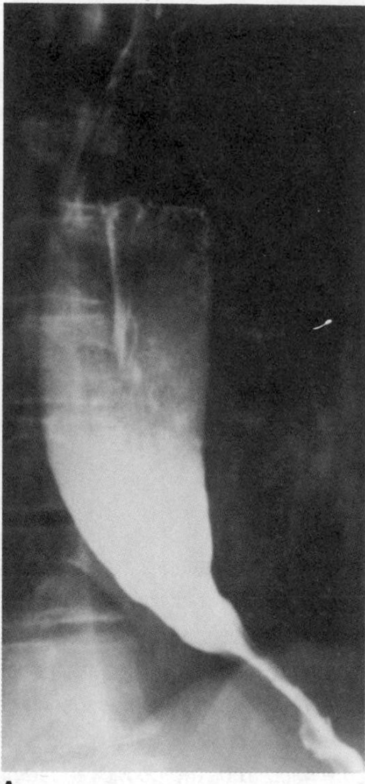

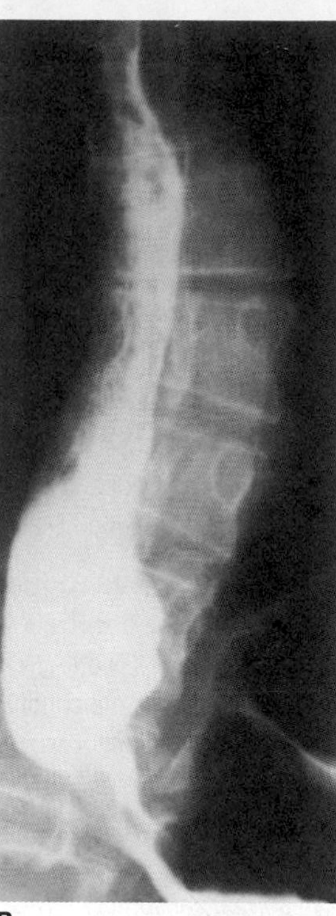

Figure 41-7 **A,** Achalasia with narrowed, elongated esophagogastric junction (rat tail sign). **B,** Widening of esophagogastric junction in patient with achalasia after balloon dilation.

and family to explore diet and lifestyle modifications that will best control it (see Patient/Family Teaching box). Patient and family teaching begins with careful assessment of the scope and severity of the dysphagia, including:

- Swallowing ability with liquids versus solids
- Response to foods of differing textures and temperatures
- Variability of the dysphagia (intermittent or constant)
- Response to stress, fatigue, and activities
- Approaches used by the patient to manage the dysphagia and the degree of success

PATIENT/FAMILY TEACHING
Strategies to Manage the Dysphagia of Achalasia

- Experiment with food types and consistencies and evaluate the effectiveness of each.
- Evaluate the effect of meal size on successful swallowing. Small, frequent, semisoft meals are usually best tolerated.
- Avoid temperature extremes that may worsen esophageal spasm. Warm liquids are usually best tolerated.
- Try changing positions during eating and evaluate the effect on swallowing.
  —Arching the back is successful for some persons.
  —Raising the arms above the head aids gravity and raises intrathoracic pressure to aid swallowing.
- Try using Valsalva's maneuver (bearing down with a closed glottis) while swallowing and evaluate its effect.
- Sleep with the head elevated on a foam wedge to reduce the risk of nighttime reflux and aspiration.
- Pay particular attention to frequent oral hygiene.

Research

Altorki N: COX-2: a target for prevention and treatment of esophageal cancer, *J Surg Res* 117:114-120, 2004.

This study reviewed the available evidence regarding the relationship between the suppression of COX-2 levels and the incidence of esophageal cancer. The role of COX-2 in the development of esophageal cancer is under investigation, since increased amounts of COX-2 are commonly found in both adenocarcinomas and squamous cell carcinomas of the esophagus. There is also significant epidemiologic evidence that regular or occasional use of aspirin or other nonsteroidal antiinflammatory inhibitors may reduce the risk of esophageal cancer. This protective influence has already been demonstrated with the incidence of colon cancer. Several studies by the American Cancer Society indicate as much as a 40% reduction in the risk of esophageal cancer for individuals using aspirin frequently (15 or more times per month).

Esophageal Carcinoma

Etiology and Epidemiology. Both benign and malignant tumors occur in the esophagus. Benign tumors, usually leiomyomas, are extremely rare and usually asymptomatic; they require no intervention unless symptoms necessitate local excision. Malignant tumors of the esophagus are relatively rare (less than 2% of all newly diagnosed cancers) but virulent, with a 5-year survival rate of just 10%.[19]

The two primary forms of esophageal cancer are squamous cell carcinoma and adenocarcinoma. They are distinctly different in terms of location, persons affected, and associated risks and are best considered as separate diseases.[3] Cancer of the esophagus typically affects men between the ages of 50 and 80 years. It occurs in men four times more often than in women, and in African-Americans four times more often than in Caucasians. The etiology of both forms is unknown (see Research box).

Squamous cell carcinoma typically arises in the middle and lower third of the esophagus. It disproportionately affects African-American men and is the fourth leading cause of cancer deaths in this population.[19] The incidence of squamous cell carcinoma has remained fairly stable. Adenocarcinoma of the esophagus, which is almost exclusively found in the distal esophagus, is rare, but its incidence has increased from 0.7 to 3.2 per 100,000 population over the past 2 decades, an increase of 350%.[19] This form of the disease primarily affects Caucasian men.

Cancer of the esophagus also shows a marked variation in incidence worldwide. Although rare in the United States, cancer of the esophagus is common in portions of China, Japan, Russia, Iran, and southern Africa, where it may account for as much as 25% of all cancer deaths.

In the United States alcohol intake and tobacco use have been identified as the primary risk factors for esophageal cancer, and there is a clear dose-response and duration-of-use relationship.[3] Heavy alcohol use increases the risk threefold even without the synergistic effect of smoking, which can drive the incidence up to six times that of the rest of the population. The carcinogenic effects are clearly cumulative. In areas of the world where esophageal cancer is

Risk Factors

Esophageal Cancer

Squamous Cell Carcinoma

Sex: higher risk in men
Ethnicity: higher risk in African-Americans
Tobacco use
Heavy alcohol use
Dietary nitrates
Poor nutrition, lack of fresh fruits and vegetables
Vitamin deficiency
Mucosal irritants

Adenocarcinoma

Sex: higher risk in men
Ethnicity: higher risk in Caucasians
Barrett's epithelium
Heavy alcohol use
Smoking
Obesity (possible link to reflux)

common, the development of the tumor is linked to high levels of nitrosamines and other contaminants in the soil and foods. Diets that are chronically inadequate in fresh fruits, vegetables, and vitamins are also implicated (see Risk Factors box).

Cancer of the esophagus is almost always fatal, particularly in the African-American population. The tumor is theoretically curable in its earliest stage but is rarely diagnosed early enough to allow for effective treatment. Disease is confined to the mucosa or submucosa in less than 10% of cases.

Pathophysiology. Tumors may develop at any point along the length of the esophagus, but the majority occur in the middle and lower two thirds. Esophageal tumors of all types appear to develop as part of a slow process that begins with benign tissue changes. The pathogenesis of the disease remains unclear, but animal studies suggest that oxidative damage occurs from factors such as smoking and reflux, causing inflammation and esophagitis that may initiate the carcinogenic process.[3] It is now generally accepted that Barrett's epithelium can progress to a dysplasia that can ultimately result in adenocarcinoma.[25] Barrett's epithelium is an acquired condition in which tissue changes occur in response to acid irritation over a period of months to 2 years. Barrett's epithelium is typically present for 20 to 30 years before malignant change occurs, but its presence increases the risk of cancer by 30 to 400 times.[24]

Local growth of the tumor is rapid and early spread is common because of the rich lymphatic supply found in the esophagus and the absence of a serosal membrane. Tumors are characteristically intraluminal and ulcerating, with a tendency to encircle the esophageal wall, as well as extend up or down its length (Figure 41-8). Spread of the carcinoma is by local invasion or through the bloodstream or lymphatics. Neoplasms of the upper and middle esophagus may extend into the pulmonary system and those of the lower esophagus into the diaphragm, vertebrae, or heart. Metastasis is present in about 80% of esophageal cancers at the time of diagnosis.

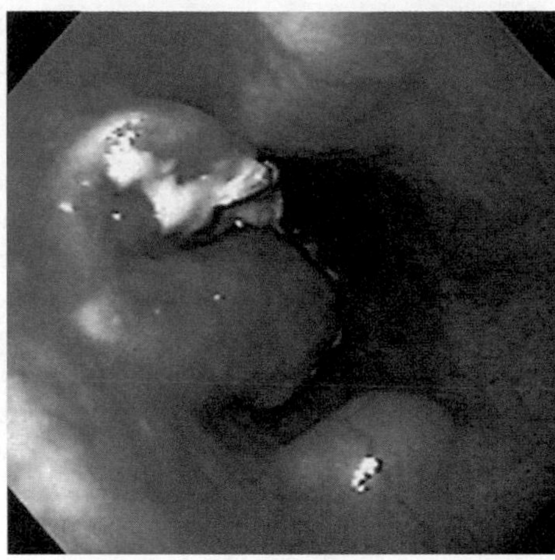

Figure 41-8 Squamous cell carcinoma of esophagus.

Ninety percent of the circumference of the esophagus is commonly involved before symptoms develop, and early diagnosis is rare. Tumors of less than 10 cm are considered small. Progressive dysphagia and abrupt weight loss are the most common presenting symptoms. Dysphagia begins with solid foods but progresses to include liquids. Pulmonary complications such as fistula formation or aspiration are common, and complete obstruction is inevitable without successful therapy. Common clinical manifestations of esophageal cancer are summarized in the Clinical Manifestations box.

COMPLICATIONS. Esophageal cancer is commonly a terminal illness, and complications are expected. Tumor regrowth and metastasis may cause recurrent dysphagia and obstruction, and dilation may be required. Weight loss may persist. Pulmonary complications are common concerns. A wide range of complications can occur after surgery, including anastomosis leakage, bleeding, and infection.

Collaborative Care Management

DIAGNOSTIC TESTS. Barium swallow with fluoroscopy and endoscopy are the two primary diagnostic tools. The barium swallow clearly outlines large masses, and endoscopy allows for direct visual inspection and biopsy for cytologic analysis. Computed tomography may be used to assess for regional and distant

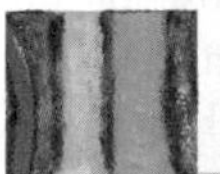

CLINICAL MANIFESTATIONS
Esophageal Cancer

- Early disease: largely asymptomatic
- Gradually progressive dysphagia
  —Usually not present until more than 90% of diameter is obstructed
  —Progresses from solids to liquids
  —Continuous, not intermittent
- Anorexia
- Weight loss: commonly up to 40 pounds in 2 to 3 months
- Odynophagia: typically a steady, dull, substernal pain
- Regurgitation: foul breath from retained food in esophagus
- Heartburn

metastasis. Endoscopic ultrasound may be used to accurately assess the depth of tumor invasion before treatment decisions are made.

MEDICATIONS. Primary treatment of esophageal cancer increasingly combines chemotherapy, radiation, and surgery. Preoperative chemotherapy has been used in an effort to eradicate metastases, shrink the tumor, and increase the success of surgical resection. Efficacy studies show contradictory results, but squamous cell tumors appear to respond more positively to preoperative chemotherapy than do adenocarcinomas.[14] Postoperative chemotherapy does not appear to offer any increased survival benefit.[27] Chemotherapy does offer some benefit in treating patients with inoperable tumors.[9] Therapy that combines chemotherapy and radiation is also used for palliation in advanced disease, but quality-of-life issues are important to consider in treatment decisions.

DIET. Maintaining adequate nutrition as the cancer progresses is the primary consideration. The diet is modified as needed as dysphagia worsens. Tube or gastrostomy feedings and short-course parenteral nutrition may all be needed at some point in the disease process. Malnutrition significantly impairs surgical healing and increases the risk of treatment complications.

TREATMENTS. External beam radiation is the primary treatment in the management of esophageal cancer. It has been used as an alternative to surgery in patients who are poor surgical candidates or who are unwilling to undergo rigorous surgery.[27] External beam radiation is extremely effective in rapidly relieving symptoms of obstruction. It reduces tumor size and gives consistent long-term symptom relief, but it can lead to debilitating stricture or stenosis, since esophageal tissue is extremely sensitive to radiation. Even though the incidence of micrometastases is high after surgery, postoperative radiation appears to offer no clear survival benefit.[4] Combining radiation and chemotherapy is thought to improve the results.[30]

Other treatment options for esophageal cancer include laser treatment, dilation of strictures, and prosthesis insertion. They are typically employed when an individual is unable or unwilling to undergo radical surgery. The focus in on symptom palliation. The neodymium:yttrium-aluminum-garnet (Nd:YAG) laser, which vaporizes a portion of the tumor, may be used to open the esophageal lumen. The treatment is performed endoscopically and offers substantial relief of obstruction in more than 90% of cases. Esophageal dilation is performed as needed throughout therapy to relieve dysphagia resulting from either tumor obstruction or radiation stricture (see the discussion under Achalasia, p. 1195). The beneficial effects are brief, however, and repeated dilations may be necessary. Metal stents are being used successfully to maintain the patency of the esophageal lumen (Figure 41-9). A semirigid prosthesis can also be inserted into the esophagus to bypass an obstruction or fistula. The procedure preserves swallowing and a patent esophagus, but it creates a significant risk of aspiration, dislodgement, or esophageal perforation. The prosthesis disrupts the function of the LES and permits free reflux of gastric contents.

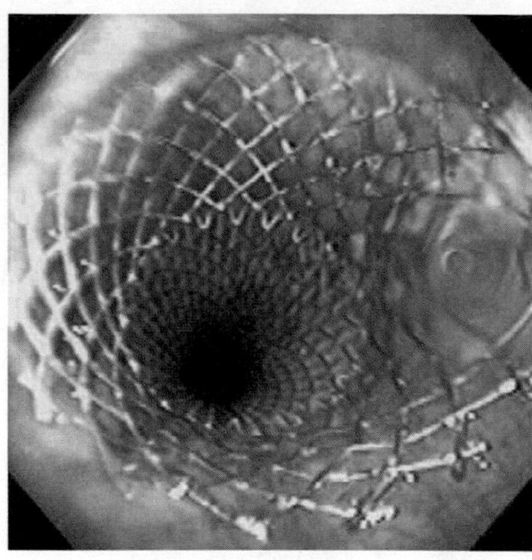

Figure 41-9 Placement of a covered self-expanding metallic stent to relieve dysphagia and obstruction.

SURGICAL MANAGEMENT. Radical surgery is the only definitive treatment for esophageal cancer, and it is the treatment of choice for otherwise healthy individuals with early-stage disease. The surgeries are extensive and have a high mortality rate, especially for patients with concurrent health problems. Subtotal or total esophagectomy is usually required; both surgeries are technically difficult. Although several options exist, the preferred surgery is the esophagectomy with either gastric pull through (esophagogastrostomy) (Figure 41-10) or colonic interposition (Figure 41-11). Colonic interposition is usually necessitated by spread of the tumor into the stomach. The surgeries are complex and may involve either a thoracic or abdominal approach or both.

The tremendous advances in laparoscopic surgery now make it technically feasible to perform esophagectomy via minimally

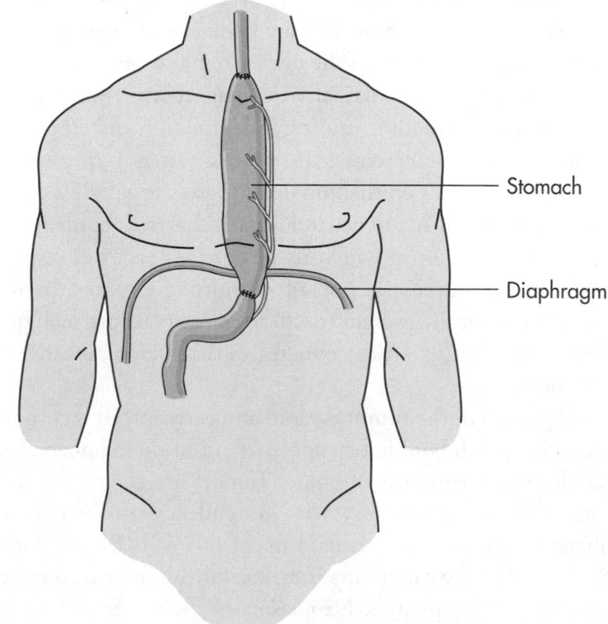

Figure 41-10 Esophagogastrostomy for esophageal cancer. Esophagectomy with gastric pull through.

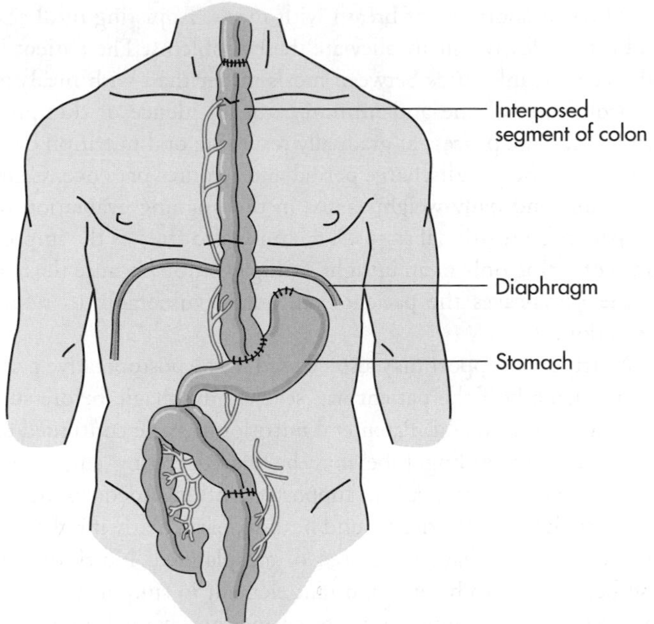

Figure 41-11 Esophagectomy with colon interposition.

invasive techniques. In skilled hands it is a safe and effective alternative to traditional open techniques.[25] It is more likely to be employed to treat Barrett's epithelium than invasive cancer, however, because of the usual need for widespread lymph node sampling and excision. The availability of minimally invasive surgery does make it possible to more strongly advocate for curative esophagectomy earlier in the process of conversion from Barrett's epithelium to dysplasia and ultimately carcinoma.[25]

In addition to the usual surgical risks of shock, hemorrhage, and infection, these procedures also create a serious risk of leakage at the site of anastomosis, particularly with colon interposition. Anastomosis leakage occurs in up to 20% of cases, and operative mortality is about 7%. Even when surgical healing is successful, the patient remains at serious risk for reflux and aspiration from the elimination of the sphincter protection of the LES.

▶ ARE You READY?

Which of the following findings in a patient's health history is considered a primary risk factor of esophageal cancer?

1. Ingestion of large amount of fruits and raw vegetables
2. Use of chewing tobacco and carbonated beverages
3. Smoking and alcohol use
4. High-fiber diet and elevated blood sugar

Nursing Management

of the Patient undergoing Esophagectomy Surgery

PREOPERATIVE CARE

The duration of preoperative preparation is largely determined by the patient's nutritional status. Nutritional support is provided as needed via tube feedings or parenteral nutrition. Most of this preparation takes place in the home setting. The nurse carefully monitors intake and output, total daily calories, and body weight. The nurse encourages the patient to perform frequent mouth care to reduce the risk of postoperative infection, since the patient may be regurgitating retained food particles, blood, or pus from the tumor. Mouthwashes can help control foul mouth odors and make oral intake more palatable. Dental problems are usually corrected before surgery, particularly if adjunctive radiation is planned.

The nurse ensures that the patient and family are knowledgeable about the planned surgery and its expected outcomes. Specific teaching includes the purpose, number, and location of all incisions, lines, and tubes. Wound drainage, chest and NG tubes, and intravenous lines may all be in place. Pulmonary hygiene is a major focus of postoperative care, and the nurse instructs the patient about the importance of turning and deep breathing regimens and other aspects of chest physical therapy. Practice time is provided. The likelihood of temporary intubation and ventilator support is also introduced. If a colon interposition procedure is planned, the nurse also performs a complete bowel preparation in the preoperative period.

The nurse encourages the patient to verbalize feelings and concerns related to this extensive surgery. It is natural for the patient to be both extremely anxious and ambivalent about the surgery. The nurse encourages family members to be involved in all teaching sessions and ensures that all caregivers are familiar with the patient's wishes as expressed through advance directives. Quality-of-life issues are extremely relevant when the prognosis is poor.

POSTOPERATIVE CARE

Protecting the Airway. Patients are typically managed in an intensive care unit setting for a day or two after surgery to allow for intensive cardiopulmonary monitoring and ventilatory support. The patient receives routine but meticulous postoperative care because the risk of complications is high. Respiratory care is the highest priority. The patient may remain intubated for the first 24 hours. The nurse assesses and documents respiratory status every 1 to 2 hours and initiates vigorous turning, deep breathing, coughing, and chest physical therapy routines. Endotracheal suctioning is avoided if possible because of the risk of disturbing the anastomosis incision.[13] Adequate analgesia is essential to the achievement of respiratory goals. The nurse helps the patient adequately splint major incisions for turning and coughing and ensures that appropriate opioid analgesia is provided, usually through patient-controlled or epidural analgesia.

The patient is placed in a semi-Fowler's or high Fowler's position to support ventilation and prevent regurgitation and reflux. Supplemental oxygen is administered, and blood gases and oxygen saturation levels are monitored. The nurse ensures the patency of any chest tubes and the water seal drainage system. Drainage should decrease gradually and be serosanguineous within a few hours. A sudden change in the color or quantity of the drainage may indicate leakage at the anastomosis site. The nurse also monitors carefully for the development of subcutaneous emphysema, which can also indicate anastomosis leakage.[13]

The presence of multiple incisions and drains significantly increases the potential for problems with wound healing. Anastomosis leakage is a serious complication that can compromise the airway and pulmonary gas exchange. The risk is highest 5 to 9 days after surgery. Prompt identification of leakage is essential. The nurse monitors for signs of inflammation, fever, or fluid accumulation. Pulmonary edema is a common problem, and fluid intake is carefully monitored. Early symptoms of shock, such as tachycardia, tachypnea, or restlessness, may be the first warning signs.

Promoting Adequate Nutrition. The patient is usually allowed nothing by mouth for 5 to 7 days until initial healing occurs and GI motility is fully reestablished. The nurse provides frequent oral hygiene to improve patient comfort. The NG tube is carefully secured and monitored to prevent movement or dislodgement, which might disrupt the sutures at the anastomosis sites. The tube is not routinely irrigated or repositioned. The initial NG drainage is bloody, but it should gradually resume a normal greenish yellow color by the end of the first postoperative day. The continued presence of blood usually indicates oozing at the anastomosis.

After this initial period of stabilization the patency of the anastomoses are assessed using fluoroscopy, and the patient is offered approximately 5 ml of water every 15 to 30 minutes throughout the day. The quantity is gradually increased as tolerated. The nurse supervises the patient during all initial swallowing efforts and ensures that an upright position is maintained. The NG tube remains in place while oral fluids are introduced because esophageal tissue is friable and bleeds easily. The surgical area needs to remain decompressed to protect the anastomoses.

The patient is slowly progressed to a pureed or semisolid diet if problems do not develop. The nurse assists the patient in determining the amount and type of foods and fluids that can be safely and comfortably swallowed. Small meals are essential because the food storage area of the stomach is drastically reduced. Initially patients may experience a feeling of fullness in the chest or shortness of breath with meals. Adjusting meal size and eating slowly usually alleviate these problems. The patient is advised to drink fluids between meals rather than with meals to control food volume and minimize the incidence of dumping syndrome. The process of gradually resuming oral nutrition continues into the postdischarge period and requires patience. Calorie counts and daily weights assist in the ongoing evaluation of the patient's nutritional status. The nurse also stresses the importance of eating only in an upright sitting position because the loss of the LES leaves the patient continually vulnerable to reflux aspiration.

Nutritional support may also be used in the postoperative period, particularly if the patient was severely dysphagic before surgery and losing weight. Parenteral nutrition may be continued or a jejunostomy feeding tube may be placed during surgery to bypass the operative area and support nutrition. Adequate nutrition is critical for effective wound healing, particularly if radiation or chemotherapy have been used or are planned. Nutrition has also been found to be an important element in supporting effective ventilator weaning and preventing nosocomial infection. Nutritional support includes attention to an adequate protein intake. Serum albumin levels should remain above 3.5 g/dl.

Promoting Coping. Despite the radical surgery, the patient with esophageal cancer still has a potentially terminal illness and dramatically shortened life expectancy. Considerable psychologic support is needed by the patient and family in their efforts to cope with the uncertain prognosis and physical limitations of the disease. The nurse encourages the patient and family to talk about the situation together, make realistic plans, and seek out supports available in the community.

Guidelines for care of the patient undergoing esophagectomy are summarized in the Guidelines for Safe Practice box.

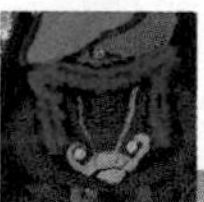

GUIDELINES FOR SAFE PRACTICE *The Patient Undergoing Esophagectomy*

Preoperative Care

Encourage improved nutritional status.
- —High-protein, high-calorie diet if oral intake is possible
- —Tube feedings or parenteral nutrition for severe dysphagia or obstruction

Assist with frequent oral hygiene to minimize breath odor.

Teach appropriate techniques for effective deep breathing and coughing and the importance of frequent pulmonary hygiene; have patient demonstrate respiratory exercises and how to splint the incision for coughing.

Teach patient about all tubes and drains that will be used postoperatively and how surgical pain will be managed.

Postoperative Care

Promote good pulmonary ventilation.
- —Hourly deep breathing and coughing if needed
- —Incentive spirometry and chest physical therapy as ordered
- —Auscultation of lung fields every 2 hours (avoiding tracheal suctioning if possible)
- —Monitoring blood gases and oxygen saturation levels

Maintain chest drainage system as prescribed.

Provide for adequate analgesia by patient-controlled analgesia or epidural catheter; monitor respiratory and neurologic response.

Maintain gastric drainage system.
- —Small amounts of blood may drain from nasogastric tube for 6 to 12 hours after surgery.
- —Do not irrigate or reposition the nasogastric tube (to prevent irritation to suture line).

Maintain nutrition.
- —Start clear fluids at frequent intervals when oral intake is permitted.
- —Introduce soft foods gradually, and slowly progress to several small meals of bland foods.

Prevent aspiration if lower esophageal sphincter is removed or disrupted.
- —Always raise the head of the bed for swallowing food or liquid.
- —Elevate the head of the bed for sleeping.

Instruct patient to avoid bending or stooping.

Keep suction apparatus available at the bedside.

GERONTOLOGIC CONSIDERATIONS

Cancer of the esophagus is usually identified in late middle age or old age. These patients have a high incidence of chronic health problems, which increase the risks that accompany such radical surgery. Postoperative complications are more common and more severe than in younger patients. Older adults are also less likely to have family and support networks to help them manage their care after discharge. Most patients with cancer of the esophagus require significant assistance after discharge. Even without major postoperative complications, the patient needs to deal with ongoing respiratory care, wound healing concerns, and nutritional support. The nurse must be vigilant in assessing the need for postdischarge assistance and initiating needed referrals. The nurse encourages the family to seek out and use supports such as those available from the American Cancer Society and makes referrals to community home care agencies as needed. Hospice referrals may be appropriate for patients needing palliative care.

? Critical Thinking

1. A 79-year-old woman has come to the medical clinic with a 6-month history of heartburn, which has been steadily increasing in both frequency and severity. She also reports frequent regurgitation of acidic fluid into the mouth. She has self-medicated with antacids and over-the-counter H_2 blockers, but they no longer control the discomfort. She is 5 feet, 4 inches tall and weighs 180 pounds. She is an avid gardener and spends long hours weeding and pruning. She laughs as you ask her to put on a gown for a physical examination, saying that it will take a few moments to get out of her corset. What specific factors in her presentation will you target to teach her how to better control esophageal reflux? What other data do you need to improve your understanding of her situation?
2. Review the *Healthy People 2010* guidelines for oral health. What services are available in your community to support achievement of these goals? Which services are lacking for indigent patients or those without health insurance?

References

1. Da Silveira EB, Rogers AI: Achalasia: a review of therapeutic options and outcomes, *Compr Ther* 28(1):15-22, 2002.
2. Devault KR: Gastroesophageal reflux: medical and surgical treatment options, *Am Fam Phys* 68(7):1305-1308, 2003.
3. Enzinger PC, Mayer RJ: Esophageal cancer, *N Engl J Med* 349:2241-2252, 2003.
4. Gibson MK, Forastiere AA: Combined-modality therapy for esophageal cancer: are we making progress? *Cancer J* 9(4):238-240, 2003.
5. Heidelbaugh JJ et al: Management of gastroesophageal reflux disease, *Am Fam Phys* 68(7): 1311-1317, 2003.
6. Hubbard PM: Update on gastroesophageal reflux disease, *Am J Nurse Pract* 6(2):9-12, 15-16, 18, 2002.
7. Karlowicz D: An endoscopic approach to GERD? *RN* 66(12):56-60, 2003.
8. Katz PO: Antireflux surgery: who needs it? *Am J Gastroenterol* 98(11):2341-2342, 2003.
9. Leonard GD, McCaffrey JA, Maher M: Optimal therapy for oesophageal cancer, *Cancer Treatment Rev* 29:275-282, 2003.
10. Levy RA, Stamm L, Meiner SE: Conservative management of GERD, *MEDSURG Nurs* 11(4):169-175, 2002.
11. Lew RJ, Kochman ML: A review of endoscopic methods of esophageal dilation, *J Clin Gastroenterol* 35(2):117-126, 2002.
12. Little AG: Gastroesophageal reflux disease, *J Surg Res* 117(1):30-33, 2004.
13. Mackenzie DJ, Popplewell PK, Billingsley KG: Care of patients after esophagectomy, *Crit Care Nurse* 24(1):17-28, 2004.
14. Markary MA et al: Multimodality treatment of esophageal cancer, *Am Surgeon* 69(8):693-700, 2003.
15. Mirowski GW, Chuang TY: Oral disease and oral cutaneous manifestations of gastrointestinal and liver diseases. In Feldman M, Friedman LS, Sleisenger MH, editors: *Gastrointestinal and liver disease,* ed 7, Philadelphia, 2002, Saunders.
16. Neville BW, Day TA: Oral cancer and precancerous lesions, *CA: Cancer J Clin* 52:195-215, 2002.
17. Oleynikow D, Oelschlager B: New alternatives in the management of gastroesophageal reflux disease, *Am J Surg* 186(2) 106-111, 2003.
18. Orlando R: Pathogenesis of gastroesophageal reflux disease, *Am J Med Sci* 326(5):274-278, 2003.
19. Pickens A, Orringer MB: Geographical distribution and racial disparity in esophageal cancer, *Ann Thorac Surg* 76:S1367-S1369, 2003.
20. Ray SW et al: Managing gastroesophageal reflux disease, *Nurse Pract* 27(5):36-38, 41-42, 44, 2002.
21. Rayhorn N et al: Understanding gastroesophageal reflux disease, *Nursing* 33(10):36-42, 2003.
22. Richter JE: Dietary advice for patients with GERD, *Medscape*, accessed April 2004 from website: www.medscape.com/viewarticle/460314.
23. Richter J: Diagnostic tests for gastroesophageal reflux disease, *Am J Med Sci* 326(5):300-308, 2003.
24. Ruol A et al: Barrett's esophagus: management of high-grade dysplasia and cancer, *J Surg Res* 117:44-51, 2004.
25. Schuchert MJ, Luketich JD: Barrett's esophagus: current status of treatment. In Feldman M, Friedman LS, Sleisenger MH, editors: *Gastrointestinal and liver disease*, ed 7, Philadelphia, 2002, Saunders.
26. Shaheen N, Provenzale D: The epidemiology of gastroesophageal reflux disease, *Am J Med Sci* 326(5):264-273, 2003.
27. Spechler SJ: Clinical manifestations and esophageal complications of GERD, *Am J Med Sci* 326(5):279-284, 2003.
28. Stylopoulous N, Rattner D: Paraesophageal hernia: when to operate? *Adv Surg* 37:213-229, 2003.
29. Swinson BD et al: Principles of management in oral cancer, *Hosp Med* 64(7):404-441, 2003.
30. Tak V, Naunheim K: Current status of multimodality therapy for esophageal carcinoma, *J Surg Res* 117:22-29, 2004.
31. Tutuian R, Castell D: Management of gastroesophageal reflux disease, *Am J Med Serv* 326(5):309-318, 2003.
32. Weinberg MA, Estefan DJ: Assessing oral malignancies, *Am Fam Phys* 65(7):1379-1384, 2002.
33. Williams H: Gastroesophageal reflux disease: clinical manifestations, *Gastroenterol Nurs* 26(5):195-202, 2003.
34. Woltman T et al: Surgical management of esophageal motility disorders, *J Surg Res* 117:34-43, 2004.

Visit the Evolve website: http://evolve.elsevier.com/Monahan/medsurg

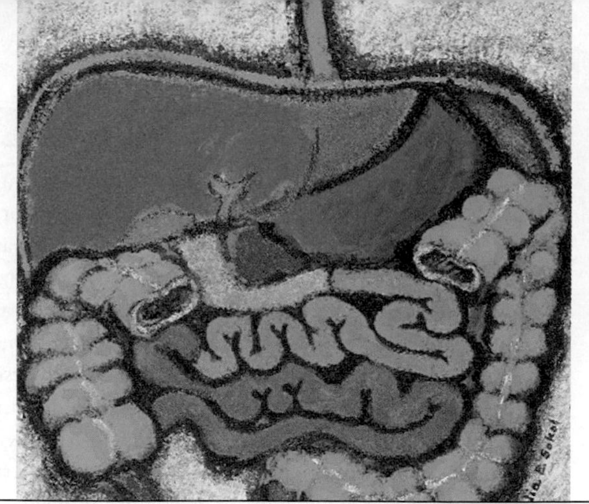

CHAPTER 42
Stomach and Duodenum Problems

by Judith K. Sands

OBJECTIVES

After studying this chapter, the learner should be able to:

1. Discuss the etiology and epidemiology of common problems affecting the stomach and duodenum.
2. Describe the mechanisms of mucosal defense and breakdown and the roles of *Helicobacter pylori,* nonsteroidal antiinflammatory drug administration, and other risk factors in the development of peptic ulcer disease.
3. Compare the advantages and disadvantages of the medical and surgical management of peptic ulcer disease and its complications.
4. Describe appropriate nursing interventions for the management of peptic ulcer disease and its complications.
5. Outline the medical and nursing management of gastric cancer.
6. Identify the essential nursing care associated with gastric surgery.
7. Discuss nursing responsibilities in the management of enteral and parenteral nutrition.

KEY TERMS

chemoreceptor trigger zone, p. 1227
Curling's ulcer, p. 1219
Cushing's ulcer, p. 1219
dumping syndrome, p. 1223
enteral nutrition, p. 1231
gastritis, p. 1205
***Helicobacter pylori*,** p. 1205
hematemesis, p. 1210
hematochezia, p. 1210
malabsorption, p. 1229
melena, p. 1210
negative nitrogen balance, p. 1230
omental patch, p. 1214
osmolality, p. 1232
parenteral nutrition, p. 1234
peritonitis, p. 1225
short-bowel syndrome, p. 1230
vagotomy, p. 1214

Problems related to the stomach are extremely common in U.S. society. Many of these problems are episodic and can easily be managed through temporary diet modification or self-medication in the home setting. Other stomach problems require aggressive medical or surgical intervention. Peptic ulcer disease (PUD) is the primary focus of this chapter. Also discussed is the management of gastric cancer and surgery, problems of nutrient absorption, and enteral and parenteral nutrition.

Dyspepsia

Etiology and Epidemiology. *Dyspepsia* is an imprecise term used to describe a variety of common upper abdominal symptoms that may accompany a range of gastrointestinal (GI) disorders, but also occur in the absence of any demonstrable pathologic condition. Common descriptions of dyspepsia include pain or discomfort, fullness, bloating, aching, belching, burning, heartburn, nausea, and anorexia. The individual often reports that the symptom pattern is chronic and recurrent. The complaint is estimated to affect as much as 25% to 40% of the population.[10,18]

In most individuals dyspepsia is more a symptom than a diagnosis, and careful clinical workup usually results in the problem being classified as gastroesophageal reflux disease (GERD) or peptic ulcer. Less frequently the symptoms can be attributed to a wide variety of medication side effects, food allergies or intolerances, or a seemingly unrelated systemic illness such as cancer or diabetes. But a supportable organic cause can only be identified in about 40% of all patients experiencing dyspepsia.[27] The remainder of the cases are eventually classified as idiopathic, functional, or nonulcer dyspepsia with no demonstrable cause. Establishing an etiology for functional dyspepsia is more a matter of ruling out other contributing factors than identifying a clearly identifiable cause. Despite extensive research, no causative link has ever been established to specific foods or spices, medications, or infection by the *Helicobacter pylori* organism.[27]

Pathophysiology. The lack of clarity over the etiology of functional dyspepsia also contributes to a poor understanding of the pathophysiology underlying the disorder. The symptoms are theorized to be caused by some complex interplay between physiologic factors in the GI tract (such as GI motility and visceral sensitivity) and the individual's psychosocial makeup (e.g., personality and stress levels).[18] Much of the explanation remains hypothetical because 50% to 70% of sufferers exhibit no significant identifiable lesion on endoscopy. Common abnormalities that have been identified in persons with dyspepsia include disorders of gastric emptying and stretch accommodation to the food bolus, hypersensitivity to distention of the stomach, and autonomic neuropathies in the stomach (particularly decreased vagal tone).[27] Functional abnormalities are frequently uncovered, but their role in symptom causation remains unproven.

Collaborative Care Management. Because the etiology and pathophysiology of functional dyspepsia remain elusive, the management is not definitive. The health care provider must use sufficient diagnostic options to rule out identifiable and treatable organic causes such as GERD and ulcer disease before falling back on a diagnosis of functional dyspepsia with empirical treatment of the patient's symptoms. GERD management is discussed in depth in Chapter 41; PUD management is discussed later in this chapter. Patients with true functional dyspepsia may be treated with a trial of proton pump inhibitors (PPIs). Some patients have a positive response to this therapy, as indicated by decreased symptoms, but it remains unclear to what extent this is a placebo response. Histamine$_2$ (H_2)-receptor antagonists and antacids have shown little benefit.[28]

PATIENT/FAMILY TEACHING. The symptoms of functional dyspepsia can negatively affect social interaction and job attendance and performance. Lack of a definitive diagnosis and treatment can be frustrating and demoralizing for the patient. The nurse carefully explains what is known about the syndrome and outlines the diagnostic alternatives. The nurse encourages the patient to experiment with diet and lifestyle changes and evaluate the effect of these changes on the frequency and severity of symptoms. The effects of coffee, caffeine, and alcohol are carefully evaluated. A variety of herbal products are available to treat dyspepsia symptoms, but they have had little formal testing[39] (see Complementary & Alternative Therapies box). A combination of peppermint and caraway oil has been the most extensively tested and appears to show greater benefit in symptom reduction than a placebo.[9] Turmeric has also been used extensively in Asia. The use of an alternative medicine practitioner may also be helpful to the patient who is willing to explore psychosocial and emotional aspects of the disease process. Physicians often prescribe low-dose antidepressants to patients with functional dyspepsia, and alternative medicine may provide the patient with a greater range of treatment options.[29]

Gastritis

Etiology and Epidemiology. The term **gastritis** refers to a diffuse or localized response of the gastric mucosa to injury or infection. The disorder is classified numerous ways based on causative mechanisms and histologic tissue changes, but none of the classifications is in universal use. Controversy even exists over whether gastritis is a histologic diagnosis or a symptom complex.

Complementary & Alternative Therapies

Herbal Products for Relieving Dyspepsia Symptoms

A variety of herbal products are available, and studies thus far have shown all of them to be more effective than placebo in relieving dyspepsia symptoms. Most studies show a strong placebo effect, which also occurs in response to conventional therapies.

Widely Used Products

Peppermint and caraway oil *(Mentha piperita* and *Carum carvi)*
Turmeric *(Curcuma longa)*

Other Reported Products

Greater celandine *(Chelidonium majus)*
Banana *(Musa sapientum)*
Indian gooseberry *(Emblica officinalis)*
Liu Jun Zi Tang
Shenxiahewining

Acute gastritis is a short-term inflammatory process that can be initiated by numerous factors such as excess alcohol ingestion, drug effects, severe physical stress or trauma, ingestion of caustic or noxious substances, radiation exposure, and bacterial contamination of food or water. Aspirin, even in low doses, and other nonsteroidal antiinflammatory drugs (NSAIDs) are the most common causes of reactive gastritis. Alcohol ingestion is also commonly implicated as it promptly triggers subepithelial hemorrhages. The combined effects of NSAIDs or aspirin and alcohol are even more powerful.[23] Acute gastritis is predominantly an erosive process and is believed to be responsible for up to 10% to 30% of all episodes of GI bleeding.

Chronic gastritis is a separate clinical entity. Although it has myriad possible causes, the most common form worldwide is caused by infection with ***Helicobacter pylori***.[13] The causal relationship has been clearly documented. Virtually all *H. pylori*–positive patients exhibit signs of gastritis in the antrum of the stomach, and treatment of *H. pylori* leads to resolution of the gastritis.[13] More than 90% of diagnosed cases of chronic gastritis show clear evidence of *H. pylori* infection.[13] The infection is usually acquired from contaminated food and water, and fecal-oral or oral-oral transmission is theorized. An estimated 30% to 50% of the U.S. population is infected with the organism, and the incidence increases with age. Caucasians are infected more commonly than other races in the United States.[23] The prevalence of *H. pylori* infection is inversely proportional to socioeconomic status, and the infection rate is more than 90% in developing countries. People typically contract *H. pylori* infection during childhood and remain infected for life unless treated. Infection with *H. pylori* also plays a pivotal role in the development of PUD. Although numerous other organisms and disease processes can cause chronic gastritis, *H. pylori* is by far the most important clinically.

Pathophysiology. Acute gastritis develops when the protective mechanisms of the stomach mucosa are overwhelmed by bacterial toxins or irritating substances. Mucus provides little protection against chemical injury. Regeneration of the gastric mucosa after injury is both prompt and efficient, however, and the disorder usually is self-limiting after the irritating agent is removed. Common symptoms, which may be severe, include anorexia, nausea and vomiting, abdominal cramping or diarrhea, epigastric pain, and fever. Painless GI bleeding may occur and is more likely if the person regularly uses aspirin or NSAIDs.

Chronic gastritis involves primarily the fundus and antrum of the stomach. Most patients with histologic gastritis are asymptomatic, and the diagnosis is established via endoscopy and biopsy. The diagnosis is challenging because the endoscopic appearance of the mucosa does not necessarily correlate with the histology. Acid secretion is slightly reduced, gastrin levels remain normal, and vitamin B_{12} absorption is rarely impaired. As the condition progresses, the mucosa atrophies, and acid secretion is reduced. The diagnosis cannot be made on the basis of symptoms because most persons are asymptomatic after the initial acute infection, but even asymptomatic persons have some evidence of gastric tissue reaction to *H. pylori.* Persons who experience symptoms report simply general dyspepsia. No apparent causal relationship exists between the presence of dyspepsia and the severity of the gastritis.

Collaborative Care Management. Most cases of acute gastritis are managed by removing the causative agent and supporting the patient while the mucosa heals itself. The person usually receives nothing by mouth (NPO) to support healing of the mucosa and then slowly advances to liquids and a normal diet. Antacids, H_2-receptor antagonists, or PPIs may be administered to reduce acid secretion and increase comfort. The nurse monitors the patient carefully for signs of bleeding.

Although chronic gastritis is caused almost exclusively by *H. pylori* infection, routine treatment of the infection remains controversial unless the person is symptomatic or develops an ulcer.[42] Treatment guidelines continue to evolve, but it is generally agreed that neither asymptomatic patients with *H. pylori*–related chronic gastritis, nor patients with dyspepsia symptoms but no evidence of ulceration, should be routinely treated. Symptomatic treatment with antacids, H_2 blockers, and over-the-counter PPIs may be an option. When ulcers are also present, current guidelines recommend treatment of the *H. pylori.* Treatment of *H. pylori* is discussed under Peptic Ulcer Disease, p. 1214.

Patient/Family Teaching. Patient and family teaching for the patient with gastritis is targeted to the etiology of the gastritis and may include counseling about alcohol use or the routine use of aspirin and NSAIDs. The nurse suggests that the patient gradually resume a normal diet, eating only foods that do not exacerbate symptoms. The nurse also encourages the patient to experiment with minor diet and lifestyle modifications that may reduce the incidence and severity of symptoms. These include reducing the intake of dietary fat to minimize postprandial bloating, eating smaller and more frequent meals, and avoiding known precipitators such as alcohol and smoking. Stress management techniques may also be helpful for some patients. The nurse emphasizes the importance of seeking prompt care if symptoms recur after treatment or if any symptoms of PUD develop.

Patients receiving treatment for *H. pylori* are instructed in the safe use of any prescribed medications and how to manage expected side effects. If antibiotic treatment is prescribed, the nurse stresses the importance of completing the entire course of medications. Relapse is common with inadequate treatment, and drug-resistant strains of *H. pylori* are already a concern.

Peptic Ulcer Disease

Etiology and Epidemiology. Peptic ulcers were initially believed to be caused by diet and stress. Over time, thinking shifted toward acid oversecretion as the primary cause, probably in response to stress and dietary factors. Thus the traditional treatment approaches emphasized diet modification and acid neutralization. The past two decades have revolutionized thinking about the etiology of PUD, and the development of effective new pharmacologic agents has enabled cure to become a reasonable goal for a traditionally chronic disease.

When *H. pylori* infection was identified in the early 1980s, attention slowly began to focus on its role in ulcer etiology. Today, *H. pylori* infection is recognized as one of the most common bacterial infectious diseases in humans,[32] and its role in ulcer etiology is widely accepted. It is estimated that 95% of persons with duodenal ulcers and 80% of persons with gastric ulcers are infected with *H. pylori.*[28] The remainder of cases are attributed to the effects of chronic NSAID use. Both *H. pylori* and NSAIDs target the mucosal defenses of the stomach and duodenum and lead to ulceration in vulnerable persons. The relationship between *H. pylori* infection and the development of ulcers is clearly causal, but current knowledge cannot explain why only a small percentage of those infected with *H. pylori* actually develop ulcers; clearly other factors influence host resistance.[41]

The causal association between NSAID use, mucosal injury, and gastric ulcers (and, to a lesser degree, duodenal ulcers) is also unequivocal.[11] The GI complications of NSAID use are increasingly recognized as one of the most common and severe drug side effects. The risk of ulcers is not predictable, however, and most low-risk NSAID users do not experience complications. The annual risk of GI complications is about 2% in low-risk individuals but increases to as much as 50% among high-risk users.[11] The risk appears to be dose related, but problems can occur with even low doses. Ulcer risk rises rapidly after age 60. The widespread use of NSAIDs in the older population has created a large high-risk pool. No causal interaction has been proven between use of NSAIDs and infection with *H. pylori*, but researchers hypothesize that the risk is additive.[15] Risk factors for PUD are presented in the Risk Factors box.

Other factors may play a secondary role in ulcer etiology. A strong positive association exists between smoking and ulcer incidence, complications, recurrence, and mortality.[28] Smoking and *H. pylori* appear to have a synergistic effect, which is related to both the amount smoked and duration. Smoking's effects are particularly significant in ulcer relapse. Alcohol is known to cause direct surface irritation of the gastric mucosa and can cause acute gastritis, but its role in ulcer development, if any, is unproven. Wine and beer are potent secretagogues for acid secretion, but no etiologic role in ulcers has been identified.

Diet was once considered to be a primary factor in ulcer etiology, but no current data support an etiologic role for diet in PUD. The role of stress in ulcer development is also unsupported. The

Risk Factors

Peptic Ulcer Disease

Major

Helicobacter pylori infection
Chronic use of nonsteroidal antiinflammatory drugs

Minor

Age
- Ulcer incidence clusters in middle age.
- Gastric ulcers are more common in older adults.

Smoking is implicated in both ulcer incidence and recurrence.
Race: Gastric ulcers are more common in African-Americans and extremely common in Hispanics.
Sex: Ulcers are more common in men than in women, but the ratio is approaching 1:1.

relationship between intense physiologic stress and acute hemorrhagic gastritis is well documented, but no "ulcer personality" plays an etiologic role in ulcer development.

Ulcer prevalence in the United States peaked in the 1950s, declined until 1980, and now appears to have stabilized. Up to 10% of the population will be affected at some point in their lives.[40] The incidence of duodenal ulcers has declined, whereas the incidence of gastric ulcers has remained fairly stable, probably related to the steady aging of the population and the high incidence of NSAID use in this population.[14]

Enormous progress has been made in treating PUD, but the disease still consumes billions of dollars annually in direct care costs, and the cost of medications has skyrocketed. The importance of the disease is reflected in the *Healthy People 2010* objective to "reduce hospitalizations caused by PUD in the United States from the baseline of 71 per 100,000 to a target of 46 per 100,000 population."[40]

Baffling changes in ulcer incidence in men and women have also occurred in the past 50 years. The incidence of duodenal ulcers in men was about four times that of women during the peak period of the 1950s. This incidence seemed to support the theory that ulcer etiology was related to social and occupational stress. The current sex ratio approaches 1:1. The ratio of duodenal to gastric ulcers has also steadily declined since the 1950s, from nearly 4:1 to almost 1:1. The prevalence of both types of ulcers increases steadily with age, peaking in the sixth decade. The overall mortality rate for ulcer is low, but it increases dramatically in persons over 75 years old. An increased incidence is found in persons with chronic systemic diseases such as chronic obstructive pulmonary disease, end-stage renal disease, and cirrhosis. Racial and cultural variations have also been noted. Gastric and duodenal ulcers occur about equally in Caucasians, but gastric ulcers are more common in African-Americans and extremely common in Hispanics.

ZOLLINGER-ELLISON SYNDROME. Zollinger-Ellison syndrome is caused by a gastrinoma (gastrin-producing tumor), commonly found in the noninsulin-producing islet cells of the pancreas. Most patients have a single tumor that eventually becomes malignant. The tumor produces an enormous quantity of gastrin, which massively overstimulates gastric acid secretion. The resulting duodenal and jejunal ulcers usually do not respond to conventional therapy, and complications are common. This rare syndrome occurs more commonly in men, usually in early or middle adulthood.

Diarrhea is a common symptom, caused by a relative lack of the pancreatic lipase needed for fat digestion. Zollinger-Ellison syndrome is differentiated from standard duodenal ulcers by radioimmunoassay measurements of high serum gastrin levels. The tumor is removed, if possible, and the ulcers are treated as outlined for PUD.

Pathophysiology. The integrity of the gastric mucosa is maintained when a balance exists between the acid-secreting and mucosal protective functions of the stomach and duodenum A peptic ulcer is diagnosed when a distinct crater is visible on the mucosa, either radiologically or endoscopically. Figure 42-1 illustrates the classic lesions of PUD.

ACID SECRETION. Acid secretion is controlled by endocrine, neural, and paracrine factors. Gastric acid is secreted by the parietal cells of the fundus of the stomach in response to (1) gastrin, which is secreted by cells in the pyloric region of the stomach; (2) acetylcholine, which is secreted by cholinergic activation of the vagus; and (3) histamine, which is found in cells throughout the gastric mucosa. The body has two types of cellular receptors to histamine. H_2 receptors are found in stomach cells and mediate the secretion of hydrochloric acid (HCl). Acid oversecretion was long assumed to be the primary factor contributing to ulcer development, but it has now been proven that acid oversecretion rarely plays a significant role. Neither *H. pylori* infection nor NSAID use significantly influences the process of acid secretion.

MUCOSAL DEFENSES. The entire stomach and duodenum are covered by a 100-μm thick layer of gel-like mucus that is 95% water and 5% glycoproteins. This layer is continuously being both broken

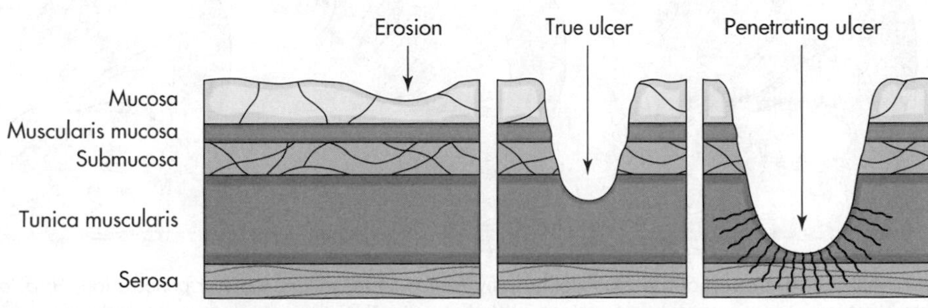

Figure 42-1 Lesions caused by peptic ulcer disease.

down and replaced. The gel protects the mucosa against shearing and mechanical injury, assists in the transport of food particles, retains water near the mucosa, and blocks the back diffusion of hydrogen ions. The epithelial cells of the stomach are densely packed and secrete bicarbonate into the mucous layer, which helps maintain a neutral pH immediately adjacent to the mucosa. The mucosa is therefore remarkably resistant to physical injury. When minor injury occurs, the epithelium is capable of quick repair. These defenses are so powerful that mucosal pH is maintained at a level greater than 6, even when the gastric luminal pH is as low as 1.5.

EFFECTS OF *HELICOBACTER PYLORI* INFECTION. *H. pylori* is a gram-negative bacterium with a spiral shape. Once in the stomach, it uses flagella to imbed itself in the mucosal layer (Figure 42-2). The most striking characteristic of the bacterium is its production of significant amounts of urease that form a cloud around the bacterium and both neutralize the gastric acid and have a toxic effect on the epithelial cells. This allows the bacterium to thrive in the extremely hostile environment of the stomach.[32] The presence of chronic *H. pylori*–related gastritis causes slow metaplastic changes in the adjacent cells of the duodenum and facilitates the movement of *H. pylori* into the duodenum.

The *H. pylori* bacterium releases cytokines that cause chronic gastritis. It is theorized that various strains of *H. pylori* differ in the virulence of their cytotoxins, which≥ could explain the relatively small number of people infected with *H. pylori* who actually develop ulcers.

EFFECTS OF NSAIDS. Most NSAIDs are weak acids that can cause local mucosal irritation and inflammation, but their primary adverse effect on the stomach involves the inhibition of cyclooxygenase (COX), an enzyme needed to produce endogenous prostaglandins. Prostaglandins are critical in maintaining normal mucosal defenses. A deficit in prostaglandins results in decreased mucus and bicarbonate secretion, decreased mucosal blood flow, and a failure to inhibit gastric acid secretion. It also prevents the formation of the mucous "cap" that supports epithelial regeneration in the event of injury.

The major elements involved in the pathophysiology of peptic ulcers are presented in Figure 42-3. Peptic ulcers usually occur at or near mucosal transition zones that are believed to be particularly vulnerable to the effects of acid, pepsin, and enzymes. Most gastric ulcers are localized in an area about 2 cm long on the antral side of the stomach along the lesser curvature, where muscle fibers are prominent and blood supply decreased. Duodenal ulcers are concentrated at the junction of the antrum and duodenum.

Symptoms reported by patients with gastric and duodenal ulcers overlap and may be nonspecific. Pain is the classic symptom associated with PUD, but its sensitivity and specificity as a disease marker are low. The pain traditionally has been attributed to the irritation of gastric acid over the eroded mucosa. During endoscopy, however, rubbing, cutting, burning, and even directly applying HCl to the mucosa produce little or no perceived pain in most individuals. Epigastric pain, described as "burning" or vague discomfort, is present in 60% to 80% of patients. The pain is episodic, lasts 30 minutes to 2 hours, and occurs 1 to 3 hours after meals. Pain that occurs at night and awakens the person from sleep is a common symptom of duodenal ulcers. The pain may radiate and often is relieved by food or antacid. A complication may be the first clinical manifestation in about 25% of persons with PUD.

Dyspepsia is also commonly reported, but because this is such a common complaint in the general population, it is not helpful in establishing the presence of an ulcer. Fewer than 30% of persons who experience chronic and severe dyspepsia are found to have ulcers on endoscopy, but many ulcer sufferers experience dyspepsia. No special features clearly distinguish gastric ulcers from duodenal ulcers, although patients with gastric ulcers, particularly older adults and NSAID users, are more likely to be asymptomatic. Clinical manifestations associated with PUD are summarized in the Clinical Manifestations box.

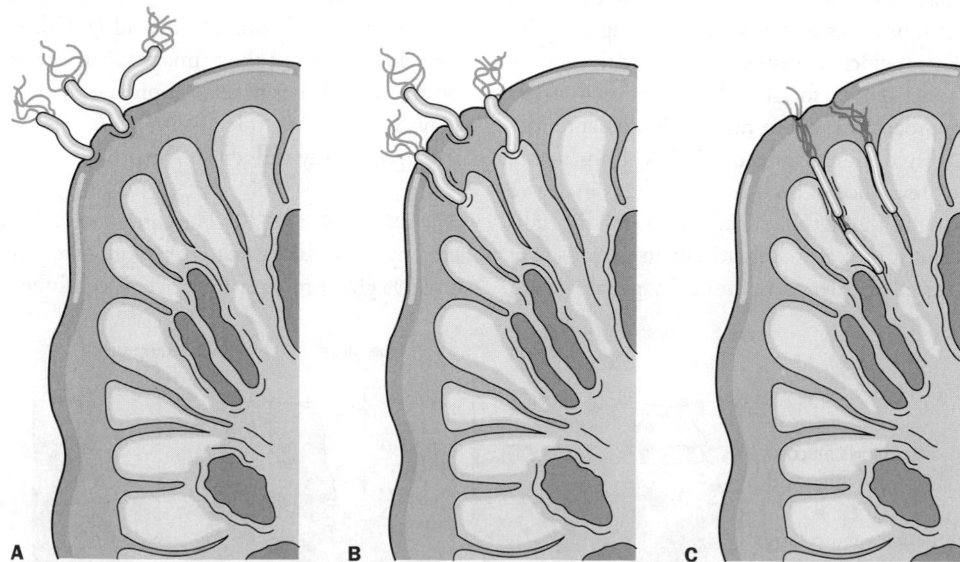

Figure 42-2 Penetration of the mucosal layer by *Helicobacter pylori*. **A,** After penetration, *H. pylori* forms clusters near membranes of surface epithelial cells. **B,** Some attach to cell membrane. **C,** Others lodge between epithelial cells.

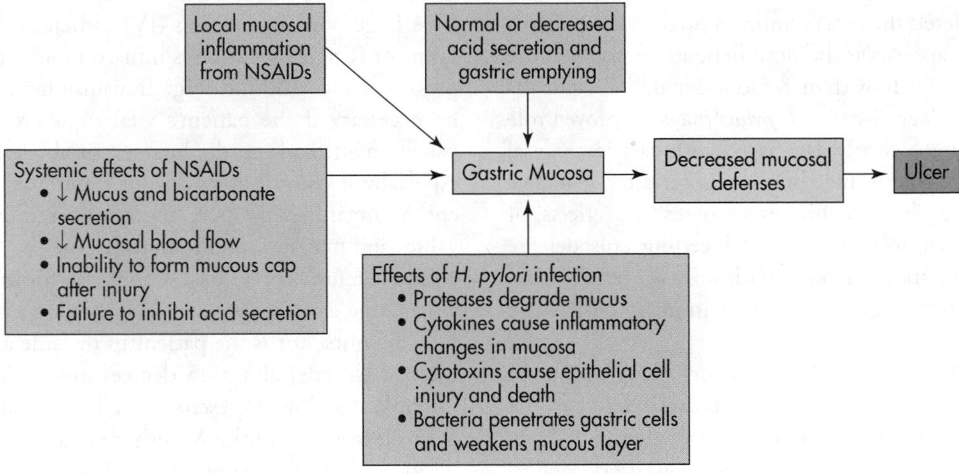

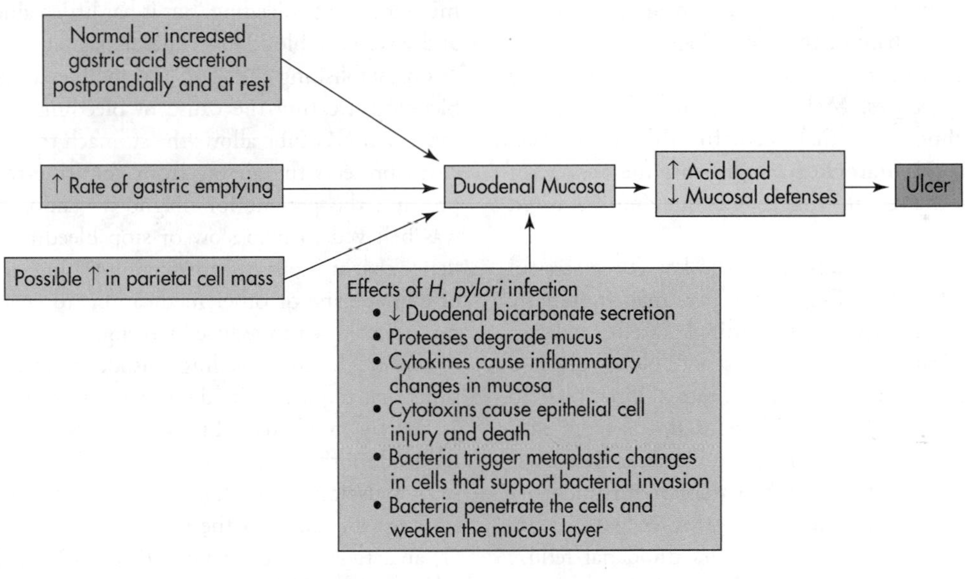

Figure 42-3 Pathophysiologic components of peptic ulcer.

COMPLICATIONS. Hemorrhage, perforation, and obstruction of the pyloric outlet are the major complications of PUD.

HEMORRHAGE. Acute upper GI bleeding results in more than 300,000 hospital admissions each year, and PUD is responsible for more than 75% of all cases.[8] The 5% to 10% associated mortality rate has remained fairly stable throughout the years despite vast improvements in treatment of both ulcer disease and bleeding.[2] Improvements in care over the past several decades appear to have been offset by the growing numbers of older patients and the fact that most upper GI bleeding–related deaths are the result of comorbid conditions and not the bleeding itself. Increasingly effective pharmacologic management of PUD has also had little if any effect on the incidence of GI bleeding, and most patients report no prior ulcer history or symptoms. Bleeding occurs from gastritis, gastric ulcers, and duodenal ulcers in approximately equal numbers.[27]

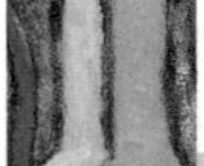

CLINICAL MANIFESTATIONS
Peptic Ulcers

- May be completely asymptomatic
- Pain:
  - —Episodic, lasting 30 minutes to 2 hours
  - —Epigastric location near midline; may radiate around costal border to back
  - —Described as dull or gnawing, burning, aching
  - —Occurs 1 to 3 hours after meals and at night (12 to 3 AM)
  - —May or may not be relieved by food or antacid
- Dyspepsia syndrome: fullness, epigastric discomfort, vague nausea, distention, and bloating
- Anorexia and weight loss

Aging is clearly the most critical risk factor, since the risk of bleeding is three to five times greater for older adults. Aspirin and NSAID use are considered the most common predisposing factors for bleeding. The risk appears to be dose dependent and is more significant for gastric bleeding than for duodenal.[35] Despite its primary role in peptic ulcer disease, *H. pylori* plays no proven role in bleeding. Alcohol use is clearly associated with gastric mucosal injury, but its causative role in bleeding is less certain.[8] Evidence does seem to indicate that alcohol exacerbates the effects of NSAIDs and aspirin. Almost 80% of all bleeding episodes are self-limiting and resolve spontaneously with only supportive care, but massive bleeding may require treatment in an intensive care unit (ICU).

The severity of ulcer bleeding ranges from slight oozing to frank, profuse hemorrhage. The term **hematemesis** refers to the vomiting of blood and usually represents a proximal upper GI site of bleeding. Emesis that is dark or of coffee-ground appearance indicates the blood has been in the stomach long enough for HCl to alter it. Bright red bleeding indicates a recent onset. Significant bleeding is almost always arterial and usually originates from a single eroded vessel in the base of the ulcer (Figure 42-4). Small arteries typically are involved, but deep erosion (more than 1 mm) may also affect larger arteries. **Melena** refers to the passage of black, tarry, foul-smelling stools that occur from the breakdown of blood in the bowel. **Hematochezia** represents the passage of bright red blood from the rectum that may or may not be mixed with stool.

Rapid assessment and resuscitation are the keys to successful treatment of upper GI bleeding. Every attempt is made to rapidly and accurately assess the severity of the bleeding. Careful vital sign assessment can yield important clues. Postural blood pressure changes of 10 mm Hg or an increase in pulse rate of more than 20 beats/min indicates at least a 20% blood loss. Clinical manifestations vary with the extent and location of the bleeding. The most common sign is hematemesis, although patients with duodenal ulcers may not exhibit any overt bleeding signs even with gastric aspiration if the pylorus successfully prevents duodenal reflux. They may experience melena. Anxiety and altered alertness may also be present. Shock will not occur until blood loss approximates 40% of the total volume, but frail older patients may exhibit signs of shock with much less significant volume losses. (See Chapter 19 for a detailed discussion of shock assessment.)

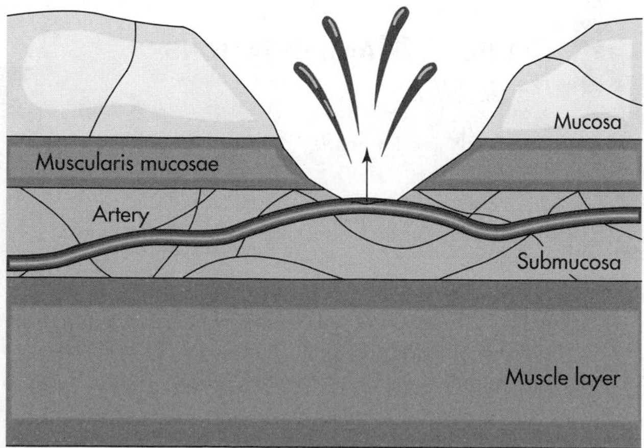

Figure 42-4 Bleeding vessel at ulcer base occurs when ulcer erodes into artery.

A large-bore intravenous (IV) catheter is inserted, and normal saline or Ringer's solution is infused rapidly to sustain the systolic pressure above 100 mm Hg. Transfusion with packed RBCs may be necessary if the patient's vital signs are unstable. Efforts are usually made to keep the hematocrit above 30% in older adults, especially if comorbid cardiac or respiratory conditions are present. Younger, healthy people can tolerate much lower hematocrit values and may not require transfusion.

Hematemesis presents a serious risk for aspiration, particularly when large clots are present. Maintaining a patent airway is critical. The nurse turns the patient to the side and keeps the head of the bed elevated about 45 degrees unless the vital signs become unstable. Suction is present at the bedside and used as needed to help clear the mouth. Mouth care after vomiting episodes is important. Supplemental oxygen is provided. Intubation may be necessary to protect the airway in the case of severe bleeding.

Nasogastric (NG) lavage has been widely used to help determine the site of bleeding, but it has little value in assessing the rate and severity of blood loss. The management of GI bleeding focuses on establishing the source of the bleeding, stopping the active bleeding, treating the cause of bleeding, and preventing recurrence. An NG tube allows the stomach to be cleared of blood and clots, protects the airway from vomiting-related aspiration, and prepares the patient for diagnostic endoscopy.[35] Gastric lavage was believed to help slow or stop bleeding, but there is no evidence that it is effective in accomplishing this goal. The addition of epinephrine or other medications to lavage solutions has also not been shown to reduce bleeding.

Although most bleeding episodes resolve spontaneously, situations that require more definitive interventions cannot always be accurately predicted. Endoscopic evaluation has dramatically reduced morbidity associated with GI bleeding and is an essential step in isolating and evaluating the bleeding site. Endoscopic findings that support the use of additional interventions include (1) an actively bleeding ulcer (Figure 42-5), (2) a nonbleeding visible vessel, and (3) an adherent clot at the base of the ulcer.[8] A clean white ulcer bed presents a very low risk of rebleeding, and most patients with this presentation can be discharged safely and monitored on an outpatient basis.[2]

Therapeutic endoscopy may incorporate thermocoagulation of the bleeding vessel, injection therapy, or both. Both approaches

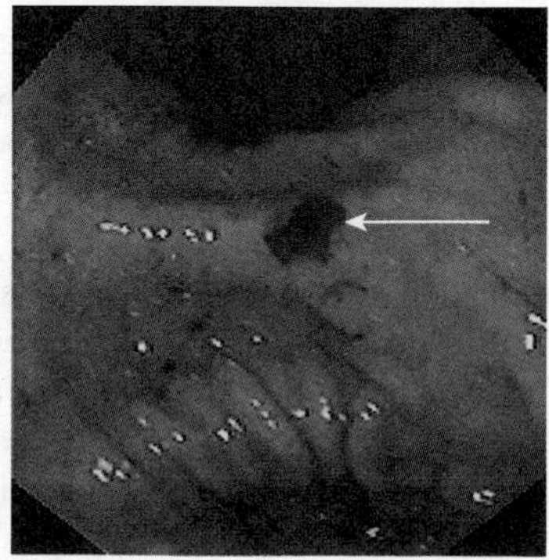

Figure 42-5 Bleeding ulcer on gastric mucosa.

are effective, and the choice is a clinical one. Thermocoagulation may be achieved through bipolar electrodes, heater probes, or laser therapy (Figure 42-6). Lasers produce excellent results, but they are expensive pieces of equipment that can rarely be brought directly to the bedside and require a highly skilled operator. Thermocoagulation with the other technologies is more efficient and cost effective.[2]

Injection therapy with epinephrine, absolute alcohol, or another sclerosing agent is the easiest and least expensive treatment approach. Injection of an epinephrine-containing solution is increasingly being combined with thermocoagulation to manage severe bleeding, and it appears to have increased effectiveness.[35] Repeat endoscopic treatment can also be employed if rebleeding occurs. Angiographic techniques that embolize the bleeding vessel with foreign materials can produce dramatic results, but the techniques require experienced and skilled angiographers.

Drug therapy during an active bleeding episode has employed antacids, H_2-receptor antagonists, and, most recently, PPIs. Neither antacids nor H_2-receptor antagonists appear to offer any therapeutic advantage during early treatment. PPIs quickly raise the gastric pH to a level that can support clotting. It is assumed that reducing the acid load promotes healing. The role and effectiveness of PPIs in healing the ulcer and preventing rebleeding appear to be even stronger, but PPIs have no proven effectiveness in managing nonulcer-related causes of bleeding. Treatment of *H. pylori* may also be appropriate once the acute bleeding has resolved, but it plays no role in controlling the initial bleeding episode.[35]

Surgery is used when nonsurgical methods have been unable to control the bleeding. However, surgical outcomes are directly linked to the promptness of the decision to operate; outcomes deteriorate rapidly when surgery is delayed. Operative mortality ranges from 30% to 40%. There is no consensus about which procedure to use. Simple oversewing of the ulcer is quick and effective, but many surgeons advocate performing an acid reduction procedure (vagotomy) at the same time to reduce the risk of future bleeding. Laparoscopic approaches have shown promise in decreasing operative mortality rates.

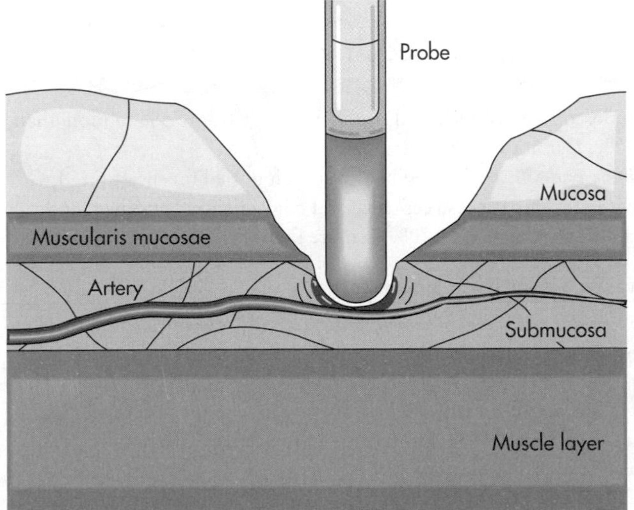

Figure 42-6 Heater probe or bipolar electrode is used first for tamponade of bleeding vessel, then to bring about coagulation.

The nursing role in the management of GI hemorrhage is largely collaborative and involves careful ongoing patient assessment, prevention of complications, and support of the patient and family. The nurse establishes IV access and implements fluid resuscitation and ongoing vital sign monitoring. The nurse may be responsible for gastric lavage. Acute bleeding can be terrifying for the patient. The nurse maintains a calm and confident approach and remains at the bedside to reassure the patient and explain all interventions. Management of the patient with GI bleeding is summarized in the Guidelines for Safe Practice box.

PERFORATION. Perforation involves the erosion of an ulcer through the muscular wall of the stomach or duodenum, with spillage of gastric secretions into the abdominal cavity. It may occur spontaneously or as a complication of therapeutic endoscopy. A chemical peritonitis quickly develops from contact with the GI contents, and a bacterial peritonitis develops within 12 hours. The clinical presentation of perforation usually is dramatic in younger adults, but it may be minimal in older persons. This typically causes delays in seeking treatment and contributes to mortality rates as high as 35% with perforation in older patients.[34] Perforations may seal spontaneously in younger adults but are less likely to do so in older persons.

The classic clinical picture of ulcer perforation includes (1) severe, sharp abdominal pain; (2) a rigid abdomen with rebound tenderness; (3) tachycardia, tachypnea, and diaphoresis; and (4) decreased bowel sounds. A perforation usually is diagnosed by the symptom pattern and the finding of subdiaphragmatic free air on abdominal x-ray film. Immediate care consists of establishing IV access to replace fluids and inserting an NG tube for drainage of the GI tract. Antibiotics are administered in anticipation of sepsis. Effective management of pain is crucial.

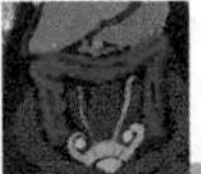

GUIDELINES FOR SAFE PRACTICE
The Patient With Gastrointestinal Bleeding

- Establish at least one large-bore intravenous (IV) access:
  —Infuse normal saline or Ringer's lactate as ordered.
  —Administer blood products as ordered.
- Monitor vital signs frequently for signs of shock.
- Start oxygen by nasal cannula as ordered (extremely important in older persons).
- Measure and record all output.
- Raise head of bed 45 degrees if vital signs remain stable.
- Turn vomiting patient on side to protect the airway.
- Maintain the patient on nothing-by-mouth status.
- Provide oral suction at bedside to help clear blood.
- Provide mouth care after vomiting episodes.
- Reassure patient and maintain a calm manner.
- Administer IV proton pump inhibitors as ordered.
- Prepare patient for therapeutic endoscopy.
- Insert nasogastric tube and institute gastric lavage if ordered:
  —Instill 250 ml room-temperature tap water.
  —Allow a 2-minute dwell time.
  —Aspirate and evaluate the returns using a piston type of syringe.

The patient is kept in a low Fowler's position to attempt to contain the escaped secretions in a limited area of the abdomen. The nurse provides the patient with emotional support and reassurance, offers comfort measures, and prepares the patient for surgery.

Surgery provides the definitive treatment for perforation. Most penetrating ulcers create pinprick holes on the anterior surface of the stomach, duodenum, or pylorus and can be readily repaired with a Graham patch, using a piece of omentum to seal the perforation.[34] Controversy exists over whether the surgery should simply repair the defect or include definitive ulcer correction. Truncal vagotomy and pyloroplasty may be performed in stable older patients in whom the risk of recurrence is believed to be high. Gastric resection is seldom the procedure of choice anymore, but it may be used in more complex cases, especially if the perforation accompanies an episode of rebleeding.

OBSTRUCTION. With improved treatment of peptic ulcers, gastric outlet obstruction has become rare. Obstruction can result from scar tissue formation, muscle obstruction, or narrowing caused by spasm and inflammatory edema. It is usually associated with longstanding PUD. The obstruction usually develops slowly, and the patient may initially experience dyspepsia symptoms, including anorexia and nausea, as the stomach fails to empty completely. Weight loss and malnutrition develop if the diagnosis is delayed, which is more likely in older persons. Vomiting occurs when the chyme is completely unable to pass into the duodenum, which usually represents a narrowing of the normally 10- to 20-mm pyloric channel to less than 6 mm.[34]

The diagnosis of obstruction can be made by aspiration of stomach contents or abdominal x-ray films that show gastric distention and large fluid levels. Endoscopy is performed to rule out an obstructing tumor and may be used to treat uncomplicated obstructions. Initial management of obstruction involves fluid and electrolyte replacement and gastric decompression with an NG tube. Aggressive therapy for the ulcer may be initiated first, since obstruction is rarely an emergent condition. The obstruction may resolve sufficiently with ulcer healing to eliminate the need for surgical intervention. When surgery is needed, vagotomy plus drainage is the procedure of choice to minimize postoperative digestive problems. Even high-risk older adults can generally tolerate this surgery if attention is paid to careful preoperative stabilization.

Collaborative Care Management

DIAGNOSTIC TESTS. The diagnosis of PUD cannot be made from the symptoms alone because they are nonspecific. A definitive diagnosis involves endoscopy with biopsy to accurately differentiate between benign ulcers and gastric cancer, which frequently initially presents as an ulcer. *H. pylori* screening is increasingly being included in the diagnostic workup for ulcers. A variety of invasive and noninvasive tests are described in Box 42-1.

MEDICATIONS. The major objectives of drug therapy for PUD are to facilitate healing, eliminate symptoms, and prevent complications and recurrences, all at reasonable cost with minimal side effects. Advances in drug therapy have dramatically changed the management of PUD. Drug therapy controls peptic ulcer symptoms effectively, often in a matter of days. It heals most ulcers completely within 8 weeks. However, ulcer relapse remains a significant problem, and long-term control is difficult. Successful ulcer treatment must also eradicate any underlying *H. pylori* infection; this is now believed to be the most important step in preventing ulcer recurrence. Common medications used to treat PUD and eradicate *H. pylori* are presented in Table 42-1.

ANTACIDS. Antacids are weak bases that neutralize free HCl to prevent irritation and permit mucosal healing. Antacids usually play a supporting role in ulcer therapy today and are used primarily for symptomatic relief; however, they can also heal ulcers, although at a slower rate than other products. The main disadvantage to antacid therapy is the frequency with which the antacids must be administered. These drugs are available over the counter.

Aluminum hydroxide antacids are the preferred preparations. In addition to neutralizing acid, they appear to decrease pepsin activity and possibly stimulate prostaglandin synthesis. Administration in tablet rather than liquid form prolongs the buffering effect slightly and is recommended. Antacids should never be given concurrently

Box 42-1 Diagnostic Tests for *H. Pylori* Screening

Noninvasive

Serology: laboratory-based ELISA: Measures immunoglobulin G (IgG) in response to *Helicobacter pylori* infection; levels remain positive for up to 1 year. More than 90% sensitivity and specificity but cannot confirm cure.

Whole blood: office-based ELISA: Again measures IgG but is less accurate. Fast, convenient, and inexpensive but sensitivity reduced to 50% to 85% and specificity to 75% to 100%.

Stool HpSA: Measures *H. pylori* antigens in the stool. Has more than 90% sensitivity and specificity and can be used to confirm cure.

Urea breath test: Measures urease activity. Has more than 95% sensitivity and specificity, although sensitivity is reduced by acid suppressive therapy. Can be used to confirm cure.

String test: Involves string being swallowed and recovered. Culture or polymerase chain reaction testing is done. A minimally invasive method of obtaining organisms for culture, but less effective than endoscopy. Sensitivity and specificity range from 75% to more than 90%. Cannot confirm cure.

Urinary and salivary ELISA: New tests being tried for measuring IgG with greater patient acceptance and convenience. Sensitivity and specificity range from 70% to more than 90%.

Invasive (Requiring Endoscopy)

Steiner's stain of biopsy specimen: Histologically identifies *H. pylori* organisms. Considered the gold standard of diagnosis. Specificity of nearly 100% and confirms cure.

Rapid urease test: Measures urease activity in a biopsy specimen. Specificity is nearly 100%, but sensitivity is reduced with bleeding and acid suppressive therapy. Can confirm cure.

Culture: Used primarily for research, since culturing the organism is technically difficult.

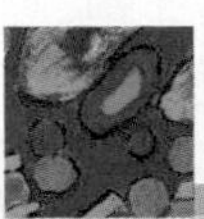

TABLE 42-1
COMMON MEDICATIONS *for Peptic Ulcer Disease*

Drug	Action	Nursing Intervention
Histamine$_2$ (H$_2$)-Receptor Antagonists		
Cimetidine (Tagamet) Ranitidine (Zantac) Famotidine (Pepcid) Nizatidine (Axid)	Inhibit HCl secretion by binding to the H_2 receptors on stomach cells and blocking the release of H_2, a potent stimulant for HCl release Acid production reduced postprandially 50%-80%	Teach patient about potential side effects, which are usually minimal. Address appropriate use of over-the-counter products.
Proton Pump Inhibitors		
Omeprazole (Prilosec) Lansoprazole (Prevacid) Pantoprazole (Protonix) Rabeprazole (Aciphex) Esomeprazole (Nexium)	Reduce 24 hr acid secretion by >90%	Teach patient safe and appropriate use and importance of not abruptly discontinuing the drug, which could trigger severe acid rebound. Address appropriate use of over-the-counter products.
Mucosal Protective Agents		
Sucralfate (Carafate)	Creates a sticky paste that coats the ulcer crater and provides barrier against irritation May increase prostaglandin synthesis	Teach patient to swallow tablet whole, not chew or crush it. Constipation is common side effect.
Misoprostol (Cytotec) Enprostil	Synthetic prostaglandin analogs that augment gastric prostaglandins in patients taking NSAIDs May have antisecretory action	Teach patient about use and side effects; abdominal discomfort and diarrhea are common. Drugs should not be used by women of childbearing years.

HCl, Hydrochloric acid; *NSAIDs*, nonsteroidal antiinflammatory drugs.

with other ulcer drugs such as H_2 blockers because they decrease drug absorption by 10% to 20%. Because aluminum hydroxide products used alone commonly cause constipation, they are usually combined with magnesium hydroxide for its laxative effect. Table 42-2 summarizes the commonly used antacids.

HISTAMINE$_2$-RECEPTOR ANTAGONISTS. H_2-receptor antagonists inhibit HCl secretion by binding to the H_2 receptors on stomach cells and blocking the release of histamine, which is a secretagogue for HCl. Basal and postprandial acid production is reduced 50% to 80%, and gastric emptying is unaffected by their use. Several different generations of H_2-receptor antagonists have been developed, with no clear evidence that one is best. They vary in potency and cost but are equally effective in healing peptic ulcers after an average of 4 weeks of therapy. Recommended dosage schedules have varied over the years. Most are now administered twice a day in divided doses or in one bedtime dose. Suppression of nocturnal acid secretion appears to support rapid healing. H_2 blockers produce few side effects and have an excellent safety record. Cimetidine (Tagamet), ranitidine (Zantac), and famotidine (Pepcid) are all available in intravenous forms to address acute and emergency situations. Several of the H_2-receptor antagonists are also now available in nonprescription strength for over-the-counter purchase.

PROTON PUMP INHIBITORS. Proton pump inhibitors (PPIs) reduce 24-hour acid production by more than 90% with a single daily dose, and they are significantly more effective than other medications in healing ulcers. With higher doses, acid secretion is virtually eliminated, and clinically significant side effects are rare. These drugs also appear to have some antibacterial effect on *H. pylori* infection and are increasingly being included in treatment protocols. Available drugs include omeprazole (Prilosec), lansoprazole (Prevacid), pantoprazole (Protonix), rabeprazole (Aciphex), and esomeprazole (Nexium). Prohibitive cost is their major drawback. Omeprazole is now available for over the counter purchase.

MUCOSAL PROTECTIVE AGENTS. Improved understanding of the etiology of peptic ulcers has shifted attention to the development and use of drugs designed to support the mucosal barrier. These include sucralfate (Carafate) and misoprostol (Cytotec).

Sucralfate is a complex of aluminum hydroxide and sulfated sucrose that is believed to coat an ulcer crater and provide a sealant barrier against acid irritation. Research indicates that it also acts as a cytoprotective agent and increases prostaglandin synthesis.[11] It neither inhibits acid secretion nor neutralizes gastric acid, but it is comparable to H_2 blockers in its ability to heal ulcers. Its only common side effect is constipation. The drug comes in a large tablet and must be taken orally several times a day, which limits its acceptability to patients. A liquid form is in use in critical care. Combining sucralfate with an acid-suppressing agent does not significantly improve healing and is not recommended.

Misoprostol and the newer enprostil are synthetic prostaglandin analogs that offer a new dimension in ulcer management. They enhance mucosal defenses by replacing gastric prostaglandins and also appear to have some antisecretory properties. In low doses they have a protective effect on the stomach but not the duodenum. They are used primarily for the prevention of gastric ulcers in high-risk older patients who need to continue to take NSAIDs.[36] The pain-relieving effectiveness of NSAIDs does not appear to be lessened by their use. Misoprostol frequently causes diarrhea and crampy abdominal pain, which are usually dose dependent. The drug can

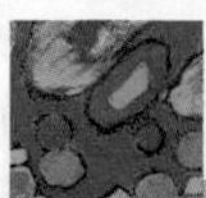

TABLE 42-2
COMMON MEDICATIONS *for Ulcer Discomfort (Antacids)*

Drug	Action	Nursing Intervention
Aluminum Products		
Amphojel AlternaGEL Alu-Cap Basaljel	All antacids act by buffering excess acidity in stomach to neutralize pH.	All aluminum hydroxide antacids are constipating. Teach patient to maintain regular bowel elimination. Teach patient to use as needed for ulcer discomfort, but not at the same time as a histamine$_2$-receptor antagonist.
Combinations of Aluminum and Magnesium		
Maalox Gaviscon Magaldrate (Riopan)	As above	As above, but nonconstipating.
Calcium Products		
Alka-Mints Tums Rolaids	As above	As above, but only for short-term use. These are often severely constipating and may cause acid rebound.
Antacids With Simethicone		
Mylanta Maalox Plus Gelusil	As above	Simethicone is non–gas forming and can be recommended to patients with gas problems. These are also nonconstipating.

NOTE: Antacid tablets have a longer duration of effect than liquids and are recommended.

induce abortion, and it is not used by women of childbearing age. The increased use of selective COX-2 NSAIDs for managing arthritis pain was expected to decrease the incidence of NSAID-related ulceration, but ongoing research has not consistently demonstrated a strong protective effect, especially in preventing recurrent bleeding.[6]

***HELICOBACTER PYLORI* DRUG TREATMENT.** *H. pylori* infection is now recognized as the main determinant of ulcer relapse, but controversy continues over exactly which patients need to be treated for the infection. Consensus is slowly emerging, however, that *H. pylori* treatment is a cost-effective way of preventing predictable ulcer reoccurrence.[32]

Drug protocols for the treatment of *H. pylori infection* continue to evolve with research and testing. Drug regimens involve three or four drugs because no single agent has proven effective, and the development of antibiotic-resistant strains of the organism is an increasing concern.[24] Treatment takes 10 days to 2 weeks and involves taking multiple pills a day with a variety of side effects. Treatment adherence is a serious concern. Box 42-2 summarizes some recommended treatment options. Treatment of the *H. pylori* infection reduces the incidence of ulcer relapse to well below 10%, and often makes maintenance therapy with PPIs or other drugs unnecessary (see Research and Evidence-Based Practice boxes).

TREATMENTS. No treatments are routinely ordered because most peptic ulcers respond to an aggressive pharmacologic approach. If an ulcer bleeds, obstructs, or perforates, however, the management shifts dramatically. Treatments for these problems are discussed under Complications.

SURGICAL MANAGEMENT. The emergence of effective drug therapy for PUD has also changed the role of surgery in disease management. Surgery is used primarily for the management of complications such as perforation and the treatment of the occasional intractable ulcer that is resistant to all standard therapy. Patients who require surgery to manage acute complications are usually older and frailer and commonly have significant comorbid conditions, which frequently compromise outcomes.[34]

The **omental patch** to close perforations and **vagotomy**, with or without drainage procedures, are the most commonly performed ulcer surgeries today. Vagotomy procedures reduce gastric acid production by decreasing cholinergic stimulation of the parietal cells and limiting the response to gastrin. The vagotomy procedure of choice is the highly selective vagotomy, which preserves the pylorus and almost abolishes the negative outcomes of dump-

BOX 42-2 *Helicobacter pylori* Treatment Options

Triple Therapy Options

1. Omeprazole or lansoprazole *plus* metronidazole or amoxicillin *plus* clarithromycin
2. Ranitidine bismuth citrate *plus* clarithromycin or metronidazole *plus* tetracycline or ampicillin

Quadruple Therapy Options

1. Bismuth subsalicylate *plus* metronidazole *plus* tetracycline *plus* a histamine$_2$-receptor antagonist
2. Bismuth subsalicylate *plus* metronidazole *plus* tetracycline *plus* a proton pump inhibitor

NOTE: Most regimens are prescribed for 10 to 14 days. Antibiotics may need to be taken up to four times daily. Combination drug packaging is increasingly available.

Research

Tomita T et al: Successful eradication of *H. pylori* prevents relapse of peptic ulcer disease, *Aliment Pharmacol Therap* 16(Suppl 2):204-209, 2002.

This study sought to validate the hypothesis that eradication of *Helicobacter pylori* infection helps prevent the recurrence of peptic ulcers. A pool of 445 patients with duodenal and gastric ulcers was randomly assigned to three groups. The first group (A) received conventional treatment with a proton pump inhibitor (PPI). The second group (B) received a PPI plus one recommended antibiotic. The third group (C) received a PPI plus two recommended antibiotics. Eradication of *H. pylori* was assessed by biopsy with endoscopy at 4 weeks and 6 and 12 months. Endoscopy screening was continued for 5 years.

Eradication rates were group A, 0%; group B, 46%; and group C, 80%. No ulcer relapse occurred in duodenal ulcer patients with successful eradication after 5 years, and relapse occurred in only 4% of gastric ulcer patients. In contrast, relapse rates were 100% and 92% for duodenal and gastric ulcer patients who did not experience eradication of *H. pylori*.

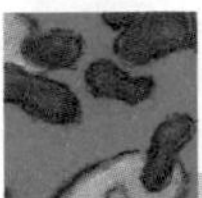

EVIDENCE-BASED PRACTICE

Topic Question: Is *Helicobacter pylori* eradication therapy more effective than antisecretory therapy in preventing recurrent bleeding from peptic ulcers?

Evidence Base: The review of evidence included seven studies with a total of 518 patients in the first meta-analysis and three studies of 470 patients in the second. All included patients who experienced peptic ulcer bleeding and were treated with various protocols of proton pump inhibitors and *H. pylori* eradication therapy.

Findings: Eradication of *H. pylori* was consistently associated with a significantly lower incidence of rebleeding from peptic ulcer disease, even with the inclusion of patients who continued to use nonsteroidal antiinflammatory drugs.

Conclusions: Treatment of *H. pylori* infection is more effective than antisecretory, noneradicating therapy (with or without long-term maintenance therapy) in preventing rebleeding from peptic ulcer. All patients with peptic ulcer bleeding should be tested for *H. pylori* and receive eradication therapy if positive for the bacterium.

Gisbert JP et al: *H. pylori* eradication therapy vs. antisecretory noneradication therapy for the prevention of recurrent bleeding from peptic ulcer, *Cochrane Library* (2):ID#CD004062, 2004.

ing syndrome, diarrhea, and bilious vomiting. More aggressive procedures that include various forms of partial gastrectomy are rarely recommended today. Vagotomy procedures are being successfully adapted for laparoscopic approaches, which appear to significantly minimize morbidity and recovery time.[37] All vagotomy procedures are highly technical, with results strongly related to the surgeon's skill and experience.[20] Figure 42-7 illustrates the various approaches to vagotomy.

DIET. The role of diet in PUD management has changed dramatically over the past 40 years. The Sippy and Hurst milk-based therapy was used for years in the belief that constantly diluting and neutralizing acid would facilitate ulcer healing. Although milk-based diets provide symptomatic relief, they do not influence healing. In fact, research has shown that the amino acids and calcium in milk act as secretagogues and increase acid secretion.[24] Current thinking is that diet plays no defined role in ulcer etiology or treatment. Bland diets do not facilitate healing; patients are simply encouraged to eliminate or restrict specific foods that cause discomfort until healing occurs.

HEALTH PROMOTION AND PREVENTION. The vast majority of ulcers are caused by *H. pylori* infection and the adverse effects of NSAID use. At present there are no recommendations for routine screening for *H. pylori* unless the individual develops ulcer-related symptoms or complications.[28] *H. pylori* infection is acquired early in life, possibly from contaminated water, and more than 90% of those infected are asymptomatic. A stronger case can be made for prevention related to NSAID use. Although the vast majority of NSAID users never develop GI problems, the risk increases with age and duration of use. Acetaminophen is the least damaging analgesic and should be used if at all possible. High-risk patients should at least be evaluated for possible misoprostol administration. Smoking cessation and alcohol moderation are other important considerations for health promotion and prevention.

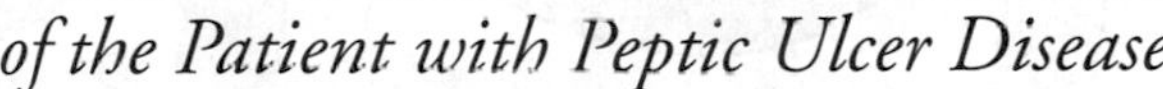

Nursing Management

of the Patient with Peptic Ulcer Disease

ASSESSMENT

Health History. Assess for:

- Pain: presence, location, severity, nature, and relationship to eating and sleeping
- Medications used (prescription, over the counter, and herbal preparations), particularly aspirin, NSAIDs, and other ulcerogenic drugs; frequency and pattern of use; effectiveness for symptom control
- Dietary habits, meal patterns, and alcohol history
- Smoking history
- General lifestyle: work, leisure, exercise, stressors, usual coping measures
- Knowledge of PUD: causes, treatment, complications

Physical Examination. Assess for:

- Evidence of GI bleeding, including occult blood in stool
- Changes in hemoglobin, hematocrit, and red blood cell (RBC) counts
- Weight loss or gain from baseline

NURSING DIAGNOSES, OUTCOMES, AND INTERVENTIONS

Nursing Diagnosis: Acute Pain

OUTCOMES. A common example of an expected outcome for the patient with a diagnosis of *acute pain* related to mucosal irritation is: Patient will:

- Describe pain as decreased, minimal, or absent.

NURSING INTERVENTIONS. Taking prescribed medications as ordered is the major strategy for relieving ulcer pain. Drug therapy

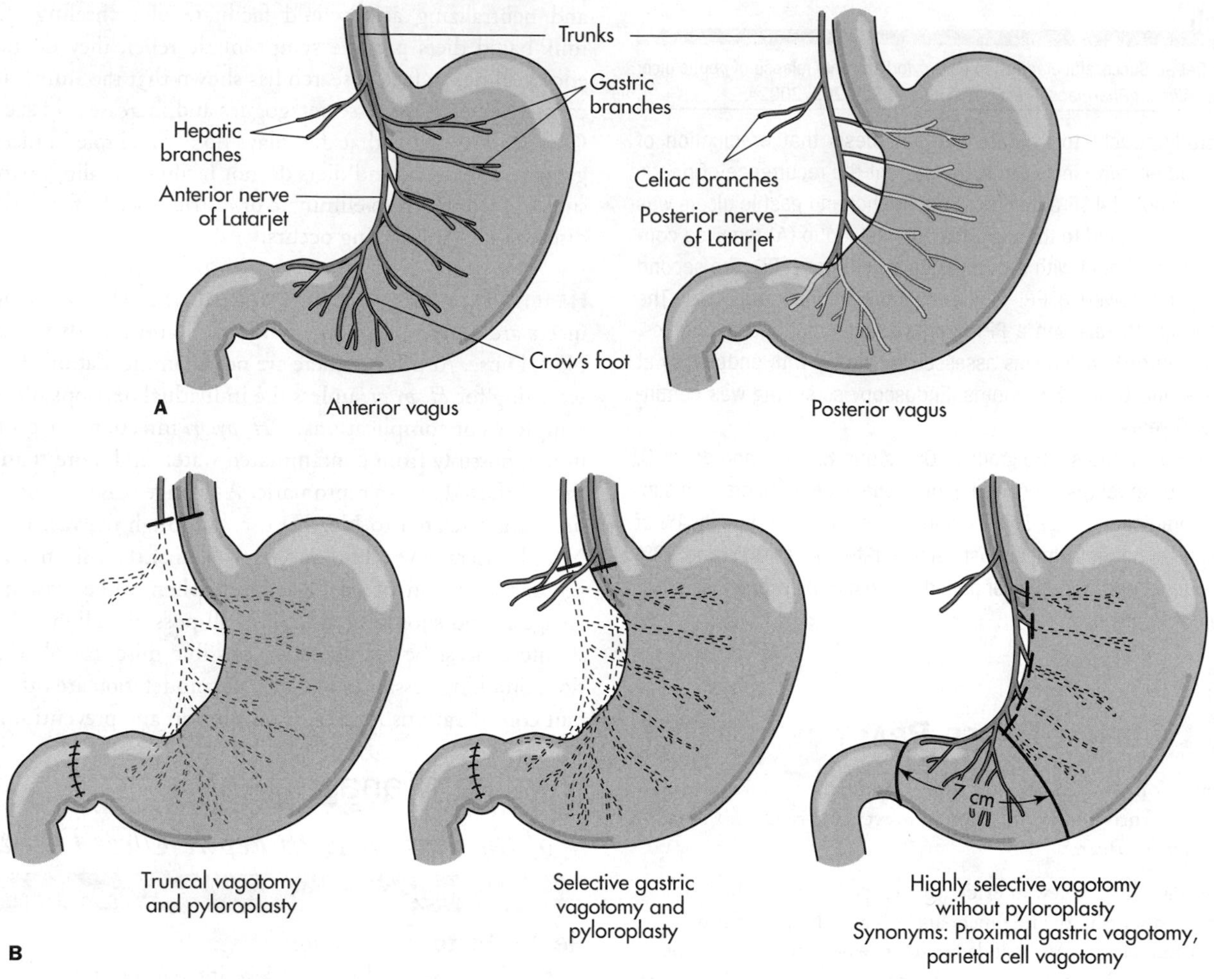

Figure 42-7 **A,** Normal vagal anatomy. **B,** Types of vagotomy with and without pyloroplasty.

controls or eliminates the pain within a few days to a week, but peptic ulcer control is a long-term process. Successful self-care depends on a clear understanding of the purpose of each drug and the importance of adherence to the complete ulcer regimen, including follow-up care. Initial treatment is likely to involve daily use of a PPI. Antacids may be used to control breakthrough discomfort or dyspepsia. Most cases of ulcer relapse can be traced to nonadherence unless the initial treatment is inadequate or does not include treatment of *H. pylori.* The nurse stresses the importance of regimen adherence from the first day of treatment.

Related NIC Interventions. Medication Administration: Oral, Medication Management, Pain Management, Teaching: Prescribed Medication

Nursing Diagnosis: Risk for Ineffective Health Maintenance

Outcomes. A common example of expected outcomes for the patient with a diagnosis of *ineffective health maintenance* is:
Patient will:

- Accurately describe the components of disease management, including:
  Medication schedule and control of side effects
  Lifestyle factors that may facilitate ulcer healing
  Symptoms that indicate complications
  Plans for follow-up care

Nursing Interventions. PUD treatment typically occurs in the home setting with patient self-management unless complications occur. Adherence issues are important. The severity of symptoms provides an initial impetus for regimen adherence, but this effect is often difficult to sustain once symptom control has been achieved. Patient education is essential for long-term success.

The nurse strongly encourages the patient to substitute the use of acetaminophen for NSAIDs in routine pain and fever management. Patients with chronic arthritis who need to continue daily NSAID use are encouraged to explore with their physician the use of misoprostol or a COX-2 inhibitor NSAID that might decrease the risk of gastric ulceration. This is particularly important for older patients.

The nurse encourages the patient to avoid any food that causes discomfort and to avoid overdistention of the stomach and binge eating. No research evidence shows that a pattern of small, frequent feedings is any more effective in ulcer healing than a standard three-meal-a-day pattern, but patients should avoid overeating. Eating slowly and chewing thoroughly prevent overdistention and reflux. Bedtime snacking may promote nighttime acid secretion and should be avoided.

The nurse may encourage the patient to limit the use of foods that have been shown to have a strong acid-stimulating effect, at least during the initial treatment period. These include coffee, tea, cola, beer, and chocolate. Direct irritants such as spices and red and black pepper also should be limited.

The role of lifestyle or psychologic stress in PUD, if any, is unclear, although mental and physical rest does appear to facilitate ulcer healing. The nurse encourages the patient to establish a pattern of regular exercise and to explore appropriate approaches to stress reduction at home and work.

The role of cigarette smoking in ulcer relapse is clearly documented, and the nurse strongly encourages the patient to quit smoking. Referral to community smoking cessation programs should be made in consultation with the health care provider about the appropriateness of the various nicotine replacement systems. The role of alcohol in ulcer relapse is less clear, but moderation is encouraged, and alcohol should never be ingested on an empty stomach because of its irritating effects on the mucosa.

A Nursing Care Plan for a patient with a peptic ulcer is found on p. 1218.

RELATED NIC INTERVENTIONS. Health Education, Risk Identification, Teaching: Disease Process

Patient/Family Teaching. The nurse teaches the patient with PUD how to take prescribed medications and discusses the management of common side effects. Patients are taught to never abruptly discontinue their antiulcer medications because of the danger of severe acid rebound. Antacids interfere with the absorption of PPIs or H_2-receptor antagonists and therefore should not be taken at the same time.

The nurse cautions the patient about the use of over-the-counter H_2-receptor antagonists once therapy is completed. The return of pain may indicate that the ulcer treatment has been inadequate or that further *H. pylori* treatment is indicated. Use of over-the-counter ulcer medications to manage symptoms could delay treatment or mask complications.

Although the initial peptic ulcer cannot usually be prevented, it is often possible to minimize the risk of relapse by effective *H. pylori* treatment. Many patients are unaware of the role of *H. pylori* in ulcer development, and the nurse teaches the patient about this and the importance of completing recommended treatment to prevent relapse. Other teaching components for effective health maintenance are summarized in the Patient/Family Teaching box.

EVALUATION

To evaluate the effectiveness of nursing interventions, compare patient behaviors with those stated in the expected patient outcomes.

RELATED NOC OUTCOMES. Client Satisfaction: Symptom Control, Comfort Level, Knowledge: Disease Process, Symptom Control

GERONTOLOGIC CONSIDERATIONS

Although the incidence of PUD in the general population has declined, the incidence in older persons has increased slightly as the population ages. Older adults are much more likely to be colonized by *H. pylori,* which contributes to an increased incidence of peptic ulcers.

Hospitalization rates for older adults with PUD also have risen steadily in the face of a continuing overall decline in hospitalization for the disease. Most of the complications and mortality associated with ulcers occur in older patients, with more than 80% of ulcer-related deaths occurring in the over-65 age-group.

Older adults experience frequent dyspepsia, which hinders the diagnosis of ulcers. They are also less likely to seek medical attention for their symptoms. The frequent use of NSAIDs in this population is another significant contributor to ulcer incidence. An estimated 1% to 2% of the total U.S. population uses NSAIDs

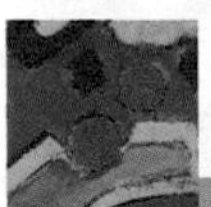

PATIENT/FAMILY TEACHING *Managing a Peptic Ulcer*

Know the symptoms of ulcer recurrence and report them promptly to your health care provider.

Medications

Know the dosage, administration, action, and side effects of all drugs in use.

Take all of prescribed drug, even when pain is relieved. It is essential to complete the full treatment to eradicate *Helicobacter pylori* and prevent recurrence.

Keep antacids available for use as needed, but do not take them at the same time as a histamine$_2$-receptor antagonist or proton pump inhibitor. Antacids should be taken 1 to 3 hours after meals, at bedtime, and as needed for pain.

Use acetaminophen for routine pain relief during treatment if needed. Avoid the use of all nonsteroidal antiinflammatory drugs (NSAIDs), including aspirin and ibuprofen.

If the treatment of arthritis or other chronic illness requires the ongoing use of NSAIDs, explore with health care provider the use of misoprostol or a COX-2 inhibitor.

Diet

Eat slowly and chew foods thoroughly. Do not overeat.

Avoid any foods that increase discomfort.

Avoid the use of alcohol during treatment if possible.

Never drink alcohol on an empty stomach.

Avoid bedtime snacking because it increases nighttime acid secretion.

Smoking

Stop smoking if possible.

Explore community supports for smoking cessation or use of nicotine withdrawal patches.

Stress Reduction

Provide for increased rest during healing.

Participate in recreation and hobbies that promote relaxation.

Participate in a moderate aerobic exercise program for promotion of well-being.

Nursing Care Plan

Patient With a Bleeding Peptic Ulcer

Data The patient is a 42-year-old man who relates a 4-year history of intermittent "stomach pain" that he self-treats with Maalox and over-the-counter cimetidine. Pertinent history includes taking aspirin on a regular basis for headaches, smoking about one and a half packs of cigarettes daily (though he has tried to quit on numerous occasions), drinking three or four beers an average of three times weekly, and working at a high-stress job.

Two days ago he was admitted to the hospital with hematemesis, tarry stools, lightheadedness, acute pain, and blood pressure of 96/54 mm Hg (baseline blood pressure of 124/84 mm Hg). Intravenous fluids were initiated and a nasogastric (NG) tube inserted for lavage. When the bleeding persisted, an endoscopic examination was performed and treatment of a duodenal ulcer started. Antacids were administered hourly through the NG tube, and *H. pylori* treatment with antibiotics and a PPI was initiated.

The patient's blood pressure is now stable, and the NG tube has been removed. He is taking oral fluids and has been started on a soft diet. He continues to receive antibiotics and a PPI. Maalox 30 ml is ordered 1 hour and 3 hours after meals as needed. The patient states that he is unaware of the nature of peptic ulcer disease, its treatment, and potential complications.

Nursing Diagnosis

Acute pain related to duodenal mucosal irritation and ulceration

Outcomes

- Patient will report pain of less than 3 on a scale of 0 to 10.
- Patient will report satisfactory control of gastric pain.

Related NOC Outcomes

- Comfort Level
- Pain Control
- Pain Level

Related NIC Interventions

- Analgesic Administration
- Pain Management

Nursing Interventions/Rationales

- Administer the PPI once daily before breakfast. PPIs reduce gastric acid secretion by greater than 90%, which supports healing and aids in eradication of *H. pylori*. *Pain is reduced as inflammation is reduced and healing occurs.*
- Administer antacids as prescribed. *Antacids neutralize HCl and quickly reduce pain; they interfere with absorption of PPIs given concurrently. They must be administered frequently because they are cleared rapidly from the stomach.*
- Monitor pain quality and duration. *To differentiate ulcer pain from perforation and to determine the effectiveness of medications.*

Nursing Diagnosis

Ineffective health maintenance related to lack of knowledge of disease process, treatment regimen, and complications

Outcomes

- Patient will verbalize understanding of disease process, treatment regimen, and potential complications.
- Patient will verbalize the need to make lifestyle modifications necessary to facilitate ulcer healing.
- Patient will adhere to prescribed medication regimen.

Related NOC Outcomes

- Health Promoting Behavior
- Knowledge: Treatment Regimen
- Participation in Health Care Decisions

Related NIC Interventions

- Health System Guidance
- Self-Modification Assistance
- Smoking Cessation Assistance
- Teaching: Disease Process

Nursing Interventions/Rationales

- Encourage patient to avoid foods that cause pain or stimulate acid formation (tea, coffee, chocolate, cola, milk). *Dietary elements do not cause and cannot heal ulcers, but they can increase discomfort.*
- Teach patient the effect of aspirin use and smoking on peptic ulcer disease. *Aspirin and ibuprofen contribute to mucosal breakdown. Smoking appears to exacerbate ulcer relapse.*
- Refer patient to community smoking cessation program. *Greater success with smoking cessation may be achieved when support systems are available and used.*
- Encourage the use of acetaminophen instead of aspirin or ibuprofen for routine pain relief. *Acetaminophen does not contribute to mucosal breakdown.*
- Avoid use of over-the-counter H_2 receptor antagonists or PPIs unless prescribed. *May mask ulcer relapse symptoms.*
- Encourage the use of stress-reduction techniques. *Ulcer recurrence is more common in patients with chronic anxiety and poor coping skills.*
- Explain side effects of prescribed medications and potential effect on bowel elimination. *Antacids may have either a cathartic or constipating effect depending on their constituents. Bowel elimination may need to be supported through dietary changes.*
- Reinforce the importance of completing *H. pylori* treatment to prevent relapse. H. pylori *drug treatment creates multiple gastrointestinal side effects that adversely affect treatment adherence. Failure to adhere contributes to drug resistance.*
- Teach patient to monitor for and report persistent epigastric pain, sudden severe abdominal pain, tarry stools, persistent vomiting, and bloody or brown vomitus. *These symptoms may indicate ulcer complications such as gastrointestinal bleeding, perforation, or obstruction.*

Evaluation

Evaluation is based on comparing the patient's outcomes with desired outcomes.

daily, and older adults are the most frequent users. From 2% to 4% of long-term NSAID users develop serious complications each year, and 30% of ulcer-related deaths can be directly attributed to NSAID use. If GI hemorrhage occurs, its seriousness is potentiated by the platelet inhibition associated with NSAID use.

PUD often manifests in an atypical manner in older adults. Symptoms tend to be more poorly defined, and the classic pain is frequently absent. If discomfort is present at all, it often is poorly localized and vague, radiating in confusing ways that overlap with the presentations of angina, gallbladder disease, and dysphagia. Because early, accurate diagnosis is rare, ulcers in older adults tend to be larger or already causing complications at diagnosis. The risk of serious complications is four times higher in older persons, and most patients are completely asymptomatic until complications develop. Older women appear to be at particular risk.

The diagnosis and treatment of PUD in older adults follow the same guidelines previously outlined. Older adults are more likely to require aggressive *H. pylori* treatment to heal the ulcer and minimize relapse, and they are more likely to need maintenance ulcer therapy. Older adults should be thoroughly assessed concerning their use of both prescription and over-the-counter NSAIDs and cautioned to eliminate use of these drugs if possible. Acetaminophen is considered a much safer alternative for occasional use than aspirin and most NSAIDs. Consideration should be given to the use of a COX-2 inhibitor NSAID or a synthetic prostaglandin such as misoprostol in this population.

▶ ARE You READY?

Which of the following statements by a patient with peptic ulcer disease indicates that dietary teaching was effective?

1. "I only have to avoid those foods that cause me to have pain after eating."
2. "I should eat six bland meals per day."
3. "I should include a milk product with each meal."
4. "It is important that I eat within 2 hours of going to bed."

Stress Ulcers

Etiology and Epidemiology. The terms *stress-related mucosal damage* and *stress ulcer* refer to a syndrome characterized by the development of multiple diffuse gastric lesions and ulceration shortly after the onset of acute illness, trauma, or sepsis. In the 1970s the incidence of stress ulcers in the critical care population was greater than 80%, and the incidence of clinically significant bleeding was nearly 20%.[1] Because GI hemorrhage in the critically ill was accompanied by a high mortality rate, aggressive prevention protocols were developed and implemented with virtually every critically ill patient. The incidence of significant bleeding has declined dramatically over the past 15 to 20 years, probably in response to significant overall improvements in the care of the critically ill. Clinically significant bleeding is now a rare event, but a mortality rate of nearly 50% is still associated with the development of upper GI bleeding after admission and continues to make the prevention of significant stress ulcer bleeding in high-risk patients a top priority.[1]

Not all ICU patients are at equal risk for stress ulcer bleeding (see Risk Factors box). Multiple studies over the past decade have confirmed the importance of two major risk factors: mechanical ventilation for more than 48 hours and coagulopathy.[38] Shock is considered a secondary risk factor, and advanced age complicates the situation. Other factors that have not proven to be statistically significant on their own include sepsis, liver failure, kidney failure, enteral feedings, and glucocorticoid administration. However, their presence may increase the risk of patients who already have a primary risk factor. Current research focuses on the effectiveness of prevention strategies in high-risk patients and the need for ongoing aggressive prevention in patients without a primary risk factor.

Pathophysiology. The major factor that causes stress ulceration is a loss of ability to maintain the integrity of the gastric mucosa. The maintenance of mucosal homeostasis is a complex process involving mucus production, mucosal blood flow, prostaglandin secretion, bicarbonate production, and maintenance of the needed pH gradient. The severe stress state decreases gastric mucosal blood flow and triggers a series of changes that can ultimately result in mucosal breakdown. The epithelial cells of the mucosa are extremely sensitive to hypoxia, and the process of cellular necrosis can begin within minutes. Drops in intramural pH appear to be the key. The incidence of bleeding increases in direct proportion as the intramural pH falls from 8 to 6. Stress ulceration cannot occur without the presence of acid and pepsin, but actual overproduction of acid is rarely the cause. In fact, acid secretion typically is diminished in the acute stress state. Mucosal resistance therefore is believed to be the key. The notable exceptions are **Cushing's ulcer** and **Curling's ulcer**, which are associated with massive increases in acid output, often exceeding 3 to 4 L/day.

Stress ulcer lesions tend to be shallower than standard peptic ulcers and develop in multiple sites rather than as a single well-defined lesion. The proximal acid-secreting areas of the stomach are the prime targets. The classic presentation of stress ulcers is the development of painless GI bleeding within 3 to 7 days of admission to a critical care unit.

Risk Factors

Stress Ulcer Bleeding

Primary

Intubation with mechanical ventilation for longer than 48 hours
Coagulopathy
Hypotension or shock (did not quite reach statistical significance in studies)

Secondary

Sepsis
Liver failure
Kidney failure

NOTE: The presence of more than one risk factor significantly increases the likelihood of bleeding. Advanced age compounds the risk.

Collaborative Care Management. Clinical management focuses on prevention because of the high mortality rate associated with significant stress ulcer bleeding. The challenge is to identify which patients to treat prophylactically and in what way. Efficacy, ease of administration, and cost are all important considerations. The traditional approach was to treat all critical care patients aggressively with antacids, acid suppressors, or sucralfate. Frequent monitoring of gastric pH is usually performed through either intermittent aspiration of gastric secretions or special NG tubes capable of continuous pH monitoring. The pH of the gastric aspirate is usually kept above 3.5, although some sources recommend a pH of at least 4.0.[17]

Authorities are increasingly recommending that only critical care patients with primary risk factors or multiple risk factors be routinely treated with the intent of preventing stress ulcer bleeding. Treatment options include antacids, H_2-receptor antagonists, PPIs, and sucralfate. Multiple clinical studies have reported contradictory conclusions, but the consensus is that antacids are the least effective choice, and their use is no longer recommended.[38] Sucralfate has shown consistent effectiveness and, in some studies, is linked with a lower incidence of ventilator-associated pneumonia; but the need to administer the drug either orally or by NG tube limits its usefulness. Less comparative data are available about the usefulness of PPIs, but the data that exist indicate PPIs are more effective than H_2-receptor antagonists.[42] The availability of IV pantoprazole rapidly expanded the use of this class of drugs in critical care. The issue has significant cost implications, especially with the increased popularity of PPIs, and continues to be studied.

Concern arose that the prophylactic neutralization of gastric secretions might be contributing to an increased incidence of pneumonia in mechanically ventilated patients. In the absence of gastric acid, nosocomial organisms can colonize the stomach within 2 to 5 days. Research is ongoing, but again the results have so far been contradictory.[19] Much remains to be learned about the origins, prevention, and treatment of stress ulcers, but clearly meticulous bedside monitoring of critically ill patients by skilled ICU nurses will continue to play an essential role. As PPIs are increasingly prescribed for the management of GERD and PUD, concern has also arisen about the pulmonary risks for long-term users in the community. The Research box presents the results of one major study.

Research

Laheij RJF et al: Risk of community acquired pneumonia and use of gastric acid suppressive drugs, *JAMA* 292(16):2013-2016, 2004.

This study used the national Integrated Primary Care Information database that is maintained in the Netherlands. It identified a study population of more than 350,000 individuals and a subset of individuals prescribed acid suppression drugs whose health was then monitored by their primary care practitioners for 1 to 7 years. In this cohort of patients the use of acid suppression drugs was associated with an increased risk of community-acquired pneumonia. The risk was most significant for persons taking proton pump inhibitors and showed a clear dose response relationship.

This study adds significant evidence to the evolving hypothesis that the use of acid suppression therapy weakens the barrier that gastric acid provides against pathogen invasion from the gastrointestinal tract and increases the risk of bacterial and viral colonization.

Patient/Family Teaching. The nurse needs to keep critically ill patients and families informed about all aspects of the care plan, including all measures aimed at the identification, prevention, or treatment of stress ulcers. The nurse is the primary liaison with the family and informs them about the rationale for all planned interventions.

Most laypersons are not familiar with stress ulcers, and the nurse needs to lay the foundation for understanding all relevant care. The stresses of the situation may make it difficult for the patient and family to hear and process information, and time for reteaching should be planned as needed.

Cancer of the Stomach

Etiology and Epidemiology. Gastric cancer was once the leading cause of cancer death worldwide; despite declining incidence in Europe, North America, and Australia, it still ranks as the second leading cause of cancer death in the world.[22] Since the 1940s, the mortality rate from gastric cancer in the United States has declined from 22.5 to 6 per 100,000 population, and the incidence declined almost 70% between 1950 and 1980.[22] The disease exhibits tremendous variation among different regions of the world; it is10 times more common in Japan, which has the highest incidence in the world. Gastric cancer primarily affects individuals over 65 years of age in the United States and is rare before age 40. The age at diagnosis in Japan tends to be at least a decade younger.[31] The male/female ratio is about 2:1.

The etiology of gastric cancer is multifactorial, and its highly erratic worldwide incidence pattern indicates a complex interplay of genetic-familial, environmental, and cultural factors. Environmental factors are clearly pivotal, since the incidence of the disease in immigrants to the United States drops sharply by the second generation. Diet has received a great deal of attention, but no single dietary element explains the great variations in incidence. High nitrate content in soil and water and diets high in smoked and salt-preserved foods are believed to be important factors. Nitrates and nitrites in foods are reduced to nitrosamines in the body, which can trigger a cascade of deoxyribonucleic acid (DNA) changes that lead to cancer. Improved access to refrigeration and fresh fruits and vegetables appears to have decreased the risk in industrialized societies despite the fact that vegetables are a major source of nitrates in some diets.

Lower temperatures reduce the rate of bacterial, fungal, and other contaminants of fresh food, as well as the bacterial formation of nitrites, but the correlation of these factors with carcinogenesis is unproven. Cultures with diets high in salt (dried, salted, and smoked foods) exhibit a 50% to 80% increase in gastric cancer risk.[22] A high intake of fresh fruits and raw vegetables has repeatedly been found to convey a protective effect against cancer of the stomach. The sharp decline in incidence rates for gastric cancer in the United States since the 1950s is largely believed to be attributable to these factors. Alcohol and caffeine have not been shown to be independent risk factors for gastric cancer, but heavy cigarette smoking clearly increases risk (see Risk Factors box).

Familial clusters are seen in gastric cancer, and individuals with a first-degree relative with the disease have a two or three times

Risk Factors

Gastric Cancer

- *Helicobacter pylori*–initiated chronic gastritis
- Diets high in smoked and preserved foods, which contain nitrites and nitrates and high levels of salt
- Diets low in fresh fruits and vegetables
- High nitrate content in the soil and water
- History of heavy smoking
- Age and sex (steadily increasing incidence after age 40; male-to-female ratio of 2:1)
- Genetic abnormalities

NOTE: Aspirin appears to have a protective effect and lowers risk.

greater risk of developing it. Researchers are increasingly identifying genetic factors, primarily related to changes affecting tumor suppressor genes.[22] COX-2 levels have also been found to be elevated in gastric cancer, and aspirin use appears to play a protective role. The role of *H. pylori* infection has received increasing attention in recent years as its causative role in PUD has been confirmed. A significant group of *H. pylori*–infected patients develop achlorhydria, and atrophic gastritis appears also to be linked to the development of gastric cancer.[31] Therefore *H. pylori* infection is now considered to be a major carcinogen for gastric cancer despite the confounding data demonstrating that the vast majority of persons infected with *H. pylori* never develop either ulcers or cancer.[5]

Pathophysiology. Most gastric cancers are primary adenocarcinomas derived from the epithelium. The disease can be divided into two main pathologic varieties. The diffuse form, which lacks glandular structure and is poorly differentiated, occurs at an earlier age and is associated with a poorer prognosis. The intestinal form, which is characterized by glandlike structures that mimic intestinal glands, is more closely linked to the environmental factors presented above and has been most responsive to the changes in diet, sanitation, and refrigeration that have occurred in the past 50 years. The intestinal form is believed to follow a multistep pattern similar to the progression of colon cancer from polyp to carcinoma (Figure 42-8).

Cancer may occur anywhere in the stomach, but about 50% occur in the antrum (Figure 42-9). A significant proximal shift has occurred over the past 30 years, with more than 40% of gastric cancers now originating in the fundus, cardia, and gastroesophageal junction.[4]

Early gastric cancer is confined to the mucosa or submucosa and exhibits a long latency period. All forms of gastric cancer develop on gastric mucosa that has been damaged by longstanding gastritis. Infection and inflammation progress to atrophy of the mucosa and replacement with an intestinal type of epithelium (metaplasia). From this initial change, dysplasia and adenocarcinoma may develop over time.[13] Gastric cancer may spread directly through the stomach wall into adjacent tissues; to the lymphatics; to the regional lymph nodes of the stomach; to the esophagus, spleen, pancreas, and liver; or through the bloodstream to the lungs or bones. Involvement of regional lymph nodes occurs early. Prognosis depends on the depth of invasion, extent of metastasis, and location. Cancer that occurs in the upper third of the stomach is associated with a poor prognosis. Three fourths of patients with gastric carcinoma have metastases at the time of diagnosis, since early diagnosis in the United States is rare.

Gastric cancer has an insidious onset; cancers that do not penetrate the muscular layer are completely asymptomatic in more than 80% of patients.[22] The patient may complain of vague, nondescript dyspeptic symptoms that overlap with multiple benign disorders, including functional dyspepsia and PUD (see Clinical Manifestations box). Pain does not usually develop until late in the disease. Significant weight loss, which occurs in advanced cancer, is frequently the first identified symptom that brings the patient to the health care provider. Some clinicians are concerned that the availability of over-the-counter H_2-receptor antagonists and PPIs may further delay diagnosis and treatment, since early ulcerative lesions frequently respond to acid reduction, at least temporarily.

COMPLICATIONS. Rapid weight loss is a common symptom of gastric cancer and patients with advanced disease often are challenged to maintain adequate nutrition. Cachexia is a common complication and is not easily treated. Tumors that intrude on the pylorus may also cause bowel obstruction. Radical surgery can produce predictable complications such as malabsorption and dumping syndrome, which are discussed on pp. 1223 and 1224.

Collaborative Care Management

DIAGNOSTIC TESTS. Upper endoscopy with biopsy has proven extremely accurate in diagnosing gastric cancer. Multiple biopsy specimens are obtained. Many gastric cancers can be located by barium contrast upper GI x-ray films, but only biopsy can confirm the diagnosis. Mass screening programs are in use in Japan that have significantly increased the identification of gastric cancer in early, treatable stages, but gastric cancer is rarely diagnosed in early treatable stages in the United States. Box 42-3 summarizes diagnostic tests that may be used.

MEDICATIONS. Medications do not play a role in the management of gastric cancer. The role of chemotherapy remains controversial and continues to be studied. Chemotherapy is the mainstay of treatment for nonresectable tumors, but gastric cancer is fairly resistant to conventional chemotherapy. The most promising approach appears to be combination chemotherapy as an adjunct to surgery. Early studies show a significantly improved 1-year survival with this protocol.[13] Hyperthermic peritoneal

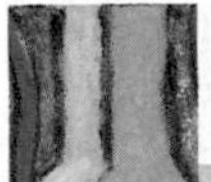

CLINICAL MANIFESTATIONS
Gastric Cancer

- Dyspepsia: early satiety, bloating, anorexia
- Epigastric pain or burning (usually mild and relieved by antacids, histamine$_2$-receptor antagonists, or proton pump inhibitors)
- Mild nausea
- Weight loss (may be rapid and severe)
- Fatigue and weakness
- Typically asymptomatic in early stages

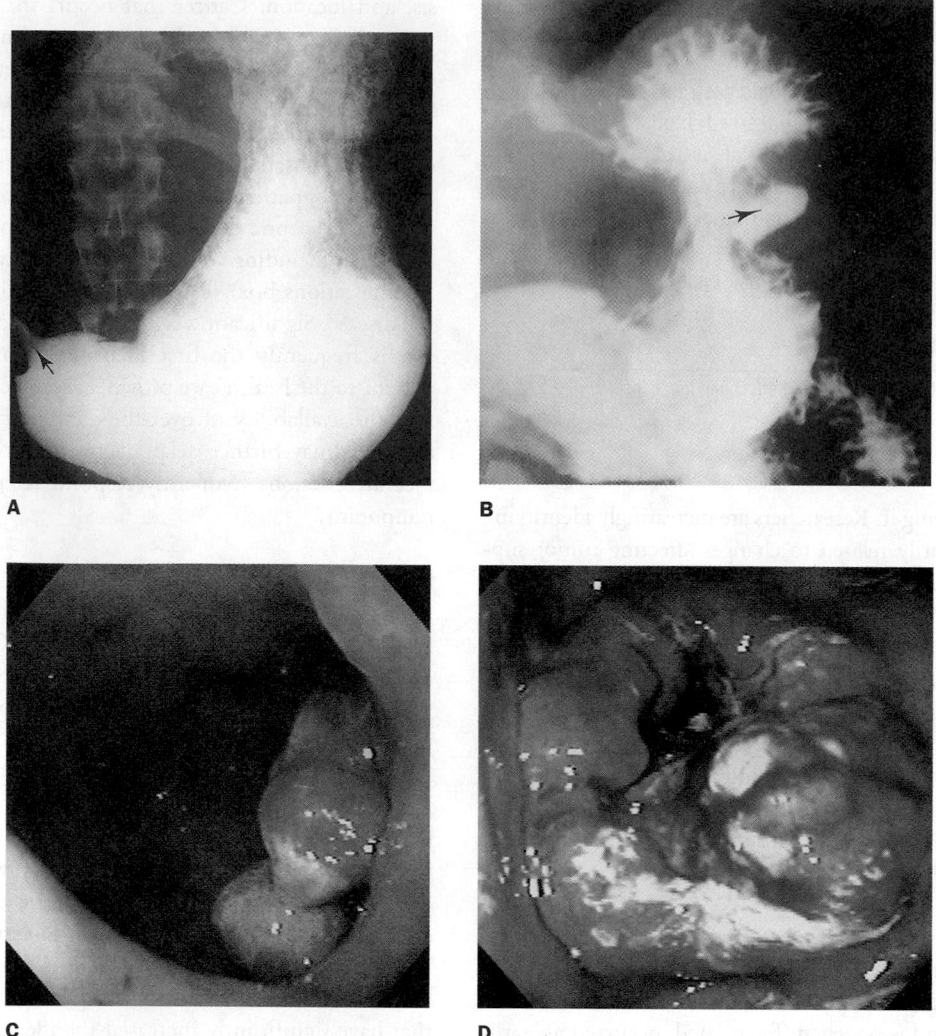

Figure 42-8 Radiographic examples of gastric cancer. **A,** Pyloric (gastric outlet) obstruction *(arrow)*. **B,** Large greater curvature ulcer within a mass *(arrow)*. **C,** Polypoid gastric cancer. Trilobed polyp at the angularis. **D,** Exophytic gastric cancer. Circumferential masslike lesion involving the gastric body and collapsing the antrum.

chemotherapy used during surgery also shows some early promise. Adjuvant chemotherapy after surgery offers no proven benefit at this time.

DIET. No specific dietary considerations exist in the treatment of gastric cancer. Patients may experience profound weight loss and cachexia and eventually require nutritional support. If a patient experiences ulcer-related pain, the standard recommendations for avoiding spicy and irritating foods are made. The patient is encouraged to work within the scope of individual preferences to maintain adequate nutrition. Patients who undergo gastric resection may develop significant problems with dumping syndrome and malabsorption.

TREATMENTS. Radiotherapy is being researched as a treatment option for gastric cancer, but at present it shows little proven effectiveness. The stomach is fairly resistant to radiation, and the proximity of other radiosensitive tissue such as the kidneys and spinal cord limits its usefulness. Intraoperative radiation is being used in Japan and shows initial promise in increasing 5-year survival rates.[4] Physicians in the United States have insufficient experience with this approach to evaluate its potential.

Endoscopic photodynamic laser therapy is being used to treat superficial gastric cancer with reports of complete remission in 80% of patients, but it is too early to know how widely useful this treatment will be. Endoscopic treatment may also be used for palliation of symptomatic unresectable or recurrent tumors, and to control bleeding and relieve obstructive symptoms.

SURGICAL MANAGEMENT. The only potentially curative treatment for gastric cancer is surgical resection. The procedure of choice depends on the location and extent of the tumor, but the value of total gastrectomy is debated today. It is no longer commonly used in the United States because of the serious digestive

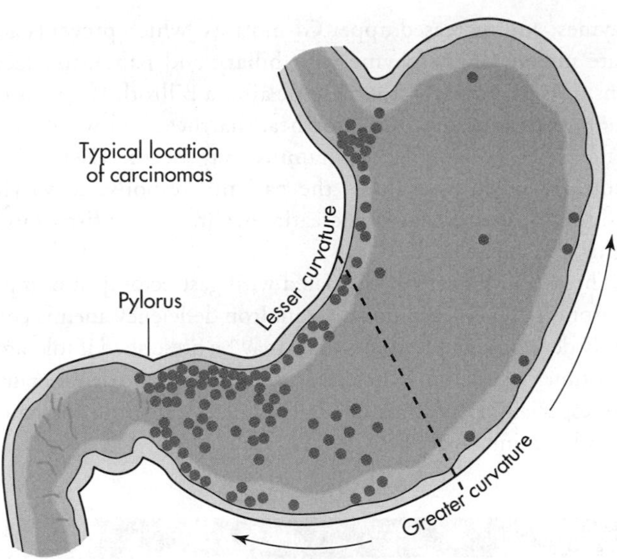

Figure 42-9 Typical sites of gastric cancer.

Box 42-3 Diagnostic Tests for Gastric Cancer

- *Endoscopy:* Diagnostic procedure of choice
- *Biopsy:* Six to eight samples taken from the ulcer edge and base
- *Upper gastrointestinal series:* Good accuracy for diagnosing advanced cancer but cannot distinguish between a benign and malignant tumor
- *Endoscopic ultrasonography:* Allows for visualization of the five layers of the gastric wall
- *Computed tomography scan:* Primarily used to identify metastases

difficulties and quality-of-life issues that may result from the surgery. Surgical procedures attempt to remove all of the tumor plus surgical margins of 5 to 10 cm beyond the cancer. No significant differences in 5-year survival or operative mortality rates have been found for subtotal versus total gastrectomy. Common procedures are illustrated in Figure 42-10. Japanese surgeons, who have extensive experience with the treatment of gastric cancer, recommend performing more extensive lymph node dissections than have been standard in the United States, but U.S. physicians have been reluctant to adopt this aggressive approach and question its applicability to the U.S. population. Tumors that are high in the cardia present more technical challenges to resection and anastomosis. Removal of other abdominal organs appears to have no positive impact on survival. The development of successful laparoscopic techniques has revolutionized gastric surgery as it has other forms of GI surgery. Most gastrectomies and lymph node dissection can now be performed laparoscopically by highly skilled surgeons.

COMPLICATIONS OF GASTRIC SURGERY. Patients who undergo gastric resection may develop a variety of complications that influence nutrition and quality of life.

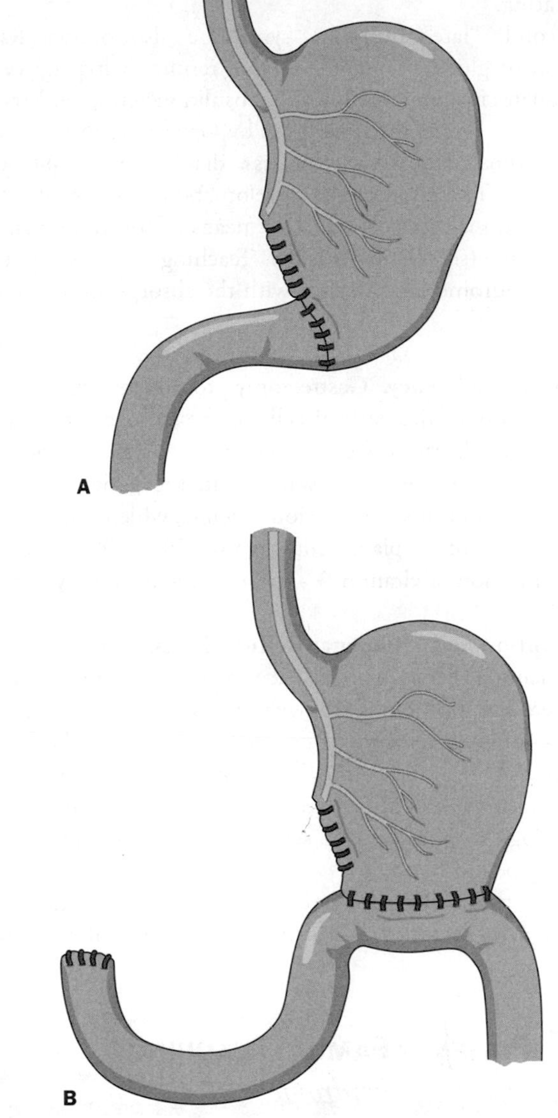

Figure 42-10 Types of gastric resections with anastomoses. **A,** Billroth I, anastomosis of gastric segment to duodenum. **B,** Billroth II, anastomosis of gastric segment to proximal jejunum.

Dumping Syndrome. Dumping syndrome is the term used for a group of unpleasant vasomotor and GI symptoms that occur after gastric resection and vagotomy surgery in as many as 50% of patients. It is a complex process with several contributing factors. One major element is the rapid entry of food boluses directly into the upper small intestine that have not first undergone the usual breakdown and dilution in the stomach. This causes distention, produces an intense feeling of fullness and discomfort, and stimulates motility that can result in diarrhea. The undiluted chyme is hyperosmolar and causes an osmotic shift of fluid from the intravascular compartment into the intestine.[34] This worsens the distention and triggers a systemic response of weakness, diaphoresis, tachycardia, and flushing. This reaction, called the early dumping syndrome, typically occurs within 15 to 30 minutes of eating.

A second, "late" dumping syndrome also occurs. Rapid absorption of glucose from the chyme results in hyperglycemia and stimulates insulin secretion. The insulin secretion outlasts the hyperglycemia, which then swings to hypoglycemia and its associated symptoms of anxiety, weakness, diaphoresis, palpitations, and faintness. These symptoms develop about 2 hours after eating. Prevention is the most effective means of controlling dumping syndrome (see Patient/Family Teaching box). Over time dumping syndrome can interfere with the absorption of essential nutrients.

Vitamin B_{12} Deficiency. Gastrectomy procedures result in a partial or total loss of the parietal cells of the stomach that secrete intrinsic factor. Intrinsic factor is essential to the absorption of vitamin B_{12} in the intestine. Without it, the patient gradually develops the symptoms of pernicious anemia, which can be fatal if not treated. Lifelong replacement therapy with a 100- to 200-mg monthly injection of vitamin B_{12} prevents the deficiency.

Malabsorption and Duodenal Reflux. Excessive reflux of duodenal or jejunal secretions may occur after gastric resection and cause severe irritation of the stomach or distal esophagus, depending on the extent of resection. Bile acids are believed to be the primary cause. Chronic abdominal pain and vomiting may result. The syndrome is difficult to treat and does not respond well to pharmacologic intervention. In severe cases a surgical bypass procedure may be indicated.

Malabsorption of fat may occur after gastric resection from decreased acid secretion; decreased availability of pancreatic enzymes; and increased upper GI motility, which prevents adequate mixing of the chyme with biliary and pancreatic secretions. It is particularly troublesome after a Billroth II operation. The patient experiences steatorrhea, diarrhea, and weight loss. Deficiencies in fat-soluble vitamins may occur. Diet adjustments are made to evaluate the patient's response to varying amounts of dietary fat. Pancreatic enzymes or antispasmodic agents may be helpful.

The digestive changes associated with gastrectomy also impair absorption of both calcium and iron. Iron deficiency anemia commonly develops, and ferrous sulfate may be prescribed if tolerated. Over time the calcium deficiency can result in bone demineralization, especially in postmenopausal women. Calcium supplementation has minimal effect.

PATIENT/FAMILY TEACHING
Dumping Syndrome

With dumping syndrome, the onset of symptoms occurs within 1 hour of eating and may recur after 2 hours. The nurse teaches the patient to monitor the occurrence of the common clinical manifestations:

- Weakness
- Dizziness
- Diaphoresis
- Tachycardia
- Palpitations
- Feeling of fullness or discomfort
- Nausea
- Diarrhea

Strategies for prevention or management include:

- Eat small frequent meals.
- Eat a moderate-fat, high-protein diet.
- Limit carbohydrates; avoid eating simple sugars.
- Drink minimal liquids with meals.
- Avoid very hot and very cold foods and beverages.
- Rest on left side for 20 to 30 minutes after eating.
- Use anticholinergic or antispasmodic medications as prescribed.

▶ ARE YOU READY?

Which of the following content should be included in the discharge teaching for a patient experiencing dumping syndrome after gastric surgery? (Choose all that apply.)

1. Eat small frequent meals.
2. Eat a high-protein diet.
3. Limit fat in diet.
4. Limit carbohydrates in diet.
5. Drink 8 ounces of fluid before each meal.
6. Avoid very hot and very cold food and beverages.

Nursing Management

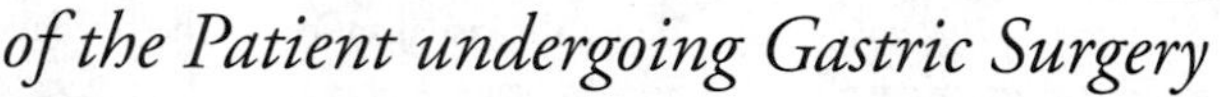

of the Patient undergoing Gastric Surgery

PREOPERATIVE CARE

Preoperative care focuses on patient teaching and ensuring that the patient is in the best nutritional state to support healing. Correction of nutritional deficits may involve short-term parenteral nutrition if the patient is severely cachectic.

A high abdominal incision is standard with gastric surgery if an open procedure is performed. This incision limits ventilation and creates a high risk of postoperative respiratory complications. The nurse focuses preoperative teaching on pulmonary hygiene and the importance of deep breathing, effective coughing, splinting the incision, frequent position changes, incentive spirometry, and chest physical therapy if indicated. These teaching interventions are even more critical if the patient has a history of smoking. The nurse also discusses planned methods for postoperative pain control. Pulmonary hygiene is still an important focus of preoperative care when laparoscopic approaches are used, but the tissue damage is minimized and pain is significantly less so it is easier for the patient to comply with recommendations.

Most patients undergoing gastric surgery have an NG tube in place for several days after surgery. The NG tube prevents trauma, reduces pressure on the suture lines, and minimizes gas and fluid accumulation from decreased postoperative peristalsis. The nurse teaches the patient about the NG tube and its purpose, the necessity for an initial nothing-by-mouth (NPO) status, and the planned use of any other wound-drainage device.

Anxiety is another important issue to address in the preoperative period. Gastric cancer carries a poor prognosis, and the threat of death affects the patient's ability to attend to teaching and participate in self-care. Accurate staging of the cancer is often not possible until surgical exploration is performed, compounding the uncertainty in an already stressful situation. The nurse provides support and encourages the patient to verbalize any concerns.

POSTOPERATIVE CARE

Maintaining a Patent Airway and Ventilation. A patient who undergoes open or conventional gastric surgery tends to lie still and breathe shallowly to limit incisional pain. Adequate pain management is essential to achieving respiratory goals and is ideally accomplished through patient-controlled or epidural analgesia. Turning, deep breathing, incentive spirometry, and ambulation are essential postoperative activities, and the nurse must ensure that the patient is comfortable enough to participate actively in them. A semi-Fowler's position assists with natural chest expansion. The nurse routinely auscultates the patient's lungs to monitor pulmonary status and encourages the patient in all pulmonary hygiene routines.

Supporting Adequate Nutrition. The patient is given nothing by mouth until peristalsis resumes and initial surgical healing occurs. Drainage from the NG tube usually contains some blood for the first 6 to 12 hours, but the presence of bright red blood, large amounts of blood, or excessive bloody drainage is reported to the surgeon at once. If the NG tube stops draining, the surgeon also is notified immediately because a buildup of gas or fluid can put pressure on the suture line, resulting in rupture or dislodgement.[26]

To protect the healing suture line, the nurse does not routinely irrigate or reposition the NG tube. Fluids are given parenterally until the tube is removed and the patient is able to drink sufficient fluids. The nurse offers or provides the patient with frequent mouth care. It is important to accurately measure and record gastric drainage and urinary output.

Oral fluids may be restricted for 12 to 24 hours after the NG tube is removed. The nurse offers small amounts of fluid frequently and observes the patient for signs of leakage, such as difficulty in breathing, pain, or a rise in temperature. Foods are added as tolerated by the patient. The dietary regimen must be adapted to the individual, since some persons tolerate increasing amounts of food and fluids better than others.

When the cardia of the stomach has been removed, the patient may experience nausea and vomiting. This problem is usually caused by irritation of the esophageal mucosa by the gastric juices or duodenal fluids that reflux into the esophagus when the patient lies down. The patient should avoid lying flat in bed, bending, and stooping.

Early satiety is a common problem after gastric surgery. Regurgitation after meals may occur from eating too fast, eating too much, or postoperative edema around the suture line that prevents the food from passing into the intestines. If regurgitation occurs, the patient is encouraged to eat more slowly and to temporarily decrease the size of each meal. The combined effects of dumping syndrome and steatorrhea can result in significant weight loss. The patient is encouraged to monitor body weight at least weekly and to experiment with food supplements as tolerated to meet nutritional needs. The ongoing involvement of a dietitian or nutritionist may be necessary.

Monitoring for Complications. Patients who undergo gastric surgery are vulnerable to a wide range of short- and long-term complications (Figure 42-11). Bleeding at the anastomosis site is a common problem that may resolve spontaneously. Major risk periods include the first 24 hours after surgery and again between the fourth and seventh days when clot breakdown occurs. The nurse carefully monitors the NG tube drainage for blood and avoids irrigating or repositioning the tube unless specifically ordered. Patients treated laparoscopically are taught the warning signs of problems with the anastomosis and the importance of calling the surgeon immediately if problems should occur.

Any of the anastomosis sites are at risk for leakage in the early postoperative period. The blind-end duodenal stump that is created with a Billroth II operation (see Figure 42-10) appears to be particularly vulnerable. The nurse monitors for and teaches the patient about classic **peritonitis** symptoms such as severe abdominal pain, rigidity, and fever. Surgical drainage and closure are often necessary.

The Guidelines for Safe Practice box summarizes the nursing care provided to a patient undergoing gastric surgery.

Patient/Family Teaching. Patients with gastric cancer may be facing a dramatically shortened life expectancy and a steady

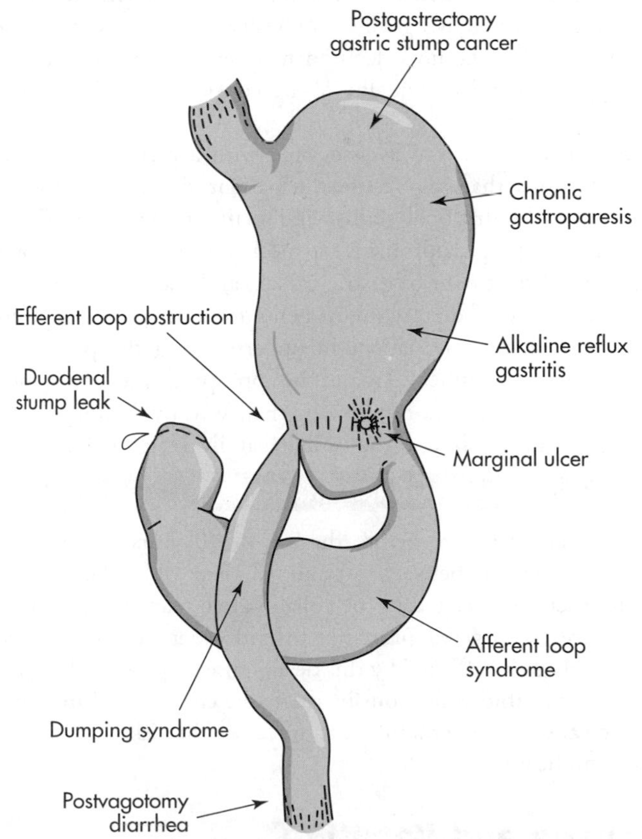

Figure 42-11 Complications of gastric surgery.

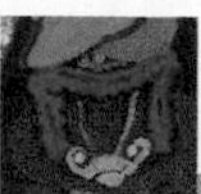

GUIDELINES FOR SAFE PRACTICE *The Patient Undergoing Gastric Surgery*

Preoperative Care

Teach deep breathing, coughing, and splinting techniques.
Explain special postoperative measures: nasogastric tube and parenteral fluids until peristalsis returns; planned method of pain control.

Postoperative Care

Promote pulmonary ventilation.
—Position patient in mid- or high Fowler's position.
—Encourage patient to turn and breathe deeply at least every 2 hours (or more frequently until ambulating well); splint or support incision with hands or folded towel during coughing if needed to clear secretions.
—Provide adequate analgesia during first few days; patient-controlled analgesia is most effective.
—Encourage ambulation.
—Provide good mouth care until oral fluids can be resumed.

Promote nutrition.
—Measure nasogastric drainage accurately; monitor for blood in drainage. Do not irrigate or reposition tube unless ordered.
—Monitor for signs of leakage of anastomosis (dyspnea, pain, fever) when oral fluids are resumed.
—Offer food in small amounts at frequent intervals until well tolerated.
—Monitor for early satiety and regurgitation.
—If regurgitation occurs, tell patient to eat less food at a slower pace.
—Report signs of dumping syndrome to physician (weakness, faintness, palpitations, diaphoresis, nausea, diarrhea).
—Monitor weight.
Provide patient and family teaching (see Patient/Family Teaching box).

decline in self-care abilities. In many cases the disease is fatal within 1 year of diagnosis, and the patient's decline can be rapid and frightening. The nurse ensures that the patient and family are aware of resources available for support in their community, particularly the services of the American Cancer Society and hospice, and makes appropriate referrals as needed. Patients are encouraged to clearly articulate their wishes for future care in the form of advance directives, living wills, and health care powers of attorney to support their family's decision making. The nurse reinforces the appropriateness of quality-of-life considerations in all treatment decisions.

Subtotal gastrectomy is associated with a variety of digestive complications that may cause the patient significant problems with eating, nutritional status, and maintaining a stable body weight. Dumping syndrome is the most common complication of the surgical treatment of gastric cancer, and the patient needs to make a variety of dietary adjustments to control its symptoms. The nurse assists the patient in understanding the physiologic basis for these complications and the appropriate diet and lifestyle modifications aimed at minimizing their severity. Major teaching points are summarized in the Patient/Family Teaching box.

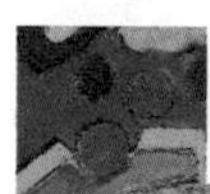

PATIENT/FAMILY TEACHING *Gastric Surgery*

After gastric surgery, the nurse instructs the patient to:
- Gradually increase the amount of food at each meal until you are able to eat three to six meals per day, if possible.
- Decrease the size of meals and the amount of fluids with meals if discomfort occurs after eating; eat slower.
- Avoid stress during and immediately after meals; plan a rest period after eating. Lie on left side.
- Elevate head when lying down (if cardia of stomach removed).
- Monitor weight regularly.
- Report signs of complications: vomiting after meals, increasing feelings of abdominal fullness or weakness, hematemesis, tarry stools, persistent diarrhea.

GERONTOLOGIC CONSIDERATIONS

Gastric cancer is rare before the age of 40 years and typically occurs in persons between 50 and 70 years old. Therefore the entire discussion related to the collaborative management of gastric cancer is targeted primarily toward older persons who are most likely to be affected by this deadly disease process. The presence of comorbid conditions increases the challenge of managing gastric cancer in older adults and increases the risk of postoperative complications.

Nausea and Vomiting

Etiology and Epidemiology. Nausea and vomiting, which often occur together but may occur independently, are common GI symptoms. They are part of the body's protective mechanisms and are usually a response to chemical, bacterial, or viral insults to the body's integrity. They are present in a wide array of disorders and, if persistent, can lead to serious consequences. Chronic problems with nausea and vomiting may develop during pregnancy, in severe metabolic imbalances associated with uremia or alcoholism, and during cancer chemotherapy. Box 42-4 presents some of the many causes of nausea and vomiting.

Pathophysiology. Nausea is a subjective sensation of an impending urge to vomit. It may be accompanied by weakness, hypersalivation, and diaphoresis. Gastric tone and peristalsis are typically slowed or absent. The neural pathways that control nausea are not well identified but probably are the same general pathways that control vomiting. Vomiting is a complex phenomenon that begins with rhythmic contractions of the respiratory and abdominal muscles and culminates in the forceful expulsion of gastric contents from the mouth. It may be accompanied by

Box 42-4 Common Causes of Nausea and Vomiting

- Infectious gastroenteritis
  —Viral (e.g., rotaviruses, adenoviruses, Norwalk virus)
  —Bacterial (e.g., staphylococci, salmonellae, clostridia, *Bacillus cereus*)
- Medications
  —Chemotherapy (e.g., cisplatin, methotrexate, nitrogen mustard)
  —Analgesics (e.g., opioids, nonsteroidal antiinflammatory drugs)
  —Antibiotics (e.g., tetracycline, erythromycin)
- Pregnancy
- Anesthesia effects
- Gastrointestinal disturbances
  —Obstruction
  —Dyspepsia
  —Gastroparesis
  —Alcohol abuse
  —Inflammations (e.g., cholecystitis, pancreatitis, appendicitis)
- Labyrinthine disorders
  —Motion sickness
  —Meniere's disease
- Central nervous system disorders
  —Increased intracranial pressure
  —Tumors
  —Meningitis
  —Migraine headache

retching or dry heaves and should be distinguished from the classic regurgitation that may accompany gastroesophageal reflux.

The vomiting center, located in the medulla adjacent to the respiratory and salivary control centers, can be stimulated directly by both the vagus nerve and sympathetic nervous system. Receptors can be found throughout the GI tract and internal organs that, when triggered by spasm or inflammation, can directly produce vomiting. Indirect stimulation can come from the **chemoreceptor trigger zone** (CTZ), which is located on the floor of the fourth ventricle and appears to respond to chemical stimuli in the blood. A wide variety of medications and other substances can act on the CTZ. The CTZ may also mediate the response to nonchemical stimuli such as radiation and motion sickness.

Strong evidence suggests that dopamine receptors in the CTZ play a role in mediating vomiting. Serotonergic pathways also play pivotal roles in mediating the effects of peripheral stimuli. Gastrointestinal serotonin is synthesized by enterochromaffin cells found throughout the abdomen, and is believed to activate 5-hydroxytryptamine 3 (5-HT_3) receptor sites on afferent vagal fibers. This pathway plays a crucial role in the severe, protracted vomiting commonly associated with chemotherapy. Activation of the CTZ causes a reflex loss in gastric tone and peristalsis, resulting in delayed gastric emptying. The CTZ may also play a role in psychogenic vomiting, which occurs in response to specific sensations and situations.

Short-term episodic nausea and vomiting are distressing, but prolonged vomiting can have serious physiologic effects. Prolonged and severe vomiting interferes with nutrition and causes fluid and electrolyte imbalances—specifically dehydration and metabolic alkalosis, with loss of potassium, chloride, and hydrogen ions. The act of vomiting strains the abdominal muscles and in postoperative patients may cause wound dehiscence. It can also result in Mallory-Weiss lacerations in the esophagus or stomach and trigger severe bleeding.

Vomiting is especially dangerous for anesthetized patients and persons with decreased alertness because they are at risk for aspiration of the vomitus. Aspiration may cause atelectasis, pneumonitis, or asphyxia, especially in older persons whose protective reflexes work less efficiently.

Collaborative Care Management. Treatment of nausea and vomiting depends on the cause and severity. Short-term problems resolve without intervention, but protracted vomiting requires intervention. Medications or other substances known to cause nausea and vomiting are discontinued if possible, and fluid and electrolyte imbalances are corrected. Fluids may be given intravenously if vomiting persists.

Antiemetic medications may be necessary. Drugs that are classified as antiemetics are theorized to act as a pharmacologic blockade to stimuli that may trigger nausea and vomiting. Most of the drugs also are believed to have some direct sedative action on the CTZ. Antiemetics are prescribed orally if the patient is able to retain the tablets, but they often need to be given by rectal, intramuscular, or IV routes. The choice of drug is governed by the specific clinical situation. Drug categories include antihistamines, anticholinergics, dopamine receptor antagonists, prokinetic agents, serotonin antagonists, and miscellaneous agents (Table 42-3). The choice of drug depends on the circumstances and severity of the problem. Antihistamines are useful in controlling motion sickness but otherwise have limited usefulness. Dopamine antagonists are effective but produce significant sedation, and their use is primarily limited to postoperative situations. The serotonin antagonists were developed to manage the debilitating nausea and vomiting associated with some aggressive chemotherapy protocols. Their use has been gradually expanded to incorporate other situations, including after surgery. They are generally regarded as the most effective drugs available for managing nausea and vomiting. Dexamethasone, a synthetic glucocorticoid, appears to increase the effect of other antiemetics when administered in combination. Its mechanism of action is unknown. Cannabis derivatives are a controversial option. Their antiemetic site of action is uncertain, but the active ingredient in marijuana is often useful in controlling chemotherapy-related nausea and vomiting. Drowsiness and dry mouth are common side effects.

Effective management of nausea and vomiting includes drug therapy but may also include complementary therapies such as acupuncture and acupressure, which produce dramatic results for some people. Prevention or correction of dehydration are important because dehydration appears to worsen the cycle of nausea and vomiting. Fluids may be needed if vomiting is protracted or severe. Guidelines for the management of nausea and vomiting are summarized in the Guidelines for Safe Practice box, p. 1229.

PATIENT/FAMILY TEACHING. Nausea and vomiting can be distressing and debilitating problems that severely interfere

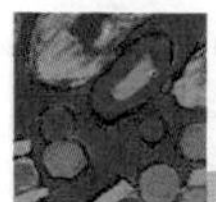

TABLE 42-3
COMMON MEDICATIONS *for Nausea and Vomiting*

Drug	Action	Nursing Intervention
Antihistamines		
Meclizine (Antivert) Diphenhydramine hydrochloride (Benadryl) Dimenhydrinate (Dramamine, Dimetabs) Hydroxyzine hydrochloride/ hydroxyzine pamoate (Atarax, Vistaril)	Act on neurons in vomiting center and vestibular pathways Used in morning sickness and motion sickness	Monitor for drowsiness. Teach patient to use caution with all activities that require alertness. Driving may be hazardous.
Promethazine (Phenergan)	Phenothiazine with strong antihistaminic activity	Same as above.
Antidopaminergics		
Prochlorperazine (Compazine) Thiethylperazine (Torecan) Droperidol (Inapsine) Chlorpromazine (Thorazine)	Antagonize dopamine receptors in CTZ; also have antihistaminic and anticholinergic effects	Monitor severity of drowsiness and sedation. Teach patient to avoid all hazardous activities and driving during use and to avoid alcohol use and sun exposure.
Prokinetic Agents		
Metoclopramide (Reglan) Domperidone (Motilium)	Complex actions in both CNS and GI tract; stimulate gastric emptying; domperidone does not cross blood-brain barrier	Monitor for side effects: diarrhea, mild sedation.
Anticholinergics		
Scopolamine (Transderm Scōp)	Reduce neuron transmission; useful in motion sickness and postoperative nausea	Teach patient to apply to dry surface behind ear and to use in advance of anticipated need.
Serotonin-Receptor Antagonists		
Ondansetron (Zofran) Granisetron (Kytril) Dolasetron (Anzemet)	Bind serotonin-receptor sites along GI tract and afferent nerves	Monitor for side effects: diarrhea, headache.
Cannabis Derivatives		
Dronabinol (Marinol) Nabilone (Cesamet)	Site of antiemetic action unknown	Teach patient to be alert to mood and behavior change. Drowsiness is common, so driving should be avoided. Warn patient to avoid concurrent alcohol use.
Miscellaneous		
Trimethobenzamide (Tigan)	Believed to act on CTZ; has weak antihistaminic action, similar to phenothiazines	Monitor for side effects: hypotension, diarrhea, irritation at injection site. Drowsiness is common.
Benzquinamide (Emete-Con)	Inhibits stimulation of CTZ; similar activity to antihistamines and phenothiazines	Monitor for side effects: drowsiness, fluctuations in blood pressure.
Corticosteroids: dexamethasone	Mechanism of action unknown; useful in combination to treat chemotherapy-induced vomiting	Monitor for side effects: mood changes.

CTZ, Chemoreceptor trigger zone; *CNS,* central nervous system; *GI,* gastrointestinal.

with quality of life. The nurse encourages the patient to explore modifications in diet, eating habits, and lifestyle in an effort to control the symptoms. Stress management and relaxation strategies are often helpful. The nurse teaches the patient that liquids are often better tolerated than solids because they exit the stomach rapidly. A liquid diet may be successful when symptoms are severe. Small, frequent feedings are suggested, and overdistention of the stomach should be avoided. The nurse encourages the patient to limit intake of creamy and milk-based liquids and foods because they are rarely well tolerated. Likewise, starches are more easily tolerated than fatty foods. Lean poultry is usually the best tolerated source of protein. The nurse also encourages the patient to relax while eating and ensure that their environment is pleasant and odor free. The nurse offers support and encouragement because rarely are there quick and easy answers to this problem.

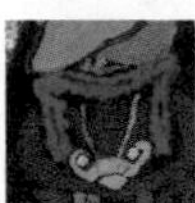

GUIDELINES FOR SAFE PRACTICE
Nausea and Vomiting

Safety and Comfort

Keep head of bed elevated and emesis basin handy.
Protect airway with suction and positioning if patient is not alert.
Provide frequent mouth care.
Control odors in room.
Reduce anxiety if possible.
Provide quiet or distraction on the basis of patient response.
Modify environmental stimuli (cool cloth, dim light), and evaluate response.
Provide ongoing patient support. Explore new strategies.

Diet Modifications

Maintain patient on nothing-by-mouth status if vomiting is severe.
Explore use of clear liquids:
—Serve liquids cool or room temperature.
—Try carbonated drinks and evaluate effect.
—Encourage adequate fluids to prevent dehydration.
Have patient avoid fatty foods, highly sweetened foods, and milk products.
Keep meals small; avoid overdistention.

Drugs

Administer medications before vomiting occurs, if possible.
Evaluate patient response to medications.
Maintain patient safety and assess for sedation or confusion.

Problems of Nutrition and Absorption

The importance of adequate sustained nutrition to the maintenance and restoration of health is increasingly recognized in health care. Adequate nutrition is critical to wound healing, resistance to infection, ventilator weaning, and organ function. Acutely and chronically ill patients may experience social and environmental problems related to food access and preparation, as well as complex problems related to the structure and function of various organs of the GI tract and related structures.

Malabsorption

Etiology and Epidemiology. The GI tract must be able to both break down ingested food and transport nutrients across the mucosa to the bloodstream. Approximately 7 to 10 L of liquid chyme move through the GI tract daily, but absorption is so efficient that all but 600 to 800 ml are reabsorbed before reaching the ileocecal valve. The term **malabsorption** refers to a heterogeneous category of disorders that share the common feature of failure to assimilate one or more essential ingested nutrients. It can result from impaired function of any of the primary or accessory organs of digestion and may be structural, involve a digestive alteration, or result from impairment of nutrient transport across the mucosa. The problem with absorption may be caused by a primary disorder such as celiac disease or lactase deficiency; or it may develop secondary to gastric or bowel surgery, inflammatory diseases, infections, or specific medications (Box 42-5).

Box 42-5 Primary and Secondary Causes of Malabsorption

Primary Causes

Lactase deficiency
Celiac disease, tropical sprue

Secondary Causes

Inflammatory bowel disease
Subtotal gastrectomy, gastric bypass
Ileal resection or bypass greater than 3 feet
Pancreatic disease: chronic pancreatitis, cancer, cystic fibrosis
Liver or biliary disease or obstruction
Bacterial, viral, or parasitic infection of the bowel
Radiation enteritis
Drug side effects: antibiotics, colchicine

Pathophysiology. Malabsorption syndrome is a group of symptoms produced by inadequate absorption of fat, protein, or carbohydrates. Fat malabsorption is the most common problem, but malabsorption can occur with any nutrient. The symptoms vary somewhat based on the specific problem. Because fat-soluble vitamins (A, D, E, and K) require fat for absorption, decreased absorption of fat also typically results in a deficiency of these vitamins.

The classic sign of fat malabsorption is steatorrhea, excess loss of fat in the stool that may be mild or severe. Fat gives the stool a greasy, bulky appearance and a foul odor. The stools float because of their low specific gravity and high gas content. The patient may pass one or multiple stools a day. Steatorrhea also causes flatulence with borborygmus (loud bowel sounds) and abdominal distention. Decreased fat absorption can lead to weight loss, weakness, fatigue, and anorexia.

Malabsorption of carbohydrates may cause abdominal cramping and bloating. A wide variety of extraintestinal symptoms such as anemia and bone loss may also accompany malabsorption disorders. Concurrent deficiencies of fat-soluble vitamins can produce bleeding (ecchymosis and hematuria), bone pain, fractures, hypocalcemia, anemia, glossitis, cheilosis, muscle tenderness, peripheral neuritis, and dermatitis. Protein deficiency results in hypoalbuminemia, edema, and loss of muscle mass. Primary malabsorption disorders in adults are described below.

GLUTEN-SENSITIVE ENTEROPATHY (CELIAC DISEASE). This familial disorder involves a permanent intolerance to fractions of gluten (wheat protein). It primarily affects Caucasians, and about 30% to 40% of those affected develop diarrhea, which is the primary symptom. Effective treatment involves the rigid and lifelong exclusion of gluten.[12]

DISACCHARIDE MALABSORPTION. Congenital lactase deficiency is the most common form of genetic deficiency syndrome in humans. It affects more than 50% of the world's population and is particularly prevalent among non-Europeans. The intolerance to milk products may be mild or severe and is treated by diet restriction, enzyme supplement, or both.[16]

SHORT-BOWEL SYNDROME. The small intestine has a tremendous functional reserve, but loss of more than 50% of its length significantly reduces the amount of mucosal surface area available for absorbing nutrients and produces a condition called **short-bowel syndrome**. The shortened bowel results in rapid intestinal transit and impaired digestion and absorption. Diarrhea and steatorrhea are the predominant symptoms, and their severity depends on the site and extent of bowel loss. A bowel length of less than 200 cm usually results in a failure of the remnant intestine to maintain nutritional balance. Treatment is complex and may involve long-term parenteral nutrition, enteral feedings, and drugs to decrease peristalsis.[25] Inflammatory bowel disease, particularly Crohn's disease, is the major cause in adults.

Secondary malabsorption problems can accompany a wide variety of GI disorders and treatments. Protein-losing gastroenteropathy involves the excess loss of serum proteins and is a common component of disorders such as inflammatory bowel disease, pancreatic disease, and cystic fibrosis.

Collaborative Care Management. Treatment for malabsorption is based on the underlying cause. The adequacy of nutrition is the priority concern, and dietary intervention is the primary approach to management. Diet modifications and supplements are often successful in compensating for the malabsorption on a daily basis, but more aggressive management with enteral or parenteral feedings may be necessary during times of illness or disease exacerbation.

PATIENT/FAMILY TEACHING. The patient with a malabsorption syndrome manages self-care at home and must be knowledgeable about the specific disease process and the recommended dietary modifications necessary to maintain adequate nutrition. The nurse helps the patient incorporate needed dietary changes into the daily lifestyle and works with the family on strategies to promote adherence. The patient must also know the warning signs of exacerbations and complications and how to prevent or treat any accompanying vitamin deficiencies. Safe administration of home-based enteral or parenteral feedings may also be part of effective disease management. The severely malnourished person may require frequent gentle mouth care to increase comfort and prevent oral inflammations, as well as skin care to prevent skin breakdown.

Protein-Calorie Malnutrition

Etiology and Epidemiology. Although malnutrition is not a widespread problem in American society, acute and chronic illness, trauma, infection, and wound healing put enormous strain on the body's nutritional reserve. A poor nutritional state is a common problem in both acute and long-term care settings, and the problem of protein-calorie (protein energy) malnutrition and its adverse effects on wound healing, immunocompetence, and ventilator weaning now reinforce the importance of supporting nutrition during illness and treatment. The actual incidence of protein-calorie malnutrition is unknown, but it is a particularly severe problem in older adults. Some authors estimate that it occurs in up to 60% of hospitalized older adults, 80% of older adults in nursing homes, and 20% of older adults living in the community. Box 42-6 identifies some of the typical causes of malnutrition in hospitalized patients.

Pathophysiology. If a diet provides adequate carbohydrates and fats, the body uses these nutrients to meet its energy needs. When intake of these nutrients is inadequate, however, the body uses its own stores. Most severely ill hospitalized adults experience a deficiency of all dietary elements, but the deficiency of protein is most significant. The process of protein synthesis occurs continuously, and although the body can synthesize certain amino acids from its stored pools, it depends on ingested protein sources for others. Dietary amino acids that are not used are excreted. **Negative nitrogen balance** occurs when more nitrogen (which is an end product of amino acid breakdown) is excreted than is ingested via dietary proteins; its presence indicates that body tissue is being broken down faster than it is being replaced.

Ongoing severe protein deficit leads to decreases in both muscle and visceral mass. Cardiac output decreases, respiratory muscles weaken, and malabsorption occurs in the GI tract. Immunocompetence is impaired, and the risk of infection increases. Loss of albumin can compromise the ability of the plasma proteins to support osmotic pressure in the blood. The greatest impairment is noted in cell-mediated immunity as the number of T cells declines. Weight loss, decreased muscle mass, and weakness are common, but the affected person may exhibit few overt signs and appear physically well nourished.

Collaborative Care Management. The foundation of malnutrition management in health care settings is identifying persons at risk; monitoring physical and laboratory parameters; and intervening with oral supplements, tube feedings, or parenteral nutrition as indicated. Weight loss typically exceeds 15% of usual body weight.

BOX 42-6 Causes of Malnutrition in Hospitalized Patients

Decreased Intake

Anorexia and nausea
Nothing-by-mouth status
Pain
Medication effects
Self-care deficits
Dysphagia
Depression

Increased Losses

Vomiting
Diarrhea
Gastrointestinal suctioning
Open wounds (NOTE: Patients can lose 50 g of protein daily through an open pressure ulcer.)

Increased Needs

Fever
Infection
Trauma
Surgery

Serial measurements of serum albumin and transferrin levels are important. Albumin is a major protein synthesized by the liver, and levels less than 3.5 g/dl indicate early malnutrition. Prealbumin levels are monitored during treatment because they provide an indication of protein changes occurring during the previous 48 hours. Serum transferrin is a beta-globulin synthesized by the liver that transports iron in the plasma. Levels lower than 100 mg/dl indicate severe depletion. The total lymphocyte count reflects a basic measure of immunity and should remain greater than 16% of the total. A nutrition support team, if available, guides decision making concerning dietary supplements or replacements.

PATIENT/FAMILY TEACHING. The nurse teaches the patient and family about protein-calorie malnutrition and its planned management. Anemia-induced fatigue is common, and the nurse provides the patient with frequent rest periods and spaces needed treatments and activities throughout the day. A high-calorie, high-protein diet is encouraged if the patient can tolerate an oral diet. The nurse ensures that the environment is conducive to eating and arranges for small, frequent feedings rather than large meals. It is essential that all nutritional planning incorporate the patient's food preferences and cultural habits as much as possible. The goal is to modify the diet enough to meet the body's needs for tissue growth and repair. The nurse keeps an accurate record of the patient's weight and records calorie counts if ordered. Care for the patient receiving tube feedings or parenteral nutrition is discussed in the next section.

Enteral and Parenteral Nutrition

Enteral Nutrition

Patients who are critically ill or experience GI diseases are prone to the development of nutritional abnormalities, and the negative impact of nutritional deficiencies on immune function, metabolic homeostasis, and healing is well established. It is now possible to adequately feed all patients who cannot or will not take in sufficient nutrients to meet physiologic needs. **Enteral nutrition** involves the delivery of nutrients directly into the GI tract via tube feeding. It can be used to either supplement or replace oral nutrition, as long as the GI tract is physically capable of receiving and absorbing nutrients. The major choices involve timing of the nutritional interventions, method of nutritional support, and composition of the feeding.

Enteral nutrition is generally accepted as being the preferred method for providing nutritional support whenever possible. It is safer and usually more cost-effective than parenteral nutrition and is also significantly less likely to cause sepsis and other serious complications. Other advantages of enteral feedings include:

- Preservation of the normal sequence of intestinal and hepatic metabolism, which supports the structural and functional integrity of the GI tract and prevents mucosal atrophy
- Maintenance of normal insulin/glucagon ratios
- Maintenance of lipoprotein synthesis by the intestinal mucosa and liver
- Stimulation of gallbladder motility, which prevents biliary sludge and cholelithiasis

Tube feedings may be delivered to the stomach (nasogastric) or to the distal duodenum or proximal jejunum (nasointestinal). Nasointestinal feedings have become increasingly popular since it was confirmed that the adynamic ileus that frequently occurs with acute illness or trauma is primarily limited to the stomach and colon. The small intestine frequently retains both motility and the ability to absorb nutrients. Early feeding after major surgery and trauma has now become routine. Long-term enteral nutrition is usually delivered with a permanent access, either into the stomach or jejunum. The choice of route is influenced by the patient's diagnosis and prognosis, patency of the GI tract, and risk of aspiration.

Enteral Feeding Tubes. A wide variety of containers, tubes, catheters, and delivery systems are available for use in enteral feedings.[3] Enteral tubes are classified according to their composition, external diameter, length, and presence or absence of a weighted tip. Most tubes are constructed of either polyurethane or silicone with a monofilament or stainless steel stylet to aid in insertion and accurate placement. The polyurethane tubes have a larger internal diameter, which facilitates fluid flow. Enteral feeding tubes vary in diameter from 8 to 10 F (small bore), to 12 to 14 F (medium bore), to 16 to 18 F (large bore) (Figure 42-12).

NG feeding tubes can be used with patients who have intact gag and swallow reflexes and a competent lower esophageal sphincter to minimize reflux. Nasointestinal tubes are preferred for patients who are at risk for aspiration or who are experiencing acute stress-related gastric ileus. They are typically small bore and have a weighted tip to help the tube move through the pylorus into the duodenum or jejunum.

GASTROSTOMY. Gastrostomy tubes are the most common method for delivering enteral nutrition to patients who are unable to take oral nutrients for long periods. The gastrostomy tube is inserted endoscopically or surgically through an incision in the abdominal wall.

The percutaneous endoscopic gastrostomy (PEG) and radiologic percutaneous gastrostomy do not require surgery and have largely replaced surgical gastrostomies in most settings. A PEG tube is placed via endoscopy with the patient under local anesthesia. A small incision is made on the skin of the abdomen, and a

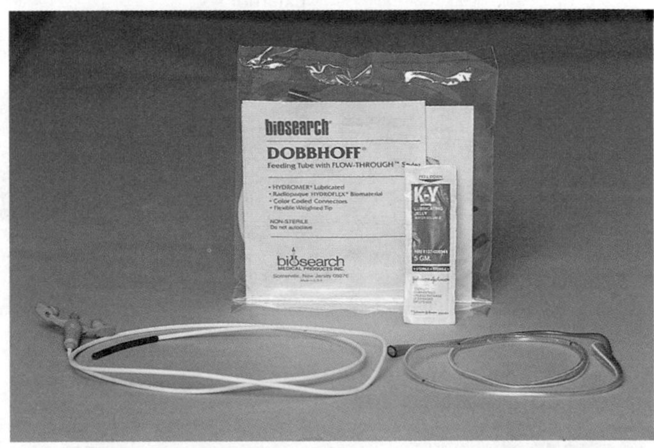

Figure 42-12 Typical small-bore feeding tube.

cannula is pushed through the abdominal and gastric walls into the stomach while the site is observed through a gastroscope (Figure 42-13). A long suture is threaded through the cannula, grasped, and pulled up through the endoscope, which is then removed. A specially prepared catheter is attached to the suture thread, and the catheter is then pulled back through the esophagus and stomach and out the abdominal wall. The tube may also be inserted through the endoscope and then "pulled" out through the abdominal wall. There is no clear advantage to one technique over the other; both are highly successful and rapidly performed.[21] Internal and external dams hold the catheter in place. A jejunostomy tube may be inserted by a similar method. Once the pathway heals, a skin-level "button" can be inserted to replace the protruding tube.

PEG tubes are 12 to 16 F in diameter and usually are anchored by a 1- to 2-inch cross-linked latex tube placed inside the stomach. A dressing is not generally used. Keeping the site open helps prevent skin breakdown and infection. The skin around the gastrostomy may be cleaned with a dilute hydrogen peroxide solution to remove crusts and rinsed with normal saline or water. The "button" gastrostomy does not require a tube and lessens the chance of complications from tube irritation or obstruction. A tube is inserted into the button just for feedings.

Enteral Feeding Solutions. A variety of feeding solutions are available to meet diverse patient needs. All enteral formulas contain the essential nutrients, but they differ in the balance of those nutrients and in the amount of digestion and absorption required to use them. Table 42-4 compares the various components of a few sample formulas.[7]

Caloric density (the number of calories per unit volume) is an extremely important consideration. High-density formulas tend to be more hypertonic and may contribute to diarrhea. Lower-density formulas require a larger volume of solution to provide needed nutrients, which may be an issue if fluids must be restricted.

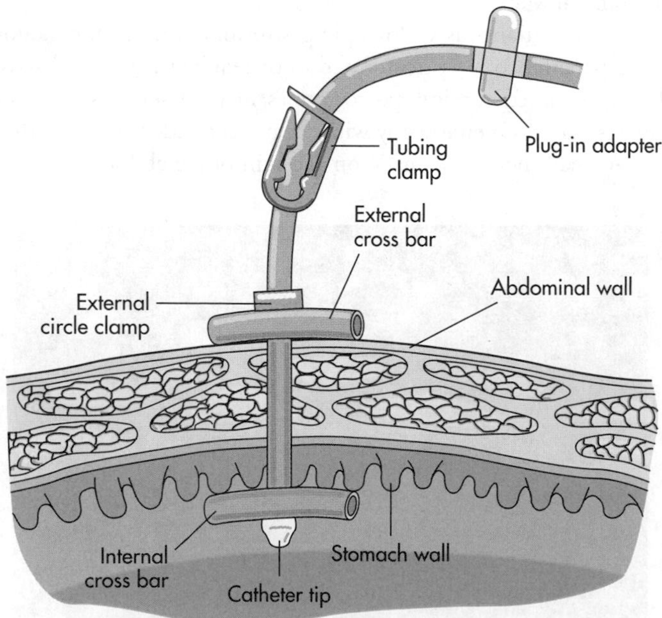

Figure 42-13 A percutaneous endoscopic gastrostomy (PEG) tube in place in the stomach.

Protein is considered the most critical component of any formula. The molecular composition of the formula may vary substantially, however, based on the patient's digestive and absorptive capabilities. Polymeric formulas contain intact proteins and are generally administered to patients with normal levels of pancreatic enzymes for adequate digestion. Oligomeric formulas contain predigested proteins (hydrolyzed protein, dipeptides and tripeptides, or some free amino acids). These formulas can be given to patients with limited or impaired digestive ability but intact GI absorption.[7] Monomeric formulas, also known as elemental diets, contain nitrogen in the form of free fatty acids. They require minimal digestive function and have been recommended for use with a variety of GI disorders, but recent research does not show them to be more effective than oligomeric formulas.[21] The fat content of monomeric formulas causes them to be very hyperosmolar, which can be a real drawback.

Osmolality is an essential consideration for all enteral solutions and varies considerably among formulas. Isotonic formulas approximate the osmolality of plasma (280 to 300 mOsm/kg body weight) and are easiest to tolerate. They can be administered at full strength with the rate adjusted to patient tolerance. Adequate amounts of hypotonic fluids such as water are also essential to maintain the desired osmolality. The osmolality of most enteral solutions is a reflection of the concentration of proteins and carbohydrates. Hypertonic formulas typically have osmolalities ranging from 400 to 1100 mOsm/kg and need to be diluted or administered at an extremely slow rate until patient tolerance increases.

The major concerns about the carbohydrate content of feeding solutions relate to total calorie needs and lactose content. Increasing awareness of the pervasiveness of partial lactose intolerance has stimulated the development of formulas without a milk base. Carbohydrates in standard formulas are easily used as long as intestinal absorption remains intact. Formula components include starch and polysaccharides, disaccharides, and monosaccharides. Effective carbohydrate use also depends on the person having adequate amounts of insulin, glucagon, norepinephrine, and vitamins. Any imbalance or deficiency in these elements can impair absorption and produce watery diarrhea.

Fats in the formula are a source of concentrated calories and essential fatty acids and serve as a carrier for fat-soluble vitamins. Fat digestion depends on pancreatic enzymes, bile salts, and normal intestinal flora. Short-, medium-, and long-chain fatty acids may be included in both saturated and polyunsaturated forms. All formulas are supplemented with substantial amounts of essential vitamins and minerals.

Enteral Feeding Techniques. Feeding schedules may be planned on a continuous, intermittent, or bolus basis. Continuous feedings are used for most short-term nutritional support because the volume of fluid delivered can be kept very low, which increases patient tolerance. This is ideal for nasointestinal delivery because the small intestine normally receives nutrients from the stomach in small volumes over several hours after each meal. Intermittent or bolus scheduling significantly increases the risk of dumping syndrome and diarrhea. When long-term support is needed, an intermittent schedule with delivery of the feeding to

TABLE 42-4 SAMPLE TUBE FEEDING COMPOSITION

Formula Type	Osmolality (mOsm/kg)	Protein (g/L)	Fat (g/L)	Carbohydrate (g/L)
OLIGOMERIC FORMULAS				
Vivonex Plus Travasorb HN Subdue Peptamen	300-650	30-94	5-68	127-221
POLYMERIC FORMULAS (LACTOSE FREE)				
Ensure Isocal Osmolite Boost HP	300-520	34-60	35-45	127-169
HIGH NITROGEN FORMULAS				
Ensure HN Osmolite HN Boost HN Promote	300-610	45-63	26-45	123-144
LOW FAT OR FAT FREE FORMULAS				
Citrosource Enlive Resource	480-700	37-41	0-2	120-152

the stomach best replicates a normal eating pattern. It also permits the patient to be free of the tube feeding for long intervals throughout the day. Clinical decisions are based on the unique patient circumstances.

Intermittent feedings are administered by gravity over 30 to 40 minutes, typically four to six times per day. The nurse checks residual volumes before each intermittent feeding and at specified intervals, usually every 4 to 6 hours, for patients receiving continuous feedings.[33] Most protocols direct that an intermittent feeding be held if the residual is greater than 100 to 150 ml. Lower parameters are set for patients with gastrostomies. With continuous feedings a residual of two times the amount of feeding delivered over the last hour would usually require notification of the physician. Consensus does not exist over whether the aspirated fluid should be refed to the patient, although this is frequently recommended. Careful review of the research suggests that principles of medical or surgical asepsis should be followed in changing or administering a tube feeding.[30] See the Guidelines for Safe Practice box.

Managing Complications

TUBE OBSTRUCTION. Feeding tube obstructions are relatively common. Pill fragments, formula residue adhering to the tube lumen, and formula-medication incompatibilities are common causes. Thoroughly flushing tubes with 30 to 60 ml of water before and after feedings and medication administration, or every 4 to 6

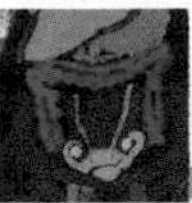
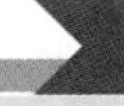

GUIDELINES FOR SAFE PRACTICE *The Patient Receiving Enteral Tube Feedings*

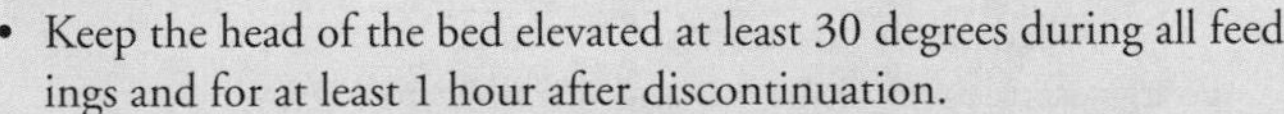

- Keep the head of the bed elevated at least 30 degrees during all feedings and for at least 1 hour after discontinuation.
  —Use high Fowler's position for intermittent feedings if permitted.
- Verify tube placement.
  —Check the length of tube that protrudes from the nose.
  —Inject 10 to 30 ml of air into the tube and auscultate over the left upper quadrant of the abdomen.
  —Aspirate secretions if possible, and check the pH of the aspirate. A pH of 1 to 5 indicates gastric contents.
  —Check the volume of the residual against ordered parameters.
  —Refeed aspirated fluid per institution protocol.
- Flush tube with 30 to 50 ml of water before initiating and at the end of the feeding or every 4 to 6 hours for continuous feedings.
- Always flush the tube before and after medication administration.
- Verify rate settings on the delivery pump.
- Ensure that the tube is properly and securely taped, and check for nasal irritation.
- Record all administered volumes and residuals, including irrigation fluids, on intake and output records.
- Cleanse delivery equipment after each use and discard per institution protocol (usually 24 to 48 hours).

Intermittent (Bolus) Feedings

1. Attach syringe to feeding tube.
2. Elevate syringe 18 inches above the patient's head.
3. Fill syringe with formula.
4. Allow feeding to empty by gravity.
5. Keep syringe filled to avoid infusion of air.

hours during continuous administration, is the best prevention. Avoiding administration of pill fragments or thick medications also helps prevent occlusion. Strategies to prevent feeding tube obstruction are summarized in the Guidelines for Safe Practice box below.

Regurgitation or Aspiration. Pulmonary complications are the most dangerous problems associated with enteral feedings. A tube of any size may enter the tracheobronchial tree on insertion or migrate there with vigorous coughing or suctioning. Patients who are obtunded and have impaired cough or gag reflexes are at particular risk. Misplacement of the tube is common in unconscious patients.

No method except chest x-ray examination is foolproof in verifying correct tube placement. Most institutions use several tests of tube placement. The tube should be properly taped to secure it in position, and the external length of the tube should be routinely verified. Instilling a small amount of air while simultaneously auscultating the abdomen is a recommended test of tube placement, even though sounds are readily transmitted throughout the abdomen so the tube may not be located where the sounds are heard. Aspirating tube contents is more accurate, and pH testing of the aspirate can help to verify accurate placement; however, small-bore tubes often collapse easily, making aspiration difficult or impossible. The head of the bed is kept elevated 30 to 40 degrees at all times if possible to decrease the risk of aspiration. The use of nasointestinal tubes with weighted tips appears to decrease the incidence of reflux in patients at high risk for aspiration.

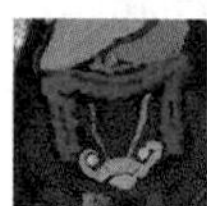

Guidelines for Safe Practice
Preventing Feeding Tube Obstruction

- Use a polyurethane feeding tube if possible.
- Flush the tube with at least 30 ml of water every 4 hours; do this before and after administering medications and before and after checking gastric residual volumes.
- Use a controller pump to maintain a steady flow.
- Administer all medications with care. Use oral route if possible.
  —Do not administer medications with the tube feeding running. Always flush first.
  —Do not administer any enteric-coated, chewable, or sublingual drugs through the tube. Obtain liquid forms of medications if possible.
  —Do not crush slow-release tablets. The beads from slow-release capsules may be flushed through the tube if size permits.
  —Crush all tablets thoroughly into a fine powder. Do not open the package before crushing. Mix with 15 to 100 ml of water before administering. Administer through a medication port.
  —Time the administration of antacids around other medications.
  —Administer each drug separately; do not combine.
  —Stop feedings for 15 to 30 minutes before administration if a drug needs to be given on an empty stomach.
- Irrigate clogged tubes with water. If this is ineffective, Viokase or a declogging stylus may be used per institution policy. There is no evidence that cranberry juice is effective, and water is as effective as cola products.

Diarrhea. Diarrhea is the most commonly encountered complication of enteral feedings, and it may be caused by a variety of factors. Formulas containing lactose, a high-fat content, or a low-fiber content have all been implicated in the development of diarrhea. High osmolality also appears to be important, particularly with severely malnourished patients. Diarrhea may also be caused by prescribed medications, such as antibiotics, H_2-receptor antagonists, and elixirs containing sorbitol. Diarrhea occurs in 30% to 50% of critically ill patients receiving tube feedings and appears to correlate most closely with the administration of antibiotics.[21] Methods of combating tube feeding–associated diarrhea include the use of bulking agents, slow delivery rates, and formula dilution during the initial administration period. It is also essential that dehydration be prevented through the administration of adequate amounts of free water. The greater the osmolality of the formula, the more water is needed. Diphenoxylate or loperamide may also be used.

Bacterial contamination is another significant cause of diarrhea. Formula can become contaminated at any point in the preparation and delivery process. Formulas with higher osmolalities appear to be less likely to support bacterial growth. The length of time the formula hangs at room temperature also is a factor. Hospital-prepared formulas that contain milk are the most vulnerable. The Guidelines for Safe Practice box below summarizes measures to reduce the risk of bacterial contamination of formula.

Parenteral Nutrition

Parenteral nutrition delivers concentrated solutions intravenously to maintain or supplement a patient's nutritional balance when oral or enteral nutrition is inadequate or not possible. Parenteral nutrition is indicated for patients whose GI tract is not functioning as a result of obstruction, acute inflammation, or malabsorption. It is also used for patients who are extremely hypermetabolic from trauma or sepsis, need to be kept NPO for more than 5 to 7 days, are unable to take adequate amounts of nutrients orally, or experience severe GI side effects from radiotherapy or chemotherapy. Parenteral nutrition is considered whenever enteral intake is, or

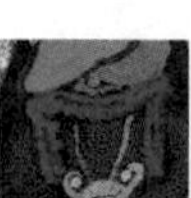

Guidelines for Safe Practice
Preventing Bacterial Contamination of Tube Feeding Formulas

- Use prefilled, ready-to-use sets if available.
- Follow aseptic technique in handling all components:
  —Good hand washing is essential.
  —Wear nonsterile disposable gloves when handling the equipment.
  —Wear a mask if you have a cold.
- Use full-strength ready-to-use formula; dilution and reconstitution increase the chances of contamination.
- Rinse the delivery set with water before adding new formula.
- Hang commercially prepared formulas for no more than 8 to 12 hours (hospital-prepared formulas for no more than 6 hours).
- Discard feeding system after 24 hours (48 hours if a closed system).
- Use systems with medication ports.
- Cover, label, and refrigerate opened or prepared formulas below 4° C and use within 24 hours.

is anticipated to be, inadequate for 7 to 10 days or more. The increased recognition of the importance of adequate nutrition for healing has resulted in physicians initiating parenteral nutrition as a therapeutic tool much earlier in the disease management process.

Parenteral nutrition is commonly administered through the central venous route, but it can be administered by peripheral vein as well. Peripheral solutions differ primarily in their glucose content, which generally does not exceed 10%. Strongly hypertonic solutions can be extremely irritating to the peripheral veins, limiting the longevity of the catheter. Peripheral solutions rely more heavily on isotonic lipid emulsions as the main nonprotein calorie source.

Home administration of parenteral nutrition has enabled thousands of patients to remain in their homes and out of the acute care setting while receiving prolonged nutritional support. Advanced inflammatory bowel disease is the most common medical indication, but acquired immunodeficiency syndrome and cancer are other common diagnoses. Cost constraints put significant pressure on patients and families to learn to safely administer the parenteral nutrition without the ongoing supervision of a home health nurse. With a well-structured teaching plan and ongoing supervision or support from a nutrition support team, most families are able to successfully provide the needed care.

Central Venous Catheters. Central venous catheters allow rapid mixing and dilution of strongly hypertonic solutions. Subclavian, tunneled, and implantable port catheters are available in single-lumen and multilumen forms. Central venous catheters and venous access devices are discussed and illustrated in Chapter 23. Infection is the primary concern related to the administration of parenteral nutrition. It is believed that catheter contamination at the point of entry into the skin and migration of bacteria along the catheter are the major sources of sepsis. Multilumen catheters carry an increased infection risk.[21]

Rigorous dressing care is essential, but institutional protocols vary widely. Research is ongoing to determine the optimal interval for dressing changes and the effectiveness of the various dressing materials. Dressings are usually changed every 48 to 72 hours, more often if they become wet or contaminated. Tubing is also changed every 48 to 72 hours, and appropriate size filters are used to administer solutions and lipids. The use of a 0.2-μm filter is recommended for administering all parenteral nutrition solutions, but if lipids are also administered, their large molecules require the use of a filter of at least 1.2 μm or larger. The effectiveness of filters in reducing the risk of bacterial contamination remains unproven, but they do trap crystals and air from the solution and tubing.

Solutions. Parenteral nutrition solutions are complex formulas that provide all known essential nutrients in quantities that will support wound healing, anabolism, weight gain or maintenance, and growth in children. All such solutions contain water, protein, carbohydrates, fat, vitamins, and trace elements. The various proportions of each element are individualized to the patient's unique clinical situation and needs.

Solutions used to deliver parenteral nutrition usually consist of 25% to 35% dextrose, 3% to 5% amino acids, electrolytes, minerals, and vitamins. Intravenous fat emulsions in 10% to 20% concentrations also may be added. Dextrose and fat are given for their caloric value. The body uses them to meet its energy needs. This permits the administered amino acids to be used for tissue building. Fat provides twice the caloric value of dextrose, exerts minimal osmotic pressure, and prevents fatty acid deficiency. Regular insulin may be added to the solution or administered subcutaneously to support glucose utilization.

Parenteral nutrition solutions provide good culture media for bacteria. Catheter-related sepsis is most commonly caused by *Staphylococcus epidermidis* and *Staphylococcus aureus*. Immunocompromised patients may be colonized by a wide variety of gram-positive and gram-negative organisms. Solutions are prepared under strict aseptic conditions in the pharmacy under a laminar airflow hood. The solutions are kept refrigerated until ready for use and are left at room temperature for 30 minutes before administration. Prepared formulas ideally should be used within 24 hours to minimize the risk of contamination, but institutional protocols may vary.

Parenteral nutrition solutions are administered slowly and the rate increased as patient tolerance permits. Blood glucose levels are checked frequently at the beginning of treatment while endogenous insulin production adjusts to the increased glucose load. An infusion pump is used to ensure a steady infusion rate. If administration needs to be interrupted for any reason, infusions of 10% dextrose are substituted to prevent rebound hypoglycemia. Parenteral nutrition administration is gradually tapered before it is discontinued to allow the body time to make the necessary metabolic adjustments. Lipid emulsions may be mixed with the solution, given through a separate peripheral IV line, or given through a Y-connector in the main IV line.

Complications. Complications of parenteral nutrition include problems with the catheter, infection, and metabolic imbalances. Correct insertion and placement of the catheter are extremely important. Proper insertion prevents most problems related to pneumothorax or hemothorax, air embolism, brachial plexus injury, and thromboembolism and also decreases the incidence of sepsis.

Catheter-related sepsis is a serious complication of parenteral nutrition that cannot always be prevented. Strict aseptic technique during catheter insertion and subsequent care is essential. The nurse monitors vital signs regularly and assesses the insertion site for tenderness, redness, and drainage. The catheter site is the most common source of infection. The onset of sepsis may be preceded by the development of unexplained hyperglycemia. Injecting an antibiotic solution (antibiotic lock) into the catheter lumen and allowing it to "sit" for about 12 hours each day shows promise in reducing catheter-related infection, but the technique appears to have no benefit in treating or preventing tunnel or skin infections.[21]

The major metabolic alteration associated with the use of parenteral nutrition is glucose intolerance. Blood glucose levels are carefully monitored through fingersticks. Insulin may be added to the solution or administered on a sliding scale if needed. Severe osmotic diuresis can result from uncontrolled hyperglycemia and can lead rapidly to dehydration. Hypoglycemia is also a potential problem when the patient is being weaned from parenteral nutrition or whenever the continuous infusion of solution is interrupted for any reason. The goal is to keep blood glucose levels between 100 and 150 mg/dl during treatment.

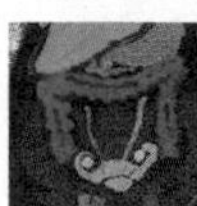

GUIDELINES FOR SAFE PRACTICE *The Patient Receiving Parenteral Nutrition*

Do not use the catheter for other purposes if possible.

Preventing Infection

Maintain strict aseptic technique.
Keep solutions cold until ready for use, but allow solution to warm to room temperature before administration; use solutions within 24 to 36 hours.
—All additions to parenteral solutions should be performed in laminar flow areas.
Change dressing according to institutional protocol.
—Follow strict aseptic technique in handling catheter, dressing, tubing, and solution. Explore use of "antibiotic lock" for high-risk patients.
Change administration sets every 24 hours or by institution protocol. Use appropriate filters on tubing.
Monitor for signs of redness, swelling, or drainage at insertion site.
Suspect sepsis if afebrile patient develops a fever.

Preventing Air Embolism

Tape all connections securely.
Clamp catheter before opening system.
Cover subclavian catheter insertion site with an air-occlusive dressing (adhesive tape) or transparent polyurethane dressing (OpSite).
Position patient as flat as possible for dressing and tubing changes.
Instruct patient to perform Valsalva's maneuver whenever catheter hub is open to the air.

Maintaining Fluid and Electrolyte Balance

Maintain a uniform infusion rate. Never abruptly discontinue solution administration.
—Use a pump for controlled delivery rates.
—Never exceed prescribed rate of administration; do not attempt to "catch up" if infusion falls behind schedule.
Monitor for signs of *overhydration* (neck vein distention, cough, weight gain):
—Weigh patient daily.
—Record accurate intake and output.
Check electrolyte values every other day.

Preventing Metabolic Imbalance

Monitor and report to physician signs of *hypoglycemia* (pallor, diaphoresis, tachycardia, hunger, trembling, behavioral changes).
—Administer 10% glucose solution if parental nutrition must be interrupted for any reason
Monitor for signs of *hyperglycemia* (nausea, weakness, thirst, headache, rapid respirations).
—Check fingerstick blood glucose as ordered (every 6 hours initially and every day once stable).
Administer sliding scale insulin as ordered.

Promoting Comfort

Provide for good oral hygiene.
Encourage ambulation and participation in activities of daily living.
Monitor for "refeeding syndrome" when parenteral nutrition is initiated (first 24 to 48 hours). Syndrome results from the abrupt shift of electrolytes from the plasma to the intracellular compartment.
Symptoms include respiratory depression, lethargy, confusion, and weakness.

Other possible complications associated with parenteral nutrition include fluid, electrolyte, and acid-base imbalances (primarily acidosis). Vitamin D deficiency and vitamin A excess also may occur. Serum electrolyte levels are monitored several times a week. Carbohydrate metabolism yields water and carbon dioxide. The increased production of carbon dioxide caused by concentrated glucose solutions can induce respiratory distress in patients with compromised pulmonary status. Abnormalities in liver function may also occur when patients receive high volumes of carbohydrate calories. The body converts the calories into intrahepatic fat, which can cause liver dysfunction. Cholelithiasis from gallbladder stasis is also a common problem.

Care of the patient receiving parenteral nutrition is summarized in the Guidelines for Safe Practice box.

Critical Thinking

1. You are having lunch with a co-worker and observe him taking an over-the-counter H_2-receptor antagonist. He tells you he's been experiencing frequent abdominal pain that often wakes him up at night. You ask him if he has seen his primary care provider and he replies that he doesn't think that is necessary. He has been watching his diet, eating bland foods, and drinking lots of milk, and he is certain the symptoms will go away as soon as he successfully meets his deadline for a major project. What other information might you want to obtain from him? What teaching will you try to provide?
2. You are a nurse in a busy medical ICU where routine stress ulcer prophylaxis is the standard of care. Design a research project to test the effectiveness of routine prophylaxis. What patient criteria would you use for selection? How will you measure your outcomes?

References

1. Abraham E: Acid suppression in a critical care environment: state of the art and beyond, *Crit Care Med* 30(Suppl 6):S349-S350, 2002.
2. Barkun A, Bardou M, Marshall JK: Clinical guidelines: consensus recommendations for managing patients with nonvariceal upper gastrointestinal bleeding, *Ann Intern Med* 139(10):843-857, 2003.
3. Bauer J: Enteral feeding pumps, *RN* 66(8):69-70, 2003.
4. Benson AB: New perspectives in the management of upper gastrointestinal malignancies, *Semin Oncol* 30(4 Suppl 11):1-31, 2003.
5. Blankfield RP et al: *Helicobacter pylori* infection and the development of gastric cancer, *N Engl J Med* 346(1):65-67, 2002.
6. Chan FKL, Leung WK: Peptic ulcer disease, *Lancet* 360(9337):933-941, 2002.
7. Collins N: What's in that feeding formula anyway? *Nursing 2001* 31(12):32hn1-32hn2, 2001.

8. Conrad SA: Acute upper gastrointestinal bleeding in critically ill patients: causes and treatment modalities, *Crit Care Med* 30(Suppl 6):S365-368, S371, S379, 2002.
9. Coon J, Ernst E: Systematic review: herbal medicinal products for non-ulcer dyspepsia, *Aliment Pharamacol Therap* 16(10):1689-1699, 2002.
10. El-Serag HB, Talley NJ: The prevalence and clinical course of functional dyspepsia, *Aliment Pharmacol Therap* 19(6):643-654, 2004.
11. El-Serag B et al: Prevention of complicated ulcer disease among chronic users of nonsteroidal anti-inflammatory drugs, *Arch Intern Med* 162(18):2105-2110, 2002.
12. Farrell RJ, Kelly CP: Celiac sprue and refractory sprue. In Feldman M, Friedman LS, Sleisinger MH, editors: *Gastrointestinal and liver disease*, ed 7, Philadelphia, 2002, Saunders.
13. Genta RM: The gastritis connection: prevention and early detection of gastric neoplasms, *J Clin Gastroenterol* 36(5)(Suppl):S44-S49, 2003.
14. Go MF: *Helicobacter pylori*: when to test and how to treat, *Medscape Gastroenterol* 5(2), accessed Sept 2003 from website: www.Medscape.com
15. Graham DY: NSAIDs, *Helicobacter pylori*, and Pandora's box, *N Engl J Med* 347(26):2162-2164, 2002.
16. Hogenauer C, Hammer HF: Maldigestion and malabsorption. In Feldman M, Friedman LS, Sleisinger MH, editors: *Gastrointestinal and liver disease*, ed 7, Philadelphia, 2002, Saunders.
17. Jamulitrat S et al: Stress ulcer prophylaxis and risk of developing ventilator-associated pneumonia, *Am J Infect Control* 32(1):52, 2004.
18. Jones MP: Evaluation and treatment of dyspepsia, *Postgrad Med J* 79(927):25-29, 2003.
19. Jung R, MacLaren R: Proton-pump inhibitors for stress ulcer prophylaxis in critically ill patients, *Ann Pharmacother* 36(12):1929-1937, 2002.
20. Khaitan L, Holzman M: Laparoscopic advances in general surgery, *JAMA* 287(12):1502-1504, 2002.
21. Klein S, Rubin D: Enteral and parenteral nutrition. In Feldman M, Friedman LS, Sleisinger MH, editors: *Gastrointestinal and liver disease*, ed 7, Philadelphia, 2002, Saunders.
22. Koh TJ, Wang T: Tumors of the stomach. In Feldman M, Friedman LS, Sleisinger MH, editors: *Gastrointestinal and liver disease*, ed 7, Philadelphia, 2002, Saunders.
23. Lee EL, Feldman M: Gastritis and other gastropathies. In Feldman M, Friedman LS, Sleisinger MH, editors: *Gastrointestinal and liver disease*, ed 7, Philadelphia, 2002, Saunders.
24. Louw JA, Marks IN: The management of peptic ulcer disease, *Medscape* 19(6):533-539, 2002.
25. Malik A, Westergaard H: Short bowel syndrome. In Feldman M, Friedman LS, Sleisinger MH, editors: *Gastrointestinal and liver disease*, ed 7, Philadelphia, 2002, Saunders.
26. Maze CDM: Nursing care of patients with gastrointestinal cancer: a staff development approach, *J Nurses Staff Devel* 18(6):327-332, 2002.
27. McQuaid K: Dyspepsia. In Feldman M, Friedman LS, Sleisinger MH, editors: *Gastrointestinal and liver disease*, ed 7, Philadelphia, 2002, Saunders.
28. Meurer LN, Bower J: Management *of Helicobacter pylori* infection, *Am Fam Phys* 65(7):1327-1336, 2002.
29. Moayyedi P et al: Pharmacological interventions for non-ulcer dyspepsia (Cochrane Review). In *Cochrane Library*, Issue 3, 2004, Chichester, UK, John Wiley & Sons.
30. Padula C et al: Enteral feedings: what the evidence says, *AJN* 104(7):62-69, 2004.
31. Parsonnet J, Forman D: *Helicobacter pylori* infection and gastric cancer—for want of more outcomes, *JAMA* 291(2):244-245, 2004.
32. Peterson W, Graham D: *Helicobacter pylori*. In Feldman M, Friedman LS, Sleisinger MH, editors: *Gastrointestinal and liver disease*, ed 7, Philadelphia, 2002, Saunders.
33. Pullen R: Measuring gastric residual volume, *Nursing 2004* 34(4):18, 2004.
34. Rege RV, Jones DB: Current role of surgery in peptic ulcer disease. In Feldman M, Friedman LS, Sleisinger MH, editors: *Gastrointestinal and liver disease*, ed 7, Philadelphia, 2002, Saunders.
35. Rockey D: Gastrointestinal bleeding. In Feldman M, Friedman LS, Sleisinger MH, editors: *Gastrointestinal and liver disease*, ed 7, Philadelphia, 2002, Saunders.
36. Rostom A et al: Prevention of NSAID-induced gastroduodenal ulcers, *Cochrane Library,* ID No. CD002296, 2005.
37. Siu WT et al: Laparoscopic repair for perforated peptic ulcer: a randomized controlled trial, *Ann Surgery* 235(3):313-319, 2002.
38. Steinberg KP: Stress-related mucosal disease in the critically ill patient: risk factors and strategies to prevent stress-related bleeding in the intensive care unit, *Crit Care Med* 30(Suppl 6):S362-S364, 2002.
39. Thompson D: Complementary healthcare practices: east meets west: the use of traditional Chinese medicine for gastrointestinal disorders, *Gastroenterol Nurs* 26(6):266-268, 2003.
40. US Department of Health and Human Services: *Healthy people 2010: understanding and improving health,* Washington, DC, 2001, The Department.
41. US Department of Health and Human Services, Public Health Service: *Helicobacter pylori* in peptic ulcer disease, *National Institutes of Health* 12(1):1-23, 2004.
42. Yildizdas D, Yapiciogulu H, Yilmaz HL: Occurrence of ventilator-associated pneumonia in mechanically ventilated pediatric intensive care patients during stress ulcer prophylaxis with sucralfate, ranitidine, and omeprazole, *J Crit Care* (17)4:240-245, 2002.

Visit the Evolve website: http://evolve.elsevier.com/Monahan/medsurg

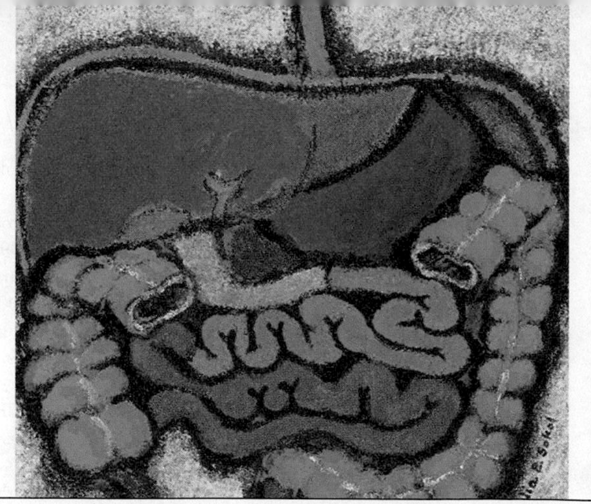

CHAPTER 43
Intestinal Problems

by Frances D. Monahan, Sharon A. Aronovitch

OBJECTIVES

After studying this chapter, the learner should be able to:

1. Discuss lifestyle modifications for the management of constipation and diarrhea and the prevention of foodborne illness.
2. Compare the common forms of intestinal inflammation and their management.
3. Describe current pharmacologic and nursing management of inflammatory bowel disease.
4. Compare the pathophysiology of hernias, cancer, and volvulus as causes of bowel obstruction.
5. Discuss the nursing management of the patient with an ostomy.
6. Differentiate among the various surgical approaches to the management of common anorectal disorders.
7. Discuss preoperative and postoperative care of the patient undergoing bowel surgery.

KEY TERMS

adynamic, p. 1269
anastomosis, p. 1257
autosomal dominant, p. 1271
borborygmus, p. 1241
chemoprotection, p. 1273
comorbidity, p. 1261
intraluminal pressure, p. 1245
McBurney's point, p. 1245
microperforations, p. 1247
molecular marker, p. 1276
promotility, p. 1271
tenesmus, p. 1241

Disorders that affect the intestines are major health problems in the United States, ranging from mild to life threatening and affecting digestion, absorption, and elimination. The categories of intestinal disorders discussed in this chapter include problems of elimination, inflammatory bowel diseases, bowel obstructions, and anorectal disorders.

Functional Bowel Disorders

Constipation

Etiology and Epidemiology. The act of defecation, which is initiated when feces enter the rectum, is voluntarily controlled by contraction of the external anal sphincter. Most people have a regular pattern of defecation, but the pattern varies widely, from three times a day to once every 3 or more days. The term *constipation* refers to an abnormal infrequency of defecation, the passage of abnormally hard stools, or both. The term lacks precise definition because it has different meanings for different people. Almost everyone experiences occasional constipation, and it is considered an almost universal problem in Western countries. It is particularly common among older adults.[42] Each year constipation accounts for millions of physician visits and millions of dollars expended on products to cause or support defecation.[34] Many of these products are unnecessary; some are even harmful.

Constipation can be a functional consequence of numerous disorders. Endocrine and neurologic diseases such as diabetes, hypothyroidism, multiple sclerosis, and Parkinson's disease are commonly associated with chronic constipation. Constipation is also a frequent side effect of the use of opioids, anticholinergics, and a wide variety of specific drugs such as anticonvulsants and calcium channel blockers. In many adults, however, occasional constipation can be attributed to physical inactivity, stress, dietary changes, lack of fluids, and failure to respond to the urge to defecate.[42] Common risk factors for constipation are summarized in the Risk Factors box.

Pathophysiology. Constipation may result from decreased motility of the colon or from retention of feces in the lower colon or rectum. The longer the feces remain in the colon, the greater the amount of water resorbed and the drier the stool becomes. The stool is then more difficult to expel. The urge to defecate

Risk Factors

Constipation

Functional Disorders

Diabetes mellitus
Hypothyroidism
Multiple sclerosis
Parkinson's disease
A wide variety of other neurogenic and collagen disorders

Medications

Aluminum- and calcium-based antacids
Opioids
Anticholinergics
Antidepressants or antipsychotics
Iron, calcium, and bismuth salts
Anticonvulsants
Calcium channel blockers

Dietary Factors

Dehydration
Lack of dietary fiber

Physical and Psychologic Factors

Immobility
Confusion, disorientation
Interruption of normal bowel routines, stress

occurs most often after meals, particularly breakfast, as a result of stimulation of the gastrocolic reflex from food entering the stomach. If the urge to defecate is not promptly heeded, it is quickly suppressed, and the feces remain in the rectum and harden.

Occasional constipation is not detrimental to health, but habitual constipation leads to decreased intestinal muscle tone, increased use of Valsalva's maneuver as the person bears down in an attempt to pass the hardened stool, and increased incidence of hemorrhoids. Fecal impaction can result from chronic constipation, especially in institutionalized older adults in whom mental confusion and immobility may complicate the effective management of elimination. The rectum overdistends and is unable to respond to normal sensory stimulation from the anus, leading to damaging cycles of impaction, rebound diarrhea, and eventually fecal incontinence.

Collaborative Care Management. The treatment of constipation begins with a careful assessment of the nature, severity, and duration of the problem. Treatment is individualized to the patient's unique needs. It generally includes dietary and fluid modifications, increased activity, establishment of regular toileting patterns, and use of fiber supplements as needed. Dietary fiber increases the water content of the stool and promotes colonic motility through bacterial degradation.

Adherence to the prescribed regimen successfully manages the problem for most individuals. Nonabsorbable saccharides (e.g., sorbitol or lactulose) may be added if needed. Numerous laxative agents are available over the counter, but the chronic use of stimulant laxatives is avoided if possible. Stool softeners are a popular option, but little concrete research supports their effectiveness.[29] Table 43-1 presents drugs commonly used in the management of constipation.

Hospitalization inevitably interferes with a person's normal patterns of exercise and eating. The nurse monitors all hospitalized patients for constipation and records all bowel elimination. For greatest success, preventive bowel programs are initiated before problems with constipation arise. Initiation of a plan to prevent constipation should be a priority for any patient on bed rest or receiving frequent doses of opioids.

PATIENT/FAMILY TEACHING. Teaching begins with ensuring patient understanding of the relationship between diet, fluids, activity, stress, and the development of constipation. The nurse encourages patients to eat a high-fiber diet and to limit highly refined foods (see Box 43-1 for the fiber content of selected foods). Bran may be used as a supplement in a limited way. Patients should attempt to drink at least 2 L of fluid daily unless their medical condition contraindicates a liberal fluid intake. Regular exercise and a planned daily time for defecation are important measures. The patient is instructed to manage occasional episodes of constipation with bulk-forming laxatives if needed and to avoid the regular use of harsh laxatives or any type of enema.

Box 43-1 Fiber Content in Common Foods

Fruits

Raspberries: 6 g/cup
Apples: 3 g each
Tangerines: 3 g each
Peaches: 1 g each

Vegetables

Carrots: 2 g each
Peeled potatoes: 2 g each
Broccoli: 1 g/½ cup
Cauliflower: 1 g/½ cup
Lettuce: 1 g/cup
Spinach: 1 g/½ cup

Starchy Vegetables

Lima beans: 4 g/½ cup
Kidney beans: 3 g/½ cup
Black-eyed peas: 4 g/½ cup

Grains

Whole-wheat bread: 2 g/slice
White rice: 1 g/cup
Brown rice: 3 g/cup
Oatmeal: 3 g/⅔ cup

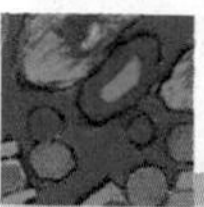

TABLE 43-1
COMMON MEDICATIONS *for Treatment of Constipation*

Drug	Action	Nursing Intervention
Bulk Formers		
Psyllium (Metamucil) Methylcellulose (Citrucel)	Polysaccharides and cellulose derivatives, which mix with intestinal fluids, swell, and stimulate peristalsis	Ensure adequate fluid intake to prevent impaction or obstruction. Instruct patient to take separately from prescribed drugs to avoid problems with absorption.
Stool Softeners (Emollients)		
Docusate sodium (Colace) Docusate calcium (Surfak)	Act as detergents in intestine, reducing surface tension, which facilitates incorporation of liquid and fat, softening stool	Explain to patients that preparations lose effectiveness with long-term use so they should not rely on this measure alone. Instruct patient to discontinue if abdominal cramping occurs.
Lubricants		
Mineral oil	Soften fecal matter by lubricating intestinal mucosa, facilitating easy stool passage If used excessively, interferes with absorption of fat-soluble vitamins A, D, E, and K, leading to deficiency	Instruct patient not to take with meals or drugs because oil can impair absorption and to swallow carefully to prevent lipid aspiration.
Hyperosmolar Laxatives		
Lactulose (Cephulac) Polyethylene glycol (GoLYTELY) Sorbitol	Nonabsorbable sugars degraded by colonic bacteria and increase stool osmolarity; fluid drawn into intestine, stimulating peristalsis	Adjust dose and frequency of administration to control side effects and regulate defecation. Monitor for fluid and electrolyte imbalance if response is severe.
Saline Laxatives		
Magnesium citrate Magnesium sulfate (Epsom salts) Magnesium hydroxide (Milk of Magnesia)	Cause osmotic retention of fluid, which distends colon and increases peristalsis Liquid preparations more effective than tablets	Instruct patient to take with full glass of water. Monitor for fluid and electrolyte imbalance if response is severe.
Stimulant or Irritant Laxatives		
Senna (Senokot) Bisacodyl (Dulcolax) Castor oil	Directly stimulate and irritate intestine, promoting peristalsis	Explain to patient that cramps and diarrhea can occur. Monitor for fluid and electrolyte imbalance if reaction is severe.

Diarrhea and Foodborne Illness

Etiology and Epidemiology. Diarrhea is a major cause of morbidity in the United States and remains a leading cause of death in developing nations, especially among infants and small children. Diarrhea involves an increase in stool number, a change to a more fluid consistency, or both. However, the diagnosis is based primarily on the consistency of the stool rather than the number of stools per day. Diarrhea is a classic sign of gastrointestinal (GI) disease and has a wide range of etiologies. These include infectious and inflammatory processes, autoimmune disease, malabsorption, and secretory diarrhea. Acute diarrhea, continuing for less than 2 to 3 weeks, is usually self-limiting, although supportive intervention may be necessary. Chronic diarrhea is usually related to changes in the GI tract that alter the transport of fluids, electrolytes, and solids. Common causes of diarrhea are listed in Box 43-2.

Acute diarrhea is by far the most frequent type and is usually caused by infectious agents. Despite improvements in sanitation, hygiene, and food-handling practices that have decreased the inci-

Box 43-2 Common Causes of Diarrhea

Infections

Bacteria (*Escherichia coli,* salmonellae, shigellae, staphylococci, *Campylobacter jejuni*)
Viruses (rotavirus, human immunodeficiency virus)
Parasites (*Giardia, Cryptosporidium,* and *Trichinella* organisms; *Entamoeba histolytica*; hookworm)

Hypersensitivity

Food allergy

Autoimmune Disease

Ulcerative colitis, Crohn's disease
Graft-versus-host disease

Effects of Cytotoxic Agents

Chemotherapy-induced mucositis
Radiation enteritis

dence of acute diarrhea in developed countries, it is still a common occurrence. According to the World Health Organization (WHO), 76 million cases of foodborne illness occur in the United States each year, leading to 325,000 hospitalizations and 5000 deaths at an annual cost of care exceeding $28 billion.[39] Raw and undercooked eggs and undercooked chicken are two of the prime sources of infection.[52] It is estimated that up to 20% of commercially sold eggs are contaminated with salmonellae.[12,16] *Campylobacter jejuni* is considered the leading cause of bacteria-induced diarrhea in the United States, and most hens are believed to be contaminated with the organism.[12] The contamination of food preparation surfaces has also been identified as a prime source of infection. Organisms proliferate rapidly when food is either inadequately cooked or inadequately refrigerated. Risk factors for infectious diarrhea are identified in the Risk Factors box, and Table 43-2 provides an overview of some of the major causes of foodborne illness.

Risk Factors

Acute Diarrhea

- Recent travel to developing nations
- Outdoor camping
- Ingestion of raw meat, seafood, or shellfish
- Eating at banquets, restaurants, picnics, or fast-food establishments
- Day care placement or employment
- Residence in institutions, nursing homes, prisons, or mental institutions
- Homosexual lifestyle
- Prostitution
- Intravenous drug abuse

Pathophysiology. Large-volume diarrhea is caused by a hypersecretion of water and electrolytes by the intestinal mucosa. This secretion occurs in response to the osmotic pressure exerted by nonabsorbed food particles in the chyme or to direct irritation of the mucosa. Peristalsis is increased, and the transit time through the intestine is significantly decreased. Increased peristalsis may also result from inflammation as mucosal cells hypersecrete water in the presence of infectious organisms. Severe abdominal cramping, **tenesmus** (persistent spasm) of the anal area, abdominal distention, and **borborygmus** (loud bowel sounds) may also occur.

Fluid and electrolyte imbalances can quickly result from diarrhea, depending on its severity. Mild diarrhea in adults can lead to

TABLE 43-2 FOODBORNE ILLNESS

Causative Agent	Clinical Manifestations	Treatment
Staphylococcus aureus	Nausea, vomiting, diarrhea, and cramps within 1-6 hr of eating	Supportive care; IV fluids if needed
Bacillus cereus enterotoxin	Watery diarrhea and cramps within 8-16 hr of eating or nausea and vomiting within 1-6 hr of eating	Supportive care
Clostridium perfringens	Diarrhea and intense cramps within 8-16 hr of eating	Supportive care; IV fluids if needed
Escherichia coli (toxigenic)	Profuse watery diarrhea, cramps, low fever, and nausea within 16-24 hr of eating	Supportive care; bismuth subsalicylate (Pepto-Bismol) sometimes helpful; IV fluids if needed
E. coli (invasive)	Cramps, fever, vomiting, and bloody diarrhea within 6-48 hr of eating	Supportive care, antibiotics
E. coli O157:H7	Cramps and bloody diarrhea within 3-5 days of eating; hemolytic uremic syndrome if fever develops	Supportive care; plasma exchange if uremic syndrome develops
Shigellae	Cramps, vomiting, fever, and diarrhea within 6-48 hr of eating	Supportive care, fluids, antibiotics
Salmonella enteritidis	Diarrhea, nausea, vomiting, cramps, and fever within 6-48 hr of eating	Supportive care, bland diet
Campylobacter jejuni	Diarrhea, cramps, fever, and nausea within 6-48 hr of eating	Supportive care, antibiotics
Vibrio cholerae	Cramps and watery diarrhea within 16-72 hr of eating	Fluid replacement, tetracycline
Vibrio parahaemolyticus	Diarrhea, cramps, nausea, vomiting, fever, and headache within 4 hr-4 days of eating	Supportive care
Clostridium botulinum	Nausea, vomiting, diarrhea, and paralysis, including respiratory failure and death, within 18-36 hr of eating	Antitoxin, mechanical ventilation

IV, Intravenous.

losses of sodium and potassium, causing metabolic alkalosis. Severe diarrhea causes dehydration, hyponatremia, hypokalemia, and metabolic acidosis from the loss of large amounts of bicarbonate. Malnourished, immunosuppressed, and older persons tolerate severe diarrhea less well than do younger or well-nourished persons. Persistent diarrhea also readily leads to skin breakdown in the perianal region.

Collaborative Care Management. The management of diarrhea focuses on preventing fluid and electrolyte imbalance, controlling symptoms, and treating the underlying cause if possible. The risk of a serious outcome or death is usually related to dehydration, and short-term hospitalization may be necessary to ensure adequate fluid replacement. Aggressive rehydration with oral replacement solutions is used if the person is alert and able to take oral fluids. Solutions such as the World Health Organization solution, Pedialyte, Resol, and Rehydralyte are preferred over fruit juices, soda, or even Gatorade because they contain a balanced electrolyte composition plus glucose.

"Bowel rest" is no longer routinely recommended in most cases of acute diarrhea, since malnutrition can develop rapidly. However, bed rest can support recovery and ease the discomfort of cramps. Clear liquids are provided along with a diet low in fiber but rich in sodium and glucose. Motility-altering drugs are rarely given in infectious diarrhea because these drugs interfere with clearance of the bacteria from the GI tract, but antidiarrheal agents may be used to manage other kinds of diarrhea (Table 43-3). Bismuth subsalicylate is usually safe and effective, but kaolin-pectin preparations are rarely helpful. Antibiotic therapy is also controversial and is reserved for patients with infections caused by specific agents (e.g., *Escherichia coli* or *Clostridium difficile*).[20] The decision is based on the nature of the causative organism.

When patients are hospitalized with acute diarrhea, the nurse maintains an accurate record of incidence and severity, estimates fluid losses, assesses for fluid and electrolyte disturbances, and promotes patient comfort. The prevention of perianal skin breakdown is an important nursing intervention. The nurse may need to assist a weakened patient in keeping the area clean and dry. Skin ointments and barriers (e.g., zinc oxide) are reapplied as needed after each episode of diarrhea. Sitz baths can be comforting when perianal skin becomes irritated.

Patient/Family Teaching. Patient teaching primarily focuses on measures related to the preventable causes of acute diarrhea. Strategies for ensuring food safety are summarized in Box 43-3. Strict cleanliness in regard to all food preparation surfaces and utensils is critical. Care should be taken in defrosting and handling uncooked meat and ensuring prompt and adequate refrigeration of all foods. Avoiding raw or undercooked meats and seafood is essential. Travelers are warned to exercise caution in consuming local water, uncooked fruits, and raw vegetables. Thorough hand washing and meticulous personal hygiene practices are helpful preventive strategies for all forms of infectious diarrhea. Reducing the incidence of food-borne illness is an important goal of *Healthy People 2010*[56] (see Healthy People 2010 box).

▶ ARE You READY?

The nurse incorporates which of the following into the standardized plans of care for patients hospitalized with acute diarrhea?

1. Bowel rest
2. Low-fiber diet
3. Motility-altering medications
4. Antibiotic therapy

Fecal Incontinence

Etiology and Epidemiology. Fecal incontinence is the involuntary release of stool. It is a complex problem with a variety of causes, including relaxation of the external or internal anal sphincters,

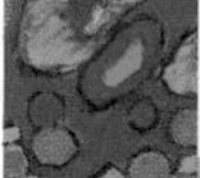

TABLE 43-3
COMMON MEDICATIONS *for Treatment of Acute Diarrhea*

Drug	Action	Nursing Intervention
Local Acting		
Bismuth subsalicylate (Pepto-Bismol)	Mechanism not known; may bind bacterial toxins	Shake liquids well before using. Inform patients that bismuth products may turn stool black.
Atta pulgite (Kaopectate)	Soothes intestinal mucosa and increases absorption of water, nutrients, and electrolytes No significant side effects	Shake liquids well before using.
Systemic Acting		
Loperamide (Imodium) Tincture of opium (paregoric) Diphenoxylate hydrochloride with atropine (Lomotil)	Act systemically to reduce peristalsis and gastrointestinal motility Part of opioid family Paregoric: potential for dependency Loperamide: few side effects and no associated physical dependency Lomotil: low potential for dependency	Monitor patient response because it can enhance bacterial invasion and prolong excretion of pathogen. Monitor for opioid side effects: central nervous system depression or respiratory depression.

Box 43-3 Prevention of Foodborne Illness

Food Buying

Do not buy cans or jars that are damaged or have bulging lids.
Refrigerate all perishable and frozen foods promptly.
Never buy raw, unpasteurized milk.
Buy eggs that are clean and without cracks.
Do not buy fish that has a strong odor, cloudy eyes, or discolored skin.

Food Handling

Wash hands before handling food and after contact with raw meat or poultry.
Do not thaw foods on the kitchen counter; keep meat, fish, poultry, mayonnaise, and cream-filled foods refrigerated.
Store eggs in the refrigerator, and use within 3 to 5 weeks; use hard-boiled eggs within a week.
Cook hamburger thoroughly.
Do not place cooked meat or poultry on counters or platters used for uncooked foods.
Make sure your refrigerator is 40° F or colder and that the freezer is 0° F or colder.
Wash vegetables and fruits thoroughly or peel off skin.
Clean the wheel of the can opener after every use.
Change dishcloths and towels frequently.
Use a meat thermometer for cooking large pieces of meat.
Avoid slow cooking.
Stuff poultry immediately before cooking, and remove stuffing after the meal.

Eating

Do not eat raw eggs in any form. Do not consume uncooked pancake, cake, or cookie batter.
Cook eggs well.
Do not eat raw fish, oysters, or clams.
Do not eat raw ground beef.
Order hamburger or meatloaf well done without a pink middle.
Verify that Caesar salad and hollandaise sauce have not been made with raw eggs.

interruption of voluntary control of defecation in the spinal cord or brain, impaired anal sensation, or structural damage. Loss of conscious control of defecation can be caused by neurologic disorders, diarrheal illnesses, trauma to the anal sphincter (e.g., from a fistula, an abscess, or surgery), loss of mobility, and psychiatric disorders. Perineal relaxation and damage to the anal sphincter often result from vaginal delivery. Relaxation of the sphincter occurs as part of the general loss of muscle tone in aging, but the normal changes that occur with aging are not sufficient to cause fecal incontinence unless other health problems are present. Statistics about incidence and prevalence of fecal incontinence are difficult to obtain because of the social stigma associated with the problem, but it is estimated that as much as 18% of the population has experienced some occurrence of fecal incontinence, and the problem is pervasive among nursing home residents.[51]

Pathophysiology. Normally the contents of the bowel are propelled by mass movements toward the rectum. The rectum stores the feces until defecation. Distention of the rectum by feces triggers stretch receptors in the walls that initiate the urge to defecate. The external sphincter then tightens to maintain continence until voluntary defecation can take place. The rectum quickly accommodates the increased volume, and the urge to defecate subsides. With voluntary defecation, relaxation of the internal anal sphincter is followed by relaxation of the external anal sphincter, and Valsalva's maneuver helps expel the stool. Voluntary control of defecation is learned in early childhood and typically lasts throughout life.

Reflex defecation continues to occur even in the presence of most upper and lower motor neuron lesions, because the musculature of the bowel contains its own nerve centers that respond to distention through peristalsis. Reflex defecation therefore often persists or can be stimulated even when motor paralysis is present. Reflex defecation occurs primarily in response to mass peristaltic movements that follow meals. Any physical, mental, or social problem that disrupts any aspect of this complex, learned behavior can result in incontinence.

Collaborative Care Management. Treatment of fecal incontinence is multifaceted and depends on the cause. Correction of the underlying problem is crucial. This may involve control of diarrheal illnesses, treatment of impaction, prevention of constipation (which can weaken the sphincter and damage the nerve plexus as a result of chronic pressure in the rectum), or correction of structural problems.

Bowel training is the major approach used with patients who have cognitive and neurologic problems resulting from stroke or other chronic diseases. If a person can sit on a toilet, it may be possible to achieve automatic defecation when a pattern of consistent timing, familiar surroundings, and controlled dietary and fluid intake can be achieved. This approach allows many patients to defecate predictably and remain continent throughout the day.

Biofeedback training is the cornerstone of therapy for patients who have motility disorders or sphincter damage that causes fecal incontinence. The patient learns to tighten the external sphincter in response to manometric measurement of responses to rectal distention. This technique has demonstrated effectiveness with alert, motivated patients.

PATIENT/FAMILY TEACHING. Bowel training requires significant time and effort on the part of the nursing staff, family, and patient. The nurse teaches the family about the training program and how they can assist and support the effort. Incontinence is a major issue in home care and often is cited as the most common reason for older persons being admitted to nursing homes.[51]

To plan the most effective approach, the nurse gathers specific information concerning the person's general physical and cognitive

Healthy People 2010

Goals and Objectives Related to Food Safety

Goal

Reduce foodborne illnesses.

Objectives

Reduce infections caused by key foodborne pathogens (e.g., *Campylobacter* species, *Escherichia coli* 0157:H7, *Listeria monocytogenes*, salmonellae, *Cyclospora cayetanensis*, *Toxplasma gondii*).

Reduce outbreaks of infections caused by key foodborne bacteria (e.g., *E. coli* 0157:H7, salmonellae, staphylococci).

Prevent an increase in the proportion of isolates of *Salmonella* species from humans and from animals at slaughter that are resistant to antimicrobial drugs.

Reduce deaths from anaphylaxis caused by food allergies.

Increase the proportion of consumers who follow key food safety practices.

Improve food employee behaviors and food preparation practices that directly relate to foodborne illnesses in retail food establishments.

Reduce human exposure to organophosphate pesticides from food.

Goal

Promote health for all through a healthy environment.

Objective

Reduce waterborne disease outbreaks arising from water intended for drinking among persons served by community water systems.

From US Department of Health and Human Services: *Healthy people 2010: understanding and improving health*, Washington, DC, 2000, The Department.

condition, ability to contract the abdominal and perineal muscles on command, and awareness of the need or urge to defecate. Data are also collected about the nature and frequency of the incontinence problem, particularly its relationship to meals or other regular activities.

The nurse teaches the family about the importance of a high-fiber diet and ensuring that the patient consumes at least 2.5 L of fluid daily. The nurse evaluates the need for a regular stool softener or bulk former. When an optimal time for defecation has been established, usually after breakfast, a glycerin suppository may be inserted to stimulate defecation.

Despite honest efforts by family members, staff, and the patient, the fecal incontinence may remain uncontrolled. Efforts then shift toward controlling odor, preventing skin breakdown, and supporting the patient's psychologic integrity. Commercially available protective pants are expensive, but they can substantially reduce the burden of care for the family and provide the patient with a sense of security and dignity. Construction of a colostomy may be a more manageable option for a small group of patients with unremitting fecal incontinence problems.

Irritable Bowel Syndrome

Etiology and Epidemiology. Irritable bowel syndrome (IBS) is one of the most common chronic disorders, affecting about 24% of women and 19% of men.[57] The disorder shows widespread variation among cultural groups but can be found worldwide. It is most common in Western countries and in the United States.[22]

The American Gastrointestinal Association defines IBS as a combination of chronic and recurrent GI symptoms, usually including abdominal pain, distention, and disturbed defecation that cannot be explained by structural or biochemical abnormalities. Because no demonstrable sign of disease can be found during a routine diagnostic workup, IBS is classified as a functional disorder. It is usually mild and annoying, but in severe cases can be incapacitating.

Pathophysiology. IBS is theorized to result from disturbances in nervous system control of the intestines that cause visceral hypersensitivity and abnormal bowel motility. The bowel wall is extremely sensitive to distention and normal motor events such as peristalsis. Patients with IBS consistently experience increased discomfort related to distention at lower volumes than do control subjects.[41] Serotonin is hypothesized to play a role in IBS and is currently being studied because it can produce a variety of mechanical and neurohormonal responses that are closely related to IBS symptoms.

Classic symptoms of IBS include abdominal pain; diarrhea, constipation, or an alternating pattern of the two; mucus in the stool; a sensation of incomplete evacuation; and relief of discomfort with defecation. Some persons also experience a wide range of general dyspepsia symptoms, including excessive gas and bloating. Psychologic stress exacerbates symptoms.

Collaborative Care Management. Because IBS has no definitive tests or biologic markers, the diagnosis is made by eliminating other potential causes of the symptoms and determining whether the patient meets one of the symptom-based criteria sets that have been developed. These include the Rome I, Rome II, and Manning criteria. The Manning criteria consist of the symptoms of abdominal pain relieved by defecation, looser stools with onset of pain, more frequent stools with the onset of pain, passage of mucus in the stool, abdominal bloating, and sensations of incomplete evacuation. Rome II criteria encompass symptoms, frequency, and duration (Box 43-4).

Nonpharmacologic treatment focuses on thorough dietary analysis and elimination of any irritating substances. Limiting gas-producing foods may be helpful, and adding fiber to the diet improves symptoms in many patients. Cognitive behavioral strategies to more effectively manage stress are also frequently helpful.

A number of pharmacologic options exist, depending on the person's symptoms. Antidiarrheal agents and cholestyramine for diarrhea, bulk-forming laxatives for constipation, and antispasmodics for pain are routine options (see Tables 43-1 and 43-3). Tricyclic antidepressants may be used for severe pain.[4] Tegaserod, a 5-hydroxytryptamine 4 (5-HT4, serotonin) receptor agonist, is used in the short-term treatment of women with constipation-predominant IBS. The serotonin 5-HT4 receptor prevents contractions when serotonin binds to it. By blocking the 5-HT4

Box 43-4 Rome II Criteria for Diagnosis of Irritable Bowel Syndrome

- At least 3 months of continuous or recurrent symptoms of the following:
  —Abdominal pain or discomfort
    —Relieved with defecation, or
    —Associated with a change in frequency of stool, or
    —Associated with a change in consistency of stool
- Two or more of the following, on at least one fourth of occasions or days:
  —Altered stool frequency (For research purposes, altered may be defined as more than three bowel movements each day or less than three bowel movements each week.)
  —Altered stool form (lumpy/hard or loose/watery stool)
  —Altered stool passage (straining, urgency, or feeling of incomplete evacuation)
  —Passage of mucus
  —Bloating or feeling of abdominal distention

From Drossman DA, editor: *Rome II: the functional gastrointestinal disorders,* ed 2, McLean, Va, 2000, Degnon Associates.

receptor and thereby preventing serotonin from binding to it, tegaserod causes an increase in intestinal contractions. This increases the speed at which digesting food passes through the intestine and reverses the constipation. Tegaserod has also been shown to reduce the sensitivity of the intestinal pain-sensing nerves and thereby reduces the perception of pain.[47] Alosetron, a 5-HT3 receptor antagonist, is currently under study for the treatment of diarrhea-predominant IBS.

PATIENT/FAMILY TEACHING. Patient teaching and reassurance are critical aspects of the care of a person with IBS. The absence of a demonstrable structural cause of the symptoms can quickly lead to suspicions of malingering. The physiologic basis of IBS is difficult to understand, but patients need reassurance that it is not "all in their head" or a symptom of some other deadly disease process. The nurse assists the person in analyzing his or her diet and lifestyle to identify factors that minimize or worsen symptoms, and also assists in designing a regimen that effectively blends pharmacologic and nonpharmacologic strategies for improved symptom control.

Acute Inflammation of Intestines

Appendicitis

Etiology and Epidemiology. The vermiform appendix is a small, fingerlike projection attached to the cecum just below the ileocecal valve (Figure 43-1). The appendix is approximately 10 cm (4 inches) long and has no clearly identified function. It is an integral part of the cecum and fills with chyme and empties by peristalsis along with the rest of the bowel.

Appendicitis, an acute inflammation of the appendix, is one of the most common surgical emergencies. Classically, appendicitis was believed to result from obstruction of the narrow lumen of the appendix, most often with a fecalith (hardened feces) or a foreign body. According to this theory, obstruction of the lumen increases **intraluminal pressure,** which leads to occlusion of the capillaries and venules, ischemia of the appendiceal wall, and subsequent bacterial invasion. Current thinking is that one of a variety of factors precipitates breakdown in the mucosal lining of the appendix and that secondary bacterial infection with normal colonic bacteria ensues. Possible precipitating factors are obstruction of the lumen of the appendix, bacterial or viral enteric infection, and trauma. This theory is based on a review of pathologic specimens in which obstruction was found in a minority of cases and well-defined superficial mucosal ulcers in the majority.[49]

Appendicitis occurs most commonly in teenagers and young adults but can occur at any age. Males are affected more commonly than females. Approximately 7% of the population is affected by the disorder at some point. Appendicitis is associated with an overall mortality of 0.2% to 0.8% primarily because of complications, not the surgical procedure. In patients over age 70, the mortality rate rises to greater than 20%.[13] Appendicitis appears to occur more commonly in Western societies, in which the diet is low in fiber and high in refined carbohydrates. The higher incidence of constipation associated with this dietary pattern is theorized to increase the chance of developing obstructive fecaliths.

Pathophysiology. The inflammatory process of acute appendicitis, which is first manifested as injection of the serosal blood vessels and edema of the wall, can involve all or part of the appendix. Mucosal ulcerations and microabscesses in the appendiceal wall or surrounding tissue may develop. Unless treated, the latter can progress to gangrene and perforation within 24 to 36 hours. If the inflammatory process develops fairly slowly, the infection may be successfully walled off in a local abscess. More rapidly developing cases have a risk of rupture and acute peritonitis.

The primary clinical manifestation of appendicitis is abdominal pain that comes in waves. The pain starts in the epigastric or umbilical region but gradually becomes localized in the right lower quadrant of the abdomen. Localization at **McBurney's point,** halfway between the umbilicus and the anterior spine of the ileum (Figure 43-2), is considered classic. The pain is intermittent at first but becomes steady and severe over a short time. Pain is often accompanied by anorexia, nausea, and vomiting. Light palpation of the abdomen elicits acute pain in the right lower quadrant. Rebound tenderness is a common finding (see Chapter 40). The abdominal muscles overlying the area of inflammation may feel tense as a result of voluntary rigidity. The person with appendicitis often lies on the side or back with knees flexed in an attempt to decrease muscle strain on the abdominal wall. Other symptoms may include some combination of mild to moderate nausea, vomiting and anorexia, temperature elevations in the range of 100.5° to 101.5° F (38° to 38.5° C), an elevation in the white blood cell (WBC) count to more than 10,000/mm^3, and a neutrophil count of more than 75%.

Some patients with appendicitis experience less well-defined local symptoms, making prompt and accurate diagnosis a challenge. This is particularly true in older patients, whose response to pain is decreased. Because appendicitis is relatively rare in this age-group and symptoms may be mild or vague, the diagnosis

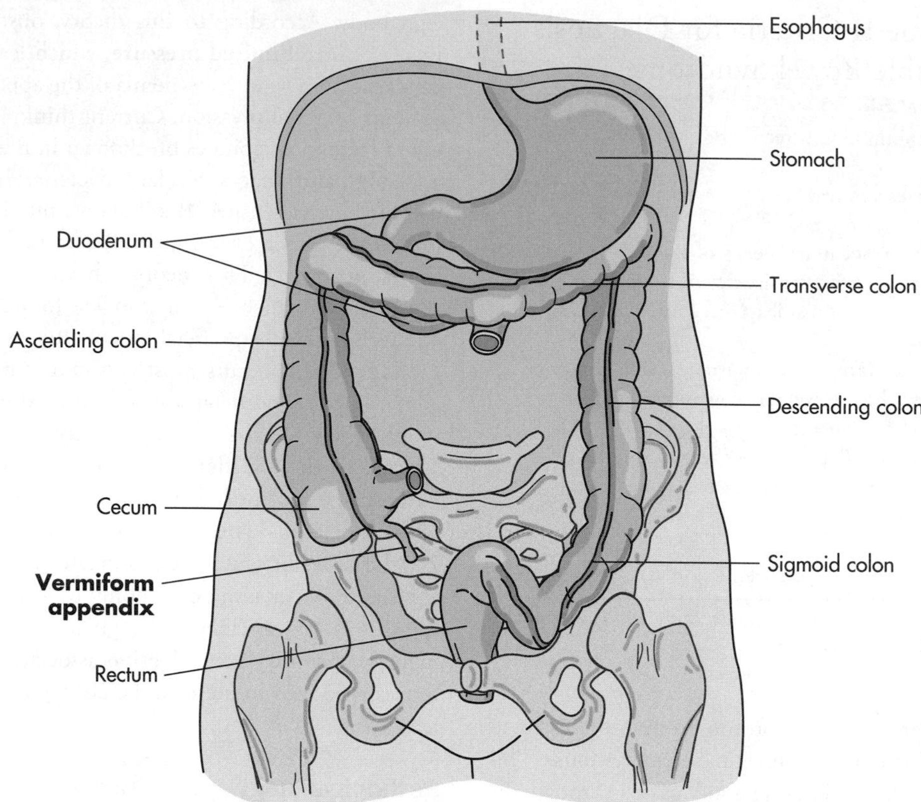

Figure 43-1 Appendix at the beginning of ascending colon.

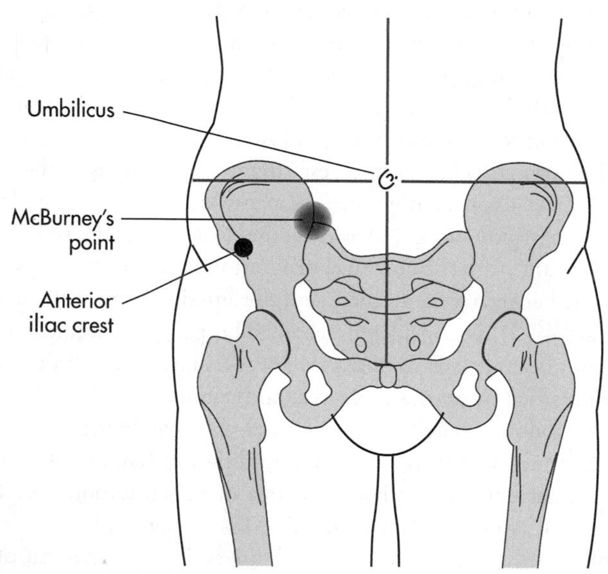

Figure 43-2 McBurney's point, located halfway between umbilicus and anterior iliac crest in right lower quadrant of abdomen.

may be delayed or missed. Delay or confusion about the diagnosis of appendicitis can lead to perforation, which is associated with substantial morbidity and mortality, particularly in children and older adults. In adults a perforation generally results in a localized abscess. Perforation is believed to occur early in the disease process in older adults, increasing the incidence of complications.

Collaborative Care Management. No single diagnostic indicator is specific to appendicitis. The diagnosis is based on a constellation of classic physical and laboratory findings. When atypical symptoms present, computed tomography (CT) scanning or ultrasonography may be used to confirm the diagnosis; current evidence suggests that CT is more sensitive and specific although not suitable for children or pregnant women.[49] A variety of other disorders that can cause symptoms similar to those of appendicitis may need to be ruled out before a positive diagnosis can be made. These disorders include ureteral stones, acute salpingitis, regional ileitis, ovarian cysts, and biliary colic.

During the diagnostic period the nurse focuses on keeping the patient as comfortable as possible, relieving anxiety, and preparing the patient for surgery. The patient is placed on bed rest and given nothing by mouth (NPO). Intravenous (IV) fluids are administered to maintain fluid and electrolyte balance, and antibiotic therapy may be initiated. To avoid masking critical changes in symptoms, pain medication is usually withheld until a definitive diagnosis of appendicitis has been made. The nurse explains the need for withholding analgesics and uses nonpharmacologic methods such as positioning and environmental management to increase the patient's comfort. Unnecessary movement, which typically increases the patient's pain, is avoided. Heat is not applied to the abdomen because the increased circulation to the appendix can lead to rupture.

The appendix is removed surgically (appendectomy) as soon as possible to prevent rupture with subsequent peritonitis. Traditional surgery involves removing the appendix through a small incision over McBurney's point or through a right paramedial incision. The incision usually heals with no need for external drainage. Drains are inserted when an abscess is discovered, when the appendix has ruptured, or when the appendix is severely edematous and surrounded by a pocket of clear fluid. Bowel function usually returns to normal soon after surgery, and convalescence is short. Appendectomies can also be successfully performed laparoscopically, but the cost is greater and the length of stay not significantly reduced. Patients may report less pain, however, and are able to return to full activity 1 week sooner than after the traditional procedure.

PATIENT/FAMILY TEACHING. The nurse provides the patient with an overview of the planned surgery and postoperative care. Postoperative nursing care after an appendectomy is similar to that provided to any surgical patient. Oral fluids and foods are restarted as tolerated, and discharge is rapid. The patient usually can resume all normal activities within 2 to 4 weeks. The nurse provides the patient with instructions concerning monitoring for wound healing, avoidance of strenuous activities and heavy lifting, and the importance of promptly reporting any symptoms indicative of complications.

▶ ARE You READY?

Which nursing action is most appropriate for the patient during the diagnostic period of suspected appendicitis?

1. Providing clear liquids only
2. Administering pain medications every 3-4 hours prn
3. Applying heat to the abdomen
4. Avoiding unnecessary changes in position

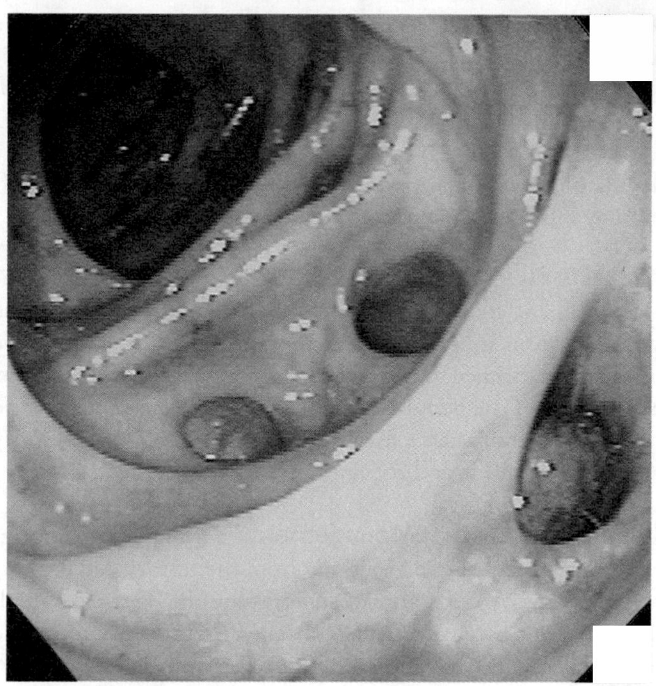

Figure 43-3 Diverticular disease.

Diverticular Disease and Diverticulitis

Etiology and Epidemiology. Diverticula are small outpouchings or herniations of the mucosal lining of the colon (Figure 43-3). Many regard them as part of the normal aging process. Thirty percent of individuals older than 50 years of age are estimated to have diverticula, and the incidence increases to about 70% in persons over 70 years of age.[19] Diverticula develop primarily in the left colon and rarely occur alone. The number of diverticula is also believed to increase with age. The vast majority of diverticula are never formally diagnosed, and the person remains completely asymptomatic. Patients typically seek medical care only if diverticulitis occurs. Diverticulitis is an episode of acute inflammation that can occur from local obstruction of a diverticulum by mucus or fecal matter. Ten percent to 25% of persons with diverticula experience an episode of diverticulitis at some point.[53]

Diverticulosis (the condition of having uninflamed diverticula) has been described as a disease of Western civilization because of its high incidence in developed countries. The disease shows wide geographic variations in incidence that are at least partly attributable to the quantity of nonabsorbable fiber in the daily diet. The increased incidence of diverticular disease parallels the changes in Western diet that have occurred since the 1850s when the refinement of grains became standard. The steady aging of the population is also reflected in these figures. Low-fiber diets have been shown to increase intraluminal pressure in the bowel, but aging also appears to change the composition of the bowel and decreases its tensile strength.

Pathophysiology. The development of intestinal diverticula is believed to be related to increased intraluminal pressure in the colon and decreased muscle strength in the colon wall. Diverticula tend to form at points in the wall where blood vessels penetrate the mucosal and muscular layers, creating points of relative weakness.

Diverticula are most often found in the sigmoid colon, where the lumen is narrowest and pressure is highest, but they can occur throughout the colon.[17] Muscle contractions in the sigmoid increase the thickness of the muscle and cause the weaker connective tissue to herniate between the circular muscle bands and form the diverticula. Diverticulitis often develops in a single diverticulum in response to irritation initiated by trapped fecal material. The blood supply to the area decreases, and bacteria proliferate in the obstructed diverticulum. The diverticular sac is a thin structure composed entirely of mucosal tissue, which is easily perforated. **Microperforations** usually quickly and effectively wall off because they are directly adjacent to the mesocolon. Larger perforations may progress to abscess formation or general peritonitis. Generalized inflammation can result in thickening and scarring of the bowel wall.

Diverticular disease is usually asymptomatic, but mild inflammation can trigger a nonspecific bowel dysfunction that resolves in a matter of hours or days. The clinical manifestations of diverticulitis reflect the inflammation of the diverticula or the development of complications. Crampy lower left quadrant abdominal pain accompanied by low-grade fever is a classic sign. The pain is triggered by muscle spasms of the sigmoid colon and is acute and persistent. Nausea, vomiting, and a feeling of bloating are also common. The inflammatory process also often involves the bladder and may cause urinary symptoms. The development of an abscess initiates the symptoms of localized peritonitis (see the following section). The traditional symptoms tend to be less pronounced or underreported by older adults.

DIVERTICULAR BLEEDING. Diverticular disease is also one of the most common causes of lower GI bleeding because the diverticula develop around a rich network of blood vessels.[53] Episodes of acute bleeding occur in 15% to 40% of persons with diverticular disease. The bleeding is abrupt and copious and not related to any identifiable precipitating event in most cases. The bleeding is self-limiting and stops spontaneously in most patients.

MECKEL'S DIVERTICULUM. Meckel's diverticulum is a congenital abnormality in which a blind tube, similar in structure to the appendix, opens into the distal ileum near the ileocecal valve. The tube may be attached to the umbilicus by a fibrous band. It occurs in about 2% of the population and is more common in men. The anomaly usually remains asymptomatic but can become grossly inflamed later in life and require surgical excision.

Collaborative Care Management. The preliminary diagnosis of diverticulitis may be made from the history and presenting symptoms. A CT scan can demonstrate the presence of both diverticula and abscesses. A barium enema can clearly reveal the classic diverticular pouches and thickened muscle layers but is usually not performed until after the inflammation subsides. A proctosigmoidoscopy may be performed to rule out other serious colon diseases such as inflammatory bowel disease and cancer.

An episode of diverticulitis is managed by resting the bowel. Hospitalization may be required in acute episodes.[53] The patient is kept NPO or restricted to clear liquids, and a regimen of IV fluids, antibiotics, and analgesics is begun. Anticholinergics (e.g., propantheline bromide [Pro-Banthine]) may be administered to reduce bowel spasm. Symptoms should subside within 48 to 72 hours. Mild cases can be effectively managed in the home.

Acute diverticulitis usually resolves with conservative medical management. However, surgical intervention may be needed to deal with complications.[58] Surgical resection of the involved part of the bowel may be necessary, particularly if abscesses need to be drained. An end-to-end anastomosis is performed if possible. A temporary colostomy is occasionally necessary.

Nursing care during an acute episode is largely supportive and focuses on patient comfort. The nurse explains the rationale for bed rest and bowel rest and the role that these interventions play in bowel healing. The nurse monitors fluid and electrolyte balance and the status of the patient's pain. The patient is regularly assessed for signs of complications.

PATIENT/FAMILY TEACHING. With asymptomatic diverticulosis, prevention of constipation is the goal. The nurse encourages the patient to maintain a liberal fluid intake of 2.5 to 3 L/day and to ingest a diet that contains soft foods high in fiber, such as fruits, vegetables, and whole grains. The American Dietetic Association recommends 20 to 35 g of fiber daily. Small amounts of bran may be added to regular foods, or bulk-forming agents may be used daily to increase stool mass and softness, increase the diameter of the colon, and prevent straining at hard stool. Patients used to be advised to avoid eating foods such as nuts or seeds, which could become trapped in the diverticula and trigger inflammation. However, no evidence exists that these foods represent actual risks for obstruction, and avoidance is no longer suggested. High-fiber foods should not be consumed when symptoms of inflammation are present because they can be highly irritating to the mucosa. The fiber content of selected foods is presented in Box 43-1. The patient is also encouraged to avoid activities that increase intraabdominal pressure. Weight loss may be recommended in an attempt to lower the resting intraabdominal pressure.

Peritonitis

Etiology and Epidemiology. Peritonitis involves either a local or generalized inflammation of the peritoneum, the membranous lining of the abdomen that covers the viscera. It can result from bacteria or intestinal contents in the peritoneal cavity. Peritonitis may be primary or secondary, aseptic or septic, and acute or chronic. Primary peritonitis has no identifiable cause. Spontaneous bacterial peritonitis is a common form of primary peritonitis. Secondary peritonitis has an identifiable cause, usually bacteria that enter the peritoneal cavity through an opening in the intestinal wall or by extension of infection through the wall of a hollow organ. Openings in the intestinal wall can result from a variety of causes, including trauma; surgical injury; a ruptured appendix; perforation associated with a peptic ulcer, diverticulitis, ulcerative colitis, or Crohn's disease; or necrosis of the intestine secondary to obstruction or malignancy. Extension of infection into the peritoneal cavity may result from pelvic inflammatory disease or urinary tract infection. Bacterial invasion may also be associated with continuous ambulatory peritoneal dialysis. Common invading organisms include *E. coli,* streptococci, staphylococci, pneumococci, gonococci, *Klebsiella* organisms, and pseudomonads.

Secondary peritonitis may also develop as a result of chemical irritation from GI secretions (gastric acid, pancreatic juice, bile) that have entered the peritoneum. This can occur with hemorrhagic pancreatitis or a leak at an internal suture line involving the stomach, liver, or pancreas.

Pathophysiology. The body creates natural barriers to attempt to control the inflammation associated with peritonitis. Adhesions form rapidly and may be successful in limiting involvement to only a portion of the abdominal cavity. The end result may be abscess development. Adhesions are more likely to develop in the lower part of the abdomen. As healing progresses, the adhesions may shrink and virtually disappear, or they may persist as constrictions that bind the involved structures together, possibly creating intestinal obstruction.

The peritoneum is a semipermeable membrane that allows the flow of water and electrolytes between the bloodstream and peritoneal cavity. When peritonitis occurs, fluid can shift into the abdominal cavity at a rate of 300 to 500 ml/hr in response to the acute inflammation.[9] The inflammatory process also shunts extra blood to the inflamed areas of bowel to combat the secondary bacterial infection, and peristalsis slows or ceases. The bowel becomes increasingly distended with gas and fluid. The circulatory, fluid, and electrolyte changes can rapidly become critical. Local reactions of the peritoneum include redness, inflammation, and the production of large amounts of fluid containing electrolytes and proteins. Hypovolemia, electrolyte imbalance, dehydration, and finally shock can develop. The loss of circulatory volume is proportional to the severity of peritoneal involvement. The fluid usually becomes purulent as the condition progresses and as the bacteria become more numerous. The bacteria may also enter the blood and cause septicemia.

The clinical manifestations of peritonitis are both local and systemic. They depend to some degree on the site and extent of the inflammation. Abdominal findings include local or diffuse pain and rebound tenderness. Guarding and rigidity are classic signs. Distention and paralytic ileus with absence of bowel sounds in all four quadrants develop as the inflammation progresses. Systemic signs may include fever (100° to 101° F [37.7° to 38.3° C]); an elevated WBC count; nausea and vomiting; and symptoms of early shock such as tachycardia, tachypnea, oliguria, restlessness, weakness, pallor, and diaphoresis. Patients are usually immobile, since any movement worsens the pain. The symptoms initially are much less severe in older persons, and the diagnosis may be overlooked until the condition is serious. Pain may even be absent in older patients, psychotic patients, patients receiving high doses of corticosteroids or analgesics, diabetic patients with advanced neuropathy, and those under the influence of alcohol.[46] The mortality rate from peritonitis is highest among older patients and those with preexisting organ failure. Mortality can be as low as 10% from a perforated ulcer or a ruptured appendix and as high as 50% from postoperative peritonitis.[46] The mortality rate has not changed in 50 years despite advances in antimicrobial therapy and clinical care.[31]

Collaborative Care Management. The diagnosis of peritonitis is made primarily on the basis of the symptom pattern, laboratory findings, and x-ray studies, which may show abnormalities in gas and air patterns in the abdomen. Free air or fluid in the abdominal cavity is indicative of perforation. Specimens of blood and peritoneal fluid are obtained for culture before the initiation of antibiotic therapy. WBC counts often are elevated to 20,000/mm^3 or higher with a shift to the left and are the single most common laboratory sign of peritonitis in immunocompetent patients. Electrolyte values are carefully monitored.

Treatment focuses on fluid resuscitation, antibiotic therapy, and surgery to correct the underlying cause and remove infected material. Surgical healing is impaired if sepsis or ischemia occurs, and complications associated with wound healing are common. Peritoneal lavage with warm saline may be performed during surgery, followed by the insertion of drainage tubes to facilitate healing. In some cases surgery is delayed until the patient's condition can be medically stabilized.

The patient with peritonitis is critically ill and requires careful monitoring of all vital parameters. Placement in a critical care environment may be indicated. The nurse monitors vital signs and intake and output and adjusts IV lines and medications as ordered. Fluid, electrolyte, and colloid replacement is the major focus of medical care. The fluid shifts that cause massive hypovolemia and shock need aggressive management. Broad-spectrum antibiotics effective against suspected organisms are administered and then adjusted as needed in response to culture and sensitivity reports. Other medications aimed at modifying bacterial adhesion or affecting the patient's cytokines may be used in an attempt to limit inflammation and infection.

A nasogastric (NG) tube is inserted to help relieve abdominal distention. Bed rest in a semi-Fowler's position is maintained to support ventilation and increase patient comfort. The nurse encourages the patient to deep breathe frequently because pain and distention can significantly impair ventilation. The nurse also promotes comfort through frequent mouth care, basic hygiene, and use of measures to reduce anxiety. Nutritional management with parenteral nutrition may be necessary when sepsis is severe and recovery is expected to be prolonged.

PATIENT/FAMILY TEACHING. Peritonitis typically develops rapidly and creates a serious and frightening situation for the patient and family. The nurse reinforces teaching about the problem and its treatment and provides ongoing support and encouragement. The nurse teaches the patient the importance of routine respiratory care and encourages ambulation when tolerated. If the abdominal involvement is extensive, the patient may have multiple drains in place, and wound healing is complex. Careful teaching about wound management is important, since recovery is often prolonged and the patient is likely to be discharged with ongoing needs for wound care support from home health care services. Careful discharge preparation and referrals are critical.

Inflammatory Bowel Disease

Inflammatory bowel disease (IBD) is an umbrella term used to describe conditions that are characterized by bowel inflammation. Crohn's disease and ulcerative colitis are the two major forms. They have distinctly different pathologies but share many overlapping features. Their management is therefore presented together.

Etiology and Epidemiology. The etiology of IBD remains unclear despite extensive research. Both Crohn's disease and ulcerative colitis are believed to occur in response to some complex interplay of genetic, immune system, and environmental factors. It appears that persons with IBD have a genetic predisposition to the disease. A positive family history is the most important risk factor for IBD.[55] First-degree relatives have a significantly increased risk of developing IBD, and familial aggregations of cases have been found. Genetic studies indicate that genes associated with IBD exist on chromosomes 5 and 6 and have clearly shown that mutations in the CARD15 gene, which modulates cell response to bacteria, are associated with some forms of Crohn's disease. All these genes are permissive (allow it to occur), not causative, of IBD.

Factors that actually trigger the development of the inflammatory response characteristic of the disease have not been definitively identified. Research has focused on potential infective, dietary, autoimmune, and environmental triggers, but findings have been inconclusive. Extensive studies of diet have not shown any dietary substance to activate the disease. Environmental factors have not been proven to play an etiologic role with one striking exception: smoking. Smokers have a two to four times greater risk of developing Crohn's disease and have more aggressive disease than nonsmokers. Nonsmokers, however, appear to be at greater risk of developing ulcerative colitis and have more severe disease than smokers.[1] These effects occur independent of the amount of smoking. Research has also failed to support a psychogenic cause of IBD. Stress and emotional factors, which once were believed to play an important etiologic role, have not been shown to trigger the disease.[26,48]

IBD is clearly multifactorial in origin.[17] Genetic factors result in a predisposition or susceptibility to the disease. Immune system dysfunction may play a role, with environmental agents acting as triggers to produce inflammation in the bowel wall. Crohn's disease probably develops as an aberrant response to normal bowel flora in genetically predisposed individuals.[17] Environmental factors may influence the disease presentation and severity, as well as the tendency for relapse.

IBD occurs worldwide with an apparent preference for industrialized nations, urban areas, and cold climates. In the United States, which along with Northern Europe has the highest incidence of IBD, approximately 1 million people deal with the disease on a daily basis. Ulcerative colitis used to be the most common form of IBD in the United States, but the incidence of Crohn's disease is now almost equal to that of ulcerative colitis. Whether this reflects an actual increase in the disease or just improved disease recognition and diagnosis is unknown.[45]

IBD is common among Americans of European descent, with the Jewish population having a prevalence four to five times greater than all others. IBD among African-Americans appears to be increasing, and it is estimated that its incidence is approaching that of Americans of European descent. The disease is less common in Native Americans and Americans of Asian and Hispanic descent, although it also appears to be increasing in the latter.[45]

No gender pattern is evident in racially mixed groups, but Caucasian women appear to be at particular risk. Although IBD can occur at any age, its peak period of onset is in young adulthood between the ages of 15 and 25 years. A second smaller peak occurs between the ages of 55 and 65 years.[55] Risk factors for IBD are summarized in the Risk Factors box.

Pathophysiology. Although inflammation is the hallmark of both Crohn's disease and ulcerative colitis, the two disorders have significantly different effects on the bowel. The diseases are distinguished largely by the nature of the inflammation, the location of lesions in the GI tract, the pattern of distribution, and the degree of mucosal penetration (Table 43-4).

Both forms of IBD are characterized by exacerbations and remissions. Despite a great deal of overlap in the presenting symptoms, ulcerative colitis and Crohn's disease have different characteristic features. There is also a great deal of overlap in the clinical picture of IBD and that of IBS.

Risk Factors

Inflammatory Bowel Disease

- Ages 15 to 25 years
- Caucasian race
- Women at slightly higher risk
- Jewish ancestry (does not apply to native-born Israelis)
- First-degree relative of person with inflammatory bowel disease
- Residence in the United States or Northern Europe
- History of smoking (Crohn's disease)
- Nonsmoking status (ulcerative colitis)
- Use of oral contraceptives (among Caucasian women)

ULCERATIVE COLITIS. Ulcerative colitis targets the bowel mucosa and creates a diffuse, continuous process of inflammation characterized by edema and shallow ulceration (Figure 43-4). It primarily affects the distal colorectal area, and about 40% to 50% of patients have disease that is confined to this region.[26] More extensive disease is described as left sided and affects 30% to 40% of patients.[26] It involves the colon up to the splenic flexure. In severe disease the inflammatory process extends all the way to the hepatic flexure or ileocecal junction. A fortunate subset of patients with ulcerative colitis develops a less virulent disease variant that is confined to the rectum and referred to as ulcerative proctitis. Although relapses are common with ulcerative proctitis, the disease rarely progresses and is associated with a low risk for the development of cancer and other long-term complications.

In ulcerative colitis the mucosa is fragile and bleeds spontaneously or in response to minimal trauma. Over time it becomes thickened and edematous. The ulceration and healing process gradually result in scar tissue formation that can cause the colon to lose its normal elasticity and absorptive capability. As normal mucosa is gradually replaced by scar tissue, the colon becomes thickened, rigid, and pipelike. The mucosa may also undergo structural changes over time, forming pseudopolyps that can become malignant.

Bloody diarrhea and abdominal pain are the classic symptoms of ulcerative colitis. The diarrhea ranges in severity from three or four times daily to hourly; it is small in volume, mushy in consistency, and liberally mixed with blood, mucus, and pus. The inflammatory exudate and mucus secretion increase both the fecal solutes and water. The diarrhea is associated with significant urgency and left-sided abdominal pain that is colicky and relieved by emptying the bowel. Severe diarrhea may result in significant losses of fluids, sodium, potassium, bicarbonate, and calcium. As scarring within the bowel occurs, the sensation of the urge to defecate can be lost, leading to involuntary leakage of stool.

CROHN'S DISEASE. Crohn's disease can affect any portion of the digestive tract with any degree of severity but is found most often in the proximal colon and ileocecal junction, making it a right-sided disease. Forty percent of patients experience disease confined to the cecum and ileum.[55] More than one site may be affected. The presentation of Crohn's disease varies depending on its location, the degree of inflammation, and the presence of intestinal complications or extraintestinal manifestations.

The inflammation of Crohn's disease is transmural, affecting all layers of the intestinal wall. It follows a "skip" or "cobblestone" pattern in which affected areas are separated by normal tissue. Mucosal granulomas, luminal narrowing, thickening of the intestinal wall, mucosal nodularity, and ulceration are characteristic features. The lesions may perforate and form fistulas that connect with the bladder, vagina, or other segments of the bowel or mesentery. Scar tissue may form as the lesions heal, preventing the normal absorption of nutrients, and stricture bands may form, causing intestinal obstruction. Figure 43-5 illustrates several of the common complications of Crohn's disease.

Diarrhea and abdominal pain are the classic features of Crohn's disease, but the pattern of symptoms varies according to the location and severity of the inflammation. The diarrhea with disease affecting the small intestine is likely to consist of three to five daily large, semi-

TABLE 43-4 **COMPARISON OF ULCERATIVE COLITIS AND CROHN'S DISEASE**

Characteristic	Ulcerative Colitis	Crohn's Disease
Usual area affected	Left colon, rectum	Distal ileum, right colon Can occur anywhere in gastrointestinal tract
Extent of involvement	Diffuse areas, contiguous	Segmental areas, noncontiguous
Inflammation	Mostly mucosal	Transmural
Mucosal appearance	Shallow mucosal ulcerations, edematous, superficial bleeding	Cobblestone effect, granulomas Thickened walls, narrowed lumen
Complications	Loss of absorption and elasticity Replacement of mucosa by scar tissue Development of pseudopolyps that may become malignant Toxic megacolon Hemorrhoids Bleeding	Fistulas Perianal disease Strictures Abscesses Perforation Anemia Malabsorption of fat and fat-soluble vitamins

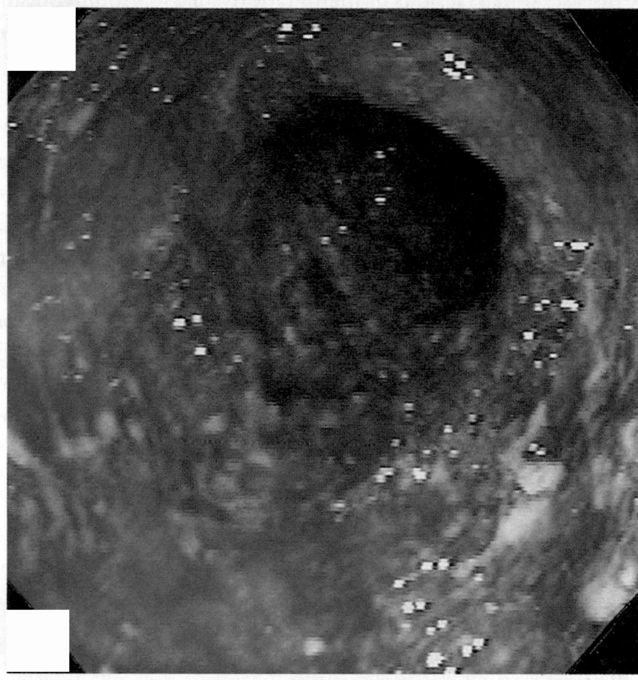

Figure 43-4 Severe ulcerative colitis.

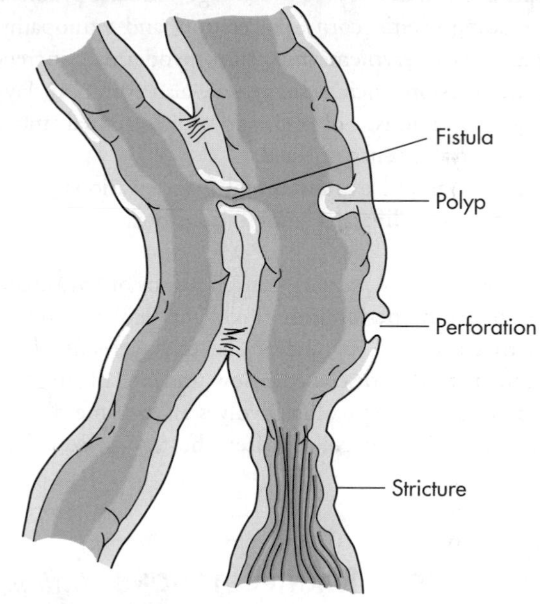

Figure 43-5 Common complications of Crohn's disease.

solid stools that contain mucus and pus but no blood. Steatorrhea may be present if the inflammation extends high into the small intestine. Fat-soluble vitamins—A, D, E, and K—may be poorly absorbed. With disease of the colon or rectum, there may be small-volume diarrhea associated with urgency and tenesmus because of scar tissue formation, which leaves the rectum unable to distend.

Colicky, severe abdominal pain that occurs after eating and tenderness that is diffuse or localized in the right lower quadrant are also characteristic of Crohn's disease. A tender mass of thickened intestine may be palpable in the area. During an acute episode the symptoms may closely resemble those of appendicitis.

SYSTEMIC AND EXTRAINTESTINAL SYMPTOMS OF INFLAMMATORY BOWEL DISEASE. Systemic and extraintestinal symptoms of IBD occur commonly and often complicate the patient's disease management. Systemic symptoms include anorexia, nausea, weakness, and malaise from the chronic inflammation. Weight loss is common and may result in nutritional deficiencies if the bowel's absorption capability is significantly impaired. Intermittent fever and leukocytosis often accompany an exacerbation, and iron deficiency anemia may develop from both chronic mucosal bleeding and poor iron absorption. Patients are often pale and thin and look chronically ill. The course of IBD is highly unpredictable and cannot be determined from the initial presentation. In most patients the course is chronic and recurrent, but occasionally patients are able to achieve and sustain long-term remissions.

Extraintestinal symptoms of IBD can involve virtually every organ system. Although it is generally accepted that extraintestinal symptoms are separate systemic disorders, their etiology is not understood. They appear to reflect some type of generalized tissue vulnerability and are considered immunologic phenomena. They may precede or accompany the underlying bowel disorder. Some extraintestinal symptoms follow the same clinical course as the bowel disease, and others follow an unrelated course.[55] A patient with one extraintestinal manifestation has an increased risk of developing others.

The most common extraintestinal manifestation of IBD is arthritis, which may take the form of colitic peripheral arthritis or ankylosing spondylitis.[55] Colitic peripheral arthritis is migratory; affects single joints in an asymmetric pattern; and primarily targets the hips, ankles, wrists, and elbows. This arthritis parallels the course of the intestinal inflammation, and successful treatment of the bowel results in improvement in the arthritis. Ankylosing spondylitis is characterized by morning stiffness, low back pain, and a stooped posture.

Extraintestinal problems also occur in the liver and biliary tract. These include pericholangitis, chronic active hepatitis, and cirrhosis. Sclerosing cholangitis is seen in ulcerative colitis and cholelithiasis in Crohn's disease. In the urinary tract, calcium oxalate renal calculi and inflammation of the ureters with obstruction and hydronephrosis can develop. A wide range of ocular problems may occur, including uveitis, corneal ulceration, and retinopathy. Skin lesions particularly erythema nodosum, pyoderma gangrenosum, and infectious lesions such as herpes, are also common. Hypercoagulability is characteristic of IBD, and strokes, retinal emboli, and pulmonary emboli are not unusual.

Classic clinical and extraintestinal manifestations of IBD are summarized in the Clinical Manifestations box.

COMPLICATIONS. The primary complications of IBD are hemorrhage, obstruction, perforation, toxic megacolon, and cellular dysplasia that can lead to cancer. The management of the first three is similar to that discussed below under Collaborative Care Management. Toxic megacolon involves an extreme dilation of a segment of the diseased colon (often the transverse colon) that results in complete obstruction. The patient is at risk for toxic megacolon during acute exacerbations. The problem may develop after bowel preparation for a barium enema or other diagnostic test, or from the negative effects of opioids and anticholinergic drugs on peristalsis. Bacteria rapidly invade the inflamed tissue, creating the acute state. The condition may respond to conservative management or require surgical correction.

The development of cellular dysplasia and eventually colorectal adenocarcinoma is significantly more common in patients with IBD than in the general population. For patients with ulcerative colitis, adenocarcinoma is 10 to 20 times more common; for those with Crohn's disease, it is four to seven times more common.[14] The longer the time since the onset of disease and the more of the colon involved, the higher is the risk of cancer. Patients who have had the disease for 8 to 10 or more years need routine surveillance with colonoscopy and multiple biopsies at 2-year intervals.[14] Colectomy eliminates the risk and may be recommended even when medical management satisfactorily controls the disease. If mass lesions or high-grade dysplasia is found on surveillance colonoscopy, colectomy usually is recommended; otherwise colonoscopy is repeated at least every 3 months.

Collaborative Care Management

DIAGNOSTIC TESTS. The diagnosis of IBD begins with a careful health history that includes the symptom pattern and its severity and duration. The clinician performs a stool culture and *C. difficile* toxin assay, as well as examination for leukocytes, parasites, blood, and culture, to rule out an infectious origin for the symptoms.[45] Laboratory tests may include a complete blood count, erythrocyte sedimentation rate, and serum albumin measurement. They may also include a serologic antibody assay to aid in the diagnosis of Crohn's disease and in differentiating Crohn's colitis from ulcerative colitis. This is a combined test

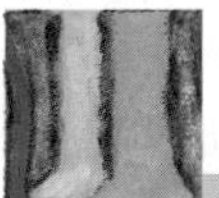

CLINICAL MANIFESTATIONS *Inflammatory Bowel Disease*

General

Anorexia, nausea, and weight loss
Weakness and malaise
Fever and leukocytosis (a high fever and white blood cell count of more than 15,000/mm^3, suggesting an abscess)
Iron deficiency anemia

Specific to Ulcerative Colitis

Profuse diarrhea (15 to 20 stools per day)
Stools containing blood, mucus, and possibly pus
Abdominal cramping possibly present before the bowel movement
Losses of fluid, sodium, potassium, bicarbonate, and calcium

Specific to Crohn's Disease

Three to five large, semisolid stools per day
Stools containing mucus and possibly pus but rarely blood
Steatorrhea if small bowel affected
Right lower quadrant cramping: may be severe and mimic appendicitis; diffuse rather than localized pain

Extraintestinal Manifestations

Arthritis (4% to 23%)
Involvement of large joints: hips, ankles, wrists, and elbows
Migratory and asymmetric incidence, nondeforming

Ocular (4% to 10%)
Uveitis, episcleritis
Serous retinopathy

Skin (3% to 6%)
Erythema nodosum: raised, red, tender nodules on anterior tibial surfaces
Pyoderma gangrenosum: painful, necrotizing ulcerations; most common on legs

Hepatobiliary (4% to 5%)
Cholelithiasis
Fatty liver, cirrhosis
Cholangitis (70% of patients with cholangitis have ulcerative colitis)

Renal (4% to 23%)
Kidney stones
Ureteral obstruction

which identifies perinuclear antineutrophil cytoplasmic antibodies (pANCA), which have been found in some patients who have ulcerative colitis; anti–*Saccharomyces cerevisiae* antibodies (ASCA), which have been found in patients with Crohn's disease; and a related antibody marker. The test is 94% sensitive in differentiating IBD from IBS.[32]

A barium enema usually is performed to evaluate the physical changes in the bowel; it provides accurate data about the structure of the colon, can be performed rapidly, and provides a permanent record for future disease comparison. The classic "string lesions" representing the typical strictures of Crohn's disease are readily visible on barium enema. They are caused by extensive bowel narrowing and are often found in the terminal ileum. These asymmetric, segmental lesions help distinguish Crohn's disease from ulcerative colitis. The cobblestone appearance of advanced Crohn's disease is also visualized. An upper GI series may be performed to evaluate small bowel involvement (see Future Watch box).

Transabdominal ultrasound is being successfully used to identify abscesses and fistulas. CT scanning provides even greater accuracy but is much more expensive. New imaging techniques using labeled leukocytes and erythrocytes are providing a noninvasive way of identifying sites of disease activity or bleeding.[48] Endoscopic procedures such as sigmoidoscopy or colonoscopy may be used to directly examine the nature and pattern of the inflammation and obtain biopsies if necessary. Major perianal complications such as abscesses and fistulas are characteristic of Crohn's disease. The classic cobblestone, skip pattern of Crohn's disease is also readily apparent on endoscopy, with focal patches of ulcerative lesions. In ulcerative colitis there is often a small zone where the mucosa makes a distinct transition back to normal, and no evidence of disease is found above this point.

MEDICATIONS. Medications are a cornerstone of the treatment of IBD and are used to relieve symptoms, induce remission, postpone the need for surgery, and improve the quality of life (Table 43-5). Since the cause of IBD remains basically unknown, the components of drug therapy are empirically based on a combination of clinical trials and practical experience. A stepped approach, in which the drug regimen is systematically progressed until a response occurs, is used. Step 1 is usually aminosalicylates; step 1a is antibiotics; step 2 is corticosteroids; step 3 consists of immunomodulatory agents, or in the case of Crohn's disease infliximab (Remicade), which is a monoclonal antibody; and step 4 involves agents that have been shown to help selected types of patients.

Future Watch

Capsule Video Endoscopy

Capsule video endoscopy is a new technology primarily designed to allow visualization of the small intestine. It uses a miniature camera incorporated into a pill that the patient swallows after fasting for 12 hours. Images are transmitted to a small receiver worn at the patient's waist and are downloaded about 8 hours later, by which time the camera has passed through the small intestine. Subsequently they are viewed as either still images or film. The capsule is expelled from the rectum in 24 to 48 hours.

AMINOSALICYLATES. Sulfasalazine (Azulfidine) was developed in the 1930s and first used for treating arthritis. Arthritis was believed to have an infectious origin, and sulfasalazine combined the proven effectiveness of aspirin with a sulfonamide antibiotic. Its use was quickly broadened to include IBD, and it has been a mainstay of treatment ever since. The exact mechanism of action of sulfasalazine is unknown, but its effectiveness is primarily attributed to its antiinflammatory effects. It successfully induces and sustains remission in most patients with mild to moderate ulcerative colitis and mild Crohn's disease affecting the colon. Sulfasalazine is split by bacteria in the colon into its two components. The first component, 5-acetylsalicylic acid (5-ASA) is poorly absorbed and thus maintains prolonged contact with the inflamed mucosa. Sulfapyridine, the second component, which is the carrier drug, has no proven effectiveness against IBD and accounts for most of the troubling side effects.

Because of the side effects, efforts have focused on developing 5-ASA products that can be delivered intact to the colon without an additional carrier drug. Options include olsalazine (Dipentum), which is poorly absorbed in the small intestine and broken down in the colon by the action of the intestinal bacteria; and mesalamine (Pentasa, Asacol), which is coated with a pH-sensitive resin that dissolves only in a pH greater than 7 in the terminal ileum and proximal colon. Sustained-release granules of this product are also available. The pH-sensitive coating allows these drugs to be delivered to the small intestine and increases their effectiveness with Crohn's disease. These drugs are generally well tolerated if prescribed in increasing doses and taken buffered with food. Toxicity appears to be minimal. The most common side effects include nausea, vomiting, and diarrhea.

Aminosalicylates can also be used topically for the 25% or more of patients with ulcerative colitis whose disease is confined to the rectal and sigmoid area. The drugs can be administered by enema, which provides for homogeneous delivery to the inflamed lower colon. Enemas provide high local concentrations of the drug, with minimal systemic absorption, and have been shown to be as effective as steroids in many situations. However, patients often find daily enemas to be unacceptable for long-term therapy, so suppository forms of the drugs have also been developed.

CORTICOSTEROIDS. Corticosteroids have played an important role in IBD management for many years. Because they are rapidly acting antiinflammatory agents, corticosteroids are used to treat acute flares of moderate to severe Crohn's disease and severe ulcerative colitis. They are not used as maintenance therapy to sustain remissions because of their widespread and severe side effects, which include fluid and electrolyte abnormalities, osteoporosis, aseptic necrosis, peptic ulcers, cataracts, neurologic and endocrine dysfunctions, infection, and occasional psychiatric problems.

Steroids can be administered intravenously, orally, or rectally. IV administration is reserved for acutely ill, hospitalized patients. Rectal administration is aimed at a topical effect, but most forms absorb readily from the rectal mucosa and also produce systemic effects. Regardless of the route of administration, the dose of steroid is tapered as soon as a clinical response to the drug occurs, usually in 1 or 2 days. Prednisone remains the most commonly prescribed steroid, but budesonide (Entocort) offers the advantages of high topical potency, poor absorption, and rapid first-pass

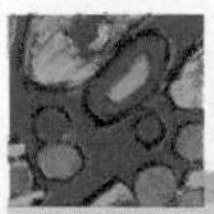

TABLE 43-5 COMMON MEDICATIONS *for Treatment of Inflammatory Bowel Disease*

Drug	Action	Nursing Intervention
Aminosalicylates (Oral)		
Sulfasalazine (Azulfidine)	Converted in colon to sulfapyridine and 5-aminosalicylic acid (5-ASA), which may exert antiinflammatory effect, possibly through prostaglandin inhibition	Assess for allergy to sulfonamides or aspirin. Monitor for common side effects: anorexia, nausea and vomiting, headache. Teach patient to: Take in divided doses. Take with full glass of fluid or with food. Maintain liberal fluid intake (2.5-3 L/day). Report skin rash or other adverse effects.
Olsalazine (Dipentum)	As above without antibacterial action of sulfapyridine	Monitor for common side effects as above and for mild to moderate diarrhea. Teach patient to: Take in divided doses. Take with full glass of fluid or with food. Maintain liberal fluid intake (2.5-3 L/day).
Balsalazide (Colazal)	Prodrug 5-ASA connected to carrier by an A20 bond Colon bacteria break bond, releasing active 5-ASA with action as above	Teach patient to: Take with a full glass of water. Stop drug and see physician if signs of allergy or worsening colitis occur. Continue taking but consult physician if headache, nausea and vomiting, fatigue, stomach, or joint pain occurs.
Mesalamine (Asacol, Pentasa)	Same as olsalazine	Teach patient to: Take in divided doses. Maintain liberal fluid intake (2.5-3 L/day). Swallow tablets whole; do not chew or break outer coating.
Aminosalicylates (Rectal)		
Mesalamine in suspension for retention enema Mesalamine suppository	As above	Administer enema while patient is positioned on left side, and teach patient to retain as long as possible.
Corticosteroids (Oral or IV)		
Prednisolone Prednisone	Potent systemic antiinflammatory action	Teach patient to: Take with food or fluid. Monitor weight gain; assess for edema. Have blood pressure checked regularly. Be alert to signs of infection and report promptly. Be aware that mood swings occur commonly. Do not change dose or schedule or abruptly discontinue drug. Maintain good personal hygiene; keep perianal area clean and dry.

metabolism. It can now also be administered in a pH-sensitive coating for delivery to the distal ileum and cecum.[47]

IMMUNE MODIFIERS. Potent immunosuppressive agents such as azathioprine (Imuran) and mercaptopurine (6-MP, Purinethol) may be used in selected patients with extensive disease who cannot be successfully weaned from steroids. These potent immunosuppressive drugs have a slow onset of action and may take up to 4 months to demonstrate effectiveness. They are not useful in acute situations but are effective in prolonging remission and are usually well tolerated. Monthly complete blood counts with differentials and platelet counts are needed for 1 year because of the risk of significant neutropenia or pancytopenia. If the patient is stable, the interval then may be lengthened. Liver function tests must be monitored regularly.

Methotrexate has been shown to improve symptoms in patients with steroid-dependent Crohn's disease, but its side effect of bone marrow depression requires careful, ongoing monitoring.

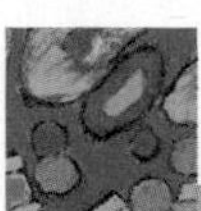

TABLE 43-5
COMMON MEDICATIONS *for Treatment of Inflammatory Bowel Disease—cont'd*

Drug	Action	Nursing Intervention
Corticosteroids (Rectal)		
Hydrocortisone Intrarectal foam (Cortifoam) Retention enema (Cortenema)	As above	As for oral or IV corticosteroids
Budesonide enema	As above; rapid presystemic metabolism minimizes absorption	Administer enema while patient is positioned on left side, and teach patient to retain as long as possible. Perform other interventions as above; side effects should be less.
Immune Modifiers		
6-Mercaptopurine (6-MP, Purinethol)	Potent systemic suppression of immune response; may take 4-6 mo for full effect	Teach patient to: Report any signs of infection. Be alert to easy bruising. Return for laboratory work as scheduled. Maintain liberal daily fluid intake (2.5-3 L/day). Take with food or after meals.
Azathioprine (Imuran)	As above	As above
Cyclosporine (Sandimmune)	As above; effects seen after several days	Oral solution may be mixed in glass and given with milk or orange juice at room temperature; avoid refrigeration. Teach patient to: Monitor blood pressure. Report hematuria or any change in urinary function.
Monoclonal Antibodies		
Infliximab (Remicade)	Binds to tumor necrosis factor-alpha, blocking its activity and decreasing inflammation	Monitor for infusion-related problems: pruritus, hypotension, dyspnea, headache, fatigue. Teach patient to promptly report any signs of infection.
Antibiotics		
Metronidazole (Flagyl)	No apparent effect on ulcerative colitis but useful in colon-based Crohn's disease; action not clear	Teach patient to: Report side effects: diarrhea, peripheral neuropathies, strong metallic taste. Avoid alcohol use; alcohol use with drug can cause disulfiram (Antabuse) reaction.

IV, Intravenous.

Cyclosporine (Sandimmune) may be tried for ulcerative colitis although its effectiveness has not been proven.

ANTIBIOTICS. Metronidazole (Flagyl) and ciprofloxacin are the two antibiotics most used for patients with IBD. In ulcerative colitis, antibiotic use is mainly perioperative because of low effectiveness and the risk of antibiotic-associated pseudomembranous colitis. For Crohn's disease, metronidazole has been effective in mild cases confined to the colon. Frequent adverse effects such as a strong metallic taste and dose-related, usually reversible peripheral neuropathy limit its use. Antibiotics are appropriate for severely ill patients at risk for infection and for situations in which bowel stricture causes stasis and bacterial overgrowth in the bowel.

MONOCLONAL ANTIBODIES. Infliximab, a monoclonal immunoglobulin G_1 antibody against tumor necrosis factor–alpha (TNF-alpha), has been shown to be effective in treating active Crohn's disease and healing fistulas.[21] TNF-alpha is an inflammatory agent found in high amounts in patients with Crohn's disease. By binding to TNF-alpha, the drug blocks its activity, leading to decreased inflammation and healing. Natalizumab is another monoclonal antibody found to be effective in active Crohn's disease.[18]

OTHER AGENTS. Fat-soluble vitamin supplements are often necessary for patients with IBD. In some patients, antidiarrheal medications, bile acid–binding agents, acid suppressants, and antispasmodics may also be used. These drugs are administered for symptomatic relief, and an accurate record of their administration and effectiveness in controlling symptoms needs to be maintained. Antidiarrheals and anticholinergics are not used in severe ulcerative colitis because of the risk of inducing toxic megacolon.

TREATMENTS. No specific treatments are indicated for IBD management. Patients with primarily rectal involvement may follow a regimen of daily enema administration. Other prescribed treatments may be related to the management of skin breakdown or excoriation accompanying severe diarrhea. With severe episodes of IBD, bed rest, NPO status, and IV rehydration are needed. Total parenteral nutrition is initiated if malnutrition is present. Hospitalization may be required for initiation of high-dose steroid or immunosuppressive therapy.

SURGICAL MANAGEMENT. Surgery plays important but different roles in the management of Crohn's disease and ulcerative colitis. Surgery is indicated for patients whose disease is refractory to medical therapy and for the management of complications. It plays a curative role in ulcerative colitis.

CROHN'S DISEASE. Surgical intervention is avoided whenever possible in Crohn's disease because of the high rate of recurrence of the disease process in the same area. Nevertheless, about 75% of patients have surgery at least once either for uncontrolled disease or to manage a complication.[48] Surgical approaches to Crohn's disease focus on sparing and conserving as much of the bowel as possible, particularly when the small bowel is involved. The loss of more than 100 cm of bowel almost inevitably results in short-bowel syndrome and persistent problems with malabsorption and diarrhea (see Chapter 42).

Segmental resection with reanastomosis has been the primary surgical approach. Surgeons typically resect the bowel 5 to 10 cm above and below the macroscopically visible disease. Symptoms have been estimated to recur at a rate of approximately 10% per year,[40] but they do not always necessitate repeat surgery. The primary indications for surgery include bowel obstruction, fistula, abscess, perforation, and hemorrhage. Laparoscopic approaches may significantly reduce the morbidity associated with these procedures.

Bowel strictures are a common complication of Crohn's disease that can cause acute bowel obstruction. The development of strictureplasty (Figure 43-6), which is analogous to pyloroplasty and can be done laparoscopically, allows release of strictures without the loss of involved bowel segments. Strictured segments tend to be fibrous rather than acutely inflamed and rarely obstruct again.

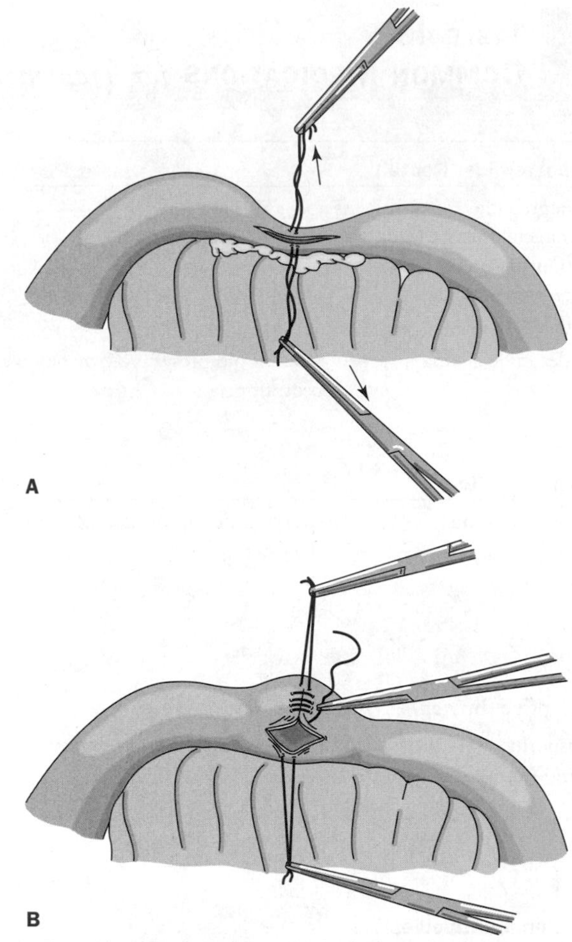

Figure 43-6 Strictureplasty. **A,** A linear incision is made at and beyond the stricture site. The site is spread open. **B,** Widened site is sutured closed.

ULCERATIVE COLITIS. Surgical intervention may be selected for patients with ulcerative colitis whose disease cannot be satisfactorily controlled with standard medical management. The procedures are curative and involve the removal of the entire colon. Surgery is also undertaken when acute complications such as hemorrhage or toxic megacolon develop or when cellular dysplasia indicates an unacceptably high risk of bowel cancer. Most patients are able to achieve a high quality of life after surgery, particularly since the successful development of continent procedures (see Research box).

Ileostomy. The Brook ileostomy procedure is the oldest colectomy procedure and the standard operation for ulcerative colitis.[55] The Brook procedure involves removal of the colon, rectum, and anus, with permanent closure of the anus. The ileostomy is created by bringing the end of the terminal ileum out through the abdominal wall to form a stoma (Figure 43-7). Any colectomy procedure decreases the bowel's ability to resorb fluid and electrolytes, and the ileostomy drainage is profuse and watery; but the terminal ileum dilates over time and assumes some of the functions of the cecum. The volume of stool decreases, although about 300 to 800 ml of fluid is still lost in the stool each day along with substantial amounts of electrolytes, particularly sodium. The per-

Research

Farouk R et al: Functional outcomes after ileal pouch-anal anastomosis for chronic ulcerative colitis, *Ann Surg* 231(6):1-11, 2000.

This study assessed long-term functional outcomes in 1450 patients who underwent ileal pouch construction for chronic ulcerative colitis between 1981 and 1994, with particular attention to the impact of aging, childbirth, and pouch failure. Functional outcomes were comparable between men and women. Stool frequency and continence were similar in both men and women. Aging was found to be related to more frequent pouch evacuation and a slightly increased risk of incontinence. Patients who were younger than 45 years of age at the time of surgery experienced increased fecal spotting as they aged, but incontinence remained uncommon.

Earlier studies had found a significantly increased risk of pouch problems after pregnancy and vaginal delivery, including anal sphincter injury, pelvic floor denervation, and incontinence. This study did not uncover any patterns of functional compromise with childbirth. Pelvic pain and soiling during intercourse were significant concerns for a small number of participants. Pelvic sepsis was the major cause of pouch failure in this population, but the incidence was low.

son experiences chronic fluid deficit as the small intestine is unable to fine-tune fluid balance, and any increase in fluid intake simply increases the volume of the ileostomy drainage.

This surgery cures the ulcerative colitis and eliminates the risk of colon cancer. However, the permanent ileostomy creates both physical and emotional challenges for the patient. Malfunctioning of the ostomy is relatively common, since poorly digested foods can easily obstruct the narrow lumen. Fears of leakage; embarrassment from noise and odor; and negative effects on self-concept, body image, and sexuality are common problems. Impotence can also occur after the surgery unless the surgeon is able to successfully dissect around the autonomic nerves in the pelvis.

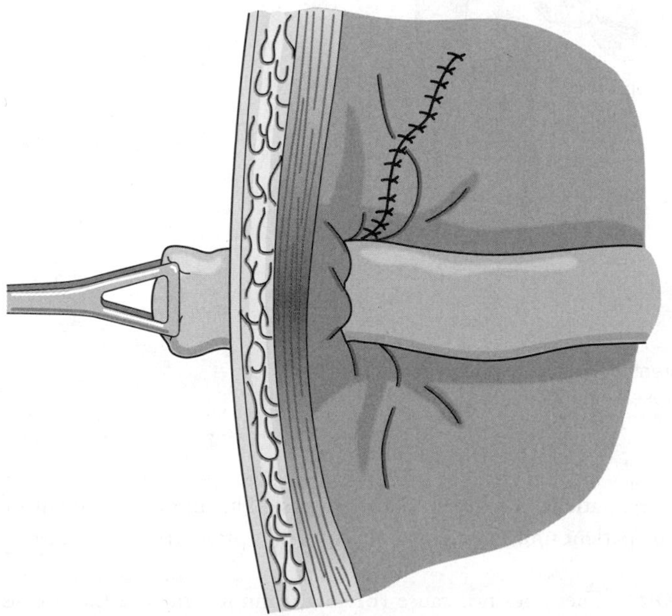

Figure 43-7 Construction of an ileostomy.

Continent Ileostomy. In the late 1960s Dr. Nils Kock developed a surgical procedure to spare patients some of the challenges of traditional ileostomy. The procedure (the Kock ileostomy) involves the creation of an abdominal reservoir from a piece of terminal ileum to store the feces. The end of the ileum is intussuscepted to form a nipple valve that lies flush with the abdomen. A catheter is used to drain the pouch, and a small dressing or adhesive bandage is worn over the stoma between emptyings. The pouch eventually can expand to hold about 500 ml of drainage. Problems with the nipple valve are common and often require surgical repair. Valve failure plus the incidence of chronic inflammation in the pouch limits the usefulness of the procedure, and it is rarely recommended any longer as a primary intervention.

Ileoanal Anastomosis (Ileorectostomy). The ileoanal anastomosis or pull-through operation was the first colectomy procedure developed that did not require any type of ileostomy. Originally it was a straight **anastomosis** in which a 12- to 15-cm rectal stump was left after removal of the colon. The small intestine was inserted inside this rectal sleeve and anastomosed (Figure 43-8). Problems with the procedure related to recurrence of the ulcerative colitis or development of cancer in the rectal stump. Advantages of the procedure are that not only is an ostomy avoided but the remaining rectum with its ability to resorb water and electrolytes results in a decreased volume of stool.

A new approach is attempting to decrease the complications of the anastomosis procedure while maintaining its benefits. The ileoneorectal anastomosis focuses on meticulous stripping of the mucosa, the target of ulcerative colitis, from the rectum. Mucosal transplantation is then performed from the disease-free ileum, and direct anastomosis can take place without the need for the sleeve. Original rectal function is preserved.[11]

Ileoanal Pouch Anastomosis. The ileoanal pouch anastomosis (IPAA), which involves the creation of a pouch from the terminal ileum that is sutured directly to the anus, is currently the procedure of choice for most patients requiring colectomy.[37] Advantages of IPAA are that it leaves the anal sphincter intact, preserving continence and the normal route of defecation; removes almost all mucosal disease because only about 1 inch of rectum is left and that is stripped of its mucosa; and limits pelvic dissection, decreasing the risk of disrupting innervation to the sexual organs.

Several different approaches to reservoir construction have been developed. A J-shaped anastomosis is commonly chosen because of its ease of construction (Figure 43-9). W- and S-shaped pouches also are used, but the S-shaped pouch is large, and the distal limb may not empty effectively. IPAA is a two-stage procedure because at the time of initial surgery a temporary loop ileostomy is created to divert bowel contents away from the suture lines until healing is complete. The loop ileostomy is then closed within 2 to 3 months.[37] Functional results continue to improve for up to 12 months after surgery, and most patients have three to eight bowel movements per day. Slight fecal incontinence is a problem—sometimes a persistent one, especially at night—but the normal manner of defecation makes this a preferred procedure. It ordinarily is not used in persons older than 55 years of age, who may experience anal sphincter deterioration related to aging.

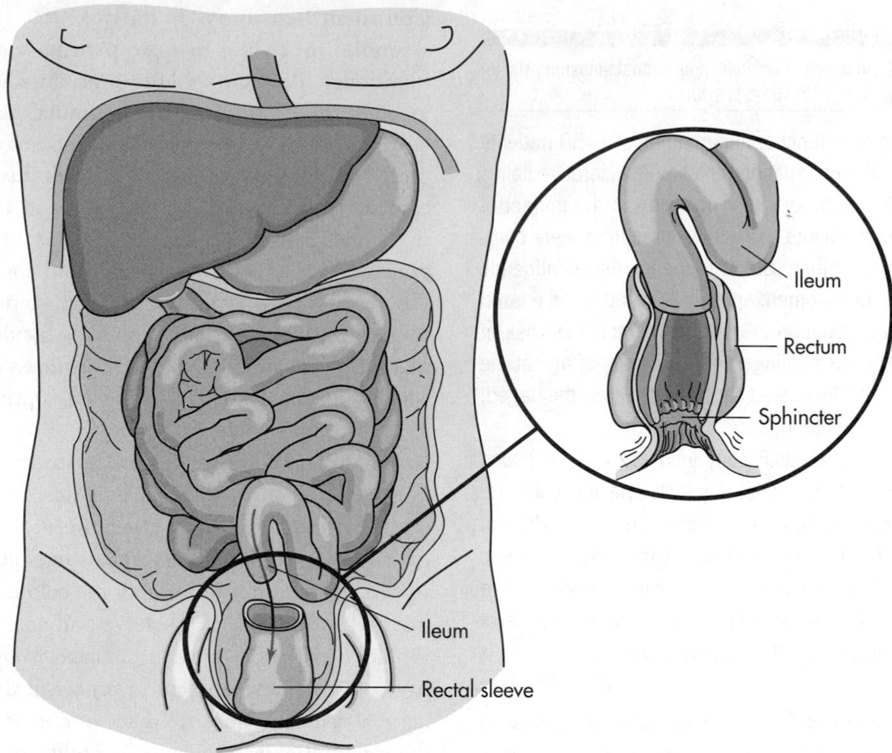

Figure 43-8 Ileoanal anastomosis. Also referred to as *ileorectostomy* or *pull-through procedure.*

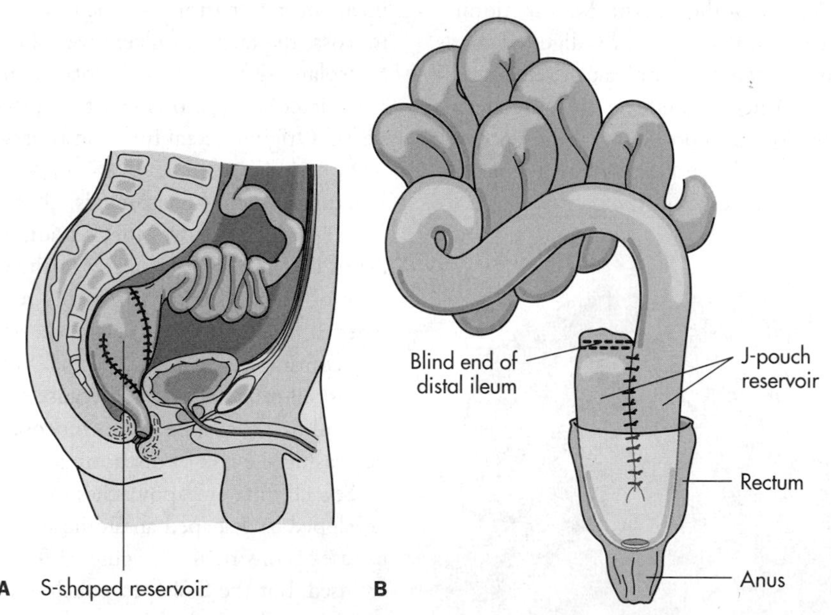

Figure 43-9 Two types of ileoanal reservoir created in ileoanal pouch anastomosis procedures. **A,** S-shaped reservoir. **B,** J-pouch reservoir.

The procedure is not without complications, and "pouchitis," acute inflammation within the reservoir, can occur.[45] Pouchitis creates discomfort, bleeding, and increased output that is similar in many ways to the original disease process. It is attributed by some researchers to faulty diagnosis of the colitis and the possibility that Crohn's disease is the primary pathologic process. Others attribute this inflammatory reaction to a general propensity of these patients for inflammatory disease. Nursing management of the patient undergoing ostomy surgery is presented on p. 1261.

DIET. Diet does not cause IBD and cannot influence the course of the disease, but diet is an important consideration in patient comfort. Nutritional concerns become important during exacerbations of the disease when diarrhea may be severe, and anorexia and nausea make it difficult for the patient to meet nutritional needs through an oral diet.

Dietary recommendations are tailored to the needs of the individual patient, but as a rule patients with diarrhea or abdominal pain are encouraged to restrict their intake of raw fruits and vegetables, as well as fatty and spicy foods. Constipation may be a problem in distal colon or rectal disease and usually can be controlled with bulk hydrophilic laxatives such as psyllium (Metamucil). The general guideline for IBD is that when patients feel well, they can eat almost anything, but when they feel sick, they should limit what they eat.[28] Bowel rest plays a role in Crohn's disease management, and elemental diets or supplements may be used. These preparations are completely digested and absorbed in the duodenum and ileum and place no demands on the large bowel. Recent attention has focused on the possible suppressive effect of fish oil on the inflammatory process. Lactose intolerance is often a problem in persons with IBD, and patients are encouraged to evaluate whether restricting dairy products has a positive effect on their symptoms.

Acute exacerbations of IBD make it difficult to maintain adequate nutrition. Short-term parenteral nutrition may occasionally be necessary to ensure minimal amounts of essential nutrients. Nutritional support is particularly important when the patient requires surgery.

COUNSELING. Although neither stress nor personality plays a role in the etiology of IBD, coping with the effects of IBD can put a tremendous strain on a person's adaptive abilities. Disease exacerbations may leave the patient particularly vulnerable to depression and even despair. The disease typically affects young adults who are just beginning their education, careers, or families. The stress of this unpredictable and potentially incapacitating disease cannot be ignored. The nurse should routinely refer patients and families to the support services of the National Foundation for Ileitis and Colitis or other organizations.

Nursing Management *of the Patient with Inflammatory Bowel Disease*

ASSESSMENT

Health History. Assess for:

- Patient's knowledge base and understanding of the disorder
- Pain location, nature, severity, frequency; relationship to eating; measures used to self-treat
- Constipation or diarrhea; frequency and character of stools
- Usual meal pattern and intake, recent weight changes, food intolerances and allergies, appetite, fatigue or weakness, nausea
- Support network; impact of illness on family, employment, lifestyle, and sexuality
- Perceived life stress and usual coping patterns
- Medications in current use: prescribed and over the counter, dosage and side effects, perceived effectiveness in managing disease and symptoms

Physical Examination. Assess for:

- Body weight
- Skin turgor and condition of mucous membranes
- Fever
- Bowel sounds: presence and character
- Condition of perianal skin
- Composition of stools: presence of blood, fat, mucus, or pus

NURSING DIAGNOSES, OUTCOMES, AND INTERVENTIONS

Nursing Diagnosis: Chronic Pain

OUTCOMES. Common examples of expected outcomes for the patient with a diagnosis of *chronic pain* are:

Patient will:

- Report decreased frequency and severity of abdominal discomfort.
- Use dietary and nonpharmacologic pain relief measures to manage pain.

NURSING INTERVENTIONS. The nurse encourages the patient to document the character and severity of the pain and to record its relationship to eating, drinking, and passing stool or flatus. Anticholinergic or antispasmodic medications such as propantheline bromide are used as prescribed to reduce the cramping. A warm heating pad applied to the abdomen often is comforting but should not be used during acute exacerbations. The nurse encourages the use of diversional activities and relaxation strategies. The nurse documents the patient's pain pattern and response to all interventions.

RELATED NIC INTERVENTIONS. Analgesic Administration, Anxiety Reduction, Environmental Management: Comfort, Pain Management

Nursing Diagnosis: Diarrhea

OUTCOMES. Common examples of expected outcomes for the patient with a diagnosis of *diarrhea* are:

Patient will:

- Experience fewer episodes of diarrhea.
- Identify dietary and activity factors that improve or worsen diarrhea.
- List the major signs and symptoms of dehydration and electrolyte imbalance.

NURSING INTERVENTIONS. Chronic diarrhea often becomes a focus of care during exacerbations of the disease process. Patients may feel trapped by the frequency and urgency of their need to defecate. The nurse encourages the person to keep accurate records of the frequency, severity, and character of each diarrheal episode, particularly if blood or pus is present.

The medication regimen is designed to control the inflammation and eventually the diarrhea, but this process may take days or weeks. Antidiarrheal agents such as loperamide (Imodium) may be used to slow peristalsis, and mucilloids such as psyllium may add bulk to the stool and help reduce the frequency of defecation. The patient is encouraged to limit activity when diarrhea is severe and to lie down for 20 minutes after meals to limit peristalsis.

Patients are encouraged to use the toilet or commode whenever possible, but a weak, acutely ill person may need to have a bedpan readily accessible. Room deodorizers may be necessary for odor control.

The anal region often becomes excoriated from the frequent stools. Painful anal fissures and fistulas may develop, and the anal area needs to be kept clean and dry. Medicated wipes (such as Tucks) and sitz baths three times a day can provide both comfort and cleanliness. Ointments such as Desitin or zinc oxide can create a barrier to protect the perianal skin.

Profuse diarrhea can lead to severe losses of fluids and electrolytes. If the patient is consuming an oral diet, the nurse encourages a liberal fluid intake (at least 2.5 to 3 L/day) and explores the patient's tolerance to solutions such as Gatorade, which can help replace lost electrolytes. It is important for the patient to understand that any increase in fluid intake will also increase output, since the bowel has a limited ability to resorb fluids. The nurse records accurate intake and output, assesses the skin and mucous membranes for signs of dehydration, and monitors the patient's weight daily.

RELATED NIC INTERVENTIONS. Diarrhea Management, Fluid/Electrolyte Management

Nursing Diagnosis: Imbalanced Nutrition: Less Than Body Requirements

OUTCOMES. Common examples of expected outcomes for the patient with a diagnosis of *imbalanced nutrition: less than body requirements* are:

Patient will:

- Follow a balanced, high-nutrient diet, avoiding foods that increase symptoms.
- Maintain desired weight or regain weight to desired goal at a rate of ½ to 1 lb/wk.
- Achieve a positive nitrogen balance as evidenced by a serum albumin level greater than 4 g/dl.

NURSING INTERVENTIONS. During acute exacerbations of IBD, the patient may be malnourished from anorexia, inflammation of the bowel, and malabsorption. The method of feeding depends on the type and extent of the disorder. With severe or extensive disease, especially when complications are present, the patient may be kept NPO, and parenteral nutrition may be instituted. Bowel rest can be helpful in Crohn's disease but has no proven therapeutic benefit in ulcerative colitis.

Elemental feedings, similar to those given in tube feedings, are started as soon as possible. These feedings are absorbed rapidly in the upper GI tract, causing minimal demand on the colon. Palatability is a problem with elemental diets, and serving the fluids chilled and offering a variety of flavors may increase patient acceptance. A low-residue, high-protein, high-calorie diet is then gradually reintroduced.

During periods of remission, patients are advised to eat a well-balanced, high-calorie diet with a liberal fluid and salt intake to compensate for daily losses. Only foods known to cause problems are restricted. The person with ulcerative colitis may need to avoid intestinal stimulants such as alcohol, caffeinated beverages, high-fat foods, and very high–fiber foods such as raw fruits and vegetables (cooked fruits and vegetables are usually better tolerated). Milk products are often poorly tolerated, since lactose intolerance is common in persons with IBD, and the nurse encourages the patient to evaluate the effect of milk product restriction on the severity of symptoms. Multivitamin and mineral supplements are used regularly.

RELATED NIC INTERVENTIONS. Diet Staging, Fluid/Electrolyte Management, Fluid Monitoring, Nutrition Management, Nutritional Monitoring

Nursing Diagnosis: Ineffective Coping

OUTCOMES. Common examples of expected outcomes for the patient with a diagnosis of *ineffective coping* are:

Patient will:

- Identify factors that increase disease-related anxiety and stress.
- Verbalize coping strategies and support mechanisms to handle problems.

NURSING INTERVENTIONS. IBD is characterized by periods of exacerbation and remission throughout the patient's adult life. It can significantly disrupt the patient's preferred lifestyle. Although emotions and stress do not play a role in disease etiology, they are believed to influence the severity and frequency of disease exacerbations. Frustration, depression, and a sense of powerlessness are common responses to the disease and may precipitate hostile or dependent behaviors. Patients often become preoccupied with their physical symptoms.

The nurse encourages the patient to become an active participant in all decisions related to disease management and to verbalize concerns and feelings related to the disease and treatment. The nurse provides the patient with information about local support groups and encourages involvement with the National Foundation for Ileitis and Colitis.

Fatigue is a common problem with IBD and can worsen the patient's psychologic response to the disease. Fatigue results from the combination of increased energy demands secondary to the inflammatory process and the decreased energy supply from inadequate nutrition, anemia, and depression. Planned rest periods should be included in daily activities. When the acute episode begins to subside, progressive activity is encouraged. During remissions, the nurse encourages the patient to participate in social activities but not to overexert to the point of fatigue. Sexual response also may be affected by IBD. Malnutrition and frequent diarrhea often lead to decreased libido, and the ileostomy may be associated with a sense of diminished sexual attractiveness. The nurse encourages the patient to express sex-related concerns and explore them openly with the spouse or partner. IBD support groups can be excellent resources for strategies to manage concerns over odor and leakage during sexual activity, particularly after a colectomy.

RELATED NIC INTERVENTIONS. Coping Enhancement, Decision-Making Support, Family Involvement Promotion, Role Enhancement, Support System Enhancement

Nursing Diagnosis: Ineffective Health Maintenance

OUTCOMES. Common examples of expected outcomes for the patient with a diagnosis of *ineffective health maintenance* are: Patient will:

- Describe the illness, prescribed therapy schedule, and side effects of all medications.
- List symptoms requiring medical attention.
- Identify plans for ongoing medical follow-up care.

NURSING INTERVENTIONS. Accurate knowledge about the disease process and therapeutic modalities can help the patient achieve a sense of control. The nurse explores the patient's existing knowledge base about the cause, course, and prognosis of the disease; treatment options; and the identification and management of complications (see Patient/Family Teaching box). Patient education materials are available from the National Foundation for Ileitis and Colitis and the National Institutes of Health. The nurse ensures that the patient understands the importance of careful adherence to the medication regimen and has a schedule for medical follow-up visits.

RELATED NIC INTERVENTIONS. Family Support, Mutual Goal Setting, Teaching: Individual

EVALUATION

To evaluate the effectiveness of nursing interventions, compare patient behaviors with those stated in the expected patient outcomes.

RELATED NOC OUTCOMES. Adherence Behavior, Bowel Elimination, Coping, Decision-Making, Fluid Balance, Knowledge: Treatment Regimen, Nutritional Status: Food & Fluid Intake, Nutritional Status: Nutrient Intake, Pain Control, Pain Level, Participation in Health Care Decisions, Role Performance, Social Support, Symptom Control

GERONTOLOGIC CONSIDERATIONS

Although both forms of IBD typically begin in young adulthood, the onset can occur after age 60 years. The presentation, clinical course, and response to treatment generally are similar in both age-groups. The disease often takes the form of proctitis in older adults, and local treatment is usually effective. Complications are more likely to be related to **comorbidity** problems than to the primary IBD, but toxic megacolon occurs often. Once the disease process is controlled, an older adult with ulcerative colitis is less likely to have a relapse, and the risk of disease-related cancer is minimal. Crohn's disease in older adults tends to be localized in the distal colon and rectum, and generalized involvement is unusual. Because both forms of IBD tend to concentrate in the distal colon and rectum, the differential diagnosis may be unclear in older patients. This is particularly true if the disease does not have an acute onset.

Surgical intervention is avoided, if possible, because older patients tend to experience an increased incidence of complications, although recurrence of Crohn's disease after surgery is not common in older adults. Sphincter-sparing colectomy procedures are used less commonly in this population because it is more difficult to achieve successful wound healing and adequate continence, particularly at night.

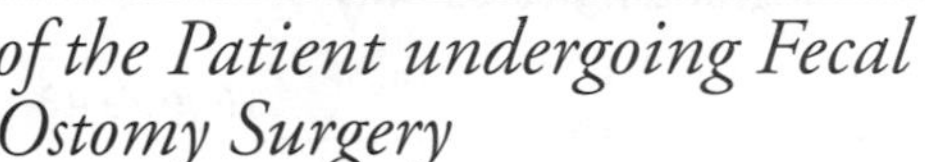

Nursing Management *of the Patient undergoing Fecal Ostomy Surgery*

The word *ostomy* refers to a surgical procedure in which an opening is created to drain either urine or feces. A fecal ostomy may be created as a temporary or permanent approach to the management of a wide variety of bowel problems. Ostomies can be created from the ileum or at various sites within the large bowel (Figure 43-10;

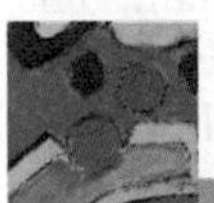
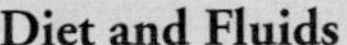

PATIENT/FAMILY TEACHING *The Patient With Inflammatory Bowel Disease*

Diet and Fluids

Eat a high-calorie, well-balanced diet.
Avoid any foods that increase symptoms (e.g., fresh fruits and raw vegetables, fatty foods, spicy foods, and alcohol).
Assess the effect of dairy products on disease symptoms, and limit use if appropriate.
Take a multivitamin or mineral supplement daily.
Ensure a liberal fluid intake—2.5 to 3 L/day:
—Drink Gatorade or other commercial products, if tolerated, during flare-ups to replace lost electrolytes.
Use salt liberally during disease flare-ups.

Elimination

Take medication as prescribed.
Keep the rectal area clean and dry; use analgesic rectal ointment or sitz baths for rectal discomfort.
Consult with physician about the appropriateness of antidiarrheal agents or bulk-forming laxatives when diarrhea is present.
Monitor weight daily during disease flare-ups.

Rest and Coping

Maintain a regular sleep schedule.
Schedule daily activities to avoid fatigue; take rest periods as necessary.
Use relaxation strategies when stress levels rise.
Discuss concerns with family or support person.
Attend a local support group for inflammatory bowel disease if available.

Health Maintenance

Report signs requiring medical attention:
—Change in pattern or severity of abdominal pain or diarrhea
—Constipation
—Change in stool character
—Unusual discharge from rectum
—Fever
Plan for regular follow-up care.

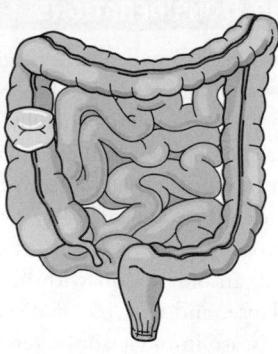

The **ascending colostomy** is done for right-sided tumors.

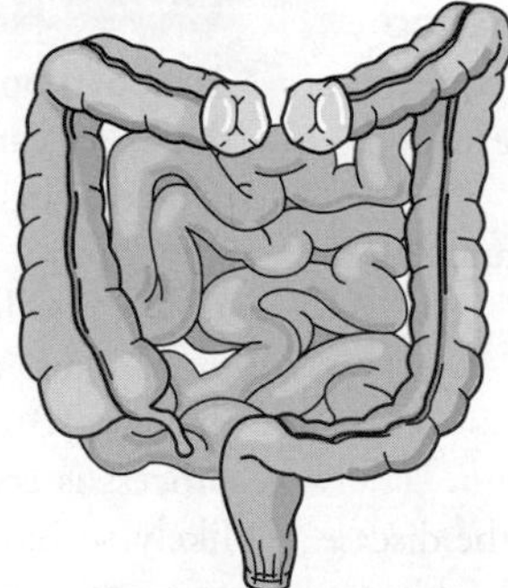

The **transverse (double-barreled) colostomy** is often used in such emergencies as intestinal obstruction or perforation because it can be created quickly. There are two stomas. The proximal one, closest to the small intestine, drains feces. The distal stoma drains mucus. Usually temporary.

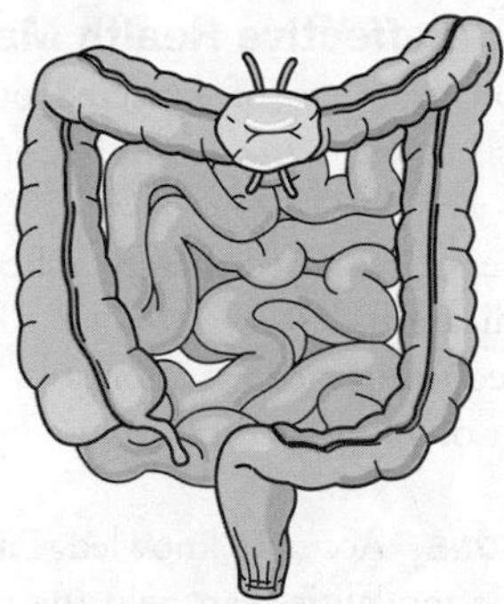

The **transverse loop colostomy** has two openings in the transverse colon, but one stoma. Usually temporary.

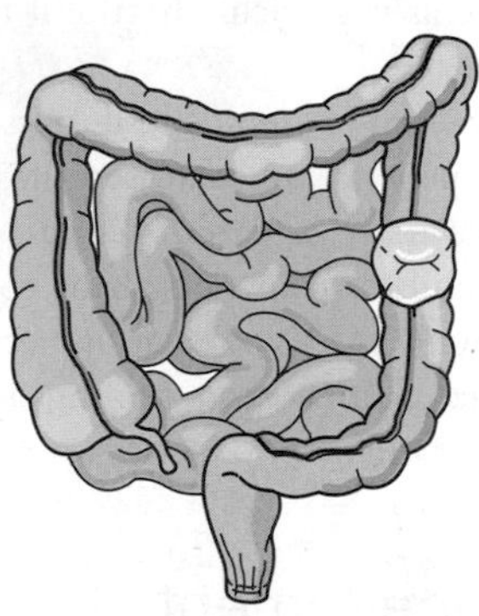

Descending colostomy

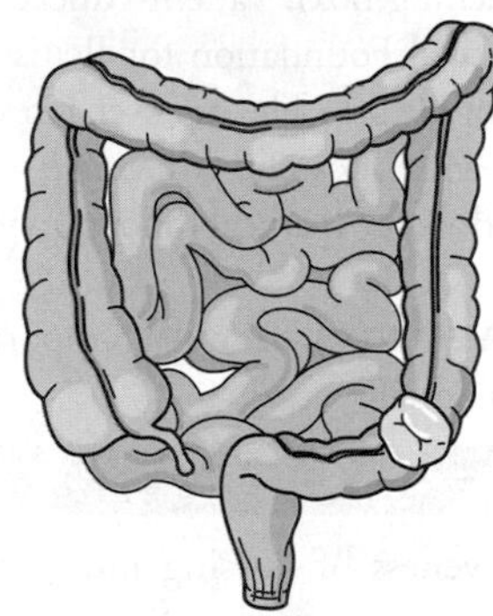

Sigmoid colostomy

Figure 43-10 Types of colostomies.

see also Figure 43-7). Loop colostomies are generally temporary and allow for easy closure at a future point. Although each type of ostomy presents its own unique management problems, all ostomies challenge patients to maintain skin integrity and achieve effective self-care.

Preoperative Care

Preoperative care focuses on patient teaching. The nurse assesses the patient's knowledge and understanding of the proposed surgery and its outcomes. This includes a brief overview of GI tract structure and function and the nature and function of an ostomy. Written materials also are provided that reinforce the teaching and outline the postoperative care plan. Comprehensive ostomy care involves a team approach and ideally includes an ostomy nurse (formerly known as an enterostomal therapy nurse), dietitian, and discharge planner in addition to the surgeon and staff nurses. Early involvement of the ostomy nurse provides structure for the teaching plan and ensures that an ostomy specialist is involved in selecting the most appropriate site for the stoma. Many common stoma complications can be avoided by appropriate site selection with consideration for the shape and contour of the skin folds of the patient's abdomen in both a sitting and an upright position.[15] The site should be visible and accessible to the patient when sitting or standing; lie within the rectus muscle; and avoid scars, bony prominences, skin folds, and the belt line. The site selected for the stoma plays a significant role in the patient's ability to maintain a good ostomy appliance seal and manage the ostomy independently after surgery.

Emotional preparation for ostomy surgery is important. The nurse encourages the patient to verbalize feelings related to this radical change in body image and function. Validating the appropriateness of these concerns lays the foundation for an effective working relationship with the patient. The patient needs to work through the grieving process, and specific factual teaching may be ineffective if the patient is in the shock and disbelief stage. The nurse accepts all feelings and reinforces the importance of open communication.

The preoperative preparation phase may include nutritional support, possibly with parenteral nutrition, if the patient's nutritional state is inadequate for surgery. The patient should know what to expect in the postoperative period. The nurse discusses the management of postoperative pain, the nature and appearance of all incisions and drains, and the purpose of the NG tube and IV lines. Thorough bowel cleansing is performed and may include the use of enemas, laxatives, and antibiotics to reduce intestinal bacterial flora.

Postoperative Care

The nurse provides general postoperative care. NG suction is usually maintained for a few days after surgery, and the patient is kept NPO to prevent distention and pressure on the suture lines. Careful attention paid to pain management ensures patient comfort and supports the patient's ability to follow the deep breathing and early ambulation protocols.

Maintaining Fluid and Electrolyte Balance. Attention to fluid and electrolyte balance is crucial for all ostomy patients, particularly those with an ileostomy. After surgery the fecal drainage from the ileostomy is liquid and may be constant. Fecal outputs range from 1000 to 1500 ml/24 hr. This amount begins to decrease slightly within 10 to 15 days as the terminal ileum absorbs more water and the stool thickens. The losses are still significant, however, and careful intake and output records are essential. The ileostomy patient becomes dehydrated easily. The stool may not thicken if the patient has had previous small bowel resections for Crohn's disease. The more intestine that has been resected, the greater the chance for a high-volume output of liquid stool. Loperamide or diphenoxylate hydrochloride–atropine (Lomotil) may be used to control the output and the fluid loss in severe cases.[15]

The pouch may initially need to be emptied every 1 to 2 hours. High-volume, liquid ileostomy effluent can best be managed using a urinary pouch attached to a urinary bedside drainage system. Once the ileostomy effluent thickens and decreases in volume, the urinary pouch is changed to a drainable pouching system used to manage stool. Volumes in excess of 1500 ml/24 hr are considered excessive. Fluid and electrolyte problems are usually not a major concern after colostomy surgery, although it may take time to reestablish a normal pattern of elimination.

Stoma Monitoring. The patient who has undergone ostomy surgery typically returns from surgery with an ostomy pouch system in place. The nurse observes the stoma regularly for color and edema. Color reflects perfusion, and the stoma should be bright red and moist. A dark, dusky, or brown-black stoma indicates ischemia and necrosis and should be reported immediately to the surgeon. A small amount of bleeding from the stoma is expected because it has a rich blood supply, but any significant bleeding should be reported to the surgeon immediately. Initial stoma edema is an expected response to surgical manipulation. Edema typically resolves in 5 to 7 days, but the stoma continues to slowly decrease in size over 6 to 8 weeks.[24] The shape of the stoma also changes slightly throughout the day in response to peristalsis, and the pouch opening must be able to accommodate the changing stoma size.

The nurse inspects the abdominal incision and the sutures anchoring the stoma for intactness. Some of the stoma mucosa may pull away from the abdominal skin before healing is complete. Superficial separations heal by granulation, but deeper separations may require packing or resuturing. The stoma drainage consists initially of mucus and serosanguineous secretion. As peristalsis returns, flatus and fecal drainage begin, usually in 2 to 4 days.

A loop colostomy may be opened during surgery or in the patient's room 48 to 72 hours later. A cautery is used to create two openings, one proximal and one distal, in the one stoma (see Figure 43-10). The nurse reassures the patient that the procedure causes no pain because the bowel has no sensory nerve endings for pain sensation. The procedure creates a distinct burning smell, however, and can be frightening. The nurse offers support and reassurance during the loop opening. The supporting rod for the loop is removed after 7 to 10 days, when adhesions prevent the stoma from retracting into the surrounding skin.

Managing a Perineal Wound. The abdominal perineal resection (formation of a permanent colostomy with removal of the rectum and anus using both an abdominal and a perineal incision) has been the gold standard for the treatment of rectal cancer for many years and is still the treatment of choice for managing highly invasive disease. Postoperative care is more complex because of the presence of a major perineal wound that may require up to 6 months to heal completely. The patient's convalescence is prolonged.

The perineal wound is created by the removal of the entire rectum and anus plus muscle and fatty tissue. The wound may be left open and loosely filled with packing. The large gap that is created gradually fills with granulation tissue. Wound irrigations and absorbent dressings are used until the wound closes. Alternatively, the perineal wound may be sutured with stab wounds formed for drainage and irrigation. The remaining pelvic organs shift slightly to fill the remaining space.

The perineal wound makes it difficult for the patient to sit or find a comfortable position. Foam pads or soft pillows may increase comfort while the patient is sitting. The nurse instructs the patient to avoid the use of air or rubber rings that separate the buttocks and put stress on the healing wound. The side-lying position is usually preferred. Phantom rectal sensations and itching may occur after healing. The origin of these sensations is unknown. Serosanguineous wound drainage initially is copious and must be effectively removed to prevent infection and abscess formation. The drainage tubes may work passively by gravity or be attached to suction. Wound irrigations, usually with normal saline, are initially done with a catheter, but the patient may progress to a handheld shower massage or Water Pik. The dressings are changed as needed. A T-binder may be useful in holding the dressings in place over the perineum. Sitz baths may be substituted for irrigations once the patient is ambulatory, but a free flow of water on the perineal wound is preferred.

Teaching for Self-Care. It is essential that the patient acquire basic ostomy self-care skills during the postoperative period. Successful self-care provides the foundation for both independence and a reintegration of body image that includes the ostomy. The nurse teaches the patient the principles of ostomy care and encourages the patient to handle, assemble, and use all equipment. Acquiring sufficient confidence and expertise to manage an ostomy effectively requires time and practice. The process can rarely be completed during the hospitalization, particularly with older persons, and the nurse initiates referrals to appropriate home health care and community ostomy services for ongoing teaching and supervision. Involvement of a family member or supportive friend can be helpful if it is acceptable to the patient. Support groups are available in most larger cities and are a good source of information about day-to-day management problems related to acquiring supplies and coping with ostomy challenges.

STOMA CARE. An ostomy appliance is placed over the new stoma at the conclusion of the surgery. Teaching begins with the first appliance change. The patient may or may not be ready to view the stoma, but the nurse gently encourages the patient to look at and touch it. The nurse briefly and factually explains each step of the procedure. The nurse reminds the patient that the stoma has no touch sensation but that the rest of the abdomen will be painful from the surgery. Surgical pain should be adequately controlled before any teaching session takes place.

A systematic plan should be in place to guide teaching of ostomy care. Teaching sessions should be spaced throughout the hospitalization to allow for repetition and assimilation. The ostomy appliance is changed more frequently than needed to allow for practice time. Written instructions and resource materials are invaluable supplements to instruction by the nurse.

Ostomy Appliance Selection. An effective pouching system protects the skin, contains stool and odor, molds to the body's contours, allows for movement, and is inconspicuous under clothing. It is the most important aspect of ostomy management. Choices are based on the ostomy type, the size and contour of the abdomen, the peristomal skin condition, financial considerations, and individual preferences.

Products for ostomy care are available in a variety of styles, shapes, and sizes. Disposable pouches are available in one- and two-piece systems, with skin barriers attached, and in a variety of materials (Figure 43-11). Reusable pouches are worn, cleaned, and worn again. Drainable pouches are easier to keep clean and are more economical than closed, nondrainable pouches. They are available in one- and two-piece systems in a variety of materials. Drainable pouches are used for both an ileostomy and colostomy and are changed every 3 to 7 days if there are no problems with leakage. The patient with an ileostomy is instructed to empty and rinse the pouch every 4 to 6 hours.

A properly applied pouching system is odor free except while changing or emptying the pouch of stool. Persistent odor is usually the result of inadequate cleansing of the drainage spout or a poor pouch seal. Pinholes in a pouch destroy its odor-proof quality and should not be used to release gas. Fecal odor is caused by the action of bacteria in the colon. Therefore the drainage from an ileostomy should not be foul smelling. A foul odor may indicate a problem such as infection or obstruction.

It is essential that the patient learn to accurately measure the stoma during each pouch change in the first weeks after surgery to ensure a proper pouch fit. The pouch should closely surround the stoma but not press or rub against it. The stoma may shrink dramatically during the first week after surgery, and it will continue to change in size slightly throughout the first several months. Cutouts of various diameters are included in the box of pouches. The skin barriers are cut approximately 1/16 to 1/8 inch larger than the stoma to accommodate stoma swelling. Once the stoma has stabilized in size, only occasional checks are needed to maintain proper fit. The pouch change procedure is outlined in the Patient/Family Teaching box.

The nurse teaches the patient to change the ostomy appliance immediately if leakage occurs and to establish a routine for changing the appliance before stool leakage occurs. The pouch should be emptied when it is one-third to one-half full. The pouch of a two-piece system or a one-piece ostomy appliance is changed during inactive times and before meals to minimize the chance of the intestine emptying during the change. The nurse instructs the

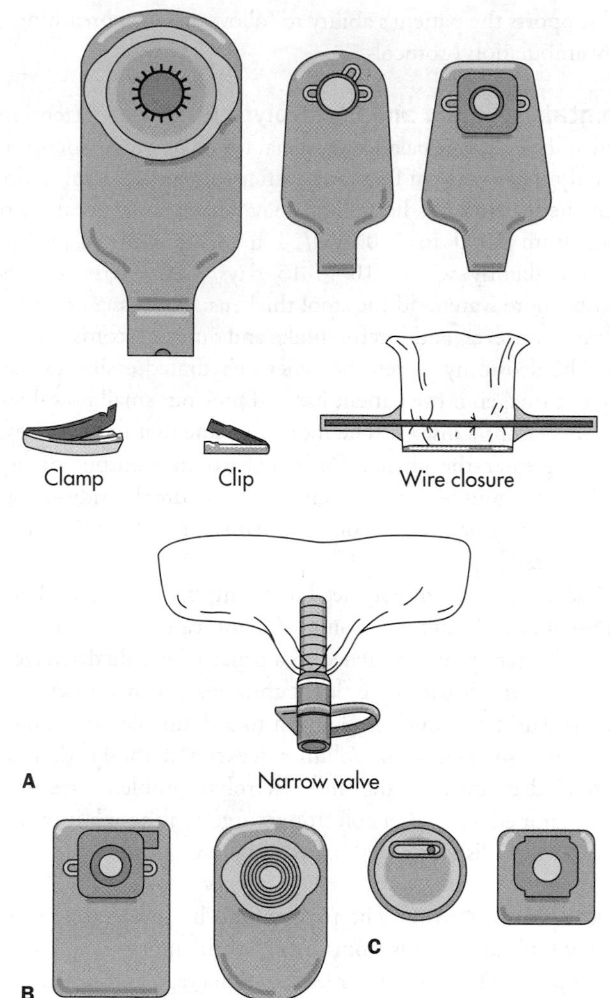

Figure 43-11 Common ostomy pouch products, closures, and patches. **A,** Drainable pouches and pouch closures. **B,** Nondrainable pouches. **C,** Patches for regulated colostomies.

patient to use each pouch or ostomy appliance change as an opportunity to carefully assess the stoma and peristomal skin.

The nurse ensures that the patient has adequate temporary supplies before discharge, a complete list of supplies needed for home management, and information about where supplies can be obtained in the local community. A prescription for supplies may be needed for Medicare or insurance reimbursement.

Skin Care. The drainage from an ileostomy is both continuous and erosive, and it is essential that the ostomy appliance be secure and properly fitted. Ileostomy drainage contains residual digestive enzymes that will break down the peristomal skin if they are allowed to make contact with it. Skin care is also important with colostomies. In addition to irritation from stool, the skin can also be damaged by an allergic reaction to the tape or skin barrier product, rough or frequent removal of pouch adhesives, or infection. The skin around the stoma should appear as healthy and normal as the remainder of the skin on the abdomen. The most common peristomal skin infection is a bright red rash with papular lesions caused by *Candida albicans.* Dryness and scaling develop if the condition persists. It can be treated by applying an antifungal powder with each pouch change.[7]

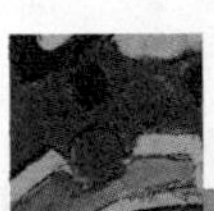

PATIENT/FAMILY TEACHING *Changing an Ostomy Appliance*

1. Gather all needed supplies.

Stoma Measurement

2. Use the measuring guide and sample diameters, and cut the ostomy appliance to fit—pattern should be ⅛ to ¼ inch larger than the stoma. It may be necessary to measure both the length and width to create a pattern for an irregularly shaped stoma.
3. Use the same procedure to prepare the skin barrier, if using a two-piece nonsnapping ostomy system. NOTE: The pouch opening is cut slightly larger (about ⅛ inch) than the skin barrier to prevent the paper from cutting the stoma.
4. Apply a ring of stoma adhesive paste to the skin barrier if needed.

Removal of Old Pouch

5. Put on clean gloves.
6. Empty the drainable pouch to prevent spills.
7. Disconnect the pouch from the skin wafer if a two-piece system is used.
8. Beginning at the top, gently peel the wafer away from the skin by pushing the skin and peeling downward. If the wafer adheres to the skin, use a moist wash cloth pressed between the wafer adhesive and skin to decrease skin irritation as the wafer is removed.

Skin Care

9. Cleanse the skin with warm water; use soap only if stool adheres to the skin. Rinse with water, and dry thoroughly.
10. Assess the peristomal skin and stoma carefully for signs of irritation or infection.
11. Thoroughly pat the peristomal skin dry.
12. Apply a layer of skin sealant and paste if needed to fill spaces.

Application of New Pouching System

13. Label the template top, bottom, right, and left.
14. Place the opening of the template over the stoma to ensure fit.
15. Center the pouch opening, if using a one-piece system, over the stoma. Tense abdominal muscles to make application easier.
16. Gently press into place, and hold for at least 30 seconds to seal.
17. If a two-part system is used, apply the pouch to the flange until it snaps in place, then apply ostomy appliance as if it is a one-piece appliance.

Prevention of skin problems is always easier and less expensive than treatment. The use of a skin barrier is an important means of protecting the peristomal skin.[43] Skin barriers come in several basic forms: powder, paste, washer, or wafer (Figure 43-12). Skin barriers include products such as karaya, Stomahesive (ConvaTec), Hollihesive (Hollister), ReliaSeal (Bard), Coloplast Skin Barrier, and Mason Colly-Seal Disc. They come already attached to the pouch for both one- and two-piece systems or as single-use items that can be used with any pouch.

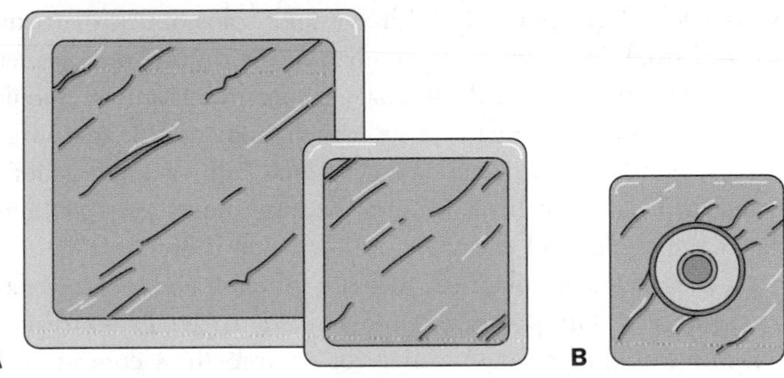

Figure 43-12 Skin barrier products. **A,** Skin barriers. **B,** Wafer.

POWDER. A pouch will not adhere to powder, cream, or ointment. If powder is applied to the skin, it must be sealed before applying the pouch. Karaya powder releases an acid that may sting irritated skin, but Stomahesive powder is well tolerated.

PASTE. Paste barriers are available for use around the stoma, to fill in creases or folds, and to extend the life of the seal. The use of paste has made it easier to keep a pouch seal intact in poor locations.

SKIN BARRIER WAFERS. Skin barrier wafers may be used with a variety of pouches and protect the skin from stool. The opening in the wafer is carefully measured so that it fits around the base of the stoma without rubbing into or onto the stoma.

SKIN SEALANTS. Skin sealants come in sprays, liquids, gels, and wipes and are used to seal in powders and coat the skin with a clear film; they are useful under pouch adhesives to avoid pulling off the stratum corneum layer of the skin when adhesive is removed from the skin.

Guidelines for skin care are summarized in the Patient/Family Teaching box, p. 1266. If the peristomal skin becomes irritated, barrier powder may be applied to help dry moist irritation. The addition of barrier powder or a wafer to the usual pouching system allows for rapid healing. An ostomy nurse should be consulted for the management of severe skin problems. The use of antacids or products that contain alcohol should be avoided because they dry the skin and alter the pH, leaving it vulnerable to infection.

MANAGING ODOR. Ostomy pouches are made of odor-proof plastic, but a leaking seal or improperly cleaned pouch can emit an unpleasant odor. The inside of the pouch is rinsed with tepid water after emptying, and the pouch outlet is wiped with toilet paper. Oral deodorizing agents exist, and deodorizing solutions and tablets may be placed in the pouch.

Attention to diet can also be helpful. The nurse encourages the patient to eat a balanced diet and to chew foods slowly and thoroughly. No special diet is required once healing has occurred; however, patients need to be informed about foods that increase gas and odor. Dairy products, highly seasoned foods, fish, and a variety of vegetables are known to increase the odor of the stool. Individual responses to gas-producing foods tend to be variable, with known exceptions such as beans, cabbage, and Brussels sprouts. The patient needs to experiment with dietary modifications that reflect individual food preferences and tolerances. Closed pouches usually have a charcoal filter at the top that releases and deodorizes gas. Pouches

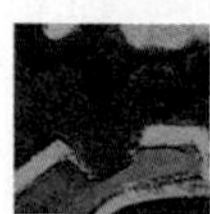

PATIENT/FAMILY TEACHING
Ostomy Skin Care

1. Empty pouch when two-thirds full to avoid leakage. Stool held against the skin can quickly cause severe skin irritation.
2. Apply clean gloves.
3. Remove pouch gently, with one hand holding the skin in place to decrease pulling.
4. Gently but thoroughly clean the skin, rinse it, and pat it dry.
5. Trim peristomal hair, but do not shave it to prevent folliculitis.
6. Use a skin barrier to protect the peristomal skin from contact with stool.
7. Use a skin sealant under all tape.
8. Encourage patient to consult an ostomy or a wound, ostomy, and continence nurse for specific care guidelines if skin irritation/breakdown occurs.

can be opened to release accumulated gas but should never be pricked. A puncture in the pouch creates a constant odor problem.

OSTOMY IRRIGATION. An ostomy irrigation is an enema given through the stoma to stimulate bowel emptying at a regular and convenient time. The procedure is no longer routinely recommended and is used only with sigmoid colostomies that expel formed stool. Irrigation is never a part of the routine management of an ileostomy because the drainage is continuous and semiliquid. A patient who uses irrigations successfully may be able to dispense with a standard pouch and wear a stoma cap—a small adhesive pouch with an absorbent dressing. Because the ostomy continues to secrete mucus and release flatus, a gas filter is desirable.

If irrigations are planned, they are initiated about 5 to 7 days after surgery. The procedure is described in the Patient/Family Teaching box, at right. A variety of equipment is commercially available, and most sets include irrigating sleeves, a cone tip for insertion into the stoma, a bag to hold the solution, and clips to close the sleeve.

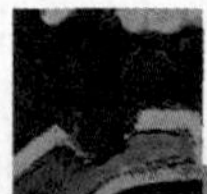

PATIENT/FAMILY TEACHING
Colostomy Irrigation

1. Assemble all equipment:
   a. Water container, irrigating sleeve, and belt
   b. Skin care items
   c. New pouch system, ready for use
2. Apply clean gloves.
3. Remove the old pouch, and dispose of it.
4. Clean the stoma and peristomal skin with water and assess.
5. Apply the irrigating sleeve and belt. Place the open end of the sleeve in the toilet.
6. Fill the irrigating container with 500 to 1000 ml of lukewarm tap water, and suspend the container at shoulder height.
7. Run water through the tubing to remove air.
8. Gently insert the irrigating cone into the stoma, and slowly start the flow of water. Catheters are inserted no more than 2 to 4 inches. Do not force. If cramping occurs, stop the irrigation and wait.
9. Allow approximately 15 to 20 minutes for stool to empty.
10. Rinse the sleeve, dry the bottom, roll it up, and close off the end. Patient should go about regular activities for 30 to 45 minutes.
11. Remove the sleeve, clean the stoma, and apply a new pouch.
12. Clean and store the irrigating equipment.

Preventing Ileostomy Complications. Excessive loss of fluid can be a serious concern after ileostomy surgery, and the nurse explains to the patient that diarrhea accompanied by nausea and vomiting can rapidly progress to dehydration. The nurse provides the patient with a list of signs of dehydration and electrolyte imbalance. Losses of sodium and potassium are of particular concern. The patient needs to know how to safely replace lost fluids and when to seek medical attention. Patients with an ileostomy also may become dehydrated if they are given laxatives in preparation for diagnostic procedures.

Enteric-coated, time-released medications or hard tablets may not be absorbed by a patient with an ileostomy and should not be used. Liquid or chewable forms of medications are preferred. Because the remaining ileum develops bacterial flora, antibiotic therapy can cause diarrhea. Supplementation of vitamins A, D, E, and K is a standard measure inasmuch as colon absorption and synthesis are eliminated.

Ileostomy patients should be aware of the potential for obstruction. Obstruction usually is caused by a large mass of undigested food that becomes lodged at a narrow point in the bowel and blocks the intestinal lumen. Dietary changes are essential. Patients are encouraged to eat a soft diet divided into six small meals a day. New foods are added gradually. Raw fruits and foods with nuts, skins, or seeds are all potential problems. Chewing all food thoroughly (20 to 25 times) is a helpful strategy. Obstructions typically manifest as crampy abdominal pain, bloating, constipation, and an inability to pass flatus (see p. 1270). Rest and a liquid diet are sufficient to resolve minor obstructions, but if the symptoms persist beyond 24 hours or become severe, the individual should contact the physician.[15] Adhesions are another common cause of obstruction. Gentle irrigation of the stoma may be successful in relieving mild obstructions related to food boluses.

Supporting a Positive Self-Concept. The formation of a stoma often is viewed as mutilating, and most patients need time and support to work through their feelings. Removal of any part of the body involves a sense of loss and grief. The nurse encourages the patient to express these feelings of loss and makes no attempt to suppress them or minimize their validity. The nurse acknowledges the work involved in grief resolution and explores the patient's usual coping strategies. The resolution of grief is not a quick or easy process, and it will not be accomplished during the hospitalization. Both the patient and the family need to be aware that grief resolution can take as much as a year or more and that grief can make a return to independent self-care more difficult.

The nurse encourages the patient to view the stoma and care for it in a matter-of-fact manner. Emotional support is incorporated into all self-care sessions, and the nurse encourages the patient to verbalize concerns and feelings about the stoma and its anticipated effects on daily life. The nurse provides positive support and reinforcement for all self-care efforts. The nurse encourages the patient to use the services of the United Ostomy Association and to involve family members in the teaching-learning process.

Patients are encouraged to gradually resume all their usual activities. No clothing restrictions are necessitated by the stoma except the avoidance of tight belts or garments directly over it. Pouches hold well in baths and showers, and normal hygiene patterns may be resumed as soon as the incision is healed. There are no specific restrictions on exercise or recreational activities.

The nurse reminds the patient to always carry ostomy supplies when traveling and to not place them in checked luggage. Traveler's diarrhea can create serious problems, and the patient is encouraged to carefully consider the quality of local water when traveling.

Preventing Sexual Dysfunction. Many patients do not directly verbalize their concerns about sexuality after ostomy surgery; thus it is usually necessary for the nurse to address the topic directly. The nurse provides the patient with specific suggestions for dealing with sexual concerns such as:

- Explore positions for sexual activity that minimize stress and pressure on the pouch.
- Empty and clean the pouch before sexual activity.
- Use a smaller-sized pouch or a pouch cover during sexual activity.
- Use a binder or special underwear to hold the pouch secure.

The nurse encourages the patient to discuss sexual concerns with his or her partner. Silence and emotional distancing are common reactions, but they can be destructive to the patient's sexual relationship. Role playing or visualizing worst-case scenarios helps some patients acknowledge their fears. The use of a community support group can be particularly helpful for getting practical advice about sexual matters. About 15% of male ostomates report a decrease in sexual activity after surgery. Female patients should be reassured that ostomy surgery does not interfere with contraception, pregnancy, or delivery; and pregnancy seldom produces stoma complications. Pamphlets on sex and the male, female, and single ostomate are available from the United Ostomy Association.

GERONTOLOGIC CONSIDERATIONS

Ostomy surgery may be required at any age, but a majority of ostomy procedures are performed on older patients as part of treatment for colorectal cancer. Adjusting to an ostomy can be particularly difficult for older adults, who may need to simultaneously cope with this radical surgery and the shock of a cancer diagnosis. Older adults can clearly learn to manage an ostomy successfully but may take longer to reach a point of readiness than can be supported by shortened hospital stays. The nurse needs to incorporate teaching and learning principles for older adults into the care plan, allowing for additional time, repeat presentation of information, and consistent caregivers if possible. Arthritis and sensory problems may make manipulation of equipment and regimen mastery more difficult. Discharge planning is particularly important for older adults, who often live alone and may not have adequate assistance in the home or community.

▶ ARE YOU READY?

In assessing the stoma of a patient in the immediate postoperative period, which of the following findings would require the nurse to immediately notify the physician?

1. Bright red, moist stoma
2. Small amount of bleeding from the stoma
3. Mild swelling of the stoma
4. Dark red, dusky-colored stoma

Obstructive Disorders

Abdominal Hernias

Etiology and Epidemiology. A hernia is a protrusion of an organ or structure from its normal cavity through a congenital or acquired defect, usually in the muscle of the abdominal wall. Hernias occur in both males and females and at any age but are more common in men and older adults. Depending on location, they may contain peritoneum, omentum, a loop of bowel, or a section of bladder and are identified as inguinal, femoral, umbilical, or incisional (Figure 43-13). Inguinal hernias, which account for a large majority of all hernias, result from primary muscular defects and are classified further as direct or indirect. Indirect inguinal hernias develop from weakness of the abdominal wall at the point where the spermatic cord emerges. Indirect hernias are the most common and are found much more often in men than in women, probably because the testes pass through the inguinal ring during fetal development. A parallel weakness is found in women from the emergence of the round ligament. The protruded bowel of an indirect inguinal hernia may rest in the inguinal canal or move down into the scrotum in men and, on rare occasions, into the labia in women.

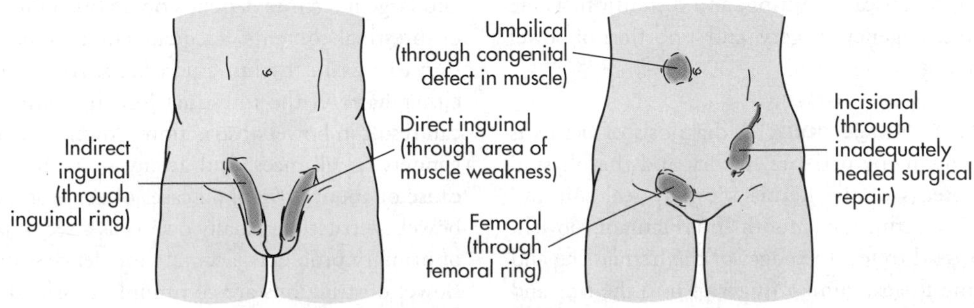

Figure 43-13 Common sites of abdominal herniation.

Direct inguinal hernias pass through the posterior inguinal wall at a point of muscle weakness. They typically are caused by increased intraabdominal pressure. These hernias occur most commonly in older men. They are technically difficult to repair and often recur after surgery.

Femoral hernias occur almost exclusively in women. They develop when a loop of intestine passes through the femoral ring and down the femoral canal. The hernia creates a round bulge below the inguinal ligament and is thought to be caused by pressure and changes in the ligaments related to pregnancy. Umbilical hernias develop at the umbilicus, and incisional hernias occur at the site of a surgical incision, usually as a complication of surgery.

Hernias are further described by terms that reflect the degree of hernia obstruction. A *sliding* hernia moves freely in and out of the hernia sac. If the protruding structure requires manipulation to return it to its proper position, the hernia is described as *reducible.* If the protruding structure cannot be returned to its proper position, the hernia is labeled *irreducible.* The term *incarcerated* is usually reserved for an irreducible hernia in which bowel obstruction occurs. The size of the defect largely determines whether the hernia can be reduced. When the blood flow to the trapped segment is compromised by pressure from the surrounding muscle ring, the hernia is said to be *strangulated.* Intestinal obstruction occurs, and gangrene of the viscera can rapidly develop.

Pathophysiology. Hernias typically form as a result of increased abdominal pressure, decreased resistance of the tissues of the abdominal wall, and presence of spaces in the abdominal cavity. Aging usually results in a loss of muscle strength and tone, and obesity increases intraabdominal pressure. The major pathologic concern associated with hernias is the risk of strangulation and bowel obstruction. Once present, hernias tend to extend, and the risk of complications increases.

The person with a hernia typically has a mass in the groin, around the umbilicus, or protruding from an old surgical incision. The mass may have always been present, or it may have appeared suddenly after coughing, straining, lifting, or other vigorous exertion. There may be no other symptoms. The protrusion usually disappears when the person lies down and reappears with standing, coughing, or lifting.

The person may perceive a vague feeling of discomfort as the hernial contents slide in and out of the abdominal defect, but little actual pain is experienced as long as the hernia is freely reducible. A "dragging" sensation or feeling of heaviness is common, especially with inguinal hernias. An irreducible hernia may become strangulated, causing severe pain and symptoms of intestinal obstruction such as nausea, vomiting, and distention. These complications require emergency surgery, and a portion of bowel may have to be resected.

Collaborative Care Management. A diagnosis of hernia is readily established through the patient's history and the physical examination. The contents of the hernia sac may feel soft and nodular to palpation (omentum) or smooth and fluctuant (bowel). Fingertip palpation is used to feel the edges of the hernia ring and its contents by inserting the examining fingertip into the ring and feeling for the surge of the intestine into the hernia sac as the person coughs.

Hernias are repaired by elective surgery if at all possible. Strangulation is an ever-present risk, and if it should occur, the surgical repair would have to be performed on an emergency basis. The herniated tissues are returned to the abdominal cavity, the hernia sac is excised, and the defect in the fascia or muscle is closed with sutures (herniorrhaphy). To prevent recurrence of the hernia and facilitate closure of the defect, a hernioplasty may be performed. This procedure uses fascia or a variety of synthetic materials to strengthen the muscle wall. Surgeons generally do not attempt to reduce strangulated hernias because of the high risk of rupture. The emergency surgery is accompanied by a high incidence of postoperative complications. Elective hernia surgery is often performed in ambulatory surgical centers with the patient under local or spinal anesthesia. The patient is discharged directly home after the repair.

Hernia repair may be performed by either open or laparoscopic methods. The results appear to be similar, although laparoscopic surgery causes less pain and allows a more rapid return to normal activities. On the other hand, laparoscopic surgery is also significantly more expensive and necessitates the use of general anesthesia. The benefits of a laparoscopic approach are less clear with hernia repair than with many other laparoscopic surgeries, and the use of this approach is not routine at this time.[36]

Recovery from hernia repair usually is rapid and without incident. Standard postoperative interventions are used, but the nurse encourages the patient to deep breathe rather than cough. Fluid and food are resumed as tolerated. Ice bags are applied after inguinal hernia repair to minimize edema, particularly in the scrotum. A scrotal support or "jockey" style underwear may make initial ambulation less painful. Fluids are encouraged, and IV infusions are continued until the patient is able to successfully empty the bladder.

PATIENT/FAMILY TEACHING. Discharge teaching focuses on the avoidance of any heavy lifting, pushing, or pulling for about 6 weeks. Driving and stair climbing are initially restricted. The nurse instructs the patient to monitor the incision for signs of infection. Postoperative ecchymosis should disappear in a few days. The use of prescribed stool softeners or bulk-forming laxatives to prevent straining at defecation is reinforced. The nurse also reassures the patient that sexual function is not affected by the surgery and that sexual activity may be resumed once healing is complete.

Bowel Obstruction

Etiology and Epidemiology. Normal function of the small and large intestines depends on an open lumen for the movement of intestinal contents, adequate circulation, and nervous innervation to sustain rhythmic peristalsis. Any factor or condition that either narrows the intestinal lumen or interferes with peristalsis can result in bowel obstruction. Bowel obstruction occurs in both genders, in all races, and at any point in the life span. It is the cause of about 20% of all cases of acute abdominal pain. Because bowel obstruction usually occurs as a secondary effect of a variety of primary problems, accurate incidence statistics are unavailable. Bowel obstructions are commonly classified as either mechanical (affecting the intestinal lumen) or nonmechanical (related to peristalsis) and can be either partial or complete.

MECHANICAL OBSTRUCTION. A wide variety of conditions and disorders can result in mechanical bowel obstruction. The problem may arise outside the bowel or within the lumen.

ADHESIONS. Adhesions, which are fibrous bands of scar tissue, are the most common cause of small bowel obstruction.[55a] Adhesions typically develop after gynecologic procedures or surgeries involving the small or large bowel. They may occur anytime after the procedure, from just a few days to 10 to 20 years. Their cause is unknown but may be related to the inflammatory response. In some persons adhesions may become massive. Adhesions can loop over bowel segments, contract with time, and compress a segment of bowel. The resultant obstruction often creates a closed loop, which is associated with strangulation (Figure 43-14, *A*).

VOLVULUS. A volvulus is a twisting of the bowel on itself, usually at least 180 degrees, that obstructs the intestinal lumen both proximally and distally (Figure 43-14, *B*). The acute obstruction can quickly result in bowel infarction and can be life threatening in the presence of bowel necrosis, perforation, and peritonitis.

HERNIAS. A hernia can result in bowel obstruction if the abdominal wall defect through which the hernia protrudes becomes so tight that the bowel segment becomes strangulated (Figure 43-14, *C*).

TUMORS. A tumor mass gradually restricts the internal lumen of the bowel from within as it enlarges. Eventually a fecal mass may be unable to pass through the constricted area, leading to partial or complete obstruction. Bowel cancer accounts for the majority of obstructions of the large intestine, with most obstructions occurring in the sigmoid colon.[55a]

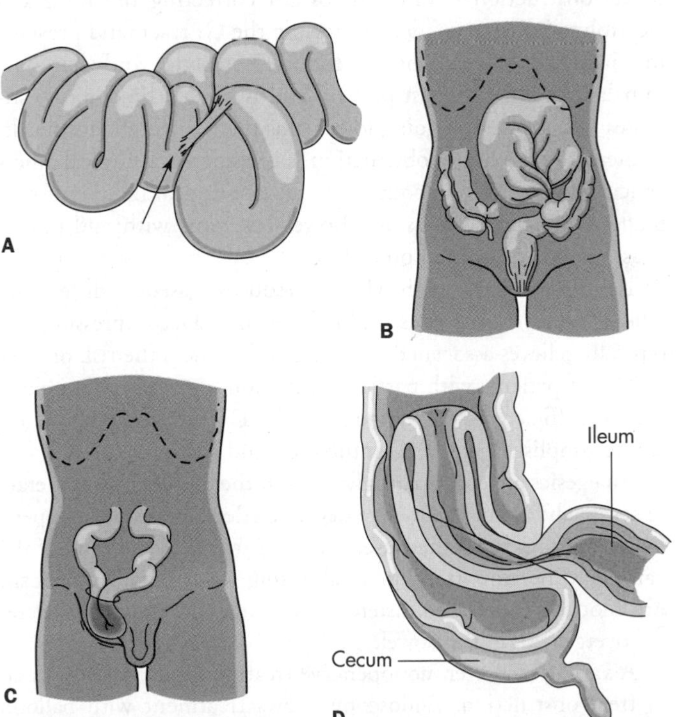

Figure 43-14 Common causes of intestinal obstruction. **A,** Constriction by adhesions. **B,** Volvulus of sigmoid colon. **C,** Strangulated inguinal hernia. **D,** Ileocecal intussusception.

INTUSSUSCEPTION. Intussusception occurs when a leading segment of bowel invaginates into an adjacent segment (Figure 43-14, *D*). In the adult the invagination is often triggered by peristalsis, which propels a bowel segment containing a tumor mass into the adjacent bowel segment. The inner walls of the trapped segment rapidly become edematous, and venous obstruction, infarction, and necrosis can occur.

OTHER CAUSES. Other possible causes of mechanical obstruction include fecal impaction, gallstones, and the strictures produced by chronic inflammatory bowel disease.

NONMECHANICAL OBSTRUCTION

ILEUS. Ileus is a state of impaired or absent peristaltic motility. Also known as **adynamic** or paralytic ileus, it is a common temporary problem after abdominal surgery, particularly if the bowel has been extensively handled. The diagnosis is an absence of peristalsis for longer than 72 hours. Conditions associated with ileus are well recognized, but the origins of the disorder remain unclear. Neurogenic impairment, drug effects, reflex inhibition, and metabolic abnormalities are all believed to play a role.[27]

OTHER CAUSES. A variety of other chronic disorders can cause a form of nonmechanical obstruction from failure to propel the intestinal contents. Most cases result from a failure of nervous innervation (e.g., multiple sclerosis, Parkinson's disease, or Hirschsprung's disease). Primary collagen or muscle disorders can affect bowel propulsion and cause obstruction. Endocrine disorders such as diabetes mellitus are commonly associated with problems of GI motility. Although constipation is the more common manifestation of all these disorders, chronic problems with bowel obstruction also may occur. Thrombosis of the mesenteric arteries is a possible complication of heart disease in older adults. It can cause an abrupt ischemic episode that may necessitate surgical intervention to remove the affected area of the bowel.

Pathophysiology. Intestinal obstruction triggers a series of GI tract events whose clinical manifestations depend largely on the location of the obstruction and the degree of circulatory compromise. Approximately 7 to 10 L of electrolyte-rich fluid is secreted into the small intestine each day. In the normal bowel all but approximately 600 to 800 ml is resorbed before the chyme enters the cecum. About 200 ml is lost daily in the stool. When obstruction occurs, this GI secretion continues, at least initially. The result is a steadily worsening imbalance between secretion and absorption with accumulation of fluid and air proximal to the site of the obstruction. The outcomes are the result of changes in blood flow, motility, bowel contents, and bowel flora. The mediators that control secretion in the presence of obstruction have not been clearly identified. Progressive distention occurs with an increase in intraluminal pressure. The bowel wall becomes increasingly edematous, and venous drainage is impeded. Increased capillary permeability allows massive amounts of isotonic fluid to move from the plasma into the distended bowel, which begins to weep fluids from its surface into the peritoneum. Gas accumulates in the bowel from both air swallowing and the action of intestinal bacteria on stagnant bowel contents. This worsens the abdominal distention.

Vascular compromise is the most serious aspect of obstruction. Closed-loop obstruction impairs blood flow and causes local mucosal ischemia. Visible changes occur in the villi within 30 to 60 minutes, and basic transport functions are impaired. Bowel ischemia breaks down the normal protective barriers, and the stagnant and distended bowel becomes increasingly permeable to bacteria. Organisms can enter the peritoneal cavity and cause peritonitis. Bacteria are normally sparse in the small bowel but accumulate rapidly during obstruction. Normal motility effectively clears both nutrients and organisms from the bowel, and tremendous bacterial overgrowth can occur in the presence of stasis.[55a] Within hours of a complete bowel obstruction, the proximal bowel contents become fetid and foul smelling from the rapid proliferation of anaerobic organisms. *E. coli* and *Klebsiella* and *Pseudomonas* organisms are particularly prevalent, and the release of toxins can result in septic shock. The ischemic process can progress to gangrene and perforation. Submucosal hemorrhage and sloughing can be a source of substantial blood loss. Adynamic ileus differs from mechanical obstruction in that the intraluminal pressure generated by adynamic ileus is rarely significant enough to impair mucosal blood flow.

The loss of extracellular fluid can range from 2 to 6 L within 2 to 3 days of a mechanical bowel obstruction. The resulting hypovolemia may be mild or severe enough to compromise renal perfusion and induce dehydration, electrolyte imbalance, and shock. The resultant concentration of the blood can even cause vascular thrombosis.

The clinical manifestations of bowel obstruction depend on the exact site and extent of the obstruction (see Clinical Manifestations box), but crampy abdominal pain, distention, and vomiting are common symptoms. Simple obstruction produces crampy and poorly localized pain. Its onset parallels an initial increase in peristalsis proximal to the obstruction that raises intraluminal pressure in an attempt to clear the blockage. Frequent, loud, high-pitched bowel sounds are often heard on auscultation. The pain intensifies as the obstruction becomes complete. Smooth muscle atony decreases peristalsis, and bowel sounds gradually diminish. The pain associated with bowel strangulation is constant and severe. Pain is much less intense with ileus than with mechanical obstruction and may be described as pressure or fullness.

Nausea and vomiting are also common features, especially with obstructions in the small intestine. Depending on the level of the obstruction, vomiting can be profuse. Vomiting temporarily relieves the pain in proximal but not distal obstructions. Abdominal distention usually develops slowly, although severe constipation is common. Rising fever usually indicates the presence of necrotic bowel. Laboratory values typically reflect the progressive nature of the dehydration and fluid losses through vomiting.

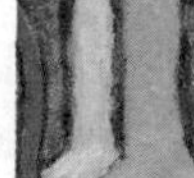

CLINICAL MANIFESTATIONS
Bowel Obstruction

- Pain
  - —Crampy
  - —Poorly localized
  - —Severe, continuous pain with strangulation of the bowel
- Nausea and vomiting
  - —Presence and severity dependent on the level of obstruction
  - —Can be profuse with proximal small bowel obstructions
  - —May have fecal odor if the obstruction is in the distal small bowel
  - —Occurs late if at all in most large bowel obstructions
- Obstipation
- Abdominal distention
  - —Usually nontender
  - —Slow to develop, especially with large bowel obstructions
- Bowel sounds
  - —Frequent and high pitched early in the obstructive process
  - —Decreased or absent late in the obstructive process
- Fever
  - —Indicates necrosis of bowel tissue
- Laboratory values reflective of dehydration and fluid shifts
  - —Decreased urinary output
  - —Hemoconcentration
  - —Hypokalemia and hyponatremia

Collaborative Care Management. Intestinal obstruction is diagnosed primarily from its clinical manifestations. In addition, abdominal x-ray films generally show clear patterns of air and fluid entrapment in the obstructed area. Obstruction cannot be ruled out, however, by the presence of apparently normal x-ray findings.

No laboratory tests can confirm or rule out a diagnosis of bowel obstruction. WBC counts and a variety of enzymes may be elevated in the presence of strangulation but otherwise are normal. Once hypovolemia becomes severe, hemoconcentration elevates the hemoglobin and hematocrit values and the serum potassium level typically falls.

Once the diagnosis has been established, the treatment of bowel obstruction is directed toward correcting the fluid and electrolyte imbalances, decompressing the GI tract, and preventing infection. Correction of fluid, electrolyte, and acid-base imbalances is the highest priority and is guided by clinical estimates of prior and ongoing losses plus daily maintenance needs. Acute complete bowel obstruction is considered a surgical emergency, and a decision about the need for surgical intervention is made as quickly as possible. Bowel resection with end-to-end anastomosis is the usual procedure.

Decompression of the bowel reduces gaseous distention, relieves pressure on organs, and reduces pain. Decompression also typically relieves associated vomiting and reduces the risk of aspiration. In patients with partial obstruction, decompression alone may be sufficient to relieve the problem. Decompression is generally accomplished with NG intubation and suction.

Analgesics are used sparingly, even in the presence of moderate to severe abdominal pain. The negative effects of opioids on peristalsis contraindicate their use, and the pattern and severity of the pain may be important in establishing an accurate diagnosis. Antibiotics may be administered to counter the significant bacterial overgrowth in the bowel.

A variety of newer, nonoperative treatments also may be used to treat obstruction. Endoscopy allows treatment with balloon catheters to dilate obstructed bowel segments, and lasers, cautery devices, or heater probes may be used to reduce or remove obstructing tumor. The gentle instillation of barium has been routinely successful in reversing sigmoid colon volvulus.

The treatment of nonmechanical obstruction and adynamic ileus is generally conservative and supportive. Temporary ileus is initially expected in the postoperative period but needs to be addressed if it persists for more than a few days. An NG tube may be inserted to decompress the stomach and relieve nausea and bloating, and careful attention is paid to restoring and maintaining the balance of fluids and electrolytes. Careful monitoring for complications is ongoing. **Promotility** drugs are most likely to be useful in treating nonmechanical obstructions.

Nursing management focuses on careful monitoring of all physical parameters. The nurse monitors the patient's vital signs, urinary output, and NG output and is alert for early signs of shock (see Chapter 19). The nurse administers IV fluids as ordered and monitors for symptoms of electrolyte imbalance. Fluid replacement is provided for all patients with intestinal obstruction because fluid losses usually are significant. Supplemental potassium is added to the IV infusions as needed to compensate for losses through vomiting and fluid shifts.

Third spacing of fluids is typical with intestinal obstruction. The nurse assesses for edema and measures abdominal girth every 2 to 4 hours. Fluid losses trigger nagging thirst, and small amounts of ice chips may be soothing.

General comfort measures include positioning the patient with the head of the bed elevated to relieve abdominal pressure and providing frequent position changes. A side-lying position often is the most comfortable. The patient may be encouraged to be out of bed and walk frequently to promote peristalsis. Oral and nasal care is offered every 2 to 4 hours to counter the drying and irritating effects of the NG tube and NPO status.

The nurse regularly assesses the patient's pain. Since analgesics are used sparingly, it is critical for the nurse to explore nonpharmacologic measures to increase the patient's comfort. If the pain increases significantly or shifts from cramping to constant pain, it should be reported promptly, since this may indicate strangulation or perforation of the bowel. A Nursing Care Plan for a patient with a bowel obstruction is found on p. 1272.

Surgical correction of mechanical bowel obstruction is often necessary after bowel decompression. Specific surgical procedures depend on the nature and location of the obstruction. Release of adhesions, bowel resection with reanastomosis, and temporary colostomy may all be used. Bowel strangulation or vascular compromise necessitates emergency corrective surgery. Postoperative care is the same as that provided to any patient who undergoes major abdominal surgery.

PATIENT/FAMILY TEACHING. The patient may be anxious during the initial treatment period. The nurse thoroughly explains all tests, procedures, and planned care. Support and reassurance are important, especially if corrective bowel surgery is planned.

The majority of large bowel obstructions affect older patients and are often related to cancer. The nurse needs to assist the patient in dealing with the discomfort and anxiety of the obstruction, as well as the diagnosis of cancer and the possible need for ostomy surgery. Both the patient and the family are likely to feel overwhelmed and need teaching and reteaching as they attempt to understand the diagnosis and treatment options.

Discharge planning is tailored to the patient's unique needs. Recovery from intestinal obstruction may be swift or prolonged, depending on the location and severity of the obstruction and whether surgery was performed. Home care issues include wound healing, reestablishing a normal diet, and restoring regular bowel habits. Teaching is provided concerning the prevention of constipation through a fiber-rich diet, adequate fluids, and exercise.

Patients who undergo colostomy surgery because of cancer or complications of obstruction need ongoing support and supervision as they adjust to new self-care patterns. The nurse initiates referrals to a home health care agency as needed.

Colorectal Cancer

Etiology and Epidemiology. Knowledge about colorectal cancer has expanded tremendously in recent years, but the precise causes remain unclear. The importance of genetics has become increasingly apparent, and the development and gradual cancerous transformation of bowel polyps and adenomas can often be traced to specific gene mutations. The incidence of bowel cancer varies substantially in different parts of the world, and these variations point to the importance of environmental factors in its etiology.

The role of genetics in bowel cancer was first recognized in a rare disorder called familial adenomatous polyposis. This **autosomal dominant** disorder causes the early development of hundreds of polyps in the colon and rectum. The incidence of bowel cancer in individuals with this disorder is nearly 100% by age 40.[14] Gardner's syndrome is one subtype of this disorder that causes osseous and soft tissue tumors. A second disorder, familial nonpolyposis syndrome, is also an autosomal dominant disorder. It causes only a small number of bowel polyps, but they demonstrate a strong tendency to undergo malignant change in affected persons at a young age. The malignant change is attributed to a mutant gene that promotes mutations in other genes. The polyposis syndromes account for only about 6% of all bowel cancers, but genetics is believed to play an important role in up to half of all the other so-called sporadic cases of colorectal cancer.[14] A person who has one first-degree relative with colorectal cancer has two or three times the normal risk of developing the disease; if two first-degree relatives have colorectal cancer, the person has five or six times the normal risk.[14]

Colorectal cancer usually develops as part of a slow, orderly change process in the bowel mucosa from polyp development to gradual malignant transformation in response to genetic signals. Most of the genetic changes involve the deletion of chromosome fragments, but the total number of mutations appears to be more significant than their specific placement or sequence. A number of the mutations have been identified, but none of them can currently be used for general screening. Although virtually all colon cancers appear to develop from polyps that gradually transform into adenomas, fewer than 5% of all colon adenomas ever become malignant.[14]

Environmental factors are believed to function as stimulants or enablers that initiate the gene mutations that result in bowel cancer. Chronic irritation of the mucosa such as that seen in Crohn's disease and ulcerative colitis is associated with a high risk of colorectal cancer. Because colorectal cancer is more common in industrialized societies, diet low in fiber and high in fat, protein, and refined carbohydrates has been considered a possible risk factor. It has been theorized that processed foods are converted into

Nursing Care Plan

Patient With a Bowel Obstruction

Data A 62-year-old woman was admitted last evening with a probable small bowel obstruction, after several hours of cramping upper abdominal pain, which steadily worsened. She complained of feeling bloated and became increasingly nauseated. Initially, she thought the episode was related to something she ate. Vomiting improved her symptoms temporarily, but the cycle continued to repeat itself. Her family became concerned and insisted she go to the emergency department. Her health history includes an appendectomy in her teens, three uncomplicated births, and a vaginal hysterectomy for dysfunctional uterine bleeding 5 years ago.

The patient's vital signs are temperature, 100° F (37.7° C); blood pressure, 110/60 mm Hg; pulse rate, 88 beats/min; and respiration, 12 breaths/min. She continues to report abdominal pain and a tight bloated feeling in her abdomen. Auscultation reveals diminished bowel sounds in the lower quadrants but high-pitched sounds in the upper quadrants. She is not passing gas per rectum and has not had a bowel movement for 2 days. She voided 90 ml of concentrated urine on admission. Abdominal x-rays show significant accumulation of gas and fluid in the intestine. Her blood work is normal except for her hematocrit, which is 40%, and for decreased sodium and potassium. Adhesions are suspected as the cause of a bowel obstruction.

An intravenous line is present for hydration and she is taking nothing by mouth (NPO) except for small amounts of ice chips. Intake and output are being strictly recorded. A nasogastric (NG) tube is in place for decompression. A decision about the need for surgery will be made within 48 hours.

Nursing Diagnosis

Acute pain related to distention of the bowel with fluid and gas

Outcomes

- Patient will report pain of less than 3 on a scale of 0 to 10.
- Patient will report satisfaction with pain control measures.

Related NOC Outcomes

- Comfort Level
- Pain Control
- Pain Level

Related NIC Interventions

- Analgesic Administration
- Coping Enhancement
- Pain Management

Nursing Interventions/Rationales

- Assess patient's pain level at least every 4 hours. *Pain presence and severity are important clues for identifying subtle changes in patient status. Worsening or unrelenting pain can indicate bowel ischemia or peritonitis.*
- Assist patient with developing a pain-related scale for evaluating changes. Record patient's pain ratings on bedside flow record. *Pain scales assist the patient in communicating pain status and enhance the nurse's ability to evaluate pain. Pain records demonstrate patterns of change over time.*
- Administer prescribed analgesics and antiemetics as ordered. *Analgesics are frequently withheld until the diagnosis is established. Aggressive comfort measures are needed to help the patient gain control of the pain. Nausea and vomiting contribute significantly to general discomfort.*
- Use nonpharmacologic comfort measures that are acceptable to the patient (hygiene and linen changes, oral care, back care and repositioning, relaxation techniques, distraction). *Analgesic administration is limited due to the adverse effect on peristalsis. Adjunct pain relief measures may therefore be beneficial.*
- Maintain patency and proper functioning of NG suction (attach to low intermittent suction as prescribed; irrigate or reposition tube as needed to maintain drainage). *Effective decompression of the gastrointestinal (GI) tract will reduce both fluid and gas distention and reduce pain.*
- Position in semi- to high Fowler's position. *An upright position relieves pressure in the abdomen and facilitates ventilation.*
- Encourage frequent position changes and ambulation once condition is stabilized. *Activity is important to help reestablish peristalsis.*
- Provide frequent oral care and lip lubrication. *NG intubation causes significant dryness and irritation of the oral mucous membranes. Oral care decreases thirst and helps relieve irritation and bad tastes.*

metabolic and bacterial end products that act as carcinogens in the bowel. Low-fiber diets have been implicated because they increase colon transit time and increase the overall time in which the bowel mucosa is in contact with carcinogenic agents. However, recent studies involving ingestion of high-fiber diets with reduced red meat content have not shown any effect on the incidence of colorectal cancer.[50] The roles of smoking and alcohol have also been extensively studied. Although it appears that neither plays a major role in colorectal cancer development, tobacco use has been associated with colorectal adenomas, and increased ethanol intake, particularly as beer, is associated with an increased risk of colorectal cancer.[14] Risk factors for colorectal cancers are summarized in the Risk Factors box.

Just as some factors increase the risk of colorectal cancer, other factors appear to decrease the risk. One of the most important of these is the long-term use of aspirin and nonsteroidal antiinflammatory drugs (NSAIDs).[6] The benefits appear to be related to cumulative use over a period of about 5 years and not to the magnitude of the daily dose. The specific nature of the protective effect is unknown but is theorized to be related to prostaglandin inhibition. Prostaglandins influence cell growth and proliferation in

Risk Factors

Colorectal Cancer

- Age over 50 years
- Family history
  - —Colon cancer in a first-degree relative
  - —Familial adenomatous polyposis syndrome
- History of ulcerative colitis
  - —Risk increased 8 to 12 years after diagnosis
- Colon polyps or adenomas
- Cigarette smoking
  - —High pack-year history important
- Diet low in fiber, high in fat
- Obesity (nature of the risk currently unknown)

Nursing Diagnosis

Risk for deficient fluid volume related to vomiting, NG suction, NPO status, and fluid shifts in the GI tract

Outcomes

- Patient will be free from signs of fluid volume deficit.
- Patient will maintain urinary output of greater than 30 ml/hr.

Related NOC Outcomes

- Electrolyte & Acid/Base Balance
- Fluid Balance
- Hydration

Related NIC Interventions

- Fluid Management
- Fluid Monitoring
- Intravenous (IV) Therapy

Nursing Interventions/Rationales

- Maintain accurate intake and output. *To provide initial data about the patient's fluid needs and degree of third spacing. Decreased urinary output is an indication of fluid volume deficit or renal compromise.*
- Maintain IV fluids at prescribed rate and flow. *Obstruction causes significant fluid and electrolyte losses from vomiting and changes in bowel permeability. Steady replacement helps prevent stressful fluid swings and decreases nausea.*
- Monitor weight daily. *Body weight is the most accurate method of assessing fluid gains and losses in the adult patient.*
- Measure abdominal girth each shift until stabilized. *Fluid and gas accumulation in GI tract can result in significant abdominal distention and subsequent pain.*

Nursing Diagnosis

Anxiety related to lack of knowledge concerning cause of bowel obstruction and uncertainty over need for surgery

Outcomes

- Patient will communicate concerns about illness and treatments.
- Patient will verbalize understanding of planned interventions.

Related NOC Outcomes

- Anxiety Level
- Coping

Related NIC Interventions

- Anxiety Reduction
- Calming Technique
- Presence

Nursing Interventions/Rationales

- Provide reassurance and comfort by spending time with the patient and family. *Communicates a feeling of empathy and willingness to support patient through crisis situation.*
- Listen attentively. *Demonstrates concern and empathy.*
- Provide simple explanations of all tests and procedures. *Correct misconceptions as needed. Accurate, understandable information reduces unnecessary fears and restores a sense of control.*
- Encourage supportive involvement of the family. *When relationships are supportive, family involvement decreases fear and increases active coping.*
- Set aside time to address family concerns. *The family can transfer their anxiety to the patient. Addressing and reducing their anxiety will help reduce the patient's anxiety.*

Evaluation

Evaluation is based on comparing the patient's outcomes with desired outcomes.

poorly understood ways and may be associated with tumor promotion. The effects appear to operate before the development of adenomas. A small protective effect has been noted among women taking estrogen and progestin postmenopausal hormone replacement.[12a,33,44] Isolated studies have also indicated small benefits associated with calcium and lutein supplementation.[5] Studies of protective factors are ongoing in the hope of developing **chemoprotection** protocols (use of natural or synthetic agents to reverse, suppress, or prevent progression or recurrence of cancer).[10]

Colorectal cancer is the third most commonly occurring cancer and the third most common cause of death from cancer in adults of both sexes. The most current American Cancer Society (ACS) study estimated 71,820 new cases will occur in men and 73,470 in women in 2006, for a total of 145,290. Of this total, the ACS estimated rectum involvement in 40,340 cases and colon involvement in 104,950. The number of deaths from colorectal cancer in 2006 is estimated to be 56,290.[2] When bowel cancer is diagnosed in its early stage, the 5-year survival rate is 90%. The 5-year survival rate decreases to 67% if regional spread to adjacent organs or lymph nodes has occurred at the time of diagnosis and is only 10% if distant metastases have occurred. These data supporting the importance of early diagnosis are reflected in the objectives presented in the Healthy People 2010 box. Between 1998 and 2001, incidence rates declined by 2.99% per year, suggesting that increased screening resulted in removal of polyps and prevented their transformation into carcinomas.[3]

The incidence of bowel cancer is clearly age related. Peak incidence is between 60 and 70 years of age, with fewer than 10% occurring before age 50.[14] All adults older than age 50 are believed to be at average risk for the disease. The incidence of colorectal cancer rose steadily throughout the second half of the twentieth century with the steady aging of the population. The incidence in Caucasians peaked in the 1980s and has since declined slightly, which is possibly related to increasingly widespread screening and removal of polyps. A similar decline in African-Americans has not occurred. Currently both incidence

Healthy People 2010

Objectives Related to Colorectal Cancer

- Reduce the colorectal cancer death rate from a baseline of 21.2 per 100,000 to a target of 13.9 per 100,000.
- Increase the proportion of adults who receive a colorectal cancer screening examination:
  –The proportion of adults 50 and over who have had a fecal blood test in the past 2 years
  –The proportion of adults 50 and over who have ever had a sigmoidoscopy

From US Department of Health and Human Services: *Healthy people 2010: understanding and improving health,* Washington, DC, 2000, The Department.

and mortality rates for colorectal cancer are higher among African-Americans than Caucasian Americans.[10] The incidence rates continue to be significantly higher in the industrialized Western world than in Asia or Africa. However, the rates in immigrant families rapidly increase to match those of the larger society, again indicating an as yet unidentified environmental link.

Figure 43-15 illustrates the pattern of incidence of colon cancer by site. A steady shift toward cancer development in the proximal colon has occurred in recent years. The decline in incidence for Caucasians has primarily been for distal colon and rectal sites. Currently almost 40% of cancers develop in the proximal colon, with about 53% developing in the distal colon and the rectum.[14] This "shift to the right" appears to be more pronounced with advancing age.[25] The development of cancer in the small intestine is extremely rare and accounts for less than 1% of all GI tract malignant tumors.

Pathophysiology. There is strong evidence that almost all bowel cancers arise from preexisting benign adenomatous colon polyps.[25] Polyps occur in about 24% to 47% of asymptomatic, average-risk adults over age 50. All adenomas are dysplastic by definition and are considered premalignant lesions even though few actually develop into cancers. The likelihood of a polyp becoming malignant is related to its size, histologic type, and degree of dysplasia. Large polyps with villous as opposed to tubular or tubulovillous histology, and severe as opposed to mild or moderate dysplasia, are most likely to undergo malignant change. This is a slow process. It is theorized that it can take 5 to 12 years for a polyp to undergo malignant transformation[25] (Figure 43-16).

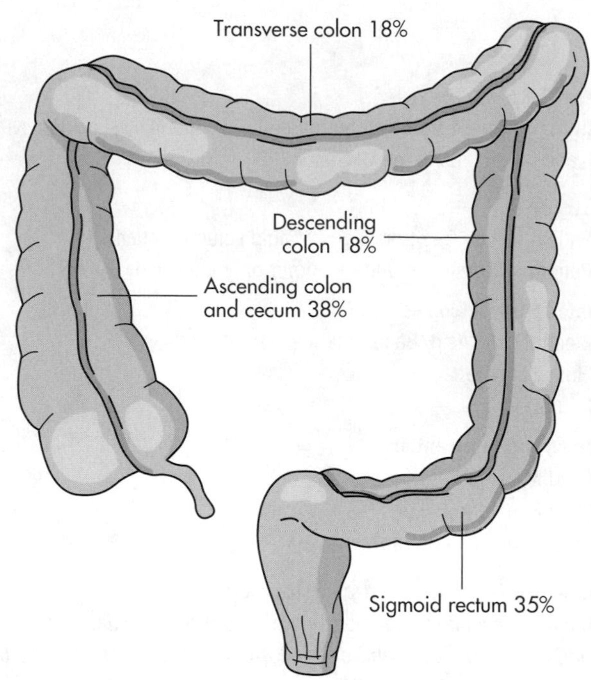

Figure 43-15 Incidence of cancer in various segments of colon and rectum.

Adenomas may be seen in various shapes and configurations (Figure 43-17). They are typically round and polypoid (sessile) but may be more elongated and have stalks (pedunculated). Infrequently they appear flat or even depressed. Over time the lesions penetrate the colon wall and extend into the surrounding tissue.

Cancer of the colon may spread by direct extension or metastasize through the lymphatic or circulatory system. It may seed at distant points in the peritoneum or the colon. The organs to which it most often metastasizes are the liver and lungs. Colorectal cancer is staged using both Dukes' and the universal TNM classifications (Table 43-6), with stage determined by the degree of invasion of the tumor and not by its size. Staging is used to determine the appropriate treatment. Persons with stage A disease have a 90% 5-year survival rate; those with stage D disease have less than a 5% 5-year survival rate.[14]

Usually colorectal cancer has no early symptoms, and the disease is often diagnosed incidentally. When symptoms do develop, they vary with the location of the tumor. Cancer in the left colon and rectum typically produces symptoms related to partial obstruction. This is because the left colon is narrower than the right and the lesions are more likely to be annular and grow cir-

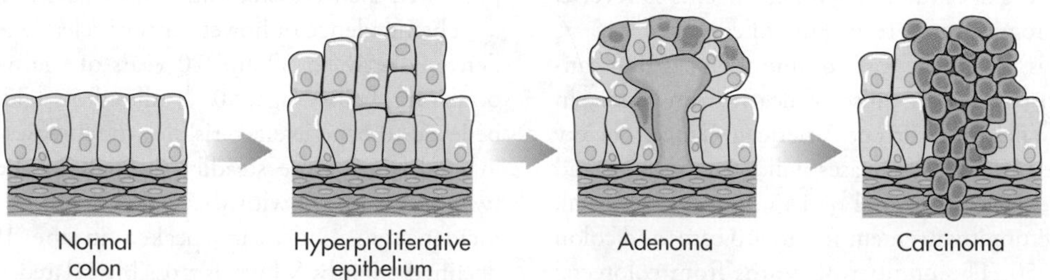

Figure 43-16 Progression to malignancy in bowel cancer.

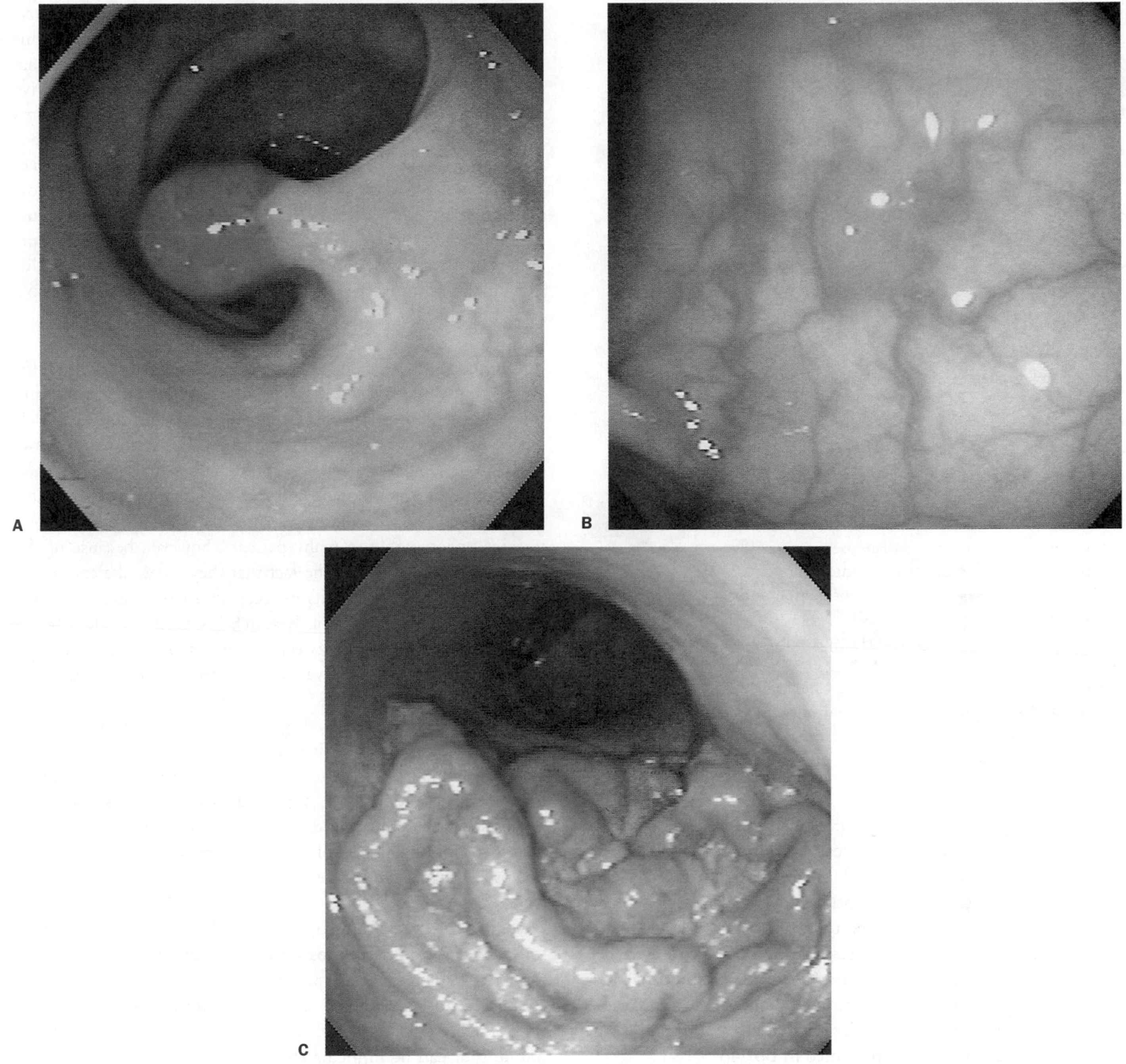

Figure 43-17 **A,** Typical polyp. **B,** Hyperplastic polyp. **C,** Villous adenoma.

cumferentially, encircling the colon wall. This results in a narrow, constricted lumen through which formed stool of normal diameter is unable to pass. This may cause a change in bowel habits; colicky abdominal pain, especially after meals; or a feeling of incomplete bowel emptying. Bright red rectal bleeding or bright red blood coating the surface of the stool is another symptom that may be present with tumors of the left colon or rectum.

Symptoms of obstruction are less likely to occur with tumors of the right colon because of its larger lumen and the semiliquid nature of the stool. Patients with these tumors may first manifest symptoms such as weakness, shortness of breath, or angina, which are due to hypochromic microcytic anemia secondary to prolonged occult blood loss from the tumor. In other cases the initial symptom may be vague abdominal discomfort, abdominal pain, a palpable mass, or mahogany stools resulting from blood admixed with stool.

Weakness, malaise, anorexia, and weight loss are nonspecific symptoms that occur often in patients with colorectal cancer. Weight loss often accompanies metastases. The tumor occasionally may perforate into the peritoneal cavity, and acute peritonitis occurs before the person notices any other signs of illness. The clinical manifestations of bowel cancer are summarized in the Clinical Manifestations box.

Collaborative Care Management

DIAGNOSTIC TESTS. Clinical evidence clearly indicates that early detection of colorectal cancer improves survival.[14] Thus the goal of

TABLE 43-6 DUKES' AND UNIVERSAL TNM CLASSIFICATION OF COLORECTAL CANCER

Dukes	TMN*	Stage	Pathology
A	T1N0M0	I	No invasion beyond submucosa
B_1	T2N0M0	I	Extension into muscularis
B_2	T3N0M0	II	Extension into or through serosa
C	TxN0M0	III	Involvement of regional lymph nodes
D	TxNxM1	IV	Distant metastases present

Adapted from DuBoss RN: Neoplasms of the large and small intestine. In Goldman L, Ausiello D, editors: *Cecil textbook of medicine*, ed 22, Philadelphia, 2004, Saunders.

*T is the depth of tumor penetration, N is lymph node involvement, and M indicates the presence of distant metastases.

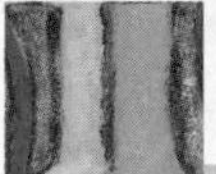

CLINICAL MANIFESTATIONS
Colorectal Cancer

- Often asymptomatic and diagnosed incidentally
- Symptoms of partial bowel obstruction
- Change in bowel habits (e.g., constipation or diarrhea)
- Pencil- or ribbon-shaped stool
- Sensation of incomplete bowel emptying
- Gas or bloating
- Occult blood in the stool or rectal bleeding
- Weakness, fatigue, malaise, and anorexia
- Weight loss
- Abdominal pain

diagnostic testing is early and accurate diagnosis to enable prompt treatment, since most bowel cancers are slow growing and easily removed in their early stages. This is an enormous challenge because some of the diagnostic options are expensive and virtually all adults over age 50 are believed to be at average risk and would need to be included in any mass screening program. Research is ongoing to attempt to determine the optimal tests and time intervals for bowel cancer screening; at this time no single approach to screening is preferred.[38] Screening guidelines endorsed by the American Cancer Society are presented in Box 43-5.

FECAL OCCULT BLOOD TEST. The use of fecal occult blood testing (FOBT) is based on the premise that evolving adenocarcinomas routinely bleed in amounts that are too small to be visible but can be readily detected in laboratory tests. The problem with FOBT is that it often produces both false-positive and false-negative results. Occult blood tests yield false-negative results by missing cancers that were not bleeding at the time of testing and yield false-positive results because many other conditions can cause blood in the stool. Diet and medication can also cause false-positive results. Accurate stool sampling requires patients to eliminate red meat, aspirin, NSAIDs, turnips, horseradish, and vitamin C from their daily diet for 2 days before and throughout the 3 days of stool sample collection. False negatives are a problem because of the missed diagnosis, and false positives are a problem because of the cost and stress associated with follow-up colonoscopy.

A newer type of FOBT, known as a *fecal immunochemical test* (FIT), detects a specific portion of a human blood protein. This test, which is done in a similar manner to the conventional FOBT, is more specific and reduces the number of false-positive results. Vitamins or foods do not affect the FIT, and some forms require only two stool specimens as opposed to three for conventional FOBT. Like the conventional FOBT, the FIT cannot detect a tumor that is not bleeding.[3a] FOBTs are included on most screening guidelines at least partly because of their relatively low cost and general acceptability to patients. The widespread acceptance of this testing despite its limitations is reflected in its inclusion in the *Healthy People 2010* objectives (see Healthy People 2010 box, p. 1274).

SIGMOIDOSCOPY. Flexible fiberoptic sigmoidoscopy allows for good endoscopic visualization of the rectum and descending colon, but it cannot visualize the proximal colon. More than half of all bowel cancers occur within the range of sigmoidoscopy, however, and the bowel preparation is milder and better tolerated than that required for colonoscopy. The cost of sigmoidoscopy is also much lower, since sedation is not required. Sigmoidoscopy remains unacceptable to many patients, however, because of the associated discomfort and the fact that they are awake and aware during the procedure, and its unacceptability decreases its usefulness as a mass screening tool. Research is ongoing to identify the appropriate time interval between screenings for low- and average-risk patients. Five-year intervals are currently recommended.

BARIUM ENEMA. High-quality double-contrast barium enemas permit screening of the entire colon and can produce results that are comparable to those of colonoscopy at a significant cost savings. Barium enemas are unpopular with patients, however, because of their significant discomfort. Barium enemas are excellent for outlining large polyps but are relatively ineffective for polyps less than 1 cm in size.

COLONOSCOPY. Colonoscopy is considered the gold standard for colorectal cancer diagnosis, but it is expensive, must be performed by highly trained professionals, requires patients to be sedated, and is associated with an uncomfortable bowel preparation. A major advantage of colonoscopy is that if small lesions are found, they can be immediately removed by a snare that is built directly into the colonoscope (Figure 43-18). Screening with FOBTs and barium enemas requires a second stage to treat any lesions that are discovered. However, at present it would be virtually impossible from a resource perspective to offer colonoscopy screening to the entire adult population. The optimal interval and frequency of screening by colonoscopy has not been proven, but the current recommendation is once every 10 years. Some authorities believe that enormous diagnostic gains could be achieved by screening the entire bowel just once or perhaps twice in a lifetime.

OTHER TESTS. Other, newer diagnostic tests for colorectal cancer include stool screening tests using molecular markers and CT or virtual colonoscopy. **Molecular marker** tests detect known deoxyribonucleic acid mutations associated with colorectal cancer. They do not require that a tumor be bleeding to be detected and are 90% accurate on initial testing. In CT or virtual

Box 43-5 American Cancer Society Guidelines for Colorectal Cancer Screening for Individuals at Average Risk

Beginning at age 50, both men and women at average risk for developing colorectal cancer should follow one of these five testing schedules:

- Yearly fecal occult blood test (FOBT)* or fecal immunochemical test (FIT)
- Flexible sigmoidoscopy every 5 years
- Yearly FOBT or FIT plus flexible sigmoidoscopy every 5 years†
- Double-contrast barium enema every 5 years
- Colonoscopy every 10 years

All positive tests should be followed up with colonoscopy. People should begin colorectal cancer screening earlier or undergo screening more often if they have any of the following colorectal cancer risk factors:

- A personal history of colorectal cancer or adenomatous polyps
- A strong family history of colorectal cancer or polyps (cancer or polyps in a first-degree relative younger than 60 or in two first-degree relatives of any age) NOTE: A first-degree relative is defined as a parent, sibling, or child.
- A personal history of chronic inflammatory bowel disease
- A family history of a hereditary colorectal cancer syndrome (familial adenomatous polyposis or hereditary nonpolyposis colon cancer)

Modified from American Cancer Society: *Cancer facts and figures 2005,* Atlanta, 2005, The Society.

*For FOBT, the take-home multiple sample method should be used.

†The combination of yearly FOBT or FIT plus flexible sigmoidoscopy every 5 years is preferred over either of these options alone.

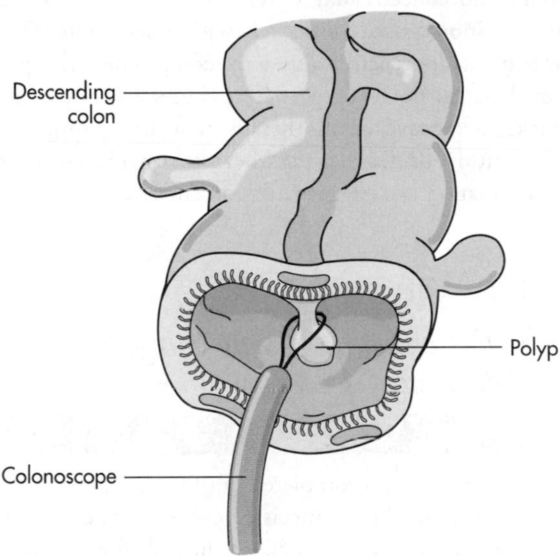

Figure 43-18 Colonoscopy allows for both diagnosis and treatment during same procedure. Built-in snare attachment can remove any polyps found during examination.

colonoscopy, air is pumped into the colon to distend it, and then a helical or spiral CT scan is done. This test requires the same bowel prep as a barium enema or colonoscopy; it appears to be more sensitive than a barium enema in visualizing very small polyps but less sensitive than a colonoscopy. Its advantages are that it is quickly done, no sedation is involved, and the cost is lower than that of colonoscopy.[30]

Digital rectal examination can detect masses in the anal canal or lower rectum. However, it is not a stand-alone test for colorectal cancer because of its limited reach.

MEDICATIONS. Chemotherapy is primarily palliative and is not used as a primary treatment modality for colorectal cancer. 5-Fluorouracil (5-FU) is the drug with the most established record of effectiveness, but this record involves only 10% to 20% of patients with advanced disease. 5-FU may be combined with leucovorin to promote binding of 5-FU to target tumor cells. This combination has been shown to improve survival in patients with stage III disease. A newer chemotherapy regimen being used for patients with metastatic disease is 5-FU with oxaliplatin followed by leucovorin. There are also two new targeted therapies for metastatic disease. One is bevacizumab (Avastin), which blocks the development of blood vessels to the tumor. The second is cetuximab (Erbitux), which blocks hormone-like factors that support tumor growth.[3b] 5-FU is also used routinely as an adjunct to the newer sphincter-sparing surgeries, and the incidence of recurrences is significantly reduced. When liver metastases are present, chemotherapy is sometimes infused directly into the hepatic artery, but it has only a small effect on survival. Chemotherapy may also be administered in combination with radiotherapy, although outcomes have so far been mixed.

TREATMENTS. Radiation is rarely used in the treatment of colon cancer, but it plays an important role in the management of rectal cancer. Anatomic constraints make the rectum less accessible surgically than the colon, and wide excision is rarely possible; therefore radiation may be used before surgery to reduce tumor size. Radiation may also be used either preoperatively or postoperatively in conjunction with 5-FU and leucovorin to decrease local recurrence and metastasis. External beam radiation or endocavitary irradiation, in which the radiation source is placed directly on the tumor, may be used. Radiation enteritis is a common complication during treatment, but the incidence of serious complications is low.

SURGICAL MANAGEMENT. Surgery is the treatment of choice for colorectal cancer. The specific type of surgery performed depends on the tumor's location and size and the patient's overall condition. It typically involves removal of the tumor, surrounding colon, and lymph nodes (Figure 43-19). When the tumor is located in the ascending, transverse, or descending colon, the surgeon can usually perform a resection with end-to-end anastomosis that

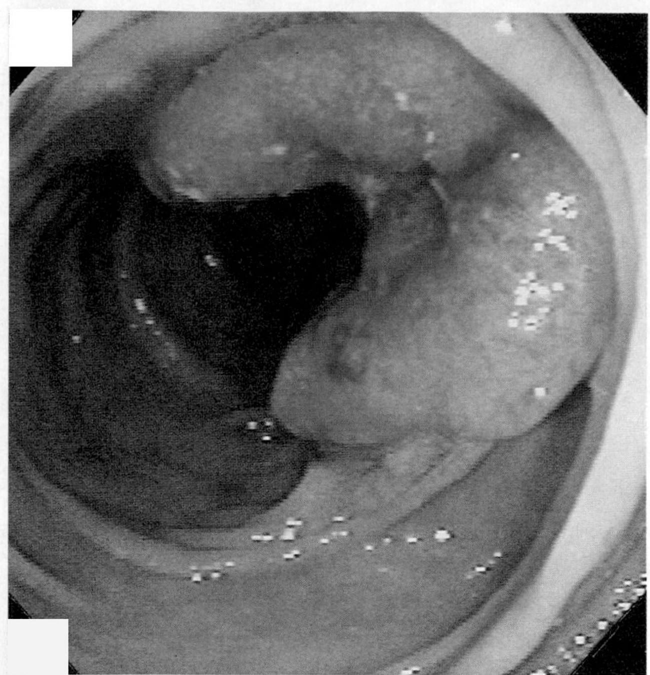

Figure 43-19 Adenocarcinoma of sigmoid colon.

preserves the natural process of defecation. Bowel resections commonly are performed laparoscopically, and outcomes, though still under study, appear to be similar to those from open surgery.

At this time no clear guidelines exist on the use of local versus wide excision and whether extensive lymph node dissection should be performed. Local excision is used for Dukes' stage A and some stage B tumors. Wide excision plus adjuvant therapy is used for more aggressive disease.

Patients with tumors in the rectum previously were managed exclusively by removing the entire rectum and anus through a dual-incision procedure called an abdominoperineal resection. The procedure necessitates a permanent colostomy and leaves a significant perineal wound that heals slowly by granulation. The anus is sutured closed. Patients with early, localized rectal cancers are now routinely offered the option of a sphincter-sparing procedure.[10] Regional rectal resection is performed, and the rectum is reconstructed with the creation of a pouch from the descending colon. The use of an anastomotic stapler has made these technically difficult procedures feasible. The surgery is performed in two stages with the creation of a temporary ileostomy while adjuvant treatments and healing are completed. The risk of rectal recurrence of the cancer is greater with this type of surgery. Therefore adjuvant therapy with chemotherapy and external beam radiation is also provided. Complications and challenges are similar to those described for patients undergoing a colectomy for ulcerative colitis.

The newer procedures have significantly reduced the need for permanent colostomies, but temporary colostomies are often created to allow for bowel rest and healing, particularly if bowel obstruction with inflammation occurred preoperatively. A palliative permanent colostomy may be needed if a tumor obstructing the bowel cannot be resected. Examples of various colostomy procedures are illustrated in Figure 43-10. General nursing care associated with abdominal surgery and ostomy management is discussed on pp. 1262 to 1267.

COMPLICATIONS OF SURGERY. Many of the surgeries are extensive, and wound complications are a real risk, particularly for older patients and those with diabetes. Complications include infection, bleeding, anastomosis leakage, and fistula development. Close monitoring is required in the initial days and weeks after surgery for signs and symptoms of these complications.

Patients who undergo extensive lymph node dissection in the pelvic region often experience difficulties with urinary control and may develop sexual dysfunction from disruption of the nerve pathways. These problems may resolve with time or cause permanent disruption in the patient's lifestyle. The use of radiotherapy as an adjuvant therapy is often accompanied by mucosal inflammation that may result in severe and protracted diarrhea. When the patient has a coloanal pouch, this inflammation can result in fecal incontinence. These problems are not easily or quickly resolved, and the patient and family need ongoing support as they attempt to address these challenges.

DIET. No special dietary restrictions are needed for patients with colorectal cancer. Anorexia and weight loss are common early symptoms, and concern may develop over the adequacy of the patient's nutritional status, especially with older adults. The standard treatment approaches also may compromise the patient's nutritional status. Bowel surgery necessitates a period of limited oral intake; aggressive chemotherapy may be accompanied by nausea, vomiting, or diarrhea; and both external beam and endocavitary irradiation can trigger radiation enteritis.

Nursing Management

of the Patient undergoing Surgery for Colorectal Cancer

PREOPERATIVE CARE

Most preoperative care is completed in the community before the patient's admission. The diagnosis of cancer adds anxiety to the preoperative period and may make it difficult for the patient to understand and retain information about the planned surgery and postoperative care.

The nurse ensures that the patient has been adequately prepared for abdominal surgery and general anesthesia. Bowel cleansing is required. This is accomplished by dietary modifications, mechanical cleansing, and pharmacologic suppression of colon bacteria that might lead to infection in the postoperative period. The patient is placed on a low-residue diet and then a clear liquid diet as surgery approaches. Boluses of vitamins K and C may be given to support clotting and wound healing in the postoperative period because the synthesis and absorption of these vitamins are impaired by the vigorous bowel preparation.

Immediate preparation of the bowel for surgery involves the use of laxatives, enemas, or both. Bowel preparation cleanses the colon and suppresses bacterial growth that might lead to infection in the postoperative period. A solution such as sodium sulfate plus polyethylene glycol (GoLYTELY) provides for an osmotic cleansing of the entire bowel. Up to 4 L is administered orally in divided doses 10 to 15 minutes apart. The cleansing usually is complete in about 4 hours. Systemic or oral antibiotics may be administered to reduce colonic bacteria. Oral neomycin is a standard preparation. If the patient is in good physical condition, bowel preparation is performed at home before admission.

Teaching is another focus of preoperative nursing care. The nurse teaches the patient about the planned surgery and its expected outcomes, including incisions, NG and wound drainage, and the need for an ostomy if applicable. Most patients are concerned about the severity of postoperative pain, and the nurse discusses the plan for postoperative pain management, including the use of patient-controlled analgesia if indicated (see Chapter 16). Pulmonary hygiene is important in the early postoperative period, and the nurse reviews the correct technique for deep breathing, splinting for effective coughing, and using an incentive spirometer. The nurse also stresses the importance of early ambulation in preventing respiratory and circulatory complications.

POSTOPERATIVE CARE

Maintaining Fluid and Electrolyte Balance. The patient is kept NPO for brief or extended periods after surgery, and NG suctioning may be in use. NG suctioning was formerly a standard intervention after any bowel surgery, but it is increasingly omitted entirely or terminated quickly, since studies have failed to demonstrate any difference in outcomes for patients who do not develop prolonged ileus (see Evidence-Based Practice box). If an NG tube is used, the nurse carefully assesses and records output from the tube and irrigates it as needed to maintain patency. The nurse evaluates intake and output balance, maintains IV fluids as ordered, records daily weight, and monitors for electrolyte imbalance. Monitoring continues as the patient is gradually advanced to a normal diet.

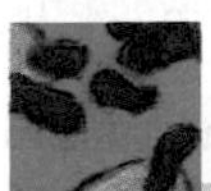

EVIDENCE-BASED PRACTICE

Topic Question: Is routine use of nasogastric (NG) decompression after abdominal surgery effective in promoting rapid return of bowel function, preventing pulmonary complications, decreasing the risk of anastomotic leakage, increasing patient comfort, and shortening hospital stay?

Evidence Base: Twenty eight studies involving 4195 patients having nonlaparoscopic abdominal operations of any type, 2108 of whom were randomly assigned to routine NG tube use and 2087 to no tube or early tube removal (in surgery, in recovery, or within 24 hours).

Findings: Patients with no tube or early removal had a significantly earlier return of bowel function (time to passage of flatus). They also showed a trend toward a decrease in pulmonary complications and an increase in wound infection and ventral hernias, although these findings were not significant. No difference in anastomosis leak was found between the groups. Data suggested that patients without an NG tube were more comfortable, had less nausea and vomiting, and had a shorter length of stay.

Conclusions: Routine NG decompression should be discontinued and replaced with selective NG tube use.

Nelson R, Edwards S, Tse B: Prophylactic nasogastric decompression after abdominal surgery, *Cochrane Database of Systematic Reviews,* Issue 3, 2004, Art. No.: CD004929.pub2. DOI: 10.1002/14651858.CD004929.pub2.

Early feeding has also become fairly standard, and patients may be kept NPO for the first 24 hours only. The success of early feeding after laparoscopic surgery has supported this change. The importance of adequate nutrition for wound healing lends support to a policy of limiting the time the patient is kept NPO. The nurse carefully assesses the adequacy of the patient's oral intake as oral feeding is resumed.

Promoting Ventilation. Incisional pain typically is severe with abdominal surgery, and pain can interfere with lung expansion. The nurse monitors the effectiveness of the patient-controlled analgesia system or ensures that adequate opioid analgesia is provided to allow for early ambulation and regular deep breathing. The nurse auscultates regularly for signs of atelectasis and encourages the use of incentive spirometry to keep the alveoli open. Deep breathing must be performed hourly in the early postoperative days to prevent pulmonary complications.

Supporting Peristalsis. Temporary ileus is an expected complication of bowel surgery resulting from manipulation of the intestines. Prolonged ileus may indicate an abdominal abscess or obstruction. The passage of gas rectally indicates the beginning return of peristalsis. The nurse auscultates the patient's abdomen for bowel sounds every 4 hours and assesses for the movement of gas or presence of distention. Ambulation facilitates the return of peristalsis, and the nurse encourages the patient to be as active as possible. The diet and activity changes plus loss of bowel tissue that accompany resection may make it difficult for the patient to resume a normal elimination pattern. Diarrhea may occur initially, but it usually is temporary and self-limiting. The nurse teaches the patient to avoid constipation through regular exercise, adequate fluids, and adjustment of the fiber content of the diet. Laxatives should be avoided if possible. Patients who undergo coloanal pouch construction, especially older patients, may experience significant problems reestablishing continence.[59]

Teaching for Follow-up Care. Long-term concerns primarily relate to the risk of disease recurrence and metastasis. Ongoing disease surveillance is an important focus of patient and family teaching. Carcinoembryonic antigen is a tumor marker produced in the body in response to cancer and secreted into the circulation. Its levels can be used to monitor for recurrence, especially when the original cancer is advanced at the time of diagnosis. Surveillance colonoscopy is typically performed at 2-year intervals unless the patient's clinical status warrants a shorter interval.[14] The prognosis is primarily related to the degree of invasiveness of the cancer at the time of diagnosis and initial treatment.

GERONTOLOGIC CONSIDERATIONS

The incidence of bowel cancer is strongly skewed toward the older adult population, and the entire discussion of the disease is targeted at that population. The issues of comorbidity and general health therefore are important. Healthy older adults can withstand the rigors of treatment well, but the concurrent existence of other chronic health problems increases the risk for postoperative complications.

Early diagnosis is often difficult in the older population. Symptoms tend to be underreported and attributed to the effects of aging. This is particularly true for symptoms related to digestion and elimination. Chronic constipation is a frequent complaint in this population, so changes in bowel habits may go unnoticed and unreported.

The challenges of learning an ostomy self-care regimen also may be more significant for older persons, who may have difficulty processing new information and learning new tasks. Arthritis or failing vision may make it difficult for older adults to acquire the psychomotor skills necessary for self-care. The teaching plan needs to address these concerns and needs to move at a slower pace. Because hospital stays are short, many older persons need additional teaching at home to master self-care. Discharge planning must begin at admission. The nurse assesses the patient's home environment and the supports that are available to meet the patient's physical and emotional needs. For older adults, particularly those who live alone, this assessment includes extended family and friendship networks. The involvement of a social worker is helpful to determine insurance and financial qualifications for home care assistance, and referral for home health follow-up or community-based services is appropriate.

Anorectal Disorders

A variety of common disorders can affect the perianal area. Persons who experience anorectal disorders typically seek medical care for symptoms such as pain, tenderness, itching, or rectal bleeding. Many of the disorders can be treated on an outpatient basis.

Hemorrhoids

Etiology and Epidemiology. Hemorrhoids are masses of dilated blood vessels that lie beneath the lining of the skin in the anal canal. They result from dilation of the superior and inferior hemorrhoidal veins, which form a plexus, or cushion, in the submucosal layer of the lower rectum. Because this cushion is a normal anatomic feature, virtually all adults are at risk for hemorrhoids; they are estimated to be present in up to 50% of the population by age 50.[17]

The exact cause of hemorrhoids remains unclear, but pregnancy is a common initiating condition. Other conditions associated with hemorrhoids include obesity, congestive heart failure, and chronic liver disease with portal hypertension. These conditions are all associated with persistent elevations in intraabdominal pressure. Sedentary occupations that involve long periods of sitting or standing also are implicated, although the exact mechanism is not known. Chronic constipation and diarrheal diseases such as IBD are also risk factors.

Hemorrhoids are classified as either internal or external. Internal hemorrhoids are those which occur above the anal sphincter. External hemorrhoids are those which occur below the anal sphincter (Figure 43-20). Internal hemorrhoids are further classified by size, since size determines both the nature and severity of symptoms and the appropriate management. Box 43-6 presents the grading scale for hemorrhoids. Individuals often have both forms of hemorrhoids at the same time. Although hemorrhoids usually are a chronic health problem, acute episodes may occur.

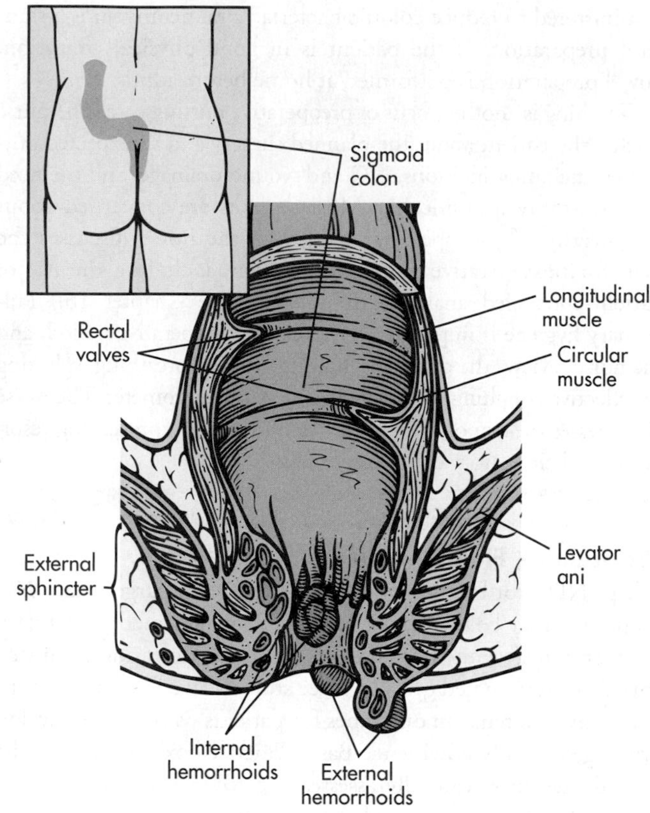

Figure 43-20 Internal and external hemorrhoids.

Pathophysiology. Hemorrhoids traditionally have been viewed as varicose veins of the rectum. The superior hemorrhoidal veins contain no valves and are vulnerable to overdistention when the person is in an upright position. Age and other predisposing factors are theorized to promote deterioration of the anchoring and connective tissue, allowing the vessels to bulge, descend, and become symptomatic.[23]

External hemorrhoids are seen most often in young and middle-aged adults and can be detected by the affected person. The classic "skin tag" consists of small lumps of fibrous tissue and folds of anal skin that have been stretched by bulging of the hemorrhoids (Figure 43-21). They rarely bleed and become truly symptomatic only when they become thrombosed or rupture subcutaneously with hematoma formation. A thrombosed external hemorrhoid may

Box 43-6 Hemorrhoidal Grading Scale

- *First degree:* The hemorrhoid bulges into the lumen of the anorectal canal but does not protrude through the anus.
- *Second degree:* The hemorrhoid prolapses out of the anus with defecation or straining but spontaneously returns to its normal anatomic position.
- *Third degree:* The hemorrhoid prolapses out of the anus with defecation or straining and requires manual reduction to return it to its normal anatomic position.
- *Fourth degree:* The hemorrhoid prolapses out of the anus, is irreducible, and is at risk for strangulation.

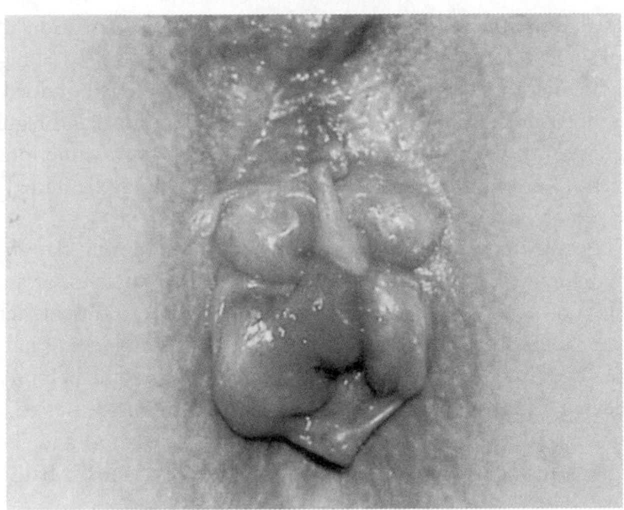

Figure 43-21 External hemorrhoids.

occur suddenly after vigorous exercise or after a severe episode of diarrhea or constipation. The intense pain accompanying thrombosis is caused by the multiple sensory nerve endings in the epithelial tissue that composes the hemorrhoid. Bluish skin-covered lumps are readily visible in the anal region, and the thrombosed hemorrhoids are quite large and may encompass the entire anus.

Internal hemorrhoids are usually asymptomatic. Excessive engorgement and prolapse occur, but painless rectal bleeding is their most common feature. The person may notice spotting on the toilet tissue or occasional spurts of blood that accompany defecation. Bleeding is almost always self-limiting but is usually what causes the person to seek treatment.[17] Although the blood loss typically is small, it can deplete iron reserves if it persists over a long period. Internal hemorrhoids can be uncomfortable but rarely cause significant pain unless strangulation and prolapse occur. These conditions interfere with the blood supply to the area and require immediate surgical correction.[35]

Hemorrhoids of both types are basically asymptomatic unless complications occur. Routinely painful defecation accompanied by rectal bleeding is more commonly associated with anal fissure than with uncomplicated hemorrhoids. Perianal itching may occur with higher-grade internal hemorrhoids, but other causes should also be explored. If the hemorrhoids cause pain or bleeding, the patient may develop constipation in an effort to limit defecation.

Collaborative Care Management. The diagnosis of hemorrhoids is fairly straightforward. The person's presenting symptoms establish the initial diagnosis, which usually can be confirmed by inspection and digital palpation. Proctoscopy or sigmoidoscopy may be used to confirm the diagnosis, and middle-aged or older patients who are experiencing rectal bleeding may undergo colonoscopy to rule out cancer. Occult blood in the stool is not associated with hemorrhoids.

Both forms of hemorrhoids can be managed conservatively if the symptoms are not severe. Conservative management includes a high-fiber diet, bulk-forming laxatives, warm sitz baths, and gentle cleansing. If severe pain, bleeding, or thrombosis is present, however, more definitive management may be indicated. A variety of treatment options are available, including sclerotherapy, cryotherapy, bipolar diathermy, rubber band ligation, and surgical hemorrhoidectomy. Currently grades 2 and 3 internal hemorrhoids are treated with rubber band ligation, and complicated grades 3 and 4 hemorrhoids are treated with surgery. Patients with thrombosed external hemorrhoids that are diagnosed promptly can be treated with surgical evacuation or excision with the patient under local anesthesia. The wound is left open to heal by secondary intention. Most thrombosed external hemorrhoids resolve spontaneously after 48 to 72 hours. Complicated prolapses may require surgery.

RUBBER BAND LIGATION. Internal hemorrhoids may be treated with ligation with latex bands. No anesthesia is required, the treatment can take place in a physician's office, and the procedure is both cost-effective and successful. The hemorrhoid is grasped with forceps and pulled down into a special instrument that slips a latex band over the hemorrhoid and onto the rectal mucosa above it (Figure 43-22). The band constricts the circulation and causes necrosis, and the tissue usually sloughs off within a week. Submucosal scarring and fibrosis prevent the development of new hemorrhoidal tissue. An enema is given before the treatment to prevent a bowel movement for the first 24 hours, thus preventing straining that could cause the band to break or slip off. Local discomfort is usually minimal and can be successfully relieved by NSAIDs or acetaminophen and sitz baths.

SCLEROTHERAPY. The injection method can be effective for treating first- and second-degree, small, bleeding internal hemorrhoids. A sclerosing solution such as 5% phenol in oil is injected into the hemorrhoidal tissue, producing an intense inflammatory reaction. Fibrous induration occurs at the site of the injection, adhering the mucosa to the underlying muscle. The procedure is palliative, not curative, and repeat injection may be required in

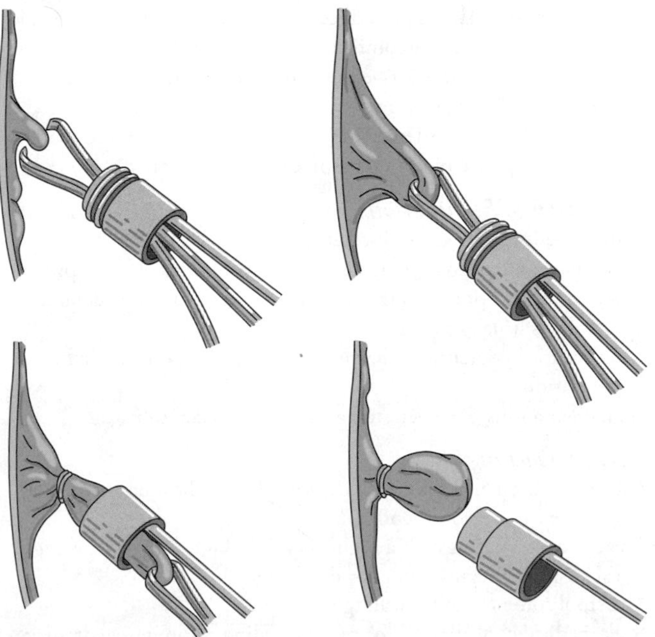

Figure 43-22 Rubber band ligation of internal hemorrhoid.

the future. However, it is economical and is rarely associated with complications, making it an appropriate choice for selected patients.

CRYOSURGERY AND PHOTOCOAGULATION. Cryosurgery and photocoagulation use a probe to expose the hemorrhoidal tissue to liquid nitrogen, radiation, or another agent. Local tissue destruction occurs, and the tissue then gradually necroses and sloughs off, causing a foul-smelling discharge for several days or more. The drainage limits the acceptability of the treatment, which is also expensive because of the complexity of the equipment.

HEMORRHOIDECTOMY. Surgical excision (hemorrhoidectomy) is the treatment used for most third-degree hemorrhoids, all fourth-degree and strangulated hemorrhoids, and other hemorrhoids that have not responded to more conservative therapy. The procedure involves the excision of all involved tissue with careful preservation of the anal sphincter. Care of the patient after anorectal surgery is summarized in the Guidelines for Safe Practice box.

PATIENT/FAMILY TEACHING. Minor problems with hemorrhoids often can be successfully managed through a combination of strict personal hygiene and prevention of constipation and straining. The nurse encourages the patient to follow a high-residue diet rich in fruit and vegetable fiber. Bran may be added to the diet to ease stool passage. A liberal intake of fluids and regular exercise also are encouraged to promote normal bowel function. If necessary, a bulk-forming hydrophilic laxative may be added to the person's daily routine.

Local treatment promotes comfort during symptom flare-ups. The patient is instructed to apply ice, warm compresses, or analgesic ointments such as dibucaine (Nupercainal) to provide temporary relief from pain and reduce the edema around external or prolapsed internal hemorrhoids. Sitz baths also are helpful in relieving pain and supporting cleanliness. The nurse stresses the importance of good personal hygiene after defecation and thorough cleansing of the bathtubs or containers used for sitz baths.

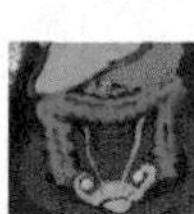

GUIDELINES FOR SAFE PRACTICE
The Patient Undergoing Anorectal Surgery

Preoperative Care

Bowel preparation is standard, but an enema may not be prescribed if rectal pain is acute.
Stool softeners may be given to promote a soft stool before surgery.

Postoperative Care

Promotion of Comfort

Administer analgesics as prescribed, especially before initial defecation (considerable rectal discomfort may be present).
Provide emotional support before and after first defecation.
Suggest a side-lying position.
Provide sitz baths as ordered (monitor for hypotension secondary to dilation of pelvic blood vessels in early postoperative period).

Promotion of Elimination

Administer prescribed stool softeners.
Encourage patient to defecate as soon as inclination occurs (prevents strictures and preserves the normal anal lumen). Considerable anxiety is usually present.
Monitor for hypotension, dizziness, and faintness during first defecation.
If an enema must be given, use a small-bore rectal tube.

Patient Teaching

Clean the rectal area after each defecation until healing is complete (a sitz bath is recommended).
Prevent constipation with a high-fiber diet, high-fluid intake, regular exercise, and regular time for defecation.
Use stool softeners until healing is complete.
Seek medical consultation for rectal bleeding, suppurative drainage, continued pain on defecation, or continued constipation despite preventive measures.

Anal Fissures, Abscesses, and Fistulas

Etiology and Epidemiology. Anal fissures, fistulas, and abscesses are relatively common problems that develop from trauma or infection in the anorectal area. An anal fissure is a painful elongated tear between the anal canal and the perianal skin, most often along the posterior midline.[35] Fissures may be primary or secondary. Most primary fissures are idiopathic and occur in young and middle-age adults. Secondary fissures are associated with chronic constipation and the passage of hard stool, trauma, or chronic ulceration from IBD. Anal abscesses result most often from feces obstructing gland ducts in the anorectal region, but they also may complicate the presence of a fissure. They occur twice as often in men, usually during the third and fourth decades. Stasis of duct contents results in acute infection that can spread to adjacent tissue. An anal fistula involves the development of an abnormal communication between the anal canal and skin outside the anus. The rupture and drainage of infected material from an abscess often causes the fistula.

Pathophysiology. Most acute anal fissures are superficial and heal spontaneously or in response to conservative therapy. If healing does not occur, however, the fissure may cause significant bleeding or become infected. Infection may be relatively minor and confined to a single rectal crypt or become widespread. Widespread infection or sepsis may develop in patients with immunodeficiencies. The development of a fistula may necessitate extensive surgical repair.

Pain is the primary problem associated with anal fissures and abscesses. It can be severe and prolonged from pressure on the somatic nerves in the perianal area. Any position can be painful, since the pain often is widespread. Constipation is inevitable because the patient attempts to avoid pain by preventing defecation. Local swelling, erythema, and acute tenderness accompany abscess development. Pruritus in the anal region often accompanies both fissures and fistulas. When a fistula is present, the patient notices periodic purulent drainage, which stains undergarments.

Collaborative Care Management. The degree of medical intervention necessary for anal fissures, abscesses, and fistulas depends on the nature and severity of the problem. Medical treat-

TABLE 43-7 TREATMENT OPTIONS FOR ANAL FISSURE, ABSCESS, AND FISTULA

Lesion	Clinical Manifestations	Medical Management
Fissure: slitlike ulceration in epithelium of anal canal	Pain with defecation; bleeding; pruritus; constipation	Stool softeners; analgesic ointments; sitz bath; sphincterotomy or fissurectomy if medical therapy ineffective
Abscess in tissue around anus	Persistent throbbing; anal pain with walking, sitting, defecation; systemic signs of infection	Incision and drainage of abscess
Fistula: hollow track leading through anal tissue from anorectal canal through skin near anus	Purulent discharge near anus; pain; pruritus	Fistulotomy or fistulectomy

ment options are outlined in Table 43-7. Prompt surgical treatment is important because of the high risk of overwhelming sepsis from an abscess. Initial nursing interventions for anal disorders focus on improving the patient's comfort level. These may include sitz baths and the local application of heat, cold, topical anesthetics, or astringent preparations such as witch hazel. Analgesics are often required. These interventions are also important if the patient is undergoing surgical excision or repair. The repair of fistulas is technically involved, and nursing interventions focus on restoring and maintaining skin integrity and ensuring adequate nutrition for healing.

PATIENT/FAMILY TEACHING. Patient education focuses on the prevention of recurrences. The nurse teaches the patient the importance of careful perianal hygiene and avoidance of constipation. All standard measures are presented, including a diet rich in fiber, the selective addition of bran to the diet, adequate intake of fluids, exercise, and the use of stool softeners or bulk-forming laxatives to prevent straining.

Critical Thinking

1. A woman has been admitted to the hospital with a diagnosis of acute diverticulitis. She has experienced mild episodes in the past, but this one is severe and has quickly led to perforation. She has developed acute peritonitis and is now extremely ill. While you are administering an antibiotic, she asks you how she became so sick. She is obviously worried that she may not get better. How could you best explain the complication of peritonitis and its treatment to her?
2. An 18-year-old first-year nursing student was recently diagnosed with ulcerative colitis. She has lost 20 pounds in the past 8 weeks from persistent, severe diarrhea, which occurs every 1 to 2 hours and causes occasional fecal incontinence at night. She is fatigued and anorexic, but she desperately wants to continue her education. What specific concerns would you anticipate that she would have about her disease and treatment regimen? What modifications would you recommend that she make in her lifestyle to attempt to meet her goal? What resources would you refer her to?
3. A 43-year-old woman has successfully managed her ulcerative colitis since its diagnosis 12 years ago. She has experienced only occasional exacerbations, which have thus far responded promptly to short courses of high-dose steroids. Her physician told her recently that it is about time for her to think seriously about having a complete colectomy. She is upset at the prospect of surgery and wants things to continue "as they are." What is the rationale for the physician's recommendation? How important is it to her future health and well-being? What alternatives, if any, exist?
4. Early diagnosis is clearly critically important in the management of colorectal cancer. Consider our current state of knowledge, and take and defend a position concerning the appropriate mass screening for adults over age 50. Consider economics, effectiveness, high-risk groups, and resources in your answer.

References

1. Achkar JP: *Inflammatory bowel disease*, accessed from website: http://www.acg.gi.org/patients/gihealth/ibd.asp.
2. American Cancer Society: *Colorectal cancer facts and figures—special edition 2005*, accessed from website: www.cancer.org.
3. American Cancer Society: *Detailed guide: colon and rectum cancer: can colorectal polyps and cancer be found early? Colorectal cancer screening*, Feb 2005, accessed from website: www.cancer.org.

3a. American Cancer Society: *How is colorectal cancer found?* Accessed February 1, 2005 from website: www.cancer.org.

3b. American Cancer Society: *New cancer drugs offered hope in 2004 improvements in treating breast, lung, colon, and prostate cancers*, accessed December 31, 2004, from website: www.cancer.org.

4. American College of Gastroenterology Functional Gastrointestinal Disorders Task Force: Evidence-based position statement on the management of irritable bowel syndrome in North America, *Am J Gastroenterol* 97(Suppl 1): 61-65, 2002.
5. Baron JA et al: Calcium supplements for the prevention of colorectal adenomas, *N Engl J Med* 340(2):101-107, 1999.
6. Baron J et al: A randomized trial of aspirin to prevent colorectal adenomas, *N Engl J Med* 348:891-899, 2003.
7. Barr JE: Assessment and management of stomal complications: a framework for clinical decision making, *Ostomy Wound Manage* 50(9):50-52, 54, 56, 2004.
8. Bernard L et al: Emerging technologies in screening for colorectal cancer: CT colonography, immunochemical fecal occult blood tests, and stool screening using molecular markers, *CA Cancer J Clin* 53:44-55, 2003.
9. Breitfeller JM: Peritonitis, *Am J Nurs* 99(4):33, 1999.
10. Bresalier RS: Malignant neoplasms of the large intestine. In Feldman M, Friedman LS, Sleisenger MH, editors: *Sleisenger and Fortran's gastrointestinal and liver disease*, ed 7, vol I, Philadelphia, 2002, Saunders.

11. Cees JHM et al: Ileoneorectal anastomosis, *Ann Surg* 230(6):757-758, 1999.
12. Cerrato PL: When food is the culprit, *RN* 62(6):52-54, 1999.
12a. Chlebowski RT et al: Estrogen plus progestin and colorectal cancer in postmenopausal women, *N Engl J Med* 350(10):991-1004, 2004.
13. Craig S: *Appendicitis: acute*, 2005, accessed May 26, 2005, from website: www.emedicine.com/emerg/topic41.htm.
14. DuBois RM: Neoplasms of the small and large intestine. In Goldman L, Asiello D, editors: *Cecil textbook of medicine*, ed 22, Philadelphia, 2004, Saunders.
15. Erwin-Toth P: Ostomy pearls: a concise guide to stoma siting, pouching systems, patient education and more, *Adv Skin Wound Care* 16(3):146-152, 2003.
16. Estimate of illnesses from *Salmonella enteritidis* in eggs, United States, 2000, *Emerg Infect Dis* 11(1):113, 2005.
17. Forbes A et al: *Atlas of clinical gastroenterology*, ed 3, St Louis, 2005, Mosby.
18. Ghosh S et al: Natalizumab Pan-European Study Group: natalizumab for active Crohn's disease, *N Engl J Med* 348(1):24-32, 2003.
19. Goroll AH: Management of diverticular disease. In Goroll AH, Mulley AG, editors: *Primary care medicine*, ed 4, Philadelphia, 2000, Lippincott.
20. Hamer DH, Gorbach SL: Infectious diarrhea and bacterial food poisoning. In Feldman M, Friedman LS, Sleisenger MH, editors: *Sleisenger and Fortran's gastrointestinal and liver disease*, ed 7, vol I, Philadelphia, 2002, Saunders.
21. Hanaauer SB et al: Maintenance infliximab for Crohn's disease: the ACCENT I randomized trial, *Lancet* 359:1541-1549, 2002.
22. Heitkemper M, Jarrett M: Irritable bowel syndrome, *Am J Nurs* 101(1): 26-32, 2001.
23. Hull T: Examination and diseases of the anorectum. In Feldman M, Friedman LS, Sleisenger MH, editors: *Sleisenger and Fortran's gastrointestinal and liver disease*, ed 7, vol II, Philadelphia, 2002, Saunders.
24. Hyland J: The basics of ostomies, *Gastroenterol Nurs* 25(6):241-244, 2002, quiz pp 244-245.
25. Itzkowitz SH: Colonic polyps and polyposis syndromes. In Feldman M, Friedman LS, Sleisenger MH, editors: *Sleisenger and Fortran's gastrointestinal and liver disease*, ed 7, vol II, Philadelphia, 2002, Saunders.
26. Jewell DP: Ulcerative colitis. In Feldman M, Friedman LS, Sleisenger MH, editors: *Sleisenger and Fortran's gastrointestinal and liver disease*, ed 7, vol II, Philadelphia, 2002, Saunders.
27. Jones MP, Wessinger S: Small bowel motility, *Current Opin Gastroenterol MAR* 21(2):141-146, 2005.
28. Klonowski E, Masoodi J: The patient with Crohn's disease, *RN* 62(3):32-37, 1999.
29. Lennard-Jones JE: Constipation. In Feldman M, Friedman LS, Sleisenger MH, editors: *Sleisenger and Fortran's gastrointestinal and liver disease*, ed 7, vol I, Philadelphia, 2002, Saunders.
30. Levin B et al: The future of colorectal cancer screening: experts examine newer early detection methods, *CA Cancer J Clin* 53:44-55, 2003.
31. Lucey MR: Diseases of the peritoneum, mesentery, and omentum. In Goldman L, Asiello D, editors: *Cecil textbook of medicine*, ed 22, Philadelphia, 2004, Saunders.
32. Maltz C: GI consult: Crohn's disease, *Emerg Med*, accessed from website: emedmag.com.
33. Meyer JU et al: Estrogen plus progestin and colorectal cancer in postmenopausal women, *N Engl J Med* 350:2417-2419, 2004.
34. National Institute of Diabetes and Digestive and Kidney Diseases: *Constipation, national digestive diseases classification*, Bethesda, Md, 2002, National Institutes of Health.
35. Nelson H: Diseases of the rectum and anus. In Goldman L, Asiello D, editors: *Cecil textbook of medicine*, ed 22, Philadelphia, 2004, Saunders.
36. Neumayer L et al: Open mesh versus laparoscopic mesh repair of inguinal hernia, *N Engl J Med* 350:1819-1827, 2004.
37. Pemberton JH: Ileostomy and its alternatives. In Feldman M, Friedman LS, Sleisenger MH, editors: *Sleisenger and Fortran's gastrointestinal and liver disease*, ed 7, vol II, Philadelphia, 2002, Saunders.
38. Pignon M et al: Screening for colorectal cancer in adults at average risk: a summary of the evidence for the US Preventive Services Task Force, *Ann Intern Med*, 127, 132-141, 2002.
39. Prier R, Solnick JV: Foodborne and waterborne infectious diseases, *Postgrad Med* 107(4):245-255, 2000.
40. Rampton DS: Management of Crohn's disease, *BMJ* 319:1480-1485, 1999.
41. Read NW: Irritable bowel syndrome. In Feldman M, Friedman LS, Sleisenger MH, editors: *Sleisenger and Fortran's gastrointestinal and liver disease*, ed 7, vol II, Philadelphia, 2002, Saunders.
42. Richards S: Constipation: a common problem, *Practice Nurse* 28(4): 953-612, 2004.
43. Rolstad BS, Erwin-Toth PL: Peristomal skin complications: prevention and management, *Ostomy Wound Manage* 50(9):68-77, 2004.
44. Rowan T et al, for Women's Health: *Estrogen plus progestin and colorectal cancer in postmenopausal women*
45. Rowe WA: *Inflammatory bowel disease*, accessed June 2004 from website: http://www.emedicine.com/MED/topic 1169.htm.
46. Runyon BA, Such J: Surgical peritonitis and other diseases of the peritoneum, mesentery, omentum, and diaphragm. In Feldman M, Friedman LS, Sleisenger MH, editors: *Sleisenger and Fortran's gastrointestinal and liver disease*, ed 7, vol II, Philadelphia, 2002, Saunders.
47. Saltiel E: Budesonide, accessed from website: medicinenet.com.
48. Sands BE: Crohn's disease. In Feldman M, Friedman LS, Sleisenger MH, editors: *Sleisenger and Fortran's gastrointestinal and liver disease*, ed 7, vol II, Philadelphia, 2002, Saunders.
49. Sarosi GA, Turnage RH: Appendicitis. In Feldman M, Friedman LS, Sleisenger MH, editors: *Sleisenger and Fortran's gastrointestinal and liver disease*, ed 7, vol II, Philadelphia, 2002, Saunders.
50. Schatzkin A et al: Lack of effect of a low-fat, high-fiber diet on the recurrence of colorectal adenomas, *N Engl J Med* 342(16):1149-1155, 2000.
51. Schiller LR: Fecal incontinence. In Feldman M, Friedman LS, Sleisenger MH, editors: *Sleisenger and Fortran's gastrointestinal and liver disease*, ed 7, vol I, Philadelphia, 2002, Saunders.
52. Schroeder C: Food-borne illness strikes at least 2 billion people a year, *Hepatitis Weekly* Nov 1, 2004, p 24.
53. Simmang CL, Shires TG: Diverticular disease of the colon. In Feldman M, Friedman LS, Sleisenger MH, editors: *Sleisenger and Fortran's gastrointestinal and liver disease*, ed 7, vol II, Philadelphia, 2002, Saunders.
54. Smith RA, Cokkinides V, Eyre HJ: American Cancer Society guidelines for the early detection of cancer, *CA Cancer J Clin* 55(1):31-44, 2005.
55. Stenson WF: Inflammatory bowel disease. In Goldman L, Asiello D, editors: *Cecil textbook of medicine*, ed 22, Philadelphia, 2004, Saunders.
55a. Turnage RH, Bergen PC: Intestinal obstruction and ileus. In Feldman M, Friedman LS, Sleisenger MH, editors: *Sleisenger and Fortran's gastrointestinal and liver disease*, ed 7, vol II, Philadelphia, 3002, Saunders.
56. US Department of Health and Human Services: *Healthy people 2010: understanding and improving health*, Washington, DC, 2000, The Department.
57. Van Norman GA: Diagnostic tests in irritable bowel syndrome. In Feldman M, Friedman LS, Sleisenger MH, editors: *Sleisenger and Fortran's gastrointestinal and liver disease*, ed 7, vol II, Philadelphia, 2002, Saunders. Update accessed from website: www.ffgastro.com.
58. Wilcox CM: Appendicitis, diverticulitis, and miscellaneous intestinal inflammatory conditions. In Goldman L, Asiello D, editors: *Cecil textbook of medicine*, ed 22, Philadelphia, 2004, Saunders.
59. Young M: Caring for patients with coloanal reservoirs for rectal cancer, *Med Surg Nurs* 9(4):193-197, 2000.

evolve Visit the Evolve website: http://evolve.elsevier.com/Monahan/medsurg

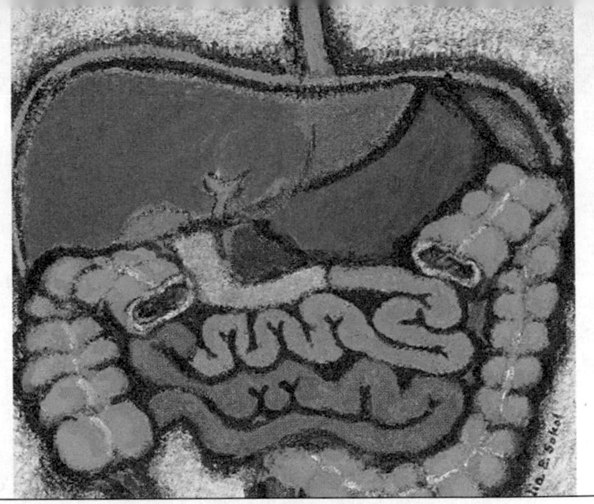

CHAPTER 44

Gallbladder and Exocrine Pancreatic Problems

by Elizabeth W. Good, Judith K. Sands

OBJECTIVES

After studying this chapter, the learner should be able to:

1. Describe the etiology, epidemiology, and pathophysiology of cholelithiasis, cholecystitis, and cancer of the biliary tract.
2. Compare treatment alternatives for biliary tract disease.
3. Describe the nursing care needs of patients with disorders of the biliary system.
4. List the causes of acute and chronic pancreatitis.
5. Explain the pathophysiologic basis for signs and symptoms of acute and chronic pancreatitis.
6. Discuss management approaches for acute and chronic pancreatitis and pancreatic tumors.
7. Develop nursing diagnoses, patient outcomes, and nursing interventions for patients who have acute or chronic pancreatitis or cancer of the pancreas.

KEY TERMS

autodigestion, p. 1291
biliary colic, p. 1286
cholecystitis, p. 1285
choledocholithiasis, p. 1285
cholelithiasis, p. 1285
extracorporeal shock wave lithotripsy, p. 1288
Murphy's sign, p. 1287
pseudocysts, p. 1292

Problems of the Gallbladder

Problems of the biliary system include obstruction, inflammation, infection, and cancer. Gallbladder disorders are extremely common and affect millions of adults every year.

Cholelithiasis, Cholecystitis, and Choledocholithiasis

Etiology and Epidemiology. Gallstones can occur anywhere in the biliary tree. The term **cholelithiasis** refers to stone formation in the gallbladder and is the most common biliary disorder. Either acute or chronic inflammation, termed **cholecystitis,** can be precipitated by the presence of stones. When stones form in or migrate to the common bile duct, the condition is termed **choledocholithiasis.** Figure 44-1 illustrates common sites for gallstones.

The prevalence of gallstones varies widely around the world and among various ethnic groups; the overall prevalence of gallstone-related disorders appears to have increased during the twentieth century.[16] Cholelithiasis is a common health problem in the United States, affecting more than 20 million Americans.[16] In the United States the disease is more common in Caucasians, Hispanics, and Native Americans, and is uncommon in African-Americans.[11] Cholelithiasis is two or three times more common in women than in men, and the incidence increases steadily with age.[11] In one striking example, more than 70% of women over 25 years old among the Pima Indians of Arizona have gallstones.

Approximately 80% of gallstones are composed of cholesterol in Western populations.[15] The remaining are pigmented stones, which are further classified as black or brown. Although the precise etiology of gallstones remains unknown, it is theorized that an imbalance in bile components that leads to supersaturation and crystallization plays a major role.[11] Because most healthy individuals experience supersaturation of the bile at various times without developing gallstones, clearly other factors such as gastrointestinal (GI) and gallbladder motility are also involved.[16] Risk factors for gallstones include various clinical states associated with changes in cholesterol formation and excretion (see Risk Factors box). The development of pigmented stones is linked to disease states such as cirrhosis, hemolytic disease, and chronic small bowel disease.

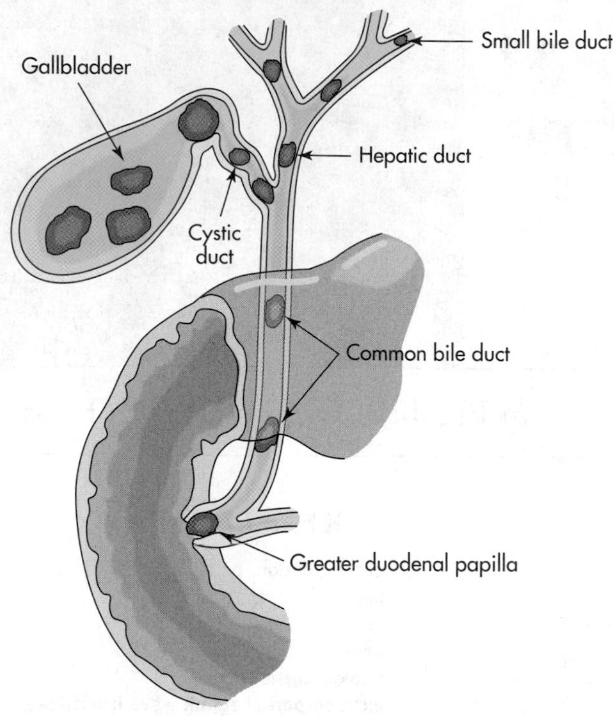

Figure 44-1 Common sites of gallstones.

Risk Factors

Cholesterol Gallstones

- Sex: two or three times more common in women
- Obesity, particularly in women
- Middle age (risk increased with age)
- Rapid weight loss (about 5 lb/wk)
- Caucasian, Native American, Hispanic race
- Pregnancy, multiparity, use of oral contraceptives
- Hypercholesterolemia, use of anticholesterol medications
- Diseases of the ileum

Although strategies to prevent gallstone disease are not well known, regular exercise, a low-carbohydrate diet, and the intake of caffeinated coffee may offer some protection.[10] The Research box presents a study describing the possible effects of nut consumption on the risk of gallbladder disease.

Symptomatic gallbladder disease is one of the most common GI disorders requiring hospitalization. Gallbladder treatment costs and hospital stays are estimated at $6.5 billion annually and include the more than 700,000 gallbladder surgeries performed each year.[16] Once the disease becomes symptomatic, the risk of complications is 1% to 3% annually.

Pathophysiology. Bile is primarily composed of water plus conjugated bilirubin, organic and inorganic ions, small amounts of proteins, and three lipids: bile salts, lecithin, and cholesterol. When the balance of these three lipids remains intact, cholesterol is held in solution. If the balance is upset, cholesterol can begin to precipitate. Cholesterol gallstone formation is enhanced by the production of a mucin glycoprotein, which traps cholesterol particles. Twenty percent of biliary cholesterol comes from new synthesis, but the association with serum cholesterol levels remains unclear. Excess secretion is associated with aging, obesity, and the effects of certain drugs and hormones.[11,16] Supersaturation of the bile with cholesterol also impairs gallbladder motility and contributes to stasis. The gallbladder has the ability to absorb excess water and concentrate bile, which further complicates the picture of supersaturation and stasis.[16]

Research

Tsai CJ et al: Frequent nut consumption and decreased risk of cholecystectomy in women, *Am J Clin Nutr* 80:76-81, 2004.

Researchers have used the large pool of female subjects identified as part of the ongoing Nurses' Health Study to explore a wide variety of nutrition and lifestyle factors over more than 20 years. This study looked at the questionnaire responses of more than 81,000 nurses to identify the potential link between varying degrees of nut consumption and the development of symptomatic gallstones requiring cholecystectomy.

Cholesterol stones form because of disproportionate amounts of cholesterol, bile acids, and phospholipids in the biliary tract. Dietary fiber is capable of lowering triglyceride levels and enhancing intestinal motility, which in turn reduces bile acid presence. Nuts are considered a good source of dietary fiber and are composed primarily of unsaturated fats.

The researchers studied the effects of eating peanuts, other nuts, and peanut butter. Women who consumed 5 or more ounces of nuts per week had a lower risk of developing symptomatic gallstone disease than those who rarely ate nuts. The unsaturated fatty acid profile of nuts likely plays a role, but other intrinsic aspects of nuts are thought to possibly contribute also. Other recent studies have also credited caffeinated coffee intake and dietary fiber intake with lowering women's risk of symptomatic gallstone disease.

Cholesterol stones are soft, yellowish green, and radiolucent. They range in size from 1 mm to 2.5 cm.[11] The stones most commonly occur in multiples but can be solitary. The process of stone formation is slow. Stones are theorized to grow steadily for 2 to 3 years and then stabilize in size. Eighty-five percent are less than 2 cm in diameter. Most are found in the gallbladder, but 15% to 60% of persons older than age 60 who undergo surgery for gallstones are also found to have stones in the common bile duct.[17]

Black stones result from an increase in unconjugated bilirubin and calcium with a corresponding decrease in bile salts. Impaired gallbladder motility may also be a factor. Black stones are very small, hard, and usually numerous. Brown stones develop in the intrahepatic and extrahepatic ducts and are usually preceded by bacterial infection.[14]

Although most persons with gallstones are asymptomatic, cholecystitis can develop at any time, usually from the stone obstructing the cystic duct or from edema and spasm initiated by the presence or passage of the stone. In acute cholecystitis the gallbladder is enlarged, tense, and inflamed. A secondary bacterial infection can occur within several days and cause most of the serious consequences of the disease.

Biliary colic is the classic clinical manifestation of symptomatic gallstones in 70% to 80% of persons.[11] It is caused by spasm of the gallbladder or transient obstruction but is not associated with inflammation of the mucosa. Biliary colic causes sudden-onset sharp pain that may occur anywhere in the upper abdomen or epigastrium. The pain steadily increases in intensity, may last for minutes or up to 6 hours, and may localize to the right upper quadrant (RUQ) or radiate to the back. It may awaken the patient at night or occur after a heavy meal. Vomiting and diaphoresis may also occur.[11,16]

Acute cholecystitis begins with stone-related obstruction in more than 90% of cases but then progresses to mucosal inflammation and damage.[11,16] The patient experiences acute pain that localizes in the RUQ, often accompanied by chills and fever. About 75% of patients experience vomiting.[10] Palpation of the abdomen causes a severe increase in pain and temporary inspiratory arrest **(Murphy's sign)**. The episode of cholecystitis usually subsides within 1 to 4 days. The clinical manifestations of biliary colic, acute cholecystitis, and choledocholithiasis are compared in the Clinical Manifestations box. Symptoms are typically milder and more subtle in older adults, who may develop bacteremia before they seek help.

Stones are found in the common bile duct in approximately 15% of patients.[5] When gallstones pass into the common bile

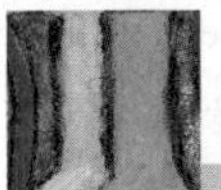

CLINICAL MANIFESTATIONS *Biliary Colic, Acute Cholecystitis, and Choledocholithiasis*

	Biliary Colic	Acute Cholecystitis	Choledocholithiasis
Pathophysiologic condition	Intermittent obstruction of cystic duct No inflammation of gallbladder mucosa	Impacted stone in cystic duct Acute inflammation of gallbladder mucosa Secondary bacterial infection in ~50% of cases	Intermittent obstruction of CBD
Symptoms	Severe, poorly localized epigastric or RUQ visceral pain growing in intensity over 15 min and remaining constant for 1-6 hr, often with nausea Frequency of attacks varies from days to months Gas, bloating, flatulence, dyspepsia *not* related to stones	75% preceded by attacks of biliary colic Visceral epigastric pain giving way to moderately severe, localized pain in RUQ, back, shoulder, or (rarely) chest Nausea with some emesis—frequent Pain lasting >6 hr suggests cholecystitis (versus colic)	Often asymptomatic Symptoms (when present) indistinguishable from biliary colic symptoms Predisposes patient to cholangitis and acute pancreatitis
Physical findings	Mild to moderate gallbladder tenderness during attack with mild residual tenderness lasting days Often completely normal examination	Febrile, usually <102° F (39° C) unless complicated by gangrene or perforation of gallbladder Right subcostal tenderness with inspiratory arrest (Murphy's sign) Palpable gallbladder in 33% of cases, especially in first attack Mild jaundice in 20%, higher frequency in older patients	Often completely normal examination if obstruction intermittent Jaundice with pain suggestive of stones; painless jaundice and palpable gallbladder suggestive of malignancy
Laboratory findings	Usually normal In patients with findings of only uncomplicated biliary colic, elevated bilirubin, alkaline phosphatase, or amylase level suggestive of coexisting CBD stones	Leukocytosis of 12,000-15,000/mm^3 with left shift common Serum bilirubin of 2-4 mg/dl; aminotransferase and alkaline phosphatase levels possibly elevated, even in absence of CBD stone or hepatic infection Mild serum amylase elevation even in absence of pancreatitis Bilirubin >4 mg/dl or amylase >1000 unit/L suggests CBD stone	Elevated serum bilirubin and alkaline phosphatase levels seen with CBD obstruction Serum bilirubin level >10 mg/dl suggestive of malignant obstruction or coexisting hemolysis Transient spike in serum aminotransferase or amylase levels suggestive of stone passage

Adapted from Horton JD, Bilhartz LE: Gallstone disease and its complications. In Feldman M, Friedman LS, Sleisenger MH, editors: *Sleisenger and Fordtran's gastrointestinal and liver disease*, ed 7, Philadelphia, 2002, Saunders

CBD, Common bile duct; *RUQ*, right upper quadrant; *WBC*, white blood cell.

duct, they may obstruct the flow of bile and cause jaundice and pruritus. Cholangitis is a serious potential complication resulting in pain, fever, chills, and rigors from bacteremia. The development of acute pancreatitis if the stone obstructs the sphincter of Oddi is also of concern.

Diagnosis of gallstones is fairly straightforward when the classic symptoms are present but is more difficult when the symptoms are milder and mimic other common GI conditions. Patients with irritable bowel syndrome or peptic ulcer disease may also have gallstones, and the exact cause of the patient's symptoms needs to be determined so that the correct clinical problem can be treated.

Cholecystitis may become chronic after several acute attacks. Chronic cholecystitis is usually the result of stone injury to the gallbladder wall that causes scarring, thickening, and possibly ulceration.[6] Bacterial infection may also be present. Patients with chronic disease often do not seek help until jaundice or other complications develop. Figure 44-2 shows the relationship between stone formation and associated outcomes in uncomplicated gallbladder disease.

Collaborative Care Management. Ultrasonography is the primary diagnostic tool for identifying cholelithiasis. This inexpensive test provides for precise visualization of the gallbladder and bile ducts and has greater than 95% accuracy in identifying all types of stones.[11] A gallbladder radionuclide scan, cholescintigraphy, may also be useful in diagnosing cholecystitis. Liver function and serum amylase tests may be ordered to evaluate the functional effects of obstruction, and endoscopic retrograde cholangiopancreatography (ERCP) is preferred for identifying and treating stones in the common bile duct.

Surgery is the treatment of choice for symptomatic gallstones. Cholecystectomy provides definitive treatment and has proved safe and effective. Laparoscopic cholecystectomy was first performed in France in 1987 and has revolutionized the care of patients with gallbladder disease,[16] rapidly becoming the standard of care for the treatment of gallstones. It offers several advantages over traditional laparotomy surgery. It is less invasive, allows a shorter healing and recuperation time, causes less scarring, and is associated with significantly less pain. The average hospital stay is less than 24 hours, and more and more patients are discharged the day of surgery.[2] Patients can return to normal activities in 2 to 3 days. An estimated 95% of patients are now considered good candidates for laparoscopic surgery. The need to revert to an open operation occurs in less than 5% of cases.[23] When the laparoscopic approach was first introduced, the ability to explore the common bile duct was limited. Surgical techniques have continued to improve, however, and laparoscopic approaches are now being successfully combined with endoscopic exploration and sphincterotomy to effectively treat patients with common bile duct stones. Open surgery is generally reserved for patients with multiple previous surgeries, extremely inflamed gallbladders, peritonitis, or gallbladder cancer.

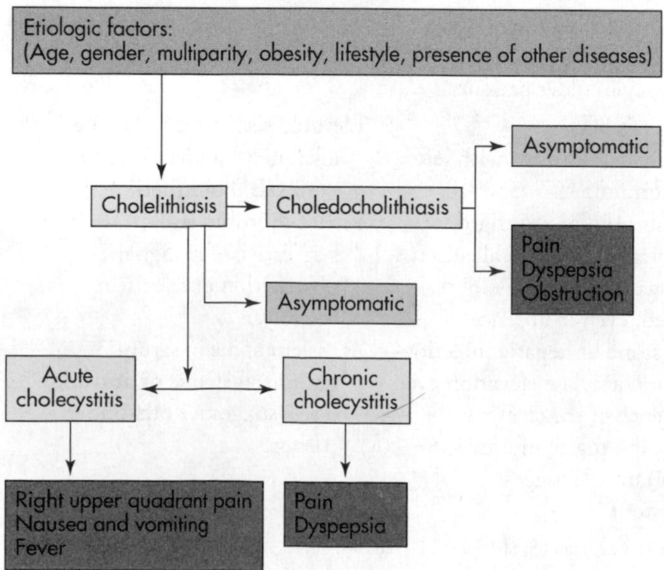

Figure 44-2 Development of uncomplicated cholecystitis.

Laparoscopic cholecystectomy is performed with the patient under general anesthesia. Four ½-inch incisions are made and 3 to 4 L of carbon dioxide gas is introduced to insufflate the abdomen and permit adequate visualization. A laser or cautery is used to dissect the gallbladder, which is deflated and removed through the umbilical incision. If problems should develop during the procedure, it can be rapidly converted to an open cholecystectomy. The skill of the surgeon is the primary determinant of outcomes.

Oral dissolution therapy with ursodeoxycholic acid (ursodiol [Actigall]) may be prescribed for patients who are poor surgical risks or who refuse surgical treatment.[4] This drug therapy has significant limitations and side effects and is used only when absolutely necessary. The drug gradually dissolves cholesterol stones by expanding the pool of bile acids and altering cholesterol metabolism. Direct dissolution therapy with methyl tert-butyl ether is occasionally used in high-risk surgical patients. The drug is instilled through a percutaneous catheter, which is monitored fluoroscopically. Multiple drug instillations are required over 12 to 24 hours, which makes the treatment both labor intensive and extremely expensive.

Extracorporeal shock wave lithotripsy, which uses shock waves to disintegrate stones, was pioneered in Germany and has been adapted to the treatment of gallstones, but few patients are candidates for this type of treatment. Oral dissolution therapy is given after the lithotripsy treatment to dissolve any residual stone fragments. Recurrence is a common problem. Endoscopic bile duct stone removal may be used in selected high-risk patients when choledocholithiasis is suspected, or sphincterotomy may be performed to allow obstructing stones to spontaneously pass into the duodenum.[19] Basket or balloon retrieval may be undertaken to trap the stones and pull them down through the bile duct (Figure 44-3).

PATIENT/FAMILY TEACHING. Laparoscopic cholecystectomy takes about 90 minutes and is more expensive than traditional open surgery, but the short hospital stay and tremendous patient satisfaction with the procedure clearly outweigh the higher surgical costs. The nurse informs the patient that mild shoulder pain may persist for up to 1 week after surgery. It is attributed to nerve irritation from distention with the carbon dioxide, but the discomfort is easily managed with mild analgesics.

Most patients have no specific care needs after discharge beyond routine management of wound healing. Normal activities can be quickly resumed. Complications are rare after laparoscopic cholecystectomy, but the nurse informs the patient that transient

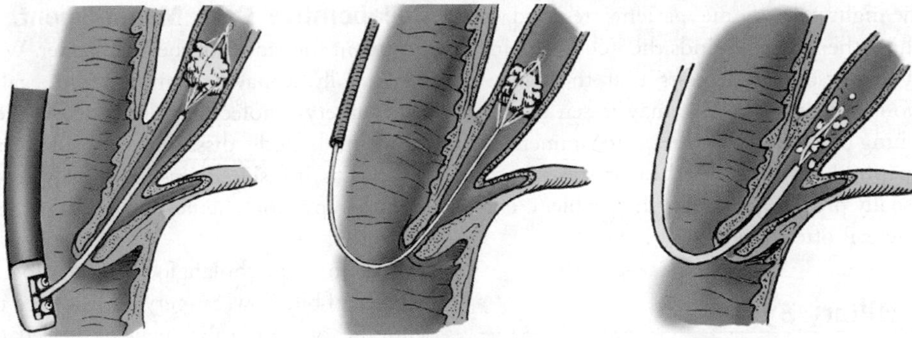

Figure 44-3 A basket contained in a flexible cord spring sheath is used to trap a stone and crush it.

mild diarrhea is occasionally reported. Chronic dyspepsia has been frequently discussed as a possible complication of cholecystectomy, but no concrete evidence has been found that the loss of the reservoir function of the gallbladder and the resulting decrease in the pool of bile salts in any way compromises digestion or increases the incidence of duodenal reflux. Some researchers suggest that these so-called complications may actually reflect situations in which the patient's original digestive symptoms were never related to the presence of gallstones.

The most common complication of the nonsurgical management of gallstone disease is recurrence, and it is clear that undiagnosed or inadequately treated gallbladder disease can result in serious and even life-threatening complications, including overwhelming sepsis and peritonitis.[4]

The nurse encourages the patient to resume a normal diet after surgery, since no diet is proven to either prevent or cause the formation of gallstones. Patients with symptomatic cholecystitis are encouraged to follow a low-fat diet and eat small meals until definitive therapy is completed.

Primary Sclerosing Cholangitis

Etiology and Epidemiology. The term *sclerosing cholangitis* refers to a variety of pathologic processes that cause bile duct injury from inflammation, fibrosis, thickening, or strictures.[10] Gallstones and infection are common causes. When no cause for the injury can be found, the process is called *idiopathic* or *primary sclerosing cholangitis (PSC).* The etiology of PSC is unknown, but genetic, immune, and infectious mechanisms are suspected. The disease occurs alone but is often associated with other disorders, most of which have a strong immunologic component. The most important link is with inflammatory bowel disease (IBD), and 3% to 5.6% of ulcerative colitis patients and 1.2% of Crohn's patients have PSC.[17] The PSC may precede the diagnosis of IBD or follow it from 1 to 20 years later. Patients with PSC are usually men, and the disease is diagnosed in early or middle adulthood, with an average age of 40.[25] PSC is the third most common reason for liver transplant in adults.

Pathophysiology. With PSC, inflammatory and fibrotic changes occur in and around the large bile ducts, gradually resulting in obstruction. Bile duct strictures can usually be found in multiple locations. The strictures alternate with normal or dilated segments of the ducts to create a beadlike appearance on x-ray examination. The disease does not usually involve the gallbladder or cystic duct. Liver biopsy documents the classic inflammation, fibrosis, proliferation, and ductal obliteration that confirm the presence of the disease. PSC is rarely diagnosed early, and in later stages biliary cirrhosis is also usually present (see Chapter 46), making the diagnosis complex.

Many patients are asymptomatic in early stages. Common complaints include fatigue, fever, jaundice, abdominal pain, and weight loss. Persistent, severe pruritus can be a particularly difficult aspect of the disease. Patients may experience recurrent attacks of cholangitis.

Collaborative Care Management. PSC is slowly progressive and difficult to diagnose. The classic symptoms overlap with those of other, more common GI disorders. PSC causes elevated liver enzymes and serum bilirubin levels, but elevation in alkaline phosphatase is considered the hallmark feature of the disease. ERCP (see Chapter 40) is used to visualize the biliary tree and reveals the characteristic structural problems of PSC.[1] Liver biopsy helps rule out other causes of the symptoms and assists in estimating the severity of the liver damage.

The prognosis of PSC largely depends on its clinical course, which is variable. The aggressiveness of the disease is influenced by the presence of infection and the development of complications related to cirrhosis and cholangiocarcinoma.[17] Survival is typically about 10 years after diagnosis unless a liver transplant is performed.

Drug therapy is aimed at reducing biliary tree inflammation and preventing the scarring that leads to obstruction. Steroids and other immunosuppressive agents have not proved effective, but the use of ursodeoxycholic acid has been shown to clearly improve the biochemical abnormalities of PSC. The mechanism of action of ursodeoxycholic acid is unknown. Endoscopic treatment to remove stones, relieve obstruction, dilate ducts, and place stent tubes is used primarily in clinical trials.[1] Liver transplantation is the only curative option.

PATIENT/FAMILY TEACHING. The uncertain course of PSC is one of its most difficult aspects. The nurse instructs patients about the disease and its possible outcomes and prepares them for the possibility of the eventual need for liver transplant. Persistent jaundice may negatively affect body image, and chronic, severe pruritus can be a daily nightmare. Some patients respond to cholestyramine resin, which theoretically binds the itch-triggering elements in the bile. The nurse also suggests that the patient experiment with common interventions that may lessen itching (see Patient/Family Teaching box). A low-fat diet is recommended to patients who develop problems with diarrhea or steatorrhea, and the fat restriction usually promptly corrects the problem. Fat-soluble vitamin replacement is often needed.

Carcinoma of the Biliary System

Etiology and Epidemiology. Primary tumors of the gallbladder are extremely rare, and their incidence may be declining because of prompt surgical intervention for gallbladder disease.[30] Their etiology is unknown. Gallbladder cancer occurs most commonly in persons older than 65 years of age and is three times as common in women. High-risk groups for gallbladder disease such as Native Americans have an increased risk of gallbladder cancer.[24] The presence of gallbladder stones is a significant risk factor for cancer. Most of the cancers of the biliary tract are primary adenocarcinomas of the bile ducts or gallbladder.

Cancer can also develop in the bile ducts and typically affects patients between 50 and 70 years of age. Cholangiocarcinoma is strongly associated with certain parasitic infections that affect small populations in various places in the world. Approximately 10% of patients with PSC develop cholangiocarcinoma.[24]

Pathophysiology. Carcinoma can occur anywhere in the biliary system. It has an insidious onset and metastasizes by direct extension and through the lymphatics and blood. Most patients have no early symptoms that are directly referable to the gallbladder; by the time the cancer produces symptoms, it is usually incurable.[30] When symptoms develop, they are similar to those seen with cholelithiasis and cholecystitis. Intermittent pain in the upper abdomen is the most common symptom. Anorexia, nausea, vomiting, weight loss, and jaundice may also be present. The patient may have a palpable abdominal mass. Signs and symptoms indicative of metastasis to the liver or pancreas may also be present. The development of jaundice indicates spread beyond the gallbladder.

PATIENT/FAMILY TEACHING
Strategies to Control Pruritus

- Avoid irritating clothing (wool or restrictive clothing).
- Use tepid water for bathing rather than hot water.
  —Experiment with nonirritating soaps and detergents.
  —Pat skin dry after bathing or showering; do not rub.
- Apply emollient creams and lotions to dry skin regularly.
- Maintain a cool environment, and ensure adequate amounts of humidity in the air.
- Avoid activities that increase body temperature or cause sweating.
- Experiment with treatments such as oatmeal baths.
- Keep the fingernails short, and consider use of cotton gloves at night to minimize skin damage from scratching.
- Use antipruritic medications as ordered.

Collaborative Care Management. Surgery is the primary treatment for cancer of the gallbladder. When the disease is found incidentally, it may be confined to the gallbladder and be curable with surgery. Cholecystectomy with wedge resection into the liver plus lymph node dissection is usually performed. Survival for those with invasive disease is usually less than 2 years. Neither radiotherapy nor chemotherapy has thus far improved patient outcomes.

Treatment of cholangiocarcinoma focuses on maintaining the patency of bile flow. Surgery may be used to divert bile flow to the jejunum, or stent tubes may be placed to attempt to maintain duct patency. When bile flow can be maintained, patients may live for several years after diagnosis.

PATIENT/FAMILY TEACHING. Nursing intervention focuses on helping the patient self-manage the symptoms and possibly care for bile drainage systems. The remainder of care and teaching are generally supportive, since the patient and family face an uncertain future and poor prognosis. General care of the cancer patient is discussed in Chapter 23.

Problems of the Pancreas

Acute Pancreatitis

Etiology and Epidemiology. Acute pancreatitis is a clinical syndrome of pancreatic inflammation with varying amounts of injury to the gland and adjacent organs.[26] The defining characteristics of the syndrome are abdominal pain and elevated pancreatic enzyme levels. The two major causes of acute pancreatitis in the United States are biliary stones and alcohol abuse. Together they account for more than 80% of all cases.[18] Other, less common causes of pancreatitis include trauma, cancer, drug toxicities, infectious diseases, and other chronic diseases of the GI tract. In more than 10% of cases no underlying cause can be identified.[26]

The incidence of acute pancreatitis has increased in recent years, but this increase may represent improved diagnostic capabilities rather than a true increase in the number of cases. The current annual incidence is estimated to be one to five cases per 10,000 population.[28] Acute pancreatitis may follow a mild, severe, or fulminant course. The overall mortality rate for acute pancreatitis remains at about 5%, rising to 20% for severe acute pancreatitis.[10] The disease may be recurrent, and repeated episodes can lead to chronic pancreatitis in approximately 10% of cases.[18]

Patients with biliary pancreatitis are likely to be 55 to 65 years of age and predominantly female, whereas patients with alcohol-related pancreatitis are usually slightly younger and predominantly male. Risk factors for acute pancreatitis are summarized in the Risk Factors box.

ALCOHOL-RELATED PANCREATITIS. The role of alcohol in the development of acute pancreatitis is well recognized clinically but remains poorly explained. Alcohol is presumed to have a direct toxic effect on the pancreas in selected persons, probably through some increased susceptibility to injury. Alcohol is theorized to interfere with pancreatic function in several ways. Alcohol both stimulates pancreatic secretions and triggers spasm in the sphincter of Oddi, a combination that can result in obstruction. Alcohol

Risk Factors

Acute Pancreatitis

Major

Biliary stones
Alcohol use or abuse

Minor

Age

55 to 65 years for biliary pancreatitis
45 to 55 years for alcohol-related pancreatitis

Sex

Female for biliary pancreatitis
Male for alcohol-related pancreatitis

Other Gastrointestinal Tract Problems

Trauma
Infectious disease
Cancer
Chronic diseases (e.g., inflammatory bowel disease)
Drug toxicities

NOTE: Ten percent of cases cannot be attributed to any identifiable risk factors.

may also change the composition of proteins secreted by the pancreas, possibly causing protein plugs to form in the small ducts. Alcohol weakens cell membranes and makes the acinar cells more vulnerable to injury and is also known to decrease the amount of trypsin inhibitor available, which increases the risk of injury. Alcohol alters both systemic and pancreatic lipid metabolism and can exacerbate hyperlipidemia.[26] All these factors are believed to contribute to the development of alcohol-related pancreatitis, but none of them adequately explains the disease.

BILIARY PANCREATITIS. Although gallstone disease is clearly linked to acute pancreatitis, only a small number of patients with gallstones ever develop the disease. It is likely that most cases of biliary pancreatitis are caused by transient obstruction of the ampulla of Vater. Stones have been recovered from the stool of 30% to 85% of patients with gallstone pancreatitis, confirming stone migration.[26] How the obstruction activates the pancreatic enzymes is not known, but the obstruction does not have to be prolonged to initiate acute inflammation. The presence of tiny gallstones (microlithiasis or biliary sludge) too small to be identified by imaging studies is believed to play a role. There is also considerable evidence that structural abnormalities that lead to narrowing at the sphincter of Oddi can cause biliary pancreatitis. It is theorized that obstruction can temporarily reverse the normal pancreatic pressure gradient and permit reflux of bile or duodenal contents into the pancreatic ducts.

Pathophysiology. The two major pathologic varieties of acute pancreatitis are (1) the acute interstitial form and (2) the acute hemorrhagic form. Either form can be fatal, but the interstitial form is often a milder disease.

In acute interstitial pancreatitis the gland is diffusely swollen and inflamed but retains its normal anatomic features. Neither hemorrhage nor necrosis is present. The interstitial spaces become grossly swollen by extracellular edema, and the ducts may contain purulent material. The acute hemorrhagic disease has a very different presentation. The gland is acutely inflamed, and both hemorrhage and marked tissue necrosis are present. Extensive fat necrosis is evident in patients with fulminant disease, not just in the pancreas but throughout the abdominal and thoracic cavities and subcutaneous tissues.[7] Necrosis of blood vessels can cause significant loss of blood, and abscesses and infection form in areas of walled-off necrotic tissue. Systemic complications such as fat emboli, hypotension, shock, and fluid overload are common. Organ failure occurs in about 50% of patients with pancreatic necrosis.[10,26] Pancreatic secretions normally contain only inactive forms of the proteolytic enzymes. The pancreas secretes a trypsin inhibitor specifically to prevent activation of these enzymes within the gland, because once trypsinogen is activated to trypsin, it can then activate the other enzymes as well. Activation of the pancreatic enzymes before they reach the duodenum has long been recognized as a major component of the disease process. The mystery of acute pancreatitis is how that pathologic sequence is initiated. The etiologic roles of alcohol and biliary disease have been discussed, but they fail to fully explain the disease process. Enzyme activation overwhelms all the normal protective mechanisms of the pancreas and initiates a massive attack on the pancreatic tissues, a process called pancreatic **autodigestion**. Other systemic effects of the activated enzymes include:

- Activation of complement and kinin, producing increased vascular permeability and vasodilation
- Increased stickiness of the inflammatory leukocytes with the formation of emboli, which plug the microvasculature
- Initiation of consumptive coagulopathy, leading to disseminated intravascular coagulation
- Increased vascular permeability, causing massive movement of fluids, which leads to circulatory insufficiency
- Release of myocardial depressant factor, which further compromises cardiac function
- Activation of the renin-angiotensin network, which impairs renal function in conjunction with circulatory insufficiency

Figure 44-4 outlines the major pathologic events that can occur in acute pancreatitis. The clinical manifestations of acute pancreatitis vary somewhat according to the severity of the attack. Acute pain in the epigastric region is the hallmark of the disease and occurs in 95% of all patients.[26] The pain is usually steady and may radiate to the lower thorax and back. It is typically worsened by lying supine, and patients may curve their backs and draw their knees up toward the body in an attempt to diminish its intensity. The classic pain is deep and visceral and may persist for hours or days. In severe cases the pain is agonizing. The pain is variously attributed to stretching of the pancreatic capsule, obstruction of the biliary tree, or chemical burning of the peritoneum by activated enzymes.

Nausea and vomiting occur in 85% of patients.[28] The severity of the vomiting varies and is typically worsened by the ingestion of food or fluid. Vomiting does not relieve the pain and may become protracted. Physical findings for patients with severe pancreatitis include abdominal tenderness and rigidity, progressive abdominal distention, and decreased bowel activity. Fever is common, but it rarely exceeds 102° F (39° C). Fulminant disease may progress to hypovolemic shock, ascites, acute tubular necrosis,

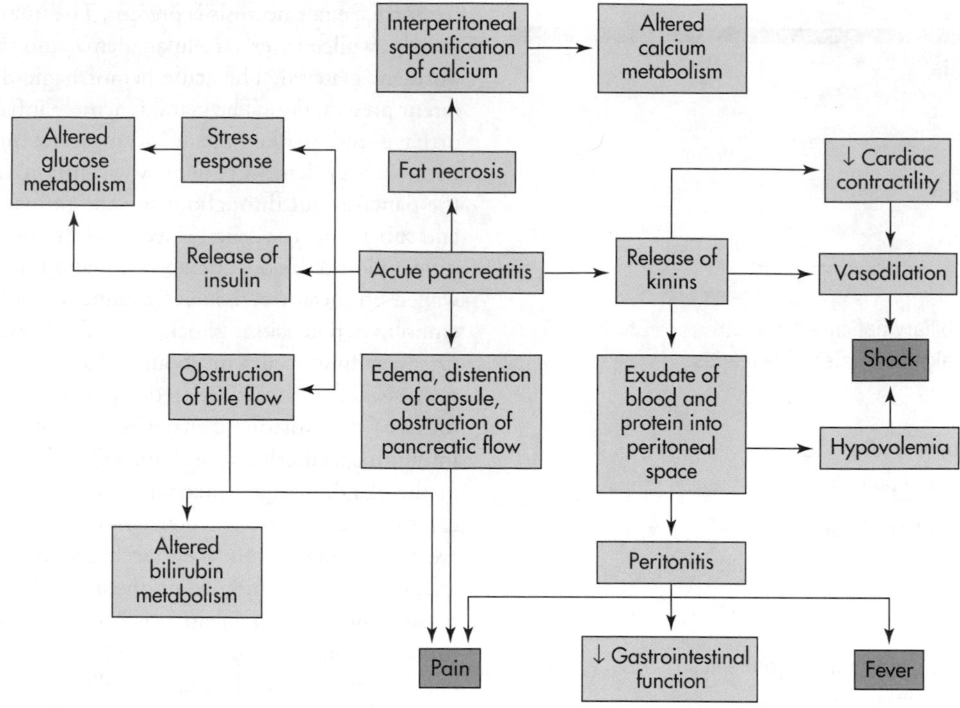

Figure 44-4 Major pathologic events that occur in acute pancreatitis.

and respiratory failure with acute respiratory distress syndrome (ARDS). The clinical manifestations of mild and severe pancreatitis are summarized in the Clinical Manifestations box.

COMPLICATIONS. The course of acute pancreatitis is not always apparent; about 25% of patients who experience acute pancreatitis develop complications, and most deaths associated with the disease occur in that group of patients. Complications may be local or systemic. The systemic complications tend to occur within the first week and have largely been discussed within the context of the fulminant disease process. These include complications such as hypovolemic shock, sepsis, renal failure, and ARDS (Box 44-1). Bedside assessment alone is often inadequate. Several clinical prognostic rating scales have been developed to help clinicians identify patients at greatest risk (Box 44-2). The Ranson scale tracks 11 separate criteria; five are evaluated at admission, and the remainder within the first 48 hours. The simplified Glasgow scale tracks just eight criteria and appears to be equally accurate.

PSEUDOCYSTS. Pseudocysts, localized collections of fluid enclosed in a fibrous capsule, occur in about 10% of all acute pancreatitis patients.[26] Pseudocysts may resolve over time, and intervention is not always warranted. However, pseudocysts can become life threatening if they obstruct neighboring structures, rupture or hemorrhage, or become infected. A "wait and see" policy, with regular monitoring, is generally followed. Progressive enlargement of the pseudocyst or signs of early infection are indications for drainage. Inflammatory exudate from the pancreas may form into an inflamed mass, which is called a phlegmon. Again, intervention is not indicated unless bleeding or infection develops. Pseudocysts and phlegmons can be drained endoscopically, percutaneously, or surgically depending on their size and location.[26]

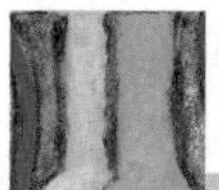

CLINICAL MANIFESTATIONS
Acute Pancreatitis

Pain

Steady and severe; excruciating in fulminant cases
Located in the epigastric or umbilical region; may radiate to the back
Worsened by lying supine; may be lessened by flexed knee, curved-back positioning

Vomiting

Varies in severity but is usually protracted
Worsened by ingestion of food or fluid
Does not relieve the pain
Usually accompanied by nausea

Fever

Rarely exceeds 102° F (39° C)

Abdominal Findings

Rigidity, tenderness, guarding
Distention
Decreased or absent peristalsis

Additional Features of Fulminant Disease

Symptoms of hypovolemic shock
Oliguria: acute tubular necrosis
Ascites
Jaundice
Respiratory failure
Grey-Turner's sign (bluish discoloration along the flanks)*
Cullen's sign (bluish discoloration around the umbilicus)*

*NOTE: These signs indicate the accumulation of blood in these areas and represent the presence of hemorrhagic pancreatitis.

BOX 44-1 Major Complications of Acute Pancreatitis

- Hypotension or shock from hypovolemia or hypoalbuminemia
- Leukocytosis from generalized inflammation or secondary infections, anemia from blood loss, disseminated intravascular coagulation from unknown causes
- Atelectasis, pneumonia, pleural effusion, acute respiratory distress syndrome
- Gastrointestinal bleeding
- Pancreatic pseudocysts, pancreatic necrosis or phlegmon, pancreatic abscesses, pancreatic ascites
- Oliguria and acute tubular necrosis
- Hyperglycemia, hypocalcemia, hyperlipidemia

BOX 44-2 Two Representative Prognostic Scoring Systems Used in Acute Pancreatitis

Ranson

Admission
Age >55 years
WBC count >16,000 cells/mm^3
LDH >350 IU/L
AST >250 IU/L
Glucose >200 mg/dl

Initial 48 Hours
Hematocrit decrease >10%
BUN increase >5 mg/dl
Calcium <8 mg/dl
Po_2 <60 mm Hg
Base deficit >4
Estimated fluid sequestration >6 L

Glasgow

Within 48 Hours of Admission
Age >55 years
WBC count >15,000 cells/mm^3
Glucose >180 mg/dl
BUN >45 mg/dl
Po_2 <60 mm Hg
Albumin <3.2 g/dl
Calcium <8 mg/dl
LDH >600 IU/L

Modified from Agarwal N, Pitchumoni CS: Assessment of severity in acute pancreatitis, *Am J Gastroenterol* 85:356, 1990; and Marshall JB: Acute pancreatitis: a review with an emphasis on new developments, *Arch Intern Med* 153:1185, 1993.

AST, Aspartate transaminase; *BUN,* blood urea nitrogen; *LDH,* lactic dehydrogenase; *Po_2,* partial pressure of oxygen; *WBC,* white blood cell.

PANCREATIC INFECTION. Pancreatic infection is the most frequent cause of serious morbidity and mortality associated with acute pancreatitis. Infection typically appears 8 to 20 days after the onset of pancreatitis and has a 100% mortality rate if untreated. Infection usually develops in the areas of necrosis created by fulminant disease and then spreads into adjacent tissue. The initial diagnosis of infection can be complicated by the fact that acute pancreatitis itself manifests with the common symptoms of inflammation and infection. Infection-related fever, however, typically exceeds 102° F (39° C), and the patient's clinical condition can deteriorate rapidly.

CT scanning allows for the accurate identification of areas of necrosis, which can then be aspirated by CT-guided needle aspiration.[22] Gram stain and culture of the aspirate can identify the specific organisms responsible for the infection. Broad-spectrum antibiotics are initiated immediately, but definitive therapy requires percutaneous drainage or surgical debridement. Attempts to prevent infection with the prophylactic use of antibiotics have not proved consistently effective, but intravenous (IV) prophylactic antibiotics do appear to reduce the incidence of complications in patients with severe disease and extensive necrosis.[26]

CHRONIC PANCREATITIS. Patients with alcohol-induced acute pancreatitis are believed to already have asymptomatic chronic disease when they experience their first acute episode. If the patient continues to drink, the likelihood of developing chronic pancreatitis is extremely high. Chronic pancreatitis is similar to acute pancreatitis in presentation, but it reflects a very different pathologic process (see p. 1296).

Collaborative Care Management

DIAGNOSTIC TESTS. The diagnosis of acute pancreatitis is based on the presence of acute abdominal pain and an elevated serum amylase level, which rises within a few hours of the onset of the disease. In mild disease amylase may remain elevated for only a few days. No apparent relationship exists between the severity of the disease and the height of the enzyme levels. Levels of urinary amylase may also be measured if the patient has adequate kidney function. Serum lipase elevations are also diagnostic and persist for up to 7 days. Lipase levels are more reliable indicators than amylase if the patient is not evaluated until several days after the onset of illness.[22] Neither amylase nor lipase elevations are exclusive to pancreatic disease, which complicates diagnosis in questionable cases. Other potential laboratory findings are included in Box 44-3.

Abdominal x-ray studies are performed on all patients with acute abdominal pain to rule out other problems such as perforation. Ultrasonography is the best noninvasive method for identifying gallstones and can reveal pancreatic edema if the gland can be visualized. However, it is often obscured by gas and ileus. Computed tomography (CT) scanning can estimate the size of the pancreas; identify cysts, abscesses, and masses; and, with a

BOX 44-3 Laboratory Tests Used in Diagnosing Acute Pancreatitis

- Serum amylase: levels elevated within a few hours of disease onset
- Serum lipase: levels remain elevated up to 7 days after disease onset
- Serum glucose: hyperglycemia of 500 to 900 mg/dl
- Serum calcium: hypocalcemia from calcium sequestering in abdomen; hypocalcemia is a poor prognostic sign
- Liver function tests: elevations commonly seen
- Urinary amylase: elevated when kidney function is adequate

contrast medium, clearly diagnose hemorrhagic disease. It is a useful tool for diagnosing acute pancreatitis, although it is usually only needed for patients with severe disease and suspected complications.

MEDICATIONS. No effective drug treatment is available for acute pancreatitis, but research is ongoing.[12] Drug therapy to reduce pancreatic secretion has not been shown to have any therapeutic effect. Pain management is the primary consideration, and patients may require substantial amounts of opioids. Synthetic opioids such as meperidine (Demerol) have traditionally been used because they do not cause spasm in the sphincter of Oddi. Morphine, however, is now believed to have minimal effects on the sphincter and is a more effective analgesic. Hydromorphone is also an option for severe pain.

TREATMENTS. There are no known treatments for pancreatitis. Most patients with mild to moderate disease receive general supportive care. Nasogastric (NG) suctioning has often been used, but it is probably not necessary unless the patient develops ileus or experiences persistent vomiting.

Fluid and electrolyte replacement is critical. Pancreatitis often leads to "third spacing," and the loss of intravascular fluid through membrane leakage averages 4 to 6 L, or more in severe cases. Prevention of hypovolemic shock necessitates aggressive fluid management. Urinary output should remain at or above 30 to 50 ml/hr. Potassium losses can also be significant in both vomitus and pancreatic fluids, and serum levels must be supported. Hypocalcemia often develops, and replacement may be initiated if the patient becomes symptomatic. Hyperglycemia may also be present, and exogenous insulin may be needed in severe disease. It is used cautiously, however, because patients with acute pancreatitis are vulnerable to severe hypoglycemia from decreased glycogen and glucagon reserves.[26] The removal of retained gallstones by ERCP reduces overall morbidity in the select group of patients in whom an obstructing stone can be identified.

Peritoneal lavage has occasionally been used in patients with severe pancreatitis in an attempt to remove toxic substances, but the effectiveness of this treatment has not been proven. More aggressive and invasive interventions are used with patients who are at high risk for complications.

SURGICAL MANAGEMENT. Surgery is not a routine part of the management of acute pancreatitis, but surgical intervention may be necessary to control related problems such as pseudocyst, or abscess. Percutaneous drainage is used most effectively with infected pseudocysts because minimal particulate matter is present that can clog the tubes. The traditional surgical approach has been to excise as much necrotic material as possible and then place multiple large-bore sump drains in the operative areas to remove infected material. Continuous saline infusion and suction are needed to maintain tube patency. Many surgeons use an open method in which the resected areas are packed, and the dressings are changed with the patient under anesthesia every 2 to 3 days until granulation is well under way. The abdomen is left open and eventually closes over an absorbable mesh barrier. A feeding tube can be placed once granulation is under way. The development of fistulas can complicate the healing process.

DIET. The patient is given nothing by mouth (NPO) until the abdominal pain has subsided and amylase levels have returned to normal. This practice, in theory, rests the pancreas and limits the secretion of enzymes. Most patients recover without complications or sequelae. Oral fluids and feedings can usually be resumed within 3 to 7 days and gradually advanced to a normal diet once peristalsis is reestablished. Hunger is a good indicator of readiness for eating.[26] There is no clinical proof of the need for a low-fat diet or any other dietary restrictions during recovery except for abstinence from alcohol. Patients recovering from severe pancreatitis may begin an oral diet even when elevations in amylase and lipase have not yet returned to normal if they are symptom free.

Total enteral or parenteral nutrition may be implemented for patients who are unable to eat for extended periods. Enteral nutrition is preferred to parenteral, although either can be used. A nasojejeunal feeding tube may be placed for enteral nutrition. Efforts are made to keep plasma albumin levels above 3.5 g/dl and total protein values above 6.5g/dl, thereby maintaining a positive nitrogen balance.

HEALTH PROMOTION AND PREVENTION. There are no proven strategies for preventing acute pancreatitis. The disease is associated with both alcohol abuse and biliary disease, however, and any measures designed to prevent either of those risk factors would indirectly reduce the risk of acute pancreatitis as well.

Nursing Management

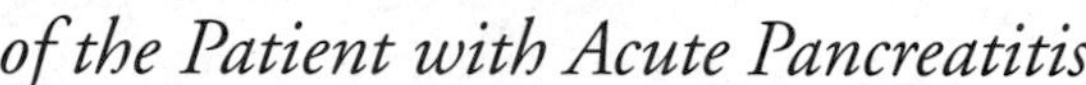

of the Patient with Acute Pancreatitis

ASSESSMENT

Health History. Assess for:

- History of gallbladder disease, treatment
- History of other GI diseases (e.g., peptic ulcer disease, IBD)
- History of alcohol use: amount and duration
- Medications in use: prescription, over the counter, and herbal preparations
- Onset and progression of symptoms such as:
  —Pain, which is often steady and severe; is located in the epigastric or umbilical region or may radiate to the back; worsens when patient is supine; is unrelieved by vomiting
  —Nausea and vomiting, which are usually severe and protracted, worsen with ingestion of food or fluid and do not relieve the pain

Physical Examination. Assess for:

- Vital sign indications of hypovolemia: tachycardia, tachypnea, normal to low blood pressure, restlessness, and anxiety
- Abdominal rigidity, distention, guarding, and tenderness to palpation
- Diminished or absent bowel sounds on auscultation
- Fever, which is generally no higher than 102° F (39° C)
- Signs of third spacing: falling urinary output, decreased skin turgor, dry or sticky mucous membranes, increased abdominal girth

- General affect: appearing distressed, lying with knees pulled toward abdomen
- Presence of Grey-Turner's or Cullen's sign: bluish discoloration on flanks or around umbilicus

NURSING DIAGNOSES, OUTCOMES, AND INTERVENTIONS

Nursing Diagnosis: Acute Pain

OUTCOMES. Common examples of expected outcomes for the patient with a diagnosis of *acute pain* are:

Patient will:

- State that pain is controlled.
- Display a relaxed, nondistressed appearance.
- Not guard or limit activity or movement.

NURSING INTERVENTIONS. Control of pain is a major priority, and either morphine or meperidine may be administered. Critically ill patients may receive a continuous IV infusion of opioids supplemented by boluses as needed for breakthrough pain. Patient-controlled analgesia is used if feasible to allow for successful pain management. The nurse frequently assesses the patient's level of pain using a scale of 1 to 10 and evaluates the patient's response to interventions. The physician is consulted for needed changes in the regimen. Epidural analgesia may be considered if the pain persists and is not relieved by routine opioid administration. Staff occasionally exhibit the attitude that patients with alcohol-induced pancreatitis are "getting what they deserve," especially on repeat admissions for recurrent disease. The nurse must serve as the patient's advocate in the system, documenting the severity of the patient's pain and ensuring that an effective plan is in place to manage it. The early involvement of a pain specialty team may be helpful in designing and implementing a comprehensive plan for pain management.

Some patients find that the pain decreases if they assume a sitting position with the trunk flexed or a side-lying position with their knees drawn up to the abdomen. Although the research is currently inconclusive, most patients are NPO to "rest" the pancreas and decrease the autodigestive process. An NG tube may be inserted to keep the stomach decompressed if vomiting persists.

The nurse also explores with the patient the use of a variety of nonpharmacologic pain relief strategies, such as distraction, imagery, massage, and back rubs. The environment is kept quiet, comfortable, and conducive to rest. These measures are used in addition to, and not in place of, opioid administration for pain control.

RELATED NIC INTERVENTIONS. Coping Enhancement, Medication Management, Pain Management

Nursing Diagnosis: Deficient Fluid Volume

OUTCOMES. A common example of an expected outcome for the patient with a diagnosis of *deficient fluid volume* is:

Patient will:

- Maintain adequate fluid volume as demonstrated by normal blood pressure, absence of orthostatic blood pressure changes, normal skin turgor, moist mucous membranes, and adequate urinary output.

NURSING INTERVENTIONS. As soon as the patient is admitted, the nurse institutes monitoring related to fluid and electrolyte status, cardiac output, and renal status. Monitoring includes intake and output; vital signs; daily weights; abdominal girth; and all routine laboratory values with particular emphasis on hematocrit, potassium, and calcium levels. The nurse also assesses for physical signs of hypokalemia and hypocalcemia (see Chapter 17). An indwelling Foley catheter may be inserted to monitor renal function, which can be impaired by poor renal perfusion from hypotension or shock. Monitoring parameters and the frequency of monitoring depend on the patient's stability.

Aggressive fluid replacement necessitates establishing and maintaining adequate IV access. Fluids, electrolytes, colloids, or blood is administered as necessary. The nurse is responsible for administering the fluids and monitoring the patient's response. The development of hypovolemic shock is of particular concern in the early days of the disease, and the nurse monitors carefully for early signs of shock (see Chapter 19). Blood glucose is checked four times a day to monitor for hyperglycemia, which can further contribute to fluid losses. If severe hyperglycemia occurs, it may be treated with insulin.

RELATED NIC INTERVENTIONS. Fluid/Electrolyte Management, Fluid Monitoring, Hyperglycemia Management, Intravenous (IV) Therapy, Surveillance

Nursing Diagnosis: Imbalanced Nutrition: Less Than Body Requirements

OUTCOMES. A common example of an expected outcome for the patient with a diagnosis of *imbalanced nutrition: less than body requirements* is:

Patient will:

- Gradually resume a normal oral diet and regain lost weight.

NURSING INTERVENTIONS. The patient is kept NPO and may have an NG tube in place. Good oral hygiene is necessary to decrease discomfort from dry mouth and irritation from the NG tube. Enteral or parenteral feedings may be used during the critical phase of the illness. When the acute symptoms subside, oral fluids and food are restarted. The patient is given clear liquids and then slowly advanced toward a regular diet. The nurse carefully monitors the patient for tolerance for oral feedings and the return of pain. Frequent small meals are usually better tolerated in the early refeeding period. The only dietary restriction after discharge is the avoidance of alcohol. Restriction of fat in the diet has no proven effect on healing.

RELATED NIC INTERVENTIONS. Enteral Tube Feeding, Nausea Management, Nutrition Therapy, Nutritional Monitoring, Total Parenteral Nutrition (TPN) Administration, Vomiting Management

Nursing Diagnosis: Ineffective Health Maintenance

OUTCOMES. A common example of an expected outcome for the patient with a diagnosis of *ineffective health maintenance* is:

Patient will:

- Adopt optimal health practices and control alcohol intake as appropriate.

NURSING INTERVENTIONS. If unhealthy lifestyle patterns such as alcoholism are a cause of acute pancreatitis, the nurse must help the patient realistically address the problem. This care is begun once the patient's condition has stabilized and before he or she leaves the hospital. See Chapter 3 for further information about promoting a healthy lifestyle. Achieving and sustaining sobriety can be extremely challenging, but a severe attack of acute pancreatitis may leave the patient ready to take steps along the path to alcohol abstinence. The nurse ensures that the patient and family have all the information and referrals they need to plan intelligently for the future.

If the patient's pancreatitis is related to biliary disease, it is important to discuss treatment for gallstones. Pancreatitis is frightening and could make the patient reluctant to undergo any further medical or surgical treatment. The nurse reinforces the etiologic role of biliary disease in acute pancreatitis and encourages the patient to follow through on recommended treatment.

RELATED NIC INTERVENTIONS. Risk Identification, Substance Use Treatment, Teaching: Disease Process

Patient/Family Teaching. Education for the patient and family is an ongoing part of nursing care. At the beginning of the hospitalization, the patient and significant others need basic information about acute pancreatitis, planned diagnostic tests, and the rationale for the proposed treatment. Because of the pain and distress that acute pancreatitis causes and the seriousness of the disease process, the patient and family may experience tremendous anxiety. Therefore explanations and instructions need to be brief and as simple as possible and may need to be repeated frequently. Support and continuity of care also help decrease anxiety.

Education is directed toward preventing future attacks and maintaining a nutritious diet. The patient must know to immediately report any return of the signs and symptoms of acute pancreatitis. The nurse explains the plan for follow-up care in detail and provides written instructions to the patient and family. Every effort is made to assist the patient and family to accept the need for alcohol treatment and cessation. The nurse ensures that the patient has all relevant information about alcohol treatment facilities and supports in the community.

A Nursing Care Plan for a patient with a diagnosis of *acute pancreatitis* is found on p. 1298.

EVALUATION

To evaluate the effectiveness of nursing interventions, compare patient behaviors with those stated in the expected patient outcomes.

RELATED NOC OUTCOMES. Comfort Level, Fluid Balance, Knowledge: Disease Process, Nausea & Vomiting Severity, Nutritional Status: Food & Fluid Intake, Pain Control, Risk Control: Alcohol Use

GERONTOLOGIC CONSIDERATIONS

Biliary disease becomes increasingly common as people age, and biliary disease–related pancreatitis is most likely to occur in the older patient. The severity of the disease is difficult to predict, but older adults with acute pancreatitis may become critically ill faster because of comorbid conditions. Older adults are also more likely to develop complications from both the pancreatitis and the disease-enforced immobility. Respiratory complications are of particular concern, and the older patient needs frequent respiratory assessment and aggressive pulmonary hygiene during the acute stage of the disease.

Infection is a common complication of pancreatitis (see discussion under Complications), and older patients are less able to withstand the stress imposed on the body by sepsis. The same is true for the development of hypovolemia and fluid shifts. These factors strain the cardiovascular system and may overwhelm the older patient's ability to adapt and respond.

Chronic Pancreatitis

Etiology and Epidemiology. Chronic pancreatitis is a separate disorder from recurrent acute pancreatitis. In acute pancreatitis the gland gradually returns to normal as the inflammation resolves. Chronic pancreatitis is characterized by persistent and progressive functional and morphologic damage to the tissue. Fibrosis and scar tissue gradually replace the normal pancreatic tissue.

Alcohol consumption accounts for 70% to 80% of cases of chronic pancreatitis in the United States.[10] Both the amount and duration of alcohol consumption appear to be contributory; it generally takes at least 5 to 10 years of heavy drinking to produce symptomatic disease. Since alcohol use is pervasive and chronic pancreatitis is rare, obviously other factors are at work as well. The actual prevalence of the disease is unknown, and subclinical pancreatic drainage may be more common than currently recognized. Other potential causes of chronic pancreatitis include obstruction, trauma, and metabolic disturbances. Twenty percent of cases are considered idiopathic. Malnutrition is the most common cause of chronic pancreatitis in developing countries. Hereditary pancreatitis is rare, making up only 1% of all cases of chronic pancreatitis.[9] The Future Watch box explores early genetic research that shows promise in increasing our understanding of the incidence of chronic pancreatitis.

Pathophysiology. The basic pathologic change of chronic pancreatitis is destruction of the exocrine parenchyma and replacement

Future Watch

Predicting Pancreatitis?

A number of genetic mutations are associated with chronic pancreatitis. The mutant trypsinogen gene (PRSS1) is linked to hereditary pancreatitis. This is an autosomal dominant trait identified on chromosome 7. Serine protease inhibitor, Kazal type 1 (SPINK1), along with the cystic fibrosis transmembrane conductance regulator (CFTR), have been shown to be associated with idiopathic chronic pancreatitis. These mutations appear to have a direct or indirect influence on chronic pancreatitis. Greater understanding of these mutations may enable researchers to develop additional approaches to test, identify, and treat chronic pancreatitis at an early stage.

Current research also continues to investigate the role and importance of these genetic mutations and their relationships to one another. The SPINK1 mutations, but not the CFTR mutations, have been identified in a portion of alcoholic pancreatitis patients. The PRSS1 mutations have been identified in some idiopathic pancreatitis patients.

with fibrous tissue. This process is associated with varying degrees of duct dilation. Scarring and fibrotic changes may occur throughout the pancreas or be limited to selected areas. Calcium salts may be deposited in both the ducts and the parenchyma; the factors that influence the solubility of calcium in the calcium-rich pancreatic secretions are not well identified. As the process becomes increasingly severe, the islets of Langerhans are gradually destroyed. The disease therefore can lead to insufficiency or failure of both the exocrine and endocrine functions of the gland.

The patient with chronic pancreatitis may exhibit symptoms that are similar to those of acute pancreatitis. Abdominal pain is again the major symptom, and it is described as severe in intensity, dull in quality, and constant. The pain is epigastric, may radiate to the back or both upper quadrants, and is immediately worsened by eating. As the disease progresses, the pain of chronic pancreatitis may persist, diminish, or even disappear. The mechanisms underlying the pain are unclear but may include nerve inflammation and increased pressure.[21]

Nausea, vomiting, anorexia, and weight loss are other common symptoms of chronic pancreatitis. Weight loss occurs primarily from decreased caloric intake related to pain, but malabsorption may also play a role.

Pancreatic insufficiency begins once the majority of the pancreatic tissue has been destroyed.[20] Diarrhea and steatorrhea develop when the secretion of pancreatic enzymes is too low to support normal digestion. Diabetes is common and may precede other clinical symptoms. Unique impairments in glucose metabolism make patients with chronic pancreatitis extremely vulnerable to hypoglycemia, and their need for insulin is smaller than expected. Oral hypoglycemic agents are not effective. Malabsorption also leads to clinical deficiencies in vitamins E and B_{12} and other fat-soluble vitamins, but patients rarely develop overt symptoms of deficiency.

Collaborative Care Management. The diagnosis of chronic pancreatitis is suggested by the history and presenting symptoms and then confirmed by diagnostic tests. Serum enzyme levels may be elevated, normal, or low. Diffuse calcification can be seen on abdominal x-ray and ultrasound studies, and CT scanning reveals dilation of the pancreatic ducts and cystic lesions. Stool analysis can quantify the severity of the steatorrhea and estimate the degree of pancreatic insufficiency.

Treatment of chronic pancreatitis is directed at pain control and the correction of malabsorption. Effective management of abdominal pain is the greatest challenge. Patients who continue to consume alcohol usually continue to experience pain, and eventually even abstinence is no guarantee of relief. Patients can usually adapt to the malabsorption and steatorrhea, but the persistent pain can be incapacitating and lead to drug dependence.

Flare-ups of chronic pancreatitis are managed similarly to the acute disease. "Bowel rest" is maintained, and attention is paid to managing the acute pain. Nonopioid analgesics are used if possible, but the pain is often severe enough to necessitate opioid administration. Octreotide is a synthetic analog of somatostatin that inhibits pancreatic secretion and may be useful for patients who do not respond to conventional pain treatment.

Ongoing care involves a low-fat diet and supplemental pancreatic enzymes. These enzymes improve absorption and help the patient gain weight, increasing the patient's general sense of well-being. The recommended diet is high in protein and carbohydrates and may provide as much as 3000 to 6000 cal/day. The use of medium-chain triglycerides to improve the patient's nutritional state is being evaluated. Fat-soluble vitamin replacement may also be indicated, and the management of diabetes often requires the use of insulin.

Chronic pancreatitis affects the small ducts of the pancreas and is usually not amenable to surgical correction. However, surgical intervention may be used to relieve ductal obstruction, bypass obstructed parts of the gland, or resect small or large parts of the diseased pancreas. Outcomes of these procedures are not predictable. A celiac plexus block is occasionally used to interrupt pain transmission.

The nurse serves as the patient's advocate in the search for comfort. Concerns about drug dependence must not be allowed to prevent the patient from receiving adequate and necessary analgesia. Health care providers can easily become frustrated with patients who are unable or unwilling to stop drinking and may begin to consider the pain of chronic pancreatitis an appropriate retribution for the patient's addiction. This attitude can seriously compromise the patient's care.

In some instances the patient has had negative experiences with pain management during previous hospitalizations and believes that analgesics are not being given because the health care team does not care about him or her. The involvement of a pain management team is appropriate if such services are available. See Chapter16 for further discussion of pain management.

PATIENT/FAMILY TEACHING. The role of alcohol in the etiology and progression of chronic pancreatitis is unequivocal, and yet many patients find themselves unable or unwilling to abstain from alcohol use. The nurse consults with a substance abuse specialist to develop a consistent and appropriate approach for the patient's care and ensures that the patient has all the information necessary to make informed decisions about his or her present and future. The nurse offers the patient current and accurate information concerning community resources for alcohol treatment. The involvement of the family is encouraged if the family dynamics are supportive. Family members and health care workers need to be helped to understand and accept that ultimately it is the patient's right to make fundamental decisions about his or her own care, even when those decisions do not appear to be in the patient's own best interests.

The patient also needs to learn how to modify the diet and use pancreatic enzyme replacement pills or capsules (pancrelipase [Creon, Viokase]) effectively to control diarrhea and maintain a stable weight. Timing of the medications is critical. The nurse teaches the patient to take the capsules 1 to 2 hours before, during, or after meals. Powders can be mixed directly with food. Patients are informed that these products often have a bad taste and may alter the taste of foods. The patient is instructed to monitor the body's response to the supplements and consistently track weight changes. The anorexia and poor eating habits commonly associated with long-term alcohol use make adherence to a high-protein, high-calorie diet difficult. The use of vitamin supplements is encouraged if recommended by the physician.

Patients who continue to drink alcohol will always be just one step away from their next flare-up or complication. The nurse

Nursing Care Plan

Patient With Acute Pancreatitis

Data A 52-year-old man underwent a laparoscopic cholecystectomy 4 weeks ago after a 2-year history of occasional intermittent abdominal pain, which was relieved by vomiting. Today he is readmitted to the hospital with complaints of acute abdominal pain that is generally localized in the midepigastric region and radiates to his back. He rates the pain as 8 in severity on a 10-point scale. He states that he has had nothing to eat or drink and has been vomiting since late yesterday afternoon. He also states that he has had large, soft, foul-smelling stools that have been increasing in frequency and severity over the past couple of weeks. He has lost 6 pounds. The patient denies alcohol intake and his wife concurs.

Acute pancreatitits is the admitting diagnosis. The patient's vital signs are blood pressure, 94/60 mm Hg; pulse, 92 beats/min; respirations, 22 breaths/min and shallow; and temperature, 99.8° F (37.6° C) orally. Testing reveals that the patient's hemoglobin is 10.2 g/dl; red blood cell count, 2.9 million/mm^3; serum potassium, 3.0 mg/dl; serum calcium, 8.2 mg/dl; and glucose, 162 mg/dl. An intravenous (IV) drip of 1000 ml 5% dextrose in 50% normal saline with 20 mEq/L potassium chloride is initiated at 125 ml/hr. The patient is placed on nothing-by-mouth (NPO) status, and nasogastric intubation with suction is prescribed if vomiting persists. Meperidine (Demerol), 100 mg, is administered intramuscularly and then set up for IV PCA administration.

Nursing Diagnosis

Acute pain related to distention of pancreatic capsule and activation of pancreatic enzymes

Outcomes

- Patient will verbalize effective control of pain by rating it as less than 3 on a scale of 0 to 10.
- Patient will use patient-controlled analgesia to maintain pain at a tolerable level (less than 3).

Related NOC Outcomes

- Comfort Level
- Pain Control
- Pain Level

Related NIC Interventions

- Analgesic Administration
- Coping Enhancement
- Pain Management

Nursing Interventions/Rationales

- Assess pain levels frequently. *To validate the nature and severity of the patient's pain experience.*
- Document pain levels on flow record. *Allows nurse to establish a pattern of pain and evaluate the effectiveness of pain control methods.*
- Encourage patient to use the analgesic PCA on a regular basis, rather than as needed. *Allows for a steady blood level to be established and better pain control.*
- Validate your acceptance of the reality of the patient's pain and its severity. *To convey empathy and understanding. A patient may not complain of pain for fear of being perceived as a drug seeker.*
- Evaluate the effectiveness of the opioid analgesic. Collaborate with physician to make adjustments in dose or drug as needed. *Acute pain can be immobilizing. Morphine may be substituted for meperidine (some patients will experience sphincter of Oddi spasms from morphine).*
- Collaborate with wife to determine which nonpharmacologic methods have helped reduce pain in the past. *Nonpharmacologic methods allow the patient a degree of control of the pain experience and may augment pharmacologic pain control methods.*
- Explore patient's experience with strategies such as distraction, massage, relaxation, and guided imagery. *These methods can be effective in reducing pain, but the patient must be open minded and willing to experiment with new strategies.*
- Position patient in a mid- to high Fowler's position with his knees flexed. *This position is theorized to reduce tension on the abdomen and reduce pain.*

Nursing Diagnosis

Risk for deficient fluid volume related to vomiting, hyperglycemia, and increased capillary permeability secondary to acute pancreatitis

Outcomes

- Patient will maintain fluid and electrolyte balance within normal limits.
- Patient will maintain stable weight.

Related NOC Outcomes

- Electrolyte & Acid/Base Balance
- Fluid Balance
- Hydration

provides the patient with written material that outlines the symptoms of complications and encourages the patient to adhere to the plan for continued follow-up care.

▶ ARE You READY?

The nurse includes which statement in the dietary teaching for a patient with chronic pancreatitis?

1. "Limit alcohol intake to 1-2 drinks per day."
2. "Limit fluids to 1 L per day."
3. "Increase protein and carbohydrates in diet."
4. "Maintain caloric intake at 2500 calories per day."

Cancer of the Pancreas

Etiology and Epidemiology. Cancer of the pancreas is a malignant disease of the exocrine pancreas, and more than 90% of cases are ductal adenocarcinomas.[8] Nearly two thirds of these adenocarcinomas develop in the head of the pancreas; the remainder occur in the body or tail of the gland. Both benign and malignant tumors can also arise from the islet cells, but these are rare.

About 32,000 new cases of pancreatic cancer are diagnosed each year in the United States.[13] Pancreatic cancer occurs more commonly in men and adults over 60 years of age. The etiology is unknown, but cigarette smoking is believed to be an important causative agent. Incidences of familial clustering of the disease

Related NIC Interventions
- Fluid Management
- Fluid Monitoring
- Intravenous (IV) Therapy

Nursing Interventions/Rationales
- Assess fluid and electrolyte status each shift. *Patient is at risk for hypovolemic shock and dehydration and may lose 4 to 14 L of fluid into the abdomen (third spacing).*
- Maintain accurate intake and output. *Urinary output of 30 to 50 ml/hr is essential to prevent acute tubular necrosis. Fluid replacement is based on fluid losses.*
- Monitor weight daily. *Body weight is the most accurate method of assessing fluid gains and losses.*
- Assess skin turgor and status of mucous membranes each shift. *Good indicators of hydration or lack of hydration.*
- Maintain IV fluids at prescribed rate and flow. *To replace fluid losses and prevent hypovolemia and dehydration. Steady replacement helps prevent stressful fluid swings and decreases nausea.*
- Measure abdominal girth each shift until stabilized. *Fluid and gas accumulation in GI tract can result in significant abdominal distention.*
- Monitor blood glucose four times daily and administer sliding-scale insulin as prescribed. *Destruction of beta cells and islets of Langerhans produces severe hyperglycemia. Because of the risk of labile hypoglycemia, insulin is not given unless glucose level continues to rise.*
- Monitor for hypokalemia (muscle weakness, cramping) and hypocalcemia (numbness and tingling in fingertips or around mouth; positive Chvostek's and Trousseau's sign). *Large amounts of potassium are lost through vomiting and in the pancreatic secretions. Calcium is believed to bind with free fats and can drop to levels that increase neural excitability.*
- Monitor cardiovascular response to fluid replacement. *Fluid replacement can overload the intravascular space and place stress on the heart.*

Nursing Diagnosis
Imbalanced nutrition: less than body requirements related to vomiting, NPO status, and malabsorption secondary to pancreatitis

Outcomes
- Patient will maintain body weight within 5 pounds of baseline.
- Patient will maintain serum albumin levels above 3.8 g/dl
- Patient will not experience vomiting.
- Patient will produce normal stools.

Related NOC Outcomes
- Electrolyte & Acid/Base Balance
- Fluid Balance
- Nutritional Status
- Nutritional Status: Nutrient Intake

Related NIC Interventions
- Fluid/Electrolyte Management
- Fluid Monitoring
- Nausea Management
- Nutrition Management

Nursing Interventions/Rationales
- Maintain NPO status and bed rest until patient's condition stabilizes. *NPO status reduces the secretion of pancreatic enzymes. Bed rest decreases the body's metabolic rate.*
- Monitor daily weight, serum albumin, and serum protein levels. *These parameters provide the best ongoing data about nutritional status.*
- Initiate total parenteral nutrition (TPN) or enteral nutrition as prescribed if NPO status is prolonged. *The rapid catabolism of the disease must be counteracted by TPN or enteral nutrition to prevent life-threatening complications.*
- Reinitiate oral feedings once abdominal pain is controlled and amylase and lipase levels stabilize. *Once pain and enzyme levels are stable, there is no contraindication to oral feeding, and the malnourishment needs to be corrected.*
- Offer small, frequent feedings to the patient's tolerance and assess patient's response. *To minimize distention and malabsorption symptoms.*
- Restrict fat in the diet if steatorrhea persists. *Malabsorption primarily affects the digestion of fats.*
- Evaluate composition and volume of stools. Adjust dose of pancreatic enzymes to achieve normal elimination. *Malabsorption manifests as large-volume, greasy, foul-smelling stools. Adequate enzyme replacement will restore the stool to near normal.*

Evaluation
Evaluation is based on comparing the patient's outcomes with desired outcomes.

point to a hereditary component. Approximately 10% of all pancreatic cancer cases are attributable to genetic factors.[8] A history of pancreatitis, particularly chronic pancreatitis, also appears to increase the risk for developing pancreatic cancer. However, despite the proven link between alcohol abuse and pancreatitis, no evidence has yet been found to link alcohol ingestion and the development of pancreatic cancer. A diet high in fresh fruits and vegetables appears to play a protective role, as does the routine use of aspirin.[3]

Pathophysiology. Pancreatic tumors are usually deeply encased in normal tissue and can vary dramatically in size at the time of diagnosis. Tissue margins are frequently poorly demarcated, and metastasis has almost always occurred before the tumor produces its first symptoms, since the pancreas has no capsule surrounding it to contain the growth and extension of the tumor. The tumor frequently causes the common bile duct and pancreatic duct to distend and obstruct, blocking the flow of digestive enzymes and bile salts. Direct extension of the lesion may cause it to spread to the posterior wall of the stomach, the duodenal wall, the colon, the common bile duct, and lymph nodes. Vital blood vessels in the area are also commonly involved.

Pain and jaundice are the most common symptoms of pancreatic cancer.[8] The pain is usually described as epigastric in location, steady, and relentlessly progressive. Jaundice is another presenting symptom in the majority of patients with cancer in the head of the pancreas. Jaundice is produced from compression and obstruction of the bile duct. Bile duct obstruction also typically results in light-colored stools and dark, frothy urine. Weight loss is another common symptom, usually as a result of pain-related anorexia or malabsorption associated with the blockage of the flow of pancreatic enzymes from the pancreatic duct to the duodenum. Diarrhea and steatorrhea occur if pancreatic duct obstruction is severe.

Collaborative Care Management. The diagnosis of pancreatic cancer is often initially made on the basis of the patient's symptom pattern and then is confirmed through multiple radiologic studies. Ultrasound, helical CT scan, and magnetic resonance imaging are the most commonly used diagnostic scans. Endoscopic ultrasound with biopsy or fine-needle aspiration are the preferred techniques for sampling the tissue of the pancreatic mass and nearby lymph nodes to aid in staging and confirming a cancer diagnosis.[29] A false-negative biopsy result is possible and does not rule out the presence of malignancy. If the presence and extent of the cancer are still uncertain after the use of these common tests, a positron emission tomography scan may be considered.[14] An immunologic blood test to check for an elevated cancer antigen 19-9 level can also be helpful in identifying the presence of pancreatic cancer.

A tissue diagnosis is not necessary before proceeding with surgery, but a diagnostic laparoscopy may be performed on patients with suggestive signs of advanced disease that has not been confirmed through imaging studies. Surgical resection is the only curative option available for pancreatic cancer at this time, but only a small percentage of patients are eligible for surgery, since many tumors are inoperable at the time of diagnosis. Cancer of the pancreas is almost universally fatal, and the median survival time after surgery is only 18 to 20 months.[8] The 5-year survival rate is about 15% but may be a bit higher for those with no lymph node involvement, negative surgical margins, and smaller and well-differentiated tumors at the time of surgery.[8]

Surgeons who attempt curative surgery typically use the Whipple procedure, or pancreatoduodenectomy (Figure 44-5). This is a complex surgical procedure that includes a partial gastrectomy; cholecystectomy; and removal of the distal common bile duct, head of the pancreas, duodenum, proximal jejunum, and regional lymph nodes. Some surgeons prefer to modify the procedure by

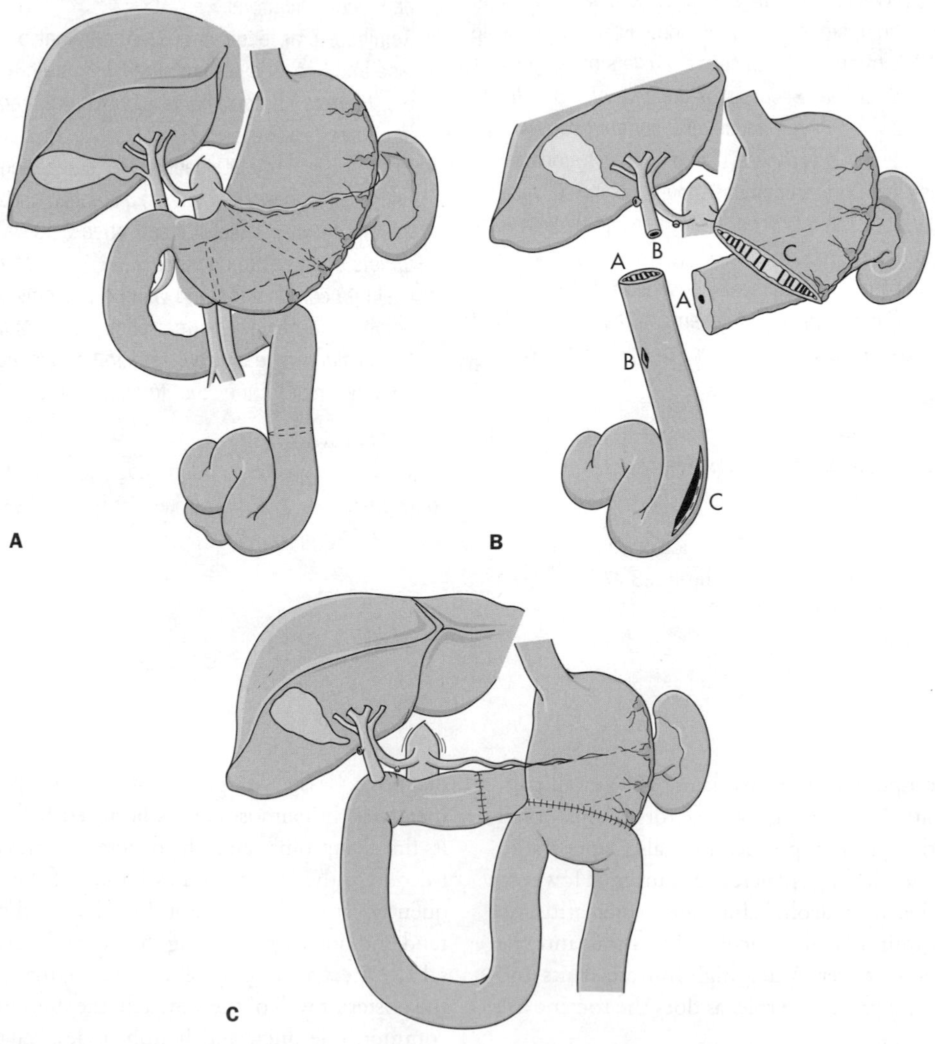

Figure 44-5 Standard Whipple operation. **A,** *Dotted lines* indicate margins for resection. **B,** Tissue has been resected. Sites for anastomoses are labeled *A, B,* and *C.* **C,** Anastomoses are complete.

preserving the stomach, pylorus, and first portion of the duodenum to maintain gastric emptying. Although the operative mortality rate associated with this surgery is now just 1% to 2% with a highly skilled surgeon, the procedure is extensive and in the best of circumstances requires a prolonged recovery. It is therefore reserved for patients whose tumors are believed to have a chance of cure.[8] Delayed gastric emptying and pancreatic leaks or fistulas are the most common complications associated with the surgery.

Obstruction is a common problem with large tumors involving the pancreatic head, and surgical bypass procedures may be necessary even when curative resection is not feasible. Options include gastrojejunostomy to bypass the duodenum, and choledochojejunostomy to relieve biliary obstruction. Endoscopic placement of stent tubes to support biliary drainage allows many patients with unresectable tumors to avoid major surgery. Stents may be placed internally or inserted for external drainage.

The success of adjuvant treatment after pancreatic cancer surgery remains uncertain. Radiotherapy, chemotherapy, or combinations of therapies continue to be studied, since none has conclusively proven to influence life expectancy. The Research box presents the results of one study using chemoradiotherapy and chemotherapy after surgical resection for pancreatic cancer. When a patient's pain is unrelenting and cannot be effectively managed with medications, a celiac plexus block may be performed.

Nursing care initially focuses on meticulous postoperative care. The extensive surgery leaves the patient vulnerable to numerous postoperative problems with nutrition, wound healing, and anastomosis leakage. Weight loss from inadequate preoperative nutrition increases the challenges for wound healing. Removal of so many components of the digestive system create the potential for ongoing problems related to digestion and absorption, which may only begin to manifest themselves before discharge, depending on the aggressiveness of postoperative feeding.[27] As discharge approaches, nursing care shifts to preparing the patient and family to provide needed care in the home setting. Nursing care of the patient undergoing pancreatic surgery is summarized in the Guidelines for Safe Practice box.

Research

Neoptolemas JP et al: A randomized trial of chemoradiotherapy and chemotherapy after resection of pancreatic cancer, *N Engl J Med* 350(12):1200-1210, 2004.

The use of adjuvant therapy after surgery for pancreatic cancer has shown at best mixed results. Effects of these therapies on patient survival have been inconclusive. This article reports the final results of the European Study Groups for Pancreatic Cancer (ESPAC) multicenter trial, which included 289 patients from 11 countries. All study patients had a diagnosis of adenocarcinoma of the pancreas and had received potentially curative surgery. Patients were randomly placed in one of four study groups: chemoradiotherapy, chemotherapy, chemoradiotherapy and chemotherapy, or observation. Survival comparisons were made between the groups.

The study showed a survival benefit for patients treated with chemotherapy (20%) versus observation alone (8%). The addition of radiotherapy to the protocol not only did not improve patient survival, it actually decreased it. The ESPAC study concluded that the current standard of care for patients with resectable and potentially curable pancreatic cancer should include both curative surgical resection and adjuvant systemic chemotherapy. Continued exploration of adjuvant therapies is recommended to improve the survival of patients with both resectable and unresectable pancreatic cancer.

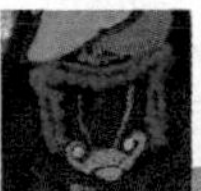

GUIDELINES FOR SAFE PRACTICE *The Patient Undergoing Pancreatic Surgery*

Preoperative Care

Provide thorough teaching about planned surgical procedure and expected postoperative care.
Monitor prothrombin time and other clotting studies; vitamin K can be administered and fresh frozen plasma given intraoperatively (rare).
Assess nutritional status. Administer nutritional support if ordered.
Administer broad-spectrum antibiotics on-call to the operating room and after surgery as ordered.

Postoperative Care

Critical care placement is not indicated for every patient. Patients with preoperative cardiac or pulmonary compromise, or health status changes during surgery, generally require close monitoring and a critical care placement immediately after surgery.
Check vital signs, intake and output, and hemodynamic parameters as ordered.
Perform blood gas, oxygen saturation, and routine blood studies as ordered.
Be alert to signs of bleeding or shock.
Maintain urinary output at 30 to 50 ml/hr.
Assess incision for signs and symptoms of infection.
Initiate pulmonary hygiene every hour with deep breathing, coughing as needed, and use of incentive spirometry.
Establish effective pain management regimen. Monitor every hour. Pain management may include a patient-controlled analgesia pump or administration via an epidural pump.
Monitor dressings and drainage tubes. Nasogastric tube, Foley catheter, and closed suction drainage tubes may be present. Keep skin clear of drainage.
Maintain nutritional support with enteral or parenteral nutrition. In the presence of delayed gastric emptying, administer medications to promote gastric motility as ordered.
- —Initiate oral feedings with clear liquids. Advance as tolerated.
- —Assess patients for pancreatic leaks once patient is on a regular diet. Milky drainage from closed suction drainage tubes and positive fluid amylase indicate a leak.
  - —Low-output versus high-output fistulas have differing consequences and home care needs.
- —Monitor blood glucose and administer insulin as ordered. Begin teaching new diabetic patients as indicated.
- —Monitor patient's weight and the development of steatorrhea.
  - —Administer pancreatic enzyme replacement as ordered.
- —Assess for signs of dumping syndrome (see Chapter 42).

Provide support for patient and family, and initiate discharge planning.
Monitor home health needs closely for patients going home with enteral tube feedings or closed suction drainage tubes.

PATIENT/FAMILY TEACHING. Pain management can be an ongoing challenge and is often the primary determinant of quality of life. The nurse serves as the patient's advocate in the health care system to establish an effective pain management protocol and continuously adapt it to changes in the patient's condition. The nurse provides careful teaching about the use of opioid analgesics and the inevitable development of tolerance, physical dependence, and associated constipation (see Chapter 16). Instruction is also provided about other expected medication side effects and their management.

The nurse also provides teaching about diet modification and other measures to support nutrition. Frequent meals and supplemental feedings are often necessary to maintain adequate nutrition. The patient is taught about the symptoms that reflect malabsorption and is encouraged to keep careful track of body weight changes. Measures to address anorexia, nausea, and vomiting are discussed. Wound healing is another ongoing concern, and the nurse instructs the patient and family in signs of wound infection to report to the surgeon.

Psychologic support is critical for both the patient and family. The nurse provides general instruction about the stages of grief and community resources available to deal with the poor prognosis. Additional general measures include those provided to any patient with invasive cancer (see Chapter 23), especially if the patient has agreed to further treatment with radiation or chemotherapy.

Palliative care services for symptom control and management, as well as comfort care initiatives, are initiated for patients with unresectable tumors and surgically treated patients who experience tumor recurrence. Pain management, depression, fatigue, and biliary or intestinal obstruction are some of the important topics addressed by palliative care specialists.

? Critical Thinking

1. You work on an acute medical unit in a large urban hospital and care for a steady stream of patients with acute and chronic pancreatitis. You are interested in studying the question of enteral versus parenteral feeding for this population. Design a clinical study to compare the efficacy and cost-effectiveness of the two approaches. How will you select your sample, and what variables will you study?
2. A woman has been diagnosed with unresectable cancer of the pancreas and has a grim prognosis. Her family is clear that they want everything possible to be done for her. She is ambivalent and expresses the desire to not pursue aggressive treatment. How will you address this quality-of-life issue? Who should be involved in the planning?

References

1. Adam A, Wilkinson M: Interventional radiology in liver disease, *Medicine* 30(12):85-87, 2002.
2. Aslar AK et al: Impact of laparoscopy on frequency of surgery for treatment of gallstones, *Surg Laparosc Endosc Percut Tech* 13(5):315-317, 2003.
3. Aspirin is found to reduce the incidence of pancreatic cancer, *Clin J Oncol Nurs* 7(2):135, 2003.
4. Bliss SJ et al: A window of opportunity, *N Engl J Med* 349(19):1848-1853, 2003.
5. Byrne MF, Mitchell RM, Baillie J: Common bile duct stones, *Emerg Med* 34(10):54, 57-58, 63, 2002.
6. Chowbey PK et al: Laparoscopic reintervention for residual gallstone disease, *Surg Laparosc Endosc Percut Tech* 13(1):31-35, 2003.
7. DiMagno EP, Chari S: Acute pancreatitis. In Feldman M, Friedman LS, Sleisenger MH, editors: *Sleisenger and Fordtran's gastrointestinal and liver disease,* ed 7, Philadelphia, 2002, Saunders.
8. Duffy JP, Reber HA: Nonendocrine tumors of the pancreas. In Yamada T, editor: *Textbook of gastroenterology,* ed 4, Philadelphia, 2003, Lippincott, Williams & Wilkins.
9. Forsmark CE: Chronic pancreatitis. In Feldman M, Friedman LS, Sleisenger MH, editors: *Sleisenger and Fordtran's gastrointestinal and liver disease,* ed 7, Philadelphia, 2002, Saunders.
10. Friedman LS: Liver, biliary tract and pancreas. In Tierney LM, McPhee SJ, Papadakis MA, editors: *Current medical diagnosis and treatment,* ed 43, New York, 2004, Lange Medical Books/McGraw Hill.
11. Horton JD, Bilhartz LE: Gallstone disease and its complications. In Feldman M, Friedman LS, Sleisenger MH, editors: *Sleisenger and Fordtran's gastrointestinal and liver disease,* ed 7, Philadelphia, 2002, Saunders.
12. Hughes E: Understanding the care of patients with acute pancreatitis, *Nurs Standard* 18(18):45-52, 54-55, 2004.
13. Jemal A et al: Cancer statistics 2004, *CA Cancer J Clin* 54:8-29, 2004.
14. Ladabaum U, Minoshima S: Positron emission tomography. In Yamada T, editor: *Textbook of gastroenterology,* ed 4, Philadelphia, 2003, Lippincott, Williams & Wilkins.
15. Lee SP, Ko CW: Gallstones. In Yamada T, editor: *Atlas of gastroenterology,* ed 3, Philadelphia, 2003, Lippincott, Williams & Wilkins.
16. Lee SP, Ko CW: Gallstones. In Yamada T, editor: *Textbook of gastroenterology,* ed 4, Philadelphia, 2003, Lippincott, Williams & Wilkins.
17. Mahadevan U, Bass NM: Sclerosing cholangitis and recurrent pyogenic cholangitis. In Feldman M, Friedman LS, Sleisenger MH, editors: *Sleisenger and Fordtran's gastrointestinal and liver disease,* ed 7, Philadelphia, 2002, Saunders.
18. Mitchell RMS, Byrne MF, Baillie J: Pancreatitis, *Lancet* 361(9367):111-112, 2002.
19. Ostroff JW, LaBerge JM: Endoscopic and radiologic treatment of biliary disease. In Feldman M, Friedman LS, Sleisenger MH, editors: *Sleisenger and Fordtran's gastrointestinal and liver disease,* ed 7, Philadelphia, 2002, Saunders.
20. Owyang C: Chronic pancreatitis. In Yamada T, editor: *Textbook of gastroenterology,* ed 4, Philadelphia, 2003, Lippincott, Williams & Wilkins.
21. Owyang C, Chotiprasidhi P: Chronic pancreatitis. In Yamada T, editor: *Atlas of gastroenterology,* ed 3, Philadelphia, 2003, Lippincott, Williams & Wilkins.
22. Powell JJ, Parks RW: Diagnosis and early management of acute pancreatitis, *Hosp Med* 64(3):150, 152-155, 2003.
23. Serralta AS et al: Prospective evaluation of emergency versus delayed laparoscopic cholecystectomy for early cholecystitis, *Surg Laparosc Endosc Percut Tech* 13(2):71-75, 2003.
24. Strasberg SM, Drebin JA: Tumors of the biliary tract. In Yamada T, editor: *Textbook of gastroenterology,* ed 4, Philadelphia, 2003, Lippincott, Williams & Wilkins.
25. Talwalkar JA, Wiesner RH: Primary sclerosing cholangitis and other cholangiopathies. In Yamada T, editor: *Textbook of gastroenterology,* ed 4, Philadelphia, 2003, Lippincott, Williams & Wilkins.
26. Topazian M, Gorelick FS: Acute pancreatitis. In Yamada T, editor: *Textbook of gastroenterology,* ed 4, Philadelphia, 2003, Lippincott, Williams & Wilkins.
27. Trujillo EB, Robinson MK, Jacobs DO: Nutrition: feeding critically ill patients, current concepts, *Crit Care Nurse* 21(4):60-71, 2001.
28. Ulodov J, Tenner SM: Acute and chronic pancreatitis, *PrimaryCare: Clin Office Pract* 28(3):607-628, 2001.
29. Varadarajulu S, Wallace MB: Applications of endoscopic ultrasonography in pancreatic cancer, *Cancer Control* 11(1):15-22, 2004.
30. Yamamoto T et al: Early gallbladder carcinoma associated with primary sclerosing cholangitis and ulcerative colitis, *J Gastroenterol* 38(7):704-706, 2003.

Visit the Evolve website: http://evolve.elsevier.com/Monahan/medsurg

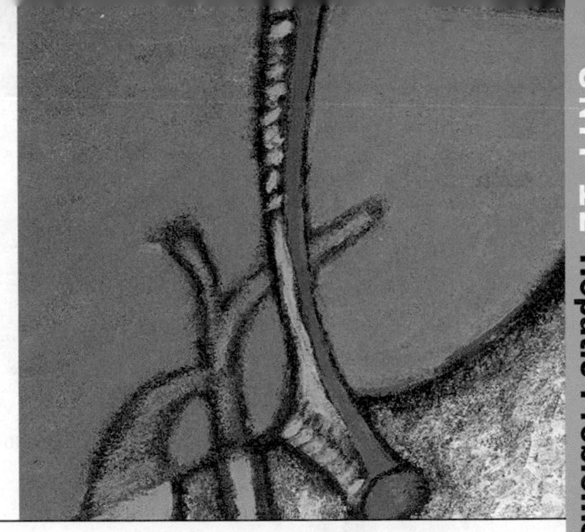

CHAPTER 45

Assessment of the Hepatic System

by Sally A. Brozenec

OBJECTIVES

After studying this chapter, the learner should be able to:

1. Describe the normal anatomy and physiology of the liver.
2. Describe the role of the liver in metabolism and maintenance of energy balance.
3. Explain the basis for data that must be collected to identify problems of the hepatic system.
4. Explain the role of laboratory and diagnostic tests in identifying pathophysiologic states of the liver.
5. Compare and contrast the radiologic and special tests used in diagnosing hepatic dysfunction.

KEY TERMS

ascites, p. 1308
bilirubin, p. 1306
clotting factors, p. 1305
gluconeogenesis, p. 1305
glycogenesis, p. 1305
glycogenolysis, p. 1305
hepatocytes, p. 1305
hepatotoxins, p. 1308
jaundice, p. 1307
Kupffer cells, p. 1304
lipogenesis, p. 1305
metabolic detoxification, p. 1306
paracentesis, p. 1313
portal hypertension, p. 1303

The liver is the largest gland in the body and has 500 identified functions. Therefore pathologic conditions in this organ can cause a variety of problems that have an impact on the entire body. Of primary importance is its role in metabolism and the maintenance of normal energy stores.

Anatomy and Physiology

Anatomy

The liver, one of the most complex organs in the body, weighs approximately 1.3 to 1.8 kg. The falciform ligament divides the liver into right and left lobes and provides attachment to the anterior abdominal wall (Figure 45-1). The round ligament is a remnant of the umbilical vein and extends from the umbilicus to the inferior surface of the liver. Glisson's capsule, a fibroelastic capsule containing blood vessels, lymphatics, and nerves, covers the liver.

Anatomically the liver extends up under the ribs and is 4 to 8 cm in height at the midsternal line and 6 to 12 cm in height at the midclavicular line. The liver normally extends from the fifth intercostal space.

The liver is served by two separate blood supplies, and at any one time contains about 13% of the total blood. Approximately 75% of the blood flow to the liver is through the portal vein, which carries nutrient-rich blood from the stomach and intestines (Figure 45-2). The remaining 25% of the blood flow is through the hepatic artery, which carries oxygenated blood from the lungs to the hepatic cells. The portal system is a venous pathway through the liver. Blood from the portal vein flows to the large capillaries, called sinusoids, which separate the layers of hepatic cells. From the sinusoids the portal blood, along with the oxygenated blood from the hepatic artery, progresses to the hepatic vein from which it is emptied into the inferior vena cava for return to the right atrium (Figure 45-3).

Pressure in the portal system is normally 3 mm Hg. **Portal hypertension,** a rise in portal pressure to at least 10 mm Hg, can be caused by any disorder that obstructs or impedes blood flow through any portion of the portal system or vena cava. Elevated pressures in the portal system cause collateral vessels to open between the portal veins and the systemic veins, avoiding the obstructed portal vessels. These collateral vessels may develop in the esophagus, anterior abdominal wall, or rectum.

The liver is innervated by the sympathetic and parasympathetic nervous systems. Sympathetic fibers innervate the hepatic artery branches and the bile ducts, whereas parasympathetic nerve fibers supply the intrahepatic and extrahepatic biliary tract system. Stimulation of the sympathetic and parasympathetic nervous systems affects both blood flow and the flow of bile within the biliary tract,

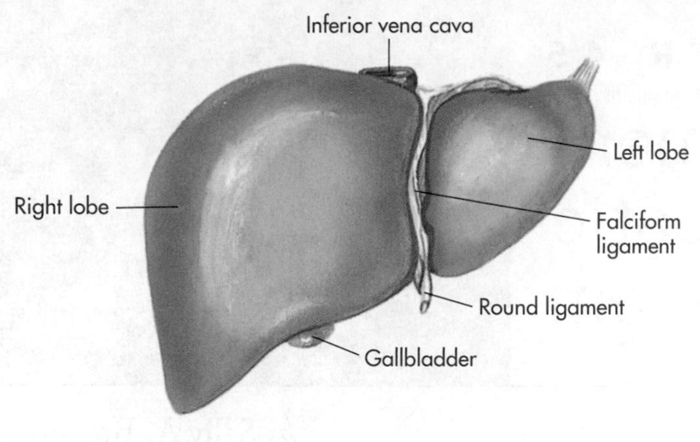

Figure 45-1 Gross structure of the liver, anterior view.

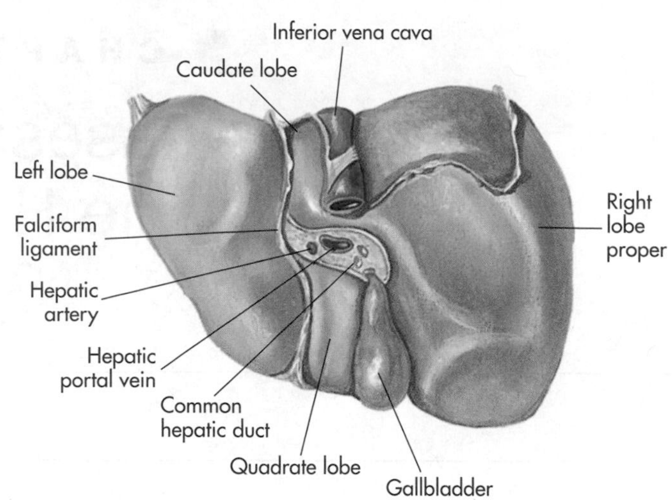

Figure 45-2 Gross structure of the liver, inferior view.

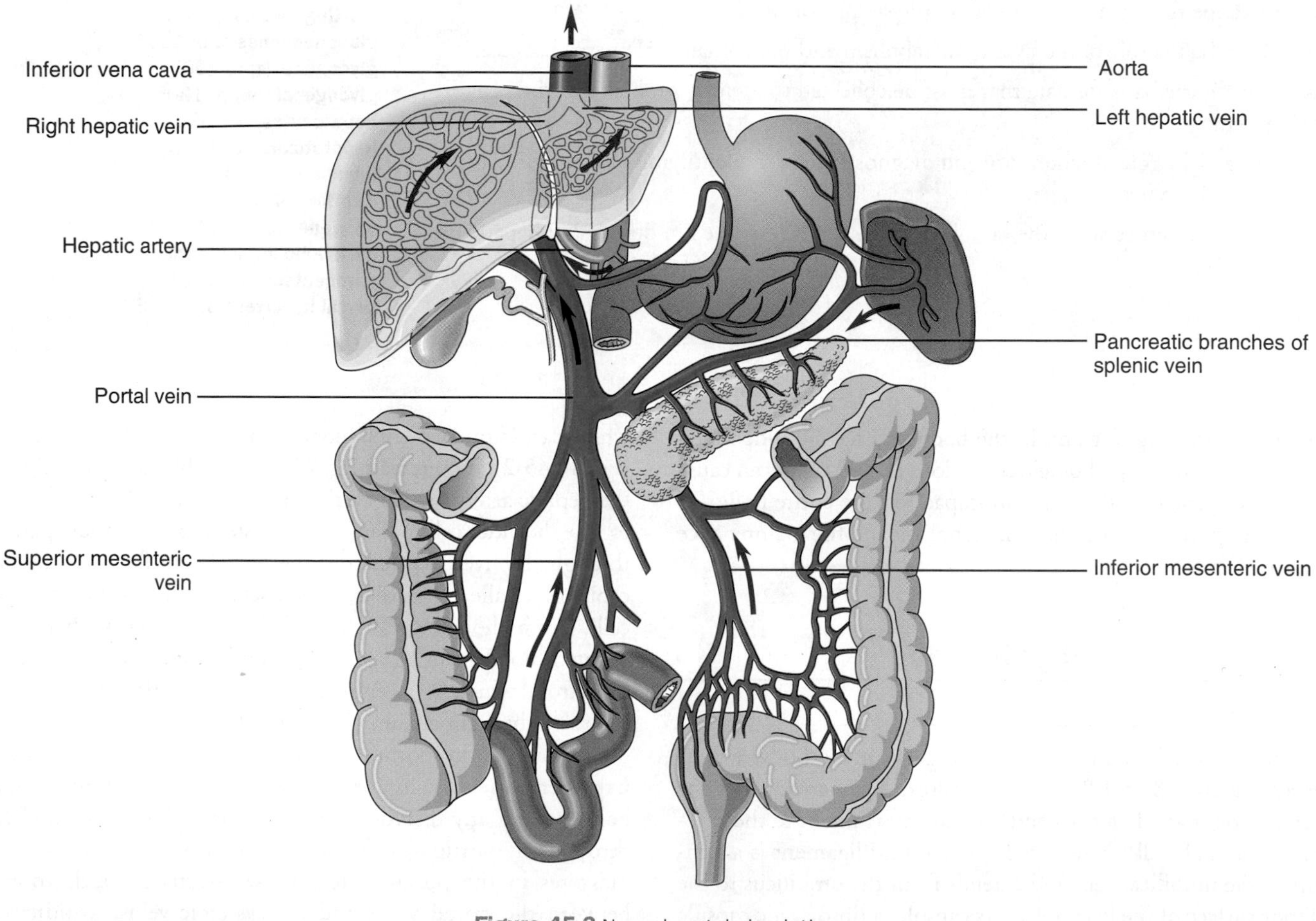

Figure 45-3 Normal portal circulation.

but it does not influence the function of the hepatic or parenchymal cells.[1]

The functional unit of the liver is the liver lobule (Figure 45-4). Each lobule is composed of multiple plates of hepatic cells. Between the individual cells of each cellular plate are bile canaliculi, which empty into the bile ducts. The terminal bile ducts join to form the hepatic duct, which merges with the cystic duct of the gallbladder to form the common bile duct. Each side of each cellular plate contains a venous sinusoid, which receives blood from branches of the portal vein and hepatic artery. As blood flows through the sinusoids, the hepatic cells and blood can exchange substances.

The sinusoids are lined with phagocytic cells of the reticuloendothelial system **(Kupffer cells)**. These cells remove bacteria and other foreign substances from the blood. Because the portal blood originates in the gastrointestinal (GI) tract, some bacteria or other

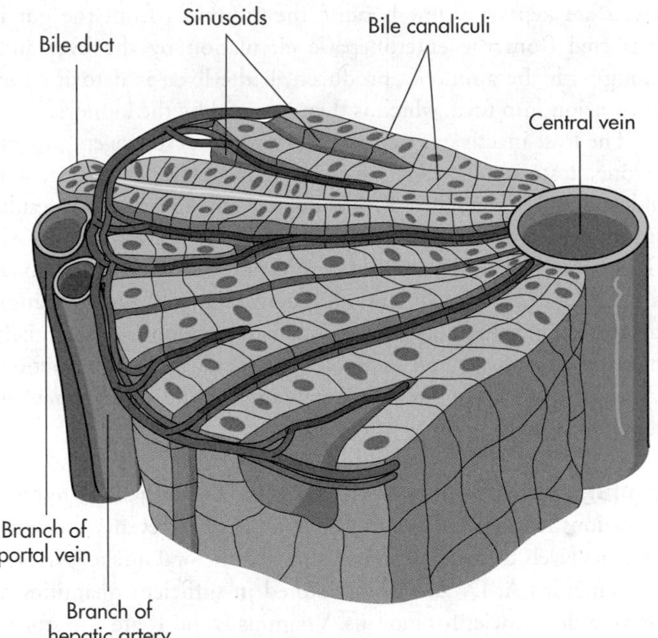

Figure 45-4 A liver lobule. A central vein is located in center of lobule with plates of hepatic cells disposed radially. Branches of portal vein and hepatic artery are located on periphery of lobule, and blood from both perfuses sinusoids. Peripherally located bile ducts drain bile canaliculi that run between hepatocytes.

foreign substances need to be removed. The blood from the venous sinusoids empties into the central vein and then into the hepatic vein. The hepatic vein empties into the inferior vena cava.

Hepatocytes are stable cells that regenerate on demand. Animal studies have shown that the liver can regenerate even after two thirds of the organ has been removed.

Physiology

The liver can be thought of as a metabolic factory and a waste disposal plant. As seen in the anatomic description of the blood and bile flow, the liver is ideally structured to carry out its multiple metabolic and waste disposal functions. The major functions of the liver are summarized in Box 45-1 and presented in more detail in the following sections.

Nutrient Metabolism. The liver has a significant role in the metabolism of each of the three major nutrients. It either oxidizes the nutrients for energy, uses them to synthesize storage forms of substances for future use, or uses them to synthesize other essential compounds.

CARBOHYDRATES. Immediately after meals, the liver extracts glucose, fructose, and galactose from the blood. These simple sugars are metabolized into glycogen **(glycogenesis)** to replenish liver stores. If the diet ingested is low in carbohydrates, the liver converts protein to glucose to replenish glycogen stores. If more carbohydrate is ingested than is needed to replenish glycogen stores or to supply energy, the excess carbohydrate is converted to fat **(lipogenesis)**. Between meals and during other fasting states, the liver assists in maintaining the blood glucose concentration by breaking down glycogen **(glycogenolysis)** or forming new glucose **(gluconeogenesis)**. The new glucose is made from amino acids, glycerol, and lactic acids. Through glycogenesis, lipogenesis, glycogenolysis, and gluconeogenesis, all of which are under hormonal control, the liver helps maintain a normal blood glucose level, preventing high levels (hyperglycemia) immediately after eating (postprandially) and hypoglycemia between meals or during other periods of fasting.

PROTEINS. The liver is vital to normal protein metabolism. It provides needed amino acids through transamination. Transamination is the process of nitrogen metabolism in which the liver transfers an amino group (NH_2) to form nonessential amino acids. The liver also is the only source of some of the major plasma proteins. One of these major proteins is albumin, which is necessary for the maintenance of a normal internal environment and for fluid and electrolyte balance. Albumin is responsible for maintaining colloid osmotic pressure and thus the proper distribution of fluids between the vascular and interstitial compartments.

The liver is the source of several **clotting factors**, which are proteins. It produces fibrinogen (factor I), prothrombin (factor II),

Box 45-1 Summary of Liver Functions

- Carbohydrate metabolism
  - —Glycogen formation and storage
  - —Glucose formation from glycogen (glycogenolysis) and from amino acids, lactic acids, and glycerol (gluconeogenesis)
- Protein metabolism
  - —Protein catabolism
  - —Protein synthesis
  - —Albumin
  - —Alpha and beta globulins
  - —Clotting factors
  - —C-reactive protein
  - —Transferrin
  - —Enzymes
  - —Ceruloplasmin
  - —Formation of needed amino acids
- Fat metabolism
  - —Oxidation of fatty acids for energy
  - —Ketone formation
  - —Synthesis of cholesterol and phospholipids
  - —Formation of triglycerides from dietary lipids and excess dietary carbohydrates and proteins
  - —Formation of lipoproteins
- Production of bile salts
- Bilirubin metabolism
- Detoxification of endogenous and exogenous substances
  - —Ammonia
  - —Steroids
  - —Drugs
- Storage of minerals and vitamins
- Blood reservoir

factor V (proaccelerin), factor VII (serum prothrombin conversion accelerator, or proconvertin), factor IX (plasma thromboplastin component, or Christmas factor), and factor X (Stuart or Stuart-Prower factor). (See Chapter 32 for information on blood clotting.) The production of factors II, VII, IX, and X requires vitamin K. Vitamin K is a fat-soluble vitamin and therefore requires adequate production and excretion of bile for its absorption. In addition to protein synthesis, the liver catabolizes proteins as necessary for energy or glucose production.

FATS. The liver is involved in multiple aspects of fat metabolism. Triglycerides in the diet are absorbed in chylomicrons. The chylomicrons are taken up by the liver and metabolized to fatty acids. These fatty acids may be (1) oxidized and used for energy by the liver and other body tissues; (2) metabolized to ketones; (3) converted to phospholipids; (4) combined with cholesterol, which is synthesized in the liver, to form cholesterol esters; or (5) reesterified to triglycerides and combined with protein, cholesterol, and phospholipids to form lipoproteins. The liver also uses fatty acids released from adipose tissue storage sites for these same processes.

Production of Bile Salts. Bile production is one of the liver's major functions. Bile is a complex compound composed of cholesterol, phospholipids, bile salts, bile pigments **(bilirubin)**, and small amounts of proteins and electrolytes; 97% of bile is water. Metabolites of drugs and other substances that need to be excreted may also be found in bile. Bile salts are necessary for the absorption of fats, cholesterol, and fat-soluble vitamins, particularly vitamin K. Bile is released from the liver and concentrated and stored in the gallbladder. The liver secretes approximately 700 ml of bile daily. The bile salts released during each meal are resorbed into the enterohepatic circulation and recycled two or three times during a meal. Bile itself is resorbed along the total intestinal tract, but the terminal ileum has a major role in its active resorption. If the terminal ileum is diseased or resected, resorption of bile does not occur and abnormal fat absorption results.

Bilirubin Metabolism. Bilirubin is a byproduct of the heme portion of red blood cells and is released when these cells are destroyed. The released bilirubin is not water soluble (unconjugated). Unconjugated bilirubin is carried in the blood bound to albumin and other proteins. The liver extracts the unconjugated bilirubin from the blood and combines it with glucuronide, creating a water-soluble form (conjugated). The conjugated bilirubin is secreted into the bile and then enters the duodenum. In the GI tract bilirubin is metabolized to urobilinogen. Urobilinogen is excreted in feces as stercobilin, which gives feces its brown color, or it is resorbed. Most of the resorbed urobilinogen is extracted from the blood by the liver and recycled; some is excreted in the urine.

Metabolic Detoxification. The liver has a prime role in **metabolic detoxification** or biotransformation of endogenous and exogenous substances. Ammonia (NH_3) is a major toxic product processed by the liver. Ammonia is produced in the gut and the liver from the deamination of amino acids (the removal of NH_2 from amino acids). Bacteria in the GI tract are responsible for the ammonia formation in the gut. Peripheral blood ammonia levels are kept very low because the ammonia from the gut is extracted from the enterohepatic circulation by the liver and, along with the ammonia produced in the liver, is detoxified by conversion into urea, which is then excreted by the kidneys.

The liver inactivates steroids and hormones (estrogen, progesterone, testosterone, corticosterone, antidiuretic hormone, and aldosterone). Liver diseases may depress this inactivation, resulting in pathologic levels of these hormones. The liver also detoxifies many drugs; it metabolizes barbiturates (except phenobarbital and barbital), amphetamines, and many sedatives. Detoxification decreases intestinal or renal tubular resorption of potentially harmful substances and facilitates intestinal or renal excretion. Pathologic states of the liver may impair the effectiveness of detoxification.

Storage of Minerals and Vitamins. The liver stores reserves of various minerals and vitamins. This storage prevents abnormal internal levels from occurring, even when the oral intake is irregular. Vitamins A, D, and B_{12} are stored in sufficient quantities to prevent deficiencies for months. Vitamins E and K are also stored. Iron in the form of ferritin is stored and can be used to resupply iron for hemoglobin formation as needed; copper is stored as well.

Blood Reservoir. The liver, because of its tremendous vascular supply and sinusoidal system, can act as a reservoir for blood. When the venous vascular volume becomes greater than can be handled by the right side of the heart, the excess blood can be stored in the liver. In the event of hemorrhage the liver can release blood to maintain systemic circulatory volume.[2]

Physiologic Changes With Aging. As the body ages, the number and size of hepatic cells decrease, which results in an overall decrease in the size and weight of the liver by about 37%. Hepatic blood flow also decreases by 35% with increasing age. Despite this, common liver function tests usually show normal results in older persons unless a pathologic condition exists.

One of the most serious concerns about the aging liver is the decreased synthesis of enzymes that assist in the metabolism of drugs, particularly anticonvulsants, psychotropic drugs, and oral anticoagulants. Research indicates that the metabolic reactions associated with drug clearance decrease 5% to 30% with age. Thus the nurse should be alert for signs and symptoms of drug toxicity even when drugs are administered in normal doses because the decreased metabolism in the liver can cause an accumulation of the drug. There is also some evidence that normal aging may adversely affect liver tissue regeneration, resulting in prolonged recovery time from injury and disease.[1]

▶ ARE You READY?

The liver's absorption of which vitamin is instrumental in normal blood clotting?

1. Vitamin A
2. Vitamin D
3. Vitamin E
4. Vitamin K

Health History

A thorough history is necessary to assess the health status of people with dysfunction of the hepatic system. Assessment focuses on comfort status; nutritional status; fluid and electrolyte status; elimination patterns; energy level; perception, motion, and cognition; potential exposure to toxins; and general living conditions and lifestyle. Information related to history of hepatic disease or family history of disease is collected.

Comfort Status

Two major sources of discomfort associated with hepatic disease are abdominal pain and pruritus (itching). The person may complain of continuous upper abdominal discomfort or a dull ache in the upper right quadrant. This discomfort does not usually alter normal function, although it can cause shallow breathing. The discomfort is most significant in that it verifies the presence of a pathologic process. General body aching may be present in cases of acute viral infections of the liver.

Pruritus, which may cause significant discomfort, is usually associated with **jaundice**. The pruritus results from a combination of two factors. One is the capillary dilation caused by the elevated serum bilirubin that occurs with jaundice. The second is the irritating effect of the bilirubin on the chemosensitive area of the skin. The history should include a description of any discomfort stated in the patient's own words, along with information about factors that worsen itching and measures that help relieve it.

Nutritional Status

People with hepatic dysfunction often experience alterations in nutritional status. Some hepatic problems result in anorexia, nausea, and vomiting. The examiner should question the patient about such episodes, including onset, precipitating factors, association with food or alcohol intake, and measures that provide relief.

Poor nutritional habits and malnutrition resulting from lifestyle patterns or food intolerances may be present. A useful method to assess the patient's nutritional status is to ask the patient what he or she has eaten in the past 24 hours and ascertain whether this is the typical eating pattern.

Alcohol use should also be explored. Alcohol exerts a toxic effect on liver cells and provides calories but no nutrition. Malnutrition, often associated with alcoholism, may aggravate the tissue injury. In the case of chronic alcohol use, muscle mass may have decreased while the overall weight remained stable. In addition, weight loss may be masked by water retention.

People with chronic problems of the hepatic system often require treatment with special diets, such as low sodium, altered protein intake, and water restriction. The history should include information about food intolerances and food preferences.

Fluid and Electrolyte Status

Hepatic dysfunction can be associated with either fluid volume deficit or excess. Fluid volume deficit can result from nausea and vomiting or from acute bleeding with cirrhosis. Fluid volume excess (edema) typically occurs in people with hepatic dysfunction as a result of peripheral vasodilation initiating renal retention of sodium and water. This expansion of the vascular space effectively decreases the circulating blood volume, which results in the release of renin, angiotensin, and aldosterone. These hormones increase sodium and water retention.

Also contributing to fluid volume excess is the hypoalbuminemia associated with liver disease. Albumin is the primary source of osmotic pressure in the vasculature; decreased albumin causes fluid to leave the vascular space and enter the interstitial space, resulting in edema or ascites. Levels of electrolytes, particularly sodium, potassium, hydrogen, and bicarbonate, can be elevated or decreased.

To assess fluid and electrolyte status, the examiner collects information about:

- Normal fluid and food intake and output
- Abnormal fluid and electrolyte losses, such as vomiting, diarrhea, or bleeding
- Changes in weight, both losses and gains
- Signs and symptoms (in addition to weight loss) of fluid or electrolyte deficit, such as weakness, dizziness, or syncope
- Signs and symptoms (in addition to weight gain) of fluid or electrolyte excess, such as edema in hands, feet, and legs or an increase in abdominal girth

Elimination Patterns

Intestinal and urinary elimination may be altered in people with liver problems. If bile flow is obstructed, the person may have grayish white or clay-colored stools and dark amber, brown, or mahogany-colored urine. Urine bilirubin levels will be elevated. Blood may be present in the urine or stools. The nurse can test for occult blood in the urine by using a reagent strip and test the stool by performing a fecal occult blood test (Hematest) or guaiac test. Nocturia or a reported decrease in urinary output may result from sodium and water retention.

Energy Level

Because of altered nutrient intake, abnormal fluid and electrolyte status, and increased metabolic needs, people with hepatic problems often report an intolerance to normal daily activities or simply fatigue and weakness. If the patient has ascites, the increased fluid in the abdomen pushes up on the diaphragm and can cause respiratory distress. As the underlying liver condition resolves, so may the fatigue and weakness; however, the patient and family must understand that the energy level may take a long time to return to normal.

Perception, Motion, and Cognition

Chronic health problems of the hepatic system can cause changes in neurologic function, particularly in relation to the peripheral nervous system and higher cognitive functions. The nurse should ask the patient about alterations in sensation in extremities, any noticeable changes in memory, episodes of forgetfulness or blackouts, and alterations in coordination or in the ability to do fine motor tasks. The onset of any alterations, pattern of changes (continuous or intermittent), and duration of any changes should be determined.

Exposure to Toxins

Hepatic dysfunction can be caused by various agents, such as alcohol, drugs, industrial chemicals, and viruses. To determine whether the patient has been exposed to these **hepatotoxins,** the nurse elicits a history of exposure to any toxins and a drug and alcohol history.

The drug history focuses on prescription, over-the-counter, and street drugs. For example, acetaminophen is often used by adolescents to commit suicide and can cause severe liver damage in doses 10 times greater than the recommended dose. The liver damage is intensified by the combination of acetaminophen and alcohol. The alcohol history should focus on the usual amount of intake and time since last intake. It is also important to assess for use of herbal preparations (see Complementary & Alternative Therapies box).

An occupational history helps identify potential toxins in the work environment such as methylene chloride solvents. An environmental and social history helps identify potential sources of viruses (Box 45-2). This history also can identify particular persons, factors, or places associated with substance abuse, if a problem exists, and can help in its long-term management.

Complementary & Alternative Therapies

Herb-Drug Interactions

Physicians are concerned that herbal products are often used by older patients in conjunction with prescription medications without the knowledge of their health care provider. Research has shown that more than 2 million individuals who use herbal medications take the preparations along with their prescription medications. Herb-drug interactions are common, especially for the medications most frequently taken by older adults for a variety of symptoms. Some herbal products may interact with prescription drugs and probably should not be used by older adults. Physicians and nurses should assess what herbal preparations their older patients are taking. Education about the potential harmful effects of combining prescription medications and herbal products is essential.

Alternative medicine: what are the risks when elderly patients combine herbal and prescription medications? *Geriatr Psychopharmacol* 8(1):1, 2004.

Box 45-2 Health History Information to Identify Exposure to Hepatitis Viruses

- Contact with persons with jaundice
- Travel or visits to environments with poor sanitation (e.g., camping trips, developing countries)
- Ingestion of shellfish or raw fish
- Recent ear or body piercing or tattooing
- Recent blood transfusions
- Intravenous drug abuse (sharing of contaminated needles)
- Occupational exposure (e.g., health service personnel with frequent blood contact, personnel in day care centers, personnel in centers of custodial care)
- History of hemodialysis
- History of multiple sex partners; male bisexual or male homosexual lifestyle

Physical Examination

To assess the function of the hepatic system, a thorough assessment of the total body is required. First, a general survey of the patient includes:

- Inappropriate general appearance
- Lethargy, restlessness, inattentiveness
- Signs of malnourishment such as thinness; poor skin turgor; sunken eyes; thinning, lifeless hair; or obesity, especially in abdominal area
- Jaundice of the skin or sclera or, in a dark-skinned person, of the palms of the hands
- Palmar erythema
- Bruises, petechiae, and spider angiomas, usually on the nose, cheeks, or upper thorax
- Muscle wasting
- Edema
- Changes in secondary sexual characteristics

After the general inspection, a detailed assessment should occur. The first area of focus is the patient's fluid status. The nurse assesses vital signs, including orthostatic changes, weight, temperature, skin turgor, mucous membrane moisture, edema, and behavior changes.

To assess energy level and nutritional status, the nurse examines the patient's total muscle mass and muscle strength and determines the patient's current and usual weight. While performing the assessment, the nurse notes the patient's mental status, affect, and alertness, as well as changes in facial expression, responsiveness, and level of consciousness. The nurse observes the patient for periods of confusion or disorientation, and notes the appropriateness of the patient's affect for the situation. Because handwriting or the ability to draw a geometric figure deteriorates with decreasing liver function, a sample may be obtained from the patient.

Next the nurse inspects the abdomen for enlargement, presence of distended or dilated periumbilical veins (caput medusae), and ascites. **Ascites** is characterized by distention of the abdomen with tight, glistening skin, protruding umbilicus, and bulging flanks. The nurse uses palpation and percussion to ascertain the presence of a fluid wave and shifting dullness, which are indicative of ascites, and to assess for hepatic tenderness, size, and consistency and the presence of hepatic masses. The spleen often is enlarged in the patient with chronic hepatic dysfunction. The nurse percusses the spleen to determine the size and location; palpation is deferred because of the fragility of the enlarged spleen. Abdominal girth is also measured. Hemorrhoids caused by prolonged elevations in portal system pressure may be present.[5]

Assessment measures and variations in normal findings relevant to the care of older adults are presented in the Gerontologic Assessment box.

Diagnostic Tests

Laboratory Tests

Multiple tests may be necessary to determine the extent and seriousness of hepatic disease. To be of benefit, many tests require serial readings. Table 45-1 summarizes the procedure, preparation, and interpretation of blood, stool, and urine studies used to evaluate liver function.[3,4] In addition to performing the nursing

Gerontologic Assessment

Monitor Effects of Medications

Older patients seem to have more problems with both the therapeutic effects of medications and drug toxicity. This may be due to the decrease in hepatic circulation that accompanies aging and to the decrease in the liver's enzyme activity.

Standard doses of medication published in a formulary may be too high for older patients. Most drug dosages are calculated for healthy white adult men.

Polypharmacy occurs when the older patient receives multiple medications from multiple prescribers.

Assess Nutritional Status

Because the liver has many functions that maintain energy stores and metabolism, the older patient may show signs of fatigue if liver function has diminished enough to limit the available energy needed to support activities of daily living.

care interventions listed in the middle column, the nurse explains the tests to the patient and answers questions.

Radiologic Tests

Radiologic tests assist in identifying the cause of hepatic dysfunction. In addition to specific liver tests, the physician may order abdominal films, barium swallow, barium enema, and gastroscopy. These tests help identify pathologic GI conditions that may cause signs and symptoms similar to those found in hepatic dysfunction.

Ultrasonography. Ultrasonography of the liver is used to assess jaundice of unknown etiology, hepatomegaly, or suspected tumors. The ultrasound provides information on liver size, shape, and location; presence of cysts or abscesses; and filling or dilation defects.

Preparation of the patient for ultrasonography of the liver is relatively simple. Usually the patient is not allowed to eat for 8 to 12 hours before the procedure, since gas in the GI tract can interfere with the test. Also any residual barium from other tests needs to be eliminated from the GI tract. Finally, the patient must be well hydrated, since dehydration can decrease the ability of ultrasonography to distinguish between the liver and surrounding tissues.

Computed Tomography. Computed tomography (CT) scanning can identify problems similar to those described under ultrasonography and, in addition, can be used with a contrast medium to intensify the appearance of vascular structures and hepatic parenchyma. The patient should take nothing by mouth for 8 to 12 hours before the test. If a contrast medium is to be used, the nurse assesses the patient for allergies to iodine or contrast media. Adequate hydration is also necessary when a contrast medium is used. Barium studies should be done at least 4 days before a CT scan or after a CT scan because the barium can interfere with test results.

Magnetic Resonance Imaging. Magnetic resonance imaging (MRI) is used to detect liver tumors. Because magnetic fields are used instead of radioactive isotopes to produce the image, no special patient preparation is necessary. It is important to inform the patient that this test is painless. The nurse instructs the patient to remove any jewelry, dentures, and partial dentures if they contain metal, or any other item that contains metal, such as hairpins or limb prostheses. The nurse assesses patients for claustrophobia before the procedure because of the enclosed nature of the testing equipment.

Radionuclide Imaging. Radionuclide imaging techniques outline the liver with selected radioisotopes given intravenously. After injection of the radioisotope, the patient is placed in the supine position, and a scintillation detector is passed over the abdomen in the area of the liver. The radiation coming from the isotopes immediately beneath the probe of the scanner is detected, amplified, and recorded. Scanning helps to differentiate nonfunctioning areas from normal tissue and to identify hepatic tumors, cysts, and abscesses. Usually a nonfunctioning area appears as an area of decreased activity. However, gallium-67 (^{67}Ga) is preferentially taken up by hepatocellular carcinomas and abscesses; hence these areas appear as areas of heavy radioactivity.

Adverse reactions to the radioisotopes used for radionuclide imaging are unusual, and the procedure is relatively safe. Discomfort is minimal. Only small amounts of radioactive material are given, and radiation precautions are not necessary. Only ^{67}Ga scanning requires special preparation. ^{67}Ga is excreted by the GI tract. To avoid absorption of the radioisotope by the GI contents, laxatives and enemas are prescribed. The toilet should be flushed twice for bowel movements after the ^{67}Ga scanning to ensure the safety of the patient and others. Ultrasonography, CT scanning, and MRI have replaced radionuclide imaging in most instances of hepatic dysfunction.

Angiography and Portal Pressure Measurements. Catheterization of the hepatic artery, portal venous system (by various routes), and hepatic vein allows injection of a contrast medium and the visualization of the vascular supply of the hepatic system. Angiography determines the patency of the system and the presence of tumors, abscesses, collateral circulation, varices, and bleeding.

Portal and hepatic vein pressure (wedge hepatic vein pressure) can be measured. These readings may be done in conjunction with angiography or as a separate study. These measurements help in determining the degree of portal hypertension.

The nurse assesses the patient's allergy to contrast media before angiography is done. After both angiography and pressure readings, the nurse observes the insertion site for bleeding and checks the patient's vital signs every 15 minutes for 1 hour, every 30 minutes for the next hour, every hour for the next 4 hours, and then, if the patient is stable, every 4 hours. Bed rest is maintained for 24 to 48 hours after the test.

Special Tests

Liver Biopsy. A liver biopsy may aid in establishing the cause of liver disease. In this procedure the physician inserts a specially

Text continued on page 1313.

TABLE 45-1 LABORATORY TESTS OF LIVER FUNCTION

Function and Test	Procedure and Preparation	Interpretation
FAT METABOLISM		
Serum total cholesterol and cholesterol esters	Venipuncture; fasting sometimes required	Desirable range is <200 mg/dl of blood; approximately 70% is cholesterol ester. In hepatocellular disease, amount of total serum cholesterol and cholesterol ester may be decreased. In obstructive biliary tract disease, total serum cholesterol is increased, but amount of esterified cholesterol is decreased. Normal cholesterol levels rise with age.
Serum phospholipids	Venipuncture; no special preparation	Normal level is 150-250 mg/dl. Serum phospholipids tend to be low in severe hepatocellular disease and high in obstructive biliary tract disease.
PROTEIN METABOLISM		
Total serum protein	Venipuncture; no special preparation	Normal level is 6-8 g/dl; test measures all serum protein. Levels may be normal in hepatocellular disease because increased serum globulin will replace decreased serum albumin; increased serum globulin is seen in chronic inflammatory disease, neoplastic diseases, and biliary obstruction.
Albumin	Venipuncture; no special preparation	Normal level is 3.5-5.5 g/dl. Albumin is made only in liver; in hepatocellular disease, serum albumin level may decline.
Protein electrophoresis	Venipuncture; no special preparation; protein fraction of blood will migrate in characteristic directions in electrical field; after separation of fractions, specimen stained, and densitometer used to measure amounts of various serum protein	Normal fractions in relation to total serum protein (100%) are albumin, 52%-68%; alpha globulins, 12%-17%; beta globulins, 7%-15%; and immune serum globulins (gamma globulins), 9%-19%. In severe hepatocellular damage, amount of albumin may be decreased; inflammatory processes of liver may produce increased amounts of alpha$_1$ globulins; neoplastic disease is associated with increased levels of alpha$_2$ globulins; some patients with obstructive biliary tract disease may have high levels of beta globulins.
Immunoglobulins (Igs)	Venipuncture; no special preparation	Five classes of antibodies are IgA, IgG, IgM, IgF, and IgD. IgA and IgG are often increased in presence of cirrhosis; IgG is elevated in presence of chronic active hepatitis; biliary cirrhosis and hepatitis A cause increase in IgM component.
Blood urea nitrogen (BUN)	Venipuncture; no special preparation	Normal is 11-23 mg/dl. In severe hepatocellular disease, if portal venous flow is obstructed, level may decrease; varies with dietary protein intake and fluid volume.
Serum prothrombin time (PT)	Venipuncture; no special preparation; reflects activity of extrinsic and common coagulation pathways, including prothrombin; fibrinogen; and factors V, VII, IX, and X	Normal PT is 12-14 sec; it is compared with a control level; the normal PT is calculated based on the institution's control and therefore may differ among institutions; it may be expressed as international normalized ratio (INR). PT reflects activity of extrinsic and common coagulation pathways, including prothrombin; fibrinogen; and factors V, VII, IX, and X. PT may be increased in hepatocellular disease because of liver's inability to produce clotting factors or in obstructive hepatic or biliary tract disease because of malabsorption of vitamin K; persistence of abnormal PT after parenteral administration of vitamin K indicates hepatocellular damage.

TABLE 45-1 LABORATORY TESTS OF LIVER FUNCTION—CONT'D

Function and Test	Procedure and Preparation	Interpretation
PROTEIN METABOLISM—CONT'D		
Serum partial thromboplastin time (PTT) and activated partial thromboplastin time (aPTT)	Venipuncture; no special preparation; reflects activity of intrinsic and common coagulation pathways	Normal PTT is 68-82 sec with standard technique; aPTT is 20-35 sec; as with the PT, the normal value may differ among institutions, depending on control used. PTT reflects activity of intrinsic and common coagulation pathways. PTT and aPTT are increased in hepatocellular disease because of inability of liver to produce clotting factors.
Blood ammonia levels	Venipuncture; may require fasting	Normal level is <75 mg/dl; may be elevated in severe hepatocellular disease because of obstruction of portal blood flow and, rarely, because of decreased urea synthesis.
BILIRUBIN METABOLISM		
Total bilirubin: Conjugated (direct) Unconjugated (indirect)	Venipuncture, no special preparation	Total serum bilirubin measures both conjugated and unconjugated bilirubin; normal total serum bilirubin values range from 0.3-1.1 mg/dl; conjugated bilirubin acts directly with diazo reagents; unconjugated bilirubin requires addition of methyl alcohol—hence the terms *direct* and *indirect*. Conjugated bilirubin increases in presence of hepatocellular or obstructive biliary tract disease; unconjugated bilirubin is elevated in presence of increased hemolysis of red blood cells or hepatocellular disease.
Urine bilirubin	Spot urine specimen; no special preparation	Normally no bilirubin is excreted in urine; urine with abnormal bilirubin is mahogany colored and has a yellow foam when shaken (foam test); unconjugated bilirubin even in excess is not excreted in urine because it is not water soluble. Conjugated serum bilirubin levels >0.4 mg/dl will lead to conjugated bilirubin being excreted in urine because it is water soluble; this indicates hepatocellular or obstructive biliary tract disease. Bilirubinuria may be present before jaundice.
Urine urobilinogen	24-hr urine collection or 2-hr afternoon collection	Normally 0.2-1.2 units/dl are found in specimen; fresh urine urobilinogen is colorless. Decreased amounts of urine urobilinogen are found in obstructive biliary tract disease; increased amounts are found in hepatocellular disease; alterations in intestinal flora by broad-spectrum antibiotics may change test.
Fecal urobilinogen	Stool specimen; no special preparation	Normal is 90-280 mg/day; presence of fecal urobilinogen (stercobilin) gives stool brown color; absence of stercobilin causes stools to become clay (grayish white) to white colored. Increased amounts of stercobilin are found with increased hemolysis of red blood cells; absence of fecal stercobilin indicates obstructive biliary tract disease.
SERUM ENZYMES		
Aspartate aminotransaminase (AST), formerly called serum glutamic-oxaloacetic transaminase (SGOT)	Venipuncture; no special preparation	Normal values vary, depending on measurement used. These enzymes are present in hepatic cells; with necrosis of hepatic cells, enzymes are released and elevated serum levels will be found. GGT is found in high levels in liver cells and kidneys; ALT is primarily present in liver cells; AST is also present in high levels in skeletal and heart muscle. LDH is also present in heart cells, kidney cells,

Continued

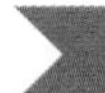

TABLE 45-1 LABORATORY TESTS OF LIVER FUNCTION—CONT'D

Function and Test	Procedure and Preparation	Interpretation
SERUM ENZYMES—CONT'D		
Alanine aminotransaminase (ALT), formerly called serum glutamic-pyruvic transaminase (SGPT) Lactate dehydrogenase (LDH) Gamma-glutamyltransferase (GGT) (gamma-glutamyl transpeptidase)		skeletal muscle cells, and erythrocytes, but in each tissue the LDH enzyme has characteristic composition: thus tissue source of elevated serum LDH levels can be determined by isoenzyme tests. With other three enzyme tests, necrosis of other organs must be ruled out; GGT is elevated early in liver disease, and elevation persists as long as cellular damage continues; GGT is routinely elevated in alcohol-induced liver disease, and increased levels are often seen before other abnormal test results occur.
Alkaline phosphatase	Venipuncture; no special preparation	Normal values vary, depending on measurement used; this enzyme originates in liver, bone, intestine, and placenta. Alkaline phosphatase is slightly to moderately elevated in hepatocellular disease but extremely elevated in obstructive biliary tract and bone disease.
Antigens and antibodies of viral hepatitis	Venipuncture; no special preparation	Normally no hepatitis antigens are found in serum or other body fluids; hepatitis A virus (HAV) can be found in stool during last part of incubation period and early prodromal phase; IgM-class anti-HAV appears in acute and early convalescent period and is used to diagnose hepatitis A; IgG-class anti-HAV becomes detectable during convalescent period and confers immunity. Hepatitis B has many associated serum particles; complete hepatitis B virus (HBV) is also called Dane particle; hepatitis B core antigen (HBcAg) can be found in liver, and its antibody (anti-HBc) can be found in blood, indicating past infection with HBV at some undefined time. Surface antigen (HBsAg) and several subtypes and antibody (anti-HBs) are also measurable; HBsAg is one of antigens measured to diagnose hepatitis B, and its presence indicates infectivity; presence of anti-HBs indicates past infection and immunity to HBV, presence of passive antibodies from hepatitis B immunoglobulin (HBIG), or immune response from HBV vaccine; hepatitis B e antigen (HBeAg) indicates high infectivity, and its antibody (anti-HBe) chronic infectivity; enzyme-linked immunosorbent assay (ELISA) has detected antibodies to hepatitis C (anti-HCV) in people who have been exposed to hepatitis C; however, antibodies do not appear in most people until at least 5 months after exposure to virus; an enterically transmitted virus that was previously related to hepatitis non-A non-B has been identified and labeled hepatitis E (HEV); anti-HEV has been detected using ELISA but is not available in United States at this time.

Data from Karnam S, Reddy R: Evaluation of the liver. In Reddy K, Long, W, editors: *Hepatology tract and pancreas*, St Louis, 2004, Mosby; and Mallory M, Lee S, Kowdley K: Abnormal liver test results on routine screening, *Postgrad Med* 115(3):53-66, 2004.

designed needle through the chest or abdominal wall into the liver, and removes a small piece of tissue for study. Liver biopsy is contraindicated for patients with infection of the right lower lobe of the lung, ascites, a blood dyscrasia, a problem with blood clotting, or an inability to cooperate by holding the breath. To prevent hemorrhage, vitamin K may be given parenterally for several days before and after the biopsy. A biopsy usually is not done if the prothrombin time is below 40% of normal.

The nurse explains to the patient the importance of holding one's breath and remaining absolutely still when the needle is introduced, since chest movement may cause the needle to slip and to tear the liver covering. Most hospitals require that the patient sign a written consent form for the procedure. In preparation for the biopsy, food and fluids may be withheld for several hours and a sedative given about 30 minutes before the procedure.

For the procedure itself, the patient lies supine, and the skin over the area selected (usually the eighth or ninth intercostal space) is cleansed and anesthetized with procaine hydrochloride. A nick is made in the skin with a sharp scalpel blade. Next the patient is instructed to take several deep breaths and then to hold his or her breath while the physician introduces a needle through the intercostal or subcostal tissues into the liver. The special needle assembly is rotated to separate a fragment of tissue and then is withdrawn. The specimen is placed into an appropriate container, which is labeled and sent to the pathology laboratory. A simple dressing is placed over the wound.

The complications of liver biopsy are accidental penetration of blood vessels, causing hemorrhage, or accidental penetration of a bile canaliculi, causing a chemical peritonitis from leakage of bile into the abdominal cavity. After the procedure the nurse assesses the patient for signs of hypovolemia and shock. The nurse monitors the patient's pulse and blood pressure every 30 minutes for the first few hours after the procedure and then hourly for 24 hours. The nurse takes the patient's temperature at least every 4 hours to determine a baseline and detect fever, which could indicate peritonitis. The physician may order pressure applied to the biopsy site to help stop any bleeding. An effective way to apply pressure is to have the patient lie on the right side with a small pillow or folded bath blanket placed under the costal margin for several hours after the biopsy. Bed rest is maintained for 24 hours after the test.

Paracentesis. A **paracentesis**, or peritoneal tap, is done to drain large volumes of ascitic fluid or to obtain a sample of peritoneal fluid (ascitic fluid) for cytologic or other laboratory studies. A paracentesis to drain fluid may be necessary with conditions such as respiratory distress, severe abdominal discomfort, or cardiac dysfunction caused by ascites. Repeated paracenteses are not the treatment of choice for controlling chronic, recurring ascites because of complications.

Paracentesis is a sterile procedure. When paracentesis is performed, the skin is cleansed, and the abdominal wall is anesthetized. The patient is assisted into an upright position, and a long aspiration needle is inserted. Fluid is aspirated for diagnostic tests, drained, or both. In preparation for the procedure, the patient receives a complete explanation and signs a consent form. Also, to diminish the risk of puncturing the bladder, the patient voids immediately before the procedure.

Complications of paracentesis include peritonitis and peritoneal bleeding resulting from trauma to blood vessels. When large amounts of fluid are removed from the peritoneal space, hypovolemia and shock can occur because additional fluid can shift from the intravascular compartment into the peritoneal cavity. (This risk is minimal in the patient with cirrhosis and edema.) The nurse monitors the patient's vital signs, including temperature, urinary output, and skin temperature and moisture, after the procedure and assesses the patient's abdomen for rigidity and pain. Observations for signs and symptoms of shock (pallor, tachycardia, decreased blood pressure, oliguria, and dyspnea) should also be made. The puncture site is assessed for evidence of persistent leakage. Serum levels of protein and potassium are monitored, since these substances are commonly lost during paracentesis.

Peritoneal Lavage. Peritoneal lavage may be used to assess damage to the liver from abdominal trauma in persons with altered states of consciousness who cannot give a satisfactory history. It may also be used in patients with abdominal trauma when unexplained hypotension is present, when physical examination results are unreliable, or when general anesthesia is required for other injuries.

Peritoneal lavage can be done by either the closed or open method. In the closed method a peritoneal dialysis catheter is inserted, and the peritoneal space is aspirated for gross blood. If no gross blood is found, lavage is carried out with normal saline. In the open method the peritoneum is exposed completely and then opened enough to allow entry of a dialysis catheter. Again, gross blood is aspirated first, and if no blood is found, lavage is carried out.

Peritoneal lavage requires a complete explanation to the patient and significant others and informed consent. The nurse inserts a nasogastric tube and Foley catheter before the procedure to prevent penetration of the intestines or bladder. In the closed method, a local anesthetic is used, whereas in the open method general anesthesia is necessary. Postprocedural nursing care of patients who have closed peritoneal lavage involves monitoring for peritonitis and bleeding. Patients who have open peritoneal lavage require general postanesthetic care.

Endoscopy

The hepatic system and gallbladder can be examined by several types of endoscopic procedures. The endoscope can be inserted directly through the peritoneum (peritoneoscopy), thus allowing direct visualization of the abdominal organs and the taking of biopsy specimens. Esophagoscopy and gastroscopy can be used to diagnose esophageal varices or to perform injection sclerotherapy. Endoscopic retrograde cholangiopancreatography (ERCP) can be done to visualize and provide radiographic examination of the liver, gallbladder, and pancreas. All these procedures require that the patient fast for at least 12 hours before the test. Before undergoing ERCP the patient is asked about allergies or sensitivities to x-ray dye. Intravenous sedation may be used during the endoscopic procedure.

After the procedure the nurse assesses the patient's ability to swallow. The patient's gag reflex may not return for 1 to 2 hours.

After ERCP the nurse monitors the patient for signs of complications, including perforation, sepsis, and pancreatitis. Vital signs are usually taken every 30 minutes for 2 hours and then hourly for 4 hours. The nurse provides emotional support before, during, and after the procedure, since the patient and family may be stressed and anxious while awaiting results.

▶ ARE You READY?

In monitoring a patient after a liver biopsy, which of the following findings would be most indicative of a complication of this procedure?

1. Decreasing blood pressure
2. Oozing of blood at the puncture site
3. Pain
4. Bile leakage from the site

References

1. Damjanov I: Hepatobiliary system. In Damjanov I, editor: *Pathology secrets,* Philadelphia, 2002, Hanley & Belfus.
2. Johnson LJ: Secretion. In Johnson LR, editor: *Essentials of medical physiology,* ed 3, San Diego, 2003, Elsevier.
3. Karnam S, Reddy R: Evaluation of the liver. In Reddy K, Long W, editors: *Hepatology tract and pancreas,* St Louis, 2004, Mosby.
4. Mallory M, Lee S, Kowdley K: Abnormal liver test results on routine screening, *Postgrad Med* 115(3):53-66, 2004.
5. Seidel HM et al: *Mosby's guide to physical examination,* ed 5, St Louis, 2003, Mosby.

evolve Visit the Evolve website: http://evolve.elsevier.com/Monahan/medsurg

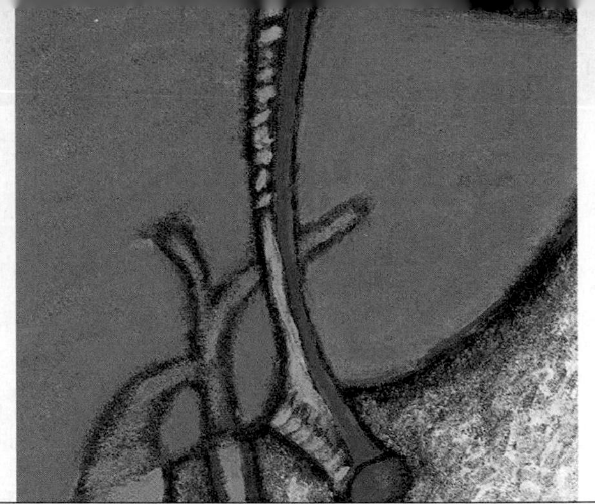

CHAPTER 46

Hepatic Problems

by Sally A. Brozenec

OBJECTIVES

After studying this chapter, the learner should be able to:

1. Explain signs and symptoms of a variety of hepatic disorders based on the pathophysiology.
2. Anticipate the nursing care needs of patients with focal hepatocellular disorders.
3. Differentiate the signs, symptoms, and treatments for hepatitis A, B, C, D, and E.
4. Differentiate among toxic, autoimmune, and viral hepatitis.
5. Describe the pathophysiologic basis for the clinical manifestations of cirrhosis and its complications.
6. Develop care plans for patients with diffuse hepatocellular disorders.

KEY TERMS

ascites, p. 1319
cirrhosis, p. 1316
encephalopathy, p. 1315
fulminant, p. 1315
hepatitis, p. 1332
hepatocellular, p. 1343
jaundice, p. 1335
paracentesis, p. 1321
peritoneovenous (PV) shunt, p. 1321
portal hypertension, p. 1317
spider angiomas, p. 1327
varices, p. 1319

Because the liver is so complex and has so many functions, it is affected in many disorders and produces a variety of physiologic and psychosocial problems for patients. The degree of illness in people with liver disease ranges from critical, requiring intensive nursing care, to chronic, requiring home care or an extended care facility. Severe liver problems can be caused by a variety of factors, including infection, neoplastic growths, toxic agents, and trauma. Regardless of the cause, clinical manifestations of liver disorders are similar and reflect alterations in normal liver function (see Clinical Manifestations box).

The most dreaded outcome of any liver disorder is liver failure. This general term implies a degree of tissue necrosis such that all liver function is lost. Researchers believe that a minimum mass of well-functioning hepatocytes is required to meet the body's basic metabolic needs, and once this critical threshold is lost, organ failure occurs. Liver failure may occur as an acute presentation or develop over time.

Acute Liver Failure

Acute liver failure (ALF), also called **fulminant** hepatic failure, is a condition in which previously healthy persons develop severe liver dysfunction evidenced by the rapid onset of **encephalopathy** and/or bleeding. It is a highly complex clinical syndrome that arises within a few days or weeks. About three fourths of patients with acute liver failure die within days of symptom onset.[53]

Etiology and Epidemiology. ALF has numerous causes, including hepatitis B infection, especially with concurrent infection with the delta virus. The major cause of ALF in persons without another liver disease is acetaminophen overdose. This may be deliberate overdose as in suicide attempts or it may be inadvertent. Individuals are at high risk for ALF if they combine acetaminophen with chronic alcohol intake, some anticonvulsants, or antituberculosis drugs.[5] In many cases of acute liver failure, the etiology is unknown. Less common causes are poisoning with mushrooms *(Amanita muscaria)* and eclampsia or preeclampsia of pregnancy.

Pathophysiology. A sudden, massive necrosis of hepatocytes results in dramatic clinical manifestations of liver failure and multiple organ dysfunction syndrome involving the kidneys, lungs, and circulatory system. Hallmarks of this disorder are clinical encephalopathy, rapid decrease in coagulation ability, cerebral edema, and multiorgan failure. The pathogenesis of multiple organ dysfunction is complex and poorly understood. In addition to the loss of hepatocyte function, key mediators such as interleukin-1, tumor necrosis factor, and others have been identified. Microvascular obstruction with cellular debris from the damaged

CLINICAL MANIFESTATIONS
Liver Disease

- *Jaundice:* When the liver is diseased, problems with the uptake, conjugation, or excretion of bilirubin may occur. This results in excess bilirubin in the blood, which is distributed to the skin, sclera, mucous membranes, and other body fluids and tissues, causing yellow pigmentation.
- *Ascites:* This accumulation of fluid in the peritoneal cavity is the result of changes in the hemodynamics of the abdominal circulation. Serous fluid moves out of the vessels into the peritoneum.
- *Portal hypertension:* The portal vascular system may become obstructed, causing increased portal venous pressure and resulting in portal hypertension.
- *Portal-systemic encephalopathy (PSE):* PSE results from several metabolic derangements. If the liver is unable to metabolize and cleanse the blood of ammonia and mercaptans, alterations in the level of consciousness, intellectual function, and neuromuscular function occur.

liver may impair tissue oxygen extraction and lead to lactic acidosis and circulatory failure. Although ammonia levels are high in ALF, the encephalopathy appears to be more related to hypoxia. Cerebral edema may result from fluid overload. Failure of the liver to manufacture the coagulation factors I, II, V, VII, IX, and X causes severe bleeding disorders, and there is also great risk of disseminated intravascular coagulation. Patients with ALF are susceptible to severe infections; cerebral edema and septicemia are the most frequent causes of death.

Typically most of the damage to the liver has been done by the time symptoms appear. A prolonged prothrombin time is characteristic and is closely related to the severity of organ damage. Values of more than 4 seconds secure the diagnosis of ALF, especially if mental status changes are also present. Jaundice is common, especially when hepatitis is the cause.[45,51]

Collaborative Care Management. The primary treatment for ALF is organ transplantation. The patient is maintained on life-support systems until a donor is found. Recent research on the use of extracorporeal liver assist devices as a support for liver function during the waiting period for transplantation has been promising. These devices, similar to hemodialysis, use hepatocytes from pigs or humans to provide liver function. They have been successful in improving neurologic parameters, liver function tests, cardiovascular status, renal function tests, and coagulation factors.[2] Dr. Jörg Gerlach, a researcher at the University of Pittsburgh, invented the machine that functions as a substitute liver by growing and sustaining liver cells using cells from livers that were not viable for transplants. This technology has kept patients in acute liver failure alive for 1 to 2 weeks while awaiting a transplant.[35]

Nursing care of the patient in ALF involves the intensive care monitoring of a patient in need of life support. The nurse monitors neurologic changes, especially increasing intracranial pressure; hemodynamic status; and cardiovascular, renal, and coagulation function. Other major concerns include the development of sepsis and shock.[48]

Chronic Liver Failure

Chronic liver failure represents the progressive, irreversible destruction of liver function over time. It is often referred to as end-stage liver disease.

Diffuse Hepatocellular Disorders

Hepatic disorders classified as diffuse are those which spread through a major portion of the liver. Disorders that are localized to one portion of the liver are classified as focal (Box 46-1).

Cirrhosis of the Liver

Cirrhosis of the liver is the term applied to chronic disease of the liver characterized by diffuse inflammation and fibrosis resulting in drastic structural changes and significant loss of liver function. The basic changes with cirrhosis are liver cell death and replacement of normal tissue by scar tissue that results in nodules of normal liver parenchyma surrounded by fibrous tissue and fat. These changes result in distortion of liver structure and loss of function.

Cirrhosis of the liver can be classified in various ways. Table 46-1 lists the major types based on a pathologic classification.

Etiology and Epidemiology. Alcoholism and malnutrition are two major predisposing factors for cirrhosis. Cirrhosis can also result from liver disease secondary to intrahepatic and extrahepatic cholestasis, viral hepatitis, and other hepatotoxins (drugs and chemicals). Primary biliary cirrhosis is less common causes, as are right-sided congestive heart failure, hemochromatosis, Wilson's disease, glycogen storage disease, cystic fibrosis, and small bowel bypass. In some patients the cause is idiopathic.[29]

The role of alcohol in the development of cirrhosis is still under study. It is known, however, that approximately 15% of all alcoholics develop cirrhosis and that the volume of alcohol rather than the type of alcohol is the important factor. Most persons with alcoholic liver disease have a history of consumption equivalent to a pint of whiskey a day for 15 years. *Healthy People 2010* indicates that sustained heavy alcohol consumption is the leading

Box 46-1 Common Liver Disorders

Diffuse Hepatocellular Disorders

Cirrhosis
Hepatitis

Sequelae of Chronic Diffuse Hepatocellular Disorders

Portal hypertension
Ascites
Esophageal varices
Portal-systemic encephalopathy
Hepatorenal syndrome

Focal Hepatocellular Disorders

Abscess
Trauma
Tumors

TABLE 46-1 TYPES OF CIRRHOSIS

Type	Etiology	Description
Laënnec's cirrhosis (nutritional or alcoholic cirrhosis)	Alcoholism, malnutrition	Massive collagen formation occurs; liver is fatty and in early hepatitis stages is large and firm; in late stage, it is small and nodular.
Postnecrotic cirrhosis	Massive necrosis from hepatotoxins, usually viral hepatitis	Liver is decreased in size with nodules and fibrous tissue.
Primary biliary cirrhosis	Inflammation of intrahepatic bile ductules resulting in biliary obstruction in liver and common bile duct; cholangitis (destruction of the intrahepatic bile ducts) possible; thought to be autoimmune disorder; 95% are women 30-60 years old	Chronic impairment of bile drainage occurs; liver is first large, then becomes firm and nodular; patient has increased skin pigmentation resembling a deep tan, jaundice, and pruritus.
Cardiac cirrhosis	Right-sided congestive heart failure (CHF)	Liver is swollen, and changes are reversible if CHF is treated effectively; some fibrosis occurs with longstanding CHF.
Nonspecific, metabolic cirrhosis	Metabolic problems, infectious diseases, infiltrative diseases, GI diseases	Portal and liver fibrosis may develop; liver is enlarged and firm.

cause of cirrhosis and that reduction in alcohol consumption over time is associated with reduction in the death rate from cirrhosis. Recent research is investigating drugs that may help those who have stopped drinking remain sober (see Future Watch box).

The death rate from cirrhosis in the United States is high, so *Healthy People 2010* set a goal to lower the rate to 3 deaths per 100,000 by 2010.[14,50] Cirrhosis as a cause of death in the United States now ranks fourth in middle-aged men and women, accounting for 350,000 deaths each year. Cirrhosis can occur in any age-group, but in the United States it is more common in 45- to 64-year-old Caucasian men and in non-Caucasians of both sexes.

Pathophysiology. In Laënnec's cirrhosis, fatty infiltration of the liver is the first alteration seen. This fatty infiltration is usually reversible if the causative factor (alcohol, malnutrition, or biliary obstruction) is halted or reversed. If the degenerative process continues, acute inflammation (alcoholic hepatitis) and cirrhosis result. Primary biliary cirrhosis is presumed to be autoimmune in origin, and there is persistent T-cell attack on the bile ducts, resulting in accumulation of toxic substances like bile acids in the liver.[26] The alterations in physiology associated with cirrhosis are usually seen late in the progression of the disease because of the liver's large reserve capacity. As much as three fourths of the liver can be destroyed before physiologic function is altered. The relationships between normal functions of the liver and alterations seen in liver disease such as in cirrhosis are presented in Table 46-2.[14,25]

A variety of signs and symptoms can be seen in persons with cirrhosis; they reflect the diminishing capacity of the liver to function normally. The patient may exhibit any or all of the signs and symptoms. Most manifestations can be directly related to the pathophysiologic changes (see Table 46-2, Figure 46-1, and Clinical Manifestations box).

COMPLICATIONS. Persons with cirrhosis frequently develop **portal hypertension,** which can result in ascites and esophageal varices; other complications include portal-systemic encephalopathy (PSE) and hepatorenal syndrome.

Future Watch

FDA Approves New Drugs for Treatment of Alcoholism

Alcohol abuse is a disease with severe, often life-threatening consequences. In addition to the individual suffering related to alcohol dependence, society bears a burden in terms of health care costs and lost wages. The U.S. Food and Drug Administration has approved the drug acamprosate (Campral) for the treatment of alcohol-dependent individuals who have stopped drinking. The drug may not be effective in patients who are actively drinking at the start of treatment or in patients who abuse other drugs.

Although the mechanism of action is not fully understood, acamprosate is thought to act on the brain pathways related to alcohol abuse. In clinical trials it proved to be superior to a placebo in maintaining abstinence, was not addicting, and was well tolerated.

FDA approves new drug for treatment of alcoholism, *FDA Talk Paper,* July 29, 2004, accessed Aug 2004 from website: www.fda.gov.

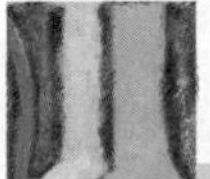

CLINICAL MANIFESTATIONS
Cirrhosis

- History of failing health
- Nausea
- Vomiting
- Anorexia
- Indigestion
- Flatulence
- Constipation
- Weight loss masked by water retention
- Malnutrition
- Abdominal pain (usually right upper quadrant)
- Late signs occurring gradually:
  - —Ascites
  - —Jaundice
  - —Edema
  - —Anemia
  - —Bleeding

TABLE 46-2 RELATIONSHIP BETWEEN NORMAL LIVER FUNCTIONS AND ALTERED FUNCTIONS WITH LIVER DISEASE

Normal Liver Functions	Altered Physiologic Functions
Maintenance of normal size and drainage of blood from gastrointestinal (GI) tract	Liver inflammation ↓ Venous congestion of GI tract → Altered GI function ↓ GI symptoms
Metabolism of carbohydrates	Increased glycogenesis and decreased glycogenolysis and gluconeogenesis ↓ Altered glucose metabolism ↓ Decreased energy
Metabolism of fats	Increased fatty acid and triglyceride synthesis and decreased fatty acid oxidation and triglyceride release ↓ Fatty liver ↓ Hepatomegaly ↓ Decreased energy production; weight loss
Protein metabolism	Decreased production of albumin→ Decreased colloidal osmotic pressure → Edema and ascites Decreased production of clotting factors ↓ Altered clotting studies ↓ Bleeding tendencies ↓ Blood loss → Anemia Decreased protein synthesis in general ↓ Alteration in immune function and alteration in healing
Detoxification of endogenous substances	Decreased metabolism of sex steroids (estrogen, progesterone, and testosterone) ↓ Male ↓ Loss of masculine characteristics and development of some feminine characteristics from excessive estrogen ↓ Female ↓ Loss of feminine characteristics and development of some masculine characteristics from excessive testosterone Decreased metabolism of aldosterone ↓ Sodium and water retention ↓ Edema, ascites ↓ Increased potassium and hydrogen excretion ↓ Hypokalemia and alkalosis Decreased metabolism of ammonia (usually resulting from blood bypassing liver rather than loss of parenchymal cell function) → Increased ammonia levels Hepatic encephalopathy ← ↓ Changes in coordination, memory, orientation; coma

PORTAL HYPERTENSION. Fibrotic changes in the liver that result from continual destruction distort the hepatic structures and result in obstruction of the splanchnic veins and portal blood flow. This obstruction causes an increase in hydrostatic pressure and can result in additional problems with fluid retention, including increasing edema, ascites, and hydrothorax. The backflow of blood caused by increased portal pressure and splanchnic venous congestion results in splenomegaly, which can cause leukopenia, thrombocytopenia, and anemia.

Portal hypertension also causes the development of collateral circulation to bypass the obstruction. These collateral vessels are most likely to form in the paraumbilical and hemorrhoidal veins (causing hemorrhoids), and at the cardia of the stomach extending into the esophagus. The collateral vessels in the upper stomach and

TABLE 46-2 RELATIONSHIP BETWEEN NORMAL LIVER FUNCTIONS AND ALTERED FUNCTIONS WITH LIVER DISEASE—CONT'D

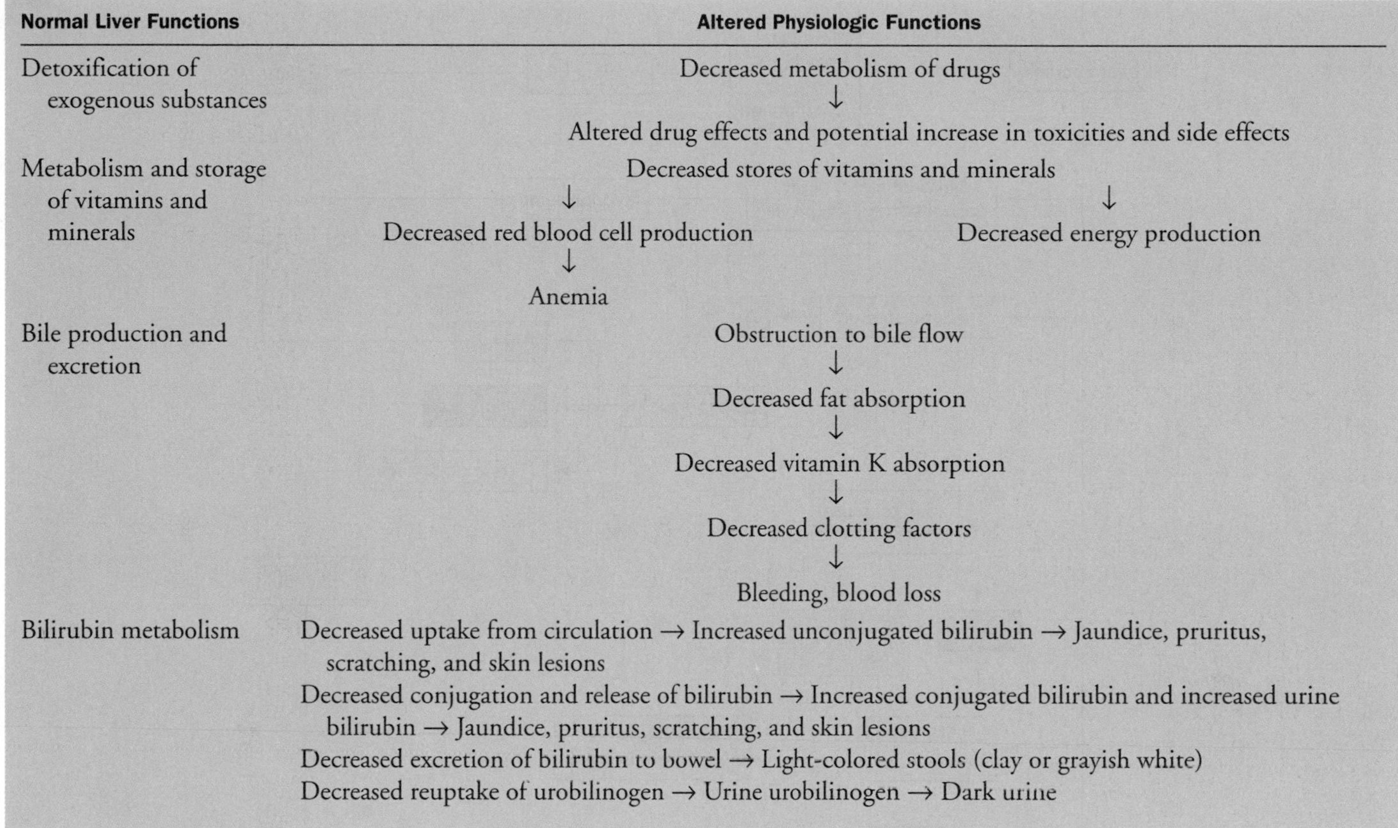

Normal Liver Functions	Altered Physiologic Functions
Detoxification of exogenous substances	Decreased metabolism of drugs ↓ Altered drug effects and potential increase in toxicities and side effects
Metabolism and storage of vitamins and minerals	Decreased stores of vitamins and minerals ↓ Decreased red blood cell production ↓ Anemia ↓ Decreased energy production
Bile production and excretion	Obstruction to bile flow ↓ Decreased fat absorption ↓ Decreased vitamin K absorption ↓ Decreased clotting factors ↓ Bleeding, blood loss
Bilirubin metabolism	Decreased uptake from circulation → Increased unconjugated bilirubin → Jaundice, pruritus, scratching, and skin lesions Decreased conjugation and release of bilirubin → Increased conjugated bilirubin and increased urine bilirubin → Jaundice, pruritus, scratching, and skin lesions Decreased excretion of bilirubin to bowel → Light-colored stools (clay or grayish white) Decreased reuptake of urobilinogen → Urine urobilinogen → Dark urine

esophagus are called **varices**; they are thin walled and fragile and have limited ability to withstand increases in pressure. This collateral circulation places the individual at high risk for a massive upper gastrointestinal (GI) bleeding episode (Figure 46-2).[23]

Figure 46-3, *A,* depicts the venous drainage of splanchnic organs, and Figure 46-3, *B,* depicts the massive ascites and gynecomastia (the enlarged breasts of this male patient, caused by failure of the liver to metabolize estrogen) that can be seen in cirrhosis.

ASCITES. **Ascites** is the accumulation of fluid in the peritoneal cavity, resulting from changes in the hemodynamics of the abdominal circulation. Increased pressure in the portal circulation from liver congestion increases capillary plasma hydrostatic pressure, and impaired production of albumin by the liver decreases capillary plasma oncotic pressure. These events combine to facilitate movement of serous fluid out of the vessels into the peritoneum. Increased levels of aldosterone and obstruction of hepatic lymph flow also contribute to the development of ascites. In addition to disrupting normal hemodynamics, ascites may cause respiratory distress from massive accumulation of fluid in the abdomen, which raises the diaphragm and decreases the space for respiratory excursion.[6,7,9]

PORTAL-SYSTEMIC ENCEPHALOPATHY. PSE, also called hepatic encephalopathy or hepatic coma, is one of the major complications of severe liver disease. The onset of the condition may be acute or chronic.

PSE results from several metabolic derangements. A major cause is the liver's inability to metabolize and cleanse the blood of ammonia and mercaptans. Ammonia is an end product of protein metabolism, whereas mercaptans are toxins produced from the metabolism of sulfur-containing compounds. These metabolic activities occur in the intestines, and the end products are normally carried to the liver where they are metabolized and excreted. The manifestations of PSE vary and may occur quickly or over the course of a few days. PSE produces alterations in the level of consciousness, intellectual function, behavior and personality, and neuromuscular function.[1]

HEPATORENAL SYNDROME. Hepatorenal syndrome is a poorly understood complication of end-stage liver disease. It is characterized by sudden kidney failure for no known cause in a patient with progressively worsening liver failure. The patient with hepatorenal failure has oliguria and azotemia. The onset of hepatorenal syndrome is a grave sign in a patient with liver failure.[12]

Collaborative Care Management. The goal for discharge of patients with cirrhosis as determined by a diagnosis-related group system is 7 days. The nurse works collaboratively with the physician for implementation of prescribed medical therapy. The nurse's major role in discharge planning and patient teaching is discussed under Nursing Management.

DIAGNOSTIC TESTS. The patient with cirrhosis has various abnormalities in blood and urine laboratory data (see Figure 46-1).

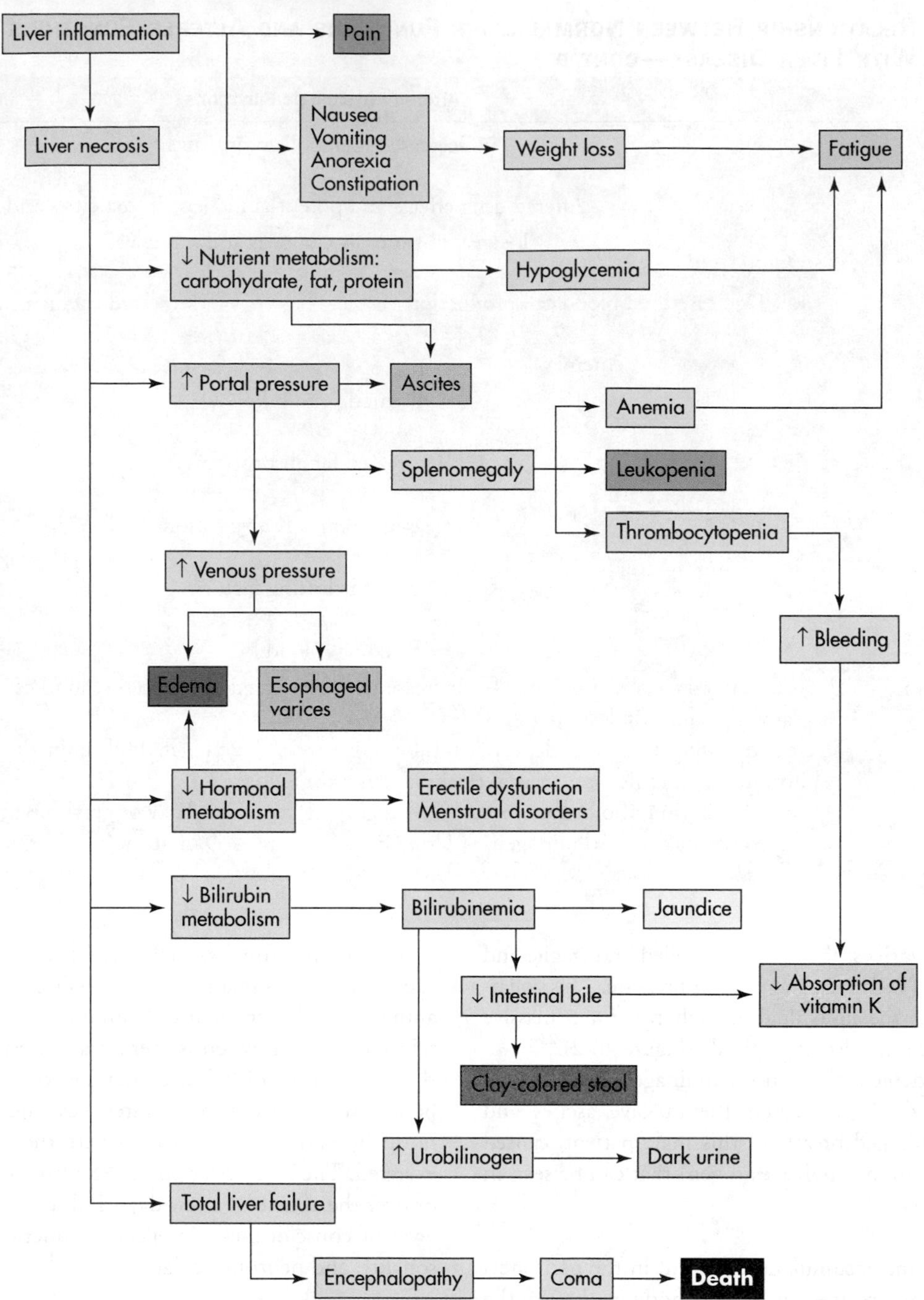

Figure 46-1 Progression of liver cell failure. Pathophysiology of signs and symptoms that occur in cirrhosis. NOTE: Process can be arrested if adequate liver regeneration occurs. Regeneration is rarely complete, and there is always some liver cell deficiency.

Other studies, such as liver biopsy, computed tomography (CT) scan, endoscopy, barium contrast, and angiography, may be done if the clinical manifestations are vague or inconsistent. The results of these later diagnostic tests depend on the complications the patient has developed.

MEDICATIONS. Drug therapy varies, depending on the signs and symptoms. The patient may be given antihistamines to alleviate pruritus from jaundice; potassium supplements to correct hypokalemia; diuretics (particularly aldosterone antagonists for edema, since the patient with cirrhosis does not catabolize aldosterone appropriately and has hyperaldosteronism); and folic acid, thiamine, and other vitamins and minerals for deficiencies and anemia. Persons with alcoholism are particularly deficient in thiamine and folic acid because these water-soluble vitamins have been depleted, and thus deficits occur rapidly with lack of intake of nutrients. Sodium and fluids are also usually restricted. Occasionally albumin may be given for hypoalbuminemia; however, its effects last only a short time.

TREATMENTS. No specific treatment exists for cirrhosis. Management is directed toward removal or treatment of causative factors

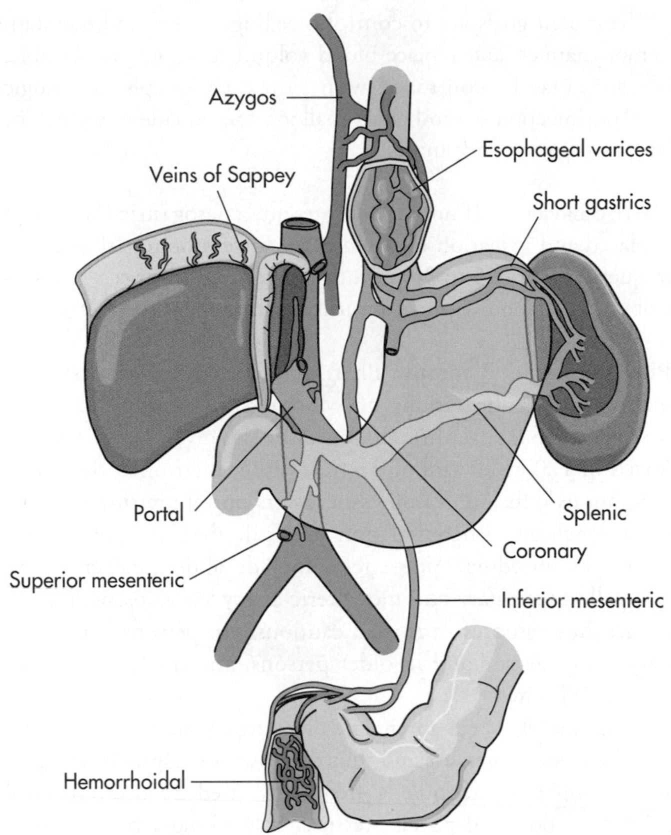

Figure 46-2 Varices related to portal hypertension. Portal vein, its major tributaries, and the most important collateral veins between portal and caval systems.

such as alcoholism, biliary obstruction, infections, and cardiac problems and toward preventing additional liver damage.

SYMPTOM MANAGEMENT

PORTAL HYPERTENSION. Nursing and medical management of portal hypertension is directed first to treating its consequences: ascites and esophageal varices. The only way to permanently lower portal pressure is surgical creation of a shunt to reduce blood flow through the obstructed part of the portal system. Because of the risks of the surgery and the frequent fatalities from liver failure after surgical treatment, these shunting procedures are used only in persons who have esophageal varices, have bleeding from the varices, and do not respond to other therapy. Surgical care is discussed later in this section.

ASCITES. Ascites, which may occur with or without peripheral edema, is one of the most frequent complications of cirrhosis of the liver. Restriction of sodium and diuretic therapy may prevent ascites. When these first-line therapies fail, **paracentesis** or shunting procedures may be necessary.

Large-Volume Paracentesis. Large volume paracentesis (LVP) is the removal of 5 L or more of ascitic fluid during a single treatment. Because this fluid loss disrupts the individual's hemodynamics, plasma expanders such as intravenous (IV) albumin are given simultaneously. Although this treatment resolves ascites in most patients, it is limited by a high frequency of recurrent ascites and the need for further paracentesis. LVP does not correct the underlying pathologic condition or improve patient survival rates.[9]

Peritoneovenous Shunt. In chronic and resistant ascites a LeVeen or Denver **peritoneovenous (PV) shunt** may be used (Figure 46-4). The shunt provides continuous reinfusion of ascitic fluid into the venous system through a silicone catheter with a one-way pressure-sensitive valve. One end of the catheter is implanted in the peritoneal cavity, and the tube is channeled through subcutaneous tissue to the superior vena cava, where the other end is implanted. The valve opens when there is a pressure differential of more than 3 mm H_2O between the peritoneal cavity and the vein in the thoracic cavity, allowing fluid to move from the peritoneal cavity into the superior vena cava. The Denver shunt is a variation of the LeVeen catheter and has a subcutaneous pump that can be compressed manually to irrigate the tubing to

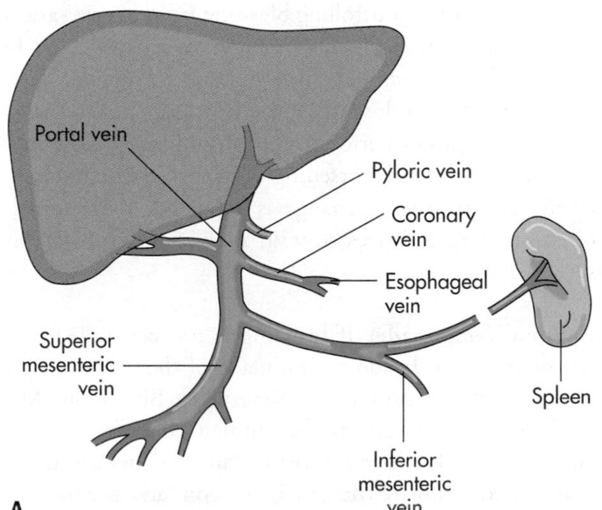

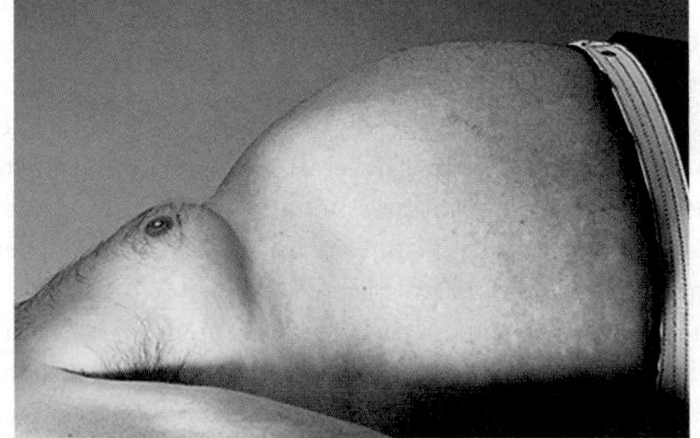

Figure 46-3 Splanchnic veins. **A,** Venous drainage of splanchnic organs. When portal hypertension develops, other vessels can become engorged, leading to stasis and hypoxia of the respective organs. **B,** Ascites and gynecomastia associated with cirrhosis of the liver. Photograph taken after a paracentesis was performed.

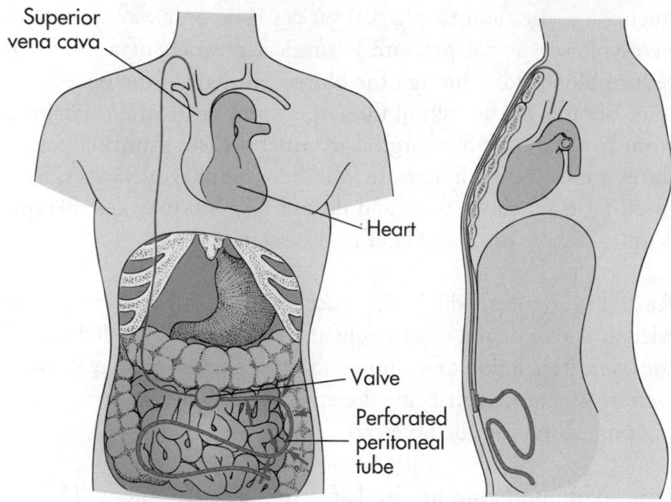

Figure 46-4 LeVeen peritoneovenous shunt, showing placement of catheter.

keep it patent. Although the efficacy of these shunts is comparable to that of LVP, they have a high incidence of thrombus formation at the venous tip of the shunt, catheter occlusion, and infections. PV shunts also do not improve survival rates.[17,43,52]

Esophageal Varices. Bleeding esophageal varices are the most dangerous complication of portal hypertension. The mortality associated with variceal hemorrhage is 50%. In portal hypertension the azygos vein and the vena cava become distended where they join the smaller vessels of the esophagus. Distention occurs because of the greater volume of blood flowing through these vessels as a result of higher pressure within the portal system. Normal portal pressure is about 9 mm Hg. The increased portal venous pressure forces the blood, which normally flows through the liver, into these other vessels (see Figure 46-3, *A,* for a diagram of the relationship between these various blood vessels). These small vessels cannot accommodate the increased blood volume, and they become tortuous and fragile. Changes in the vessels' structure predispose them to injury whenever intraabdominal pressure is increased as a result of coughing, vomiting, sneezing, or straining during defecation (Valsalva's maneuver). Bleeding may also be initiated by mechanical trauma from ingestion of coarse foods and acidic pepsin erosion.

Primary prophylaxis should be initiated for any patient diagnosed with cirrhosis. A screening endoscopy is done and repeated every 2 to 3 years. If large varices or other signs of increased risk of bleeding are found, treatment with nonselective beta-blockers should be initiated. Propranolol (Inderal) and nadolol (Corgard) have been used to reduce portal pressure and successfully prevent the first episode of bleeding. Nitrates are also used if the patient does not respond to beta-blockers alone.

The first priority in the medical management of an active bleeding episode is to establish the source of bleeding. Esophagoscopy is the major diagnostic tool; if this is not possible, angiography is used. If severe hemorrhage is not present, barium studies or scans may be used. It must be remembered that in patients with cirrhosis, bleeding may be from other causes such as peptic ulcers or gastritis.[21]

Treatment goals are to control bleeding, restore and maintain hemodynamics, and replace blood volume as rapidly as possible. Bleeding may be controlled with gastric lavage, pharmacologic therapy, injection sclerotherapy, balloon tamponade of varices, or surgery (ligation and shunts).

Gastric Lavage. If not already present, a nasogastric (NG) tube is placed and irrigation initiated. The nurse monitors the patient frequently, every 15 to 30 minutes, since the patient can lose several units of blood within 1 hour if hemorrhage is severe.

Pharmacologic Therapy. Pharmacologic therapy is started, including administration of vasopressin, propranolol, and octreotide (Sandostatin). Vasopressin is given intravenously mixed in 120 to 200 ml of dextrose either intermittently or as a continuous infusion. Vasopressin lowers portal pressure by causing splanchnic vasoconstriction and can thus stop or control esophageal bleeding. Side effects include abdominal cramping and pallor. Coronary and mesenteric artery vasoconstriction can occur; thus vasopressin is used cautiously in persons with coronary artery disease and in older persons, and the length of this therapy is limited.

Propranolol, a beta-adrenergic blocking agent, has been shown to reduce portal pressure and thus decrease esophageal bleeding in some people. Octreotide is frequently used to decrease total splanchnic flow and portal pressure. It is a long-acting octapeptide that mimics the action of the hormone somatostatin and is administered subcutaneously.

Endoscopic Sclerotherapy. Endoscopic sclerotherapy is the first-line treatment for active variceal bleeding. The surgeon passes a fiberoptic endoscope into the esophagus, identifies the bleeding site, and injects a sclerosing agent (morrhuate sodium, 5 ml) into the varices. This agent causes thrombosis and sclerosis of the vessel and should result in hemostasis in 3 to 5 minutes. If hemostasis does not occur, a second injection may be given. The procedure may be repeated as necessary and can be performed while the varices are bleeding or as an elective procedure. Endoscopic therapy is ineffective in controlling bleeding from gastric varices. Endoscopic variceal ligation, an alternative to sclerotherapy, has fewer complications and similar efficacy in controlling bleeding.[21,42]

As after any endoscopic procedure, the nurse monitors the patient for signs of perforated esophagus, aspiration pneumonia, pleural effusion, and worsening of ascites. Respiratory support to ensure adequate air exchange is provided. Retrosternal pain is often present and is treated with analgesics; fever is common for several days.

Balloon Tamponade. If bleeding is not controlled by the preceding methods, balloon tamponade of the varices may be instituted. Esophagogastric tubes (Sengstaken-Blakemore, Minnesota, or Linton) are three- or four-lumen tubes with two balloon attachments. One lumen serves as an NG suction tube, the second is used to inflate the gastric balloon, and the third is used to inflate the esophageal balloon (Figure 46-5). The Minnesota esophagogastric tamponade tube has a fourth lumen used for esophageal aspiration, and is currently used most often. The physician passes the tube through the nose into the stomach with

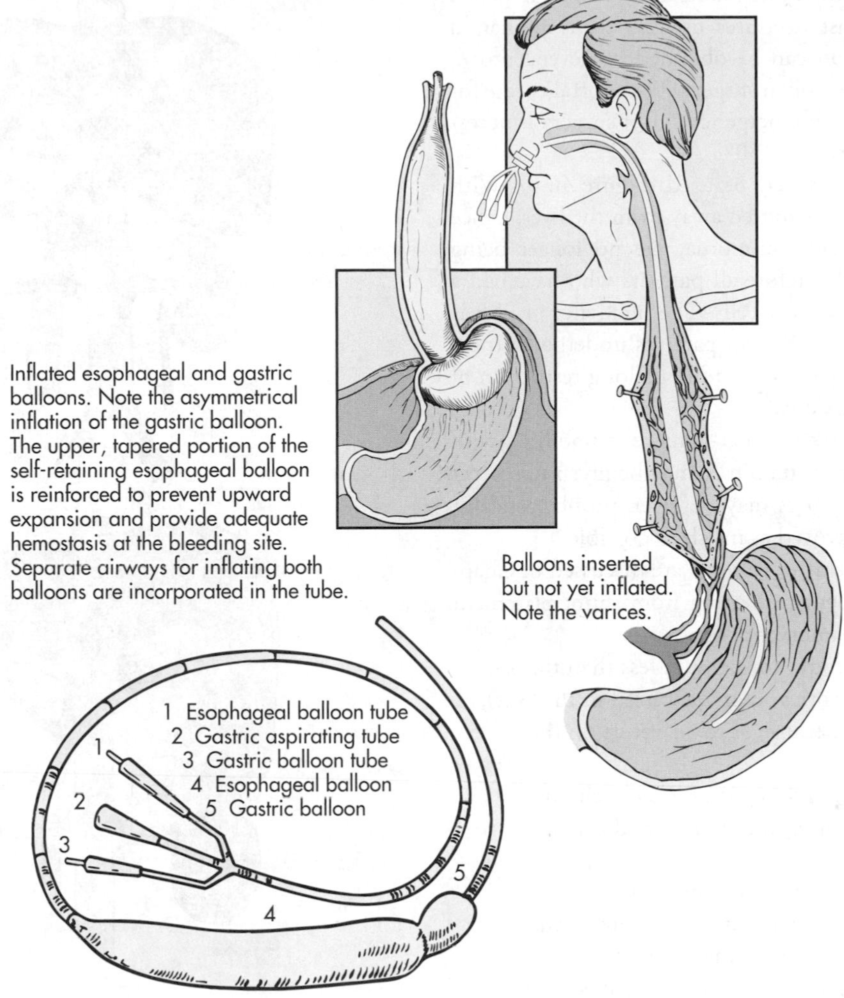

Inflated esophageal and gastric balloons. Note the asymmetrical inflation of the gastric balloon. The upper, tapered portion of the self-retaining esophageal balloon is reinforced to prevent upward expansion and provide adequate hemostasis at the bleeding site. Separate airways for inflating both balloons are incorporated in the tube.
Balloons inserted but not yet inflated. Note the varices.
1 Esophageal balloon tube
2 Gastric aspirating tube
3 Gastric balloon tube
4 Esophageal balloon
5 Gastric balloon

Figure 46-5 Esophageal tamponade accomplished with a Sengstaken-Blakemore tube.

the balloons deflated. When the tube is in the stomach, the physician inflates the gastric balloon with 250 to 300 cc of air, clamps the lumen, and pulls the tube out slowly so that the balloon is held tightly against the cardioesophageal junction. Traction may be applied. The esophageal balloon is inflated to 25 to 45 mg Hg, and both remaining lumens are then attached to low intermittent suction. It is important to remove all blood from the stomach, since it may precipitate PSE from ammonia produced from the digestion of protein in the blood.

The esophageal balloon can be left inflated for up to 48 hours without causing tissue damage. The fully inflated gastric balloon with traction compresses the stomach wall between the balloon and the diaphragm, and can cause ulceration of the gastric mucosa and severe discomfort. To offset the possibility of necrosis, the physician may release traction on the gastric balloon and deflate the gastric balloon pressure periodically. If the gastric balloon ruptures (and the patient is not intubated), the entire tube may move and obstruct the airway. If this occurs, the tube is immediately removed. The major complication in the use of these tubes is esophageal ulceration.[21,42]

Nursing care of the patient with esophageal tamponade includes maintenance of the proper position of the tube; care of the mouth and nares; frequent oral suctioning, since the patient is unable to swallow even saliva; and provisional comfort measures, both physical and psychologic, to patient and family.[47]

Balloon tamponade should be reserved as a lifesaving, temporary measure until the patient can undergo transjugular intrahepatic portosystemic shunt (TIPS) or surgical shunting.

Shunts

Transjugular Intrahepatic Portosystemic Shunt. TIPS is a procedure in which, using radiography guidance, the surgeon creates a shunt between the hepatic and portal veins and keeps it open by the placement of a metal stent. This decompresses the portal system and reduces portal hypertension enough to control active bleeding in most patients. Because TIPS is associated with long-term complications, it is primarily used as rescue therapy when pharmacologic and endoscopic treatment of an acute bleed has failed. These complications include stent dysfunctions, such as thrombosis or stenosis, and right-sided heart failure. The advantage of TIPS is that it is relatively noninvasive and does not require anesthesia for a patient with a failing liver. TIPS may also be used as a prophylactic treatment for portal hypertension; however, the benefits of this procedure over other methods are debatable. TIPS procedures are often performed while the patient awaits liver transplantation.[10,21]

Surgical Shunts. Surgery to shunt blood away from the portal circulation is one of the last measures used to treat esophageal varices. Portal decompression can be obtained by several procedures, most of them requiring open surgery. The mortality rate for shunt surgery is 5% to 15%; if emergency shunt surgery is necessary, the mortality rate increases to 50%.

Various surgical procedures may be used (Figure 46-6). With all of them the portal blood is shunted away from the liver; hence toxins in the blood, especially ammonia, are no longer being metabolized and excreted. Therefore all patients who have had a portosystemic shunt are at risk for PSE. The incidence of PSE is reportedly as high as 25% to 100% in patients undergoing these shunting procedures. Some patients require lifelong restriction of protein to limit ammonia toxicity.[22]

Before surgery the patient's vascular volume is stabilized with fluids and blood as necessary. Vitamin K may be given to correct coagulation problems, antibiotics may be given prophylactically, and nutritional status is improved as much as possible.

General needs of postoperative patients are discussed in Chapter 15. In addition, the patient recovering from shunt placement needs the following nursing interventions:

- Administration of narcotics for pain (at less than the usual dosage, since most narcotics are metabolized in the liver); avoidance of sedatives because of toxic effects on the diseased liver
- Careful observation for early signs of PSE (including mental confusion, slowness in response, and generally inappropriate behavior)
- Monitoring for hemorrhage and signs of shock
- Monitoring for signs of thrombosis at the site of anastomosis (pain, distention, fever, and nausea)
- Encouragement of activity within the prescribed limits; initiation of leg and arm exercises on the first postoperative day
- Monitoring of the lower extremities for signs of edema; elevation of the lower extremities if ordered to prevent edema formation from the sudden increase of blood flow into the inferior vena cava

In addition, other nursing care responsibilities for the patient with bleeding esophageal varices include:

- Administration of fresh whole blood and IV infusions. Use of fresh blood avoids the increased ammonia and citrate of stored blood; fresh blood also has relatively more coagulation factors.
- Administration of saline cathartics through the NG lumen of the esophagogastric tube or through an NG tube to hasten expulsion of blood from the GI tract and to prevent an increase in the production of ammonia. Enemas may also be ordered to decrease gut content and bacterial action on the blood.
- Administration of lactulose or neomycin to prevent or decrease PSE.

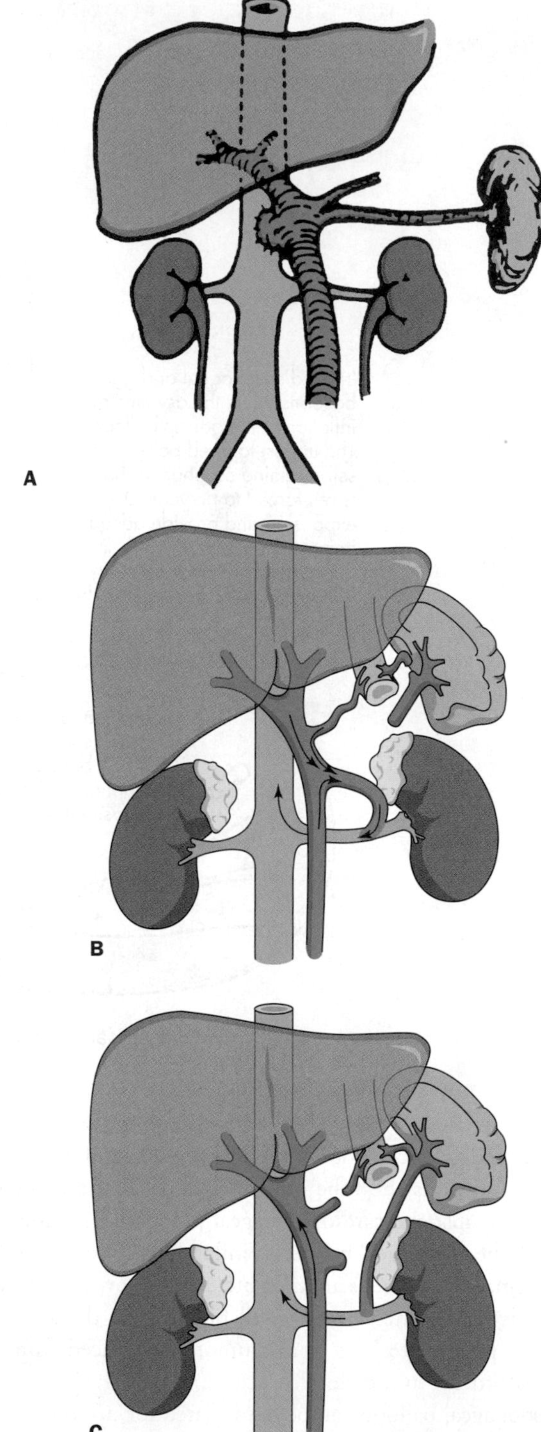

Figure 46-6 Decompression procedures for portal hypertension. **A,** Side-to-side portacaval shunt. **B,** Splenorenal shunt. **C,** Distal splenorenal shunt.

PORTAL-SYSTEMIC ENCEPHALOPATHY. PSE is a major complication of cirrhosis, the result of rising levels of toxic substances normally metabolized and excreted by the liver. Thirty percent of patients diagnosed with cirrhosis die in hepatic coma. Common factors that precipitate PSE are summarized in Box 46-2. The manifestations of PSE vary and may occur quickly or gradually over the course of a few days. PSE results in alterations in the state of consciousness, intellectual function, behavior and personality, and neuromuscular function. These changes have been graded in four stages (Table 46-3).

Box 46-2 Common Factors Associated With Portal-Systemic Encephalopathy

Factors Depressing Central Nervous System or Liver Function

Hypoxia
- —Secondary to hemorrhage and hypovolemic shock
- —Secondary to morphine and other sedatives

Infections
Exercise
In patients with chronic liver disease and impending coma:
- —Sedatives
- —Abdominal paracentesis resulting in reduction of plasma volume

Factors Increasing Level of Ammonia

Gastrointestinal (GI) ammonia (old blood in bowel from GI hemorrhage)
High protein intake
Transfusions, especially with stored blood, since it contains more ammonia
Hypokalemia
- —Secondary to thiazide diuretics
- —Secondary to potassium loss from the bowel

Alkalosis secondary to hyperventilation or hypokalemia
Shunting of blood into systemic circulation without passing through hepatic sinusoids
Natural collateral bypass of liver
Surgical bypass of liver
Constipation

Medical management of PSE involves identifying and treating precipitating factors such as hypokalemia, hemorrhage, and hypoxia; reducing serum ammonia levels; and providing supportive care. An elevated serum ammonia level provides the definitive diagnosis of PSE, but it does not occur in all patients with PSE. Therefore treatment is determined by the signs and symptoms and not the serum ammonia levels.

Lactulose and neomycin are given to decrease the serum ammonia levels. Lactulose is a synthetic disaccharide degraded by bacteria in the lower intestines. It is given either orally or by retention enema and promotes the excretion of ammonia in the stool by decreasing the pH of the bowel. Ammonia remains in its ionized state, which facilitates its movement from the blood to the stool. Bacterial growth is discouraged by the acidic environment. Lactulose also causes diarrhea, which helps eliminate blood from the GI tract in patients with bleeding esophageal varices.[1]

Neomycin is a broad-spectrum antibiotic that destroys the normal flora of the bowel. Bacteria in the bowel normally break down protein, including blood protein in the GI tract, producing ammonia. Therefore neomycin decreases the protein breakdown by bacteria in the bowel.[1]

A low-protein diet may be prescribed, but this practice is controversial. Some researchers have found that increasing the calories and protein in patients with alcoholic liver disease does not worsen the encephalopathy.

Nursing management focuses on four goals: (1) providing continual, regular monitoring of patients at high risk for PSE; (2) assisting with the therapeutic regimen; (3) providing supportive care; and (4) providing long-term care

As can be seen from a review of Table 46-3, the early indications of PSE are subtle and can easily be missed if regular, objective assessments are not made. The nurse must (1) be as consistent and descriptive as possible; (2) assess skills such as handwriting or the ability to draw a circle, box, or square; and (3) maintain continuity of care so that the staff becomes familiar with the patient's behavior. Early detection of symptoms allows for more rapid treatment and consequently improves the patient's chance of recovery.

Monitoring also focuses on the patient's vital signs and overall status to detect deterioration of baseline function. The onset of fever or worsening results of laboratory studies (e.g., serum enzyme [alanine aminotransaminase (ALT) and aspartate aminotransaminase (AST)] levels, prothrombin time, and bilirubin and albumin levels), and subtle mental status changes can indicate the onset of PSE.

If encephalopathy is present, a major focus of nursing is to implement the prescribed regimen. Treatment is directed toward eliminating the causes of PSE, such as GI bleeding or hypokalemia, if known. The patient is protected from injury, since altered mental

TABLE 46-3 STAGES OF PORTAL-SYSTEMIC ENCEPHALOPATHY

Stage	Consciousness	Intellect, Personality	Neurologic Status	Ammonia Levels	Electroencephalogram
Subclinical	N	N	Some impaired psychomotor testing	N	N
1	Insomnia, disturbed sleep	Confusion, forgetfulness, agitation	Tremor, apraxia, uncoordination	↑	Slight abnormalities
2	Lethargy	Disorientation, bizarre behavior	Asterixis, ataxia	↑↑	Slowing of triphasic waves
3	Somnolent; may be arousable	Disorientation, aggression	Asterixis, hyperreflexia, positive Babinski's sign	↑↑↑	Same as above
4	Coma, no response	Coma	Decerebrate	↑↑↑↑	Slow waves, 2-3 per second

N, Normal.

status increases the risk. Other interventions focus on reducing ammonia levels and include:

- Eliminating or restricting protein intake
- Increasing carbohydrate intake to decrease metabolism of endogenous proteins
- Administering oral cathartics or enemas to empty the bowel and decrease ammonia formation
- Administering intestinal antibiotics such as neomycin to kill bacteria in the GI tract
- Administering lactulose
- Hemodialysis

The patient with PSE is very ill and requires care for the prevention of respiratory problems. Ventilatory support may be required. Coughing is prohibited if the patient has esophageal varices. The patient also needs care to prevent skin breakdown that may be worsened by malnutrition, pruritus, ascites, and frequent stools or incontinence. Infection must be prevented. If PSE progresses to hepatic coma, nursing care is similar to that of any unconscious patient.

Many patients with PSE die of kidney failure secondary to inadequate circulating blood volume (hypovolemia). In some patients, renal function progressively deteriorates without any apparent cause (hepatorenal syndrome). Treatment of PSE requires a careful balancing of fluid administration to maintain adequate perfusion of the kidney without creating an excessive load on the cardiovascular system. To monitor renal function adequately, an indwelling catheter is inserted, especially if the patient is being maintained on IV fluids. Frequently central venous pressure is also monitored to determine fluid volume status.

Because most narcotics and sedatives must be detoxified by the liver, their use is contraindicated in patients with impaired liver function. If a sedative must be used, drugs such as chlordiazepoxide (Librium), barbital, or phenobarbital, which are excreted by the kidney, are prescribed. If any sedatives, analgesics, or hypnotics are used, they should be given in less than normal doses, and the patient's response should be evaluated carefully.

The patient and family need instructions regarding dietary restrictions and how to take medications. They also must be taught to be alert for subtle changes in the patient's behavior that indicate worsening or onset of PSE and to seek medical attention immediately if the patient shows any of these behaviors.[48]

▶ ARE YOU READY?

What is the rationale for administering neomycin to a patient with portal-systemic encephalopathy?

1. Protect against infection due to malnourishment
2. Enhance vitamin K absorption from the bowel to decrease bleeding
3. Increase excretion of ammonia through the bowel
4. Decrease protein breakdown by bacteria in the bowel

HEPATORENAL SYNDROME. The sudden onset of oliguria and azotemia in a patient with end-stage liver disease is a grave sign. The blood pressure may be elevated or decreased. The patient complains of anorexia, fatigue, and weakness. Fluid retention leads to hyponatremia and a decrease in urine osmolality. The continual accumulation of waste products and alterations in fluid and electrolytes cause neurologic changes that can resemble those of PSE. Blood pressure continues to drop. Hepatorenal syndrome has a poor prognosis, and its onset suggests impending death.

Management begins with determining whether the oliguria is caused by decreased cardiac output, hepatorenal syndrome, or acute tubular necrosis. Any of these processes can occur in the person with cirrhosis. Once the diagnosis of hepatorenal syndrome is made, management is designed to improve hepatic function and support renal function. Fluid and electrolytes are given to maintain hemodynamic status. Potentially nephrotoxic drugs such as neomycin are stopped. Some patients have shown improvement after a portacaval shunt has been performed. Liver transplantation is the major intervention for most patients with hepatorenal syndrome; however, these patients are poor surgical risks. Hemodialysis has been successful in treating hyperkalemia and fluid overload and thereby improving symptoms. It does not improve the hepatorenal syndrome itself, since the basic problem is in the liver, not the kidney.[11]

DIET. Because alcoholism and malnutrition are major factors in the development of cirrhosis, supplying an adequate diet (well-balanced with normal nutrients) and helping the patient control alcohol intake are important. Vitamin supplements are usually prescribed. In the presence of ascites, a low-sodium diet is recommended. Daily intake of sodium may be limited to 500 to 1000 mg. Fluids may be restricted to avoid exacerbating fluid volume excess. Providing good oral hygiene; maintaining a pleasant, clean environment; and serving small, attractive meals can help increase appetite. A low-protein (20 to 40 g/day) diet may be prescribed when signs of PSE are seen. Dietary or IV supplements that provide selected branched-chain amino acids, which are metabolized in the muscle instead of the liver, may be used. Both oral and IV preparations are available commercially; these also contain carbohydrates. Vitamins and minerals are added as necessary.

HEALTH PROMOTION AND PREVENTION. The goal of *Healthy People 2010* is to reduce the number of deaths from cirrhosis to no more than 3 per 100,000 people, with African-American men, Native Americans, and Alaskan Inuits being targeted populations. Even though cirrhosis among African-American and Native-American men has declined in the past few years, the death rate for non-Caucasian men is 70% higher than for Caucasian men.[50]

In the United States programs aimed at the prevention of cirrhosis are designed primarily to control the ingestion of alcohol. The loss of time from work related to alcoholism is estimated to cost billions of dollars annually. Many large corporations have programs to help employees control their alcohol intake.

Since research has shown that the combination of acetaminophen and alcohol can impair liver function and increase the risk of cirrhosis, all over-the-counter acetaminophen must carry a warning label that reads "Alcohol Warning: If you consume three or more alcoholic drinks every day, ask your doctor whether you should take acetaminophen or other pain reliever/fever reducers. Acetaminophen may cause liver damage."[51]

Early detection of cirrhosis is difficult because three fourths of the liver can be destroyed before signs of cirrhosis become evident. For this reason, cessation of alcohol intake is the focus of secondary prevention.

Nursing Management of the Patient with Cirrhosis

ASSESSMENT

Health History. Assess for:

- Recent temperature elevations, frequent infections
- Changes in color of skin or sclera; skin marks such as bruising and hematomas; changes in secondary sex characteristics (external genitalia, body hair distribution, or breast tissue); increase in abdominal girth (belt size); edema; complaints of itching; muscle wasting
- Social habits: drug and alcohol use, amount, factors that precipitate use, any attempts to quit, limitations on success, reasons for failure; last time patient had a drink; work environment
- Nutritional history: daily 24-hour intake for past 1 to 3 days; recent change in appetite, anorexia, or weight loss
- Nausea, vomiting, anorexia, indigestion, flatulence, or abdominal tenderness
- Changes in amount or color of urine, in bowel movements, or in color of feces
- Weakness or fatigue; decreased ability to do work; changes in memory or coordination; tremors
- Erectile dysfunction, decreased libido (men and women), or change in menstrual patterns

Physical Examination. Assess for:

- Elevated temperature, weight changes, orthostatic hypotension
- Jaundice, bruises, hematomas, petechiae, **spider angiomas**, palmar erythema, dilated vessels on upper body or lower extremities, loss of chest hair (men), gynecomastia, edema of lower extremities, and lesions from scratching
- Abnormal breath sounds and presence of dullness in right lower lobe
- Hypoactive bowel sounds, abdominal distention or guarding, ascites (fluid wave or shifting dullness), increased abdominal girth, increased liver size, hepatic bruits, enlarged spleen, and dilated veins on abdomen (caput medusae)
- Muscle wasting, decreased muscle strength, deficits in memory or coordination, tremors, asterixis, exaggerated deep tendon reflexes, changes in orientation, behavior or emotional changes, apraxia
- Decreased urinary output, changes in color of urine and stools, testicular atrophy

NURSING DIAGNOSES, OUTCOMES, AND INTERVENTIONS

Nursing Diagnosis: Ineffective Breathing Pattern

OUTCOMES. Common examples of expected outcomes for the patient with a diagnosis of *ineffective breathing pattern* are:
Patient will:

- Have normal breath sounds and normal chest x-ray films.
- Be free from any increase in dullness on percussion of the thorax.

NURSING INTERVENTIONS. A high Fowler's position may assist respiratory exchange. The patient for whom bed rest is prescribed should be encouraged to turn frequently and to take deep breaths to prevent stasis of secretions. Hydrothorax is sometimes treated with thoracentesis (see Chapter 26). The nurse prepares the patient for this procedure, assists with the procedure, and monitors the patient's response during and after the procedure.

A sample Nursing Care Plan is on p. 1328.

RELATED NIC INTERVENTIONS. Airway Management, Oxygen Therapy, Respiratory Monitoring

Nursing Diagnosis: Fatigue

OUTCOMES. Common examples of expected outcomes for the patient with a diagnosis of *fatigue* are:
Patient will:

- Demonstrate a gradual increase in activities.
- Meet self-care needs.
- Walk an increased amount each day.

NURSING INTERVENTIONS. Patients with cirrhosis have various levels of fatigue. The amount and type of activity encouraged depend on the individual's energy level, level of consciousness and coordination, and any complications. If the patient has severe fluid excess and ascites or signs and symptoms of other complications, bed rest is usually required. In this case special attention to skin care is necessary, particularly if the patient also has severe peripheral edema. Alternating pressure mattresses or flotation pads may be helpful. If bed rest is not required, the patient should be walked within the room or hall as tolerated. Level of tolerance is based on the patient's statement about the level of fatigue, on pulse changes, or both. The pulse rate should not increase by more than 10 beats/min above baseline with activity.

RELATED NIC INTERVENTIONS. Energy Management, Nutrition Management, Sleep Enhancement

Nursing Diagnosis: Excess Fluid Volume

OUTCOMES. Common examples of expected outcomes for the patient with a diagnosis of *excess fluid volume* are:
Patient will:

- Have a urinary output that is greater than fluid intake.
- Demonstrate a daily decrease in weight.
- Demonstrate a resolution of edema and decrease of abdominal girth.
- Demonstrate a return of electrolyte values to normal.

NURSING INTERVENTIONS. Potassium replacement for hypokalemia is usually given orally, and the nurse should monitor the patient's serum potassium values to verify that the patient is not developing hyperkalemia. This is important because some patients with cirrhosis develop hepatorenal syndrome and have decreased renal function, which impairs the excretion of potassium, possibly resulting in hyperkalemia.

Sodium imbalance and ascites are treated in several ways. The basis for determining the amount of dietary restriction necessary to reduce sodium and water retention may initially be a collection of urine for 24 hours to determine sodium loss. Sodium is generally

Nursing Care Plan

Patient With Cirrhosis

Data A 55-year-old man with portal hypertension is admitted to the hospital with upper gastrointestinal tract bleeding. Abnormal physical findings include slight jaundice of the skin and sclera, ascites, 2+ pitting edema of both lower extremities, and thin legs and arms with poor musculature. His vital signs are blood pressure, 116/60 mm Hg; pulse, 60 beats/min; respirations, 32 breaths/min; and temperature, 99.4° F (37.4° C) orally. He complains of fatigue, anorexia, and itching. He also states that he has participated in Alcoholics Anonymous (AA) for 1 year and has been sober since joining.

Endoscopy reveals enlarged esophageal and upper gastric veins and a bleeding ulcer. One unit of packed red blood cells is immediately administered, and the patient is placed on protein (20 g/day) and sodium (1000 mg/day) restrictions, fluid restriction (1000 ml/day), neomycin (1 g every 4 hours), thiamine (1 ml intramuscularly), vitamin K subcutaneously daily, and spironolactone (25 mg twice daily).

Nursing Diagnosis

Fatigue related to muscle wasting, blood loss, and anemia secondary to cirrhosis

Outcomes

- Patient will report decreased fatigue on a scale of 1 (no fatigue) to 10 (severe fatigue).
- Patient will demonstrate a gradual increase in ability to perform activities without assistance.

Related NOC Outcomes

- Activity Tolerance
- Endurance
- Energy Conservation

Related NIC Interventions

- Energy Management
- Sleep Enhancement
- Teaching: Prescribed Activity/Exercise

Nursing Interventions/Rationales

- Ensure or maintain bed rest as prescribed during the acute phase of illness or relapse. *Bed rest decreases metabolic rate, oxygen consumption, and energy demands.*
- After acute phase, encourage increasing activity interspersed with rest periods as tolerated. *Resting between activities allows greater energy availability for performing tasks. Activities can be increased as nutritional status and energy level are restored.*
- Intervene if patient shows fatigue after or during visits by family and friends. *Patients often feel they must entertain visitors and expend more energy than is available to do so.*
- Encourage intake of well-balanced diet within prescribed restrictions. *To help restore nutritional balance and increase energy.*

Nursing Diagnosis

Imbalanced nutrition: less than body requirements related to anorexia and flulike symptoms secondary to cirrhosis

Outcomes

- Patient will ingest adequate nutrients and calories daily as evidenced by weight gain.
- Patient will maintain (or regain) weight to within 5 pounds of baseline (or ideal) weight.

Related NOC Outcomes

- Nutritional Status
- Nutritional Status: Food & Fluid Intake
- Nutritional Status: Nutrient Intake

Related NIC Interventions

- Nutrition Management
- Nutrition Therapy
- Nutritional Monitoring

Nursing Interventions/Rationales

- Assess nutritional needs. *Baseline data are needed to plan effectively for nutritional needs.*
- Encourage intake of well-balanced, high-carbohydrate, low-protein diet with adequate vitamins. *Food intake within prescribed limitations can influence liver regeneration.*
- Decrease dietary roughage. *To prevent irritation and possible bleeding of esophageal varices.*
- Encourage use of salt substitute or alternative seasonings. *To decrease sodium intake without discouraging food intake.*
- Administer antiemetics as prescribed and mouth care if nausea is present. *To increase comfort and reduce nausea so that dietary intake is possible.*
- Encourage six small meals daily. *Large meals are overwhelming. Small meals encourage intake without producing distention or fatigue.*
- Use measures to encourage eating (clean environment, meals served after patient has rested). *To increase the likelihood that the patient will intake sufficient food to meet dietary needs.*
- Support continuation in AA activities while patient is hospitalized. *To avoid breaking continuity of support system. Allow AA representative to see patient as condition permits.*

Nursing Diagnosis

Excess fluid volume related to impaired metabolism of aldosterone

Outcomes

- Patient will experience daily decreases in weight and abdominal girth.
- Patient will be free from peripheral edema.

Related NOC Outcomes

- Electrolyte & Acid/Base Balance
- Fluid Balance
- Nutritional Status: Food & Fluid Intake

Related NIC Interventions

- Fluid Management
- Fluid Monitoring
- Hypervolemia Management

Nursing Interventions/Rationales

- Monitor weight daily, blood pressure every 4 hours, edema every shift, and abdominal girth daily. *To provide a baseline for comparisons to determine effectiveness of treatment interventions.*
- Monitor intake and output on every shift until excess fluid is excreted. *Diuresis in cirrhosis is undertaken slowly using conservative measures because of the contracted intravascular fluid volume. Excessive diuresis can compromise renal perfusion and precipitate portal-systemic encephalopathy.*
- Teach patient the rationale for sodium restriction when able to comprehend teaching. *Understanding the basis for interventions increases the likelihood of compliance.*
- Provide bed rest until ascites is relieved. *To decrease metabolism and energy consumption.*
- Restrict fluids as prescribed and distribute those fluids throughout the 24 hours. *To prevent further fluid excess. Taking small amounts of fluid throughout the day increases the patient's comfort.*

Nursing Diagnosis

Ineffective breathing pattern related to ascites, immobility, and stasis of secretions

Outcomes

- Patient will achieve clear lung sounds.
- Patient will verbalize decreasing dyspnea.

Related NOC Outcomes

- Immobility Consequences: Physiological
- Respiratory Status: Airway Patency
- Respiratory Status: Gas Exchange

Related NIC Interventions

- Fluid Management
- Respiratory Monitoring

Nursing Interventions/Rationales

- Monitor respirations and lung sounds every 4 hours and more frequently if indicated. *To detect changes that require intervention.*
- Position patient in high Fowler's position. *This position relieves pressure on diaphragm, allowing for maximal ventilation and prevention of stasis of secretions.*
- Encourage frequent position changes and deep breathing exercises. *To prevent complications such as atelectasis.*
- Encourage ambulation when appropriate. *To prevent muscle weakness and complications such as atelectasis.*

Nursing Diagnosis

Risk for impaired skin integrity related to immobility, edema, poor nutrition, and pruritus

Outcomes

- Patient will remain free from skin breakdown or excoriation.
- Patient will verbalize relief from itching.
- Patient will experience decreasing peripheral edema when compared with baseline.

Related NOC Outcomes

- Fluid Balance
- Immobility Consequences: Physiological
- Tissue Integrity: Skin & Mucous Membranes
- Tissue Perfusion: Peripheral

Related NIC Interventions

- Exercise Promotion: Joint Mobility
- Pressure Ulcer Prevention
- Pruritus Management
- Skin Surveillance

Nursing Interventions/Rationales

- Assess patient's skin daily for signs of breakdown or excoriation from scratching. *Patient has several risk factors for skin breakdown, including itching from jaundice and immobility. Early identification of potential or actual skin breakdown leads to early intervention.*
- Use measures such as flotation mattress and routine turning schedule. *To prevent skin breakdown by preventing pressure over bony prominences.*
- Keep skin clean and well moisturized. *Dry skin is predisposed to cracking and excoriation. Unclean skin promotes bacterial growth, which predisposes patient to skin breakdown.*
- Keep finger and toenails short and clean. *To prevent accidental scratches or cuts. Jaundice can be irritating and lead to scratching.*
- Elevate extremities when feasible to reduce peripheral edema. *Aids in venous return of fluids from the periphery.*
- Avoid heat and heavy clothing; provide cool environment. *To reduce itching and promote comfort.*
- Apply antipruritic lotion as prescribed as needed. *To reduce itching and promote comfort.*
- Administer prescribed antihistamines. *Blocks the release of histamine to reduce itching.*
- Offer diversional activities such as music or television if acceptable to patient. *Distraction is often useful in blocking the perception of discomfort.*
- If patient must scratch, provide a soft cloth. Itching may be intense. *Use of a soft cloth will protect the skin from excoriation.*
- Use tepid water for bathing. *Tepid water does not generally exacerbate itching to the extent that hot water does.*

Continued

Nursing Care Plan—cont'd

- Monitor for signs of localized skin infection. *Scratching can result in infection, which is characterized by redness, swelling, warmth, and tenderness.*

Nursing Diagnosis

Risk for infection related to immunocompromise secondary to chronic illness

Outcomes

- Patient will be free from systemic infection (fever, chills, lethargy).
- Patient will be free from localized infection (redness, warmth, swelling, pain).
- Patient will maintain white blood cell (WBC) count within normal limits.

Related NOC Outcomes

- Immune Status
- Risk Control

Related NIC Interventions

- Infection Control
- Infection Protection
- Surveillance

Nursing Interventions/Rationales

- Monitor for indications of infection every shift (fever, chills, lethargy, increased WBC count). *To detect early signs of infection so treatment can be implemented. Infections in a patient with cirrhosis can be life threatening, since they can result in sepsis and liver failure.*
- Use sterile technique for all invasive procedures. *To decrease the risk of introduction of microorganisms and resultant infection.*
- Encourage pulmonary hygiene, such as turning and deep breathing every 2 hours. *To prevent stasis of secretions and increased risk for atelectasis and pneumonia.*
- Restrict exposure to persons with infection. *To decrease risk of transmitting infections to the immunocompromised patient.*

Nursing Diagnosis

Ineffective coping related to health crisis

Outcomes

- Patient will use coping strategies such as relaxation to deal with health crisis.
- Patient will show interest in diversional activities.
- Patient will participate in decision making about health when physically able.

Related NOC Outcomes

- Coping
- Decision-Making
- Information Processing

Related NIC Interventions

- Coping Enhancement
- Decision-Making Support
- Distraction

Nursing Interventions/Rationales

- Assess patient's perception of health and present illness. *The nurse's perception of the illness may differ considerably from the patient's or family's perception. Misunderstandings can be corrected when the patient's perceptions are known.*
- Identify and support the patient's successful coping strategies (prayer, music, conversation). *Coping strategies that have been effective in the past are likely to be effective in new situations.*
- Listen actively if patient expresses feelings of powerlessness, fears, or spiritual distress. Plan times for active listening. *To demonstrate caring and empathy and improve patient's ability to cope.*
- Assess and facilitate family support. Meet with the family and significant others on a scheduled basis. *The family must feel secure to provide support to the patient.*

Evaluation

Evaluation is based on comparing the patient's outcomes with desired outcomes.

restricted to 1 g/day. The sodium restriction along with bed rest may relieve the ascites and edema.[4] If not, diuretics may be used. Spironolactone A (Aldactone A), which inhibits the resorption of sodium in the distal tubules and promotes potassium retention by inhibiting the synthesis and renal effects of aldosterone, is frequently used. The therapy is adjusted on an individual basis. Sometimes furosemide (Lasix) or another diuretic is used with spironolactone. Because furosemide causes potassium excretion, the nurse monitors the serum potassium level frequently and observes the patient for signs and symptoms of hypokalemia such as abdominal distention, nausea, vomiting, anorexia, decreased bowel sounds, weakness, or irregular pulse. Removal of ascitic fluid through the kidneys has the advantage of preventing the loss of essential body proteins, which can occur when fluid is removed from the abdominal cavity by paracentesis. However, diuretic therapy may cause serious side effects for the patient with cirrhosis. An extremely rapid diuresis can precipitate oliguria and uremia as a result of the rapidly diminished blood volume. Ascites should not be mobilized at rates greater than 500 ml/day or approximately 1 lb/day. Fluid losses in excess of 500 ml/day can result in the loss of nonascitic extracellular fluid. Infusions of albumin in 25-g units, which promote retention of an adequate vascular volume, may be given to prevent azotemia and encephalopathy by maintaining adequate perfusion of the kidneys and the brain and to promote diuresis. Administration of salt-poor albumin may expand the blood volume rapidly, and the patient should be monitored carefully for signs of congestive heart failure and pulmonary edema during and after administration.

Fluids are restricted if hyponatremia is caused by fluid retention. Fluid restriction is monitored closely because it may lead to decreased output and the hepatorenal syndrome. When fluids are restricted, the nurse must work with the patient to select fluids that are tolerated best and to spread the allotted fluids throughout the total 24 hours. Fluids must be distributed so that some are available at each meal and for required medications. Some fluids should be given on all three shifts while the patient is hospitalized. At home the patient should distribute fluids over the waking hours.[17]

To further evaluate the effectiveness of therapy, daily weighing is required. Measurements of abdominal girth assist in determining the gross amount of abdominal swelling. Patients need to be taught the importance of monitoring and reporting weight gain or a rapid increase in abdominal girth after discharge. When ascites is intractable to the therapies mentioned, other procedures such as a PV shunt may be used.[45]

RELATED NIC INTERVENTIONS. Electrolyte Monitoring, Fluid Management, Hypovolemia Management

Nursing Diagnosis: Risk for Injury

OUTCOMES. Common examples of expected outcomes for the patient with a diagnosis of *risk for injury* are:
Patient will:

- Have no falls or injuries.
- Have no serious bleeding episodes.

NURSING INTERVENTIONS. Neurologic impairment associated with cirrhosis may place the patient at risk for falls. The patient's environment should be kept clear of objects that can cause a fall. If necessary, the patient should have assistance with ambulation, using devices such as a cane or a walker.

The patient with cirrhosis is at great risk for bleeding because of poor vitamin K absorption, impaired production of clotting factors, and thrombocytopenia. Esophageal varices and hemorrhoids can easily rupture, causing excessive bleeding. Nursing care should focus on monitoring for bleeding and instituting measures that decrease the risk of bleeding from trauma or injury to varices (see Guidelines for Safe Practice Box and Patient/Family Teaching box).

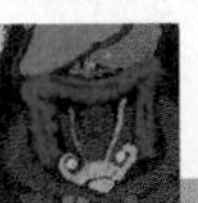

GUIDELINES FOR SAFE PRACTICE
Monitoring for Bleeding in the Patient With Cirrhosis

- Monitor urine and stool for blood.
- Check the patient's body daily for purpura, hematomas, and petechiae.
- Check mouth, especially gums, carefully for signs of bleeding.
- Check vital signs at least every 4 hours.
- Monitor prothrombin time, partial thromboplastin time, and thrombocyte count frequently.

RELATED NIC INTERVENTIONS. Bleeding Precautions, Fall Prevention, Teaching: Disease Process

Nursing Diagnosis: Imbalanced Nutrition: Less Than Body Requirements

OUTCOMES. Common examples of expected outcomes for the patient with a diagnosis of *imbalanced nutrition: less than body requirements* are:
Patient will:

- Eat food from all food groups (unless restricted) in adequate amounts to meet caloric needs.
- Demonstrate a decrease in signs of muscle wasting.

NURSING INTERVENTIONS. Most patients with cirrhosis require a well balanced, high-calorie, high-carbohydrate diet with adequate vitamins to provide nutrients for repair of the liver. Protein intake may need to be limited. This is determined by liver function tests. When nausea is a problem, antiemetics should be given 30 minutes before meals to help increase food tolerance. Sodium restriction is

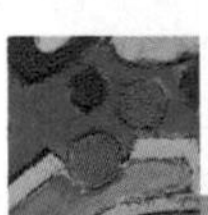

PATIENT/FAMILY TEACHING *Cirrhosis*

The nurse is responsible for teaching the patient to:

- Avoid further hepatic damage.
  —Abstain from alcohol.
  —Abstain from any drugs not prescribed by physician, including over-the-counter drugs such as analgesics or cold remedies.
  —Avoid exposure to hepatotoxins in the work and home environments.
- Eat a well-balanced diet that includes foods high in protein such as milk, eggs, fish, and poultry. (There may be sodium or protein restrictions.)
- Maintain fluid restriction if required by spreading intake of the total allowable fluids throughout the day.
- Report signs and symptoms requiring immediate follow-up care: weight gain; increased abdominal girth; recurrence of edema, fever, or bleeding (blood in urine, stool, or vomitus; epistaxis; cuts that continue to bleed); change in mental function or behavior.
- Take medications (diuretics, potassium, and antihistamines) as ordered, reporting any problems with drug regimen.
- Plan activities to allow adequate rest.
- Use measures that help control pruritus.
- Practice measures that lessen chance of bleeding:
  —Avoid all intramuscular and subcutaneous injections, if possible, but if necessary ask provider to use the smallest-gauge needle possible when giving an injection. Be sure pressure is applied to injection sites and venous puncture sites for at least 5 minutes and to arterial puncture sites for at least 10 minutes.
  —Use a soft-bristled toothbrush or cotton swabs for oral hygiene.
  —Do not strain on defecation, and avoid vigorous blowing of nose or coughing.
  —Avoid foods (e.g., spicy, hot, or raw) that can traumatize esophageal varices.
  —Ask for assistance to avoid falls.
  —Keep room free of clutter, keep floors dry, and wear shoes or slippers to avoid injuries.

frequently necessary, and this restriction can make finding a palatable diet difficult. Salt substitutes and information on alternative seasonings may help.

Frequent oral hygiene and a pleasant environment are provided to help increase food intake. The patient's food preferences are incorporated into the diet. Food is served in small, frequent amounts. Because persons with cirrhosis need increased calories but often have poor appetites, measures to increase calories without increasing the volume of food are used. These measures include use of butter as a seasoning, adding dry milk to appropriate foods, and using gravies and sauces. The patient with cirrhosis has the same nutritional needs after discharge, and the person who shops and cooks for the patient must be included in the teaching. The patient's economic situation should be assessed to determine his or her ability to purchase the food required for the prescribed diet. A social service referral may be necessary to help the patient obtain financial assistance. For the person who eats out frequently, instruction about selecting appropriate meals from a restaurant menu is necessary. If the patient's meals are obtained through a service such as Meals on Wheels, arrangements can be made for special dietary requirements.

Related NIC Interventions. Nutrition Management, Nutrition Therapy, Nutritional Counseling

Evaluation

To evaluate the effectiveness of nursing interventions, compare patient behaviors with those stated in the expected patient outcomes.

Related NOC Outcomes. Electrolyte & Acid/Base Balance, Energy Conservation, Fall Prevention Behavior, Fluid Balance, Knowledge: Personal Safety, Nutritional Status, Respiratory Status: Ventilation, Safe Home Environment, Sleep

Gerontologic Considerations

Blood flow to the liver decreases with aging. This physiologic change may worsen the effects of hypotension on the liver. An episode of severe hypotension in the older patient may result in shock liver. Patients with preexisting right-sided heart failure may experience severe liver complications with a hypotensive episode. Shock liver results from ischemia of hepatic tissues and elevated liver enzymes, progressing to liver failure. Lactic acid levels increase and clotting factors decrease, creating increased risk of metabolic imbalance and hemorrhage. Patients should be monitored closely to avoid episodes of hypotension. The aging liver has decreased ability to metabolize drugs; therefore treatment with such drugs as diuretics and vasopressin should be carefully adjusted or avoided in the elderly.[12]

Control of pruritus is especially important in the older patient because of skin changes associated with aging. The older person's skin is more fragile, and lesions may develop as a result of scratching. As the disease progresses, complications such as esophageal varices, ascites, and encephalopathy may develop. The older patient with anemia is at even greater risk from bleeding.

Encouraging a nutritionally adequate diet is an important intervention for the older patient. A low-fat diet and vitamin supplements are recommended. Strict dietary restrictions such as a low protein intake should be avoided in the elderly because they may be undernourished to start. Severe salt restrictions may inhibit appetite, since food may be less palatable.

Hepatic encephalopathy can be confused with senile dementia syndromes because of some similar symptoms. Careful assessment of neurologic status is critical in the older person with cirrhosis.

The incidence of primary biliary cirrhosis increases with age and peaks at age 50; the disease progresses until most patients are 60 to 70 years old and thus is a serious problem in older adults. Early symptoms are vague or absent. Late symptoms include jaundice, diarrhea, bone pain, bruising, night blindness, and gradual weight loss. Many symptoms are attributed to malabsorption of vitamins and nutrients. Skin manifestations, including thickening and darkening of the skin and pruritus, are common. Because of the absence or vagueness of early symptoms, diagnosis may be made in the last stage of the disease when the prognosis is poor because of the complications associated with cirrhosis. Liver transplantation is considered for persons with primary biliary cirrhosis when liver failure occurs. Advanced age is no longer an absolute contraindication for transplantation, but it is certainly controversial. Death usually results from bleeding, ascites, or encephalopathy.

Emotional support is necessary to assist the older patient in living with a chronic liver disease. An assessment of the patient's support system and coping methods can assist the nurse in formulating a plan to reduce the patient's anxiety.

▶ ARE You READY?

The nursing diagnosis *ineffective breathing pattern* related to accumulation of fluid in the peritoneal cavity (ascites) is related to:

1. Hypoaldosteronism
2. Hypoalbuminemia
3. Elevated serum ammonia
4. Elevated serum glucose

Hepatitis

Hepatitis is any acute inflammatory disease of the liver. Although the term *hepatitis* is most often used in conjunction with viral hepatitis, the disease can also be caused by bacteria, toxic injury, and autoimmune liver cell destruction. Some differences exist in the pathologic and clinical phenomena of these various causes of hepatitis, but the clinical management is similar. Almost any form of hepatitis can result in postnecrotic cirrhosis, unless the hepatitis responds to treatment.

Toxic Hepatitis

Etiology and Epidemiology. Because the liver has a primary role in the metabolism of foreign substances, many agents, including drugs, alcohol, industrial toxins, and plant poisons, can cause toxic hepatitis (Table 46-4). Many health care workers are concerned about hepatic injury caused by adverse drug reactions from the drugs they handle (especially those needing to be mixed from powder).

As many as 25% of all cases of acute hepatic failure are the result of adverse drug reactions, and drugs are responsible for 2%

TABLE 46-4 SELECTED HEPATOTOXINS

Hepatotoxin	Source or Effect
AGENTS	
Carbon tetrachloride and other chlorinated hydrocarbons	Dry-cleaning fluid
Chlorophenothane	Insecticide
Toluene	Glue
Yellow phosphorus	Rat poison, firecrackers
PLANT POISONS	
Mushrooms	*Aminita phalloides*
Pyrrolizine alkaloids	Bush teas, comfrey
Guaiaretic acid	Guaiacum trees
DRUGS	
Acetaminophen	Causes liver cell necrosis
Acetylsalicylic acid	Elevates liver serum enzyme levels
Allopurinol	Causes cholestatic jaundice
Chlorpromazine	Impairs secretion of bile
Clorpropamide	Hepatotoxic
Diazepam	Long-term use alters liver function by unknown mechanisms
Erythromycin	Hepatotoxic
Isoniazid	Symptoms mimic viral hepatitis
6-Mercaptopurine	Hepatotoxic
Nitrofurantoin	Causes cholestatic jaundice
Oral contraceptives	May interfere with bile secretion
Phenobarbital	Lowers serum bilirubin levels
Phenytoin	May cause hepatitis

to 5% of all hospital admission for jaundice in the United States.[5] Some plant sources used as alternative therapy also have been found to be hepatotoxic.[3,46]

The agents that produce hepatic injury are categorized into two major groups: predictable (intrinsic) and nonpredictable (idiosyncratic) hepatotoxins. The predictable hepatotoxins are further divided into two subgroups: direct and indirect (Box 46-3). Most drugs, including some antibiotics, monoamine oxidase inhibitors, anticonvulsants, and antitubercular medications,[8] are nonpredictable hepatotoxins; however, acetaminophen produces a predictable hepatotoxic reaction. Studies are being conducted to determine an individual's susceptibility to drug-induced liver injury (see Future Watch box).

Pathophysiology. The morphologic changes produced in the liver by the toxins vary, depending on the specific hepatotoxin. For example, carbon tetrachloride, tetracycline, and ethanol cause fatty infiltration or necrosis. Oral contraceptives, cholecystographic dyes, and chlorpromazine produce cholestasis and portal inflammation. A major cause of toxic hepatitis is the use of acetaminophen, especially in conjunction with alcohol and other medications such as anticonvulsants and antituberculosis drugs. Regardless of the cause, some alteration in liver function occurs. The alteration may result in only minimal manifestations of altered liver function, such as slightly elevated serum enzymes, or in major manifestations associated with acute liver failure (see Clinical Manifestations box).

BOX 46-3 Classification of Hepatotoxins

- *Predictable hepatotoxins:* Agents cause toxic hepatitis with predictable regularity and produce injury in a high percentage of persons exposed to them; occurrence of toxic hepatitis is dose dependent.
- *Nonpredictable hepatotoxins:* Agents produce hepatic injury only in unusually susceptible persons and in only a small percentage of persons exposed to them; occurrence is not dose dependent.
- *Direct predictable hepatotoxins:* Agents have direct effect on hepatic cells and organelles, producing structural changes that lead to metabolic defects.
- *Indirect predictable hepatotoxins:* Agents first interfere with normal metabolic function, and this alteration in metabolic function produces structural changes.

Future Watch

Drug-Induced Liver Injury

Drug-induced liver injury (DILI), although rare, can be life threatening, resulting in death if the search for a donor liver for transplantation is unsuccessful. To increase understanding of this problem, the National Institutes of Health recently established the Drug-Induced Liver Injury Network, a consortium of five academic medical centers. A major goal of this network is to better define the genetic factors that predispose certain individuals to severe liver injury from drugs so that DILI can be prevented in the future. A study of DILI will ensue, enrolling individuals older than 2 years of age who had an episode of DILI caused by one of four drugs: isoniazid (INH), valproic acid (Depacon), phenytoin (Dilantin), or clavulanic acid–amoxicillin (Augmentin).

American Liver Foundation: *Drug induced liver studies,* accessed Aug 2004 from website: www.liverfoundation.org.

Collaborative Care Management. Attention focuses on identifying the toxic agent and removing or eliminating it. Gastric lavage and cleansing of the bowel may be indicated to remove the hepatotoxin from the intestinal tract. In some instances, a specific treatment is available for a particular hepatotoxin. For example, acetylcysteine, a mucolytic agent, can be given within 16 hours (immediately is preferred) of ingestion of an acetaminophen overdose. The drug may be given orally or intravenously, although only the oral form has been approved for use in the United States. However, in most instances of toxic hepatitis, medical treatment is supportive and focused on particular manifestations, such as treatment of cirrhosis, PSE, or kidney failure.

Nursing care for the person with toxic hepatitis is supportive. In the acute care setting the nurse promotes comfort, maintains normal fluid and electrolyte balance, promotes a well-balanced diet

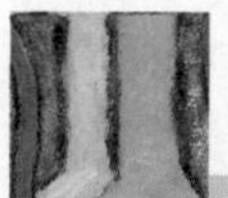

CLINICAL MANIFESTATIONS
Toxic Hepatitis

Early Manifestations

Anorexia
Nausea and vomiting
Lethargy
Elevated alanine aminotransaminase and aspartate aminotransaminase levels

Later Manifestations

Jaundice
Hepatomegaly
Hepatic tenderness
Dark urine
Elevated serum bilirubin level
Elevated urine bilirubin level

(when food and fluid are allowed), and promotes rest, as discussed in the section on viral hepatitis. Preventive education is also an important nursing responsibility (see Patient/Family Teaching box).

Autoimmune Hepatitis

Autoimmune hepatitis is a chronic necroinflammatory liver disorder associated with circulating autoantibodies and high serum globulin levels.

Etiology and Epidemiology. The etiology of autoimmune hepatitis is unknown, although it is associated with a genetic predisposition to autoimmunity. It develops after exposure to some environmental agent. Familial studies have not proven whether there is a genetic basis for this response, or whether the autoantibodies are an indicator of disease susceptibility. Autoimmune hepatitis is less common than chronic viral hepatitis, but its diagnosis is often missed because of vague early symptoms. It may occur at any age, but is most prevalent in girls and women between 15 and 40 years old.

Pathophysiology. The autoimmune response is directed at liver antigens and causes progressive necrosis and inflammation of hepatocytes. Fibrosis and cirrhosis result. Clinical manifestations range from mild to those of clinically advanced cirrhosis. Some patients are asymptomatic. Early diagnosis is important, since this form of hepatitis responds well to corticosteroid therapy.[16]

Collaborative Care Management. No single diagnostic test is available for autoimmune hepatitis. Diagnosis is made by obtaining a detailed history and physical examination to rule out other causes of liver disease, and analyzing laboratory and biopsy results. The presence of circulating autoantibodies such as antinuclear antibodies, antimitochondrial antibodies, and others is useful, although it is not clear what role these antibodies play in the pathologic condition. Corticosteroids are the mainstay of treatment for autoimmune hepatitis, and azathioprine (Imuran) has also proven useful. Medications such as cyclosporine, 6-mercaptopurine, and methotrexate are under investigation.[31]

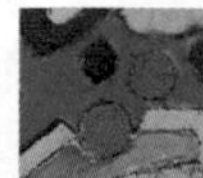

PATIENT/FAMILY TEACHING
Toxic Hepatitis

It is important that patients understand the potential for toxic hepatitis from improper use of chemicals at home, exposure to chemicals in the work environment, or injudicious use of drugs or other materials. The nurse teaches the patient and family that:

- Cleaning agents, solvents, and related substances sometimes contain products that are harmful to the liver.
- Labels need to be read carefully and directions followed explicitly. For example, dry-cleaning fluids may contain carbon tetrachloride, which can cause liver injury if inhaled. If these fluids are used inside the home, windows should be open, the fluids should be used quickly, and the user and others should vacate the premises as soon as possible.
- Many solvents used to remove paint and plastic material and to stain and finish woodwork contain injurious substances and should be used outdoors. Cleaning agents and car finishes should be applied outdoors or in an open garage.
- Industrial hazards such as nitrobenzene, tetrachloroethane, carbon disulfide, and dinitrotoluene are dangerous and can cause liver damage if used improperly.
- Some drugs can interfere with liver function or cause damage if used improperly. Over-the-counter drugs must be used judiciously.
  —Some prescription drugs reach the market before dangers of their uses are conclusively ruled out. The prescription drug chlorpromazine, a tranquilizer, was marketed and then found to cause bile stasis and liver damage.
  —Acetaminophen in large doses or when taken with alcohol can cause liver damage.

Nursing care of the patient with autoimmune hepatitis centers around symptom management and varies, depending on the presentation of the disease. Of primary importance is patient, family, and community education. Any individual who experiences chronic malaise, abdominal discomfort, or arthralgias should seek health care and not wait until the more obvious manifestations of liver disease (jaundice, ascites) appear. Clinicians also need to improve their understanding of autoimmune hepatitis. Often nurses are the first to be "consulted" about health care problems.

Patients diagnosed with autoimmune hepatitis require follow-up care every 3 to 4 weeks to evaluate response to treatment. Once clinical and serologic responses are normalized, reevaluation should occur every 3 months. The nurse informs the patient and family about the need for this continuous care and evaluation.[24]

Viral Hepatitis

Viral hepatitis is by far the most important liver infection and is a major health problem in the United States and in many other countries. The term *viral hepatitis* is used to refer to several clinically similar but etiologically and epidemiologically distinct infections.

Etiology and Epidemiology. Five major categories of viruses have been identified as causing viral hepatitis: hepatitis A (HAV), hepatitis B (HBV), hepatitis C (HCV), hepatitis D (HDV or delta virus), and hepatitis E (HEV). Two other forms of hepatitis,

F and G, have been identified but occur rarely. Table 46-5 summarizes the modes of transmission for each viral type.

Viral hepatitis is a reportable disease in all states in the United States. It is one of the most frequently reported infectious diseases in the country. Native Americans and Native Alaskans have a high rate of endemic disease. The most common type of hepatitis worldwide is HAV, which causes 40% of the reported cases of hepatitis.

The incidence of HBV infection has stayed steady at about 5% of the world's population. Approximately 60% of the reported cases of HBV infection in the United States occur in heterosexuals with multiple sex partners, homosexual men, and IV drug users. The incidence of HBV infection in health care workers is about 3% of all reported cases.

Of all cases of viral hepatitis reported to the CDC, 20% are caused by HCV infection, and 50% to 80% of these persons develop chronic hepatitis. HDV is endemic among persons with HBV in areas around the Mediterranean and Middle East. HEV is extremely rare in the United States but occurs in epidemic proportions in areas of India. Cases of HEV have also been reported in Mexico, Asia, and Africa. The mortality rate is low, except for pregnant women, in whom it reaches 20%.

Hepatitis in the vast majority of patients seen clinically is caused by HAV or HBV. Most cases of all types of hepatitis occur in young adults. Factors such as the viral agent, transmission, and high-risk groups vary for the five types of hepatitis.[37,50]

Pathophysiology. Viral hepatitis causes diffuse inflammatory infiltration of hepatic tissue with mononuclear cells and local, spotty, or single cell necrosis. The liver cells may be swollen. With typical acute viral hepatitis, there is no collapse of lobules, no loss of lobular architecture, and minimal or no fibrosis. Inflammation, degeneration, and regeneration occur simultaneously, distorting the normal lobular pattern, creating pressure within and around the portal vein areas, and obstructing the bile channels. The pathologic changes in the hepatocytes are not always related to the effects of the virus itself, but rather to the injurious response of the body's own immune system attempting to clear the virus. These changes are associated with elevated serum transaminase levels, prolonged prothrombin time, slightly elevated serum alkaline phosphatase level, and elevated bilirubin level.

Most patients recover from acute viral hepatitis, with normal liver function and no residual hepatic necrosis. Although chronic hepatitis can occur with all types of hepatitis, it is virtually unseen with HAV and HEV. Chronic hepatitis is defined as the presence of serum viral antigens 6 months after the acute episode. Persons with chronic hepatitis are carriers of the virus and remain contagious. Chronic hepatitis has been classified into active and persistent categories based on symptoms and histologic tissue changes on liver biopsy. However, the latest recommendation is to use terms that include the etiology and degree of hepatic injury, regardless of symptoms. Mild, moderate, or marked chronic presentations indicate the degree of hepatic damage and the risk of progression to cirrhosis or liver cancer. The patient with chronic hepatitis may be asymptomatic, except for minimal abnormalities in serum transaminase levels, or have mild to severe symptoms of liver disease. There is strong evidence of an association between chronic hepatitis B and the development of hepatocellular cancer. Chronic hepatitis C is the most common chronic liver disease in the United States and the leading indication for liver transplant (see Research box).[36,41]

The clinical manifestations of the various forms of acute viral hepatitis are generally not distinct. The shorter incubation period of HAV infection results in a more abrupt onset and shorter duration of symptoms. Clinical manifestations of viral hepatitis, including abnormal values in diagnostic tests, fall into three phases: preicteric, icteric, and posticteric (see Clinical Manifestations box). **Jaundice,** a common clinical manifestation of hepatitis, is caused by a disturbance in bilirubin metabolism. (See Chapter 45 for an explanation of bilirubin metabolism.) When the liver is diseased, problems with the uptake, conjugation, or excretion of bilirubin may occur, resulting in increased serum bilirubin levels (both conjugated and unconjugated). This excess bilirubin in the blood is distributed to the skin, mucous membranes, sclerae, and other body fluids and tissues, causing a yellow pigmentation. Because conjugated bilirubin is water soluble and is excreted in urine, darkening of the urine may also be seen. The presence of bilirubin in the skin causes pruritus in about 20% to 25% of patients who have jaundice.

Research

Kim WR: The burden of hepatitis C in the United States, *Hepatology* 36(5):S30, 2002.

According to the Third National Health and Nutrition Survey, 3.9 million U.S. citizens have been infected with the hepatitis C virus (HCV), and 74% (2.8 million) of these have been diagnosed as chronic. Between 1990 and 2000 there was a fivefold increase in the annual number of patients with HCV who underwent liver transplantation, and currently more than one third of liver transplant candidates have HCV. Researchers predict a fourfold increase between 1990 and 2015 in persons at risk for chronic liver disease, suggesting a continued rise in the burden of HCV in the foreseeable future.

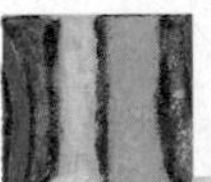

CLINICAL MANIFESTATIONS
Viral Hepatitis

Preicteric Phase

- Nonspecific complaints of fatigue, anorexia, nausea, cough, joint pain, loss of appetite
- Laboratory values indicating elevated serum alanine aminotransaminase and aspartate aminotransaminase and elevated urine bilirubin levels
- Presence of viral antibodies, antigens, or virus particles

Icteric Phase

- Appearance of jaundice and darkening of urine; stools clay colored because of decreased urobilinogen
- Preicteric symptoms subsiding, although appetite remains poor
- Right upper quadrant pain and increasing pruritus
- Laboratory studies showing elevated direct bilirubin levels

Posticteric Phase

- Decreasing jaundice, return of normal color to urine and stool, improvement of appetite
- Laboratory values returning to normal
- Fatigue continuing

TABLE 46-5 CHARACTERISTICS OF VIRAL HEPATITIS

Hepatitis A	Hepatitis B	Hepatitis C	Hepatitis D	Hepatitis E
TRANSMISSION				
Fecal-oral	Parenteral, sexual, perinatal	Parenteral, sexual, perinatal	Superinfection or coinfection with chronic HBV	Fecal-oral
INCUBATION PERIOD				
2-6 wk	4-24 wk	2-20 wk	4-24 wk	2-8 wk
VIRUS TYPE				
RNA picornavirus	DNA hepadnavirus	RNA flavins	Defective RNA virus	Unclassified RNA virus
DIAGNOSTIC SEROLOGIC TESTS				
Acute phase: IgM anti-HAV	Acute phase: HBsAg, anti-HBc IgM, HBeAg	Acute phase: anti-HDV	Acute phase: anti-HCV	None
Lifetime: IgG anti-HAV	Lifetime: anti-HBs; anti-HBc	Lifetime: anti-HCV		
SECRETIONS FOUND TO CONTAIN INFECTIVE AGENT				
Feces, blood	Blood and serous fluids, saliva, semen, urine, nasopharyngeal washings, feces, pleural fluid	Blood, semen	Blood	Feces
INDICATION OF PROTECTIVE IMMUNITY				
IgG anti-HAV	anti-HBs, total anti-HBc	None	None	None
CHRONICITY				
None	90% infants, 6%-10% adults	50%-80%	2%-70%	None
MORTALITY RATE				
<1%	1%-2%	1%-2%	2%-20%	1%-2% (as high as 20% in pregnant women)
HIGH-RISK GROUPS				
Travelers to developing countries; staff and patients in custodial care institutions (prison, day care, nursing homes)	Household and sexual partners of HBV carriers; immigrants from HBV-endemic areas; IV drug users; patients and staff in custodial care institutions; sexually active gay men; patients on hemodialysis; health care workers with frequent contact with blood	Travelers to endemic areas; people receiving frequent blood transfusions; IV drug users; persons with tattoos; organ transplant recipients; 40% report no risk factors	Same as for HBV	Immigrants and travelers to HEV-epidemic and HEV-endemic areas
VACCINE AVAILABLE				
Yes	Yes	No	No	No

HAV, hepatitis A virus; *DNA,* deoxyribonucleic acid; *HBc,* hepatitis B core (antigen); *HBeAg,* hepatitis B e antigen; *HBs,* hepatitis B surface (antigen); *HBsAg,* hepatitis B surface antigen; *HCV,* hepatitis C virus; *HBV,* hepatitis B virus; *HDV,* hepatitis D virus; *HEV,* hepatitis E virus; *IgG,* immunoglobulin G; *IgM,* immunoglobulin M; *IV,* intravenous; *RNA,* ribonucleic acid.

Jaundice may also result from hemolysis (increased destruction of red blood cells) or obstruction of extrahepatic and intrahepatic biliary ducts. Table 46-6 compares the different types of jaundice. Clay-colored (grayish white) stools indicate that bile is not reaching the intestines and suggest extrahepatic obstruction. Frequent causes of extrahepatic obstruction are gallstones lodged in the common bile duct, pancreatitis, and carcinoma of the head of the pancreas (see Chapter 44). The level of jaundice does not correlate with disease severity in hepatitis, but in persons with cirrhosis, jaundice suggests a poorer prognosis.

Potential complications of viral hepatitis include chronic hepatitis and cirrhosis, liver failure, or hepatocellular cancer.

Collaborative Care Management

DIAGNOSTIC TESTS. Blood tests are checked for viral antibodies and antigens and for actual viral particles (see Table 46-5). Elevations in the serum liver enzymes ALT and AST are present in hepatitis A and B. Liver function tests are monitored until normal.

MEDICATIONS. Because most medications are metabolized in the liver, only essential drugs should be given to patients with hepatitis. Vitamin K may be necessary if the prothrombin time is prolonged. Analgesics are given sparingly. Patients with chronic hepatitis C are treated with interferon, with some success. Combinations of interferon with antiviral drugs such as ribiviron are being studied. These medications have not worked well with chronic hepatitis B.[15]

TREATMENTS. Most persons infected with hepatitis are not hospitalized. Rest is advised, but complete bed rest is not necessary. Persons requiring hospitalization include those with serum bilirubin concentrations of 10 mg/dl, or more than 10 times the normal, and those with acute liver failure. Although some evidence suggests that alternative medicines may be beneficial in some types of hepatitis, health care providers need to be aware of potential complications (see Complementary & Alternative Therapies box, Research box, and Evidence-Based Practice box, p. 1338).[18,38,46,49]

DIET. If liver function is not impaired, a well-balanced diet is adequate. A low-fat, high-carbohydrate diet may be better tolerated. Protein and sodium are restricted if liver function is compromised. These decisions are based on laboratory values. Abstinence from alcohol is essential.

HEALTH PROMOTION AND PREVENTION

HEPATITIS A. Preexposure prophylaxis with the vaccine for HAV is recommended for persons traveling to HAV-endemic countries, persons with occupational risk of infection (such as those who work with HAV-infected primates or with the virus in a laboratory), persons with chronic liver disease, chronic IV drug users, and persons who engage in anal sex. Other high-risk groups are Native Americans and Native Alaskans. Postexposure prophylaxis with serum immunoglobulin (gamma globulin), given within 2 weeks of exposure, is recommended for selected people who have had contact with a person known to be positive for HAV; this includes close household and sexual contacts of people with HAV; staff and attendees of daycare centers, custodial care centers, and hospitals who have close contact with patients with HAV; people exposed to a common source of infection (infected food or water), if identified within 2 weeks of exposure; and food handlers working with a handler in whom hepatitis A has been diagnosed.[19]

HEPATITIS B. Hepatitis B is a vaccine-preventable disease. HBV vaccine is given as a series of three intramuscular injections (deltoid in adults and children; anterolateral thigh muscles in

TABLE 46-6 TYPES OF JAUNDICE

Category	Pathology	Possible Findings
Obstructive		
Intrahepatic	Suppression of bile flow in canaliculi or small biliary ductiles (cholestasis)	Direct* bilirubin elevated; alkaline phosphatase elevated; no enlargement of bile ducts seen on scan or ultrasound
Extrahepatic (bile duct obstruction)	Obstruction of bile flow in large bile ducts, as in gallbladder disease	Direct bilirubin elevated; alkaline phosphatase elevated; enlargement of bile ducts documented by scan, ultrasound; absence of urobilinogen in urine
Hepatocellular	Hepatocyte injury from toxins (toxic hepatitis), from viruses (viral hepatitis), from cancer, or as part of syndrome of cirrhosis (all types)	Transaminases (ALT, AST) elevated 10- to 15-fold; both direct and indirect† bilirubin may be elevated (direct more than indirect); prolonged prothrombin time
Hemolytic	Excessive amounts of bilirubin are released from red blood cells as would be seen in sickle cell anemia or other hemolytic anemias; liver is unable to excrete bilirubin as rapidly as it forms	Usually mild elevation of total bilirubin (indirect more than direct)

ALT, Alanine aminotransaminase; *AST,* aspartate aminotransaminase.
*"Direct" measures conjugated bilirubin.
†"Indirect" measures unconjugated bilirubin.

Complementary & Alternative Therapies

Alternative Therapy for Hepatitis

Natural therapies can be of great benefit in treating hepatitis. Several nutrients and herbs have been shown to inhibit viral reproduction, improve immune system function, and stimulate regeneration of the damaged liver cells. During the acute phase of hepatitis, the focus should be on replacing fluids through consumption of vegetable broths, diluted vegetable juices, and herbal teas. Solid foods are restricted to brown rice, steamed vegetables, and moderate intake of lean protein sources. Vitamin C in high doses (40 to 100 g orally) has been known to diminish acute viral hepatitis in 2 to 4 days, including the clearing of jaundice.

In chronic cases a diet largely consisting of plant foods has been shown to increase elimination of bile acids, drugs, and toxic substances from the system. Liver extracts are said to promote hepatic regeneration and are especially useful in treatment of chronic hepatitis. Orally administered bovine thymus extracts have been used in both acute and chronic cases, with decreases in liver enzyme studies, elimination of the virus, and a higher rate of formation of antibody to hepatitis B e antigen (anti-HBe). Plant medicines used in the treatment of hepatitis include milk thistle (silymarin) and *Glycyrrhiza glabra* (licorice).

Milk Thistle

The seeds from the plant *Silybum marianum*, a member of the daisy and thistle family, exert hepatoprotective and antihepatoxic action over liver toxins, including the deadly mushroom *Amanita phalloides*. Silymarin alters the outer liver membrane cell structure so that toxins cannot enter the cell. It also stimulates ribonucleic acid polymerase A, which results in activation of the liver's regenerative capacity. It has been reported to be useful as an antidote for ingestion of poisonous mushrooms, viral hepatitis (both acute and chronic), and cirrhosis.

Glycyrrhiza glabra

Glabra is derived from the roots of the licorice plant. Its main effect is to potentiate endogenous steroids. It has been useful in the treatment of hepatitis by enhancing the immune system, potentiating interferon, and promoting the flow of bile and fat to and from the liver.

Pizzorno JE, Murray MT, Joiner-Bey H: *Clinician's handbook of natural medicine*, St Louis, 2001, Elsevier.

infants and neonates), with the second and third doses given 1 and 6 months after the first dose. The vaccine has shown an efficacy of 85% to 95%. The effect of the vaccine on the developing fetus is not known; however, pregnancy should not be considered a contraindication to its use in protecting the mother. Because HBV vaccine has no benefits for HBV carriers and because of the cost of the vaccination, prevaccination serologic screening for antibodies to hepatitis B core antigen (anti-HBc) and surface antigen (anti-HBs) may be done to identify both carriers and previously infected noncarriers who have adequate immunity. The cost of screening is weighed against the cost of unnecessary but harmless vaccination to identify whether screening should be performed.

Preexposure vaccination against hepatitis B is recommended for everyone, with highest priority to occupationally exposed workers, IV drug users, heterosexuals with multiple partners, and those who engage in anal sex. Remember that health care workers include medical technologists, phlebotomists, nurses, physicians (especially surgeons), pathologists, dialysis unit staff, dentists, oral surgeons, dental hygienists, laboratory and blood bank technicians, emergency medical technicians, and morticians. Those who

Research

Strader DB et al: Use of complementary and alternative medicine in patients with liver disease, *Am J Gastroenterol* 97(9):2391, 2002.

Forty-two percent of the U.S. population uses complementary and alternative medicine (CAM); however, its specific use by patients with chronic liver disease has not been defined. This study surveyed 989 patients in six geographically diverse liver disease clinics in the country.

The study found that 39% of the patients surveyed admitted to using some form of CAM at least once during the previous month. Predictive variables included female gender, young age (less than 50 years old), college education, and higher income. Although those surveyed described general use of herbals or botanicals such as milk thistle, garlic, ginseng, green tea, gingko, echinacea, and St. John's wort, the only herbs taken specifically for liver disease were milk thistle and licorice root.

Seventy-four percent of patients stated they informed their physician or medical care provider about their use of alternative methods. Forty percent indicated that their primary source of information about CAM was families or friends. Another 36% learned about CAM from magazines and books.

The fact that 26% of patients did not tell their primary care provider about the use of CAM underscores the importance of proper assessment about this usage. Another important point is that 2.5% of the patients were taking potentially hepatotoxic substances. Health care providers need to be knowledgeable about herbal medications, their usefulness, and the possible complications.

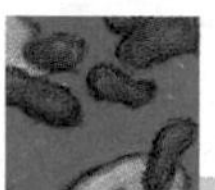

EVIDENCE-BASED PRACTICE

Topic Question: Are medicinal herbs beneficial for hepatitis C virus (HCV) infection?

Evidence Base: Researchers examined controlled trials registered in the Cochrane Library and Hepato-Biliary Group, reported in MEDLINE, and found in Chinese and Japanese databases. They compared medicinal herbs with placebos, no interventions, and other proven medical treatments for HCV infection.

Findings: In 10 random trials using patients with chronic HCV infection, 10 different herbal products were evaluated and compared with control groups using no interventions, placebos, or interferon. None of the herbs showed positive results compared with the placebo group. Two herbs showed a slight positive effect in one of the studies analyzed.

Conclusions: The evidence is insufficient to determine that medicinal herbs are effective for the treatment of HCV.

Liu JP et al: *Medicinal herbs for hepatitis C infection* (Cochrane Review). In Cochrane Library, Issue 3, 2004, Chichester, UK, John Wiley & Sons, accessed July 2004 from website: www.cochrane.org.

are frequently exposed to blood products, such as hemophiliacs and patients on hemodialysis, are also at high risk.

Postexposure prophylaxis involves the injection of hepatitis B immunoglobulin (HBIG), which contains high amounts of anti-HBs. HBIG should be given within 24 hours of exposure, followed by the routine three-dose vaccination for HBV. Babies born to mothers with hepatitis B should receive HBIG and the first dose of the vaccination series at birth. If the exposed person has been vaccinated, he or she is checked for anti-HBs and given HBIG immediately plus a booster dose of HBV vaccination.

Postexposure prophylaxis should be considered for persons who have been exposed to hepatitis B surface antigen (HBsAg)–positive blood, those who have sexual contact with HBsAg-positive persons, and infants younger than 12 months old exposed to a primary caregiver who has acute hepatitis B.[28,30]

HEPATITIS C AND E. Prophylaxis for HCV and HEV infections is not as effective as that for HBV. For travelers to countries where HEV is endemic, preventive health teaching is the best prophylactic measure. The value of immunoglobulin in this situation is unknown. For postexposure prophylaxis in persons exposed through breaks in the skin to blood from a patient with HCV, immunoglobulin may be given, but its value is questionable.

HEPATITIS D. HDV requires the presence of HBV to be active; thus the preexposure and postexposure prophylaxes that are recommended for HBV should suffice to prevent delta hepatitis. Currently, no method exists for preventing HDV infection in HBV carriers except health teaching.

***HEALTHY PEOPLE 2010* GOALS.** Vaccination against hepatitis A and B is the mainstay of these recommendations, especially the Vaccines for Children Program. Until the goal of universal vaccination of newborns is achieved, it is important to find targeted high-risk populations and provide vaccination services. A goal of *Healthy People 2010* is to increase the proportion of international travelers who receive recommended preventive services for hepatitis A. Studies have pointed to missed opportunities for the vaccination of individuals at high risk for hepatitis B, 70% of whom were seen in settings such as drug treatment clinics, correctional facilities, or clinics for the treatment of sexually transmitted diseases, which could be used for hepatitis B vaccination programs. Although hepatitis C has no vaccine, an important preventive strategy is to identify infected individuals.[26] This provides an opportunity for counseling to prevent further transmission of the HCV, vaccination against HAV and HBV to prevent additional liver damage, possible antiviral therapy, and counseling to avoid potential hepatotoxins. Community teaching about the spread of all types of hepatitis and the lifestyle changes that can reduce this spread are essential in the prevention of hepatitis[50] (see Healthy People 2010 box).

Healthy People 2010

Viral Hepatitis: Midcourse Review and Revisions

Reduction in Viral Hepatitis

	1997 Baseline (per 100,000 adults)	2010 Target (per 100,000 adults)
Hepatitis B	59.0	11.3
Hepatitis A (new cases)	11.3	4.4
Hepatitis C (new cases)	2.4 (1996)	1

Special Population Targets With Hepatitis B

	1997 Baseline (number of cases)	2010 Target (number of cases)
Injecting drug users	7232	1808
Heterosexually active people	15,225	1240
Men who have sex with men	7232	1808
Occupationally exposed workers	249	62
Infants and young children	1682 (1995)	400

From US Department of Health and Human Services: *Healthy people 2010: understanding and improving health*, Washington, DC, 2000, The Department.

Nursing Management

of the Patient with Viral Hepatitis

ASSESSMENT

Nursing assessment focuses on identifying changes related to viral hepatitis and sources of transmission that are controllable.

Health History. Assess for:

- Length of time since onset of symptoms
- Headache, right upper abdominal quadrant tenderness, arthralgia, and pruritus
- History of weight change, anorexia, nausea, vomiting, dyspepsia, chills, fever, or adenopathy
- Changes in food or fluid intake
- Weakness or malaise that is not relieved by rest
- Potential previous exposure to hepatitis in work environment; during international travel; or through recent blood transfusion, contaminated food or water, IV drug abuse, or sexual contact
- Knowledge or understanding about the disease

Physical Examination. Assess for:

- Elevated temperature or weight changes
- Poor skin turgor, petechiae, bruises, lesions, and jaundice in skin or sclera
- Enlarged lymph nodes
- Enlarged or tender liver
- Guarding in upper right quadrant
- Changes in muscular strength or ability to perform daily activities

NURSING DIAGNOSES, OUTCOMES, AND INTERVENTIONS

Nursing Diagnosis: Imbalanced Nutrition: Less Than Body Requirements

OUTCOMES. Common examples of expected outcomes for the patient with a diagnosis of *imbalanced nutrition: less than body requirements* are:

Patient will:

- Maintain present weight or gain weight.
- Increase food intake until adequate in amount and content for body weight.

Nursing Interventions. During the acute phase of the illness, the patient needs 3 L/day of fluids because of the febrile illness and vomiting. Fluid can usually be given orally if nausea and vomiting are not severe. When nausea and vomiting are severe, IV infusions are given. The nurse monitors intake, output, and weight to assess the adequacy of intake. Fluids such as fruit juices and carbonated beverages that provide both volume and nutrients are encouraged. No special dietary restrictions are required in most patients. The diet should be well balanced and provide adequate nutrients and calories based on the patient's size and age. Most calories should be from carbohydrate sources. The diet should be planned with the patient so that it is appealing. Frequent, small meals are usually better tolerated than larger meals. Fats are usually restricted, since they are poorly tolerated. Alcoholic beverages should be avoided because they cause direct damage to the liver.

Related NIC Interventions. Fluid Management, Fluid Monitoring, Nutrition Management, Nutrition Therapy, Nutritional Monitoring

Nursing Diagnosis: Pain

Outcomes. Common examples of expected outcomes for the patient with a diagnosis of *pain* are:
Patient will:

- Rate the pain as 3 or less on a scale of 0 (no pain) to 10 (severe pain).
- Verbalize that pain is controlled.

Nursing Interventions. During the early phase of illness the patient may have headaches and arthralgia. General comfort measures—relaxing baths; backrubs; fresh linen on the bed; and a quiet, dark environment—may ease the patient's discomfort. During the icteric phase of the illness, the presence of bile pigments in the skin may cause severe pruritus. Pruritus can be exhausting and demoralizing to the patient. The major aim of care is to prevent scratching with resultant injury to the skin. It is impossible for people with pruritus not to scratch. Sometimes the person may be given a soft cloth with which to rub the skin. The patient's fingernails should be kept short and the hands clean to decrease the likelihood of excoriation or infection, if scratching occurs. Use of soothing lotions and emollients may help.

Related NIC Interventions. Analgesic Administration, Anxiety Reduction, Coping Enhancement, Distraction, Environmental Management, Pain Management, Patient-Controlled Analgesia (PCA) Assistance, Positioning

Nursing Diagnosis: Activity Intolerance

Outcomes. Common examples of expected outcomes for the patient with a diagnosis of *activity intolerance* are:

Patient will:

- Report a decrease in fatigue as evidenced by a lower rating on a scale of 1 to 5, with 2 indicating no fatigue.
- Slowly increase activity until former activity level is achieved.

Nursing Interventions. The patient with hepatitis needs considerable rest during the acute phase of the illness. The level of physical activity allowed is individually determined based on the amount of fatigue and severity of the disease. Rest periods should be interspersed throughout the day, and patient care should be scheduled to allow uninterrupted periods for napping and relaxation. The nurse instructs the patient to increase activity slowly as tolerated. A nutritionally complete diet provides needed energy for increasing activity. If hepatic enzyme levels increase with resumption of near-normal activities, activity limitations are imposed.

Related NIC Interventions. Energy Management, Environmental Management, Teaching: Prescribed Activity/Exercise

Patient/Family Teaching. Patient and family teaching for the patient with viral hepatitis is presented in the Patient/Family Teaching box.

Evaluation

To evaluate the effectiveness of nursing interventions, compare patient behaviors with those stated in the expected patient outcomes.

Related NOC Outcomes. Activity Tolerance, Comfort Level, Endurance, Energy Conservation, Nutritional Status: Food & Fluid Intake, Nutritional Status: Nutrient Intake

Gerontologic Considerations

Some types of hepatitis have a higher incidence in the older adult population in some areas of the United States. Because of the depressed immunity of some of these individuals, mortality rates may increase. Nurses in long-term care facilities need to be astute in their initial and ongoing assessment of the residents, observing for early signs of viral hepatitis.

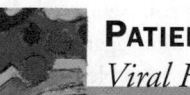

Patient/Family Teaching
Viral Hepatitis

The nurse should provide an open, honest environment for frank discussions about dangerous sexual practices and drugs. The nurse should inform the patient and family about:

- Methods to avoid transmission of viral hepatitis
- Risk of contracting viral hepatitis through multiple sex partners
- The dangers of sharing intravenous drug equipment and alternatives such as local treatment programs
- Importance and availability of immunizations for close contacts
- Appropriate preexposure and postexposure prophylaxis

Focal Hepatocellular Disorders

Liver Abscess

Etiology and Epidemiology. Liver abscesses may result from a variety of organisms. *Escherichia coli* and *Klebsiella pneumoniae* are the most common; *Staphylococcus, Streptococcus, Pseudomonas,* and *Proteus* organisms may also be found. Patients with depressed immune function, such as those with neutropenia or leukemia, may develop systemic candidiasis with multiple hepatic abscesses. Many people with abscesses have multiple bacteria involved.

Hepatic abscesses are uncommon in the United States but are associated with a high mortality rate. Amebic liver abscesses are common worldwide, particularly in countries with tropical and subtropical climates. In the United States, amebic abscesses occur occasionally in the temperate regions and in people who have traveled to tropical climates.

Pathophysiology. Pyogenic abscesses can occur as either a single large abscess or multiple small or microscopic abscesses. Amebic liver abscesses are typically large and singular and are usually a secondary site of infection. Pyogenic organisms originating in various areas of the body reach the liver through the biliary, vascular, or lymphatic systems. In addition, pyogenic organisms may be introduced by penetrating injuries to the liver or by direct continuous extension. The organisms cause necrosis of the liver tissue and abscess formation. In amebic abscesses the vegetative form of the organism moves from the gut to the small portal vessels and into the hepatic tissue, where it becomes activated.

If liver abscesses are not identified, they continue to grow and can perforate the pleural, peritoneal, or pericardial cavity. Fistulas from the abscess to other abdominal organs or through the abdominal wall may also develop. The major manifestations of liver abscess are caused by the infection rather than by changes in hepatic function (see Clinical Manifestations box). The patient with pyogenic abscesses, particularly multiple small or microscopic abscesses, may have clinical manifestations of sepsis and septic shock. Fever and constitutional symptoms such as malaise, anorexia, and weight loss are common. The patient with amebic abscesses may have signs and symptoms of intestinal amebiasis or give a history of intestinal signs and symptoms such as bloody, mucoid diarrhea; generalized abdominal pain; rectal tenesmus; dehydration; and hypotension. However, many patients with amebic abscess report no history of intestinal signs and symptoms.[27,44]

Collaborative Care Management. Diagnostic tests usually reveal leukocytosis and an elevated erythrocyte sedimentation rate caused by the infection, accompanied by moderate elevation of serum alkaline phosphatase and minimal elevation of serum transaminases (AST and ALT) from liver cell damage. Hyperbilirubinemia and hypoalbuminemia result from impaired liver function (see Chapter 45). In patients with amebic liver abscesses, serologic laboratory tests such as immunoglobulins against antigens, indirect hemagglutination titers, complement fixation tests, and latex agglutination tests are highly diagnostic. Hepatic radioisotope scans, ultrasonic scanning, and CT scans can reveal abscesses and are used in diagnosis and follow-up evaluation. Scanning is also useful for guided drainage procedures.

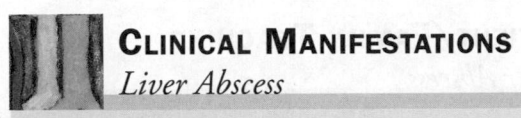

CLINICAL MANIFESTATIONS
Liver Abscess

Infectious Process

Fever and chills (temperature between 102° and 106° F [38.8° and 41.1° C])
Cough
Diaphoresis
Difficulty breathing
Abnormal breath sounds from pleural involvement
Right upper quadrant abdominal pain and tenderness
Anorexia
Nausea and vomiting
Clinical manifestations of peritonitis (see Clinical Manifestations box, p. 1342)

Hepatic Dysfunction

Hepatomegaly
Jaundice and pruritus
Splenomegaly
Abdominal distention and ascites

Empiric antimicrobial therapy is used initially for pyogenic abscesses with the specific type of antibiotic determined from the culture and sensitivity of the aspirate of the abscess. Metronidazole (Flagyl), chloroquine, and dehydroemetine or emetine are the drugs of choice for amebic abscesses. Acetaminophen is used to control fever, and fluid and electrolyte replacement is initiated as supportive therapy when needed.

For pyogenic abscesses, surgical drainage or needle aspiration may be necessary because the necrotic tissue walls off the abscess from the healthy liver tissue and makes it more difficult for antimicrobial therapy to reach the infection. Drainage is usually attempted only for a single pyogenic abscess. After locating an abscess by ultrasound, arteriography, or CT scan, the surgeon can attempt percutaneous aspiration, usually under ultrasound guidance. After the application of a local anesthetic agent, the surgeon inserts a large-bore needle into the abscess and aspirates the contents. Complications of this procedure are similar to those of a liver biopsy, with hemorrhage being the most common. In the case of amebic abscesses, aspiration is not usually indicated because medications alone are effective.

Patients with liver abscesses commonly complain of abdominal pain in the right upper quadrant or, more rarely, the shoulders. The patient may report nausea, vomiting, and anorexia. There may be few objective signs of a liver abscess. Fever is common. A palpable mass in the right upper quadrant may be felt in some patients. Weight loss may result from the nausea, vomiting, and anorexia and the increased metabolic needs. Some patients exhibit dyspnea and pleural pain if the diaphragm is involved.[44]

The first priority of care is management of fluid volume deficit or shock, if present. Subsequently, nursing care focuses on provision of adequate fluids and nutrition, provision of comfort, and patient teaching for self-management (see Patient/Family Teaching box).

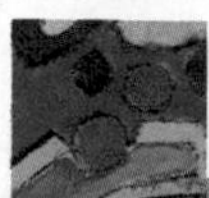

PATIENT/FAMILY TEACHING
Liver Abscess

Patient education for long-term care is a major nursing responsibility. The nurse should instruct the patient and family:

- To continue adherence to the medication regimen. In some cases medication may need to be continued for several weeks or months.
- To notify the health care provider if any of the following signs or symptoms occurs:
  - —Chills, fever, diaphoresis (recurring infection)
  - —Worsening abdominal pain or increased difficulty breathing (spread of infection)
  - —Jaundice or ascites (deterioration of liver function)
- About the side effects of the medications, and to report any side effects to the health care provider
- About the need for continued follow-up care

At first the patient may tolerate only IV fluids or require IV fluids to replace deficits. The effectiveness of these measures is evaluated by monitoring the patient's daily weight and skin turgor and assessing laboratory values for hemoconcentration or dilution. Food should be given in small amounts, with the patient's preferences considered to help overcome anorexia. Frequent oral hygiene (at least once every 2 hours) is necessary because fever and fluid loss dry the mucous membranes and may worsen anorexia. The environment should be clean, free of odors, and relaxed.

Comfort measures are essential because of the high temperature, episodes of chills and diaphoresis, pruritus, anorexia, and abdominal pain. During periods of chills, adequate blankets to provide comfort without increasing temperature are necessary. Cool sponge baths may help lower the temperature. The gown and bed linens should be changed if the patient is diaphoretic. Pruritus can be controlled with cool sponge baths, use of soft linens, prevention of dry skin, and cool environmental temperatures.

Liver Trauma

Etiology and Epidemiology. Because of its location and size, the liver is frequently subjected to trauma, which may be either penetrating (gunshot wound or stab wound) or blunt (collision with steering wheel during an automobile accident or the impact of a fall). If the injury is severe, the liver may rupture, with severe internal hemorrhage.

Pathophysiology. The pathophysiology depends on the type of liver injury. Injuries vary from a laceration and capsular tear with minimal parenchymal damage to liver rupture with extreme parenchymal damage and damage to the retrohepatic vasculature. Stab wounds often make a relatively superficial incision and may do no more damage than a needle biopsy. Gunshot wounds and blunt trauma can result in severe hemorrhage leading to hypotension, shock, and peritonitis. Bile may also leak from the bile canaliculi and contaminate the peritoneal cavity, causing peritonitis. Less severe blunt trauma may just result in a subcapsular hematoma.

The clinical manifestations of liver trauma also vary with type of injury (see Clinical Manifestations box). If peritoneal contamination from hemorrhage or bile has occurred, signs and symptoms of peritonitis may be present (see Clinical Manifestations box).

Late complications of liver trauma may include:

- Severe hemorrhage resulting from disseminated intravascular coagulation, which often accompanies shock
- Degeneration and sloughing of liver segments that have had disrupted circulation with resultant hemorrhage and microvascular damage
- Intrahepatic cyst or abscess formation
- Infections of other areas of body after the trauma
- Subphrenic abscess formation
- Biliary fistulas

The mortality rate for liver trauma has decreased over the years. It depends on the type of injury (highest for blunt trauma because of a larger portion of liver being damaged and because of other associated injuries), the severity of the injury (highest for those requiring resection of a large amount of liver), and associated injuries (increasing mortality with each additional injury to another organ).[34]

Collaborative Care Management. In some instances the only sign of hepatic trauma is blood in peritoneal lavage fluid. Useful diagnostic tools include CT and ultrasonography of the abdomen. Laboratory studies may reveal a decreasing hematocrit and hemoglobin from blood loss and leukocytosis from peritoneal infection and inflammation.

The immediate medical management for patients with suspected liver trauma is the same as that for any patient with intraabdominal trauma. Most penetrating abdominal injuries

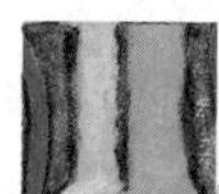

CLINICAL MANIFESTATIONS
Liver Trauma

Signs of Shock

Pale, cool, clammy skin
Diaphoresis
Hypotension
Tachycardia
Mental confusion

Penetrating Trauma

Entry and sometimes exit wounds

Blunt Trauma

Abdominal pain exacerbated by breathing
Shoulder pain indicating diaphragmatic irritation

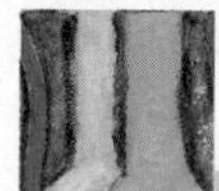

CLINICAL MANIFESTATIONS
Peritonitis

- Abdominal tenderness
- Rebound tenderness
- Muscle rigidity or spasms
- Decreased or absent bowel sounds
- Sometimes a fluid wave
- Fever
- Tachycardia
- Tachypnea
- Nausea
- Vomiting

require surgical exploration to detect abdominal hemorrhage, trauma to the liver or other organs, necrotic tissue, or bile drainage. Management of the blunt hepatic injury, in which there is no abdominal penetration, has changed over the past 10 years. Studies have indicated that approximately 85% of all patients with blunt hepatic trauma are hemodynamically stable, and non-operative management significantly improves outcomes compared with surgical management. These outcomes include decreased incidence of abdominal infection, decreased need for transfusions, and decreased length of hospital stay. Surgery remains the treatment of choice for individuals with blunt injury who are hemodynamically unstable. Other medical interventions relate to the stabilization of airway, fluid and electrolyte status, blood replacement, laboratory assessments, and the prevention or treatment of shock and peritonitis.[20,32]

Nursing care for the patient with suspected liver trauma consists of a systematic assessment of cardiovascular, fluid volume, and neurologic status, along with observations for signs and symptoms of peritonitis (see Guidelines for Safe Practice box). This assessment is required from the moment the patient is first seen through the postoperative period. The nurse should anticipate the possibility of surgery and prepare the patient and family accordingly. Because of the unexpectedness of trauma and the circumstances involved, helping the patient and family control their anxiety is essential. The nurse provides simple explanations about care to be administered, answers all questions, and provides information about spiritual or other resources as appropriate.

Liver Tumors

Liver neoplasms or tumors may be either benign or malignant. Benign lesions include hemangioma, cysts, and rarely adenoma. Most benign tumors are asymptomatic, but occasionally they enlarge enough to become symptomatic. In such cases surgical intervention may be required. This section focuses on malignant neoplasms.

Etiology and Epidemiology. The incidence of primary liver cancer is increased in people with chronic liver disease, particularly those with chronic hepatitis B or C. Any chronic inflammatory liver disease has the potential to induce hepatocellular cancer, but the pathologic condition most commonly associated with the disease is cirrhosis. The risk of developing hepatocellular cancer is approximately 40 times greater in persons with alcohol-induced cirrhosis compared with the general population. Certain environmental and hereditary causes of cirrhosis also have a strong correlation with hepatocellular cancer. However, a direct carcinogenic effect of alcohol on the liver has not been proved.

Hepatocellular cancer is one of the most common cancers in the world and is also the most deadly, with a 5-year survival rate of less than 5% without treatment. The incidence bears marked geographic differences, with rates in Africa and Asia 20 times higher than in the United States. This disparity is probably related to endemic rates of viral hepatitis and nutritional deficits in these areas. Recently, however, the incidence of hepatocellular cancer in the United States has begun to rise.[4,40]

Metastatic liver tumors occur 20 times more frequently than primary tumors. They rank second only to cirrhosis as a cause of fatal liver disease in the United States.

Pathophysiology. The liver is highly vascular and is a common site for metastasis from the cancers of the GI tract, lungs, breasts, and kidneys and also malignant melanomas. Primary liver tumors arise in the liver cell **(hepatocellular)** or the bile duct cell (cholangiocellular), or they can be of mixed origin. The lesions are multiple or singular, are diffuse or nodular, and involve a lobe or the entire liver. The cancerous cells compress the surrounding normal liver cells and invade the portal vein branches. Some cells infiltrate the gallbladder, mesentery, peritoneum, and diaphragm by direct extension. Primary cancers also tend to cause hemorrhage by extension into the vascular tissue of the liver and necrosis by depriving normal hepatic tissue of adequate circulation. The most common site for metastasis of the primary liver lesion is the lung, but metastasis can occur to the adrenal glands, spleen, vertebrae, kidneys, ovaries, or pancreas. Primary lesions grow rapidly, sometimes without signs or symptoms, and often the patient lives only a short time after diagnosis.

Metastatic carcinoma of the liver varies from a few small nodules to large growths. Adjacent nodules may eventually fuse and compress the surrounding liver tissue. Usually different parts of the liver are uniformly involved; thus liver biopsy may be a useful diagnostic aid.

The signs and symptoms of liver cancer depend on the size and extent of the tumor, the amount of hepatocellular damage, and the presence of liver failure (see Clinical Manifestations box, p. 1344). Patients with liver tumors often experience epigastric fullness, fatigue, weight loss, and abdominal pain early in the course of their illness. Later the fatigue becomes more pronounced, and patients may report weakness and anorexia. As the disease progresses, the patient may become jaundiced, have ascites, and show signs of liver failure, including variceal bleeding and PSE. The disease is often clinically silent until it is well advanced.[33,39]

COMPLICATIONS. The poor prognosis associated with liver cancer is partially due to the late onset of definitive signs of disease and hence advanced disease at the time of diagnosis. If the cancer is untreated, death usually occurs within 6 to 8 weeks of diagnosis.

GUIDELINES FOR SAFE PRACTICE

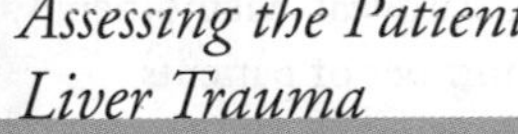

Assessing the Patient with Suspected Liver Trauma

- Respiratory status (rate, breath sounds, pulse oximetry, and blood gases)
- Vital signs every 15 minutes (blood pressure, pulse)
- Mean arterial pressure every hour
- Other hemodynamic monitoring such as intraarterial pressure monitoring and cardiac output measurements as ordered
- Urinary output and other fluid losses documented hourly
- Intake documented hourly
- Serum and urinary electrolytes and osmolality at least daily
- Hematocrit and hemoglobin daily
- Neurologic checks for responsiveness and motion every hour
- Consciousness monitored every hour using Glasgow Coma Scale
- Skin temperature, color, and moisture checked every hour
- Bowel sounds, pain, and abdominal tenderness

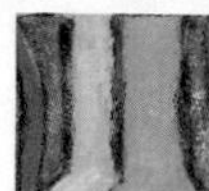

CLINICAL MANIFESTATIONS
Liver Cancer

Early Signs
Right upper quadrant mass
Epigastric fullness
Pain
Fatigue
Weight loss
Changes in liver function tests

Later Signs
Fatigue
Ascites
Liver failure
Fever
Hepatic bruits
Jaundice
Variceal bleeding

Metastatic Liver Tumors
Fatigue
Anorexia
Weakness
Weight loss followed by weight gain resulting from ascites
Hepatomegaly
Hepatic bruits
Jaundice
Portal-systemic encephalopathy

Nearly 50% of persons with hepatic cancer have distant metastases to the lungs, bone, adrenal glands, and brain. Tumors spread rapidly within the liver, and occlusion of the portal vein, which can lead to necrosis, rupture, and hemorrhage, is common. As the cancer progresses, multiple body systems are affected and complications arise. The cause of death in approximately 50% of patients with liver cancer is liver failure and hemorrhage. Other causes of death include pneumonia, malnutrition, and thromboemboli.

Care for persons with advanced liver cancer is primarily supportive. Persons with advanced disease often experience liver failure, ascites, infection, bleeding, pain, weight loss, anorexia, vomiting, weakness, and pneumonia. Both the patient and family should be informed about treatment plans and be assured that care will focus on promoting comfort.

Collaborative Care Management

DIAGNOSTIC TESTS. Diagnostic tests include blood studies and other tests to locate or determine type of lesions (Table 46-7). The blood studies may show an increased erythrocyte sedimentation rate associated with generalized inflammation of the liver; anemia resulting from increased metabolism and decreased food intake; hyperbilirubinemia; elevated alkaline phosphatase, AST, and ALT; decreased blood glucose; and hypoalbuminemia. The number of abnormalities depends on the severity of hepatocellular damage. A special test that is useful in the diagnosis of primary liver carcinoma is serum concentrations of alpha-fetoprotein (AFP). AFP in concentrations of 500 ng/ml to 5 mg/ml is considered positive. High levels that occur in any adult without obvious GI tract tumors strongly suggest primary liver cancer. The sensitivity of an elevated AFP is only 60%.

MEDICATIONS. Increasingly, chemotherapy is being used to treat primary and metastatic tumors of the liver. Chemotherapy is often the treatment of choice when hepatic resection is not an option. It may be given systemically or by infusion directly into the hepatic artery. This direct arterial infusion allows more drug to be delivered directly to the tumor and decreases systemic side effects. Direct hepatic arterial infusion can be accomplished by one of two methods. In the first method, a percutaneous catheter is inserted into the hepatic artery using fluoroscopy. The catheter is attached to an external infusion pump (Figure 46-7) that is filled with the appropriate chemotherapeutic agent and programmed to deliver the agent over a desired period. The catheter is removed after each drug treatment cycle.

In the second method a catheter is surgically inserted into the hepatic artery and connected to an implanted infusion pump (Figure 46-8). The implanted pump can be filled with the correct amount of drug and programmed to deliver the chemotherapeutic agent over a desired time (generally up to 14 days) and at a desired dosage. In chemotherapy-free intervals, the pump is filled with a heparin solution to maintain patency of the hepatic artery catheter. The chamber should be adequately filled to avoid complete emptying.

The implanted infusion pump allows the patient to be treated at home. The patient comes into an outpatient site at prescribed times for addition of drugs or heparin solution and a recheck of pump flow rate. The patient needs physical care before and after surgery similar to that for any patient having surgery and instructions regarding self-care needs related to the chemotherapeutic agent being used. The nurse also is involved in refilling the pump at the prescribed intervals.

High-dose chemotherapy, usually 5-fluorouracil and fluorodeoxyuridine, has been used to induce regression in primary and metastatic tumors. Intraperitoneal chemotherapy has been used successfully in a limited number of patients.

TABLE 46-7 DIAGNOSTIC TESTS FOR LIVER TUMORS OR CANCER

Test	Purpose
Computed tomography scan and/or magnetic resonance imaging	To locate lesions
Liver biopsy	To assess cellular type; determine definitive diagnosis of cancer
Radioisotope scans	To diagnose lesions and location
Serum alpha-fetoprotein (AFP)	Can suggest primary liver cancer if concentration is 500 ng/ml to 5 mg/ml (Sensitivity of elevated AFP is only 60%.)
Ultrasonography	To locate tumors

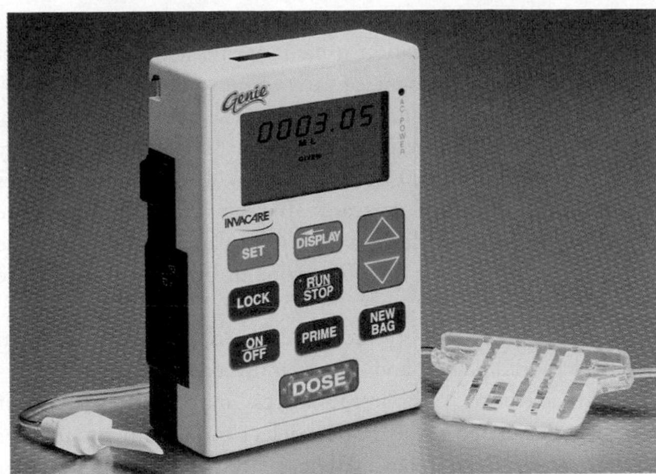

Figure 46-7 External infusion pump. Lightweight, battery-operated infusion pump for ambulatory patient. Flow rate is adjustable; power pack operates for 7 days before needing recharging.

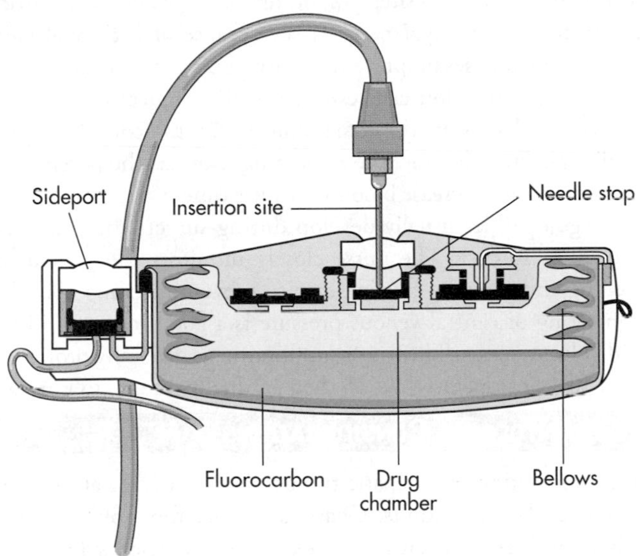

Figure 46-8 Implantable infusion pump (Infusaid pump).

DIET. A special diet is necessary only if signs and symptoms of cirrhosis occur.

TREATMENTS. Radiotherapy may be used to control pain, but it does not improve survival rates. Ligation of the hepatic artery decreases the oxygen delivered to the tumor and may help control the pain and diminish the tumor mass.

SURGICAL MANAGEMENT. For solitary primary tumors and some solitary metastatic tumors, surgery may be performed. The liver has remarkable regenerative capacity, which allows for as much as 90% resection. Orthotopic transplantation (removal of the recipient's liver and replacement with a graft liver) has been performed for patients with primary liver tumors with varying success. In the United States, liver transplantation for hepatocellular carcinoma is indicated only for patients with unresectable tumors, focal tumor recurrence after resection, or kidney failure.

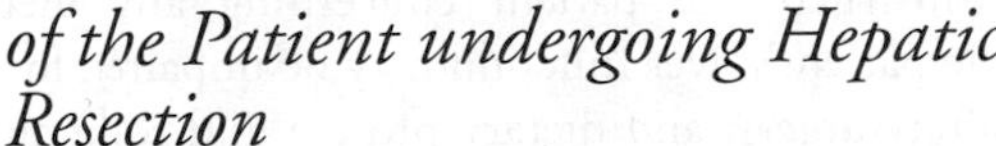

Which clinical manifestation is an early sign of liver cancer?

1. Jaundice
2. Right upper quadrant mass
3. Anorexia
4. Fever

Nursing Management

of the Patient undergoing Hepatic Resection

PREOPERATIVE CARE

For the patient having a surgical resection of a hepatic tumor (hepatic resection), skilled perioperative care is necessary. The nurse teaches about the preoperative preparation, the procedure itself, and postoperative care (see Chapters 13 to 15). The patient may need vitamin K for defects in clotting factors, as well as other vitamins if deficits are present. Preparation of the bowel is the same as for intestinal surgery (see Chapter 43). If a blood volume deficit is present, blood is given. The goal is to make the patient's physical condition as stable as possible before surgery. Sometimes, preoperative total parenteral nutrition is initiated to improve the patient's status.

POSTOPERATIVE CARE

After surgery the patient requires close monitoring for complications, especially sepsis and hypovolemia from blood loss. The nurse monitors vital signs every 15 minutes until the patient is stable and then every hour, checks dressings for oozing or bleeding, monitors intake and output every 4 to 8 hours, and records weights daily. Assessment of the cardiorespiratory system (cardiac rhythm, breath sounds, and pulse oximetry) is also necessary. Temperature should be monitored at least every 4 hours. Laboratory values for serum electrolytes and complete blood count with hematocrit and hemoglobin levels are carefully monitored.

Assessment also includes monitoring for decreased liver function. The nurse checks liver enzymes, blood glucose, coagulation status, serum albumin levels, and neurologic status at regular intervals. The nurse should anticipate the possibility of administering glucose, albumin, and blood.

To promote turning and deep breathing, the nurse must ensure adequate pain control by giving the patient medications as ordered, splinting the incision, and positioning the patient properly (upright). Patient-controlled analgesia may be used to manage postoperative pain. Because most analgesics, narcotic and nonnarcotic, are metabolized in the liver, no "safe" analgesic exists for the patient with liver dysfunction, and the nurse should monitor closely for signs of toxicity.

The patient has nothing by mouth for several days after surgery and has an NG tube attached to suction. Mouth care every 2 hours and monitoring of the suction device are indicated. Oral intake is started on approximately the fifth postoperative day. Initially ice chips and clear liquids are given, and then the diet is advanced as tolerated based on appetite and bowel function. The patient needs adequate calories, protein, vitamins, and minerals. Adequacy of intake may be monitored by daily calorie counts. The patient's tolerance to protein nitrogenous waste products must be monitored. If the patient cannot metabolize protein adequately because of loss of liver tissue, a low-protein diet is necessary. If the patient can adequately detoxify ammonia, a high-protein diet is given.

After surgery the patient initially dangles on the side of the bed and is out of bed by the first postoperative day. Close monitoring of vital signs, tolerance for activity, and respiratory status are required. Care of the patient undergoing hepatic resection is summarized in the Guidelines for Safe Practice box.

The nurse instructs the patient concerning any dietary restrictions. The patient's liver function may be impaired for up to 6 months after surgery, and dietary protein and sodium are restricted accordingly. Corticosteroids may be given to enhance regeneration and prevent fibrosis. If steroids are to be continued after discharge, the nurse gives the patient written and verbal instructions regarding dosage, purpose, administration, side effects, and what to report to the prescriber. The patient's activity tolerance gradually increases. Activities such as heavy lifting (more than 5 to 10 pounds) are avoided. Usually the patient relies on feelings of fatigue and tiredness as indicators of what can or cannot be done. The patient is unable to assume all activities of daily living immediately because of fatigue, and the nurse assesses whether the family and patient can meet self-care and home care needs or require outside help. Referrals for home health care should be made if necessary.

Jaundice is common after surgery, usually as a result of the inability of the remaining liver to use bile. Other causes of jaundice include multiple transfusions, vascular occlusion, and anoxia of hepatocytes during surgery. Jaundice usually resolves in about 10 days. If it persists, obstruction should be suspected.

Major postoperative complications after hepatic resection include hemorrhage; biliary fistula; infection; subphrenic abscess; respiratory complications such as pneumonia, atelectasis, and respiratory failure; portal hypertension; and clotting defects.

Hemorrhage is common because of the liver's vascularity. This potentially fatal complication usually occurs within 24 hours of surgery and must be recognized early to prevent death.

After hepatic resection, a T tube (in the common bile duct) and subhepatic drain are usually in place. The T tube normally drains approximately 400 ml of bile daily. If the drain becomes dislodged, the drainage decreases. Excessive drainage from the subhepatic drain can indicate a biliary fistula leaking bile into the subhepatic space. Other manifestations of biliary fistula include fever and pain.

Infection following hepatic resection is associated with an increased mortality rate and occurs more commonly in persons who have cirrhosis. Subphrenic abscess may result because of insufficient drainage of the surgical defect and usually occurs later in the postoperative course. The placement and output of drainage tubes should be closely monitored in the postoperative period. An acute onset of sharp, piercing, right upper quadrant pain with low-grade fever and the presence of adventitious sounds in the lung bases suggest a subphrenic abscess.

Respiratory complications can arise because of the anatomic location of the surgical site. Patients are often reluctant to participate in pulmonary hygiene exercises because of incisional pain. Nursing care focuses on preventing any respiratory complications.

Portal hypertension can result from the surgical alteration of venous blood flow in the remaining liver. This complication is usually transitory because the remaining liver has the potential to compensate and increase blood flow over time.

Coagulopathies usually develop during surgery, but may also occur after surgery. The nurse closely monitors the patient for bleeding and provides nursing care to prevent bleeding episodes. Monitoring of central venous pressure is a good indicator of the fluid volume status. The prothrombin time is generally prolonged in the first postoperative week, then gradually returns to normal.

GERONTOLOGIC CONSIDERATIONS

Surgical resection of a hepatic tumor poses a risk for all persons, but especially older adults. Changes in liver function associated with aging include decreased blood flow, decreased synthesis of

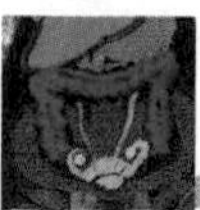

GUIDELINES FOR SAFE PRACTICE *The Patient Undergoing Liver Resection*

Preoperative Care

Explain special postoperative procedures (nasogastric intubation and parenteral fluids for several days).
Teach deep breathing exercises, leg exercises, and the use of side rails to facilitate turning in bed without exerting pull on the abdominal muscles.
Prevent hemorrhage.
Give prescribed vitamin K.
Complete bowel preparation.

Postoperative Care

Promote oxygenation.
—Encourage turning and deep breathing exercises.
—Encourage activity and ambulation as ordered.
Maintain fluid and electrolyte balance.
—Check dressings for oozing or bleeding.
—Maintain prescribed rate of parenteral fluids.
—Monitor for signs of fluid imbalance (daily weight changes, hematocrit, lung congestion, and dry skin and mucous membranes).
Maintain patency of gastrointestinal tube.
Promote comfort.
—Give analgesics on a regular basis during the first 48 hours to minimize severe pain.
—Give frequent oral hygiene until oral fluids are resumed.
Promote appropriate nutrition.
—Explain menu choices for a low-protein diet.
—Reinforce information about a low-sodium diet.

cholesterol, and reduced ability to regenerate. These normal changes may be more evident with destruction of liver tissue associated with tumors. The older adult is also susceptible to drug toxicity. Patients with impaired liver function should be monitored for toxic and adverse effects, which may indicate a need for a reduced dosage of certain drugs, particularly chemotherapeutic agents. Fatigue and weakness, which are common symptoms associated with hepatic cancer, may be increased in older patients as a result of aging and coexisting chronic disease.

Liver Transplantation

Etiology and Epidemiology. The first liver transplantation was performed in 1963. It is now a therapeutic option for both adults and children with liver failure. Liver transplantation is used to treat biliary atresia, fulminant hepatic failure, cirrhosis, hepatitis, metabolic disorders, and primary hepatic malignancy[13,54] (see Research box, p. 1335). If the damage from these diseases is severe enough, transplantation may be necessary. A transplant may allow a patient with a previously life-threatening illness to keep up with the demands of a full, active life. Cirrhosis of the liver is the major pathologic condition in adult patients seeking transplantation, and the importance of abstinence from alcohol creates unique dilemmas in the selection procedures for liver transplant recipients. The use of transplantation to treat liver cancer is controversial because of the high rate of recurrence, even with no evidence of disseminated disease.

Bilirubin concentrations of more than 10 mg/dl, serum albumin concentrations of less than 2.5 mg/dl, and prothrombin times of more than 5 seconds beyond the control value are clinical features predictive of the need for liver transplantation. Other criteria include incapacitating encephalopathy, recurrent variceal bleeding not controlled by sclerotherapy, intractable ascites that does not respond to diuretic therapy or paracentesis, and recurrent spontaneous bacterial peritonitis.

The patient must meet the criteria to receive the donor liver. The patient's condition, donor condition, organ condition, compatibility, and transplant center factors are all considered before the transplantation surgery. Liver donors may be live (living donor liver transplants), donating a right lobe; or deceased, donating the whole liver or a lobe.

Collaborative Care Management. Once a patient has been selected for a liver transplant, a constant vigil begins to keep the patient in the best health possible for the surgery. Waiting for a liver transplant can trigger a patient and family's stress and anxiety. To help manage the stress, the nurse should advise the patient to:

- Eat right, take prescribed medications, and follow a daily exercise program.
- Continue activities of daily living and usual social activities as much as possible.
- Seek counseling, relaxation therapy, or any other diversional activity to reduce the constant pressure of the "waiting time."
- Share feeling with family, friends, and others as necessary.

Once the patient receives the call that a donor liver is available, he or she is admitted to the hospital and undergoes usual preoperative measures (see Chapter 13). A liver transplant takes 8 hours or more and involves the removal of the recipient's diseased liver followed by implantation of the donor liver allograft. The diseased liver is removed en bloc. A venovenous bypass system may be used to maintain normal hemodynamic values while the recipient is without a liver. This bypass system helps prevent venous hypertension, circulatory instability, and excessive bleeding. The liver transplant procedure is the most technically complex of the solid organ transplants because of the intricate vascular and biliary anastomoses that are required (Figures 46-9 and 46-10).

The major postoperative complications include rejection, infection, and occlusion of vessels. The liver is less susceptible to acute rejection than the kidneys, but adequate immunosuppressive therapy is still a high priority. The extensive surgery combined with the preoperative liver failure significantly increases the patient's risk for postoperative complications (see Clinical Manifestations box).

Initial care of the liver transplant recipient is challenging and complex; therefore the postoperative patient is admitted to an intensive care setting. Constant monitoring of the patient's hemodynamic status and liver function is critical. Bed rest is maintained for several days. The patient should expect to have some

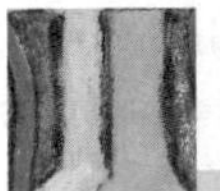

CLINICAL MANIFESTATIONS
Liver Transplant Rejection

- Fever
- Flulike symptoms
- Jaundice
- Itching
- Abdominal pain
- Back pain
- Elevated liver enzymes

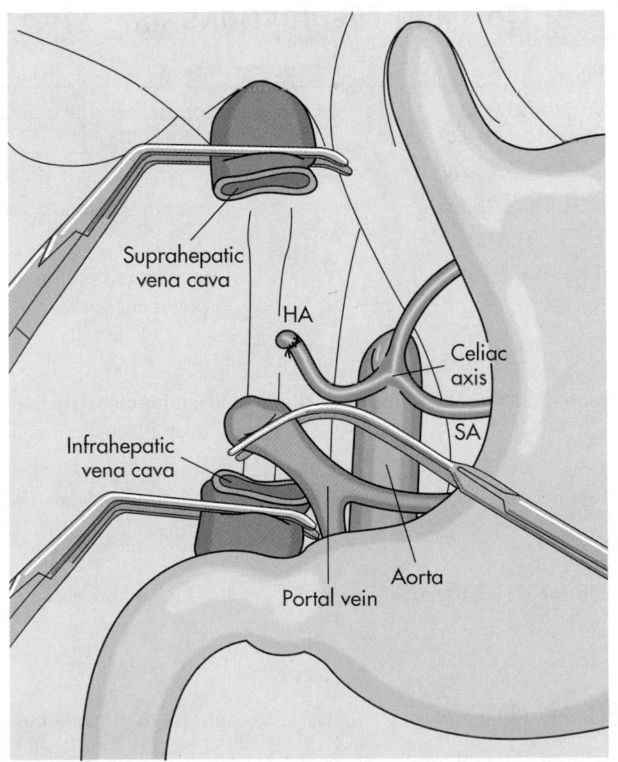

Figure 46-9 Vascular anastomosis of liver transplant. *HA*, Hepatic artery; *SA*, splenic artery.

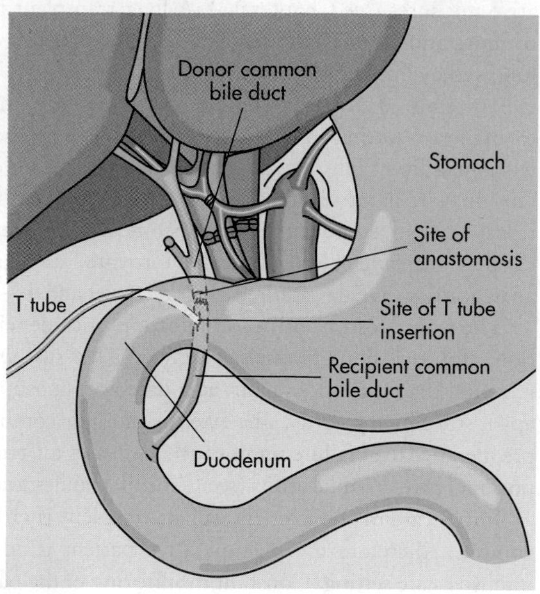

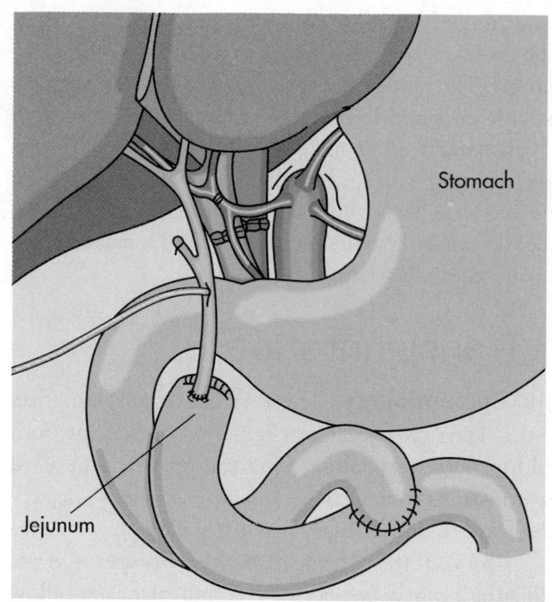

Figure 46-10 Biliary anastomoses of liver transplant. **A,** Choledochocholedochostomy. **B,** Choledochojejunostomy.

pain and general discomfort. An NG tube in usually in place to keep the stomach empty. Usual postoperative care such as turning and coughing is instituted (see Chapter 15). IV therapy is continued for several days. Drains are placed in or near the incision during surgery and are usually removed 5 to 7 days after surgery. The patient's liver function tests, including serum transaminases, bilirubin, albumin, and clotting factors, often show improvement within 24 hours if complications do not occur.

Immunosuppressive therapy is started before surgery and continued on a regular schedule after the procedure (Table 46-8).[23] The

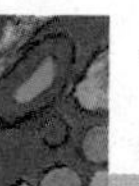

TABLE 46-8
COMMON MEDICATIONS *after Liver Transplant*

Drug	Action	Nursing Intervention
Acyclovir (Zovirax)	Decreases severity of infections; inhibits DNA replication	Monitor side effects. Teach patient it is not a cure but used to manage and reduce symptoms.
Azathioprine (Imuran)	Immunosuppression to prevent rejection of new liver	Tell patient to observe for bruising or bleeding; must take for life.
Ganciclovir (Cytovene)	Decreases severity of infections; inhibits DNA polymerases	Monitor side effects. Tell patient that drug therapy should not be interrupted and to avoid persons with known infections.
Muromonab-CD3 (Orthoclone OKT)	Given immediately to prevent rejection of new liver; blocks action of T cells	Monitor side effects. Tell patient oral care is important and to avoid persons with known infections.
Mycophenolate mofetil (CellCept)	Immunosuppression by decreasing number of white cells	Monitor side effects. Tell patient to take on empty stomach and to avoid persons with known infections.
Prednisone (Deltasone)	Immunosuppression	Monitor side effects, including fluid retention. Tell patient not to stop abruptly for any reason (contact physician) and to avoid persons with known infections.
Sirolumus (Rapamune)	Immunosuppression to prevent rejection of new liver; inhibits T cell activation and proliferation	Monitor side effects. Tell patient to refrain from taking with grapefruit juice and to avoid persons with known infections.

DNA, Deoxyribonucleic acid.

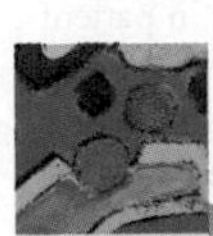

PATIENT/FAMILY TEACHING
When to Call the Physician After Liver Transplantation

After liver transplantation but before discharge, the nurse should teach the patient and family to notify the transplant physician if the patient:

- Is unable to take the prescribed medications because of illness
- Has a change in health status, weight, or eating habits
- Develops diarrhea, nausea, or vomiting
- Changes prescription medications from the primary provider
- Is taking cold medicines, acetaminophen, or other pain relievers
- Experiences any unusual symptoms
- Plans to have any dental work done
- Is unsure or has questions about the prescribed regimen

patient may also take antibiotics, antifungal agents, and nutritional supplements. Worsening liver function, fever, swelling, and tenderness of the liver are all warning signs of a complication. Infection is a crucial concern and can be bacterial, viral, or fungal. The risk of infection is greatest during the first 3 months after surgery. High blood pressure, rejection, and diabetes are also common complications.[13] The patient with alcoholic cirrhosis is counseled that ongoing involvement with a chemical dependency program is an essential strategy to prevent disease recurrence from relapse.

PATIENT/FAMILY TEACHING. Patient and family teaching is presented in the Patient/Family Teaching box.

Critical Thinking

1. Mrs. Smith, age 40, works in a homeless shelter. She has never been immunized for hepatitis B. She is exposed to HBV through a needlestick from an infected patient. What are the possible treatments that the nurse in the emergency department should inform Mrs. Smith about? If Mrs. Smith refuses any treatment, what should the nurse say to her? Is there anything else the nurse should do?
2. What diets are most appropriate for patients with hepatic disorders? What should you teach the patient and family about the importance of the special diet?

References

1. Abou-Assi S, Vlahevic Z: Hepatic encephalopathy, *Postgrad Med* 109(2): 52-70, 2001.
2. Adham M: Extracorporeal liver support: waiting for the deciding vote, *ASAIO J* 49(6):621-632, 2003.
3. Alexander D, Schaffer S, Leilman C: Noninfectious liver disorders: assessment and diagnosis, *Nurse Pract* 28(12):12-24, 2003.
4. American Cancer Society: *Facts and figures 2004,* accessed June 2004 from website: http://www.cancer.org.
5. American Liver Foundation: *Drug induced liver injury studies,* accessed June 2003 from website: http://www.liverfoundation.org.
6. Anadon M, Arroyo V: Ascites and spontaneous bacterial peritonitis. In Schiff ER, Sorrell MF, Maddrey WC, editors: *Schiff's diseases of the liver,* ed 9, Philadelphia, 2002, Lippincott-Raven.
7. Anand BS: Drug treatment of the complications of cirrhosis in the older adult, *Drugs & Aging* 18:575, 2001.
8. Arguedas MR, Fallon MB: Prevention in liver disease, *Am J Med Sci* 321:145, 2001.
9. Arroyo V: Pathophysiology, diagnosis and treatment of ascites in cirrhosis, *Ann Hepatol* 1(2):72-79, 2002.
10. Bilbao JI, Quiroga J, Benito A: Transjugular intrahepatic portosystemic shunt (TIPS): current status and future possibilities, *Cardiovasc Intervent Radiol* 25(4):251-269, 2002.
11. Briglia AE, Anania FA: Hepatorenal syndrome: definition, pathophysiology and intervention, *Crit Care Clinics* 18(2):345-373, 2002.
12. Buffum M, Buffum JC: Geropharmacology. In Ebersole P, Hess P, Luggen A, editors: *Toward healthy aging,* ed 6, St Louis, 2004, Mosby.
13. Chung-Mao L: Lessons learned from 100 right lobe living donor liver transplants, *Ann Surg* 240(1):151, 2004.
14. Disarthy S, McCullogh A: Alcoholic liver disease. In Schiff ER, Sorrell MF, Maddrey WC, editors: *Schiff's diseases of the liver,* ed 9, Philadelphia, 2002, Lippincott-Raven.
15. Dougherty AS, Heyward MD: Hepatitis C: current treatment strategies for an emerging epidemic, *Med Surg Nurs* 10:9, 2001.
16. Flynn M: Noninfectious liver disorders: adult autoimmune hepatitis, *Nurse Pract* 28(12):28-33, 2003.
17. Garcia N, Sanyal AJ: Minimizing ascites, *Postgrad Med* 109:91, 2001.
18. Giese LA: Complementary healthcare practices, *Gastroenterol Nurs* 24(1): 38-40, 2001.
19. Goldrick BA: Emerging infections: hepatitis A, *Am J Nurs* 104(3):27, 2004.
20. Gur S et al: Surgical treatment of liver trauma, *Hepato-Gastroenterol* 50(54):2109-2111, 2003.
21. Hegab AM, Luketic VA: Bleeding esophageal varices: how to treat this dreaded complication of portal hypertension, *Postgrad Med* 109:75, 2001.
22. Henderson JM: Surgical management of portal hypertension. In Schiff ER, Sorrell MF, Maddrey WC, editors: *Schiff's diseases of the liver,* ed 9, Philadelphia, 2002, Lippincott-Raven.
23. Hoffman RL, Roesch T: Update on transplant pharmacology, *Dimens Crit Care Nurs* 23(2):69, 2004.
24. Janotha B: Autoimmune hepatitis, *Adv Nurse Pract* 9:79, 2001.
25. Kaplan MM: Primary biliary cirrhosis: past, present, and future, *Gastroenterology* 123(4):1392-1394, 2002.
26. Kim WR: The burden of hepatitis C in the United States, *Hepatology* 36(5 Suppl):S30-S34, 2002.
27. Kershenobich D, Torre-Delgado A, Olivera-Matinez MA: Liver abscesses. In Schiff ER, Sorrell MF, Maddrey WC, editors: *Schiff's diseases of the liver,* ed 9, Philadelphia, 2002, Lippincott-Raven.
28. Lavanchy D: Hepatitis B virus epidemiology, disease burden, treatment and current and emerging prevention and control measures, *J Viral Hep* 11(2):97-107, 2004.
29. Levy C, Lindor KD: Current management of primary biliary cirrhosis and primary sclerosing cholangitis, *J Hepatol* 38(Suppl 1):S24-S37, 2003.
30. Lin KW, Kirchner JT: Hepatitis B, *Am Fam Phys* 69(1):75-82, 2004.
31. Luxon B: Autoimmune hepatitis: making sense of all those antibodies, *Postgrad Med* 114(1):85-88, 2003.
32. Oller DW, Udekwu PO: Liver trauma: a victory for conservative approaches, *Current Surgery* 61(1):21-24, 2004.
33. Omata M, Yoshida H: Prevention and treatment of hepatocellular carcinoma, *Liver Transplantation* 10(2 Suppl 1):S111-S114, 2004.
34. Ong A, Cohn S: Trauma of the liver. In Schiff ER, Sorrell MF, Maddrey WC, editors: *Schiff's diseases of the liver,* ed 9, Philadelphia, 2002, Lippincott-Raven.
35. Organ transplants cells from usable livers extend life, *Nursing* 33(9):35, 2003.
36. Patel K, McHutchison J: Current treatment for chronic hepatitis C, *Postgrad Med* 114(1):48-62, 2003.
37. Piasecki B, Forman L: Acute and chronic viral hepatitis. In Reddy K, Long W, editors: *Hepatology tract and pancreas,* vol 3, St Louis, 2004, Mosby.
38. Pizzorno JE, Murray MT, Joiner-Bey H: Hepatitis. In *The clinician's handbook of natural medicine,* St Louis, 2001, Elsevier-Churchill Livingstone.
39. Pons-Renedo F, Llovet J: Hepatocellular carcinoma: a clinical update, *Medscape Gen Med* 5(3), 2003, accessed June 2004 from website: http://www.medscape.com.
40. Porter S, Reddy K: Hepatocellular carcinoma. In Reddy K, Long W, editors: *Hepatology tract and pancreas,* vol 3, St Louis, 2004, Mosby.

41. Purow D, Jacobson I: Slowing the progression of chronic hepatitis B, *Postgrad Med* 114(1):65-76, 2003.
42. Rosemurgy AS, Zervos EE: Management of variceal hemorrhage, *Current Probl Surg* 40(6):263-343, 2003.
43. Rosemurgy AS et al: TIPS versus peritoneovenous shunt in the treatment of medically intractable ascites, *Ann Surg* 239(6):883-889, 2004.
44. Saeian K: Non-viral hepatic infections. In Reddy K, Long W, editors: *Hepatology tract and pancreas,* vol 3, St Louis, 2004, Mosby.
45. Schiodt FV, Lee WM: Fulminant liver disease, *Clin Liver Dis* 7(2):331-349, 2003.
46. Seeff LB et al: Complementary and alternative medicine in chronic liver disease, *Hepatology* 34(3):595-603, 2001.
47. Stacy KM, Lough MF: Gastrointestinal disorders. In Urden LD et al, editors: *Thelan's critical care nursing,* ed 4, St Louis, 2002, Mosby.
48. Starr S, Hand H: Nursing care of chronic and acute liver failure, *Nurs Standard* 16(40):47-56, 2002.
49. Strader DB et al: Use of complementary and alternative medicine in patients with liver disease, *Am J Gastroenterol* 97(9):2391-2397, 2002.
50. US Department of Health and Human Services: *Healthy people 2010: understanding and improving health,* Washington, DC, 2000, The Department.
51. US Food and Drug Administration: *Acetaminophen*, accessed July 2004 from website: http://www.fda.gov.
52. US Food and Drug Administration: *FDA approves new drug for treatment of alcoholism,* accessed July 2004 from website: http://www.fda.gov.
53. Williams R, Riordan S: Fulminant hepatic failure. In Schiff ER, Sorrell MF, Maddrey WC, editors: *Schiff's diseases of the liver,* ed 9, vol 1, Philadelphia, 2002, Lippincott-Raven.
54. Zaina FE, Lopes RW, Souza MRD: A comparison of nutritional status in three time points of liver transplant, *Transplant Proc* 36(4):949, 2004.

Visit the Evolve website: http://evolve.elsevier.com/Monahan/medsurg

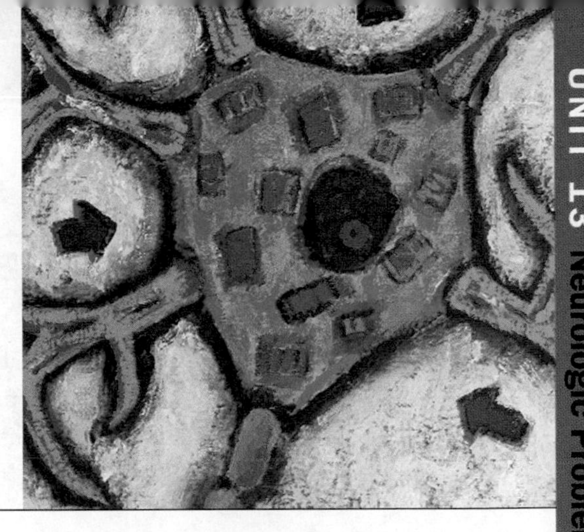

CHAPTER 47

Assessment of the Nervous System

by Shelley Yerger Huffstutler

OBJECTIVES

After studying this chapter, the learner should be able to:

1. Explain the four general functions of the nervous system.
2. Describe the normal anatomy and physiology of the nervous system.
3. Analyze health history and physical examination data essential for assessment of the nervous system.
4. Describe age-related physiologic changes that occur in the nervous system.
5. Explain the rationale for common tests used in diagnosing neurologic diseases.
6. Discuss the rationale for the nursing interventions provided after various common neurologic tests.

KEY TERMS

anosmia, p. 1369
aphasia, p. 1366
apraxia, p. 1367
ataxia, p. 1372
circle of Willis, p. 1358
conjugate movement, p. 1370
dermatome, p. 1368
diplopia, p. 1370
dysarthria, p. 1366
gait, p. 1372
gnosia, p. 1367
homonymous hemianopia, p. 1370
nystagmus, p. 1370
paresthesias, p. 1365
ptosis, p. 1370
reflex arc, p. 1361
stance, p. 1372
vertigo, p. 1365

The ability to conduct an accurate neurologic assessment depends on the nurse's knowledge of neuroanatomy and neurophysiology along with skill in recognizing and interpreting subtle deviations from normal. This chapter includes an overview of neurologic anatomy and physiology, essential components of a neurologic assessment, and common neurologic diagnostic tests.

Anatomy and Physiology

The nervous system, like an electrical conduction system, coordinates and controls all activities of the body. It accomplishes this by means of four general functions:

1. Receiving stimuli or information from the internal and external environments over varied afferent, or sensory, pathways
2. Communicating information between distant parts of the body (periphery) and the central nervous system (CNS)
3. Computing, or processing, information received at various reflex (spinal cord) and conscious (higher brain) levels to determine appropriate responses to situations
4. Transmitting information rapidly over varied efferent, or motor, pathways to effector organs for body action, control, or modification

Macroscopically, the nervous system is divided into two major divisions: (1) the CNS and (2) the peripheral nervous system (PNS). The CNS consists of the brain and spinal cord. The PNS includes the 12 pairs of cranial nerves, 31 pairs of spinal nerves, and autonomic nervous system (ANS).

Neuron

The single neuron is the basic structural and functional unit of the nervous system. It shares all the basic biologic and biochemical properties of other body cells and is highly specialized and differentiated. The single neuron acts as a miniature nervous system and has properties specialized for its electrical function. Neuroglial cells serve as adjuncts to the neurons, providing nourishment, support, and protection. They make up almost half of the microscopic structures of the brain and spinal cord. Four different types of neuroglial cells have been identified, each with different

TABLE 47-1 NEUROGLIAL CELLS

Type of Cell	Function
Astrocyte	Maintain chemical environment for conduction and transmission of impulses
Ependymal cell	Produce cerebrospinal fluid
Microglial cell	Part of phagocytosis process
Oligodendroglial cell	Produce lipid-protein complex that forms myelin

functions (Table 47-1). Neuroglial cells divide and multiply by mitosis and can be a source of tumors of the nervous system.

Microscopically the neuron consists of a cell body, or soma, and two extensions that project from it: a dendritic tree and an elongated cylindric axon. The cell bodies are the primary components of the gray matter of the CNS. A cell membrane encloses the soma, dendrites, and axon and creates a large surface area that enables the neuron to receive multiple synaptic contacts at one time (Figure 47-1). The axon is designed to transmit information along its extension away from the cell body to adjacent neurons; the dendrite or dendrites are designed to receive information from axon terminals at special sites called synapses and conduct impulses to the cell body. The word *axon* is used in various ways and may describe the extension of one cell or the extension of several cells making up a nerve. Figure 47-2 depicts several types of neurons.

Cell Membrane. Many of the most important functional properties of the neuron lie within the cell membrane. Structurally, the membrane is made up of lipids and proteins and has the ability to translocate materials across itself. The membrane exhibits differential permeability. For example, the membrane is permeable to oxygen, carbon dioxide, and certain inorganic ions, but impermeable to organic compounds (proteins) and other inorganic ions. This differential permeability results in a characteristic ion distribution. The inside of the neuron contains a high concentration of proteins and potassium, whereas the outside of the cell is high in sodium. This unequal distribution, or gradient, of potassium and sodium across the membrane is supported by the presence of an active sodium-potassium pump within the membrane. The pump requires metabolic energy for rapid movement of sodium and potassium across the membrane, and this produces an electrical potential difference, or charge, between the inside and the outside of the cell. The magnitude of the potential difference is a function of the ratio of charged particles on opposite sides of the membrane and is called the resting membrane potential (resting potential). Thus in the resting state all neurons possess a potential for action and are polarized. This resting potential is small, 260 mV, with the inside of the cell being electrically negative compared with the outside of the cell.

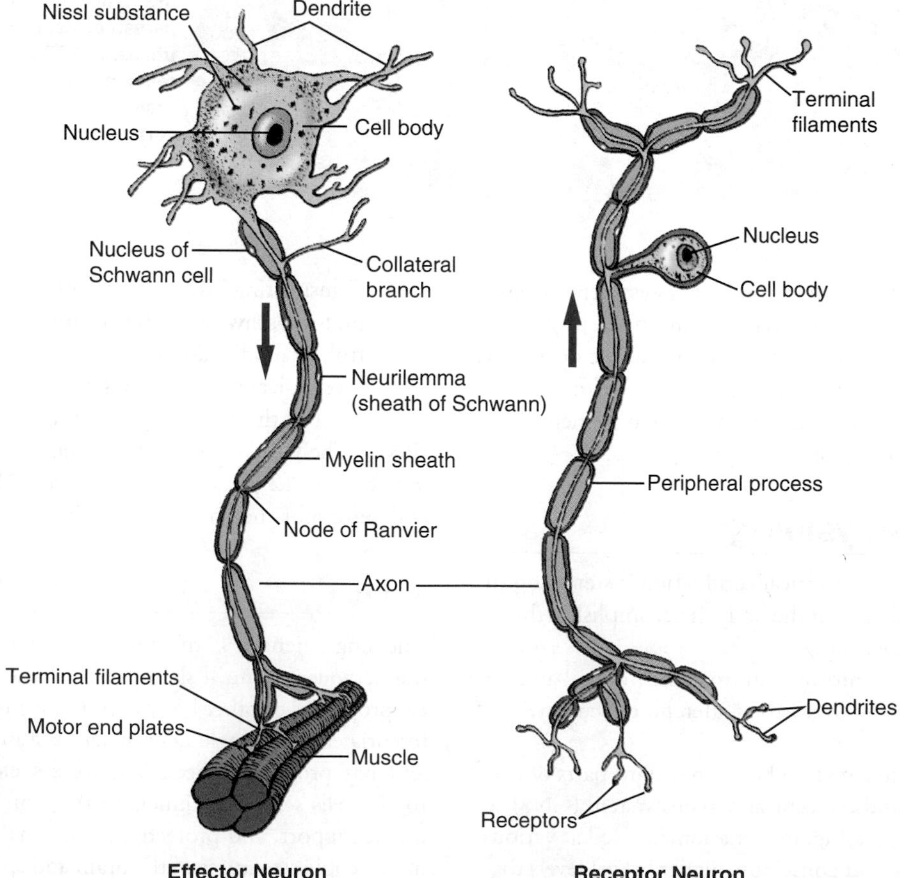

Figure 47-1 Motor (effector) neuron and sensory (receptor) neuron. *Arrows* indicate direction of impulse conduction.

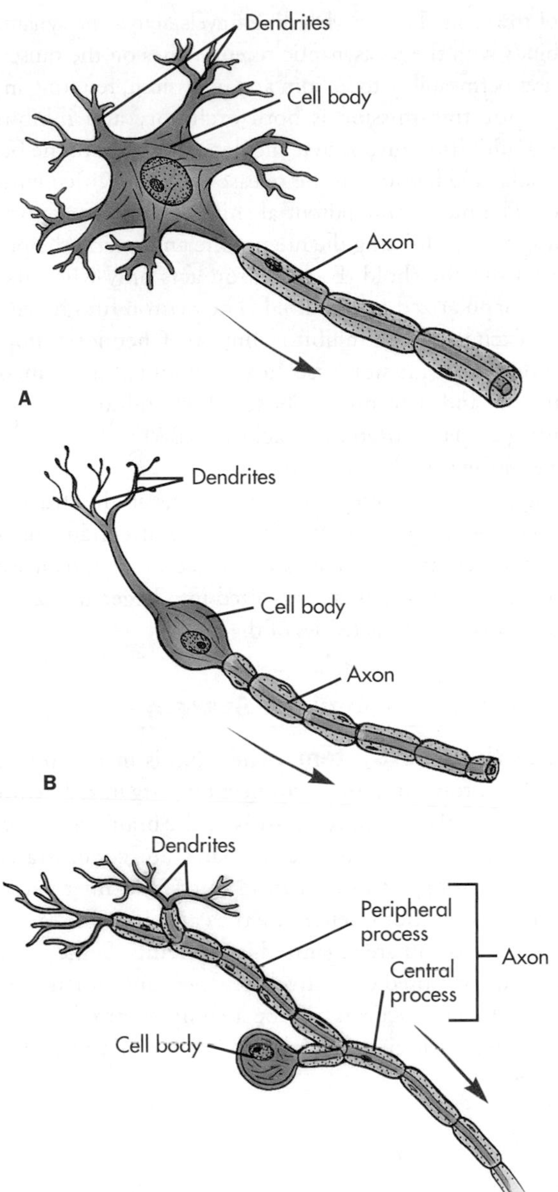

Figure 47-2 Structural classification of neurons. **A,** Multipolar neuron: neuron with multiple extensions from cell body. **B,** Bipolar neuron: neuron with exactly two extensions from cell body. **C,** Unipolar neuron: neuron with only one extension from cell body. Central process is an axon; peripheral process is modified axon with branched dendrites at its extremity. *Arrows* show direction of impulse travel.

Excitability. The neuron also exhibits the property of *excitability,* which means that the resting potential is unstable under certain conditions. For example, a neuronal membrane becomes unstable when subjected to stimulation, application of chemicals, or mechanical damage. This instability gives rise to the generation of action potentials (APs), which is a capacity unique to excitable cells. APs transmit information within the nervous system and, therefore, are the basic phenomena underlying all nervous system functions.

An AP occurs when a neuron is stimulated, resulting in a significant increase in membrane permeability to sodium. Sodium quickly moves to the inside of the membrane through membrane pores or channels. The sodium ions carry a sufficiently large positive charge to overwhelm the normal resting potential. A positive state develops within the cell, and depolarization occurs (Figure 47-3).

Almost instantaneously the membrane pores return to being virtually impermeable to sodium while potassium moves to the outside of the cell. Active transport then returns the sodium and potassium back to their original state. These mechanisms result in the disappearance of the internal positive state and a return to the normal resting potential, a phase called repolarization. These two phases together form the AP. An entire AP occurs within 1 to 2 ms.

When an AP is generated, it proceeds automatically to completion, independent of the property of the stimulus that initiated the depolarization. In other words, a strong stimulus does not give rise to a larger AP; the AP proceeds to completion in an "all-or-none" fashion. The AP is also spread, or propagated, over the entire membrane without a decrease in its velocity. The propagation velocity is related to the size of the axon (the larger the diameter, the higher the velocity) and to the presence or absence of myelin.

Myelin. Myelin is an excellent insulator of axons and makes up the white matter of the CNS. The myelin sheath is deposited around the axons by Schwann cells, and this sheath may be as thick as the axon itself. Myelin prevents almost all ion flow across the axon and its membrane. However, at distances approximately

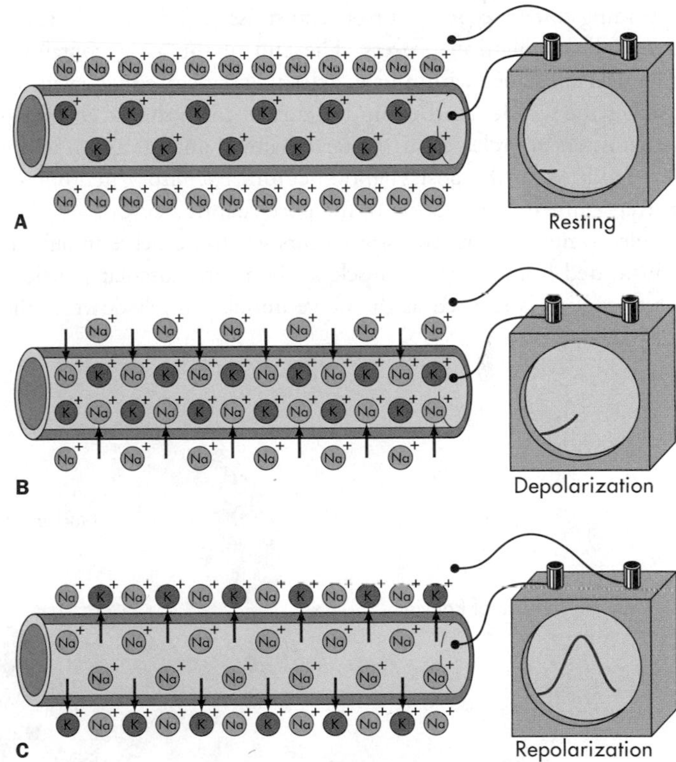

Figure 47-3 Depolarization and repolarization. **A,** Resting membrane potential results from excess of positive ions on outer surface of cell membrane. More sodium (*Na*$^+$) ions are on outside of the membrane than potassium (*K*$^+$) ions are on the inside. **B,** Depolarization of membrane occurs when Na$^+$ channels open, allowing Na$^+$ to move to area of lower concentration (and more negative charge) *inside* the cell—reversing polarity to inside-positive state. **C,** Repolarization of a membrane occurs when K$^+$ channels then open, allowing K$^+$ to move to area of lower concentration (and more negative charge) *outside* the cell—reversing polarity back to inside-negative state. Each voltmeter records changing membrane potential as a red line.

1 mm apart, the sheath is interrupted by nodes of Ranvier. At these small, uninsulated areas, ions can flow easily between the extracellular fluid and the axon. The concept of conduction of nerve impulses from node of Ranvier to node of Ranvier is termed *saltatory conduction* (Figure 47-4).

Axons with myelin are called large fibers, and the myelin creates their white appearance. Axons without myelin are called small fibers. Large fibers have a greater conduction velocity because (1) the jumping effect allows depolarization to proceed quickly, and (2) energy is conserved, since only the nodes depolarize.

Many neuron APs originate in a receptor neuron where internal and external stimuli are normally received. A receptor is similar to a transducer in that it can change one form of energy into another form. A receptor, however, responds (or depolarizes) to only one type of stimulus. For example, the retina of the eye responds only to the stimulus of light. Thus the receptor neuron may initiate depolarization but only in response to a specific stimulus. The receptor neuron obeys the all-or-none principle, although a strong stimulus makes the receptor neuron fire more APs per unit of time than does a weak stimulus.

Synapse. Neurons make functional contact with one another at specialized sites called synapses. Whenever an AP is generated in a neuron synapse, a sequence of processes results in the AP spreading to the second neuron. Transmission across a synapse is essentially a chemical process. The end of the axon contains a chemical substance within its vesicles that is released when an AP reaches the vesicle. As the impulse travels down the axon, neurotransmitters are released at the terminal end and are taken up by the dendrites of the postsynaptic neuron. Excitatory neurotransmitters cause depolarization of the postsynaptic neuron.

Neuromuscular transmission occurs when the nerve impulse is transmitted from nerve to muscle at the neuromuscular junction. Acetylcholine is released as the nerve impulse travels down to the end of the axon. The acetylcholine travels across the synaptic cleft and binds with the postsynaptic receptor sites on the muscle. This increases permeability to sodium and potassium, resulting in an AP.

Synaptic transmission is both excitatory and inhibitory in nature. Inhibition means that the dendritic membrane becomes hyperpolarized because of the release of the specific neurotransmitter. The membrane potential shifts toward potassium equilibrium, thus stabilizing the membrane and taking the potential further from threshold. Each neuron acts only when its membrane is depolarized to threshold. The neuron fires based on the sum of excitatory and inhibitory inputs. Chemicals supporting excitatory transmission are acetylcholine, norepinephrine, dopamine, and serotonin. Those which inhibit transmission include gamma aminobutyric acid (GABA) in brain tissue and glycine in the spinal cord.

In summary, each single neuron contains all the structural and functional building elements of an electrical conduction system that also makes interconnections with adjacent neurons at synapses. Collectively, the neurons are organized into larger and larger units that coordinate all the activities of the body.

Divisions of the Nervous System

Central Nervous System. The CNS is made up of collections of neurons and their connections organized within the brain and spinal cord. Specific areas of the brain and spinal cord can be distinguished where cell bodies are concentrated into nuclei, and groups of axons run in tracts that interconnect the parts. The connections determine the capabilities of each collection of neurons and are organized into circuits. Some circuits are simple and composed of relatively few neurons; others are highly complex. A single neuron may be a component of a number of different neuronal circuits and thus play a role in a variety of functions.

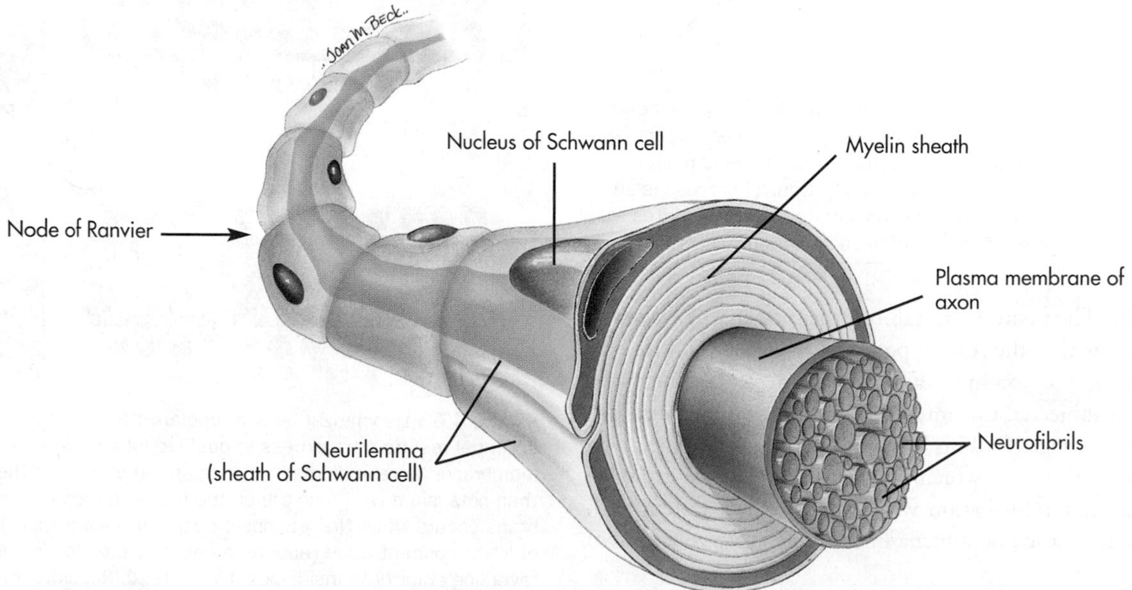

Figure 47-4 A nerve fiber and its coverings. This myelinated axon is located outside the central nervous system. Myelin is produced in concentric layers by the Schwann cell. Neurilemma is the outer sheath of the Schwann cell and is indented by successive nodes of Ranvier.

Structurally the brain and spinal cord are continuous and are protectively housed within the skull and vertebral column. When injured, centrally located neuron cell bodies are unable to reproduce or repair themselves. However, nerve endings can regenerate because of the presence of the neurilemma, which covers all peripheral nerves and is believed to contain openings through which axonal regrowth can occur.

A blood-brain barrier in the nervous system limits the free movement of substances from the blood to the brain tissue. The myelin sheath and capillaries with thickened basement membranes slow the process of diffusion between the blood and the brain. The barrier is selective, allowing entry of fluid, gases, small molecular substances, and lipid-soluble drugs, while preventing the entry of toxic substances, plasma proteins, large molecules, and most water-soluble drugs.

MENINGES. The meninges are the coverings of the nervous tissue in the brain and spinal cord. The three coverings (dura mater, arachnoid, and pia mater) help support, protect, and nourish the brain and spinal cord (Figure 47-5). The outermost layer is the dura mater, a tough membrane consisting of two layers. Four segments of the dura mater extend deep into the brain to form fibrous compartments that separate and support portions of the brain. These segments are the falx cerebri, the tentorium cerebelli, the falx cerebelli, and the diaphragma sellae.

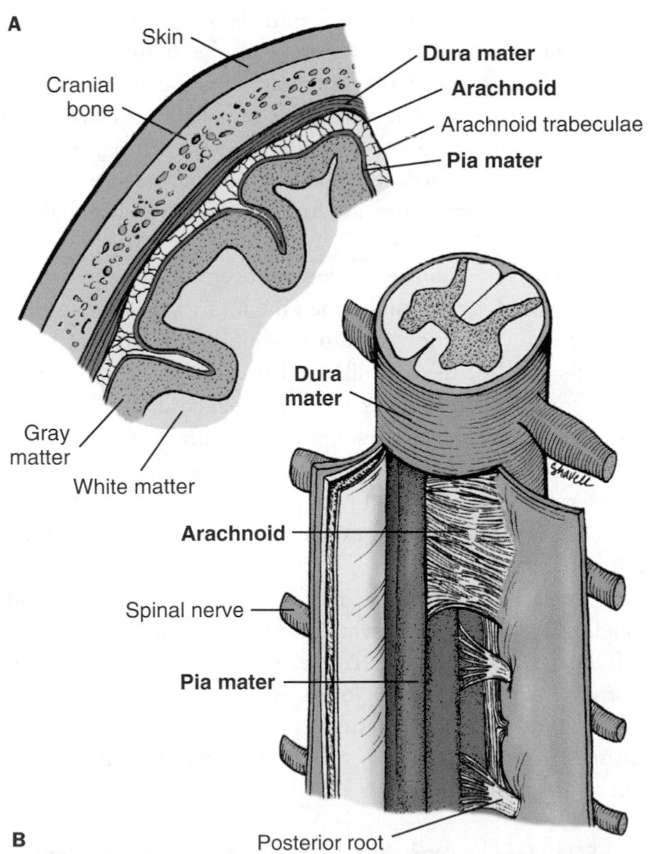

Figure 47-5 The three meninges, or membranes, that cover **A,** the brain and **B,** spinal cord. Dura mater is of leathery consistency and is outermost of the three membranes. Arachnoid, which is loose, vascular, and like a spider web, is the middle membrane. Pia mater is thin, delicate, and closely adherent to brain and spinal cord.

The arachnoid, the delicate membrane lying beneath the dura, covers the brain more loosely. Projections called the arachnoid villi extend into the overlying dura. The pia mater, innermost of the meninges, is a vascular membrane having many small plexuses of blood vessels. The pia mater follows the course of the penetrating blood vessels as they dip into the substance of the brain. These three meningeal layers give rise to three potential spaces. The spaces are epidural, external to the dura; subdural, between the dura and arachnoid; and subarachnoid, between the arachnoid and pia mater.

These three meningeal layers are also found in the spinal cord. The spinal cord arachnoid expands to surround the cauda equina; thus the subarachnoid space ends at S2 in the adult and is widest caudally. The spinal cord pia mater is thicker and less vascular than that of the brain.

BRAIN. The brain (encephalon) is grossly divided rostrally to caudally into four main areas: the cerebrum, diencephalon (thalamus, hypothalamus), brainstem (midbrain, pons, and medulla), and cerebellum (Figure 47-6). Each area carries out unique functions.

CEREBRUM. The cerebrum, or cerebral cortex, is composed of two frontal lobes, two parietal lobes, two temporal lobes, and two occipital lobes. Each cerebral lobe is named for its overlying cranial bones (Figure 47-7) and carries out one or more functions (Table 47-2). The cortex of the cerebrum is approximately 0.25 inch thick. It controls more than 14 billion neurons, receives and analyzes all impulses, controls voluntary movement, and stores knowledge of all impulses received. The cerebral cortex is divided into right and left hemispheres, which have convoluted surfaces with many peaks, known as gyri (singular, gyrus); and valleys or indentations, known as sulci (sulcus). The hemispheres are connected at the bottom by the corpus callosum, a thick structure of nerve fibers that directly links corresponding areas of each hemisphere to one another.

Each of the hemispheres is further divided into the respective lobes by fissures, or sulci. The frontal lobe is separated from the

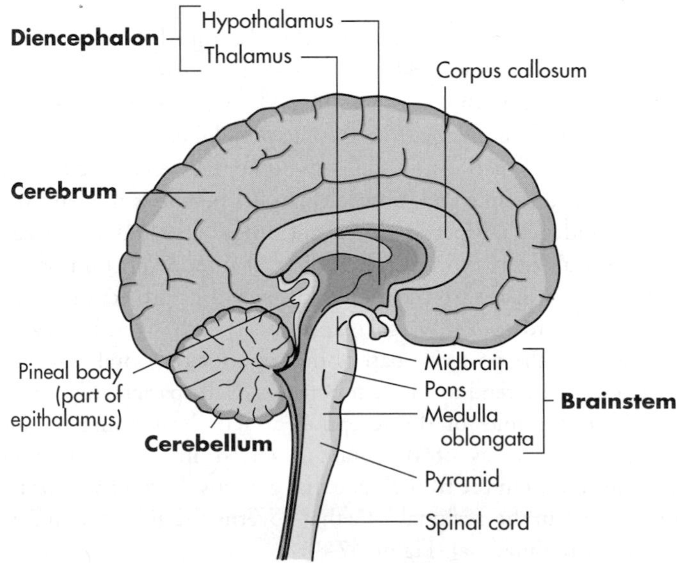

Figure 47-6 Major structures of the brain.

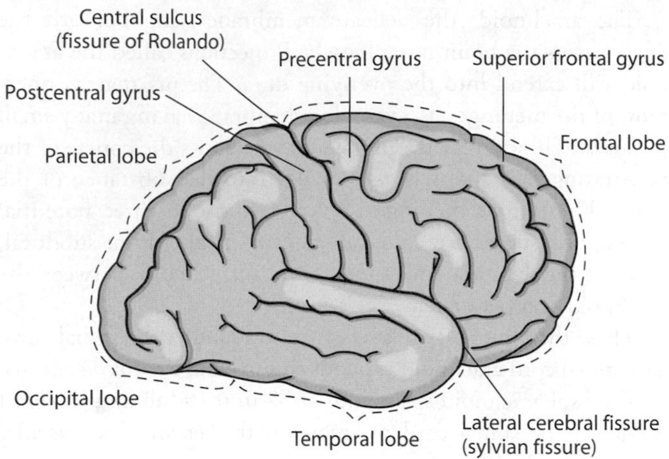

Figure 47-7 Lobes, sulci, and gyri of the brain.

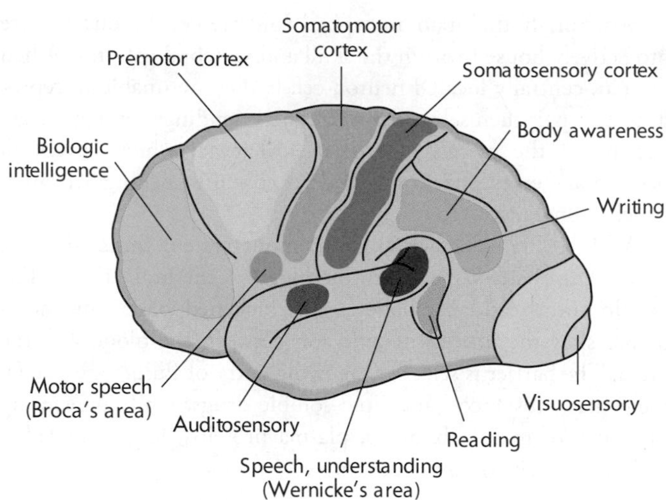

Figure 47-8 Lateral view of cerebral cortex with identification of major cortical areas.

TABLE 47-2 SPECIFIC FUNCTIONS OF CEREBRAL CORTEX

Lobe	Function
Frontal	Conceptualization Abstraction Motor ability Judgment formation Ability to write words
Parietal	Integrative and coordinating center for perception and interpretation of sensory information Ability to recognize body parts Left versus right
Temporal	Memory storage Integration of auditory stimuli
Occipital	Visual center Understanding of written material

parietal lobe by the fissure of Rolando (also called the central sulcus) and from the temporal lobe by the sylvian fissure; the temporal lobe lies below the sylvian fissure. The parietooccipital fissure separates the frontal lobe from the occipital lobe.

Speech is a function of the dominant hemisphere, which for all right-handed people and most left-handed people is the left side. The two identified speech centers are Broca's area and Wernicke's area. Broca's area is located in the lateral inferior portion of the frontal lobe adjacent to the motor cortex and its projections. This area appears to control verbal, expressive speech. Wernicke's area is located in the posterior part of the superior temporal convolution and may extend to adjacent portions of the parietal lobe. This area is responsible for the reception and understanding of language. Other areas of the brain involved in communication include an area in the frontal lobe that governs the ability to write, and an area in the occipital lobe that governs the ability to understand written material (Figure 47-8).

Deep within the cerebrum are structures called the basal ganglia. These masses of gray matter (cell bodies) include such structures as the caudate nucleus, putamen, and globus pallidus. In general, the basal ganglia function as part of the extrapyramidal system and are responsible for postural adjustments and gross voluntary muscle movements.

DIENCEPHALON. The diencephalon consists of the hypothalamus, thalamus, subthalamus, and epithalamus. It surrounds and includes most of the third ventricle of the brain. The diencephalon often is called the interbrain because it lies directly beneath the cerebrum. The thalamus composes four fifths of the diencephalon and acts as a relay station for some sensory impulses while interpreting others. See Table 47-3 for a more detailed explanation of the structures and functions of the diencephalon.

BRAINSTEM. The brainstem is located deep in the center of the hemispheres and is not visible when the intact brain is viewed. It includes a series of sections that make connections with the spinal cord at the level of the medulla, and it contains all nerve fibers passing from the hemispheres and the spinal cord. Twelve cranial nerves connect to the undersurface of the brain (Figure 47-9), mostly on the brainstem. The brainstem is made up of several structures, including the midbrain, pons, and medulla oblongata. See Table 47-3 for a detailed explanation of brainstem structures and functions.

Of special importance is the core of tissue that extends throughout the entire brainstem called the reticular activating system (Figure 47-10). This interconnected network of cells contains important integrating centers for respiration, cardiovascular function, afferent and motor systems, and state of consciousness. Increased stimulation leads to wakefulness, and decreased stimulation results in sleepiness.

CEREBELLUM. The cerebellum is located in the posterior cranial fossa, just below the posterior cerebrum, and contains short and long tracts. The short tracts act as connections between nuclei within the cerebellum; the long tracts enter and exit through three peduncles, the inferior, middle, and superior. The inferior peduncle connects the cerebellum with the medulla, the middle peduncle

TABLE 47-3 DIENCEPHALON AND BRAINSTEM STRUCTURES AND FUNCTIONS

Structure	Function
DIENCEPHALON	
Thalamus	Synapse of all sensory fibers for final relay to appropriate portion of sensory cortex Perceives general sensation (meaning and locality imparted by cortex) Houses pain threshold
Epithalamus	Contains pineal body, or epiphysis (thought to be endocrine gland whose secretion retards sexual development and growth)
Subthalamus	Receives fibers from globus pallidus; is part of efferent descending pathway
Hypothalamus	Contains cell bodies mediating most autonomic functions, endocrine functions, and emotional responses; regulates appetite, sexual arousal, sleep-wake cycle, and visceral-somatic activities; contains stalk of pituitary
BRAINSTEM	
Midbrain	Relays impulses from cerebral cortex above and subcortical structures below Origin of righting and postural reflex located here
Pons	Connects medulla, midbrain, and cerebrum Contains pneumotaxic center—controls rhythmic quality of respirations
Medulla	Connects with central canal of spinal cord Contains vital centers of cardiac, respiratory, and vasomotor control, as well as swallowing and hiccuping; gag and cough reflexes

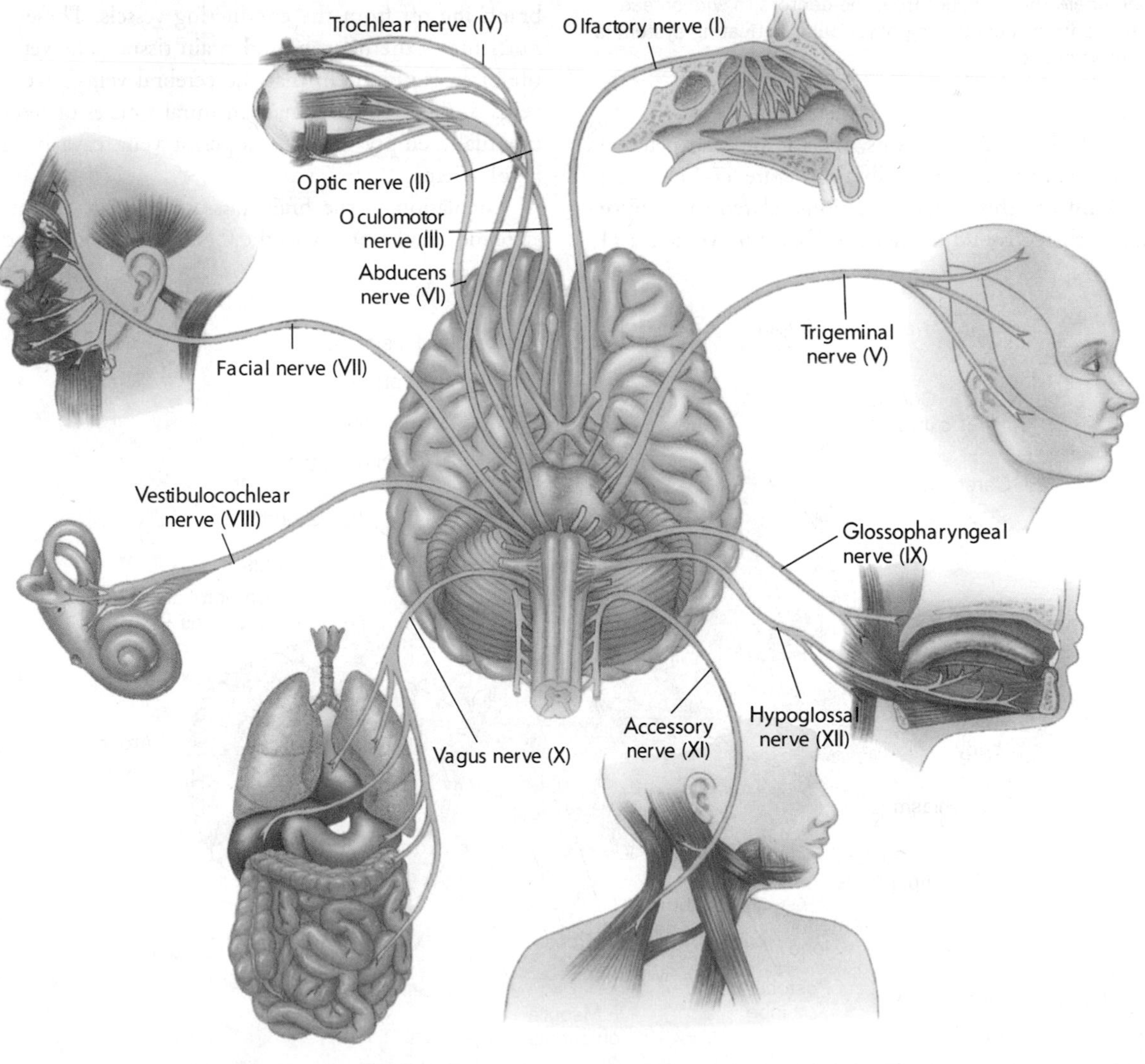

Figure 47-9 Ventral surface of brain showing attachment of cranial nerves.

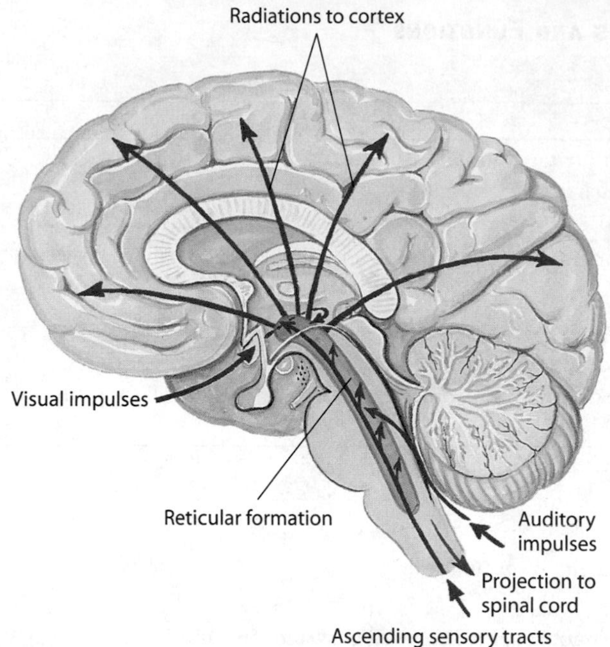

Figure 47-10 Reticular activating system consists of centers in the brainstem reticular formation plus fibers that conduct to the centers from below and fibers that conduct from the centers to widespread areas of cerebral cortex. Functioning of reticular activating system is essential for consciousness.

connects the cerebellum with the pons, and the superior peduncle connects the cerebellum with the midbrain (Figure 47-11).

The cerebellum has three main functions related to monitoring and making corrective adjustments of body movements: (1) keeping the body oriented in space and maintaining truncal equilibrium, (2) controlling antigravity muscles, and (3) checking or halting voluntary movements.

Circulation of the Brain and Spinal Cord. The blood supply for the brain derives from the aortic arch via the right innominate, left common carotid, and left subclavian arteries (Figure 47-12) and includes both conducting and penetrating vessels. The two conducting arteries are (1) the internal carotids, which supply most of the cerebral hemispheres, basal ganglia, and the upper two thirds of the diencephalon; and (2) the vertebral arteries, which supply the brainstem, the lower one third of the diencephalon, the cerebellum, and the occipital lobes. These two systems anastomose at the **circle of Willis**, which is formed by the interconnection of the internal carotid, anterior cerebral, anterior communicating, and posterior communicating arteries (Figure 47-13). The circle of Willis ensures equal circulation to both sides of the brain and helps compensate for alterations in blood flow and blood pressure. If blood flow through one side of the circle of Willis is inadequate, the other side supports blood flow to the area normally supplied by the damaged side. The specific parts of the brain supplied by each of these vessels are listed in Table 47-4.

The penetrating vessels enter the brain at right angles after branching off from the conducting vessels. These vessels supply nutrients to the neurons and brain tissue. The venous system of the brain is unique in that the cerebral veins have no valves. All veins of the brain terminate in dural sinuses or reservoirs, which eventually empty into the superior vena cava by means of the jugular veins.

Circulation in the brain possesses special characteristics. The systemic circulation favors the CNS over all other body parts. This

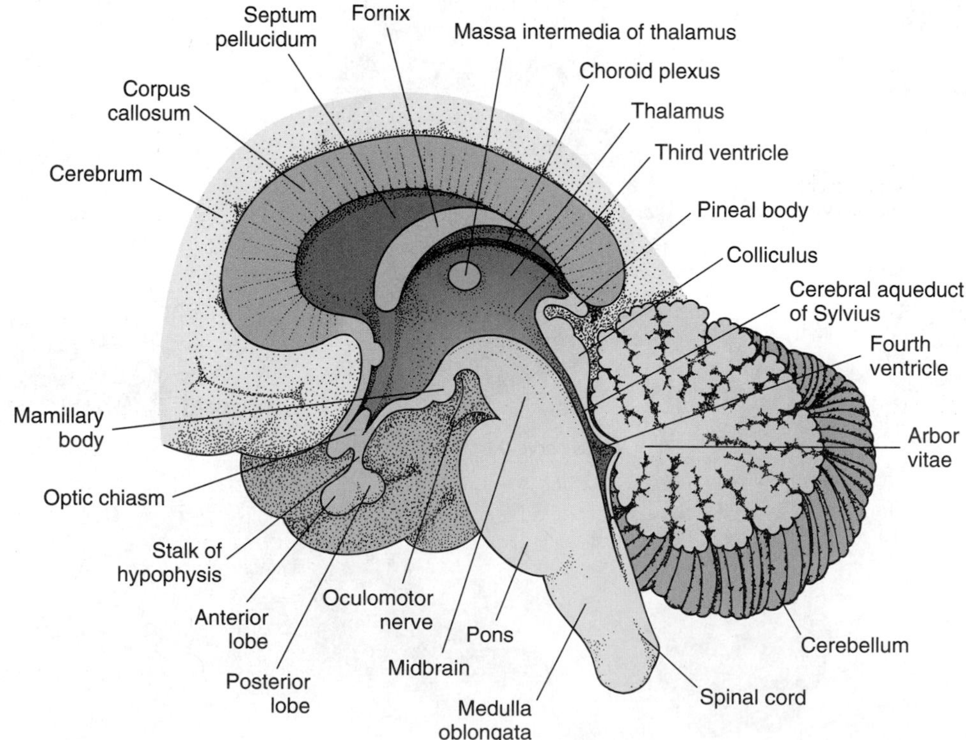

Figure 47-11 Sagittal section through midline of brain showing continuity of brain and spinal cord.

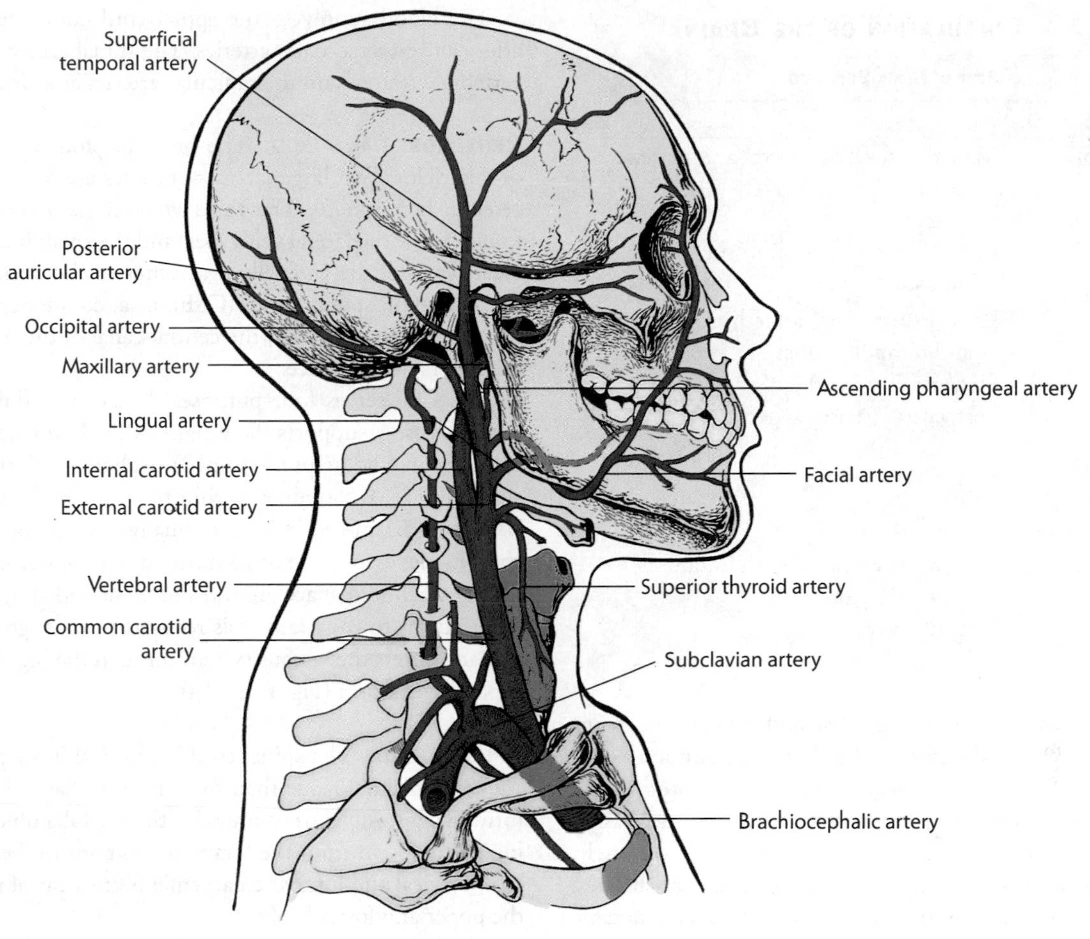

Figure 47-12 Major arteries of head and neck.

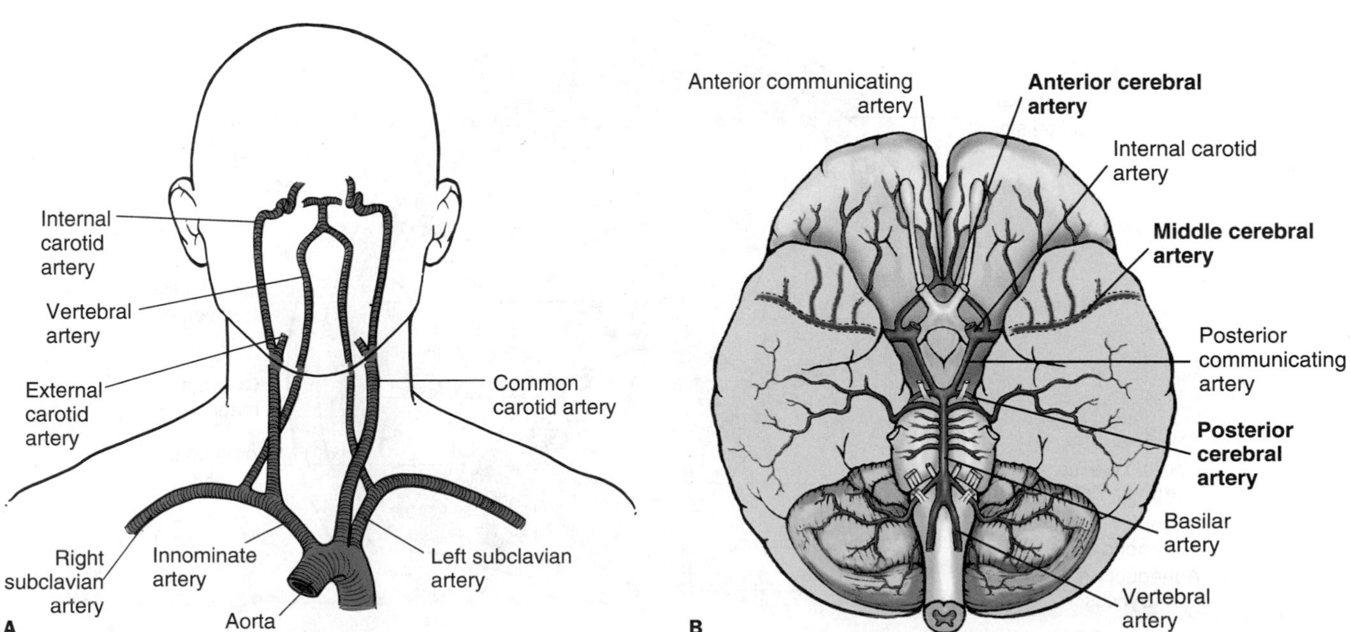

Figure 47-13 A, Major arteries supplying blood to brain. **B,** Circle of Willis. Note anterior, middle, and posterior cerebral arteries, which are major pairs of arteries supplying cerebrum.

TABLE 47-4 CIRCULATION OF THE BRAIN

Vessel	Part of Brain Supplied
INTERNAL CAROTID ARTERIES	
Anterior cerebral	Medial surface of frontal and parietal lobes Basal ganglia Parts of internal capsule and corpus callosum
Middle cerebral	Lateral surface of parietal, frontal, and temporal lobes Precentral (motor) gyri Postcentral (sensory) gyri
VERTEBRAL ARTERIES	
Basilar	Brainstem Cerebellum
Posterior cerebral	Parts of temporal and occipital lobe Vestibular organs Cochlear apparatus

helps provide a constant supply of glucose and oxygen to nervous tissue. The brain's vessels also possess the ability to maintain a constant blood flow through autoregulation. In the presence of increased blood pressure, cerebral vessels constrict, decreasing blood flow and preventing possible tissue damage. Conversely, cerebral vessels can dilate in the presence of biochemical changes. Elevated carbon dioxide content in the blood causes notable vasodilation of cerebral vessels; hypoxia and elevated hydrogen ion concentration also cause vasodilation. These autoregulatory mechanisms become less responsive with increasing age and in the presence of arteriosclerosis.

The blood supply to the spinal cord comes from the spinal artery and two radicular arteries. The spinal artery arises from the vertebral arteries, and the radicular arteries arise from the aorta.

CEREBROSPINAL FLUID. The brain has four fluid-filled spaces, or ventricles. Two large lateral ventricles are located within each cerebral hemisphere. The third ventricle is a thin fluid pocket found below the lateral ventricles, and the small fourth ventricle is located where the cerebellum attaches to the back of the brainstem. Cerebrospinal fluid (CSF) is a colorless, odorless fluid found in these ventricles, the central canal of the spinal cord, and the subarachnoid space.

The CSF serves four purposes. It acts as a fluid cushion for nervous tissue, supports the weight of the brain, carries nutrients to the brain, and helps to remove metabolites. Normally, the total amount of CSF contained within the adult brain and spinal cord is 90 to 150 ml. CSF is continually formed by vessels of the choroid plexus at a rate of 18 ml/hr and is constantly circulated in the subarachnoid space around the brain and spinal cord. As the CSF returns to the brain, it is reabsorbed through the arachnoid villi and enters the venous system through the jugular veins to the superior vena cava (Figure 47-14).

SPINAL CORD. The spinal cord is elliptical in shape and appears wider from side to side than from front to back. The spinal cord forms a continuous structure with the medulla oblongata extending 42 to 45 cm from the foramen magnum to the lumbar vertebra. Cervical and lumbar enlargements are areas of nerve origin to the upper and lower limbs.

The spinal cord structurally includes H-shaped central gray matter, which is composed of nerve cell bodies surrounded by white matter that is divided into three columns, or funiculi, named according to their location: anterior (ventral), lateral, and

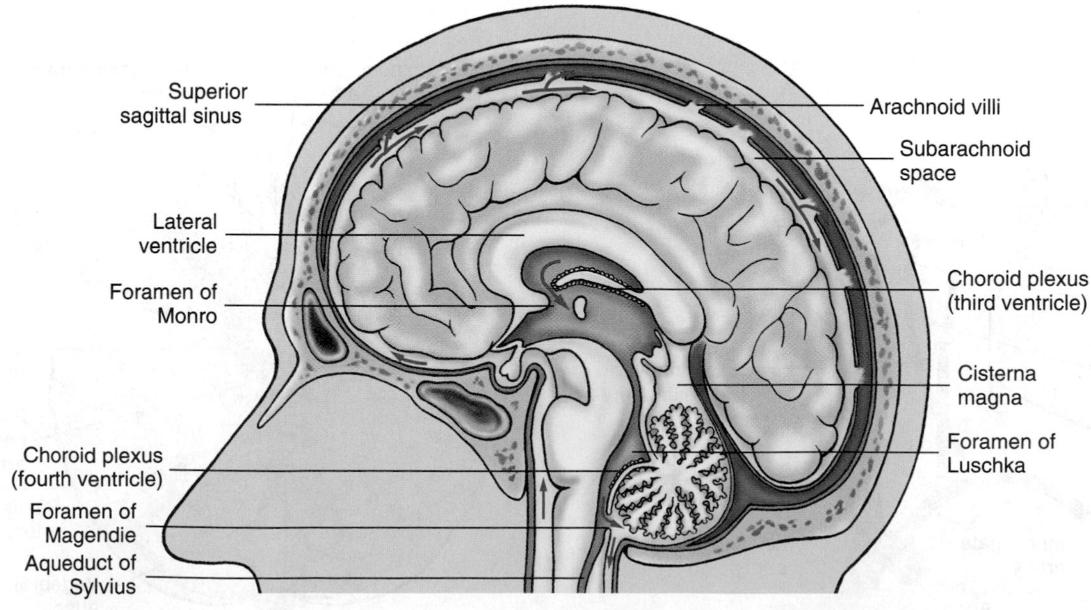

Figure 47-14 Cerebrospinal fluid circulation. Cerebrospinal fluid is produced by choroid plexus in lateral ventricles and flows around brain and spinal cord until it reaches arachnoid villi, from which it is absorbed into venous circulation. *Arrows* indicate major pathway of cerebrospinal fluid flow.

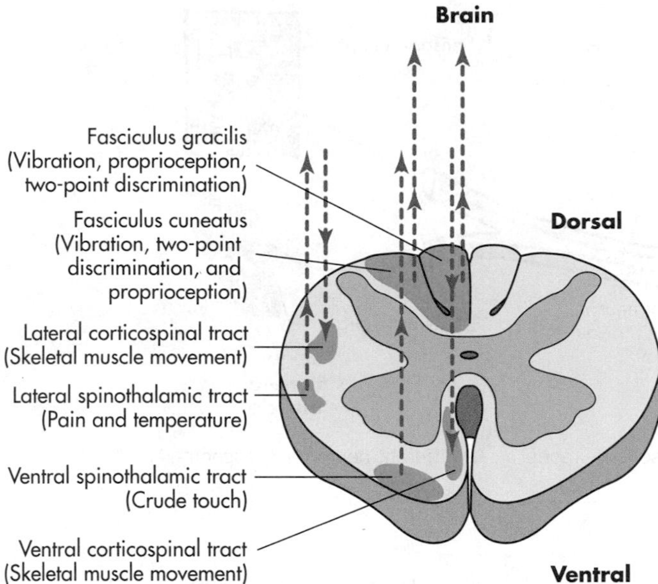

Figure 47-15 Nerve pathways arise from white matter of spinal cord. Impulses travel to and from spinal cord and brain along these pathways.

posterior (dorsal) columns. Each column contains both ascending and descending tracts that connect different segments of the spinal cord to one another and connect the spinal cord with the brain (Figure 47-15). The tracts are named with the first part of the name indicating the point of origin and the last part of the name indicating the end point (Table 47-5).

The spinal cord is also the site of reflex pathways. Reflexes are an example of the simplest neuronal circuit and do not require relay to the brain for action. A reflex consists of a specific motor response to a sensory stimulus. The response may involve skeletal muscle movement or glandular secretion. A reflex may involve only two neurons, as in the simple monosynaptic **reflex arc** that occurs with the knee jerk reflex. A brisk tap over a partially stretched knee tendon stimulates sensory nerve endings within the tendons; the stimulus travels over a sensory nerve fiber within a peripheral nerve toward the spinal cord where it synapses with a central motor neuron (anterior horn cell). The impulse is then transmitted down the motor nerve (over the anterior nerve root of the spinal nerve or peripheral nerve) and across the neuromuscular junction to stimulate the muscle to contract. Figure 47-16 illustrates a classic monosynaptic reflex arc. A reflex may involve only one spinal cord level, as in the knee jerk reflex; a few spinal cord levels (segmental reflexes); or structures in the brain that influence the spinal cord (supraspinal reflexes).

Peripheral Nervous System. The PNS is basically a set of communication channels located outside the CNS and is divided into the somatic and autonomic nervous systems. The somatic nervous system innervates skeletal (striated) muscles. Its neuronal cell bodies lie in groups within the CNS, and its axons exit the spinal cord at all levels. These fibers continue without synapse until they reach skeletal muscle cells. A small cleft exists between the nerve and the muscle. Vesicles containing acetylcholine are located at the end of the nerve terminal, and as the impulse moves down the nerve, the acetylcholine is released and crosses the cleft

TABLE 47-5 TRACTS OF THE SPINAL CORD

Tract	Direction	Function
ANTERIOR COLUMN		
Ventral corticospinal	Descending	Voluntary motion
Vestibulospinal	Descending	Balance reflex
Tectospinal	Descending	Sight and vision reflex
Reticulospinal	Descending	Muscle tone
Ventral spinothalamic	Ascending	Pressure and simple touch
Spinoolivary	Ascending	Proprioception reflex
LATERAL COLUMN		
Lateral corticospinal	Descending	Voluntary movements
Rubrospinal	Descending	Synergy and muscle tone
Olivospinal	Descending	Reflex
Dorsal spinocerebellar	Ascending	Reflex proprioception
Ventral spinocerebellar	Ascending	Reflex proprioception
Lateral spinothalamic	Ascending	Pain and temperature
Spinotectal	Ascending	Reflex
POSTERIOR COLUMN		
Fasciculus interfascicularis	Descending	Integration and association
Septomarginal fasciculus	Descending	Integration and association
Fasciculus gracilis	Ascending	Vibration, proprioception, and two-point discrimination
Fasciculus cuneatus	Ascending	Vibration, proprioception, and two-point discrimination

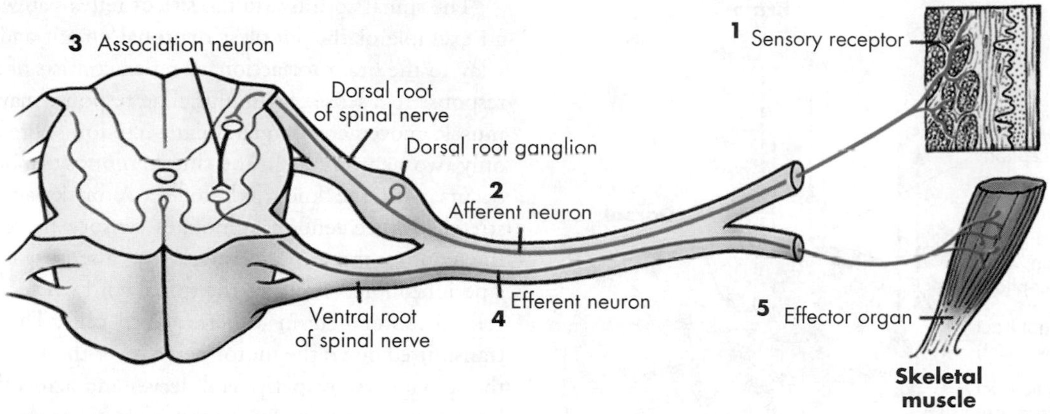

Figure 47-16 Basic diagram of a reflex arc, including *(1)* sensory receptor, *(2)* afferent neuron, *(3)* association neuron, *(4)* efferent neuron, and *(5)* effector organ.

to the muscle, causing a muscle contraction. The muscle contraction is stopped by acetylcholinesterase, which is released from the muscle and inactivates the acetylcholine.

The ANS regulates automatic body functions, usually in an effort to preserve homeostasis. The ANS is further divided into the sympathetic nervous system (adrenergic), which functions to maintain homeostasis and to provide defense against stressors, and the parasympathetic nervous system (cholinergic), which is responsible for conserving and restoring vegetative functions (Table 47-6).

Fibers of the ANS synapse once after leaving the CNS and before arriving at the neuroeffector junction. The site of this synapse is called a ganglion, and its neurotransmitter is acetylcholine. Fibers leaving the ganglia finally synapse at the effector organ. The neurotransmitter at the effector site of the parasympathetic nervous system is acetylcholine; the neurotransmitter at the effector site of the sympathetic nervous system is norepinephrine.

Peripheral nerves are bundles of individual nerves that are sensory, motor, or mixed (having both sensory and motor fibers). Structurally, the PNS consists of 12 pairs of cranial nerves and 31 pairs of spinal nerves. The cranial nerves carry impulses to and from the brain. They originate mainly in the brainstem, except for the first nerve (olfactory), which arises in the olfactory bulb. (See Table 47-9, p. 1368, for an explanation of the functions of each cranial nerve.)

Spinal nerves are composed of a dorsal and ventral root. They correspond to the spinal cord segment from which they arise: 8 cervical, 12 thoracic, 5 lumbar, 5 sacral, and 1 coccygeal. The first pair of cervical spinal nerves comes off the cord above C1. From L3 to S5, the spinal nerves branch out to form the cauda equina (Figure 47-17).

Peripheral nerves that transmit information toward the CNS are afferent, or sensory, in nature; peripheral nerves that transmit information away from the CNS are efferent, or motor, in nature. The sensory and motor nerves usually travel together in the periphery, but they separate at the level of the spinal cord into a posterior, or sensory, root and an anterior, or motor, root.

Sensory System Pathways. Sensation is initiated by stimulation of receptor neurons located throughout the body. Receptor

TABLE 47-6 PARASYMPATHETIC AND SYMPATHETIC NERVOUS SYSTEM INFLUENCE

Organ System	Parasympathetic Influence	Sympathetic Influence
Heart	Decreases rate	Increases rate
Blood vessels	Dilates visceral and brain vessels	Constricts
Lungs	Constricts bronchi	Dilates bronchi
Gastrointestinal	Increases peristalsis	Decreases peristalsis
Gastric and salivary secretions	Increases	Decreases
Anal sphincter	Opens	Closes
Liver	Not applicable	Stimulates glycogenesis and glycogenolysis
Adrenal medulla	Not applicable	Stimulates production of epinephrine
Bladder	Contracts bladder Opens sphincter	Relaxes bladder Closes sphincter
Eyes	Constricts pupil Accommodates for near vision	Dilates pupil Accommodates for far vision
Skin	Not applicable	"Goose flesh"

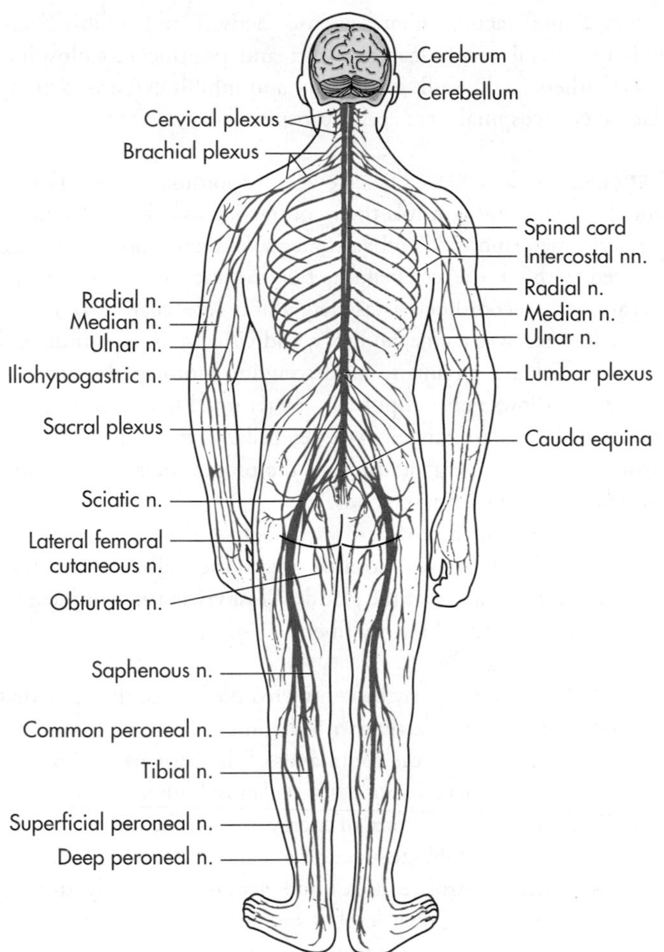

Figure 47-17 Central and peripheral divisions of the nervous system. Central nervous system consists of brain and spinal cord. Peripheral nervous system is composed of cranial and spinal nerves.

neurons provide the brain with information about the condition and composition of both the internal environment (e.g., position [*proprioception*] and action [*interoception*] of body parts) and the external environment (*exteroception*). The latter is achieved through the eyes, ears, nose, skin, and tongue. The general sensory system by which this information is conveyed includes (1) receptor neurons responsive to special stimuli from both the internal and external environments, (2) posterior roots of the peripheral or afferent sensory nerves carrying nerve impulses toward the CNS, (3) ascending or sensory tracts within the spinal cord and upper brain centers, and (4) sensory areas of the cerebral cortex where stimuli are perceived and localized.

From the receptor neuron, the sensory impulse travels to the spinal cord along the afferent fibers, enters the spinal cord through the posterior root, and proceeds along either the spinothalamic tracts or the posterior columns. The pathway followed is specific to the sensation. For example, nerve fibers conducting the sensations of pain and temperature pass into the posterior horn of the spinal cord, synapse with a secondary sensory neuron, cross immediately to the contralateral side of the cord, and continue upward as the lateral spinothalamic tract. These fibers arrive at the thalamus, synapse with a third sensory neuron, and terminate in the appropriate area of the sensory cortex.

Sensations for simple touch follow a similar pathway but ascend the spinal cord as the ventral spinothalamic tract. Impulses travel to the thalamus where they synapse with a third sensory neuron and terminate in the appropriate area of the sensory cortex. Sensations of fine touch, deep touch and pressure, vibration, and proprioception arrive at the spinal cord and are conducted by the posterior columns (fasciculus gracilis or fasciculus cuneatus) to the level of the medulla before synapsing with a second neuron, crossing over to the contralateral side, and continuing to the thalamus. At this location, they synapse with a third sensory neuron that terminates at the appropriate area of the sensory cortex (Figure 47-18).

MOTOR SYSTEM PATHWAYS. Motor impulses travel by one of three descending motor pathways: the corticospinal (pyramidal) system, the extrapyramidal system, and the cerebellar system.

CORTICOSPINAL (PYRAMIDAL) SYSTEM. The corticospinal system is primarily concerned with skilled voluntary skeletal muscle movements of the distal extremities. Fibers that combine to form the corticospinal tracts arise from the upper motor neurons. Their cell bodies are located in the primary motor area of the cerebral cortex in the precentral gyrus of the frontal lobe and in the premotor cortex in the frontal lobe.

Motor fibers leave the cerebral cortex, descend through the internal capsule through the basilar portion of the pons, and then collect into discrete bundles within the medulla. The majority of

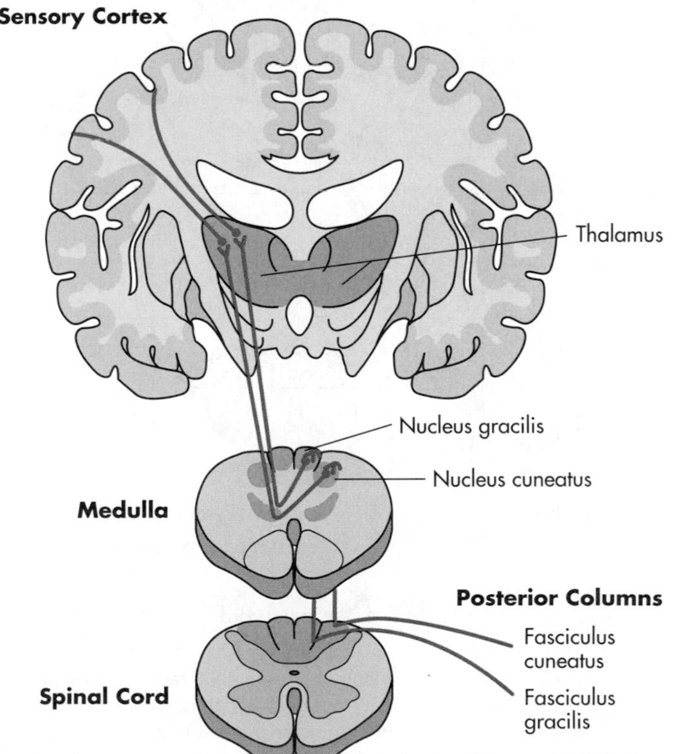

Figure 47-18 Pathways for fine touch, deep touch and pressure, vibration, and proprioception. Note how stimuli entering through dorsal route (posterior) travel on same side as posterior columns to medulla, where they cross to opposite side, ascend to thalamus, and end in the somasthetic area where perception occurs.

the fibers cross over, or decussate, to the opposite side of the medulla and become the lateral corticospinal tract, which passes to all spinal cord levels in the lateral funiculus (Figure 47-19). The remaining motor fibers descend directly from the medulla (do not decussate) and synapse with motor neurons in the spinal cord. This pathway is known as the anterior corticospinal tract. The left cerebral motor area controls muscular movement on the right side of the body, and vice versa.

Motor fibers synapse with large anterior horn cells in the spinal cord. These cells are the lower motor neurons and are responsible for providing the final direct link, or common pathway, with the muscles. Thus skeletal muscle activity is the result of the net influence of upper motor neurons on the motor neurons through the anterior horn cells (lower motor neurons) in the spinal cord.

Extrapyramidal System. The extrapyramidal tracts are complex and provide separate pathways between the cortex, basal ganglia, brainstem, and spinal cord. Extrapyramidal tracts (the name indicates that they do not pass through the medulla) include all descending motor pathways other than the corticospinal tract. These tracts are named for their points of origin and termination. The extrapyramidal tracts collectively assist in maintaining muscle tone and the control of gross automatic skeletal muscle movements. Some tracts facilitate extensor activity and inhibit flexor activity (lateral vestibulospinal tract and pontine reticulospinal tract); others facilitate flexor activity and inhibit extensor activity (lateral corticospinal tract and rubrospinal tract).

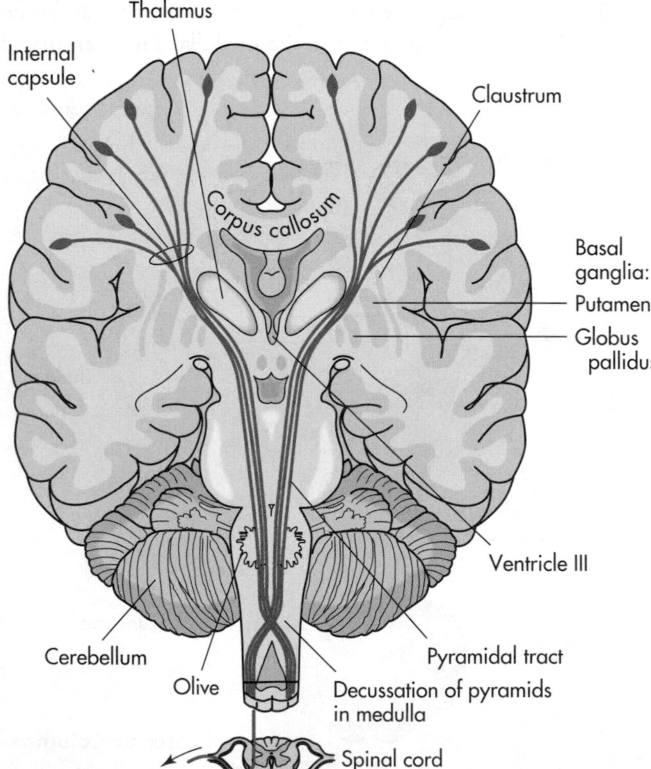

Figure 47-19 Crossed corticospinal (pyramidal) tracts. Axons that compose pyramidal tracts come from neuron cell bodies in cerebral cortex. After they descend through internal capsule of cerebrum and white matter of brainstem, about three fourths of the fibers decussate (cross over from one side to the other) in the medulla, as shown. Then they continue downward in lateral corticospinal tract on opposite side of cord. Each crossed corticospinal tract, therefore, conducts motor impulses from one side of brain to interneurons or anterior horn motor neurons on opposite side of cord. Therefore impulses from one side of cerebrum cause movements of opposite side of body.

Cerebellar System. The cerebellum coordinates the action of muscle groups and controls their contractions so that movements are performed smoothly and accurately. Voluntary movements can proceed without the cerebellum, but the movements would be clumsy and uncoordinated (asynergia and cerebellar ataxia). The cerebellum receives tactile, auditory, and visual sensory stimuli and contains feedback circuits to all descending motor pathways. The cerebellum allows nerve impulses to be returned to the same region from which they originated. The cerebellar cortex can detect any errors in muscle synergy and return the proper messages to adjust muscular control within the body.

Visceral efferent motor pathways mediate the action of involuntary, or smooth, muscles located within the walls of tubes, hollow organs, the heart, and the glands. Most viscera are supplied by both excitatory and inhibitory fibers.

Effectors. Effectors may be considered the cells of the body that "do something" by interacting with the internal and external environments and following the commands of the nervous system. The two classes of effectors are muscles and glands; both are transducers, capable of converting one form of energy into another. Effectors, like nerve tissue, are excitable tissues and are able to generate APs. The nervous system controls muscles and glands by directly turning them on or by altering their level of spontaneous activity through a neuron-to-effector chemical communication system.

Physiologic Changes With Aging

Changes in the nervous system occur with normal aging. However, normal aging is not associated with either senility or Alzheimer's disease. The healthy older person continues to function mentally at a high level into advanced age.

Physiologic changes in the nervous system associated with aging include the loss of brain cells with actual loss of brain weight. The nerve cell loss usually is diffuse and gradual. The gyri of the brain surface also atrophy, causing widening and deepening of the spaces between the gyri. Blood flow to the brain decreases, and the brain's ability to autoregulate its blood supply declines with increased age.

The ANS control over various body functions remains intact as a person ages but becomes more labile and unpredictable. In addition, the velocity of nerve impulses decreases, which slows sensory and motor conduction; sensory conduction decreases faster than motor and is more pronounced in peripheral nerves.

Health History

The nature and extent of the neurologic health history depends on the patient's condition and the urgency of the situation. The patient may be ambulatory, alert, and oriented, or may be experiencing an altered level of consciousness (LOC) with neurologic deficits. In the latter situation the nurse conducts the health history in phases over time. The interview not only provides a mechanism for gathering data and dispensing information but also serves as a tool for establishing a working relationship with the patient and family. The nurse explores the patient and family history along with classic neurologic symptoms such as headache, dizziness, vertigo, weakness, paresthesia, and pain.[7]

Patient History

Patients often state they are having difficulty performing their usual activities but are unable to associate the changes in function with a neurologic disorder. The nurse always questions the patient about chronic diseases; use of prescription, over-the-counter, herbal, and recreational drugs; and patterns of alcohol consumption, since these factors may contribute to the current problem or affect the patient's performance during the neurologic assessment. Other important areas to explore as part of the medical history include previous trauma or injury to the CNS; diagnoses affecting the neuromuscular system such as strokes, seizures, multiple sclerosis, or Parkinson's disease; and neurosurgical procedures performed, along with outcomes.[2]

Family History

An accurate and thorough review of the patient's family history can help establish the diagnosis and guide the management of a patient experiencing a neurologic alteration. The nurse asks the patient about relevant illnesses in the family. These include those of a neurologic origin and diseases of other body systems that can affect neurologic status. Examples of the latter include hypertension, diabetes mellitus, renal disease, and peripheral vascular disease. Any history of a family member experiencing a stroke, seizure, CNS tumor, migraine headaches, or neuropathic disorder is thoroughly explored.[7]

Headache

The nurse questions the patient about headaches, which can be associated with a variety of conditions. Associated signs and symptoms such as nausea, vomiting, auras, tinnitus, lacrimation of the eyes, and vertigo are explored. Transient headaches may occur after a diagnostic test such as a lumbar puncture.

Dizziness and Vertigo

The nurse must differentiate between dizziness and vertigo by questioning the patient carefully about these symptoms. Patients who describe a feeling of lightheadedness or experience a syncopal (fainting) episode are experiencing dizziness that is probably related to decreased cerebral blood flow. In contrast, descriptions of the room spinning around or the sensation that one is spinning indicates **vertigo** and may be related to neurologic dysfunction or a problem with the inner ear.

Weakness and Paresthesia

The nurse also thoroughly explores any description of a sudden or gradual onset of weakness or paresthesia. Weakness may be associated with a neuromuscular disorder such as myasthenia gravis or multiple sclerosis; however, the weakness may also be attributable to a nutritional deficiency or hematologic disorder such as anemia. **Paresthesias** (abnormal sensations perceived as burning, tingling, prickling, etc.) may be associated with a diabetic neuropathy or other arterial insufficiency. The numbness and tingling may also be due to a PNS disorder such as a herniated disc or nerve impingement that can manifest itself in the upper or lower extremity.

Pain

Pain is a highly subjective symptom that nurses attempt to quantify using a pain scale of 0 to 10. Pain may be a symptom of a variety of disorders in other body systems such as angina, toothache, or pleuritic-type pain. Pain also can indicate pressure on a sensory nerve as is frequently the case with low back pain caused by trauma or injury. Individuals have different pain thresholds, and nurses attempt to accurately record the pain experience from the patient's perspective (see Chapter 16).

Physical Examination

The sequence of the neurologic examination varies with the examiner, but the nurse attempts to ensure completeness without exhausting the person being examined. The neurologic examination depends largely on inspection and palpation with occasional use of percussion. Auscultation may be used to detect related vascular abnormalities.[5] Functions may first be tested in a general way, followed by definitive testing of any identified abnormality. Box 47-1 lists equipment commonly used in a neurologic examination.

Assessment measures and variations in normal findings relevant to the care of older adults are presented in the Gerontologic Assessment box, p. 1366. Also identified are disorders common in older adults that may be responsible for abnormal assessment findings.

Box 47-1 Equipment Needed for Neurologic Examination

- Cotton applicators
- Diagram of dermatomes
- Flashlight
- Miscellaneous items of varied shapes and sizes (coin, key, marble)
- Ophthalmoscope
- Otoscope
- Colored pencil
- Pins with sharp and blunt ends
- Printed page
- Reflex hammer
- Tape measure
- Tongue depressors
- Tuning fork
- Snellen chart
- Stoppered vials containing:
  —Peppermint, oil of cloves, coffee, soap (smell)
  —Sugar, salt, vinegar (taste)
  —Cold and hot water (temperature)
- Watch with second hand

Gerontologic Assessment

- Reaction time increases with age.
- Noticeable age-related effects on cognitive abilities include a slight, gradual decline in some intellectual abilities such as short-term memory.
- Age-related changes in vision include a decrease in visual acuity, diminished peripheral vision, increased sensitivity to glare, and difficulty adapting to dark and light.
- Hearing loss for high-frequency sound is a common finding.
- Tactile sensation decreases; there is difficulty in temperature discrimination and performing fine motor tasks.
- Both taste perception and olfactory sensation decline.
- Deep tendon reflexes are less brisk. Ankle jerks are commonly lost; those in the upper extremities are usually present. Older adults often have difficulty relaxing their limbs; the examiner should always support the limb when eliciting reflexes.
- Loss of the sensation of vibration at the ankle malleolus is common after age 65. Position sense in the big toe may be absent, but this is less common.
- Gait may be slower and more deliberate. Also, the gait may deviate slightly from a midline path because of decreased coordination.
- A decrease in muscle bulk often occurs and is most apparent in the hands. The hand muscles appear wasted; however, grip strength remains relatively good.
- Senile tremors occasionally occur and are considered benign.
- Common disorders in older adults include strokes, aneurysms, falls, Alzheimer's disease, and dementia.

Mental Status

The nurse carefully observes and assesses the patient's mental function, since specific difficulties or abnormalities can be significant in identifying organic brain disease. Changes in LOC can be the most sensitive indicator of a person's level of neurologic function. The functional components of consciousness are arousal (alertness) and awareness (content) of self and environment. Arousal is mainly controlled by brainstem activity, including the reticular activating system. Awareness requires an intact cerebral cortex and association fibers.[4] Thus the state of consciousness depends on successful interaction between the brainstem and cerebral hemispheres.

Eye opening is a crucial component of arousal. The patient should spontaneously open the eyes when the examiner speaks to him or her. If eye opening does not occur in response to verbal and auditory stimuli, the nurse can apply a painful stimulus to determine whether the arousal mechanism is intact (see p. 1368). Evaluating a patient's orientation to self and the environment assesses awareness. Assessment of person, place, and time (day, month, year) is the most effective method to evaluate awareness.

The mental examination also includes an assessment of mood and behavior, since particular mood changes may be associated with specific diseases. For example, emotional lability, where the mood shifts easily and quickly from one extreme to the other, is often seen in bilateral (diffuse) brain disease. The nurse determines whether the person's mood is appropriate to the situation and topic of conversation.[1] Personality changes (e.g., the appearance of a violent temper and aggressive behavior) may occur with destructive lesions of the inferior frontal parts of the limbic system. Family and friends are the best sources of information about behavioral changes.

The nurse tests the individual's knowledge and vocabulary by referring to current events, tests the ability to think abstractly by asking the person to explain the meaning of a proverb, and tests calculation by asking the person to serially subtract 7 from 100. Dyscalculia is the inability to solve simple problems because of brain injury or disease. Recent memory loss is more common in brain disease than is remote memory loss. The findings of these gross tests may indicate the need for more definitive tests of mental function.

Language and Speech

Language ability is distributed across a variety of areas of the cortex, including parts of the temporal lobe, the temporoparietal-occipital junction, the frontal lobe of the dominant (usually the left) hemisphere, and the occipital lobe. Lesions in any of these areas can impair language ability.

To assess language and speech, the nurse carefully distinguishes between aphasia and dysarthria. **Aphasia** is a general term used to describe an impairment of language function; it represents a disorder of symbolic language. **Dysarthria**, on the other hand, causes problems with word articulation or enunciation from interference with the peripheral speech mechanisms (e.g., the muscles of the tongue, palate, pharynx, or lips). Gross assessment of speech and language is made while the history is being taken.

Aphasia. Three major types of aphasia have been identified: (1) motor (expressive), (2) sensory (receptive), and (3) global (Table 47-7). Although one type often predominates, one or more of the other types is commonly present to some degree. Aphasic problems can be detected by assessing spontaneous speech and by asking the patient to follow simple commands, written and oral; to read and interpret newspaper stories; or to write down thoughts.

Dysarthria. The nurse carefully assesses the person's ability to produce speech and observes for weakness or incoordination of the muscles used in articulating speech. Limitations may be observed during cranial nerve testing, particularly in cranial nerves V, VII, IX, X, and XII. Impairment of the motor component of these nerves may produce alterations in phonation, resonance, and articulation. The nurse asks the individual to produce different speech sounds to help localize the problem.

Dysarthrias are usually noticed during ordinary conversation or by having the person repeat a difficult phrase such as "Methodist Episcopal" or "third riding artillery brigade." Dysarthrias may be manifested by a single alteration or a variety of alterations, and characteristic changes accompany particular diseases. For example, in cerebellar disease, speech is often thick with a prolongation of speech sounds occurring at intervals (scanning). In parkinsonism, speech is characterized by a decrease in volume and a change in vocal emphasis patterns that makes sounds seem monotonous.

TABLE 47-7 TYPES OF APHASIA

Type	Definition	Site of Lesion
Motor (Expressive)	Impairment of ability to speak and write; still able to understand written and spoken words	Insula and surrounding region, including Broca's motor area
Anomic	Inability to name objects, qualities, and conditions although speech is fluent	Area of angular gyrus
Fluent	Speech well articulated and grammatically correct but lacking in content and meaning	
Nonfluent	Problems in selecting, organizing, and initiating speech patterns May also affect writing	Motor cortex at Broca's area
Sensory (Receptive)	Impairment of ability to understand written or spoken language	Disease of auditory and visual word centers
Wernicke's	As above	Wernicke's area of left hemisphere
Mixed aphasia	Combined expressive and receptive aphasia deficits	Damage to various speech and language areas
Global aphasia	Total aphasia involving all functions that make up speech and communication Few if any intact language skills	Severe damage to speech areas

Perception

Sensation is integrated and interpreted in the sensory cortex, especially in the parietal lobe. It is important for the nurse to recognize perceptual problems, since they can be more difficult to deal with than changes in the patient's ability to move or sense. Disorders of perception commonly involve spatial-temporal relationships or the perception of self.

The ability to recognize objects through any of the special senses is known as **gnosia**. Lesions involving a specific association area of the cortex produce a specific type of agnosia (absence of this ability). One frequently tested ability is stereognosis, the ability to perceive an object's nature and form by touch. This is assessed by asking the person to identify familiar objects that are placed in the hand one at a time with the eyes closed. **Apraxia** is another common perceptual problem and involves the inability to perform skilled, purposeful movements in the absence of motor, sensory, or coordination losses (Table 47-8).

Sensory Status. Accurate assessment of sensory function depends on the person's cooperation, alertness, and responsiveness. The person should be relaxed and keep the eyes closed during all portions of the sensory examination to avoid receiving visual clues. Sensation is tested on both sides and distally to proximally.

TABLE 47-8 APRAXIA

Type	Impairment Produced	Lesion Site
Constructional	Impairment in producing designs in two or three dimensions; involves copying, drawing, or constructing	Occipitoparietal lobe of either hemisphere
Dressing	Inability to dress accurately; making mistakes, as putting clothes on backward, upside-down, or inside-out or putting both legs in same pant leg	Occipital or parietal lobe, usually in nondominant hemisphere
Motor	Loss of kinesthetic memory patterns, which results in inability to perform a purposeful motor task although it is understood	Frontal lobe of either hemisphere, precentral gyrus
Idiomotor	Inability to imitate gestures or perform a purposeful motor task on command; may be able to do task spontaneously	Parietal lobe of dominant hemisphere, supramarginal gyrus
Ideational	Inability to carry out activities automatically or on command because of inability to understand the concept of the act	Parietal lobe of dominant hemisphere or diffuse brain damage as in arteriosclerosis

Both superficial and deep sensation is tested on the trunk and extremities. Areas of sensory loss or abnormality are mapped out on a body diagram according to the distribution of the spinal dermatomes and peripheral nerves (see Figure 47-17). A **dermatome**, or skin segment, may be thought of as the area of skin supplied by one dorsal root of a cutaneous nerve. An area in which sensation is absent (anesthesia) is differentiated from areas in which sensation is intensified (hyperesthesia) or lessened (hypesthesia or hypoesthesia). Paresthesia is an abnormal sensation that is perceived as burning, prickly, or itching.

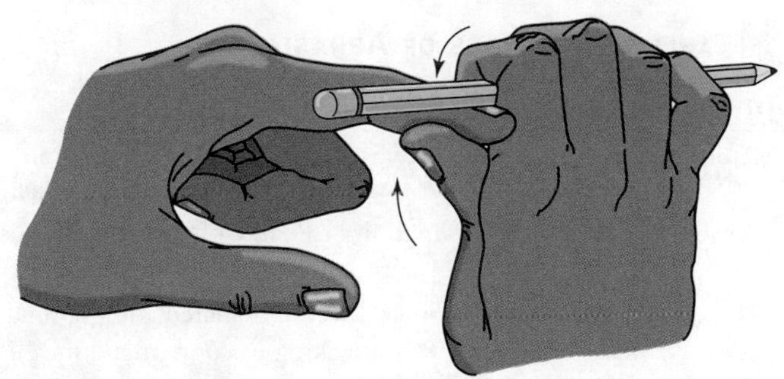

Figure 47-20 Nail bed pressure stimulation using pencil.

Pain, Temperature, and Touch. The nurse assesses superficial pain perception by lightly stroking or pricking an area with a pin and asking the person when discomfort is perceived. Sharp and dull objects can be alternated for increased discrimination. Deep pain can be assessed by multiple means, some of which have the potential of causing tissue injury. Assessing deep pain is necessary only when the person has a decreased LOC. Deep pain is assessed by applying pressure over the nail beds (Figure 47-20), supraorbitally, or over bony areas such as the sternum. Deep pain may also be elicited by squeezing the trapezius muscle. Pinching may damage tissues and is avoided whenever possible.

The nurse assesses perception of crude touch by having the patient close his or her eyes and then lightly touching an area with a cotton ball and requesting the person to indicate when the touch is felt. Temperature is assessed by touching areas of the body with warm to hot, and cool to cold, objects in a random fashion; the person states whenever a sensation is felt. Because pain and temperature sensations use the same nerve pathway (lateral spinothalamic), testing for temperature can be eliminated in the routine examination if the tests for pain perception are normal.

Motion and Position. Proprioceptive fibers (fasciculus gracilis and fasciculus cuneatus) transmit sensory impulses from muscles, tendons, ligaments, and joints. These impulses create an awareness of the position of one's limbs in space (kinesthetic sense). The nurse grasps the sides of the person's distal phalanx and moves it up and down to test proprioception. If proprioception is intact, the person reports correctly the direction in which the joint is being moved. Proprioceptive abilities can also be assessed by

TABLE 47-9 CRANIAL NERVES AND THEIR FUNCTIONS

Cranial Nerves	Function
Olfactory (I)	Sensory: smell reception and interpretation
Optic (II)	Sensory: visual acuity and visual fields
Oculomotor (III)	Motor: raise eyelids, most extraocular movements Parasympathetic: pupillary constriction, changes in lens shape
Trochlear (IV)	Motor: downward, inward eye movement
Trigeminal (V)	Motor: jaw opening and clenching, chewing and mastication Sensory: sensation to cornea, iris, lacrimal glands, conjunctiva, eyelids, forehead, nose, nasal and mouth mucosa, teeth, tongue, ear, facial skin
Abducens (VI)	Motor: lateral eye movement
Facial (VII)	Motor: movement of facial expression muscles except jaw; closing eyes; labial speech sounds (b, m, w, and rounded vowels) Sensory: taste—anterior two thirds of tongue, sensation to pharynx Parasympathetic: secretion of saliva and tears
Vestibulocochlear (VIII)	Sensory: hearing and equilibrium
Glossopharyngeal (IX)	Motor: voluntary muscles for swallowing and phonation Sensory: sensation of nasopharynx, gag reflex, taste—posterior one third of tongue Parasympathetic: secretion of salivary glands, carotid reflex
Vagus (X)	Motor: voluntary muscles of phonation (guttural speech sounds) and swallowing Sensory: sensation behind ear and part of external ear canal Parasympathetic: secretion of digestive enzymes; peristalsis; carotid reflex; involuntary action of heart, lungs, and digestive tract
Spinal accessory (XI)	Motor: turn head, shrug shoulders, some actions for phonation
Hypoglossal (XII)	Motor: tongue movement for speech sound articulation (l, t, n) and swallowing

From Seidel HM et al: *Mosby's guide to physical examination,* ed 5, St Louis, 2003, Mosby.

Romberg's test, in which the person is asked to stand erect with the feet together and eyes closed. A positive test, when the person loses balance, indicates a pathologic condition.

Vibration is assessed by placing the base of a low-frequency tuning fork on a distal bony prominence, such as the finger or toe, of one extremity at a time. The person indicates to the nurse when the vibration is initially felt and when it stops.

Cranial Nerves

The 12 cranial nerves are tested in either numbered sequence (Table 47-9) or by grouping cranial nerves with similar function, such as voluntary motor function, visceral motor function, and special sensory or general sensory functions. Note, however, that some cranial nerves have both motor and sensory functions.

Cranial Nerve I (Olfactory). The function of cranial nerve I is purely sensory, namely, smell. Special receptors within the superior (or uppermost) part of each nasal chamber transmit neural impulses over the olfactory bulbs to the olfactory nerves in the area of the central cortex concerned with olfaction. When testing this cranial nerve, the nurse asks if the patient smells an odor. If the answer is yes, the patient is asked to name the odor. Awareness of an odor must be differentiated from the ability to name a specific substance. **Anosmia** (absence of smell) or hyposmia (decreased sensitivity of the sense of smell) is often associated with complaints of lack of taste, even though tests may demonstrate that sense to be intact. Varied lesions involving any part of the olfactory pathways can cause anosmia.

Cranial Nerve II (Optic). The function of cranial nerve II is also purely sensory, that is, sight or vision. When the retina is stimulated, nerve impulses are transmitted over the optic nerves (extending from the optic disc to the chiasm) and the optic tracts with the radiations terminating in the visual cortex of the occipital lobes. As shown in Figure 47-21, the medial (nasal) fibers of each optic nerve cross at the chiasm to the opposite side of the brain, whereas the lateral (temporal) fibers remain uncrossed. Thus fibers of the left optic tract contain fibers from only the left half of each retina and carry impulses to the left occipital lobe; fibers of the right optic tract contain fibers from only the right half of each retina and carry impulses to the right occipital lobe.

Optic nerve function is assessed in relation to visual acuity, visual fields, and the appearance of the fundus. Each eye is tested separately.

VISUAL ACUITY. The cones of the retina mediate visual acuity. Reading newspaper print grossly tests central vision. Distance visual acuity is assessed through the use of the Snellen chart (see Chapter 60). Individuals with vision impairment are tested to determine light perception, hand movement, and finger count.

VISUAL FIELDS. Field of vision is defined as the range in which objects are visible when vision is fixed in one direction. The field

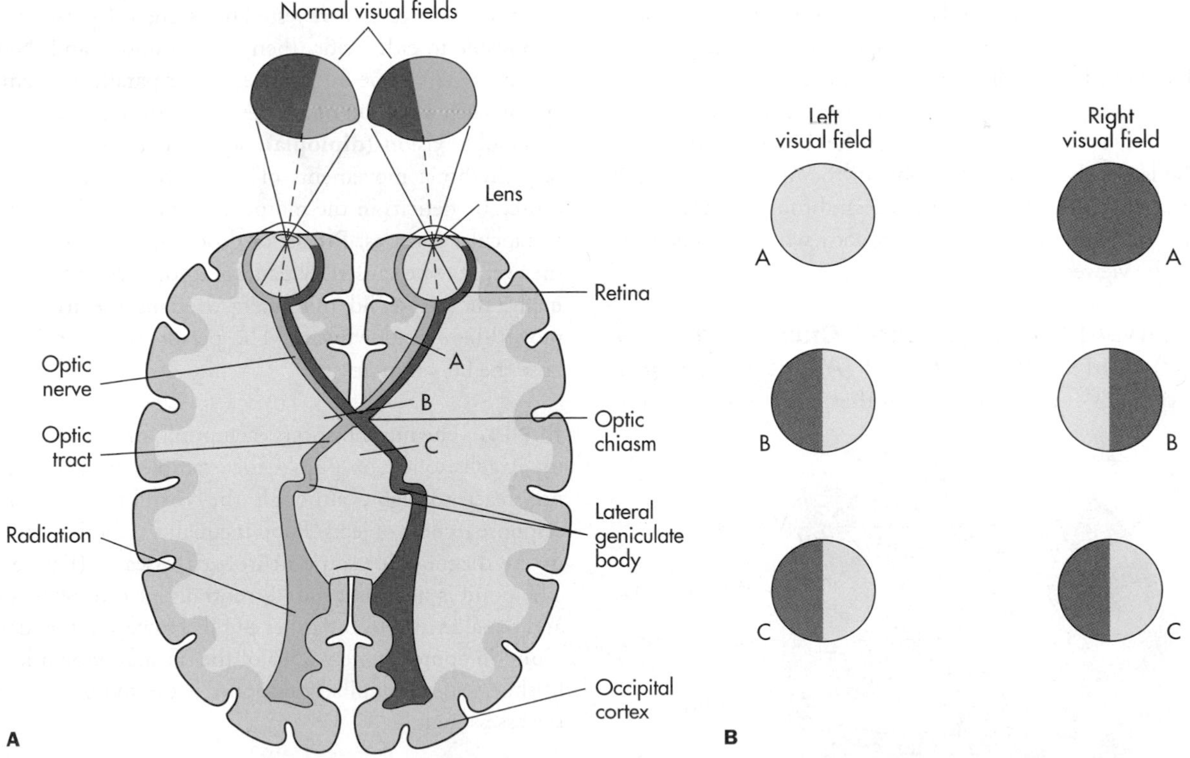

Figure 47-21 **A,** Visual pathways showing partial decussation of optic chiasm. Normal visual fields show reversal of light rays from temporal and nasal sides to receptors in retina. **B,** Abnormal visual fields. *A,* Normal left field of vision with loss of vision in right field as a result of complete lesion of right optic nerve. *B,* Loss of vision in temporal half of both fields as a result of lesion of optic chiasm (bitemporal hemianopia). *C,* Loss of vision in nasal field of right eye and temporal field of left eye caused by lesion of right optic tract (homonymous hemianopia).

of vision thus relates to peripheral vision, or indirect vision. Full visual fields depend on the intactness of all parts of the visual pathway of the eye. The visual fields are tested grossly by confrontation techniques where an object is moved into the periphery of each of the quadrants of the eye. The person is instructed to cover one eye, fix the other eye on a point straight ahead, and report when the moving object is first detected at the edge of each visual field. The nurse's finger may be used as the moving object.

Visual fields may be altered in a variety of CNS diseases, such as neoplasia and vascular disease. Glaucoma is a major cause. Damage to one optic nerve anterior to the chiasm affects only the field of the involved eye. Lesions at the chiasm or posterior to it produce a variety of bilateral visual field defects (see Figure 47-21). For example, compression of the optic chiasm damages the crossing fibers from the nasal retina and causes bitemporal hemianopia, or the loss of vision in the temporal halves of each eye. Loss of vision in the corresponding halves of both visual fields produces **homonymous hemianopia**, which can be further designated as right or left.

Ocular Fundus. The ocular fundus is that portion of the interior of the eyeball that lies posterior to the lens. It includes the optic disc, blood vessels, retina, and macula and is examined by means of an ophthalmoscope. The funduscopic examination begins with the optic disc (papilla), the area where the blood vessels and nerve fibers enter and exit the eyeball (Figure 47-22). The disc is normally the most prominent structure visible and is examined in detail to assess its size, shape, margins, and color (Box 47-2). Either excessive pallor or redness may be present, as well as swelling, or papilledema, which can be caused by active inflammation or passive congestion. Papilledema that results from passive congestion or increased ICP is also called a choked disc. Optic atrophy indicates partial or complete destruction of the optic nerve and is associated with decreased visual acuity and a change in the color of the disc to a lighter pink or gray. The largest blood vessels visible in the fundus, the central retinal artery and central retinal vein, branch throughout the retina. The retina is the only site in the human body where the microcirculation can be viewed directly.

Cranial Nerve III (Oculomotor), Cranial Nerve IV (Trochlear), and Cranial Nerve VI (Abducens).

Cranial nerves III, IV, and VI are motor nerves that arise from the brainstem and innervate the six extraocular muscles attached to the eyeball. These muscles function as a group to provide the coordinated movement of each eyeball in the six cardinal fields of gaze, giving the eye both straight and rotary movement. The four straight, or rectus, muscles are the superior, inferior, lateral, and medial rectus muscles. The two slanting, or oblique, muscles are the superior and inferior.

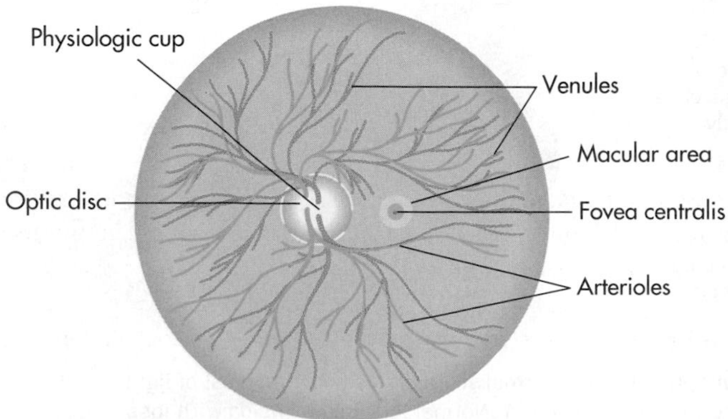

Figure 47-22 Structures of left eye as visualized through ophthalmoscope.

Box 47-2 Normal Characteristics of the Optic Disc

- *Size:* 1.5 mm
- *Shape:* Flat round or vertically oval
- *Margins:* Sharply defined
- *Color:* Creamy red with a small whitish depression in the center (physiologic cup)

The action of each muscle is coordinated with one in the other eye, thus ensuring that the axes of the two eyes always remain parallel **(conjugate movement)**. Parallel axes are important in a binocular system to present the brain with only one visual image. A single image is possible because the eyes move as a pair.

Extraocular Movements. Eye movements are tested by instructing the patient to cover one eye and follow the nurse's finger through all fields of gaze. Limitation of movement in any direction is noted, as well as actual paralysis (ophthalmoplegia). If one of the extraocular muscles is paralyzed, the eye is unable to move fully into the corresponding field of gaze. Conjugate movements of the eyes also are tested by asking the person to look as far as possible to either side, then up and down, and then obliquely (Figure 47-23). The nurse observes for parallel movements of the eyes in each direction or any deviation from normal.

Double vision **(diplopia)**, squint (strabismus), and involuntary rhythmic movements of the eyeballs **(nystagmus)** may be caused by deficits in the motor nerves that cause weakness in the extraocular muscles. **Ptosis**, or drooping of the upper eyelid over the eye, may be caused by damage to the oculomotor nerve. Normally, the upper lid minimally overlaps the iris as the person moves the eyes downward. The person with ptosis is unable to raise the lid voluntarily.

Pupils. The nurse inspects each pupil for size, shape, and equality. Argyll Robertson pupils, for example, are constricted and do not react to light, although they exhibit accommodation in response to near objects. Pupil inequality, or anisocoria, may assist in the diagnosis of some neurologic diseases (Figure 47-24, *A*). The pupil is normally round, centrally placed, regular in outline, and equal in size to the other pupil. However, unequal pupils are found in approximately 25% of the normal population. Thus the briskness of the pupillary response is the more important part of the assessment.

Direct Light Reflex. The nurse darkens the room and focuses a small beam of light directly into each pupil. Normally the pupil constricts quickly when a light is focused on the retina. Constriction is reported to be especially brisk in young people and those with blue eyes. After a head injury, a dilated and fixed

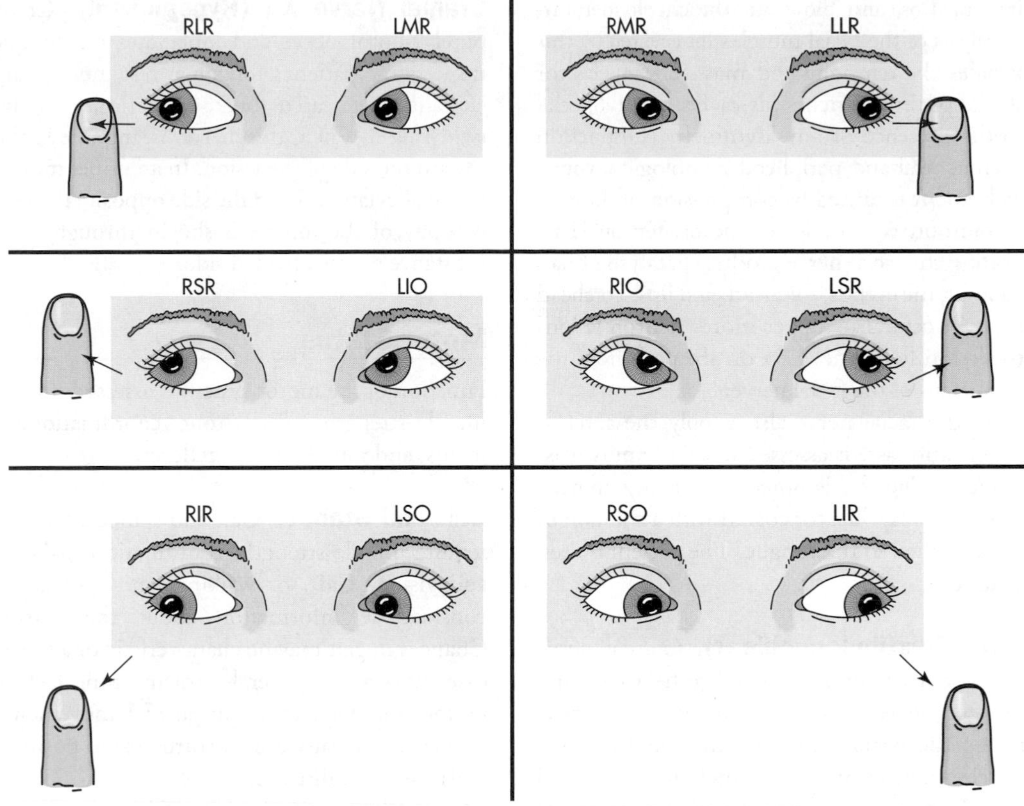

Figure 47-23 Examination of extraocular muscles. Note that two muscles are involved in each cardinal direction. *R*, Right; *L*, left; *LR*, lateral rectus; *MR*, medial rectus; *SR*, superior rectus; *IO*, inferior oblique; *IR*, inferior rectus; *SO*, superior oblique.

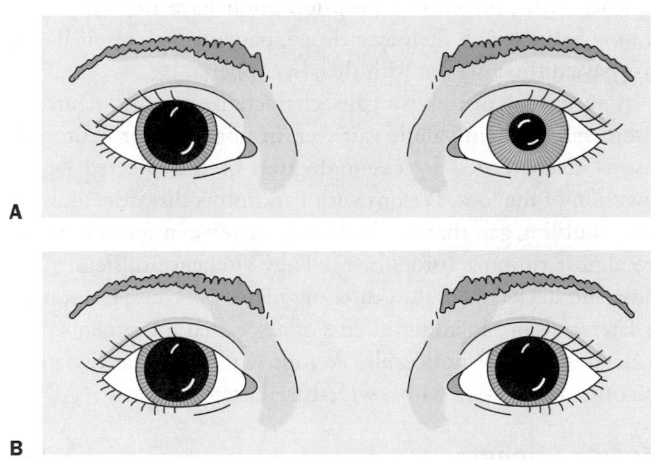

Figure 47-24 **A,** Unequal pupils, also called anisocoria. **B,** Dilated and fixed pupils, indicative of severe neurologic deficit.

pupil may be observed on the side of the injury (Figure 47-24, *B*). A pupil is described as slow or sluggish if it contracts slowly or imperfectly and then relaxes immediately.

CONSENSUAL LIGHT REFLEX. When one pupil is directly stimulated by light, the pupil of the other eye also constricts. This consensual response is the result of the decussation (crossing) of nerve fibers both in the optic chiasm and in the pretectal area, causing both the homolateral and contralateral pupil to react to light.

Cranial Nerve V (Trigeminal). Cranial nerve V is a mixed nerve with both motor and sensory components and is the largest cranial nerve. The motor portion innervates the temporal and masseter muscles; the sensory part supplies the cornea, face, head, and mucous membranes of the nose and mouth.

The motor portion of the nerve is tested through jaw movement. If muscle weakness is present, the opened jaw tends to deviate to the side opposite the weakened muscles. The sensory components supplying the face are tested for touch, pain, and temperature. Bilateral corneal reflexes may also be assessed. Normally the person blinks bilaterally when a wisp of cotton is brought in from the side and lightly touched to the cornea (not to an eye with a contact lens in place). This is an especially important reflex to assess in persons with a decreased LOC because the absence of the blink reflex can result in corneal damage.

Sensation in the face is assessed by both light and deep touch. The three branches of the trigeminal nerve, which include the ophthalmic, maxillary, and mandibular, are tested using a cotton ball for light touch and a blunt object such as a paper clip for deep touch. The nurse touches each of the three areas with the object in a random fashion while the patient's eyes are closed; the patient responds on experiencing the sensation. The procedure is performed on each side of the face.

Cranial Nerve VII (Facial). Cranial nerve VII is also a mixed nerve concerned with facial movement and sensation. The inability to smile, close both eyes tightly, look upward, wrinkle the forehead, show the teeth, purse the lips, and blow out the cheeks demonstrates weakness or paralysis of the facial muscles innervated by this nerve. The nurse palpates the temporal and masseter muscles for strength and mass as the patient clenches his or her teeth. Special attention is given to the presence of any asymmetry. Distinction must be made between central and peripheral neurologic involvement. Peripheral involvement is caused by compression of this cranial nerve and is a common type of lower motor neuron facial paralysis. Lesions affecting the facial nerve produce paralysis of half of the entire face, including the eyelids, forehead, and lips. Forehead function remains intact in central or upper motor neuron lesions and indicates that the lesion lies somewhere on the path from the cerebral cortex to the nucleus of the facial nerve.

Sensory branches of the facial nerve also supply the anterior two thirds of the tongue, and taste is assessed when the nurse suspects a facial nerve injury. The test is otherwise usually omitted from the assessment. A cotton applicator coated with a solution of sugar, salt, or vinegar is applied to the tongue. The patient is then asked to identify the taste.

Cranial Nerve VIII (Vestibulocochlear). Cranial nerve VIII is composed of a cochlear division related to hearing and a vestibular division related to equilibrium. The cochlear part is tested grossly by having the person listen to and identify whispered words. A more complete examination, including bone and air conduction of sound, involves assessment with a tuning fork and audiometric testing; Rinne's test and Weber's test are the most commonly used (see Chapter 62). The vestibular function of the nerve is evaluated by assessing balance through Romberg's test, as discussed below under Gait and Stance. A positive Romberg's test suggests an inner ear or cerebellar problem.

Cranial Nerve IX (Glossopharyngeal) and Cranial Nerve X (Vagus). Cranial nerves IX and X are tested together. The chief function of cranial nerve IX is to provide sensation to the pharynx and taste to the posterior third of the tongue. Both nerves supply the posterior pharyngeal wall; normally, when the wall is touched, the muscles on both sides promptly contract, with or without gagging. The test is thus unreliable for evaluating either nerve alone. Because cranial nerve X is the chief motor nerve to the muscles of the soft palate, pharynx, and larynx, assessment includes testing voice and cough. In unilateral involvement of the motor portion of the vagus nerve the voice is harsh and nasal. When the person says "Ah," the soft palate does not stay in the midline but deviates to the intact side. Bilateral involvement produces more severe speech problems; swallowing is difficult (dysphagia), and fluids regurgitate through the nose because of palatal and pharyngeal muscle impairment. Sensory function of the vagus usually is not tested.

Cranial Nerve XI (Spinal Accessory). Cranial nerve XI is a motor nerve that supplies the sternocleidomastoid muscle and the upper part of the trapezius muscles. To assess the muscles for weakness and paralysis, the nurse inspects the muscles on each side for equality of size, places a hand against each side of the patient's face in turn and asks the patient to turn the head against this resistance, and places hands on the patient's shoulders and asks the patient to shrug against the resistance.

Cranial Nerve XII (Hypoglossal). Cranial nerve XII is a purely motor nerve and innervates the tongue. The nurse first inspects the patient's tongue at rest, noting any asymmetry, unilaterality, decreased bulk, deviations, or fasciculations (fine twitching). When this nerve is impaired, the tongue deviates toward the side of the lesion. In an upper motor neuron lesion the tongue deviates toward the side opposite the lesion (contralateral). Atrophy of the tongue is shown through wrinkling and loss of substance on the affected side.

Motor Status

Function of the motor system is assessed through gait and stance, muscle strength, muscle tone, coordination, involuntary movements, and muscle stretch reflexes.

Gait and Stance. Gait and stance are complex activities that require muscle strength, coordination, balance, proprioception, and vision. **Gait**, or walking, and associated movements give considerable information about the person's motor status. Changes in gait may be characteristic of a specific neurologic disease. **Ataxia** is a general term meaning lack of coordination in performing a planned, purposeful movement such as walking. Ataxia can be caused by disturbance of position sense or by cerebellar or other diseases.

To evaluate gait, the nurse asks the person to walk freely and naturally and then walk heel to toe in a straight line, since this exaggerates any abnormalities. To evaluate **stance**, the nurse asks the person to perform Romberg's test by standing still with the feet close together, first with eyes open and then with eyes closed. Patients with problems of proprioception have difficulty maintaining balance with their eyes closed; patients with cerebellar disease have difficulty even with their eyes open.

A variety of distinctive gaits characterize specific neurologic disorders. The hemiparetic gait seen in upper motor neuron disease is characterized by circumduction of the affected leg and inversion of the foot. Persons with Parkinson's disease walk with a slow, shuffling gait that may gradually increase in speed until they are almost running (propulsive). They also have difficulty stopping, and deviation in the center of gravity can cause retropulsion or lateropulsion. In addition, loss of associated movements of the arms in walking is noticeable. Persons with cerebellar disease, on the other hand, walk with a wide-based, staggering gait.

Muscle Strength. Muscle strength, or power, is assessed systematically, including the trunk and extremity muscles. One common assessment of muscle strength involves asking the patient to grasp the nurse's hands and squeeze them simultaneously. The nurse compares the squeezing ability of one hand with that of the other. Muscle strength in the feet can be assessed by asking the patient to plantar flex and dorsiflex the feet. During manual testing of these and other muscle groups, the person attempts to resist the force applied by the nurse in moving the muscles. If an impaired muscle is identified, the nurse documents the extent and degree of muscle weakness.

The nurse may also test the patient for drift by asking him or her to hold the arms straight out for 20 to 30 seconds with palms up and eyes closed. Hemiparesis (weakness or incomplete paralysis) is suggested when there is pronation of one forearm or a downward drift of the arm.

Muscle Tone. Resting skeletal muscles have a certain number of fibers that are always partially contracted because of continuous stimulation of receptors in certain reflex arcs, especially the stretch reflex. The minimal degree of contraction exhibited by a muscle at rest is called muscle tone. When some of the lower motor neurons or afferent fibers innervating neuromuscular spindles are injured, stimulation of a muscle is reduced, with a concomitant loss of tone referred to as hypotonia. In contrast, increased muscle tone is referred to as hypertonia. A wide variety of disorders in muscle tone may accompany neurologic diseases.

To test muscle tone, the nurse passively moves the person's limbs through a full range of motion. A skilled examiner can readily differentiate hypertonic from hypotonic muscles. Hypertonic extremities tend to stay in fixed positions and feel firm; hypotonic extremities assume a position governed by gravity. Hyperextension and hyperflexion are found in hypertonia; an initial resistance to passive movement may increase rapidly and then suddenly give way to spasticity, or *clasp-knife rigidity.* A steady, passive resistance throughout the full range of motion is characteristic of *parkinsonian rigidity*; the combination of passive resistance and parkinsonian tremor with small, regular jerks is called *cogwheel rigidity.* In *decorticate rigidity* the upper limbs are flexed and pronated and the lower limbs are extended. In *decerebrate rigidity,* however, the upper limbs are extended.

Coordination. Coordination of muscle movements, or the ability to perform skilled motor acts, may be impaired at any level of the motor system. The cerebellum is primarily responsible for coordinating movements so that they are smooth and precise. Thus disturbances in cerebellar function may result in ataxia, difficulty in controlling the range of muscular movement (dysmetria), and an inability to alternate rapid and successive movements on opposite sides (adiadochokinesia). The nurse evaluates simple motor activities by asking the person to perform rapid, rhythmic movements, such as the nose-finger-nose test, which requires the individual to alternately touch his or her nose and then the tip of the nurse's finger; or the knee pat (pronation-supination). For the latter, the patient places the palms of the hands on his or her knees, lifts the hands, turns them over, and touches the knees with the backs of the hands.

Involuntary Movements. The nurse also assesses and documents involuntary movements during the neurologic examination. It is important to observe the location of muscles involved, amplitude of movement, speed of onset, duration of contraction and relaxation, and rhythm. The nurse determines the effects of posture, rest, sleep, distraction, voluntary movements, and emotional stress on involuntary movements. Emotional stress usually increases involuntary movements, which may subside during sleep. Abnormal movements may be the result of organic disease or may be psychosomatic in origin.

Tremor consists of rhythmic to-and-fro movements, usually of small amplitude. These movements are the result of alternating contractions of opposing groups of muscles, are continuous while the patient is awake, and may or may not be present during sleep. Chorea refers to short, sharp, rapid, irregular movements, usually of small excursion, which occur in different parts of the body and persist during sleep. Hemiballismus is a variation of chorea in which movement is confined to one side of the body and primarily affects the limbs. Athetosis consists of slow, sinuous, and more sustained movements that may be of considerable amplitude; these movements occur in the neck and trunk, as well as the extremities. Myoclonus refers to irregular, abrupt, and arrhythmic contractions of a muscle or a group of muscles in the extremities, trunk, or face.

Reflexes. A reflex is a predictable response that results from a stimulus that initiates a reflex arc. The term *reflex* is typically used to describe involuntary responses. Although all muscles can be made to undergo reflex contraction, most are not tested clinically.

The stretch (myotatic) reflex is a two-neuron (monosynaptic) reflex arc. A well-known example is the knee jerk reflex, or patellar reflex, which is produced by tapping the patellar tendon of the relaxed quadriceps femoris muscle (Figure 47-25). Such a reflex is described as ipsilateral because the response occurs on the same side of the body and spinal cord where the stimulus is received. Tapping on the patellar tendon elicits a stretching of the quadriceps tendon and its muscles along with some neuromuscular spindles within the muscle and generates nerve impulses. Afferent fibers convey these nerve impulses to the L2-L3 level of the spinal cord. The afferent neurons synapse with the lower motor neurons, which are large spinal neurons. Axons carry the impulse rapidly to the motor end plates of the quadriceps muscle, stimulating contraction and extension of the lower leg.

Assessment of reflexes requires an experienced examiner, a reflex hammer, and a relaxed patient. The reflex is elicited by striking the hammer onto the muscle's insertion tendon. Comparison of right and left sides should reveal equal responses. Some of the more common diagnostic reflexes tested are listed in Table 47-10. The reflex response is graded on a subjective, four-point scale that requires clinical practice to use accurately (Table 47-11). If the reflex response fails to appear on the first attempt, the nurse encourages the person to relax by varying position or increases the strength of the hammer blow.

Any abnormal reflex response may indicate a disorder of the nervous system. For example, Babinski's reflex, or plantar reflex, is abnormal and may indicate pyramidal tract disease. To test this reflex, the nurse strokes the lateral aspect of the sole of the foot from the heel to the ball using the end of the handle on the reflex hammer. The expected finding is plantar flexion of all toes; a response of extension of the great toe along with fanning of the other toes is abnormal. Hyporeflexia occurs when a reflex is less responsive than normal resulting from a lesion of the lower motor neurons; hyperreflexia, a reflex more responsive than normal, occurs from lesions in upper motor neuron pathways.

▶ ARE You READY?

Damage to the reticular activating system results in which of the following?

1. Depressed arousal
2. Impaired speech
3. Decreased vision
4. Impaired mobility

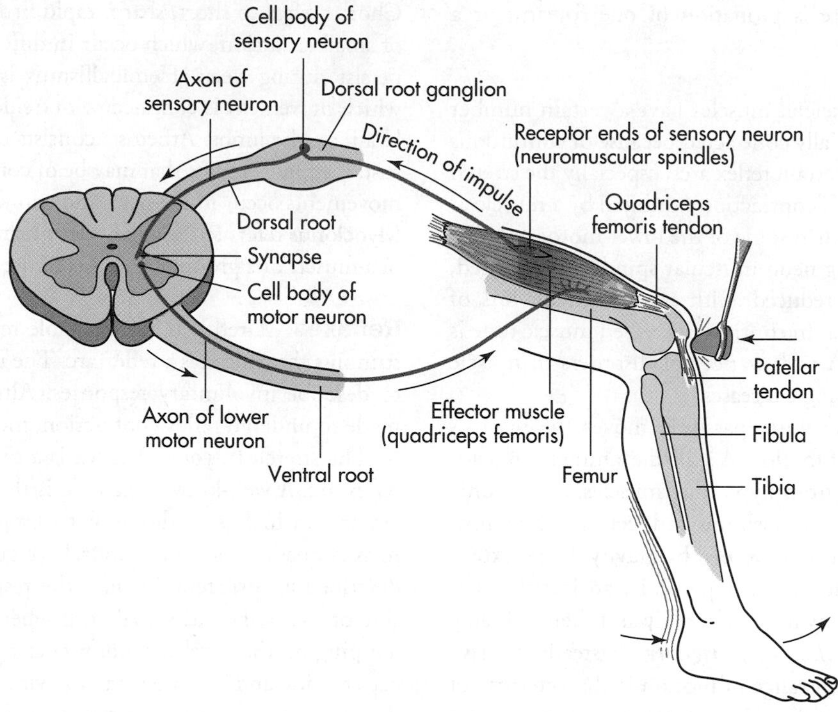

Figure 47-25 The two-neuron patellar reflex, or knee jerk reflex.

TABLE 47-10 Some Diagnostic Reflexes of the Central Nervous System

Reflex	Description	Indication
Abdominal reflex	Anterior stroking of sides of lower torso causes contraction of abdominal muscles.	Absence of reflex indicates lesions of peripheral nerves or in reflex centers in lower thoracic segments of spinal cord; may also indicate multiple sclerosis.
Achilles reflex (ankle jerk)	Tapping of calcaneal (Achilles) tendon of soleus and gastrocnemius muscles causes both muscles to contract, producing plantar flexion of foot.	Absence of reflex may indicate damage to nerves innervating posterior leg muscles or to lumbosacral neurons; may also indicate chronic diabetes, alcoholism, syphilis, subarachnoid hemorrhage.
Biceps reflex	Tapping of biceps tendon in elbow produces contraction of brachialis and biceps muscles, producing flexion at elbow.	Absence of reflex may indicate damage at C5 or C6 vertebral level.
Brudzinski's sign	Forceful flexion of neck produces flexion of legs, thighs.	Reflex indicates irritation of meninges.
Kernig's sign	Flexion of hip, with knee straight and patient lying on back, produces flexion of knee.	Reflex indicates irritation of meninges or herniated intervertebral disc.
Patellar reflex (knee jerk)	Tapping of patellar tendon causes contraction of quadriceps femoris muscle, producing upward jerk of leg.	Absence of reflex may indicate damage at the L2, L3, or L4 vertebral level; may also indicate chronic diabetes, syphilis.
Plantar reflex	Stroking of lateral part of sole causes toes to curl down; if corticospinal damage, great toe flexes upward and other toes fan out (Babinski's reflex).	Reflex indicates damage to upper motor neurons; normal in children less than 1 year old.
Triceps reflex	Tapping of triceps tendon at elbow causes contraction of triceps muscle, producing extension at elbow.	Absence of reflex may indicate damage at C6, C7, or C8 vertebral level.

TABLE 47-11 GRADING OF MUSCLE STRETCH REFLEXES

Scale	Interpretation
0	Areflexia
1+	Hyporeflexia
2+	Normal
3+	Brisker than normal
4+	Hyperreflexia

Diagnostic Tests

Relevant diagnostic tests provide an important source of data for diagnosing neurologic disease. A variety of laboratory, radiologic, and special tests are available to assist in the diagnostic process.

Laboratory Tests

Blood. Blood screening is an important component of the neurologic assessment. Screening usually includes electrolytes and a complete blood count. Serology screening is used to rule out syphilis, which in its tertiary form may cause neurologic symptoms. Arterial blood gases offer valuable information regarding oxygen and carbon dioxide levels. Additionally, drug levels may be drawn to provide information about the person's adherence to a medication regimen and the way the individual metabolizes the drug. Abnormalities in a variety of blood studies may indicate neurologic disease (Table 47-12).

TABLE 47-12 BLOOD ABNORMALITIES

Element	Abnormality Seen	Possible Reason
Sodium	Decreased	Syndrome of inappropriate antidiuretic hormone
Potassium	Decreased	Poor dietary intake
Red blood cells	Increased	Dehydration
	Decreased	Anemia
Hematocrit and hemoglobin	Increased	Dehydration
	Decreased	Anemia
White blood cells	Increased	Infection such as meningitis
		Common steroid effect
Po_2	Decreased	Increased intracranial pressure
Plasma cortisol	Increased	Acute head injury
Anticonvulsant drug	Increased	Toxicity or patient overdose
	Decreased	Patient not taking drug

Urine. Urinary output and electrolyte excretion are easily disturbed by cranial surgery and trauma, especially if the pituitary gland is involved. Both diabetes insipidus and the syndrome of inappropriate secretion of antidiuretic hormone are frequently encountered problems (see Chapter 48). See Table 47-13 for possible alterations in urinary tests.

Cerebrospinal Fluid. CSF is a clear fluid that is formed in the third, fourth, and lateral ventricles of the brain. Samples are obtained through either a lumbar or cisternal puncture and examined for any increase or decrease in its normal constituents and for foreign substances such as pathogenic organisms and blood.[8] Spinal fluid is normally under slight positive pressure of 75 to 180 mm H_2O. The pressure is measured with a manometer when a lumbar puncture is performed.

Normally each milliliter of spinal fluid contains up to eight lymphocytes. An increase in the number of lymphocytes can occur with both bacterial and viral infection. CSF is naturally clear but can become cloudy as a result of an increase in polymorphonuclear leukocytes from pyogenic infections. Bacterial infections can also alter the components of CSF. For example, tuberculosis and meningitis lower CSF glucose and chloride levels. A culture of CSF may assist in organism identification in an ill patient. Degenerative diseases and tumors usually cause an increased protein level in the CSF. See Table 47-14 for normal values of CSF. The colloidal gold test is another test of CSF that is useful in diagnosing neurosyphilis or multiple sclerosis. CSF testing for syphilis is important because serologic blood tests are often negative in the presence of neurologic involvement, whereas CSF tests are positive. CSF abnormalities are present in about 90% of patients with multiple sclerosis, including CSF pleocytosis and abnormal gamma globulins as demonstrated by electrophoresis.

Blood in the spinal fluid indicates bleeding into the ventricular system. It may be caused by a fracture at the base of the skull that has torn blood vessels or from the rupture of a blood vessel (e.g., with an aneurysm). Occasionally the first specimen of CSF obtained during a lumbar puncture contains blood from the

TABLE 47-13 URINE ABNORMALITIES

Element	Abnormality Seen	Possible Reason
Urinary output	Decreased	Metabolic problem
	Increased	Kidney failure
		Diabetes insipidus
Specific gravity	Decreased	Diabetes insipidus
	Increased	Dehydration
Glucose and acetone	Present	Steroid effect—possibly chemical diabetes
Sodium	Increased	Syndrome of inappropriate antidiuretic hormone
		Diabetes insipidus

TABLE 47-14 NORMAL VALUES OF CEREBROSPINAL FLUID

Element	Normal Range
Pressure	75-180 mm H_2O
Glucose	50-80 mg/dl
Chloride	700-750 mg/dl
Protein	12-50 mg/dl
Gamma globulin	3%-9%
White blood cells	0-5/mm^3

trauma of the test. Therefore the specimens of CSF are numbered and the first vial is not used for the cell count.

Radiologic Tests

Multiple radiologic procedures of the brain and spinal cord may be performed, including plain radiographs, carotid Doppler studies, computed tomography (CT), and special contrast studies of the ventricular system and the cerebral vessels.

Routine or Plain Radiographs. Plain radiographs of the skull and spinal column are commonly used diagnostic tests because they are safe and readily available. They can detect developmental, traumatic, or degenerative bone abnormalities.

Carotid Doppler Studies. Carotid Doppler studies use a Doppler instrument that emits ultrasound waves to evaluate carotid arterial blood flow. Moving red blood cells reflect ultrasound waves back to the Doppler instrument; the velocity of the blood flow influences the reflection of the ultrasound waves. Velocity of blood flow is measured through an audible sound and a series of images for visualization. Stenosis, or occlusion of the carotid arteries, can be detected as the instrument is moved over the common carotid artery to the bifurcation of the internal and external carotid arteries. The test is noninvasive, painless, and accurate. No specific nursing care is required before or after the procedure.

Computed Tomography. CT scans can provide 100% more information about the brain than conventional radiographs, and they provide enhanced image detail. A series of x-rays studies is taken, scanning in successive layers with a narrow beam of x rays so that each image is derived from a specific layer of brain tissue. Data are collected in x-ray and printout form, and information is also stored for future comparison. By comparing tissue densities found on the CT scan with norms, the clinician can detect abnormalities, including tumor masses, infarctions, and displacements of bone and ventricles. The CT scan is particularly efficient in detecting brain tumors and cerebrovascular lesions.

No special physical preparation is required. The nurse informs the patient that the CT scan is painless except for insertion of an intravenous access before the procedure if a contrast medium is used, in which case patients are carefully assessed for allergies. The procedure takes 30 to 60 minutes depending on whether a contrast medium is used. The person is supine during the scan, with the head positioned in a rubber head holder. After the scan, the nurse monitors the patient for signs of increased ICP if dye was used. If the person becomes disoriented as a result of the test, the nurse provides reassurance and protection from injury.

Brain Scan. The brain scan is a relatively safe and painless procedure that uses radioactive isotopes and a scanner to detect cerebral pathologic conditions. The patient is given an intravenous injection of a radionucleotide, and then the radioactivity is traced with a gamma scintillation camera or scanner, which converts the rays into images displayed on an oscilloscope screen. The underlying principle of the brain scan is that the radionucleotide can penetrate the brain only through a disruption in the blood-brain barrier and subsequently collects in abnormal brain tissue.

Nursing care primarily centers on the patient's educational needs. The nurse informs the patient that the injection of radioactive material causes burning at the insertion site, but no dangers are associated with its administration. The nurse explains that the scanner oscillates around the head during the scan and creates some loud noises. The patient removes all jewelry and metal objects before the procedure, which typically takes about 45 minutes.

Myelography. Myelography is performed by introducing either a gas or a radiopaque liquid into the spinal subarachnoid space after a lumbar or cisternal puncture. The flow of dye is monitored fluoroscopically as it moves through the subarachnoid space, and radiographs are taken to help identify lesions in the intradural or extradural compartments of the spinal canal. Water-based dyes such as metrizamide (Amipaque) are absorbed into the bloodstream and require no special considerations. Less frequently used oil-based dyes are removed at the completion of the test while the person remains upright to prevent the dye, which would cause meningeal irritation, from flowing above the level of the spine.

Before the procedure food and fluids are restricted for approximately 4 to 8 hours. The nurse assesses for any history of allergies to iodine or dyes, then asks the person to sign a consent form and remove all jewelry and metal objects. A sedative may be given to relax the person immediately before the procedure.

After the procedure the person must lie supine for several hours if an oil-based dye was used. In contrast, the person assumes a semirecumbent position with the head elevated 30 to 60 degrees for 12 hours if a water-based dye was injected. These interventions attempt to decrease the incidence of headache, nausea, vomiting, and seizures in the posttest period. Complaints of neck stiffness or pain with neck flexion are immediately reported to the physician because these symptoms could indicate meningeal irritation. Other nursing interventions include monitoring vital signs and encouraging fluid consumption of 2400 to 3000 ml during the initial 24 hours. A normal diet can be resumed after 4 hours. Phenothiazine drugs are withheld for 48 hours after the procedure to decrease the risk of seizures.

Cerebral Angiography (Angiogram). Cerebral angiography involves the injection of a contrast medium into the cerebral arterial circulation to assist in determining the cause of strokes, seizures, headaches, and motor weakness. A catheter is inserted into the femoral artery (the most common entry site) and advanced to the carotid and cerebral vessels. Serial films are taken as the dye circulates throughout the cerebral circulation.

Before the procedure the nurse informs the person that the procedure typically takes 1 to 2 hours and that a feeling of warmth often occurs after the dye is injected. The nurse carefully assesses for any allergies to iodine, seafood, or contrast medium. The person is given nothing by mouth for 6 to 10 hours before the procedure. Informed consent is required and jewelry, dentures, and hearing aids are removed. A sedative may be ordered before the test.[6]

After the procedure the person typically remains on bed rest for 12 to 24 hours; however, the duration of bed rest varies among institutions. The nurse monitors neurologic status, vital signs, distal pulses, intake and output, and hemostasis at the insertion site. The puncture site is immobilized for approximately 8 hours, and ice may be applied at the site to decrease the incidence of hemorrhage and edema.

Potential complications from cerebral angiography include allergic reactions to the radiopaque dye, vasospasm, hemorrhage, hematoma, embolism, or stroke. These complications usually manifest as motor, sensory, or language dysfunction.

Digital Subtraction Angiography. Digital subtraction angiography (DSA) is a method of radiographically studying blood vessels and is particularly useful when the area of study is blocked by bone. Intravenous DSA is often preferred over standard cerebral angiography because DSA uses less radiation, is less expensive, and has a lower incidence of serious complications.

The nurse carefully assesses the patient for potential allergy to the contrast medium and informs him or her of the importance of lying completely still during the procedure. Images of target areas are taken before and after injection of the dye. Pictures are digitized, stored, and compared in a computer that subtracts anything common between the before (mask) and after (contrast) images. After the procedure the nurse encourages fluid intake, monitors the insertion site for bleeding, and performs neurovascular checks based on institution protocols.

Special Tests

Lumbar Puncture. The lumbar puncture (LP) is performed to measure pressure and obtain CSF for examination. The needle is inserted below the level of the spinal cord at the L4-L5 or L5-S1 interspaces (Figure 47-26). After removal of the inner needle, CSF is collected and pressures are measured with a manometer. Queckenstedt's test is routinely performed to assess for subarachnoid blockage by compressing each jugular vein one at a time for approximately 10 seconds while monitoring for changes in spinal fluid pressures. Any pressure greater than 200 mm H_2O is considered abnormal. LP is not typically performed in the presence of increased ICP because of the risk of brainstem herniation into the foramen magnum.

No dietary or fluid restrictions are required before the test. A consent form is signed, and a sedative may be ordered. The person is encouraged to empty the bowel and bladder and is helped either to assume a fetal position near the edge of the bed or to sit upright on the side of the bed with the chest and head extended toward the knees. Local anesthesia is used, but the patient may still experience sensations of pressure or brief pain as the spinal needle is inserted.

The person is encouraged to lie in a prone position with a pillow under the abdomen after the procedure to increase intra-abdominal pressure and help seal the puncture site.[3] A period of bed rest is encouraged, but no specific duration is ordered. Nursing interventions include monitoring the insertion site for

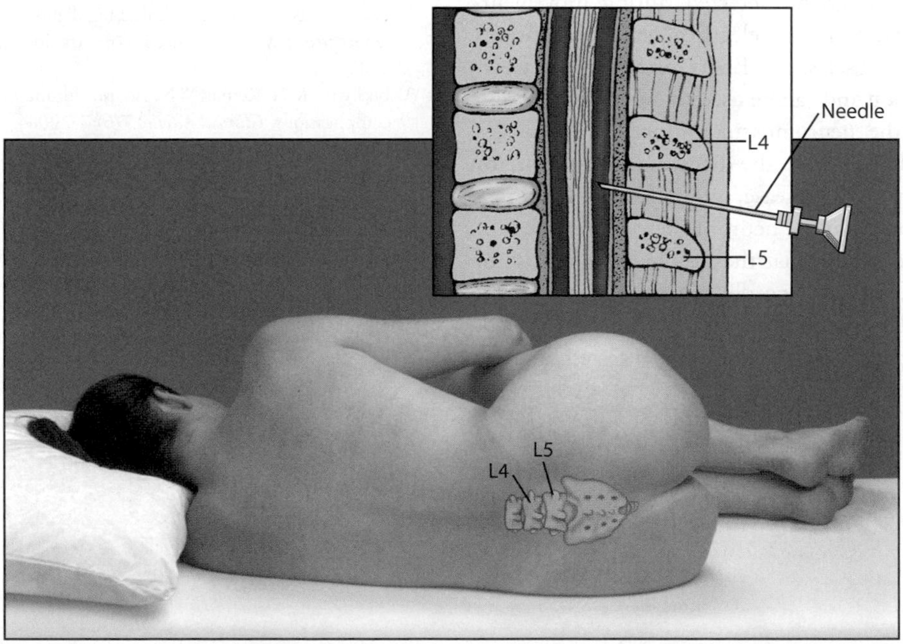

Figure 47-26 Lumbar puncture. With the patient in flexed position to maximize the space between vertebrae, the lumbar puncture needle is inserted between L4 and L5 to gain entry to the subarachnoid space. (During actual procedure patient would be gowned and draped to protect privacy.)

swelling, redness, and drainage. Signs of complications such as neck stiffness, irritability, and changes in LOC or vital signs are reported immediately to the physician. A postlumbar puncture headache can occur as a result of leakage of CSF at the puncture site and traction on the meninges. The headache may occur a few hours to several days after the procedure and is typically described as a throbbing in the frontal or occipital area. The headache may be severe but is not serious and is treated with analgesics along with bed rest in a quiet, darkened room.

Electroencephalography. The electroencephalogram (EEG) amplifies and records the electrical activity of the brain (brain waves) as they are transmitted by electrodes attached to the scalp. Any spikes, slowed activity, or asymmetric rhythms on the EEG are considered abnormal. Electroencephalography is indicated for all patients who experience unexplained confusion, loss of consciousness, or seizure activity. The EEG is also used to establish brain death.

The nurse reassures the patient that the test is painless and is not a form of shock therapy. Cola, tea, and coffee are avoided the morning of the EEG because they produce a stimulating effect. The person's hair should be clean and free of hair sprays, gels, and lotions. EEG recordings may be altered by slight movements; therefore the person is instructed to rest quietly and avoid movement during the test. Medications are usually not withheld before the test, but protocols may vary.

Electromyography. The electromyogram (EMG) measures the electrical activity of muscles and records the variations of electrical potential (voltage) detected by a needle electrode inserted into skeletal muscles. The electrical activity can be heard over a loudspeaker and simultaneously viewed on both an oscilloscope and a graph. No electrical activity can be detected in muscles at rest, but action potentials can be detected during movement. However, in motor disease abnormal electrical activity of various types appears in resting muscles. An EMG provides direct evidence of motor dysfunction and can be used to detect dysfunction in the motor neuron, the neuromuscular junction, or muscle fibers. This is particularly helpful in the detection of lower motor neuron disease, primary muscle disease, and defects in the transmission of electrical impulses at the neuromuscular junction.

The nurse assures the patient that the needle poses no risk of electrocution, but the sensation of needle insertion is painful and similar to an intramuscular injection. Informed consent is required. After the procedure the person may be encouraged to rest, and the nurse observes for bleeding at the insertion sites.

Magnetic Resonance Imaging. Magnetic resonance imaging (MRI) uses a powerful electromagnet to detect radio frequency pulses from the alignment of hydrogen protons in the magnetic field. Computers convert the electromagnetic echo into images, which provide excellent visualization of tissue even without the use of contrast media. The MRI demonstrates an increased sensitivity to tissue variations and can often detect lesions such as brainstem tumors and brain abscesses that are not identifiable by CT scans.

The MRI requires no special preparation. The nurse informs the patient that the MRI is painless but requires the patient to assume a supine position and to lie still. The nurse prepares the patient for the confining narrow space of the machine, especially if there is any history of claustrophobia. The machine produces a "beating" noise, and earplugs are offered if the noise becomes bothersome. Jewelry is removed before the test; it is important to ascertain whether the person has any surgical or orthopedic clips, heart valves, or a pacemaker because the MRI can cause displacement.

▶ ARE YOU READY?

Nursing care of a patient after an oil-based myelogram includes which of the following?

1. Maintaining patient in a semi-recumbent position with head elevated 30 to 60 degrees
2. Maintaining patient in a supine position for several hours
3. Limiting fluids to 1000 ml in first 24 hours
4. Administering phenothiazine medications to decrease risk of seizures

References

1. Auerbach S, Karow CM: Neurobehavioral assessment of mood and affect in patients with neurological disorders, *Semin Speech Lang* 24(2):131-143, C1-C6, 2003.
2. Bauer J: RN news watch: clinical highlights—women, more than men, report stroke symptoms that are "nontraditional," *RN* 66(1):20, 22, 76, 2003.
3. Beckwith MG, Kernan WN: Advisor forum: how to avoid lumbar puncture complications, *Clinical Advisor* 7(6):75, 2004.
4. Crimlisk JT, Grande MM: Neurologic assessment skills for the acute medical surgical nurse, *Orthopaedic Nurs* 23(1):3-11, 2004.
5. Martin J, Hauser S: Approach to the patient with neurologic disease. In Brauwald E et al, editors: *Harrison's principles of internal medicine,* accessed Oct 2004 from website: http://harrisons.accessmedicine.com.
6. McDaniel J: Code gray case studies, *Crit Care Nurs Q* 26(4):303-315, 2003.
7. Robinson K, Merrill R: Relation among stroke knowledge, lifestyle, and stroke-related screening results, *Geriatr Nurs* 24(5):300-305, 2003.
8. Seehusen DA, Reeves MM, Fomin DA: Cerebrospinal fluid analysis, *Am Fam Phys* 68(6):1103-1012, 2003.

Visit the Evolve website: http://evolve.elsevier.com/Monahan/medsurg

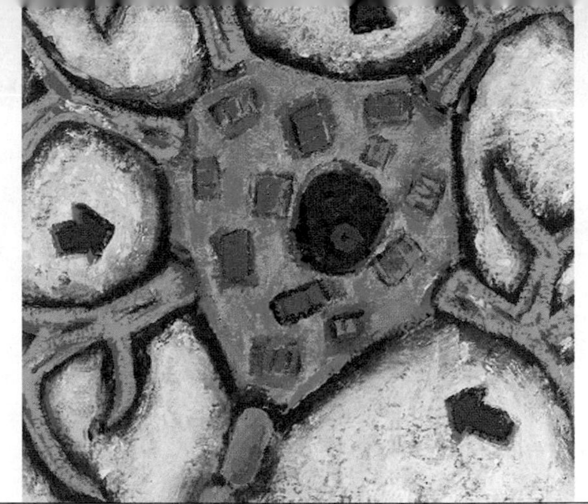

CHAPTER 48

Traumatic and Neoplastic Problems of the Brain

by Lisa W. Forsyth, Janet C. Garnett

OBJECTIVES

After studying this chapter, the learner should be able to:

1. Identify at least four causes of altered level of consciousness.
2. Describe three assessment parameters for the person with an altered level of consciousness.
3. Outline four nursing strategies to prevent increases in intracranial pressure.
4. Explain the significance of cerebral perfusion pressure in the patient with increased intracranial pressure.
5. Describe nursing assessment of the patient with a head injury.
6. Develop a care plan for the patient with a severe head injury.
7. Outline preoperative and postoperative nursing care for the patient undergoing craniotomy for a brain tumor.
8. Differentiate among migraine, cluster, and tension headaches.
9. Differentiate between partial and generalized seizures.
10. Describe the emergent management of status epilepticus.
11. Design a care plan for a patient with meningitis or encephalitis.

KEY TERMS

aura, p. 1394
autoregulation, p. 1389
brain death, p. 1380
cerebral perfusion pressure, p. 1389
decerebrate posturing, p. 1382
decorticate posturing, p. 1382
generalized seizure, p. 1398
herniation, p. 1390
hydrocephalus, p. 1402
ictal, p. 1398
intracranial pressure, p. 1389
locked-in syndrome, p. 1380
nuchal rigidity, p. 1417
orientation, p. 1381
partial seizure, p. 1398
persistent vegetative state, p. 1380
postictal, p. 1398
primary headache, p. 1394
stereotactic radiation, p. 1405

This chapter discusses the care of persons with traumatic, neoplastic, and related problems of the brain. The initial presentations of altered level of consciousness and increased intracranial pressure apply to the management of multiple neurologic conditions. The remaining sections present specific disease processes such as headache, epilepsy, intracranial tumors, craniocerebral trauma, and infections and inflammations of the nervous system.

Altered Level of Consciousness

Etiology and Epidemiology. Consciousness and coma exist at opposite ends of a spectrum. Full consciousness is a state of awareness and ability to respond optimally to one's environment. Coma is the opposite, a state of total absence of awareness and ability to respond even when stimulated. A wide range of awareness and responsiveness exists between these two extremes (Figure 48-1). The labels used to identify the various points along the continuum are arbitrary and do not reflect any universal agreement as to the nature of consciousness. Terms such as *lethargy* or *stupor* may be interpreted differently by different health care professionals. Box 48-1 provides common definitions for terms used to describe level of consciousness (LOC).

Consciousness has two primary components: arousal and content. Arousal is a function of the brainstem pathways that govern wakefulness, particularly the reticular activating system (RAS). Content is the sum of multiple interconnected cerebral hemisphere functions, including thought, behavior, language, and expression.[12] Disruptions in arousal, content, or both can alter the individual's LOC.

Two general categories for causes of altered LOC are structural and metabolic (Box 48-2). Structural causes include physical lesions such as tumors that interrupt neuronal pathways in the cortex or brainstem. Metabolic causes, such as hypoglycemia or hypoxia, alter the cellular environment and affect the function of neurons. The number of people experiencing altered LOC is not known, but its multiple causes indicate that it is a commonly

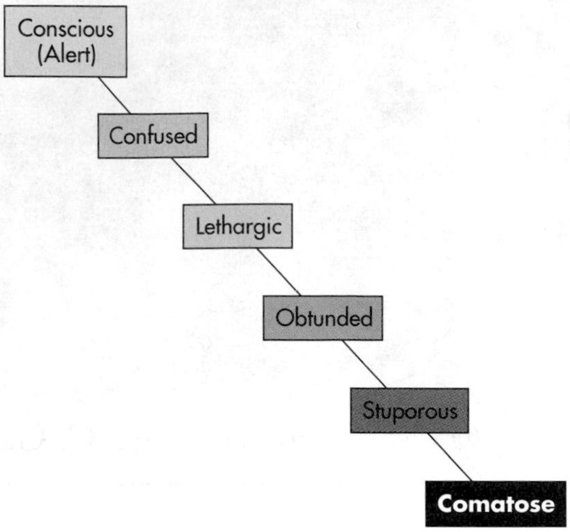

Conscious (Alert)
Confused
Lethargic
Obtunded
Stuporous
Comatose

Figure 48-1 Continuum of consciousness.

Box 48-1 Altered Level of Consciousness Terminology

- *Alert:* Attends to the environment; responds appropriately to commands and questions with minimal stimulation
- *Confused:* Disoriented to surroundings; may have impaired judgment; may need cues to respond to commands
- *Lethargic:* Drowsy; needs gentle verbal or touch stimulation to initiate a response
- *Obtunded:* Responds slowly to external stimulation; needs repeated stimulation to maintain attention and response to the environment
- *Stuporous:* Responds only minimally with vigorous stimulation; may only mutter or moan as a verbal response
- *Comatose:* No observable response to any external stimuli

encountered problem in clinical practice. Patients of all ages may experience altered LOC—for brief periods or long term.

Three unique conditions of altered LOC illustrate the complexity of the physiology of consciousness. A **persistent vegetative state** is a condition that can develop after a severe brain injury. Patients in this state demonstrate eye opening and sleep-wake cycles that indicate arousal, but they exhibit no cognitive function.[19] In other words, these patients possess intact "vegetative" functions of the brainstem, such as respiratory drive, brainstem reflexes, and some functions of the RAS, but have no cognitive functions to enable them to interact voluntarily with their environment.

Locked-in syndrome is a condition in which the motor pathways in the brainstem are destroyed but the RAS and higher cognitive functions remain intact. In this state, patients are unable to move or speak because of destruction of the motor pathways that control those functions, but they are capable of interacting with their environment. The motor functions of blinking and extraocular movements are usually spared because those pathways lie above the level of the pons. Locked-in patients therefore can communicate with eye movements and are capable of full arousal and understanding.

Box 48-2 Possible Causes of Decreased Level of Consciousness

Structural Causes

Trauma (concussion, contusion, traumatic intracerebral hemorrhage, subdural hematoma, epidural hematoma, cerebral edema)
Vascular disease (infarction, intracerebral hemorrhage, subarachnoid hemorrhage)
Infections (meningitis, encephalitis, abscess, acquired immunodeficiency syndrome)
Neoplasms (primary brain tumors, metastatic tumors)

Metabolic Causes

Systemic metabolic derangements (hypoglycemia, diabetic ketoacidosis, hyperglycemic nonketotic hyperosmolar states, uremia, hepatic encephalopathy, hyponatremia, myxedema)
Hypoxic encephalopathies (severe congestive heart failure, chronic obstructive pulmonary disease with exacerbation, severe anemia, prolonged hypertension)
Toxicity (heavy metals, carbon monoxide, and drugs—especially opiates, barbiturates, and alcohol)
Extremes of body temperature (heatstroke, hypothermia)
Deficiency states (Wernicke's encephalopathy)
Seizures

Brain death is the third unique alteration in LOC with specific physiologic features. Severely brain-injured patients are considered brain dead when they meet strict criteria set forth by state law. The laws governing brain death may vary by state, but most include criteria such as[5]:

- A known cause of coma so that reversible causes, such as drug overdose or hypothermia, can be ruled out
- Unresponsiveness to external stimuli
- Absent brainstem reflexes
- Absent respiratory effort in the presence of hypercapnea

These criteria are crucial because they do not include the classic layperson's criterion for death—an absent heartbeat. The definition of brain death becomes particularly important in situations involving tissue and organ donation.

Pathophysiology. Full consciousness is a product of many delicate interactions within the nervous system. Arousal is a function of the RAS.[1] Fibers from the upper brainstem, thalamus, and hypothalamus receive input from sensory pathways in the brain and peripheral nervous system. The RAS fibers stimulate the cerebral hemispheres to initiate and maintain arousal. When a person is aroused, or awake, he or she is ready to respond to the environment. The cerebral cortex also provides feedback to the RAS to modulate and regulate the information sent to the cortex. See Chapter 47 for further description of RAS.

The ability to consciously respond to the environment is a function of the cerebral hemispheres. The cerebral cortex, diencephalon, and upper brainstem act together to control voluntary motor functions, language, memory, and emotion. These higher-level cognitive functions represent the content portion of consciousness. A person needs both arousal, or wakefulness, and content to be considered fully conscious.

Disruptions to the nervous system controlling consciousness can be structural or metabolic (see Box 48-2). Structural lesions, such as a tumor or stroke, disrupt the pathways of nerve transmission and produce specific, localized neurologic deficits that reflect the location of the lesion. Metabolic causes, such as hypoglycemia or drug overdose, affect the biochemical environment of the brain and alter cellular function. Altered LOC resulting from metabolic changes usually produces more global, nonlocalized neurologic deficits.

Patients with selected sensory-perceptual alterations also may experience altered LOC. Patients experiencing hallucinations, agitation, and delirium are often found to have underlying metabolic problems such as hypoxia, infection, or medication interactions that disturb the brain's metabolic environment. Classic clinical manifestations, including sensory-perceptual alterations, associated with altered LOC are presented in the Clinical Manifestations box.

COMPLICATIONS. Patients experiencing a change in LOC are vulnerable to a wide variety of complications because of their inability to fully and appropriately interact with the world and protect themselves from injury. The more profound the change in LOC, the more vulnerable the patient becomes to injury in virtually every body system. Many complications are related to immobility or the inability to meet basic care needs. Specific complications of altered LOC are discussed under the individual disease processes.

Collaborative Care Management

DIAGNOSTIC TESTS. Diagnostic evaluation of altered LOC includes searching for the structural or metabolic cause of the changes. The workup includes a detailed history, extensive neurologic examination, radiologic examination, and laboratory testing (Box 48-3). In the emergency setting, diagnostic tests can be subdivided into those tests which explore the possibility of structural lesions and those which evaluate possible metabolic causes of altered LOC. Interventions to protect the airway and support breathing and circulation are initiated while further diagnostic testing is done. A trial dose of naloxone (Narcan) may be administered to any patient in whom opioid overdose is suspected.

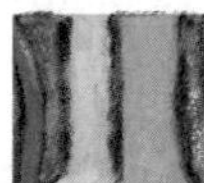

CLINICAL MANIFESTATIONS
Altered Level of Consciousness

- Decreased wakefulness
- Decreased attention to environment
- Confusion
- Disorientation
- Agitation
- Poor memory
- Decreased ability to carry out activities of daily living
- Decreased mobility
- Incontinence
- Hallucinations: subjective sensory perceptions that occur in the absence of relevant external stimuli; may be auditory, visual, tactile, or somatic
- Delusions: false, fixed, personal beliefs that are not shared by others
- Illusions: misinterpretations of real external stimuli

BOX 48-3 Diagnostic Tests for Altered Level of Consciousness

Laboratory Tests

Complete blood count
Blood glucose
Electrolytes
Liver function studies, blood urea nitrogen
Cardiac enzymes
Serum osmolarity
Arterial blood gases
Toxicology screens for opiates, alcohol, barbiturates, antidepressants
Urinalysis
Lumbar puncture and cerebrospinal fluid analysis

X-Rays and Scans

Skull x-ray films
Computed tomography scan of head
Magnetic resonance imaging of head
Electroencephalogram
Cerebral angiogram
Evoked potentials

While diagnostic tests are being scheduled or test results are pending, a detailed history and thorough physical examination are performed. The neurologic examination provides the most important data for evaluating alterations in LOC. (See Chapter 47 for details of a complete neurologic examination. The items discussed here are specific to the evaluation of altered states of consciousness.) The initial examination may be performed by a physician or advanced practice nurse and then repeated on an ongoing basis by the bedside nurse.

The mental status examination includes an overall assessment of consciousness and the patient's ability to remain awake and participate in the examination. Orientation, cognitive function, and language are thoroughly assessed. Subtle changes in **orientation** are often the first indications of altered LOC, and patients may be disoriented to varying degrees. The patient is asked about the day, month, and year. If a patient cannot name a specific date, the examiner may ask about the season or recent holidays to obtain a more general response. Orientation to place is also assessed. If a patient cannot name the exact current location, the examiner asks what kind of place he or she is in (e.g., a hospital, hotel, grocery store). If the patient cannot correctly answer a question about place, he or she is considered disoriented with an impaired ability to reason and use information. Significant cognitive or language impairment is typically present when patients are unable to state or respond to their names. It is important to clarify what name the patient is used to responding to; this name should be used during interactions.

The patient's LOC may fluctuate, and practitioners must use clear communication and documentation of each assessment so they can recognize changes and trends in the patient's condition. Thorough documentation of a patient's LOC includes both the patient's response and the stimulation needed to obtain the response. This objective information about the patient's response to a specific stimulus allows other practitioners to reproduce the same results. For example, "Patient opens eyes and answers questions when his name is called" provides clearer and more useful information than simply writing, "Patient is lethargic." It is also important to remember that orientation is only a small part of the overall mental status examination. Assessment of altered LOC also includes attention, a component of mental status not often covered in the standard neurologic examination. The examiner assesses the patient's ability to focus, or concentrate, and observes for distractibility, irritability, restlessness, and boredom, since these may all be signs of cerebral dysfunction.

The time frame associated with the altered LOC can be important in differentiating between delirium and dementia. Delirium develops over a short period, and its duration is usually brief. Because delirium is usually caused by an underlying organic disease process, the altered LOC often resolves when the disease is successfully treated. Dementia is not associated with reduced arousal or wakefulness, but it impairs intellectual function, memory, orientation, and self-care. Dementia develops slowly; is usually progressive; and is a chronic, irreversible state.

Next the examiner performs a motor examination, assessing the patient's muscle strength and coordination, as well as the reflexive or pathologic responses of the motor system. When patients have marked reductions in LOC, the examiner may need to use a noxious stimulus to elicit a response. The examiner begins with verbal stimuli, such as calling the patient's name or asking the patient to follow a simple command. A slightly stronger stimulus would involve touching the patient's shoulder and gently tapping or shaking the patient while calling his or her name. Some patients can respond only to a painful stimulus. Pressing on the sternum, squeezing the trapezius muscle at the junction of the shoulder and neck, applying supraorbital ridge pressure, and applying pressure to the fingernail beds are common examples of painful stimuli. Both the stimulus used and the patient's response are carefully recorded so the next examiner can duplicate the examination and accurately assess for changes in the patient's status. The patient who reacts to a painful stimulus and attempts to push the examiner away is said to "localize to pain." If the patient grimaces or demonstrates nonpurposeful movement, he or she is said to "withdraw to pain."

Lesions in the cerebral hemispheres below the primary motor cortex can cause pathologic motor responses and abnormal flexor or extensor posturing (Figure 48-2). Abnormal flexion of the arms at the elbows, wrists, and hands with concurrent extension of the legs is called **decorticate posturing**. Lesions in the motor pathways of the midbrain or upper pons may cause abnormal extension of the arms with hyperpronation of the forearms, which is called **decerebrate posturing**.

The sensory part of the neurologic examination is conducted to reveal deficits that affect a cognitively impaired patient's ability to function. Patients with a sensory-perceptual deficit after a stroke may neglect, or not attend to, the affected side of the body.

The last part of the neurologic examination is the cranial nerve examination. Several specific cranial nerve reflexes are particularly important in assessing altered LOC. Protective reflexes, including gag, corneal, and cough, are checked to assess the patient's ability to protect himself or herself from injury and aspiration (see Chapter 47).

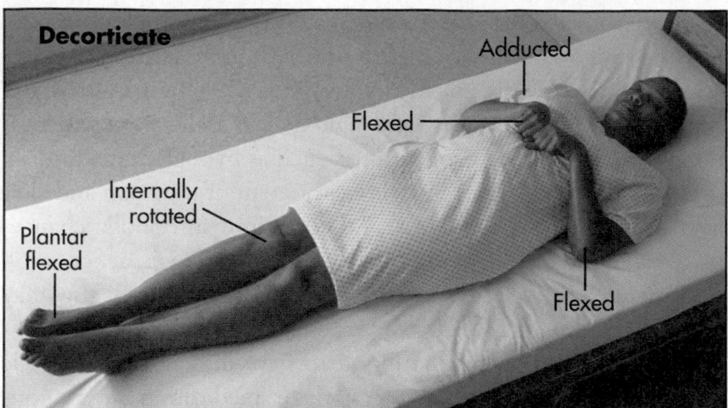

A

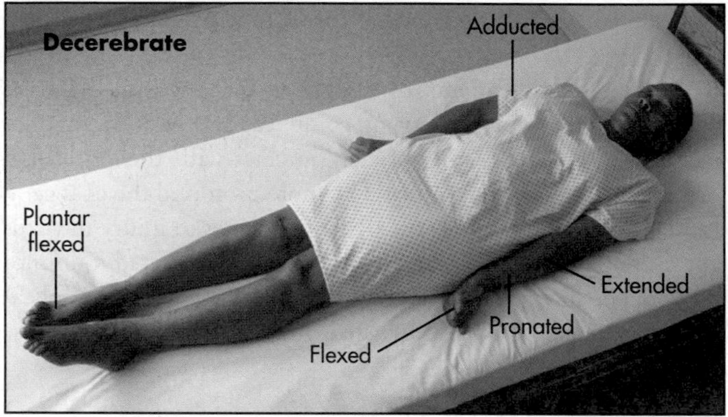

B

Figure 48-2 Types of posturing. **A,** Decorticate. **B,** Decerebrate.

The oculocephalic and oculovestibular reflexes are not part of a standard neurologic examination but are performed to assess the extent of a pathologic condition in the brainstem. They are an integral part of the determination of brain death. The oculocephalic reflex (doll's eyes) is tested by holding the person's eyelids open and rotating the head quickly, first to one side and then to the opposite side. When the brainstem is intact, the eyes move in the opposite direction to the head turning. This is considered a positive or normal response (Figure 48-3). If a person has a brainstem lesion, the eyes passively follow the head movement.

The oculovestibular reflex (calorics) may be tested in a nonresponsive patient. The patient is positioned supine with the head of the bed elevated 30 degrees, and the patient's eyelids are held open while the ear canals are irrigated with 50 ml of ice water, stimulating the semicircular canals. A normal response involves conjugate eye movements toward the side being irrigated, followed by rapid nystagmus to the opposite side (Figure 48-4); this indicates intact functioning of cranial nerves III, VI, and VIII. Absent or dysconjugate eye movements indicate brainstem damage.

A detailed neurologic examination provides the foundation for the initial assessment of patients with altered LOC, but a variety of standardized scales are also used for the ongoing evaluation of patient function. The Glasgow Coma Scale (GCS) was developed specifically to evaluate head-injured patients, but it can also be effectively used with a wide variety of other neurologic problems (Box 48-4).[9,24] The patient's total score is a sum of scores from three scales: eye opening, verbal response, and motor response.

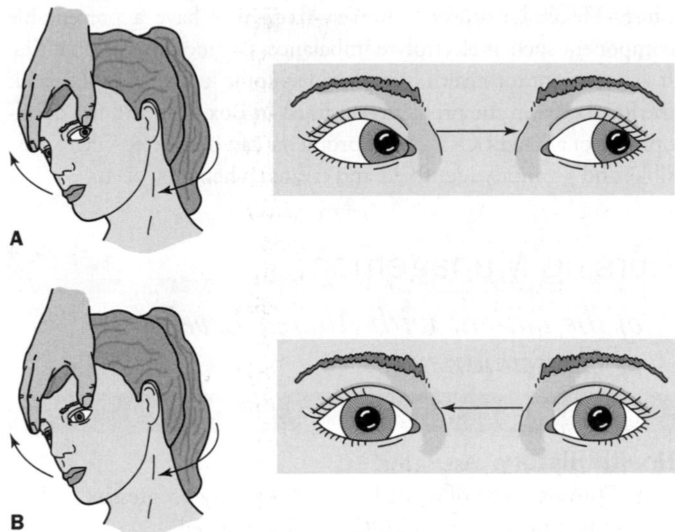

Figure 48-3 Oculocephalic reflex testing. **A,** Normal response: eyes move to the left as head is briskly rotated to the right. **B,** Abnormal response: eyes do not move as head is turned, but passively follow the head.

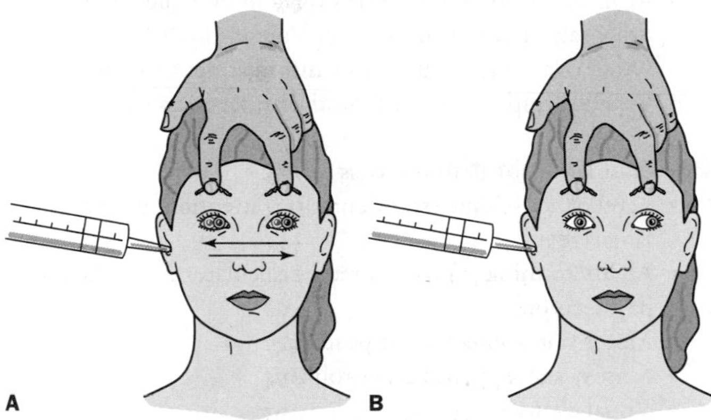

Figure 48-4 Test for oculovestibular reflex response (caloric ice water test). **A,** In normal response, individual's eyes slowly move toward side being irrigated, followed by rapid conjugate eye movements to opposite side. **B,** Dysconjugate, or asymmetric, eye movements would be abnormal.

Box 48-4 Glasgow Coma Scale

Eye Opening

4 Spontaneously open
3 Open to verbal request
2 Open with painful stimuli
1 No opening

Best Verbal Response

5 Oriented to time, place, person; converses appropriately
4 Converses, but confused
3 Words spoken, but conversation not sustained
2 Sounds made, no intelligible words
1 No response

Best Motor Response

6 Obeys commands
5 Localizes to painful stimulus
4 Withdraws to painful stimulus
3 Abnormal flexion to pain (decorticate posturing)
2 Abnormal extension to pain (decerebrate posturing)
1 No response

Box 48-5 Levels of Cognitive Functioning (Rancho Los Amigos Scale)

I. No response: Patient is completely unresponsive to any stimuli.
II. Generalized response: Patient reacts inconsistently and nonpurposefully to stimuli in nonspecific manner.
III. Localized response: Patient reacts specifically but inconsistently to stimuli.
IV. Confused—agitated: Patient is in heightened state of activity with severely decreased ability to process information.
V. Confused—inappropriate: Patient appears alert and is able to respond to simple commands fairly consistently.
VI. Confused—appropriate: Patient shows goal-directed behavior but depends on external input for direction.
VII. Automatic—appropriate: Patient appears appropriate and oriented within hospital and home setting, goes through daily routine automatically with minimal to absent confusion, and has shallow recall of actions.
VIII. Purposeful—appropriate: Patient is alert and oriented, is able to recall and integrate past and recent events, and is aware of and responsive to culture.

From Malkmus D et al: *Rehabilitation of the head-injured adult: comprehensive cognitive management,* Downey, Calif, 1980, Professional Staff Association of Rancho Los Amigos Medical Center, Adult Brain Inquiry Service.

Numbers are assigned to the patient's best response in each area, and notations are made if a scale is not able to be evaluated, such as "eyes swollen shut" or "intubated; unable to test verbal response." The GCS does not take the place of a comprehensive neurologic examination, but the cumulative results can be graphed and used to identify trends in the patient's overall function and predict outcomes.

The Rancho Los Amigos Levels of Cognitive Functioning was developed as a behavioral rating scale to aid in the assessment and treatment of brain-injured persons. It assesses the progressive recovery of cognitive abilities as demonstrated through behavioral change and is most commonly used in subacute and rehabilitation settings (Box 48-5).

A third tool is the Mini-Mental State Examination (MMSE). This classic, brief examination assesses orientation, registration, attention, recall, and language and can also be used to follow trends in the patient's level of functioning.[9] Box 48-6 shows examples of assessment questions and tasks from the MMSE.

Vital signs can also provide important information regarding a patient's altered LOC. Blood pressure and heart rate may reflect cardiac dysfunction affecting blood flow to the brain. The patient's respiratory rate and pattern can help localize lesions in the central nervous system. Figure 48-5 provides examples of abnormal respiratory patterns that can result from neurologic problems.

Box 48-6 Mini-Mental State Examination (Sample Items)

Orientation to Time

"What is the date?"

Registration

"Listen carefully, I am going to say three words. You say them back after I stop. Ready? Here they are ... HOUSE (pause), CAR (pause), LAKE (pause). Now repeat those words back to me." (Repeat up to five times, but score only the first trial.)

Naming

"What is this?" (Point to a pencil or pen.)

Reading

"Please read this and do what it says." (Show examinee the words on the stimulus form.) CLOSE YOUR EYES

MEDICATIONS. Medications are used in the treatment of altered LOC to correct the underlying disease process or to control specific symptoms. Naloxone may be given to reverse the effects of opioid overdose. Flumazenil is a benzodiazepine antagonist used to reverse the effects of overdoses of drugs such as diazepam (Valium) or lorazepam (Ativan). If seizures are the cause of decreased LOC, anticonvulsants are administered to treat actual seizures and prevent future ones. A variety of other medications (see p. 1392) may be administered to treat increased intracranial pressure (ICP), a common cause of altered LOC.

TREATMENTS. There are no specific treatments for patients with altered LOC. Common interventions used are discussed in the section on Nursing Management.

SURGICAL MANAGEMENT. If the cause of the patient's altered LOC is a space-occupying lesion, surgical removal of the mass may improve the patient's condition. For example, a patient with a subdural hematoma becomes more alert and able to follow commands after the hematoma is evacuated. If the lesion has been present long enough to damage the surrounding tissue, however, some residual deficits may remain. See sections on Craniocerebral Trauma and Intracranial Tumors for further discussion of surgical management of neurologic problems.

DIET. A patient's swallowing ability is carefully assessed before any decision is made about diet. Patients with decreased gag and cough reflexes, oral motor weakness, or decreased LOC may be candidates for placement of an enteral feeding tube to more safely deliver nutrients and medications.

HEALTH PROMOTION AND PREVENTION. No specific measures can be recommended to prevent altered LOC that has a structural cause. Metabolic causes, however, frequently have a preventable component such as electrolyte imbalances or glucose abnormalities. It is important for health care providers to be knowledgeable about the link between the problems outlined in Box 48-2 and the development of altered LOC so that problems can be averted where possible, and promptly identified and treated when they occur.

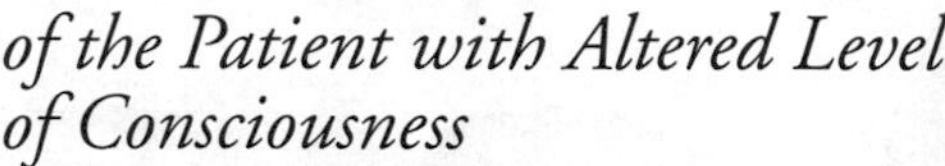

Nursing Management

of the Patient with Altered Level of Consciousness

ASSESSMENT

Health History. Assess for:

- Date and type of onset (sudden or slowly progressive)
- When the change in LOC was first noticed
- Patient's and family's awareness and understanding of the symptoms; health history from the patient when possible but also from family members, significant others, prehospital care providers, and home care providers as appropriate
- Recent history of falls, infection, or other trauma
- Medications in use—prescription and over-the-counter drugs, alcohol, nutritional supplements, herbal preparations
- Other comorbid health problems, treatment regimen
- Related symptoms—pain, headache, fever, nausea

Physical Examination. Assess for:

- Level of consciousness, orientation, attention, use of language
- Ability to think, think abstractly, calculate, and make everyday decisions
- Motor status, presence of posturing
- Sensory status, perceptual problems
- Visual changes
- Protective reflexes, alterations in cranial nerve responses
- Breathing pattern
- Oxygenation status
- Laboratory results (see Box 48-3)
- Drug levels (opiates, sedatives, anticonvulsants)

NURSING DIAGNOSES, OUTCOMES, AND INTERVENTIONS

Nursing Diagnosis: Ineffective Breathing Pattern

OUTCOMES. One common example of an expected outcome for the patient with a diagnosis of *ineffective breathing pattern* is: Patient will:

- Maintain an effective breathing pattern and adequate ventilation.

NURSING INTERVENTIONS. Patients with decreased LOC may not be able to turn themselves or cough effectively to mobilize pulmonary secretions or prevent atelectasis. They may require assistance in keeping the airway clear, including the use of suctioning when warranted. The nurse closely monitors the patient's breathing patterns and positions the patient on either side, keeping the head of the bed elevated at least 30 degrees to facilitate an open airway. The nurse helps the patient turn, encourages deep

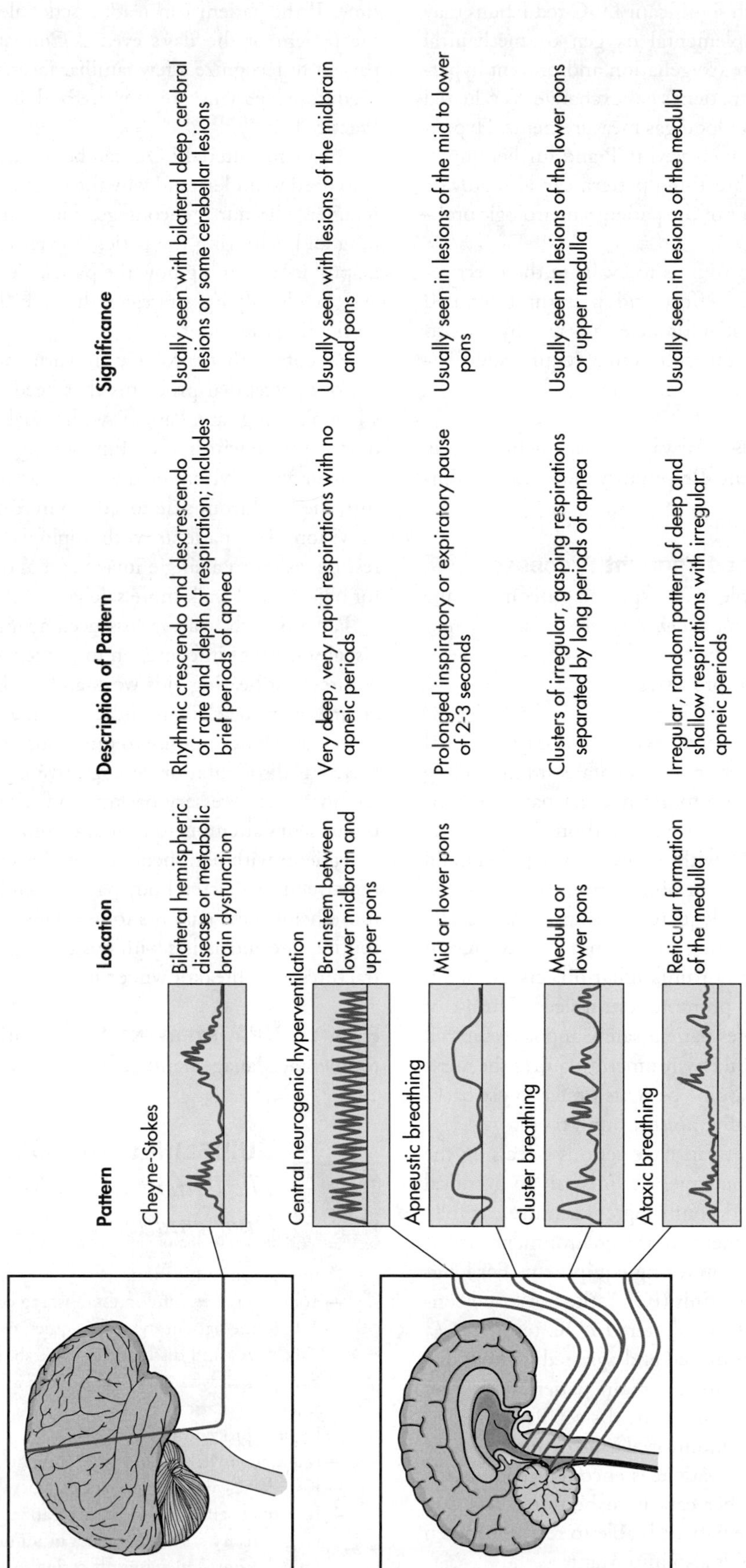

Pattern
Location
Description of Pattern
Significance
Cheyne-Stokes
Bilateral hemispheric disease or metabolic brain dysfunction
Rhythmic crescendo and descrescendo of rate and depth of respiration; includes brief periods of apnea
Usually seen with bilateral deep cerebral lesions or some cerebellar lesions
Central neurogenic hyperventilation
Brainstem between lower midbrain and upper pons
Very deep, very rapid respirations with no apneic periods
Usually seen with lesions of the midbrain and pons
Apneustic breathing
Mid or lower pons
Prolonged inspiratory or expiratory pause of 2-3 seconds
Usually seen in lesions of the mid to lower pons
Cluster breathing
Medulla or lower pons
Clusters of irregular, gasping respirations separated by long periods of apnea
Usually seen in lesions of the lower pons or upper medulla
Ataxic breathing
Reticular formation of the medulla
Irregular, random pattern of deep and shallow respirations with irregular apneic periods
Usually seen in lesions of the medulla

Figure 48-5 Abnormal respiratory patterns with corresponding level of central nervous system activity.

breathing every hour, and encourages the use of incentive spirometers when feasible. Patients with significant LOC reductions may hypoventilate and require supplemental oxygen or mechanical ventilation to maintain adequate oxygenation and prevent hypercapnea. The effectiveness of the patient's gas exchange is evaluated with pulse oximetry and arterial blood gas measurements. Hypoxia or hypercapnea may result in increased ICP and further impair the patient's LOC. Changes in breathing pattern can also provide insight into the nature and extent of the patient's neurologic problems (see Figure 48-5).

The nurse auscultates breath sounds to evaluate the effectiveness of the patient's respiratory effort and pattern. Decreased breath sounds indicate the potential for atelectasis and hypoventilation. Patients with swallowing difficulties may require additional precautions to prevent aspiration at mealtimes.

RELATED NIC INTERVENTIONS. Airway Management, Airway Suctioning, Cough Enhancement, Respiratory Monitoring, Ventilation Assistance

Nursing Diagnosis: Disturbed Thought Processes

OUTCOMES. A common example of an expected outcome for the patient with a diagnosis of *disturbed thought processes* is:
Patient will:

- Maintain coherent thought processes.

NURSING INTERVENTIONS. Patients with sensory-perceptual alterations can easily misinterpret environmental stimuli, leading to confusion. The nurse takes care to arrange the patient's environment to minimize confusion or altered thought processes. Large-print calendars and clocks within view can help maintain time orientation. Familiar pictures or objects from home provide a link to family and friends. Adequate lighting helps visually impaired patients see who is entering the room and may prevent the misinterpretation of shadows or unfamiliar objects. At night, lights are kept to a minimum to promote restful sleep. The use of low-wattage night lights promotes patient safety and access to call bells. The need for a quiet, restful environment requires the nurse to eliminate unnecessary noise. Some patients prefer to use background music to "drown out" other noise around them.

The critical care environment can have serious effects on the patient with altered LOC. An emergent admission to a critical care unit can be frightening and confusing. The nurse carefully explains all of the unfamiliar elements in the environment such as infusion pumps or beeps from monitoring equipment. For long-term patients in the intensive care unit (ICU), the noise and constant stimulation can lead to a type of altered LOC termed *ICU psychosis.* The patient becomes confused and agitated without discernible physiologic cause. The nurse alters the patient's care plan to include adequate periods of uninterrupted sleep at night, and meaningless stimulation such as monitor alarms or intercom use is eliminated when possible. The patient is encouraged to decide how and when some of his or her care is to be done, and care activities are grouped so that the patient is able to rest in between activities. Adequate pain control is also important.

Communicating with a confused patient requires patience and consistency. The nurse speaks quietly and slowly, using simple sentences or phrases to explain all care. It is important to speak to patients before touching them and to request only one action at a time. If the patient can read, a schedule of activities can remind the patient of the day's events. Consistent caregivers allow the patient to recognize a few familiar faces. Guidelines for caring for a confused patient are summarized in the Guidelines for Safe Practice box.

A patient's altered LOC can be frightening to family members, who need to understand why the patient is behaving in a confused manner. The nurse encourages the family to participate in planning and delivering the patient's care. Family members are often helpful in explaining how the patient reacts to unfamiliar settings and in identifying strategies that are likely to be successful in reorienting the patient.

Patients with neurologic impairments may have a variety of sensory-perceptual problems that need to be taken into account when planning care. Patients with visual field deficits need to have objects placed within their functioning field of vision and learn to compensate for visual field losses. The nurse instructs patients to turn the head from side to side to maximize the functional range of vision. For patients with diplopia, alternating eye patches restore vision to a single image and allow patients to read, reach for objects, and walk more safely.

Patients with hearing loss need adaptive devices or additional visual sources of information to participate in self-care. The nurse ensures that hearing aids work and are fitted properly. Notations are made on the chart to indicate that a patient is hard of hearing so that a lack of response to questions or instructions is not interpreted as disorientation or cognitive impairment. The nurse also eliminates unnecessary background noise that can interfere with the patient's attempts to hear and communicate.

Patients with peripheral sensory losses such as hemiparesis may not attend to affected body parts, a condition termed *neglect.* The nurse helps these patients to use their affected extremities during routine care and assists with positioning the limbs to prevent contractures, skin breakdown, or injury.

RELATED NIC INTERVENTIONS. Delirium Management, Environmental Management: Safety; Reality Orientation

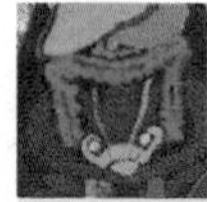

GUIDELINES FOR SAFE PRACTICE

The Patient With Confusion or Disorientation

- Promote communication.
  —Touch may be useful in establishing communication.
  —Talk to the patient in a calm, quiet, unhurried voice.
  —Talk slowly and distinctly and use short sentences.
  —Face patient when talking and stay within conversational range.
- Promote orientation.
  —Explain procedures in advance.
  —Maintain a well-lighted environment.
  —Keep large calendar and clock in view.
  —Introduce self when caring for patient.
  —Keep sensory stimulation to a minimum.
  —Provide consistency in staff caring for patient.
  —Keep decision making to a minimum.
- Support family.

Nursing Diagnosis: Risk for Injury

OUTCOMES. Common examples of expected outcomes for the patient with a diagnosis of *risk for injury* are:

Patient will:

- Avoid injury.
- Maintain body temperature within normal limits.
- Maintain highest possible degree of mobility with the use of assistive devices and the assistance of others.

NURSING INTERVENTIONS. Numerous nursing activities are geared toward providing a safe environment for the patient experiencing altered LOC. The nurse inspects the patient's environment for equipment that may present a hazard. Call signals are left within reach, and the patient is instructed on how to use them. Adaptive call signals are available for patients with limited motor abilities. Seizure precautions may be appropriate for patients with a history or risk of seizures.

Patients with severely reduced LOC are unable to communicate that they are too cold or too warm, so the nurse must ensure the patient maintains a stable body temperature. Patients with neurologic impairment can experience fever and/or hypothermia as a result of damage to the hypothalamus. If a patient becomes hypothermic, the nurse carefully uses heat lamps, warmed blankets, and increased room temperature to help restore the patient's temperature to the normal range. Management of fever may involve antipyretics, tepid baths, lowered room temperature, and careful assessment for physical sources of infection.

Patients with limited mobility face other safety risks. The nurse positions patients who are unable to move themselves and performs range-of-motion exercises to prevent contractures and other musculoskeletal complications. Helping patients change position at least every 2 hours enhances circulation and venous return. The nurse ensures that clothing, bed linens, and body position do not constrict circulation. Immobile patients develop impaired circulation at dependent sites. Passive or active range-of-motion exercise is implemented to support blood flow and restore circulation to pressure-occluded or dependent sites. Intermittent compression sleeves may be applied to prevent venous pooling and thrombus formation in the legs.

Changes of position also help patients who are unable to move themselves to mobilize pulmonary secretions. Getting patients out of bed and assisting them with ambulation supports weight bearing on the long bones and slows the bone demineralization associated with bed rest. An upright posture also improves the patient's ability to interact with the environment. The physical therapist may recommend specific activities to promote mobility and supply adaptive equipment, such as walkers, canes, or wheelchairs, that can increase the patient's independence.

The bed is kept in a low position. Some patients may need a "seat belt" or slide cushion to prevent them from slipping or falling out of chairs. Confused patients may attempt to climb out of bed or wander off, but physical restraints are used only as a last resort. Restraints have been consistently shown to increase patient agitation and actually increase the risk of injury.

The nurse provides regular opportunities for patients to meet elimination needs. Helping patients remain out of bed as much as desired may prevent them from trying to get up on their own. This behavior cannot always be prevented but is sometimes a response to muscle aches, thirst, the need to urinate, or simple loneliness. Frequent visits and monitoring are essential. Simple reorientation and reassurance can be calming for agitated or confused patients. The nurse uses touch therapeutically with patients who respond positively to it. For the patient who wanders, electronic monitoring systems can alert the staff when the patient moves outside the monitored area.

Patients with altered LOC are prone to skin breakdown. Agitated patients may accidentally abrade their skin or bruise themselves if not protected. Skin must be kept clean and free of excess moisture but well lubricated to prevent dryness. Patients on prolonged bed rest or with actual skin breakdown are placed on special pressure relief mattresses. Adequate nutrition and hydration contribute greatly to the maintenance of skin integrity. The nurse carefully assesses the patient's skin during hygiene activities and protects the skin from friction and shearing forces when helping the patient change positions or get out of bed. The nurse gives special attention to the skin in the axilla and perineal area and any skin folds that might retain moisture, such as under the breast. These areas are particularly vulnerable to breakdown and infection with yeast and other organisms.

Patients with altered LOC may be unable to meet their own self-care needs. Some patients may require simple assistance with activities of daily living (ADLs), such as supervision or verbal cueing during bathing or dressing. Others require the complete support of the nursing staff to complete hygiene activities. Engaging in self-care is an important part of rehabilitation. This may include bathing, hair shampooing, mouth care, eye care, and nail care.

RELATED NIC INTERVENTIONS. Environmental Management: Safety; Fall Prevention; Positioning; Skin Surveillance; Surveillance: Safety

Nursing Diagnosis: Imbalanced Nutrition: Less Than Body Requirements

OUTCOMES. A common example of an expected outcome for the patient with a diagnosis of *imbalanced nutrition: less than body requirements* is:

Patient will:

- Consume adequate balanced nutrients to maintain a stable body weight.

NURSING INTERVENTIONS. Decreased LOC makes it difficult for patients to meet their ongoing nutritional needs, particularly if they also have swallowing difficulties. Adequate nutrition is essential to prevent infection and protect tissue integrity. The nurse keeps records of the patient's food and fluid intake so that accurate assessments can be made. The nurse works with the dietitian to determine the best diet to meet patient needs. The patient may simply need reminders to take small bites and swallow carefully, but if the patient is unable to maintain an adequate oral intake without aspiration, enteral feedings may be started. Nasogastric tubes can be used for short-term feeding. If long-term nutritional support is anticipated, a gastrostomy, percutaneous endoscopic gastrostomy, or jejunostomy tube is placed (see Chapter 42). Daily or weekly weights are obtained to monitor the patient's status.

Sensory loss on the face can affect the patient's ability to chew and swallow. Food or medications can unknowingly become pocketed in the cheek and later cause choking or aspiration. The nurse carefully checks the patient's mouth after meals and medication administration and removes any pocketed material.

RELATED NIC INTERVENTIONS. Enteral Tube Feeding, Nutrition Management, Nutritional Monitoring

Nursing Diagnosis: Risk for Constipation

OUTCOMES. A common example of an expected outcome for the patient with a diagnosis of *risk for constipation* is:
Patient will:

- Pass soft formed stool without straining, daily or every other day.

NURSING INTERVENTIONS. Patients with altered LOC need to be started on a bowel program, especially if they are on bed rest, which increases the risk of constipation or impaction. The nurse uses preventive measures such as stool softeners, fiber added to tube feedings or diet, and additional hydration to prevent constipation. The patient is offered the bedpan or placed on a commode at times close to the patient's usual time for elimination, such as in the morning after breakfast. If constipation is suspected, the nurse checks the patient for impaction and gently removes the stool if needed. Mild laxatives or suppositories can also be used to treat constipation, but enemas are used only as a last resort because they can seriously disrupt the normal elimination pattern.

The need for communication among the nursing staff about the patient's bowel function is especially important. Bowel movements are carefully recorded as to time, amount, and consistency to enable the nurse to make appropriate judgments about the need for timely intervention to support elimination.

RELATED NIC INTERVENTIONS. Constipation/Impaction Management, Medication Management

Nursing Diagnosis: Risk for Impaired Urinary Elimination

OUTCOMES. A common example of an expected outcome for a patient with a diagnosis of *risk for impaired urinary elimination* is:
Patient will:

- Maintain a regular pattern of urinary elimination without evidence of infection.

NURSING INTERVENTIONS. Indwelling catheters may be used in the acute care setting if frequent monitoring of urinary output is required, but they are avoided for long-term management, if possible, because of the high risk of chronic infection. A condom catheter can be used for incontinent male patients, but female patients may require the ongoing use of an indwelling catheter. Some neurologic conditions cause urinary retention and necessitate the use of either an indwelling catheter or an intermittent catheterization program. When patients are able to communicate their needs, the nurse attempts to establish a regular schedule for bladder emptying that eliminates the need for catheters or diapers.

RELATED NIC INTERVENTIONS. Urinary Elimination Management, Urinary Incontinence Care

Patient/Family Teaching. Altered LOC may leave patients with motor, sensory, or cognitive deficits that create safety concerns and significantly interfere with their ability to be independent and resume their normal lifestyle. Patient and family teaching is ongoing throughout the patient's hospitalization and intensifies as the time approaches for discharge home or to an extended care facility.

The nurse explains the hospital routines and surroundings to the patient and family to make the environment seem less foreign. The family is directed to a quiet place where they can sit, make phone calls, and wait while the patient is being cared for. When family members are in the patient's room, the nurse provides chairs and encourages them to touch and talk to the patient. Some institutions encourage families to participate in care delivery.

The patient's educational background and current cognitive abilities affect his or her ability to be involved in the education process. The patient and family need education about the diagnostic process and results, treatment options, and how the treatment plan will be carried out. As care is delivered, the nurse updates the patient and family on the progress of the treatments and any changes in the care plan. Patients with altered LOC may be unaware of the severity of their situation, but the family is acutely aware and thus often anxious and stressed. The family may also need to make decisions about the patient's care, for which they may feel unprepared. The nurse listens to family members' concerns and assesses their ability to cope. The nurse clarifies which family member will assist the patient with health care decisions and what information can and should be shared with other family members. The nurse explores what information the family needs to make current decisions and asks whether the patient has a living will or advance directive that can be used to guide decision making.

It is also important to find out what resources the family uses for support, including extended family, neighbors, co-workers, and friends. The nurse ensures that the family is aware of other available resources, such as chaplains, social workers, and community groups appropriate to the patient's illness. Discharge planning involves identifying community resources and making appropriate referrals to ensure continuity of care. If the family will be providing home care, the nurse develops a teaching plan to ensure that they have adequate knowledge and skills before discharge. Arranging needed services takes time, and the nurse must anticipate discharge to allow sufficient time for planning, teaching, and referral. Contact names and phone numbers are provided to ensure the family has ready access to needed supports.

EVALUATION

To evaluate the effectiveness of nursing interventions, compare patient behaviors with those stated in the expected patient outcomes.

RELATED NOC OUTCOMES. Bowel Elimination, Cognitive Orientation, Falls Occurrence, Neurological Status: Consciousness; Respiratory Status: Airway Patency, Respiratory Status: Ventilation; Risk Control, Urinary Elimination

GERONTOLOGIC CONSIDERATIONS

The healthy older adult should not experience memory loss, dementia, depression, or any decrease in LOC. All these changes are unexpected and should be investigated and treated just as they would be in a younger individual. Older adults do experience a reduction in the speed of their reflexes, and they are prone to decreases in vision and hearing that may affect their ability to interact with those around them. These sensory losses are usually treatable and need to be addressed so the patient can continue to participate fully in education and self-care activities.

The older adult is more likely to experience comorbid medical problems and therefore is more likely to be taking multiple medications. Medication interactions or sensitivity to side effects are potential causes for some alterations in cognition and awareness.

Increased Intracranial Pressure

Etiology and Epidemiology. An increase in **intracranial pressure** (ICP) is a pathologic process common to many neurologic conditions (Box 48-7). The intracranial volume is composed of brain tissue (85%), intracranial blood (5%), and cerebrospinal fluid (CSF) (10%). An increase in the volume of any of these contents, singly or in combination, results in an increase in ICP because the cranial vault is rigid and nonexpandable. Any lesion that increases one or more of the intracranial contents is considered a space-occupying lesion.[15] Increased ICP is a common concern with a number of neurologic conditions, but no data are available concerning its incidence or distribution.

Pathophysiology. The cranial vault is a rigid, closed compartment. The intracranial contents of brain, blood, and CSF fully occupy the vault and exist in a dynamic equilibrium under normal conditions. The Monro-Kellie hypothesis states that conditions that increase one or more of the intracranial contents must cause a reciprocal decrease in the remaining contents or ICP will increase.[1] As the intracranial volume increases, compensatory mechanisms take place. CSF-filled spaces can be compressed and CSF redistributed to the lumbar cistern to reduce intracranial CSF volumes. Intracranial blood vessels, especially the veins, can be compressed by surrounding brain tissue and reduce intracranial blood volume.

These compensatory mechanisms initially are able to accommodate a growing intracranial volume without significant increases in ICP, but when the volume within the skull overwhelms the compensatory mechanisms, ICP begins to rise. The volume-pressure curve in Figure 48-6 shows that small changes in volume initially cause only small increases in pressure. However, as compensatory mechanisms fail, continued increases in volume cause dramatic increases in ICP. A normal ICP is between 0 and 15 mm Hg; pressures over 20 mm Hg are considered "increased."

As pressure within the skull increases, the cerebral arteries and veins become increasingly compressed, which reduces cerebral perfusion. Inadequate perfusion initiates a vicious cycle, causing the partial pressure of carbon dioxide (PCO_2) to increase and the partial pressure of oxygen (PO_2) and the pH to decrease.[17] Cerebral arterioles have the ability to autoregulate, dilating or constricting as needed to maintain a constant blood supply to the brain. The increasing PCO_2 or decreasing pH associated with decreased perfusion causes vasodilation of the cerebral blood vessels and increases the intracranial blood volume, which contributes to further increases in ICP.

Cerebral perfusion pressure (CPP) is a parameter used to monitor the adequacy of blood flow to the brain in the face of increased ICP. The systemic blood pressure needs to be high enough to overcome the ICP and deliver adequate amounts of oxygen and glucose to brain tissues. The CPP is measured by subtracting ICP from the mean arterial pressure (MAP):

$$CPP = MAP - ICP$$

The CPP is kept above 70 mm Hg to prevent cerebral ischemia. **Autoregulation** is operative as long as the MAP is between 50 and 150 mm Hg and the brain's metabolic environment is normal. Severe anoxia and hypotensive states cause a failure in autoregulation, allowing the brain's blood supply to experience the wide variations characteristic of systemic blood pressure. Autoregulation

Box 48-7 Common Causes of Increased Intracranial Pressure

- Edema from surgery, infarction, lesion, or injury
- Subdural or epidural hematoma
- Intracerebral or subarachnoid hematoma
- Brain tumor
- Abscess or infection
- Hydrocephalus
- Head trauma
- Status epilepticus

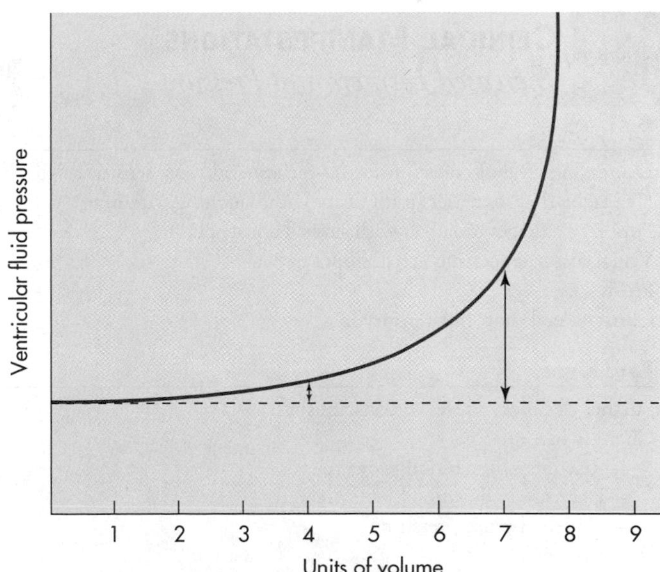

Figure 48-6 Intracranial volume-pressure curve. Note that for the addition of any given unit of volume *(horizontal axis)*, a markedly different rise in pressure occurs, depending on location on the curve (flat or steep portion). Thus adding 1 unit of volume at second arrow results in nearly four times the increase in pressure from same volume at first arrow.

fails at high ICP ranges because the vessels cannot effectively dilate against the pressure of the surrounding brain tissues.

The actual brain structures can also be affected by increased ICP. The dura mater surrounds the brain and divides it into compartments within the skull. Edema or space-occupying lesions may cause brain tissue to shift or herniate. Subfalcial, or cingulate, **herniation** occurs when the brain is forced under the falx cerebri that separates the cerebral hemispheres. Uncal herniation occurs when the uncal portions of the temporal lobes shift over the edge of the tentorium cerebelli. Transforaminal herniation occurs when the brainstem is forced downward through the foramen magnum.

Increased ICP produces multiple signs and symptoms (see Clinical Manifestations box), but decreased LOC is the earliest and most sensitive sign. Altered blood flow and an altered cerebral metabolic environment reduce the brain's ability to respond to stimuli (see earlier discussion of altered LOC). Headache is often an early nonspecific symptom of increased ICP. It is thought to result from tension on intracranial blood vessels. Vomiting may occur, but it is more common in children.

Pupillary responses are controlled by the oculomotor nerve (cranial nerve III), which carries the motor fibers for pupil constriction and eyelid opening. The oculomotor nerve becomes severely compressed when herniation of the uncal portion of the temporal lobe occurs or is imminent. If the nerve is only moderately compressed or stretched, pupil dilation with slowed constriction may be seen. A pupil that is fixed and dilated sometimes is referred to as a blown pupil. Dilation of the ipsilateral pupil occurs when the herniation is limited to one hemisphere. If ICP continues to rise and both hemispheres herniate, bilateral pupil dilation and fixation occur.

The optic nerve attaches to the eye at the optic disc. The meninges surround both the optic nerve and its attachment to the eye. As ICP increases, the resulting pressure is transmitted to the eyes through the CSF in the subarachnoid space and to the optic disc, causing papilledema (choked disc). This may be a late sign of increased ICP. Other visual acuity changes are related to pressure on or shifting of optic pathways within the brain.

The effect of ICP on blood pressure and pulse is variable. Ischemia in the vasomotor center excites vasoconstrictor fibers throughout the body, causing an increase in systolic blood pressure. The vasomotor center also sends parasympathetic impulses via the vagus nerve to slow the heart rate. A rising systolic blood pressure, widened pulse pressure, and slow heart rate are referred to as Cushing's response and are classic indicators of increased ICP. If the pressure on the brainstem is severe, the vasomotor center is no longer able to function. A drop in blood pressure and an increase in heart rate are seen as the patient's condition continues to deteriorate.[15]

Herniation also produces respiratory dysrhythmias that correspond to the level of brainstem compression (see Figure 48-5). An irregular respiratory pattern or periods of apnea are particularly significant. Cushing's triad adds the symptom of slowed respirations to the bradycardia and rising systolic blood pressure that are already present.[20] Patients with decreasing LOC may have difficulty keeping the airway clear and exhibit shallow respirations that worsen the hypoxia or hypercarbia, which, in turn, worsens the cycle of vasodilation and increased ICP.

Failure of the thermoregulatory center is a late sign of increased ICP. The most common manifestation of this failure is a fever without a clearly identifiable source of infection. Hyperthermia, in turn, increases the metabolic needs of the compromised brain tissues and further increases ICP.

The rising pressure compresses the motor and sensory tracts between the primary motor and sensory areas in the frontal and parietal lobes and leads to contralateral loss of motor and sensory function. When disruptions to motor pathways become severe, the patient may exhibit posturing (see p. 1382). Motor inhibitory fibers from the frontal lobes are blocked, resulting in hyperactive deep tendon reflexes. Damage to the corticospinal tracts also causes a positive Babinski's reflex.

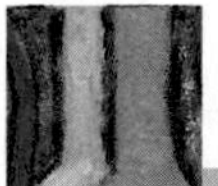

Clinical Manifestations
Increased Intracranial Pressure

Early Signs

Decreasing level of consciousness—earliest and most sensitive sign
Headache that increases in intensity with coughing, straining
Pupillary changes: dilation with slowed constriction
Visual disturbances such as diplopia
Ptosis
Contralateral motor or sensory losses

Late Signs

Further declines in level of consciousness
Changes in vital signs
- Rise in systolic blood pressure
- Decrease in diastolic blood pressure
- Widened pulse pressure
- Slow pulse
- Respiratory dysrhythmias
  - Shallow, slowed respirations
  - Irregular patterns or periods of apnea

Hiccups
Fever without a clear source of infection
Vomiting (more common in children)
Decerebrate or decorticate posturing

ARE YOU READY?

What is the cerebral perfusion pressure of the patient with blood pressure of 140/80 mm Hg, mean arterial pressure of 100 mm Hg, and intracranial pressure of 20 mm Hg?

1. 40 mm Hg
2. 80 mm Hg
3. 120 mm Hg
4. 140 mm Hg

Collaborative Care Management. The nature of the underlying disease process largely determines the outcome for a patient with increased ICP. The collaborative care of the patient is aimed at controlling and reducing the increased ICP and preventing neurologic damage. A computed tomography (CT) scan of the head can demonstrate the structural changes associated with increased ICP and locate space-occupying lesions and sites of edema or bleeding. A reduction in the size of the cisterns, CSF-filled spaces located at the base of the skull, indicates that CSF is being shunted out of the skull as a compensatory mechanism. Any herniation of brain tissue can also be readily identified on CT scans.[20]

The diagnosis of increased ICP is most accurately made when the pressure is measured by one of several available devices. However, the diagnosis can also be made through careful neurologic examination and ongoing assessment. Several methods have been developed to directly measure ICP (Figures 48-7 and 48-8). An intraventricular catheter, also known as a ventriculostomy, can be inserted through the brain and directly into one of the lateral ventricles by means of a small hole drilled into the skull. The catheter is connected to a sterile drainage system with a three-way stopcock

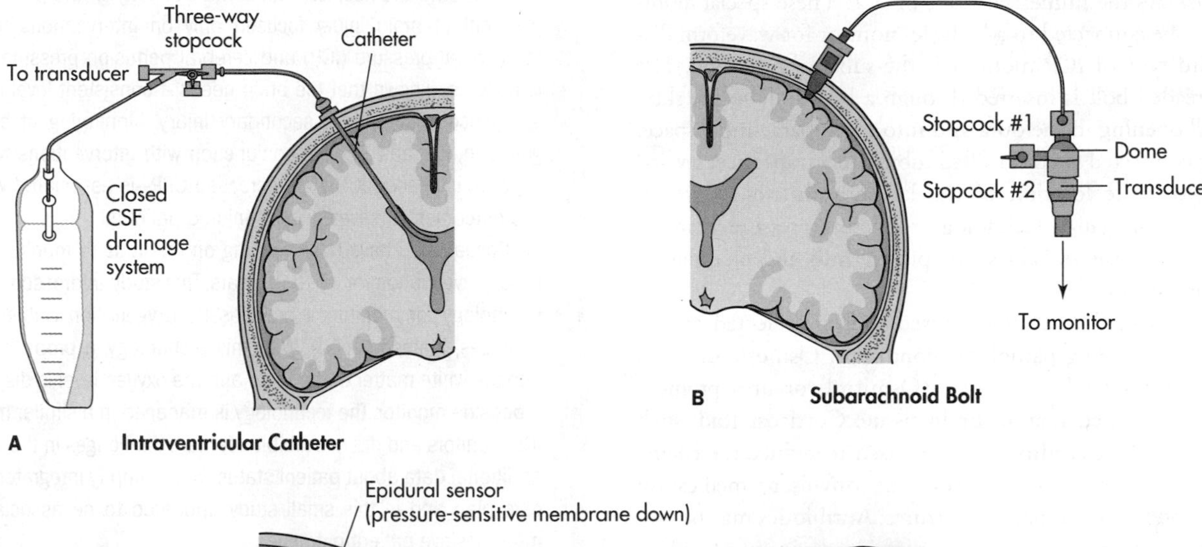

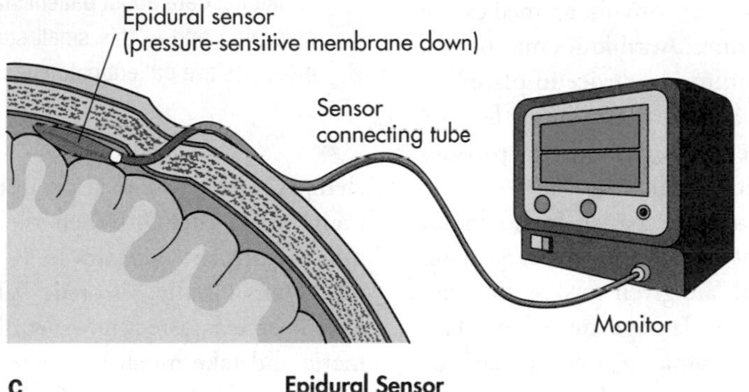

Figure 48-7 **A,** Intraventricular catheter monitoring system with a closed cerebrospinal fluid *(CSF)* drainage system. **B,** Subarachnoid bolt monitoring system. **C,** Epidural monitoring system.

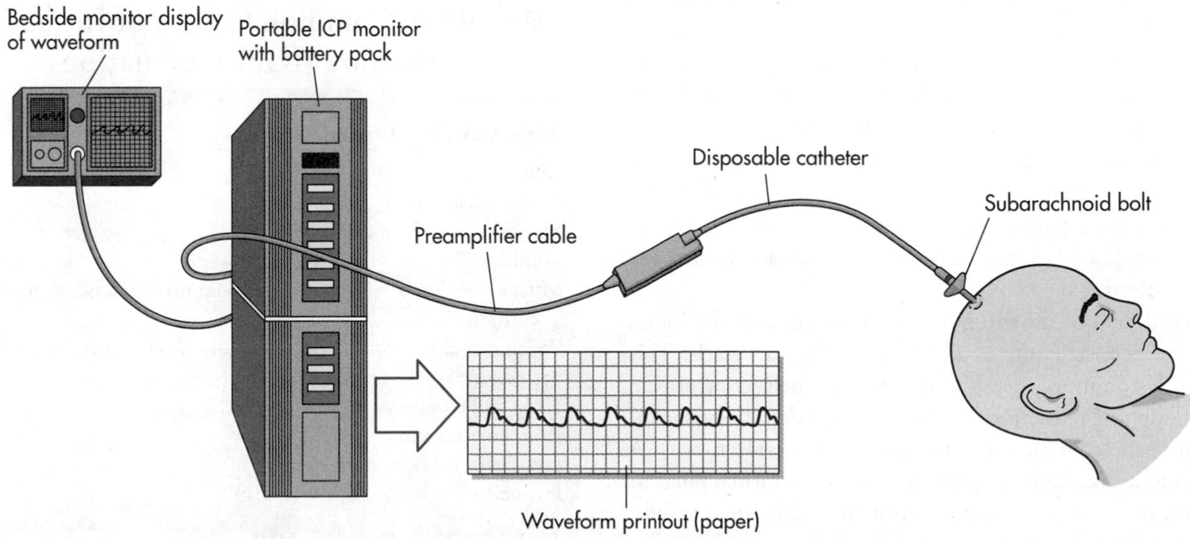

Figure 48-8 Fiberoptic monitoring system using subarachnoid bolt *(patient)*, disposable catheter connected to preamplifier cable with continuous visual intracranial pressure *(ICP)* waveform display on bedside monitor *(upper left)*, and continuous digital readout of ICP *(lower monitor)* with ICP waveform printout.

that allows simultaneous drainage of CSF and monitoring of pressures via a transducer connected to a bedside monitor. Another approach uses a fiberoptic monitor. The fiberoptic device measures changes in the amount of light reflected from a pressure-sensitive diaphragm in the catheter tip. This device can be placed directly into the brain parenchyma, subarachnoid space, epidural space, or ventricle. The fiberoptic cable is connected to a precalibrated monitor that displays the numerical value of ICP. These special monitors can also be connected to a bedside monitor for waveform display. A third type of ICP monitor is the subarachnoid bolt. The hollow, threaded bolt is inserted through a burr hole in the skull into a small opening in the dura and into the subarachnoid space. The bolt is connected via fluid-filled tubing to a transducer leveled at the approximate location of the lateral ventricles. A fourth device uses strain gauge technology to detect pressure changes. Thin, pressure-sensitive cables are placed into the epidural or parenchymal spaces.

Medications used to treat increased ICP are selected on the basis of the underlying pathologic condition. Osmotic diuretics such as intravenous (IV) mannitol (Osmitrol) or urea promote fluid removal from edematous brain tissue. Corticosteroids such as dexamethasone (Decadron) may be used to reduce the edema associated with tumors or abscesses. Anticonvulsant medication may also be prescribed to prevent seizures. Antibiotics may be prescribed if the patient has an ICP monitoring device in place.[15,20] Opioids and sedative medications are used cautiously because they have respiratory depressant effects and may alter the patient's ability to cooperate with a neurologic examination.

Barbiturate coma is occasionally used for patients who do not respond to conventional management of elevated ICP. Large doses of barbiturates, usually pentobarbital, are given to slow the cerebral metabolic rate and minimize the damage caused by ICP-induced ischemia. The barbiturate coma is accompanied by numerous side effects, such as hypotension, that may require vasoactive drug treatment (e.g., dopamine infusion).[15] The high doses of barbiturate also obscure the accuracy of any neurologic assessment for the duration of the coma.

Surgical interventions are also designed to correct the underlying cause of the increase in ICP. Mass lesions such as tumors, abscesses, or hematomas are surgically removed if possible. Excess CSF can be removed with a surgically placed ventriculostomy. If hydrocephalus becomes a chronic problem, a shunt from the lateral ventricle to the peritoneum can be placed for long-term CSF drainage. On rare occasions a decompressive craniectomy may be performed to remove part of the skull and allow the edematous brain to expand. The bone can be replaced at a later date after the edema has resolved.[1]

Hyperventilation of the intubated patient decreases the $PaCO_2$ and causes vasoconstriction of the cerebral blood vessels. This intervention is commonly used to temporarily help control ICP. However, if ongoing reductions in $PaCO_2$ are needed, the vasoconstriction can lead to brain tissue ischemia (see Research box). A balance is sought that keeps the $PaCO_2$ in the low-normal range of 30 to 35 mm Hg to prevent hypercapnea and subsequent vasodilation without reducing the $PaCO_2$ to a level that results in vasoconstriction-induced brain ischemia.[17]

Control of activity plays an important role in the treatment of increased ICP. The pressure inside the skull is dynamic and changes in response to shifts in blood flow, CSF movement, and brain tissue edema. When the compensatory mechanisms are intact, transient increases in ICP are brief and baseline normal values are rapidly restored. When compensatory mechanisms have been exhausted, however, the rise in ICP may be more dramatic and take much longer to return to normal. The patient's ICP response to any and all activities and treatments is therefore monitored, and activities are restricted as needed. Box 48-8 lists common causes of ICP fluctuations.

Research

Littlejohns LR, Bader MK, March K: Brain tissue oxygen monitoring in severe brain injury, part I, Research and usefulness in critical care, *Crit Care Nurse* 23(4):17-22, 24-25, 2003.

Each year about 1.5 million cases of traumatic brain injury are reported in the United States. Of those, 50,000 persons die and 80,000 leave the hospital with some disability. In the past the management of brain injury focused only on interventions to control intracranial pressure (ICP) and cerebral perfusion pressure (CPP). It is now also known that the brain needs a consistent level of oxygen and glucose to prevent secondary injury. Monitoring of brain oxygenation, ICP, and CPP—in conjunction with interventions to prevent hypoxia, increased ICP, and decreased CPP—is associated with positive outcomes for severely head-injured patients.

Researchers have been working on methods to monitor for brain tissue oxygenation for 15 to 20 years. This study addressed the LICOX technology for monitoring brain tissue oxygenation (Integra NeuroSciences, Plainsboro, NJ). With this technology, a probe is inserted into the white matter of the brain and the oxygen level is displayed on a bedside monitor. The technology is managed in a similar manner to ICP monitors and did not exhibit new care challenges in the study. The additional data about patient status was promptly integrated into the care plan and in this small study appeared to be associated with more positive patient outcomes.

Box 48-8 Common Causes of Intracranial Pressure (ICP) Fluctuations

Activities That Increase ICP

- Coughing
- Airway obstruction, suctioning
- Valsalva's maneuver, defecation
- Vomiting
- Muscle exertion or tension: range-of-motion exercise, isometric exercise
- Position changes (prone, Trendelenburg, neck flexion, acute hip flexion)
- Stress and emotional upset
- Pain, noxious stimuli
- Hypercapnia (PCO_2 over 45 mm Hg)
- Hypoxia (PO_2 less than 50 mm Hg)

Activities That Decrease ICP

- Inspiration
- Central nervous system depressant medications

Nurses carefully time and coordinate the patient's care to prevent prolonged increases in ICP. Activities such as bathing and position changes may need to be alternated with rest periods to allow time for the patient's ICP to return to baseline.[15] Endotracheal suctioning contributes to increases in ICP because of increases in intrathoracic pressure and changes in oxygen and carbon dioxide levels. Preoxygenation and hyperventilation before suctioning the ventilated patient with increased ICP helps minimize this problem (see Guidelines for Safe Practice box).

The patient's neck is kept in proper alignment to promote venous drainage through the jugular veins (see Research box).[20] In some cases a cervical collar may be used to maintain the alignment. The head of the bed may also be elevated to promote venous drainage from the skull.[15] Activities that increase intrathoracic or intraabdominal pressure, such as coughing, straining to have a bowel movement, or moving in bed, may also increase ICP by interfering with venous drainage from the brain. These activities are prevented or avoided if possible. Involuntary patient responses such as shivering, vomiting, agitation, or abnormal posturing also contribute to increased ICP. If increases in ICP become severe during these activities and do not promptly return to baseline, the patient may need to be sedated to decrease activity.

PATIENT/FAMILY TEACHING. The presence or risk of ICP creates a frightening and confusing situation for both patients and families. Patients are more likely to cooperate with the frequent neurologic checks and activity restrictions if the nurse explains the reason for them. Patient and family teaching includes information

Research

Fan J: Effect of backrest position on intracranial pressure and cerebral perfusion pressure in individuals with brain injury: a systematic review, *J Neurosci Nurs* 36(5):278-288, 2004.

Head elevation is a common procedure used by nurses to reduce intracranial pressure (ICP) for brain-injured patients in neurologic intensive care units. Raising the head of the bed promotes intracranial venous return and increases cerebrospinal fluid drainage from the head. However, raising the head of the bed for patients who have experienced prolonged flat bed rest can be detrimental, since prolonged supination can impair cerebral autoregulation. Impaired cerebral autoregulation is commonly associated with conditions such as traumatic brain injury. Because of this concern, nurses are questioning the appropriateness of this common procedure to reduce ICP.

This study reviewed current literature addressing the effects of changing the back rest position, and the degree of elevation, on ICP and cerebral perfusion pressure (CPP) in brain-injured patients. The study found that patients with multisystem involvement (other injuries, such as fractures or pneumothorax in addition to brain injury) required vigilant monitoring of ICP and CPP during head elevation. The review of the literature revealed two clinical suggestions for back rest positioning: increasing the head of the bed up to 30 degrees to significantly reduce the ICP, and monitoring CPP during the head-elevation positioning, since head elevation may decrease CPP by decreasing the mean arterial blood pressure. The study recommends future studies to evaluate the effect of the side-lying lateral position on ICP and CPP, especially for brain-injured patients with multisystem involvement.

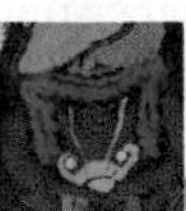

GUIDELINES FOR SAFE PRACTICE *The Patient With Increased Intracranial Pressure*

- Avoid hypotension (systolic blood pressure less than 90 mm Hg) and hypoxia ($Pa{O_2}$ less than 60 mm Hg).
- Elevate head of bed (check to see if spine films have been done and cleared before raising head of bed).
- Avoid jugular venous outflow obstruction. (Keep neck midline, cervical collar or endotracheal tube tape not too tight; check collar frequently when edema is developing.)
- Prevent or instruct patient to avoid coughing, Valsalva's maneuver, hip flexion, high levels of positive end-expiratory pressure.
- Maintain normothermia. Work up and treat fever promptly.
- Prevent seizures. Phenytoin is used to prevent early posttraumatic seizures. Fosphenytoin is a prodrug of phenytoin that causes fewer side effects when given intravenously and may be given in some circumstances.
- Prevent or treat agitation. Search for causes of agitation, such as hypoxia or pain. Sedation with short-acting agents allows for neurologic monitoring. Pharmacologic paralysis may be used if sedation alone is inadequate in controlling agitation that contributes to increased intracranial pressure (ICP).
- Monitor ICP to serve as an indicator of mass effect, to calculate cerebral perfusion pressure (CPP), and to assess effectiveness of interventions. Treatment for high ICP usually begins at 20 mm Hg. Ventriculostomies may be used if the patient has intraventricular blood or hydrocephalus.
- Calculate CPP if an ICP monitor is in use. (CPP = Mean arterial pressure − ICP.) The CPP should be kept above 70 mm Hg to prevent cerebral ischemia. Maintain adequate CPP by using fluid resuscitation, lowering the ICP, or adding vasopressor support to the systemic blood pressure.
- Give mannitol, an osmotic diuretic, to treat cerebral edema. This is usually given in bolus doses of 0.25 to 1.0 g/kg body weight. Monitor for serum osmolarity of greater than 310 to 320 mOsm/L and for the effect of fluid and electrolyte shifts. Mannitol can contribute to dehydration and to decreased blood pressure and CPP.
- Surgical evacuation of hematomas or skull fracture repair may be necessary. On rare occasions a piece of skull may be removed and left off to allow the brain more room to swell (craniectomy).
- Hyperventilation may be used initially in resuscitation when information about ICP is not readily available, and it may be used acutely for herniation. In general, ventilated patients have their settings adjusted to keep Pco_2 between 30 and 35 mm Hg. Hyperventilating (and hyperoxygenating) patients before, during, and after endotracheal suctioning is still recommended to reduce the adverse effects of sudden rises in ICP with coughing and suctioning.
- Barbiturates may be used but have significant complications. They work by reducing cerebral metabolic needs and cerebral blood flow. Monitoring of electroencephalogram burst suppression is suggested.

Adapted from Bullock MR, Povlishock JT: Guidelines for the management of severe head injury, *J Neurotrauma* 17(6/7):463-469, 2000.

about the underlying disease process and its relationship to increased ICP. As treatments and medications are introduced, the nurse explains their purpose. When patients are unable to care for themselves, the nurse includes the family in providing care and encourages them to touch and speak quietly with the patient.

Headache

Etiology and Epidemiology. Headache is a common symptom of many neurologic conditions and is also a unique disease process. The National Headache Foundation estimates that more than 45 million Americans suffer from headache.[26] For most people headache is an occasional annoyance, but for a smaller group of persons chronic headaches can be debilitating and seriously compromise activities of daily living and quality of life. Headaches trigger more than 10 million physician office visits each year, and billions of dollars in sick time and lost wages are attributed to headaches.[1]

The International Headache Society classifies headaches as primary or secondary.[15] **Primary headaches** are not associated with any known pathologic cause. Examples of primary headaches include migraine, tension, and cluster headaches. Although the etiology of primary headaches remains unclear, they are believed to result from a complex interplay of muscles, nerves, blood vessels, and pain-producing substances in the brain. Secondary headaches are caused by a known pathologic condition such as meningitis, tumors, or subarachnoid hemorrhage. Another classification system describes headaches as vascular or nonvascular. Migraine and cluster headaches are the major forms of vascular headache, whereas tension headaches are nonvascular.

Migraines, the most common form of headache, occur more often in women than in men. They typically develop in adolescence and young adulthood, and their incidence decreases with aging. Migraines are estimated to affect 18% of women and 6% of men in the United States, with the highest prevalence in the 35- to 45-year-old age-group.[26] They demonstrate a strong hereditary pattern, but no specific genetic link has been identified. Tension headaches can occur at any age and are typically associated with muscle tension and stress. Cluster headaches, one of the most severe forms of head pain, seem to primarily affect young men, often in association with alcohol use.[13] They appear in cycles lasting from 7 days to 12 months with periods of remission between clusters of attacks.

Pathophysiology. The pathophysiology of headache is not fully understood. Although some structures of the head are incapable of sensing pain, the skin, muscles, periosteum of the skull, eyes, ears, nasal cavities and sinuses, meninges, cerebral blood vessels, and sensory cranial nerves are all capable of perceiving and transmitting pain. Headache pain is caused by traction, stretching, or movement of structures or by vasodilation of blood vessels. Serotonin, a powerful vasoconstrictor, is the primary neurotransmitter found in the pathways involved in headache, but its role is not fully understood. Migraines are believed to be caused when cerebral blood vessels initially narrow and blood flow is reduced to some areas of the brain. This initial vasoconstriction is followed by significant vasodilation and neurogenic inflammation of the blood vessels, which triggers release of serotonin and causes the headache. The disturbance appears to be localized in the hypothalamic and limbic systems.[39]

Cluster headaches are thought to be similar to migraines, but the episodes are brief, usually lasting 45 minutes or less. They occur in "cluster" periods of weeks or months. Tension headaches are the result of stress-induced muscle tension over the neck, scalp, and face. Table 48-1 compares the three major types of primary headaches. Specific clinical manifestations vary considerably with the type of headache involved.

Some migraines are preceded by prodromal signs and symptoms, or **auras**. The aura occurs 10 to 30 minutes before the acute attack and may include visual field defects such as flashing lights, photophobia, confusion, and speech or motor-sensory symptoms. Auras typically last an hour or more. These symptoms are associated with the reduction in cerebral blood flow that precedes the vasodilation of the migraine.[13]

Collaborative Care Management. The diagnosis of headache is made primarily from the patient's history. Careful questioning can help rule out secondary headaches caused by other illnesses. Headache caused by subarachnoid hemorrhage is sudden, severe, and generalized. Meningitis headaches are also generalized and severe and may radiate down the neck. Brain tumors can also cause headaches, usually as a result of increased ICP. These headaches may occur more often with straining, coughing, exertion, or sudden movement. Imaging studies such as CT and magnetic resonance imaging (MRI) are not usually performed unless symptoms suggestive of other neurologic processes are present.[7]

Assessment parameters for headache are outlined in Box 48-9. The International Headache Society has developed specific criteria for the diagnosis of primary headache that include an aura, nausea or vomiting, frequency, duration, location, aggravating factors such as exercise, severity of pain, and photophobia.[1,7] Characteristic migraine symptoms include headaches that are preceded by an aura, are slow in onset, and build in intensity. Migraines are also often accompanied by other symptoms such as nausea and vomiting or photophobia (see Table 48-1).

The patient may be asked to keep a headache diary to record the events surrounding the occurrence of headache, such as food intake, sleep pattern, stressful events, stage of the menstrual cycle, and medication use. By providing clues to headache triggers, the diary aids in the design of an individualized care plan to prevent future attacks.[36]

Medications for the treatment of headache fall into two broad categories: symptomatic relief and prevention (Table 48-2). Symptomatic relief for mild, infrequent headache pain can usually be found with analgesic drugs such as ibuprofen (Motrin), propoxyphene (Darvon), or codeine. Triptans, drugs that bind to serotonin receptors on the cranial arteries and cause vasoconstriction, are first-line drugs for treating a migraine headache. They can be given by mouth or subcutaneously and are administered at the first sign or symptom of the attack.[14] Ergot alkaloids are other drugs used to cause cerebral vasoconstriction and abort the attack.[29] Opioids are rarely used for headache pain because of concerns over drug dependency. Antiemetics such as promethazine (Phenergan) or metoclopramide (Reglan) may be given to relieve associated symptoms of nausea and vomiting.

A wide range of other drugs are also used to attempt to prevent migraines. Beta-blockers inhibit vasodilation of cerebral blood vessels and inhibit the reuptake of serotonin. Tricyclic antidepressants may be used to block the uptake of catecholamines and sero-

TABLE 48-1 COMPARISON OF MIGRAINE, CLUSTER, AND TENSION HEADACHES

Onset	Frequency and Duration	Pattern	Prodromal and Associated Symptoms	Treatment
MIGRAINE HEADACHES				
Prevalence highest between 35 and 45 yr Strongly familial More common in women than in men More common in Caucasians	Episodic; tend to occur with stress or hormone changes Last hours to days	Progress slowly, with pain becoming severe; one side of head affected more than other	Prodromal: visual field defects, confusion, paresthesias Associated: nausea, vomiting, fatigue, irritability, photophobia, phenophobia	Ergotamine tartrate Propranolol Nonopioid analgesics Relaxation techniques
CLUSTER HEADACHES				
Early adulthood; precipitated by alcohol or nitrate use Most common in young men, often associated with alcohol use	Episodes clustered together in quick succession for few days or weeks with remissions that last weeks or months Last minutes to a few hours	Intense, throbbing, deep, often unilateral pain; begins in infraorbital region and spreads to head and neck One of most severe neurologic pain syndromes	Prodromal: usually none Associated: flushing, tearing of eyes, nasal stuffiness, sweating, swelling of temporal vessels	Opioid analgesics during acute phase, often given intramuscularly
TENSION HEADACHES				
Often begin during adolescence; related to tension or anxiety No family history Most common type of headache	Episodic; vary with stress Duration variable; can be constant	Dull, constant, aggravating pain; varies in intensity; usually bilateral and involves neck and shoulders; pain may be poorly defined	Prodromal: usually none Associated: sustained contraction of head and neck muscles Not aggravated by activity	Nonopioid analgesics Relaxation techniques Amitriptyline (Elavil)

BOX 48-9 Headache Assessment

- *Headache characteristics:* Time of onset, location, frequency, severity, duration, quality (deep, superficial, steady, throbbing, stabbing, burning); situations or activities that make the headache better or worse
- *Presence of an aura:* Duration, relation to onset of pain
- *Associated symptoms occurring before, during, or after a headache:* Nausea, vomiting, photophobia, visual disturbances, dizziness, incoordination, redness of the eye, facial symptoms (sweating, paleness, flushing), fatigue or sleepiness, mood swings, weakness, paresthesia
- *Potential precipitating factors:* Change in eating pattern, dietary substances (e.g., tyramine, nitrates), relationship to menstrual cycle, sexual intercourse, pregnancy, menopause, psychosocial stressors, change in sleep pattern, weather changes, hot or cold wind, altitude, lights, smog
- *Activities of daily living patterns:* Eating, sleeping, exercise, relaxation
- *Drug history:* Over-the-counter and prescribed headache medications, other medications (nitroglycerin, reserpine, birth control pills, vitamin A, indomethacin, hormone replacement), alcohol and drug use, smoking history
- *Medical history:* Asthma; peptic ulcer; motion sickness; head injury; seizure disorder; sleepwalking; Raynaud's disease; irritable bowel syndrome; infertility; skin problems; pain in neck, head, or throat; abdominal distress; anxiety; depression; insomnia
- *Family history:* History of headache and other medical problems

NOTE: A headache daily diary must include a complete description of each headache, precipitating events, associated symptoms, and, in women, the relationship to the menstrual cycle.

Adapted from Barker E: *Neuroscience nursing,* St Louis, 2002, Mosby.

tonin.[14] Diuretics may be given in low doses to prevent fluid retention, which can lead to migraines.

Other treatments for headache also attempt to prevent the attack or provide symptomatic relief. Patients with migraine or tension headaches can frequently be helped with biofeedback, relaxation techniques, or other behavioral therapy.[16] Massage is also receiving increased attention in headache management (see Research box).[33] For patients who already have a headache, lying quietly in a darkened room and getting additional sleep may offer some relief from pain. Chronic headache is often self-treated using

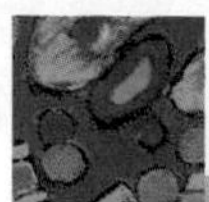

TABLE 48-2
COMMON MEDICATIONS *for Headache*

Drug	Action	Nursing Intervention
Symptomatic Treatment		
Mild analgesics: Aspirin NSAIDs Acetaminophen	Block peripheral prostaglandins, pain transmission	Use only for mild headache pain.
Ergot alkaloids: Ergotamine (Ergostat SL) Ergotamine tartrate plus caffeine (Cafergot) Dihydroergotamine (D.H.E. 45)	Cause cerebral vasoconstriction Decrease pulsation of cranial arteries	Instruct patient to take as soon as migraine symptoms begin. Nausea is common side effect; patients may also need antiemetics. Ergots have cumulative effect; use sparingly and monitor for signs of ergotism—numbness and tingling, weakness, muscle pain. Do not use during pregnancy or for patients with cerebral, coronary, or peripheral vascular disease.
Triptans: Sumatriptan (Imitrex) Naratriptan (Amerge) Zolmitriptan (Zomig)	Serotonin receptor agonist; cause vasoconstriction	Drugs are contraindicated during pregnancy or for those with coronary artery disease. Teach patient to take drug at first sign of headache.
Isometheptene (Midrin)	Weaker vasoconstrictor than the ergots	Use for mild to moderate migraine. Do not use with monoamine oxidase inhibitors or patients with coronary disease.
Prophylaxis		
Beta-blockers: Propranolol (Inderal) Nadolol (Corgard) Atenolol (Tenormin) Timolol (Betimol) Metoprolol (Lopressor)	Inhibit vasodilation and serotonin uptake; propranolol first drug of choice for prophylaxis of migraines	Drugs may cause cardiac dysfunction; monitor for bradycardia, orthostatic hypotension, lethargy, depression.
Tricyclic antidepressants: Amitriptyline (Elavil) Methysergide (Sansert)	Block uptake of serotonin and catecholamines Most effective for migraine-associated tension headaches Alternative if beta-blockers are not tolerated Used for migraine prophylaxis	Drugs may cause dry mouth, drowsiness, and urinary retention. Instruct patients to avoid driving if drowsiness occurs and to maintain a liberal fluid intake.

alternative and complementary therapies, and it is important for the nurse to carefully explore these practices during the patient assessment (see Complementary & Alternative Therapies box).

Once the patient has kept a headache diary, the nurse may be able to help identify specific foods that trigger headache and should be reduced or eliminated from the diet. Diet is believed to be an important trigger. Headache triggers can be confirmed by excluding them from the diet and monitoring the patient for the recurrence of symptoms. Foods that have been shown to cause cerebrovasodilation in migraine patients include nitrites, nitrates, tyramines, alcohol, and monosodium glutamate. Eating small, frequent meals also helps prevent fluctuations in glucose and serotonin levels. Fasting increases serotonin turnover in the brain, which can lead to vasodilation and trigger a headache. Nicotine has also been associated with an increased incidence of headache, despite its vasoconstrictive effects, and the nurse advises the patient to quit smoking, initiates referral to a smoking cessation program, and cautions the patient to avoid the use of nicotine gum or patches. A high salt intake may lead to fluid retention, which is a problem

Research

Quinn C, Chandler C, Moraska A: Massage therapy and frequency of chronic tension headaches, *Am J Pub Health* 92(10):1657-1661, 2002.

Massage therapy is a natural option for treatment of tension headaches. This study looked at the effect of massage therapy on chronic tension headache. Patients received structured massage therapy treatment specifically directed at the muscles of the neck and shoulders. Patients were then monitored, and the frequency, duration, and intensity of their headache experiences were evaluated. The study found that this structured massage therapy triggered an almost immediate reduction in headache frequency that continued for the remainder of the study period. Duration of headaches also tended to decline during the treatment period, but the intensity of headaches was unchanged. Massage therapy was deemed to be a safe nonpharmacologic option for the management of tension headaches.

Complementary & Alternative Therapies

Chronic Headache

Complementary and alternative medicine (CAM) use by people experiencing chronic headache is extremely common, especially among the 30% or so who do not achieve satisfactory pain control with traditional pharmacologic treatment. The literature today suggests that behavioral therapies predominate. These include relaxation (progressive muscle relaxation, autogenic training, meditation), biofeedback, and stress management techniques. A study sponsored by the Agency for Healthcare Research and Quality reviewed a series of controlled trials and found that some combination of behavioral therapies yielded a 35% to 55% reduction in migraine activity, especially in children and adolescents, and was considered a low-risk alternative during pregnancy. One study found equal preventive effect from behavioral therapies and pharmacologic agents.

Other CAM therapies being researched for headache include supplementation with magnesium and riboflavin (vitamin B_2). Aggressive treatment with magnesium produced good responses in 50% of headache sufferers shown to have low serum and tissue levels of magnesium. Riboflavin has also shown benefit, but the effects are delayed, not appearing until after several months of therapy.

Herbals are also being studied, although most of the current work is anecdotal. At present some research evidence supports the potential benefits of feverfew *(Tanacetum parthenium)* and guarana, although the high caffeine content of the latter has been associated with some rebound headache.

Holroyd KA, Mauskop A: Complementary and alternative treatments, *Neurology* 60(7):S58-S62, 2003.

for some women who experience migraines around the time of their menstrual cycle. Migraine sufferers should not use oral contraceptives because of a correlation between oral contraceptive use and an increase in migraine incidence.[1]

Vigorous activity can also trigger migraine headaches. However, moderate exercise should not act as a trigger. Exercise clearly lowers stress and contributes to an overall sense of well-being. During the actual headache, patients benefit from rest until medications and other treatments take effect.

PATIENT/FAMILY TEACHING. Headache management is largely self-management once pharmacologic options have been determined. Patients with headache commonly worry that it is a symptom of some other serious disease. The nurse encourages the patient to accurately report all signs and symptoms and provides education that helps the patient and family prevent and treat headaches. Identification of triggers is just a first step. The patient must then make lifestyle changes to avoid these triggers. The nurse teaches the patient how to appropriately use all medications. Drugs prescribed to prevent migraine need to be taken on a regular schedule, without missing doses. Drugs prescribed to treat headache symptoms need to be available and taken as soon as the patient becomes aware of symptoms or an aura.

The nurse may refer the patient to a dietitian if the patient needs guidance regarding dietary changes to prevent headache. Referrals may also be made for biofeedback or relaxation training to prevent stress-induced headache. In addition, local support groups can help headache sufferers. The National Headache Foundation is a good source of consumer health information for persons with headache.

Epilepsy

Etiology and Epidemiology. Epilepsy is a chronic disorder surrounded by many myths and misconceptions. Recent advances in the understanding and treatment of epilepsy have improved societal attitudes toward this condition, but the diagnosis still represents a social stigma for many patients. A seizure is an abnormal, paroxysmal electrical discharge from the cerebral cortex, and epilepsy is defined as recurrent, stereotypic seizures.[8] Seizures are seen clinically as alterations in sensation, behavior, movement, perception, or consciousness. Symptoms are related to the area of the cortex involved.

Any condition that causes cerebral irritation or alters the biochemical environment of the brain can result in seizures. The risk of having an isolated seizure during one's lifetime is thought to be about 10%.[8] Seizures can occur as a result of a wide range of metabolic derangements that affect the central nervous system; if the underlying condition is corrected, the seizures do not recur. These episodic seizures are not the same as epilepsy.

An estimated 2 million people in the United States have epilepsy, and approximately 125,000 new cases are diagnosed each year. Thirty percent of newly diagnosed patients are under 18 years of age. The prevalence of epilepsy in persons over 65 years of age is 1%. When no identifiable cause for epilepsy can be found, the seizures are considered idiopathic; idiopathic epilepsy accounts for 70% of all cases.[4] Genetics clearly plays a role in some forms of epilepsy. The remaining 30% of cases are related to a known cause, such as structural lesions in the central nervous system. Risk factors for developing epilepsy in adulthood include lesions within the central nervous system (e.g., traumatic brain injury), meningitis or encephalitis, cerebral tumors, and stroke.[9] Initial seizures in children are often fever related (see Risk Factors box).

Pathophysiology. A seizure can be caused by any process that disrupts the cell membrane stability of a neuron. A seizure starts

Risk Factors

Epilepsy

- Anoxia
- Cerebral palsy
- Perinatal problems (toxemia, difficult delivery, low birth weight, hypoxia)
- Congenital central nervous system defects
- Mental retardation
- Febrile conditions
- Family history of epilepsy
- Head trauma
- Central nervous system infections
- Central nervous system tumors
- Cerebrovascular disease
- Alcohol or drug abuse
- Metabolic disturbances
- Exposure to toxins
- Degenerative diseases (Alzheimer's disease)

when a tiny cluster of brain cells begins to emit rapid, repetitive, highly synchronized electrical discharges. The discharges may remain localized or rapidly spread to involve the entire brain. The point at which the cell membrane becomes destabilized and uncontrolled electrical discharge begins is known as the *seizure threshold*. Some people have lower seizure thresholds than others and are therefore more prone to seizures.

In 1981 the International League Against Epilepsy proposed a revised classification for seizures (Table 48-3). The major categories are **partial** (focal) and **generalized seizures**. Further subdivisions within the categories are based on the person's clinical behaviors during the ictal and interictal times. **Ictal** refers to the time during a seizure. *Interictal* refers to the time between seizure activity. **Postictal** refers to the time immediately after a seizure as the patient recovers.

Partial seizures do not always affect consciousness. Simple partial seizures have less motor, sensory, and consciousness involvement because they are limited to a smaller area of the brain. The wider the area of cerebral cortex affected, the more clinical symptoms are seen. With simple partial seizures a patient may experience uncontrolled movement of an extremity or a portion of the face. He or she is able to interact with others during the seizure and remembers the event afterward. Complex partial seizures affect consciousness. Patients may recall an aura, a warning sensation that occurs before the seizure, and often exhibit automatisms (automatic behaviors) such as lip smacking, chewing, rubbing, or picking at clothes. These behaviors are not voluntary because consciousness is impaired. Some complex partial seizures spread to larger areas of the cortex and become generalized tonic-clonic seizures, but these are different from true tonic-clonic seizures, in which the initial seizure behavior is generalized.

Generalized seizures impair consciousness from the start. Absence seizures do not include motor signs and may last less than 1 minute, making them difficult to detect. These seizures are often seen in children and may initially be thought of as "daydreaming." There is no postictal state, and absence seizures can occur many times a day.

Tonic-clonic seizures have a tonic phase, during which the muscles become rigid, and then a clonic phase, which involves rhythmic muscle jerking. As the muscles of the trunk and diaphragm

TABLE 48-3 CLASSIFICATION OF SEIZURES

Type of Seizure	Effect on Consciousness	Signs and Symptoms	Postictal State
PARTIAL SEIZURES			
Simple partial (focal)	Not impaired	Focal twitching of extremity Speech arrest Special visual sensations (e.g., seeing lights) Feeling of fear or doom	No
Complex partial (formerly psychomotor or temporal lobe seizures)	Impaired	May begin as simple partial and progress to complex Automatic behavior (e.g., lip smacking, chewing, or picking at clothes)	Yes
Complex partial progressing to generalized tonic-clonic	Impaired	Begins as complex partial as above, then progresses to tonic-clonic as described below	Yes
GENERALIZED SEIZURES			
Absence (formerly petit mal)	Impaired	Brief loss of consciousness, staring, unresponsiveness	No
Tonic-clonic (formerly grand mal)	Impaired	Tonic phase involving rigidity of all muscles, followed by clonic phase involving rhythmic jerking of muscles, and possibly tongue biting and urinary and fecal incontinence May be any combination of tonic and clonic movements	Yes
Atonic	Impaired for only a few seconds	Brief loss of muscle tone, which may cause patient to fall or drop something; referred to as drop attacks	No
Myoclonic	Impaired for only a few seconds or not at all	Brief jerking of a muscle group, which may cause patient to fall	No

become rigid, the air moving past the vocal cords creates a "cry." Once the diaphragm is contracted, the patient is unable to breathe. If the seizure lasts long enough, the patient may become cyanotic. Bladder and bowel muscles are also affected, and the patient may experience incontinence.

Other generalized seizures include myoclonic and atonic types. Myoclonic seizures cause one or several muscles to jerk, often causing the patient to fall. Atonic seizures cause a brief loss of tone in one or more muscles, causing the patient to drop things or fall. They cause only a brief loss of consciousness and no postictal state. The patient is able to get up right away unless he or she is injured from the fall. A seizure is not generally fatal but creates a risk for injury from falls and other environmental problems.

Postictal states represent periods of recovery from the seizure. The brain must recover from the intense burst of electrical activity. The length of the postictal period varies from patient to patient. Patients may have some degree of confusion, lethargy, or an inability to follow commands or speak clearly during this period. In rare cases the patient may experience Todd's paralysis, which is prolonged weakness involving one or more extremities. Although not permanent, the paralysis may persist beyond the postictal period of confusion or fatigue.

Status epilepticus is an episode of seizure activity lasting at least 30 minutes, or repeated seizures without full recovery between each seizure. Seizures cause a marked increase in cerebral metabolic activity and demands. Oxygen consumption typically increases by 60% and cerebral blood flow by as much as 250%.[28] These demands may outpace the delivery of oxygen and nutrients from the cerebral blood flow, and prolonged seizures can lead to cellular exhaustion and destruction and even death if not effectively interrupted.

Collaborative Care Management. The diagnosis of epilepsy begins with a detailed health history. A thorough description of the seizure experience itself is also obtained, including:

- Description of the aura, if any (preseizure sensation or feeling)
- Precipitating factors, if any, such as lack of sleep, alcohol intake, emotional stress, excess caffeine, time of day, menses
- Description of the patient's behavior from the beginning of the seizure to the end, especially if the motor signs started in one part of the body and spread to another part (jacksonian march)
- Length of the seizure
- Length of the postictal recovery period and behavior during this phase
- Incidence of incontinence
- Frequency of the seizures (if more than one) and interval between them

A physical examination is performed to identify possible neurologic disease that could cause seizures and is supplemented by selected diagnostic tests such as a CT or MRI scan to check for structural lesions. Laboratory tests, including electrolytes, creatinine, blood urea nitrogen, arterial blood gases, and toxicology screens, are done to rule out metabolic causes for seizures.

An electroencephalogram (EEG) may be ordered to help identify the location, or foci, of the seizures and their pattern of spread, if any, over the cortex. The EEG may be recorded during a brief outpatient visit, overnight, or after 12 to 24 hours of sleep deprivation.[2] However, an EEG can only identify a seizure if one occurs during the test. A normal EEG does not rule out the possibility of a past or future seizure. In some cases patients may be monitored for several days as inpatients.

Antiepileptic drugs (AEDs), also referred to as anticonvulsants, are the primary treatment for seizures. A vast array of medications are used in the management of epilepsy (Table 48-4). Different types of epilepsy respond differently to specific drugs, and patients vary significantly in their response to and toleration of the drugs. The process of finding the best match is often one of trial and error.[37] Once control of the seizures is established, drug levels are monitored to ensure that the patient maintains a therapeutic level. Although specific therapeutic ranges have been established for commonly used drugs, the appropriate dose for any patient is one that prevents seizures but does not cause excessive side effects or toxicity, even if the blood level is higher or lower than the established norm.[39] In the past, patients were maintained on anticonvulsant therapy for life. Today physicians often attempt to wean patients from the medication if the patients remain seizure free for 1 to 2 years. A common side effect of most AEDs is drowsiness or other mental status changes. These side effects may interfere with the patient's social life or work. Multiple changes in drug or dose may be needed before the best seizure control with the fewest side effects is achieved.

Because of the critical nature of status epilepticus, benzodiazepines are used to rapidly terminate seizure activity while a loading dose of anticonvulsants is administered, since anticonvulsants take longer to achieve a therapeutic blood level (see Guidelines for Safe Practice box and the Nursing Care Plan).

Nurses need to act quickly when a patient has a seizure. The nurse makes careful observations to document the seizure accurately and reassures the patient that help is nearby if it is needed. If the seizure generalizes or begins as a generalized seizure, the

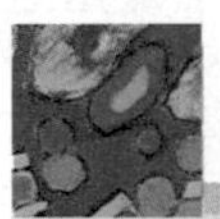

TABLE 48-4 COMMON MEDICATIONS *for Seizures*

Seizure Type	Drugs of First Choice	Other Options
Partial Seizures		
Simple or complex partial	Carbamazapine (Tegretol) Phenytoin (Dilantin) Oxcarbazepine (Trileptal)	Valproic acid (Depakene) Phenobarbital (Luminal) Primidone (Mysoline)
Generalized Seizures		
Tonic-clonic	Valproic acid	Phenytoin Carbamazepine Phenobarbital Primidone
Myoclonic	Valproic acid Clonazepam (Klonopin)	Phenobarbital
Absence	Ethosuximide (Zarontin) Valproic acid	Lamotrigine (Lamictal) Felbamate (Felbatol)

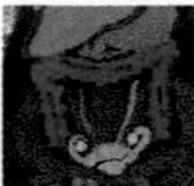

Guidelines for Safe Practice
The Patient in Status Epilepticus

- Protect airway and provide oxygen. Position patient on side to prevent aspiration. Place an oral airway if the teeth are not clenched. Administer oxygen by mask. If respiratory depression occurs from seizures or medication used to control seizures, intubation may be necessary.
- Establish intravenous access for medication delivery and fluids.
- Draw blood for measuring electrolytes and arterial blood gases and for toxicology screening to rule out metabolic causes for seizures.
- Administer benzodiazepines, usually lorazepam (Ativan), 4 to 8 mg over 2 to 4 minutes, or diazepam (Valium), 5 to 20 mg over 5 to 10 minutes, to stop seizures. These drugs are fast acting and will control seizures until anticonvulsant drugs reach therapeutic levels.
- Administer anticonvulsants, usually phenytoin (Dilantin), 15 to 20 mg/kg body weight in normal saline at 50 mg/min maximum rate, at the same time as the benzodiazepines to begin establishing therapeutic levels. Dilantin can cause significant hypotension and cardiac dysrhythmias. Place patient on a monitor during loading doses.
- Continue search for an underlying cause of seizures.

nurse acts promptly to protect the patient from injury. No attempt is made to restrain the patient, since this could cause injury. The nurse protects the patient from hitting his or her extremities or head on furniture or bed rails by moving them or padding obstructions. Nothing is forced into the patient's mouth. Patients having a tonic-clonic seizure will not have effective air exchange during the seizure, but a patient cannot "swallow" his or her own tongue. However, patients may occlude their airway by flexing their neck or clenching their jaw. After the seizure the nurse gently clears oral secretions, positions the patient to open the airway, and administers oxygen if needed. After securing the airway, the nurse assesses the patient for injuries such as abrasions, bruises, or tongue biting that might have occurred during the seizure. The duration of the postictal phase is assessed and documented, including the time from the end of the seizure until the patient can follow commands and answer questions. The nurse arranges for someone to remain with the patient until he or she becomes fully responsive to the surroundings.

The nurse also institutes seizure precautions to protect the patient from injury if the patient's seizures are not well controlled or if the patient has a new illness or injury that predisposes him or her to a lower seizure threshold. In most hospitals, seizure precautions include keeping side rails up and padded if the patient has tonic-clonic seizures, ensuring that suction is available at the bedside, disabling the locks on bathroom and room doors, and avoiding the use of oral thermometers. Helmets may be used to prevent head injury in patients who are permitted to be up and walking.

Most patients with epilepsy can achieve satisfactory control of their disease through the use of pharmacologic agents. More aggressive interventions may be necessary, however, if the patient's epilepsy remains unresponsive to standard treatment. Surgery may be performed to remove the epileptogenic focus in patients experiencing intractable epilepsy.

Patient/Family Teaching. Patients with epilepsy and their families must learn to cope with a chronic illness that greatly affects their everyday life and independence. General health promotion can play an important role in preventing seizures. The nurse encourages patients to plan for adequate rest and sleep and to manage life stress as effectively as possible.[35] The intake of alcohol is known to lower the seizure threshold, and the nurse encourages the patient to use alcohol only in moderation if at all.

No specific dietary restrictions are prescribed for the patient with epilepsy. If the patient can identify certain foods that trigger seizures, these foods are eliminated from the diet. Common examples include caffeine and chocolate. The Research box presents information on the use of the Atkins diet with patients experiencing uncontrolled epilepsy. Alternative therapies are also being explored for potential benefit in the control of seizures.

The Epilepsy Foundation of America is a patient-focused organization providing education and support for patients and their families. Local chapters can provide information about services available in the community, and the nurse encourages the patient to use this important resource.

The nurse educates the patient and family about the causes of epilepsy in an effort to dispel the myths that epilepsy represents "possession" or is a "mark of the devil." Attitudes toward epilepsy have gradually changed, but old prejudices persist, and the disease can still carry a stigma. With adequate pharmacologic control, the patient with epilepsy can lead a normal life, and the nurse helps the patient understand the importance of adhering to the medication regimen and avoiding precipitating factors.[35] Self-care is an ongoing challenge. Medications are prescribed and adjusted to achieve the best control of seizures without excessive side effects or toxicity. The timing of doses can be altered to fit the patient's lifestyle and prevent missed doses.

The nurse stresses the importance of carrying some form of identification with information about the seizure disorder and all

Research

Kossoff EH et al: Efficacy of the Atkins diet as therapy for intractable epilepsy, *Neurology* 61(12):1789-1791, 2003.

This small study tracked a group of patients with epilepsy that had proven resistant to standard antiepileptic drug (AED) therapy. The patients ranged in age from 7 to 52 years. They were started on the Atkins diet and maintained moderate to large ketosis for periods from 6 weeks to 24 months. Half the patients experienced a reduction in their seizure activity and were able to reduce the level of AEDs. Although limited in size and scope, the study gives additional support to anecdotal evidence that strict diet modification may be a useful strategy to reduce the frequency and severity of seizure activity in patients whose epilepsy has proven resistant to conventional pharmacologic therapy. The authors recommend additional study to gain more insight into appropriate patient choice and other variables that may be associated with successful outcomes from a ketogenic diet.

Nursing Care Plan

Patient With Status Epilepticus

Data The patient is a 29-year-old man with a history of seizures. He experiences complex partial seizures that occasionally generalize to tonic-clonic seizures. His seizures are controlled by phenytoin (Dilantin), 300 mg once a day at bedtime, and carbamazepine (Tegretol), 200 mg three times a day. Despite good compliance with medications, he experiences four or five seizures a year.

This morning, after he mowed his lawn in hot weather, the patient's wife found him having a tonic-clonic seizure, which lasted about 2 minutes. Within 5 minutes he began to seize again so his wife called for emergency assistance. By the time the patient arrived at the emergency department, he had seized for 25 minutes. Oxygen was started by mask. An intravenous infusion of 0.9% saline was initiated. Blood was drawn for electrolytes, toxicology, and anticonvulsant drug levels. Lorazepam, 2 mg, was administered intravenously every 4 minutes for four doses for a total of 8 mg. Phenytoin, 1000 mg in saline, was infused over 1 hour. After the fourth dose of lorazepam, the seizure stopped. His postseizure respiratory rate was 6 breaths/min, oxygen saturation was 85%, and blood pressure was 85/50 mm Hg. Therefore he was intubated, ventilated and admitted to the intensive care unit (ICU).

It is now 1 hour after his admission to the ICU. He is responding to painful stimuli but not following commands. His phenytoin bolus has infused, and his blood pressure has increased to 110/70 mm Hg, with a respiratory rate of 8 breaths/min, but he is not breathing above the ventilator. Breaths sounds are clear bilaterally, and his oxygen saturation is 99% on 40% Fio_2.

Nursing Diagnosis

Risk for injury related to seizure activity

Outcomes

- Patient will remain free from injury.

Related NOC Outcomes

- Neurologic Status
- Risk Control
- Symptom Control

Related NIC Interventions

- Artificial Airway Management
- Seizure Management
- Seizure Precautions
- Surveillance: Safety

Nursing Interventions/Rationales

- Implement seizure precautions (side rails up and padded, bed in low position). *To minimize environmental risks when seizures occur. Restraining the patient is contraindicated, since injury can occur from restraints during seizure activity.*
- Ensure rapid access to oxygen, suction, and other emergency equipment. *To maintain a patent airway, ensure adequate oxygenation, and prevent respiratory compromise or arrest during or following seizure activity.*
- Administer antiseizure medications as prescribed. *Aggressive drug therapy is the key to halting seizures.*
- Monitor patient response to medications. *To determine the effectiveness of treatment or the need for additional or different interventions.*
- Insert nasogastric tube to administer carbamazepine if needed. *Carbamazepine cannot be administered intravenously and may be needed. Oral medications cannot be administered during seizure activity because of the risk for aspiration from inability to swallow.*

Nursing Diagnosis

Risk for deficient fluid volume related to altered mental state

Outcomes

- Patient will maintain balanced intake and output.

Related NOC Outcomes

- Fluid Balance
- Hydration

Related NIC Interventions

- Fluid Management
- Fluid Monitoring
- Hypovolemia Management
- Intravenous (IV) Therapy

Nursing Interventions/Rationales

- Assess and monitor for adequacy of fluid volume (blood pressure, heart rate, urinary output, skin turgor, mucous membranes). *Patient may be dehydrated from working in heat. The sooner fluid volume deficiency is identified, the quicker fluid balance can be reestablished.*
- Maintain nothing-by-mouth status until patient is fully awake. *Aspiration is a risk until the patient is fully alert with protective reflexes intact.*
- Administer prescribed intravenous fluids. *To replace fluid losses and prevent hypovolemia.*
- Monitor vital signs every hour or more frequently if needed. *Phenytoin increases the risk of hypotension.*
- Monitor intake and output. Intake should approximate output. *Monitoring helps identify fluid deficits.*

Evaluation

Evaluation is based on comparing the patient's outcomes with desired outcomes.

prescribed medications in case strangers must provide first aid in the event of a seizure or accident. If the patient feels comfortable sharing the information, a colleague at work or school can be informed about the disease and instructed what to do in the event of a seizure. This strategy can help prevent unnecessary trips to the emergency department.

Safety is a primary consideration for the patient with epilepsy. Activity is not generally restricted unless it puts the patient at risk for injury should a seizure occur. However, a history of epilepsy does limit the patient's options in terms of employment, since employers must consider their own liability in case of seizure activity on the job. Each state also has laws defining driver's licensing for persons with a seizure history. Driving may be permitted once a patient has been seizure free on medication for a designated period, often as much as 1 to 2 years.

▶ ARE You READY?

Which medication is administered to stop seizure activity in the patient experiencing status epilepticus?

1. Phenytoin
2. Lorazepam
3. Diprivan
4. Propranolol

Intracranial Tumors

Etiology and Epidemiology. Primary intracranial tumors arise from the support cells of brain tissues rather than from the neurons. As they grow, these tumors invade or displace brain tissue and lead to neurologic symptoms. Although no clear cause has been identified, brain tumors are generally believed to be the result of a change in the genetic control of cellular growth, leading to abnormal cell mutations and loss of organized cell growth.[15] Genetic, familial, and environmental factors are all under investigation. Both benign and malignant tumors occur, although this differentiation has less meaning for intracranial tumors than for other types of tissue. A histologically "benign" tumor can be surgically inaccessible, continue to grow, and cause increasing dysfunction ranging from increasing ICP to death.

The incidence of primary brain tumors is about 20,000 to 30,000 cases per year.[1] Brain tumors affect people of all ages with two peak periods of incidence: early childhood and the fifth to seventh decades of life. Children are primarily affected by infratentorial tumors of the posterior fossa such as medulloblastomas. Adults are most commonly affected by the various forms of gliomas. Gliomas and neuromas are more common in males, whereas meningiomas and pituitary adenomas are more common in females.

Secondary brain tumors originate elsewhere in the body and metastasize to the brain. Primary sites in the lung and breast are most common. As cancer diagnosis and treatment in general have continued to improve, the incidence of secondary brain tumors has risen significantly, exceeding 100,000 cases per year.[25] Primary brain tumors, however, rarely metastasize systemically because the brain does not have a lymphatic drainage system. Brain tumors of all types are the second leading neurologic cause of death after stroke.

Pathophysiology. Brain tumors are named for the tissues from which they arise. The more common ones are gliomas, meningiomas, pituitary adenomas, and acoustic neuromas (Table 48-5). Gliomas account for about 45% of all brain tumors and arise from the connective tissue, the glial cells, of the brain.[1] Gliomas primarily infiltrate the tissues of the cerebral hemispheres and are not encapsulated, making them difficult to excise. They grow rapidly, and most persons do not survive longer than a few years after diagnosis.

Some intracranial tumors are graded from I to IV, reflecting the nature of the cellular changes. The more abnormal and anaplastic the tumor cells are, the higher the grade.[25] Highly malignant grades III and IV astrocytomas are the most common types of brain tumors in adults. The less malignant gliomas are low-grade astrocytomas and oligodendrogliomas. Ependymomas arise from cells lining the ventricular system. The most malignant and rapidly growing forms of gliomas are the glioblastoma mulitiforme and medulloblastoma. Gliomas may start as one grade and rapidly become more malignant, especially if left untreated.[1]

The meningiomas, which account for 15% of all primary brain tumors, arise from the meningeal coverings of the brain. They occur most commonly in the meninges over the cerebral hemispheres in the parasagittal region along the ridge of the sphenoid bone and in the anterior fossa near the olfactory groove or sella turcica. When located in the posterior fossa, they arise from the cerebellopontine angle, from the tentorium, or rarely from the region of the foramen magnum. Meningiomas are usually benign and slow growing, but they may undergo malignant changes or be located in a place that makes surgery impossible without causing significant neurologic damage. These slowly growing tumors can reach a remarkable size as long as the highly plastic brain is able to gradually accommodate their presence (Figure 48-9).

Acoustic neuromas constitute about 7% of all primary brain tumors. These tumors grow from the sheath covering the eighth cranial nerve, and the patient exhibits symptoms such as hearing loss or balance disturbance if the vestibular portion of the nerve is compressed. If the tumor becomes large, surrounding structures such as the trigeminal and facial nerves may also be involved, causing additional neurologic symptoms.

Pituitary adenomas make up another 7% of brain tumors. These tumors are considered benign but may be difficult to completely remove because of their location in the sella turcica and their proximity to the pituitary gland. They frequently produce symptoms reflecting hormonal changes, such as acromegaly from increased growth hormone production.[11] Visual symptoms may develop if the tumor expands beyond the sella turcica and compresses the optic chiasm, which crosses above the pituitary gland.

Brain tumors produce a wide range of neurologic symptoms depending on their size, location, and invasive qualities (see Clinical Manifestations box). Locally the tumor invades, displaces, and destroys brain tissue, producing symptoms related to the functions of that particular site. Brain tumors also exert direct pressure on nerve structures, causing degeneration and interference with local circulation. They interfere with the blood brain barrier and create cerebral edema, which can elevate ICP and interfere with nerve transmission. Some tumors displace the structures of the ventricular system as they expand, leading to partial obstruction of the flow of CSF. The accumulation of CSF causes the ventricles to dilate and exert outward pressure on the brain. ICP rises, and hydrocephalus may result.

Tumors occurring above the tentorium may disrupt brain function and lead to seizures. If the tumor is small and has not caused other symptoms, a seizure may be the first symptom that causes the person to seek medical attention.

COMPLICATIONS

HYDROCEPHALUS. Any obstruction of the normal flow of CSF can result in **hydrocephalus**. Hydrocephalus can be caused by an obstructing tumor but is also a potential complication of surgery to remove the tumor. When the obstruction occurs between the

TABLE 48-5 TYPES OF BRAIN TUMORS OCCURRING IN ADULTS

Type	Pathology
GLIOMAS	
Astrocytomas (grades I to III) Glioblastoma multiforme (also called astrocytoma grade IV) Oligodendroglioma (grades I to III) Ependymoma (grades I to IV) Medulloblastoma	Nonencapsulated, tend to infiltrate brain tissue; arise in any part of brain connective tissue; infiltrate primarily cerebral hemisphere tissue; not well outlined so difficult to excise completely; grow rapidly—most persons live months to years after diagnosis; tumors assigned grade from I to IV, with IV being most malignant
TUMORS FROM SUPPORT STRUCTURES	
Meningiomas	Arise from meningeal coverings of brain; usually benign but may undergo malignant changes; usually encapsulated, and surgical cure possible; recurrence possible
Neuromas (acoustic neuroma, schwannoma)	Arise from Schwann cells inside auditory meatus on vestibular portion of eighth cranial nerve; usually benign but may undergo cellular change and become malignant; will regrow if not completely excised; surgical resection often difficult because of location
Pituitary adenoma	Arise from various tissues; surgical approach usually successful; recurrence possible
DEVELOPMENTAL (CONGENITAL) TUMORS	
Dermoid, epidermoid, craniopharyngioma	Arise from embryonic tissue in various sites in brain; success of surgical resection dependent on location and invasiveness
Angiomas	Arise from vascular structures; usually difficult to resect
METASTATIC TUMORS	
	Cancer cells spreading to brain via circulatory system; surgical resection difficult; even with treatment, prognosis poor; survival beyond 1-2 yr uncommon

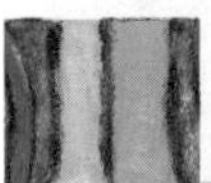

CLINICAL MANIFESTATIONS
Intracranial Tumors

Symptoms can be generalized or specific to the tumor location and the structures of the brain that are compressed.

- Pressure headaches (generalized or periorbital)
- Nausea and vomiting unrelated to food intake
- Symptoms of increased intracranial pressure
- Visual changes:
  - —Blurred vision
  - —Diplopia (with third, fourth, and sixth nerve compression)
  - —Visual field alterations (with tumor compression of the optic chiasm or optic pathways)
  - —Enlarged blind spot related to papilledema
- Seizures
- Weakness or hemiparesis (when tumor affects the motor cortex)
- Aphasia
  - —Expressive (with frontal lobe tumor affecting the language area in the dominant hemisphere)
  - —Receptive (with temporal lobe tumor)
- Alterations in level of consciousness (with a midbrain tumor)
- Personality changes from subtle to obvious psychosis (with frontal lobe tumors)
- Inappropriate affect (with frontal lobe tumors)
- Sensory-perceptual deficits (with parietal lobe tumors)

ventricles, the CSF cannot flow out of the ventricular system and move through the brain and spinal cord. This is called *noncommunicating hydrocephalus.* When the obstruction prevents the CSF from being reabsorbed via the arachnoid granulations in the sagittal sinus, the resulting condition is called *communicating hydrocephalus.* The arachnoid granulations can become obstructed by blood or proteins produced by infection in the CSF.

Acute hydrocephalus may require immediate intervention via a ventriculostomy. A small catheter is placed into the lateral ventricle via a frontal opening, or burr hole, in the skull. The catheter is connected to an external drainage system that monitors ICP and allows for drainage of CSF. The tubing and drainage system must be kept closed and sterile. If drainage appears to stop, the neurosurgeon is notified immediately. Ventriculostomies are left in place for only a few days to minimize the risk of infection. If the patient requires ongoing drainage of CSF, a shunt replaces the external drain (Figure 48-10). The different types of shunts are named for their points of origin and termination and include ventriculoperitoneal, lumboperitoneal, ventriculojugular, and cyst-peritoneal.

When a shunt is placed, excess CSF is diverted away from the central nervous system and into either the peritoneal cavity or, occasionally, the venous system, where it is reabsorbed. Shunts may include special valves or access reservoirs at the point where

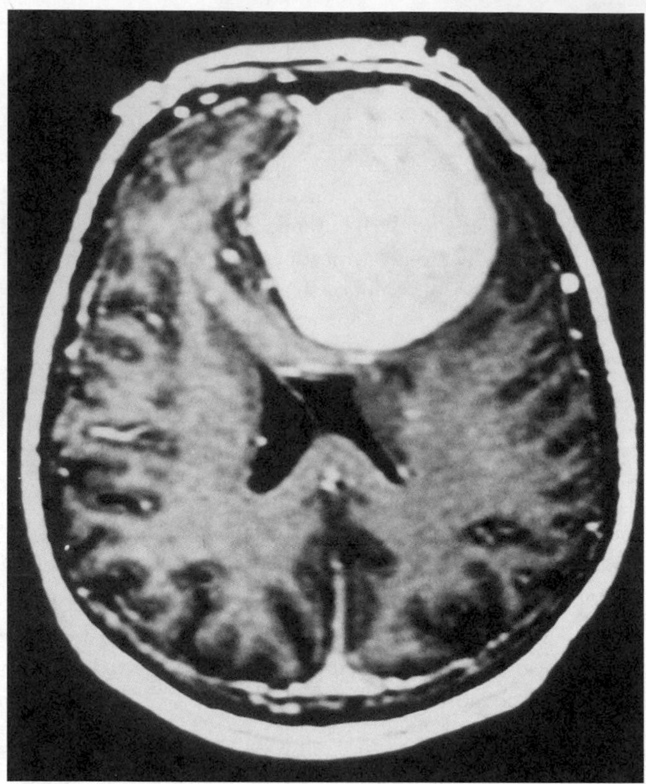

Figure 48-9 Preoperative magnetic resonance imaging view of meningioma.

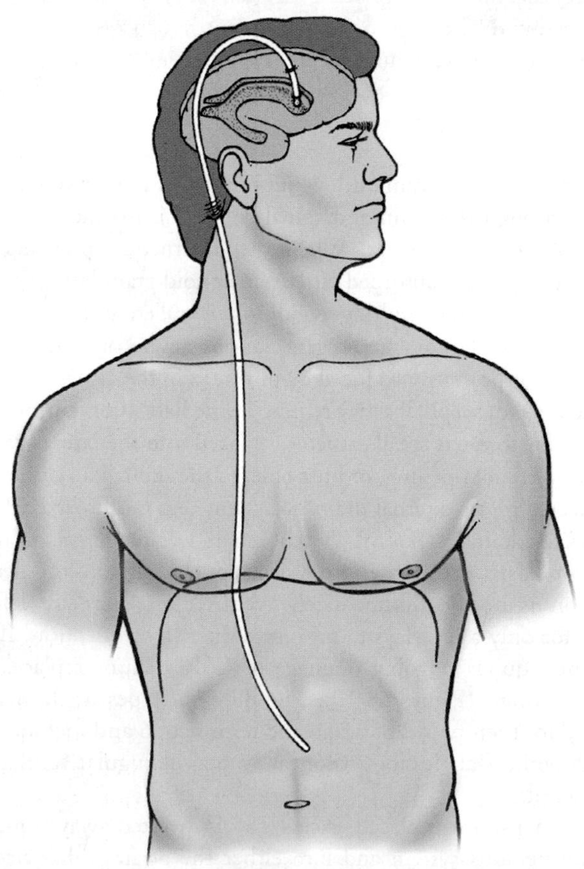

Figure 48-10 Ventriculoperitoneal internal shunt.

the catheter leaves the skull. These valves or reservoirs help control the volume and pressure of CSF leaving the ventricular system. Care of the patient undergoing shunt placement is summarized in the Guidelines for Safe Practice box.

Diabetes Insipidus and Syndrome of Inappropriate Antidiuretic Hormone. Patients undergoing surgery in the pituitary region are at risk for diabetes insipidus (DI), since antidiuretic hormone (ADH) is made and stored in this area. Surgery, trauma, or cerebral edema from almost any neurologic condition can disrupt the delicate balance of this essential fluid regulatory mechanism.[11]

DI occurs when there is insufficient ADH to cause the renal tubules to reabsorb water. Large quantities of dilute urine are excreted, and the patient is at risk for severe dehydration. Serum sodium levels and osmolarity rise from the loss of fluid (Table 48-6). Treatment involves fluid replacement and administration of synthetic ADH in the form of desmopressin acetate (DDAVP) or aqueous vasopressin. The condition is usually self-limiting but can become chronic.

The syndrome of inappropriate antidiuretic hormone (SIADH) is a direct contrast to DI and can occur as a complication of intracranial surgery or almost any central nervous system disorder, damage to the hypothalamus, and a variety of other factors (see Chapter 38). In this syndrome too much ADH is secreted, causing the renal tubules to reabsorb excess amounts of water. The patient's

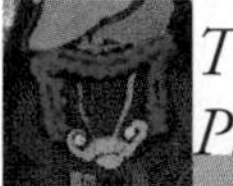

Guidelines for Safe Practice

The Patient Undergoing Shunt Placement

- Perform monitoring.
  - —Assess neurologic status frequently for any decrease in mental status.
  - —Observe for symptoms of subdural hematoma, one of the possible side effects of the surgery.
  - —Monitor for symptoms of overdrainage, as evidenced by headache, especially when patient is sitting upright or standing.
  - —Assess degree and character of drainage.
    - —Amount of drainage and bleeding should be minimal.
    - —Reinforce dressing as needed.
    - —Incisional areas may be left open to air after several days.
- Maintain gastrointestinal status.
  - —Check frequently for signs of paralytic ileus; manipulation of the bowel that occurs during placement of the shunt's peritoneal segment can predispose patient to ileus.
  - —Patient usually is given nothing by mouth for the first day, and then clear liquids are started.
  - —Regular diet is resumed as soon as active bowel sounds are present and patient tolerates liquids.
- Maintain comfort.
  - —Patient may need frequent pain medication because of involvement of abdominal area.
  - —Keep pressure off incisional sites.
- Promote mobility.
  - —Turning to either side is permitted.
  - —Raise head of bed gradually when mobilizing patient.
  - —Patient is encouraged to walk as much as possible to encourage adaptation to decreased intracranial pressure.

TABLE 48-6 LABORATORY PARAMETERS AND TREATMENT OF DIABETES INSIPIDUS AND SYNDROME OF INAPPROPRIATE ANTIDIURETIC HORMONE

Parameters	Diabetes Insipidus	Syndrome of Inappropriate Antidiuretic Hormone
Urine specific gravity	1.001-1.005	1.030 or more
Serum osmolarity	High	Low
Serum sodium	High	Low
Urinary output	Very high	Low
Treatment	Fluid replacement Desmopressin, 0.1-0.4 ml intranasally every 12-24 hr Aqueous vasopressin, 5-10 unit subcutaneously every 3-4 hr	Fluid restriction Furosemide (Lasix) for diuresis Demeclocyline, 300 mg 4 times daily

urinary output is low, generalized weight gain occurs, and the patient's serum sodium and osmolarity are low as a result of the dilutional effects of water retention (see Table 48-6). The treatment for SIADH is fluid restriction, often to 1500 ml of fluid per day or less. If the patient is receiving IV fluids, normal saline is given to provide additional sodium. On rare occasions 3% hypertonic saline may be administered under close monitoring. The problem is usually self-limiting. In severe cases the drug demeclocycline (Declomycin) may be given to suppress the effects of ADH on the renal tubule.

GASTRIC ULCERATION. Neurosurgical procedures predispose the patient to gastric ulceration, commonly known as Cushing's ulcers. The underlying pathologic condition is not well understood but is thought to represent a massive stress response. The use of steroids after surgery is also believed to increase gastric secretions and can contribute to gastric irritation and ulceration. Patients are usually given a histamine$_2$ blocker or proton pump inhibitor as a preventive measure. If a nasogastric tube is in place, the pH of the gastric secretions can be monitored and proton pump inhibitors or sucralfate (Carafate) administered to protect the gastric mucosa. See Chapter 42 for a discussion of stress ulcer.

Collaborative Care Management

DIAGNOSTIC TESTS. The CT scan is the most commonly used test to diagnose and evaluate brain tumors and their effect on surrounding brain tissue. A cerebral angiogram may be performed if the tumor is situated near major blood vessels and information is needed about vessels that might be feeding the tumor. MRI is also used, particularly to help visualize tumors of the posterior fossa, where MRI can provide greater detail than CT.

MEDICATIONS. Drug therapy is used in the management of brain tumors for both adjuvant treatment of the tumor and symptom management. A wide variety of chemotherapeutic agents are used, typically in combination protocols, although malignant gliomas have proven highly resistant to chemotherapy. Chemotherapy can be delivered by the standard IV route, but the tight junctions of the blood-brain barrier make it difficult for therapeutic levels of the drugs to reach the brain tumor. Intrathecal administration delivers the drug directly into the central nervous system, but the distribution of the drug to the tumor is still uneven. The use of an Ommaya reservoir allows for the delivery of drugs directly into the lateral ventricle (Figure 48-11). Controlled-release polymer "wafers" can also be used to allow the chemotherapy to diffuse directly into the tumor cavity. The wafers are implanted in the cavity when the tumor is resected and are left in place to gradually degrade after the drug has been delivered (Figure 48-12).[1]

Drug therapy also plays a significant role in symptom management. Most patients receive a corticosteroid such as dexamethasone (Decadron) to help control cerebral edema around the tumor site. The effects are temporary, and steroids are usually tapered after about a month. A histamine receptor antagonist or proton pump inhibitor may be administered along with the steroid to decrease the risk of peptic ulcer formation. Anticonvulsant medications are also initiated to prevent the development of seizures. Phenytoin (Dilantin) is the drug of choice, since carbamazepine (Tegretol) is known to cause bone marrow suppression.

DIET. No special diet is prescribed for the patient with a brain tumor. Rather, the patient's diet is modified as needed to reflect the patient's LOC and ability to swallow and protect the airway. A speech pathologist may be consulted if the patient is experiencing swallowing difficulties.

TREATMENTS. Radiotherapy is also commonly used in the management of brain tumors, especially when the tumor cannot be completely resected. Radiation is usually administered after surgical resection of the tumor; however, it may be used as the primary therapy if the tumor is surgically inaccessible.[25] Metastatic lesions and medulloblastomas are the most responsive to radiation. Radiation is also used after surgery in the treatment of most gliomas because the infiltrative nature of these tumors makes them extremely difficult to completely remove.

Most patients respond well to radiotherapy, but some patients experience severe radiation-induced cerebral edema that is not controllable with steroids. These patients may exhibit symptoms of compromised brain function. Most brain tumors are invasive, and the radiation has to be administered to a large area of the brain, increasing the risk of collateral cell damage and necrosis in the surrounding brain tissue. Brachytherapy introduces a radioisotope directly into the tumor bed to deliver high doses of radiation to a small area. Both radioisotope seeds and liquids instilled via balloon are in use.[1]

Stereotactic radiation, or Gamma Knife therapy, is an alternative form of radiotherapy available at selected centers. It is used to noninvasively treat deep-seated tumors that are inaccessible to

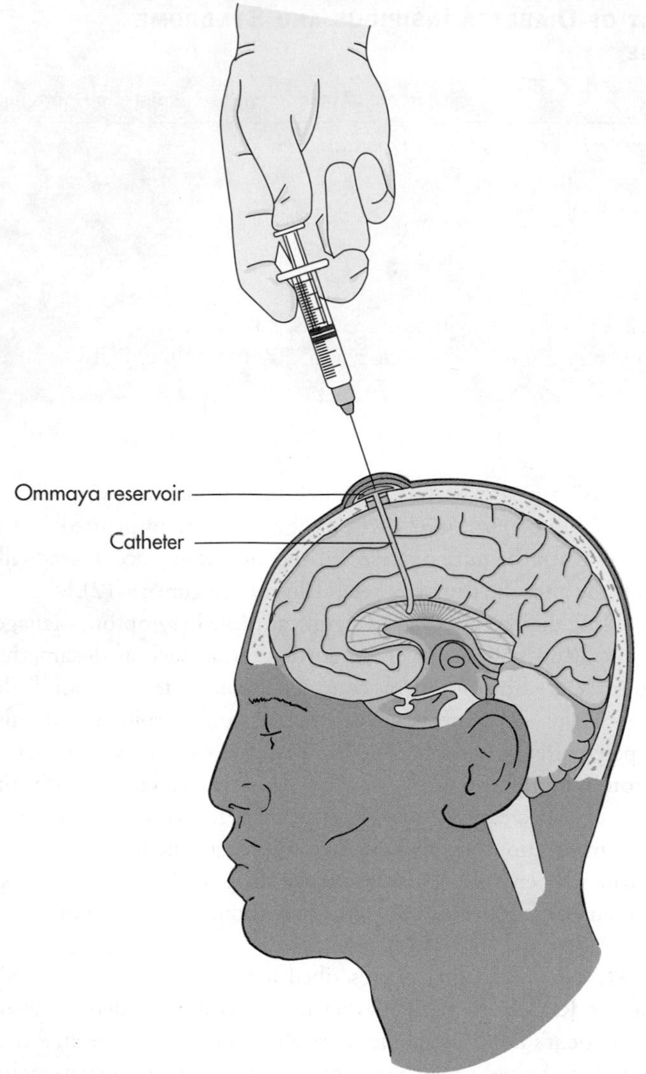

Figure 48-11 Ommaya reservoir, a mushroom-shaped device with attached catheter that is implanted into lateral ventricle through a burr hole. A silicone injection dome rests over the burr hole under the scalp. Drugs can be injected directly into reservoir with a syringe.

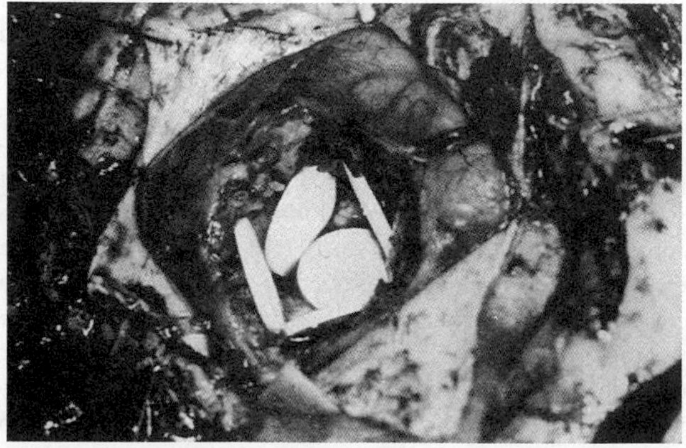

Figure 48-12 Intraoperative view of chemotherapy-impregnated polymers implanted in tumor bed after tumor resection.

conventional surgery. Using a stereotactic frame fixed to the patient's head, the surgeon directs concentrated beams of radiation at small areas of brain tissue known to be malignant. This minimizes the radiation damage to surrounding normal brain tissue. The final effects of treatment are not known for several weeks because the irradiated area responds slowly to the treatment.[21]

Another adjunct to surgical treatment for brain tumors is the neuroradiologic procedure referred to as embolization. A cerebral angiogram is performed to identify the feeding blood vessels of a tumor, usually a meningioma. These vessels are then embolized by introducing a material that blocks blood flow through the vessel. Reduced blood flow to the meningioma enables the surgeon to resect the tumor with less blood loss.[25] Similar treatments are used in preparation for surgery to remove or repair aneurysms and arteriovenous malformations.[15]

Surgical Management. Surgery is the treatment of choice for most intracranial tumors. Surgery is used to establish the histologic tissue diagnosis and to either debulk or completely resect the tumor if possible. If the tumor is slowly growing, the surgical procedure may keep the patient symptom free for years, even when complete resection is not possible. Surgery may also be used emergently to deal with obstructions to the flow of CSF, which can cause increased ICP and hydrocephalus.

Surgical treatment of brain tumors typically involves a craniotomy, a surgical opening through the skull that allows access to brain tissue. The procedure is also used to repair the effects of trauma and to treat aneurysms and the effects of stroke. Preoperative preparation and postoperative care are virtually the same, regardless of the underlying condition.

The possibility of neurologic deficits after surgery must be considered, and the surgeon discusses this possibility with the patient and family. The location of the lesion and the overall health of the patient are important considerations in evaluating the patient's risks. A clear discussion of risks, presented in lay terms, is a necessary component of the process of informed consent.

The surgical site depends on the anatomic location of the lesion. The incision is usually made behind the hairline so the scar will be hidden once the patient's hair grows back. A portion of the skull bone is removed, placed aside during the surgery, and replaced at the end of the procedure (Figure 48-13). On rare occasions the bone is not replaced, such as with depressed skull fractures or a brain that is severely swollen after trauma. If the bone is left off, the procedure is referred to as a craniectomy. If possible, the bone is saved, stored in a bone bank, and replaced at a later date. Repair of the cranial defect may be performed with stored bone or with substitute acrylic bonelike materials. Once the bone is off, the dura mater is opened, allowing access to the brain. At the end of the surgery the dura is carefully closed with sutures to prevent CSF from leaking while healing takes place.

Tumors involving the pituitary gland that do not extend outside the sella turcica may be removed by a transsphenoidal approach. An incision is made either beneath the nose under the upper lip, or through the nose, and access to the sella turcica is gained through an opening at the rear of the sphenoid sinus (see Figure 38-3 and the discussion in Chapter 38). After the surgery, packing is placed in the nose and a fat graft from the abdomen is

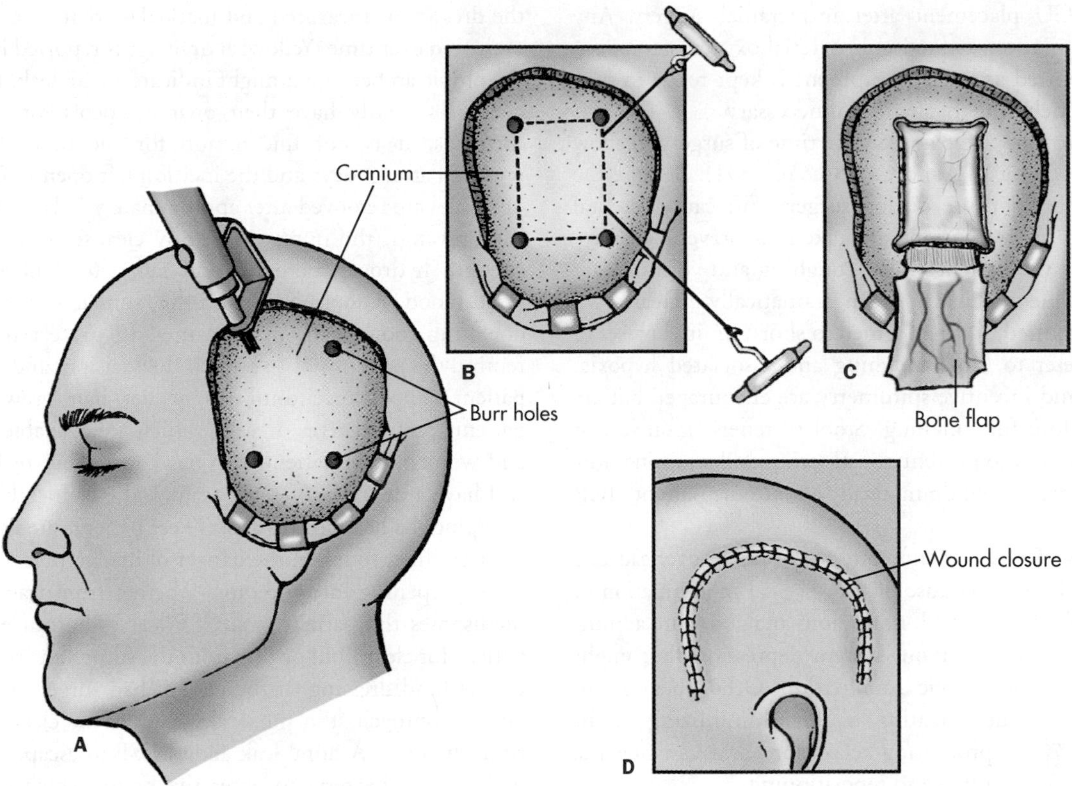

Figure 48-13 Craniotomy procedure. **A,** Burr holes are drilled into skull. **B,** Skull is cut between burr holes with a surgical saw. **C,** Bone flap is turned back to expose cranial contents. **D,** After surgery, bone flap is replaced and wound is closed.

used to close the defect in the dura.[34] Recovery is rapid, tissue damage in the brain is minimized, and the patient has no loss of hair or visible incision.

Nursing Management

of the Patient undergoing Intracranial Surgery

PREOPERATIVE CARE

A baseline neurologic assessment is performed and documented before surgery. The nurse involves both the patient and the family in all preoperative teaching to address their natural fears and concerns related to the surgery, postoperative care, a permanent change in appearance or behavior, dependency, or death. Psychologic support for the patient and family is a priority nursing intervention. The nursing staff provides sufficient time for the family to ask questions and allay their fears. The patient or family may wish to see a spiritual counselor before surgery.

The nurse carefully explains all treatments and procedures to the patient even if he or she does not seem to fully understand. The operative site is usually shaved in the operating room. Long hair is saved in case the patient wishes to have a wig made. Some surgeons prefer to shave only the area directly around the surgical site; other surgeons shave the entire head. To avoid depressing the patient's LOC, preoperative sedatives and opioids are rarely administered.

Family members need to know where to wait during surgery, approximately how long the surgery will take, and where the patient will receive care after surgery. If the patient is going to be in an ICU after surgery, the patient or family may want a brief tour of the unit. The nurse also prepares the family for the patient's appearance after surgery. A bulky head dressing is typically in place, and significant facial and periorbital edema may develop. The patient's LOC is also likely to be initially compromised.

POSTOPERATIVE CARE

Monitoring Vital Functions. In the immediate postoperative period the nurse performs frequent monitoring for subtle changes in the patient's neurologic status that might indicate complications requiring immediate management. The nurse assesses the patient regularly for signs of increased ICP. The frequency of assessment depends on the patient's condition.

Any changes in the patient's vital signs, LOC, cranial nerve examination, or motor examination are reported at once to the surgeon. Subtle changes in behavior, such as restlessness, can indicate increased ICP or bleeding into the surgical site that might require immediate corrective surgery. Respiratory arrest may occur after posterior fossa surgery as a result of edema in the brainstem and the inability to protect the airway with the cough or gag reflex. Respiratory monitoring is one of the major reasons for temporary ICU placement after intracranial surgery. Any irregularity of respiration, reduction in arterial oxygen saturation, or dyspnea is reported at once. Equipment is kept ready to support ventilation, including intubation, if necessary

An ICP monitor may be placed at the time of surgery to allow for direct monitoring of ICP and CPP (see p. 1391). Because the manipulation of brain tissue during surgery can cause cerebral edema after surgery, precautions are taken to prevent activity-related changes in the patient's ICP. Coughing and vomiting are prevented, if possible, because they can dramatically increase ICP. If suctioning is required, it is performed in short, limited passes of the suction catheter to limit coughing and associated hypoxia. Deep breathing and incentive spirometry are encouraged but are not followed by forceful coughing. Stool softeners, laxatives, or suppositories are given to prevent constipation and straining during defecation, which could dramatically elevate the patient's ICP.

Promoting Comfort. Patients often complain of headache after intracranial surgery because of the surgical manipulation of the coverings of the brain. Mild, nonopioid analgesics are administered to prevent central nervous system depression that might obscure the patient's neurologic examination. Other measures to promote comfort include treating nausea; minimizing bright lights and loud noises; promoting relaxation; and assisting the patient with hygiene, turning, and repositioning.

Preventing Injury. Most patients are started on anticonvulsant therapy preoperatively to prevent postoperative seizures. Seizure precautions are maintained during the immediate postoperative period, and the nurse checks blood levels of the anticonvulsant frequently. Care is taken to protect confused or agitated patients from injuring themselves by pulling at catheters, ICP monitors, or head dressings. Ventricular catheters are taped securely or wrapped in bulky dressings, and a stockinette can be loosely tied under the patient's chin to keep a head dressing in place. As a last resort, and with a physician's order, the nurse may apply restraints, using the least restrictive devices possible because struggling against restraints increases the patient's ICP. Commercially available hand mittens prevent patients from picking at dressings or tubes but still allow arm movement and enable the nurse to adequately assess the patient's skin and circulation.

Positioning of the patient during intracranial surgery may present the risk of corneal abrasions. Trauma, dysfunction, or surgery in the area of the seventh cranial nerve, which controls the ability to close the eyes, also predisposes the patient to this complication. The nurse inspects the patient's eyes for redness and the ability to blink and keeps the eyes moist. If the corneal reflex is absent, lubricating eyedrops or eye ointment is used to keep the eyes moist. Patients may need teaching to continue this intervention after discharge. Preventive eye care is extremely important with patients experiencing severe impairments of LOC. Corneal abrasion is a serious complication that can rapidly progress to severe eye infection.

Caring for the Incision. The craniotomy incision is usually covered with gauze dressings that are wrapped securely around the head. The nurse regularly inspects the head dressing for the presence, type, and amount of drainage. Serosanguineous drainage on the dressing is measured and marked so that it can be accurately evaluated over time. Yellowish drainage is reported immediately to the physician because it might indicate a CSF leak. Individual surgeons frequently have their own protocols for changing head dressings. It is not uncommon for the head dressing to be removed after 3 days and the incision left open to the air. Sutures or staples are removed after approximately 7 days. After removing the dressings, the nurse can gently cleanse the scalp with half-strength hydrogen peroxide and saline to remove any residual dried blood. A loose head covering, similar to the caps worn by operating room staff, may be used to protect the incision, to remind the patient not to scratch the incision, and to improve the patient's appearance until his or her hair grows back. Some patients prefer scarves or wigs, which are available for both men and women. The patient who has had a piece of bone removed will have a depression in the scalp and is vulnerable to injury by bumping the head in this area. These patients are usually provided with a helmet to lessen the danger of inadvertent brain injury.

Any opening into the dura, whether from trauma or surgery, predisposes the patient to a CSF leak. The nurse monitors the patient for clear fluid oozing from the suture line or clear drainage on the head dressing. If the patient had surgery via a transsphenoidal approach, the nurse also checks for clear fluid draining from the nose. A dural leak allows CSF to escape and provides a pathway for bacteria to enter the brain, which could result in meningitis.

CSF leaks usually heal spontaneously and do not require surgical intervention. The head of the bed is kept elevated to reduce CSF pressure at the site of the leak. Occasionally a lumbar drain is placed to remove small amounts of CSF and further reduce CSF pressure at the leak site.[39] The patient is instructed not to blow his or her nose and to restrict activities that would increase ICP and force CSF out of the leak. Antibiotics are administered until the leak is resolved.

Promoting Fluid Balance. Although fluids are carefully monitored until the patient's ICP has stabilized, fluids can usually be resumed as soon as the patient has active bowel sounds; is alert; and has adequate protective gag, swallow, and cough reflexes to drink without aspiration. IV fluids are used to supplement oral intake until the patient can drink 2000 to 2500 ml/day. An oral diet is resumed if the patient remains alert and does not experience nausea or vomiting.

Urinary output is monitored with an indwelling catheter for the first day or two postoperatively. The specific gravity of the urine is checked at least twice a day to rule out the presence of diabetes insipidus (DI). Although DI occurs most commonly after pituitary surgery, it can also occur after head trauma or other intracranial surgery (see Chapter 37).

Promoting Mobility. The postcraniotomy patient may be allowed out of bed on the first postoperative day. If the patient has been on bed rest for more than a few days, some deconditioning is expected. The nurse helps the patient to sit on the edge of the bed and dangle his or her legs. The nurse monitors the patient for postural hypotension or difficulty maintaining balance in the sitting position. Patients with motor or sensory deficits require additional support getting up to a chair or walking the first few times.

Early mobility prevents the complications associated with bed rest and helps the patient return to normal activity before discharge. Guidelines for care of the person after intracranial surgery are summarized in the Guidelines for Safe Practice box.

Patient/Family Teaching. The diagnosis of a brain tumor is frightening for the patient and family, and all aspects of the diagnosis and treatment are overwhelming and usually completely foreign. The nurse integrates teaching into all aspects of care, from explaining procedures and equipment to reassuring family members about the possible slow pace of recovery and rehabilitation. Many brain tumors carry a poor prognosis, which adds considerable stress to the patient's and family's attempts to cope and to plan for the future.

The nurse instructs the patient and family in the care of the incision and signs and symptoms indicating complications. The nurse ensures that they know how to safely use and monitor all medications, and explores their current and anticipated needs for assistance. The nurse provides written information about community resources for ongoing care and support, including the services of the American Cancer Society and hospice. Brain tumor associations can also be excellent sources of information and support.

The nurse also ensures that the patient and family know and understand the plans for follow-up care, including radiotherapy or chemotherapy if appropriate. The nurse ensures that initial appointments are scheduled and that they have accurate knowledge about anticipated side effects or complications of all planned care.

GERONTOLOGIC CONSIDERATIONS

Older adults undergoing intracranial surgery have special needs, both before and after surgery. It is important to differentiate between deficits related to the brain tumor and those related to other disease processes. For example, the patient may have underlying weakness from a prior stroke or unrelated orthopedic problem. The older patient may have underlying cardiac or pulmonary dysfunction that requires special preparation before surgery and meticulous monitoring during the postoperative period. The patient with a significant medical history may spend more time in the ICU for close monitoring.

Older patients may be slower to recover after surgery. Patients with significant cerebrovascular disease are at greater risk for hemorrhage or ischemic stroke as a result of intracranial vessel manipulation. Cerebrovascular disease can also compromise collateral circulation and cause ischemic damage during or after intracranial surgery. Slower postoperative recovery rates may necessitate planning for a short-term stay in a rehabilitation facility.

▶ ARE YOU READY?

Which statement by the patient diagnosed with a glioblastoma multiforme indicates the need for further teaching?

1. "I will have radiation therapy after surgery."
2. "This surgery will not cure my tumor."
3. "I will be taking anti-seizure medications after surgery."
4. "I am glad the surgeon will take the entire tumor out."

Craniocerebral Trauma

Etiology and Epidemiology. Craniocerebral trauma, or traumatic brain injury (TBI), causes death and serious disability in persons of all ages. Each year an estimated 2 million Americans sustain a TBI, and approximately 50,000 of these injuries result in death.[1] Serious TBIs have a devastating effect, making this diagnosis the leading cause of disability in the United States. Costs to society from TBI exceed $30 billion a year.[3] Motor vehicle accidents cause about 50% of TBIs, falls cause 21%, assaults and violence cause 12%, and sports-related injuries make up

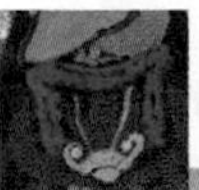

GUIDELINES FOR SAFE PRACTICE *Care of the Patient After Intracranial Surgery*

- Perform monitoring.
  - —Assess neurologic status, including ability to move, level of orientation and alertness, and pupil responses.
  - —Assess degree and character of drainage.
    - —Amount of drainage and bleeding should be minimal.
    - —Initial head dressing can be reinforced as necessary.
    - —Often incision is left open to air after first several days.
- Promote mobility.
  - —Turning to either side is permitted.
  - —If supratentorial surgery was performed, keep the head of the bed elevated at least 30 degrees.
  - —Early ambulation is encouraged to prevent complications of bed rest. Observe carefully for signs of postural hypotension; raise head of bed gradually; patient should always sit on side of bed before standing.
- Promote decreased intracranial pressure.
  - —Space nursing activities to allow patient to rest between them.
  - —Coughing and vomiting should be avoided.
  - —Perform suctioning only as necessary, and then gently and cautiously.
- Protect patient from injury.
  - —Use soft hand restraints if restraints are necessary.
  - —Use mittens as alternative to restraints. Change mittens every 4 hours; perform range-of-motion exercises with hand at this time.
  - —Keep side rails up at all times.
- Promote fluid and electrolyte balance.
  - —Perform accurate intake and output and specific gravity measurements. Do frequent testing for blood glucose.
  - —Have patient resume oral diet as soon as possible; assess for difficulty in swallowing or absence of gag reflex.
  - —Monitor electrolytes for evidence of abnormalities.
- Promote comfort.
  - —Medicate for comfort with codeine sulfate or nonopioid analgesic.
  - —Ice cap for headache may be helpful.

10%; alcohol is implicated in a significant percentage of all injuries.[15] Both morbidity and mortality rates are higher in males, and TBI is the major cause of death in persons between ages 1 and 35 years.[10] Research into the effects of helmet laws and requirements for protective gear for young athletes is ongoing as prevention of TBIs becomes an ever higher priority (see Research box).

Craniocerebral trauma may result from injury to the scalp, skull, and brain tissues, either singly or collectively. Variables that influence the extent of the injury to the head include (1) status of the head at the time of impact (moving or still), (2) location and direction of the impact, (3) rate of energy transfer, and (4) surface area involved in the energy transfer. Injuries vary from minor scalp wounds to open skull fractures with severe brain injury. The amount of visible external damage does not necessarily reflect the seriousness of the injury. Serious craniocerebral damage can occur in the absence of any apparent external injury.

The initial injury from head trauma is regarded as the primary trauma. Primary head injuries include scalp lacerations, concussions, contusions, skull fractures, and penetrating injuries. The effects of the initial trauma are typically compounded by subsequent secondary trauma, which represents the body's response to the initial injury. Examples of secondary injuries include edema, hematoma formation, hydrocephalus, and infection.

Pathophysiology. Primary head trauma results from three general types of injury: deformation, acceleration-deceleration, and rotation (Figure 48-14). Deformation results from the direct or indirect transmission of energy to the skull. If the force is sufficient, the skull is deformed or fractured. Acceleration-deceleration injuries typically occur when the accelerating skull, moving in a motor vehicle, suddenly decelerates when it hits an immobile object such as the steering wheel or windshield. The brain injury that results is often termed *coup–contra coup* because the brain first strikes the skull in the direction of movement and then rebounds and strikes the inner surface of the skull in the opposite direction. The damage from such injuries varies, depending on the speed of acceleration and deceleration. Rotational forces also distort the brain and can cause tension, stretching, and diffuse shearing of brain tissues. Often the forces of acceleration-deceleration and rotation occur together, affecting both the brain and the spinal cord.

Contusions, abrasions, and lacerations of the scalp may also occur. Lacerations of the scalp bleed profusely because of the scalp's rich blood supply and the poor vasoconstrictive abilities of these vessels. Hematomas that form under the surface of the scalp may obscure underlying skull fractures. Penetrating injuries cause direct destruction of brain tissue, vessel laceration, bleeding, and

Research

Coffman S: Bicycle injuries and safety helmets in children: review of research, *Orthopaed Nurs* 22(1):9-15, 2003.

This study reviewed the literature on the effects of social policy and custom in regard to bicycle helmet use and the incidence and severity of head injury in children. The problem is significant, since bicycle injuries are the most common cause of serious head injury in children and the most prevalent cause of pediatric trauma deaths, at 10%. Used correctly, helmets are believed to reduce the risk of severe head trauma by 68% to 88%.

A large national parent survey found wide state-to-state variation in estimated helmet use, ranging from 9.3% to 62.8%. The rates are consistently lowest in older adolescents and held at 3.8% in the late 1990s. Comprehensive standards for helmet quality have been developed and approved, and by 2001, 17 states and the District of Columbia had enacted mandatory helmet legislation, but the gains in rates of use have been modest. Several studies found that legislation is the most cost-effective way to increase helmet usage, paralleling the experience with car safety belts. Ample evidence now exists that use of helmets is directly linked to reductions in injury, hospital admissions, and injury severity. It remains to be seen whether the federal government will actively pursue a 50-state helmet requirement policy.

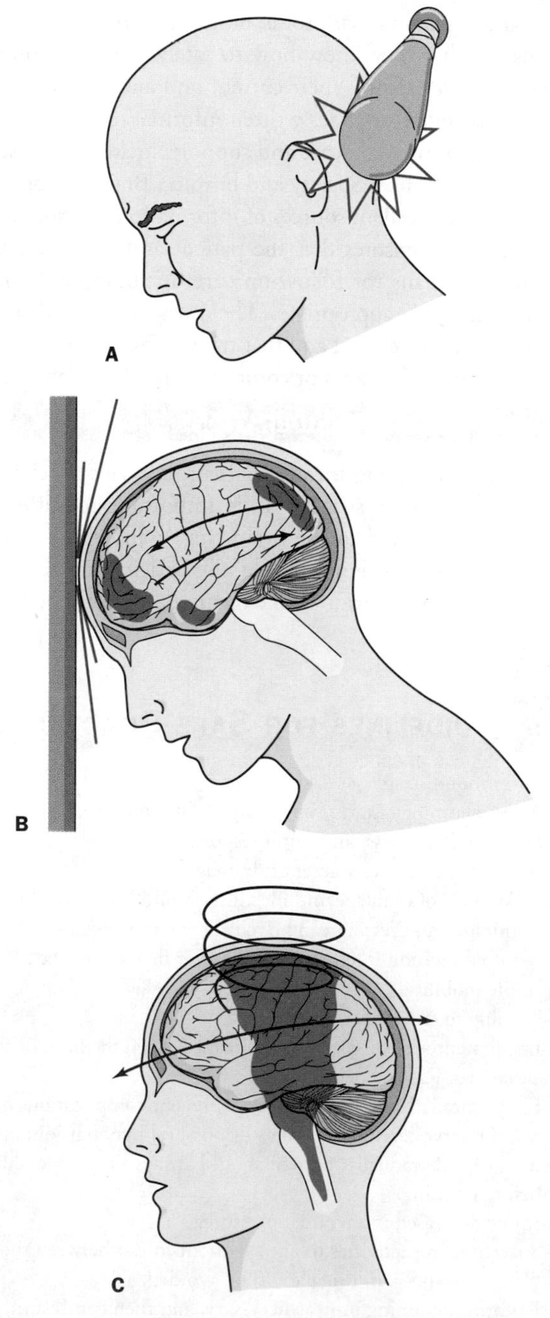

Figure 48-14 Mechanisms of injury. **A,** Deformation. **B,** Acceleration-deceleration. **C,** Rotation.

hematoma formation. Gunshot wounds are by far the most common cause.

Another primary brain injury is a concussion, which is characterized by an immediate and transient impairment of neurologic function induced by mechanical force. An instant or delayed loss of consciousness may occur, but usually the person recovers rapidly and the injury is classified as mild. A person who exhibits any alteration in consciousness after a blow to the head is closely observed after the injury, since the extent of the damage is not always immediately apparent. Postconcussion symptoms may develop, including headache, dizziness, fatigue, impaired memory, and impaired concentration. Although no structural neurologic changes are evident, current research indicates that the concussion of minor head injury may be correlated with subsequent cognitive impairments.[31] Diffuse axonal injury is caused by rapid movement of the brain during which delicate axons are stretched and damaged. This damage interferes with nervous transmission and can cause extensive diffuse deficits.[27] The effects of concussion are being carefully studied in the population of young athletes[23] (see Research box).

A contusion is a structural alteration characterized by the extravasation of blood into the brain. It can be likened to bruising without tearing of tissues. The contusion may be at the site of impact or on the opposite side—a *coup–contra coup* type of injury. Contusions often damage the cerebral cortex. Laceration of the brain and its blood vessels can occur with severe contusions and may be caused by a sharp fragment or a shearing force. On CT scanning, small, petechia-like areas of bleeding are seen.

Research

McCrea M et al: Acute effects and recovery time following concussion in collegiate football players, *JAMA* 290(19):2556-2563, 2003.

Guskiewicz KM et al: Cumulative effects associated with recurrent concussion in collegiate football players, *JAMA* 290(19):2549-2555, 2003.

The incidence and long-term effects of the chronic minor head trauma that occurs in sports has gotten increasing attention over the past decade. The National Collegiate Athletic Association (NCAA) in particular has taken an aggressive approach to exploring and tracking the effects of concussion in collegiate athletes. These two studies report findings from two parts of the ongoing NCAA Concussion Study, targeted at football players.

The first study looked at acute effects of concussion, considering symptom severity, cognitive impairment, and balance problems, and compared the findings with preseason baseline test results. Players experiencing concussion demonstrated symptoms in all areas with symptoms subsiding on average by day 7. Balance symptoms subsided first in 3 to 4 days, and cognitive impairment persisted for 5 to 7 days, by which point most players were actively involved in practice and playing again.

The second study looked at the association between prior concussion and the likelihood of experiencing another. The findings were striking. A strong positive association was found between a concussion history and the likelihood of experiencing an additional concussion. In addition, players who had experienced concussion in the past demonstrated a much slower recovery to baseline than those with no prior history. Headache was the most common persistent recognizable symptom reported by the players. Headache typically persisted for about 82 hours after injury.

Skull fractures are another common form of primary craniocerebral trauma. Fractures of the skull may be linear, comminuted, depressed, or basilar (Figure 48-15). Linear skull fractures appear as a fine line on skull x-ray studies. If the fracture crosses the path of the meningeal artery, arterial bleeding above the dura can occur, creating a medical emergency. Comminuted or depressed skull fractures involve bone displacement, sometimes down into the brain tissue itself. If the dura is torn, a CSF leak may occur.

Basilar skull fractures are particularly serious because the vital respiratory and vasomotor centers, cranial nerves, and major nerve pathways may be permanently damaged. If the injury creates a direct communication between the cranial cavity and the middle ear or the sinuses, meningitis or a brain abscess may develop. Bleeding from the nose and the ears suggests a basilar fracture. Serosanguineous drainage from the ears or nose may contain CSF. Any drainage is routinely tested for glucose, and positive results are reported to the physician immediately.[34] Drainage can also be blotted on a gauze pad. CSF, if present, will form a ring, or halo, as it dries. Other signs suggestive of basilar skull fracture include hemotympanum (a hemorrhagic exudate in the middle ear), bruising over the mastoid process (Battle's sign), and periorbital ecchymosis (raccoon eyes) (Figure 48-16). The latter two signs may not be evident for the first 24 hours after injury.

SECONDARY INJURY. Secondary injury results from the body's response to the initial trauma and includes cerebral edema, increased ICP, and hematoma formation. The brain becomes edematous in response to local injury, bleeding, and disturbances in the circulation that result in hypoxia. Cell damage and hypoxia increase cell membrane permeability, leading to cytotoxic edema. The damaged capillaries also become more permeable and allow fluid to leak out into the interstitial space. The fluid leak creates a condition called vasogenic edema that contributes to increased ICP. Most deaths from head injury occur from the effects of increased ICP rather than from the injury itself.

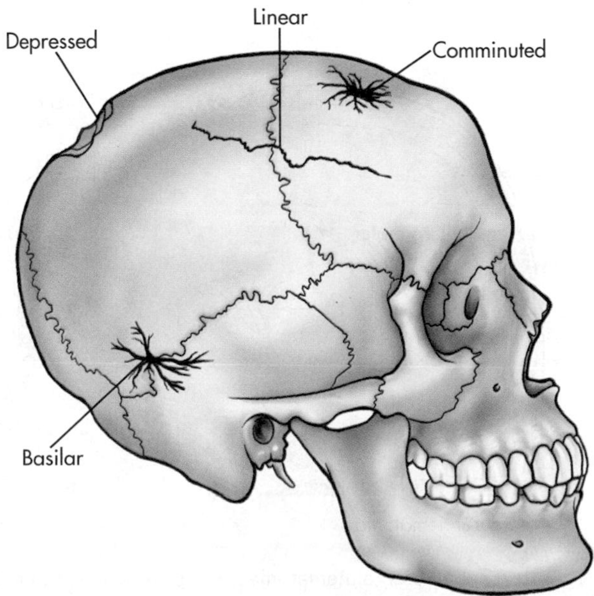

Figure 48-15 Types of skull fractures.

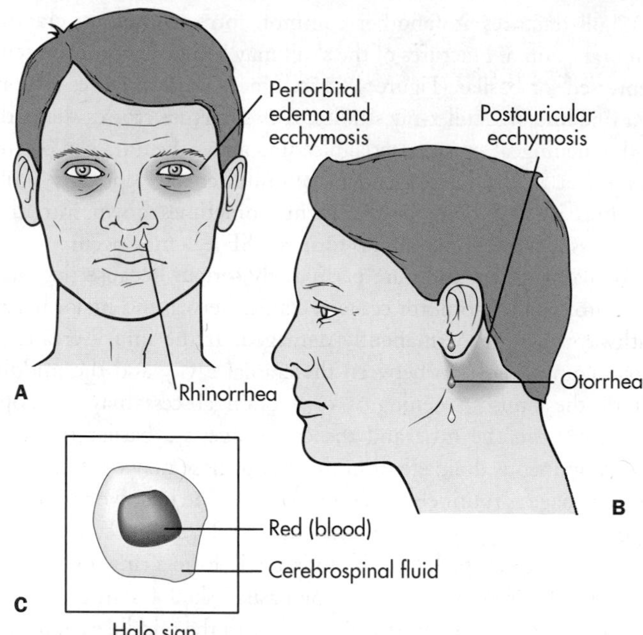

Figure 48-16 **A,** Raccoon eyes and rhinorrhea. **B,** Battle's sign (postauricular ecchymosis) with otorrhea. **C,** Halo, or ring, sign. Drainage containing cerebrospinal fluid forms a ring, or halo, as it dries on gauze pad.

Hematoma formation is another form of secondary injury (Figure 48-17). An *epidural hematoma* forms as blood collects between the dura and the skull. Because bleeding in this area is usually caused by laceration of the middle meningeal artery, the hematoma forms rapidly. The bleeding must be controlled promptly and the blood evacuated, or life-threatening neurologic deterioration occurs. Epidural hematomas often accompany basilar and temporal skull fractures. The nurse assesses frequently for signs of epidural hematoma (sudden deterioration in level of consciousness, signs of increasing ICP) when injuries occur in these sites.

A *subdural hematoma* forms when venous blood collects below the dural surface but above the brain. Because the bleeding is venous, the hematoma forms relatively slowly. However, the accumulating clot puts pressure on the brain surface and eventually displaces brain tissue if it becomes large enough. Subdural hematomas are subdivided into acute, subacute, and chronic varieties. Acute subdural hematomas develop within 48 hours of injury and have an organized clot. Subacute subdural hematomas develop within 3 days to 2 weeks after injury. The clot may become more fluid as the body attempts to break it down and remove it. Chronic subdural hematomas can produce symptoms from about 3 weeks to several months after the injury. The damaged area is filled with fluid rather than an organized clot. Acute and subacute hematomas present a greater threat to neurologic function because of the rapidity of their development. Chronic subdural hematomas evolve over a longer time, and the symptoms are typically less acute.

A third type of hematoma, the *intracerebral hematoma*, is common after a hemorrhagic stroke or aneurysm rupture. The blood collects within the brain parenchyma itself, and the symptoms are related to the specific area of the brain where the clot forms.

Complications. A wide range of complications can occur after head injury. Some patients develop seizures and need lifelong anticonvulsant therapy. Other patients develop obstructions to CSF flow and need to be treated for hydrocephalus. Autonomic responses to the injury may increase stomach acid production and cause peptic ulcers. The nurse works collaboratively to identify possible complications and develop plans for prevention and treatment. Neurobehavioral changes after head injury are well documented and present numerous challenges to the rehabilitative process.[27]

Complications during the treatment period are related to immobility, including atelectasis, pneumonia, cardiovascular deconditioning, skin breakdown, muscle atrophy, and constipation. Patients are also at risk for infection from breaks in the body's natural defenses

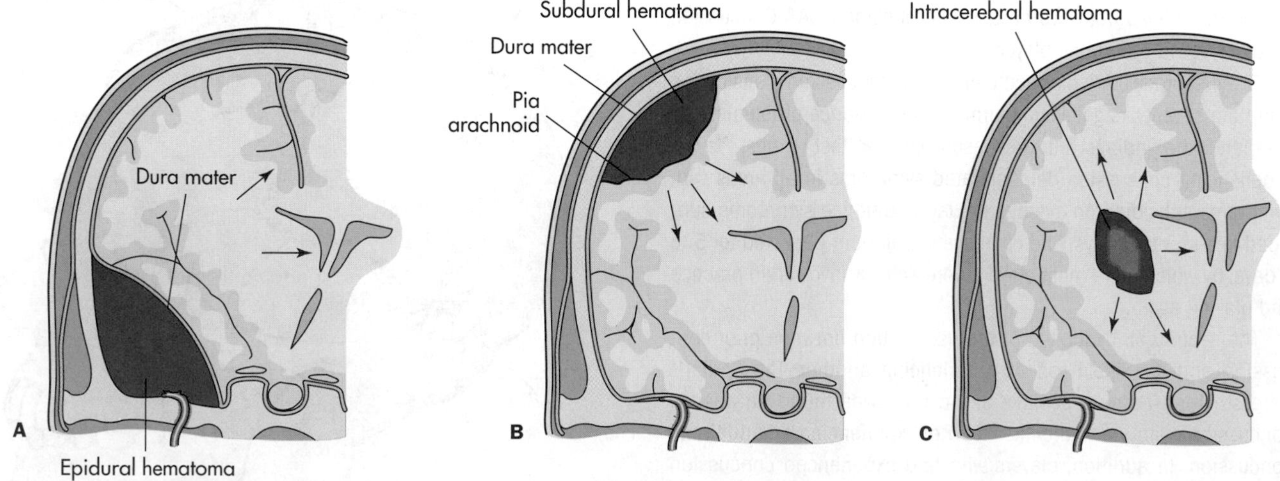

Figure 48-17 Cerebral hematomas. **A,** Epidural hematoma. **B,** Subdural hematoma. **C,** Intracerebral hematoma. *Arrows* indicate direction of pressure generated by the hematoma.

caused by invasive monitoring devices, IV lines, urinary catheters, and endotracheal tubes. If the patient has a skull fracture with a dural tear, meningitis is also a risk.

Collaborative Care Management

DIAGNOSTIC TESTS. Diagnostic procedures used to evaluate the nature and extent of head injury include CT scans, skull x-ray studies, and possibly cerebral angiography. The CT scan assesses for hematomas, edema, or damage related to skull fractures. X-ray films reveal skull or facial fractures. Cerebral angiography may be used to assess for injury to blood vessels or to determine if blood found within the skull is the result of trauma or a stroke.

Laboratory tests performed during the emergent care period include arterial blood gases, blood alcohol levels, and toxicology screens to rule out other potential contributors to any altered LOC.[30] Hemoglobin and hematocrit levels are drawn to establish a baseline for evaluating occult blood loss.

MEDICATIONS. Medications for the treatment of a head injury depend on the nature and severity of the injury. Medications may include drugs to reduce ICP, prevent seizures, or provide analgesia. Antibiotics are administered to any patient with a penetrating injury or evidence of a CSF leak.

TREATMENTS. Treatments for head injury depend on the presenting symptoms, the severity of the injury, and the presence of other systemic injuries. Multiple injuries are frequently present. The patient may be intubated to protect the airway, undergo surgery to treat internal injuries, or be immobilized to correct concurrent musculoskeletal injuries.

Initial management of a head injury focuses on resuscitation and stabilization, as well as prompt identification of rising ICP and other complications. The patient's ICP is monitored and treated as necessary. Ventilatory support is maintained and then gradually withdrawn as the patient recovers from his or her injuries. As the patient becomes more stable, less invasive monitoring is required and the patient is encouraged to participate more fully in ADLs.

SURGICAL MANAGEMENT. If the head injury causes hematoma formation, surgical intervention may be necessary. Craniotomies are performed to evacuate both epidural and subdural hematomas and repair the source of bleeding. If severe edema is present, the dura is closed surgically, but the overlying bone may be temporarily removed to allow room for anticipated brain swelling.[6] The bone is replaced when the edema subsides. Patients with depressed skull or facial fractures also undergo surgery to repair the injury and relieve pressure on the brain or other structures.

DIET. No special diet is prescribed for the patient with a head injury. The diet is determined largely by the patient's condition. If, after several days, the patient is unable to take in sufficient nutrients by mouth, enteral or parenteral nutrition may be initiated.

HEALTH PROMOTION AND PREVENTION. Traumatic head injuries can often be prevented. The importance of prevention is reflected in the objectives presented in the Healthy People 2010 box.[38]

Healthy People 2010

Objectives Related to Head Injury

- Reduce hospitalization for nonfatal head injuries to 45 per 100,000 persons.
- Reduce deaths caused by motor vehicle crashes to no more than 0.8 per 100 million vehicle miles traveled and 9.2 per 100,000 persons.
- Increase the use of safety belts to 92% of the total population.
- Reduce deaths from falls and fall-related injuries to no more than 3.0 per 100,000 persons.

From US Department of Health and Human Services: *Healthy people 2010: understanding and improving health,* Washington DC, 2000, The Department.

Primary prevention focuses on reducing the incidence of head injury through improved environmental safety and increased use of safety devices by all populations. Public health and information campaigns focus on specific strategies such as:

- Using seat belts, passive restraints, and air bags in automobiles
- Using helmets when riding motorcycles, snowmobiles, bicycles
- Practicing firearm safety and gun control
- Avoiding excess consumption of alcohol and drugs
- Avoiding driving after using drugs or drinking alcohol
- Improving home environmental safety features (e.g., securing throw rugs, removing clutter on stairs, installing grab bars in bathrooms, and increasing lighting)

Nurses have multiple opportunities to participate in primary prevention efforts with professional and community organizations through the schools, senior centers, bike clubs, and civic groups.

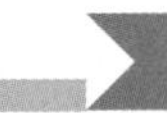

Nursing Management *of the Patient with Craniocerebral Trauma*

ASSESSMENT

Health History. Assess for:

- Details related to the nature of the injury—how it happened, treatment to date
- Any change in or loss of consciousness, duration
- Bleeding from the ears, nose, eyes, or mouth
- Patient's understanding of the injury and resulting pathologic consequences
- Patient's ability to understand
- Comorbid health conditions and current treatment regimen
- Medications in use: prescription, over the counter, and herbal
- Pattern of alcohol or drug use: type and amount
- Living situation, availability of family and social support

Physical Examination. Assess for:

- Adequacy of ventilation (patency of the airway, ability to cough, need for intubation)

- Adequacy of oxygenation (arterial blood gases, oxygen saturation)
- Changes in vital signs
- Signs of increased ICP (see Clinical Manifestations box, p. 1390)
- LOC, alertness, orientation
- Headache, nausea, or vomiting
- Pupil size, equality, reactivity
- Diplopia or other visual problems
- Movement and strength of extremities
- Sensory status, presence of unusual sensations (paresthesias, ringing in the ears)
- Speech pattern abnormalities
- Bleeding
- Battle's sign (ecchymosis behind the ears; indicates a basilar skull fracture)
- Raccoon eyes (ecchymosis and swelling around the eyes; indicates a possible orbital fracture)
- Discharge from the ears or nose

NURSING DIAGNOSES, OUTCOMES, AND INTERVENTIONS

Nursing Diagnosis: Risk for Impaired Spontaneous Ventilation

OUTCOMES. Common examples of expected outcomes for the patient with a diagnosis of *risk for impaired spontaneous ventilation* are:

Patient will:

- Demonstrate regular unlabored respirations.
- Maintain adequate ventilation as indicated by pulse oximetry reading above 90%, respiratory rate less than 20 breaths/min, and blood gas values within normal range.
- Maintain adequate cerebral perfusion and exhibit no signs or symptoms of increased ICP.

NURSING INTERVENTIONS. The nurse carefully monitors blood oxygen levels after any head injury. Pulse oximetry may be used to monitor oxygenation if the patient remains alert and awake. Alert, cooperative patients are encouraged to deep breathe frequently, but not to cough because of the risk of increasing ICP. Suctioning is used only if absolutely necessary to ensure a patent airway, and the nurse carefully hyperventilates and hyperoxygenates the patient before suctioning to minimize the adverse effects on ICP.[24] Arterial blood gases and pH are checked frequently when the patient's respiratory exchange or alertness is compromised.

Respiratory failure is a common complication of severe head injury. The patient with respiratory failure may develop dyspnea, hypoxia, hypercapnia, and hypotension. Each of these problems results in adverse consequences for the injured brain, and intubation and mechanical ventilation are often necessary. Cerebral anoxia is a leading cause of death among head-injured patients.

The nurse's role is primarily collaborative. Ongoing monitoring frequently necessitates admission to a critical care unit. Effective management of the patient's ventilatory status is carefully balanced with efforts to minimize any rise in ICP. Increased ICP is a major concern in patients with head injury; bedside neurologic checks and vital signs assessments are performed frequently until the patient's condition stabilizes. Patients with head injury are at immediate risk for increased ICP but may have also experienced trauma to other body systems and are at risk for shock. Specific interventions for increased ICP are discussed on pp. 1390 to 1394.

RELATED NIC INTERVENTIONS. Airway Management, Airway Suctioning, Mechanical Ventilation, Respiratory Monitoring

Nursing Diagnosis: Risk for Imbalanced Fluid Volume

OUTCOMES. A common example of an expected outcome for the patient with a diagnosis of *risk for imbalanced fluid volume* is:

Patient will:

- Maintain balanced fluid intake and urinary output, specific gravity within normal limits, normal electrolyte values, and stable body weight.

NURSING INTERVENTIONS. The nurse carefully measures and records intake and output, along with urine specific gravity if DI or SIADH is suspected. Fluid balance may be evaluated hourly when the patient's condition is unstable. Fluids are prescribed according to the patient's need for blood pressure support, for replacement of gastrointestinal losses from suctioning, or for balancing urinary output. Fluids are usually given parenterally but may be administered by feeding tube or by mouth, depending on the patient's condition. The nurse uses caution in administering fluids orally because the patient may have difficulty swallowing or may vomit and aspirate. The patient's urinary output is also carefully monitored if an osmotic diuretic such as mannitol is administered to help reduce cerebral edema and ICP. An indwelling catheter is inserted when mannitol is given because of the large amounts of urine produced and the need to measure output accurately. The catheter increases the risk of urinary tract infection and is removed as soon as possible.

Careful monitoring of electrolytes is also necessary. Several types of sodium imbalances are known to occur after head injury. Natriuresis, or increased urinary excretion of sodium, frequently occurs and is attributed to an increased plasma level of ADH resulting from SIADH. This causes hyponatremia and hypoosmolarity, which aggravate cerebral edema. Hypernatremia, or sodium retention, also may occur and has equally negative consequences for cerebral function. Plasma cortisol levels also tend to be elevated after an acute head injury.

RELATED NIC INTERVENTIONS. Cerebral Edema Management, Electrolyte Monitoring, Fluid/Electrolyte Management, Fluid Monitoring, Intravenous (IV) Therapy

Nursing Diagnosis: Risk for Infection

OUTCOMES. A common example of an expected outcome for the patient with a diagnosis of *risk for infection* is:

Patient will:

- Remain free from infection.

NURSING INTERVENTIONS. The nurse carefully observes the patient's ears and nose for blood or serous drainage, which may indicate that the meninges have been torn (common in basilar skull fractures) and that cerebrospinal fluid is escaping. Drainage from the nose can be tested for glucose to help differentiate CSF from mucus. Drainage can also be blotted on a gauze pad, since

CSF forms a halo on the gauze as it dries. No attempt should be made to clean the nose or ears or to block the drainage.[24] Usually the leak of CSF subsides spontaneously, but there is a risk of meningitis whenever a tear in the dura allows communication between the nasal cavity, the ears, and the brain. Antibiotics are started immediately if a patient is believed to be at risk.

If a leak is suspected, nurse instructs the patient not to cough, sneeze, or blow the nose. These activities may, in addition to contributing to the development of meningitis, enable air to enter the cranial cavity and increase ICP. Nasal suctioning is not used to remove secretions, and neither nasogastric nor nasotracheal tubes are inserted with any patient suspected of having a leak because of the risk of causing further damage or introducing infection.

Patients who develop fever undergo an immediate workup to identify the specific source of infection. Once cultures are obtained, the patient may be treated with empiric antibiotics and antipyretics to increase comfort. Fever may reach life-threatening levels if the brain's thermoregulation system fails, and tepid sponge baths or other more aggressive measures of reducing body temperature, such as cooling blankets, are used as a last resort.

The Guidelines for Safe Practice box summarizes the major foci for nursing care of the person who has experienced a closed head injury.

RELATED NIC INTERVENTIONS. Infection Control, Infection Protection

Nursing Diagnosis: Risk for Compromised Family Coping

OUTCOMES. Common examples of expected outcomes for the family with a diagnosis of *risk for compromised family coping* are: Family will:

- Verbalize concerns about effects of injury and ability to provide needed care.
- Explore methods to strengthen coping resources and utilize available community support services.

NURSING INTERVENTIONS. The duration of convalescence following head injury depends on how much damage has been done and how rapidly recovery progresses. Patients are usually encouraged to resume normal activities as soon as possible. The patient with a head injury may lose cognitive function and memory and develop behavioral problems associated with restlessness and a lack of judgment. Headache and occasional dizziness may be present for several months but gradually resolve. Loss of memory and initiative may also be present. Neuropsychologic testing can be used to identify subtle cognitive deficits and help guide rehabilitation.

Emotional support is important for both the patient and family caregivers, since both are likely to experience significant frustration. Patients need firm but gentle care and specific guidelines for appropriate behavior. If the patient with neurologic disease experiences severe personality changes, aphasia, or seizures, the family may even be afraid of the patient or may make tactless remarks in front of the patient. The nurse carefully assesses the family's response and reinforces teaching concerning head injury and its many possible consequences. Some persons require intensive physical rehabilitation, and others fail to make a satisfactory recovery and are left with serious functional deficits. Complete recovery from head injury is most likely to occur in persons younger than 20 years of age. Persons between the ages of 20 and 50 years who remain in a coma longer than 2 weeks rarely recover.

The nurse encourages the patient and family to focus on short-term gains rather than long-term goals to avoid becoming discouraged with the slow pace of recovery. Head injury support groups can be extremely helpful as the family learns to cope with the patient's behavior and deficits. The nurse also reinforces the importance of regular respite time for family caregivers.

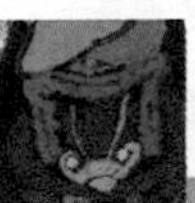
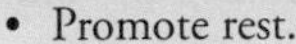

GUIDELINES FOR SAFE PRACTICE *The Patient With a Closed Head Injury*

- Promote rest.
  - —Provide a quiet environment.
  - —Observe patient frequently.
  - —Administer anticonvulsants as ordered.
  - —Medicate for pain as necessary.
- Maintain temperature.
  - —Give tepid sponge baths if patient is hyperthermic.
  - —Administer antipyretics as ordered.
  - —Use hypothermia blanket if ordered.
  - —Reduce or increase temperature in patient's room as needed.
- Promote adequate respiration.
  - —Suction only as necessary to provide adequate airway. Do not use nasal suctioning if CSF leak is suspected.
  - —Elevate head of bed to 30 degrees.
  - —Administer supplemental oxygen if ordered.
  - —Place patient in side-lying position.
- Observe for drainage from ears or nose.
  - —Make no attempt to clean out orifice.
  - —Do not suction nose if drainage is present.
  - —Have patient avoid coughing, sneezing, or blowing nose.
  - —Test drainage for presence of cerebrospinal fluid and report immediately if present.
- Control cerebral edema.
  - —Administer diuretics as ordered.
  - —Elevate head of bed to 30 degrees.
  - —Perform neurologic checks as ordered.
- Maintain electrolyte balance.
  - —Observe for syndrome of inappropriate antidiuretic hormone or diabetes insipidus.
  - —Monitor electrolytes.
- Maintain elimination.
  - —Keep accurate intake and output record.
  - —Monitor urine specific gravity.
  - —Restrict fluid if ordered.
  - —Remove catheter as soon as possible.
- Provide emotional support.
  - —Give specific guidelines for appropriate behaviors.
  - —Give positive feedback.
  - —Allow patient adequate time to complete tasks.

Patient/Family Teaching. A patient with a mild head injury may be evaluated in the emergency department but not admitted to the hospital. The families of these patients need very specific teaching about how to monitor for complications during the first 24 hours (see Patient/Family Teaching box). The person who has suffered a mild head injury can still experience long-term effects. These most often include cognitive problems such as difficulty with concentration and loss of memory. Recovery of full intellectual function often is delayed, and the deficits may manifest in the inability to keep a job or manage the challenges of daily living.

Patients with moderate head injuries may be discharged home to continue their rehabilitation on an outpatient basis. Hospital-based nurses assist families to identify appropriate resources in the local community. Resource selection is based on the patient's ability to perform self-care and the family's capabilities for providing the needed care and support.

Patients with severe head injuries and their families require a great deal of support during the critical care period. Trauma is unexpected, and families need to cope with sudden changes in their lives and the possibility of losing a loved one. Helping a family cope during the crisis phase is a major nursing responsibility in the ICU and continues throughout the patient's recovery. Research has found that the families of the critically ill list their most important needs as information about the patient's condition and access to the patient.[15] Family members may have severe emotional reactions and need a counselor's assistance to come to terms with the injury and its consequences. Sometimes neither the patient nor the family can grasp the enormity of the diagnosis and may need weeks or months to adjust to the patient's losses.

Patients with more severe head injuries may need long-term care either at a rehabilitation facility or at home. This care is often more supportive than restorative. The care needs of head-injured patients can be enormous, involving physical, psychologic, and cognitive challenges. It is imperative that the family participate actively in all long-term planning for the patient. Families need physical, social, and emotional support when providing this level of care long term. Teaching for the head-injured patient who is left with deficits is targeted to the patient's and family's unique strengths and deficits. The rehabilitation principles used are similar to those discussed in Chapters 49 and 50 for patients with stroke, spinal cord injury, or degenerative neurologic diseases.

PATIENT/FAMILY TEACHING

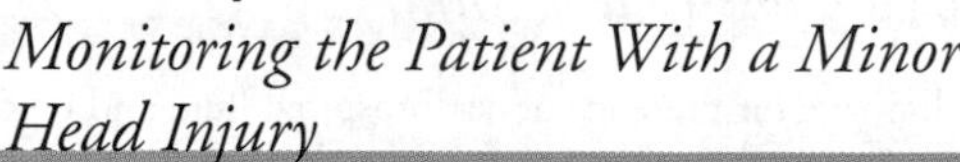

Monitoring the Patient With a Minor Head Injury

The patient should be awakened periodically through the first 24 hours to be sure he or she can wake up easily. Also, for the first 24 to 48 hours the family should watch carefully for the following warning signs:

- Vomiting, often with force behind it
- Unusual sleepiness, dizziness and loss of balance, or falling
- Complaint of seeing two of everything or blurry objects; jerking movements of the eyes
- Bleeding or discharge from nose or ears
- A headache that worsens, with the patient complaining of feeling worse while moving about (A slight headache may be expected.)
- Seizures—any twitching or movements of arms or legs that the patient is not able to control
- Any behavior or symptom that is not normal for the individual
- Change in speech or ability to converse

Call a physician at once if any of these signs is observed. Call either your personal physician or emergency services.

EVALUATION

To evaluate the effectiveness of nursing interventions, compare patient behaviors with those stated in the expected patient outcomes.

RELATED NOC OUTCOMES. Caregiver Emotional Health, Caregiver-Patient Relationship, Electrolyte & Acid/Base Balance, Family Coping, Fluid Balance, Neurological Status: Consciousness, Respiratory Status: Ventilation, Risk Control, Thermoregulation

GERONTOLOGIC CONSIDERATIONS

The older patient may have preexisting conditions that contributed to the head injury. Altered gait, balance, and reflexes make the older patient more prone to falls. Osteoporosis increases the risk, frequency, and severity of fractures of the skull and face. Syncope, hypotension, and cardiac dysrhythmias can also lead to falls. Patients receiving anticoagulant therapy are more likely to develop hematomas after falls.

Older patients with significant medical histories, especially problems with hypertension or cerebrovascular disease, have less physiologic reserve to survive the acute period following a moderate to severe head injury.[6] The assessment of patients with a known degenerative disorder such as Alzheimer's disease is complicated by the need to differentiate between pretrauma abnormalities and those related to the trauma itself. Patients with sensory losses related to aging, such as vision or hearing losses, may have difficulty participating in therapy. An older patient who was barely independent before a nervous system trauma may not be able to regain independence even when the residual deficits are minor.

Nurses educate patients and families in ways to keep the older population safe from injuries that rob them of their independence and health. Environmental modifications to remove hazards and the use of mobility aids, sensory enhancement aids, and structured exercise can help the older patient retain strength and mobility.

Infections and Inflammation

The nervous system may be attacked by a variety of bacteria and viruses that reach the nervous system by various routes. Chronic otitis media, sinusitis, mastoiditis, and fracture of any bone adjacent to the meninges can be a source of infection. Some organisms, such as the tubercle bacillus, reach the nervous system by means of the blood or lymph system. Infection can also occur as a complication of invasive procedures such as lumbar puncture. The exact route by which some infectious agents reach the central nervous system is not known. The infection may wall off and create an abscess, or the meninges and sometimes the brain itself may become involved. Two of the more common central nervous system infections—meningitis and encephalitis—are discussed here.

Meningitis

Etiology and Epidemiology. Meningitis can be caused by bacteria, viruses, and fungi. The infection targets the arachnoid and pia layers of the meninges (leptomeminges) and the CSF. Bacterial meningitis usually develops acutely and can cause serious morbidity and mortality. Bacterial meningitis was fatal in more than 70% of cases before the development of antibiotics and still carries a mortality rate of about 25%.[1] The incidence of meningitis is fairly constant throughout the year, but declines somewhat during the summer months. It targets the very old and very young and affects males more often than females.[32] About 3000 new cases are diagnosed each year. The bacterial causative organisms vary substantially throughout the life span (Box 48-10). Most of the infecting organisms can routinely be found in the oropharnyx. Viral meningitis, also known as aseptic meningitis, is usually a more benign and self-limiting disease. It is commonly caused by enteroviruses and mumps organisms and usually does not require extensive treatment.

Pathophysiology. Bacteria in the nasopharynx can enter the bloodstream during an upper respiratory tract infection; once organisms reach the brain, both the CSF in the subarachnoid spaces and the pia-arachnoid membrane can become infected. The infection then spreads rapidly throughout the meninges and eventually can invade the ventricles. Most organisms create a purulent exudate that clings to the meningeal layers and clogs the CSF. It tends to accumulate at the base of the brain and progress rapidly to vascular congestion and obstruction. Cranial nerve dysfunction occurs as the inflammatory exudate coats the nerve sheath. Pathologic alterations include hyperemia of the meningeal blood vessels; edema of brain tissue; increased ICP; and a severe, generalized inflammatory reaction accompanied by massive exudation of white blood cells into the subarachnoid spaces. Acute hydrocephalus may result when this exudate blocks the small passages between the ventricles. Seizures occur in up to 50% of patients.

Meningitis can manifest as a medical emergency. The onset is usually sudden and characterized by severe headache, stiff neck **(nuchal rigidity)**, fever, irritability, malaise, and restlessness. Nausea, vomiting, delirium, and complete disorientation may develop quickly. The patient's LOC may decline rapidly from drowsiness to coma. Kernig's sign (an inability to extend the leg at the knee when the thigh is flexed) usually is present, and Brudzinski's sign (the hip and knee flexing when the patient's neck is flexed) may also be present (Figure 48-18).

Box 48-10 Causes of Bacterial Meningitis

- *Haemophilus influenzae*
  —Most common form in young children
  —Usually follows an upper respiratory tract infection
  —Neurologic complications in 30% to 50% of those infected
- *Neisseria meningitidis* (meningococcal)
  —A common form; rapidly progressive and serious
  —Affects primarily children and young adults
  —Epidemics in winter and spring
  —Petechial rash in 50% of those infected
- *Streptococcus pneumoniae* (pneumococcal)
  —Seen primarily in children and older adults
  —High mortality despite antibiotics
  —Deafness and mental retardation common complications
- Group B streptococci
  —Commonly seen following other group B strep infections
- Staphylococci
  —Associated with infected shunts, septicemia
- Gram-negative organisms (enteric bacilli, e.g., *Escherichia coli*, *Enterobacter* and *Serratia* organisms)
  —Usually a nosocomial infection
  —Associated with neurotrauma or neurosurgery

Collaborative Care Management. Rapid, accurate diagnosis of bacterial meningitis is critical, since the patient's condition can deteriorate quickly. Definitive diagnosis requires culturing the CSF, which is obtained by lumbar puncture or from a ventriculostomy. The causative organism can usually be isolated from the spinal fluid, which is cloudy if a pyogenic organism is present. The CSF pressure and protein level are also usually elevated, whereas glucose content is usually decreased.[18] A CT scan may also be performed to rule out other pathologic conditions.

Treatment for bacterial meningitis consists of antibiotic therapy targeted at the specific causative organism. Parenteral antibiotics are given for at least 10 days and may be administered directly into the spinal canal (intrathecally). Respiratory isolation is required with meningococcal infections until the pathogen can no longer be cultured from the nasopharynx, usually after 24 hours of antibiotic therapy. Isolation is not needed with other forms of the disease. Hyperosmolar agents or steroids may be administered to control cerebral edema, and anticonvulsants may be given to prevent or control seizures. If the patient develops hydrocephalus as a result of the meningitis, a shunt may need to be inserted to facilitate the flow of CSF.

Treatment includes supportive care to control and reduce fever, balance fluids and electrolytes, and promote comfort. The headache can be severe, and the patient's fever may remain high throughout the illness. Acetaminophen (Tylenol) is typically given to reduce the fever and relieve the headache. Ice packs may increase the patient's comfort. The nurse monitors the patient frequently, avoiding unnecessary stimulation and touching. Seizure precautions are instituted, and tepid baths may be necessary to control the patient's fever. Patients who experience photophobia are more comfortable in a darkened room. Lights and noise are minimized.

The course of viral meningitis is typically much less severe, and the patient is less obviously ill than with bacterial meningitis. However, there is no effective treatment, and both the patient and family need to understand the nature of supportive care.

PATIENT/FAMILY TEACHING. The patient and family are often anxious and have many questions regarding how the disease started and the plan for treatment. The extent and severity of symptoms vary greatly from patient to patient. Some patients are only mildly affected and simply need supportive care. Others are acutely ill and need critical care monitoring and support. The nurse keeps the family fully informed about the patient's status and prognosis and helps them to understand that the disease can cause permanent neurologic impairment and occasionally death.

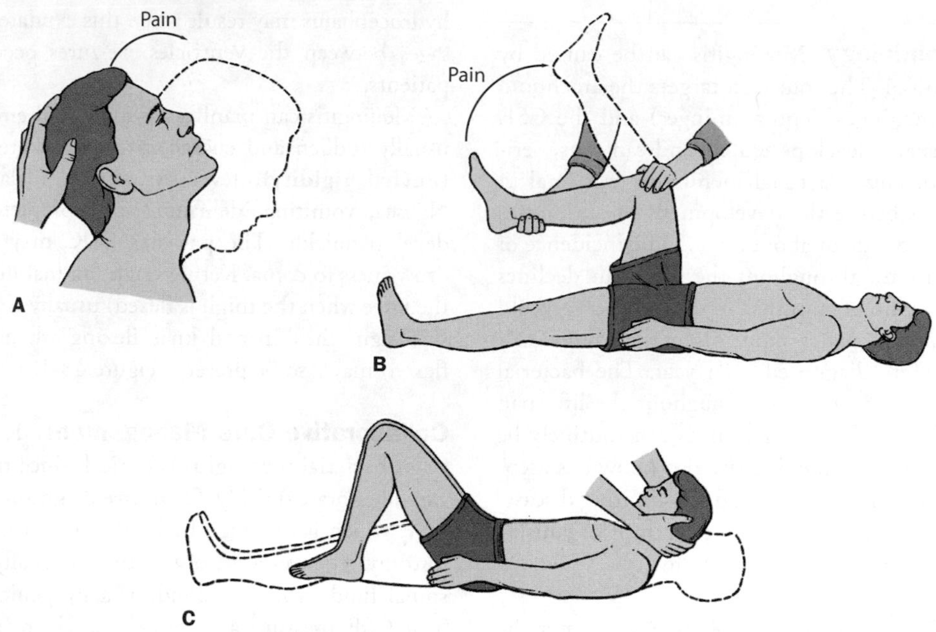

Figure 48-18 Signs of meningeal irritation. **A,** Nuchal rigidity. Neck is held extended and immobile. Attempts to flex the neck cause pain. **B,** Positive Kernig's sign: inability to extend leg from position of 90-degree flexion at the hip. Attempts to extend leg cause pain and spasms in hamstrings. **C,** Brudzinski's sign: passive flexion of head and neck causes flexion of thighs and legs.

Parents of young children in particular need ongoing teaching and support.

Encephalitis

Etiology and Epidemiology. Encephalitis is an acute infection of the brain parenchyma and meninges that can be caused by bacteria, viruses, or fungi. Viral infections are by far the most common and are typically caused by the arboviruses or herpes simplex. A wide variety of viruses, indigenous to various geographic areas, are capable of causing the disease if they gain access to the brain. The St. Louis virus is the most common. Encephalitis has often appeared in epidemics. The most significant outbreak in the United States followed the influenza epidemic of 1918 and involved von Economo's disease. This particular form of encephalitis has not reappeared since 1926.

West Nile virus has brought renewed attention to the problem of encephalitis in the United States. The illness first appeared in New York in the late 1990s and has been steadily and slowly spreading to other areas of the country.[22] The disease is found in the bird population, particularly in crows, and is transmitted to humans via mosquitoes. West Nile virus is a form of flavovirus and has proven fatal in older, debilitated patients.[18]

Pathophysiology. Encephalitis causes widespread inflammation of the meninges and brain parenchyma, resulting in congestion and swelling. This triggers degenerative changes in the myelin and nerve cells. Symptoms vary significantly, depending on the causative organism, but often include the abrupt onset of fever, headache, stiff neck, seizures, and a declining LOC that can progress from lethargy and restlessness to coma. A variety of local neurologic signs can also be present. The mortality rate for encephalitis also varies substantially with the causative organism, but is as much as 20% for those who are hospitalized. Most patients who recover are left with some degree of residual deficit, including decreased cognitive functioning, personality changes, paralysis, and dementia. Patients can also be left deaf and blind.

Collaborative Care Management. Encephalitis is diagnosed primarily from the clinical picture, serology assays, and MRI. Treatment is largely supportive and symptomatic because no effective antiviral treatment is available for most forms of the disease. Acyclovir has demonstrated effectiveness against herpesvirus infections if treatment is initiated promptly, reducing the mortality rate from as much as 80% to less than 28%.[15] Culture of the CSF is much less helpful with viral encephalitis than with bacterial disease.

Analgesics may be prescribed for the headache and neck pain that accompany the disease. Steroids are administered to suppress inflammation, and anticonvulsants are used to control seizures. In severe cases dramatic increases in ICP can result in brainstem herniation or widespread areas of cell necrosis.

Patient/Family Teaching. The needs of the patient and family for education and support are similar to those outlined for patients with meningitis, particularly when the patient is seriously ill. The fear associated with the disease and its uncertain outcome necessitate frequent interventions and ongoing support from the nurse. It is essential that the nurse include the family in all decisions about the patient's care and keep them honestly apprised of the patient's status.

Preparing for Practice

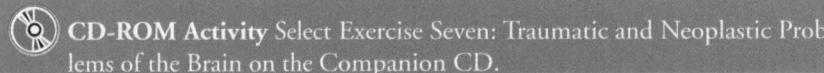

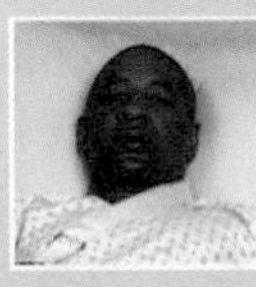

Patient: *David Ruskin,* **Room 303**

David Ruskin is a 32-year-old African-American man who suffered a closed head injury, fractured humerus, and scalp lacerations after being struck by an automobile while bicycling.

Assessment

View the patient's **Report**.

Open the patient's **Medical Record** to familiarize yourself with his care. Specifically, click on the following areas as part of your review: History & Physical (focus on the Emergency Department Report), Physicians' Orders, and Nurses' Notes.

Conduct a **Patient Interview**. As you conduct your interview, focus primarily on data that will be helpful in planning care for this patient. Record the data you collect.

Nursing Diagnoses, Outcomes, and Interventions

1. What are the four variables that directly influence the extent of traumatic brain injury (or craniocerebral trauma) sustained by a patient?
2. What is the description of David Ruskin's head injury in the chart? What other data are important to note with regard to the accident and the events that immediately followed?
3. To what extent does David Ruskin fit the profile of the typical patient admitted to the emergency department with traumatic brain injury? *Hint:* Note the discussion under Etiology and Epidemiology for craniocerebral trauma on pp. 1409 and 1410.
4. Review the mechanisms of traumatic brain injury in Figure 48-14. Note the picture that represents the type of injury experienced and briefly describe why it applies to David Ruskin.
5. What is the Glasgow Coma Scale? What are its three categories, and how is it scored?
6. What were David Ruskin's Glasgow Coma Scale scores in the emergency department? What interpretation can you make about his neurologic status based on these scores?
7. What documentation did you find in the Nurses' Notes related to neurologic status?
8. Mr. Ruskin is admitted to your unit. What nursing actions should you implement to promote optimal outcomes in this patient with closed head injury? *Hint:* Refer to the Guidelines for Safe Practice box, p. 1415, for help. Describe the rationale for each of your actions.

Critical Thinking

1. A 34-year-old woman is admitted after having a tonic-clonic seizure. She has never experienced a seizure before. What would you assess during her postictal phase? Once she is completely alert, what areas would you explore as part of a detailed health history?
2. Does your state or community have helmet laws for motorcycle and bicycle riders? Prepare a teaching plan concerning the prevention of head injury to use with school-age children. How would you modify the plan to address adolescents? Older adults?

References

1. Barker E: *Neuroscience nursing: a spectrum of care,* ed 2, St Louis, 2002, Mosby.
2. Barkley GL, Baumgartner C: MEG and EEG in epilepsy, *J Clin Neurophysiol* 20(3):163-178, 2003.
3. Bellner J et al: Diagnostic criteria and the use of ICD-10 codes to define and classify minor head injury, *J Neurol Neurosurg Psychiatry* 74(3):351-352, 2003.
4. Benbadis SR, Tatum WO, Gieron M: Idiopathic generalized epilepsy and choice of antiepileptic drugs, *Neurology* 61(12):1793-1795, 2003.
5. Booth CM et al: The rational clinical examination: is this patient dead, vegetative or severely neurologically impaired? *JAMA* 291(7):870-879, 2004.
6. Bulgar EM et al: Management of severe head injury, *Crit Care Med* 30(8):1870, 1876, 2002.
7. Cady R, Dodick DW: Diagnosis and treatment of migraine, *Mayo Clin Proc* 77(3):255-261, 2002.
8. Chabolla DR: Characteristics of the epilepsies, *Mayo Clin Proc* 77(9):981-990, 2002.
9. Cheung RTF, Zou L: Use of the original, modified, or new intracerebral hemorrhage score to predict mortality and morbidity after intracerebral hemorrhage, *Stroke* 34(7):1717-1722, 2003.
10. Donders J, Callahan CD: Moderating factors in rehabilitation outcome, *J Head Trauma Rehab* 18(2):105-195, 2003.
11. Elovic EP: Anterior pituitary dysfunction after traumatic brain injury, part 1, *J Head Trauma Rehabil* 18(6):541-543, 2003.
12. Erlanger DM et al: Development and validation of a web based screening tool for monitoring cognitive status, *J Head Trauma Rehabil* 17(5):458-476, 2002.
13. Evans RW, Olesen J: Migraine classification, diagnostic criteria, and testing, *Neurology* 60(7 Suppl S2):S24-S30, 2003.
14. Goadsby PJ, Lipton RB, Ferrari MD: Migraine: current understanding and treatment, *N Engl J Med* 346(4):257-270, 2002.
15. Hickey JV: *The clinical practice of neurological and neurosurgical nursing,* ed 5, St Louis, 2003, Lippincott.
16. Holroyd KA, Mauskop A: Complementary and alternative therapies, *Neurology* 60(7):S58-S62, 2003.
17. Huynh T et al: Positive end-expiratory pressure alters intracranial and cerebral perfusion pressure in severe traumatic brain injury, *J Trauma: Injury Infect Crit Care* 53(3):488-493, 2002.
18. Jeha LE et al: West Nile virus infection: a new acute paralytic illness, *Neurology* 61(1):55-59, 2003.
19. Jennett B: The vegetative state, *J Neurol Neurosurg Psychiatry* 73(4):355-357, 2002.
20. Josephson L: Management of increased intracranial pressure: a primer for the non-neuro critical care nurse, *Dimens Crit Care Nurs* 23(5):194-207, 2004.

21. Kanan A, Gasson B: Brain tumor resections guided by magnetic resonance imaging, *AORN J* 77(3):583, 585-586, 588-589, 2003.
22. Katz LM, Bianco C, Morse DL: West Nile virus: not a passing phenomenon, *N Engl J Med* 349(19):1873-1874, 2003.
23. Kaut KP et al: Reports of head injury and symptom knowledge among college athletes, *Clin J Sports Med* 13(4):213-221, 2003.
24. LeJeune GM, Howard-Fain T: Nursing assessment and management of patients with head injuries, *Dimens Crit Care Nurs* 21(6):226-231, 2002.
25. Lemke DM: Epidemiology, diagnosis, and treatment of patients with metastatic cancer and high grade gliomas of the central nervous system, *J Infusion Nurs* 27(4):263-269, 2004.
26. Lipton RB, Newman LC: Epidemiology, impact, and comorbidities of migraine headaches in the United States, *Neurology* 60(7 Suppl 2):S3-S8, 2003.
27. Machamer JE, Temkin NR, Dikmen SS: Neurobehavioral outcome in persons with violent or nonviolent traumatic brain injury, *J Head Trauma Rehabil* 18(5):387-397, 2003.
28. Manno EM: New management strategies in the treatment of status epilepticus, *Mayo Clin Proc* 78(4):508-518, 2003.
29. Matchar DB: Acute management of migraine: highlights of the US Headache Consortium, *Neurology* 60(7 Suppl 2):S21-S23, 2003.
30. Mateo MA: Evaluation of patients with mild traumatic brain injury, *Lippincott's Care Manage* 8(5):203-207, 2003.
31. McKeag DB: Understanding sports related concussion: coming into focus but still fuzzy, *JAMA* 290(19):2604-2605, 2003.
32. Parini SM: The meningitis mind bender, *Nurs Manage* 33(8 part 1):21-26, 2002.
33. Quinn C, Chandler C, Moraska A: Massage therapy and frequency of chronic tension headache, *Am J Pub Health* 92(10):1657-1661, 2002.
34. Schlosser RJ, Bolger WE: Nasal cerebrospinal fluid leaks: critical review and surgical considerations, *Laryngoscope* 114(2):255-265, 2004.
35. Shackleton DP: Living with epilepsy: long term prognosis and psychosocial outcomes, *Neurology* 61(1):64-70, 2003.
36. Silberstein SD, Freitag FG: Preventive treatment of migraine, *Neurology* 60 (7 Suppl 2):S38-S44, 2003.
37. Sirven JI: Antiepileptic drug therapy for adults: when to initiate and how to choose, *Mayo Clin Proc* 77(12):1367-1375, 2002.
38. US Department of Health and Human Services: *Healthy people 2010: national health promotion and disease prevention objectives,* Washington, DC, 2000, The Department.
39. Welch KM, Curter FM, Goadsby PJ: Migraine pathogenesis: neural and vascular mechanisms, *Neurology* 60(7 Suppl 2):S9-S14, 2003.

evolve Visit the Evolve website: http://evolve.elsevier.com/Monahan/medsurg

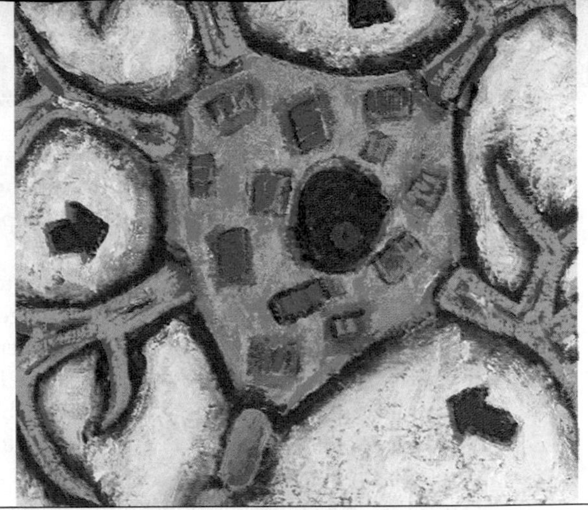

CHAPTER 49 Vascular and Degenerative Problems of the Brain

by Jeanne Flannery, Susan Bulecza

OBJECTIVES

After studying this chapter, the learner should be able to:

1. Identify the major risk factors for ischemic and hemorrhagic stroke.
2. Correlate stroke pathology with its major clinical manifestations.
3. Compare neurologic and behavioral findings associated with right versus left hemisphere strokes.
4. Develop specific assessment strategies for identifying the primary communication and sensory-perceptual deficits of stroke.
5. Discuss the rationale for antiplatelet therapy, reperfusion therapy, and carotid endarterectomy in the management of cerebrovascular disease and stroke.
6. Develop nursing interventions to assist patients in regaining self-care independence after stroke.
7. Describe nursing interventions to prevent the musculoskeletal and nutritional complications of stroke.
8. Develop a patient and family teaching plan to manage the communication, cognitive, behavioral, and emotional outcomes of stroke.
9. Compare the treatment options for aneurysms and arteriovenous malformations.
10. Compare the major degenerative and autoimmune neurologic disorders in terms of incidence, populations affected, and primary pathologic condition.
11. Describe the pharmacologic management of myasthenia gravis and Parkinson's disease.
12. Compare the major nursing interventions used to manage mobility, self-care, nutrition, bowel and bladder elimination, and safety concerns for each of the major degenerative and autoimmune neurologic disorders.

KEY TERMS

demyelination, p. 1441
dopaminergic neurons, p. 1445
hemiparesis, p. 1426
hemiplegia, p. 1426
hemorrhagic, p. 1422
ischemic, p. 1422
neurologic deficits, p. 1424
neurotoxins, p. 1444
neuromuscular junction, p. 1449
reperfusion, p. 1424

This chapter presents the management of selected vascular, degenerative, and autoimmune disorders affecting the brain. Stroke is by far the most important of these disorders because of its incidence and its extensive residual deficits, which challenge patients, families, and health care providers. All the common autoimmune and degenerative disorders presented here have complex associated care needs, which share the common goal of maximizing the patient's independence in self-care for as long as possible and supporting overall coping. These disorders are managed by a multidisciplinary team, but the nurse is commonly called on to serve as the case manager, coordinating needed services.

Cerebrovascular Disease

The term *cerebrovascular disease* refers to any pathologic process involving the blood vessels of the brain. Cerebrovascular disease is the most common neurologic disorder in adults and is the third leading cause of death in the United States, after heart disease and cancer. The heterogeneous category of cerebrovascular disease encompasses two major types of disorders—**ischemic** and **hemorrhagic**—each of which can produce either temporary or permanent deficits in neurologic functioning.

Major ischemic or hemorrhagic problems create a syndrome of neurologic deficits that reflect impairment of oxygenation to a specific area of the brain. This syndrome is usually referred to as a brain attack or stroke. A stroke is a group of sudden focal neurologic deficits resulting from interruption of cerebral blood flow. It is called a syndrome rather than a disease because it has more than one cause. A synonym used in the past is cerebrovascular accident, but a stroke is frequently caused by an underlying cerebrovascular disorder and is therefore no accident. The term *stroke* is preferred for this reason. More recently, however, as research increases our understanding of the metabolic cascade of alterations that follow the initial insult, health care givers are promoting the term *brain attack*. In this text the term *stroke* is generally used because it is more common; in the future *brain attack* will likely be the preferred term.

The outcome of a stroke depends on how rapidly treatment can be started,[19] since it is not an "all-or-nothing" event but instead produces progressive cellular changes. The whole approach in caring for the patient with ischemic stroke will change in the future. Education for all health care providers, from paramedics at the scene, to hospital personnel receiving the patients, will focus on neuroprotection within the tight window of time available. These patients need to be viewed as class A emergencies, just like persons with heart attacks.

Although strokes can have either an ischemic or a hemorrhagic origin, the following discussion is primarily directed toward the management of ischemic strokes, which are by far the most common form.[31] Hemorrhagic strokes are discussed later in the chapter under Cerebral Aneurysm and Arteriovenous Malformation.

Box 49-1 Causes of Ischemic Strokes

- *Atherosclerotic:* Atherosclerosis affects both the large extracranial and the intracranial arteries. The lumen of the vessel narrows and can be a target site for thrombus formation. Transient ischemic attacks occur in about half of patients before the stroke.
- *Small penetrating artery thrombosis, lacunar:* Thrombosis of a small penetrating brain artery causes a small damaged area of tissue in the deep white matter structures of the brain, called a lacuna. Lacunae typically occur in the basal ganglia, internal capsule, pons, or thalamus.
- *Cardiogenic embolic:* Most of these strokes are the result of emboli, usually of cardiac origin, that break off and travel in the arterial circulation until they reach a vessel that is too narrow to allow further passage. Atrial fibrillation is the most common cause of the emboli.
- *Other causes:* Ischemic strokes can also result from arteritis vasospasm; inflammation; coagulation disorders; and the effects of drug abuse, particularly cocaine.
- *Idiopathic:* No identifiable cause is established in up to 30% of all ischemic strokes.
- *Global hypoperfusion:* Cardiac arrest or pulmonary embolism lead to devastating reduction of cerebral blood flow and cerebral perfusion pressure.

Brain Attack (Stroke)

Etiology. A brain attack is a focal neurologic deficit that has a sudden onset as a consequence of a disturbance in circulation or cerebral ischemia that lasts for more than 24 hours; it may cause irreversible brain injury. Global cerebral ischemia develops when the blood flow is inadequate to meet the metabolic requirements of the brain, as in cardiac arrest followed by resuscitation. Ischemic strokes account for an estimated 83% of the total, and this percentage can be further broken down into atherothrombotic strokes (40%), global hypoperfusion (18%), and embolic strokes (25%)[6] (Box 49-1).

Hemorrhagic strokes are typically classified by the location of the bleeding. Subarachnoid hemorrhagic strokes (about 7% of all strokes) occur from bleeding into the subarachnoid space, and intracerebral hemorrhagic strokes (about 10% of all strokes) occur from bleeding into the brain tissue itself. Subarachnoid bleeding is usually the result of the rupture of a cerebral aneurysm or arteriovenous malformation, whereas intracerebral bleeds result from the rupture of a small artery, often a deep penetrating vessel, and are often related to poorly controlled hypertension.

Both modifiable and nonmodifiable risk factors are associated with stroke. The nonmodifiable risks of age, gender, sex, and race are discussed under Epidemiology and summarized in the Risk Factors box. In addition, hypertension, cardiac disease, diabetes mellitus, and blood lipid abnormalities can all increase the risk of stroke, particularly when they are present in combination. Atherosclerosis elsewhere in the body is presumed to also involve the cerebral vessels. Patients who have preexisting heart disease have a clearly increased risk, as do patients with diabetes mellitus, which accelerates the processes of atherosclerosis and arteriosclerosis. The reduction of modifiable risk factors such as hypertension, hyperlipidemia, tobacco use, and inactivity has been shown to reduce the incidence and recurrence of stroke.

Epidemiology. In the United States, someone has a stroke every 45 seconds. Although a significant decrease in stroke incidence and mortality has occurred over the past 2 decades, stroke remains the third leading cause of death in the United States. An estimated 500,000 first-time strokes occur each year. The mortality rate has declined about 15% since 1988,[2] but stroke leaves about 30% of its victims with mental or physical disabilities that require ongoing assistance with activities of daily living (ADLs).[1] This creates a pool of more than 1 million people who are currently partially or totally disabled from stroke, and this number is expected to rise as the population continues to age. The importance of stroke as a national health concern is reflected in the *Healthy People 2010* goal "to reduce stroke deaths to no more than 48 per 100,000 people."[42]

Stroke has profound social and economic consequences for the person, family, and community. Direct and indirect costs for stroke management and ongoing care are estimated at $56.8 billion.[1] The obvious economic impact of stroke is reflected in the rapid proliferation of clinical pathways for case management of stroke patients. These pathways delineate the specifics of care to be provided at each stage of rehabilitation. The social and emotional tolls are more difficult to quantify but are readily apparent to anyone whose family has been touched by stroke.

Risk Factors

Stroke

Nonmodifiable

Age: About 88% of stroke deaths occur in persons over 65 years of age; risk doubles with each decade after age 55.
Sex: Although men have almost twice the incidence of stroke as women, more deaths occur in women. Also, men are more likely to have a second stroke within 5 years.
Race: African-Americans have almost twice the risk of stroke and twice the mortality rate when compared with Caucasians.
Other factors: Other nonmodifiable risk factors are heredity and history of stroke or cardiovascular disease.

Modifiable

Hypertension: Hypertension is a major risk factor for stroke. Individuals with blood pressure below 120/80 mm Hg reduce the lifetime risk of stroke by half.
Heart disease: Heart disease is a major contributor to stroke, primarily from atrial fibrillation, which causes a fivefold increase in risk.
Diabetes: Diabetes is associated with an accelerated rate of microvascular and macrovascular changes that contribute to atherosclerosis.
Other factors:
- Cigarette smoking
- Oral contraceptive use (especially if also a smoker)
- Alcohol intake
- Obesity*
- Sedentary lifestyle*
- Elevated serum cholesterol and triglycerides*

*These factors are less well studied but are believed to contribute to stroke.

About 88% of all strokes occur in persons over 65 years of age. Strokes are slightly more common in men than in women. African-Americans are two times more likely to experience ischemic strokes and three times more likely to experience hemorrhagic strokes than Caucasians. It is unclear whether this increased incidence is directly related to racial factors or reflects generally poorer diagnosis and treatment of hypertension, heart disease, and diabetes in this population—especially African-American men. Some variations in incidence and mortality have also been noted worldwide, particularly in Japan. The meaning of these differences is not clear.[1]

Pathophysiology. The brain must receive a steady supply of nutrients from the blood because it has no capacity to store either oxygen or glucose. It is supplied with blood from two major pairs of arteries: the internal carotids and the vertebrals. The carotids supply the anterior portions of the brain, including most of the cerebral hemispheres except for the occipital lobes (Figure 49-1). The vertebrals join together to become the basilar artery and supply the posterior portions of the brain, including the cerebellum, brainstem, and occipital lobes. The circle of Willis is the region of the brain in which the branches of the basilar and internal carotid arteries join, creating a circular network, which in theory allows

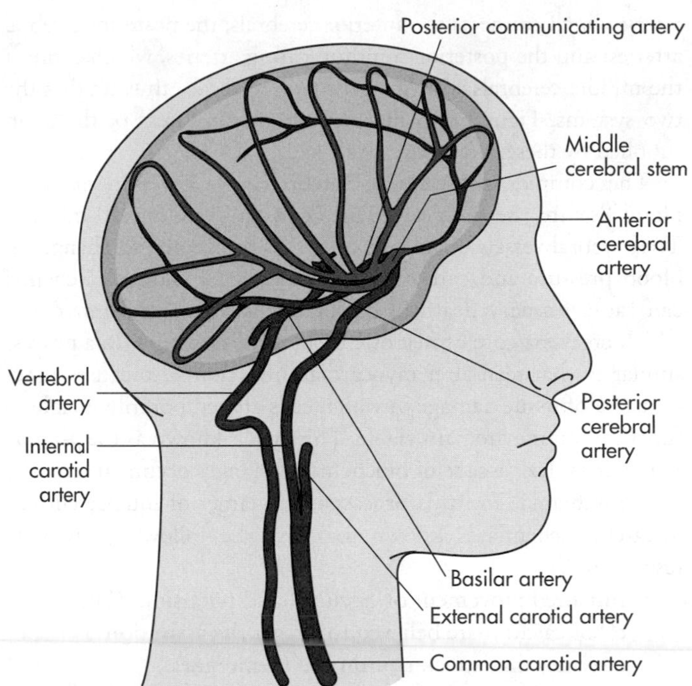

Figure 49-1 Major arteries that supply the brain. Internal carotids branch to supply anterior portions of the brain. Vertebral arteries supply posterior portions.

blood to circulate from one hemisphere to the other and from the anterior to the posterior portions of the brain (Figure 49-2). Functionally, however, the circulations of the two hemispheres usually remain separate. The circle is composed of the middle cerebral arteries; the anterior cerebral arteries; the anterior communicating

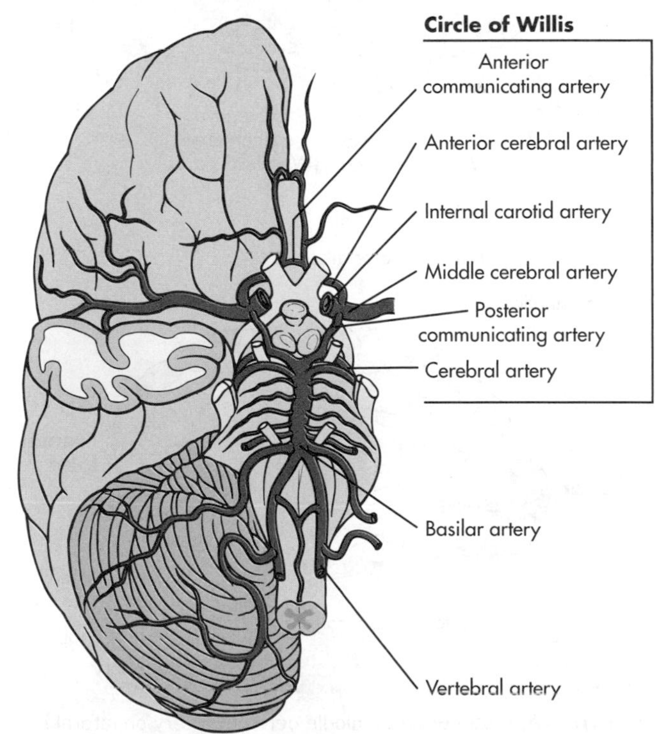

Figure 49-2 Circle of Willis as seen from below the brain.

artery, which connects the anterior cerebrals; the posterior cerebral arteries; and the posterior communicating arteries, which connect the middle cerebrals with the posterior cerebrals, thus uniting the two systems. Figure 49-3 illustrates the major areas of the brain supplied by these cerebral vessels.

The complex processes of cerebral autoregulation maintain blood flow to the brain at a fairly constant rate of 750 ml/min. The cerebral vessels dilate and constrict in response to changes in blood pressure and carbon dioxide tension. Prolonged ischemia can cause primary death of cerebral cells or cerebral infarction, which creates a core of necrotic tissue. The ischemia, in a process similar to that seen after myocardial infarction, also causes a second area of tissue damage in which cells are temporarily unable to function but may remain viable. This area is known as the *penumbra*. A complex cascade of biochemical changes occurs in response to the ischemia, and this process is the target of intense current research. Ischemia is known to cause the following disparate responses[20]:

- Impaired movement of calcium[5] and potassium (High levels of calcium are believed to trigger the activation of enzymes that attack neuron cell membranes.)
- Accumulation of oxygen free radicals, which further disrupt calcium metabolism

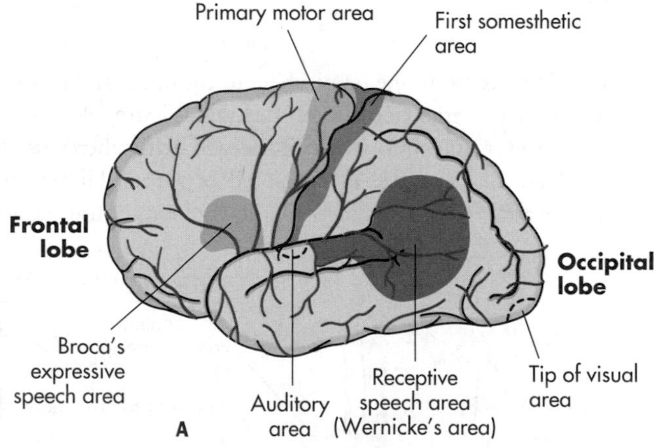

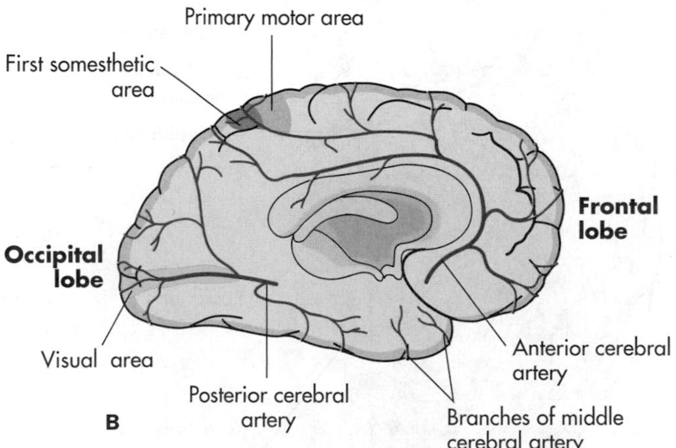

Figure 49-3 **A,** Distribution of middle cerebral artery on lateral surface of the brain. **B,** Distribution of anterior and posterior cerebral arteries on medial surface of the brain.

- Enhanced lactate production from the presence of glucose in low perfusion areas, which worsens cellular damage and acidosis
- An influx of fluid-activated white blood cells and coagulation factors that further clog the microcirculation

If **reperfusion** to the core can be provided within 1 to 3 hours, blood flow and metabolism in the stunned cells in the penumbra may be normalized. Because hypoperfusion and hyperperfusion may be occurring simultaneously in adjacent areas, a "low flow" state that occurs actually worsens the ischemic area. This hyperperfusion zone may steal blood intended for the core, and produce an infarction. This event is called *reperfusion injury,* manifested by an increase in **neurologic deficits**.[4]

Additionally, a secondary injury that occurs after ischemia includes (1) disruption of the blood-brain barrier from the toxic oxygen free radicals released from the damaged tissue; (2) cell membrane destruction from intravascular chemicals, which leads to increased interstitial edema; (3) disturbance in autoregulation, which causes vasodilation; and (4) acidosis.

Once infarction (necrosis or cellular death) occurs, damage is irreversible. Ischemia leads to cellular edema, and the capillaries are compressed by the swollen cells, further impeding the blood supply. The overall effect of cerebral edema may peak by 72 hours after infarction and remain present for 2 weeks. This condition may exacerbate neuronal damage and increase the risk of death if not controlled.[4]

Brain attacks related to ischemia from thrombi are classified according to four developmental processes: transient ischemic attack, reversible ischemic neurologic deficit (RIND), stroke in evolution, and completed stroke.

TRANSIENT ISCHEMIC ATTACK. A transient ischemic attack (TIA) is a relatively brief episode of neurologic deficit that resolves without any residual effect. The episode may last for seconds, minutes, or hours, but the average duration is 10 minutes, and the vast majority resolve within an hour. By definition, the symptoms must resolve within 24 hours. When multiple TIAs recur with the same symptoms, a thrombotic origin is suggested. The recurrence with different symptoms implies embolic origin. TIAs are generally thought to be warning signs of an impending ischemic problem and usually reflect advanced atherosclerotic disease. A person who has had a TIA is more than nine times as likely to have a stroke as a person without a TIA, and so should be aggressively evaluated and treated before a stroke occurs. The risk of recurrence without treatment is 30% at 3 months, 60% at 6 months, and 80% at 1 year.

Some researchers theorize that TIAs may be caused by microemboli that break off from atherosclerotic plaque lesions. However, TIAs can also be triggered by events that temporarily decrease blood flow to the affected area of the brain, such as vasospasm or hypotension. TIAs may recur over days, weeks, and even years without progressing to stroke. The unique symptoms produced by the TIA are specific to the vessel involved and can usually be traced to involvement of the carotid supply or the vertebral arteries. A wide range of symptoms are possible (see Clinical Manifestations box).

REVERSIBLE ISCHEMIC NEUROLOGIC DEFICIT. This condition may also be called small stroke. Reversal usually occurs within 48

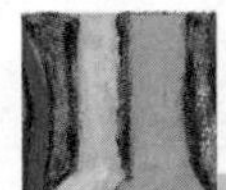

CLINICAL MANIFESTATIONS
Transient Ischemic Attacks

Symptoms Related to Carotid Artery Involvement

Visual disturbances
- —Temporary blindness in one eye
- —Blurred vision

Motor disturbances
- —Hemiparesis
- —Localized motor deficits in face or extremities

Sensory disturbances
- —Hemianesthesia
- —Sensory deficits in face or extremities

Symptoms Related to Vertebral Artery Involvement

Motor disturbances
- —Ataxia
- —Dysarthria
- —Dysphagia
- —Unilateral or bilateral weakness

Visual disturbances
- —Diplopia
- —Bilateral blindness

Other
- —Brief lapses in level of consciousness
- —Sensory disturbance
- —Dizziness, vertigo
- —Tinnitus

NOTE: Clinical manifestations are brief in duration and reversible.

hours, but may extend up to 3 weeks. A person may have multiple RINDs over a period of years, but they commonly involve the same area of the brain, usually as a result of arteriosclerotic carotid artery stenosis.

STROKE IN EVOLUTION. Stroke in evolution may also be called progressive stroke. The deficit occurs in a stepwise pattern. If the problem involves the carotid artery distribution, the progression does not usually extend beyond 24 hours, but if it involves the vertibrobasilar distribution, it can progress up to 72 hours. The patient may remain at home during this evolutionary phase, which may include 24 hours after the first symptom, and come to the hospital only when the symptoms continue to worsen or do not resolve.

COMPLETED STOKE. Most completed strokes produce a stable syndrome of neurologic deficits within an hour, but some may take more than 72 hours because of secondary injury or cerebral edema. Approximately 60% of thrombotic strokes occur during sleep, with the full effect evident on awakening. This may be related to the decline in baseline blood pressure that occurs at rest or to increases in blood viscosity that develop during sleep periods. Symptoms may develop abruptly or progress over a period of hours, depending on how much blood is able to move through the obstructed vessel lumen.

CEREBRAL INFARCTION CAUSED BY EMBOLI. These strokes occur suddenly, often during waking activities, and the patient remains conscious during the event. If the embolus arises from the heart, as 14% of strokes do, it may fragment and move. Symptoms clear, but the fragments occlude smaller branches, providing new symptoms. Patients with embolic strokes are four times as likely as other stroke patients to die within 30 days, have more severe deficits at time of the event, and have poorer functional outcomes. Many patients experience recurrent strokes if the underlying cause is not corrected.

HEMORRHAGIC BRAIN ATTACKS. This type of stroke is commonly related to a ruptured vessel caused by hypertension and typically occurs during waking hours. If a small hemorrhage of 1 to 2 ml from an arteriole occurs, it usually is walled off in a cystic formation called a lacuna. These may be multiple. When the hemorrhage is extensive or massive, it forms a hematoma, causing disruption of the blood-brain barrier and increased intracranial pressure (ICP). A massive hemorrhage (50 ml or less) probably will be fatal. Initially the patient experiences direct destruction of tissue from the space-occupying hematoma, brain tissue displacement, and the toxic effects of the blood components. Then in addition to local ischemia, hyperemia, global ischemia, disruption of the autoregulation and the blood-brain barrier, and cerebral edema quickly follow (increased ICP). Hemorrhagic stroke has a higher mortality rate than ischemic stroke. The pathophysiologic process of increased ICP is described in Chapter 48.

COMPLICATIONS. The list of possible complications of stroke is almost endless. Stroke may result in death or profound neurologic injury. With less severe strokes, the initial acute period may be complicated by respiratory problems related to aspiration and atelectasis. Other disuse-related complications include skin breakdown, deep venous thrombosis, muscle atrophy, and joint contractures. Urinary tract infections often result from the use of Foley catheters, and both constipation and impaction may result from immobility. Stroke patients are at high risk for environmental injury from a variety of physical and cognitive impairments, and the consequences of communication impairments can isolate the patient from full and active participation in the world. Furthermore, for each complication the patient experiences, additional problems may develop for the family and support network. Prevention of these multiple complications is addressed in the Collaborative Care Management and Nursing Management sections.

CLINICAL MANIFESTATIONS. The specific neurologic deficits produced by stroke reflect the location and severity of the ischemia and the adequacy of the collateral circulation in the region. The term *stroke* commonly evokes a classic mental picture of specific disabilities, but a wide variety of presentations can occur. Commonly encountered symptoms are summarized in the Clinical Manifestations box, p. 426. Many of the features overlap with other forms of brain injury. A number of specific syndromes have been identified that reflect the involvement of specific vessels and the areas of the brain that they serve (Box 49-2), but in clinical practice it is unusual to see these syndromes in their pure forms. The two vessels affected most commonly are the middle cerebral artery and the internal carotid artery. Each of the major types of stroke is associated with a fairly typical onset and course of symptoms.

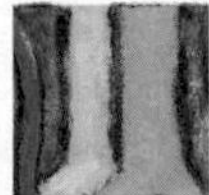

CLINICAL MANIFESTATIONS *Stroke*

Specific symptoms reflect the site and severity of ischemic damage. The following is a general listing of common deficits. See also Box 49-2 for specific deficits associated with ischemia in individual cerebral vessels.

Motor

Hemiparesis or hemiplegia of the side of the body opposite the site of ischemia
—Initially flaccid, progressing to spastic
Dysphagia; possible impairment of swallowing reflex
Dysarthria

Bowel and Bladder

Frequency, urgency, and urinary incontinence
—Potential for bladder retraining good if patient cognitively intact
Constipation; related more to immobility than to the physical effects of stroke

Language

Nonfluent aphasia (also known as motor or expressive aphasia): difficulty or inability to express self verbally
Fluent aphasia (also known as sensory or receptive aphasia): difficulty or inability to comprehend speech
Alexia: inability to understand the written word
Agraphia: inability to express self in writing

Sensory-Perceptual

Diminished response to superficial sensation (touch, pain, pressure, heat, and cold)
Diminished proprioception (knowledge of position of body parts in the environment)
Visual deficits
—Decreased acuity
—Diplopia
—Homonymous hemianopia (see Figure 49-4)
Perceptual (see Box 49-3)
—Unilateral neglect syndrome
—Distorted body image
—Apraxia: inability to carry out learned voluntary acts
—Agnosia: inability to recognize familiar objects through sight, sound, or touch; inability to recognize faces
—Anosognosia: inability to recognize or denial of a physical deficit
—Possible deficits in:
—Telling time
—Judging distance
—Right-left discrimination
—Memory of locations, objects

Cognitive-Emotional

Emotional lability and unpredictability
—Socially inappropriate behavior (e.g., crying jags, swearing)
Depression
Memory loss
Short attention span, easy distractibility
Loss of reasoning, judgment, and abstract thinking ability

Box 49-2 Characteristics of Major Stroke Syndromes

Middle Cerebral Artery Syndrome (Most Common Occlusion)

If blockage of the main stem of the middle cerebral artery (MCA) occurs, the infarction can affect most of the hemisphere, since the MCA accounts for about 80% of the blood supply to the cerebral hemispheres. Characteristics include:

- Contralateral hemiparesis or hemiplegia (arm affected more severely than the leg)
- Contralateral sensory impairment over same area affected by hemiplegia (proprioception, touch)
- Unilateral neglect or inattention (if nondominant hemisphere)
- Aphasia (if dominant hemisphere)
- Contralateral homonymous hemianopia

Internal Carotid Artery Syndrome

The symptoms of MCA and internal carotid artery strokes are almost identical, but if blockage of the main stem of the MCA occurs (see above), the deficits can be profound, since cerebral edema is usually extensive. Characteristics of internal carotid artery strokes include:

- Contralateral hemiparesis or hemiplegia
- Contralateral sensory losses
- Aphasia (if dominant hemisphere)

Vertebrobasilar Artery Syndromes

Occlusion of the vessels in this system creates unique symptoms that reflect the perfusion of the cerebellum and brainstem:

- Ataxia, clumsiness
- Dysphagia and dysarthria
- Dizziness and nystagmus
- Bilateral motor and sensory deficits
- Facial weakness and numbness

MOTOR DEFICITS. Motor symptoms are the most widely recognized clinical manifestations of stroke. Compromise of the motor pathways can affect the initiation of movement, strength of movement, integration of movement, muscle tone, and reflex activity. The classic symptoms are **hemiparesis** or **hemiplegia** on the side of the body opposite the site of cerebral ischemia. Most patients are initially hyporeflexic and then progress to hyperreflexia and spasticity as recovery progresses. The upper and lower extremities may be affected to different degrees. Motor deficits also commonly impair swallowing and produce weakness in the muscles of speech.

BOWEL AND BLADDER DEFICITS. Frequency, urgency, and incontinence are common problems in the initial days after stroke, but the reflex arc remains intact, as does at least a partial sensation of bladder filling. The stroke lesion usually affects only half of the motor and sensory control of the bladder, which makes effective continence rehabilitation a reasonable goal. If extended indwelling catheterization can be avoided, bladder retraining has a good chance of success. The problems that develop with bowel elimination are more related to cognitive losses and immobility than to the physical effects of the stroke. Constipation is the most common problem.

COMMUNICATION DEFICITS. The ability to communicate is a complex process that involves receiving and effectively processing the written or spoken word and being able to express one's self appropriately both verbally and in writing. The left hemisphere is dominant for language in all right-handed and many left-handed individuals. Broca's area, which is located at the inferior gyrus of the frontal lobe, is critical for the motor control of speech. Wernicke's area, which is located in the temporal lobe on the superior temporal gyrus, is responsible for auditory association (see Figure 49-3). When the dominant hemisphere is affected, stroke can create aphasia, a language disorder that can be subdivided and classified in several ways. Expressive (or motor) aphasia is primarily a motor disorder involving Broca's area. Patients have difficulty expressing thoughts because Broca's area contains the memory for motor patterns of speech. The deficits range from difficulty finding the desired word to oral communication that is restricted to single-word responses. The ability to understand language usually remains intact, although many patients with aphasia have mixed patterns of abilities and disabilities. Agraphia, the inability to express ideas in writing, may or may not be present.

Receptive aphasia is primarily a sensory disorder involving Wernicke's area. The patient may speak fluently but be unable to comprehend speech. The patient's use of language is often full of errors, although automatic social responses such as yes, no, and fine are used appropriately. Either agraphia or alexia, the inability to understand the written word, may also be present. Global aphasia reflects damage to both regions of the brain and may result in the inability to either understand or use language. The presence of dysarthria can complicate the picture of aphasia.

SENSORY-PERCEPTUAL DEFICITS. Perception is a complex process of recognizing and interpreting environmental stimuli. The right side of the brain (particularly the parietal lobe) plays a significant role in perception. Sensory-perceptual deficits are common after stroke and can take a variety of forms. Straightforward sensory losses manifest as a diminished response to superficial sensations such as touch, temperature, heat, and cold. These create a substantial risk for injury.

Visual deficits may complicate environmental management and commonly occur because the visual pathways pass through most of the cerebral hemispheres. These may manifest as decreased visual acuity or diplopia but more commonly involve some degree of homonymous hemianopia—loss of vision in a portion of the visual field of each eye. Figure 49-4 compares the visual deficits created by ischemic damage at different portions of the visual pathway.

The more subtle perceptual problems that occur with stroke may initially be overlooked but can be profoundly disturbing to the family because of their bizarre manifestations. Proprioceptive knowledge of the position of body parts in the environment may be affected, which contributes to the potential for injury. Distortions of body image; lack of ability to accurately judge spatial relationships; apparent denial of the physical effects of the stroke (anosognosia); and the loss of ability to identify or use familiar objects correctly (apraxia), particularly to complete tasks essential for self-care, can all be present to some degree (Box 49-3).

COGNITIVE-EMOTIONAL DEFICITS. Patients commonly demonstrate a loss of control over their emotions after a stroke. Their emotional responses can be exaggerated, flattened, or inappropriate and are often unpredictable. Most patients experience depression, compounded by frustration over the losses in functional abilities and communication. It is often difficult to distinguish between normal emotional responses and those related to emotional lability. Uncontrolled anger or tears can be frightening symptoms for families. Stress and fatigue may increase the unpredictability and severity of the patient's emotional responses.

Memory and judgment are also commonly compromised by stroke, although these losses may not be apparent in the early days of recovery. A short attention span with easy distractibility may be present, which interferes with self-care learning. The ability to reason and think abstractly may be significantly altered, which can deepen the depressive response to stroke, since patients must come to terms with the extent of their losses.

EFFECTS OF LATERALITY. As our understanding of the functions of each side of the brain continues to increase, some predictions about the effects of stroke injury to each hemisphere are possible. The effects of left hemisphere versus right hemisphere stroke for individuals who are left hemisphere dominant (all

BOX 49-3 Perceptual Deficits Caused by Stroke

- *Unilateral neglect syndrome:* A distortion in body image in which the patient ignores the affected side of the body
- *Anosognosia:* Apparent unawareness or denial of any loss or deficit in physical functioning
- *Loss of proprioceptive skills:* Lack of awareness of where various body parts are in relationship to each other and the environment
- *Agnosia:* Inability to recognize a familiar object by use of the senses
  —Visual agnosia
  —Auditory agnosia
  —Tactile agnosia
- *Apraxia:* Loss of ability to carry out a learned sequence of movements or use objects correctly when paralysis is not present
  —Constructional: Inability to sequence a planned act necessary for activities of daily living (e.g., dressing, brushing teeth, combing hair)
- *Spatial relationships*
  —Loss of ability to judge distance or size or localize objects in space
  —Impaired right-left discrimination

Visual Pathways

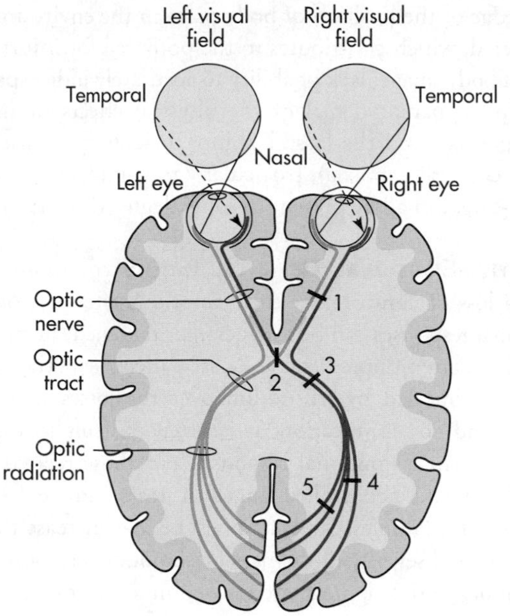

Left visual field | Right visual field | Temporal | Temporal | Nasal | Left eye | Right eye | Optic nerve | Optic tract | Optic radiation | 1 | 2 | 3 | 4 | 5

Visual Fields | Blackened Field Indicates Area of No Vision

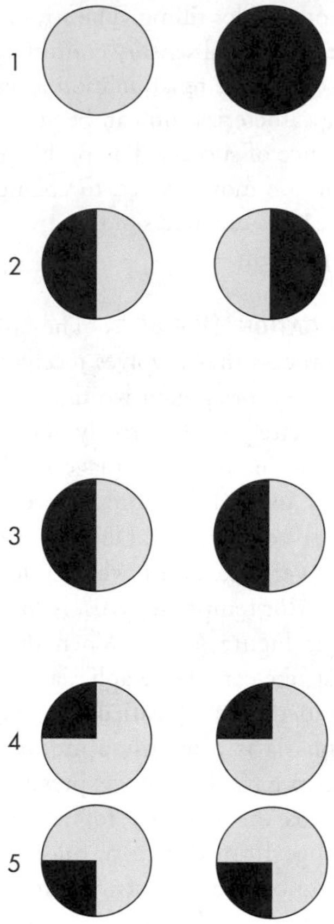

1 **Blind Right Eye (Right optic nerve)** A lesion of the optic nerve produces unilateral blindness.

2 **Bitemporal Hemianopia (Optic chiasm)** A lesion at the optic chiasm may involve only those fibers that are crossing over to the opposite side. Because these fibers originate in the nasal half of each retina, visual loss involves the temporal half of each field.

3 **Left Homonymous Hemianopia (Right optic tract)** A lesion of the optic tract interrupts fibers originating on the same side of both eyes. Visual loss in the eyes is therefore similar (homonymous) and involves half of each field (hemianopia).

4 **Homonymous Left Upper Quadrantic Defect (Optic radiation, partial)** A partial lesion of the optic radiation may involve only a portion of the nerve fibers, producing, for example, a homonymous quadrantic defect.

5

Figure 49-4 Visual field defects produced by selected lesions in visual pathways.

right-handed individuals and many left-handed persons) are summarized in Box 49-4.

▶ ARE YOU READY?

Which of the following are clinical manifestations of left hemisphere stroke? (Choose all that apply.)

1. Motor deficits on left side
2. Motor deficits on right side
3. Poor judgment
4. Intellectual impairment
5. Distractibility
6. Language deficits

Collaborative Care Management

DIAGNOSTIC TESTS. A stroke is initially diagnosed by means of a careful history and physical examination. Aggressive early intervention to attempt reperfusion of the ischemic portions of the brain necessitates a rapid differentiation between ischemic and hemorrhagic strokes, and this may be accomplished by either a computed tomography (CT) scan or magnetic resonance imaging (MRI). A CT scan is used to rule out bleeding; the extent of infarction will not be visible on CT scanning for 24 hours, but it detects 90% of subarachnoid hemorrhage within that time. The

Box 49-4 Left Hemisphere Versus Right Hemisphere Stroke

Left Hemisphere* Stroke

Motor deficits on right side
Language deficits
—Expressive, receptive, or global aphasia
—Agraphia or alexia
Right visual field deficits
Slow and cautious behavior
Severe anxiety before attempting new skills
Intellectual impairment
High level of frustration, depression over losses

Right Hemisphere Stroke

Motor deficits on left side
Left visual field deficits
Spatial perceptual deficits
Denial or unawareness of deficits
Poor judgment, overestimation of abilities
Impulsiveness, distractibility
Apparent unconcern over losses

*Dominant hemisphere for most persons.

MRI can demonstrate the ischemic zone within the first few hours after stroke, but its high cost and limited accessibility usually make MRI the second diagnostic option.

A variety of other tests may be used to identify other problems that may have contributed to the stroke. These might include a cardiac workup to rule out the possibility of cardiogenic emboli. Carotid Doppler or duplex ultrasonography may be performed to rule out or evaluate the degree of carotid stenosis. Cerebral angiography may be used to localize and evaluate a bleeding site if a hemorrhagic stroke has occurred, or to evaluate the extent of arterial occlusion. Magnetic resonance angiography can be used for clot visualization and more detailed information about plaque composition. Other studies include blood flow studies, such as single-photon emission CT, positron emission tomography, xenon CT, and electrocardiogram. No laboratory tests confirm the presence of stroke, but routine blood work, such as complete blood count, blood glucose, serum cholesterol, lipids, platelets, prothrombin time, partial thromboplastin time, sedimentation rate, serum homocysteine, electrolytes, and coagulation studies, may be performed to assess the patient's baseline status and provide a framework for anticoagulation if needed.

MEDICATIONS

ANTIPLATELET AGENTS. Platelet aggregation inhibitor drugs are the mainstay of drug therapy, primarily for the prevention of recurrence of TIA or stroke. Aspirin, the most extensively used antiplatelet drug, has been proven to decrease platelet aggregation. It can be used in the management of TIAs, strokes in evolution, or ischemic strokes. Aspirin has been shown to reduce recurrence after an initial stroke.[24] Even in low doses, however, some patients are unable to tolerate the long-term use of aspirin, and its use increases the risk of peptic ulcer disease. Several alternative antiplatelet drugs, including ticlopidine (Ticlid), clopidogrel (Plavix), and dipyridamole (Persantine), have been shown to be effective for secondary stroke prevention, but these agents are more costly than aspirin, and patients must be monitored for drug-specific side effects. Patients may be given a combination of these drugs, adding to the concern about side effects. The U.S. Food and Drug Administration recently approved a new combination of low-dose aspirin and extended release dipyridomole, Aggrenox, with the goal of increased effectiveness without increased side effects.

NEUROPROTECTANTS. These agents, in active clinical trials, take different approaches to protecting the brain from secondary injury by interfering in the various steps of the ischemic cascade and reperfusion injury. Those under consideration include acid-sensing ion channel blockers, sodium channel blockers, calcium channel antagonists, oxygen free radical scavengers, neuronal cell membrane stabilizers, glutamate receptor antagonists, gamma-aminobutyric acid agonists, and monoclonal antibodies that interrupt the inflammatory process.[4]

In addition, the physical effects of hypothermia in reducing oxygen consumption, thereby reducing the release of oxygen free radicals and excitatory amino acids, have been shown to improve outcomes through neuroprotection.

ANTICOAGULANTS. Intravenous (IV) anticoagulation may be used during acute management of a progressing ischemic or embolic stroke or to prevent progression of a TIA. Anticoagulation with heparin and enoxaporin (Lovenox) has not been effective in acute stroke and is not routinely recommended. Although the low-molecular-weight heparinoids cause fewer bleeding complications, they are not recommended in patients with large infarcts or with greater than 130 mm Hg mean arterial pressure because of the possibility of hemorrhagic transformation of the infarct or death.[38]

Long-term oral anticoagulation therapy (warfarin) is started the first day of IV heparin therapy in the patients appropriate for this therapy. Heparin is discontinued in 4 days with an international normalized ration (INR) of 2.0, and oral therapy is monitored closely to maintain this therapeutic level.

OTHER AGENTS. Patients with severe hypertension may require pharmacologic intervention, but hypertension is not treated in the emergent phase to avoid reducing perfusion pressure in the brain. Blood pressure control is usually initiated for patients with hemorrhagic strokes, who also commonly require control of elevated ICP.

TREATMENTS

THROMBOLYTICS. The use of tissue plasminogen activator (t-PA), which digests fibrin threads and fibrinogen and lyses the clot, was approved in 1996 in the United States for acute ischemic strokes (see Future Watch box below). It is the first drug to reverse the effects of stroke, but it must be given in a 3-hour treatment window, measured from onset of the first symptom.[37] The risk of cerebral hemorrhage is still a concern, but the incidence is low when the exclusionary criteria are followed in selection of patients and it is not administered beyond the 3-hour window, when risk for hemorrhagic transformation of the infarct or hemorrhage in vessels beyond the stroke is greater (see Future Watch box, p. 1429).

In patients who have missed the 3-hour treatment window, another method of dissolving the clot is through direct access to the clot. This procedure must be done within a 6-hour window from onset of symptoms in an ischemic stroke. The patient receives the treatment in the radiology department under the guidance of cerebral angiography. A size 6 F catheter is placed in the common carotid artery proximal to the clot and advanced slowly until the tip is in the clot. The thrombolytic, such as t-PA or urokinase, is administered slowly by manual push with frequent control angiograms; then a follow-up angiogram is done to determine the success of recanalization.

Future Watch

Fibrinogen-Depleting Agents

Fibrinogen-depleting agents such as Ancor are under investigation in the United States for use in the treatment of patients with acute ischemic stroke. These agents have the potential to improve blood flow to the affected areas of the brain by helping to remove obstructing thrombi and by decreasing blood viscosity. This in turn should improve patient outcomes following stoke and, in fact, review trials conducted in other countries involving the use of fibrinogen-depleting agents started within 14 days of stroke found that the proportion of patients dead or disabled at the end of the follow-up period was moderately reduced.

Lium et al: Fibrinogen-depleting agents for acute ischemic stroke, *Stroke* 36:173-174, 2004.

Future Watch

Stroke Treatment

Clinical trials of several new devices aimed at improving stroke treatment and patient outcomes are currently ongoing. One trial involves tiny wire-mesh tubes and microcatheters that are used as expandable stents in the arteries of the brain. These devices would be an option for patients at risk for recurrent stroke because of plaque deposits who have not responded to drug therapy. A carotid artery stent, accompanied by a filter to collect loose debris, has been developed to prevent stroke from narrowed or occluded carotid arteries or clots that travel to the brain. Another device, shaped like a corkscrew, can extract blood clots directly, more quickly than clot-dissolving drugs can work. Because the brain is deprived of oxygen for a shorter time, use of this device could lessen brain damage.

American stroke month highlights major cause of death and disability: medical technology innovation helps lower stroke mortality, *Med Technol Innovation* 5(11), May 12, 2004, accessed from website: http://.www.advanced.org/newsroom/mti.

Hypervolemic-Hyperdilution Therapy. Maintaining adequate and stable cerebral perfusion is an essential goal of early stroke management. Systolic pressure is usually maintained at about 150 mm Hg after stabilization. The hypervolemic-hemodilution therapy helps maintain the cerebral perfusion pressure (CPP) by lowering blood viscosity and maintaining a slightly elevated blood pressure. The hematocrit is reduced to 33 to 35 mg/dl, and dilution is accomplished through the use of normal saline and albumin. This treatment arguably supports a sustained blood pressure and promotes vasodilation of the cerebral vessels, theoretically maximizing perfusion to the brain. Hypervolemic-hyperdilution therapy has been successfully used to treat vasospasm after subarachnoid hemorrhage, but its efficacy in acute ischemic stroke is unproven.

Surgical Management. Carotid endarterectomy is the primary surgical intervention used in stroke management.[29] It is targeted at stroke prevention primarily for patients with symptomatic carotid stenosis. Endarterectomy involves careful removal of the plaque after the artery has been clamped both above and below the obstruction (Figure 49-5). Circulation to the brain on the affected side is maintained through the vertebrobasilar arterial system with supplemental flow through a temporary bypass shunt. Despite these precautions, the greatest risks associated with the procedure relate to compromised cerebral blood flow, especially if carotid stenosis is present on both sides. Embolization of plaque and microthrombi resulting from the surgical manipulation increase the risk of additional strokes and are the primary postoperative concerns. Intervention is usually reserved for patients with more than 70% carotid blockage.

A primary focus of care in the postoperative period relates to blood pressure instability, which usually persists for about 12 to 24 hours and can cause both hypertension and hypotension. The sudden restoration of blood flow through a significantly obstructed carotid artery can in itself result in hemorrhage, and the increased perfusion may initially overwhelm the brain's ability to autoregulate. In appropriate surgical candidates, carotid endarterectomy significantly reduces the risk of stroke. The major nursing care

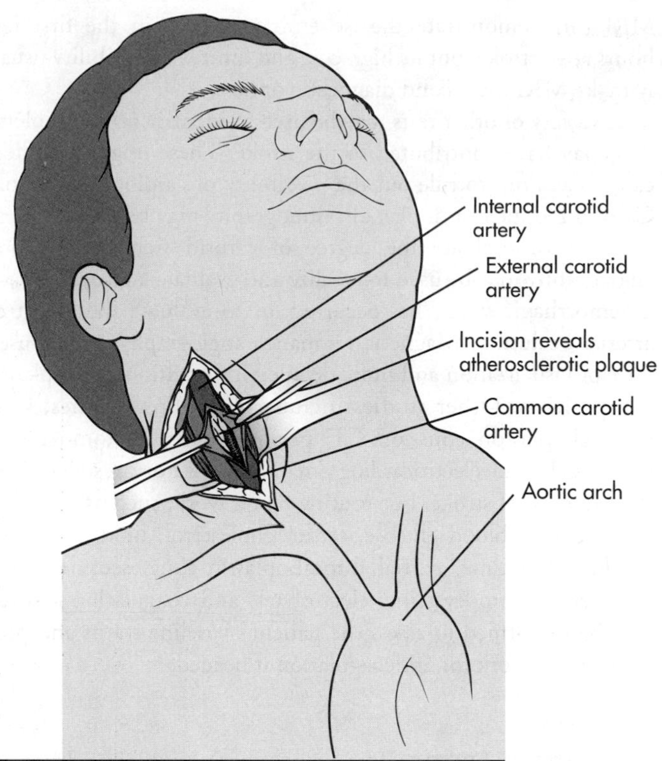

Figure 49-5 Carotid endarterectomy. Atherosclerotic plaque is removed from internal carotid artery.

considerations for patients undergoing carotid endarterectomy are listed in the Guidelines for Safe Practice box.

An alternative to carotid endarterectomy is carotid stenting.[36] This procedure is particularly useful for patients who are not good candidates for an open surgical procedure. Stenting is contraindicated for patients allergic to antiplatelet drugs since this type of therapy is necessary for 3 to 4 weeks after stenting. Other con-

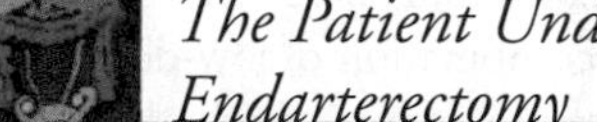

Guidelines for Safe Practice
The Patient Undergoing Carotid Endarterectomy

Postoperative nursing care focuses on monitoring vital signs and the early identification of potential complications.

Vital Signs

Monitor vital signs every 1 to 2 hours.
—Anticipate blood pressure instability in the first 12 to 24 hours.
—Immediately report blood pressure fluctuations above or below established parameters.

Complications

Monitor neurologic status through frequent neurologic checks.
—Evaluate cranial nerves, particularly facial and vagus.
Monitor for dysrhythmias and chest pain.
Monitor for signs of reperfusion injury, including:
—Worsening or recurring stroke symptoms
—Signs of increasing intracranial pressure
Monitor incision site for patency, drainage.
Maintain head of bed as prescribed by physician.

traindications include ischemic stroke in the past 2 weeks, severe renal disease, and characteristics of blood vessels that interfere with the procedure. Postprocedure care requires groin checks to assess the femoral access site and monitoring for hypotension, which can persist for up to 3 days. If the access site is stable, ambulation is encouraged, and discharge may be on the same day.

DIET. The patient is usually placed on nothing-by-mouth status on admission until a thorough evaluation of swallowing can be performed. Protecting the airway from aspiration of food, fluid, and secretions is the primary concern. Intact gag and swallow reflexes are essential prerequisites for oral feedings, and their presence and strength are closely monitored. The process of swallowing is complex and requires the coordination of several structures and muscle groups. If the patient is unable to ingest an oral diet, tube feedings may be initiated to prevent excessive catabolism and resultant malnutrition. A nasogastric route is initially used for either continuous or intermittent tube feedings. The standard concerns relate to formula hyperosmolality and problems with dehydration and diarrhea (see Chapter 42). A percutaneous gastrostomy may be needed for long-term nutrition management. Nutritional concerns are discussed further in the Nursing Management section.

ACTIVITY. Patients who have experienced an intracerebral hemorrhage require bed rest until the risk of rebleeding is minimized and ICP stabilizes. Patients who have experienced an ischemic stroke are mobilized into active rehabilitation as soon as the stroke has stabilized, usually within 48 hours. A multidisciplinary team of physical and occupational therapists and nurses then collaboratively plan the patient's self-care rehabilitation. Preventing immobility-associated problems (which can include pneumonia, urinary incontinence or urinary tract infection, pressure ulcers, deep venous thrombosis, and pulmonary embolus) is a major focus of collaborative in-hospital care.[3] Prophylactic measures against deep venous thrombosis, which occurs in up to 50% of hemiplegic stroke patients, may include the use of elastic hose, pneumatic compression stockings, or subcutaneous heparin injections.

Care of the patient with a stroke is truly a multidisciplinary collaborative effort.[10] It is complex and frequently can involve ethical issues for the stroke team (see Ethical Alert box).

HEALTH PROMOTION AND PREVENTION. Increased attention to high blood pressure diagnosis and control has been successful in reducing the mortality and morbidity of stroke. Outreach efforts concerning hypertension control need to expand, especially for the African-American and Hispanic populations and for the very old.

Ethical Alert

Issues Related to Stroke

Stroke teams frequently encounter the following ethical issues:

- Resource allocation in relation to stroke services versus other services
- Do-not-resuscitate decisions
- Advance directives
- Patient choice in relation to hospital stay and institutionalization
- Withholding or withdrawing life-sustaining therapies

Reducing cardiac risk factors, including lowering cholesterol through statin therapy,[33] normalizing body weight, promoting smoking cessation, and controlling diabetes can all positively affect stroke statistics. High-risk patients are usually given antiplatelet agents, as are most patients who experience TIAs. Compliance with these medication regimens can reduce stroke incidence. All patients who experience TIAs are encouraged to undergo a workup to establish whether their symptoms are attributable to carotid stenosis that could be surgically reversed. Current public health education efforts are teaching individuals to consider stroke as a form of "brain attack," viewed as a corollary of heart attack, in which early intervention can be critical in limiting the extent of ischemic damage and reducing poststroke disability.

Nursing Management 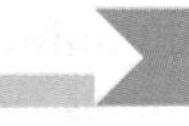

of the Patient with Stroke

ASSESSMENT

Health History. Assess for:

- Baseline level of function
- History of hypertension and its management, coronary artery disease, diabetes, and TIA (symptoms, frequency, workup, and treatment, if any) or previous stroke
- Medications in use: prescription, over-the-counter drugs, herbal preparations
- Smoking history, and history of alcohol or other drug use
- Circumstances surrounding the stroke
- Onset, nature, location, severity, and duration of symptoms
- Headache: nature and location
- Visual acuity, diplopia, blurred vision, field cuts
- Ability to concentrate and follow commands, memory
- Emotional and affective response
- Family and social support network, current living situation, financial and insurance status

Physical Examination. Assess for:

- Change in vital signs using an arterial line, if needed, for close monitoring of blood pressure and arterial blood gases
- Level of consciousness, orientation, and response to tactile stimuli (A change in status indicates need for monitoring every 15 minutes.)
- Presence and severity of paresis or paralysis on left or right side
- Coordination: gait, balance
- Ability to communicate (speak and understand speech)
- Cranial nerve function, including gag and swallow reflexes, facial movement, tongue movement, eye blink, eye movement, and pupillary response
- Bowel and bladder function
- Awareness of disorder (anosognosia)

NURSING DIAGNOSES, OUTCOMES, AND INTERVENTIONS

Nursing Diagnosis: Ineffective Tissue Perfusion (Cerebral)

OUTCOMES. A common example of expected outcomes for the patient with a diagnosis of *ineffective cerebral tissue perfusion* is:

Patient will:

- Maintain cerebral perfusion as indicated by stable vital signs, stable or improving level of consciousness, stable or improving neurologic deficits, and the absence of signs of increased ICP.

Nursing Interventions. Immediately after admission, nursing care focuses on monitoring the patient's neurologic status and preventing complications while simultaneously assessing the severity of the stroke. Maintaining a patent airway is essential to support oxygenation and cerebral perfusion. The patient is placed on bed rest with the head of the bed elevated about 30 degrees and is positioned to prevent the tongue from falling back and partially obstructing the airway. Supplemental oxygen may be administered. The nurse performs vital signs and neurologic checks frequently to monitor for stroke in evolution and to rule out increasing ICP. The environment is kept as quiet and restful as possible, and all activities that are known to increase ICP, such as coughing, straining, lying prone, isometric muscle contraction, emotional upset, and abrupt head or neck flexion, are avoided or minimized.

See Chapter 48 for a more thorough discussion of the management of changes in ICP and Chapter 47 for a thorough review of neurologic assessment.

Related NIC Interventions. Cerebral Perfusion Promotion, Neurologic Monitoring, Peripheral Sensation Management

Nursing Diagnosis: Risk for Disuse Syndrome

Outcomes. Common examples of expected outcomes for the patient with a diagnosis of *risk for disuse syndrome* are:

Patient will:

- Remain free from the complications of disuse as evidenced by full range of motion and intact skin.
- Use adapted equipment and strategies to regain independence in ADLs.
- Transfer independently or with standby assistance from bed to chair or wheelchair.

Nursing Interventions

Positioning. Appropriate positioning is fundamental to preventing complications such as contractures and skin breakdown. The challenge of positioning is increased by the presence of sensory impairments, flaccidity or spasticity of muscle groups, and the need to minimize the time the patient spends lying on the paralyzed side. The nurse helps the patient change position every 2 hours and encourages him or her to move independently in bed as soon as possible. The affected arm is positioned with the hand elevated above the wrist and the wrist above the elbow to support venous return and minimize edema. Special care must be taken to avoid excess pressure or pull on the affected shoulder joint, which is extremely vulnerable to joint subluxation and adduction contractures. The shoulder is positioned in a neutral position with support as needed from positioning devices. Pillows, rolled towels, and sandbags are used to support normal body alignment, with particular attention to preventing external rotation of the hip. The heels are elevated off the mattress to avoid pressure injury, and foot-positioning aids such as boots and high-top sneakers may be used to decrease the incidence of footdrop. The use of a footboard to position the feet is no longer recommended because it is believed to stimulate plantar flexion.

The same principles apply to the affected hand. Resting splints are often necessary to prevent contractures in the hand when spasticity is present, but rolled washcloths are avoided because they stimulate the grasp reflex. Firm hand splints are preferred (Figure 49-6). Skin under the splint must be assessed frequently.

The supine position is avoided for any patient who has a diminished or absent gag reflex to minimize the risk of aspiration. A side-lying position with the head of the bed elevated 10 to 20 degrees is preferred.

Skin care is another essential aspect of positioning. Use of pressure reduction devices such as 4-inch foam mattresses and elbow and heel protectors is standard. The nurse assesses the patient for signs of pressure, shearing, or friction damage during each repositioning. Once the patient is out of bed, attention shifts to pressure reduction in chairs and preventing injury related to dragging and pulling on the affected extremities. Arm and shoulder supports are important when the patient is out of bed.

Massage can be an important part of skin care and has also been shown to promote physical and emotional comfort. Older stroke patients who received 10 minutes of slow-stroke back massage at bedtime each evening for a week reported decreased anxiety and pain and had a lowered blood pressure and heart rate.[30]

Exercise. The rehabilitation plan incorporates active physical therapy, but the nurse needs to follow through with the plan over the whole 24 hours. The foundation of the plan is range-of-motion exercise for all joints. The exercise is initially passive but progresses as soon as possible to active exercise of the unaffected side and assisted exercise of the affected side. The return of motor impulses is significant for the future use of the affected part, but it

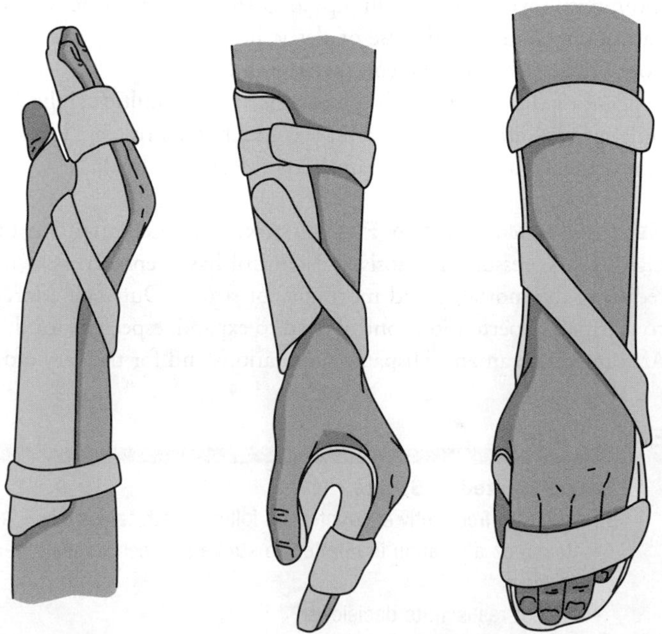

Figure 49-6 Volar resting splint provides support to wrist, thumb, and fingers of a patient after a stroke, maintaining them in position of extension.

also presents new challenges. Most stroke patients are initially flaccid on the affected side (stage 1) but within a few days begin to exhibit signs of muscle spasticity (stage 2). If flaccidity persists, the chances of return of function decrease substantially.

Preventive measures, such as resistive exercises and on-off splinting to prevent contractures, must be implemented as part of the plan. Muscles that draw the limbs toward the midline become very active because the adductor and flexor muscles are stronger than opposing muscles. The arm may be held inward and adducted to, or beyond, the midline. Without regular preventive exercise, the heel cord shortens, the heel may be lifted off the ground, and the knee becomes bent. In the upper extremity the elbow flexes into a bent position, the wrist is flexed, and the fingers curl into palmer flexion.

Strengthening exercises must be implemented to improve residual weakness. Synergy, the third stage of recovery, develops after several weeks. In synergy the flexion of a single muscle group results in simultaneous flexion of a broader group of muscles such as the elbow, wrist, hand, and fingers. Over time, synergy can resolve into a nearly normal pattern of movement, although residual muscle weakness is almost always present. The patterns of recovery are unpredictable, however. The arm and hand recover sooner than the leg but rarely to the same extent. Recovery may also stop at any stage and progress no further. Frequent reminders and assistance to sit straight and focus on maintaining a balanced posture are essential, as is balance training. Patients may experience problems with proprioception, dizziness, and sensory-perceptual deficits that make it difficult to control movement even when they have adequate muscle strength and coordination. Voluntary muscles lose tone rapidly with bed rest, which makes fatigue an additional challenge during early rehabilitation.

Learning to make safe transfers to a chair or wheelchair is the next step. The chair is placed next to the patient's unaffected side. The patient stands and faces the chair, places the unaffected arm on the distant chair arm, and then turns and sits down. The nurse stands on the patient's affected side during transfers and can use a safety or transfer belt around the patient's waist to provide needed support and stability without grasping or pulling on the affected arm. If the patient's knees buckle, the nurse can quickly move in front of the patient and block the unaffected knee so that it locks in position. The chair should provide firm support and have a high back and arms. A lapboard, pillow, or other device can provide additional support to the affected arm and shoulder. As strength and balance improve, the hemiplegic patient can be taught to transfer independently (Figure 49-7).

The same basic principles guide the gradual move to ambulation. Early ambulation promotes vasomotor tone and has strong positive psychologic effects on both the patient and family. Correct walking patterns must be established early because incorrect patterns are difficult or impossible to change. A sideward shuffle should be prevented. A walker, crutch, or four-point cane may be helpful, and the affected arm can be placed in a sling for support during ambulation. Ambulation retraining begins between the parallel bars in physical therapy, but on-unit practice time provides essential reinforcement. The use of a safety belt enables the nurse or therapist to provide additional support and stability.

In some rehabilitation settings the Bobath neurodevelopmental technique has been useful in stroke rehabilitation.[21] This approach seeks to normalize muscle tone, posture, and movement and promote bilateral function. Therapy seeks to redirect short-term memory toward an appreciation of normal movement on the paralyzed side. When a Bobath approach is used, transfers are made to the affected and unaffected sides to promote bilateral functioning. Other principles of Bobath rehabilitation are presented in Box 49-5.

RELATED NIC INTERVENTIONS. Energy Management, Exercise Therapy: Ambulation, Exercise Therapy: Balance, Exercise Therapy: Joint Mobility

Nursing Diagnosis: Self-Care Deficit (Feeding, Bathing/Hygiene, Toileting)

OUTCOMES. Common examples of expected outcomes for the patient with a diagnosis of *comprehensive self-care deficit* are:

Patient will:

- Participate in feeding self, with guidance, adaptive equipment, and assistance, until independence can be achieved.
- Participate as much as possible in decision making about bathing, grooming, and dressing, and will assist in self-care activities.
- Participate in toileting activities, with assistance, until independence can be achieved.

NURSING INTERVENTIONS. The physical, occupational, and speech therapists design a rehabilitation plan, which is then implemented by the nursing staff and family. The plan is developed after thorough assessment of the patient's motor skills and deficits, as well as the cognitive and sensory-perceptual issues that will support or complicate rehabilitation. Rehabilitation seeks to help patients relearn lost skills and compensate for temporary or permanent losses.

Each new skill is demonstrated, and then the patient practices with ongoing support and encouragement from the nursing staff and family. Families need to be incorporated into all teaching so they understand how to support independence rather than dependence. Providing extra time for activities is essential. Most motivated patients with moderate impairments can relearn the skills needed to complete basic ADLs.

Assistive devices play a major role in regaining self-care independence, since accomplishing basic tasks with only one hand is both challenging and frustrating. A wide variety of devices can assist patients with eating and dressing, and the nurse helps the patient

Box 49-5 Application of Bobath Rehabilitation Principles

- The use of both sides of the body is emphasized during activities of daily living and other activities.
- Weight bearing on the affected side is encouraged during sitting and standing.
- Movement toward the affected side is encouraged.
- Positioning is accomplished in opposition to the patterns of spasticity.
- The patient is consistently encouraged to straighten the trunk and neck to normalize body tone and posture.

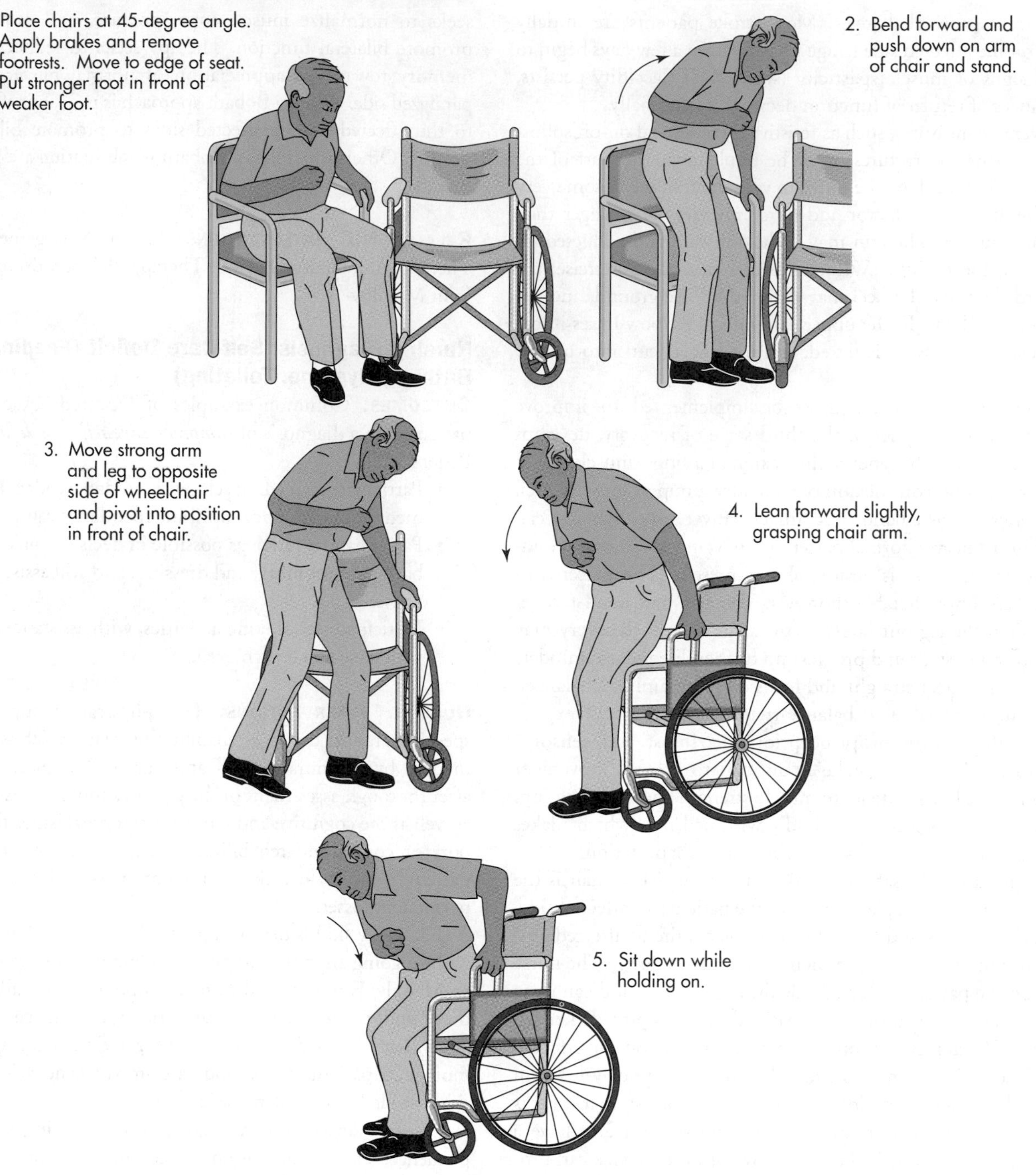

1. Place chairs at 45-degree angle. Apply brakes and remove footrests. Move to edge of seat. Put stronger foot in front of weaker foot.
2. Bend forward and push down on arm of chair and stand.
3. Move strong arm and leg to opposite side of wheelchair and pivot into position in front of chair.
4. Lean forward slightly, grasping chair arm.
5. Sit down while holding on.

Figure 49-7 Doing a standing transfer from chair to wheelchair.

and family think of simple modifications that can promote independence, such as slip-on shoes, Velcro closures, loose pullover shirts, and elastic-waist pants (Figure 49-8). The nurse encourages patients to dress in simple workout-type clothes rather than pajamas and gowns as soon as active rehabilitation is started (Figure 49-9).

Related NIC Interventions. Bathing, Environmental Management, Feeding, Self-Care Assistance: Bathing/Hygiene, Self-Care Assistance: Feeding, Self-Care Assistance: Toileting

Nursing Diagnosis: Impaired Swallowing

Outcomes. Common examples of expected outcomes for the patient with a diagnosis of *impaired swallowing* are:

Patient will:

- If able to tolerate food and fluid without choking or aspiration, ingest sufficient nutrients to maintain a stable weight and meet the body's baseline nutritional needs.
- If unable to take food and fluids by mouth, tolerate tube feeding to meet nutritional needs.

Nursing Interventions. The protective swallowing and gag reflexes usually return within a few days after the stroke, but the patient may have ongoing problems managing the complex act of swallowing. A number of cranial nerves are involved in this process. The presence of facial drooping or asymmetry, drooling, and a weak voice are strong indicators of swallowing difficulties.

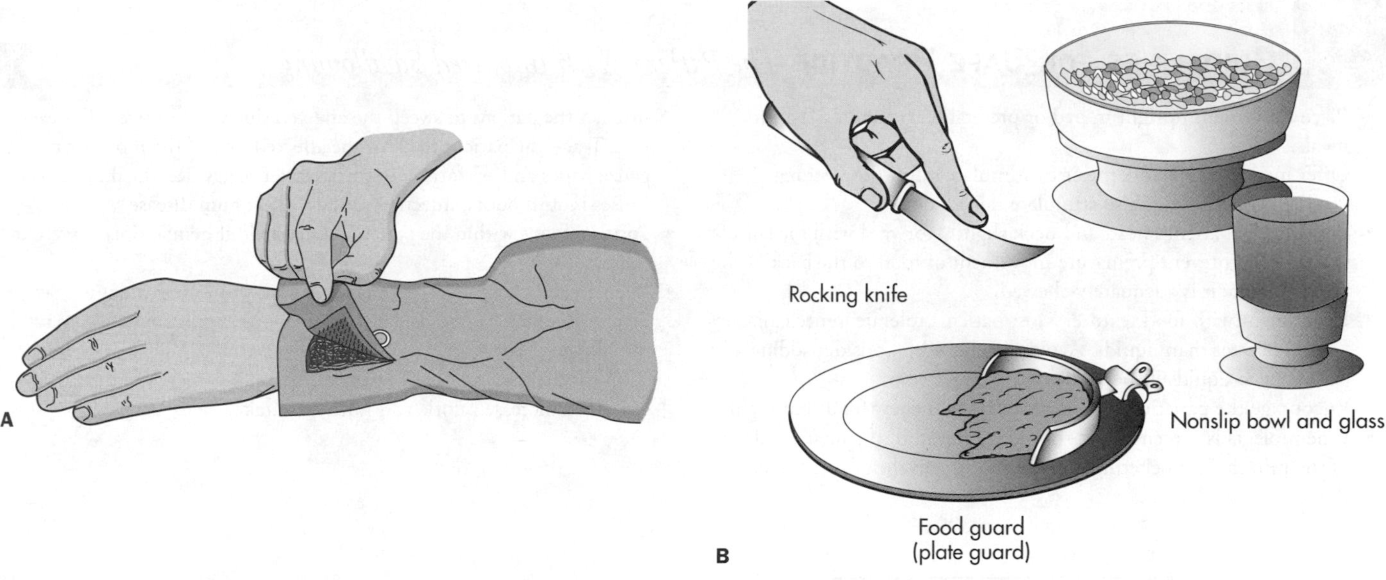

Figure 49-8 Assistive devices for self-care. **A,** Velcro closure on shirtsleeve. **B,** Assistive devices for eating.

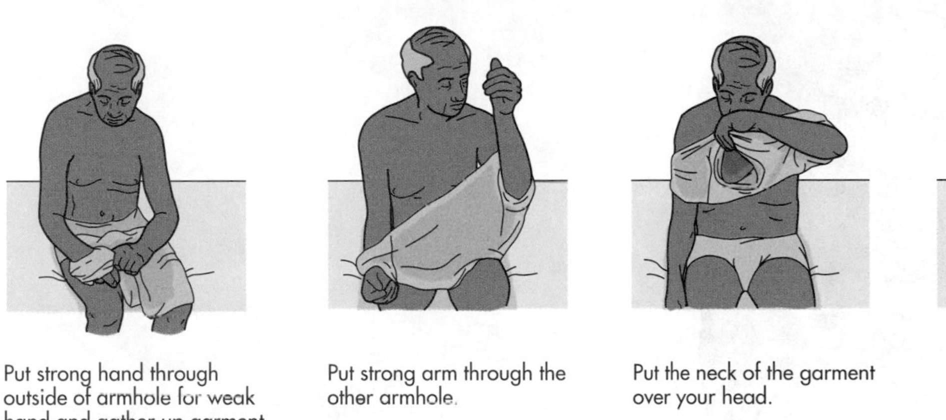

Put strong hand through outside of armhole for weak hand and gather up garment with strong hand. Then pull weak hand and arm through the inside of garment and out the armhole.
Put strong arm through the other armhole.
Put the neck of the garment over your head.
Pull down and adjust.

Figure 49-9 Putting on a pullover garment.

The gag and swallow reflexes are carefully assessed, and a speech therapist may be consulted to establish a management plan. A modified barium swallow may be recommended to further assess swallowing function and the risk of aspiration. Even if swallowing is intact, the patient may still be at risk for aspiration because of easy distractibility.

At the bedside, the act of swallowing can be grossly assessed by placing the thumb and index finger on either side of the patient's larynx and feeling for symmetric elevation when the patient attempts to swallow. The nurse should never give anything by mouth to a patient whose swallowing has not been thoroughly evaluated because the patient can aspirate without the usual accompanying coughing or choking if protective reflexes are not intact. It should be noted that up to 40% of stroke patients with dysphagia experience silent aspiration.

A quiet environment for eating where the patient can concentrate on effective swallowing is recommended. Specific strategies for approaching the problems of swallowing and nutrition in stroke patients are presented in the Guidelines for Safe Practice box, p. 1436.

RELATED NIC INTERVENTIONS. Aspiration Precautions, Swallowing Therapy

Nursing Diagnosis: Impaired Verbal Communication

OUTCOMES. Common examples of expected outcomes for the patient with a diagnosis of *impaired verbal communication* are: Patient will:

- Use alternative methods of communication to communicate needs effectively.
- Actively participate in speech therapy and continue to practice speaking without feeling stressed about performance.

NURSING INTERVENTIONS. A speech therapist is an integral part of the patient's rehabilitation plan, but the nurse can reinforce that learning and help the family be an active part of the

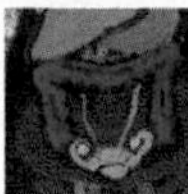

GUIDELINES FOR SAFE PRACTICE *The Patient With Impaired Swallowing*

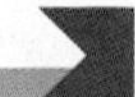

- Place the patient upright in bed or preferably sitting in a chair for meals.
- Offer mouth care before meals to stimulate saliva flow. Strong-tasting or salty liquids also stimulate saliva flow.
- Position the patient's head and neck slightly forward with the chin tucked in to prevent premature movement of food to the back of the mouth before it is adequately chewed.
- Experiment with food texture. Most patients tolerate a mechanically soft diet better than liquids. Avoid thin liquids. Consider adding a thickener to liquids if they are poorly tolerated.
- Encourage the patient to take small bites and chew food thoroughly.
- If hemiplegia is present, food should be placed in the unaffected side of the mouth. If "pocketing" of food occurs on the affected side, instruct the patient to sweep the affected side with a finger after each bite. Teach the patient to clean the affected side of the mouth with gauze wipes and perform mouth care after meals. Retained food causes mouth odors, infection, and tooth or gum disease.
- Position foods within the patient's visual field if hemianopia is present (Figure 49-10).
- Keep an accurate intake and output record until the patient is drinking sufficient liquids daily. Intravenous supplementation may initially be needed.
- Monitor the patient's weight weekly. Add supplements to diet or liquids to increase caloric and nutrient intake.

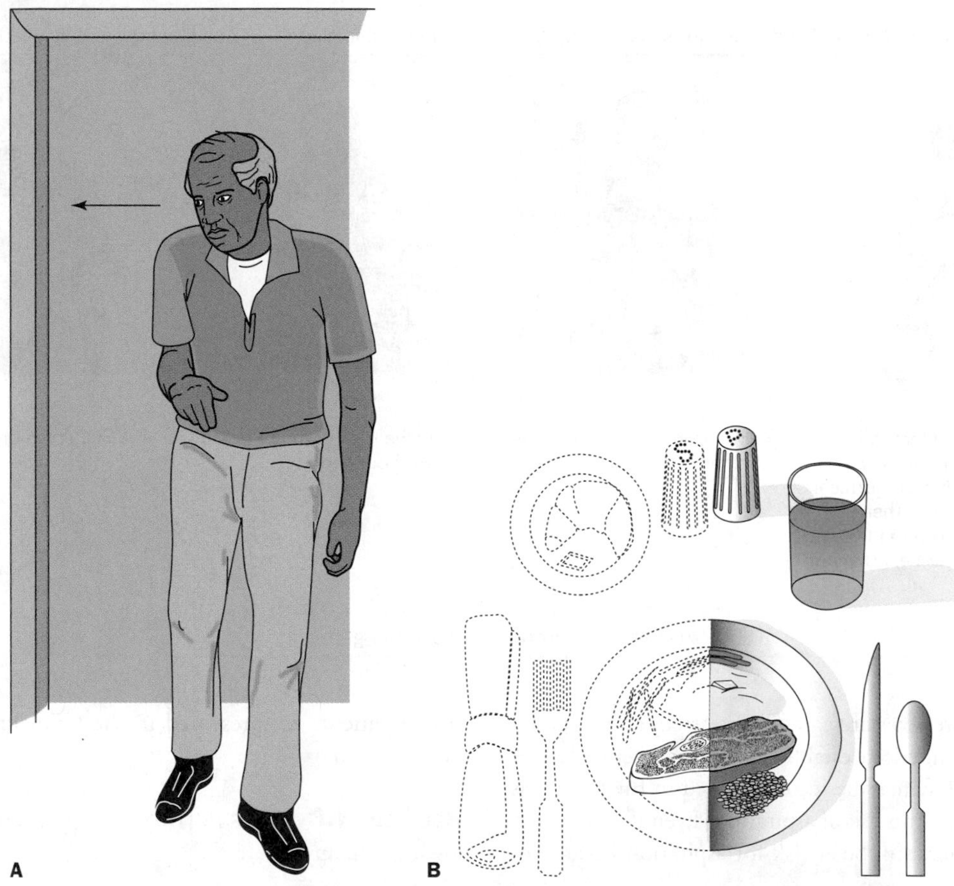

Figure 49-10 Spatial and perceptual deficits in stroke. **A,** Patient is instructed to look toward affected side when walking to avoid bumping into things. **B,** With homonymous hemianopia, patient is unable to see left side of tray and may ignore items on that side.

rehabilitation team. The patient needs frequent and meaningful communication and ample time to practice speaking in a nonstressful environment.

Communication problems after stroke may include both aphasia and dysarthria. Each person reacts to language problems differently, but anger and frustration are common. Some patients become discouraged when they encounter problems and may refuse to speak. This can progress to complete withdrawal from social interactions, even with family and close friends. The nurse must assess each patient's unique needs and provide support.

Family members may be at a loss as to how to respond to the patient's problems and may even encourage the patient to avoid frustration by not trying to communicate. Embarrassment at the person's attempts at speech is common. The nurse can model for

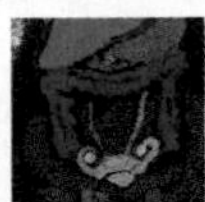

GUIDELINES FOR SAFE PRACTICE *The Patient With Aphasia*

Expressive Aphasia

Allow the patient adequate time to respond. Establish an unhurried atmosphere.

Be supportive and encouraging of the patient's efforts to communicate.

Use open-ended questions at intervals to assess spontaneous communication ability.

Involve the family or significant other in exercises to name objects used for routine self-care.

Express understanding and support for behavioral responses to frustration, such as tears or anger. Remind the patient that speech skills will improve.

If the aphasia is severe, a picture board or book may be necessary to communicate needs. Encourage the patient to communicate by whatever means are successful (e.g., pointing, pantomime). Anticipate the patient's needs when appropriate, and verify your interpretation of the patient's meaning.

Receptive Aphasia

Face the patient and speak slowly and distinctly. Do not increase your volume; hearing is not the problem.

Break instructions into component parts and give them one at a time. Repeat as needed.

Use gestures appropriately to support your verbal messages.

Involve the family in planning and implementing all strategies.

Provide support and encouragement when the patient becomes frustrated.

General

Provide practice at times when the patient is rested and not fatigued.

Offer liberal praise and reinforcement for efforts. Remind the patient and family that small gains can still be made months into the rehabilitation process.

the family strategies to help the patient and, at the same time, ease the family's discomfort.

Patients with receptive forms of aphasia may have baffling abilities to sing, recite poetry or Bible verses, or swear creatively. These actions can be troubling to family members, who need to understand the organic basis of the behavior. Specific strategies for assisting patients with aphasia are summarized in the Guidelines for Safe Practice box above.

RELATED NIC INTERVENTIONS. Communication Enhancement: Speech Deficit, Presence

Nursing Diagnosis: Disturbed Sensory Perception (Visual, Tactile)

OUTCOMES. Common examples of expected outcomes for the patient with a diagnosis of *disturbed sensory perception* (visual, tactile) are:

Patient will:

- Compensate for visual and spatial perception impairments and remain free from injury.
- Attend to affected side, touching limbs and skin to be sure of location and safety.

NURSING INTERVENTIONS. A wide variety of sensory-perceptual deficits may be present after stroke, particularly strokes involving the right hemisphere. These deficits make it more difficult for patients to react appropriately to their environment. Deficits that involve proprioception and depth and distance perception can present serious risks of injury as the patient becomes more active. These deficits are of particular concern when a patient also denies the stroke limitations and approaches activities with impulsive self-confidence. Until the exact nature and severity of the deficits are determined, the nursing staff provides increased supervision during all activities to ensure patient safety. The room should be kept as free of clutter as possible, but familiar personal objects from home can often help the patient remain oriented.

Frequent verbal cuing helps patients with a right hemisphere stroke stay focused on the task at hand. Showing pictures and demonstrating actions may assist the patient with a left hemisphere stroke. A mirror can be used to enable the patient to see the position of his or her body and maintain posture.

Consistent caretakers improve ongoing assessment and evaluation and support implementation of a consistent care plan. Accurate documentation is important in evaluating outcomes and planning for future services. Specific interventions to address the major sensory-perceptual deficits are presented in the Guidelines for Safe Practice box, p. 1438.

RELATED NIC INTERVENTIONS. Communication Enhancement: Visual Deficit, Environmental Management, Peripheral Sensation Management

Patient/Family Teaching. The greatest challenges for the patient and family occur after the patient has survived the initial acute stroke period. Married couples often express the view that the stroke has happened to both of them because the threat to their established way of life is so profound. The patient and family need to be included in all explanations of interventions and procedures, as well as be provided with realistic appraisals of the patient's future status and deficits. Most people have a basic understanding of stroke and its classic manifestations, but this knowledge is rarely sufficient to understand the unique challenges they face. The nurse uses every opportunity for teaching (see Research box) and encourages the family to be involved in the patient's actual care within the scope of their comfort level.

The acute care phase of stroke management is brief, and the family needs assistance to make decisions about the next phases of care. A social service referral is usually helpful. A lifetime of family dynamics and history complicate the efforts to make reasonable and rational decisions about bringing a patient home or seeking long-term nursing home placement. The financial consequences of either decision can be devastating. Ongoing and

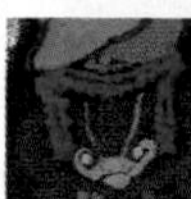

GUIDELINES FOR SAFE PRACTICE *The Patient With Sensory-Perceptual Deficits*

Hemianopia (Loss of Vision in a Portion of the Visual Field)

Approach the patient from the side of intact vision.
Position the patient in the room so that his or her intact visual field faces the door, if possible.
Teach the patient to move the head from side to side (scan) to compensate for diminished visual fields. Scanning is also important with meals (see Figure 49-10).
Place objects needed for self-care within the patient's intact visual fields.

Denial or Neglect and Body Image Distortions

Encourage the patient to look at and touch the affected side. Remind the patient to check the position and safety of the affected side during activity; help the patient through doorways to avoid bumping.
Lightly touch and stimulate the affected side during care.
Provide gentle but consistent reminders to include the affected side in care (e.g., bathing, dressing).
Monitor the affected side for injuries when the patient is out of bed. A sling may be used to protect the affected arm during ambulation.
Use a full-length mirror to assist the patient in reintegrating an intact body image and to assist with posture and balance.
Help the family understand the patient's behavior.
After the acute phase, approach the patient from the affected side and place frequently used objects on that side to stimulate it.

Agnosia or Apraxia

Encourage the patient to use all senses to compensate for problems in object recognition.
Practice the recognition and naming of commonly used objects and encourage the family to participate in the relearning process.
Encourage the patient to participate in self-care.
Correct the misuse of any object or task, guiding the patient's hand if necessary.
Continue to cue the patient verbally about the correct use of any objects or self-care tasks.
Be aware that memory deficits may make frequent reteaching necessary.
Explain all deficits to the family.

Research

Nir Z, Zolotogorsky Z, Sugarman H: Structured nursing intervention versus routine rehabilitation after stroke, *Am J Phys Med Rehab* 83:522-529, 2004.

The purpose of this study was to determine whether specific structured nursing interventions during the rehabilitation of stroke patients would enhance psychologic and physical recovery. The study's 155 participants were divided into control and intervention groups using stratified random sampling. Nursing students delivered the structured interventions using a guidebook prepared by the researchers and were closely monitored. The guidebook was based on Orem's model of self-care and focused on common topics after a stroke. Interventions were tailored to meet the needs of the patients, and each topic contained specific outcome goals. Topics focused around three domains: affective, cognitive, and instrumental (self-care skills). The interventions were provided weekly for 1 to 2 hours over a 12-week period.

Participants were assessed at 3- and 6-month intervals after intervention for effect. The tools used for data collection were FIM Instrument, Instrumental Activities of Daily Living Scale (IADL), Dietary Habits, Self-Perception of Health, Short Geriatric Depression Scale, Internal-External Locus of Control Scale, and Rosenberg Self-Esteem Scale. Baseline data were also collected using the same tools.

The study findings show significant short- and long-term effect on both functional and emotional variables of rehabilitation as a result of the structured nursing interventions. Further, this effect was over and above any attributed to time alone or neurorecovery. This study provides further support for making structured nursing interventions a key element of stroke rehabilitation.

sometimes severe deficits are common after stroke, and most patients require some degree of supervision and assistance. The effects of stroke are usually life altering and can be devastating to the patient and family. Depression and despair are normal responses to stroke. In addition, the patient may experience significant difficulty in responding to situations with appropriate emotions. The patient's tolerance to stress is usually diminished, and significant emotional lability may be present. The patient may be extremely emotional and cry easily, which may differ significantly from his or her behavior before the stroke.[13]

These emotional changes are distressing and commonly embarrassing to the spouse and family. The nurse helps families understand that these emotional responses are outcomes of the stroke and not volitional acts by the patient. Distraction and shifting the patient's attention can help the patient regain control. The nurse teaches the family not to become sidetracked by attempting to explain or interpret the behavior and to avoid feeling responsible for causing it. Emotional responses typically become more stable with time.[13] Problems with mood show potential for improvement with complementary therapies (see Complementary & Alternative Therapies box). This support may be needed on a temporary or permanent basis. Stroke support groups and resources such as the American Heart Association and National Stroke Association can be useful sources of information and referral services.

Recent years have seen an increased emphasis on aggressive stroke rehabilitation, but this can increase the pressure on the family to attempt to manage the patient's care at home. Decision making about care is difficult, and the nurse attempts to support all parties, facilitate communication, and ensure that the family has all the information they need. Involvement in the patient's daily care may help the family have a more realistic picture of the patient's needs for assistance and their ability to provide such support at home. Chapter 7 provides additional information about the challenges of rehabilitation. The nurse may need to remind the family to incorporate regular respite for caregivers into the overall plan.

EVALUATION

To evaluate the effectiveness of nursing interventions, compare patient behaviors with those stated in the expected patient outcomes.

Complementary & Alternative Therapies

Effects of Back Massage on Pain and Anxiety in Older Stroke Patients

This experimental study was guided by a conceptual framework combining the gate control theory of pain and Selye's physiologic stress theory. Based on power analysis, 118 stroke patients, ages 65 and older, who were experiencing shoulder pain were selected and randomly assigned to experimental or control groups. The experimental group received 10-minute slow-stroke back massages for 7 consecutive days, while the control group had no intervention. Both groups completed the State Anxiety Inventory before and after intervention and again 3 days after intervention. At the same times, blood pressure and heart rate were measured, and patients rated their pain on the Vertical Visual Analogue Scale. The experimental group completed a questionnaire on the third day after the intervention.

The study showed no change in the control group on the tested variables from time 1 to times 2 and 3. However, the experimental group showed significant reduction in systolic and diastolic blood pressure, heart rate, shoulder pain rating, and anxiety from time 1, before intervention, to time 2, after seven massages, and also 3 days after the last massage. Further, their questionnaire responses were positive about the experience. Also, significant differences were found in these five variables between the control and experimental posttests, indicating the intervention was effective. Thus this alternative adjunct to pharmacologic treatment reduced shoulder pain and anxiety in older stroke patients and, from their own responses, helped them sleep better.

Mok E, Woo C: The effects of slow-stroke back massages on anxiety and shoulder pain in elderly stroke patients, *Compl Therapies Midwifery* 10:209-216, 2004.

RELATED NOC OUTCOMES. Communication, Communication: Expressive, Nutritional Status, Nutritional Status: Food & Fluid Intake, Nutritional Status: Nutrient Intake, Self-Care: Activities of Daily Living (ADL), Self-Care: Bathing, Self-Care: Dressing, Self-Care: Eating, Self-Care: Hygiene, Sensory Function: Proprioception, Sensory Function: Vision, Tissue Perfusion: Cerebral, Mobility: Transfer

GERONTOLOGIC CONSIDERATIONS

The majority of all strokes affect the older population, and the incidence is likely to continue rising as the population ages. It is difficult to overestimate the impact of a stroke on an older adult's ability to maintain an independent lifestyle. The burdens for the spouse and family can be sudden and completely overwhelming. Even a mild stroke may require the complete restructuring of daily living patterns. In more severe strokes long-term institutionalization is commonly necessary. Even when physical consequences are limited, the cognitive, emotional, and behavioral effects of stroke may still change the patient in significant ways.

The nature and scope of stroke rehabilitation are usually prescribed within the managed care framework. The nurse plays a crucial role in helping patients gain access to needed services and move appropriately through the established care pathway. Stroke care for older adults necessitates multidisciplinary collaborative management and strategies to address the multiple areas of concern and provide high-quality, cost-effective care.

Cerebral Aneurysm and Arteriovenous Malformation

Etiology and Epidemiology. A cerebral aneurysm is a thin-walled outpouching or dilation of an artery of the brain. Aneurysms typically develop at points of bifurcation of the blood vessels, and the vessels of the circle of Willis are affected most often. If the aneurysm ruptures, bleeding into the subarachnoid space usually ensues. This is termed *subarachnoid hemorrhage*. Aneurysms can be classified by both their shape and size:

- Shape:
  - Berry (saccular): berry shaped with a neck or stem; most common type
  - Fusiform: an outpouching of the vessel wall without a stem
  - Dissecting: the intimal layer of the artery pulling away from the medial layer, allowing blood to be forced between the layers
- Size:
  - Small: up to 10 mm
  - Medium: 10 to 15 mm
  - Large: 15 to 25 mm
  - Giant: 25 to 50 mm
  - Supergiant: more than 50 mm

An estimated 10 million to 15 million people in the United States have cerebral aneurysms, but most of these aneurysms are extremely small and remain asymptomatic throughout the person's life. Approximately 30,000 persons experience subarachnoid hemorrhage each year related to aneurysmal bleeding, and the outcome for these individuals remains poor. From 20% to 40% die at the time of rupture. Subarachnoid hemorrhage primarily affects the 35- to 60-year-old age group and is more common in women than in men by a ratio of 3:2.[20]

A congenital developmental weakness in the artery has long been believed to play a major role in the etiology of aneurysms. Research also suggests that aneurysms develop as a result of degenerative vascular disease of the intima. Hypertension may predispose a person to aneurysm development; head trauma, bacterial and fungal infections, and atherosclerosis are all clearly implicated. Because multiple aneurysms are occasionally found in family groups, a genetic factor is being explored.

Arteriovenous malformations (AVMs) are also commonly diagnosed for the first time when the patient has signs of acute cerebral bleeding, but the nature of the problem is different. AVMs are among the more common developmental cerebrovascular malformations and are composed of a tangled mass of arteries and veins that lack a capillary network. Blood is directly shunted from the arteries to the veins. AVMs may form anywhere in the brain but are commonly found in the distribution of the middle cerebral artery. Most patients develop symptoms for the first time between the ages of 20 and 40 years. The annual incidence of AVMs is about 3 per 100,000, which represents 9% of all intracerebral hemorrhages and 1% of all strokes.[20]

Pathophysiology. When a cerebral aneurysm ruptures, blood at high pressure is forced out into the tissue, usually into the subarachnoid space. However, in some situations blood is forced into the brain substance itself, resulting in an intracerebral hemorrhage. The amount of blood lost is usually small because acute vasoconstriction occurs in adjacent vessels, and rising tissue pressure helps seal the bleeding site while fibrin and platelets initiate clot formation.

AVMs develop over time. The lack of a capillary network between the arteries and veins results in lower resistance in the arteries and the need for the veins to continually expand to handle the additional blood flow. Brain tissue within the AVM suffers degenerative changes. The patient may become more symptomatic over time or have an active intracerebral hemorrhage.

Many patients are completely asymptomatic before the hemorrhage of either an aneurysm or AVM. The classic symptom is a sudden violent headache, usually described as the "worst headache of my life." Immediate loss of consciousness may occur from the abrupt rise in ICP, and focal or widespread symptoms of an acute stroke develop. In addition, the blood itself irritates the blood vessels, meninges, and brain as it hemolyzes. Arterial spasms are triggered by the blood and the release of vasoactive substances, which can further decrease cerebral perfusion. AVMs also commonly manifest first as an acute hemorrhage, but some patients experience warning signs such as persistent unilateral headache or seizures.

Collaborative Care Management. The diagnosis of cerebral aneurysms and AVMs is usually made from the symptom pattern and the findings of CT scanning, which demonstrate bleeding. Once the diagnosis is made, cerebral angiography is used to visualize the major cerebral vessels, identify the specific characteristics of the aneurysm or AVM, and determine the presence and severity of vasospasm.

Surgical repair is the treatment of choice if anatomically and technically feasible. The surgery is performed as soon as possible after an initial period of stabilization and workup. Patients whose aneurysms are graded I to III by an aneurysm classification system are the best candidates for early surgical intervention (Box 49-6).

The surgical approach depends on the location and size of the aneurysm. A berry aneurysm is usually clipped or ligated around the stem, whereas other types of aneurysms may be wrapped to support the weakened vessel and induce scarring around the wrapping (Figure 49-11). Balloon therapy involves the insertion and inflation of a small silicone catheter with a balloon to occlude either the aneurysm or the parent vessel. These latter procedures are still considered experimental.

Box 49-6 Grading System for Symptoms and Neurologic Deficit After Subarachnoid Hemorrhage

- *Grade I—minimal bleed:* Asymptomatic or minimal headache, slight nuchal rigidity
- *Grade II—mild bleed:* Moderate to severe headache, nuchal rigidity, minimal neurologic deficits
- *Grade III—moderate bleed:* Drowsiness, confusion, mild focal neurologic deficits
- *Grade IV—moderate to severe bleed:* Stupor, moderate to severe hemiparesis, early decerebrate posturing
- *Grade V—severe bleed:* Deep coma, decerebrate rigidity, disruption of vegetative functions

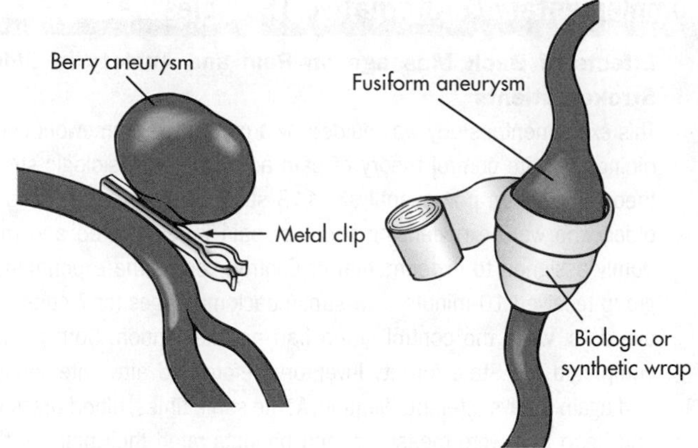

Figure 49-11 Clipping and wrapping of aneurysms.

Surgery for AVMs is extremely difficult from a technical perspective and may involve ligation or occlusion of feeder vessels. Surgery may be preceded by attempts to embolize feeder vessels with liquid polymerizing agents, Gelfoam particles, and microcoils. These treatment techniques progressively reduce the blood flow to the AVM. Gamma Knife surgery may be used for certain inaccessible lesions (see Chapter 48).

Rehabilitation for patients with aneurysms and AVMs is similar to that previously discussed for ischemic stroke. However, initial management focuses on stabilizing the patient and minimizing the risk of rebleeding. Medical management is directed toward maintaining a stable CPP by sustaining systolic blood pressure in the 150 mm Hg range and intervening to prevent rebleeding and manage vasospasm.

Vasospasm complicates the course of significant numbers of persons who survive initial aneurysm hemorrhage. Symptomatic vasospasm occurs in about 30% of patients and peaks in incidence at 4 to 15 days after the aneurysm. Treatment is directed at increasing cerebral perfusion by administering crystalloid and colloid solutions to expand the intravascular volume and keep the vessels dilated. A calcium channel blocker is also routinely given to enhance collateral blood flow. Steroid use is widespread but remains controversial.

Nursing care involves careful patient monitoring and implementation of aneurysm bleeding precautions to maintain a stable perfusion pressure. The rigor of aneurysm precautions has decreased in recent years because of concern over the development of sensory deprivation and related behavioral and cognitive impairments. Basic principles of care are outlined in the Guidelines for Safe Practice box and are similar to those used for the management of increased ICP. Care after neurosurgery is described in Chapter 48.

PATIENT/FAMILY TEACHING. Aneurysm or AVM bleeding creates a sudden and potentially life-threatening crisis for the patient and family. The nurse plays an essential role in explaining all needed care routines, especially in a critical care environment. Fear and anxiety can easily overwhelm the family's ability to learn and retain information. Participating in informed consent concerning high-risk surgical interventions can be particularly overwhelming. The nurse bridges the gap between the neurosurgical team and the patient and family, providing concrete explanations

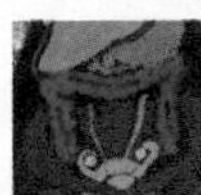

GUIDELINES FOR SAFE PRACTICE
The Patient on Aneurysm Precautions

- Place the patient in a quiet, private room without a telephone.
- Maintain bed rest with the head of the bed elevated about 30 degrees. Some surgeons now permit bathroom privileges for selected patients. If the patient is allowed out of bed, stress the importance of not bending over (e.g., to pick up slippers or dropped objects).
- Restrict visitors to close family or significant others and keep visits short. Prevent contact with visitors who upset or excite the patient.
- Encourage quiet, restful activities such as reading or listening to quiet music. Television may be permitted if it does not excite the patient.
- Keep the room slightly darkened and avoid bright, artificial light.
- Use stool softeners to prevent straining at stool.
- Discourage isometric contraction and use of Valsalva's maneuver (e.g., coughing, dragging self up in bed by the elbows, holding the breath during painful interventions such as venipuncture). Avoid the use of restraints.
- Provide gentle assistance with all needed care.
- Administer analgesics as needed for headache.
- Monitor the patient carefully for any changes in alertness or mental status.

and support as needed. The nurse carefully explains the rationale for all treatments and restrictions and incorporates the family into the patient's care whenever it is safe and feasible to do so. Referral for social service and spiritual support may also be appropriate.

▶ ARE You READY?

The nurse admits a patient after a ruptured cerebral aneurysm. Which of the following physician's orders should be questioned?

1. Admit patient to private room
2. Laxative of choice prn
3. Elevate head of bed to 30 degrees
4. Encourage isometric exercises

Degenerative Diseases

Degenerative neurologic disease includes a wide variety of disorders involving breakdown or progressive dysfunction of nerve cells. This section discusses only the most common of these disorders. Alzheimer's disease is not presented here because, although it is an organic brain disorder, it is primarily seen and managed in nursing homes and long-term psychiatric care facilities. Conversely, Guillain-Barré syndrome is discussed, even though it is not strictly a degenerative problem, because it shares many care concerns with the other disorders presented.

Patients with degenerative neurologic diseases are primarily managed in the community setting. Care focuses on effectively managing symptoms and supporting independence. This requires an interdisciplinary approach to care, with treatment decisions resting with the patient and family in close collaboration with medicine, nursing, physical therapy, occupational therapy, and social services.

Degenerative diseases typically cause a slowly progressive loss of independence. The care team helps the patient maintain a balance between the goal of independent self-care and acceptance of appropriate self-help aids and devices or direct assistance. Patients and families are forced to adjust constantly to changes in the patient's health status and cope with declining abilities. The patient's and family's psychosocial responses to these losses are often as important as the physical challenges of the disease process. The nurse's role is one of ongoing patient education and support. Being knowledgeable about the disease process and treatment options allows the patient to manage his or her environment effectively and plan appropriately for the future. Nurses support the patient's and family's coping resources and remain alert and sensitive to quality-of-life issues as they arise. Community support groups can be extremely helpful to patients and their families in dealing with today's challenges and future crises.

Multiple Sclerosis

Etiology and Epidemiology. Multiple sclerosis (MS) is a chronic degenerative neuromuscular disease that is characterized by inflammation, **demyelination**, and scarring of the myelin sheath. The cause of MS is unknown. MS is an autoimmune disorder possibly originating from environmental triggers such as virus or bacteria, as well as genetic susceptibility. However, few experts believe a single agent is the cause, and genetic research has found that multiple genes are involved with development of MS.

An estimated 250,000 to 350,000 persons in the United States have MS. The highest incidence is in young adults, with 70% to 75% of cases diagnosed in women. Average age of onset is 30 years old, and Caucasians are affected more than any other race. Epidemiologic studies consistently demonstrate a higher incidence in colder northern latitudes.[9]

MS is typically discussed as a single disease process, but it actually assumes a variety of patterns and in a significant minority of patients causes little or no disability. Sclerotic lesions are even discovered on autopsy or by incidental scanning in completely asymptomatic individuals. Patients with more aggressive forms of the disease are obviously more likely to be hospitalized and have come to symbolize the disease for many health care professionals. MS is classified into four types[4]:

1. *Relapsing-remitting disease* (85% of all cases): Disease exacerbations occur over several days and then gradually resolve over several weeks, usually returning the patient to baseline or near-baseline functioning. This continues over a 10-year period with minimal increase in deficits. In 50% to 70% of patients, it progresses to secondary-progressive type.
2. *Primary-progressive disease:* This is a gradually progressive disease in which exacerbations occur but the patient does not return to baseline and is left with increasing residual disability. This type will have spinal cord involvement.
3. *Secondary-progressive disease:* The disease starts as relapsing-remitting and becomes progressive after 2 decades. Individuals who have been living with relapsing-remitting type have difficulty adjusting to the progressive worsening of deficits.

4. *Progressive-relapsing disease:* This occurs in about 5% of patients. A progressive decline in ability follows symptom onset with progression during remission phases. It includes periods of acute relapse.

Pathophysiology. MS causes scattered demyelination of the myelin sheath. Although the exact etiology remains unclear, research evidence suggests that viral infection initiates an autoimmune response that results in demyelination. In MS, activated T cells, antibodies, and macrophages attack the fatty myelin sheath and the oligodendrocytes that produce it. The central nervous system damage is thought to be caused by a delayed type of hypersensitivity, a cell-mediated immune response.

The acute inflammation reduces the thickness of the myelin sheath that surrounds the axons and nerve fibers, and impulse conduction is slowed or blocked (Figure 49-12). Astrocytes or scavenger cells then remove the damaged myelin, and scar tissue forms over the affected areas. Natural healing may restore some of the myelin's function, or the lesions may continue to interfere with nerve conduction. This partial healing accounts for the transitory early disease symptoms. Eventually the nerve fibers may become permanently damaged, increasing the person's overt disabilities.

The course of MS is highly variable and unpredictable. Sites of inflammatory demyelination can occur virtually anywhere in the brain and spinal cord, producing a wide range of signs and symptoms (see Clinical Manifestations box). Classic symptom categories include sensory, motor, cerebellar, and neurobehavioral. Visual problems and fatigue are common early symptoms. Events that can precipitate a relapse include emotional stress, fatigue, infection, fever, and hot and humid weather. Viral infections are again implicated in disease exacerbations. Early relapses may last just a day or two but typically become more prolonged as the disease progresses. Clinically silent relapses can also occur and are evident on MRI scans even in the absence of overt clinical symptoms.

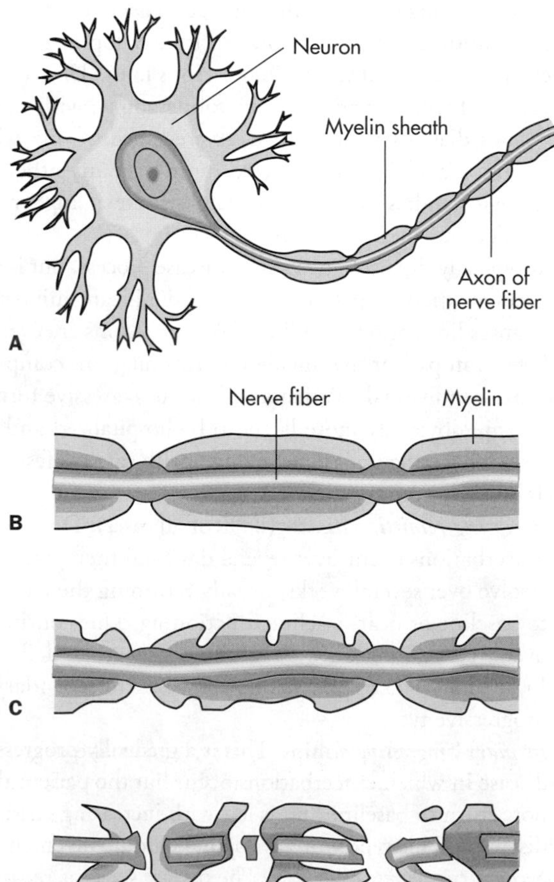

Figure 49-12 Process of demyelination. **A** and **B,** Normal nerve cell and axon with myelin. **C** and **D,** Slow disintegration of myelin, resulting in disruption in axon function.

Collaborative Care Management. The wide variety of initial symptoms and their transitory nature make the diagnosis of MS a challenge. MS has no single reliable diagnostic test, and diagnosis often requires more than one episode of symptoms. MRI is extremely sensitive to white matter lesions and is useful in identifying specific sites of demyelination. When gadolinium is administered during the MRI, it is even possible to distinguish between old and new lesions. Nevertheless the diagnosis of MS remains a clinical one established by ruling out other neurologic causes of the symptoms.

Laboratory testing shows an increase in activated T4 lymphocytes and immunoglobulin G (IgG) content. Oligoclonal bands of IgG are commonly isolated from the cerebrospinal fluid (CSF). Myelin basic protein, which is found in the myelin sheath, is liberated during an acute attack and can be measured by radioimmunoassay. Finally, visual, auditory, and somatosensory evoked potentials are performed to assess nerve conduction.

Drug therapy is used in the management of MS to treat an acute attack, decrease the number and frequency of relapses, and support symptom management. The basic goal of all drug therapy is to decrease the inflammation and destruction of the myelin sheaths. Some patients fail to respond to or respond poorly to drug therapy, and most approaches remain part of ongoing disease research studies. Drug therapy that is aimed at reducing the frequency and severity of relapses is summarized in Box 49-7. The development of recombinant forms of interferon-beta has offered patients with relapsing-remitting forms of MS a new drug therapy. Interferons have the ability to "interfere" with viral infections, but their mode of action in MS is not clear. Studies suggest that interferon-beta inhibits the number of lymphocytes migrating to the central nervous system and suppresses production of macrophages. These are the first drugs proven to decrease the frequency and severity of MS exacerbations. A wide variety of additional drugs may be used for symptom management, including drugs to reduce tremor, spasticity, bladder dysfunction, and depression (Box 49-8).

The goal of all collaborative interventions for MS is to keep the patient as independent as possible for as long as possible. Care is managed in the community and home setting except for short-term hospitalizations to treat disease exacerbations. A multidisciplinary team approach to care is essential, and the nurse commonly acts as the case manager. Physical therapy plays a crucial role. Range-of-motion and muscle-strengthening exercises are important in maintaining the function of uninvolved nerves. Gait retraining is essential when spasticity or ataxia is present, and the patient may need to be fitted with assistive or supportive devices for safety. Stretching exercises are useful in compensating for mild

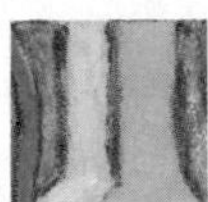

CLINICAL MANIFESTATIONS *Multiple Sclerosis*

Sensory Symptoms

*Numbness and tingling** on the face or extremities
Decreased proprioception
Paresthesias (burning, prickling)
Decreased sense of temperature, vibration, and depth

Motor Symptoms

Weakness or a feeling of heaviness in the lower extremities
Paralysis
Spasticity
Diplopia
Bowel and *bladder dysfunction* (retention or urge incontinence)
Intolerance to heat resulting in motor function decline

Cerebellar Symptoms

Spasticity
Incoordination, ataxia
Intentional tremor in upper extremities
Slurred speech, dysarthria
Scanning speech (slow, with pauses between syllables)
Nystagmus
Dysphagia

Neurobehavioral Symptoms

Emotional lability, euphoria, *depression* (occurs in 30% to 50% of patients)
Difficulty learning new information
Short attention span
Poor judgment, inability to problem solve effectively
Loss of short-term memory
Decreased concentration

Other

Optic neuritis (visual clouding, visual field deficits)
Impotence, sexual dysfunction
Fatigue (extremely common, ranges from mild to disabling)

*Commonly occurring symptoms are highlighted in italics.

Box 49-7 Principles of Drug Therapy for Multiple Sclerosis: Reducing Frequency or Severity of Relapses

Acute Exacerbations

Short course of high-dose corticosteroids
- —Methylprednisolone (Medrol) by IV infusion daily for 3 to 7 days, which may or may not be followed by tapered doses of oral prednisone
- —Oral prednisone tapered over 2 to 4 weeks
- —Corticotropin (ACTH) by IV infusion or IM injection, gradually tapered over 2 to 4 weeks

Long-Term Treatment

Interferon beta-lb (Betaseron) by SC injection
Interferon beta-1a (Avonex; Rebif) by IM injection
Glatiramer acetate (Copaxone; formerly known as copolymer 1), an injectable synthetic copolymer with immunologic similarities to myelin basic protein
Mitoxantrone (Novantrone) by IV infusion; limited number of doses can be given

ACTH, Adrenocorticotropic hormone; *IM,* intramuscular; *IV,* intravenous; *SC,* subcutaneous.

Box 49-8 Common Medications for Managing Symptoms of Multiple Sclerosis

Spasticity

Baclofen (Lioresal)
Dantrolene (Dantrium)
Diazepam (Valium)

Tremors

Propranolol (Inderal)
Isoniazid (INH)
Clonazepam (Klonopin)
Primidone (Mysoline)

Spastic Bladder and Urge Incontinence

Oxybutynin (Ditropan)
Propantheline (Pro-Banthine)

Urinary Retention

Bethanechol chloride (Urecholine)

Antidepressants

Amitriptyline (Elavil)
Imipramine (Tofranil)
Trazodone (Desyrel)
Fluoxetine (Prozac)
Paroxetine (Paxil)
Sertraline (Zoloft)

Fatigue

Amantadine (Symmetrel)

Constipation

Stool softeners
Laxatives

spasticity. Range-of-motion exercise assumes greater importance as the need to prevent contractures develops.

PATIENT/FAMILY TEACHING. MS challenges patients and their families with its unpredictability and uncertainty. The threat of relapse and loss of function is always present. These threats assume even greater magnitude for patients in their young or middle adult years at their height of productivity. Enormous pressure is placed on the patient to maintain normal daily activities, pursue a career, establish relationships, marry, and make responsible reproductive decisions. Patient and family education plays a critical role in helping them to understand the disease process and how to prevent or minimize relapses if possible.

MS is a debilitating rather than a fatal disease process, and patients and families need to cope with disease challenges over many years. The nurse assumes major responsibility for coordinating patient education. The goal is to help the patient effectively manage self-care and minimize both recurrences and the need for hospitalization. The nurse encourages MS patients to maintain a general health-promoting lifestyle. This includes remaining active in normal daily activities to the limits of their energy tolerance and balancing activity with adequate rest to effectively manage fatigue. The nurse stresses the use of energy conservation techniques, and an occupational therapist may be consulted about the use of appropriate self-help devices and aids. Chronic fatigue can be one of the disease's most debilitating features, and patients must become skilled at interpreting their body's responses and avoiding overexertion.

The nurse instructs the patient on the importance of maintaining optimal nutrition. Patients with MS should eat a well-balanced diet that includes all major food groups. Natural fiber is encouraged to promote bowel regularity. Some researchers advocate diets that limit the consumption of animal fat because the body uses some polyunsaturated vegetable fatty acids to produce myelin.

Patients with sensory losses need instruction about environmental safety. They need to compensate for their losses by using their eyes if possible to protect their extremities from trauma related to heat, cold, and pressure. Patients with diplopia often find that an eye patch is helpful. The nurse teaches the patient about the effect of heat, especially moist heat, on symptoms. When body temperature rises, the nerves may decrease or cease transmission, and disease symptoms can escalate dramatically. The patient should avoid hot baths, showers, hot tubs, steam baths, and saunas. Fever, stress, and infection can have the same effect. Chilling can also exacerbate symptoms. Female patients should be informed that pregnancy often exacerbates the disease, but they should be supported in their decision making about childbearing.

Bladder problems are extremely common in progressive disease. Drug therapy can be helpful in controlling symptoms, and the nurse instructs the patient about the effective use of prescribed medications. Urinary tract infection is a common cause of morbidity in MS and cannot always be prevented. A high daily fluid intake is important, and the nurse instructs the patient about the symptoms of infection that need to be reported to the health care provider. An intermittent catheterization program can be helpful for some patients with severe bladder problems. Bowel problems are best managed by the intake of adequate fluids and a high-fiber diet to establish regular elimination.

If the patient progresses to permanent disabilities, a variety of additional interventions may be necessary. Referral to support groups such as the Multiple Sclerosis Association of America and the National Multiple Sclerosis Society can be helpful to both patients and families. Resources for coping need to expand to adapt to the challenges posed by the steady loss of self-care abilities. Multiple changes may be required in family, occupational, and social roles. Changes in sexual patterns and abilities for couples should not be ignored. Families also need ongoing support to deal with the cognitive and behavioral changes that may accompany MS (see Research box). They need to understand that these symptoms, although often troubling and frightening, are organic and disease related.

Research

Fraser C, Stark S: Cognitive symptoms and correlates of physical disability in individuals with multiple sclerosis, *J Neurosci Nurs* 35(6):314-320, 2003.

The purpose of this study was to look at perceived cognitive impairment in individuals with secondary-progressive and relapsing-remitting multiple sclerosis (MS), and to assess the relationship between level of disability, age, and years with MS and self-reported cognitive symptoms. Of the 447 participants, the majority had relapsing-remitting MS. Participants were mailed a data collection booklet containing sociodemographic data sheets, three psychologic scales, the Performance Scales (to measure disability), and a consent form.

Eighty-three percent of individuals with secondary-progressive MS and 82% of those with relapsing-remitting MS reported having cognitive disability ranging from minimal to total disability. Although no significant differences were found in cognitive symptoms, there were significant differences between total disability scores. A significantly higher level of disability was reported by those with secondary-progressive MS. Also significant positive relationships were found in both groups between fatigue, sensory symptoms, vision, hand function, bladder or bowel symptoms, spasticity, and cognitive symptoms. No relationship was found in either group between cognitive symptoms and age or years with MS.

Since this study found the perception of cognitive deficits to be more prevalent than previous reported, it is important that health care providers initiate early screening for cognitive impairment and intervene appropriately.

Parkinson's Disease

Etiology and Epidemiology. Parkinson's disease (PD) is a chronic degenerative disorder that primarily affects the neurons of the basal ganglia. First described in 1817 by James Parkinson, PD is the second most common neurodegenerative disease, after Alzheimer's disease. An estimated 16 persons per 100,000 in the United States, or about 40,000 new cases, are diagnosed annually. About 1.5 million persons are currently living with the disease in the United States.

About 2% of those over 65 years of age and 3% of those 95 and over have PD. In autopsy studies, 10% of 70 year olds show evidence of PD. Slightly more men than women (3:2) are at risk. All races are affected similarly, but Asians and African blacks have a lower incidence than African-Americans and especially Caucasians. The mean age of onset of PD is 58 to 62; however, the incidence of younger persons has been growing, with 10% of these younger people under the age of 40.[4]

A number of theories of causation for PD (including viral, vascular, metabolic, and environmental) are being tested, but the cause remains unknown.[18] Recent research has supported the existence of a genetic component. Secondary types, called parkinsonism, may be linked to a variety of causes.[16,34] Symptoms of parkinsonism may develop in response to the use of antipsychotic, antihypertensive, or neuroleptic agents or illicit drug use; following an encephalitis infection; in response to brain trauma, tumors, hydrocephalus, or ischemia; in association with rare metabolic disorders; and in response to arteriosclerosis. **Neurotoxins** such as cyanide, manganese, carbon monoxide, and certain pesticides and herbicides have also been proposed as possible causes of the disorder.[14] Most cases are primary idiopathic PD. Smoking and caffeine consumption, on the other hand, have been studied for their neuroprotective effects modulating the risk for PD. Primary, or sporadic PD, which is the most common type, still remains idiopathic, but may be associated with a combination of genetic and environmental factors.[39,40]

Pathophysiology. The primary pathology of PD involves degenerative changes in several areas within the basal ganglia. The major degeneration occurs in the nigrostriatal pathway in the midbrain, which depletes the inhibitory neurotransmitter, dopamine, normally provided to the basal ganglia by the pigmented neurons in the substantia nigra. Loss of the pigmented neurons is greatest, but cells are also lost in the caudate, putamen, and globus pallidus ganglia at the base of the brain, as well as in the locus ceruleus in the midbrain and, to some extent, the dorsal vagal nucleus and sympathetic and parasympathetic ganglia. These and other nuclei are an integral portion of the extrapyramidal system of motor control, which regulates posture and intentional movements at the subconscious level, providing tone and fluidity.[6]

Destruction of the **dopaminergic neurons** in the substantia nigra significantly reduces the amount of available striatal dopamine. Dopamine and excitatory acetylcholine are the primary neurotransmitters responsible for controlling and refining motor movements, and they have opposing effects. The impairment produced in the extrapyramidal system produces loss of inhibition of the gross intentional movements, which lead to tremor; loss of tone, which leads to rigidity; and changes in posture, which leads to abnormal gait and equilibrium. When the excitatory activity of acetylcholine is inadequately balanced by dopamine, an individual has difficulty controlling or initiating voluntary movements.

In addition, in primary PD, Lewy bodies (cytoplasmic eosinophilic inclusions) are found in the remaining neurons in the substantia nigra; this finding differs from parkinsonism from known causes. Atrophy and neuronal loss are also found in the cerebral cortex in more than 50% of patients with PD, particularly in the later stages, causing dementia and an endogenous depression. Lewy bodies are found diffusely in neocortical neurons as well. As the disease progresses, dopamine receptors in the basal ganglia are significantly reduced, which could partially explain the decreased responsiveness to dopaminergic drug treatment after about 5 years.

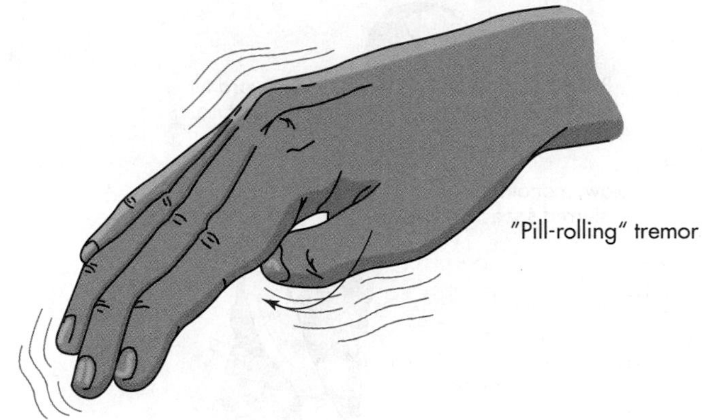

Figure 49-13 Classic tremor of Parkinson's disease. Movement of thumb across the palm gives it a "pill-rolling" appearance. Tremor is present at rest and may be relieved by movement.

Clinical manifestations of PD do not usually occur until about 70% of the targeted neurons are destroyed, and 60% to 90% depletion of striatal dopamine occurs. The disease begins insidiously and usually progresses so slowly that the person is seldom able to recall its onset. A faint tremor is a common early symptom that may be attributed to the aging process (Figure 49-13). The mnemonic TRAP is often used to describe the four major disease manifestations: tremor, rigidity, akinesia or bradykinesia, and postural instability. The disease is often categorized according to the nature and severity of the patient's symptoms and staged I to V, based on disability. The major disease manifestations are described in more detail in the Clinical Manifestations box and illustrated in Figure 49-14.

PD also has numerous secondary disease manifestations (Box 49-9). Patients usually experience generalized weakness and fatigue, difficulty with fine motor movements, loss of facial expression, difficulty chewing and swallowing, and voice changes. Many

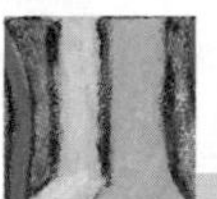

CLINICAL MANIFESTATIONS *Parkinson's Disease*

Tremor

Most recognized and least disabling symptom; usually first symptom
Present in 75% of patients
Nonintentional; present at rest but usually not during sleep
Characterized by rhythmic movements of 4 or 5 cycles/sec
Movement of the thumb across the palm gives a "pill-rolling" character (see Figure 49-13)
Tremor also seen in limbs, jaw, lips, lower facial muscles, and head

Rigidity

Muscles stiff and require increased effort to move
Discomfort or pain perceived in muscle when rigidity is severe
"Cogwheel" rigidity: ratchetlike rhythmic contractions of the muscle that occur when the limbs are passively stretched

Akinesia or Bradykinesia

Poverty of or absence of active movement
Difficulty initiating movement, slowness of movements, "freezing"
Often the most disabling symptom; interferes with activities of daily living and predisposes patient to complications related to constipation, circulatory stasis, skin breakdown, and other related complications of immobility

Postural Instability

Changes in gait
—Tendency to walk forward on the toes with small, shuffling steps
—Once initiated, movement sometimes accelerates almost to a trot
—Festination, which propels the patient either forward or backward propulsively until falling is almost inevitable
Changes in balance
—Stooped-over posture when erect (see Figure 49-14)
—Arms semiflexed and do not swing with walking
—Difficulty maintaining balance and sitting erect
—Cannot "right" or brace self to prevent falling when balance is lost

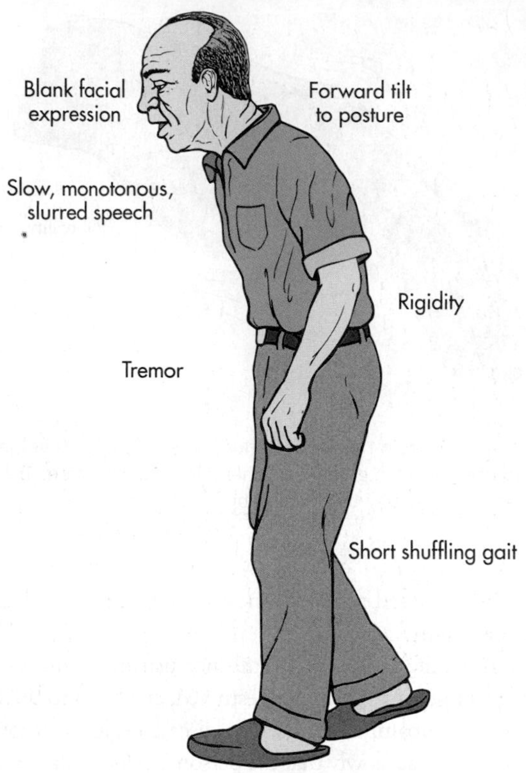

Figure 49-14 Characteristic appearance of a patient with Parkinson's disease.

patients, particularly older adults, also experience memory loss, problem-solving difficulties, and visual-spatial deficits.[32] Many persons with PD remain cognitively intact despite major clinical manifestations of the disease. Many other signs and symptoms, primarily related to autonomic nervous system dysfunction, may also be present. All symptoms typically worsen with stress and fatigue.

Collaborative Care Management. The diagnosis of PD is made clinically from the patient's history and symptoms. No definitive diagnostic test exists, and the diagnosis may be confirmed primarily from the patient's response to medication.

PD can be neither stopped nor cured, but developments in drug therapy over the past 40 years have resulted in enormous progress in symptom control. In addition, general supportive care and education are provided to assist the patient in effectively managing disease manifestations in the home setting. Supportive care is primarily directed at supporting independence in self-care, developing coping resources, and ensuring safety. Multidisciplinary involvement of specialists such as physical, occupational, and speech therapists can help create a daily regimen that is effective in slowing the rate of disability.

MEDICATIONS. Drug therapy for PD involves the potential use of six different classes of drugs (Table 49-1). Each patient's drug program is individually designed, taking into account age, symptoms, symptom severity, and lifestyle. All treatment decisions are made collaboratively with the patient and family, who need to be carefully instructed about the advantages, disadvantages, and predicted side effects of each option.

LEVODOPA. Levodopa is a precursor of dopamine that is able to cross the blood-brain barrier. Once present in the brain, it is converted to dopamine by the action of the enzyme dopa decarboxylase. This enzyme is also found outside of the central nervous system and acts on the levodopa wherever it is encountered. Most patients are therefore given Sinemet, which is a combination of levodopa and carbidopa. Carbidopa blocks the conversion of levodopa in the peripheral tissues. This ensures that more levodopa reaches the brain and increases its effectiveness. Combining levodopa and carbidopa usually permits a reduction in the dose of levodopa, which helps control its multiple and sometimes disabling side effects.

Box 49-9 Secondary Manifestations of Parkinson's Disease

Facial Appearance

Expressionless (masklike)
Eyes staring straight ahead

Speech Problems

Low volume
Slurred, muffled, tremulous
Monotone
Difficulty with starting speech and word finding

Visual Problems

Blurred vision
Impaired upward gaze
Blepharospasm: involuntary, prolonged closing of the eyelids
Decreased blinking

Fine Motor Function

Micrographia: handwriting progressively decreasing in size
Decreased manual dexterity
Clumsiness and decreased coordination
Decreased capacity to complete activities of daily living

Autonomic Disturbance

Constipation (hypomotility and prolonged gastric emptying)
Urinary frequency or hesitancy, retention
Orthostatic hypotension (dizziness, fainting, syncope)
Dysphagia (neuromuscular incoordination)
Drooling (results from decreased swallowing)
Oily skin, seborrhea
Excessive perspiration

Cognitive, Behavioral

Depression in about 50% of patients (endogenous)
Slowed responsiveness
Memory deficits
Visual-spatial deficits
Dementia in more than 50% of patients

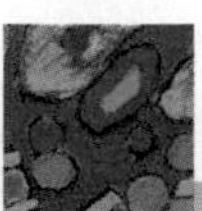

TABLE 49-1
COMMON MEDICATIONS *for Parkinson's Disease*

Drug	Action	Nursing Intervention
Anticholinergics		
Trihexyphenidyl (Artane) Benztropine (Cogentin) Biperiden (Akineton) Orphenadrine (Norflex) Procyclidine (Kemadrin)	Antagonize transmission of acetylcholine in central nervous system; most effective in decreasing rigidity; selective action but still have systemic anticholinergic effects	Monitor incidence and severity of side effects: dry mouth, constipation, urinary retention, dysarthria, blurred vision, changes in memory, confusion.
Indirect Agonist		
Antivirals: amantadine (Symmetrel)	Blocks reuptake and storage of catecholamines, allowing accumulation of dopamine	Positive effects may not last beyond 3 mo. Monitor for effectiveness and severity of side effects (e.g., mental confusion, visual disturbances).
Levodopa		
Carbidopa-levodopa (Sinemet), immediate or controlled release	Restores deficient dopamine to brain; carbidopa blocks peripheral conversion of levodopa	Monitor for side effects (e.g., nausea and vomiting, orthostatic hypotension, dry mouth, constipation, sleep disturbances, confusion, hallucinations). See teaching guidelines in Patient/Family Teaching box, p. 1448.
Dopamine Receptor Agonists		
Bromocriptine (Parlodel) Pergolide (Permax) Pramipexole (Mirapex) Ropinirole (Requip)	Directly stimulate dopamine receptors and increase effect of levodopa; minimize fluctuations in drug response	Monitor for side effects, which are similar to those of levodopa. Mental dysfunction is common.
Monoamine Oxidase B Inhibitor		
Selegiline (Eldepryl, Deprenyl)	Blocks metabolism of dopamine; may slow underlying disease process	Monitor for orthostatic hypotension. Do not exceed prescribed dose. May give this in combination with levodopa as disease progresses.
Catechol *O*-Methyltransferase (COMT) Inhibitors		
Tolcapone (Tasmar) Entacapone (Comtan)	Increase availability of levodopa by inhibiting COMT, an enzyme that metabolizes levodopa in gut, thus increasing available central nervous system dopamine; may allow for decrease of levodopa dose or improve effect	Monitor for side effects (e.g., orthostatic hypotension, diarrhea, nausea and vomiting, liver failure). Monitor for elevated liver enzymes, electrolyte changes with diarrhea.

The effectiveness of levodopa gradually decreases over time, which may necessitate gradual increases in the dose to sustain its beneficial effects. However, sensitivity to drug side effects increases, however, which limits the ability to continue to increase the dose. Some patients experience unpredictable responses to levodopa, including an "on-off" phenomenon. Motor function can fluctuate in a matter of minutes from active and ambulatory to severe motor freeze-ups. Some authorities recommend "drug holidays" for patients receiving prolonged levodopa therapy. Patients are admitted to the hospital and completely withdrawn from their medication. Although symptoms dramatically worsen, it is usually possible to restart the levodopa after about a week at a much lower dosage. Guidelines for the safe use of levodopa are summarized in the Patient/Family Teaching box, p. 1448.[4]

ANTICHOLINERGICS. These drugs are typically used in conjunction with levodopa or for patients who cannot tolerate levodopa. They have been used in the treatment of PD for almost a century. They antagonize the excitatory effects of the cholinergic neurons, are most effective for treatment of tremor, and have some effect in relieving muscle rigidity. Although somewhat selective in action, they still produce widespread anticholinergic side effects and may not be well tolerated. Trihexyphenidyl (Artane) and benztropine mesylate (Cogentin) are two traditional drugs in this category.

ANTIVIRAL AGENTS. Amantadine hydrochloride (Symmetrel) is an antiviral agent with known antiparkinsonian action. It blocks the reuptake of catecholamines, which allows dopamine to accumulate at synaptic sites. The drug's effectiveness is usually limited to about 3 months, and drug holidays do not prolong sensitivity to the drug's effects.

DOPAMINE AGONISTS. Dopamine agonists stimulate dopamine receptors in the brain. They help prevent or minimize the fluctuations in motor response that occur in PD. Bromocriptine (Parlodel) and pergolide (Permax) are two forms in use.

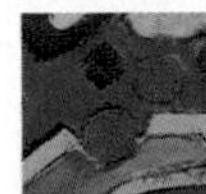

PATIENT/FAMILY TEACHING *Guidelines for the Safe Use of Levodopa*

- Levodopa is best absorbed on an empty stomach. If nausea occurs, it can be taken with food.
- Dry mouth is a common side effect. Chewing gum and hard candy can counter this effect.
- Depression and mood swings may occur. Report these or other cognitive-behavioral changes such as insomnia, agitation, or confusion to the health care provider.
- Avoid the use of alcohol or minimize alcohol intake. It is believed to antagonize the effects of levodopa.
- Avoid protein ingestion near the times for medication administration. Some protein amino acids are believed to inhibit the absorption of levodopa. A pattern of a low-protein breakfast and lunch with a high-protein dinner has improved symptoms in selected patients.
- Be alert to the possibility of orthostatic hypotension. Change positions slowly. Avoid steam baths, saunas, and hot tubs. Experiment with the use of support stockings to support venous return.
- Avoid vitamin supplementation with products that contain vitamin B_6 (pyridoxine). Pyridoxine increases the conversion of levodopa in the liver, which decreases the amount available for conversion to dopamine in the brain.
- Consult with the primary care provider and pharmacist about the use of all other drugs. Levodopa has multiple adverse drug interactions.

MONOAMINE OXIDASE B INHIBITORS. Selegiline (Eldepryl) may be used in the early stages of PD to block the metabolism of dopamine and delay the need for levodopa therapy. This drug directly targets the disease process and not just its symptoms.

CATECHOL *O*-METHYLTRANSFERASE INHIBITORS. Tolcapone (Tasmar) is a relatively new drug that inhibits catechol *O*-methyltransferase (COMT), an enzyme that breaks down levodopa in the body. Given together with levodopa, COMT inhibitors can increase the availability of dopamine in the central nervous system. Because of the risk of significant side effects, including fatal liver dysfunction, tolcapone is reserved for patients who have failed other drug therapy.[44]

SURGICAL MANAGEMENT. A variety of experimental approaches have been tried in the management of PD. Stereotactic surgery was used in the 1960s before levodopa became readily available. It is again being used in the management of severe tremor and rigidity. Thalamotomy and pallidotomy are procedures in which selected portions of the thalamus or basal ganglia are destroyed to relieve intractable tremors or dyskinesias. Case histories demonstrate positive outcomes in severe cases, but the risk of complications remains high. Experimental treatment approaches also have included autotransplantation of tissue from the adrenal medulla, where dopamine is produced peripherally, in hopes that the transplanted tissue would produce dopamine in the brain. Because of high mortality rate, this procedure has been all but abandoned in the United States. Experimental human and porcine embryonic tissue transfer has also been performed and continues to be used.

The Food and Drug Administration has approved the use of thalamic, or deep brain, stimulation to treat tremor. Electrodes are implanted into bilateral subthalamic nuclei and are connected to an external pulse generator, which is similar to a pacemaker and is implanted under the skin of the chest. Clinical results of this surgery have been promising in patients with disabling tremor.[11] Prevention of lead breakage has improved with anchoring of the lead extension at the level of the skull.

PATIENT/FAMILY TEACHING. PD is primarily managed in the community and home setting, and the nurse's role is to educate the patient and family effectively for the challenges of self-care. Patients and families need a thorough understanding of the disease process, appropriate self-care strategies, and signs that indicate medication failure or toxicity. The purpose of all interventions is to keep the patient as independent as possible in the face of a progressive decline in function. Teaching, support, and encouragement are needed throughout the course of the disease. A Nursing Care Plan for the patient with PD follows on p. 1450.

The nurse teaches the patient and family about the management of rigidity. Activity and exercise promote independence and reduce the risks of injury and complications. A physical therapist should be consulted to establish an initial activity plan and teach the patient and family range-of-motion exercises. These exercises are performed several times each day to relieve stiffness and prevent joint contractures.

Massage and muscle stretching are also effective strategies for reducing rigidity. The nurse can also teach strategies for managing gait problems and preventing injury during ambulation. A wide-based stance helps maintain balance for ambulation. Holding the hands clasped behind the back when walking may help the patient keep the spine erect and counter the postural problems created by the arms hanging stiffly at the sides.

The nurse emphasizes the importance of correct posture. Lying on a firm bed without a pillow during rest periods may help prevent the spine from bending forward, and lying in the prone position at intervals is also helpful. The use of assistive devices to prevent injury and support mobility is also explored. Patients with severe resting tremor may find that holding an object or placing the hands firmly along the arms of a chair when sitting may reduce its severity.

Environmental safety is an ongoing concern. The nurse can help the patient and family evaluate the home environment for fall risks posed by scatter rugs, clutter, or poor lighting. Simple home adaptations such as raised toilet seats and grab bars in the bathroom can significantly improve patient safety. Episodes of akinesia (freeze-ups) are more difficult to manage. The nurse reminds the patient to change positions frequently. The use of firm, supportive chairs with arms and rocking movements to initiate large movements such as rising from a chair can be helpful for some patients.

Patients with PD may face a wide variety of other daily disease-related challenges. General teaching guidelines are summarized in the Patient/Family Teaching box, p. 1449. Patients and families need ongoing support and encouragement because the burden of caregiving is heavy and will become more severe as the patient's condition worsens. They may profit from referral to the National

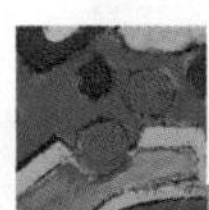

PATIENT/FAMILY TEACHING *Parkinson's Disease*

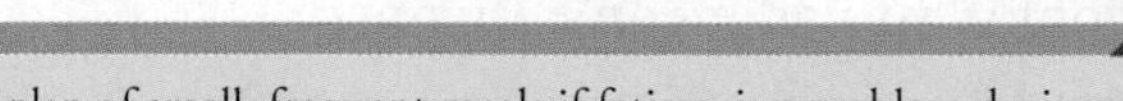

Activity and Exercise

Perform range-of-motion exercise to all joints three times daily.
Massage and stretch muscles to reduce stiffness.
Use a broad base of support when walking. Consciously lift and place the feet.
Pay attention to posture. Try walking with the hands clasped behind the back.
Explore the use of assistive devices.
Avoid staying in one position for prolonged periods. Alter position regularly.
Rest without a pillow and lie prone frequently to deter flexed posture.

Safety

Examine the home environment for risks of injury.
Modify the environment to improve lighting and remove hazards.
Consider installing devices such as raised toilet seats and grab bars.
Change position slowly if orthostatic hypotension develops.
Be alert to the effects of heat, stress, and excitement on symptom severity.

Nutrition

Monitor weight once a week.
Evaluate dysphagia and modify diet to increase ease of chewing and swallowing if appropriate.
Practice swallowing and take small bites.
Provide an unhurried atmosphere and allow additional time for meals.
Follow a plan of small, frequent meals if fatigue is a problem during meals.
Avoid eating high-protein meals at times of medication administration.
Do not use vitamin supplements containing pyridoxine (vitamin B_6).
Ensure adequate fiber and fluid intake to prevent constipation.
Manage drooling problems with soft cloths.

Elimination

Monitor bowel elimination pattern.
Use diet, exercise, and fluids to ensure regularity if possible.
Use stool softeners if needed.
Keep a urinal or commode at the bedside.
Respond promptly to the urge to urinate, and be sure to empty the bladder at least every 2 to 4 hours. Bradykinesia can result in episodes of incontinence.

Cognitive, Behavioral

Monitor for depression. Report its presence to the health care provider.
Monitor for changes in sleep pattern; disordered thoughts; and the development of agitation, confusion, or hallucinations. Report these symptoms promptly.

Communication

Exercise the voice regularly by singing or reading aloud.
Attempt to project the voice and alter volume and pitch.
Consult a speech therapist if vocal problems are severe.

Parkinson Foundation, American Parkinson Disease Association, and local support groups. All persons involved with caring for an individual with PD should be aware of the possibility of cognitive changes and deterioration, as well as the frequency with which patients develop severe depression. Pharmacologic intervention to treat depression may be necessary.

Myasthenia Gravis

Etiology and Epidemiology. Myasthenia gravis (MG) is a chronic disease that affects the **neuromuscular junction**. Although its exact cause is unknown, MG results from an autoimmune response that destroys a variable number of acetylcholine receptors (AChRs) at the neuromuscular junction. This results in the classic disease features of weakness and fatigue of selected voluntary muscles. It is estimated that the incidence of MG in the United States is 5 in 100,000 people. MG can occur at any age, affecting women more than men in a 3:2 ratio. It tends to affect women 20 to 30 years of age and men 60 to 70 years of age. There is a familial incidence of 5% to 7%. Infants of affected mothers may exhibit symptoms at birth, but the symptoms generally disappear within a few weeks. The thymus gland has long been believed to play a role in the autoimmune process of MG, since thymic hyperplasia is seen in as many as 80% of MG patients, and 10% have thymic tumors. However, the exact role of the thymus gland in the disease is not understood.[4]

Pathophysiology. Effective muscle contraction is contingent on adequate amounts of acetylcholine (ACh), a neuromuscular transmitter, being available at the postsynaptic membrane to generate an action potential that can spread along the length of the muscle and culminate in muscle contraction. Mitochondria in the motor nerve axons synthesize ACh, which is released when the nerve is stimulated. The ACh crosses the neuromuscular junction and binds with an AChR on the postsynaptic membrane to initiate the action potential (Figure 49-15).

Acetylcholinesterase (AChE) is also released into the synaptic cleft. The AChE breaks down the ACh, which limits the duration of the muscle contraction. The number of AChR sites is significantly reduced in persons with MG as a result of the destructive effects of an antibody-mediated autoimmune attack that specifically targets the AChR sites. As a result, the stimuli may lack sufficient amplitude to trigger an effective action potential in some muscle fibers. The strength of muscle response is diminished, and with repeated stimuli the amount of ACh steadily decreases, resulting in profound muscle fatigue.

The severity of MG is directly related to the number of AChR sites involved. Muscle biopsy can demonstrate the normal number of sites being reduced by as much as two thirds. The disease can be classified on the basis of either the severity of the clinical symptoms or the course of the disease (Box 49-10). The onset of MG is usually gradual, and the disease may elude diagnosis for a prolonged period. The course of the disease is also highly variable, as is typical of autoimmune disorders.

SIGNS AND SYMPTOMS. Early findings in 80% of patients are diplopia and ptosis, the hallmarks of MG. In 15% to 20% the disease is confined to the ocular muscles (ocular myasthenia). After eye muscles, next usually to become affected are those muscles

Nursing Care Plan

Patient With Parkinson's Disease

Data A 75-year-old retired man was diagnosed with Parkinson's disease 3 years ago. Over the past year he has developed tremors; a mask-like appearance; slow, monotonous speech; difficulty swallowing; and a shuffling, unsteady gait. He has experienced two falls within the past month. The patient's health history includes laparoscopic gallbladder surgery 8 months ago but no serious health problems. He lives with his wife in a two-story house.

Nursing Diagnosis

Ineffective airway clearance related to disease process (truncal muscle rigidity and resultant dysphagia, impaired cough mechanism, and decreased automatic swallowing)

Outcomes

- Patient will maintain a patent airway.
- Patient will remain free from aspiration.

Related NOC Outcomes

- Aspiration Prevention
- Respiratory Status: Airway Patency

Related NIC Activities

- Airway Suctioning
- Aspiration Precautions
- Respiratory Monitoring

Nursing Interventions/Rationales

- Elevate head of bed by at least 30 degrees. *Elevated position helps with gravitational flow of food and fluids into stomach, decreasing the risk for aspiration.*
- Encourage swallowing of secretions if gag reflex is intact. *Increased salivation and decreased cough reflex increases the patient's risk of aspirating.*
- Remove excess secretions with tissue or by suctioning. *To remove excess secretions that cannot be swallowed or expectorated and may produce coughing or choking.*
- Encourage deep coughing every hour when sedentary. *Facilitates oxygenation and the removal of secretions from the lungs.*
- Monitor respiratory status (lung sounds, respiratory rate and effort, altered level of consciousness). *To detect the flow of air and any adventitious lung sounds.*
- Assess ability to cough, gag, and swallow. *To determine existing deficits.*
- Avoid thin, warm liquids when cough and gag reflexes are intact. Thicken liquids as needed. *Thickened foods such as pudding are more easily swallowed than thin food because of their weight, which decreases the risk for aspiration.*
- Institute aspiration precautions (check gag reflex before feeding, elevate head of bed to 90 degrees, keep suction equipment at bedside). *Precautions are essential to prevent aspiration and resultant respiratory compromise.*

Nursing Diagnosis

Risk for injury related to decreased postural reflexes, orthostatic hypotension, rigidity, and retropulsive gait

Outcomes

- Patient will remain free from falls and injuries.

Related NOC Outcomes

- Neurological Status
- Risk Control
- Symptom Control

Related NIC Interventions

- Environmental Management: Safety
- Fall Prevention
- Surveillance: Safety

Nursing Interventions/Rationales

- Assess for drop in blood pressure or dizziness immediately after patient changes to upright position. *To detect orthostatic hypotension in response to position change. Orthostatic hypotension can result in fainting or falling.*
- Instruct patient to change positions slowly when orthostatic hypotension is present. *Reduces sudden drop in blood pressure, which can cause dizziness and place the patient at increased risk for falling.*
- Encourage patient to use side bars in bathrooms, hand rails in hallways, and chairs with back and arm rests. Use gait belt for assisted transfers. *Use of safety devices decreases the risk of falls and injury.*
- Encourage patient to choose a clear path for walking, avoiding crowds, narrow doorways, fast turns, uneven surfaces, and area rugs. *Environmental hazards can contribute to falls.*
- Encourage use of closed-heeled, supportive shoes or slippers. *Decreases the risk for shoes slipping from feet and patient falling.*
- Repeatedly remind patient to maintain upright position when walking. *Patients have tendency to flex excessively at knees and hop, which increases risk of falls.*
- Encourage patient to stop occasionally to slow walking speed (festinating gait). *To prevent falls.*
- Repeatedly remind patient to maintain wide-based gait (12 to 15 inches). *Provides greater support and decreases the risk of falls.*
- Place call light, telephone, etc., within patient's reach. *To prevent leaning, which may result in falling.*

Nursing Diagnosis

Impaired communication (verbal and written) related to micrographia and decreased ability to speak

Outcomes

- Patient will communicate his needs effectively.

Related NOC Outcomes
- Communication
- Communication: Expressive

Related NIC Interventions
- Active Listening
- Communication Enhancement: Speech Deficit

Nursing Interventions/Rationales
- Assess patient's ability to speak, read, and write. *Patients with Parkinson's disease have limited movement of facial muscles, tremors, and rigidity, which cause micrographia, decreased speech tone, and decreased volume. Accurate assessment of patient's abilities allows for selection of the most effective means to assist with communication.*
- Reduce environmental noise. *To reduce distractions that interfere with communication.*
- Encourage patient to speak slowly and pause to breathe between words. *Assists the patient with articulation of words and decreases frustration from not being able to communicate needs.*
- Watch patient's lips for clues and ask patient to repeat unclear words. *Aids the patient with communicating his needs accurately.*
- Teach patient to express ideas in short phrases or sentences. *Aids in articulation of words and communication of needs.*
- Do not interrupt patient while he is trying to communicate. *Spontaneous speech may take time. Interrupting the patient increases anxiety and decreases the ability to articulate.*
- Encourage patient to use facial expressions when speaking. *This exercise aids with word articulation.*
- Encourage patient to talk for 10 to 15 minutes each day or sing. *To help maintain facial muscle tone to enhance ability to speak.*
- Encourage writing when antiparkinsonian medications are at their peak effectiveness. *Patient may experience less frustration by writing rather than trying to speak.*
- If speech cannot be understood, encourage patient to use alternative methods to communicate needs (communication board or list of words). *To enhance patient's ability to communicate needs when speaking or writing is not possible.*

Nursing Diagnosis
Risk for constipation related to decreased fluid intake, decreased peristalsis, and decreased mobility

Outcomes
- Patient will maintain normal pattern of bowel elimination.

Related NOC Outcomes
- Bowel Elimination
- Hydration
- Mobility

Related NIC Interventions
- Bowel Management
- Exercise Promotion
- Fluid Management

Nursing Interventions/Rationales
- Assess patient's bowel regularity. *Consider patient's usual pattern of bowel elimination. A bowel movement every 2 or 3 days may be normal. Design interventions to reinstitute patient's usual bowel elimination pattern.*
- Increase fluid intake to 2 to 3 L/day if not contraindicated. *Adequate fluid is necessary to prevent hard, dry stool formation.*
- Encourage consumption of high-fiber foods. *Fiber coupled with adequate fluid stimulates peristalsis and elimination.*
- Encourage regular bowel elimination schedule. *A regular schedule aids with bowel elimination. The gastrocolic reflex may be helpful in stimulating bowel movement after meals.*
- Provide ample time for defecation. *Some patients take longer than others. Rushing the patient increases anxiety and prevents relaxation, which is necessary for normal elimination.*
- Use bathroom or bedside commode instead of a bedpan when possible. *Proper positioning allows gravity and abdominal muscles to promote stool elimination.*
- Implement bowel training program aided by suppositories. *May be necessary when regularity cannot be established through diet and exercise.*
- Avoid use of laxatives and enemas unless absolutely necessary. *Patient may become laxative or enema dependent and unable to establish normal bowel elimination patterns.*

Nursing Diagnosis
Imbalanced nutrition: less than body requirements related to decreased gag reflex, dysphagia, and difficulty chewing

Outcomes
- Patient will maintain weight within 5 pounds of baseline (or gain weight to attain ideal weight for height).

Related NOC Outcomes
- Nutritional Status
- Nutritional Status: Food & Fluid Intake
- Nutritional Status: Nutrient Intake

Related NIC Interventions
- Nutrition Management
- Nutrition Therapy
- Nutritional Monitoring

Nursing Interventions/Rationales
- Provide small, frequent, high-calorie meals. *Patients who have difficulty chewing and swallowing become frustrated when they must eat large amounts of food. Small, frequent meals provide the same nutrients and are less tiring to consume.*

Continued

Nursing Care Plan—cont'd

- Allow adequate time for eating. *Rushing the patient creates anxiety and frustration and may result in the patient refusing to eat or not eating an adequate amount of food.*
- Provide thick, cold foods (ice cream, shakes, frozen liquid supplements). *These foods are easier to swallow than hot or thin foods and are less likely to result in choking and aspiration.*
- Provide oral care before and after meals. *A clean mouth and pleasant taste simulate eating. A bad taste can discourage eating.*
- Assess daily caloric intake. *To determine if patient is consuming adequate calories to meet metabolic demands.*
- Record weight at least every third day. *To identify pattern of weight gain, loss, or stability.*
- Schedule medications so that peak time coincides with meals. *Medications control symptoms that interfere with the patient's ability to self-feed and swallow.*
- Encourage family to bring patient's favorite meals from home. *Consumption of adequate nutrients is more likely to occur if the patient enjoys the foods that are served.*

Nursing Diagnosis

Self-care deficit (feeding, bathing, grooming) related to akinesia, decreased reflexes, and tremor

Outcomes

- Patient will perform self-care independently with use of self-help aids.

Related NOC Outcomes

- Self-Care: Activities of Daily Living (ADL)
- Self-Care: Bathing
- Self-Care: Dressing
- Self-Care: Eating
- Self-Care: Hygiene

Related NIC Interventions

- Bathing
- Dressing
- Feeding
- Self-Care Assistance

Nursing Interventions/Rationales

- Obtain adaptive equipment for feeding (padded utensils and plate guards), bathing (sponge mitts), and dressing (Velcro straps), and teach patient correct use. *These devices aid the patient with completing self-care tasks, which increases self-confidence and allows some control over the situation.*
- Encourage use of chairs and commodes with elevated seats. *To aid the patient with sitting and prevent falls from loss of balance.*
- Provide unhurried atmosphere and allow time for completion of tasks. *Many patients can remain independent if they are allowed adequate time to complete tasks. Hurrying patients makes them frustrated and impedes their ability to function.*
- Foster independence and provide encouragement if problems arise. *Patients may become easily frustrated. Rewarding small successes provides encouragement for continued independence.*
- Perform active or passive range-of-motion exercises to all extremities. *Muscle rigidity can quickly progress to joint contracture.*
- Encourage patient to actively swing arms when walking. *Improves balance and decreases tremor, which facilitates movement.*
- If patient becomes "stuck" while walking, face patient and either hold patient's hands or have patient hold your shoulders or waist with both hands. Gently and slightly rock the patient from side to side. *Bradykinesia is a classic sign of Parkinson's disease. With episodes of akinesia or freeze-up, the patient cannot initiate movement. Gentle rocking helps unfreeze the patient so he can continue walking.*

Evaluation

Evaluation is based on comparing the patient's outcomes with desired outcomes.

innervated by the cranial nerves: facial, masticator, speech, swallowing, and neck muscles. Mobility of the face is decreased, leading to a blank expression; an attempt to smile produces a classic MG snarl (Figure 49-16). Dysphagia, aspiration, and dysarthria may result. The voice becomes nasal and weak.

Generalized weakness occurs in 85% of patients. When proximal muscles are involved, the patient has difficulty raising the arms over the head or climbing stairs. Weakness of the arm and hand muscles may first become apparent during self-care activities such as shaving or combing the hair. Weakness of neck extensors allows the head to fall forward. Symptoms develop rapidly, but early in the course of the disease they are relieved easily with rest. As the disease progresses, fatigue becomes evident with less and less exertion. Involvement of the muscles of the trunk and lower limbs may create difficulties with walking and even sitting. The distal muscles are rarely affected as severely as the proximal muscles. During a disease exacerbation, muscle weakness of the intercostal muscles and diaphragm may become so severe that myasthenia crisis results, with reduced static pressures and forced vital capacity. Intubation and ventilation may be required. Exacerbations of the disease can be triggered by upper respiratory tract infection, emotional stress, secondary illness, trauma, surgery, pregnancy, and even menstruation. There is no accompanying sensory loss in the affected areas.

Collaborative Care Management. The diagnosis of MG is first established presumptively from the patient's history and symptoms and is then confirmed through laboratory testing. A positive Tensilon test is considered diagnostic. In this test, edrophonium (Tensilon), a short-acting anticholinesterase, is administered intravenously. A patient with MG experiences a brief but significant increase in muscle strength in previously weakened muscles in response to the drug, and this response is considered a positive result.[41] AChR antibody titers are elevated in the vast majority of patients with MG, and electromyogram (EMG) results are believed to be 99% sensitive in diagnosing MG. The

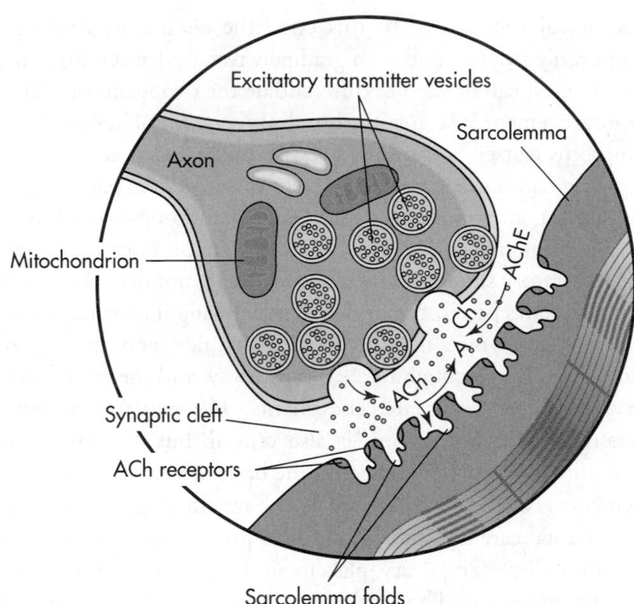

Figure 49-15 Normal neuromuscular junction. Acetylcholine *(ACh)* released from nerve initiates muscle contraction. Acetylcholinesterase *(AChE)* breaks down ACh, limiting duration of contraction.

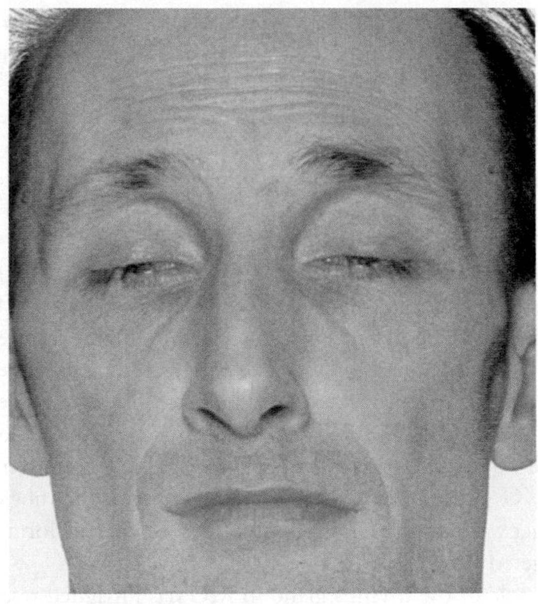

Figure 49-16 Facial appearance in myasthenia gravis. Note ptosis, lack of expression, and wrinkled brow.

Box 49-10 Classification System for Myasthenia Gravis

- *Type 1:* Ocular myasthenia
- *Type 2A:* Mild, generalized
- *Type 2B:* Moderately severe; bulbar paralysis
- *Type 3:* Fulminating, acute; respiratory crisis
- *Type 4:* Chronic, late severe; progressive over 2 years

EMG can detect transmission delay or failure in muscle fibers that are repetitively stimulated. A thoracic MRI may be performed to evaluate thymus gland involvement.[26]

MG has no known cure, but drug therapy is effective in managing symptoms in most patients. Individual responses vary tremendously, however, and an individualized treatment plan needs to be developed collaboratively for each patient. The management of MG primarily takes place in the community, and it is essential for patients to be well informed about self-care management of their disease. Patients may require hospitalization in rare circumstances to manage disease crises, but the bulk of care and treatment takes place in the home.

Drug therapy with anticholinesterase drugs is the cornerstone of MG treatment, but these drugs do not reverse the actual disease process.[35] With the action of AChE being blocked in the neuromuscular junction, more ACh is available for receptor site binding. Pyridostigmine (Mestinon) is the most commonly used drug. Its use is associated with multiple side effects (Box 49-11), and an individualized dosage schedule needs to be established that allows the patient to receive maximal benefit from the drug while keeping side effects within tolerable limits. The drug effect peaks in about 2 hours, and its duration of effect is 3 to 6 hours, so its administration must be carefully timed to support specific muscle group activities such as chewing and swallowing at mealtimes. Atropine is the antidote for pyridostigmine and should be available to treat adverse side effects. The patient may be permitted to adjust the dosage and time of administration slightly within stated parameters to meet the fluctuating needs of daily living.

Other treatment approaches for MG target the disease process itself. Long-term immunosuppression with corticosteroids, azathioprine (Imuran), or cyclosporine may be prescribed for patients who do not respond well to cholinesterase inhibitors or develop disabling ocular or generalized MG. The potential benefits of this treatment must be carefully weighed against the risks of long-term immunosuppression. Prednisone is the drug of choice and produces improvement in 70% to 80% of patients, but it is often difficult to sustain these improvements when the drug is tapered. It may be used for 1 to 3 months. Azathioprine has been shown to reduce the number of circulating AChR antibodies, but improvement may not

Box 49-11 Side Effects of Pyridostigmine (Mestinon) Therapy

Muscarinic Effects (Effects on Smooth Muscle and Glands)

Gastrointestinal distress, heartburn
Nausea and vomiting
Increased peristalsis, abdominal cramping, diarrhea
Bradycardia
Increased bronchial secretions, bronchoconstriction or bronchospasm
Excessive salivation, tearing
Sweating
Miosis, blurred vision
Involuntary micturition

Nicotinic Effects (Effects on Skeletal Muscle)

Muscle twitching (fasciculations) and spasms
Profound muscle weakness

be noticed for months. It is gradually discontinued after 1 to 2 years of improvement. Cyclosporine acts by decreasing T cell function and also decreases circulating AChR antibodies; a response is usually seen within weeks. These drugs may also be used in conjunction with plasmapheresis to treat a serious disease exacerbation. Tacrolimus given for up to 2 years to patients with generalized MG has also been shown to improve patient status without serious side effects.[25]

Plasmapheresis or intravenous immunoglobulin (IVIG) administration provides for short-term immunomodulation. During plasmapheresis the patient's plasma is removed and replaced with albumin or fresh frozen plasma. The AChR antibodies are removed in the process.[45] Improvements can be dramatic but are often temporary. IVIG is also used to treat disease exacerbations; although its action is not understood, it has produced dramatic improvement in some MG patients. It is theorized that human immunoglobulins may react with antigens in the plasma and decrease the formation of the targeted antibodies.

The role of the thymus gland in MG has intrigued researchers for years. A thymectomy results in symptom remission in about 40% of patients. It appears to be most effective when performed in patients under 40 years of age who have had symptomatic MG for less than 5 years.

Myasthenic and Cholinergic Crises. Patients with MG are vulnerable to two crisis situations that may result in dramatic symptom exacerbation and the need for acute ventilatory support. A myasthenic crisis represents an acute exacerbation of the disease process and may occur in response to stress, trauma, or infection. Problems with breathing and swallowing can rapidly progress to life-threatening levels, and intubation is usually performed when the patient's vital capacity drops below 1 L. Mechanical ventilation is continued until the patient shows signs of returning muscle strength. Cholinesterase inhibitor drugs are gradually restarted in an effort to again find an effective balance.

A cholinergic crisis represents a toxic response to medication. The muscarinic side effects develop slowly, but as toxic levels are reached, severe nicotinic effects can rapidly appear. The patient experiences profound weakness, copious respiratory secretions, and respiratory failure, which again may require intubation and mechanical ventilation. In this crisis the cholinesterase drug is temporarily stopped and then gradually restarted and retitrated. A Tensilon test can be used to differentiate the two forms of crisis. If no improvement is seen with the administration of Tensilon, or if symptoms worsen, a cholinergic crisis can be assumed.

Acute care nurses are most likely to encounter patients with MG during an episode of disease exacerbation or crisis. Nursing care involves meticulous neurologic and respiratory monitoring and respiratory support. The nurse regularly monitors the severity of the patient's ptosis, the degree of swallowing impairment, hand strength, and voice quality. Respiratory rate and quality, the patient's ability to cough to clear the airway, and the use of accessory muscles are standard assessments. The patient's subjective assessment of breathlessness is also crucial, but decisions about intubation are generally made on the basis of vital capacity measurements. Patients who are weak enough to require intubation require total care and interventions to prevent the complications of immobility. Temporary placement in an intensive care unit may be necessary. The crisis is extremely frightening for the patient, who needs ongoing support and reassurance. Patients and families dealing with any stage of the disease may profit from referral to the Myasthenia Gravis Foundation of America.

Patient/Family Teaching. Self-care is the foundation of MG management, and education of the patient and family is its most critical component. Respiratory complications are the most serious disease threat, and knowledgeable self-care can positively affect their frequency and severity. The medication regimen is also commonly adjusted by the patient within preset parameters, and the patient needs to be knowledgeable about safe drug administration and the management of side effects. Box 49-11 outlines the major side effects associated with the use of pyridostigmine, and principles of patient teaching for MG are summarized in the Patient/Family Teaching box.

Amyotrophic Lateral Sclerosis

Etiology and Epidemiology. Amyotrophic lateral sclerosis (ALS) is a chronic and rapidly progressive motor neuron disease that eventually weakens and paralyzes the respiratory muscles,

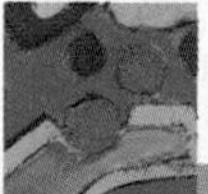

Patient/Family Teaching *Myasthenia Gravis*

- Use pyridostigmine (Mestinon) safely and appropriately.
  - —Take drug with food or fluid.
  - —Take drug before meals to permit maximum effect for chewing and swallowing.
  - —Adjust drug dosage and time of administration within set parameters in response to your individual pattern of weakness.
  - —Do not take any other medication, including over-the-counter products, without prior approval of the health care provider or pharmacist. Many drugs (e.g., local anesthetics, aminoglycosides, beta-blockers, and calcium channel blockers) can compromise neuromuscular transmission and will worsen disease symptoms.
- Modify diet as needed in response to swallowing problems.
  - —A soft diet is usually well tolerated.
  - —Eat slowly and take small bites.
- Balance rest and activity throughout the day in response to weakness.
  - —Plan for additional rest periods.
  - —Seek out energy conservation strategies for routine activities.
- Keep Medic-Alert identification with you at all times.
- Know the symptoms of cholinergic and myasthenic crisis and contact physician promptly.
- Be alert to disease response to periods of stress, infection, temperature extremes, and hormonal swings (e.g., menstruation or pregnancy).
- Wear sensible shoes for ease in walking and balance maintenance.
- Avoid stress, extreme heat, or extensive exposure to ultraviolet light.

resulting in death. It is also referred to as Lou Gehrig's disease after the New York Yankees baseball player who died from the disease.

ALS is a rare disease that occurs in 1 or 2 persons per 100,000 annually. Men have a higher incidence of ALS than women. The peak age at onset is around 50 years. The cause is unknown, but there are many theories. Some researchers believe that there is a defect in the processing of glutamate, which is an excitatory neurotransmitter. Others believe free radicals cause oxidative stress, which results in cell damage. Still others believe that autoimmune destruction results in cytoskeletal, mutated and damaged neurofilaments. Approximately 10% of ALS patients inherit an autosomal dominant gene that is associated with the disease.[6]

Pathophysiology. The term *amyotrophic* refers to the weakness and atrophy that occur from the degeneration of the alpha or lower motor neurons. Lower motor neurons originate in the anterior horn of the spinal cord, and their axons connect the central nervous system with the voluntary muscles. They are essential for motor function and innervate the voluntary skeletal muscles. The term *lateral sclerosis* refers to the scarring of the corticospinal tract in the lateral column of the spinal cord and refers to upper motor neuron involvement. ALS involves degeneration of both upper and lower motor neurons of the final pathway. Upper motor neurons originate in the upper regions of the brain. The neurons of the brainstem are primarily affected by ALS. The axons of the upper motor neurons synapse in the descending corticospinal or pyramidal tract to the lower motor neurons.

ALS causes progressive degeneration of both the upper and lower motor neurons from demyelination and scar tissue formation. The disease gradually destroys motor pathways but leaves sensation and mental status intact. Lower motor neurons are usually affected first, resulting in muscle weakness and atrophy. The muscles of the upper body are affected much earlier than those of the legs. Patients may notice that they drop items or have a decreased ability to perform tasks that require fine motor skills. Other early symptoms include muscle atrophy, fasciculations and fibrillations of the muscles, and decreased tendon reflexes. Muscle cramping and generalized fatigue are also common. The disease is relentlessly progressive and eventually involves the upper motor neurons, which causes increased weakness and spasticity in affected muscles. Hyperactive reflexes, jaw clonus, tongue fasciculations, and a positive Babinski's reflex may be present. As the muscles of the neck, pharynx, and larynx become increasingly involved, slurring of the voice occurs, which gradually progresses to dysarthria and dysphagia. Paralysis is inevitable, and death usually results from pneumonia and respiratory failure within 5 years of diagnosis.

Collaborative Care Management. ALS is diagnosed by a process of elimination because no definitive diagnostic test exists. Muscle biopsies may be performed to determine the source of muscle weakness, and an EMG will show muscle denervation, fibrillation, and fasciculation, which are closely associated with ALS. Blood studies typically show elevations in creatine phosphokinase.

ALS has no cure, and treatment is primarily directed toward symptom relief. Riluzole (Rilutek) is the only drug currently approved for use in ALS treatment. Its action is unknown, but it is believed to have a neuroprotective effect and to extend the lives of ALS patients by several months. Specific interventions are directed at managing complications as they arise. Nursing care focuses on supporting the patient's self-care abilities and the family's coping resources. General interventions are targeted at maintaining good health, supporting nutrition, promoting adequate sleep, appropriately balancing activity and rest, and introducing the use of self-help devices as they become appropriate. Physical therapy targets both the muscle weakness and spasticity, and occupational therapy assesses the need for adapted equipment and assistive devices.[20]

As ALS progresses, it is increasingly important to help the patient maintain a patent airway. Aspiration is a common concern and makes it increasingly difficult to meet the patient's nutritional needs with oral feedings. A gastrostomy may be created to support nutrition.

PATIENT/FAMILY TEACHING. Both the patient and the family need specific teaching concerning airway protection. The patient is taught to use a tucked-chin position while eating or drinking to encourage more effective swallowing and to always sit in an upright position for meals. If the patient's cough is weak, it may be necessary to keep suction equipment at the bedside during meals to assist in clearing the mouth. The patient is taught how to manage oral suctioning independently if possible.

Disease education is an important ongoing nursing responsibility. The patient remains alert throughout the course of the disease, and most patients experience significant fear and anxiety over both the reality of today and the uncertainty of the future. Health care providers assist patients and families in making decisions about the types of interventions that will be used as the disease progresses. One of the most difficult decisions involves the use of a ventilator as respiratory muscles weaken. Death commonly results from aspiration, infection, or respiratory failure, and decision making in this area is essential. The issues need to be addressed before a respiratory crisis occurs, and the participants need to receive nonjudgmental support for whatever decision they make. Patients also need to know that they can change their minds as the reality of their situation becomes apparent. Long-term ventilatory support may be accepted and incorporated into daily care or completely rejected. The nurse clearly communicates the inevitability of complete dependency. Referral to local or regional support groups for ALS patients and families may be helpful. Respite care for families who are caring for ALS patients at home needs to be addressed and legitimized, since the burden of caregiving can be overwhelming. Involvement with hospice services can be of tremendous aid to both patients and families. The nurse plays an important role in helping patients and families to deal with loss and grief (see Chapter 8).

Guillain-Barré Syndrome

Etiology and Epidemiology. Guillain-Barré syndrome (GBS) is an acute inflammatory polyneuropathy characterized by varying degrees of motor weakness or paralysis. It primarily affects the motor component of the cranial and spinal nerves and is known by a variety of other names, including acute inflammatory demyelinating polyradiculopathy, postinfectious polyneuritis, and idiopathic polyneuritis. It is a rare disorder with an incidence of 1 to 2 per 100,000 population. GBS affects all races and age-groups, with a male-female ratio of 2:1. Incidence increases with age, peaking at 70 to 80 years. The actual frequency may be understated.[23]

The etiology of the disorder is unknown; however, it is recognized as an autoimmune disorder that commonly (in 60% to 70% of cases) occurs a few days after a viral or bacterial infection, usually respiratory or gastrointestinal. The most commonly associated organism (in 26% to 40% of patients) is *Campylobacter jejuni*, found in eggs and poultry. Other organisms that may be involved include herpesvirus, Epstein-Barr virus, and cytomegalovirus. Additionally, the triggering event may be surgery, transplantation, immunization, or an immune disorder such as human immunodeficiency virus infection or Hodgkin's disease. Studies of the large outbreak following the 1976 swine flu immunization may link the eggs used for the serum to *C. jejuni*.[17] The syndrome usually develops over days to weeks, is rapidly progressive, and can advance to full paralysis. Ninety percent of patients are weakest by the third week. The mortality rate is approximately 2% to 12%. Full recovery occurs in 67% to 80% of cases; between 5% and 10% experience significant disability.

Pathophysiology. In GBS an immune-mediated response triggers destruction of the myelin sheath surrounding the peripheral nerves, nerve roots, root ganglia, and spinal cord. Collections of lymphocytes and macrophages are believed to be responsible for the myelin stripping. Demyelination occurs between the nodes of Ranvier, which impairs or blocks the transmission of impulses from node to node. The nerve axons are generally spared, and recovery may eventually take place, although the process of remyelination occurs slowly. In severe forms of the disease, wallerian degeneration occurs that involves the axons, making recovery slower and more difficult. In a small percentage of patients the disease does not resolve and becomes chronic or recurrent.

The four major forms of GBS reflect different degrees of peripheral nerve involvement:

1. Ascending GBS is the most common form. Weakness and numbness begin in the legs and progress upward. Fifty percent of patients experience respiratory insufficiency. Sensory involvement is also usually present.
2. Pure motor GBS is similar to the ascending form, but without sensory involvement. It is usually a milder form of the disease.
3. Descending GBS begins with weakness in the muscles controlled by the cranial nerves and then progresses downward. The respiratory system is quickly impaired. Sensory involvement is present.
4. Miller Fisher syndrome, a variant of GBS, is rare and primarily involves the eyes, loss of reflexes, and severe ataxia.

The patient with GBS has symmetric muscle weakness and flaccid motor paralysis. The paralysis usually starts in the lower extremities and ascends upward to include the thorax, upper extremities, and face. Cranial nerves may also be affected, particularly the fifth cranial (facial) nerve. When the seventh, ninth, and tenth cranial nerves are involved, the patient may have difficulty swallowing, speaking, and breathing.

Pain and paresthesias are present when sensory nerves are involved. Tingling or a pins-and-needles sensation is common. Either numbness or a heightened sensitivity to touch may occur, and about 25% of patients experience pain. The pain is usually a cramping in the extremities but can become severe enough to require analgesics.

Autonomic dysfunction is now recognized as a common problem with GBS and may include dysrhythmias, blood pressure instability, tachycardia or bradycardia, flushing, sweating, urinary retention, and paralytic ileus. GBS does not affect the patient's level of consciousness, alertness, or cognitive functioning. The patient is alert and aware throughout the course of the disease and is acutely vulnerable to sensory deprivation problems from the decrease in environmental stimuli.

GBS generally progresses through three stages. The initial period lasts from 1 to 3 weeks and ends when no further physical deterioration occurs. A plateau period follows, which lasts from a few days to a few weeks. The recovery period can last from 6 months to well over 1 year. The remyelination of damaged nerves occurs during the recovery phase. Permanent deficits may remain, although complete recovery is the norm.

Collaborative Care Management. The diagnosis of GBS is made from the clinical presentation supported by a history of recent viral or bacterial infection, elevations in the levels of protein in the CSF, and the results of EMG studies. Collaborative management of GBS is largely supportive and aimed at preventing complications until the recovery process can begin. Respiratory support is always the priority intervention. Corticosteroid therapy may be used to attempt to reduce the autoimmune inflammation, but steroids have not been conclusively proven to be of benefit in GBS. Positive outcomes have been achieved with the use of plasmapheresis during the first 1 to 2 weeks after disease onset. With plasmapheresis, plasma is removed and filtered of antibodies, immunoglobulins, fibrinogens, and other proteins. The filtered plasma is then mixed with an isotonic solution or fresh frozen plasma and returned to the patient. IVIG is also used to treat GBS. IVIG is as expensive as plasmapheresis, but it is easier to administer and is more readily available.

Respiratory failure from neuromuscular weakness is common in GBS, and 10% to 30% of patients require ventilatory support.[8] The nurse performs frequent monitoring of vital capacity, tidal volume, or minute volume, and intubation with mechanical ventilation is generally initiated when the patient's vital capacity falls below a preset level, usually about 1.0 to 1.5 L for an average-size adult. The need for long-term ventilatory support may necessitate a tracheostomy. Atelectasis and pneumonia are common complications. Intensive care placement may be necessary for weeks, and meticulous supportive care is needed. Rigorous assessment of motor, sensory, and cranial nerve status is ongoing.

Patients can lose weight rapidly with GBS, and nutritional support is a priority concern, especially for patients who will need to be weaned from mechanical ventilation. Complete immobility can cause a rapid loss of muscle mass. Tube feedings may be used, but if the patient also experiences autonomic dysfunction and paralytic ileus, parenteral nutrition may need to be implemented.

Supportive care also addresses the range of concerns related to partial or total immobility and loss of self-care abilities. Interventions include standard measures for preventing skin breakdown and maintaining range of motion in all joints. The risk of deep venous thrombosis and pulmonary embolus is high, and low-dose anticoagulant therapy may be initiated. A regular bowel program is established, and either indwelling or intermittent catheterization is implemented to address bladder dysfunction. A thorough rehabilitation plan is established as soon as the patient begins to recover.

It is critical to remember that the patient remains alert, aware, and cognitively intact throughout the course of GBS. Sleep disturbances are common and can contribute to sensory deprivation or overload symptoms in patients who are cared for in an intensive care unit for protracted times. The patient needs meaningful stimulation and communication and should be included in care decisions as much as possible even if eyebrow raising or eye blinks are the full extent of the patient's ability to communicate. Family members are also encouraged to participate in care activities to their level of comfort.

PATIENT/FAMILY TEACHING. GBS is an alarming and unsettling disease process for the patient and family. It is often difficult to convince the patient and family that recovery is not just possible but expected. Teaching about the disease and its management is an important nursing responsibility. Reteaching of basic principles is commonly necessary. The nursing staff also needs to encourage the patient and family to remain optimistic about the future. Each stage of GBS, particularly the need for intubation, increases the anxiety level of an alert patient. It is difficult for patients to communicate their needs for position changes, pain relief, and restful sleep. The slow pace of recovery may be discouraging. Once patients are moved from the intensive care unit setting, they lose the constant support and care of the critical care nurses and may become extremely anxious about the ability of nurses on less acute units to adequately meet their needs. The patient's care manager needs to carefully coordinate all needed services to ensure that transitions are as smooth and anxiety free as possible. Referral for community-based care and rehabilitation may also be needed.

▶ ARE You READY?

The nursing diagnosis *impaired physical mobility related to destruction of acetylcholine receptors* is most appropriate for the patient with which of the following?

1. Myasthenia gravis
2. Guillain-Barré syndrome
3. Multiple sclerosis
4. Amyotrophic lateral sclerosis

Critical Thinking

1. You are caring for a patient who was admitted 2 days ago with a left hemisphere ischemic stroke. You were told during report that the patient has "some aphasia." What kinds of assessment activities would you plan to thoroughly evaluate the nature and extent of the communication problems?
2. A patient has experienced a right hemisphere stroke, and you suspect that sensory-perceptual deficits may be present. How would you assess the presence and severity of problems such as hemianopia, unilateral neglect, or agnosia? What effects might the right-sided stroke have on your plan for compensating for these deficits?
3. The nursing diagnosis of Risk for Altered Nutrition: Less Than Daily Requirements might apply to patients with PD and MG. How would your nursing interventions related to nutrition be the same for patients with these two disorders? How would your interventions differ?
4. A patient is admitted for an acute exacerbation of MG. You gave a dose of pyridostigmine at 11:30 AM, before lunch. It is now 1 PM, and the patient is reporting dramatically increased weakness, cramping, gastrointestinal upset, and difficulty swallowing saliva. Is this likely to be a myasthenic or a cholinergic crisis? Support your answer. How could the two forms of crisis be differentiated?

References

1. American Heart Association: *Heart disease and stroke statistics—2005 update,* Dallas, 2005, The Association.
2. American stroke month highlights major cause of death and disability: medical technology innovation helps lower stroke mortality, *Med Technol Innovation* vol 5, issue 11, 2004.
3. Aminoff M: Nervous system. In Tierney L, McPhee S, Papadakis M, editors: *Current medical diagnosis and treatment,* New York, 2005, Lange Medical Books/McGraw-Hill.
4. Barker E: *Neuroscience nursing: a spectrum of care,* ed 2, St Louis, 2002, Mosby.
5. Benveniste M, Dingledine R: Limiting stroke-induced damage by targeting an acid channel, *N Engl J Med* 325(1):85-86, 2005.
6. Boss B: Alterations of neurologic function. In McCance K, Huether S, editors: *Pathophysiology: the biologic basis for disease in adults and children,* ed 4, St Louis, 2002, Mosby.
7. Calne S, Kumar A: Nursing care of patients with late-stage Parkinson's disease, *J Neurosci Nurs* 35(5):242-251, 2003.
8. Cheng BC et al: Predictive factors and long-term outcome of respiratory failure after Guillain-Barré syndrome, *Am J Med Sci* 327(6):336-340, 2004.
9. Courtney SW: *All about multiple sclerosis,* ed 2, Cherry Hill, NJ, 2003, Multiple Sclerosis Association of America.
10. Duncan PW et al: Adherence to postacute rehabilitation guidelines is associated with functional recovery in stroke, *Stroke* 33(1):167-177, 2002.
11. Erikson S et al: Bilateral subthalamic nucleus stimulation for the treatment of Parkinson's disease: results of six patients, *J Neurosci Nurs* 35(4):223-231, 2003.
12. Fahn S et al: Levodopa and the progression of Parkinson's disease, *N Engl J Med* 351(24):2498-2508, 2004.
13. Flannery J: *Rehabilitation nursing secrets,* St Louis, 2005, Mosby.
14. Friedrich MJ: Parkinson disease studies yield insights, *JAMA* 293(4): 409-410, 2005.
15. Geleijns K et al: The occurrence of Guillain-Barré syndrome within families, *Neurology* 63:1747-1750, 2004.
16. Gispert S et al: Failure to find a-Synuclein gene dosage changes in 190 patients with familial Parkinson disease, *Arch Neurol* 62:96-98, 2005.
17. Haber P et al: Guillain-Barré syndrome following influenza vaccination, *JAMA* 292(20):2478-2481, 2004.
18. Hampton T: Parkinson disease registry launched, *JAMA* 293(2):149, 2005.
19. Hanley D, Hacke W: Critical care and emergency medicine neurology in stroke, *Stroke* 36:205-207, 2004.
20. Hickey J: *The clinical practice of neurological and neurosurgical nursing,* ed 5, Philadelphia, 2003, Lippincott/Williams & Wilkins.
21. Hoeman SP: Movement, functional mobility, and activities of daily living. In Hoeman S, editor: *Rehabilitation nursing: process, application, and outcomes,* ed 3, St Louis, 2002, Mosby.
22. Keegan B, Noseworthy J: Multiple sclerosis. In Johnson R, Griffin J, McArthur J, editors: *Current therapy in neurologic disease,* ed 6, St Louis, 2002, Mosby.
23. Khan F: Rehabilitation in Guillain Barré syndrome, *Austral Fam Phys* 33(12):1013-1017, 2004.
24. Kieseier BC, Hartung HP: Therapeutic strategies in the Guillain-Barré syndrome, *Semin Neurol* 23:159-166, 2003.

25. Konishi T et al, Japanese FK506 MG Study Group: Long-term treatment of generalized myasthenia gravis with FK506 (tacrolimus), *J Neurol Neurosurg Psychiatry* 76:448-450, 2005.
26. Lauriola L et al: Thymus changes in anti-MuSK-positive and -negative myasthenia gravis, *Neurology* 64:536-538, 2005.
27. Leonardi-Bee J et al: Dipyridamole for preventing recurrent ischemic stroke and other vascular events: a meta-analysis of individual patient data from randomized controlled trials, *Stroke* 36(1):162-168, 2005.
28. Liu M et al: Fibrinogen-depleting agents for acute ischemic stroke, *Stroke* 36:173-174, 2004.
29. Marchak BE: Carotid endarterectomy. In Mohr JP et al: *Stroke pathophysiology, diagnosis, and management,* ed 4, Philadelphia, Churchill Livingstone.
30. Mok E, Woo C: The effects of slow-stroke back massages on anxiety and shoulder pain in elderly stroke patients, *Compl Therap Midwifery* 10: 209-216, 2004.
31. Mohr JP: Classification of ischemic stroke. In Mohr JP et al: *Stroke pathophysiology, diagnosis, and management,* ed 4, Philadelphia, Churchill Livingstone.
32. Nagano-Saito A et al: Cerebral atrophy and its relation to cognitive impairment in Parkinson disease, *Neurology* 64:224-229, 2005.
33. Ovbiagele B, Kidwell S, Saver J: Expanding indications for statins in cerebral ischemia: a quantitative study, *Arch Neurol* 62:67-72, 2005.
34. Racette BA et al: Prevalence of parkinsonism and relationship to exposure in a large sample of Alabama welders, *Neurology* 64:230-235, 2005.
35. Risak R: Myasthenia gravis. In Johnson R, Griffin J, McArthur J, editors: *Current therapy in neurologic disease,* ed 6, St Louis, 2002, Mosby.
36. Roubin GS et al: Carotid stenting. In Mohr JP et al: *Stroke pathophysiology, diagnosis, and management,* ed 4, Philadelphia, Churchill Livingstone.
37. Saver J: Acute ischemic stroke. In Johnson R, Griffin J, McArthur J, editors: *Current therapy in neurologic disease,* ed 6, St Louis, 2002, Mosby.
38. Schmidt W et al: Determinants of IV heparin treatment in patients with ischemic stroke, *Neurology* 63:2407-2409, 2004.
39. Schwartzschild MA, Chen J, Ascherio A: Parkinson's disease: caffeinated clues and the promise of adenosine A(2A) antagonists in PD, *Neurology* 58(8):1154-1160, 2002.
40. Scott WK et al: Family-based case-control study of cigarette smoking and Parkinson disease, *Neurology* 64:442-447, 2005.
41. Thanvi BR, Lo TCN: Update on myasthenia gravis, *Postgrad Med* 80: 690-700, 2004.
42. US Department of Health and Human Services: *Healthy people 2010: national health promotion and disease prevention objectives,* Washington, DC, 2000, The Department.
43. Vincent A et al: Seronegative myasthenia gravis, *Semin Neurol* 24:125-133, 2004.
44. Wilson B, Shannon N, Stang C: *Nurses drug guide,* Upper Saddle River, NJ, 2005, Prentice Hall.
45. Wolfe GI, Gross B: Treatment review and update for myasthenia gravis, *J Clin Neuromusc Dis* 6:54-68, 2004.
46. Zaja-Milatovic S et al: Dendritic degeneration in neostriatal medium spiny neurons in Parkinson disease, *Neurology* 64:545-547, 2005.

Visit the Evolve website: http://evolve.elsevier.com/Monahan/medsurg

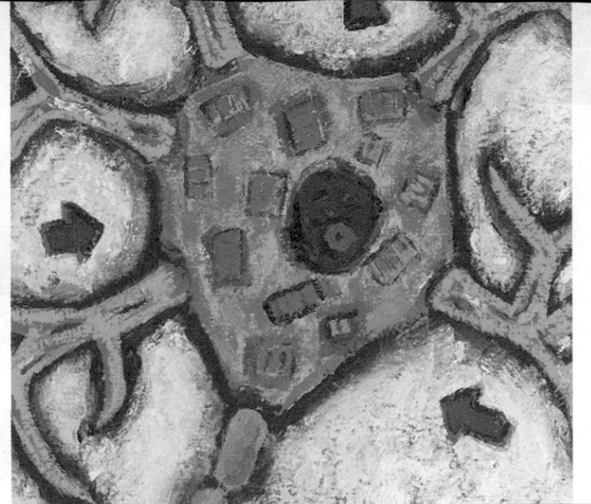

CHAPTER 50

Spinal Cord and Peripheral Nerve Problems

by Dea Mahanes, Judith K. Sands

OBJECTIVES

After studying this chapter, the learner should be able to:

1. Discuss the demographics of spinal cord injury (SCI) and the major targets for prevention.
2. Describe how the process of secondary injury extends the damage resulting from SCI.
3. Link the clinical manifestations of spinal shock, neurogenic shock, and autonomic hyperreflexia with the specific physiologic consequences of SCI.
4. Discuss the options for medical and surgical management of SCI.
5. Describe the impact of SCI on bowel, bladder, and sexual functioning.
6. Describe the nursing management of the patient with SCI with a focus on prevention of secondary complications and patient and family education.
7. Outline a standard protocol for preventing and treating autonomic hyperreflexia.
8. Contrast the care provided to patients with SCI with that required by patients with spinal tumors.
9. Compare the clinical manifestations and treatment of the patient with trigeminal neuralgia versus Bell's palsy.

KEY TERMS

autonomic hyperreflexia, p. 1469
flaccid, p. 1466
lower motor neuron, p. 1466
neurogenic bladder, p. 1463
neurogenic shock, p. 1463
neuropathic pain, p. 1469
paraplegia, p. 1463
paresthesias, p. 1476
secondary injury, p. 1462
spasticity, p. 1469
spinal shock, p. 1462
tetraplegia, p. 1463
upper motor neuron, p. 1466
wallerian degeneration, p. 1487

This chapter presents an overview of the collaborative management of problems involving the spinal cord and peripheral nerves, particularly the multidisciplinary challenges of spinal cord injury (SCI). SCI is not a common problem, but its complexity and impact on the patient's life make it an enormous management concern in all phases of care. The pathophysiology of spinal cord and peripheral nerve injuries is complex, and the reader is referred to Chapter 47 for a review of neurologic anatomy and physiology.

Spinal Cord Injury

Etiology and Epidemiology. The spinal column consists of stacked vertebrae separated by intervertebral discs. The individual vertebrae are held in place by ligaments and muscles with multiple articulations that allow for a wide range of head and neck movements. The spinal cord runs through the center of the spinal column in a canal formed by the ring-shaped vertebrae. When the canal is penetrated by bone, disc material, or a foreign object, the spinal cord and its blood supply are at risk for injury. The close anatomic proximity of the spinal cord to the vertebrae, muscles, and ligaments increases the chance that injury to any of these supporting structures will also injure the cord itself. The cervical spine is most at risk for injury because the vertebrae in this region are more mobile and smaller, and the supporting structures are not as strong as in other areas of the spinal column.[27] Most SCIs are the result of sudden and often violent external trauma, but persons who have chronic conditions that affect the vertebrae, such as stenosis, arthritis, or osteoporosis, are also at increased risk of SCIs.

SCI is commonly associated with events that cause abrupt, forceful acceleration and deceleration, such as vehicular accidents. Specific mechanisms of injury include the following:

- *Hyperflexion* injuries (Figure 50-1) are frequently the result of sudden deceleration as might occur in a head-on collision. The head and neck are forcibly hyperflexed and then may be snapped backward into forced hyperextension.

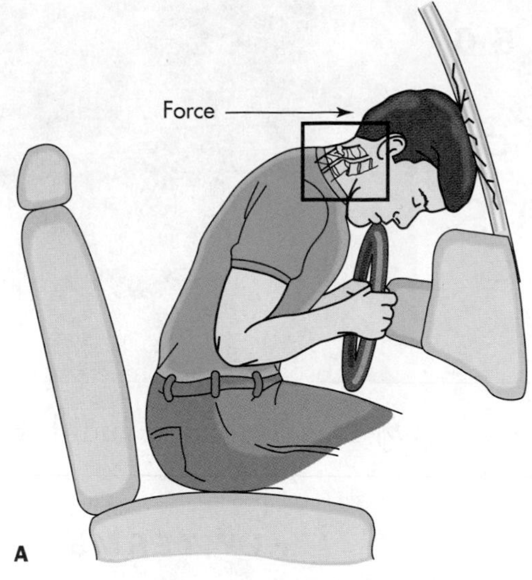

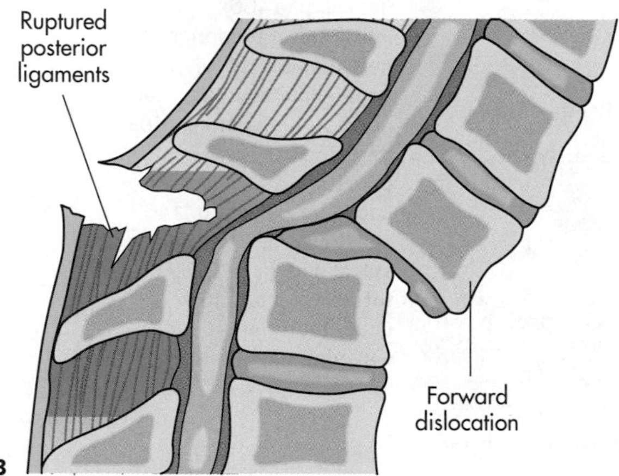

Figure 50-1 Hyperflexion injury. **A,** If hyperflexion occurs in cervical spine, **B,** it can result in tearing or rupture of posterior ligaments with resulting fracture or dislocation in anterior spine.

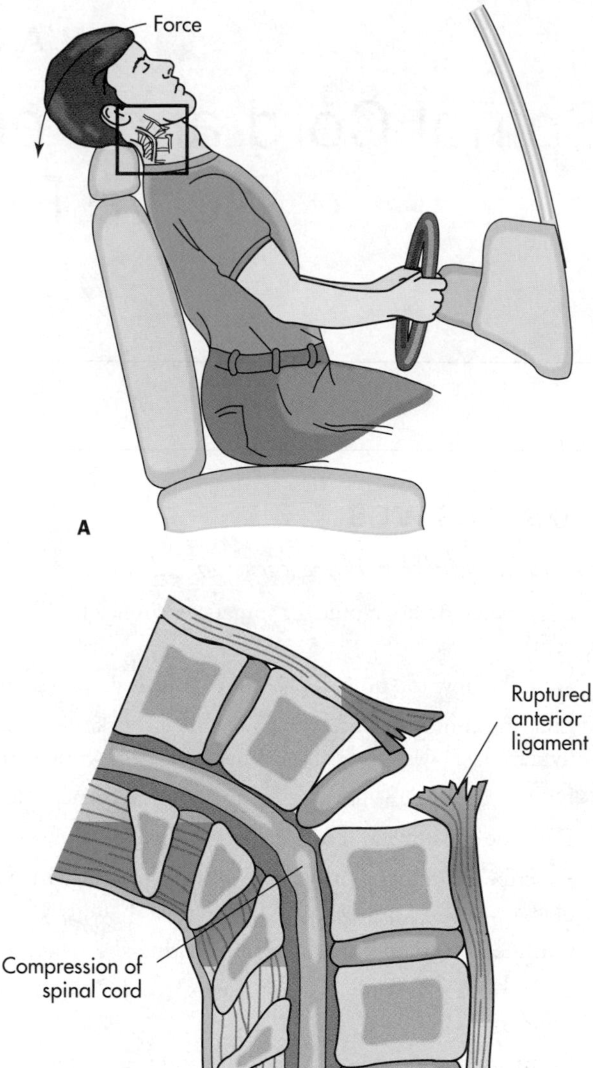

Figure 50-2 Hyperextension injury. **A,** If hyperextension occurs in cervical spine, **B,** it can result in rupture or tearing of anterior ligaments with dislocation or compression in posterior spine.

These injuries are typically seen in the C5-C6 area of the cervical spine. Hyperflexion may result in fracture or dislocation of the vertebra and/or tearing of the posterior ligaments.

- *Hyperextension* injuries (Figure 50-2) are frequently acceleration injuries such as those associated with rear-end collisions or falls in which the chin is forcibly struck. These injuries tend to cause significant damage because of the pronounced downward and backward arc of the head. The middle to lower portions of the cervical spine are most commonly affected.
- *Compression* injuries result from extreme vertical force, which causes the vertebra to shatter or burst (Figure 50-3). The cervical and thoracolumbar regions of the spine are most frequently affected. Blows to the top of the head and forceful landing on the feet or buttocks can result in compression injury.
- *Rotational* injuries are caused by extreme lateral flexion or twisting of the head and neck (Figure 50-4). Dislocation, fracture, and/or tearing of ligaments can result in a highly unstable spine. Soft tissue damage often complicates the primary injury. Many SCIs involve more than one type of directional force (e.g., both hyperextension and rotation).
- *Penetrating* injuries occur as the result of direct contact with the spinal cord by an object such as a knife or bullet. Gunshot wounds typically cause more injury than knife wounds because of the higher velocity of impact to the cord.

SCI was long considered to be an untreatable injury, and the associated mortality rate was as high as 85% until the 1940s. The multitude of injuries produced by World War II stimulated a tremendous upsurge in research into SCI management. Life expectancy has increased in recent years but remains somewhat less than that of individuals without SCI and varies widely depending on age at injury and functional level. Mortality rates are highest during the first year after injury. Currently, approximately 11,000 new spinal cord injuries occur each year in the United States, roughly 40 per 1 million people, and about 222,000 to 285,000 individuals are currently living with SCI. More than 50% of injuries occur in the cervical spinal cord, and about 80% of all SCIs occur in males.[22] SCI is reflected in the

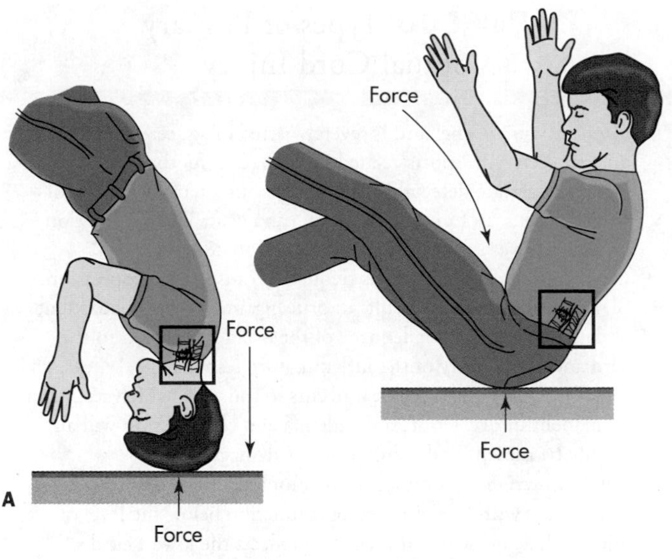

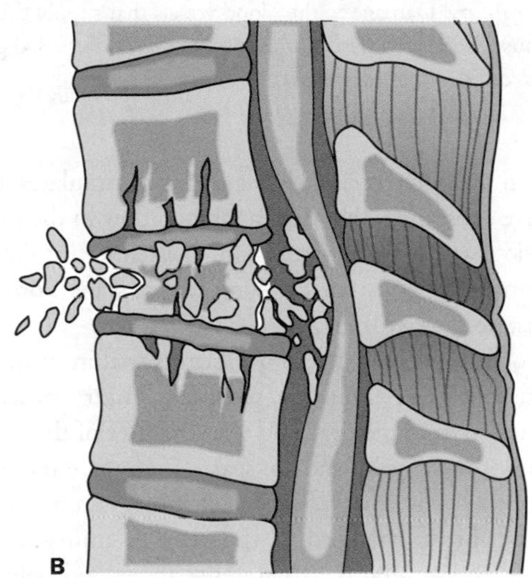

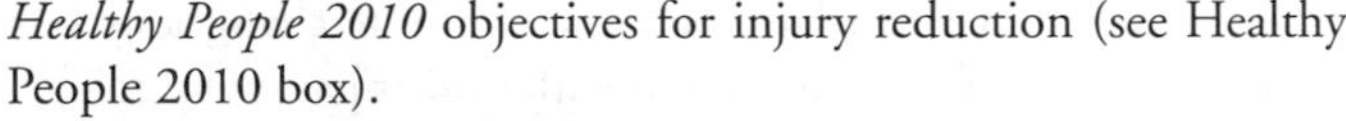

Figure 50-3 Compression injury. **A,** Excessive direct force to either cervical or lumbar spine can **B,** result in shattering of vertebra.

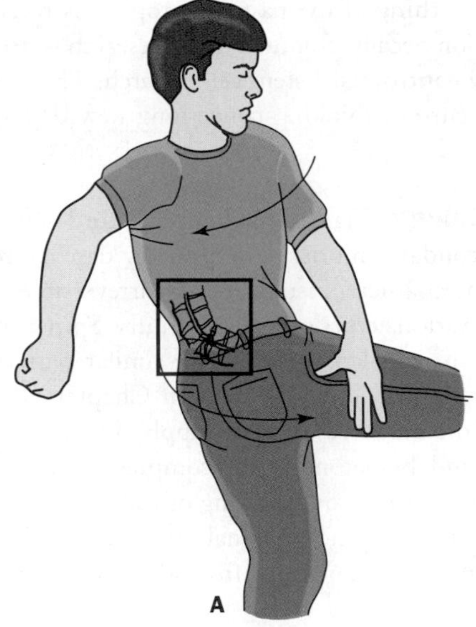

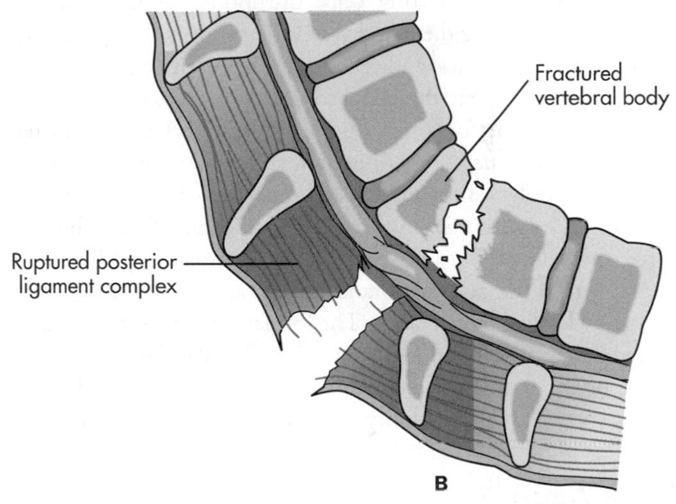

Figure 50-4 Rotational injury. **A,** When rotational force occurs, it is frequently accompanied by **B,** fracture and/or tearing of ligaments.

Healthy People 2010 objectives for injury reduction (see Healthy People 2010 box).

Although SCI continues to primarily affect young adults, the average age at injury has risen from 28.6 years to 38.0 years since the 1970s. The percentage of individuals older than 60 years at the time of injury has increased significantly and presents unique management challenges. The most common cause of SCI is motor vehicle crashes (50.4%) followed by falls (23.8%), acts of violence (11.2%), and sports-related injuries (9%).[22] Alcohol or drug use is a factor in a large number of accidents resulting in SCI, and failure to use safety equipment such as seatbelts significantly increases risk.[8] Falls are a common cause of SCI in older adults. Risk factors for SCI are summarized in the Risk Factors box.

Recent advances in our understanding of the spinal cord's ability to repair itself have raised the hope that irreversible SCI may

Healthy People 2010

Objective Related to Injury Reduction

- Reduce hospitalizations for nonfatal spinal cord injuries from the baseline of 4.5 per 100,000 population to a target of 2.4 per 100,000 population.

From US Department of Health and Human Services: *Healthy people 2010: understanding and improving health,* Washington, DC, 2000, The Department.

Risk Factors

Spinal Cord Injury

- *Age:* More than 50% of spinal cord injuries (SCIs) occur in persons 16 to 30 years of age. Older persons experience the most fall-related injuries.
- *Sex:* Males are affected four times more often than females.
- *Race:* Some reports indicate a higher incidence of SCI among African-Americans.
- *Alcohol use:* Alcohol is a factor in many motor vehicle accidents that result in SCI, as well as in many other accidents, diving incidents, and episodes of violent trauma.

eventually be a thing of the past. The topic has received a great deal of attention because so much of the research is deeply imbedded in highly controversial stem cell research. The Future Watch box presents current thinking concerning new directions in the treatment of SCI.

Pathophysiology. Trauma to the spinal cord causes both primary and secondary injuries. The primary damage results from the initial mechanical insult and is irreversible. Box 50-1 describes the various types of primary injury. Spinal cord concussion, contusion, and laceration follow similar patterns to those described for traumatic brain injury in Chapter 48. Tearing or laceration of the blood vessels that supply the cord may result in hemorrhage and hematomas that compress surrounding nerve cells. Complete transection, severing of the spinal cord, is a relatively rare initial outcome of spinal trauma, but physiologically complete transection can result from the process of **secondary injury**.

The primary injury creates an ischemic environment by destroying neurons and supporting cells, disrupting nerve tracts, and stretching or shearing the blood vessels that supply the spinal cord. A cascade of biochemical and cellular changes then occurs, resulting in secondary damage to the spinal cord. Research into the process of secondary injury is ongoing, but identified mechanisms include electrolyte shifts, the release of excitatory amino acids, and inflammation. Electrolyte shifts and the accumulation of excitatory neurotransmitters cause a buildup of calcium inside the cell. This buildup affects the cell's ability to use energy and perform vital functions. Breakdown of the cell membrane and intracellular swelling occur, eventually leading to cell death. The formation of free radicals causes lipid peroxidation and results in further cellular destruction. The release of inflammatory mediators in response to injury leads to increased capillary permeability and edema, which create additional compression and ischemia. Cellular hypoxia stimulates the release of vasoactive substances that decrease blood flow in the microcirculation and may induce vasospasm. Systemic insults such as hypotension and hypoxia further compromise spinal cord perfusion and increase secondary injury.[28]

The process of secondary injury begins within minutes of the original insult. With time, the secondary injury process causes structural changes in the gray and white matter of the spinal cord, destruction of the myelin sheath, scarring of nerve tissue, and the formation of a cystic cavity. Secondary injury can destroy the full thickness of the spinal cord at the level of injury and further extend its effects several cord segments above and below. Extensive research focuses on identifying all the factors that are operational during secondary injury and determining which of these cellular processes can be slowed or interrupted.

The terms *spinal shock* and *neurogenic shock* refer to physiologic sequelae of SCI. These terms are often used interchangeably but in fact describe different conditions with similar pathophysiology. Virtually all SCI patients experience spinal shock, whereas neurogenic shock occurs in patients with injuries to the cervical or high thoracic spine.

Spinal shock refers to the temporary suppression of reflexes below the level of injury. Normal function of the spinal cord (including spinal reflex activity) depends on a constant, low-level, axonal stimulation from the higher centers in the brain, which keeps the cord neurons in a state of excitability or readiness. SCI interrupts this stimulation, causing a drastic reduction in the resting excitability of the cord. Over time the spinal neurons gradually regain their excitability, which ends the period of spinal shock. An SCI has long-term effects on body functions such as sensation and voluntary movement that require transmission of nerve impulses from the area above to the area below the injury. Functions controlled by spinal reflex arcs, however, do not depend on communication with the brain, and the impact of injury on these functions is limited to the period of spinal shock. The gradual

Future Watch

Spinal Cord Repair: Are We Getting Closer?

Spinal cord injury (SCI) was once considered irreparable, but new advances bring hope that function can be restored. High-profile sports and entertainment figures have directed the nation's attention to the problem of SCI, and basic research has expanded exponentially. Major areas of research include limiting the damage caused by secondary injury (neuroprotection), promoting regeneration of surviving neurons, and encouraging surviving nerve cells to perform new functions (synaptic plasticity). Specific examples include the use of mild hypothermia, administration of growth factors, transplantation of nerve tissue, and functional neuromuscular stimulation. Most experts believe that a cure for SCI will involve a combination of strategies aimed at neuroprotection, regeneration, and plasticity. Although these techniques are promising, they are still in the experimental phase and require additional research before they are a realistic option for most individuals with SCI.

Nurses who care for individuals with SCI will be asked about experimental therapies by patients and families. Although many legitimate therapies exist, it may be difficult to differentiate these therapies from so-called fringe treatments that do not undergo scientific scrutiny. One reliable source of information is a website sponsored by the National Institutes of Health, www.clinicaltrials.gov.

Box 50-1 Types of Primary Spinal Cord Injury

- *Cord concussion:* The cord is severely jarred or squeezed, as is frequently seen with sports-related injuries (e.g., football). No pathologic changes are detectable in the cord, but a temporary loss of motor or sensory function, or both, can occur. The dysfunction usually resolves spontaneously within 24 to 48 hours.
- *Cord contusion:* This injury is frequently caused by compression. Bleeding into the cord results in bruising and edema. The extent of damage reflects the adequacy of the overall perfusion to the cord and the severity of the inflammatory response.
- *Cord laceration:* An actual tear occurs in the cord, which results in permanent injury. Contusion, edema, and compression will all usually be present and complicate the damage.
- *Cord transection:* A complete or incomplete severing of the spinal cord occurs with loss of neurologic function below the level of injury. The cord segment identified reflects the lowest cord segment in which neurologic function is preserved.
- *Vascular injury:* Damage to the blood vessels that supply the spinal cord causes decreased perfusion and ischemia. If decreased perfusion persists, cell death results in permanent injury.

reappearance of reflex activity signals the resolution of the spinal shock period. The reported duration of spinal shock varies among sources from hours to weeks, perhaps in part because of confusion regarding terminology.

Neurogenic shock refers to the hemodynamic instability caused by the loss of innervation from the brain to the sympathetic nervous system. Injury above the thoracic outflow of the sympathetic nervous system (T6-T7) disconnects the sympathetic nervous system from control by higher centers in the brainstem and results in a loss of autoregulatory control of blood pressure. Vasoconstrictive messages from the medulla cannot be transmitted, and sympathetic tone is lost. This lack of a functional sympathetic nervous system causes widespread venous pooling in the lower extremities and splanchnic circulation, which results in hypotension. The unopposed parasympathetic stimulation of the vagus nerve causes bradycardia, which worsens hypotension. The presence of bradycardia helps to distinguish neurogenic shock from hypovolemic shock, which is also commonly associated with trauma. Peripheral vasodilation causes the skin to feel warm and dry and also permits significant heat loss to occur. The peak effects of neurogenic shock are most evident in the days immediately after injury, and then gradually taper off and stabilize over 10 days to 2 weeks.

The functional manifestations of SCI depend on the extent of cord damage (complete or incomplete), the level of cord injury, and the type of nerve tracts involved (upper or lower motor neurons). SCI is termed *complete* when there is a total loss of sensory and voluntary motor function below the level of the injury. An *incomplete* lesion is one in which some motor or sensory function is preserved below the level of the injury because some spinal cord tracts remain intact. The potential for at least some recovery of motor and sensory ability is higher with incomplete injury.[10] The extent of SCI is classified into one of five grades using the American Spinal Injury Association (ASIA) Impairment Scale (Figure 50-5). Accurate determination of complete versus incomplete injury cannot be made before spinal shock is resolved.

Several unique syndromes can occur after incomplete SCI. They represent specific types of localized damage, although it is unusual to see any of these syndromes in their pure form. Incomplete SCI syndromes include:

- *Central cord syndrome.* This syndrome is caused by damage that primarily affects the central part of the spinal cord (Figure 50-6), often as a result of hemorrhage or edema. This fairly common syndrome usually occurs in older adults who experience a hyperextension injury in the cervical region. Motor weakness occurs that is more severe in the arms than in the legs. The amount of sensory impairment is highly variable, but is also more apparent in the arms. Bowel and bladder function may or may not be affected. Recovery varies, but many patients improve over time.
- *Anterior cord syndrome.* This syndrome typically results from injury or infarction involving the anterior spinal artery, which perfuses the anterior two thirds of the spinal cord (Figure 50-7). It can also result from tumors and acute disc herniation. Loss of strength and loss of pain and temperature sensation occur below the level of the injury. Position, vibration, and light touch sensation remain intact.
- *Posterior (dorsal) cord syndrome.* This is an extremely rare syndrome in which damage to the posterior columns of the spinal cord cause loss of position and vibration sense. Movement, pain, and temperature sensation remain intact.
- *Brown-Séquard syndrome.* This syndrome typically results from a penetrating injury that involves half the spinal cord (Figure 50-8). There is a resulting loss of motor ability, touch, pressure, and vibration sensation on the same side as the injury with a contralateral loss of pain and temperature sensation.
- *Conus medullaris syndrome.* This syndrome is caused by injury to the cone-shaped termination of the spinal cord at the L1-L2 level (Figure 50-9) as a result of fractures or disc herniation. Common sequelae include urinary retention, loss of anal sphincter tone, constipation, and impotence. Motor weakness is usually minimal, and sensory loss is characterized by "saddle anesthesia," or loss of sensation to the perineum and areas of the thighs and buttocks.
- *Cauda equina syndrome.* Damage to the lumbar and/or sacral nerve roots that comprise the cauda equina (see Figure 50-9) results in cauda equina syndrome. Asymmetric weakness, numbness, and pain along the nerve roots are common presenting symptoms. **Neurogenic bladder** and bowel dysfunction may also occur.

The level of SCI, described by the terms *tetraplegia* (previously called quadriplegia) or *paraplegia,* also has important implications for functional potential. **Tetraplegia** refers to a lesion in the cervical spinal cord with loss of function in the arms, legs, trunk, bowel, and bladder. **Paraplegia** indicates a lesion in the thoracic, lumbar, or sacral segments of the spinal cord, resulting in loss of function affecting the legs, bowel, and bladder. The functional losses and residual abilities that characterize injuries at specific spinal segments are summarized in Figure 50-10. The sparing of even one spinal segment can have significant impact on the patient's self-care potential, particularly when injuries affect the cervical spine.

Respiratory function after SCI varies with the level of injury and is particularly affected by cervical injury. All ventilatory muscles receive their innervation from the spinal cord. The diaphragm (C3-C5), the accessory muscles (C2-C8), the intercostal muscles (T1-T7), and the abdominal muscles (T6-T12) may all be affected by SCI and in turn affect respiratory function. The diaphragm is controlled by the phrenic nerve, which is innervated by the C3-C5 nerve roots. Complete injury above the level of C3 results in immediate cessation of breathing. Individuals with injuries at C3-C4 typically have markedly decreased inspiratory volumes. Individuals with SCI between the levels of C5 and T1 can initiate breaths normally but may experience hypoventilation because of loss of intercostal and accessory muscle strength. Vital capacity and inspiratory force are greatly decreased. The intercostal muscles below the level of injury are flaccid and collapse inward with inspiration, decreasing the capacity of the thorax and contributing to hypoventilation and atelectasis. The sitting position allows the abdomen to protrude and thus accentuates these paradoxical respirations. Many patients initially breathe more effectively in the supine position, although abdominal binders can be used to improve respiratory function when the patient is upright. Over a period of weeks to months, spasticity develops in the muscles of

ASIA IMPAIRMENT SCALE

- ☐ **A** = **Complete:** No motor or sensory function is perserved in the sacral segments S4-S5.
- ☐ **B** = **Incomplete:** Sensory but not motor function is preserved below the neurological level and includes the sacral segments S4-S5.
- ☐ **C** = **Incomplete:** Motor function is preserved below the neurological level, and more than half of key muscles below the neurological level have a muscle grade less than 3.
- ☐ **D** = **Incomplete:** Motor function is preserved below the neurological level, and at least half of key muscles below the neurological level have a muscle grade of 3 or more.
- ☐ **E** = **Normal:** Motor and sensory function are normal.

CLINICAL SYNDROMES

- ☐ Central cord
- ☐ Brown-Séquard
- ☐ Anterior-cord
- ☐ Conus medullaris
- ☐ Cauda equina

Figure 50-5 ASIA scale for assessment of spinal cord injury.

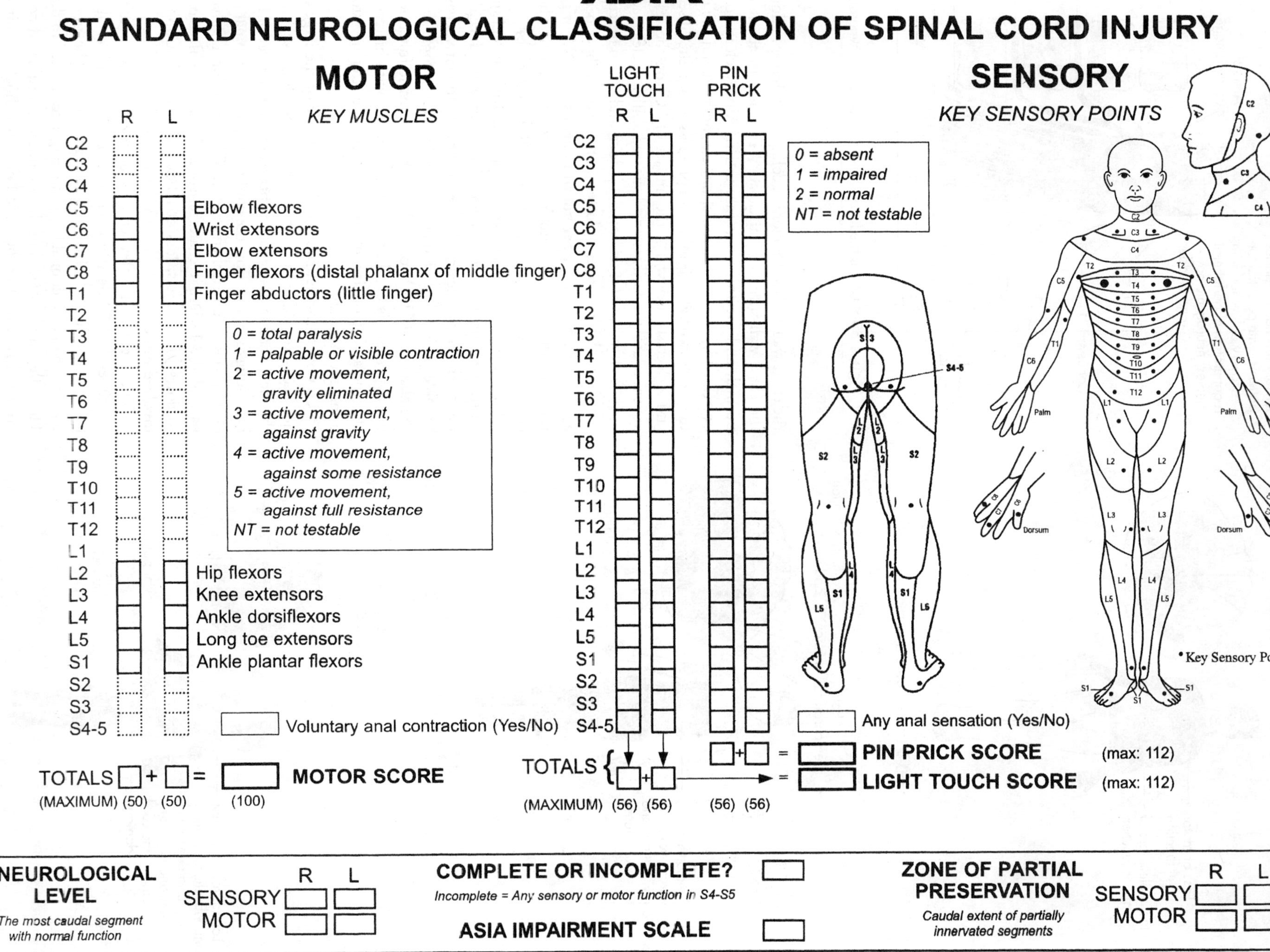

ASIA

STANDARD NEUROLOGICAL CLASSIFICATION OF SPINAL CORD INJURY

MOTOR

KEY MUSCLES

	R	L	
C2			
C3			
C4			
C5			Elbow flexors
C6			Wrist extensors
C7			Elbow extensors
C8			Finger flexors (distal phalanx of middle finger)
T1			Finger abductors (little finger)
T2			
T3			
T4			
T5			
T6			
T7			
T8			
T9			
T10			
T11			
T12			
L1			
L2			Hip flexors
L3			Knee extensors
L4			Ankle dorsiflexors
L5			Long toe extensors
S1			Ankle plantar flexors
S2			
S3			
S4-5			

0 = total paralysis
1 = palpable or visible contraction
2 = active movement, gravity eliminated
3 = active movement, against gravity
4 = active movement, against some resistance
5 = active movement, against full resistance
NT = not testable

Voluntary anal contraction (Yes/No)

TOTALS ☐ + ☐ = ☐ MOTOR SCORE
(MAXIMUM) (50) (50) (100)

	LIGHT TOUCH R	LIGHT TOUCH L	PIN PRICK R	PIN PRICK L
C2				
C3				
C4				
C5				
C6				
C7				
C8				
T1				
T2				
T3				
T4				
T5				
T6				
T7				
T8				
T9				
T10				
T11				
T12				
L1				
L2				
L3				
L4				
L5				
S1				
S2				
S3				
S4-5				
TOTALS				
(MAXIMUM)	(56)	(56)	(56)	(56)

SENSORY

KEY SENSORY POINTS

0 = absent
1 = impaired
2 = normal
NT = not testable

Any anal sensation (Yes/No)

☐ + ☐ = ☐ PIN PRICK SCORE (max: 112)

☐ + ☐ = ☐ LIGHT TOUCH SCORE (max: 112)

NEUROLOGICAL LEVEL
The most caudal segment with normal function

	R	L
SENSORY		
MOTOR		

COMPLETE OR INCOMPLETE? ☐
Incomplete = Any sensory or motor function in S4-S5

ASIA IMPAIRMENT SCALE ☐

ZONE OF PARTIAL PRESERVATION
Caudal extent of partially innervated segments

	R	L
SENSORY		
MOTOR		

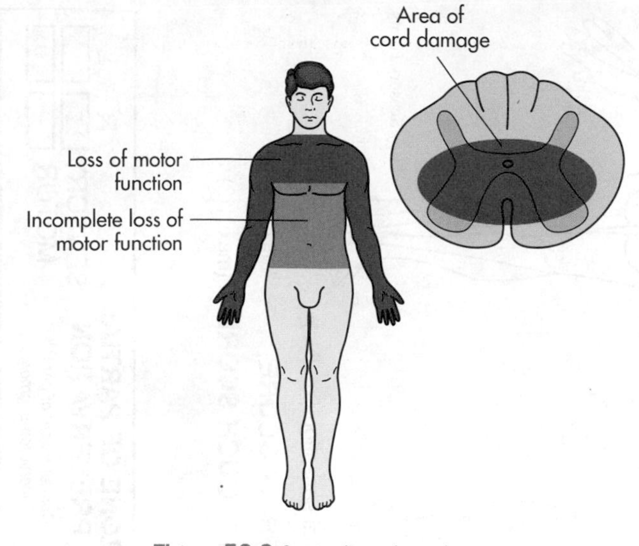

Figure 50-6 Central cord syndrome.

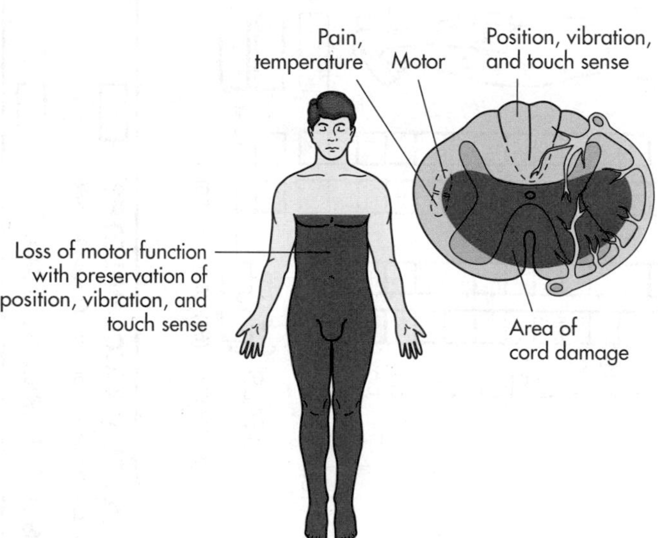

Figure 50-7 Anterior cord syndrome.

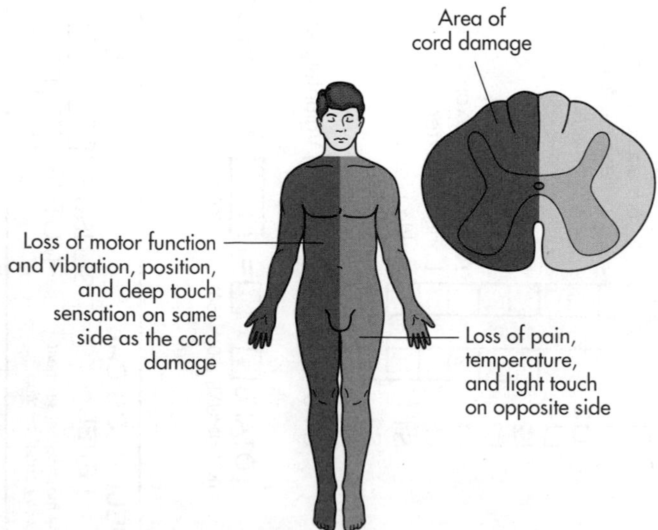

Figure 50-8 Brown-Séquard syndrome.

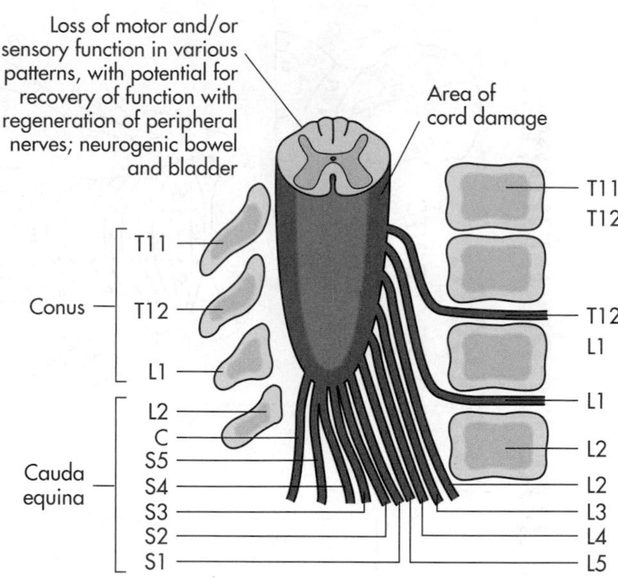

Figure 50-9 Conus medullaris and cauda equina syndrome.

the chest wall so that it no longer collapses with inspiration. Once the chest wall stiffens, vital capacity increases to about 60% of normal, and breathing becomes easier.[5] Airway clearance is also decreased by loss of abdominal muscle function and the inability to take deep breaths, leading to a progressive buildup of secretions and atelectasis. Below T1, the impact of SCI on the respiratory system relates primarily to the decreased ability to clear secretions.

The effects of SCI on bowel, bladder, and sexual function vary based on whether upper or lower motor neurons have been damaged (Figure 50-11). **Upper motor neurons** (UMNs) originate in the brain and synapse with lower motor neurons in the spinal cord. Any lesion that destroys UMNs or interferes with their influence over LMNs is called an upper motor neuron injury. Initially, the muscles affected by a UMN injury are **flaccid** (hypotonic) and hyporeflexic. This period of hypotonicity persists for a variable period, but gradually the reflex arcs become reactive in the absence of UMN control. Voluntary muscle function is lost, but hyperreflexia of all cord segments occurs with increased muscle tone and spasticity in response to muscle stretch, autonomic, or noxious stimuli.

Lower motor neurons (LMNs) consist of the large anterior horn cells located in the anterior gray matter of the spinal cord or the motor cranial nuclei of the brainstem. Each anterior horn cell has a long axon that exits the cord via the anterior spinal root and extends out to a peripheral nerve. When a lesion involves some part of the LMN, it characteristically results in flaccid muscle weakness or paralysis, loss of reflex activity, and atrophy of the involved muscles.

The micturition reflex center is located in the conus medullaris at the level of S2-S4 (vertebral level T12-L2). Injury above this level affects the UMN control of micturition. The micturition center remains functional but is no longer connected to the brain. The reflex arc is intact but the voluntary coordinated control of urination is lost. After the period of spinal shock, as spinal reflex activity resumes, a spastic automatic bladder develops. The person is unable to sense bladder fullness or an urge to void. Spontaneous

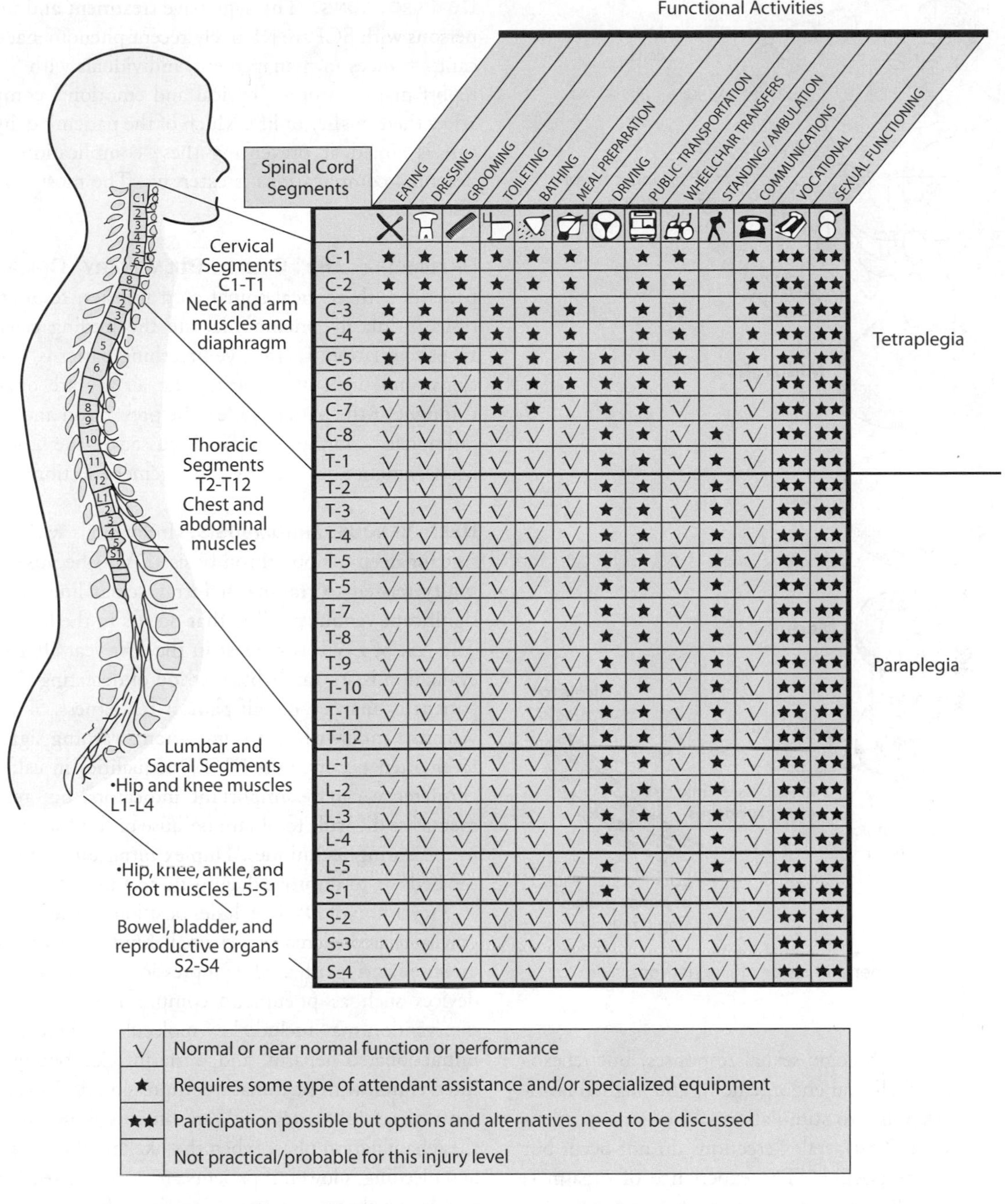

	EATING	DRESSING	GROOMING	TOILETING	BATHING	MEAL PREPARATION	DRIVING	PUBLIC TRANSPORTATION	WHEELCHAIR TRANSFERS	STANDING/ AMBULATION	COMMUNICATIONS	VOCATIONAL	SEXUAL FUNCTIONING
C-1	★	★	★	★	★	★		★	★		★	★★	★★
C-2	★	★	★	★	★	★		★	★		★	★★	★★
C-3	★	★	★	★	★	★		★	★		★	★★	★★
C-4	★	★	★	★	★	★		★	★		★	★★	★★
C-5	★	★	★	★	★	★	★	★	★		★	★★	★★
C-6	★	★	√	★	★	★	★	★	★		√	★★	★★
C-7	√	√	√	★	★	√	★	★	√		√	★★	★★
C-8	√	√	√	√	√	√	★	★	√	★	√	★★	★★
T-1	√	√	√	√	√	√	★	★	√	★	√	★★	★★
T-2	√	√	√	√	√	√	★	★	√	★	√	★★	★★
T-3	√	√	√	√	√	√	★	★	√	★	√	★★	★★
T-4	√	√	√	√	√	√	★	★	√	★	√	★★	★★
T-5	√	√	√	√	√	√	★	★	√	★	√	★★	★★
T-5	√	√	√	√	√	√	★	★	√	★	√	★★	★★
T-7	√	√	√	√	√	√	★	★	√	★	√	★★	★★
T-8	√	√	√	√	√	√	★	★	√	★	√	★★	★★
T-9	√	√	√	√	√	√	★	★	√	★	√	★★	★★
T-10	√	√	√	√	√	√	★	★	√	★	√	★★	★★
T-11	√	√	√	√	√	√	★	★	√	★	√	★★	★★
T-12	√	√	√	√	√	√	★	★	√	★	√	★★	★★
L-1	√	√	√	√	√	√	★	★	√	★	√	★★	★★
L-2	√	√	√	√	√	√	★	★	√	★	√	★★	★★
L-3	√	√	√	√	√	√	★	★	√	★	√	★★	★★
L-4	√	√	√	√	√	√	★	√	√	★	√	★★	★★
L-5	√	√	√	√	√	√	★	√	√	★	√	★★	★★
S-1	√	√	√	√	√	√	★	√	√	√	√	★★	★★
S-2	√	√	√	√	√	√	√	√	√	√	√	★★	★★
S-3	√	√	√	√	√	√	√	√	√	√	√	★★	★★
S-4	√	√	√	√	√	√	√	√	√	√	√	★★	★★

√	Normal or near normal function or performance
★	Requires some type of attendant assistance and/or specialized equipment
★★	Participation possible but options and alternatives need to be discussed
	Not practical/probable for this injury level

Figure 50-10 Spinal cord injury functional activity chart.

voiding occurs, often at low volumes, but the bladder may not empty completely. In contrast, an LMN injury directly affects the micturition center. The reflex arc is no longer intact, resulting in an autonomous, flaccid bladder. Urinary retention with overflow incontinence is common.

The spinal defecation reflex center is also located at S2-S4. Injuries affecting the UMNs cause a loss of voluntary control over the anal sphincter. In addition, the person cannot feel rectal fullness or the urge to defecate because ascending impulses to the brain are blocked. The anal sphincter is flaccid during spinal shock but then regains tone. Evacuation of the bowel may occur in response to stimulation of the reflex arc. Injuries below the level of the spinal defecation reflex center create flaccid bowel dysfunction as a result of LMN damage. The bowel and sphincter are flaccid. Both constipation and incontinence can occur. Compared with patients with UMN injury, patients with LMN bowel dysfunction report increased frequency of bowel movements, more incontinence, increased need for oral medications, and more time each week spent on bowel care.[33]

The sexual reflex center is also located at the level of S2-S4. The reflex center controls erection in males and labial-clitoral engorgement and vaginal lubrication in females. Injury above the level of

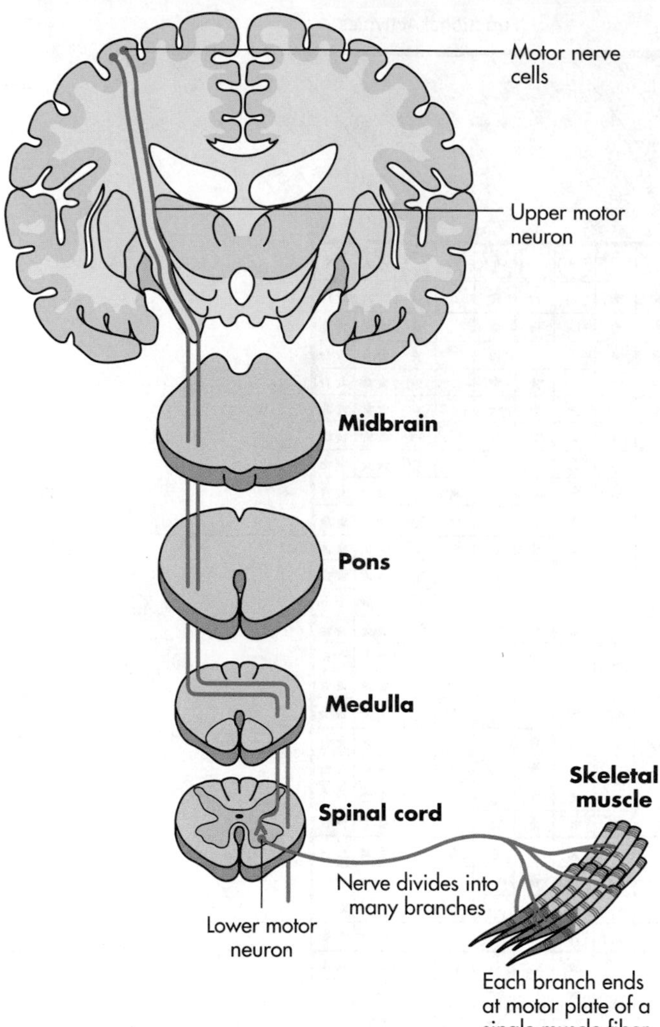

Figure 50-11 Upper and lower motor neurons.

the reflex arc prevents psychologic sexual responses, but reflexogenic erection, labial and clitoral engorgement, and vaginal lubrication may occur in response to stimulation. When injury affects the sacral spinal nerves (S2-S4), reflex erections do not occur but psychogenic erections are possible. The experience of orgasm is altered after SCI, but both men and women with SCI can experience fulfilling sexual activity with creativity and a willing partner. Fertility is also a concern for individuals with SCI. Ejaculation is rare, but options for semen retrieval exist. Fertility is decreased in males because of poor sperm quality, but remains intact in females once the menstrual cycle is reestablished. Box 50-2 provides an overview of the impact of SCI on sexual function.

ARE YOU READY?

Respiratory arrest in a patient with a complete injury above C3 is primarily related to the loss of:

1. Intercostal muscle innervation
2. Abdominal muscle innervation
3. Diaphragmatic innervation
4. Accessory muscle innervation

COMPLICATIONS. The aggressive treatment and rehabilitation of persons with SCI are relatively recent phenomena; despite significant advances in management, individuals with SCI continue to report major chronic physical and emotional complications that affect their quality of life. Much of the patient's daily self-care routine is aimed at preventing these complications. The range of potential complications is extensive. The most common are presented here.

PNEUMONIA AND OTHER PULMONARY COMPLICATIONS. In patients with cervical spinal cord injuries, respiratory complications, primarily pneumonia, are the leading causes of death.[22] Hypoventilation, ineffective breathing patterns, pooling of secretions, and difficulty clearing the airway are ongoing concerns throughout the patient's life. The prevention and management of pulmonary complications is discussed in the Collaborative Care Management and Nursing Management sections.

DEEP VENOUS THROMBOSIS. Individuals with SCI are at high risk for deep venous thrombosis (DVT) because of the vascular injury related to trauma or intravascular line insertions and the significant venous pooling that occurs in the lower extremities.[1,2] The risk of DVT is highest in the first year after injury. Clinical evaluation is an unreliable method of detecting DVT because the patient is unaware of calf pain or tenderness. Skin discoloration, warmth, and swelling are important warning signs. A low-grade fever often occurs with DVT. Inequalities in calf and thigh circumference can be important indicators, but reliable measurements are difficult to obtain because of fluid shifts and differences in measuring techniques. Duplex ultrasound can also be used at the bedside to improve diagnostic accuracy.

Prevention of DVT includes positioning the extremities to avoid gravity-related edema or pressure behind the knee, range-of-motion exercise, and graduated compression stockings and mechanical devices such as pneumatic compression sleeves. Pharmacologic intervention may include low-molecular-weight heparin, low-dose unfractionated heparin, and warfarin. Combining pharmacologic intervention with pneumatic compression devices appears to be the most successful strategy.[26] Warfarin is typically reserved for use in the rehabilitation phase when the likelihood of invasive procedures and bleeding is lower. If patients are unable to receive anticoagulant prophylaxis because of other injuries, a filter may be placed in the inferior vena cava to prevent clots from traveling to the lungs and causing a pulmonary embolism. DVT prophylaxis is continued for about 3 months after injury unless the patient has other risk factors.

PAIN. An estimated 60% to 80% of individuals with SCI develop pain.[7,30] Chronic pain syndromes can develop after SCI and become extremely difficult management issues. Chronic pain negatively affects participation in exercise, work, household chores, and other daily activities, and also causes sleep disruption.[32]

Pain after SCI can be classified as musculoskeletal, visceral, or neuropathic.[7,12,23] Musculoskeletal pain is described as dull or aching and commonly increases with movement.[7] It is common in the initial stages of SCI, but may also occur later due to added stress on nerves, muscles, or joints. Nonsteroidal antiinflammatory drugs, muscle relaxants, or opioids may bring relief.[12,23] Muscle relaxants are often effective if spasticity is contributing to pain.

Box 50-2 Sexual Function After Spinal Cord Injury

Men

Most men with spinal cord injuries (SCIs) are not able to experience psychogenic erections (those which occur in response to sexual thoughts), but they are usually capable of reflexogenic erections. Reflexogenic erections occur from direct stimulation of the genitalia, but may also result from stroking the inner thigh, rectal stimulation, or manipulation of a urinary catheter.

The ability to ejaculate is usually not present or may occur in a retrograde fashion; but orgasm, with a perceived release of tension, is possible.

Both urinary catheterization and bowel emptying should be completed before intercourse to prevent the possibility of reflex emptying.

Men with indwelling catheters can either remove the catheter just before sexual activity or fold it back on the penis and use the catheter to provide extra support for the erection.

A variety of resources are available for men whose reflex erections are not sufficient for sexual activity. These include oral medications, implants, injections, and vacuum pumps (see Chapter 57).

Most men with SCI experience infertility or low sperm counts, but this needs to be verified by laboratory analysis before sterility can be assumed. Sperm harvesting, artificial insemination, and in vitro fertilization offer couples the hope of successful pregnancy.

Women

Both urinary catheterization and bowel emptying should be completed before intercourse to prevent the possibility of reflex emptying.

Women who have indwelling catheters can leave them in place if desired.

Women with SCIs typically retain their ability to conceive. The menstrual cycle is interrupted by the injury, but usually resumes after about 4 to 6 months, reestablishing fertility. Birth control counseling is essential.

Pregnancy can proceed safely after SCI, and infants can be successfully delivered vaginally, although there is an increased incidence of urinary tract infections and autonomic hyperreflexia during both pregnancy and labor.

Visceral pain is described as dull or cramping and is caused by complications affecting the abdominal or pelvic organs, including renal calculi or urinary tract infection. Treatment of visceral pain focuses on eliminating the cause.

Neuropathic pain is often considered the most difficult type of pain to treat. It can occur above, below, or at the level of injury and is typically described as burning, sharp, or shooting.[1] The area where pain occurs may also be described as hypersensitive.[29] Neuropathic pain appears to be more responsive to antidepressants and anticonvulsants than traditional analgesics. Other management strategies include the use of nerve blocks and local anesthetics (transdermal lidocaine).[19,25] If pain control remains elusive, surgical options are explored.

SCI pain is a complex problem, and patients often benefit from the involvement of an interdisciplinary pain management team. The patient needs reassurance that caregivers accept the reality of the pain and will work collaboratively to find acceptable management strategies. Nonpharmacologic therapies, such as physical activity or exercise and massage, are also useful for some patients.[31]

SPASTICITY. Spinal reflex activity begins to reappear with the resolution of spinal shock, and muscle spasticity can become a serious concern for patients. The appearance of spinal reflex activity is not an indication of returning function because the muscle movement is not under voluntary control, but it can give false hope to patients. As **spasticity** develops, heightened muscle responsiveness adds resting tone to the flaccid muscles and may make it easier to move the patient and prevent muscle wasting. However, spasticity also creates safety concerns and heightens the risk for contractures. Contractures limit a patient's rehabilitation and self-care potential and must be prevented. Both sustained (tonic) and intermittent (clonic) spasticity can occur. Most patients experience a peak of spasticity within the first year after injury, and it stabilizes within about 2 years. Spasticity may increase in frequency and severity when other complications, such as urinary tract infection, are present.

Positioning and exercise are the two primary interventions for managing spasticity. The frequency of passive range-of-motion exercise is increased to at least four times a day, since general muscle stiffness tends to worsen the spasticity. The nurse limits the amount of incidental tactile stimulation that occurs while providing care and handles the patient's limbs in a gentle yet firm manner. The patient's position is changed at least every 2 hours, and the joints are carefully positioned to support function. Splints may be needed to support optimal positioning in vulnerable joints such as the fingers. Physical and occupational therapists establish an appropriate exercise plan for the patient and design effective splinting devices. Spasticity that does not respond to these general measures may require the use of muscle relaxant medications such as baclofen (Lioresal), diazepam (Valium), tizanidine (Zanaflex), or dantrolene (Dantrium).[7] Long-term implantable delivery systems may be used if symptoms persist.[10] In severe cases surgical intervention with rhizotomy (section of the spinal nerve roots) or a similar procedure may be necessary.

AUTONOMIC HYPERREFLEXIA. Autonomic hyperreflexia (previously autonomic dysreflexia) is an exaggerated sympathetic response that occurs in patients with cord injuries at T6 or above, after spinal shock has resolved. It is unique to SCI. The spinal nerves that innervate the sympathetic nervous system emerge from the thoracic and lumbar regions of the spine, with the thoracic chain having primary control over vasoconstriction. When injuries affect the upper cord at or above the level of T6, the sympathetic nervous system below the level of injury can still respond but is shut off from the inhibitory control of higher centers in the brain. Therefore a stimulus from below the level of injury produces afferent impulses that ascend the cord but are blocked when they reach the area of injury. The stimulus then acts on the thoracic chain and triggers a massive sympathetic discharge, causing profound vasoconstriction and paroxysmal hypertension. The abrupt rise in blood pressure distends the baroreceptors in the carotid sinus and aortic arch. These baroreceptors stimulate the vagus nerve to slow

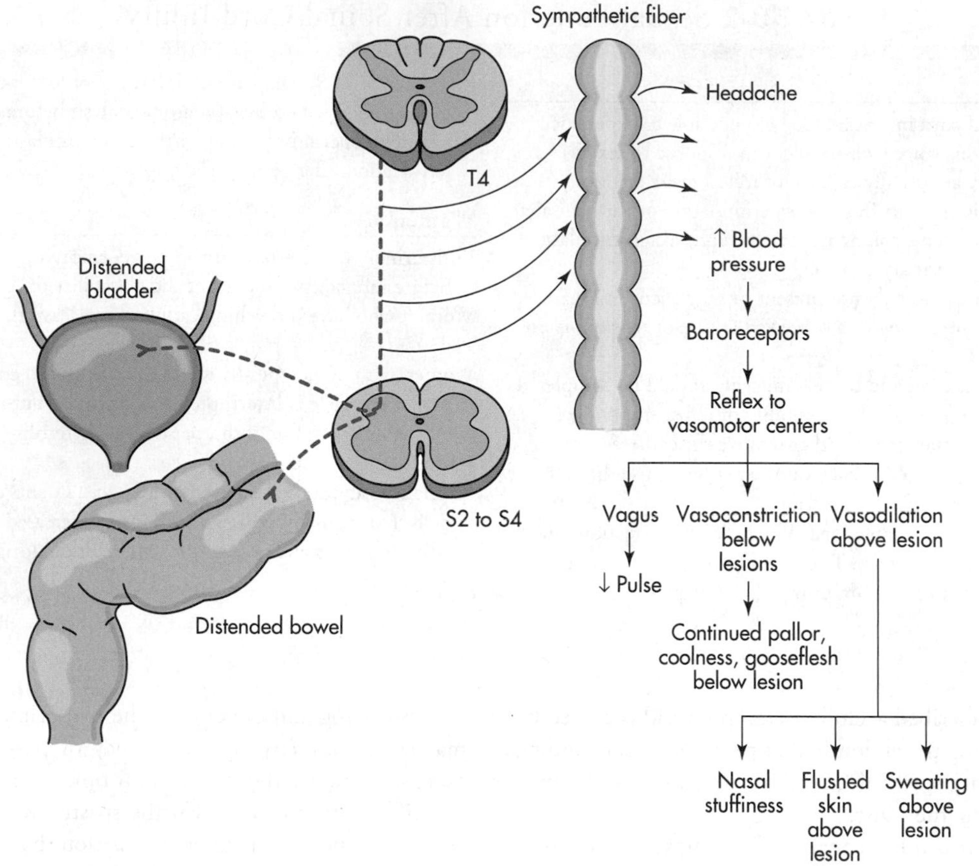

Figure 50-12 Causes of autonomic hyperreflexia and results.

the heart and induce vasodilation in the vessels above the level of the cord injury in an attempt to reduce blood pressure. The intense sympathetic response continues below the level of the injury, however, because the inhibitory impulses from the higher centers of the brain cannot reach the thoracic chain. The majority of the blood vessels remain constricted, and hypertension persists (Figure 50-12). Patients become vulnerable to autonomic hyperreflexia only after the period of spinal shock has resolved. An overdistended bladder is the most common cause, although any stimulus below the level of injury can trigger autonomic hyperreflexia (Box 50-3).

The clinical manifestations of autonomic hyperreflexia are summarized in the Clinical Manifestations box. The classic defining feature is paroxysmal hypertension, often accompanied by a pounding headache, nausea, and blurred vision. Vasodilation above the injury level results in skin flushing and profuse perspiration in those areas. The continuing vasoconstriction in areas below the injury level causes cool, pale skin and piloerection (goosebumps).

Autonomic hyperreflexia is a medical emergency that can result in stroke, blindness, or death. The major goal is to prevent episodes by maintaining effective regimens for bladder emptying and bowel evacuation to prevent overdistention. If the syndrome occurs, prompt treatment is essential (see Guidelines for Safe Practice box).

Altered Thermoregulation. The control of body temperature is significantly altered by SCI at or above the T6 level. Loss of sympathetic stimulation causes widespread vasodilation with an ongoing associated heat loss through the skin. Loss of UMN control by the thermoregulatory center of the brain means that the body can neither sweat nor shiver below the level of the injury to raise or lower body temperature. The nurse carefully monitors the patient's temperature and tries to minimize temperature variations in the care environment, since the body gradually assumes the ambient temperature. Extra blankets or environmental cooling are employed as needed to keep the patient's temperature around 98.6° F (37.0° C). The inability to regulate temperature persists beyond the initial acute care period, and the nurse instructs the

Box 50-3 Precipitating Factors for Autonomic Hyperreflexia

- Bladder distention (80% of all cases)
- Bowel distention
- Local pressure or irritation (especially to the penis, groin, or sacrum); pressure ulcers
- Constrictive clothing
- Catheterization of bladder; digital stimulation of rectum or anus
- Abdominal or pelvic stimulation or irritation
  - —Menstruation
  - —Urinary tract infection
  - —Urinary calculi
  - —Sexual activity, ejaculation
  - —Gastritis, peptic ulcers, or gallstones
  - —Labor contractions
  - —Colonoscopy or cystoscopy

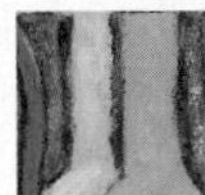

CLINICAL MANIFESTATIONS
Autonomic Hyperreflexia

- Elevated blood pressure
- Pounding headache
- Visual changes
- Nasal congestion
- Bradycardia or other arrhythmia
- Profuse sweating, flushed skin, or chills above the level of injury
- Cool, pale or mottled skin, or piloerection (goosebumps) below the level of injury

NOTE: Patients experience different manifestations of autonomic hyperreflexia. Most patients become able to recognize their own unique pattern of symptoms.

patient and family about the risks of both chilling and overheating in extreme temperatures.

GASTROINTESTINAL PROBLEMS. Patients with SCI are at risk for a variety of gastrointestinal complications, especially during the acute hospitalization. These complications include adynamic ileus and gastrointestinal bleeding or ulcers. Ileus develops after SCI because of the loss of autonomic innervation to the gastrointestinal tract. Abdominal distention caused by ileus may impair respiratory status and increase the risk for vomiting and aspiration. An orogastric or nasogastric tube may be inserted to reduce abdominal distention. In most cases, adynamic ileus resolves within 3 to 7 days.

SCI is a significant risk factor for the development of gastric ulcers, and this risk is further increased by the use of high-dose steroids. Prophylaxis against gastric ulcers typically includes a histamine$_2$ receptor antagonist or proton pump inhibitor. The nurse closely monitors the patient for signs of gastric bleeding such as bloody or coffee ground emesis or aspirate from the gastric tube or occult blood in the stool.

ORTHOSTATIC HYPOTENSION. Loss of sympathetic tone after SCI causes blood to pool in the lower extremities and causes a drop in blood pressure that worsens when the patient is upright. The drop in blood pressure may be accompanied by dizziness, visual disturbances, or syncope. Management of orthostatic hypotension includes applying graduated compression stockings, wrapping the legs with elastic bandages, and applying an abdominal binder before sitting the patient up. The nurse monitors blood pressure and assesses the patient for dizziness while the head is slowly raised. If orthostatic hypotension persists and cannot be managed with these nonpharmacologic measures, sodium chloride tablets or the mineralocorticoid fludrocortisone (Florinef) is sometimes given to raise blood pressure by increasing intravascular volume. Sympathomimetic medications may also be prescribed.

URINARY COMPLICATIONS. Common genitourinary complications include urinary tract infection and renal calculi from the use of an indwelling catheter, overdistention of the bladder, large postvoid residuals, and bladder outlet obstructions.[9] Prevention focuses on adequately draining and emptying the bladder, avoiding the use of indwelling catheters when possible, and ensuring adequate hydration. Bladder management strategies are further discussed on pp. 1478 and 1479.

MUSCULOSKELETAL COMPLICATIONS. Musculoskeletal complications include the development of spasticity (described above), osteoporosis, and heterotopic ossification. Osteoporosis occurs due to loss of calcium from the bone matrix with an increased risk of pathologic fracture. Heterotopic ossification is the formation of bone within connective tissue, causing inflammation and decreased

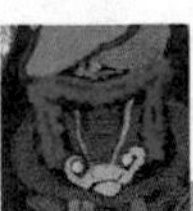

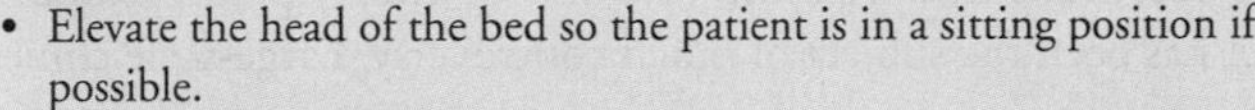

GUIDELINES FOR SAFE PRACTICE *The Patient With Autonomic Hyperreflexia*

- Elevate the head of the bed so the patient is in a sitting position if possible.
- Loosen clothing and any constrictive devices, including antiembolism compression stockings, elastic wraps, abdominal binders, and pneumatic compression devices. This action encourages venous blood to pool in the abdomen and legs to decrease blood pressure.
- Monitor the blood pressure and pulse every 2 to 5 minutes until the episode resolves and the effect of any antihypertensives given has subsided. Hypotension may occur after resolution of hyperreflexia.
- Investigate for bladder distention:
  —Check the patency of the indwelling catheter, if present. Ensure that it is not kinked or plugged. Remove and replace the indwelling catheter if not patent. Follow institutional protocols regarding the instillation of anesthetic gel before catheterization.
  —Catheterize immediately if an indwelling catheter is not in place. Follow institutional protocols regarding the instillation of anesthetic gel before catheterization.
- If hyperreflexia persists, check for bowel impaction:
  —Apply dibucaine (Nupercaine) or another anesthetic ointment to the rectum and anal area and monitor response. The use of anesthetic ointment is important to prevent triggering another visceral stimulus and worsening the hyperreflexia.
  —Remove stool gently after application of anesthetic ointment.
- If hyperreflexia continues, initiate drug therapy per unit protocol and promptly notify the physician. Medications are chosen on the basis of a rapid onset and short duration. Nifedipine, captopril, and hydralazine are among the medications used.
- Bladder and bowel problems are the most common causes of autonomic hyperreflexia. If no cause can be identified:
  —Assess the skin carefully for signs of irritation or breakdown (apply topical anesthetic to areas of skin irritation).
  —Change the patient's position.
  —Send a urine specimen for culture and sensitivity.
- Remain with the patient to provide support, reassurance, and explanations of care.

NOTE: Some experts recommend control of hypertension and physician notification before checking for bowel impaction. Follow institutional guidelines.

range of motion in the affected joint. Treatment with medications or surgery may be required.

SYRINGOMYELIA. A cystlike cavity, or syrinx, may form in the damaged spinal cord as areas of hemorrhage and cell death break down and liquefy. The cavity may ascend or descend over time, causing a decline in motor or sensory function. Syringomyelia is suspected in patients who experience delayed worsening of neurologic function after SCI. Surgical treatment consists of shunt placement to drain fluid from the syrinx into the subarachnoid, pleural, or peritoneal space.

ANXIETY AND DEPRESSION. Anxiety and depression are common after SCI, both immediately after injury and long term. The incidence of depression among individuals with SCI exceeds that of the general population. Psychologic complications are a common cause of rehospitalization after SCI. In one study, 28% of individuals with SCI were treated for depression during the first 6 years after injury.[11] Depression affects self-care abilities and thus increases the risk for complications such as skin breakdown. Depression may also affect pain perception.

Patients with high cervical cord injuries frequently question their motivation to continue living, and this can create great tension and distress for caregivers who are committed to supporting patient autonomy in decision making and self-determination. The Ethical Alert box discusses this important ethical dilemma for nurses and other health care professionals working with spinal cord–injured patients.

▶ ARE You READY?

Which of the following is seen in the patient with autonomic hyperreflexia?

1. Elevated heart rate
2. Elevated blood pressure
3. Piloerection above the level of injury
4. Profuse perspiration below the level of injury

Collaborative Care Management

DIAGNOSTIC TESTS. The diagnosis of SCI is fairly straightforward. A preliminary diagnosis is established from the patient's neurologic assessment. Standard x-ray examinations can demonstrate fracture or dislocation of the vertebral bodies or spinal processes. Additional diagnostic tests are used to evaluate the stability and alignment of the vertebral column and make initial decisions regarding the next steps of treatment.

Spine injuries can be classified as stable or unstable. A stable injury is one in which the vertebrae are in alignment and remain in alignment with position changes and activity. Unstable injuries are those in which the vertebrae move in relation to each other. The greatest concerns for spinal instability exist with injuries to the cervical spine, which is capable of extensive movement. Instability is also a concern with injuries from T11-L2. Individuals with unstable injury to the spinal column require a procedure to keep the spinal vertebrae in alignment as the bones heal. A computed tomography (CT) or magnetic resonance imaging (MRI) scan may be used to add detail and resolution to the diagnostic process. Box 50-4 summarizes common diagnostic tests used with patients with SCI.

Ethical Alert

Decision-Making Autonomy Among Patients With Spinal Cord Injury

Patients with spinal cord injury (SCI) retain the ability to make their own decisions regarding treatment, unless they are compromised by an injury or condition external to SCI (such as traumatic brain injury or medication effects). Decision making is complicated when the patient is receiving mechanical ventilation, since communication may be limited. The patient is unable to speak, and loss of upper extremity function limits the use of common alternative communication techniques (writing, the use of letter boards). Concerns about communication and capacity for independent decision making are compounded when the decision in question involves continuation of life support. Some patients, when faced with a lifetime of disability and ventilator dependence, may choose not to proceed with continued ventilation or tracheostomy placement. Even if this decision reflects the patient's longstanding values, it may create conflict among the health care team and cause significant moral distress. Resources such as ethics consult teams, psychiatrists, and palliative care teams may be useful in ensuring that the patient truly understands the implications of his or her decision and is psychologically able to make this choice. If the decision is made to proceed with withdrawal of mechanical ventilation, the palliative care team can be a valuable resource in ensuring that the patient is comfortable throughout the process.

MEDICATIONS. Drug therapy after SCI is targeted at supporting hemodynamic function and suppressing the physiologic processes that cause secondary injury. Methylprednisolone (Solu-Medrol) is commonly administered after SCI, provided it can be started within 8 hours of injury. Protocols suggest a 30 mg/kg body weight bolus, followed by a 5.4 mg/kg/hr infusion for a total of 24 hours if initiated within 3 hours of injury. A 48-hour infusion is used if treatment is initiated between 3 and 8 hours after injury. If treatment is not begun within 8 hours, methylprednisolone is not recommended. Recently the use of methylprednisolone in SCI has been the subject of much controversy. Large-scale clinical

Box 50-4 Diagnostic Tests for Spinal Cord Injury

- *Standard radiographs (x-rays):* Standard x-ray films can reveal fracture or dislocation of the vertebral bodies or spinal processes. Several x-ray films are taken to provide more than one view of the vertebrae.
- *Computed tomography (CT):* CT scans can reveal the exact anatomy of any bony injury and sometimes cord compression. CT is used to further evaluate areas of the spine that may be injured but cannot be adequately visualized on standard x-ray examinations.
- *Magnetic resonance imaging (MRI):* MRI shows bone poorly but provides excellent visualization of the spinal cord and nerve roots. It is useful in the diagnosis of ligamentous injury, which can be present without obvious abnormalities visible on standard x-ray or CT. It can also identify hemorrhage, contusion, or compression of the cord.

trials have reported significant improvements in neurologic recovery with the use of methylprednisolone, but these studies have been criticized as methodologically flawed. Guidelines published by the American Association of Neurological Surgeons and the Congress of Neurological Surgeons in March 2002 recommend the use of methylprednisolone as an option with the recognition that the risk of significant side effects may outweigh potential benefits.[3] The recommended dose of methylprednisolone is very large, and careful attention must be paid to side effects. The most common side effects are gastrointestinal bleeding, hyperglycemia, and infection.

Ongoing management may involve the administration of drugs to prevent gastric ulceration, promote bowel function, prevent urinary tract infection, and control spasticity. Common medications used in SCI management are summarized in Table 50-1.

TREATMENTS. Treatment of SCI begins at the scene of the accident with prehospital care providers. SCI is initially suspected on the basis of the mechanism of injury and presenting clinical symptoms. The focus is on spine stabilization to prevent further damage, cardiac and respiratory support, and rapid transport to a specialty care center. A rigid cervical collar (Figure 50-13) and long backboard are standard interventions before transport. Immobilization continues in the emergency department. All trauma patients are suspected of having an SCI until ruled out clinically or through diagnostic testing.

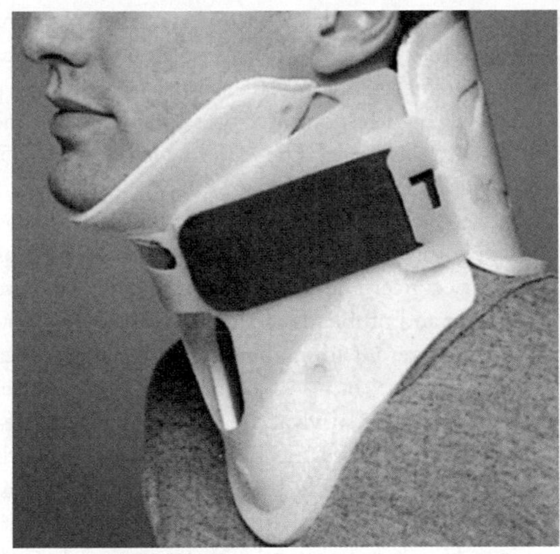

Figure 50-13 Rigid cervical collar.

The initial assessment roughly establishes the extent of injury and provides a baseline for evaluating symptoms related to secondary injury. Systematic assessment of the movement and strength of all major muscle groups is performed and documented. A digital rectal examination is performed to determine whether the injury appears to be "complete." Any voluntary contraction or sensation in

TABLE 50-1
COMMON MEDICATIONS *for Spinal Cord Injury*

Drug	Action	Nursing Intervention
Enoxaparin (Lovenox)	Anticoagulant used to decrease risk of deep venous thrombosis	Give subcutaneously in abdomen. Do not rub injection site.
Dibucaine (Nupercaine)	Topical anesthetic	Apply to rectum before bowel program if SCI at or above T6, to decrease risk of autonomic hyperreflexia.
Bisacodyl (Dulcolax)	Stimulant suppository often used as part of bowel program	Use dibucaine ointment before administering bisacodyl if SCI is at or above T6. For some patients, glycerin suppository or digital stimulation alone is sufficient to trigger bowel elimination.
Gabapentin (Neurontin)	Anticonvulsant used in treatment of neuropathic pain	Give with or without food. Monitor for side effects, including dizziness, somnolence, and visual changes.
Baclofen (Lioresal, Lioresal Intrathecal)	Muscle relaxant used in treatment of spasticity	Abrupt discontinuation can cause withdrawal syndrome. Monitor for signs and symptoms, including muscle rigidity; increased spasticity; high fever; altered mental status; and (rarely) rhabdomyolysis, multisystem organ failure, and death. For severe spasticity, administer baclofen via an intrathecal pump.
Tizanidine hydrochloride (Zanaflex)	Muscle relaxant used in treatment of spasticity	Monitor for side effects, including somnolence, dizziness, mild hypotension, asthenia (loss of strength or energy), and abnormal liver function tests.
Dantrolene sodium (Dantrium)	Muscle relaxant used in treatment of chronic muscle spasticity	Be aware of potential for hepatic toxicity. Monitor liver function tests.

SCI, Spinal cord injury.

the perianal area indicates that some nerve fibers remain intact (sacral sparing). This represents an incomplete injury and carries a more favorable prognosis. A complete sensory evaluation of proprioception, pinprick, and response to light touch is performed and recorded for each dermatome. The ASIA scale (see Figure 50-5) is widely used in the assessment of acute SCI.

The impact of SCI on pulmonary function can be substantial and requires ongoing assessment throughout the course of treatment. Respiratory concerns after SCI can be divided into problems of hypoventilation and problems of airway clearance. Hypoventilation is the most dangerous immediate outcome of a cervical SCI. Patients with complete injuries above C3 require immediate mechanical ventilation for survival. Individuals with injuries at C3 or C4 almost always require mechanical ventilation during the acute phase but may eventually be able to breathe unassisted, at least for short periods. Patients with middle to lower cervical SCI are often able to initiate breaths and maintain adequate respiratory function for a period of hours to days, but may become unable to compensate for decreased tidal volume and airway clearance. They may require mechanical ventilation temporarily, but most can be gradually weaned from the ventilator. Pulmonary management for patients with thoracic SCI focuses on airway clearance techniques unless the patient has an accompanying lung injury that requires mechanical ventilation.

A baseline respiratory assessment is performed on admission. The nurse then assesses unstable patients hourly and apparently stable patients at least every 4 hours. The nurse closely monitors the patient's vital capacity, tidal volume, or both. Maximum inspiratory force may also be measured. A vital capacity of less than 10 to 15 ml/kg body weight indicates respiratory insufficiency and the potential need for intubation and mechanical ventilation. Because of the need to provide cervical spine immobilization in the patient with known or suspected SCI, it is preferable to intubate the patient in a controlled manner before respiratory fatigue becomes severe. Blood gas changes are often late indicators of respiratory failure in SCI patients. Patients with chronic pulmonary diseases or lung injury have a higher risk of pulmonary complications.

Hypotension caused by neurogenic shock compromises spinal cord perfusion. Acute management of neurogenic shock first focuses on differentiating neurogenic shock from the hemorrhagic shock that may be caused by associated trauma. A high index of suspicion for other injuries is essential, since signs and symptoms may be masked by sensory-motor losses and neurogenic shock. An intravenous (IV) line is established and IV fluids administered. Hypotension (systolic blood pressure of less than 90 mm Hg) is prevented or promptly corrected.

Neurosurgical organizations recommend maintaining a mean arterial blood pressure between 85 and 90 mm Hg for the first 7 days after acute SCI, but definitive studies of the impact of this intervention on outcomes are not yet available.[2] The goal is to decrease secondary injury by improving spinal cord perfusion. Blood pressure is supported as needed by the use of inotropic and chronotropic agents. Bradycardia is common and may occasionally become profound or progress to asystole, especially in patients with high cervical injuries. Profound bradycardia and asystole most often occur during suctioning or when the patient is being moved (e.g., from bed to chair). Treatment includes atropine or (in rare cases) a pacemaker. Patients who experience bradycardia during suctioning of an artificial airway may require manual ventilation with supplemental oxygen during the procedure.

Reduction of spinal fractures and realignment of the spinal column prevent ongoing cord compression by restoring the diameter of the spinal canal, thus creating more room for the cord. Decompression and stabilization procedures may need to take place on an emergency basis if deterioration in neurologic status is noted. Both surgical and nonsurgical approaches to realignment and stabilization are available.

Closed reduction is accomplished by applying axial traction to the spinal column using tongs (Crutchfield or Gardner-Wells) or a halo ring attached to weights. IV pain medications and sedatives are often required for traction placement, and the patient is monitored continuously for cardiorespiratory compromise or change in neurologic function. The tongs or halo ring is attached to the skull by pins after local anesthesia is injected. Tongs require the use of two pins, one on each side of the head, whereas the halo ring is attached to the skull by two anterior and two posterior pins. In-line traction is then applied to the spine using progressively heavier weights, with alignment checked using either x-rays films or fluoroscopy before additional weight is added. Assessment of motor and sensory function is performed before and after the addition of each weight.

Tongs are used only for reduction and realignment, but the halo ring is sometimes used as part of a stabilization system after appropriate alignment has been achieved. External vertical rods attach the halo ring to a body vest (Figure 50-14). The device provides complete external immobilization of the head and neck without flexion, extension, or rotation movements while the vertebrae and supporting ligaments heal (usually 6 weeks to 3 months). Patients with halo vests can be managed in standard hospital beds and be mobilized into active rehabilitation as soon as they are hemodynamically stable and x-rays have confirmed that no movement of the spinal

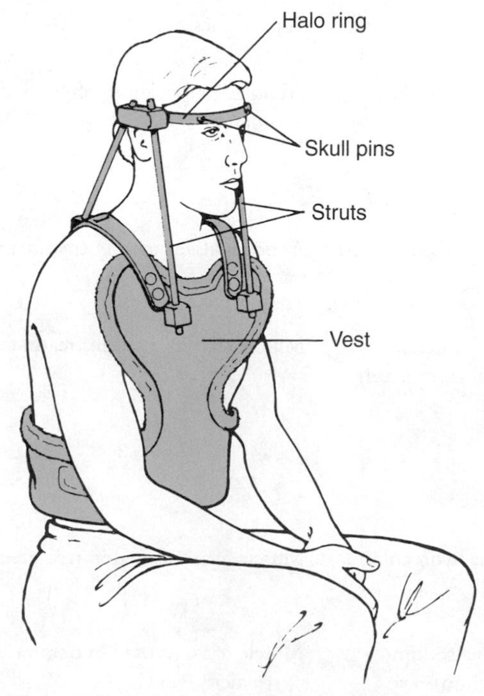

Figure 50-14 Halo vest.

column occurs when the patient is upright. Care of the patient in a halo device is summarized in the Guidelines for Safe Practice box. Until the spine is definitively stabilized (e.g., surgically or with a halo vest), the patient must be log-rolled using three or four people. Specialty beds that rotate while maintaining in-line stabilization can be used in conjunction with traction. The weights must hang freely for traction to be effective.

Bed rest alone may be sufficient to provide initial immobilization for lower thoracic and lumbar injuries. The thoracolumbar area cannot be stabilized with traction. Braces, corsets, or specially made orthotic devices may be used to provide support during healing, but unstable fractures usually require surgical repair.

SURGICAL MANAGEMENT. Surgical intervention is used to relieve compression, correct alignment, and improve the stability of the spine so the patient can be mobilized and participate in rehabilitation. Patients and families must understand that surgery cannot repair the spinal cord itself. Immediate surgery is performed if realignment cannot be attained through nonsurgical management or if unrelieved cord compression compromises function. In some patients, surgery may be delayed to allow for improvement in cardiorespiratory status or reduction of edema in the affected area. An MRI scan can help determine the need for immediate surgical decompression. Although some studies show improved outcomes and shorter hospital stays with early surgical intervention, definitive proof is lacking.[18,24] Decompression of the cord may be achieved by removing bone fragments or a portion of the vertebral ring. Stabilization and fusion are achieved with some combination of plates, rods, screws, wiring, and bone grafts. Postoperatively, a cervical collar, halo vest, or other brace may be ordered to provide external stabilization until the bones fuse. X-ray films may be ordered to check vertebral alignment with the patient upright.

Following either operative or nonoperative stabilization, the patient is aggressively mobilized and rehabilitation efforts are started. The ultimate goal of aggressive multidisciplinary rehabilitation after SCI is to help the patient achieve the maximal self-care potential and return to the home environment. In the current world of managed care, the patient's acute care hospital stay is likely to be brief. The patient is transferred to an acute rehabilitation setting as soon as he or she is hemodynamically stable and the problems of spinal instability and misalignment have been resolved. Social services and community resources are contacted soon after the patient's admission to allow adequate time for thoughtful planning about placement and the acquisition of needed equipment for patient care in the home or community. Social services are also essential to assist the family in dealing with the maze of financial costs and insurance coverage. Discharge planning must truly begin at admission, even though the patient's and family's shock over the consequences of the injury make it difficult for them to play an active role in early planning.

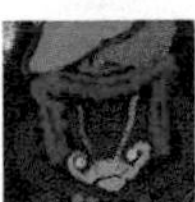

GUIDELINES FOR SAFE PRACTICE
The Patient in a Halo Vest

- Know how to remove the vest to gain access to the patient in the event of a cardiac arrest or other emergency. Some vests incorporate a specially constructed break-away front panel, whereas others require the use of a wrench. Follow manufacturer guidelines, and always keep the appropriate size wrench at the bedside.
- Inspect the pins and pin sites each shift. Be sure that all pins are tight.
- Provide pin care with soap and water each shift.
- Do not allow anyone to use the halo bars to move the patient.
- Inspect the margins of the vest for signs of skin irritation.
- Provide skin care to all areas affected by the halo and vest. Avoid the use of soap, powders, or lotions.
- Support the vest when the patient is in bed.
- Adjust the patient's diet to compensate for swallowing difficulties and discomfort.
- Ensure patient comfort by providing analgesics and frequent repositioning.
- Implement standard measures to minimize the complications of immobility:
  —Bowel and bladder care
  —Deep breathing and coughing
  —Skin care
  —Prevention of deep venous thrombosis

DIET. SCI produces a hypermetabolic, catabolic state in the acute phase, leading to a negative nitrogen balance, weight loss, and a loss of muscle mass. The patient is at risk for malnutrition and its accompanying negative effects on immune system functioning and wound healing. Nutritional support is provided as soon as feasible after injury, usually within 4 days. Enteral nutrition is preferred to parenteral. Patients with high cervical SCI may be unable to take in sufficient nutrients orally to meet their needs, and may require the temporary placement of a feeding tube. The nutritionist is consulted early in the patient's hospital stay.

In the posthospitalization stage, individuals with tetraplegia usually expend less energy and have reduced caloric requirements. Energy expenditure and caloric needs vary widely among patients with paraplegia depending on their activity level. Although weight loss is common in the acute phase after injury, individuals with chronic SCI often gain weight. Maintaining a stable weight is an important care goal, since excessive weight gain places additional strain on the cardiovascular and musculoskeletal systems, increases the risk of skin breakdown, and makes it more difficult for the individual to perform transfers and activities of daily living.

HEALTH PROMOTION AND PREVENTION. Primary prevention efforts are directed at decreasing the incidence of traumatic SCIs through public education and legislative action directed at improving bicycle and vehicle safety, improving workplace safety, reducing violence, and increasing access to specialty care. Health promotion and the prevention of complications also play a significant role in the care of patients after injury. Health promotion begins in the acute care setting. Interventions that decrease the feelings of powerlessness that often accompany SCI improve the patient's sense of self-worth and encourage personal responsibility for health (see the Nursing Management section).

Kidney failure was the leading cause of death among persons with SCI for many years, but improvements in urologic management have dramatically altered that scenario. Although mortality related to urologic complications has declined, urinary tract infections and other urologic problems are common causes of hospital

Research

Phillips VL et al: Telehealth: reaching out to newly injured spinal cord patients, *Pub Health Rep* 116(Suppl 1):94-102, 2001.

This study was designed to evaluate the impact of telehealth interventions on rehospitalization, depressive symptoms, and health-related quality of life among newly injured patients with spinal cord injury (SCI) after discharge from acute rehabilitation. One hundred and eleven patients with SCI were randomly assigned to three groups: video (n=36), telephone (n=36), and standard care (n=39). Patients assigned to the video and telephone groups participated in educational sessions with a certified rehabilitation nurse once a week for 5 weeks, then once every 2 weeks for an additional month. Educational sessions focused on skin care, nutrition, bowel and bladder routines, psychosocial issues, and equipment needs. The standard care group was advised to call the rehabilitation center help line with any questions before a routine follow-up visit scheduled for 2 months after discharge.

No significant differences were found in health-related quality of life at the end of the intervention period (9 weeks), but at 1 year the participants in the video and telephone groups reported significantly higher health-related quality of life than those individuals receiving standard care. Mean annual hospital days also varied among groups: 3.00 for individuals who received the video intervention, 5.22 for the telephone intervention, and 7.95 for the standard care group. Although this is a preliminary study, it shows that the potential impact of telehealth interventions can be significant.

readmission.[20] Annual urologic evaluation is recommended initially, then every 1 to 2 years throughout the patient's life.

Since 1973, pulmonary problems such as pneumonia, emboli, and septicemia have had the greatest impact on life expectancy for individuals with SCI.[22] Individuals with SCI are also at increased risk for cardiovascular disease. The reason for this increased risk is unclear, but it may be attributable to altered autonomic function or decreased physical activity. Weight control is important not only because of the impact of obesity on cardiovascular risk, but because of the effect of excess weight on the skin and musculoskeletal system. Skin breakdown is a major contributor to morbidity and decreased quality of life after SCI. Regular screening for anxiety, depression, and substance abuse is also recommended.

Several barriers limit access to recommended health care for individuals with SCI. Health care providers in the community are frequently unfamiliar with the special needs of SCI patients; transportation problems and lack of insurance coverage may also limit access to health care for many patients.[13] The use of telehealth shows promise in addressing some of these barriers and improving health maintenance and health promotion (see Research box).

Nursing Management

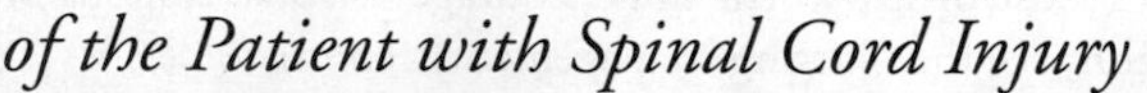

of the Patient with Spinal Cord Injury

Assessment

Health History. Assess for:

- The nature of the injury and its circumstances
- History of loss of consciousness
- Patient's understanding of the injury and the resulting deficits
- Comorbid conditions, treatment, and medications
- Family and social resources
- History of smoking, substance abuse
- Preinjury weight, usual dietary pattern
- Time of last urination and defecation

Physical Examination. Assess for:

- Level of consciousness
- Positioning and alignment of head, neck, and spine
- Baseline respiratory status; rate, pattern
- Dyspnea: presence and severity
- Tidal volume and vital capacity
- Abdominal breathing, use of accessory muscles
- Baseline vital signs, heart rate, blood pressure, and temperature
- Baseline motor evaluation: level of injury, motor strength, and movement
- Presence or absence of spinal reflexes
- Presence or absence of anal wink (contraction of anal sphincter in response to pinprick stimulation of perineum)
- Baseline sensory evaluation
- Dermatome assessment: pain, touch, temperature, pressure, proprioception
- Presence of **paresthesias**, other abnormal sensation
- Baseline skin assessment: signs of redness, pressure, or breakdown
- Presence and activity of bowel sounds
- Presence of stool in rectum
- Presence and severity of bladder distention
- Presence of priapism (an erection caused by unopposed parasympathetic tone)

Nursing Diagnoses, Outcomes, and Interventions

Nursing Diagnosis: Ineffective Airway Clearance

Outcomes. Common examples of expected outcomes for the patient with a diagnosis of *ineffective airway clearance* are:

Patient will:

- Effectively expel secretions using assisted coughing.
- Have clear breath sounds to auscultation.

Nursing Interventions. Deep breathing is a critical intervention for patients who do not require intubation. The nurse helps the patient use an incentive spirometer every 1 to 2 hours while awake to expand the alveoli and support adequate gas exchange. Adequate humidity and hydration are provided to keep the secretions thin. Chest physical therapy, including chest percussion and postural drainage, may be necessary to help the patient expel secretions and keep the alveoli open. The nurse monitors oxygen saturation levels and administers supplemental oxygen as needed.

The patient is turned at least every 2 hours. If positioning limitations exist before the stabilization of the spine, a specialty bed may be used such as the kinetic treatment bed, which turns the patient through a maximal arc of about 120 degrees while maintaining proper spinal alignment (Figure 50-15).

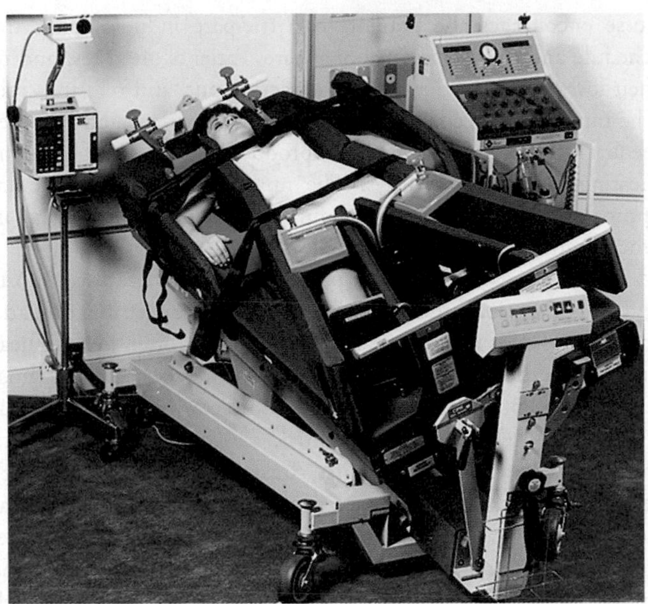

Figure 50-15 The Rotorest kinetic treatment table. This rotating bed keeps patient's spine in proper alignment while turning patient through maximum arc of approximately 120 degrees.

Early tracheostomy may be performed in patients with high cervical injury who require mechanical ventilation to facilitate airway clearance and increase comfort. Endotracheal suctioning is performed as needed. A moist but unproductive cough clearly indicates the need for more aggressive airway clearance. Suctioning can trigger a vasovagal response in patients with SCIs and result in profound bradycardia, especially in patients with high cervical injuries. Prevention and management of this response focus on providing adequate oxygenation and ventilation.

The nurse uses assisted cough techniques to improve airway clearance. The most commonly used techniques are manually assisted coughing ("quad coughing") and mechanically assisted coughing using the In-Exsufflator Cough Machine. Manually assisted coughing involves placing the hands above the patient's umbilicus, but well below the xyphoid, and pushing vigorously inward and upward as the patient exhales. Careful attention to hand placement is necessary to avoid damaging internal organs. When mechanically assisted coughing is used, the In-Exsufflator delivers a deep breath using positive pressure and then quickly applies negative pressure to imitate a normal cough. Most patients use the manually assisted cough for secretion clearance once they return to the community, and the nurse teaches this technique to the patient and family.

RELATED NIC INTERVENTIONS. Airway Management, Cough Enhancement, Mechanical Ventilation, Mechanical Ventilatory Weaning

Nursing Diagnosis: Risk for Powerlessness

OUTCOMES. Common examples of expected outcomes for the patient with a diagnosis of *risk for powerlessness* are:

Patient will:

- Verbalize belief in ability to influence current and future situations and outcomes.
- Make decisions regarding care and treatment.
- Participate in care at the highest level possible.
- Share appropriate information and feedback to care providers.

NURSING INTERVENTIONS. The psychologic impact of SCI on the patient and family is tremendous and must be understood by all members of the multidisciplinary team. Roles and relationships are abruptly and often permanently altered by the injury, and the family's sense of the future is shattered. While each individual with SCI reacts differently, most patients go through a similar series of emotions. The nurse needs to be aware of the range of possible responses to crisis and be skilled in assisting patients and families to progress toward effective coping.

Initially, the patient may feel numb and express relief simply to be alive. The nurse supports the patient by providing basic explanations of care and addressing specific concerns. The nurse answers questions honestly and allows the patient to dictate the pace at which information is shared. Patients commonly ask about their potential to walk again and may ask about sexual function. They may ask questions repeatedly, especially if they are receiving opioid pain medication or sedatives. As the patient experiences disbelief and denial regarding the injury and functional sequelae, he or she may ask the same question of multiple caregivers, in search of a more acceptable answer regarding potential abilities. Consistency among care providers helps establish trust. It is important not to mislead patients with SCI about functional status, but the patient benefits from maintaining realistic hope for the future.

Grief, sometimes overwhelming, occurs as the patient moves past denial and realizes the extent of his or her losses. Feelings of guilt may also surface, especially if the injury was preventable. Grief is a natural response and is expressed differently by each individual. The individual may become withdrawn or tearful. During this time, patients are typically unable to learn new information and require significant support. The nurse focuses on the present while acknowledging the loss that the patient has suffered. Access to support systems is crucial. Coping mechanisms such as diversional activities may be useful. Grief over functional losses may also be expressed as anger or manipulative behavior. Limit setting regarding acceptable behavior may become necessary.

Coping evolves over time, and it may take years for the patient to reach the stage of grief resolution. Gradually the patient begins to seek information and becomes an active participant in care. Educational efforts have the greatest impact during this stage. The eventual goal is successful integration of the injury into the sense of self, but not all patients achieve this goal. Psychologic adaptation to SCI frequently takes months to years, and the process is not linear. Individuals may return to a previous stage of adaptation. For example, grief may resurface throughout the patient's life, typically in response to life events that refocus the patient's attention on the losses caused by the SCI (e.g., when a daughter gets married and the father is unable to walk arm in arm with her down the aisle). The Research box on p. 1478 describes the results of research investigating components of quality of life for individuals living with SCI.

Attention to family concerns is crucial in the care of the individual with SCI. Family members grieve for the lost potential of

Research

Manns PJ, Chad KE: Components of quality of life for persons with a quadriplegic and paraplegic spinal cord injury, *Qual Health Res* 11(6):795-811, 2001.

This study was designed to identify key factors affecting quality of life in individuals with spinal cord injury (SCI). The participants were 15 patients who had been living with SCI for 3 to 30 years. This qualitative research study used semistructured interviews to identify themes that contributed to quality of life. Key factors identified include physical function and independence (to be as independent as possible given physical limitations), access to the environment, relationships and social function, stigma, spontaneity, emotional well-being (coping, adjustment), physical well-being (freedom from medical complications), meaningful work (whether paid, volunteer, or homemaking), and financial resources. Health care providers can integrate these findings into the development of treatment approaches that maximize quality of life.

the injured person and the loss of the family unit as it was before the injury. Each person moves through the stages of grief at a different pace. Family members are often so focused on being positive and supportive for the patient that they fail to acknowledge their own needs. Family members are challenged to assume significant caregiving roles. The impact on both physical and emotional intimacy can adversely affect relationships with partners. The nurse plays a pivotal role in helping each family member deal openly and honestly with these complex feelings, and encourages family members to meet their own needs as well.

The nurse can use multiple strategies to structure the care environment in ways that foster coping and a sense of control. Providing consistent staffing assists in the development of trust and ensures that care is provided in a consistent, predictable manner. Loss of function and dependence on others leads to fear and anxiety. The nurse can create an environment in which the patient feels safe by explaining all equipment in use and ensuring that the patient has an accessible means of contacting staff. Adaptive call signal equipment, such as mouth-operated call bells and touch pad devices, that patients can operate within the limits of their functional abilities is crucial. Many patients require anxiolytic medications at some point during the acute hospitalization. Nonpharmacologic relaxation strategies can be introduced once the initial state of panic has subsided.

If the patient is mechanically ventilated and unable to speak, the nurse provides an alternative communication method. Alphabet boards and lipreading are commonly used, but can be very frustrating for both patient and staff. Effective communication can be facilitated by providing consistent care providers and creating individualized lists of commonly used words and phrases (e.g., "Turn off the light," "I need to be suctioned," "Is my wife here?"). Devices are available that can spell words in response to eye gaze, but they are extremely expensive at this time. As the patient's pulmonary status improves, a speaking valve may be fitted to the tracheostomy tube to enable better communication.

The nurse offers the patient choices whenever possible to increase his or her sense of control while remaining clear and consistent about nonnegotiable aspects of care. For example, frequent turning is not negotiable, but which side to turn to often is. The nurse encourages the patient to participate in developing the schedule and routine for personal care. Patients often respond to their loss of control through anger, acting out, and refusing care. The nurse often needs to set limits with the patient and provides feedback about productive and unproductive methods of communicating needs and feelings. The nurse uses a nonjudgmental approach while consistently encouraging the patient to engage in rehabilitation and self-care activities.

The nurse works with the patient to establish realistic short- and long-term goals and answers all questions concerning care and the prognosis for recovery of function. Patients often need to hear questions addressed multiple times, and the nurse clarifies any misconceptions, provides accurate and complete information about the patient's rehabilitation potential, and explains strategies to increase independence. The nurse constantly assesses the patient's readiness to learn and teaches new concepts as appropriate. Educational efforts initially focus on providing basic explanations of care, then progress to include more detailed information about the injury and its impact. The nurse encourages the patient to ask questions, since lack of knowledge contributes to powerlessness.

The nurse explores the patient's preinjury coping strategies and support systems and seeks out new resources that may be helpful in addressing the challenges of SCI. Resources may include peer counselors, mental health practitioners, social work professionals, and chaplains. Teaching patients the use of stress management techniques such as relaxation strategies, visual imagery, and structured problem solving can help to expand their coping skills. The nurse offers encouragement and positive feedback for any progress made toward the established goals. Family members are encouraged to bring in personal items, such as pictures, music, or a pillow. When appropriate, the patient can be encouraged to wear his or her own clothes. Makeup and jewelry may also improve self-image for female patients.

RELATED NIC INTERVENTIONS. Coping Enhancement, Decision-Making Support, Emotional Support, Family Support, Self-Esteem Enhancement

Nursing Diagnosis: Impaired Urinary Elimination

OUTCOMES. Common examples of expected outcomes for the patient with a diagnosis of *impaired urinary elimination* are:
Patient will:

- Establish a bladder management program that provides functional continence.
- Identify methods of integrating the bladder management program into lifestyle.
- Exhibit no signs of urinary tract infection.

NURSING INTERVENTIONS. In the immediate postinjury period, an indwelling catheter frequently is inserted to prevent overdistention of the bladder and allow close monitoring of urinary output. Once the patient has stabilized and consistent intake is established, the nurse initiates an individualized bladder management program. In most cases the indwelling catheter is removed and a program of intermittent catheterization (IC) is started. Strict aseptic technique is followed while the patient is hospitalized, although a clean technique may be taught for use at home.

The nurse performs IC every 3 to 4 hours; if more frequent catheterization is required, an indwelling catheter is a more realistic option and IC can be reattempted at a later date. The goal is to establish a schedule of IC that keeps the urine volume per catheterization at less than 400 ml for women and 500 ml for men.[9] If the urine volume at any single catheterization exceeds 400 to 500 ml, the interval between catheterizations is decreased. If high volumes persist, an indwelling catheter is reinserted and the reason for the high volumes (increased intake, diuretic administration) is explored. If the urine volume per catheterization remains consistently less than 400 to 500 ml, the nurse slowly increases the time between catheterizations. Any urine volume greater than 400 to 500 ml requires a return to the previous schedule. Most patients stabilize at a 4- to 6-hour interval between catheterizations. IC may be required more often at night because of fluid shifts.

If the patient's bladder dysfunction is related to an LMN injury, voiding can sometimes be induced by Valsalva's maneuver or Credé's maneuver (manually pushing on the lower abdomen to compress the bladder). However, voiding induced by these maneuvers is often incomplete, and incontinence is common. Many patients with LMN injury rely on IC for bladder management. Most of these patients have intact arm and hand function and can therefore independently maintain a program of IC.

If the patient's bladder dysfunction is related to a UMN injury, the reflex arc that controls voiding remains intact and a reflexive voiding capability will likely return once spinal shock resolves. Individuals with UMN injury may then void spontaneously in response to stimulation of the bladder wall (tapping the suprapubic area, pulling on the pubic hair). This phenomenon is called "triggering" or "kicking off." If the patient begins to experience reflexive voiding, the nurse checks postvoid residuals using IC. Most patients void only a small amount of urine initially, leaving a large residual volume in the bladder. Once the residual volume drops to about 100 ml, it may be possible to discontinue the IC regimen. Male patients may be able to combine reflexive voiding with the use of an external collection device (condom catheter). This approach is less realistic for females because an adequate external collection device is not available.

The nurse monitors the patient carefully for signs of urinary tract infection such as hematuria, clouding, increased sediment, or mucus in the urine, and teaches the patient to recognize these signs as well. Urologic follow-up monitoring is strongly recommended. If none of the approaches discussed above is successful, other options exist for long-term bladder management. For example, a suprapubic catheter may be placed. Functional electrical stimulation (FES) has recently been used to manage UMN bladder dysfunction.[21] Electrodes are surgically placed on the sacral spinal nerves, and a stimulator is implanted under the skin. An external control unit is used to activate the stimulator. This causes the bladder to contract and the urethral sphincter to relax, and voiding occurs. FES requires surgery and is not used in the acute care of patients with SCI, but may be an option for long-term bladder management.

RELATED NIC INTERVENTIONS. Urinary Catheterization, Urinary Catheterization: Intermittent, Urinary Elimination Management

Nursing Diagnosis: Risk for Constipation

OUTCOMES. Common examples of expected outcomes for the patient with a diagnosis of *risk for constipation* are:
Patient will:
- Have a soft, formed bowel movement every day or every other day.
- Experience no episodes of bowel incontinence.

NURSING INTERVENTIONS. As soon as the patient is stabilized, the nurse initiates a bowel program and performs it at least every other day to prevent constipation. Planning an appropriate bowel program begins with a careful assessment of the patient's preinjury bowel elimination patterns, diet, and lifestyle. The bowel program must be designed so that it can be integrated into the individual's daily routine.

The nurse works with the patient to establish an acceptable and consistent time for bowel elimination, such as in the morning after breakfast or in the evening after dinner. Timing the bowel program for approximately 30 minutes after a meal takes advantage of the gastrocolic reflex. Drinking warm fluids may also stimulate this reflex. Even if the patient is receiving continuous tube feedings, it is still important for the nurse and patient to establish a consistent time for elimination. A successful routine increases the patient's sense of control and sets the stage for successful long-term bowel management. Ensuring privacy is an important component for success.

A successful bowel program incorporates a balance of fiber, fluids, positioning, suppositories, and digital stimulation. The nurse establishes appropriate levels of fluid and fiber intake based on the individual's needs and response. Fluid intake must also take into consideration the needs and restrictions of the bladder program. Patients are typically started on 5 to 25 g of fiber per day. Stool softeners or bulk-forming agents may be incorporated into the program but require a physician's order in most inpatient settings. Once acceptable levels of fiber and fluid are established, the nurse instructs the patient and family on appropriate dietary modifications to use at home.

The nurse gently performs digital rectal examination to evaluate for fecal impaction, using anesthetic ointment for individuals whose SCI is at or above T6 to decrease the risk of autonomic hyperreflexia. A stimulant suppository is administered, if ordered, again using anesthetic ointment for individuals with SCI at or above T6. The bowel program is best performed with the patient in a sitting position. If the patient is unable to sit, the nurse positions him or her in a left side-lying position. Pressure can be applied to the abdominal wall during defecation, either manually or with an abdominal binder, to help compensate for the loss of abdominal muscle tone.

Twenty to 30 minutes after suppository administration, digital stimulation may be used to stimulate reflex defecation in patients with UMN bowel dysfunction. The nurse gently inserts a lubricated, gloved index finger into the patient's rectum and moves the finger in a circular motion. Anesthetic ointment is used in patients with injury at or above T6 to prevent autonomic hyperreflexia. If the individual has an LMN injury, no reflex emptying is possible and the nurse performs manual removal of stool daily.

The nurse monitors stool frequency and consistency during the establishment of the bowel program to evaluate the effectiveness of the various components. Once a regular pattern of elimination has been established, digital stimulation alone, combined with careful management of diet and fluids, may be sufficient to maintain regular bowel elimination for patients with UMN injury. Once a successful bowel program has been established, the nurse carefully instructs the patient and family about the program components, including the use of any assistive devices. If the patient is not functionally able to perform the bowel program, it is still important that he or she be able to accurately direct caregivers in its performance.

RELATED NIC INTERVENTIONS. Bowel Management, Fluid Management, Nutrition Management

Nursing Diagnosis: Risk for Impaired Skin Integrity

OUTCOMES. Common examples of expected outcomes for the patient with a diagnosis of *risk for impaired skin integrity* are:

Patient will:

- Perform pressure relief or weight shifts every 15 to 20 minutes (using adaptive equipment or caregiver assistance if needed).
- Perform skin inspection twice daily (using adaptive equipment or caregiver assistance if needed).
- Maintain intact skin without pressure ulcers or other breakdown.

NURSING INTERVENTIONS. Skin protection begins immediately after the injury. Pressure-related injury occurs when capillaries are compressed and occluded, leading to tissue hypoxia. Microscopic tissue changes related to local ischemia can occur in less than 30 minutes. Venous pooling and decreased tissue perfusion during the acute phase of injury further compromise the skin. Pressure injury is frequently initiated when the patient is strapped to a rigid backboard. It is critical that bony prominences be effectively padded to reduce the chance of pressure injury in the patient who must remain on the backboard for an extended period for transport or diagnostic scanning.

Skin breakdown is a common complication of SCI due to the loss of sensory input and restricted mobility. Direct pressure-related skin injury is the primary concern but shearing forces are also important. The primary cause of pressure-related injury is prolonged time in one position. The nurse repositions the patient at least every 2 hours while in bed. Pressure-relieving mattresses are used once the patient's spine is stabilized. Care is taken to keep the patient's heels off of the bed surface. The patient's weight is distributed as evenly as possible across the bed surface. Keeping the head of the bed low can accomplish this objective, but the nurse must balance the need to limit pressure with the need to elevate the head of the bed to reduce the risk of aspiration and promote interaction with the environment.

Shearing injury occurs when layers of tissue slide over each other in different directions such as occurs when the patient slides down in bed or is pulled up in bed without using a lift sheet. The nurse avoids shearing forces by using lift sheets and adequate personnel to move the patient up in the bed or transfer the patient to a chair. A pressure reduction cushion is used whenever the patient is sitting. The nurse slowly increases the amount of daily sitting time (1 hour is an appropriate starting point for most patients) and carefully inspects the patient's skin after sitting. If no redness occurs, sitting time can be gradually increased, provided adequate pressure relief is ensured.

Pressure relief is critical whenever the patient is out of bed and is performed every 15 to 20 minutes when the patient is sitting. Depending on the patient's mobility limitations, strategies for pressure relief include wheelchair pushups to relieve pressure on the buttocks, leaning over alternate sides of the wheelchair to shift weight, or brief rest periods with the wheelchair in a fully reclined position. The nurse encourages the patient to take responsibility for his or her own skin health. Patients who are unable to independently perform skin protection activities (weight shifts, skin inspections) are taught to monitor the plan and contact caregivers for assistance or intervention at appropriate times. Skin breakdown significantly impacts quality of life, and skin protection is a lifetime management concern for individuals with SCI. Early patient involvement provides the best basis for long-term health maintenance.

The nurse inspects the patient's skin carefully after position changes, while the patient is in bed, and after sitting time, checking for evidence of erythema and blanching. Reddened areas that do not blanch within 20 to 30 minutes are serious warning signs of pressure damage. Bony prominences covered by minimal soft tissue are at highest risk for breakdown. These include the occiput, sacrum, ischium, trochanters, heels, and elbows. The affected areas are not rubbed or massaged to avoid damaging capillaries and increasing tissue injury. The nurse teaches the patient to perform frequent skin inspection with the use of mirrors and caregiver assistance.

The nurse uses a variety of other strategies to support the health of the skin and works with the patient to incorporate

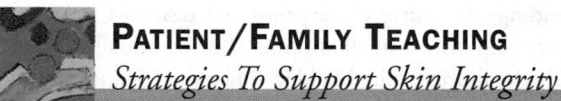

PATIENT/FAMILY TEACHING

Strategies To Support Skin Integrity

- Consume a liberal amount of fluid each day, staying within the guidelines of the bladder and bowel program.
- Ensure that the daily diet is high in protein with adequate vitamins and minerals.
- Use a mild soap for skin care that does not dry skin or alter the pH. Dry the skin carefully, especially in folds and creases.
- Keep the skin well lubricated.
- Apply a protective barrier to the perineal area if incontinent.
- Avoid the use of incontinence pads that trap moisture next to the skin.
- Avoid any use of heating pads or ice packs in areas where skin sensation is altered or absent.
  —Monitor the temperature of bath water carefully.
- Follow the guidelines from physical and occupational therapists about the duration of use for assistive devices.
  —Monitor the skin under splints for signs of redness or irritation.
  —If redness occurs, remove the splint and notify the therapist.
- Change positions at least every 2 hours.
- Keep weight evenly distributed in the bed or chair.
- Adhere to established guidelines for safe sitting times.
- Engage in pressure relief strategies every 15 to 20 minutes while sitting.

appropriate strategies into the daily routine (see Patient/Family Teaching box, p. 1480).

RELATED NIC INTERVENTIONS. Pressure Management, Pressure Ulcer Prevention, Skin Surveillance

Patient/Family Teaching. Important educational components for the patient with SCI and his or her family are discussed under each nursing diagnosis and summarized in the Patient/Family Teaching box below.

EVALUATION

To evaluate the effectiveness of nursing interventions, compare patient behaviors with those stated in the expected patient outcomes.

RELATED NOC OUTCOMES. Bowel Elimination, Depression Self-Control, Family Participation in Professional Care, Health Beliefs: Perceived Control, Participation in Health Care Decisions, Respiratory Status: Airway Patency, Respiratory Status: Gas Exchange, Respiratory Status: Ventilation, Tissue Integrity: Skin & Mucous Membranes, Urinary Elimination

GERONTOLOGIC CONSIDERATIONS

SCI is a devastating and life-altering process at any age. Although most SCIs occur in young adults, the incidence of SCI in older adults (over 65 years old) is increasing. These injuries are usually the result of falls and often reflect the weakening of vertebrae related to osteoporosis. The challenges of SCI can be overwhelming for the older person, who is more likely to have comorbid conditions like heart disease, pulmonary disease, or diabetes.[16] These conditions complicate the management of neurogenic shock and have significant implications for respiratory management and skin care. The mortality rate for geriatric patients is higher than for younger patients during hospitalization and at 60 days after injury.[16] The functional losses of SCI are also often more severe for older adults. Concurrent health problems contribute to increased complications and reduce self-

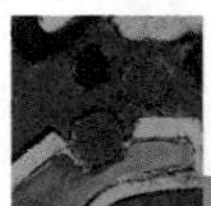

PATIENT/FAMILY TEACHING *Spinal Cord Injury*

The content of patient and family teaching varies widely based on the type of injury, treatment provided, and functional impact. Basic education begins during acute hospitalization and continues at a more detailed level in rehabilitation. Many handbooks and other instructional aids are available for patients with spinal cord injury (SCI) and their families and can be used as a supplement to the teaching provided by the nurse. The following list includes a wide range of topics that are important in patient and family education, but it is not all inclusive and should be adapted to meet individual patient needs:

- Function of the spinal cord
- Relationship of the vertebrae to the spinal cord
- Specific motor-sensory level and anticipated functional outcomes
- Role of health care team members, including physicians, nurses, physical therapist, occupational therapist, and respiratory therapist
- Stabilization devices (cervical collar, halo vest, thoracic shell, or other device as appropriate to patient)
  —Purpose
  —When device must be worn, if removable
  —Skin care and hygiene
- Pulmonary care
  —Effect of positioning on respiratory function
  —Use of incentive spirometer or deep breathing exercises
  —Assisted cough techniques
  —Signs and symptoms of respiratory infections (fever, cough, change in sputum production, change in breathing pattern or sound)
- Bladder routine
  —Intermittent catheterization or other bladder management technique, as appropriate for patient
  —Fluid intake
  —Signs and symptoms of a urinary tract infection (foul-smelling urine, cloudy urine, fever, chills, autonomic hyperreflexia)
- Bowel routine
  —Bowel training program
  —Fluid and fiber intake as appropriate to individual
- Mobility
  —Active and passive range of motion (performed at least twice daily)
  —Splinting and positioning equipment
  —Bed mobility
  —Transfer techniques
  —Orthostatic hypotension
- Skin care
  —Surveillance by self or another twice daily
  —Technique and timing of pressure relief while in wheelchair
  —Use of wheelchair cushion
  —Turning schedule (at least every 2 hours)
- Sexuality
  —Changes in sexual function related to injury
  —Importance of sexuality
  —Fertility implications based on gender
- Autonomic hyperreflexia
  —Prevention
  —Signs and symptoms
  —Interventions (including when to seek help from a health care provider)
- Coping strategies
  —Visual imagery, distraction, and other relaxation technique
  —Knowledge of support mechanisms throughout the continuum of care, including social work, chaplaincy, and local and national SCI organizations
- Discharge planning
  —Most patients discharged from acute care to an inpatient rehabilitation hospital
  —Most ultimately return home, but some require placement in a long-term care facility if sufficient resources (financial and family support) are not available for home care.

care potential. The demands on families can be overwhelming and are compounded by distance, career, and nuclear family responsibilities.

Tumors of the Spinal Cord

Etiology and Epidemiology. Both primary and metastatic tumors affect the spinal cord, typically in individuals between 20 and 60 years of age. The thoracic spine is the most common site. Primary tumors arise from the substance of the cord and meninges or from the surrounding bone or blood vessels. In adults, primary tumors are often benign but can cause significant deficits in function because they compress the cord. The majority of primary spinal tumors are extramedullary, arising in the extradural or intradural space outside the actual spinal cord (Figure 50-16). Common examples include schwannomas, meningiomas, and neurofibromas. Examples of intramedullary primary spinal tumors include astrocytomas and hemangioblastomas.

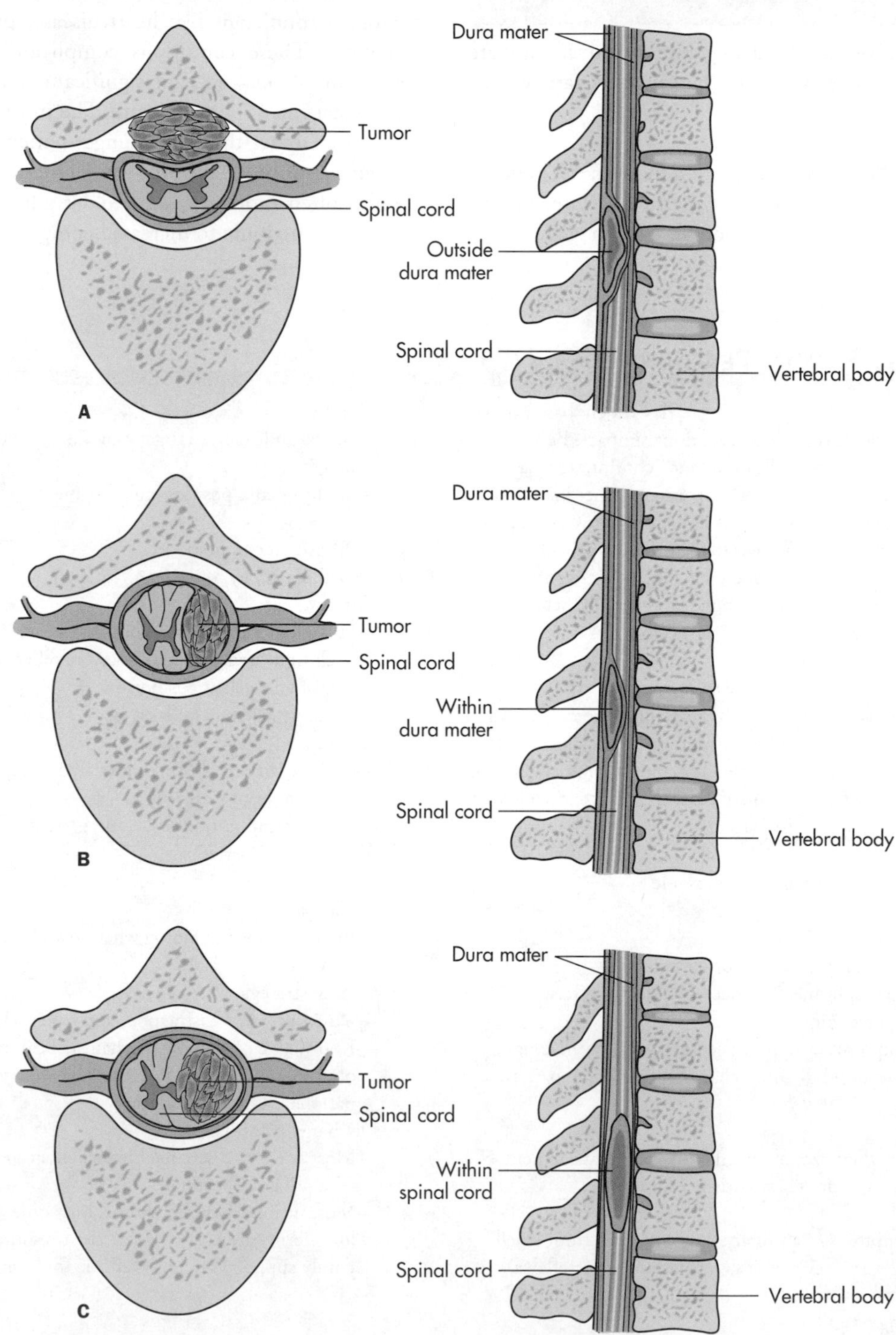

Figure 50-16 Spinal tumors. **A,** Extradural tumors—outside the dura mater. **B,** Subdural tumors—within the dura mater. **C,** Intramedullary tumors—within the spinal cord.

Metastatic spinal cord tumors are more common than primary spinal tumors and can be traced to primary tumors in other organs, especially the lungs, breast, and prostate. Most metastatic tumors are located in the extradural space of the thoracic spine and affect the richly vascular vertebral body or paravertebral tissue. Erosion of the vertebrae may occur, increasing the risk of fracture and spine instability.

Pathophysiology. The pathologic consequences of both primary and metastatic spinal tumors are primarily related to the effects of cord compression. Infiltration and invasion of the cord itself occur much less commonly. Pressure can irritate the spinal nerve roots, displace the cord, interrupt perfusion, cause ischemia and edema, and obstruct the flow of cerebrospinal fluid. The combined effects of pressure and edema cause the typical symptoms of pain, weakness, and motor and sensory loss. The exact symptoms relate to the specific level of the spine affected by the tumor. The rate of tumor growth is important. Slowly growing tumors allow time for the spinal cord to initially adapt and may produce few symptoms until advanced. A rapidly growing tumor, particularly one composed of dense tissue, causes significant amounts of edema and early symptoms.

Pain, with or without accompanying neurologic deficits, is the first symptom in the majority of patients with spinal tumors. The pain may be localized or radiate along the path of the involved spinal nerve root (radicular pain). The pain varies in intensity from mild to severe. Sensory losses reflect the exact anatomic location of the compression within the cord and may be accompanied by weakness or paralysis in the same nerve distribution. Problems with bladder, bowel, or sexual function frequently occur, but the onset of these symptoms is usually preceded by pain or motor-sensory losses unless the lesion is in the lumbar spine or cauda equina.

Collaborative Care Management. The diagnosis of a spinal cord tumor begins with a detailed history and neurologic examination. The diagnostic test of choice is the MRI with contrast administration. CT and myelography are sometimes used, especially in patients who are unable to undergo MRI scanning. MRI clearly visualizes tumors in the vertebral bodies and within the cord itself.

Treatment is aimed at tumor removal or control, pain relief, and preservation of neurologic function. Corticosteroids, most often dexamethasone (Decadron), are administered to treat edema and thus decrease cord compression. Further treatment varies based on tumor type and location and the rate of symptom development. Surgical intervention is the treatment of choice for most primary spinal tumors. The surgery is often technically complex, especially when the blood supply is involved. Surgery for metastatic tumors usually focuses on decompression of the spinal cord and debulking of the tumor to improve the patient's quality of life. Radiotherapy is a common treatment for many metastatic tumors and all tumors that exhibit invasive growth patterns that make complete surgical excision impossible. Radiation is an effective palliative strategy for relieving pain in patients with advanced disease. Administration of steroids is frequently combined with radiotherapy to minimize spinal cord edema. Chemotherapy has little documented effectiveness in the management of spinal tumors, although adjunctive hormonal treatment may be useful when the primary cancer site is the breast or prostate gland.

Immobilization is a priority if the spine is unstable. Immobilization may involve simple bed rest with the patient in correct body alignment or the use of cervical collars, thoracic braces, and shells. Surgical stabilization may be necessary. Many of the nursing care priorities for patients with spinal tumors are similar to those discussed under SCI, with an emphasis on restoring independence and preventing complications.

PATIENT/FAMILY TEACHING. Patient and family education varies based on the patient's unique functional deficits, tumor type (primary versus metastatic), and medical treatment plan. For patients with metastatic spinal cord tumors who are in an advanced stage of a complex battle against cancer, care focuses on successfully managing pain and minimizing the impact of functional deficits on quality of life. The nurse assesses the needs of both patient and family and initiates appropriate referrals for community-based services and support. Both the patient and family may require extensive teaching and support to adequately address each major area of concern. A hospice referral may be appropriate.

Cranial Nerve Diseases and Disorders

The three classic disorders affecting the cranial nerves are Meniere's disease, trigeminal neuralgia, and Bell's palsy. Meniere's disease is presented in Chapter 63 because of its primary effects on the auditory and vestibular systems. Trigeminal neuralgia and Bell's palsy are discussed here.

Trigeminal Neuralgia (Tic Douloureux)

Etiology and Epidemiology. Trigeminal neuralgia is a chronic condition affecting one or more branches of the fifth cranial nerve (trigeminal). It causes intense paroxysmal pain along the nerve pathway. No cause has been clearly identified, although a variety of associated factors are recognized. The most widely accepted theory of disease etiology involves vascular compression of the nerve root resulting in irritation and demyelination. Other potential causes include trauma or infection in the teeth or jaw and pressure on the trigeminal nerve from an aneurysm or tumor.

Trigeminal neuralgia can occur at any age but is most common in middle-aged and older individuals. Women are affected more often than men. The disease typically follows a pattern of exacerbation and remission, with the patient experiencing pain episodes over a period of weeks or months and then undergoing a spontaneous remission of variable length. The length of remissions tends to shorten over time, while exacerbations increase in frequency and severity. Trigeminal neuralgia is the most common facial neuralgia syndrome and is believed to be one of the most painful of all conditions. The severity of the pain has a significant negative impact on the patient's quality of life and even on the ability to maintain self-care and adequate nutrition.

Pathophysiology. The trigeminal nerve exits the pons and merges into the gasserian ganglion before it separates into its three major branches (Figure 50-17). The trigeminal nerve is the largest of the cranial nerves and has both motor and sensory fibers. The pain syndrome of trigeminal neuralgia primarily

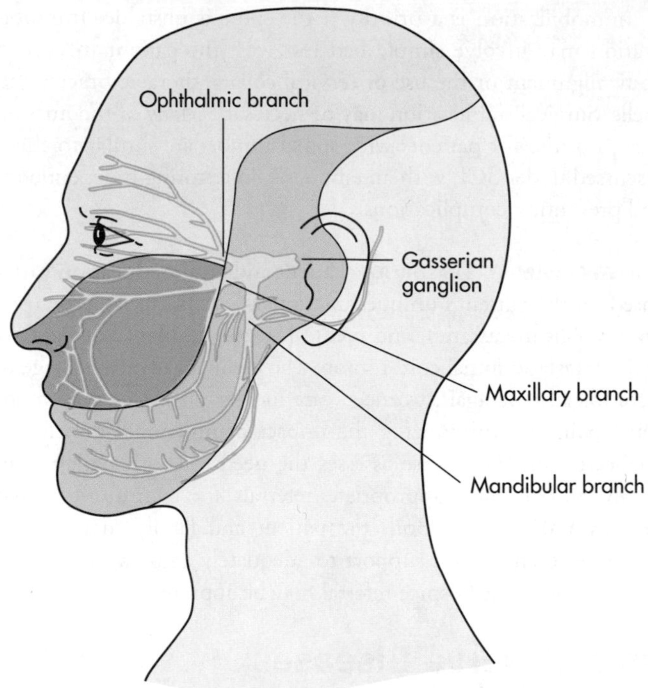

Figure 50-17 Pathway of trigeminal nerve and facial areas innervated by each of its three main divisions.

affects the maxillary or mandibular branch of the nerve. Involvement of the ophthalmic branch is rare. The pain typically affects the right side of the face for no known reason. The pain occurs abruptly and lasts from a few seconds to a few minutes. Typically described as intense, piercing, burning, or "like a lightening bolt," the pain affects only one side of the face, and there are no identifiable motor or sensory deficits in the regions innervated by the involved branch. The classic pain pattern is the only diagnostic feature of trigeminal neuralgia, and the diagnosis is made by excluding other possible causes of facial pain. A head CT may be performed to rule out an intruding lesion, and an MRI can be useful in identifying vascular compression or widespread demyelinating disease (such as multiple sclerosis).

Significant pathologic changes are frequently found in the myelin sheath of the trigeminal nerve, which predispose the nerve to erratic and hyperexcitable firing. Most patients are able to identify specific trigger points along the course of the nerve where the slightest stimulus can initiate pain. Chewing, talking, smiling, brushing teeth, touching the face, and even a draft of air can trigger the pain. Patients typically go to great lengths to avoid a triggering stimulus. It is not uncommon for patients to socially isolate themselves or neglect routine personal hygiene such as washing the face, brushing the teeth, or shaving in an effort to avoid pain. Significant weight loss can occur if chewing is a triggering stimulus.

Collaborative Care Management. Treatment options for trigeminal neuralgia include both medical and surgical interventions. The goal of intervention is to reduce the intensity or duration of pain episodes in the most minimally invasive way. The first treatment tried is usually drug therapy. Eighty percent of patients respond positively to treatment with anticonvulsants, at least initially. The drug of choice is carbamazepine (Tegretol), a sodium channel blocker that inhibits transmission of impulses that are perceived as pain. It usually lessens the frequency and duration of the pain episodes, but it may not be able to eliminate them and symptoms may worsen again over time. Patients taking carbamazepine require regular blood work to monitor for myelosuppression. Many other medications, including gabapentin (Neurontin), phenytoin (Dilantin), lamotrigine (Lamictal), topiramate (Topamax), clonazepam (Klonopin), or baclofen (Lioresal), may also be prescribed. Some practitioners advocate the use of multiple medications to target several different pain mechanisms and decrease side effects of the individual drugs.

In patients with refractory disease, surgical treatment may be indicated. Three types of procedures may be performed: neurodestructive procedures, stereotactic radiosurgery, and microvascular decompression.[6] Neurodestructive procedures relieve pain by destroying nerve tissue, resulting in partial facial numbness and potential loss of innervation to the cornea. These procedures are performed using a percutaneous approach with no surgical incision. Nerve tissue is destroyed using an injection of glycerol, balloon compression, or radio frequency thermocoagulation. Pain relief is often immediate, but recurrence rates are significant. Stereotactic radiosurgery (Gamma Knife surgery) provides relief using highly targeted radiation of the trigeminal nerve. Pain relief takes 4 to 6 weeks to achieve but occurs in most patients, and loss of normal facial sensation is rare. Microvascular decompression is an increasingly used surgical option in which the surgeon performs a craniotomy to adequately visualize the trigeminal nerve and then dissects away the compressing vessel. Teflon felt may be placed between the artery and nerve. The mortality rate after microvascular decompression is 0.3%.[17] Because microvascular decompression requires a craniotomy, postoperative monitoring differs from that provided for the other procedures, and the patient may be admitted to the intensive care unit overnight.

PATIENT/FAMILY TEACHING. Patients with trigeminal neuralgia face multiple daily living challenges during the diagnostic and pharmacologic treatment period, and the nurse provides support and guidance as the patients explore lifestyle changes and pain management strategies (see Patient/Family Teaching box).

Neurodestructive procedures may result in diminished or lost sensation. This is of particular concern when the loss of sensation affects the eye. The nurse instructs the patient to avoid rubbing the eye on the affected side and to monitor the eye regularly for signs of irritation or infection. Regular dental care is also essential because the protective pain warning signs associated with dental disease are often absent. A Nursing Care Plan for a patient with trigeminal neuralgia follows on pp. 1486 and 1487.

Bell's Palsy

Etiology and Epidemiology. Bell's palsy is an acute disorder of cranial nerve VII, the facial nerve, resulting in the loss of motor, sensory, and parasympathetic function on one side of the face. It affects approximately 40,000 people per year in the United States. The cause of the disease is believed to be the herpes simplex virus in most cases. The disease usually affects adults between 20 and 60 years of age, and the incidence in men and women is about equal. About 80% of patients recover over a period of a few weeks. Most

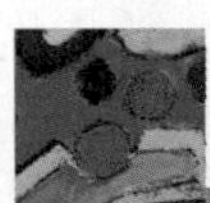

PATIENT/FAMILY TEACHING *The Patient With Trigeminal Neuralgia*

Patient and family education about trigeminal neuralgia focuses on pain management, avoidance of pain triggers, good oral hygiene, medications, and treatment options. Specific teaching points include:

- Take prescribed medications at the time they are due to maintain a steady blood level of medication. Take analgesics at the first sign of pain, since they work more effectively if taken before pain reaches severe levels.
- Nonpharmacologic strategies such as relaxation and imagery may be helpful in augmenting the pain control effects of medications.
- Monitor and record weight at least weekly, and discuss any weight loss with a health care practitioner.
- Explore dietary modifications to increase nutrient intake without worsening pain (softer consistency, liquid supplements, adding skim milk or powders to foods). Eat small, frequent meals to increase caloric intake and minimize pain. Chew on the unaffected side of mouth.
- Avoid empty calories. Because eating triggers pain, all foods ingested should be nutritious and of sufficient value to meet metabolic needs. Drink fluids with nutritional value (supplements, juices) to avoid dehydration.
- A liquid multivitamin supplement may be added to food or fluid to ensure adequate intake of vitamins in case of insufficient intake. Discuss this with your health care provider.
- If regular oral care (toothbrushing, flossing) triggers pain, use soft swabs, mouthwashes, or a water-powered toothbrush. Perform frequent oral care during pain-free intervals.
- Rinse the mouth carefully after eating to reduce mouth odor from retained food particles.
- See your dentist regularly (at least every 6 months).

patients experience no residual effects, although complete recovery may take as much as 6 to 12 months.

Pathophysiology. The facial nerve is primarily composed of motor nerves that innervate the muscles of expression on the face. The sensory branches supply the anterior two thirds of the tongue. Bell's palsy is characterized by a rapid weakening or paralysis of the facial muscles on one side of the face, which creates a masklike appearance (Figure 50-18). Taste may be diminished, and the patient may complain of increased sensitivity to sound on the affected side. The onset of facial paralysis is sometimes preceded by pain behind the ear or a feeling of facial stiffness. Symptoms are the result of rapid demyelination of the nerve, which completely interrupts its function. The person is unable to blink on the affected side, so the eye appears to tear constantly. Difficulty swallowing is another common complaint. Symptoms typically develop over 24 to 36 hours but can also be fully present when the individual wakens from sleep. The diagnosis is one of exclusion and is established from the history and classic presenting symptoms. Complications include corneal abrasions and permanent facial weakness.

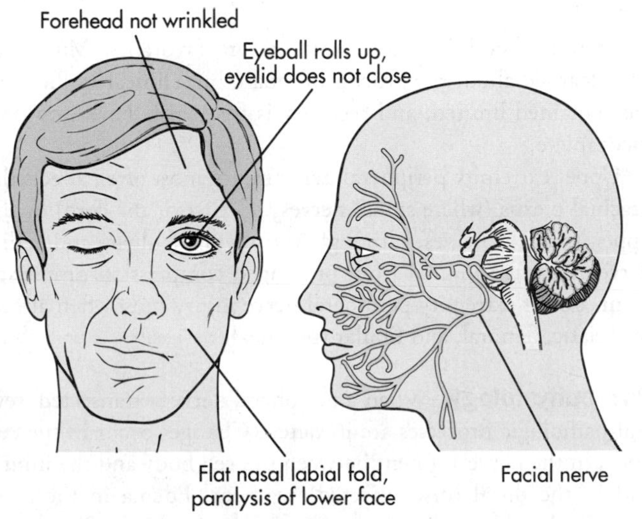

Figure 50-18 Bell's palsy.

Collaborative Care Management. Treatment with steroids is generally believed to improve outcomes in persons with Bell's palsy.[13] Combined treatment with corticosteroids and antiviral agents may further improve outcomes.[4,15] Nursing care focuses on the prevention of complications. Eye care is essential because the patient is unable to blink or close the eyelid on the affected side. Injury prevention and airway protection are also priorities for care.

PATIENT/FAMILY TEACHING. Patients with Bell's palsy require repeated reassurance about the temporary nature of this frightening syndrome, which may literally appear overnight. Teaching focuses on self-care and injury prevention strategies, since the patient will need to maintain this care at home during the weeks or months that may elapse before recovery is complete (see Patient/Family Teaching box on p. 1486).

▶ ARE You READY?

Bell's palsy is related to dysfunction of which cranial nerve?

1. CN II
2. CN III
3. CN V
4. CN VII

Peripheral Nerve Trauma

Etiology and Epidemiology. The peripheral nerves are vulnerable to injury from athletic injuries, vehicular accidents, mechanical and equipment injury, falls, and acts of violence. Chronic nerve compression and entrapment can also result in nerve damage. Well-known syndromes such as carpal tunnel are described in Chapter 53. The mechanisms of injury in peripheral nerve trauma include partial or complete transection, contusion, compression, ischemia, avulsion, stretch trauma, and electrical or thermal burns. Peripheral nerves possess the potential to

Nursing Care Plan

Patient With Trigeminal Neuralgia

Data The patient is a 56-year-old woman in whom trigeminal neuralgia was diagnosed 3 years ago after a severe tooth infection. Her initial episode was short and followed by an extended period of remission, but over the past year the attacks occurred more frequently and lasted longer each time. Treatments have included trials of gabapentin (Neurontin) and carbamazepine (Tegretol). Although she dislikes the drowsiness that occurs from carbamazepine, it seems to control her pain best. She has difficulty eating because of pain and is losing weight. She was forced to take disability retirement this year because of incapacitating pain. She has a generally unkempt appearance and a foul odor to her breath. She states that she rarely leaves her house except for clinic appointments.

Her physician has suggested surgery as the next logical step in her care. She is reluctant to agree to microsurgery despite the incapacitating nature of her pain episodes because she fears it will not be successful.

Nursing Diagnosis

Chronic pain related to activation of trigger zones along the trigeminal nerve pathway

Outcomes

- Patient will report satisfactory control of pain by rating it as less than 3 on a scale of 0 to 10.

Related NOC Outcomes

- Pain Control
- Pain: Disruptive Effects
- Pain Level

Related NIC Interventions

- Analgesic Administration
- Coping Enhancement
- Pain Management

Nursing Interventions/Rationales

- Assess current pain management strategies and their effectiveness (pharmacologic and nonpharmacologic). *To establish a baseline for measuring effectiveness of new pain control strategies and to determine if other measures need to be considered.*
- Assess patient's knowledge of specific trigger activities for pain (chewing, talking, smiling or laughing, heat or cold, drafts, pressure, grooming, or mouth care). *To identify factors that can be manipulated by pain control interventions to reduce pain without compromising the patient's ability to talk, perform oral care, or eat.*
- Explore acceptability of cognitive and behavioral strategies to use in pain management (relaxation, imagery, distraction). *The patient must believe that nonpharmacologic strategies can be effective adjuncts to pain management.*
- Consult with pain management service regarding options for drug therapy. *Chronic pain necessitates a concentrated approach to management, which may be multidisciplinary.*
- Encourage patient to take medication at regular intervals and to use analgesics at the first sign of pain. *Steady blood levels increase drug effectiveness, and analgesics work more effectively if administered before pain reaches severe levels.*

Nursing Diagnosis

Imbalanced nutrition: less than body requirements related to fear of triggering pain with eating

Outcomes

- Patient will maintain weight within 5 pounds of baseline.

Related NOC Outcomes

- Nutritional Status
- Nutritional Status: Nutrient Intake
- Pain Control

Related NIC Interventions

- Nutrition Management
- Nutritional Monitoring
- Pain Management

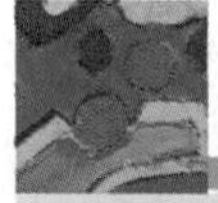

PATIENT/FAMILY TEACHING
The Patient With Bell's Palsy

Most patients with Bell's palsy can be adequately managed in the community setting, and the nurse focuses on offering support and educating the patient and family about the disease process. Teaching points include:

- Protect the affected eye from injury and infection. Use artificial tears during the daytime and patch or tape the eye shut when outdoors and at night to protect it from abrasion, wind, and light damage.
- Eat and drink only in an upright position. The consistency of foods may need to be altered so swallowing is easier.
- Massage of the affected side may be useful.
- As nerve function begins to return, facial exercises may be done to help regain facial muscle tone.

regenerate after injury if conditions are favorable. Much has been learned about the process of repair, but clinical application has remained limited, and recovery is frequently both slow and incomplete.

Upper extremity peripheral nerve injury most often affects the brachial plexus (where spinal nerves C5-T1 exit the cord) or the upper thoracic nerves, although the median, ulnar, and radial nerves are often injured from prolonged compression or entrapment. Lower extremity peripheral nerve injury most often affects the sciatic, femoral, and fibular (peroneal) nerves.

Pathophysiology. When a peripheral nerve is transected, several pathologic processes are initiated. Changes occur in the cell body, in the nerve segment between the cell body and the injury, and in the distal (disconnected) segment. Edema in the axon fibers leads to demyelination and degeneration of the fibers, progressing proximally back toward the nerve cell body. At the same

Nursing Interventions/Rationales

- Complete 24-hour recall assessment of dietary intake. *Provides objective data to determine adequacy of diet.*
- Explore dietary modifications to increase dietary intake without exacerbating pain (consistency, texture, liquid supplements, adding skim milk powder to foods). *An inadequate diet can be supplemented with powders and formulas to increase nutrient intake without increasing volume substantially.*
- Avoid empty calories. *Since eating triggers pain and pain affects the amount of food eaten, all foods ingested must be nutritious and of sufficient value to meet metabolic needs.*
- Add liquid multivitamin supplement to food or fluid. *To ensure adequate intake of vitamins in case of insufficient intake in the diet.*
- Ensure adequate fluid intake. *To prevent dehydration, since patient is reluctant to drink.*
- Help patient explore ways to avoid pain while eating (mechanically soft foods, well-balanced liquid supplements). *Success in avoiding pain will allow patient to consume more nutrients.*
- Place food on the unaffected side of the mouth. *May reduce pain sensation, which will allow greater consumption of food.*
- Involve dietitian in planning. *Dietitian has expert knowledge about community access to appropriate supplements.*
- Teach patient to weigh self weekly and maintain weight record. *Helps track progress in meeting nutritional goals.*

Nursing Diagnosis

Impaired oral mucous membrane related to inadequate oral hygiene secondary to fear of pain

Outcomes

- Patient will maintain health of teeth and gums without exacerbating pain.

Related NOC Outcomes

- Oral Hygiene

Related NIC Interventions

- Oral Health Maintenance
- Oral Health Promotion

Nursing Interventions/Rationales

- Inspect oral tissue on each visit. *Provides baseline for evaluation of progress or problems.*
- Assess patient's current practice for oral care and evaluate effectiveness. *Provides baseline for planning interventions.*
- Explore alternatives for oral care with patient (swabs, Water Pik, mouthwashes). *Provides alternatives to patient for achieving mouth care goals.*
- Encourage patient to carefully rinse mouth after eating. *Helps reduce mouth odor from retained food particles and destruction of tooth enamel from plaque accumulation.*
- Encourage patient to perform thorough oral hygiene between pain episodes. *Allows patient to take advantage of pain-free intervals for performing more thorough mouth and teeth care.*
- Refer patient to dentist for regular assessment and care. *Infection in teeth or mouth is a common trigger for increased pain episodes. Frequent dental assessments help identify early infections so they can be treated.*

Evaluation

Evaluation is based on comparing the patient's outcomes with desired outcomes.

time the distal nerve also degenerates and retracts (**wallerian degeneration**). The axon and its myelin sheath break down, and the debris is cleared by an aggressive phagocytic process. A gap occurs in the nerve axon, and motor and sensory functions are lost distal to the injury. The body attempts to repair the damage through two major processes. Schwann cells in the neurilemma proliferate from both ends of the injury to form neurilemmal cords, which act as guidewires for the regenerating axon (Figure 50-19). The axon cylinder generates multiple tiny buds or sprouts at its tip, and if some of the sprouts are successful in using the neurilemmal cords to cross the transected gap, they achieve union with the distal stump. Nerve fibers regenerate at a rate of about 1 to 4 mm/day, and major injuries require months to repair.

Like SCI, peripheral nerve injury may be described as complete or incomplete. With complete injury, all the neurons at the site of injury are disrupted, resulting in loss of all distal motor and sensory function. Residual motor or sensory activity distal to the injury indicates that some neurons remain intact, and the injury is incomplete. When the nerve has been completely transected, the axons have no pathway to follow as they regenerate, and natural recovery is often poor. With incomplete transection, the surviving axons provide a path for the regenerating axons to follow, and natural recovery is more likely.

The clinical manifestations of peripheral nerve injury depend on the location of the trauma and the specific function(s) of the involved nerve or nerves. Because peripheral nerves contain both sensory and motor components, deficits frequently exist in both functions distal to the site. Motor alterations include LMN signs such as flaccid paralysis and muscle wasting. Sensory symptoms include pain, burning, and abnormal sensations in response to stimuli. Autonomic changes may also be present after injury. Damage to sympathetic fibers creates an initial warm phase in which the affected area is dry and warm to the touch and flushed

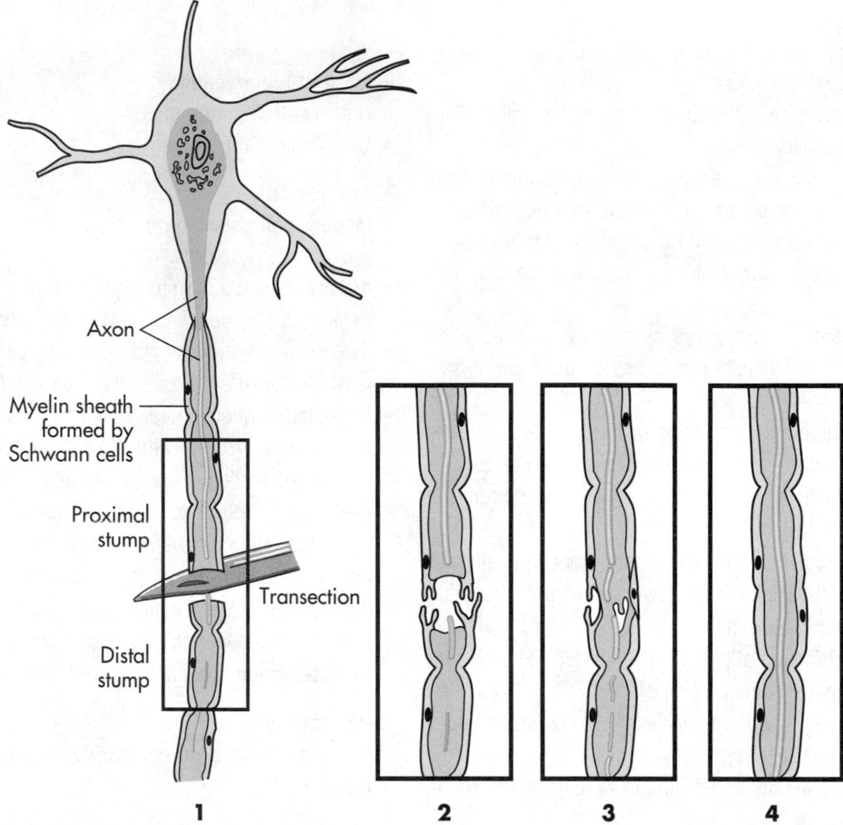

Figure 50-19 Process of repair and regeneration of a peripheral nerve. *1,* After nerve transection, degeneration and retraction of the distal stump occur within 24 hours. *2,* Healing begins as Schwann cells of the neurilemma proliferate from both proximal and distal stumps, forming neurilemmal cords that will guide the regenerating axon. *3,* Some unmyelinated axon sprouts that are generated from the proximal stump find their way to the distal stump, guided by the neurilemmal cords. *4,* The axon regrows and remyelinates.

in appearance. A cold phase may follow in several weeks in which the extremity becomes cold and cyanotic.

Collaborative Care Management. Peripheral nerve injury is suspected on the basis of the injury history and presenting symptoms. Diagnostic tests include standard x-ray films to evaluate for fractures or other bony changes, myelogram, CT, and MRI. Electromyography and nerve conduction studies may be used to determine the presence and extent of any residual connection between the nerve and muscle.

Microsurgical techniques now allow skilled surgeons to successfully explore the injury and perform decompression and repair, with the goal of improved motor function. Early surgical intervention is performed when the ends of the nerve are sharply transected to realign the proximal and distal portions of the nerve and encourage regeneration. Successfully realigned nerves remyelinate and regrow to nearly their former size. The conduction velocity of regenerated nerves is typically about 80% of normal, and the chances for functional return are good. If nerve injury appears incomplete, surgery is often delayed for 3 to 6 months to allow for natural recovery. Surgery is also performed if the nerve is entrapped or compression is ongoing.

Physical and occupational therapy are initiated as soon as possible after the injury because the loss of innervation quickly causes

PATIENT/FAMILY TEACHING

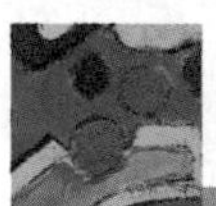

The Patient With Peripheral Nerve Injury

In addition to instruction about the type of peripheral nerve injury and the individualized treatment plan, teaching points for the patient with peripheral nerve injury include:

- Monitor the affected area closely. Protect the affected area from temperature extremes, such as cold weather or a hot bath.
- Inspect the skin over the affected area frequently for evidence of breakdown. Cleanse the skin gently and dry thoroughly. Lanolin creams or cocoa butter may be used to counteract dryness and scaling.
- Weakness and sensory loss may limit your ability to perform activities of daily living. The nurse and therapists will instruct you on the use of assistive devices or techniques.
- The rehabilitation process after peripheral nerve injury is prolonged, and recovery is not guaranteed. Careful protection of the affected area is important to optimize your chance for recovery.

Preparing for Practice

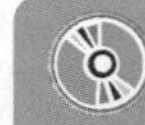

CD-ROM Activity Select Exercise Eight: Spinal Cord and Peripheral Nerve Problems on the Companion CD.

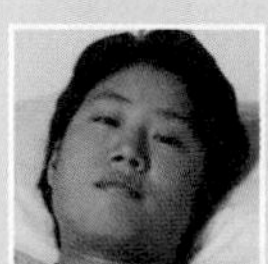

Preparing for Practice

Patient: *Andrea Wang,* **Room 310**

Andrea Wang, a 20-year-old Asian-American woman, suffered a spinal cord injury in a diving accident.

Assessment

View the patient's **Report**.
Open the patient's **Medical Record** to familiarize yourself with her care. Specifically, review the following areas: History & Physical, Physicians' Orders, and Nurses' Notes.
Conduct a **Patient Interview**. As you conduct your interview, focus primarily on data that will be helpful in planning care for this patient. Record the data you collect.

Nursing Diagnoses, Outcomes, and Interventions

1. What diagnostic studies were done in the emergency department (ED)? What did the results of these tests reveal?
2. According to the ED documentation, what was Andrea Wang's mechanism of injury?
3. What type of spinal injury did Andrea Wang experience: hyperflexion, hyperextension, or compression?
4. What concerns emerge from the Nurses' Notes?
5. What type of changes in reflexes should you expect Andrea Wang to exhibit immediately after spinal trauma? What changes are expected as cord edema subsides? What intervention was done in the emergency department that is associated with loss of function?
6. What are the six types of syndromes associated with incomplete spinal cord injury? Which of these is Andrea Wang experiencing?
7. How long should spinal shock last; and how can you determine whether it is resolving?
8. Based on your assessment findings and your knowledge of spinal cord injury, identify two high-priority nursing diagnoses for Ms. Wang. What nursing actions would you implement, and how will you measure the effectiveness of your interventions?

the muscles to atrophy. Physical therapy includes range of motion, resistive exercise, splints and braces to support proper positioning and immobilization, and possibly electrical nerve stimulation to the affected muscles to minimize atrophic changes. The flaccid muscles are unable to successfully balance their opposing muscles (i.e., flexors versus extensors), and the risk of contracture is high. Positioning in neutral or counter positions is essential to help prevent joint deformities. If the associated tendons are allowed to shorten, the contracture will be permanent.

PATIENT/FAMILY TEACHING. Patients with peripheral nerve injuries need extensive teaching and reteaching about the injury and its effects, as well as any planned treatment. Recovery is slow, and it is important for patients to understand the importance of following all positioning and activity restrictions during the months after the injury (see Patient/Family Teaching box).

Critical Thinking

1. A 19-year-old man with a C6 SCI was injured 5 weeks ago. He has recently developed muscle spasticity, which is becoming increasingly severe. His family is optimistic that the spasms are an indication he will eventually walk again. How would you respond to them? What nursing interventions can you implement to reduce the spasticity?
2. What services exist in your community or region to care for patients with SCIs? Is there a specialty neurotrauma unit? Who offers acute specialty SCI rehabilitation? Do they accept patients without health insurance? If a family cannot provide care for a ventilator-dependent person with a C3 level injury, what choices are available for long-term care? Do any home health agencies offer services for this type of patient? What would this level of care cost per month?

References

1. Ahn SH et al: Gabapentin effect on neuropathic pain compared among patients with spinal cord injury and different durations of symptoms, *Spine* 28(4):341-346, 2001.
2. American Association of Neurological Surgeons, Congress of Neurological Surgeons, Section on Disorders of the Spine and Peripheral Nerves: Blood pressure management after acute spinal cord injury, *Neurosurgery* 50 (3 Suppl):58-62, 2002.
3. American Association of Neurological Surgeons, Congress of Neurological Surgeons, Section on Disorders of the Spine and Peripheral Nerves: Pharmacological therapy after acute cervical spinal cord injury, *Neurosurgery* 50 (3 Suppl):63-72, 2002.
4. Axelsson S, Lindberg S, Stjernquist-Desatnik A: Outcome of treatment with valacyclovir and prednisone in patients with Bell's palsy, *Ann Otol Rhinol Laryngol* 112(3):197-201, 2003.
5. Baydur A, Adkins RH, Milic-Emili J: Lung mechanics in individuals with spinal cord injury: effects of injury level and posture, *J Appl Physiol* 90(2):405-411, 2001.
6. Brown C: Surgical treatment of trigeminal neuralgia, *AORN J* 78(5): 744-758, 2003.
7. Burchiel KJ, Hsu FPK: Pain and spasticity after spinal cord injury, *Spine* 26(Suppl 24):146-160, 2001.
8. Burke DA et al: Incidence rates and populations at risk for spinal cord injury: a regional study, *Spinal Cord* 39(5):274-278, 2001.
9. Burns AS, Ditunno JF: Establishing prognosis and maximizing functional outcomes after spinal cord injury, *Spine* 26(Suppl 24):137-145, 2001.
10. Burns AS, Rivas DA, Ditunno JF: The management of neurogenic bladder and sexual dysfunction after spinal cord injury, *Spine* 26(Suppl 24):129-136, 2001.
11. Dryden DM et al: Utilization of health services following spinal cord injury: a 6-year follow-up study, *Spinal Cord* 42(9):513-525, 2004.
12. Finnerup NB et al: Treatment of spinal cord injury pain, *Pain: Clin Updates* 9(2), 2001, accessed from website: www.iasp-pain.org/PCU01-2.
13. Groah SL et al: Spinal cord injury medicine, part 5, Preserving wellness and independence of the aging patient with spinal cord injury: a primary care approach for the rehabilitation specialist, *Arch Phys Med Rehabil* 83 (Suppl 1):82-89, 2002.
14. Grogan PM, Gronseth GS: Practice parameter: steroids, acyclovir, and surgery for Bell's palsy (an evidence-based review), *Neurology* 56(7): 830-836, 2001.

15. Hato N et al: Efficacy of early treatment of Bell's palsy with oral acyclovir and prednisolone, *Otol Neurotol* 24(6):948-951, 2003.
16. Irwin ZN et al: Variations in injury patterns, treatment, and outcome for spinal fracture and paralysis in adult versus geriatric patients, *Spine* 29(7):796-802, 2004.
17. Kalkanis SN et al: Microvascular decompression surgery in the United States, 1996 to 2000: mortality rates, morbidity rates, and the effects of hospital and surgeon volumes, *Neurosurgery* 52(6):1251-1262, 2003.
18. La Rosa G et al: Does early decompression improve neurological outcome of spinal cord injured patients? Appraisal of the literature using a meta-analytical approach, *Spinal Cord* 42(9):503-512, 2004.
19. Levendoglu F et al: Gabapentin is a first line drug for the treatment of neuropathic pain in spinal cord injury, *Spine* 29(7):743-751, 2004.
20. Middleton JW, Keast JR: Artificial autonomic reflexes: using functional electrical stimulation to mimic bladder reflexes after injury or disease, *Auton Neurosci* 113(1-2):3-15, 2004.
21. Middleton JW et al: Patterns of morbidity and rehospitalisation following spinal cord injury, *Spinal Cord* 42(6):359-367, 2004.
22. National Spinal Cord Injury Statistical Center: *Spinal cord injury: facts and figures at a glance*, accessed Aug 2004 from website: www.spinalcord.uab.edu.
23. Nicholson BD: Evaluation and treatment of central pain syndromes, *Neurology* 62(5 Suppl 2):30-36, 2004.
24. Papadopoulos SM et al: Immediate spinal cord decompression for cervical spinal cord injury: feasibility and outcome, *J Trauma* 52(2):323-332, 2002.
25. Putzke JE et al: Long-term use of gabapentin for treatment of pain after traumatic spinal cord injury, *Clin J Pain* 18(2):116-121, 2002.
26. Rogers FB et al: Practice management guidelines for the prevention of venous thromboembolism in trauma patients: the EAST practice management guidelines work group, *J Trauma* 53(1):142-164, 2002.
27. Sekhon LHS, Fehlings MG: Epidemiology, demographics, and pathophysiology of acute spinal cord injury, *Spine* 26(Suppl 24):2-12, 2001.
28. Stevens RD et al: Critical care and perioperative management in traumatic spinal cord injury, *J Neurosurg Anesthesiol* 15(3):215-229, 2003.
29. To TP et al: Gabapentin for neuropathic pain following spinal cord injury, *Spinal Cord* 40(6):282-285, 2002.
30. Turner JA et al: Chronic pain associated with spinal cord injuries: a community survey, *Arch Phys Med Rehabil* 82(4):501-508, 2001.
31. Warms CA et al: Treatments for chronic pain associated with spinal cord injuries: many are tried, few are helpful, *Clin J Pain* 18(3):154-163, 2002.
32. Widerström-Noga EG, Felipe-Cuervo E, Yezierski RP: Chronic pain after spinal cord injury: interference with sleep and daily activities, *Arch Phys Med Rehabil* 82(11):1571-1577, 2001.
33. Yim SY et al: A comparison of bowel care patterns in patients with spinal cord injury: upper motor neuron bowel vs lower motor neuron bowel, *Spinal Cord* 39(4):204-207, 2001.

evolve Visit the Evolve website: http://evolve.elsevier.com/Monahan/medsurg

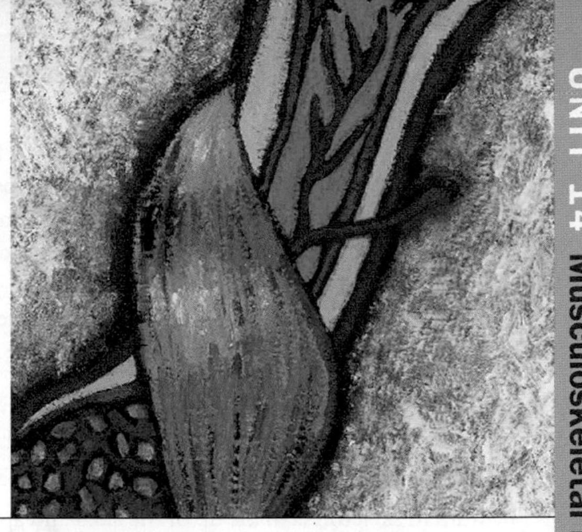

CHAPTER 51 Assessment of the Musculoskeletal System

by Jane F. Marek

OBJECTIVES

After studying this chapter, the learner should be able to:

1. Describe the structure and function of the different tissues that compose the musculoskeletal system.
2. Analyze the interrelationship of the tissues of the musculoskeletal system with overall function of the system.
3. Discuss the physiologic changes that occur in the musculoskeletal system as a result of the aging process.
4. Describe components of the nursing assessment of the musculoskeletal system, including the health history and physical examination.
5. Explain the diagnostic tests indicated for the person with a musculoskeletal problem, the rationale for each test, and appropriate nursing responsibilities associated with each test.
6. Synthesize a care plan for a person with a musculoskeletal problem, using relevant subjective and objective data and results of diagnostic tests.

KEY TERMS

arthroscopy, p. 1521
articular, p. 1500
callus, p. 1496
cancellous, p. 1492
contracture, p. 1512
cortical, p. 1492
crepitus, p. 1512
diaphysis, p. 1492
diarthrodial, p. 1503
epiphysis, p. 1492
haversian system, p. 1493
metaphysis, p. 1492
osteoblasts, p. 1493
osteoclasts, p. 1493
osteocytes, p. 1493
synovium, p. 1501

People often take the ability to move about freely in the environment for granted. Movements as simple as making a fist or as complex as a ballerina performing a cabriole depend on the structure, function, and integrity of the musculoskeletal system. The musculoskeletal system is one of the body's largest systems and accounts for more than 50% of the body's weight. This dynamic system is made up of bones, joints, muscles, and supporting structures, all the components working together to produce movement and to supply structure and support to the body. Any disturbance in this well-integrated system results in musculoskeletal dysfunction. Problems can develop as a result of disease or trauma to the system or surrounding structures. Problems arising outside of the musculoskeletal system, such as endocrine or neurologic disease, may also directly affect the system, resulting in some degree of disability.

Musculoskeletal problems affect hundred of millions of people worldwide, with a huge economic burden to society. Musculoskeletal disability affects persons across the life span, from skeletal and developmental abnormalities in children to crippling joint disease and osteoporotic fractures in older adults. In the United States, musculoskeletal problems are the leading cause of physician office visits, with more than 130 million visits annually, and are a leading cause of disability. One in three Americans is affected by musculoskeletal problems.

As a result of these concerns, the World Health Organization initiated the Bone and Joint Decade in 2000. More than 50 countries and 750 health organizations have endorsed the initiative. President George W. Bush declared 2002 to 2011 the U.S. Bone and Joint Decade, and each October, National Awareness Week is celebrated to educate the public about prevention of musculoskeletal disease. More information is available at www.boneandjointdecade.org and www.usbjd.org. The goals of the Bone and Joint Decade are to:

- Increase public awareness of the growing burden of musculoskeletal disorders on society and persons worldwide
- Empower patients to participate in their own health care and treatment
- Increase global funding for research on disease prevention and treatment strategies
- Promote cost-effective prevention and treatment

Planning appropriate interventions for individuals with alterations in musculoskeletal functioning requires a careful and thorough assessment based on the nurse's knowledge of the anatomy and physiology of the musculoskeletal system. The patient's reaction to the disability and implications of diagnostic studies must also be considered. This chapter discusses the anatomy and physiology of the musculoskeletal system, methods and rationale for collecting subjective and objective data from the patient and family, and the relevance of selected diagnostic studies.

Anatomy and Physiology

Bones

The human skeleton is made up of the axial and appendicular skeletons, which consist of 206 bones (Figure 51-1). The *axial* skeleton consists of 80 bones—the hyoid bone and those of the skull, vertebral column, and thorax. The remaining 126 bones comprise the *appendicular* skeleton, which contains the bones of the upper and lower extremities, pectoral girdle, and pelvic girdle (os coxae). The skeleton makes up 14% of the weight of the adult body.

Types. Bones are divided into four types, according to their shape: (1) long (femur, humerus); (2) short (carpals), which are often cuboidal; (3) flat (skull); and (4) irregular (vertebrae). Each bone is composed of **cancellous** (spongy) and **cortical** (compact) bone. In the long bones the cancellous portions are found in the ends of the bones, and cortical bone is in the shaft. The short and irregular bones have an inner core of cancellous bone with an outer layer of cortical bone. Flat bones have two outer plates of cortical bone with an inner layer of cancellous bone. Cancellous bone is also found in the ends of long bones and in the iliac crests, tibiae, and sternum.

Long bones (Figure 51-2) are made up of a diaphysis, a metaphysis, and an epiphysis. The **diaphysis** (midportion) is made of thick cortical bone and contains the medullary cavity, where the marrow is stored. The diaphyseal cavity is composed primarily of fatty tissues and contains yellow marrow, which is not capable of hematopoiesis except in times of stress. The endosteum is a layer of connective tissue that lines both yellow and red marrow cavities. The marrow cavity of the diaphysis connects to the cancellous bone of the **metaphysis,** or broad neck, of the long bone. The **epiphysis,** or broad end, of the bone contains the red marrow, which is responsible for hematopoiesis. The epiphysis is made up of spongy bone covered with a thin layer of cortical bone. The broad end allows weight to be distributed over a greater surface area. A cartilaginous growth plate, or *epiphyseal plate,* separates the metaphysis from the epiphysis in children. The epiphysis and metaphysis merge after puberty when the epiphyseal plate calcifies. This growth plate, easily seen on x-ray examination in children, is undetectable in adults (see Figure 51-2).

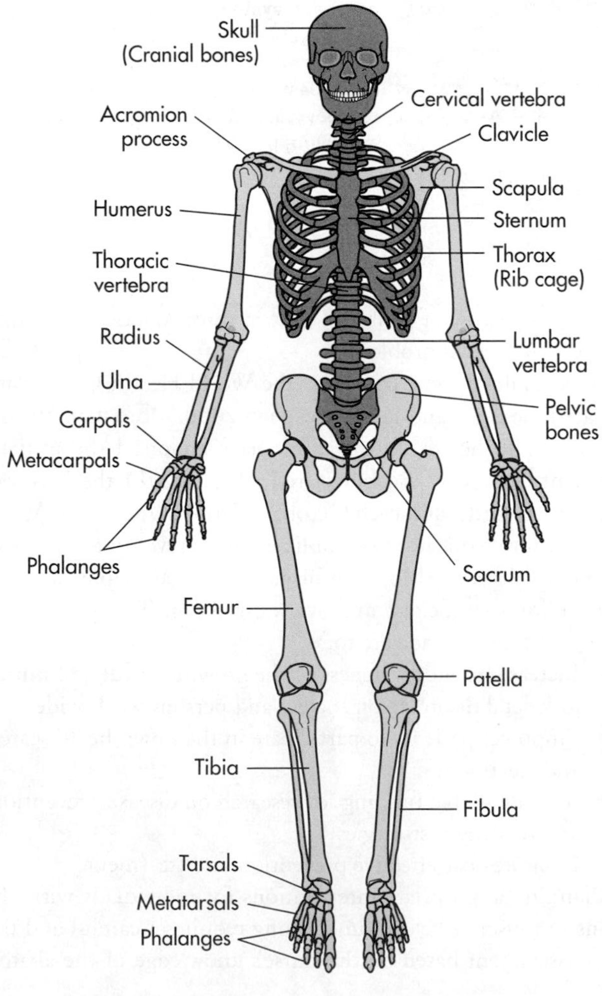

Figure 51-1 Axial and appendicular skeleton.

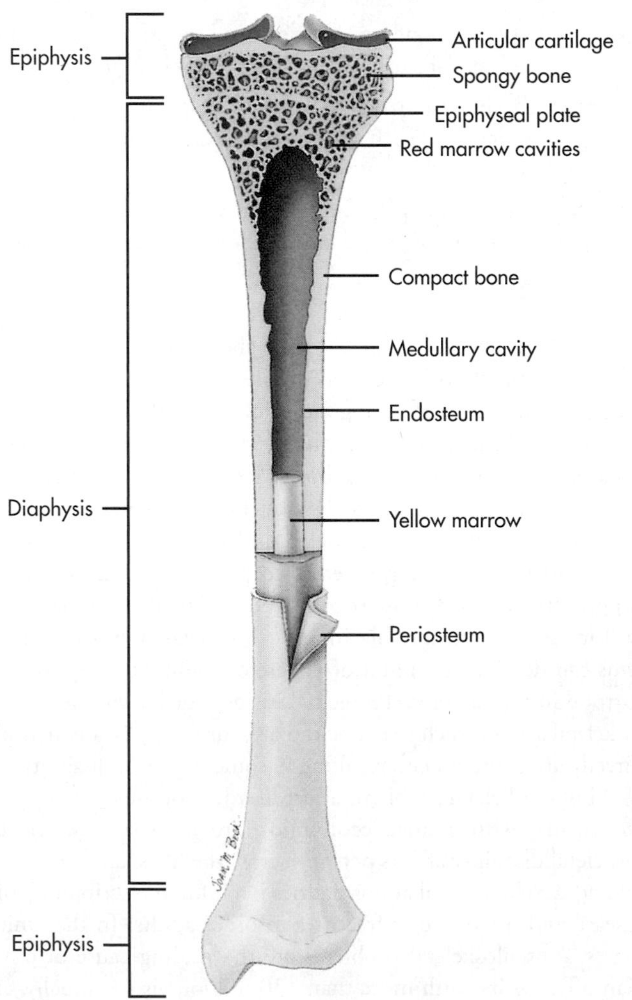

Figure 51-2 Cross section of a long bone.

Structure. Bone, like other connective tissue, is made up of cells, fibers, and ground substance. Unlike other connective tissue, bone also contains crystallized minerals, which give it rigidity (Table 51-1). Bone is a dynamic substance, continuously synthesizing and resorbing bone tissue. Bone cells allow growth, repair, and remodeling. Bone formation begins in the fetal stage as cartilage formation and continues throughout life. In the mature individual the first step in bone formation is the initiation of an organic matrix by the bone cells. Next, mineralization takes place as minerals are bound to collagen fibers, providing support and tensile strength to bone.

Three types of bone cells are found in the body. **Osteoblasts**, or bone-forming cells, are responsible for laying down new bone. They produce type I collagen and respond to changing levels of parathyroid hormone (PTH). New bone is formed as the osteoblasts produce osteoid and mineralize the bone matrix. Once this is accomplished, osteoblasts become **osteocytes** and are trapped in the mineralized bone matrix. Osteocytes maintain the mineral content and organic elements of bone. The third type of bone cell, **osteoclasts**, resorbs bone during growth and repair. They are able to resorb bone by secreting citric and lactic acid and collagenases, which dissolve minerals and break down collagen.

Bone is primarily composed of organic matrix and calcium salts. Collagen fibers account for 90% to 95% of the organic matrix; ground substance makes up the remainder. The collagen fibers extend along the lines of tensional force and give bone its great tensile strength. The ground substance functions as a medium for the diffusion of nutrients, oxygen, minerals, and wastes between bone tissue and blood vessels. Ground substance contains extracellular fluid and proteoglycans, particularly chondroitin sulfate and hyaluronic acid, which help control the deposition of calcium salts. The bone morphogenic proteins, important substances responsible for inducing cartilage formation, are also found in the bone matrix. The glycoproteins found in the matrix play a role in the calcification, resorption, and metabolism of bone. The minerals contained in the matrix are primarily calcium and phosphate. Hydroxyapatite, the primary bone salt, is formed as a result of the mineralization and crystal formation of calcium and phosphate. Mineralization is the final step in the process of bone formation.

Both cancellous and cortical bone contains the same structural elements, but they differ in the organization of the bone matrix (Figure 51-3). Concentric layers of bone matrix are called lamellae.

The basic unit of cortical bone is the **haversian system**. At the center of this arrangement of concentric rings is the haversian canal, which runs through the long axes of bones. This canal contains blood vessels (capillaries, arterioles, or venules), nerve fibers, and lymphatics. Blood vessels in the canal communicate with blood vessels in the periosteum. Lacunae are small spaces between the rings of the lamellae and contain osteocytes. Canaliculi, very small canals that connect the lacunae and the haversian canal, run parallel to the long axis of the bone. This connection allows the osteocytes access to the nutrient supply. Haversian units (lamellae, haversian canal, lacunae, canaliculi) fit closely together in cortical bone. The hardness and density of cortical bone give it strength and rigidity.

In contrast, cancellous bone lacks haversian systems. The lamellae are arranged not in concentric layers but in connecting plates or bars called trabeculae, which form an irregular meshwork. The pattern of the trabecular bone depends on the direction of stress in the

TABLE 51-1 STRUCTURAL ELEMENTS OF BONE

Structural Element	Function
BONE CELLS	
Osteoblasts	Synthesize collagen and proteoglycans; stimulate osteoclast resorptive activity
Osteocytes	Maintain bone matrix
Osteoclasts	Resorb bone; assist with mineral homeostasis
BONE MATRIX	
Collagen fibers	Lend support and tensile strength
Proteoglycans	Control transport of ionized materials through matrix
Bone morphogenic proteins: BMP-1, BMP-2A, BMP-3, BMP-7	Induce cartilage and bone formation
Glycoproteins	
Sialoprotein	Promotes calcification
Osteocalcin	Inhibits calcium-phosphate precipitation; promotes bone resorption
Laminin	Stabilizes basement membranes in bones
Osteonectin	Binds calcium in bones
Albumin	Transports essential elements to matrix; maintains osmotic pressure of bone fluid
Alpha-glycoprotein	Promotes calcification
Minerals (elements)	
Calcium	Crystallizes to lend rigidity and compressive strength
Phosphate	Regulates vitamin D and thereby promotes mineralization

From McCance KL, Huether SE: *Pathophysiology: the biologic basis for disease in adults and children*, ed 4, St Louis, 2002, Mosby.

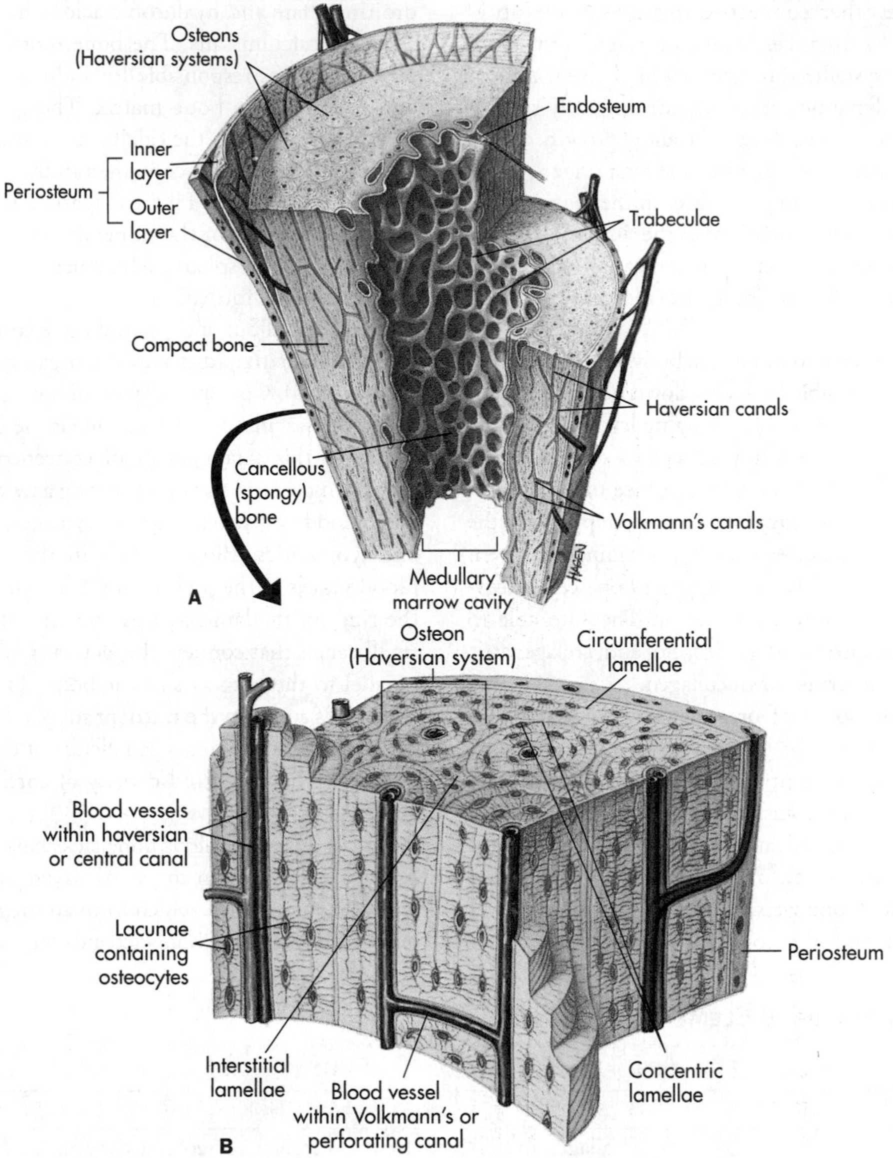

Figure 51-3 Structure of compact and cancellous bone. **A,** Longitudinal section of a long bone showing both cancellous and compact bone. **B,** Magnified view of compact bone.

particular bone. Red marrow fills the spaces between the trabeculae. Lacunae, rich in osteocytes, are distributed among the trabeculae and connected by canaliculi. Capillaries flowing through the marrow provide nutrients to the osteocytes. The fine, thready structure of trabecular bone provides strength to cancellous bone while reducing its weight.

The outer, nonarticulating surfaces of long bones are covered with a white fibrous membrane called the periosteum. The outer layer of the periosteum contains blood vessels and nerves that reach the inner bones through Volkmann's canals. Nutrient arteries in the periosteum communicate with the haversian system. Collagenous fibers (Sharpey's fibers) anchor the inner layer of the periosteum to the bone.

The surfaces of bones contain grooves or ridges for nerves and blood vessels, prominences for muscular attachments, and openings for blood vessels and muscles. Articulating surfaces are covered with hyaline cartilage (Figure 51-4).

Blood supply to bone is maintained through the haversian canals, periosteal vasculature, and vessels located in the marrow and ends of bones. Bones are supplied with sensory nerve endings in the periosteum that connect with the central nervous system.

Function. Bones have five functions:

1. *Support:* The skeletal framework supports body tissues and gives form and shape to the body.
2. *Protection:* The bones protect body organs; for example, the bony casing of the skull protects the brain, and the bones of the thorax and pelvis protect the heart, lungs, and reproductive organs.
3. *Movement:* Bones allow for movement by muscular attachments to bone and by joint movement.
4. *Hematopoiesis:* The marrow of some bones has a hematopoietic function. Normally after birth, red blood cell (RBC) production occurs only in the bone marrow

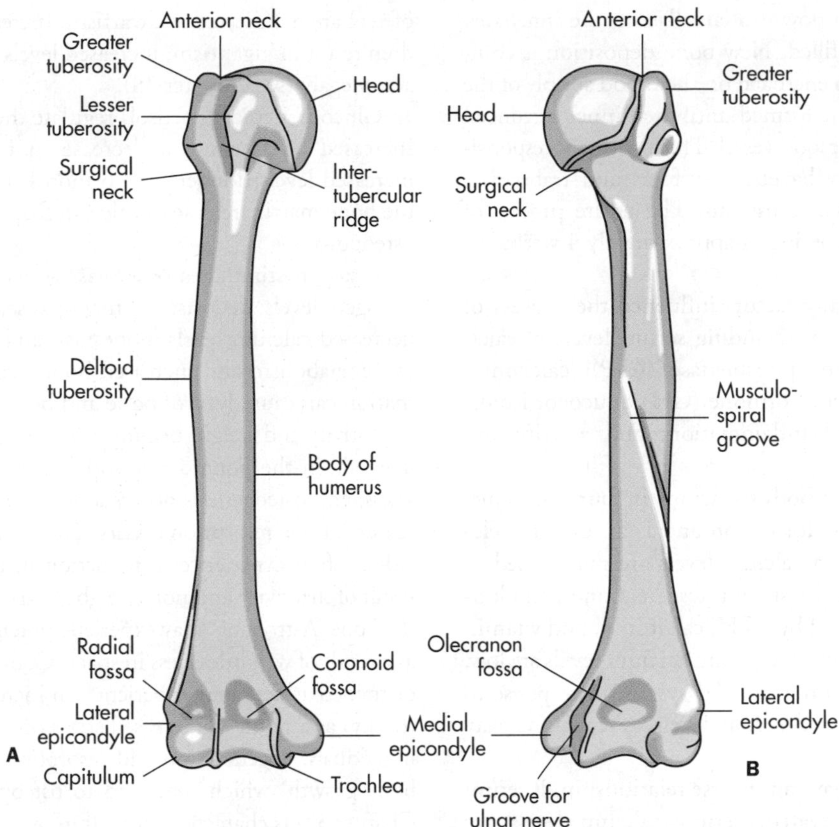

Figure 51-4 A, Anterior view of right humerus. **B,** Posterior view of right humerus. Note groove for ulnar nerve and tuberosities for muscular attachments.

(medullary hematopoiesis). Extramedullary hematopoiesis is usually a sign of disease. In adults the marrow in the bones of the skull, vertebrae, ribs, sternum, shoulders, and pelvis produces RBCs. The hematopoietic function of bone continues throughout life. Blood cells are produced to replace those lost through disease, bleeding, and cellular aging. An increase in RBC production can be triggered by anemia, hemorrhage, infection, stress, and other disorders that deplete their stores. Medullary hematopoiesis is accomplished by conversion of yellow marrow to red, increased differentiation of daughter cells, and increased growth of stem cells.

5. *Mineral homeostasis:* Bones store calcium, phosphate, carbonate, and magnesium, which are necessary for normal cellular function; approximately 99% of the body's calcium is stored in the skeleton.

Bone Growth and Remodeling. Longitudinal growth of the long bones emanates from the epiphyseal cartilage, which thickens because of rapid proliferation of the cartilage and undergoes ossification (endochondral ossification). Growth in the diameter of the bone is accomplished as osteoblasts in the periosteum produce new bone on the outside of the bone (intramembranous ossification). Bone reaches maturity after puberty.

Bone is continuously being deposited by osteoblasts and resorbed by active osteoclasts. In the adult, osteoblastic activity occurs on approximately 4% of all surfaces of living bone, resulting in a constant state of bone formation. In contrast, osteoclastic activity is present on less than 1% of the bony surfaces of a normal adult.[1]

Except in growing bones, the rate of bone deposition equals the rate of bone destruction until approximately 35 years of age. Thus the total mass of bone remains constant. The equilibrium between bone destruction and formation fulfills some physiologically important functions. Most important, bone responds to the amount of stress to which it is subjected; bone thickens and strengthens itself in response to a heavy load. Second, bone can also be reshaped in response to alterations in its mechanical function. These responses are in accordance with Wolff's law. Wolff, a German anatomist (1836-1902), stated: "Every change in form and function of bones or their function alone is followed by definite changes in their external configuration in accordance with mathematical laws." Finally, in old bone the organic matrix degenerates and the bone becomes weak and brittle; new organic matrix is necessary to maintain the strength and toughness of bone.

Remodeling is the process by which existing bone is resorbed and new bone replaces the old. In the first phase (activation), bone cell precursors form osteoclasts in response to a stressor or stimulus. In phase 2 (resorption), masses of osteoclasts form a cutting cone and begin to eat away at the bone for approximately 3 weeks, creating a tunnel or cavity 0.2 to 1 mm in length.[1,3] In cancellous bone this tunnel is parallel to the trabeculae; in cortical bone it follows the longitudinal surface of the haversian system. In phase 3 (formation), the tunnel is then invaded by osteoblasts, and new bone (secondary bone) is laid down in lamellae on the inner surface of the tunnel until it is filled. New bone deposition is complete when the bone begins to encroach on the blood supply of the area. Subsequently, lamellae are formed until the tunnel is reduced to a haversian canal around a blood vessel. This process is responsible for the formation of new haversian systems and trabeculae. Areas of new bone are known as osteons. The entire process of remodeling takes place over a period of approximately 4 weeks.

INFLUENCING FACTORS. Many factors influence the process of bone formation and resorption, including serum levels of calcium, phosphorus, and alkaline phosphatase (ALP); calcitonin; vitamin D levels; PTH; growth hormone (GH); glucocorticoids; sex hormones; infection and inflammation; and activity and weight bearing.

Approximately 99% of the body's calcium is found in bone. Calcium is necessary for bone formation and is an essential element in bone structure. Serum calcium levels are maintained in homeostasis by the actions of the small intestine, bones, and kidneys. These organs are regulated by PTH, calcitonin, and vitamin D_1, an inactive form of vitamin D. If serum calcium levels are low, the bone releases calcium into the vascular system in response to stimulation by PTH. Decreased serum levels of calcium delay bone formation.

Phosphorus and calcium have an inverse relationship. If serum levels of phosphorus are elevated, serum calcium levels are decreased. Phosphorus is found in bone and skeletal muscle and, like calcium, is controlled by PTH. Increases in PTH cause a decrease in serum phosphorus levels and increased excretion of phosphorus by the kidney. Bone resorption results in the release of phosphorus into the extracellular fluid.

The enzyme ALP is found in osteoblasts. It is excreted via the biliary tract and is necessary for the use of mineral salts and bone formation. Levels of ALP rise in response to increased osteoblastic activity in the bones (e.g., during fracture healing).

Calcitonin is a hormone produced and secreted primarily by the thyroid gland. Calcitonin inhibits bone resorption, inhibits calcium absorption from the gastrointestinal tract, and increases calcium and phosphorus excretion from the kidneys.

Vitamin D is derived from the action of ultraviolet light on provitamins found in the skin and from vitamin D–enriched foods. Vitamin D is activated in the liver and kidneys through the action of PTH. The activated form, calcitriol, is a hormone necessary for calcium absorption. Activated vitamin D elevates calcium and phosphate levels in the plasma by increasing intestinal absorption of calcium and phosphate and by increasing the release of calcium from bone into the blood. Vitamin D deficiencies can manifest themselves as rickets in children and osteomalacia in adults.

PTH, produced by the parathyroid gland, controls serum calcium and phosphorus levels. Decreased serum calcium levels are the stimulus for release of more PTH to keep the serum calcium levels normal. In conjunction with vitamin D, PTH works to stimulate absorption of calcium and phosphorus by the intestinal mucosa. It also causes mobilization of calcium from the bones by promoting osteoclastic activity and bone resorption.

GH is secreted by the anterior lobe of the pituitary gland and promotes the growth of bone and other tissues. Decreased levels of GH are manifested as dwarfism. Increased levels of GH in children result in gigantism; increased levels of GH in adults result in acromegaly (see Chapter 38).

Glucocorticoids (cortisol) regulate the metabolism of proteins. Increased levels cause a decrease in protein stores. Prolonged increased levels (longer than 6 months) may result in damage to the bone matrix, release of calcium from the bone, and eventually osteoporosis.

Estrogen stimulates osteoblast activity and inhibits PTH. As estrogen levels decrease at menopause, women are at risk for decreased calcium levels, bone loss, and osteoporosis. Androgens cause anabolism and increased bone mass. Infection and inflammation can cause lysis of bone and bone resorption.

Activity and weight bearing affect the structure of bone. Trabeculae within the bone develop and align themselves along lines of stress, and osteogenesis occurs along these lines. If the bone is not stressed, bone resorption occurs. The paraplegic or tetraplegic individual often experiences a reduction in bone mass (atrophy) as a result of inactivity and non–weight-bearing status (lack of stress) on the bone. Astronauts may experience a temporary loss of bone mass as a result of weightlessness in space. Conversely, a marathon runner or trained athlete may experience an increase in bony mass (hypertrophy) as a result of increased stress on bones. In older or inactive individuals, degeneration and resorption occur more rapidly than bone growth, which may lead to osteoporosis. Osteoporosis (see Chapter 53) is characterized by thin, weakened cortices and trabeculae, which render the bone more susceptible to fracture.

PHYSIOLOGY OF BONE HEALING. The process of bone healing is known as callus formation. Fractures and surgical disruption of bone both heal by the same process. Callus formation proceeds in five general stages (Figure 51-5):

1. *Hematoma formation.* Because bone is highly vascular, bleeding occurs at both ends of the fractured bone. Increased capillary permeability permits further extravasation of blood into the injured area. Blood collects in the periosteal sheath or adjacent tissues and fastens the broken ends together.
2. *Fibrin meshwork formation.* Fibroblasts invade the hematoma, forming a fibrin meshwork. White blood cells (WBCs) wall off the area, localizing the inflammation.
3. *Invasion by osteoblasts.* As osteoblasts invade the fibrous union, making it firm, blood vessels develop from capillary buds, establishing a supply for nutrients to build collagen. Granulation tissue, or *procallus*, is formed. Collagen strands become longer and begin to incorporate calcium deposits, and cartilage begins to form. The bone morphogenic proteins, enzymes, and growth factors are active in this stage of bone healing.
4. *Callus formation.* Osteoblasts form woven bone, known as **callus**. Osteoblasts continue to lay the network for bone buildup as osteoclasts destroy dead bone and help synthesize new bone. Collagen strengthens and becomes further impregnated with calcium. Calcium and phosphate are deposited as mineral salts. Lamellar or trabecular bone continues to replace the callus.
5. *Remodeling.* Excess callus is resorbed, and trabecular bone is laid down along lines of stress in accordance with

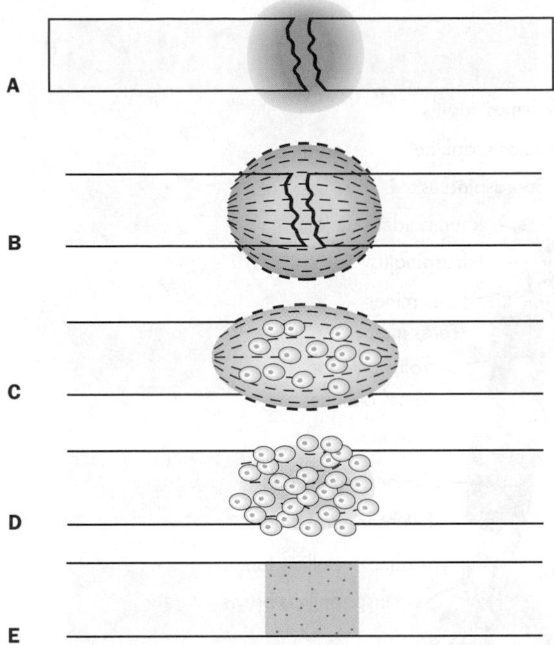

Figure 51-5 Bone healing (schematic representation). **A,** Bleeding at broken ends of bone with subsequent hematoma formation. **B,** Organization of hematoma into fibrous network. **C,** Invasion of osteoblasts, lengthening of collagen strands, and deposition of calcium. **D,** Callus formation: new bone is built up as osteoclasts destroy dead bone. **E,** Remodeling is accomplished as excess callus is resorbed and trabecular bone is laid down.

Wolff's law. Remodeling is an important stage because bone that has not undergone remodeling lacks the mechanical properties necessary for weight bearing.

Factors impeding callus formation include (1) inadequate reduction of the fracture; (2) excessive edema at the fracture site impeding the supply of nutrients to the area of injury; (3) excessive bone loss at the time of injury, which prevents sufficient bridging of the broken ends; (4) inefficient immobilization; (5) infection at the site of injury; (6) bone necrosis; (7) anemia or other systemic conditions; (8) endocrine imbalance; and (9) poor nutritional status. If callus formation does not occur normally and efficiently, the result is nonunion, or an ununited fracture (see Chapter 52).

Muscles

Types. The body has three major types of muscle: visceral, cardiac, and skeletal. Visceral muscle, also known as smooth or involuntary muscle, is found in the blood vessels, stomach, and intestines. Visceral muscle is innervated by the autonomic nervous system and is not under voluntary control. The cardiac muscle, found in the myocardium, has the properties of automaticity, rhythm, and conductivity. The cardiac conduction system and the autonomic nervous system exert control over cardiac muscle.

The primary focus of this chapter is skeletal muscle (Figures 51-6 and 51-7), also known as striated, voluntary, or extrafusal muscle. Skeletal muscle accounts for 45% to 50% of an average adult's body weight and contains 75% water, 20% protein, and 5% organic and inorganic compounds. Muscle contains 32% of all protein stores necessary for energy and metabolism.[3] Skeletal muscle is innervated by nerve fibers from the cerebrospinal system and can be controlled by will.

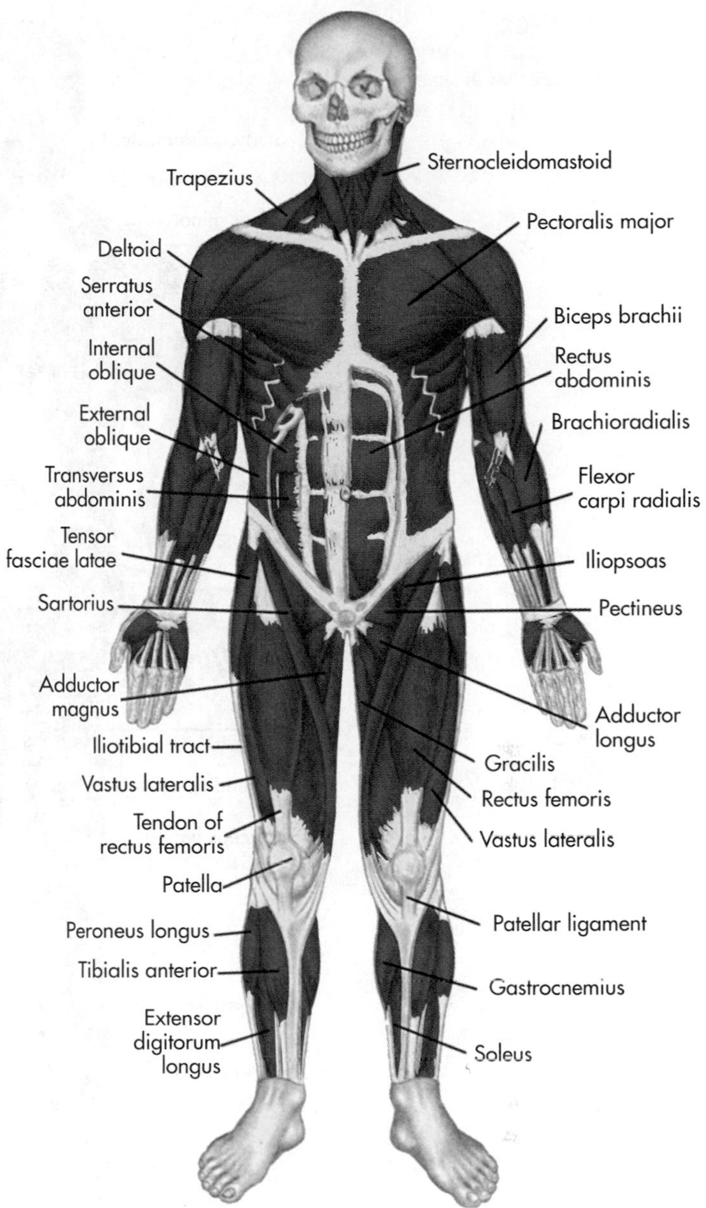

Figure 51-6 Skeletal muscles of body, anterior view.

The body has approximately 350 skeletal muscles, most in pairs. Muscle length varies greatly, from 2 to 60 cm. The function of a muscle determines its shape. Fusiform muscles are elongated and run from one joint to another (e.g., the quadriceps, which extends the knee). The deltoid is an example of a pennate muscle, which is characteristically broad and flat. The muscle fibers run obliquely to the muscle's long axis.

Structure. Each skeletal muscle is covered with a layered connective tissue called fascia. The epimysium, or outer layer, tapers at each end to form the tendon, which allows joint mobility. The middle layer, or perimysium, divides the muscle fibers into fascicles, or bundles of connective tissue. The endomysium, or inner layer, is the smallest unit of fibers and surrounds the fascicles (Figure 51-8).

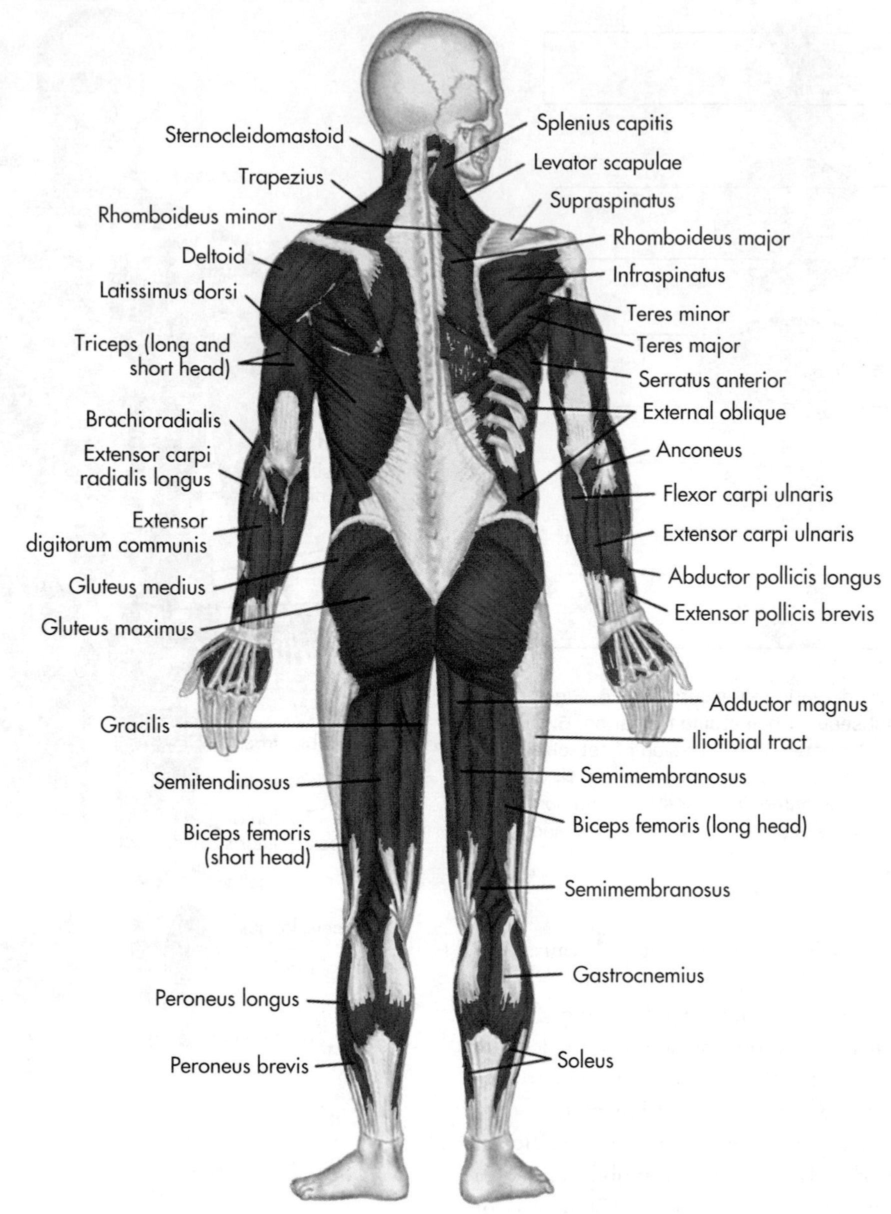

Figure 51-7 Skeletal muscles of body, posterior view.

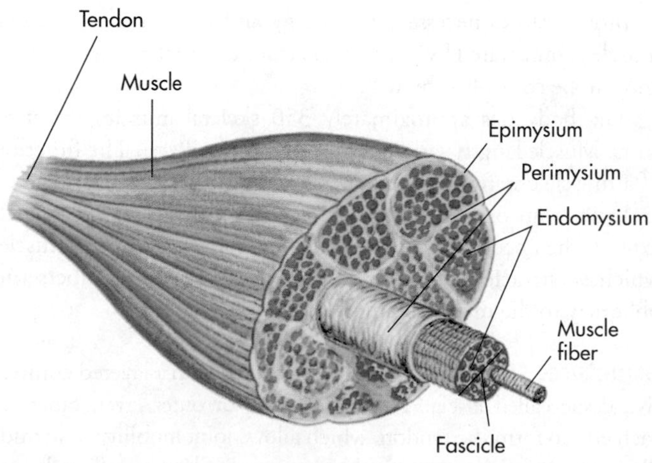

Figure 51-8 Cross section of skeletal muscle showing muscle fibers and their coverings.

Skeletal muscle fibers (cells) are contained within a membrane, the sarcolemma, which contains the sarcoplasm or cytoplasm. The sarcolemma transmits electrical impulses and plays a role in protein synthesis and nutrient supply. Sarcoplasm is similar to cytoplasm and contains proteins and enzymes necessary for the cell's energy production, protein synthesis, and oxygen storage. Small, closely packed fibers (called myofibrils) within the sarcoplasm alternate light and dark horizontal stripes and produce the striated appearance that lends this type of muscle its name (Figure 51-9). The myofibril is the functional unit of muscle contraction. The dark stripes are A bands, and the light stripes are I bands. Light bands crossing the middle of the dark stripes constitute the H band, and dark lines crossing the middle of the light stripes are called Z lines. Myofibrils consist of several sections, called sarcomeres, which contain the contractile proteins actin and myosin. Each sarcomere is a section that extends from one Z line of a myofibril to the next. Bundles of muscle fibers (cells)

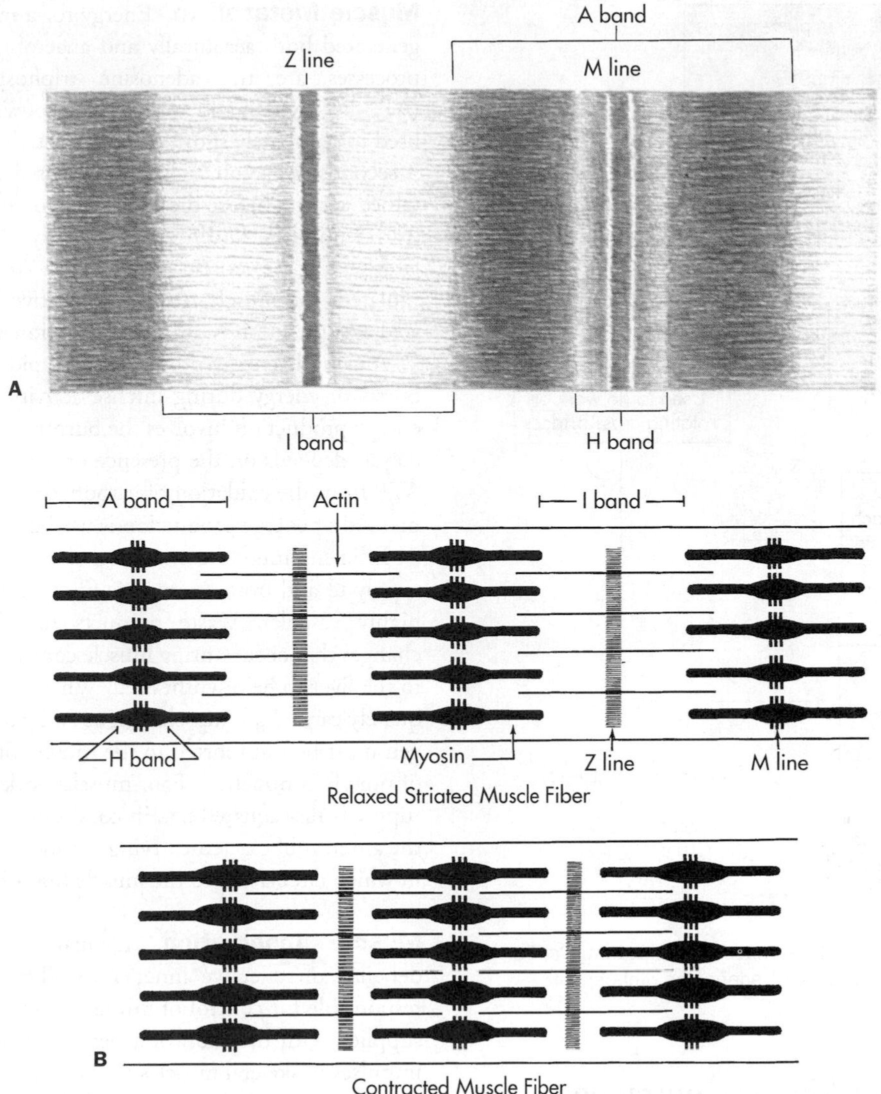

Figure 51-9 Muscle fibers. **A,** Lines and bands in striated muscle. **B,** Relationships of bands, actin, myosin, and lines in relaxed and contracted muscle fibers.

make up the muscle itself. Glycogen is present in muscle as an energy source.

Function. Skeletal muscle provides controlled movement and maintains posture. Movement is accomplished by muscle contractions and work production. Muscular contraction is a complex process triggered by nerve impulses arriving at the muscle fiber (Figure 51-10). Calcium ions, released when the impulse is received, bind to troponin (an inhibitor of the molecular myosin-actin interaction). Once troponin is bound, the myosin-actin interaction takes place and the sarcomeres of the myofibrils contract. This is known as the cross-bridge theory, which replaced the sliding filament theory described by Huxley.[5] The energy for muscle contraction is supplied by the breakdown of adenosine triphosphate (ATP), a substance that muscle cells produce by combining adenosine diphosphate with creatine phosphate. Relaxation of the muscle occurs when the calcium separates from the troponin.

Muscle cells obey the "all or none" law; that is, they contract fully or not at all. This does not mean that the entire muscle contracts fully. Only those individual cells that receive the nerve impulse contract. Oxygenation affects muscle contraction; adequately oxygenated muscle fibers contract more forcefully than those inadequately oxygenated.

Types of Contractions. The arrangement of the fibers within the muscle determines the capacity of the forceful contraction of the muscle. Skeletal muscles contract only if they are stimulated. There are many types of contractions (Box 51-1).

Mechanism of Muscle Movement. Movements of the body are produced by muscles pulling on bones; the bones serve as levers, and the joints serve as fulcrums for the levers. Most movements depend on several muscles acting in a coordinated manner. To produce movement, a muscle acts as a prime mover, or agonist, as its reciprocal muscle, or antagonist, relaxes. Synergistic muscles contract at the same time as the prime movers, either to produce the movement or to stabilize a body part so that contraction of the prime movers is more efficient.

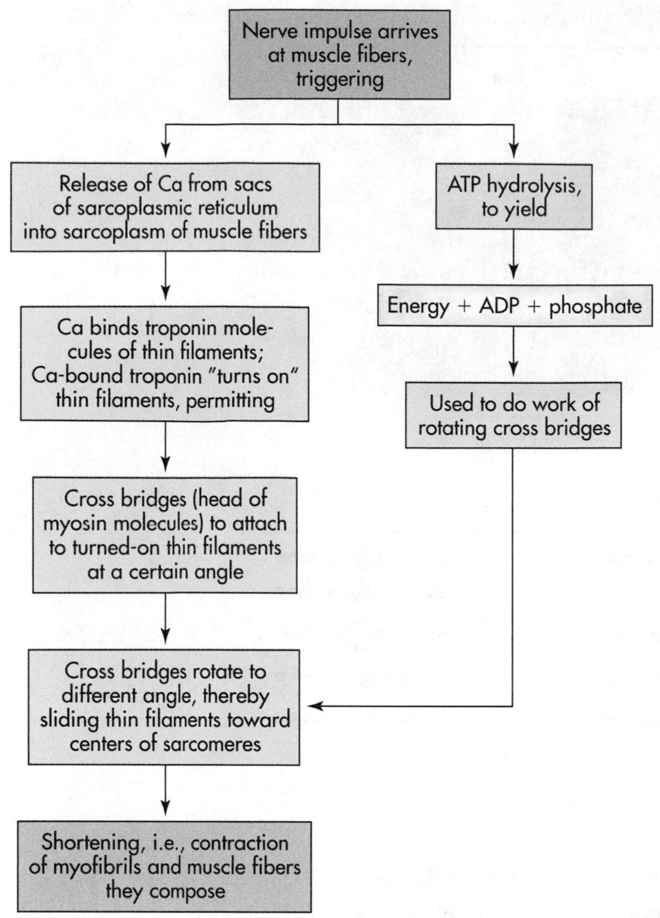

Figure 51-10 Mechanism of skeletal muscle contraction. *Ca*, Calcium; *ATP*, adenosine triphosphate; *ADP*, adenosine diphosphate.

Box 51-1 Types of Muscle Contractions

- *Tonic:* A continual partial contraction that is vital in the maintenance of posture.
- *Clonic:* Alternating, repetitive contraction and relaxation.
- *Isotonic:* A contraction in which tension within the muscle is constant but the length of the muscle changes. It can either shorten (concentric contraction) or lengthen (eccentric). Examples of concentric contractions include lifting weights or climbing stairs; going down stairs and putting down a weight are examples of eccentric contractions. Eccentric contraction uses less energy and results in pain and stiffness after unaccustomed exercise.
- *Isometric (static or holding):* Tension within the muscle increases, but the muscle does not shorten. Postoperative leg exercises are examples of isometric contractions.
- *Twitch:* A jerky reaction to a single stimulus.
- *Tetanic:* A more sustained contraction than the twitch, produced by a series of stimuli in rapid succession.
- *Spasm:* An involuntary contraction caused by stimulation of an entire motor unit.
- *Treppe:* Stronger twitch contractions in response to regularly repeated, constant-strength stimuli.
- *Fibrillation:* A synchronous contraction of individual fibers.
- *Convulsive:* Abnormal, uncoordinated tetanic contractions occurring in varying groups of muscles.

Muscle Metabolism. Energy for a muscle contraction can be generated both aerobically and anaerobically. The two anaerobic processes are the adenosine triphosphate–phosphocreatinine (ATP-PC) system and anaerobic glycolysis. The ATP-PC system is used for extremely short, explosive activities lasting no longer than 3 seconds. Anaerobic glycolysis is used at the beginning of sustained activity before the onset of aerobic metabolism and lasts for 2 to 3 minutes. During anaerobic glycolysis, lactic acid accumulates within the muscle. When 60 to 70 g of lactic acid has accumulated, the muscle reaches exhaustive levels. The rate of lactic acid accumulation is directly proportional to exercise intensity.

Anaerobic energy production is rapid and is valuable for quick bursts of energy during intense activity. The aerobic method of energy production involves the burning of foodstuffs. Aerobic glycolysis depends on the presence of oxygen and the production of ATP from the oxidation of carbohydrates, fats, and proteins. This method of energy production is used during prolonged activity.

Efficient muscle contraction depends on an adequate blood supply to and from the muscle fibers. Therefore skeletal muscle is highly vascular. Waste products resulting from the chemical changes that occur during muscle contraction must be transported to the liver to be resynthesized. When waste products are not adequately carried off, muscle fatigue and pain result. Conversely, oxygen must be transported to the muscle fibers to support the work of muscle contraction. Poor muscle work occurs when the oxygen supply is inadequate (e.g., in conditions such as anemia, in which the amount of oxygen-carrying hemoglobin is reduced, or trauma, in which circulation to the muscle fibers is interrupted).

Muscle Innervation. Adequate muscle contraction also depends on effective innervation. The cerebellum is primarily responsible for control of muscle movement. Every muscle cell is supplied with the axon of a nerve cell. Nerve cells that transmit impulses to skeletal muscles are known as somatic motor neurons. The neuron and the muscle cell it activates are called a motor unit. The number of motor units per muscle varies significantly. The motor units, made up of lower motor neurons, extend to the skeletal muscle. The axon of one somatic motor neuron may be divided into any number of branches and therefore innervates a like number of muscle cells. The fewer muscle cells innervated, the more precise (or fine) are the resultant movements.

The actual contraction of the muscle is set off by the release of acetylcholine, a chemical contained in small vesicles in the axon terminal. When acetylcholine makes contact with the sarcolemma, it stimulates the contraction. This reaction takes place across a structure known as the motor end plate or neuromuscular junction, where the muscle and the nerve are in contact. Damage to

▶ ARE You READY?

Which area of the brain is largely responsible for control of muscle movement?

1. Cerebrum
2. Cerebellum
3. Brain stem
4. Hypothalamus

the nervous system at the cerebrospinal level or at any point in the nerve's course through the local motor neuron level will result in muscular dysfunction.

Cartilage

Cartilage is composed of fibers embedded in a firm gel. Structurally cartilage is a strong but flexible material. Another important characteristic, particularly of **articular** cartilage, is its avascularity. Nutrients reach the cartilage cells by diffusion through the gel from capillaries located in the perichondrium (fibrous covering of the cartilage) or, in the case of articular cartilage, through the synovial fluid.

The number of collagenous fibers found in the cartilage determines its type: fibrous, hyaline, or elastic. Fibrous cartilage (or fibrocartilage) composes the intervertebral discs. The amount of fibrous cartilage increases with age; the transformation of hyaline cartilage into fibrous cartilage is a sign of aging. Hyaline, the most common type of cartilage, is composed of chondrocytes (cartilage cells), type II collagen fibers in the matrix, and protein polysaccharide complexes and water between the matrix and fibers. The composition of hyaline cartilage is responsible for its spongy and elastic qualities, which are crucial to preventing injury to the bone during weight bearing. Articular cartilage is hyaline cartilage that covers the articulating surface on the ends of bone, reducing friction and evening weight distribution in the joint. The amount or thickness depends on the type of bone and amount of weight and shearing force to which the joint is subjected.

Articular cartilage contains 60% to 80% water and does not contain any blood vessels, lymph tissue, or nerves. As a result, it is insensitive to pain and does not easily repair itself after injury. Regeneration occurs at the junction of the synovial membrane and cartilage because of the adjacent blood supply and nutrients supplying the synovial membrane.

Yellow, or elastic, cartilage has the fewest fibers. Elastic cartilage may be found in areas such as the external ear and epiglottis.

Ligaments

Ligaments are parallel bands of flexible, dense fibrous connective tissue. Their primary function is to connect the articular ends of bones and provide stability. Ligaments permit movement in some directions but limit movement in others, preventing joint injury, as in the knee and hip joints (Figure 51-11). The medial and lateral collateral ligaments of the knee provide mediolateral stability to the knee joint; the anterior and posterior cruciate ligaments within the joint capsule of the knee provide anteroposterior stability. Ligaments may also attach to soft tissue to suspend structures (e.g., the suspensory ligament of the ovary that passes from the tubal end of the ovary to the peritoneum).

Tendons

Tendons are bands of dense, fibrous tissue that form the origin and insertion of muscle to bone (Figure 51-12). The longitudinal arrangement of fibers provides tensile strength while preventing injury to the tendon. The tendon is an extension of the fibrous sheath that envelops each muscle and is continuous with the periosteum at its other end. Tendon sheaths are tubular structures of connective tissue that enclose certain tendons, especially in the wrist and ankle. These sheaths are lined with a synovial membrane, which provides lubrication (synovial fluid) for each movement of the tendon. Ligaments and tendons may add extra stability to the joint capsule. The synovial membrane, or **synovium**, lines the

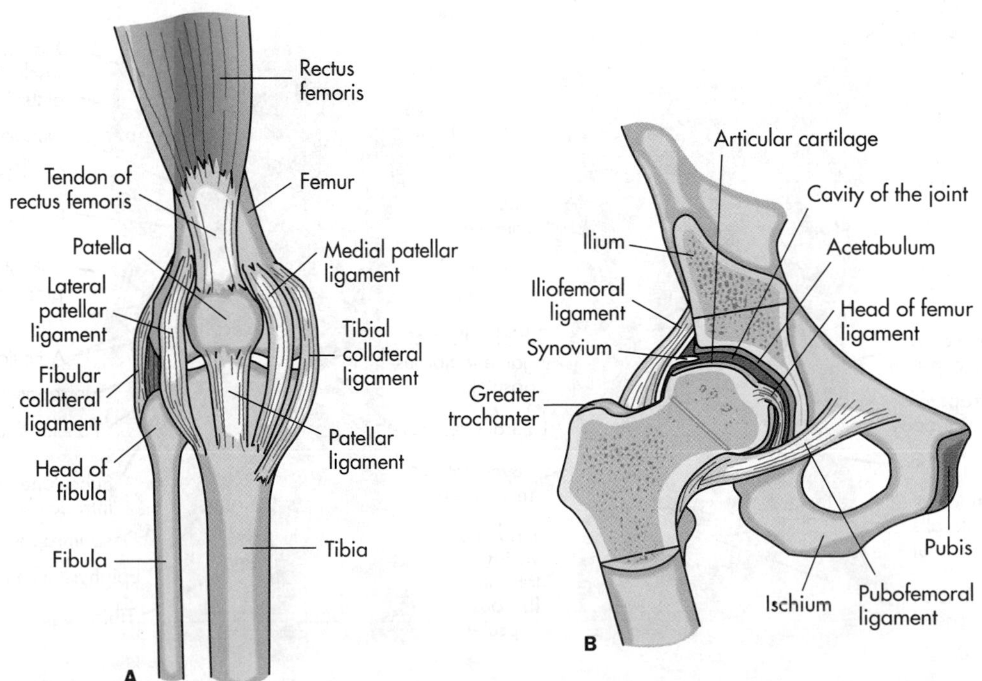

Figure 51-11 **A,** Ligaments of knee joint. **B,** Ligaments of hip joint.

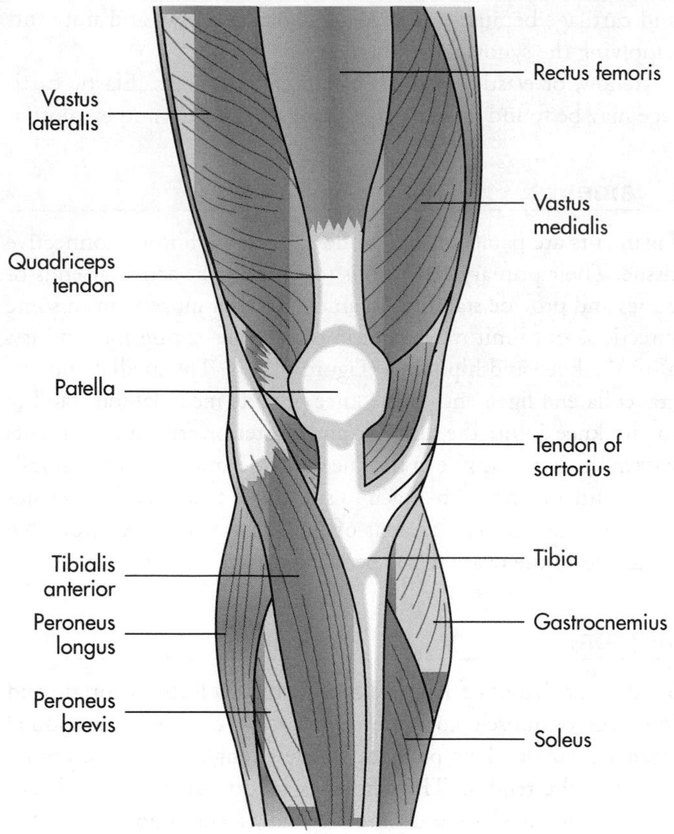

Figure 51-12 Anterior view of tendons around knee joint.

nonarticulating surfaces of the joint capsule. The synovium is capable of repair because of its rich blood and lymph supply. The synovial membrane secretes synovial fluid into the joint capsule for lubrication (Figure 51-13). Synovial fluid is plasma derived from blood vessels in the synovium. In addition to joint lubrication, synovial fluid provides nourishment to articular cartilage and contains leukocytes that have a phagocytic action on bacteria and debris in the joint. A decrease in synovial fluid can lead to destruction of the articular cartilage.

Fascia

Fascia is a sheet of loose connective tissue that may be found directly under the skin as superficial fascia or as a sheet of dense, fibrous connective tissue making up the sheath of muscles, nerves, and blood vessels. The latter is known as deep fascia.

Bursae

Bursae are small sacs of connective tissue located wherever pressure is exerted over moving parts. They may occur between skin and bone, between tendons and bone, or between muscles. Bursae are lined with synovial membrane and contain synovial fluid and serve as cushions between moving parts. One such bursa, the olecranon bursa, is located between the olecranon process and the skin. New bursae can develop as a result of prolonged or increased pressure or friction, often resulting in pain. The shoulder bursa (subacromial) is a common site of bursitis (Figure 51-14).

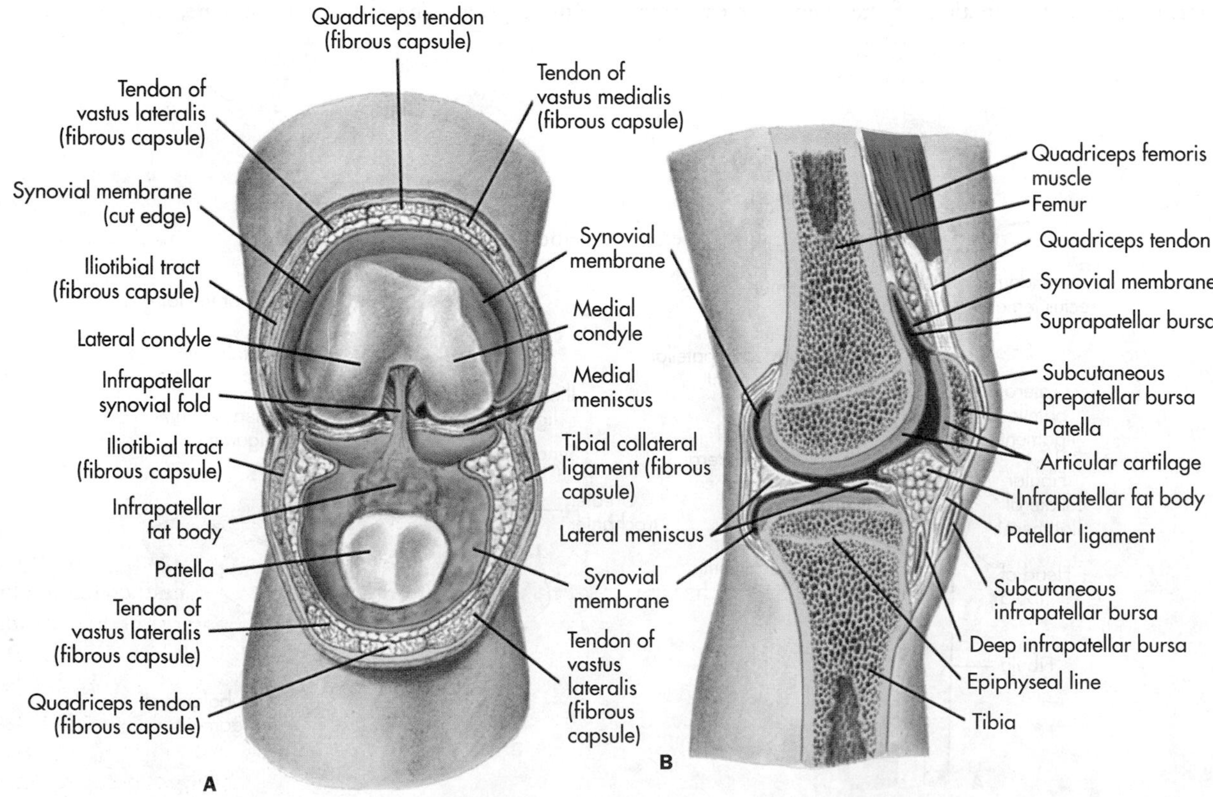

Figure 51-13 Knee joint (synovial joint). **A,** Frontal view. **B,** Lateral view.

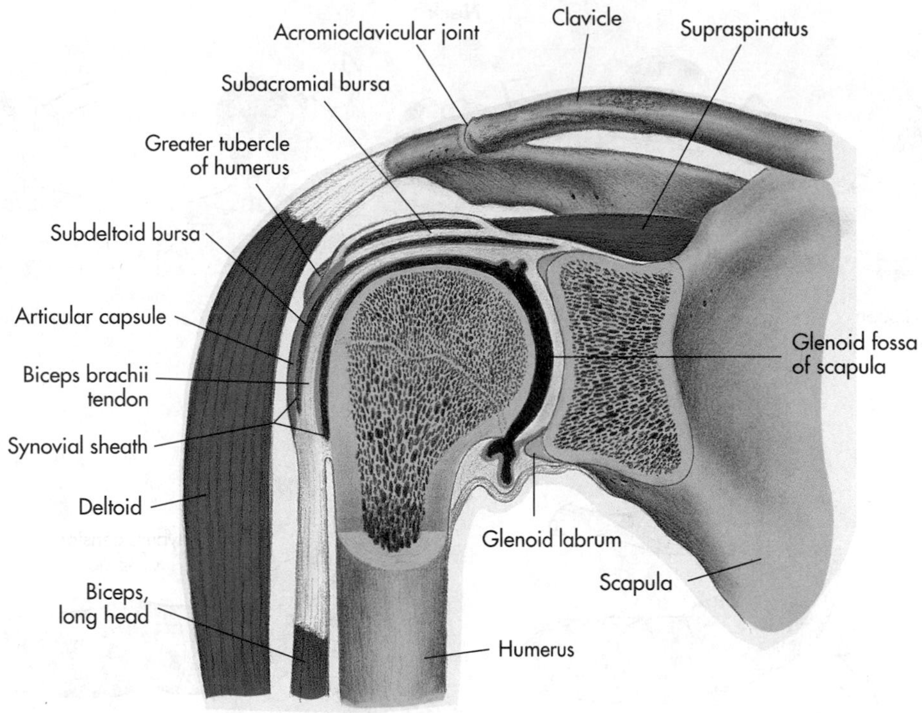

Figure 51-14 Shoulder joint bursae.

Joints

Movement would be impossible without flexibility within the skeletal framework. This flexibility is provided by the joints, or places where the bones come together and articulate. The shape of the joint determines the amount and type of movement possible. Joints are classified by the amount of movement they allow and by the type of connective tissue that joins them.

Types. There are three major types of joints:

1. *Synarthroses or fibrous*: Allow no movement and are exemplified by the sutures of the skull. Sutures bind bones tightly together with a thin layer of dense, fibrous tissue.
2. *Amphiarthroses or cartilaginous*: Allow little movement and are exemplified by the intervertebral joints and symphysis pubis. A syndesmosis is a type of amphiarthrosis joint that is joined by a ligament or membrane, such as the radioulnar joint and the tibiofibular joint.
3. *Diarthroses or synovial*: Allow free movement and are exemplified by the hip, knee, shoulder, and elbow.

The synarthroses and amphiarthroses may be classified together as synarthroses, since both lack a joint cavity. Fibrous, cartilaginous, or osseous tissue grows between their articular surfaces. Because diarthroses are the joints that permit movement, they are discussed in the most detail.

Structure of Diarthrodial Joints. Each **diarthrodial** joint contains a small space, or joint cavity, between the articulating surfaces of the bones that make up the joint. Articular hyaline cartilage covers the articulating surfaces of both bones, allowing for the smooth, gliding motion of the joint. A joint capsule, or sleeve of fibrous tissue, encases the joint (see Figure 51-13).

Small pieces of dense cartilage may also be interposed between the articulating surfaces. These are crescent–shaped structures (menisci) that provide additional cushioning of the joint. Examples include the medial and lateral menisci of the knee joint.

Function of Diarthrodial Joints. Joints provide the skeleton with both stability and mobility. In addition to the joint types already described, diarthrodial joints are further classified by the shape of their surface and the type of movement they permit. Examples include ball and socket (shoulder, hip), hinge (elbow, knee), pivot (atlas, axis), condyloid (wrist), saddle (first metacarpal, trapezium), and gliding (intervertebral discs).

Each joint has its own range and direction of movement. Diarthrodial joints permit one or more of the following movements: flexion, extension, abduction, adduction, rotation, circumduction, supination, pronation, inversion, and eversion (Figures 51-15 to 51-17).

Physiologic Changes With Aging

Physiologic changes occur in the musculoskeletal system throughout a person's life span (Table 51-2). Childhood and adolescence are a time of rapid growth and development of the musculoskeletal structures. However, with maturity and aging, tissue strength and integrity begin to decline as the total number of body cells decreases. Connective tissues, particularly the articular cartilage of the joints and the intervertebral discs of the spine, lose some of their elasticity and resilience. Cartilage becomes more rigid because of increased cross-linking of collagen and elastin and decreased water content in the ground substance. As the amount

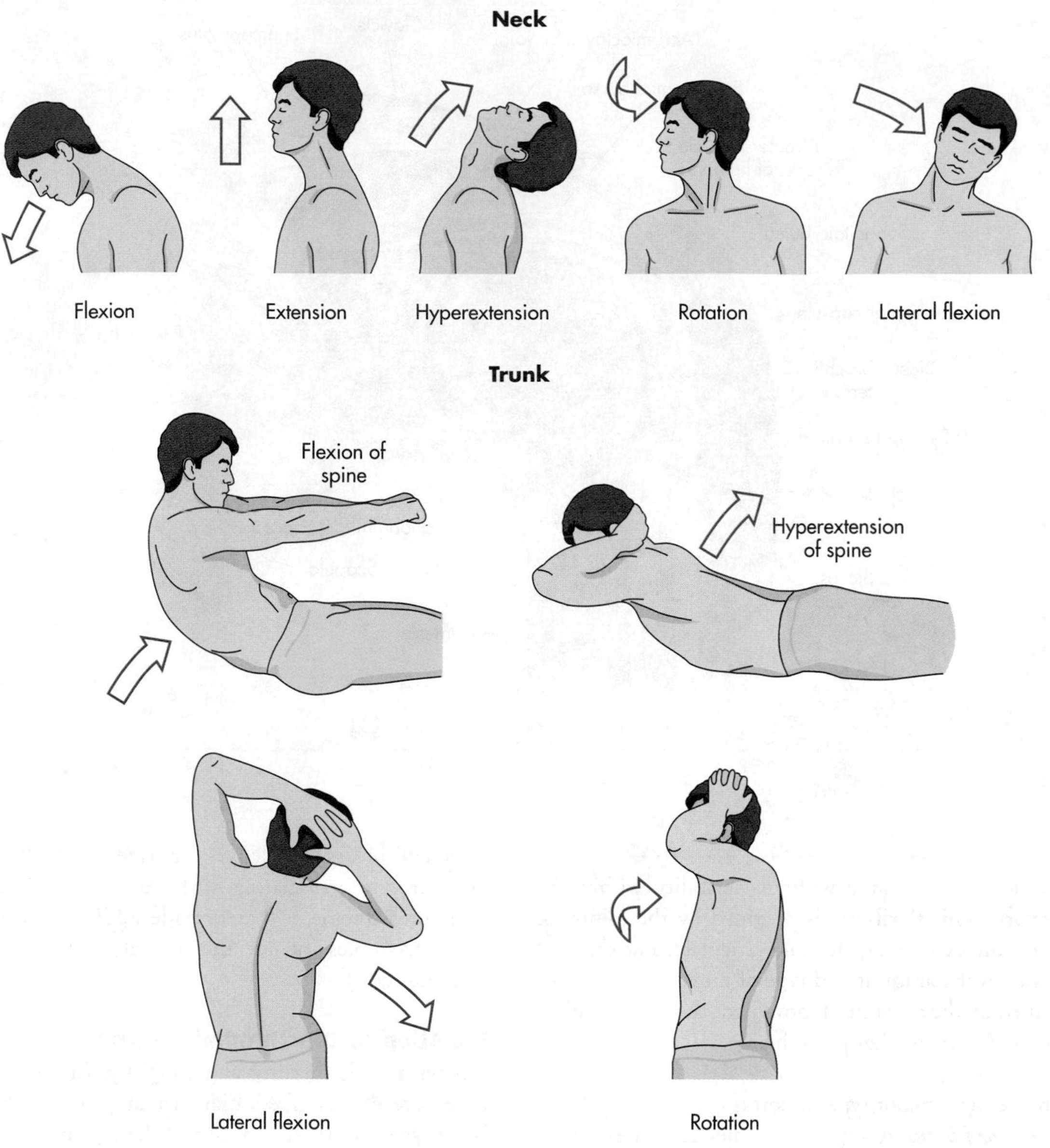

Figure 51-15 Range of motion for neck and trunk.

of vigorous activity an individual engages in decreases, muscles lose bulk, tone, and strength.

Bone resorption takes place more rapidly than bone growth, and, particularly in postmenopausal women, calcium is lost from the bone. A universal effect of aging is impaired osteoblastic activity. Women in particular experience loss of bone density and increased osteoclastic bone resorption with the aging process. By age 70 a woman has lost approximately 50% of her peripheral cortical bone mass.[2] In contrast, men experience bone loss later and at a slower rate than women. In addition, men initially have 30% more bone mass than women. African-Americans have denser bones than Caucasians, Asians, and Native Americans.

Muscle strength reaches a peak at 25 to 30 years, is maintained through the fifth decade, and then declines noticeably after 70 years of age. Lean muscle mass decreases with aging; the term *sarcopenia* refers to age-related skeletal muscle loss. The aging process results in a decrease in the number of muscle fibers and decreased enzymatic reactions in the mitochondria, affecting muscle contraction and function. Lack of use (disuse atrophy) leads to muscle wasting and decreased elasticity of the ligaments and tendons.

The age-related changes in the musculoskeletal system are manifested in several ways. With age, the shoulders may become stooped and narrowed. The knees and hips may be slightly flexed when standing or walking because of pain associated with joint degeneration. Posture becomes stooped as the body attempts to compensate for changes in the center of gravity caused by lower extremity joint flexion and forward thrusting of the head, neck, and shoulders. With these changes, height can decrease by 6 to 10 cm. Gait may become unsteady because of loss of muscle strength and coordination, and the individual is more susceptible to falls. An estimated one third of persons 65 years of age and older experience falls annually; an estimated 50% of nursing home residents fall each year. Falls are the leading cause of accidental death in older adults. Assessments of fall risk and fall prevention are important nursing interventions.

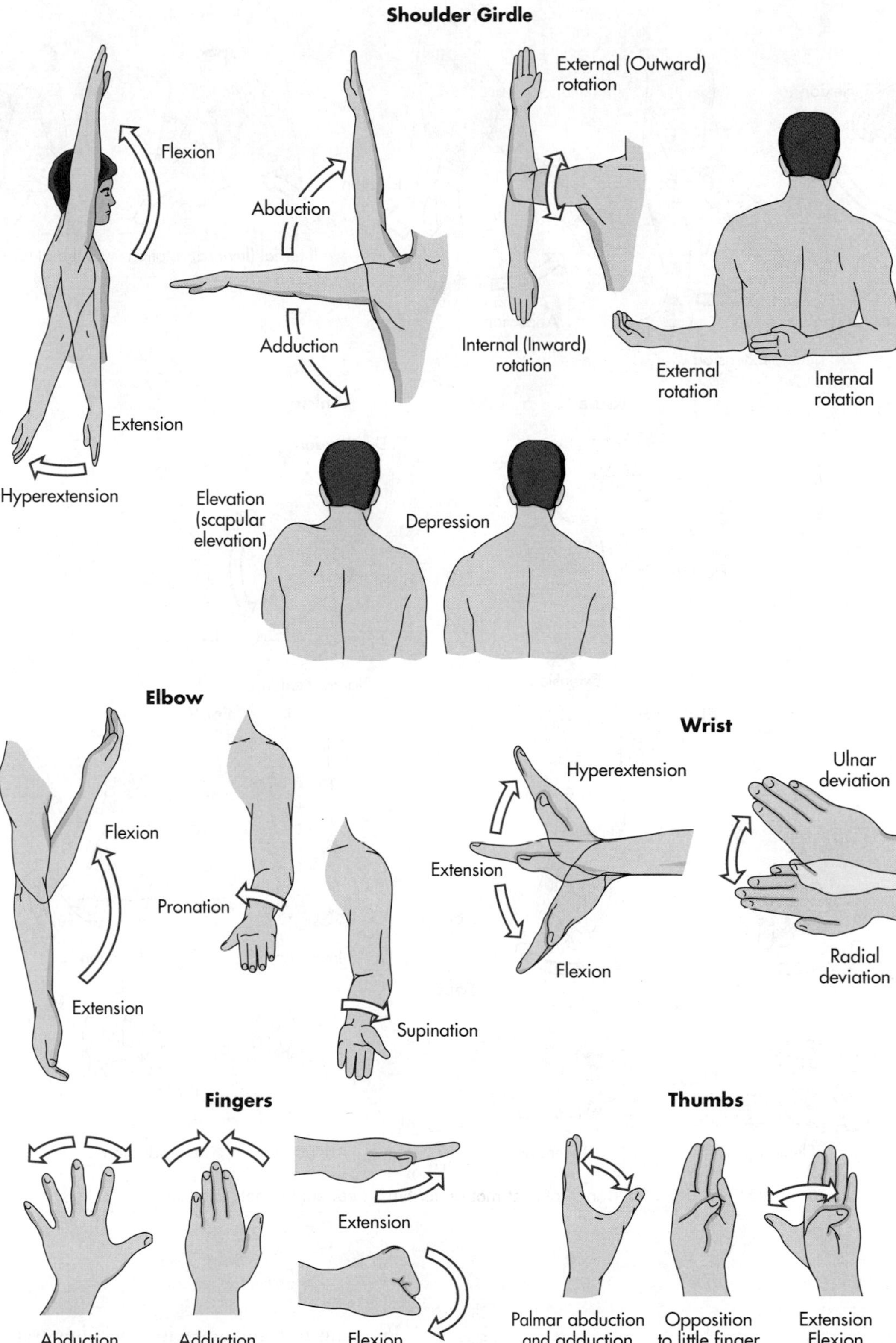

Figure 51-16 Range of joint motion for shoulder girdle, elbow, forearm, wrist, fingers, and thumbs.

Arthritis is common in older persons, causing chronic joint pain and decreased mobility. Independence and the ability to perform activities of daily living (ADLs) are commonly affected. Although diseases of the musculoskeletal system are not usually fatal, they have significant impact on the individual and family because of chronic pain and disability. However, complications arising as a result of a musculoskeletal problem can be fatal. An example is pneumonia or pulmonary embolus developing in an older patient recovering from surgical fixation of a hip fracture.

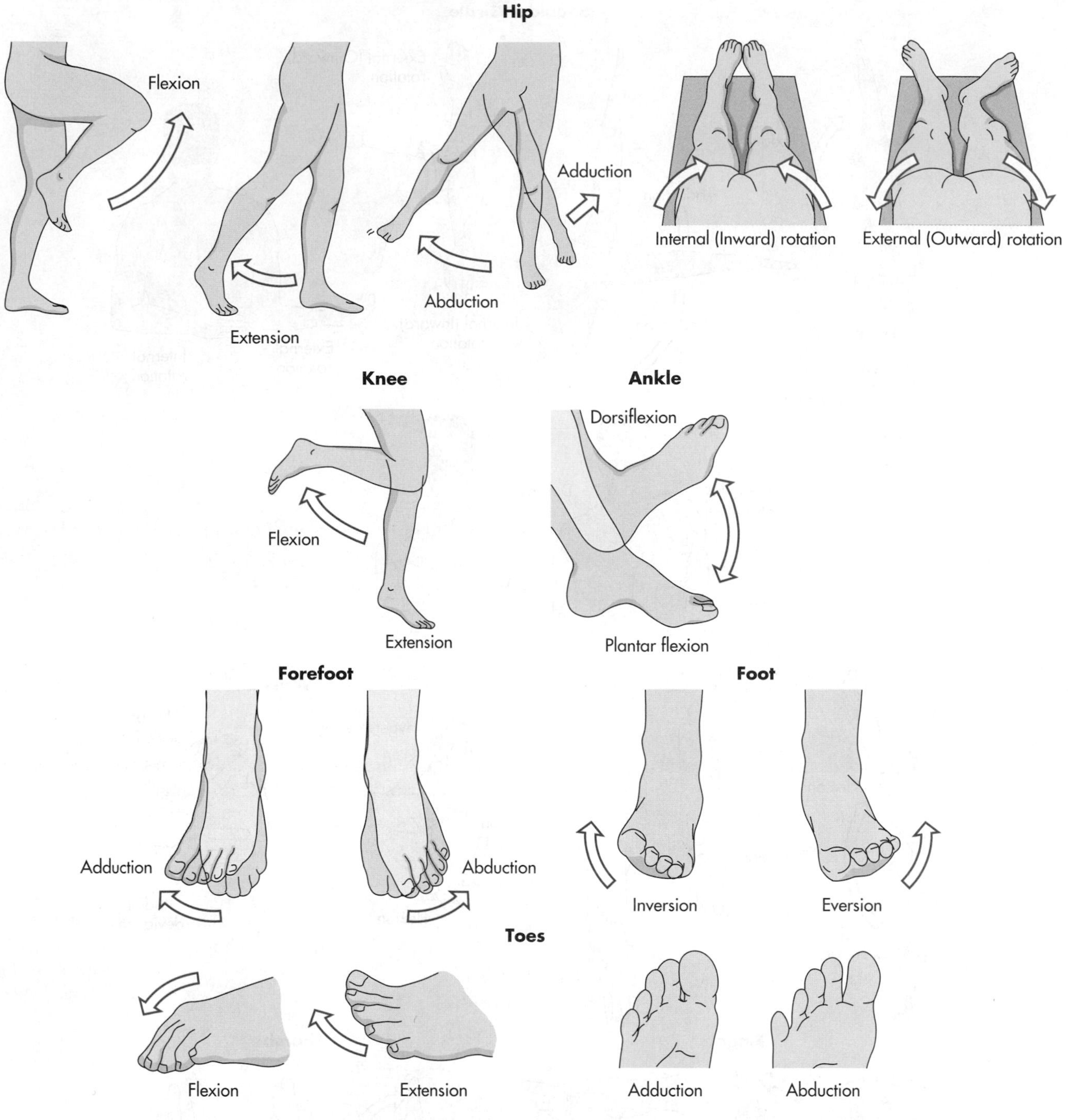

Figure 51-17 Range of joint motion for hip, knee, ankle, foot, and toes.

> **▶ ARE You READY?**
>
> Which of the following is an age-related change of the musculoskeletal system?
>
> 1. Increased water content in articular cartilage of joints
> 2. Declining muscle strength in the fourth decade
> 3. Bone density increases in men
> 4. Fifty percent loss of bone mass in women by age 70

Programs of regular exercise (including weight-bearing activities) and resistive muscle strengthening can decrease or prevent some of the age-related changes in the musculoskeletal system. A nutritionally adequate diet is also beneficial.

Health History

Nursing care for the individual with a musculoskeletal problem is based on a systematic assessment of needs, capabilities, and resources. A thorough assessment includes subjective data gath-

TABLE 51-2 PHYSIOLOGIC CHANGES WITH AGING

Tissue	Change	Potential Problem
Bone	Decreased total bone mass Impaired osteoblastic activity Resorption exceeding growth Erosion of haversian systems Cortical bone changing to cancellous bone Porous cortical bone	Osteoporosis, pathologic fracture, delayed healing
Muscles	Decline in strength past 70 years Decline in number of muscle fibers Decrease in muscle mass Atrophy of muscle cells	Weakness; incoordination; disuse atrophy; slow, unsteady gait; poor posture; falls; contractures
Joints	Decreased elasticity of cartilage Increased susceptibility to tears in cartilage	Arthritis, decreased range of motion, contractures

ered from patient and family interviews. Information to obtain and areas to explore include:

- Age, which can be a predictor of common problems associated with a particular age-group (For example, older adults are susceptible to falls, older women have an increased risk for osteoporosis, and young men are at a higher risk for trauma.)
- Height and weight: any changes in weight and whether they were intentional; the person's ideal weight and body mass index; any loss of height, particularly in older adults
- Nutrition: dietary intake of calcium, vitamin D, minerals, total calories, fad diets
- Occupation (past, present): sedentary, standing, repetitive movements, safety factors, lifting, ergonomic environment
- Exercise regimen: type, frequency, duration, weight-bearing activity, safety equipment, type of shoes, warm-up and cool-down activities
- Ability to perform ADLs, including type and amount of assistance required, use of assistive or adaptive device
- Transfer ability
- Psychosocial factors such as marital status, support systems, methods and effectiveness of coping with stress, role changes, leisure activities, and cultural beliefs
- Availability of transportation
- Physical layout of home: steps, accessibility; assessment of risk for injury
- Reliance on community services: past, present; usefulness of services
- Exposure to environmental irritants, radiation
- Allergies: any reaction to iodine, shellfish
- Medications: use of aspirin, nonsteroidal antiinflammatory drugs, steroids, anticoagulants, hormones, vitamins, or analgesics; include frequency, duration, indications, and effectiveness
- Smoking, alcohol, and recreational drug use
- Dominant hand
- Childbearing history (Nulliparity is a risk factor for osteoporosis.)
- Age at menopause

Family History

Taking a family history includes finding about any genetic disorders or abnormalities; congenital abnormalities; and musculoskeletal disorders such as arthritis, scoliosis, and ankylosing spondylitis.

Medical and Surgical History

The medical and surgical history includes information on developmental abnormalities; childhood diseases, illnesses, and trauma; chronic illnesses or hospitalizations; and past surgeries, recovery, complications, and rehabilitation.

Review of Systems

The examiner obtains data regarding history of integumentary, ophthalmic, auditory, hematologic, immunologic, respiratory, cardiovascular, gastrointestinal, genitourinary, endocrine, neurologic, or psychologic problems that may have relevance to the presenting problem.

History of the Current Problem

The nurse elicits the following information:

- Circumstances surrounding the onset of the problem: any precipitating or associated events or injuries, time of onset, duration
- Patient's perception of the problem and its impact on his or her lifestyle and ability to carry out ADLs and enjoy leisure activities
- Any efforts to treat the problem and their effectiveness
- Adherence to treatment programs
- Trauma, mechanism of injury, sensations or sounds at the time of injury
- Any history of paresthesias, paralysis, swelling (location and timing), locking, "giving way"
- Unilateral or bilateral joint involvement
- Reasons for seeking and expectations of current treatment

TABLE 51-3 PHYSICAL EXAMINATION DATA

Observations	Finding
GENERAL APPEARANCE	
Race	Caucasian and Asian race: risk factor for osteoporosis
Posture	May be characteristic of a specific problem (e.g., scoliosis; kyphotic posture in ankylosing spondylitis; guarding of head, neck, and shoulders after whiplash)
Overweight	May indicate diminished ability to perform regular exercise or activity; increases stress on joints
Underweight	May indicate inability to secure or prepare nutritious meals or to carry out feeding activities adequately; women with thin build at risk for osteoporosis May relate to specific systemic condition causing anorexia, nausea, vomiting, or malabsorption of food
SKIN	
Turgor	Thin, papery skin indicative of aging, systemic connective tissue disease, or long-term steroid use; skin easily broken
Texture	Thick, leathery patches over forearms, hands, chest, and face indicative of scleroderma; skin ulcerating easily, especially over joints
Integrity: breaks in skin, ulcerations, reddened areas	Individuals with limited mobility subject to skin breakdown and pressure ulcers from pressure over bony areas, which interferes with circulation; possibility of shearing forces against sheets, chair surfaces, bedpans, or other surfaces tearing or abrading skin
Temperature	Warmth, especially over painful joints, indicative of inflammatory or infectious process within joint
Erythema over joints	Indicates inflammation and need to keep joint at rest May be present in systemic connective tissue disorders (psoriasis, scleroderma, dermatomyositis); initial observations useful as baseline to determine effectiveness of treatment
Color change on exposure to cold	Change from white (resulting from arteriolar spasm) to blue (cyanosis caused by stagnation of blood) to red (warming and reactive vasodilation) indicative of some connective tissue disorders (Raynaud's phenomenon)
Bruising	Often present after trauma and consequent to long-term treatment of connective tissue disease with corticosteroids; anticoagulant use

Discomfort Associated With the Problem

Many musculoskeletal problems are marked by pain or discomfort. Questions about pain or discomfort include its nature, location, and duration; radiating or referred pain; an evaluation of the pain, using pain-rating scale; measures the patient has taken to alleviate pain or discomfort and the effectiveness of these measures; the effect on daily or leisure activities; and associated or precipitating events.

Physical Examination

The nurse makes observations regarding general appearance, skin, nails, and hair (Table 51-3). In addition, data are collected regarding deformities, muscle strength and range of motion, ability to transfer and ambulate, and a complete functional assessment.

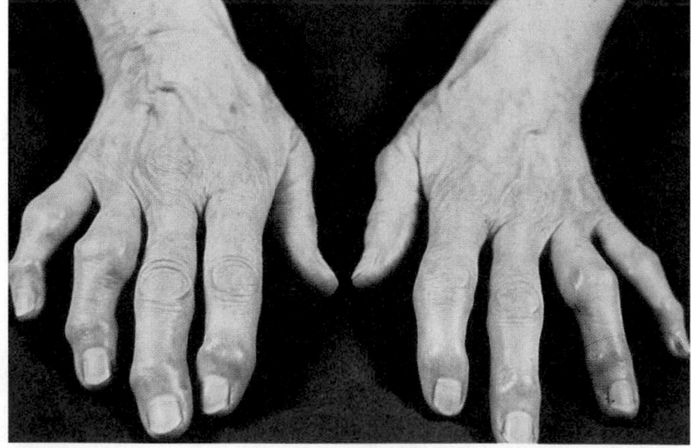

Figure 51-18 Heberden's nodes at distal interphalangeal joints and Bouchard's nodes at proximal interphalangeal joints.

Inspection

Much information can be gathered even before the physical examination begins. The nurse observes the patient's gait as he or she enters the examining room and notes the person's ability to stand, sit, and rise from a chair. The nurse notes whether the patient uses assistive devices for ambulation or transferring, and whether the devices are being used properly. At the same time that patient privacy is ensured, the nurse assesses the person's ability to dress and undress. These data are useful in determining the individual's functional status. The nurse observes the person's posture while standing erect and notes any abnormal curvatures of the spine. A gentle lordotic (concave) curve in the lumbar spine is normal, and

TABLE 51-3 PHYSICAL EXAMINATION DATA—CONT'D

Observations	Finding
SKIN—CONT'D	
Swelling of extremities or joints	In extremities, may denote prolonged dependent position, lack of activity, circulatory or renal impairment In joints, may indicate effusion (serous, purulent, or bloody fluid in joint capsule); inflamed synovium (feels boggy): indication of need to rest joints involved
Bony enlargements	Indicative of disease process; for example, Heberden's nodes in osteoarthritis (hard, irregular swellings over distal interphalangeal joints of fingers) or Bouchard's nodes (cartilaginous or bony enlargement of proximal interphalangeal finger joints) (Figure 51-18)
Subcutaneous nodules	Indicative of rheumatoid arthritis: hard, mobile swellings commonly found in subolecranon area
Bursal swelling	Indicative of bursal inflammation: palpated as soft swelling over bursa
Synovial cyst	Indicative of hypertrophy of synovial tissue (e.g., Baker's cyst—swelling in popliteal area, often extending into calf)
Tophaceous deposits	Indicative of gout: hard translucent swellings over joints or in cartilage such as that of ear
Tenderness: may be elicited by direct pressure and graded by amount of pressure required to produce discomfort	Degree of tenderness usually in direct proportion to severity of inflammation or trauma (e.g., in joint inflammation or injured soft tissue or overlying fracture)
General hygiene: evidence of uncleanliness of body, clothing	May indicate inability to adequately carry out hygienic requirements (Because this may be embarrassing for patient, plan to introduce self-help devices or provide assistance in ways that will not be demeaning.)
NAILS AND HAIR	
Poorly kept or diseased nails	May indicate lack of strength or inability to reach nails to care for them Change in nail structure possibly indicative of connective tissue disease
Poorly kept hair	May indicate inability to lift arms to comb hair
Alopecia, scaling of scalp	May indicate connective tissue disease, side effect of medications

a gentle kyphotic (convex) curve in the thoracic spine is also normal (Figure 51-19). Any exaggeration of these normal curves, such as a lateral curvature or scoliotic curve of the spine, is considered abnormal.

A person's gait is his or her manner or style of walking (Box 51-2). An altered gait pattern indicates a pathologic process. Having the patient walk 20 to 25 feet is usually adequate to make an accurate assessment of gait. During observation of ambulation, the nurse notes the presence and type of any limp, involved joints, the ability to bear weight, balance, and the degree of any deformity in the lower extremities. Deformity of the lower extremities (e.g., genu varum, talipes varus) may not be as apparent when the joint is examined at rest as when weight-bearing forces are exerted across the joint. Furthermore, in persons with significant upper extremity involvement, some consideration must be given both to the amount of weight bearing that might be expected from the arms and hands and to the appropriate type of assistive device. For example, the individual with severe rheumatoid involvement of the hands might need a device that permits weight bearing on the forearms.

Other problems, such as cardiovascular disease, respiratory impairment, or anemia, may also affect ambulatory ability and must be considered during the assessment of ambulation. Assessment of transfer and ambulatory ability helps determine a suitable

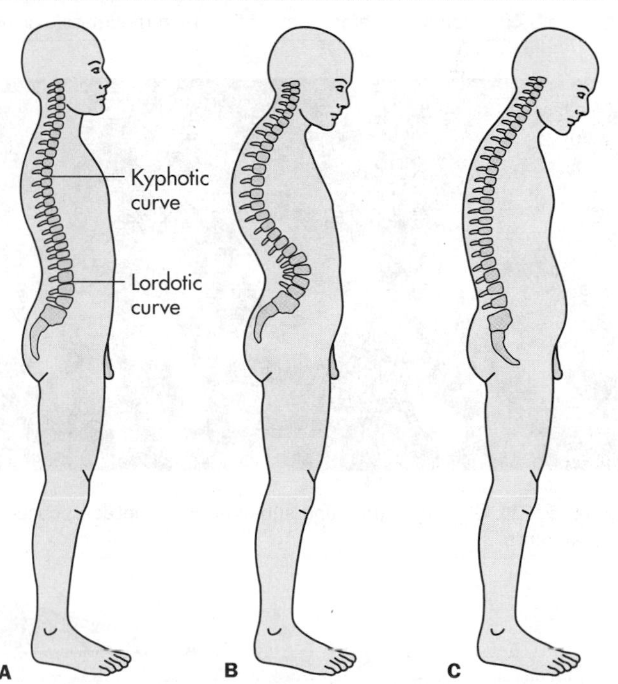

Figure 51-19 **A,** Curves of spine in good posture. **B,** Curves of spine in slumping posture. **C,** Obliteration of spinal curves, as in early spondylitis.

Box 51-2 Normal Gait Cycle

- *Stance phase:* Begins with heel strike and ends with toe-off
- *Swing phase:* Begins with toe-off and continues through heel strike
- *Double support:* Brief period when both feet are on ground

level of activity for the patient. The nurse observes all extremities for overall muscle mass, deformities, asymmetry, and masses. Box 51-3 lists common musculoskeletal deformities.

Palpation

In a head-to-toe fashion, the nurse palpates all bones, joints, and soft tissue for temperature, swelling, tenderness, pain, crepitus, or

Box 51-3 Common Musculoskeletal Deformities

- *Swan-neck deformity:* Flexion contracture of the metacarpophalangeal joints, hyperextension of the proximal interphalangeal joints, and flexion of the distal interphalangeal joints of the fingers (Figure 51-20), found in advanced rheumatoid arthritis
- *Ulnar deviation or drift:* Fingers deviating at the metacarpophalangeal joints toward the ulnar aspect of the hand (Figure 51-21)
- *Valgus deformities:* Distal arm of the angle of the joint pointing away from the midline of the body
  —*Hallux valgus:* Great toe turning toward the other toes
  —*Genu valgum:* "Knock-knees" (Figure 51-22)
  —*Talipes valgus:* Eversion of the foot
- *Varus deformities:* Distal arm of the angle of the joint pointing toward the midline of the body
  —*Genu varum:* Bowing of the knees
  —*Talipes varus:* Inversion of the foot
- *Scoliosis:* Lateral curvature of the spine
- *Kyphosis:* Thoracic spinal curvature, the convexity of the curve being posterior
- *Atrophy:* Reduction in size of an extremity or body part (e.g., wasting of muscles so that they appear to lack the bulk of normal muscle); can result from lack of use or disease process (e.g., polymyositis)
- *Hypertrophy:* Abnormal enlargement of an organ or body part; may be associated with limitation of function
- *Pes planus:* Flatfoot (Figure 51-23, *A*)
- *Pes cavus:* High instep (Figure 51-23, *B*)

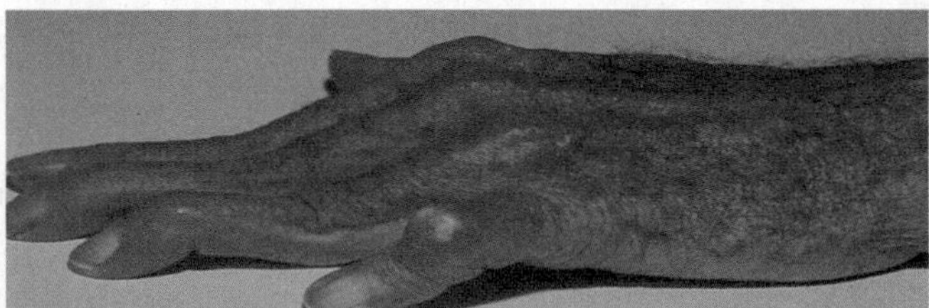

Figure 51-20 Swan-neck deformities of fingers in rheumatoid arthritis.

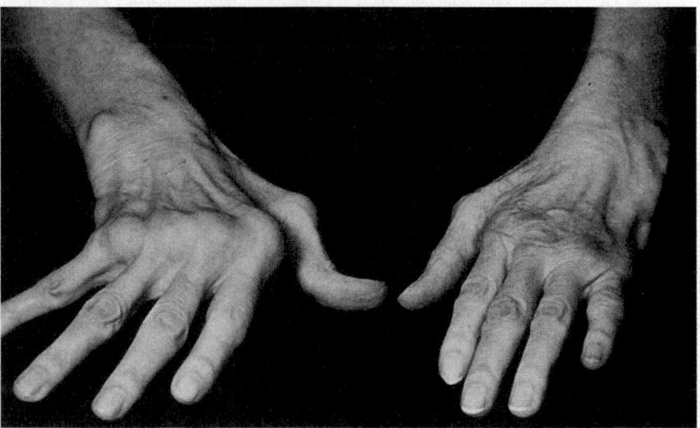

Figure 51-21 Ulnar deviation and subluxation of metacarpophalangeal joints.

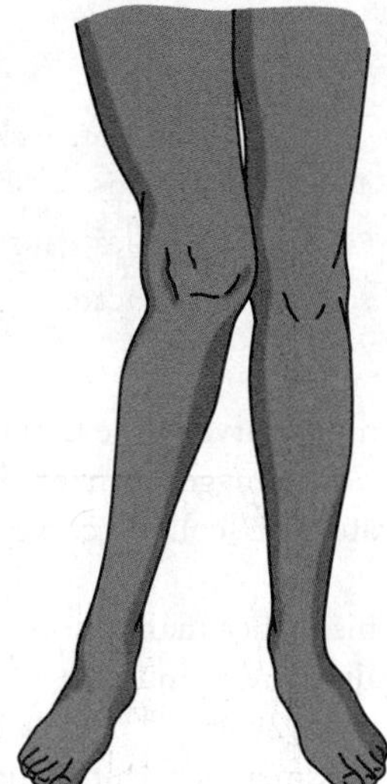

Figure 51-22 Valgus deformity of right knee.

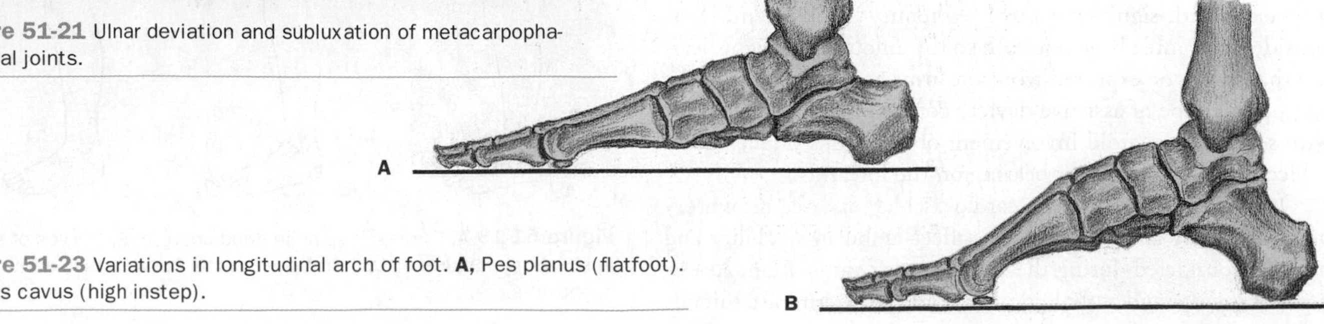

Figure 51-23 Variations in longitudinal arch of foot. **A,** Pes planus (flatfoot). **B,** Pes cavus (high instep).

masses. The spinous processes and intervertebral spaces are also palpated for tenderness.

Assessment of Sensory Function

To evaluate sensory innervation, the nurse assesses the person's ability to discern light touch, gentle pressure, pain, and temperature. Each test is performed bilaterally, and results are compared. Sensation in the dermatomes is checked to detect abnormalities in spinal nerve innervation (Figure 51-24). The nurse also evaluates the person's sense of proprioception (position sense) in the extremities.

Deep Tendon Reflex Activity

Decreased or absent reflexes may indicate neuropathy or a lower motor neuron lesion, whereas brisk reflexes indicate an upper motor neuron lesion. After checking reflexes, the nurse compares bilateral responses. Figure 51-25 shows the location of tendons and their corresponding spinal level, and Figure 51-26 illustrates the documentation of deep tendon response. The grading of responses is shown in Table 51-4.

Range of Motion

The term *range of motion* refers to the normal arc of movement provided for by the structure of a joint. Active range of motion is motion performed independently. Passive range of motion is accomplished with the assistance of someone else or with a mechanical device.

Before testing the muscle strength or range of motion of a joint, the nurse assesses the position of the person's extremities. Sudden changes from normal may indicate the presence of fractures, dislocations, or ruptures of supporting structures. Typical of this kind of sudden change is the marked external rotation and shortening of the leg after a hip fracture; the inability to extend a "dropped" finger after rupture of an extensor tendon in the hand; or postoperative footdrop, a complication that may occur after surgical procedures on the back, hip, or knee because of pressure on or stretching of the sciatic or peroneal nerve.

The nurse should also note subluxation, or partial dislocation of a joint. This is often a chronic problem, as in the shoulder of the hemiplegic person or in the wrist of the arthritic person. It is usually accompanied by some loss of function or need for support. Subluxation of the shoulder may be detected by examination; a

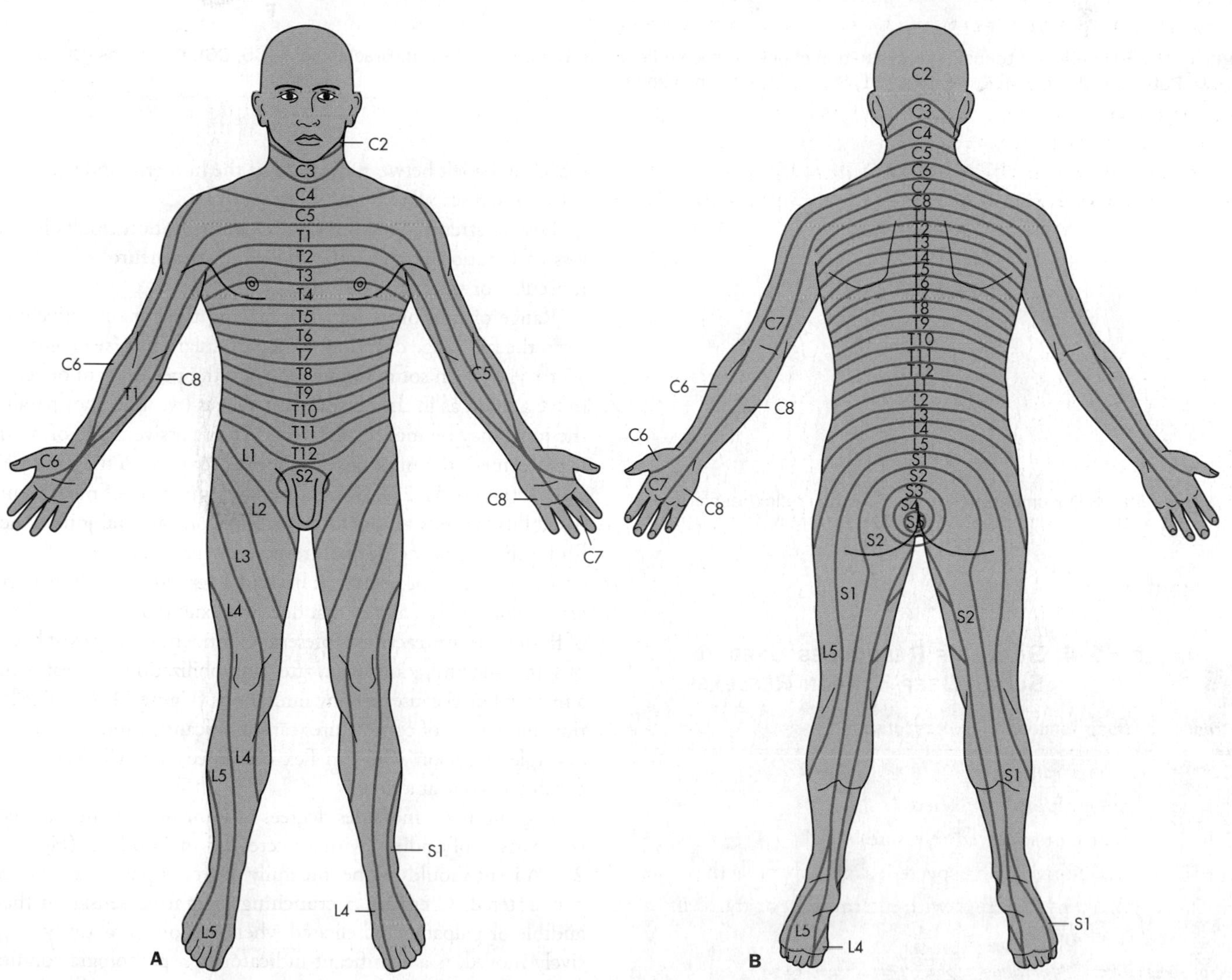

Figure 51-24 A, Dermatomes, anterior view. **B,** Dermatomes, posterior view.

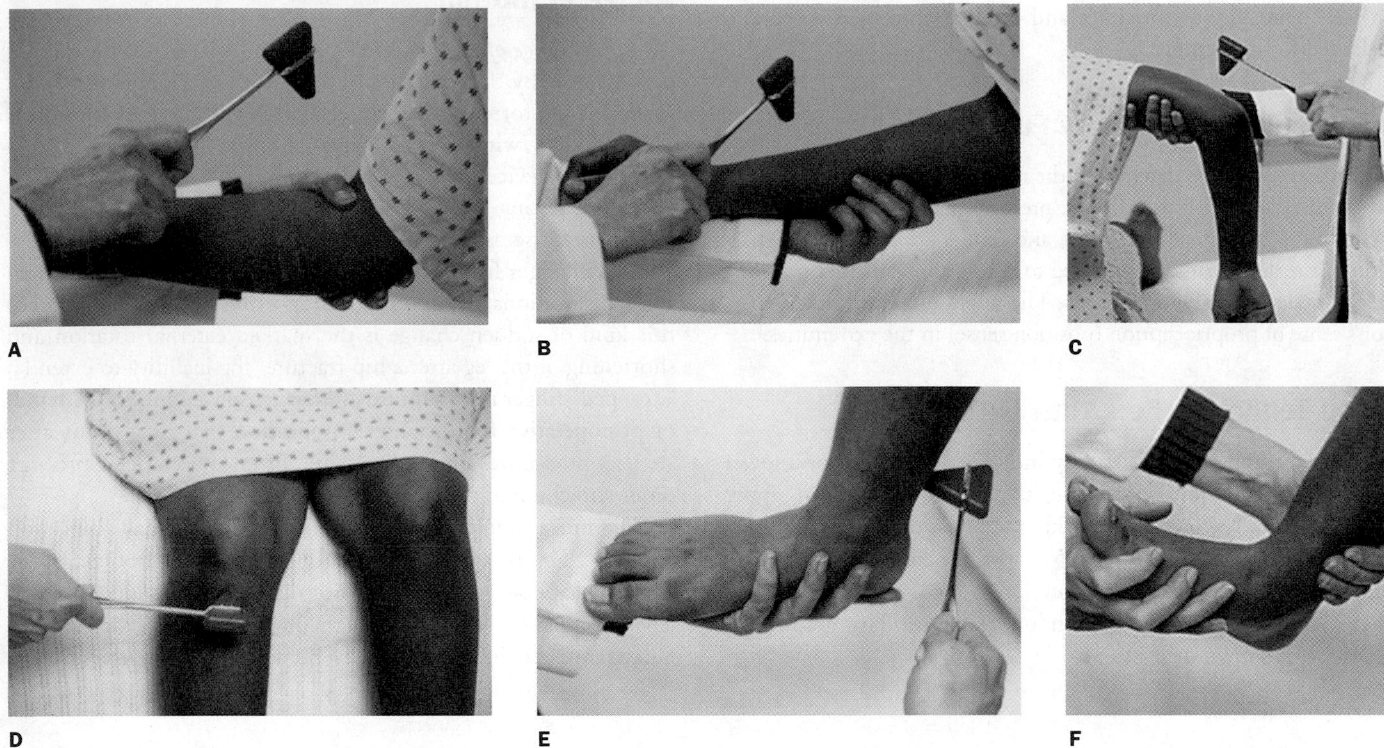

Figure 51-25 Location of tendons for evaluation of deep tendon reflexes. **A,** Biceps (C5, C6). **B,** Brachioradial (C5, C6). **C,** Triceps (C6, C7, C8). **D,** Patellar (L2, L3, L4). **E,** Achilles (S1, S2). **F,** Evaluation of ankle clonus.

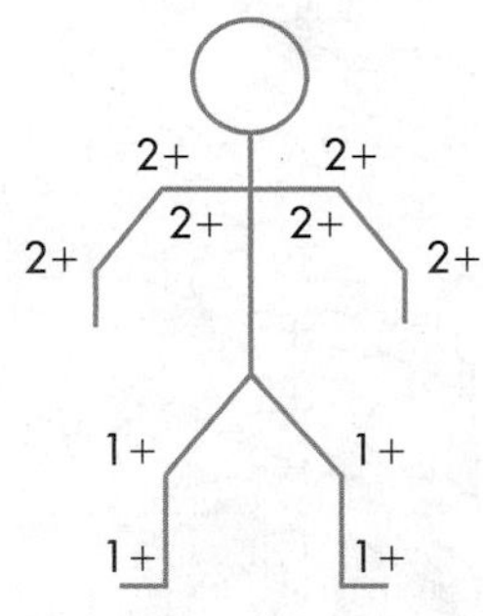

Figure 51-26 Documentation of deep tendon reflex response.

TABLE 51-4 SCALE OF RESPONSES USED TO SCORE DEEP TENDON REFLEXES

Grade	Deep Tendon Reflex Response
0	No response
1+	Sluggish or diminished
2+	Active or expected response
3+	More brisk than expected, slightly hyperactive
4+	Brisk, hyperactive, with intermittent or transient clonus

From Seidel HM et al: *Mosby's guide to physical examination,* ed 5, St Louis, 2003, Mosby.

space can be felt between the head of the humerus and the glenoid cavity of the scapula.

Loss of strength or limitation of joint motion results in some loss of function and may be the result of a neurologic, skeletal, muscular, or traumatic disorder.

Range of motion is tested by having the person actively perform the full range of motion of a particular joint (see Figures 51-15 to 51-17). In some instances, when the person cannot actively move a joint, as in the person with paresis (weakness) or paralysis, the joint may be moved passively. When passive range of motion is performed, the nurse gives support proximal to the joint being moved (Figure 51-27). Comparing the limitation of movement or instability present in one joint with its contralateral joint is helpful in differentiating normal from abnormal findings.

If a joint cannot be moved beyond a certain point in its normal arc of motion (e.g., a knee that does not extend beyond 130 degrees of flexion), a **contracture** is present. Contractures may exist because of soft tissue limitations (e.g., after immobilization for treatment of a fracture) or because of bony limitations (Figure 51-28). The location and nature of contractures can significantly limit function. For example, a person who can flex one knee only 15 degrees must climb stairs one at a time.

A goniometer measures degrees of joint movement and allows comparison of findings with expected normal findings (Figure 51-29). A joint should not be forcefully moved if pain or resistance is encountered. **Crepitus**, a crunching or grating sensation that is audible or palpable and elicited when the joint is actively or passively moved, is a significant indicator of a pathologic condition within the joint. This sensation can also be palpated or heard if the ends of a broken bone move against one another. In the pres-

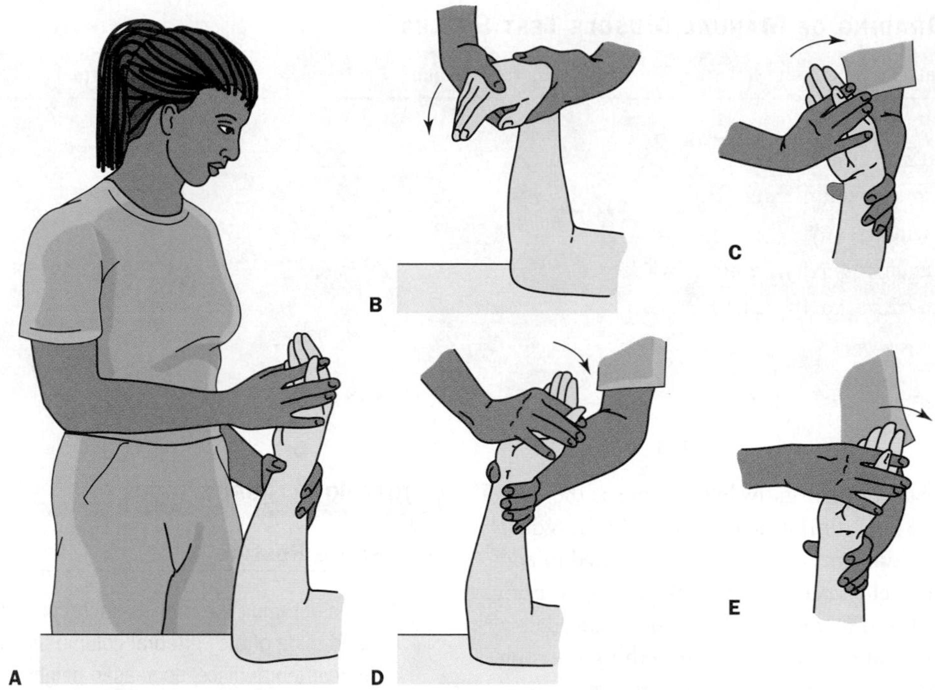

Figure 51-27 Techniques of passive range of motion. With patient in supine position, upper arm is supported on bed. **A,** Forearm is supported with nurse's hand; hand is supported with nurse's other hand. **B,** Wrist is flexed forward. **C,** Wrist is extended. **D,** Wrist is moved to ulnar side. **E,** Wrist is moved to radial side.

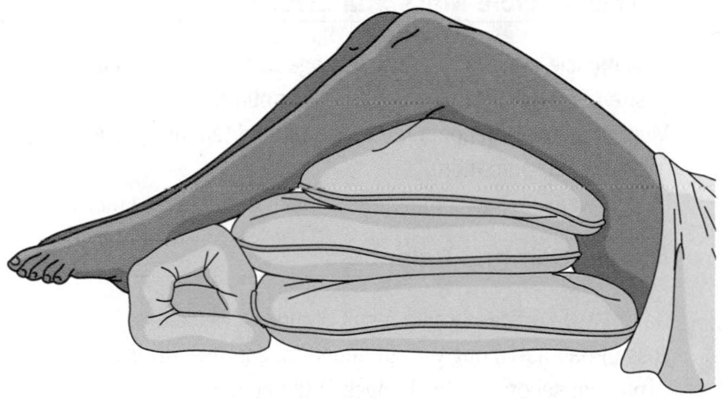

Figure 51-28 Contractures of hips and knees in patient with rheumatoid arthritis caused by continuous use of pillows to support knees in flexed position.

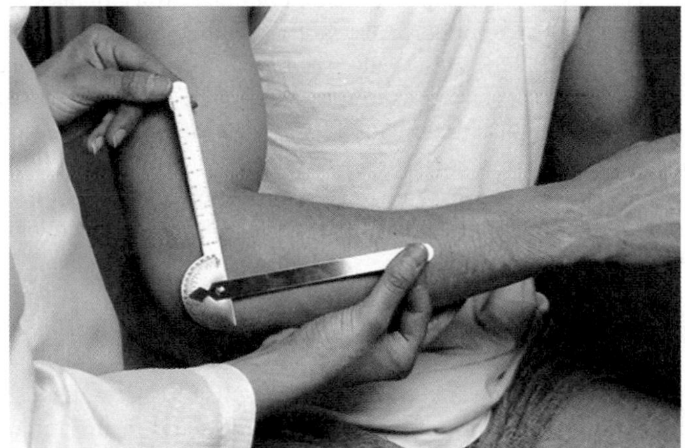

Figure 51-29 Measurement of joint motion with a goniometer.

ence of a possible fracture, no attempt should be made to elicit crepitus.

Muscle Strength

The nurse performs the manual muscle test (MMT) to determine the degree of muscular weakness resulting from disease, injury, or lack of use. The MMT rates the strength of muscles by their performance in relation to gravity and manually applied resistance. Factors such as gravity, stabilization of the tested part, proper positioning, amounts of resistance, range of the joint, pain, and abnormal muscle tone may influence the accuracy of the MMT.

Muscle strength can be assessed by asking the person to contract a certain muscle group and resist while the examiner exerts an opposing force. Responses are compared bilaterally. If pain occurs, the joint is not forced past the point of pain. The examiner notes the presence of spasms and evaluates muscles for flaccidity (lack of tone), hypotonicity (decreased tone), or hypertonicity (increased tone). Atrophy or hypertrophy of muscle mass is also noted. Findings are documented using a standard scale of measurement (Table 51-5).

The preceding tests of strength, dexterity, and range of motion are simple to perform; however, pain (rather than weakness, lack of coordination, or joint limitation) may limit the person's ability to perform the movement. It is often difficult to differentiate the cause of the deficit. The patient may have actual muscle weakness because of chronic pain and consequent disuse of muscles.

TABLE 51-5 GRADING OF MANUAL MUSCLE TEST SCALES

Muscle Functional Level	Grade	Percentage of Normal	Lovett Scale
No evidence of contractility	0	0	0 (zero)
Slight contractility, no movement	1	10	T (trace)
Full range of motion, gravity eliminated*	2	25	P (poor)
Full range of motion with gravity	3	50	F (fair)
Full range of motion against gravity, some resistance	4	75	G (good)
Full range of motion against gravity, full resistance	5	100	N (normal)

From Seidel HM et al: *Mosby's guide to physical examination,* ed 5, St Louis, 2003, Mosby.
*Passive movement.

Although the effect of pain is quantitatively the same as the effect of weakness or limitation (i.e., diminished function), pain is qualitatively different, and requires treatment measures geared to pain relief rather than to muscle strengthening. When performing these tests, the nurse must remember not to move the person beyond the point of pain. Pain indicates that something is wrong. Injudicious testing techniques can produce untoward results (e.g., the fracture of an osteoporotic bone).

The desired result of diagnostic testing is the establishment of a baseline of strength, motion, and dexterity from which interventions to assist the person in gaining strength, regaining lost motion, and increasing functional capacity may be planned and evaluated. Many specialized physical examination techniques aid in the diagnosis of abnormalities of the musculoskeletal system (Table 51-6). These are usually performed by advanced practice nurses, physician's assistants, or physicians. The reader is referred to a text on physical examination for a more in-depth description and illustration of these tests.

Assessment measures and variations in normal findings relevant to the care of older adults are presented in the Gerontologic Assessment box.

Gerontologic Assessment

Assess Posture

In the older adult the trunk is short compared with the extremities; shortening of the vertebral column as a result of thinning of the intervertebral discs, decreased height of individual vertebrae from osteoporosis, and, with advanced age, osteoporotic vertebral collapse result in loss of height.

Stooped posture (kyphosis) with a compensatory backward head tilt is common as a result of change in the center of gravity caused by lower extremity joint flexion.

Assess Muscle Mass and Strength

Total muscle mass decreases with age because of a decrease in size of some muscles and atrophy of others.

Muscle contours become more evident and tendons are more distinct on palpation.

Muscle weakness is common as a result of decreased mass.

Assess Gait and Balance

Gait may be unsteady as a result of muscle weakness.

Loss of balance along with the need for assistive devices may be present secondary to changes in the center of gravity.

Assess Bones and Joints

Flexion of the knees and hips accompanies joint degeneration.

Pain on palpation of spinous processes can indicate a compression fracture.

Enlarged, deformed joints occur with osteoarthritis and rheumatoid arthritis.

Tenderness and erythema of a joint is indicative of inflammation.

Diagnostic Tests

As with other illnesses, diagnostic test results offer data useful in diagnosing a patient's musculoskeletal illness and formulating a treatment plan. Elements of the patient's care may depend on the outcome of diagnostic studies. Some of the principal studies used for the person who has a musculoskeletal problem are described here.

Laboratory Tests

Laboratory tests consist of two major categories: serologic and urinary (Tables 51-7 and 51-8).

Radiologic Tests

Bones and Joints. Radiologic tests of bones and joints are imperative for the identification and treatment of fractures. They are also helpful in determining the presence of disease (e.g., rheumatoid arthritis, spondylitis, avascular necrosis, and tumor) and effects of treatment on these disorders. Consult a specialized text for further discussion of specific radiologic tests.

Many patients are unable to lie on x-ray examination tables for long periods. In particular, persons with arthritis develop joint stiffness and pain if their ability to move is restricted. Radiologic examinations for individuals with rheumatic diseases are often extensive, but few of these patients can tolerate having all the required views of all the involved joints taken in a single session.

TABLE 51-6 SPECIAL ASSESSMENT TECHNIQUES FOR THE MUSCULOSKELETAL SYSTEM

Assessment Technique	Description	Abnormality Detected
Limb measurement	Measure (in cm) extremities from a major landmark.	Asymmetric limb length may indicate pelvic obliquity or hip deformities; discrepancies in circumference may indicate atrophy or paresis of muscle groups; 1-cm discrepancy is normal in most people.
Ballottement	Compress suprapatellar pouch, which is normally snug against femur.	Fluid wave indicates excess fluid in knee (effusion).
Bulge sign	Stroke medial aspect of knee, then tap lateral side of patella; if fluid is present, a fluid wave or bulge will appear.	Fluid wave indicates effusion, excess fluid in suprapatellar pouch.
McMurray's test	Apply external rotation and valgus stress to knee while leg is held flexed at knee and hip (patient is lying supine); normally there is no pain or sound.	"Click" or pain indicates meniscal tear.
Drawer test (anteroposterior and mediolateral)	With patient supine and knee flexed, push forward and backward on tibia at joint line; with patient supine and knee extended, stabilize femur and ankle while attempting to abduct and adduct knee; normally there is little or no movement—assess symmetry of responses.	Laxity or movement suggests instability of anterior or posterior cruciate ligaments or medial or lateral collateral ligaments of knee.
Lachman's test	The patient is supine, heel on table, knee flexed 10-15 degrees. The examiner places one hand above the knee to stabilize the femur; he places the other hand around the proximal tibia and pulls the tibia anteriorly.	Increased laxity >5 mm compared with the unaffected side indicates injury to the anterior cruciate ligament.
Straight leg raising test (Lasègue's sign)	With patient supine, raise leg straight with knee extended; normally there is no pain.	If maneuver reproduces sciatic pain, it is considered positive and suggests a herniated disc.
Trendelenburg's test	While patient stands on one foot and then the other, both iliac crests should appear symmetric.	Asymmetry suggests hip dislocation.
Thomas test	With patient lying supine and one leg fully extended and the other flexed on chest, observe patient's ability to keep extended leg flat on table.	Inability to keep leg extended suggests hip flexion contracture in extended leg that may be masked by increased lumbar lordosis.
Phalen's test	Flex both wrists together to 90 degrees and hold for 60 seconds; normally this produces no symptoms.	Numbness, tingling, or burning in median nerve distribution suggests carpal tunnel syndrome.
Tinel's sign	Tap over median nerve where it passes through carpal tunnel in wrist; normally this does not produce any symptoms.	Tingling along median nerve distribution is associated with carpal tunnel syndrome.
Drop arm test	Raise affected arm to 90 degrees of flexion, then have patient slowly adduct arm to side.	Inability to lower arm slowly or smoothly is associated with disruption of rotator cuff mechanism of shoulder.
Scoliosis screening, "forward bend" test	Have patient bend forward; observe symmetry and height of scapulae, shoulders, iliac crests, rib cage.	Asymmetry of scapulae or shoulder height, "winged" iliac crests, demonstrable curve of spine, or rib hump indicate scoliosis.

Instead, 1 or 2 days of rest between shorter sessions may be required. Analgesics or local heat applications for relief of joint pain after x-ray examinations may be necessary.

Systemic Radiologic Studies. Systemic radiologic studies such as the barium enema, upper gastrointestinal series, and intravenous pyelogram are helpful in determining the extent of involvement of various internal organs (bowel, kidneys) in systemic rheumatic diseases. These examinations are discussed in Chapters 34 and 40.

Myelography. A myelogram is a radiologic examination of the spinal canal. Any portion of the spine (cervical, thoracic, or lumbar) can be examined. A radiopaque solution or, less commonly, air is injected into the subarachnoid space. Myelography is used to identify lesions such as herniated nucleus pulposus, nerve root

TABLE 51-7 SEROLOGIC TESTS

Test	Rationale for Performing Test
Serum muscle enzymes: Aspartate transaminase (AST; serum glutamatic-oxaloacetic transaminase [SGOT]) Aldolase Creatine phosphokinase (CPK) isoenzymes MM (CK_3-MM)	Enzymes can be elevated in presence of primary myopathic (muscle) diseases. Elevated levels may result from muscle fiber degeneration or from diffusion through a muscle membrane that has increased permeability. Enzyme levels are index of both progress of myopathic disorder and effectiveness of treatment. Aldolase levels are most commonly used to diagnose and monitor treatment of muscular dystrophy. NURSING PRECAUTION: Avoid intramuscular injections when these enzymes are being monitored. *Normal values:* AST 5: 8-20 unit/L Aldolase: 3-8.2 unit/dl CK_3-MM (muscle): percentage of total CK 90%-97%
Serologic test for syphilis (STS)	False-positive STS results occur in 10%-15% of persons with connective tissue diseases, so test may aid diagnosis.
Fluorescent treponemal antibody absorption (FTA-ABS)	FTA-ABS excludes presence of syphilis.
Rheumatoid factor or latex fixation (reaction of rheumatoid factor antibodies with IgG 7S gamma globulin)	Rheumatoid factor antibodies are found in sera (50%-95%) of individuals with rheumatoid arthritis. Test is considered positive if rheumatoid factor is found in titrations of 1:40 or greater. Test may be positive in persons with systemic lupus erythematosus (SLE). CAUTION: Rheumatoid factor may be found in other conditions (e.g., aging, scleroderma, acute pulmonary tuberculosis, hepatitis).
Antinuclear antibodies	Circulating antibodies, which are composed of protein material and called antinuclear antibodies, react with cellular nuclei and various individual constituents of cellular nuclei, and can be identified by fluorescent techniques using antihuman gamma globulin labeled with fluorescein. Positive tests are used in diagnosing Sjögren's syndrome, scleroderma, and SLE. Pattern of nuclear staining varies with different diseases. Poor positive predictive value for SLE and other rheumatic diseases.
Serum complement	Protein substances that are found in serum and synovial fluid are associated with immune and inflammatory mechanisms; low levels often occur in SLE and rheumatoid arthritis.
Erythrocyte sedimentation rate (ESR)	Increased rate of settling of erythrocytes is important index of inflammation. *Normal values:* men, <15 mm/hr; women, <20 mm/hr

involvement, spinal stenosis, tumor, or other lesions that may encroach on the spinal canal. Myelography has largely been replaced by magnetic resonance imaging (MRI) and computed tomography (CT) in the diagnosis of spinal disorders. However, myelograms may be used in conjunction with CT, particularly if the results of the CT scan are inconclusive. Other indications for myelography include obesity and postoperative spinal surgery.

The contrast medium used is either an oil- or a water-based solution. The viscosity of the oil-based solution (iophendylate [Pantopaque]) provides a good contrast medium for visualization of the spinal structures. However, its major disadvantage is that it must be removed as completely as possible after the examination or it may cause arachnoiditis, encephalopathy, or severe headaches.

Because of these limitations, water-soluble, nonionic solutions such as metrizamide (Amipaque) and iohexol (Omnipaque) are primarily used. Water-based dyes are less viscous and fill the canal and narrow spaces easily, allowing good visualization of the structures. They are absorbed into the cerebrospinal fluid (CSF) and excreted by the kidneys, and need not be removed after the procedure. Major adverse effects are seizures, nausea, headache, and vomiting after the procedure. Iohexol has a lower risk of neurotoxicity and seizures than metrizamide. Emergency medications and equipment should be immediately available in case of allergic response to the contrast medium. Informed consent is necessary before the procedure.

Patient education is vital. A thorough explanation of events before, during, and after the procedure may help allay fears and clarify any misconceptions regarding myelography.

Myelography is an outpatient procedure done in the radiology department by a radiologist with the assistance of a radiology technician. The patient should be instructed to fast, usually for 4 hours before the procedure. A careful history should be taken, noting any previous allergic reactions to other contrast agents, iodine, or shellfish. If a water-based solution is used, the patient may not take amphetamines, phenothiazines, or tricyclic antidepressants for 12 hours before the procedure because these drugs lower the seizure threshold.

If necessary, a sedative may be prescribed before the procedure. In the radiology department the patient is transferred to the x-ray table. The patient is placed in either a lateral or a sitting position and local anesthetic is injected before the lumbar puncture (see Chapter 47). The myelogram is performed with the patient in the prone position. Approximately 10 ml of CSF is withdrawn and sent to the laboratory for analysis. The contrast medium is then

TABLE 51-7 SEROLOGIC TESTS—CONT'D

Test	Rationale for Performing Test
Hematocrit	Individuals with systemic connective tissue disease often have normocytic (normal RBC count), normochromic (normal amount of iron carried by RBCs) anemia in absence of any abnormal bleeding. Individuals who suffer trauma or undergo major surgery to musculoskeletal system sustain significant blood loss. Symptoms of anemia (e.g., extreme tiredness, fatigue, weakness) are experienced when hematocrit drops quickly; acute symptoms may be absent if anemia develops gradually or is chronic. Individuals with acute anemia should not be physically stressed. *Normal values:* men, 45-50 vol/dl; women, 40-45 vol/dl
Calcium	Immobility and bone demineralization (bone cancers, multiple myeloma) will show increase in serum levels. Rickets, vitamin D deficiency, will show decrease in levels. Malnutrition also results in decreased levels. *Normal values:* total 9-10.5 mg/dl; ionized 4.5-5.6 mg/dl
Alkaline phosphatase (ALP)	Bone tumor and infections, fractures, Paget's disease, rickets, and other conditions that cause increase in osteoblastic activity will cause increase in ALP levels. Also used to monitor response to treatment for osteoporosis. In hypophosphatasia (characterized by defect in bone formation), levels are decreased. *Normal value:* 30-85 ImU/ml; slightly higher in older adults
Phosphorus	Together with calcium, plays vital role in bone metabolism. Conditions that cause increase in calcium levels will cause decrease in serum phosphates. *Normal value:* 2.5-4.5 mg/dl
Anti-DNA antibody	Antibodies to DNA are present in serum of 60%-80% of persons with SLE and can be used in diagnosis of SLE or to monitor response to treatment.
C-reactive protein	C-reactive protein is used as a nonspecific indicator of infection and inflammation, is commonly used to aid in diagnosis of rheumatoid arthritis, and may also be used to monitor responses to antibiotics or antiinflammatory medication.
LE prep	This is used in diagnosis and treatment of SLE. Antinuclear factor in SLE is LE factor; LE test detects antinuclear antibodies, but many patients with SLE have negative results.

DNA, Deoxyribonucleic acid; *IgG,* immunoglobulin G; *LE,* lupus erythematosus *RBC,* red blood cells.

TABLE 51-8 URINARY TESTS

Diagnostic Test	Rationale for Test
24-hr urine for creatine/creatinine ratio	In presence of muscle disease, ability of muscle to convert creatine decreases, amount of creatine excreted by kidneys increases, and ratio of urinary creatine to creatinine increases. Periodic studies are helpful in diagnosis and evaluation of progress of treatment of primary myopathies.
Urinary uric acid levels (24-hr collection)*	This is helpful in diagnosis and decisions regarding treatment modalities for gout. *Normal value:* <900 mg uric acid excretion per day
Urine for deoxypyridinoline (first morning void) routine collection	Deoxypyridinoline (Dpd) cross-links assay provides quantitative measurement of Dpd, which is excreted unmetabolized in urine during bone resorption. Used to monitor effectiveness of antiresorptive therapies. *Normal value:* 2.3-7.4 nmol Dpd/mmol creatinine

*NOTE: 24-hr urine collections must be accurate to facilitate proper diagnosis and treatment.

injected, and the x-ray table is moved and tilted, allowing the dye to fill the canal as films are taken. The procedure may take up to 1 hour. Commonly a CT scan follows the myelography.

After myelography, fluids are encouraged to replace the removed CSF and to aid in the excretion of the contrast medium. If an oil-based dye was used, the patient is kept flat in bed for approximately 8 hours. If a water-soluble dye was used, bed rest is maintained, with the head of the bed elevated 30 degrees for 6 to 8 hours. If air was used, the head of the bed should be kept lower than the trunk for up to 48 hours.

Contrast material has a diuretic effect. The nurse teaches the patient to monitor output for at least 8 hours after the test. The patient's diet is resumed as tolerated, and fluids are encouraged, regardless of the dye used. The nurse observes the patient for any reactions to the contrast agent. Headaches, nausea, and vomiting are the most common side effects. Neurologic checks are performed hourly. The lumbar puncture site is covered with a small adhesive strip and observed for any bleeding. The patient can be discharged the afternoon of the procedure. Patients should continue with bed rest at home and then gradually resume normal activities. They should avoid lifting or strenuous activity for 24 hours.

The nurse teaches the patient to check the puncture site for drainage, swelling, or signs of infection. Anticonvulsants or other medications withheld before the procedure may be resumed in 48 hours. The patient is instructed to contact the physician if persistent nausea or vomiting develops.

Myelography is contraindicated for persons with multiple sclerosis. Allergy to contrast material or renal impairment affects the choice of contrast medium.

Bone Densitometry. Bone densitometry measures bone density to aid in the diagnosis of osteoporosis, predict fracture risk, and monitor the effectiveness of treatment protocols. The most widely used method is dual-energy x-ray absorptiometry (DEXA or DXA scan). This noninvasive radiologic test measures bone mass and density in the lumbar spine, proximal femur, and wrist. DEXA scans can measure bone mineral density (BMD) and bone mineral concentration with results in a few minutes. Two photon energy beams are emitted by an x-ray machine. A digital imaging device that scans the fingers is also available. The two types of scanners are the pencil-beam and the fan-beam. The fan-beam produces images with better resolution in less time. Both emit low-dose radiation, approximately 1 to 3 mrem, compared with 20 to 50 mrem for a chest x-ray film. The duration of the procedures varies from 30 seconds per site to 4 minutes per site. No special preparation or aftercare for this test is needed. A certified x-ray technologist performs the tests.

The hip, spine, wrist, finger, tibia, or heel may be used to measure BMD. The patient's results are compared against two norms: the T score and the Z score. The T score or "young normal" compares the patient's results with the peak bone density of a 30-year-old healthy adult. The Z score or "age-matched" score compares the patient with the peak bone density expected in a healthy adult of the same age, sex, and race. T scores show the number of standard deviations the patient differs from the normal scores of a 30-year-old person. Z scores are the number of standard deviations the patient differs from age-matched normals. Scores within 1 standard deviation of the norm are considered as normal bone density by the World Health Organization.[6] Scores below the norm are given in negative numbers. Standard deviations of negative one (−1) represent a 12% reduction in bone mass.

Treatment is generally initiated for persons with BMD results 2.5 SD below the T score. The American Association of Clinical Endocrinologists recommends that all women 65 years and older have screening BMD; women under 65 years should have BMD testing if they are at risk for osteoporosis.[4] BMD testing is also recommended for all men over 65 years of age. Younger persons may need BMD testing if they have additional risk factors for osteoporosis (glucocorticoid-induced osteoporosis). BMD should be reassessed every 2 years for most persons.

Other methods to assess bone density include single x-ray absorptiometry (SXA), quantitative ultrasonography, and qualitative computed tomography (QCT). Bone ultrasonography is best used as a screening tool and measures the bone density in the calcaneus, assessing for osteoporosis and risk of fracture. The test estimates the BMD of the heel. Results represent the quantitative ultrasound index and are reported as T scores; the lower the T score, the greater the risk of fracture. QCT has the capacity to measure true bone mineral values, but its use is limited due to cost and the amount of ionizing radiation exposure.

Arthrography. Arthrography permits visualization of structures within the joint that are not normally seen on routine radiographic films. An arthrogram is usually performed on the knee or shoulder for evaluation of persistent pain or preoperative assessment. The elbow, wrist, hip, and temporomandibular joints may also be visualized with arthrography.

The joint cavity is injected with radiopaque dye, air, or both. When both are used, the test is referred to as a double-contrast arthrogram. The dye or air serves as a contrast medium against which the outlines of soft tissue components of the joint may be seen. Tears of the menisci and internal derangement of the joint such as ligament disruption and synovial cysts can be diagnosed with the aid of arthrograms.

Before the examination the nurse checks the patient for allergies to iodine or seafood. Patients may experience pain while the joint is expanded by the dye or air, and local anesthetic may be injected before the examination. Analgesics are prescribed after the examination. The nurse instructs the patient to watch for redness, edema, or unusual pain in the joint after the procedure.

Radioisotope Bone Scans. Radioisotope bone scans are performed primarily to demonstrate the presence of metastatic disease, tumors, infection (osteomyelitis), and other conditions with increased bone activity. This nuclear scanning test can also be used to diagnose the cause of undetermined bone pain and assess the healing of fractures. Intravenously injected sodium pertechnetate technetium 99m (^{99m}Tc) is the isotope most commonly used in this study. The ^{99m}Tc concentrates in areas of osteoblastic activity involved in the exchange of calcium.

Technetium, a bone-seeking radioisotope, is taken up by the bone in areas of adequate blood supply and metabolic activity. "Hot spots" on the scan indicate areas of increased bone turnover, as in fractures, bone healing, and inflammatory responses. "Cold spots," or areas of decalcified bone, indicate no bone activity, as in lytic lesions. Lesions may be visualized on bone scans as early as 3 to 6 months before they are evident on routine x-ray films. Bone scans are commonly used to rule out bony metastases from the prostate, breast, and lung.

Technetium scans are also of some use in determining the degree of parotid gland involvement in Sjögren's syndrome. The uptake, concentration, and excretion of the isotope by the major salivary glands are measured by a technique known as sequential scintigraphy.

Persons being prepared for these procedures should know that the procedures are not painful and the isotopes will not harm them. However, the patient may have to remain quietly in one position for an hour or more. The nurse assesses the patient for iodine or seafood allergies and encourages the patient to drink fluids before the examination. The bladder should be emptied just before the scan to avoid interference with visualization of the pelvis. The radioisotope is injected intravenously about 2 hours before scanning. Procedures using barium or iodine are not scheduled before the bone scan, since these substances interfere with scanning. The kidneys excrete the radioisotope in the urine within 6 to 24 hours. Fluids are encouraged after the scan to aid in excretion of the isotope.

Computed Tomography. Tomography is an x-ray technique by which detailed images of "slices" of tissue are obtained by focusing x-ray beams at predetermined planes or depths of the tissue being studied. Clear and detailed images of the structures at that level are produced, and details of structures surrounding that level are blurred or eliminated. CT scanning is tomography employing a computer to compose a picture of the tissue being studied. A series of x-ray beams is rotated, 1 degree at a time, around the specific area being examined. With each rotation a picture is generated that depicts the difference in tissue density. CT may be used in conjunction with intravenous or oral contrast media to allow better visualization of structures.

The scan picks up disruptions in normal structures. The procedure can be used in diagnosing spinal pathologic conditions and tumors and in evaluating the hip before custom joint replacement. The procedure is noninvasive and does not require repositioning of the patient, as does conventional tomography. Disadvantages of CT include poor depiction of intraspinal processes and poor differentiation between disc herniation and postoperative scar tissue. CT is commonly done after myelography in diagnosing spinal pathologic conditions. Patients who are claustrophobic may have difficulty tolerating the procedure because they must lie in a cylindric metal scanner for up to 1 hour.

Diskography. Diskography is a radiologic procedure that uses a contrast medium to evaluate the integrity of the intervertebral discs. Diskography is performed on an outpatient basis in the operating room or radiology department with the use of fluoroscopy. The patient is placed in the prone position, and local anesthetic is administered. The patient may require additional sedation, since the procedure can be uncomfortable. Needle position is confirmed by fluoroscopy; contrast medium and saline are then injected into the disc space. If a pathologic condition is present, injection of the saline reproduces the patient's back or leg pain. Despite the accuracy of myelography, CT, and MRI, the diskogram is still a useful diagnostic tool because the ability to reproduce the patient's symptoms may aid the surgeon in differential diagnosis, especially when several vertebral levels are involved. However, this technique is less specific than myelography.

▶ ARE YOU READY?

In providing preprocedure teaching for a patient undergoing arthrography, the nurse states which of the following?

1. "You may not eat or drink anything for 12 hours before the procedure."
2. "You will receive general anesthesia."
3. "You will have air or contrast dye injected into your joint."
4. "Your joint will need to be immobilized for 6 to 8 hours after the procedure."

Special Tests

Magnetic Resonance Imaging. Magnetic resonance imaging (MRI) is a scanning technique that produces tomographic images using magnetic forces rather than x-ray beams. The patient lies on a nonmagnetic scanning table that slides, head first, into a large cylindric magnet. The magnet causes the body's atomic protons to line up and spin in the same direction. A radio frequency signal is beamed into the magnetic field, causing the protons to move out of alignment. When the signal stops, the protons move back into alignment and release energy. A receiver coil measures the energy released by the movement of the protons and the time it takes for the protons to return to their aligned position. These measurements provide information regarding the type of tissue in which the protons lie, as well as the condition of the tissue. A computer uses this information to construct an image on a television screen, showing the distribution of protons of hydrogen atoms; the television image may also be recorded on film or magnetic tape. The images produced by MRI are more accurate than those produced by CT or myelography.

Patients undergoing an MRI should know that the procedure is painless and requires no special preparation. However, because a magnetic field is used, the patient is asked to remove any metallic objects, such as jewelry, hairpins, credit cards, and nonpermanent dentures. Patients who have cardiac pacemakers or intracranial vascular aneurysm clips are excluded from MRI. Persons who have metal implants cannot have that area scanned.

As with CT scanning, patients who are claustrophobic may have difficulty being placed in the scanner. Scanning time is usually 30 to 90 minutes. Sometimes medication such as diazepam (Valium) is prescribed to help the patient relax. "Open-air" MRI scanners allow the patient to feel less confined but still obtain high-quality images. These scanners are an option for some patients. During the scan the patient hears the hum of the machine, a loud thump when the radio waves are turned on and off, and other machinelike noises. The thumping can be annoying or even frightening if patients were not warned about it. Many facilities offer earplugs to reduce noise while in the scanner.

Contrast media may be used with MRI to enhance the quality of the images. For example, gadolinium-DPTA differentiates recurrent disc herniation from epidural scarring.

Electromyography. An electromyogram (EMG) is a recording of the variations of electrical potentials (voltage) detected by a needle electrode inserted into skeletal muscle. An EMG, an electrophysiologic test, differentiates between myopathies (muscle diseases) and neuropathies (nerve diseases). The electrical activity can be heard over a loudspeaker and viewed on an oscilloscope and graph at the same time. No electrical activity can be detected in normal muscles at rest, but during volitional movement, action potentials can be detected. In both primary myopathic and neuropathic disorders, specific variations exist in the size of individual motor unit potentials. In neurogenic atrophy, fibrillations may be present in the resting muscle. An EMG provides direct evidence of motor dysfunction and can be used to some extent to detect a dysfunction located in the motor neuron, the neuromuscular junction, or the muscle fibers. Thus it is particularly helpful in the diagnosis of lower motor neuron disease, primary muscle disease, and defects in the transmission of electrical impulses at the neuromuscular junction, such as those occurring in myasthenia gravis. However, electromyography cannot be used to differentiate specific disease entities in either the myopathic or neuropathic categories.

No special preparation is required for this procedure. The patient may fear that insertion of electrode needles will be painful or that electrical stimulation of the needles will cause severe shock. Although the patient may be reassured that the procedure is not dangerous, some individuals do experience mild to moderate discomfort. Therefore nurses preparing patients for this test should not refer to the test as "painless."

Biopsy. Biopsies of tissue from a variety of organs are helpful in the diagnosis of disease or disorders affecting the musculoskeletal system. Table 51-9 lists the tissues that may be biopsied, the tests performed, the significance of results, and nursing considerations for patients undergoing biopsy.

Joint Aspiration. Joint aspiration (arthrocentesis) is performed to obtain a sample of synovial fluid from within the joint cavity. This procedure (performed by introducing a needle into the joint cavity and withdrawing fluid) helps determine the presence of an

TABLE 51-9 TYPES OF BIOPSIES

Organ Tested	Tests Performed	Positive Results	Nursing Considerations
Skin (punch biopsy)	Immunofluorescent staining—tissue washed with solution of fluorescein-labeled antihuman gamma globulin antibody	Band of immunofluorescence at epidermal-dermal junction, indicating presence of rheumatic disease (e.g., scleroderma, systemic lupus erythematosus, psoriatic arthritis)	Keep biopsy site clean and dry with small adhesive bandage until scab develops; patient experiences only mild discomfort.
Muscle (operative procedure)	Histochemical staining	Tissue reveals features of lower motor neuron disease, degeneration, inflammatory reaction as in polymyositis, or involvement of specific fibers indicating primary myopathic disease	Instruct patient and prepare for surgery; monitor patient per postanesthesia routine (local or general); patient experiences mild to moderate pain and stiffness in biopsy area; routine activity encouraged within 24 hr to avoid undue stiffness; change dressings as necessary.
Synovium (closed—performed with needle; open—performed in surgery)	Histologic examination—synovial fluid obtained at same time; may be cultured to determine presence of infection	Differentiates various forms of arthritis	Instruct patient about procedure; patient may require postanesthesia monitoring; strict asepsis is observed throughout procedure and in caring for wound; apply small compression dressing to joint; rest joint for 24 hr to prevent hemorrhage or effusion.
Buccal mucosa (punch biopsy)	Histologic examination of tissue from inside lower lip	Helpful in diagnosing Sjögren's syndrome	Instruct patient about procedure; patient generally experiences minor discomfort; diet is altered to avoid rough and hot foods (they will irritate surgical site).
Bone (operative procedure)	Microscopic analysis	Can confirm presence of infection or neoplasm	Instruct patient and prepare for surgery; monitor patient per postanesthesia routine; patient may experience mild to severe discomfort; activity restrictions depend on location and extent of surgical procedure; change dressings as necessary.

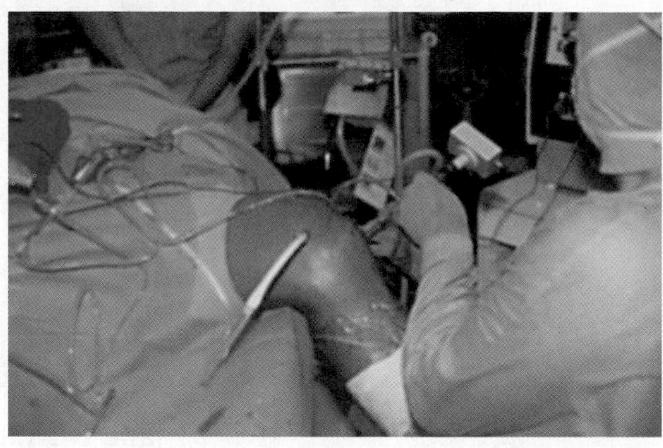

A

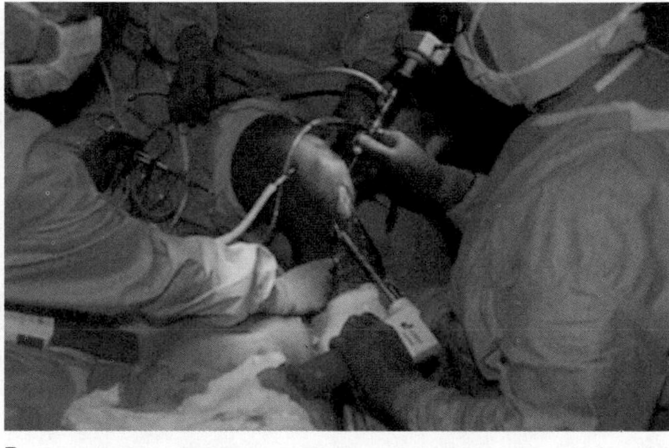

B

Figure 51-30 **A,** Arthroscopy of knee. **B,** Arthroscopically aided reconstruction of anterior cruciate ligament.

aseptic inflammatory process such as rheumatoid arthritis or a septic process such as bacterial arthritis. Samples of synovial fluid are cultured and examined both microscopically and chemically.

The synovial fluid is normally straw colored and clear; the viscosity resembles that of clean motor oil. In the presence of inflammation the fluid becomes turbid and watery. The mucin clot test is performed by mixing synovial fluid with glacial acetic acid. Normal synovial fluid forms a white, ropy mucin clot. When inflammation is present, the clot breaks apart easily and becomes flaky (flocculent). The degree of flocculence increases with the degree of inflammation. Also, when inflammation is present, the WBC count, the protein content, and the number of polymorphonuclear cells in the synovial fluid are increased and the glucose content is decreased.

A local anesthetic is usually administered before the procedure. Strict asepsis is observed. After the procedure the joint is often wrapped in a small compression (elastic) dressing. The joint may be rested for 8 to 24 hours.

Endoscopy

Arthroscopy (visualization of a joint) is performed in the operating room, usually in an ambulatory surgical center, with the patient under local or regional anesthesia. A specially designed endoscope (arthroscope) is inserted through a small incision into the joint cavity, enabling the physician to visualize the structure and contents of the joint (Figure 51-30). Most arthroscopic procedures are performed on the knee, although the wrist, ankle, hip, shoulder, and temporomandibular joint are also examined and treated using this technique.

The procedure is used to diagnose and treat such conditions as chondromalacia of the knee, ligamentous disruption, meniscal tears, carpal tunnel syndrome, osteoarthritis, rheumatoid arthritis, and impingement syndrome. Endoscopy is also used in minimally invasive surgical procedures.

Analgesics are prescribed after the procedure. The nurse instructs the patient to observe the operative site for swelling and signs of infection. The time the joint is rested and the use of any immobilizing devices depend on the location and extent of the procedure. To avoid damaging the joint, the surgeon is consulted regarding the activity the patient is permitted after the procedure.

References

1. Guyton AC, Hall JE: *Textbook of medical physiology,* ed 10, Philadelphia, 2001, Saunders.
2. Maher AB, Salmond SW, Pellino TA: *Orthopaedic nursing,* ed 3, Philadelphia, 2002, Saunders.
3. McCance KL, Huether SE: *Pathophysiology: the biologic basis for disease in adults and children,* ed 4, St Louis, 2002, Mosby.
4. Morgan A: The basics of bone density testing, *Clin Adv* 44(4):76, 2002.
5. Thibodeau GA, Patton KT: *Anatomy and physiology,* ed 5, St Louis, 2003, Mosby.
6. WHO Scientific Group: *Prevention and management of osteoporosis,* Report of a WHO Scientific Group, Who Technical Report Series, No 921, Geneva, 2003, author.

evolve **Visit the Evolve website:** http://evolve.elsevier.com/Monahan/medsurg

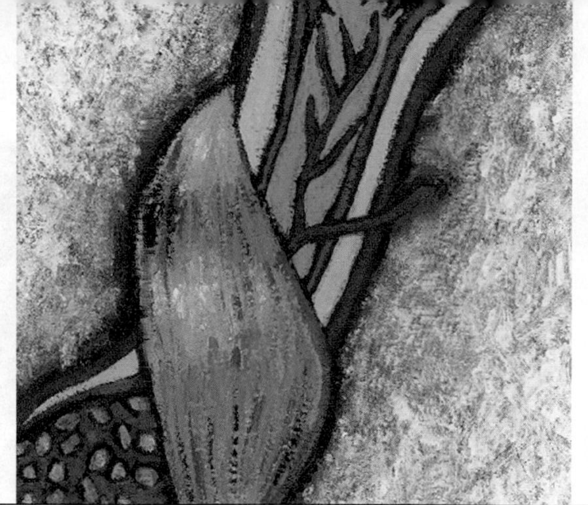

CHAPTER 52

Trauma to the Musculoskeletal System

by Jane F. Marek

OBJECTIVES

After studying this chapter, the learner should be able to:

1. Describe measures to promote bone health and prevent fractures.
2. Explain various treatment modalities for fracture healing.
3. Correlate complications of fractures with the available treatment regimens.
4. Explain the nursing role in the management of fractures and prevention of complications.
5. Develop a nursing care plan for a person who has undergone surgical repair of a hip fracture.
6. Compare the nursing care required by a person with a prosthetic implant for a hip fracture with that required by a person who has received an internal fixation device.
7. Delineate the special nursing considerations in caring for the patient with a spinal fracture.
8. Analyze the various types of soft tissue trauma and joint injuries.
9. Discuss the nursing care of patients who have sustained soft tissue trauma and joint injuries.
10. Discuss the special care considerations of the patient who has sustained multiple injuries.

KEY TERMS

abduction, p. 1546
alignment, p. 1523
callus formation, p. 1523
comminuted, p. 1523
cortex, p. 1523
displaced fracture, p. 1523
hemiarthroplasty, p. 1543
heterotopic bone formation, p. 1526
immobilization, p. 1523
internal fixation, p. 1523
nonunion, p. 1525
open fracture, p. 1523
open reduction, p. 1526
pathologic fracture, p. 1522
pseudarthrosis, p. 1525
subluxation, p. 1550

The person with musculoskeletal trauma has sustained an interruption in the integrity of one or more components of the system. Musculoskeletal trauma is most commonly manifested as a bone fracture, but it may include injury to soft tissue or to a muscle, ligament, meniscus, tendon, or joint. The National Center for Health Statistics estimates that annually an average of 1 in 10 persons suffers acute injury to the musculoskeletal system. The most common injuries are fractures, dislocations, and sprains.

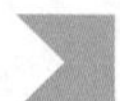

Trauma to Bone

Fracture

Etiology. A fracture is a disruption in the continuity of a bone, usually as a result of a blow to the body, a fall, or another accident. The amount of force or stress required to break the bone depends on several factors, including the size and density of the bone involved, the type and amount of stress applied, and the patient's age. A fracture results when the bone is unable to absorb stress.

Although most fractures occur as a result of an accident or injury, stress fractures occur as a result of normal activity or after minimal injury. There are two types of stress fractures: fatigue and insufficiency related. *Fatigue* fractures are more common in young, healthy persons and are caused by repeated stress and impact, usually from sports-related activities. The fracture begins as a small area of cortical infarct and progresses with continued stress. An *insufficiency-related* fracture, also called **pathologic fracture,** occurs as a result of normal weight bearing or minimal activity; the bone is unable to absorb the stress and recover. These types of fractures typically occur to bones weakened by disease, such as primary or metastatic cancer, metabolic disorders, or osteoporosis. Another type of fracture, avulsion fracture, occurs when a strong ligamentous or tendinous attachment pulls a fragment of bone away from the rest of the bone.

Epidemiology. Fractures occur in all age-groups, but the highest incidence is in young men, 15 to 24 years of age, and in older adults, particularly women, 65 years of age and older. Tibial fractures are the most common long bone fracture and are usually a result of motor vehicle accidents. Neuromuscular instability is an important contributing factor to the risk of falls, which commonly precede a fracture in the older population. Wrist, hip, and vertebral fractures are most common in older adults. The incidence of fatigue stress fractures is higher in athletes than in the general population. The higher incidence of stress fractures in female athletes with menstrual irregularities is thought to be a result of decreased estrogen levels, which cause decreased bone density. Persons in high-risk occupations (e.g., steelworkers, race car drivers) and persons with chronic degenerative or neoplastic diseases are also at higher risk for injury.

This section discusses fractures in general. Later the chapter addresses complications of fractures and hip and spinal fractures.

Pathophysiology

TYPES OF FRACTURES. A fracture is a complete or partial interruption of osseous tissue. *Complete* fractures penetrate both cortices, producing two bone fragments; in *incomplete* fractures only one **cortex** is broken. The part of the bone nearest the center of the body is referred to as the *proximal fragment*; the part more distant from the center is called the *distal fragment*. The proximal fragment is also called the *uncontrollable fragment* because its location and muscular attachments prevent it from being moved or manipulated in an attempt to bring the separate fragments into **alignment**. The distal fragment is called the *controllable fragment* because it can usually be moved to bring it into correct relationship to the proximal fragment. Fractures in long bones are designated as being in the proximal, middle, or distal third of the bone.

If the skin over the fracture is intact, the fracture is classified as *simple*, or *closed*. A fracture is classified as *compound*, or *open*, when there is direct communication between a skin wound and the fracture site. An **open fracture** has a high risk of contamination, which is an important factor in treatment. Open fractures can be classified into three categories based on the severity of the fracture and the degree of soft tissue involvement. Type 3 fractures are the most severe and are further subdivided into three subtypes (Box 52-1).[10]

When the two bone fragments are in proper alignment with no change from normal position despite the break in continuity of bone, the fracture is referred to as a *nondisplaced* fracture. A **displaced fracture** occurs when the bone fragments are separated at the point of fracture. The degree of displacement varies with the type of injury and the condition of the bone and soft tissues. The position of the bone fragments depends on the mechanism of injury. The type, direction, and strength of the force and pull of the attached muscles determine the position of the bone fragments. Bone fragments that slide over each other are referred to as *overriding* fragments.

The line of fracture as revealed by x-ray film or fluoroscopy is usually classified according to type (Figure 52-1 and Box 52-2). Fractures may be classified as a *greenstick* fracture, with splintering on one side of the bone (this occurs most often in older adults and in young children); *transverse*, with the break being straight across the bone; *oblique*, with the line of the fracture at an oblique angle to the bone shaft; or *spiral*, with the fracture lines partially encircling the bone. The fracture may be referred to as *telescoped*, or *impacted*, if the distal fragment is forcibly pushed against and into the proximal fragment. This occurs most often with compression and force applied to the distal fragment. If the fracture has several bone fragments, it is referred to as **comminuted.**

Because bones are more rigid than their surrounding structures, any force severe enough to fracture a bone may also injure adjacent muscles, nerves, connective tissue, and blood vessels. The force that causes the fracture is dissipated through the surrounding soft tissue, and small fragments of bone may become embedded in muscle, blood vessels, or nerves.

Box 52-1 Classifications of Open Fractures

Type 1

Length of wound less than 1 cm
Low-energy injury

Type 2

Length of wound greater than 1 cm
More energy absorbed during fracture

Type 3

Length of wound greater than 10 cm
Comminuted fracture with extensive soft tissue damage
High-energy injury typically from gunshot wounds, motor vehicle accidents, farming accidents

Type 3A

Does not require major reconstructive surgery for closure

Type 3B

Major soft tissue defects requiring reconstructive surgery for closure

Type 3C

Vascular and neural compromise
Require major reconstructive procedures

HEALING OF FRACTURES. A fracture disrupts the cortex, periosteum, and adjacent soft tissues. Bleeding occurs at the broken ends of the bone and surrounding soft tissues. Important considerations in fracture healing are the blood supply to the fracture site and adequate **immobilization.** Once immobilization is accomplished, the bone heals by the process of **callus formation** (see Chapter 51). Immobilization of the fracture is vital for proper healing and may be accomplished in one of three ways:

1. Physiologic splinting, a naturally occurring phenomenon related to pain in the affected area that causes guarding, muscle spasm, and avoidance of use, as well as a desire to rest the whole body until some repair has occurred
2. External orthopedic splinting with devices such as casts, plaster splints, and braces
3. **Internal fixation** with screws, plates, or rods to hold the opposing ends of the fracture in place

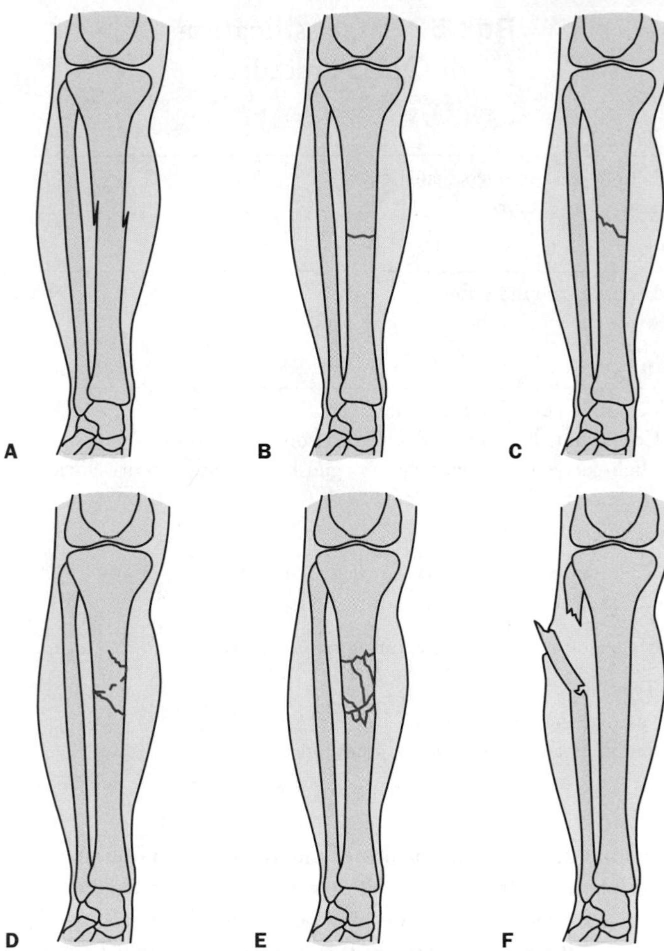

Figure 52-1 Types of fractures. **A,** Greenstick. **B,** Transverse. **C,** Oblique. **D,** Spiral. **E,** Comminuted. **F,** Open.

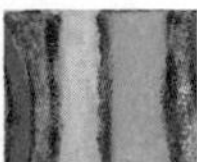

Clinical Manifestations
Fractures

- Pain (caused by swelling at site, muscle spasm, damage to periosteum)
  - —Immediate
  - —Severe
  - —Aggravated by pressure at site of injury
  - —Aggravated by attempted motion
- Loss of normal function (injured part incapable of voluntary movement)
- Obvious deformity resulting from loss of bone continuity
- Excessive motion at site (i.e., motion where it does not usually occur)
- Crepitus or grating sound if limb is moved gently*
- Soft tissue edema in area of injury resulting from extravasation of blood and tissue fluid
- Warmth over injured area resulting from increased blood flow to the area
- Ecchymosis of skin surrounding injured area (may not be apparent for several days)
- Impairment or loss of sensation or paralysis distal to injury resulting from nerve entrapment or damage
- Signs of shock related to severe tissue injury, blood loss, or intense pain
- Evidence of fracture on x-ray film

*No attempt should be made to elicit this sign when a fracture is suspected because it may cause further damage and increase pain.

The clinical manifestations of fractures differ, depending on the location and type of fracture and associated soft tissue injuries (see Clinical Manifestations box). Characteristics of most fractures include pain, impairment or loss of function, deformity, abnormal or excessive motion, swelling, altered sensation, and radiologic evidence of fracture. The immediate pain associated with a fracture is usually severe. Attempts at movement increase the pain. Factors contributing to the pain are associated soft tissue injuries, muscle spasms, and overriding of fracture fragments. Alterations in sensation are caused by pressure, pinching, or severing of nerves from the trauma or from bone fragments.

Fracture healing begins with hematoma formation 24 to 72 hours after the injury. The healing time required for fractures depends on many factors, including the patient's age and the type of bone fractured. Adults require a longer healing time than children.

Box 52-2 Types of Fractures

Typical Complete Fractures

Closed (simple) fracture: Noncommunicating wound between bone and skin
Open (compound) fracture: Communicating wound between bone and skin
Comminuted fracture: Multiple bone fragments
Linear fracture: Fracture line parallel to long axis of bone
Oblique fracture: Fracture line at 45-degree angle to long axis of bone
Spiral fracture: Fracture line encircling bone
Transverse fracture: Fracture line perpendicular to long axis of bone
Impacted fracture: Fracture fragments pushed into each other
Pathologic fracture: Fracture at a point in the bone weakened by disease (e.g., by tumor or osteoporosis)
Avulsion fracture: Fracture in which a fragment of bone connected to a ligament breaks off from the main bone
Extracapsular fracture: Fracture close to the joint but outside the joint capsule
Intracapsular fracture: Fracture within the joint capsule

Typical Incomplete Fractures

Greenstick fracture: Break on one cortex of bone with splintering of inner bone surface
Torus fracture: Buckling of cortex
Bowing fracture: Bending of the bone
Stress fracture: Microfracture
Transchondral fracture: Separation of cartilaginous joint surface (articular cartilage) from main shaft of bone

From McCance KL, Huether SE: *Pathophysiology: the biologic basis for disease in adults and children,* ed 4, St Louis, 2002, Mosby.

Osteoporotic bone, commonly found in older adults, requires additional healing time.

The objective of healing is to restore the normal anatomy and function of the fractured bone. A fracture is considered united when radiographic evidence demonstrates a bony bridge at the fracture site. Other evidence of healing includes lack of motion at the fracture site, a nontender fracture site, the ability to resume normal function, and pain-free weight bearing (in lower extremity fractures).

In general, cancellous bone fractures heal faster than cortical bone fractures because of the rich blood supply, especially when fracture fragments remain in direct contact. Midshaft fractures of the humerus, ulna, and tibia usually heal slowly because of poor blood supply. An adequate blood supply enables the bone to bleed with the injury, allowing adequate hematoma formation, which is the first stage of bone healing. A greenstick fracture takes only a few weeks to heal, in contrast to an open, comminuted fracture, which may take up to 2 years for complete healing. Articular fractures are technically difficult to treat and are slower to heal; the fibrinolysin in synovial fluid is thought to slow the first stage of healing.[10] Factors conducive to fracture healing include close approximation of fracture fragments, an adequate blood supply, a surrounding muscular envelope, absence of infection, and adequate immobilization. Once immobilization is achieved, weight bearing stimulates healing and bone repair. Factors that impede bone healing include inadequate reduction, immobilization, or blood supply; systemic disease; and infection (Table 52-1).

Failure of a fracture to consolidate in the expected time is termed *delayed union,* and failure to form a stable union after 6 months is termed **nonunion**. The incidence of nonunion in tibial fractures is higher than the incidence in other long bones, especially when the fracture occurs as a result of a high-energy injury, such as a motor vehicle accident. Certain bones are more likely to result in nonunion, regardless of proper fracture management. The distal tibia, carpal navicular, and proximal fifth metatarsal have the highest incidence of nonunion.[18]

Malunion refers to healing with angulation or deformity. If a fracture is nonunited, excessive mobility occurs at the fracture site, creating a false joint, or **pseudarthrosis**.

COMPLICATIONS. Complications can arise as a result of the initial trauma, the treatment, or the resulting loss of mobility. Systemic complications usually are a result of immobility or surgical intervention (see Chapter 15) and include cardiovascular, respiratory, gastrointestinal, and urinary complications.

Complications of fractures affect the patient's recovery and functional outcome. Early recognition and treatment of complications is extremely important. Fracture blisters, fat embolism syndrome, and compartment syndrome are discussed later. Deep venous thrombosis (DVT) and pulmonary embolism are also complications of fracture and are discussed in Chapters 15, 26, and 31.

Impaired fracture healing may result in malunion or nonunion and pseudarthrosis. These complications are generally treated with revision of the reduction. Posttraumatic arthritis and refracture may also occur. Posttraumatic arthritis occurs mainly in weight-bearing joints; severe cases may require joint replacement surgery. Of persons with tibial fractures, 5% to 40% have complications, including osteomyelitis, nonunion, compartment syndrome, and delayed union.[10]

Infection, which is the leading cause of delayed union and nonunion, occurs primarily in open fractures. Most symptoms of

TABLE 52-1 MAJOR FACTORS THAT IMPEDE BONE HEALING

Factor	Effect on Bone
Inadequate immobilization	Movement of fragments
Poor approximation of fracture fragments	Inaccurate reduction or malalignment of fracture fragments Excessive bone loss at time of fracture, preventing sufficient bridging of broken ends Excessive fragmentation of bone, allowing soft tissue to be interposed between bone ends Inability of patient to comply with restrictions imposed by immobilization and fixation device(s), resulting in movement of fragments
Compromised blood supply	Damage to nutrient vessels Periosteal or muscular injury Severe comminution Avascularity (type of fracture, result of internal fixation device)
Excessive edema at fracture site	Tissue swelling impeding supply of nutrients to area of fracture
Bone necrosis	Injury to blood vessels impeding supply of nutrients to involved bone
Infection at fracture site	Infection disrupting normal callus formation
Metabolic disorders or diseases (cancer, diabetes, malnutrition, immunodeficiency, Paget's disease)	Retardation of osteogenesis
Soft tissue injury	Disruption of blood supply
Medication use (e.g., steroids, anticoagulants)	Steroids causing osteoporosis, avascular necrosis; long-term use of heparin causing osteoporosis

infection occur within 4 weeks of the injury. Pain is the primary symptom, followed by erythema and edema. Infections after open fractures commonly result in osteomyelitis (infection of the bone), which is discussed in Chapter 53.

Heterotopic bone formation is the formation of bone in soft tissue and occurs as a result of trauma in approximately 10% of cases and may cause pain and restricted joint motion. Evidence of heterotopic ossification is detectable by x-ray examination as early as 1 to 2 months after injury. Persons with head injuries are more prone to heterotopic bone formation. Treatment consists of surgical resection and, in some cases, low-dose radiation.

Two types of complex regional pain syndrome (CRPS) can occur as complications of a fracture. These pain syndromes are progressive and potentially disabling chronic conditions, both recognized by the International Association for the Study of Pain.[12] Although they typically occur in a distal extremity, symptoms are systemic. CRPS I, or reflex sympathetic dystrophy, occurs in 5% to 30% of persons with fractures or bone or soft tissue injury. This condition is characterized by pain, hyperalgesia, edema, sweating, weakness, flushing or pallor (thought to be a result of sympathetic nervous system dysfunction), and skin changes.[10] Anxiety may exacerbate the symptoms.

The precipitating event for CRPS II is injury to a nerve. CRPS II, or causalgia, has symptoms similar to those of CRPS I. Symptoms are progressive and include severe, burning pain; restricted joint motion; osteopenia; muscle atrophy; and joint fibrosis. Treatment goals are preservation of limb function and pain relief. Modalities include gabapentin and adjuvant medications, physical therapy, nerve blocks, electrical stimulation, and physical therapy.[13]

▶ ARE You READY?

Which of the following findings in a patient with a midshaft fracture of the left humerus would require immediate intervention?

1. Cool, pale left hand and fingers
2. Grating sound when arm is moved
3. Severe pain
4. Ecchymosis

Collaborative Care Management

DIAGNOSTIC TESTS. Diagnosis is confirmed by x-ray examination. Other studies, including computed tomography (CT) and magnetic resonance imaging (MRI), may be indicated if multiple injuries or complex fractures have been sustained. Healing progress may be documented by x-ray examination; stress films may be needed in some cases.

MEDICATIONS. A fracture results in pain. Pain is managed by opioid and nonopioid analgesics and adjuvant drugs. Alternatives to nonsteroidal antiinflammatory drugs (NSAIDs) should be considered in persons with fractures, since as these medications diminish bone healing, bone formation, and remodeling.[5,17,20] Skeletal muscle relaxants may be prescribed in addition to analgesics. Antibiotics are given when an open fracture has occurred or surgical intervention is necessary. Tetanus toxoid may be necessary in the case of an open fracture. If prolonged immobilization or bed rest is necessary for treatment, anticoagulants may be prescribed as prophylaxis for DVT and pulmonary embolism. Vitamin and iron supplements may be prescribed to prevent or treat anemia.

TREATMENTS. The primary objectives of management are to reduce the fracture by realigning the fracture fragments, to maintain the fragments in correct alignment through immobilization, and to restore function and prevent excessive loss of joint mobility and muscle tone. Thus immediate treatment of the injury consists of:

1. Maintaining the airway and assessing for signs of shock
2. Splinting the fracture to prevent movement of the fracture fragments and further injury to the soft tissues by bony fragments (Splinting and immobilization also decrease pain.)
3. Maintaining correct body alignment
4. Elevating the injured body part to decrease edema
5. Applying cold packs (during the first 24 hours) to reduce hemorrhage, edema, and pain
6. Observing for changes in color, sensation, circulation, movement, or temperature of the injured part

Subsequently, simple fractures are reduced (replacing bone fragments in their correct anatomic position) and immobilized. Simple fractures can be reduced through manual manipulation (also known as closed reduction) in which bone fragments are moved into position by applying manual traction and pressure to the distal fragment; through the use of traction; or through **open reduction**, which is a surgical intervention that may incorporate an internal fixation device.

The secondary management of compound fractures includes surgical debridement; irrigation of the wound to remove dirt, foreign material, devitalized tissue, and necrotic bone; and wound culture. The wound is packed and observed for signs of osteomyelitis, tetanus, and gas gangrene. The wound is closed when there is no sign of infection. The fracture is reduced and immobilized. In some cases of nonunion, bone growth stimulators that use low-voltage electrical impulses are used to enhance healing.

The purpose of immobilization is to hold the broken bone fragments in contact with each other (or in close approximation) until healing takes place. Immobilization can be accomplished externally with external fixation devices (cast, splint, brace, cast brace), traction, or external fixators, or internally with metal plates, pins, screws, and nails, alone or in combination with bone grafts or prosthetic implants. Both external and internal methods can be combined. The appropriate period of immobilization must be maintained to prevent nonunion or malunion.

METHODS OF EXTERNAL FIXATION

Casts. The most common external fixation device is the cast. Materials used for casts include plaster of Paris, fiberglass, and plastic. All these materials are available as rolled bandages and are applied over the body part to be immobilized in much the same manner as an elastic bandage. Plaster, which has to be moistened before application, dries slowly, is heavy, and loses its strength and integrity if it becomes wet after the initial drying. If a plaster cast requires revision, it usually must be removed and a new one applied. However, plaster is less expensive than fiberglass or plastic. Fiberglass and plastic dry quickly, are lightweight, and may be immersed in water without losing their strength. Plastic casts may be reheated and remolded if revision is necessary. Some types of fiberglass require drying under special ultraviolet lights, and persons wearing fiberglass or plastic casts may suffer maceration of the skin unless they dry the skin thoroughly with a warm air dryer after bathing or showering. Specific advantages or disadvantages of various cast materials are discussed in orthopedic texts.

A cast may enclose (1) all or part of an extremity (Figure 52-2), (2) all or part of the trunk and cervical area, or (3) all or part of the trunk with all or a portion of one or more extremities. The latter type of cast is called a spica cast (Figure 52-3). Splints are made from cast material, but they may be thought of as half-casts because they do not wholly enclose a body part. They can be applied anteriorly, posteriorly, medially, or laterally and usually are wrapped in place with an elastic bandage. Cast braces are made of two separate casts, applied above and below the involved joint and joined by metal or heavy polyethylene hinges incorporated into the cast material. Cast braces permit the patient joint mobility below the fracture while still providing immobilization for the fracture fragments.

Casts are applied over skin that has been cleansed and assessed for potential areas of infection or breakdown. Before the cast is applied, skin lesions may be treated with tincture of benzoin and

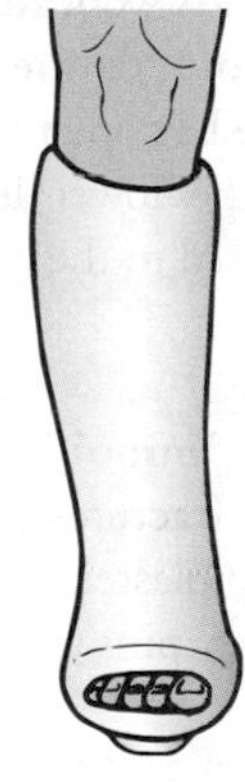

Figure 52-2 Short leg walking cast.

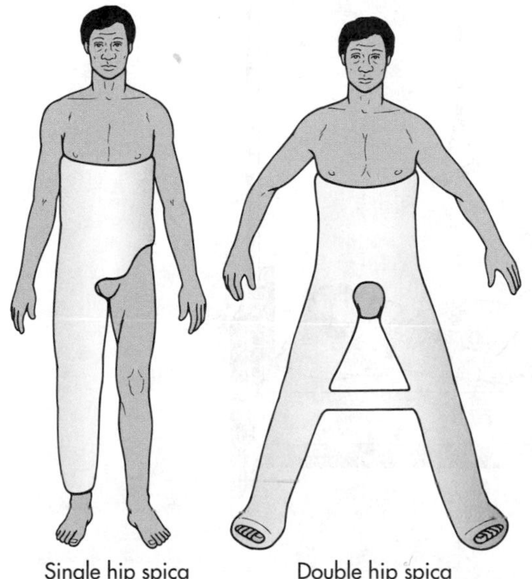

Figure 52-3 Hip spica casts.

wrapped with cotton padding or stockinette. Bony prominences are padded with sheet wadding or felt to prevent pressure points. For specific techniques of cast application, consult specialized texts.

Traction. Traction is the mechanism for exerting a steady pull on a part or parts of the body. Traction may be used to reduce a fracture, maintain correct alignment of bone fragments during healing, immobilize a limb while soft tissue healing takes place, overcome muscle spasm, stretch adhesions, or correct deformities.

Countertraction is a force that counteracts the pull of traction. The patient's body may provide the countertraction, in which case the patient's feet should not rest on the foot of the bed. Buck's extension is an example of using the patient's body as countertraction.

Suspension is the use of traction equipment, such as frames, splints, ropes, pulleys, and weights, to suspend but not exert a "pull" on a body part. To suspend the part correctly and continuously, the suspension must be balanced by weights. Suspension, also referred to as balanced suspension, is often used in conjunction with traction to allow the patient to move about more freely and easily in bed.

Two types of traction are used: skin traction and skeletal traction. Skin traction is achieved by applying wide bands of moleskin, adhesive, or commercially available devices directly to the skin and attaching weights. The pull of the weights is transmitted indirectly to the involved bone or other connective tissue. Buck's extension and Russell traction are the two most common forms of skin traction for injury to the lower extremities.

Buck's extension is the simplest form of skin traction and provides for straight pull on the affected extremity (Figure 52-4). It is

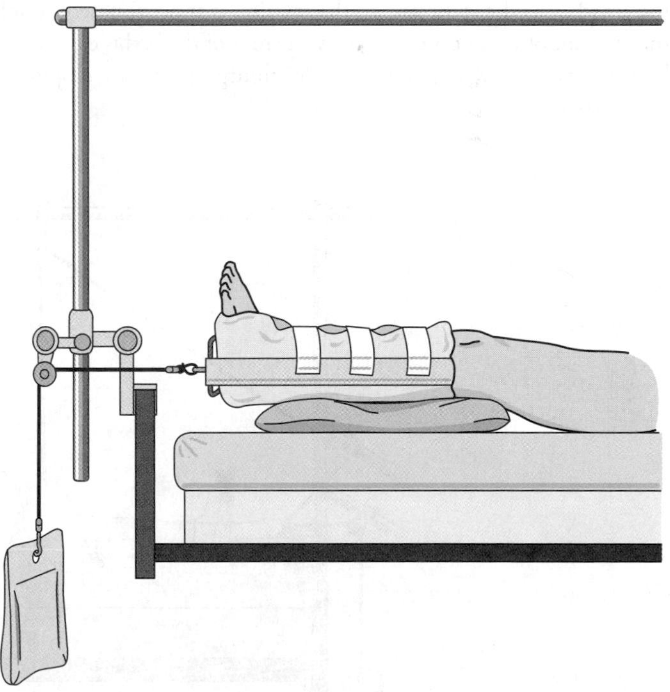

Figure 52-4 Buck's extension. The heel is supported off the bed to prevent pressure on the heel; the weight hangs free of bed, and toot is well away from footboard of bed. The limb should lie parallel to the bed unless prevented, as in this case, by a slight knee flexion contracture.

often used to relieve muscle spasm and to immobilize a limb temporarily (e.g., to treat a hip fracture before open reduction and internal fixation [ORIF]). If adhesive substances are to be used, the leg is shaved and tincture of benzoin applied to protect the skin. Adhesive tape or moleskin is then placed on the lateral and medial aspects of the leg and secured with a circular gauze or elastic bandage. The adhesive material should not cover the malleoli because of the risk of skin breakdown over these bony prominences. The tapes are attached to a spreader bar wide enough to pull the tapes away from the malleoli. Rope is attached to the spreader, passed through a pulley on a crossbar at the foot of the bed, and suspended with weights. The maximum weight that should be applied by skin traction is 2 to 4 kg (4.5 to 9 pounds); more weight can cause skin damage. Commercial foam rubber Buck's extension splints are widely used and are applied with Velcro straps. Contraindications to placing a patient in Buck's extension are stasis dermatitis, arteriosclerosis, allergy to adhesive tape, severe varicosities or varicose ulcers, diabetic gangrene, or marked overriding of bone fragments that would require more than 3.6 kg of weight to reduce the fracture.

Russell traction is sometimes used because it permits the patient to move somewhat freely in the bed and permits flexion of the knee joint (Figure 52-5). An overhead frame is attached to the bed and the leg is prepared as for Buck's extension. A footplate with pulley attachments is used instead of a spreader bar. The knee is suspended in a sling with an attached rope. The rope is directed up to a pulley placed on the overhead frame directly above the tibial tubercle of the affected extremity. The rope is then passed down through a pulley on a crossbar at the foot of the bed, back through a pulley on the footplate, back again to another pulley on the crossbar, and then suspended with weights. This arrangement places a double pull from the crossbar to the footplate, so the traction is approximately double the amount of weight used. Usually the foot of the bed is elevated on blocks (or the bed is put in Trendelenburg's position) to provide countertraction.

Russell traction is used in the treatment of an intertrochanteric fracture of the femur when surgery is contraindicated. Either bilateral Russell traction or Buck's extension may be used to treat back pain, since both partially immobilize the patient and reduce muscle spasm.

Skeletal traction is traction applied directly to bone. With the patient under local or general anesthesia, a Kirschner wire or Steinmann pin is inserted through bone distal to the fracture; the site of insertion varies with the type of fracture. The pin protrudes through the skin on both sides of the extremity, and the ends of the pin are covered with cork or metal protectors. Small sterile dressings are usually placed over the entry and exit sites of the pin, or pin sites may be left uncovered for easier observation. A U-shaped metal spreader or bow is attached to the pin, and the rope on which the traction weights are hung is tied onto the spreader. Skeletal traction can be used for fractures of the tibia, femur, humerus, and cervical spine. Skeletal traction applied to the cervical spine is achieved through the use of tongs applied to the skull (Figure 52-6).

When a balanced suspension apparatus is used in conjunction with skin or skeletal traction, the patient is able to move about in bed more freely without disturbing the line of pull of the traction. A full- or half-ring Thomas or Hodgen splint is commonly used for suspension of the lower extremity (Figure 52-7). Straps of canvas, muslin, or synthetic lamb's wool are placed over the splint and secured to provide a support for the leg. The areas under the popliteal space and heel are left open to prevent pressure. If knee flexion or movement of the lower leg is desirable, a Pearson attachment is clamped or fixed to the Thomas splint at the level of the knee.

Other Types of External Immobilization. Other devices for external immobilization of fractures include (1) braces made of rigid plastic material and (2) plaster or plastic braces that incorporate metal struts attached to pins inserted into bone, such as a halo brace (Figure 52-8).

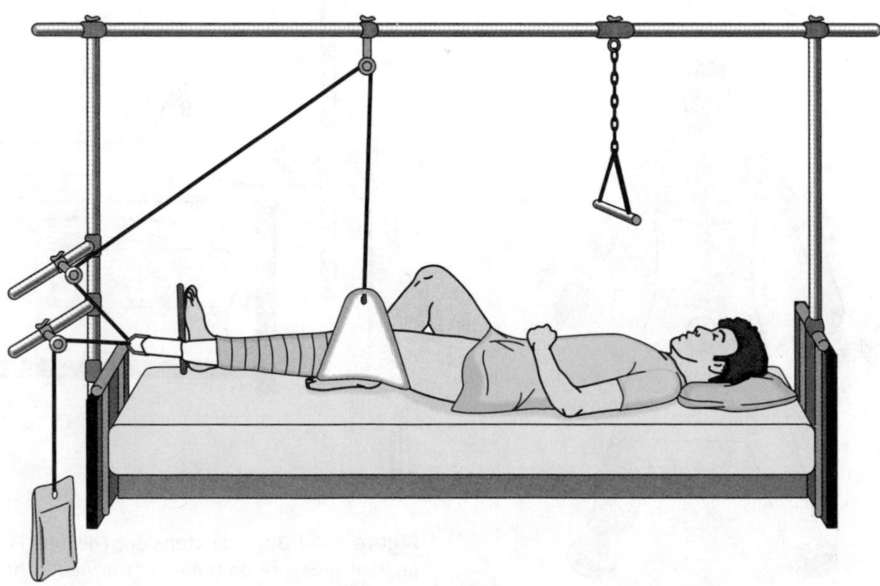

Figure 52-5 Russell's traction. Hip is slightly flexed. Pillows may be used under lower leg to provide support and keep heel free of the bed.

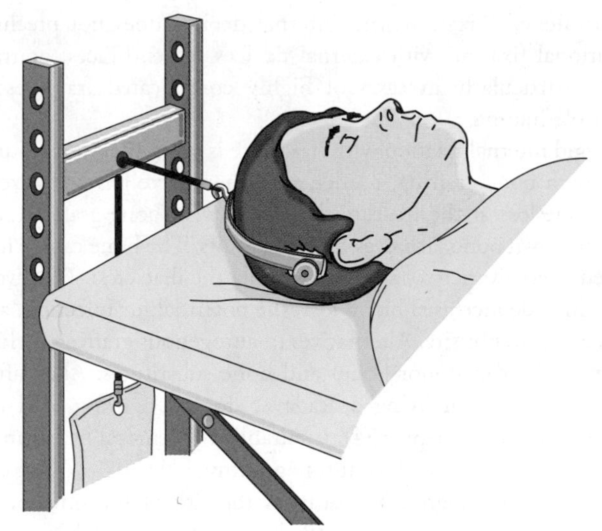

Figure 52-6 Traction to cervical spine can be maintained through use of Crutchfield tongs inserted into skull.

SURGICAL MANAGEMENT. A variety of procedures and materials exist for operative fracture fixation. The materials selected and type of procedure performed depend on the individual patient, the surgeon, and the location and type of fracture. Materials selected for internal fixation must be strong and flexible. Two common materials are titanium alloy and stainless steel. Both these materials provide adequate strength and fatigue resistance to allow healing of the fracture. Both may be contoured to fit irregularities in bone surfaces.

One method of fracture fixation is the *external fixator,* which consists of metal struts attached to pins inserted into bone (Figure 52-9). Advantages of external fixators include access to soft tissue injuries, management of complex comminuted fractures, alignment of fracture fragments, and early mobilization. External fixators such as the Hoffmann or Synthes device may be used alone or in conjunction with plaster. All these devices provide extremely rigid fixation while allowing the patient some degree of mobility. The patient with an external fixator on the lower leg can be out of bed in a wheelchair and can walk without bearing weight on the affected leg. As healing progresses, progressive weight bearing is allowed. The potential for infection is a major concern with the use of external fixators. In cases of severely comminuted fractures, bone grafting may be needed to promote healing.

The Ilizarov external fixator was developed in the Soviet Union in 1951 (Figure 52-10). It can be used to treat fractures, nonunions, osteomyelitis, deformities, and bony defects (caused by resection of malignancies) and to lengthen limbs. The basic principle of the Ilizarov technique is to achieve new bone growth by performing *corticotomies* (osteotomies through the cortex) and through the application of distraction (separation of bone surfaces using force without loss of alignment). The corticotomy creates a "pseudo" growth plate without disrupting the medullary cavity, thereby preserving blood supply and allowing new bone to fill in the distraction gap. The application of gentle traction on the bone stimulates growth. Weight bearing, which also stimulates new bone growth, is usually encouraged.

Open reduction with internal fixation (ORIF) of fractures has the advantage of allowing visualization of the fracture and surrounding tissues. ORIF is indicated for unstable or open fractures and those with significant soft tissue injuries. Other indications include failed closed reduction and displaced or intraarticular fractures. Advantages include solid fixation and early mobilization. Internal fixation is carried out under the most vigorous aseptic conditions, and patients may receive a course of perioperative prophylactic intravenous antibiotics. Tibial fractures often open because of the close proximity of bone to skin and often require ORIF.

A variety of internal fixation devices are available, including plates and nails, intramedullary rods (Figure 52-11), transfixion screws (Figure 52-12), and prosthetic implants (Figure 52-13). Hip implants are indicated for fractures through or immediately below the femoral head, when blood supply to the femoral head

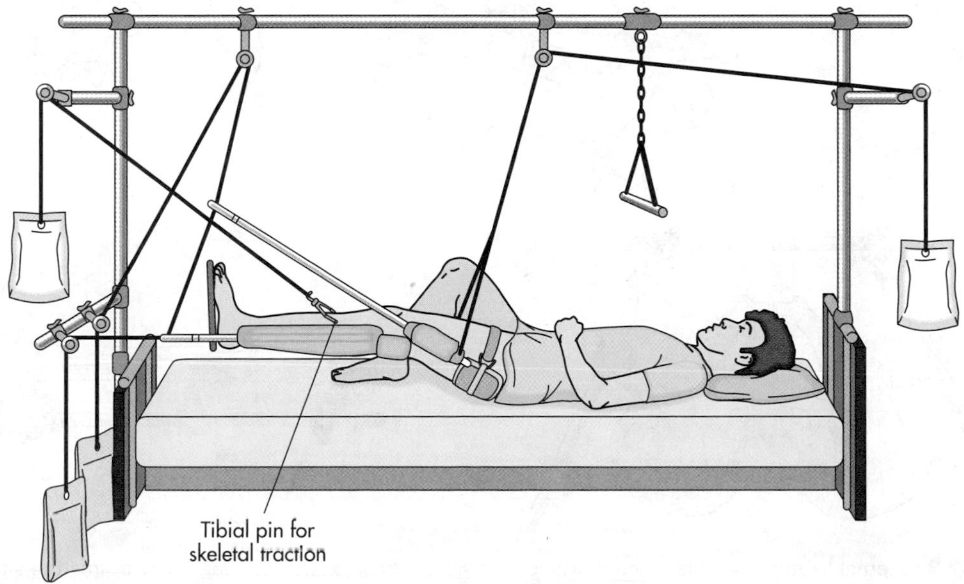

Figure 52-7 Balanced suspension with Thomas splint and Pearson attachment. This apparatus can be used alone or, as in this case, with skeletal traction.

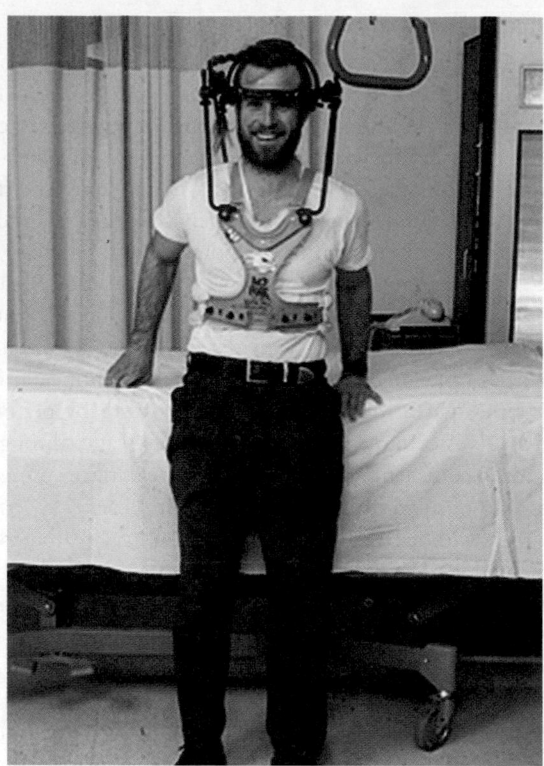

Figure 52-8 Halo vest. Note rigid shoulder straps and encompassing vest. Various vest sizes are available prefabricated. The halo ring, superstructure, and vest are magnetic resonance imaging compatible.

is threatened. Fixation with internal devices does not preclude additional fixation with external devices (casts, braces, or traction), particularly in cases of highly complicated fractures or multiple trauma.

Rigid internal fixation with hardware is often used in conjunction with bone grafting, particularly when there has been excessive bone loss at the fracture site. *Autogenous* bone grafting (the patient's own bone) achieves the best results. The bone can be harvested from a variety of sites, commonly the iliac crest. Disadvantages include increased blood loss, the potential for infection, and pain at the donor site. Alternatives to autogenous grafting include *allograft* (human donor bone) and bone substitutes. Allograft is bone derived from living or cadaver donors. During total hip arthroplasty (see Chapter 54), if suitable, the femoral head can be harvested and processed for future grafting.

The use of allograft bone carries the risk of transmission of blood and tissue-borne disease. Before use, bone bank bone must undergo processing. Methods of processing the bone differ. Immunogenicity, sterility, mechanical properties, and bone stimulation potential depend on the method of collection and processing. Bone that carries the highest risk of viral and bacterial contamination is cadaveric bone collected by sterile technique and used without further processing. However, cadaveric bone also contains the most bone growth factors, and thus it has the greatest potential to stimulate new bone formation. Ethylene oxide, a sterilizing agent, is not able to penetrate large pieces of allograft; therefore large grafts must be secondarily sterilized with gamma radiation.

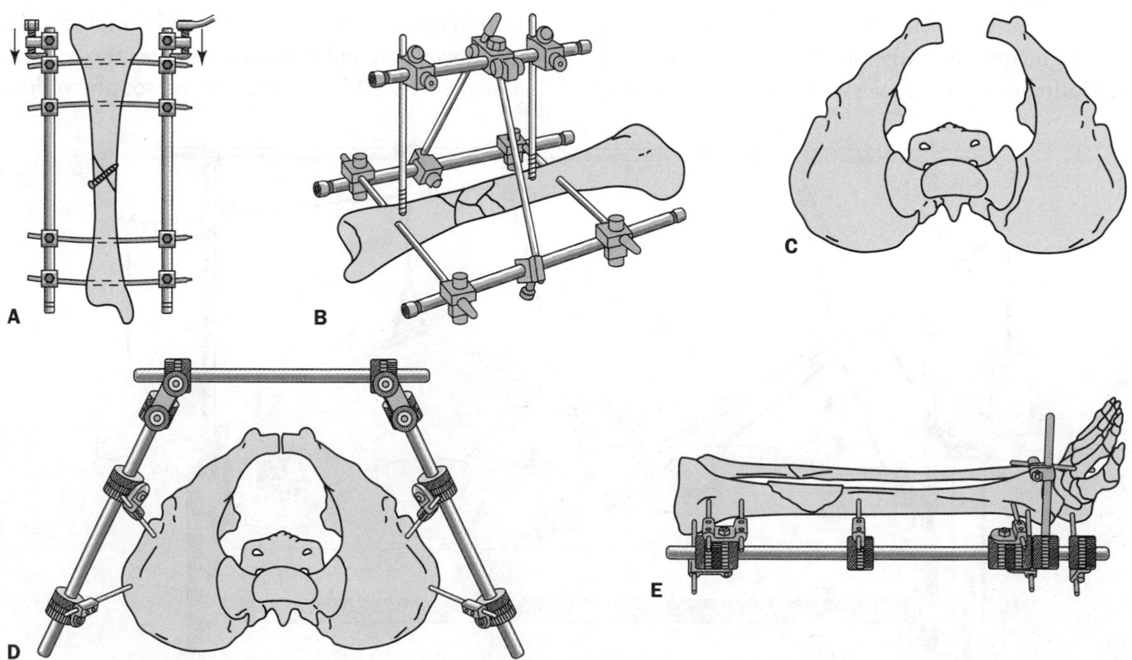

Figure 52-9 External fixators. **A,** Tibial fracture with simple AO external fixation with lag screw at fracture site. **B,** AO (Synthes) external fixator with three-dimensional or triangular fixation of comminuted fracture of tibia. **C,** Pelvic diastasis (dislocation). **D,** Hex-Fix external fixator in place, showing reduction of pelvic fracture. **E,** Hex-Fix external fixator used to treat tibial fracture. Immobilization of ankle and foot allows soft tissue healing.

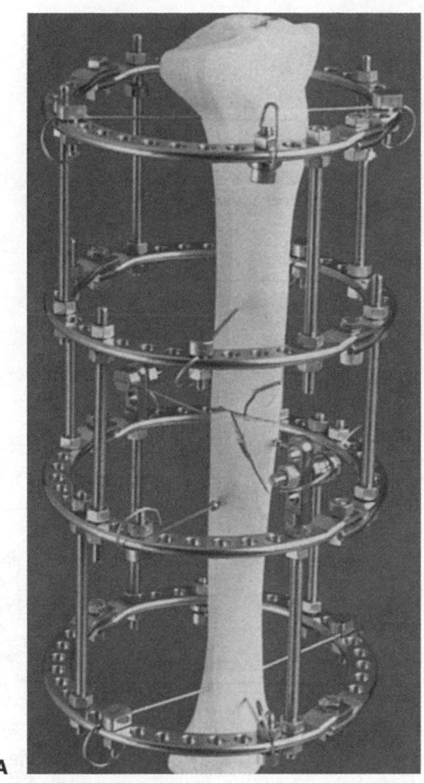

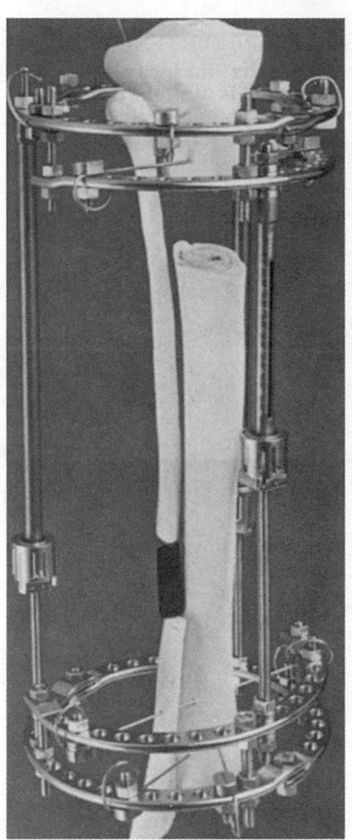

Figure 52-10 **A,** Ilizarov device in place to treat comminuted fracture. **B,** Ilizarov device assembly for lengthening of tibia.

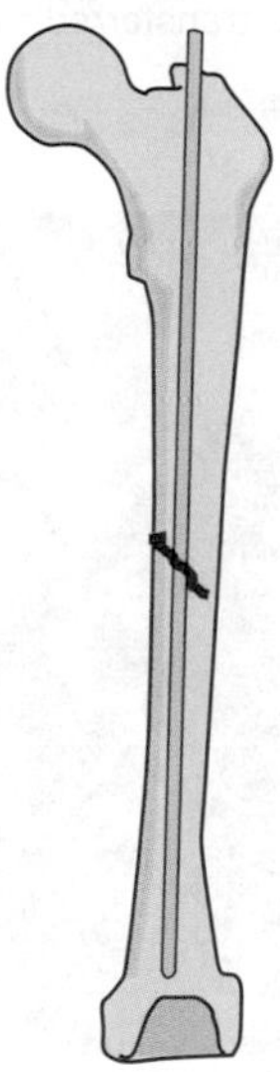

Figure 52-11 Intramedullary rod used to repair midshaft femoral fractures.

Another alternative for grafting is the use of hydroxyapatite or similar materials. Hydroxyapatite, a material derived from coral, is useful for filling bone defects but does not stimulate bone growth. Other materials, including synthetics and combinations of collagen, tricalcium phosphate, and hydroxyapatite, also require autogenous bone grafting to stimulate bone growth. The biomechanical and structural properties of these bone substitutes differ greatly from those of bone. In general, their structural properties are inferior to those of human bone. Augmenting bone substitutes with a human bone graft may improve their structural properties, particularly elasticity.[23] These bone "pastes" can be injected directly into the fracture site and harden in about 10 minutes. Twelve hours later, they are as strong as normal human bone. Ideally, as with a human bone graft, the body eventually resorbs the graft material and transforms it into bone mineral.

In general, the major objective of care is to protect the fixation until healing takes place. Metal, which can fatigue and break, cannot be expected to substitute for intact bone. If the fixation device breaks, healing of the fracture is disrupted. However, mobilization of patients who have had internal fixation is usually much faster than that for patients who have had external fixation.

Special consideration must be given to prevent infection in open fractures. Management protocols that include administration of antibiotics in addition to irrigation, surgical debridement, and stabilization reduce the incidence of early infection in open fractures of the extremities.[7] Severe open fractures can be treated with antibiotic "beads" placed directly in the wound. Antibiotic-impregnated (usually tobramycin) beads of bone cement (polymethylmethacrylate) are placed temporarily in the wound, and the wound is covered with a porous, transparent dressing. This method, first used in total hip arthroplasty, is effective in reducing infection.

DIET. Inadequate nutrition can retard bone healing. Adequate intake of proteins, vitamins, and minerals, particularly calcium, vitamins C and D, zinc, and phosphorus, is essential for fracture healing and health promotion. Avoiding smoking and limiting alcohol consumption is encouraged to promote bone health. Maintaining optimal body weight to avoid excess stress on bones and joints is another important consideration. Weight loss or gain may affect the fit of a cast or molded brace; if a significant change in weight occurs, the immobilizing device may need to be refitted.

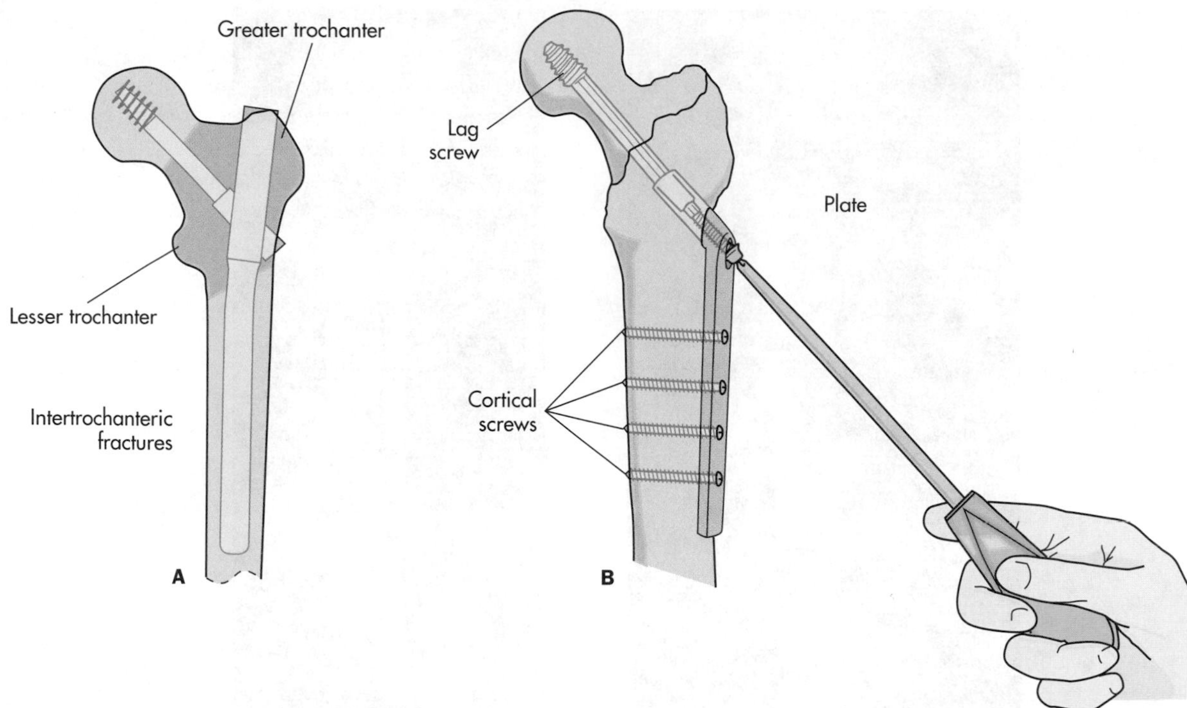

Figure 52-12 **A,** Richards intramedullary hip screw used for proximal femur fractures. Shown here for management of intra-trochanteric fracture *(shaded area).* The device consists of an intramedullary nail, lag screw, compression screw, centering sleeve, and set screw. **B,** Richards compression screw and plate for hip fractures. The compression screw *(shown at end of screwdriver)* threads into distal end of lag screw and draws fracture fragments together. The sliding feature of the nail and plate assembly reduces risk of acetabular penetration and allows weight-bearing forces to be transferred to the bone, rather than to the device.

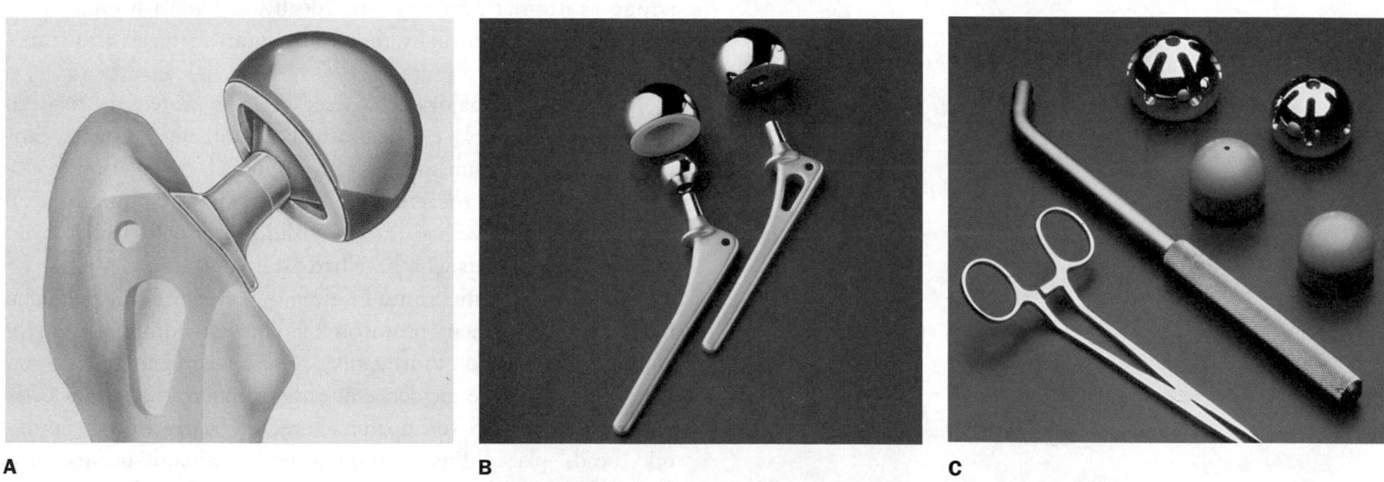

Figure 52-13 **A,** Bipolar modular prosthesis commonly used to replace femoral head and neck in hip fractures when vascular supply to femoral head may be compromised. **B,** Bipolar *(left)* and unipolar *(right)* hip prostheses for hip fractures. In unipolar prostheses the femoral head attaches directly to the femoral stem. In bipolar prostheses the femoral head consists of two components. **C,** Instrumentation used for hip prostheses. Trial components used for sizing actual implant.

If mobility is restricted, catabolic activity is accelerated, producing a rapid breakdown of cellular materials, leading to protein deficiency and a negative nitrogen balance. In addition, metabolic needs are increased during healing. Decalcification and demineralization of bone take place during immobility, regardless of the quantity of calcium intake. Therefore increasing dietary calcium above normal requirements is not recommended, since the excess calcium cannot be used. However, a diet high in protein (150 to 300 g/day) is indicated to overcome protein deficiency and to return the body to a state of positive nitrogen balance. Patients who have had fractures have increased needs for iron, protein, and vitamins if bone repair is to progress normally.

Patients with fractures, particularly if immobilized, are at risk for developing bladder infections and renal stones. Dietary interventions to decrease these risks include increasing fluid intake and decreasing intake of calcium and citrus fruits and juices. Adequate fluid intake also aids in preventing urinary stasis, which contributes to the development of urinary tract infection. Constipation is a complication of immobility. Fluids (2 to 3 L/day) and fiber should be encouraged to promote bowel elimination.

HEALTH PROMOTION AND PREVENTION. Because most fractures occur as a result of accidents or injuries, prevention is a key intervention. Education should be targeted at high-risk groups, including children, young men ages 15 to 24 years, and older adults. These latter two groups have an increased incidence of motor vehicle–related deaths. Each day more than 400 persons in the United States die as a result of motor vehicle accidents, guns, falls, and other injuries.[6] Nurses can be instrumental in providing education to prevent accidents and fractures.

Public education regarding prevention should include:

- Dangers of driving while impaired
- Importance of using seat belts and air bags in motor vehicles and adhering to speed limits
- Need for safety precautions when climbing ladders and using power tools or heavy equipment
- Recommended use of protective clothing (e.g., steel-toed shoes and hard hats for hazardous work at home or on the job)
- Need for proper protective clothing while engaging in sports (e.g., protective padding, helmets, and properly fitting running shoes)

Safety measures and fall prevention are particularly important for older adults. In the home, grab bars, handrails, nonskid floor and tub surfaces, night lights, and an obstacle-free environment can help prevent falls and injury. Individuals who must use ambulatory devices and wheelchairs should be instructed on how to use them properly. Knowledge of the patient's medication history, with attention to drugs that may cause dizziness, sedation, or orthostatic hypotension, may alert the family or caregivers to the risk of falls. A third approach to prevention is education regarding prevention of osteoporosis (see Chapter 53).

HEALTHY PEOPLE 2010. Injury and violence are the leading health indicators related to fracture; objectives include reducing deaths caused by motor vehicle crashes. Other *Healthy People 2010* objectives related to osteoporosis are discussed in Chapter 53 in the section on osteoporosis.

Nursing Management

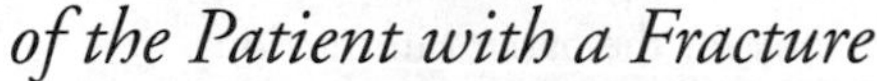

of the Patient with a Fracture

ASSESSMENT

Health History. Assess for:

- Mechanism of injury and events leading up to injury
- Pain
- Loss of sensation or movement of the affected part
- Medication use
- History of drug or alcohol use
- Ability to perform activities of daily living (ADLs); amount of assistance required
- Medical and surgical history (Chronic diseases may affect the healing process.)
- Previous musculoskeletal injuries and surgical procedures
- Nutritional history (The patient's nutritional status will affect the healing process.)
- Support of family and significant others; coping skills
- Expectations of treatment

Physical Examination. Assess for:

- Warmth, edema, or ecchymosis over and surrounding the injured part
- Obvious deformity; changes in normal alignment
- Crepitus
- Loss of normal function in the injured part
- Status of the immobilization device
- Neurovascular status (Table 52-2)
- Skin condition
- Indicators of pain, anxiety

NURSING DIAGNOSES, OUTCOMES, AND INTERVENTIONS

Prevention of infection is an important nursing intervention, particularly for patients with open fractures or those who have undergone ORIF of the fracture. If injuries are extensive or prolonged immobilization or bed rest is required for treatment, Risk for Disuse Syndrome is an appropriate diagnostic choice. This comprehensive diagnosis guides the nurse in planning care to prevent multisystem complications associated with immobility.

Nursing Diagnosis: Impaired Physical Mobility

OUTCOMES. Common examples of expected outcomes for the patient with a diagnosis of *impaired physical mobility* are:
Patient will:

- Demonstrate maximal mobility within prescribed activity and weight-bearing limits.
- Demonstrate proper use of adaptive or assistive devices.
- Participate in a program of progressive activity.

NURSING INTERVENTIONS. One objective in the care of the patient who has sustained a fracture is to prevent loss of mobility and muscle tone. This is true for the fractured part, as well as for the rest of the body. The patient should be as active as possible within the restrictions of the fracture reduction and the immobilizing devices. When permissible, weight bearing is encouraged, since it stimulates bone healing.

An initial assessment of the patient's strength, range of motion (ROM), transfer ability, and functional status is useful in planning outcomes and measuring progress. Before the patient begins physical activity, the nurse assesses his or her response to and tolerance of activity, since prolonged immobilization may result in physical deconditioning. Management of pain is another important consideration before beginning activity to avoid reluctance to move or exacerbation of pain.

The nurse encourages the patient to perform ROM and isometric exercises at least twice daily to prevent contractures, maintain joint mobility, and increase circulation and muscle tone. Another benefit of exercise is that it promotes a sense of well-being. The nurse performs passive ROM exercises for immobile

TABLE 52-2 SIGNS AND SYMPTOMS OF NEUROVASCULAR IMPAIRMENT*

Signs and Symptoms	Interpretation
Pallor	Decreased arterial blood supply
Cyanosis	Venous stasis and poorly oxygenated tissue
Prolonged capillary refill	Decreased arterial blood supply
Edema	Fluid accumulating in tissues; poor venous return
Tissue cold or cool to touch	Decreased arterial blood supply
Patient unable to move parts distal to injury or external fixation device; paralysis or paresis	Pressure on nerves that innervate parts distal to injury or underlie external fixation device
Patient report of extreme pain unrelieved by elevation, analgesic, or repositioning	Pressure on nerves that innervate parts distal to injury or underlie external fixation device; ischemia
Patient report of heightened or decreased sensation or paresthesia in parts distal to injury or underlying external fixation device	Pressure on nerves that innervate parts distal to injury or underlie external fixation device
Diminished or absent pulses	Arterial injury; vascular compromise secondary to tissue edema

*Tissue should be compared with uninvolved limb to determine extent of deviation from normal.

patients. A physical therapy consult may be initiated for specific exercises, weight training, and progressive ambulation. If appropriate, the nurse encourages the use of walkers, crutches, walking belts, or wheelchairs to increase mobility. The patient should be encouraged to be as independent as possible in self-care activities. Occupational therapy can provide assistive devices to aid in self-care. An overhead trapeze can increase the patient's mobility in bed and increase upper body muscle tone.

RELATED NIC INTERVENTIONS. Bed Rest Care, Exercise Promotion: Strength Training, Exercise Therapy: Ambulation, Exercise Therapy: Joint Mobility

Nursing Diagnosis: Pain

OUTCOMES. Common examples of expected outcomes for the patient with a diagnosis of *pain* are:

Patient will:

- Verbalize that pain is controlled.
- Rate pain at 4 or below using a scale of 0 to 10 (where 0 equals no pain and 10 is the most severe pain imaginable).

NURSING INTERVENTIONS. The person with a fracture often has severe pain at the fracture site, pressure from edema in the damaged soft tissues adjacent to the fracture, and spasm of the muscles in the fracture area. If the fracture is repaired by ORIF, the patient also has operative pain. Continued pain and muscle spasm can put undue stress on the fracture fragments and retard efforts to reduce and to maintain reduction of the fracture. Patients in severe pain may resist measures designed to prevent complications.

Effective pain management requires a team approach and the involvement of the patient in the treatment plan. Both pharmacologic and nonpharmacologic methods are used in treating pain. Depending on the severity of pain, opioids and/or nonopioid analgesics are prescribed. The patient's self-report is the most reliable indicator of pain. Adjuvant drugs may be added, including muscle relaxants or anxiolytics.

Methods of administration include around-the-clock dosing, as-needed dosing, and patient-controlled analgesia. If opioids are used, the nurse assesses the patient's level of consciousness, respiratory status, sedation level, and pain intensity at least every 4 hours. The nurse instructs the patient and family regarding the pain management plan and evaluates the effectiveness of the treatment at regular intervals. As pain subsides, reduction in the strength or frequency of analgesic administration should be negotiated with the patient.

In addition to pharmacologic methods, nonpharmacologic interventions are effective in managing pain. The nurse assesses the patient's previous experiences with these methods, including guided imagery, distraction, and relaxation. Application of ice also decreases pain by reducing swelling.

The patient must be repositioned frequently within the prescribed position or activity limitations to avoid prolonged pressure over bony prominences and to prevent stiffness. Repositioning promotes comfort, provides for adequate ventilation and mobilization of pulmonary secretions, enhances circulation, and relieves pressure on vulnerable skin areas. To safely reposition a patient, the nurse must know the location and type of fracture, reduction techniques used, and any special activity or positioning restrictions.

The nurse should use the following guidelines for positioning the patient with a fracture:

- Maintain the alignment of the fracture.
- Maintain the direction of pull of traction (see Guidelines for Safe Practice box for the patient in traction).
- Maintain the integrity of the cast (see Guidelines for Safe Practice box for the patient in a cast, p. 1536).
- Maintain positioning, activity, and weight-bearing restrictions of an internal fixation device (see Guidelines for Safe Practice box for the patient with an internal fixation device, p. 1537).

Generally, nurses should avoid changing the position of patients with unreduced, unsplinted fractures. Manipulation of fracture fragments, particularly long bones, may cause release of fat into the

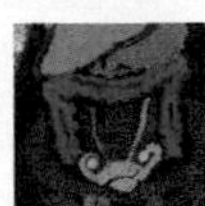

GUIDELINES FOR SAFE PRACTICE *The Patient in Traction*

- Patient education
  - —Explain traction in relation to the fracture and the physician's plan of treatment.
  - —Explain the amount of movement permitted and how to achieve it (e.g., how the trapeze can be used to assist with movement).
  - —Explain correct body positioning. Ensure that patient maintains proper body alignment.
- Maintenance of continuous traction, unless indicated otherwise
  - —Inspect the traction apparatus frequently to ensure that the ropes are running straight and through the middle of the pulleys, that the weights are hanging free, and that nothing impinges on the traction apparatus.
  - —Check ropes frequently to be sure they are not frayed.
  - —Avoid releasing weights or altering the line of pull of the traction.
  - —Avoid adding weight to the traction.
  - —Check the position of the Thomas splint frequently; if the ring slides away from the groin, readjust the splint to its proper position without releasing traction.
  - —Avoid bumping into or jarring the bed or traction equipment.
  - —Be certain weights are securely fastened to their ropes.
  - —Avoid manipulation of pins.
- Maintenance of countertraction
- Skin care
  - —Encourage the patient to turn slightly from side to side and to lift up on the trapeze to relieve pressure on the skin of the sacrum and scapulae; have the patient lift up for routine skin care to prevent friction and shearing forces.
  - —Avoid padding the ring of the Thomas splint, since this will create dampness next to the skin. Bathe the skin beneath the ring, dry it thoroughly, and powder the skin lightly.
  - —Inspect the skin frequently to be certain it is not being rubbed, contused, or macerated by traction equipment; readjust splints or the extremity in the splint to free the skin from pressure.
  - —Keep skin areas around pin sites clean and dry. Data are inconclusive to support the best practice for pin site care.[19] Use institutional protocol or physician order regarding pin care frequency and method.
- Toileting
  - —Use a fracture pan with a blanket roll or padding as support under the small of the back.
  - —Protect the ring of the Thomas splint with waterproof material.
- Prevention of neurovascular problems
  - —Perform neurovascular checks every hour for the first 24 to 48 hours; notify the physician of changes from baseline status.
  - —Monitor for signs of deep venous thrombosis, pulmonary embolism, and fat embolism syndrome (if applicable).

vasculature (see discussion under Fat Embolism Syndrome). Once the parameters for safe positioning are defined, the nurse should assist the patient in changing position at least every 2 hours until the patient can do so independently.

RELATED NIC INTERVENTIONS. Analgesic Administration, Cast Care: Maintenance, Positioning, Splinting, Traction/Immobilization Care

Nursing Diagnosis: Risk for Peripheral Neurovascular Dysfunction

OUTCOMES. Common examples of expected outcomes for the patient with a diagnosis of *risk for peripheral neurovascular dysfunction* are:

Patient will:

- Maintain tissue perfusion.
- Maintain intact peripheral neurovascular status in all extremities.

NURSING INTERVENTIONS. The nurse monitors for neurovascular compromise every hour in the initial stages of a fracture. Damage to blood vessels or nerves may occur at the time of the fracture or after reduction. Some swelling of a fractured extremity may be expected and is often well controlled by elevating the extremity. However, unrelieved swelling of an extremity that is confined in a cast or compression dressing causes undue pressure on vessels and nerves and can result in circulatory or neurologic impairment or skin breakdown. The nurse evaluates the affected extremity frequently for signs of compression and reports evidence of impaired circulation or sensation to the physician immediately. The frequency of neurovascular checks can usually be reduced if there is no evidence of compromise within 48 hours of the fracture or reduction (see Table 52-2). Observations of the involved extremity should be compared with observations of the uninvolved extremity to validate deviations from the patient's baseline status.

Monitoring neurovascular status of the injured part includes (1) palpating for warmth, (2) observing color, (3) assessing capillary refill time, (4) questioning the patient about pain and paresthesias in the injured part, (5) assessing the patient's ability to discriminate sensation, and (6) observing the patient's ability to voluntarily move the body part distal to the fracture.

Immobility is a risk factor for the development of DVT. Ambulation should begin as soon as possible to help prevent clot formation. Isometric leg exercises help promote venous return and decrease venous stasis. Other interventions that have proved effective in decreasing the incidence of DVT include the use of graduated compression elastic stockings, intermittent compression devices, and prophylactic anticoagulants. The nurse monitors frequently for signs of DVT, which include redness, swelling, tenderness, pain, and a palpable cord in the involved leg. Homans' sign is not a reliable indicator for the presence of DVT. The most common presentation is pain and swelling in the affected extremity. The nurse measures calf and thigh circumferences daily and reports differences greater than 2 cm between the legs to the physician. The affected extremity is elevated for the first 48 hours; thereafter the extremity is elevated when the patient is at rest.

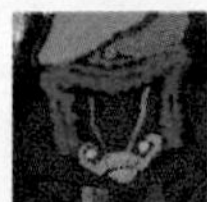

GUIDELINES FOR SAFE PRACTICE *The Patient in a Cast*

- Patient education
  —Before cast application, explain why and how the cast will be applied.
  —Advise the patient that the plaster cast will feel warm as it dries.
  —Explain the extent to which the patient will be immobilized.
  —After cast application, explain care of the cast and expectations after discharge.
  —Instruct the patient not to insert sharp objects (coat hangers or pencils) under the cast, since these may abrade the skin and lead to infection.
  —Before cast removal, explain that the saw used for removal is noisy but will not harm the skin.
- Handling the new cast
  —Support the wet cast with the flat of the hands or on pillows to avoid indentations that will cause pressure on the underlying skin.
  —Place cotton blankets or other absorbent material under the cast to aid the drying process.
  —Expose the cast to air as much as possible to aid the drying process.
  —Turn the patient frequently to aid the drying process.
  —Use a fan to circulate air over the cast.
  —Instruct the patient not to apply anything to the cast; plaster is a porous material that allows air to circulate to the skin.
- Skin care and prevention of infection
  —Inspect the skin at the edges of the cast and underlying the cast for redness or irritation; apply petal-shaped strips of adhesive tape or moleskin around the rough edges of the cast.
  —Instruct the patient to report any drainage, foul odor, or increased pain, which may indicate infection, bleeding, or skin irritation. Circle existing drainage with a marker to detect increases.
  —Remove plaster crumbs from the skin with a washcloth moistened with warm water.
  —Use creams and lotions sparingly, since they may soften the skin and cause the cast to stick to the skin.
  —Apply waterproof material around the perineal area to prevent skin irritation and soiling of and damage to the cast.
  —Attend to the patient's report of pain under the cast, particularly over bony prominences, since this may indicate pressure on the skin. If discomfort is not relieved by repositioning, report to the physician. Cast pressure may need to be relieved by windowing or bivalving (cutting the cast in half).
  —After cast removal, provide skin care to remove built-up exudate of secretions and dead skin. Mineral oil and warm water soaks are helpful.
- Turning
  —Turning to any position is generally permitted, as long as the integrity of the cast is not compromised and the patient is comfortable.
- Toileting (for a long leg or hip spica cast)
  —Use a fracture pan with a blanket roll or padding as support under the small of the back.
  —Elevate the head of the bed if permitted, or place the bed in reverse Trendelenburg's position.
- Abdominal discomfort
  —Spica cast may be "windowed" (cut an opening into cast) to provide relief of abdominal distention or as a port for checking bladder distention.
- Mobilization
  —The physician will prescribe the amount of weight bearing permitted.
  —A cast shoe or a walking heel incorporated into a lower extremity cast will permit weight bearing without damaging the cast.
- Prevention of neurovascular problems
  —Perform neurovascular checks every hour for at least 24 hours after cast application to detect difficulty from swelling or pressure of the cast on nerves or vessels. Notify the physician of changes in color, changes in pulse quality, or alterations in sensation or motion unrelieved by position change; the cast may need to be bivalved to relieve pressure.
  —Elevate the affected extremity on pillows until the danger of swelling is over (usually 24 to 48 hours).
  —After mobilization of the patient with a lower extremity or upper extremity cast, avoid keeping the extremity in a dependent position for prolonged periods.
  —After a lower extremity cast is removed, encourage the patient to wear an elastic stocking and elevate the affected leg at rest until full mobility is regained. Encourage isometric exercises to prevent circulatory complications.

RELATED NIC INTERVENTIONS. Circulatory Precautions, Circulatory Care: Arterial or Venous Insufficiency, Pressure Management

▶ ARE YOU READY?

Which of the following is an indication of deep vein thrombosis in the right calf?

1. Homans' sign
2. Turner's sign
3. Circumference of right calf 2.5 cm greater than left calf
4. Decreased distal pulses in left foot

Nursing Diagnosis: Risk for Impaired Skin Integrity

OUTCOMES. Common examples of expected outcomes for the patient with a diagnosis of *risk for impaired skin integrity* are:

Patient will:

- Maintain skin integrity.
- Demonstrate behaviors to prevent skin breakdown.

NURSING INTERVENTIONS. When determining interventions to maintain skin integrity, the nurse must consider ways to prevent skin breakdown and promote wound healing. A risk assessment tool such as the Braden Scale can be used on admission and at regular intervals thereafter. The nurse monitors the skin at least daily for signs of pressure, which include color changes (redness or pallor), warmth or coolness, induration, and nonblanchable areas. Bony prominences (heels, sacrum, elbows, scapulae, ischial tuberosities) are at increased risk for breakdown. Skin over bony prominences should not be massaged, since massage can trauma-

GUIDELINES FOR SAFE PRACTICE
The Patient With an Internal Fixation Device

- Patient education
  —Prepare the patient for anesthesia.
  —Explain the surgical procedure and general perioperative care.
  —After surgery explain the limits of motion and weight bearing to the affected part.
- Promoting mobility
  —Consult with the physician regarding activity, range-of-motion, and weight-bearing limits.
  —Instruct and help the patient to turn, transfer, and walk within the prescribed limits (mobilization may begin as early as the day of surgery).
  —Instruct and help the patient to use an appropriate ambulatory aid if lower extremity fracture.
- Prevention of neurovascular problems
  —Perform neurovascular checks every hour for the first 24 to 48 hours; notify the physician of any change from preoperative status, since this may indicate pressure from swelling, constricting bandages, or damage to nerves or vessels during surgery.
  —Keep the affected extremity elevated.
  —Monitor for signs of deep venous thrombosis, pulmonary embolism, and fat embolism syndrome, if applicable.
- Maintenance of immobilization of fracture
  —Considerations for care are the same as for patients in cast or traction.

tize the underlying deep tissues. Patients with sensory deficits are at increased risk for skin breakdown.

Because moisture contributes to the development of skin breakdown, the nurse helps the patient keep the skin clean and dry, especially under casts, slings, and traction apparatus. Skin care should be performed after toileting. If the patient is incontinent, exposure to urine and feces should be minimized to prevent breakdown. Skin areas in contact with cast edges or traction apparatus should be assessed frequently, and measures taken to eliminate moisture, chafing, or pressure in those areas.

If permissible, the nurse turns the patient every 2 hours, using a turn sheet to reduce friction and shearing forces. During transferring or positioning of the patient, friction and shearing forces should be eliminated or reduced. Foam wedges, pressure-relieving devices, sheepskin, pillows, and heel and elbow pads can be used to relieve pressure. In some instances a special bed or mattress or a turning frame may be required. When sitting in a chair, the patient should perform weight shifts at least every 2 hours.

RELATED NIC INTERVENTIONS. Positioning, Pressure Management, Skin Surveillance

Patient/Family Teaching. Teaching for the patient with a fracture and his or her family is presented in the Patient/Family Teaching box.

EVALUATION

To evaluate the effectiveness of nursing interventions, compare patient behaviors with those stated in the expected patient outcomes.

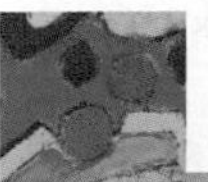

PATIENT/FAMILY TEACHING
The Patient With a Fracture

Treatment of the acute fracture is usually carried out in the hospital's emergency department or in the operating room before the patient is admitted to the general hospital unit. Patients may have little or no opportunity to become oriented to the hospital or to the care they will receive. In addition, they are probably frightened or overwhelmed by what has happened to them, may be in pain, and may be groggy from pain medication or anesthesia. Careful and repeated explanations and directions are necessary. The nurse must give patients time to adjust to their situations before they can begin to understand how to cooperate in their care. Teaching should include information regarding:

- Expected course of treatment
- Skin and wound care
- Pain management
- Medication use
- Activity and weight-bearing restrictions
- Signs of complications
- Ambulation and positioning techniques
- Use of assistive devices
- Care of immobilization devices
- Range-of-motion exercises
- Safety measures
- Fall prevention

RELATED NOC OUTCOMES. Bone Healing, Mobility, Pain Control, Pain Level, Risk Control, Tissue Integrity: Skin & Mucous Membranes, Tissue Perfusion: Peripheral

GERONTOLOGIC CONSIDERATIONS

Older persons who sustain fractures often incur some loss of functional ability. Older adults are prone to fractures for many reasons, including osteoporosis, neoplasms, sensorimotor deficits, and falls. Falls are the most common cause of fractures in the elderly. Bones most commonly fractured are the proximal femur (hip), distal radius (Colles' fracture), vertebrae, and clavicle. Colles' fractures usually occur as a result of placing an outreached hand to break a fall, most commonly in women with osteoporosis. Treatment usually consists of closed reduction and immobilization. The majority of clavicular fractures in older adults are sustained in a manner similar to that with a Colles' fracture. The fracture usually occurs in the medial third of the clavicle. The patient exhibits swelling, point tenderness, local deformity, and crepitus. Treatment consists of closed reduction and immobilization with a sling or cast. Vertebral fractures are usually pathologic and are a result of osteoporosis. The fracture is usually a compression fracture of the vertebral body.

Fracture Blisters

Etiology and Epidemiology. Fracture blisters are skin bullae and blisters representing areas of epidermal necrosis with separation of the stratified squamous cell layer by edema fluid. They are associated with fractures, twisting types of injuries, and joint trauma. Fracture blisters may also develop as a result of compartment syndrome, as the body attempts to relieve rising tissue pressures. The development of blisters is also influenced by the interval between time of fracture and immobilization.

The presence of fracture blisters predisposes the patient to infection, delays in treatment, nonunion, impaired healing, and ultimately a longer hospital stay and increased costs. Wound complications can result in serious infection. Delaying surgery until swelling has lessened may decrease the risk of wound infection. The highest incidence of fracture blisters occurs in the ankle, elbow, distal tibia, and foot, which are anatomic areas with tight skin constraints and little muscle or surrounding fascia, characteristics that contribute favorably to the formation of fracture blisters.

Pathophysiology. After the acute injury, severe tissue edema and swelling develop as a result of damage to bone, ligaments, tendons, and surrounding soft tissues. The vasculature and lymphatic drainage are disrupted, which causes the epidermis to separate from the dermis. Detachment of the epidermis results in disruption of its blood supply, causing necrosis of the epidermal layers. The edema and venous stasis that occur after the injury cause collapse and thrombosis of the affected blood and lymph vessels, which increase circulatory problems. Blisters may result from the local tissue hypoxia. Deep tissue damage may result, necessitating later full-thickness skin grafting. The time for reepithelialization is an estimated 4 to 21 days.

Collaborative Care Management. Preventive nursing measures include identifying persons at risk and early and frequent assessment of the skin. In addition to fractures associated with a greater incidence of blisters, other risk factors include diabetes, hypertension, peripheral vascular disease, smoking history, alcohol use, and lymphatic obstruction. Initial treatment measures that may decrease the development of blisters include early immobilization and elevation to limit edema formation, both of which help maintain normal blood and lymphatic circulation.

If the patient develops a fracture blister, a dry dressing is recommended for protection. "Popping" the blister is not recommended, since the blister covering provides a biologic dressing. A ruptured blister provides an excellent environment for infection; it is moist, provides nutrients (serum), lacks initial phagocytic activity, and has few coexisting microorganisms. If blister rupture occurs, a hydrocolloid dressing is helpful to maintain a moist wound environment. Despite treatment, a ruptured blister may result in a full-thickness loss. Intravenous antibiotics are recommended if the wound culture reveals *Staphylococcus aureus*. Anticoagulants may be prescribed to prevent thrombus formation.

PATIENT/FAMILY TEACHING. Education for the patient with a fracture blister is similar to that for the patient with a fracture (refer to the Patient/Family Teaching box in the preceding section).

Fat Embolism Syndrome

Etiology and Epidemiology. Fat embolism syndrome (FES) is a potentially fatal complication associated with fractures, multiple crush injuries, total hip arthroplasty, and total knee arthroplasty. Fat emboli may lead to acute respiratory distress syndrome (ARDS), with an associated mortality rate of 50%, especially if the onset is more than 5 days after trauma. The onset of symptoms of FES usually occurs within 12 to 24 hours after injury.

FES is most common after multiple trauma and pelvic and long bone fractures. Persons with total hip and knee arthroplasties are at risk for FES because of surgical reaming of the intramedullary canal to allow seating of the prosthesis and pressurizing of the medullary canal during sizing and cementing of the prosthesis, which may cause fat to enter the venous system. Cerebral microemboli have occurred during total hip arthroplasty, with both cemented and uncemented prostheses. Increased serum glucose and beta-lipoprotein levels may increase the incidence of FES. Morbidity, although difficult to determine, is estimated at 12% to 87%.[8]

Pathophysiology. On autopsy, fat globules have been found in the lungs of a number of patients with long bone fractures. After a fracture, fat globules and tissue thromboplastin are released from the bone marrow and local tissue into the circulation, increasing clotting and blood viscosity. The fat molecules enter the venous circulation, travel to the lungs, and embolize the small capillaries and arterioles. Lipase is produced to break down fat molecules into fatty acids. These chemical changes irritate pulmonary tissue and result in deterioration of lung surfactant, increased permeability of the alveolocapillary membrane, interstitial hemorrhage, edema, and atelectasis. Eventually, hypoxemia and ARDS may develop. Fatty acids attract red blood cells and platelets, forming an aggregate, which can lead to disseminated intravascular coagulation and emboli to the brain and other vital organs. Retinopathy as a result of FES may also occur. Other complications include pneumonia, coma, kidney failure, and congestive heart failure.

Symptoms of FES include hypoxemia, tachypnea, tachycardia, petechiae, fever, lipuria, chest pain, and altered mental status. Alteration in mental status and changes in arterial blood gas readings (primarily hypoxemia) are early clinical indicators of FES. Approximately 75% of persons with FES develop significant neurologic symptoms, which may manifest as restlessness, confusion, lethargy, or coma. Petechiae, considered a classic symptom of FES, occur in only 50% to 60% of patients. They are usually found on the conjunctivae, axillae, chest, and neck and are thought to be caused by capillary occlusion with fat and fibrin. Other causative factors include capillary fragility and platelet defects. The rash does not blanch with pressure but usually disappears within 48 hours of onset. Unexplained fever, especially when accompanied by a change in mental status and petechiae, should alert the caregiver to the possibility of FES. This is a medical emergency, and the physician should be notified immediately.

Collaborative Care Management. Diagnosis is confirmed by a decrease in arterial Po_2, an increase in systemic Pco_2, infiltrates on chest x-ray films, petechiae, and mental confusion in persons at risk. A drop in the hemoglobin level because of sequestration of red blood cells in fat and a platelet count of less than 150,000/ml is considered diagnostic of FES.[8] Thrombocytopenia occurs as a result of hemodilution, the clotting process, and platelet attraction to fat globules. The platelet count usually returns to normal within 1 week. Prothrombin and partial thromboplastin times increase. Pathologic examination of the lungs reveals fat globules diffusely distributed throughout the pulmonary vasculature.

Arterial blood gases are obtained to determine the degree of hypoxemia. Fat may be found in the blood and urine. However, lipuria is a normal finding after a fracture and therefore is not of clinical significance in the diagnosis of FES. Chest x-ray films detect changes related to a fat embolus in only one third of patients. If ARDS develops, chest films will show areas of consolidation. A lung scan (ventilation-perfusion scan) may be used to rule out a pulmonary embolus (Table 52-3).

The most important nursing interventions are the recognition of patients at risk for developing FES and careful monitoring for early detection of clinical indicators of FES. Careful handling of the fractured extremity, especially when turning and positioning the patient, decreases manipulation of the fracture site, thus decreasing the risk of fat emboli.

As stated earlier, medical management is the same as for a person with ARDS (see Chapter 26). Adequate hydration to prevent kidney failure and to flush out fatty acids is an important intervention. Corticosteroids have been effective in reducing morbidity but must be used cautiously because of side effects. Steroids are beneficial in reducing cerebral edema, restoring capillary permeability, and decreasing capillary leakage. Hemodynamic monitoring is usually indicated. Other treatments include packed red blood cells to restore volume and decrease hypoxemia and low-dose dopamine to increase cardiac output and renal perfusion. Preventive measures include early stabilization (within 24 hours of injury) of patients with long bone fractures. Patients who undergo early stabilization of fractures experience shorter hospital stays and fewer respiratory complications than those with late stabilization of fractures (more than 48 hours after injury).

Early recognition of symptoms, including respiratory insufficiency, decreased oxygenation, mental status changes, unexplained drop in hemoglobin, thrombocytopenia, and fat in the urine or sputum, should alert the caregiver to the possibility of a fat embolus.

PATIENT/FAMILY TEACHING. Because the onset of FES is acute, the patient and family may not be prepared to deal with the severity of the situation. Early education of high-risk patients is an important intervention. Education regarding the rationales for treatment and emotional support while the patient is in the critical care environment are essential. If complications develop, the patient and family will require long-term support.

▶ ARE You READY?

Which of the following patients does the nurse monitor most closely for fat embolism syndrome?

1. Patient with spinal fracture
2. Patient with pelvic fracture
3. Patient with chest trauma
4. Patient with joint trauma

Compartment Syndrome

Compartment syndrome is usually a complication of trauma in which increased pressure within a limited anatomic space compromises the circulation, viability, and function of the tissues

TABLE 52-3 COMPARISON OF FAT EMBOLISM AND PULMONARY EMBOLISM

Characteristic	Fat Embolism	Pulmonary Embolism
Pathophysiology	Fat globules released from marrow after fracture(s) enter bloodstream and obstruct pulmonary circulation	Deep vein thrombus dislodges and obstructs pulmonary circulation
Onset of symptoms	Usually 12-24 hr after injury	Usually 4-10 days after trauma or development of thrombophlebitis but can occur much later
Signs and symptoms	Altered mental status Dyspnea Tachypnea Tachycardia Petechial rash Fever Restlessness Agitation	Dyspnea Chest pain Apprehension Anxiety Cough Hemoptysis Tachypnea Tachycardia Fever
Risk factors	Hypovolemia Shock Delayed immobilization of fracture Multiple fractures Crush injuries	Venous stasis Immobility Obesity Trauma Major surgery History of heart disease Age over 40 yr History of deep venous thrombosis, pulmonary embolism

within that space. Compartment syndrome was recognized over 100 years ago. Volkmann described an upper-extremity ischemic contracture resulting from trauma, swelling, and restrictive dressings (Figure 52-14). This complication may occur after fracture, soft tissue injury, or orthopedic surgery. If unrecognized, compartment syndrome can lead to loss of function, deformity, and possibly amputation. Failure to recognize compartment syndrome is a common cause of medical litigation in the United States.

Compartment syndrome can be either acute or chronic. Acute compartment syndrome is usually a complication of trauma. Chronic compartment syndrome commonly occurs in persons who are active in sports such as long-distance running, cycling, dancing, and cross-country skiing. Increased pressure results in ischemia and pain. Muscle mass may be increased by 20% with repeated muscle contraction during exercise; chronic compartment syndrome may occur as a result of the accumulated metabolic wastes produced during exercise.[1] Symptoms usually resolve with rest and rarely result in tissue damage. If exercise continues despite pain, chronic compartment syndrome may lead to acute compartment syndrome, requiring treatment.

Crush syndrome (rhabdomyolysis) is also a form of compartment syndrome. Trauma from extensive soft tissue and muscle damage has multisystemic effects. Protein breakdown from the damaged cells results in myoglobinuria, release of potassium from the cells, and an inflammatory reaction; third-space fluid loss, kidney failure, acidosis, and shock may ensue. The following sections pertain to acute compartment syndrome.

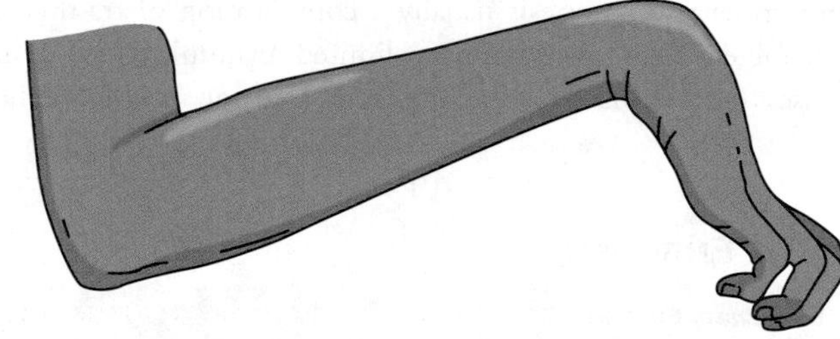

Figure 52-14 Volkmann's ischemic contracture.

Etiology and Epidemiology. For compartment syndrome to occur, there must be a space-limiting sleeve surrounding the tissue and increased tissue pressure. The space-limiting sleeve can be a restrictive dressing, a splint, a cast, fascia, or epimysium. Increased pressure within the compartment results from anything that either increases the contents of the compartment or decreases its size. Compartments consist of muscles, nerves, and blood vessels surrounded by a nonelastic covering. The body contains 46 compartments; 36 of these are in the extremities and are the most vulnerable to compartment syndrome. The most common sites are the four compartments of the lower leg (deep posterior, superficial posterior, lateral, and anterior) (Figure 52-15), the dorsal and volar compartments of the forearm, and the interosseous compartments of the hand. Persons with tibial shaft fractures are at increased risk for compartment syndrome. Older adults may have a lower risk of compartment syndrome because of increased tolerance for higher tissue pressures as a result of relatively higher blood pressures; smaller muscle mass may also be a factor.[9]

Although compartment syndrome usually occurs as a result of trauma, it has several other causes (Box 52-3). Fracture blisters may be an early warning sign of increased intracompartmental pressure.[9] Shock can also increase the risk of compartment syndrome.

Pathophysiology. After trauma, fluid accumulates in the compartment, and fascia cannot expand to accommodate the excess fluid, causing compartmental pressure to rise. Increases in tissue and venous pressures result in a decreased arteriovenous gradient. The end result is decreased blood supply and tissue hypoxia. In an attempt to correct the hypoxia, histamine is released, causing vasodilation and increased capillary permeability, which causes compartmental pressure to continue to rise. Rising pressures lead to tissue ischemia and eventually to necrosis. Peripheral muscle

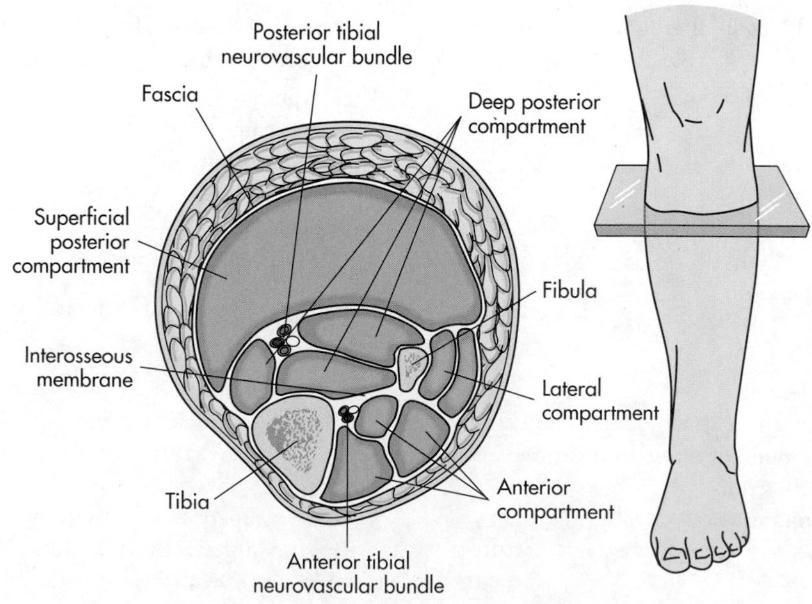

Figure 52-15 Compartments of lower leg.

Box 52-3 Causes of Compartment Syndrome

- Bleeding
  - —Vascular injury
  - —Coagulation defect (hemophilia, anticoagulant therapy)
- Nephrotic syndrome
- Excessive muscle use
  - —Exercise
  - —Seizures
  - —Tetany
  - —Eclampsia
- Trauma
  - —Fractures
  - —Crush injuries
  - —Hypothermia, frostbite
  - —Burns
  - —Snake or spider bites
- Infiltrated infusions
- Surgery
- External pressure
  - —Positioning (lying on limb)
  - —Surgical tourniquets
  - —Military antishock trousers (MAST)
  - —Circumferential restrictive dressings
  - —Tight cast
  - —Splints
- Decreased compartment size
  - —Excessive traction
  - —Closure of fascial defects

tissue undergoes ischemic changes within 6 hours of injury. Necrotic muscle cannot regenerate and is eventually replaced by dense, fibrous scar tissue. Peripheral neuropathy can develop within 24 hours, and contracture (ischemic paralysis) development begins within 4 to 12 hours of ischemia. If extensive ischemic muscle damage occurs, myoglobinuria may occur, leading to systemic complications that include kidney failure, metabolic acidosis, hyperkalemia, and sepsis.

Normal tissue compartmental pressure is 0 to 10 mm Hg; pressure in excess of 20 mm Hg is abnormal. Sustained pressure readings of 30 to 40 mm Hg usually require prompt treatment with fasciotomy, but this varies with the individual patient. Pressures of 65 mm Hg in the forearm and 55 mm Hg in the calf can cause complete cessation of circulation, resulting in avascular tissues.[1]

Early recognition of symptoms and prompt treatment may preserve the function of the limb. Pain is the most common symptom of compartment syndrome. The patient may report severe, unrelenting pain, unrelieved by analgesia and increased by elevation of the extremity. The pain is usually more intense than that expected for the extent of the injury. As pressures increases, so does the pain. Passive movement or stretching of the digits increases pain. It is important to note that epidural analgesia may mask the onset of compartment syndrome.

Motor and sensory function is also affected. It may be helpful to remember the six Ps: pain, pallor, paresthesia, pressure, paralysis, and pulselessness. Hypoesthesia, paresthesia, and muscular weakness or paralysis are common. Skin color, temperature, capillary refill, and the quality of peripheral pulses are not reliable early clinical indicators of compartment syndrome. If pallor, coolness, slow capillary refill, and diminished or absent pulses are present, extensive and potentially irreversible damage has probably already occurred.

Laboratory data supporting the diagnosis of compartment syndrome include an elevated white blood cell count and erythrocyte sedimentation rate as a result of the inflammatory response; hyperkalemia caused by cell damage; myoglobinuria; elevated creatine phosphokinase, lactate dehydrogenase, and aspartate aminotransferase levels, indicative of muscle damage; and a decreased serum pH. An elevated temperature may occur as a result of ischemia or infection.

Collaborative Care Management. Goals of treatment include (1) decreasing tissue pressure, (2) restoring blood flow, and (3) preserving limb function. Removal of external compression devices by splitting dressings or bivalving casts may alleviate early compartment syndrome. If conservative measures fail, surgical intervention may be indicated. Decompressive fasciotomy is performed along the complete length of the compartment to open the affected compartments, decrease pressure, and restore normal perfusion. Epimysiotomy, in which the outermost sheath of connective tissue is removed from the skeletal muscle, also may be necessary. Necrotic tissue is debrided to prevent infection. Postoperatively the wound is covered with wet saline dressings, and the extremity is splinted in a position that avoids stretching of the tissues (functional position). Further debridement may be necessary until secondary closure is possible. If extensive damage or infection occurs, the limb may require amputation.

If contractures develop, splints and physical and occupational therapy may be indicated. In some cases additional surgery such as joint fusion, tenotomy, or tendon transfers may be performed.

As mentioned earlier, recognition of early signs and symptoms may lead to prompt diagnosis and treatment. In an unconscious patient or one with sensory deficits, pain and changes in neurovascular status may be difficult to assess. Therefore, if compartment syndrome is suspected, invasive measurement of compartmental pressures can be performed. A variety of systems are available either for one-time use or for continuous monitoring (Figure 52-16). Compartmental pressure readings should always be evaluated in relation to the clinical picture, including the patient's blood pressure. To maintain compartmental perfusion, the diastolic pressure minus the compartmental pressure must be at least 30 mm Hg. Maintaining adequate compartmental perfusion may eliminate the necessity of surgical decompression.[9]

Segmental limb blood pressures and Doppler-derived ankle-brachial indices are sometimes used to evaluate compartment syndrome. Nerve conduction studies may be performed to evaluate nerve function. Venograms or arteriograms may be ordered to rule out DVT or vascular injury.

Nursing management of the patient with or at risk for developing compartment syndrome focuses on maintaining neurovascular integrity of the extremities. Careful monitoring of the neurovascular status of the extremities is crucial in the detection and prevention of compartment syndrome. The nurse performs baseline and ongoing assessments on both extremities to compare the findings.

Knowledge of the innervation to the extremities is useful when assessing for deficits. The nurse performs and records hourly assessments, noting any reports of increased pain, pain that occurs with passive stretching, and alterations in sensory or motor function. Assessments of the patient's ability to detect touch, ability to determine the difference between sharp and dull, and two-point discrimination are important nursing interventions to detect neurovascular dysfunction. The patient with upper extremity involvement should be assessed for the ability to extend, flex, abduct, adduct, and oppose the fingers and thumbs and flex the wrist. If

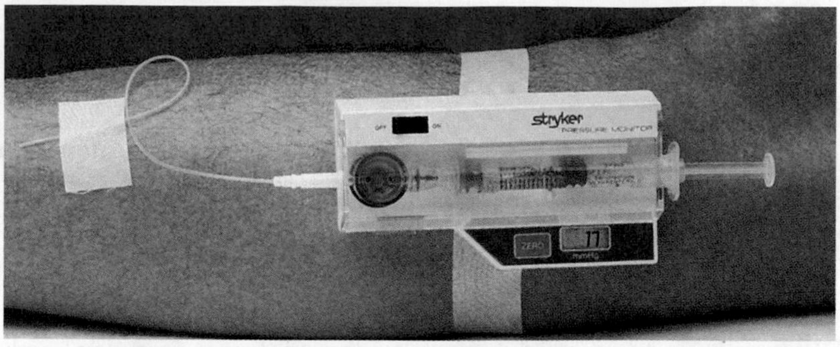

Figure 52-16 Compartmental pressure monitor.

the lower extremities are involved, the nurse assesses the ability to extend and flex the toes, perform plantar flexion and dorsiflexion, and invert and evert the foot.

If compartment syndrome is suspected, the physician is notified and restrictive dressings are loosened. To reduce edema, the extremity should be elevated to heart level, but not above, since that would compromise arterial flow. If ice packs are being used, they are removed because the application of cold and elevation of the limb may further impair the circulation. The nurse checks dressings, splints, and casts for excessive pressure; monitors and records compartmental pressures; assesses for pain; and monitors the effectiveness of pain relief measures. Any significant changes are reported to the physician.

PATIENT/FAMILY TEACHING. Teaching for the patient with compartment syndrome is presented in the Patient/Family Teaching box.

PATIENT/FAMILY TEACHING
The Patient With Compartment Syndrome

The nurse teaches persons at risk to recognize the signs of compartmental pressure and to report them immediately. Perioperative teaching is necessary if fasciotomy is performed. Patients with extensive tissue damage, neurologic deficits, or amputation require a referral for rehabilitative care. Return to normal activities is gradual and depends on the type of injury. Teaching should include information about:

- Pain management
- Treatment
- Surgical complications of fasciotomy: malunion, delayed union, bony necrosis, fracture instability, wound infection, recurrence of compartment syndrome
- Exercises
- Use of assistive devices
- Wound care
- Signs of infection
- Prognosis

Hip Fracture

Etiology and Epidemiology. Hip fractures are a leading cause of morbidity and mortality in the older population. The incidence of hip fracture increases with age; an estimated one of every five women older than 80 years of age will suffer a hip fracture. Currently more than 350,000 hip fractures occur annually, accounting for 30% of fracture-related hospitalizations.[14] The number of hip fractures will increase dramatically as the population ages; by the year 2040, the number of persons over age 65 is expected to double.[14] Ninety percent of persons suffering a hip fracture are 65 years or older; repair of a hip fracture is probably the most common surgical procedure for persons over age 85.

Risk factors commonly associated with hip fractures include osteoporosis (see Chapter 53), advanced age, being female and Caucasian, decreased estrogen levels (because of postmenopausal changes or bilateral oophorectomy), prior hip fractures, Alzheimer's dementia, institutional residence, and sedentary lifestyle. Other risk factors include an inadequate dietary intake of calcium and vitamin D, excessive dietary protein, caffeine intake, smoking, alcohol use, and use of psychotropic drugs. Although the incidence of hip fracture is most commonly associated with women, the risk of hip fractures in elderly men has increased as well. African-Americans older than 45 years of age are less likely to experience hip fractures than Caucasians because of increased mineral content and increased bone mass.

The hospital stay of older patients with hip fractures is often complicated and prolonged and may result in chronic disability, transfer to an extended care facility, or death. The older the individual, the lower the chance of regaining prefracture functional status. Factors that negatively influence recovery and increase the risk of mortality following a hip fracture include being male, preexisting medical problems, cognitive impairment, and postoperative complications.

Pathophysiology. A hip fracture is a fracture of the proximal femur and may be classified as follows (Figure 52-17):

1. *Intracapsular* (femoral neck): within the hip joint and capsule
   a. Subcapital
   b. Transcervical
   c. Basal neck
2. *Extracapsular or intertrochanteric*: outside the hip joint and capsule to an area 5 cm (2 inches) below the lesser trochanter
3. *Subtrochanteric*: below the lesser trochanter

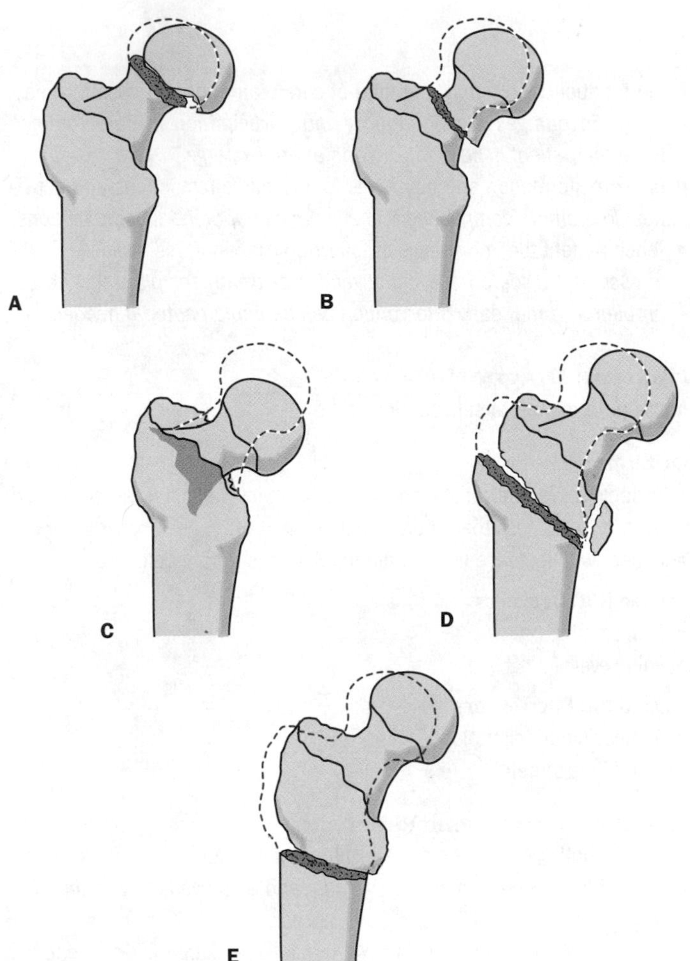

Figure 52-17 Fractures of the hip. **A,** Subcapital fracture. **B,** Transcervical fracture. **C,** Impacted basal neck fracture. **D,** Intertrochanteric fracture. **E,** Subtrochanteric fracture.

The location of the fracture is an important consideration in predicting healing. Intracapsular fractures, especially displaced fractures, can disrupt the blood supply to the femoral head (Figure 52-18). They are associated with an increased incidence of nonunion and avascular necrosis of the femoral head. Intertrochanteric fractures occur in the well-nourished vascular metaphyseal region of the hip and do not generally interfere with the blood supply of the proximal femur. Complications associated with intertrochanteric fractures include malunion and shortening of the affected extremity. Intertrochanteric and femoral neck fractures account for approximately 90% of all hip fractures, and subtrochanteric fractures account for approximately 10%.

Signs and symptoms of a hip fracture are severe pain at the fracture site, inability to move the leg voluntarily, shortening and external rotation of the leg, and other signs and symptoms consistent with those of any fracture.

Collaborative Care Management. Surgical intervention is the standard of care unless the patient's general medical condition precludes that option. Conservative management (Buck's extension) involves prolonged immobility with the associated complications, including DVT, pulmonary embolism, pneumonia, and skin breakdown. The goals of management are to return the

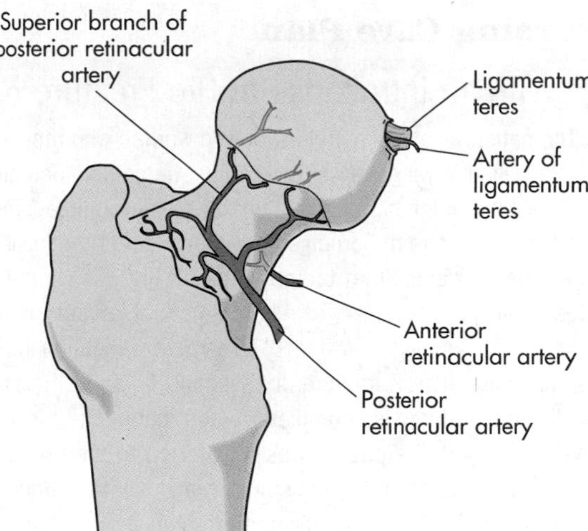

Figure 52-18 Posterior view of blood supply to head of femur.

patient to prefracture functional ability and to prevent any further disability.

Surgery involves reduction and stabilization of the fracture and insertion of an internal fixation device. The choice of fixation device depends on the fracture's location, the potential for avascular necrosis of the femoral head, and the individual patient. An impacted intracapsular fracture without displacement may be treated only with bed rest. Other surgical options include a compression screw and plate, a fixed or sliding nail and plate, percutaneous pinning, and a prosthetic implant. A **hemiarthroplasty** (usually a bipolar prosthesis), which replaces only the femoral head, or a total hip arthroplasty (see Chapter 54) (replacement of both articular surfaces of the joint) is also an option. The weight-bearing limitation (up to 2 months) and positioning restrictions vary with the type of implant and type of fixation used. Cemented prostheses often allow immediate full weight bearing, which may make compliance easier for older adults, especially those with impaired cognition.

Improving the general medical condition of the older patient before surgery, which includes stabilizing preexisting medical problems and correcting fluid and electrolyte imbalances, increases the chances for functional recovery. Factors influencing postoperative outcomes include age, gender, prefracture status, mental status, depression, operative risk, and fracture type. Nursing interventions include those to prevent the most common postoperative complications, such as thromboembolism, pneumonia, alterations in skin integrity, and voiding dysfunction (see Chapter 15 and the Nursing Care Plan).

Nursing management includes those interventions already noted for general care of patients with fractures, with specific attention given to interventions for persons with internal fixation. Pain management is an important consideration in both the acute care and rehabilitation settings (see Research box, p. 1546). Undertreatment of pain is a problem for residents in long-term care facilities.

Patients begin physical therapy in the hospital and continue in the rehabilitation unit. Positioning and weight-bearing limitations after hemiarthroplasty or total arthroplasty generally require the patient to:

- Avoid hip flexion beyond 60 degrees for up to 10 days.

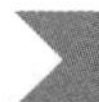

Nursing Care Plan

Patient With an Intracapsular Hip Fracture

Data The patient is a 71-year-old widowed woman who tripped and fell on an icy step when leaving her niece's home. She complained of immediate, severe pain in her left hip and was unable to move her leg. The patient was immediately taken to the emergency department of the local hospital. Initial assessment revealed that the patient's left leg was shorter than her right and externally rotated. Her vital signs were stable, and the neurovascular status of the left leg was intact. An x-ray examination revealed an intracapsular femoral neck fracture. Intravenous fluids were initiated. An electrocardiogram, urinalysis, complete blood count, and serum electrolytes were obtained. The patient was transferred to the orthopedic unit with physician's orders for morphine sulfate via patient-controlled analgesia (PCA) pump, bed rest, pneumatic compression devices bilaterally, and diet as tolerated. Five pounds of Buck's extension was applied to the left leg. Informed consent was obtained for surgical repair of the fracture. The patient will undergo a hemiarthroplasty (prosthetic replacement of the femoral head and neck) in the morning. She states that she is afraid because she has never undergone surgery before. Her niece is present and supportive.

Nursing Diagnosis

Deficient knowledge related to lack of previous experience with surgery and treatment protocols

Outcomes

- Patient will express decreased anxiety regarding impending surgery.
- Patient will actively participate in plan of care.

Related NOC Outcomes

- Knowledge: Disease Process
- Knowledge: Medication
- Knowledge: Prescribed Activity

Related NIC Interventions

- Teaching: Disease Process
- Teaching: Preoperative
- Teaching: Procedure/Treatment

Nursing Interventions/Rationales

- Assess need for teaching and provide as needed. *Teaching needs vary among patients. Assessment helps individualize teaching. Understanding of surgery and treatments reduces fear related to the unknown.*
- Provide written materials if available. *Patients often want to review material later or may not remember specifics.*
- Review preoperative and postoperative care with patient and family before the surgery; provide examples of prostheses if available. *Understanding the surgical procedure and postoperative care lessens anxiety and promotes participation in postoperative routines.*
- Evaluate patient's understanding of information taught and reinforce learning as needed. *To determine the need for further teaching. Reinforcement of information improves retention and promotes patient compliance.*
- Keep patient and family informed of care plan and rationales for treatment. *Encourages family support and participation in care routines while the patient is hospitalized and after discharge.*
- Provide information and rationales for discharge restrictions and activities. *To promote compliance and avoidance of potential complications.*
- Teach patient the importance of follow-up examinations. *Follow-up care is essential to determine effectiveness of treatment plan and detect problems so that early intervention can be implemented if needed.*

Nursing Diagnosis

Acute pain related to surgical procedure

Outcomes

- Patient will report satisfaction with pain relief measures as evidenced by rating pain less than 3 on a scale of 0 to 10.
- Patient will decrease use of pain medications before discharge.

Related NOC Outcomes

- Pain Control
- Pain Level

Related NIC Interventions

- Analgesic Administration
- Pain Management

Nursing Interventions/Rationales

- Assess patient's pain before and after comfort interventions. *To determine the degree of postoperative pain and effectiveness of pain relief measures.*
- Apply ice to operative site for 48 hours after surgery. *Cold reduces swelling by decreasing the blood supply to the area. Reducing swelling reduces pain.*
- Encourage use of PCA before pain becomes severe. *Milder pain is more readily controlled than severe pain. The ability to self-medicate allows the patient control over her pain.*
- Monitor use and effectiveness of PCA. *PCA avoids peaks and valleys associated with intermittent use of analgesics. It also allows the patient greater control over her pain.*
- Encourage use of nonpharmacologic pain relief measures if acceptable to the patient. *Relaxation, repositioning, and distraction are helpful for reducing and controlling pain; however, the patient must believe they will help.*

Nursing Diagnosis

Impaired physical mobility related to pain secondary to surgical repair and placement of prosthesis

Outcomes

- Patient will use assistive devices correctly to aid with mobility.
- Patient will remain free from complications of immobility.
- Patient will perform prescribed exercises.
- Patient will maintain prescribed limitations.

Related NOC Outcomes
- Ambulation
- Pain Control
- Pain Level

Related NIC Interventions
- Analgesic Administration
- Exercise Therapy: Ambulation
- Pain Management

Nursing Interventions/Rationales
- Perform neurovascular checks every 2 hours for the first 24 to 48 hours and notify physician of changes from preoperative status. *To detect signs of neurovascular compromise as quickly as possible so that correct interventions can be initiated.*
- Encourage performance of active dorsiflexion, plantar flexion, isometric quadriceps and gluteal exercises, and active range of motion of unaffected limbs every 12 hours until ambulatory. *Exercising promotes venous return, prevents thrombus formation, and helps maintain muscle tone.*
- Maintain prescribed limits of motion and weight bearing. *Positioning restrictions are designed to prevent dislocation of the prosthesis.*
- Turn patient from back to nonoperated side every 2 hours and as needed. Avoid positioning patient on operative side, and observe flexion restrictions when elevating the head of the bed. *Frequent turning and repositioning promote circulation, respiratory effort, and muscle activity. Maintaining prescribed positioning restrictions prevents dislocation of the prosthesis.*
- When turning the patient, hold the opposite leg in abduction, using pillows to maintain 30-degree abduction. *Prevents adduction of leg and dislocation of the prosthesis.*
- Encourage sitting when patient demonstrates sufficient control of the affected leg to sit within flexion restrictions. *Prepares patient for discharge while ensuring that patient functions safely within prescribed flexion limits.*
- Elevate sitting surface with pillows to keep angle of hip within prescribed limits. *To prevent hip flexion beyond 90 degrees, which may cause dislocation of the prosthesis.*
- Assist patient with walking on second postoperative day and increase the frequency and distance of ambulation as tolerated. *To hasten recovery and prevent postoperative complications related to immobility.*
- Reinforce use of assistive devices provided by physical or occupational therapy. *Assistive devices aid with mobility while helping prevent injuries.*
- Teach patient and family that for the first 2 to 3 months hip flexion is limited to less than 90 degrees, adduction beyond midline and extreme internal or external rotation are prohibited, and partial weight bearing with the aid of a walker is maintained. *To aid with healing and prevent dislocation of the prosthesis.*

Nursing Diagnosis
Risk for impaired home maintenance related to lack of previous experience

Outcomes
- Patient and family will express satisfaction with arrangements made for rehabilitation facility or self-care management at home.
- Patient and family will verbalize understanding of prescribed medications.
- Patient will correctly self-administer prescribed medications.
- Patient and family will verbalize need for keeping follow-up appointments.

Related NOC Outcomes
- Compliance Behavior
- Participation in Health Care Decisions

Related NIC Interventions
- Discharge Planning
- Family Support
- Home Maintenance Assistance
- Mutual Goal Setting

Nursing Interventions/Rationales
- Assess patient's and family's perception of problems that may occur with management of self-care at home. *To identify actual or perceived needs and obstacles to the patient caring for herself at home.*
- Determine the type of equipment needed (e.g., crutches, walker, elevated toilet seat) and obtain any needed equipment. *To facilitate the patient and family's ability to successfully care for the patient at home.*
- Assess the home environment for needed changes (e.g., stairs, proximity of bathroom to bedroom). *To facilitate the patient's recovery at home and the patient and family's ability to provide that care.*
- Teach patient and family regarding anticoagulant use and potential side effects. *Bleeding and thrombocytopenia are side effects of some anticoagulants. Patients need to be taught how to monitor for bruising and bleeding, which indicate excessive anticoagulation.*
- Teach patient and family the need for monitoring coagulation studies as prescribed. *To determine drug effectiveness and to prevent excessive anticoagulation.*
- Encourage patient to participate in decisions about rehabilitation and self-care at home. *Involving the patient in decision making increases the likelihood of compliance with the prescribed treatment and rehabilitation plan.*

Evaluation
Evaluation is based on comparing the patient's outcomes with desired outcomes.

- Avoid hip flexion beyond 90 degrees from day 10 to 2 months.
- Avoid adduction of the affected leg beyond midline for 2 months.
- Maintain partial weight-bearing status for approximately 2 months (varies with the type of prosthesis and method of implantation [cement versus bony ingrowths]).

The nurse carefully instructs the patient on the limits of motion to observe and provides nursing care within those constraints (Figure 52-19). Generally, positioning the patient on the operative side is avoided, although this can depend on the surgeon's preference. The patient is helped to maintain hip **abduction** using an A-shaped abduction pillow or bed pillows (Figure 52-20). Maintaining hip abduction requires that the nurse carefully monitor the patient's position during transferring. A chair with armrests and a firm, no reclining seat should be provided; the sitting surface is elevated as necessary with pillows or foam cushions to keep the angle of the hip within the prescribed limits when the patient is sitting. In general, patients who have had any kind of internal fixation for a fractured hip should avoid elevation of the operative leg when sitting in a chair because this puts excessive strain on the fixation device.

Research

Feldt KS, Gunderson J: Treatment of pain for older hip fracture patients across settings, *Orthop Nurs* 21(5):63-70, 2002.

After a hip fracture, as many as 50% of older adult patients become partially dependent and one third require long-term care. Most patients recovering from hip fracture are discharged from the acute care setting to a rehabilitation or skilled nursing facility to continue with physical therapy. Problems with pain management, musculoskeletal function, emotional stability, and medication management for older patients continue after discharge from the hospital. Older adults recovering from hip fracture may be cognitively impaired. Disparity exists in the pain management of cognitively intact and cognitively impaired older patients. Effective pain management across settings is an important aspect of nursing care for all patients recovering from hip fracture.

This retrospective review compared the amount of analgesia administered to two groups—cognitively intact and cognitively impaired—of older patients recovering from surgical fixation of hip fracture. The amount of analgesia administered during the last 24 hours in the hospital was compared with amount given in the first 24 hours in the nursing home or rehabilitation facility (NHR). Study participants received significantly less analgesia in the first 24 hours in the NHR than in the hospital. More than 37% of patients received no opioids and 18% received no analgesia at all during the first 24 hours in NHR. The most common medications given in both settings were acetaminophen with codeine and propoxyphene napsylate. Cognitive status did not affect medication administration; the only significant factor affecting analgesic administration was the setting. Because this was a secondary analysis, no data were available on patients' report of pain severity.

Information regarding effective pain management strategies should be communicated to the NHR staff as patients are discharged from the hospital to ensure continuity of care. Postoperative pain management should be included in NHR staff education.

PATIENT/FAMILY TEACHING. Teaching for the patient with a hip fracture is presented in the Patient/Family Teaching box.

Fracture of the Spine

Etiology and Epidemiology. Spinal or vertebral fractures occur as a result of falls, motor vehicle or diving accidents, or blows to the head or body by heavy objects. With increasing frequency, fractures of the spine are also occurring as a result of osteoporosis (see Chapter 53) and metastatic lesions of the spine. A spinal fracture can occur at any age.

Pathophysiology. A vertebral fracture may occur with or without displacement. Displaced fracture fragments may place pressure on spinal nerves or injure the spinal cord itself. Such pressure results in partial or complete dysfunction of the body parts innervated by nerves at the level of injury. Depending on the extent of injury to the nervous system, dysfunction may be permanent or temporary.

A fracture can occur at any level of the spine, from the occipital through the sacral. Signs and symptoms of a vertebral fracture include pain at the site of injury, partial or complete loss of mobility or sensation below the level of injury, and evidence of a fracture or fracture dislocation on routine x-ray examination, a CT scan, or an MRI scan.

Collaborative Care Management. Long-term goals of treatment are stabilization and reduction of the fracture and decompression (i.e., removal of pressure from spinal nerves or the spinal cord). Immediate management objectives are (1) immobilization of the patient with a backboard and cervical collar and (2) immediate transport to a hospital.

Objectives of surgical management are:

- Decompression of nerve structures through laminectomy (see Chapter 53) or appropriate reduction of the fracture and removal of fracture fragments
- Reduction of the fracture through operative procedures or, in some cases, traction (e.g., cervical traction through application of tongs to the skull)
- Stabilization of the fracture with bone grafting or internal fixation devices such as pedicle screws and plates or rods
- Maintenance of stabilization with external fixation devices such as casts, corsets, or braces as necessary

Nondisplaced compression fractures without neurologic compromise may be treated with bed rest until the patient's pain subsides. The patient is then gradually mobilized, sometimes with stabilization by a corset or brace.

Many of the nursing interventions required by the patient with a spinal fracture are identical to those outlined for the patient with spinal cord injury in Chapter 50. Of special concern are interventions designed to (1) maintain the stability of the fracture fixation, (2) prevent neurovascular problems, and (3) promote psychologic comfort.

To maintain stability of the fracture fixation, the head of the bed should not be elevated beyond the prescribed level, which is usually only 30 degrees. In the absence of an elevation order, the bed is maintained in a flat position. When the patient is in a side-lying position, pillows are placed between the patient's legs and

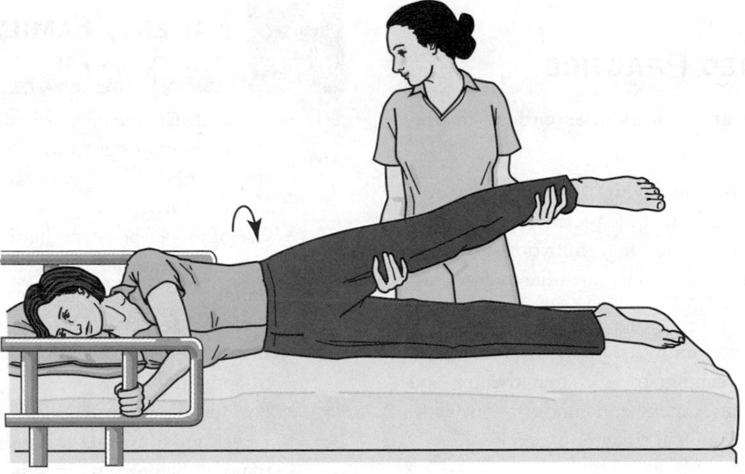

Figure 52-19 Assisting patient with turning while maintaining abduction of the hip. The leg is supported at the thigh and just above the ankle to avoid putting undue stress on the hip. An abduction pillow may also be used.

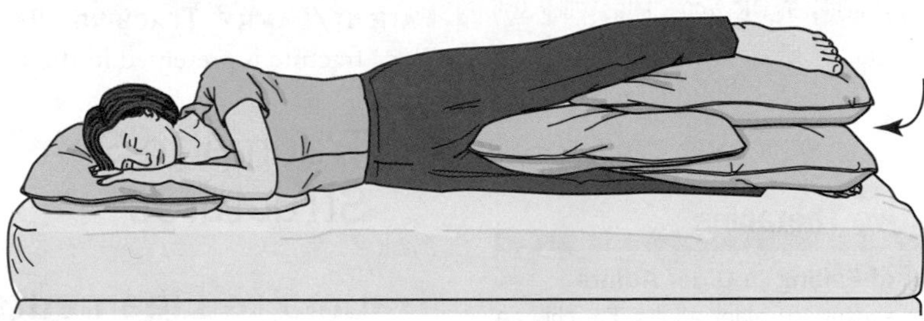

Figure 52-20 Pillows are staggered in a wedge-shaped arrangement to maintain abduction of hip.

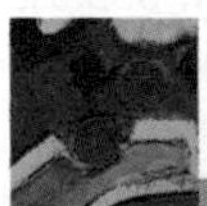

PATIENT/FAMILY TEACHING *The Patient With a Hip Fracture*

Most patients are discharged to a rehabilitation facility, typically after a 4- to 5-day stay in the hospital. The nurse reminds the patient and family that complete recovery might take as long as 6 months. Recovery is generally measured by the patient's ability to regain prefracture functional status. The patient and family need reassurance that the process of healing and recovery is gradual. Discharge instructions and information include:

- Medication instruction. Many patients are prescribed anticoagulants for as long as 3 months postoperatively. Deep venous thrombosis may occur in as many as 70% of patients after a hip fracture. The patient and family should be familiar with medication administration (the patient may be prescribed subcutaneous injections of low-molecular-weight heparin).
- Positioning and weight-bearing restrictions.
- Ambulation techniques with assistive devices.
- Use of adaptive equipment for the home, such as an elevated toilet seat, grab bars for the bath, long-handled reachers, and an elevated chair with armrests.
- Signs and symptoms of complications.
- Prevention of future falls. Falls are a major cause of hip fracture (see Evidence-Based Practice box). A Clinical Falls Assessment should be included for high-risk patients.[14]
- Prevention or control of osteoporosis.
- Importance of adequate dietary intake of calcium and vitamin D to decrease bone loss and prevent fractures.
- Need for regular weight-bearing exercise to maintain bone mass and reduce the risk of hip fractures. Thirty minutes of exercise daily is recommended. Exercise has the added benefit of reducing the risk of falling in older adults (see Complementary & Alternative Therapies box).

behind the back to prevent back strain. Changes of position are best accomplished using special beds that rotate 45 degrees from side to side; the literature indicates that in persons with unstable spine fractures, logrolling and turning frames are contraindicated because they can stress the fracture site. When logrolling the patient, the nurse must pay strict attention to avoid twisting the spine and placing stress at the fracture site. If a corset or brace is ordered, it should be applied before getting the patient out of bed.

To prevent neurovascular problems, the nurse performs neurovascular checks every hour for the first 24 to 48 hours postoperatively. Any decrease in neurovascular function must be reported to the physician, since this may indicate displacement

EVIDENCE-BASED PRACTICE

Topic Question: How effective are various interventions to prevent falls in older adults?

Evidence Base: In randomized trials involving 21,668 participants, interventions to reduce the risk for falls included screening programs, muscle strengthening and balance retraining, nutritional supplements, home hazard modification, and medication adjustment. Outcomes measured the number of falls.

Findings: Effective interventions were multidisciplinary, multifactorial, health and environmental risk screening; muscle strengthening and balance retraining; home hazard assessment and modification; withdrawal of psychotropic medication; and t'ai chi' group exercise.

Conclusions: Effective interventions to reduce the number of falls in older people are available, but little is known about their effectiveness in preventing fall-related injuries. More research is needed to study the interventions found to be of unknown effectiveness.

Gillespie LD et al: *Interventions for preventing falls in elderly people* (Cochrane Review). In *Cochrane Library*, Issue 3, Chichester, UK, 2004, John Wiley & Sons.

Complementary & Alternative Therapies

T'ai Chi' May Reduce Risk of Falling in Older Adults

Falls are a major cause of hip fracture in older adults. T'ai chi', an ancient Chinese exercise form, may be an effective intervention to reduce the risk of falls in this population. This review of 31 controlled experimental studies and clinical trials examined the physiologic responses and effects on general health and fitness of t'ai chi' in 2216 older men and women. T'ai chi' is considered moderate exercise and does not demand more than 55% of maximum oxygen intake. Data analysis revealed that t'ai chi' has positive effects on cardiorespiratory, immune, and musculoskeletal functioning. In addition to reducing the incidence of falls in older persons, t'ai chi' improved their flexibility, balance, posture, and mental control.

Li JX, Hong Y, Chan KM: Tai chi: physiological characteristics and beneficial effects on health, *Br J Sports Med* 35(3):148-156, 2001.

or pressure at the fracture site. Passive ROM to involved extremities is performed at least three times daily to maintain joint motion, and the patient is encouraged to perform active ROM to noninvolved extremities hourly to maintain joint motion and promote circulation.

Promotion of psychologic comfort begins with recognizing that the patient may have feelings of powerlessness, anger, or fear about the situation, particularly if there is a sensorimotor deficit. The nurse encourages the patient to express his or her feelings and arranges for a counselor if indicated. The patient also is prepared for long-term care in a rehabilitative facility if needed.

Other nursing interventions are similar to those for any patient who has a fracture, including interventions for individuals in casts or traction, which are discussed earlier in this chapter.

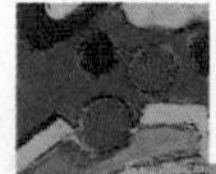

PATIENT/FAMILY TEACHING
The Patient With a Spine Fracture

The nurse instructs the patient and family on the following:

- Recognition of signs and symptoms of neurologic impairment (pain, paresthesias, weakness, paralysis, bowel or bladder impairment)
- Use of proper body mechanics and lifting techniques to avoid strain on the spine; the need to avoid lifting more than 5 to 10 pounds
- Protocol for exercises to strengthen back and abdominal muscles
- Instructions regarding skin care and care of the brace or corset (if applicable)
- Postoperative instructions (if applicable)
- Prevention of further injury if the fracture was a result of trauma; the need for extreme caution when engaging in contact sports

PATIENT/FAMILY TEACHING. Teaching for the patient with a spine fracture is presented in the Patient/Family Teaching box.

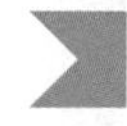

Trauma to Soft Tissue Structures

Trauma to Ligaments and Tendons

Etiology and Epidemiology. Trauma to ligaments and tendons is usually seen in connection with injury to a joint caused by a blow, twisting, or severe stretching. The most common site of ligament damage is the knee, often from a sports injury, because of the anatomy, location, and complex motions of the joint. The Achilles tendon is susceptible to partial or complete tears, usually caused by a sports injury. Shoulder and ankle injuries are common, particularly sports injuries. Ankle sprains are the most common injury seen in emergency departments.[21] Sports-related injuries account for 500,000 visits to health care providers annually.[22] Many of these injuries are to the musculoskeletal system (Table 52-4).

This section contains a general discussion of ligamentous and tendon injuries. A more detailed discussion of anterior cruciate ligament trauma and rotator cuff trauma follows.

Pathophysiology. The most common ligamentous or tendon injuries are partial or complete tears. Injury to the knee may include damage to the medial, lateral, and posterior ligaments and to the anterior and posterior cruciate ligaments (see Clinical Manifestations box). Injuries may be classified as:

- Mild (class I): stretching of ligament without obvious tear
- Moderate (class II): several ligament fibers torn with a partial loss of function; partial tear
- Severe (class III): severe or complete disruption of the ligament with resulting instability

Signs and symptoms of class I injuries are mild pain and swelling. Class II injuries are associated with moderate pain and

TABLE 52-4 COMMON SOFT TISSUE INJURIES

Mechanism of Injury	Symptoms	Treatment
MENISCAL		
Medial and lateral tears usually occur with rotary or extension or flexion injuries of knee	Joint pain Swelling "Locking"	Splint, bracing, or cast Surgical treatment by meniscectomy via arthroscopy or arthrotomy
ANTERIOR CRUCIATE LIGAMENT (ACL)		
Valgus stress applied to knee while in hyperextension and external rotation Associated with deceleration and changes in direction	Audible "pop" or "snap" Pain Joint effusion Hemarthrosis Joint deformity Joint instability "Giving way" of knee Positive anterior drawer test	Treatment depends on patient's age and lifestyle: Conservative treatment: quadriceps and hamstring strengthening, bracing, and avoidance of high-risk activities Surgical reconstruction of ACL, either open or arthroscopically aided, using autologous or synthetic graft followed by extensive rehabilitation program
ROTATOR CUFF		
Strain or tear of rotator cuff muscles or tendons of shoulder (supraspinatus, infraspinatus, teres minor, subscapularis) Usually results from falling on outstretched hand, throwing objects (baseball pitchers), or chronic or excessive use	Severe pain with loss of ability to flex and abduct shoulder Positive drop arm test	Rest, sling and swath for immobilization, physical therapy, NSAIDs Surgical repair for complete rupture, disability, or chronic pain; followed by physical therapy
ANKLE SPRAIN		
Represent approximately 75% of all ankle injuries; 25% of injuries occur in running and jumping sports Higher incidence in sports (basketball, soccer); also can occur while walking on uneven surfaces; lateral ligaments more susceptible to injury Usually results from inversion and plantar flexion force on ankle (95% as result of inversion) Severity of injury affected by position of foot, type of sport, directional changes, joint laxity, and magnitude of force	Swelling Tenderness Reluctance to bear full weight, perform full range of motion Deformities Ecchymoses	Rest, ice, elastic compression, elevation for grades I, II sprains Grade II sprains: immobilization by cast or bracing, gradual resumption of activity Aggressive treatment sometimes includes primary surgical repair or ankle stabilization procedure

NSAIDs, Nonsteroidal antiinflammatory drugs.

swelling, and class III injuries with severe pain, swelling, joint instability, and disability or loss of function.

Collaborative Care Management. Immediate first-aid measures for soft tissue injuries of the musculoskeletal system can be easily remembered by the mnemonic RICE:

- *R*est of the injured part
- *I*ce for at least 48 to 72 hours to decrease bleeding and edema
- *C*ompression with elastic bandages, splints, or casts (Be sure to monitor for signs of compartment syndrome.)
- *E*levation of the extremity to slightly above the level of the heart to increase venous return and decrease edema

Diagnosis is based on evaluation of the patient history and physical examination, including specialized tests to detect ligamentous instability. It is especially important to elicit a complete history of the specific mechanism of injury, which aids in differential diagnosis. X-ray films are used to rule out a fracture. Arthrography and arthroscopy may be performed to visualize the extent of the injury.

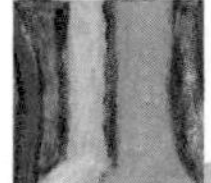

CLINICAL MANIFESTATIONS
Knee Trauma

- Tenderness
- Swelling, effusion (usually within 2 to 4 hours of injury)
- Pain
- Hematoma
- Disability; "knee gives way"
- Abnormal motion at joint
- Audible pop

Treatment varies with the extent of injury. For mild injuries, rest and a compression dressing are used. Moderate injuries are also treated with rest but may require aspiration of excess fluid. The compression dressing controls swelling and further effusion, and support is provided with a splint or a brace. Strengthening exercises are needed.

In cases of severe injury, surgical repair is done to prevent disability and instability, via arthroscope, open, or arthroscopically aided procedures. A modified compression dressing is applied to prevent effusion, and the joint is immobilized for a prescribed time. Joint remobilization may include a continuous passive motion machine and physical therapy for strengthening exercises. The use of crutches is necessary for lower extremity injuries.

Medications used for pain relief depend on the severity of discomfort. Choices include opioids and nonopioids. Skeletal muscle relaxants may be used to relieve pain and spasm. Relaxation of hypertonic muscles promotes healing and decreases pain.[3]

Postoperative nursing interventions for the patient with a ligamentous or tendon tear include the same considerations as for the partially immobilized patient after fracture reduction and application of an external fixation device.

PATIENT/FAMILY TEACHING. If surgery was performed, the nurse gives the patient general perioperative instructions, including the correct use and application of the immobilization device (brace, cast, splint), activity or weight-bearing restrictions, medication use, symptoms of complications, and the plan for follow-up care. Methods to prevent future injury are stressed. Patients need to understand that repetitive injuries may result in posttraumatic degenerative arthritis and that safety equipment, proper footwear, and warm-up and cool-down exercises should be a part of any sport.

Trauma to the Anterior Cruciate Ligament

Etiology and Epidemiology. Trauma to the anterior cruciate ligament (ACL) is the most common ligamentous injury to the knee; more than 250,000 injuries are diagnosed annually.[2,22] It is also the knee injury most often treated surgically; the cost of ACL reconstruction surgery is approximately $17,000. Annual costs for ACL injury total $1.5 billion, with the majority of costs associated with female high school and collegiate sports injuries.[4] Ninety percent of all injuries occur in the middle third of the ligament. The highest incidence is in persons 15 to 44 years of age who participate in pivoting sports; the incidence is also higher in women than in men.[4]

The anatomy and function of the knee make it vulnerable to injury because of the stresses of motion and load bearing on the joint. The knee joint moves in six independent directions and depends on the quadriceps, hamstrings, and gastrocnemius muscles for stabilization and functioning. Mechanism of injury includes both contact and noncontact motions. Injury usually occurs when the knee is hyperextended and the femur is externally rotated on a fixed tibia. Injuries commonly occur during soccer, football, skiing, and basketball, with the affected leg firmly planted on the ground. The patient usually sustains a twisting type of injury and typically reports a "pop" as the injury occurs. Contact injury often involves multiple structures, for example, O'Donoghue's triad, tearing the ACL, medial collateral ligament, and the medial meniscus.[4]

Pathophysiology. The ACL provides support to the knee joint. It is paired with the posterior cruciate ligament to stabilize the knee joint. The ligament originates from the posteromedial aspect of the lateral femoral condyle and crosses (hence the name *cruciate*) the knee joint obliquely. The insertion is on the anteromedial aspect of the tibial plateau. The ACL functions primarily to prevent anterior displacement of the tibia, hyperextension, and excessive internal rotation of the knee. Lesser functions include decreasing varus and valgus stresses to the knee while in flexion.

The patient usually reports the knee "giving way" and severe swelling and pain. Effusion usually occurs 2 to 4 hours after the injury. Ruptured blood vessels are the cause of hemarthrosis, which is particularly indicative of ACL injury. Examination of the patient is often difficult because of the pain.

Chronic injury occurs as a result of a missed diagnosis, failure to seek treatment, or unsuccessful conservative treatment of an acute injury. The knee becomes increasingly unstable anteriorly and "gives way" more frequently. Muscle weakness and decreased activity are common.

Collaborative Care Management. Diagnosis is made on the basis of the history and physical examination. The drawer test and Lachman's test are both done to determine the degree of anterior displacement of the tibia and the amount of laxity of the knee (see Chapter 51). The pivot shift maneuver also detects anterolateral stability of the knee. It is important to evaluate both knees for comparison. Radiographs and MRI scans confirm the diagnosis. Although x-ray films are not useful in diagnosing ACL tears, they are essential to rule out a fracture or avulsion of the ACL from its insertion site.

The patient's age, activity level, type of job and leisure activities, and general medical condition are factors to consider before determining the type of treatment. Options are physical therapy and rehabilitation or surgical intervention and rehabilitation. If meniscal damage is also present, surgical treatment is highly recommended because the resultant degenerative arthritis is difficult to treat. The goals of treatment are to prevent further damage to the knee (traumatic arthritis and meniscal tears) and allow the patient to return to his or her former level of functioning.

Conservative management usually consists of NSAIDs; application of ice and heat; electrical stimulation; rest and immobilization for a few days, followed by physical therapy to restore muscle strength; ROM exercises; and weight bearing as quickly as possible. A brace and activity modification to avoid further injury are recommended. If the patient is not willing to modify activity, surgical repair should be considered.

The goal of surgical reconstruction is elimination of anterior **subluxation** of the tibia. Surgical options include repair with or without augmentation of the ligament and reconstruction using various types of grafts. The procedure is often performed with the aid of arthroscopy, limiting the need to open the joint surgically. A popular reconstructive technique involves the use of a patellar tendon graft with a bone block at both ends; the graft is passed through to the origin and insertion sites of the ligament. Hamstring tendons and the Achilles tendon may be substituted. Both autograft and allograft can be used for the patellar tendon. Autograft options include bone–patellar tendon–bone, quadriceps tendons, semitendinosus/gracilis; allograft options include Achilles tendon and anterior or posterior tibialis tendons.[13]

Controversy surrounds the ideal time between injury and surgical repair. Patients undergoing reconstruction of a chronic ACL tear may actually attain more joint ROM than those who have had acute injuries repaired. Early reconstruction is indicated for high-performance athletes and persons who wish to remain active in vigorous sports.

The surgical procedure is generally performed on an outpatient basis. The degree of pain control is usually the main determinant of the hospital length of stay. Newer techniques are aimed at minimizing the amount of postoperative pain and facilitating early discharge (see Research box). Intraarticular injection of bupivacaine in the operating room provides pain relief for up to 4 hours. Intraarticular morphine also shows promise in reducing postoperative knee pain for as long as 3 to 6 hours after injection. Cryotherapy, or the use of cooling pads, is another method of controlling pain and swelling, which contributes to pain.

Research

Pulido PA et al: The efficacy of continuous bupivacaine infiltration for pain management following orthopaedic knee surgery: anterior cruciate ligament reconstruction and total knee arthroplasty, *Orthop Nurs* 21(1):31-36, 2002.

Although pain management is a national health care goal, undertreatment of pain remains a problem. Pain management in the orthopedic patient population is especially challenging. Multimodal or balanced analgesia (combining different analgesics at reduced doses) is recommended for postoperative pain management because it minimizes the adverse effects associated with any one single agent. Two drug classes often used in balanced analgesia are opioids and local anesthetics.

In these two studies the researchers examined the effectiveness of a postoperative pain regimen combining continuous low-dose infiltration of local anesthetic and opioids. Study participants were recovering from either total knee arthroplasty (TKA) or endoscopic anterior cruciate ligament (ACL) reconstruction.

In the ACL study, all participants received a bolus injection of 5 mg of morphine and 25 cc of 0.25% bupivacaine injected via a subcutaneous catheter into the patellar tendon graft site. For 48 hours after the bolus dose, the experimental group received a continuous subcutaneous infusion of bupivacaine; the control group received normal saline.

TKA participants received a single bolus dose of 30 cc of 0.25% bupivacaine with 1:200,000 epinephrine injected into the suprapatellar pouch of the knee joint. For 48 hours after the bolus injection, the experimental group received a continuous infusion of 0.25% bupivacaine and 1:200,000 epinephrine; the control group received a normal saline infusion. Both TKA groups had patient-controlled analgesia available.

Participants receiving the bupivacaine infusion in the ACL and TKA studies used fewer opioids than the controls. Pain scores were lower in the ACL experimental group, but showed no significant differences among the TKA groups. No adverse effects were associated with the bupivacaine infusion in any group. Limitations of these studies include a small sample size and heterogeneity of the ACL and TKA participants. Further research is needed to support the use of continuous bupivacaine infusion for postoperative pain control.

Postoperative complications include nausea, infection, DVT, pulmonary embolism, graft failure, and recurrent laxity.[2] Depending on protocol, the patient may be seen in the office the next day for a dressing change and evaluation of the knee for hemarthrosis. Approximately 10% of patients require joint aspiration for hemarthrosis.[2]

PATIENT/FAMILY TEACHING. If surgical repair is performed, patient education focuses on postoperative activity restrictions, exercises, weight-bearing limits, brace instruction, crutch walking, and recognition of signs and symptoms of complications. The goals of rehabilitation are to protect the graft, restore ROM, promote early weight bearing, and return the patient to preinjury activity levels. The amount of permissible weight bearing depends on the surgeon's protocols. Generally, touching down or weight bearing as tolerated is prescribed after surgery.

Physical therapy sessions usually begin 1 to 4 weeks after surgery. The rehabilitation process can take as long as 1 year. Ankle pumps, quadriceps and hamstring isometrics, and straight leg raises are taught before discharge. The patient is cautioned against overdoing exercise too early in the rehabilitation process. The graft often takes up to 12 months to revascularize and up to 24 months to attain preinjury strength.[2]

The nurse instructs the patient and family to call the physician if the patient experiences fever, chills, increased swelling, increased wound drainage, or pain unrelieved by analgesics. The nurse also instructs the patient and family regarding the appropriate use of prescription pain medication.

Overuse and Traumatic Injuries of the Shoulder

Etiology and Epidemiology. The shoulder is the third most commonly injured joint, after the knee and ankle. Injury commonly occurs during athletic activities. Sports injuries are associated with direct trauma and overuse (as with throwing motions), which causes overloading of the shoulder's supporting structures. Overhead arm motion can stress the soft tissues surrounding the glenohumeral joint, causing injury over time. The large head of the humerus and the comparatively shallow glenoid fossa allow the shoulder to be the most mobile joint in the body. Because of the mobility of the shoulder joint, it has fewer structural restraints to prevent potentially damaging movements. Chronic overuse is insidious and usually results in impingement syndrome. Acute trauma may result in a partial or complete tear of the rotator cuff, dislocation, subluxation, separation, or fracture. Acromioclavicular separation is one of the most common shoulder injuries. Injuries to the rotator cuff usually result from chronic impingement in persons over the age of 40.

Pathophysiology. The rotator cuff is composed of subscapularis, supraspinatus, infraspinatus, and teres minor muscles and tendons. The rotator cuff functions to stabilize the humeral head in the glenoid fossa while the arm is raised. Primary movements of these muscles are abduction, external rotation, joint stabilization, and (to a lesser extent) internal rotation. The term *impingement syndrome* refers to the impingement of the rotator cuff by the acromion, coracoacromial ligament, and acromioclavicular joint. The syndrome occurs as the arm is abducted past 90 degrees and the greater tuberosity of the humerus compresses the rotator cuff against the acromion. The impingement causes microtrauma to the cuff, edema, hemorrhage, and cuff shortening. A poor blood supply to the tendons results in decreased potential for healing. Fibrosis, tendinitis, bony changes, a rotator cuff tear, or a biceps tendon rupture may progressively result. Symptoms of impingement are limited movement, increased pain on external rotation and abduction, weakness on manual muscle testing, muscle atrophy, and point tenderness over the insertion of the rotator cuff. Differentiating the pain occurring from impingement from the pain that occurs as a result of a rotator cuff tear is difficult.

Collaborative Care Management. Treatment is based on the following principles: decrease the inflammatory response by administering an NSAID or applying ice, alleviate pain, immobilize or limit motion in the joint, and rehabilitate the patient to achieve maximal functional outcome. Rehabilitation begins with isometrics, passive ROM progressing to active ROM exercises, and exercises to strengthen the rotator cuff and surrounding muscles. Subacromial cortisone injections, activity modifications to avoid repetitive overhead motions, heat, and electrical stimulation are also prescribed to decrease inflammation and promote healing. The use of cortisone injections should be limited because repeated injections into the cuff may weaken it and predispose the tissues to tearing.

Surgical intervention is indicated if conservative methods fail to improve functioning within 6 months to 1 year. Extremely active persons or athletes may opt for immediate surgical treatment, without a trial of conservative therapy. Most procedures can be performed arthroscopically, which offers the advantage of less discomfort, less chance of infection, and quicker return to overhead activities, usually within 6 to 8 weeks. Laser surgery can also be used for rotator cuff repair and relief of impingement. Rehabilitative exercises are prescribed after surgery, in the same progression as described earlier (Figure 52-21).

Patient/Family Teaching. Teaching for the patient with overuse or traumatic injury to the shoulder is presented in the Patient/Family Teaching box.

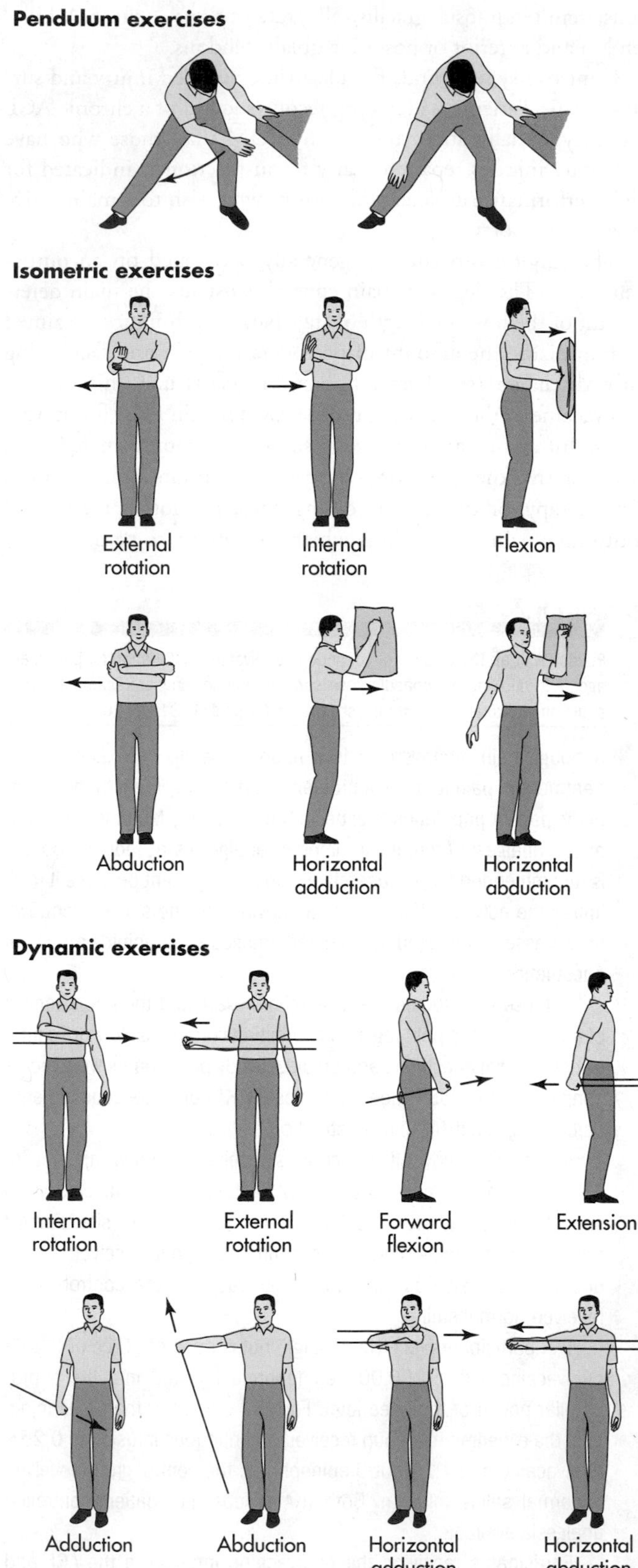

Figure 52-21 Rehabilitative exercises of the shoulder.

Cumulative Trauma Disorders

Cumulative trauma disorder (CTD) and *repetitive strain injury* are relatively new terms for a group of upper extremity soft tissue musculoskeletal disorders. Less commonly used terms are *work-related upper extremity disorder* and *occupational overuse syndrome.* As these names imply, these disorders are caused by cumulative trauma and overuse of the neck and upper extremities in the workplace. The widespread use of computers in the home and workplace for both recreational and occupational purposes has been cited as a major factor in the development of CTD.

The impact of CTDs on society is significant. CTD claims are more costly than the average traumatic injury claim and are the basis of a large number of lawsuits filed against employers by data processors, telephone operators, and keyboard operators. More time is lost from work because of CTD than any other musculoskeletal disorder, including lower back pain. The National Insti-

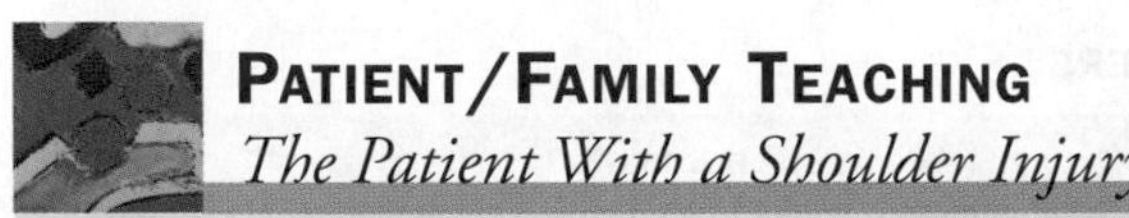

PATIENT/FAMILY TEACHING
The Patient With a Shoulder Injury

Surgical repair of shoulder injuries is performed on an outpatient basis or requires a short hospitalization. Discharge instructions focus on:

- Wound care
- Hygiene methods
- Medication instruction
- Signs of infection
- Activity restrictions
- Signs of complications: decreased sensation in the affected arm, increased pain, unusual swelling, increased drainage from the wound (if applicable), and coolness of the extremity

The patient should be familiar with the proper application of any immobilization devices (slings, splints) and how to inspect the skin for signs of irritation. The patient is taught passive range-of-motion (ROM) techniques in addition to prescribed exercises. A physical therapist provides the initial instruction, which is then reinforced by the nurse. The amount of active ROM and shoulder movement permitted varies, depending on the type of injury and treatment.

tute for Occupational Safety and Health (NIOSH) has named occupational musculoskeletal disorders, including CTDs, one of the top 10 priority work-related conditions. The goal of NIOSH is to promote a better understanding of the incidence, presentation, prevention, treatment, and rehabilitation of these common disorders. The Occupational Safety and Health Administration has proposed ergonomic standards to address work-related disorders. Adoption of such standards would require employers to make efforts to reduce workplace exposure to CTD. *Healthy People 2010* also addresses repetitive motion disorders (see Healthy People 2010 box).

CTD can occur in any muscle group that is used repeatedly for long, uninterrupted periods with the body in a relatively fixed posture. Women are affected twice as often as men. Most sources cite repetitive motion as the predominant risk factor for the development of a CTD. Other risk factors include obesity; excessive, forceful movements; poor tool design; ergonomic factors in the workplace; vibration exposure; extremes of flexion or extension; and static positioning. The most common CTDs include carpal tunnel syndrome, medial and lateral epicondylitis, thoracic outlet syndrome, and de Quervain's tenosynovitis (Table 52-5). Symptoms are primarily those of entrapment neuropathies, including pain and paresthesias.

Healthy People 2010

Objective Related to Repetitive Motion Disorders

- *Objective:* Reduce the rate of injury and illness cases involving days away from work because of overexertion or repetitive motion.
- *Target:* 338 injuries per 100,000 full-time workers
- *Baseline:* 675 injuries per 10,000 full-time workers from overexertion or repetitive motion reported in 1997
- *Target setting method:* 50% improvement

Data source: Annual Survey of Occupational Injuries and Illnesses. From US Department of Health and Human Services: *Healthy people 2010: understanding and improving health,* Washington, DC, 2000, The Department.

Carpal Tunnel Syndrome

Etiology and Epidemiology. Carpal tunnel syndrome (CTS) is caused by pressure exerted on the median nerve of the wrist. The condition occurs most commonly in women 30 to 50 years of age and usually affects the dominant hand. Many conditions can cause an increase in pressure in the carpal tunnel, thereby producing symptoms of median nerve compression. Symptoms are usually consistent, regardless of etiology. CTS is considered a CTD because the cause is often repetitive hand or wrist motions. CTS is closely related to computer use.

As with all other CTDs, the cause is not always repetitive motion. Inflammatory processes such as rheumatoid arthritis, flexor tenosynovitis, and gout can cause thickening of the flexor synovium, which leads to elevated pressure in the carpal tunnel. Patients receiving long-term hemodialysis for chronic kidney failure may be at risk for developing CTS because of synovial edema and amyloid deposits. Previous trauma may also contribute to the development of CTS. Burns, fractures, and dislocations of the wrist can constrict the tunnel by the formation of contractures, scarring, or bony deformities.

Work-related CTS is a CTD caused by job-related tasks that involve certain motions or actions: forceful grasping or pinching of objects (e.g., tools), awkward positions, direct pressure over the carpal tunnel, repetitive motions, and use of vibrating handheld tools.

Other conditions that contribute to CTS include diabetes, myxedema, pregnancy, abnormalities of the median artery and flexor muscles, ganglions, and lipomas. Alcoholism has also been associated with CTS. Certain occupations put workers (typists, computer operators, assembly line workers, and truck drivers) at risk for developing the syndrome.

Pathophysiology. The median nerve passes through a tunnel bounded by the carpal bones on the dorsal surface and by the transverse carpal ligament on the volar surface (Figure 52-22). In addition to the nerve, nine flexor tendons pass through this tunnel. The median nerve provides sensation to the radial aspect of the palm and volar surfaces of the thumb, index finger, middle finger, and radial half of the ring finger. The median nerve also innervates the muscles of the anterior forearm and thenar (the padded area of the palm below the base of the thumb) muscles of the thumb and supplies sensation to the skin of the thumb, index finger, middle finger, and half of the ring finger. Any narrowing within this canal leads to compression of the medial nerve and CTS.

Initially pressure on the median nerve causes temporary blockage of the myelinated nerve fibers, which results in numbness of and pressure on the hand and fingers. Continued pressure causes ischemia, resulting in axonal death, muscular atrophy, and pain. The severity of symptoms varies. Mild manifestations include intermittent paresthesias, tingling, and pain in the median nerve distribution. The pain may awaken the patient at night; symptoms persist and increase if the condition is not treated. More

TABLE 52-5 COMMON TYPES OF CUMULATIVE TRAUMA DISORDERS

Disorder	Manifestations	Etiology	Treatment
de Quervain's tenosynovitis	Pain with thumb and wrist movement; pain radiating to forearm; aching over dorsal thumb surface; swelling; decreased pinch-grip strength	Inflammation of abductor pollicis longus and extensor pollicis brevis tendons in first dorsal compartment of wrist, at base of thumb; first described in 1895 as "washerwoman's strain" from wringing clothes; workers at risk include operating room personnel, housekeepers, musicians, and butchers (repetitive pinching and forearm rotation)	Wrist and thumb spica splint, gentle active range-of-motion exercises, joint protection, and ergonomically designed workplace and tools; surgical treatment (release of first dorsal compartment) only if conservative measures fail
Thoracic outlet syndrome	Pain; paresthesias; swelling; temperature changes; weakness of forearm, shoulder, arm	Compression of brachial plexus, subclavian artery, and subclavian vein; mechanical compression; posture of head, neck, shoulders; cervical rib; overhead activities	Physical therapy; patient education about posture, workstation dynamics, ergonomics, physical activity; surgical resection if compression is due to cervical rib
Lateral epicondylitis (tennis elbow)	Microscopic tears in extensor carpi radialis brevis tendon, which originates at lateral epicondyle of elbow; repetitive activities	Pain over lateral epicondyle and extensor muscle mass; increased pain with elbow extension and forceful grip; persons at risk include construction workers, assembly line workers, tennis players (only 5% of identified cases), swimmers, golfers, and carpenters (hammering)	Reduce elbow extension; splinting; cold compresses followed by stretching; electrical stimulation, heat, and ultrasound; patient education about avoidance of aggravating movements or postures, tool or handle modification; surgical intervention to lengthen and repair tendon if conservative measures fail

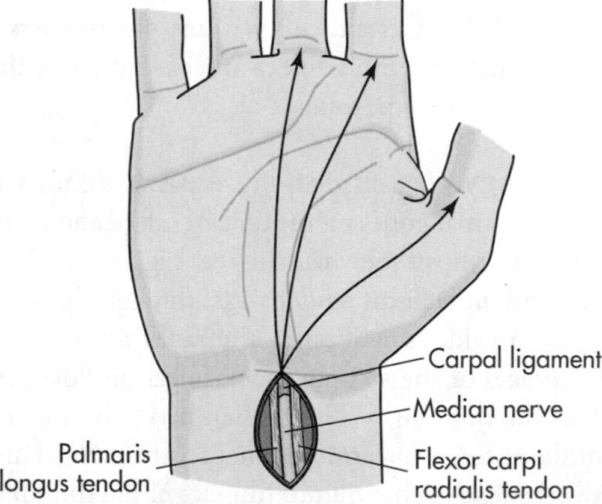

Figure 52-22 Carpal tunnel syndrome. Volar aspect of wrist retracted to demonstrate position of median nerve. Distribution of median nerve is to thumb and first two fingers.

severe cases of CTS include symptoms of hypoesthesia, awkwardness, and loss of dexterity and pinch strength. The patient may complain of dropping things or changes in handwriting. Symptoms may be worse at night, perhaps as a result of sleeping with the wrists in a flexed position. Complaints usually increase when there has been forced flexion of the wrist for long periods, as with knitting or typing. The patient may describe the hand as "swollen" and may complain of clumsiness. Pain referred to the upper extremity and base of the neck is common. Longstanding CTS may manifest with pronounced thenar atrophy, chronic pain, and major functional impairment secondary to axonal death. The prognosis at this stage is poor, regardless of treatment.

Collaborative Care Management. Diagnosis is based on the patient history, physical examination, and evaluation of diagnostic tests. Other conditions with similar symptoms must be eliminated, including cervical radiculopathy, brachial plexopathy, de Quervain's tenosynovitis, arthritis, and thoracic outlet syndrome. Symptoms can be reproduced by tapping the median nerve at the wrist (positive Tinel's sign). Phalen's test is also used to diagnose CTS. The examiner holds the wrists in acute flexion for 60 seconds; if symptoms are reproduced or increased, the test is considered positive. Direct compression of the median nerve at the wrist for 30 seconds will also reproduce or increase symptoms in the presence of CTS. Nerve conduction studies and electromyography are also used to evaluate nerve function and muscle abnormalities.

Effective conservative therapies for CTS include local and oral steroid administration, splinting, ultrasound, yoga, and carpal bone mobilization.[11,15] Medical management of the patient with CTS begins with rest and splinting to maintain the wrist in a neutral position. Splinting is most effective if begun within 3 months of the onset of symptoms. NSAIDs are used for pain relief. Short-term use of diuretics may be prescribed to reduce fluid volume in the carpal tunnel, and oral vitamin B_6 may be prescribed, since pyridoxine deficiency has been noted in some persons with CTS. If inflammation is prominent, local steroid injections may be given.

Surgical decompression of the median nerve is done if conservative treatment fails or symptoms are longstanding. This surgery involves open or endoscopic release and decompression. Endoscopic release is associated with decreased postoperative pain, reduced scarring, and decreased recovery time. This approach is contraindicated in patients with rheumatoid arthritis and flexor synovitis.

Nursing care of patients having a surgical decompression procedure includes teaching regarding rest and splinting of the wrist, as well as general preoperative instructions (see Chapter 13). The nurse obtains an occupational history and obtains referrals for job counseling or retraining if occupational factors such as wrist flexing and repetitive tasks contributed to the condition.

Postoperative care focuses on promotion of circulation, comfort, and the prevention of complications. The affected hand and arm are elevated for 24 hours, and ice is used to reduce swelling and pain. The fingers are checked for circulation, sensation, and movement every 1 to 2 hours for 24 hours. Active thumb and finger motion is encouraged within the limits imposed by the dressing. The nurse administers analgesics as prescribed and assesses their effectiveness.

Discharge instructions include directions for recognizing and reporting symptoms of neurovascular compromise and directions for care of the splint, which usually is maintained for 2 to 3 weeks after surgery. The patient is also scheduled for follow-up wound assessment and a dressing change in the physician's office within 1 week. The nurse explains the need for this follow-up care and for lifestyle modification if repetitive motions (workplace or leisure) contributed to the disease process. Referral to physical therapy for ROM and strengthening exercises is initiated.

PATIENT/FAMILY TEACHING. Because of the increasing incidence of cumulative trauma–related injuries in the workplace, it is important for nurses to recognize persons at risk and to teach preventive measures. As a result of the number of lawsuits against employers filed by employees, many businesses have initiated programs to prevent the development of CTD. These programs include redesign of the workplace with the focus on ergonomics, stress reduction techniques, and classes to teach proper mechanics and body awareness and to reduce computer stress. Nurses are in an ideal position to promote wellness and reduce the risks associated with the development of CTS and other CTDs.

Proper body position at the computer terminal is sitting erect and leaning slightly forward while using the keyboard. The arms should be elevated with the wrists straight to reduce pressure on the nerves, tendons, and muscles of the arms and hands. The forearms and palms should be angled toward each other while typing to reduce fatigue. The keyboard height should be modified to avoid placing the wrists into hyperextension, which stretches the muscles and ligaments. Foam pads on which to rest the wrists while typing are available commercially. When keystroking, avoid rapid, prolonged finger movements, which can cause pain. Avoid long fingernails, which cause awkward positioning of the fingers and wrists during keystroking.

Trauma to Joints and Joint Structures

Injuries to joints and joint structures may occur as a sprain (tearing of the capsule or ligaments surrounding a joint, including disruption of the synovial membrane), meniscal tear, joint dislocation, or joint subluxation.

Trauma to ligaments and tendons and principles of patient management are discussed earlier in the chapter. This section discusses joint dislocation. The shoulder is susceptible to traumatic dislocation. Closed reduction, followed by rehabilitative exercises, is the first choice of treatment. Chronic instability may necessitate surgical stabilization.

Traumatic Hip Dislocation

Etiology and Epidemiology. Traumatic hip dislocation usually occurs as a result of a motor vehicle accident, especially if frontal impact is sustained. This type of force can drive the victim's knees into the dashboard, forcibly dislocating the hip. Traumatic hip dislocation is considered an orthopedic emergency because of the risk of avascular necrosis of the femoral head. Prompt treatment is critical; reduction within 6 hours of injury decreases the risk of persistent pain, decreased ROM, and avascular necrosis. Traumatic dislocations occur most commonly in persons under 50 years of age unless an underlying disease is present, such as a neuromuscular disease or rheumatoid arthritis.

Pathophysiology. As the hip is forcibly dislocated, the blood supply to the femoral head can be disrupted (see Figure 52-18). Damage to the sciatic nerve is also possible and can result in partial to complete motor and sensory loss in the affected extremity (see Clinical Manifestations box). Sciatic nerve injury is present in 10% to 20% of persons with a posterior dislocation. Another potential problem is fracture of the femoral head, acetabulum, or pelvis. The articular surface of the femoral head may be eroded by bone fragments. Most dislocations of the femoral head occur posteriorly with the thigh in flexion. The femoral head cannot be completely displaced from the acetabulum unless the ligamentum teres is torn or

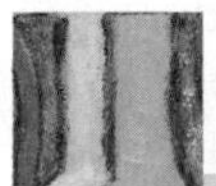

CLINICAL MANIFESTATIONS
Traumatic Hip Dislocation

- Pain
- Deformity
- Decreased range of motion
- Decreased sensation
- Diminished or absent pulses
- Anterior dislocation: hip in extension and external rotation; palpable femoral head
- Posterior dislocation: hip in flexion and internal rotation; shortening; may be a visible leg length discrepancy when compared with unaffected leg

ruptured. Anterior dislocations occur with the hip in extension and external rotation. The femoral head may be palpable anteriorly below the inguinal area. Complications of dislocation include avascular necrosis, infection, malunion, posttraumatic arthritis, and sciatic nerve injury. Avascular necrosis may occur as late as 2 years after the injury. Residual neuropathy occurs in approximately 20% of persons who sustained sciatic nerve damage.

Collaborative Care Management. Diagnosis is made on the basis of the history, physical examination, and evidence of dislocation on x-ray films. If possible, the hip is reduced immediately. The patient is given intravenous sedation, and the physician uses manual traction to relocate the hip (closed reduction). If closed reduction is not feasible, or in the presence of an acetabular or pelvic fracture, skeletal traction may be used to reduce the hip until surgery is possible. If there is no fracture, open reduction is accomplished by opening the hip capsule and relocating the head. For pelvic and acetabular fractures, internal fixation devices are usually used; a pelvic external fixator may also be used. If avascular necrosis results, prosthetic replacement of the hip is required.

Nursing management of the patient with a traumatic hip dislocation is the same as that for the patient with a hip fracture. The major emphasis is on keeping the limb in alignment by proper positioning. In addition, some patients have a brace applied either in surgery (if an orthotist is available) or the next day.

Patient/Family Teaching. If surgical intervention is necessary, teaching is similar to that following surgical repair of a hip fracture. After closed reduction the patient begins active and passive ROM exercises. Teaching also includes prevention of further injury and the use of assistive devices. Crutches or a walker is usually required until the patient has progressed to full weight bearing, generally in 4 to 6 weeks.

Multiple Trauma

Etiology and Epidemiology. The leading cause of death in the United States for persons under the age of 45 is trauma. Causes include falls, crush injuries, vehicular (including airplane) accidents, and gunshot wounds. The injuries sustained in trauma are often extensive, involving multiple organ systems and multiple sites of injury. Approximately 50% of trauma deaths occur at the scene of injury, before medical help can arrive. Death usually results from brainstem trauma, spinal cord injury, hemorrhage, or major organ injuries. The second peak of trauma deaths occurs within 2 hours of injury, as a result of hemorrhage or head, chest, or abdominal injuries. Death during the third peak occurs within days to weeks of the initial injury, usually because of sepsis or multisystem failure.

More than 60 million persons per year survive major trauma.[16] Survival rates are related to care at the accident scene, quick methods of transport to hospitals, and advances in the fields of emergency medicine and nursing. Regional trauma centers allow transfer of patients to facilities equipped to manage complex care needs of the victim of polytrauma. Personnel in any hospital should be prepared to treat a multiply injured patient. Often the patient is stabilized and then airlifted to a trauma center.

The most common orthopedic injuries that occur as a result of multiple trauma are pelvic fractures and crush injuries. Approximately 30% of persons with multiple injuries sustain a pelvic fracture. Fractures of the pelvis usually occur as a result of motor vehicle accidents, falls, and crush injuries. Depending on the type of fracture and coexisting injuries, closed pelvic fractures have an associated mortality rate of 8% to 15%, and open pelvic fractures have an associated mortality rate of 30% to 50%.[16] Hemorrhage is usually the cause of death. Shearing forces from the impact of trauma rupture blood vessels surrounding the pelvic ring, causing hemorrhage and hypotension. Damage to internal organs, especially urogenital injuries, can occur from shearing forces, bone fragments, and compression. The retroperitoneal space can accommodate up to 4 L of blood before tamponade results. Coagulopathy is a significant problem because of loss of clotting factors and because of continued bleeding at the fracture site. Pelvic fractures are classified by the mechanism of injury and degree of instability.

Crush injuries (see discussion under Compartment Syndrome) may result from falls, motor vehicle accidents, and blunt trauma, such as being trapped under heavy fallen objects. Multiple fractures and internal bleeding may result, with hemorrhage being the usual cause of death. Crush syndrome follows crush injury and is characterized by muscle necrosis, hypovolemia, compartment syndrome, rhabdomyolysis, fluid and electrolyte imbalance, coagulopathy, and kidney failure. The development of kidney failure increases the mortality rate. Fluid and electrolyte imbalances commonly seen in crush syndrome include hypocalcemia, hyperphosphatemia, hyperkalemia, edema, and third spacing.

Collaborative Care Management. Treatment of victims of multiple trauma is based on the ABCs of airway management with cervical spine control, breathing, and circulation (see Chapters 9 and 10). The pelvis and abdomen must be evaluated for fractures and hemorrhage (Box 52-4). Rib fractures and spinal fractures may cause life-threatening neurologic and cardiovascular injuries.

Obvious fractures are immobilized and splinted, and sterile dressings are applied to open fractures until surgical reduction is feasible. The management goals are to correct or stabilize any life-threatening problems (e.g., obstructed airway, pneumothorax, bleeding) and then to reestablish the continuity of injured tissues. Musculoskeletal injury may require reduction of fractures and repair of related soft tissue injuries. Because life-threatening problems must be addressed first, musculoskeletal injuries are usually not repaired until the patient has been stabilized. However, sites of fractures or potential fractures must be splinted or otherwise protected until reduction can be effected.

The principles of nursing management are:

1. Before reduction, all actual or potential sites of fractures must be protected by maintaining splints, traction, or positioning precautions; manipulation of fracture fragments must be avoided; and the patient must be monitored for hemorrhage and other complications.
2. After reduction, all the previously discussed principles of nursing management of the patient with a fracture must be observed.

BOX 52-4 Pelvic Fractures

Signs and Symptoms

Pain with compression of iliac crests
Asymmetry of iliac crests
Abnormal rotation of femurs
Leg length discrepancy
Lacerations of perineum, vagina, or rectum
Hematuria
Neurologic deficits
Hypotension

Diagnostic Tests

X-ray study
Computed tomography scan*
Peritoneal lavage to determine presence of intraabdominal bleeding*
Arteriogram: intravenous pyelogram (if patient is stable) to determine extent of internal injury

Management

Pelvic sling
Skeletal traction
Spica cast
Open reduction and internal fixation
External fixators: the treatment of choice

Associated Injuries

Vascular
Genitourinary
Abdominal
Intestinal and rectal

*Controversial.

Preparing for Practice

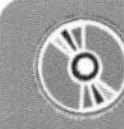

CD-ROM Activity Select Exercise Nine: Trauma to the Musculoskeletal System on the Companion CD.

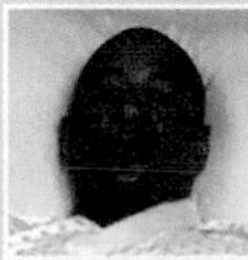

Patient: *David Ruskin,* **Room 303**

David Ruskin, a 32-year-old African-American man, suffered a closed head injury, fractured humerus, and scalp lacerations after being struck by an automobile while bicycling.

Assessment

View the patient's **Report**.

Open the patient's **Medical Record** to familiarize yourself with his care. Specifically, click on the following areas as part of your review: History & Physical (focus on the Emergency Department Report), Diagnostics, and Nurses' Notes.

Conduct a **Patient Interview**. As you conduct your interview, focus primarily on data that will be helpful in planning care for this patient. Record the data you collect.

Nursing Diagnoses, Outcomes, and Interventions

1. Review the Emergency Department report to find the injuries sustained by this patient. List the injuries cited in the report in the order of priority for nursing assessment and management. Describe how each of the other injuries may affect assessment of the fractured humerus.
2. On admission, in what stage of bone healing is David Ruskin? What factors could affect healing of his fractured humerus? *Hint:* Refer to p. 1523.
3. Note the type of fracture that is documented in the Diagnostics report, AP/Lateral right humerus x-ray, that was done before David Ruskin's surgery. Identify the illustration in Figure 52-1 that depicts this type of fracture and describe its character.
4. Develop a care plan related to Mr. Ruskin's fracture. In light of Mr. Ruskin's other injuries, keep in mind any barriers or special considerations in implementing certain aspects of care related to the humoral fracture. *Hint:* Consider pain management in the head-injured patient.

The challenge for the nurse is to devise a care plan that takes into account the demands of the variety of fixation techniques, fracture sites, and mobilization or immobilization requirements for the patient. The psychosocial needs and the rehabilitation requirements for individuals who have sustained multiple injuries are often long term and extensive. Rehabilitation requirements must be considered early in the patient's hospital course and be reviewed frequently (see Chapter 7).

PATIENT/FAMILY TEACHING. Nurses can play a role in the prevention of multiple trauma by promoting safety awareness among all persons, especially those at risk. Promoting safety in the work environment may prevent industrial or on-the-job accidents. Public awareness of the dangers of driving while intoxicated and the importance of wearing seat belts may help decrease the number of motor vehicle accidents and the injuries sustained in them.

Persons who have sustained multiple injuries may have residual deficits and require an extensive rehabilitative process. Teaching focuses on adaptive techniques and measures to prevent further disability.

Critical Thinking

1. Compare and contrast the nursing care for a patient undergoing an open reduction of a fracture with that for a person undergoing a closed reduction.

2. Discuss nursing interventions and rationales for the care of a patient after open reduction of a midshaft femoral fracture. What are potential complications? Discuss the essential assessment parameters the nurse uses to detect systemic complications of a bone fracture.
3. Develop a health promotion plan for a group of office workers to prevent repetitive motion disorders.
4. Describe nursing interventions for a 24-year-old man who suffered a pelvic and femoral fracture in a motor vehicle accident. What are potential complications of his injury? What preventive nursing measures are indicated?

References

1. Altzier A: Compartment syndrome, *Orthop Nurs* 23(6):391-396, 2004.
2. Bach BR, Boonos CL: Anterior cruciate ligament reconstruction, *AORN J* 74(2):152-164, 2001.
3. Barnett R et al: A patient oriented approach to the management of musculoskeletal injury, *Therap Bull Suppl Clin News* 6(2):1-8, 2002.
4. Childs SG: Pathogenesis of anterior cruciate ligament injury, *Orthop Nurs* 21(4):35-40, 2002.
5. Dahners LE, Mullis BH: Effects of nonsteroidal anti-inflammatory drugs on bone formation and soft-tissue healing, *J Am Acad Orthop Surg* 12(3): 139-143, 2004.
6. Doheny MO, Deucher MJ: Healthy people 2010: implications for orthopaedic nurses, *Orthop Nurs* 20(4):59-65, 2001.
7. Gosselin RA, Roberts I, Gillespie WJ: Antibiotics for preventing infection in open limb fractures (Cochrane Review). In *Cochrane Library*, Issue 3, Chichester, UK, 2004, John Wiley & Sons.
8. Hager CA, Brncick N: Fat embolism syndrome: a complication of orthopedic trauma, *Orthop Nurs* 17(2):41-46, 1998.
9. Harvey C: Compartment syndrome: when it is least expected, *Orthop Nurs* 20(3):15-25, 2001.
10. Maher AB, Salmond SW, Pellino TA: *Orthopaedic nursing*, ed 3, St Louis, 2002, Mosby.
11. Marshall S, Tardiff G, Ashworth N: Local corticosteroid injection for carpal tunnel syndrome (Cochrane Review). In *Cochrane Library*, Issue 3, Chichester, UK, 2004, John Wiley & Sons.
12. McCaffery M, Pasero C: *Pain: clinical manual*, ed 2, St Louis, 1999, Mosby.
13. Miller SL, Gladstone JN: Graft selection in anterior cruciate ligament reconstruction, *Orthop Clin North Am* 33(4):675-683, 2002.
14. National Consensus Conference on Improving the Continuum of Care for Patients with Hip Fracture: Conference report, *Orthop Nurs* 21(1):16-21, 2002.
15. O'Connor D, Marshall S, Massy-Westropp N: Non-surgical treatment (other than steroid injection) for carpal tunnel syndrome (Cochrane Review). In *Cochrane Library*, Issue 3, Chichester, UK, 2004, John Wiley & Sons.
16. Parsons LC, Krau SD, Ward KS: Orthopedic trauma: managing secondary medical problems, *Crit Care Clin North Am* 13(3):433-442, 2001.
17. Simon AM, Manigrasso MB, O'Connor JP: Cyclo-oxygenase 2 function is essential for bone fracture healing, *J Bone Miner Res* 17(6):963-976, 2002.
18. Skinner HB: *Current diagnosis and treatment in orthopedics*, ed 3, Norwalk, Conn, 2003, Appleton & Lange.
19. Temple J, Santy J: Pin site care for preventing infections associated with external bone fixators and pins (Cochrane Review). In *Cochrane Library*, Issue 3, Chichester, UK, 2004, John Wiley & Sons.
20. Thaller J et al: The effect of nonsteroidal anti-inflammatory agents on spinal fusion, *Orthopedics* 28(3):299-305, 2005.
21. Unger J, Selfridge-Thomas J: Common sports injuries, part 1, Ankle injuries. In *Nursing contact hours for nurse practitioners*, Atlanta, 2001, American Health Consultants.
22. Unger J, Selfridge-Thomas J: Common sports injuries, part 2, Knee and shoulder injuries. In *Nursing contact hours for nurse practitioners*, Atlanta, 2001, American Health Consultants.
23. Verdonschot N et al: Time dependent mechanical properties of HA/TCP particles in relation to morsellized bone grafts for use in impaction grafting, *J Biomed Mater Res* 58(5):599-604, 2001.

Visit the Evolve website: http://evolve.elsevier.com/Monahan/medsurg

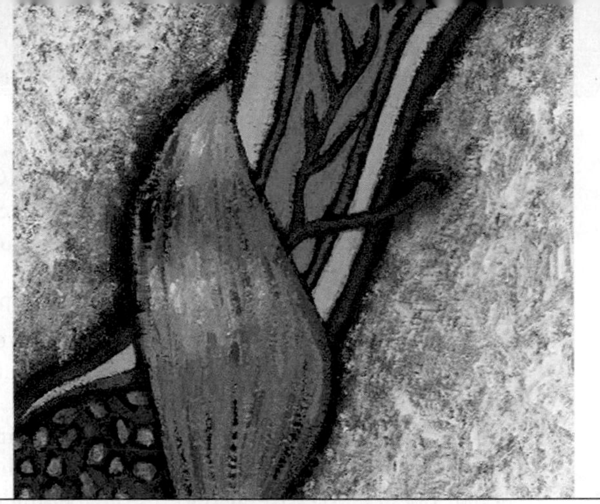

CHAPTER 53

Degenerative Disorders

by Jane F. Marek

OBJECTIVES

After studying this chapter, the learner should be able to:

1. Correlate the pathophysiology with the collaborative care for persons with inflammatory and degenerative disorders affecting the joints.
2. Compare the pathophysiology and collaborative care of the different types of degenerative and inflammatory processes affecting bones.
3. Discuss the incidence, pathophysiology, and clinical manifestations of osteoporosis.
4. Describe the collaborative care management of persons with osteoporosis.
5. Develop a teaching plan for persons at risk for osteoporosis, including preventive measures.
6. Relate the pathophysiology and clinical manifestations to the collaborative care of persons with a degenerative disease of the spine.
7. Correlate the pathophysiology with collaborative care strategies for persons with scoliosis.
8. Describe the etiology, pathophysiology, and treatment for common tumors of the musculoskeletal system.
9. Explain the medical, surgical, and nursing management for persons with osteosarcoma.
10. Compare potential complications after limb salvage surgery with those following amputation.
11. Discuss the etiology, epidemiology, pathophysiology, and clinical manifestations of disorders affecting the soft tissues of the musculoskeletal system.
12. Explain the medical and nursing interventions used in the care of persons with soft tissue disorders of the musculoskeletal system.

KEY TERMS

arthropathy, p. 1563
Brodie's abscesses, p. 1591
compression, p. 1579
creeping substitution, p. 1597
debridement, p. 1591
involucrum, p. 1591
kyphoplasty, p. 1582
radiculopathy, p. 1594
remodeling, p. 1577
resorption, p. 1575
sequestrum, p. 1591
spinal stenosis, p. 1594
spondylitis, p. 1564
tophi, p. 1560

The essence of nursing care for patients with musculoskeletal problems lies in helping them make the physiologic and psychosocial adaptations necessary to cope with a temporary or permanent disability. Inflammatory and degenerative processes can affect all structures in the musculoskeletal system and are often chronic and disabling. Pain and impaired mobility are major problems that must be considered when planning nursing care. Nursing interventions focus on helping the patient maximize independent functioning and teaching methods of joint protection, energy conservation, and prevention of further disability.

Disorders Affecting the Joints

Gout

Etiology and Epidemiology. Gout is a clinical syndrome resulting from the deposition of urate crystals in the synovial fluid, joints, or articular cartilage. Most cases are idiopathic; genetic defects in purine metabolism have been identified. Considered a metabolic disorder, gouty arthritis develops as a result of prolonged hyperuricemia (elevated serum uric acid) caused by problems in the synthesis of purines or by poor renal excretion of uric acid.

Gout must be distinguished from pseudogout, which occurs as a result of calcium pyrophosphate dihydrate (CPPD) crystals. Pseudogout resembles gout, with intraarticular calcium deposits and CPPD crystals in synovial fluid, and primarily affects older adults. Articular cartilage, menisci, and adjacent tendinous or ligamentous structures are affected by pseudogout. Persons with previous joint trauma or a history of meniscectomy are prone to developing pseudogout. Both disorders resemble rheumatoid arthritis (RA).

Gout primarily affects adult men; less often it occurs in postmenopausal women. Risk factors include familial history, male gender, obesity, excessive alcohol use, hyperlipidemia, hypertension, renal insufficiency, diuretic use, and lead exposure.[56] Persons who have received organ transplants have a higher incidence of gout, secondary to the use of diuretics and cyclosporine.[56]

Pathophysiology. Gout is classified as primary or secondary. Primary gout is the result of a genetic error in purine metabolism, which leads to either retention or overproduction of uric acid. Undersecretion, which can be caused by decreased tubular secretion, increased tubular absorption, or a combination of both, accounts for approximately 90% of all cases of primary gout.

Secondary gout results from an overproduction of uric acid secondary to increased purine catabolism or impaired excretion of uric acid, which occurs in association with another disease or as a result of medication. Secondary gout usually occurs in the acute care setting (Box 53-1).

Urate crystals form in the synovial tissue, causing severe inflammation. The inflammatory process is extremely rapid, occurring over a few hours. Acute symptoms are extreme pain, swelling, and erythema of the involved joints. Typically, the first metatarsophalangeal joint of the great toe is involved (50% of patients), but other joints, such as the ankle, heel, knee, or wrist, may also be affected. Pain is so severe that the patient may not tolerate even the weight of a sheet over the joint. Renal damage may occur, especially if recurrent uric acid stones are present. Between attacks of gout the patient may be asymptomatic, but attacks can recur with gradually increasing frequency if the disease is untreated. Patients with gouty symptoms may develop **tophi**, or deposits of monosodium urate, in their tissues. These consist of a core of monosodium urate with a surrounding inflammatory reaction. Patients with tophaceous deposits (Figure 53-1) tend to have more frequent and more severe episodes of gouty arthritis.

Box 53-1 Causes of Secondary Gout

Overproduction of Uric Acid

Paget's disease
Cancer
Polycythemia vera
Multiple myeloma
Chronic myelocytic and lymphocytic leukemia
Hemolytic anemias
Cytotoxic drugs

Underexcretion of Uric Acid

Chronic renal insufficiency
Ketoacidosis
Lactic acidosis
Drug ingestion (diuretics, cyclosporine, levodopa, pyrazinamide, low-dose salicylates)

Unknown Etiology

Hyperparathyroidism
Hypoparathyroidism
Hypothyroidism
Adrenal insufficiency

Collaborative Care Management. Laboratory studies typically indicate an elevated serum uric acid level and a normal or increased urinary uric acid level over a 24-hour period, as well as the presence of monosodium urate monohydrate crystals in the synovial fluid and in the tophi. Hyperuricemia is not necessary for the diagnosis of gout. Uric acid levels are controlled by diet, purine metabolism, and renal clearance. Treatment focuses on control of acute attacks, prevention of recurrent attacks, and long-term uricosuric therapy to prevent the formation of tophi. Results are best when therapy is initiated shortly after the onset of symptoms.

Colchicine, because of its ability to inhibit phagocytosis of urate crystals by neutrophils, was once considered the mainstay of treatment, but is used less often now for management of acute attacks because of the distressing side effect of diarrhea. Colchicine is not effective once an attack has been present for several days. However, in persons who are able to recognize the symptoms of an acute attack, one or two 0.6-mg tablets of colchicine may be taken to thwart the attack. Colchicine, 0.6 mg, is given orally every 1 to 2 hours until diarrhea develops (to a maximum of 10 mg).[56,60] Joint inflammation usually subsides within 48 hours.

For persons with adequate renal function and no other contraindications, nonsteroidal antiinflammatory drugs (NSAIDs) are a good choice for reducing the acute inflammation. Patients at risk for NSAID toxicity include older adults and those with a history of peptic ulcer disease or gastrointestinal (GI) hemorrhage, renal disease, hypertension, congestive heart failure, inflammatory bowel disease, or anticoagulant use. Most patients have complete resolution of symptoms within 8 days of initiating NSAID therapy.[60] Although any NSAID may be prescribed, indomethacin has been successful in the treatment of gout. For persons in whom NSAIDs

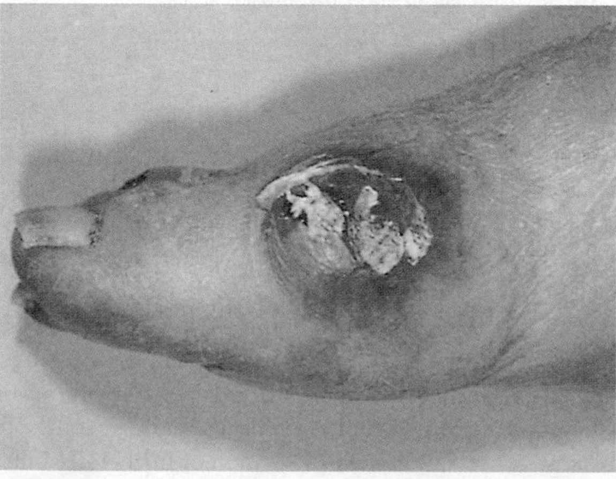

Figure 53-1 Gouty tophus on right first metatarsophalangeal joint.

are contraindicated, corticosteroids are effective. Intraarticular injections or systemic therapy can be used for treatment of acute attacks.

The recurrence rate is approximately 60% within the first year, increasing to 90% by 5 years.[60] Long-term pharmacologic prophylaxis is indicated when recurrent attacks affect the patient's lifestyle or the patient is at risk from complications from medications used to treat the acute episode. Future attacks of acute gout can be prevented by the administration of colchicine, allopurinol, or sulfinpyrazone. Therapy with allopurinol, which lowers uric acid levels, should not be started during an acute attack, since it may prolong symptoms. Initially, the frequency of acute attacks may be increased with allopurinol therapy; it may take as long as 3 to 4 months for the medication to be effective in preventing acute attacks. During this time, colchicines or NSAIDs may be used as prophylaxis or treatment.

Identifying and correcting the cause of hyperuricemia may help prevent future gouty attacks. Medications can be given that inhibit the synthesis of urate or increase its secretion. Some causes of hyperuricemia may require lifelong medication to decrease serum levels. Attention should concentrate on factors that increase uric acid levels: regular alcohol consumption, obesity, and a high-purine diet. Patients with gout should avoid alcohol because it not only increases production of uric acid but also prevents its excretion.

Rest and joint immobilization are recommended until the acute attack subsides. Local application of cold can relieve pain. Application of heat should be avoided, since it will increase the inflammatory process.

PATIENT/FAMILY TEACHING. Teaching for the patient with gout is described in the Patient/Family Teaching box.

PATIENT/FAMILY TEACHING
The Patient With Gout

Most persons with gout are cared for at home; patient education should focus on prevention of further attacks and complications. Instructions should include information regarding:

- Medication use and possible side effects
- Diet: reducing or eliminating alcohol intake and avoiding excessive intake of purines (sweetbreads, yeast, heart, herring, herring roe, and sardines)
- Fluid intake: in the absence of renal or cardiac disease, drinking 3 L/day to eliminate uric acid and prevent renal calculi
- Monitoring intake and output; signs of decreasing kidney function
- Skin care: daily assessment for tophi formation, use of emollients for softening, and positioning for comfort
- Importance of properly fitting shoes to decrease skin irritation and increase comfort
- Use of ice for pain relief
- Pain management: during acute attacks, immobilizing affected joint to decrease pain until inflammation subsides; use of a foot cradle to keep sheets off the feet
- Follow-up care, including monitoring of serum uric acid levels

Bacterial or Septic Arthritis

Etiology and Epidemiology. Bacterial arthritis is the result of invasion of the synovial membrane by microorganisms, most often *Neisseria gonorrhoeae,* meningococci, streptococci, *Staphylococcus aureus,* coliform bacteria, salmonellae, and *Haemophilus influenzae.* Less common causes include viruses, tuberculosis, and fungi. Viral diseases may have an associated arthralgia, which usually resolves spontaneously. The two major types of bacterial arthritis are nongonococcal and arthritis resulting from *Neisseria* bacteria. Incidence of bacterial arthritis is increasing with the spread of resistant strains of microorganisms.

Bacteria can enter the joint by hematogenous spread, direct inoculation, or extension from an adjacent infection. The most common cause of bacterial arthritis is hematogenous infection (e.g., from an upper respiratory tract infection or otitis media). Infection usually involves one joint, most commonly the knee in the adult. Other joints affected are the ankle, elbow, and small joints of the hand and wrist. Persons with an underlying medical illness are at greatest risk. Advanced age, immunodeficiency, chronic disease, intravenous drug abuse, local joint surgery or trauma, intraarticular injections, and RA increase the risk for developing bacterial arthritis.

A septic joint is an orthopedic emergency. The mortality rate for nongonococcal bacterial arthritis is 5% to 15%, with a 25% to 60% rate of chronic joint damage and disability.[51] Complications include avascular necrosis, osteoarthritis, and osteomyelitis.

Pathophysiology. Bacteria usually invade the joint from a distant portal of entry. Synovial tissues respond to bacterial invasion by inflammation. The joint cavity may become involved, and pus develops in the synovial membrane and synovial fluid. Polymorphonuclear leukocytes release enzymes that can digest hyaline cartilage within 24 hours. If allowed to progress, the infection causes abscesses in the synovium and subchondral bone, eventually destroying cartilage and resulting in ankylosis of the joint.

The onset of symptoms is usually acute, but exact presentation depends on the joint involved. The patient reports pain, swelling, decreased range of motion, and tenderness of the joint. The ability to bear weight may be affected. Systemic symptoms include fever and chills. Gonococcal arthritis has different presenting symptoms: skin lesions on the extremities or trunk, dermatitis, fever, polyarthralgia, and tenosynovitis. Genitourinary symptoms may also be present.

Collaborative Care Management. Prompt diagnosis and treatment can save the joint from destruction. A health history is obtained and physical assessment done to identify risk factors for joint infection and possible portals of entry. Joint aspiration is performed to identify the causative organism and determine treatment. Strict aseptic technique must be followed to avoid introducing additional bacteria into the joint. White blood cell counts are high, and the glucose content of synovial fluid may be reduced. X-ray films taken days to weeks after the onset of infection may reveal loss of joint space and lytic changes in bones.

The results of treatment depend on the infecting organism, duration of infection before treatment, and host defenses. Treatment starts immediately with appropriate antibiotic therapy and rest or immobilization of the joint. If infection does not respond to antibiotic therapy, or if osteomyelitis is present, surgical drainage by needle aspiration, arthroscopy, or arthrotomy is done. Needle aspiration of purulent exudate may be required daily until drainage ceases. Infections of the hip joint must be drained immediately to prevent necrosis of the femoral head. When infection subsides and motion can be tolerated, active range of motion (ROM) is resumed.

Nursing management focuses on promoting rest of the affected joint, administering antibiotics on time and as prescribed to maintain blood levels, and administering prescribed pain medication as necessary. The nurse also encourages the patient to participate in self-care to the extent possible within restrictions of prescribed rest for the joint.

PATIENT/FAMILY TEACHING. Teaching for the patient with bacterial arthritis is described in the Patient/Family Teaching box.

Lyme Disease

Etiology and Epidemiology. Lyme disease (LD) is caused by the tick-borne spirochete *Borrelia burgdorferi*. The disease was discovered in Lyme, Connecticut, in 1976 and declared a nationally notifiable disease by the Centers for Disease Control and Prevention (CDC) in 1991; in 2002 more than 23,000 cases were reported to the CDC.[57] For surveillance purposes, the presence of an erythematous migrans (EM) rash 0.5 cm in diameter or laboratory documentation of infection with evidence of musculoskeletal, neurologic, or cardiovascular disease confirms the diagnosis of LD. LD is transmitted by ticks, present most commonly on deer, mice, dogs, cats, raccoons, cows, and horses. Deer ticks are responsible for 95% of cases of LD.[3] Birds help spread infected ticks by their migratory flights. The tick bite is usually painless, and the patient may not remember being bitten.

The disease has been reported in most European countries, throughout Asia, and in 49 states and the District of Columbia in the United States. LD is the number one vector-borne disease in the United States. The disease is prevalent in the Northeastern, North-Central, and Mid-Atlantic regions. LD affects all ages, although the highest incidence is in children under 15 years of age and adults over 29 years of age; those living in endemic areas with outdoor exposure are at risk. The peak months for early clinical manifestations of the disease are June through October. Increased public awareness, increasing deer populations, and the trend toward use of farmlands and forest that increases contact between humans and vectors are responsible for the increasing rates of the disease. Humans can be exposed to the ticks in wooded areas and in well-landscaped areas in endemic regions. Transmission of the disease from the tick to humans requires some time. A minimum of 24 to 48 hours is necessary for effective transmission of the spirochete; the tick usually must feed for 72 hours to effectively transmit enough spirochetes to infect a human.[48,57] The incubation period from exposure to the onset of symptoms is usually 7 to 14 days but may be 3 to 30 days.[57]

Pathophysiology. LD has been called the "great imitator" because it mimics other diseases such as influenza, RA, multiple sclerosis, chronic fatigue syndrome, amyotrophic lateral sclerosis, fibromyalgia, lupus erythematosus, and Alzheimer's disease. Infection with *B. burgdorferi* stimulates inflammatory cytokines and autoimmune mechanisms, which results in Lyme arthritis. Primarily an extracellular organism, *B. burgdorferi* is thought to invade some cells and cross the blood-brain barrier, resulting in the neurologic manifestations of LD.

An EM rash is usually the first sign of infection, beginning at the site of a tick bite. The rash appears after a delay of 3 to 31 days. Lesions may develop on other areas of the body; the rash may develop a clear center as it enlarges, resulting in a bull's eye appearance. Infection with *B. burgdorferi* can be divided into three stages. Not all patients develop all stages. The early manifestations of the disease are usually self-limiting, and the late manifestations can become chronic (see Clinical Manifestations box).

The arthritis associated with LD is either monoarticular or oligoarticular, affecting the knee and other large joints. Inflammation is a result of immune complex deposition in the synovium. Chronic and recurrent arthritis develops, possibly as a result of genetic factors or an autoimmune process.

Collaborative Care Management. The varied signs and symptoms, coupled with the fact that most persons do not remember the tick bite, make diagnosis difficult. Laboratory testing can confirm a difficult diagnosis. Serologic tests used to diagnose LD include enzyme-linked immunosorbent assay (ELISA), Western blot, and indirect immunofluorescence assay. In endemic areas, diagnosis may be made by the presence of the EM rash alone or by one organ system involvement and positive serology.[57] Less than 50% of persons with stage I disease have detectable antibodies; in stage II disease the percentage rises to 70% to 90%. Both serum and cerebrospinal fluid should be tested to diagnose LD. Synovial fluid may be sampled if arthritic symptoms are present. An electrocardiogram should be done for patients with cardiac symptoms.

Treatment of LD is usually successful if therapy is initiated early with penicillins, cephalosporins, macrolides, or tetracy-

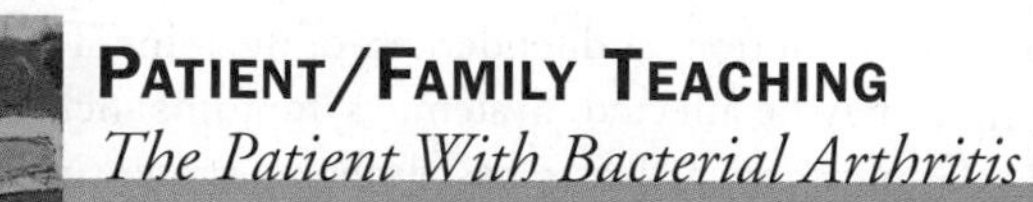

PATIENT/FAMILY TEACHING

The Patient With Bacterial Arthritis

Patient and family education is important to preserve joint function. Teaching includes:

- Importance of adhering to prescribed antibiotic regimen (Antibiotic therapy may be prescribed for 2 to 6 weeks. Encourage the patient to comply with treatment to ensure eradication of infection.)
- Sources of infection
- Methods to reduce risk of infections, including sexually transmitted disease
- Joint rest
- Joint protection
- Pain management
- Use of crutches or assistive devices
- Cast or splint care
- Range-of-motion exercises
- Signs and symptoms of recurring joint infection
- Recognizing complications
- Follow-up care

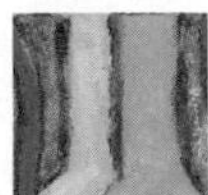

CLINICAL MANIFESTATIONS *Lyme Disease*

Stage I (Early Localized Infection)

Symptoms usually appear 7-14 days after tick bite but may occur after a delay of 30 days.
Erythema migrans in 80% of patients; resolves spontaneously in a few weeks
Fatigue
Headache
Lethargy
Myaliga, arthralgia
Lymphadenopathy

Stage II (Secondary, Early Disseminated Infection)

Symptoms occurring weeks to month after tick bite

Cardiac Symptoms
Carditis
Dysrhythmias
Heart failure
Pericarditis
Palpitations
Dyspnea

Neurologic Symptoms
Meningitis
Encephalitis
Cranial and peripheral neuropathy
Myelitis

Musculoskeletal Symptoms
Arthralgia, myalgia
Fibromyalgia

Other Symptoms
Conjunctivitis, optic neuropathy
Hepatomegaly, hepatitis
Generalized lymphadenopathy

Stage III (Tertiary, Late Infection)

Symptoms occurring months to years after tick bite
Monoarticular or oligoarticular arthritis
Chronic arthritis
Acrodermatitis chronica atrophicans (bluish red, doughy lesions)
Lyme encephalitis, encephalomyelitis
Ataxia
Spastic paresis
Periventricular lesions
Memory loss
Behavioral changes

clines. Empiric treatment with doxycycline or amoxicillin is indicated for patients with the EM rash and a high probability of having LD. For patients with allergies or inability to tolerate doxycycline or amoxicillin, cefuroxime is an alternative therapy.[3,48] Patients in stage I disease should be treated with amoxicillin or doxycycline to prevent further symptoms. During stages II and III, intravenous therapy is indicated, usually ceftriaxone (which crosses the blood-brain barrier), cefotaxime, or penicillin.

The nurse monitors the patient for the development of cardiac and neurologic sequelae. Persons with musculoskeletal symptoms resulting in impaired mobility may require physical therapy (PT), occupational therapy (OT), and analgesics to relieve joint pain. Nursing care is similar to interventions for patients with RA. All confirmed cases of LD must be reported to community health officials.

The vaccine for LD was withdrawn from the market. A single dose of doxycycline, 200 mg, may be given after a tick bite if there is significant risk of LD.

PATIENT/FAMILY TEACHING. *Healthy People 2010* has named prevention of LD as a priority. Goals include decreasing the overall incidence of LD in endemic regions. Education is the best prevention against LD (see Patient/Family Teaching box, p. 1564).

Seronegative Arthropathies

The term *seronegative arthropathies* is used to describe a group of diseases characterized by arthritis **(arthropathy)** in which the rheumatoid factor is not present in the serum. Another commonality is the absence of rheumatoid nodules. Approximately 2 million persons in the United States have seronegative arthropathies, including Reiter's syndrome (reactive arthritis), psoriatic arthritis, enteropathic arthritis (accompanying ulcerative colitis and Crohn's disease), and ankylosing spondylitis (AS) (Table 53-1). In many instances symptoms overlap and do not meet the diagnostic criteria, so these patients are often diagnosed with the disease given the more general term *spondyloarthropathy.*[29] The majority of persons with AS and Reiter's syndrome have a specific gene, HLA-B27, which is found in 8% of North American Caucasians.[29] Common clinical features include inflammatory spinal pain and asymmetrical, lower extremity synovitis.

The spondyloarthropathies are also known as *spondylarthritides* and have several characteristics in common, including:

- Axial arthritis (sacroiliitis and spondylitis [inflammation of the vertebrae characterized by stiffness and pain])
- Peripheral inflammatory arthritis, usually asymmetric and oligoarticular
- Enthesitis (inflammation at tendon attachment sites to bone)
- The cell marker HLA-B27
- Extraarticular manifestations, including ocular inflammation (conjunctivitis, uveitis), skin and nail lesions, aortitis, and ulceration of the GI and genitourinary tracts

Ankylosing Spondylitis

Etiology and Epidemiology. AS (Marie-Strümpell disease) is the most common chronic inflammatory disorder of the axial skeleton, affecting primarily the sacroiliac joints and spine. The etiology is unknown. The course of the disease is marked by remissions and exacerbations.

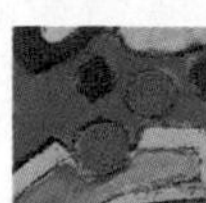

PATIENT/FAMILY TEACHING *The Patient With Lyme Disease*

To prevent Lyme disease, the nurse instructs patients to:

- Avoid tick-infested areas and sitting directly on the ground. Stay on paths while hiking.
- When outdoors in high-risk areas, wear long sleeves and long pants in light colors (to easily see ticks). Tuck shirt into pants and pants into shoes or socks.
- Wear closed shoes when hiking.
- Use Environmental Protection Agency–approved tick repellents on skin and clothing. Wash off repellent thoroughly when returning inside. Avoid spraying repellents directly on the skin of small children.
- Check frequently for ticks; check pets also.
- Have pets wear tick collars; do not allow outdoor pets on furniture or bedding.
- If a tick is found, use fine-pointed tweezers to grasp the tick at the point of attachment; gently pull the tick straight out. Place the tick in a sealed jar, and have it tested by a local veterinarian or health department. Do not squeeze the tick; doing so may release infected fluids.
- Wash the tick site thoroughly with soap and warm water, apply antiseptic, and disinfect the tweezers. Wash hands. Wash clothes thoroughly.
- Ticks are susceptible to dehydration. Reduce humidity by pruning trees, clearing brush, and mowing the lawn on your property.
- Do not have bird feeders or birdbaths in your yard; these attract animals that may have ticks.
- Keep woodpiles away from the house.
- Keep children's play areas away from wooded areas.
- See a physician or nurse practitioner if flulike symptoms or a rash develops.

For persons with the disease, the nurse provides information on:

- Signs and symptoms and complications of later disease
- Joint protection and energy conservation techniques
- Referral to Lyme Disease Foundation

The incidence of AS in the Caucasian population ranges from 0.02% to 23%, affecting men more than women by a 3:1 ratio.[29,32] The disease may be underdiagnosed in women because of milder symptoms and delayed onset.[32] The onset of disease is usually early adulthood. The genetic marker HLA-B27 is present in 95% of persons with AS; it is questionable whether bacterial infection triggers the disease.[29]

Pathophysiology. **Spondylitis** means inflammation of the spine. As a result of inflammation, the bones of the spine grow together and ankylose (fuse). The primary site of pathologic findings is the enthesis, where ligaments, tendons, and the joint capsule insert into bone. In AS, fibrous ossification and eventually fusion of the joint occur. The joint capsule, articular cartilage, and periosteum are invaded by inflammatory cells that trigger the development of fibrous scar tissue and growth of new bone. The bony growth changes the contour of the vertebrae and forms a new enthesis, or syndesmophyte, on top of the old one. As the spinal ligaments undergo progressive calcification, the vertebral bodies lose their original contour and appear square, which gives the spine the classic bamboo appearance of AS. Inflammation usually begins around the sacroiliac joints and progresses up the spine, eventually resulting in fusion of the entire spine. As the inflammatory process involves the costosternal and costovertebral cartilage, it causes chest pain, which is worse on inspiration.

Initial symptoms may include lower back pain (LBP) or aching; pain and swelling of the hips, knees, or shoulders; mild fever; loss of appetite; and fatigue. LBP flares and subsides intermittently. Over time, pain subsides and motion of the back becomes restricted. Fusion of the sacroiliac joints and spine up through the cervical vertebrae may occur over 10 to 20 years. As a result of rigidity, fractures may develop at multiple sites. The spine loses its normal lordotic curve, and the patient may have either a "poker back" deformity or a kyphosis at the cervicodorsal junction (Figure 53-2). The knees are flexed as the person attempts to move the head upright.

Extraarticular manifestations include iritis, uveitis, pulmonary fibrosis, and aortic insufficiency. One third of persons develop uveitis, which can cause tearing, photosensitivity, and ocular pain. Involvement is typically unilateral.

Collaborative Care Management. Differential diagnosis should include other causes of LBP. Diagnosis is made primarily by the patient history and radiographic findings. The erythrocyte sedimentation rate is usually elevated, but this is not specific for diagnosis. X-ray films show the presence of syndesmophytes and "bamboo" spine. Ankylosis of peripheral joints may be seen. Computed tomography (CT) scans and magnetic resonance imaging (MRI) may show changes before they are visible on plain films. Testing for HLA-B27 is not useful for diagnosis.

Goals of treatment are to relieve pain and stiffness, achieve and maintain the best possible alignment of the spine, strengthen the paraspinal muscles, and prevent complications. Antiinflammatory medications (aspirin or NSAIDs) are given to control pain and inflammation, but they do not retard disease progression. NSAIDs shown to be beneficial in treating AS include indomethacin, diclofenac, naproxen, piroxicam, meloxicam, and celecoxib.[32] Protection against GI toxicity is advised in older persons or those with a history of GI bleeding, peptic ulcers, or dyspepsia.[32] If treatment with NSAIDs is ineffective, short-term treatment (6 weeks or less) with oral steroid therapy may be prescribed. Intraarticular or periarticular steroid injections are another alternative. Infliximab and etanercept are used for persons with disease unresponsive to treatment, but there are no protocols for their use.[32] Pamidronate and thalidomide have been used in some cases; use of thalidomide is contraindicated in women with childbearing potential. If pain is unrelieved, additional analgesia should be added to the regimen (acetaminophen, opioids, or adjuvants).

Exercise (e.g., swimming in a warm pool) is an important component of treatment. Rest should be discouraged unless a fracture is present. PT is recommended to maintain mobility and

TABLE 53-1 SERONEGATIVE ARTHROPATHIES

Disorder	Etiology	Signs and Symptoms	Collaborative Management
Reiter's syndrome (reactive arthritis)	Sexually transmitted organisms or intestinal bacteria Precipitating event commonly urethritis Common organisms: *Chlamydia, Salmonella, Shigella*	Classic triad: arthritis, urethritis, and conjunctivitis (present in 33% of patients)[29] Acute onset of monoarthropathy or oligoarthropathy Fatigue, fever, generalized aching, joint stiffness, and back pain Arthritis usually affecting knees, ankles, feet, or toes: upper extremity involvement (sausage digits) with long-term disease Oral or genitourinary lesions; cutaneous lesions on soles and palms	Goals: alleviate pain, maintain joint mobility, and relieve systemic symptoms Medications: antibiotics for underlying infection, NSAIDs, sulfasalazine, methotrexate, ocular or topical steroids PT referral may be indicated; application of heat or cold for comfort Patient education regarding the disease No cure; exacerbations in one third of persons
Psoriatic arthritis	Complication of psoriasis (occurs in 7% of persons with psoriasis) May result from abnormal immune response to streptococci that collect in psoriatic skin lesions	Distal interphalangeal joints of fingers, toes (sausage digits) Spondyloarthropathy similar to ankylosing spondylitis Sacroiliac joint involvement Skin lesions Nail changes (see Chapter 65)	Similar to treatment for rheumatoid arthritis
Enteropathic arthritis	Develops in 9%-20% of persons with inflammatory bowel disease, specifically ulcerative colitis and Crohn's disease (see Chapter 43) May result from immune response to intestinal bacteria	Arthritis in multiple joints, particularly knees, ankles, and wrists Spine, hips, and shoulders also affected Occurs during exacerbations of bowel disease and disappears when bowel symptoms subside In persons with spondylitis, symptoms not correlated with bowel symptoms	Similar to treatment for rheumatoid arthritis

NSAIDs, Nonsteroidal antiinflammatory drugs; *PT,* physical therapy.

reduce the severity of deformity; for example, ROM exercises and lying prone (extension) may be done three or four times per day for 15 to 30 minutes, and deep breathing exercises may be performed to promote maximal chest expansion (rib cage mobility is decreased) (Figure 53-3). Surgery is indicated for persons with unrelieved pain and mobility problems. Procedures may include spinal osteotomy (usually cervical) and fusion and hip replacement.

PATIENT/FAMILY TEACHING. Patient/family teaching for the patient with AS is described in the Patient/Family Teaching box, p. 1566.

Autoimmune Connective Tissue Diseases

Several autoimmune disorders affect the joints. These diseases are of unknown origin and are similar to RA, affecting the skin and other organs. These disorders include systemic lupus erythematosus, scleroderma, CREST syndrome (*c*alcinosis cutis, *R*aynaud's phenomenon, *e*sophageal motility disorder, *s*clerodactyly, and *t*elangiectasia), and Sjögren's syndrome (Table 53-2).

Sjögren's syndrome is the most common autoimmune disorder among women; 90% of affected persons are female, white, and middle-aged.[35,47] Sjögren's affects 2 million to 4 million persons in the United States; the mean age at diagnosis is 50 years.[17,42] Nursing care for the person with musculoskeletal symptoms is similar to the care for the person with RA. Lupus is discussed in the following section.

Systemic Lupus Erythematosus

Etiology and Epidemiology. Lupus is classified as discoid (see Chapter 65), systemic, or drug induced. Systemic lupus erythematosus (SLE), which means "red wolf," refers to a chronic inflammatory disease of autoimmune origin that affects primarily the skin, joints, and kidneys, although the disease may affect virtually

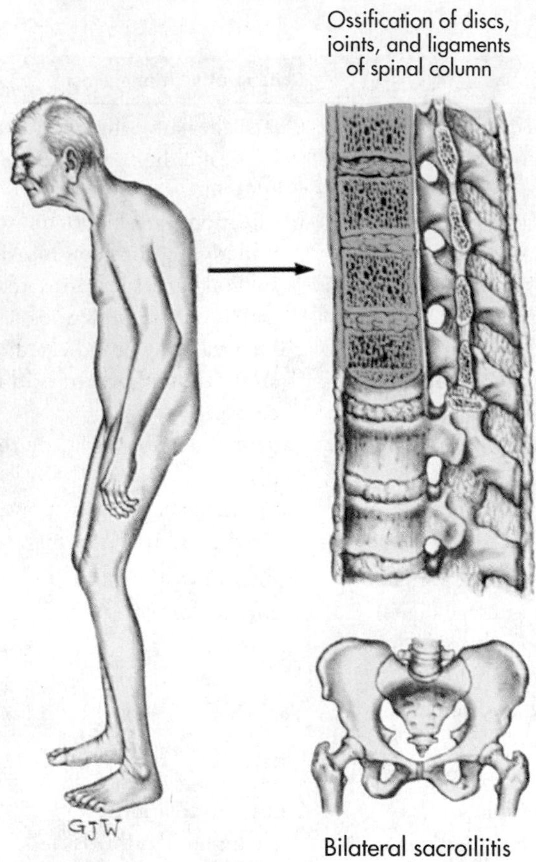

Figure 53-2 Characteristic posture and sites of ankylosing spondylitis.

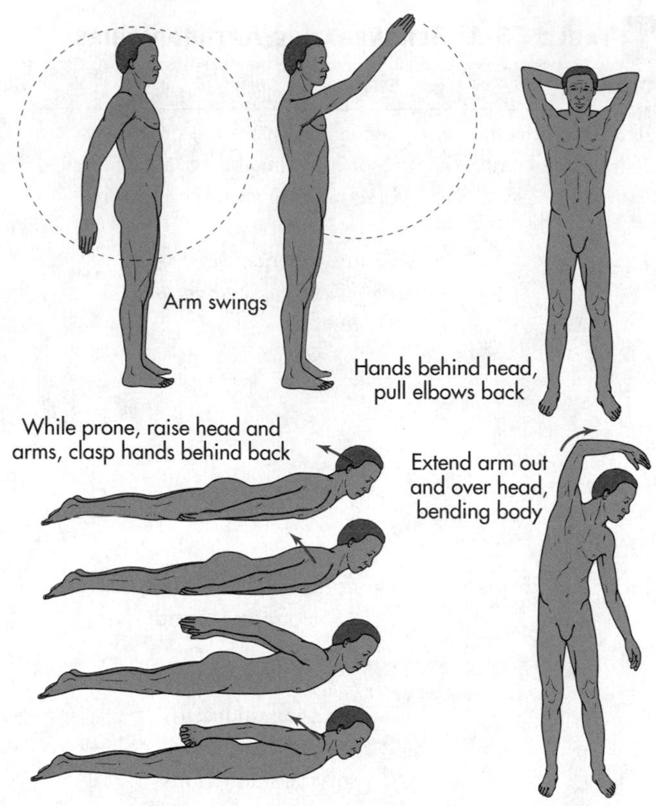

Figure 53-3 Typical chest cage stretching and deep chest breathing exercises for ankylosing spondylitis.

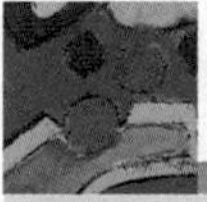

PATIENT/FAMILY TEACHING *The Patient With Ankylosing Spondylitis*

Patient teaching focuses on:
- Nature and course of the disease
- Therapy regimen
- Medications
- Pain management
- Signs and symptoms of complications
- Follow-up care

Specific information includes:
- Exercises to maintain mobility and reduce the severity of deformity. Stretching and extension exercises for the spine are beneficial. Heat and hydrotherapy can help with stiffness and pain relief as an adjunct to exercise.
- Regular deep breathing and chest expansion exercises to optimize respiratory function. If respiratory complications occur, promoting adequate oxygenation is a priority of care. Include smoking cessation techniques if applicable.
- Energy conservation techniques.
- Workplace design. Proper sitting and standing posture to decrease spinal flexion are important in the workplace and at home. Making ergonomic modifications to the work area and changing positions frequently can increase comfort and decrease stiffness.
- Use of firm mattress or a bedboard. Lying with the head flat helps maintain spine extension; sleeping with pillows causes cervical extension.
- Physical therapy or occupational therapy referrals to maximize participation in ADLs.
- Support and acceptance for persons with changes in appearance and body image. Clothing may be difficult to fit if significant spinal deformity is present.

every organ of the body. The disease was named after the characteristic erythematous butterfly rash over the nose and cheeks, which resembles a wolf's snout.

Although the cause is unknown, genetic, hormonal (disturbances in estrogen metabolism), and immune factors have been identified. As many as 20 genes may be responsible for predisposing an individual to SLE.[53] Drugs, including procainamide, isoniazid, and hydralazine, are known to induce lupuslike syndromes. Persons with drug-induced lupus usually do not develop renal and neurologic disease. The symptoms usually resolve after the drug is discontinued.

SLE affects women, particularly of childbearing years. The incidence is estimated to be 40 to 50 per 100,000 women and is higher in African-American women.[39,53] The incidence is also higher among Native Americans, Asians in Hawaii, and Chinese persons. Lupus has been seen in some men with Klinefelter's syndrome.[53] Menses and pregnancy can exacerbate the disease. The risk for developing SLE drops significantly after menopause in women but remains constant throughout the life span in men. There is no cure, but the course of SLE can usually be controlled. Although it is potentially fatal, 85% of persons with SLE survive 15 years or longer.[39] Mortality is usually a result of lesions affecting major organs or of secondary infections.

Pathophysiology. The exact mechanism of pathogenesis is unknown. However, several alterations in the immune system are associated with SLE. Numerous cellular antibodies have been identified in persons with the disorder. Antinuclear antibodies, antibodies to deoxyribonucleic acid (DNA), antihistones, and antibodies to ribonucleoprotein (Sm antigen) are all strongly associated with SLE.

Abnormalities in both B cells and T cells also have been identified in persons with the disease. The appearance of B cells is thought to cause an increase in the production of antibodies to self and nonself antigen. These antibodies are responsible for the tissue injury seen in SLE. Most visceral lesions are mediated by type III hypersensitivity, and antibodies against red blood cells are mediated by type II hypersensitivity. An acute necrotizing vasculitis can occur in any tissue. Most lesions are found in the blood vessels, kidney, connective tissues, and skin.

Because of the multisystem involvement and characteristic remissions and exacerbations, the clinical manifestations of SLE can be overwhelming. The initial manifestation is often arthritis, typically a nonerosive synovitis without deformity. Ninety-five percent of persons with SLE develop arthritis and arthralgias. Joint deformity occurs without bony erosion and resembles that of persons with RA. Contractures may also develop. In many instances the joint symptoms are migratory and transient and

TABLE 53-2 AUTOIMMUNE CONNECTIVE DISEASES

Disorder	Pathophysiology	Clinical Manifestations	Treatment
Scleroderma (systemic sclerosis)	Most common in middle-aged women Causes microvascular damage and fibrous degeneration of tissue in skin, GI tract, heart, lung, kidneys; excess collagen causing fibrosis and malfunction of involved organ	Raynaud's phenomenon GI: dysphagia, gastroesophageal reflux disease (GERD), diarrhea, malabsorption Renal: hematuria, proteinuria, renal crisis, hypertension Cardiopulmonary: pericarditis, dysrhythmias, pulmonary hypertension, fibrosis Dermatologic: hardening, tightening, and thickening of skin; edema, pallor, deepened pigmentation Musculoskeletal: muscle atrophy, rheumatoid arthritis, tightening of tendons, flexion contractures	Dependent on amount of organ involvement Avoidance of cold; protective clothing Thoracic sympathectomy for Raynaud's phenomenon Metoclopramide, proton pump inhibitors, and esophageal dilation for GI symptoms ACE inhibitors for renal symptoms Doppler evaluation of palmar circulation; thrombolytics if needed Cyclophosphamide for alveolitis; calcium channel blockers or epoprostenol for pulmonary hypertension; lung transplant for persons with end-stage lung disease Skin care for ulcers NSAIDs, PT, OT, exercises to maintain joint mobility Splints for contractures and deformities Heat and cold as needed
CREST syndrome (limited cutaneous scleroderma)	Variant of scleroderma, classified by extent of skin thickening More favorable prognosis and less organ involvement	Calcinosis (result of chronic vascular insufficiency); intracutaneous or subcutaneous calcifications on digital pads, periarticular tissues, extensor surfaces of forearms, olecranon, and prepatellar bursae	Treat as for scleroderma Surgical removal of calcium deposits

Continued

TABLE 53-2 AUTOIMMUNE CONNECTIVE DISEASES—CONT'D

Disorder	Pathophysiology	Clinical Manifestations	Treatment
CREST syndrome—cont'd		*R*aynaud's phenomenon *E*sophageal dysmotility *S*clerodactyly *T*elangiectasia Pulmonary involvement in many patients	
Sjögren's syndrome	Primary disease: inflammation and dysfunction of exocrine glands, particularly lacrimal and parotid glands, which results in dryness of mouth, eyes, and mucous membranes Lymph nodes, bone marrow, and organ involvement Rheumatoid arthritis in 50% of patients Secondary disease: individual with connective tissue disorder (RA, SLE, polymyositis) developing sicca symptoms	Xerostomia, xerophthalmia (dry mouth and dry eye, known as sicca syndrome) Enlarged parotid glands Oral candidiasis (complication of xerostomia) Dyspareunia Gritty sensations in eyes Dysphagia Dental caries Cough Rheumatoid and antinuclear antibody factors positive in most patients Anemia	Artificial tears Vaginal lubrication or estrogen creams Surgical punctual occlusion Saliva substitutes; pilocarpine to promote salivary and lacrimal flow Increased fluid intake, especially with meals Good dental and oral hygiene, especially after meals Avoidance of respiratory infections and smoking Increased humidity in home and work environment Antimalarials NSAIDs for arthritic symptoms Steroids, immunosuppressants for renal, lung symptoms

ACE, Angiotensin-converting enzyme; *GI,* gastrointestinal; *NSAIDs,* nonsteroidal antiinflammatory drugs; *PT,* physical therapy; *OT,* occupational therapy; *RA,* rheumatoid arthritis; *SLE,* systemic lupus erythematosus.

respond to treatment. Avascular necrosis, particularly of the femoral head, may occur; high-dose prednisone treatment is a risk factor. Osteoporosis is common, and steroid treatment may worsen bone density loss.

Vague symptoms such as weakness, fatigue, depression, myalgia, and weight loss may be present. The patient may report photosensitivity, a rash, and at times fever or arthritis on exposure to sunlight. Erythema, usually in a butterfly pattern, appears over the cheeks and bridge of the nose. These lesions have bright red margins and may extend beyond the hairline with partial alopecia above the ears. Lesions may also occur on the exposed part of the neck. Lesions spread slowly to the mucous membranes and other tissues of the body, or they may originate there. These lesions do not ulcerate but cause degeneration and atrophy of tissues.

Depending on the organs involved, the clinical manifestations of SLE vary (see Clinical Manifestations box). Renal and neurologic manifestations are among the more serious complications of the disease.

Collaborative Care Management. The American College of Rheumatology developed criteria for the diagnosis of SLE (Table 53-3). Diagnosis is made after evaluation of the patient history, physical examination, and laboratory tests.

The immunofluorescence test for antinuclear antibodies (ANA) is positive in more than 95% of patients with SLE; the higher the titer, the more likely the diagnosis of SLE. However, the diagnosis of SLE cannot be made solely on the basis of a positive ANA result, because it is also positive in many other autoimmune disorders, such as systemic sclerosis (both CREST syndrome and diffuse sclerosis), Sjögren's syndrome, and polymyositis. Positive results are also found among older adults and pregnant women or secondary to many prescription medications. As mentioned earlier, antibodies against double-stranded DNA and anti-Sm antigen are positive in 20% to 60% of patients with SLE. The LE cell test is positive in 70% of patients with SLE. The LE cell is any phagocytic leukocyte that has engulfed the nucleus of an injured cell.

Kidney failure is the most common cause of death in persons with lupus. Cyclophosphamide, either orally or by intravenous pulse therapy, is effective in treating lupus nephritis but is associated with significant toxicity. Dexamethasone and ondansetron can be given to improve tolerance of side effects. Treatment with azathioprine is an alternative to cyclophosphamide, especially for those who wish to preserve reproductive function. Renal symptoms are often silent; urinalysis and renal function tests should be done at regular intervals. Renal biopsy may be indicated to evaluate the condition of the parenchyma.[11]

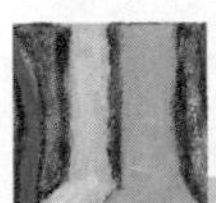

CLINICAL MANIFESTATIONS *Systemic Lupus Erythematosus*

General

Fatigue
Malaise
Episodic fever

Musculoskeletal

Arthralgia
Arthritis
Morning stiffness
Joint deformities

Skin

Photosensitivity
Butterfly rash
Discoid lesions of skin and mucous membranes
Alopecia
Telangiectasia

Neurologic

Neuropathy
Stroke
Headache
Seizures

Pulmonary

Cough
Dyspnea
Pleurisy
Pneumonitis

Cardiovascular

Pericardial effusion
Myocarditis
Coronary artery disease
Valvular disease
Thrombophlebitis
Raynaud's phenomenon
Vasculitis

Hematologic

Anemia
Leukopenia
Thrombocytopenia
Lymphadenopathy
Splenomegaly
Antibodies to clotting factors

Renal

Nephritis
Glomerulonephritis
Urinary tract infection

Gastrointestinal

Dysphagia
Nausea
Vomiting
Pancreatitis
Elevated liver function tests

Psychiatric

Anxiety
Depression
Psychosis

Dialysis or a transplant may be needed for patients with uncontrolled lupus nephritis.

Arthritis and arthralgia are the most common presenting symptoms of SLE; avascular necrosis may develop as a result of the disease or steroid therapy. Orthopedic surgery may be required for persons with severe arthritic manifestations of SLE. Pharmacologic management of arthritic symptoms is similar to treatment for RA. NSAIDs are first-line treatment, but patients with SLE are prone to developing NSAID-induced hepatitis and should be monitored carefully. Renal function should be monitored regularly; NSAIDs are contraindicated with renal impairment. Hydroxychloroquine sulfate to suppress synovitis is indicated for those unresponsive to NSAIDs. Corticosteroids and methotrexate are used if other medications are ineffective in controlling symptoms. If methotrexate is used, folic acid should be given to decrease side effects, and blood and liver function studies should be monitored.

Antimalarials are also effective in treating skin lesions, serositis, fever, and fatigue. Topical corticosteroids are prescribed for less extensive skin lesions. Corticosteroids are also effective in treating neurologic, cardiac, or hematologic effects. Because of the side effects associated with systemic steroids, their use should be limited to persons with severe, life-threatening complications (severe hemolytic anemia, thrombocytopenia, pulmonary hemorrhage) or those unresponsive to other, less toxic therapies.

During exacerbations, persons with SLE are acutely ill, and nursing care depends on the symptoms manifested. The nurse monitors the patient for the effects of medications and for renal dysfunction. The patient's neurologic status must be assessed frequently for the development of cognitive dysfunction. Seizures may occur in 15% to 20% of persons with SLE; psychosis may develop as a result of steroid therapy or the disease process.[11,52]

PATIENT/FAMILY TEACHING. Teaching for the patient with SLE is described in the Patient/Family Teaching box.

Polymyositis and Dermatomyositis

Polymyositis (PM) and dermatomyositis (DM) are considered both rheumatic connective tissue diseases and idiopathic inflammatory myopathies. Both may occur alone or in combination with other rheumatic diseases, most notably scleroderma, SLE, and Sjögren's syndrome.

TABLE 53-3 AMERICAN COLLEGE OF RHEUMATOLOGY: CRITERIA FOR CLASSIFICATION OF SYSTEMIC LUPUS ERYTHEMATOSUS*

Criterion	Definition
1. Malar rash	Fixed erythema, flat or raised, over malar eminences, tending to space nasolabial folds
2. Discoid rash	Erythematous raised patches with adherent keratotic scaling and follicular plugging; atrophic scarring may occur in older lesions
3. Photosensitivity	Skin rash as result of unusual reaction to sunlight, by patient history or physician observation
4. Oral ulcers	Oral or nasopharyngeal ulceration, usually painless, observed by physician
5. Arthritis	Nonerosive arthritis involving two or more peripheral joints, characterized by tenderness, swelling, or effusion
6. Serositis	a. Pleuritis—convincing history of pleuritic pain or rub heard by physician or evidence of pleural effusion, *or* b. Pericarditis—documented by electrocardiogram or run or evidence of pericardial effusion
7. Renal disorder	a. Persistent proteinuria greater than 0.5 g/dl or greater than 3+ if quantitation not performed, *or* b. Cellular casts—may be red blood cell, hemoglobin, granular, tubular, or mixed
8. Neurologic disorder	a. Seizures—in absence of offending drugs or known metabolic derangements (e.g., uremia, ketoacidosis, or electrolyte imbalance), *or* b. Psychosis—in absence of offending drugs or known metabolic derangements (e.g., uremia, ketoacidosis, *or* electrolyte imbalance)
9. Hematologic disorder	a. Hemolytic anemia—with reticulocytosis, *or* b. Leukopenia—less than 4.0×10^9 L (4000/mm^3) total on 2 or more occasions, *or* c. Lymphopenia—less than 1.5×10^9 L (1500/mm^3) on 2 or more occasions, *or* d. Thrombocytopenia—less than 100×10^9 L (100×10^3/mm^3) in absence of offending drugs
10. Immunologic disorder	a. Positive lupus erythematosus cell preparation, *or* b. Anti-DNA antibody to native DNA in abnormal titer, *or* c. Anti-Sm—presence of antibody to Sm nuclear antigen, *or* d. False-positive serologic test for syphilis known to be positive for at least 6 mo and confirmed by negative *Treponema pallidum* immobilization or fluorescent treponemal antibody absorption test
11. Antinuclear antibody	Abnormal titer of antinuclear antibody by immunofluorescence of equivalent assay at any point in time and in absence of drugs known to be associated with drug-induced lupus syndrome

Data from Tan EM et al: The revised criteria for the classification of systemic lupus erythematosus, *Arthritis Rheum* 25:1271, 1982.
DNA, Deoxyribonucleic acid.
*The classification is based on 11 criteria. For the purpose of identifying patients in clinical studies, a person shall be said to have systemic lupus erythematosus if any 4 or more of the 11 criteria are present, serially or simultaneously, during any interval of observation.

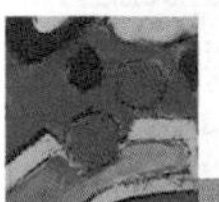

PATIENT/FAMILY TEACHING *The Patient With Systemic Lupus Erythematosus*

Instructions for joint protection, pain management, energy conservation, and self-care are similar to those for the patient with rheumatoid arthritis (see Chapter 54). The patient and family may need help in coping with a chronic systemic disease with an unpredictable course. Compliance may be an issue, particularly since strict adherence to the treatment regimen does not necessarily prevent exacerbation. Additional information includes:

- Signs and symptoms of complications
- Medication use, including signs of adverse effects
- Signs and symptoms of infection
- Importance of reducing exposure to sources of infection, since infection exacerbates symptoms
- Skin care: avoiding drying soaps or powders, harsh chemicals; taking cool baths to decrease skin discomfort
- Importance of avoiding sun exposure and applying sunscreen (sun protection factor 15 or higher) liberally when outdoors, since sun exposure exacerbates skin and systemic manifestations; when skin manifestations are present, keeping the lesions clean to avoid secondary sources of infection; use of hypoallergenic cosmetics on the face
- Use of wigs to mask hair loss
- Stress reduction techniques
- Methods to cope with changing body image resulting from physical changes, such as rash, alopecia, or joint deformities
- Planning pregnancy in consultation with an obstetrician who treats high-risk patients, since 25% to 30% of pregnancies in patients with systemic lupus erythematosus result in miscarriage[53]; carefully considering the safety of medications used for treatment during pregnancy
- Availability of support groups such as the Lupus Foundation of America or Arthritis Foundation

Etiology and Epidemiology. PM is a chronic, acquired, systemic connective tissue disease characterized by chronic inflammation of skeletal muscle. When a characteristic skin rash is present, the disorder is referred to as DM. The cause of both disorders is unknown, but abnormal reactions of the immune system have been implicated, perhaps triggered by a virus. Autoantibodies are found in the serum of affected individuals. The incidence of both disorders is estimated to be 1 per 1 million population; PM and DM are the most common inflammatory muscle diseases.[4] PM occurs twice as often in women as in men. Another type of idiopathic inflammatory myopathy is inclusion body myositis, which is more common in men than women and typically affects persons over age 50. Inclusion body myositis is characterized by an insidious onset of progressive proximal and distal muscle weakness. Myositis may also occur in association with cancer or other connective tissue disease, such as RA, SLE, or scleroderma; this type is known as myositis overlap syndrome.

Pathophysiology. Both PM and DM are characterized by inflammation of muscle fibers and connective tissue, resulting in extensive tissue necrosis and destruction of muscle fibers. Both cell-mediated and humoral immune mechanisms are associated with the diseases. Inflammatory cells at the perimysial and perivascular sites contain B cells and helper T cells in DM. Less vascular involvement occurs in PM, and B and T cells are found surrounding the muscle fibers and fascicles.

Results of histologic studies of muscle biopsy are variable, but the pathologic alterations, in order of frequency, are:

- Primary degeneration of muscle fibers, either focal or extensive
- Basophilia of some fibers with central migration of the sarcolemmal nuclei
- Necrosis of parts or entire groups of muscle fibers
- Inflammation of blood vessels supplying the muscles
- Interstitial fibrosis varying in severity with the duration and, to some extent, the type of disease
- Variation in the cross-sectional diameter of fibers

The initial symptoms of both disorders are similar to those associated with any inflammatory response: fever, swelling, malaise, and fatigue. Criteria used to diagnose both disorders are outlined in Box 53-2[41]; not all criteria must be present to confirm diagnosis. A dusky red lesion may be found in the periorbital region (heliotrope rash), along with periorbital edema in persons with DM. This rash may extend over the face, forehead, neck, upper shoulders, chest, and upper back. Scaly, erythematous lesions over the metacarpophalangeal (MCP) or interphalangeal (IP) joints, knees, elbows, or medial malleoli are known as Gottron's papules. Scaly, erythematous macules occur over the MCP and IP joints (Gottron's sign). Calcinosis can also occur in DM.

The diseases, which run a course of exacerbations and remissions, are usually first noted in proximal muscles, particularly the pelvic and shoulder girdles. The weakness is symmetric. Climbing stairs, rising from a chair, and other activities that involve lifting the body become increasingly difficult or impossible, as does lifting the arms or combing the hair. Other muscles such as the neck flexors and the muscles of swallowing may also become involved. Muscle pain or tenderness is sometimes present in the early stages.

Box 53-2 Diagnostic Criteria for Polymyositis and Dermatomyositis

- Progressive, systemic proximal muscle weakness
- Characteristic changes in electromyography
- Elevated serum levels of muscle enzymes
  - —Creatine kinase
  - —Aldolase
  - —Lactate dehydrogenase
  - —Transaminases
- Chronic inflammation on muscle biopsy
- Characteristic rashes
  - —Gottron's papules
  - —Gottron's sign
  - —Heliotrope rash

The weakness of myositis, if it persists, can lead to contractures and atrophy.

Systemic clinical manifestations common to both PM and DM include photosensitivity, dysphagia, delayed gastric emptying and reflux, decreased esophageal motility, cardiomyopathy, dyspnea, atelectasis, vasculitis, and Raynaud's phenomenon. Older adults with DM seem to have a greater chance of malignancy than the population at large, although the frequency ranges from 6% to 45%. Women with DM have a higher frequency of ovarian cancer than those without the disease.

Collaborative Care Management. Diagnosis is based on:

- The patient history and physical examination, including manual muscle tests to delineate weakness in specific muscles
- An electromyogram to delineate a specific pattern of findings to differentiate PM from other types of muscle disease
- Muscle biopsy to define specific pathologic changes in muscle
- Elevated serum enzymes in the presence of active disease
- A 24-hour urine test to determine an abnormal creatine/creatinine ratio

Treatment goals include decreasing inflammation, relieving symptoms, and increasing endurance and muscle strength. High-dose corticosteroid therapy (prednisone, up to 60 mg/day) is used for patients with PM or DM. Serial muscle testing helps document response to treatment. With clinical improvement and the normalizing of serum creatinine kinase, the steroid dosage should be slowly tapered. With exacerbations, high-dose steroid therapy is resumed.

If steroids are contraindicated or ineffective, methotrexate, azathioprine, intravenous gamma globulin, cyclosporine A, cyclophosphamide, and anti–tumor necrosis factor agents are options. Hydroxychloroquine may improve the rash in persons with DM.

PT is important to maintain ROM and prevent contractures during periods of active disease. Exercise, in increasing intensity, can be initiated during disease remission. Nursing interventions focus on maintaining the patient's strength, ROM, and level of function. Measures to prevent falls from muscle weakness include using assistive devices for ambulation, performing strengthening exercises, and evaluating the home and work environment for safety. Because osteoporosis may develop as a result of steroid therapy, prevention of falls and fractures is an important intervention. ROM exercises should be performed regularly to prevent contractures. Sitting surfaces may need to be elevated to facilitate transfer; a firm chair with arm rests is best; an elevated toilet seat and handrails can be added to the commode.

PATIENT/FAMILY TEACHING. Teaching for the patient with PM or DM is described in the Patient/Family Teaching box.

Fibromyalgia Syndrome

Although fibromyalgia syndrome (FMS) is considered a generalized pain syndrome, it is discussed here because of its association with RA, SLE, PM, and Sjögren's syndrome. Other generalized pain syndromes affecting the musculoskeletal system include polymyalgia rheumatica, which can be accompanied by a destructive, inflammatory arthritis and often occurs with giant cell arteritis (Table 53-4).

Etiology and Epidemiology. FMS, one of the most common musculoskeletal disorders, is associated with chronic pain and disability. The disorder affects an estimated 3 million to 6 million persons in the United States and 2% to 10% of the population in industrialized countries.[13,63] The typical age of onset is between 30 and 60 years; 90% of persons with FMS are women.[2,52] FMS has been described since antiquity; however, some practitioners are reluctant to recognize this syndrome as a legitimate diagnosis, perhaps because of the nonspecific pain and unknown mechanism of disease.[13] This disabling disease is characterized by widespread pain and tenderness to palpation at anatomically defined tender points. Both myofascial pain syndrome and chronic fatigue syndrome share similar features with FMS.

The cause is unknown, but it is associated with sleep disturbance and lack of exercise. Fibromyalgia-like symptoms have occurred in persons deprived of sleep or exercise; specific exercise prescriptions effectively treat symptoms. FMS often is found in persons with RA, lower back pain, SLE, Sjögren's syndrome, inflammatory bowel disease, restless leg syndrome, and osteoarthritis.

Theories of pathogenesis include a low pain threshold, malfunction in supraspinal processing of external stimuli, and hypoactivity of the autonomic nervous system and hypothalamic-pituitary-adrenal axis.[13] Possible triggers include stress, viral infection (parvovirus, Epstein-Barr), hormonal alterations, hypothyroidism, and LD. A familial pattern of disease prevalence has been identified.

Pathophysiology. FMS is considered in the differential diagnosis of RA, SLE, AS, polymyalgia rheumatica, myositis, neuropathies, and hypoparathyroidism. The pathophysiology of FMS is not completely understood. Several abnormalities in muscle have been documented in persons with FMS, including lower adenosine triphosphate and adenosine diphosphate levels, higher adenosine monophosphate levels, and changes in the number of capillaries and fiber area.

A general hypothesis is that increased muscle tenderness is caused by generalized pain intolerance, perhaps as a result of central nervous system (CNS) abnormalities (Figure 53-4). Central sensitization, an increase in sensory impulses within the CNS, is a key feature of FMS. Characteristics of central sensitization include an exaggerated response to a peripheral stimulus, pain response following a normally nonpainful stimulus, persistence of pain, greater intensity of pain, or wider distribution of pain than originally stimulated.[2] Sleep disorders, primarily sleep apnea and restless leg syndrome, are common in persons with FMS. Decreased levels of serotonin and tryptophan and low levels of growth hormone may be responsible for the sleep dysfunction and weight gain experienced by many persons with FMS.

Collaborative Care Management. The American College of Rheumatology defined diagnostic criteria for FMS in 1990 (Box 53-3 and Figure 53-5). Palpation of the tender points should reproduce pain, not tenderness or pressure. A pressure threshold meter can be used for objectivity. Excessive or inadequate pressure can lead to false-positive or false-negative results. Tender points must be present bilaterally, above and below the waist, and in the midline.

The characteristic symptom of fibromyalgia is a generalized chronic pain, which may be described as "burning or gnawing." Common symptoms include chronic aching, nonrestorative sleep, morning stiffness, and fatigue. Patients with FMS demonstrate loss of functional abilities similar to that in patients with RA, yet no radiographic changes in articular structures are found. Depression is a common finding. Headaches, sensitivity to extreme temperatures,

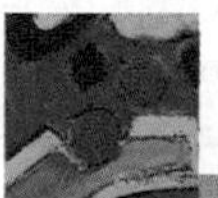

PATIENT/FAMILY TEACHING *The Patient With Dermatomyositis or Polymyositis*

Patient and family teaching focuses on:

- Knowledge of disease process and treatment plan. The patient should be aware of the need for serial laboratory and clinical examinations. Remissions and exacerbations are characteristic of this disease.
- Medications: side effects associated with long-term steroid therapy (see Chapter 38). The nurse should stress the importance of following the medication regimen and not altering dosages or frequency.
  —Abrupt cessation of steroid therapy may result in adrenal crisis.
  —Osteoporosis, fluid retention, gastrointestinal bleeding, diabetes mellitus, and avascular necrosis are all associated with long-term steroid therapy.
  —Steroid therapy increases the risk of infection.
  —Patients should wear a Medic-Alert bracelet or identification card indicating that they are receiving steroid therapy.
- Recognition of signs of systemic disease and complications.
  —Prevention of aspiration caused by dysphagia or pulmonary involvement
- Skin care, limiting sun exposure, and use of sunscreen.
- Energy conservation techniques.
- Fall and injury prevention.
- Muscle strengthening and range-of-motion exercises.
- Use of assistive devices for activities of daily living.
- Home health services during acute phases of illness because of muscle weakness.

TABLE 53-4 POLYMYALGIA RHEUMATICA

Epidemiology	Etiology	Clinical Manifestations	Treatment
Peak incidence: Caucasians older than 50 yr Twice as many women as men 10% of persons with PR develop GCA; 50% of persons with GCA have PR[66]	Unknown cause Theories include trauma to cell-mediated response; immune process; genetic predisposition or environmental influences such as infectious agents, drugs, and toxins[46] Studies suggest single causative agent for PR and GCA	ESR: 50 mm/hr Anemia, thrombocytosis Elevated C-reactive protein and elevated alkaline phosphatase Creatine kinase normal and rheumatoid factor negative Acute or insidious onset of symptoms Morning stiffness lasting over 30 min classic symptom Bilateral aching in shoulders, neck, and pelvic girdle Knees, elbows, wrists, and metatarsophalangeal joints also affected No radiologic evidence of bone erosion Fever, anorexia, night sweats, apathy, depression, weight loss, and malaise Diagnosis of GCA confirmed by temporal artery biopsy	Steroid therapy, typically prednisone, in lowest dose to control symptoms for shortest period of time (PR: 15-20 mg/day, then tapered; GCA: 40-60 mg/day, then tapered); NSAIDs for discomfort after steroids discontinued Baseline bone density and antiresorptive therapy with long-term steroid therapy Possibility of disease recurrence within 18 mo of cessation of prednisone Patient teaching about signs and symptoms of disease and medications Adequate rest and regular exercise

PR, Polymyalgia rheumatica; *GCA*, giant cell arteritis; *ESR*, erythrocyte sedimentation rate; *NSAIDs*, nonsteroidal antiinflammatory drugs.

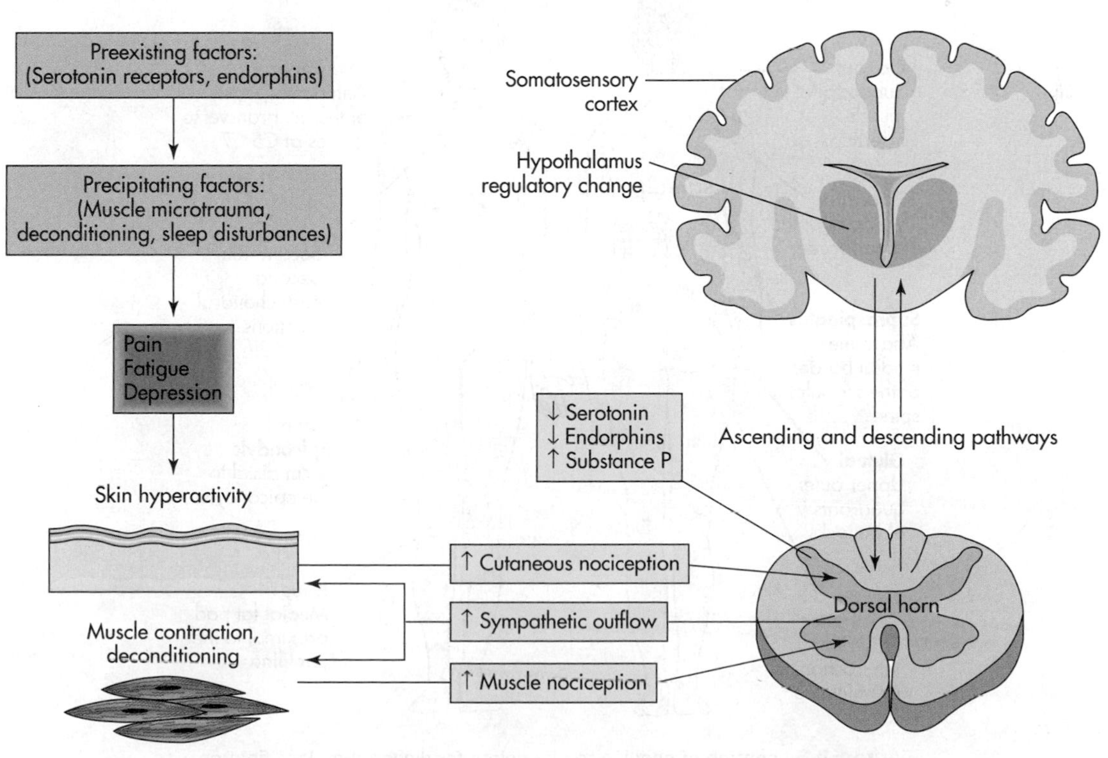

Figure 53-4 Theoretic pathophysiologic model of fibromyalgia.

Box 53-3 Diagnostic Criteria for Fibromyalgia Syndrome

- Patient history of chronic (lasting longer than 3 months) widespread pain in all four quadrants of the body
- Pain in 11 of 18 specific tender point sites when palpated with 4 kg of palpation pressure
- Bilateral tender point sites:
  —Occiput
  —Low cervical
  —Trapezius
  —Supraspinatus
  —Second rib
  —Lateral epicondyle
  —Gluteal
  —Greater trochanter
  —Knee

Data from Clauw DJ: Elusive syndromes: treating the biologic basis of fibromyalgia and related syndromes, *Cleve Clin J Med* 68(10):830-839, 2001; and Arslan S, Yunnus MB: Fibromyalgia: making a firm diagnosis, understanding its pathophysiology, *Consultant* 43(10):1233-1243, 2003.

abdominal pain, paresthesias, menstrual irregularities, irritable bowel, temporomandibular dysfunction, and difficulty concentrating may be reported. There are no visible signs of FMS.

There is no cure for FMS. Goals of therapy are to restore sleep and reduce pain. Persons with sleep apnea may need continuous positive airway pressure or surgery. A multidisciplinary approach to managing the person with FMS is most effective. Medications used to treat FMS include tricyclic antidepressants (amitriptyline or nortriptyline) to increase non–rapid eye movement sleep. Cyclobenzaprine, which has both antidepressant and muscle relaxant qualities, and selective serotonin reuptake inhibitors (SSRIs) are also used effectively. A combination of a tricyclic antidepressant at bedtime and an SSRI in the morning may be effective in restoring adequate sleep and reducing fatigue. Tramadol and gabapentin have been used successfully for pain control. NSAIDs also may be used for pain control. *S*-adenosylmethionine (SAMe) has been used in small randomized trials with mixed results.[1]

Exercise is an important treatment modality for persons with FMS (see Research box). Stretching exercises, PT, and massage can aid in relaxation, reduce fatigue, and improve overall conditioning. Other relaxation techniques such as biofeedback, deep breathing, and meditation can be useful adjuncts to pharmacologic therapies. Stress management techniques should be included in treatment. Other treatments that may be effective include acupuncture; acupressure; biofeedback; hypnotherapy; massage; and heat in the form of whirlpools, moist packs, or a hot shower.[1]

Support of the patient and family is an important nursing responsibility. FMS affects not only the patient but also the entire family. The patient may have considerable anxiety, especially if diagnosis of the disorder was difficult, and may need reassurance that she or he is not crazy. Because of the lack of objective signs of illness, others may doubt its reality. Some patients may require psychologic counseling. Reassurance and validation of the patient's reports of symptoms are important. The nurse should encourage the patient and family to discuss their feelings.

PATIENT/FAMILY TEACHING. Patient/family teaching is described in the Patient/Family Teaching box.

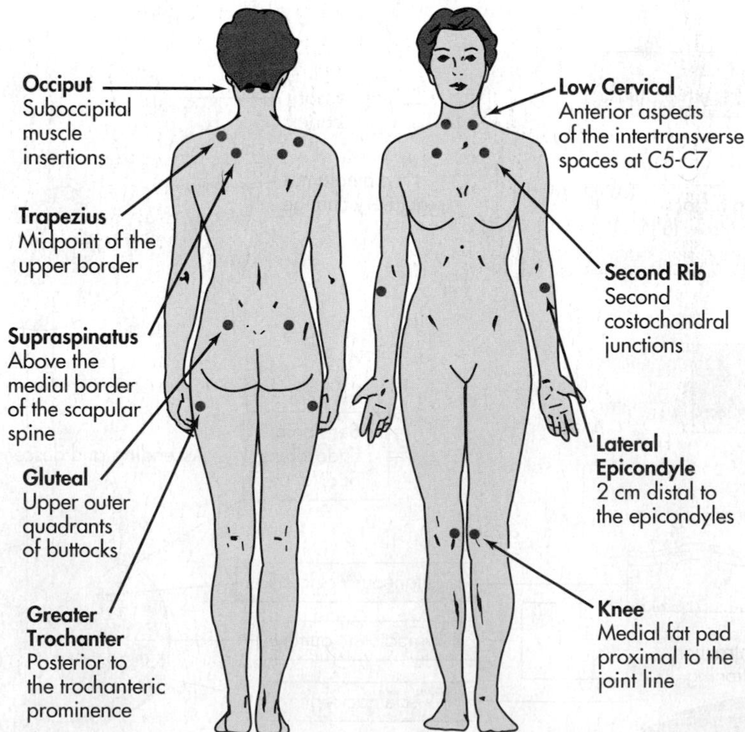

Figure 53-5 Location of specific tender points for diagnostic classification of fibromyalgia.

Research

Taggart HM et al: Effects of t'ai chi' exercise on fibromyalgia symptoms and health-related quality of life, *Orthop Nurs* 22(5):353-360, 2003.

Pharmacologic therapy is ineffective alone in treating the symptoms of fibromyalgia syndrome (FMS). Exercise is known to be an effective adjunct for treating the chronic pain, sleep disorders, fatigue, and functional disabilities associated with FMS.

The purpose of this study was to explore the effectiveness of t'ai chi' exercise in reducing symptoms and enhancing the health of persons with FMS. Thirty-seven participants with FMS attended biweekly 1-hour t'ai chi' classes for 6 weeks. FMS symptoms and health-related quality of life were measured before and after the t'ai chi'; intervention. Results supported the hypothesis that t'ai chi' is an effective intervention in reducing FMS symptoms and improving health-related quality of life. Additional benefits included weight loss. Some participants continued with t'ai chi' after the study concluded. The small sample size limits generalization of findings.

The National Association of Orthopaedic Nurses has named knowledge of interventions that enhance the health of persons with musculoskeletal problems a priority. T'ai chi' involves slow, gentle movements; requires no special equipment; and is a practical intervention to implement. More research is needed to validate the findings of this pilot study.

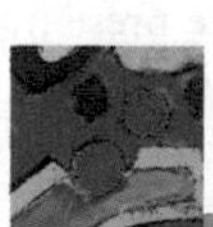

PATIENT/FAMILY TEACHING
The Patient With Fibromyalgia Syndrome

Teaching should include information about the disease and rationales for treatment, as well as:

- Exercise and rest. The patient should be taught the relationship between exercise and sleep and other factors that may disturb sleep (alcohol, stress, noise, and pain). Making a lifetime commitment to regular exercise can decrease symptoms and improve well-being. Time management and balancing work and leisure activities can improve symptoms and reduce stress.
- Diet. Certain foods are thought to trigger exacerbation of fibromyalgia syndrome (FMS) symptoms; these include dairy products, caffeine, wheat and corn cereal, citrus fruits, and yeast.[26]
- Coping skills. Nurses can provide support to individuals trying to cope with chronic disease. The principles of therapeutic communication are important when listening to patients' reports of illness and exploring methods to effectively cope with a disabling illness. Support groups are available for patients with FMS. The Arthritis Foundation is an excellent resource for exercise programs in the community. Other resources are the Fibromyalgia Network and the American Fibromyalgia Syndrome Association.

Disorders Affecting the Bones

Metabolic Bone Diseases

Metabolic bone diseases, such as Paget's disease and osteoporosis, affect the normal homeostatic function of the skeletal system. The etiology of metabolic bone diseases includes hormonal, genetic, and dietary factors.

Paget's Disease

Etiology and Epidemiology. Paget's disease, also referred to as osteitis deformans, is characterized by an excess of bone destruction and unorganized bone formation and repair. It is the second most common metabolic bone disorder in the United States, following osteoporosis. The cause of Paget's disease is unknown; however, a genetic predisposition has been identified in 10% of patients, most probably with autosomal dominant inheritance.[31] Research suggests that a slow viral infection of the osteoclasts triggers the disease in genetically predisposed individuals. Other causative theories include autoimmune dysfunction, vascular disorders, vitamin D deficiency in childhood, and mechanical stressors to bone.

Paget's disease is a common disorder in Northern Europe, including the United Kingdom, where the incidence is 5% of the population older than 55 years of age,[31]North America, Australia, and New Zealand but is relatively uncommon in other parts of the world. The average age at diagnosis is 50 to 60 years; the incidence of symptomatic disease increases with age. The disorder is relatively rare in Scandinavian countries, China, Japan, and the Middle East and among aboriginal Australians.[31]

Paget's disease usually affects the axial skeleton, particularly the vertebrae and skull, although the pelvis, femur, and tibia are other common sites of disease. Many persons with mild disease are asymptomatic, and diagnosis is incidental.

Pathophysiology. Initial changes in Paget's disease involve an increase in osteoclast-mediated **resorption** of cancellous bone, along with an increase in osteoblast-mediated bone formation. The new bone is structurally weak and enlarged. Bone resorption and formation are increased, resulting in a mosaic-like mix of abnormal woven and normal lamellar bone. Mineralization may encroach into the marrow, and excessive bone formation usually occurs around partially resorbed trabeculae, causing thickening and hypertrophy. Vascularity is increased in affected portions of the skeleton. Lesions may occur in one or more bones, but the disease does not spread from bone to bone.

Deformities and bony enlargement often occur. Bowing of the limbs and spinal curvature may occur in persons with advanced disease. Bone pain is the most common symptom of Paget's disease. Degenerative arthritis may occur at adjacent joints. Microfractures, cortical swelling, and lytic bone lesions contribute to the pain. Pain is usually worse with ambulation or activity but may also occur at rest. Involved bones may feel spongy and warm as a result of the increased vascularity. Weight-bearing bones such as the tibia and femur may become deformed, and the person's gait is affected (Figure 53-6).

Skull involvement is usually accompanied by headache, warmth, tenderness, and enlargement of the head. Flattening of the base of the skull *(platybasia)* may result in serious complications of obstructive hydrocephalus or brainstem compression. Facial bone involvement may cause deformity or, less often, affect the airway. Conductive or sensorineural hearing loss and vertigo may develop secondary to otosclerosis or neurologic abnormalities. With extensive skeletal involvement, cardiac involvement may develop as a result of increased vascularity and increased cardiac output. Other cardiac complications include atherosclerosis and endocardial and valvular calcification.[44]

Figure 53-6 Paget's disease with bilateral tibial deformities.

Pathologic fractures are a problem for persons with Paget's disease. Because of the increased vascularity of the involved bone, bleeding is a potential danger. Long bones with lytic lesions are the most susceptible to fracture. Longstanding disease may lead to malignant transformation, usually osteosarcoma. Symptoms include increased pain and swelling of affected bones. The most common sites for malignancy are the pelvis, femur, and humerus.

Alkaline phosphatase levels are usually markedly elevated as a result of osteoblast activity. Serum calcium levels are usually normal except with generalized disease or immobilization. Kidney stones are a potential complication if immobility is prolonged. Calcium deposits may also occur in the joint spaces. There is the risk of developing secondary hyperparathyroidism in persons with normal serum calcium levels and increased levels of serum alkaline phosphatase. Gout and hyperuricemia may develop as a result of increased bone activity, which causes an increase in nucleic acid catabolism.

Collaborative Care Management. Radiographs of individuals with Paget's disease reveal radiolucent areas in the bone, typical of increased bone resorption. Deformities and fractures may also be present. A bone scan is indicated at the time of diagnosis to determine the extent of disease. A CT scan may be indicated if malignancy or neural compression is suspected. Urinary pyridinoline cross-links (see Chapter 51), a marker of bone turnover, can be followed to determine the effectiveness of treatment.

Goals of treatment are to relieve pain and prevent fracture and deformity. Asymptomatic patients generally do not require treatment. Pharmacologic agents, including the bisphosphonates and calcitonin, are used to suppress osteoclastic activity. The third-generation biphosphonates (alendronate, risedronate, and pamidronate) are the drugs of choice for symptomatic disease.[62] These drugs directly inhibit the abnormally rapid osteoclastic bone resorption. The bisphosphonates and calcitonin are effective agents to decrease bone pain and bone warmth and may also relieve neural compression, joint pain, and lytic lesions. Neurologic deficits are relieved as the bone mass decreases along with vascularity. Deformity or hearing loss does not improve with pharmacologic treatment.

Plicamycin is not approved for treatment of Paget's disease but has been used parenterally to treat persons with severe disease or neurologic symptoms. Dexamethasone may be used in combination with plicamycin in the case of spinal cord compression. Some individuals may require surgical decompression.

Other treatments include the use of analgesics and NSAIDs. Assistive devices, including canes and walkers, may be needed. A shoe lift may be required for persons with deformities resulting in leg length discrepancy. Deformities may also be corrected by surgical intervention (osteotomy). Open reduction and internal fixation may be necessary for fractures. In some cases total joint arthroplasty may be indicated for severe degenerative arthritis.

The patient may benefit from a PT referral. Local application of ice or heat may alleviate pain. However, application of heat may increase the warmth associated with increased vascularity, which some patients find uncomfortable. Massage may be effective in some patients.

PATIENT/FAMILY TEACHING. The nurse provides the patient and family information regarding the course of disease, complications, and treatments, including instructions for taking medications. The patient should understand the need for follow-up medical care and monitoring for complications. A regular exercise program should be maintained; walking is best. Patients should avoid extended periods of immobility to avoid hypercalcemia. A nutritionally adequate diet is recommended. Because of the pathologic fractures, safety precautions are important to avoid falls or other injuries. The patient may need assistance in learning to use canes or other ambulatory aids. If deformities are present, the patient may need support in dealing with changes in body image. The Arthritis Foundation and the Paget Foundation are useful resources for patients and their families.

ARE You READY?

Which of the following laboratory results is seen in a patient with Paget's disease?

1. Elevated phosphorus
2. Elevated alkaline phosphatase
3. Decreased calcium
4. Decreased uric acid

Osteoporosis

Etiology and Epidemiology. Osteoporosis is the most common bone disorder in the Western world and is second only to arthritis as a cause of musculoskeletal morbidity in the older population. The initial definition of *osteoporosis,* which means "porous bone," was "too little bone in the bone."[59] Although the exact cause of osteoporosis is unknown, several risk factors have been identified (see Risk Factors box). Important risk factors are a low peak bone mass at skeletal maturity, aging, and accelerated postmenopausal bone loss. Researchers have identified the gene controlling bone density, which may have significant implications for the prevention of osteoporosis.[55]

Osteoporosis is classified in several ways: postmenopausal (women up to age 65 years), senile (any sex over 65 years), or idiopathic. It is also categorized as type I and type II forms (Table 53-5). In some persons the two types of osteoporosis overlap. Osteoporosis can be further classified as primary or secondary. Primary osteoporosis, the more common form, has no underly-

Risk Factors

Osteoporosis

- Aging
- Female
- Caucasian or Asian race
- Nulliparity
- Family history
- Postmenopausal status (surgical or natural)
- Chronic calcium deficiency
- Vitamin D deficiency
- Sedentary lifestyle
- Small frame, low body weight (less than 127 pounds)
- Smoking
- Diet high in protein and fat
- Chronic alcohol use
- Excessive caffeine intake
- History of fracture in first-degree relative[6]
- History of fracture after age 50

ing pathologic condition. Secondary osteoporosis results from another cause or medical condition, such as glucocorticoid-induced osteoporosis[37] (Box 53-4). Treatment of secondary osteoporosis focuses on removal of the underlying cause.

Low bone mass is a critical element in the diagnosis of osteoporosis. The World Health Organization has classified bone mass as[38]:

- *Normal skeletal status:* bone mineral density (BMD) values of no more than 1 standard deviation (SD) below the young adult woman (30 to 40 years of age) mean value (T score above 1)
- *Osteopenia (low bone mass):* BMD values between 1 and 2.5 SDs below the young adult mean value (T score between 1 and 2.5 SD); increased risk for future osteoporosis
- *Osteoporosis:* BMD values 2.5 or more SDs below the young adult mean value (T score at or below 2.5 SD)
- *Severe osteoporosis:* BMD values 2.5 or more SDs below the young adult mean value and the presence of one or more pathologic (fragility) fractures

These definitions are used in reference to BMD values determined by dual-energy x-ray absorptiometry (DEXA or DXA) of the hip or spine. They are not applicable to bone density measurements at all sites or with all types of measuring devices. Another disadvantage is that the young adult "normal" reference range used for comparison is Caucasian women's scores; criteria are needed for men and women of diverse racial backgrounds.[34]

Decreased bone mass and susceptibility to fracture with little or no trauma are hallmarks of the disease. At age 50, the lifetime risk of hip, spine, and forearm fracture is 40% in Caucasian women and 13% in Caucasian men.[15,45,49] The mortality risk for osteoporotic fracture in women is 2.8%, or equal to that for breast cancer.[45] BMD decreases with aging, as rapidly as 5% every 5 years after age 65.[45] As bone density decreases by 1 SD, the risk of fracture increases 2.6 times.[45]

Osteoporosis is usually asymptomatic until fracture occurs. With the advent of bone densitometry, the ability to safely and easily measure bone density allows identification of persons at risk for fracture before fracture occurs (see Chapter 52). Early intervention can prevent or decrease further bone loss and decrease the risk of fractures.

Bones are constantly undergoing **remodeling**. The remodeling process is a complex and highly integrated activity that strategically balances the forces of resorption with the process of bone formation. The osteoblastic forces predominate throughout childhood and young adulthood, until peak bone mass is reached at about age 35. After a variable period of relative balance, the resorptive breakdown forces begin to predominate. High rates of bone turnover and progressive loss persist throughout aging. In osteoporosis the bone is essentially normal, but there is not enough of it to withstand mechanical stresses. Simple bone mass is the major determinant of bone strength and accounts for about 75% to 85% of its variance.

Other factors associated with the development of osteoporosis relate to hormonal balance. The loss of natural estrogen at menopause appears to dramatically increase the process of bony resorption, although the exact mechanism is not well understood. Chronic calcium deficiency is a common problem in the aging population, and adequate calcium is essential for bone production. The mechanism of intestinal absorption of calcium becomes less efficient with advancing age, increasing the demand for calcium. Diets high in fat appear to decrease calcium absorption, and excess protein ingestion—particularly animal protein—increases the

TABLE 53-5 TYPES OF OSTEOPOROSIS

	Type I: Postmenopausal	Type II: Senile
Age of onset	Postmenopausal women (natural or surgically induced), 55-75 yr	Women: >70 yr Men: >80 yr
Sex	F:M = 6:1	F:M = 2:1
Pathology	Osteoclast mediated Increased resorption	Osteoblast mediated Decreased bone formation
Rate of bone loss	Rapid	Slow
Type of bone lost	Predominantly trabecular Associated with vertebral (compression-type) and distal radial fractures; hip fracture possible	Cortical and trabecular Associated with vertebral (wedge), proximal humerus, tibia, and hip fractures
Bone density	>2 SD below normal	Low normal

SD, Standard deviation.

Box 53-4 Causes of Secondary Osteoporosis

Endocrine Disorders
Diabetes
Cushing's syndrome
Hyperparathyroidism
Parathyroidism
Hypogonadism
Hyperprolactinemia and acromegaly
Hyperthyroidism

Drug-Induced
Glucocorticoids
Heparin (long-term use)
Chronic use of phosphate-binding antacids
Loop diuretics
Anticonvulsants
Barbiturates
Thyroid medication
Lithium
Chemotherapy
Cyclosporine

Disuse
Prolonged immobilization (prolonged bed rest, immobilization of limb by casting or splinting)
Paraplegia
Tetraplegia
Lower motor neuron disease

Chronic Illness
Sarcoidosis
Cirrhosis
Renal tubular acidosis

Cancer
Multiple myeloma
Lymphoma
Leukemia

Alterations in Gastrointestinal and Hepatobiliary Function
Biliary sclerosis
Sclerosing cholangitis
Alcoholic cirrhosis
Inflammatory bowel disease
Celiac disease
Malabsorption syndrome
Anorexia nervosa
Prolonged parenteral nutrition

Other
Amenorrhea in premenopausal women
Organ transplantation
Renal disease
Rheumatoid arthritis

excretion of calcium by the kidney. Alcohol may be toxic to osteoblasts, and chronic use usually results in malnutrition. Alcohol and possibly caffeine also increase calcium excretion. Both a history of smoking and current smoking affect bone remodeling and appear to lower estrogen levels and block calcium absorption. Current smokers have a 4.3% lower BMD than nonsmokers; BMD scores for persons with a history of smoking are 1.7% lower than those of nonsmokers.[49]

Lack of exercise is another causative factor. In accordance with Wolff's law (see Chapter 51), bone is a dynamic substance that responds to stressors and weight-bearing forces. Chronic immobility is accompanied by well-documented increases in bone resorption. In normal daily lifestyles, this translates into an increased risk of osteoporosis for individuals with small frames, low body weight, and a sedentary activity pattern.

The use of steroids for treatment of persons with chronic illness is widespread. However successful it is in controlling conditions such as RA or asthma, steroid use is associated with many side effects, including osteoporosis. Glucocorticoids interfere with calcium metabolism, reduce the synthesis of proteins by osteoblasts in the bone matrix, and may interfere with calcium absorption in the gut and renal tubule.[33] A reduction in serum sex hormone levels has also been noted, particularly in men and postmenopausal women. The rate of bone loss is greatest during the first few months of steroid therapy. The amount of bone lost during the first year of therapy has been reported to be as high as 20%.[33] Fracture risk increases significantly with steroid use: the risk for hip fracture in persons receiving prednisone increases 77% to 127%; higher risk is associated with higher daily doses.[15]

Characterized by decreased bone mass and increased susceptibility to fracture, osteoporosis has become a major health problem. The prolonged longevity of the American population is expected to increase the number of persons affected by osteoporosis. By 2020, one in two Americans over age 50 will be at risk for osteoporosis if current trends continue.[12]

Ten million persons (8 million women) in the United States over age 50 have osteoporosis, and an additional 34 million are at risk for developing the disease.[6,12] Considered primarily a women's disease, osteoporosis in men is now gaining increasing attention. More than 5 million men in the United States have or are at risk for developing osteoporosis (see Risk Factors box).[65] One in eight men and half of all women are affected by osteoporosis.[16]

More than 1.5 million fractures occur annually as a result of osteoporosis; direct costs for care of osteoporotic fractures are estimated at $18 billion annually.[24] Hip fracture and its sequelae are of major concern. Proximal hip fractures are associated with a significant mortality rate. Approximately 20% of older persons with hip fracture die within 1 year; 20% are admitted to a nursing home within the year.[12] The age-related increase in fractures begins about 10 years later in men than in women; the mortality rate after hip fracture is greater in men than in women. BMD of the hip in men decreases by 1% each year, regardless of hormonal status.[9] Interventions to prevent or decrease bone loss in both sexes is well warranted.

The racial distribution of osteoporosis is influenced by differences in bone mass, rather than rates of bone loss. African-Americans have approximately 10% greater bone mass than do Caucasians and consequently are at less risk of developing osteo-

Risk Factors

Osteoporosis in Men

- Hypogonadism (majority prostate cancer)[9,16]
- Alcoholism
- Smoking history
- Liver disease
- Renal tubular acidosis
- Hypercalciuria
- Hyperparathyroidism
- Hyperthyroidism
- Mastocytosis
- Hyperprolactinemia
- Vitamin D deficiency
- Gastrointestinal disease (postgastrectomy)[65]
- Glucocorticoid therapy

porosis. Asians and persons of Northern European or Scandinavian ancestry are at greatest risk of developing osteoporosis.

Pathophysiology. In the process of normal bone remodeling, bone formation equals bone resorption. An osteoporotic state develops if bone resorption exceeds bone formation. Trabecular bone accounts for approximately 20% of the skeletal mass; cortical bone accounts for the remaining 80%. Age-related bone loss begins in both sexes at approximately age 40 years. In women the most significant bone loss begins after menopause as a result of decreased levels of estrogen. Once menses cease, the rate of bone loss increases by 7.[20] During the first 5 to 10 years of menopause, women can lose up to 15% of cortical bone and 30% of trabecular bone. This loss can be prevented by estrogen therapy. The skeleton continues to lose bone mass in the hip and appendicular skeleton, even after the age of 80 years.

Two processes of bone loss have been identified: rapid bone loss and gradual bone loss. Rapid bone loss occurs during menopause and is osteoclast mediated, whereas gradual bone loss is osteoblast mediated and occurs after menopause. The time required to complete one cycle of bone remodeling in a healthy adult is about 4 months; that time is increased to almost 2 years for individuals with osteoporosis.

The remodeling process consists of the following steps: clusters of bone precursor cells respond to a stimulus (drug, hormone, or physical stressor) to activate the remodeling process and form osteoclasts. Osteoclasts form a cutting cone and begin to resorb bone, leaving a resorption cavity. In cortical bone, osteoblasts line the cavity and begin laying down layers (lamellae) of new bone until a haversian canal results (see Chapter 51). Trabeculae are formed in cancellous bone. If this process of remodeling is disrupted, osteoporosis may result. A decrease in the number of bone precursor cells or in the rate of bone formation, an increase in the rate of bone resorption, or an increase in the number of stimuli that activate the process can all result in osteoporosis. Osteoporosis also occurs if the whole process is not completed in entirety. Interference in the bone's vascular system results in a decreased number of bone precursor cells, which may also cause osteoporosis.

Cortical thinning begins at age 40 years, increases with age, and almost ceases late in life. After menopause women lose cortical bone at a rate of 2% to 4% per year, returning to normal levels approximately 10 years after menopause.[20] In contrast, trabecular bone loss begins earlier in both sexes and is lost in greater amounts. After menopause the rate of trabecular bone loss is as high as 8% annually.[20] There are fewer and smaller trabeculae, with large spaces between them, decreasing the bone density. The compressive strength of trabecular bone is related to its density; as the density decreases, so do its compressive force and ability to withstand mechanical stressors. The bones most susceptible to fracture are those rich in trabecular bone, particularly the vertebrae, proximal femur, and distal radius. Cortical bone undergoes osteoporotic changes as well, becoming thin and porous and thus susceptible to fracture. Collapse and deformity may occur as a result of the bone's decreased density.

Osteoporosis has been called the "silent thief" and "the silent disease" because most persons affected have no outward manifestations. Previously the disease was not diagnosed unless fracture occurred. Many fractures related to osteoporosis occur without the patient's knowledge, although some are associated with excruciating pain. The earliest manifestation of osteoporosis may be an acute onset of back pain in the middle to lower thoracic region as a result of vertebral fracture, occurring at rest or with minimal activity. Vertebral fracture can involve the entire vertebrae **(compression)** or a portion, usually the anterior section (wedge). Motion of the spine is restricted, especially forward flexion. Anterior compression fractures of the thoracic vertebrae may cause a "dowager's hump," or thoracic kyphosis (Figure 53-7). Loss of height and a protruding abdomen (because of pressure on abdominal viscera) are associated with this condition. Eventually the lower rib cage may rest on the iliac crests. Paravertebral muscle spasm often occurs, but neurologic deficits are rare with spontaneous vertebral compression fractures.

These postural changes may affect exercise and food tolerance. The patient reports early satiety. Vertebral compression fracture can result in decreased mobility, decreased quality of life, difficulty sleeping, altered body image, increased pulmonary complications, increased risk of subsequent fracture, and a 23% increased mortality rate.[19]

Distal radial fractures (Colles' fractures) usually occur after a fall on an outstretched hand. Fractures of the proximal femur are associated with considerable morbidity and mortality (see Chapter 52). Osteoporotic hip fracture often occurs after little or no trauma. Intracapsular hip fracture is caused by bone loss, and intertrochanteric fracture is caused by both cortical and trabecular bone loss.

COMPLICATIONS. Complications of osteoporosis are primarily fractures (see Chapter 52). An estimated one in two women and one in four men over age 50 will have an osteoporosis-related fracture in their lifetimes. Osteoporosis is responsible for more than over 1.5 million fractures annually, including 300,00 hip fractures, 700,000 vertebral fractures, and 250,000 wrist fractures.[43]

Collaborative Care Management

DIAGNOSTIC TESTS. The risk for fracture can be assessed by identifying the patient's risk factors and history and measured precisely with noninvasive diagnostic tools. Measurements of BMD and biochemical markers of bone resorption are the basic tools for diagnosis of osteoporosis. Diagnostic techniques can assess the

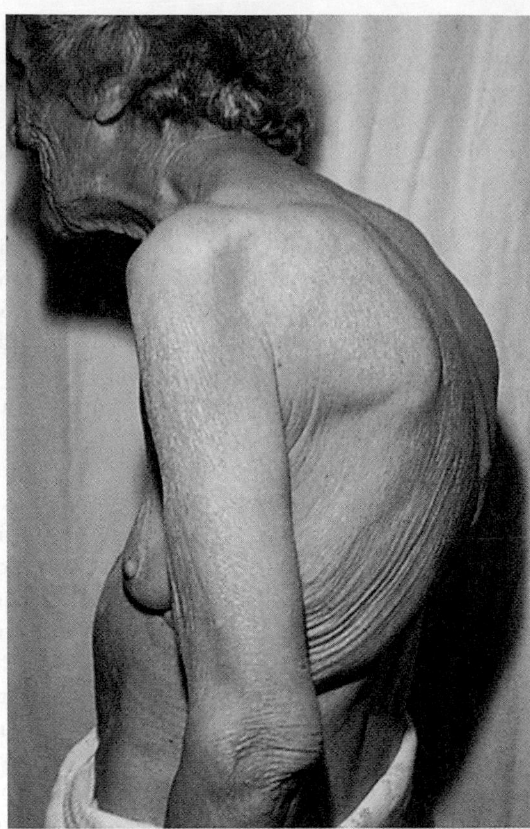

Figure 53-7 Kyphosis. This elderly woman's condition was caused by a combination of spinal osteoporotic vertebral collapse and chronic degenerative changes in the vertebral column.

extent of disease, effects of treatment, progression of disease, and, perhaps most important, risk of fracture. A variety of techniques are used to measure bone density at various parts of the skeleton (Table 53-6), and the accuracy of predicting fracture risk measuring the BMD of the finger is being studied.[15] Once the diagnosis of osteoporosis is established, BMD studies should be performed every 1 to 2 years to determine response to treatment.

Biochemical markers of bone turnover (bone formation [bone alkaline phosphatase, serum osteocalcin] and bone resorption [urine deoxypyridinolines, urine pyridinium cross-links]) are easily assessed by either a blood or a urine sample; their effectiveness in predicting fracture risk and in monitoring therapy continue to be tested.[20] These studies are most often used in conjunction with BMD and may be helpful in monitoring response to treatment.

Guidelines for screening are controversial. Medicare provides reimbursement for BMD testing for women over 65 years of age who are at clinical risk for osteoporosis. The National Osteoporosis Foundation (NOF) recommends BMD screening for persons under 65 years of age who have one or more risk factors for osteoporosis (in addition to menopause) and for all women over 65 years of age, regardless of associated risk factors.[36] Men over age 55 who have lost 2 or more inches in height should be screened for osteoporosis.[6] Acceptable height loss over a lifetime is 2 inches for men and 1.5 inches for women.[6] NOF suggests that height loss of one inch or more may be indicative of osteoporosis-related vertebral fracture (see Research box).

The U.S. Preventive Services Task Force (USPSTF) concluded there is insufficient evidence to warrant routine BMD testing of all postmenopausal women.[7] The USPSTF recommends the use of two screening tools to assess risk for osteoporosis (Box 53-5).[7] Both tools use a scoring system to calculate risk in women ages 60 to 64. Patients are referred for BMD testing based on the scores.

TABLE 53-6 METHODS OF MEASURING BONE MINERAL DENSITY

Method	Site	Advantages and Disadvantages
Single-photon and x-ray absorptiometry (SPA, SXA)	Radius, calcaneus	Inexpensive, easy to use Lengthy time required for results
Dual-photon absorptiometry (DPA)	Lumbar spine, proximal femur, total body	Reasonably precise, inexpensive Lengthy examination times; largely replaced by DEXA
Dual-energy x-ray absorptiomety (DEXA or DXA)	Lumbar spine, proximal femur, proximal radius, distal radius, calcaneus, whole body	Accurate, gold standard; DEXA most widely used; allows precise measurement of hip and spine with low radiation exposure
Quantitative computed tomography (QCT)	Spine, radius (both cortical and trabecular)	Rapid results, widely available, able to assess trabecular content of spine Higher exposure to radiation than other methods; expensive
Quantitative ultrasound (QUS)	Calcaneus, tibia	Inexpensive, portable, no radiation exposure, questionable value in predicting fracture risk[20]; persons identified at risk should be referred for DEXA

Research

Thornton MJ, Sedlak CA, Doheny MO: Height change and bone mineral density revisited, *Orthop Nurs* 23(5):315-320, 2004.

Early detection and diagnosis of osteoporosis results in decreased probability of fractures and an improved quality of life. Screening at risk persons is necessary for early diagnosis.

Osteoporosis can affect the spine; the loss in bone density in the vertebrae can result in pathologic fracture, kyphosis, and height loss. Although height loss is associated with normal aging process, excessive loss may be indicative of vertebral fracture. Women over 45 years old may lose 0.09% of their height annually. The National Osteoporosis Foundation (NOF) suggests that height loss of more than 1 inch may be a result of vertebral fracture. Height and height change are not routinely documented on physical assessments of women at risk for osteoporosis. The purpose of this study was to explore the relationship between bone mineral density (BMD), height change, and osteoporosis risk factors.

This study was a secondary analysis of data; 168 healthy postmenopausal women ages 50 to 65 years made up the convenience sample. The researchers evaluated the participants' height change; BMD; and osteoporosis risk factors, including calcium intake, weight-bearing exercise, amount of smoking, and amount of caffeine and alcohol intake. The results did not support a significant relationship among the variables. The mean height loss of the sample (− 0.187 inches) was less than the 1-inch parameter suggested by the NOF as indicative of osteoporosis. The women did not have the recommended daily intake of calcium or minimum weight-bearing exercise.

The lack of significant relationships between the variables may be attributed to the percentage of women with normal BMD and no height loss (44%). Homogeneity of the sample was another limitation of the study. Although height loss should not be used as a sole measure of risk for osteoporosis, it should be part of the comprehensive assessment. Further research is needed to explore the relationship between height loss and risk for osteoporosis.

DEXA scanning of the proximal femur or spine is usually done. BMD testing of the proximal femur is recommended as the best predictor of hip fracture and is preferred in older persons because degenerative changes in the spine may mask decreases in bone density of the vertebral bodies.

MEDICATIONS. The goals of pharmacologic therapy for persons with osteoporosis are to prevent further bone loss and to decrease the risk of fracture. Relieving symptoms associated with skeletal deformity and fracture and maximizing functional capacity are other goals of treatment. Medications used to treat osteoporosis either decrease bone resorption or increase bone formation (Table 53-7). Alendronate has been approved to treat osteoporosis in men; androgen replacement may be beneficial in treating androgen-deficient men with osteoporosis but is associated with significant adverse effects.[9]

Estrogen therapy has been a mainstay of osteoporosis treatment since the 1940s. The results of the Women's Health Initiative trial caused the Food and Drug Administration to issue warnings that estrogen-progestin therapy increased the risk of breast cancer, myocardial infarction, stroke, and thromboembolic events. Results from this study raised serious questions about the use of long-term hormone replacement therapy (HRT) for disease prevention. The American College of Obstetricians and Gynecologists supports the use of estrogen therapy or estrogen-progestin therapy (EPT) as an antiresorptive agent to prevent bone loss. Medium-dose estrogen and biphosphonates have been found to be as effective. Discontinuation of therapy is not advised, since rapid bone loss and increased fracture risk can occur.[67] The lowest dose of estrogen to prevent osteoporosis (as measured by BMD) is advised; concomitant use of calcium and vitamin D is recommended.[67] HRT is not recommended for women with, or at risk for, heart and vascular disease.[38,67]

HRT therapy should only be prescribed after evaluating the individual's risk/benefit ratio. When prescribed, HRT should be in the lowest effective dose for the shortest duration.[21] Transdermal HRT may have fewer side effects than oral preparations, but further research is needed to evaluate the long-term effects of low-dose and transdermal HRT.[21]

Other drugs used to treat osteoporosis, including fluorides, growth factors, calcitonin, anabolic steroids, and parathyroid hormone analogs, are under investigation. Mild analgesics are used to relieve pain associated with muscular aches and spasms.

Box 53-5 Screening Tools for Osteoporosis

Osteoporosis Risk Assessment Instrument (ORAI)

Age in years
Weight in kilograms
Current estrogen use

Simple Calculated Osteoporosis Risk Estimation (SCORE)

Ethnicity
Presence of rheumatoid arthritis
History of fracture
Age
Weight
Estrogen use

TREATMENTS. Osteoporosis is easier to prevent than to treat. Diet, medications, exercise, and prevention of falls and fractures are the foundations of preventive therapy. No specific treatments are available for persons with osteoporosis. Chapter 52 discusses treatments for persons with fractures. Wrist fractures are usually treated by closed reduction and immobilization. Treatment for acute vertebral fractures is bed rest for 1 to 2 days and analgesics. Persons who have sustained a vertebral fracture as a result of osteoporosis may benefit from a corset (fitted by an orthotist) to provide support. Rigid bracing should be avoided, since complete immobilization results in bone loss. Pain usually subsides after 6 to 12 weeks as the fracture heals. Activity is essential during the healing period to avoid chronic back symptoms. Calcitonin has been effective in relieving the pain after vertebral fracture. Ultrasound, massage, and local application of heat or cold may alleviate pain and muscle spasms. Assistive or adaptive devices may be needed in the home or work environment. Persons who have had one fracture are at risk for subsequent fractures.

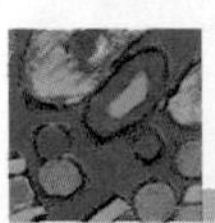

TABLE 53-7
COMMON MEDICATIONS *for Osteoporosis*

Drug	Action	Nursing Intervention
Calcium	Necessary for bone formation High calcium intake may retard bone loss; insufficient alone to prevent or treat osteoporosis	Daily recommended dose for adults over age 65 is 1200 mg, taken in divided doses of 600 mg twice a day for maximal absorption. Observe for signs of hypercalcemia. Calcium is contraindicated with severe renal disease.
Vitamin D: calcitrol, calcifediol	Necessary for bone formation and calcium absorption from gastrointestinal (GI) tract	Effectiveness of therapy depends on adequate calcium intake. Monitor for effects of hypercalcemia.
Hormone replacement therapy (HRT)	Improves calcium balance Inhibits osteoclastic bone resorption; positive effect on calcium balance; protects against postmenopausal osteoporosis	Inform patient of benefits and risks (myocardial infarction, breast cancer, stroke, thromboembolic events). Use lowest effective dose for shortened duration.
Estrogen therapy (ET)	Prevents cortical and trabecular bone loss	Do not give to persons with or at risk for cardiovascular disease.
Estrogen-progestin therapy (EPT)	EPT increases bone mineral density (BMD) and reduces fracture risk	Estrogen when given without progestin increases risk of endometrial cancer.
Selective estrogen receptor modulator (SERM): raloxifene (Evista)	Mimics effects of estrogen in some, but not all, tissues Blocks estrogen's cancer-promoting effects in other tissues Reduces rate of bone resorption and decreases rate of overall bone turnover Increases bone density, lowers blood lipid levels, does not increase high-density lipoprotein level Does not adversely affect breast, uterine tissue; studies being done to determine effect on breast cancer risk in younger women FDA approved for prevention of osteoporosis in postmenopausal women Inconclusive data regarding decreasing fracture risk; has been shown to decrease vertebral fracture risk in older women with postmenopausal osteoporosis	These present risk of venous thromboembolic events, similar to risks associated with HRT. Avoid use in women with history of blood clots. Inform patient of side effects, including hot flashes and leg cramps. Advise patient to avoid smoking while taking SERMs. Caution women of childbearing potential to avoid pregnancy. Risk of breast cancer increases with long-term use.[7]
Bisphosphonates: etidronate, pamidronate, alendronate (Fosamax), risedronate, tiludronate	Inhibit osteoclast-mediated bone resorption Also used in treatment of Paget's disease Increase bone resorption, increase BMD, and prevent fractures in postmenopausal women with osteoporosis (alendronate) Given once weekley, prevents bone loss in men with prostate cancer receiving androgen deprivation therapy (alendronate)[43b]	Use as alternative for HRT. Administer on empty stomach (at least 1 hour before any food or medications) with full glass of water because of poor absorption. Take vitamins, calcium, and antacids at a different time of day. Monitor BMD during therapy

SURGICAL MANAGEMENT. Surgical intervention is necessary to repair some fractures. However, vertebral fractures without neurologic deficits usually do not require surgical intervention. Severe kyphotic deformities and vertebral compression fracture can be treated with minimally invasive kyphoplasty and percutaneous vertebroplasty. Both procedures are performed with fluoroscopy to identify the fracture site. **Kyphoplasty** is performed for vertebral compression fractures; methylmethacrylate is injected into the vertebrae for stabilization and relief of pain. Both procedures reduce deformities and relieve pain. Kyphoplasty also restores vertebral height. Complications associated with vertebroplasty include rib fracture, radiculopathy, and extravasation of the cement possibly resulting in nerve compression, infection, and pulmonary embolus.[25]

Wrist fractures may need open reduction for the person to achieve maximal functional results. Almost all hip fractures are managed surgically (see Chapters 52 and 54, including the section on hip arthroplasty). The choice of procedure and fixation depends on the individual patient, the location of the fracture, and the vascular supply to the femoral head. As with all types of fractures, the principles of management are to mobilize the patient as quickly as possible to prevent the complications of immobility and to restore the patient to the maximal level of functioning.

DIET. Adequate nutrition is essential throughout life for a healthy skeleton. Calcium and vitamin D intake should be adequate from childhood through maturity to develop peak bone mass before menopause, thus protecting against osteoporosis later in life.

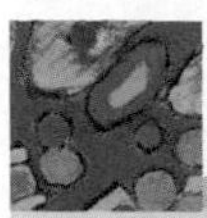

TABLE 53-7
COMMON MEDICATIONS *for Osteoporosis—cont'd*

Drug	Action	Nursing Intervention
Bisphosphonates—cont'd	Protect against bone loss during long-term steroid therapy (risedronate)	To decrease risk of esophagitis and GI side effects, have patient remain standing or upright for 30 min after administration. Patient should not take within 1 hr of calcium-containing foods, beverages, or medications. Alendronate is poorly absorbed with food; instruct patient to fast evening before and 30 min after administration. It has convenience of once-weekly dosing. Etidronate: for maximum absorption, patients should not eat or drink 2 hr before and after administration.
Ibandronate sodium (Boniva)	Treatment and prevention of osteoporosis in postmenopausal women; increases BMD and reduces vertebral fracture risk by 52% when compared to placebo	Available in either 2.5 mg daily or 150 mg once monthly dosing. Intravenous infections administered every 2-3 months are available for persons unable to tolerate oral drug.[43a] Contraindicated in persons unable to remain upright for 60 minutes after administration and in persons with uncorrected hypocalcemia. Instruct patient to maintain adequate vitamin D and calcium intake. Side effects include dyshpagia, esophagitis, gastric and esophageal ulcers, diarrhea, and pain in extremities. Cautious use in persons taking ASA or NSAIDs because of increased risk of gastric irritation and in persons with impaired renal function.
Calcitonin (human or salmon): intranasal (Miacalcin)	Opposes effect of parathyroid hormone in bone and kidneys Inhibits bone resorption; decreases fracture risk Increases bone mass in persons with steroid-induced osteoporosis Analgesic effect with osteoporotic fractures	Use is limited to parenteral or intranasal administration; side effects with subcutaneous injection include nausea, flushing, and local inflammatory reaction; administering dose at bedtime may decrease adverse effects. Monitor for hypocalcemia. Assess for allergy. Teach importance of reading labels; many over-the-counter products contain calcium. Few systemic effects occur with intranasal use.

ASA, Aspirin; *FDA,* Food and Drug Administration; *NSAIDs,* nonsteroidal antiinflammatory drugs.

Healthy People 2010 named inadequate calcium intake as a priority nutritional problem in the United States; inadequate dietary calcium often indicates a nutritionally poor diet.[30] The importance of adequate calcium intake increases with aging. Vitamin D and calcium absorption are gradually impaired as a result of the aging process. The daily recommended intake of calcium for adults older than 51 years of age is 1200 mg (Table 53-8).[18] Persons with osteoporosis should have a daily intake of calcium of 1500 mg. If the person is unable to take in adequate calcium in the form of dairy products, supplements are needed. Single doses of calcium should not exceed 600 mg/dose. Calcium-enriched juices and breads, which contain approximately 300 mg of calcium (equal to one glass of milk), are available. Foods rich in calcium include dairy products, green vegetables, and tofu (Table 53-9).

Vitamin D is necessary for calcium absorption and stimulates bone formation. Deficiencies of vitamin D are common in persons with osteoporosis, strict vegetarians, and those living in northern latitudes with restricted sunlight exposure. The recommended daily allowance of vitamin D is 400 IU. Persons with vitamin D deficiencies may require supplements, but persons with sun exposure throughout the year usually do not. Foods rich in vitamin D include milk, fish, and eggs.

Dietary phytoestrogens, isoflavones found in soy foods, may contribute to bone health. A diet high in soy protein is associated with greater bone density and decreased bone resorption. Reports from the World Health Organization indicate osteoporosis is less common in Asian women, despite their smaller bone structure and lower calcium intake when compared with Western women.

TABLE 53-8 RECOMMENDATIONS FOR DAILY CALCIUM INTAKE

Age (yr)	Daily Recommendation (mg)	Servings*
1-3	500	2
4-8	800	3
9-18	1300	4
19-50	1000	3
51+	1200	4

*1 serving is equal to 1 cup whole, reduced-fat, fat-free, or flavored milk; 1 cup yogurt; 1½ oz natural cheese; 1 cup pudding made with milk.

Soy intake is estimated to be 8 to 10 g/day in Asia, compared with less than 5 mg/day in the West.[27] More research is needed to identify the role of soy on bone health in postmenopausal women. The three major isoflavones, genistein, daidzein, and glycitein, are found primarily in soybeans, textured vegetable protein, and tofu. Phytoestrogens are also available as a dietary supplement. The use of plant estrogens, both dietary and by supplement, has increased as an alternative to HRT.

Another dietary recommendation for persons with osteoporosis is avoidance of excessive intake of alcohol and caffeine, both of which are risk factors for osteoporosis. For persons with fractures, a diet adequate in proteins and vitamin C is necessary to promote wound and tissue healing.

HEALTH PROMOTION AND PREVENTION. Teaching should include health promotion techniques, especially for persons at risk of developing osteoporosis. To decrease the risk of osteoporosis, all persons should consume a diet adequate in calcium and vitamin D and perform regular weight-bearing exercise, beginning in childhood, to accumulate peak bone mass at skeletal maturity. Education pertaining to bone health should begin in childhood and adolescence. Older adults, including older men, are another at-risk target population. Premenopausal women benefit from an explanation of the effects of estrogen on bone mass and strategies to prevent osteoporosis before the need arises. Osteoporosis is one of the targeted initiatives for *Healthy People 2010* (see Healthy People 2010 box). Screening for BMD should be done for persons at risk of developing osteoporosis or before beginning treatment to determine baseline levels to monitor the effectiveness of treatment.

The NOF, an excellent resource for information about osteoporosis, publishes a quarterly newsletter regarding advances in treatments and offers *Boning Up on Osteoporosis*, a guide to the treatment and prevention. National Osteoporosis Week is held in May each year; U.S. Surgeon General R.H. Carmona named May as national Bone Health Month. Dr. Carmona published the "People's Piece" for the American people, a free booklet offers information to improve bone health. Copies are available by calling 800-624-BONE.

Other resources include the National Institutes of Health's Osteoporosis and Related Bone Diseases National Resource Center. Many tools and teaching materials are available over the Internet at government-sponsored sites.

TABLE 53-9 MAJOR DIETARY SOURCES OF CALCIUM

Food	Quantity	Calcium (mg)
MILK		
Skim	1 cup (240 ml)	302
1%	1 cup	300
2%	1 cup	297
ICE CREAM		
Hard	1 cup	176
Soft	1 cup	236
ICE MILK (VANILLA)		
Hard	1 cup	176
Soft	1 cup	274
CHEESE		
Cheddar	1 oz	204
Swiss	1 oz	272
American	1 oz	150
Cottage	1 cup	155
BEANS (COOKED)		
Pinto	1 cup	86
Soy	1 cup	131
Navy	1 cup	95
Green	1 cup	80
VEGETABLES		
Turnip greens (cooked)	1 cup	249
Broccoli (cooked)	1 cup	90
Tofu	4 oz	108
FISH AND SHELLFISH		
Oysters (raw)	1 cup	226
Salmon (canned)	3 oz	167
YOGURT		
Plain (low fat)	8 oz	415
Fruit (low fat)	8 oz	343
Frozen (fruit)	8 oz	240
Frozen (chocolate)	8 oz	160

COMPLEMENTARY AND ALTERNATIVE THERAPIES. Complementary therapies for osteoporosis include t'ai chi' and yoga to improve muscle strength and flexibility. Isoflavones (discussed previously) may play a role in improving bone density. Dietary supplements rich in phytoestrogens include dong quai, gingko biloba, black cohash, and ginseng. Collard greens, rich in vitamin K, may have protective effect for bone and reduce risk of fracture.

Healthy People 2010

Goals Related to Osteoporosis

- Reduce the number of adults with osteoporosis.
- Increase the number of culturally competent community health prevention programs.
- Increase the number of persons who meet dietary requirements for calcium intake.
- Increase the number of adults who engage in physical activities that promote flexibility, muscular strength, and endurance.
- Reduce the number of adults hospitalized for osteoporosis-related vertebral fractures.

From US Department of Health and Human Services: *Healthy people 2010: understanding and improving health,* Washington, DC, 2000, The Department.

▶ ARE YOU READY?

Which of the following foods is a good source of vitamin D?

1. Citrus fruits
2. Raw green vegetables
3. Shellfish
4. Poultry

Nursing Management *of the Patient with Osteoporosis*

The nursing management section pertains to persons with osteoporosis but without fractures. The nursing management of persons with fractures is discussed in Chapter 52.

ASSESSMENT

Health History. Assess for:

- Risk for osteoporosis: diet (calcium, vitamin D, soy protein intake, history of anorexia or bulemia, exercise habits, amount of caffeine and alcohol consumption, amount and frequency of sunlight exposure)
- Medications used, including over-the-counter drugs
- Nutritional and dietary supplements
- Family history of osteoporosis or bone diseases
- Gynecologic history for females: menstrual history, including history of amenorrhea; pregnancies; onset of menopause; history of HRT
- History of prostate cancer in men
- BMD results
- Any changes in height or posture
- Fracture history
- Falls
- Previous treatments
- Pain
- Expectations of treatment
- Ability to perform activities of daily living (ADLs)
- Layout of home, number of stairs
- Any disturbances in self-esteem because of loss of independence or functional ability
- Depression

Physical Examination. The nurse performs a complete physical examination focusing on the musculoskeletal and neurologic system. Assess for:

- Height and weight
- Size of frame and build
- Gait and balance
- Posture
- Sensory status
- Kyphosis (If present, a complete respiratory and GI assessment is required, since the deformity may cause decreased respiratory excursion, respiratory compromise, abdominal distention, ileus, and constipation.)
- Tenderness with palpation over intervertebral body spaces
- ROM
- Muscle strength

NURSING DIAGNOSES, OUTCOMES, AND INTERVENTIONS

Nursing Diagnosis: Impaired Mobility

OUTCOMES. Common examples of expected outcomes for the patient with a diagnosis of *impaired mobility* are:
Patient will:

- Maintain maximal level of mobility and functioning.
- Participate in regular, weight-bearing exercise to increase muscle strength and increase bone density.

NURSING INTERVENTIONS. The nurse monitors the patient's ROM and muscle strength and documents limitations in mobility. The nurse also monitors the patient's pain level, since unrelieved pain may interfere with mobility. Analgesics should be given as needed, especially before planned activities. Active ROM should be encouraged daily; if the patient is unable to perform active ROM, the nurse performs passive ROM.

If the patient has a vertebral fracture, a corset may be prescribed to provide support and increase mobility while the fracture heals. The nurse encourages maximal mobility and weight-bearing exercises while the fracture heals to avoid bone loss from immobility. In addition, strengthening exercises increase circulation to both bone and muscle. A PT referral is an option for teaching weight-bearing and resistive exercises. OT can provide the patient with adaptive devices to assist in ADLs. The nurse encourages participation in ADLs to maintain independence, allowing the patient adequate time to complete self-care.

Affected parts of the body can be supported with slings or pillows as needed, especially during rest. Uninterrupted periods of rest throughout the day can increase energy and prevent fatigue. Fatigue is common among persons with musculoskeletal impairments. The nurse encourages the patient's family and friends to participate in care, since they can assist the patient in managing problems associated with immobility.

Exercise is an often-prescribed intervention for the prevention and treatment of osteoporosis (see Evidence-Based Practice box). Benefits of exercise include increased muscle tone and muscle

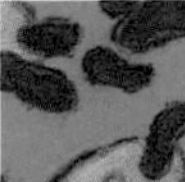

EVIDENCE-BASED PRACTICE

Topic Question: Is exercise effective in preventing bone loss and fractures in postmenopausal women?

Evidence Base: Reports of 18 randomized controlled trials were reviewed. Relative risk of fracture was calculated using fixed effects model. For bone mineral density (BMD), weighted mean differences were calculated to evaluate change from the baseline.

Findings: Walking is effective in increasing the BMD of the hip and spine; aerobic exercise is effective in increasing BMD of the wrist. This meta-analysis found poor quality in reporting the trials, particularly regarding concealment and blinding.

Conclusions: Aerobic, weight bearing, and resistance exercise are all effective in increasing the BMD of the spine in postmenopausal women.

Bonaiuti D et al: Exercise in preventing and treating osteoporosis in postmenopausal women (Cochrane Review). In *Cochrane Library*, Issue 3, Chichester, UK, 2004, John Wiley & Sons.

mass, which may improve balance and flexibility and thus prevent falls. In addition to the benefits of overall well-being and cardiovascular effects, impact-loading exercise seems to be effective in maintaining bone mass. Regular weight bearing or bone stressing (weight training and resistance exercises) is necessary to maintain bone mass in both children and adults. The effects of exercise on peak bone mass are most significant during the years of skeletal growth and have less significance in older adults. Premenopausal women who exercise regularly and have regular menstrual cycles have the greatest bone mass; amenorrhea leads to bone loss.

The ideal amount and type of exercise needed to maintain bone mass have not been determined. Research has shown positive effects of exercise on BMD in postmenopausal women. Resistance training strengthens muscles, increases BMD, and reduces fractures.[28,64] A basic resistance training program consists of five or six weight-bearing exercises done two or three times per week; results are usually seen in 4 to 6 weeks.[64]

Recommendations for all adults should include a daily (or at least five times per week) program of weight-bearing and mild weight-training exercises. Thirty minutes a day is recommended. Brisk walking or low-impact aerobics are good choices for the older adult. Extension exercises of the spine are beneficial for posture and flexibility, but flexion exercises may contribute to fracture. Jogging may also precipitate vertebral fracture. Walking outdoors has the added benefit of sunlight exposure, essential for vitamin D formation. Swimming or water exercises have no direct effect on bones but are good choices for an aerobic workout.

RELATED NIC INTERVENTIONS. Exercise Promotion: Strength Training, Exercise Therapy: Ambulation, Exercise Therapy: Joint Mobility, Positioning

Nursing Diagnosis: Risk for Injury

OUTCOMES. Common examples of expected outcomes for the patient with a diagnosis of *risk for injury* are:

Patient will:

- Be free from injury.
- Experience no falls or fractures.
- Identify factors that increase the risk of injury and steps to correct the situation or modify the environment.

NURSING INTERVENTIONS. Pathologic fracture can result from minor trauma in the individual with osteoporosis. Falls commonly result in hip fracture, a significant cause of mortality in the older adult. The environment should be modified to protect the patient from accidental harm or injury.

The nurse monitors the patient for level of consciousness, ability to make judgments, motor strength, coordination, balance, and sensory deficits. Many medications may cause weakness, drowsiness, or dizziness, which pose an additional risk for injury. If adverse effects occur, the nurse should consult the physician for alternatives. Electrolyte imbalances are common in older adults and may manifest as mental status changes or weakness. Blood chemistry results should be evaluated for abnormalities.

The nurse provides instructions about the proper technique for transferring from bed to chair, bending, and lifting. Proper body mechanics can protect the patient from back injuries (Figure 53-8). Excessive flexion of the spine may contribute to compression fracture of the vertebrae. Kyphosis may alter the patient's center of gravity and diminish vision. The nurse encourages the patient to maintain an upright posture to improve ambulatory ability and also to enhance respiration. Assistive devices and ambulatory aids may be necessary for some persons. A PT referral may be needed to teach the patient the proper technique for using a walker or cane to provide support and decrease the risk for falls.

The environment should be kept as hazard free as possible while the patient is hospitalized. The nurse should keep the bed in a low position and assess the need for side rails, particularly for confused persons or those receiving sedation. Careful monitoring of the patient is crucial, since some persons may attempt to climb over the rails and sustain a fall. The call light should be within reach, and the nurse should instruct the patient in its use. Nonskid shoes or slippers can also help prevent falls. Environmental hazards such as equipment, electrical cords, and slippery floors should be eliminated. The home environment should also be assessed for safety hazards (see Patient/Family Teaching box).

Exercise is an important intervention for preventing falls. Regular exercise increases energy, muscle tone, strength, flexibility, and coordination, which may help in fall prevention. ROM exercises should be included in the program to maintain joint mobility.

RELATED NIC INTERVENTIONS. Fall Prevention, Surveillance: Safety

Nursing Diagnosis: Situational Low Self-Esteem

OUTCOMES. Common examples of expected outcomes for the patient with a diagnosis of *situational low self-esteem* are:

Patient will:

- Manifest positive self-esteem.
- Participate in desired activities to fullest level.

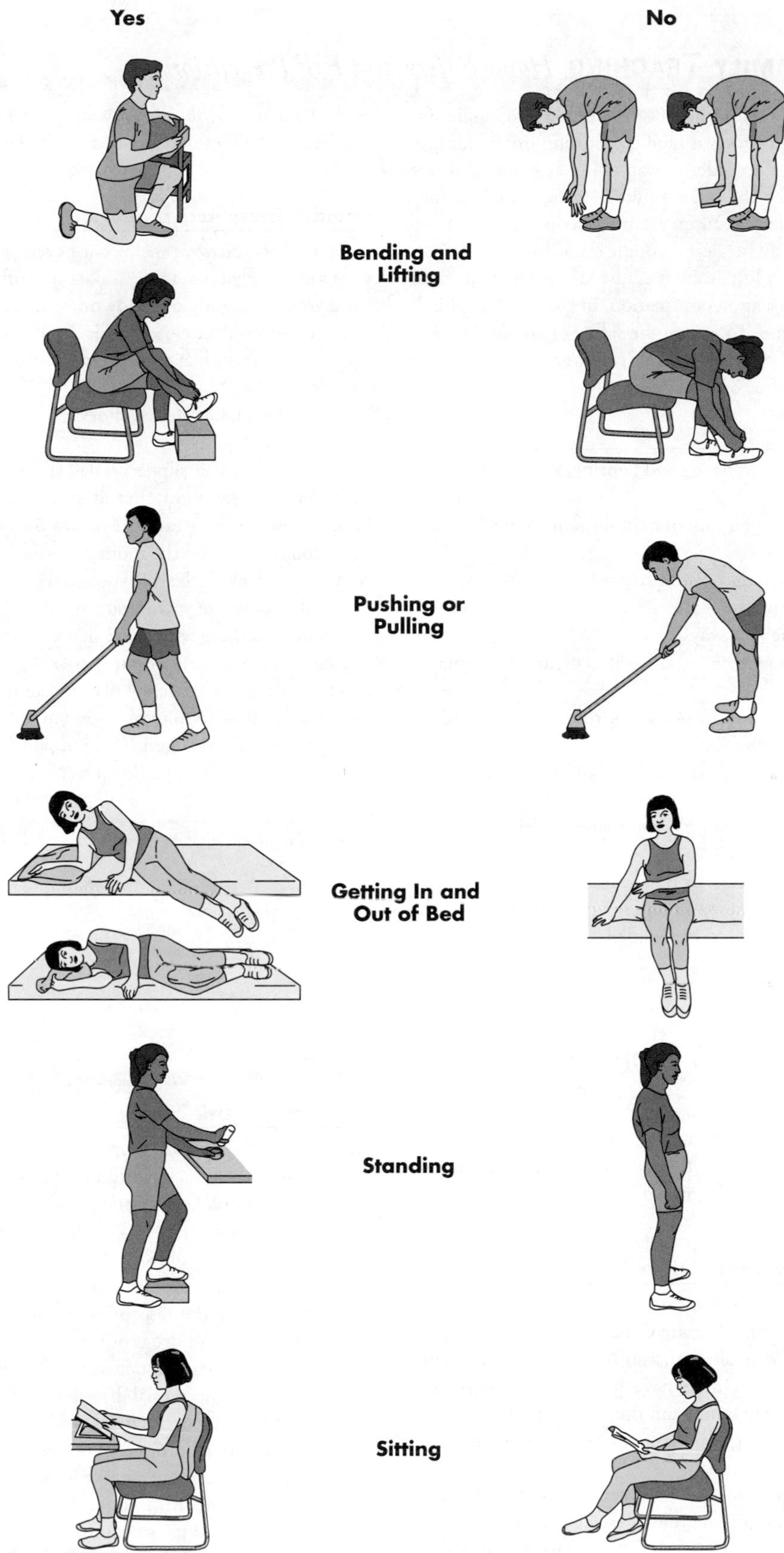

Figure 53-8 Proper body mechanics.

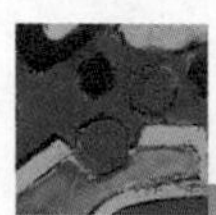

PATIENT/FAMILY TEACHING *Home Safety and Fall Prevention*

Unintentional injury is the third leading cause of death and disability for persons older than 65 years of age. A disability resulting from an injury may end the independence of an older person living at home. Falls are the leading cause of injury for the older adult. Because the bones may become more brittle with aging, a fall may cause a serious injury. A hip fracture secondary to a fall may be a catastrophic event for an older person. Most falls in the older adult occur because of an environmental hazard, loss of muscle strength and coordination, impaired sense of balance, and slowed reaction time. To ensure the safety of an older person and to help prevent falls and other injuries, it is important to make the person's living space safe and free of hazards.

Environmental Safety

Steps should be highly visible and have good lighting, nonskid treads, and handrails.

A strong banister running along all indoor and outdoor steps is essential.

Clearly mark and light the top and bottom steps.

Use bright lighting in the living space.

Remove all floor clutter in the walkways.

Remove slippery floor coverings such as polished linoleum, small mats, and area or throw rugs.

Use nonskid floor wax, wall-to-wall carpeting, or rubber-backed rugs. Tack down the corners of area rugs.

Install nonskid mats and handrails in the bathtub and near the toilet and bed.

A bedside lamp or low-wattage night light should be available in the bedroom.

Secure electrical cords along the walls or baseboards.

Store frequently used dishes, clothes, and other items within easy reach; climbing on a stool or chair should be avoided.

Set the temperature on the hot water heater to no hotter than 130° F, or have a mixing valve installed on the bathtub faucet to prevent burns.

Personal Safety Activities

If you need glasses, wear them, but never walk around with glasses that are meant only for reading. Take them off before moving around.

If you are even slightly unsteady on your feet, use a cane. Do not hesitate to use a walker either inside the house or outdoors.

Always turn lights on and use adequate-wattage lightbulbs to brighten the room.

Wear wide-based, low-heeled shoes with corrugated soles to help prevent slips and falls.

Do not wear flimsy or slippery-soled shoes or slippers.

When getting up at night, first sit on the edge of the bed to make sure you are awake and steady, then turn on a light before walking to the bathroom or around the room.

Do not ever smoke in bed. If you are sleepy, don't light up a cigarette regardless of where you are sitting.

Always wear clothing with short sleeves when you are cooking. Never reach over a hot burner on the stove.

If you live alone, have a safety plan to call for help or to get assistance.

If you take a medication that makes you dizzy or weak, discuss these symptoms with your health care provider. Being dizzy or weak when you get up to walk or go down stairs may increase your risk of falling.

From *Mosby's patient teaching guides: update 3,* St Louis, 1997, Mosby.

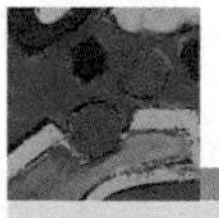

PATIENT/FAMILY TEACHING *What Is Osteoporosis?*

Osteoporosis is the most common metabolic bone disease. It results from the loss of calcium in the bones, causing the bones to become brittle and susceptible to breaking. The term *osteoporosis* means "porous bone." The disease is usually not diagnosed until the person suffers a fracture or broken bone.

Why Are Women Affected More Often Than Men?

One out of four women and half the women older than 65 years of age have osteoporosis to some extent. Most are Caucasian women who have gone through menopause. Generally, African-Americans have greater bone mass than Caucasians, and men have greater bone mass than women. Petite women with small bones and thin bodies have very small bone masses. Thus women are at greater risk of developing osteoporosis if they are Caucasian, Asian, or petite.

Osteoporosis is also caused by low estrogen levels that occur in women after menopause. Although the role of estrogen is not clear, it is linked to the processes of bone formation and resorption. Estrogen is thought to reduce bone resorption, to reduce calcium loss through the kidneys, and to increase calcium absorption in the digestive tract. Estrogen protects women who have had an inadequate intake of calcium in their growing years. However, when estrogen levels drop after menopause, bone resorption in women increases greatly.

What Are the Risk Factors?

Two major risk factors for osteoporosis are lack of exercise and inadequate intake of calcium, vitamin D, and protein. Osteoporosis caused by calcium and vitamin D deficiencies affects men and women over age 50. Other risk factors contributing to the disease are:

- A family history of osteoporosis
- Smoking and consuming too much alcohol and caffeine, which interfere with the absorption of calcium
- Prolonged use of drugs or medications such as steroids, magnesium-based antacids such as Maalox, and heparin
- Diseases and hormonal disorders such as rheumatoid arthritis, liver disease, certain cancers, and an overactive thyroid gland
- Poor calcium absorption in the intestines

Although osteoporosis primarily affects middle-aged or older adults, it can occur in young adults. Injuries that result in paralysis or long periods of immobility can lead to osteoporosis.

From *Mosby's patient teaching guides: update 3,* St Louis, 1997, Mosby.

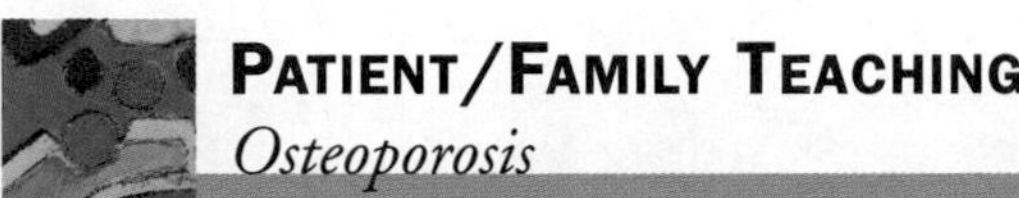

PATIENT/FAMILY TEACHING
Osteoporosis

Understanding the disease process is essential. Many resources about osteoporosis are available in print and on the Internet. Information for patients and families includes:

- Awareness of risk factors and strategies to decrease risk
- Medications: use, administration, possible adverse effects
- Body mechanics
- The need to engage in regular weight-bearing exercise (see Figure 53-9)
- The need to maintain healthy body weight
- The importance of preventing falls and fractures
- Ways to modify the home environment to prevent falls and injury
- Adequate dietary calcium and vitamin D (The average adult under 50 needs 200 IU of vitamin D. Vitamin D is produced by the skin in response to sun exposure. One cup of fortified milk contains 302 mg of calcium and 50 IU of vitamin D. Dietary supplements are also available.)
- Limiting alcohol and caffeine consumption
- Smoking cessation
- Managing pain

NURSING INTERVENTIONS. Osteoporosis, in addition to the effects on musculoskeletal functioning, also significantly affects an individual's social and emotional functioning. Changes in the body and body function may cause anxiety. Deformities such as kyphosis, the onset of menopause, or decreased mobility as a result of musculoskeletal disease may be difficult changes for the patient to assimilate. With spinal curvature and changes in body contours, finding attractive clothing to fit, particularly without alterations, may be problematic. This may compound changes in body image. Depression is not an uncommon reaction to an altered body image and functional limitations.

If respiratory involvement from kyphosis is significant, the patient may experience activity intolerance and inability to pursue desired activities. Dissatisfaction with appearance may cause a patient to avoid going out and pursuing social activities, leading to feelings of dependency and isolation. Patients who experienced previous falls often fear falling again. Explaining the process of aging, menopause, and the effects on bone can help reassure patients that aging and menopause are normal events. Knowledge of the treatment and preventive strategies for protecting bone mass can alleviate patients' fears. Nurses can provide support and help patients adapt to change and maintain a positive outlook.

The social support of family and friends is essential for assisting a patient in dealing with the dependency that results from pain, disability, and physical deformities. Spouses, friends, or family can assist the patient with household tasks. Social contacts should continue, and outings that do not pose hazards to the person can be arranged. Walking with friends outdoors or in a mall can foster social support and fulfill the need for exercise. The woman with osteoporosis can continue to perform as many aspects of her usual role as possible, perhaps with some adaptations. Clothing can be purchased or altered to decrease the prominence of back deformities, thus ameliorating embarrassment or negative self-image.

RELATED NIC INTERVENTIONS. Body Image Enhancement, Coping Enhancement, Self-Esteem Enhancement

Patient/Family Teaching. Teaching for the patient with osteoporosis is described in the Patient/Family Teaching boxes. Also refer to Figure 53-9.

EVALUATION

To evaluate the effectiveness of nursing interventions, compare patient behaviors with those stated in the expected outcomes.

RELATED NOC OUTCOMES. Ambulation, Falls Occurrence, Mobility, Risk Detection, Risk Control, Safe Home Environment

GERONTOLOGIC CONSIDERATIONS

Many patients with osteoporosis are elderly. Osteoporosis is an asymptomatic disease, until fractures occur. A typical patient is an older woman admitted for a hip fracture, unaware that she has osteoporosis. Education and lifestyle modification are essential elements in preventing the disease and reducing morbidity associated with fractures in older adults. Regular exercise may pose a problem for some frail older persons or those with limited resources.

Infectious Bone Disease

Osteomyelitis

Etiology and Epidemiology. Although the development of osteomyelitis is often precipitated by a traumatic event or is a complication of trauma, it is included with the degenerative disorders because of its chronic and debilitating aspects. Osteomyelitis is an infection of the bone, most often of the cortex or medullary portion. It is usually caused by bacteria but can also be caused by fungi, parasites, and viruses.

The two types of osteomyelitis are classified by the pathogen's mode of entry. *Contiguous focus* or *exogenous osteomyelitis* is caused by a pathogen from outside the body or by the spread of infection from adjacent soft tissues. The most common offending organism is *S. aureus.* Examples include pathogens from an open fracture or surgical procedure, particularly a joint replacement or procedure involving instrumentation. *Staphylococcus epidermidis* is associated with implant-related infection. The infection can also be caused by human or animal bites and by fist blows to the mouth. The most common organism found in human bites is *S. aureus;* the most common organism found in animal bites is *Pasteurella multocida.* The infection spreads from the soft tissues to the bone. Risk factors for developing exogenous osteomyelitis are chronic illness or diabetes, alcohol or drug abuse, and immunosuppression. In persons with diabetes or vascular disease, osteomyelitis occurs most often in the feet. Pain may be absent as a result of neuropathy. The onset is insidious: initially cellulitis progressing to the underlying bone.

Hematogenous osteomyelitis is caused by bloodborne pathogens originating from infectious sites within the body. Examples

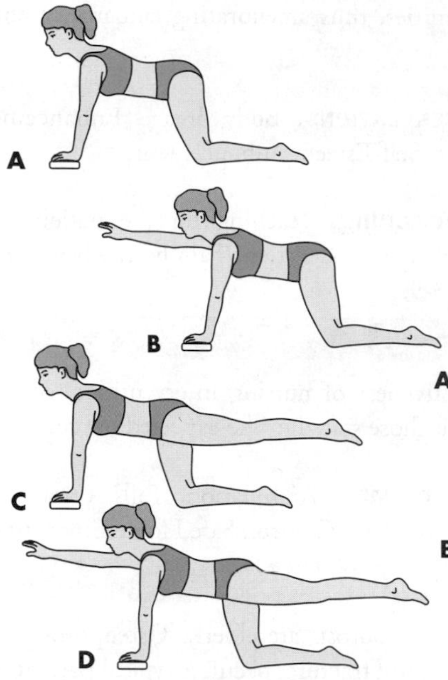

All Fours Arm/Leg Lifts
Position yourself on your hands and knees, with your hands directly under your shoulders and your knees directly under your hips **(A).** Your back should be flat or slightly arched. Lift one arm and hold for 3 seconds **(B).** Repeat with the other arm. Then lift one leg and hold for 3 seconds **(C).** Repeat with the other leg. If you can do these exercises comfortably, try lifting your right arm and left leg simultaneously **(D),** and then your left arm and right leg.

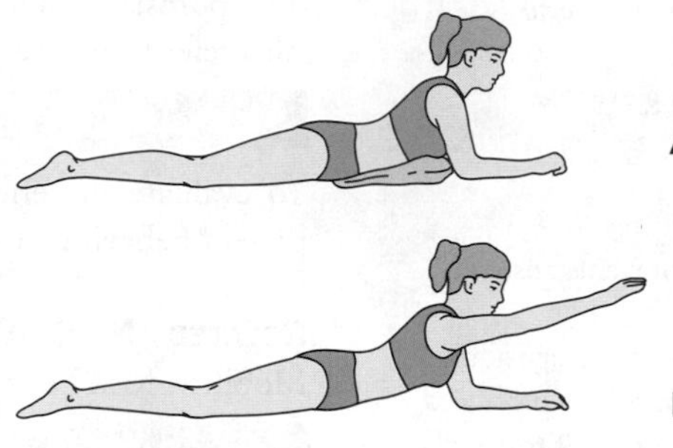

The Elbow Prop
Lie on your stomach with your elbows holding the weight of your upper body **(A).** Stay in this position for 5 minutes the first day; gradually increase the time to half an hour. You may be more comfortable if you put a pillow under your stomach. The elbow prop position helps reverse the effects of bad posture by passively decompressing the vertebrae and discs. To exercise the back as well, reach the right arm forward **(B),** then the left, and repeat.

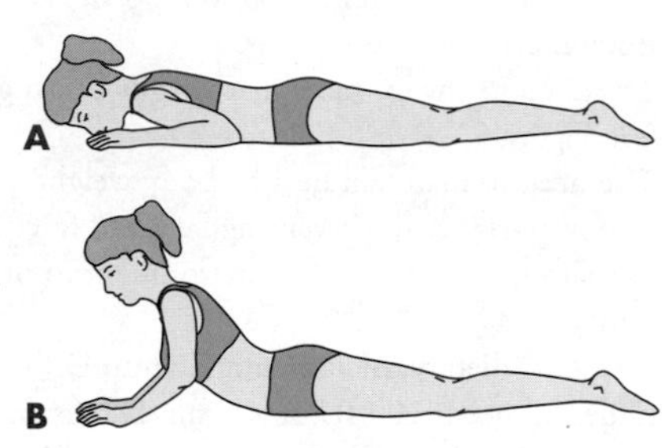

Prone Press-ups with Deep Breathing
Start out in a conventional "push-up" position **(A).** Arch your back, pinching your shoulder blades together **(B).** As you push up, inhale; as you lie down, exhale. Keep elbows partially bent to protect the back. Make sure you don't lift your pelvis.

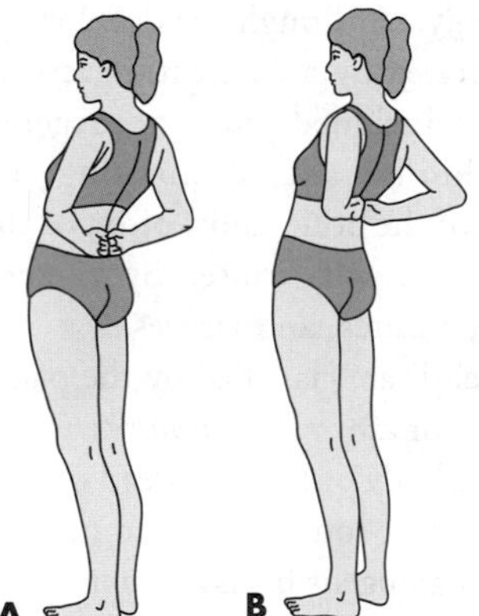

Standing Back Bend
Put your fists on your lower back. Arch backwards slowly while taking a deep breath **(A).** Relax and put your arms down, then repeat, this time with the fists on the middle back **(B).**

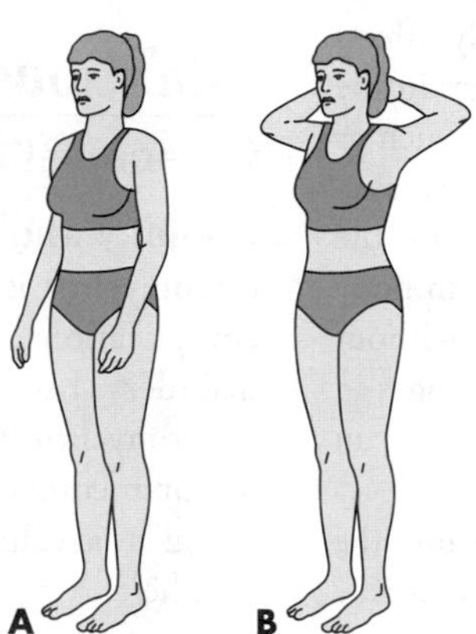

Isometric Posture Correction
Stand as tall as you can, with your chin in, not up **(A).** Place your palms against the back of your head. Simultaneously push your hands against your head while pinching your shoulder blades together **(B).** Hold for 3 seconds, then relax for 3 seconds. Maintain an erect posture throughout the exercise.

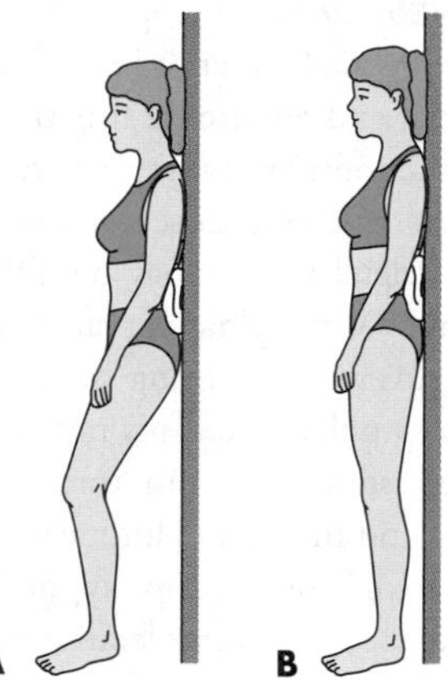

Standing and Pelvic Tilt
Stand with your feet about a foot from the wall, with your knees slightly bent and your back straight **(A).** Use a towel to support your lower back. Slide up and down, keeping the back straight and the stomach muscles contracted. You should be able to plant your feet closer to the wall as you improve **(B).**

Figure 53-9 Exercises for prevention of osteoporosis.

include sinus, ear, dental, respiratory, and genitourinary infections. In hematogenous osteomyelitis the infection spreads from the bone to the soft tissues and can eventually break through the skin, becoming a draining fistula. This type of osteomyelitis is more common in infants, children, and older adults. Among older adults, men are more commonly affected than women. Again, *S. aureus* is the most common causative organism. Other responsible organisms include streptococcus B, *H. influenzae,* salmonellae, and gram-negative bacteria. Salmonella is linked with sickle cell anemia, and gram-negative organisms are associated with infections occurring in older and immunocompromised individuals. Acute osteomyelitis left untreated or unresolved after 10 days is considered chronic osteomyelitis. Osteomyelitis of long bones can also be categorized by the stages of infection (Box 53-6).[58]

Pathophysiology. Pathologic mechanisms of osteomyelitis are inflammation and destruction of bone, bone necrosis, and formation of new bone. Necrotic bone is the distinguishing feature of chronic osteomyelitis. In hematogenous osteomyelitis the organisms reach the bone through the circulatory and lymphatic systems. The bacteria lodge in the small vessels of the bone, triggering an inflammatory response. Blockage of the vessel causes thrombosis, ischemia, and necrosis of the bone. The femur, tibia, humerus, and radius are commonly affected. Infections of the pelvic organs often spread to the pelvis and vertebrae. The pathophysiology of osteomyelitis is similar to that of infectious processes in any other body tissue.

Bone inflammation is marked by edema, increased vasculature, and leukocyte activity. Exudate seals the bone's canaliculi, extends into the metaphysis and marrow cavity, and finally reaches the cortex. New bone, laid down over the infected bone by osteoblasts, is referred to as **involucrum**. Openings in the involucrum allow infected material to escape into soft tissues. The infectious process weakens the cortex, thereby increasing the risk of pathologic fracture. **Brodie's abscesses** are characteristic of chronic osteomyelitis. These are isolated, encapsulated pockets of microorganisms surrounded by bone matrix, usually found in long bones. These pockets of virulent organisms are capable of reinfection at any time. The microscopic channels found in bone allow bacteria to proliferate without being affected by the body's defenses.

In patients with exogenous osteomyelitis the infection begins in the soft tissues, disrupting muscle and connective tissue, and eventually forming abscesses. Signs and symptoms associated with soft tissue infection are most common.

Chronic osteomyelitis is difficult to treat. Recurrent infection, areas of dead bone **(sequestrum)**, and scar tissue are contributing factors to its resistance to treatment. Complications of chronic osteomyelitis include sepsis, nonunion, draining fistulas, shortening of the affected extremity, and eventually amputation.

The clinical manifestations of osteomyelitis vary with the individual, type of responsible organism, precipitating event, and type of infection (acute or chronic). The patient may report fever, malaise, anorexia, and headache. The affected body part may be erythematous, tender, and edematous. There may be a fistula draining purulent material.

Box 53-6 Classification of Long Bone Osteomyelitis by Cierny-Mader System

- *Stage 1: Medullary*—Necrosis limited to medullary canal and endosteal surfaces
- *Stage 2: Superficial*—Bone necrosis only on exposed surface
- *Stage 3: Localized*—Bone stable; sequestrum through one cortex; well-marginated infection
- *Stage 4: Diffuse*—Unstable bone, infection all around bone, through both cortices

Collaborative Care Management. Blood tests reveal an increase in white blood cells, erythrocyte sedimentation rate, and C-reactive protein levels. A culture and sensitivity test of the drainage reveals the causative organisms, allowing identification of appropriate antibiotic therapy. Blood cultures determine the presence or absence of septicemia. MRI and a radionuclide bone scan may be performed. Pathologic changes are visible after the infection has been present for 7 to 10 days.

Treatment is difficult and costly. The goals are complete removal of dead bone and affected soft tissue, control of infection, and elimination of dead space (after removal of necrotic bone). Treatment depends on the area of bone involved, causative organism, ability to maintain a functional limb, and expected outcomes. Other considerations include ensuring adequate soft tissue coverage and restoring blood supply.

Debridement surgery to remove necrotic tissue is the foundation of management for osteomyelitis. Debridement involves removal of sequestrum and surrounding granulation tissue. Surgical excision of the bone must be adequate to ensure eradication of the causative organism. Debridement often results in a bony defect or dead space. Techniques to fill the dead space include flaps, antibiotic beads, and bone grafts. The goal is to replace necrotic bone and scar tissue with vascularized tissue. Wound closure is done whenever possible; healing by secondary intention is avoided because of the risk of decreased vascular supply to scar tissue.[58]

Irrigation and drainage systems, once popular for management, are not recommended because of the high incidence of nosocomial infection.[58] Temporary placement of polymethylmethacrylate antibiotic beads in the wound can be used to stabilize and temporarily maintain dead space.[58] Agents commonly used include vancomycin, tobramycin, and gentamicin. An implantable pump can also be used to deliver antibiotics directly to the wound. Placement of antibiotic beads offers higher drug levels at the infection site than with systemic administration. The wound is closed and covered; the beads are usually removed after 2 to 4 weeks, and then reconstruction is performed. Soft tissue defects can be repaired with a split-thickness skin graft; larger defects may require flaps and vascularized muscle flaps.

Other options include the use of allograft bone and stabilization by external or internal fixation. The Ilizarov technique (see Chapter 52) can be used for difficult cases, nonunion, and large bone defects. Prevention of infection is crucial. The Papineau technique consists of removal of infected and necrotic bone, immobilization (usually achieved by an external fixator [see Chapter 52]), delayed cancellous bone grafts, and, finally, soft tissue closure. This technique is used to treat osteomyelitis in the diaphysis of long bones and has been highly successful in the treatment of chronic osteomyelitis.

Revascularization procedures, including local pedicle flaps and myocutaneous flaps, are commonly performed for recurrent osteomyelitis. Hyperbaric oxygen treatments have been used for gas gangrene and chronic osteomyelitis and should be an adjunct to surgical and antibiotic therapy.[58]

The choice of antibiotic therapy depends on the causative organism, which is verified by culture and sensitivity. Most treatment involves 2 to 4 weeks of intravenous therapy, followed by 4 weeks of oral medication. Antibiotic-resistant organisms present a challenge to treatment. Three to 6 months of therapy may be necessary for infections related to orthopedic implants.[58]

Essential to the nursing management of the patient with osteomyelitis is the use of aseptic technique during dressing changes. The nurse observes the patient for signs and symptoms of systemic infection, and administers antibiotics on time and as prescribed. The nurse also administers prescribed analgesics and antipyretics and monitors the patient for their effectiveness. Rest of the affected joint or limb is promoted, and the affected extremity is handled carefully to avoid pathologic fracture. Splints are often used for immobilization.

The nurse encourages ROM exercises to prevent contractures and flexion deformities; promotes participation in ADLs to the fullest extent possible; and instructs the patient in the correct use of assistive devices as needed.

Patient/Family Teaching. If home-going antibiotic therapy is prescribed, the nurse teaches the proper administration of medications. A peripherally inserted central catheter or implanted vascular access device allows for long-term venous access. The nurse instructs the patient and family in care of the insertion site and catheter, discusses drug side effects, and teaches aseptic technique. Long-term antibiotic therapy can be performed at home with the help of a home health nurse. The patient and family can also administer antibiotics with periodic visits by the nurse. Dressing changes may also be performed at home.

Persons with total joint implants need instruction regarding the signs and symptoms of infection and how to avoid sources of infection. The patient with an acute infection is instructed to avoid the use of heat and exercise, which increase circulation and may spread infection. The nurse offers information regarding follow-up care.

If surgery is performed, the nurse provides perioperative instructions. Persons with radical resections, flaps, external fixators, or amputations need emotional support in accepting body image changes and decreased mobility and independence. The patient and family need support in coping with a chronic illness, which may lead to depression. The patient and family may need support and referrals for financial assistance, particularly if they lack insurance or have insufficient coverage.

Disorders Affecting the Spine

Lower Back Pain

Etiology and Epidemiology. LBP is one the most common conditions a nurse encounters in any practice setting. Although a common disorder, LBP is also a challenge to health care professionals. Ninety percent of Americans have at least one episode of LBP in their lifetime.[10] Second only to the respiratory problems in the number of primary care office visits and time lost from work, LBP is also a major cause of permanent work disability.[10,14] LBP is the major cause of disability in persons under 45 years.

LBP is a challenge to the health care professional because it is a symptom that is not usually attributable to a specific cause or disease. Eighty percent of cases of LBP are idiopathic. Indeed, in approximately 80% of persons with LBP without neurologic symptoms, the pain resolves within 4 to 6 weeks without specific treatment.[22] However, 15% to 20% of patients develop pain resulting in functional limitations.[22] LBP may be attributable to a specific cause, including a herniated disc, spinal stenosis, compression fracture, systemic disease related to the spine, and systemic disease unrelated to the spine.

Common systemic conditions related to LBP include malignancy and infection. Persons in whom a systemic cause of LBP should be suspected include those younger than 20 years of age or older than 50 years of age and those with a history of cancer, fever or chills, and unexplained weight loss. Other symptoms that require immediate attention include severe pain, significant neurologic deficit, sensory loss in the saddle area, abdominal pain, and trauma.

LBP affects the area below the ribs and gluteal muscles, often radiating to the thigh, and can be acute or chronic. The most common cause is a lumbar strain after lifting or twisting. More men than women are affected by back pain; postmenopausal women have a higher incidence than premenopausal women.[40] Risk factors associated with LBP include occupational hazards (repetitive motions, prolonged exposure to vibrations, and forward bending and twisting motions of the spine), smoking, osteoporosis, and hyperthyroidism.

Pathophysiology. The pathophysiology of common causes of back pain, including herniated disc, spinal stenosis, and spondylolisthesis, is discussed in the following sections. If disc herniation is the cause of back pain, the pain comes from the irritated dura and spinal nerves, since the nucleus pulposus lacks intrinsic innervation. Pain can arise from the joint capsule, ligaments, or muscles in the lumbar spine. The ligamentous structures of the lumbar spine are richly supplied with pain receptors and are susceptible to tears, sprains, and fracture. Muscle sprains and strains are also common causes of back pain. See Chapter 16 for a discussion of the theories of pain.

Back pain may be accompanied by radicular symptoms or sciatica. Radicular pain is caused by compression of a nerve root. Differentiating radicular pain from LBP and referred pain is important in establishing a diagnosis and treatment plan.

Collaborative Care Management. A detailed history and complete physical examination are required for accurate diagnosis and treatment of the person with LBP. The nurse asks the patient about any associated symptoms, any neurologic deficits, and any loss of bowel or bladder control. Bowel or bladder symptoms should alert the health care provider to the possibility of *cauda equina syndrome,* which requires emergency surgical intervention. Cauda equina syndrome is compression of the caudal sac by herniated disc material. Abdominal pain may suggest an abdominal aortic aneurysm.

The physical examination should include neurologic assessment, ROM, and muscle testing. The nurse evaluates the lower extremities for any asymmetry in neurologic function. Calf and thigh circumference are measured; inequality may indicate muscle atrophy caused by neurologic deficit. Limits in forward flexion are commonly found, with localized pain in the lumbosacral area. The nurse should also screen for malignancy. Specialized tests, including straight leg raising (see Chapter 51) and crossed leg raising, are incorporated into the examination. The nurse performs a complete assessment of the pain. The patient's descriptors are important in determining the effect of pain on his or her lifestyle.

Routine laboratory examinations are not indicated. Controversy exists regarding the appropriateness of ordering x-ray studies at the first visit. Federal guidelines recommend a conservative approach. Many cases of back pain resolve; hence delaying diagnostics may avoid unnecessary expense and radiation exposure. Plain films are recommended only for persons over age 50, those with symptoms suggestive of systemic disease, and persons with radiculopathy.[10] CT scans and MRI are indicated for persons with neurologic compromise, surgical candidates, or those in whom malignancy or fracture is suspected.[10]

Most persons with LBP respond well to conservative therapy. Only 1% to 2% of patients require surgical intervention.[40] A multidisciplinary approach is necessary. Patients benefit from an early return to work and physical activity. Prolonged bed rest and missed work are actually harmful, reinforcing the concept of illness and disability. Bed rest is limited to 2 or 3 days for patients with radiculopathy. For those without neurologic symptoms bed rest is not recommended, or at most is recommended for 1 or 2 days. Management strategies using the least amount of analgesics and fewest activity restrictions have been shown to have the best outcomes.[10]

Back exercises to strengthen lumbar musculature are indicated for treatment of LBP. Stretching and extension exercises have shown positive results, whereas flexion exercises are of little benefit. A PT referral is beneficial to instruct patients in proper performance of exercises.

The application of heat or cold within 48 hours of the onset of symptoms or heat for symptoms persisting over 48 hours is effective in reducing pain. Massage therapy provides temporary relief for some patients. Traction, transcutaneous electrical nerve stimulation, acupuncture, and ultrasound have not been proven effective in clinical trials.[10,61] Other treatments include trigger-point therapy and spinal manipulation. Chiropractic treatment is contraindicated for patients with radiculopathy. See Chapter 16 for other nonpharmacologic methods of pain control.

Pharmacologic treatments include NSAIDs, analgesics, and adjuvants. Muscle relaxants may be used in combination with NSAIDs.[10] Topical medications for local pain relief may be effective for some persons. Steroid injections have also been used with some success. Implantable pumps to deliver intrathecal or epidural opioids have been used for persons with chronic pain, who are usually managed by a chronic pain specialist.

Interventions addressing psychosocial needs are important in the management of persons with LBP. Some persons are motivated by secondary gain, making treatment difficult. Depression and substance abuse are common and should trigger a referral to a psychologist or counselor for additional therapy. Persons whose pain has persisted for longer than 3 months may need referral for management of chronic pain. Cognitive coping strategies have been used effectively by patients with chronic pain. Their positive perceptions of their self-efficacy may assist them in implementing strategies to relieve pain and cope with a chronic pain condition. Reassurance that most persons with back pain respond favorably to conservative treatment and are able to return to work and leisure activities can help decrease anxiety about the long-term effects of pain.

PATIENT/FAMILY TEACHING. The patient and family need education about the pathogenesis of back pain, particularly if no specific cause is found. If appropriate, the nurse gives information about lifestyle changes such as cessation of smoking, weight loss, and regular exercise. Body weight should be maintained within 10% of the ideal body weight. If environmental conditions such as occupational hazards are contributing to the LBP, perhaps the work environment can be modified. In some cases employment retraining may be indicated. Ergonomics should be incorporated into the design of the worksite.

Providing information about proper body mechanics and methods to avoid back injury is important. The nurse instructs the patient on the proper way to sit, stand, bend, and lift objects to prevent further injury (see Figure 53-8). When seated, the patient should have the feet flat on the floor or stool. The knees should be higher than the hips with the arms supported. When lifting, the patient should bend the knees, not the back, and lift objects no higher than the level of the elbows. While sleeping supine, the patient should place a pillow under the knees and use a firm mattress or bedboard for adequate support.

Information to prevent further episodes of back pain allows patients to take responsibility for managing their pain. Many back pain clinics have a "back school," where patients are taught principles of body mechanics, posture, and exercises. They should do regular aerobic exercise in addition to back-strengthening exercises (Figure 53-10) for at least 30 minutes five times per week. Walking and swimming are good choices. Some persons may believe that exercise will do further harm to the back; they need reassurance and encouragement to participate in a regular exercise program.

Support groups may help the individual with LBP. Exercising at community centers provides companionship. For persons with chronic pain, a referral to a pain support group may be indicated. Information can be obtained from the American Pain Society.

Degenerative Disorders of the Spine

A number of degenerative disorders that affect the cervical, thoracic, and lumbar portions of the spine are treated by surgical intervention. The collaborative care and nursing management sections pertain to persons with any of these disorders.

Etiology and Epidemiology. Degenerative disease of the spine is a common but difficult problem. The spine has 23 intervertebral disc joints and 46 posterior facet joints (Figure 53-11), all of which are subjected to stresses and strains in holding the human body upright and moving it about. The vertebrae in the spinal column are articulated in a series of "couplets" that are able to move through an intervertebral disc joint and two posterior facet joints. The intervertebral discs are composed of an outer

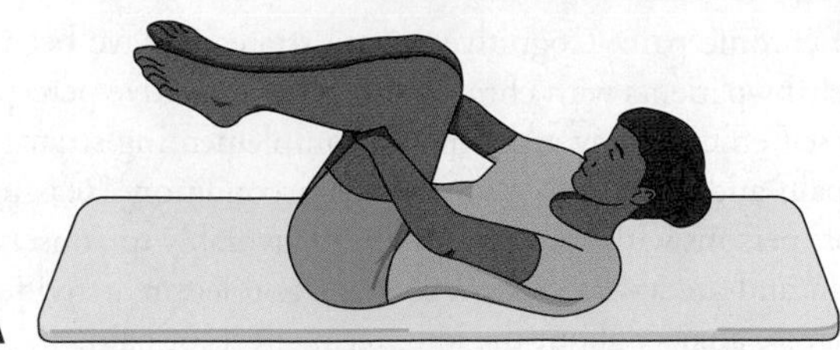

Back Roll

The back roll stretches your back, buttocks, and neck muscles. Lie on your back on the floor, relax, and bring your knees to your chest. Clasp your hands behind your knee and rock back and forth, from your buttocks to your neck. Slowly return to the starting position. Repeat 5 to 10 times.

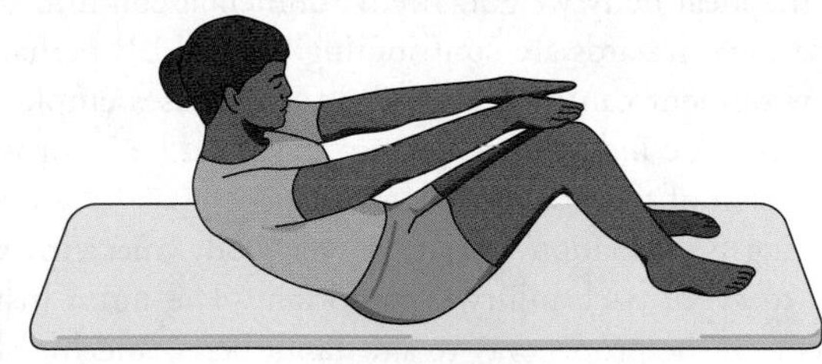

Partial Sit-ups

Partial sit-ups strengthen your abdominal muscles. Lie flat on your back on the floor with your knees bent and feet flat on the floor. Tuck in your chin and tighten your abdomen. Slowly raise your head and neck while reaching out with your hands to touch your knees. Hold your knees for a count of five and slowly return to the starting position. Repeat 5 to 10 times.

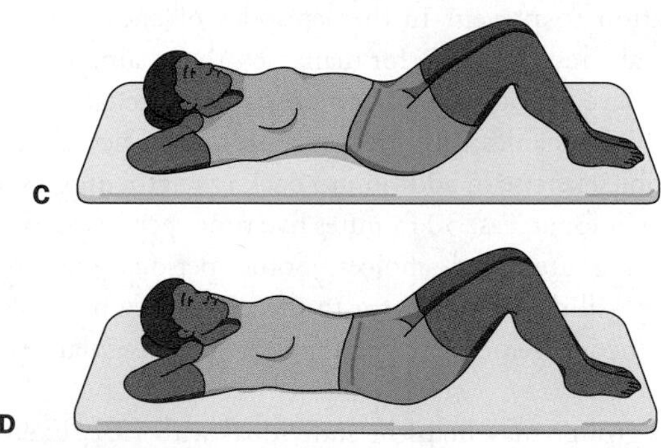

Pelvic Tilt

The pelvic tilt strengthens your abdominal and back muscles. Lie flat on your back on the floor with your knees bent and feet flat on the floor. Join your hands behind your head. Firmly tighten your buttock and abdominal muscles, pressing your lower back flat against the floor. Hold for a count of five and relax muscles. Repeat 5 to 10 times.

Figure 53-10 Exercises for lower back pain. **A**, Back roll. **B**, Partial sit-ups. **C** and **D**, Pelvic tilt.

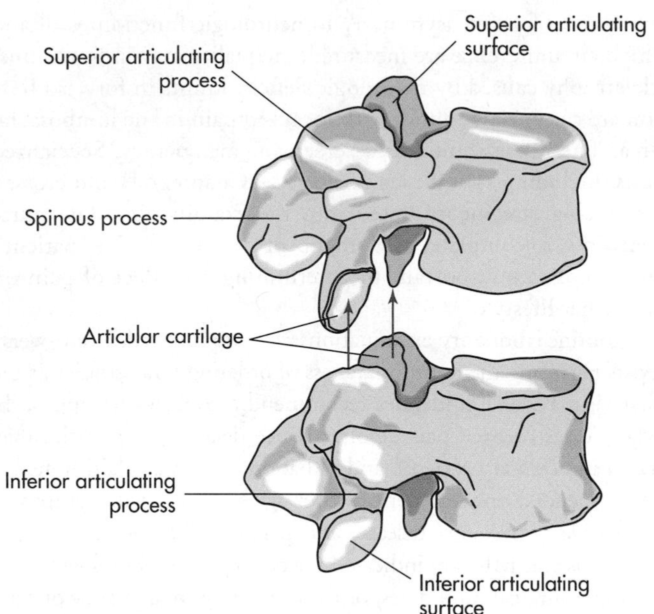

Figure 53-11 Posterior facet joints of lumbar vertebrae. Each vertebra has four surfaces—two on its superior aspect and two on the inferior—by which it articulates with adjacent vertebrae. Superior articulating surfaces are medially located; inferior articulating surfaces are laterally located. These joints are diarthrotic, having a joint capsule with a synovial lining.

layer of cartilage called the annulus fibrosus and an inner layer called the nucleus pulposus. Several common problems arise with these structures in degenerative disease of the spine. These include degenerative disc disease, herniated intervertebral disc, spinal stenosis, spondylolisthesis, and spondylosis.

Degenerative disc disease develops as a result of biochemical and biomechanical changes in the intervertebral discs. The gelatinous mucoid material of the nucleus pulposus is replaced with fibrocartilage as a result of aging. The disc's water content also decreases with aging.

Spinal stenosis occurs as a result of aging, degenerative disc disease, spondylosis, osteophyte formation, or a congenital condition. The disc space is narrowed and less resilient and may be unstable at the affected levels. Smoking is a risk factor for the development of disc degeneration and herniation. Other identified risk factors include a sedentary lifestyle and extensive motor vehicle driving.

Spondylosis is degeneration of the vertebrae; it may occur in the cervical, thoracic, or lumbar spine. It is often accompanied by arthritic changes, including osteophyte formation, ligamentous disruption, and subluxation.

Degenerative disorders of the spine develop most commonly in persons over 50 years of age. Cervical spondylosis is generally found in persons over 55 years of age. Disc herniation is seen in persons of all ages, but the peak incidence is between 35 and 45 years of age.

Pathophysiology. Pathophysiologic changes associated with degenerative disc disease include spinal stenosis (narrowing of the spinal canal), spondylosis (degeneration and stiffness of the vertebral joints), subluxation, and vertebral degeneration. Initial disc changes are followed by facet arthropathy, osteophyte formation, and ligamentous instability. Myelopathy and **radiculopathy** (disease involving a spinal nerve root) may follow. The degenerative process usually involves synovitis, which causes cartilage erosion, leading to the formation of osteophytes. Disc degeneration begins with water loss from the nucleus pulposus, resulting in loss of disc height.

Herniated intervertebral disc is a protrusion of the nucleus pulposus through a tear or rupture in the annulus. Herniation can occur anteriorly, posteriorly, or laterally. Extrusion of the disc material may impinge on a nerve root or on the spinal cord (Figure 53-12). Herniation may occur as a result of trauma, a sharp or sudden movement, or degeneration. In the cervical spine, herniation usually occurs at the more mobile segments—C5-C6, C6-C7, and C4-C5. Most lumbar herniations occur at the L5-S1 and L4-L5 levels.[59] Herniation of thoracic discs is less common. Symptoms may develop immediately or take years to manifest. The location and size of the herniation determines the signs and symptoms associated with it (see Clinical Manifestations box). Pain associated with disc herniation may be caused by direct pressure of disc fragments on the nerve root, by breakdown products from a degenerated nucleus pulposus, or by an autoimmune reaction. The nurse's knowledge of dermatomes and spinal nerve innervation aids in the assessment of a patient with a herniated intervertebral disc (Table 53-10). Another consideration is the size of the patient's spinal canal. A slight herniation may cause significant symptoms in an individual with a congenitally narrow canal.

Spinal stenosis is a narrowing of the spinal canal, intervertebral foramina, or nerve root canal at any level of the spine, creating pressure on the involved nerve root(s), resulting in neurologic symptoms. The narrowing may occur at single or multiple levels. Spinal stenosis results from hyperplasia and cartilaginous changes in the ligamentum flavum, laminae, and facet joints. Anatomic abnormalities may also contribute to spinal stenosis. The condition can be congenital, acquired, or a combination. Osteophyte formation may cause neuroforaminal stenosis, resulting in joint instability and subluxation.

Spondylolisthesis is an anterior or posterior slippage of one vertebral body on another. It can be a congenital abnormality or caused by degenerative changes, trauma, or bone disease. Spondylolysis or a structural defect in the lamina is often the cause. The pars interarticularis (between the superior and inferior articular facets) is usually the site of the defect. The degree of spondylolisthesis is graded on a scale of 1 to 4, depending on the percentage of slip that is shown on x-ray films of the spine. Grades 3 and 4 are usually treated surgically. Spondylolisthesis usually occurs at L5-S1. The forward slip of the vertebra can cause nerve impingement, manifested by motor and sensory deficits at the level(s) involved, such as pain, weakness, or bowel and bladder involvement. The slip may be detected when the spinous processes are palpated.

Cauda equina ("horse's tail") syndrome may occur after trauma, spinal stenosis, fracture, tumor, or disc herniation. Pressure on the

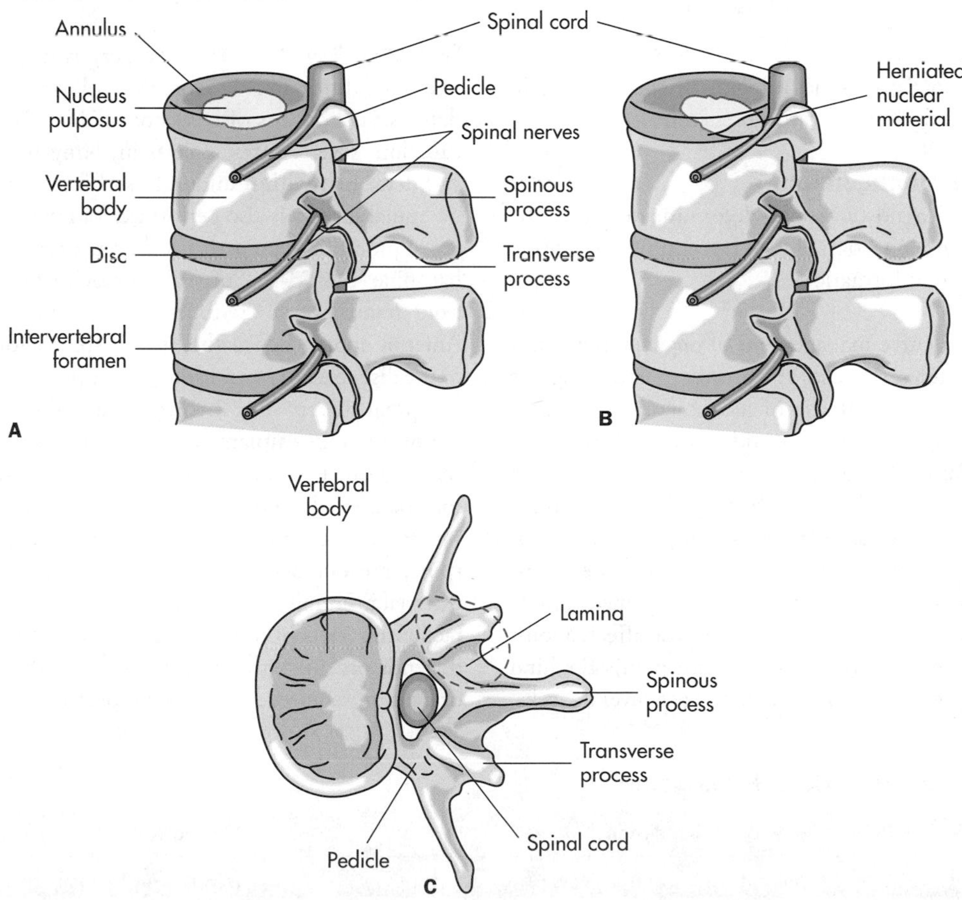

Figure 53-12 Compression of spinal cord and nerve root. **A**, Discs, composed of a cartilaginous outer layer (anulu fibrosus) and a gel-like inner layer (nucleus pulposus), lie between vertebral bodies. Spinal nerves exit spinal cord laterally just above pedicle. **B**, Laminae compose posterior portions of vertebrae. Each pedicle joins with a lamina; transverse and spinous processes project from laminae. **C**, When nucleus pulposus herniates posteriorly through its fibrous covering and the posterior longitudinal ligament, it may compress the spinal cord and trap the nerve root. The surgical approach to relieve this compression is through lamina *(dotted line)*, posterior to transverse process.

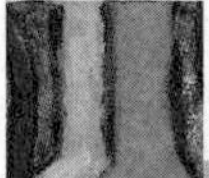
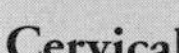

CLINICAL MANIFESTATIONS
Herniated Intervertebral Disc

Cervical

Decreased range of motion of cervical spine
Paresthesias of upper extremities, depending on nerve root involved
Weakness or atrophy of upper extremity musculature, depending on level involved
Pain in affected nerve root distribution
Abdominal reflex activity
Possible motor or sensory disturbances in lower extremities

Lumbar

Sciatica in 40% of persons
Tenderness or pain with palpation of disc spaces and sciatic notch
Pain or decreased range of motion of lumbar spine
Motor and sensory impairment in affected nerve root distribution (possible discrepancies in calf circumference, weakness in lower extremity muscle groups, pain and numbness in dermatomal distribution)
Decreased or absent reflexes
Bowel or bladder impairment
Positive straight leg raising (Lasègue's sign): straight leg raising with opposite leg flat producing leg pain or radicular symptoms
Pain radiating down leg in dermatomal distribution
Pain relieved by lying down

cauda equina nerve roots causes neurologic deficits, varying in intensity, depending on the degree of compression.

Collaborative Care Management

DIAGNOSTIC TESTS. Diagnostic tests to determine defects in the spine include x-ray films, myelography, CT scanning, and MRI. See Chapter 51 for more information.

MEDICATIONS. Conservative management of degenerative problems of the spine includes the use of antiinflammatory agents (usually NSAIDs). Concomitant use of alcohol or aspirin may increase GI irritation and bleeding tendencies and therefore should be avoided. Pain relief is usually noted after 1 week of therapy. If not, opioids should be prescribed. Oral corticosteroids are useful for treating pain for short periods; long-term use is not recommended. Steroids may also be prescribed for acute symptoms of cauda equina syndrome. Antiinflammatory medications or local anesthetics may be injected directly into the affected joint or structure (epidural space to relieve nerve root pain). Epidural steroid injections are given in a series of three over several weeks. The use of steroid injections should be limited because of adverse effects on tissue healing.

Skeletal muscle relaxants may also be prescribed. The nurse cautions the patient against driving or engaging in potentially hazardous activities because of drowsiness, a frequent side effect of muscle relaxants. The nurse also informs the patient that alcohol or other CNS depressants will increase the effects of the muscle relaxant. Muscle relaxants often cause dry mouth, and the nurse instructs the patient in measures to counteract this side effect.

DIET. Although a special diet is not indicated for the treatment of degenerative disorders of the spine, weight reduction may be advised. The patient should try to attain or maintain ideal body weight to decrease the mechanical stressors on the back, as well as other joints. If surgical intervention is necessary, obesity adds risks to the perioperative period, including delayed wound healing and increased risk of thrombophlebitis.[8]

TREATMENTS. Conservative treatment is implemented initially (see discussion under Lower Back Pain). Pain control and return to functioning are the goals of treatment. Conservative management is given a trial before surgical intervention is considered, unless neurologic deficits are present. Corsets or braces are sometimes prescribed to provide external support to the spine, especially during physical activity. Braces and corsets are fitted by an orthotist.

SURGICAL MANAGEMENT. Surgery is indicated when conservative modalities fail or for the following reasons: neurologic deficits, such as loss of bowel or bladder control or loss of motor function; severe, intractable pain; bony instability; and progressive deformity with resultant loss of function.

Spinal surgery is also performed for fractures and tumors. A variety of procedures are performed on the cervical, thoracic, and lumbar spine (Box 53-7). Surgical approaches to the spine include anterior, transthoracic, retroperitoneal, and posterior approaches. Anterior approaches to the lumbar spine allow direct visualization of the disc space. The transthoracic approach involves thoracotomy.

Spinal surgery may involve the use of instrumentation. A variety of different implants are available, using rods, cables, plates, screws, pedicle screws, metal cages, and hooks. Instrumentation may be used alone or with bone graft or bone substitutes. Instrumentation can maintain correction of deformity, stabilize the spine, prevent neurologic damage, enhance bony fusion, avoid external immobilization, and allow for early mobilization, thereby facilitating rehabilitation. The type of instrumentation used depends on the pathologic condition, individual patient, degree of fixation required, and surgeon preference.

TABLE 53-10 Lumbar Disc Herniation

Level of Herniation	Nerve Root	Reflex	Sensation	Muscle Testing
L3-L4	L4	Patellar	Medial aspects of leg and foot	Inversion of foot (tibialis anterior)
L4-L5	L5	—	Lateral aspect of leg and dorsal surface of foot	Extension of toes (extensor hallucis longus)
L5-S1	S1	Achilles	Lateral aspect of foot	Eversion of foot (peroneus longus, brevis)

Box 53-7 Types of Spinal Surgery

- *Laminectomy:* Removal of a portion of the lamina, the posterior arch of the vertebra, to gain access to the disc and spinal canal
- *Diskectomy:* Removal of all or part of a herniated intervertebral disc; performed via open incision, microdiskectomy, or endoscopic approach
- *Foraminotomy:* Widening of the intervertebral foramen to allow free passage of the spinal nerve
- *Spinal fusion:* Stabilization of two or more vertebrae by insertion of bone grafts with or without the addition of hardware (rods, plates, screws, cages, or disc prostheses) to achieve vertebral stability
- *Decompression:* Release of pressure or impingement on spinal nerve roots by removal of osteophytes, bone, or soft tissue

When bone grafts are used, they function as a form of scaffolding into which osteogenic cells grow and/or as a means of mechanical support. Autograft, allograft, or bone substitute may be used for grafting. The success of the bone graft depends partially on the type of fixation of the graft and the site and condition of the host recipient.

Both cortical and cancellous bone can serve as graft material. Allogeneic and autologous cortical grafts both initially act as weight-bearing struts to provide support until the host bone has incorporated and remodeled the graft and is able to bear weight. Freshly implanted autografts are capable of osteogenesis, the process of bone synthesis by graft or host cells. Cancellous bone, because of its larger surface area, has greater potential for osteogenesis than does cortical bone. Host bone is produced by osteoconduction, a process in which mesenchymal cells of the host differentiate into osteoblasts.

Initially all types of bone graft are partially resorbed. Incorporation of the bone graft takes place in overlapping stages. It begins by **creeping substitution** (gradual resorption of the graft) and finally results in replacement of the graft by new bone. Both autografts and allografts produce an acute inflammatory response within the first week, followed by the formation of fibrous granulation tissue and an increase in osteoclastic activity. This is followed by osteoinduction, which is probably regulated by bone morphogenic protein, which promotes new bone production by the host. Bone morphogenic protein is present in fresh autografts and in modified allografts, but autoclaving for sterilization destroys it. Osteoinduction is followed by osteoconduction, characterized by capillary growth and infiltration of the graft by perivascular tissue and osteoprogenitor cells of the host. This process may last for several months in cancellous autografts and for years in cortical autografts or allografts. Cancellous grafts are eventually completely replaced, whereas cortical grafts remain a mixture of necrotic graft bone and viable host bone. As remodeling takes place, the graft is resorbed and replaced by living bone, subject to Wolff's law.

Advantages of autografts are tissue compatibility and low cost. Disadvantages include a limited supply of bone, a weakened donor site with a potential for fracture, and an added surgical site that can cause considerable pain. The most common sites for graft harvesting are the iliac crests and the fibulae.

Advantages of allografts are fewer surgical sites and thus less pain. Allografts also come in a variety of sizes and shapes. Disadvantages include a limited and costly supply and a high graft failure rate. Allografts trigger local and systemic immune responses that may affect their failure rate. Freezing and freeze-drying implants have decreased rejection rates.

Surgical techniques have evolved to replace the traditional open approach to spinal surgery and instrumentation. Total disc arthroplasty is a new procedure performed for degenerative disc diseases (see Future Watch box). Microdiskectomy involves a surgical incision, but one that is much smaller than that with the open approach. The use of MRI and other imaging techniques allows direct access to the disc through a very small incision. Decompression and disc removal can be accomplished with less exposure and thus less pain and a shorter hospital stay. The surgeon must have considerable experience to perform the procedure with limited exposure. The success rates for open diskectomy and microdiskectomy are equal.

Endoscopic approach to spine surgery is a minimally invasive technique allowing the surgeon to perform diskectomy, decompression, and fusion through endoscopic portals. These procedures are most commonly performed on the thoracic or lumbar spine. Procedures performed without fusion can usually be done on an outpatient basis. Patients undergoing endoscopic fusions can expect a 1- to 3-day hospital stay. Persons with multilevel disease or previous spinal surgery may not be candidates for these techniques.

COMPLICATIONS. Complications associated with general anesthesia are important considerations after surgery. These include

Future Watch

Total Disc Replacement Arthroplasty

Degenerative disc disease (DDD) is traditionally treated conservatively. Patients who have neurologic deficits or are unresponsive to conservative treatment are usually treated with spinal fusion with or without instrumentation. Although fusion is usually effective in relieving pain, there is loss of motion at the fusion site and an increased risk of developing DDD above or below the fused levels.

An alternative is total disc arthroplasty for disease of the cervical and lumbar spine. The Food and Drug Administration approved the Charité artificial disc for treatment of lumbar DDD at L4 to S1; other designs are in clinical trials in the United States and Europe. A prosthetic disc is implanted at the level of disc disease, allowing more natural function and motion. A variety of prostheses are available: Aeroflex, SB Charité, ProDisc II, Flexcore, and the Maverick Disc. Although long-term data are not available, researchers believe these alternatives pose less risk of developing disease in adjacent levels.

The surgical approach is anterior, transperitoneal, or retroperitoneal for lumbar replacements. Postoperative care is similar to that following anterior interbody fusion, although rehabilitation differs significantly. Motion of the spine is encouraged within 2 weeks of the surgery, and exercises are initiated as soon as the incision is healed. Patient satisfaction is reportedly high following this new procedure.

From Rodts MF: Total disc replacement arthroplasty, *Orthop Nurs* 23(3):216-218, 2004.

atelectasis, paralytic ileus, and urinary retention. Infection is a complication associated with the operative procedure. When instrumentation is used, the risk for infection increases. There is also a risk for hardware failure.

Posterior approaches to the spine are performed using a variety of frames and positioning devices, with the patient in the prone position. Potential complications from positioning techniques and lengthy procedures include pooling of blood in the lower extremities; pressure areas on the knees, forehead, chest, and other bony prominences; and neuropathies as a result of local ischemia caused by prolonged pressure.

Complications of the procedure and the postoperative period include dural tear and cerebrospinal fluid leakage, blood loss, hypovolemia and decreased cardiac output, hematoma formation, infection, instrumentation or graft failure, pseudarthrosis, loss of correction of deformity, persistence of pain or deficits, neurologic impairment or loss, deep venous thrombosis (DVT), pulmonary embolism, fluid volume overload, and fat embolism.

Monitoring of sensory evoked potentials is a common method of reducing injury to the neural elements intraoperatively. Before surgery begins, electrodes are placed on the patient's scalp and extremities. Baseline data are collected, and impulse transmissions through the posterior columns of the spinal cord are monitored throughout the procedure. Any changes indicate possible injury, and the patient is given a "wake-up test." The level of anesthesia is lightened sufficiently to allow the patient to follow commands to move the extremities. Inability to do these tasks is considered indicative of neurologic impairment. This monitoring technique allows the surgeon to explore, ascertain, and possibly correct the cause of neurologic loss before closing the incision.

A complication often occurring in the postoperative period of patients undergoing spinal fusion is the syndrome of inappropriate antidiuretic hormone (SIADH). Contributing factors include decreased blood volume, the use of anesthetic agents and analgesics, and physical and emotional stressors. Postoperative monitoring of spinal fusion patients should include accurate measurement of intake and output. SIADH should be suspected if the patient has decreased hemoglobin and hematocrit values (which should be normal 2 to 4 days postoperatively) and the blood pressure and pulse remain within the patient's normal range.

Complications associated with approaches to the cervical spine include injury to the blood vessels and laryngeal nerve because of their proximity to the surgical site. Complications associated with surgical correction of thoracic spine disorders include those associated with thoracic surgery (see Chapter 26), since the thoracic cavity is entered through an anterior approach to the thoracic spine.

Complications of fusion include graft failure, infection, and pseudarthrosis. The use of hardware is associated with potential complications, including hardware failure or loosening, infection, damage to neurovascular structures, and adverse reactions to implant materials. Nonunion rates are higher in smokers because smoking retards bone formation by interfering with metabolism and revascularization. Perioperative use of NSAIDs should be avoided in persons having spinal fusion, since their use delays bone formation.[8]

Endoscopic procedures, although less invasive, are also associated with complications, including visceral injury; bleeding; instrument breakage or failure; oxygen retention in the abdomen, chest, or vasculature; hypoxia to local tissues; infection; carbon dioxide absorption; and scar tissue formation.

Nursing Management

of the Patient undergoing Spinal Surgery

Preoperative Care

Preoperative nursing care is similar for persons undergoing all types of spinal surgery. Persons undergoing elective spinal surgery are admitted on the morning of their surgery. Preoperative teaching and testing are completed and evaluated before admission. Depending on the patient's condition, preoperative evaluation may include complete history and physical examination; laboratory work, including complete blood count; urinalysis, blood chemistry, prothrombin time, and partial thromboplastin time; type and screen or cross-matching of blood; chest x-ray films; electrocardiogram; and diagnostic tests related to the spine, such as x-ray films, myelography, CT scans, and MRI. If significant blood loss is expected, autologous donation should be discussed with the patient.

If postoperative bracing is required, an orthotist fits the patient for the brace, fabricates it, and gives instructions for its use before the surgery. Many types of braces are available, depending on the type of procedure performed. Some examples are cervical four-poster braces, a thoracolumbosacral orthosis, and soft corsets.

The nurse provides general preoperative teaching for the patient and family (see Chapter 13). Many patients are curious about the types of implants to be used. If a sample of the instrumentation is available, it may be helpful to show it to the patient. The patient should also be informed about the location and extent of the surgical incision(s). If a spinal fusion with autologous graft is planned, the nurse explains the donor site location and degree of postoperative pain. The patient should also be informed if allograft bone is to be used.

The nurse instructs the patient in performing logrolling technique, isometric exercises, incentive spirometry, and coughing and deep breathing. Instructions are also given regarding general postoperative care, such as postanesthesia care, care of intravenous lines and catheters, vital signs routines, and pain management.

Postoperative Care

Postoperative care of the patient recovering from spinal surgery includes interventions to prevent or minimize complications (see Chapter 15; Nursing Care Plan, p. 1600). If an anterior or lateral approach was used, general care of the patient is as described in Chapters 26 and 43.

Prevention of DVT and pulmonary embolism is an important nursing intervention after surgery. The use of elastic stockings and pneumatic sleeves applied in the operating room is continued after surgery. The nurse instructs patients to perform isometric exercises hourly while awake and administers anticoagulants as prescribed as prophylaxis against DVT and pulmonary embolism. Ambulation is encouraged as soon as possible. The patient is evaluated daily for signs of DVT.

Monitoring of hemoglobin and hematocrit levels is important, especially if the patient experienced extensive blood loss during surgery. The nurse assesses the surgical site and dressing for signs of infection and hemorrhage. Clear drainage may indicate leakage of cerebrospinal fluid and should be reported to the surgeon.

After any spinal procedure, careful monitoring of neurologic function and comparison with baseline function is vital. The nurse performs neurovascular checks of the extremities every hour in the immediate postoperative period and less frequently thereafter. The nurse tests the patient's ability to detect touch and distinguish sharp from dull. Motor strength in the extremities is evaluated, and any changes are reported to the surgeon. Neurologic changes can occur up to 72 hours after surgery. If neurologic deficits were present before surgery, improvement in sensation may not be immediately evident after surgery. Careful assessment to monitor sensation and motor function is essential to detect changes from baseline. Drainage from surgical drains should be assessed and measured. Drains are usually removed after 24 to 36 hours. If a fusion has been done, the nurse assesses the donor site for bleeding.

Urinary retention is common after spinal surgery. If the patient does not have an indwelling catheter, he or she should be assessed for the ability to void. Lying flat in bed can make voiding difficult, particularly for male patients. Patients who have not undergone fusion are usually allowed out of bed the evening of surgery, which may facilitate the ability to void. The physician may order that the patient be catheterized if the patient is unable to void after 8 hours.

Correct positioning of the patient after spinal surgery is important. When turning, patients should be logrolled to keep the spinal column straight. If bracing is required postoperatively, the patient may be in bed without the brace, but must wear it while walking. The patient should sit in a straight-backed chair to avoid twisting the back.

Because of shortened lengths of stay, much of the recovery from spinal surgery takes place at home. Modification of the home environment should be considered if potential hazards exist. Falls and injury can cause neurologic injury or graft displacement.

The patient and family should understand the indications for the prescribed medications and, if opioid analgesics are taken, the precautions associated with administration.

A follow-up appointment with the surgeon (usually 6 weeks after surgery) is necessary to evaluate progress. Before that, a home care nurse may visit in 7 to 10 days to remove any sutures or staples. The patient or family member should evaluate the incision for signs of infection and healing. Dressing changes should be done daily or as needed until the wound is free of drainage, then the incision may remain open to air. Any excessive or purulent drainage should be reported to the physician. A nutritionally adequate diet is recommended to promote wound healing. The patient may require some assistance with meal preparation until energy reserves are restored. Cigarette smoking is not recommended and actually delays bone healing.

Depending on the degree of mobility restrictions, the patient may require assistance with ADLs. Clothing should be loose fitting, especially if worn under a brace. The patient may benefit from long-handled reachers and sponges if back flexion is limited. The occupational therapist can supply these and other assistive devices before discharge. An elevated toilet seat should be obtained. Bathing may be easier if a shower chair is used. If the patient does not have a shower, a sponge bath is best until activity restrictions are lifted.

If bracing is used, the patient and family should be able to demonstrate the proper technique of applying and removing the brace. The nurse teaches the patient to assess the skin for evidence of pressure or breakdown. A cotton T-shirt is worn under the brace.

Once healing is progressing, the nurse recommends an exercise program. Walking is a safe and effective exercise for patients recovering from back surgery. Low-heeled walking shoes with a nonskid sole are a good choice. The patient should resume activities gradually, allowing adequate time for rest and sleep. Driving is usually not permitted until cleared by the surgeon at the 6-week appointment. If a cervical collar is needed, the patient may not drive until the collar is removed. Driving with a halo vest is illegal in most states. When riding in a car as a passenger, the patient should comply with seat belt laws. To avoid injury, proper body mechanics are required for getting in and out of an automobile. The nurse encourages the patient to comply with recommendations for activity and mobility restrictions to prevent dislodging the graft if a fusion was performed. The patient should avoid physical activities that involve bending, twisting, and lifting until cleared by the surgeon. Lifting is generally restricted to objects lighter than 10 pounds. For reference, a gallon of milk weighs about 9 pounds. Parents with small children may require assistance with child care in the early postoperative period.

Symptoms to report immediately to the surgeon include increased temperature, new onset of neurologic deficit, bleeding from the incision(s), or new onset of pain. The nurse reminds the patient that numbness and tingling present before surgery do not always abate immediately after surgery. Resolution of symptoms may take months or years, and occasionally symptoms never completely resolve.

Most persons can return to work after 6 weeks. The work environment should be modified to include proper body mechanics and ergonomic design. The patient should avoid staying in one position for prolonged periods, taking frequent breaks to get up and move about. If the patient's job involves heavy manual labor, vocational retraining may be an option.

Lumbar Spine Surgery. The length of stay for persons undergoing lumbar spine surgery varies. Patients undergoing endoscopic disc removal may go home the same day; persons undergoing fusions may be hospitalized for up to 4 days (see Guidelines for Safe Practice box, p. 1602).

Cervical Spine Surgery. Persons undergoing cervical spine surgery may require tongs, halo traction, or a halo brace. Edema of the throat is present in the early postoperative period, requiring careful assessment of the airway and ability to swallow (see Guidelines for Safe Practice box, p. 1603). The estimated length of stay is 1 to 3 days.

Thoracic Spine Surgery. Mobility restrictions are more prolonged for thoracic spine surgery than for lumbar surgery, since the thoracic spine is more mobile and the risk of dislodging grafts through improper motion is greater (see Guidelines for Safe Practice box, p. 1603).

Nursing Care Plan

Patient Undergoing Cage Spinal Fusion

Data A 68-year-old woman has been treated conservatively for about 12 years for degenerative disc disease and resultant spinal stenosis at L5-S1. Within the past 2 years the patient has developed progressive, unrelenting pain; weakness; and early neurologic deficits, not controlled by medications, braces, or physical therapy. After extensive diagnostic evaluation, the physician and patient decide that the best course of action is surgical stabilization by fusion cage. The patient's history is positive for cigarette smoking and occasional alcohol use. She lives with her husband, who will be her primary caregiver. Her primary concerns are pain and possible loss of bowel and bladder control if the surgery is unsuccessful.

Nursing Diagnosis

Deficient knowledge related to lack of experience with spinal surgery and treatment protocols

Outcomes

- Patient will express decreased anxiety regarding impending surgery.
- Patient will actively participate in care plan.

Related NOC Outcomes

- Knowledge: Disease Process
- Knowledge: Medication
- Knowledge: Prescribed Activity

Related NIC Interventions

- Teaching: Disease Process
- Teaching: Preoperative
- Teaching: Procedure/Treatment

Nursing Interventions/Rationales

- Reassure patient regarding positive outcomes from cage fusion. *Intervertebral cage fusion procedures have a high success rate. They are less invasive and promote a faster recovery with fewer complications than other spinal procedures. Providing such information may reduce the patient's fears regarding recovery.*
- Assess need for teaching regarding cage fusion and provide as needed. *Teaching needs vary among patients. Assessment helps individualize teaching to specific patient needs. Understanding of surgery and treatments reduces fear related to the unknown. An interbody cage fusion involves the use of a hollow threaded fiber cylinder to fuse two intervertebral bodies together and provide spinal stability. The patient's diseased disc is removed, and cages are placed in the opening. The cages are then filled with bone graft, which grows through the holes in the cages and fuses the vertebrae.*
- Provide written materials if available. *Patients often want to review material later or may not remember specifics.*
- Review preoperative and postoperative care with patient and family before the surgery; provide examples of prostheses if available. *Understanding the surgical procedure and postoperative care lessens anxiety and promotes participation in postoperative routines.*
- Evaluate patient's understanding of information taught and reinforce learning as needed. *To determine the need for further teaching. Reinforcement of information previously taught improves retention and promotes patient compliance.*
- Keep patient and family informed of care plan and rationales for treatment. *Encourages family support and participation in care routines while the patient is hospitalized and after discharge.*
- Teach patient signs and symptoms that need to be reported immediately. *Cage procedures have fewer complications than other spinal fusion procedures. However, the patient needs to be taught to promptly report paresthesias, paralysis, escalating pain, weakness, or changes in bowel and bladder function.*
- Teach patient the importance of follow-up examinations. *Follow-up care is essential to determine effectiveness of treatment plan and detect problems so that early intervention can be implemented if needed.*

Nursing Diagnosis

Acute pain related to surgical procedure

Outcomes

- Patient will report satisfaction with pain relief measures as evidenced by rating pain less than 3 on a scale of 0 to 10.
- Patient will decrease use of pain medications before discharge.

Related NOC Outcomes

- Pain Control
- Pain Level

Gerontologic Considerations

Degenerative disc disease and spinal stenosis primarily affect the elderly population. Disc degeneration that occurs with aging causes the facet joints and posterior ligamentum flavum to hypertrophy in an attempt to stabilize the posterior elements of the spine. These anatomic changes result in a narrowed spinal canal. Consequently, nerve roots may not receive an adequate blood supply and nutrition, depending on the diameter of the person's spinal canal. The onset of spinal stenosis is usually insidious, and physical symptoms may take years to manifest. Care must be taken to differentiate spinal stenosis from peripheral vascular disease, since the claudication (leg pain and weakness after walking) symptoms are similar. In persons with spinal stenosis, the pain in the legs is reproduced by walking and relieved by resting. Back pain often accompanies the leg pain, probably as a result of facet arthritis and degenerative disc disease.

Are You Ready?

Which of the following findings in a patient 24 hours after lumbar spine surgery would require immediate notification of the surgeon?

1. Clear fluid drainage from surgical site
2. Swelling at the surgical site
3. Bruising at the surgical site
4. Numbness and tingling consistent with preoperative presentation

Related NIC Interventions
- Analgesic Administration
- Pain Management

Nursing Interventions/Rationales
- Assess patient's pain before and after comfort interventions. *To determine the degree of postoperative pain and effectiveness of pain relief measures.*
- Encourage use of patient-controlled analgesia (PCA) before pain becomes severe. *Milder pain is more readily controlled than severe pain. The ability to self-medicate allows the patient to have control over her pain.*
- Monitor use and effectiveness of PCA. *PCA avoids peaks and valleys associated with intermittent use of analgesics. It also allows the patient greater control over her pain and its elimination.*
- Encourage use of nonpharmacologic pain relief measures if acceptable to patient. *Relaxation, repositioning, and distraction are helpful for reducing and controlling pain; however, the patient must believe that they will help.*

Nursing Diagnosis
Risk for impaired home maintenance related to lack of experience

Outcomes
- Patient will verbalize understanding of prescribed medications.
- Patient will verbalize need for keeping follow-up appointments.

Related NOC Outcomes
- Compliance Behavior
- Participation in Health Care Decisions

Related NIC Interventions
- Discharge Planning
- Home Maintenance Assistance

Nursing Interventions/Rationales
- Assess patient and family's perception of problems that may occur with management of self-care at home. *To identify actual or perceived needs and obstacles to the patient caring for herself at home.*
- Encourage patient to participate in decisions about rehabilitation and self-care at home. *Involving the patient in decision making increases the likelihood of compliance with the prescribed treatment and rehabilitation plan.*
- Encourage patient to enter a smoking cessation program. *Cigarette smoking is a contributing factor to degenerative disc disease. Further spinal degeneration can occur if the patient continues to smoke.*

Evaluation
Evaluation is based on comparing the patient's outcomes with desired outcomes.

Scoliosis

Etiology and Epidemiology. Scoliosis, or lateral curvature of the spine, can be classified as nonstructural or structural. Nonstructural scoliosis is also described as postural or functional and is caused by posture, pain, leg length inequality, and other factors. This form of scoliosis is usually easily corrected, either by exercise or by removing the underlying cause. An important distinction is the absence of vertebral rotation. However, untreated nonstructural scoliosis can progress to structural scoliosis.

Structural scoliosis involves a rotational deformity of the vertebrae. It is further divided into three major categories:

1. *Congenital* scoliosis occurs as a result of vertebral malformations in fetal life and accounts for 15% of structural scoliosis cases.
2. *Neuromuscular* scoliosis is a consequence of several diseases and represents approximately 15% of cases. Curves generally appear early and progress rapidly.
3. *Idiopathic* scoliosis has no known cause, but genetic factors have been linked to the development of disease. It accounts for approximately 65% to 80% of cases and affects about 1% of all children, mostly preadolescents and adolescents.[50] Idiopathic scoliosis is further divided into three groups, depending on the age of onset (Box 53-8). Girls and boys are affected equally; however, curvatures in girls are usually more progressive.[50]

Pathophysiology. Scoliosis may develop in localized areas of the spinal column or involve the whole spinal column. Curvatures

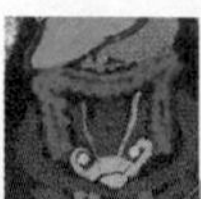

GUIDELINES FOR SAFE PRACTICE *Postoperative Care of the Patient Who Has Undergone Lumbar Spine Surgery*

- Positioning
  —Encourage the patient to logroll to change position from side to back to side.
  —Use a turning sheet until the patient can assist with turning.
- Neurovascular checks to assess circulatory status and motor and sensory function
  —Monitor the patient for signs of neurologic deficit, deep venous thrombosis, and pulmonary embolism. Prophylactic anticoagulants may be prescribed.
- Wound care (drains placed in wound to prevent hematoma formation, if necessary)
  —Maintain constant suction through drains as required.
  —Maintain drains free of contamination.
  —Monitor for excessive output from drains. Output ranges from 20 to 250 ml/8 hr for the first 24 hours; it tapers for 12 hours postoperatively, and the drains usually are removed 24 to 36 hours postoperatively. Drains that allow reinfusion of serous drainage may be used.
  —Inspect surgical area frequently for evidence of excess drainage or hematoma formation (bulging of tissues surrounding the surgical site).
  —If a spinal fusion with autologous graft has been done, inspect donor site (usually iliac crest) for drainage, hematoma.
- Promoting comfort
  —Reposition patient frequently.
  —Administer opioids; change from intravenous route to oral route as tolerated, transition to nonopioids as patient tolerates. Monitor respiratory status and effectiveness of pain management.
  —Monitor use and effectiveness of the patient-controlled analgesia pump, if ordered.
  —Use a fracture bedpan.
- Promoting mobility
  —Activity out of bed varies depending on whether fusion was done. Bed rest may be ordered if the dura was damaged intraoperatively.
  —Transfer patient out of bed with as little time spent in the sitting position as possible.
    —Start the transfer with the patient in a side-lying position at the edge of the bed.
    —Have patient push off the bed with the upper hand and the lower elbow.
    —One person assists by guiding the patient's trunk, and another helps the patient's legs over the side of the bed.
    —Reverse the process for return to bed.
  —Permit the patient to walk as much as tolerated, with an assistive aid if necessary.
  —Braces or corsets, if prescribed, are applied before the patient gets out of bed.
  —Encourage patient to participate in activities of daily living within prescribed limits of mobility.
- Discharge instructions
  —Do not lift or carry anything heavier than 5 pounds.
  —Do not drive a car until permitted by the surgeon.
  —Avoid twisting motions of the trunk.
  —Report any signs of infection or neurologic deficit to surgeon.

may be S shaped or C shaped (Figure 53-13). The earliest pathologic changes begin in the soft tissues. Muscles and ligaments shorten on the concave side of the curve, progressing to deformities of the vertebrae and ribs. In skeletally immature persons, vertebral deformation occurs as asymmetric forces are applied to the epiphysis by the shortened and tight soft tissue structures on the concave side of the curve. The Scoliosis Research Society has devised a method of classifying curves: by magnitude, direction, location, and etiology. Curve direction is designated by the convex side of the curve.

The degree of rotation of the curve is important because it determines the amount of impingement on the rib cage. The amount of vertebral compression and twisting depends on the position of the vertebrae in the curve. The forces of compression are greatest on the apical vertebrae, which become the most deformed. Deformity progresses quickly during skeletal growth

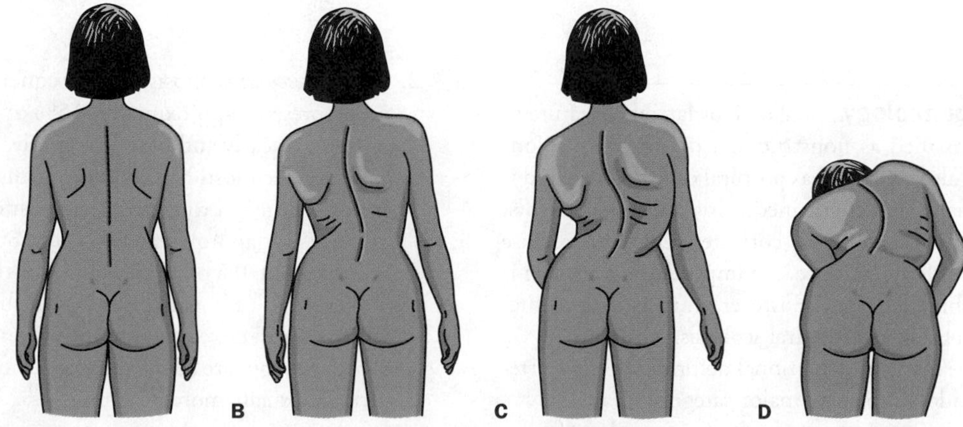

Figure 53-13 Normal spinal alignment and abnormal spinal curvatures associated with scoliosis. **A**, Normal. **B**, Mild. **C**, Severe. **D**, Rotation and curvature of scoliosis.

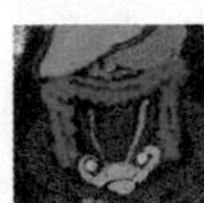

GUIDELINES FOR SAFE PRACTICE *Postoperative Care of the Patient Who Has Undergone Cervical Spine Surgery*

- Positioning
  - —Keep head of bed elevated 30 to 45 degrees, particularly if an anterior surgical approach was used, to decrease swelling in the throat and facilitate respiration.
  - —If the patient is in a cervical brace, position is not restricted except by the patient's tolerance.
  - —If the patient is in cervical traction, the patient may be turned side to back to side, as tolerated.
- Promoting safety
  - —Assess the airway and respiratory function frequently. Swelling may compromise the airway.
  - —Provide suction equipment and a tracheotomy set in the patient's room until swelling in the throat subsides and the patient is swallowing and breathing normally.
  - —Check adjustment screws and straps frequently to ensure the brace is not loosening.
  - —Advise physician or orthotist of loosening of the brace consequent to a decrease in edema so the brace can be readjusted.
- Wound care
  - —Inspect surgical area frequently, including the iliac crest donor site, for evidence of excess drainage or formation of a hematoma. Apply an ice bag to the donor site for comfort.
  - —If a tong or halo traction is used, pin care may be required (see Chapter 51).
- Promoting comfort and relieving pain
  - —Provide ice chips to soothe sore throat.
  - —Make progressive diet changes slowly; the patient will have difficulty swallowing and will be afraid of choking. Full liquids or semisolids (ice cream, custards, gelatin, nectars) are often better tolerated than clear juice or broth; however, milk products may increase mucus production.
  - —Administer analgesics as for any patient undergoing spinal surgery. The donor site often causes more discomfort than the neck incision.
  - —The patient may require aerosol treatments or humidification of air to loosen mucus secretions or make breathing more comfortable.
- Promoting mobility
  - —If the patient is in traction, encourage patient to perform ankle dorsiflexion–plantar flexion exercises and quadriceps setting on a regular basis to promote circulation and maintain leg strength. Monitor the patient for signs of deep venous thrombosis and pulmonary embolism.
  - —If the patient is in a brace, out-of-bed activity, including walking, may begin as soon as the patient tolerates.
  - —Provide for temporary use of a walker if the donor site pain restricts mobility.
  - —Encourage patient to participate in activities of daily living to the greatest extent possible.
- Discharge instructions
  - —Wear the brace at all times.
  - —Report any difficulty with the brace to the physician immediately.
  - —Do not drive a car during the period that the brace must be worn.
  - —Report symptoms of graft dislodgement (dysphagia and a feeling of "fullness" in the throat), infection, or neurologic deficit.

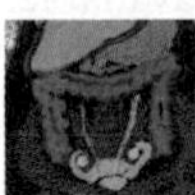

GUIDELINES FOR SAFE PRACTICE *Postoperative Care of the Patient Who Has Undergone Thoracic Spine Surgery*

The care is the same as for lumbar surgery with the following additions and exceptions:

- Positioning
  - —The head of the bed may often be elevated to 30 degrees.
- Wound care
  - —If the pleural cavity is entered, a chest tube will be inserted and must be managed after surgery (see Chapter 26).
- Promoting comfort
  - —Help patient splint the chest while coughing.
- Promoting mobility
  - —Encourage and assist the patient in performing vigorous pulmonary hygiene measures.
  - —Encourage dorsiflexion–plantar flexion and gluteal and quadriceps exercises hourly while awake. Monitor the patient for signs of deep venous thrombosis and pulmonary embolism. Prophylactic anticoagulants may be prescribed.
  - —Keep spine in alignment; help patient logroll.
  - —A brace is routinely prescribed and must be applied before the patient is allowed out of bed.
  - —Permit patient to perform whatever activities are comfortable within the limitations of the brace.
  - —Encourage patient to participate in activities of daily living within prescribed limits of mobility.
- Discharge instructions
  - —Apply and remove brace before getting out of bed.
  - —Wear the brace whenever out of bed; assess the skin under the brace.
  - —Use proper body mechanics; avoid lifting more than 5 to 10 pounds.
  - —Report symptoms of infection or neurologic deficit to surgeon.

and slows later in life, but the greatest increase in curvature may occur in adult life. Gravity and an increase in upper body weight may increase the deformity in adulthood. Curves greater than 60 degrees have a significant effect on pulmonary function.

Initially the individual may have slight, mild, or severe deformity. Early deformity may not be obvious except on specific examination. In the early stages individuals may note that clothing does not fit correctly or hang evenly, since the height of the shoulders is uneven. Pain is not usually an accompanying factor. Persons affected with structural scoliosis may exhibit asymmetry of hip height; pelvic obliquity (tilting of the pelvis from the normal horizontal position); inequalities of shoulder height; scapular

Box 53-8 Classification of Scoliosis

Congenital

Neuromuscular Causes

Cerebral palsy
Charcot-Marie-Tooth disease
Syringomyelia
Spinal cord injury
Poliomyelitis
Myelomeningocele
Muscular dystrophy
Neurofibromatosis
Marfan's syndrome

Idiopathic

Infantile: 0 to 3 years of age
Juvenile: 4 to 10 years of age
Adolescent: older than 10 years of age

prominence; rib prominence; and rib humps, which is a posterior, unilateral prominence of the rib cage visible on forward bending. In severe cases cardiopulmonary and digestive function may be affected by compression or displacement of internal organs. Total lung capacity, vital capacity, and maximum voluntary ventilation may be decreased. Cardiac output may also be compromised. Significant deviations in balance of the curve may affect gait patterns.

Right thoracic, right thoracic and left lumbar, and right thoracolumbar curves are most common in idiopathic scoliosis. A compensatory curve may develop, allowing the head to be centered over the pelvis. In general, compensatory curves are of a lesser degree, are more flexible, and are less rotated.

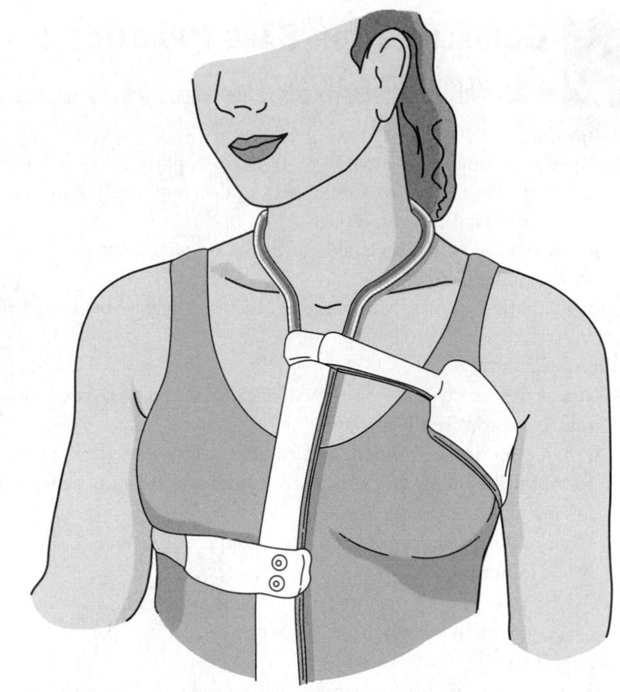

Figure 53-14 Milwaukee brace.

Collaborative Care Management. A complete radiologic examination of the spine is performed. Curve angles, flexibility, and the degree of vertebral rotation are calculated. Radiographs may also be done to determine skeletal maturity. In patients with severe thoracic scoliosis, pulmonary function studies may be completed to evaluate the degree of restrictive lung disease.

Treatment depends on the individual patient and the degree of lateral curvature. Early or postural scoliosis may be amenable to postural exercise or exercise combined with traction. Cottrell's traction, which is a combination of a cervical head halter with 5 to 7 pounds and pelvic traction with 10 to 20 pounds, may be used. When the curve is flexible (less than 40 degrees) and the patient is cooperative, bracing, in combination with exercise, may be sufficient to correct the deformity (e.g., Milwaukee brace [Figure 53-14], Risser jacket, or halofemoral or halopelvic traction).

Maintaining ideal weight can help reduce stress on the spine. The patient should be advised against weight gain, especially if bracing is prescribed, because the brace is specifically fitted and contoured to the individual. The brace can usually accommodate a 10-pound gain or loss. Transcutaneous electrical muscle stimulation may be used to stimulate the muscles on the convex side of the curve. Repeated stimulation strengthens the muscles and pulls the spine into alignment. The patient typically uses the stimulator at night.

Surgery is indicated for patients when conservative management fails to halt curve progression; for those with severe, progressing curves, intractable pain, or compromised pulmonary function; or for cosmesis. Many patients with neuromuscular scoliosis are unable to walk. Surgical correction can facilitate the ability to transfer or increase sitting ability or tolerance. Surgical correction is usually performed when curves are greater than 45 degrees[50] (Figure 53-15).

Surgical correction usually involves a posterior approach to the spine with instrumentation and bony fusion. Patients with severe, rigid curves and pelvic obliquity often require a staged procedure. A transthoracic or retroperitoneal approach to the spine is performed first, followed by a posterior procedure in 1 to 2 weeks. Many types and combinations of instrumentation are available. The type used is based on the individual patient and surgeon preference. Complications of scoliosis fusion are similar to those described under Nursing Management of the Patient Undergoing Spinal Surgery. The interventions described in that section are also applicable to the patient with a scoliosis fusion. Particular attention should be paid to assessment of respiratory function, pain management, and acceptance of changes in body image.

Patient/Family Teaching. Teaching for the patient with scoliosis is described in the Patient/Family Teaching box, p. 1606.

Disorders Affecting the Hands and Feet

Dupuytren's Contracture

Etiology and Epidemiology. Dupuytren's contracture is a progressive condition marked by hypertrophic hyperplasia of the palmar fascia that results in a flexion deformity of the distal palm and fingers (Figure 53-17). The cause of Dupuytren's contracture is unknown. A familial tendency has been noted. Dupuytren's contracture appears most commonly in persons of Northern European ancestry, between 40 and 60 years of age. Caucasian men, middle aged or older, are more frequently affected. Women with Dupuytren's contracture seem to experience only mild deformity. Dupuytren's deformity is associated with diabetes, epilepsy,

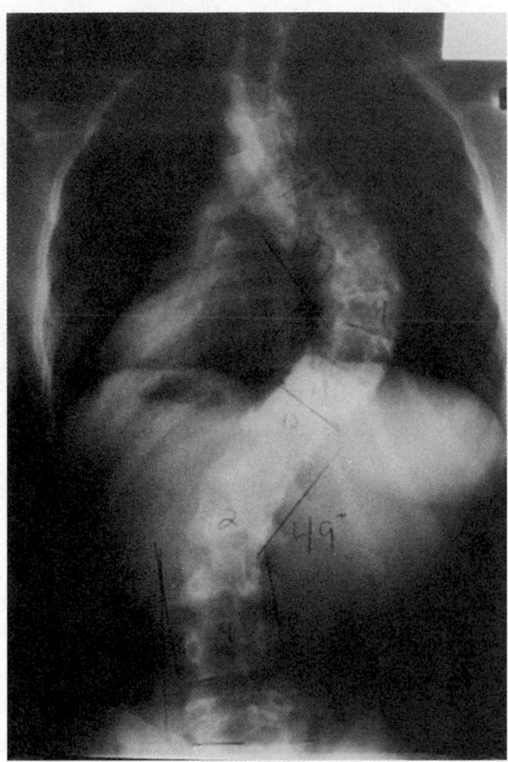

A

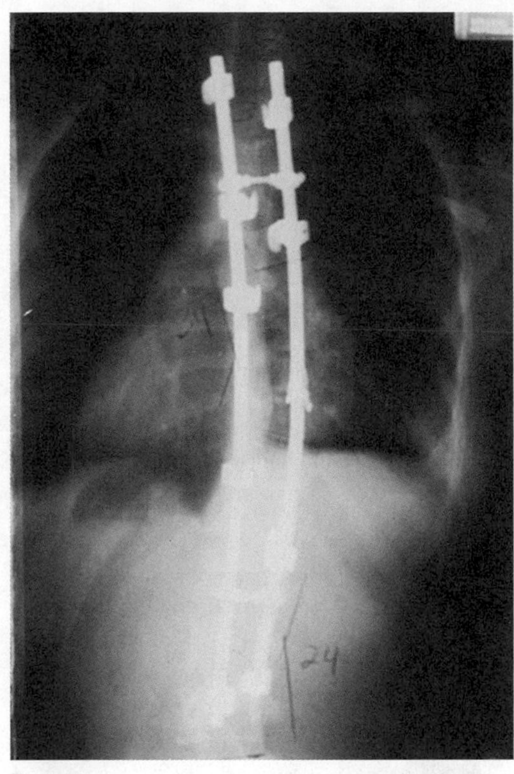

B

Figure 53-15 **A**, Preoperative radiograph of adult with idiopathic scoliosis. **B**, Postoperative film showing correction of curve with Cotrel-Dubousset instrumentation in place.

alcoholism, penile lesions (Peyronie's disease), and hyperplasia of the plantar fascia (Ledderhose's disease).

Pathophysiology. Deformity results from changes mediated by the myofibroblasts, which is not completely understood. The anatomy of the palmar fascia is distorted. Dupuytren's contracture may take up to 20 years to reach maximal deformity. It often occurs bilaterally and symmetrically. Hyperplasia and progressive fibrosis of the palmar fascia on the ulnar side of the band cause progressive shortening of the pretendinous bands of the ring and small fingers. The bands shorten, and the MCP joints are drawn into flexion contractures. Web space contractures and scissoring of the fingers develop from ligamentous contracture. The proximal IP joint may also be involved. The skin of the palm is drawn down, forming tight puckers and nodules.

Depending on the severity of the deformity and hand dominance, the patient may have difficulty grasping objects. Burning pain may accompany attempts at grasping. Usually, the main complaints are deformity and mild interference with hand function.

Collaborative Care Management. Surgery is the preferred method of treatment. Persons with fixed flexion contractures of 30 degrees or more at the MCP or proximal interphalangeal (PIP) joints are candidates for surgical intervention. Surgical repair involves regional fasciectomy or subtotal palmar fasciectomy to allow the patient full motion. Recurrence of disease is common. More advanced cases may require joint fusion or amputation if neurovascular structures are involved. Splints worn at night may decrease residual flexion contractures of the digits. After surgery referrals for PT and OT are necessary for exercises to regain ROM and splinting.

Surgical repair is performed as an outpatient procedure. The most common postoperative complications are hematoma and inadequate skin closure. Nursing management focuses on postoperative care, including pain management, neurovascular assessment of the fingers, care of the dressing or splint, and promotion of self-care.

PATIENT/FAMILY TEACHING. The inability to flatten the fingers and palm against a hard surface ("flat hand" test) usually indicates a deformity significant enough to warrant surgery. Postoperative instructions include care of the dressing and splint. The hand should be elevated for comfort and to decrease swelling. A sling may be worn. The nurse instructs the patient to contact the surgeon if the fingers become cool, pale, or painful or if paresthesias or decreased movement is experienced. The splint should be maintained until the follow-up visit.

Analgesics are prescribed as needed. If the dominant hand is affected, the patient may need assistance in ADLs. The patient can generally return to work in a few days. A PT referral is indicated for postoperative ROM exercises. The patient and family should understand the signs and symptoms of recurrent disease.

Hallux Valgus

Etiology and Epidemiology. Foot problems are a significant source of pain, deformity, and disability. Hallux valgus is the lateral angulation of the proximal phalanx on the metatarsal head of

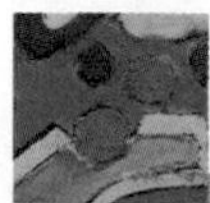

PATIENT/FAMILY TEACHING *The Patient With Scoliosis*

Persons who have undergone spinal fusion need teaching as described in the section on spinal surgery. When conservative interventions are used, the patient's and family's understanding of the treatment plan is important for achieving the desired outcomes. Bracing will only be successful if the patient complies with the treatment plan.

Focus areas include:

- Disease process.
- Rationales for treatment.
- Proper use of traction (if applicable) and prescribed exercises.
- Bracing (Figure 53-16): how to apply, remove, and care for the brace. Wearing a brace need not restrict normal or desired activities. A cotton T-shirt can be worn underneath the brace. The skin should be inspected frequently for signs of irritation. Wearing loose-fitting, front-buttoning, elastic waisted clothing that conceals the brace may be important to women and adolescents. Radiographs will be taken after a short period in the brace, then as indicated.
- Support groups: the Scoliosis Association and the National Scoliosis Foundation.

The Scoliosis Research Society recommends annual screening of all children ages 10 to 14 years. Scoliosis screening is mandated by law in some states; others have voluntary screening programs. The U.S. Preventive Services Task Force has insufficient evidence to recommend either for or against routine screening of asymptomatic adolescents.

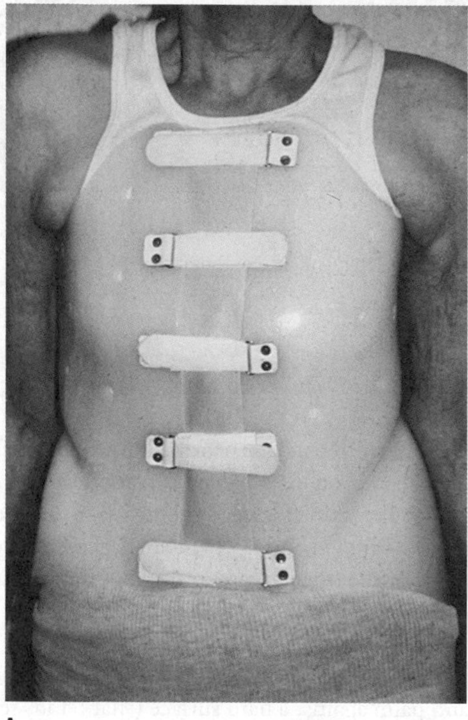

A

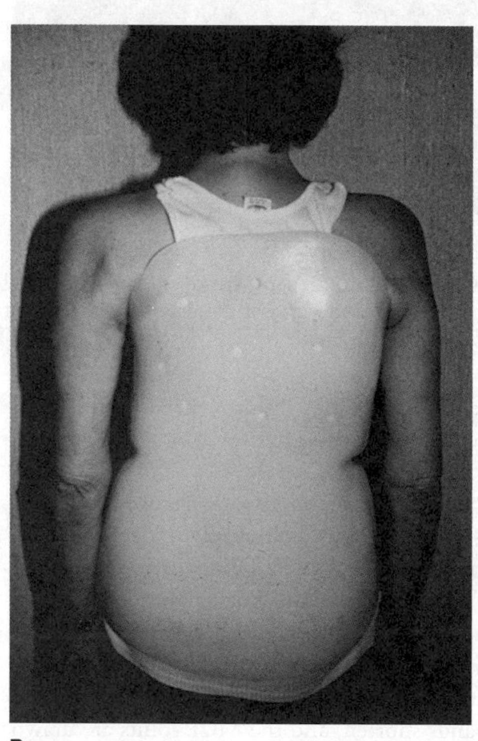

B

Figure 53-16 **A**, Anterior view of thoracolumbosacral orthosis (TLSO). **B**, Posterior view of TLSO. Note cotton shirt worn under brace.

the great toe. This common foot problem is often bilateral (Figure 53-18). Depending on the degree of angulation, prominence of the medial eminence may occur, resulting in bunion deformity (Figure 53-19).

Women develop hallux valgus deformity 10 times more often than men. There is a familial tendency. Wearing improper shoes, such as pointed-toe shoes that cause crowding and angulation of the toes, also contributes to the development or worsening of the deformity. Other associated factors include pes planus (flatfoot), chronic tightening of the Achilles tendon, spasticity, and RA.

Pathophysiology. Lateral deviation of the proximal phalanx causes pressure on the medial metatarsal head and attenuation and contracture of the joint capsule. The adjacent sesamoid bones, anchored by the adductor tendon and transverse metatarsal ligament, become subluxed. The flexor and extensor hallucis longus, which insert at the base of the distal phalanx, also deviate laterally, increasing the deformity. The medial eminence of the metatarsal head becomes prominent, and a protective bursa forms as it rubs against the shoe. The great toe may cause crowding and deformity of the second toe.

Collaborative Care Management. Diagnosis is made by the patient history and physical examination. The type of shoes worn, occupation, and amount of exercise are important points to include in the history. The gait and neurovascular status of the feet are

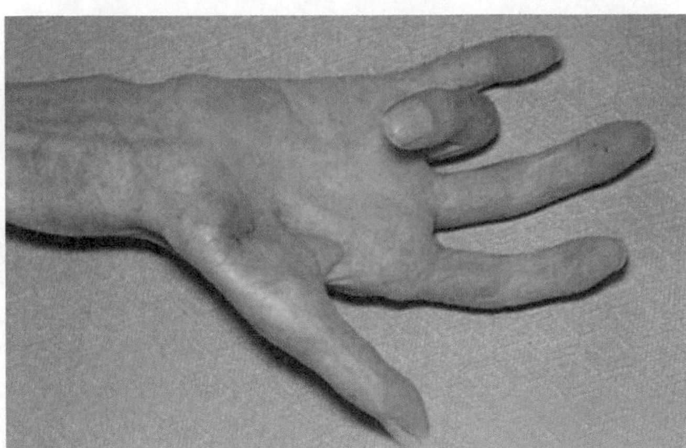

Figure 53-17 Dupuytren's contracture.

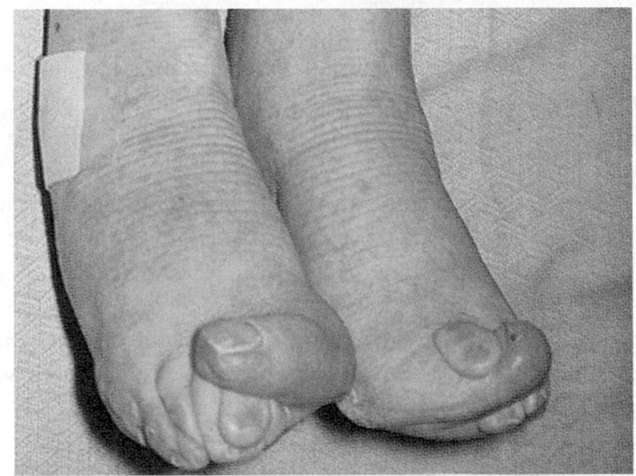

Figure 53-18 Bilateral hallux valgus.

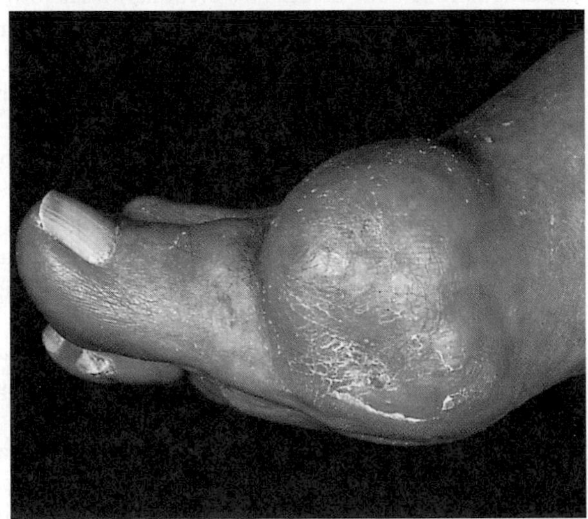

Figure 53-19 Bunion deformity.

important points of the objective examination. Corns and calluses may also be present, and the patient may have flatfoot. Radiographs confirm the diagnosis and define the severity of the deformity.

Conservative treatment includes encouraging the patient to wear properly fitting shoes of the correct size and shape to allow room for the toes; this alone may alleviate the problem. Shoes should be wide enough to accommodate the medial eminence. A protective pad can be taped under the metatarsal head to change the weight-bearing pressure. Insoles can be purchased to cushion the foot. A pad can be placed over the corn or bunion to decrease pain and pressure. Medications such as NSAIDs or acetaminophen can prescribed for pain relief.

If conservative treatment fails or the patient is reluctant to change footwear, surgical intervention may be indicated. Several surgical procedures, including osteotomy and fusion, can correct hallux valgus and bunions (Figure 53-20). Pain relief, correction of deformity, and a functional foot are the goals of surgical correction. Before consenting to surgery, the patient should be completely informed of the risks and benefits of the procedure. After bunion surgery, it is not always possible to wear whatever type of shoes is desired. The surgical procedure is not indicated for cosmesis, but to correct a structural deformity.

After surgery the foot is wrapped in a soft, bulky dressing, and in some patients a splint or cast is applied. The patient wears a postoperative cast shoe and walks with crutches or a walker until full weight bearing is permitted.

PATIENT/FAMILY TEACHING. Bunion surgery is performed as an outpatient procedure, and the patient and family need discharge instructions regarding pain management, signs of infection, and postoperative care. The cast shoe is worn for approximately 2 weeks or until the splint or cast is removed. Activity and weight bearing should be limited during this time. Two to 4 weeks after surgery, round-toed, lacing shoes or sandals can be worn. A bunion splint is worn at night for approximately 6 weeks. At 6 weeks full activity can be resumed. The nurse teaches the patient about wearing properly fitting shoes and avoiding pointed-toe and high-heeled shoes, which alter the weight-bearing pressure on the feet. A PT referral may be required for some patients. A podiatry consult for custom shoes may be required for patients with severe deformity. The nurse also teaches about proper foot care (see Patient/Family Teaching box, p. 1608).

Emotional support in accepting body image changes associated with the appearance of the feet may be needed. Because bunions often occur bilaterally, the patient should be taught to assess the other foot for signs of beginning deformity.

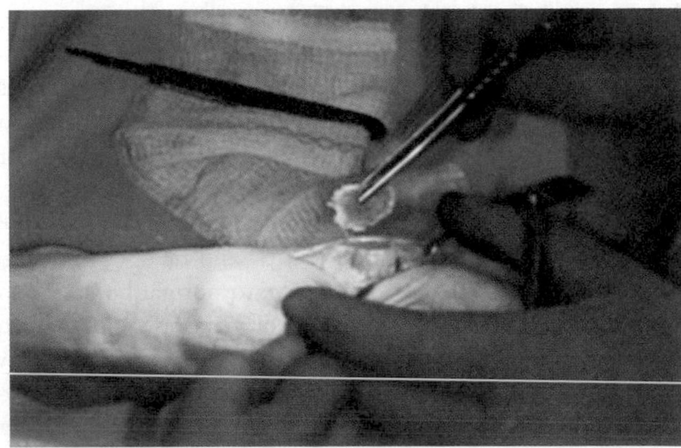

Figure 53-20 Surgical correction of bunion and hallux valgus. Medial eminence is removed.

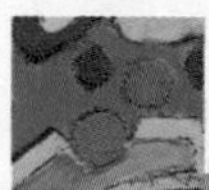

PATIENT/FAMILY TEACHING
Foot Care

In addition to recognizing common problems, you can take many steps to promote healthy feet and prevent problems. Follow these guidelines:

- Walk regularly. This will improve circulation, increase flexibility, and encourage bone and muscle development. Walking is important for maintaining overall foot health.
- Always wear comfortable shoes that provide proper support. The shoes should be sufficiently wide and have low enough heels so that you feel no leg fatigue, leg or foot cramps, or pain.
- Massage your feet at least daily to improve circulation and promote relaxation of the feet.
- If you have bunions, wear shoes that are extra long or wide. This will ease pressure on your toes. In addition, use donut-shaped bunion cushions or moleskin to take pressure off of the joints.
- Wear heel pads or cushions in the bottom of your shoes to protect your heels if you walk on hard surfaces for long times.
- Wash your feet every day in warm water. Dry them by blotting with a towel, rather than rubbing.
- If your feet perspire a lot, dust your feet with talc or a hygienic foot powder. You may also sprinkle some powder into your shoes. Do not use cornstarch because it may lead to a fungal infection.
- Trim your nails shortly after you have taken a bath or shower, while they are soft. Cut the nails straight across with toenail clippers.
- Do not go barefoot outdoors, especially if you are in an area that is not your own yard. A foreign body may cut or puncture your foot.
- Inspect your feet every day for cuts, blisters, and scratches. Provide care as needed and observe for proper healing.

From *Mosby's patient teaching guides: update 3,* St Louis, 1997, Mosby.

Tumors of the Musculoskeletal System

Etiology and Epidemiology. Tumors may arise from any of the structures of the musculoskeletal system (Tables 53-11 and 53-12). The type of tumor is determined and classified by the tissue of origin (Figure 53-21). Tumors can be benign or malignant and can affect both adults and children. Musculoskeletal tumors constitute 3% of all malignant tumors.

Generally, malignant tumors tend to cause more bone destruction, invasion of the surrounding tissues, and metastasis. Benign bone tumors tend to be less destructive to normal bone, do not invade soft tissues, and are not capable of metastasis. The cause of bone tumors is unknown. A tumor can be defined as a new growth or hyperplasia of cells. This growth may be in response to inflammation or trauma. Other tumors result from a spontaneous, rapid, poorly differentiated proliferation of cells.

The incidence of bone tumors varies with age. Adults 30 to 35 years of age have a low incidence of bone tumors. Adolescents and adults over age 60 years have the highest incidence of bone tumors; the higher incidence in the older adult is related to metastatic tumors. Osteosarcoma is the most common type of primary bone tumor, representing 20% of all cases.[23,54]

TABLE 53-11 Common Tumors of Musculoskeletal System*

Type	Benign	Malignant
Bone	Osteoma	Osteosarcoma
Cartilage	Osteochondroma Enchondroma Periosteal Chondroblastoma	Chondrosarcoma
Fibrous	Fibroma	Fibrosarcoma
Bone marrow	Giant cell	Ewing's sarcoma Myeloma
Uncertain cell	Unicameral bone cyst Aneurysmal bone cyst	

*See also Table 53-12.

Other factors that increase the risk of bone tumors include a history of Paget's disease or radiotherapy. Bone tumors can also occur as a result of metastases from other primary sites of neoplasia. Cancers of the breast, prostate, kidney, thyroid, and lungs often metastasize to bone. Common sites for metastases include the spine, ribs, pelvis, hip, and proximal long bones. Survival rates for those with metastatic disease depend on the primary tumor site.

Pathophysiology. Bone tumors commonly cause bone destruction and erosion of the cortex. Benign bone tumors have a controlled growth rate, normally compressing and displacing rather than invading normal bone tissue. This eventually leads to weakening of the normal bone. Other malignant types of tumors destroy normal bone by either resorption or disruption of the blood supply to the bone. Three patterns of bone destruction have been identified[59]:

1. *Geographic*: These are characterized by slowly growing or benign tumors, with an identifiable margin between the normal and abnormal bone.
2. *Moth eaten:* Margins are less defined. This type of destruction characterizes rapidly proliferating tumors and malignancies.
3. *Permeative:* Tumor and normal bone are meshed with no perceivable margins—a characteristic of rapidly growing malignant tumors.

A staging system developed for bone tumors classifies malignancies according to their growth patterns and sites of metastases (Table 53-13). Common tumors of the musculoskeletal system, their characteristics, and treatment are described in Table 53-14.

OSTEOSARCOMA. Osteosarcoma exhibits a moth-eaten pattern of bone destruction with poorly defined margins (Figure 53-23). Osteoid and callus produced by the tumor invade and resorb normal cortical bone. The tumor erodes through the cortex and periosteum and eventually invades soft tissues. Metastasis to the lungs is common.

TABLE 53-12 MUSCLE TUMORS

Tumor	Characteristics	Treatment
Leiomyoma	Affects smooth muscle, usually uterus Palpable mass Tenderness	Surgical excision
Rhabdomyoma	Affects striated muscle Rare Tenderness	Surgical excision
Leiomyosarcoma	Affects smooth muscle, usually uterus, stomach, or small bowel Radical growth	Surgical excision with wide margins Radiation Chemotherapy
Rhabdomyosarcoma	Affects striated muscle, usually in inguinal, popliteal, or gluteal areas Slow-growing mass Tenderness	Radiation Surgical excision Chemotherapy

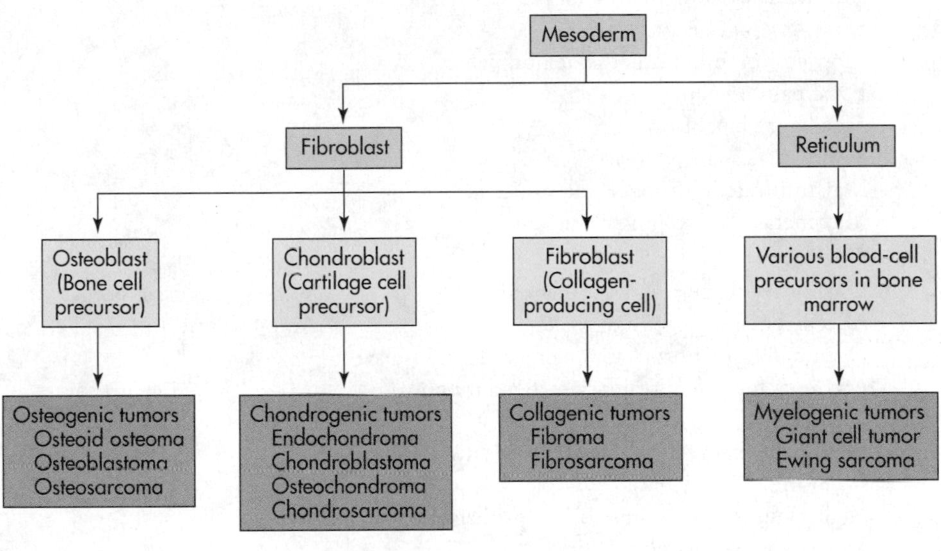

Figure 53-21 Derivation of bone tumors.

TABLE 53-13 SURGICAL STAGING SYSTEMS FOR BONE TUMORS

Stage	Grade	Site (T)	Metastasis (M)
IA	Low (G1)	Intracompartmental (T1)	None (M0)
IB	Low (G1)	Extracompartmental (T2)	None (M0)
IIA	High (G2)	Intracompartmental (T1)	None (M0)
IIB	High (G2)	Extracompartmental (T2)	None (M0)
IIIA	Low (G1)	Intracompartmental or extracompartmental (T1 or T2)	Regional or distant (M1)
IIIB	High (G2)	Intracompartmental or extracompartmental (T1 or T2)	Regional or distant (M1)

Data from Simon SR, editor: *Orthopaedic basic science*, Chicago, 1994, American Academy of Orthopaedic Surgeons.

Ninety percent of osteosarcomas occur in the metaphyses of long bones, especially the distal femur and proximal tibia.[23] The initial pain is often described as dull, aching, and intermittent, but the pain rapidly increases in intensity and duration. Night pain is common. Other frequent complaints include swelling, generalized malaise, anorexia, and weight loss.

Two types of lesions are seen with metastatic tumors. Bone destruction exceeds bone formation in lytic lesions, which are commonly seen in lung metastases. Tumors in which bone formation exceeds bone destruction, as seen in prostate metastases, are called blastic lesions. Bone lysis generally occurs with metastatic disease and hypercalcemia. Pathologic fractures pose a significant

TABLE 53-14 OTHER COMMON TUMORS OF MUSCULOSKELETAL SYSTEM

Tumor	Characteristics	Treatment
Osteochondroma	Exostosis (bony outgrowth) composed of osseous and cartilaginous substance Develops during growth periods at metaphysis of bone Also appears in tendons May limit joint motion May recur	Surgical excision
Enchondroma	Destroys cancellous bone Usually occurs in humerus or finger Can cause pathologic fractures May become malignant, especially in long bone or pelvis	Surgical excision with wide margins Amputation
Chondrosarcoma	Usually affects persons 50-70 yr old Accounts for 20% of all bone tumors Affects males more than females Slow growing, insidious onset Most common in humerus, femur, pelvis Local pain, swelling May have palpable mass Severe, persistent pain May infiltrate joint space and soft tissue May metastasize to lung tissue May recur	Surgical excision Amputation
Fibrosarcoma	Usually affects persons 30-50 yr old Affects females more than males Occurs in bony fibrous tissue of femur and tibia Accounts for 4% of primary malignant bone tumors May result from radiotherapy, Paget's disease, or chronic osteomyelitis Night pain, swelling, possible palpable mass May cause pathologic fractures May metastasize to lungs	Wide surgical excision Amputation
Giant cell tumor (Figure 53-22)	Usually affects persons ages 20-40 yr Affects females more than males Accounts for 4%-5% of all benign bone tumors Appears in epiphyseal area; destroys bone matrix; can invade soft tissues Commonly found in femur, tibia, or humerus Dull, aching night pain Limitation of motion Swelling High incidence of recurrence	Wide excision May require bone graft Amputation

risk to persons with metastatic bone lesions and can occur with any activity.

Collaborative Care Management. Bone biopsy is used to confirm the diagnosis. Because of the rapid growth rate of osteosarcomas, the prognosis is poor. Death, usually from pulmonary complications as a result of metastases, may occur within 2 years of diagnosis if the tumor is left untreated.

X-ray films, CT scans, MRI, and bone scans show tumor location and size. X-ray films have limited use, since 50% of trabecular bone must be destroyed before lesions are visible. Blood tests reveal an elevated serum alkaline phosphatase level. Chest x-ray films confirm the presence of metastases.

Treatment options for the patient with metastatic disease include radiation, hormonal therapy, chemotherapy, surgical excision, surgical repair (with prostheses or hardware), and palliative

TABLE 53-14 OTHER COMMON TUMORS OF MUSCULOSKELETAL SYSTEM—CONT'D

Tumor	Characteristics	Treatment
Myeloma, multiple myeloma (multifocal)	Poor prognosis Common in persons over 40 yr old Affects males more than females Accounts for 27% of bone tumors Higher incidence in African-Americans Neoplastic proliferation of plasma cells Causes cortical and medullary bone lysis and infiltrates bone marrow Aching, intermittent pain in spine, pelvis, ribs, or sternum Pain increased with weight bearing May cause weight loss, malaise, or anorexia Causes pathologic fractures	Palliative treatment Radiation Chemotherapy
Osteoma	Usually affects persons 10-20 yr old Accounts for 20% of benign bone tumors Slow growth	Treatment only if symptomatic, then excision

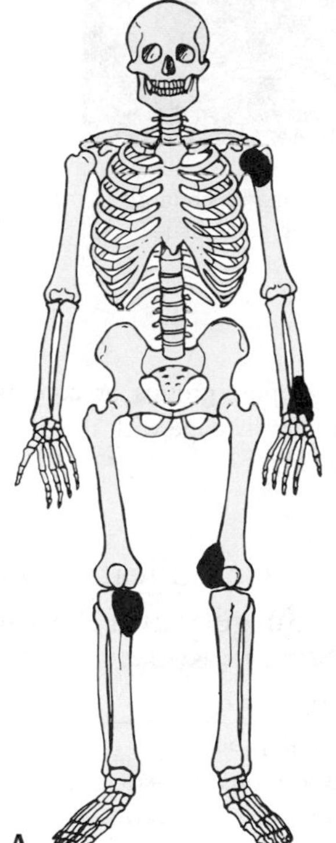

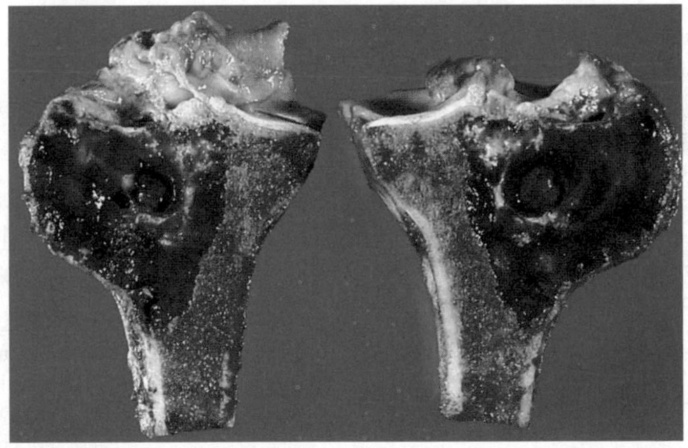

Figure 53-22 Giant cell tumor. **A**, Common skeletal locations. **B**, Gross picture of cell tumor on bone (epimetaphysis).

measures. Treatment modalities may be combined to improve outcomes. Radiation is effective in relieving pain, especially from fracture and nerve compression. Treatment for primary lesions depends on the size and location of the tumor; the presence of metastases; and the patient's age, general health, lifestyle, and preferences. Surgical management includes excision of the lesion, resection, amputation, and limb salvage procedures (Figures 53-24 and 53-25). The extent of the procedure varies from wide resection to more radical procedures, including hemipelvectomy and hip disarticulation.

Historically, the treatment of choice for high-grade bone sarcomas has been amputation. Advances in chemotherapy, diagnostic techniques, and surgical techniques led to the development of a less radical treatment option: limb salvage surgery (LSS). Disease-free survival rates after LSS are similar to those after amputation. With current adjuvant chemotherapy protocols, the disease-free

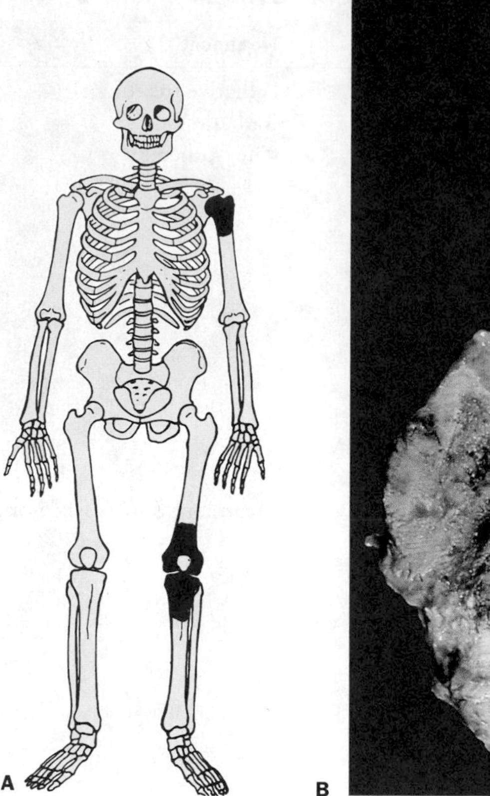

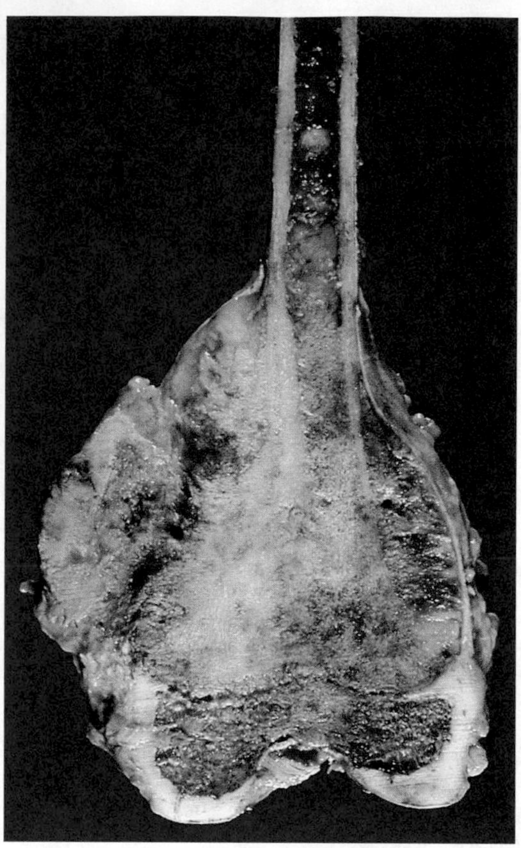

Figure 53-23 Osteosarcoma. **A,** Common skeletal locations. **B,** The femur has a large mass involving metaphysis of bone; tumor has destroyed cortex, forming soft tissue component.

survival rate for osteosarcoma is 40% to 70%.[23,54] With tumor recurrence, amputation is usually indicated (in the absence of metastases).

LSS has no histologic contraindications. In addition to treatment of osteosarcoma, LSS is used to treat patients with Ewing's sarcoma, chondrosarcoma, giant cell tumor, and other tumors. Preoperative chemotherapy has allowed more persons to be considered for LSS. Contraindications to LLS include a large invasive tumor; involvement of the neurovascular bundle; inability to achieve tumor-free margins; or a technically difficult surgical approach, such as a tumor in the distal tibia. Complications of amputation and LSS are summarized in Box 53-9.

Patient/Family Teaching. Nursing care for the patient undergoing tumor resection surgery is challenging. The patient and family, who may still be trying to cope with the diagnosis of cancer, are now faced with difficult decisions regarding treatment options. Nursing interventions focus on education, support, and clarification of information. The nurse ensures that the patient and family are fully informed regarding expected treatment outcomes, risks, and benefits. A full explanation of the possible side effects associated with chemotherapy and radiotherapy, as well as interventions to reduce their incidence, is important. Depending on the type of surgical resection, alterations in body image and function may result. Providing support and promoting acceptance of body image and role changes are important nursing interventions. Referrals to support groups or community services may help the patient and family cope with the diagnosis of cancer and changes in function.

Box 53-9 Complications of Limb Salvage Surgery and Amputation

Limb Salvage Surgery

Local recurrence of tumor
Wound and skin necrosis (may necessitate extensive soft tissue flaps)
Deep infection (risk possibly increased by the immunosuppressant action of chemotherapy)
Neurovascular complications
Deep venous thrombosis
Nonunion
Hemorrhage
Implant or graft failure
Arthritis (long term)

Amputation

Infection
Wound necrosis
Phantom limb pain
Contractures
Skin breakdown

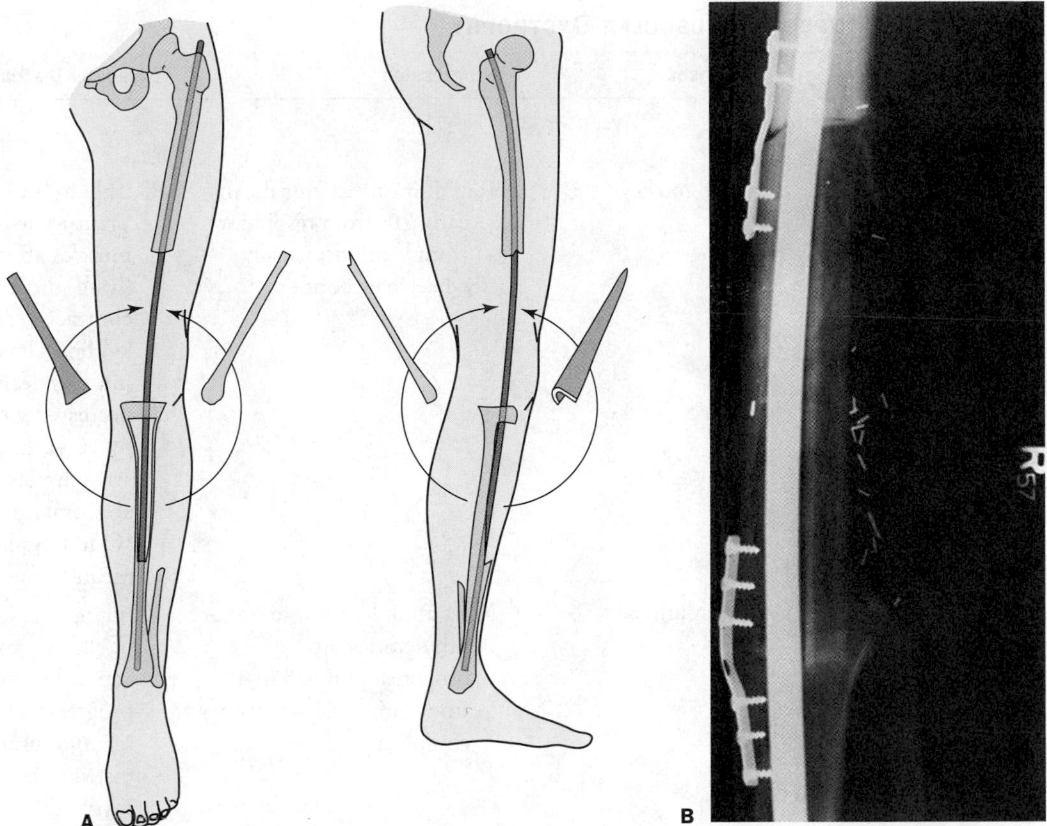

Figure 53-24 **A**, When distal femur has been resected and arthrodesis is desired, anterior one third of tibia and proximal fibula may be used to span the defect. Extremity is stabilized with long, fluted intramedullary rod. When proximal tibia is resected, anterior one third of distal femur and a segment of fibula are used to span the defect. Iliac bone graft is added to improve strength of reconstruction. Allograft segments also have proved successful in filling defects. **B**, Postoperative radiograph of patient who had resection arthrodesis for stage IIB tumor in distal femur. He uses no external aids and is fully active.

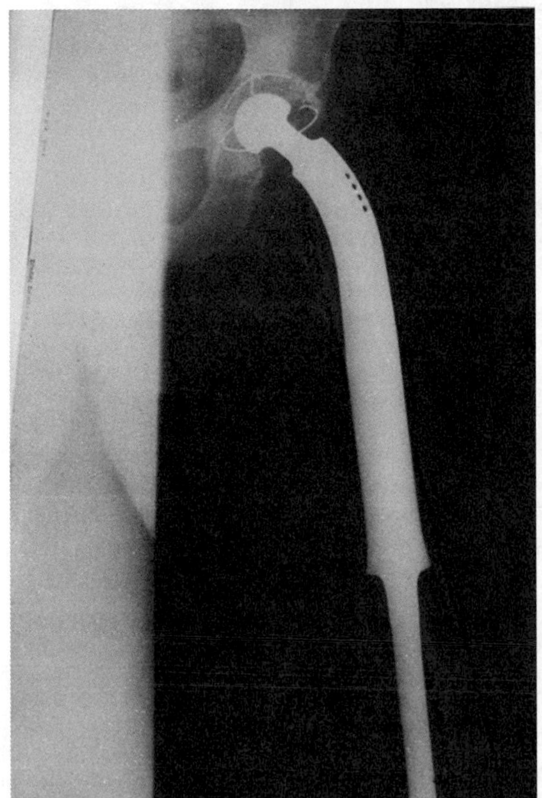

Figure 53-25 This custom-made total hip was used to replace proximal femur and hip joint of a 50-year-old woman with chondrosarcoma. She has had no recurrence of tumor and walks with modest limp while using a cane, but has no active abduction of hip.

TABLE 53-15 COMMON TYPES OF MUSCULAR DYSTROPHY

Type	Genetics	Onset	Progression	Muscular Distribution
X linked	Mutation of dystrophin at Xp21			
Duchenne's		18 mo-3 yr	Rapid; most patients die in early 20s from respiratory complications; usually wheelchair bound by 12 yr	Unable to lift head fully against gravity; proximal muscles affected early (limb-girdle pattern); joint contractures, kyphoscoliosis; respiratory muscles decline with decreased vital capacity by 10 yr; heart failure and arrhythmias late in disease; abnormal ECG; average IQ in boys below normal mean
Emery-Dreifuss		Childhood	Most ambulatory into 3rd or 4th decades; slow progression, death in 40s from cardiac or respiratory complications	Triad of 1: early contractures of elbows, ankles, posterior cervical muscles; 2: progressive weakness in scapulohumeroperoneal distribution; 3: cardiomyopathy with atrial conduction defects
Becker's		5-15 yr	Wheelchair needed usually by age 30 yr	Pattern of weakness resembles Duchenne's, but less severe; calf hypertrophy
Limb-girdle	Majority autosomal recessive; at least 10 subtypes identified	Variable, 2nd or 3rd decade	Variable, shortened life span, severe disability by 15-20 yr after disease onset	Pelvic and shoulder girdle, neck muscles
Congenital	Autosomal-recessive	Rapid with CNS involvement; without CNS involvement usually nonprogressive course, patients may walk independently	Occurs with and without CNS involvement (mental retardation, seizures, and visual loss); death by age 10-12 yr for those with CNS involvement	Onset of hypotonia and proximal weakness in infancy; joint contractures of elbows, hips, knees, and ankles (arthrogryposis)

Disorders Affecting the Muscles

Muscular Dystrophy

Etiology and Epidemiology. The muscular dystrophies (MDs) are a group of familial disorders characterized by varying degrees of skeletal muscle weakness and degeneration, leading to disability and deformity. Classification has traditionally been by phenotype, mode of inheritance, rate of progression, and distribution of involvement. Genetics has allowed the identification of the mutation and abnormal gene product for many of these inherited myopathies. Major types are outlined in Table 53-15.

Duchenne's MD affects 1 in 3500 male births.[5] Becker's MD is also an X-linked recessive disease but is less common than Duchenne's. Other types of MD seen in adults can occur in either sex. Children with MD rarely live past 25 years of age. Genetic theories include defects in muscle cell membranes and biochemical abnormality.

Pathophysiology. The genetic abnormality in MD causes a defect in the intracellular metabolism of the muscle fibers. Defects in

TABLE 53-15 COMMON TYPES OF MUSCULAR DYSTROPHY—CONT'D

Type	Genetics	Onset	Progression	Muscular Distribution
Facioscapulohumeral	Autosomal dominant; linked to chromosome 4q35	Childhood or adult	Variable; some may require wheelchair	Early involvement of facial muscles, then affects scapular muscles, upper arm, and anterior leg
Distal Welander	Autosomal dominant	Late onset, 4th to 6th decade	Progressive, may eventually involve proximal muscles and loss of ambulation	Weakness of forearm extensor, hand intrinsics, then anterior leg and foot muscles
Myotonic	Autosomal dominant	Most common type; variable, but most common onset in 2nd or 3rd decade	Variable, some remain symptom free for life	Facial weakness, balding, ptosis, and neck weakness; extremity weakness beginning distally and progressing proximally to limb-girdle muscles; affects skeletal and smooth muscle and other systems, including respiratory involvement, intellectual impairment, sleep apnea, cataracts, dysphagia, cardiac conduction defects, and insulin resistance

ECG, Electrocardiogram; *IQ,* intelligent quotient; *CNS,* central nervous system.

TABLE 53-16 TREATMENT FOR COMMON TYPES OF MUSCULAR DYSTROPHY

Type	Treatment
Duchenne's	Function of unaffected muscles maintained; muscle fiber breakdown hastened by strenuous exercise Physical therapy (PT) for range of motion (ROM) Orthoses, braces, use of wheelchair Surgical release of contractures Spinal fusion Respiratory exercises
Becker's	Surgical release of contractures, tenotomies Ambulation maintained as long as possible Monitor for cardiac complications
Limb-girdle	PT for ROM; contracture development rare; patient usually ambulatory up to 20 yr after diagnosis
Facioscapulohumeral	PT for exercises Orthoses Preserve ambulation Wheelchair for distance Surgical stabilization to prevent winged scapulae Arthrodesis of scapulae to ribs
Myotonic	Monitor for cardiac and endocrine disorders Aspiration precautions for dysphagia Decreased esophageal motility; feeding tube may be necessary Cataract surgery Pemoline or methylphenidate for somnolence

creatine metabolism and intracellular enzymes in the glycolytic system have been identified. Muscle cells exhibit phagocytosis and necrosis, with dissolution of myofilaments. The striation of the fibers is altered, and the fibers are either hypertrophied or atrophied. Eventually, muscle fibers are replaced with fat and connective tissue, causing fatty infiltration and fibrosis. Serum creatinine kinase is either elevated or normal. There is no pattern of the involved muscle fibers. Mental retardation occurs in some types of MD.

Collaborative Care Management. Diagnosis is made by the patient history and physical examination. Laboratory and diagnostic data include muscle biopsy, electromyography, and serum muscle enzyme levels. Ninety-percent of persons with Duchenne's MD have abnormal electrocardiograms. Creatine kinase levels are elevated during infancy and before the onset of weakness.

There is no cure for any of the MDs. Treatment varies with the type of disorder (Table 53-16). Genetic counseling is important. Steroids and immunosuppressants have been used with some success. Nursing care of the person with MD is supportive. Because of the severity of the disability and the multiple manifestations, a multidisciplinary approach is necessary. Referrals to PT and OT can assist the patient and family in dealing with ADLs and problems with mobility. Monitoring for cardiac and other system involvement is important.

PATIENT/FAMILY TEACHING. The patient and family should be aware of the signs, symptoms, and possible complications of MD. Prevention of the complications associated with immobility is vital. Medication teaching is necessary if the patient is receiving steroids or immunosuppressants. Emotional support is vital, especially for parents of children with MD. The family may need help coping with feelings such as grief and guilt about disease transmission. Genetic counseling should be offered to appropriate individuals. Encouraging ambulation and mobility to the fullest extent should be balanced with ensuring adequate rest and sleep to prevent fatigue. Family members need instruction about transfer techniques for wheelchair-bound patients. A lift may be necessary if the family members are unable to assist with transfers. Caregiver relief may be an issue for family members. The Muscular Dystrophy Association, with chapters in all states, is a good resource for patients and families of persons with MD.

? Critical Thinking

1. You are asked to speak to a group of perimenopausal women at a local community center. The topic is "healthy bones." Describe essential components of your presentation.
2. A 45-year-old woman is admitted for surgery to correct scoliosis. She has decreased respiratory function as a result of severe spinal curvature. What preoperative assessments are necessary to plan her care? Describe priority interventions for postoperative care.
3. A 65-year-old man with type 2 diabetes is seen in the clinic for a draining wound on the great toe. He is diagnosed with osteomyelitis. What assessment data are needed to plan his care? Describe essential components of his teaching plan.

References

1. Alper BS: What treatments work for fibromyalgia? *Clin Adv* 7(3):125-126, 2004.
2. Arslan S, Yunus MB: Fibromyalgia: making a firm diagnosis, understanding its pathophysiology, *Consultant* 43(10):1233-1243, 2003.
3. Aucott JN, Sigal LH, Smith RP: Lyme disease: the debate continues, *Patient Care Nurse Pract* 26(6):38-54, 2001.
4. Barohn RJ: Inflammatory and other myopathies. In Goldman L, Bennett JC, editors: *Cecil textbook of medicine,* ed 22, Philadelphia, 2004, Saunders.
5. Barohn RJ: Muscular dystrophies. In Goldman L, Bennett JC, editors: *Cecil textbook of medicine,* ed 22, Philadelphia, 2004, Saunders.
6. Becker M: Osteoporosis: essentials for diagnosis and management, *Am J Nurse Pract* 8(2):49-57, 2004.
7. Berg AO: Screening for osteoporosis in postmenopausal women: recommendations and rationale, *AJN* 103(1):73-81, 2003.
8. Best JT: Understanding spinal fusion, *Orthop Nurs* 21(3):48-55, 2002.
9. Birge SJ: Osteoporosis. In Rakel RE, Bope ET, editors: *Conn's current therapy,* Philadelphia, 2004, Saunders.
10. Birrer R, Jepson KK: Low back pain: a focused approach, *Consultant* 43(8):993-996, 2003.
11. Callen JP: Connective tissue disorders. In Rakel RE, Bope ET, editors: *Conn's current therapy,* Philadelphia, 2004, Saunders.
12. Carmona RH: Bone health and osteoporosis: a report of the surgeon general, accessed May 2005 from website: http://www.surgeongeneral.gov/library/bonehealth/docs/full_report.pdf.
13. Clauw DJ: Elusive syndromes: treating the biologic basis of fibromyalgia and related syndromes, *Cleveland Clin J Med* 68(10):830-839, 2001.
14. Connelly C: Low back pain: management of the psychosocial component, *Consultant* 43(1):84-87, 2003.
15. Curry LC, Hogstel MO: Osteoporosis, *Am J Nurs* 102(1):26-33, 2002.
16. Davidson M, DeSimone ME: Osteoporosis update, *Clin Rev* 12(4):76-82, 2002.
17. DeNisco, Ferro L: Sjögren's syndrome: recognizing and treating an autoimmune disease, *Am J Nurse Pract* 8(5):9-19, 2004.
18. Dowd R: Role of calcium, vitamin D, and other essential nutrients in the prevention and treatment of osteoporosis, *Nurs Clin North Am* 36(3):417-429, 2001.
19. Erikson K, Baker S, Smith J: Kyphoplasty: minimally invasive vertebral compression fracture repair, *AORN J* 78(5):766-773, 2003.
20. Finkelstein JS: Osteoporosis. In Goldman L, Bennett JC, editors: *Cecil textbook of medicine,* ed 22, Philadelphia, 2004, Saunders.
21. Freeman SB: Lower-dose hormone therapy for postmenopausal women, *Am J Nurse Pract* 8(3):9-19, 2004.
22. Garfin SR, Vives MJ: Low back pain. In Rakel RE, Bope ET, editors: *Conn's current therapy,* Philadelphia, 2004, Saunders.
23. Gibs CP, Weber K, Scarborough MT: Malignant bone tumors, *J Bone Joint Surg Am* 83A(11):1727-1745, 2001.
24. Goulding PM: Osteoporosis: the brittle bone disease, Course 5006, *National Center for Continuing Education,* 4-26, Lakeway, Tex, 2003.
25. Gross KA: Vertebroplasty: a new therapeutic option, *Orthop Nurs* 21(1):23-29, 2002.
26. Handel BL: Inflammatory disorders. In Zychowicz ME, editor: *Orthopedic nursing secrets,* Philadelphia, 2003, Hanley & Belfus.
27. Harkness L: Soy and bone: where do we stand? *Orthop Nurs* 23(1):12-16, 2004.
28. Hertel KL, Trahiotis MG: Exercise in the prevention and treatment of osteoporosis, *Nurs Clin North Am* 36(3):441-450, 2001.
29. Inman RD: The spondyloarthropathies. In Goldman L, Bennett JC, editors: *Cecil textbook of medicine,* ed 22, Philadelphia, 2004, Saunders.
30. Jerzak LA: The role of dietary calcium in promoting health and preventing disease across the lifespan, *Am J Nurse Pract* 9(3):21-28, 2005.

31. Kanis JA: Paget's disease of bone. In Goldman L, Bennett JC, editors: *Cecil textbook of medicine,* ed 22, Philadelphia, 2004, Saunders.
32. Keat A: Ankylosing spondylitis. In Rakel RE, Bope ET, editors: *Conn's current therapy,* Philadelphia, 2004, Saunders.
33. Lacasey B: Corticosteroid-induced osteoporosis, *Nurs Clin North Am* 36(3):455-464, 2001.
34. Lappe JM: Pathophysiology of osteoporosis and fracture, *Nurs Clin North Am* 36(3):393-398, 2001.
35. Lash AA: Sjögren's syndrome: pathogenesis, diagnosis, and treatment, *Nurse Pract* 26(8):50-58, 2001.
36. Licata A: Clinical uses of ultrasound, *Osteoporosis: Clinical Updates,* III(1), Washington, DC, 2002, National Osteoporosis Foundation,
37. Licata A: The many faces of secondary osteoporosis, *Osteoporosis: Clinical Updates,* III(3), Washington, DC, 2002, National Osteoporosis Foundation.
38. Licata AA: An updated look at therapies for osteoporosis, *Clin Adv* 6(2): 10-19, 2003.
39. MacDonald PA: Autoimmune and inflammatory disorders. In Maher AB, Salmond SW, Pellino TA, editors: *Orthopaedic nursing,* ed 3, Philadelphia, 2002, Saunders.
40. McCaffery M, Pasero C: *Pain: clinical manual,* ed 2, St Louis, 1999, Mosby.
41. Miller FW: Polymyositis and dermatomyositis. In Goldman L, Bennett JC, editors: *Cecil textbook of medicine,* ed 22, Philadelphia, 2004, Saunders.
42. Naguwa S, Gershwin ME: Sjögren's syndrome. In Goldman L, Bennett JC, editors: *Cecil textbook of medicine,* ed 22, Philadelphia, 2004, Saunders.
43. National Osteoporosis Foundation: *Fast facts,* accessed 2005 from website: http://www.nof.org/osteoporosis/diseasefacts.htm.
43a. Newsline: A better way to give Boniva? *Clin Advisor* 8(12):23, 2005.
43b. Newsline: Biphosphonate prevents male bone loss, *Clin Advisor* 8(12):22, 2005.
44. Nivens AS: Paget's disease: a case in point, *Orthop Nurs* 23(6):355-360, 2004.
45. Paduchi-Hyde L: Assessment of risk factors for osteoporosis and fracture, *Nurs Clin North Am* 36(3):401-406, 2001.
46. Paget SA: Polymyalgia rheumatica and temporal arteritis. In Goldman L, Bennett JC, editors: *Cecil textbook of medicine,* ed 22, Philadelphia, 2004, Saunders.
47. Petruzzi LM, Vivino FB: Sjögren's syndrome: implications for perioperative practice, *AORN J* 77(3):612-624, 2003.
48. Re VL et al: Identifying the vector of Lyme disease, *Am Fam Phys* 69(8):1935-1967, 2004.
49. Rizzoli R, Schaad MA, Uebelhart B: Osteoporosis in men, *Nurs Clin North Am* 36(3):467-477, 2001.
50. Rodts MF: Disorders of the spine. In Maher AB, Salmond SW, Pellino TA, editors: *Orthopaedic nursing,* ed 3, Philadelphia, 2002, Saunders.
51. Salmond SW, Fine C: Infections of the musculoskeletal system. In Maher AB, Salmond SW, Pellino TA, editors: *Orthopaedic nursing,* ed 3, Philadelphia, 2002, Saunders.
52. Schoen RT: Bursitis, tendonitis, myofascial pain, and fibromyalgia. In Rakel RE, Bope ET, editors: *Conn's current therapy,* Philadelphia, 2004, Saunders.
53. Schur PH: Systemic lupus erythematosus. In Goldman L, Bennett JC, editors: *Cecil textbook of medicine,* ed 22, Philadelphia, 2004, Saunders.
54. Scully SP et al: Pathologic fracture in osteosarcoma: prognostic importance and treatment implications, *J Bone Joint Surg Am* 84A(1):49-57, 2002.
55. Searle T, Baughn P, editors: Researchers find bone-density gene, *Campus News* (Case Western Reserve University) 13(31):1, 4, 2001.
56. Sedlak CA, O'Doheny MO: Metabolic conditions. In Maher AB, Salmond SW, Pellino TA, editors: *Orthopaedic nursing,* ed 3, Philadelphia, 2002, Saunders.
57. Selius BA, Alper BS: Lyme disease: stat consult, *Clin Advisor* 7(7):85-87, 2004.
58. Septimus E: Osteomyelitis. In Rakel RE, Bope ET, editors: *Conn's current therapy,* Philadelphia, 2002, Saunders.
59. Skinner HB: *Current diagnosis and treatment in orthopedics,* ed 3, Norwalk, Conn, 2003, Appleton & Lange.
60. Thompson AE, Reid GD: Gout and hyperuricemia. In Rakel RE, Bope ET, editors: *Conn's current therapy,* Philadelphia, 2004, Saunders.
61. van Tulder MW et al: Acupuncture for low-back pain (Cochrane Review). In *Cochrane Library,* Issue 3, Chichester, UK, 2004, John Wiley & Sons.
62. Wallach S: Paget's disease of bone. In Rakel RE, Bope ET, editors: *Conn's current therapy,* Philadelphia, 2004, Saunders.
63. Wassem R, Beckham N, Dudley W: Test of a nursing intervention to promote adjustment to fibromyalgia, *Orthop Nurs* 20(3):33-43, 2001.
64. Whyte JJ, Marting RN: Osteoporosis prevention: what kind of exercise is best? *Consultant* 44(7):1002-1007, 2004.
65. Wildauer JM: Men and osteoporosis, *Adv Nurse Pract* 9(4):31-35, 2001.
66. Wimmer TG, Bridges SL: Polymyalgia rheumatica and giant cell arteritis. In Rakel RE, Bope ET, editors: *Conn's current therapy,* Philadelphia, 2004, Saunders.
67. Woodward J: Hormone therapy in menopause: review of evidence-based guidelines, *Clin Rev* 15(4):46-52, 2005.

evolve Visit the Evolve website: http://evolve.elsevier.com/Monahan/medsurg

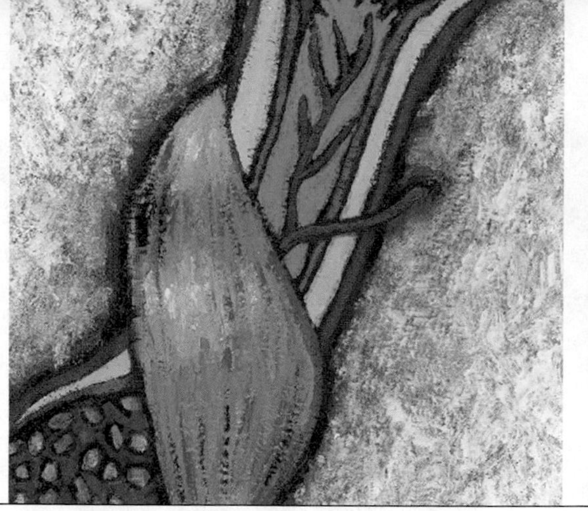

CHAPTER 54

Osteoarthritis and Rheumatoid Arthritis

by Jane F. Marek

OBJECTIVES

After studying this chapter, the learner should be able to:

1. Differentiate the etiology, epidemiology, pathophysiology, and clinical manifestations of osteoarthritis and rheumatoid arthritis.
2. Compare the collaborative care management of osteoarthritis and rheumatoid arthritis.
3. Correlate the pathophysiology with the collaborative care management for persons with degenerative and inflammatory disorders affecting the joints.
4. Develop a care plan for a person undergoing joint replacement surgery.

KEY TERMS

ankylosis, p. 1640
arthrodesis, p. 1625
arthroplasty, p. 1625
articular cartilage, p. 1619
cytokines, p. 1640
effusion, p. 1619
Heberden's nodes, p. 1618
hyaluronan, p. 1623
intraarticular, p. 1621
osteophytes, p. 1619
pannus, p. 1640
proteoglycans, p. 1618
rheumatoid nodules, p. 1641
subluxation, p. 1619

Arthritis (inflammation of a joint) is a common disorder of the musculoskeletal system that causes joint pain and stiffness. Although there are more than 100 arthritic conditions, osteoarthritis and rheumatoid arthritis are the two main types. Found worldwide, arthritis is the major cause of disability in the United States.[40]

Osteoarthritis

Etiology. Osteoarthritis (OA), also known as degenerative joint disease (DJD), hypertrophic arthritis, osteoarthrosis, or senescent arthritis, results from a series of cellular, biochemical, and biomechanical factors affecting cartilage, subchondral bone, and soft tissues of diarthrodial joints. The cause of primary OA is unknown, but several genetic and acquired risk factors have been identified. The quantity and quality of **proteoglycans** decrease with the aging process and predispose the cartilage to break down and degenerate. Genetic factors suggest a mutation of the gene that directs the formation of type II collagen.

Epidemiology. OA is the most common form of arthritis; by age 55, more than 80% of the population have radiographic evidence of the disease, although the percentage of those with clinical symptoms is much lower. OA affects an estimated 20 million Americans and accounts for approximately 3.7 million hospital admissions annually.[11,40] The number of persons affected by OA is projected to increase, and by the year 2020, an estimated 59 million Americans will have OA.[19]

The pattern of joint involvement is affected by age, gender, and occupation. Advancing age is a major risk factor for OA; men usually develop symptoms before 45 years of age; women usually do not develop symptoms until after age 55. Before age 55 little difference exists in joint involvement by gender. Older women usually develop OA in the hands (particularly proximal interphalangeal [PIP] joints and thumbs) (Figure 54-1) and knees, whereas men typically develop OA in the hips, knees, and spine. **Heberden's nodes** are more likely to develop in women than in men; a familial tendency has also been noted.

Racial background also influences the development of OA; compared with Caucasian women, African-American women have a higher incidence of OA of the knee, a lower incidence of Heberden's nodes, and a lower prevalence of distal interphalangeal joint (DIP) disease. OA of the hip has a relatively low incidence among Chinese, black Africans, and Jamaicans.[2,19]

An important modifiable risk factor for developing OA is weight. Obesity increases the risk of disease and disease progression. This is an important consideration, in view of the fact that

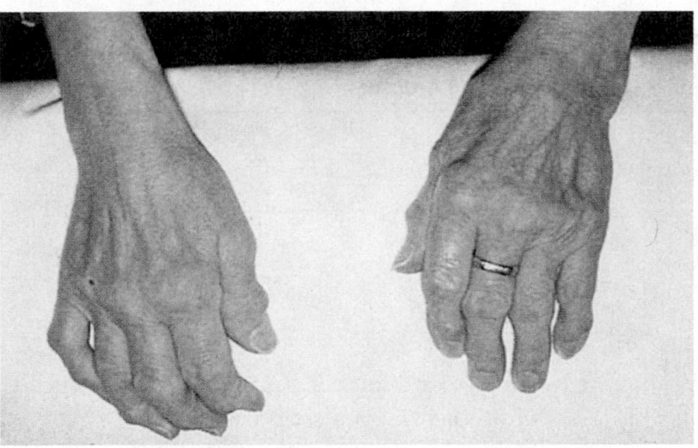

Figure 54-1 Osteoarthritis of hands.

more than 50% of Americans are overweight (as defined as body mass index over 25). Obesity significantly increases the risk of OA of the knee in women[4,28,40] Weight loss has been shown to slow progression of knee OA.

The joints most commonly affected by OA are the PIP, DIP, and first carpometacarpal joints; hips; knees; and cervical and lumbar spine. The two forms of OA are primary (idiopathic) and secondary. Primary joint disease is the most common type of noninflammatory joint disease. Primary DJD is distributed throughout the central and peripheral joints of the body, usually affecting the hand, wrist, neck, lumbar spine, hip, knee, and ankle. Secondary joint disease is caused by any condition that damages cartilage, subjects the joints to chronic stress, or causes joint instability. Causes of secondary joint disease include previous joint infection, inflammation, trauma, surgery, and certain occupations or activities. Persons with occupations involving heavy lifting, frequent crawling or squatting, and repetitive motions are at increased risk for OA.

Other causes include endocrine disorders (acromegaly or hyperparathyroidism); neurologic disorders (pain and proprioceptive responses are altered, thereby increasing the risk of abnormal movement or weight bearing); skeletal deformities; and hemophilia (bleeding into the joints). Regular moderate exercise does not appear to cause or increase existing DJD in normal joints.[19,35] Injury to the joint is a significant risk factor for later development of OA.

▶ ARE You READY?

In planning a staff development workshop on osteoarthritis (OA), the nurse includes which of the following? (Choose all that apply.)

1. Racial background is unrelated to the development of OA.
2. By age 55 over 80% of the population have x-ray evidence of OA.
3. Incidence of OA decreases with age.
4. Older women usually develop OA in the hands.
5. Men usually develop symptoms before age 45.
6. Men usually develop OA in the hips and spine.

Pathophysiology. Despite the name *osteoarthritis*, this disorder does not involve a significant inflammatory component. A small amount of low-grade inflammation is observed, and mechanical abnormalities in the joints irritate surrounding soft tissues and can cause inflammation. OA is generally termed *noninflammatory* to distinguish it from rheumatoid arthritis (RA) (Table 54-1). Both primary and secondary DJDs affect the **articular cartilage**. Characteristic pathologic changes include erosion of articular cartilage, thickening of subchondral bone, and formation of osteophytes.

Normal articular cartilage is white, translucent, and smooth. When affected by DJD, it becomes yellow and opaque. Areas of cartilage soften, and the surface becomes rough, frayed, and cracked. This process is thought to occur as a result of digestion of the cartilage by enzymes and alteration of the nutrition of the cartilage. Eventually the cartilage is destroyed, and the underlying subchondral bone goes through a remodeling process. **Osteophytes**, or bone spurs, appear at the joint margins and at the sites of attachment of supporting structures. These may break off and appear in the joint cavity as "joint mice."

Symptoms vary, depending on the joints involved and degree of disease (see Clinical Manifestations box). Pain is the primary feature and is usually described as a deep aching in the joint. Weather changes and increased activity tend to increase the pain; rest usually provides relief. In contrast to RA, joint stiffness typically lasts less than 1 hour. Decreased joint motion may be caused by the loss of articular cartilage, muscle spasms, shortening of ligaments, and osteophytes; loss of articular cartilage and subchondral bone can lead to joint **subluxation** and deformity. As the joint degenerates, the person may report decreased mobility and the sensation of grinding and catching. Joint laxity may also develop as a result of **effusion** and remodeling of tendinous and ligamentous insertions.

Arthritic changes in the hip cause an antalgic gait, and pain is usually felt on the outer aspect of the hip and in the groin, buttocks, inner thigh, and knee. Patients with OA of the knee are most likely to report pain with motion, stiffness after inactivity, and decreased flexion. A varus deformity is common (Figure 54-2 and Box 54-1). OA of the spine is the most common cause of lower back pain.

CLINICAL MANIFESTATIONS
Osteoarthritis

- Pain: worse with weight bearing; improves with rest; may be accompanied by paresthesias
- Swelling and joint enlargement: may be from inflammatory exudate or blood entering joint capsule, causing an increase in synovial fluid, or from fragments of osteophytes entering synovial cavity
- Decreased range of motion: depends on amount of destroyed cartilage
- Muscular atrophy: from disuse, joint instability, and deformity
- Crepitus: may be present on movement
- Joint stiffness: worse in morning (morning stiffness of less than 1 hour) and after a period of rest or disuse

TABLE 54-1 DISTINGUISHING FEATURES OF OSTEOARTHRITIS AND RHEUMATOID ARTHRITIS

	Osteoarthritis	Rheumatoid Arthritis
Etiology	Primary: unknown, genetic component Secondary: mechanical stress, trauma, hormonal	Unknown Theories: overstimulation of inflammatory process; autoimmune, genetic, antigen-antibody reaction, viral
Onset	45-55 yr Insidious	After age 30 Average age 55 yr Insidious or acute
Pathophysiology	Disease of articular cartilage Biochemical changes leading to deterioration and loss of cartilage Reactive new bone formation Changes in articular surface Areas of exposed bone possible Formation of osteophytes No systemic manifestations	Inflammatory disease of joints, connective tissue with systemic manifestations Inflammatory process destroying joint components Formation of pannus Cartilage erosion Soft tissue changes causing joint subluxation and dislocation Formation of rheumatoid nodules
Joint involvement	Asymmetric, monoarticular, or polyarticular DIP joints (Heberden's nodes) PIP joints (Bouchard's nodes) First CMC, first MTP Hips, knees, lumbar and cervical spine	Symmetric, polyarticular PIP joints MCP joints MTP joints Cervical spine Large joints (hip, knee; more common in older adults)
Clinical manifestations	Joint enlargement Crepitus Pain increased with weight bearing, relieved with rest Limitation of joint motion Noninflammatory joint effusion Morning stiffness <1 hr Joint stiffness or laxity	Fever Weight loss Fatigue Night pain Pain with rest Morning stiffness >1 hr Joint "boggy" on palpation, tender, erythematous Inflammatory joint effusion Subluxation, dislocation Rheumatoid nodules
Diagnostic data	No laboratory abnormalities Radiographic evidence of joint space narrowing, osteophytes, bony sclerosis	Rheumatoid factor positive in 75%-80% of patients; elderly onset positive in 90% of persons[24,28] Elevated ESR Radiographic evidence of joint space narrowing, bone erosion, osteopenia

CMC, Carpometacarpal; *DIP,* distal interphalangeal; *ESR,* erythrocyte sedimentation rate; *MCP,* metacarpophalangeal; *MTP,* metatarsophalangeal; *PIP,* proximal interphalangeal.

Patients may report pain, stiffness, and occasionally neurologic symptoms. Neurologic symptoms can be caused by osteophytes, foraminal stenosis, disc protrusion, or subluxation.

Collaborative Care Management. Objectives in management include relief of pain, restoration of joint function, and prevention of disability or further progression of the disease.

DIAGNOSTIC TESTS. Diagnosis is based on evaluation of the patient history and physical assessment and the results of radiologic studies. Serologic and synovial fluid examinations are essentially normal. Synovial fluid is noninflammatory and pale yellow or clear with a low leukocyte count—500 to 2000 cells/mm^3. Leukocyte counts in excess of 2000 to 3000 cells/mm^3 are indicative of inflammation; a workup for RA, gout, lupus, and other inflammatory arthropathies should follow. Bloody effusions are usually the result of trauma, fractures of osteophytes or subchondral bone, or synovial or ligamentous tears. Arthroscopy is not necessary for diagnosis of OA, but it allows direct visualization of articular surfaces and detection of early disease. X-ray films reveal

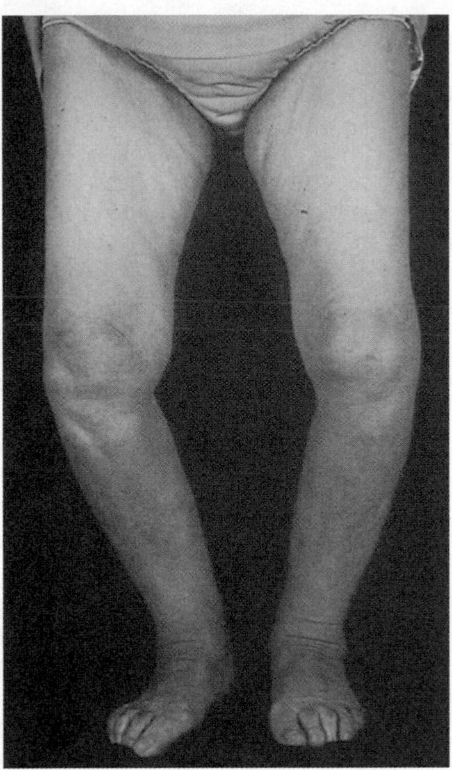
Figure 54-2 Typical varus deformity of knee osteoarthritis.

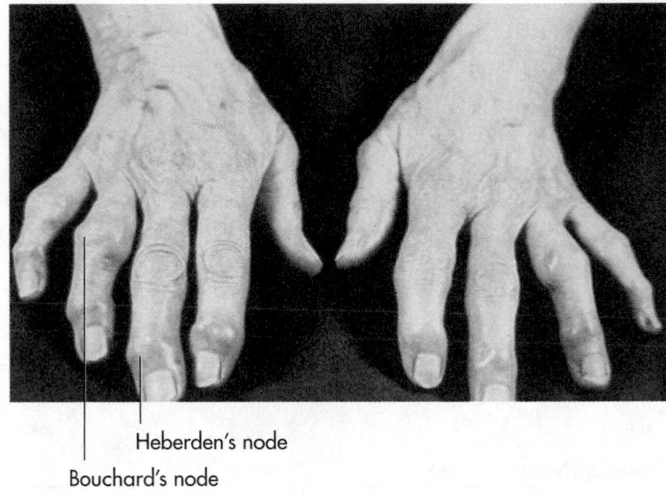

Figure 54-3 Heberden's and Bouchard's nodes.

narrowing of the joint space, osteophyte formation, and eburnation (sclerosis) of subchondral bone. Almost 50% of patients with evidence of OA on x-ray studies are asymptomatic.

MEDICATIONS. Analgesics, nonsteroidal antiinflammatory drugs (NSAIDs), and **intraarticular** corticosteroids are the mainstays of pharmacologic treatment of OA (Table 54-2). The objective of treatment is symptomatic relief of pain; benefits such as improved mobility and function have not been established. Glucosamine and chondroitin are common nutritional supplements used alone or in combination with medications for the treatment of OA (see Complementary & Alternative Therapies box, p. 1624).

Expert opinion is divided over the use of acetaminophen and NSAIDs as first-line agents in the treatment of OA. NSAIDs have the potential for serious side effects, including cardiovascular, gastrointestinal (GI), and renal toxicities; acetaminophen in doses greater than 2 g/day is associated with a risk of serious upper GI toxicity.[28,37] NSAIDs have been shown to be superior to acetaminophen in improving knee and hip pain in persons with OA, but are less effective in improving function [28,37] Another important prescribing consideration is patient preference; 60% to 80% of patients prefer NSAIDs to acetaminophen for treatment of OA.[28]

The American College of Rheumatology recommends acetaminophen as a first-line drug therapy for OA to reduce the gastrophy associated with NSAIDs.[28] Dosages up to 4 g/day may be given in the absence of hepatic or renal disease; many patients get relief with dosages of 2 g/day. The nurse must instruct the patient to read labels of other over-the-counter medications to avoid concurrent use of other products containing acetaminophen. Liver function studies must be done at regular intervals while the patient is receiving therapy. Constant pain is best relieved by dosing at regular intervals; intermittent pain may be relieved by "as needed" dosing. Moderate to severe pain can also be managed by opioids or adjuvant drugs if nonopioids and NSAIDs are ineffective. Other analgesics include tramadol (Ultram) and carisoprodol. Tramadol has a dual action of binding to mu-opioid receptors and also blocking reuptake of norepinephrine and serotonin. The American Pain Society's guidelines for treating OA recommend tramadol for persons who do not receive relief with acetaminophen or for those at risk for adverse effects associated with NSAIDs.[40] A combination drug tramadol and acetaminophen (Ultracet) is available, which minimizes adverse effects and maximizes the analgesic effects.[40]

If acetaminophen is contraindicated because of a history of heavy drinking or liver or renal disease, NSAIDs are the next choice for therapy. As mentioned earlier, a small degree of inflammation may be present; thus NSAIDs have the advantage of having an antiinflammatory effect. No convincing evidence supports the hypothesis that NSAIDs retard articular cartilage degeneration or alter the course of the disease.

NSAIDs act by preventing the formation of prostaglandins, which play a major role in pain and inflammation; most inhibit both cyclooxygenase-1 (COX-1) and COX-2 enzyme formation. Many nonselective NSAIDs are available; all demonstrate similar efficacy in treating OA in groups of patients, but a specific

Box 54-1 Characteristic Changes or Symptoms in Certain Joints

- *Knee involvement:* varus (see Figure 54-2), valgus (knocked knees), flexion deformity; crepitus; limited range of motion
- *Heberden's nodes:* bony protuberances on the dorsal surface of the distal interphalangeal joints of the fingers (Figure 54-3)
- *Bouchard's nodes:* bony protuberances on the proximal interphalangeal joints of the fingers (see Figure 54-3)
- *Coxarthrosis* (degenerative joint disease of the hip): pain in the hip on weight bearing, with pain progressing to include groin and medial knee pain and limited range of motion

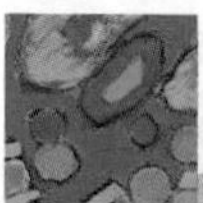

TABLE 54-2
COMMON MEDICATIONS *for Osteoarthritis*

Drug	Action	Nursing Intervention
Analgesic		
Acetaminophen (1-4 g/day)	Analgesic for mild to moderate pain; first-line treatment for patients with minimal inflammation	Drug provides low cost, good safety profile. Monitor liver function at beginning of therapy and every 6-12 mo while patient is taking medication. Do not give to persons with liver disease or regular high intake of alcohol because of risk of liver toxicity. Instruct patient not to exceed 4 g/day and to carefully read OTC medication labels, since many contain acetaminophen. Nausea is most common side effect.
NSAIDs (Nonselective)		
Diclofenac (Voltaren, Cataflam) Diflunisal (Dolobid) Etodolac (Lodine) Fenoprofen (Nalfon) Ibuprofen (Motrin) Indomethacin (Indocin) Naproxen (Naprosyn) Oxaprozin (Daypro) Piroxicam (Feldene) Sulindac (Clinoril) Tolmetin (Tolectin) Diclofenac sodium and misoprostol (Arthrotec)	Analgesic and antiinflammatory; prevent formation of prostaglandins	Studies show NSAIDs do not provide superior pain relief to acetaminophen.[2,9] Prescribe with caution because of side effects (cardiovascular events, nausea, heartburn, GI bleeding, platelet dysfunction, renal and liver dysfunction, congestive heart failure). Prescribe in lowest effective dose, shortest duration, and with prophylactic gastroprotective drug. NSAIDs increase fluid overload and blood pressure. Monitor blood pressure, renal and liver function, and signs of GI bleeding. Avoid concomitant use of other NSAIDs, steroids, anticoagulants, and alcohol.
NSAIDs (COX-2 Selective Inhibitor)		
Celecoxib (Celebrex)	Analgesic and antiinflammatory; selectively inhibits prostaglandin synthesis by inhibiting COX-2 Uncertainty about benefit in reducing risk of serious GI bleeding compared with non-selective NSAIDs[8]	Do not prescribe immediately after CABG surgery. Do not give to persons with allergies to aspirin, other NSAIDs, sulfonamides; renal and hepatic dysfunction; asthma; or pregnancy. Monitor for renal and hepatic function, signs of bleeding. Use extreme caution in persons with cardiovascular disease, congestive heart failure, or hypertension. Lowest effective dose should be prescribed.

NSAID may be more effective in individual patients.[28] The popularly prescribed COX-2 inhibitors valdecoxib and rofecoxib were withdrawn from the market in 2004 and 2005, respectively, after clinical trials demonstrated an increased risk of serious cardiovascular events when compared with placebo.[15] Celecoxib is still currently available. If prescribing celecoxib, providers are cautioned to weigh the benefits and risks and other treatment options; the Food and Drug Administration (FDA) recommends prescribing the lowest effective dose for the shortest duration of use.[8] Persons at high risk for GI bleeding and those in whom nonselective NSAIDs are not tolerated or are ineffective for pain relief may be candidates for celecoxib.

NSAIDs have the risk of causing serious, potentially fatal GI side effects, including bleeding, ulceration, and perforation of the stomach or intestines; older patients are at greater risk. All NSAIDs have the potential for causing renal and hepatic dysfunction; kidney and liver function studies should be monitored for persons receiving long-term therapy. The FDA has proposed labeling changes for all NSAIDs, both prescription and over the counter.[15] Recommendations include a boxed warning summarizing the potential for cardiovascular and potentially fatal GI bleeding. The labeling for celecoxib would contain a warning regarding the increased risk of serious cardiovascular events. Packaging inserts would contain warnings that NSAID use is contraindicated for in patients immediately following coronary artery bypass graft surgery.

Cardiovascular risks associated with the use of NSAIDs include thrombotic events, myocardial infarction, and stroke; risk increases with duration of use. Studies have shown that NSAIDs increase blood pressure by 5 mm Hg in normotensive and hypertensive persons.[39] Hypertensive effects are increased in persons taking angiotensin-converting enzyme inhibitors, diuretics, and beta blockers. The risk of developing side effects is increased with a history of ulcers, GI bleeding, congestive heart failure, cirrhosis,

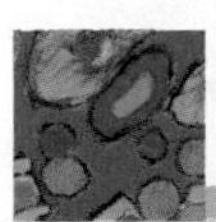

TABLE 54-2
COMMON MEDICATIONS *for Osteoarthritis—cont'd*

Drug	Action	Nursing Intervention
Opioid Analgesics		
Tramadol (Ultram) (synthetic opioid) Codeine Oxycodone (may be combined with acetaminophen [Percocet] or aspirin [Percodan]) Propoxyphene (Darvon) (may be combined with acetaminophen [Darvocet])	Bind with receptors in CNS to produce analgesia; relief of moderate to severe pain when acetaminophen or NSAIDs are ineffective in relieving pain	Causes CNS depression, respiratory depression; side effects include nausea, dizziness, constipation, sedation. Use cautiously in persons with renal or hepatic disease. Monitor for signs of toxicity. Teach patient to avoid hazardous activity when taking medication; institute safety precautions. Monitor bowel function; patient may take stool softener to prevent constipation. Be alert for potential for drug dependence and tolerance.
Intraarticular Steroid Injection		
Triamincinolone (Kenalog) Methylprednisolone (Depo-Medrol)	Antiinflammatory; used in cases of inflammation or knee infusion	Be alert for potential adverse effects on connective tissue. Limit injections to 2 or 3 per year per joint.
Viscosupplementation		
Intraarticular hyaluronan, hylan G-F 20 (Synvisc) Sodium hyaluronate (Hyalgan; Nuflexxa [non-avian derived]) Hyaluranon (Orthovisc)	Glycosaminoglycan; simulates synovial fluid; mode of action poorly understood; substitutes for naturally produced hyaluronic acid, which lubricates joint and acts as shock absorber	Drugs require a series of injections and are expensive. Pain relief begins 5-9 wk after completing injections and may last up to 6 mo. Pain may occur at injection site; be aware of risk of infection, few local reactions; systemic reactions rare. Rate of response is less in persons with advanced disease; it may benefit those awaiting joint replacement. Synvisc is made from chicken combs and is contraindicated in persons with poultry allergy.
Topical Agents		
Capsaicin NSAIDs (salicylate, benzydamine, diclofenac, ibuprofen) OTC preparations (Icy Hot, Aspercreme)	Provide pain relief and/or antiinflammatory action; capsaicin, derived from pepper plant, acts as substance P inhibitor; others may contain local anesthetics	These agents are relatively safe and inexpensive and have fewer side effects with short-term use of topical agents than with systemic NSAIDs. Avoid contact with mucous membranes.

OTC, Over-the-counter; *NSAIDs,* nonsteroidal antiinflammatory drugs; *GI,* gastrointestinal; *COX-2,* cyclooxygenase-2; *CABG,* coronary artery bypass graft; *CNS,* central nervous system.

diabetes, and NSAID intolerance; with concomitant use of steroids or anticoagulants; in older person; and in persons in poor general health.[2,9] Certain NSAIDs are available in cream or gel form for topical application.

Intraarticular injection of steroids may be needed if analgesics and NSAIDs are ineffective or as an adjunct to therapy. Unstable or infected joints should never be injected. Steroid injections are effective in controlling pain and improving function. However, repeated injections may actually accelerate joint degeneration. To prevent articular cartilage damage, a joint should not be injected more than three or four times per year. Other complications include infection and cutaneous atrophy.

Viscosupplementation, developed in the 1960s, is based on the fact that synovial fluid in persons with OA is less elastic and less viscous than normal synovial fluid. The objective of treatment is to restore the normal elasticity and viscosity of the synovial fluid and restore the normal balance of hyaluronan within the fluid. **Hyaluronan** (hyaluronic acid) is a glycosamine polysaccharide found in high concentrations in normal synovial fluid. In persons with OA the concentration of hyaluronan is decreased, and the amount of synovial fluid is increased. Hyaluronan exerts an antiinflammatory effect, by suppressing prostaglandin release, similar to NSAIDs, but acts locally in the joint. Evidence supports hyaluronan's effectiveness as an analgesic and in inhibiting joint degradation.[10] Persons with complete joint space collapse and no articular cartilage are not candidates for viscosupplementation. Viscosupplementation is proven to be an effective and long-lasting nonsurgical treatment option with few side effects; it may be used in combination with other medications for treatment of OA.

TREATMENTS. A variety of treatments and therapies are available for the person with OA. These include traditional and alternative treatments (see Future Watch box). Alternative therapies are used alone or in conjunction with traditional therapy[12,32,33]

Complementary & Alternative Therapies

Glucosamine and Chondroitin

Both glucosamine and chondroitin are classified as nutritional supplements and are not approved by the Food and Drug Administration for the treatment of osteoarthritis (OA). Both products are available over the counter and are widely used to relieve mild pain and stiffness associated with OA. Glucosamine has been used successfully in Europe for more than 25 years.

Glucosamine (glucosamine hydrochloride and sulfate) occurs naturally in the body and, when taken as a supplement, is derived from chitin in the shells of shrimp, crab, and lobster. It is available as a tablet, cream, or beverage and has been shown to be effective in reducing pain and possibly in improving the health of cartilage by contributing to cartilage repair.[2] Most studies demonstrating the effectiveness of glucosamine have involved glucosamine sulfate. The few known side effects include nausea, rash, and possible allergic reactions in persons with shellfish allergy. Glucose metabolism, particularly in persons with diabetes, should be monitored, since glucosamine is a derivative of glucose. The usual dosage is 1500 mg/day (2000 mg/day for persons weighing more than 200 pounds); at least 2 months of therapy is necessary to determine effectiveness.

Chondroitin sulfite is a component of human cartilage; when taken as a supplement, it is derived from the trachea of cattle. The recommended dosage is 1200 mg/day in two divided doses. It is available in pills, capsules, lotion, or liquid and is often sold in combination with glucosamine. Studies have shown chondroitin to be effective in relieving pain and stiffness associated with OA, with few or no adverse effects. There is no evidence to support topical use of chondroitin. Persons taking warfarin should not use chondroitin, since it interferes with warfarin levels. As with glucosamine, it may take 2 months or longer to determine effectiveness of therapy. Monthly costs for both substances average $30 to $45.

The American College of Rheumatology believes that more studies are indicated to prove the efficacy of these agents in the treatment of OA. The National Institute of Arthritis and Musculoskeletal and Skin Diseases, the National Institutes of Health, and the National Center for Complementary and Alternative Medicine are conducting studies to evaluate the effectiveness of both these substances.[27] Nurses should be prepared to discuss the benefits and precautions regarding the use of these nutritional supplements for treatment of OA.

(see Complementary & Alternative Therapies box at right). An estimated 20,000 products are available for arthritis, and as many as 79% of patients report using alternative therapies.[12] Many of these products have not been evaluated in controlled clinical studies, and nurses should help the arthritis patient evaluate the risk and benefits of alterative therapies.

Treatment early in the course of DJD can make a significant improvement in the person's quality of life and may alter the course of the disease. Three foci of therapy are relief of pain, joint protection, and physical therapy (PT) to stabilize joints and prevent deformity.

To protect joints, appropriate nutritional intake is encouraged to maintain ideal body weight and avoid weight gain. Weight gain places an unnecessary stress on joints, particularly the hips and knees. Exercise is a cornerstone of joint protection for persons with DJD. Emphasis is placed on unloading the stress on painful weight-bearing joints through the use of canes, walkers, or crutches; range-of-motion (ROM) exercises to prevent deformities and contractures; and muscle-strengthening exercises to increase or maintain muscle tone and strength.

Benefits of exercise are well known and include reduced pain, increased strength and mobility, decreased fatigue, improved gait, reduction of cardiovascular risk, improved lipid management, increased bone mass, and improved sense of well being.[41] In persons with advanced disease, exercise may exacerbate symptoms.

Future Watch

Leech Therapy for Osteoarthritis of the Knee

Leeches have been used since medieval times for medicinal purposes. Leeches are classified as medical devices by the Food and Drug Administration. Leeches' saliva contains substances that have antiinflammatory, anesthetic, and analgesic effects; one identified substance is hirudin, a potent anticoagulant. Researchers are studying morphine-like effects associated with leech therapy.

A study is under way at Beth Israel Medical Center, New York, where patients will receive leech therapy for osteoarthritis of the knee. This program is based on results of a German study of 51 patients with knee OA. In the German study, participants received either one local application of four to six leeches or a 28-day regimen of topical diclofenac (control group). Pain, function, and stiffness were measured for 91 days after the intervention. These parameters improved for the duration of the study in the leech therapy group. Pain scores were not significantly different among the two groups after day 7. More research is needed to compare leeches with other traditional therapies for OA and to increase understanding of the pharmacologic properties of leech saliva.

Michalsen A et al: Effectiveness of leech therapy in osteoarthritis of the knee: a randomized, controlled trial, *Ann Intern Med* 139(9):724-730, 2003.

Complementary & Alternative Therapies

Osteoarthritis

- Acupuncture (for pain relief)
- Low-level laser therapy
- Antiinflammation diet: omega-3 fatty acids
- Green-lipped mussel extract
- Shark cartilage
- Herbal supplements: alfalfa, devil's claw, yucca root, saw palmetto
- *S*-adenosylmethionine (SAMe) (may have chondroprotective action)
- Methylsulfonylmethane sulfur powder (MSM) (may have chondroprotective action)
- Magnets (may reduce pain and improve functional ability)
- Copper bracelets
- Massage
- Meditation
- Reflexology
- T'ai chi'
- Yoga

Rest relieves most joint pain but should be avoided for prolonged periods, since immobility promotes joint stiffness.

Weight loss, another benefit of regular exercise, can be beneficial in easing the pain of arthritis. Obesity, a risk factor for knee OA, increases joint pain and disability. Results from the Arthritis, Diet, and Activity Promotion Trial, a long-term clinical trial of older, obese adults with knee OA, demonstrated that weight loss as little as 5% to 6%, when combined with moderate exercise, decreased arthritis pain by 30% and improved functioning.[23]

Essential elements of an exercise program for the person with OA include stretching, strengthening, and aerobic exercise. It is important to prevent deconditioning of the muscles that stabilize joints and to promote overall fitness while protecting the joints. Recommendations include exercising for at least 30 minutes per day, five times per week. *Healthy People 2010* recommends exercise as an effective self-management strategy for persons with OA.[41]

Muscle strength can be maintained by engaging in regular exercise. An appropriate warm-up and cool-down program is essential to prevent muscle strain and damage. ROM exercises should be performed daily. Isometric and isotonic exercises, which do not stress the joint, are an excellent starting point. As strength and endurance increase, progressive, resistive exercises can be added to the regimen. Low-impact aerobic exercise improves cardiovascular function, increases well-being, and helps with weight reduction if needed. Swimming and water exercises, which decrease stress on joints, are good choices. In general, persons with OA should avoid high-impact activities and exercises, which can increase symptoms, especially if weight-bearing joints are involved. The Arthritis Foundation offers exercise classes at many community centers. Other resources include the National Institute on Aging and the American College of Rheumatology.

Heat applied before exercise can be helpful in relaxing the muscles, increasing blood flow to the region, and decreasing pain. Moist heat is generally preferred. Application of cold after exercise or during periods of acute inflammation decreases pain and swelling. For the patient with decreased function because of DJD, adaptive aids, PT, and pain relief medications can be prescribed. Adaptive devices may be beneficial for completing activities of daily living (ADLs) for persons with DJD of the hands. (See section on treatments for RA for information on assistive and adaptive devices and joint protection techniques.)

SURGICAL MANAGEMENT. Persons with advanced DJD, severe pain, or severe limitations in function or mobility may be candidates for surgical management of their disease. Surgical management of the person with OA is indicated to relieve pain, improve function, or correct deformity. Surgical procedures include those which preserve or restore articular cartilage and those which realign, fuse, or replace joints. Surgical management usually provides the patient with excellent results; however, the patient is at risk for developing surgical complications, including infection, nerve and blood vessel injury, deep venous thrombosis (DVT), and pulmonary or fat embolism. Surgery is performed when medications and PT have failed. However, surgery should be performed before severe deformity, joint instability, contracture, or severe muscle atrophy develops, all of which can compromise the outcome and place the patient at a higher risk for complications.

Procedures to restore or preserve articular cartilage include joint debridement (via arthroscopy), abrasion chondroplasty (abrasion of subchondral bone to stimulate growth of cartilage), and replacement of articular cartilage with grafts. These procedures are not indicated for patients with advanced DJD, because they usually produce only short-term results. An alternative therapy is the transplantation of healthy cartilage cells (autologous cartilage implantation) into the knees of persons with traumatic arthritis or other cartilage defects. Chondrocytes are harvested, cultured in the laboratory, and injected into the knee. Young persons with small areas of damaged cartilage are the ideal candidates for cartilage transplantation; the patient must be committed to a 12-month rehabilitation program.

An osteotomy is a surgical incision through a bone. Osteotomy may be thought of as a surgical or intentional fracture, whose purpose is to realign a joint or bone or to redistribute the load-bearing surface of a joint to a region that has more articular cartilage (Figure 54-4). Osteotomy is useful for correcting angulation or rotational deformities. The patient is treated much like a patient who has suffered a fracture. Persons with stable joints, functional ROM, adequate musculature, and some remaining articular cartilage benefit the most from osteotomy.

Arthrodesis, or joint fusion, is performed to relieve pain and to restore stability and alignment. Joint fusion, as the term implies, results in lost motion; hence this procedure has limited application. The fusion of one joint increases the load bearing of adjacent joints, which may accelerate degeneration of those joints. Arthrodesis is most commonly performed on the cervical and lumbar spine, interphalangeal joints, first metatarsal joints, and wrist and ankle.

Joint replacement, or **arthroplasty**, has been a mainstay of treatment for OA since the 1960s. More than 200,000 total hip replacements are performed annually in the United States.[3,31] Although arthroplasty procedures of the hip and knee are the most common (Figures 54-5 and 54-6), the procedure can also be performed on the shoulder, elbow, ankle, and finger joints.

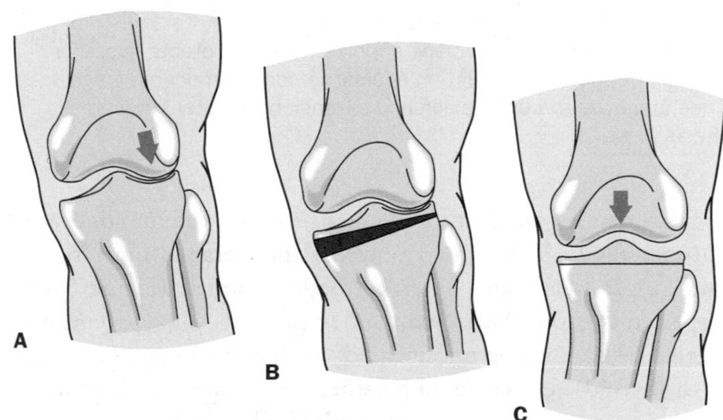

Figure 54-4 Osteotomy of tibia for genu valgum (valgus deformity); anterior view of left knee. **A,** Weight-bearing force is concentrated on one compartment of knee. **B,** Wedge of bone is removed from tibia. Amount of bone removed is determined by how much correction in angulation is necessary. **C,** Distal portion of tibia is swung to proximal portion. Correction of angulation obtained allows weight-bearing forces to be more evenly distributed through both compartments of knee.

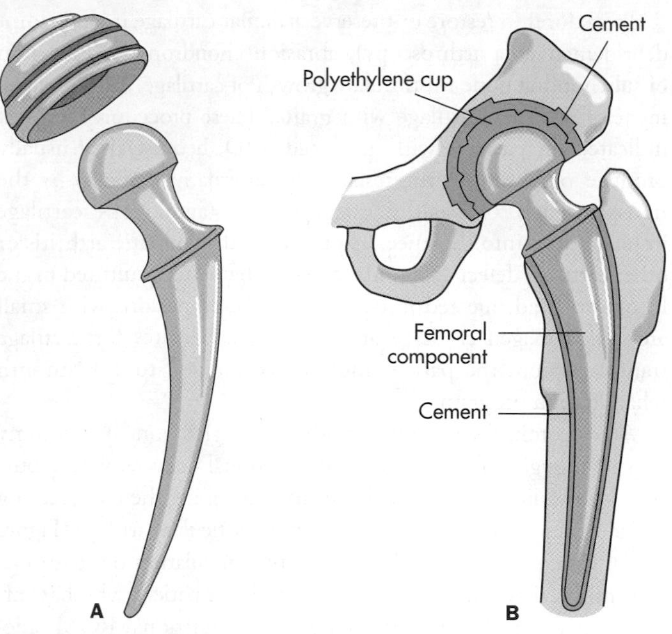

Figure 54-5 **A**, Acetabular and femoral components of total hip prosthesis. **B**, Total hip prosthesis in place.

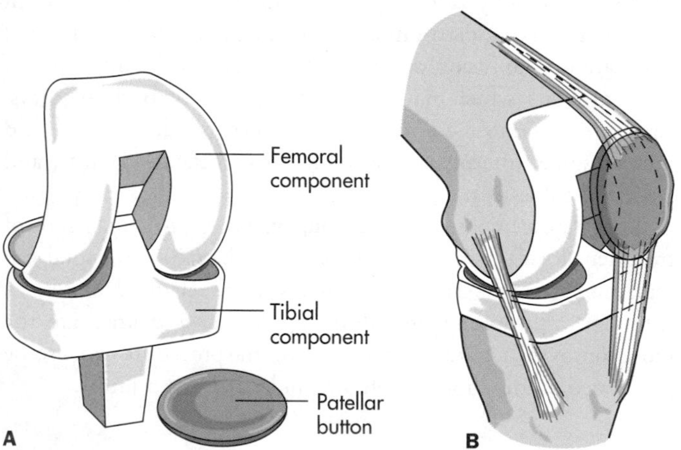

Figure 54-6 **A**, Tibial and femoral components of total knee prosthesis. A patellar button, made of polyethylene, protects posterior surface of patella from friction against femoral component when knee is moved through flexion and extension. **B**, Total knee prosthesis in place.

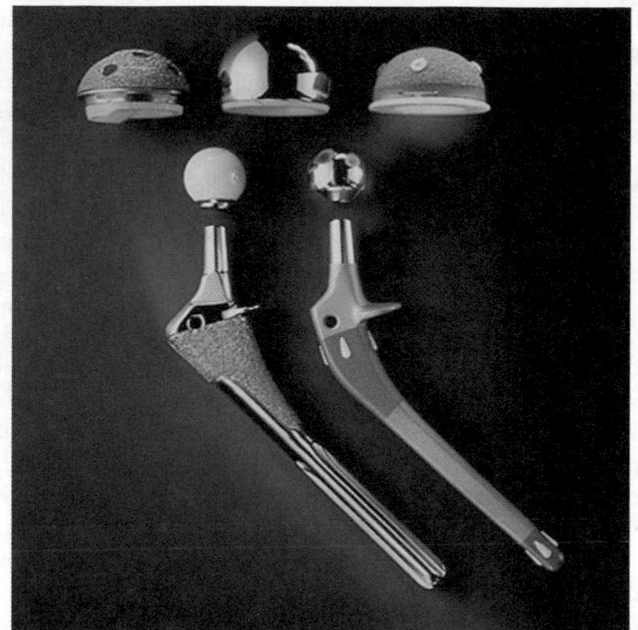

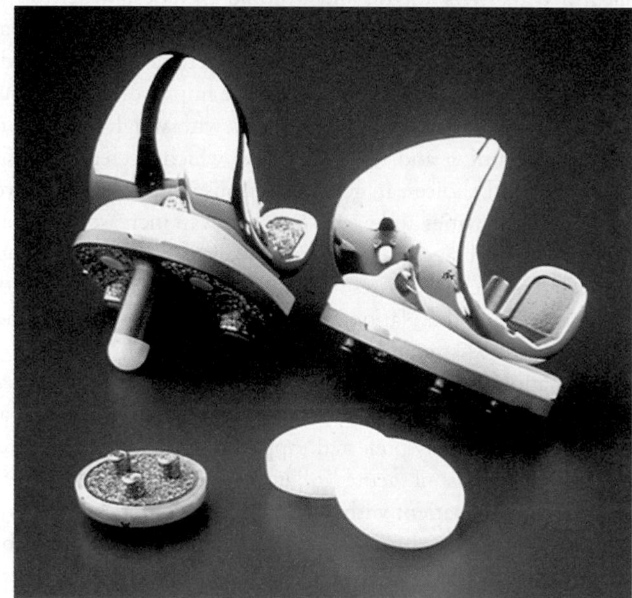

Figure 54-7 **A**, Hip prostheses. *Left:* Porous ingrowth acetabular cup and femoral stem, ceramic femoral head. *Middle:* Bipolar head for hemiarthroplasty (component fits on top of femoral head component). Used with either cemented or uncemented femoral stems. *Right:* Cemented femoral stem and cemented acetabular cup. **B**, Knee prostheses. *Left:* Porous ingrowth femoral and tibial components; porous ingrowth patellar button. *Right:* Hybrid: cemented femoral component and patellar button; porous ingrowth tibial component.

Materials for prosthetic implants are metal (titanium or cobalt-chrome alloy), high-density polyethylene, ceramic (low friction and longer wear), and other synthetic materials (Figure 54-7). Replacement prostheses may be implanted with polymethylmethacrylate, may be uncemented, or may be a combination of both (hybrid). Uncemented prostheses are treated with a porous coating that promotes bony ingrowth (see Figure 54-7).

Surgical approaches for hip arthroplasty include anterolateral, lateral, transtrochanteric, or posterolateral. The posterior and direct lateral are most commonly used. The posterior approach is technically easier, has less risk of gait disturbance postoperatively, but is associated with an increased risk of dislocation. The lateral approach decreases the risk of dislocation and injury to the sciatic nerve, but is associated with an increased risk of postoperative limp. No evidence is available to determine which is the optimal approach.[16]

Minimally invasive total hip arthroplasty is performed through an incision that is less than 10 cm long.[18] Many procedures are done through two 5 cm incisions; muscles and tendons are avoided or separated in this approach. Traditional total hip arthroplasty requires one 20- to 30-cm incision, and muscles and tendons are surgically cut. The major disadvantage of minimally invasive hip replacement is decreased visualization of the operative field; long-term results are not known, since the procedure is relatively new.[18] Advantages are less soft tissue trauma, preservation of muscle and ligament strength, and faster recovery and rehabilitation time. Robotically aided surgery is also being developed for joint replacements.

The decision whether to use cement depends on such factors as the individual patient, including his or her bone stock, age, and ability to comply with weight-bearing restrictions after surgery. Uncemented components are thought to last longer, since the bony growth lessens the likelihood of the prosthesis loosening, which is a consideration with cemented joints. Loosening of the components may lead to implant failure. In addition, uncemented (press fit) joints are usually easier to replace and revise than cemented joints. Some cementless prostheses have a calcium hydroxyapatite coating to promote bone growth and enhance component fixation. Many surgeons prefer the hybrid technique, using a press fit porous acetabulum and a cemented femoral stem.[3]

Total knee (medial and lateral femorotibial and patellar-femoral) arthroplasty (TKA) is a technically more difficult procedure than total hip replacement, because of the complex movements of the knee joint. The patella may or may not be replaced in total knee surgery. A unicompartmental or unicondylar knee arthroplasty (UKA) replaces the medial or lateral compartment of the femorotibial joint. The majority of persons undergoing UKA have anteromedial OA.[13] Indications for UKA include single compartmental OA with an intact anterior cruciate ligament, lack of ligamentous laxity, weight less than 90 kg (200 pounds), osteoporotic bone, varus or valgus deformity greater than 15 degrees, and flexion contractures greater than 15 degrees.[13] Advantages of UKA are greater ROM, preservation of bone stock, faster rehabilitation time, and fewer complications.[13] The UKA is more technically challenging surgical technique than tricompartmental TKA, which is a disadvantage at centers that do not perform large numbers of these procedures.[13]

All joint components have a finite life span. When originally developed in the 1970s, joint prostheses were expected to last about 10 years; then revision surgery was indicated. Today approximately 80% of hip joint implants will last 20 years; 10-year success rates for TKA nears 98%.[3,31] Advances in prosthetic components, surgical technique, bearing surfaces, and methods of fixation have resulted in increased implant survival rates. The prosthetic implants are subject to fatigue, wear, breakage, and failure. A particular risk associated with total joint arthroplasty is infection, which usually necessitates removal of the prosthesis. Most revisions are done because of component loosening; infection and implant failure are other reasons for revision. Revision surgery typically lasts longer, involves more blood loss, and results in less joint function than the primary procedure.

Total shoulder arthroplasty (TSA) involves replacement of both the glenoid and humeral component; hemiarthroplasty involves replacement of the humeral component only. Relief of pain is the most common indication for shoulder replacement surgery; restoration of motion and strength are lesser considerations, particularly in persons with damage to the rotator cuff.[31] The surgical procedure is challenging because of the dynamic structure and movements of the joint. The shoulder joint lacks a true socket and depends on surrounding soft tissue structures for its stability. Instability accounts for nearly 38% of TSA complications.[31] Other complications include infection, dislocation, and lack of motion.

Total elbow replacements are primarily performed to relieve the pain and disability associated with RA, not OA. The patient must have adequate bone stock and ligamentous structures to provide stability to the implanted joint. Both components are usually cemented in place.

Ankle fusion has traditionally been the procedure of choice for surgical treatment of ankle OA. Fusion provides pain relief and durable fixation but results in lost motion, which may result in arthritis of the hindfoot. Joint replacement offers the benefit of pain relief and ankle motion. Disadvantages of ankle arthroplasty include problems with wound healing, loosening of components, and higher complication rates.[6] The ankle joint is formed by the tibia, talus, and fibula. Both two- and three-component prostheses are available; currently all are the bony ingrowth type. Wound healing has historically been a major problem with ankle replacement; more long-term data are needed to evaluate newer prostheses and surgical techniques.[6]

Another type of joint replacement is the interposition arthroplasty, in which the joint surface on one or both sides is replaced with metal, inert material (polyethylene), fascia, or tendon. Interposition arthroplasty is usually performed on the wrist or metacarpophalangeal (MCP) joints of the fingers.

Preventing infection is a priority of care with all joint replacement surgery. Revision surgery carries a higher risk of infection because of the longer operating time. Sources of infection in the operating room include direct contamination of the wound and contamination of the sterile field or personnel. The rate of infection in patients with total hip replacements is approximately 1%; the rate is higher in knee and shoulder replacements.[31] The majority of infections originate in the operating room by direct wound contamination. Measures taken to prevent surgically acquired infection include the use of laminar airflow systems, body exhaust systems for scrubbed and circulating personnel (Figure 54-8), limited traffic in the operating room and use of an outside circulating nurse, skin preparation, and strict adherence to sterile technique.

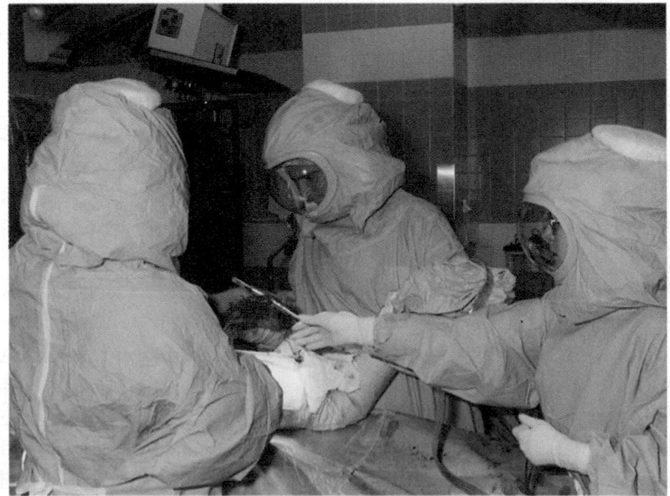

Figure 54-8 Body exhaust system during total joint replacement surgery.

Other techniques include antibiotic-impregnated cement and prophylactic perioperative antibiotics.

COMPLICATIONS. Complications associated with total joint replacement include wound infection (superficial or deep), thrombophlebitis or DVT, pulmonary embolism, fat embolism, dislocation of the prosthesis, and mechanical failure of the components. Other complications associated with the surgical procedure include urinary tract infection (if an indwelling catheter is used) and pneumonia.

Infection is a potentially severe complication after joint replacement. Deep infection may necessitate removal of the prosthesis. More than 50% of hip infections occur more than 3 months after surgery. Infections that develop within the first 3 postoperative months are usually superficial or suprafascial infections (stage I). Deep or subfascial infections are commonly seen within 3 to 24 months after surgery (stage II). Infections occurring later than 24 months after surgery are usually attributed to hematogenous spreading from other locations in the body (stage III).

Stage II infections are attributed to direct contamination of the wound in the operating room. Symptoms associated with mechanical loosening of the prosthesis resemble those of stage II infections; however, loosening rarely occurs in the first year after replacement. A patient's report of new pain in the operative site should be immediately investigated. Conditions such as diverticulitis; cellulitis; abscesses; or seeding resulting from dental procedures, GI procedures, or any surgery can be a source of stage III infections.

Once an infection occurs, several treatment options exist, depending on the patient's condition and the causative organism. Surgical debridement, resection arthroplasty, arthrodesis, amputation, antibiotic therapy, and reimplantation are all options for treating persons with infected total joints. If infection necessitates removal of the prosthesis, first the area is debrided and then the appropriate antibiotics are administered on the basis of culture and sensitivity results. Reimplantation of the joint is done between 6 weeks and 1 year later, depending on the causative organism and the patient's condition. Antibiotics are continued for several weeks.

Intraoperatively, antibiotic-treated cement can be used for susceptible organisms during reimplantation. If it is not possible to replace the prosthesis in a patient with a total hip replacement, a "girdlestone" hip results. Fibrous scar tissue replaces the hip joint, but the patient can still walk. In the case of a TKA that cannot be replaced, the patient can undergo an arthrodesis, resulting in an immobile knee joint. Patients with severe systemic infection, intractable pain, or extensive bone loss may eventually require an amputation.

Persons with RA are more likely to develop major wound complications as a result of immunosuppressive medications used to treat RA. Patients with diabetes are also at an increased risk for developing infections after total joint replacement.

Dislocation of the prosthesis is a particular concern for persons with hip replacements. Dislocation can result in significant morbidity and possibly an additional surgical procedure. Dislocation often occurs during transfers. Safety precautions and education of patients and personnel are necessary during the acute care and rehabilitation phases. Box 54-2 lists other complications of total joint arthroplasty.

Nursing Management

of the Patient undergoing Joint Replacement Surgery

A Nursing Care Plan for a patient undergoing joint replacement is found on p. 1630.

PREOPERATIVE CARE

As described in Chapter 13, preoperative data are usually gathered at a preadmission appointment or surgeon's office. Many institutions have joint replacement classes, brochures, videos, and other teaching aids to enhance preoperative instruction and decrease anxiety (see Research box). Preoperative education is beneficial in decreasing anxiety in patients undergoing hip and knee replacements.[21] The nurse assesses the patient for risk factors that may influence perioperative care. Nursing interventions focus on providing the patient accurate information on the perioperative experience.

Infection is a contraindication to joint replacement surgery. Infection causes loosening of the prosthetic components and may progress to osteomyelitis. Respiratory conditions may delay surgery. Persons with severe chronic obstructive pulmonary disease or pneumonia are at particular risk perioperatively, since methylmethacrylate (bone cement) is excreted through the lungs, which may cause pneumonitis or worsen a preexisting respiratory condition.

The nurse teaches the patient and family about potential complications and preventive measures after joint replacement surgery. Persons having knee or hip joints replaced are at risk for DVT and pulmonary or fat embolism. A history of DVT or bilateral knee or hip replacement surgery increases the patient's risk. Without prophylactic anticoagulation, the frequency of DVT in

Research

Thomas K et al: Impact of a preoperative education program via interactive telehealth network for rural patients having total joint replacement, *Orthop Nurs* 23(1):39-43, 2004.

Preoperative teaching programs are beneficial and positively affect patient outcomes. Traditional programs are done individually or in groups at the hospital or surgeon's office. Rural patients may experience difficulty traveling to the medical center before the scheduled surgery date. A multidisciplinary group in central Kentucky developed a preoperative education program for total joint replacement patients and their families to be delivered via an interactive telehealth network. Objectives of the program were to provide necessary information regarding the perioperative experience, decrease patient and family anxiety, and decrease length of stay. In addition to the telehealth session, written materials were delivered to the patients' homes.

The telehealth network was successful in reaching patients who may otherwise have been unable to attend a teaching session. Participants expressed satisfaction with the method of education. Participation in preoperative education programs increased since implementing the telehealth network. The average length of stay for joint patients has decreased since the telehealth intervention, but this may be due to other variables. More research is needed to explore the use of technology in patient teaching.

Box 54-2 Complications of Total Joint Arthroplasty

Hip

Dislocation
Infection
Deep venous thrombosis
Pulmonary embolism
Fat embolism
Leg length discrepancy
Altered gait
Pneumonia
Footdrop (secondary to nerve damage)

Knee

Infection
Deep venous thrombosis
Pulmonary embolism
Fat embolism
Acute compartment syndrome
Instability
Loosening of prosthesis
Patellar fracture
Poor patellar tracking
Vascular injury (intraoperative) and hemorrhage
Reflex sympathetic dystrophy
Nerve damage

Shoulder

Infection
Loosening of prosthesis
Glenohumeral instability
Dislocation, subluxation
Intraoperative fracture
Rotator cuff tears
Deltoid dysfunction
Nerve damage
Impingement syndrome
Pulmonary embolism

Elbow

Infection
Dislocation
Deep venous thrombosis
Pulmonary embolism
Loosening of prosthesis
Delayed wound healing

Ankle

Infection
Problems with wound healing or skin closure
Residual pain
Impingement
Loosening of prosthesis

persons undergoing hip replacement surgery is as high as 50% to 60% and up to 80% in persons undergoing knee replacement surgery.[25,36] Persons with recurrent embolism or those in whom anticoagulant therapy is contraindicated may require a more invasive approach to prevention of thromboembolism, including placement of an inferior vena cava filter.[31]

The high incidence of DVT in patients with a hip replacement may be related to occlusion of the femoral vein, which occurs during the operative procedure. The femoral vein may become twisted, damaging the endothelium during disarticulation of the femoral head from the acetabulum. These factors, in addition to postoperative immobility and hypercoagulability, place the patient at a significant risk for DVT. Length of surgery in excess of 30 minutes is the most documented risk factor for DVT. Any joint replacement surgery takes longer than 30 minutes; revision surgery may last as long as 4 or more hours. Proximal DVTs are more likely to occur because of the surgical technique. Persons undergoing a total knee replacement are at an increased risk for DVT because of surgical technique. Intraoperatively, the extremity is wrapped in an elastic bandage, and a pneumatic tourniquet is inflated to reduce blood loss. The use of the tourniquet and elastic wrap may damage the endothelial lining of the vein, attracting platelets and causing aggregation and possibly thrombus. In addition, the use of bone cement, which produces release of heat, may cause local venous damage and an increased risk of DVT.[36] Reaming of the intramedullary canal and seating of the femoral component may result in a fat embolus.

Prophylaxis for DVT may begin preoperatively or intraoperatively using low-molecular-weight heparin (LMWH), heparin, or warfarin. Other protocols begin anticoagulation postoperatively. Following institutional or surgeon protocol, the nurse advises the patient to discontinue any NSAIDs, aspirin, anticoagulants, or steroids at the prescribed interval before surgery. Steroid therapy needs to be tapered and may take several weeks to discontinue; aspirin and NSAIDs are generally discontinued 7 to 10 days before surgery. Results of coagulation studies should be within the normal range before surgery. Despite prophylactic steps, the incidence of pulmonary embolism in postoperative total hip patients is estimated at 2%.[3]

Persons undergoing major orthopedic surgery often have significant perioperative blood loss; persons undergoing total hip replacement may lose 1000 to 2000 ml. Depending on the procedure performed and expected blood loss, either type and screen or type and cross-match is ordered. Autologous donation (see Chapter 13) is another alternative. The patient should be informed about this option in sufficient time to allow donation. Preoperative autologous donation decreases the patient's hemoglobin and hematocrit levels before surgery and can exacerbate anemia. An iron supplement is usually prescribed if the patient opts for autologous donation. Erythropoietin-alpha given before surgery is effective in stimulating erythropoiesis and reducing the need for allogeneic transfusion. In cases where anticipated blood loss is significant, intraoperative and postoperative blood salvage techniques may be used to allow for reinfusion either intraoperatively

Nursing Care Plan

Patient With a Total Knee Replacement

Data A 59-year-old man has osteoarthritis of the left knee. Over the past 8 months he has experienced increased pain with only minimal relief from nonsteroidal antiinflammatory drugs (NSAIDs). He now walks with a cane when his pain is severe. He is no longer able to participate in many activities he once enjoyed because of pain and limited mobility. On the advice of his physician, he has elected to undergo total knee replacement. His nursing history reveals that he lives with his wife in a two-story house. Their bedroom is upstairs. He plans to return home after his hospitalization where he will remain during his 1-month leave from work. He has no preexisting medical problems and takes only NSAIDs.

He and his wife attended a total knee replacement class 2 weeks before his admission as part of his preadmission screening. He stopped taking NSAIDs 1 week ago.

Nursing Diagnosis

Deficient knowledge related to lack of previous experience with total knee replacement surgery

Outcomes

- Patient will verbalize understanding of impending surgery and need for continued follow-up care.
- Patient will participate in postoperative rehabilitation care and exercises.
- Patient will verbalize understanding of prescribed home medications.

Related NOC Outcomes

- Knowledge: Disease Process
- Knowledge: Medication
- Knowledge: Prescribed Activity

Related NIC Interventions

- Teaching: Disease Process
- Teaching: Preoperative
- Teaching: Prescribed Activity/Exercise
- Teaching: Prescribed Medication

Nursing Interventions/Rationales

- Assess need for teaching and provide as needed. *To individualize teaching to specific patient needs.*
- Review preoperative instructions with patient and caregiver. Provide written materials, videos, anatomical model of knee, and sample knee prostheses if available. *To help the patient and caregiver understand the surgical procedure, decrease anxiety, and increase postoperative compliance with treatment plan. Written materials reinforce verbal teaching and are available for review at later times. Models or videos better demonstrate the procedure than do oral descriptions.*
- Evaluate patient's understanding of information taught and reinforce learning as needed. *To determine the need for further teaching. Reinforcement of information previously taught improves retention.*
- Keep patient and family informed of care plan and rationales for treatment. *Encourages family support and participation in care routines while the patient is hospitalized and after discharge.*
- Have patient demonstrate independent transfer and ambulation with appropriate ambulatory aid before discharge. *To assess patient's ability to walk and determine the need for further teaching or assistance.*
- Have patient demonstrate exercises to be performed at home (straight leg raising and active flexion). *To determine the need for further teaching or assistance.*
- Provide information and rationales for discharge restrictions and activities. *Understanding the rationale for activities and restrictions may promote compliance and possible avoidance of complications.*
- Assess the caregiver's ability to assist with home care. *To determine the need for further support.*
- Assess layout of home, number of stairs, proximity of bathroom to bedroom, and potential safety hazards. *Home environment may need to be arranged to increase patient's independence and decrease potential for injury.*
- Teach patient the importance of follow-up examinations. *To determine effectiveness of treatment plan and detect problems for early intervention.*
- Have patient verbalize the need for maintaining lifelong activity restrictions. *Jogging and high-impact activities should be avoided to reduce stress on the prosthesis.*

Nursing Diagnosis

Acute pain related to surgical incision and joint replacement

Outcomes

- Patient will report decrease or absence of pain within 30 minutes of pain interventions.
- Patient will report satisfaction with pain relief measures by rating pain less than 3 on a scale of 0 to 10.
- Patient will decrease use of pain medications before discharge.

Related NOC Outcomes

- Pain Control
- Pain Level

Related NIC Interventions

- Analgesic Administration
- Pain Management

Nursing Interventions/Rationales

- Assess patient's pain before and after comfort interventions. *To determine the degree of postoperative pain and effectiveness of pain relief measures. Alternative pain relief measures may be needed if current measures are ineffective.*
- Apply ice or cooling pad to operative site for 48 hours after surgery as prescribed. *Ice reduces blood flow to the operative area, which decreases swelling. Swelling contributes to pain.*
- Encourage use of patient-controlled analgesia (PCA) before pain becomes severe. *Milder pain is more readily controlled than severe pain. PCA allows the patient control over his pain status.*

- Encourage use of PCA before exercise periods. *Patient can better perform exercises if pain is manageable.*
- Monitor use and effectiveness of PCA. *PCA avoids peaks and valleys associated with intermittent use of analgesics. It also allows the patient greater control over his pain.*
- Encourage use of nonpharmacologic pain relief measures if acceptable to patient. *Relaxation, repositioning, and distraction are helpful for reducing and controlling pain; however, the patient must believe that they will help.*

Nursing Diagnosis

Impaired physical mobility related to pain secondary to total knee replacement

Outcomes

- Patient will regain mobility within prescribed limitations by discharge.

Related NOC Outcomes

- Joint Movement: Knee
- Mobility
- Transfer Performance

Related NIC Interventions

- Exercise Promotion: Strength Training
- Exercise Therapy: Ambulation
- Exercise Therapy: Joint Mobility
- Positioning

Nursing Interventions/Rationales

- Turn patient from side to back to side every 2 hours and as necessary while on bed rest. *Frequent turning and repositioning promote circulation, respiratory effort, and muscle activity.*
- Elevate operative leg on pillows when in bed and up in chair for first 24 to 48 hours, avoiding passive flexion of the knee. *Elevating limb enhances venous return. Avoiding flexion prevents flexion contracture.*
- Assist patient with transfer out of bed on first postoperative day, allowing weight bearing on the operative leg with assistive device only. *To prevent complications of immobility. Weight-bearing restrictions depend on the method used to implant the prosthesis.*
- Encourage patient to perform active dorsiplantar flexion, isometric quadriceps setting exercises, and straight leg raises (after drain is removed) every 2 hours until fully ambulatory, then four times per day. *Exercising the lower extremities prevents venous stasis and promotes muscle strengthening.*
- Help the patient walk using the appropriate ambulatory aid, increasing the distance walked each day. *Hastens recovery and prevents postoperative complications related to immobility.*
- Encourage patient to sit up in chair as tolerated, especially for meals. *To encourage movement to prevent complications from immobility.*
- If continuous passive motion machine is used, patient's leg should be in the machine a minimum of 8 to 12 hr/day up to 22 hr/day if tolerated. *To prevent excessive swelling and bruising at the site of surgery, and promote even healing of the involved joint tissues.*
- Begin active flexion exercise of the knee on second postoperative day and encourage flexion four times per day. *Promotes return of function. It is desirable that the patient achieves approximately 90 degrees of active flexion before discharge from the hospital.*
- Encourage use of knee exerciser. *Promotes return of function.*
- Advise patient that a knee immobilizer may be worn at night as a resting splint. *Helps prevent painful muscle spasms by supporting the knee at rest.*

Nursing Diagnosis

Risk for ineffective therapeutic regimen management related to perceived barriers to self-care at home

Outcomes

- Patient will assume gradual responsibility for self-care.
- Patient will use assistive devices correctly to aid with mobility.
- Patient will perform prescribed exercises correctly.
- Patient will maintain prescribed limitations.

Related NOC Outcomes

- Compliance Behavior
- Participation in Health Care Decisions

Related NIC Interventions

- Discharge Planning
- Family Support
- Home Maintenance Assistance
- Mutual Goal Setting

Nursing Interventions/Rationales

- Assess patient's and caregiver's perception of problems that may occur with management of self-care at home. *To identify actual or perceived needs and obstacles to the patient caring for himself at home.*
- Determine the type of equipment needed (e.g., crutches, walker, elevated toilet seat) and obtain any needed equipment. *To enhance the patient's and caregiver's ability to successfully care for the patient at home.*
- Assess the home environment for needed changes (e.g., arranging for first floor sleeping arrangements). *To facilitate the patient's recovery at home and the patient's and caregiver's ability to provide that care.*
- Encourage patient to participate in decisions about rehabilitation and self-care at home. *Involving the patient in decision making increases the likelihood of compliance with the prescribed treatment and rehabilitation plan.*

Evaluation

Evaluation is based on comparing the patient's outcomes with desired outcomes.

or after surgery. A pneumatic tourniquet is used intraoperatively during knee replacement surgery to reduce blood loss.

Preoperative diagnostics depend on the patient's age and medical condition (see Chapter 13). The results of the examinations and laboratory testing should be evaluated before the patient's admission to the hospital, in case additional studies are needed or abnormal results require medical intervention. Objective data to be gathered regarding the musculoskeletal system include joint ROM; presence of deformities such as varus, valgus, or flexion; leg length discrepancies; condition of joints, enlargement, erythema, crepitus, and asymmetry; gait; and ability to perform ADLs.

The nurse also instructs the patient about the perioperative routine, including respiratory and leg exercises (see Chapter 13). The patient may have a PT evaluation before surgery and be measured for crutches, a walker, or a cane. Persons with arthritis involving the joints of the upper extremity may be fitted with a platform walker, which distributes most of the upper body weight on the forearms during ambulation. Platform walkers are particularly beneficial to persons with RA, who typically have wrist and finger joint involvement. The nurse informs the patient about the adaptive equipment needed on discharge. Postoperative pain control is usually achieved with the use of patient-controlled analgesia (PCA) pumps. Both epidural and intravenous pain control are used for patients with joint replacement surgery. At the preoperative interview, the nurse shows the patient the pump and gives instructions regarding its use.

The patient is instructed to take nothing by mouth after midnight on the day preceding surgery and is admitted to the hospital on the day of surgery. Intravenous antibiotics are begun at least 30 minutes before the incision time to establish a therapeutic level; antibiotics are usually continued for 24 to 48 hours after surgery. The lowest rate of infection occurs when antibiotics are given no more than 2 hours before incision time.

Discharge planning is also begun at the preadmission interview. The length of hospital stay varies with the joint replaced and the individual patient's condition. Most patients admitted for hip or knee replacement are discharged after 4 days, usually to a rehabilitative facility or subacute division for continued therapy. The nurse assesses the patient's and family's resources and preferences at the preadmission interview to begin planning for transfer after discharge.

Postoperative Care

Routine postoperative nursing care for the patient recovering from total joint replacement surgery includes monitoring vital signs and level of consciousness, assisting with coughing and deep breathing, monitoring and recording intake and output (including suction drains at the operative site), providing adequate nutrition and hydration, managing pain, assessing the surgical site for drainage and signs of infection, maintaining the position of the operative extremity to prevent dislocation of prostheses, performing frequent neurovascular checks, providing skin care, encouraging progressive ambulation, preventing infection, teaching, and monitoring for signs of complications. See Chapter 15 for general postoperative care.

Priorities of care include interventions to prevent the complications associated with immobility, including constipation, urinary retention, respiratory complications, altered skin integrity, and venous stasis. Nursing interventions specific to the joint replaced are discussed separately following this section.

DVT is a common complication after both hip and knee replacement. Generally, a combination of treatments is implemented to reduce the incidence of DVT, including prophylactic anticoagulation, graduated elastic stockings, leg exercises, pneumatic compression devices, and early mobilization. The threat of DVT and pulmonary embolism continues 4 to 6 weeks after surgery. Proximal DVT is most often associated with pulmonary embolism.

Depending on the individual patient and surgeon preference, patients are given heparin, low-dose heparin, LMWH (enoxaparin or dalteparin), or warfarin for prophylactic anticoagulation. LMWH has a longer half-life than standard heparin and does not require laboratory testing for twice-daily dosing. LMWH has been shown to be more effective than standard heparin in reducing the incidence of proximal DVT but showed no difference in preventing distal DVT.[30] LMWH is usually administered subcutaneously twice daily for 7 to 14 days and is highly effective in reducing the incidence of proximal and distal DVT after total hip and knee replacement. Low doses of warfarin can be administered daily on the basis of the patient's daily prothrombin time or international normalized ration (INR) results. The goal is to maintain a prothrombin time of 15 seconds and a control of 1.5 seconds.

To prevent DVT, in many institutions pneumatic compression devices are applied intraoperatively and are continued until the patient is fully ambulatory. The venous foot pump is an alternative method of decreasing venous stasis and thus the risk of DVT. This device has been shown to be as effective as natural weight bearing in producing adequate pumping action to increase venous return. Nurses should encourage the patient to perform isometric leg exercises every 1 to 2 hours, with 10 repetitions per session. The use of antiembolism hose should be continued until the patient is fully ambulatory. Some institutions include ultrasound or other diagnostic testing to rule out DVT as part of the postoperative protocol.

Early ambulation is a safe and inexpensive method of preventing venous stasis. Most patients are helped out of bed on the first postoperative day, with progressive ambulation and PT sessions daily to follow. Activity and weight-bearing restrictions vary, depending on the joint replaced, whether cement was used, and surgeon protocol. The nurse should help and encourage the patient to perform active and passive ROM exercises, isometrics, and other exercises prescribed by the physical therapist to increase muscle strength and decrease the complications of mobility.

While the patient is receiving anticoagulants, the nurse is responsible for monitoring for signs of bleeding. The stool, urine, and sputum are monitored for blood; a soft-bristled toothbrush is used; dental floss is avoided; electric razors are used in place of razor blades; and needle punctures are kept to a minimum. The nurse assesses the suction drain and dressing for excessive drainage and monitors the patient's coagulation studies and complete blood count (CBC) daily.

Closed wound drainage systems are surgically placed at the time of closing of the incision to prevent hematoma formation and are left in place 24 to 48 hours after surgery. Because of intraoperative blood loss, the patient may require a transfusion after surgery. An alternative is an autotransfusion drain, a closed drainage system that collects and filters the blood, which can then be reinfused intravenously into the patient. Used alone, postoperative salvage and reinfusion have been shown to reduce the amount of autologous blood needed postoperatively. The blood obtained through intraoperative and postoperative salvage methods has several advantages over homologous banked blood. Platelets and clotting factors remain intact in the salvaged blood, the pH of the blood is identical to the patient's, red blood cells are viable, reinfused blood has a greater affinity for oxygen, and the risk of transfusion reaction or transmission of bloodborne diseases is less.

In addition to monitoring the drain and dressing site for excessive bleeding, the nurse monitors the patient's hemoglobin and hematocrit daily. Output from the surgical drain is generally less than 300 ml per shift. Patients are often given an iron supplement postoperatively to increase blood counts.

Preventing infection is a nursing priority for any patient who has undergone total joint replacement. A postoperative wound infection can lead to prolonged hospitalization with significant cost increase, permanent disability, and removal of the prosthesis with a decreased chance for success in subsequent replacements. Infection rates for persons undergoing elbow replacement surgery are significantly higher than for other joint replacement procedures because of the superficiality of the joint and poor skin coverage for closure.

Gram-positive organisms are responsible for 60% to 65% of all joint infections; *Staphylococcus aureus* and *Staphylococcus epidermidis* are the most often cultured organisms from hip and knee wounds. The patient's skin has been identified as the major source of infection; airborne bacteria in the operating room are another major source of pathogens. Bone and joint infections are particularly difficult to treat because of the multiple channels in bone that may harbor organisms for long periods. The use of prophylactic antibiotics in the perioperative period has been effective in reducing the incidence of postoperative infection in patients undergoing hip or knee replacement. Antibiotics should be given as prescribed to maintain therapeutic blood levels.

The nurse monitors the patient for any signs of infection, including elevated temperature; elevated white blood cell (WBC) count; and erythema, edema, or drainage from the wound. Dressing changes are performed using aseptic technique. A report of a dull aching pain or unusual or persistent pain may be indicate joint infection and should be reported to the physician for further evaluation. The nurse teaches the patient and family to recognize the signs and symptoms of infection. Discharge instructions include methods of avoiding sources of infection, including the necessity for prophylactic antibiotics when undergoing dental or genitourinary procedures or other invasive procedures and for instances of systemic bacterial infections. Many institutions provide patients wallet-sized cards with antibiotic prophylaxis information.

Pain management is an important aspect of nursing care for patients after total joint replacement. Many patients with arthritis have endured years of chronic pain as a result of degenerative changes in the joint. Total joint replacement may offer relief from that pain. However, postoperative pain is different from that associated with arthritis. Use of pharmacologic and nonpharmacologic methods may enhance pain management in the postoperative patient (see Research box). Many institutions use intravenous or epidural PCA with opioid analgesics (morphine, fentanyl, hydromorphone) for pain control. Epidural PCA may include a local anesthetic with the opioid for enhanced pain control. The PCA pump is usually continued for up to 48 hours postoperatively; then oral analgesics are ordered as needed.

The nurse monitors the patient for bowel function because of the side effects of the medication and immobility after surgery. Ice is applied to the incision area for the first 48 hours to prevent swelling and to decrease pain. Ice also helps alleviate pain after PT sessions. The nurse should consider the patient's PT schedule and make sure the patient is adequately medicated before going to therapy.

Because of the shortened length of stay (4 to 5 days for total hip replacement), most patients are discharged to a subacute facility or rehabilitative center for PT. Those who decide to be discharged directly to home need a referral for home PT or need to arrange for outpatient PT. A home health nurse visit should be scheduled for suture or staple removal.

The nurse informs patients and their families that the rehabilitative phase after joint replacement lasts at least 1 year. At 1 year most patients have achieved approximately 90% of functional return. Patients and families should be reminded that cooperation in the rehabilitative process is necessary for success. Daily exercise is an important component of the recovery process.

The follow-up appointment with the orthopedic surgeon is usually at 6 weeks after surgery. After this time patients are allowed a little more flexibility in activity; at 6 to 8 weeks, they can usually resume sexual activity, although persons with joint revisions may need additional time. Nurses should discuss the safe time for resuming sexual activity with patients, preferably at the preoperative visit, but certainly before discharge. Once intercourse is resumed, appropriate positioning of the affected extremity is a key consideration. Persons with hip replacements should follow positioning guidelines to avoid dislocating the prosthesis.

The nurse cautions the patient against driving without consulting the surgeon. Patients with total hip replacements generally

Research

Antall GA, Kresevic D: The use of guided imagery to manage pain in an elderly orthopaedic population, *Orthop Nurs* 23(5):335, 2004.

Uncontrolled pain after joint replacement surgery may negatively affect long-term joint function and rehabilitation. The purpose of this pilot study was to evaluate the effectiveness of guided imagery as an adjunct therapy to control pain after joint replacement surgery. Study participants were adults with osteoarthritis ages 55 and older recovering from either hip or knee replacement surgery. The control group received usual postoperative care, including pain management and a tape of relaxing music. The experimental group received the usual care and a guided imagery audiotape. Outcomes were measured using pain and anxiety scores, and use of pain medications and health services.

The experimental group demonstrated decreased length of stay, decreased anxiety, less opioid use, and lower pain scores as measured by nursing. Limitations of this study include the small sample size (N=13) and homogeneity of sample (all men). Further research is needed to generalize findings to a larger population. Guided imagery is an easy, low-cost intervention that may enhance usual postoperative regimens to manage pain.

have sufficient muscle strength to resume driving a car with an automatic transmission at 6 to 8 weeks; driving while using pain medication is contraindicated.

When the patient has regained maximal strength, he or she may resume low-impact activities such as walking, swimming, golfing, biking, bowling, and tennis. High-impact activities and exercises that place an increased load on the joints are not recommended, since they decrease the longevity of knee and hip prostheses.

Teaching includes information about home-going medications, particularly anticoagulants. The patient and family should be aware of the purpose, side effects, dosage, and method of administering prescribed medications. The patient and family should be knowledgeable about the signs and symptoms of complications, such as prosthesis dislocation, infection, DVT, fat embolism, and pulmonary embolism.

Temporary rearrangement of the home environment may be necessary, especially if the patient returns directly home. It is easiest if the bathroom and the patient's bedroom are on the same floor, although a bedside commode or urinal can be used temporarily if necessary. For persons recovering from lower-extremity joint replacements, the bed should be arranged so that the patient can exit the bed on the opposite side of the operative leg. The floors and doorways should be free of any obstructions. Throw rugs should be removed. A firm chair with armrests is necessary for persons recovering from total hip or knee surgery. Adding pillows can raise the height of the seat. The room can be arranged with commonly used items within close reach of the patient. A tote bag can be attached to the patient's walker to carry the phone, reachers, or other necessary items. A raised toilet seat is needed for persons with total knee and hip replacements. For bathing, a long-handled sponge will allow the patient to wash his or her legs. A walk-in shower is best, and a chair can be added for safety. If the patient has a tub, a sponge bath may be easier for the first few weeks. If the patient has pets, a friend or family member may need to help care for them, since dogs or cats can trip a person using a walker, cane, or crutches. The patient should be instructed to wear comfortable, well-fitting, nonskid, walking shoes. Regular follow-up appointments are continued for the first year and as necessary thereafter.

Total Hip Arthroplasty. In addition to general postoperative care, there are some important considerations for care after total hip arthroplasty (see Guidelines for Safe Practice box, p. 1636). Positioning restrictions protect the prosthesis and depend on the surgical approach and technique and type of prosthesis. The positioning restrictions outlined pertain to the posterolateral approach to the hip, which is commonly used. Patients undergoing an anterolateral approach are able to tolerate sitting upright with 90 degrees of flexion but should avoid active abduction, external rotation, and extension of the operative leg.

Dislocation of the prosthesis is a serious complication that may require additional surgery or anesthesia to relocate the prosthesis. Signs of possible dislocation include a sudden pain unrelieved by medication, a "popping" sensation associated with movement, loss of movement, leg length discrepancy, and deformity. The affected extremity may be either externally or internally rotated, depending on the direction of the dislocation, and the head of the femoral prosthesis may be palpable.

Extremes of flexion, adduction, or rotation should be avoided because these motions may cause dislocation (Figure 54-9). Flexion is generally limited to 60 degrees for 6 to 7 days and then to 90 degrees for 2 to 3 months. When the patient is supine or lying on the side, the legs should be kept in abduction; pillows or an abduction splint can be used (Figure 54-10). Positioning the patient on the operative side is usually avoided to prevent adduction of the operative limb. Positioning restrictions are maintained until the hip capsule is well healed and the risk of dislocation has passed. Bone growth around the prosthesis begins in approximately 10 days.

Most patients have some restriction on weight bearing, which limits the distraction force on the prosthesis. The surgeon prescribes the amount of weight bearing allowed. Patients with cemented prostheses are usually allowed weight bearing as tolerated. With the help of physical therapists, the goal is for the patient to accomplish safe transfer from bed to chair and toilet; perform prescribed exercises independently; and ambulate with the appropriate weight-bearing restrictions using a walker, cane, or crutches. The patient should also be taught to ascend and descend stairs safely.

Assistive devices to aid the patient in completing ADLs are usually obtained through the occupational therapy (OT) department. The patient is instructed about the use of an elevated toilet seat, which prevents extreme hip flexion; long-handled reachers; and devices that aid in donning shoes and stockings; these items are used after discharge as well.

Total Knee Arthroplasty. Postoperative management of persons with total knee replacement may include the use of a continuous passive motion (CPM) machine (Figure 54-11). The CPM machine supports the operative extremity while passively moving it within preset limits of flexion and extension. Use of the CPM machine reduces postoperative swelling, prevents adhesions, decreases pain, and facilitates early mobility. The CPM is usually applied in the operating room or postanesthesia care unit, and patients are encouraged to use the machine while in bed as tolerated (up to 22 hr/day). Increases in the amount of knee flexion are ordered by the physician; the goal is usually 90 degrees. If the CPM is not used, a knee immobilizer is often placed over the bulky dressing and kept in place until the dressing is reduced. Other surgical protocols call for the use of a knee exerciser, which is attached to the overhead frame of the bed and allows the patient to exercise the knee while in bed. The physician determines when active flexion exercises may begin.

There are no real positioning restrictions, although the patient should adhere to the physician's orders regarding the amount of weight bearing and knee flexion permitted. Kneeling is usually discouraged. Flexion is increased at intervals. While in bed, the patient is cautioned against having a pillow under the knee, which may cause the knee to remain in a flexed position (see Guidelines for Safe Practice box, p. 1637).

Total Shoulder Arthroplasty. Priorities of care for the patient after total shoulder arthroplasty are pain management, assessment of neurovascular status, promotion of self-care and mobility, and prevention of complications. Nerve damage is uncommon, but the brachial plexus can be injured intraoperatively or as a result of positioning. Motor, sensory, and vascular assessment of the opera-

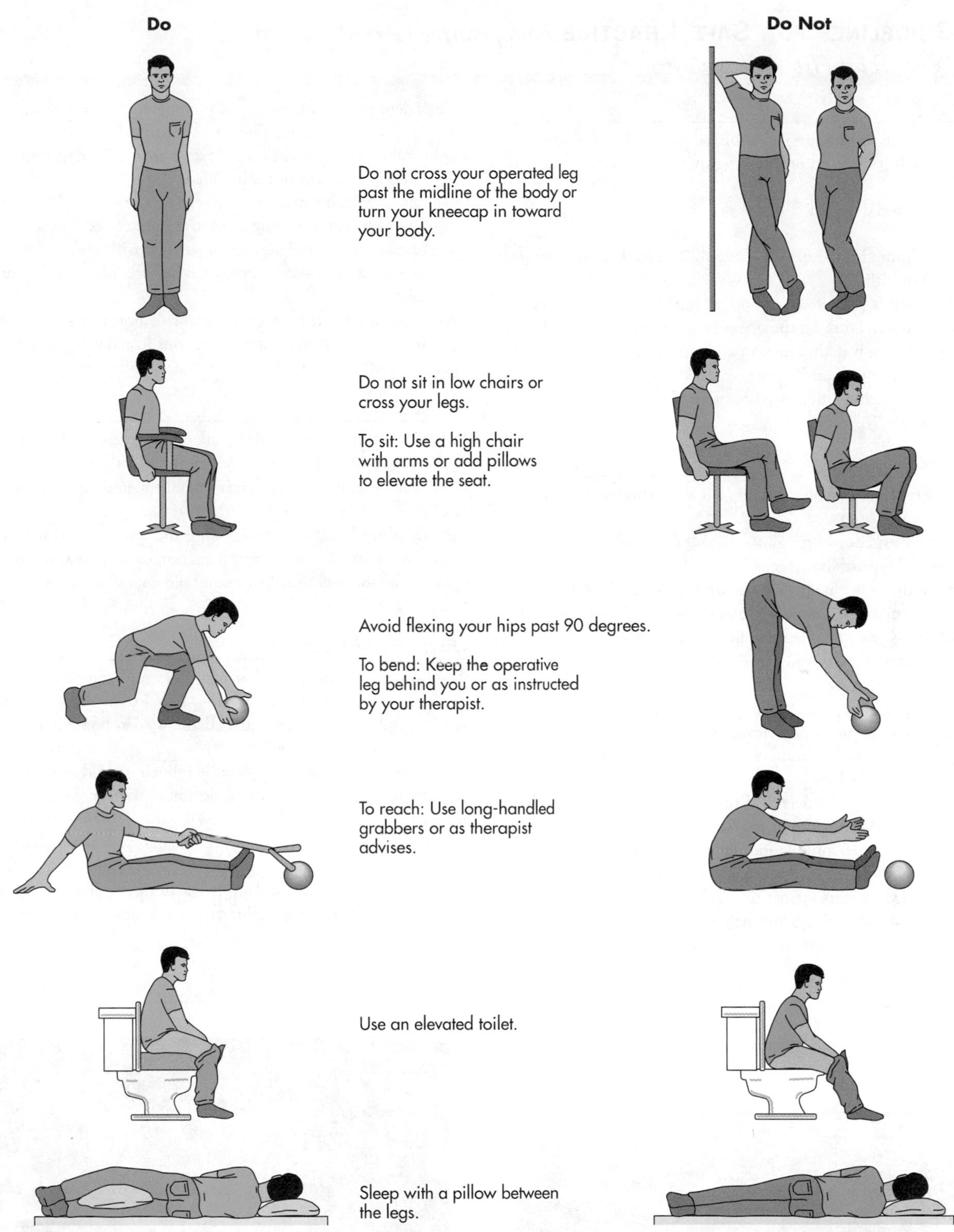
Do
Do Not
Do not cross your operated leg past the midline of the body or turn your kneecap in toward your body.
Do not sit in low chairs or cross your legs.
To sit: Use a high chair with arms or add pillows to elevate the seat.
Avoid flexing your hips past 90 degrees.
To bend: Keep the operative leg behind you or as instructed by your therapist.
To reach: Use long-handled grabbers or as therapist advises.
Use an elevated toilet.
Sleep with a pillow between the legs.

Figure 54-9 Home-going instructions illustrating *do's* and *do not's* for patients with a total hip replacement. Patients are to avoid extreme flexion (past 90 degrees), adduction, and internal rotation of operated hip—any of which may cause dislocation of the prosthesis.

tive extremity should be done every 4 hours, and the findings compared with the patient's preoperative baseline. After total shoulder replacement, the operative extremity is placed in an immobilizer, which is kept in place for 1 or 2 days (Figure 54-12). The sling is then worn at night and for comfort during the day. Passive exercises are initiated immediately after surgery, and pendulum exercises are begun 1 to 10 days after surgery (see Chapter 52). Shoulder CPM machines may be used for passive ROM exercises. Isometric exercises are started the second week. The patient is cautioned to limit the amount of external rotation. Patients undergoing total

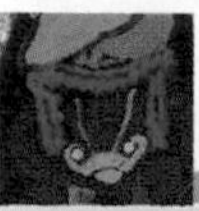

GUIDELINES FOR SAFE PRACTICE *Postoperative Care of the Patient With Total Hip Arthroplasty*

Positioning

Positioning depends on the surgical approach and technique, method of implantation (cemented or bony ingrowth prosthesis), and prosthesis design.

Restrictions to avoid dislocation of the prosthesis usually include the following:

—Flexion is limited to 60 degrees for 6 to 7 days, then to 90 degrees for 2 to 3 months.

—No adduction is permitted beyond midline for 2 to 3 months; therefore no side lying on the operative side unless ordered by the surgeon. The leg is maintained in abduction when the patient is lying supine or on the nonoperative side.

—No extreme internal or external rotation is permitted (see Figure 54-9).

Wound Care

Drains are inserted in the wound to prevent a hematoma and left in place for 24 to 48 hours.

Maintain constant suction through a self-contained suction device.

Note amount and type of drainage.

After the initial dressing change, change dressing once daily and as needed, using aseptic technique. Observe incision line for signs of infection. The wound may be left open to air if there is no drainage. Staples or sutures are removed 7 to 10 days after surgery.

Activity

Observe flexion restrictions when elevating the head of the bed.

Encourage periodic elevation and lowering of the head of the bed to provide motion at the hip.

Instruct patient in use of the overhead trapeze to shift weight and lift for the bedpan and change of linen.

Encourage active dorsiflexion–plantar flexion exercise of the ankles and quadriceps and gluteal setting exercises to promote venous return, prevent thrombus formation, and maintain muscle tone (see Chapter 15). Gluteal sets also help strengthen the muscle around the hip joint capsule, which will decrease the risk of dislocation.

The patient may be turned to the nonoperative side with the operative leg maintained in abduction and extension.

Begin ambulation as early as the first postoperative day, if tolerated. Physical therapy consult is initiated.

—Observe flexion and adduction restrictions.

—Observe weight-bearing restrictions prescribed by the surgeon (usually partial weight bearing assisted with a walker or crutches).

—Increase amount of walking each day according to the patient's tolerance.

Patient can begin sitting when he or she demonstrates sufficient leg control to sit within flexion restrictions (usually requires elevation of sitting surfaces, including use of a raised toilet seat).

Medications

Prophylactic anticoagulant drugs are usually prescribed to decrease the risk of thrombus formation. Monitor patient for signs of deep venous thrombosis, pulmonary embolism, and fat embolism syndrome.

Initially control pain with positioning and opioid analgesics (usually patient-controlled analgesia); transition to oral opioids, nonsteroidal antiinflammatory drugs, or nonopioid analgesics according to the patient's tolerance.

Discharge Instructions

The patient must use an ambulatory aid, avoid adduction, and limit hip flexion to 90 degrees for about 2 to 3 months.

A raised toilet seat is to be obtained and used at home until flexion restrictions are removed.

The patient may need a long-handled shoehorn and reacher to facilitate activities of daily living within flexion restriction.

Instruct patient on the lifelong need for antibiotic prophylaxis when undergoing invasive procedures or dental work to protect the prosthesis from bacteremic infection.

Inform patient that the implant may activate metal detector alarms. Provide a wallet identification and information card if available.

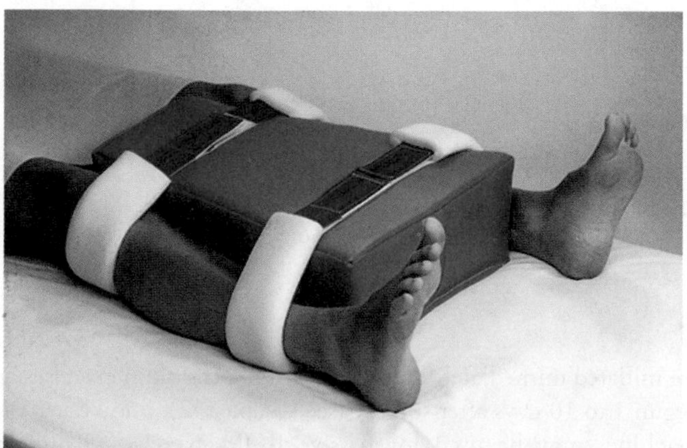

Figure 54-10 Abduction splint for postoperative hip arthroplasty.

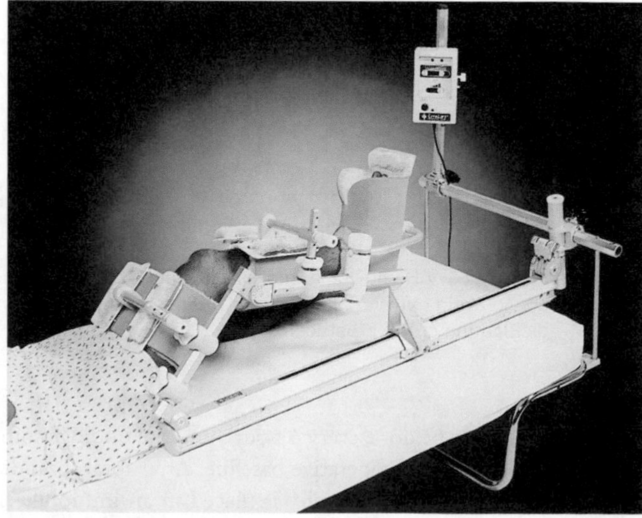

Figure 54-11 Example of continuous passive motion machine.

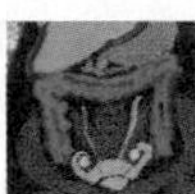

GUIDELINES FOR SAFE PRACTICE *Postoperative Care of the Patient With Total Knee Arthroplasty*

Positioning

Elevate the operative leg(s) on pillows to enhance venous return for the first 48 hours. Pillows are placed with care to avoid flexing to the knee(s). It is becoming more common for patients to have bilateral total knee replacements done at one time.

The patient may be turned from side to back to side.

Wound Care

Care of drains is as for total hip replacement.

Assess the patient for systemic evidence of loss of blood (hypotension, tachycardia) if a bulky compression dressing is used, since it may hold large quantities of drainage before drainage is visible.

Remove bulky dressings before the patient begins active flexion.

Assess wound for healing and signs of infection. Perform a dry sterile dressing change once the bulky dressing is discontinued. Leave incision open to air if there is no drainage.

Activity

Passive flexion is provided in a continuous passive motion (CPM) machine within prescribed flexion-extension limits. The patient's leg may remain in the CPM machine as much as tolerated (up to 22 hr/day) to facilitate even healing of tissue.

Encourage the patient to perform active dorsiflexion–plantar flexion of the ankles, gluteal and quadriceps setting, and (after drains are removed) straight leg raising exercises.

The patient begins active flexion exercises three or four times per day on about the second to third postoperative day.

Partial weight bearing with an assistive device may be started as early as the first postoperative day and increased as the patient tolerates. Physical therapy consult initiated.

Sitting in a chair with the leg(s) elevated may be started on the first postoperative day.

The patient may be encouraged to wear a resting knee extension splint (immobilizer) on the operative extremity until able to demonstrate quadriceps control (independent straight leg raising).

Medications

Prophylactic anticoagulants are usually prescribed to decrease the risk of thrombus formation. Monitor the patient for signs of deep venous thrombosis, pulmonary embolism, and fatty embolism syndrome.

Initial control of pain is with opioid analgesics (usually patient-controlled analgesia [PCA]) and positioning; after PCA is discontinued, oral opioids, nonsteroidal antiinflammatory drugs, or non-opioids are given as needed.

Ice is usually prescribed to be applied to the knee to reduce swelling and pain.

Encourage the patient to apply ice to the knee(s) for 20 to 30 minutes before and after active flexion exercise.

Discharge Instructions

The patient must observe partial weight-bearing restrictions and use an ambulatory aid for approximately 2 months after discharge. Kneeling should be avoided indefinitely.

The patient should continue active flexion and straight leg raising exercises at home.

The patient must be made aware of the lifelong need for antibiotic prophylaxis before invasive procedures or dental work.

Inform patient that the implant may activate metal detector alarms. Provide a wallet identification or information card if available.

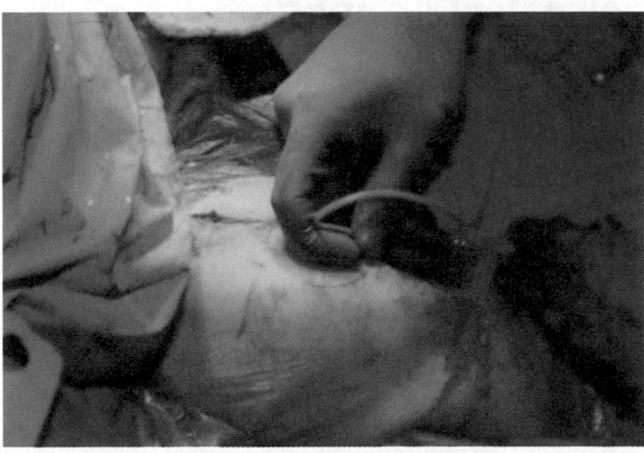

Figure 54-12 Total shoulder arthroplasty with postoperative immobilization. Note Hemovac drain.

shoulder replacement may require only overnight hospitalization. Lifelong precautions include prevention of infection and avoidance of contact or load-bearing activities.

Total Elbow Arthroplasty. Damage to the ulnar nerve is a possible complication of elbow replacement surgery. Frequent neurovascular checks, focusing on assessment of ulnar nerve function, are important interventions. Edema and hematoma formation may cause alterations in sensation or motion. Knowledge of the patient's preoperative function is important for making comparisons. The surgeon should be notified of any changes in the patient's neurovascular status.

After total elbow replacement the operative extremity is placed in a plaster splint and bulky dressing (Figure 54-13). The splint may be flexed up to 90 degrees. The arm should be elevated, and ice applied. Active ROM of the fingers is encouraged to maintain mobility and decrease edema. The drain is removed within 24 to 36 hours, and the bulky dressing is reduced. Elbow flexion and extension exercises are begun after the dressing is removed. Activity restrictions include limiting lifting to no more than 1 pound for 3 months and less than 5 pounds long term. The patient should avoid contact sports for life.

Total Ankle Arthroplasty. Total ankle replacement is performed most often for patients with RA. Neurovascular assessment is important to evaluate intraoperative damage to the neurovascular bundle. A drain is placed to decrease hematoma formation; elevation helps reduce swelling.

After surgery the extremity is placed in a soft compression dressing and plaster splint. The operative extremity should be kept elevated, with ice applied. The dressing is removed, and a

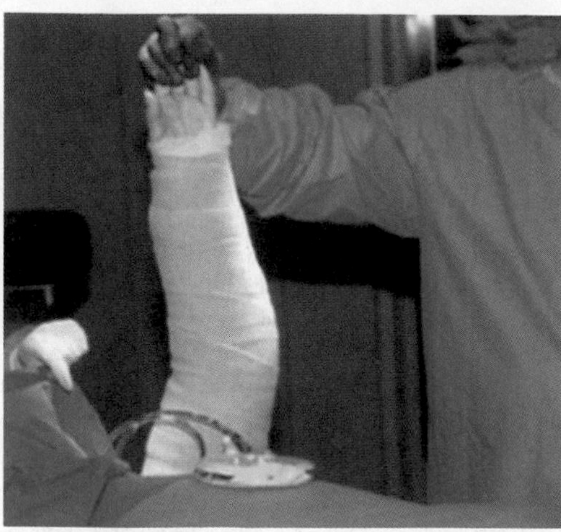

Figure 54-13 Total elbow arthroplasty with postoperative splint and dressing. Elbow is in full extension.

short leg walking cast is applied for 2 to 3 weeks. Nursing care is similar to care for the person with a fracture (see Chapter 52). PT and exercises are begun after cast removal. Preventing infection and promoting wound healing are key interventions to avoid serious complications with skin closure and healing.

Gerontologic Considerations

Arthritis is a common problem among the older population and may affect their ability to perform ADLs and to enjoy leisure activities. OA is the most common form of arthritis in the older adult. More than 40% of women over age 60 have OA. Joint involvement is typically symmetric, and the onset of pain is insidious, progressing to more persistent pain, unrelieved by rest (see Guidelines for Safe Practice box).

PT is an important treatment for older adults with OA. Exercise and PT can improve the quality of life and maintain independence. Resting the affected joint typically provides pain relief but can contribute significantly to contractures, atrophy of disuse, and osteoporosis. Thus the nurse advises the older adult to maintain a constant level of physical activity, even in the presence of active arthritis. The patient should perform passive and active exercises to maintain ROM and muscle tone. Swimming and walking are good choices for regular exercise.

Assistive and adaptive devices can improve the quality of life and allow the patient independence in ADLs. Orthoses (braces) and special shoes for foot problems can help maintain alignment and provide support for diseased joints.

Medications to treat OA should be chosen carefully for older patients. The health care provider should be aware of any other medications the patient is taking because of the possibility of drug interactions. Kidney and liver function should be evaluated before a pharmacologic regimen is prescribed. Acetaminophen in doses up to 4 g per day is a good choice for older patients without renal or hepatic disease. If NSAIDs are prescribed, a CBC, urinalysis, and liver and kidney function tests should be performed before treatment and at 1- to 3-month intervals thereafter. Increased age has been identified as a significant risk factor for the development of side effects associated with NSAIDs.[2] All NSAIDs should be used with caution in older adults; piroxicam should be avoided because of its long half-life.[20] A chronic pain management program should include nonpharmacologic modalities as well.

Many older patients with OA require or elect surgical intervention to relieve pain or to improve mobility. Any coexisting disease such as heart disease, hypertension, diabetes, or kidney problems must be stabilized before elective surgery. See Chapters 13 to 15 for perioperative considerations for the older patient.

After surgical intervention the older patient may be discharged to a rehabilitative facility to continue with PT and to attain independence in ADLs, transfers, and ambulation. If the patient is transferred directly to home, a family member, friend, or home health care referral will be necessary to assist in care.

Rheumatoid Arthritis

Etiology. RA is a chronic systemic inflammatory disease affecting primarily the diarthrodial joints and surrounding soft tissues. The disease process is characterized by inflammation of the con-

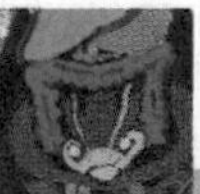

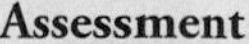

Guidelines for Safe Practice *The Elderly Patient With Arthritis*

Assessment

Assess all older adults for muscle strength and tone, gait, sensory deficits, painful joints or muscles, contractures, deformities, and foot problems that may interfere with ambulation and activities of daily living (ADLs).

Assess availability, condition, and use of assistive aids, such as walkers, canes, or crutches.

Assess environmental factors conducive to falls, since older adults are at high risk for falls.

Intervention

Order assistive aids to foster independence and to increase ambulation, such as a walker, cane, lift, and bedside commode.

Encourage an exercise program to maintain baseline muscle and joint function.

Assist in active and passive range-of-motion exercises for older patients needing bed rest.

Obtain orders for progressive ambulation as early in hospitalization as possible.

Position extremities in proper body alignment to prevent contractures.

Teach good foot care and the importance of well-fitted shoes.

Request physical therapy for patients with gait or mobility problems.

Request occupational therapy for problems with ADLs and fine-motor coordination.

Teach older patients how to transfer and walk safely.

Initiate a fall prevention program that identifies risk factors and promotes an individualized plan for each patient, depending on his or her abilities and tendency to fall.

Be sure the environment is free of clutter, the bed is kept in lowest position, and a night light illuminates the floor.

nective tissues throughout the body. Systemic manifestations include pulmonary, cardiac, vascular, ophthalmologic, dermatologic, and hematologic effects. Mortality is associated with the extraarticular manifestations of RA and may shorten the individual's life expectancy by 3 to 18 years.

The cause of RA is not known, but several theories have been postulated regarding its pathogenesis. The stimulus that triggers the inflammatory process remains unknown. RA is thought to be an autoimmune process, specifically the interaction of immunoglobulin G with rheumatoid factor, which appears to perpetuate the rheumatoid inflammation. A genetic predisposition has also been identified in relation to certain human leukocyte antigens. Another theory postulates that the disease occurs as an altered immune response to an unknown antigen. Possible causative antigens include *Helicobacter pylori*, Epstein-Barr virus, human T-lymphotrophic virus 1, parvovirus B19, bacteria, and mycoplasma.[29,38] Environmental factors, including cigarette smoking and caffeine consumption, have also been thought to trigger the inflammatory response.[29,38] Prolonged exposure to the antigen causes normal antibodies (immunoglobulin) to become autoantibodies and attack host tissues (self-antigen). These autoantibodies, called *rheumatoid factors,* bind with self-antigens in the blood and synovial membrane to form immune complexes (Figure 54-14).

Epidemiology. RA affects 1% to 2% of the U.S. population, altering the socioeconomic and mobility status of those affected.

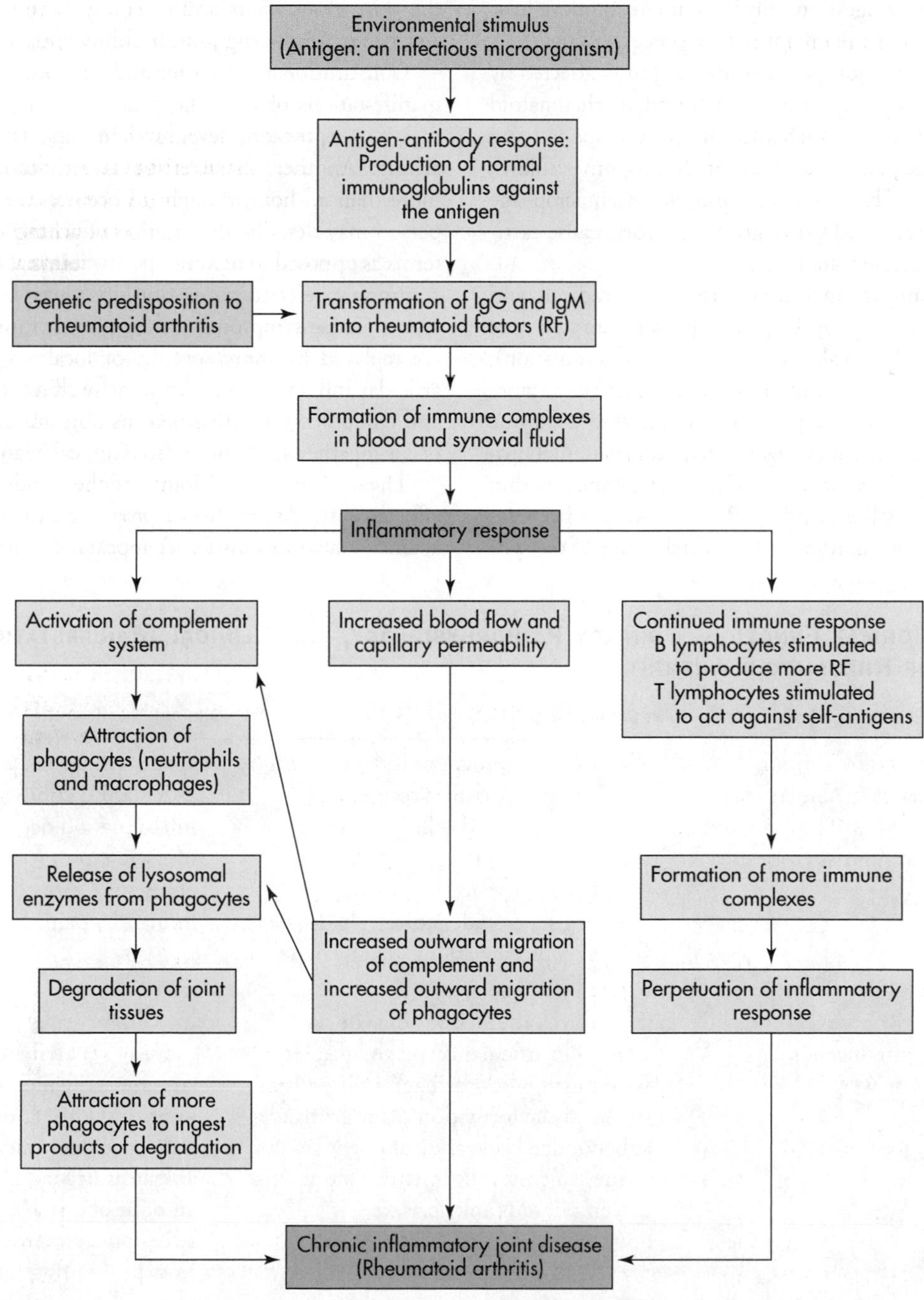

Figure 54-14 Probable pathogenesis of rheumatoid arthritis. *IgG,* Immunoglobulin G; *IgM,* immunoglobulin M.

A diagnosis of RA can be associated with a 35% drop in household income; almost all patients experience pain and loss of function.[1,38] Women are two to three times more likely to be affected by RA than men. The age of onset is between 20 and 50 years, with women usually diagnosed in later childbearing years; onset in men before age 45 is uncommon.[26] There is a higher incidence of RA among Chippewa and Pima Native Americans.[26,38]

Pathophysiology. Key pathologic features of RA are proliferation of the synovial membrane and erosion of articular cartilage and subchondral bone. These processes result in destruction of intraarticular and periarticular structures and joint deformity.

The stimulus that triggers the inflammatory process is unknown. The disease begins in the synovial membrane within the joint. Edema, vascular congestion, fibrin exudate, and cellular infiltrate occur as a result of the inflammatory process. Activated T cells, not present in normal joints, are found in joints affected by RA. Macrophages and monocytes are also found in rheumatoid joints and produce **cytokines**, which affect immune responses and inflammatory reactions. The cytokines, including interleukins, tumor necrosis factor (TNF)–alpha, granulocyte-macrophage colony-stimulating factors, and other growth factors, cause cartilage destruction and increase inflammation.

WBCs release chemicals (including superoxide radicals and hydrogen peroxide) that destroy both the bacteria and normal cells. Prostaglandins (chemicals that mediate inflammation), leukotrienes (producers of inflammation), and digestive enzymes are released. Particularly damaging to joint tissue is the enzyme collagenase, which breaks down collagen, the main structural protein of connective tissue. The presence of these substances within the joint attracts more WBCs, and in RA the process becomes chronic. Continued inflammation leads to thickening of the synovium, particularly where it joins the articular cartilage. At these junctures fibrin develops into a granulation tissue, known as **pannus**, that covers the cartilage surface. The pannus also invades subchondral bone and interferes with the normal nutrition of the articular cartilage, causing necrosis. Pannus formation leads to adhesions between the joint surfaces, and a fibrous or bony union **(ankylosis)** develops. Destruction of cartilage and bone, in addition to some weakening of tendons and ligaments, may lead to subluxation, or dislocation, of joints. Invasion of the subchondral bone may cause eventual regional osteoporosis (Table 54-3).

Pain occurs as a result of cartilage degeneration. Areas of bone exposed because of cartilage erosion may develop fissures or bone cysts. These cysts, caused by an excessive amount of inflammatory exudate, may develop into draining fistulas, communicating with the skin. Bone spurs and osteophytes (outgrowth of bone) may also occur, decreasing joint mobility and increasing pain.

Constitutional symptoms and new onset of joint pain are early manifestations of RA. The patient may report lymphadenopathy, malaise, depression, fever, weight loss, fatigue, and generalized aching. Another characteristic is early-morning stiffness lasting more than an hour, thought to occur as a result of synovitis. The person may describe the location of aching and stiffness in general terms as opposed to naming specific joints. This kind of discomfort, commonly referred to as fibrositis, may be the patient's earliest report. These symptoms may be present for some time before they are replaced by more specific, or localized, problems (i.e., frank articular inflammation with joint swelling, pain, redness, warmth, and tenderness). In other persons fibrositis and joint inflammation occur together at the onset (see Clinical Manifestations box).

The PIP and MCP joints of the hands and fingers are often affected early. As the disease progresses, the fingers develop a characteristic tapering (fusiform) appearance with a classic ulnar devia-

TABLE 54-3 NORMAL FUNCTION, PRIMARY PATHOPHYSIOLOGY, AND CLINICAL MANIFESTATIONS OF RHEUMATOID ARTHRITIS

Normal Function	Pathophysiology	Clinical Manifestations
Synovial tissue secretes synovial fluid, which contains leukocytes, mucin, fat, albumin, and electrolytes. This provides joint lubrication and nourishment to articular cartilage.	Proliferation of synovium: inflammation causes edema, vascular congestion, fibrin exudate, and cellular infiltrate to build up around synovium. White blood cells move into synovium, releasing superoxide radicals, hydrogen peroxide, prostaglandins, leukotrienes, and collagenase.	Synovium thickens, particularly at articular junctions. Symptoms of inflammation occur within and overlying joint (pain, swelling, erythema, warmth). Joint mobility is limited by pain.
Articular (hyaline) cartilage covers ends of articulating bones to reduce joint friction and distribute weight-bearing forces in joint.	Pannus forms at junctions of synovial tissue and articular cartilage, interfering with nutrition of cartilage and resulting in scar tissue formation. Pannus invades subchondral bone and supporting soft tissue structures (ligaments, tendons), causing fibrous ankylosis.	Joint pain increases at rest and with movement. Destruction of soft tissue structures (ligaments, tendons) causes joint to sublux or dislocate. Fibrous tissue becomes calcified, and bony ankylosis occurs. Depending on amount of articular cartilage destroyed, adhesions can develop and joints can fuse, prohibiting joint motion. Atrophy of soft tissues adjacent to involved joint may result.

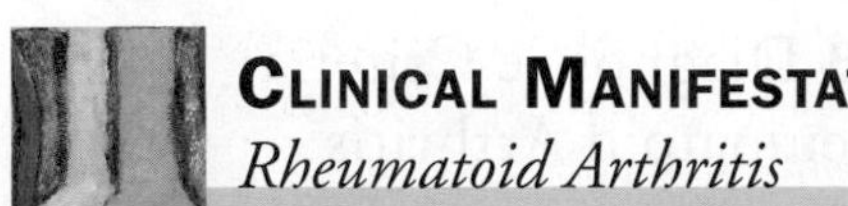

CLINICAL MANIFESTATIONS
Rheumatoid Arthritis

Early Symptoms

Fatigue
Weight loss
Fever
Malaise
Morning stiffness
Pain at rest and with movement, night pain
Edematous, erythematous, "boggy" joint

Late Symptoms

Pallor
Anemia
Color changes of digits (bluish, rubor, pallor)
Muscle weakness, atrophy
Joint deformities
Paresthesias
Decreased joint mobility
Contractures (usually flexion)
Subluxation
Dislocation
Increasing pain

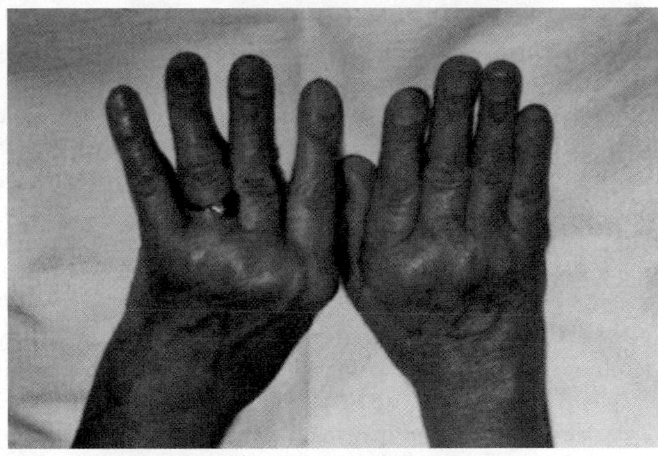

Figure 54-15 Rheumatoid arthritis of hands.

tion of the hand (Figure 54-15). Virtually all joints can become involved, but most commonly involved are the joints of the hands, wrists, ankles, elbows, and knees. Shoulder and hip involvement occurs later. Joint involvement usually occurs in a bilaterally symmetric pattern. Joint swelling is caused by inflammation of the synovial membrane, new bone formation, and tissue hyperplasia. The joint feels warm and boggy on palpation and may be erythematous.

Eventually all joints may be affected by RA. Involvement of the temporomandibular joint (TMJ) may limit the person's ability to open the mouth. Spinal involvement is usually limited to the cervical spine, particularly the first and second vertebrae. Subluxation of the cervical vertebrae may result in death or paralysis. Both TMJ and cervical spine pathologic conditions should be assessed before the use of general anesthesia.

Inflammation of the tendon sheaths, particularly in the wrist, may occur. Muscle spasms contribute to the deformity of involved joints. Muscle atrophy may occur as a result of disuse secondary to pain. **Rheumatoid nodules** are an aggregate of inflammatory cells around a center of cellular debris and may develop near joints, over body prominences, or along extensor surfaces in the subcutaneous tissues. Twenty percent of persons with RA develop rheumatoid nodules.[7]

RA may also affect other body systems, and rheumatoid nodules may form in the heart, lungs, and spleen (Table 54-4). Glaucoma may result from rheumatoid nodule formation on the sclerae. Other manifestations of the multisystem involvement of RA include pleuritis, pulmonary fibrosis, pericarditis, aortic valve disease, lymphadenopathy, and splenomegaly. Acute necrotizing vasculitis, also common in other autoimmune disorders, may result in myocardial infarction, stroke, kidney damage, or Raynaud's phenomenon.

The course and severity of RA is unpredictable and is marked by periods of exacerbation and remission. However, in most patients narrowing of the joint space and bony erosion progress most rapidly during the first 2 years of disease.[29] Individuals with seropositive rheumatoid disease (positive rheumatoid factor) tend to have a chronic progressive pattern of disease. In a few patients, the disease may be rapidly progressive, marked by unremitting joint destruction and diffuse vasculitis. This form of the disease is referred to as malignant rheumatoid disease.

TABLE 54-4 SYSTEMIC MANIFESTATIONS OF RHEUMATOID ARTHRITIS

Body System	Clinical Manifestations
Cardiovascular	Pericarditis, valvular lesions, myocarditis, vasculitis, Raynaud's phenomenon
Pulmonary	Pleurisy, rheumatoid nodules on lungs, pneumoconiosis (Caplan's syndrome), interstitial pneumonitis, pulmonary fibrosis, pulmonary hypertension
Neurologic	Compression neuropathy, peripheral neuropathy, cervical myelopathy
Hematologic	Anemia, leukopenia (Felty's syndrome when accompanied by hepatosplenomegaly)
Renal	Rheumatoid nodules on kidney
Dermatologic	Rheumatoid nodules, brown lesions on skin caused by ischemia, ulcers, draining fistulas
Ophthalmologic	Scleritis, sicca syndrome (keratoconjunctivitis); Sjögren's syndrome (keratoconjunctivitis, xerostomia, vaginal dryness), glaucoma, scleromalacia
Other	Fever, malaise, weakness

The length of time between exacerbations varies with individuals. Physiologic and psychologic stress can contribute to exacerbations of the disease.

Increased morbidity and mortality are associated with more severe active cases of the disease. Remission is unlikely after 3 years of sustained disease activity. If untreated, RA tends to relapse and recur in a more severe form. Even with careful management, approximately 10% of patients with RA develop a severe, crippling form of the disease.

COMPLICATIONS. Complications associated with RA are usually a result of systemic manifestations. Pericarditis occurs in approximately 40% of patients with RA.[29] Pulmonary complications are usually asymptomatic but may manifest as infiltrates, nodules, or interstitial pneumonitis. Pulmonary complications may also result from treatment of RA with methotrexate and gold.

Compression neuropathy may develop in the form of carpal and tarsal tunnel syndrome and ulnar nerve palsy. Atlantoaxial (C1 and C2) subluxation is a potentially fatal complication in persons with RA. Cervical subluxation occurs in approximately 15% of persons with RA within 3 years of the onset of disease; patients with RA should be carefully screened for cervical subluxation, particularly if they are undergoing general anesthesia. Any patient with a new onset of neck pain or myelopathy should be evaluated for cervical subluxation.

Rheumatoid vasculitis, inflammation and blockage of small blood vessels, is another potentially severe complication of RA. The extremities are most commonly affected, but involvement of the heart, abdominal organs, muscle, and nerves is possible. Treatment for internal organ involvement is usually high-dose corticosteroids and cyclophosphamide. The initial manifestation of vasculitis may be 1- to 3-mm brown spots on the fingers and fingernails, resulting from small areas of skin infarction. Eventually skin ulcers may form, which may be difficult to heal. Concomitant treatment with corticosteroids or other immunosuppressants may compound the problem.

Collaborative Care Management

DIAGNOSTIC TESTS. The American Rheumatism Association has devised a system for the diagnosis of RA; four of the seven criteria must be present (Box 54-3).[26,29] The American College of Rheumatology has proposed criteria defining remission of disease, which must be present for at least 2 consecutive months (Box 54-4).[26] Diagnostic tests results usually include:

- Elevated erythrocyte sedimentation rate (ESR), although up to 40% of patients have normal ESR on presentation[28]
- Positive C-reactive protein test during acute phases
- Positive antinuclear antibody test, present in 30% to 40% of cases
- Mild leukocytosis or normal WBC count; possibility of eosinophilia in persons with severe disease
- Anemia (hypochromic, normocytic in the range of 30% to 35%); low serum iron and iron-binding capacity
- Positive rheumatoid factor or latex fixation test (present in 50% to 90% of patients, depending on disease duration and severity)
- Narrowing of the joint space and erosion of articular surfaces on x-ray examination; subluxation, dislocation of joints; radiographic changes proportional to the degree of inflammation and disease activity; in persons with early RA, magnetic resonance imaging possibly showing focal bone changes undetectable by plain x-ray films
- Inflammatory changes in synovial tissue obtained by biopsy
- Synovial fluid analysis: poor mucin clot test, elevated WBC count, immune complexes present, increased turbidity and decreased viscosity of fluid

Box 54-3 Diagnostic Criteria for Rheumatoid Arthritis

- Morning stiffness lasting more than 1 hour and at least 6 weeks' duration
- Soft tissue swelling of three or more joints for at least 6 weeks
- Swelling of wrist, metacarpophalangeal, or proximal interphalangeal joints for at least 6 weeks
- Symmetric soft tissue swelling
- Rheumatoid nodules
- Positive serum rheumatoid factor test
- Radiographic changes (bone erosion or decalcification) in hand or wrist joints

Box 54-4 Diagnostic Criteria for Remission of Rheumatoid Arthritis

- Duration of joint stiffness less than 15 minutes
- Absence of fatigue
- No joint pain (per history) and no joint pain or tenderness with motion
- Absence of soft tissue swelling in joints or tendon sheaths
- Erythrocyte sedimentation rate less than 30 mm/hr in women; less than 20 mm/hr in men

MEDICATIONS. The purposes of pharmacologic therapy are relief of pain, control of inflammation, and prevention of bone erosion (Table 54-5). Minimization of drug side effects is also desirable. Early aggressive drug therapy is recommended to prevent irreversible changes in articular cartilage that typically occur within 2 years of disease onset.[26,29] The American College of Rheumatology uses criteria to evaluate the effectiveness of treatment with disease-modifying antirheumatic drugs (DMARDs) (Box 54-5). These criteria are evaluated as improvement from the patient's baseline and are often used in clinical trials.[14]

The goal of medication management for RA has changed from alleviating pain, swelling, and stiffness to slowing the destruction of cartilage and bone.[14] Disease management and improved quality of life are now realistic goals for the person with RA.[14] Complete remission of symptoms may be obtained in some patients.[28]

The use of NSAIDs and aspirin were traditionally the first line of treatment (see Table 54-2). However, in addition to the risk of adverse effects associated with the COX-2 selective and nonselective NSAIDs, these drugs do not prevent long-term joint damage in persons with RA. NSAIDs, including salicylates, modify the inflammatory process by inhibiting prostaglandin synthesis but do nothing to prevent bony erosion and alone are usually ineffective in the management of RA. Thus NSAIDs should not be used as monotherapy, but may be used in combination with DMARDs and steroids. Some patients still take NSAIDs or diclofenac coated with misoprostol for GI protection, usually on an as needed basis. The American College of Rheumatology recommends that before initiation of therapy with NSAIDs, baseline values be obtained for CBC; blood urea nitrogen, creatinine, liver enzymes, and potassium levels; and urinalysis.[26]

The primary medications for treating RA are the DMARDs or slow-acting antirheumatic drugs, which are effective in preventing joint damage and suppressing symptoms. DMARDs are classified as methotrexate, glucocorticoids, small molecules, and biologic agents. The use of DMARDs has been shown to result in less functional disability, less pain, less joint tenderness and swelling, and lower ESRs than in persons using NSAIDs. Monitoring begins in 1 to 3 months after initiation of therapy, then at 3- to 12-month intervals thereafter. GI side effects can be controlled with the addition of an H_2 blocker, proton pump inhibitor, or sucralfate. Misoprostol has been effective in reducing the incidence of gastric ulcers and hemorrhage and should be considered in high-risk persons (those with a history of ulcers, older adults, smokers, and those who are receiving concomitant steroid therapy).

DMARDs are introduced early in the disease to preserve joint function and improve outcomes. DMARDs "modify" the disease by preventing erosions. Most drugs in this class demonstrate the ability to stop or slow the radiographic progression of RA.[26] Most persons with moderate or severe RA are started on a regimen of methotrexate. Long-term studies have demonstrated the safety and effectiveness of methotrexate, especially when prescribed with folic acid.

The effectiveness of DMARDs may not be evident until after weeks to months of therapy. Disadvantages of DMARD therapy include the high cost, toxic effects, and long onset of action. DMARDs are continued at low dosages even after disease control is achieved because of the risk of a rebound effect after drug

TABLE 54-5
COMMON MEDICATIONS *for Rheumatoid Arthritis*

Drug	Action	Nursing Intervention
DMARDs		
Methotrexate (Rheumatrex), oral or intramuscular	Rapid onset of action inhibiting degradation of folic acid, which inhibits DNA synthesis of inflammatory cells; effective for long-term therapy; concomitant use with folic acid 1 mg/day decreases toxicity without decreasing effectiveness	Evaluate renal function before therapy; monitor patient for hepatic and pulmonary toxicity, leukopenia, thrombocytopenia, anemia. Explain to patient that nausea, diarrhea, and stomatitis are common. Advise patient to use birth control while taking medication. Check for drug interactions that may increase toxicity risk. Perform liver function tests every 4-8 wk. Teach patients signs and symptoms of pneumonitis, a serious side effect.
Prednisone (oral) Hydrocortisone (intraarticular)	Antiinflammatory Limited disease-modifying potential	Use as bridge therapy or with DMARD. Long-term use is appropriate only for persons with aggressive joint disease unresponsive to other agents; use smallest dose possible (prednisone 5-10 mg every other day) when necessary. Instruct patient to take with food or milk and to abruptly discontinue medication. Monitor patient for fluid and electrolyte balance, glucose levels, hypertension, skin thinning, skin lesions (purpura), decreased healing potential, cataract formation. Encourage adequate calcium and vitamin D intake to retard osteoporosis. Advise osteoporosis screening and possible prophylaxis with antiresorptive agents.[14] Teach patient to avoid sources of infection. Systemic effects are rare with intraarticular use; avoid more than 3 injections per joint per year.

Continued

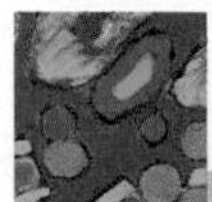

TABLE 54-5
COMMON MEDICATIONS *for Rheumatoid Arthritis—cont'd*

Drug	Action	Nursing Intervention
Small Molecules		
Hydroxychloroquine (Plaquenil)	Mechanism of action unclear; acts on DNA synthesis, antiinflammatory Usually ineffective as single agent	Inform patient of need for eye examination before therapy and every 6 mo thereafter (retinal edema may result in blindness). Monitor patient for hematologic toxicity, GI irritation, and hypertension; evaluate renal function.
Sulfasalazine (Azulfidine)	Unknown, antiinflammatory Single agent, or in combination	Assess for sulfa allergy. Monitor patient for neurologic and GI toxicity, leukopenia, anemia, and Stevens-Johnson syndrome. Educate patient about need for CBC and liver function tests throughout therapy.
Gold compounds: gold salts (Myochrysine), auranofin (Ridaura), aurothioglucose (Solganal), oral and intramuscular	Antiinflammatory mechanism unclear; effect not noted until several months of therapy	Monitor patient for renal and hepatic damage, dermatitis, and mouth ulcerations. Inform patient of need for CBC and urinalysis before and at intervals throughout therapy. Stress need for oral hygiene; therapy may cause metallic taste in mouth. Oral gold has fewer side effects than intramuscular.
Azathioprine (Imuran)	Unknown, immunosuppressant	Monitor patient for blood dyscrasias, hepatitis, and pancreatitis. CBC is necessary as baseline and throughout treatment.
D-Penicillamine (Depen, Cuprimine)	Unknown	Monitor patient for fever, rash, GI upset, blood dyscrasias, and delayed wound healing; assess for penicillin allergy. Inform patient of potential for dysgeusia (taste alteration). Food interferes with absorption. Rare side effects include polymyositis and Goodpasture's syndrome. Urinalysis and CBC are required before and at intervals during therapy.

Box 54-5 American College of Rheumatology: Criteria for Evaluating Clinical Response

- Subjective evaluation of pain
- Number of tender or swollen joints
- Improvement as measured by health assessment questionnaire
- Provider evaluation of global arthritis activity
- Measurement of C-reactive protein or erythrocyte sedimentation rate

From Hoffman KL: Medical management of rheumatoid arthritis, *Clin Rev* 13(3):47-54, 2003.

discontinuation. Careful monitoring is required to prevent the development of toxic effects. Most adverse effects are reversible after the drug is discontinued. Many physicians prescribe two or more DMARDs in combination. Failure to respond to multiple DMARDs is associated with a poor prognosis.

Steroid therapy, oral and intraarticular, is also used in the management of RA. Monotherapy with glucocorticoids should be avoided, but they can be used as bridge therapy until DMARDs are effective, or as combination therapy.[26] An important consideration is prophylaxis against osteoporosis. The many side effects associated with steroid use rarely occur with intraarticular injections. More than three injections in the same joint per year are not recommended. The use of low-dose (5 to 7.5 mg) prednisone can significantly reduce the incidence of side effects; dosages in excess of 10 mg/day are rarely indicated. Supplemental calcium (1200 to 1500 mg/day) and vitamin D or antiresorptive agents can be prescribed to reduce steroid-induced osteoporosis.

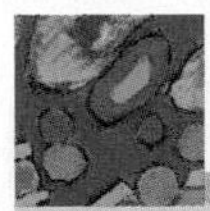
TABLE 54-5
COMMON MEDICATIONS *for Rheumatoid Arthritis—cont'd*
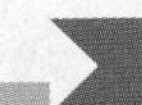

Drug	Action	Nursing Intervention
Leflunomide (Arava)	Immunosuppressant Pyrimidine antagonist, immunomodulator, antiinflammatory; inhibits activated T lymphocytes	Begin with loading dose followed by maintenance dose. Use caution with patients with renal or hepatic disease. Drug has few toxic effects; monitor liver function tests. Dosages over 25 mg/day are associated with increased incidence of side effects, including alopecia, weight loss, and elevated liver enzymes. Educate patient regarding use of contraception while taking medication.
Cyclophosphamide (Cytoxan)	Immunosuppressant Suppresses synovitis; retards bony erosions	Monitor patient for toxic effects, including GI distress, bone marrow suppression, alopecia, and hemorrhagic cystitis. Inform patient of possible long-term effects, including bladder fibrosis and cancer, infections, sterility, and hematologic malignancies. Inform patient of need for monitoring CBC and urinalysis during therapy. Teach patient to increase fluid intake to ensure frequent bladder emptying.
Biologic Agents		
Anakinra (Kineret)	Recombinant human interleukin-1 (IL-1) receptor antagonist; counteracts effects of IL-1, decreasing inflammation, bone erosion, and cartilage destruction; also relieves pain; given alone or in combination with other DMARDs; contraindicated for use with etanercept and infliximab	Administer daily by subcutaneous injection. Most common adverse effect is pain at injection site (rotating sites is recommended). Other adverse effects are rare and include neutropenia, neoplasia, and infection. Refrigerate medication and protect from light.
Etanercept (Enbrel)	Recombinant TNF-alpha antagonist; originally developed for use with methotrexate, now used as monotherapy	Use in patients with severe disease unreceptive to other disease-modifying agents. Cost is high, and biweekly subcutaneous injections are required.

Continued

Newer agents include human TNF-alpha antagonists, which have been shown to retard radiographic progression of disease. Disadvantages include the high cost and paucity of data regarding safety and efficacy of long-term use. Because of cost, most insurance companies require proof that other agents have been ineffective in retarding disease progression before approving the use of these agents. Anakinra blocks interleukin-1, a protein present in excess in persons with RA. The use of anakinra is recommended for persons unresponsive to other DMARDs. Adalimumab (Humira) is a human-derived antibody made from recombinant deoxyribonucleic acid, which blocks TNF-alpha, controlling rheumatoid symptoms. Adalimumab may be used in combination with methotrexate to retard joint deterioration.[17,22]

Other pharmacologic therapies used to treat RA include cytokines, cytokine agonists, cyclosporine, antibiotics (minocycline, tetracycline), and monoclonal antibodies. These therapies are reserved for use in persons who do not respond to conventional therapy. Adjuvant drugs to control chronic pain and to improve sleep quality are also used. Tricyclic antidepressants are commonly prescribed; patients should be monitored for side effects, including sedation and dry mouth.

TREATMENTS. The goals of therapy for persons with RA are to relieve symptoms, prevent joint destruction, maintain joint and muscle function, and promote independence and quality of life. For management of systemic manifestations of RA, the reader is referred to the appropriate section of the text.

In addition to pharmacologic therapy, OT and PT are mainstays of treatment to preserve joint mobility and promote independence. An exercise program, designed with the physical therapist, is important for maintaining mobility and preventing muscle atrophy. Ample evidence supports the fact that exercise can improve the individual's sense of well-being, which is helpful in trying to cope

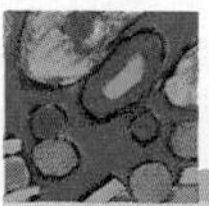

TABLE 54-5
COMMON MEDICATIONS *for Rheumatoid Arthritis—cont'd*

Drug	Action	Nursing Intervention
Biologic Agents—cont'd		
Etanercept (Enbrel)—cont'd		No data are available regarding long-term use; it is contraindicated in pregnancy, lactation, malignancy, and sepsis. Avoid vaccinations (particularly live) while taking drug. Side effects include pain at injection site, respiratory infections.
Infliximab (Remicade)	TNF-alpha monoclonal antibody and immunoglobulin G1 antibody that neutralizes TNF-alpha; administered intravenously; used with methotrexate	Side effects include headache, rash, hypotension, respiratory and urinary tract infections, and local infusion site reactions. Administer intravenously every 2 mo.
Adalimumab (Humira)	Human monoclonal anti-TNF antibody Monotherapy or with methotrexate	Administer 40 mg subcutaneously every other week. Patient may have pain at injection site. Monitor for upper respiratory tract infections, congestive heart failure, optic neuritis, increased risk of infection, development of autoantibodies. Limited long-term data are available.

DMARDs, Disease-modifying antirheumatic drugs; *DNA,* deoxyribonucleic acid; *GI,* gastrointestinal; *CBC,* complete blood count; *TNF-alpha,* tumor necrosis factor–alpha.

with a chronic, disabling disease. T'ai chi' has proven to be beneficial to persons with RA, improving ROM of the lower extremity, particularly the ankle.[34]

Splints and orthoses are prescribed by the physician and fitted by a physical therapist, occupational therapist, or orthotist. The purposes of splints and braces are to (1) stabilize or support a joint, (2) protect a joint or body part from external trauma, (3) mechanically correct a dysfunction such as footdrop by supporting the joint in its functional position, and (4) assist patients in exercising specific joints.

Splints and braces (Table 54-6) are designed to be as lightweight and cosmetically acceptable as possible. Many splints are made of plastic, which can be molded to fit. In many instances plastic has replaced metal and leather braces, which are often obvious, even under loose-fitting clothing. Shoes may be modified or corrective shoes prescribed to provide special support for the feet. Braces can be fitted to the patient's own shoes.

Many assistive devices are available for individuals who have impaired upper or lower extremity function (Table 54-7). These devices are obtained by referring the patient to an occupational therapist.

Supportive devices or ambulatory aids (walkers, canes, and crutches) are usually recommended for persons who cannot bear weight on one or more joints of the lower extremities. Other indications for use include instability, loss of balance, or pain on weight bearing. The physical therapist evaluates the patient to determine the specific device that matches the patient's needs and abilities. Nurses are expected to supervise patients in their use of these devices and encourage patients to use their walking aids correctly. Table 54-8 presents advantages and disadvantages of different aids and the techniques of walking with each.

Other treatment modalities for the person with RA include the application of hot and cold packs to the affected joints. Heat may be applied by means of:

- Hydrocollator packs (packs containing chemical filler that expands in water and retains heat; may be heated in a pot of water or special machines that maintain a constant temperature of 80° C [176° F])

TABLE 54-6 TYPES AND FUNCTIONS OF SPLINTS AND BRACES

Type	Function
Spring-loaded braces	Oppose action of unparalyzed muscles and act as partial functional substitutes for paralyzed muscles (Figure 54-16)
Resting splints	Maintain limb or joint in functional position while permitting muscles around joint to relax (Figure 54-17)
Functional splints	Maintain joint or limb in usable position to enable body part to be used correctly
Dynamic splints	Permit assisted exercise to joints, particularly after surgery to finger joints (Figure 54-18)

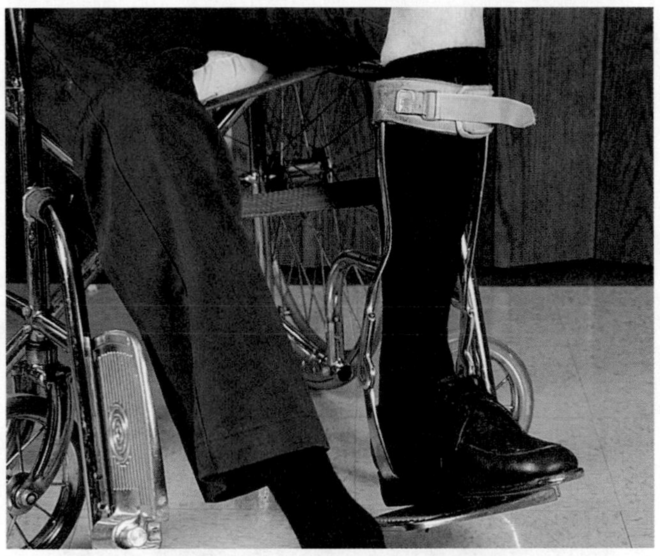

Figure 54-16 Leg brace.

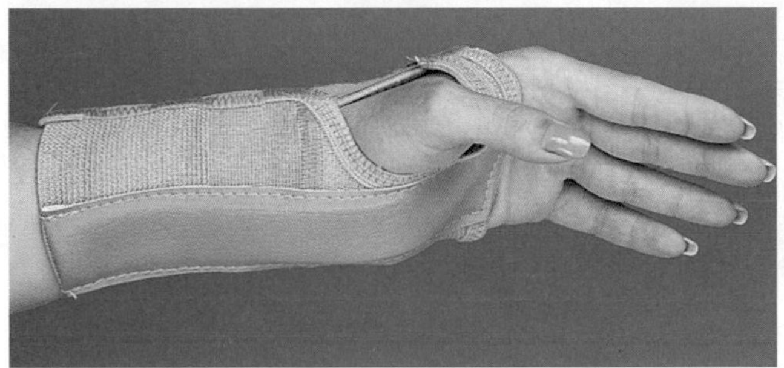

Figure 54-17 Wrist splint.

- Paraffin baths
- Electric heating pads that are approved for use with moist towels
- Electric heating pads that produce moisture
- Warm soaks, tub soaks, or showers

Application of cold or ice packs is helpful in reducing or preventing swelling (especially after trauma), reducing pain, and relieving stiffness. Cold packs may take the form of plastic bags containing ice, commercially available gel packs that can be refrozen and reused, or large bags of frozen vegetables (especially for home use).

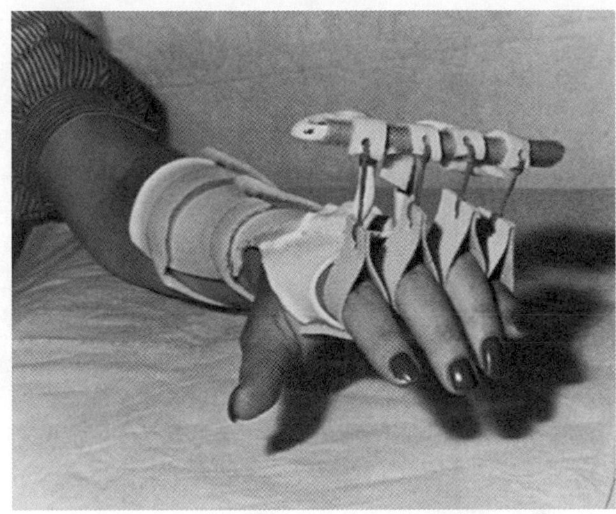

Figure 54-18 Dynamic hand splint.

Heat or cold are left on for 15 to 20 minutes to achieve maximal effect. Cold packs and moist heat packs are wrapped in protective towels to prevent burns to the skin, and the skin is checked 5 minutes after application for any evidence of tissue damage. Heat or cold should be applied with caution to any individual with decreased sensation, because of the risk of injury.

SURGICAL MANAGEMENT. Referral to an orthopedic surgeon is indicated if conservative therapies are ineffective. Surgery is indicated for the prevention or correction of deformity, relief from pain, and restoration or maintenance of function. If loss of function or permanent deformity is not preventable, the patient's powers of compensation and adaptation must be developed.

Before performing surgery, the orthopedist considers the procedure best suited to achieve the desired objectives for the individual patient. It is important that those caring for the patient understand the expected outcomes so that care may be adapted to achieving them.

A description of commonly performed surgical procedures is found in Table 54-9. Synovectomy is performed early in the disease to decrease pain and retard the degenerative changes in the joint. Osteotomy and joint arthroplasty are performed in advanced disease.

TABLE 54-7 ASSISTIVE DEVICES FOR PERSONS WITH MOTOR IMPAIRMENTS

Patient Limitation	Assistive Device
Cannot adequately close hand	Utensil with built-up handle (Figure 54-19)
Loss of opposition of thumb	Utensil with cuffed handle
Loss of only one hand	Combination knife-fork
Unable to grasp regular cup handle	Mug with special handle
Unable to bend to reach feet; hip flexion limitation	Long-handled shoehorn (Figure 54-20)
Unable to stoop or reach; hip flexion limitation	Long-handled reacher (to reach for or pick up objects) (Figure 54-21)
Unable to reach feet; hip flexion limitation	Stocking guide (Figure 54-22)

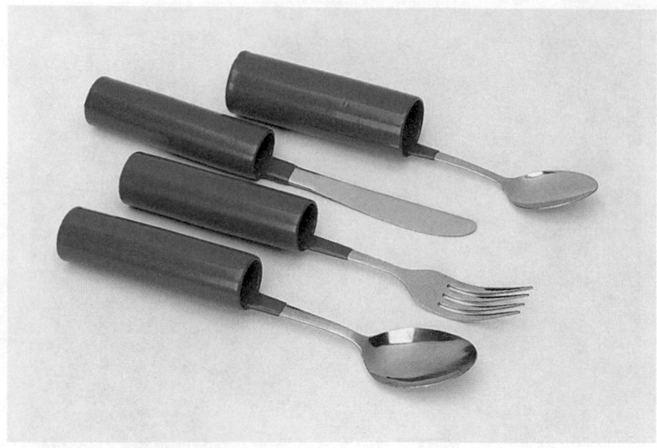

Figure 54-19 Utensils with special handles.

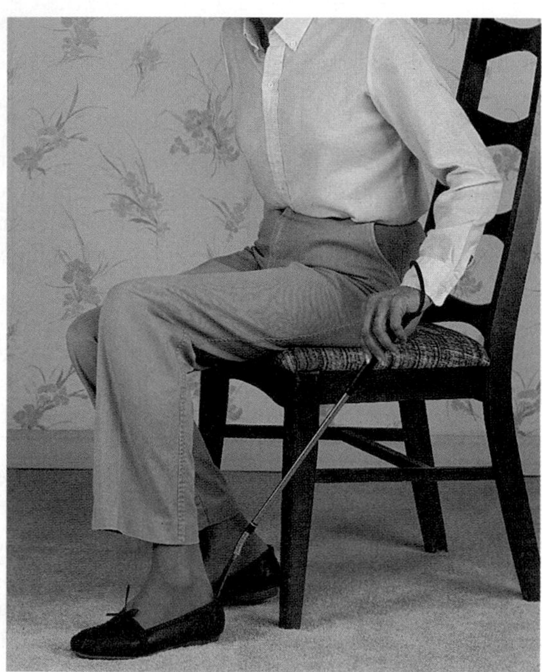

Figure 54-20 Long-handled shoehorn.

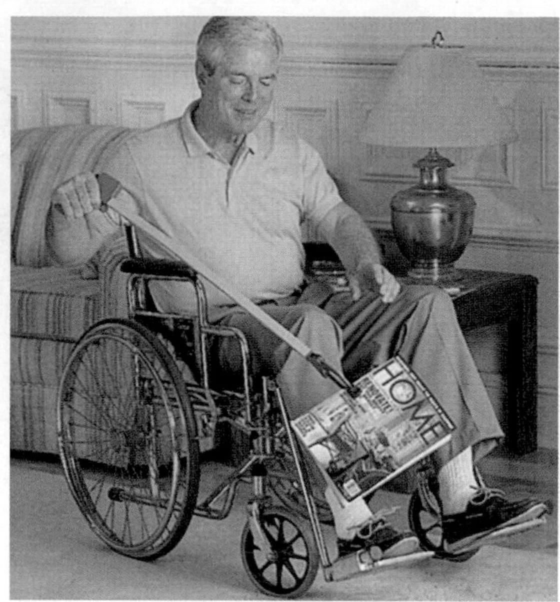

Figure 54-21 Long-handled reachers.

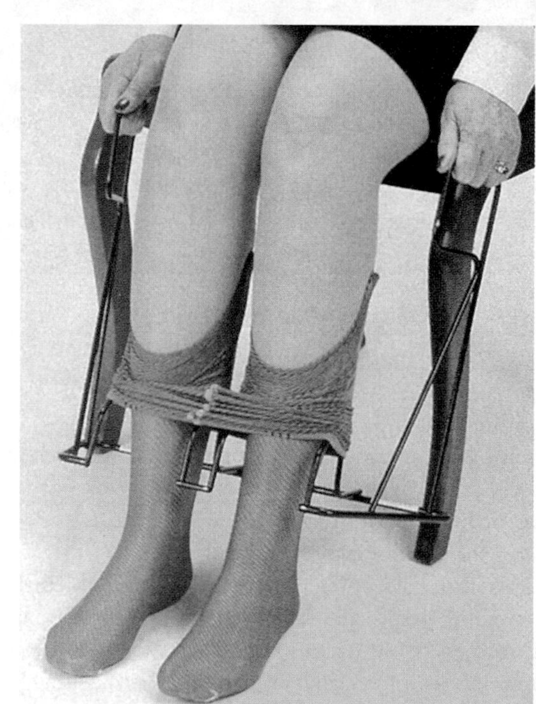

Figure 54-22 Stocking helper.

Diet. Evidence suggests that ingestion of fish oil (a type of omega-3 polyunsaturated fat) as a dietary fat is beneficial to persons with RA. Benefits include a decrease in the number of swollen joints, decrease in the duration of morning stiffness, and overall improvement in function. How fish oil produces a therapeutic effect is unknown, but it does suppress inflammatory mediator (prostaglandins, leukotrienes, and cytokines) production. More research is needed to determine the optimal effectiveness of fish oil in the diet.

Persons with RA often have anemia. A diet containing iron-rich foods (liver, oysters, clams, organ meat, lean meat, whole grains, legumes, and leafy green vegetables) is recommended to decrease anemia. Calcium and vitamin D supplements can reduce bone resorption.

Fatigue and malaise are common in persons with RA. A diet containing adequate calories and balanced nutrition is necessary to prevent fatigue and increase energy. Malnourishment also increases susceptibility to infection, which can exacerbate symptoms. If the patient is being treated with an immunosuppressant, the risk for infection is intensified. If the patient is overweight, a weight reduction diet, combined with exercise, is recommended to decrease the strain on weight-bearing joints.

TABLE 54-8 COMPARISON OF AMBULATORY AIDS

Device	Advantages and Disadvantages	Gait*
Single-support device: cane, quad cane, single crutch	Less cumbersome than crutches or walkers Less effective in unloading weight than double support	Device is held in hand opposite involved leg. Device and involved leg are advanced first, followed by uninvolved leg.
Double-support device	Provides solid support	
Walker	Can be used by individuals with loss of balance Limits speed of ambulation Hazardous on stairs or uneven ground	Walker is advanced first, then involved extremity, then uninvolved extremity.
Crutches	Require dexterity and good sense of balance Permit faster ambulation than a walker Can be used on stairs	3-point gait—same as walker gait 4-point gait—crutch, opposite leg, opposite crutch, other leg 2-point gait—both crutches, both legs (one leg may be non–weight bearing)

*NOTE: Climbing stairs is accomplished by moving the uninvolved leg first, then the device and the involved leg; to descend stairs, the involved leg and device are moved first, then the uninvolved leg. The device and the involved leg always move together.

TABLE 54-9 SURGICAL MANAGEMENT OF RHEUMATOID ARTHRITIS

Procedure	Definition	Indication
Arthroscopy	Endoscopic examination of a joint	Diagnosis Synovectomy Chondroplasty Removal of bone spurs, osteophytes, and "joint mice"
Arthrotomy	Opening of joint	Exploration of joint Drainage of joint Removal of damaged tissue
Arthroplasty	Reconstruction of joint	Restore motion Relieve pain Correct deformity Avascular necrosis
Interposition	Replacement of part of joint with prosthesis or with soft tissue	
Hemiarthroplasty	Replacement of one articulating surface	
Replacement (total joint)	Replacement of both articulating surfaces of joint with prosthetic implants	
Synovectomy	Removal of part or all of synovial membrane	Delay progress of rheumatoid arthritis
Osteotomy	Cutting bone to change its alignment	Correct deformity (varus or valgus) Alter weight-bearing surface of diseased joint to relieve pain
Arthrodesis	Surgical fusion of joint by removal of articular hyaline cartilage, introduction of bone grafts, and stabilization with internal or external fixation devices	Stabilize joint Relieve pain
Tendon transplants	Moving tendon from its anatomic position	Substitute one tendon for another that is not working Realign tendon function (e.g., for stability)

Health Promotion and Prevention. Several objectives in *Healthy People 2010* are related to arthritis treatment strategies and the effect of a chronic disease on daily functioning (see Healthy People 2010 box).

Health promotion and teaching are integral to the treatment of the patient with RA. The nurse can teach the patient and family joint protection techniques and energy conservation measures, as well as clarify myths and claims for instant cures. Each year it is estimated that hundreds of millions of dollars are spent on gadgets, programs, and "medicines" that allegedly cure arthritis. Persons with RA and other chronic diseases are particularly susceptible to claims of "cures" and nontraditional therapies. For example, acupuncture and electroacupuncture are commonly used by rehabilitation specialists to decrease pain and symptoms of RA, but there is inconclusive clinical evidence to support their effectiveness.[5] The patient should be educated to evaluate carefully risks and benefits before trying any of these remedies (see Complementary & Alternative Therapies box).

In some instances the disease and associated disability may progress despite all efforts to control the disease process; this is extremely discouraging for the patient, family, and members of the health care team. However, many persons are able to live reasonably normal, productive lives while managing their arthritis. Their ability to do so partially depends on their knowledge of the disease and its treatment.

Helping the patient to cope with any loss of function or change in role is an important aspect of nursing care. The nurse may need to refer the patient to a counselor or religious leader for additional support if the patient is having difficulty coping with dependency or loss of control. The patient may benefit from involvement in the Arthritis Foundation or community group. The Arthritis Foundation is an excellent resource; it publishes the magazine *Arthritis Today* and offers the "Arthritis Self-Help" course to help individuals manage pain, fatigue, and stress and to develop individualized exercise programs.

Healthy People 2010

Objectives Related to Arthritis and Other Rheumatic Conditions

- Increase the mean number of days without severe pain among adults who have chronic joint symptoms.
- Reduce the proportion of adults with chronic joint symptoms who experience a limitation in activity because of arthritis.
- Reduce the proportion of all adults with chronic joint symptoms who have difficulty performing two or more personal care activities, thereby preserving independence.
- Increase the proportion of adults ages 18 years and older with arthritis who seek help in coping if they experience personal and emotional problems.
- Increase the employment rate among adults with arthritis in the working-age population.
- Eliminate racial disparities in the rate of total knee replacements.
- Increase the proportion of adults who have seen a health care provider for their chronic joint symptoms.
- Increase the proportion of persons with arthritis who have had effective, evidence-based arthritis education as an integral part of the management of their condition.

From US Department of Health and Human Services: *Healthy people 2010: understanding and improving health,* Washington, DC, 2000, The Department.

Complementary & Alternative Therapies

Rheumatoid Arthritis

Myriad supplements are available that claim to provide relief from pain and inflammation and other symptoms associated with rheumatoid arthritis (RA). Pharmacologic treatment often causes adverse side effects, so many patients may be tempted to try "natural remedies." Nurses caring for patients with RA should be familiar with the most common products so they can provide information necessary to make informed decisions. The Arthritis Foundation has identified the following supplements as potentially beneficial for persons with RA. Before trying these products, patients should discuss their safety and efficacy with the health care provider.

- *Dehydroepiandrosterone* (DHEA) is a naturally occurring hormone compound; when used as a supplement, it is derived from chemically treated yams. It is purported to relieve pain and inflammation and reduce fatigue; it may increase bone density. DHEA is currently under review by the Food and Drug Administration as a treatment for lupus. As a hormone, it has potentially serious side effects, including acne, abdominal pain, hypertension, hair growth, and menstrual irregularities. This supplement should be used only under medical supervision.
- *Fish oil* derived from cold-water fishes contains omega-3 fatty acids that have been shown to decrease the inflammation and pain associated with RA. It may increase the blood-thinning effects of anticoagulants and nonsteroidal antiinflammatory drugs. Fish oil may be taken as a supplement or by eating cold-water fish two or three times weekly.
- *Flaxseed (Linum usitatissimum)* is derived from meal or oil of the flax plant. It is available as a pill, meal, flour, or oil. Flaxseed is also a source of omega-3 fatty acids, which are effective in reducing inflammation. Flaxseed is also a laxative, so gastrointestinal side effects may occur.
- *Gamma-linoleic acid* (GLA) is found in black currants, borage oil, and evening primrose oil. It is available as a capsule or oil. Claims include relief from inflammation and stiffness and symptoms of Sjögren's syndrome and Raynaud's phenomenon. Some studies support its efficacy in reducing pain and inflammation, but none support topical use for aching joints. Side effects include increased action of anticoagulants and, with evening primrose oil use, gastrointestinal symptoms.
- *Green tea (Camellia sinensis)* supposedly relieves pain and inflammation, but no human studies support this claim. Green tea contains polyphenols, which are antioxidant compounds that may relieve inflammation. Green tea has been used medicinally in Asia for years; when taken as a beverage in moderate amounts, it is considered safe.

Horstman J: *Arthritis Today's* supplement guide, *Arthritis Today,* July-Aug 2001, pp 34-49.

Nursing Management of the Patient with Rheumatoid Arthritis

ASSESSMENT

Health History. Assess for:

- Fatigue
- Aching and joint stiffness, especially in the morning
- Loss of strength
- Loss of mobility, ROM
- Difficulty with ADLs
- Pain
- Changes in appetite, anorexia
- Weight loss
- Paresthesias

Physical Examination. Assess for:

- Joint deformity
- Joint tenderness or pain
- Joint swelling and warmth
- Decreased ROM
- Joint contractures
- Joint nodules
- Crepitus
- Fever
- Muscle atrophy
- Decreased muscle strength
- Decreased or altered sensation in extremities
- Changes in posture
- Altered gait
- Use of assistive devices, ambulatory aids
- Transfer ability
- Cervical spine tenderness, loss of motion
- Difficulty opening the mouth, pain with chewing

NURSING DIAGNOSES, OUTCOMES, AND INTERVENTIONS

Nursing Diagnosis: Chronic Pain

OUTCOMES. Common examples of expected outcomes for the patient with a diagnosis of *chronic pain* are:

Patient will:

- State that joint pain is decreased.
- Verbalize ways to control pain.

NURSING INTERVENTIONS. The nurse performs a complete pain assessment (see Chapter 16). Patients with RA have both chronic and acute pain. The challenge to the nurse is managing pain control while promoting mobility. Exercise and movement are difficult when a person is in pain; weight bearing increases stress on inflamed joints, possibly causing more pain. Both pharmacologic and nonpharmacologic methods should be used to manage the pain associated with RA.

Medications are used to decrease the pain and inflammation associated with exacerbations of symptoms. The nurse provides the patient with information regarding prescribed medications, adverse and therapeutic effects, dosage, and administration. Additional interventions to control pain include the application of heat or cold, relaxation techniques, proper body alignment, joint protection and rest, and ROM exercises to decrease stiffness. A warm shower or tub bath may be effective in reducing pain and stiffness, whereas cold can reduce pain and decrease swelling. Transcutaneous electrical nerve stimulation may be prescribed as an adjunct for pain relief.

RELATED NIC INTERVENTIONS. Heat/Cold Application, Medication Management, Pain Management

Nursing Diagnosis: Impaired Mobility

OUTCOMES. Common examples of expected outcomes for the patient with a diagnosis of *impaired mobility* are:

Patient will:

- Maintain active joint ROM within limits of disease to strengthen muscles and prevent injuries.
- Demonstrate improved ability to perform self-care activities and participate in usual activities.

NURSING INTERVENTIONS. Exercise is prescribed to preserve joint mobility (active and passive ROM), maintain muscle tone (active ROM and isometrics), and strengthen selected muscle groups (resistive exercises performed against resistance provided by another person or by weights).

Interventions to promote joint mobility begin with a baseline assessment of functional abilities and joint motion. The nurse encourages active and, if necessary, passive ROM exercises at least twice daily. Controversy exists regarding performing ROM exercises during exacerbations of acute inflammation; periods of joint rest may be prescribed. Complete bed rest should be avoided because of the significant risk of complications associated with immobility. Activity should be balanced with rest.

Exercise may be facilitated by the application of heat or cold or the administration of an analgesic before the exercise period. Exercise is contraindicated in the presence of acute joint or muscle inflammation. Until the inflammatory process subsides, patients with acute joint or muscle inflammation may benefit from an aquatic exercise program, which reduces stress on joints.

Exercise programs should be tailored to the patient's specific needs and capabilities. Nurses need to be aware of the specific exercise program the patient is following and be prepared to provide assistance in performing the exercises as needed and reinforcing the purpose, technique, frequency, and duration of the exercises.

Most people want to live their lives independently. However, persons with musculoskeletal problems may be unable to manage one or more activities for themselves. Assistive devices (e.g., button hook or Velcro closures) are available to increase independence in ADLs. An OT referral may be necessary to evaluate the patient for appropriate assistive devices. Overhead trapezes, handrails, tub rails or shower chairs, grooming aids, elevated toilet seats, and shoes with Velcro fasteners may assist the patient in performing self-care. The patient should allow extra time for completing ADLs; frequent rest periods may be needed because of pain or fatigue.

The patient can use safety devices to enhance function and prevent accidents when normal function, balance, or dexterity is compromised. Examples of safety devices include safety arms around toilets, grab bars mounted at tubs or showers, elevated toilet seats, adhesive strips on tub or shower floors, handrails along staircases, and nonskid wax applied to floors. Nurses need to be familiar with the various devices available and help patients learn to use them.

Splints may be prescribed to provide joint rest or proper alignment. The patient must avoid positions that may lead to contractures. For example, when the patient is supine, pillows should not be placed under knees or under the head, forcing the neck into forward flexion. It is important that the patient wear properly fitted footwear with nonskid soles for safety. The nurse should discuss with the patient or family ways to improve the safety of the home environment to prevent falls and injury.

Adaptations to the home environment may be necessary. Elevated toilet seats and safety equipment for the bathroom can be installed in the home. Doorways should be wide enough to accommodate a walker or wheelchair if necessary. A ramp can be added for access to the front door. Countertops and cupboards can be lowered to accommodate the person who is wheelchair bound. These modifications may be costly.

Patients with severe RA are disabled and may need the assistance of a family member or friend to complete ADLs; if that is not feasible, a home health aide may be needed. Meals on Wheels may help provide nutritious meals for those unable to independently prepare meals.

RELATED NIC INTERVENTIONS. Energy Management, Exercise Therapy: Joint Mobility, Self-Care Assistance: IADL, Teaching: Prescribed Activity/Exercise

Nursing Diagnosis: Fatigue

OUTCOMES. Common examples of expected outcomes for the patient with a diagnosis of *fatigue* are:

Patient will:

- Report reduced fatigue.
- State factors that lead to fatigue and how fatigue might be avoided.

NURSING INTERVENTIONS. Persons with RA commonly report fatigue; the patient may experience overwhelming exhaustion and an inability to complete his or her usual activities. The nurse can use an intensity scale (0 to 10) to evaluate the severity of fatigue and to establish a baseline assessment. Inadequate nutrition and poor quality or amount of sleep can contribute to fatigue. Dietary counseling and methods to enhance sleep and rest may help decrease fatigue.

The nurse should encourage the patient to discuss factors that cause fatigue, identify times of greatest fatigue, and structure activities accordingly. The nurse can help the patient set small, attainable goals and use energy conservation techniques (Box 54-6). Rest is often prescribed for persons with RA and is beneficial in reducing fatigue and decreasing the systemic inflammatory response. Resting specific joints or immobilization may also be prescribed.

Activity must be balanced with adequate rest. Individuals who have pain and stiffness with or after certain activities must learn to recognize their tolerances and adapt their ADLs accordingly. This does not mean stopping all activity; it means modifying activity. Some tasks may be delegated to family or friends, and the patient may need to temporarily limit social or work responsibilities. Referral to a support group can help the individual deal with body and role changes. A regular aerobic exercise program, if permitted by the physician, may reduce fatigue.

BOX 54-6 Joint Protection and Energy Conservation Techniques

- Maintain good standing and sitting posture and proper body alignment.
- Avoid keeping joints in flexion for prolonged periods.
- Avoid twisting motions with small joints, such as turning a jar lid.
- Change positions frequently.
- Use the strongest joints and muscles when performing activities.
- When working at a desk, stand up and walk about for a few minutes every half hour.
- Use the knees, not the back, when lifting heavy objects.
- Push a door open with the shoulder, not the wrist.
- Use a shoulder strap, not a handheld strap, to carry a heavy bag or purse.
- Avoid reaching or bending when another approach would work as well.
- Work at a comfortable height.
- Avoid trying to accomplish difficult tasks in a single period.
- Take breaks during work periods.
- Slide rather than lift objects.
- Use a wheeled cart to move objects from one place to another.

RELATED NIC INTERVENTIONS. Energy Management, Exercise Promotion

Nursing Diagnosis: Situational Low Self-Esteem

OUTCOMES. Common examples of expected outcomes for the patient with a diagnosis of *situational low self-esteem* are:

Patient will:

- Demonstrate self-esteem.
- Verbalize acceptance of abilities and changes in functioning.

NURSING INTERVENTIONS. A major problem faced by many individuals who have musculoskeletal problems is that the disorder may be disfiguring in addition to being disabling. Not only must they adapt to functional disability, but they also may have to adapt to "looking different" from other people. Loss or alteration of function or the need to use an assistive device or prosthesis can also cause patients to view themselves as different from others. Depending on the nature and strength of pressures from family, social, or work situations and the individual's self-confidence, he or she may attempt to cover up the disability so as not to lose support, respect, or a livelihood. If the disability cannot be concealed, some persons may withdraw or limit their contact with others. Feelings of loneliness or social isolation may result. Maintenance of social supports and continued participation in social and recreational activities are necessary to prevent social isolation and depression.

Nursing interventions to enhance self-esteem include establishing a trusting relationship with the patient and family members, encouraging expression of feelings regarding the disease process and personal appearance, supporting positive coping mechanisms, and conveying respect and nonjudgmental acceptance. The nurse provides positive feedback and helps the patient perform a self-appraisal, identifying strengths and weaknesses and a realistic approach to achieving desired goals. If necessary, the nurse makes referrals to self-help groups, support groups, or counseling services.

RELATED NIC INTERVENTIONS. Coping Enhancement, Self-Esteem Enhancement

Patient/Family Teaching. Teaching for the patient with RA is presented in the Patient/Family Teaching box.

EVALUATION

To evaluate the effectiveness of nursing interventions, compare patient behaviors with those stated in the expected patient outcomes.

RELATED NOC OUTCOMES. Activity Tolerance, Adaptation to Physical Disability, Comfort Level, Energy Conservation, Mobility, Pain Control, Self-Care: Activities of Daily Living (ADL), Self-Esteem

GERONTOLOGIC CONSIDERATIONS

Early manifestations of RA, such as fatigue and myalgia, are vague and can be attributed to a number of other conditions, such as hypothyroidism, a common condition in the elderly population. The older patient with rheumatic disease probably has at least one other comorbid condition. Care must be taken to ensure that the arthritic symptoms are not a result of a comorbid condition. The older patient may not exhibit the typical symptoms associated with RA. In contrast to the usual presentation, the larger joints are usually affected in the older adult, and the onset is usually acute.

An important factor when considering treatment of RA in older adults is the choice of drug therapy. Altered drug metabolism is a physiologic event of aging, and the dosage of many drugs needs to be decreased in older patients. The older adult is more sensitive to the toxic and therapeutic effects of analgesics. Even with reduced dosages, drug toxicity occurs more often and is more serious in the older patient. The use of NSAIDs is a particular concern. Serious adverse effects include cardiovascular events and GI and renal toxicity. Renal function may already be impaired in the older adult, and drug dosage should depend on age and renal function. Concomitant use of misoprostol and lower NSAID dosages has been effective in reducing the incidence of GI side effects. Medications such as methotrexate and steroids, which are associated with serious adverse effects, may be safer and more effective than the use of NSAIDs in treating RA in elderly patients. NSAIDs are not known to modify disease progression.

Older adults with RA need modifications of the home environment to meet their needs. Mobility impairments induced by RA, coupled with changes associated with aging (hearing loss, decreased vision, loss of balance, and loss of muscle mass), are potential obstacles to preserving independence and function. Raised toilet seats, support bars in the bathroom, handrails, avoidance of scatter rugs, and other modifications to prevent injury may allow the person to remain at home and avoid relocation to an extended care or assisted living facility. Prevention of falls is an important intervention for the older person with RA to avoid fractures and the possible associated complications.

Coping with a chronic and potentially disabling condition, in addition to pain and alterations in body image and role performance, may result in depression in the older adult. Nurses are in an ideal position to provide support and counseling to patients. If depression is suspected, a referral for evaluation is indicated.

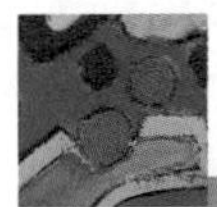

PATIENT/FAMILY TEACHING
The Patient With Rheumatoid Arthritis

Teaching is perhaps the most important aspect of nursing care of patients with rheumatoid arthritis. The patient has to evaluate the response to and effectiveness of the prescribed therapy. Patient teaching should include information about:

- Balance of rest and activity
- Joint protection and energy conservation methods
- Medication use
- Exercise programs
- Proper use of walking aids or assistive devices
- Use and care of splints or braces
- Safety measures
- Falls prevention
- Follow-up care

▶ ARE You READY?

Which of the following is a feature of rheumatoid arthritis and not of osteoarthritis?

1. Elevated erythrocyte sedimentation rate
2. Morning stiffness for less than one hour
3. Pain relieved with rest
4. Crepitus

Critical Thinking

1. A patient is admitted to the hospital with systemic manifestations of RA. The patient remarks, "I thought I just had arthritis. How did this happen?" Develop a teaching plan for this patient.
2. A 70-year-old patient is admitted 6 months after a right knee replacement with right knee pain, an elevated temperature, and general malaise. What are probable causes for his symptoms? What treatment might you expect? Develop a discharge teaching plan for this patient.
3. A 73-year-old woman has undergone left hip revision arthroplasty. She has a history of dislocation. Devise a teaching plan for her to prevent further dislocation of the prosthesis.

References

1. Anderson DL: TNF inhibitors: a new age in rheumatoid arthritis treatment, *AJN* 104(2):60-69, 2004.
2. Baird C: First-line treatment for osteoarthritis, *Orthop Nurs* 20(5):17-26, 2001.
3. Branson JJ, Goldstein WM: Primary total hip arthroplasty, *AORN J* 78(6):947-969, 2003.

4. Brunton S: The use of analgesics in the management and treatment of osteoarthritis, *Rheumatology Express Report*, 2002, Millennium Medical Publications & University of Medicine & Dentistry of New Jersey.
5. Casmiro L et al: Acupuncture and electroacupuncture for the treatment of RA (Cochrane Review). In *Cochrane Library*, Issue 3, Chichester, UK, 2004, John Wiley & Sons.
6. Cook RA, O'Malley MJ: Total ankle arthroplasty, *Orthop Nurs* 4:(21):30-37, 2001.
7. Crowther CL, Mourad LA: Alterations of musculoskeletal function. In McCance KL, Huether SE, editors: *Pathophysiology: the biologic basis for disease in adults and children*, ed 4, St Louis, 2002, Mosby.
8. Food and Drug Administration: *FDA alert for healthcare professionals: celecoxib (marketed as Celebrex)*, accessed April 2005 from website: http://www.fda.gov/cder/drug/infopage/celebrex_hcp.pdf.
9. Freeman S: Diagnosis and management of osteoarthritis, *Am J Nurse Pract* 5(8):9-24, 2001.
10. Geier KA et al: Viscosupplementation: a new treatment option for osteoarthritis, *Orthop Nurs* 21(5):25-32, 2002.
11. Grober JS, Thethi AK: Osteoarthritis: practical nondrug steps to successful therapy, *Consultant* 43(1):53-60, 2003.
12. Grober JS, Thethi AK: Osteoarthritis: when are alternative therapies a good alternative? *Consultant* 43(2):197-202, 2003.
13. Hall VL et al: Unicompartmental knee arthroplasty (alias uni-knee): an overview with nursing implications, *Orthop Nurs* 23(3):163-171, 2004.
14. Hoffman K: Medical management of rheumatoid arthritis, *Clin Rev* 13(3):48-54, 2003.
15. Jenkins JK, Seligman PJ: *Analysis and recommendations for agency action regarding nonsteroidal anti-inflammatory drugs and cardiovascular risk*, Food and Drug Association, April 6, 2005, accessed from website: http://www.fda.gov/cder/drug/infopage/COX2/NSAIDdecisionMemo.pdf.
16. Jolles BM, Bogoch ER: Posterior versus lateral surgical approach for total hip arthroplasty in adults with osteoarthritis (Cochrane Review). In *Cochrane Library*, Issue 3, Chichester, UK, 2004, John Wiley & Sons.
17. Kagen LJ: An update on the newer therapies for rheumatoid arthritis, *Clin Adv* 7(1):10-16, 2004.
18. Kohler SE: Minimally invasive total hip arthroplasty, *AORN J* 79(6): 1244-1258, 2004.
19. Ling SM, Bathon JM: Osteoarthritis. In Rakel RE, Bope ET, editors: *Conn's current therapy*, Philadelphia, 2004, Saunders.
20. McCaffery M, Pasero C: *Pain: clinical manual*, ed 2, St Louis, 1999, Mosby.
21. McDonald S, Hetrick S, Green S: Pre-operative education for hip or knee replacement (Cochrane Review). In *Cochrane Library*, Issue 3, Chichester, UK, 2004, John Wiley & Sons.
22. Medication update: rheumatoid arthritis treatment approved, *Nurse Pract* 28(4):51, 2003.
23. Miller GD et al: The arthritis, diet, and activity promotion trial (ADAPT): design, rational, and baseline results, *Controlled Clin Trials* 24(4):462-480, 2003.
24. Mochan E: Rheumatoid arthritis: clues to early diagnosis, *Consultant* 45(5):545-552, 2005.
25. Morris B: Nursing implications for deep vein thrombosis prophylaxis: pragmatic timing of administration, *Orthop Nurs* 23(2):142-147, 2004.
26. O'Dell JR: Rheumatoid arthritis. In Goldman L, Bennett JC, editors: *Cecil textbook of medicine*, ed 22, Philadelphia, 2004, Saunders.
27. O'Rourke M: Determining the effectiveness of glucosamine and chondroitin for osteoarthritis, *Nurse Pract* 26(6):44-52, 2001.
28. Pincus T: Managing the patient with musculoskeletal pain: a practical approach to the patient with chronic musculoskeletal pain, *Clin Adv* (Suppl), May 2005, pp. 3-20.
29. Pincus T, Sokka T: Rheumatoid arthritis. In Rakel RE, Bope ET, editors: *Conn's current therapy*, Philadelphia, 2004, Saunders.
30. Rice KL, Walsh E: Minimizing venous thromboembolic complications in the orthopaedic patient, *Orthop Nurs* 20(6):21-27, 2000.
31. Roberts D: Degenerative disorders. In Maher AB, Salmond SW, Pellino TA, editors: *Orthopaedic nursing*, ed 3, Philadelphia, 2002, Saunders.
32. Roberts D: Alternative therapies for arthritis treatment, part 1, *Orthop Nurs* 22(5):335-341, 2003.
33. Roberts D: Alternative therapies for arthritis treatment, part 2, *Orthop Nurs* 22(6):412-418, 2003.
34. Robinson HA et al: Tai chi for treating rheumatoid arthritis (Cochrane Review). In *Cochrane Library*, Issue 3, Chichester, UK, 2004, John Wiley & Sons.
35. Schnitzer TJ, Lane NE: Osteoarthritis. In Goldman L, Ausiello D, editors: *Cecil textbook of medicine*, ed 22, Philadelphia, 2004, Saunders.
36. Skinner HB: *Current diagnosis and treatment in orthopedics*, ed 3, Norwalk, Conn, 2003, Appleton & Lange.
37. Towheed TE et al: Acetaminophen for arthritis (Cochrane Review). In *Cochrane Library*, Issue 3, Chichester, UK, 2004, John Wiley & Sons.
38. Trebelo S: Rheumatoid arthritis: making the diagnosis, *Clin Rev* 13(2): 58-64, 2003.
39. Unger J, Selfridge-Thomas J: *The role of COX-2 inhibitors in inflammatory arthritis and common pain syndromes*, Atlanta, 2001, Nursing Contact Hours for Nurse Practitioners.
40. Vallerand AH: Treating arthritis pain, *Nurse Pract* 28(4):7-17, 2003.
41. Whyte JJ, Marting RN: Exercise programs for your arthritis patients: a quick guide, *Consultant* 45(3):341-349, 2005.

evolve Visit the Evolve website: http://evolve.elsevier.com/Monahan/medsurg

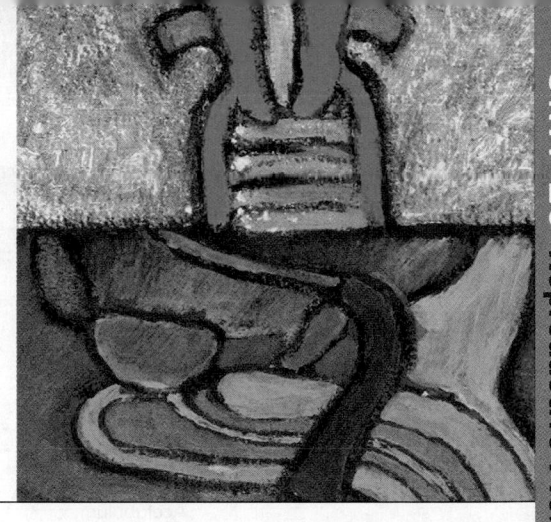

CHAPTER 55

Assessment of the Reproductive System

by Grace Newsome, Kim Hudson

OBJECTIVES

After studying this chapter, the learner should be able to:

1. Describe the structures and functions of the female and male reproductive systems.
2. Explain the functions of the major hormones that control the reproductive systems.
3. Describe age-related changes in the reproductive systems.
4. Identify data related to the reproductive system and sexuality that should be obtained from a patient history.
5. Describe the physical examination components of the reproductive system.
6. Discuss patient preparation and related nursing interventions for diagnostic and laboratory tests used in identifying reproductive tract problems.

KEY TERMS

androgens, p. 1661
ejaculation, p. 1662
estrogen, p. 1665
genitalia, p. 1655
libido, p. 1669
menarche, p. 1665
menopause, p. 1665
ovulation, p. 1665
spermatozoa, p. 1662

Conditions affecting healthful functioning of the reproductive systems of men and women take a high toll in loss of life and acute and chronic physical and emotional stress. The nurse assists in general health education, refers patients for appropriate health care, and uses knowledge of the usual treatments available and nursing care needed when disease develops. A basic knowledge of the structure and function of the reproductive system is important for accurate assessment and planning.

Anatomy and Physiology

Pelvis

The pelvis is the weight-bearing structure of the upper body and trunk. The pelvic bones consist of the innominate bones, the sacrum, and the coccyx (Figure 55-1). Each of the two innominate bones is made up of the pubic bone, ilium, and ischium. Anteriorly, the pubic bones join at the symphysis pubis. The inferior borders of the pubic bones and symphysis form an inverted V, called the pubic arch. The sacrum and coccyx come together at the sacrococcygeal joint, which is movable.

The pelvis is divided into the true and the false pelvis by a bony ridge called the pelvic brim (Figure 55-2). The false pelvis is the broad, expanded portion above the pelvic brim. The narrow part below the pelvic brim is the true pelvis. The true pelvis has an inlet and an outlet. The inlet is located at the pelvic brim, and the outlet is at the base of the pelvis. The iliac spines mark the midpoint between the inlet and the outlet. The distances between the bones of the true pelvis have special significance during childbirth, since the baby must pass through this bony canal to be born.

There are four basic pelvic types: gynecoid, anthropoid, android, and platypelloid. The gynecoid, or typical female pelvis, occurs in the majority of women. It is wide and shallow and well suited for childbirth. The android, or typical male pelvis, is heart shaped and characterized by a narrow subpubic angle and straight sacrum. These pelvic types vary by age, race, and gender. True pelvic types are rare; most pelves are a combination of two types, for example, gynecoid and android. The major differences between the pelves of men and women are in the contour of the pelvis and thickness of the bones.

Female Genital System

External Structures. The external **genitalia** (Figure 55-3), known collectively as the vulva or pudendum, consist of the mons pubis (mons veneris), labia majora, labia minora, clitoris, prepuce, frenulum, vestibule, urethral meatus, Skene's (paraurethral) ducts, vaginal orifice, hymen, fossa navicularis, Bartholin's (vulvovaginal) ducts, fourchette, perineum, and escutcheon. The escutcheon

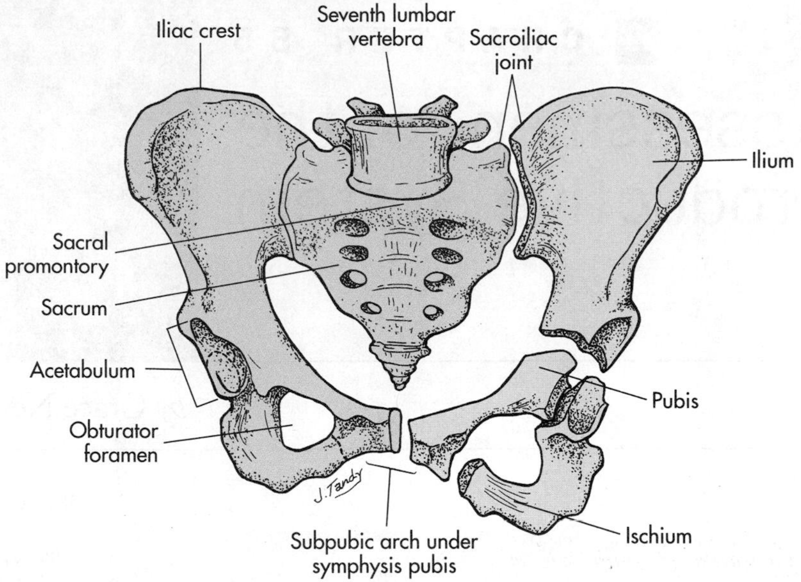

Figure 55-1 Adult female pelvis.

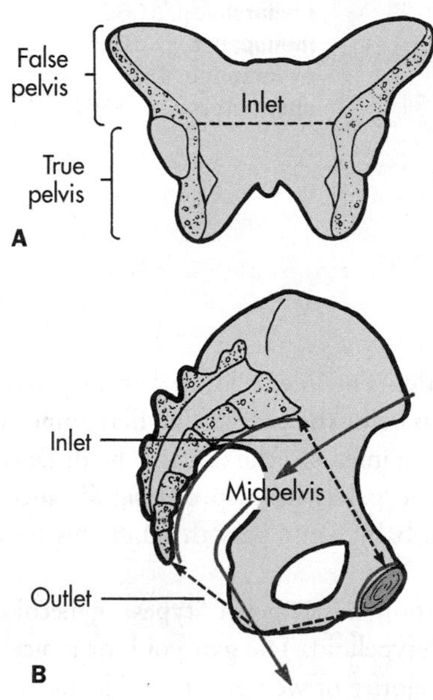

Figure 55-2 Female pelvis. **A,** Cavity of false pelvis is a shallow basin above the inlet; true pelvis is a deeper cavity below the inlet, which is completely surrounded by bone. **B,** Cavity of the true pelvis is an irregularly curved canal *(arrows).*

is the triangular pubic hair pattern from the upper portion of the pubic bone to the lateral areas of the labia majora. The mons pubis is the rounded area in front of the symphysis pubis. It consists of a collection of fatty tissue beneath the skin and is covered with hair after puberty.

The labia majora are two prominent, longitudinal folds of tissue extending back from the mons pubis. The labia are thicker in front, gradually become thinner as they extend back, and appear to flatten out as they merge with the adjacent tissues in the area of the perineum. The labia majora have two surfaces. The outer surface is covered by a thin layer of skin containing hair follicles and sebaceous and sweat glands. The inner surfaces are smooth, lack hair, and are supplied with many sebaceous follicles. The labia are homologous to the male scrotum and serve as protection for the inner structures of the vulva.

The labia minora are two smaller folds of tissue inside and parallel to the labia majora. In sexually active women and in women who have borne children, the labia minora may project beyond the labia majora. The labia minora join near the prepuce, which covers the clitoris, extend backward to enclose the urethral and vaginal orifices, and merge with the labia majora in the perineum. The labia minora are made up of connective and elastic tissue and contain little fatty tissue. Sweat glands and hair follicles are absent from the labia minora, but sebaceous glands are present. The labia minora increase in size and deepen in color in response to sexual stimulation.

The clitoris is situated near the anterior folds of the labia minora. The glans of the clitoris is a small, rounded area consisting of erectile tissue enclosed in a layer of fibrous membrane. The physiologic functions of the clitoris are the initiation and elevation of sexual tension levels. Sexual stimulation initiates a process whereby the clitoris becomes enlarged, erect, and very sensitive to stimuli. Female orgasm can occur from stimulation of the clitoris and other sites sensitive to touch.

The vestibule is a boat-shaped fossa formed between the labia minora, clitoris, and fourchette. The fossa navicularis is a small depression between the fourchette and hymen. The vaginal and urethral orifices can be seen inside the labia minora.

The hymen is a thin membrane that partially covers the vaginal orifice, or introitus. It can be broken or avulsed by coitus, digital examination, tampon use, vigorous exercise, or surgery. Remnants of the hymen called caruncles remain after avulsion and form an irregular border around the vaginal orifice.

The paraurethral, or Skene's, ducts are located on either side of the urethral meatus and drain the multiple urethral glands. The greater vestibular glands (Bartholin's glands) and their ducts are located near the vaginal orifice on either side of the labia. These glands secrete lubricating mucus needed for intercourse. The paraurethral or the greater vestibular glands or their ducts are usu-

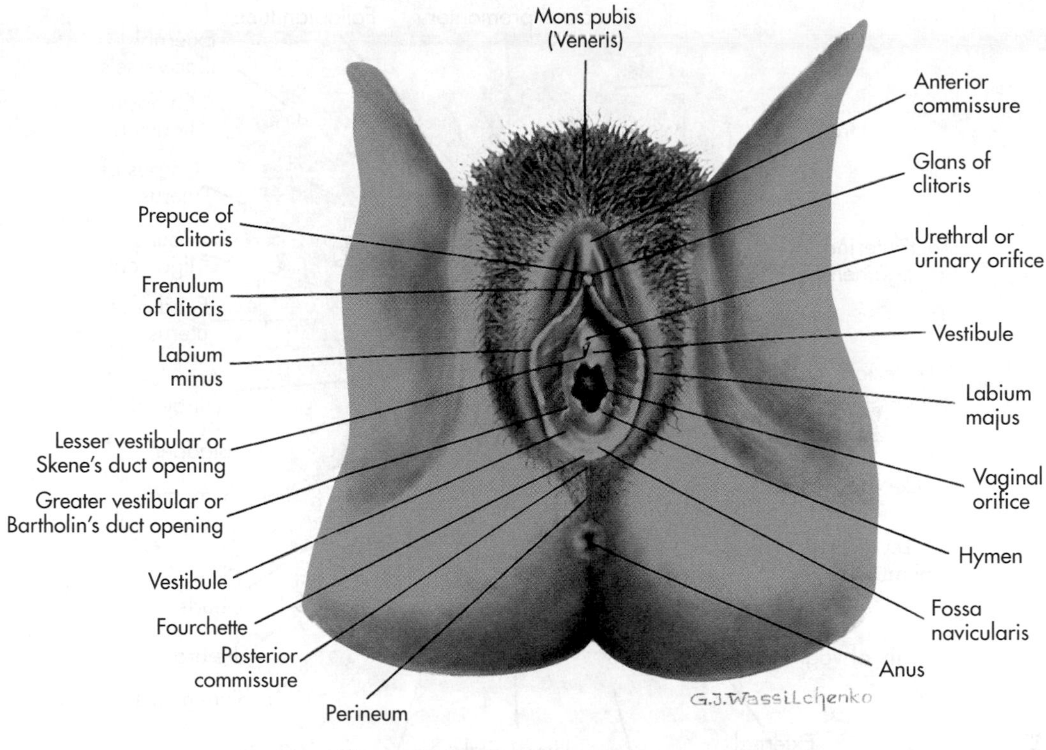

Figure 55-3 External female genitalia.

ally not visible or palpable unless infected. If infected, they are enlarged, erythematous, and painful.

The perineum, the area between the vagina and anus, is composed of muscles and subdermal and dermal tissue. It is the site for an episiotomy incision that is sometimes needed during labor and delivery.

Appearance of the external genitalia varies with age and development and can be quantified using the five-stage Tanner scale. Before puberty, there is no pubic hair, and the labia minora are larger than the labia majora. Sexual maturation in girls usually begins between 8½ and 13 years of age. Thelarche, breast bud development, is the first physical sign of puberty following the adolescent's growth spurt. The mean age for thelarche is 10.9 years. Adrenarche, pubic hair growth, is the second physical sign of adolescence and has a mean age of 11.2 years for its onset. Menarche, onset of menstruation, is the final physical sign of pubertal development and has a mean age of 12.7 for onset. Physical changes progress through Tanner's staging until adult proportions and distribution are established. With the onset of menopause and gradual withdrawal of hormones, the external genitalia atrophy, and the pubic hair begins to thin. In older women, the mons pubis is thinner secondary to the loss of the fat pad, and the clitoris and labia become smaller. See p. 1667 for reproductive physical changes related to aging.

Internal Structures. The female internal reproductive organs (Figures 55-4 and 55-5) are located in the true pelvis and remain there unless altered by a disease process, pregnancy, or sexual stimulation.

VAGINA. The vagina is a soft, tubular structure that extends upward and back from the vaginal orifice to connect the vulva with the cervix and uterus. Located between the rectum and urethra, the vagina permits discharge of the menstrual flow, accommodates the penis during intercourse, contracts during orgasm, and is the passageway for childbirth. The length of the vaginal canal varies, and the posterior wall is longer (8 to 9 cm) than the anterior wall (6 to 8 cm).

The vagina is lined with pink mucous membrane arranged in transverse folds called rugae. The rugae make it possible for the vagina to distend and stretch during coitus and childbirth. The rugated appearance of the vaginal canal is prominent during adolescence and tends to disappear with multiparity and menopause. The length of the vagina shortens after menopause, and the vaginal mucosa becomes thin and dry because of the decrease in estrogen.

The external os of the cervix projects into the upper vagina, creating a cup shape, and the vaginal walls end in a blind pouch around it called the fornix. The vaginal squamous epithelium is continuous with the epithelium of the cervix. The cervix has the same pink color as the vaginal epithelium, but is smoother. In early puberty the columnar epithelium of the cervical canal extends outward onto the surface of the cervix. The point where the squamous and columnar epithelium meet is referred to as the squamocolumnar junction (SCJ). Once the hormonal changes of adolescence occur (onset of ovulation with the production of estrogen and progesterone), the vaginal environment becomes more acidic. The SCJ slowly recedes into the cervical canal to protect columnar cells from the acidic environment. The SCJ is the site of "normal metaplasia" and is therefore vulnerable to the effects of viruses such as the human papillomavirus and bacteria. Because of this inherent vulnerability, this site is included in the Pap test sample. The position of the cervix varies somewhat and can be influenced by the position of the uterus. In the nonpregnant woman the cervix is normally

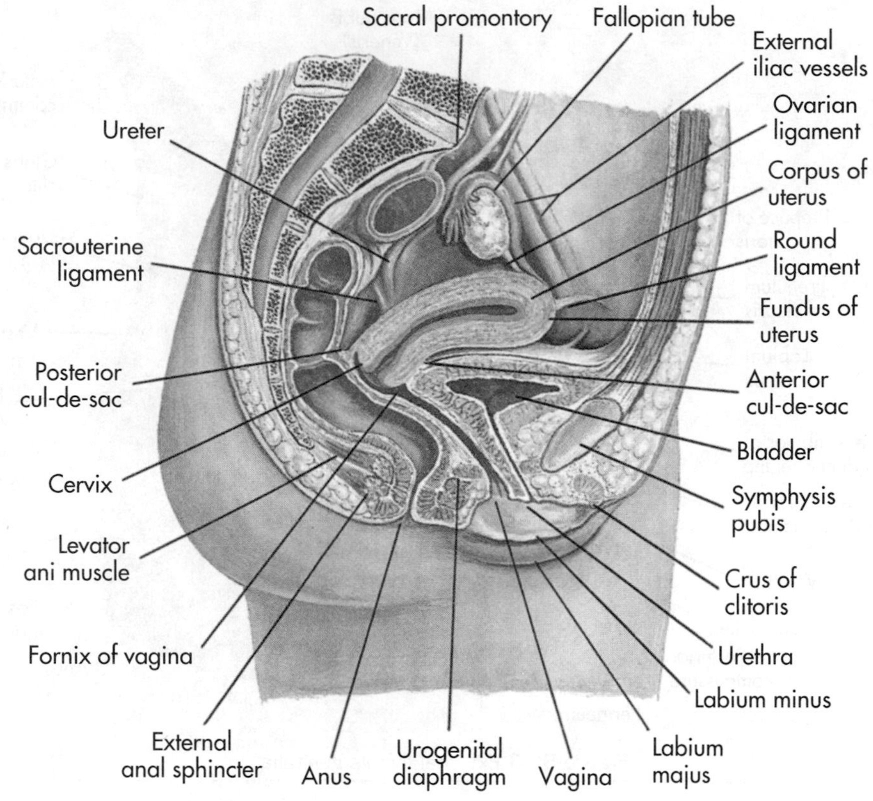

Figure 55-4 Midsagittal view of female pelvic organs.

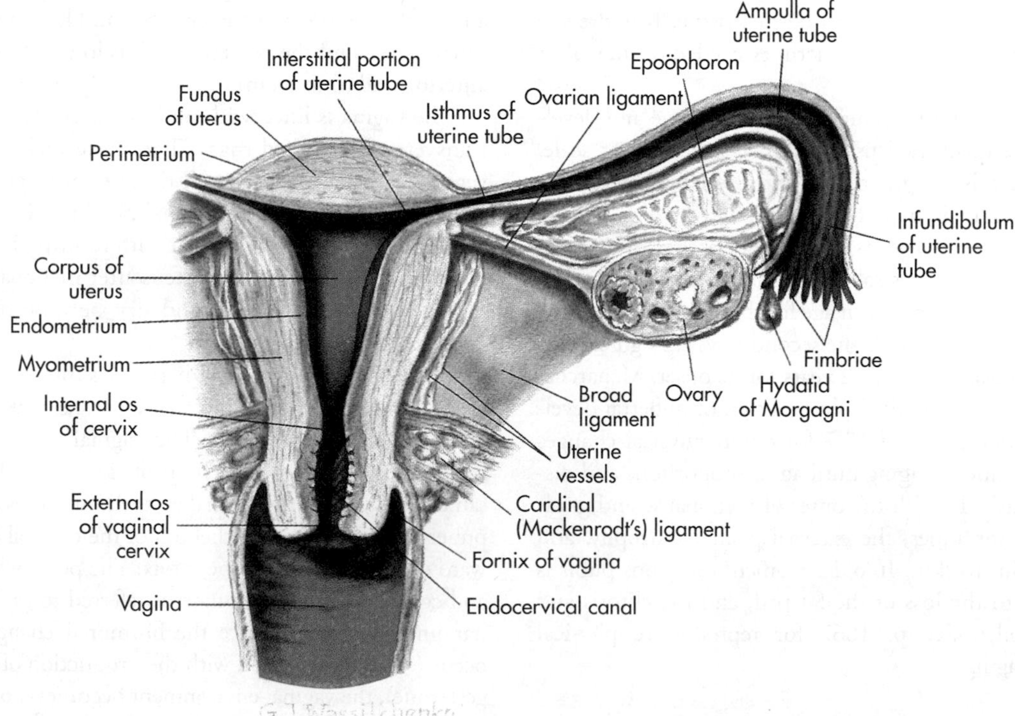

Figure 55-5 Cross section of uterus, adnexa, and upper vagina.

round and firm (consistency of the end of the nose) with a central indention called the os.

The vagina is lubricated by transudation from its own cells and by secretions from the cervix and Bartholin's ducts. Before puberty the vaginal pH tends to be neutral (7.0). With the onset of puberty, the pH drops to 4.0 to 5.0. The vaginal secretions remain acidic throughout the reproductive years and become even more strongly acidic during pregnancy. Neutral or alkaline values are normally found in postmenopausal women. Acidity is strongly influenced by the estrogen concentration, which controls the glycogen levels of the cells. The normal vaginal flora, Döderlein's bacilli, interacts with the secreted glycogen to produce lactic acid and maintain an acid pH.

The vaginal pH can be influenced by personal hygienic measures such as douches, deodorant tampons, and bubble baths or by pathogenic bacteria. Any increase in vaginal pH lessens the natural vaginal defenses and increases the risk of infection. See Table 55-1 for additional physical changes that occur at puberty and at menopause.

UTERUS. The uterus is a hollow, muscular organ located between the urinary bladder and rectum. Its three sections are the fundus, corpus (body), and cervix. The fundus is the thick muscular region above the insertion of the fallopian tubes. The corpus is the main portion of the uterus joined to the cervix by an isthmus of constricted tissue. The cervix is the narrow lower segment. The external os extends into the vagina. The size of the uterus decreases from the fundus to the cervix, creating a triangular, pear-shaped appearance. The size of the uterus varies among women, ranging from 5.5 to 9 cm long, 3.5 to 6 cm wide, and 2 to 4 cm thick in nonparous women. All dimensions may be 2 to 3 cm larger in multiparous women.

The position of the uterus is subject to considerable variation. The uterus is usually anteverted and slightly anteflexed, although it may be retroverted, retroflexed, or in midposition. The body of the uterus is positioned over the bladder so that the fundus is behind the symphysis pubis. The uterus is in direct contact with the bladder and may also touch the rectum, sigmoid colon, and small intestines. The cervix curves forward. With sexual excitation, the uterus elevates into the false pelvis and contracts during orgasm. During pregnancy the uterus changes in size, shape, structure, and position; it returns to its prepregnancy state within 6 to 8 weeks after delivery.

The outer surface of the uterus is covered by peritoneum, which is reflected from the abdominal wall. The anterior and posterior reflections of the peritoneum join at the sides to enclose the fallopian tubes and ovaries. Reflection of the peritoneum over the top of the pelvic organs creates spaces between the uterus and bladder anteriorly and the uterus and rectum posteriorly. The posterior space of the pelvic cavity is known as Douglas' cul-de-sac and is a common entry site of entry into the pelvic cavity for culdoscopy, colpotomy, and surgical drainage.

The uterus has three functional layers. The perimetrium is the peritoneal and fascial outer layer that supports the uterus within the pelvis. The myometrium is the middle muscular layer, which prevents the backflow of menstrual fluids, supports the developing fetus, and moves the term fetus toward the cervix during labor. The endometrium is the inner lining of the uterus and responds to cyclic levels of estrogen and progesterone. The cavity of the uterus is continuous with the cervical canal and has an average fluid capacity of 3 to 8 ml. Near the fundus, the uterus opens into the lumen of the fallopian tubes. Thus a direct route exists from the vagina through the cervix, uterus, and fallopian tubes to the peritoneum.

The cervix is firm, smooth, and round. It is primarily made up of elastic and fibrous connective tissue and smooth muscle. The external os is located in the center of the vaginal portion of the cervix. Extending upward from the external os is the cervical canal, which averages 2 to 3 cm long. The cervical canal terminates as it joins the corpus. The junction of the cervical canal and

TABLE 55-1 REPRODUCTIVE SYSTEM PHYSICAL CHANGES THAT OCCUR AT PUBERTY AND MENOPAUSE

	Puberty	Menopause*
Breasts	Tissue increases	Tissue decreases, less elastic
Nipple and areola	More pronounced	Smaller, flatter
Mons pubis	More prominent, fat deposits	Thinner, loss of fat deposits
Pubic hair	Increases in texture and amount	Sparse, gray
Clitoris	More erectile	Smaller
Labia majora	Enlarges, thickens	Smaller
Labia minora	Enlarges	Thinner
Vaginal opening	1 cm	Smaller
Vaginal epithelium	Layers thicken	Thin, pale, fragile
Vaginal secretions	More acidic, increase	Less acidic, decrease
Vagina	Lengthens	Shortens
Uterus	Increases in size	Decreases in size
Endometrial lining	Thickens	Thins
Ovaries	Increase in size	Shrink to 1-2 cm, no longer palpable

*Changes may be influenced by hormone replacement therapy.

the corpus is called the internal cervical os. The cervix provides a channel for discharge of the menstrual flow, secretes mucus to facilitate the transport of sperm, and dilates during labor for the passage of the fetus.

FALLOPIAN TUBES. The term *adnexa* refers to the fallopian tubes, ovaries, and supporting tissues. The fallopian tubes are two narrow, muscular canals ranging from 8 to 14 cm long. They function as the site for fertilization and transport of the ovum to the uterus. The fallopian tubes extend outward from the corpus near the fundus and are enclosed in the folds of the broad ligaments. The tubes are divided into four sections. The interstitial section lies within the myometrium. The isthmus is the narrow section extending from the fundus. The ampulla is the longer, middle section where fertilization usually occurs. The distal section is the infundibulum, which terminates in the fimbriae (see Figure 55-5). The wavelike motion of the fimbriae encourages the ovum to enter the infundibulum. The walls of the fallopian tubes contain smooth muscles that possess peristaltic properties and are lined with a mucous membrane that contains cilia. At the time of ovulation, both peristaltic and ciliary actions facilitate ovum transport.

OVARIES. The ovaries are endocrine glands as well as reproductive organs. The ovaries store primordial follicles; produce mature ova; and produce and secrete estrogen, progesterone, and androgens. The two almond-shaped ovaries, which are 3 to 4 cm long, 2 cm wide, and 1 to 2 cm thick, lie near the fimbriae of the fallopian tubes. They are partly enclosed by the broad ligaments. The innermost portion of the ovary is the medulla, which contains nerves and blood vessels.

The cortex, which is the outer layer of the ovary, is where primordial follicles are stored. Each follicle contains an undeveloped ovum that has the capacity to respond to stimulation by pituitary hormones. Each ovary contains an estimated 500,000 primordial follicles at birth. Unlike sperm, which are produced constantly, only one ovum normally matures at a time, and the process of ovum maturation requires an average of 28 days. When the ovum reaches maturity, it leaves the ovary by the process of ovulation. Many primordial follicles disintegrate before puberty, and the process of disintegration continues throughout the childbearing years. Few if any primordial follicles are found in the ovaries after menopause.

The ovaries undergo physical changes in position, size, and shape during the life span. At birth the ovaries are very small and are located in the false pelvis. Between infancy and puberty, the ovaries increase in size and descend into the true pelvis. During the childbearing years the ovaries appear long and flat and have a nodular surface caused by follicles. During pregnancy, the ovaries are lifted out of the pelvis by the enlarging uterus, but they descend back into the pelvis after childbirth. After menopause the ovaries undergo rapid, regressive changes, decrease in size, and become wrinkled. In most postmenopausal women the ovaries are so small that they cannot be palpated during vaginal examination.

▶ ARE YOU READY?

Which of the following patients is at greatest risk for an infection based on vaginal pH?

1. 12-year-old at onset of puberty
2. 24-year-old on birth control pills
3. 32-year-old who is 4 months pregnant
4. 64-year-old who is postmenopausal

Pelvic Ligaments and Muscles

The internal and external reproductive structures are maintained in their positions by groups of ligaments and muscles. In the female, the broad, round, cardinal, ovarian, infundibulopelvic, pubocervical, and uterosacral ligaments support the uterus, ovaries, cervix, and vagina (see Figure 55-5).

The levator ani and external anal sphincter muscles comprise the pelvic diaphragm or pelvic floor. The muscles of the perineum, located between the anus and vagina, commonly called the perineal body, reinforce the support provided by the levator ani muscles.

Blood, Lymph, and Nerve Supply

In males and females the organs of reproduction are supplied with blood from the aorta as it branches and divides into the internal iliac (hypogastric) artery with branches to the uterus and genitalia. The ovarian arteries branch off the aorta to furnish the ovaries with blood. The venous drainage empties into the vena cava. In both males and females, lymphatic drainage of the external and internal reproductive organs is extensive, structurally follows much of the blood supply network, and includes the inguinal area.

Nerve supply is derived from both sympathetic and parasympathetic fibers of the autonomic nervous system. In the female the pudendal nerve and its branches supply the majority of the motor and sensory fibers of the muscles and skin of the vulvar region. The pudendal nerve arises from the second, third, and fourth sacral roots. In the male the motor segment of the pudendal nerve innervates the urinary sphincter, and the sensory portion supplies the glans penis and urethra.

Breasts

The paired female breasts, or mammary glands, are accessory structures of the reproductive system meant to nourish the infant after birth (Figure 55-6). They are located between the second and sixth ribs, the edge of the sternum, and the midaxillary line. They develop in response to hormonal stimulation from the hypothalamus, pituitary gland, and ovaries.

The tissue of the breast has three primary components: an interconnected network of glandular and ductal tissue, fibrous tissue, and fat. The proportion of each tissue is a reflection of the individual woman's genetic makeup, age, obstetric history, and weight. The breast is supported by Cooper's suspensory ligaments, which attach to the underlying muscles.

The nipple is the primary external structure of the breast. It arises from the center of the pigmented areola and consists of erectile tissue responsive to sexual stimulation. Montgomery's glands are sebaceous glands that appear as small, round elevations on the areola. They are believed to secrete a fatty substance that offers some protection to the nipple during breastfeeding.

Internally each mature breast is composed of 15 to 25 lobes arranged radially around the breast and separated from each other

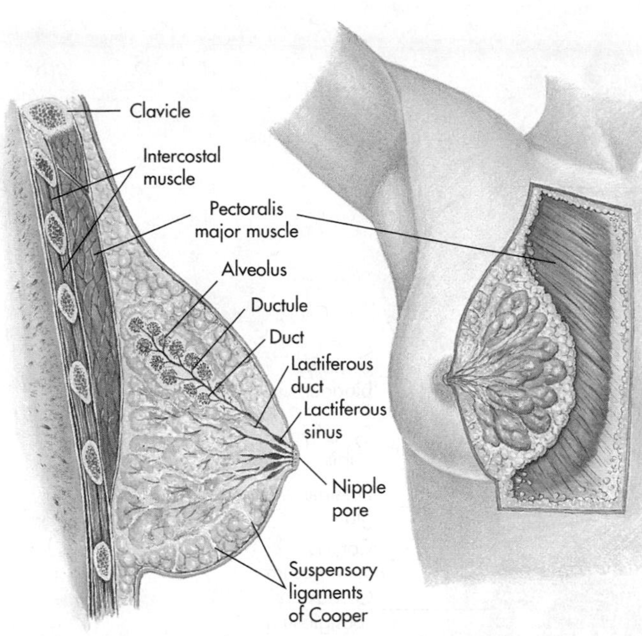

Figure 55-6 Anatomy of the breast, showing position and major structures.

by fatty tissue. Each lobe is composed of several lobules, which in turn are composed of numerous alveoli. Each alveolus is connected by a duct to a larger lactiferous duct from the lobule; the lactiferous ducts join to form one duct from each lobe and then converge at the nipple. Just before the nipple, the ducts expand into sinuses, which serve as reservoirs. The epithelial linings of the alveoli synthesize and secrete the components of breast milk in response to stimulation by prolactin from the pituitary.

The breasts receive an abundant blood supply from the internal mammary and lateral thoracic arteries. Their venous drainage connects to the superior vena cava. They contain an extensive lymphatic drainage network originating within the breast and draining radially into the axillary and subclavian nodal system. Drainage from the axillary region empties into the jugular and subclavian veins. This short and direct route assumes significance in the metastasis of breast cancer (Figure 55-7).

Many women experience noticeable changes in their breasts in response to the menstrual cycle. The breasts may enlarge and become tender or nodular in the premenstrual period in response to the increasing levels of estrogen and progesterone. The cellular growth regresses after menstruation, and water retention is relieved.

Male Genital System

The male reproductive organs and associated structures are shown in Figure 55-8. The Tanner stages of sexual development are also used to determine the level of development in males. In boys the initial changes occur in the testicles and begin at an average age of 12 years old. A physical growth spurt occurs after the beginning of testicular changes. Penile growth and the growth of pubic hair both begin before the appearance of facial hair. The male reproductive organs produce sperm, suspend the sperm in a liquid, and deliver the sperm into the vagina to fertilize an ovum. They also secrete male hormones, the **androgens**. The male genitalia include the penis, scrotum, testes, epididymis, vas deferens, spermatic cord, seminal vesicles, prostate gland, and Cowper's glands.

External Structures

PENIS. The penis is a conduit for elimination of ejaculate and urine through the urethral orifice. It includes the pendulous

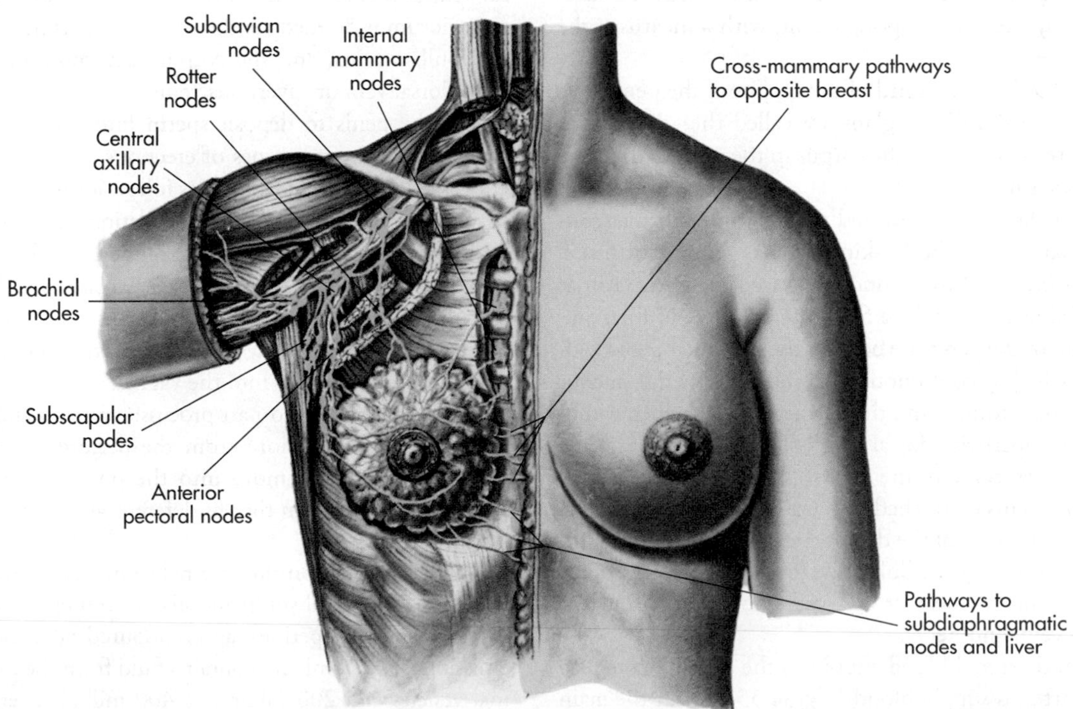

Figure 55-7 Lymphatic drainage of breast.

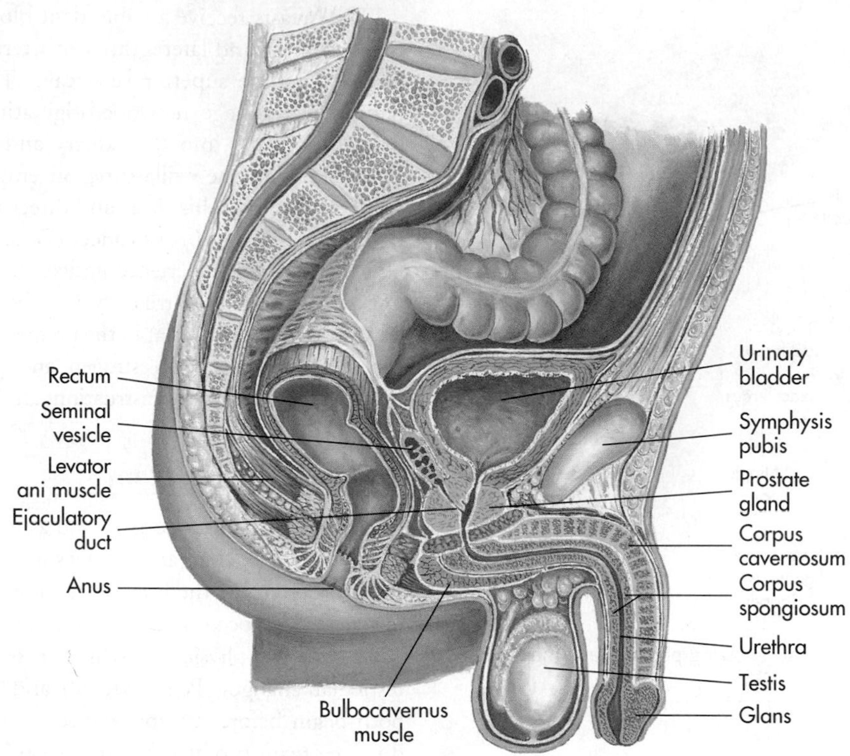

Figure 55-8 Male reproductive system: internal and external genitalia.

portion, or corpus, and the perineal portion, or radix (root). The penis consists of three erectile columns of cavernous tissue. The two corpora cavernosa form the dorsum and sides of the penis. The corpus spongiosum forms the ventral side. In the root of the penis the spongiosum is bulbous and is called the bulb of the penis. The corpus spongiosum continues distally and expands at the end of the penis to the glans, or balanus. The urethra is encircled by the corpus spongiosum, with a meatus at the distal end.

The glans covers the distal third of the corpus of the penis. The dorsum and lateral sides of the glans are called the corona. The dorsal surface of the glans meets the corpus in the neck of the penis or (retroglandular) sulcus.

The corpus of the penis is covered with a thin skin that contains no fat, is darker than body skin, and has redundant tissue, which allows for erection. In an uncircumcised male, the skin at the glans is folded over on itself to form the prepuce, or foreskin.

Under the skin of the penis the body of the penis is covered with the dartos layer, which is continuous with the fascia of the anterior abdominal wall, the scrotum, and the perineum. Contained within this layer are the superficial dorsal veins. The deep fascia of the penis, or Buck's fascia, contains the neurovascular bundle.

The root of the penis is attached to the abdominal wall through a thickening and extension of the dartos and Buck's fascia. In addition, the root is covered by the bulbocavernous muscle. This muscle also contains the perineal artery, vein, and nerve, and the pudendal artery, vein, and nerve.

The venous and arterial blood supply to the penis is complex. Several pairs of arteries supply blood (Figure 55-9), but the main arterial source is the internal pudendal artery, which branches to form the cavernous, bulbar, urethral, and dorsal arteries. These arteries continue to branch to form the vascular complex of the corpora cavernosa.

The venous drainage includes the superficial dorsal veins in the dartos tunic, the deep dorsal vein under Buck's fascia, and the deep or cavernous veins of the corpus cavernosum. The deep dorsal vein branches to form multiple circumflex veins. The corpus spongiosum is drained via the emissary veins through the urethral and bulbar veins, and the corpora cavernosa drain through the deep dorsal vein or cavernous veins.

For the penis to deposit sperm into the vagina, an erection must occur. The two types of erections are reflexogenic and psychogenic. Reflexogenic erections follow local stimulation, whereas psychogenic erections follow stimulation of erotic centers in the brain. Erection and ejaculation are mediated by the sympathetic nervous system, but the exact mechanism is unknown. During erection, the corpora cavernosa and the corpus spongiosum vascular spaces fill with blood, which transforms the penis into a firm organ permitting entry into the vagina.

Ejaculation is a two-part process: emission and ejaculation. In the first phase, secretions from the periurethral glands, seminal vesicle, and prostate move into the posterior urethra. Through peristalsis, sperm from the vas deferens also moves into the posterior urethra.

During ejaculation the internal sphincter of the bladder closes, the external urethral sphincter relaxes, and ejaculate is expelled by contraction of the perineal and bulbourethral muscles. The typical emission is 3 to 4 ml and contains fluid from the prostate and seminal vesicles and 200 million to 400 million **spermatozoa**. After ejaculation the penis returns to a flaccid state in 1 to 2 minutes.

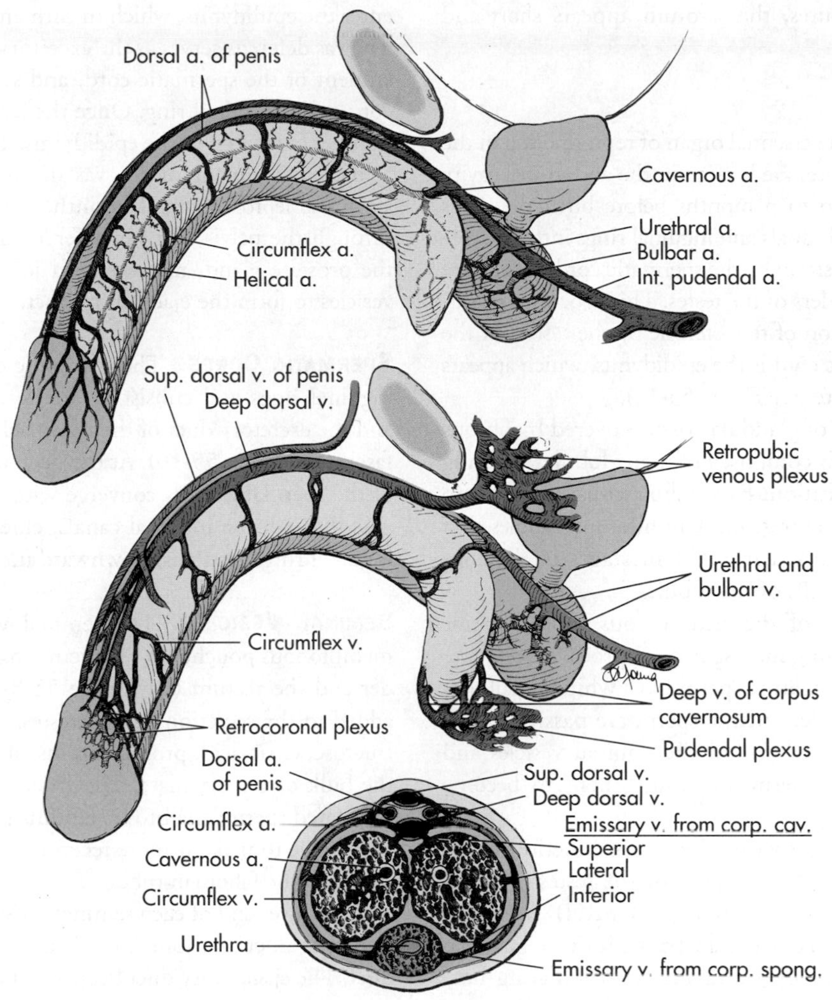

Figure 55-9 Vasculature of penis. *a,* Artery; *v,* vein; *int.,* internal; *sup.,* superior; *corp. cav.,* corpus cavernosum; *corp. spong.,* corpus spongiosum.

SCROTUM. The scrotum is a cutaneous pouch that covers and protects the testes and spermatic cords (Figure 55-10). Because the testes are surrounded by serous membrane and are suspended in the cavity of the scrotum, the testes are capable of being moved about readily. The ease of movement within the scrotum protects the testes from injury.

The skin of the scrotum is thin, more deeply pigmented than other skin areas, and elastic because it contains rugae. Because of the rugae, the scrotum distends readily and may become greatly enlarged when edema is present. The scrotal skin is covered by thinly scattered hair and contains sebaceous follicles. The surface of the scrotum is divided into two halves by a ridge (raphe) that extends anteriorly to the undersurface of the penis and posteriorly along the midline of the perineum to the anus. Internally, a septum divides the scrotum into two halves, each containing a testis and its epididymis and portion of spermatic cord. The left side of the scrotum normally hangs lower than the right side because the left spermatic cord is longer.

The external appearance of the scrotum varies under different conditions. In warm temperatures and in older or debilitated men, the scrotum becomes elongated and flat. In young, healthy

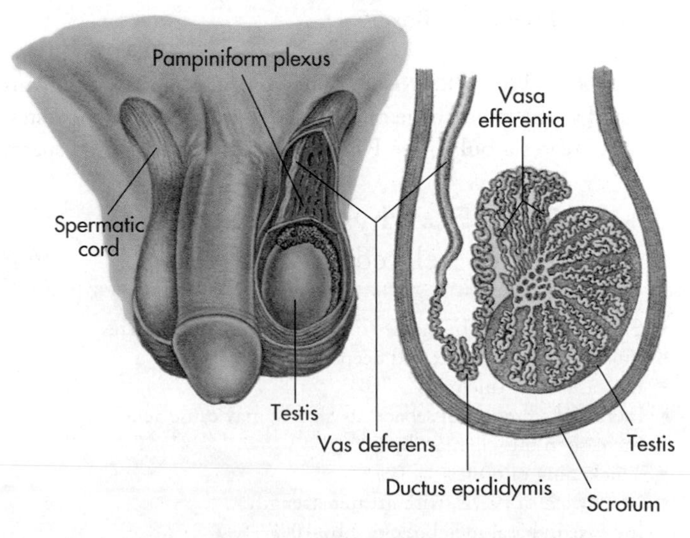

Figure 55-10 Scrotum and its contents.

men and in cool temperatures, the scrotum appears short and more wrinkled.

Internal Structures

TESTES. The oval testis is the essential organ of reproduction in the male. During fetal life the testes are located in the abdominal cavity behind the peritoneum. Two to 3 months before birth the testes descend through the inguinal canals and inguinal rings into the scrotum and are suspended in position by the spermatic cords, which are attached to the posterior borders of the testes. This process is stimulated by the increased secretion of testosterone by the testes. At the lateral edge of each spermatic cord is the epididymis, which appears as a narrow, flattened structure (see Figure 55-10).

The testes are composed of glandular tissue covered by fibrous tissue. The glandular tissue is composed of many lobules differing in size according to their location. Each lobule consists of 600 to 1200 small, convoluted structures, the seminiferous tubules that produce the sperm; spermatozoa in different stages of development can be seen along the cells of the tubules.

After puberty the lining of the seminiferous tubules forms sperm continuously. In a young man sperm are produced at a rate of 120 million per day. Each mature sperm has a whiplike tail that makes free movement possible, but the sperm are passive within the testes. The fluids produced within the seminal vesicles and prostate gland suspend the sperm and cause them to become active and motile.

In addition to producing sperm, the testes function as an endocrine gland. Production of androgens by the testes is stimulated by gonadotropin-releasing hormone (GnRH) from the hypothalamus. GnRH stimulates the anterior pituitary gland to secrete luteinizing hormone (LH) and follicle-stimulating hormone (FSH). LH stimulates testosterone production in the testes. FSH stimulates sperm development. The testes produce testosterone, dihydrotestosterone, and androstenedione. Testosterone is produced in much greater amounts than the other hormones and is therefore considered the most important testicular hormone.

Increased testosterone production at puberty causes several changes in the male body. These include an increase in the size of the penis and scrotum, hair growth on the pubis and face, and a deepening of the voice (Box 55-1).

EPIDIDYMIS, VAS DEFERENS. The comma-shaped epididymis is located at the lateral edge of the posterior segment of the testes, where it creates a bulge (see Figure 55-10). Newly formed sperm enter the epididymis, which in turn empties into the vas deferens. The vas deferens serves as the excretory duct of the testes, is a constituent of the spermatic cord, and separates from the spermatic cord at the inguinal ring. Once the testes form the sperm, a small number are stored in the epididymis. The majority is stored in the acidic environment of the vas deferens and, although inactive, stays viable for about 1 month. After taking a complex path through the pelvis, the vas deferens descends, enters the base of the prostate gland, narrows, and joins the ducts of the seminal vesicles to form the ejaculatory duct.

Box 55-1 Physical Changes in Males Related to Testosterone

- Eightfold increase in the size of penis, scrotum, and testes
- Enlargement of larynx and deepening of voice
- Increased skin thickness
- Increased secretion of sebaceous glands; may cause acne
- Increase in muscle mass by 50%
- Thickening of bones
- Narrowing of pelvis, with greater strength
- Increase in basal metabolic rate by 10%
- Increase in red blood cells

SPERMATIC CORDS. The spermatic cords extend from the deep inguinal rings and consist of arteries, veins, lymphatics, nerves, and the excretory duct of the testes held together by the spermatic fascia (see Figure 55-10). At the deep inguinal rings the structures of the spermatic cords converge with the structures of the testes, pass through the inguinal canals, emerge through the superficial inguinal rings, and pass downward into the scrotum.

SEMINAL VESICLES. The seminal vesicles are two lobulated, membranous pouches, 5 to 10 cm long, located between the bladder and the rectum (see Figure 55-8). They secrete fluid that is added to the secretions of the testes. This alkaline fluid contains fructose, citric acid, prostaglandins, and fibrinogen, which add to the bulk of the ejaculate. The fructose provides nutrients to the ejaculated sperm; the prostaglandins react with cervical mucus in the female to make it more receptive and probably help to propel sperm to the fallopian tubes.

The lower end of each seminal vesicle becomes constricted into a straight duct and joins the vas deferens to form the ejaculatory duct. The ejaculatory duct begins at the base of the prostate gland, runs posteriorly and downward, and enters the prostate gland in the midline. In the prostate gland, the ejaculatory duct opens into the prostatic portion of the urethra.

PROSTATE GLAND. The prostate gland is located below the internal urethral orifice, behind the symphysis pubis, and close to the rectal wall, extending around the beginning of the urethra (see Figure 55-8). Enveloped in a firm, adherent capsule, the prostate gland grows to the size and shape of a walnut during puberty and weighs about 20 g. Internally, the prostate gland is partly muscular and partly glandular. The glandular substance consists of numerous follicular pouches that open into long canals and join to form 12 to 20 small excretory ducts. Prostatic ducts open into the prostatic portion of the urethra, thus adding the prostatic secretion to the seminal fluid. The prostatic secretion is a thin, white fluid that helps raise the pH of the fluid from the vas deferens and enhance motility and fertility of the sperm. Another substance secreted by the prostate gland is acid phosphatase.

COWPER'S (BULBOURETHRAL) GLANDS. Cowper's (bulbourethral) glands are two small, round bodies located at the sides and to the back of the membranous portion of the urethra. Each gland has an excretory duct that opens into the urethra. The main excretory duct of a Cowper's gland represents the joining of many ducts from its internal glandular tissue. Cowper's glands secrete an alkaline substance into the semen to counteract vaginal and urethral acidity.

Endocrine Functions

Male Hormones. In males andrenarche refers to the increased secretion of the androgenic hormones at puberty, which results in the appearance of secondary sex characteristics and production of mature sperm. Testosterone is the androgen most closely related to reproduction, since it specifically stimulates maturation of sperm and is responsible for maintaining the reproductive organs in a functional state. Testosterone secretion is closely related to pituitary gland function. The rate of secretion of testosterone is determined by levels of LH in the blood. Testosterone levels show temporary elevations during the fetal and neonatal periods with peak levels seen during adolescence.

Female Hormones. The major hormones produced by the ovaries are estrogen and progesterone. The ovaries produce three different forms of **estrogen**. Estriol (E3) is produced during pregnancy. Estradiol (E2) is produced in the ovulatory follicle and is the primary estrogen of premenopausal women. The third form, estrone (E1), is a by-product of the metabolism of estradiol and is also produced and held in adipose tissue. Estrogen is responsible for the development of secondary sex characteristics at puberty. After puberty estrogen primarily causes development of the endometrium in preparation for implantation of a fertilized ovum. Progesterone enhances the action of estrogen on the endometrium. The ovaries depend on stimulation from the pituitary hormones FSH and LH to fulfill their functions.

Menarche. **Menarche** is the term used to designate the onset of menstruation, and it reflects the time when reproduction is first possible. The onset of menarche varies with age, heredity, general health, weight, and nutritional status and cannot be accurately predicted. The average age at menarche has decreased significantly over the past 100 years and is now 12.5 years, with a normal range from 10.5 to 14.5 years. It is believed that a percentage of body fat (17%) must be attained for the average girl to reach menarche.

MENSTRUAL CYCLE. The menstrual cycle includes a complex series of uterine and ovarian cyclic changes that result in menstruation. The uterine cycle includes the menstrual, proliferative, and secretory phases that correspond to specific phases of the ovarian cycle (Figure 55-11). These phases together require an average of 28 days. The first day of menstrual flow is considered to be the first day of the menstrual cycle. Normal variation exists in the intervals between menstrual periods, but most cycles occur within a range of 26 to 36 days and last for 3 to 7 days. The greatest variance typically occurs during the perimenarchal and perimenopausal years. The smooth functioning of the menstrual cycle depends on complex relationships among the hypothalamus in the central nervous system, anterior pituitary, ovaries, and uterus.

MENSTRUATION. During menstruation the endometrium breaks down and is shed. The production of estrogen and progesterone stops before the onset of menstrual flow, which results in rupture of uterine capillaries and necrosis of endometrial tissue. The menstrual phase of the cycle lasts an average of 4 days. Menstrual fluid does not clot unless it is retained in the uterus or vagina for a prolonged time. It is believed that the endometrium produces an anticoagulant that prevents the clotting of blood in the uterus.

PROLIFERATIVE PHASE. When menstruation ceases, the proliferative phase begins, extends until day 14 of the ovarian cycle, and ends with ovulation. During the proliferative (ovarian follicular) phase, the hypothalamus releases GnRH, which signals the pituitary gland to secrete increasing amounts of FSH, which stimulates a primordial follicle to develop into a mature graafian follicle containing a mature ovum. The graafian follicle produces estrogen, so FSH is essential for estrogen production. While increasing in size, the graafian follicle moves toward the surface of the ovary, where it appears as a blisterlike structure. Finally, the graafian follicle ruptures **(ovulation)**, allowing the ovum to enter the fallopian tube and be carried in the direction of the uterus.

As the graafian follicle matures, it secretes increasing amounts of estrogen. Estrogen causes the endometrium to become thicker and softer as it prepares for implantation of a fertilized ovum. Estrogen also causes the cervical mucus to increase in quantity and attain a clear, elastic state that permits sperm to enter the cervix more readily. The high level of estrogen also suppresses pituitary release of FSH and triggers release of LH. A sharp rise in LH levels occurs 12 to 24 hours before ovulation, followed by a peak level about 8 hours after ovulation.

On the day of ovulation about 25% of women experience pain in the lower abdomen on the side of ovulation. This pain, referred to as mittelschmerz, is probably a result of peritoneal irritation from follicular fluid or blood released from the ovary with the ovum.

SECRETORY PHASE. The proliferative phase ends with ovulation and the secretory phase begins, lasting for approximately 10 to 14 days. The secretory (ovarian luteal) phase is the least variable part of the menstrual cycle. Irregular menstrual cycles are usually related to variations in the menstrual or proliferative phases.

Under the influence of LH, the corpus luteum forms in the ovary at the site of the ruptured graafian follicle and produces progesterone. Progesterone further alters the endometrium by stimulating growth of cells and circulation of blood to the uterus. With these additional endometrial changes, the uterine environment is prepared for implantation of a fertilized ovum.

If pregnancy occurs, the corpus luteum remains secretory by the action of human chorionic gonadotropin (HCG), which the placental cells produce within 1 week of conception. By 6 to 8 weeks after conception, the placenta is developed and assumes the function of secreting progesterone to maintain the endometrium. If pregnancy does not occur, the corpus luteum degenerates in about 10 days, progesterone secretion drops significantly, and the endometrium degenerates; menstruation results, and the cycle begins again.

MENOPAUSE. The medical term **menopause** refers to a single, specific physical event in a woman's life—the occurrence of the final menstrual period; however, research on menopause has expanded to include the entire perimenopausal period, which may extend from age 35 to as old as 60 years of age. This is the period in which physical changes can be clearly linked to altered levels of hormones. Natural menopause may occur in women between the ages of 35 and 60 years of age. The average age is 51 years in Western societies. This average has remained stable over time, despite fairly significant changes in the average age of onset

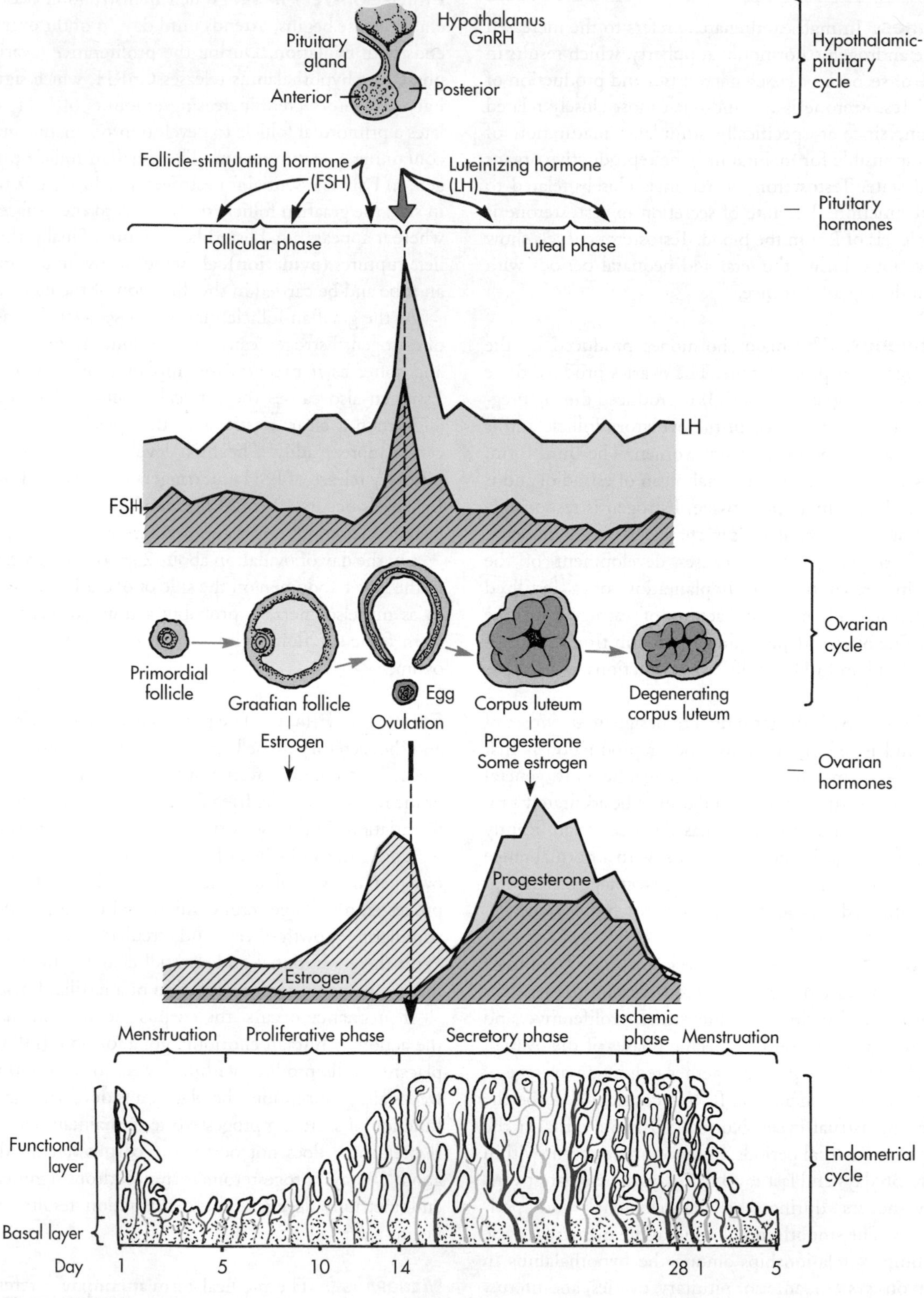

Figure 55-11 Menstrual cycle: hypothalamic-pituitary, ovarian, and endometrial. *GnRH*, Gonadotropin-releasing hormone.

for menstruation: 25% of all women experience menopause before age 45, 50% between 45 and 50 years of age, and 25% after age 50. Factors influencing the onset of menopause include genetic differences in the estrogen receptors and current smoking status. Menopause may be artificially induced by surgical removal or irradiation of the ovaries, severe infections, and the effects of alkylating chemotherapeutic agents. The removal of the uterus, or hysterectomy, results in cessation of menses but does not itself result in menopause, as long as the ovaries are left intact.

Changes during the perimenopausal period are primarily related to a gradual decline in ovarian production of estrogen. Over a period of years the menses become more scanty and may become irregular or spaced further apart until they eventually stop. Estrone is the primary postmenopausal estrogen and has a potency only one-tenth that of estradiol. Cellular estrogen receptors are found in organs throughout the body, so a decline in estrogen triggers a wide variety of potential symptoms. The intensity of symptoms is thought to be related to the rapidity of changes in estrogen level and may be mediated somewhat by the fat content of the body. Women with higher fat stores in their bodies retain a storage pool of estrogen to buffer them through the early transition period. Commonly reported symptoms of the perimenopausal period are summarized in Box 55-2.

ARE YOU READY?

Which of the following changes is related to increased testosterone that occurs with puberty?

1. Increase in size of mammary glands
2. Increase in muscle mass
3. Decrease in red blood cell count
4. Decrease in sebaceous gland secretions

Physiologic Changes With Aging

The major physiologic changes that occur in the female reproductive tract with aging are related to the process of menopause. When ovulation ceases, the production of progesterone is halted, and estrogen levels decrease. These two primary hormone changes are responsible for most aging-related changes in the uterus, ovaries, and vagina. The ovaries begin to atrophy around age 40 and become nonpalpable within 3 to 5 years of menopause. The uterus decreases in size. The vagina decreases in width and length, and the entrance narrows. The mucosal lining becomes thinner, and vaginal secretions are diminished. Externally the mons pubis decreases in fullness and the labia majora and minora decrease in size. Pubic hair becomes thinner and turns gray or white. Muscle weakness in the pelvis can lead to cystocele, rectocele, uterine prolapse, or stress incontinence. The woman's capacity for sexual response, however, remains intact.

The primary changes in the male reproductive tract during the climacteric are also related to variations in hormone level. After peaking in adolescence, testosterone levels decline throughout adulthood and appear to level off around age 60. This causes a decrease in the size and firmness of the penis and testes. The scrotum is more pendulous and has fewer rugae. Although some spermatogenesis continues throughout life, the seminal fluid decreases in amount and force of ejaculation decreases. The prostate gland typically hypertrophies and creates problems with urinary retention. The pelvic muscles decrease in strength, and the pubic hair thins and turns gray or white. The capacity for sexual response remains intact in healthy men, and fertility, although diminished, does continue.

Health History

Assessment of the reproductive system can be uncomfortable for both the nurse and patient. It is important to examine one's own attitudes about the various ways people express their sexuality so that personal beliefs and prejudices do not interfere with patient care. As with any nursing history, the nurse should ask questions in a nonjudgmental manner, using open-ended and focused questions. Attention to supportive nonverbal communication is also important. The interview should take place before the patient undresses for the physical examination.

Box 55-2 Common Perimenopausal Symptoms

Vasomotor

Hot flashes
Hot flushes
Perspiration
Palpitations

Vaginal

Dryness
Vulvar itching or burning
Dyspareunia

Menstrual

Irregular uterine bleeding
Shorter or longer cycles
Missed periods

Urinary

Frequency or urgency
Stress incontinence
Urinary tract infections

Psychologic

Sleep disorders, insomnia
Irritability
Mood swings
Depression
Anxiety

Other

Weight gain
Skin changes
Sensory changes
Osteoporosis
Joint pain
Headache

Chief Complaint

Information may be organized through a review of systems or by a history of the chief complaint with a system review. For example, a sexually transmitted disease (STD) can mimic a urinary tract infection; therefore information about both the urinary and reproductive systems is important. The nurse begins the interview with open-ended questions and records the chief complaint in the patient's own words. The nurse then follows up with focused questions to assess the critical characteristics of the symptoms, including onset, duration, location, character and quality, quantity and severity, timing, setting, aggravating or relieving factors, associated factors, and the patient's perception of the problem.

Sexuality and Sexual Activity

It is best to incorporate questions about intimate relationships and sexual activity into the genitourinary and gynecologic portions of an annual health assessment or during evaluation of specific complaints in these areas. Open-ended questions that can be helpful include, "What concerns do you have about your sexual functioning?"; "What changes have you experienced in your sexual relationships in the past 6 months?"; and, if appropriate, "How has your illness affected your sexual relationship?" More focused questions include, "What is your sexual preference?" and "How satisfied are you with your sexual relationships?" The nurse determines whether a patient is currently sexually active, practices safer sex behaviors, or has recently changed sexual partners. The nurse records the number of current and past sexual partners to determine risk status for STDs. Although the risk of exposure to STDs certainly increases with the number of partners, sexual activity with one partner in a nonmonogamous relationship also carries risk.

Screening for childhood or adult sexual abuse or sexual assault needs to be a routine part of the health history, since the incidence is estimated to range from 12% to 40%. Screening questions and tools should be a part of all documentation systems. Survivors of childhood sexual abuse can have a variety of symptoms related to the reproductive system, including chronic pelvic pain and sexual dysfunction such as dyspareunia, nonspecific vaginitis, vaginismus, fear of intimacy, lack of enjoyment, and compulsive promiscuity. Having a vaginal, pelvic, or prostate examination may be especially traumatic for adult survivors of sexual abuse. Including questions about abuse in assessment tools ensures that these issues are not excluded or missed. See Box 55-3 for sample abuse assessment questions, which can be adapted for use with male patients. Document any areas of injury on a body map in the patient record.

Female Genitourinary Status

Genitourinary health histories for women generally include data about the patient's menstrual and reproductive status and urinary system function. The menstrual and reproductive history includes information about the onset and pattern of menses and the last menstrual period (LMP); sexuality; sexual activity and contraceptive use; number of pregnancies, abortions, and deliveries and associated problems; reproductive surgeries and procedures; and genitourinary function. This history may be gathered as a part of a complete health history or during an episodic examination and must be tailored to the patient's age. For example, middle-aged women can be questioned about perimenopausal symptoms, whereas older women should be screened for postmenopausal bleeding and incontinence.

Because acute and chronic illnesses and many medications can affect reproductive function, the nurse should obtain detailed information about these areas. The nurse should ask patients directly about use of complementary and alternative medicines, which are frequently used and often not considered medications. Family history is also important. For example, diethylstilbestrol (DES) use during pregnancy by the mothers of female patients may predispose the patients to vulvar cancer, and the presence of the BRCA1 and BRCA2 genes in the patient's immediate family may lead to breast cancer.

History of contraception focuses on method, whether it is properly used, the patient's satisfaction, and indications of common complications or serious side effects. Although not part of the reproductive system, breast health is usually assessed during a routine gynecologic visit. The following outline summarizes the interview items, symptoms, and health promotion activities to be included in the assessment.

Box 55-3 Sample Abuse Screening

1. Have you ever experienced unwanted touching or sexual experiences in childhood?
   Yes ☐
   No ☐
2. Have you ever been forced or pressured to have sex when you did not want to?
   Yes ☐
   No ☐
3. Have you ever been hit, kicked, slapped, pushed, or shoved by your boyfriend, husband, or partner?
   Yes ☐
   No ☐

Female Breast and Genitourinary History

Current breast health
Problems with breasts
- —Pain or tenderness
- —Lumps
- —Skin dimpling
- —Lesions or changes in the skin
- —Discharge from the nipples

Current genitourinary health
Urinary symptoms, including infections and voiding dysfunction
- —Dysuria
- —Frequency
- —Urgency
- —Hematuria
- —Nocturia
- —Lower abdominal pain
- —Urge incontinence (urge and frequency resulting from detrusor dysfunction)
- —Stress incontinence (loss of urine with increased abdominal pressure because of sphincter dysfunction)

Menstrual history
- —Age at menarche (first menses)
- —LMP
- —Interval or frequency; regular or irregular
- —Duration
- —Menstrual flow: light, medium, or heavy (number of pads or tampons used in a specified period)
- —Hypermenorrhea (increased amount or duration of flow)

—Dysmenorrhea (pain with menstruation): frequency and severity
—Bleeding between periods
—Postcoital bleeding (bleeding after intercourse)
—Postmenopausal bleeding (essential to screen for endometrial cancer)
—Premenstrual syndrome or premenstrual dysphoric disorder: irritability, anxiety, anger, depression, fatigue, insomnia, weight gain, headaches, breast tenderness, and breast swelling

Obstetric history
—Number of pregnancies (gravida)
—Pregnancy outcomes
Term: number of births between 37 and 42 weeks of pregnancy
Premature: number of births before 37 weeks of pregnancy
Abortions: spontaneous or elective
Living: number of living children
Types of deliveries: vaginal, forceps, vacuum, or cesarean
Complications of pregnancies

Perimenopausal symptoms
—Hot flashes or flushes
—Headaches
—Night sweats
—Vaginal dryness
—Mood swings
—Numbness and tingling
—Insomnia

Vulvovaginal problems
—Discharge: color, amount, and odor
—Vaginal itching
—Vulvodynia
—Lesions or lumps
—Dyspareunia (pain with intercourse)
—Vaginismus (spasms of muscles around vagina)
—History of STDs

Sexual health
—Sexually active: monogamous versus multiple partners; male, female, or both
—Types of sexual activity
—Satisfaction with or problems related to sexual activity
—Changes in ability to engage in sex: vaginal dryness, loss of **libido**, female sexual arousal disorder, inhibited orgasm, or dyspareunia

Health promotion practices
—Contraceptive choice, barrier protection, proper use of method, satisfaction, and side effects
—Pelvic examinations: date of last Pap test and results
—Breast self-examination (technique and frequency)
—Vulva self-examination
—Date of last mammogram and results
—Nutritional patterns, intake of folic acid
—Personal hygiene: douche, bubble baths, tampons, feminine sprays
—Smoking cessation efforts
—Use of complementary and alternative products or practices
—Immunization status

Family history
—Breast cancer
—Cervical, ovarian, or endometrial cancer
—History of exposure to DES

Male Genitourinary Status

A male genitourinary history includes current health status and medical history. The interview can be tailored to screen for specific age-related problems. For example, prostate enlargement occurs in older men, and therefore it is necessary to screen for factors such as urinary retention, straining, and hesitancy. The nurse collects data about the bladder, kidney function, the penis and testes, possible hernias, sexual health, and health promotion activities. The following outline summarizes symptoms and health-promotion behaviors to be included in the assessment.

Male Genitourinary History

Current genitourinary health status
Urinary symptoms relating to infections, voiding dysfunction, or prostate problems
—Dysuria (pain with urination)
—Frequency
—Urgency
—Hematuria
—Nocturia
—Urinary retention
—Straining
—Hesitancy
—Change in force or caliber of stream
—Dribbling
—History of prostate problems
—History of urinary tract infections

Incontinence
—Urge
—Stress

Problems with the penis such as skin lesions, cancer, or STDs
—Pain
—Lesions or sores
—Discharge
—History of STDs

Problems with testes such as torsion, cancer, or infection, and problems with the scrotum such as hydrocele, hernia, or varicocele
—Lump or swelling in testes
—Bulge or swelling in scrotum
—Change in size of scrotum
—History of hernia

Sexual health
—Sexually active: monogamous versus multiple partners; male, female, or both

—Types of sexual activity
—Satisfaction with or problems related to sexual activity
—Changes in ability to engage in sex: erectile dysfunction, premature ejaculation, loss of libido

Health promotion practices
—Contraceptive choice, barrier protection, proper use of method, satisfaction, and side effects
—Prostate examination: date of last examination and results
—Testicular self-examination (technique and frequency)
—Smoking cessation efforts
—Use of complementary and alternative products or practices
—Immunization status

Physical Examination

Physical examination of the breasts and genitourinary system may cause embarrassment for the patient. Before the examination it is important to inquire whether the patient has previously had an examination of this nature. The nurse explains the procedure and answers any questions before the patient is undressed and on the examination table. If this is the first breast, pelvic, testicular, or prostate examination, ignorance about the process may also cause fear. The nurse should take time to explain the process, review normal anatomy, and teach self-examination of the breasts or testes. Pictures, three-dimensional anatomic models, and examples of equipment such as a speculum aid in the educational process. Models of the pelvic organs and pamphlets assist with the presentation of information about the purpose of the pelvic or prostate examination, what is done, and what to expect.

Assessment measures and variations in normal findings relevant to the care of older adults are presented in the Gerontologic Assessment box. Also identified are disorders common in older adults, which may be responsible for abnormal assessment findings.

Breast Examination

Female Breast. In a menstruating female the ideal time to examine the breasts is 7 days after menstruation when they are less tender and nodular. In nonmenstruating females the timing of the examination is less important. Examination of the breasts begins with inspection of the skin and areola. The examination should be performed in both the sitting and supine position (Figure 55-12). Currently, the American Cancer Society (ACS) recommends clinical breast examinations every 3 years for women ages 20 to 39 and annually for women 40 and older. Yearly mammograms are recommended beginning at age 40. Breast self-examinations are optional for women of all ages; however, it is recommended that women be advised of the benefits of breast self-examination.

With the woman's hands at her sides, the examiner inspects the breasts for symmetry and the skin for dimpling, puckering, scaling, scars, or discharge from the nipples. A dimple, pucker, or retraction in breast tissue may indicate an underlying chest wall lesion. Scaly skin or nipple tissue can be seen in eczema of the breast or Paget's disease. While the woman slowly raises her hands over her head, the breasts are observed for signs of retractions. The woman is asked to put her hands on her waist and flex her shoulders and elbows while the breasts are observed for puckering or retractions and for symmetric movement. Women with large breasts should lean forward. The breast should move smoothly without signs of adhesions to the chest wall.

The breasts and axilla can be palpated in both sitting and supine positions. Bimanual palpation of large breasts is easily accomplished while the patient is sitting. It should be repeated in a supine position. Before the patient lies down, the examiner pal-

Gerontologic Assessment

Assessment

Determine meaning of sexuality to patient, level of sexual satisfaction, and any problems engaging in sexual intercourse.
–Personal beliefs and social mores influence attitudes toward sexuality. Disability or disease can interfere with sexual satisfaction.

Inquire about the use of complementary or alternative therapies.
–Complementary or alternative therapies, which are in common use today, can interact positively or negatively with conventional therapies and must be considered when planning care.

For Women

Determine frequency of regular gynecologic examinations, mammography, and breast self-examination.
–Some women are not aware that these examinations should be continued after menopause.

Assess for signs of vaginitis (vaginal pruritus and discharge).
–Older women are at risk for vaginitis because of changes in hormone levels and the resultant thinning of the vaginal epithelium and rise in vaginal pH.

Assess for signs of cystocele or rectocele (urinary incontinence and lower back pain).
–Cystocele and rectocele are common findings in older women as a result of longstanding childbirth injuries and decline in muscle tone and strength.

For Men

Inquire directly about problems urinating.
–Benign prostatic hypertrophy (BPH) is common in older men. The classic symptoms are frequency, nocturia, hesitancy, dribbling, and a feeling of being unable to empty the bladder. Dysuria and hematuria are present if cystitis develops.

Assess knowledge and understanding of common prostate problems.
–Prostatitis, BPH, and prostatic cancer affect large numbers of older men and are responsible for significant morbidity and mortality. Early diagnosis and effective treatment depend on understanding the problem and the need for screening and intervention.

Common Reproductive Disorders in Older Adults

Vaginitis
Uterine prolapse
Cystocele, rectocele
Erectile dysfunction
Hernias
Cancer of cervix, uterus, breast, prostate

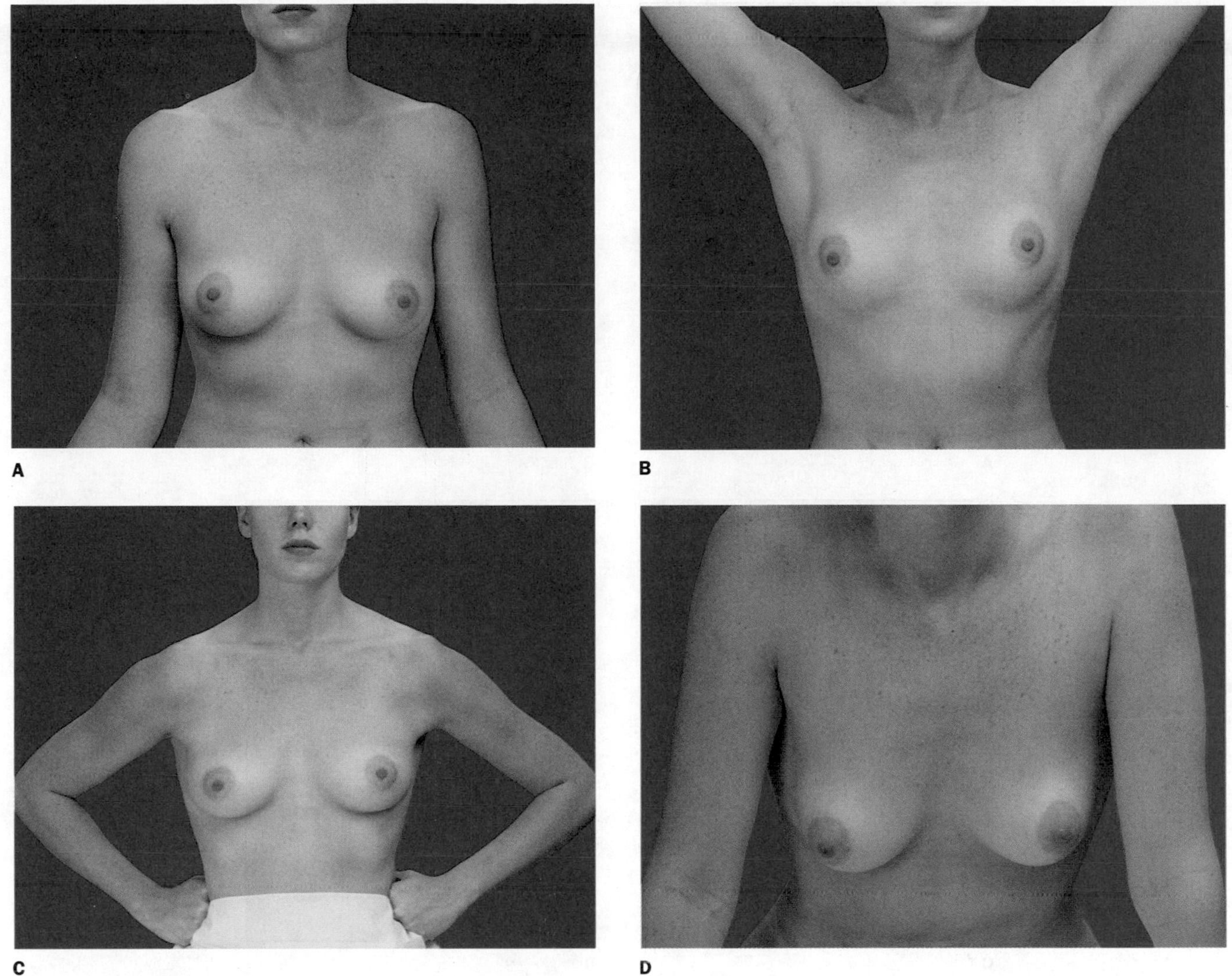

Figure 55-12 Patient positions during breast self-examination. Note distribution of breast tissue in different positions. **A,** Patient position at start of examination: sitting with arms at sides. **B,** Arms over head position. **C,** Patient with arms lowered and hands pressed against hips. **D,** Forward leaning position, typically used for patient with large, pendulous breasts.

pates the supraclavicular and axillary lymph nodes for size, shape, mobility, or tenderness. The majority of the breast lymphatics drain toward the axilla.

When the patient is supine, a small pillow or towel is placed under the shoulder of the breast to be examined. The examiner asks the woman to raise her arm over her head, since this helps flatten the breast tissue. The breast can be palpated in a circular, spokes of a wheel, vertical, or horizontal pattern (Figure 55-13). The breast tissue is systematically palpated at three different depths using the pads of three fingers. It is important to palpate the entire breast, including the tail of Spence in the upper outer quadrant near the axilla. The examiner notes the consistency of the breast tissue and the presence of any tenderness, lumps, or nodules. If a nodule is identified, the examiner notes its location, size in centimeters, shape, and consistency. When the examination is completed, the woman can be instructed in breast self-examination.

The nipple is palpated for underlying masses or tumors, and is gently squeezed to check for masses or discharge. A milky discharge may be related to pregnancy, lactation, hormones, or drugs. A nonmilky discharge may indicate a pathologic condition. The process is then repeated on the opposite breast.

Male Breast. The male breast can be easily and quickly examined during a routine physical examination. Although rare, breast cancer does occur in males, most frequently in the areolar area. The examination is initiated with inspection of the skin and areolae. Any swelling, retractions, or lesions are noted. The breast, areola, and axilla are then palpated for masses.

Abdominal Examination

Physical assessment of the reproductive organs includes a standard assessment of the lower abdomen (see Chapter 40). Any localized areas of prominence are noted, since these may indicate enlargement of the reproductive organs or adjacent structures. The skin of the abdomen and pubic area is inspected for amount, distribution, and character of hair; abnormal pigmentation; and lesions.

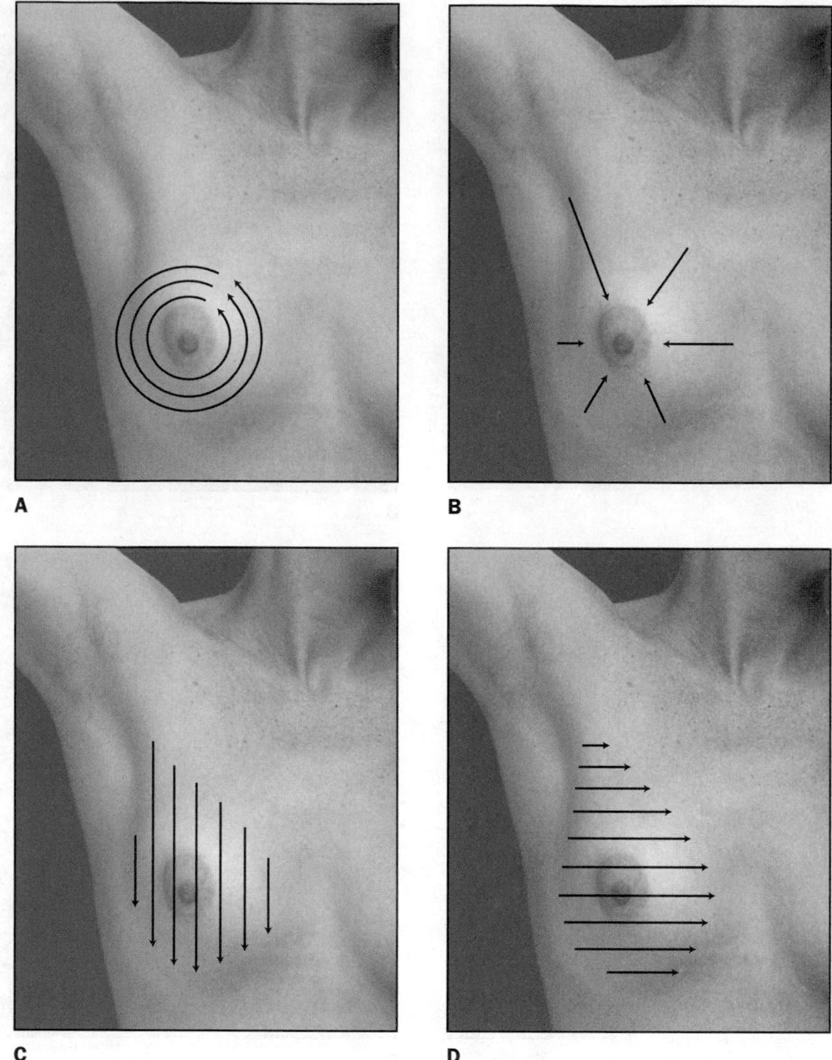

Figure 55-13 Different patterns used in palpation of the breasts. **A,** Spiral. **B,** Spokes of a wheel. **C,** Vertical lines. **D,** Horizontal lines.

Abdominal muscle tone is assessed by having the patient cough or raise the head.

Auscultation of the abdomen for bowel sounds and bruits should precede palpation. After auscultation, the examiner completes percussion of the abdomen to identify any enlarged organ, tumor, or masses. A tumor, such as an ovarian cyst or uterine myoma, produces a dull, flat, tone. Because the reproductive organs in the female are normally situated in the pelvic cavity, they are usually not palpable through the abdominal wall unless enlarged with pregnancy. Abdominal palpation is performed to rule out or discover abnormalities. If an abdominal mass is felt, the examiner describes its position, size, shape, consistency, contour, tenderness, movability, and relationship to any pelvic or abdominal organ.

Enlargement of the uterus is detected by palpating in the midline of the lower abdomen. Palpation starts just below the umbilicus and continues in the direction of the symphysis pubis. In contrast with a full bladder, which feels soft, an enlarged uterus feels firm and may be round or asymmetric. A firm, isolated area of enlargement may be caused by a tumor of the uterus.

Enlargement of the fallopian tubes and ovaries may be detected by palpation of the right and left lower quadrants. Even when enlarged, these organs are not always palpable through the abdominal wall. However, enlargement is often associated with pain or tenderness on palpation of the lower quadrants.

Physical Examination of the Female Genitalia

The external genitalia are examined before performing the internal examination. Self-examination of the vulva can be simultaneously explained to the patient with the use of a mirror and good lighting. Before each step of the examination, the examiner informs the patient of what he or she plans to do. For example, "First I am going to examine the vulva. You will feel me touching the labia (or skin) around the vagina." The examiner inspects the mons pubis, labia, and perineum for nits, lesions, swelling, inflammation, altered pigmentation, or discharge. Small painful vesicular lesions may indicate genital herpes, whereas condylomata acuminata appear as warty lesions. The labia are gently separated and the clitoris, urethral orifice, and vagina are inspected. Next, Bartholin's glands are palpated between the index finger and thumb if swelling is seen. Any discharge from the glands is noted and cultured. If urethritis or inflammation of the Skene's glands is suspected, the examiner milks the urethra by inserting a finger into the vagina and gently stroking the urethra in a downward motion. Any discharge is cultured and noted.

The pelvic examination is frequently a stressful event for the patient. The nurse can help the woman overcome pain, embarrassment, and anxiety by establishing a relaxed, positive atmosphere and addressing the woman's questions and concerns. Women who are scheduled for pelvic examination should be advised to avoid douching, sexual intercourse, using tampons, and applying any vaginal preparations (medicinal or deodorant) for at least 48 hours before examination. A Pap test should not be performed if there is significant menstrual bleeding, since this makes interpretation of the test difficult. Patients should void and defecate, if needed, immediately before examination because an empty bladder and lower bowel make palpation of the pelvic organs easier, decrease patient discomfort, eliminate possible distortion of the position of pelvic organs caused by a full bladder, and obviate the risk of incontinence during examination.

Positioning. The most common position for the pelvic examination is the lithotomy position. This position may need to be modified for a woman with poor mobility or arthritis (Figure 55-14). The older woman is assisted to a position of comfort for pelvic examination if lithotomy position is not possible. The stirrups can be adjusted depending on the woman's age. The head of the examination table can be raised for comfort, and so that the woman can see the examiner. The woman may or may not prefer to be draped with a sheet. In addition, a mirror can be offered to the woman if she desires to watch the examination. This also provides an excellent teaching opportunity. Encourage the older woman to change positions slowly after pelvic examination, since orthostatic hypotension may occur.

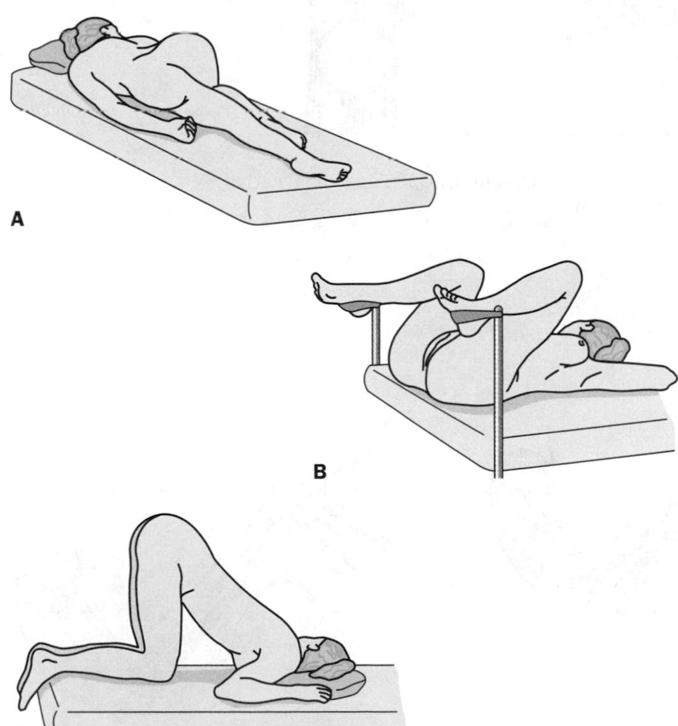

Figure 55-14 Various positions that can be assumed for examination of rectum and vagina. **A,** Sims' (lateral) position. Note position of left arm and right leg. **B,** Lithotomy position. Note position of buttocks on edge of examining table and support of feet. **C,** Knee-chest (genupectoral) position. Note placement of shoulders and head.

Inspection of the Vagina and Cervix. Before insertion of the speculum, the examiner separates the labia majora and minora with the nondominant gloved hand. The appropriately sized speculum is gently inserted into the vagina at an oblique angle along the natural plane of the vagina. The speculum is rotated to a horizontal plane, and the blades are opened (Figure 55-15). The cervix is visualized at the tip of the speculum. The examiner notes the cervical color; location of the os; and characteristics such as lesions, nodules, or discharge.

Vaginal samples for pH and wet mount are obtained first, followed by the Pap test. Currently there are two acceptable methods of obtaining cervical samples. Cervical specimens can be obtained with a plastic or wooden ectocervical spatula followed by an endocervical brush (Figure 55-16) or with a broomlike device. Some facilities use a cotton-tipped swab for the endocervical sample, which should be moistened with sterile saline before specimen collection to avoid cell trapping.

In the first method, with the long end of the spatula in the os, the examiner rotates the spatula circumferentially around the entire cervical os. The endocervical brush is inserted into the endocervical os and rotated just 180 degrees to limit bleeding. A similar process is followed when a broom is used. Regardless of the method, examiner should obtain the specimen from the entire transformational zone of the cervix, since the majority of cervical cancers develop at the junction of the squamous epithelium and the columnar epithelium of the endocervix. The presence of endocervical cells on the Pap test is considered the gold standard for an adequate Pap test. The specimens are then "rolled" onto a glass slide and fixed immediately with a spray or alcohol solution. A newer method, approved by the U.S. Food and Drug Administration, of transporting cervical cells in liquid suspension is rapidly replacing the conventional glass slide method. With this technology the sample is immediately placed in the liquid preservative after each collection. It is important to swirl the spatula or brush or broom several times to release the maximal number of cervical cells into the preservative.[4] After transport to the laboratory, cells are filtered and plated in a thin layer on a slide. After collection of the cervical sample, the examiner collects cultures for chlamydia and gonorrhea with the appropriate swabs.

Bimanual examination follows the Pap test. The examiner inserts the middle and forefinger of the dominant hand into the vagina canal and evaluates the size, shape, and consistency of the ovaries and uterus. The ovaries are normally slightly tender to palpation and are not always palpable, especially in obese women. When palpable, healthy ovaries feel smooth and oval. Any irregular, firm palpable mass in the area of the fallopian tubes and ovaries indicates a possible deviation from normal. Because the ovaries atrophy during menopause, any mass felt in the areas of the ovaries in postmenopausal women is usually a sign of a problem. The uterus should feel smooth and about the size of a pear in

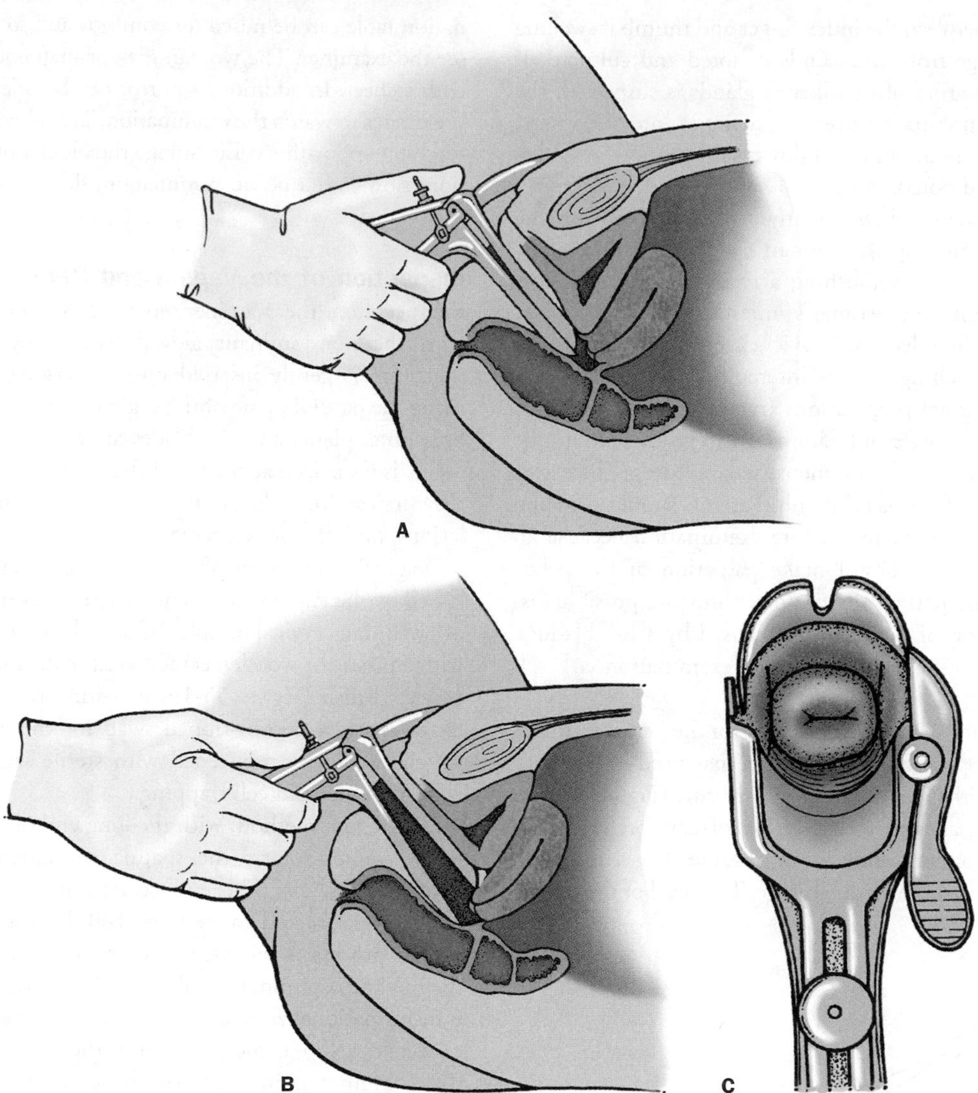

Figure 55-15 Speculum examination of cervix. **A,** Insertion of a speculum. **B,** Open speculum within vagina. **C,** Examiner's view of the cervix through open speculum.

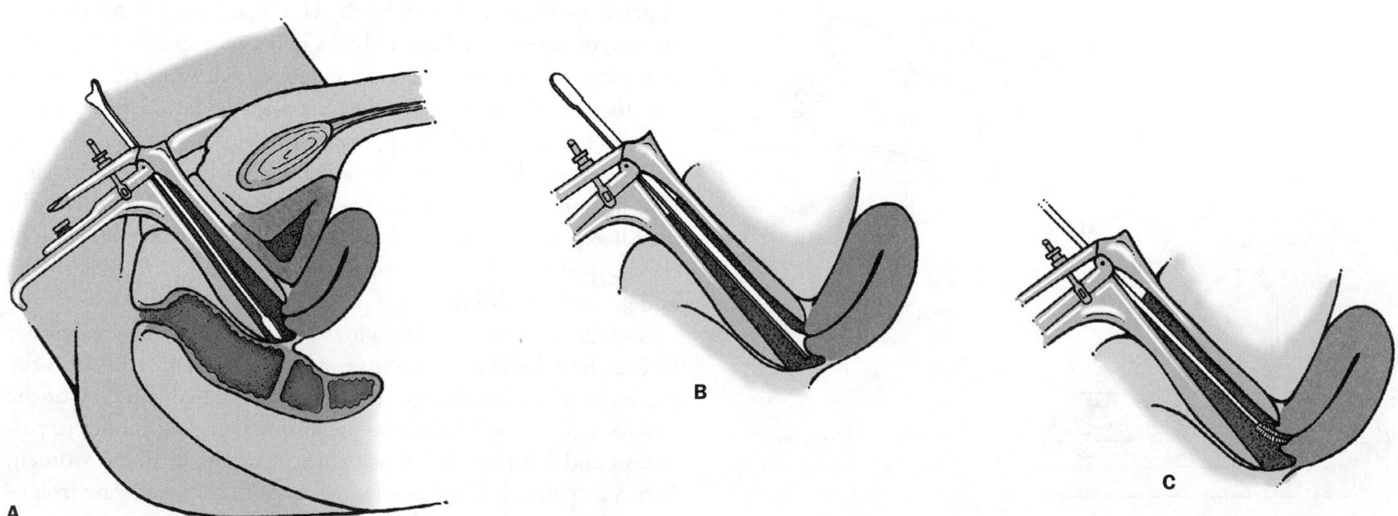

Figure 55-16 Method of obtaining specimen for Pap test. **A,** Blunt end of Ayre spatula used to scrape specimen from posterior fornix. **B,** Most pointed tip of bifid end of an Ayre spatula inserted into the cervical os and rotated 360 degrees to obtain specimen from the squamocolumnar junction. **C,** Cytobrush inserted into cervical os and rotated 360 degrees to collect specimen from endocervix. A glass pipette or cotton swab may also be used.

the nonpregnant patient. Irregular shapes or consistencies of the uterus are noted. The cervix should be gently moved between the fingers of the examining hand for evaluation of cervical motion tenderness.

The rectovaginal examination is performed to confirm uterine position, reassess the adnexal areas, follow up on complaints of pain or bleeding, and determine rectal sphincter tone. The woman is told that it may be uncomfortable, and she may feel as though she has to have a bowel movement. Hemorrhoids, fistulas, or fissures are noted. Stool for occult blood is obtained.

After the pelvic examination, a woman may need assistance removing lubricating jelly or discharge from her genitalia, removing her legs from the stirrups, and getting down from the table. If a bloody discharge is present, a sanitary pad is provided. Older women merit assistance after pelvic examination because positions such as the knee-chest and lithotomy positions may alter the normal circulation of blood sufficiently to cause blood pressure changes or faintness.

Physical Examination of the Male Genitalia

Physical examination of the male genitalia includes inspection, auscultation, and palpation of the lower abdomen; inspection and palpation of the external genitalia; and palpation of the prostate gland by rectal examination.

Positioning. Depending on the patient's age, the external genitalia can be examined after the abdominal examination with the patient supine or standing. However, the patient should be in a standing position to evaluate hernias. The examiner inspects the inguinal and femoral areas for any bulges or masses and asks the patient to bear down as the area is reinspected. A bulge while straining may indicate a femoral hernia. Straining is preferred over coughing as a method of assessment, since it causes more sustained pressure in the lower abdomen. After auscultation of the abdomen and palpation of the upper abdomen, the examiner palpates the inguinal and femoral areas for enlarged lymph nodes and hernias. Once again the patient is asked to bear down and the inguinal region is palpated. A bulge will be felt with a direct hernia.

Penis. The examiner inspects the skin of the penis for swelling, inflammation, or lesions caused by chancres, genital warts, herpes, or penile cancer. Pubic hair should be inspected for nits, lice, or scabies. The uncircumcised patient is instructed to retract the foreskin while the glans is inspected for lesions. Normally the foreskin, or prepuce, retracts easily and the glans is smooth. Smegma, a cheesy white substance that collects under the prepuce, is a normal finding.

The examiner notes the location and color of any discharge from the urethral meatus. The urethral meatus is usually centrally located on the glans. Congenital displacement of the meatus can occur on either the ventral surface (hypospadius) or dorsal surface (epispadius) of the penis. The examiner asks the patient to compress the glans and collect any discharge for culture and smear. If the patient has complained of discharge but none is seen, the patient can milk the penis from the base to the glans. Cultures for gonorrhea and chlamydia can be collected by inserting a swab 2 to 4 cm into the urethra. This is an uncomfortable procedure and should be performed at the end of the examination. Last, the penis is palpated for masses and tenderness.

Scrotum and Testes. The examiner inspects the scrotum for size, symmetry, swelling, inflammation, and lesions. The left testis is lower than the right, which causes the scrotum to appear asymmetric under normal conditions. Scrotal size is also determined by room temperature and age. In warm temperatures the dartos muscles relax, and the testes are more pendulous. Likewise, with age the dartos muscles atrophy, which also causes a pendulous appearance. Marked asymmetry can be caused by an undescended testicle, indirect hernia, hydrocele, tumor, or edema.

Palpation of the scrotum is necessary to distinguish between enlargement caused by a mass and swelling caused by the collection of fluid. The size, shape, and consistency of the testes are noted by palpating the testes between the thumb and first two fingers. The testes feel smooth and firm, are oval, and move freely. Any painless, hard nodule should be further investigated, since it may indicate testicular cancer. The epididymis and spermatic cord are palpated from the testes to the inguinal ring. At this time, the examination for hernia is repeated by invaginating the scrotal skin with the index finger to the external inguinal ring (Figure 55-17). The examiner asks the patient to strain; the presence of a hernia will produce a bulge or tap. A load test can be done at this time if the hernia is not palpated despite complaints of hernia symptoms. Finally, transillumination of the scrotum with a flashlight may be attempted to differentiate the cause of scrotal swelling. Serous fluid will transilluminate and produce a red glow. Tissue and blood will not transilluminate.

Prostate. Rectal examination is the most important step in the diagnosis of prostatic disease, especially carcinoma. Cancer of the

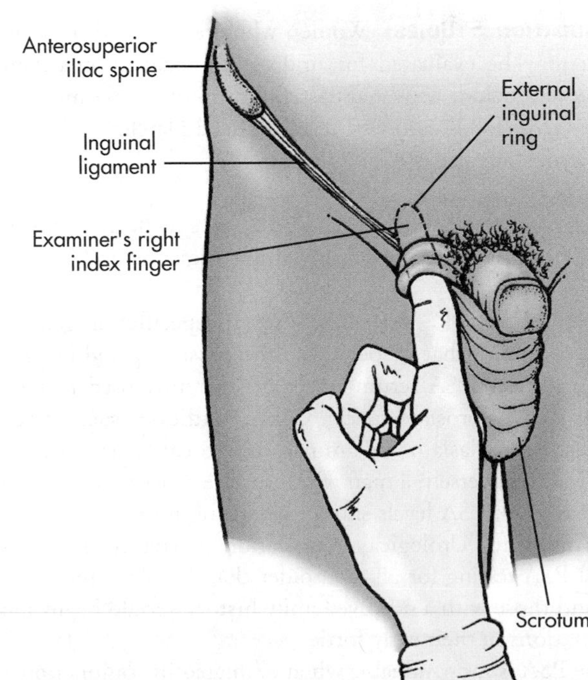

Figure 55-17 Palpating for inguinal hernia at the right inguinal ring.

prostate gland may start as a localized, hard nodule, which is palpable on rectal examination, before proceeding to an advanced stage. For this reason, it is recommended that all men, especially those older than 50 years of age, have a rectal examination at least once a year.

Examination of the prostate can be stressful for the patient. The nurse can help the man overcome pain, embarrassment, and anxiety by establishing a relaxed, positive atmosphere and addressing the man's questions and concerns. The prostate gland is palpated by means of a rectal examination with the patient standing with hips flexed over an examination table or in a side-lying position (Figure 55-18). Before the examination the man is advised that he may feel as though he needs to have a bowel movement. The patient is asked to bear down while a lubricated index finger is gently inserted into the anal canal and then the rectum. The examiner palpates the prostate and seminal vesicles, noting the size, shape, and consistency of the lobes and median sulcus of the prostate. The normal prostate is 2.5 × 4 cm, smooth, heart shaped, rubbery, and nontender.

Diagnostic Tests

Many diagnostic tests are useful in providing data about the reproductive system. They include blood tests, urine tests, cytologic tests, radiologic tests, biopsies, and endoscopic procedures.

Laboratory Tests

Blood Tests

ENDOCRINE TESTING. Because the endocrine system is so closely related to reproductive function, almost any study of endocrine function may be ordered, including determination of estrogen levels and thyroid hormones in women and 24-hour urine collections for ketosteroids and pituitary gonadotropins in both sexes. Endocrine system tests are presented in Chapter 37.

COAGULATION STUDIES. Women who are seen with hypermenorrhea may be evaluated for underlying coagulation disorders. Tests could include activated partial thromboplastin time, platelet count, factor levels, and ristocetin-induced platelet agglutination assay, which are discussed in Chapter 32.

HUMAN IMMUNODEFICIENCY VIRUS TESTING. Assessment of human immunodeficiency virus status is presented in Chapter 22.

PROSTATE-SPECIFIC ANTIGEN. Prostate-specific antigen (PSA) is a glycoprotein that is specific to the prostate gland but not to prostate cancer. PSA serum levels are currently used to identify men at risk for prostate cancer. Other conditions such as benign prostatic hyperplasia or inflammation also can cause an elevated PSA level. Conversely, a man with prostate cancer can have a normal PSA level. PSA levels should be 4.0 ng/ml or less. The ACS and American Urological Association currently recommend annual PSA testing for all men older than 50. African-American men and those with a positive family history should begin annual examinations in their early forties.

The PSA is most valuable when evaluated in conjunction with the patient's symptoms, a family history of prostate cancer, and the findings of the digital rectal examination. Men who are believed to be at risk for prostate cancer are further evaluated by transrectal ultrasound or biopsy. The PSA is also valuable in evaluating the efficacy of treatment and in detecting recurrence of prostate cancer. Contrary to previous belief, blood for the PSA test does not have to be drawn before the rectal examination. PSA levels can be increased after recent ejaculation; cycling; infection; and prostate massage, needle biopsy, or ultrasound.[5]

PROSTATIC ACID PHOSPHATASE. Another glycoprotein used in the evaluation of prostate cancer is prostatic acid phosphatase (PAP). PAP is found in the epithelium of the prostate, and persistently elevated levels may indicate metastasis, although metastasis can also be present with a normal PAP level. Although useful in following the course of prostate cancer, the test is not a practical for screening because of the high rate of false-positive results. An elevated PAP level can occur after a rectal examination or with either prostatitis or benign prostatic hyperplasia.

SYPHILIS STUDIES. Serologic testing can also be used to detect syphilis, since two identifiable antibodies appear in the blood 1 to 4 months after syphilis is contracted. Two types of tests, treponemal and nontreponemal, are currently available. The tests differ in the type of antibody measured and in the antigen used to detect antibodies.

The nontreponemal tests, typically called serologic tests for syphilis (STS), measure an antibody-like substance called reagin. Blood samples are obtained by venipuncture. The VDRL (Venereal Disease Research Laboratory) and the rapid plasma reagin (RPR) screening tests are the most common syphilis tests and typically are used for routine premarital and prenatal screening. The RPR screening test has replaced the VDRL in many institutions.

Syphilitic reagin is thought to form from tissue breakdown products resulting from the interaction of the organism and body tissues. STSs are usually reported as nonreactive, weakly reactive, or reactive. If any degree of reactivity is found, a quantitative test is also performed. Quantitative reactions are reported in ratios and reflect the highest dilution at which the serum reacts.

Reactive STSs are confirmed by alternate serologic tests because hypersensitivity reactions, acute bacterial and viral infections, and chronic systemic diseases such as tuberculosis or collagen disease can all trigger reactivity without exposure to syphilis. It is important, therefore, not to tell patients they have syphilis based on STS alone. The microhemagglutination assay–*Treponema pallidum* (MHA-TP) has replaced the fluorescent treponemal antibody absorption (FTA-ABS) test as the most often used serologic test to confirm reactive STS. A positive MHA-TP or FTA-ABS test must be obtained to confirm the diagnosis of syphilis.

The serologic tests in use today do not always indicate an active syphilitic infection; they only detect the presence of antibodies. There is an urgent need for a specific, rapid method of detecting infection caused by syphilis. Until new tests are developed, the patient's history, clinical symptoms, and serologic testing are the best available tools for diagnosis.

OTHER SERUM TUMOR MARKERS. Alkaline phosphatase is monitored in men with metastatic prostate cancer. Alphafetoprotein and HCG can be elevated in men with metastatic testicular cancer.

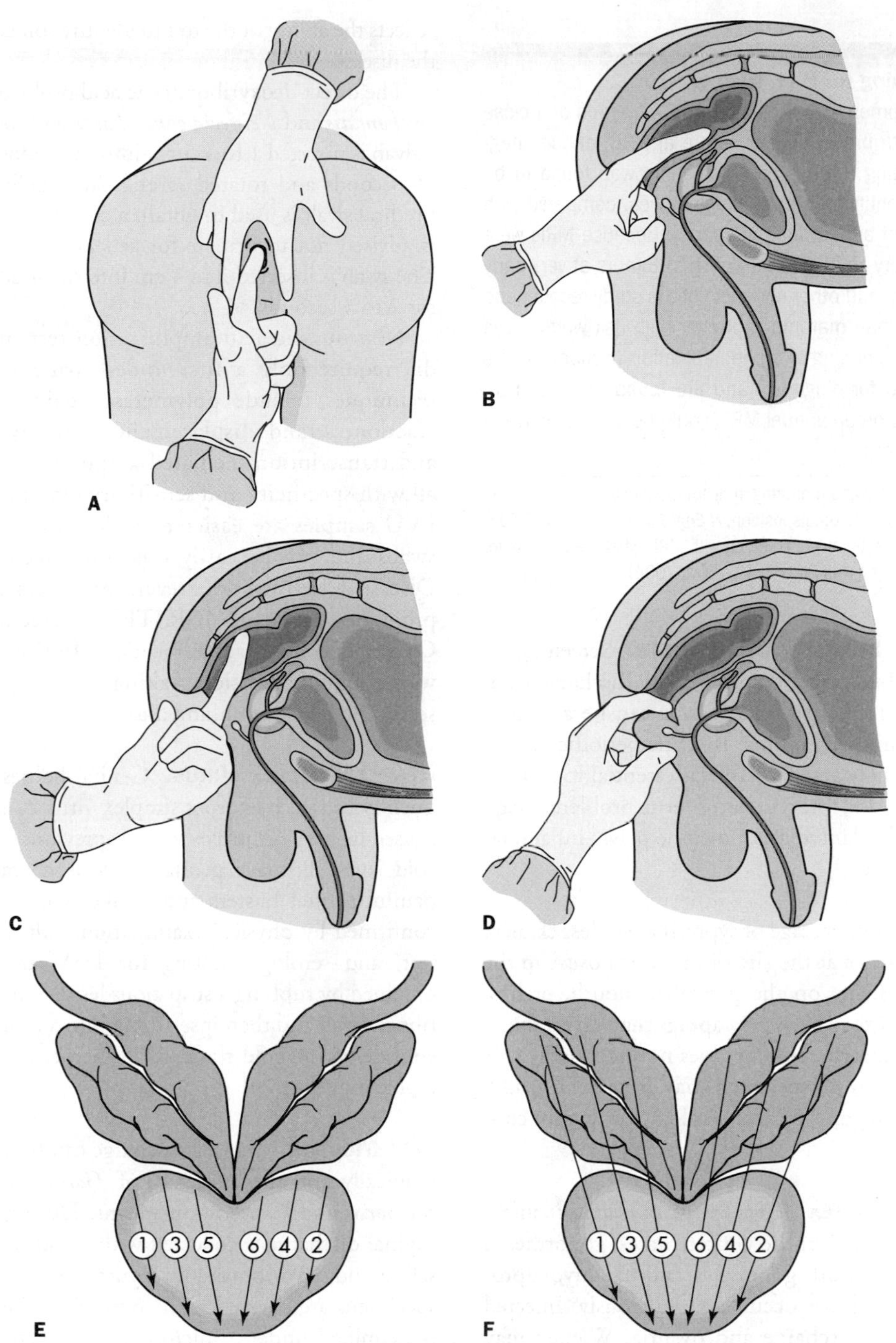

Figure 55-18 Rectal examination. **A,** Introduction of protected, well-lubricated finger. **B,** Palpation of prostate gland and seminal vesicles, lateral view. **C,** Palpation of anterior surface of sacrum and coccyx. **D,** Palpation of Cowper's glands. **E,** Massage of prostate gland for specimen collection or treatment; order of strokes is indicated by gradually working toward center (verumontanum). **F,** Massage of seminal vesicles and prostate gland.

Genetic Testing. Genetic testing for the general population is not recommended; however, the American Society of Clinical Oncology recommends that women who have an increased risk of breast or ovarian cancer be offered genetic testing for mutations in the tumor suppressor genes BRCA1 and BRCA2. Such women include those with three or more first- or second-degree relatives who develop the disease, cancer diagnosis before age 45, family members with known BRCA1 or BRCA2 mutations, family history of ovarian cancer, breast cancer in male relative, Ashkenazi Jewish descent, and breast or ovarian cancer history.[3] Genetic testing should be conducted only within the context of a pretesting and posttesting counseling program. Women with the BRCA1 or BRCA2 gene mutations should be screened earlier than the recommendations for low-risk women (see Future Watch box) and may consider other options such as prophylactic surgery or chemoprevention.[1]

Future Watch

MRI Breast Screening for High Risk Women

In a study of 1909 women with BRCA1 or BRCA2 genes or a close relative diagnosed with breast cancer before age 30, annual magnetic resonance imaging (MRI) breast screening was found to be 79.5% effective in identifying breast malignancies, compared with 33.3% effectiveness of annual mammography. Because MRIs were better at identifying very small (10 mm or less) tumors at very early stages, the researchers and other reviewers of the study recommend MRI screening rather than mammography for high-risk women. The disadvantage of MRI screening is the identification of many tumors that must be biopsied for diagnosis and are found to be benign. However, for high-risk women annual MRIs could be an alternative to prophylactic mastectomy.

Kriege M et al: Efficacy of MRI and mammography for breast cancer screening in women with a familial or genetic predisposition, *N Engl J Med* 351(5):427-437, 2004; and Liberman L: Breast cancer screening with MRI—what are the data for patients at high risk?, *N Engl J Med* 351(5):497-500, 2004.

Scrapings, Cultures, Smears, Urine Tests. Screening for STDs can be done by obtaining a culture of any discharge from the male and female reproductive tract. STDs can be asymptomatic or produce only mild symptoms. Routine periodic screening for STDs among sexually active persons is essential to identify asymptomatic infections and prevent long-term problems (e.g., the sequelae of untreated chlamydia can include pelvic inflammatory disease and infertility).

SYPHILIS. During the primary stage of syphilis a painless chancre develops within 1 to 3 weeks at the site of initial exposure to the *T. pallidum* organism, usually on the genitalia, mouth, or lips. Dark field examination of the chancre scrapings may reveal the *T. pallidum* spirochete. A negative scraping does not necessarily rule out syphilis, however, since the specimen may have been inadequate. The later stages of syphilis require serologic testing for confirmation (discussed above).

CHLAMYDIA AND GONORRHEA. *Chlamydia trachomatis* infection is the most common STD in the United States; gonorrhea is the second most common. Both gonorrhea and chlamydia produce similar symptoms and can occur simultaneously. Infected men complain of urethral discharge and dysuria. Women may note postcoital bleeding or an increase in vaginal discharge or have mucopurulent cervicitis. Testing for *C. trachomatis* has evolved in recent years to include direct antigen detection and nucleic acid amplification techniques using either polymerase or ligase chain reactions, as well as cultures, which used to be the gold standard.

Nonculture testing for chlamydia is not as specific as the culture method, but it is cheaper and easier to complete. Direct fluorescent antibody detection uses visualization of chlamydia elementary bodies, whereas enzyme immunoassay uses spectrophotometry to identify color changes in the elementary bodies. These tests require a cervical specimen and have a sensitivity of about 60% and a specificity of about 96% to 99%.[3] The sensitivity reflects the ability of the test to identify someone who has the disease, and the specificity reflects the ability of the test to identify someone who does not have the disease.

The direct deoxyribonucleic acid probe test screens for both *C. trachomatis* and *Neisseria gonorrhoeae* with one culture. In women, a swab is inserted 1 to 1.5 cm into the endocervical canal for 10 to 30 seconds and rotated several times before removal. A smaller urethral swab is used to obtain a culture in men. The male patient is advised not to urinate for at least 2 hours before the culture. The swab is inserted 2 to 4 cm into the urethra and rotated gently for 2 to 3 seconds.

New nucleic acid amplification tests for detecting chlamydia require only a first-voided urine sample (FVU). These techniques include polymerase chain reaction, ligase chain reaction, strand displacement assay, hybrid capture system, and transcription-mediated amplification of ribonucleic acid, all with specificity and sensitivity ranging from 82% to 100%. FVU samples are easier to collect than cervical and urethral swabs and can be easily used for screening. The Centers for Disease Control and Prevention offers clinicians a software program called SOCRATES (Screening Optimally for Chlamydia: Resource Allocation, Testing and Evaluation Software) to guide decision making regarding the most appropriate screening tests for chlamydia.[3]

HERPES SIMPLEX VIRUS. Genital herpes is an STD most frequently caused by herpes simplex virus 2, although it can also be caused by herpes simplex virus 1, previously thought to cause only cold sores. Primary genital HSV is characterized by multiple, painful genital blisters and flulike symptoms. Diagnosis can be confirmed by physical examination, culture for herpesvirus, Pap test, and serologic testing for HSV antibodies. A culture is obtained by rubbing a suspicious lesion with a cotton- or Dacron-tipped swab and then inserting it into a transport medium. This is considered the gold standard for herpes diagnosis. A final culture report may take 7 days.

WET MOUNTS. Vaginal discharge can be easily examined microscopically for the presence of *Gardnerella vaginalis* and *Trichomonas* and *Candida* organisms. During a pelvic examination vaginal discharge is collected with a cotton swab and mixed with saline and 10% potassium hydroxide on two clean slides. The specimens are covered with cover slips. The saline-prepared slide is examined under a microscope for bacteria, white blood cells, "clue" cells (stippled epithelial cells), and trichomonads. The potassium hydroxide slide is examined for *Candida* organisms and a positive whiff test. Potassium hydroxide causes the epithelial cells to lyse and, in cases of yeast infections, release hyphae. In bacterial vaginosis, vaginal discharge that is mixed with potassium hydroxide produces a fishy smell, or positive whiff test. See Table 55-2 for interpretation of wet mounts.

PROSTATIC SMEAR. For a prostatic smear the prostate is first massaged during a digital rectal examination and any discharge from the penis is collected. If no discharge is expressed, the first urine sample after the examination is collected. Although some cases of tuberculosis and cancer can be detected by this method, the use of the prostatic smear has declined in recent years. Find-

TABLE 55-2 WET MOUNT INTERPRETATIONS

	Normal	Bacterial Vaginosis	Candida	Trichomonas	Atrophic
Symptoms	None	Thin, gray-white discharge Malodorous Pruritus can be present	Thick, white, curdlike discharge Pruritus	Increased, thin, frothy, yellow-green discharge Pruritus	Vulvar and vaginal dryness
pH	3.5-4.1	>4.5	<4.5	>4.5	7.0
Microscopic findings	Lactobacilli	Clue cells	Budding yeast	Increased WBCs Trichomonads	Increased WBCs Parabasal and intermediate cells
KOH	No findings	Positive whiff test (fishy odor)	Budding yeast Pseudohyphae	No findings	No findings

WBCs, White blood cells; *KOH,* potassium hydroxide.

ings from the digital rectal examination, PSA levels, and biopsy are used to diagnose prostate cancer.

Cytology: Pap Test. The Pap test is a screening test for abnormal cervical cells, including cancer. It is designed to determine who needs further evaluation and the type of evaluation needed. Pap tests can also identify vaginal infections such as *Trichomonas* and human papillomavirus, as well as evaluate hormone status.

The accuracy of the Pap test depends on the quality of the sample and the reliability of the laboratory interpreting the test. Results of 10% to 40% of tests are estimated to be reported as false negative partly as a result of inadequate specimens or misdiagnosis on the part of the cytologist. Several new systems have been developed to improve the reliability of Pap test samples and thereby reduce the incidence of false-negative results. The speculoscopy has been shown to improve the identification of abnormal cervical lesions during a pelvic examination. In speculoscopy, a chemiluminescent light is attached to the blade of a speculum. Once the Pap test is obtained, the cervix and vagina are washed with 5% acetic acid. Using 4003 magnification, the examiner inspects the cervix for distinct acetowhite areas, which indicate cervical pathologic changes.[7] The use of speculoscopy, combined with Pap tests, identifies more cervical lesions than Pap tests alone.

The preparation of the Pap test slide or specimen can also lead to false-negative results. Traditionally, Pap test samples are rolled or scraped across a slide and sprayed with a fixative. The thin-layer preparation is the most current slide preparation method developed to reduce the effects of air-drying distortion, excessive blood or mucus, or a thick layer of cells.[6] After obtaining the Pap test sample, the examiner rinses the collection device in a bottle of preservative solution. A slide is prepared from the suspended cells and screened by a cytologist in a conventional manner. The ThinPrep slides produce an evenly distributed sample without obscuring artifacts, which is easier to interpret. The ThinPrep method is associated with an increase in the number of cervical lesions identified and with better Pap samples.

A system has also been developed to rescreen Pap tests initially reported as negative or normal. The AutoPap 300 QC computer is a high-speed image processing computer with the ability to analyze the specimen for size, shape, density, and color of cells. Any Pap test with abnormalities is reexamined by a cytologist. The misinterpretation of Pap tests should decline with this process.

The ACS recommends that all women who are, or have been, sexually active or who are at least 18 years of age have an annual Pap test for 3 consecutive years and then every 3 years until middle age. A woman should not douche, take a bath, use vaginal medications or deodorants, or have sexual intercourse for at least 24 hours before the test. Some physicians request a 48-hour delay before the test. Pap tests are preferably obtained 5 or 6 days after menstruation, since menses makes interpretation difficult and may camouflage atypical cells. Infections can also interfere with hormonal cytology. Pap tests should be delayed for at least 1 month after use of topical antibiotics, which produce rapid, heavy shedding of cells. Many women experience slight vaginal bleeding after a Pap test. They should be advised that this is expected, but to report to the health care provider any bleeding in excess of spotting.

The results of Pap tests are reported using the Bethesda System. The Bethesda System evaluates the adequacy of the sample (e.g., satisfactory or not satisfactory for interpretation) and provides a general classification of normal or abnormal and a descriptive diagnosis of the Pap test. The descriptive diagnosis indicates whether the cells were atypical squamous cells of undetermined significance, low-grade squamous intraepithelial lesions, high-grade squamous intraepithelial lesions, or glandular cells.[2] It is important to monitor Pap tests and ensure proper follow-up care, including treatment of vaginal infections and colposcopy if necessary (see Research box).

Radiologic Tests

Diagnostic radiographic studies, including computed tomography (CT), magnetic resonance imaging (MRI), ultrasonography of the male and female reproductive system, and mammography or xeromammography, are used to identify soft tissue and bony abnormalities, to diagnose tumors and masses, and to diagnose infertility problems. Patient preparation and aftercare associated with the use of CT and MRI tests are similar to those described for other body systems and are not repeated here.

Ultrasonography. Ultrasonography (ultrasound) has become a useful diagnostic tool for persons with reproductive system

Research

Khanna N, Phillips MD: Adherence to care plan in women with abnormal Papanicolaou smears: a review of barriers and interventions, *J Am Board Fam Pract* 14(2):123-130, 2001.

The purpose of this paper was to evaluate interventions that increase adherence to follow-up care for abnormal Pap tests. Cervical cancer is the ninth leading cause of death for American women. Therefore effective prevention is essential. Prevention measures include appropriate use of the Pap test and patient adherence to a care plan. Common barriers to follow-up of abnormal Pap tests include lack of understanding about the purpose of colposcopy; fear of cancer; forgetting appointments; and lack of time, money, and child care. Focused intervention strategies to increase adherence to follow-up care include personalized reminders to patients by their primary care provider, educational brochures, incentive vouchers, and case management. Studies revealed that patients in the intervention control compared with the control group adhered to a higher rate of follow-up (72% to 75%) than those who were in the control group without interventions (30% to 64%). The most effective strategies for improved adherence were case management and personalized reminders to patients from their primary health care provider.

problems. It can be used to locate pelvic masses, intrauterine devices, ectopic pregnancies, and prostatic neoplasms. Abdominal ultrasounds require the patient to have a full bladder. Transvaginal ultrasonography provides improved picture clarity of the immediate area compared with transabdominal sonography. Transvaginal sonography is currently being used to inspect and assess the uterus, ovaries, fallopian tubes, and extragenital structures (Box 55-4).

The patient is asked to void before the procedure and then assisted into the lithotomy position. A female staff member should be available to provide emotional support for the woman during the procedure. Vaginal probes are lubricated with coupling gel and inserted into a condom or latex glove before insertion. The clinician uses one hand placed on the patient's abdomen to assess organ mobility. Additional assessments of pain and size of masses are obtained. The transvaginal probe is also used to guide procedures involving needle puncture, such as ova retrieval for in vitro fertilization. Transvaginal color Doppler sonography adds information on the quality of blood flow for the assessment of pelvic masses. Ultrasound is also used to determine whether a breast mass is fluid filled or solid.

Transrectal ultrasonography (TRUS) may be used as part of a workup for benign prostatic enlargement or prostate cancer. The procedure is preceded by a rectal examination and possibly an enema. A transrectal probe is inserted 8 to 9 cm into the rectum. TRUS is valuable in evaluating the size of the prostate, determining the response of a prostate tumor to treatment, and guiding placement of needles for biopsy. However, TRUS is not sensitive enough to be used alone for the diagnosis of cancer because of the high number of false-negative and false-positive results.

Hysterosalpingography. Hysterosalpingography involves radiographic visualization of the uterine cavity and fallopian tubes after the injection of contrast material through the cervix. The test is useful in the evaluation of uterine tumors, tubal obstructions, and abnormalities. The procedure is usually performed in the radiology department, and the patient is placed in a lithotomy position on a fluoroscopy table. A plastic speculum rather than a metal one is inserted into the vagina to allow for better visualization. A cannula is filled with a water-soluble contrast material, which is injected slowly under direct fluoroscopy. The hysterosalpingogram has largely replaced the older Rubin test, which was associated with numerous false-negative and false-positive results.

Before the test the nurse assesses the patient for allergy to iodine dye or shellfish, although allergic reactions are rare, since the contrast material is not injected intravenously. The bowel may be cleansed with laxatives, suppositories, or enemas, but no food or fluid restrictions are needed. The patient may be given a sedative or antispasmodic agent before the test. The patient is advised that she may feel menstrual-type cramping and that she may experience shoulder pain caused by subphrenic irritation from the dye as it leaks into the peritoneal cavity.

After the procedure the nurse assesses the patient for nausea, faintness, and discomfort. Analgesics may be prescribed. The patient is instructed to apply a perineal pad, since vaginal drainage may occur for 1 or 2 days after the test, and the radiopaque dye may stain clothing. The patient should report any signs of infection such as fever, increased pulse rate, or pain to the health care provider.

Box 55-4 Uses of Transvaginal Sonography

Uterus

Size, position
Inspection of myometrium and endometrial lining
Detection of malformations
Identification of small fibroids
Early pregnancy determination
Early fetal heartbeats

Ovaries

Size, texture, location
Monitoring of follicular growth
Evaluation of ovulation
Identification of corpus luteum
Identification of tumors and structural deformities
Follicular aspiration

Fallopian Tubes

Diagnosis of tubal pathologic changes
Detection of tuboovarian abscess
Early recognition of tubal pregnancy

Extragenital Structures

Evaluation of free pelvic fluid
Detection of pelvic blood clots

Mammography, Xeromammography. Mammography is a radiologic study of the breast used to evaluate differences in the density of tissue, particularly small or poorly defined masses or nodules. It is capable of detecting many breast cancers that are too small to be palpated on physical examination. Mammograms are most effective in older women who have a higher percentage of fatty tissue in their breasts, which creates a greater contrast density on x-ray film. The density of benign cysts and malignant tumors may be similar, but their appearance is usually different. Suspicious lesions may be referred for needle aspiration or biopsy.

Recommendations for mammography screening are under constant evaluation and revision (see Future Watch box, p. 1678). Currently, the ACS recommends that a woman have annual routine screening beginning at age 40.

No special preparation is required before a mammogram, but the woman should be instructed to avoid using deodorant, cream, or powder, which can mimic calcium clusters on x-ray film. Pretest teaching is critical, since most women are anxious about the examination and the possibility of breast cancer. The woman is positioned standing next to the x-ray machine, and one breast at a time is placed between the platform and film plate. Most women experience some discomfort from the breast compression. At least two views of each breast are taken.

Aftercare involves providing clear information concerning how and when the results of the test will be communicated to the patient. Most centers use this opportunity to reinforce skill and understanding of the purpose, technique, and timing of breast self-examination as well.

The xeromammogram provides an x-ray image with a much lower dose of radiation than that required for a traditional mammogram. The images are recorded on paper rather than film. The technique has become increasingly popular because the high-contrast result is easier to read and may be more accurate.

Special Tests

Pregnancy Tests. Most of the frequently used pregnancy tests are based on the fact that HCG is present in the blood and urine of pregnant women. Results are obtained within minutes to 2 hours. The newer tests can detect as little as 25 mIU/ml of HCG as early as 3 or 4 days after implantation. First morning urine specimens provide the best sample. Do-it-yourself pregnancy tests, available over the counter, are sensitive and easy to perform.

The radioreceptor assay test for pregnancy is rapid and reliable. It is extremely accurate, and serial blood samples may be used to determine the viability of the pregnancy or identify molar or ectopic pregnancies. Serum HCG levels double approximately every 2 days until the tenth week of pregnancy. In men and nonpregnant women the normal HCG level is less than 5 mIU/ml. At 2 weeks' gestation the value is 50 to 500 mIU/ml. In ectopic pregnancies the level increases at a slower rate.

Schiller's Test. Schiller's test is a simple test that reveals the presence of atypical cervical cells. A solution of 3.5% iodine or Lugol's solution is applied to the cervix. Atypical cells, both malignant and benign, do not contain glycogen and will fail to stain. Early cancerous lesions and benign lesions, such as cervicitis, may appear as glistening areas of a lighter color than surrounding tissue. Biopsies can then be obtained from these targeted areas. The test is used infrequently because colposcopy is a more accurate method of obtaining the same information.

Biopsies

CERVICAL BIOPSY. A cervical biopsy is performed to obtain a tissue specimen for pathologic examination. It is almost always performed with colposcopic direction. Although bleeding is minimal, the biopsy is ideally performed shortly after the menses when the cervix is less vascular. A punch biopsy can be safely performed as an office procedure without the use of anesthesia because the cervix has few pain receptors. The woman is instructed to leave the packing or tampon in place for 8 to 24 hours and report excessive bleeding.

CONIZATION OF CERVIX. Conization of the cervix may be performed as a diagnostic or therapeutic measure. It is typically performed in an outpatient setting with the woman under local anesthesia. A cone-shaped portion of the cervix containing the suspected malignant or infected tissue is removed. Bleeding from the site of conization is greater than that occurring from punch biopsy. If the bleeding is excessive or if hemorrhage seems likely, the cervix is sutured to control blood loss. Oozing is controlled by packing, which is kept in place for 24 to 48 hours. The patient is instructed to rest and avoid heavy lifting for at least 3 days. She should be informed that her next two or three menstrual periods may be heavy and prolonged.

ENDOMETRIAL BIOPSY. Although an ideal method for screening for endometrial cancer has not been developed, a variety of methods are now in use. Less than half of women with uterine cancer have an abnormal Pap test at diagnosis. Cells rarely exfoliate from the endometrium in the early stages of the cancer, making this an unsatisfactory method of screening and diagnosis. The best results are obtained when cervical aspiration is performed as part of the Pap test. It is important to ensure the woman is not pregnant before performing the procedure. A paracervical block or local anesthetic may be used.

Endometrial cells obtained by aspiration test show malignant changes 75% to 90% of the time when uterine cancer exists. A small cannula is inserted through the cervix into the uterine cavity, and suction is applied by means of a syringe attached to the cannula. The specimen obtained is prepared as for a Pap test.

Endometrial biopsy can be used to diagnose cancer; evaluate bleeding, polyps, or inflammatory conditions; and determine whether ovulation has occurred by assessing the effects of estrogen or progesterone on the endometrium. It is performed by introducing a small curette into the uterus and obtaining several strips of endometrial tissue. The specimens are taken from several sites in the uterine cavity to increase the chances of obtaining malignant cells. The biopsy method is considered to be about 90% accurate in diagnosing endometrial cancer.

Complications include perforation of the uterus, uterine bleeding, interference with early pregnancy, and infection. Any temperature elevation after the biopsy should be reported to the physician because this procedure may activate pelvic inflammatory disease. The patient is advised to wear a pad after the procedure because some vaginal bleeding is expected. If excessive bleeding occurs, the physician should be notified. The nurse advises the patient to avoid douching and intercourse for 72 hours after the biopsy; to rest over the next 24 hours; and to avoid heavy lifting to prevent uterine hemorrhage.

Breast Biopsy. It is widely accepted that most breast masses need to be evaluated for cancer. Biopsy can differentiate fibrocystic lesions, fibroadenomas, and intraductal papillomas. Three major approaches are in use. An excisional biopsy removes the mass for pathologic evaluation, an incisional biopsy samples some of the tissue from the mass, and an aspiration biopsy removes fluid or tissue from the mass through a large-bore needle. The aspiration method is in widespread use. Bloody fluid aspirated from the mass indicates the possibility of cancer. If nothing can be aspirated, the mass is considered solid and needs to be evaluated via the incisional route.

Breast biopsies are usually performed in ambulatory settings with the patient under local anesthesia. It is crucial that the woman clearly understand what procedure is planned, the anesthesia to be used, and the sensations she may experience during the procedure. Aftercare is straightforward. The nurse assesses the incision site for bleeding, edema, or infection. Mild analgesics are provided for discomfort. Numbness at the biopsy site may persist for months.

Needle Biopsy of Prostate. A needle aspiration biopsy of the prostate is performed to retrieve cells for histologic study. The procedure is usually performed at the same time as cystoscopy but can also be done as an office procedure with the patient under local anesthesia. Either a transrectal or a transperineal approach is used.

A transrectal approach uses guided ultrasound to identify biopsy sites (Figure 55-19). Before the procedure a digital rectal examination is performed to locate the suspicious lesions. A condom-covered ultrasound transducer is inserted into the rectum, and tissue samples are collected from suspicious lesions and other areas of the prostate.

Aspiration may be repeated several times in different locations to sample the tissue adequately. This method is thought to be slightly more accurate than the transperineal approach, which involves insertion of the needle through the perineum into the prostate using the examiner's finger, which is placed in the rectum, as a guide.

Patient preparation for prostatic biopsy may include bowel cleansing if a rectal approach is used. Sepsis is a rare but potentially life-threatening complication. Prophylactic antibiotics are usually prescribed before and after the procedure. The patient may also experience transient hematuria and rectal bleeding. The patient should be advised to promptly report a temperature of greater than 100° F (37.7° C), chills, or difficulty voiding.

Open Perineal Biopsy. To obtain a specimen of tissue by open perineal biopsy, the clinician makes a small incision in the perineum between the anus and scrotum. This technique gives the greatest accuracy because the suspicious lesion can be clearly identified, and multiple specimens can be taken from the prostate gland. The procedure requires regional or general anesthesia.

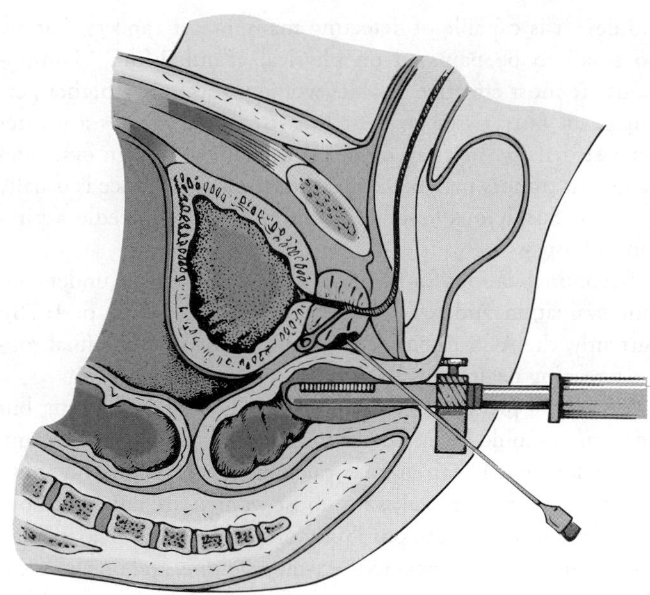

Figure 55-19 Transrectal biopsy with transrectal ultrasound.

A dressing is applied to the biopsy site and can be held in place for about 24 hours with a two-tailed binder. The nurse instructs the patient to wipe from front to back after defecation to avoid contaminating the incision. Perineal irrigation is sometimes advised for both cleanliness and comfort. Unless the physician prescribes a solution, warm water can be poured from front to back over the incision. After the sutures are removed, sitz baths can add much to the patient's general comfort. The man is instructed to promptly report any signs of infection to the physician.

Testicular Biopsy. Smears or biopsy specimens from the testes can be obtained by the needle method or by an incision made through the scrotum. Most often an incision is used. After a local anesthetic has been administered, a small incision about 2.5 cm long is made, and a small piece of the testis is removed. A dressing is applied, and postoperative management is similar to that after open perineal prostatic biopsy. Testicular biopsy specimens are sometimes used to evaluate fertility. If sperm are present in the biopsy tissue but are absent from the semen, the infertility is often the result of stricture of the tubal system beyond the testes.

Dilation and Curettage. Dilation and curettage (D&C) may be performed for a variety of purposes, including evaluating infertility, treating bleeding, and inducing abortion. Because the entire uterine cavity is "scraped," a large tissue sample is obtained. This minimizes the likelihood of missing malignant cells. Most of the procedures used to diagnose endometrial cancer require some dilation of the cervix to introduce instruments into the uterus. Vacuum curettage applies suction to the entire uterine cavity to obtain tissue specimens.

For a D&C, metal dilators of graduated sizes are inserted into the cervical canal. Once the cervix is dilated, sharp curettes are used to remove endometrial tissue. The major complications of a D&C are hemorrhage and perforation of the uterus. Postoperative care is summarized in the Guidelines for Safe Practice box.

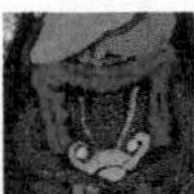

GUIDELINES FOR SAFE PRACTICE
After Dilation and Curettage

1. Apply a perineal pad to absorb the expected drainage.
2. Take vital signs every 15 minutes until stable.
3. Monitor bleeding every 15 minutes for 2 hours; if active bleeding continues, monitor every hour for about 8 hours.
4. Record each pad change and amount of blood loss in estimated milliliters (60 ml saturates a perineal pad).
5. Monitor urinary output.
6. Give mild analgesics as prescribed; report immediately any abdominal pain that is continuous, sharp, and not relieved by analgesics (may indicate perforation of uterus).
7. Encourage ambulation when patient is awake and vital signs are stable.

Most women are discharged on the day of the procedure and resume normal daily activities, but vigorous exercise is discouraged. Sexual intercourse may be resumed when the woman feels comfortable. The menstrual cycle usually is not disturbed by a D&C, and all vaginal bleeding should disappear in a week to 10 days. Women are advised to report the recurrence of bright-red blood or the development of a vaginal discharge with an unpleasant odor.

Infertility Tests. The purposes of an infertility evaluation are to establish the cause of infertility; give a prognosis for future fertility; provide a basis for medical or surgical treatment; and help the couple accept their diagnosis, treatment, and future options. The assessment and intervention can be physically painful as well as emotionally and economically stressful.

A full description of an infertility workup is beyond the scope of this discussion. Both the man and woman undergo a thorough physical examination to rule out any undetected medical problems. Specific diagnostic studies used in infertility evaluation include determination of ovulation status of the woman by assessing basal temperature, LH levels, and serum progesterone. A biopsy of the endometrium may be done to assess barriers to implantation. A hysterosalpingogram can determine if the fallopian tubes are scarred or blocked. The man's semen is examined to determine adequacy of sperm counts.

Endoscopy

The pelvic organs and surrounding tissues can be visualized directly by endoscopy. The procedures by which this can be accomplished are colposcopy, culdoscopy, laparoscopy (peritoneoscopy), hysteroscopy, and falloposcopy (Box 55-5). Most of the procedures can be performed on an outpatient basis even if general anesthesia is used.

Colposcopy is used to augment a detailed examination of the vagina and cervix or to guide cervical biopsy. The associated care is the same as that for other types of cervical biopsy. The use of culdoscopy is declining because laparoscopy has become a standard diagnostic and treatment intervention. Hysteroscopy is routinely performed as part of a D&C to allow the physician to inspect the inside of the uterus before scraping or treatment. In the male, cystoscopic examination allows the physician to inspect the condition of the urethra and bladder mucosa and to detect prostatic encroachment on the urethra (see Chapter 34).

Laparoscopy (pelvic endoscopy or peritoneoscopy) may be used to inspect the outer surface of the uterus, fallopian tubes, and ovaries. A laparoscope is inserted through the abdominal wall through a small incision in the subumbilical area. The peritoneal cavity is filled with 3 to 4 L of carbon dioxide to separate the abdominal wall from the viscera and increase visualization. The laparoscope is then inserted to conduct the planned procedure. Laparoscopy may also be used for tubal sterilization, for lysis of adhesions, for biopsy, and in various infertility procedures. Conscious sedation may be used in office settings; however, general anesthesia is typically used for more extensive procedures. At the end of the procedure, the carbon dioxide is removed, but referred pain to the shoulder from gaseous irritation of the diaphragm and phrenic nerve often occurs. Air may enter the abdominal cavity during the procedure and cause discomfort; a prone position with a pillow under the abdomen may increase the woman's comfort. Complications such as hemorrhage and infection are rare, but

Box 55-5 Procedures for Visualization of Pelvic Organs

- *Colposcopy:* Visualization of vagina and cervix under low-power magnification
- *Culdoscopy:* Insertion of culdoscope through posterior fornix into Douglas' cul-de-sac for visualization of fallopian tubes and ovaries
- *Falloposcopy:* Transcervical endoscopic examination of fallopian tubes
- *Hysteroscopy:* Insertion of hysteroscope through cervix for visualization of inside of uterus
- *Laparoscopy:* Insertion of laparoscope (with patient under local or general anesthesia) through small incision in abdominal wall (inferior margin of umbilicus), which is insufflated with carbon dioxide; permits visualization of all pelvic organs

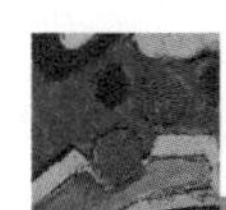

PATIENT/FAMILY TEACHING
Discharge Instructions After Routine Laparoscopy

- Rest for 24 hours before resuming normal activities.
- Avoid sexual intercourse until after postoperative visit with physician.
- Discomfort may be experienced in shoulder and upper abdominal area. Take oral pain medications as prescribed.
- Call the physician if abdominal pain increases; if temperature rises; if abnormal vaginal bleeding occurs; or if there is increased redness, swelling, soreness, or foul drainage at wound sites before the first postoperative visit.
- Wound dressings may be removed in 24 hours, and showering is permitted.
- Resume regular diet and drink plenty of fluids.

women are cautioned to report fever or pain in the lower abdomen. Discharge instructions are summarized in the Patient/Family Teaching box.

References

1. American Cancer Society: *American Cancer Society recommendations for early breast cancer detection*, 2003, accessed July 2004 from website: http://www.cancer.org/.
2. Apgar BS, Zoschnick L: The 2001 Bethesda System terminology, *Am Fam Phys* 68(10):1992-1998, 2003.
3. Heise A: The clinical significance of HPV, *Nurse Pract* 28(10):8-21, 2003.
4. Newman DK, Palmer MH, editors: The state of the science on urinary incontinence, *Am J Nurs* 3(Suppl):1-58, 2003.
5. US Preventive Services Task Force: Screening for cervical cancer: recommendations and rationale, *Am Fam Phys* 67(8):1759-1766, 2003.
6. US Preventive Services Task Force: Screening for prostate cancer: recommendations and rationale, *Am Fam Phys* 67(4):787-792, 2003.
7. The Regent Group: Medical policy, speculoscopy, 2003, accessed November 2005 from website: www.regence.com/trqmedpol/medicine/med106.html.

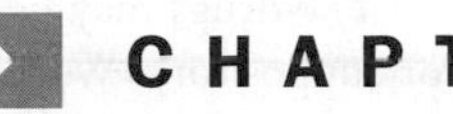 Visit the Evolve website: http://evolve.elsevier.com/Monahan/medsurg

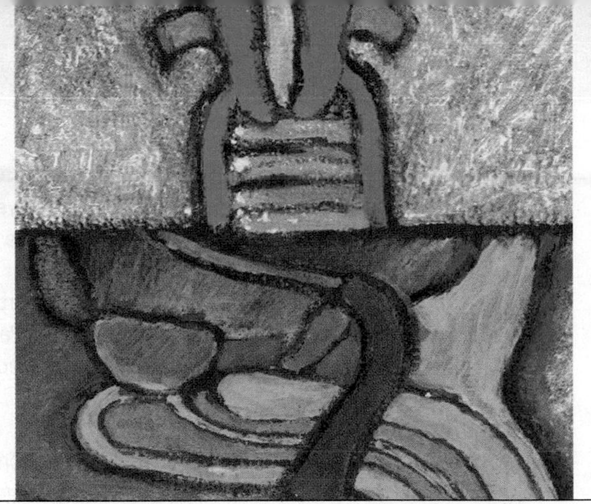

CHAPTER 56
Female Reproductive Problems

by Jeanne Linhart

OBJECTIVES

After studying this chapter, the learner should be able to:

1. Discuss the collaborative management of common infectious diseases of the female reproductive tract.
2. Discuss the management of various disorders of menstruation.
3. Adapt preoperative and postoperative care for women undergoing hysterectomy.
4. Discuss nursing management for women undergoing intracavitary radiotherapy to the female reproductive tract.
5. Discuss options for couples considering sterilization or experiencing problems with fertility.
6. Identify anticipatory guidance for promoting reproductive health in women.

KEY TERMS

anovulatory cycle, p. 1691
cryosurgery, p. 1686
dysplasia, p. 1698
endometrium, p. 1711
intracavitary implant, p. 1700
normal flora, p. 1685
Pap tests, p. 1697
perineal hygiene, p. 1689
prostaglandins, p. 1689

Diseases and disorders of the female reproductive system impair the physical and emotional health of millions of women each year. Infectious processes and disorders of menstruation are common and pervasive problems. Malignant neoplasms destroy childbearing potential and end numerous lives each year. Disorders affecting the female reproductive system are important national health concerns and are reflected in the *Healthy People 2010* goals, as summarized in the Healthy People 2010 box.

Infectious Processes

Vaginitis

Etiology and Epidemiology. Although the vulva and vagina are relatively resistant to infection, vaginitis is one of the most common problems for which women seek medical care. The most commonly involved organisms are *Candida albicans, Trichomonas vaginalis,* and *Gardnerella vaginalis*. Bacterial vaginosis is the most common cause of symptomatic vaginal discharge.[3] It occurs from an overgrowth of **normal flora** in the vagina, usually *G. vaginalis,* primarily in women who are sexually active (see Chapter 59).

Pathophysiology. Disturbances in the flora of the normally acidic vaginal environment result in a variety of symptoms, including vaginal discharge, vulvar pruritus, tissue irritation and inflammation, and burning. Different organisms are associated with specific types of discharge and symptom patterns, but pruritus is an extremely common symptom, regardless of the cause, and commonly is severe.

If the pH of the vaginal mucosa is altered or the woman's resistance is decreased by aging-related changes, stress, or disease, her risk of vaginitis increases. Specific factors that increase this risk include the use of antibiotics, which destroy the normal protective flora of the vagina; diseases causing immunocompromise, such as human immunodeficiency virus (HIV) infection; diseases altering carbohydrate metabolism, such as diabetes mellitus; the use of steroids or other immunosuppressants; and tissue injury from mechanical irritation by foreign objects such as tampons or by chemical irritation from douches, which makes tissues more susceptible to invasion by organisms. Because many organisms proliferate in a more alkaline environment, postmenopausal women are at increased risk for vaginitis because of the decrease in normal vaginal secretions and a rise in vaginal pH caused by a decline in estrogen levels. Risk factors for vaginitis are listed in the Risk Factors box.

Collaborative Care Management. The diagnosis of vaginitis is based on the history, physical examination, and laboratory testing. Abnormal vaginal discharge is evaluated using a wet

Healthy People 2010

Objectives Related to Female Reproductive Problems

- Cervical cancer deaths: Reduce the death rate from cancer of the uterine cervix to 2 per 100,000 women.
- Pap tests: Increase to at least 97% the proportion of women ages 18 and older who have ever received a Pap test and to at least 90% the proportion of those who received a Pap test within the preceding 3 years.
- Chlamydial infection
  –Increase the proportion of sexually active women ages 25 and younger who are screened annually for genital *Chlamydia trachomatis* infection.
  –Reduce the proportion of adolescents and young adults with *C. trachomatis* infection to 3% of those attending family planning and sexually transmitted disease (STD) clinics.
- Pelvic inflammatory disease (PID): Reduce the proportion of women who have ever required treatment for PID to 5%.
- Fertility problems: Reduce the proportion of childless women with fertility problems who have had an STD or who have required treatment for PID to 15%.
- Smoking cessation by adults
  –Reduce cigarette smoking by adults to 12%.
  –Increase smoking cessation attempts by adult smokers to 75%.

From US Department of Health and Human Services: *Healthy people 2010: understanding and improving health,* Washington, DC, 2000, The Department.

preparation, potassium hydroxide test (whiff test), and pH analysis. Serologic testing and urine culture may also be used. The management of vaginitis is primarily pharmacologic. Antifungal oral and topical agents are used for candidiasis; antianaerobic oral and intravaginal preparations are used for bacterial vaginitis (Table 56-1). Many of these drugs are available as over-the-counter preparations, but women are advised to seek diagnosis from their primary health care provider for an initial episode of vaginitis if symptoms do not subside after one course of over-the-counter treatment.

Risk Factors

Infections of the Vulva and Vagina

- Pregnancy
- Age—premenarche and postmenopause
- Low estrogen levels
- Dermatologic allergies
- Diabetes mellitus
- Oral contraceptive use
- Inadequate hygiene
- Douching
- Treatment with broad-spectrum antibiotics
- Use of vaginal contraceptives—foams, inserts
- Sexual intercourse with infected partner
- Frequent sexual intercourse with multiple partners
- Tight, nonabsorbent, and heat-retaining clothing

The drugs may be administered orally or by ointment, cream, or suppository. Women are informed that the use of metronidazole (Flagyl) turns the urine dark reddish brown. It also causes numerous gastrointestinal (GI) side effects that may be reduced by taking the drug with meals. The use of alcohol can trigger a disulfiram (Antabuse)–like reaction of severe nausea, vomiting, and abdominal distress and should be avoided during treatment and for 48 hours after completing the medication. The Centers for Disease Control and Prevention guidelines point out that vaginal clindamycin treatment for bacterial vaginosis may be less effective than the metronidazole regimen.[3] Complementary therapies with *Lactobacillus acidophilus* or with yogurt douches have not shown efficacy in randomized clinical trials.[17]

Patient/Family Teaching. Women have self-managed vaginitis for generations, and a number of alternative treatments are in common use. The nurse explores the woman's use of alternative therapies; ensures that the treatment is not contraindicated for the specific causative organism; and provides specific instructions about the safe and appropriate use of soaks, irrigations, and douches in vaginitis treatment.

Prevention of reinfection is an important consideration because vaginitis can easily become a recurrent problem. Thus the nurse discusses various lifestyle modifications that can reduce the incidence of vaginal infection (see Patient/Family Teaching box).

Cervicitis

Etiology and Epidemiology. The term *cervicitis* is used for a number of conditions characterized by inflammation and infection of the cervix. Risk factors include early initiation of sexual intercourse, oral contraceptive use, and multiple partners. When cervicitis is associated with human papillomavirus (HPV), it increases the risk of cervical cancer.

Pathophysiology. *Chlamydia trachomatis* is the most common offending organism, along with *Neisseria gonorrhoeae,* herpes simplex virus, HPV, and trichomonas. Leukorrhea is the most common sign, but the amount may not be significant. On examination, the cervix is grossly erythematous and edematous with or without erosion. There is usually a mucopurulent discharge, but the amount may be so small that the patient does not notice it. The woman commonly has no subjective signs but may report backache, lower abdominal pain, or painful sexual intercourse. Urinary frequency and urgency may also be present. It is important to rule out a cancerous lesion.

Collaborative Care Management. The cervix is cultured and appropriate pharmacologic therapy initiated. See Chapter 59 for a thorough discussion of the treatment of sexually transmitted diseases (STDs). If the woman's cervicitis does not respond to antibiotics or if she has significant cervical erosion, **cryosurgery**, electrocauterization or loop electrosurgical excision procedure (LEEP), or laser therapy may be necessary.

Patient/Family Teaching. The prevention of cervicitis includes those measures outlined in the Patient/Family Teaching box, since many cases of cervicitis develop from vaginal infection. If the cervici-

TABLE 56-1 COMMON CAUSES, SIGNS AND SYMPTOMS, AND TREATMENT OF VAGINITIS

Cause	Signs and Symptoms	Treatment
Bacterial vaginosis *(Gardnerella vaginalis)*	Pruritus Thin, "fishy" vaginal discharge pH <4.5, clue cells, positive potassium hydroxide test	Antibiotics with anaerobic activity (oral or intravaginal) Metronidazole Clindamycin
Fungal infections *(Candida albicans)*	Pruritus Vulvar burning and erythema Thick, white drainage Presence of yeast buds on wet-mount preparation	Antifungal agents (oral or intravaginal) Clotrimazole Miconazole Fluconazole
Protozoan infections *(Trichomonas vaginalis)*	Copious, foul-smelling discharge pH >4.5, leukocytes and flagellated organisms on wet-mount preparation "Strawberry cervix"	Antibiotics (oral) Metronidazole
Estrogen deficiency	Dryness and burning	Estrogen (oral or topical)

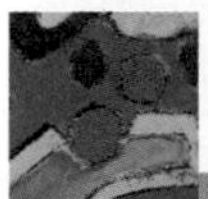

PATIENT/FAMILY TEACHING *Preventing and Treating Vaginal Infections*

Patient teaching should include information about the disease and prescribed medications and the following instructions.

Preventing Vaginal Infection

Cleanse genital area thoroughly with mild soap and water daily.
Wipe genital area from front to back after bowel movements.
Avoid use of vaginal irritants (e.g., harsh deodorant and perfumed soap, deodorant sprays, douches).
Avoid routine douching, which can alter the vaginal pH.
Use underwear with a cotton crotch and change panties daily; avoid any clothing that is tight in the crotch or thighs. Avoid wearing underpants while sleeping.
Assess sexual partners for any sign of infection (e.g., discharge, lesions, reddened areas on genitalia).
Use a barrier method of contraception.
Avoid any sexual practice that is painful or abrasive.
Avoid anal-genital intercourse.
Cleanse genital area of self and partner and void before and after sexual intercourse.
Change tampons or napkins frequently during menstruation.
Treat athlete's foot and "jock itch" with over-the-counter antifungals.
Consider taking vitamin C, 500 mg orally twice a day, to increase the acidity of vaginal secretions.
Recognize the signs of infection and respond promptly.

Managing an Existing Infection

Wash hands carefully before and after treatment.
Cleanse the genital area thoroughly with soap and water and dry well before applying any medication.
Remain recumbent for 30 minutes after insertion of a suppository or cream to facilitate absorption and prevent loss from the vagina.
Avoid use of tampons during treatment.
Wear a minipad if vaginal drainage is present.
Take sitz baths for comfort.
Refrain from sexual intercourse while the infection is being treated, and have male partner use a condom until all symptoms of inflammation have resolved.

tis was caused by an STD, then the patient's sexual contacts should receive appropriate treatment. Most treatment failures are actually reinfection from an untreated sexual partner.[4] If surgical intervention is needed, it is generally performed as an outpatient procedure, and patients are instructed accordingly. Women are told that a watery discharge is common, especially after cryosurgery, but that it resolves in several weeks. Healing is usually complete within 6 weeks. The patients are also told that they may experience mild to moderate cramping during the procedure.

Bartholinitis (Bartholin's Cysts)

Etiology and Epidemiology. Bartholin's cysts are one of the most common disorders of the vulva. They result from obstruction of a duct and may become infected. Thickened mucus, stenosis, or mechanical trauma may initiate the process.

Pathophysiology. The infection usually is unilateral but can be bilateral. *N. gonorrhoeae* is the most common infecting organism. The secretory function of the gland continues, and the duct fills up with fluid, producing severe inflammation, enlargement of the gland, and tissue edema. The area becomes tender, and even walking may be difficult. The pain is constant, and dyspareunia can be severe. The abscess may rupture, resulting in temporary symptom relief, but it usually reforms. Occasionally, the acute inflammation resolves, leaving scar tissue that can form a cyst. The cyst usually is nontender but may interfere with ambulation or sexual intercourse.

Collaborative Care Management. Cultures are taken, and the woman is treated for any underlying infectious process with broad-spectrum antibiotics. If the cysts are symptomatic, incision and drainage may be performed. The cysts tend to recur, and a permanent opening for drainage of the gland may need to be constructed by placing a tiny catheter through a stab wound into the cyst cavity. The catheter remains in the cyst for 4 to 6 weeks until healing occurs and a new duct forms. The catheter is assessed weekly. Bathing is permitted for hygiene and comfort.

PATIENT/FAMILY TEACHING. Nursing interventions focus on comfort. Mild analgesics and sitz baths help relieve pain. Because most procedures are performed on an outpatient basis, the nurse instructs the woman on home care and reinforces the need to report any signs of infection.

Pelvic Inflammatory Disease

Etiology and Epidemiology. *Pelvic inflammatory disease* (PID) is a general term that refers to acute, subacute, recurrent, or chronic infection of the reproductive organs, pelvic peritoneum, veins, or connective tissue. The infection may be confined to just one structure or be widespread. Sexually active adolescents are at greatly increased risk of contracting PID, which causes a significant number of hospitalizations for women. PID occurs in women using intrauterine devices (IUDs) more often than in women using other forms of contraception.

The risk factors for PID are the same as those for STDs: low socioeconomic status, early onset of sexual activity, multiple sex partners, vaginal douching, lower educational level, and ethnicity. Chlamydial infection and gonorrhea are frequent causes; therefore sexually active women should be screened for the organisms causing these infections in an effort to prevent PID. Surgery on the reproductive organs, childbearing, and abortion all lower the woman's resistance to infection and provide portals of entry for pathogens.

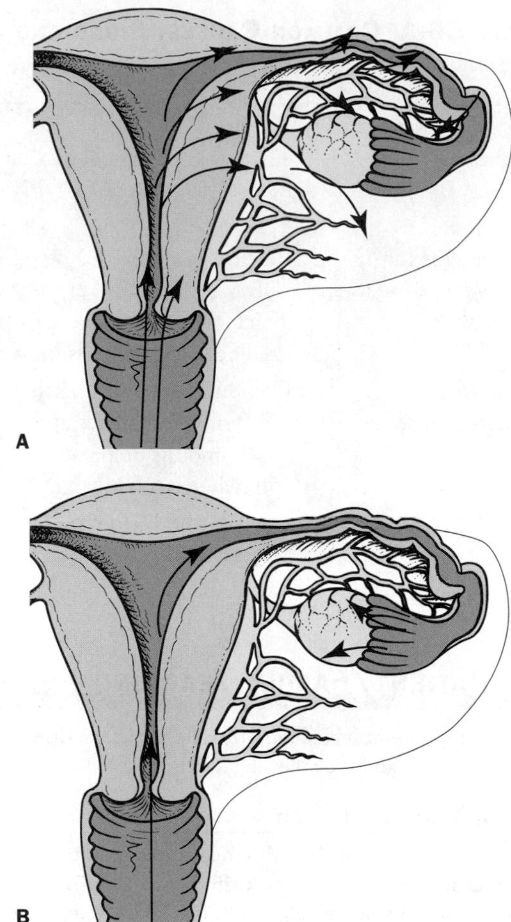

Figure 56-1 Common routes of spread of pelvic inflammatory disease. **A,** Direct spread of bacterial infection other than *Neisseria gonorrhoeae*. **B,** Direct spread of *N. gonorrhoeae*.

Pathophysiology. The routes of pelvic infection are illustrated in Figure 56-1. Pathogenic organisms usually are introduced from outside the body and pass up the cervical canal into the uterus. Common causative organisms include gonococci, chlamydiae, *Haemophilus* organisms, and streptococci. The causative organisms invade the pelvis by way of the fallopian tubes or through the uterine veins or lymphatics. Many of the pathogens lodge in the fallopian tubes and create an acute or chronic inflammatory reaction. Purulent material collects in the tubes; adhesions and strictures form; and sterility, one of the most serious consequences of PID, may occur. Partial obstruction of the tubes may predispose a woman to ectopic pregnancy because the fertilized ovum cannot reach the uterus. Inflammatory adhesions become so severe that surgical removal of the uterus, tubes, and ovaries may be necessary. The infection usually remains localized in the lower abdomen and pelvis, although abscesses may form.

Clinical manifestations of acute PID include severe abdominal pain, lower abdominal cramping, intermenstrual bleeding, dyspareunia, fever and chills, malaise, nausea, and vomiting. A sensation of pelvic pressure and back pain may also be present. A foul-smelling vaginal discharge is copious and commonly purulent and may cause pruritus and excoriation. Physical examination usually reveals abdominal tenderness on palpation and, on bimanual examination, adnexal tenderness and cervical motion tenderness (chandelier sign). Masses may be felt, indicating enlargement of the fallopian tubes or ovaries or the presence of an abscess. However, it is also possible to be asymptomatic and have normal laboratory values.

Collaborative Care Management. Diagnostic studies include white blood cell counts, C-reactive protein, erythrocyte sedimentation rate, and culture of any purulent secretions. Laparoscopy may be ordered to visualize pelvic structures, drain abscesses, and lyse obstructing adhesions. Transvaginal sonography may be used to evaluate masses and structural thickening.

Treatment is aimed at eradicating the infection and preventing complications. Hospitalization may be necessary if the woman is acutely ill. Broad-spectrum antibiotics are used until drug sensitivities are determined. If the woman has an IUD, it is generally removed 24 to 48 hours after antibiotic therapy is started.

Nursing interventions are largely supportive. Bed rest in a semi-Fowler's position is recommended to assist with pelvic drainage. Heat applied to the abdomen may be comforting, but tub or sitz baths should be avoided during active infection. Naproxen can be used for pain management. Adequate oral fluids are encouraged. Other nursing measures include managing fever, monitoring vital signs, monitoring intake and output, and providing emotional support.

PATIENT/FAMILY TEACHING. The nurse instructs the woman to cleanse the perineal region every 3 to 4 hours and maintain scrupulous hygiene after urination and defecation. Tampons should not be used, and drainage pads should be changed frequently. A minimum of 2000 ml of fluids daily is recommended. Women treated as outpatients are reminded of the importance of completing the antibiotic regimen and seeking appropriate follow-up care, since PID can have serious consequences for fertility. Patients should avoid sexual activity until the infection is adequately treated. Partner notification, treatment, and counseling should be done. The nurse stresses the importance of using condoms to prevent reinfection or future infections, along with the risk factors for PID.

▶ ARE You READY?

Which of the following interventions would the nurse question if ordered for a patient with pelvic inflammatory disease?

1. Bed rest in semi-Fowler's position
2. Sitz baths twice daily
3. Heat applied to abdomen
4. Naproxen 250 mg orally twice daily

Toxic Shock Syndrome

Etiology and Epidemiology. Toxic shock syndrome (TSS) is a severe disease that, in most cases, is caused by strains of staphylococci that produce a unique epidermal toxin. It can occur in any situation in which staphylococcal organisms can be harbored. TSS has occurred in infants, children, and men and has been associated with a variety of surgical procedures, including gynecologic, urologic, and orthopedic procedures. However, it is most common in women during menstruation, particularly women who use tampons. Women at increased risk include those who use superabsorbent tampons, insert tampons with their fingers, or have chronic vaginal infections or herpes genitalis. The overall incidence has decreased dramatically with the awareness of appropriate use of tampons. Mortality rates for patients with streptococcal TSS range from 30% to 70% despite treatment with antibiotics and supportive care.[5]

Pathophysiology. The exact mechanism by which staphylococcal toxins gain access to the circulatory system is unknown. The role of tampons also remains unclear. They may cause mucosal damage, but it is theorized that superabsorbent tampons obstruct the vagina and cause retrograde menstruation with peritoneal absorption of bacteria or toxins. The use of a diaphragm during menstruation creates a similar risk. Tampons may also cause an increase in aerobic bacteria from oxygen trapped in the interfibrous spaces. The longer a tampon is left in place, the greater the risk for TSS.

The onset of symptoms is usually abrupt, with fever, vomiting, watery diarrhea, headache, and myalgia. The patient appears acutely ill, with a fever near 102° F (39° C) or higher, and the syndrome can progress to hypotensive shock within hours. An erythematous sunburn-like rash develops over the face, proximal extremities, and trunk, followed by desquamation of the skin. Systemic symptoms often include vomiting, watery diarrhea, severe myalgia, and inflamed mucous membranes (oropharyngeal, conjunctival, or vaginal). Muscle and abdominal tenderness commonly are present. Signs of central nervous system irritation may be present. Prompt diagnosis is critical, and these symptoms occurring in a menstruating woman using tampons are thoroughly explored. If the woman is wearing a tampon, it is removed immediately.

Collaborative Care Management. Diagnostic tests for TSS include a complete blood screen and cultures of the blood, throat, urine, vaginal secretions, and possibly cerebrospinal fluid. Vaginal cultures usually show penicillinase-producing *Staphylococcus aureus*. The cornerstone of medical care is beta-lactamase–resistant antibiotics such as nafcillin, methicillin, and oxacillin. Penicillinase-resistant agents, antistaphylococcal agents, and corticosteroids may all be used. Aggressive fluid and electrolyte management is indicated if the patient shows signs of shock. Mechanical ventilation may be necessary if acute respiratory distress syndrome develops. The management of shock is discussed in detail in Chapter 19. Nursing care revolves around careful monitoring and supportive care similar to that provided for any critically ill patient (see Chapter 10).

PATIENT/FAMILY TEACHING. Approximately 30% of women who develop TSS experience recurrences. The greatest risk for recurrence is during the first three menstrual periods after treatment. Recurrent episodes are usually less severe than the initial one. Women can almost entirely eliminate the risk of TSS by avoiding tampon use. In addition to providing this information, the nurse instructs women about the importance of careful **perineal hygiene**, avoiding douching, and limiting the use of a contraceptive diaphragm to no more than 24 hours at one time. The use of tampons requires thorough hand washing before insertion. This is essential, especially for health care workers in hospital settings.

Disorders of Menstruation

Almost all women experience a problem with their menstrual cycle at some point in their reproductive years. Problems produce a variety of symptoms that may be related directly or indirectly to the pelvic organs. Most problems are self-managed and are rarely brought to a physician's attention unless they become severe or persistent.

Dysmenorrhea

Etiology and Epidemiology. Dysmenorrhea, pain during menstruation, affects 40% to 50% of menstruating women and has been cited as the most common cause of regular absenteeism among young women. Primary dysmenorrhea is not associated with pelvic pathologic conditions and occurs in the absence of any organic disease. Its severity usually declines after pregnancy or by age 30. Secondary dysmenorrhea occurs in response to organic disease such as PID, endometriosis, or leiomyomas (uterine fibroids) and to IUD use.

Pathophysiology. Dysmenorrhea is related to the high levels of **prostaglandins** that the uterus produces during menses. What causes some women to have excess prostaglandins or increased sensitivity to them remains in question, but women with dysmenorrhea have been found to have concentrations up to four times higher than those in women without pain. Prostaglandins increase uterine contractility and decrease uterine artery blood flow, causing ischemia. The end result is the painful sensation of cramps.

The pain of primary dysmenorrhea typically occurs on the first or second day of the menses. It is usually described as colicky, cramping pain in the lower abdomen that may be perceived as minor, controllable with mild analgesics, or incapacitating. Backache and other systemic symptoms, particularly involving the GI tract, may also occur.

Collaborative Care Management. Primary dysmenorrhea treatment includes nonsteroidal antiinflammatory drugs (NSAIDs), such as ibuprofen and naproxen. Oral contraceptives, which block ovulation, are also used. Vitamin E is a mild prostaglandin inhibitor and may help relieve menstrual discomfort. Treatment of secondary dysmenorrhea is aimed at correcting the underlying organic cause. Options include both pharmacologic and surgical interventions.

PATIENT/FAMILY TEACHING. Women rarely seek professional help for mild primary dysmenorrhea. However, women who are consistently unable to engage in normal activities because of menstrual pain should be encouraged to seek medical care. The nurse instructs the patient that NSAIDs are most effective when taken at the onset of menses before pain becomes severe, and can be buffered with food or antacid if GI irritation occurs. The nurse also encourages the woman to ensure adequate rest, nutrition, and exercise. Constipation should be avoided. If pain occurs, the nurse can suggest that the woman use local heat, which helps dilate the blood vessels and relieve ischemia. Massage can also soothe aching muscles and promote relaxation and blood flow.

Amenorrhea

Etiology and Epidemiology. Amenorrhea is the absence of menstruation. Primary amenorrhea exists if the first menses has not occurred by age 16. Secondary amenorrhea exists when an established menses, of longer than 3 months, ceases. Skipping an occasional single period is normal. Pregnancy is the most common cause of secondary amenorrhea. Amenorrhea can result from anatomic abnormalities, genetic conditions, hypothalamic or pituitary dysfunction, or ovarian failure.

Pathophysiology. Anatomic abnormalities include congenital absence of the uterus, ovaries, or vagina; congenital obstruction; or imperforate hymen. Hypothalamic dysfunction can be related to marked weight loss, excessive exercise, and severe prolonged stress. Pituitary dysfunction can result from disease and tumors of the pituitary that cause changes in many hormones that the pituitary gland manufactures. Sheehan's syndrome, head trauma, and cancer may also cause hypopituitarism. Ovarian failure can be related to genetic disorders such as Turner's syndrome. Other causes of ovarian failure include radiation exposure, chemotherapy, viral infection, and surgical removal of the ovary.

Collaborative Care Management. The diagnostic workup for amenorrhea includes a detailed history and careful examination of the reproductive system. Laboratory analysis of levels of follicle-stimulating hormone, prolactin, thyroid-stimulating hormone, cortisol, calcium, and autoantibodies, as well as assessment of karyotype, may be indicated. Pregnancy should be ruled out as a possible cause. The treatment depends on the cause. An organic problem is corrected, if possible, through surgery or hormone replacement.

PATIENT/FAMILY TEACHING. The nurse teaches the woman about the problem, its causes, and the diagnostic studies planned. Teaching may include information about weight gain, stress reduction, and the energy drain of strenuous exercise. Women may need counseling and support to deal with feelings of threat to their self-concept and concerns over fertility related to the amenorrhea.

Premenstrual Syndrome

Etiology and Epidemiology. The term *premenstrual syndrome* (PMS) has been given to a cluster of distressing physical and behavioral symptoms that occur in the second half of the menstrual cycle and are followed by a symptom-free period. Premenstrual dysphoric disorder (PMDD) is an official psychiatric diagnosis used to describe severe mood swings and physical symptoms that begin 7 to 14 days before menses and interfere with social and role functioning. PMDD is considered a severe form of PMS distinguished by the severity of its emotional component. Estimates suggest that up to 80% of women experience physical or emotional changes premenstrually, but only 20% to 40% of these women have problems as a consequence. An even smaller number, 2.5% to 5%, think that the changes jeopardize their work, home life, and relationships.[9]

The cause of PMS is unknown, although there are many theories to explain it. Researchers currently speculate that PMS is related to serotonin, since serotonin levels in women with PMS fall after ovulation.[9]

Pathophysiology. Symptoms of PMS are many and varied and range in severity from mild to severe. The symptoms are not well defined and involve multiple body systems. The lack of a proven cause makes it difficult to track a cause-and-effect relationship for physiologic changes and observed or reported symptoms. The symptoms appear only in the luteal phase of the menstrual cycle and disappear completely with menopause. Symptoms include affective and somatic complaints, including depression, irritability, anger, confusion, anxiety, social withdrawal, breast tenderness, abdominal bloating, headache, acne, swelling, cravings for sweets, constipation, vertigo, and possibly migraines. The physical symptoms of PMDD are identical to those of PMS, but the affective symptoms are more serious. For example, a feeling of sadness and mild depression is often characteristic of PMS, whereas hopelessness and significant depression are characteristic of PMDD.

Collaborative Care Management. No objective means of diagnosing PMS exists, so the diagnosis is primarily established by exclusion. A careful clinical history is critical. The woman is asked to keep an accurate diary during her menstrual periods of the occurrence, nature, and severity of symptoms. A woman is considered to have PMS if her symptoms interfere with activities of daily living. Symptoms that occur in the 5 days preceding menses for two consecutive cycles confirm the diagnosis. Women who have menstrual symptoms have a significantly lower health status compared with women who report none (see Research box).

Numerous treatments have been suggested, including both pharmacologic and nonpharmacologic strategies, but no treatment has proved effective in all cases. In severe cases treatment focuses on lifestyle changes and natural approaches. Pharmacologic treatments include vitamin supplementation, diuretics, and prostaglandin inhibitors. For a woman who is not planning a pregnancy, the use of oral contraceptives is often useful.

PATIENT/FAMILY TEACHING. The nurse helps the woman and her family understand the possible causes of the syndrome and the rationale for any planned treatments. Simple lifestyle modifications can reduce symptoms and improve the woman's overall wellbeing. Regular aerobic exercise is strongly recommended, since exercise results in a release of endorphins, which can elevate the mood. The nurse encourages the woman to avoid fatigue, because it exaggerates the symptoms of PMS. This is particularly important in the premenstrual period. Dietary supplements may help relieve symptoms of PMS (see Complementary & Alternative Therapies box). Stress management techniques are also recommended. The Patient/Family Teaching box summarizes patient teaching related to PMS. The nurse can refer interested patients and families to the National Women's Health Information Center (http://www.4woman.gov) or the National PMS Society.

Dysfunctional Uterine Bleeding

Etiology and Epidemiology. Dysfunctional uterine bleeding (DUB) is abnormal vaginal bleeding that occurs during menstrual cycles in which ovulation does not take place. The term *dysfunctional uterine bleeding* should only be used for anovulatory bleeding.[10] DUB is a diagnosis of exclusion, which means that it is

Research

Barnard K et al: Health status among women with menstrual symptoms, *J Women's Health* 12(9):911-919, 2003.

Menstrual symptoms (including irregular menses, hypermenorrhea, dysmenorrhea, and premenstrual syndrome) are common, but little is known about their impact on health status. A study was done to determine the prevalence of menstrual symptoms and the degree to which these symptoms affect health status as measured by the Medical Outcomes Study's Short Form 36. The women in the study were a randomly selected sample of veterans who had made at least one ambulatory visit to a Veterans Administration facility.

The results were that the veterans who reported one or more menstrual symptoms had significantly lower health status compared with those reporting none. Health care providers who are caring for women should be attuned to the potential impact of menstrual symptoms on the lives of their patients.

Complementary & Alternative Therapies

Premenstrual Syndrome

Here is what is currently known about the effectiveness of some of the more common complementary dietary supplements used to soothe the symptoms of premenstrual syndrome (PMS):

- *Calcium:* Consuming 1200 mg/day of dietary and supplemental calcium may reduce the physical and psychologic symptoms of PMS.
- *Magnesium:* Consuming 200 mg/day of magnesium may help reduce fluid retention, breast tenderness, and bloating.
- *Vitamin E:* This vitamin, taken dosages of in 400 IU/day, may ease PMS symptoms by reducing the production of prostaglandin hormone-like substances that cause cramps and breast tenderness.

All patients should check with their health care provider before taking any dietary supplements.

From Mayo clinic staff: *Premenstrual syndrome,* accessed Jan 2004 from website: www.mayoclinic.com.

determined only after ruling out other causes of abnormal vaginal bleeding such as systemic disease, medications, early pregnancy disorders, eating disorders, gynecologic infections, structural anomalies, tumors, or polyps (Table 56-2).

Pathophysiology. **Anovulatory cycles** are common for the first year after menarche and later in life as a woman approaches menopause. The exact cause of an anovulatory cycle is not known, but it may represent a dysfunction of the hypothalamic-pituitary-ovarian axis that results in continuing estrogen stimulation of the endometrium. The endometrium outgrows its blood supply, partially breaks down, and is sloughed in an irregular manner. Anovulation may result from other endocrine disorders.

Collaborative Care Management. The diagnostic workup for DUB begins with a thorough history of the frequency, amount, and duration of bleeding. Pelvic examination is done to detect gross abnormalities, which are further evaluated by pelvic or transvaginal ultrasound, hysteroscopy, or endometrial biopsy.

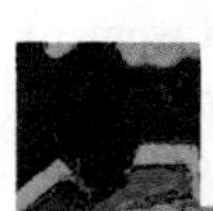

PATIENT/FAMILY TEACHING
The Patient With Premenstrual Syndrome

Patient teaching should include information about the disease, prescribed medications, and various relaxation techniques and the following instructions:

- Avoid stressful activities during the premenstrual period.
- Ensure adequate rest, especially during the premenstrual period. Fatigue exaggerates symptoms.
- Take medications as prescribed (explain rationale).
- Reduce or eliminate smoking and alcohol consumption.
- Follow a regular exercise program.
- Eat a well-balanced diet with complex carbohydrates and a reduced intake of salt and refined sugars.
- Incorporate stress-reducing strategies into daily lifestyle.
- Use relaxation techniques regularly.

TABLE 56-2 CAUSES OF ABNORMAL UTERINE BLEEDING DURING CHILDBEARING AND POSTMENOPAUSAL YEARS

Type	Cause
Hypermenorrhea (menorrhagia): prolonged, profuse menstrual flow during regular period	Submucous myomas, pregnancy complications, adenomyosis, endometrial hyperplasias, malignant tumors, hypothyroidism, von Willebrand's disease
Metrorrhagia: bleeding between periods	Endometrial polyps, endometrial and cervical cancer, exogenous estrogen administration
Polymenorrhea: increased frequency of menstruation	Anovulation, shortened luteal phase
Cryptomenorrhea: unusually light menstrual flow	Hymenal or cervical stenosis, Asherman's syndrome (uterine synechiae), oral contraceptives
Menometrorrhagia: bleeding at irregular intervals	Any condition causing intermenstrual bleeding; sudden onset indicates malignant tumors or complications of pregnancy
Oligomenorrhea: menstrual periods more than 35 days apart	Anovulation from endocrine causes (pregnancy, menopause) or systemic causes (excessive weight loss); estrogen-secreting tumors
Dysfunctional uterine bleeding: abnormal bleeding	Anovulation possibly caused by problem in hypothalamic-pituitary-ovarian axis

Laboratory tests may include blood counts to estimate blood loss, pregnancy tests, endocrine studies, ovulation tests, and coagulation studies.

The cause of the bleeding guides medical care. In the absence of an organic cause the preferred treatment is usually conservative. The goals of treatment are to control bleeding, prevent or treat anemia, prevent hyperplasia of the endometrium, and restore the quality of the women's life. Pharmacologic options to stop heavy bleeding or reduce future blood loss in subsequent menstrual cycles include the use of estrogens, progestins, NSAIDs, antifibrinolytic agents, and gonadotropin-releasing hormone (GnRH) agonists such as danazol. Dilation and curettage (D&C), endometrial ablation, or hysterectomy may be necessary for those women whose bleeding cannot be controlled with hormones.

PATIENT/FAMILY TEACHING. Because most care for DUB is provided in the outpatient setting, the nursing role is largely educational. The impact of chronic excessive bleeding on a woman's lifestyle can be profound. The nurse teaches the woman to accurately assess the amount of bleeding in terms of number of pads or tampons, type of pad or tampon, and degree of saturation. The nurse helps the woman set up and maintain a diary to accurately record the bleeding. The nurse also encourages the woman to express her concerns and fears. Anxiety related to infertility or fear of cancer can be intense but remain unexpressed.

Endometriosis

Etiology and Epidemiology. Endometriosis is a condition in which endometrial cells that normally line the uterus are seeded throughout the pelvis. Endometriosis typically affects women during their childbearing years; it affects approximately 10% to 15% of the female population and often causes pelvic pain. The cause of endometriosis remains unknown. Proposed causative factors include retrograde menstrual flow of the endometrium, physiologic disturbance after gynecologic surgery or cesarean birth, hereditary tendency, and an immunologic defect.

Pathophysiology. With each menstrual period the seeded endometrial cells are stimulated by ovarian hormones and bleed into the surrounding tissues, causing an inflammatory response. Encased blood may lead to palpable masses known as chocolate cysts. Occasionally the cysts rupture and spread endometrial cells deeper into the pelvis. Repeated inflammation and healing may create adhesions severe enough to fuse pelvic organs or cause bowel or bladder strictures.

The ovaries are the most common site of involvement, and the process is usually bilateral (Figure 56-2). The pelvic peritoneum; the anterior and posterior cul-de-sac; and the uterosacral, round, and broad ligaments are other common sites.

Endometriosis progresses gradually and usually does not produce symptoms until the woman is 30 to 40 years of age. The classic feature is menstrual pain or discomfort that becomes progressively worse. Other possible symptoms include abdominal pain, dyspareunia, irregular menses, bowel problems, and urinary dysfunction. Pelvic examination often reveals a fixed, retroverted uterus that is enlarged, tender, and nodular. Occasionally, the disease is far advanced but causes no symptoms, and it may first be diagnosed as part of a workup for infertility. Researchers are investigating the possibility that women with endometriosis lack specific molecules in the uterus that allow the embryo to attach to the uterus (see Future Watch box).

Collaborative Care Management. Laparoscopy is the only definitive method of diagnosing endometriosis. The endoscopy is used to carefully map and describe the extent of disease involvement. Biopsies of suspicious tissue can be obtained during the procedure.

Because the cause of endometriosis is not understood, treatment is highly individualized. In rare cases endometriosis disappears

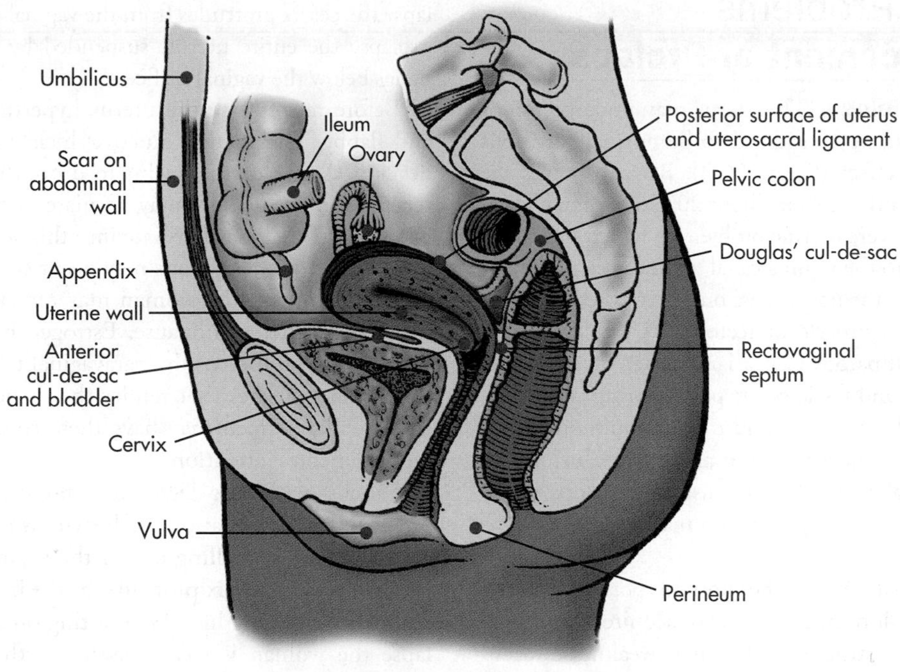

Figure 56-2 Common locations for endometriosis.

Future Watch

Endometriosis

Researchers at the National Institutes of Health report that some women who experience infertility as a result of endometriosis lack molecules in the uterus that allow the embryo to attach to the uterine wall. The researchers report that a number of genes present in the uteri of endometriosis patients appear to be functioning inappropriately. The researchers' data support the theory that having certain genes in the incorrect amount contributes to the development of endometriosis. It may also create an inhospitable environment for an embryo to attach to the uterus. The findings add weight to the hypothesis that the endometrium of women with endometriosis is abnormal. These findings might lead to a new way to screen for the disease. Currently, diagnosis requires a laparoscopy or laparotomy. This new research may one day enable scientists to develop a less invasive test, based on the detection of abnormal gene activity.

Researchers identify a possible cause of infertility in some women with endometriosis, *NIH News*, June 17, 2003, accessed from website: www.nih.gov/news/pr/jun2003/nichd-17.htm.

spontaneously. Pregnancy appears to slow the progression of the condition, since menstruation is halted during pregnancy and lactation. Some women remain asymptomatic after pregnancy. A couple may be encouraged to attempt pregnancy if children are desired, because the fertility rate of women with endometriosis is low and continues to deteriorate with time. Mild cases may be managed with NSAIDs and regular monitoring.

Hormonal treatment with agents such as danazol, medroxyprogesterone, oral contraceptives, and GnRH agonists has been effective in reducing the pain of endometriosis. Oral contraceptives with minimal estrogen and high levels of progestins may be used to produce endometrial atrophy. Disadvantages to this approach include irregular bleeding and symptoms such as nausea, fatigue, and depression.

Drugs with antigonadotropic action, such as danazol, may be used to suppress ovarian activity. Danazol stops endometrial proliferation, prevents ovulation, and produces atrophy of the ectopic endometrial tissue. The major drawbacks to the treatment are its high cost and common side effects such as hot flashes, depression, and weight gain. GnRH agonists are even more expensive. These drugs induce a hypoestrogenic state and result in amenorrhea. Side effects mimic the symptoms of menopause. A steady loss in bone density limits the duration of possible treatment.

Surgical intervention may be necessary if the disorder does not respond to drug therapy. Conservative approaches that attempt to preserve the woman's fertility include lysis of adhesions and destruction of pockets of implanted endometrial tissue by means of laparoscopic laser surgery. More radical surgery involves the removal of the uterus, tubes, and possibly the ovaries. Ovarian function is preserved if at all possible. The onset of menopause halts the disorder.

PATIENT/FAMILY TEACHING. Because most care for women with endometriosis is delivered in the community, the nurse's role is largely educational and supportive. The nurse reassures the woman that endometriosis can be treated. The nurse teaches about the prescribed drugs, the management of side effects, and strategies to manage chronic pain. The importance of ongoing follow-up care is reinforced. Referral to support groups may be beneficial, particularly for women with infertility related to the endometriosis. Two excellent organizations are the Endometriosis Association (http://www.endometriosisassn.org) and RESOLVE: The National Infertility Association (http://www.resolve.org).

Structural Problems

Uterine Displacement or Prolapse

Etiology and Epidemiology. The uterus may undergo minor displacement in ways that are considered to be normal variations with little or no clinical effect (Figure 56-3). Retroversion is the most common variation and occurs in about 20% of women. Uterine prolapse represents a severe uterine problem in which the uterus is displaced downward into the vaginal canal, even to the point that the cervix and the body of the uterus pass outside of the body. It is usually associated with a cystocele or rectocele. Uterine prolapse occurs most often in multiparous Caucasian women as a response to injuries to the muscles and fascia of the pelvis during childbirth. Systemic conditions, such as obesity and chronic pulmonary disease, and local conditions, such as ascites and uterine or ovarian tumors, are other potential causes. Prolapse usually develops gradually, suggesting that the effects of aging play a major role.

Pathophysiology. Variations in the normal position of the uterus or prolapse can result from congenital or acquired abnormalities of the pelvic support structures. Acquired weaknesses occur after childbirth, surgery, and closely spaced pregnancies and in response to obesity and the loss of tissue elasticity with aging. The severity of the prolapse is designated by degree. In a first-degree prolapse the cervix is still within the vagina. In a second-degree prolapse the cervix protrudes from the vaginal orifice. In a third-degree prolapse the entire uterus, suspended by its stretched ligaments, hangs below the vaginal orifice.

Before menopause the uterus hypertrophies and is engorged and flabby. The vaginal mucosa thickens, and stasis ulcers may develop. As the uterus begins to drop, the vaginal walls become relaxed and the bladder may herniate into the vagina (cystocele), or the rectal wall may herniate into the vagina (rectocele) (see Figure 56-3). Both conditions may occur simultaneously. Cystoceles are common, and the woman may remain completely asymptomatic until after menopause. Estrogen helps maintain adequate blood flow and tone of the paravaginal tissues, and its loss results in atrophic changes that render the tissues more subject to prolapse. Older women may have these conditions for years before seeking medical attention.

Patients with first-degree prolapse experience few symptoms but may report sensations of heaviness or fullness and a feeling that something is falling out of the vagina. In more severe prolapse, when the cervix protrudes at the introitus, the patient may complain of feeling like she is sitting on a ball. With severe prolapse the woman is clearly aware of the mass. Leukorrhea or menometrorrhagia may develop in premenopausal women with prolapse as a result of uterine engorgement. After menopause, discharge and bleeding with prolapse usually result from infection and ulceration.

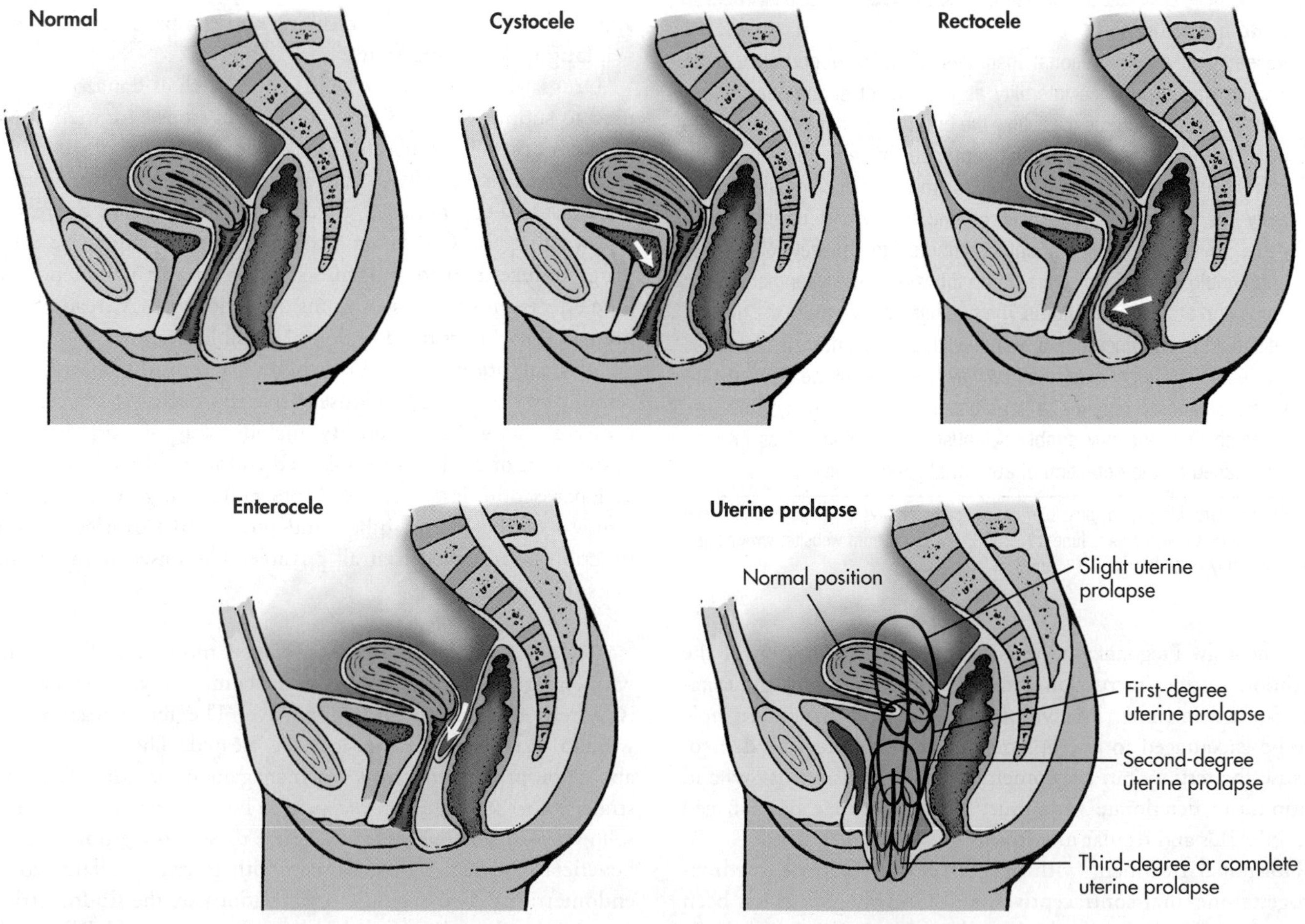

Figure 56-3 Types of uterine displacement.

The woman with a cystocele may complain of urinary incontinence accompanying any activity that increases intraabdominal pressure, such as coughing, laughing, or lifting. She may also experience frequent urinary tract infections. The patient with a rectocele may complain of chronic constipation and develop hemorrhoids.

Collaborative Care Management. Uterine prolapse can be readily identified on pelvic examination. If a cystocele is present, the vaginal outlet is relaxed with a thin-walled, smooth, bulging mass present in the anterior vaginal wall below the cervix. The mass descends when the patient is asked to bear down. If a rectocele is present, palpation of the vaginal area reveals a thin-walled rectovaginal septum projecting into the vagina. Many women are found to have both a cystocele and a rectocele.

A first-degree prolapse in a postmenopausal woman is treated with estrogen therapy to maintain the tone and integrity of the pelvic floor muscles. Exercise therapy is suggested for all women. (Exercises for the pelvic floor are discussed under Patient/Family Teaching.) If pain or bleeding occurs, the uterus may be manually repositioned and supported by the insertion of a vaginal pessary (Figure 56-4). Pessaries are devices made of hard rubber or plastic that maintain the uterus in a forward position by exerting pressure on the ligaments attached to the posterior wall of the cervix.

Conservative treatment with estrogen, exercise, and a pessary may also be employed for a cystocele or rectocele if the woman experiences only mild symptoms. Surgery to repair cystoceles, rectoceles, and more advanced prolapses is undertaken when symptoms significantly interfere with the patient's lifestyle or threaten other organ function, such as the kidney if repeated urinary tract infections are present. The procedures designed to tighten the vaginal wall are referred to as anterior and posterior colporrhaphy. They are often combined with hysterectomy. Cystocele repair may be done abdominally and combined with a urethrovesical suspension procedure, called a Marshall-Marchetti-Krantz procedure, to correct stress incontinence.

PATIENT/FAMILY TEACHING. Exercise teaching is an important nursing intervention for any patient with a uterine displacement or prolapse. Kegel perineal exercises are the mainstay. The woman is instructed to tighten the muscles of the perineum as if to stop the flow of urine, maintain the tension for 5 seconds at a time, and repeat the exercise in sets of 10. The exercise is repeated 10 to 12 times daily. Knee-chest exercises are used less often but may be ordered to stretch or strengthen the pelvic ligaments. Corrective exercises for poor posture may also be prescribed.

The nurse encourages obese patients to lose weight to reduce intraabdominal pressure. Chronic cough and chronic constipation are also corrected, since these conditions contribute to weakness of the muscular wall.

Women fitted with a pessary need to be taught how to insert it and withdraw it if the device becomes displaced or uncomfortable. Pessaries are removed and cleaned once every few weeks or months as recommended by the physician. If the pessary is neglected, it can cause infection or fistula. Women who undergo anterior colporrhaphy are instructed to refrain from heavy lifting, straining, and strenuous exercise for 3 months. Sexual intercourse may be resumed after about 3 weeks (see Guidelines for Safe Practice box).

Fistulas

Etiology and Epidemiology. A fistula is an abnormal tunnel-like opening between hollow internal organs or between an organ and the exterior of the body. Fistulas can develop from a variety of causes but are usually the result of surgery, childbirth, trauma, or radiotherapy.

The name of the fistula indicates the connecting structures. Fistulas can develop between the vagina and the rectum (rectovaginal), bladder (vesicovaginal), or urethra (urethrovaginal) (Figure 56-5). Vesicovaginal fistulas are the most common, followed by rectovaginal fistulas.

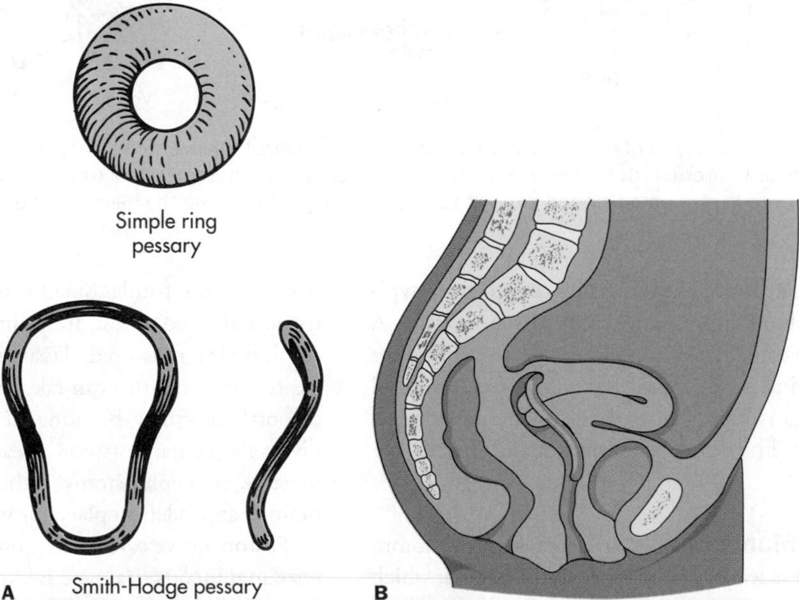

Figure 56-4 **A,** Examples of pessaries (simple ring, Smith-Hodge). **B,** Pessary in place to hold posterior vaginal fornix and, with it, attached cervix wall backward and upward in pelvis.

GUIDELINES FOR SAFE PRACTICE *The Patient Undergoing Vaginal Surgery*

- Provide perineal care after each voiding or defecation.
  —Pour sterile normal saline over vulva and perineum.
  —Cleanse perineum as needed with sterile cotton balls; cleanse away from vagina toward rectum.
  —Dry perineum as needed with sterile cotton balls.
- Encourage sitz baths after sutures are removed.
- If douches are ordered during immediate postoperative period:
  —Use sterile equipment and sterile solution.
  —Insert douche nozzle very gently.
- Prepare patient for discharge by instructing her to:
  —Take daily douches and tub baths as prescribed.
  —Avoid straining at stool.
  —Use stool softeners and laxatives as prescribed.
  —Avoid lifting for 6 weeks.
  —Avoid sexual intercourse until physician gives permission (usually about 6 weeks).
  —Avoid jarring activities.
  —Avoid prolonged standing, walking, or sitting.
  —Continue leg exercises for 6 weeks.
  —Recognize that vaginal sensation may be lost for several months after surgery, but sensation will return.
  —Eat a high-fiber diet, and drink 3000 ml of fluids daily.

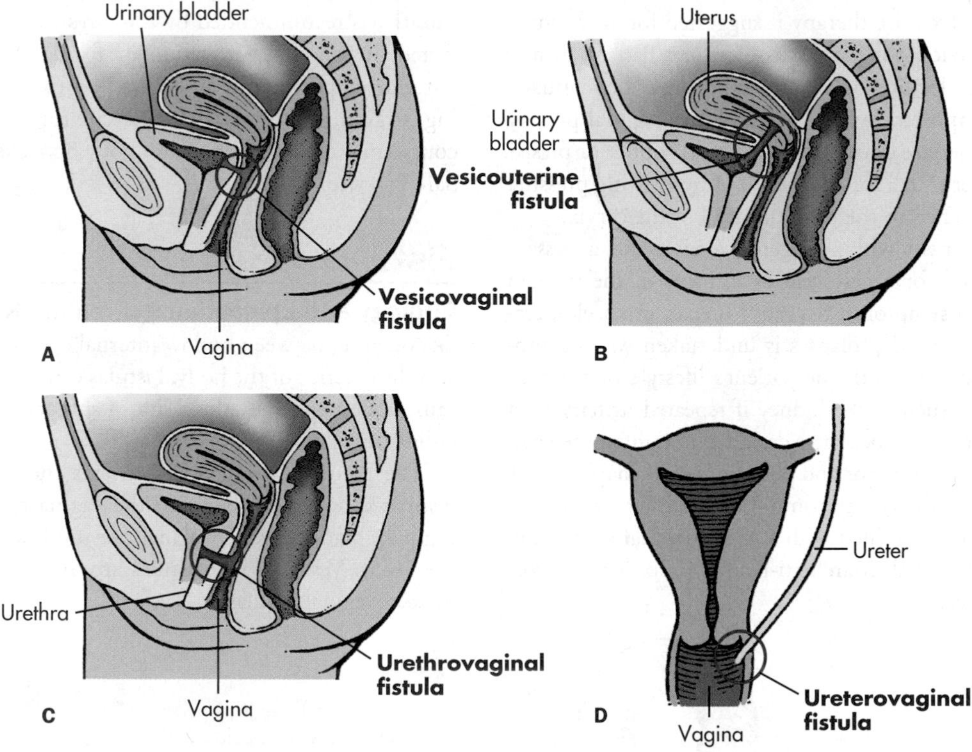

Figure 56-5 Types of genitourinary fistulas. **A,** Vesicovaginal (bladder to vagina). **B,** Vesicouterine (bladder to uterus). **C,** Urethrovaginal (urethra to vagina). **D,** Ureterovaginal (ureter to vagina). Fistulas range in size from tiny and difficult to locate to large, disfiguring the base of the bladder.

Pathophysiology. Conditions that cause fistulas to form typically compromise the blood supply and cause tissue damage. A passageway between the vagina and the bladder or rectum results in a constant leak of urine or escape of flatus and fecal material through the vagina. This is highly distressing to the patient and creates an offensive odor. The drainage excoriates and irritates the vaginal and vulvar tissue.

Collaborative Care Management. The primary symptom of a genitourinary fistula is leakage of urine into the vagina, which can be a source of embarrassment for the woman. Fistulas are diagnosed primarily through pelvic examination with the patient in the knee-chest position. A fistulogram, which involves the injection of dye into the vagina, may be used to assess the exact location and severity of the fistula. Small fistulas may heal spontaneously if the tissue is allowed to rest. If healing does not occur within 6 months, surgical closure is used. Tissue inflammation and edema must be treated first, and this can take months. Either anterior or posterior colporrhaphy may be done. It may be necessary to temporarily divert the urinary or fecal stream in complex situations. A Foley, ureteral, or nephrostomy catheter is used to keep the area well drained and is left in place for weeks in some patients.

Postoperative care focuses on tissue healing. A small amount of serosanguineous drainage is expected, but the patient is carefully monitored for continued fecal or urinary drainage. Douches may be ordered, and the nurse administers them gently and at low pressure to protect healing tissue. Bed rest is often enforced for several days.

If the fistula is being conservatively managed, nursing intervention focuses on comfort and the prevention of infection. Sitz baths and careful cleansing with mild soap and water are helpful. Although protective pads may be worn, the nurse stresses that cleansing must be repeated at regular intervals to prevent skin breakdown and odor.

Surgical repair is not always successful, and repeat procedures may be needed. The risk of infection is constantly present, and the nurse anticipates that the patient may become anxious and depressed about her situation. The nurse encourages the patient to verbalize her concerns and seek support from family and friends.

Benign and Malignant Neoplasms of the Female Reproductive Tract

Neoplasms of the Cervix

Cervical Polyps

Etiology and Epidemiology. Cervical polyps are relatively common. The two main types are (1) endocervical from the canal in the opening of the cervix and (2) ectocervical from the lower portion of the cervix that protrudes into the vagina. Endocervical polyps tend to occur in middle-aged multiparous women. Ectocervical polyps are found most often in postmenopausal women. Polyps are thought to arise from hyperplasia, possibly in response to chronic inflammation, abnormal responses to hormonal stimulation, or localized vascular congestion. Hyperestrogenism is thought to play a major role. Although most cervical polyps are benign, some cervical cancers manifest as a polypoid mass.

Pathophysiology. Most polyps are asymptomatic and discovered on routine pelvic examination. Endocervical polyps are usually reddish purple to cherry red, smooth, soft growths that may vary from a few millimeters to 2 or 3 cm in diameter and length. They are usually attached to the mucosa by a narrow pedicle and may be single or multiple. Ectocervical polyps are pale or flesh colored, round or elongated, and often attached with a broad pedicle. Polyps are usually vascular. The classic symptom is intermenstrual bleeding, particularly after sexual intercourse or douching. Leukorrhea may be present. The chronic irritation and bleeding can lead to cervicitis, endometritis, or even salpingitis.

Collaborative Care Management. Cervical polyps are usually diagnosed by direct inspection and can be removed safely in a physician's office through clamping or incision. The procedure causes minimal bleeding, but if bleeding should occur, it can be controlled by electrical or chemical cautery. All the excised tissue is sent for pathologic examination.

PATIENT/FAMILY TEACHING. The nurse encourages the woman to rest and avoid strenuous activity after polyp removal. A perineal pad can be provided to absorb drainage. The nurse instructs the woman to report any significant bleeding or signs of infection. The nurse also instructs the woman to avoid tampon use, douches, and sexual intercourse for about a week while healing takes place.

Cancer of the Cervix

Etiology and Epidemiology. An estimated 10,370 diagnosed cases of cervical cancer and 3710 deaths from the disease were expected to occur in the United States in 2005.[1] Virtually all squamous cell cervical carcinomas contain one of 18 types of HPV.[14] Risk factors for cervical cancer include multiple sex partners, first sexual intercourse before age 16, and ethnicity (see Risk Factors box). A recent study suggests that women who are overweight are more likely to die of cervical cancer.[12] Another study states smoking may double cervical cancer risk.[15] Yet another study found an increased risk by more than 50% after 5 years of oral contraceptive use.[16]

Immunosuppression also increases the risk of cervical cancer, and studies indicate that women positive for HIV are at high risk for cervical cancer and have a poorer disease prognosis. STDs are also linked with atypical cell transformation. Dietary factors include deficiencies of vitamins A and C and derangement in folic acid metabolism.

Cervical cancer screening through **Pap tests** has significantly reduced the mortality rate associated with cervical cancer in the United States. Cancer of the cervix is the leading cause of cancer deaths among women in developing countries with inadequate cervical screening programs.

The incidence of cervical cancer in the United States has generally declined, although the overall incidence of Pap test abnormalities has risen rapidly over the past 2 decades. Cervical carcinoma in situ, a precancerous noninvasive stage, is now the most common form diagnosed and peaks in incidence between the ages of 25 and 35. Preinvasive lesions seem to occur in some populations at an

Risk Factors

Cervical Cancer

Risk Factors

- Human papillomavirus infection
- Cigarette smoking
- Low socioeconomic status
- Early age at first coitus
- Multiple sexual partners
- History of sexually transmitted diseases
- High-risk male partner
- Compromised immunity, including human immunodeficiency virus infection
- Early age at first pregnancy
- Multiparity, especially for African-Americans, Hispanic-Americans, and Native Americans
- Prostitution

Potential Risk Factors

- Heavy use of talc
- Use of oral contraceptives
- Deficiencies of vitamins A and C
- Derangement of folic acid metabolism
- Intrauterine exposure to diethylstilbestrol
- Diabetes
- Nulliparity
- Frequent douching

early age, perhaps related to the sexual practices of teenagers. The incidence of invasive cervical cancer increases with age. Women need to be informed of and supported in their efforts to reduce their modifiable risk factors for cervical cancer. Patient teaching relative to the prevention of cervical cancer is presented in the Patient/Family Teaching box.

Pathophysiology. Ninety-five percent of all cervical cancers are squamous cell, arising from the epidermal layer of the cervix. Cell **dysplasia** indicates the presence of a precursor lesion, typically called cervical intraepithelial neoplasia (CIN), which has been divided into three stages:

- CIN I: mild to moderate dysplasia
- CIN II: moderate to severe dysplasia
- CIN III: severe dysplasia to carcinoma in situ

Women diagnosed with dysplasia may experience disease regression, persistence, or a progression to carcinoma. Usually no signs or symptoms are related to dysplasia, and the diagnosis is based on cytologic findings. Early detection is important to ensure positive outcomes. Routine Pap screening begins within 3 years of the onset of sexual activity or at age 21 (Box 56-1).[6] Undertested groups, including ethnic minorities and older women, need special encouragement to have routine Pap screening. Abnormal tests should be followed up with colposcopy and biopsy to further investigate cellular change.

Cervical cancer spreads through the blood, by direct extension, and by lymph invasion. As the lymph nodes grow larger, venous flow is obstructed, and leg edema, ureteral obstruction, or hydronephrosis may occur. Distant organ metastasis to the lung, liver, or bone can occur in the advanced stage. Prognosis is based on the stage of the disease, depth of invasion, and vascular involvement of the tumor (Table 56-3).

Cervical cancer is asymptomatic in the early stages. As the disease progresses, the woman may experience a slight watery vaginal discharge and occasional bloody spotting, especially after sexual intercourse. With advanced disease, a foul-smelling discharge may develop from sloughing of the epithelial tissue. Pain is usually a late sign and can involve the pelvis, flank, lower back, and abdomen. The growing tumor may place pressure on the rectum and bladder, causing irritation and discharge. Hemorrhage is possible with advanced infiltrative tumors, which may also erode the walls of adjacent organs and create fistulas. The signs and symptoms of cervical cancer are summarized in the Clinical Manifestations box.

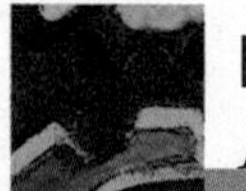

Patient/Family Teaching
Prevention of Cervical Cancer

- Reinforce importance of condom use during sexual intercourse to limit transmission of sexually transmitted diseases and genital viruses.
- Encourage adolescent girls to delay the onset of sexual activity and limit the number of their sex partners.
- Teach importance of prompt and effective treatment of vaginal or cervical infections.
- Stress importance of following American Cancer Society guidelines for Pap screening (see Box 56-1).
- Implement Agency for Healthcare Research and Quality guidelines on tobacco cessation. Ask about smoking status and exposure to environmental sources. Advise about quitting; ask if woman is ready to set quit date. Support smoking cessation efforts and plan follow-up support.

Box 56-1 New Guidelines on Pap Tests

New cervical cancer screening guidelines issued by the U.S. Preventive Services Task Force (USPSTF) and the American Cancer Society (ACS) are noteworthy because they call for less screening of adolescents, older women, and women who have had a hysterectomy. They also address the role of new and emerging testing technologies. Major changes in both guidelines are:

- *Starting screening:* Both guidelines say that screening with cervical cytology should begin within 3 years of the onset of sexual activity or at age 21, whichever comes first. Previous guidelines recommended starting screening at age 18 or at the onset of sexual activity.
- *Screening intervals:* Once they have begun screening, women should be tested annually until age 30. If results are normal for 2 or 3 years in a row and the patient has no new risk factors, screen every 2 or 3 years thereafter. (The ACS recommends screening annually until age 30 if performing a conventional Pap test or every 2 years if using a liquid-based Pap test.)
- *Posthysterectomy patients:* Both sets of guidelines advise discontinuing screening for women who have had a total hysterectomy for benign conditions. However, screening should continue for the small number of women (less than 1%) who retain their cervix after undergoing a hysterectomy.
- *Ending screening:* Both guidelines recommend against routinely screening women after ages 65 to 70 if they have received regular screening with normal results three times in a row. Continue screening patients over 65 who have other risks for cervical cancer (such as human immunodeficiency virus infection or immune system disorders) or a history of high-grade lesions.

From American College of Physicians Observer, April 2003, accessed from website: www.acponline.org/journals/news/apr03/pap_guides.htm#overview.

Complications. Recurrence and metastasis of the cancer are the primary concerns. The diagnosis can compromise the woman's body image, sexuality, and fertility. Implant therapy results in radiation-induced menopause, which adds to the challenge of keeping the vagina dilated, supple, and lubricated for sexual intercourse. Prolonged vaginal discharge does not promote the resumption of sexual activity, and the couple's relationship can deteriorate as a result of communication problems between the partners. The woman must also cope with odor and drainage that can compromise her image of herself as a desirable sexual being. Physical complications such as fistula formation, tissue fibrosis, and inflammatory bowel problems are addressed in the discharge teaching, but the woman typically finds herself at home, dealing with the changes alone. The nurse again stresses the importance of social support.

Collaborative Care Management

Diagnostic Tests. Women with CIN are monitored closely with repeat Pap tests. Colposcopy is used to examine cervical lesions and to direct cervical biopsies. Cervical conization can also

TABLE 56-3 CLINICAL STAGES IN CARCINOMA OF THE CERVIX UTERI (FIGO SYSTEM)

Stage	Involvement
0	Carcinoma in situ, cervical intraepithelial neoplasm (CIN)
I	Carcinoma strictly confined to cervix (extension to corpus should be disregarded)
Ia	Preclinical carcinoma of cervix diagnosed only by microscopy
Ia1	Stroma invasion of 3 × 7 mm
Ia2	Stroma invasion of 5 × 7 mm
Ib	Lesions of cervix or preclinical lesions larger than Ia
II	Involvement of vagina but not lower third, or infiltration beyond cervix but not into wall
IIa	Involvement of up to upper two thirds of vagina but no evidence of parametrial involvement
IIb	Infiltration of parametrium but not out to sidewall
III	Involvement of lower third of vagina or extension to pelvic sidewall; includes all cases with a hydronephrosis or nonfunctioning kidney, unless they are known to be attributable to other cause
IIIa	Involvement of lower third of vagina but not out to pelvic sidewalls
IIIb	Extension onto pelvic sidewall or hydronephrosis or nonfunctional kidney
IV	Extension outside reproductive tract
IVa	Involvement of mucosa of bladder or rectum
IVb	Distant metastasis or disease outside true pelvis

From National Cancer Institute: Screening for cervical cancer, *PDQ Summary,* 2004, accessed from website: www.nci.gov.
FIGO, International Federation of Gynecology and Obstetrics.

CLINICAL MANIFESTATIONS
Cervical Cancer

Early Symptoms

Thin, watery vaginal discharge
Bloody spotting after coitus or douching
Metrorrhagia
Postmenopausal bleeding
Polymenorrhea

Late Symptoms

Dark, foul-smelling vaginal discharge
Pelvic, abdominal, or back pain
Flank pain
Weight loss
Anorexia
Anemia
Leg edema
Dysuria
Rectal bleeding

be used therapeutically to remove the entire lesion and remains a valuable tool for preserving a woman's fertility (Figure 56-6).

Chest x-ray films, intravenous pyelography, skeletal x-ray films, and barium studies of the lower GI tract are used to stage the cancer. Additional procedures used in staging include cystoscopy, proctoscopy, and endocervical curettage. During the staging workup the nurse ensures that the woman understands the tests and their rationale. Anxiety is typically high until the extent and invasiveness of the cancer can be determined.

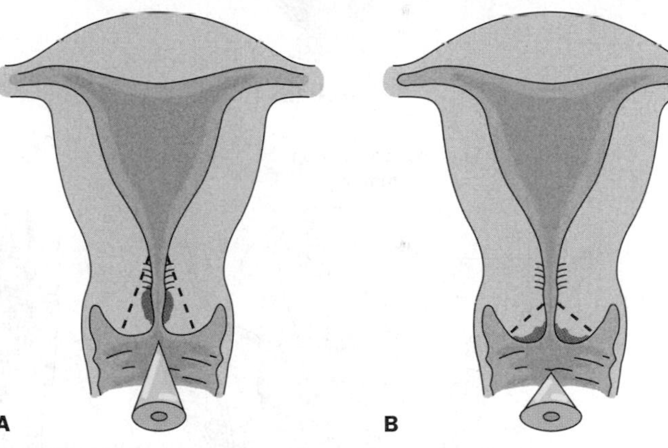

Figure 56-6 **A,** Cone biopsy for endocervical disease. Limits of lesion were not seen on colposcopy. **B,** Cone biopsy for cervical intraepithelial neoplasia of exocervix. Limits of lesion were identified on colposcopy.

MEDICATIONS. Chemotherapy has not played a significant role in the management of most cervical cancer. Squamous cell cancers tend to be relatively unresponsive to drug treatment. Recurrent cancers tend to reappear in areas previously irradiated where the tissue is fibrotic and relatively avascular, making it difficult to obtain high tissue concentrations of the drugs. For more advanced stages of cervical cancer, cisplatin-based chemotherapy treatment combined with radiation appears to improve survival. Nursing care related to chemotherapy is discussed in Chapter 23.

TREATMENTS. Cervical cancer is treated according to the stage of the disease. Figure 56-7 illustrates the extent of anatomic involvement represented by each stage. Carcinoma in situ may be treated

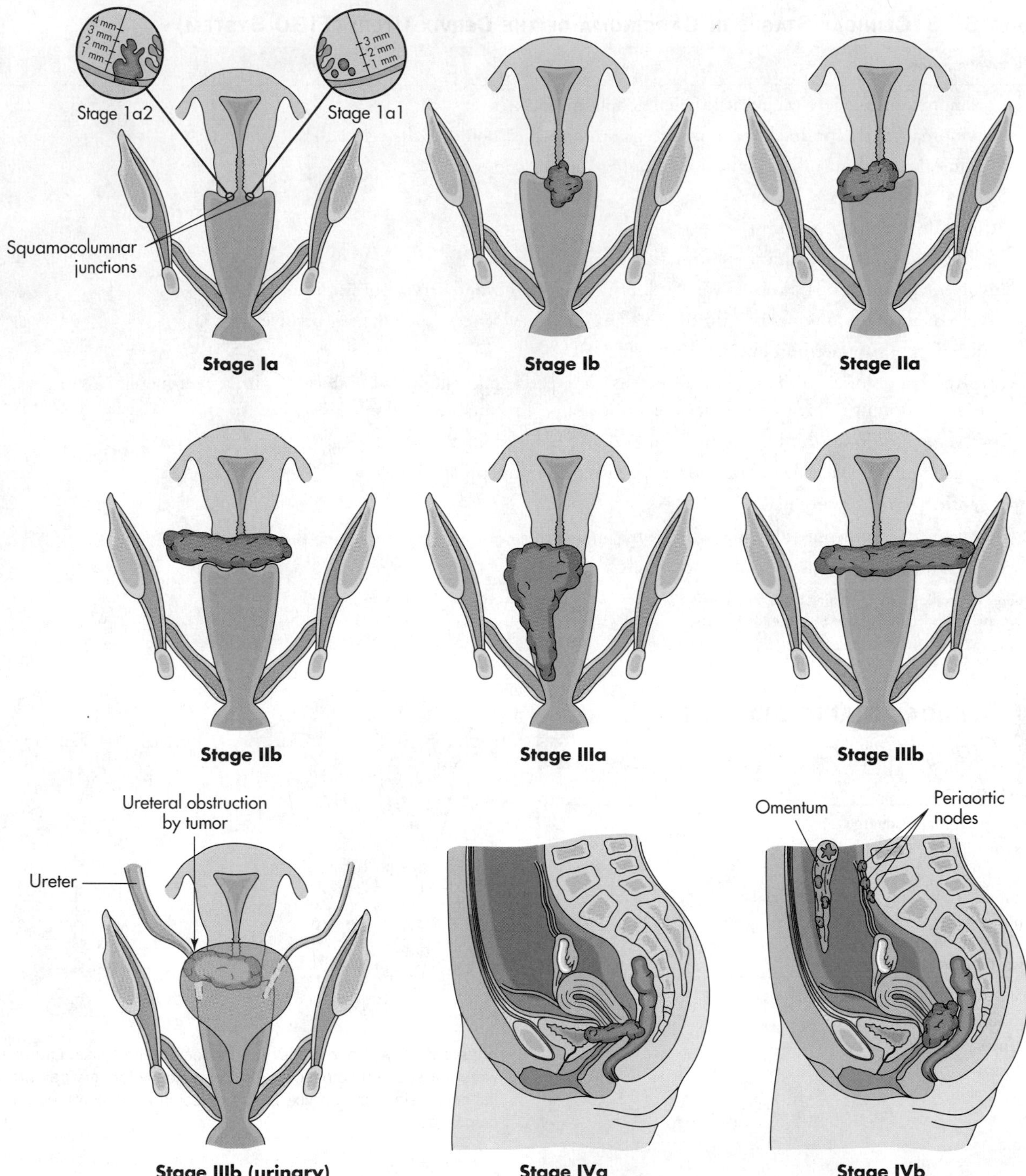

Figure 56-7 International Federation of Gynecology and Obstetrics staging and classification of cancer of cervix.

by excisional conization, LEEP, cryosurgery, or laser surgery, particularly if the woman wants to have more children. Hysterectomy may be chosen if fertility is not an issue. More invasive cancer is treated with increasingly extensive surgical procedures or radiotherapy. Table 56-4 summarizes the major treatment options for various stages of cervical cancer and their associated long-term survival projections.

RADIOTHERAPY. When radiotherapy is used in the treatment of cervical cancer, it may consist of external pelvic irradiation or **intracavitary implants** (Figure 56-8). Intracavitary implants are usually left in place for 24 to 72 hours. The use of radiotherapy as a cancer treatment is discussed in detail in Chapter 23.

During treatment with an intracavitary implant, it is important that all untreated tissues remain in their normal positions and not come in close contact with the radioactive substance. The bowel is cleansed before therapy, and the woman is maintained on a low-residue diet during treatment to prevent bowel distention with feces. A Foley catheter is typically inserted to keep the bladder small and decompressed. Gauze packing may be used in the

TABLE 56-4 TREATMENT OPTIONS FOR CERVICAL CANCER

Clinical Stage	Treatment Options	5-Year Survival (%)
0 (CIN)	Loop electrosurgical excision procedure Cryosurgery Conization Laser surgery Hysterectomy for postreproductive women	Nearly 100
Ia	Total hysterectomy Conization Radical hysterectomy Intracavitary radiation alone	95-100
Ib	Radiotherapy Radical hysterectomy and bilateral pelvic lymphadenectomy Postoperative total pelvic irradiation plus chemotherapy with subsequent radical hysterectomy and bilateral pelvic lymphadenectomy Radiotherapy and cisplatin-based chemotherapy	85-95
IIa	Radiotherapy	75-80
	Radical hysterectomy and bilateral pelvic lymphadenectomy	60
	Postoperative total pelvic irradiation plus chemotherapy with subsequent radical hysterectomy and bilateral pelvic lymphadenectomy	45
	Radiotherapy and cisplatin-based chemotherapy	18
IIb	Radiotherapy and cisplatin-based chemotherapy	
III	Radiotherapy and cisplatin-based chemotherapy	
IVa	Radiotherapy and cisplatin-based chemotherapy	
IVb	Radiotherapy, chemotherapy clinical trials of other agents such as paclitaxel, ifosfamide, and irinotecan	Palliation
Recurrent cervical cancer	Radiotherapy with chemotherapy (fluorouracil with or without mitomycin) Pelvic exenteration	40-50
	Palliative chemotherapy	32-62

From National Cancer Institute: Cervical cancer treatment, *PDQ Summary,* 2001, accessed from website: www.nci.gov.
CIN, Cervical intraepithelial neoplasm (carcinoma in situ).

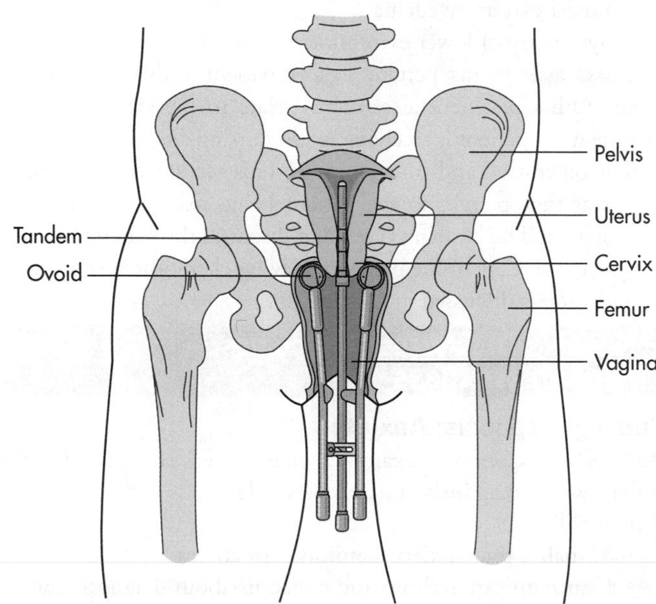

Figure 56-8 Placement of tandem and colpostats before vaginal packing.

vagina to support the rectum and bladder away from the treatment field. The woman is kept flat in bed during treatment to prevent dislodgement of the radioactive substance. The exact position of the implants can be verified by x-ray film.

The presence of the implant in the cervix may stimulate uterine contractions that may become severe. A foul-smelling vaginal discharge develops from the destruction and sloughing of cells. The woman may also develop symptoms of radiation syndrome, with nausea, vomiting, anorexia, and malaise. Local reactions include cystitis, proctitis, and acute radiation enteritis. After treatment, the catheter is removed, and an enema may be administered to restore bowel function. The vaginal discharge persists for weeks, and the woman may need to douche regularly at home to control odor. Slight vaginal bleeding may occur for 1 to 3 months after treatment. The woman can usually be discharged within 1 day after removal of the applicators.

External pelvic radiation treatments are usually given over a course of 5 to 6 weeks. General care for the patient receiving external radiotherapy is presented in Chapter 23; the nursing care of patients receiving intracavitary implants is discussed on p. 1706.

CHEMOTHERAPY. Both the National Cancer Institute and the American College of Obstetricians and Gynecologists recommend the concurrent administration of cisplatin chemotherapy for women with cervical cancer who require radiotherapy to treat their disease.

SURGICAL MANAGEMENT. Simple or radical hysterectomy is the most commonly recommended surgical procedure for treating stage I and stage II cervical cancer. A radical hysterectomy removes the uterus, supporting tissues, distal vagina, and pelvic lymph nodes (Figure 56-9). In some patients the cancer may be locally advanced but still confined to the pelvis. In these situations a pelvic exenteration procedure may be considered (Figure 56-10). The surgery is controversial, but it can be lifesaving in certain malignancies, particularly advanced or recurrent cervical cancer. The procedure involves removal of all the pelvic viscera, including the bladder, rectosigmoid colon, and all reproductive organs. Five-year survival rates after this radical surgery range from 20% to 62%. The procedure is contraindicated if the disease has spread beyond the pelvis. Improved operative techniques support the possibility of reconstructive surgery to create a neovagina at the time of surgery or as a second surgery later (Figure 56-11).

Nursing care of the patient undergoing hysterectomy is presented on pp. 1709 and 1710. Women undergoing exenteration receive this standard care and care for an abdominal-perineal resection of the bowel and an ileoconduit or a continent urinary diversion. The extensive nature of the surgery usually necessitates at least a short stay in a critical care unit. Clear and honest teaching is a prerequisite for this surgery. Women need to be fully aware of the nature and consequences of the procedure in terms of both body appearance and function. Complications are numerous, occurring in 25% to 50% of all patients, and usually involve the urinary and GI systems. Fistula formation is a common problem.

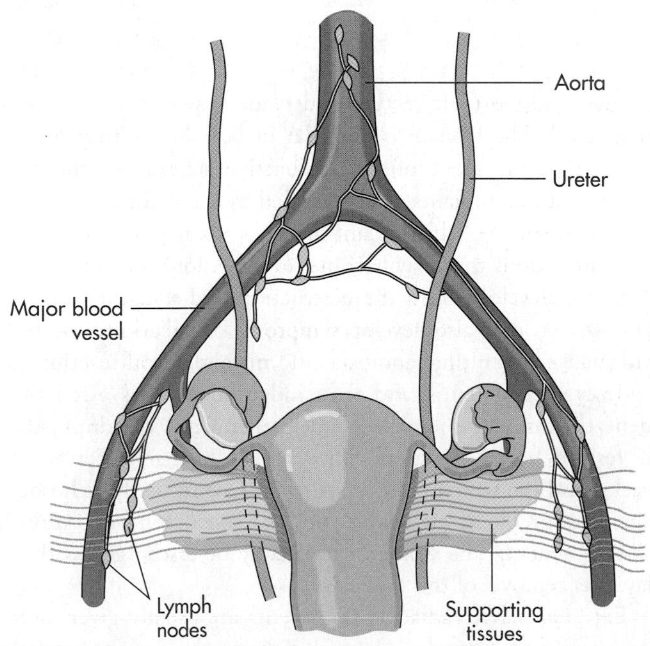

Figure 56-9 Radical hysterectomy includes removal of uterus, nearby supporting tissues, uppermost part of vagina, and pelvic lymph nodes.

DIET. No special diet is required for a patient who has cancer of the cervix. Any change in diet is usually made in response to the side effects of radiation, chemotherapy, or surgical interventions.

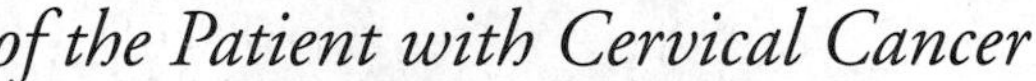

▶ ARE YOU READY?

Which of the following is one of the earliest signs of cervical cancer?
1. Foul-smelling vaginal discharge
2. Pelvic pain
3. Increased menstrual flow
4. Occasional bloody spotting

Nursing Management
of the Patient with Cervical Cancer

ASSESSMENT

Health History. Assess for:
- Foul-smelling discharge
- Spotting or intermittent metrorrhagia
- Increased amount or duration of menstrual flow
- Generalized pain or pain limited to the back, pelvis, flank, or leg
- Dyspareunia
- Changes in bowel or bladder habits
- Weight loss
- Fatigue
- Anorexia

Physical Examination. Assess for:
- Foul-smelling discharge
- Enlarged or barrel-shaped cervix with a smooth surface
- Cervical consistency hard on palpation
- Muscle guarding or rigidity on abdominal examination
- Rectal bleeding or lesions
- Lower extremity edema
- Symmetry of lower extremities

These assessments pertain to any patient with cancer of the cervix. Other pertinent assessments relate to the specific type of treatment the patient is receiving, as do nursing diagnoses, expected patient outcomes, and interventions. This section discusses these factors as they pertain to the patient being treated with internal radiotherapy. The Nursing Care Plan discusses the patient having a hysterectomy. Care of the patient receiving chemotherapy or external radiation is discussed in Chapter 23.

NURSING DIAGNOSES, OUTCOMES, AND INTERVENTIONS

Nursing Diagnosis: Anxiety

OUTCOMES. Common examples of expected outcomes for the patient with a diagnosis of *anxiety* include:

Patient will:
- Verbalize that anxiety is minimal or absent.
- Communicate feelings and concerns about diagnosis and treatment to staff or partner.
- Explain rationales for precautions followed by visitors and staff.

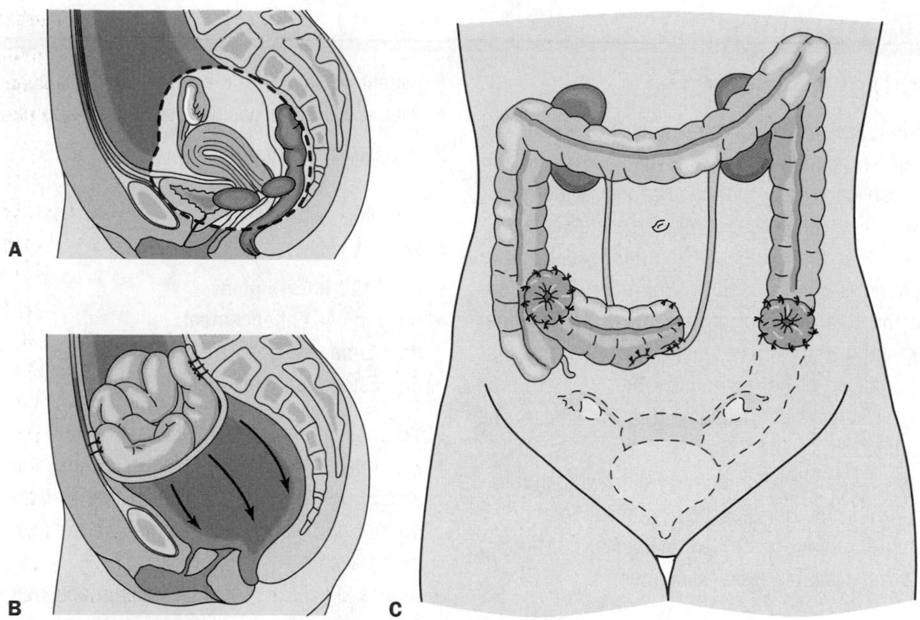

Figure 56-10 **A,** Lateral view of recurrent cancer involving cervix and upper vagina with extension into bladder and rectum. Stippled area is tissue to be removed by exenteration. **B,** Lateral view after pelvic viscera have been removed. An omental "carpet" is used to keep intestines out of pelvis during immediate postoperative period. With time, the omental "carpet" descends into pelvis and adheres to pelvic floor. **C,** Urinary conduit and colostomy diversion after exenteration. *Dotted areas* of sigmoid colon, bladder, and internal genitalia have been removed.

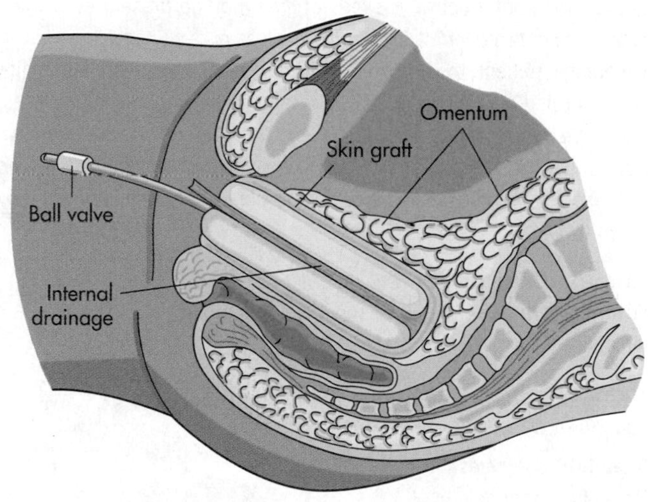

Figure 56-11 Vaginal reconstruction with skin graft. Omentum is placed in pelvis and sutured to rectum posteriorly and to sigmoid colon laterally to create a "pocket" for the neovagina. Two split-thickness skin grafts are harvested, sutured together over a Heyer-Schulte stent, and inserted into newly created pelvic space.

NURSING INTERVENTIONS. A cancer diagnosis can produce a barrage of negative feelings that commonly escalate during the diagnostic and staging period. The nurse establishes a trusting relationship and encourages the woman to talk about her feelings and concerns. The nurse supports the need to ventilate emotions through anger or crying. As anxiety is controlled, effective teaching can begin concerning the condition, treatment options, and expected side effects. The nurse should assess the meaning of the diagnosis to the patient and her significant others, clarify misconceptions, and provide reliable information to enhance their understanding. The patient and her significant others need to understand the grief response and how it may affect the woman's responses during treatment and recovery.

Careful teaching takes place before the insertion of the implant so that the woman understands the sensations she will experience. The woman and her family need to understand the rationale for all restrictions and safety measures (see Guidelines for Safe Practice box, p. 1706). It is particularly important to review the precautions related to the implant itself (Box 56-2). The cesium implant is a source of high-dose ionizing radiation to all who come into its range, and these risks must be minimized to the extent possible. The radiation hazard is clearly marked on the door to the room, and a radiation safety officer is available in the institution to deal with questions and concerns.

RELATED NIC INTERVENTIONS. Anxiety Reduction, Body Image Enhancement, Coping Enhancement, Sexual Counseling

Nursing Diagnosis: Risk for Loneliness

OUTCOMES. Common examples of expected outcomes for the patient with a diagnosis of *risk for loneliness* are:
Patient will:

- Verbalize that loneliness and boredom are manageable.
- Interact with staff and visitors within the established safety guidelines.
- Engage in appropriate diversional activities.

NURSING INTERVENTIONS. The woman receiving intracavitary radiation often feels alienated and depressed. The nurse spends

Nursing Care Plan

Patient After Abdominal Hysterectomy

Data A 42-year-old woman consulted her gynecologist 2 weeks ago because of bleeding between her periods and after sexual intercourse. Her Pap test was positive, and a cervical biopsy confirmed cancer of the cervix, stage I. She was admitted yesterday for total abdominal hysterectomy.

Admission notes indicate that the patient is married and has two teenaged children. Her husband is with her and is supportive. Her preoperative concerns center on the total removal of the cancer and whether hysterectomy will affect her relationship with her husband. She states that she feels like she is being deprived of her femininity. The nurse explores the patient's knowledge of the surgery and explains that the surgery will not physically affect sexual function.

The patient returned from postanesthesia recovery alert with an intravenous infusion and stable vital signs. Her dressing is dry and intact. She is receiving morphine sulfate per patient-controlled analgesia (PCA) pump at 1 mg/hr and a bolus of 1 mg available every 8 minutes.

Nursing Diagnosis

Acute pain related to abdominal incision

Outcomes

- Patient will report pain as less than 3 on a scale of 0 to 10 within 30 minutes following pain control interventions.

Related NOC Outcomes

- Pain Control
- Pain Level

Related NIC Interventions

- Pain Management
- Progressive Muscle Relaxation

Nursing Interventions/Rationales

- Assess duration and intensity of pain. *To monitor effectiveness of pain control measures. If pain control measures fail to sufficiently control pain, other measures should be considered.*
- Maintain analgesic infusion so that medication is delivered on a regular basis for first 24 hours. *Provides more effective pain control because it prevents severe pain, which is more difficult to control.*
- Encourage frequent changes of position in bed and early ambulation. *Activity decreases pain by increasing circulation and reducing muscle tension. Ambulation encourages peristalsis, decreasing intensity of gas pains and encouraging passage of flatus.*
- Assess adequacy of pain relief every 2 to 4 hours. *To determine if prescribed analgesia is effective or a change is needed.*
- Encourage use of PCA bolus to maintain comfort. *Allows patient control over her pain. Prevents pain from becoming severe, which is more difficult to control.*
- Encourage use of nonpharmacologic pain relief measures (massage, relaxation, music, distraction). *May work with analgesics to provide better pain control.*

Nursing Diagnosis

Risk for situational low self-esteem related to loss of uterus and concern about sexuality

Outcomes

- Patient will actively plan for resuming usual role.
- Patient will verbalize fears and concerns.
- Patient will make positive statements about self.

Related NOC Outcomes

- Body Image
- Identity
- Self-Esteem

Related NIC Interventions

- Body Image Enhancement
- Role Enhancement
- Self-Esteem Enhancement

Nursing Intervetions/Rationales

- Provide patient opportunities to express feelings and concerns about loss of uterus. *Patient may feel free to talk about her concerns if the opportunity is provided. Identification of patient feelings helps direct care plan.*
- Assess significant other's concerns and perceptions of body changes. *Helps patient and significant other verbalize doubts and resolve concerns. Provides the nurse with opportunities to correct misconceptions.*
- Provide factual information regarding anticipated bodily changes; include significant other if possible. *Provides accurate information and corrects misconceptions.*
- Be empathetic about patient's feelings, which may include grief, guilt, shame, or remorse. *Many emotions may be expressed when grieving over the loss of a body part. Expression of feelings helps the patient progress through the grief process. Feelings of grief may be present even when there is no outward indication of physical loss or dysfunction.*
- Encourage patient to continue activities associated with femininity, such as fixing her hair, wearing own apparel, applying makeup. *Expressions of femininity emphasize that the patient herself has not changed.*
- Help patient make plans for resumption of former activities. *If her life patterns are reestablished, her thoughts about her body changes may diminish.*

Nursing Diagnosis

Risk for constipation related to surgical manipulation of bowel and pain medications

Outcomes

- Patient will pass soft-formed stools.

Related NOC Outcomes

- Bowel Elimination
- Hydration

Related NIC Interventions

- Bowel Management
- Constipation/Impaction Management

Nursing Interventions/Rationales

- Monitor stool characteristics and frequency. *To identify need for treatment plan and evaluate effectiveness of that plan.*
- Encourage ambulation every 4 hours. *Ambulation promotes peristalsis, which facilitates bowel movements.*
- Assess abdomen for presence and quality of bowel sounds. *Peristalsis may be decreased from handling of pelvic viscera; helps determine flatus buildup.*

- Encourage oral fluids when permitted. *Adequate hydration promotes soft stool formation and prevents constipation and impaction.*
- Teach patient to avoid straining at stool. *Increases abdominal pain and can induce postoperative bleeding.*

Nursing Diagnosis

Impaired urinary elimination related to loss of bladder tone, pain with muscle contraction, and discomfort from urination position

Outcomes

- Patient will void spontaneously and empty bladder completely.
- Patient will remain free from urinary bladder distention.

Related NOC Outcomes

- Urinary Elimination

Related NIC Interventions

- Urinary Catheterization: Intermittent
- Urinary Elimination Management
- Urinary Retention Care

Nursing Interventions/Rationales

- Monitor urinary output until patient reestablishes her normal voiding pattern. *Urinary retention can occur from handling of bladder during surgery, which decreases bladder tone postoperatively.*
- Encourage patient to void every 2 hours. *Promotes optimal bladder tone and prevents distention.*
- Monitor for urinary bladder distention above symphysis pubis and for lower abdominal discomfort other than incisional pain every 4 hours. *Detects bladder distention and degree of bladder fullness.*
- Provide privacy during attempts to urinate. *Allows patient to relax, which facilitates urination.*
- Catheterize for residual urine as ordered. *Residual urine in bladder provides good medium for bacterial growth and infection.*
- Teach patient good perineal care. *Helps prevent urinary tract infection.*

Nursing Diagnosis

Risk for ineffective tissue perfusion related to pelvic venous stasis from surgery

Outcomes

- Patient will remain free from thrombus, emboli, or leg and thigh pain.
- Patient will maintain negative Homans' sign.
- Patient will perform leg exercises to prevent venous stasis.

Related NOC Outcomes

- Circulation Status
- Tissue Perfusion: Peripheral

Related NIC Interventions

- Circulatory Care: Venous Insufficiency
- Embolus Precautions

Nursing Interventions/Rationales

- Assess lower extremities every 8 hours. *Discomfort in legs and thighs, sudden dyspnea, positive Homans' sign, and coolness or blanching of lower extremities indicate impaired circulation. Early detection allows for early treatment of complications resulting in decreased tissue perfusion.*
- Encourage patient to lie completely flat in bed for short periods every 4 hours for 24 hours or until walking well. *To help promote blood return from pelvic veins and prevent stasis.*
- Encourage leg exercises and frequent turning in bed until walking well. *Exercise promotes venous return via muscle pumps.*
- Avoid elevating knees or placing pillows under knees. Encourage patient to keep knees flat when lying in bed and minimize use of high Fowler's position. *Pressure on popliteal veins or sharp knee flexion may increase venous stasis.*
- Provide antiembolic stockings or apply intermittent pneumatic compression stockings. *To help prevent venous stasis. Patients with varicose veins are at increased risk for phlebothrombosis.*
- Encourage ambulation. *Promotes venous return by contracting muscles to compress veins.*

Nursing Diagnosis

Risk for ineffective therapeutic regimen management related to lack of knowledge concerning postoperative self-care after discharge from hospital

Outcomes

- Patient will increasingly participate in self-care.
- Patient will comply with prescribed treatment plan, restrictions, and follow-up recommendations.

Related NOC Outcomes

- Adherence Behavior
- Knowledge: Treatment Regimen
- Participation in Health Care Decisions

Related NIC Interventions

- Family Support
- Mutual Goal Setting
- Teaching: Individual

Nursing Interventions/Rationales

- Teach patient when activities can be resumed. *Activities are resumed gradually to permit healing; heavy lifting and strenuous activities are avoided for 6 to 8 weeks postoperatively.*
- Teach patient the signs of phlebothrombosis to be monitored and reported. *Phlebothrombosis may occur 7 to 10 days postoperatively, after the patient goes home.*
- Teach patient the signs of vaginal bleeding to be reported. *Excessive or persistent bleeding indicates impaired healing.*
- Teach patient that bathing and light activity are permitted after hospital discharge. *Bathing maintains hygiene, and light activities prevent complications related to immobility.*
- Teach patient the importance of follow-up care. *Follow-up care is essential to evaluate the patient's progress or lack thereof.*
- Include significant other in teaching when possible. *Promotes compliance with discharge teaching.*
- Reinforce the preoperative explanations of the surgery and effect on sexual function, including significant other when possible. *Preoperative anxiety may have decreased her awareness. Hysterectomy does not interfere with satisfactory sexual function.*

Evaluation

Evaluation is based on comparing the patient's outcomes with desired outcomes.

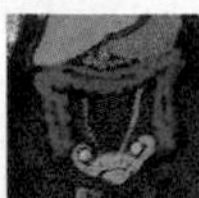

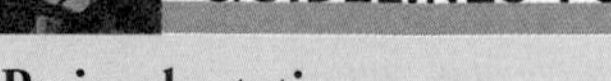

GUIDELINES FOR SAFE PRACTICE *The Patient Undergoing Internal Radiotherapy*

Preimplantation

Care before the insertion of the radioactive implant usually includes:

- Provide cleansing enema to empty the bowel.
- Insert Foley catheter to keep the bladder empty and small during treatment.
- Provide povidone-iodine (Betadine) douche and shave pubic area if ordered.

Implantation Period

Care during the 24 to 72 hours of treatment includes:

- Maintain strict bed rest.
- Elevate head of bed no more than 20 degrees. Keep patient as flat as possible.
- Assist patient in turning from side to side as needed for comfort.
- Provide low-residue diet and possibly antimotility agents to prevent bowel distention.
- Administer analgesics as needed for uterine cramping, which can be severe.
- Perform routine perineal cleansing if drainage is present; provide room deodorizer if discharge is foul smelling.
- Ensure a minimum fluid intake of 2500 ml/day.
- Visit patient frequently from the room doorway for emotional support.
- Provide diversional activities appropriate to activity restrictions.
- Monitor implant for proper placement; keep long-handled forceps and lead-lined container in the room in case of dislodgement.
- Monitor for complications.
  —Infection: increased vaginal redness or swelling; increasingly dark, foul-smelling drainage; cloudy urine; fever
  —Thrombophlebitis: painful leg swelling; positive Homans' sign

Box 56-2 Radiation Precautions for Internal Radiotherapy

- Time at the bedside is limited—each contact should last no more than 30 minutes.
- Children and pregnant women (including staff) should not visit during treatment.
- Staff members should wear a dosimeter during every patient contact to monitor radiation exposure.
- A lead shield may be installed at the side and foot of the bed.
- Staff should use the principles of distance, time, and shielding in all contacts with the patient.
- The implant is always handled by means of long-handled forceps, never with the hands. A lead-lined container is present in the room for use if the implant dislodges.
- A sign that clearly identifies the radiation hazard is posted on the room door.
- A contact number for the radiation safety officer of the institution is posted on the warning sign.

time talking with the patient but must remain at a safe distance and observe time restrictions for safety. Family members are also encouraged to visit, following the same precautions. Alternative communication methods for children or pregnant women should be used, since visitation is contraindicated for them. Strict bed rest rapidly becomes boring and uncomfortable for the patient. The nursing staff should maintain frequent contact, checking on the patient at least hourly and ensuring that the call signal is within easy reach. The nurse attempts to create a pleasant, odor-free environment with diversional activities such as reading materials, music, telephone, and television.

RELATED NIC INTERVENTIONS. Socialization Enhancement, Visitation Facilitation, Coping Enhancement

Nursing Diagnosis: Effective Therapeutic Regimen Management

OUTCOMES. Common examples of expected outcomes for the patient with a diagnosis of *effective therapeutic regimen management* are:

Patient will:

- Comply with the treatment regimen.
- Demonstrate competency in care skills such as vaginal dilation and perineal cleaning.
- Describe the components of home care and the need for follow-up monitoring.
- Identify the signs and symptoms of complications.

NURSING INTERVENTIONS. The hospitalization period for intracavitary radiotherapy is short, and the patient is discharged soon after removal of the implant. The woman must learn several self-care skills for home management and be aware of the signs and symptoms of potential complications. Radiotherapy causes fatigue, vaginal stenosis, loss of vaginal lubrication, and induced menopause. The nurse discusses energy management strategies that will allow the patient to reduce fatigue and build endurance.

The vaginal discharge often continues for weeks, and the woman may need to douche at least twice daily as long as the discharge and odor persist. The nurse cannot assume that the woman has experience with douching and reviews the technique and precautions in detail. Some vaginal bleeding may also persist for a few months after treatment, and the physician should instruct the patient about acceptable amounts of bleeding. Medication management of hormone replacement therapy may be necessary.

The cesium implant causes vaginal narrowing and fibrosis. Regular vaginal dilation is essential to minimize these effects. If the woman has a spouse or sexual partner, regular sexual intercourse, usually at least three times a week, is one method of minimizing stenosis. The woman may prefer to use a manual obturator to dilate the vagina. The nurse explains the importance of this intervention to the woman who is not sexually active: even routine pelvic examination can become difficult or almost impossible if the vagina becomes severely stenosed. Dilation should be performed at least three times a week for 1 year after treatment. The nurse informs the patient that slight bleeding may occur after dilation for up to 1 year. The obturator is lubricated before use and washed with soap and water after each use. A vinegar and water douche may be ordered after treatment.

Other self-care teaching focuses on gradually increasing activity, maintaining a liberal fluid intake to prevent urologic problems, and adjusting diet to prevent bowel problems. Either constipation or diarrhea may occur in response to radiation, and these problems may persist for months after treatment. The nurse also teaches the patient about symptoms that indicate complications. The woman should promptly report unusually heavy discharge, foul-smelling urine, low-grade fever, persistent bowel problems, or pain. Radiotherapy can cause fistulas in the pelvis, both in the early posttreatment period and in the future.

RELATED NIC INTERVENTIONS. Anticipatory Guidance, Learning Readiness Enhancement, Learning Facilitation

Nursing Diagnosis: Impaired Urinary Elimination

OUTCOMES. Common examples of expected outcomes for the patient with a diagnosis of *impaired urinary elimination* are:
Patient will:

- Drink a wide variety of oral fluids (2500 to 3000 ml/day).
- Void a minimum of 50 ml/hr.
- Report diminished burning and frequency on follow-up visits.

NURSING INTERVENTIONS. Urinary catheterization is necessary during treatment and is followed by urinary elimination management before discharge. Patients may develop symptoms of radiation syndrome that alter nutrition and elimination. An adequate fluid intake is essential to maintain fluid and electrolyte balance and prevent irritation of the bladder. The nurse encourages the patient to maintain a fluid intake of 2500 to 3000 ml/day, even in the face of anorexia and nausea, and administers antiemetics as needed.

RELATED NIC INTERVENTIONS. Bladder Irrigation, Urinary Elimination Management, Urinary Retention Care

Nursing Diagnosis: Self-Care Deficit: Bathing/Hygiene, Toileting

OUTCOMES. Common examples of outcomes for the patient with a diagnosis of *self-care deficit (bathing/hygiene and toileting)* include:
Patient will:

- Explain self-care bathing, hygiene, and toileting restrictions.
- Adapt self-care tasks to activity restrictions.
- Accept assistance as needed.

NURSING INTERVENTIONS. The patient must carefully follow the activity restrictions outlined in the Guidelines for Safe Practice box to prevent accidental dislodgement of the device or movement of the implant that endangers normal tissue. To promote adherence to the treatment plan, the woman must understand the rationale for all restrictions. The nurse provides bed rest care and ensures that all needed articles are kept within reach, but assistance may be necessary, since the woman must maintain the supine position. Hourly turning is encouraged, and back rubs may relieve some of the discomforts of bed rest. The foul-smelling vaginal discharge may be both irritating and embarrassing. The nurse assists with frequent perineal hygiene and provides a room deodorizer.

Thrombophlebitis is another concern during bed rest; therefore embolus precautions are instituted. The nurse teaches the patient range-of-motion and isometric exercises that support venous return and encourages her to perform them 10 times each hour. The patient wears elastic or compression stockings, which are removed for 15 to 20 minutes every 8 hours.

RELATED NIC INTERVENTIONS. Bathing, Self-Care Assistance

Patient/Family Teaching. The nurse provides extensive teaching, with full understanding that the anxiety associated with the diagnosis of cancer and its treatment will make it difficult for the woman to process much of the information. Repeat sessions and written reference materials are critical. The woman's partner is included in teaching sessions if possible, since the disease and treatment have significant potential impact on the couple's sexual activities, at least in the short term. The nurse ensures that the woman has the name and telephone number of all appropriate support groups and services available in her home community.

EVALUATION

To evaluate the effectiveness of nursing interventions, compare patient behaviors with those stated in the expected patient outcomes.

RELATED NOC OUTCOMES. Anxiety Level, Body Image, Coping, Self-Care: Activities of Daily Living (ADLs), Self-Care: Bathing, Self-Care: Hygiene, Sexual Function, Urinary Elimination, Communication, Knowledge: Treatment Regimen, Adherence Behavior, Social Support

GERONTOLOGIC CONSIDERATIONS

Cancer of the cervix occurs in women of all ages. Early diagnosis is critical and is an ongoing challenge in older women. After the childbearing years many women stop having gynecologic examinations. Symptoms are often discounted or attributed to the multiple effects of aging on the reproductive system. Therefore it is less likely that cervical cancer will be detected in the early and curable stages. Older women are less able to withstand the rigors of radical surgery, are more prone to complications of treatment, and often experience exaggerated tissue responses to radiotherapy. It is critical that teaching and outreach be provided to this population about the ongoing importance of Pap test screening for cancer in women who have risk factors, since the incidence and mortality rates for cervical cancer in the United States are highest among older women.[1]

Neoplasms of the Uterus

Uterine Leiomyomas (Fibroids)

Etiology and Epidemiology. Leiomyomas (myomas) are benign tumors of muscle cell origin that contain varying amounts of fibrous tissue. The etiology of leiomyomas is not completely understood. The stimulus for growth is unclear but is thought to be related to estrogen, since leiomyomas are rare before menarche and often decrease in size after menopause. The tumors often enlarge during pregnancy and with the use of oral contraceptives. Women who smoke tend to be relatively estrogen deficient and have been found to have a lower incidence of leiomyomas. The tumors can reach enormous proportions, weighing as much as 50 pounds. Malignant transformation is rare.

Leiomyomas are the most common type of pelvic tumor, developing in 25% to 58% of women.[11] Leiomyomas occur more often in African-American women and account for more than 50% of hysterectomies. Leiomyomas are more common in women who are obese. The frequency increases during the perimenopausal period.

Pathophysiology. Leiomyomas originate in the myometrium and are classified by their anatomic location (Figure 56-12). The tumor is the result of overgrowth of a single muscle cell influenced by estrogen and progesterone-stimulated growth factors. Submucous myomas lie just beneath the endometrium and compress it as they grow. They can develop a pedicle and protrude into the uterine cavity or even through the cervical canal. Intramural myomas lie within the uterine muscle, and subserosal tumors lie at the serosal surface of the uterus or may bulge outward from the myometrium. These external tumors also tend to become pedunculated. They occasionally are found in the fallopian tubes or round ligament, and approximately 5% originate from the cervix.

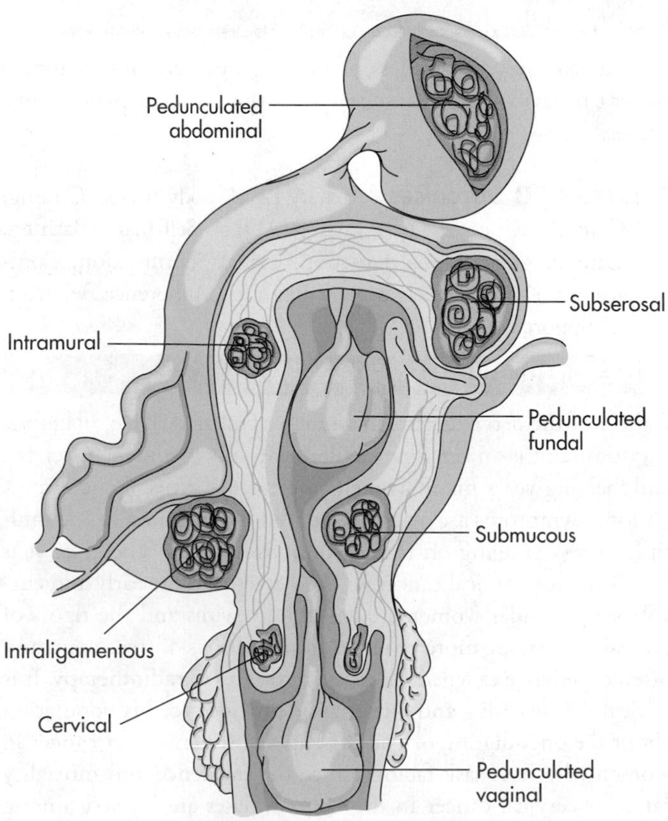

Figure 56-12 Leiomyomas of uterus.

Most leiomyomas are asymptomatic and may go undetected. The symptoms depend on the location, size, and condition of the tumor. Hypermenorrhea is the most common symptom. Bleeding can result from distortion and congestion of surrounding vessels or from ulceration of the overlying endometrium. Bleeding usually takes the form of premenstrual spotting or prolonged light bleeding after the menses. Metrorrhagia is associated with venous thrombosis or necrosis on the surface of the tumor, particularly if it extrudes through the cervix.

Pain is not a characteristic symptom, although it can result from tumor degeneration or myometrial contractions that attempt to expel the myoma from the uterus. If the pedicle stalk becomes twisted, it can cause sudden, severe pain. Women often report a sensation of pressure in the pelvis or a "bearing down" feeling, especially with large tumors. The tumor may cause pelvic circulatory congestion and create backache, constipation, or dysmenorrhea. The woman may even notice an increase in abdominal girth.

Leiomyomas interfere with fertility by blocking the opening of the fallopian tubes, inducing spontaneous abortion, or obstructing the cervical canal, making delivery hazardous. Sudden growth of a myoma after menopause is considered a classic sign of leiomyosarcoma, which necessitates hysterectomy.

Leiomyomas increase the risk of complications during pregnancy, including placental abruption and malpresentation. Anemia is associated with chronic blood loss, but women may also exhibit polycythemia secondary to erythropoietin produced by the myometrium. The signs and symptoms of leiomyomas are summarized in the Clinical Manifestations box.

Collaborative Care Management

Diagnostic Tests. Myomas often can be detected by routine pelvic examination when the uterus is displaced and irregular nodules are felt on the uterine surface. Diagnosis is confirmed through the use of magnetic resonance imaging (MRI), computed tomography (CT) scanning, pelvic sonography, and hysterography or hysteroscopy. These tests are used to determine the size and placement of the tumor(s) and to evaluate the degree of urologic compression.

Medications. GnRH agonists may be used to reduce the level of circulating estrogens and to shrink the tumor by as much as 90%, but their effect is temporary. These drugs may be used in

Clinical Manifestations
Leiomyomas

- Abnormal bleeding
- Abdominal mass
- Pressure in the pelvis
- Iron-deficiency anemia
- Sudden-onset pain, indicating a complication

Note: Most leiomyomas are asymptomatic.

perimenopausal women to avoid the need for surgery because the tumors are known to regress after menopause. The GnRH agonists are also prescribed preoperatively to reduce the incidence and severity of postoperative bleeding. Reducing the tumor size also may permit the use of a vaginal, rather than an abdominal, approach for the hysterectomy and decrease recovery time. Antiprogestins are being studied for possible use in both treatment and prevention.

TREATMENTS. Small, asymptomatic myomas are simply monitored. The myomas tend to shrink as estrogen levels begin to decline. If a patient is experiencing bleeding, an endometrial biopsy may be performed to verify the diagnosis and rule out cancer. Submucous myomas may be resected via the cervical canal using the hysteroscope and laser therapy as an outpatient procedure.

SURGICAL MANAGEMENT. Leiomyomas are the most common indication for hysterectomy. The decision to undergo surgery depends on the woman's age, symptom severity, and desire to preserve her childbearing ability. Asymptomatic leiomyomas are not treated with a hysterectomy until the uterus reaches the size of a 12-week pregnancy. Myomectomy can be performed if the tumor is near the outer wall of the uterus, leaving the muscular walls of the uterus relatively intact. Abdominal and vaginal hysterectomies are illustrated in Figure 56-13. Various gynecologic surgical procedures are defined in Box 56-3. Myolysis is a procedure that involves delivering an electric current to the leiomyoma at the time of laparoscopy, to destroy the fibroid tissue, and cryomyolysis uses liquid nitrogen to do the same.

RADIOLOGIC ALTERNATIVE. Uterine artery embolization is a radiologic alternative to surgery. It involves partial blocking of the uterine artery, thus decreasing blood flow to the myoma. Uterine fibroid embolization is a minimally invasive procedure that has been shown to shrink fibroid tumors an average of 50% to 75%, thereby relieving bleeding and other symptoms. The procedure is usually done with local or epidural anesthesia. The uterine arteries are accessed via a catheter introduced into the femoral artery; an arteriogram is done to outline the uterine arteries; and particles of embolization material such as gelfoam are injected with radiologic guidance to block arteries bringing blood to the fibroids. A second arteriogram is done to verify that blood flow to the fibroids is blocked. Cramping and nausea may be problematic for 4 to 6 hours following the procedure, and in some cases vaginal discharge, severe pain, bleeding, infection, or hematoma may occur. Because the procedure is so new, effects on pregnancy and the menstrual cycle are unclear.[11a]

BOX 56-3 Surgeries of the Female Reproductive System

- *Oophorectomy:* Removal of an ovary
- *Salpingectomy:* Removal of a fallopian tube
- *Bilateral salpingo-oophorectomy* (BSO or Bil S&O): Removal of both ovaries and fallopian tubes
- *Total hysterectomy:* Removal of the entire uterus, including the cervix; may be referred to as a total abdominal hysterectomy (TAH); can be done vaginally or abdominally
- *Subtotal hysterectomy:* Removal of the uterus except for the cervix; rarely done today
- *Hystero-oophorectomy:* Removal of the uterus and an ovary
- *Hysterosalpingectomy:* Removal of the uterus and a fallopian tube
- *Total abdominal hysterectomy and bilateral salpingo-oophorectomy* (TAH-BSO): Removal of the entire uterus and both fallopian tubes and ovaries; previously referred to as *panhysterectomy*
- *Radical hysterectomy* (Wertheim's operation): TAH-BSO, partial vaginectomy, and dissection of the lymph nodes in the pelvis

Nursing Management of the Patient undergoing Hysterectomy for Leiomyoma

PREOPERATIVE CARE

Hysterectomy is used as a treatment for a variety of reproductive tract problems in addition to leiomyoma, including cancer of the cervix, uterus, and ovaries, as well as structural problems such as severe prolapse. Vaginal, abdominal, and laparoscopic approaches are used. Women desire information on their options, including differences in symptom relief, length of stay, cost, and quality of life.

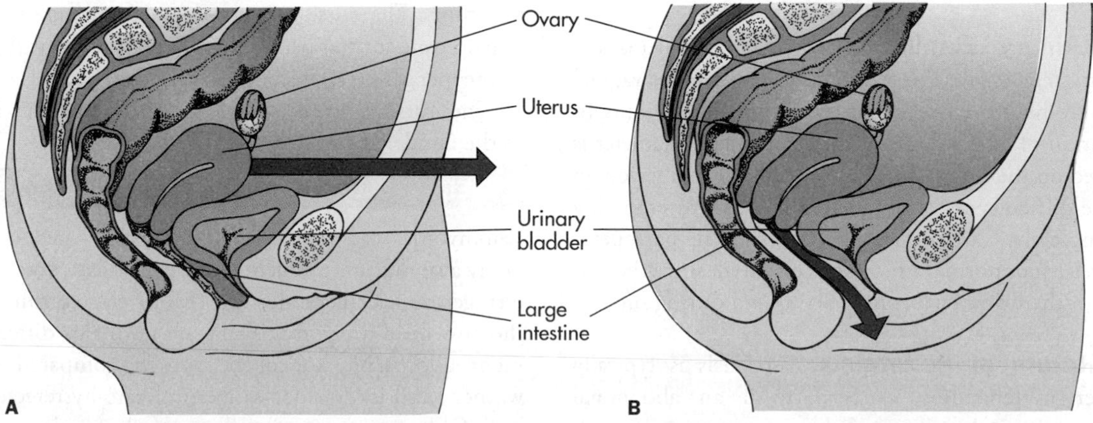

Figure 56-13 **A,** Abdominal hysterectomy. Uterus is removed through abdominal incision. **B,** Vaginal hysterectomy. Uterus is removed through vagina, and there is no abdominal incision.

Preoperative teaching is essential and usually is initiated in the physician's office or by the preadmissions team. Women who smoke should receive counseling and support for smoking cessation before surgery and at discharge. Most women are familiar with the term *fibroid* but have little real understanding of the development, treatment, or relationship of fibroids with estrogen levels. The nurse verifies that teaching has been provided and that the woman can accurately describe the planned surgery and associated care. The nurse then clarifies and reinforces that teaching as needed, thoroughly discussing the plans for pain management and the importance of early and frequent ambulation.

Physical preparation for surgery typically includes an enema or laxative the day before the procedure to empty and cleanse the bowel. An antiseptic douche may also be prescribed, or the physician may order the woman to insert an antiseptic-soaked tampon 12 hours before the surgery. Ferrous sulfate therapy may be prescribed several weeks before surgery if the woman is anemic from chronic blood loss.

Postoperative Care

Much of the postoperative care provided after hysterectomy is similar to that provided after any major surgery and includes assessment for hemorrhage and pulmonary embolism (see Chapter 15). Unique aspects of care are addressed here.

Promoting Activity. Ambulation begins on the day of surgery or the first postoperative day, and the nurse encourages regular, brief periods of ambulation throughout the day. Ambulation supports oxygenation through natural deep breathing, assists in the prompt elimination of residual anesthetic, stimulates the return of peristalsis, and supports venous return. Venous pooling and pelvic congestion are common complications after hysterectomy because of the inflammatory response to the trauma of surgery. This is particularly true if the lithotomy position was used during surgery. The risk of thromboembolism is significant, and the physician may order prophylactic subcutaneous heparin injections. Routine interventions include applying compression stockings or external devices, encouraging leg and foot flexion and extension exercises every 2 hours, and avoiding positioning the patient with the knees bent. Elevating the legs at intervals throughout the day may be helpful also. Routine monitoring for pain or swelling in the calf is included in the ongoing assessment.

Supporting Urinary Elimination. Urinary problems are common after hysterectomy. The woman who undergoes vaginal hysterectomy may have a catheter left in place for 24 hours to allow for resolution of edema around the urethra. The catheter is typically removed on the first postoperative day, but many women experience some difficulty in voiding spontaneously or emptying the bladder completely. Careful assessment during the postoperative period for return of normal function is essential, since the delicate structures of the urinary tract may be injured during surgery.

Supporting Return of Peristalsis. Peristalsis is typically suppressed after hysterectomy, particularly if an abdominal approach with extensive handling of the GI organs was used. Gaseous distention is one of the most common and troublesome postoperative complaints. The woman typically receives nothing by mouth until bowel sounds return, and intravenous fluids are continued until she is taking oral fluids well. If problems do not occur, the patient moves quickly from a liquid to a regular diet. When paralytic ileus is severe, a nasogastric tube may be placed to relieve gaseous pressure. Frequent ambulation is encouraged as the most reliable means of stimulating peristaltic activity. The woman's potassium level is monitored to ensure that hypokalemia does not contribute to the ileus. Ileus can be an ongoing problem, and patients are instructed to contact their physician if abdominal distention, nausea, or vomiting develops after discharge.

Promoting Sleep. Sleep pattern disturbance is commonly reported by women after hysterectomy and may be related to the surgical procedure and hospital environment. Efforts to promote normal sleep-wake patterns need to be balanced with the need for frequent monitoring.

Providing Emotional Support. Hysterectomy may be accompanied by emotional upset and ambivalence concerning the loss of reproductive ability, but this is not always the case. Many women are equally concerned about the effects of the surgery on femininity and sexuality. After surgery almost all women experience some degree of depression for several days and may be inexplicably tearful. Grieving for losses is both appropriate and important, and the nurse encourages the woman to deal honestly with her emotions. Family members need to be informed about these expected responses, and partners may need to be encouraged to offer the patient specific reassurance and understanding during this time. Depression resulting from hormonal changes may respond to postoperative hormone replacement therapy in women who also undergo oophorectomy.

Women are instructed to avoid sexual intercourse until the vaginal vault is satisfactorily healed. This usually takes about 6 weeks. Satisfactory sexual relations can then be reestablished and often are improved. Women need to adjust to changes in the nature of pelvic sensations and stimuli during sex. Open communication between the woman and her partner is essential. Alternative methods of expressing affection can be encouraged during the postoperative period.

Managing Fatigue. Persistent fatigue related to pain and sleep pattern disturbance is a frequent complaint of women after hysterectomy. The nurse encourages patients to use social support to free up time for rest periods throughout the day. A gradual return to preoperative responsibilities is needed.

The nursing care for the hysterectomy patient is summarized in the Guidelines for Safe Practice box.

Gerontologic Considerations

Leiomyomas typically develop in middle-aged women and are rarely a significant problem in postmenopausal women. However, estrogen replacement therapy (ERT) will continue to stimulate the growth of a myoma. There are no major differences in treatment approaches for older women compared with younger women, and most older women tolerate hysterectomy extremely well. Older patients need to be carefully monitored because complications are more common in this age-group, especially after abdominal surgery.

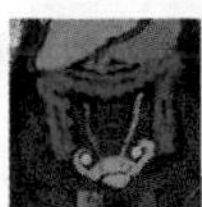
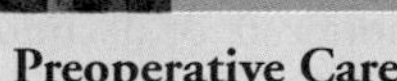

GUIDELINES FOR SAFE PRACTICE *The Patient Undergoing Hysterectomy*

Preoperative Care

Verify patient understanding of the procedure and anticipated care.
Administer prescribed enemas, laxatives, and douches.
Verify completion of prescribed skin preparation.
Promote circulation and oxygenation.
—Apply antiembolic stockings.
—Teach deep breathing, effective coughing, use of incentive spirometer, how to splint abdomen, and how to change positions.
—Teach leg and foot exercises.
Teach how to use patient-controlled analgesia (PCA) for pain control.
Encourage expression of feelings and concerns.

Postoperative Care

Promote comfort.
—Administer analgesics and encourage PCA use.
—Administer antiemetics as needed.
Promote circulation and oxygenation.
—Encourage turning, deep breathing, coughing, and use of incentive spirometer.
—Encourage leg and foot exercises every hour while in bed.
—Maintain use of antiembolic stockings as ordered.
—Encourage frequent ambulation.
—Monitor for signs of thromboembolism.
Accurately record all output and drainage.
Promote elimination.
—Monitor effectiveness of bladder emptying after catheter removal. Catheterize for residual urine if ordered.
—Monitor for signs of returning peristalsis.
—Encourage frequent ambulation and a liberal fluid intake.
—Teach diet modifications to prevent constipation.
Provide discharge teaching regarding medications and therapeutic regimens.
—Reinforce importance of and support for continued smoking cessation in those women who smoked before surgery.
—Teach signs of urinary tract infection.
—Provide teaching regarding incision care.
—Instruct patient to avoid heavy lifting, prolonged sitting, and long car rides.
—Tell patient to refrain from coitus for about 6 weeks and not to douche unless prescribed by her physician. Vaginal bleeding or discharge may persist for up to 6 weeks.
—Help patient anticipate mood swings and emotional lability during healing.

Cancer of the Endometrium

Etiology and Epidemiology. Cancer of the **endometrium** (uterine corpus) is the most common form of gynecologic cancer. It is highly curable and primarily affects women over 50 years of age. Endometrial cancer is the fourth most common cancer in women.[18]

Multiple risk factors have been identified in addition to age. These include obesity, diabetes, nulliparity, late menopause (after age 52), use of ERT, and use of tamoxifen for breast cancer. The risk of endometrial cancer among women taking ERT appears to be limited to unopposed estrogen products. Adding progesterone to the therapy appears to eliminate the risk, and women receiving combined estrogen-progesterone products actually have a lower total risk of endometrial cancer than do women who are not receiving ERT.

Pathophysiology. Uterine hyperplasia is somewhat analogous to dysplasia of the cervix. Some lesions revert to normal, some persist as hyperplasia, and a few progress to endometrial adenocarcinoma. Unfortunately, unlike cervical dysplasia, no reliable, widely available screening method for endometrial hyperplasia exists. Most women with this condition are diagnosed when they seek medical care for abnormal uterine bleeding. The diagnosis of endometrial hyperplasia can be made only by pathologic examination of uterine tissue.

Endometrial cancer is an excellent example of an estrogen-dependent lesion. The underlying pathologic process involves overgrowth of the uterine endometrium in response to an estrogen-dominant hormonal environment. Abnormal vaginal bleeding is the most common symptom. Occasionally women have a purulent, blood-tinged discharge.

Collaborative Care Management. Cancer of the endometrium is a slow-growing form of cancer and is very responsive to treatment if detected early. High-risk women may have endometrial tissue samples taken periodically. Tissue samples may be acquired in a variety of ways, as outlined in Table 56-5.

Endometrial cancer is treated according to its stage (Table 56-6). The most common treatment is simple hysterectomy and bilateral salpingo-oophorectomy. After complete surgical staging, if disease is limited to the uterus, most patients need no further treatment. The one exception is patients with a poorly differentiated, deeply invasive cancer. Studies suggest that pelvic radiation in this group may prevent both local and distant recurrence; in all other instances radiation does not appear to be of benefit.[18]

TABLE 56-5 METHODS OF DETECTION OF ENDOMETRIAL CANCER

Method	Effectiveness (%)
Endometrial aspiration	70-80
Endometrial washings	80-90
Dilation and curettage (fractional)	85-90
Pap test	45-50
Combination of above	90

TABLE 56-6 STAGES OF CANCER OF THE ENDOMETRIUM

Stage	Involvement
I	Confined to corpus
II	Involves corpus and cervix
III	Extends outside corpus but not outside pelvis (vaginal wall but not bladder or rectum)
IV	Involves bladder, rectum, or tissue outside pelvis

Postoperative brachytherapy does not appear to be efficacious in most surgical stage I cancers. Lymphadenectomy can be therapeutic in patients with true stage II disease. In patients with stage III and IV disease treatment is usually a combination of surgery and radiation. The use of chemotherapy and hormones in patients with advanced disease has not proven to be efficacious.[18]

PATIENT/FAMILY TEACHING. The nursing care associated with hysterectomy and radiotherapy was discussed previously. Nurses play a major role in health teaching about the importance of careful evaluation of all abnormal uterine bleeding in the postmenopausal population. This single factor is the most important strategy for reducing the death rate by identifying endometrial cancer in a treatable stage.

Gestational Trophoblastic Neoplasia

Etiology and Epidemiology. *Gestational trophoblastic neoplasia* (GTN) is the term used to describe choriocarcinoma and related diseases such as hydatidiform mole and invasive mole. The cause of GTN is not thoroughly understood. The hydatidiform mole often precedes malignant diseases. The risk of hydatidiform mole varies significantly in different regions of the world, being more prevalent in Asia than in the United States. Deficiencies of protein and carotene may contribute its development. There is an increased risk of molar pregnancy for women older than 40 years and at the lower end of the reproductive range.[13]

Pathophysiology. GTN is an abnormal pregnancy characterized by a degeneration, or abnormal growth, of the trophoblastic tissue of the placenta, usually in the absence of an intact fetus. It produces a serum marker, human chorionic gonadotropin (HCG), whose levels are directly related to the number of tumor cells. Early stages of GTN may be similar to normal pregnancy. As the disease progresses, most women experience uterine bleeding. Rapid uterine growth occurs, often accompanied by nausea and vomiting.

Despite widespread metastasis, these tumors are responsive to treatment, and reproductive function can be preserved in most women.[13]

Collaborative Care Management. The diagnosis of GTN usually involves pelvic examination, blood chemistries, ultrasound, chest x-ray films, and analysis of HCG levels. Suction curettage is the most common method for evacuation of a molar pregnancy. Hysterectomy may be considered for women who have completed childbearing. Weekly HCG levels are monitored in all women until normal levels are maintained for 6 months. Women are advised to use a reliable contraceptive method and avoid pregnancy. Should HCG levels rise in the absence of pregnancy, prophylactic chemotherapy with methotrexate or dactinomycin is added, usually with excellent results. Women with malignant GTN are evaluated for the extent of disease and treated with chemotherapy and possibly surgery and radiation.

PATIENT/FAMILY TEACHING. Patient and family teaching includes an overview of this rather strange disease process, implications for future pregnancies, the effect of chemotherapy on future children, and the need for effective contraception during the first year after diagnosis.

Neoplasms of the Ovaries

Ovarian Cysts

Etiology and Epidemiology. Many types of benign tumors affect the ovaries; 80% are classified in the epithelial group, which includes serous, mucinous, endometrial, and mesonephroid lesions. Epithelial tumors are composed of supporting connective tissue and ovarian stroma but have the capacity to alter the woman's hormonal status. Other types of ovarian neoplasms include simple cysts and nonneoplastic cysts originating in the graafian follicle. Nearly 80% of ovarian tumors are discovered during routine pelvic examination and are asymptomatic. Women between ages 45 and 60 years are at greatest risk. Each of the various tumor types tends to affect a different age-group and behave in a different way.

Pathophysiology. Benign cysts and tumors develop from a variety of physiologic imbalances. Elevated levels of luteinizing hormone may cause hyperstimulation of the ovaries. Follicular cysts depend on gonadotropins for growth and generally occur during the menstrual years and resolve spontaneously. Simple cysts occur commonly during menopause. Box 56-4 summarizes the characteristics of various common types of ovarian cysts and tumors.

Most ovarian tumors are asymptomatic for long periods or produce only nonspecific symptoms. Menstrual irregularities may be present when hormonal imbalance exists. Dull, unilateral, lower quadrant pain may occur, especially as the cyst grows in size, but overt pain is an unusual symptom. Fatigue or a sense of heaviness in the pelvis also may occur. Ascites and increasing abdominal girth have been reported in slender women. Large tumors may cause symptoms of pelvic pressure, such as urinary frequency and constipation.

Collaborative Care Management. Palpation of the reproductive organs during pelvic examination commonly reveals any mass or enlargement of the ovary (Figure 56-14). Any mass palpated in a postmenopausal woman requires further investigation because the ovaries normally atrophy after menopause.

Ultrasonography may be used to distinguish functional from neoplastic cysts. A CT scan is capable of distinguishing solid tumors, cysts, and ascites, but laparoscopy may be performed to confirm the diagnosis.

BOX 56-4 Characteristics of Various Types of Benign Ovarian Cysts and Tumors

Cysts

Follicular Cysts
Most common form of cysts
Often multiple; range in size from a few millimeters to as large as 15 cm in diameter
Depend on gonadotropin for growth
Occur during menstrual years and usually resolve spontaneously
May cause menstrual irregularities if blood estrogen elevated

Corpus Luteum Cysts
Less common variety
Associated with normal ovarian function or elevated progesterone
Average diameter: 4 cm
May appear purplish red from bleeding within corpus luteum
May cause delayed menstrual bleeding from progesterone secretion; hypermenorrhea common

Theca-Lutein Cysts
Least common variety
Usually bilateral and produce significant ovarian enlargement, up to 30 cm in diameter
Develop from prolonged or excessive stimulation by gonadotropins
Associated with hydatidiform mole 50% of the time and with choriocarcinomas 10% of the time

Epithelial Tumors

Serous Tumors
Found in all age-groups
Can be extremely large, filling pelvis or abdomen

Mucinous Tumors
Occur in second to third decade of life
May be bilateral
Can reach spectacular size; largest form

Endometroid Tumors
Small, purplish blue lesions
Large tumors called "chocolate cysts" because they contain brownish fluid
Very low malignancy potential

Mesonephroid Tumors
Usually multifocal
Involve peritoneal surfaces and may cause intestinal or urinary tract complications
Characterized by papillary proliferations without mitotic activity

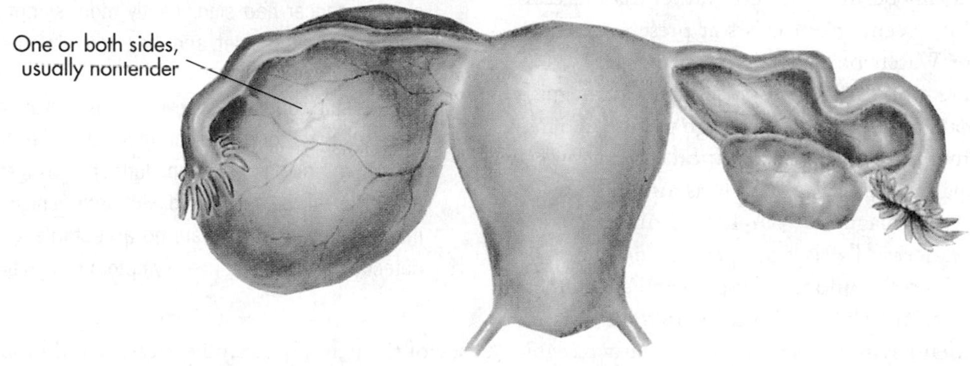

Figure 56-14 Ovarian cyst.

Many ovarian cysts resolve spontaneously. If the cyst does not decrease in size, oral contraceptives may be prescribed to shrink it. Surgery is usually recommended only when the cyst is larger than 8 cm or occurs after menopause or before puberty. A cystectomy rather than oophorectomy is performed if possible.

PATIENT/FAMILY TEACHING. The woman is reminded of the importance of follow-up care to continue to monitor the tumor's size. Most women are extremely anxious concerning the effects of the tumor on fertility and should be reassured that even oophorectomy does not reduce childbearing potential as long as the second ovary is healthy. If both ovaries are removed, the woman undergoes surgical menopause and needs to receive information concerning ERT.

Cancer of the Ovary

Etiology and Epidemiology. Malignant neoplasms of the ovaries occur at all ages, including infancy and childhood. Cancer of the ovary is a common cancer in women in the United States and has the highest mortality rate of the gynecologic cancers. More than 25,580 new cases are expected yearly in the United States. Ovarian cancer accounts for nearly 4% of all cancers among women and ranks second among gynecologic cancers, following cancer of the uterus corpus.[1]

The cause of ovarian cancer is not understood, but it appears to be associated with several factors. Family history is the most important risk factor. Increasing age, nulliparity, early menarche, late menopause, use of hormone replacement therapy, and a history of breast cancer add to the risk of ovarian cancer. Women with a family history of breast cancer are also at an increased risk of ovarian cancer. Mutations in BRAC1 or BRAC2 have been observed in some of these families. Another genetic syndrome, hereditary nonpolyposis colon cancer, also has been associated with endometrial and ovarian cancer.[1] Protective effects include using oral contraceptives long term; completing at least one pregnancy; breastfeeding; having a tubal ligation, hysterectomy, or oophorectomy; and avoiding agents such as talc, fertility drugs, and a high-fat diet. Survival rate is highest when the disease is diagnosed and treated early but decreases dramatically for advanced forms of the disease.

Pathophysiology. *Ovarian cancer* is a broad term, and ovarian neoplasms can be divided into many categories, depending on the cell type of origin. The major histologic types occur in distinctive age ranges. The four main types are described in Table 56-7. Malignant epithelial cell tumors are the most common and are seen in women over age 50. Malignant germ cell tumors are more uncommon and are seen primarily in women under age 20.

The clinical manifestations of advancing disease include pelvic discomfort, lower back pain, weight change, abdominal pain, nausea and vomiting, constipation, and urinary frequency. Any ovarian enlargement should be evaluated for malignancy. Palpable ovaries in premenarchal or postmenopausal women are abnormal physical findings.

Collaborative Care Management. The early diagnosis of an ovarian neoplasm usually occurs by chance rather than successful screening. No useful screening test exists at present for widespread use (see Future Watch box). Even ultrasonography, CT scanning, and MRI are not sufficiently specific to distinguish between benign and malignant tumors. Although the use of transvaginal ultrasonography improves the recognition of early malignancies, both abdominal and transvaginal ultrasound are usually inadequate to confirm the diagnosis. CA-125, a tumor marker produced by ovarian cancer cells, is not specific enough to be diagnostic, although it is used to monitor response to chemotherapy. A variety of other tests may be used in the search for metastasis. Listening to the patients symptoms is crucial for early recognition (see Research box).

Laparotomy is the primary tool for both diagnosis and staging. Table 56-8 presents the staging system. Surgery is also the primary therapeutic approach and usually involves total abdominal hysterectomy with bilateral salpingectomy-oophorectomy. Ascitic fluid or washings are submitted for cytologic analysis. All the tissue of the pelvis is carefully assessed, and biopsy specimens of any suspicious tissue are sent for analysis.

Adjuvant therapy is often employed, depending on the stage of the disease. Chemotherapy is typically used for stage I disease, and various combinations of agents are under investigation. Patients with stage II disease may be treated with instillation of radioactive phosphorus (^{32}P) into the peritoneum, external irradiation, or

Future Watch

Protemic Patterns May Be Useful in Screening for Ovarian Cancer

Currently no effective screening test is available for ovarian cancer, which is commonly identified only after it is far advanced. Investigators postulated that profiling low-molecular-weight serum proteins might identify peptides that are unique to this cancer. Molecular biology provides new and exciting approaches to screening for ovarian cancer.

Petricoin EF et al: Use of protemic patterns in serum to identify ovarian cancer, *Lancet* 359:572-577, 2002.

Research

Goff BA et al: Symptom pattern may support ovarian cancer, *JAMA* 291:2705-2712, 2004.

Many women with ovarian cancer report symptoms before diagnosis, but distinguishing symptoms that merit investigation is difficult. To address this problem, researchers administered a symptom survey to women attending a primary care clinic and to women awaiting surgery for a pelvic mass. They compared the frequency, severity, and duration for symptoms reported by women with ovarian cancer and benign masses with those reported by women seeking primary care. The symptom pattern of bloating, increased abdominal size, and urinary symptoms were reported by 43% of women with ovarian cancer but only 8% of the overall primary clinic population. Women with ovarian cancer had significantly more symptoms of higher severity and more recent onset, and they typically experienced symptoms 20 to 30 times per month.

This study adds further evidence that ovarian cancer is not a "silent disease." Symptoms that are more severe or frequent than expected and of recent onset warrant further investigation because they are more likely to be associated with both benign and malignant ovarian masses. Because there are no acceptable screening approaches to detect early ovarian cancer, symptom recognition is crucial.

TABLE 56-7 CLASSIFICATION OF OVARIAN NEOPLASMS

Neoplasm	Examples
Epithelium	Serous, mucinous, endometrioid
Germ cell	Teratoma (mature and immature), dysgerminoma
Gonadal stroma	Granulosa (theca, Sertoli's cells, Leydig's cells)
Mesenchyme	Fibroma, lymphoma, sarcoma

TABLE 56-8 STAGES OF CANCER OF THE OVARY

Stage	Involvement
I	Limited to ovaries
II	Involving 1 or both ovaries with pelvic extension
III	Involving 1 or both ovaries with intraperitoneal metastasis outside pelvis or positive lymph nodes
IV	Involving 1 or both ovaries with distant metastasis (e.g., liver, lungs)

combined chemotherapy. Patients with stage III or IV disease undergo surgical attempts to remove as much tumor as possible. This intervention appears to be directly related to survival. Surgery is followed by aggressive combination chemotherapy with such agents as cisplatin, paclitaxel, and cyclophosphamide.

PATIENT/FAMILY TEACHING. Teaching concerning diagnosis, surgery, and adjuvant therapy for ovarian cancer is an integral aspect of nursing care. Support and education are offered to the patient and family throughout each aspect of diagnosis and treatment. Genetic testing may involve several members of the family. Cancer of the ovary carries a poor prognosis, and the woman and her family need ongoing support.

Neoplasms of the Vulva

Cancer of the Vulva

Etiology and Epidemiology. Vulvar cancer is rare, with invasive disease accounting for just 5% of malignancies of the female genital tract. It is a disease that primarily affects older women. Preinvasive disease (vulvar carcinoma in situ) is occurring more commonly in younger women, possibly because of factors such as exposure to HPV and HIV. Among women who have a history of genital warts, smoking increases the risk of developing vulvar cancer.[2] Three times as many Caucasians are affected as African-Americans. Parity does not seem to play a role in the incidence. Survival rates are high with early detection of noninvasive disease but drop to 50% when lymph nodes are positive.

The exact cause of cancer of the vulva is still unknown. Etiologic factors are believed to include STDs involving the vulva and the use of tight-fitting apparel or nylon undergarments, perineal deodorants, smoking, and trauma. Herpes, syphilis, and genital warts have all been associated with the development of carcinoma.

Pathophysiology. Ninety percent of vulvar cancers are squamous in origin.[2] The initial lesion often arises from an area of intraepithelial neoplasia, which can eventually form a firm nodule and ulcerate. The diagnosis of vulvar cancer can be made only by biopsy and histologic tissue examination. The lesion can develop anywhere on the vulva, but 70% of lesions arise on the labia. The lesion is usually localized and well demarcated. Common clinical manifestations include vulvar itching and burning.

Collaborative Care Management. Because early detection is important in the management of carcinoma of the vulva, all women should be taught the importance of regular vulva self-examination (see Patient/Family Teaching box). Treatment of carcinoma of the vulva varies significantly, depending on the location and extent of the disease. Preinvasive disease is usually treated surgically, with laser therapy, or with skinning vulvectomy. Carcinoma in situ may also be treated nonsurgically with topical 5-fluorouracil (1% Efudex) applied daily; the response rate is 50% to 60%. The standard treatment for invasive carcinoma has been radical vulvectomy, although the procedure has been modified for women with certain types of lesions to make it less mutilating. Radical vulvectomy involves excision of the mons pubis, terminal portion of the urethra, and vagina; excision of portions of the round ligaments and saphenous veins; and selected lymph node dissection (Figure 56-15). Radical surgery achieves an 80% to 90% 5-year survival rate for stage II lesions. Radiation treatment after surgery is used in stage III disease. Chemotherapy is used for recurrent disease.

PATIENT/FAMILY TEACHING
Vulva Self-Examination

Patient teaching about vulva self-examination involves the following instructions:

- Perform once a month between menses. If a history of vulvar disease exists, perform every 2 weeks or more frequently.
- Sit in comfortable, well-lit location.
- Hold a mirror in one hand, and use the other to expose and separate parts of the vulva. (Alternatively, you may place a mirror on the floor and squat over it.)
- Inspect and palpate all areas of the vulva, looking for areas of discoloration (white, red, or dark) or pain, warts, sores, bumps, swelling, or other lesions above or below the surface.
- Beginning with the mons pubis, use the index finger to palpate. Proceed to the clitoris and the surrounding area. Continue with the right and left labia minora and majora, palpating by running the tissue between your thumb and fingertips. End with inspection and palpation of perineum and area around the anus.
- Report any abnormal findings to your health care provider.

Complications related to radical vulvectomy include wound infection and disruption because the wounds are typically left open to heal by secondary intention. Delayed complications include stenosis of the vagina from scar tissue formation, pelvic muscle relaxation leading to stress incontinence, and swelling of the legs from obstructive lymphangitis.

Postoperative care focuses initially on comfort. Because of the widespread tissue destruction, the inguinal suture line is very tight and extremely uncomfortable. The woman needs frequent

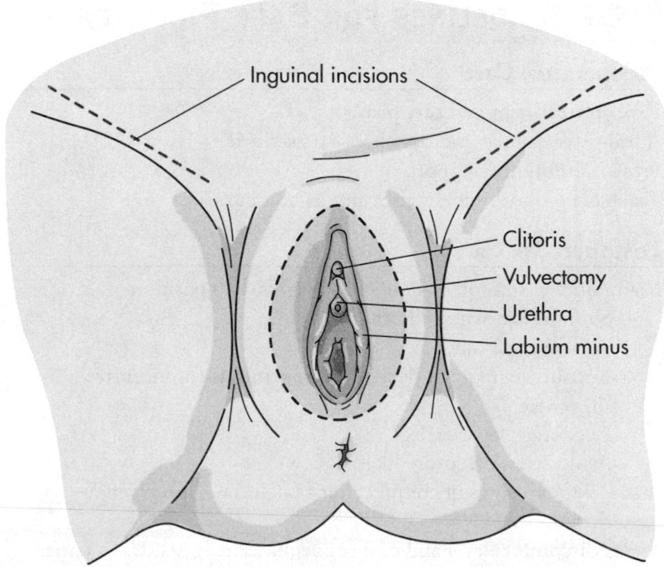

Figure 56-15 Vulvectomy with operative incision lines shown. Note groin incisions.

assistance to achieve a comfortable position. Wound breakdown is often a problem. The vulvar wound is usually left open, and sitz baths, whirlpool therapy, and topical agents may be used to support healing.

Today, the importance of sexuality to a woman's quality of life is well recognized. It has been established that, when cancer is detected early, it is not necessary to remove so much surrounding healthy tissue to achieve a cure. In addition, the sentinel node biopsy procedure avoids removing lymph nodes if the cancer has not spread.[2]

PATIENT/FAMILY TEACHING. The nurse teaches the patient that, even with meticulous care, the wounds heal slowly and complications may occur. The nurse encourages the woman to express her feelings concerning this difficult and disfiguring surgery. The woman is reassured that sexual intercourse usually can be resumed after complete wound healing has occurred—usually at least 6 weeks. Lymphedema in the legs is treated with compression stockings for at least 6 months after surgery. The warning signs of other complications are discussed with the woman before discharge. The Guidelines for Safe Practice box summarizes nursing care for patients experiencing radical vulvectomy.

Sterilization

Etiology and Epidemiology. Voluntary sterilization is the most commonly used method of fertility control for married couples over 30 years of age and is the most widely used contraceptive method worldwide. In the United States about 1 million sterilization procedures are performed annually. The primary reasons given are the desire to limit family size and the desire to be free of the risk of pregnancy with advancing age.

About 1% of sterilized women subsequently request reversal. Successful reversal is more likely in those cases where the method of sterilization used has a higher failure rate. Microsurgical techniques are used and typically involve an end-to-end anastomosis of the ligated tubes.

Pathophysiology. Tubal sterilization terminates a woman's ability to bear children but does not alter ovarian hormone secretion or menstrual function. Artificial menopause is not induced, and the ability to enjoy sexual intercourse should not be impaired. Women appear to have little regret after the surgery if they understand what to expect during and after the procedure and are able to express their feelings and have their questions answered before surgery. Occasionally, however, women who are ambivalent about the choice or have preexisting self-esteem issues develop psychologic problems after sterilization.

Collaborative Care Management. Tubal sterilization was first performed in 1823, and since that time more than 200 different techniques for the procedure have been developed. Most methods involve the mechanical removal of a part of the female reproductive system so that the sperm and ovum cannot unite. Table 56-9 summarizes available methods of sterilization. Minilaparotomy and laparoscopy are by far the most common methods.

In minilaparotomy a small (2- to 3-cm) transverse abdominal incision is made about 3 cm above the pubis, and the peritoneal cavity is entered. The fallopian tubes are located, and a portion of each tube is elevated and ligated at the base. The free ends may be tied off or cauterized. Minilaparotomy is an ambulatory procedure performed with the patient under local anesthesia.

Laparoscopic tubal sterilization is more common and requires only a small subumbilical incision for insertion of the laparoscope. A segment of each tube is coagulated by application of an electric current. Clips or rings may also be applied to the tube. The procedure is brief and safe and is performed with the patient under local anesthesia.

Essure is a method of permanent sterilization that is performed without general anesthesia. A springlike device is

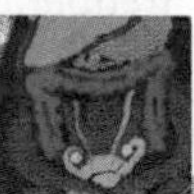

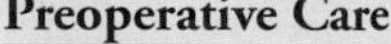

GUIDELINES FOR SAFE PRACTICE *The Patient Undergoing Radical Vulvectomy*

Preoperative Care

Explain treatment and care plan.
Administer enemas and douches as prescribed.
Provide emotional support.
Teach deep breathing exercises and leg exercises.

Postoperative Care

Maintain bed rest for 72 hours in semi-Fowler's position.
- —Support legs with pillows.
- —Turn every 2 hours.
- —Encourage frequent deep breathing and use of incentive spirometer.
- —Encourage leg exercises.
- —Avoid stress on suture lines.
- —Assess for signs of complications (atelectasis, deep venous thrombosis).

Assess discomfort level and ensure adequate analgesia. Use a patient-controlled analgesia pump, if possible, to allow patient to control dosage.

Monitor wound healing.
- —Provide perineal hygiene and give sitz baths when ordered; keep perineum dry.
- —Cleanse wound twice a day and after defecation.

Maintain patency of the Foley catheter.
Provide a low-residue diet.
Provide diversional activities.
Encourage expression of feelings.

Discharge Teaching

Instruct patient to use support hose for 6 months and to elevate legs frequently.
Patient can resume sexual activity in 4 to 6 weeks.
Discuss possible need for lubrication and position changes with coitus; genital numbness may be present.
Instruct patient to avoid straining with defecation.
Discuss signs and symptoms of complications to report to physician.
Note the possible altered directional flow of urine.

TABLE 56-9 METHODS OF TUBAL STERILIZATION FOR WOMEN

Description	Comments
ABDOMINAL	
Minilaparotomy: ligation or cutting of fallopian tubes under direct vision through small abdominal incision or near umbilicus	Complications: wound infection, hematoma, bladder injury Advantages: good chance for sterility reversal
Laparoscopy: electrocoagulation of segment of fallopian tubes by laparoscopy through small abdominal incision near umbilicus	Local anesthesia Advantages: minimal discomfort, short procedure
VAGINAL	
Culpotomy: ligation or cutting of fallopian tube through small incision in Douglas' cul-de-sac	Local, spinal, or general anesthesia Higher complication rate than with laparoscopy (infection, hemorrhage)
Culdoscopy: electrocoagulation of segment of fallopian tubes by culdoscope through small incision in Douglas' cul-de-sac	Local anesthesia Higher complication rate than with laparoscopy Local or general anesthesia
Essure: springlike devices placed in fallopian tubes via the vagina	Advantages: no surgical incision, no general anesthesia

threaded via the vagina into the uterus and then into the fallopian tubes. Eventually a benign tissue response is produced and the tubes become occluded. Because the scarring of the tubes takes time, another form of birth control should be used for 3 months after the procedure.

The laws governing sterilization vary from state to state and have undergone many changes over the years. In general, the surgery may be performed if written, informed consent is given by a woman capable of giving permission. Patients using federal funds for payment must be at least 21 years of age, and there may be a prescribed waiting period for patients using Medicaid funds.

PATIENT/FAMILY TEACHING. Patient teaching is the foundation of nursing care. The discussion of sterilization methods should be based on the federal government's informed consent guidelines (see Legal Alert). The nurse confirms that the woman understands the nature and consequences of the surgical procedure. The facts concerning reversibility, including current success rates, are discussed. Many people equate sterilization with a loss of femininity, and even women who know the difference may appreciate reassurance.

After surgery the woman is instructed to rest for 24 to 48 hours and avoid all heavy lifting and strenuous exercise for 1 week. The nurse instructs the woman to abstain from sexual intercourse until the wound is completely healed and to report any signs of fever, incisional bleeding, or persistent abdominal pain to the physician. Care of the woman after a laparoscopic procedure is discussed in Chapter 55.

Legal Alert

Informed Consent Guidelines (Federal) Relating to Sterilization

- The patient makes the choice. No pressures are placed on patient (e.g., loss of welfare benefits, wrath of health care provider).
- The health care provider describes the benefits and risks of sterilization.
  Benefits: permanent, no further costs or decision making
  Risks: usual surgical risks, possibility of future pregnancy (i.e., not 100% effective)
- The health care provider describes alternative contraceptive methods.
- The patient is encouraged to ask questions.
- The patient may withdraw from using the method without penalty.
- The health care provider gives explanations about the entire sterilization procedure, costs, and possible side effects (effects of hormones, weight changes, menstrual changes, sexual response).
- Written instructions and risk factors are given to patient.
- A written consent to the procedure is signed by patient and witnessed.

Infertility

The term *infertility* refers to the inability to achieve a pregnancy within a stipulated period of time, usually 1 year. The problem may be considered primary if the couple has never conceived or secondary if conception was successfully achieved in the past.

Etiology and Epidemiology. Approximately 15% of all couples in the United States are infertile. Infertility is most often attributed to women, but about 40% of cases result from male infertility.[8] More couples today are seeking infertility treatment, despite its high costs. The majority of couples who undergo assessment and treatment for infertility do successfully conceive.

From 80% to 90% of all women become pregnant within 1 year when they practice unprotected sexual intercourse. Fertility in women is low during the early teenage years, peaks in the mid-twenties, and declines after age 30. Approximately 33% of women who delay pregnancy until after age 35 experience problems with infertility. This rate increases to 60% after age 40. Fertility in men also peaks in the mid-twenties and subsequently declines, but the decrease is much less significant than in women. The frequency of coitus is another recognized variable in fertility, since increased frequency appears to enhance sperm motility. Other risk factors for infertility include a history of STDs and occupational and environmental hazard exposure.

Box 56-5 Causes of Infertility

Female

Developmental: uterine abnormalities
Endocrine: pituitary, thyroid, and adrenal dysfunctions; ovarian dysfunctions (inhibit maturation and release of ova)
Diseases: pelvic inflammatory disease (especially from gonococci); fallopian tube obstructions; diseases of cervix and uterus that inhibit passage of active sperm
Other: malnutrition, severe anemia, anxiety

Male

Developmental: undescended testes, other congenital anomalies (inhibit development of sperm)
Endocrine: hormonal deficiencies (pituitary, thyroid, adrenal) (inhibit development of sperm)
Diseases: testicular destruction from disease, orchitis from mumps, prostatitis
Other: excessive smoking, fatigue, alcohol, excessive heat (hot baths), marijuana use

Both Female and Male

Diseases: sexually transmitted diseases, cancer with obstructions (inhibit transport of ovum or sperm)
Other: immunologic incompatibility (inhibit sperm penetration of ovum), marital problems, diethylstilbestrol exposure in utero (suggested but not proved as a cause of male infertility)

Pathophysiology. Three basic categories of infertility account for most reproductive dysfunction: anovulation, anatomic defects of the female genital tract, and abnormal sperm production. Common causes of infertility in men and women are presented in Box 56-5. In 11.2% of cases no cause can be found.[8]

Ovulatory dysfunction is a leading cause of infertility. It can result from a malfunction at any point in the hormonal feedback system. Fallopian tube obstruction is a common structural defect. Acute salpingitis from gonorrhea or chlamydial infection is the most common cause of this obstruction. Pelvic infections, use of IUDs, and endometriosis can also cause fallopian tube obstruction.

Infection may destroy the glands that secrete the thin, watery mucus essential for sperm survival and migration. Estrogen deficiency may decrease the volume and quality of the cervical mucus. Anomalies of the uterus, including leiomyomas, may interfere with successful implantation.

A number of studies suggest that tobacco may be a causal factor in infertility. Nicotine appears to adversely affect tubal transport and implantation. Mycoplasmas, which cause cervicitis, may contribute to infertility, and the role of other infectious agents is under investigation. Dietary deficiencies are known to adversely affect secretion of pituitary gonadotropins, and strenuous exercise, such as running more than 10 miles per week, has been implicated in infertility, either through its caloric demands or the effects of endorphins on the pituitary gland.

Infertility can produce profound psychologic effects. When couples find themselves unable to have children, the trauma can affect every aspect of their lives and marriage. The experience of diagnosis and treatment can be an emotional roller-coaster of raised expectations and dashed hopes.

Collaborative Care Management. The purposes of an infertility evaluation are to establish the cause of infertility and provide a basis for determining medical or surgical treatment options. The process can be physically painful, as well as emotionally and economically stressful. The various diagnostic tests used in the diagnosis of infertility are discussed in Chapter 55 and summarized in Table 56-10.

Artificial insemination is a simple, safe, inexpensive, and highly successful infertility treatment when male infertility is the cause. Semen may be deposited by a cervical-vaginal, intracervical, or intrauterine route. A few drops of semen are injected as close to the

Table 56-10 Diagnostic Testing for Infertility

Gender	Tests	Purpose
Male	Semen analysis	Determine presence, number, and motility of sperm.
	Testicular biopsy if sperm count low or absent	Check for presence of sperm, which indicates obstruction of vas deferens.
Female	Basal body temperature chart	Determine that ovulation is occurring.
	Postcoital test of cervical secretions	Measure ability of sperm to penetrate cervical mucus and remain active; determine quality of mucus.
	Endometrial biopsy	Determine whether ovulation is occurring (if in question).
	Laparoscopy	Examine pelvis and determine patency of fallopian tubes.
	Hysterosalpingography (x-ray film after insertion of contrast media)	Determine patency of uterus and fallopian tubes.
Male and female	Hormonal tests	Determine whether problem is hormonal.

Ethical Alert

Gender Selection

Since 1995, the MicroSort method has been used to sort sperm. This method is based on the fact that X chromosomes are bigger than Y chromosomes, so when sperm are soaked in a fluorescent dye, the X chromosome soaks up more of the dye and glows brighter. The sperm is sorted according to brightness. This technique is 88% effective for couples desiring a girl and 73% effective for those desiring a boy. The only sure way to select the sex is to test the embryo before implanting. Preselecting embryos began as a way for families who have histories of sex-linked genetic diseases to avoid conceiving a child with the disease. This method costs about $15,000. Ethical questions include: Should only those who can afford this procedure be able to benefit from it? Should families without sex-linked diseases be able to choose the sex of their child?

time of ovulation as possible. Treatment may use the partner's semen (homologous) or donor semen (heterologous). The fertility of donors is carefully determined, and the sperm are screened for HIV. This can be an emotional topic for some couples and may induce strong reactions.

In the past decade a virtual explosion of reproductive technology has occurred. These procedures, known as assisted reproductive technologies, are expensive and raise ethical issues regarding parenting (see Ethical Alert). There is a movement to mandate insurance coverage for nonexperimental methods of treating infertility, since many insurance companies do not provide coverage for fertility treatment. Box 56-6 summarizes other, less commonly employed approaches to infertility.

The correction of structural problems is undertaken first if feasible. Transcervical balloon tuboplasty may be performed to correct blocked or scarred fallopian tubes. A modified cardiovascular balloon is passed into the fallopian tube and inflated to clear the occlusion.

A variety of drugs can be used to induce or support ovulation. Clomiphene citrate (Clomid, Serophene) is used for women with intact pituitary function. Follicle-stimulating and luteinizing hormones, such as menotropins (Pergonal), are used when patients have pituitary dysfunction.

Recombinant deoxyribonucleic acid–origin gonadotropins, such as follitropin-beta (Follistim) and follitropin-alfa (Gonal-F), are also used. HCG may be given to trigger the release of mature follicles, and progesterone preparations may be used for luteal phase support. The drugs may also be used in combination.

Multiple births can occur with ovulatory induction therapy. The onset of lower abdominal pain can indicate the development of an ovarian cyst or cyst rupture. The woman is informed of the multiple-drug side effects, which include hot flashes, emotional lability and depression, fatigue, nausea, and bloating.

Problems of sperm production are addressed by first eliminating alterations of thermoregulation. Optimal sperm production occurs at temperatures approximately 1° to 3° F below body temperature. The man is instructed to avoid sitting for long periods in hot tubs, wearing tight clothes that pull the testicles against the body, and sitting for long periods with poor heat dispersion. Medications (clomiphene citrate, HCG, menotropins, and a GnRH pump) can also be used to treat male infertility.

Traditional drug therapy may be combined with intrauterine insemination. This approach has achieved a success rate comparable with that of in vitro fertilization—approximately 20%.

PATIENT/FAMILY TEACHING. Infertility can produce profound psychologic effects. The nurse is challenged to help couples be active participants in the entire infertility workup and treatment plan, carefully exploring the limits they wish to set on the attempt to become pregnant. Sexual dysfunction often occurs, as this formerly pleasurable and spontaneous private activity becomes a public process to be dissected and often used as a measure of their success or failure concerning pregnancy. The nurse encourages the

Box 56-6 Alternative Approaches to Fertility Management

In Vitro Fertilization and Embryo Transfer

One or more ova are recovered from the ovarian follicles and fertilized with the partner's sperm in a Petri dish. Oocyte retrieval is performed by means of ultrasound-guided needle aspiration. The cleaved ova are placed in the patient's uterus through a small catheter about 48 hours after retrieval. Pregnancy rates are related to the number of embryos placed and vary from 18% to 30%.

Gamete Intrafallopian Transfer (GIFT)

Oocytes aspirated from follicles are mixed with washed sperm and placed in the uterine tube via laparoscopy. This approach appears to achieve a higher pregnancy rate than in vitro fertilization. The preembryo travels toward the uterus, following the natural timetable for implantation in 4 days.

Zygote Intrafallopian Transfer (ZIFT) and Tubal Embryo Transfer (TET)

ZIFT procedures are similar to GIFT, except transfer to the fallopian (uterine) tubes occurs at the zygote stage, about 16 to 18 hours after oocyte insemination. TET involves transfer of embryos into the fallopian tube around 40 to 48 hours after oocyte insemination.

Surrogate Mothers

Surrogate mothers are women who contract to conceive by artificial insemination and give the baby to the semen donor (or to the couple who arranged for the conception) after delivery. Many social and legal implications with the process have received recent attention through some extremely public lawsuits over custody of the child.

Ovum Transfer

A donor provides the ovum, which is fertilized with the partner's sperm. The embryo is transferred to the infertile woman's uterus after about 5 days via a small catheter. Pregnancy rates have been as high as 25% to 50%.

honest expression of feelings and provides time for dealing with the couple's intense feelings during treatment. Anticipatory guidance regarding side effects of medications is provided to improve tolerance.

Nurses also play an important role in promoting fertility. Patient teaching aimed at preventing infection of the pelvic organs, particularly gonorrhea and chlamydial infection, is critical. Salpingitis is often the first overt sign of gonorrhea and can result in obstruction of the fallopian tubes. Early diagnosis and effective treatment of all vaginal and cervical infections is critical. The nurse encourages the use of barrier contraceptives, which help reduce the risk of infection, and encourages the woman to limit the number of sexual partners. Women with ovarian and hormonal problems commonly experience symptoms such as menstrual irregularities. Many of these problems can be successfully managed with hormone therapy if identified early, before problems with infertility develop.

Critical Thinking

1. You have been asked to speak to a group of high school students about women's health issues. Outline how you would address the relationships among the development of pelvic inflammatory disease, cervical cancer, and infertility.
2. A patient is completing intracavitary radiation treatment for early cervical cancer. You are beginning her discharge teaching related to vaginal fibrosis when she breaks into tears. She says, "How will we ever resume sexual intercourse? I stink, this drainage is disgusting, and my husband will never find me attractive again." How will you respond?

References

1. American Cancer Society: *Facts and figures 2004,* accessed from website: www.cancer.org.
2. American Cancer Society: *Vulvar cancer 2004,* accessed from website: www.cancer.org.
3. Centers for Disease Control and Prevention: Sexually transmitted diseases treatment guidelines, *Morbid Mortal Weekly Rep* 51(RR-6):1-78, 2002.
4. Chandran L: *Cervicitis,* Jan 2004, accessed from website: www.emedicine.com/ped/topic361.htm.
5. Darenberg J et al: Intravenous immunoglobulin G therapy in streptococcal toxic shock syndrome: a European randomized, double-blind, placebo-controlled trial, *Clin Infect Dis* 37:333-340, 2003.
6. Darves B: New Pap guidelines reduce screening but raise concerns about compliance, *Am Coll Phys Observer,* April 2003.
7. Reference deleted in proofs.
8. Garcia JE, Nelson LM: *Infertility,* updated May 23, 2005, from website http://www/eMedicine.com/med/top3535.htm.
9. Hudson T: Premenstrual syndrome, part I, *The Female Patient* 27(5):47-49, 2002.
10. Johnson M: *Abnormal vaginal bleeding,* accessed May 2004 from website: www.medical-library.org.
11. Johnson M: *Alternatives to hysterectomy in management of fibroids,* accessed May 2004 from website: www.medical-library.org.

11a. Kessenich CR: UFE can spell relief from uterine fibroid misery, *NY/NJ Nurs Spectrum* pp. 21-22, September 26, 2005.

12. Lacey J: Obesity linked to cervical cancer, *Cancer* 98(4):814-821, 2003.
13. Moore LE, Ware D: *Hydatidiform mole,* updated June 24, 2005, from eMedicine.com, topic 104.
14. Munoz N et al: Epidemiologic classification of HPV types associated with cervical cancer, *N Engl J Med* 348:518-527, 2003.
15. Plummer M et al: Smoking may double cervical cancer risk, *Cancer Causes Control* 14(9):805-814, 2003.
16. Smith J: Cervical cancer and use of hormonal contraceptives, *Lancet* 361(9364):1159-1167, 2003.
17. Van Kessel K et al: Common complementary and alternative therapies for yeast vaginitis and bacterial vaginosis: a systemic review, *Obstet Gynecol Surv* 58:351-358, 2003.
18. Winter WE, Gosewehr JA: *Uterine cancer,* updated November 24, 2004, from website: eMedicine.com/top2832.

 Visit the Evolve website: http://evolve.elsevier.com/Monahan/medsurg

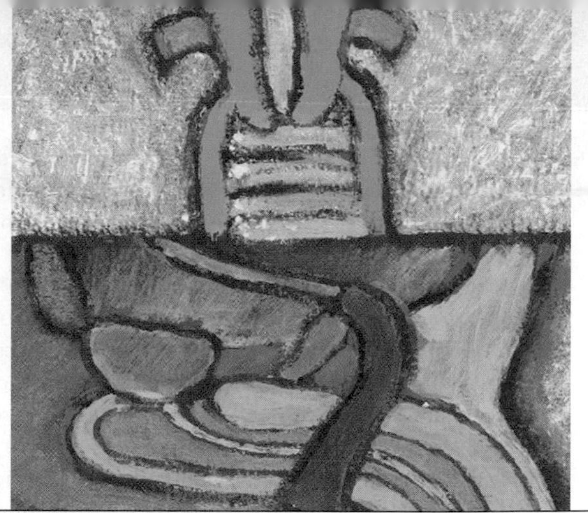

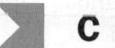

CHAPTER 57
Male Reproductive Problems

by Margaret K. Warshaw

OBJECTIVES

After studying this chapter, the learner should be able to:

1. Describe the process of infectious diseases specific to men's reproductive health.
2. Compare the nursing care associated with benign and malignant neoplasms that are specific to men's reproductive health.
3. Describe expected patient outcomes for each condition discussed.
4. Identify teaching needs for various treatments of male reproductive problems.
5. Compare the common causes of impotence, both physical and psychologic.
6. Discuss nursing interventions related to the structural and infectious problems presented in the chapter.
7. Identify the common complications related to the different problems of the male reproductive system.

KEY TERMS

alpha-fetoprotein, p. 1725
atrophy, p. 1723
continence, p. 1731
gonadal, p. 1723
hypertrophy, p. 1726
lymph node dissection, p. 1725
reflux, p. 1722
spermatogenesis, p. 1722
sterilization, p. 1747

Men's reproductive health care is one dimension of an emerging specialty area of nursing practice, men's health. Traditionally problems of the male reproductive system have been viewed only as problems related to aging or lifestyle choices. Often the health care system has minimized the complexity of the male reproductive system and the patient's multiple psychosocial needs. Consequently, men often do not seek medical care until symptoms are well advanced. Also, myths and knowledge deficits related to the specifics of sexual function are common in the male population. It is important to provide health care that is sensitive, accurate, and timely for this population. This chapter focuses on the most common health problems of the male reproductive system, particularly common infections, problems of the prostate gland, and impotence. Sexually transmitted diseases (STDs) are presented in Chapter 59. Figure 55-8 illustrates the male reproductive organs and associated structures.

Problems of the Testes and Related Structures

The scrotal sac contains the testes; epididymis; part of the spermatic cord; and other associated structures, including nerve, lymphatic, and vascular networks (see Figure 55-10). These structures are responsible for the production and storage of sperm and provide the pathway for ejaculation. The testes are also involved in the production of hormones, primarily testosterone. Consequently, any disorders related to these structures have the potential to affect male fertility adversely, as well as interfere with testosterone production.

Pathologic conditions of these structures include problems with swelling, twisting of cords, trauma, and carcinomas. The testes are particularly sensitive to changes in scrotal environment. Fluctuations in temperature and blood flow often have a negative affect on fertility. Infection is another common problem. Accurately differentiating between pathologic conditions related to infection versus structural problems or neoplasms can facilitate timely therapy and improve the patient's prognosis.

Epididymitis

Etiology and Epidemiology. The epididymis is a convoluted tubular structure within the scrotal sac that acts as a reservoir for sperm. While in this structure, sperm mature and become fertile and mobile. Epididymitis is an acute inflammatory process within the epididymis and is one of the most common intrascrotal inflammations. In the United States epididymitis accounts for more than 600,000 visits per year to health care providers.[11] This inflammation is rarely seen in children and occurs infrequently in the older adult man. The highest prevalence is in young men 19 to 35 years of age, although the incidence among sexually active adolescent males is increasing.[9]

Inflammation of the epididymis most often is caused by an ascending infection via the ejaculatory duct through the vas deferens into the epididymis. Such infections can occur in three ways. First, infection may be introduced when surgical or diagnostic procedures are performed. This occurs more frequently among boys less than 15 years old and in men over 45 years old. The most common organism of contamination in these age-groups is *Escherichia coli.* Second, structural malformations or developmental structural insufficiencies in the child may contribute to problems of urinary **reflux**. Reflux of infected urine can cause infection; reflux of sterile urine causes a chemical irritation in the epididymis and is another common cause of inflammation.

Finally, in the man between the ages of 19 and 35, sexual transmission is the most common means of infection. The pathogens most likely to cause epididymitis in heterosexual men are *Chlamydia trachomatis* and *Neisseria gonorrhoeae.*[9] In homosexual men the most common pathogens are the ones that would be found in the anal canal: *E. coli* and *Haemophilus influenzae.*

Pathophysiology. Epididymitis is an inflammation of the epididymis and scrotal sac. Fluid accumulates in the scrotal sac as a result of the process. Excess fluid loss into the interstitial space of the scrotal sac can lead to diminished blood flow, nerve damage, and resultant pain and swelling. Inflammatory fluids also can form pockets of pus called abscesses. Heat generated from the inflammatory process can negatively affect the testicular function of **spermatogenesis**. Consequently, complications of epididymitis include testicular infarction, chronic pain from nerve damage, abscess formation, and infertility.

The most common clinical manifestations are severe tenderness, pain in the scrotal area, and noticeable swelling of one or both sides of the scrotum. The onset of pain is usually gradual, increasing over hours or days. Scrotal swelling can cause pain on ambulation and discomfort that is exacerbated by wearing restrictive clothing. Elevation of the scrotum often relieves the pain of epididymitis (Prehn's sign) and may help differentiate epididymitis from testicular torsion. The diagnosis of epididymitis is supported by the presence of fever, general malaise, dysuria, and urethral discharge.[9]

Collaborative Care Management. Assessment of the patient with symptoms of epididymitis should include a sexual history. For young children, it should include questions to determine possible sexual abuse and any history of recent urinary examinations or instrumentation. In older men questions focus on history or symptoms of urinary obstruction or recent urinary examinations.

Prompt diagnosis is essential to decrease the risk of complications. Urinalysis is used to differentiate epididymitis from emergency conditions such as testicular torsion (see later discussion). With epididymitis, the urinalysis usually shows an increased white blood cell (WBC) count and bacteria. Urine and urethral cultures are used to determine the specific causative organism and its sensitivity to various antibiotics to provide information for needed drug therapies.

Other diagnostic tests to detect epididymitis focus on changes in blood flow to the inflamed scrotum. An initial increase in blood flow to the area would indicate inflammation or infection, whereas other conditions resulting in swelling might impede blood flow. Scrotal ultrasound is a noninvasive diagnostic measure used on adults when urinalysis and cultures are not conclusive. Ultrasound for this condition is usually done serially and, if possible, by comparing the unaffected scrotum to the affected side. Any indication of reduced blood flow to the affected side usually indicates a more serious condition or a complication of epididymitis. Radionuclide scanning can also be performed when the diagnosis is questionable. These scans are more sensitive than ultrasound and generally show increased blood perfusion to the affected side of the scrotum if epididymitis is present.

The nurse assesses the patient's pain, including whether the pain is bilateral or unilateral, whether it is of sudden onset or developed over hours or days, and whether it is relieved by elevating the scrotum. Any symptoms of dysuria are documented, such as burning, frequency, urgency, fever, and general malaise. A recent history of urethral discharge or change in the discharge is important to help determine the type of causative organism. The nurse documents the color, consistency, and amount of any discharge.

The patient is also observed for the classic "waddle," or a somewhat rolling gait, indicating an attempt to protect the scrotum. The nurse documents swelling of the scrotum and whether it is on the left, right, or both sides. Palpation of the scrotum at this time is generally deferred to avoid causing severe pain. The nurse instructs the patient to obtain a urine sample using the *first* voiding (not midstream) to help differentiate urinary contamination from the urethra, rather than the bladder.

Treatment of epididymitis usually consists of pain management, medications to treat the infection, and supportive care. Nonsteroidal antiinflammatory drugs (NSAIDs) such as ibuprofen may be used to decrease the inflammation and relieve the discomfort and swelling. Narcotic analgesics may be prescribed if the pain is severe. Stool softeners are given to prevent constipation and reduce straining on defecation, which may cause severe pain in the inflamed scrotum.

Eradication of the infection generally is accomplished by giving oral antibiotics. Most antibiotics prescribed are broad spectrum. Oral quinolones or cephalosporins are frequently the antibiotics of choice.[11] These antibiotics may be prescribed for a course of 14 to 30 days depending on the disease's chronicity. The nurse instructs the patient to take these medications for the entire time they are prescribed to avoid recurrence of the disease. If STDs are present, antibiotics are prescribed. The patient's sexual partners should be treated at the same time.

Measures to reduce swelling, prevent traction on the spermatic cord, and improve venous drainage are implemented. Bed rest with the scrotum elevated on a towel, application of ice packs, and the use of scrotal supports when the swelling is less severe decrease the discomfort caused by the heavy sensation resulting from the enlarged scrotum (Figure 57-1).

Unless high fever and the potential for complications are present, most men with epididymitis can be treated as outpatients.

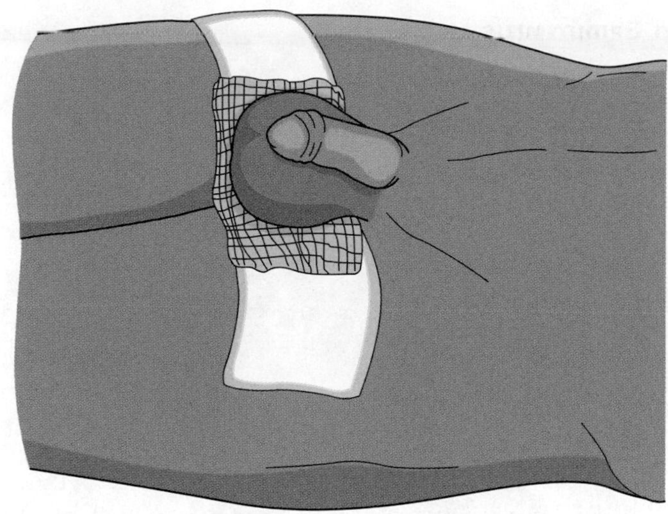

Figure 57-1 A simple scrotal support.

Frequent return appointments are indicated if swelling does not resolve in a few weeks. Because this condition can be associated with other pathologic conditions of the scrotum, a more comprehensive palpation of scrotal structures is performed after the swelling has resolved. The examination incorporates such diagnostic tests as ultrasound, magnetic resonance imaging (MRI), and aspiration of fluid from the scrotum.

PATIENT/FAMILY TEACHING. Patient education initially focuses on information about the disorder and measures to reduce the swelling of the scrotum. Bed rest is recommended until the patient is pain free. The patient is instructed to avoid work, sexual arousal, and other activities that strain the lower abdomen and scrotal area and to wear a scrotal support for approximately 6 weeks. Because STDs are the most common causes of epididymitis, it is important for the patient to be educated about prevention. Patient teaching stresses the importance of using condoms and maintaining good hygiene. (Methods of preventing STDs are discussed more completely in Chapter 59.)

Orchitis

Etiology and Epidemiology. Inflammation or infection of the testicle is known as orchitis. Orchitis may be caused by pyogenic bacteria, gonococci, tubercle bacilli, or viruses (e.g., paramyxovirus, the agent responsible for mumps), or it may follow any septicemia. Orchitis often occurs after epididymitis. Orchitis occurs as a complication of mumps in approximately 20% of all cases contracted after puberty. Symptoms may develop 4 to 6 days after the onset of parotitis. If the case of mumps is mild, there may be no symptoms until the onset of orchitis.

Pathophysiology. Inflammatory fluid seeps from the testicle into the serous membrane lining the epididymis and the testicle to create unilateral or bilateral swelling. Hydrocele (a collection of fluid within the tunica vaginalis testis) is frequently associated with orchitis. The signs and symptoms of orchitis are the same as those of epididymitis. However, because orchitis is caused by a systemic infectious process rather than a localized infection, more systemic symptoms are present, including nausea, vomiting, and pain radiating to the inguinal canal.

As a result of inflammation and fibrosis, some degree of testicular **atrophy** occurs in 20% to 50% of patients. Atrophy of the testes may lead to sterility; however, unless both testes are severely involved, infertility is rare.

Collaborative Care Management. Any postpubertal boy or man who is exposed to mumps may be given gamma globulin immediately unless he has already had mumps or been vaccinated for the disease. Gamma globulin may not prevent mumps, but the disease is usually less severe and less likely to cause complications. Bacterial orchitis is treated with broad-spectrum antibiotics. Antiinflammatory medication is given to help reduce pain and swelling.

PATIENT/FAMILY TEACHING. Patient education focuses on measures to reduce discomfort from **gonadal** swelling and alleviate systemic symptoms. During the acute phase of gonadal swelling, the scrotum may be supported as described for the patient with epididymitis. Warm or cold compresses may be applied to help reduce swelling and increase comfort. Rest and increased fluid intake are encouraged for all patients.

Testicular Torsion

Etiology and Epidemiology. Testicular torsion results from twisting of the spermatic cord and testicle that creates a loss of blood flow, producing ischemia and pain. The onset of pain may be associated with trauma or physical exertion; however, in most cases there is no precipitating event. The pain may awaken the patient at night. A risk factor for testicular torsion is a congenital defect known as "bell clapper" deformity. Occurring in approximately 12% of males, this anomaly is characterized by the inappropriate attachment of the testicle and spermatic cord. This allows the testicle to twist spontaneously on the spermatic cord one or more times, causing the torsion. As a result of its longer spermatic cord, the left testicle is more likely to be involved.[9]

Testicular torsion occurs in neonates and adolescents, but incidence peaks in patients age 14, with 60% of cases occurring in patients between the ages of 12 and 18.[9]

Pathophysiology. Torsion interrupts the blood supply to the testis, leading to ischemia and severe unrelieved pain that may be aggravated by manual elevation of the affected side. The scrotum is swollen, tender, and red. The affected side is usually elevated because the twisting and shortening of the cord pull up the testicle. The cremasteric reflex, elicited by stroking the inner aspect of the thigh to cause reflex retraction of the testicle, is usually absent on the side of the suspected torsion. Although the scrotum appears infected because of the swelling and redness, both urinalysis and blood tests are typically normal. Fever is rarely present. Absence of pain after a time may indicate infarction and necrosis. Gangrene may be a serious sequela.

TABLE 57-1 COMPARISON OF TESTICULAR TORSION AND EPIDIDYMITIS

	Torsion	Epididymitis
Age	Neonate to adolescence	Adolescence and later
Onset	Acute	Gradual
Pain		
Prehn's sign	Negative	Positive
Dysuria	Absent	Present
Fever	Rare	Common
Urinalysis	Normal	Pyuria common
Urethral discharge	None	Often present
Physical examination	Testis may be elevated with abnormal lie; testis is swollen and tender; epididymis also may be tender.	Epididymis is firm, tender, and swollen; testis may be normal or swollen.
Cremasteric reflex	Usually negative	Usually positive

Testicular viability following torsion is directly related to the duration of the torsion episode. Testicular torsion *must* be treated within 6 hours to salvage the testis. Preservation of the testis beyond 12 hours is unlikely.[9] Table 57-1 lists assessment criteria to help differentiate torsion from epididymitis.

Collaborative Care Management. Diagnostic studies for testicular torsion may include color Doppler ultrasound to help identify reduced blood flow. Doppler ultrasound also allows imaging of the structures that can help determine risk factors such as "bell clapper" deformity or rule out associated problems such as trauma.

Detorsion (a process of untwisting the spermatic cord) can be attempted manually. If detorsion is unsuccessful, surgical intervention is imperative within 6 to 12 hours to maintain viability of the testis. Even so, the testis may atrophy. Unless gangrenous, the testis is not excised, since it may still produce hormones, even if spermatogenesis is destroyed. The testis is fixed surgically to the scrotal wall (orchiopexy) to prevent recurrence. The contralateral testis is usually fixed prophylactically at the same time.

If the testicle is gangrenous or found to be nonviable after surgical detorsion, an orchiectomy (removal of the testicle) is carried out. If orchiectomy is performed, a testicular prosthesis is usually inserted. Nursing care after orchiopexy and orchiectomy is similar. Ice bags and scrotal elevation may be ordered to reduce swelling. The nurse continues to monitor the patient for signs of testicular necrosis and fever in the case of orchiopexy. A small Penrose drain may be placed in the scrotum, which will necessitate dressing changes.

PATIENT/FAMILY TEACHING. Instructions for self-care after scrotal surgery are found in the Patient/Family Teaching box. Because body image disturbances may result from castration, raising fears of loss of masculinity and issues relating to sterility and impotence, the nurse also provides specific information about the physiologic changes resulting from testicular atrophy or surgical removal of the testicle. Men are still able to have an erection after trauma or surgery to the testicles. Fertility may or may not be affected if there is still a remaining healthy testicle. If necessary, counseling on alternative means of conception may be suggested. The patient is reminded that the appearance of the scrotum will not be altered if a testicular prosthesis is inserted after orchiectomy.

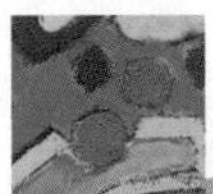

PATIENT/FAMILY TEACHING
Self-Care After Scrotal Surgery

The nurse should instruct the patient to:

- Take sitz baths as needed to relieve discomfort.
- Wear a scrotal support for at least 3 weeks to control edema.
- Limit stair climbing to two flights for 4 weeks to prevent strain on scrotal tissues.
- Avoid lifting or carrying objects weighing more than 5 pounds for 4 weeks to prevent strain on scrotal tissues.
- Refrain from sexual activity for 6 weeks to prevent strain on scrotal tissues.

Testicular Cancer

Etiology and Epidemiology. The causes of testicular cancer are still unknown. A wide range of genetic and environmental causes are being explored. Chemical carcinogens, trauma, and orchitis are all theorized to initiate malignant changes. Because the incidence of testicular cancer is greater for men who live in rural areas, environmental triggers are also suspected. Possible congenital causes include familial predisposition, genetic diseases such as Klinefelter's and Turner's syndromes, and cryptorchidism (failure of the testis to descend at birth).[7,26] There is a 20% to 40% greater risk of testicular cancer in men who have a history of cryptorchidism.[7]

Cancer of the testis is a relatively uncommon disease, accounting for only 1% of neoplasms in men. It is, however, the most common malignancy in males between the ages of 15 and 35. For unknown reasons the incidence of testicular cancer in the United States has nearly doubled since the 1930s and continues to rise. Although very treatable if detected early, testicular cancer would cause an estimated 390 deaths in 2005,[4a] up from 360 in 2004.[4] American Caucasian men have a rate four times that of African-

American men. If detected and treated early, testicular cancer has a 90% to 100% chance of cure. Unfortunately, approximately half the cases are found in advanced stages. Common areas of metastasis are the spine, peritoneum, and lung.[7]

Pathophysiology. Testicular neoplasms are divided into two classifications: germinal and nongerminal. Germinal cancers make up 90% to 95% of all testicular neoplasms and are further divided into two groups: seminomatous (40%) and nonseminomatous (NSGCT) (60%) tumors. In addition, tumors with mixed cell types can occur and are managed as nonseminomas.[7,18]

The determination of cell type helps to focus treatment. The diagnostic workup includes chest x-ray studies, ultrasound imaging, computed tomography (CT), intravenous pyelogram (IVP), skeletal surveys if the patient's alkaline phosphatase is elevated, and lymphangiography. Biopsy of the testis is contraindicated because of the highly metastatic character of testicular carcinoma. Manipulation and invasion of the cancer could cause it to seed to other areas. Laboratory tests include evaluation of **alpha-fetoprotein** (AFP), the beta subunit of human chorionic gonadotropin (beta-HCG), and lactate dehydrogenase (LDH). AFP is considered a marker that indicates the presence of nonseminomatous disease. It is never elevated with seminomas. LDH is elevated in 50% of all patients with testis tumors. LDH is not specific to any one tumor category.[7] No one combination of elevated and normal markers specifically indicates testicular neoplasm. However, changes in the laboratory values of these markers help to monitor the effectiveness of therapeutic interventions.

Clinical manifestations of testicular cancer are often subtle and go unnoticed until the man notices a feeling of heaviness or dragging in the lower abdomen and groin area. A lump or swelling may be present, which is usually nontender and painless. Other symptoms are nonspecific, such as back pain, weight loss, fatigue, and sometimes breast tenderness. Some testicular tumors may grow rapidly, doubling in size within weeks.[19]

Collaborative Care Management. In any suspected case of testicular cancer the testis is usually removed immediately. Men who are at higher risk for testicular cancer as a result of cryptorchidism may be encouraged to undergo orchiectomy as a prophylactic measure. Radical inguinal orchiectomy is performed to excise the spermatic cord, the contents of the inguinal canal, and the testis with the tunicae attached. The adjacent area is explored for metastases. The specimens are then examined to determine the cancer cell type. If NSGCT is found, then a nerve-sparing retroperitoneal **lymph node dissection** is usually done at the time of orchiectomy. Staging of the disease (Box 57-1) and pathologic findings determine the course of treatment.

Box 57-1 Staging of Testicular Neoplasia

Stage I	No metastasis; confined to testis
Stage II	Metastasis to retroperitoneal lymph nodes or other subdiaphragmatic areas
Stage III	Metastasis to mediastinal or supraclavicular nodes or supradiaphragmatic areas like lung and liver

Of the two major types of testicular cancer, seminoma is highly responsive to radiotherapy. For stage I seminoma, irradiation is administered to the retroperitoneal nodes. In stage II, irradiation of the mediastinal and supraclavicular nodes may be added. Chemotherapy may be done for both stages II and III.[19] If tumor markers are present or elevated after irradiation, nonseminomatous involvement must be suspected. Seminoma can metastasize into a different type of cancer. A second primary lesion can develop in the remaining testis. The prognosis in that case is the same as if it were the first lesion.

Nonseminomatous neoplasms are radioresistant. Therefore retroperitoneal lymphadenectomy or radical node dissection is performed at the time of orchiectomy. Chemotherapy is given for clinical, radiologic, or tumor marker evidence of metastasis. If the lymph node dissection is positive, the patient has stage II disease. Cyclic combination chemotherapy is administered for stages II and III. Drugs used in combination chemotherapy include cisplatin, etoposide, and bleomycin.

Nongerminal testicular tumors are rare. Treatment consists of various combinations of the four modes of treatment (orchiectomy, radiation, lymphadenectomy, chemotherapy) used in germinal neoplasms. Table 57-2 lists treatments and 5-year survival rates for testicular cancer for each tumor type.

PATIENT/FAMILY TEACHING. Patient teaching focuses on the planned treatment and its expected side effects. Radiotherapy and chemotherapy are discussed in Chapter 23. Low-dose radiation is used for the seminomatous tumors and has a lower incidence of side effects than the dose given for NSGCT. Although the normal testis is shielded during external radiation, it is exposed to radiation scattered from the abdomen and thighs. The nurse explains that depending on the scatter dose, sperm counts fall after radiation, but may recover in 1 to 2 years. As with chemotherapy, some men report having children after radiation treatment of seminoma. The children do not appear to have a high risk of congenital malformations.[18]

The nurse explains the effects of orchiectomy on fertility. Orchiectomy alone does not result in infertility if the contralateral testis is normal. The remaining testis undergoes hyperplasia, producing sufficient testosterone to maintain sexual function, drive, and characteristics.

After a radical node dissection, there is danger of hemorrhage. Vigorous movement may be contraindicated, since nodes may have been resected from around many large abdominal vessels. The patient should not do any lifting or driving for 10 to 14 days after surgery. Pain and swelling of the scrotum are treated with pain medications, elevation of the scrotum when the patient is supine, and scrotal support during ambulation. Application of a warm or cool compress may also provide comfort and decrease swelling.

Even though prosthetic testes are used to lessen the change in the scrotum's physical appearance, the patient is usually aware of the loss of a sexual organ. The nurse needs to explore the emotional effect this loss has on the patient and provide support and possible referral for counseling.

After a retroperitoneal lymphadenectomy, 90% of patients experience decreased ejaculatory ability, which results from a disruption of the sympathetic nervous system pathways. The nurse

TABLE 57-2 TESTICULAR CANCER: TUMOR TYPE, TREATMENT, AND 5-YEAR SURVIVAL RATE

Stage	Histology	Treatment	5-Year Survival Rate
I	Seminoma	Orchiectomy, radiation	97%
	Nonseminoma	Orchiectomy, retroperitoneal lymph node dissection (RPLND), surveillance for 1 yr	95%
II	Seminoma	*Nonbulky tumor* (<5 cm): orchiectomy and radiation	90%
		Bulky tumor (>5 cm): orchiectomy and combination chemotherapy (cisplatin-based regimen) or radiation	70%
	Nonseminoma	Orchiectomy, RPLND, followed by combination chemotherapy	95%
III	Seminoma	Orchiectomy and multidrug chemotherapy	60%-85%
	Nonseminoma	Orchiectomy and multidrug chemotherapy	50%-70%

Data from National Cancer Institute: *Testicular cancer (PDQ)*, accessed August 2004 from website: www.nci.nih.gov/cancertopics/pdq/treatment/testicular/healthprofessional.

informs the patient that ejaculation is independent of other sexual functions and that erection and orgasm are still possible. The sexual partner should also be invited to learn about these changes in function.

Follow-up visits are often scheduled monthly for the first year after surgery to have serum tumor markers drawn, chest x-ray films, and possibly a CT scan. The interval between visits increases to 2 months for 2 more years to continue monitoring for signs of cancer recurrence. The nurse also teaches the patient how to perform monthly testicular self-examination (see Patient/Family Teaching box below and Figure 57-2). All males should perform testicular self-examination starting at puberty. Because men are at greatest risk for testicular cancer between the ages of 18 and 38 years, teaching needs to be targeted to this age-group.

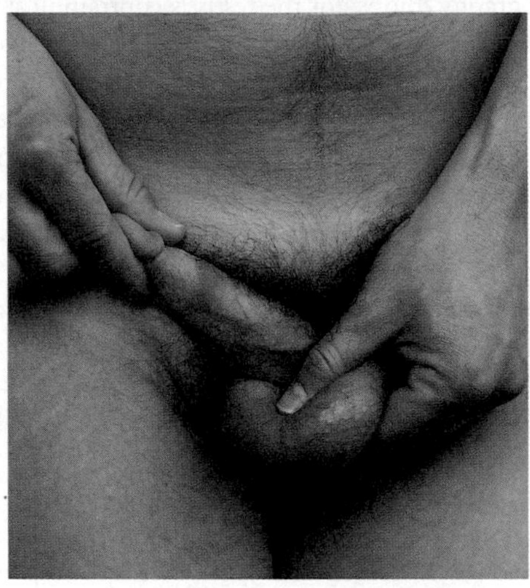

Figure 57-2 Testicular self-examination. Examination is performed after a shower when testicles are relaxed, descended, and easier to palpate. The man thoroughly palpates each testicle. Lumps are usually painless and circumscribed.

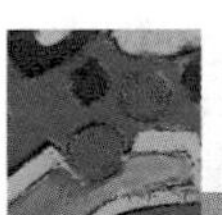

PATIENT/FAMILY TEACHING
Testicular Self-Examination

- The nurse explains the importance of regular testicular self-examination (TSE):
  —A small pea-sized palpable mass on the side or front of the testicle is most often the first sign of testicular cancer.
  —Testicular cancer is highly curable if detected and treated early.
- The nurse instructs the patient in the TSE procedure:
  —Perform TSE every month after a warm bath or shower to relax the scrotal skin and make detection of any abnormality easier.
  —Standing naked in front of a mirror, observe the scrotum for swelling or any other abnormality.
  —Find the epididymis, a cordlike structure on the top and back of the testicle, which should be soft and slightly tender to touch. By learning what the epididymis feels like, you will not mistake it for an abnormal lump.
  —Use both hands to examine each testicle. Hold your scrotum in the palm of your hands so your thumbs and index and middle fingers are free. With the thumbs on top of the testicle and the fingers below, roll each testicle between them. The testicles should both feel smooth, though one may normally be larger than the other.
  —Contact your health care provider immediately if you find a lump or abnormality.

▶ ARE You READY?

Which of the following is a clinical manifestation of testicular cancer?

1. Increased urinary frequency
2. Painful lump at base of penis
3. Red, warm scrotum
4. Heaviness in groin area

Problems of the Prostate

The prostate is a walnut-sized gland that is located below the bladder and surrounds the urethra. The gland is composed of cells that depend on male hormone to maintain its growth and size. The gland provides fluid that supports the viability and motility of sperm and modifies the pH of the vagina to help protect the sperm. The most common disorders of the prostate gland are prostatitis (inflammation of the prostate), benign prostatic **hypertrophy** (benign enlargement of the prostate), and cancer of the prostate.

Prostatitis

Etiology and Epidemiology. Prostatitis is one of the more common inflammations of the male reproductive system. It is most often seen in young and middle-aged men. The two types of prostatitis are bacterial and nonbacterial. Nonbacterial prostatitis is the most common type. *C. trachomatis* has been suspected as the cause in many cases of nonbacterial prostatitis, but frequently the infective organism cannot be identified.[15] In other cases nonbacterial inflammations may be attributed to allergic or antibody-antigen reactions. Chemical irritation from urate in noninfected urine can reflux into the prostate, also causing inflammation.

Bacterial prostatitis can be acute or chronic. It is often caused by the same bacteria that cause urinary tract infections (UTIs), such as *E. coli* and *Pseudomonas* organisms. Ascending UTIs or reflux of infected urine may be the route of bacterial contamination. Urethral instrumentation is another source of bacterial infection, as are sexually transmitted organisms.

Pathophysiology. The prostate gland becomes swollen, inflamed, and painful because of either a bacterial infection or another inflammatory process. The prostate surrounds the urethra and, when swollen, can compress the urethra and cause urinary obstruction. Prostatic abscess may also form in severe cases. Men with prostatitis typically complain of changes in voiding patterns, such as difficulty starting the stream or the need to strain on urination. Lower back pain, pelvic pain, and perineal pain are other common symptoms. Pain during or after ejaculation may also be experienced. In addition, the patient with bacterial prostatitis frequently complains of symptoms of UTIs, including urgency, frequency, painful urination, and hematuria. Bacterial infection of the prostate typically causes fever, chills, and general fatigue. Symptoms of acute bacterial prostatitis are often severe, whereas symptoms of nonbacterial prostatitis are usually vaguer.

Collaborative Care Management. Urine cultures are usually obtained to determine the organism causing bacterial prostatitis. Cultures of prostatic secretions can verify a diagnosis of bacterial infection. Patients with nonbacterial prostatitis usually have negative urine cultures. Treatment is conservative and consists of antibiotics for 30 days to prevent chronic infection, forced fluids, physical rest, stool softeners to decrease irritation of the prostate from hard feces, and local application of heat by sitz baths. Prompt treatment of prostatitis may prevent edema and resultant urinary obstruction. Urethral straight or indwelling catheterization is avoided if possible because of the risk of epididymitis. Suprapubic drainage is established if necessary. Prostatic massage may be used to eliminate residual pus pockets, but it is contraindicated during the acute phase because of the risk of bacteremia.

Recurrent episodes of acute prostatitis may cause fibrotic tissue to form. The fibrosis causes a hardening of the prostate, which may initially be confused with carcinoma. In the granulomatous form of prostatitis, the enlargement may take 3 to 6 months to resolve.

Inadequate treatment of acute infection can result in chronic prostatitis. A subacute infection may also develop into a chronic prostatitis that remains asymptomatic. Therefore prostatic secretions should be examined routinely to detect infection and to prevent complications such as acute or chronic cystitis, pyelonephritis, or epididymitis. It is believed that inflammation permits entry of antibiotics that normally do not diffuse into the prostatic fluid. They can be used during an acute infection but are ineffective in a chronic condition. Antibiotics that may diffuse into the prostatic fluid and be helpful include trimethoprim-sulfamethoxazole, carbenicillin, and ciprofloxacin.[15] Occasionally prostatic abscesses complicate the clinical course and may have to be drained surgically. If prostate calculi are present, they also may be infected. Antibiotics are ineffective against infected calculi, and surgical excision is required. Prostatectomy may be necessary to eradicate the infection.

PATIENT/FAMILY TEACHING. Patient teaching related to prostatitis is found in the Patient/Family Teaching box below.

Benign Prostatic Hypertrophy (Hyperplasia)

Etiology and Epidemiology. Benign prostatic hypertrophy (hyperplasia, BPH) is an enlargement and change in the tissue consistency of portions of the prostate. Parts of the gland may atrophy, whereas other parts become large and nodular. These changes usually occur in the transitional zone of the prostate, which is near the inner core that surrounds the urethra. The changes that take place can eventually cause problems with urination and compromise kidney function. During puberty, prostatic growth is rapid, but it tapers off by age 30. The next changes in the size and firmness of the gland occur after age 50 and commonly produce the signs and symptoms of BPH. The size of the prostate does not consistently correlate with the severity of the symptoms experienced.[31]

Changes in the size and shape of the prostate are attributed to increased tissue mass resulting from cellular proliferation. Cell growth is stimulated by an increase in the hormones androgen and estrogen and an increase in the enzyme 5-alpha reductase. This enzyme converts testosterone to dihydrotestosterone, which is 10 times more active than testosterone, thus further stimulating prostate growth.[30] The relationship of increased hormonal activity to prostate enlargement is considered significant in that males castrated before puberty do not develop BPH. If the testicles are

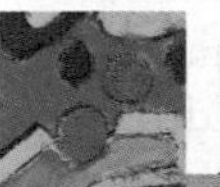

PATIENT/FAMILY TEACHING
Prostatitis

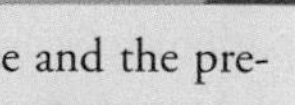

Patient teaching includes information about the disease and the prescribed medications and the following instructions:

- Take warm sitz baths.
- Take antiinflammatory medications as prescribed.
- Take entire course of antibiotics even if symptoms have been relieved.
- Refrain from sexual activity until the antibiotic has had time to work, approximately 2 weeks.
- "Flush" the prostate by means of regular ejaculation starting 2 weeks after antibiotic therapy is begun.
- Avoid use of alcohol and over-the-counter drugs such as decongestants, which can exacerbate urinary obstruction.
- Take a stool softener to decrease irritation of the inflamed prostate during defecation.

removed after BPH develops, the prostate begins to shrink.[17] Other changes occur in the prostate capsule and bladder neck, which are rich in smooth muscle and alpha-receptors. Stimulation of alpha-receptors causes muscle contraction that increases the resistance to urine flow at the bladder neck and prostatic urethra.[31]

BPH is the most common problem of the male reproductive system. It occurs in at least 50% of all men over 60 years old and 75% of men over 70 years. Symptomatic disease typically occurs in men in their mid-sixties, although not all men with enlarged prostates develop symptoms, and symptomatic disease can occur as early as age 30. An estimated 30% of men with symptomatic disease eventually need surgery.[30,31] BPH does not appear to predispose a man to the development of cancer in the gland. BPH most often develops in the inner portions of the gland, whereas cancer typically arises in the outer portions.

Pathophysiology. BPH creates bladder outlet obstruction in several ways. When the enlarged nodular tissue in the transitional zone of the prostate impinges on the urethra, the urethra elongates and compresses, obstructing urinary flow. The urine stream becomes weak, causing the man to strain to empty his bladder.[8] This can result in compensatory hypertrophy of the bands of bladder muscles. Trabeculation (contouring) of the bladder wall increases, providing pockets for urinary retention. These trabeculated areas show up on ultrasound. Because of the muscular thickening, the bladder has less capacity and is less compliant, leading to increased pressure in the bladder during filling. Prolonged exposure to high bladder pressures can adversely affect the upper urinary tract, causing hydronephrosis and kidney atrophy. Bladder muscle tone can diminish over time. Consequently, the bladder cannot empty completely at each voiding (residual urine); the urine becomes alkaline from stasis and is a fertile medium for bacterial growth.

These urethral and bladder changes can result in symptoms of urinary obstruction and irritation. Often the symptoms of obstruction are gradual and characterized by exacerbations and remissions. Consequently the patient often doesn't notice the symptoms until acute urinary retention occurs. Symptoms of gradual obstruction include a decrease in the urinary stream with less force on urination and often dribbling at the end of voiding. Other related symptoms include hesitancy, or difficulty starting the stream; intermittency; and inability to maintain a constant stream. The patient may also complain of a sense of incomplete emptying of the bladder. Straining and urinary retention are the symptoms that often convince the patient to seek medical attention.

Symptoms of irritation often accompany the obstructive problems. Nocturia from incomplete emptying is common. Dysuria, urgency, and urge incontinence are symptoms associated with loss of muscle tone in the bladder and changes in the angle of the bladder neck. The patient also may have symptoms of UTI, which occurs because of incomplete emptying and the increased risk of infection. As the prostate enlarges, so do the blood vessels, and when straining takes place, these vessels may break and cause hematuria. Urinalysis and culture and sensitivity tests are routinely done to screen for blood and possible UTIs. The typical signs and symptoms of BPH are summarized in the Clinical Manifestations box.

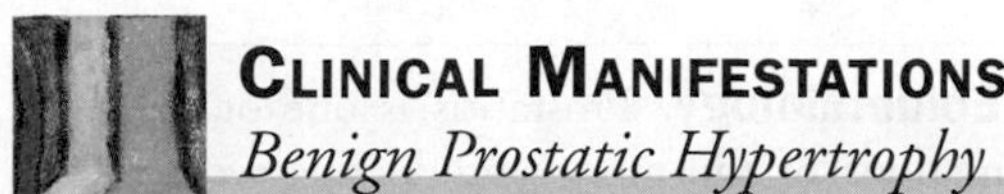

CLINICAL MANIFESTATIONS
Benign Prostatic Hypertrophy

- Straining to urinate
- Hesitancy in starting urine flow
- Decreased force of urine stream
- Postvoid dribbling
- Nocturia
- Dysuria
- Hematuria
- Urgency
- Frequency
- Incomplete emptying of bladder

COMPLICATIONS. Common complications are kidney disorders caused by pressure and backflow of urine. Urinary retention can lead to recurrent UTIs, pyelonephritis, and sepsis. Anemia may also occur as a result of severe blood loss or secondary renal insufficiency.

Collaborative Care Management

DIAGNOSTIC TESTS. Diagnostic tests for BPH include tests of renal function. Blood tests monitor changes in WBC, blood urea nitrogen (BUN), and creatinine levels, and urine tests measure specific gravity and detect the presence of proteinuria and hematuria. Other diseases that result in outflow obstruction need to be ruled out. Prostate cancer, bladder neck contracture, urethral stricture, bladder calculi, bladder cancer, inflammatory prostatitis, and neurogenic bladder are all problems that have similar symptoms. Prostate-specific antigen (PSA), a blood test, is often performed on men 50 years and older. It provides a rough estimate of the volume of the prostate. The PSA blood test is divided into free PSA and combined PSA, resulting in the total PSA score. A lower percentage of free PSA is associated with prostate cancer. Men who have 18% or greater free PSA are more likely to have BPH than prostate cancer[14] (see further discussion under Cancer of the Prostate).

Besides the urinary and blood tests already mentioned, cystoscopic procedures may be performed. Cystourethroscopy is used to assess for outflow obstruction, measure the length of the urethra, and visualize the extent of bladder involvement. Uroflowmetry is a noninvasive procedure that can evaluate bladder emptying. Urodynamics is a computerized test that measures bladder pressures and can diagnose obstruction and bladder decompensation. An IVP can be performed to outline the urinary tract. Sequential x-ray films are taken to assess the anatomy of the upper urinary tract, check for calculi (stones), and evaluate the degree of bladder emptying. IVPs are not routinely ordered for evaluation of BPH unless hematuria is present. Measuring postvoid residual urine using a catheter is an easy but invasive technique that can also assess bladder emptying. Use of a bladder ultrasound is a noninvasive method of estimating postvoid residuals.

MEDICATIONS. Medications used to treat BPH are aimed at either reducing the size of the prostate gland or relaxing the bladder neck to open the internal urethral sphincter. Finasteride (Proscar) inhibits the activity of 5-alpha-reductase so that it cannot turn testosterone into dihydrotestosterone; consequently finasteride can reduce the prostate size.[31] Often the therapeutic effects of finasteride are not noticed for several months because of the time required to demonstrate an appreciable difference in the size of the prostate. Even though this drug actually changes the size of the prostate, it may not always help the symptoms of urinary retention. The urethra may remain compressed because the nodular growth in that immediate area may not shrink sufficiently to improve the flow of urine. Finasteride seems to be most effective in the treatment of large prostates. Adverse drug effects include decreased libido, impotence, and ejaculation disorders. Finasteride can interfere with PSA monitoring by lowering the PSA levels by 50%.

Other drugs are used to relax muscles and reduce straining on urination. These drugs tend to be effective in treating prostate glands of any size. Drugs include selective or nonselective alpha-blockers. Alpha-receptors are found in the bladder neck and, when stimulated, help store urine. Blocking these receptors promotes voiding. The most selective alpha-blocker for the bladder is tamsulosin (Flomax). This drug has fewer side effects and does not need to be titrated like other alpha-blockers. Other less selective blockers are prazosin (Minipress), doxazosin (Cardura), and terazosin (Hytrin). The main side effects of most of these drugs are orthostatic hypotension and fatigue. They are usually taken in the evening to reduce side effects. Alternative medicine approaches are also being used to both prevent and treat BPH. Dietary supplements such as lycopene and the use of herbal extracts such as saw palmetto are reported to reduce prostate size and decrease the symptoms of BPH.[13] Research is ongoing.

Certain medications can exacerbate the symptoms of urinary retention because of their effects on the muscles of the bladder and urethral sphincter and should be avoided. Drugs that affect muscle function include anticholinergics such as decongestants, tranquilizers, and antidepressants.

TREATMENTS. Patients who have mild BPH may be managed through regular checkups known as *watchful waiting*. They should be advised to avoid over-the-counter cold medications and antihistamines that can exacerbate symptoms. They should also be encouraged to maintain a low-fat diet and avoid coffee and alcohol, especially after dinner. A complete physical examination, American Urological Association BPH Symptom Index (Figure 57-3), and laboratory testing should be done annually. Laser and microwave techniques are options for patients for whom drug treatment has not been effective or who are not candidates for surgery. Both procedures use heat to destroy tissue adjacent to the urethra to create a larger lumen. Although laser surgery generally requires hospitalization, it causes little blood loss and allows for

	Never	Less than 1 time in 5	Less than half the time	About half the time	More than half the time	Almost always
1. Over the past month or so, how often have you had a sensation of not emptying your bladder completely after urinating?						
2. Over the past month or so, how often have you had to urinate again less than 2 hours after you finished urinating?						
3. Over the past month or so, how often have you stopped and started again several times when you urinated?						
4. Over the past month or so, how often have you found it difficult to postpone urination?						
5. Over the past month or so, how often have you had a weak urinary stream?						
6. Over the past month or so, how often have you had to push or strain to begin urination?						
7. Over the last month, how many times did you usually get up to urinate from the time you went to bed at night until the time you got up in the morning?	Never	1 time	2 times	3 times	4 times	5 times or more
Symptom Score: 1-7 Mild, 8-19 Moderate, 20-35 Severe						

Figure 57-3 The American Urological Association BPH Symptom Index Questionnaire is used to determine the severity of BPH. The patient's answer to each of the seven symptom-related questions is scored from 0 for never to 5 for almost always. The recorded numbers are then summed to arrive at a total symptom score. A total score of 0 to 7 indicates mild BPH, 8 to 19 moderate BPH, and 20 to 35 severe BPH.

quicker recovery than conventional transurethral resection of the prostate (TURP). A Foley catheter may need to stay in place for several weeks instead of a few days. Microwave thermotherapy can be done on an outpatient basis without general anesthesia. It is an excellent option for patients receiving anticoagulants. It cannot, however, be used for patients who have hip replacements, pacemakers, or implanted defibrillators. The overall long-term effectiveness of these procedures continues to be evaluated.[6]

Surgical Management. For patients with recurrent and obstructive problems caused by BPH, surgery is often the treatment of choice. The decision for surgery is based on the severity of urinary symptoms, persistent UTIs, and the degree of physiologic change. Surgery removes the nodular gland tissue but leaves the capsule of the prostate gland intact. Men who undergo this treatment are typically symptom free for at least 8 years, after which there is a 5% to 15% retreatment rate.

Transurethral Prostatectomy. TURP is performed when the major glandular enlargement exists in the medial lobe that directly surrounds the urethra. A relatively small amount of tissue must require resection so that excess bleeding will not occur and the time required to complete the surgery will not be prolonged. TURP may be performed with the patient under general or spinal anesthesia.

A resectoscope (an instrument similar to a cystoscope but equipped with a cutting and cauterization loop attached to an electric current) is passed through the urethra. The bladder and urethra are continuously irrigated during the procedure. Tiny pieces of tissue are cut away, and the bleeding points are sealed by cauterization (Figure 57-4). Patients can develop water intoxication, known as transurethral resection (TUR) syndrome, as a result of excessive irrigating solution being absorbed during surgery. Cerebral edema may result, which creates a medical emergency. Confusion and agitation may be the first signs of this condition.[6] (See Research box.)

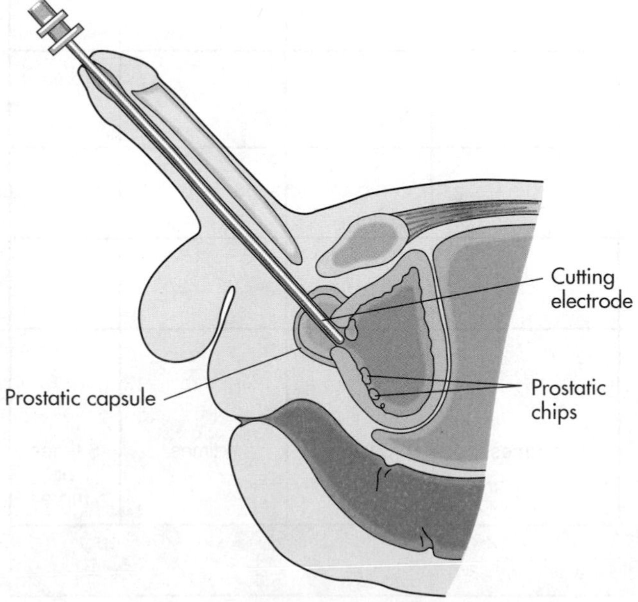

Figure 57-4 Transurethral resection of prostate gland by means of resectoscope. Note enlarged prostate gland surrounding urethra and tiny pieces of prostatic tissue that have been cut away.

After a resectoscope TURP, a large three-way Foley catheter is inserted into the bladder if a significant amount of bleeding is expected. A large catheter is used to maintain urethral patency and facilitate removal of clots from the bladder. Once the retention balloon of the catheter is inflated, the catheter is pulled down so that the balloon rests in the prostatic fossa and supports hemostasis. Traction may be applied to the Foley catheter to increase pressure on the operative area to control bleeding. Because the catheter balloon exerts pressure on the internal sphincter of the bladder, the patient may continually feel the urge to void. If the catheter is draining properly, the strongest of these sensations usually passes momentarily. Attempting to void around the catheter causes the bladder muscles to contract and results in a painful "bladder spasm." As the nerve endings become fatigued, the frequency and severity of spasms decrease. This usually occurs within 24 to 48 hours.

Constant bladder irrigation may be used to prevent excessive clotting or clot retention. This irrigation is usually performed via a three-way Foley and intravenous drip apparatus and uses a genitourinary irrigating solution. The color of urine that drains changes from bright red initially, to pink, and then to normal amber color. Constant bladder irrigation after resectoscope TURP usually is discontinued within 24 to 48 hours if no clots are draining from the bladder.

Research

Bishop P: Bipolar transurethral resection of the prostate: a new approach, *AORN J* 77:979-983, 2003.

Performance of a traditional monopolar transurethral resection of the prostate (TURP) is limited by the size of the prostate and consequently the procedure time. The limitations are set to avoid potential risk of transurethral resection (TUR) syndrome. A monopolar electrical current flows from the active electrode (wire loop) to a ground. Electrical energy that is not absorbed by tissue travels through the patient. To avoid conduction of this electrical energy to surrounding tissues, a nonconductive irrigating fluid, glycine, is used. This fluid can be absorbed through open capillaries into the bloodstream, resulting in a hypervolemic dilutional hyponatremic state, or TUR syndrome. Cerebral edema and seizures may result. The longer the surgery lasts, the greater the risk for TUR syndrome.

A new bipolar method delivers electricity using a bipolar generator. Both the active and return electrodes are contained within the instrument, so no electricity passes through the patient. In contrast to monopolar energy delivery, the bipolar technique *requires* an electrolytic medium for conduction. Saline conducts electrical current so it is used as irrigation for bipolar TURP. Performing TURP with saline eliminates the possibility of TUR syndrome, so the limitations of gland size and procedure time are also eliminated.

In a study done at Cleveland Clinic Urological Institute, preliminary conclusions are that the bipolar method for transurethral resection of the prostate is safe and efficient; eliminates concern for hemolysis, hyponatremia, or glycine toxicity; and causes little or no bleeding. Understanding TUR syndrome and new approaches for its prevention can help perioperative nurses revise standard care plans for patients undergoing TURP.

Inability to void after removal of the catheter may be a problem because of urethral edema. When this occurs, the catheter may need to be reinserted. **Continence** is carefully assessed because the internal and external sphincters lie above and below the prostate, close to the operative area, and may have been damaged during surgery.

About 2 weeks after TURP, when desiccated tissue is sloughed off, a secondary hemorrhage can occur. The patient, who is home at this time, must contact the physician immediately if bleeding occurs.

Persistent bladder discomfort, bladder spasms, or failure of a catheter to drain properly usually signifies one of the following serious complications, which require immediate medical attention: (1) hemorrhage and clot retention, (2) displacement of the catheter, or (3) unsuspected perforation of the bladder during surgery. Long-term complications of TURP include urethral stricture (1% to 29%), bladder neck contracture, impotence (5% to 10%), retrograde ejaculation (50%), and urinary incontinence. Fertility can be affected by retrograde ejaculation, which affects sperm viability.[30]

DIET. Alcohol can exacerbate urinary retention and overflow incontinence and should be avoided. Dietary supplements of zinc and vitamin E are sometimes recommended if the patient has deficiencies. These nutritional supplements are thought to help reduce nocturnal urinary symptoms. Saw palmetto, a palm extract that inhibits the effect of dihydrotestosterone on the prostate gland, is being researched as an herbal approach to reducing the size of the prostate. It is given in a pill form and at present is considered an over-the-counter dietary supplement.

Nursing Management

of the Patient undergoing Transurethral Resection of the Prostate

PREOPERATIVE CARE

A thorough preoperative assessment of the patient undergoing TURP enables the nurse to anticipate problems that increase the risk of complications. The nurse documents a baseline description of the patient's presurgical symptoms. This information is used to compare symptoms before and after surgical intervention and to monitor long-term improvement. See Figure 57-3 for a standardized format for collecting important assessment information.

Medication information is of particular importance in assessing the patient undergoing surgery on the vascular prostate gland, since bleeding is a common postoperative problem. The nurse documents information on the patient's use of over-the-counter medications that impair clotting, such as acetylsalicylic acid and NSAIDs; prescription NSAIDs and anticoagulants, such as warfarin (Coumadin); and herbal supplements. The nurse also carefully assesses the patient for a history of problems such as anemia that can affect clotting times.

Bowel elimination also is assessed before surgery. Constipation and hard stool can significantly increase the patient's discomfort in the postoperative period, and straining during defecation can cause pressure and pain to the prostate gland and exacerbate bleeding. If the patient is laxative dependent before surgery, he will need some form of stool softener or laxative to prevent constipation after surgery.

The nurse assesses the patient's knowledge of the purpose of surgery and its effects on urinary elimination, sexual functioning, and fertility. Teaching about the effects of local or general anesthesia is provided before surgery (see Chapter 13). In addition, the nurse informs the patient about the three-way Foley catheter and bladder irrigation system that may be used after surgery. The patient is informed that his urine may appear red or pink for several days after the procedure, and that this is a normal result of the manipulation of the prostate. Pain management is always a concern with surgical patients, and the nurse instructs the patient about the discomfort associated with bladder spasms and the presence of a large catheter and how this discomfort will be managed. Without an external incision of any kind, the TURP procedure is not associated with any significant incisional discomfort.

Older patients withstand surgical intervention well and do not have a significantly increased rate of problems postoperatively if they are in good general health. New developments in treatment, which have decreased the invasiveness and length of the procedures, have also clearly benefited older patients.

POSTOPERATIVE CARE

Nursing management of the patient after traditional resectoscope surgery is discussed here and in the Nursing Care Plan.

Promoting Adequate Urine Elimination. The first 24 to 48 hours after prostatectomy surgery are critical in maintaining patency of the catheter or restoring spontaneous voiding. The chance of blood clots forming and interfering with the flow of urine is greatest at this time. If bladder irrigation is being used, the flow rate of the irrigation must be set so that the urine remains free from clots and remains light red to pink. If a dark red color is noted, the flow of the fluid needs to be increased. The nurse is responsible for regulating the flow of the irrigation in response to the color and consistency of the urinary output. If bleeding persists despite the increased rate of irrigation, the physician is notified promptly.

The intake and output record documents the urinary output compared with the flow of the irrigation solution. The output should be at least 50 ml/hr greater than the hourly flow of irrigation. Less urinary output indicates a possible obstruction. The nurse checks all tubing first for patency; if no equipment problem can be determined, manual irrigations using a 50-ml syringe may be ordered to help clear the catheter of clots.

Because irrigation solutions may be used in large quantities, there is a potential risk for water intoxication. The patient may absorb excess amounts of the irrigation fluid, and problems of hyponatremia and other electrolyte imbalances may occur. The nurse assesses the patient for symptoms of elevated blood pressure, decreased pulse rate, confusion, and nausea. The nurse treats the hyponatremia as ordered by the physician. This often includes infusions of hypertonic saline and the use of diuretics such as furosemide (Lasix).

Controlling Discomfort From Bladder Spasms and Straining. Narcotics may be given to lessen the pain sensation

Nursing Care Plan

Patient After Transurethral Resection of the Prostate for Benign Prostatic Hypertrophy

Data The patient is a 67-year-old married, retired automobile mechanic who was diagnosed with benign prostatic hypertrophy. The patient has undergone medical examinations on an outpatient basis, but this is his first admission to a hospital since he was a child. Physical examination on admission was unremarkable except for slight obesity and blood pressure of 140/90 mm Hg. He has not been treated for hypertension. He takes over-the-counter acetaminophen for occasional headaches but denies use of any other medications. He is a nonsmoker. He underwent a transurethral resection of the prostate (TURP) this morning to relieve urinary retention.

Nursing Diagnosis

Risk for impaired urinary elimination related to surgical procedure

Outcomes

- Patient will maintain urinary output greater than 50 ml/hr.
- Patient will remain free from urinary bladder distention.

Related NOC Outcomes

- Urinary Elimination

Related NIC Interventions

- Bladder Irrigation
- Urinary Elimination Management
- Urinary Retention Care

Nursing Interventions/Rationales

- Monitor urinary output and characteristics. *To determine adequacy of urinary elimination and detect complications such as bleeding or infection.*
- Maintain constant bladder irrigation as prescribed during first 24 hours. *To ensure urinary drainage and prevent formation of clots.*
- Maintain patency of indwelling urinary catheter. *To ensure bladder emptying. Clots may obstruct urinary flow and must be detected early.*
- Encourage high fluid intake (2500 to 3000 ml/day). *To promote increased urinary flow, prevent urinary stasis, and decrease the risk for infection.*
- After catheter is removed, monitor for signs of retention or infection. *Initiation of the urinary stream may be difficult after catheter removal because of swelling. Fever, chills, and pain on urination, coupled with retention or frequency, may indicate infection.*

Nursing Diagnosis

Acute pain related to bladder spasms

Outcomes

- Patient will report satisfaction with pain control.
- Patient will report pain of less than 3 on a scale of 0 to 10 after pain control interventions.

Related NOC Outcomes

- Hydration
- Pain Control
- Pain Level

Related NIC Interventions

- Analgesic Administration
- Fluid Management
- Pain Management

Nursing Interventions/Rationales

- Maintain patency of urinary catheter. *Bladder distention from inadequate emptying may exacerbate bladder spasms.*
- Encourage patient to avoid trying to urinate around catheter. *A catheter can produce the feeling of the need to urinate, which may result in the patient attempting to force urination around the catheter. Forced voiding encourages bladder spasms and increases pain.*
- Monitor patient's pain status at regular intervals for 48 hours after surgery. *To identify early signs of bladder spasms so that pain relief can be implemented early.*
- Administer prescribed analgesics and antispasmodics. *Antispasmodics may offer best relief by reducing or eliminating painful spasms.*
- Reassure patient that spasms will decrease in intensity and frequency within 24 to 48 hours. *May reduce patient's anxiety about long-term effects of urinary surgery.*

Nursing Diagnosis

Risk for infection related to surgical removal of prostate gland

Outcomes

- Patient will maintain body temperature within normal limits.
- Patient will maintain white blood cell count within normal limits.
- Patient will remain free from infection.

Related NOC Outcomes

- Immune Status
- Risk Control

Related NIC Interventions

- Infection Protection
- Surveillance

Nursing Interventions/Rationales

- Monitor vital signs and report signs of infection. *Fever, chills, tachycardia, and excessive lethargy are associated with systemic infection.*
- Monitor appearance of urine. *Cloudy, frothy urine with a foul odor is associated with infection. Persistent bright red color is associated with active bleeding.*
- Maintain strict asepsis of urinary drainage system, and irrigate catheter only when essential. *To prevent introduction of microorganisms into urethra and urinary bladder.*
- Encourage high fluid volume intake. *Flushing the urinary bladder prevents excessive growth of bacteria and reduces the risk for infection.*
- Teach patient to avoid Valsalva's maneuver and avoid rectal thermometers, rectal examinations, and enemas for at least 1 week. *To prevent prostatic bleeding, which makes the patient more susceptible to infection.*

Nursing Diagnosis

Risk for stress (or urge) urinary incontinence related to catheter use and prostatic surgery

Outcomes

- Patient will be free from urinary dribbling or incontinence when coughing, laughing, or sneezing.

Related NOC Outcomes

- Urinary Continence
- Urinary Elimination

Related NIC Interventions

- Pelvic Muscle Exercise
- Urinary Elimination Management
- Urinary Incontinence Care

Nursing Interventions/Rationales

- Assess patient for dribbling after catheter is removed. *Dribbling may occur after TURP because of trauma and use of catheter but should resolve quickly. Continued dribbling indicates the need for further interventions to reestablish continence.*
- Reassure patient that dribbling is common and continence is possible. *To relieve patient's anxiety about loss of continence.*
- Teach patient how to perform perineal exercises and encourage their use. *Perineal exercises strengthen sphincter tone and enhance continence.*
- Explain use of devices and pads for temporary incontinence. *To protect patient from embarrassment and possible skin breakdown associated with incontinence.*

Nursing Diagnosis

Anxiety related to fear of sexual dysfunction after prostate surgery

Outcomes

- Patient will freely discuss fears and concerns about loss of sexual function.
- Patient will identify anxiety-reducing strategies that have been effective in the past.

Related NOC Outcomes

- Anxiety Level
- Body Image
- Coping
- Sexual Functioning

Related NIC Interventions

- Anxiety Reduction
- Body Image Enhancement
- Coping Enhancement
- Sexual Counseling

Nursing Interventions/Rationales

- Provide opportunities for patient to discuss feelings about possible effects of prostatectomy on sexual functioning. *Patients are often reluctant to discuss their concerns regarding sexuality, which is a private issue. Providing privacy and opportunities for such discussions facilitates communication and helps the nurse identify the patient's fears and concerns so that appropriate interventions can be implemented.*
- Reassure patient that the majority of patients eventually return to their former level of sexual function. *Reassures the patient that impotence is most likely temporary, which may reduce his anxiety.*
- Explain retrograde ejaculation to the patient and that it may occur the first few times he ejaculates. *So that patient will not be alarmed if his first voiding after intercourse has a milky appearance.*
- Teach patient the need for avoiding sexual intercourse for 3 to 4 weeks after surgery. *To prevent bleeding or infection.*

Nursing Diagnosis

Deficient knowledge regarding activity restrictions and prevention of complications related to lack of previous experience with surgical procedure

Outcomes

- Patient will accurately describe activity restrictions and need for follow-up care.
- Patient will verbalize understanding of self-care and signs and symptoms that need to be reported.

Related NOC Outcomes

- Knowledge: Health Promotion
- Knowledge: Prescribed Activity
- Knowledge: Treatment Regimen

Related NIC Interventions

- Teaching: Individual
- Teaching: Prescribed Activity/Exercise

Nursing Interventions/Rationales

- Teach patient to avoid heavy lifting and vigorous activities for 3 to 4 weeks. *To prevent postoperative bleeding.*
- Encourage use of stool softeners or laxatives if needed for 4 to 6 weeks after surgery. *To prevent straining during defecation, which can stimulate postoperative bleeding.*
- Encourage increased intake of fluids. *Drinking 10 or more 8-ounce glasses of fluid per day decreases the risk of constipation and straining at stool.*
- Maintain prescribed activity restriction. *To prevent fatigue, bleeding, and other postoperative complications.*
- Teach patient to be alert for possible postoperative bleeding occurring about 2 weeks after surgery. *Tissue sloughing occurs about 2 weeks after surgery, which increases the risk for bleeding.*
- Teach patient to report bleeding immediately should it occur. *So that treatment can be immediately implemented to prevent hemorrhagic shock and possible urinary obstruction from blood clots.*

Evaluation

Evaluation is based on comparing the patient's outcomes with desired outcomes.

of bladder spasms, but they are frequently unnecessary. Belladonna and opium suppositories are most often prescribed to reduce bladder spasm. These soft suppositories do not cause pain or damage to the fragile tissue around the rectum, which may have been involved in the surgical procedure. Encouraging fluids, at least 8 to 10 full glasses of fluid per day, helps flush the system and reduce irritation that causes spasms. Frequent voiding after the catheter has been removed also decreases irritation that causes spasms.

To prevent straining during defecation, which can put pressure on the recently traumatized tissues of the perineum, the nurse encourages the patient to take stool softeners or mild laxatives and maintain a well-hydrated state.

Preventing Infection. Intravenous antibiotics or oral antibiotics often are administered in the first few days after surgery. The patient is again encouraged to increase his fluid intake to promote flushing of the system, help prevent urinary stasis, and decrease the chances of infection. The nurse reviews the symptoms of UTI (fever higher than 37.6° C [99.8° F], chills, painful urination, back or flank pain, and general malaise) which the patient should report to his physician.

Relieving Anxiety. The nurse explains to the patient that bloody urine is common after surgery and that small pieces of tissue or clot may appear in the urine for up to 2 weeks. The nurse also informs the patient that most men have some temporary difficulty with continence after any type of prostatectomy. The man should understand that this is normal but will improve. Teaching perineal exercises such as Kegel exercises (see Chapter 56) can be helpful in controlling voiding. Frequent voiding can help reduce problems of dribbling. The nurse provides specific suggestions about absorptive devices and specialty underwear products that can be used for the temporary control of incontinence as needed.

Surgical procedures used to treat BPH do not usually affect a man's ability to have an erection. The patient needs to be reassured that infertility is different from impotence. Depending on the amount of prostate removed, fertility can be minimally or greatly reduced. Also, if the patient has continued retrograde emission of prostatic fluid after several months, fertility will remain diminished.

The nurse must not assume that because men with BPH routinely are older, fertility is not an issue. Even if the man is not planning to have children, he may associate fertility with sexuality. The nurse may need to provide opportunities for the patient to express these concerns. Reminding the patient that the ability to have an erection is unchanged is often helpful. The ability to experience orgasm is also intact. The patient is cautioned that he may still be fertile, and use of birth control may still be necessary to prevent unwanted pregnancies.

Preventing Abdominal and Perineal Pressure. After any prostatectomy surgery, there is a risk of bleeding associated with increased abdominal or perineal pressure. For this reason patients are instructed to avoid factors that can increase this pressure. The nurse instructs the patient to avoid sitting for long periods of time, lifting anything weighing more than 5 lbs, and engaging in strenuous exercise and sports activities for 6 weeks.

The patient should not climb more than two flights of stairs, should avoid sexual activity for at least 3 weeks, and should not drive for 2 weeks. He should also avoid constipation and straining at stool by maintaining a nonalcoholic fluid intake of 2 to 2.5 L/day and eating a well-balanced diet that includes fresh vegetables, fruits, whole grains, and bran. If constipation does occur, it should be reported early to the surgeon, and no enemas or suppositories should be used.

The nurse instructs the patient to watch for and report any sign of infection. The patient should also watch for blood or clots in the urine, any change in the urine stream, and physical activities that create excessive abdominal or perineal pressure.

▶ ARE You READY?

The nurse is monitoring the bladder irrigation in a patient 12 hours after a transurethral resection of the prostate and notes that the urinary output is dark red in color. The nurse should *first*:

1. Notify the physician.
2. Stop the irrigation.
3. Increase the rate of irrigation.
4. Manually deflate and reinflate the catheter balloon.

Cancer of the Prostate

Etiology and Epidemiology. Cancer of the prostate is the most common cancer in adult American men, with 232,090 new cases and 30,350 deaths expected in 2005, up from 230,110 new cases and 29,900 deaths in 2004. One man in six will be diagnosed with prostate cancer during his lifetime, but only 1 in 32 will die of this disease. Prostate cancer accounts for about 10% of cancer-related deaths in men.[3] The incidence and death rate in African-American men is 70% greater than in Caucasian American men.[17]

Although research is ongoing, the risk factors for prostate cancer are mostly either unknown or unavoidable. Age is thought to be the strongest risk factor. The disease is rare in men younger than 45, but the chance of acquiring it rises sharply with advancing age. Seventy percent of all prostate cancers occur in men over the age of 65. Hormonal influence has been proved clinically to be a risk factor, since men castrated before puberty do not develop prostate cancer. High intake of dietary fat has been shown to increase serum androgen levels and therefore is seen as a risk factor. Studies have demonstrated a direct relationship between a country's prostate cancer mortality rate and average total calories from fat consumed. Native Japanese, whose diets are very low in fat, have the lowest risk of prostate cancer. First generation Japanese-Americans, however, have an intermediate risk, and subsequent generations have a risk comparable to that of the U.S. population. Inherited or genetic factors are considered risk factors in that approximately 15% of men with a diagnosis of prostate cancer have a first-degree male relative (brother or father) with prostate cancer (see Future Watch box). Race and nationality are credible factors. African-American men have the highest incidence of prostate cancer in the world. Although Caucasian men in America have a lower incidence than African-American men, they have a higher rate than men in the rest of the world.[17] This fact notwithstanding, 98% of all men, regardless of the severity of the prostate cancer, survive at least 5 years.[3]

Environmental exposure to substances such as cadmium and dioxin (Agent Orange) is still being studied. Research also continues regarding the association between vasectomy, sexual activity

Future Watch

Gene Abnormality Related to Prostate Cancer

Researchers have found changes in chromosome arrangement and a specific gene fusion in over 75% of prostate cancer samples examined and not in samples of benign prostate tissue. They believe the chromosomal rearrangement triggers the gene fusion, which in turn causes overexpression of cancer, causing genes and growth of cancerous prostatic tumors. The specific fusion identified is between the regulatory region of the *TMPRSS2* gene, which is an androgen-regulated protease gene primarily found in prostate tissue, and a gene encoding an ETS transcription factor, either *ERG* or *ETV1*. This finding helps explain why androgen inhibition therapy is useful in the management of prostate cancer and also suggests the possibility of development of new methods of diagnosis and treatment. Since this gene fusion is unique to prostate cancer, development of a test to detect it or its protein products in blood or urine could provide a more accurate diagnosis than is available with the PSA test currently used for screening. The finding also suggests that treatment that would inhibit the overexpression of *ERG* or *ETV1* might be possible.

Tomlins SA et al: Recurrent fusion of TMPRSS2 and ETS transcription factor genes in prostate cancer, *Science* 310:(5748):644-648, October 28, 2005.

and/or sexually transmitted diseases, and prostate cancer. Most studies have not found these to produce increased risks.[3]

Population studies have shown that men who eat large amounts of foods containing lycopene, a plant-derived caretenoid, have a lower risk of prostate cancer than those who do not. Lycopene, which provides the red color to tomatoes and is found in smaller amounts in grapefruit, papaya and, watermelon, acts as an antioxidant, protecting cells against damage from free radicals. Studies of the effect of lycopene on already established prostate cancers are beginning.[16a]

Pathophysiology. Cancer of the prostate, which is most often an adenosarcoma, typically starts as a discrete, localized, hard nodule in an area of senile atrophy. In all, 70% of prostate cancers arise in the peripheral zone (outer area of gland, contiguous with the capsule), 20% in the transitional zone (midportion of gland), and 10% in the central zone surrounding the urethra. Because the growth is generally on the outer portion of the gland, compression of the urethra and subsequent voiding symptoms are not common until late in the disease. Nonurinary symptoms, if present, are often so ambiguous that the disease is not diagnosed until it is well advanced.

The cancer can readily spread outside the capsule boundaries and be disseminated through the lymphatic and vascular systems. The most common sites of metastasis are the bones of the pelvis, lumbar and thoracic spine, femur, and ribs. Involvement of organs such as lung, liver, and kidneys usually is not seen until the late stages of the disease.

Because the posterior of the prostate gland is adjacent to the rectal wall, the tumor may be detected by rectal examination before symptoms appear. On physical examination prostate cancer may present as a discrete or diffuse area of increased firmness. Unfortunately, a number of cancers arise anterior to the midline of the prostate gland and consequently cannot be felt on rectal examination.

Blood screening for PSA measures the elevation of a glycoprotein secreted by the prostate and is used to help identify possible cancers. Factors that can influence PSA levels are identified in Box 57-2. Epithelial cells in the ductal system of the prostate gland also secrete acid phosphatase. Elevated serum acid phosphatase usually indicates that prostatic cancer has spread beyond the capsule of the gland.

Prostate cancer can spread slowly or aggressively. The biologic aggressiveness of malignant tumors depends at least in part on the degree of differentiation of the cells. It is frequently difficult to determine the severity or extent of the tumor because multiple tumor sites may be present with varying degrees of cell differentiation.

Clinical manifestations of prostate cancer may include complaints of stiffness, back pain, hip pain, and occasionally pathologic fractures. Symptoms may also mimic those of BPH, with urinary outflow obstruction or severe bladder irritation with no signs of infection. Often there are no symptoms in the initial stages of prostate cancer (see Clinical Manifestations box).

Collaborative Care Management

DIAGNOSTIC TESTS. Because symptoms are often ambiguous, regular screening for prostate cancer is important. A combination of diagnostic tests is now used to improve the accuracy of prostate cancer detection. Blood screens, rectal examination, and ultrasound techniques all help in early detection (Box 57-3). All men over the age of 50 are advised to have an annual PSA blood test and a rectal examination (see Research box, p. 1736). Hard, nodular areas felt on the prostate during the digital rectal examination are often indicative of cancer. PSA screening is performed in conjunction with a digital rectal examination. Knowledge of prostate size, along with PSA levels, provides a more definitive diagnosis than PSA alone.

Box 57-2 Factors That Affect Prostate-Specific Antigen Levels

- *Race:* African-Americans have higher prostate-specific antigen (PSA) levels than Caucasians.
- *Age:* Older adults have increased PSA levels.
- *Benign prostatic hypertrophy:* Prostatic hypertrophy and prostatitis increase the gland volume and the PSA level.
- *Manipulation of the prostate:* Manipulation, such as instrumentation or digital rectal examination, elevates PSA level.
- *Ejaculation:* Ejaculation within 48 hours elevates PSA level.
- *Medications:* Tamsulosin (Flomax), finasteride (Proscar), and saw palmetto lower PSA.

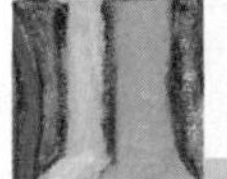

CLINICAL MANIFESTATIONS
Prostate Cancer

- Often no symptoms if cancer is confined to the gland
- Symptoms of urinary obstruction
- Symptoms of urinary tract infection
- Lower back pain, malaise, aching in legs, and hip pain if cancer has metastasized

The normal blood range for PSA is 0 to 2.5 ng/ml. Men whose PSA is between 1.0 and 2.0 ng/ml should have yearly retesting. An increase in PSA of more than 0.70 ng/ml/yr (PSA velocity) is associated with prostate cancer, and a biopsy should be done. When prostate cancer develops, the PSA level usually goes above 4 ng/ml. A patient with a level between 4 and 10 ng/ml carries a 25% chance of having prostate cancer. If the level goes above 10 ng/ml, the chance of prostate cancer is more than 67%, a chance that increases as the PSA level increases. The PSA test can be divided into two scores: a bound PSA and a free PSA. If the patient has a high percentage of free PSA, this tends to indicate BPH rather than prostate cancer.[14] The nurse needs to be aware of the fact that PSA screening itself often produces anxiety for both men and their partners.[10]

Transrectal ultrasound (TRUS) aids in the screening of nonpalpable tumors. It may also help direct the physician in biopsy of firm, palpable tumors so that these tumors can be graded and staged. TRUS allows greater accuracy than digital rectal examinations in localizing the tumor and placing the biopsy needle. Biopsy of any firm or nodular area is necessary to confirm the diagnosis of prostate cancer. The biopsy procedure may be done in an office setting or minor surgery operating rooms, with the patient under local anesthesia or light general anesthesia. If the biopsy is combined with ultrasound, a probe is placed in the rectum; otherwise, the surgeon uses a digital technique to guide the procedure. The needle biopsy can be performed by either a transperineal or transrectal route, depending on the physician's choice.

Patient preparation for prostate biopsy focuses on providing an optimal environment for visualization, preventing complications, and gathering baseline data for follow-up care. Rectal cleansing by enema or oral laxative is often done before the procedure as a means of preventing potential infection. Preprocedural antibiotics are used and may be continued for several days after the procedure. The patient may be on a nothing-by-mouth regimen or permitted to eat a light breakfast before the biopsy. The extreme vascularity of the prostate gland increases the risk of bleeding, and coagulation profiles usually are drawn before the procedure. Anticoagulants and drugs such as aspirin are discontinued at least 48 hours before the test.

Research

Weinrich SP et al: Barriers to prostate cancer screening, *Cancer Nurs* 41(2):117-121, 2000.

Getting men to participate in prostate screening has always been difficult. Even though African-American men are at greater risk for prostate cancer, they are less likely to participate in prostate screening programs than Caucasian American men. This study used univariate and multivariate logistic regression models to evaluate barriers to prostate cancer screening. African-American men for this study were recruited from 11 counties in South Carolina. Sampling sites included churches, meal sites, barber shops, and work sites. An instrument was developed to measure perceived barriers to prostate screening and used in two pilot studies to establish content validity. This 15-item questionnaire was then administered, and the men asked to check the items that would make it difficult for them to be screened. Analysis of the data found that cost and lack of knowledge were major barriers to prostate screening.

Furthermore, this study found that, even with free prostate screening and educational programs on the reason for prostate screening, barriers still remained. A follow-up phone survey revealed that barriers to screening were a lack of knowledge related to specific sites for screening and lack of transportation or the ability to "take off work" for screening purposes.

The nursing implication of this study is that education needs to be individualized. It is important for the nurse to provide information that includes addresses, directions, and office hours to promote participation in health screening programs.

STAGING. A common system of staging prostate cancer is the TNM (tumor-nodes-metastasis) system. This documents the location of the tumor, whether it has spread to the lymph nodes,

Box 57-3 Diagnostic and Staging Tests for Prostate Cancer

Examinations and Visualizations

Digital rectal examination (DRE): A procedure in which a health care provider inserts a gloved, lubricated finger into the rectum to feel the prostate

Chest x-ray film: An image that can show whether cancer has spread to the lungs or other structures such as the ribs

Bone scan: A picture that can show whether cancer has spread to the bone

Transrectal ultrasonography (TRUS): A procedure in which an instrument is inserted into the rectum and produces sound waves directed at the prostate; from these sound waves, a picture is created.

Computed tomography (CT): A picture produced by a computer from x-rays, showing the prostate and other nearby parts of the body

Intravenous pyelogram (IVP): An x-ray of the kidneys, ureters, and bladder that is taken after the patient has been injected with a special dye

Magnetic resonance imaging (MRI): A picture produced by a computer and a high-powered magnet that shows the prostate and other nearby parts of the body

Blood Tests

Prostate-specific antigen (PSA): A test useful both in diagnosis and follow-up of prostate cancer that detects a blood substance that often increases in cases of prostate cancer and other prostate diseases

Percent free-PSA ratio: A newer type of PSA test that measures how much PSA is unbound and how much is bound to other proteins in the blood; a low percent free-PSA ratio combined with a borderline PSA can help confirm a diagnosis of prostate cancer.

Tissue Samples

Prostate biopsy: The removal and microscopic examination of a small sample of the prostate to determine whether it contains cancer cells

Pelvic node dissection (lymphadenectomy): A procedure used to help determine whether prostate cancer has spread—typically done during surgery to remove the prostate and any evidence of metastasis. The extent of tumor spread is assigned a number (0-4) and a letter (a-d). For example a tumor that is confined to the prostate gland, spread to a single lymph node, but with no evidence that the cancer has metastasized to distant areas would be staged as T2aN1M0 (Box 57-4). Stages confined to the prostatic capsule have a good prognosis. Stages with higher numeric values, or with additional letter values of c or d attached to the numbers, have a poorer prognosis. Staging helps determine prognosis and provides the basis for treatment recommendations.

Treatment decisions are based on both the results of the staging and the score on the Gleason grading scale. The Gleason system of grading has total scores ranging from 2 to 10; 2 to 4 indicates well-differentiated tissue, 5 to 7 moderately differentiated tissue, and 8 to 10 poorly differentiated tissue. Two biopsy sites from areas with the most cancer are used in testing, and the scores of each, which can range from 1 to 5, are added to obtain the total score. The lower the score, the less aggressive the cancer and the better the prognosis.

MEDICATIONS. When cancer of the prostate is inoperable, or when signs of metastasis occur after surgery, pharmacologic treatment is given. Some patients experience dramatic improvement with hormonal therapy that may last for 10 years or more. Usually the response is good for about 1 year, and then the patient's condition begins to deteriorate. Because a large portion of the growth in prostate cancer is testosterone dependent, medication is used to block the production or action of this hormone. The testicles produce testosterone when stimulated by the release of hormones from the pituitary gland. Therefore drugs that inhibit the release of these pituitary hormones are often first-choice therapies. Hormone analogs such as leuprolide (Lupron) and goserelin (Zoladex) are given every 1 to 3 months, depending on the preparation, by intramuscular injection.

In conjunction with drugs that inhibit the production of testosterone, antiandrogenic drugs may be given to inhibit the action of testosterone produced by the adrenal glands. These regimens of combination hormonal therapy are called *maximal androgen blockade* (or combined androgen blockade). Examples of antiandrogen drugs include flutamide (Eulexin) and bicalutamide (Casodex). Side effects of both of these classes of drugs can include impotence, hot flashes, nausea, vomiting, chemical hepatitis, and diarrhea.

BOX 57-4 Prostate Cancer Staging

Physicians use the TNM (tumor-nodes-metastasis) system to stage prostate cancer. This system focuses on tumor anatomy by looking at first the tumor itself, then at the regional lymph nodes, and finally at the metastasis.

T: Primary Tumor

Evaluates whether the cancer has spread
Tx: Tumor cannot be assessed
T0: No evidence of tumor
T1: Tumor is not clinically apparent, is not palpable, cannot be visualized with imagining devices
T2: Tumor is confined to the prostate
T3: Tumor has broken through the prostatic capsule
T4: Tumor has invaded or affixed itself to adjacent tissue (other than the seminal vesicles)

N: Lymph Nodes

Evaluates whether the cancer has begun to spread to the local lymph glands
Nx: Cannot be assessed
N0: No evidence of spread to regional lymph nodes
N1: Spread to a single lymph node
N2: Larger spread to a single lymph node, or to more than one node
N3: Larger spread to a regional lymph node

M: Metastasis

Evaluates whether the cancer has spread to distant parts of the body
Mx: Cannot be assessed
M0: No evidence of spread to distant areas
M1: Spread to distant areas

From Prostate Health Resources: http://www.prostate90.com/book/p12.html

TREATMENTS. Radiation can be used to treat localized tumors confined to the inside of the prostate capsule. It is also used if a patient cannot tolerate or chooses not to undergo surgery. Radiation may be delivered by external beam or by implant (brachytherapy). The testes are shielded during external radiation. The external beam radiation is usually given in short sessions, once a day for several weeks. Internal retropubic prostatic implantation may be used initially or after failure of external radiotherapy. Brachytherapy is often done as an overnight or same day surgery. Small radioactive seeds are inserted into the prostate and remain in the patient. The patient gives off minimal radiation immediately adjacent to the prostate gland and then is not "radioactive" after the seeds have encapsulated into the gland (approximately 1 week) because the area of radiation from the seeds is confined to the prostate. The patient is asked to refrain from ejaculation for a week until the seeds can encapsulate into the gland. He should also avoid strenuous activity.

Complications of seed implantation include blood loss from multiple needle punctures during implantation, deep venous thrombosis, pulmonary emboli, hematomas, and abscesses. Impotence from radiation develops over time as a result of scar tissue formation. Fortunately, the majority of patients with brachytherapy-induced erectile dysfunction respond favorably to sildenafil citrate (Viagra).[27] The risk of complications increases if radioactive implants are used after external beam radiation. Irritability of the bladder caused by radioactive implants can produce urinary symptoms of frequency, urgency, and nocturia.

The use of radiotherapy in combination with androgen suppression therapy is currently being investigated (see Future Watch box).

SURGICAL MANAGEMENT. A radical resection of the prostate gland usually is curative for patients with low-grade and confined prostate cancer. The entire prostate gland, including the capsule and the adjacent tissue, is removed. The remaining urethra then is anastomosed to the bladder neck. The surgery is accomplished using a suprapubic, retropubic, or perineal approach. The suprapubic and retropubic approaches use a low midline incision, and the perineal approach uses a perineal incision. The patient has a

Future Watch

Radiation Plus Short-Term Hormonal Blocking as Treatment of Prostate Cancer

Two hundred and six men with nonmetastatic prostate cancer as evidenced by negative physical examination and imaging tests, but with high blood levels of PSA and high Gleason scores, were randomly assigned to treatment with radiation only or radiation plus an overlapping 6-month course of androgen suppression therapy (AST). Six patients receiving radiation only died of prostate cancer and 46 had evidence of recurrence. In the radiation plus AST group, no patients died and 21 had recurrence. The short-term use of AST with radiation had the same survival benefit as long-term use but without the negative side effects.

D'Amico A et al: Radiation and hormone therapy for prostate cancer, *JAMA* 292(7):821-827, 2004.

Foley catheter in place for a period of days to several weeks, depending on the approach used and whether the patient is at risk for delayed healing because of previous radiotherapy. Table 57-3 compares the different surgical methods, and Figure 57-5 illustrates the placement of drains and incisions.

SUPRAPUBIC PROSTATECTOMY. In the suprapubic resection the prostate gland is removed from the urethra through the bladder; this type of resection is performed when a large mass of tissue must be resected. Some type of hemostatic agent is placed in the prostatic fossa, and urine is drained by Foley catheter, cystotomy tube, or both.

Hemorrhage is a possible complication, and the precautions are the same as those taken after TURP. Since some oozing of blood from the prostatic fossa occurs, continuous bladder irrigations may be ordered for the first 24 hours.

Cystotomy tubes are usually removed 3 or 4 days after surgery; urethral catheters generally remain until the suprapubic wound is well healed. After the urethral catheter has been removed, the nursing care of the patient is similar to that for the patient undergoing TURP. If the suprapubic wound should reopen and drain, a urethral catheter is usually reinserted.

RETROPUBIC PROSTATECTOMY. In a retropubic prostatectomy a low abdominal incision similar to that used for suprapubic prostatectomy is made, but the bladder is not opened. The bladder is retracted and the prostatic tissue removed through an incision in the anterior prostatic capsule. A large-diameter Foley catheter is inserted. Hemorrhage and infection are potential complications, but the sphincter muscles are not damaged, and the patient rarely has difficulty voiding. Nerves that control the ability to achieve erections may be spared with this procedure.

PERINEAL PROSTATECTOMY. The perineal approach results in a draining incision in the perineal area. Often a Penrose drain is placed to help direct the serous drainage from the wound site. The bladder remains intact during this surgery. Nerves that control urinary continence and penile erection may be damaged. Also, muscles and nerves around the rectal sheath can be traumatized. Consequently these patients may have difficulty with bladder and bowel continence and impotence. Nerve-sparing approaches are being successfully used with perineal approaches as well, but the surgery is technically difficult.

ORCHIECTOMY. When testosterone suppression is necessary, one of the methods is a bilateral orchiectomy (castration). This procedure is technically minor and is often performed using local anesthesia, but it may cause the patient considerable emotional distress. The man's permission for sterilization must be obtained. If he is married, he is usually urged to discuss the procedure with his wife. This surgery eliminates the testicular source of male hormones and seems to cause regression of the cancer or at least slow its growth. Very rarely, a hypophysectomy (removal of the pituitary gland, which secretes a testosterone-stimulating hormone) may be performed to further reduce hormonal stimulation.

DIET. No therapeutic diet exists for patients with prostate cancer. There is some evidence that diet can play a role in preventing or slowing the growth of prostate cancer. A high-fiber, low-fat diet is recommended because men from countries where they routinely eat this type of diet typically have a lower incidence of prostate cancer. Vitamin E, selenium, and lycopene may also protect men from prostate cancer.[17] Diets are routinely modified if the patient is to have surgery. Increasing fluid intake after prostate surgery helps prevent problems with constipation.

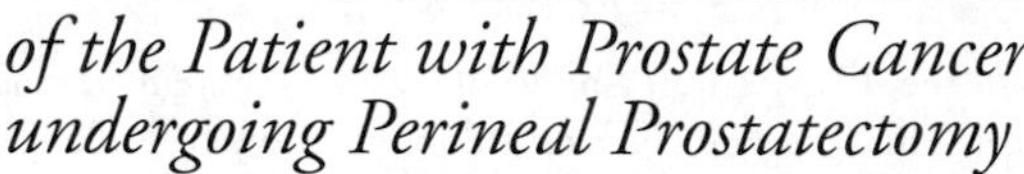

Nursing Management

of the Patient with Prostate Cancer undergoing Perineal Prostatectomy

PREOPERATIVE CARE

If the patient is to have a perineal approach in surgery, he is given a bowel preparation, which may include enemas, cathartics, and sulfasalazine (Azulfidine) or neomycin before surgery and only clear fluids the day before surgery to prevent fecal contamination of the operative site. The remainder of the preoperative care is similar to that described under Benign Prostatic Hypertrophy.

POSTOPERATIVE CARE

Caring for the Perineal Wound. Care of the perineal wound consists of monitoring for possible urine leaks, hemorrhage, and signs of infection. Drains may be placed in the incision, and the wound may be left partially open to heal by secondary intention. Often the patient wears a Fuller Shield or briefs underwear to support the dressing on the perineal incision. Open wounds may drain copious amounts, and frequent dressing changes are usually necessary. The use of rectal thermometers, rectal tubes, and suppositories is avoided to prevent injury to the fragile perineal area.

When solid food is permitted, a low-residue diet may be given until wound healing is well advanced. Diphenoxylate hydrochloride with atropine sulfate (Lomotil) may be prescribed to inhibit bowel action in the first postoperative week to prevent contamination of the incision.

Restoring Urinary and Bowel Continence. A large amount of urinary drainage on the perineal dressing for a number of hours is not unusual. This can be managed by the use of an

TABLE 57-3 COMPARISON OF TYPES OF PROSTATE SURGERY

Reason for Surgery	Location of Incision	Drainage Tubes	Bladder Spasms	Dressing	Complications
TRANSURETHRAL RESECTION					
Enlargement of medial lobe surrounding urethra—benign prostatic hypertrophy; may be palliative for advanced prostate cancer	No incision; removal by way of urethra	Three-way Foley catheter with 30 ml balloon in urethra; constant irrigation 1-24 hr	Yes	None	Hemorrhage, water intoxication, incontinence, obstruction
SUPRAPUBIC RESECTION					
Extremely large mass of obstructing tissue—prostate cancer	Low midline abdominal incision through bladder to prostate gland	Cystotomy tube or drain through incision; Foley catheter with 30 ml balloon in urethra	Yes	Abdominal dressing easily soaked with urinary drainage	Hemorrhage, obstruction, wound infection, impotence, sterility
RETROPUBIC RESECTION					
Large mass located high in pelvic area—prostate cancer	Low midline abdominal incision into prostate gland (bladder not incised)	Foley catheter with 30 ml balloon in urethra, constant irrigation for 24 hr	Few	Abdominal dressing; no urinary drainage	Hemorrhage, obstruction, wound infection, impotence, sterility
PERINEAL RESECTION					
Large mass located low in pelvic area—prostate cancer	Incision between scrotum and rectum	Foley catheter with 30 ml balloon in urethra; perineal drain	Few	Perineal dressing; no urinary drainage	Hemorrhage, obstruction, wound infection, impotence, sterility, incontinence
RADICAL PERINEAL RESECTION					
Mass extends beyond capsule; includes lymph node dissection—prostate cancer	Large perineal incision between scrotum and rectum	Foley catheter with 30 ml balloon in urethra; drain in incision	Few	Perineal dressing; no urinary drainage	Urinary incontinence, wound infection, impotence, sterility

ostomy bag around the dressing. The urinary drainage should decrease rapidly. The amount of bleeding in the urine should be less than after suprapubic prostatic surgery. Because the catheter is not being used for hemostasis, the patient usually experiences fewer bladder spasms. The catheter is used both for urinary drainage and as a splint for the urethral anastomosis; therefore the nurse must ensure that it does not become dislodged or blocked. Clinically, the risk of blockage from clots is greatest during the first hour. The catheter may be irrigated intermittently or continuously as ordered by the physician. The catheter is usually left in the bladder for at least 2 to 3 weeks.

Temporary urinary incontinence is usually a problem with patients who have had any type of radical prostatectomy. The patient needs to be encouraged, and provisions should be made to keep him dry so that he can be up and socialize with others without fear of incontinence.

Because perineal surgery causes relaxation of the perineal musculature, the patient may also have problems with fecal incontinence. It is disturbing to the patient, and sometimes can be avoided by starting perineal (Kegel) exercises within a day or two after surgery. Control of the rectal sphincter usually returns readily. Perineal exercises should be continued even after rectal sphincter control returns, since the exercises also strengthen the bladder sphincters, and unless the bladder sphincters have been permanently damaged, the patient will regain urinary control more readily on removal of the catheter.

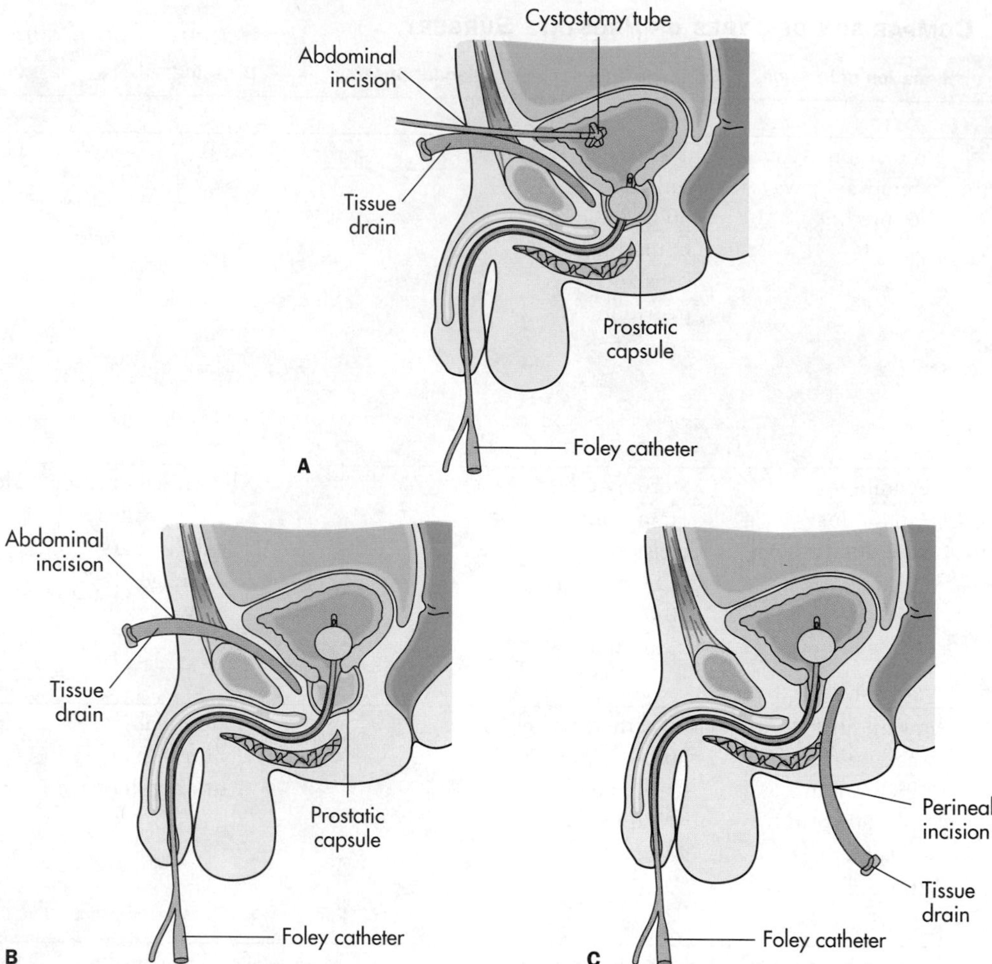

Figure 57-5 Three types of prostatectomies. **A,** Suprapubic: note placement of inflated Foley catheter in prostatic fossa. **B,** Retropubic. **C,** Radical perineal: note tissue drain placed in incision between scrotum and rectum.

Promoting Sexual Function. Total prostatectomy that includes bilateral pelvic lymphadenectomy can result in physiologic sexual dysfunction as a result of disruption of genital innervation. The patient may be impotent for several months even after a nerve-sparing prostatectomy. The patient needs to know that return of erectile capability may be delayed but it will gradually occur and he can still experience orgasm but will not ejaculate semen.

The patient and his spouse or partner should understand the sexual consequences of prostatectomy. Acknowledging the effect of surgery and radiation on intimate relationships, the nurse should encourage discussion of complications specific to prostate surgery. Sexual dysfunction and incontinence need to be addressed in a timely and sensitive manner.[24]

Dealing With Grief. Patients who have low-grade and low-stage prostate cancer have an excellent survival rate. It is important to remind patients that prostate cancer is different from many other forms of cancer, since even men with higher grades of prostate cancer often have a long survival rate. Prostate cancer is usually slow growing, and many older men do not die of their prostate cancer but of other causes. The nurse must acknowledge the fear of cancer, however, and allow the patient time and encouragement to express these fears. If surgery has resulted in impotence, the patient needs to be supported through his grief over the loss of sexuality. For more information on the grieving process related to cancer, see Chapter 23.

Postoperative care for patients undergoing any type of prostatectomy is summarized in the Guidelines for Safe Practice box.

Complications. Complications of radical prostatectomy for prostate cancer include hemorrhage, urinary and bowel incontinence, infertility, impotence, and leakage at the anastomotic site of the urethra and bladder. Prostate cancer may metastasize to local organs such as the lymph nodes, bowel, and bladder and to bony areas such as the pelvis and spine. Sites of distant metastasis include the liver and lungs.

Gerontologic Considerations

Because prostatic cancer is often slow growing, treatment options for older patients may be palliative. Radical prostatectomies do not necessarily prolong life for these patients. Consequently, radiation or measures to decrease the size of the prostate (e.g., TURP) to relieve symptoms of urinary obstruction may be the treatment of choice rather than radical prostatectomy.

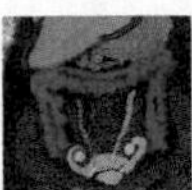

GUIDELINES FOR SAFE PRACTICE *Postoperative Care for the Patient Undergoing Prostatic Surgery*

- Maintain patency of catheter system.
- Monitor appearance of urine: red to light pink (24 hours) to amber (3 days).
- Monitor for signs of water intoxication after transurethral resection of the prostate (confusion; agitation; warm, moist skin; anorexia; nausea; vomiting).
- Instruct patient not to try to void around catheter; explain feeling of needing to void from pressure of catheter.
- Instruct patient in aseptic care of catheter and leg bag.
- Avoid use of enemas and rectal thermometers.
- Give prescribed medications (analgesics, antispasmodics) as needed; tell patient spasms will decrease in intensity and severity within 24 to 48 hours.
- After catheter removal:
  —Monitor for signs of urinary retention.
  —Monitor for continence; teach perineal exercises if dribbling occurs.
  —Encourage increased fluids and frequent voiding.
- Change dressings frequently around suprapubic wounds after suprapubic prostatectomy to prevent skin maceration.
- Give patient opportunities to discuss feelings about sexuality and possible incontinence.
- Teach patient to:
  —Avoid vigorous exercise, heavy lifting (over 20 pounds), and sexual intercourse for at least 3 weeks.
  —Avoid driving for 2 weeks.
  —Avoid straining with defecation; use stool softeners or mild laxatives if needed.
  —Drink at least 2500 ml of fluids per day to prevent urinary stasis and infection and to keep stools soft.
  —Notify physician if urinary stream diminishes or if bleeding occurs.

If surgery is performed, healing times may be prolonged. The perineal muscles of the older patient are weaker, and problems of urinary and bowel incontinence may take longer to resolve. Perineal muscle exercises may be started before surgery to help the older patient regain muscle tone sooner.

Problems of the Penis

Structural problems of the penis typically involve the head of the penis or the foreskin. The head of the penis is susceptible to problems caused by irritation, cancer, and trauma. The foreskin is the source of structural difficulties that can affect urination, cause pain, and interfere with blood flow to the penis. Functional problems of the penis primarily involve disorders of erection. Impotence is discussed later in the chapter. The anatomy of the penis is illustrated in Figure 57-6.

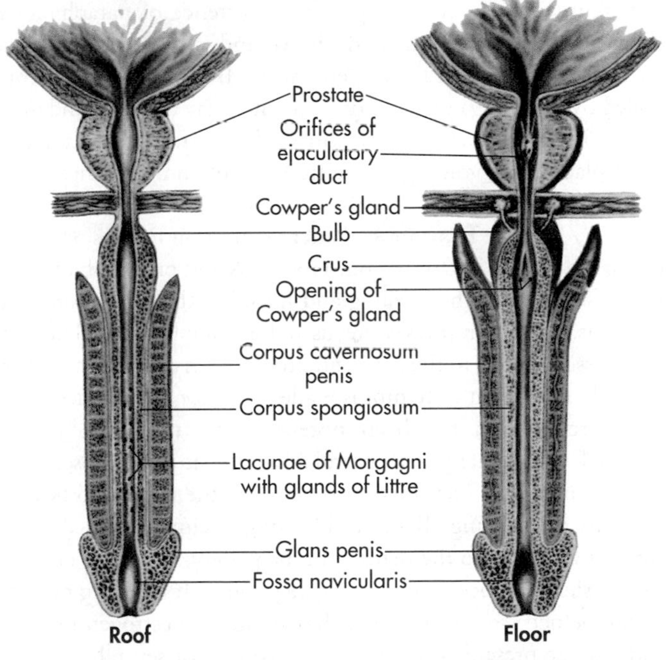

Figure 57-6 Anatomy of the penis.

Phimosis and Paraphimosis

Etiology and Epidemiology. Phimosis is a condition in which the opening of the prepuce, or foreskin, is unable to be retracted behind the glans (Figure 57-7, *A*). The condition may be congenital or acquired as a result of inflammation or infection. Paraphimosis, conversely, is a condition in which the prepuce is retracted over the glans and forms a constriction at the base of the glans (Figure 57-7, *B*). This is usually a result of manipulation of the foreskin over the glans and failure to return it to cover the glans. This condition is most often seen in children or in men with changes in mental status that predispose them to memory loss or with decreased sensation in the penis.

Pathophysiology. The inability to retract the foreskin may interfere with adequate hygiene. Consequently, urine and smegma (mucuslike drainage) may be trapped in the preputial sac, resulting in irritation and predisposing the glans to infection. Chronic irritation may be a cause of penile carcinoma. Healing of the irritation or infection causes scar tissue formation, which can worsen the acquired phimosis. If the constriction of the foreskin at the head of the penis is severe enough, it causes urinary obstruction and painful urination.

Constriction is also a major problem with paraphimosis. The constriction at the base of the glans usually results in swelling of the glans. If the swelling is not reduced, blood vessels to the glans are compressed, reducing flow. Inadequate blood flow can result in necrosis of the glans.

Collaborative Care Management. Treatment for severe cases of phimosis may consist of incisions in the foreskin to reduce

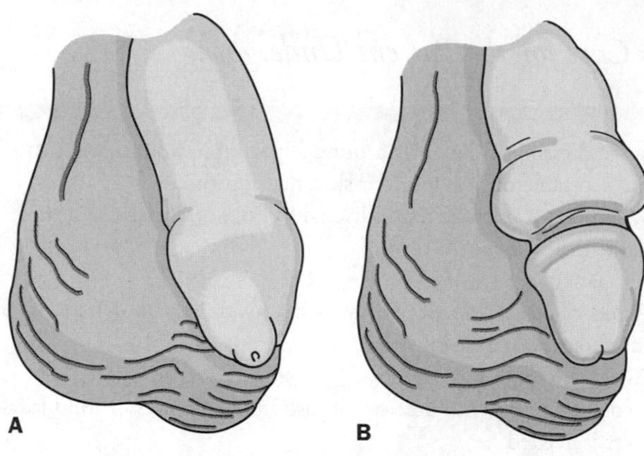

Figure 57-7 **A,** Phimosis: note pinpoint opening of foreskin. **B,** Paraphimosis. Foreskin is retracted but has become a constricting band around penis.

the contracture and widen the opening. Congenital phimosis may be successfully treated by gentle repeated stretching of the foreskin over the glans. Circumcision may be performed if the foreskin cannot be satisfactorily retracted.

Circumcision is done to prevent recurrence of paraphimosis. When the penis is circumcised, the wound is covered with gauze generously impregnated with petrolatum. Bleeding usually is controlled by applying a pressure dressing that may be bulky and must be removed before the patient can void. It is removed cautiously and replaced after voiding with a fresh petrolatum dressing.

Patient/Family Teaching. Patient education focuses on strategies to reduce the inflammation. Hot soaks and oral antibiotics are often used to treat the swelling and infection that can result from phimosis. Cool compresses are used for paraphimosis. The cool compress is applied to the penis, and the penis is elevated for a short period before a gentle attempt is made to reduce the prepuce.

If circumcision has been necessary, the nurse teaches the patient how to change the petrolatum dressing and observe for signs of infection. The nurse also instructs the patient to be alert for signs of bleeding. If severe bleeding occurs, a firm dressing should be applied to the penis, and the patient should be taken to the physician's office or the emergency room. If bleeding persists, it may be necessary to resuture the wound. An estrogen preparation may be prescribed for the adult patient for several days after surgery to prevent painful erections.

Cancer of the Penis

Etiology and Epidemiology. Penile cancer is very rare in North America and Europe. In the United States it accounts for about 0.2% of cancers in men and 0.1% of all cancer deaths in men. The incidence is much higher in some parts of Asia, Africa, and South America, where it is responsible for 10% to 20% of cancers in men. Most cases of the disease are diagnosed in men over age 50, but about 22% occur in men younger than 40.[22] The overall 5-year survival rate for all stages of penile cancer is about 50%.[2]

The incidence of penile cancer depends greatly on hygienic standards and cultural and religious practices. It almost never occurs in a male who was circumcised at birth. Circumcision after puberty does not decrease the risk of cancer when compared with the incidence among uncircumcised males. Circumcision removes the prepuce, or foreskin, which provides a haven for bacteria. The bacteria act on desquamated cells, producing smegma, which is irritating to the tissue of the glans penis and the prepuce. This chronic irritation is considered to be carcinogenic. Therefore adequate hygiene theoretically is sufficient prophylaxis against penile cancer, making circumcision unnecessary. A continuing focus of research is the association of human papillomavirus with malignant lesions of the penis.[22] Box 57-5 lists the stages of penile cancer.

Pathophysiology. Penile cancer starts as a small lesion usually on or under the prepuce and extends until the entire glans and shaft are involved. The initial lesion may appear as a small bump, resemble a pimple or wart, or as a nonhealing ulcer with the edges rolled inward. The latter is associated with earlier metastases and a poorer 5-year survival rate.

The most common (95%) type of malignancy is squamous cell carcinoma. Phimosis, which is present in 25% to 75% of patients with penile cancer, may obscure the lesion. The lesion may then cause erosion through the prepuce, resulting in a foul odor and discharge. Bleeding may or may not be present. Urethral and bladder involvement are rare. Eventually the disease can become autoamputative. If left untreated, death occurs in 2 to 3 years.

Clinical manifestations of penile cancer include weakness, fatigue, malaise, and weight loss. Men may complain of itching and burning under the prepuce and an occasional foul discharge. A 1-year delay before seeking treatment occurs in 15% to 50% of cases. Biopsy is performed to establish the diagnosis; however, benign penile lesions occur infrequently.

Metastasis usually occurs at the regional femoral and iliac nodes and is associated with a significantly worse prognosis. Late in the course of the disease metastasis to retroperitoneal nodes, liver, lung, and brain can occur.[22]

Collaborative Care Management. Treatment is usually surgical. Radiotherapy is indicated only in patients who have small superficial lesions and strongly desire to preserve sexual function. If the lesion is confined to the prepuce, circumcision may be adequate. If the lesion is on the glans, partial penectomy is required. If the shaft of the penis is involved, total amputation may be necessary. The decision is based on the amount of penis remaining after excision with an adequate tumor-free margin. The remaining penis must be long enough for the patient to void in a standing position and direct the urinary stream. If this is possible, sexual function will probably be retained. If total amputation is required, a perineal urethrostomy is performed, in which the urethra is redirected to an opening between the scrotum and the

Box 57-5 Stages of Penile Cancer

Stage I	Lesions confined to glans or foreskin
Stage II	Shaft or corpora cavernosa invaded by tumor
Stage III	Shaft involvement; lymph nodes involved but operable
Stage IV	Shaft involvement; lymph nodes inoperable; metastases to distant sites

anus. With spread of the cancer to the scrotum, radical removal, either hemipelvectomy or hemicorporectomy, is required.

Approximately one third of men with penile cancer have metastatic nodal disease at the time of initial diagnosis. Radiotherapy is used as adjuvant therapy at all stages. Brachytherapy has yielded positive results as an effective organ-sparing treatment modality.[21] Lymphadenectomy is indicated for lymph node involvement. Accurate detection of metastases is difficult, since enlarged lymph nodes may be free of cancerous tissue, whereas normal-size lymph nodes may contain metastatic lesions.

Chemotherapeutic agents have been used with some success. Agents include high-dose methotrexate, bleomycin, vincristne, and cisplatin. Because of the rarity of the disease, large-scale clinical studies to evaluate chemotherapeutic agents are lacking. If the disease is confined to the penis, 5-year survival is 80% to 85% with amputation. With metastasis to the lymph nodes, it is only 20%.

PATIENT/FAMILY TEACHING. The nurse teaches the patient about the potential side effects of radiation in the perineal area. Radiation in this location can cause the skin to become dry, itchy, and sensitive. Special gels that are safe to use during radiation may be applied to the affected area. Urethral strictures can develop several months to years after radiotherapy. The nurse informs the patient of symptoms of urethral stricture, which include difficulty starting or stopping the urine flow, frequent UTIs, and nocturia. Bowel patterns may change during radiotherapy and for up to several weeks. Effects of chemotherapy and nursing interventions are discussed in Chapter 23.

The emotional devastation of a diagnosis of penile cancer is difficult to overestimate. The proposed surgery may be unthinkable to the patient, who is frequently in a state of shock. The scope of support and sexual counseling needed by this patient is beyond the expertise of most nurses. The patient is referred for sexual counseling with experts who can clearly explain his options. Some patients with a urethrostomy have experienced orgasm and ejaculation after stimulation of the perineal, scrotal, and testicular regions.

Impotence and Erectile Dysfunction

Etiology and Epidemiology. Impotence is the inability of a man to have an erection firm enough or to sustain an erection long enough for satisfactory intercourse. The term *satisfactory* is defined by the couple involved and may vary from couple to couple. The ability to have an erection depends not only on a healthy psychologic state, but also on adequately functioning neurologic, vascular, and hormonal systems. The brain is the controlling organ for sexual arousal. The brain perceives sexual stimuli and controls the physiologic changes that occur during arousal. The two fundamental causes of impotence are physical and psychologic.

Physical causes include changes in blood flow to the penis and neurogenic dysfunctions. Diseases such as diabetes mellitus, BPH, lupus, and rheumatoid arthritis can damage blood vessels and cause obstruction of blood flow in the penis. Anemia and dehydration can cause insufficient blood volumes to maintain an erection. Cardiovascular disease, hypertension, and antihypertensive drugs can interfere with the capillary blood pressure.[20] Trauma to the peritoneum can cause scarring and reduce blood flow.

A wide variety of disorders that affect neurologic functioning (e.g., spinal cord injury, diabetes, renal failure, multiple sclerosis, and Parkinson's disease) can interfere with erectile function. Changes in testosterone levels can affect the male sex drive. Aging affects the level of testosterone, and sexual function usually declines somewhat with advancing age. Surgical procedures such as TURP or radical prostatectomy and prior radiation to the abdomen or pelvis can interfere with both blood engorgement and neurogenic innervation of the penis.[12]

Other significant risk factors for erectile dysfunction include chronic drug and alcohol abuse and the use of antidepressants, tranquilizers, antihistamines, and appetite suppressants. Smoking is considered a major risk factor, as is a sedentary lifestyle.[20] Exercising vigorously at least 3 hours a week has been found to significantly reduce the risk of erectile dysfunction.[25]

Psychologic impotence can be attributed to many factors, such as long-term stressors, fears, anxiety, anger, and frustrations. "Performance anxiety," a fear of not performing well during sexual intercourse, is common, often resulting in diminished self-esteem (see Risk Factors box).

Most men occasionally experience impotence. Short-term impotence can be caused by fatigue, stress, anxiety, or the use of alcohol or other drugs. Until recently, psychologic problems were considered to be the cause of 90% of impotence cases. Now, physical causes have been found in 85% of cases. About 5% of 40-year-old men and between 15% and 25% of 65-year-old men experience erectile dysfunction, but it is not an inevitable part of aging.[20] The tremendous anxiety produced by occasional or chronic impotence worsens the problem, even when the underlying disorder is physical.

Pathophysiology. The brain's inability to respond to sexual stimuli can interrupt the signals to the parasympathetic nervous system that release a transmitter substance causing the small arteries in the penis to dilate. The result is insufficient blood flow to fill the network of sinusoids inside the corpora cavernosa (erectile chambers) that cause the penis to enlarge and become firm. When the blood volume in the erectile chambers is inadequate, they cannot create enough pressure to block blood return. Blood drains from the penis, and an erection cannot be maintained.

Risk Factors

Impotence

- Stress
- Fatigue
- Drug effects (e.g., antihypertensive agents, beta-blockers, or alcohol)
- Diabetes mellitus
- Vascular disease (e.g., hypertension or peripheral vascular disease)
- Neurologic disorders (e.g., multiple sclerosis or spinal cord injury)
- Effects of colorectal, cystectomy, or selected prostatectomy procedures
- Trauma to the perineal area
- Psychologic factors

The sympathetic nervous system controls both orgasm and ejaculation. These two functions therefore can occur without an erection. After ejaculation, or when sexual stimulation diminishes, the arteries in the penis constrict, reducing blood flow, and the veins expand to allow disengorgement.

Collaborative Care Management

DIAGNOSTIC TESTS. Diagnostic tests for impotence include complete blood count, urinalysis, BUN, creatinine, and fasting blood sugars. These tests help rule out entities such as anemia, renal disease, and diabetes as possible causative factors. Other blood tests include cholesterol levels and hormonal studies.

Nocturnal monitoring of penile tumescence is also performed. This test involves the man wearing a device around the penis at night that can gauge normal nocturnal engorgement of the penis. Results indicate the ability of the penis to enlarge and become firm. A penile ultrasound may be done after injecting the penis with alprostadil to induce an erection, thereby providing the ability to detect circulatory blockages.[12] Invasive studies are ordered only when other testing measures are inconclusive. Arteriograms and cavernosometry, which measures pressures and blood vessel responses in the erectile chambers, are sometimes performed.

Psychologic testing is also performed, which ideally also includes the man's partner.

MEDICATIONS. The first line of treatment for impotence is oral medication. Phosphodiesterase type 5 (PDE5) inhibitors prescribed include sildenafil (Viagra), vardenafil (Levitra), and tadalafil (Cialis). These drugs enhance smooth muscle relaxation within arteries and arterioles, thereby promoting local vasodilation and thus an erection. Sildenafil and vardenafil have half-lives between 4 and 6 hours. Tadalafil has a substantially longer half-life of 16 to 18 hours, allowing for a longer period during which erection can be achieved.[16] All oral agents still require sexual stimulation for the patient to achieve an erection. PDE5 inhibitors can lower the blood pressure significantly, which has resulted in cardiac arrest in a few cases when taken in combination with nitrates. Other side effects include headache and gastrointestinal disturbances, nasal congestion, and flushing.

Oral testosterone has been used to treat erectile dysfunction in some men with low levels of natural testosterone. It is seldom prescribed because it is often ineffective, has numerous undesirable side effects, and may cause liver damage.[20]

Second-line therapy for men who do not respond to PDE5 inhibitors includes topical, injectable, and intraurethral agents that induce smooth muscle relaxation, thereby causing an erection. Topical agents such as nitroglycerin ointment are occasionally used to enhance venous congestion of the penis. These drugs can support an erection over a period of hours. Vasodilators can induce penile erections by means of increased arterial blood flow, sinusoidal relaxation, and increased venous resistance. The drugs generally used are a papaverine and phentolamine combination injected by the patient into the corpus cavernosum of the penis or inserted into the tip of the penis via suppository. Drug combinations also may include prostaglandin E (alprostadil). Once the drug is injected or inserted, the penis becomes turgid within 5 to 20 minutes, and the erection lasts about 1 hour.[20] Injection therapy has proven effective in most patients regardless of the cause of their dysfunction. Test doses are given initially to determine the appropriate drug dosage for each patient. Side effects include dizziness, facial flushing, hypotension, and priapism (an erection that lasts longer than 4 to 6 hours; Box 57-6).

Often routine medications taken daily by patients have side effects that inhibit erectile function. Modifying the dosage, changing the brand, or trying an alternative medication can prove helpful to many patients.

TREATMENTS. External vacuum devices are sometimes used to achieve an erection for a short time. These devices are cylinders that fit over the penis and use a suction pump to pull blood into the penis. A band is applied to the proximal aspect of the penis when an erection is achieved to impede the venous return. The erection may be maintained for approximately 30 minutes. The devices can be used daily and have minimal side effects if used properly. These devices are contraindicated for patients with bleeding disorders, sickle cell anemia, and severe circulatory compromise.

Counseling and sexual therapy classes may be suggested for patients who have identified psychologic impotence. They may also be suggested for men dealing with the problem of impotence and the need to find alternative measures for sexual fulfillment.

SURGICAL MANAGEMENT. Surgery to repair arteries can reduce erectile dysfunction caused by obstructions that block the flow of blood. The best candidates for such surgery are young men with discrete arterial blockage resulting from an injury to the crotch or fracture of the pelvis. This procedure is almost never successful in older men with widespread blockage. Surgery to block off veins can reduce the leakage of blood that diminishes the rigidity of the penis during erection. Experts question the long-term effectiveness of this procedure and it is rarely done.[20]

A penile prosthesis may be implanted to treat organic erectile dysfunction. There are two types of penile prostheses. One type consists of two sponge-filled silicone rods, which are implanted in the corpora cavernosa. They support the penis in a constant semierect position. Another method, which more closely simulates an actual erection, is the inflatable penile prosthesis (Figure 57-8). This consists of two inflatable rods inserted into either side of the

Box 57-6 Priapism

Priapism is a painful condition, characterized by prolonged erection (more than 4 to 6 hours). Penile ischemia can result, causing permanent impotence or necrosis of the penis.

Etiology

Caused by either prolonged venous occlusion or arterial blood engorgement
Possible side effect of some impotence therapies

Treatment

Treatment directed at the specific cause
Options: administration of alpha-agonists directly into the corpora cavernosa, and intravenous therapy to reestablish acid-base balance
Pain management a high priority

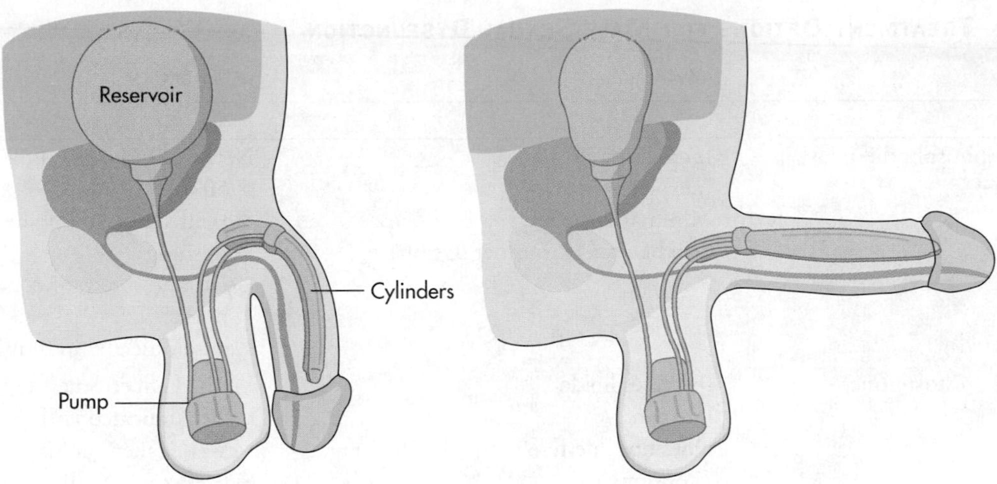

Figure 57-8 The Scott inflatable prosthesis has both erect and flaccid positions designed to mimic normal erectile function.

penis. The rods are connected to a reservoir that allows fluid to flow in or out of them when the man presses on a pump device inserted in the thigh or scrotum.

Both types of prostheses are implanted surgically and do not interfere with normal urinary elimination. The silicone implants are inserted through perineal or penile incisions and the inflatable prostheses through perineal and abdominal incisions. Penile edema is minimal, but scrotal edema may occur with the inflatable type. Pain may be severe during the first week, and mild pain may continue for several weeks after surgery. Patients with any type of penile prosthesis should be cautioned about engaging in any contact sport where a groin injury could potentially damage the prosthesis.[23] As with any prosthetic device, the man needs to integrate the device successfully into his body image and sexual relationship. Table 57-4 compares treatment options for erectile dysfunction.

Nursing Management

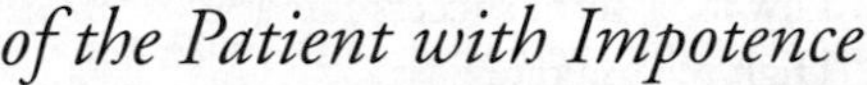

of the Patient with Impotence

ASSESSMENT

Health History. Assess for:

- Physical diseases, especially vascular and neurogenic
- Surgeries, especially TURP and prostatectomy
- Medications, especially beta-blockers and antidepressants
- Alcohol consumption, smoking, drug use
- Degree of comfort of patient and partner in discussing problem
- Current and past sexual practices and degree of satisfaction
- History of sexual dysfunction
- Length of time sexual dysfunction has been a problem
- Ability to have and maintain an erection
- Presence of psychosocial stressors
- Treatment approaches tried to alleviate problem

Physical Examination. Assess for:

- Any obvious deformity or structural defects of sexual organs
- Sensorimotor ability: manual dexterity and visual acuity needed for many treatment options

NURSING DIAGNOSES, OUTCOMES, AND INTERVENTIONS

Nursing Diagnosis: Sexual Dysfunction (Impotence)

OUTCOMES. Common examples of expected outcomes for the patient with a diagnosis of *sexual dysfunction* (impotence) are:

Patient will:

- Identify alternative methods of sexual intimacy that will provide a positive sexual interaction.
- Demonstrate effective use of devices to obtain an erection.

NURSING INTERVENTIONS. Helping the patient choose sexual therapy options by providing accurate and up-to-date information is an important part of nursing care for the patient with impotence. Myths and erroneous information are common obstacles in sexual rehabilitation. The nurse informs the patient of the physiologic and psychologic aspects of erectile function. The nurse reviews the use of external devices and medications, including their modes of action, side effects, and contraindications. Early referral to advanced practice nurses and other specialists is usually appropriate.

PENILE INJECTIONS. The nurse may be responsible for teaching the patient to administer penile injections. These patients need to be evaluated in an office or clinic on a regular basis. Systemic complications of the injections include orthostatic hypotension and dizziness. Local complications include pain, hematoma, edema, decreased glandular sensation, fibrosis, and priapism (prolonged, uncontrolled erection not associated with tactile stimulation or sexual desire). Priapism may be reversed by application of ice, manual masturbation, injection of epinephrine, or the use of antihistamines. If priapism persists longer than 4 to 6 hours, the patient should notify his physician.

Injection sites are to the lateral sides of the penis and should be rotated, and injection into the urethra should be avoided. Applying pressure to the injection site can help decrease the possibility

TABLE 57-4 TREATMENT OPTIONS FOR MALE SEXUAL DYSFUNCTION

Treatment	Advantages	Disadvantages
NONSURGICAL		
Oral medications (phosphodiesterase type 5 inhibitors)	Increase libido Inexpensive Minimal side effects Can be used with other options	Newly released and still in trials; 50%-70% effective Side effects including headache, diarrhea, flushing Contraindicated for concurrent use with nitrates Contraindicated in retinitis pigmentosa
Hormonal therapy (testosterone)	Increases libido Inexpensive Does not interfere with other treatment options Widely available	Limited effectiveness (10%-15%) Contraindicated with prostate cancer Must be taken on long-term basis Side effects including fluid retention, liver damage
External vacuum devices	Easy to understand Inexpensive Safe, reversible Can be used with other treatment options	Require preparation Long-term effects not known Side effects including bruising, pain Require manual dexterity Cumbersome Inhibit spontaneity
Counseling	Involves partner Can be used with other treatment options May improve other psychosocial issues	Limited effectiveness Longstanding problems sometimes difficult to treat
Penile injections or suppositories	Use only when desired Produces rapid, natural-appearing erections Can be used with other treatments Minimal pain	Require close monitoring May create syncope, hypertension Moderately expensive Not effective with severe blood flow problems Side effects including priapism, fibrosis Aversion to needles or insertion device in some patients
SURGICAL		
Vascular reconstructive surgery	Possibility of restoration to normal function Natural appearance	Expensive Technically difficult surgery Low long-term success rate (30%-50%) High relapse rate
Inflatable prosthesis	Natural-looking erection No preparation time Use as desired Increases girth of penis No concealment problem	Device failure Requires manual dexterity May require removal or reimplant Expensive Risk of infection, erosion
Self-contained inflatable prosthesis	Natural-looking erection No preparation time Use as desired No concealment problem Simpler surgery than that for full inflatable prosthesis	Device failure Requires manual dexterity May require removal or reimplant Expensive Risk of infection, erosion Does not increase girth
Semirigid or malleable prosthesis	Simple surgery No mechanical parts Least expensive implant Use as desired	May be difficult to conceal Does not increase length or girth of penis Expensive Risk of infection Higher risk of erosion May require removal or reimplant

of fibrosis. The nurse instructs the patient not to use injections more than twice a week. Liver enzyme levels should be monitored about every 3 months. If liver function studies are elevated or fibrosis is noted on the penis, the physician usually recommends that the injections be discontinued. The drug should be kept in the refrigerator to avoid degeneration of the solution. Dosages can be altered if initial results are not satisfactory.

EXTERNAL VACUUM DEVICES. Vacuum devices come in one size with ring seals at the end that are different diameters to accommodate individual erection size. The nurse teaches the patient to use the device and make sure that the seals are the appropriate size to ensure sufficient vacuum to the penis. The vascular ring is applied once the penis is engorged and should be left on only for approximately 30 minutes to prevent possible vascular damage. The nurse involves both partners in the teaching session if possible. Couples need to discuss in advance how sexual activity may be modified comfortably with the use of the device.

The vacuum device may be used every day if desired. Complications include pulling of scrotal tissue, hematoma, inability to achieve or maintain the erection, and discomfort with the vascular ring. These complications can usually be managed by adjusting the procedure or switching to a different product. Blocked or retrograde ejaculation may also occur. Orgasm should not be affected. The patient is encouraged to schedule ongoing medical support to help him cope with this altered sexual pattern.

PENILE IMPLANTS. Infection rates are generally low with penile implant surgery. Antibiotics may be administered a few days before surgery and for a week after surgery to prevent infection. The patient also may be told to perform a Hibiclens prewash before surgery to decrease the chance of infection. The nurse instructs the patient to take all antibiotics and report any symptoms of infection, such as unusual swelling, redness, excessive pain, or drainage around the incision sites.

To prevent the device from eroding through the penile skin, the nurse instructs the patient to avoid sexual intercourse for at least 6 to 8 weeks after surgery. When sexual activity resumes, the patient is instructed to use a water-soluble lubricant. The patient needs to avoid wearing tight-fitting clothing and sitting with the legs crossed or in other positions that put pressure on or cause friction to the penis.

The nurse explains to the patient that his erections will not necessarily be any larger than before surgery, that the implant will not affect sex drive or interfere with penile sensation, and that he should be able to have an orgasm and ejaculate with the implant in place. Patients with inflatable implants need to be instructed on how to inflate and deflate the prosthesis. The patient's partner is included in teaching sessions if possible.

RELATED NIC INTERVENTIONS. Anticipatory Guidance, Sexual Counseling

Nursing Diagnosis: Anxiety

OUTCOMES. A common example of expected outcomes for the patient with a diagnosis of *anxiety* is:

The patient will:

- Demonstrate a relaxed, positive attitude about sexual performance.

NURSING INTERVENTIONS. Sexual counseling usually is offered in conjunction with other forms of treatment for the impotent patient. The nurse is often the person to encourage the patient to avail himself of counseling opportunities. The nurse helps the patient understand his needs and explains the general nature of sexual counseling, since patients often have misconceptions concerning the treatment. The nurse provides some specific examples of exercises used during sexual counseling and explains how partner communication can be enhanced.

RELATED NIC INTERVENTIONS. Anxiety Reduction, Calming Technique, Emotional Support, Presence

EVALUATION

To evaluate the effectiveness of nursing interventions, compare patient behaviors with those stated in the expected patient outcomes.

RELATED NOC OUTCOMES. Acceptance: Health Status, Anxiety Self-Control, Body Image, Coping

GERONTOLOGIC CONSIDERATIONS

The nurse should not assume that older adults do not have sexual needs. Impotence in the older patient is often caused by narrowing of the blood vessels and consequently decreased blood flow to the penis. Most healthy men can obtain an erection even at an advanced age. Often the older man needs more intense and prolonged stimulation than his younger counterpart to have an erection. The nurse can inform patients and their partners of the need for longer foreplay with the older man.

Vasectomy: Male Sterilization

Etiology and Epidemiology. Voluntary **sterilization** has become increasingly acceptable to both men and women as a method of preventing pregnancy. It is the most frequently used method of fertility control for married couples over 30 years old and is the most widely used contraceptive method worldwide, protecting approximately 100 million couples. It has been estimated that more than 13.7 million adults have been sterilized in the United States and 100 million worldwide. Each year, 500,000 to 1 million American men have vasectomies.[5]

The primary reason given by both men and women for seeking sterilization is a desire to limit family size. More frequently than women, men also cite a desire for effective contraception that does not interfere with sexual pleasure. Also, men express concern over the health of their sex partners. Some men believe that the "pill" is actually or potentially harmful to the woman.

Laws governing sterilization vary from state to state and have undergone many changes. In general, if the surgery does not violate specific state provisions and if written informed consent is given by a man or woman legally capable of giving permission, the surgery can be performed. Because sterilization is a permanent method of contraception, informed consent is absolutely necessary before the procedure.

Pathophysiology. Bilateral vasectomy is the surgical procedure used for male sterilization. Vasectomy interrupts the continuity of the vas deferens and prevents sperm from being ejaculated with other components of the semen. However, sperm still are produced, and the ejaculate is not noticeably diminished in amount. Residual fertility may be present for a variable period because of existing sperm in the semen beyond the point of occlusion of the vas deferens. Sperm gradually disappear from the ejaculate; thus conception is possible in the immediate postoperative period.

After vasectomy, antibodies to sperm develop in about 50% to 66% of men. No relationship has been found in humans between the presence of sperm antibodies and any systemic pathologic condition. It is hypothesized that antisperm antibodies may result in circulating immune complexes that exacerbate atherosclerosis, but this has not been proven in human studies.

Collaborative Care Management. At least 11 different techniques for vasectomy exist. Bilateral partial vasectomy is the surgical method used most often. Because of its safety and simplicity, the procedure can be performed on an outpatient basis using a local anesthetic. A small incision is made in the scrotum to expose the sheath of the vas deferens. The sheath is opened, and a 0.63 to 1.27 cm segment of the vas deferens is removed. The severed ends of the vas deferens are then ligated or coagulated to ensure sterility. The incision is then sutured closed.

Complications after vasectomy are rare and usually minor. Bruising, mild edema, and mild discomfort are common and usually subside without treatment. Infection of the wound occurs in about 3% of patients. Hematoma, epididymitis, and granuloma formation can occur. The incidence of failure as a result of recanalization (reanastomosis) is reported to be 0% to 6%. The cause of spontaneous recanalization is unknown, but duplication of the vas deferens has occasionally occurred. A preoperative specimen of semen is examined to serve as a baseline for monitoring sperm disappearance after surgery.

Research is ongoing concerning techniques to reverse vasectomy and restore fertility. A vasovasostomy attempts to rejoin the severed ends of the vas deferens. Success is measured by the presence of sperm in semen specimens after reconstruction. Reports of success in restoring fertility average 84%.[28] The Food and Drug Administration has recently approved the Vasclip, a device the size of a grain of rice that atraumatically locks around the vas deferens to halt the flow of sperm. It eliminates all cutting, suturing, and cauterizing. Postoperative complications so far are extremely rare.[1]

PATIENT/FAMILY TEACHING. Patient education focuses on ensuring that the patient has made a careful and informed decision concerning sterilization. Teaching is based on the federal government's informed consent guidelines (see Chapter 56). The nurse explains the nature and consequences of the surgery to the patient, emphasizing that the sterilization procedure does nothing to increase or decrease sexual performance or enjoyment, but simply removes the risk of pregnancy. Visual aids and models can be of great value in explaining the surgery.

Every effort is made to ensure that the decision for sterilization is not based on a lack of knowledge concerning other options for contraception. Most patients are satisfied with the results of vasectomy, but some may experience emotional difficulties, since sterilization affects both partners.[29]

The nurse discusses the facts concerning reversibility, including current success rates. The chance of recanalization and return of fertility should be pointed out. The man or couple must also be informed that sterility occurs progressively rather than immediately after vasectomy, and alternate methods of contraception need to be used until sterility is achieved. Men are taught to expect slight swelling of the scrotum, minor pain, and a small amount of bleeding after surgery. Ice to the scrotal area, sitz baths, and rest will ameliorate these discomforts. Any signs of infection should be reported promptly to the physician for evaluation and treatment.

It is important for the man to schedule follow-up semen analysis. A sperm count usually is taken 4 weeks after vasectomy. Two consecutive sperm-free specimens are necessary before the man can be considered sterile. Reanastomosis of the vas deferens is suspected if sperm fail to disappear from the ejaculate, if there is an increase in sperm in the semen after two successive sperm counts, or if motile sperm are found in the semen 3 months after vasectomy.

Critical Thinking

1. As a community health nurse in an industrial company, you are designing a program to teach men in the company about reproductive health. Develop an outline depicting the priority diseases and preventive measures to teach.
2. A 59-year-old man is admitted to the hospital complaining of difficulty urinating. The emergency room physician orders routine urinalysis, complete blood count, and chemistry profile. Outline questions designed to help differentiate the cause of these symptoms.

References

1. Alternative to vasectomy cleared by FDA, *Nurs Pract* 29(2):47, 2004.
2. American Cancer Society: *What are the key statistics about penile cancer?* accessed June 2003 from website: www.cancer.org/docroot/CRI.
3. American Cancer Society: *What are the key statistics about prostate cancer?* accessed from website: www.cancer.org/cocroot/CRI/content/CRI.
4. American Cancer Society: *What are the key statistics for testicular cancer?* accessed March 2004 from website: www.cancer.org/docroot/CRIcontent/CRI.

4a. American Cancer Society: Cancer facts and figures 2005, Atlanta, 2005, ACS.

5. Amundsen GA, Kalyanakrishnan R: A vasectomy: a seminal analysis, *Southern Med J* 97(1):54-58, 2004.
6. Bishop P: Bipolar transurethral resection of the prostate—a new approach, *AORN J* 77: 982, 2003.
7. Brown CG: Testicular cancer: an overview, *MedSurg Nurs* 12(1):39-40, 2003.
8. Chambers A: Home study program: transurethral resection syndrome—it does not have to be a mystery, *AORN J* 75(1):163, 2002.
9. Cole FL, Vogler R: The acute, nontraumatic scrotum: assessment, diagnosis, and management, *J Am Nurse Pract* 16(2):54, 2004.
10. Cormier L: Impact of prostrate cancer screening on health-related quality of life in at-risk families, *Urology* 59(6):901, 2002.

11. Dufour J: Assessing and treating epididymiris, *Nurs Pract* 26(3):23, 2001.
12. Dunbar C: Men's health—treating erectile dysfunction, *Nurs Spect* 16(12):10-11, 2004.
13. Gordon A, Shaughnessy A: Saw palmetto for prostate disorders, *Am Fam Phys* 67(6):1282, 2003.
14. Hanson K: Continuing education: laboratory studies in the evaluation of urologic disease, part I, *Urolog Nurs* 6(23):401, 2003.
15. Henderson SO: *Prostatitis,* accessed Sept 2002 from website: www.emedicine.com/emerg/topic488.htm.
16. Lewis J: Erectile dysfunction—a panel's recommendations for management, *AJN* 103(10):48-56, 2003.

16a. National Cancer Institute: *Lycopene,* accessed November 2005 from website: www3.cancer.gov/prevention/agents/lycopene.html.

17. National Cancer Institute: *Prostate cancer (PDQ): prevention,* accessed October 2003 from website: www.cancer.gov/cancertopics/pdq/prevention/protocol.
18. National Cancer Institute: *Testicular cancer (PDQ): treatment*, accessed Oct 2003 from website: www.cancer.gov/cancertopics/pdq/treatment/testicular.
19. National Cancer Institute: *Testicular cancer treatment—stage I testicular cancer, stage II testicular cancer, stage III testicular cancer,* accessed Oct 2003 from website: www.cancer.gov/cancertreatment/testicular/HealthPro.
20. National Institute of Diabetes and Digestive and Kidney Diseases: *Erectile dysfunction*, accessed from website: http://kidney.niddk.nih.gov/kudiseases/pubs/impotence.
21. Newman L: Brachytherapy for penile cancer may salvage organ, *Urology Times,* vol 10, May 2002.
22. Pow-Sang M et al: Cancer of the penis, *Cancer Control* 9(4):301-302, 2002.
23. Quallich S, Ohl D: Penile prosthesis: patient teaching and perioperative care, *Urolog Nurs* 22(2):81-90, 2002.
24. Riechers E: Including partners into the diagnosis of prostrate cancer: a review of literature to provide a model of care, *Urolog Nurs* 24(1):29, 2004.
25. RN newswatch: frequent, vigorous exercise can reduce the risk of erectile dysfunction, *RN* 66(10):18, 2003.
26. Small EJ, Torti FM: Testis. In Dollinger M et al, editors: *Everyone's guide to cancer therapy*, ed 4, Kansas City, 2003, Andrews McMeel.
27. Stipetich R et al: Nursing assessment of sexual function following permanent prostate brachytherapy for patients with early-stage prostate cancer, *Clin J Oncol Nurs* 6(5):273, 2002.
28. Study finds vasectomy highly effective, even after 15years, *Womens Health Weekly* 132, March 11, 2004.
29. Stump B, Taber A, Drozd S: Are you ready for a vasectomy? *Men's Health* 16(10):112, 2001.
30. Thorpe A, Neal D: Benign prostatic hyperplasia, *Lancet* 361:1359, 1363, 2003.
31. Wehle MJ, Lisson SW: Benign prostatic hypertrophy, *Phys Sportsmed* 30: 41-42, 2002.

evolve **Visit the Evolve website:** http://evolve.elsevier.com/Monahan/medsurg

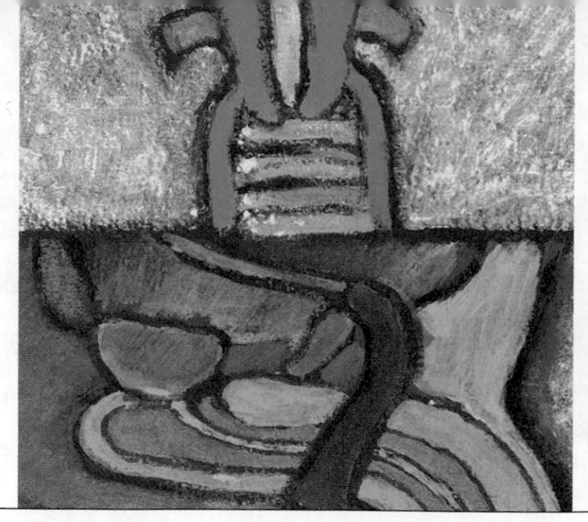

CHAPTER 58

Problems of the Breast

by Angela Sammarco

OBJECTIVES

After studying this chapter, the learner should be able to:

1. Describe the differences between benign and malignant breast conditions.
2. Identify the risk factors for developing breast cancer.
3. Describe early detection methods and diagnostic tests for breast evaluation.
4. Discuss the advantages and disadvantages of surgery, chemotherapy, radiotherapy, and hormonal therapy in the treatment of breast cancer.
5. Identify the high-priority care needs of women treated for breast cancer.
6. Explain nursing measures that meet the needs of breast cancer patients.
7. Identify special considerations for gerontologic patients treated for breast cancer.
8. Discuss issues related to the psychosocial adjustment to breast cancer.
9. Compare the treatments for common benign breast conditions.

KEY TERMS

adjuvant therapy, p. 1759
bioassay, p. 1761
cytologic examination, p. 1758
hereditary, p. 1751
in situ, p. 1752
ionizing radiation, p. 1752
lactation, p. 1752
metastasis, p. 1754
mutation, p. 1751

Breast disease, although it occurs in men, is predominantly a problem of women. Most breast disease is benign, but nonetheless breast cancer is the most commonly occurring cancer in women, with one out of seven expected to develop it during her lifetime. Because breast disease is so prevalent, breast cancer centers have been established across the United States to care for women with breast problems, whether benign or malignant. Major goals of breast cancer centers include educating the public about risk-factor reduction; providing breast examinations; instructing women in breast self-examination (BSE) techniques; initiating referrals for screening, diagnosis, and treatment; and increasing the detection of breast cancer in its early localized stage. The empowerment and education of women to take an active role in promoting their own personal breast health care is a positive outgrowth of breast cancer centers and a major component of the nursing role.

Malignant Conditions of the Breast

Etiology and Epidemiology. Breast cancer is the most common cancer among women. The incidence of breast cancer continues to increase, partly as a result of the steady aging of the population, and partly because of improved diagnostic technology. The mortality rates associated with breast cancer were relatively stable between 1950 and the late 1980s. Since 1989, the rate of breast cancer mortality has declined annually. This reduction in mortality has been attributed to improvements in breast cancer treatments and the benefits of mammography screening.[1] The underlying cause of breast cancer is still unknown, but a number of risk factors have been identified (see Risk Factors box).

Risk Factors

Age and Gender. Breast cancer is almost exclusively a disease affecting women. Only 1,690 of the 212,930 new cases of breast cancer estimated in 2005 were predicted to involve men.[1] As with most malignant conditions, the incidence of breast cancer increases with age.[1] Breast cancer is diagnosed most frequently in women older than 50 years. One reason for this age-related finding may be an increased probability of mutagenic changes occurring over a longer life span.

Heredity. Inherited breast cancer accounts for up to 10% of all breast cancer cases in Western countries. The presence of inherited

Risk Factors

Breast Cancer

Risk Factors

Female gender: Ninety-nine percent of all breast cancers occur in women and 1% in men.

History of previous breast cancer: The risk of developing cancer in the opposite breast is five times greater than for the average population at risk.

Age over 40 years: Incidence increases with age and peaks in the fifth decade.

Early menarche, late menopause, or both: The risk of breast cancer rises as the interval between menarche and menopause increases; shortening the interval by oophorectomy reduces the risk, especially in women younger than 35 years old.

Reproductive history: Childless women have an increased risk, as do women who bear their first child near or after age 30 years.

Family history: Risk increases two or three times if a mother or sister had breast cancer and is further increased if the relative was diagnosed during the premenopausal state and if the cancer was bilateral.

Ionizing radiation: Women who received ionizing radiation exposure, particularly during adolescence, demonstrate a markedly increased breast cancer risk.

Benign breast disease: Biopsy-proven atypical hyperplasia is associated with an increased risk.

Possible Risk Factors

Diet: Animal data and descriptive epidemiology of breast cancer incidence strongly suggest an association of dietary factors, specifically a high-fat diet, with an increased risk of breast cancer. The National Academy of Sciences recommends decreasing total fat intake to 30% of available calories.

Alcohol: A suggested small increase in risk with moderate alcohol consumption has been reported, although limitations in methodology have been cited, and results require confirmation.

Obesity: Obesity and increased body mass index have been reported to be associated with an increased risk of breast cancer.

Exogenous hormones: Several studies report no link between replacement hormones and breast cancer, and those which do report such a link appear to identify only subsets of patients at risk: those who have taken replacement estrogens for long periods and those who have taken large cumulative doses.

No Increased Risk

Benign breast disease: Fibrocystic breast disease is not associated with breast cancer.

Oral contraceptives: There is no evidence yet to suggest a causal relationship between oral contraceptives and incidence of and survival from breast cancer.

Adapted from Boyle P, Maisonneuve P, Autier P: Update on cancer control in women, *Int J Gynecol Obstet* 70:263-303, 2000; and McPherson K, Steel CM, Dixon JM: ABC of breast diseases: breast cancer—epidemiology, risk factors, and genetics, *Br Med J* 321(9):624-628, 2000.

breast cancer is demonstrated by the incidence in first-degree relatives, which include mother, daughter, or sister. A woman's risk of breast cancer is two or more times greater if a first-degree relative developed the disease before the age of 50, and the younger the first-degree relative at the time of breast cancer development, the greater the risk.[23,36] Additional **hereditary** risk factors include a family history of bilateral breast cancer, a combination of breast cancer and another epithelial cancer, and a combination of atypical hyperplasia and a family history of breast cancer. Most breast cancers that occur before age 65 are attributed to a genetic **mutation**.[23,36]

An important breakthrough in understanding breast cancer risk factors occurred with the discovery of mutations in the BRCA1 and BRCA2 genes in high-risk families. These genes are located on the long arms of chromosomes 17 and 13, respectively, and are transmitted through an autosomal dominant pattern of inheritance. This means that the abnormal gene can be inherited through either parent and that some family members may transmit the abnormal gene without developing cancer themselves.[36] It is thought that mutations in BRCA1 and BRCA2 genes play a role in approximately 30% to 70% of all inherited breast cancer cases and may account for 5% to 10% of all ovarian cancers.[45] Ongoing genetic research will provide more definitive data on inherited breast cancer and how to treat and counsel families about this sensitive and serious health problem. The characteristics of inherited breast cancer are listed in Box 58-1.

The development of noninherited breast cancer is considered to be a two-step process. The first step involves a change in cell structure or function, followed by a second event that promotes another change in the cell and causes it to become malignant. In hereditary breast cancer the inherited cell may already be in an altered state (first step) and require only one event to change it to a cancer cell.

MENSTRUAL AND REPRODUCTIVE HISTORY. The risk of breast cancer is increased when menstruation begins before age 12 and extends to a late menopause after age 55. Women who have a natural menopause after the age of 55 have twice the risk of developing breast cancer as do women who experience menopause before the age of 45.[23] The probability of mutagenic changes taking place from an intermediate phase to a malignant phase is greater when the menstrual cycle spans more than 30 years.

Women who have never been pregnant (nulliparity) or who have their first child after the age of 30 are at an increased risk of

Box 58-1 Characteristics of Inherited Breast Cancer

- Occurs at an early age (premenopausal)
- Incidence of bilateral disease increased
- First-degree relative (mother, daughter, sister) with breast and ovarian cancer
- Ashkenazi Jewish heritage
- Family history of male breast cancer

Adapted from Nogueria S, Appling S: Breast cancer genetics, risks, and strategies, *Nurs Clin North Am* 35(3):663, 2000.

breast cancer. Women ages 30 to 35 years in their first full-term pregnancy are at greater risk for breast cancer than women who deliver for the first time at 18 years of age or younger. The implication is that a full-term pregnancy at an early age promotes changes in breast development that protect the breast from cancer. However, pregnancies that do not end with the birth of a viable fetus do not reduce the risk of breast cancer.[36] **Lactation** and breast-feeding have historically been viewed as protective against breast cancer, but this position is controversial; now the protection is thought to be related to parity rather than breast-feeding alone.[23]

Hormones and Oral Contraception. Postmenopausal hormone replacement therapy remains controversial because of the increased risk of breast cancer associated with prolonged estrogen exposure. Postmenopausal women who receive hormone replacement therapy exhibit an increase in breast cancer risk, although not all studies support these findings.[14] Overall the incremental risk is small, but evidence suggests breast cancer risk increases with long-term use. Breast cancers diagnosed in women taking hormone replacement therapy were found to be less advanced clinically compared with those found in women who have not used hormone replacement therapy.[22,25] In addition, current research findings suggest that hormone replacement therapy does not increase breast cancer mortality.[14]

While women are taking oral contraceptives and for 10 years thereafter, the risk of developing breast cancer is slightly increased, according to current studies. Factors that appear to affect risk include age at first use of contraceptives, duration of use, dose, and type of hormone in the contraceptive agent. Research findings suggest that women who begin use of oral contraceptives before the age of 20 and take them a long time have a higher risk of breast cancer.[3,14]

Diet and Body Weight. Evidence suggests a link between high dietary fat intake and an increased risk of breast cancer.[36] For example, the incidence of breast cancer is lower in countries in which a diet low in fat is the norm.[23] Although a high-fat diet is not thought to cause breast cancer, dietary fat intake may indirectly support increased serum estrogen levels.[36]

Among postmenopausal women the risk of breast cancer appears to rise as body mass index (BMI) increases. A possible explanation for this finding is that in the postmenopausal woman, androgens in adipose tissue can be converted to estrogen, which could stimulate cancer growth and spread.[5,22] A number of studies have found a reduced risk of breast cancer in former college athletes and ballet dancers. This suggests that physical activity and reduced body weight around menarche, in early adolescence, or throughout life may be important factors associated with decreased risk.[5] Until further research can support the association between fat intake, obesity, and breast cancer, women should be advised to limit dietary fat intake and maintain optimal body weight.

Benign Breast Disease. The risk of breast cancer is four or five times higher in women with severe atypical hyperplasia (increased cellular proliferation) than in women who have no proliferative changes in their breasts. Women with atypical hyperplasia and a first-degree relative with breast cancer have a ninefold increase in risk. Women with palpable cysts, complex fibroadenomas, ductal papillomas, sclerosing adenosis, and moderate or florid epithelial hyperplasia have a slightly higher, but clinically insignificant, risk of breast cancer than women without these changes.[25]

Ionizing Radiation. **Ionizing radiation** has been shown to significantly increase the risk of breast cancer. A high incidence of breast cancer has been found among women who survived the atomic bomb explosions in Japan during World War II. Particularly high risk for breast cancer is associated with exposure of the breast to radiation around menarche. It is postulated that breast tissue is especially vulnerable to the effects of ionizing radiation during adolescence, which is a period of rapid breast development. In addition, women who have had repeated fluoroscopic examinations of the chest, mantle radiation for Hodgkin's lymphoma, or radiation as a treatment for mastitis have demonstrated a markedly increased risk of breast cancer later in life.[5,22,25]

Incidence and Mortality Rates. A comparison of the estimated cancer incidence and death rate figures reveals that breast cancer accounts for about one third (32%) of all cancers detected in women and 15% of all cancer-related deaths.[2] The mortality rate for women with breast cancer has decreased an average of 2.2% per year between 1990 and 1997, with most notable decreases observed among Caucasian women and younger women. Researchers predict that, as more breast cancers are detected **in situ** or at earlier stages of invasive disease, the mortality rate will continue to decline.[1] The cancer death rates in females by site are shown in Figure 58-1.

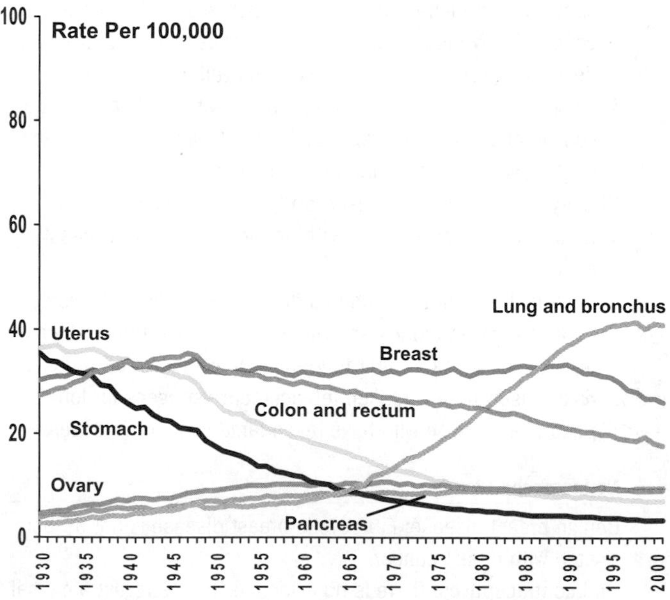

Figure 58-1 Age-adjusted cancer death rates: females by site, United States, 1930-2001.
*Rates are per 100,000 and are age-adjusted to the 2000 U.S. standard population.
†Uterus cancer death rates are for uterine cervix and uterine corpus combined. Note: As a result of changes in ICD coding, numerator information has changed over time. Rates for cancers of the uterus, ovary, lung and bronchus, and colon and rectum are affected by these coding changes.

Incidence and mortality rates for breast cancer are highest in the United States and Western Europe. The reason for this is debatable. One theory is that these countries are highly industrialized and therefore more economically and socially advantaged than some developing countries. As a consequence of this affluence, prevailing dietary patterns and lack of exercise promote obesity, which may be a contributing factor (see preceding discussion of diet and obesity). Although this theory is merely speculative, it is known that when women emigrate from developing countries and Asia to the United States and other Western countries, their breast cancer incidence rises, possibly because of changes in eating patterns.

In the United States Caucasian women have an overall higher incidence of breast cancer than do African-American women. However, African-American women younger than 40 years old are more likely to develop breast cancer than are Caucasian women of the same age, and at almost every age African-American women have a higher mortality rate from breast cancer than do Caucasian women[1] (Figure 58-2). African-American women are more likely to first be seen with advanced stages of breast cancer, have poorer survival within each stage category, are less likely to have estrogen-progesterone receptor (ER-PR)–positive tumors, and have more aggressive tumor cancer compared with Caucasian women.[17] In other racial and ethnic subgroups in the United States, breast cancer incidence rates vary widely. A high rate of breast cancer incidence and a more advanced stage at diagnosis have been observed among Native Hawaiian women. A more advanced stage at diagnosis has also been observed in Hispanic, Native American, and Filipino-American women. The lowest incidence rates have been found among Korean-American, New Mexico Native American, Vietnamese-American, and Chinese-American women.[3] Incidence rates intermediate to these groups have been found among Japanese-American, Alaska native, Filipino-American, and Hispanic women.[16]

Healthy People 2010, a federal initiative to promote health and prevent illness, disability, and premature death,[44] has objectives that specifically relate to breast cancer (see Healthy People 2010 box).

Healthy People 2010

Objectives to Reduce Breast Cancer Mortality

- Reduce breast cancer deaths to no more than 22.3 per 100,000 women by the year 2010.
- Increase, to at least 70%, the proportion of women 40 years old and older who have received a mammogram within the preceding 2 years.

From US Department of Health and Human Services: *Healthy people 2010: understanding and improving health*, Washington, DC, 2000, The Department.

PROGNOSTIC FACTORS. Overall prognosis at the time of diagnosis of breast cancer is based on several factors, including whether the tumor is noninvasive or invasive, its grade, lymph node involvement, tumor size, tumor proliferation and deoxyribonucleic acid (DNA) analysis, estrogen-progesterone markers, and genetic influence.

INVASIVE VERSUS NONINVASIVE. Breast cancer may be categorized as noninvasive or invasive. Noninvasive cancers include ductal carcinoma in situ and lobular carcinoma in situ. These cancers are completely contained in the ductal and lobular systems of the breast and are unable to reach the bloodstream or invade adjacent tissues and organs. They are rarely life threatening and have excellent prognoses.[35] The majority of primary invasive cancers are adenocarcinomas, of which infiltrating ductal carcinoma is a variant.

GRADE. An indicator of a tumor's invasive or metastatic potential can be found in its histologic differentiation or similarity compared with normal breast tissue. Differentiation or grade is determined using the Scarff-Bloom-Richardson system, which grades tumors based on the cellular factors of tubule formation, nuclear features, and mitotic index. Tumors graded with low numbers are considered well differentiated, whereas higher numbers indicate poorer differentiation.[35]

Race/Ethnicity	In Situ Cases*	%	Invasive Cases*	%	Deaths*	%
White	46,200	82.9	173,300	82.0	31,700	79.6
African American	5,400	9.7	20,000	9.5	5,700	14.3
Hispanic	2,200	3.9	11,000	5.2	1,600	4.0
Asian or Pacific Islander	1,800	3.2	6,500	3.1	700	1.8
Native American/Alaska Native	50	0.1	500	0.2	100	0.3
Total	55,700		211,300		39,800	

*Rounding to nearest hundred except Native American/Alaska Natives.
Percentages may not exactly total 100%, due to rounding.
Estimates of new cases are based on incidence rates from 1979 to 1999.

Figure 58-2 Estimated female breast cancer cases and deaths by race/ethnicity, United States, 2003.

Lymph Node Involvement. The presence of cancer cells in axillary lymph nodes is considered the most important prognostic factor, and the number of positive lymph nodes is directly proportional to the risk of breast cancer recurrence.[40] Nodal involvement is found in approximately 40% of women diagnosed with breast cancer. Those patients who have histologically negative lymph nodes have a 70% to 80% chance of remaining disease free.

There are four categories of lymph node status: 0 lymph nodes or negative involvement, 1 to 3 positive nodes, 4 to 9 positive nodes, and 10 or more positive nodes. Progressively greater nodal involvement implies worsening survival rates.[35]

Tumor Size. The tumor size is also directly related to the risk of breast cancer recurrence. Among node-negative patients, with tumors less than 1 cm, the recurrence rate is approximately 1% to 10%; with tumors measuring 1 to 3 cm, the recurrence rate is approximately 30%; and with tumors larger than 3 cm, the recurrence rate is more than 50%.[40] Tumor size is obtained by a three-way measurement of the gross tumor, with the largest dimension used for staging determination. When tumors display mixed invasive and noninvasive components, only the invasive component is measured to obtain a more accurate prognostic indicator.[35]

Tumor Proliferation and DNA Analysis. Flow cytometry is used to measure tumor proliferation through determination of the fraction of tumor cells in the synthesis (S) phase of cell division. The S phase is a sign of DNA activity. Designating the DNA activity provides information regarding the ability of breast cancer to proliferate.[35] A high S phase is associated with a fast-growing tumor and a short disease-free survival time. Ploidy status refers to the amount of DNA contained in tumor cells. Diploid tumors have the same amount of DNA as found in normal cells. Aneuploid tumors have more than the 46 normal chromosomes. Shorter survival is associated with aneuploid tumors.[35] (See Chapter 23 for a more detailed discussion on cell kinetics.)

Estrogen-Progesterone Markers. ER and PR are well-recognized predictors of long-term survival in women with breast cancer. These receptors are proteins present in and on the surface of cancer cells that bind with estrogen and progesterone and subsequently influence DNA activity and cell growth. A tumor that contains receptors that bind with estrogen or progesterone is ER positive or PR positive, respectively. Approximately 60% of all breast cancers are ER positive.[35] Tumors that are hormone receptor positive are more responsive to hormonal therapy than tumors that are negative for hormone receptors.

Genetic Influence. Approximately 30% of breast and ovarian cancers are associated with overexpression of the proto-oncogene c-erB-2/HER-2/neu. In breast cancer this overexpression and gene amplification are directly related to early **metastasis** and poor prognosis. Women with overexpression of this gene are noted to have aggressive breast cancers that are resistant to standard therapy regimens.[23] The National Comprehensive Cancer Network (NCCN) and the American Society of Clinical Oncology recommend that HER-2 status be determined for all primary breast tumors either at time of diagnosis or at tumor recurrence.[21]

Staging of Breast Cancer. Staging of breast cancer incorporates the primary tumor, regional nodes, and metastasis (Box 58-2). Treatment decisions are based on the stage of the breast cancer, as well as on those factors already discussed.

Pathophysiology. Tumors of the breast arise in the epithelial cells of either ductal or lobular tissue and are referred to as carcinomas. The breast is divided into four quadrants (Figure 58-3). A majority of breast tumors occur in the left breast and in the upper outer quadrant, but they can appear in any area of the breast.

Box 58-2 Staging of Breast Cancer

T: Primary Tumor Size

Tx	Primary tumor cannot be assessed
T0	No evidence of primary tumor
Tis	Carcinoma in situ: intraductal carcinoma, lobular carcinoma in situ, or Paget's disease of the nipple with node
T1	Tumor 2 cm or less in greatest dimension
T2	Tumor more than 2 cm but not more than 5 cm in greatest dimension
T3	Tumor more than 5 cm in greatest dimension
T4	Tumor of any size with direct extension to chest wall or skin

Note: Paget's disease associated with a tumor is classified according to the size of the tumor

N: Regional Lymph Nodes

Nx	Regional lymph nodes cannot be assessed (e.g., previously removed)
N0	No regional lymph node metastasis
N1	Metastasis to movable ipsilateral axillary lymph node(s)
N2	Metastasis to ipsilateral axillary lymph node(s) fixed to one another or to other structures
N3	Metastasis to ipsilateral internal mammary lymph node(s)

M: Distant Metastasis

Mx	Presence of distant metastasis cannot be assessed
M0	No distant metastasis
M1	Distant metastasis (includes metastasis to ipsilateral, supraclavicular lymph node[s])

Stage Grouping

Stage 0	Tis	N1	M0
Stage I	T1	N0	M0
Stage IIa	T0	N1	M0
	T1	N1	M0
	T2	N0	M0
Stage IIB	T2	N1	M0
	T3	N0	M0
Stage IIIA	T0	N2	M0
	T1	N2	M0
	T2	N2	M0
	T3	N1	M0
	T3	N2	M0
Stage IIIB	T4	Any N	M0
	Any T	N3	M0
Stage IV	Any T	Any N	M1

Adapted from McCready T: Management of patients with breast cancer, *Nurs Stand* 17(41):45, 2003.

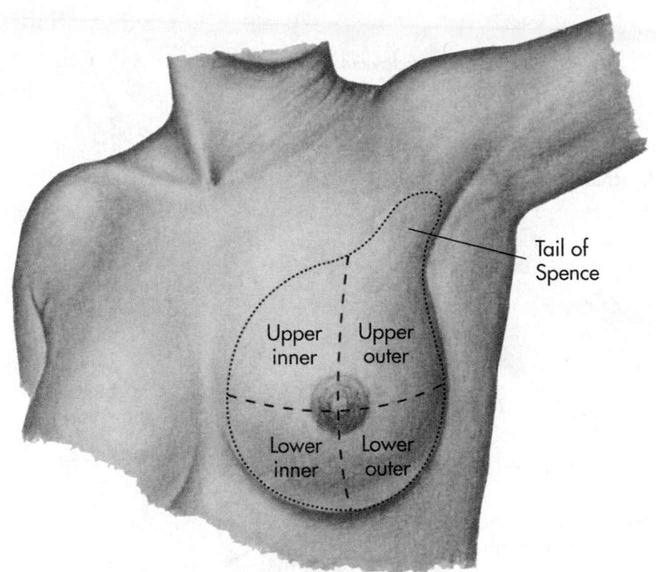

Figure 58-3 Quadrants of left breast and axillary tail of Spence. Most tumors develop in upper outer quadrant.

When the tumor is confined within a duct or a lobule and has not invaded surrounding tissue, it is considered localized or in situ carcinoma of the breast. Infiltrative ductal or lobular carcinomas are tumors that have spread directly into surrounding tissue and may have distant metastases if they have penetrated the axillary or internal mammary nodes or the systemic circulation. Of the invasive breast tumors, infiltrating ductal carcinoma is the most prevalent histologic cell type, followed by infiltrating lobular carcinoma. Subtypes of each of these histologic cell types comprise the remainder of breast tumors. Table 58-1 reviews selected histologic types of breast cancer and their characteristics.

The breast is served by an extensive lymphatic drainage system: central axillary, pectoral (anterior), subscapular (posterior), and lateral nodes. The ipsilateral axillary nodes drain up to 75% of lymph from the breast. Additional drainage flows upward to the infraclavicular and supraclavicular lymph nodes. The normal lymphatic system and directional flow are shown in Figure 58-4.

CLINICAL MANIFESTATIONS. Early-stage breast cancer is symptomless and can be detected only by physical examination of the breast, mammography, or magnetic resonance imaging (MRI). It is difficult to differentiate early-stage cancer from benign tumors, whereas more advanced cancers have a variety of distinguishing signs and symptoms (see Clinical Manifestations box). Benign tumors generally have well-defined edges, are encapsulated, and are freely movable. Malignant tumors have shapes that are more difficult to define and are less mobile on palpation, usually because of the tumor becoming "fixed" and adhering to the chest wall. As the tumor infiltrates into surrounding tissue, it can cause retraction of the overlying skin and create dimpling. The nipple also may be retracted or deviated at an odd angle from the same growth pattern. A peau d'orange breast sign, in which the breast resembles an orange peel with large, prominent pores, indicates lymphatic obstruction from tumor growth with resulting edema. These signs are ominous and usually reflect advanced disease.

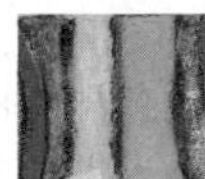

CLINICAL MANIFESTATIONS
Breast Cancer

- Lump that is:
  - —Irregular, star shaped
  - —Firm to hard in consistency
  - —Fixed, not mobile
  - —Poorly defined or demarcated
  - —Usually not tender, but can occasionally cause discomfort
  - —Single
- Presence of skin or nipple retraction
- Nipple discharge
- Peau d'orange appearance of the skin

NOTE: Many breast tumors identified by mammography lack discernible symptoms.

TABLE 58-1 SELECTED HISTOLOGIC TYPES OF BREAST CANCER

Type	Characteristics
Infiltrating ductal carcinoma	Solid mass; hard and firm on palpation
Medullary carcinoma	Characterized by a prominent lymphocyte infiltrate; frequently seen in younger patients; can reach large size
Mucinous, or colloid, carcinoma	Slow growing; mucus producing
Invasive lobular carcinoma	Multicentricity common; may involve both breasts; has ill-defined margins
Paget's disease	Scaly, eczematoid nipple with burning, itching, discharge; usually unable to palpate mass beneath nipple
Inflammatory breast cancer	Diffuse edema, skin and breast redness, firmness of underlying tissue, tenderness, pain, nipple retraction
Carcinoma in situ (ductal or lobular)	Proliferation of malignant cells within ducts and lobules, without invasion into surrounding tissue; ductal carcinoma in situ appearing as clustered microcalcifications on mammography

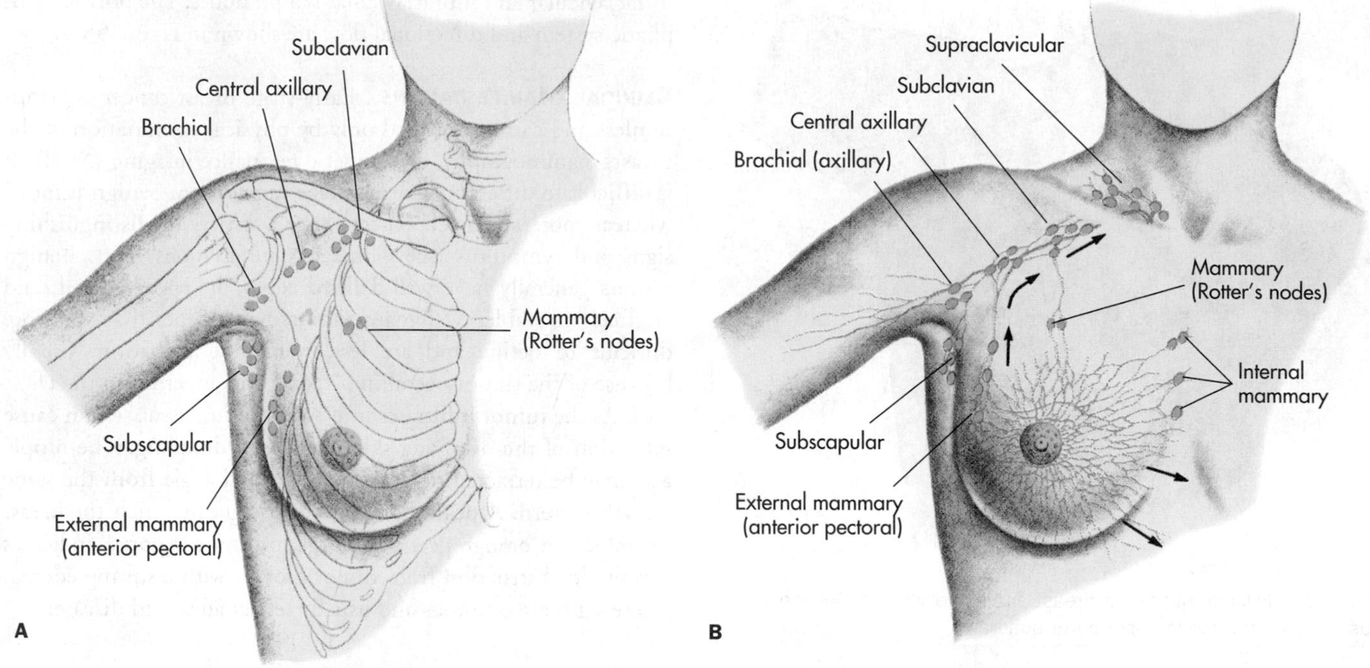

Figure 58-4 **A,** Lymph nodes of the axilla. **B,** Lymphatic drainage of the breast.

Paget's disease is an eczema-like inflammatory process affecting the nipple and areola. It may progress from an epidermal condition to an intraductal carcinoma of the breast. It may be accompanied by burning, itching, discharge, and a palpable lump.

Collaborative Care Management. Management of breast cancer is both complex and controversial. Treatment options are ever changing and influenced by new and better surgical techniques, new cytotoxic drug combinations, and more accurate knowledge of breast cancer growth and dissemination (see Future Watch box).

Diagnostic Tests. When a breast lump has been found, the exact nature of the lesion must be determined. The presence of a benign lesion, such as a fibroadenoma, cyst, or fibrocystic breast disease, must be ruled out. Most breast lesions are benign; however, only histologic examination of tissue from the lesion can determine the true nature of the disease process.

Future Watch

Blood Test for Early Prediction of Effectiveness of Breast Cancer Therapy?

A new technologic development, the CellSearch System, counts cancer cells in the patient's blood. Using it in a study of women with metastatic breast cancer, researchers found that women with high levels of malignant cells in their blood survived an average of 10.1 months, whereas those with low cell counts survived an average of more than 18 months. Monitoring levels of malignant cells in the blood has the potential to indicate early in the course of treatment whether the prescribed anticancer regimen is working and allows treatment to be changed to meet individual patient needs. Yet to be determined is the effectiveness of the system with less aggressive breast cancers and other cancers that do not readily metastasize via the bloodstream.

Cristofanilli M et al: Circulating tumor cells, disease progression, and survival in metastatic breast cancer, *N Engl J Med* 351(8):781-791, 2004.

Noninvasive Diagnostic Tests. The American Cancer Society (ACS) recommends monthly BSE as an early detection method. The goal of periodic BSE is to detect palpable tumors in the breast and to increase awareness of normal breast composition so that changes in composition may be discovered early.[42] With increasing tumor size, the likelihood of local and distant metastasis increases, and long-term survival rates become poorer. Women who choose to do BSE should be properly instructed and have their technique observed for accuracy during a periodic health examination.[42] Barriers such as lack of skill, fear, anxiety, and embarrassment may prevent women from practicing BSE.[9] Thus educating women about the importance of regular monthly self-examination and teaching the proper technique are essential to early detection and intervention (see Patient/Family Teaching box and Evidence-Based Practice box).

At present, mammography is the best diagnostic tool for breast cancer screening, especially in older women. Mammography may have limitations for those with dense breast tissue or women using hormone replacement.[42] Nevertheless, a mammogram can detect breast lesions before they become palpable on physical examination (1 cm) or before they can be seen on conventional x-ray film. Figure 58-5 compares the average size of a lesion discovered by a woman on BSE and one capable of being detected on mammogram.

The recent increase in breast cancer incidence has been at least partially attributed to the increased use of mammography and its detection of cancer in an earlier, localized stage. Many women, especially those of ethnic minorities, continue to have low adherence rates for mammographic examination (see Research box, p. 1758).

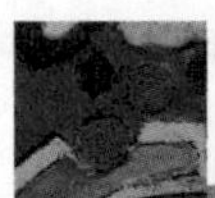

PATIENT/FAMILY TEACHING *American Cancer Society Guidelines for Breast Self-Examination*

- Examine your breasts right after your period, when they are not tender or swollen. If you do not have regular periods, sometimes skip a month, or are postmenopausal, do it on the same day of every month.
- Lie down and put a pillow under your right shoulder. Place your right arm behind your head.
- Use the finger pads of your three middle fingers on your left hand to feel for lumps or thickening in your right breast. Your finger pads are the top third of each finger.
- Press firmly enough to know how your breast feels. If you're not sure how hard to press, ask your health care provider. Or try to copy the way your health care provider uses the finger pads during a breast examination. Learn what your breast feels like most of the time. A firm ridge in the lower curve of each breast is normal.
- Move around the breast in a set way. You can choose either the circle, the up and down, or the wedge. Do it the same way each month. It will help you to make sure that you've gone over the entire breast area and to remember how your breast feels.
- Now examine your left breast using the right hand finger pads.
- Repeat the examination of both breasts while standing, with one arm behind your head. The upright position makes it easier to check the upper and outer parts of the breasts (toward your armpit). You may want to do the standing part of the breast self-examination (BSE) while you are in the shower. Some breast changes can be felt more easily when your skin is wet and soapy.
- For added safety, check your breasts for any dimpling of the skin, changes in the nipple, redness, or swelling while standing in front of a mirror right after your BSE each month.

From American Cancer Society: *How to perform a breast self-examination,* December 14, 1999, accessed from website:www.cancer.org/docroot/NWS/content /NWS_2_1x_How_to_Perform_a_Breast_Self_Examination.asp.

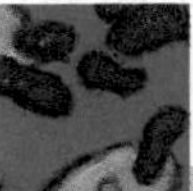

EVIDENCE-BASED PRACTICE

Topic Question: How effective are different strategies for increasing the participation rate of women invited to community (population-based) breast cancer screening activities or mammography programs?

Evidence Base: The findings were based on 16 studies that measured attendance in response to a mammogram invitation. All the studies involved women who were invited to a community breast screening activity or program and were randomized to an intervention group or a control group with no active intervention.

Findings: Evidence supported the use of letters of invitation, mailed educational material, letters of invitation plus phone call, phone call, and training activities plus direct reminders for the women. Home visits did not prove to be effective, nor did a letter of invitation to multiple screening examinations plus educational material.

Conclusions: Most active recruitment strategies for breast cancer screening programs examined were more effective than no intervention. Combinations of effective interventions can be successful. Some costly strategies were not effective.

Bonfill X et al: Strategies for increasing the participation of women in community breast cancer screening (Cochrane Review). In *The Cochrane Library,* Issue 3, Chichester, UK, 2004, John Wiley & Sons.

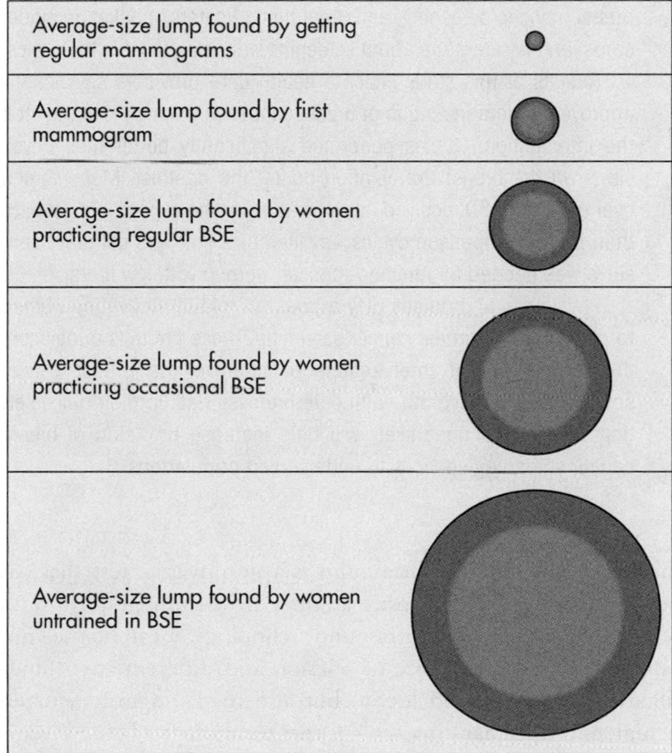

Figure 58-5 Relative sizes of tumors detected by various detection methods, as reported by the Breast Health Program of New York. *BSE,* Breast self-examination.

Economic hardship, lack of access to transportation, fear, ignorance of available community services, and modesty are factors that contribute to poor mammography compliance in underserved populations such as African-American and Hispanic/Latina women.[18]

For a mammogram to be accurate, two views of sufficiently compressed breast tissue are needed. Compression is required to decrease breast thickness, separate mammary structures, and eliminate motion, thus resulting in a more accurate image with less radiation scatter. When accurately performed and read by an experienced radiologist, a mammogram can detect a lesion 2 to 4 years before it is large enough to be detected by conventional x-ray film or palpated on physical examination. The major limitation of mammography is its inability to differentiate between malignant and benign lesions. Figure 58-6 shows a mammogram with a malignant lesion.

The U.S. Food and Drug Administration (FDA) has recently approved digital mammography, which uses a detector that emits an electronic signal in response to an x-ray exposure. This signal can be stored and processed on a computer for use later on film or

Research

Coleman EA et al.: The delta project: increasing breast cancer screening among rural minority and older women by targeting rural healthcare providers, *Oncol Nurs Forum* 30(4):669-676, 2003.

The purpose of this study was to test a multimethod intervention designed for rural health care providers in their clinics to increase breast cancer screening activities among a patient population that experiences higher mortality rates than the general population, namely, low-income, African-American, and older women. A 2-year experimental pretest and posttest with random assignment by group design was employed. The sample consisted of 224 nurses, physicians, and mammography technicians.

The main research variables were health care providers' knowledge and attitudes as measured by survey responses, providers' skills as measured by a checklist filled out by standardized patients, and the provision of breast cancer screening as measured by data from mammography centers. The standardized patients were trained to observe and record health care providers' performances of screening methods. The study provided direct feedback and newsletters to health care professionals providing up-to-date information about breast cancer screening and treatment. Posters, pocket reminder cards, and lay literature about screening were also used in the clinics.

Results of this study indicate health care providers significantly improved in demonstration of breast cancer screening practices after the intervention. Nurses performed significantly better than physicians on the breast examination during the posttest. More women over the age of 50 received mammograms in the experimental clinics than in the comparison clinics. Lay literature that was culturally sensitive was needed for African-American women with low literacy.

Physicians and nurses play a powerful role in motivating women to participate in breast cancer screening. These findings underscore the importance of interventions to improve the breast cancer screening knowledge of health care professionals in their office settings. These practices likely will help increase provision of breast cancer screening services to underserved populations.

display on a monitor. Ultrasound is a noninvasive test that has become a valuable diagnostic adjunct to mammography. With recent improvements in ultrasound technology, it can be used not only to determine the size of a lesion and differentiate a fluid-filled cyst from a solid lesion, but also to distinguish between benign and malignant masses.[42] Other technologies being investigated as useful diagnostic adjuncts to mammography include MRI, scintimammography, positron emission tomography, and electrical impedance imaging (see Future Watch box, p. 1678). The value of these adjunctive technologies as screening modalities has yet to be determined by clinical testing.[42] The ACS has recommended guidelines for breast cancer screening (see Guidelines for Safe Practice box).

INVASIVE DIAGNOSTIC TESTS. Most breast tumors are not malignant; however, an accurate diagnosis cannot be made until tissue from the tumor is examined for histologic cell type. Therefore, when a tumor mass is discovered, whether on physical examination or mammogram, an invasive procedure such as needle biopsy or excisional or incisional biopsy is required.

Fine-needle aspiration can differentiate cysts from other solid tumor masses. The contents of a cyst range from clear aspirate to bloody or even black fluid. The fluid generally is sent for **cytologic examination** and may be helpful in identifying histologic cell type.

A wide-needle biopsy is used to obtain a small piece of tissue from a breast mass. This tissue sample undergoes cytologic examination for cancer cells. Needle biopsies are performed using local anesthetics and can be done in an outpatient setting. If the needle biopsy shows cancer cells, a surgical biopsy is done to remove tissue for examination. A cytologic examination is never used alone as a diagnostic tool for cancer because of the chance of both false-positive and false-negative results.

Technologic advances in breast biopsy systems enable the removal of mammographic densities with or without calcifications that measure up to 20 mm. These techniques, which combine digital stereotactic imaging and a minimally invasive biopsy system, are used to locate and remove tissue specimens for diagnostic purposes.

Excisional or incisional biopsies can be performed with the patient under local anesthesia in an outpatient department or a physician's office. Biopsies of deep lesions in a large breast are better performed in an operating suite. A needle-wire localization procedure done under mammographic, sonographic, or stereotactic visualization may be performed before the excisional biopsy to locate suspicious but nonpalpable areas of the breast tissue.

Tissue specimens obtained from excisional or incisional biopsies are examined for cell type. If the lesion is malignant, the ER and PR status should be determined at the same time. This information is important because it helps determine treatment choices.

OTHER DIAGNOSTIC TESTS. Breast cancer has a tendency to metastasize to bones; therefore a bone scan and bone marrow biopsy may be ordered. Positive findings on these tests indicate widespread disease and a poorer prognosis. A liver scan may be indicated when results of liver function tests are abnormal. A chest x-ray film is obtained to check lung status before any surgical intervention and to check for metastases.

MEDICATIONS. The purpose of systemic drug therapy (chemotherapy and endocrine therapy) in the treatment of breast cancer is to either eradicate or impede the growth of micrometastatic disease.

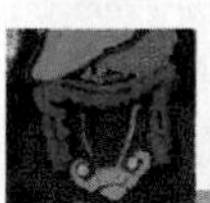

GUIDELINES FOR SAFE PRACTICE
Early Breast Cancer Detection

Women 40 Years of Age

Annual mammography
Monthly breast self-examination
Annual clinical breast examination

Women 20 to 39 Years of Age

Monthly breast self-examination
Clinical breast examination at least every 3 years

From Smith RA et al: American Cancer Society guidelines for breast cancer screening: update 2003, *CA Cancer J Clin* 53(3):141, 2003.

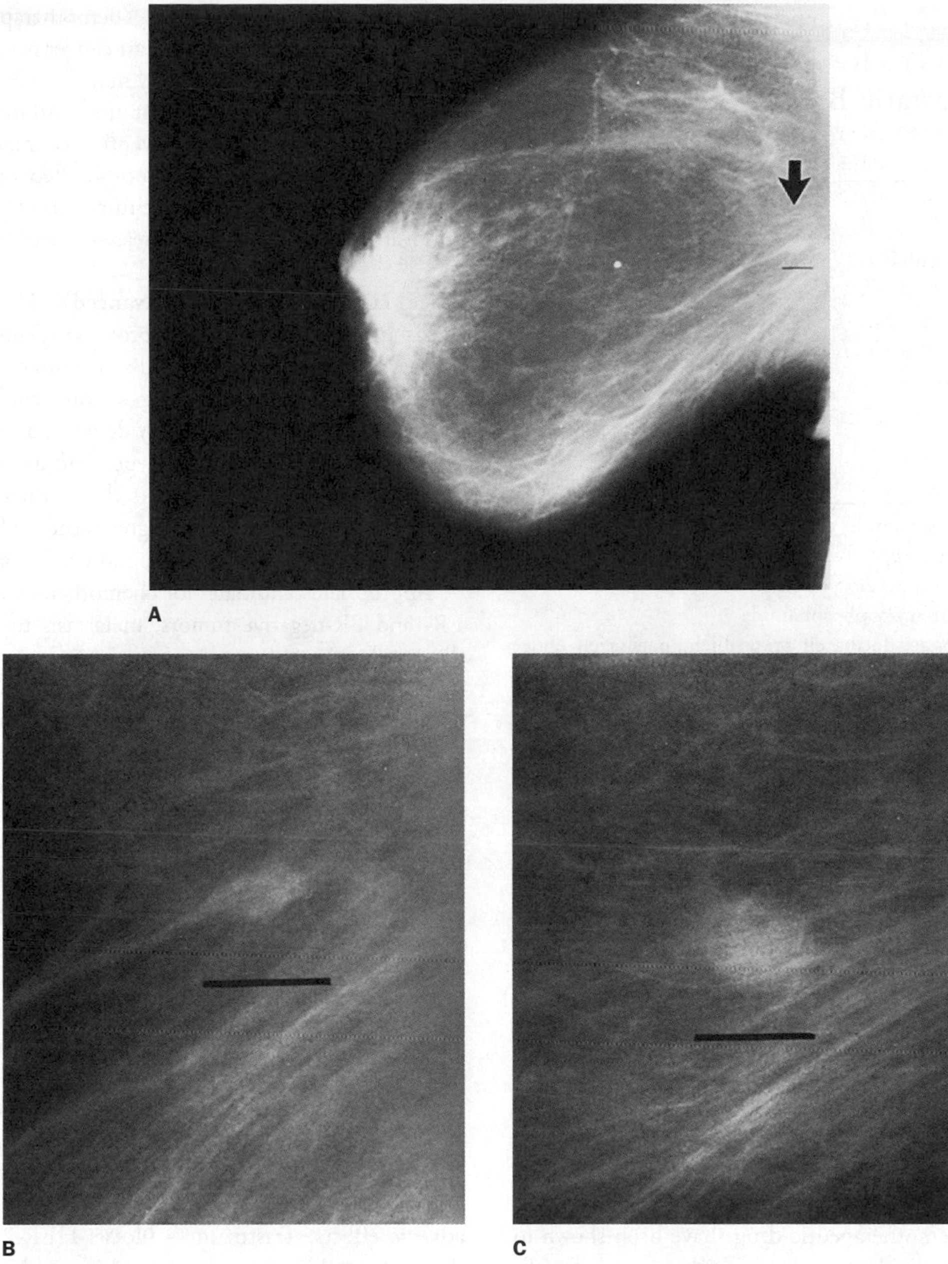

Figure 58-6 Mammogram of patient with area of density indicating carcinoma. A small nodule *(arrow)* in a large, fatty breast (**A**) was oval with ill-defined margins (**B**). The nodule increased in size over a 12-month interval (**C**). *Black line* represents 10-mm measure.

CHEMOTHERAPY

Stages I and II Disease (Localized). As a result of improved diagnostic tests, breast cancer is being discovered earlier and in a more localized stage, frequently without nodal involvement. It is estimated that more than 90% of women with tumors 1 cm or less and without nodal involvement can be expected to achieve long-term disease-free survival. However, because the tumor cells of breast cancer are heterogeneous—that is, the cells have no uniformity and are subject to changes with each cell generation—even localized, node-negative tumors can and frequently do recur. Micrometastasis may be undetected at the time of initial treatment. When micrometastasis is present, changes (mutations) can occur in the tumor cells, making them resistant to chemotherapeutic agents even though tumor sensitivity to drug therapy is greatest when the tumor burden is small. Thus it is not always possible to predict with confidence that all tumors 1 cm or less without node involvement can be "cured" with initial local or regional treatment. Therefore early introduction of systemic **adjuvant therapy** is advocated based on the estimated risk of tumor recurrence in certain subsets of women with node-negative disease. Research findings suggest that adjuvant chemotherapy improves survival. Box 58-3 lists chemotherapeutic agents and drug regimens most commonly used in the treatment of node-positive and node-negative breast cancer.

Box 58-3 NCCN Preferred Chemotherapy Regimens for Recurrent or Metastatic Breast Cancer

Preferred Single Agents

Doxorubicin
Epirubicin*
Pegylated liposomal doxorubicin
Paclitaxel
Docetaxel
Capecitabine
Vinorelbine
Gemcitabine
Albumin-bound paclitaxel

Preferred Combinations

CAF/FAC	Cyclophosphamide, doxorubicin, fluorouracil
FEC	Fluorouracil, epirubicin, cyclophosphamide
AC	Doxorubicin, cyclophosphamide
EC	Epirubicin, cyclophosphamide
AT	Doxorubicin, docetaxel; doxorubicin, paclitaxel
CMF	Cyclophosphamide, methotrexate, fluorouracil
	Docetaxel, capecitabine
GT	Gemcitabine, paclitaxel

Other Active Agents

Cisplatin
Carboplatin
Etoposide (po)
Vinblastine
Fluorouracil continuous infusion

NOTE: All recommendations are category 2A unless otherwise indicated. Clinical Trials: NCCN believes that the best management of any cancer patient is in a clinical trial. Participation in clinical trials is especially encouraged.

Combinations of chemotherapeutic drugs have been shown to be more effective than individual agents, with the greatest benefit demonstrated in women under 50 years of age.[15,23] Also various combinations of drugs (see Box 58-3) have proven beneficial in improving tumor cell sensitivity to drug therapy by reducing drug resistance. Another approach is to administer the prescribed chemotherapeutic agents at their maximal safe dosage levels while providing a "rescue" for the bone marrow. Most chemotherapeutic drugs have an adverse effect on the bone marrow's ability to produce vital cellular components (white blood cells, red blood cells, and platelets). Therefore hematopoietic growth factors such as granulocyte colony-stimulating factors and granulocyte-macrophage colony-stimulating factors are given. Bone marrow transplantation may be performed to stimulate bone marrow recovery after high-dose therapy. This approach remains controversial, however, since research suggests it does not improve survival.[24] Additional side effects of chemotherapy include hair loss, fatigue, lethargy, nausea and vomiting, oral mucositis, and ovarian suppression with loss of fertility.[23] See Chapter 23 for a more detailed discussion of chemotherapy and related nursing care.

Administering preoperative chemotherapy to patients with operable stage I and stage II breast cancer has many potential benefits. Preoperative chemotherapy may decrease drug resistance arising from ongoing cellular mutation. Additionally, preoperative chemotherapy can enhance prevention of micrometastasis that can occur with primary tumor removal. Preoperative chemotherapy also can render larger inoperable tumors more amenable to surgical removal and may permit an increased rate of breast conservation.[15]

Stages III and IV Disease (Advanced). The goals of therapy for metastatic breast cancer are prolonging life without reducing quality of life, offering maximal symptom control with low treatment toxicity, and preventing serious complications.[21,28] The choice of optimal chemotherapy depends on a variety of variables, the most important being the type of adjuvant therapy previously administered. Additional factors that influence the chemotherapeutic regimen include the aggressiveness of the disease, site or sites of metastasis, patient's age, and profile of toxicity.[21]

Appropriate candidates for chemotherapy are women that have ER- and PR-negative tumors, metastasis to visceral organs, and disease that is refractory to hormone therapy. First-line therapy includes anthracyclines such as doxorubicin and its derivative, epirubicin. The taxanes paclitaxel (Taxol) and docetaxel (Taxotere, a semisynthetic toxoid) have been the most effective agents for patients with metastatic breast cancer.[21] The combination regimen known as CMF (cyclophosphamide, methotrexate, and 5-fluorouracil) has also shown high efficacy. The administration of this combination regimen has been simplified by the development of capecitabine (Xeloda), an oral chemical precursor of 5-fluorouracil that has been approved for treatment of metastatic breast.[21] Chemotherapeutic agents that are used for second-line therapy depend primarily on the first-line regimen; a number of drugs are currently in clinical trials for this use.[21]

Another drug developed for use in advanced breast cancer is the recombinant, humanized monoclonal antibody trastuzumab. Researchers have recognized that cancer cells have specific molecular properties that differ from those of normal cells, and targeting those properties generally spares normal cells with limited adverse effects. Trastuzumab blocks HER-2 activation and has shown favorable response rates when used in combination with conventional chemotherapeutic agents. In two large, randomized clinical trials, patients with early-stage HER-2 positive invasive breast cancer who were treated with trastuzumab (Herceptin) in addition to chemotherapy had half the risk of breast cancer recurrence than did patients treated with chemotherapy alone.[29a]

The use of chemotherapy continues to generate many unanswered questions, such as optimal drug combinations, optimal dosage, and length of treatment. These are just a few of the concerns currently being addressed in clinical trials.

HORMONAL THERAPY

Stages I and II Disease. Hormonal therapy has been a useful treatment modality for breast cancer for many decades. In the early stages of breast cancer, hormonal therapy is used as systemic adjunctive therapy to surgery, radiation, and chemotherapy. Whereas chemotherapy acts on rapidly dividing cells to achieve its effects, hormonal therapy targets cells that depend on estrogen for growth. The underlying reason for the success of hormonal therapy was not known until the development of **bioassay** methods that revealed estrogen receptors on the tumor cell surface. Before this discovery it was known only that surgical removal of the ovaries interfered in some way with breast cancer growth. Research revealed that tumors that are ER rich (more than 10 receptors) grow in response to stimulation by estrogen and are classified as ER positive. It was theorized that if the level of circulating estrogen was removed or decreased, the growth of ER-positive tumors could be impeded, and disease-free interval and survival time increased. However, estrogen ablation through oophorectomy also induced menopause, since the primary source of estrogen is the ovaries. Hot flashes, vaginal dryness, a rise in plasma lipids, atherosclerosis, and osteoporosis resulted.

To counteract the menopausal effects, antiestrogen drug research led to the development of the ER modulators tamoxifen and, more recently, raloxifene (Evista). Tamoxifen and raloxifene are nonsteroidal drugs that compete for the estradiol-binding site on ER-positive cell, thus removing the stimulus (estrogen) for tumor growth. They are most effective against ER-positive breast tumors. A 5-year course of tamoxifen has been the hormonal therapy of choice for women with ER-positive tumors regardless of menopausal status.[30] The use of hormonal therapy alone or in addition to chemotherapy is determined by factors such as tumor size, grade, nodal status, and menopausal status.[30] ER modulators can produce side effects such as hot flashes, night sweats, altered libido, vaginal dryness, and weight gain. Women taking tamoxifen have also demonstrated an increased risk of endometrial cancer.[23]

The nonsteroidal aromatase inhibitors anastrozole (Arimidex) and letrozole, and the steroidal aromatase inhibitor exemestane, have shown efficacy in postmenopausal women with hormone receptor–positive breast cancer. Aromatase inhibitors block the extraovarian conversion of the androgen androstenedione to estrogen. Another drug that has shown efficacy in postmenopausal women is the steroidal ER antagonist fulvestrant, which may be an effective treatment in tamoxifen-resistant breast cancer.[21]

Stages III and IV Disease. Hormonal therapy is a mainstay of treatment for advanced breast cancer. The therapy is well tolerated and offers the possibility of temporary tumor remission or inhibition of tumor growth. Ideal candidates for endocrine therapy include women with advanced disease with ER-positive tumors, who had a long prior disease-free interval, had a prior response to hormonal treatment, or lack rapidly progressing disease. Hormonal therapies in premenopausal women include luteinizing hormone–releasing hormone (LHRH) agonists (groserelin), surgical or radiographic oophorectomy, progestins (megestrol acetate), and androgens (fluoxymesterone). In postmenopausal women, hormonal therapies include selective nonsteroidal aromatase inhibitors, steroidal aromatase inhibitors, pure antiestrogens (fulvestrant), progestins, and androgens.[30]

The usefulness of tamoxifen for preventing breast cancer in high-risk women has been underinvestigated. Results of clinical trials indicate that patients at high risk for breast cancer who received tamoxifen were significantly less likely to develop breast cancer than those receiving placebo. These findings provide compelling evidence of the usefulness of tamoxifen for the reduction of breast cancer risk in high-risk women, and the FDA has approved this use of tamoxifen.[36]

TREATMENTS: RADIOTHERAPY

STAGES I AND II DISEASE. Radiation to the breast after preservation surgery (lumpectomy) is a standard therapy for early-stage breast cancer. Radiation to the breast eradicates tumor cells left behind after manipulation and handling of the tumor during surgery. Radiation is recommended after wide local excision or quadrantectomy. Radiotherapy is also considered for patients who have had a mastectomy and are at high risk for local recurrence, patients with muscle involvement, and patients with axillary lymph node involvement.[23]

The whole breast is irradiated at a dose of 4500 to 5000 cGy.[29] A booster dose of 6000 to 6600 cGy is often given to the tumor bed and, if nodal involvement is present, to the supraclavicular area.[30] The booster dose is delivered with the use of either external beam or interstitial irradiation (Figure 58-7).[29] The risk of local recurrence is minimal after this protocol. Although tumors of less than 1 cm generally are not treated with radiation after breast preservation surgery, research has shown that ipsilateral recurrence occurs with enough frequency that women with tumors less than 1 cm may benefit from radiotherapy. Of course, individual patient and tumor characteristics must be evaluated in this situation.[7] Although radiation after conservative surgery is widely used, some large breast tumors may be irradiated before surgery to facilitate surgical removal. Close medical follow-up care is important after conservative surgery and radiation. Recommended guidelines include a breast physical examination every 3 to 6 months for years 1 to 3, every 6 months for years 4 and 5, and then yearly. A mammogram is recommended 6 to 9 months after radiation and then annually.[29]

When the breast is irradiated, the side effects include skin reactions (redness, dryness, and itching), edema, mild tenderness, and fatigue. Fatigue is the result of bone marrow suppression from radiation to the thorax, since the adult sternum, ribs, and thoracic vertebrae contain more than one third of the total body bone marrow (sternum 3%, ribs 16%, and thoracic vertebrae 16%). Patient instruction for managing the side effects of anemia and increased vulnerability to infection is vital to achieve patient compliance in completing treatment with the total prescribed radiation dose.

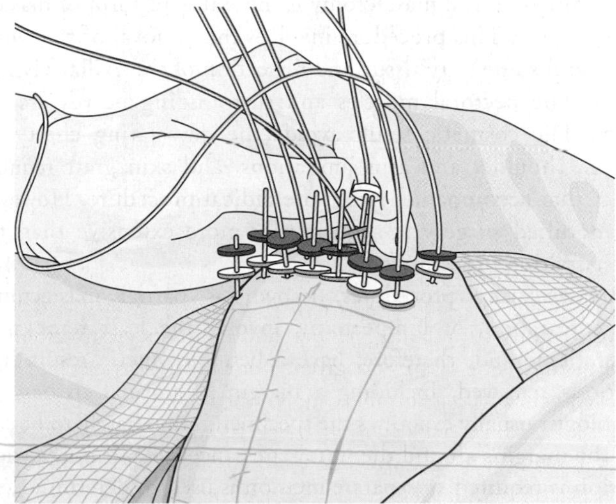

Figure 58-7 Interstitial "booster" radiotherapy for breast cancer using iridium needles.

STAGES III AND IV DISEASE. The role of radiotherapy in advanced breast cancer usually is palliative. Radiation is used to alleviate pain from bone metastases, which can result in pathologic fractures of the spinal vertebrae, causing compression of nerve roots and the spinal cord. Radiotherapy can also be used to treat metastases to the lung or liver and lesions that cause lymphatic obstruction and may result in pleural effusion. When radiation is prescribed, the patient requires information and instruction on the rationale for the therapy and any specific care measures that will be necessary during treatment. It is important that the patient be aware that the radiation treatments will not cure the disease but can provide pain relief and improve quality of life. (See Chapter 23 for a more thorough discussion of radiotherapy in the treatment of cancer.)

SURGICAL MANAGEMENT

STAGES I AND II (LOCAL DISEASE). Surgery is the initial treatment of early-stage breast cancer, especially when the disease is localized without distant metastasis. The surgical removal of breast cancer has evolved over the past 100 years from the mutilating radical mastectomy to the more conservative surgical approaches in use today. Halsted introduced the radical procedure (removal of the entire breast, skin, chest wall muscles, and axillary lymph nodes) in the mistaken belief that, as a breast tumor grows, it spreads in an orderly manner from the tumor core outward to all adjacent tissue and lymph nodes in its path. This surgical procedure became the standard form of treatment up until the early 1970s. Today, after years of clinical trials, less extensive tissue removal is now the rule.

When primary, localized breast cancer (less than 2 to 4 cm and no metastasis) is diagnosed, two surgical options may be offered: modified radical mastectomy, with or without breast reconstruction, or breast-sparing (lumpectomy) procedures. The goals of both modified radical mastectomy and lumpectomy are to control local and regional disease, to accurately stage the disease to identify patients at high risk for recurrence, to provide the best chance for long-term survival, and to achieve the best cosmetic result. The overall long-term survival rates for the two surgical methods are approximately the same.[29]

Modified radical mastectomy is the standard form of mastectomy surgery. This procedure involves the removal of the whole breast and some fatty tissue and dissection of the axillary lymph nodes. The pectoral muscles and surrounding nerves are left intact. The cosmetic result avoids the devastating chest wall defects, shoulder and arm limitations, and skin graft requirements that accompanied the more radical procedure. However, the modified surgery is significantly more extensive than the breast-sparing procedures.

Breast-sparing procedures, known as partial mastectomy, wedge resection, or lumpectomy, involve the least removal of breast tissue and, therefore, have a better cosmetic result. The tumor is removed, including a margin of normal tissue. The pathologist usually examines the specimen immediately to be sure that the margins around the tumor are cancer free. If not, a wider excision is required. A separate incision is used to determine axillary node involvement. Breast-sparing treatment for local disease is followed in 2 to 4 weeks by radiotherapy when wound healing is complete. Breast-sparing surgery is not advised for all stage I and II disease (Box 58-4).

Box 58-4 Contraindications for Use of Breast-Sparing Procedures

- Pregnancy: radiotherapy precluded in first and second trimesters
- Locally advanced or inflammatory breast cancer
- Multiple lesions located in separate quadrants of the breast or diffuse malignant or indeterminate-appearing microcalcifications
- Prior irradiation of the breast
- History of collagen-vascular disease, which is recognized as having poor tolerance to the effects of radiotherapy
- Tumor size: large tumor in a small breast, which will not allow adequate resection of tumor
- Breast size: large pendulous breasts, which are difficult to irradiate; small breasts, which may result in an unacceptable cosmetic outcome

From Morrow M et al: Standard for breast conservation therapy in the management of invasive breast carcinoma, *CA Cancer J Clin* 52(5):277, 2002.

Both modified radical mastectomy and lumpectomy may include axillary lymph node dissection, since metastatic dissemination takes place primarily through these nodes. Axillary node status is a significant prognostic indicator in breast cancer and provides valuable information to determine adjuvant therapy.[30] Low axillary dissection (level I) is the removal of an entire block of nodes in the area from the latissimus dorsi muscle laterally to the medial pectoralis muscle. Levels II and III dissection remove nodes en bloc, from the middle to the entire axillary node chain, respectively (Figure 58-8). Approximately 80% of axillary nodes are found within a level I to II dissection, with the remainder in level III. When axillary nodes are negative for cancer, a level I to II dissection is adequate. If nodes are positive for disease, a complete level III dissection is advised.

Sentinel lymph node dissection (SLND) is an important technique that helps identify axillary node involvement before axillary dissection. This procedure is based on the concept that a certain

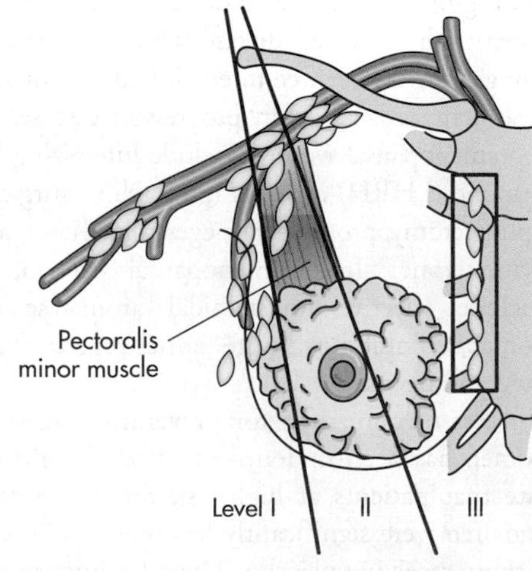

Figure 58-8 Regional axillary lymph nodes demonstrating levels I, II, and III node dissection.

anatomic region renders all its lymphatic drainage into one or two lymph nodes in the regional nodal basin. The sentinel node can reflect the tumor status of the entire nodal basin and thus reduce the number of unnecessary lymph node dissections in negative patients.[23]

For SLND, a radioisotope is injected around the tumor site or biopsy cavity on the day of surgery. Then a lymphoscintigram is obtained to identify the pathways of lymphatic drainage and the approximate location of the sentinel node. After this, isosulfan blue dye is injected around the tumor or biopsy cavity. The dye is expected to travel via the lymphatics and become trapped in the sentinel node. After an axillary incision is made, a gamma probe is used to help locate the sentinel node(s), which are identified by the blue dye. After excision of all identifiable sentinel nodes, the axilla is examined for residual radioactivity that may indicate additional sentinel nodes remaining, thus requiring further exploration. All sentinel nodes are sent for frozen section analysis, during which time the surgeon proceeds with any additional surgery that may be required (e.g., lumpectomy or mastectomy). If the sentinel node is positive for metastatic cells or not identified, the surgeon performs a standard axillary lymph node dissection. If the sentinel node is negative for metastatic cells, the lymph node dissection is omitted.[30] When performed by an experienced team consisting of surgeon, radiologist, nuclear medicine physician, and pathologist, according to exacting standards, SLND can be successfully done in more than 90% of eligible breast cancer patients.[30] In addition, the tumor status of the sentinel node can accurately predict the tumor status of all axillary nodes in more than 95% of cases.[23]

STAGES III AND IV DISEASE. Surgery for advanced breast cancer includes mastectomy in combination with systemic chemotherapy or hormonal therapy. Patients who develop a local recurrence and were initially treated by mastectomy undergo surgical resection as appropriate. Patients who were initially treated by breast-conserving therapy and develop a recurrence undergo a total mastectomy.[30] After local treatment, chemotherapy and hormonal therapy are considered as previously discussed.

BREAST RECONSTRUCTION. The goal of breast reconstruction is to create a symmetric breast mound that approximates the appearance of the opposite breast.[12] Two types of procedures are available for breast reconstruction: implants and autogenous tissue flaps (Figure 58-9).

Implants, in their simplest form, are soft sacs filled with saline or silicone gel that are placed in a pocket beneath the pectoralis major muscle and held in place by the pectoralis major, anterior serratus, and upper rectus abdominis muscles. The size and shape of the implant are matched to those of the remaining breast. Some surgeons prefer to first use a tissue expander. This expandable implant is placed in the manner just described and progressively filled with sterile saline over a period of weeks or months to stretch the skin until the desired size of breast is reached. The sterile saline is added to the expander sac through a needle inserted into a subcutaneous access port. The expander is then replaced by a permanent implant, either saline or silicone gel filled, during a second operation.[31] No activity restrictions are necessary during the expansion period, and pain and discomfort are usually easily controlled.

The use of implants is not without complications or controversy. Complications include fibrous capsular contractions around the implant causing pain, tenderness, and fixation of the implant to the chest wall. Infection is a rare cause for implant removal.[32] As a result of questions and concerns about the safety of silicone implants, the FDA has restricted the use of silicone implants to women undergoing breast reconstruction for cancer under strictly controlled clinical trials. This restriction has been in place since 1992, awaiting more definitive data on the safety of silicone implants. Research in this area is ongoing.[26]

Nipple reconstruction, using tissue obtained from the opposite nipple-areola complex or skin grafted from the upper part of the inner thigh, requires another surgical procedure about 3 to 6 months after breast reconstruction. The use of a dermal tattoo that can match normal breast pigment is an alternative method of nipple formation.[39]

The use of autogenous tissue flaps is a second means of breast reconstruction that can be performed at the time of mastectomy or at a later date. Tissue flaps eliminate the need for an implant unless insufficient tissue is available to form a breast of dimensions equal to the remaining normal breast. Flaps used include latissimus dorsi musculocutaneous tissue from the upper portion of the back or transverse rectus abdominis myocutaneous (TRAM) tissue from the lower portion of the abdomen. The latissimus dorsi flap leaves a scar on the upper back that may be visible with certain types of clothing. A TRAM flap uses tissue that is similar in elasticity to normal breast tissue and is available in sufficient quantity to construct a new breast equal in size and shape to the uninvolved breast. The scar from a TRAM flap on the lower abdomen is easily concealed beneath clothing. Nipple reconstruction is performed in the same manner as already described.[39]

The reconstruction procedure appropriate for an individual patient depends on numerous physical and emotional factors such as BMI, smoking history, previous surgeries at the donor site, circulatory conditions, and personal preferences and expectations.[32] Whether breast reconstruction surgery is performed immediately or at a later date depends on various factors. These include the type of tumor, need for radiation or chemotherapy, and the patient's wishes. Immediate breast reconstruction offers better adjustment to the loss of the breast, a better quality of life, and chest tissue undamaged by radiation or scarring, while avoiding the cost and distress of an additional hospitalization and surgery.[32] Delayed reconstruction gives the woman more time to consider all options, and some surgeons believe that a wait of 3 to 6 months is beneficial before reconstruction surgery to permit sufficient recovery of tissue integrity.[32]

When mastectomy without breast reconstruction is the chosen option, a breast prosthesis is generally used (Figure 58-10). Some women may not view this as a problem. Others find the need for prostheses an uncomfortable nuisance and a constant reminder of their breast cancer experience. Some women describe feeling "out of balance" when wearing the prosthesis compared with the weight of the opposite normal breast. They also may feel confined in their choice of clothing or participation in physical activities. These kinds of concerns may prompt women to undergo breast

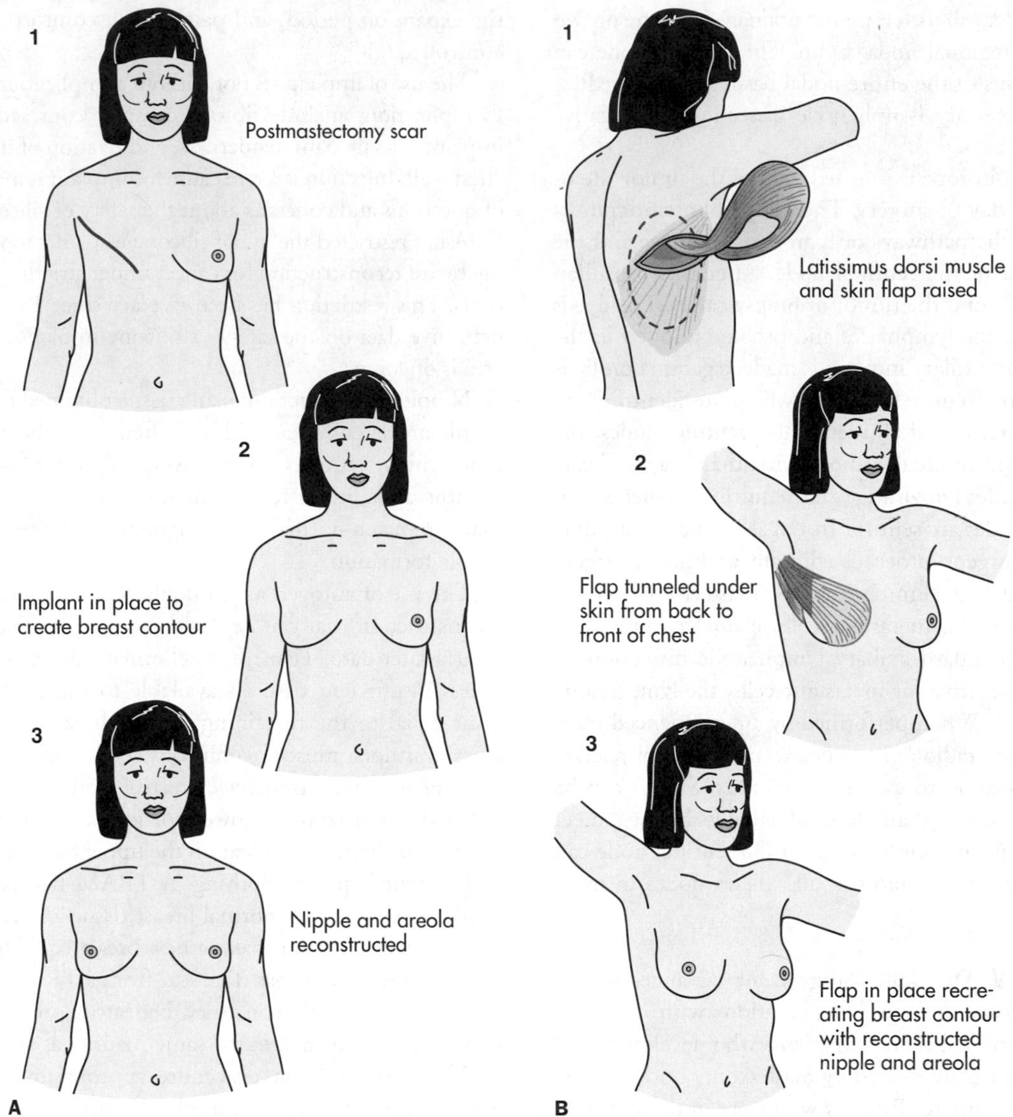

Figure 58-9 Three types of breast reconstruction procedures. **A,** Simple implant placement. **B,** Latissimus dorsi reconstruction.

reconstruction many months or years after selecting mastectomy alone.

DIET. Maintenance of good nutrition is essential for all patients with cancer. Dietary requirements include an increase in calories, carbohydrate, and protein. Body energy demands are known to increase with cancer, and more energy is necessary to withstand the potentially debilitating side effects of treatment. A diet high in calories and carbohydrates spares body protein, necessary for tissue and wound repair, from being broken down for energy needs.

Good dietary management and patient education are especially important for the person with breast cancer. This diagnosis can evoke great emotional stress, and its treatment can affect appetite and nutrition in many ways. Additionally, all the prescribed treatment options—surgery, radiotherapy, chemotherapy, and hormonal therapy, as well as adjunct medication and activity restrictions—affect body nutritional needs and maintenance to some degree. Table 58-2 provides an overview of nutritional problems generated by various cancer treatment options and the interventions commonly used to treat them.

COMPLICATIONS. The woman who has undergone treatment for breast cancer will always live with the fear of recurrent disease even when the cancer was found and treated in an early, localized stage. Local recurrence of breast cancer usually occurs within 2 to 8 years after the initial diagnosis and treatment. Approximately 80% of recurrences happen within 3 years. Generally, early recurrence suggests a graver prognosis. Thus it is important that all women, regardless of age or stage of disease, be reminded to report symptoms such as bone pain or changes at the incision site, which could indicate disease recurrence or distant metastasis. When recurrence follows conservative surgery and radiotherapy, mastectomy alone or with adjuvant systemic therapy is recommended.[30]

Tissue subjected to radiotherapy at a dose intended for a "cure" does not respond well to repeated radiation exposure. This is because of the changes that occur in the vascular bed after initial

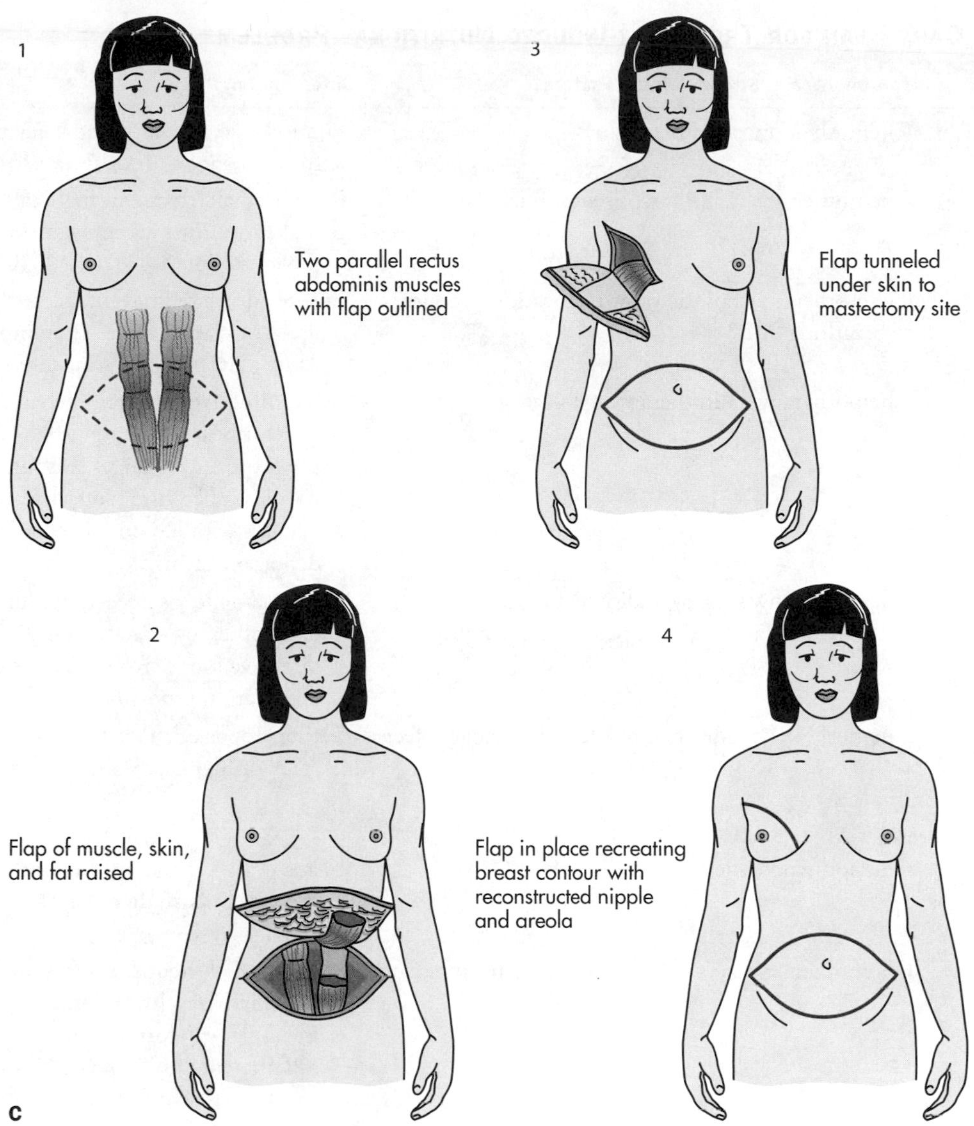

Figure 58-9 (cont'd). **C,** Rectus abdominus reconstruction.

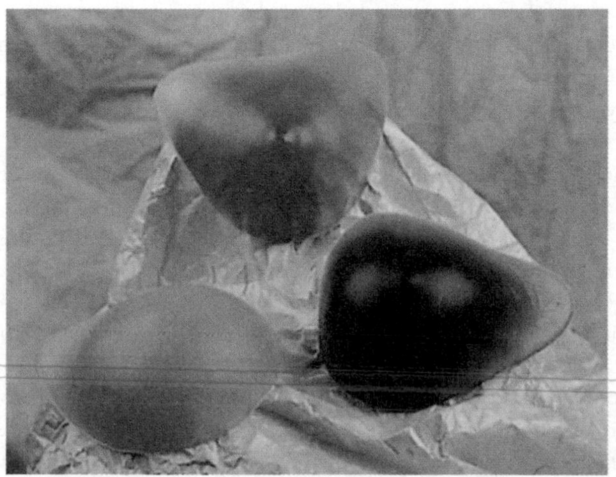

Figure 58-10 Examples of common silicone breast prostheses.

radiation treatment, which results in a reduced blood and oxygen supply to the irradiated tissue. Radiotherapy works best on tissue with a good blood supply and high oxygen saturation content. Complications of repeated radiotherapy include fibrotic changes to the lung, tissue necrosis, and rib fractures.

In addition to recurrence, the development of lymphedema is a complication of breast cancer treatment. Deformity, disability, discomfort, and recurrent episodes of lymphangitis and cellulitis can occur.[33] Lymphedema is a serious problem that requires a physician's evaluation for the institution of a proper treatment regimen. Nurses can assist women with finding treatment centers by contacting the National Lymphedema Network and the ACS.

The threat of trauma and infection after mastectomy and node dissection is ever present and requires that the woman comply with the arm precautions described under Nursing Management. If signs and symptoms of trauma or infection occur, the woman is advised to inform her physician immediately so that appropriate measures can be instituted.

TABLE 58-2 CARE PLAN FOR TREATMENT-INDUCED NUTRITIONAL PROBLEMS

Nutritional Problem	Treatment- and Stress-Related Factors	Intervention
Stomatitis (mouth sores)	Chemotherapy, radiotherapy	Eliminate acidic, salty, and spicy foods; abstain from alcohol and tobacco; use good oral hygiene.
Anorexia	Chemotherapy, radiotherapy, emotional distress	Provide small, frequent, high-caloric, bland meals; make mealtime an enjoyable occasion; avoid noxious odors.
Xerostomia (dry mouth)	Chemotherapy, radiotherapy, medications, mouth breathing	Ensure adequate fluid intake; suck on hard candies; use artificial saliva; moisten mouth with water, using a dropper or syringe if necessary.
Abnormal taste	Chemotherapy, radiotherapy, medications	Avoid offensive foods; mask bad taste by adding wine or beer to soups and sauces; marinate meats; use more and stronger seasonings; serve cold or room-temperature food; drink more liquids; add tartness with lemon juice or vinegar; remedy dental problems.
Nausea and vomiting	Chemotherapy, surgery, radiotherapy, narcotics, behavioral factors (anticipatory vomiting)	Use antiemetics as needed; withhold food before chemotherapy or radiation treatment; eliminate offensive foods; avoid noxious odors; avoid food preparation if possible.
Dysphagia (difficulty swallowing), odynophagia (painful swallowing)	Chemotherapy, radiotherapy, neuromuscular defects	Eat soft foods or foods processed in a blender; avoid spicy or highly seasoned foods.
Constipation	Chemotherapy, medications, inactivity	Increase fluid intake (prune juice, water, coffee); increase bulk in diet; use bran cereal; increase activity level.
Diarrhea	Chemotherapy, medications, radiotherapy, infection	Provide small, frequent meals high in protein and carbohydrates, low in residue. Avoid bowel-irritating, gas-forming, fatty, and lactose- and caffeine-containing foods. Avoid smoking.

ARE YOU READY?

Which of the following is a clinical manifestation of a malignant breast tumor?

1. Tumor with well-defined edges
2. Encapsulated mass
3. Nipple retraction
4. Darkening of areola

Nursing Management

PREOPERATIVE CARE

Assisting With Treatment Decisions. The discovery of a breast lump elicits one of the most powerful and distressing emotional reactions that a woman of any age can experience. Anxiety and stress levels are high. Nurses caring for patients during this critical time (discovering the tumor, undergoing diagnostic tests, making treatment decisions) need to be cognizant of the impact these events have on a woman's normal coping abilities and decision-making processes. The nurse must be ready to provide emotional support in a caring, informative manner.

Once a definitive diagnosis of breast cancer has been established, a complete explanation of treatment options must follow. Most patients come to this situation with some prior knowledge about breast cancer, either from media exposure or through friends or relatives who have had breast cancer. Their knowledge base may be accurate or laden with misconceptions and false information. Because treatment of breast cancer is constantly evolving, it is essential for the nurse, in conjunction with the physician, to determine what the patient knows and to provide accurate information so an informed treatment choice can be made. Inclusion of family and especially the spouse or partner in all discussions about treatment is vital to a successful outcome.

The physician discusses the stage of the disease and the treatment options in detail so that the patient is aware of the advantages and disadvantages of each, as well as the immediate and long-term outcome expectations. The information is often complex and confusing even to the most intelligent and well-informed patient. Women are no longer pressured to select a surgical procedure without knowledge of the final biopsy report. Delay between breast biopsy and definitive treatment provides time in which to consider the options and choose the one most personally suitable. The nurse should plan to be present, if possible, when treatment options are discussed with the patient. This allows assessment of patient and family understanding and an opportunity to clarify misinformation and misconceptions. It is important for the nurse to recognize potential barriers to accessing information, especially in older patients, such as sensory loss, medication-induced fatigue or somnolence, illiteracy, and memory loss. Patients should be encouraged to have another family member, friend, or patient advocate attend information sessions with them for information reinforcement and emotional support.[41]

During the period of diagnosis and treatment, the patient may be referred to breast cancer specialists such as surgeons and medical or radiation oncologists. The rationale for the referrals should be thoroughly discussed with the patient and her family. If breast reconstruction is to be performed at the time of mastectomy, a plastic surgeon will evaluate the patient to determine which procedure can be most easily performed and will best meet her needs. When radiotherapy or chemotherapy is part of the treatment plan, a referral to an expert in these areas is common practice. Often the woman herself initiates a referral or consultation to obtain a second opinion regarding her breast cancer diagnosis and treatment. Second opinions should be encouraged and names of appropriate medical experts provided. This ensures the patient peace of mind and confidence that the diagnosis and prescribed treatment are appropriate.

Financial concerns also can influence treatment decisions. If the patient has health insurance, generally costs for both mastectomy and breast reconstruction surgery are covered. However, concerns about treatment-related problems and out-of-pocket costs might lead some women to choose less intense treatment regimens.[11]

Assisting With the Grieving Process. The diagnosis of breast cancer is extremely traumatic, but contrary to common belief, most women cope well with surgery and the loss of a breast. Most women state that they are not concerned about body image or sexuality when deciding on a surgical procedure (lumpectomy versus mastectomy). Their most immediate concern is to have the cancer eradicated from the body. It may not be until after the mastectomy surgery that issues related to body image and sexuality arise. Therefore, during the presurgical phase of treatment, it is essential for the nurse and physician to determine what impact breast cancer and total or partial loss of a breast will have on the patient's self-esteem and perceived sexuality.

The loss of a breast can engender feelings similar to those caused by limb amputation. Reactions include anger, depression, denial, and withdrawal. Grieving for the lost body part is normal, and the patient should be permitted time to work through her grief. The nurse offers reassurance that the expression of grief is accepted and understood by staff members and is therapeutic for the patient. The nurse ensures family members are aware of the grieving process and encourages them to provide emotional support to the woman for as long as it is needed.

Promoting Patient Participation in the Treatment Plan. During the preoperative period the nurse provides information about what the patient can expect after surgery. Instruction for the patient undergoing mastectomy and lymph node dissection includes a review of the expected incision line and the type of dressing, drains, and drainage collection device anticipated. If breast reconstruction is to be performed immediately, the location of the donor tissue is indicated (upper back area or lower abdomen). The use of pictures or diagrams, similar to those shown in Figure 58-9, will facilitate patient understanding. If an implant is to be inserted, the nurse clarifies position and placement guidelines. The patient is informed that movement of the arm and shoulder on the affected side will be limited for the first 24 hours and that the arm and hand will be elevated on a pillow to facilitate lymphatic and venous drainage. A return demonstration of breathing exercises and turning techniques prepares the patient to actively participate in postoperative recovery.

POSTOPERATIVE CARE

The focus of postoperative care after breast surgery is to enhance physical comfort, maintain nutritional support, prevent complications, and prepare the patient for discharge and successful home management. The length of hospital stay varies from 24 hours to 7 days, depending on type of procedure, any complications, and whether simultaneous reconstruction was performed. In the case of a shortened hospital stay, nurses are often pressed to meet the patient's informational needs. Adequate information must be provided so that the patient has full understanding of each intervention and the degree of participation required of her to make a successful transition from hospital to home management.

Managing Pain. Surgical pain after breast surgery varies depending on the procedure. A lumpectomy may produce mild discomfort at the incision site. The pain after a mastectomy results from the transverse incision that usually extends from the sternum to the axilla. In addition, discomfort may result from either trauma to or transection of thoracic and intercostal nerves and from fluid collection in the chest wall. Both procedures may also involve pain along the axilla at the site of lymph node dissection. If the patient has had immediate breast reconstruction using the TRAM flap procedure, abdominal pain is another factor to consider in pain management.

Pain relief is managed after surgery by the administration of prescribed analgesics and comfort measures. The amount of discomfort experienced varies with the individual patient and her degree of pain tolerance. Most patients are relatively pain free by the time of discharge, requiring only a mild analgesic. Thorough assessment of the patient's pain level and prompt administration of analgesics ensure both pain relief and adequate sleep and rest. Patient-controlled analgesia (PCA) can be an effective intervention. Maintaining physical comfort also helps diminish the high stress level seen in the immediate postoperative period. Medicating the patient before activities such as turning or getting out of bed for the first time is advisable.

The patient who has had a mastectomy should be instructed to get out of bed from the unaffected side. This lessens pain and tension on the operative site. Providing support to the affected side for the first few days after surgery is necessary, since movement of the affected arm and shoulder is restricted for at least 24 hours. The patient is informed that she may feel "out of balance" initially because of the weight of the dressing and the presence of the drainage collection apparatus. Temporary use of a sling on the affected arm during ambulation, if approved by the physician, provides comfort and support by lessening strain on the shoulder and prevents dependent lymphatic and venous stasis.

Abdominal pain after a TRAM flap procedure is managed using PCA. Oral analgesics are started by the third postoperative day as tolerated.[39] The patient should maintain a semi-Fowler's position with the knees flexed and elevated to reduce pressure on the abdomen. An abdominal binder may be ordered to provide added support during ambulation.[39] Abdominal drainage devices are checked at least every 1 to 2 hours for proper function and for the amount and type of drainage. Excessive bright red drainage may indicate hemorrhage, whereas little to no return may indicate obstruction of the drain or drainage apparatus. The occurrence of either is promptly reported to the physician.

When nerves are cut or traumatized within the operative field, the patient may experience sensory changes such as numbness, tingling, changes in skin sensitivity of the chest wall, and even phantom breast sensations. The patient is informed that these changes are common and expected outcomes after surgery. The nurse can assure the patient that nerve-related discomforts gradually decrease and usually cease within a few months.

If breast reconstruction is done with the placement of a tissue expander, the patient will probably experience pulling and stretching sensations of the overlying muscles. This discomfort is caused when the expander pouch is filled with 100 to 300 ml of saline solution during surgery. Discomfort gradually subsides as the muscles adjust to their new length.[32]

Preventing Infection. Fluid collection in the chest wall or at the axillary node dissection site can be a source of infection. The buildup of lymphedema can be a secondary source. Lymphedema usually is a transitory event until collateral lymph channels are formed. When measures are not implemented to increase lymphatic flow, fibrosis can occur within the system, and lymphedema becomes an irreversible condition. The chronic collection of fluid and any subsequent injury to the involved extremity can result in infection.[6]

After the initial dressing change by the physician, the nurse performs wound care and dressing changes as needed, noting the condition of the wound and observing for signs of infection (redness, swelling, drainage, odor, increased discomfort, and fever). Proper placement of drains and drainage collection devices can prevent fluid collection and stasis. The nurse assesses the devices (Hemovac, Jackson-Pratt) for placement and for the amount and type of drainage. When the drain and drainage-collection device are functioning properly, the amount of fluid around the incision is minimal. The patient is instructed to avoid touching the dressing and drainage device, unless changing the dressing or measuring output.

When immediate breast reconstruction is performed, the hospital stay is between 2 and 7 days, depending on the extent of reconstruction (simple implant, tissue expander, or autologous tissue reconstruction). If reconstruction involves the use of a tissue flap, such as a TRAM flap, it is important to observe for tissue perfusion, flap color, temperature, and capillary refill for the first 3 days after surgery.[39]

Teaching Wound Care Management. Having the patient perform wound care before discharge is a major nursing goal. Instruction focuses on aseptic technique, care of drains, the signs and symptoms of infection, and frequency of dressing change. Because hospital stay is limited and is generally a time of high stress and anxiety, all verbal teaching should be accompanied by simple, clearly written instructions. At least one return demonstration of the care is necessary to ensure that the patient understands the procedure and performs it correctly. Additional repetitions, when possible, reinforce the patient's learning.

Dressing change is necessary at least once a day to examine the incision site for signs of infection and to ensure that the drainage device is working satisfactorily. The wound should be kept dry because infection is more likely to develop in a warm, moist environment. The nurse instructs the patient that, once the sutures and drains are removed, usually in 7 to 10 days, the physician will indicate whether the incision requires any further dressing.

Promoting Mobility of the Arm and Shoulder. One of the high-priority nursing interventions after mastectomy surgery is to maintain elevation of the affected arm and hand on pillows so that they are higher than the elbow and the elbow is higher than the shoulder. This position must be maintained while the patient is in bed or sitting in a chair to prevent venous and lymphatic pooling. The nurse monitors for lymphatic and venous stasis by measuring the circumference of the affected arm 6 inches above and below the elbow and comparing results with a preoperative baseline measurement and with measurements of the unaffected arm. The affected arm is kept relatively immobile for 24 hours to decrease any strain on the incision line. Hand exercises to facilitate lymphatic flow may be started, consisting of squeezing a ball, opening and closing the fist, and flexing and extending the wrist and elbow several times each hour. More rigorous range-of-motion exercises for the arm and shoulder are initiated at the discretion of the physician (Box 58-5).

At the time of discharge the patient still has restrictions on the type and amount of exercise permitted for the affected arm and shoulder. Squeezing a ball and bending and flexing the wrist and elbow of the affected arm are continued at home. The more rigorous exercises meant to restore full range of motion to the shoulder are delayed until the drain and sutures are removed. The physician then prescribes a gradual increase in the amount and type of exercises to be performed (such as wall climbing or combing hair). Some of these exercises are described in Box 58-5. Performing these exercises several times daily helps restore full range of motion to the arm and shoulder, thus preventing a "frozen shoulder" from lack of normal movement. The exercises also facilitate the development of collateral lymphatic channels and help prevent lymphedema.

If the patient has had breast reconstruction with simple implants, she is cautioned to avoid heavy lifting (more than 5 pounds) for 4 to 6 weeks. This time frame ensures that complete healing has occurred and minimizes strain on the incision line.[32] The patient who had a TRAM flap procedure should be cautioned to avoid arm abduction reaching exercises until permitted by the physician. However, the patient should be encouraged to use the affected arm in front of the body (as in eating or washing the face) to prevent joint stiffening. A well-fitted, nonwire brassiere provides support and normal alignment of the newly formed breast.[39]

Box 58-5 Breast Surgery Arm and Shoulder Exercises

Wand Exercise

1. Lie on your back with knees and hips bent, feet flat.
2. Hold a broom handle, yardstick, or similar object in both hands with palms facing up.
3. Lift the wand up over your head as far as you can, using your unaffected arm to help lift the wand, until you feel a stretch in your affected arm.
4. Hold for 5 seconds.
5. Lower arms and repeat five to seven times.

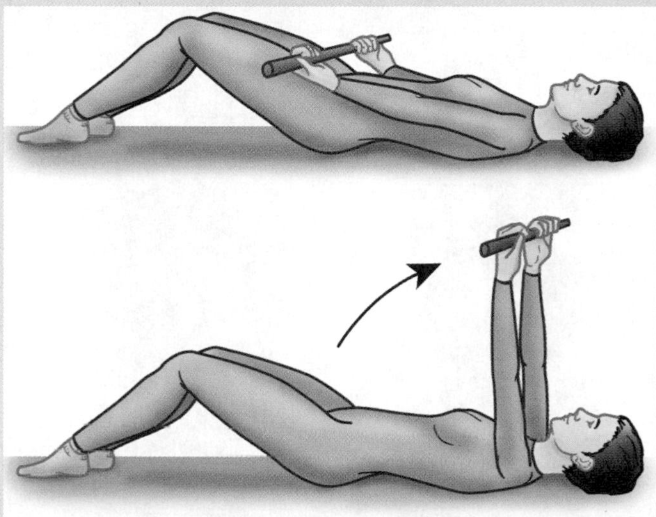

Elbow Winging

1. Lie on your back with knees and hips bent, feet flat.
2. Clasp your hands behind your neck with your elbows pointing toward the ceiling.
3. Move your elbows apart and down toward the bed (or floor).
4. Repeat five to seven times.

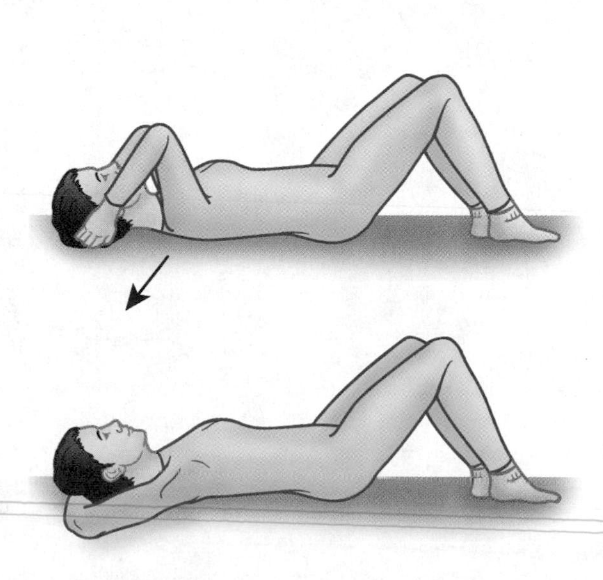

Shoulder Blade Stretch

1. Sit in a chair very close to a table with your back against the chair back.
2. Place uninvolved arm on the table with elbow bent and palm down, do not move this arm during the exercise.
3. Place affected arm on the table, palm down with elbow straight.
4. Without moving your trunk, slide affected arm toward the opposite side of the table. You should feel your shoulder blade move as you do this.
5. Relax your arm and repeat five to seven times.

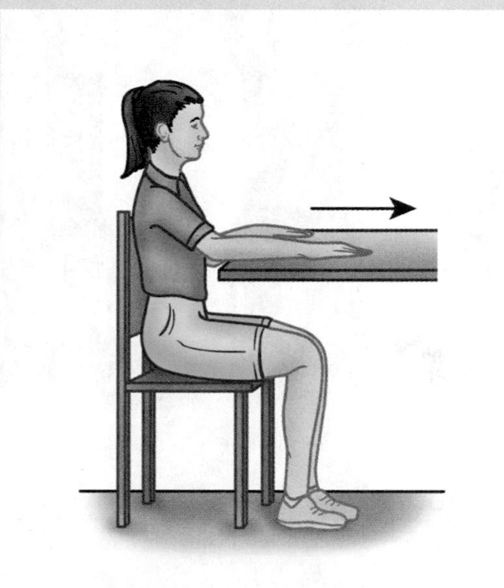

Shoulder Blade Squeeze

1. Facing straight ahead, sit in a chair in front of a mirror without resting against the back of the chair.
2. Arms should be at your sides with elbows bent.
3. Squeeze shoulder blades together, bringing your elbows behind you. Keep your shoulders level as you do this exercise. Do not lift your shoulders up toward your ears.
4. Return to the starting position and repeat five to seven times.

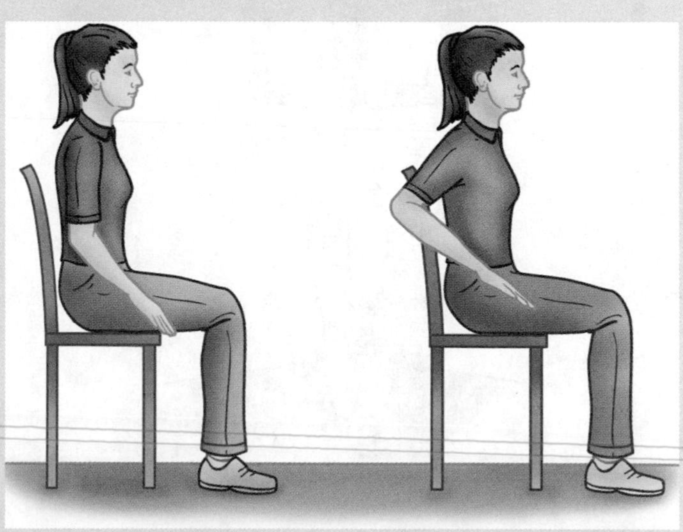

Continued

Box 58-5 Breast Surgery Arm and Shoulder Exercises—cont'd

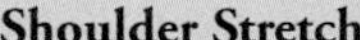

Side Bending

1. Clasp hands together in front of you and lift your arms slowly over your head, straightening your arms.
2. When arms are over your head, bend your trunk to the right while bending at the waist and keeping your arms overhead.
3. Return to starting position and bend to the left.
4. Repeat the cycle five to seven times.

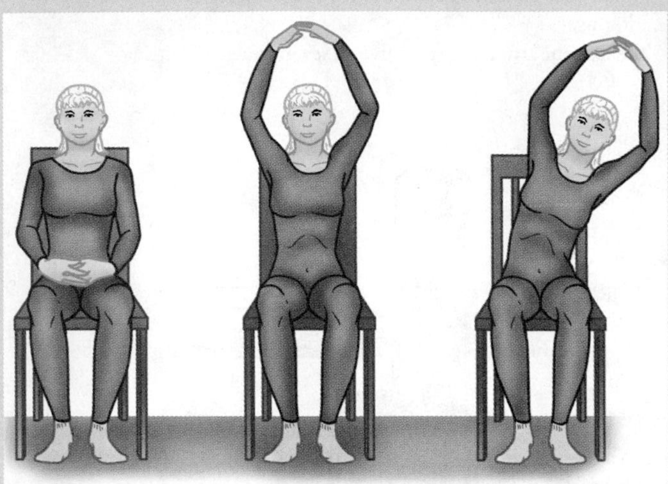

Chest Wall Stretch

1. Stand facing a corner with toes approximately 8 to 10 inches from the corner.
2. Bend elbows and place forearms on the wall, one on each side of the corner. Elbows should be as close to shoulder height as possible.
3. Keep arms and feet in position and move chest toward the corner.
4. You will feel a stretch across your chest and shoulders.
5. Return to starting position and repeat five to seven times.

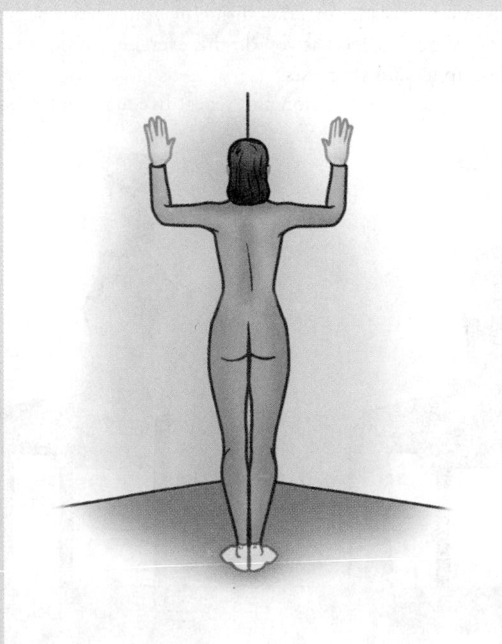

Shoulder Stretch

1. Stand facing the wall with toes approximately 8 to 10 inches from the wall.
2. Place your hands on the wall. Use your fingers to "climb the wall," reaching as high as you can until you feel a stretch.
3. Return to starting position and repeat five to seven times.

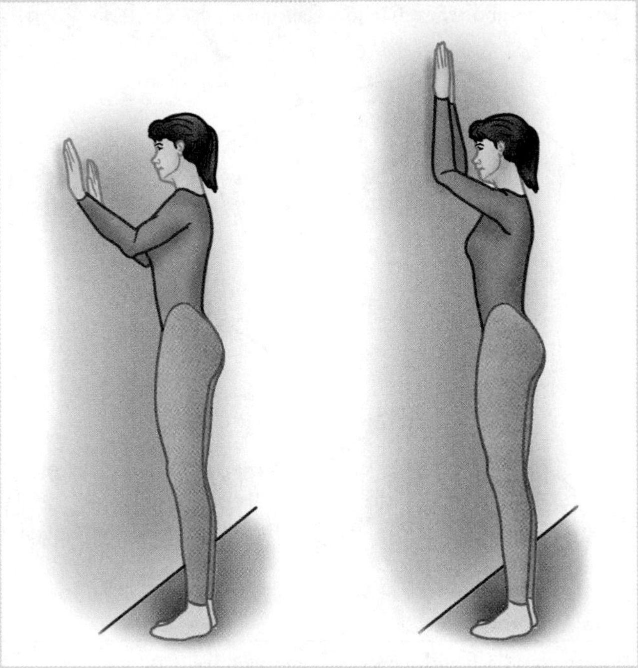

When the patient has sensory changes because of transection or trauma to nerves at the time of surgery, these may persist well after discharge. Although most sensory problems resolve within 1 year, some may continue and can cause atrophy of muscles that move the shoulder on the affected side. The patient should be alert to any signs and symptoms of impaired shoulder mobility and report them immediately.

Assessing and Managing Lymphedema. Instructions on how to assess for lymphedema and how to avoid its occurrence are important. The nurse teaches patients to observe for signs of numbness, heaviness, tightness, swelling, pain, decreased strength, decreased mobility, and infection.[6,13,33] The nurse stresses the importance of the prescribed rehabilitative exercises and teaches the patient to avoid placing the affected extremity in a dependent position for extended periods. Compliance with these instructions helps prevent the chronic form of lymphedema, which can occur soon after discharge or many months afterward. Some edema may be present at discharge, especially if lymph node dissection was performed. The greater the number of nodes removed, the greater the chance of edema. As the wound heals and the prescribed exercises are performed, the edema usually subsides.

Demonstration of the proper technique to measure arm circumference and a method to record arm measurements enables the patient to quickly recognize a problem and report it immediately. Although there is no standard degree of enlargement that constitutes lymphedema, the most common definition is a 2-cm difference in arm circumference between the affected and unaffected arm.[13] When edema is present, the patient is instructed to keep the affected extremity elevated as much as possible. If edema persists or increases, the physician should be notified. Treatment regimens may include application of a compression garment, extremity elevation, massage, exercise, skin care, manual decompression, and external compression.[6,8,13]

Strategies to Prevent Trauma and Infection. The patient who had breast surgery with a level II or III lymph node dissection must be vigilant in avoiding trauma and infection to the affected arm. Protecting the arm and hand is essential because lymphatic circulation has been compromised by removal of axillary lymph nodes. Radiotherapy is also known to interfere with the ability of the lymph nodes to remove foreign substances and destroy bacteria. Thus node dissection and radiotherapy can both lead to lymphatic dysfunction. Infectious agents can easily enter the lymphatic system from cuts, scratches, or burns.[33] Special instructions to avoid these complications are listed in the Guidelines for Safe Practice box. The patient must understand that these precautions need to be followed for the rest of her life.

Patient/Family Teaching. Before discharge, the nurse instructs the patient about wound care management, exercise guidelines and sensory change precautions, assessment and management of lymphedema, and prevention of trauma and infection (see Patient/Family Teaching box). Women who will receive additional treatment with radiation or chemotherapy are informed about when and where treatment will begin and why it is necessary to keep all follow-up appointments. If a tissue expander was used for breast reconstruction, the nurse informs the patient about the timing of subsequent injections of saline solution into the implant. The nurse advises the woman that the procedure is uncomfortable because the muscle overlying the expander is stretched immediately after each injection. Once the muscle has been stretched to the desired size, the expander may be removed or left in place over the implant. If an autogenous tissue flap was created, nipple reconstruction may be planned after the operative site has healed.

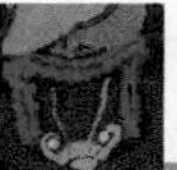

GUIDELINES FOR SAFE PRACTICE
Arm Precautions After Mastectomy

- Ensure that the affected arm is never used for blood pressure readings, injections, or venipunctures.
- Wear no constricting clothing or jewelry, including wristwatch, on affected arm.
- Do not carry heavy objects (pocketbook, packages) in affected arm.
- Wear rubber gloves when washing dishes.
- Use unaffected arm when removing items from hot oven, or protect by wearing a padded glove pot holder.
- Use a thimble when sewing; wash needlepricks and cover as necessary.
- Take care when trimming fingernails and cuticles; avoid using scissors for this task.
- Use softening lotions or creams to keep skin in soft, supple condition.
- Outdoor activities:
  —Wear gloves when gardening.
  —Avoid sunburn—wear protective clothing or use sunscreen liberally.
  —Use insect repellent in areas with biting or stinging insects.
  —Tend to cuts and scratches immediately by washing and applying protective covering.

Adapted from Ridner SH: Breast cancer lymphedema: pathophysiology and risk reduction guidelines, *Oncol Nurs Forum* 29(9):1285, 2002.

Breast cancer may recur or develop in the remaining breast. Therefore the nurse should determine the patient's knowledge and skill in the performance of BSE. If necessary, the nurse demonstrates the proper procedure and provides a pamphlet on BSE. Because breast cancer has a tendency to recur at the incision line, the nurse teaches the patient how to assess this area. Follow-up mammograms and clinical breast examinations are an integral part of long-term care. The necessity for these examinations cannot be overstressed.

The ACS is an important resource for all cancer patients. Reach to Recovery volunteers—women who have had breast cancer and undergone successful surgery and rehabilitation—are available to meet with patients after discharge to answer questions about rehabilitation; provide pamphlets and equipment for the prescribed rehabilitative exercises; accompany the patient in purchasing a permanent prosthesis and brassiere; and talk about quality of life issues and address concerns. Other ACS volunteer groups, such as I Can Cope, can help persons who need support in coping with life after cancer. Family members frequently find needed support from this group as well.

PROMOTING QUALITY OF LIFE. The impact of breast cancer and its treatment on the quality of life of breast cancer survivors and

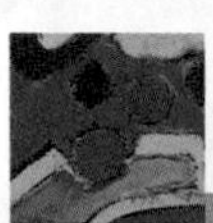

PATIENT/FAMILY TEACHING *Discharge Instructions After Mastectomy*

Dressings

Incision

A dry gauze dressing will be over the incision when you leave the hospital. It is not necessary to change this dressing until you return to see the doctor.

Drain Site

A small dry dressing will be around the site where the drain is placed. Often there is some leakage of fluid around the drain. Check the gauze dressing for drainage and change if soiled.

Some leakage is normal, but if the dressing becomes soaked more than once a day, call your doctor.

Drains

Your nurse has shown you how to empty the reservoir from your drain and how to measure the volume of drainage. You should empty the drain twice a day and record the measurements.

Drains are generally removed when drainage is about 30 ml/24 hr.

Drains are often removed at the same time as the stitches, generally 7 to 10 days after surgery.

Bathing

Take sponge baths or tub baths, making certain that the area of the drain and incision stay dry. You may shower after the stitches and drains are removed.

Hand and Arm Care

You can begin using your arm for normal activities such as eating or combing your hair.

Exercises involving the wrist, hand, and elbow such as flexing your fingers, circular wrist motions, and touching hand to shoulder are very good. More strenuous exercises can usually be resumed after the drains have been removed.

Comfort

Some discomfort or mild pain is expected after surgery. Within 4 to 5 days most women have no need for medication or require something only at bedtime.

Numbness in the area of the surgery and along the inner side of the arm from the armpit to the elbow occurs in virtually all patients. It is a result of injury to the nerves that provide sensation to the skin in those areas.

Women have described sensations such as heaviness, pain, tingling, burning, and "pins and needles." These sensations change over the months and usually resolve by 1 year.

Support and Information

Pamphlets on exercises, hand and arm care, and general facts about breast cancer are available from your nurse or volunteer visitor.

The American Cancer Society has volunteers who have had surgery similar to yours and are available to visit you.

their families is an area of ongoing concern. Breast cancer sequelae distinctive to the psychosocial life stage of the breast cancer survivor may emerge and affect quality of life well into survivorship (see Research box). The nurse should explore quality-of-life issues with patients and their families and develop strategies to assist each family member in coping with the disease.

Surgery, chemotherapy, and hormone therapy often affect sexual drive and function. Symptoms of treatment-related sexual problems most often experienced by breast cancer survivors are listed in Box 58-6. Breast cancer survivors who experience sexual dysfunction should be referred for treatment. Depending on the specific dysfunction, patients may be treated with counseling or pharmaceutical interventions such as megesterol acetate and venlafaxine for hot flashes, a vaginal lubricant (K-Y Jelly or Replens), or an estradiol vaginal ring for vaginal dryness.[43] Women with or without partners may benefit from referral to a support group of women similar to themselves.[37] Advancing age does not exempt a woman from concerns over self-esteem and sexuality, and older adults should be included in all interventions and referrals for assistance. Spouses or partners should be present, if at all possible, during all discussion about sexual concerns so that their anxieties can be addressed as well.

A Nursing Care Plan for a patient with breast cancer undergoing mastectomy and immediate breast reconstruction with a TRAM flap can be found on p. 1774.

▶ ARE You READY?

Which of the following should be included in discharge teaching about arm precautions after mastectomy? (Choose all that apply.)

1. Avoid use of sunscreen.
2. Wear gloves when gardening.
3. Wear long sleeves at all times.
4. Do not allow blood pressure to be obtained on affected side.
5. Use sharp scissors when cutting finger and toe nails.
6. Use softening lotions to maintain supple skin.

GERONTOLOGIC CONSIDERATIONS

A high incidence of breast cancer occurs in women over 65 years of age. Although breast cancer in older women tends to have less aggressive characteristics than in younger women, older women are more likely to develop metastatic disease or are more often diagnosed with advanced-stage disease.[19] Older women may not be aware of their increased vulnerability to cancer, especially breast cancer, nor know the suspicious signs and symptoms that they should report to the physician. Situations such as comorbidities, decreased physical functioning, cognitive impairment, depression, and lack of social support can interfere with early diagnosis and treatment options.[38]

Changes occurring in the breast as a result of aging such as fibrosis, calcification, shrinkage, and loss of subcutaneous fat may cause confusion regarding changes that are normal for aging and those which may indicate a possible malignant condition. Women with arthritis may have difficulty performing BSE and may discontinue the practice altogether.

Other factors that affect early diagnosis of cancer and successful treatment may relate to the socioeconomic status of older

Research

Sammarco A: Perceived social support, uncertainty, and quality of life among younger breast cancer survivors, *Cancer Nurs* 24(3):212, 2001.

Research has demonstrated that younger women are particularly vulnerable to the physical and psychosocial sequelae of breast cancer, suffering greater stress in their personal and social lives and poorer adjustment compared with their older counterparts. This study investigated the relationship between perceived social support, uncertainty, and quality of life among younger breast cancer survivors. Proposed hypotheses were a significant positive correlation between perceived social support and quality of life, and a significant negative correlation between uncertainty and quality of life. The researchers also hypothesized that perceived social support and uncertainty, considered together, would explain more of the variance of quality of life than either variable considered independently.

A mailed survey method was used in which a sample of 101 breast cancer survivors below age 50 completed the Social Support Questionnaire, the Mishel Uncertainty in Illness Scale-Community Form, and the Ferrans and Powers Quality of Life Index-Cancer Version. Data were analyzed using descriptive statistics, Pearson product-moment correlation, and stepwise multiple regression.

Findings supported all study hypotheses. Additional findings revealed significant positive correlations between perceived social support and size of support network, and between size of support network and the socioeconomic domain of quality of life. Significant negative correlations were found between perceived social support and uncertainty and between size of support network and uncertainty.

Results of the study suggested that perceived social support, especially in the area of family, was important in influencing the quality of life in this sample. Also, lower levels of uncertainty especially in the health and functioning area, enhanced quality of life in this sample. Nurses who interact with younger breast cancer survivors are in a prime position to undertake actions to decrease patient uncertainty and increase social support, which may in turn improve quality of life. Strategies can include providing referrals to age-specific support groups or counseling, facilitating tangible aid, encouraging family and spiritual support, and ensuring positive supportive interactions with younger breast cancer survivors.

Box 58-6 Symptoms of Treatment-Related Sexual Problems

- Absence of sexual desire
- Decreased libido
- Anorgasmy
- Lubrication difficulties
- Dyspareunia
- Premature menopause

From Thors CL, Broeckel JA, Jacobsen PB: Sexual functioning in breast cancer survivors, *CancerControl* 8(5):442, 2001.

adults. Retirement with reduced financial resources and a lack of health insurance beyond Medicare/Medicaid may deter older women from seeking medical care for a breast lump. Financial concerns about ability to pay for long-term chemotherapy or radiotherapy may cause them to terminate treatment. Becoming a burden, both physically and financially, on their families is frequently a concern of older patients with breast cancer.[38]

The nurse must encourage older women to participate in cancer screening and detection programs, have a yearly mammogram, and perform monthly BSE. The nurse should also act as a patient advocate when treatment options are being presented and advised.

Nonmalignant Conditions of the Breast

Benign breast disease is common and accounts for about 90% of all breast problems. Because no universally accepted classification system exists for benign disorders, the term *fibrocystic disease* has been used as an umbrella category into which most benign disorders are placed. This has resulted in confusion in diagnosing and treating patients with benign conditions.

Cystic Breast Disease

Etiology and Epidemiology. The underlying cause of cystic breast disease is not fully known. Changes in the breast are cyclic and thought to be caused by hormonal imbalance or the exaggerated response of breast tissue to ovarian hormones. Breast tenderness is more pronounced during or before menstruation. Cystic breast disease is most common in nulliparous women between the ages of 40 and 50 years but can occur at any age. Occurrence is least frequent after menopause.

Pathophysiology. A number of commonalities are seen in cystic disease, regardless of the diagnostic name used. Changes once thought to be abnormal such as microcysts, apocrine change, adenosis, fibrosis, and varying degrees of hyperplasia are now recognized as aberrancies of the involutional process of the breast. These changes include lumps of varying size, nipple discharge, and breast pain (mastodynia).[27] Cystic lesions are soft, well demarcated, and freely movable. The process is almost always bilateral, with most lesions located in the left breast. The cysts may contain clear, milky, straw-colored, or yellow to dark brown fluid. Occasionally the contents may be blood tinged. The common clinical manifestations of fibroadenomas and fibrocystic disease of the breast are compared in Table 58-3.

Collaborative Care Management. The woman who discovers a mass or masses in her breast should seek the advice of a health care provider who, after clinical breast examination, will decide whether to perform aspiration or biopsy. An ultrasound or, if necessary, a needle aspiration generally confirms the presence of a cyst. Because nodular tissue in the breast makes the early detection of malignant lesions more difficult, some physicians suggest periodic mammograms to detect any changes. There is no evidence to suggest that cystic disease predisposes women to the development of a malignant lesion; however, women with hyperplasia, papilloma, or gross cyst are at increased risk.[27]

The traditional treatment of fibrocystic disease consists of diuretics and restrictions in fluid and salt intake. The limitation or exclusion of methylxanthines (a class of chemicals found in coffee, tea, cola, and chocolate) is frequently recommended as a means of controlling cystic disease.

Nursing Care Plan

Patient With Breast Cancer Undergoing Mastectomy and Immediate Breast Reconstruction With TRAM Flap

Data A 53-year-old woman is admitted to the surgical unit with the diagnosis of cancer of the left breast. She had her annual mammogram 1 week before admission, at which time a 2-cm lesion was revealed. Tissue reports following needle biopsy confirmed the presence of infiltrative ductal carcinoma. Treatment options were discussed. Since the lesion was small and in a localized stage (stage I to II), the patient elected to undergo mastectomy and immediate reconstruction using the transverse rectus abdominis myocutaneous (TRAM) flap procedure. Construction of a new areola and nipple are planned for after surgical healing has been achieved.

In addition to routine surgical preparation, the nurse assessed the patient's understanding of the impending surgical procedure; addressed concerns and fears not previously discussed; and gave preoperative teaching regarding turning and breathing techniques, indwelling urinary catheter, incentive spirometry, antiembolism stockings, patient-controlled analgesia (PCA), nutrition plan, and positioning and mobility after surgery. The nurse also initiated a referral to Reach to Recovery for a visit by a volunteer who had had TRAM flap reconstruction.

Nursing Diagnosis

Deficient knowledge related to lack of experience with physical and cosmetic changes following mastectomy and TRAM flap reconstruction

Outcomes

- Patient will accurately discuss location of donor site, length of recovery, and rehabilitation.
- Patient will accurately describe appearance of new breast mound.
- Patient will maintain activity and mobility restrictions.
- Patient will display receptiveness to visit from Reach to Recovery volunteer.

Related NOC Outcomes

- Knowledge: Prescribed Activity
- Knowledge: Treatment Procedure(s)
- Knowledge: Treatment Regimen

Related NIC Interventions

- Teaching: Individual
- Teaching: Prescribed Activity/Exercise
- Teaching: Prescribed Procedure/Treatment

Nursing Interventions/Rationales

- Clarify location of TRAM flap from site of lower abdomen and fact that removal of muscle flap will result in some abdominal weakness and an abdominal scar. *Enables fuller understanding of the procedure so that patient will not be surprised or frightened.*
- Reinforce that surgery will take about 7 hours to complete, hospitalization will be 6 or 7 days, and employment can be resumed in about 6 weeks. A second surgery will be required to reconstruct areola and nipple. *To prepare patient for the need to continue therapy on an outpatient basis after discharge from hospital.*
- Show pictures of breast mound. Indicate that mound will have feelings of sensation and pressure. Breast size will be similar if adequate abdominal tissue is available. *Provides realistic expectation of appearance and feel of reconstructed breast.*
- Teach patient to expect a gradual increase in exercise and activities over a 3-month period. *Activities and exercises are increased as strength and endurance return.*
- Initiate referral to American Cancer Society Reach to Recovery program for visit from a volunteer who had undergone mastectomy with TRAM flap reconstruction. *Provides support from a woman with the same diagnosis, surgical reconstruction, and concerns.*

Nursing Diagnosis

Risk for ineffective tissue perfusion to affected arm related to compromised circulation and lymphatic drainage after TRAM flap breast reconstruction

Outcomes

- Patient will maintain good capillary refill in affected limb.
- Patient will maintain full sensation in affected limb.

Related NOC Outcomes

- Risk Control
- Tissue Integrity: Skin & Mucous Membranes
- Tissue Perfusion: Peripheral

Related NIC Interventions

- Neurologic Monitoring
- Positioning
- Skin Surveillance

Nursing Interventions/Rationales

- Assess flap every hour for the first 24 hours, then every 2 to 4 hours, for capillary refill, color, warmth, edema, and decreased sensation. Use Doppler if necessary. *To monitor viability of flap and adequacy of blood supply.*
- Perform neurovascular checks to affected arm every hour for the first 24 hours, then every 2 to 4 hours. Teach patient how to perform checks when able to participate. *Lymphedema may be present with axillary node dissection. Lymphedema causes pressure on peripheral nerves, leading to cool, pale extremity; diminished pulse; and poor movement.*
- Check drainage devices at TRAM flap and axillary area for patency, amount, color, and consistency each shift. Document changes and report to physician. *Decreased drainage may indicate the drain is improperly placed or obstructed, leading to lymphedema or impaired circulation at flap.*

Nursing Diagnosis

Acute pain related to surgical procedure (graft and mastectomy)

Outcomes

- Patient will report pain of less than 3 on a scale of 0 to 10 within 30 minutes of pain interventions.
- Patient will decrease use of analgesics.

Related NOC Outcomes

- Pain Control
- Pain Level

Related NIC Interventions

- Pain Management

- Positioning
- Progressive Muscle Relaxation

Nursing Interventions/Rationales

- Assess duration and intensity of pain. *To monitor effectiveness of pain control measures and provide alternative pain control methods if needed.*
- Administer prescribed analgesics to provide maximal level of comfort. If using PCA pump, assess ability to use correctly. *Freedom from pain promotes patient cooperation and compliance with care plan. PCA pump allows patient control over pain management.*
- Elevate affected arm on pillow as directed. Position in semi-Fowler's position with knees flexed and elevated on a pillow when in bed. *Promotes lymphatic and venous return and helps prevent lymphedema, which increases pain.*
- Assist with turning and ambulation. *To promote mobility without increasing pain.*
- Restrict upper extremity exercise and activity until permitted by physician. *Reduces strain on incision and helps prevent lymphedema.*
- Secure drainage devices properly (two at breast and two in abdominal wound). Check function every 2 hours. *Prevents hematoma or seroma formation, pressure on incision line, and infection. Drainage becomes clear as healing progresses.*

Nursing Diagnosis

Risk for infection related to surgery, axillary node dissection, abdominal wound, and invasive equipment (intravenous [IV] lines, catheter, drains)

Outcomes

- Patient will remain free from systemic infection.
- Patient will remain free from wound redness, warmth, swelling, tenderness, or purulent drainage.

Related NOC Outcomes

- Immune Status
- Infection Severity
- Risk Control

Related NIC Interventions

- Infection Protection
- Surveillance
- Wound Care

Nursing Interventions/Rationales

- Assist with performing deep breathing, turning every 2 hours, and incentive spirometry. Splint abdomen for coughing. Encourage early ambulation as permitted. *To prevent inadequate respiratory efforts and pooling of secretions that can result in pneumonia or atelectasis.*
- Assess for signs and symptoms of infection (elevation of temperature, redness, swelling, pain, and purulent drainage). *These are signs of localized and systemic infection. Early recognition allows for early intervention when infection is present.*
- Teach patient signs and symptoms of infection. *So the patient can recognize and report infection to ensure early treatment.*
- Perform drain care using sterile technique. Teach patient how to perform drain care before discharge and the need for good hand washing. *Promotes patient involvement and self-care before discharge. Decreases the risk for infection.*
- Monitor invasive equipment as a cause of infection. Document and report findings. *Provides for early detection and treatment if needed.*
- Post sign in room alerting staff not to use affected arm for blood pressure measurements, injections, venipuncture, and IV lines. Inform patient of guidelines to follow to protect self from infection. *Lymph node dissection disrupts lymphatic function. An inflated blood pressure cuff can obstruct lymph flow through channels and increase damage. Injections and venipunctures cause breaks in skin and provide a source for infection.*

Nursing Diagnosis

Ineffective therapeutic regimen management related to lack of knowledge regarding long-term recovery and rehabilitation

Outcomes

- Patient will accurately describe prescribed exercises, wound care, and activity limits.
- Patient will adhere to therapeutic regimen.
- Patient will progressively assume self-care without difficulty.
- Patient will participate in care planning and goal setting.

Related NOC Outcomes

- Adherence Behavior
- Knowledge: Treatment Regimen
- Participation in Health Care Decisions

Related NIC Interventions

- Family Support
- Mutual Goal Setting
- Teaching: Individual

Nursing Interventions/Rationales

- Teach wound care and care of drainage devices (if present) following discharge and have patient do return demonstration. *Demonstration, return demonstration, and written instructions give the patient and family confidence in their ability to carry out therapeutic regimen accurately.*
- Teach patient activity limitations and the need to protect the reconstructed breast from pressure until healed. *To prevent complications and ensure full recovery and rehabilitation.*
- Reinforce breast self-examination technique and compliment patient's past adherence. Discuss the need to continue breast self-examinations and mammograms on new and remaining breast. *To detect recurrence of breast cancer. Complimenting the patient's past adherence to breast examination increases self-confidence and reinforces future adherence.*

Evaluation

Evaluation is based on comparing the patient's outcomes with desired outcomes.

TABLE 58-3 CLINICAL MANIFESTATIONS OF FIBROADENOMAS AND FIBROCYSTIC DISEASE OF THE BREAST

	Fibroadenoma	Fibrocystic Disease
Likely age	15-20, can occur up to 55	30-55, decreases after menopause
Shape	Round, lobular	Round, lobular
Consistency	Usually firm, can be soft	Firm to soft, rubbery
Demarcation	Well demarcated, clear margins	Well demarcated
Number	Usually single	Multiple usually, may be single
Mobility	Very mobile, slippery	Mobile
Tenderness	Usually none	Tender, increases before menses
Risk to health	None	None
Pattern of growth	Grows quickly and constantly	Size may increase or decrease rapidly
Skin retraction	None: benign; must diagnose by biopsy	Benign, although general lumpiness may mask other cancerous lumps

From Jarvis C: *Physical examination and health assessment,* ed 4, Philadelphia, 2003, Saunders.

Vitamin A, E, and B complex and evening primrose oil have been helpful in relieving the discomfort of cystic breast disease.[4] Danazol and bromocriptine have been tried for symptom relief, but ineffectiveness and unpleasant side effects have precluded their use.[27]

PATIENT/FAMILY TEACHING. The nurse's role in the care of patients with benign breast disorders is primarily that of educator and facilitator. The nurse should be knowledgeable about benign conditions; understand their medical management; provide and clarify information; and support the patient, emotionally and physically, through diagnosis and treatment.

Hospitalization is seldom required for the treatment of cystic breast disease. The nurse teaches BSE to those women who are not familiar with it and stresses its use every month. Women are taught to recognize through touch their normal breast tissue and the location and size of any lesions present. They should report significant changes that differ from the normal cyclic fluctuations or that appear at a different time in the menstrual cycle. Using a mild analgesic and wearing a firm, supportive brassiere may provide comfort and reduce pain on movement. Warm, moist heat also may help relieve aching pain. Eliminating caffeine consumption and decreasing salt content before menstruation to relieve bloating and weight gain can be recommended. The woman is advised to consult her health care provider before using vitamin E as a therapeutic intervention, so any beneficial effects can be professionally monitored. Side effects of vitamin E use are few.

Fibroadenoma

Etiology and Epidemiology. Fibroadenomas, or adenofibromas, are the most common benign breast neoplasms. The tumors occur most often in women younger than 25 years old; some lesions become evident by age 15. Fibroadenomas usually are firm, rubbery, round, freely movable, nontender, and encapsulated; they may be multiple and bilateral. Tumor size ranges from 1 to 3 cm. A giant fibroadenoma is the most common lesion seen in the adolescent breast.

Pathophysiology. Fibroadenomas are estrogen-dependent tumors of fibroblastic and epithelial origin, usually associated with menstrual irregularities. Fibroadenomas are slow growing and often are stimulated by pregnancy and lactation. Regression may occur after delivery. At menopause they tend to regress and become hyalinized. Giant fibroadenomas grow rapidly to 10 to 12 cm in diameter but are not more prone to malignant change than smaller lesions. Dimpling or nipple retraction is not associated with fibroadenomas.

Collaborative Care Management. Surgical removal is the standard treatment for fibroadenomas. Many can be removed with the patient under local anesthesia in an outpatient setting. Although the tumor is examined for definitive pathologic characteristics, the association between fibroadenomas and cancer is weak.

PATIENT/FAMILY TEACHING. When the woman discovers a breast mass, her primary concern is whether the mass is cancer. The nurse should avoid reassuring the patient that most breast lesions are not malignant. Only the final pathology report will provide this reassurance. Before the surgical removal of the fibroadenoma, the nurse prepares the woman for the type of surgery to be performed, what to expect during the procedure, and how to care for the incision afterward. The nurse should encourage practice of BSE and the reporting of any unusual changes found during the examination.

Inflammatory Lesions

Mammary Duct Ectasia

Etiology and Epidemiology. Mammary duct ectasia, also referred to as plasma cell mastitis, is a benign condition of unknown etiology. Some investigators believe an anaerobic bacteria may be implicated. Another causative factor may be bacterial infection that results from stasis of fluid in the large ducts of the breast. Age is the primary risk factor for duct ectasia, with a mean age ranging from 45 to 55 years. Breast pain and a palpable mass are typical symptoms in premenopausal women, whereas nipple discharge predominates in perimenopausal women. In postmenopausal women, nipple retractions secondary to periductal fibrosis are more often noted.

Pathophysiology. Mammary duct ectasia involves inflammation of the ducts behind the nipple, duct enlargement, and a collection of cellular debris and fluid in the involved ducts. As the inflammatory response resolves, the ducts become fibrotic and dilated. Nipple discharge usually is bilateral and ranges from serous to thick, sticky, or pastelike. Drainage may be green, greenish brown, or blood stained. Nipple itching, suggestive of Paget's disease, may accompany transient pain in the subareolar and inner quadrants of the breast. On palpation the areolar area may feel wormlike; the nipple may be red and swollen or flat and retracted. The condition is not associated with breast-feeding.

Collaborative Care Management. Treatment varies, depending on the severity of the problem. Because of the chronic nature of this problem, most women are monitored with routine physical examination of the breast. The symptoms of mammary duct ectasia may elicit the fear of malignant disease. Once the benign nature of this chronic condition is affirmed, fears generally are dispelled and most women are able to deal with their symptoms. Although mammary duct ectasia has no cure, antibiotics are prescribed for acute inflammatory episodes, such as the development of an abscess. If the woman can no longer tolerate the chronic discharge, surgical excision of the retroareolar ducts is performed.

PATIENT/FAMILY TEACHING. The nurse must be cognizant of the chronic yet benign nature of this condition and offer support and understanding care. The nurse teaches the woman how to cleanse the breast to minimize the risk of infection. Good hand washing and personal hygiene measures are stressed. Wearing a supportive yet nonconfining brassiere padded with sterile gauze and changing the brassiere daily or as necessary helps prevent abscess formation. The nurse teaches the woman the signs and symptoms indicative of abscess that should be reported immediately.

Acute Mastitis and Abscess

Etiology and Epidemiology. There are two forms of mastitis: acute and chronic. The acute form is a rare condition almost always found in breast-feeding mothers during the first 4 months of lactation. It occurs most frequently from *Staphylococcus aureus* or *Staphylococcus epidermidis* infection that spreads from a break in the skin surface of the nipple to underlying breast tissue. It may be confined to only one quadrant of the breast. Symptoms include a fissured nipple, fever, chills, localized tenderness, and erythema. Purulent discharge from the nipple is usually not observed.

The chronic form of mastitis can follow acute mastitis or have a slow, insidious onset. Both acute and chronic mastitis are caused by the same bacterial agents. The chronic form occurs more often in older women, and the symptoms can mimic inflammatory breast cancer. The infection usually arises in the sweat or sebaceous glands and spreads to the breast. Symptoms of chronic mastitis include a painful breast mass that involves the nipple and areola and a low-grade fever.

Pathophysiology. In both acute and chronic mastitis there is edema and congestion of the periductal and interlobular stomata. The ducts are distended from the accumulation of neutrophils and retained secretions. If an abscess forms, its central core may be necrotic and contain creamy, yellow exudate. Fibrosis of the involved tissue can develop after treatment. Both the acute and chronic forms of mastitis should be investigated for inflammatory breast carcinoma, but recent lactation usually excludes the acute form from the need for further evaluation.

Collaborative Care Management. Acute mastitis is easy to diagnose in a nursing mother. Treatment with antibiotics resolves the infectious process. In older women, because the condition has similarities to inflammatory breast carcinoma, incision and drainage of the inflammatory exudate are performed to determine the cause. Antibiotics can then be prescribed.

PATIENT/FAMILY TEACHING. When acute mastitis is the result of an infection during lactation, most women immediately stop breast-feeding. The nurse should inform them that discontinuing breast-feeding is not always necessary or advisable. The infant is not affected by sucking on the involved breast, and symptoms are usually relieved within 48 hours of antibiotic treatment. Continued breast-feeding is believed to reduce the pain and lessen the volume of milk that can be a source for bacterial growth. If breast-feeding is discontinued, the woman is instructed to keep her breasts as empty as possible by pumping. If the breast is not emptied, it becomes engorged, and pain increases.

The woman is instructed to complete the entire course of antibiotics and not discontinue them when symptoms are relieved. Because the infection generally does not originate in the breast, teaching about personal hygiene measures is important. The older woman with mastitis may be anxious about a diagnosis of cancer. Emotional support and frank discussion of her concerns are provided until the aspiration biopsy results are known.

Both acute and chronic mastitis resolve with antibiotic therapy, rest, and the application of local heat. Discomfort generally is relieved by analgesics.

Male Breast Problems

Gynecomastia

Etiology and Epidemiology. Gynecomastia is a common disorder of the male breast. This condition is estimated to occur in up to 65% of pubertal boys during the time of rapid testicular growth between the ages of 12 and 15 years. Symptoms include a firm, circular, disklike, circumscribed, tender mass beneath the areola, usually bilateral at onset. In adolescent boys the condition is transient and lasts for approximately 12 to 24 months. Gynecomastia is seen again in men ages 45 years and older, with 40% of elderly men having some degree of the condition.[34] Gynecomastia is seen in obese men because obesity increases the rate of conversion of androgens to estrogen and in patients with cirrhosis of the liver, because of the incomplete hepatic clearance of estrogen. Gynecomastia may develop in men who are receiving drugs such as estrogen, cimetidine, certain antibiotics (isoniazid), antihypertensive agents (reserpine and methyldopa), calcium channel blockers, and digoxin.[34]

Pathophysiology. Gynecomastia is caused by hormonal imbalance. As a result of excess estrogen, hyperplasia (overdevelopment) of the stomata and ducts in the mammary glands occurs. The primary cause of gynecomastia in older men is the aging process. As men age, the plasma testosterone concentration declines at the same time that the plasma testosterone-estrogen level increases. Thus less free testosterone is available.

Collaborative Care Management. When gynecomastia occurs and the condition cannot be attributed to rapid testicular growth (as may be seen in teenaged boys), treatment with estrogen therapy (middle-aged men), or hepatic dysfunction, a human chorionic gonadotropin-beta subunit (HCG-beta) level should be obtained. This finding assists in ruling out a malignant testicular germ cell condition, which can manifest with gynecomastia and an elevated HCG-beta level. Chest and mediastinal x-ray films and a careful testes examination are included in the evaluation. In older men the physician may suggest obtaining a breast biopsy specimen because this age-group is more prone to male breast cancer.

Treatment of gynecomastia may involve correction of a systemic disorder, withdrawal of an offending drug, or observation for spontaneous regression. However, treatment may not be effective especially if disease duration has been lengthy and fibrosis has occurred. Surgery would then be used for cosmesis in these circumstances.[34] Patients who are treated with hormonal therapy for prostate cancer should be warned that gynecomastia is one of the side effects of treatment. Similarly, patients on medication that increase breast size should be forewarned of this side effect.

Most men are intensely embarrassed about gynecomastia because enlarged breasts constitute a serious assault on the male self-image. The condition is visible whenever the man removes his shirt for work or recreation and frequently results in taunts and jokes. Similar problems exist for the man who undergoes mastectomy for breast cancer and is visibly asymmetric. The problems and needs of these patients have not been fully recognized.

Male Breast Cancer

Etiology and Epidemiology. Male breast cancer is a rare disease and often is seen late with a poor prognosis. It accounts for approximately 1% of breast cancer incidence and mortality.[3] The epidemiology and clinical features of the disease generally parallel those of female breast cancer. Men with breast cancer tend to be older and have subareolar tumors, and their disease is found in more advanced stages compared to women with breast cancer. A family history places men at increased risk for breast cancer, as does prior exposure to radiation, exogenous estrogen therapy, and Klinefelter's syndrome. Gynecomastia is not considered a significant risk factor.[10]

Pathophysiology. Approximately 81% of breast cancers in men are ER positive, with ductal infiltrating carcinoma being the predominant histologic cell type.[10] Bioassay for the presence of ER and PR is performed at the time of biopsy. Tumor staging is based on the TNM system. Physical examination, mammography, fine-needle aspiration, and incisional or excisional biopsy are standard diagnostic procedures. The presence of advanced disease at the time of initial diagnosis is common, largely because of delays in seeking medical evaluation.[10]

Gynecomastia caused by drug, alcohol, or hormone ingestion can be differentiated from a malignant lesion by both physical examination and mammogram. Fine-needle aspiration of the lesion may also be used to differentiate gynecomastia from a malignancy. Gynecomastia generally is bilateral, whereas a malignant lesion generally occurs in a single breast.

The symptoms commonly seen at the time of diagnosis include a firm mass directly beneath the nipple in the subareolar area, most frequently in the left breast. The upper outer quadrant is the next most frequent location for tumor growth. Bloody nipple discharge with nipple inversion is common. Evidence of Paget's disease of the nipple (eczema), itching, ulceration, and local tenderness also may be present. Metastasis may occur to bone, the lungs, and the liver.

Collaborative Care Management. Treatment for a primary localized tumor is modified radical mastectomy with node dissection. Breast-sparing procedures are not often used because the male breast has sparse amounts of tissue. In addition, the typical location of the lesion in the subareolar area requires that the nipple be removed along with a tumor-free margin of tissue. Thus breast-preservation procedures cannot be safely used. Radiotherapy may be prescribed before or after surgery for control of micrometastasis or to prevent local recurrence, but radiation has not been shown to significantly increase long-term disease-free survival time.[10] When axillary nodes are involved in the disease process, systemic adjuvant therapy (chemotherapy or hormonal) is advised.

Recurrent or advanced disease is highly amenable to palliative therapy with hormonal manipulation inasmuch as most tumors are ER positive. Tamoxifen is the treatment of choice for metastatic disease. Additional hormonal agents that may be used include progestins, LHRH agonists, and aminoglutethimide. Chemotherapeutic protocols such as cyclophosphamide, methotrexate, and 5-fluorouracil (CMF), and 5-fluorouracil, Adriamycin (doxorubicin), and cyclophosphamide (FAC), may be prescribed.[10]

PATIENT/FAMILY TEACHING. Nursing management of the man with breast cancer reflects the basic principles outlined earlier in the chapter. However, a man in whom breast cancer is diagnosed faces unique psychosocial stressors that the nurse needs to address on an individual basis. The long delays in diagnosis may reflect in part a basic disbelief that this "female problem" can be occurring. A subtheme of embarrassment needs to be identified, if present, and acknowledged. The threats of cancer remain, however, and the treatment is aggressive. The use of tamoxifen has reduced the need for palliative surgeries such as orchiectomy, with their accompanying assault on male self-concept and body image. The male patient treated for breast cancer is an uncommon occurrence; however, the nurse will need to be sensitive to his unique needs and tailor the standard surgical care routines to the individual situation.[20]

Critical Thinking

1. A 78-year-old widow is recovering from a modified radical mastectomy for stage II ductal carcinoma. She has a history of osteoarthritis and hypertension. She is undergoing chemotherapy and tamoxifen therapy. Discuss the issues that may affect this patient's quality of life as a result of her age, diagnosis, treatment regimen, treatment side effects, and psychosocial needs. What interventions should you plan for her?
2. Use the research information presented in the chapter to discuss the importance of BSE and mammography as diagnostic tools for breast cancer. What nursing strategies would be helpful in encouraging earlier breast cancer detection in underserved populations?

References

1. American Cancer Society: *Breast cancer facts and figures 2005,* New York, 2005, The Society.
2. American Cancer Society: *Cancer facts and figures 2004,* New York, 2004, The Society.
3. Baquet CR, Commiskey P: Socioeconomic factors and breast carcinoma in multicultural women, *Cancer* 88(5 Suppl):1256, 2000.
4. Berry JA: Breast pain: all that hurts is not cancer, *Am J Nurs Pract* 5(4):9, 2001.
5. Boyle P, Maisonneuve P, Autier P: Update on cancer control in women, *Int J Gynecol Obstet* 70:263, 2000.
6. Davis BS: Lymphedema after breast cancer treatment, *Am J Nurs* 101(4):26, 2001.
7. Fisher B et al: Tamoxifen, radiation therapy, or both for prevention of ipsilateral breast tumor recurrence after lumpectomy in women with invasive breast cancers of 1 centimeter or less, *J Clin Oncol* 20(20):4141, 2002.
8. Forchuk C et al: Postoperative arm massage: a support for women with lymph node dissection, *Cancer Nurs* 27(1):25, 2004.
9. Gasalberti D: Early detection of breast cancer by self-examination: the influence of perceived barriers and health conception, *Oncol Nurs Forum* 29(9):1341, 2002.
10. Giordano SH, Buzdar AU, Hortobagyi GN: Breast cancer in men, *Ann Intern Med* 137(8):678, 2002.
11. Hadley J, Mitchell J, Mandelblatt J: Medicare fees and small area variations in breast conserving surgery among elderly women, *Med Care Res Rev* 58(3):334, 2001.
12. Harcourt D, Rumsey N: Psychological aspects of breast reconstruction: a review of the literature, *J Adv Nurs* 35(4):477, 2001.
13. Harris SR et al: Clinical practice guidelines for the care and treatment of breast cancer, 11, Lymphedema, *CMAJ-JMAC* 164(2):191, 2001.
14. Hindle WH: Breast cancer prevention and surveillance, *Clin Obstet Gynecol* 45(3):778, 2002.
15. Hindle WH: Treatment of invasive breast carcinoma, *Clin Obstet Gynecol* 45(3):767, 2002.
16. Hunter CP: Epidemiology, stage at diagnosis, and tumor biology of breast carcinoma in multiracial and multiethnic populations, *Cancer* 88(5 Suppl): 1193, 2000.
17. Joslyn SA, West MM: Racial differences in breast cancer survival, *Cancer* 88(1):114, 2000.
18. Kelley MA, Comley A: Breast cancer among minority women: current knowledge and efforts in early detection programs, *Am J Nurs* 101(Suppl): 13, 2001.
19. Kurtz JE, Dufour P: Strategies for improving quality of life in older patients with metastatic breast cancer, *Drugs Aging* 19(8):605, 2002.
20. Loerzel VW, Dow KH: Male breast cancer, *Clin J Oncol Nurs* 8(2):191, 2004.
21. Major MA: Clinical trials update: medical management of advanced breast cancer, *Cancer Nurs* 26(Suppl 6S):10S, 2003.
22. Martin AM, Weber BL: Genetic and hormonal risk factors in breast cancer, *J Natl Cancer Inst* 92(14):1126, 2000.
23. McCready T: Management of patients with breast cancer, *Nurs Stand* 17(41):45, 2003.
24. McGinn K, Moore J: Metastatic breast cancer: understanding current management options, *Oncol Nurs Forum* 28(3):507, 2001.
25. McPherson K, Steel CM, Dixon JM: ABC of breast diseases: breast cancer—epidemiology, risk factors, and genetics, *Br Med J* 321(9):624, 2000.
26. McSpedon C: Silicone safety, *Am J Nurs* 102(4):31, 2002.
27. Miers M: Understanding benign breast disorders and disease, *Nurs Stand* 15(50):45, 2001.
28. Morrow M, Gradishar W: Breast cancer, *Br Med J* 324:410, 2002.
29. Morrow M et al: Standard for breast conservation therapy in the management of invasive breast carcinoma, *CA Cancer J Clin* 52(5):277, 2002.

29a. National Cancer Institute: *Clinical trials: Herceptin,* accessed October 24, 2005, from website: www.cancer.gov/clinicaltrials/digestpage/herceptin.

30. National Comprehensive Cancer Network: *Clinical practice guidelines in oncology: breast cancer*, version 1.2004, accessed June 2004 from www.nccn.org.
31. Osuch J: Breast health and disease over a lifetime, *Clin Obstet Gynecol* 45(4):1140, 2002.
32. Resnick B, Belcher A: Breast reconstruction: options, answers, and support for patients making a difficult personal decision, *Am J Nurs* 102(4):26, 2002.
33. Ridner SH: Breast cancer lymphedema: pathophysiology and risk reduction guidelines, *Oncol Nurs Forumr* 29(9):1285, 2002.
34. Rohrich RJ et al: Classification and management of gynecomastia: defining the role of ultrasound assisted liposuction, *Plast Reconstr Surg* 111(2):909, 2003.
35. Rosenzweig MQ, Rust D, Hoss J: Prognostic information in breast cancer care: helping patients utilize important information, *Clin J Oncol Nurs* 4(6):271, 2000.
36. Sakorafas GH: The management of women at high risk for the development of breast cancer: risk estimation and preventative strategies, *Cancer Treat Rev* 29:79, 2003.
37. Sammarco A: Perceived social support, uncertainty, and quality of life among younger breast cancer survivors, *Cancer Nurs* 24(3):212, 2001.
38. Sammarco A: Quality of life among older survivors of breast cancer, *Cancer Nurs* 26(6):431, 2003.
39. Sandau K: Free TRAM flap breast reconstruction, *Am J Nurs* 102(4):36, 2002.
40. Shuster TD et al: Multidisciplinary care for patients with breast cancer, *Surg Clin North Am* 80(2):505, 2000.
41. Simpson JK: Treatment considerations for the elderly person with cancer, *AACN Clin Issues Adv Pract Acute Crit Care* 13(1):43, 2002.
42. Smith RA et al: American Cancer Society guidelines for breast cancer screening: update 2003, *CA Cancer J Clin* 53(3):141, 2003.
43. Thors CL, Broeckel JA, Jacobsen PB: Sexual functioning in breast cancer survivors, *CancerControl* 8(5):442, 2001.
44. US Department of Health and Human Services: *Healthy people 2010: understanding and improving health,* Washington, DC, 2000, The Department.
45. Zimmerman VL: BRCA gene mutations and cancer, *Am J Nurs* 102(8):28, 2002.

Visit the Evolve website: http://evolve.elsevier.com/Monahan/medsurg

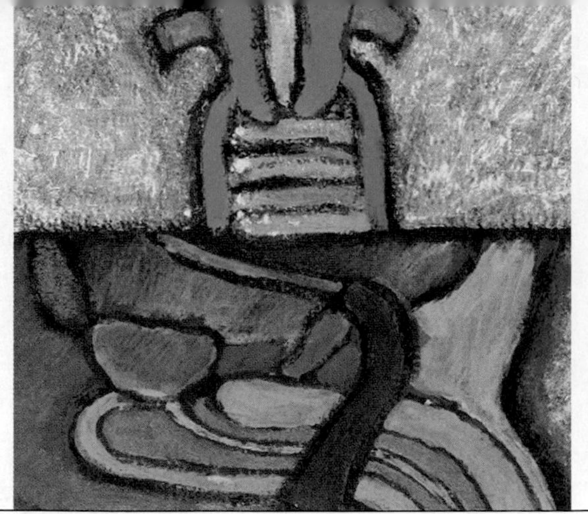

CHAPTER 59
Sexually Transmitted Diseases

by Margaret K. Warshaw

OBJECTIVES

After studying this chapter, the learner should be able to:

1. Define sexually transmitted disease (STD).
2. Describe the transmission, prevention, and control of STDs and urovaginal infections.
3. List the causative agent, incubation period, signs and symptoms, medical therapy, and long-term effects of gonorrhea, chlamydia, syphilis, genital herpes, and human papillomavirus infections.
4. Identify the information to be collected from a person suspected of having any STD or urovaginal infections.
5. Write a teaching plan for a unit on the prevention of STDs for a sexuality education course for adolescents.

KEY TERMS

abstinence, p. 1784
condom, p. 1783
congenital, p. 1780
incubation period, p. 1785
monogamous relationships, p. 1784
viral shedding, p. 1791

Etiology and Epidemiology. Sexually transmitted diseases (STDs) or sexually transmitted infections (STIs), once called venereal diseases, are among the most common infectious diseases in the United States today. STDs are infections that can be transmitted from one person to another through sexual contact. It is important to note that sexual contact includes more than vaginal or anal intercourse. Sexual contact also includes kissing, oral-genital or oral-anal contact, and use of sexual toys such as vibrators.[21]

There are some notable exceptions to sexual transmission. If a mother has syphilis during pregnancy, the fetus may become infected in utero by placental transmission, and the neonate may acquire **congenital** syphilis or be stillborn. Infants of mothers with gonorrhea or chlamydia may contract an infection of the eyes (ophthalmia neonatorum) during birth; unless treated, the infection can lead to permanent blindness. Chlamydia present at birth is a common cause of subacute, afebrile pneumonia occurring in the infant between 1 and 3 months old.

Venereology today encompasses not only the five venerable venereal diseases (gonorrhea, syphilis, chancroid, lymphogranuloma venereum, and granuloma inguinale) but also a growing number of other diseases that may be considered the new generation of STDs. Many of these newer STDs such as chlamydia, genital herpes, and human papillomavirus (HPV) have, like gonorrhea, become epidemic in nearly all countries of the world over the past 2 decades. More than 20 STDs have been identified. These diseases can be classified either by their etiologies or their clinical manifestations.[22] Table 59-1 lists an etiologic classification of the most common STDs.

Acquired immunodeficiency syndrome (AIDS) was first reported in the United States in 1981 and has since been identified as a major STD. It is caused by the human immunodeficiency virus (HIV), which destroys the body's ability to fight off infection. Because of the profound effect of AIDS on the immune system, Chapter 22 is devoted to its discussion.

In every state syphilis, gonorrhea, chlamydia, and AIDS are reportable to the Centers for Disease Control and Prevention (CDC). HIV infection and chancroid are reportable in many states. Genital herpes, trichomoniasis, and HPV infection are not nationally reportable. The requirements for reporting other STDs differ by states, and it is important that clinicians are familiar with local reporting requirements.[28]

TABLE 59-1 ETIOLOGIC CLASSIFICATION OF SEXUALLY TRANSMITTED DISEASES

Organism	Disease
BACTERIA	
Neisseria gonorrhoea	Gonorrhea
Chlamydia trachomatis	Chlamydia
Treponema pallidum	Syphilis
Haemophilus ducreyi	Chancroid
Calymmatobacterium granulomatis	Granuloma inguinale (Donovanosis)
VIRUS	
Herpes simplex virus 1 (HSV-1)	Oral herpes
Herpes simplex virus 2 (HSV-2)	Genital herpes
Hepatitis A, B, C	Acute hepatitis
Cytomegalovirus	Congenital infection, birth defects, infant mortality
Human immuno-deficiency virus (HIV)	Acquired immunodeficiency syndrome (AIDS)
Human papillo-mavirus (HPV)	Condylomata acuminata (genital warts)
Molluscipoxvirus organisms	Molluscum contagiosum (genital warts)
PROTOZOA	
Trichomonas vaginalis	Trichomoniasis
FUNGI	
Candida albicans	Vulvovaginitis
ECTOPARASITES	
Phthirus pubis	Pubic lice
Sarcoptes scabiei	Scabies

It is estimated that approximately 19 million new cases of STDs occur each year in the United States, of which almost half are among persons ages 15 to 24. The annual estimated direct medical cost of these STDs is $13 billion.[6a]

Although most STDs are treatable, the toll that these diseases take on American youth, especially females, is formidable. The complications facing many infected with an STD include pelvic inflammatory disease (PID), infertility, sterility, ectopic pregnancy (can be fatal) that is a precursor to cancer, increased susceptibility to other diseases, fetal deformities and mental retardation, and death.[3] Many reasons have been cited for the rising incidence of STDs, including:

- Failure of clinicians to ensure that the sexual partners of patients with STDs are examined and treated.[22]
- Earlier sexual activity among young people coupled with later marriage. Divorce is also more common. The result is that sexually active people are more likely to have multiple sex partners during their lives, increasing their risk for developing STDs.
- Normal tendency for risk-taking behaviors among 15 to 24 year olds.
- Increased use of birth control pills, which has reduced the use of barrier contraceptive methods that offer some protection against disease.
- Absence of recognizable symptoms of many STDs, particularly in women. A person who is infected may unknowingly transmit the disease to a sex partner.
- Vagueness of symptoms of STDs, which may be confused with those of other diseases not transmitted through sexual contact. Again, the disease may be unknowingly transmitted.
- Poor implementation of treatment guidelines despite wide dissemination. Females, particularly adolescents, are often not examined and treated with STDs as a possibility.[8]
- Widespread use of antibiotics for several decades, which has led to organisms developing a resistance to them over time, thereby decreasing their effectiveness.
- Diminished focus on STD prevention education for young people, men who have sex with men, and other high-risk populations since bioterrorism, West Nile virus, and severe acute respiratory syndrome have become greater problems.

Pathophysiology. Although many persons with STDs are clinically asymptomatic, others commonly have genital lesions, genital itching or burning, changes in vaginal discharge, lower abdominal pain, penile discharge, or pain with intercourse.

Collaborative Care Management

DIAGNOSTIC TESTS. Specific diagnostic tests are used to establish the diagnosis of each of these diseases. Diagnostic tests for selected diseases are presented in Table 59-2.

MEDICATIONS. Treatment depends on the causative organisms identified through the history, physical examination, and diagnostic tests, as discussed in the following section. It is not unusual for an individual to harbor two or more organisms simultaneously. See Table 59-2 for standard treatment modalities for gonorrhea, chlamydia, syphilis, HPV (condylomata acuminata), and genital herpes.

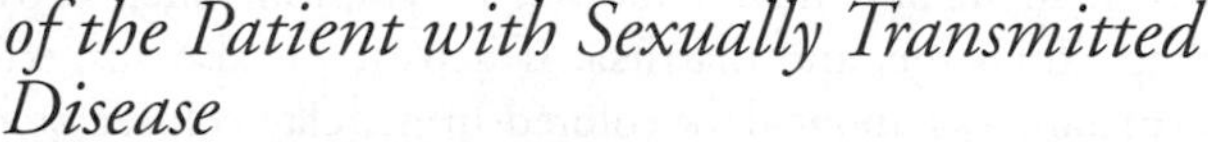

Nursing Management *of the Patient with Sexually Transmitted Disease*

ASSESSMENT

Health History. Assess for:

- Exposure to STD contact, including HIV
- Prior STD history, treatment
- Sexual orientation: heterosexual, homosexual, bisexual

TABLE 59-2 DIAGNOSIS AND TREATMENT OF SEXUALLY TRANSMITTED DISEASES

Disease	Diagnostic Test	Medical Treatment
Gonorrhea	**Nucleic acid test:** Identifies strand of bacterial DNA Done on urine or sample of secretion from potentially infected area (urethra, cervix) *Not* done on rectum or throat Highly sensitive and specific **Gram stain test:** Smear from secretions (urethra, cervix) placed on slide, stained, bacteria identified microscopically Results available during visit Results reliable for men, not reliable for women **Culture test:** Swab inserted into cervix, rectum, urethra, throat Culture plate incubated 24-72 hr Highly specific, highly reliable	Ceftriaxone, 125 mg IM in a single dose; cefixime, 400 mg PO in a single dose; ciprofloxacin, 500 mg PO in a single dose; or ofloxacin, 400 mg PO in a single dose, plus azithromycin,1 g PO in a single dose, or doxycycline, 100 mg PO bid for 7 days (individuals with gonorrhea concurrently treated for chlamydia) Quinolone therapy *not* indicated for those who contract gonorrhea in California or Hawaii; also not indicated for men who have sex with men
Syphilis	**Darkfield microscopy**: Material from chancre examined under special darkfield microscope to identify organisms **Nontreponemal blood tests (nonspecific for organisms, only antibodies)** VDRL (Venereal Disease Research Laboratory) RPR (rapid plasma reagent) Treponemal blood tests (confirm positive results of nontreponemal tests) FTA-ABS (fluorescent treponemal antibody absorption test) MHA-TP (microhemagglutination–*Treponema pallidum*)	Penicillin G benzathine, 2.4 million units IM
Genital herpes	**Viral culture:** Lesion swabbed, sample added to culture of healthy cells, examined in 2 days; changes in healthy cells indicate growth of herpes virus	Herpes primary occurrence: acyclovir, 400 mg PO tid, for 7-10 days, or 200 mg PO 5 times a day for 7-10 days; or famciclovir, 250 mg PO tid for 7-10 days; or valacyclovir, 1 g PO bid, for 7-10 days

- Relationship of onset of symptoms to last sexual intercourse
- Number of sexual partners in the past 6 months
- Travel history, self and partner(s)

Women are questioned about last menstrual period, vaginal discharge (color, odor, amount), vulvar itching, dysuria, urinary urgency, lower abdominal pain, rectal symptoms, sore throat, genital lesions, and skin rashes or itching. Men are questioned about urethral discharge, dysuria, genital lesions, skin rashes, itching, testicular pain, and sore throat. Women and gay and bisexual men are also asked about rectal symptoms such as pain, bleeding, discharge, and diarrhea. If hepatitis is also suspected, the clinician asks about dark-colored urine, clay-colored stools, fatigue, and jaundice.

Physical Examination. Assess for:

- Lesions of the skin or mucous membrane
- Erythema or other color change of genitalia
- Edema of genitalia
- Evidence of vaginal or penile discharge
- Odor
- Nits on hair shafts[11]

These assessments require inspection and palpation of the integumentary system, reproductive system, and anorectal area. Therefore the physical examination of the patient suspected of having an STD includes:

- Inspection of skin of lower abdomen, inguinal area, hands, palms, and forearms
- Inspection of pubic hair
- Inspection and palpation of external genitalia, including perineum and anus
- Speculum examination of vagina and cervix in women
- Bimanual examination of the uterus and adnexa in women
- Pregnancy test for all women of childbearing age
- Inspection of the penis, including the meatus, with retraction of the foreskin and "milking" of the urethra in men
- Palpation of the scrotum in men
- Palpation for inguinal and femoral lymphadenopathy
- Inspection of mouth and throat, including tonsils
- Inspection of the anorectal area in women and homosexual or bisexual men
- Anoscopic examination if there are rectal symptoms in women and homosexual or bisexual men

TABLE 59-2 DIAGNOSIS AND TREATMENT OF SEXUALLY TRANSMITTED DISEASES—CONT'D

Disease	Diagnostic Test	Medical Treatment
Genital herpes—cont'd	**Serum antibodies:** Blood test—does not determine if infection is active; does not distinguish HSV-1 from HSV-2 **POCkit rapid test:** Finger prick for capillary blood; instant results for HSV-2 only **ELISA kit/immunoblot kit:** Blood drawn, results 1-2 wk; determines HSV-1 and HSV-2; >99% accuracy **Herpes western blot:** Blood drawn, results in 2 wk; determines HSV-1, HSV-2; >99% accurate	Recurrence: acyclovir, 400 mg PO tid, for 5 days Suppression: acyclovir, 400 mg PO bid, for 1 yr; or famciclovir, 250 mg PO bid; or valacyclovir 0.5-1.0 g/day PO
Chlamydia	**Culture test** (direct DNA probe): Secretions placed on plate and incubated; 100% specificity **Nonculture tests** Direct fluorescein antibody (DFA): Visualization of elementary bodies on smears; takes 30-40 min EIA (enzyme immunoassays): Detects chlamydial antigens; takes 3-4 hr Rapid (STAT) test (kit): Takes 30 min Nucleic acid amplification test: FVU (first voided urine); specificity and sensitivity 82%-100%	Azithromycin, 1 g PO in a single dose, or doxycycline, 100 mg PO bid, for 7 days
Human papillomavirus	Most often diagnosed on the basis of clinical presentation; suspicious lesions are biopsied	Patient-applied: podofilox, 0.5% solution bid for 3 days, then 4 days of no therapy, repeat up to 4 cycles; or imiquimod, 5% cream qhs, 3 times a week for up to 16 wk Provider applied: 80%-90% trichloroacetic-bichloroacetic acid; intralesional interferon; surgical treatment (laser, cryotherapy, electrocautery, or loop electrosurgical excision procedure)

DNA, Deoxyribonucleic acid; *IM,* intramuscular; *PO,* by mouth; *bid,* twice a day; *HSV,* herpes simplex virus; *tid,* three times a day; *qhs,* once a day at bedtime.

NURSING DIAGNOSES, OUTCOMES, AND INTERVENTIONS

Nursing Diagnosis: Ineffective Health Maintenance

OUTCOMES. Common examples of expected outcomes for the patient with a diagnosis of *ineffective health maintenance* are:

Patient or patient and partner will:

- Explain the etiology and factors contributing to the STD.
- Describe resources necessary to achieve health.
- Identify personal strengths and weaknesses.
- Participate actively and appropriately in health maintenance activities.

NURSING INTERVENTIONS

PATIENT/FAMILY EDUCATION. The nurse's first responsibility in STD control is to educate persons who have an STD or may develop one. Nurses must be knowledgeable about the most prevalent diseases, the signs and symptoms, methods used in diagnosis, treatments used, and where individuals can obtain help and information. Nurses also can influence the knowledge and attitudes of their colleagues and peers toward STD and its control. Nurses can exert influence in the community by taking an active role in education programs. The best way to reduce the risk of STD is for every person who is sexually active to limit the number of sexual partners. Sexual activity with different partners increases the risk of infection. Using a **condom** is recommended but is no guarantee against passing on or acquiring an STD. Proper use of a condom is found in Box 59-1.

The person with an STD is often young, fearful of pain, and unaccustomed to being in a clinic or physician's office. Young people especially fear that their families and friends may learn they have an STD. For adolescents, contracting an STD and securing help means they must admit to sexual activity, which may cause guilt. People with STDs may feel their self-esteem is threatened by what has happened to them. They may express anger. Persons with an STD have not only physical and social problems but also perhaps economic problems (paying for the treatment) and emotional problems dealing with the diagnosis. They need constructive and comprehensive help. Before nurses can be effective in working with persons who have STDs, they must confront their own feelings and attitudes about STDs. The nurse must maintain a nonjudgmental approach and create an

Box 59-1 Recommendations from Centers for Disease Control and Prevention for the Use of Condoms

Condoms must be used consistently and correctly to be highly effective in preventing sexually transmitted diseases (STDs). The following recommendations ensure the proper use of male condoms:

- Use a new condom with each act of sexual intercourse (i.e., oral, vaginal, anal).
- Do not use condoms lubricated with spermicides such as nonoxynol-9. They are no more effective against transmission of human immunodeficiency virus (HIV) and other STDs than other lubricated condoms. Also, they cost more, have a shorter shelf life, and may cause urinary tract infections in young women.
- Carefully handle the condom to avoid damaging it with fingernails, teeth, or other sharp objects.
- Put the condom on after the penis is erect and before any genital contact with the partner.
- Use only water-based lubricants (e.g., K-Y Jelly, Astroglide, Aqua Lube, and glycerin) with latex condoms. Oil-based lubricants (e.g., petroleum jelly, shortening, mineral oil, massage oils, body lotions, and cooking oil) can weaken latex.
- Ensure adequate lubrication during intercourse, with the use of exogenous lubricants if necessary.
- Hold the condom firmly against the base of the penis during withdrawal, and withdraw while the penis is still erect to prevent slippage.

From Workowski K, Levine W: Sexually transmitted diseases treatment guidelines—2002, *Morbid Moral Week Rep* 51(RR06):4-5, 2002, accessed from website: www.cdc.gov/mmwr.

atmosphere of trust in which the person feels free to discuss all aspects of the problem.

Once the diagnosis, tentative or conclusive, is made, focus is placed on obtaining a cure and preventing complications and reinfection. Because some of the diseases respond to penicillin or other antibiotics, many people believe that all genital infections can be cured easily, but this is not so. Some people believe that antibiotics not only cure an infection but also produce immunity against reinfection. The nurse informs patients receiving an antibiotic or other medications of the drug's action, duration of effectiveness, side effects, chances of cure, and the need for follow-up care. The nurse advises them that treatment failures do occur and that reinfection rates are high. Return visits for follow-up care are encouraged when necessary.

Persons treated for STDs need information about self-care. To understand their therapy and to responsibly engage in self-care, they must be informed about the sexual nature of the infection, how it is transmitted, and the possibility of reinfection and infection of their sexual partner or partners. Patients need to know that it is important that sexual partners be notified and checked for signs of infection, to be advised of what the signs are, and to be tested for asymptomatic infection. The nurse advises patients to abstain from intercourse until they and their partners are cured. The use of condoms must be stressed to prevent infection or reinfection if patients persist in engaging in intercourse even when advised not to do so.

Teaching about hygiene and personal health practices is beneficial in reducing the chances of reinfection or secondary infection. Frequent bathing and hand washing are indicated. Soap and water destroy many of the organisms causing STDs. For women, douching at any time is inadvisable, since this may disturb the vaginal and cervical environments and predispose the woman to infection.

If the lesions are present on body surfaces, the person should be instructed in their care. Both men and women are advised to wear cotton underwear, and women should avoid wearing pantyhose, since they tend to trap moisture and prevent circulation of air to the genitalia. Unless lotions, creams, or ointments are specifically prescribed as local medications, the patient should not apply them to any of the lesions associated with an STD.

Genital self-examination is important for sexually active persons. The nurse recommends that they inspect skin, mouth, genitalia, and perianal areas for lesions and discharges. Self-inspection helps the person become educated about the signs and symptoms of STDs and how to look for them. In addition, people can learn to casually inspect their partners during the initial period of lovemaking to identify any signs of STDs. Urinating after sexual activity can be helpful in cleansing the urethra of organisms.

Opportunities for promoting healthy attitudes about sexual activity and STDs frequently arise. The nurse approaches these topics tactfully and with consideration of the person's feelings. Adolescents especially require an approach that indicates understanding balanced with the ability to help them set limits. They need to understand that they are responsible for their own bodies, and they do not have to give in to sexual pressures. It is well documented, however, that the strongest influence on teenagers comes from their peer group. For this reason, discussion with groups of teenagers about their sexual responsibilities may be helpful. In the climate of the twenty-first century there should be no doubt that **abstinence** is the only absolute way to prevent STDs. If a teen elects to be sexually active, he or she needs to understand that the consequences of unprotected sex may include unwanted pregnancy, an STD, or possibly cervical cancer. **Monogamous relationships** and the proper use of condoms should be stressed for those who are sexually active.

HEALTH PROMOTION AND PREVENTION. Prevention and control measures for STDs include three levels of prevention. Primary prevention is directed at preventing the disease. This includes educating uninfected persons so they can take responsibility for their own health and not expose themselves to an infected person; identification and treatment of exposed persons who are asymptomatic; interviewing persons with infection for identification, examination, and preventive treatment of contacts; educational programs for the public; and active involvement of professionals in programs of control. The goal of these efforts includes eradication of the reservoir of disease in the population. Secondary prevention is directed toward screening, early diagnosis, and treatment. Tertiary prevention focuses on preventing complications and supporting and counseling infected persons to receive treatment.

In the prevention and control of STDs, young people often fear that their parents and the parents of the sexual partner(s) will find out about their infection. Minors need to know that, in most cases, they can obtain treatment without parental consent. Currently most states permit health care providers to treat minors for STDs without obtaining parental consent, and several states are proposing changes in existing legislation that restricts treatment of minors.

The nurse interviews the patient about his or her contacts at the time of the initial visit in case the patient does not return for follow-up care. It is probably best that this interview take place after the patient is examined, the type of infection is determined, and the treatment is prescribed. If assessment is accompanied by patient education, the person will be better informed about STDs and how they are treated and be more willing to give information about sexual contacts. People may perceive reporting of STDs as a threat from an official agency and may hesitate to name their contacts out of a sense of protection if they do not know that no punishment is involved.

Because one focus of STD control is increasing self-referrals, the patient is asked to inform her or his sexual partner(s) (partner notification) to come in for examination and treatment. Confidentiality is stressed. Because of the understandable reluctance of many people to name their sexual partner(s), the patient may be given the responsibility of informing the contacts and advising them of their need for treatment. Local health departments cooperate in locating, examining, and treating contacts when necessary.

Whenever possible, the sexual partners of the infected person are advised to have an examination and tests as soon as possible. If the sexual partner or partners do not have symptoms of infection at the time of the first examination, treatment is still instituted. Giving preventive treatment to contacts who have no clinical evidence of infection is common practice in the United States; this same approach is used in management of patients with "minor" STDs.

Healthy People 2010 built on the goals attained by *Healthy People 2000* and established several goals related to the reduction of STDs to be achieved by the year 2010 (see Healthy People 2010 box). The special population targets for objective 1 appear in Table 59-3. To support the achievement of these important goals, *Healthy People 2010* identified leading health indicators. Those for the area of STDs are: (1) responsible adolescent sexual behavior, and (2) condom use by adults.

RELATED NIC INTERVENTIONS. Discharge Planning, Health Screening, Health System Guidance, Risk Identification, Support System Enhancement

EVALUATION

To evaluate the effectiveness of nursing interventions, compare patient behaviors with those stated in the expected patient outcomes.

RELATED NOC OUTCOMES. Health Promoting Behavior, Health Seeking Behavior, Self-Direction of Care, Social Support

Healthy People 2010

Goal and Objectives Related to Reduction of Sexually Transmitted Diseases

Goal

Promote responsible sexual behaviors, strengthen community capacity, and increase access to high-quality services to prevent sexually transmitted diseases (STDs) and their complications.

Objectives

Reduce the proportion of adolescents and young adults with *Chlamydia trachomatis* infections.

Reduce gonorrhea.

Eliminate sustained domestic transmission of primary and secondary syphilis.

Reduce the proportion of adults with genital herpes infection.

Reduce the proportion of persons with human papillomavirus infection.

Reduce the proportion of females who have ever required treatment for pelvic inflammatory disease (PID).

Reduce the proportion of childless women with fertility problems who have had an STD or required treatment for PID.

Increase the proportion of adolescents who abstain from sexual intercourse or use condoms if currently sexually active.

Increase the number of positive messages related to responsible sexual behavior during weekday and nightly prime-time television programming.

From US Department of Health and Human Services: *Healthy people 2010: understanding and improving health,* Washington, DC, 2000, The Department.

Gonorrhea

Etiology and Epidemiology. Gonorrhea, sometimes referred to as GC or "the clap" by laypeople, is caused by *Neisseria gonorrhoeae.* Gonorrhea is of great concern, because persons with it often have another STD such as chlamydia or HIV. There is a possibility for a high reinfection rate and serious residual effects. The **incubation period** is 3 to 30 days in men and 3 days to an indefinite period in women.[5]

The CDC estimates that more than 700,000 persons in the United States acquire new gonococcal infections each year. From 1975 to 1997 the national gonorrhea rate declined following the implementation of a national gonorrhea control program. After a small increase in 1998, the gonorrhea rate has decreased slightly since 1999. In 2002 the rate of reported gonorrheal infections was 125 per 100,000 persons, or 351,852 cases[6]; and in 2004, 330,132 cases were reported[6a] (Figure 59-1). Men and women are almost equally affected (Figure 59-2).

The incidence of gonorrhea is highest in high-density urban areas among persons under 24 years of age (Figure 59-3) who have multiple sex partners and engage in unprotected sexual intercourse. Significant increases in gonorrhea prevalence have been noted since 1993 among men who have sex with men.

Southern states continue to have the highest gonorrhea rates of any region. Young African-American women and men have the highest incidence of gonorrhea and remain at extremely high risk[6]

TABLE 59-3 *HEALTHY PEOPLE 2010* GOALS TO REDUCE SEXUALLY TRANSMITTED DISEASES

Disease	Population	Baseline	Goal
Chlamydia	Females 15-24 yr attending family planning clinics Females 15-24 yr attending STD clinics Males 15-24 yr attending STD clinics	5.0% (1997) 12.2% (1997) 15.7% (1997)	Expand *Healthy People 2000* and track percent positivity among women ages 15-24 who attend STD clinics in addition to family planning clinics. Expand *Healthy People 2000* to include men ages 15-24 yr who attended STD clinics with positive results.
Gonorrhea		123 cases per 100,000 (1997)	Reduce gonorrhea (targets not yet specified).
Syphilis (primary and secondary)		3.2 cases per 100,000 (1997)	Eliminate sustained domestic transmission of primary and secondary syphilis.
Genital herpes	Adults 20-29 yr	17% (1988-1994)	Modify *Healthy People 2000* to track proportion of persons with positive laboratory test for herpes simplex virus 2.
Human papillomavirus	15-44 yr	Operational definition does not yet exist	Propose reducing number of HPV cases to minimize prevalence of subtypes 16 and 18 and other subtypes associated with cervical cancer.

STD, Sexually transmitted disease; *HPV*, human papillomavirus.

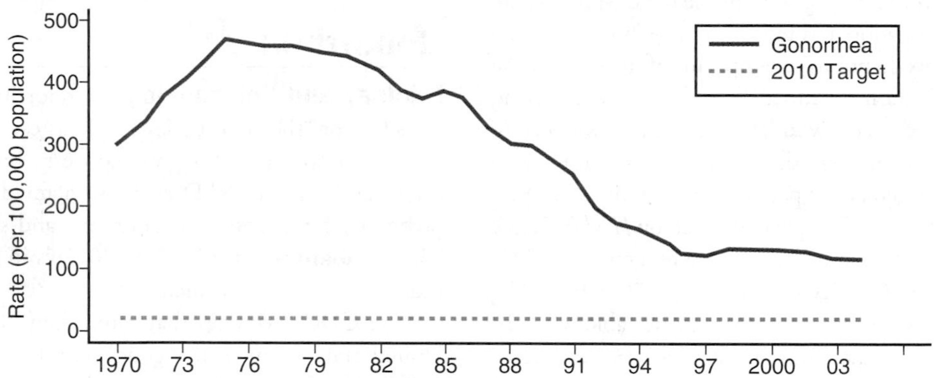

Figure 59-1 Gonorrhea rates: United States, 1970-2004, and the *Healthy People 2010* target. The *Healthy People 2010* target is 19 cases per 100,000 population.

(Figure 59-4). When considering these statistics, it is important to remember that only about half the cases treated are reported to the CDC, so the actual number of cases is much larger.

Asymptomatic persons are an important reservoir for infection because they usually remain untreated. Women are more likely to be asymptomatic than men, but suffer more severe complications from unrecognized early infections. Among men rectal infections result from penetration by an infected penis and are followed by symptomatic proctitis in half of cases. Rectal infection is found in a small number of women with cervical infections.

It is estimated that the total cost of gonorrhea in the United States is several billion dollars yearly. Women and their offspring suffer the major physical, emotional, and economic burden. PID occurs in 10% to 20% of women with gonorrhea. Even when treated, these women are likely to suffer from recurrent salpingitis, ectopic pregnancy, infertility, and menstrual abnormalities and may face surgical removal of the pelvic organs, as well as fetal loss.

Pathophysiology. The most common signs and symptoms of gonorrhea are listed in the Clinical Manifestations box. In men

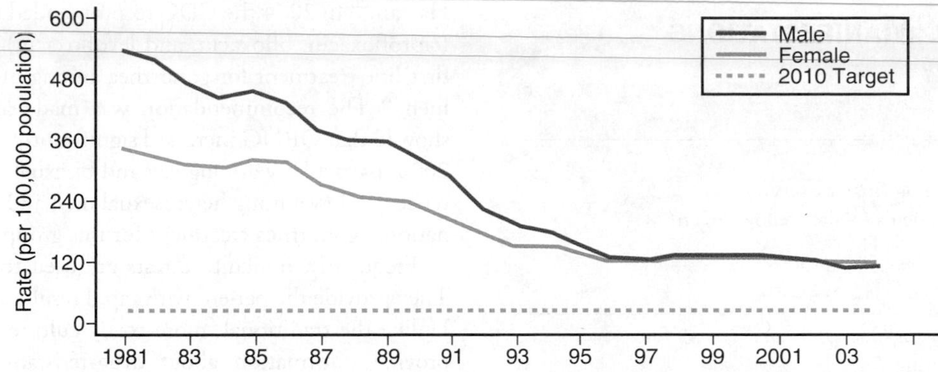

Figure 59-2 Gonorrhea rates by sex: United States, 1981-2004, and the *Healthy People 2010* target.

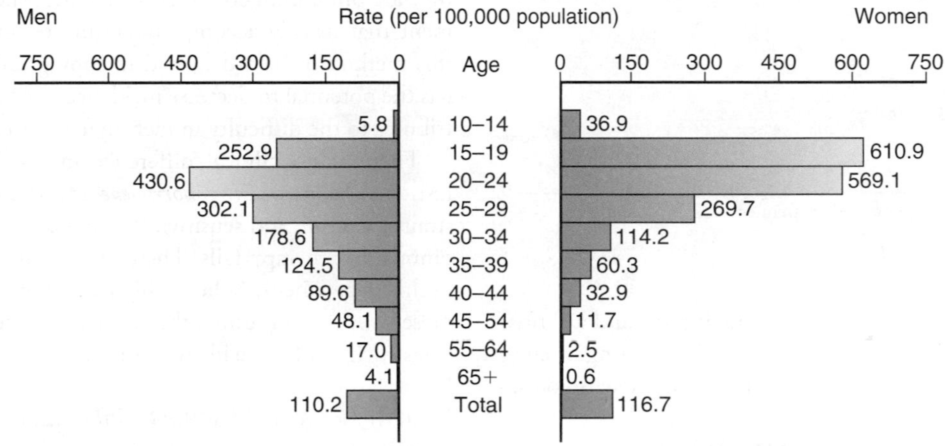

Figure 59-3 Gonorrhea age- and sex-specific rates: United States, 2004.

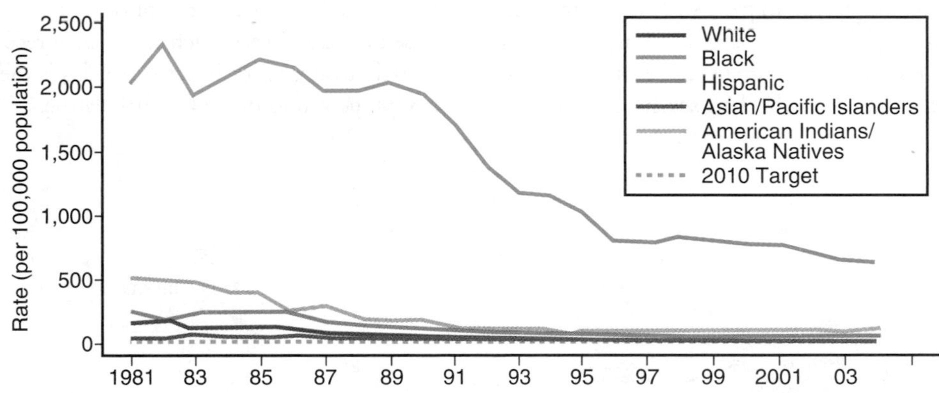

Figure 59-4 Gonorrhea rates by race and ethnicity: United States, 1981-2004, and the *Healthy People 2010* target.

the gonococcus is introduced into the anterior urethra during sexual activity. Because most men are diagnosed and treated early, complications and residual effects of gonorrhea are uncommon. Sterility from orchitis or epididymitis can occur as a rare residual effect. The incidence of asymptomatic gonorrhea in men is believed to be low; however, men with asymptomatic infection are an important factor in the transmission of gonorrhea. Some men have been found to have no symptoms of infection despite positive tests for gonorrhea 2 weeks after exposure.

Gonorrhea in women most often first results in asymptomatic cervicitis. The infection can be present for extended periods without causing noticeable signs, hence the high number of infected, asymptomatic women. These women do not receive treatment unless gonorrhea is diagnosed through screening or is identified by a sexual partner who comes in for treatment. Complications are commonly the first indicators of gonorrhea in women. In cases of untreated gonorrhea, the consequences are serious (Figure 59-5). Other complications of untreated gonorrhea in both men

CLINICAL MANIFESTATIONS
Gonorrhea

Men

Urethritis
Dysuria, frequency, burning (may be severe)
Purulent discharge from penis (white, yellow, green)
Painful, swollen testicles

Women

Vaginal discharge (yellow or bloody)
Dysuria, frequency, burning
Vaginal bleeding with intercourse
Vague feeling of fullness or discomfort in pelvis and/or abdomen

Men and Women

Rectal gonorrhea
—Anal pruritus
—Painful bowel movement
—Occasional blood in stool
Pharyngeal gonorrhea
—Occasional red, sore throat

NOTE: Persons infected with gonorrhea are frequently asymptomatic.

and women include dermatitis, carditis, meningitis, and arthritis. The incidence of these complications is higher among women because of the prolonged period of infection without symptoms.

Collaborative Care Management. Although fluoroquinolones are the treatment of choice (see Table 59-2), some *N. gonorrhoeae* strains resistant to fluoroquinolones have been reported sporadically and are more widespread in parts of Asia. Quinolone-resistant *N. gonorrhoeae* (QRNG) has also been noted in the United States. The CDC has recommended that quinolone antibiotics not be given to anyone who had sex in California or Hawaii.[28] In 2004 the CDC recommended that fluoroquinolones (ciprofloxacin, ofloxacin, and levofloxacin) no longer be used as first-line treatment for gonorrhea among men who have sex with men.[6a] The recommendation was made after preliminary data showed that QRNG increased significantly in the United States in 2003, particularly among gay and bisexual men. Since the occurrence was low among heterosexual men and women, no change in national gonorrhea treatment for this group was recommended.

Frequently, nonculture tests are used to diagnose gonorrhea. They provide the patient with rapid results at a relatively low cost. Unlike the traditional, more costly culture, however, they fail to provide information about drug-resistant strains. Nationwide monitoring of drug resistance is a difficult job. Nonculture kits are used in the field at point of service for young people in many areas of the country. Young people are treated immediately, since they are often unlikely to return for the follow-up care and treatment that usually accompany culture testing. It is believed that this method of field-delivered therapy greatly improves care and has the potential to decrease incidence.[23] At the same time, it contributes to the difficulty in identifying resistance.

There is no clinical difference in the infections caused by resistant strains of *N. gonorrhoeae* and those caused by sensitive strains. Culture and sensitivity testing is performed when the recommended therapy fails. These failures are reported to the local health department. When a high number of resistant strains are present in a community, the sequelae of acute gonococcal infections such as PID are likely to increase.

PATIENT/FAMILY TEACHING. Prevention of gonorrhea and its complications can be achieved in three stages. Primary prevention of the disease is the first and most crucial stage. Secondary prevention involves prevention of complications of the disease such as PID. Tertiary prevention entails reversal of the damage caused by the disease, such as by tubal reconstruction.

Early treatment of infected persons is the most effective way to prevent new infection of sexual partners. Treatment of choice is

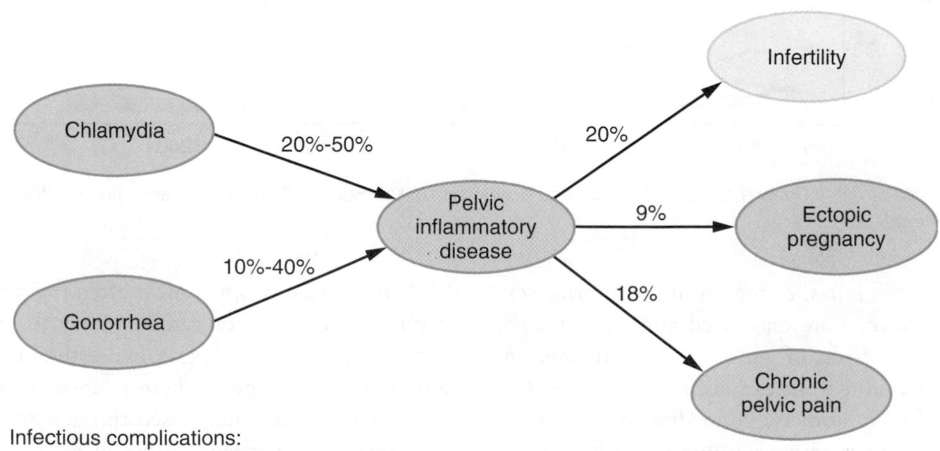

Figure 59-5 Consequences of chlamydia and gonorrhea. *HIV,* Human immunodeficiency virus.

ciprofloxacin, 500 mg orally in a single dose, or ceftriaxone, 125 mg intramuscularly (IM) in a single dose. Mechanical barrier methods such as condoms may reduce the risk of transmission but do not guarantee prevention of gonorrhea. Education to acquaint people with the symptoms of gonorrhea, the efficacy of condoms, and the availability of diagnostic and treatment resources is important. Early detection through partner notification and screening can reduce serious complications of gonorrhea, especially in women.

Most health care providers recommend that all persons with gonorrhea be treated for chlamydia even if there are no signs or symptoms because coinfection frequently occurs and treatment is often less costly than a chlamydia test.[1] All patients with gonorrhea should be offered testing and counseling for HIV and other STDs.

▶ ARE You READY?

Which of the following medications is the drug of choice to treat gonorrhea?

1. Ciprofloxacin
2. Penicillin
3. Gentamycin
4. Metronidazole

Syphilis

Etiology and Epidemiology. Syphilis is an STD caused by a spiral-shaped bacterium, *Treponema pallidum,* commonly called a *spirochete.* The organism is transmitted from open lesions of infected persons to the mucous membrane or abraded skin of sexual partners through vaginal, oral-genital, or genital-anal contacts. Syphilis may also be transmitted from an infected pregnant woman to her fetus after the fourth month of pregnancy via placental blood. The incubation period for syphilis is usually 3 weeks. However, symptoms can appear as early as 9 days or as long as 3 months after exposure. The organism requires a warm, moist environment for survival. It is readily destroyed by physical and chemical agents, including heat, drying, and soap and water. Syphilis is curable but, if untreated, can progress through several stages of development, leading to a number of severe complications. The complications of late syphilis can include damage to heart, eyes, brain, nervous system, bones, joints, or almost any other part of the body. Mental illness, blindness, and death may result.

The rate of primary and secondary (P&S) syphilis reported in the United States decreased during the 1990s and in 2000 was the lowest since reporting began in 1941. However, the number of cases of P&S syphilis increased 2.1% between 2000 and 2001 and further increased by 12.4% between 2001 and 2002. In 2004, 7980 cases of P&S syphilis were reported to CDC, an increase of 11.2% over 2003[6a] (Figure 59-6). Increases in cases from 2000 to 2002 were observed only among men and were associated with reports in several cities of syphilis outbreaks among men who have sex with men. These outbreaks have been characterized by high rates of HIV coinfection and high-risk sexual behavior. The number of P&S syphilis cases among women and among African-Americans has decreased every year from 1990 to 2003, and the number of P&S syphilis cases declined 19% among women and 10.3% among African-Americans.[7] Between 2003 and 2004 it remained unchanged at 0.5 cases per 100,000 women but increased by 453 or 16.9% in African-Americans, with all but 1% of the increase being among men.

Despite continued national progress toward elimination in these groups, syphilis remains an important problem in the South and, increasingly, in urban areas of the country that have large populations of homosexual and bisexual men. Rates in all regions of the country exceed the *Healthy People 2010* objective of 0.2 cases per 100,000 persons.[7]

Untreated syphilis during pregnancy results in perinatal death in up to 40% of cases; if acquired during the 4 years preceding pregnancy, it leads to infection of the fetus in more than 70% of cases. From 1992 to 2002, the average yearly percentage decrease in the rate of P&S syphilis reported among women was 21.2%, and the average yearly percentage decrease in the congenital syphilis rate was 19.2%. Among the 529 cases of congenital syphilis reported in 2000, 82% occurred because the mother had no documented treatment of syphilis before or during her pregnancy.[4] Between 2003 and 2004 congenital syphilis declined from 10.7 to 8.8 cases per 100,000 live births.[6a]

Pathophysiology. The signs and symptoms of the four stages of syphilis are listed in Table 59-4. If syphilis is adequately diagnosed and treated during the primary stage, the other stages can be prevented.

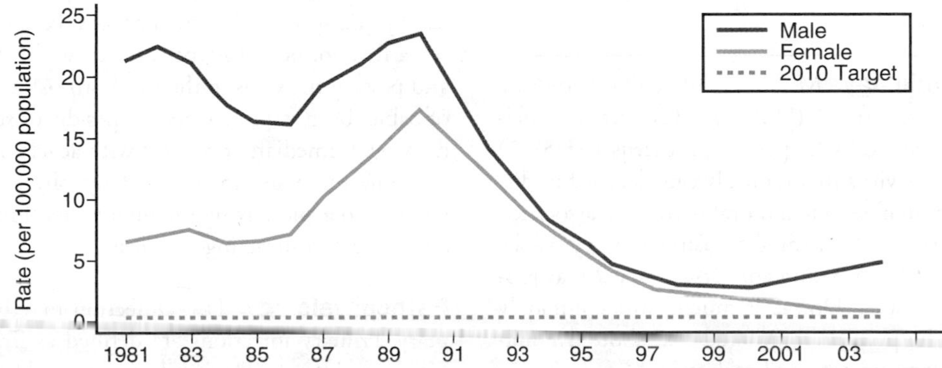

Figure 59-6 Primary and secondary syphilis rates by sex: United States, 1981-2004, and the *Healthy People 2010* target. The *Healthy People 2010* target for primary and secondary syphilis is 0.2 case per 100,000 population.

TABLE 59-4 STAGES OF SYPHILIS

Primary	Secondary	Latent	Late
DURATION			
2-8 wk	Appears 2-4 wk after chancre appears; extends over 2-4 yr	5-20 yr	Terminal if not treated
SIGNS AND SYMPTOMS			
Hard sore or pimple on vulva or penis that breaks and forms painless, draining chancre; may be single chancre or groups of more than 1; may be present also on lips, tongue, hands, rectum, vagina, cervix, or nipples; chancre heals, leaving almost invisible scar	Depends on site; low-grade fever; headache; anorexia; weight loss; anemia; sore throat, hoarseness; reddened and sore eyes; jaundice with or without hepatitis; aching of joints, muscles, long bones; sores on body or generalized fine rash, particularly on palms and soles; condylomata lata on rectum or genitalia; lymphadenopathy; patchy alopecia	No clinical signs	Tumorlike mass (gumma) on any area of body; damage to heart valves and blood vessels; meningitis; paralysis; lack of coordination; paresis; insomnia; confusion; delusions; impaired judgment; slurred speech; tabes dorsalis
COMMUNICABILITY			
Exudates from lesions and chancre highly contagious	Exudates from lesions highly contagious; blood contains organisms	Contagious for about 2 yr; not contagious to others after that; blood contains organisms; may be transmitted via placenta to fetus	Noncontagious; spinal fluid may contain organisms

Collaborative Care Management. As with gonorrhea, three levels of prevention are important. Primary prevention involves finding and treating those with the disease so that they cannot spread it to others. Treatment of choice for syphilis is penicillin G benzathine (2.4 million units IM). Secondary prevention is directed at early treatment of cases to prevent late syphilis or congenital syphilis. In tertiary prevention, efforts are made to treat the complications of syphilis when they occur. Contact investigation is necessary as for all STDs, and HIV testing is mandated for anyone with syphilis because of the high coprevalence.

Genital Herpes

Etiology and Epidemiology. Most cases of genital herpes are caused by herpes simplex virus 2 (HSV-2). However, the incidence of genital herpes caused by herpes simplex virus 1 (HSV-1) is increasing. HSV-1 is the virus that typically causes orolabial disease, or cold sores. Although genital and oral herpes are associated with different herpesviruses, oral-genital transmission is possible. Type 1 may affect the genital area, and conversely type 2 may produce a sore in the mouth area. HSV-2 is much more commonly associated with genital herpes. It is estimated that about 1.7 million new HSV-2 infections are acquired each year.[16]

Among Caucasians, 15% of men and 20% of women are HSV-2 seropositive. Among African-Americans, 35% of men and 55% of women are seropositive. Herpes is more common in women than men, infecting approximately one out of four women and one out of five men.[5] It is common in both rural and urban areas of the United States. Over the past 2 decades, rates of HSV-2 have risen quickly among adolescents and young adults.[17]

Herpes is a lifelong disease often punctuated by recurrent outbreaks. The disease may be transmitted by penile-vaginal, oral-genital, genital-anal, or oral-anal contact. It can be extremely severe in those with suppressed immune systems. Regardless of the severity of symptoms, genital herpes frequently causes psychologic distress in people who know they are infected.

Those with weakened immune systems can experience long-lasting and severe episodes of herpes. Pregnant women experiencing a first episode of herpes are at risk for delivering prematurely and passing the virus to their unborn babies. Approximately 50% of babies born with neonatal herpes die or suffer severe neurologic damage. Immediate treatment with acyclovir greatly improves the outcome for many infants.[5] Many physicians perform cesarean sections to avoid having the infant pass through the vaginal canal and thereby contracting the virus.

Pathophysiology. HSV infection may be primary or nonprimary. Primary infections are defined as first infection ever with HSV-1 or HSV-2. The incubation period for genital herpes is 3 to 7 days. Physical manifestations range from completely asymptomatic to severe disease. Herpes can masquerade as many other disorders or STDs. Typical initial symptoms are internal and external itching, nonspecific vaginal or urethral discomfort, dull perineal pain, or tissue feeling raw or irritated. Many women come in for treatment of yeast infection symptoms. Often symptoms may be so mild people do not seek medical attention. When they do, herpes frequently is not suspected, thus accounting for the vast underdiagnosis of genital herpes.

Some constitutional signs and symptoms that may occur are local inflammation; pain; enlargement of inguinal lymph nodes; generalized signs of infection such as photophobia, headache, and flulike symptoms of chills, fever, and malaise; dysuria; and urinary retention.

The typical picture of a primary outbreak is the appearance of a lesion that appears as a vesicle on the external genitalia in men and on the vagina, cervix, or external genitalia in women. Thighs and buttocks may be affected, and those who have engaged in anal intercourse may develop eruptions in and around the anus. Following primary herpes, the virus persists in a latent or unrecognized form. It is believed that the latent virus is localized in the ganglia of sensory nerves to the genitalia. When the host factors favor it, the latent infection becomes clinically apparent as recurrent herpes.

Cervical infection can accompany external lesions, and often the cervix may be the only infected site. In a primary infection, genital lesions often worsen during the first 10 to 15 days but usually heal within 3 to 4 weeks. These symptoms usually lead the individual to seek medical attention.

Vaginal discharge is common among women with primary or recurrent infections, and discharge from the urethra is usual in men who have primary infections. Urinary tract involvement may occur and is reflected in symptoms of dysuria or urinary retention. The lesions can cause severe pain, requiring hospitalization for parenteral analgesia or urinary catheterization.

Collaborative Care Management. Antiviral medications such as acyclovir, famciclovir, and valacyclovir have improved the quality of life for those infected with HSV. To decrease the severity and duration of future outbreaks, treatment should begin within 1 day of the reappearance of symptoms. Those who experience six or more recurrences per year are frequently placed on suppressive therapy. This also decreases the asymptomatic **viral shedding** between outbreaks and may be continued for up to 2 years with famciclovir or valacyclovir and up to 6 years with acyclovir.[3]

PATIENT/FAMILY TEACHING. Patients who have genital herpes should be aware of the potential for recurrent episodes and asymptomatic viral shedding. They must inform future partners before initiating a sexual relationship. Sex partners should be advised that they might be infected even if they have no symptoms. The risk for neonatal HSV infection should be explained to all patients, including men.

After the virus has finished being active, it travels to the nerves at the end of the spine where it resides in an inactive state. Reactivation of the virus results in periodic outbreaks as frequently as monthly or several times a year to only one or two times in a lifetime. Recurrences tend to be less frequent over time and are generally less severe. New sores appear near the site of the initial infection.[5] Sometimes the virus can become active but not cause any visual symptoms. Virus is still shedding at these times, and any sex partner can become infected. Recurrences may be signaled by the prodromal symptoms of tingling and itching, which may or may not be followed by skin or mucous membrane eruptions.

Outbreaks may be triggered by any of the following: stress, anxiety, depression, exposure to sunlight or cold, poor nutrition, being overtired or run down, acidic foods, menstruation, or trauma to the area usually affected by lesions.

During active herpes episodes the patient should avoid touching the sores, keep the infected area clean and dry to prevent other infections from developing, and wash hands after any contact with lesions. Sexual contact should be avoided from the first sensation of symptoms until the sores are completely healed, no scabs are present, and new skin has formed where the lesion was located.

In addition, it is important for those with HSV-2 to understand that their risk of acquiring HIV is doubled.[16] Also, genital lesions facilitate HIV shedding in the genital tract of infected individuals, thereby increasing the likelihood of transmission to HIV-negative partners.

Persons with herpes should abstain from sexual contact from the onset of prodromal signs to complete healing of lesions. Risk of transmission during asymptomatic periods exists due to viral shedding; therefore the person is advised to always use condoms to prevent transmission of the disease. A person with a primary infection should be screened for other STDs, especially HIV.[27]

Because genital herpes is a recurrent disease with no cure, persons infected with the virus require considerable emotional support. Some infected persons withdraw from an active social life rather than face the possibility of making a commitment that will require them to share knowledge of their disease with another person. For this reason, in some communities support groups have been formed for persons who have genital herpes.

A nationwide study is under way to determine if an experimental vaccine, in the final stages of testing, is safe and effective in preventing genital herpes in young women.[26]

Chlamydial Infection

Etiology and Epidemiology. Chlamydia is caused by the gram-negative bacterium *C. trachomatis.* Chlamydia is the most frequently reported bacterial sexually transmitted disease in the United States. In 2004, 929,462 chlamydial infections were reported to CDC[6a] (Figure 59-7). An estimated 2.8 million Americans are infected with chlamydia each year.[18] Of this number, 1.5 million are young people between the ages of 15 and 24 years. Chlamydia has been a reportable disease since 2000; however, underreporting is substantial because most people with chlamydia are not aware of their infections and do not seek testing. The estimated annual medical cost of this disease is more than $374 million. The consequences of this infection to the health of women and neonates are devastating, as can be seen in Figure 59-5.

Since 1984, the number of cases reported in both men and women has steadily increased. Prevalence, however, has declined in areas of the country where large-scale screening programs have been implemented.[15] Recently, the CDC and U.S. Preventive Services Task Force published recommendations that advised screening for (1) all sexually active females ages 15 to19 years, at least annually; (2) all sexually active women ages 20 to 25 years annually; and

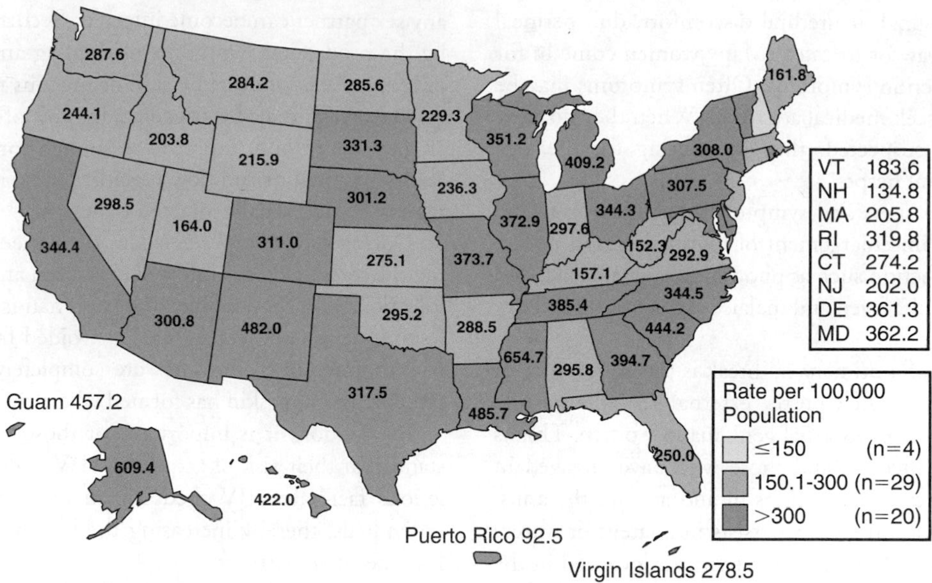

Figure 59-7 Chlamydia rates by state: United States and outlying areas, 2004. The total rate of *Chlamydia* for the United States and outlying areas (Guam, Puerto Rico, and Virgin Islands) was 316.7 per 100,000 population.

(3) sexually active women over 25 years old with risk factors (e.g., new sex partner or multiple sex partners).[17]

Pathophysiology. *C. trachomatis* is an obligate intracellular parasite once thought to be a virus. Because of the bacterium's unique developmental cycle, it was taxonomically classified in a separate order and can be found with the other well-known intracellular parasites, rickettsiae. *Chlamydia* has 15 different serotypes that cause four major diseases in humans: endemic trachoma (caused by serotypes A and C), sexually transmitted and inclusion conjunctivitis (caused by serotypes D and K), and lymphogranuloma venereum (caused by serotypes L1, L2 and L3).

The organism has two stages in its life cycle. In stage 1, the infective stage, the elementary body attaches to the host cell and is ingested by phagocytosis. In stage 2, the metabolic phase, the elementary body undergoes metamorphosis to become a reticulate or initial body. The initial body duplicates by binary fission and changes into the elementary body. The host cell, which contains the elementary bodies, undergoes lysis, liberating infectious organisms that are capable of reinfecting new cells.[10]

Chlamydia is transmitted through infected secretions only. It infects mainly mucosal membranes, such as those of the cervix, rectum, urethra, throat, and conjunctiva. It is primarily spread via sexual contact. The bacterium is not easily spread among women, so the STD is mainly transmitted by heterosexual or male homosexual contact. However, infected secretions from the genitalia to the hands and eventually to the eyes can cause trachoma. Symptoms from this contact are variable. In fact, 75% of women and 25% of men with chlamydia show no symptoms at all. In women, symptoms include increased vaginal discharge, burning during urination, irritation of the area around the vagina, bleeding after sexual intercourse, lower abdominal pain, and abnormal vaginal bleeding. Infection in women usually begins at the cervix. In men, nongonococcal urethritis is the main symptom. This includes clear, white, or yellow discharge from the urethra; burning and pain during urination; and tingling or itching sensations.[18]

Collaborative Care Management. The treatment of choice for chlamydial infections is azithromycin, 1 g orally in a single dose, or doxycycline, 100 mg twice a day for 7 days.

PATIENT/FAMILY TEACHING. It is important that the patient encourage sexual partner(s) to seek care as soon as possible to avoid reinfection of self and complications in the partner. The nurse should advise patients who are sexually active to always wear condoms. Social and emotional support of these patients is important, as it is with any person with a STD. HIV testing and screening for other STDs should be offered.

Lymphogranuloma Venereum

Etiology and Epidemiology. Lymphogranuloma venereum is a systemic STD caused by serotypes L1, L2, and L3 of *C. trachomatis*. The disease is contracted by vaginal, anal, or oral intercourse; primary inoculation with the organism may occur at any site involved in close contact. The incubation period is 3 to 30 days. Lymphadenitis of regional lymph nodes draining the site of primary infection occurs, and the disease spreads by way of the lymphatic system.

Lymphogranuloma venereum is most prevalent in the tropics. It is endemic in parts of Africa, Southeast Asia, India, the Caribbean, and Central and South America.[14] It is very rare in the United States, about 200 cases per year.

Pathophysiology. Although other serotypes of *C. trachomatis* are limited to superficial infection of mucous membranes, serotypes L1, L2, and L3 are more invasive and virulent, tending to cause systemic disease. The organism travels through the lymphatics to multiply within macrophages in regional lymph nodes. The incubation period is anywhere from 3 days to 6 weeks.[14]

The primary stage is characterized by a painless genital papule, which disappears in a few days. Most typically, papules occur on the glans penis or vaginal wall. There may be mucopurulent discharge from the urethra in men and the cervix in women. These symptoms resolve spontaneously.

Two to six weeks after the papules have healed, male patients tend to come into the physician's office with painful, usually unilateral lymphadenopathy in the groin or inguinal area. Women or those who engage in rectal intercourse may complain of lower abdominal or back pain because the vagina and rectum drain toward the deep iliac or perirectal nodes.[20]

Inguinal lymphadenopathy, far more common in men, leads to inflamed and enlarged tender lymph nodes (buboes) that contain the infective organism. One third of the inguinal buboes become fluctuant and rupture, whereas the remaining two thirds involute to form a hard, nonsuppurative inguinal mass. Extensive scarring and obstruction of the lymphatics may lead to chronic edema, infection, and ulceration.[20]

Women and men who engage in receptive anal intercourse are more likely to seek attention with the complications of the tertiary stage of the disease. These include proctocolitis, perirectal abscess, fistulas, strictures, and hyperplasia of the intestinal and perirectal lymphatics. In rare instances the end result can be esthiomene (elephantiasis of the female genitalia characterized by fibrotic labial thickening) or elephantiasis and deformation of the penis in men.

Collaborative Care Management. Lymphogranuloma is treated with doxycycline, 100 mg orally twice a day for 21 days, or erythromycin base, 500 mg orally four times a day for 21 days.

PATIENT/FAMILY TEACHING. These patients may require much counseling and teaching as they deal with their disease. Because the fluctuant lymph nodes may disturb the patient's self-image, social and emotional support is extremely important.

Chancroid

Etiology and Epidemiology. Chancroid is an STD caused by a gram-negative bacillus, *Haemophilus ducreyi.* The peak incidence of chancroid occurred in 1987 when 5035 cases were reported to the CDC. The number of cases has declined steadily since then, with 30 cases reported in 2004.[6a]

Although it is found worldwide, chancroid is most prevalent in tropical and semitropical areas in Asia, the West Indies, and sub-Saharan Africa. In areas where it is endemic, chancroid is often transmitted by prostitutes. Many women have minimal symptoms and usually are seen only with dyspareunia or dysuria.[1] However, men usually develop severe symptoms and seek treatment because of pain and the appearance of an ulcer that causes them to cease sexual activity.

The disease is particularly prevalent among non-Caucasian, uncircumcised, sexually promiscuous men with a mean age of 30 years. Because the causative organism is difficult to culture, chancroid is probably substantially underdiagnosed and underreported. The incubation period varies from 3 to 7 days.[9]

Chancroid is a cofactor for HIV transmission. A high rate of HIV infection among people with chancroid has been reported in the United States and other countries. As many as 10% of people with chancroid may be coinfected with *T. pallidum.*[28]

Pathophysiology. The initial lesions are acutely tender genital ulcers, typically with ragged and irregular borders. They are highly infectious, and autoinfection may occur, resulting in multiple lesions. The ulcers appear excavated; have a granulating, purulent surface; and are painful. Often, edema of the surrounding tissues is present.

Lymphadenopathy and tender buboes appear about 1 to 2 weeks after the primary lesion. Involvement of the inguinal lymph nodes occurs in about 50% of all cases. The buboes are most often unilateral, painful, and spherical; the skin over the buboes is inflamed. The buboes may suppurate and lead to abscesses. These abscesses in turn may suppurate and rupture, further spreading the infection. Generalized symptoms of infection usually appear when inguinal abscesses form.

In men the most common site of infection is the foreskin, but lesions may also occur on the shaft, glans, or meatus. In women ulcers most commonly occur on the labia majora, but may be seen on the labia minora, thighs, perineum, or cervix.[9]

Collaborative Care Management. Chancroid is treated with azithromycin, 1 g orally in a single dose; ceftriaxone, 250 mg IM in a single dose; ciprofloxacin, 500 mg orally twice a day for 3 days; or erythromycin base, 500 mg orally three times a day for 7 days. Successful treatment for chancroid cures the infection, resolves the clinical symptoms, and prevents transmission to others. Follow-up evaluation is essential. If treatment is successful, ulcers improve symptomatically within 3 days. If treatment fails, reasons need to be explored.

PATIENT/FAMILY TEACHING. The nurse teaches the patient to report any signs or symptoms that persist or worsen during treatment and to abstain from sexual activity until all lesions are healed. The individual needs to be screened for HIV. Proper use of a condom should also be stressed (see Box 59-1).

Granuloma Inguinale (Donovanosis)

Etiology and Epidemiology. Granuloma inguinale, or granuloma venereum, is believed to be most often transmitted by sexual contact, although nonsexual transmission has been reported. The infection is caused by a gram-negative bacillus, *Calymmatobacterium (Donovania) granulomatis,* widely referred to as *Donovan bacillus.*

Donovanosis is endemic in western New Guinea, the Caribbean, southern India, South Africa, Southeast Asia, Australia, and Brazil. In the United States fewer than 100 cases are reported annually, many of which are associated with foreign travel. The disease is more common in men, especially homosexual men, than in women. The incubation period varies from 1 week to 3 months.[2]

Pathophysiology. Lesions appear on the genitalia and in the perianal area. They are painless, are highly vascular (beefy red appearance), and bleed easily on contact. Hypertrophic, necrotic, or sclerotic lesions may also appear. These lesions may develop secondary bacterial infection or may be coinfected with another sexually transmitted pathogen. Involvement of the lymph nodes is uncommon but can occur and produce occlusion of the lymphatics, resulting in elephantiasis.[2]

Collaborative Care Management. Granuloma inguinale is treated with trimethoprim-sulfamethoxazole (Bactrim DS), orally twice a day for a minimum of 3 weeks, or doxycycline, 100 mg orally twice a day for a minimum of 3 weeks. Therapy should be continued until all lesions have healed completely.

Patient/Family Teaching. Clinician follow-up care of anyone diagnosed with granuloma inguinale is extremely important because of the possibility of treatment failure. All persons should be advised to abstain from sexual activity until all sexual partners complete a course of treatment and all lesions are healed. Relapse can occur 6 to 18 months after apparently effective therapy.

Human Papillomavirus

Etiology and Epidemiology. HPV is the most common STD in the United States, with an estimated 24 million Americans infected.[13] Approximately 6.2 million new infections occur annually.

It is estimated that 50% to 75% of sexually active men and women will acquire genital HPV infection at some point in their lives. A recent estimate suggests that 80% of women will have acquired genital HPV by age 50. Also, HIV-infected women are four times more likely to be infected with HPV than women without HIV. An estimated 9.2 million sexually active adolescents and young adults 15 to 24 years of age are currently infected with HPV.[6] The majority of those infected are asymptomatic; however, in some, the virus is manifested in genital warts.

Pathophysiology. There are more than 70 types of HPV. All HPVs have an affinity for squamous epithelium, but they also tend to be site specific according to the virus type (Table 59-5). About 30 strains of the virus affect the genital tract. Most of these are low risk, resulting in mild Pap test abnormalities and genital warts. The most common strains, 6 and 11, cause the external warts but rarely result in malignancy.[12]

Four high-risk types exist: numbers 16, 18, 31, and 45. These are associated with high-grade cervical dysplasia and are more likely to develop into cancer. Clinical studies confirm that HPV is the cause of essentially all cervical, penile, and anal cancers, and is detected in approximately 50% to 80% of vaginal and 50% of vulvar cancers.[13]

Genital warts, sometimes called condylomata acuminata, are soft, moist, flesh-colored bumps that may appear weeks or months after infection. They can be raised or flat, small or large, and sometimes grouped in clusters that are cauliflower-shaped. The warts occur in or around the vulva, vagina, cervix, perineum, anal canal, urethra, and glans penis. People who have visible genital warts can be infected simultaneously with multiple HPV types. The warts can enlarge during pregnancy and may cause difficulty with birth. Most HPV infections appear to be temporary and probably are cleared by the body's immune system. However, reactivation is possible after a period of up to decades. Reinfection is also possible.[5]

Table 59-5 Clinical Association of Human Papillomaviruses

Disease Location and Type	Predominant HPV Type
Skin	
Deep plantar wart	1
Common wart	2, 4
Flat wart	3, 10
Mucosa	
Genital warts	6, 11
Cervical cancer	
High risk	16, 18, 31, 45
Intermediate risk	33, 35, 39, 51, 52, 56, 58, 59, 68
Low risk	6, 11, 42, 43, 44
Vulvar cancer	16
Penile cancer	16
Oropharyngeal cancer	16
Respiratory papillomas	6, 11

From Heise A: The clinical significance of HPV, *Nurse Pract* 28(10):8-19, 2003.
HPV, Human papillomavirus.

Collaborative Care Management. Treatment options depend on the extent, anatomic location, and state of the disease. No single treatment is ideal for all patients or all warts. Home treatment by patients may include local application of podofilox, 0.5% solution or gel twice a day for 3 days, followed by 4 days with no therapy, repeating for four cycles; or imiquimod, 5% cream applied at hour of sleep 3 times a week for 16 weeks. Provider therapies may include cryotherapy, application of trichloroacetic acid (TCA) and bichloracetic acid (BCA), intralesional interferon injections, or laser surgery. Although treatments are aimed at removing the warts, none actually eliminates the virus.

Patient/Family Teaching. Because a diagnosis of HPV has been linked to an increased risk for cervical cancer, the sexually active woman of any age is advised to have an annual Pap test. More frequent Pap tests are recommended when abnormal Pap tests develop. Malignant changes may not develop for 5 or more years. Patients who smoke should be encouraged to stop. Through a direct carcinogenic action, smoking may advance infected cells toward a neoplastic process and increase the risk for cervical cancer once a patient is infected with the HPV virus.[13,28]

After visible genital warts have cleared, follow-up care is not mandatory; however, the patient is advised to watch for recurrences. Recurrences occur most frequently in the first 3 months after treatment. People with HPV infections need to understand that they might remain infectious even though the warts are gone. The use of condoms may reduce, but does not eliminate, the risk of transmission. As with all STDs, HIV and other STD testing should be offered.

Prevention of HPV should be stressed. It includes (1) abstaining from intercourse, (2) avoiding sexual relationships with persons in known high-risk groups, (3) using latex condoms for sexual intercourse, and (4) avoiding anal intercourse.

▶ ARE You READY?

Which of the following statements from a patient with HPV indicates the need for further teaching?

1. "I may have recurrences within the first 3 months."
2. "I can spread infection even if I do not have visible warts."
3. "Using latex condoms does not eliminate the risk of spreading the infection."
4. "I am required to have mandatory testing every 6 months."

Trichomoniasis

Etiology and Epidemiology. A single-celled protozoan parasite, *Trichomonas vaginalis,* causes trichomoniasis. The parasite commonly exists in vaginal and cervical secretions and in seminal fluid. Although no national surveillance data exist, it is estimated that 7.4 million new cases of trichomoniasis occur annually in this country, with 25%, or 1.9 million, cases occurring among persons ages 15 to 24.[5] The parasite is sexually transmitted through penis-to-vagina intercourse or vulva-to-vulva contact with an infected partner. Unsubstantiated data indicate possible spread via fomites. Women can acquire the disease from infected men or women, but men usually contract it from infected women. Women are more frequently infected than men and are more likely to exhibit symptoms, which usually appear within 5 to 28 days of exposure.[5]

Pathophysiology. Typical symptoms experienced by women include profuse, foul-smelling, frothy yellow or gray-green vaginal discharge; vaginal itching; dysuria; and dyspareunia. When men have symptoms, they most commonly include urethral discharge, urgency, and slight burning after urination or ejaculation. Untreated trichomoniasis has been linked to an increased risk for HIV infection. Infected pregnant women are at risk for premature birth, low-birth-weight infants, and infection or rupture of the placenta. Prostatitis and cystitis are associated with trichomoniasis in men.

Collaborative Care Management. Trichomoniasis is usually treated with metronidazole, 2 g orally in a single dose taken with food. Alternatively the person may take metronidazole, 500 mg twice a day for 7 days.

PATIENT/FAMILY TEACHING. Even though symptoms in men usually resolve spontaneously within a few weeks, an asymptomatic man can still spread the infection to sex partners. Therefore it is important that both partners be treated simultaneously with oral metronidazole to prevent reinfection. The partners should be cautioned against drinking alcohol while taking the drug. The drug is known to cross the placental barrier, but does not cause teratogenic effects; therefore it is deemed safe to give in the first trimester, a recent treatment change. Condom use is advised. HIV and all other STD testing should be offered.

Bacterial Vaginosis

Etiology and Epidemiology. Bacterial vaginosis describes an imbalance in the normal vaginal flora characterized by a decrease in lactobacilli and an increase in *Gardnerella, Mycoplasma,* and anaerobic bacteria. Bacterial vaginosis is the most common vaginal infection among women of childbearing age in the United States. It has been associated with having multiple sex partners; using an intrauterine device for contraception; and frequent douching, which reduces lactobacilli. Studies have consistently shown a relationship between bacterial vaginosis and adverse pregnancy outcomes, including preterm delivery, premature rupture of membranes, spontaneous abortion, preterm labor, and postpartum endometriosis.[25]

Pathophysiology. Bacterial vaginosis infection is characterized by a small amount of homogeneous gray or grayish white discharge. The discharge usually has a disagreeable odor, and because it is less irritating than discharges caused by other organisms, pruritus is mild or absent. On inspection the vaginal walls are slightly reddened, and the discharge appears to adhere to the mucosal lining. Screening criteria for bacterial vaginosis include vaginal pH level greater than 4.5, amine odor on the application of potassium hydroxide (a positive whiff test), and presence of clue cells on microscopic examination of a wet mount.[25]

Collaborative Care Management. Bacterial vaginosis can be treated with metronidazole, 500 mg orally twice a day for 7 days, or with clindamycin cream 2%, one full applicator at bedtime for 7 days, or with metronidazole gel 0.75% (Metrogel), one full applicator vaginally at bedtime for 7 days.

PATIENT/FAMILY TEACHING. Women need to understand that bacterial vaginosis increases their susceptibility to other STDs such as chlamydia, gonorrhea, and HIV infection. Therefore the use of condoms is of utmost importance for 4 to 6 weeks after diagnosis, and douching should be eliminated. A woman with both HIV and bacterial vaginosis has greater chance of transmitting HIV to a partner.

Hepatitis B Virus

Etiology and Epidemiology. Hepatitis B virus (HBV) is a deoxyribonucleic acid virus that causes acute hepatitis and is a major cause of chronic liver disease, which may lead to cirrhosis, hepatocellular cancer, and death. About 5000 deaths occur each year from chronic HBV-related liver disease.

In the United States transmission of HBV is primarily through blood or intimate contact (usually sexual). In 2002, 7996 new cases were reported, a drop of more than 65% since 1990.[6] This remarkable decrease is attributed to nationwide efforts that included (1) screening of all pregnant women; (2) postexposure prophylaxis of neonates and others having contact with the infection; (3) routine vaccination of infants, children, and adolescents; and (4) immunization of all high-risk persons such as prostitutes, health care workers, homosexuals, residents of correctional or long-term care facilities, those living with or having sexual contact with a person who has active HBV infection, and those being treated for other STDs.

Pathophysiology. The hepatitis caused by HBV has the same symptoms seen in other types of hepatitis. The liver is inflamed, and the patient may have jaundice, anorexia, slight fever, and gastrointestinal upset. For more information see Chapter 46.

Collaborative Care Management. Treatment of HBV is described in Chapter 46. Recent CDC guidelines now include hepatitis C as an STD, although the numbers infected in this manner are very low.

Other Sexually Transmitted Diseases

In addition to the diseases already discussed, molluscum contagiosum, pediculosis pubis, and scabies are considered to be STDs.

Molluscum contagiosum is a viral infection manifested by wartlike lesions on the abdomen, thighs, and genitals. Although molluscum contagiosum may be transmitted via fomites, its transmission in adults is primarily sexual. Diagnosis is often made on sight of the characteristic lesion. A punch biopsy may be used for diagnostic evaluation if visual diagnosis is uncertain. There is no effective medical treatment. Most often patients are advised to allow the lesions to resolve spontaneously. If only a few lesions are present, the core of the lesions may by surgically excised. Multiple lesions may be treated with cryotherapy. Imiquimod 5% cream is approved for treating genital warts. It is applied three times per week, left on the skin for 6 to 10 hours, then washed off. A typical course of treatment lasts from 4 to 16 weeks.[24]

For information on pediculosis pubis and scabies, see Chapter 65.

Critical Thinking

1. You have been asked to give a presentation on STDs to several health education classes at a local high school. What information should you be prepared to discuss? If you are limited to 45 minutes, what information do you think is most important to cover and why?
2. Explain why the incidence of STDs is high among American teens. How might the care of a teenager who has an STD differ from that of an adult with the same disease?

References

1. American Social Health Association: *Facts and answers about STDs: information to live by: gonorrhea*, accessed July 2004 from website: www.ashastd.org/stdfaqs/gonorrhea.
2. Boucher KW, Manders SM: *Granuloma inguinale (donovanosis)*, accessed Aug 2003 from website: www.emedicine.com/derm.
3. Brevet D, Wiggins M: Preventing and treating STDs, *Adv Nurses* 4(23): 15-18, 2002.
4. Centers for Disease Control and Prevention: Primary and secondary syphilis—United States, 2002, *Morbid Mortal Week Rep* 52(46):1119, 2003, accessed from website: www.cdc.gov/mmwr.
5. Centers for Disease Control and Prevention: *CDC fact sheet: bacterial vaginosis, chlamydia, genital herpes, genital HPV infection, ghonorrhea, syphilis and MSM, trichomoniasis*, accessed July 2004 from website: www.cdc.gov/std.
6. Centers for Disease Control and Prevention: *Chlamydia, gonorrhea, other sexually transmitted diseases: sexually transmitted disease surveillance 2002*, Division of STD Prevention, accessed July 2004 from website: www.cdc.gov/std.

6a. Centers for Disease Control and Prevention: *STD Surveillance 2004, Trends in reportable sexually transmitted diseases in the U.S*, National Surveillance Data for Chlamydia, Gonorrhea, and Syphilis, accessed from website: www.cdc.gov/std/stats/trends2004.html..

7. Centers for Disease Control and Prevention: Summary of notifiable diseases—United States 2002, *Morbid Mortal Week Rep* 51(53):1-84, accessed July 2004 from website: www.cdc.gov/mmwr.
8. Clinical rounds: care for teenagers falls short, *Nursing 2004* 34(6):34, 2004.
9. Crowe M, Hall M: *Chancroid*, accessed July 2004 from website: www.emedicine.com.
10. DeMets A: *Chlamydia trachomatis*, Bacteriology at University of Wisconsin Madison, accessed Nov 2003 from website: www.bact.wisc.edu.
11. Flinders D, DeSchweinitz P: Pediculosis and scabies, *Am Fam Phys* 69(2):344, 347, 2004.
12. Heise A: The clinical significance of HPV, *Nurs Pract* 28(10):8-9, 2003.
13. Likes W, Itano J: Human papillomavirus and cervical cancer: not just a sexually transmitted disease, *Clin J Oncol Nurs* 7(3):271-276, 2003.
14. Lorek J: *Lymphogranuloma venereum*, accessed Nov 2001 from website: www.emedicine.com.
15. Lyss SB et al: *Chlamydia trachomatis* among patients infected with and treated for *Neisseria gonorrhoeae* in sexually transmitted disease clinics in the United States, *Ann Intern Med* 139(3):183, 2003.
16. Mark H, Hanahan A, Stender S: Herpes simplex virus type 2: an update, *Nurs Pract* 28(11):34, 2003.
17. Mosure D: *Epidemiology of chlamydia in the United States*, Centers for Disease Control and Prevention, Division of STD Prevention, presentation, March 8, 2004.
18. National Institute of Allergy and Infectious Diseases: *Chlamydia*, accessed July 2004 from website: www.niaid.nih.gov.
19. *Perspectives on sexual and reproductive health* 36(1):9, Jan 2004.
20. Roberts R: *Sexually transmitted diseases: lymphogranuloma venereum (LVG)*, Weill Medical College of Cornell University, accessed 2004 from website: http://edcenter.med.cornell.edu/Patho-physiology_cases/STDs.
21. *Sexually transmitted disease*, Epigee Birth Control Guide, accessed July 2004 from website: http://www.epigee.org/guide/stds.
22. *Sexually transmitted diseases*, Weill Medical College of Cornell University, accessed 2004 from website: http://edcenter.med.cornell.edu/Pathophysiology_cases/STDs.
23. Steiner K et al: Field-delivered therapy increases treatment for chlamydia and gonorrhea, *Am J Pub Health* 93(6):882, 2003.
24. Stulberg D, Hutchinson AG: Molluscum contagiosum and warts, *Am Fam Phys* 67(6):1233-1234, 2003.
25. US Preventive Services Task Force: Screening for bacterial vaginosis in pregnancy: recommendations and rationale, *Am Fam Phys* 65(6):1148-1149, 2002.
26. Vaccine in final phase of testing, *Womens Health Wkly* 64, July 1, 2004.
27. Wald A, Warren T: *Importance of asymptomatic shedding in the prevention and treatment of genital herpes* (archived web conference), accessed May 2004 from website: www.medscape.com/viewprogram/3096.
28. Workowski K, Levine W: Sexually transmitted diseases treatment guidelines—2002, *Morbid Mortal Week Rep* 51(RR06):1-80, 2002, accessed from website: www.cdc.gov/mmwr.

evolve Visit the Evolve website: http://evolve.elsevier.com/Monahan/medsurg

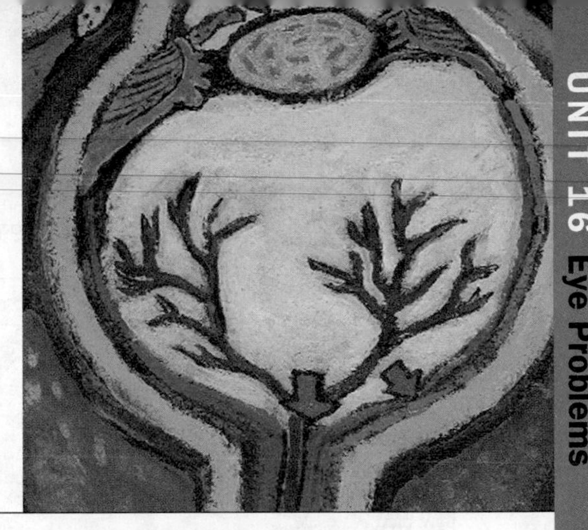

CHAPTER 60

Assessment of the Visual System

by Heather G. Boyd-Monk

OBJECTIVES

After studying this chapter, the learner should be able to:

1. Describe the structure and function of the eye.
2. Identify the normal physiologic and anatomic ocular changes that occur with aging.
3. Identify the subjective and objective data that should be obtained when assessing the eye.
4. Discuss the nursing interventions and patient teaching associated with common ocular diagnostic tests.

KEY TERMS

constriction, p. 1800
convergence, p. 1799
intraocular, p. 1798
ophthalmoscope, p. 1806
photoreceptors, p. 1797

Orientation to our world is primarily visual. We learn much about our environment and ourselves through our eyes. Practically every behavior is affected by the visual sense. A noise prompts us to look in the direction of the sound. Something touches our body, and we look to see what it was. Vision contributes meaning and pleasure to the human experience.

Assessment of the visual system is an integral part of the nurse's role. Visual screening is conducted with persons of all ages and in all settings; most eye disorders are identified by nurses and physicians in schools, industry, outpatient clinics, emergency rooms, or ophthalmologists' offices. Hospital admission is usually limited to medical or surgical treatment that cannot routinely be accomplished on an outpatient basis.

Because most people with eye problems are managed as outpatients, visual impairment is usually not the major diagnosis of the person for whom the nurse is providing care. However, visual impairment is frequently present and may be undiagnosed. Therefore nurses should routinely assess visual ability, especially in persons who have systemic diseases that affect vision or who are taking medications with known visual side effects.

Anatomy and Physiology of the Eye

Layers of the Eye

The eyeball has three main coats or layers (Figure 60-1). The tough outer layer consists of the opaque sclera (white) and the transparent cornea, which initially bends (refracts) light entering the eye. These structures are joined at the corneoscleral sulcus or limbus. The middle vascular layer or uvea is composed of three parts: the iris (with its central opening called the pupil), the muscular ciliary body delineated by the ora serrata, and the pigmented vascular choroid.

The retina, the third and innermost layer of the eye, extends from the optic disc to the ora serrata. In embryology the retina develops in two parts: a sensory portion and a layer of pigmented epithelium. The sensory portion contains the **photoreceptors** (rods and cones). These photoreceptors synapse in the retina with bipolar neurons and then with ganglion neurons, and these become the fibers of the optic nerve that pass visual information to the brain.

The cones, less numerous than the rods, are concentrated in the macula region of the retina, which is temporal to the optic disc (Figure 60-2). They are the receptors for bright daylight and color vision and allow us to see sharp images. The rods, found mostly in the retinal periphery, are receptors for dim or night vision. Rods contain rhodopsin, a photosensitive protein that rapidly becomes depleted in bright light. The slow regeneration of rhodopsin, which depends on the presence of vitamin A, explains the time needed to adjust from a bright to a dim light.

Chambers of the Eye

The eyeball's interior is divided into two segments: anterior and posterior. The anterior segment includes the space from the back of the cornea to the lens, and the posterior compartment is the space from the posterior surface of the lens to the retina.

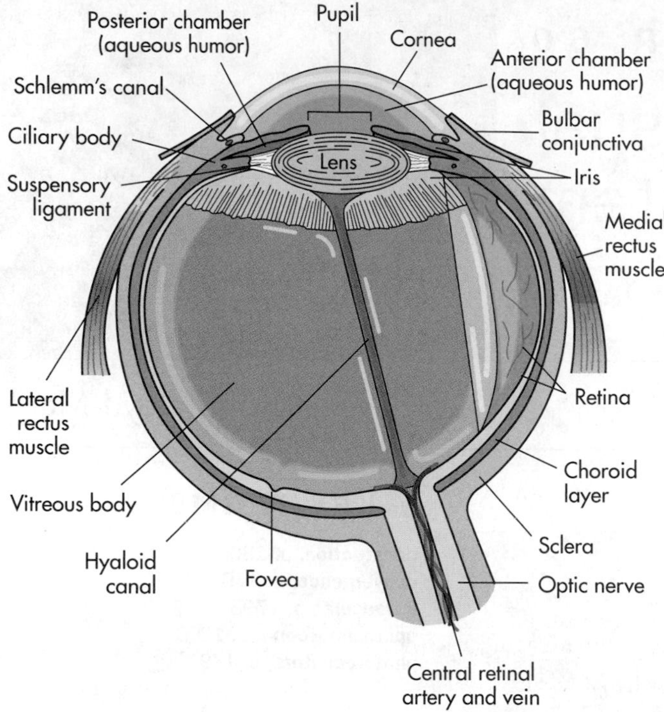

Figure 60-1 Horizontal section through the eye.

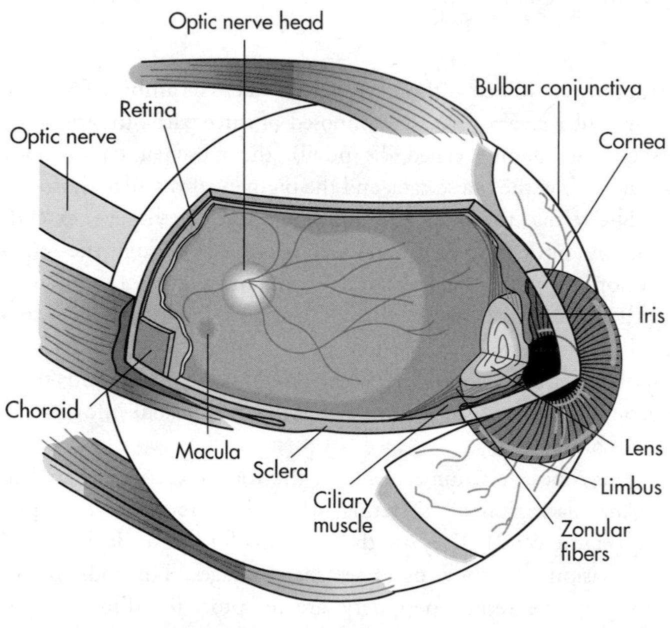

Figure 60-2 Cutaway section of the eye.

The anterior segment is further subdivided into an anterior chamber (between the cornea and the iris) and a posterior chamber (between the iris and the lens). This potential space is filled with a clear liquid called aqueous humor, whose purpose is to nourish and bathe the lens and posterior cornea and maintain the hydrostatic **intraocular** pressure. Produced by the ciliary body in the posterior chamber, aqueous humor flows through the pupil into the anterior chamber and exits via the trabecular meshwork filtration structures at the junction of the iris and cornea (anterior chamber angle). Aqueous humor then drains into Schlemm's canal, which is an encircling tubular channel. Schlemm's canal has several exit channels that empty into the scleral and episcleral veins. Aqueous humor passes through these exit channels and eventually is absorbed into the venous circulation (Figure 60-3).

The larger posterior segment is filled with a clear, gelatinous substance called the vitreous humor. The structure of the vitreous humor can be pictured as fine collagen fibers crossing one another to form scaffolding that helps maintain the shape of the eyeball. This fibrous network increases in density toward the outermost portion of the vitreous humor, particularly in the areas of strong attachment between the vitreous humor and retina. These attachments occur at the anterior edge of the retina, the optic disc, the equator of the eye, and the macula. The vitreous humor's clarity allows transmission of light posteriorly to the retina.

Lens

The lens is a transparent, biconvex structure located directly behind the iris and pupil. It is enclosed in a clear capsule and attached to the ciliary body by multiple suspensory ligaments called zonules. The lens is the fine-focusing mechanism for the eye. It refines the refracted light rays entering the eye so that they focus on the retina, producing a clear image.

Eye Muscles

The eye has two types of muscles: extrinsic and intrinsic. The six extraocular muscles are extrinsic voluntary muscles that control the extraocular movements of each eye (Table 60-1 and Figure 60-4). The lateral and medial rectus muscles control out-turning (abduction) and in-turning (adduction), respectively, with the remaining four muscles. The superior and inferior rectus muscles move the eye up and down and toward the nose, whereas the oblique muscles also control up and down movement plus movement toward the ear. The brain controls the simultaneous, integrated actions of the muscles of each eye.

The intrinsic involuntary muscles within the eye are the ciliary body muscles, which control the shape of the lens, and the iris's

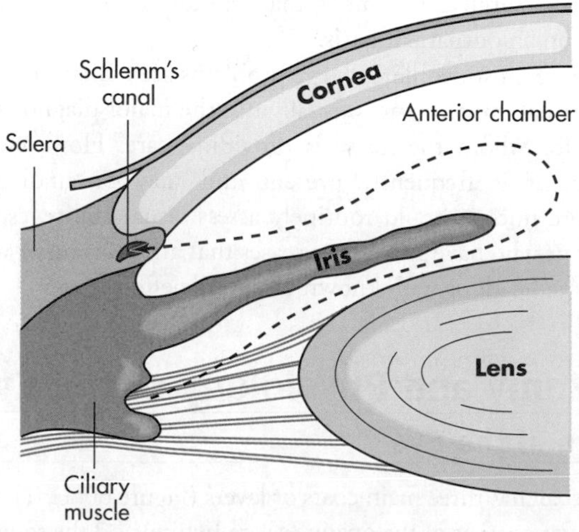

Figure 60-3 Flow of aqueous humor. Aqueous humor is produced by ciliary processes in posterior chamber; it flows into anterior chamber and leaves the eye through Schlemm's canal.

TABLE 60-1 EXTRAOCULAR MUSCLES

Name	Function
Superior rectus	Rotates eye upward and toward nose
Inferior rectus	Rotates eye downward and toward nose
Lateral rectus	Moves eye toward temporal side
Medial rectus	Moves eye toward nose
Inferior oblique	Rotates eye upward and toward temporal side
Superior oblique	Rotates eye downward and toward temporal side

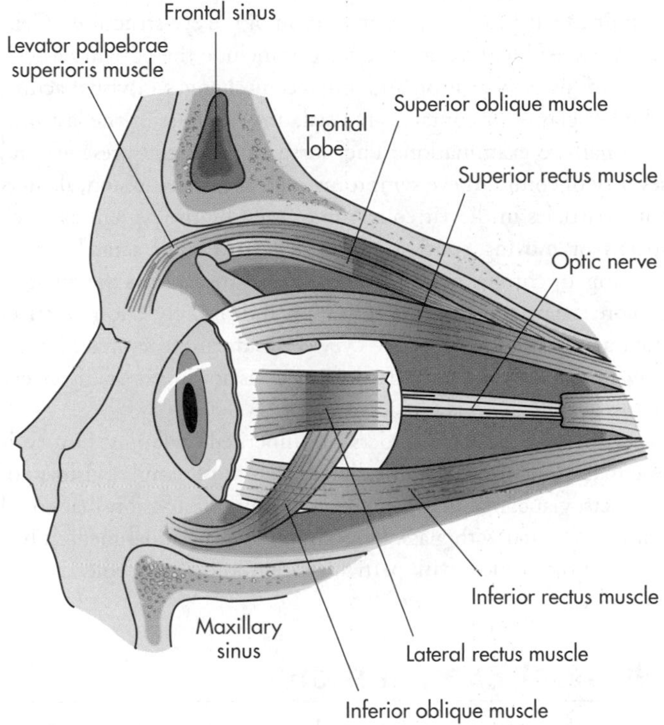

Figure 60-4 Extrinsic muscles of the eye. Both oblique muscles insert behind the equator of the globe. The inferior oblique muscle passes inferiorly to the body of the inferior rectus muscle but beneath the lateral rectus muscle.

sphincter and dilator pupillae muscles, which control pupil size and consequently the amount of light that enters the eye.

Eyelids and Conjunctiva

The eyelids (palpebrae) are made up of thin layers of skin, muscle, fibrous tissue, and mucous membrane. The main purposes of the eyelids are to protect the eye from external irritation, spread tears over the eye's external surface, and interrupt and restrict the amount of light entering the eye. The conjunctiva, a mucous membrane lining the eyelid (palpebral conjunctiva) extends from the limbus over the anterior sclera (bulbar conjunctiva), folds on itself, then extends to the lid margin. Conjunctival blood vessels provide nutrients, antibodies, and leukocytes to the avascular cornea. Conjunctival goblet cells secrete mucus, whereas the eyelid's sebaceous glands secrete the oily film that decreases friction when the lids close.

Lacrimal System

The lacrimal system consists of the lacrimal gland (which produces the aqueous [watery] portion of the tear film) and a tear drainage system (Figure 60-5). The tears flow across the eye's surface and enter the lacrimal drainage system nasally. Each time the eye blinks, tears are pumped by the blinking action across the eye's surface to drain through small openings in the eyelids (puncti) and ducts (canaliculi) to the lacrimal sac. They then drain into the nasolacrimal duct through the opening of the inferior meatus of the nasal cavity. Tears keep the surface of the eye (cornea and conjunctiva) moistened and lubricated. Tears also contain lysozyme, which functions as an antibacterial agent.

Orbit

The eye rests within the confines of the bony orbit. This orbit is a cone-shaped cavity formed by the union of cranial and facial bones. The eyeball itself occupies only about one fifth of the space of the orbit. The remainder is filled with the lacrimal gland, muscles, blood vessels, nerves, and fatty tissue. This fatty tissue serves as a protective cushion for the eye. The optic nerve exits the orbit posteriorly, transmitting visual information from the eye to the brain.

Physiology of Vision

Light rays entering the eye are refracted as they pass over the curved surfaces of the cornea and through the various clear internal structures of the eye (aqueous humor, lens, and vitreous humor) to focus on the retina. The cornea provides the major refractive change for light entering the eye, with the lens providing the fine focus for light transmitted onto the retina.

The eye can adjust to seeing objects at various distances by the flattening or thickening of the lens. Near vision (accommodation) requires contraction of the ciliary body muscles. This contraction allows the ciliary muscle to move forward and relaxes the zonules attached to the lens. The bulging lens then bends the light to focus the rays more acutely on the retina. **Convergence** of the

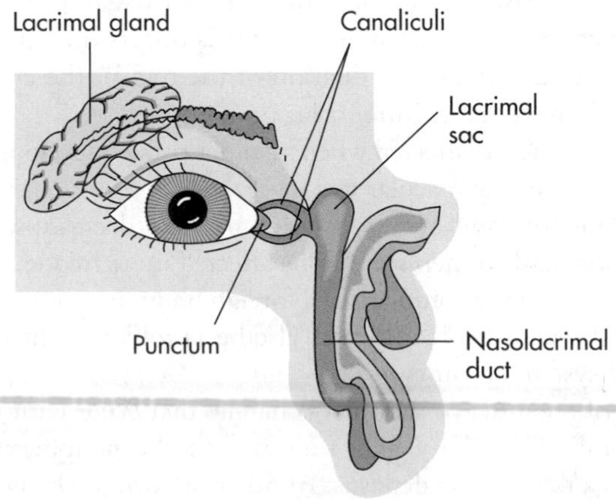

Figure 60-5 Lacrimal system.

eyes and **constriction** of the pupils further facilitate accommodation for near vision. The pupils also constrict with bright lights to protect the retina from intense stimulation.

Light rays are absorbed by the retinal photoreceptors, changed to electrical activity, and transmitted via the optic nerve to the brain's visual cortex for processing. The fibers of the optic nerve (cranial nerve II; see Chapter 47) divide at the optic chiasm; the medial portion of each nerve crosses to the opposite side and synapses at the lateral geniculate body. Some pupillary fibers go to the midbrain, whereas impulses from crossed and uncrossed fibers are transmitted to the visual cortex in the occipital lobe of the brain. Visual information received by each eye is then transmitted simultaneously to the visual cortex. Binocular vision creates depth perception.

Physiologic Changes With Aging

Physiologic and anatomic aspects of aging also affect visual function. Decrease in lens transparency begins to appear in the fifth decade of life. The lens density increases as more fibrils are laid down within the lens capsule. Presbyopia (decreased ability to see objects that are near) is the first noticeable visual change. The compression of lens fibers and protein changes all play a part in the resultant opacity of the lens or cataract formation. This in turn also may affect the older person's color vision. Bright colors become muted or even indistinguishable. Cumulative lifetime exposure to ultraviolet B radiation is also associated with lens opacities, supporting the practice of wearing sunglasses or a hat to shield the eyes.[8]

Another symptom of lens opacity is glare, which is more severe at nighttime and often causes people to seek the ophthalmologist's attention when night driving becomes impaired. Glare can also be related to increased light scatter caused by corneal edema. Glare is a veil-like luminance superimposed on the retinal image, which masks and reduces the brightness of objects in the visual field.

The visual field may be decreased in older people by such anatomic aberrations as drooping eyelids (blepharoptosis) and decreased pupillary size. A smaller pupil (senile miosis) also affects the amount of light that reaches the peripheral retina and inhibits the person's ability to adapt to dim light and darkness. As a result, the older person has impaired night vision. A disease like glaucoma also results in peripheral visual field loss. Aqueous humor production drops off sharply in the sixth decade. However, the increase in lens size contributes to shallowing of the anterior chamber, and as long as no crisis occurs (i.e., trauma to the lens capsule or sudden dilation of the pupil), the eye maintains a relatively stable intraocular pressure.

Central vision is affected when an older person develops retinal degeneration in the macular region of the eye.

The quantity and quality of tears may also decrease with age. Postmenopausal women seem to be affected more frequently than men. A person may complain of a foreign body sensation, scratchiness, and even pain. Tearing may also be a problem if the lacrimal drainage system becomes less efficient.

One of the more common eye changes that occur with aging is arcus senilis. This hazy gray ring around the periphery of the cornea is a result of fat deposits. Another important change in the cornea is its change in shape. It tends to flatten, resulting in an irregular curvature in the corneal surface. As a result, light entering the eye tends to be refracted at varying angles, leading to a distorted and blurred image (astigmatism).

▶ ARE You READY?

Which of the following is the first noticeable visual change related to physiologic changes of aging?

1. Decreased sensitivity to light
2. Decreased lacrimal secretions
3. Decreased ability to see near objects
4. Decreased ability to distinguish colors

Health History

A complete visual assessment consists of a careful patient history combined with a physical examination of the eye structures. General areas explored during the history include the patient's assessment of his or her vision and any recent changes in visual acuity, whether glasses or contacts are used, and the date of the last professional eye examination. The nurse explores the presence and severity of common eye symptoms such as blurred vision, floaters (tiny particles in the vitreous humor seen by the patient as black specks or moving spots in the visual field), dry scratchy eyes, burning, or chronic headache. The history also allows the nurse to explore the person's health promotion and risk reduction practices such as the use of protective eyewear and care of contact lenses. Any history of head trauma, loss of consciousness, or direct eye trauma or infection is important.

Because some eye disorders are inherited, a family history is essential. Questions specifically address any family history of cataracts, glaucoma, diabetes, hypertension, poor vision that could not be corrected with glasses, or blindness. A personal medical history is also obtained, with particular attention to all medications in current use.

Physical Examination

Because the eye's cornea, lens, and vitreous are transparent structures, abnormalities are easily detectable. Ocular manifestations of systemic disease also can be identified. In addition, the retinal vascular system and the optic nerve head (optic disc) can be visualized on fundus examination. Physical examination includes inspection of the external structures and assessment of visual acuity. A physician performs the fundus examination. In specific retinal diseases, specially trained nurses or technicians perform electrophysiologic tests for diagnostic purposes. A basic assessment of the eye and vision is summarized in Table 60-2.

Assessment measures and variations in normal findings relevant to the care of older adults are presented in the Gerontologic Assessment box. Also identified are disorders common in older adults, which may be responsible for abnormal assessment findings.

Inspection of External Structures

The nurse first inspects the general appearance of the patient's face and eyes. An abnormal protrusion of an eye is called exophthalmos. In older adults the eyes tend to sink into the orbit (enophthalmos), primarily as a result of the loss of orbital fat.

TABLE 60-2 BASIC ASSESSMENT OF THE EYE AND VISION

Area Assessed	Findings
Facial and ocular expression	Prominence of eyes; alert or dull expression
Eyelids and conjunctiva	Symmetry, edema, ptosis, itching, redness, discharges, blinking, equality, growths
Lacrimal system	Tears, swelling, growths
Sclera	Color
Cornea	Clarity
Anterior chamber	Depth, presence of blood or half moon of white cells
Iris and pupils	Irregularities in color, shape, size
Pupillary reflex	
Light	Constriction of pupil in response to light in that eye (direct light reaction); equal amount of constriction in other eye (consensual light reaction)
Accommodation	Convergence of eyes and constriction of pupil as gaze shifts from far to near object
Lens	Transparent or opaque
Visual acuity with and without glasses	Ability to read newsprint, clocks on wall, and name tags and to recognize faces at bedside and at door
Peripheral vision	Ability to see movements and objects well on both sides of field of vision
Supportive vision or cosmetic aids	Glasses, contact lenses, prosthesis

The nurse assesses the eyelids for color, texture, mobility, and position. The lids should be able to close completely to prevent drying of the conjunctiva and cornea. Any swelling, redness, or discharge is noted. If one upper lid seems to be lower than the other, or "droops," ptosis of the eyelid may be present. Extreme ptosis can interfere with vision by covering the pupil. Ptosis of one or both eyes may occur as a result of a neurologic or neuromuscular disease. It may also be seen in an extremely debilitated person.

As the person ages, the eyelids become thinner and less elastic, and positional defects may occur. Ectropion is eversion of the lower lid. It may be unilateral or bilateral, and symptoms include tearing and irritation. Entropion is the turning in of the eyelids. The person experiences a foreign body sensation caused by the eyelashes rubbing against the cornea. Dermatochalasis is a redundancy of upper or lower lid tissues. This occurs from loss of elasticity and results in wrinkles and drooping folds in the lids.

The nurse examines the conjunctiva of the lower lid by pulling downward on the lid as the person looks upward (Figure 60-6). To examine the conjunctiva of the upper lid, the lid must be everted (Figure 60-7).

The lacrimal gland normally is not observable. Enlargement of the gland may occur in certain disorders that cause inflammation of the eye. This may be most evident when the upper lid is everted. Small blood vessels normally are visible in the conjunctiva. The sclera beneath the transparent conjunctiva has a shiny, porcelain-like appearance. Dilation of conjunctival blood vessels (injection) may indicate conjunctival, corneal, or intrinsic ocular disease. Subconjunctival hemorrhages may occur in the normal eye after trauma or in conjunction with hypertension. A yellow discoloration of the sclera indicates jaundice but must be distinguished from the normal yellow tinge that may be present in dark-skinned individuals.

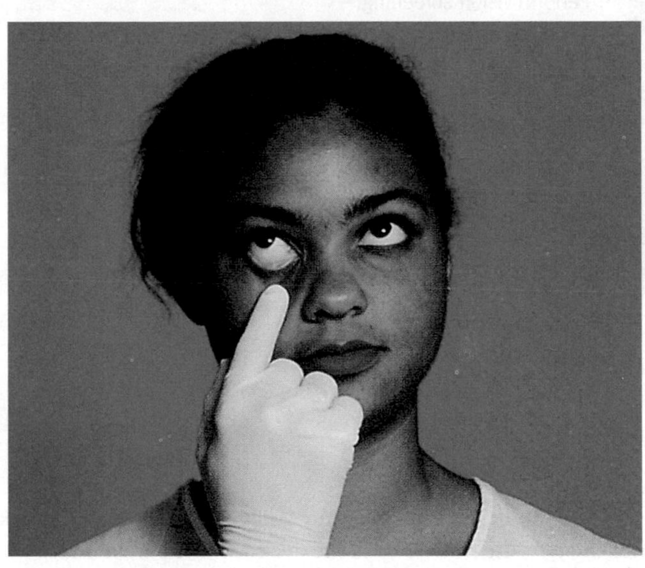

Figure 60-6 Eversion of lower eyelid by drawing margin downward as subject looks upward.

The cornea, which is normally invisible except for surface reflections, must be smooth and transparent for good vision. It should look shiny and bright when examined with a penlight. Moving the light and directing it from the side, the nurse looks for abrasions and opacities. The iris and pupil should be visible through the clear cornea.

Corneal epithelium defects may be demonstrated with the use of topical dyes. Contact lenses should be removed before dye instillation because the dye tends to stain soft lenses. The dye is put on the conjunctiva by drops or by touching the conjunctiva with a moistened strip of filter paper that has been impregnated with the dye. Injured tissue absorbs the dye, allowing visualization

Gerontologic Assessment

- Inspect the general appearance of the face and eyes.
  - –Loss of orbital fat and decreased muscle tone may cause the eyes to sink into the orbit.
- Examine the upper and lower eyelids.
  - –Loss of elasticity creates wrinkles and folds; redundant lid tissue is called dermatochalasis.
  - –Check extraocular muscles in cardinal positions of gaze.
- Examine the cornea.
  - –Irritation and scratchy sensations may result from decreased tear production.
  - –Fat deposits may create a hazy gray ring around the periphery (arcus senilis).
  - –Corneal disease creates a clouding of the cornea.
- Examine the size of the pupil.
  - –Pupillary size typically decreases with age.
- Examine the lens.
  - –Yellow discoloration may be present, which can progress to cataract formation.
- Examine the retina with an ophthalmoscope.
  - –The effects of diabetes, hypertension, and macular degeneration are often evident in hemorrhages, exudates, and abnormal areas of pigmentation.
- Perform vision screening.
  - –Normal aging is associated with refractory changes, senile miosis, and decreased visual acuity.
- Explore the impact of any change in vision or color perception on the patient's ability to perform activities of daily living and engage in desired pursuits.

Common Disorders in Older Adults

Cataract
Glaucoma
Diabetic retinopathy
Macular degeneration or macular hole
Corneal dystrophy

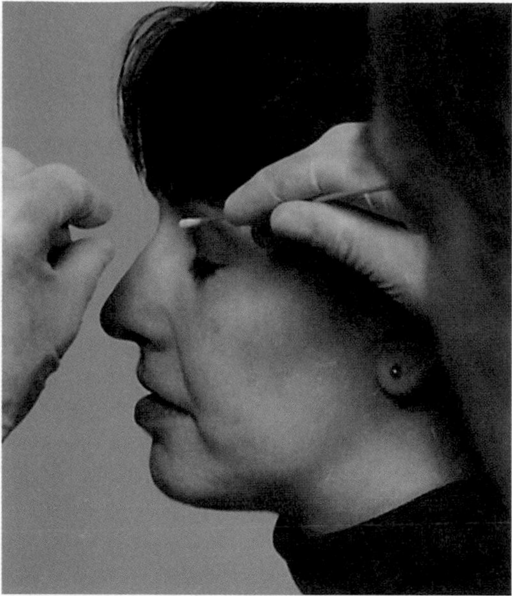

A

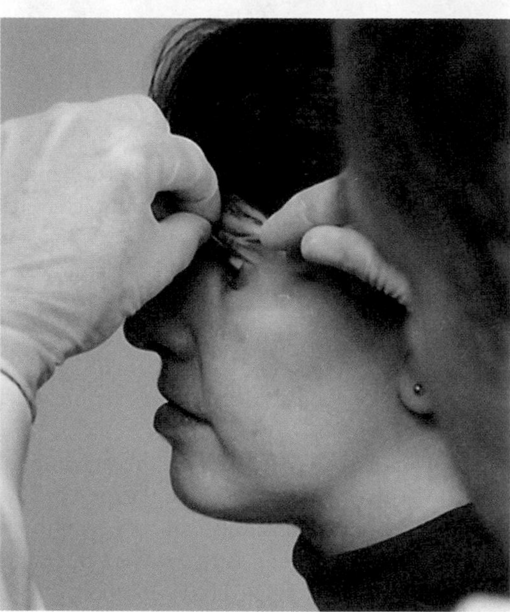

B

Figure 60-7 Eversion of upper eyelid. Patient is instructed to look downward, and lashes of upper eyelid are grasped between thumb and index finger. **A,** Cotton-tipped applicator is placed at level of tarsal fold. **B,** Eyelid is folded back on applicator while patient continues to look downward.

of foreign bodies, abrasions, and inflammation of the cornea. After the test, the nurse cleans the dye from the patient's face with a moist tissue.

When dry eyes are suspected, the nurse may perform Schirmer's test to verify abnormal tear production. The nurse explains the procedure to patients and informs them that the test may be uncomfortable but is not painful. The nurse measures the quantity of tears with a strip of filter paper, folded and hooked over the lower lid and left in place for approximately 5 minutes. The extent to which the filter paper is soaked with tears is then measured.

Next the nurse inspects the anterior chamber (the segment between the cornea and the iris) with the aid of a penlight and the "naked" eye or with the use of slit lamp magnification. The aqueous humor in the anterior chamber should be clear or transparent. After trauma, blood (hyphema) may be present. If the aqueous appears hazy or opaque, white cells are probably present, which is termed a *hypopyon.* The cells may be sterile or infectious.

The irises of the eyes are compared for color, pattern, and shape. When looking through the pupillary opening with an ophthalmoscope, the nurse should be able to visualize the red retinal fundus reflex. If the nurse looks nasally (toward the patient's nose) with the ophthalmoscope or has the patient look outward, the nurse should be able to see the optic nerve head (optic disc). Opacity of any of the clear ocular structures—cornea, lens, or vitreous—precludes clear visualization of the retina.

Pupillary Reflexes

The mnemonic PERRLA reminds the examiner that the *p*upils normally are *e*qual, *r*ound, and *r*eact to *l*ight and *a*ccommodation. When assessing the pupillary reflexes, the nurse approaches from the side and quickly shines a light into one eye, causing constriction of the pupil in that eye (direct light reaction). The pupil of the other eye should constrict the same amount (consensual light reaction). The nurse then tests the other eye in the same manner.

A light shining into a blind eye will not produce a pupillary response; however, a light shining into a normal eye will produce a pupillary response in the blind eye by consensual reaction if the oculomotor nerve is intact.[2]

Having the person focus on an object that is moved directly toward the nose tests the accommodative reflex. When the person focuses on the near object, the pupils of both eyes should constrict (near reaction or accommodation). The nurse looks for a response and notes whether the response is equal in both eyes. Loss of pupillary reflexes when sight is present is caused by neurologic disease.

Assessment of Vision

Visual acuity means acuteness or sharpness of vision and includes measurement of distance and near vision. Visual acuity can vary with attention, intelligence, and physical conditions such as lighting.[6]

Distance Vision. Distance vision usually is determined by the use of a Snellen chart (Figure 60-8, *A*), with the person positioned 20 feet (6 m) from the chart. The chart consists of rows of letters, numbers, or other characters arranged with the larger ones at the top and the smaller ones at the bottom. The uppermost letter on the chart is scaled so that it can be read by the normal eye at 200 feet, and the successive rows are scaled so that they can be read at 100, 70, 50, 40, 30, 20, 15, and 10 feet. Visual acuity is expressed as a fraction, and a reading of 20/20 is considered normal. The upper figure refers to the distance of the person from the chart, and the lower figure indicates the distance at which a normal eye can read the line. Each eye is tested separately, using a piece of stiff

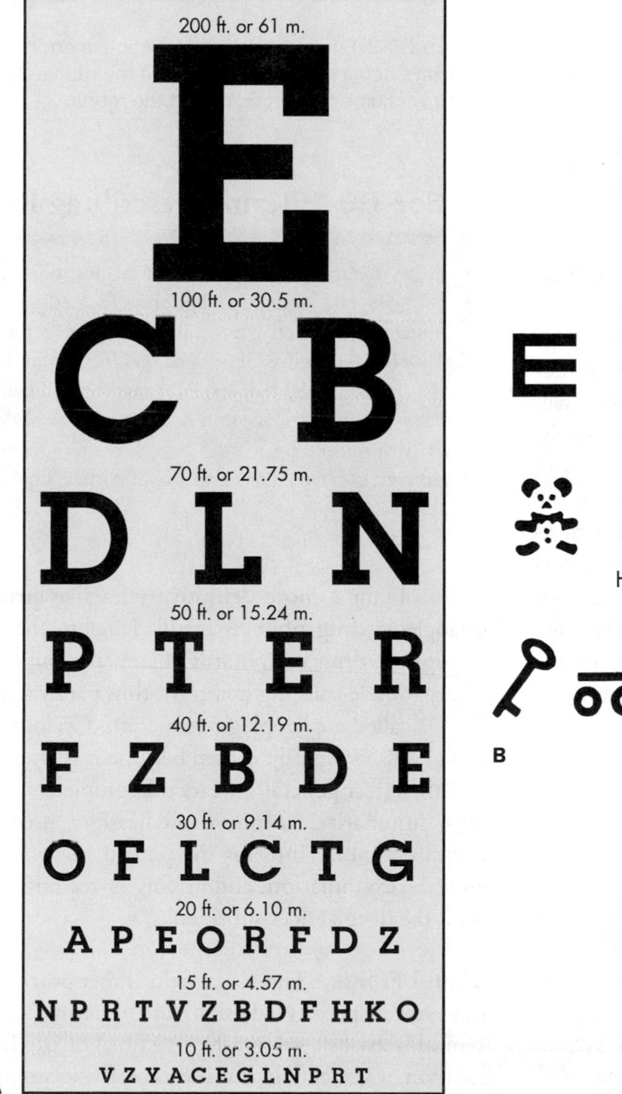

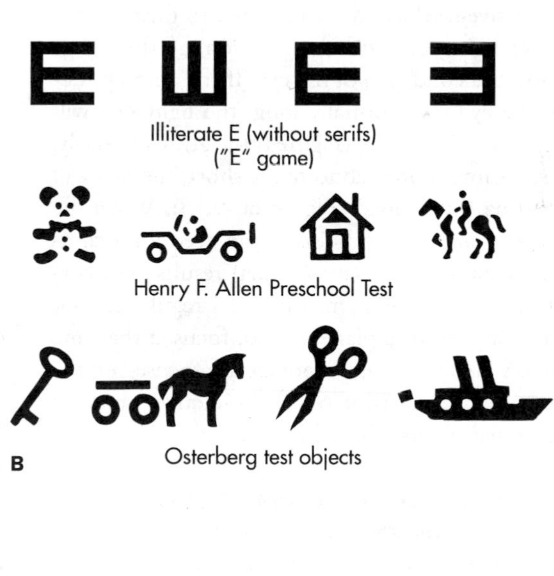

Figure 60-8 **A,** Snellen chart used in vision screening. **B,** Modified Snellen chart used in testing distance vision in children and illiterate adults.

paper or a plastic occluder to cover the eye not being tested. The person is tested with and without distance lenses, and the results are recorded. The right eye is always tested first to avoid confusion.

For preschool children, illiterate adults, and others unable to read the English alphabet, a modified Snellen chart may be used. A block E is shown in varying positions, and the person is asked to indicate in which direction the "legs" or "fingers" of the E point (Figure 60-8, *B*).

Near Vision. Near vision can be tested with the use of a Jaeger chart or newsprint. The Jaeger chart is a card containing varying sizes of print that is held 14 inches (35 cm) from the eye. The score obtained can be expressed in Jaeger or Snellen equivalent. For example, J1 is equal to Snellen 20/25; J2 = Snellen 20/30, J16 = Snellen 20/200.

For persons without sufficient vision to read letters, visual acuity can be assessed by asking them to count the number of the nurse's fingers that they can see held in front of their eyes. Some persons may not be able to count fingers but can see hand movement. Still others may be able to only tell the direction from which light is coming (light projection) or respond to light flashed in their eyes (light perception).[4] Table 60-3 presents examples of visual acuity measurements and their meanings. Any person with vision less than 20/30 OD (right eye) or OS (left eye) or with a two-line difference between eyes should be referred to an ophthalmologist for further testing and treatment, since the Snellen, block E, and Jaegar chart examinations provide only basic screening test data.

Refraction. Light rays entering the eye pass through the various transparent refractive media and are refracted to focus on the retina. The bending light rays and the location of the image depend on the shape and condition of the eye. If the anteroposterior dimension of the eye is abnormally long, the light rays will focus in front of the retina (myopia) (Figure 60-9, *A*). Conversely, if the anteroposterior dimension is abnormally short, the rays will focus behind the retina (hyperopia) (Figure 60-9, *B*). When the lens becomes less elastic and responds less to the need for accommodation, blurring of near objects (presbyopia) results. The curvature of the cornea also may be asymmetric or irregular so that rays in the horizontal and vertical planes do not focus at the same point (astigmatism). When the image is not clearly focused on the retina, refractive error is present (Box 60-1). Refractive errors are the most common impairments of good vision.

TABLE 60-3 EXAMPLES OF VISUAL ACUITY MEASUREMENT

Measurement	Meaning
20/20	Normal
20/40-2	Missed two letters of the 20/40 line
10/400	At 10 ft, reads line that normal eye sees at 400 ft
CF/2 ft	Counts fingers at 2 ft
HM/1 ft	Sees hand movement at 1 ft
LP/Proj.	Light perception with projection
NLP	No light perception

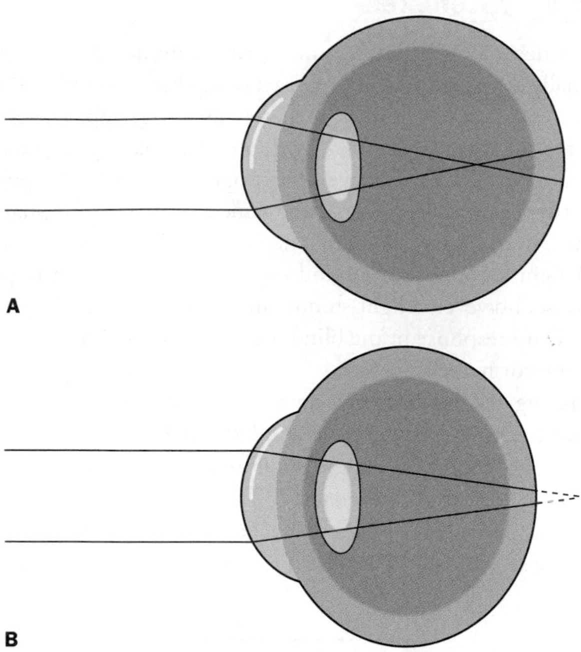

Figure 60-9 Two major types of refractive errors. **A,** Myopia. Parallel light rays come to a focus in front of the retina. **B,** Hyperopia. Parallel light rays come to a focus behind the retina.

Box 60-1 Terms Describing Refraction

- *Accommodation:* Ability to adjust for near objects
- *Emmetropia:* Normal eye; light rays focused on retina
- *Ametropia:* Refractive error; light rays not focused on retina
- *Myopia:* Nearsightedness; light rays focused in front of retina
- *Hyperopia:* Farsightedness; light rays focused behind retina
- *Presbyopia:* Loss of accommodation because of decreased lens elasticity in middle age
- *Astigmatism:* Irregular curvature of cornea; light rays not focused at same point

To obtain a more definitive refractive error measurement, a cycloplegic drug often is instilled before the examination. The cycloplegic drug temporarily dilates the pupil and paralyzes the ciliary muscle (placing it at rest), thus paralyzing accommodation. This is called a cycloplegic refraction. Cyclopentolate (Cyclogyl), 1% or 2%, ordinarily is used because it is effective in 30 minutes, and the effect generally wears off completely after 6 hours. Table 60-4 summarizes common medications used for eye examinations. The nurse informs the patient that vision will be blurred after the examination, and driving or reading will not be possible until the drug's effect subsides.

Visual Fields. The visual field is that portion of the world that the eye can perceive. Lesions of the retina, optic pathways, and central nervous system affect sections of the field of vision. The location of visual field loss indicates the location of the lesion. For instance, glaucoma decreases peripheral vision, indicating damage to the optic nerve at its head or the optic disc.

A rough measurement of the visual fields can be made with the confrontation test (see Chapter 47). If there appears to be any

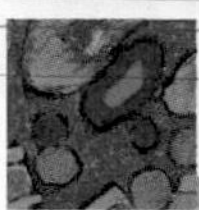

TABLE 60-4
COMMON MEDICATIONS *for Diagnostic Eye Tests*

Drug	Action	Nursing Intervention
Mydriatics (eyedrops): Phenylephrine hydrochloride (Neo-Synephrine, Mydfrin)	Pupil dilation by blocking responses to sphincter muscle of iris from cholinergic stimulation	Evaluate effectiveness (dark-eyed individuals usually require more drops to achieve dilation required). Use is contraindicated in patients with history of narrow or closed anterior chamber angles, since it may precipitate an increase intraocular pressure or angle-closure attack. Monitor for temporary blurred vision; caution patients about driving or operating machinery until vision improves. Monitor for photophobia, and instruct patient to wear dark glasses in sunlight or brightly lit rooms as needed.
Cycloplegics (eyedrops): atropine sulfate, cyclopentolate hydrochloride, homatropine hydrobromide, tropicamide	Pupil dilation, but also blocks accommodation by paralyzing ciliary muscles	Same as for mydriatics

abnormality in the field of vision, more precise testing is performed by an ophthalmologist or a specially trained nurse or technician. The patient's peripheral vision can be precisely plotted using the perimeter, an instrument that measures the visual fields in degrees of arc. The tangent screen (though seldom used) is the simplest perimeter, in which peripheral vision is plotted as a test object is moved against a black screen. Various automated and computer-assisted perimeters are more commonly used to measure visual fields.

The central portion of the visual field can also be measured with the Amsler grid, a 20-cm square divided into 5-mm squares with a dot in the center (Figure 60-10). The grid is used to detect and follow a central area of blindness (scotoma). It most commonly is used at home by the patient to detect progression of macular disease. With glasses on and one eye closed, the person holds the grid at the customary reading distance (12 inches). While fixating on the central dot, the person describes or outlines any area of distortion or absence of the grid. Distortions of the lines or blank areas imply dysfunction of the central retina (macula) or diseases of the optic nerve.

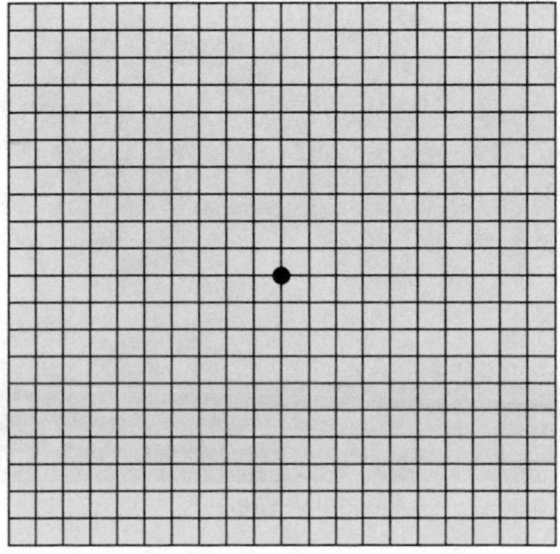

Figure 60-10 Amsler grid.

Color Vision Testing. Color vision testing is not always part of the normal eye examination. It is used most frequently to test for color blindness in persons seeking motor vehicle licenses or jobs for which color discrimination is important. Color vision deficiencies occur as a hereditary defect in both men (7%) and women (0.5%). Nutritional deficiencies, drug toxicities, and various disorders of the optic nerve and fovea centralis also can alter color perception.

There are both gross and sensitive measures of color vision. A common test consists of color plates on which numbers are outlined in primary colors and surrounded by confusion colors. The person with a color vision problem is unable to recognize the figure. The more sensitive tests involve hue discrimination. One such test consists of 84 chips of color that are ordered in terms of increasing hue.

Assessment of Ocular Movements

The nurse should observe the eyes for alignment and for movement of the eyes together in all fields of gaze.[7] Any limitation should be further investigated to detect extraocular muscle imbalance or cranial nerve disorder.

To test ocular muscles, the nurse and patient sit facing each other. The patient looks straight ahead, and the nurse shines a penlight on the cornea. The corneal light reflex should be in exactly the same position on each pupil. The nurse then evaluates the individual extraocular muscles; muscle testing is performed in six cardinal positions of gaze, as well as straight ahead. Chapter 47 presents more detailed information about assessment of ocular movements.

If a muscle weakness or deviation is found, the nurse then covers one of the subject's eyes and asks the person to look at the light. When the cover is quickly removed, the nurse notes whether the eye moves to regain fixation on the light. A movement drift of the eye behind the cover indicates a muscle imbalance.

Inspection of Ocular Structures

Slit Lamp Examination. The anterior segment of the eye is examined with a slit lamp, an instrument that combines a microscope and a light source. By adjusting the focus and light, the examiner can check for such problems as corneal abrasions and foreign bodies, anterior chamber cells, and lens changes. Vitreous and retinal changes are best examined with an ophthalmoscope.

Estimation of Intraocular Pressure. An instrument known as a tonometer is used to measure intraocular tension and is helpful in detecting early glaucoma. Goldmann's applanation tonometer is the most accurate way of estimating intraocular pressure; it is attached to the slit lamp (Figure 60-11). With this instrument a small area of the cornea is flattened to counterbalance a spring-loaded measuring device, and the pressure is measured directly.

The Schiøtz tonometer is the most common instrument in general use worldwide. The procedure is performed with the patient lying down or in the chair with the head back and looking upward at some fixed point. A topical anesthetic eye drop is give before the tonometer is placed on the cornea (Figure 60-12). The instrument's scale indicates the amount of indentation it makes in the cornea. This reading is converted using a chart to determine the intraocular pressure. Readings over 22 mm Hg (Schiøtz) suggest glaucoma, but tests usually are repeated because temporary increases sometimes are caused by factors such as emotional stress.

A relatively new tonometer, the Tono-Pen (Figure 60-13), is widely replacing the Schiøtz in the Western World. The instrument is handheld perpendicular to the cornea. Gentle tapping over the central cornea enables several readings to be taken and averaged. A digital LED screen displays the final reading.

Ophthalmoscopy. The ocular fundus is examined with a handheld instrument called an **ophthalmoscope**, which magnifies the intraocular view so that the vitreous, retina, optic disc, blood vessels, and macula can be seen through the pupil (Figure 60-14). The examiner may use either the direct (Figure 60-15) or the indirect (Figure 60-16) method of ophthalmoscopic examina-

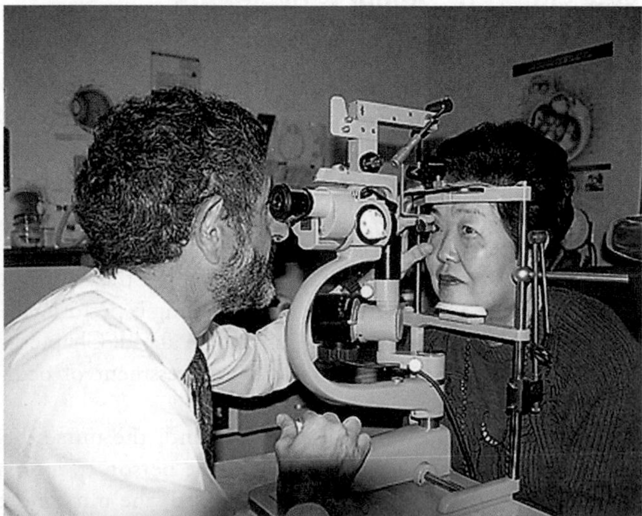

Figure 60-11 Measurement of intraocular pressure with applanation tonometer attached to a slit lamp.

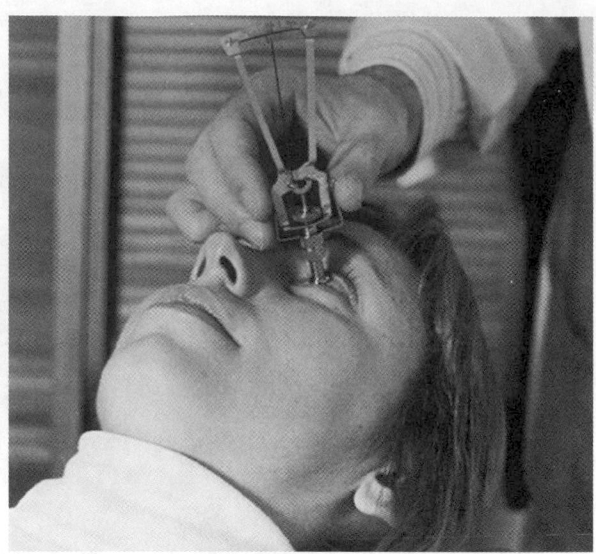

Figure 60-12 Measurement of intraocular pressure with Schiøtz tonometer.

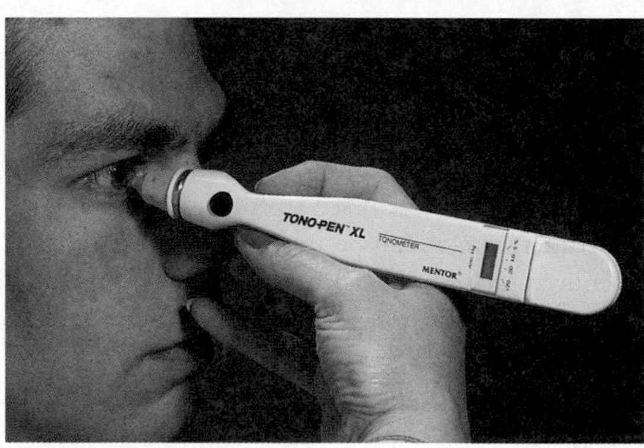

Figure 60-13 Tono-Pen tonometer.

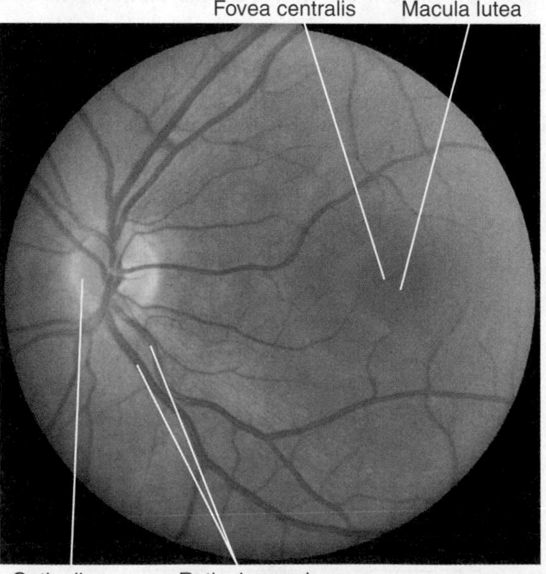

Figure 60-14 Normal right fundus seen through a direct ophthalmoscope.

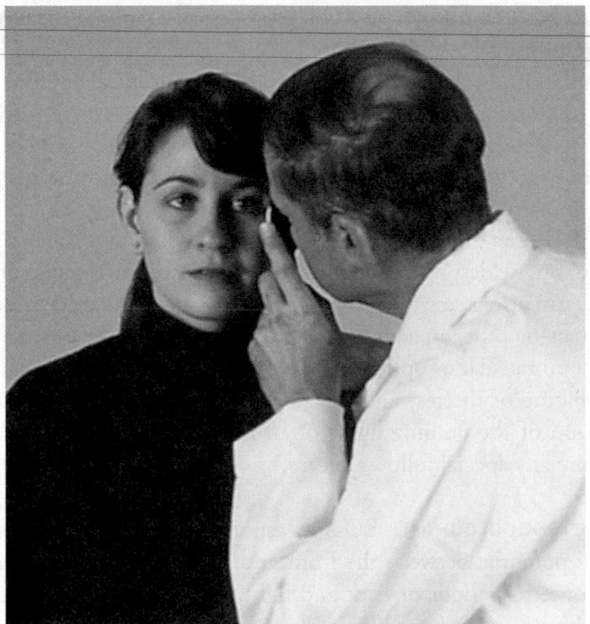

Figure 60-15 Direct method of ophthalmoscopic examination.

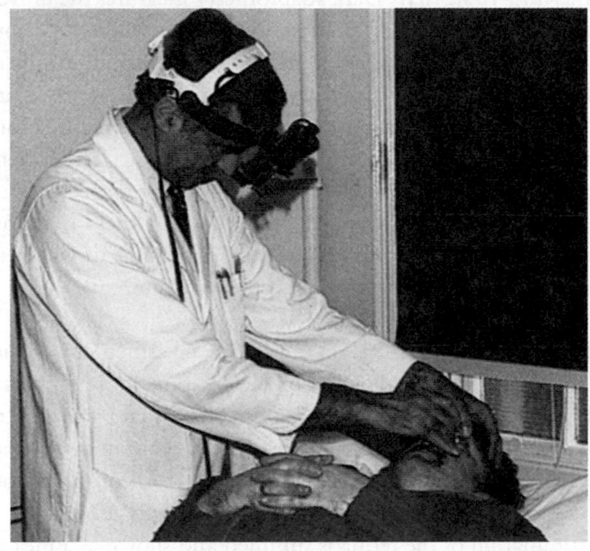

Figure 60-16 Indirect method of ophthalmoscopic examination.

tion. The indirect ophthalmoscope permits the examiner to view the retina stereoscopically, thus allowing a wide-angle, three-dimensional view. This method provides visualization of the ocular fundus as far as the ora serrata (anterior margin of the retina). The indirect method, which requires a great degree of skill, normally is performed by an ophthalmologist. Nurses trained to perform an ophthalmoscopic examination use the direct method, the more common approach. Because the entire retina cannot be visualized at one time, the examiner moves the ophthalmoscope until the entire fundus is visualized.

Difficulty in visualizing the fundus may be caused by interference with the light penetrating the eye as a result of corneal clouding, cataract, or intraocular inflammation. Data obtained from fundus examination may indicate eye disease (cupping of the disc in glaucoma) or systemic disease (arteriosclerosis or hypertension). Hemorrhages in deep retinal layers occur in advanced hypertension, severe renal disease, certain collagen diseases, advanced diabetes, and blood dyscrasias.

Diagnostic Tests

Laboratory Tests

A blood glucose test, drawn for a complaint of blurred vision, may reveal diabetes mellitus. An erythrocyte sedimentation rate is used to diagnose and monitor the disease process of temporal arteritis. Urine tests play no significant role in the evaluation of ocular problems.

Radiologic Tests

Several radiologic procedures aid in the diagnosis of ocular conditions. These include plain x-ray films, computed tomography (CT) scans, and magnetic resonance imaging (MRI).

Plain X-Ray Films. Plain x-ray films of the orbit assist in the diagnosis of orbital fractures and tumors. Right and left oblique views and a lateral view of the affected side usually provide the needed information.

Computed Tomography Scan. The CT scan is a rapid, safe, and noninvasive technique for investigating serial sections of the orbit and eye. The globe, lens, vitreous humor, optic nerve, extraocular muscles, visual pathway, and brain can all be evaluated. The CT scan is valuable in the diagnosis of orbital disease, retrobulbar tumors, intraocular masses, and intracranial disease and can be augmented by the injection of contrast material that increases the density of inflammatory or vascular lesions.[6] The nurse's primary responsibilities relate to careful pretest patient teaching.

Magnetic Resonance Imaging. MRI is a noninvasive technique that uses a high magnetic field to evaluate the brain, orbit, and eye. MRI provides better definition of tissues and fluids in the brain and eye than can be achieved with a CT scan. It is particularly helpful in identifying edema.[9] The nurse explains the procedure and carefully prepares the patient for the noises and sensations experienced during the test.

Special Tests

Ultrasonography. Ultrasonography is a noninvasive test that uses high-frequency sound waves to outline and detect intraocular and orbital structures and measure the distance between them.[5] This test can easily delineate various abnormalities, such as choroidal and retinal masses and detachments, intraocular foreign bodies, and changes in the orbit. Two types of ultrasonography, A-scan and B-scan, are used in ophthalmology. The A-scan is useful in differentiating tumors and measuring the axial length of the eyeball, a value that is needed to calculate the power of an intraocular lens for implantation after a cataract extraction. The B-scan provides a two-dimensional image that helps visualize tumors, retinal detachments, swollen muscles, or inflamed tissue.

In both scans the examiner places a probe on either the cornea or the closed eyelid, sound waves are delivered, and measurements are recorded on the screen of the oscilloscope. The test is not uncomfortable, although anesthetic drops may be instilled if the probe is applied directly to the eye. The nurse gives the patient information about the procedure itself and any sensory effects.

Fluorescein Angiography. Fluorescein angiography is a specialized procedure used in the diagnosis, monitoring, and treatment of eye diseases. After mydriatic eyedrops are instilled to dilate the pupils, thereby facilitating visualization of the fundus, fluorescein dye is injected into a vein in the antecubital fossa of the patient's arm. The retinal and ciliary arteries transmit the dye into the eyes, and the retinal arteriovenous circulation is visualized. The dye reaches the retinal arteries 10 to 16 seconds after the injection, and the veins are filled within 25 seconds. To provide a permanent record of this circulation, photographs are taken with a specially designed camera called a fundus camera. The camera is equipped with an optical system for viewing the retina and a light flash system for illumination and is mounted on a stand similar to that for a slit lamp. The patient sits in a chair with the chin placed in the chin rest and the forehead against a bar while a rapid series of photographs is taken to capture the movement of the dye through the retinal arteriovenous circulation. This test may take as long as 1 hour to complete. When the photographs are assessed, they provide definitive information about any avascular obstruction, the growth of new vessels (neovascularization), microaneurysms, abnormal capillary permeability, and defects in the pigmented layer of the retina.

Fluorescein angiography is a relatively safe procedure with few untoward effects. The patient is assessed for any allergies or previous reaction to dye. Those with a history of hay fever or asthma may be given a small test dose before the entire dose is injected.[1] A severe allergic reaction, although rare, can occur.

The nurse explains the procedure, obtains an informed consent, and explains the need to keep the head still during the test. The nurse warns the patient that a dazzle effect may occur from the frequent camera flashes and may take several minutes to resolve after the test. Some patients experience transient nausea or vomiting as the dye is injected. The nurse also informs the patient that yellowing of the skin, especially in persons with fair complexions, and a fluorescent orange or green discoloration of the urine usually is present for 24 hours. Patients are encouraged to drink increased amounts of fluids to promote excretion of the dye. The pupils remain dilated for a few hours, and the patient should avoid bright light and wear sunglasses when outdoors until the pupils return to normal.

Electrophysiology Examinations. Four electrophysiology examinations are performed in ophthalmology: electroretinogram (ERG), electrooculogram (EOG), dark adaptometry, and visual evoked potential (VEP). The main purpose of these examinations is to assess the function of the visual pathway from the photoreceptors of the retina to the visual cortex of the brain. Electrophysiologic testing is useful in diagnosing retinal vascular occlusions, toxic drug exposure, inherited retinal diseases, and intraocular foreign bodies.[3]

ELECTRORETINOGRAM. ERG is a process of graphing the electrical response from the retina that occurs as a consequence of light stimulation. In this test the pupil is dilated, a topical anesthetic is applied, and a corneal electrode is placed on the cornea using a contact lens. A grounding electrode is placed on the ear. Lights at various intensities and intervals are then flashed and the nervous response graphed.

ERG tests the function of the rods and cones and is helpful in evaluating widespread retinal disease such as retinitis pigmentosa. ERG can also assess the visual potential of an eye that has a dense cataract or other opacification. However, normal results do not rule out macular or optic nerve disease. The nurse tells the patient the nature of the test and the steps of the procedure. A demonstration of the flashing lights often is helpful. The test does not require any special follow-up care.

ELECTROOCULOGRAM. EOG measures the difference in the electrical potential between the front and back of the eye (retina) in response to periods of dark and light. Skin electrodes are placed on the lateral and medial canthi of both eyes. Corneal contact lenses are not required.

DARK ADAPTOMETRY. Dark adaptometry measures the universal phenomenon of dark adaptation. Normally, when a person is placed in a room and the lights are suddenly turned out, the eyes gradually become more sensitive and vision in the darkness improves over time. For this test, the patient is placed in a totally darkened room with a dark adaptometer machine. The patient is then exposed to a standardized level of light for a specified time. The light is gradually dimmed until total darkness is restored. Patients respond to the various intensities of light to which they are exposed by pushing a button on the machine.

VISUAL EVOKED POTENTIAL. VEP is a measurement of visual function monitored at the level of the occipital cortex with scalp electrodes that evaluate the integrity of the visual pathways from the optic nerve to the occipital cortex. Stimulation of the retina with light changes the electrical activity of the cortex. Through various computer processes, the electrical activity associated with this stimulation of the retina is summed and shown as a measurable electrical wave. Optic neuritis, demyelinating disease, and optic atrophy can alter this wave. For these electrophysiologic tests, the nurse explains the procedures, indicating that they are pain free and require no special follow-up care.

▶ ARE YOU READY?

Which of the following should be included in patient teaching after fluorescein angiography?

1. Keep affected eye covered for the first 24 hours.
2. Increase fluid intake.
3. Avoid nose blowing for 24 hours.
4. Avoid lying flat for 8 hours.

References

1. Anand R: Fluorescein angiography, part 1, Technique and normal study, *J Ophthalmol Nurs Technol* 8:48, 1989.
2. Bickley LS et al: *Bates' guide to physical examination and history taking,* ed 8, Philadelphia, 2003, Lippincott, Williams & Wilkins.
3. Follmer BA, Smith SC: Electrophysiology testing and the ophthalmic registered nurse, *Insight* 19(4):1, 1994.
4. Leasia S, Monahan FD: *A practical guide to health assessment,* ed 2, Philadelphia, 2002, Saunders.
5. Mrochuk J: Introduction to diagnostic ophthalmic ultrasound for nurses in ophthalmology, *J Ophthalmol Nurs Technol* 9:234, 1990.
6. Newell F: *Ophthalmology: principles and concepts,* ed 8, St Louis, 1996, Mosby.
7. Riordan-Eva P, Vaughan D, Asbury T: *General ophthalmology,* ed 16, Los Altos, Calif, 2004, Lange.
8. West S: Ultraviolet B exposure and lens opacities: a review, *J Epidemiol* 9(Suppl 6):97, 1999.
9. Wirtschafter JD, Berman EL, McDonald CS: *Magnetic resonance imaging and computed tomography: clinical neuro-orbital anatomy,* San Francisco, 1992, American Academy of Ophthalmology.

evolve Visit the Evolve website: http://evolve.elsevier.com/Monahan/medsurg

CHAPTER 61

Problems of the Eye

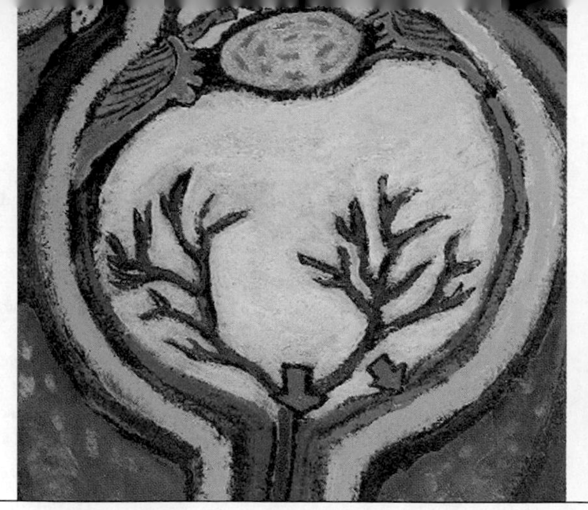

by Heather G. Boyd-Monk

OBJECTIVES

After studying this chapter, the learner should be able to:

1. Discuss the etiology and management of common forms of visual impairment.
2. Compare the pathophysiology of common eye inflammations and infections.
3. Describe the emergency treatment of eye injury.
4. Discuss the collaborative management of glaucoma.
5. Compare the preoperative and postoperative care of patients undergoing surgery for cataracts and retinal detachment.
6. Outline the effects of diabetes, hypertension, and acquired immunodeficiency syndrome on the eye.

KEY TERMS

cross-contamination, p. 1816
cycloplegic, p. 1826
hyperemia, p. 1815
microsurgical techniques, p. 1827
miotic, p. 1819
neovascularization, p. 1812
peripheral vision, p. 1814
refractive errors, p. 1810

According to the World Health Organization, an estimated 50 million people worldwide are blind. Another 150 million people suffer from blinding eye diseases. In the United States 100 million people are visually disabled without corrective lenses, and 1.5 million people have severe visual conditions not corrected by glasses. This chapter discusses the major causes of visual impairment, common eye infections and injuries, and the management of major eye disorders such as cataracts and glaucoma. The nurse plays a significant role in the collaborative care of patients experiencing eye disorders and also has an important role in educating the public about primary and secondary prevention strategies to maintain eye health.

Visual Impairment

Etiology and Epidemiology. Visual impairment ranges in severity from diminished visual acuity to total blindness. Legal blindness is defined in the United States as (1) a visual acuity, with maximal correction, of 20/200 or less; and/or (2) a visual field reduction to a range of 20 degrees (compared with a normal range of about 180 degrees). This is an arbitrary definition that was established early in the century to identify individuals who would need public assistance to function in society. This definition is not accepted or used worldwide.

An estimated 1.1 million persons in the United States are legally blind, and most of these persons are older than 65 years of age. Almost 80 million Americans suffer from potentially blinding eye disease in one or both eyes, and this figure does not include the additional millions of persons with straightforward **refractive errors** who require the use of corrective lenses to participate fully in daily activities. These figures make visual impairment one of the most common disorders affecting adults in this country.

Uncorrected vision problems have a negative impact on school and work performance. Loss of vision limits the individual's interaction with the environment and reduces the range and variety of experiences available. Personal care, home maintenance, social interaction, and interpersonal communication are all affected.

Visual impairment has numerous causes, and preventable blindness is a major worldwide health problem. Refractive errors are the most common problem, but numerous other nutritional, infectious, metabolic, and systemic disorders adversely affect the eye's function. Nutritional deficiencies are a major global health concern. A lack of adequate vitamin A and B complex can cause changes within the retina, cornea, and conjunctiva. Night blindness is a classic outcome of vitamin A deficiency, and optic neuritis can result from deficits of vitamin B, especially in persons with alcoholism. Infection (e.g., trachoma) is another common cause of visual impairment or blindness in millions of persons in developing countries. Macular degeneration, a disease of the aging retina, is the leading cause of blindness in older adults,[5] affecting 20% to 30% of persons between 75 and 85 years of age. The leading causes of visual impairment or blindness in the United States include cataracts, glaucoma, diabetic retinopathy, and macular degeneration.

The eye can also be adversely affected by a variety of systemic diseases (Table 61-1). The exophthalmos associated with Graves' disease is one of the most visible examples, and visual field defects (e.g., hemianopia—half the visual field missing) are common outcomes of stroke. An early symptom of the demyelination associated with multiple sclerosis may be a change in color vision followed by unilateral optic neuritis with loss of vision. Retinopathy is a complication of vascular disease, in particular uncontrolled hypertension, and is often both progressive and irreversible. Cytomegalovirus retinopathy is a serious complication associated with the severe immunocompromise of acquired immunodeficiency syndrome (AIDS). Diabetic retinopathy—despite the effectiveness of laser treatment in its early stages—commonly results in a steady progression toward blindness in diabetic patients with uncontrolled or brittle disease (see Chapter 39).

Pathophysiology

REFRACTIVE DISORDERS. Refractive disorders include irregularities of the corneal curvature, length, and shape of the eye, as well as the focusing ability of the lens. There are three main types of refractive disorders (Figure 61-3). The major symptoms of all three disorders include blurred vision and headache.

Myopia, or nearsightedness, occurs when parallel rays of light focus in front of the retina as the person looks at a distant object. Hyperopia, or farsightedness, occurs when light rays focus in back of the retina as the individual looks at a near object. A shortened eyeball may contribute to the problem. Astigmatism is caused by an unequal curvature of the cornea. Light rays are bent unevenly and do not focus on a single spot on the retina. Presbyopia is a common problem associated with aging. The lens loses elasticity, making it more difficult to focus on near objects.

AGE-RELATED MACULAR DEGENERATION. The pathologic changes of this chronic degenerative condition occur primarily in the retinal pigment epithelium, Bruch's membrane, and the choriocapillaris (small vessel layer of the choroid) beneath the macular

TABLE 61-1 EYE MANIFESTATIONS OF SYSTEMIC DISEASES

Disorder	Effect on Eyes
VASCULAR DISORDERS	
Hypertension	Persistent, uncontrolled hypertension can cause hemorrhage, edema, and exudates in retina. Retinal arteries narrow, causing degenerative changes.
Stroke	Depending on location of stroke, patient may experience hemianopia or blindness.
Sickle cell disease	This can cause neovascularization, arterial occlusions, or retinal hemorrhage.
NEUROLOGIC DISORDERS	
Multiple sclerosis	Demyelination can result in optic neuritis, diplopia, and nystagmus.
ENDOCRINE DISORDERS	
Graves' disease	Accumulation of fat and fluid in extraocular tissue can produce exophthalmos (protrusion of eye) and lid retraction.
Diabetic retinopathy	Retinal capillary walls thicken and develop microaneurysms. Retinal veins bead and become tortuous, leaking fluid and lipid (Figure 61-1). Small hemorrhages occur, which leave scars that decrease vision. As disease worsens, neovascularization occurs, and new vessels grow into vitreous humor. These vessels are vulnerable to both obstruction and rupture. Vision decreases, and "floaters" are perceived in eye.
CONNECTIVE TISSUE DISORDERS	
Rheumatoid arthritis, systemic lupus erythematosus	Neovascularization and inflammation of cornea, sclera, or uveal tract occur.
AIDS-RELATED DISORDERS	
Herpes zoster ophthalmicus	Herpes can invade cornea and create ulceration that is potentially blinding.
Cytomegalovirus (CMV)	CMV affects an estimated 20% of AIDS patients. It spreads rapidly through cells of retina and blood vessels and can totally destroy retina (Figure 61-2).
Kaposi's sarcoma	Lesions of Kaposi's sarcoma can affect skin of eyelids and conjunctiva or orbit itself.

AIDS, Acquired immunodeficiency syndrome.

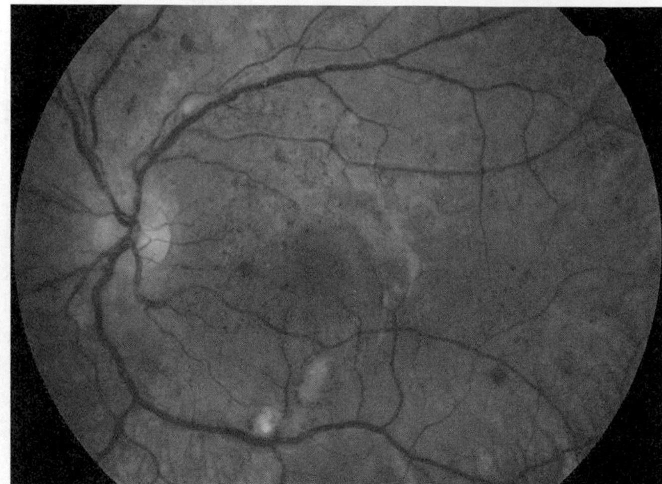

Figure 61-1 Diabetic retinopathy with cotton wool spots (exudates) below macula.

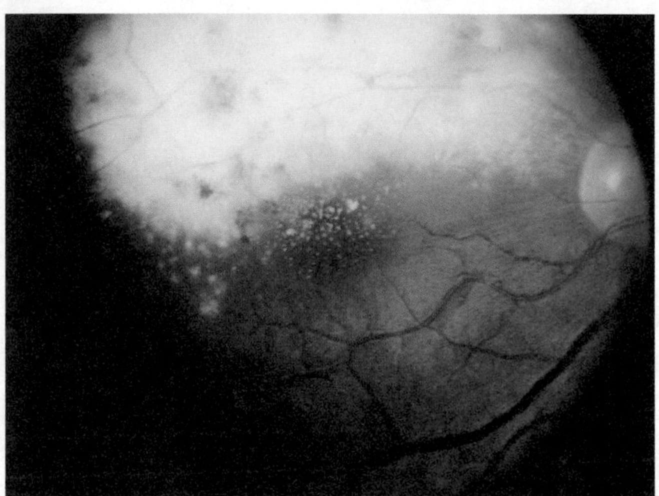

Figure 61-2 Cytomegalovirus retinitis infiltrating superior retina.

region. Both neovascular (exudative, or wet) and nonneovascular (dry) forms occur. In neovascular degeneration a sudden proliferation of new, fragile blood vessels in the normally avascular macular area tend to leak and damage the macula. A painless decrease of central vision may occur rapidly over days or weeks. Although only 5% to 10% of all patients have wet macular degeneration, it is responsible for about 80% of the severe loss of vision attributed to the disease. Degeneration occurs from the deposit of waste products and slow atrophy of the choroid and retinal pigment epithelium.

Macular degeneration causes a variety of symptoms, including initial visual blurring and distortion, some degree of central vision loss, and a decreased ability to distinguish colors. Early signs and progression of the disease can be detected with the use of the Amsler grid (see Chapter 60). The individual perceives missing areas (e.g., in a book's page) and distorted, wavy lines. Intravenous fluorescein angiography may be used to visualize or confirm the extent of **neovascularization** if macular edema is suspected.

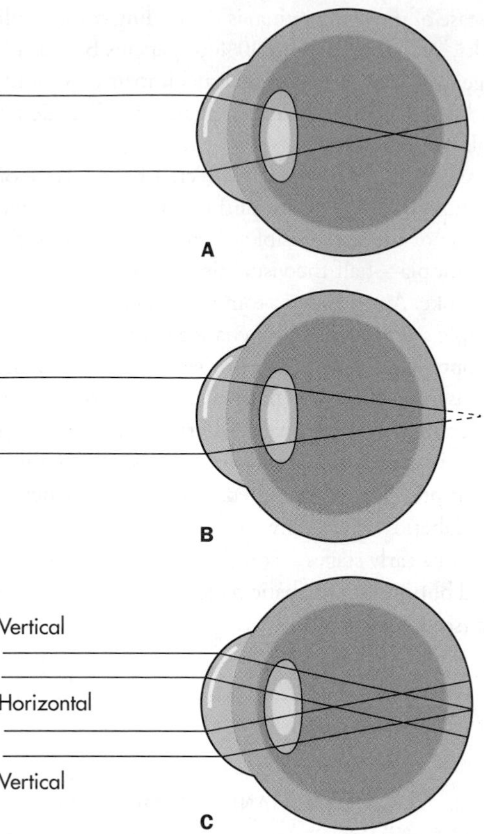

Figure 61-3 Three types of refractive errors. **A,** Myopic eye. Parallel rays of light are brought to focus in front of retina. **B,** Hyperopic eye. Parallel rays of light come to focus behind retina in unaccommodative eye. **C,** Astigmatism. Light rays entering eye are bent at different meridians, preventing a sharp focus on the retina.

Collaborative Care Management

Refractive Disorders

Corrective Lenses. Visual impairments caused by refractive errors are usually diagnosed as part of a routine eye examination. The person may initiate the diagnostic process in response to chronic headache or blurred or failing vision. Eyeglasses and contact lenses are widely used to correct common refractive errors and restore visual acuity. Federal law requires that all prescription glasses be made with impact-resistant lenses. Plastic lenses are lightweight but scratch easily. Hardened and safety lenses have been tempered to make them extremely resistant to breakage.

Contact lenses are made of various types of thin plastic that fit over the cornea. Their popularity is primarily cosmetic, but some people achieve better vision correction with contact lenses than with glasses. Contact lenses may be rigid or soft. In addition to standard hard and soft lenses, the rigid category includes gas-permeable lenses, and the soft category includes extended-wear and disposable lenses. Rigid (hard) lenses are easy to care for, are relatively inexpensive, and correct vision efficiently. However, rigid lenses that are not gas permeable are generally uncomfortable and require a prolonged period of adaptation. Wearing time generally does not exceed 12 hours. Gas-permeable lenses have the optical quality of other hard lenses but are permeable to oxygen and other gases and are generally more comfortable for the wearer.

Soft lenses are flexible and can often be used successfully by persons who cannot tolerate hard lenses. They cost more and require frequent replacement. Disposable soft contact lenses are similar to standard soft contact lenses, but they can be inexpensively manufactured and are discarded after a set period of use, thus eliminating cleaning and disinfecting. Extended-wear soft contact lenses can be left in place for as long as a month, but their use is generally limited to 1 week, at which time they are removed for cleaning and disinfection. Some physicians are concerned that use of any extended-wear contact lens increases the risk of ulcerative keratitis (inflammation of the cornea). Extended-wear contact lens users were found to have a 5 to 15 times higher risk of developing ulcerative keratitis than wearers who removed and cleaned their lenses every day.[1] Newer hyperoxygen lenses that do not cause corneal hypoxia are thought to be safer. However, all contact lenses can cause problems, and careful attention to recommended regimens for cleaning and disinfection are important for success.

REFRACTIVE SURGERY. Refractive surgery, defined as any operative procedure performed for the purpose of eliminating a refraction error, has become an increasingly viable alternative to glasses and contact lenses for persons with visual impairment related to refraction errors. The most common procedure, photorefractive keratectomy (Figure 61-4), uses an excimer laser to reshape the surface of the cornea. Thin sections of outer cornea can also be removed to correct higher degrees of myopia. Recent advances have added the ability to correct hyperopia and the age-related condition presbyopia.

The most recent innovation in refractive procedures is the implantation of two semicircular plastic rings called Intacs. Intacs are placed within the layers of the cornea but do not involve the optical center. They may be removed, if necessary, which reverses the effect. They are currently available only to treat low levels of myopia.

These procedures are usually performed in ambulatory surgery centers. Careful preoperative teaching about the goals and limitations of the surgery and the expected postoperative course is essential. Patients are permitted to gradually resume activities and usually experience a slow improvement of vision over a period of weeks or months. Analgesic pain management and infection control with antimicrobial eyedrops are implemented by the nurse in the immediate postoperative period.

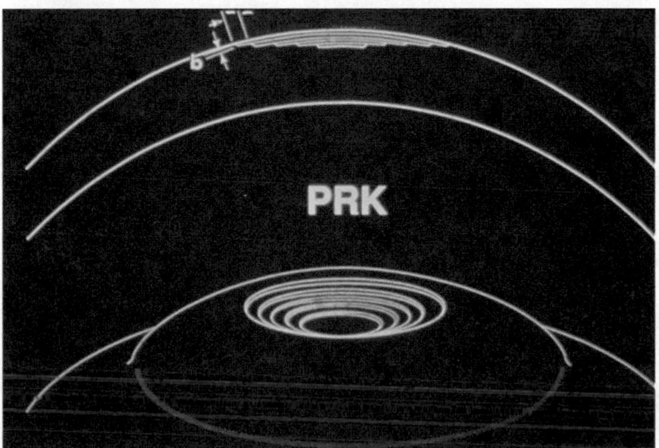

Figure 61-4 Photorefractive keratectomy *(PRK)* showing raised flap of corneal epithelium with stromal layer to be ablated with excimer laser.

MACULAR DEGENERATION. No adequate treatment is currently available for the dry (nonneovascular) form of age-related macular degeneration (AMD). A small percentage of patients with wet (neovascular) AMD may benefit from laser therapy to coagulate the abnormal vessels, or from photodynamic therapy (PDT) with intravenously injected verteporfin (Visudyne). PDT uses low-level laser light to activate the drug within the abnormal blood vessels, rendering them inactive and subsequently temporarily stabilizing central vision. Patients usually require multiple treatments spaced at least 90 days apart to obtain the desired result. Vision is not improved with either type of laser intervention; however, additional loss of central vision is often spared.

Results of the Age-Related Eye Disease Studies (AREDS), two randomized, multicenter clinical trials funded by the National Eye Institute, concluded that persons older than 55 should have dilated eye examinations to determine their risk of developing advanced AMD. The ophthalmologist looks for drusen (subretinal hyaline deposits); if these are present, the patient should consider taking a supplement of antioxidants plus zinc to prevent progression of AMD.[6]

PATIENT/FAMILY TEACHING. Some forms of visual impairment are preventable, and most forms can be slowed or treated with early diagnosis and appropriate therapy. Regular eye examinations by a competent professional are an important health promotion measure throughout life, especially as a person ages. Early identification of eye disorders such as glaucoma is essential to prevent loss of vision. Appropriate intervention for cataracts can restore useful vision, and the rigorous control of systemic diseases such as diabetes and hypertension can minimize the adverse visual consequences.

Multiple opportunities exist for education and intervention with patients and families regarding preserving visual function and promoting eye health. The importance of this area is reflected in the *Healthy People 2010* goals,[8] one of which is to improve the nation's visual health through prevention, early detection, treatment, and rehabilitation.

Maintaining eye health is an important teaching intervention for all patients, not just those experiencing eye problems. The eye is a remarkably resilient organ. The external surface (cornea and conjunctiva) is constantly cleansed by the tears that contain lysozyme (a bacteriostatic enzyme) washing over it. As a consequence, normal healthy eyes do not need special care or cleaning. Rubbing the eyes can introduce bacteria onto the surface and therefore should be avoided.

Adequate nutrition is as important for healthy eyes as it is for maintaining other body functions. Vitamin A deficiency can result in night blindness and corneal damage. Optic atrophy and neuropathy have been associated with vitamin B complex and other nutritional deficiencies. Although a sufficient vitamin intake is necessary, an excessive amount is wasted and may actually do more harm than good.

It is difficult to predict the course of any progressive visual impairment, and patients rightly fear becoming blind. The nurse ensures that the patient has accurate information about the specific disease, type of vision loss, and prognosis. Opportunities to express fears and frustrations related to declining vision could be helpful to the patient and family. Social support is a key factor in the patient's adjustment to visual impairment. The nurse can also provide referrals for the patient to the numerous community agencies that provide support services to visually impaired persons as they incorporate their changing vision status into their daily lives. Integration of declining vision or blindness into one's self-concept can take a long time. A social stigma related to blindness still exists, and patients need ongoing support and understanding.

Persons with visual impairment must make a major life adjustment, both to the initial impact of the loss and the subsequent changes in their life. Over time most patients learn new ways or adapt their present ways of carrying out normal activities. Most recognize that there are some things that they will never be able to do again or that they can do only with help. The dependence on others and the need to ask for help can be difficult. Fluctuating vision leads to frustration and difficulties in planning or implementing tasks.

The nurse ensures that the patient has any visual aids that may be useful, including magnifying glasses and high-intensity reading lights. Patients with progressive macular degeneration need to learn how to optimize their **peripheral vision** as their central vision deteriorates. Adjustment is an ongoing process, and time is a key variable. Time is needed to grieve for the lost sight, to come to terms with the implications of the loss, and to master many of the difficult tasks related to a visual impairment. Figure 61-5 and the Guidelines for Safe Practice boxes, below and p. 1814, provide useful strategies for assisting the visually impaired person.

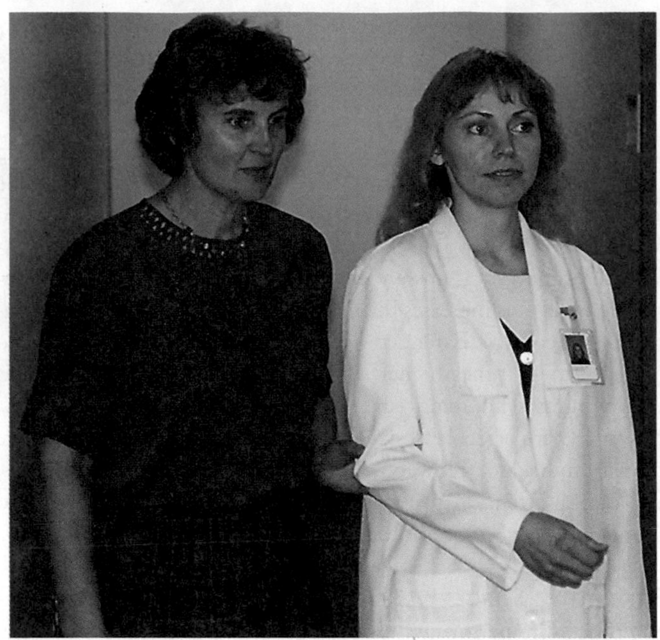

Figure 61-5 Helping a visually impaired person to walk. Note that the woman is holding the nurse's arm and is led without being held.

▶ ARE YOU READY?

Deficiency of which vitamin can result in night blindness and corneal damage?

1. Vitamin A
2. Vitamin C
3. Vitamin E
4. Vitamin K

Infections and Inflammation

Infections and inflammation can occur in any of the eye structures and may be caused by microorganisms, mechanical irritation, or sensitivity to some substance. Inflammation of the eye is the most common acute condition affecting the eye. Conjunctivitis represents about two thirds of the total cases of inflammation. Table 61-2 summarizes the common eye infections and inflammations and their management. Conjunctivitis is discussed in the following section. Box 61-1 summarizes ophthalmic drugs used to treat inflammation and infection.

Conjunctivitis

Etiology and Epidemiology. Conjunctivitis can be infectious or inflammatory. Staphylococci, streptococci, or *Haemophilus influenzae* are the most frequent causes of infections. Two sexually transmitted agents that cause conjunctivitis are *Chlamydia trachomatis and Neisseria gonorrhoeae.* Acute mucopurulent bacterial conjunctivitis (often called pinkeye) is the most common form of conjunctivitis. It is prevalent in school-age children but can occur at any age. It is highly infectious, especially in crowded environments such as schools and nursing homes. It is usually self-limiting and causes no permanent damage.

Viral agents that cause conjunctivitis include the herpes simplex viruses and most human adenovirus strains, which can also occur in highly contagious epidemic forms involving the cornea, known as epidemic keratoconjunctivitis (EKC). Inflammation may be caused by mechanical trauma (eyelashes rubbing against

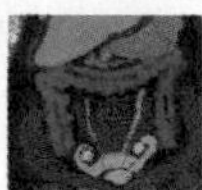

GUIDELINES FOR SAFE PRACTICE *Facilitating Independence in Activities of Daily Living for Visually Impaired Patients*

- Place clothing in specific and consistent locations in drawers and closets.
- Place food and cooking utensils in specific and consistent locations in cupboards and the refrigerator.
- Encourage use of a cane when walking.
- Keep furniture and household objects in specific and consistent places.
- When walking with a blind person, let the person take your arm (see Figure 61-5).
- Provide descriptions of food on the plate using clock placement of food; for example, put the peas at "7 o'clock." Cut food as appropriate.
- Always permit blind persons to pull out their own chairs and seat themselves.

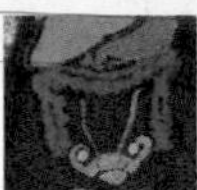

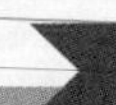

GUIDELINES FOR SAFE PRACTICE *Communicating With the Visually Impaired Patient*

- Talk in a normal tone of voice.
- Do *not* try to avoid common phrases in speech, such as "See what I mean?"
- Introduce yourself with each contact (unless well known to the patient). If in a hospital, knock on the door before entering.
- Explain any activity occurring in the room or what you will be doing.
- Announce when you are leaving the room so that the patient is not put in the position of talking to someone who is no longer there.

the conjunctiva) or by an allergy to an external irritant (e.g., pollen or cosmetics).

Pathophysiology. The symptoms of conjunctivitis vary in severity. **Hyperemia** and burning are common initial symptoms that progress rapidly to a mucopurulent exudate, which crusts on the base of the eyelashes and is easily transferred to the uninfected eye. Viral infections produce excessive tearing, and a preauricular node can be palpated. The conjunctiva is grossly injected (reddened). Invasion of the cornea can result in ulceration and even perforation, usually in response to virulent organisms such as *N. gonorrhoeae.* Involvement of the cornea, although rare, is extremely serious and can even result in loss of the eye. The corneal ulcer is usually identified on slit lamp examination and may be outlined with the use of sterile fluorescein dye.

Collaborative Care Management. Treatment of bacterial conjunctivitis includes careful cleansing of the eyelids and lashes and the use of topical antibiotics. Warm, moist compresses may be used to gently remove firm, adherent crusts from the eyes, especially in the morning (see Guidelines for Safe Practice box, p. 1816). Cold compresses are used for relief in viral EKC. Because the drainage material is infectious, it should be disposed of carefully.

Common ophthalmic antibiotics include polymixin B, bacitracin, and ciprofloxacin in ointment or eyedrop form (see Box 61-1). Ophthalmic ointments remain in contact with the eye

TABLE 61-2 EYE INFECTION AND INFLAMMATION

Disorder	Description	Collaborative Management
Blepharitis	Inflammation of eyelids; often begins in childhood and recurs, causing redness and scaling of upper and lower lid at lash borders	Perform daily facial cleansing and shampooing to remove scales. Local antibiotics may be helpful.
Hordeolum (stye)	Common infection of small glands of lid margins; caused by staphylococci; creates tender, swollen pustule that gradually resolves or ruptures	Apply warm compress 3-4 times per day. Use antibiotic ointment if severe. Make incision of pustule if it does not resolve spontaneously.
Chalazion	Granulomatous inflammation of the lid margins' meibomian gland; lump either external or internal, putting pressure on eye and possibly affecting vision	Apply warm compresses to open up lumen of gland at lid margin. Use antibiotic ointment if infected. Perform surgical excision and curettage if it does not resolve spontaneously.
Corneal abrasion	Superficial epithelial damage, causing extreme pain, photophobia, and tearing; if infected, can lead to corneal ulcer	Minor abrasions heal spontaneously without scarring. Comfort measures are critical, since pain can be severe. Give antibiotic eyedrops to prevent secondary infection.
Keratitis	Inflammation of cornea; can be superficial or deep, acute or chronic; corneal ulcer commonly caused by *Staphylococcus* and *Streptococcus* bacteria and herpes simplex viruses; pain, photophobia, and blepharospasm evident; left untreated, corneal ulcer leading to loss of vision	Administer steroids to control inflammation unless caused by active virus infection. Give antibiotics for bacterial cause, antifungal agents for fungal infection, and cycloplegics to rest the eye. Corneal transplant may be necessary. Use fluorescein dye initially to outline corneal ulcer.
Trachoma	Chronic infectious form of conjunctivitis caused by *Chlamydia trachomatis;* common in Africa and Asia; one of leading causes of blindness worldwide	This can be effectively treated early in disease with antibiotics, but is hard to eradicate once chronic.
Uveitis	Acute inflammation of uvea from infection, allergy, toxic agents, and systemic disorders; causes eye pain, swelling, photophobia, and visual impairment	Uveitis may be self-limiting. Treat underlying cause plus give cycloplegics to rest the eye and steroids to decrease inflammation and increase comfort.

Box 61-1 Ophthalmic Drugs Used to Treat Infection and Inflammation

Antibiotics and Antiviral Drugs

Polymyxin B, bacitracin (Polysporin)
Polymyxin B, neomycin, bacitracin (Neosporin)
Bacitracin
Erythromycin, ciprofloxacin hydrochloride, norfloxacin, ofloxacin, tobramycin, gentamicin, chloramphenicol
Vidarabin, trifluridine, idoxuridine

Steroids

Prednisone
Prednisolone acetate
Methylprednisolone (Depo-Medrol)
Triamcinolone (Aristocort)
Dexamethasone (Decadron, Maxidex)
Fluorometholone (FML)

Cycloplegic and Mydriatic Action

Atropine sulfate (Atropisol, Isopto Atropine)
Cyclopentolate hydrochloride (Cyclogyl)
Homatropine hydrobromide (Isopto Homatropine)
Scopolamine hydrobromide (Isopto Hyoscine)
Tropicamide (Mydriacyl)
Mydriatic action only: Phenylephrine hydrochloride

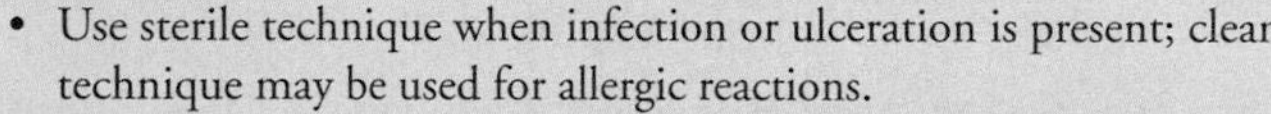

GUIDELINES FOR SAFE PRACTICE
Applying Warm, Moist Compresses to the Eye

- Use sterile technique when infection or ulceration is present; clean technique may be used for allergic reactions.
- Use separate equipment for bilateral eye infections.
- Wash hands before treating each eye.
- The temperature of the compress should not exceed 120° F (49° C).
- Change compresses frequently—every 5 minutes or as ordered.
- Do not exert pressure on the eyeball.
- If sterility is not required, apply moist heat by means of a clean facecloth.
- Wash hands at completion of treatment.

much longer, providing a prolonged effect. Eye ointments produce a film on the cornea that blurs the vision. No antiviral ophthalmic drugs are available except for the treatment of the herpesviruses.

PATIENT/FAMILY TEACHING. The nurse instructs the patient on the infectious nature of conjunctivitis, stressing the need to prevent **cross-contamination** of the other eye by keeping the hands away from the face. To prevent spread to others, patients should use only their own towels and face cloth and wash their hands before cleansing the eye with warm compresses and after administering eye medications.

The nurse instructs the patient about how to correctly instill the ophthalmic ointment. The procedure is similar to that used for eyedrops. The ointment is gently placed directly onto the exposed conjunctiva from the inner to the outer canthus, being careful to avoid the eyelashes or any part of the eye that would contaminate the tip of the tube (Figure 61-6). The nurse warns the patient about the possible blurring of vision. If both eyedrops and ointments are used, the ointment is applied last. Treatment at bedtime minimizes the adverse effects of blurred vision caused by the instillation of the ointment.

Eye Trauma and Injury

Etiology and Epidemiology. Accidental eye injury is one of the leading causes of visual impairment in the United States, with approximately 1 million eye injuries occurring each year. According to the U.S. Eye Injury Registry, about 43 percent of eye injuries occur in the home. An estimated 40,000 sports-related eye injuries occur each year in the United States, many of which could have been prevented with the appropriate use of sports-specific eyewear.[3]

Two other major injury categories are burns and mechanical trauma. Chemical burns can occur in the home, school, and industrial setting and may involve either an acid or an alkali substance. Prompt treatment is essential to prevent permanent eye damage. Ultraviolet burns may occur from excessive sun exposure (skiing, outdoor work, or sunbathing) or the use of heat lamps and tanning beds. Thermal burns (e.g., from fireworks) are less common but may destroy the eyelids and necessitate skin grafting.

Blunt trauma can cause laceration of the eyelids and direct injury to the eye itself. Contusions can cause bleeding into the anterior chamber (hyphema). Corneal lacerations and perforations are extremely painful and threaten vision because of the introduction of bacteria into the eye or the scarring that results from healing. Conjunctival and corneal foreign bodies are the most common eye injuries, but intraocular foreign bodies also occur.[2]

Pathophysiology. The eye's natural protective mechanisms both prevent and minimize minor eye injury. The heavy orbital bone protects the eye from most blunt mechanical injuries. Tears, the eye's natural lubricating system, help flush away chemicals and other foreign bodies, and the blink reflex protects the eye from most low-impact forces.

Chemical burns with acid coagulate the cornea, which produces significant local trauma but actually prevents the substance

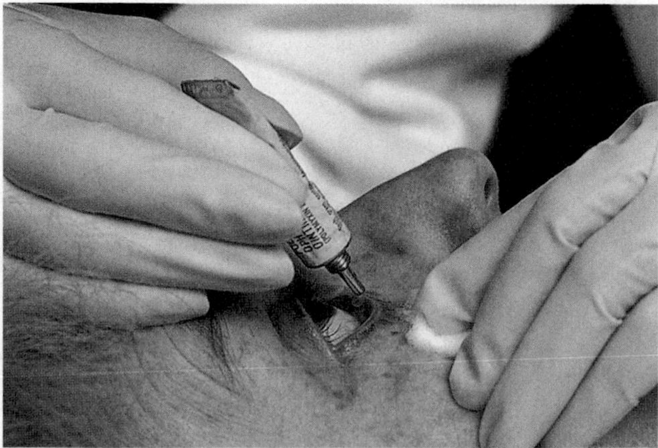

Figure 61-6 Ophthalmic ointment is squeezed onto conjunctiva of lower lid.

from penetrating and damaging the deeper structures of the eye. Alkaline substances, however, penetrate the corneal epithelium and release proteases and collagenases that can cause corneal necrosis and perforation.

Penetrating injuries or retained foreign bodies can result in sympathetic ophthalmia, a serious inflammation of the ciliary body, iris, and choroid that occurs in the uninjured eye. The cause of the acute inflammation is unknown, but it is considered an autoimmune response. The uninjured eye becomes inflamed, painful, and photophobic with a decline in visual acuity. Prompt, aggressive steroid treatment of eye injuries has decreased the incidence of this rare disorder that can result in loss of the "good" eye.

Collaborative Care Management. Prompt professional evaluation and care are the most important aspects of management of eye injuries and may protect the eye from serious visual impairment. Assessment should include a history of loss of consciousness or trauma such as cervical spine injury to rule out more extensive damage than the eye complaint.[2] First aid measures for eye injury should be widely taught and posted clearly in all settings in which eye injury is a significant risk. Chemical burns are immediately treated with copious flushing of the eye with water (see Guidelines for Safe Practice box and Figure 61-7). Irrigation should be continued for at least 15 minutes before the patient is transferred for professional medical evaluation and treatment. This simple measure may preserve eye function. Litmus paper applied to the conjunctiva will determine the pH if the substance is unknown and thus help determine the type and extent of injury. Further treatment may include topical antibiotics, steroids, and antiglaucoma agents to reduce intraocular pressure (IOP). Actinic (ultraviolet) burns are treated with cool compresses, analgesics, and anesthetics.

Blunt trauma also requires prompt professional care and evaluation, since there is risk of both infection and losing the eye. Antibiotic drops may be used to reduce the risk of infection and support healing. Cycloplegic agents, cold compresses, and wound suturing

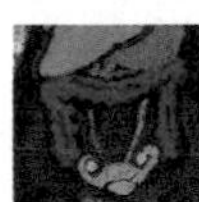

GUIDELINES FOR SAFE PRACTICE
Eye Irrigation

Purpose

Remove chemical irritants, foreign bodies, and secretions.
Cleanse.

Procedure

1. Prepare solution. Physiologic solutions of sodium chloride or lactated Ringer's solution are most commonly used.
2. Position patient comfortably on one side so that fluid cannot flow into other eye.
3. Use appropriate means (e.g., kidney basin, large towel) to catch irrigating fluid.
4. Use appropriate amounts of solution.
   a. If small amounts are needed (to cleanse the eye postoperatively), use sterile cotton balls moistened with solution.
   b. If moderate amounts of fluid are needed (i.e., for removing secretions), use a plastic squeeze bottle to direct irrigating fluid along the conjunctiva and over the eyeball from the inner to the outer canthus.
   c. If copious amounts of fluid are needed (i.e., for removing chemical irritants), use bags of solution such as intravenous bags along with tubing to direct the flow into the eye.
5. Avoid directing a forceful stream into the eye.
6. Avoid touching any eye structures with the irrigating equipment.
7. If there is drainage, wrap a piece of gauze around the index finger to raise the lid and ensure thorough cleansing.

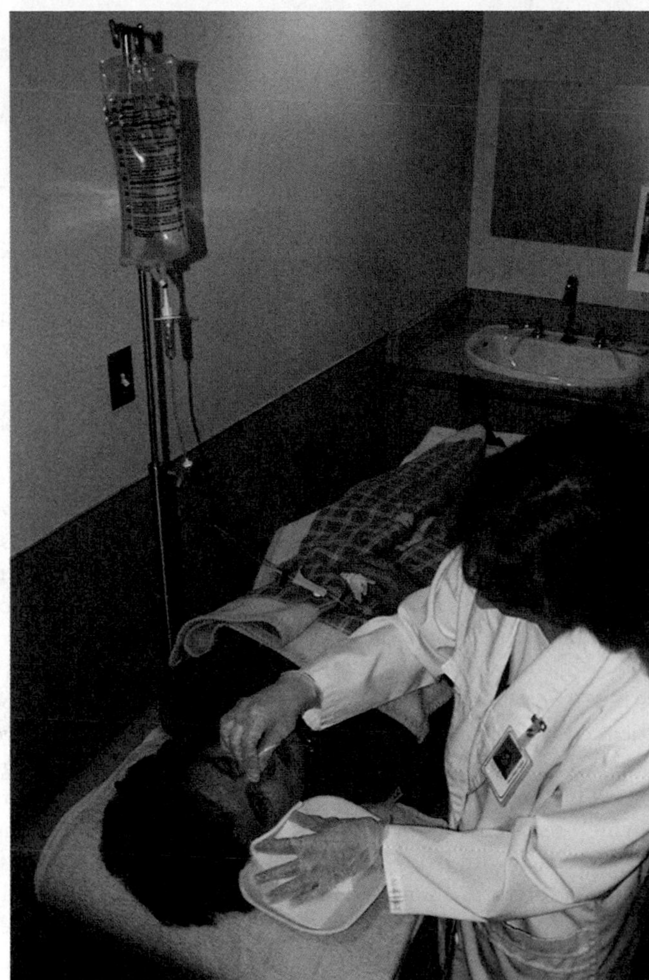

A

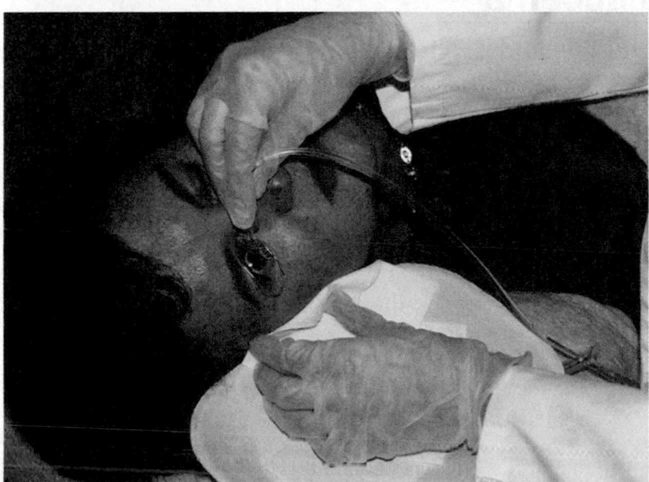

B

Figure 61-7 **A,** Eye irrigation using intravenous bag and tubing. **B,** Note lid speculum in place.

TABLE 61-3 FIRST AID FOR EYE INJURIES

Injury	Intervention
Burns: chemical, flame	Flush eye immediately for 15 min with cool water or any available nontoxic liquid. Seek medical assistance.
Loose substance on conjunctiva: dirt, insects	Lift upper lid over lower lid to dislodge substance and produce tearing. Irrigate eye with water if necessary; do not rub eye. Obtain medical assistance if above interventions fail.
Contact injury: contusion, ecchymosis, laceration	Apply cold compresses if no laceration is present; cover eye if laceration is present. Seek medical assistance.
Penetrating objects	Do not remove object. Place protective shield over eye (e.g., paper cup); cover uninjured eye to prevent excess movement of injured eye. Seek medical assistance.

are all possible interventions, depending on the injury. Table 61-3 outlines the basic first aid for common eye injuries. Significant damage can be done by well-intentioned efforts to remove a foreign body from the eye. The eye should be kept closed and loosely covered during transport to prevent further injury until definitive treatment can be provided. Sterile fluorescein solution may be instilled to help outline the foreign body for removal.

Contusions are treated with rest and the application of cold compresses to reduce swelling. Extensive laceration, termed *ruptured globe,* or penetrating eye injuries can result in blindness or loss of the eye. Surgical repair is performed whenever possible. When penetrating injuries occur, no attempt is made to remove the object or to clean the eye. Professional management is essential.

PATIENT/FAMILY TEACHING. The nurse is often responsible for patient education efforts concerning eye safety and first aid for eye injuries. The body's natural eye defenses can be appropriately augmented by the use of goggles, shields, and safety lenses for sports and high-risk activities. Children need to be taught about the risks associated with BB guns, slingshots, and even rubber bands. The use of protective sunglasses may also be important, depending on the patient's occupational and leisure time sun exposure. General guidelines for eye safety are summarized in Box 61-2.

Glaucoma

Etiology and Epidemiology. Glaucoma is a group of eye diseases (Table 61-4), with features that can include IOP too high for the health of the eye, damage to the optic nerve, and permanent loss of peripheral vision. Some people have a normally high IOP and, for them, elevated IOP is no longer a defining characteristic of glaucoma. The two major forms of glaucoma discussed here are open-angle glaucoma (OAG) and angle-closure (formerly referred to as closed-angle) glaucoma. The disease is primary when its cause is unknown and secondary when it results from another eye disorder, such as a forward shift of the iris, pupillary blockage, or contracture of the fibromuscular membrane in the anterior chamber.

Glaucoma is a major cause of visual impairment and blindness worldwide. In the United States glaucoma is the second leading cause of blindness in the general population and the leading cause among African-Americans.[4] The prevalence rate among African-Americans is six to eight times higher than that of Caucasians. In the population older than 40 years an estimated 1 million persons have been diagnosed with OAG, and 1 million more have undiagnosed disease. The incidence is expected to continue to rise as the population ages. Age, race, myopia, and a family history of glaucoma are the only identified risk factors. Angle-closure glaucoma is more prevalent in Asians.

Box 61-2 Rules of Eye Safety

- Spray aerosols away from eyes.
- Wear protective glasses during active sports such as racquetball.
- Slowly release steam from ovens, pots, pressure cookers, and microwave popcorn bags.
- Gaze at solar eclipses only through adequate filters.
- Wear safety goggles whenever you are doing hazardous work or if you are in a workplace area where such hazards exist.
- Fit all machinery with safeguards.
- Keep dangerous items and chemicals away from children.
- Store sharp objects safely.
- Pick up rocks and stones before mowing the yard.

Pathophysiology. The normal balance of production and drainage of aqueous humor allows the IOP to remain relatively constant within the normal range of 10 to 21 mm Hg with a mean pressure of 16 mm Hg. Normal diurnal variations are limited to about 5 mm Hg. Obstruction in any part of the outflow channels for aqueous humor results in a backup of fluid and an increase in IOP (Figure 61-8). A sustained elevation gradually damages the optic nerve and impairs vision. In primary OAG, which represents 90% of all cases, the changes occur slowly and damage is insidious. The process can occur more rapidly in response to injury or infection or as a complication of surgery. Signs and symptoms of glaucoma are summarized in the Clinical Manifestations box. Figure 61-9 shows the progressive loss of peripheral vision that can occur with glaucoma.

COMPLICATIONS. Loss of vision is the primary complication of glaucoma, and preventing vision loss and blindness is the ultimate goal of all therapy. Most patients with glaucoma can be successfully managed with routine pharmacologic therapy. Selected patients may require surgical intervention, and in rare instances, when the disease cannot be successfully controlled, severe visual impairment or blindness results. Glaucoma-related blindness remains a major international health concern.

TABLE 61-4 TYPES OF GLAUCOMA

Type	Description
Primary open-angle (chronic, simple)	Most common type (90%) Usually caused by obstruction in trabecular meshwork
Secondary open-angle	Can occur from abnormality in trabecular meshwork or increased intraocular pressure
Primary angle-closure (narrow angle, acute)	Outflow impaired as result of narrowing or closing of angle between iris and cornea Intermittent attacks—pressure normal when angle open; if persistent, acute ocular emergency
Secondary angle-closure	Can result from ocular inflammation, neovascularization, trauma
Congenital	Abnormal development of filtration angle; can occur secondary to other systemic eye disorders

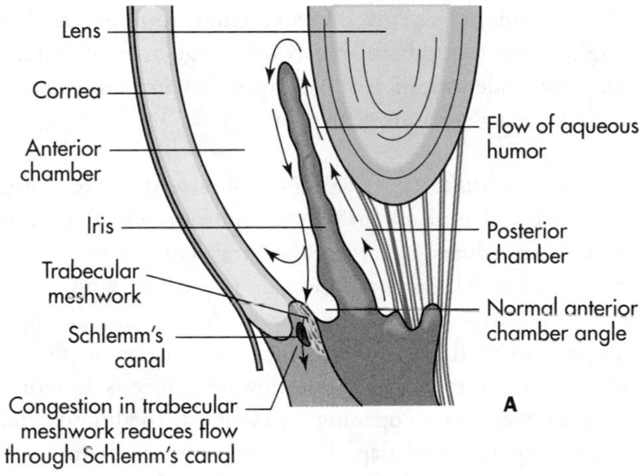

Figure 61-8 A, Chronic open-angle glaucoma. Congestion in trabecular meshwork reduces outflow of aqueous humor. **B,** Acute angle-closure glaucoma. Angle between iris and anterior chamber narrows, obstructing outflow of aqueous humor.

CLINICAL MANIFESTATIONS
Glaucoma

Open-Angle Glaucoma

Often no signs or symptoms in early stages
Intraocular pressure (IOP) typically elevated to more than 24 mm Hg
Slow, progressive loss of peripheral vision (see Figure 61-9)
Cupping of the optic disc on ophthalmoscopic examination
Tunnel vision
Persistent, dull brow pain
Difficulty adjusting to darkness
Failure to detect color changes

Angle-Closure Glaucoma

Acute: ocular pain severe enough to cause nausea and vomiting; vision decreased; pupil enlarged and fixed, colored halos around lights seen, conjunctiva red, cornea steamy
IOP dramatically elevated; may exceed 50 mm Hg
Permanent blindness if marked increase in IOP for 24 to 48 hours

Congenital Glaucoma

Hazy cornea, lacrimation, photophobia, blepharospasm, enlargement of eye

Collaborative Care Management

DIAGNOSTIC TESTS. Several diagnostic tests are used to diagnose and monitor glaucoma. These include[7]:

- Tonometry: measurement of IOP
- Tonography: estimation of the resistance in the outflow channels by continuously recording the IOP over 2 to 4 minutes
- Ophthalmoscopy: evaluation of the color and configuration of the optic cup
- Perimetry: measurement of visual function in the central field of vision
- Gonioscopy: examination of the angle structures of the eye, where the iris, ciliary body, and cornea meet

MEDICATIONS. Drug therapy is the foundation of treatment for most forms of glaucoma. The goal of treatment is to lower the individual's IOP and keep it at a level that prevents loss of vision. Drug therapy is administered topically or systemically to lower the IOP by either increasing the outflow of aqueous humor or decreasing the production of aqueous humor. Drug options include beta-adrenergic blockers and carbonic anhydrase inhibitors, which decrease aqueous humor formation; prostaglandin agonists, which increase the uveoscleral outflow of aqueous humor; and **miotic**

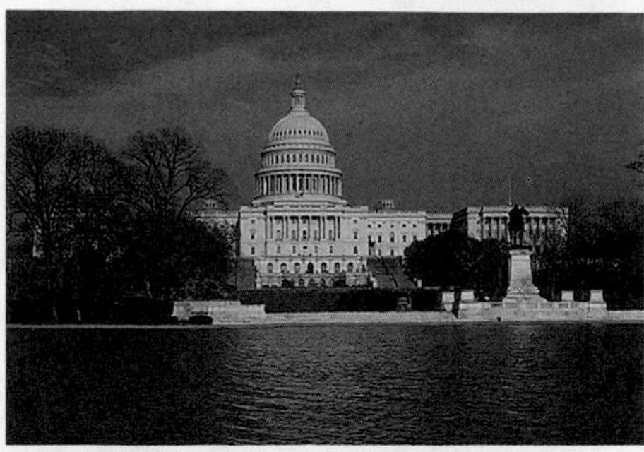

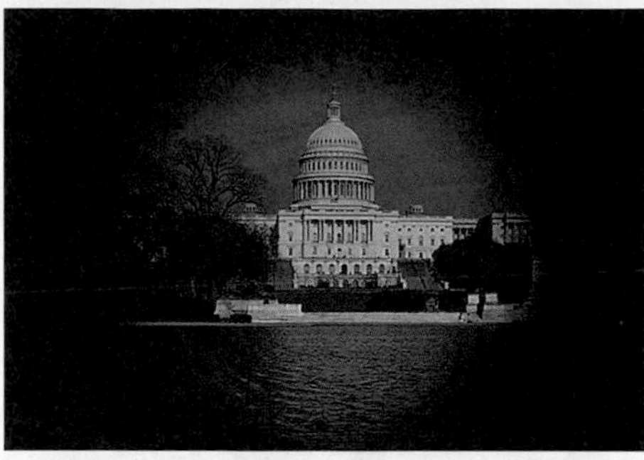

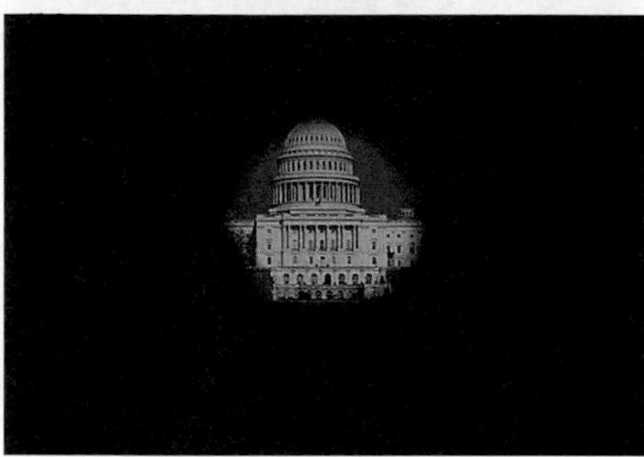

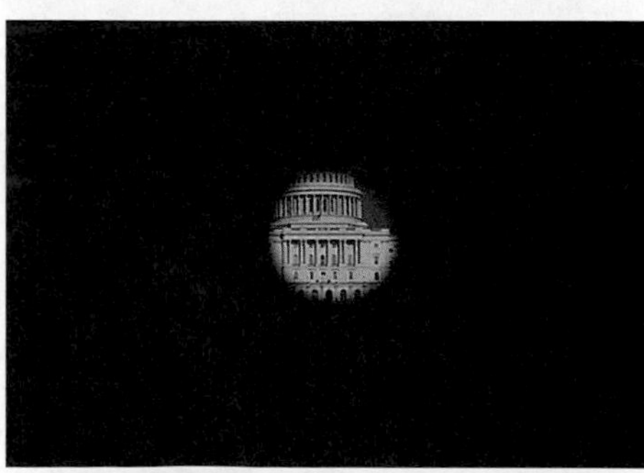

Figure 61-9 Glaucoma causes progressive loss of peripheral vision. Changes may be so insidious that extensive irreversible damage occurs before the problem is recognized.

agents, which constrict the pupil and increase the drainage of aqueous humor.

Miotic drugs, once the mainstay of glaucoma treatment, are being used less frequently because the pupil constriction adversely affects the patient's night vision and adaptation to dark places. These have been replaced by more efficient, longer-lasting eye medications that do not affect the pupil.

Table 61-5 presents the medications commonly used in the treatment of glaucoma. Once initiated, drug therapy is continued for the rest of the patient's life.

Angle-closure glaucoma usually requires more aggressive management because it represents an emergency situation with the threat of permanent loss of vision if the pressure is not controlled promptly. Intravenous carbonic anhydrase inhibitors may be given in combination with osmotic agents that draw fluid from the intraocular spaces, together with topical beta-blockers and miotics. Topical steroids are also given in an attempt to minimize damage to the iris and the trabecular network. Regular ophthalmic care often permits identification of patients with narrow angles and the potential for angle-closure glaucoma.

SURGICAL MANAGEMENT. Surgical intervention is indicated when conservative treatment fails to control the IOP. Two of the common procedures are argon laser trabeculoplasty (ALT) and trabeculectomy. ALT uses a laser beam to produce a nonpenetrating thermal burn on the trabecular meshwork that changes the configuration of the meshwork, increases tension in the meshwork, and leads to increased outflow of aqueous humor. Trabeculectomy creates an opening, or fistula, at the limbus under a partial-thickness scleral flap. The new opening circumvents the obstruction, and aqueous humor flows into the subconjunctival spaces. However, fibrosis can occur at the site of the scleral flap and interfere with drainage, causing the IOP to rise again. Antimetabolites such as 5-fluorouracil and mitomycin C may be given to inhibit fibrosis. Releasable sutures and laser suture lysis can also be used to support drainage at the site. ALT can usually be performed on an outpatient basis, whereas trabeculectomy occasionally requires an overnight hospital stay.

IOP control is achieved in about 85% of all patients, but most (75%) continue to require medications to treat glaucoma. Nursing care for the person after trabeculectomy is summarized in the Guidelines for Safe Practice box, p. 1822.

Seton implants (e.g., Baerveldt, Ahmed, Krupin, and Molteno implants) provide an alternative for patients with glaucoma that is resistant to other forms of surgery. In implant surgery a polymethylmethacrylate plate is implanted against the sclera. A tube is then surgically inserted directly into the anterior chamber. The aqueous humor drains out of the eye through the tube and collects under the plate posteriorly. The plate is designed to block scar tissue formation that could affect aqueous resorption or physically block the outflow tube. Overdrainage of aqueous humor is a potential complication that can increase the risk of retinal detachment and choroidal and vitreous hemorrhage.

Cyclodestructive procedures such as cyclocryotherapy and YAG (yttrium, aluminum, and garnet) or diode laser thermal procedures attempt to lower the IOP by permanently damaging the ciliary body. The results of these procedures are unpredictable, and repeat treatment may be necessary. Patients require

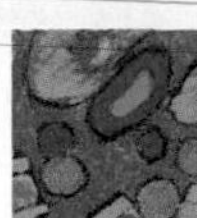

TABLE 61-5
COMMON MEDICATIONS *for Glaucoma*

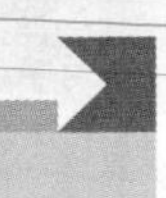

Drug	Action	Nursing Intervention
Beta-Adrenergic Antagonists		
Timolol maleate (Timoptic) Betaxolol (Betoptic) Levobunolol (Betagan) Carteolol hydrochloride (Ocupress) Metipranolol (OptiPranolol)	Decrease aqueous humor production and increase outflow, thereby decreasing IOP	Evaluate effectiveness. Do not administer nonselective beta-blockers if history of asthma is positive, since they can cause bronchospasm.
Carbonic Anhydrase Inhibitors		
Acetazolamide (Diamox) Ethoxzolamide (Cardrase) Dichlorphenamide (Daranide) Methazolamide (Neptazane) Dorzolamide (Trusopt)	Decrease aqueous humor production and increase outflow, thereby decreasing carbonic anhydrase (enzyme necessary to produce aqueous humor) in ciliary processes	Evaluate effectiveness. Monitor for tingling sensation in extremities, tinnitus, gastric upset, or hearing dysfunction. Monitor for hypokalemia.
Alpha-Adrenergic Agonists		
Apraclonidine (Iopidine) Brimonidine (Alphagan) Epinephryl borate (Eppy/N, Epinal) Epinephrine hydrochloride (Glaucon) Epinephrine bitartrate (Epitrate) Dipivefrin (Propine)	Reduce aqueous humor formation and increase outflow	Evaluate effectiveness. Do not use if discolored brown. Monitor for side effects: headache, brow ache, blurred vision, tachycardia.
Prostaglandin Agonist		
Latanoprost (Xalatan)	Increases outflow of aqueous humor; used primarily with patients intolerant to or unresponsive to other glaucoma agents	Teach patient about adverse side effects (e.g., burning on administration). Iris might change color in light-eyed patients.
Miotics		
Cholinergics: Pilocarpine hydrochloride (Pilocar, Isopto Carpine) Carbachol (Isopto Carbachol)	Constrict pupil (miosis) by directly stimulating sphincter muscle Increase outflow of aqueous humor by ciliary muscle pull on trabecular meshwork	Evaluate effectiveness. Monitor frequency of use. Inform patient that blurred vision and poor night vision may occur because of a small pupil. Brow ache, and conjunctival reddening also occur.
Cholinesterase Inhibitors		
Physostigmine (Eserine) Demecarium bromide (Humorsol) Echothiophate iodide (Phospholine Iodide)	Constrict ciliary muscle and iris sphincter; iris pulled away from anterior chamber angle, allowing drainage of aqueous humor and lowering of IOP	Use of cholinesterase inhibitors is contraindicated during pregnancy. Occlude puncta to prevent systemic absorption. These drugs also cause miosis and therefore have same side effects as miotic agents.
Osmotic Agents		
Glycerin (Osmoglyn) Mannitol (Osmitrol)	Remove water from intraocular structures, resulting in a marked ocular hypotonic effect, thereby decreasing IOP	Evaluate effectiveness. Advise patients they will feel more comfortable once they have emptied their bladder. Monitor electrolytes for depletion if more than 1 unit is given. Oral drugs can cause hyperglycemia. Monitor glucose levels in patients with type 2 diabetes.

IOP, Intraocular pressure.

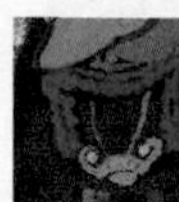

GUIDELINES FOR SAFE PRACTICE
The Patient Undergoing Trabeculectomy

Nursing care for the patient after trabeculectomy includes:
- Routine postanesthesia care
- Protection of the operative eye with a shield
- Patient seated with head elevated to have any postoperative hyphema in dependent position
- Assistance with ambulation immediately postoperatively
- Maintaining comfort in the operative eye
- Assessment, as appropriate, of the intraocular pressure, appearance of the bleb, and anterior chamber depth
- Administration of medications such as cycloplegics and a combination antibiotic and steroids

close follow-up monitoring because of an increased risk of retinal detachment, hemorrhage, and severe inflammation in the treated eye.

Acute angle-closure glaucoma is treated medically initially to reduce IOP then with either a laser peripheral iridotomy (YAG or argon) or a surgical peripheral iridectomy. This passage through the iris permanently connects the anterior and posterior chambers of the eye, preventing the iris from occluding the anterior chamber.

DIET AND ACTIVITY. Diet does not play a role in the management of glaucoma. However, patients experiencing acute angle-closure glaucoma may develop nausea and vomiting from the acute eye pain, and this may require temporary dietary adjustment.

Activity does not need to be restricted for the treatment of OAG. Patients are, however, instructed to avoid heavy lifting, isometric exercises, and constipation that would cause straining,[9] and to avoid wearing tight collars. The loss of peripheral vision that can result from the disease and the blurred vision and loss of night vision that are common side effects of several of the medications do create safety risks that may need to be addressed through a modification in activity, particularly driving.

HEALTH PROMOTION AND PREVENTION. Early diagnosis and treatment of glaucoma are essential to prevent permanent destruction of fibers on the optic disc. All persons with a family history of glaucoma should have their eyes examined, including measurement of IOP, every 2 years after the age of 40. Mass screening programs are important for detecting glaucoma in persons who do not have periodic medical eye examinations, since the permanent loss of vision glaucoma causes is usually preventable.

Once the diagnosis has been made, regular medical follow-up visits are essential to evaluate the effectiveness of treatment. Follow-up visits every 2 to 3 months may be necessary initially until it is clear that the patient's IOP is under control. Adherence to treatment and regular monitoring are the best means to prevent loss of vision from progressive disease activity. Patients with loss of vision may benefit from referrals to the National Federation of the Blind (www.nfb.org) and the National Eye Care Project (800-222-3937).

▶ ARE YOU READY?

The primary action of a beta-adrenergic blocker in a patient with glaucoma is to:
1. Increase outflow of aqueous humor.
2. Increase resorption of aqueous humor.
3. Decrease aqueous humor production.
4. Decrease viscosity of aqueous humor.

Nursing Management *of the Patient with Glaucoma*

ASSESSMENT

Health History. Assess for:
- Sudden onset of severe pain in the eye
- Acute blurring of vision
- Halos around lights
- Nausea and vomiting, which can be so severe with acute angle-closure glaucoma that an acute abdomen can be mistakenly diagnosed

Remember that patients with OAG are typically asymptomatic in the early stages of the disease and may remain asymptomatic if they receive adequate treatment.

Physical Examination. In patients with acute angle-closure glaucoma, assess for:
- Mid-dilated and fixed pupil
- Hazy, bluish appearance of the cornea
- Sharp elevation in IOP (may be over 50 mm Hg)
- Late findings:
  - Constriction of visual fields on perimeter
  - Optic cup enlargement identified on ophthalmoscopic examination of the disc

NURSING DIAGNOSES, OUTCOMES, AND INTERVENTIONS

Nursing Diagnosis: Acute Pain

OUTCOMES. Common examples of expected outcomes for the patient with a diagnosis of *acute pain* are:

Patient will:
- Rate pain as 3 or less on a scale of 0 (no pain) to 10 (severe pain).
- Verbalize that pain is controlled.

NURSING INTERVENTIONS. Aggressive pharmacologic intervention is required to control the IOP and the patient's pain. The nurse carefully explains all interventions and assesses the patient's pain level frequently. The nurse administers analgesics as needed to control the pain and carefully evaluates their effectiveness. A quiet environment enhances the patient's comfort and gives the medication time to take effect.

RELATED NIC INTERVENTIONS. Analgesic Administration, Environmental Management: Comfort

Nursing Diagnosis: Risk for Ineffective Therapeutic Regimen Management

OUTCOMES. Common examples of expected outcomes for the patient with a diagnosis of *risk for ineffective therapeutic regimen management* are:

The patient will:

- Report using glaucoma medications as prescribed.
- Have IOP maintained in normal range.
- Have no decline in visual status.

NURSING INTERVENTIONS. Glaucoma is a chronic disease that can be controlled through lifelong management but not cured. Vision that has been lost to elevated IOP cannot be restored, but further loss of vision can be prevented with careful adherence to the pharmacologic regimen and ongoing follow-up care. A normal lifestyle is possible with minimal restrictions. The nurse instructs the patient about all prescribed medications, including adverse side effects of the drugs, such as the stinging or burning sensation and temporary blurred vision. The nurse also teaches the patient how to correctly administer topical eyedrops. Frequency of eyedrops depends on the absorption rate of the medication prescribed. Guidelines for self-administration of eyedrops are summarized in the Patient/Family Teaching box. The nurse advises the patient to keep a reserve bottle of the medication available, if possible, in case the drug is lost or spilled. Eye medications should always be carried in a pocket or purse when traveling and never packed in luggage. A Medic-Alert or other information card indicating that the patient has glaucoma and takes a specific medication is a recommended safety precaution in case the person is involved in an accident.

Patients need both professional and family support to adhere to the treatment regimen, especially when an absence of disease symptoms makes the disease process seem tenuous, since the treatment can seem worse than the previously unsuspected disease.

RELATED NIC INTERVENTIONS. Teaching: Disease Process, Behavior Modification

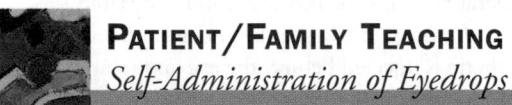

PATIENT/FAMILY TEACHING
Self-Administration of Eyedrops

1. Wash hands thoroughly before administering the medication.
2. Tilt head back and look up toward the ceiling.
3. Pull lower lid gently down and out to expose the conjunctiva and create a sac.
4. Bring dropper from the side and apply the eyedrops. Avoid touching the eyelashes, conjunctiva, or surface of the eye with the dropper. Resting the lower part of the thumb on the forehead can help stabilize the hand.
5. Close both eyes gently. Do not squeeze them tightly, or the medication will be expelled.
6. Apply slight pressure at the inner canthus of the eye to decrease systemic absorption of the medication.
7. If more than 1 drop is to be administered, wait 2 to 5 minutes before administering the second drop.

Nursing Diagnosis: Risk for Injury

OUTCOMES. A common example of expected outcomes for the patient with a diagnosis of *risk for injury* is:

Patient will:

- Remain free from injury.

NURSING INTERVENTIONS. Practical suggestions such as reducing clutter and adding extra lighting in the home may be helpful safety hints. Patients with peripheral vision loss should carefully evaluate their night driving ability.

RELATED NIC INTERVENTIONS. Environmental Management: Safety, Fall Prevention

EVALUATION

To evaluate the effectiveness of nursing interventions, compare patient behaviors with those stated in the expected patient outcomes.

RELATED NOC OUTCOMES. Pain Control, Pain Level, Knowledge: Treatment Regimen, Compliance Behavior

GERONTOLOGIC CONSIDERATIONS

The incidence of glaucoma increases with aging. Screening initiatives for glaucoma therefore need to be targeted to the older adult population, since the disease is often undiagnosed until irreversible loss of vision has already occurred. Adherence issues are particularly challenging in this population. Fixed incomes can make the purchase of any medications difficult. The fact that most patients with glaucoma are asymptomatic can make it difficult for the patient to accept these medication purchases as essential. Compliance is difficult when the regimen does not make the patient feel better and eyedrops compromise night vision skills. Mobility and dexterity may be impaired by arthritis or other physical problems, so learning correct self-administration of eyedrops becomes a challenge. In addition, older patients may be dealing with some degree of visual impairment, which affects their ability to drive, especially at night. This in turn creates a significant safety risk for individuals who are already struggling to remain independent.

The issues for older patients are challenging, and the nurse can neither solve nor eliminate them. Honest acknowledgment can be helpful, however, as the nurse helps the patient anticipate areas of difficulty and develop strategies for addressing these problems.

Cataract

Etiology and Epidemiology. A cataract is a clouding or opacity of the lens that leads to gradual painless blurring and eventual loss of vision (Figure 61-10). Cataracts are generally classified as congenital (present at birth), senile (associated with aging), traumatic (associated with injury), or secondary (occurring after other eye or systemic diseases).

Congenital cataracts resulting from the mother's exposure to rubella virus during the first trimester of pregnancy can be prevented by vaccination as a public health measure. Senile cataracts are associated with the aging process and are not preventable.

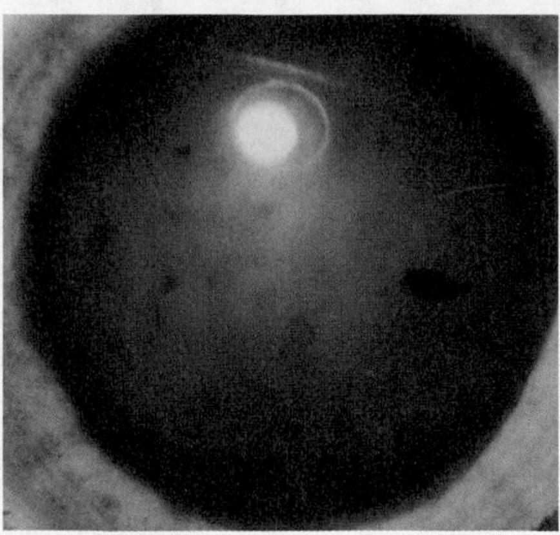

Figure 61-10 Mature senile cataract viewed through dilated pupil.

Some evidence indicates that exposure to ultraviolet radiation may significantly contribute to cataract formation, but a cause-and-effect relationship has not been proved.

Eye injury is the next most common identifiable cause of cataracts. Lens transparency may be destroyed by either a penetrating wound or a contusion. Most traumatic cataracts are preventable through adherence to standard eye safety precautions (see Box 61-2). Cataracts may result from the ingestion of injurious substances such as dinitrophenol or naphthalene. Cataracts may also occur secondary to eye diseases, such as uveitis, or with systemic diseases, such as diabetes mellitus, galactosemia, or sarcoidosis.

Cataracts are the leading cause of preventable blindness in the United States, and their incidence increases steadily with age. Visible lens changes are present in 42% of the 52- to 64-year-old population, and 5% of this age-group demonstrate some degree of visual impairment related to the cataract. Among those older than 65 years of age, 60% to 90% have visible lens changes, and between 25% and 45% have some degree of related visual impairment. A higher incidence of cataracts is found among people residing in warm, sunny climates. Risk factors for cataract formation are summarized in the Risk Factors box.

Pathophysiology. Senile cataracts occur because of a decrease in protein, an accumulation of water, and an increase in sodium content that disrupts the normal fibers of the lens. The cause of these pathologic changes is unknown. Cataracts usually develop bilaterally, but at different rates.

The primary symptom of cataracts is a progressive decrease in vision. The degree of loss depends on the location and extent of the opacity. Persons with an opacity in the center portion of the lens can generally see better in dim light when the pupil is dilated. The person with presbyopia may find that reading without glasses is possible in the early stage of cataract formation because the greater convexity of the lens creates an artificial myopia.

Signs and symptoms of a cataract are summarized in the Clinical Manifestations box.

Risk Factors

Cataract

- Age (incidence dramatically increased after age 65)
- Sex (slightly more common in women)
- Ultraviolet light exposure
  - —More common in persons living in warm, sunny climates
  - —More common in persons who have worked outdoors extensively
- High-dose radiation exposure
- Drug effects from corticosteroids, phenothiazines, and selected chemotherapeutic agents
- Poorly controlled diabetes mellitus resulting in accumulation of sorbitol (by-product of glucose)
- Trauma to the eye

Collaborative Care Management

Diagnostic Tests. The diagnosis of cataracts is made by direct inspection of the lens with an ophthalmoscope after pupil dilation. The progression of the cataract is monitored over time. Before surgery, A-scan ultrasonography, keratometry, B-scan ultrasonography, endothelial cell counts, and potential acuity meter (PAM) tests may be performed. The A-scan measures the length of the eye to help estimate the power of the intraocular lens (IOL) that will be needed. Keratometry measures the curvature of the cornea and is also used to determine the power of the IOL. A B-scan may be performed to evaluate the health of the retina if a dense cataract obscures visualization through an ophthalmoscope. Endothelial cell counts indicate the health of the cornea and its ability to withstand surgery. The PAM test enables the surgeon to ensure that cataract surgery will be beneficial in increasing the patient's visual acuity by preoperatively measuring functional retinal response.

Medications. Medications do not play a role in the management of cataracts. Antiinflammatory agents and antibiotics are used after surgery to facilitate healing and promote patient comfort.

Surgical Management. Surgery is the definitive treatment for cataracts, and it can be used safely and effectively with older adults. The success rate is between 90% and 95%. It was previously believed that a cataract had to "ripen," or mature, before it could be successfully removed. Currently, cataracts are removed when the visual impairment interferes with the individual's daily activities. The person's general health is the most important variable.

Cataract removal is performed with the patient under local anesthesia. The anesthetic is injected behind the eye and in and around the eyelids. The most popular method of cataract removal is the extracapsular cataract extraction (Figure 61-11). In this procedure only the anterior portion of the lens capsule and the lens cortex are removed, using techniques such as irrigation and aspiration or phacoemulsification (ultrasonic vibration to break up the lens).

Clinical Manifestations

Cataract

- Gradual, painless blurring and decrease of vision
- Glare at night an initial symptom when driving
- Vision often improved when pupil dilates at night
- Inability to discriminate between hues
- Cloudy, white opacity behind pupil

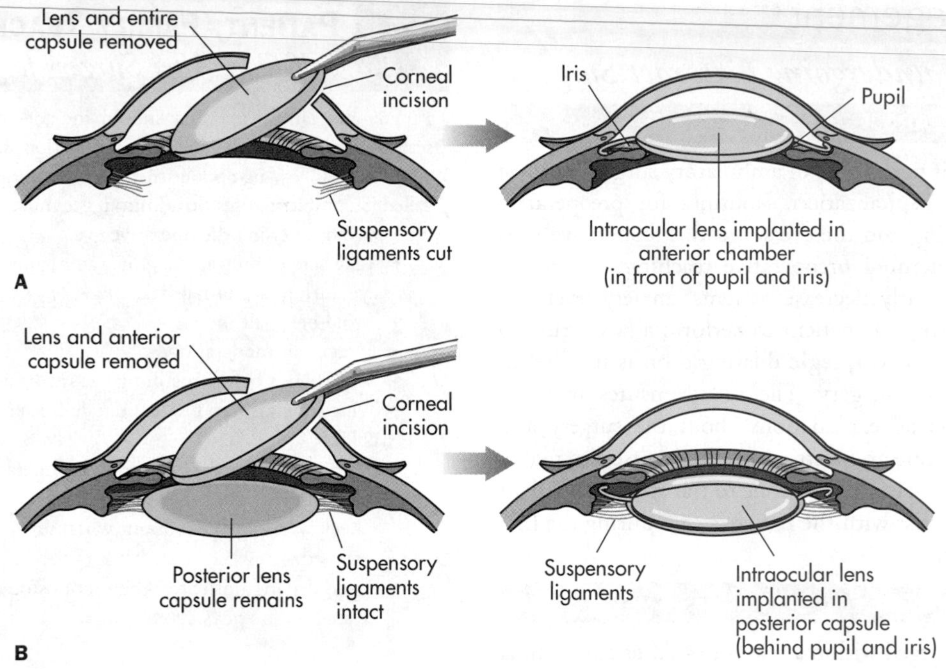

Figure 61-11 **A,** Intracapsular cataract extraction with removal of entire lens and capsule. **B,** Extracapsular cataract extraction leaving posterior lens capsule intact.

Phacoemulsification is performed in about 80% of all cataract patients in North America. This procedure uses a smaller (⅛ inch) incision that promotes healing and decreases postoperative inflammation. Other surgical innovations include making the incision on the sclera rather than the cornea and using a single stitch to close the incision, or even no stitch. These innovations are all attempts to facilitate healing and decrease the incidence of postoperative astigmatism.

Extracapsular extraction leaves the posterior lens capsule intact, which avoids disruption of the vitreous humor and facilitates the placement of a lens implant (see Figure 61-11). Cataracts can also be removed with intracapsular extraction, which involves the removal of the entire lens and its surrounding capsule using a freezing probe that adheres to the surface of the lens. This once popular technique is rarely used anymore.

An IOL implant is the preferred method for replacing the focusing power of the lens. A posterior chamber lens made of polymethylmethacrylate or silicone is placed behind the iris at the time of surgery and is supported by the posterior portion of the lens capsule that was left in place (see Figure 61-11). This type of implant is not dependent on the pupil or iris for support and rarely moves out of position. It is the most commonly used type of lens implant, since the lens position most closely approximates that of the natural lens and magnification is minimized.

Vision can be restored to near 20/20. The field of implants is rapidly evolving. Foldable implants can be folded for insertion into the eye, which allows for an even smaller surgical incision. However, most patients still need reading glasses for near vision because they lose the ability to accommodate. New multifocal and bifocal implants are now becoming available.

If an IOL is not inserted during surgery, the person must wear an external lens. Cataract glasses are the least desirable option but are used if the person cannot tolerate contact lenses. Cataract glasses tend to magnify objects about 25%, making them appear closer than they actually are. The person's field of vision is also narrowed, and a circular blind area (ring scotoma) may occur at the edge of the glasses because the glasses bend the light rays so much that they do not enter the eye. Objects tend to "pop" in and out of the person's visual field as the eyes move away from the center of the glasses. An accurate prescription cannot be made for several months until the person's vision stabilizes after surgery.

Contact lenses correct some of the problems encountered with cataract glasses, but not all of them. The extended-wear soft contact lens is commonly used. Interruption of the nerve supply to the cornea from surgery usually facilitates the wearing of a contact lens, but persons with rheumatoid arthritis in the hands or any other form of impaired mobility may be unable to insert and maintain contact lenses.

COMPLICATIONS. Infection, bleeding, and elevated IOP are the major complications of cataract surgery. The nurse instructs the patient to promptly report any drainage, excessive tearing, or decline in visual acuity. Irritation and discomfort are expected after surgery, but acute, unrelieved pain would indicate a complication that should be reported immediately. When severe pain occurs, it often indicates that there has been an acute rise in IOP. This may require immediate medical treatment and later surgical correction to preserve the patient's vision. Long-term aphakic (without a lens), myopic patients may be susceptible to retinal detachment.

Nursing Management
of the Patient undergoing Cataract Surgery

PREOPERATIVE CARE

Most cataract surgery is performed in ambulatory surgery centers; few patients require hospitalization. Routines for preoperative care vary with the setting and the eye surgeon. Preoperative routines may include structured preoperative teaching, which has been shown to significantly decrease patients' anxiety level (see Research box), and asking the patient to perform a face scrub on admission. In all cases a **cycloplegic** dilating drop is instilled in the operative eye before surgery. The nurse ensures that the patient has understood all explanations about the surgery and expected postoperative care and restrictions. The nurse also makes certain that plans are in place for someone to transport the patient home and, ideally, to assist with the patient's care during the first few postoperative days.

POSTOPERATIVE CARE

Most patients are discharged within a few hours. After any cataract operation a dressing is applied to the eye and covered with a metal or plastic shield to protect the eye from injury. The dressing is usually removed the day of or a day after surgery, but an eye shield is worn at night for 2 to 3 weeks until the eye is healed to avoid accidental bumping or pressure on the eye during sleep. Most patients have no restrictions on bending and are encouraged to resume normal self-care activities at their discretion. The exception is when a larger incision was made at surgery, in which case the nurse clarifies with the surgeon what restrictions are necessary. All discharge instructions are provided to the patient and family in writing for easy reference (see Patient/Family Teaching box).

GERONTOLOGIC CONSIDERATIONS

IOL insertion during cataract surgery in most cases changes the patient's life for the better because of improved vision. Activity limitations are all but eliminated after this type of surgery. However, on assessment the nurse should identify the patient's support system for eye care after discharge. Administration of eyedrops will be required, and the nurse should teach the patient methods of complying with the medication regimen and nighttime shield application, especially if the patient's manual dexterity is impaired. Only when no IOL is used are cataract glasses or contacts for the aphakic patient prescribed. With this method of correction, distortion of peripheral vision and the absence of depth perception (if there is some vision in the unoperative eye) may contribute to missteps when climbing stairs or stepping up on a curb.

Research

Morrel G: Effects of structured preoperative teaching on anxiety levels of patients scheduled for cataract surgery, *Insight* 26(1):4-9, 2001.

Structured preoperative instruction has clinical significance on anxiety levels and blood pressure. A significant difference was found between the anxiety scores of the control group and those of the experimental group after preoperative teaching. A positive correlation was also evident between blood pressure and structured preoperative teaching.

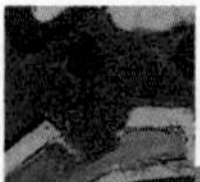

PATIENT/FAMILY TEACHING
Self-Care After Surgery for Cataracts

Patient and family teaching should include information about prescribed medications and their administration, safety precautions, time and date of follow-up appointment, and a contact phone number to be called if a problem arises. In addition, the nurse instructs the patient to:

- Avoid touching the operative eye.
- Take care to prevent soap or water from entering the operative eye during face or hair washing.
- Avoid heavy lifting.
- Exercise in moderation.
- Wash hands before instilling eye medications.
- Wear sunglasses to prevent dazzle from bright lights and colors.
- Wait 2 to 5 minutes between administration of different eye medications. Administer eye ointments last.
- Check with physician about when sexual activity can be resumed.
- Avoid driving until after the first postoperative visit or until cleared by the physician.

Anticipatory planning can reduce the patient's dependence on others. Items needed for self-care (e.g., slippers, pet supplies) can be temporarily relocated for easy access. Having the patient's hair washed before surgery delays the need to wash it in the immediate postoperative period. Meals can be prepared ahead and frozen for easy access. Frail older patients without strong family or social supports may need a brief admission to an assisted living facility.

Retinal Detachment

Etiology and Epidemiology. Retinal detachment occurs when the outer pigmented layer and the inner sensory layer of the retina separate (Figure 61-12). A primary cause is myopic degeneration; secondary causes include trauma, inflammation,

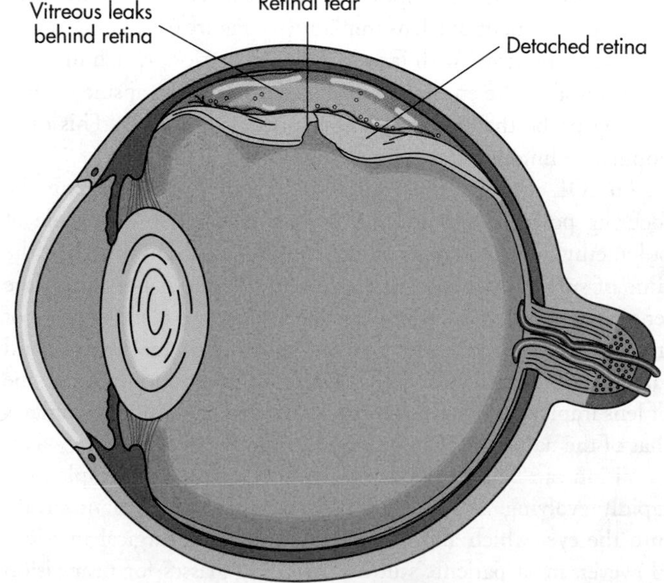

Figure 61-12 Retinal detachment.

and bleeding from a damaged or fragile blood vessel (as seen in diabetic retinopathy). Before **microsurgical techniques** for cataract extraction, retinal detachment was also seen as a complication in aphakic eyes.

Pathophysiology. The retina is a smooth, unbroken, multilayered surface. Degenerative retinal holes or tears allow liquefied vitreous humor to pass through and split the retina (rhegmatogenous detachment). The presence of an inflammatory mass, blood clot (exudative detachment), or tumor (solid detachment) can also separate the retinal layers. Vitreous also undergoes some deterioration with aging and can contract (shrink), causing a vitreous detachment. Traction detachments are most often seen when vitreous bands form in diabetic retinopathy or after trauma.

Retinal detachment may occur suddenly or develop slowly. Symptoms include showers of floating spots before the eyes, flashes of light, and progressive loss of vision in one area. The so-called floaters are cells that are freed at the time of the retinal tear, casting shadows on the retina as they drift about the eye. The flashes of light are caused by vitreous traction on the retina. The area of vision loss depends entirely on the location of the detachment. If the detachment extends to include the macula, blindness results. When the detachment is extensive and occurs quickly, the patient may have the sensation that a curtain has been drawn before the eyes. No pain is associated with a detachment.

Collaborative Care Management. The diagnosis of detached retina is established by ophthalmoscopic examination of the fundus to identify the location and extent of the retinal tear. B-scan ultrasonography may be necessary to facilitate diagnosis if the vitreous is opaque. Minor tears and retinal holes are often identified as part of a routine eye examination, and sealing degenerative holes by laser or cryopexy (cold) can prevent a retinal detachment.

Detachments that compromise vision are repaired surgically if possible. Surgery has a 90% success rate in reattaching the retina. Several different surgical techniques may be used. First, subretinal fluid is drained to return the retina to its normal position. The tear is then sealed using cryopexy to produce an inflammatory reaction that results in adhesions between the margins of the break and the choroid, thus forming a chorioretinal adhesion. In cryopexy or cryotherapy, subfreezing nitrous oxide or carbon dioxide is applied to the sclera in the area of the tear or hole to produce the inflammatory reaction. Laser photocoagulation can also provide the energy source to trigger the chorioretinitis.

Cryopexy is done before the scleral buckling procedure in which the sclera is indented (buckled) over the sealed break by placing various sizes and shapes of silicone on the outside of the eyeball. Then an encircling band of silicone may also be placed around the eye (Figure 61-13). These procedures ensure that the choroid remains in contact with the tear during healing and reduces the traction pull of any vitreous adhesions. The hole is thereby closed, and a watertight intraretinal space is reestablished.

Pneumatic retinopexy may also be used to repair a detachment, particularly for small holes in the superior portion of the retina. The instillation of an expandable gas, such as sulfur hexafluoride (SF^6) or perfluoropropane (C^3F^8), provides internal tamponade and supports the healing retina. The gas is gradually absorbed within the vitreous. Laser demarcation is performed 1 or 2 days later to provide additional support to the retina. Patient compliance with positioning is vital to the success of this procedure.

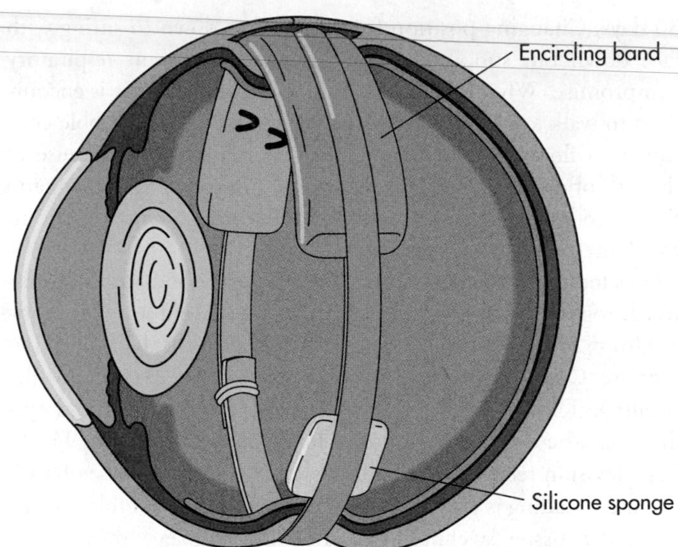

Figure 61-13 Band of silicone is placed around eye to ensure that choroid and retina remain in close contact during healing. A sponge is placed directly over the tear to depress the sclera.

A pars plana vitrectomy is performed in selected cases for repair of rhegmatogenous retinal detachments, including giant tears, macular holes, and intraocular foreign body removal. This procedure involves a three-port system in which sclerotomy incisions are made 3.0 mm posterior to the limbus. The superior port is used for the basic salt infusion, whereas the other two are used for the handheld instruments with which the vitreous is removed. A gas bubble is used to tamponade the retina. In severe cases silicone oil is used to hold the retina in place, but must usually be surgically removed after 3 months.

The location and severity of the retinal detachment guide the patient's preoperative care. With small tears in the inferior retina, the patient may be permitted to continue normal activities until the tear can be sealed. When the detachment is large, however, or the macula is threatened, the patient is encouraged not to make any jerky movements that might further detach the retina. Surgery takes place as soon as possible. This is an extremely stressful time for the patient, who needs careful teaching about the planned procedure and postoperative care. This surgery is usually an outpatient procedure, and only occasionally is anyone required to stay overnight in a hospital for IOP monitoring and initial positioning.

The eye is patched in the immediate postoperative period, and the patch may or may not be removed after discharge home depending on the surgeon's preference. The location and severity of the detachment govern the patient's specific activity restrictions in the postoperative period. Surgical removal of the vitreous (vitrectomy) may be done at the same time as the scleral buckling procedure (see Figure 61-13). If a gas bubble (as well as the basic salt solution) has been injected into the eye to reinforce the repair, the patient is positioned face down using pillows and head supports, so that the gas rises in the eye and presses against the repair. Lying prone can be extremely difficult for patients to maintain, and assisting them in achieving this position is a nursing challenge. Positioning restrictions may be in place for as long as 4 to

30 days. Changing position from lying face down to sitting with face down but supported on a table helps prevent respiratory compromise. When the patient is out of bed, he or she is encouraged to walk keeping the head down, so that the gas bubble continues to float upward. Coughing is contraindicated because of the risk of elevating the IOP. Moderate eye pain is expected, and the nurse keeps the patient comfortable through carefully monitored analgesic administration.

Cycloplegic eyedrops to rest iris and ciliary body are administered, together with a combination corticosteroid and antibiotic eyedrop. An alpha-agonist is given to ensure the IOP does not increase. Cold compresses provide comfort and help reduce ocular swelling. The light sensitivity that occurs after surgery and eyedrops can be combated with dim lights and dark glasses. Watching television relieves boredom but is a challenge because of positioning. Reading is permitted, but is often uncomfortable because of ocular tissue swelling and uncomfortable eye movements. Because the threat of permanent loss of vision can be frightening for both patient and family, support is important. Although the nurse cannot predict the visual outcome of surgery, the 90% surgical success rate can be offered as encouragement. Care of the patient after repair of a retinal detachment is presented in the Nursing Care Plan and postoperative teaching guidelines in the Patient/Family Teaching box.

Strabismus

Etiology and Epidemiology. Strabismus is an ocular misalignment that results from an imbalance in the intraocular muscles. The eyes may be misaligned in any direction (i.e., esotropia [turning in], exotropia [turning out], hypertropia [turning up], or hypotropia [turning down]). Strabismus is usually associated with childhood, but it can be a lifelong disorder. Adult strabismus can occur after an eye injury, but is also associated with brain tumor, head trauma, stroke, and thyroid ophthalmopathy. An estimated 2% to 3% of the general population have some degree of strabismus.

Pathophysiology. The six muscles that attach to each eye move the eyes and align them with each other (see Chapter 60). When they do not work in a coordinated fashion, the result is loss of alignment, or *strabismus.* A child who does not see as well out of one eye tends to suppress the vision in that eye rather than have double vision. The eye then deviates, and binocular vision and depth perception are no longer evident. Adults with new-onset strabismus are rarely able to compensate for their double vision. Children under the age of 2 years who suddenly develop strabismus should be examined to rule out an intraocular tumor.

Collaborative Care Management. Strabismus is diagnosed by noting that the corneal light reflex is not in the same place on each cornea. A cover-uncover test is then done, and prisms are used to see just how much deviation is evident. A variety of treatment options exist. Glasses with prisms may successfully realign the eyes and restore binocular vision. Patching the good eye to strengthen the poorer seeing (amblyopic) eye is an initial treatment of choice. Eye exercises prescribed for patients with strabismus to "strengthen" the weak muscles have not proved effective. Surgical correction is the standard treatment. Strabismus surgery is performed as an outpatient procedure, with the patient under either local or general anesthesia. The extraocular muscles are selectively weakened (recession), tightened (resection), or physically shifted (transposition) to achieve balanced eye movement. Adjustable sutures can be used to achieve an even more accurate alignment. A slip knot is attached during surgery. Once the anesthetic has worn off, the patient's ocular alignment is checked, and minor corrections can be made by tightening or loosening the knot.

Postoperative care focuses on careful monitoring and preparation of the patient or parent for home care. The eyes are seldom patched after surgery, even when an adjustable suture is used. Serosanguineous tears may be present and should be gently wiped from the patient's cheek with clean gauze or cotton. Conjunctival injection is expected. Irritation may necessitate a mild analgesic for comfort.

Drug therapy with botulinum neurotoxin A (Botox) may eliminate the need for surgery or be used in conjunction with surgery. Botox is injected into the extraocular muscle and interferes with the release of acetylcholine at the neuromuscular junction. The toxin appears to strengthen the antagonist muscle and weaken the injected muscle over a period of weeks to months.

PATIENT/FAMILY TEACHING. If amblyopic strabismus is the cause of the deviation, the nurse stresses parent or child compliance with patching or wearing glasses. If surgery is performed, parents are instructed to allow the child to rest at home postoperatively. They are further instructed to monitor the eye for healing and to promptly report any sign of infection.

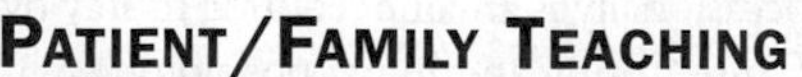

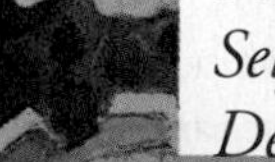

PATIENT/FAMILY TEACHING
Self-Care After Surgery for Retinal Detachment

Patient and family teaching should include information about:

- Prescribed medication
- Correct procedure for eyedrop administration
- Positioning to maintain the intraocular gas bubble or silicone in place if applicable
- Equipment that can be rented to facilitate positioning if needed
- Need to wear an eye shield during sleep for about 2 weeks
- Importance of contacting the surgeon immediately if acute eye pain develops, eye discharge increases, or symptoms of retinal detachment recur

Corneal Transplant

Etiology and Epidemiology. Corneal transplants, also called corneal grafts and penetrating keratoplasty (PK), are the most successful of all the tissue transplants, with a 95% to 98% success rate. Each year in the United States 45,000 corneal grafts are performed. Cadaver corneal tissue must be obtained and the eye enucleated within 12 hours of death. In the United States certain media such as MK and K-Sol are available in which donor corneas can be preserved for up to 7 days, while a corneal transplant is planned. A PK may be recommended for a patient who has corneal clouding as a result of an infection (corneal ulcer), injury (lacerated cornea, chemical burns), or inherited corneal thinning (keratoconus) or who has inherited corneal clouding (Fuch's dystrophy), all of which cause visual loss.

Pathophysiology. The symptoms of keratoconus may start with an increased, progressive myopia as the cornea thins and cones. Keratoconus patients are usually young, and the vision changes are exacerbated at puberty. Corneal ulcers may start with a feeling of a foreign body sensation, which does not resolve, and even after treatment a scar within the cornea's deeper structures results, which decreases vision. Traumatic corneal injuries may be successfully repaired, but a scar in the center of the cornea will affect vision. Fuch's corneal dystrophy is usually slow and progressive as the endothelial cells' pumping action fails. Other causes of corneal clouding include rare disorders such as pemphigoid, an autoimmune condition, and Stevens-Johnson syndrome, which results from a severe allergic response.

Collaborative Care Management. Vision can be restored in an eye so long as the retina is intact. Therefore replacing the cloudy cornea with clear tissue permits the light rays to reach the retina once again so that the patient can see. Most patients who undergo corneal transplant have cared for a chronic eye disorder, so they are familiar with eye medications and are usually optimistic that their vision will be restored.

CORNEAL HARVESTING. Eye banks play an important part in obtaining the corneal tissue that will be used to restore vision. An empathetic nurse can help obtain corneas from recently deceased patients by approaching relatives and requesting consent for removal of the corneas to give the "gift of sight" to another person. Donor corneas are screened for any viral diseases (e.g., human immunodeficiency virus; hepatitis; rabies; or any other disease that might be transmitted through tissue transplant, such as Creutzfeldt-Jakob disease). Donors with fever of unknown origin and ocular malignancy are not used for transplantation. Corneal age is also a factor in transplantation, since the new corneal button must last for the expected lifetime of the recipient. So young recipients and donors are matched whenever possible.

SURGICAL MANAGEMENT. Once the donor cornea is screened and had an endothelial cell count to establish that it is viable material for transplantation, it is soaked in the preserving solution until a recipient is ready for the procedure. The procedure is performed under sterile conditions in a surgicenter or hospital-based operating room. The ambulatory patient is admitted, prepared and draped, and given local or general anesthesia. The donor cornea, which has a rim of sclera around it, is prepared using an instrument called a trephine (like a cookie cutter). A central "button" is cut from the cornea. It is 0.5 mm larger than the recipient's corneal button. It is then placed in a Petri dish, endothelium side up, and covered with MK or K-Sol solution until it is ready to be transplanted.

Using the same technique, but a new sterile trephine, the surgeon next removes the patient's diseased cornea and immediately replaces it with the donor cornea. Initially four sutures are placed—superiorly, inferiorly, and one on each side—to hold the new cornea in place. The 10-0 sutures (which are finer than a hair) can then be interrupted, running, or a combination. These sutures remain in place for as long as a year, and sometimes even longer. After the anterior chamber is reformed with basic salt solution and the suture line is checked with fluorescein dye to ensure there are no leaks, the eye is patched for 24 hours. Steroid and antibiotic drops are prescribed for the patient to administer at home.

Occasionally, in the case of severe corneal injury (e.g., chemical burns), corneal stem cells are obtained from a "living" donor (usually a relative) and introduced before the transplant is initiated. Unlike fetal stem cells, corneal stem cells can only produce corneal cells. Corneal transplants for chemical burns have only a 25% success rate without this new technique.

Because the cornea is an avascular, slow healing tissue, no change in vision is realized in the immediate postoperative period. Visual improvement occurs gradually as the transplant flattens out. Postoperatively, the eye must be protected at all times: shield at night and glasses during the day. Activities are restricted initially, with prohibitions on anything that will stress the sutures by raising the IOP (e.g., straining at stool, heavy lifting). Once the patient has recovered from the anesthesia, he or she is free to go home.

PATIENT/FAMILY TEACHING. The nurse instructs the patient and family about protecting the eye, activity restrictions, and the proper use of prescribed eye medications. The nurse also discusses the importance of a follow-up visit and schedules the appointment.

Eye Tumors

Both benign and malignant tumors may affect the eye and related structures. They may originate within the eye or metastasize from another primary site. Benign neoplasms include lymphomas, hemangiomas, and mucoceles from the sinuses. Malignant tumors threaten the patient's vision and life, since extension commonly involves vital structures within the brain. The eyelids are vulnerable to any of the standard tumors that affect the skin, including nevi, and to xanthelasma (lipid deposits often seen on the eyelids near the nose). Positive treatment outcomes often require early diagnosis and prompt treatment. Treatment usually involves surgical excision but may also include various forms of radiotherapy.

Malignant Melanoma and Retinoblastoma

Etiology and Epidemiology. Metastatic breast and lung tumors are the most common ocular lesions. Retinoblastoma is the most common primary, congenital, intraocular tumor; it is diagnosed in childhood and may occur in one or both eyes. An intraocular malignant melanoma, which usually occurs unilaterally, is a rare primary tumor of the eye.

Pathophysiology. Retinoblastoma arises from the retina. About one third of all patients have bilateral retinoblastomas, and this form of the disease is hereditable. In some cases the retinoblastoma gene has been identified on the long arm of chromosome 13.

Malignant melanomas occur in the choroid (Figure 61-14), ciliary body, and iris, all vascular structures. Vision changes may be the first symptom. Small tumors may lie dormant for several years before sudden active changes occur. The tumor may be a

Nursing Care Plan

Patient With Retinal Detachment

Data A 56-year-old male warehouse clerk visits his practitioner with complaints of decreasing vision in his left eye over the past few days. He states that he began to notice spots floating in front of his eye about 2 weeks ago and flashes of light out of the corner of his eye. He was not concerned because he thought his symptoms were due to his age. Today, however, he felt like a curtain was draped over his eye. Examination of his left eye revealed a superior retinal detachment with inferior visual loss.

The patient underwent an emergency scleral buckling (retinal reattachment surgery). Postoperatively, he has a patch over his left eye and is restricted to bed rest. He is experiencing eye discomfort, which he rates as a 6 on a scale of 0 to 10. Both he and his wife have little understanding of what happened to his eye or the surgery that repaired it. They are concerned about whether he will regain his vision in that eye and whether the same thing will happen to the right eye.

Nursing Diagnosis

Acute pain related to inflammation and increased intraocular pressure (IOP) secondary to retinal detachment and scleral buckle procedure

Outcomes

- Patient will report satisfaction with pain control methods by rating pain as less than 3 on a scale of 0 to 10.
- Patient will require decreasing amounts of analgesic medications to control pain.

Related NOC Outcomes

- Pain Control
- Pain Level

Related NIC Interventions

- Analgesic Administration
- Pain Management

Nursing Interventions/Rationales

- Assess patient's level of discomfort, including the duration and quality. *Postoperative discomfort is expected, but severe pain suggests increased IOP or hemorrhage.*
- Apply cool, moist compresses to left eye. *Reduces swelling and promotes comfort.*
- * Administer prescribed analgesics. *Pain medication may be needed to decrease pain so that patient can comply with prescribed activity restrictions.*
- Teach patient to avoid rapid head movements and bending head below waist (when ambulatory). *Prevents pain and increasing IOP.*

Nursing Diagnosis

Anxiety related to fear of unknown outcome of surgical procedure

Outcomes

- Patient will be free from physical signs of anxiety (tachycardia, restlessness, increased blood pressure).
- Patient will verbalize fears and concerns.
- Patient will identify past successful strategies for coping with anxiety.

Related NOC Outcomes

- Anxiety Self-Control
- Coping

Related NIC Interventions

- Anxiety Reduction
- Coping Enhancement

Nursing Interventions/Rationales

- Provide patient and wife an opportunity to explore concerns about possible loss of vision in left eye. *Identification of specific fears helps direct the plan of action. Talking about one's fears frequently relieves anxiety and allows the nurse to correct misconceptions.*
- Answer all questions honestly. *Information decreases uncertainty and helps the person gain control and feel less anxious.*
- Encourage realistic hope about maintaining vision. *Helps relieve anxiety.*
- Explore patient's understanding of disorder and therapy. *To correct misunderstandings that may be contributing to the patient's fears and anxiety.*

Nursing Diagnosis

Risk for injury: falls related to sensory deficit and anxiety

Outcomes

- Patient will ask for assistance during ambulation.
- Patient will adhere to activity restrictions as prescribed.
- Patient will remain free from injury.

Related NOC Outcomes

- Fall Prevention Behavior
- Risk Control: Visual Impairment

Related NIC Interventions

- Environmental Management: Safety
- Fall Prevention
- Surveillance

Nursing Interventions/Rationales

- Orient patient to physical surroundings. *Increases the patient's awareness of potential hazards.*
- Keep bed in lowest position and side rails up on left side. *To ensure patient's safety while eye is patched and vision is reduced.*
- Assist patient when initially ambulating after surgery. *To ensure safety. Patient may experience dizziness or altered proprioception from having one or both eyes patched.*
- Instruct patient to avoid sneezing, coughing, and vomiting. Administer cough medication or antiemetic if required. *To avoid increasing IOP.*
- Instruct patient to wear eye shield at night or when taking a nap for 2 weeks after surgery. *To prevent accidental bumping of eye while resting or sleeping.*
- Teach the importance of maintaining prescribed activity and position restrictions. *Restricted eye movement helps increase adherence of the scleral buckle and decreases the risk of another detachment.*

- Place bedside table within patient's reach without need to turn head. *To decrease head movement, since gravity helps keeps the retina in its proper position.*
- Assist with activities of daily living (ADLs) as necessary. *To prevent excessive head movement while allowing patient to assume his usual routines as much as possible.*
- Approach patient from unaffected side and place bed so that patient is facing away from the wall. *Allows patient to see who is approaching, offsets isolation, and aids with orientation to new environment.*
- Encourage diversional activities such as radio and conversation. *Provides sensory input and encourages feelings of normalcy.*

Nursing Diagnosis

Risk for infection related to surgical repair of retina

Outcomes

- Patient will remain free from purulent drainage, swelling, or increased pain of eye.

Related NOC Outcomes

- Immune Status
- Infection Severity

Related NIC Interventions

- Infection Protection
- Surveillance

Nursing Interventions/Rationales

- Assess for signs and symptoms of infection (purulent drainage, increased eye pain, swelling, warmth, increased white blood cell count, fever). *To identify infection so that treatment can be initiated during the early stages. Infection increases the risk for permanent loss of vision.*
- Use sterile technique when performing eye care and changing dressings. *To prevent the introduction of microorganisms that can cause infection.*
- Administer antibiotic eyedrops as prescribed. *To prevent infection or treat existing infection.*

Nursing Diagnosis

Deficient knowledge related to lack of previous experience with surgery, postoperative care, and self-care

Outcomes

- Patient will accurately describe retinal detachment and corrective surgery.
- Patient will accurately describe activity restrictions and need for keeping follow-up appointments.
- Patient will participate in self-care within prescribed restrictions.

Related NOC Outcomes

- Knowledge: Disease Process
- Knowledge: Prescribed Activity
- Knowledge: Treatment Regimen

Related NIC Interventions

- Teaching: Disease Process
- Teaching: Individual
- Teaching: Prescribed Activity/Exercise

Nursing Interventions/Rationales

- Teach about the eye and the role of the retina in vision. Explain symptoms associated with detached retina. *To increase understanding of disease process and promote cooperation with postoperative routines and treatment regimen.*
- Explain the importance of following prescribed postoperative activities. *To prevent increased IOP or another detachment.*
- Teach patient that he may engage in activities as long as they do not precipitate eye pain (climbing stairs, watching television, reading, ADLs). *To allow more freedom of activity without increasing risk of increased IOP or another detachment.*
- Encourage patient to avoid driving, heavy house or yard work, or sporting activities until released by physician to do so. *To prevent increased IOP or another detachment.*
- Suggest ways the patient can make himself comfortable if he must maintain a specific position (e.g., facedown). *If a gas bubble is injected to cover the retinal hole, a specific position will be required to ensure its success (usually prone).*
- Demonstrate and have patient return demonstrate correct technique for hand washing and cleansing his eye from inner to outer canthus using clean cotton ball for each wipe. *To reduce the risk of introducing microorganisms into the operated eye.*
- Demonstrate and have patient return demonstrate correct technique for self-administering eyedrops and ointments and for applying eye shield. *To ensure he receives the prescribed dose of medication without increasing the risk of contamination of the eye.*
- Instruct patient to notify the physician immediately if he experiences new flashing lights, floaters or shadows, severe or persistent eye pain, increased redness of the eye or lid, or increased quantity or change in color of eye drainage. *May indicate IOP or infection, which necessitates immediate intervention.*

Evaluation

Evaluation is based on comparing the patient's outcomes with desired outcomes.

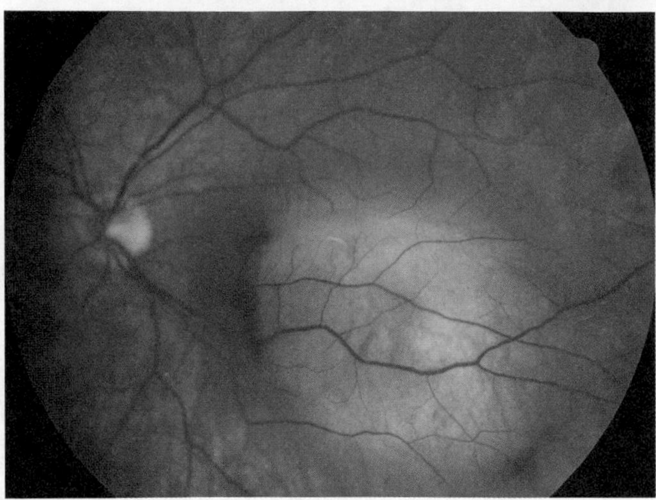

Figure 61-14 Large choroidal melanoma.

pigmented or nonpigmented mass. It may appear nodular, and if it breaks through Bruch's membrane, mushroomed shaped.

Collaborative Care Management. The first symptom usually reported by a patient with an ocular tumor is a change in vision. On slit lamp and ophthalmoscopic examination, a tumor may be identified. Fluorescein angiography documents the vascular involvement of the tumor. Ultrasonography establishes the tumor's depth and width in the choroid, and fundus photography documents its location. A fine needle biopsy may be performed to establish the diagnosis.

Retinoblastoma is often discovered when a parent notices a white "cat's eye" reflex in a child when the pupil is dilated. A certain percentage of children develop strabismus as the first symptom. Enucleation (surgical removal of the entire eyeball, including the sclera) is treatment of choice if the tumor is unilateral. In bilateral tumors the worst eye is enucleated, and the child undergoes chemotherapy to shrink the tumor in the remaining eye, followed by brachytherapy in an attempt to save vision.

Treatment for an intraocular melanoma is based on the size, shape, and location of the tumor. The patient's vision is preserved wherever possible. Patients are advised of all the options. Photocoagulation may be all that is necessary initially. Small iris tumors may be successfully treated with surgical iridectomy, which sometimes includes a portion of the ciliary body as well. Small and medium-sized tumors are successfully treated with iodine 125 radioactive plaques (brachytherapy) sutured onto the sclera, over the intraocular tumor, so that the base of the tumor is irradiated for about 4 days. External beam radiation is also used occasionally. Depending on Nuclear Regulatory Commission regulations for the state in which treatment is performed, radioactive plaque therapy may mean confinement to a room for the duration of treatment. After plaque removal the patient's eye is patched for 48 hours, after which antibiotic-steroid and cycloplegic eyedrops must be instilled.

Large choroidal melanomas are usually treated with enucleation of the eye. If there is extraocular extension of the tumor, then an exenteration (removal of the eyeball and all other soft tissues in the bony orbit) may be necessary.

When enucleation is undertaken, good cosmesis with ocular movements has been achieved using a hydroxyapatite (coral) or synthetic Medpor ball implant. Hydroxyapatite ball implants are wrapped in either fascia lata or cadaver sclera, so that four of the extraocular muscles can be attached to it. The Medpor has the muscles attached directly to it. Both ball implants are porous, and eventually blood vessels invade the implant, making it permanent. The implant is held in place by the conjunctiva. A plastic conformer is placed between the lids to maintain the integrity of the eyelids. The patient is sent home with a pressure dressing, which is left in place for 2 to 4 days to decrease edema. Headaches or pain on the operative side may be evident during the first 24 to 48 hours. Prophylactic antibiotic eyedrops are prescribed once the pressure patch is removed to prevent infection.

A custom-made prosthetic eye can be used as soon as healing is complete and edema has disappeared. Healing is usually complete 4 to 8 weeks after surgery. Today artificial eyes are made of plastic instead of glass and can be made in shades that closely match the normal eye.

Patient/Family Teaching. The diagnosis of eye malignancy, along with the need to undergo treatment, creates a crisis situation for the patient and family. The fact that the ocular malignancy can be life threatening adds urgency to the need for treatment so patients have little time to prepare themselves either physically or emotionally for therapy. Thus teaching must be combined with support and counseling if it is to be effective (see Patient/Family Teaching box).

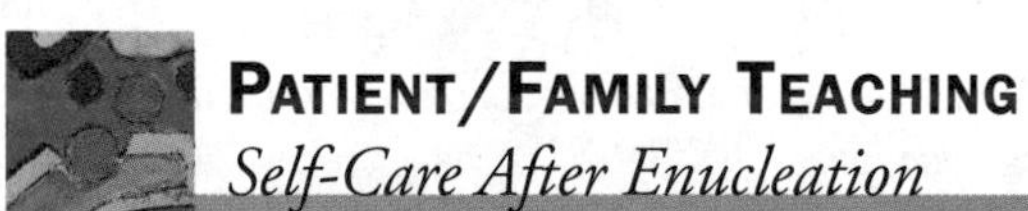

Patient/Family Teaching
Self-Care After Enucleation

Patient teaching should include information about:

- The disease
- Prescribed medications
- Procedure for replacing the conformer should it dislodge after the eye patch is removed and the swelling goes down
- Importance of protecting the remaining eye
- Change in depth perception resulting from loss of binocular vision and the adjustments needed to carry out normal activities (For example, when driving, a one-eyed person must learn to pan like a camera and leave more distance between the car in front. The nurse should stress that, with patience and practice, almost all activities are possible.)
- Technique of instilling eyedrops or ointment by raising the upper lid to prevent the conformer from coming out of the socket
- Care of the prosthetic eye: remove, wash with tap water every 3 months, and one or two times per year follow up with an oculist who will clean and polish the prosthesis to remove salt and protein buildup

Critical Thinking

1. How would you teach a visually impaired person who is using three different types of eyedrops to identify the correct drops?
2. What approaches might you consider for a person with glaucoma who refuses to administer eyedrops four times a day as prescribed by the physician?
3. A 20-year-old woman has a foreign object floating on the surface of her left eye. The nurse has her lie on her right side and begins irrigating the left eye with a syringe filled with normal saline. She directs the fluid from the outer to the inner canthus. Critique this irrigation procedure.

References

1. American Academy of Ophthalmology: *Extended-wear of contact lenses,* accessed August 30, 2004, from website: www.aao.oraleducation/library/statements/contact_lenses.cfm.

1a. American Society of Ophthalmic Registered Nurses: *Ophthalmic procedures: a nursing perspective—operating room and ambulatory surgery center,* rev ed. Dubuque, Iowa, 2003, Kendall/Hunt.

2. Boyd-Monk H: Eye injuries, *Adv Nurses* 4(16):31-32, 2002.
3. Eye MD Association: *Important facts about eye injuries,* San Francisco, 2002, American Academy of Ophthalmology.
4. Eye MD Association: *Elevated risk of glaucoma among African Americans,* San Francisco, 2003-2004, American Academy of Ophthalmology.
5. National Eye Institute: *Age-related macular degeneration,* accessed March 2004 from website: www/nei.nih.gov.
6. A randomized, placebo-controlled, clinical trial of high-dose supplementation with vitamins C and E, beta carotene, and zinc for age-related macular degeneration and vision loss: AREDS report no. 8, *Arch Ophthalmol* 119(10):1417-1436, 2001.
7. Stein HA, Slatt BJ, Stein RM: *The ophthalmic assistant: a guide for ophthalmic medical personnel,* ed 7, St Louis, 2000, Mosby.
8. US Department of Health and Human Services, U.S. Public Health Service: *Healthy people 2010: understanding and improving health* and *Objectives for improving health,* 2 vols, Washington, DC, 2001, The Department.
9. Whitaker RJ et al: Glaucoma: what the ophthalmic nurse should know, *Insight* 24(3):86-90, 1999.

Visit the Evolve website: http://evolve.elsevier.com/Monahan/medsurg

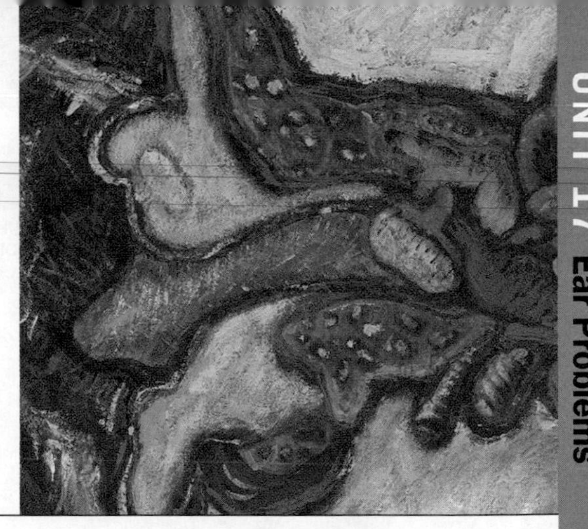

CHAPTER 62

Assessment of the Auditory System

by Frances D. Monahan

OBJECTIVES

After studying this chapter, the learner should be able to:

1. Describe the basic structure and function of the temporal bone and ear.
2. Use behavioral clues to detect loss of hearing and balance.
3. Describe anatomic and physiologic age-related changes in the auditory and vestibular systems.
4. Recognize normal assessment findings related to the ear and its functions.
5. Identify specific diagnostic tests for hearing and balance and their associated nursing interventions.

KEY TERMS

air conduction, p. 1838
audiometry, p. 1843
binaural hearing, p. 1835
bone conduction, p. 1838
eustachian tube, p. 1836
otoscope, p. 1840
tuning fork, p. 1842
tympanic membrane, p. 1835

The two major functions of the ear relate to hearing and balance, both of which play an important role in the activities of daily living. Hearing helps us interact with the environment. It is essential for the normal development and maintenance of speech, provides warning of danger, and adds a dimension of aesthetic pleasure to life. The organs of balance contained within the ear relay information about the body's position to the brain and thus are critical to the ability to function within the environment.

Nurses are involved in all aspects of patient care related to auditory and vestibular problems: prevention, detection, and treatment. In fact, the nurse is frequently the first member of the health care team to be approached by patients regarding problems with hearing and balance. Therefore every nurse needs to be skillful in examining the outer ear and grossly assessing the patient's hearing and equilibrium.

Anatomy and Physiology

The ears are a pair of complex sensory organs located in the middle of both sides of the head at approximately eye level. The position of the ears is important because the use of both ears simultaneously produces **binaural hearing**, allowing a person to detect the direction of sound and maintain equilibrium. A person detects the direction from which a sound comes by the time lag between the sound entry into one ear compared with the sound entry into the other ear and by the intensity of sound in each ear.

The ears are housed in the temporal bones, which form part of both the base and the lateral walls of the skull. The temporal bones, the hardest bones in the human body, protect the organs of hearing and balance.

Each ear is divided into three parts: the external ear, the middle ear, and the inner ear (Figure 62-1).

External Ear

The external ear consists of the pinna, or auricle, and the external auditory canal. The pinna is primarily composed of cartilage covered by skin. It is attached to the side of the head at approximately a 10-degree angle. In the adult the external auditory canal extends in an inward, forward, and downward path from the concha, which is the deepest part of the pinna, to the tympanic membrane. The canal is irregular and constricts about midway and again near the tympanic membrane. Skin lines the canal and covers the tympanic membrane. The supporting wall of the first half of the external auditory canal is cartilaginous and that of the second half is osseous. The skin lining this bony portion of the canal is thin and highly sensitive and contains fine hairs and sebaceous glands.

Ceruminous glands, which are modified sweat glands found in the external auditory canal, produce cerumen, or ear wax. Cerumen has a protective function in that its sticky consistency, along with the fine hairs of the ears, help cleanse the auditory canal of foreign matter.

The funnel shape of the external ear collects sound and channels it toward the tympanic membrane, which is thin and semitransparent. The **tympanic membrane** protects the middle ear and conducts

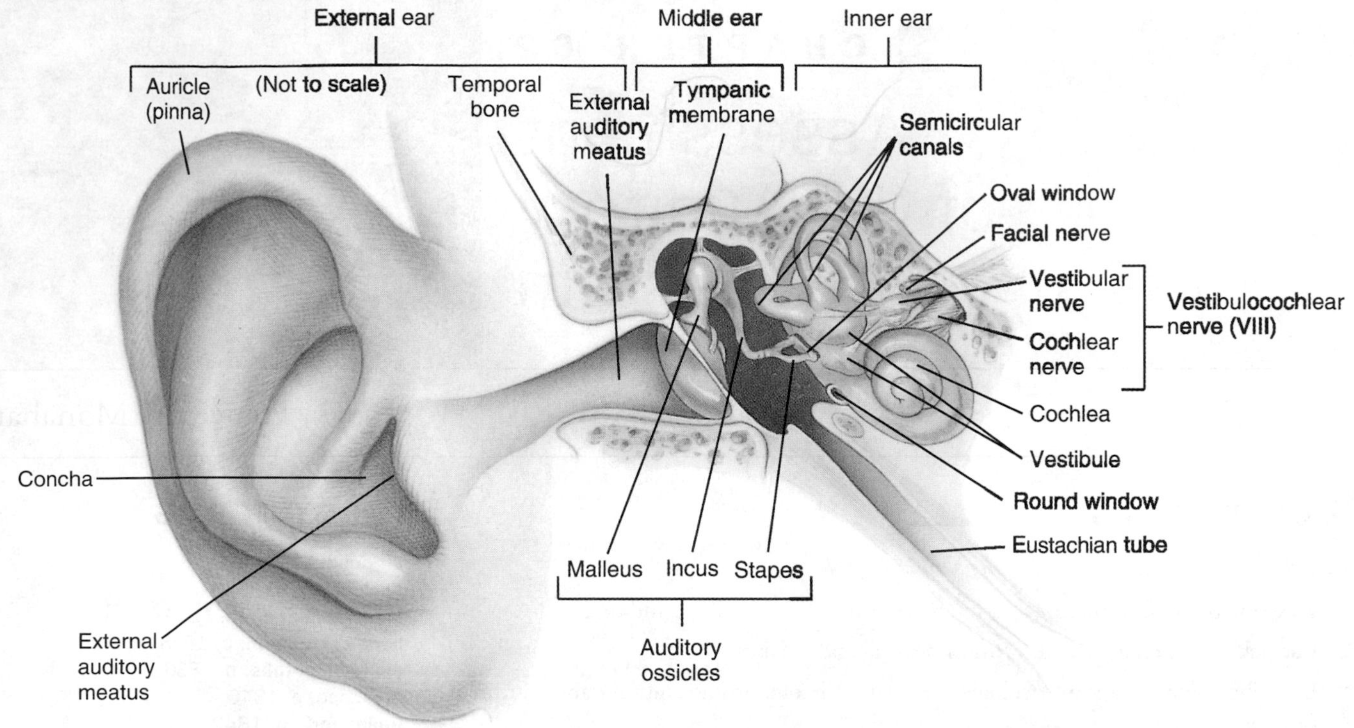

Figure 62-1 Structures of external, middle, and inner ear. (Anatomic structures not drawn to scale.)

sound vibrations from the external ear to the ossicles. It is approximately 9 mm in diameter, nearly oval, obliquely directed downward and inward, and pearly gray. Distinguishing landmarks of the normal tympanic membrane include the annulus, the thickened border that attaches the tympanic membrane to the temporal bone; the umbo, the most depressed point where the first ossicle attaches to the tympanic membrane; the pars flaccida, a small triangular area above the short process of the malleus; and the largest portion, the pars tensa (Figure 62-2).

The tympanic membrane is composed of three layers: an outer skin layer continuous with the skin of the external auditory canal, a fibrous middle layer, and an inner mucosal layer continuous with the lining of the middle ear.[1] The pars flaccida is composed of only two layers. The absence of the fibrous middle layer makes the pars flaccida more vulnerable to negative pressure and resulting disorders.

Middle Ear

The middle ear consists of an air-filled cavity and its contents: the ossicles, the oval and round windows, and the opening of the eustachian tube.

The ossicles—the malleus (hammer), the incus (anvil), and the stapes (stirrup)—are the three smallest bones in the body. The ossicles have been given these common names because of their appearance. The ossicles are joined together in a movable chain, which connects the tympanic membrane to the labyrinth. They are held in place by muscles, ligaments, and joints. The ossicles function to mechanically transmit sound vibrations and also protect the inner ear from loud sounds by means of a dampening mechanism. The ossicles provide an efficient means by which the moving air molecules of sound in the external ear can be transferred to the fluid molecules that circulate in the inner ear. Liquids offer more resistance than air and need more force to produce movement; the ossicular chain produces this force against the inner ear fluids.[1]

The oval window, which is covered by the footplate of the stapes, is the opening into the inner ear where sound vibrations enter. The round window is a true window and provides an exit for sound vibrations from the inner ear.

The **eustachian tube** is a channel approximately 35 mm (1½ inches) long that connects the middle ear with the nasopharynx. The tube is composed of bone, cartilage, and fibrous tissue lined with mucous membrane. The eustachian tube allows air to enter and leave the middle ear and is responsible for both ventilation and pressure regulation, which are necessary for normal hearing.

Only a small segment of the eustachian tube remains open permanently; otherwise the walls are in direct contact with each other. This prevents the sound of normal nasal respiration and one's own voice from passing up the eustachian tube into the middle ear. The tube can be forcibly opened by increasing nasopharyngeal pressure ("popping the ears").

The mastoid includes the mastoid bone (part of the temporal bone); the mastoid process, which can be felt as a bony protuberance behind the lower portion of the pinna; the mastoid cavity, a large cavity that is continuous with the middle ear; and the mastoid air cells that branch off the mastoid cavity. The cavity and system of air-filled cells contained within the mastoid bone aid the middle ear in adjusting to changes in pressure and lighten the weight of this protective bony structure.

Inner Ear

The inner ear is a complex system of intercommunicating chambers and connecting tubes located in the petrous part of the temporal bone (Figure 62-3). The two major structures of the inner

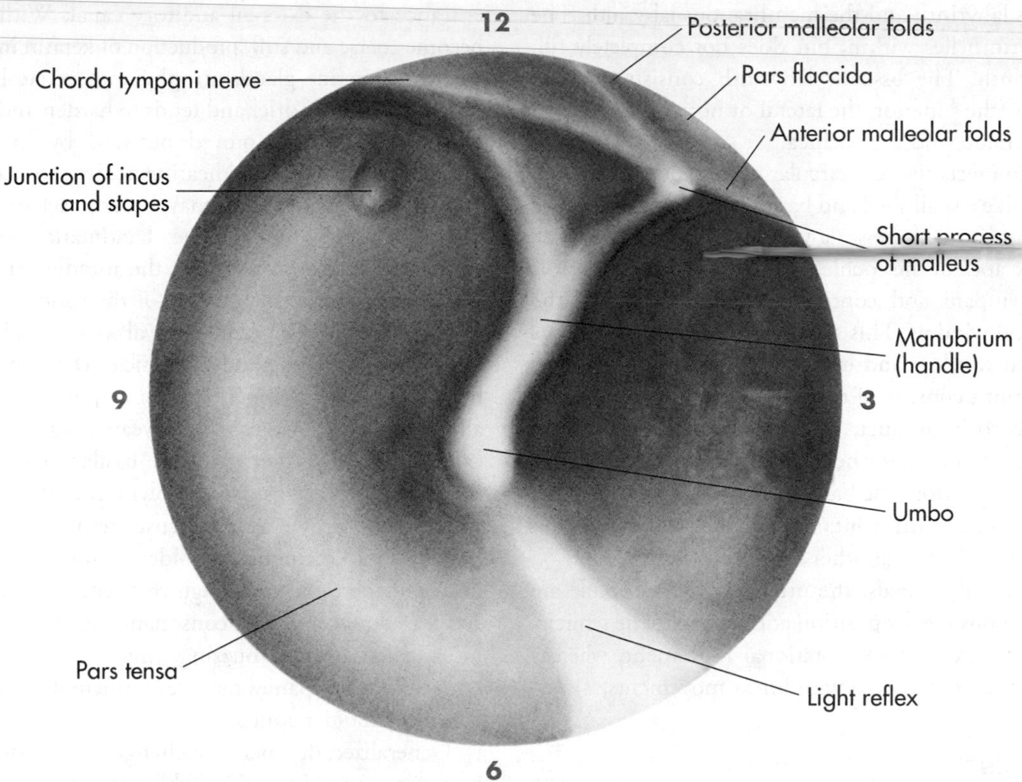

Figure 62-2 Structural landmarks of tympanic membrane in relationship to a clock face.

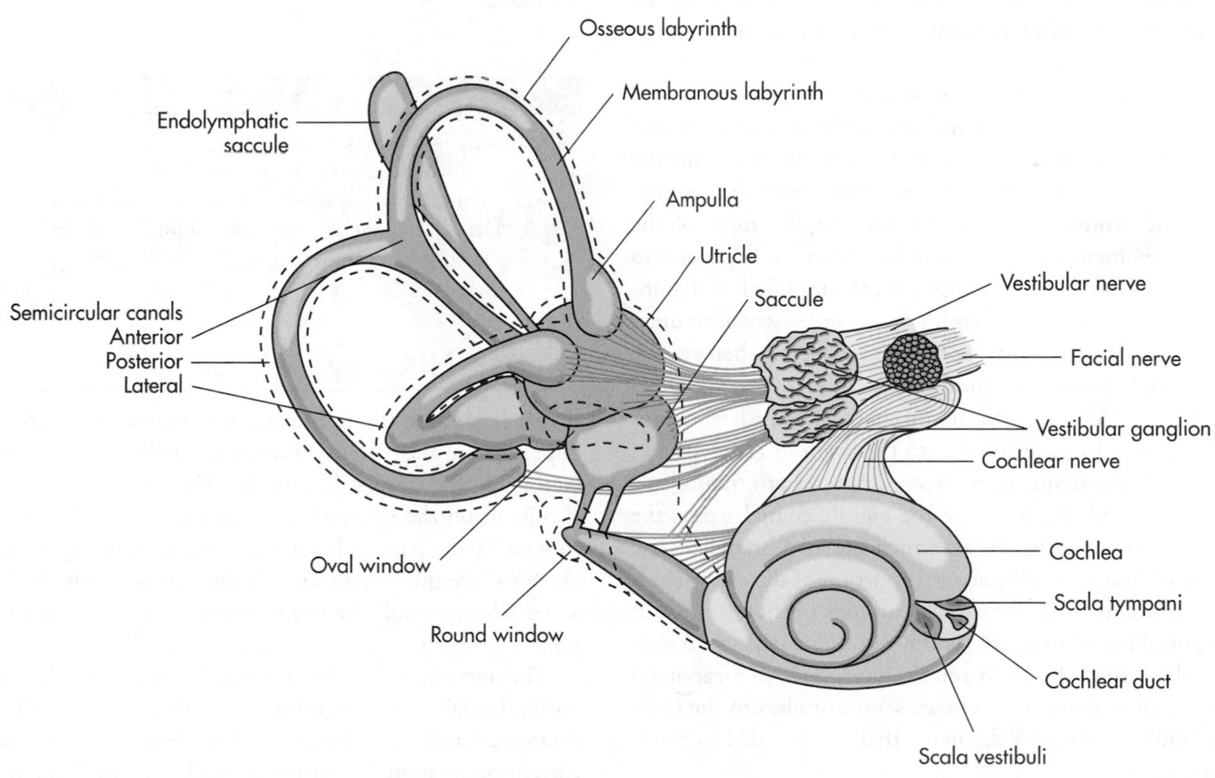

Figure 62-3 Structures of the inner ear.

ear are the osseous labyrinth and the membranous labyrinth. The membranous labyrinth lies within, but does not completely fill, the osseous labyrinth. The osseous labyrinth consists of three semicircular canals (the superior, the lateral or horizontal, and the posterior), the vestibule, and the cochlea.

The vestibule connects the semicircular canals and the cochlea. The cochlea looks like a snail shell and has two compartments. The upper compartment is called the scala vestibuli and leads from the oval window to the apex of the cochlea. The lower compartment is called the scala tympani and continues from the apex of the cochlea to the round window. This system allows sound vibrations to enter at the oval window and exit at the round window. The membranous labyrinth consists of the utricle, saccule, three semicircular ducts, the cochlear duct, and the organ of Corti. The organ of Corti, the end organ for hearing, is located on the basilar membrane and stretches from the base to the apex of the cochlea.

The membranous labyrinth contains a fluid called endolymph and is continuously bathed in another fluid, called perilymph.

The three semicircular canals, the utricle, and the saccule are the sense organs responsible for position and balance. The semicircular canals are arranged to sense rotational movement, whereas the utricle and saccule are involved with linear movements.

Sound Transmission

Sound is transmitted from the external ear to the inner ear by two routes, air conduction and bone conduction. **Air conduction** transmits sound vibration through the middle ear to the inner ear, whereas **bone conduction** transmits sound vibrations through the skull to the inner ear.

In air conduction the tympanic membrane conducts sound vibrations to the ossicles and then through the oval window into the perilymph. The pressure exerted by the vibrations on the stapes in the oval window is 22 times greater than the pressure exerted on the tympanic membrane because the force of the sound vibrations increases with transmission from a larger area to a smaller area. From the perilymph, these amplified vibrations travel through the vestibular membrane, enter the cochlear duct, and cause movement of the basilar membrane.[3] They then exit the inner ear through the round window.

The organ of Corti transforms mechanical sound vibrations into neural activity for transmission to the brain. It also separates sound into different frequencies. Nerve impulses are transmitted between the ear and the brain by the eighth cranial nerve, the vestibulocochlear (acoustic) nerve, which has two branches. The cochlear branch innervates the acoustic portion of the ear, whereas the vestibular branch innervates the vestibular portion of the ear. Electrochemical impulses travel via the vestibulocochlear nerve to the temporal cortex of the brain and are interpreted as meaningful sound. In a similar way the inner ears send impulses to the brain via the vestibular portion of the nerve that are decoded to maintain normal balance.[3]

Physiologic Changes With Aging

A variety of changes occur in the ear as a result of normal aging. The auricle enlarges and loses its elasticity. The lobe enlarges and becomes pendulous. A tuft of wiry hair frequently develops at the entrance to the external auditory canal. Within the canal, cilia become coarse and stiff, production of keratin in the skin increases, and the apocrine glands atrophy and secrete less cerumen. As a result, cerumen is drier and tends to harden and accumulate, since it is not efficiently moved outward by the cilia. Ultimately impaction and decreased hearing acuity can occur. The tympanic membrane atrophies and may become sclerotic. It appears dull white or cloudy, and opaque. Landmarks are more prominent because of retraction. Within the middle ear muscles and ligaments stiffen, and calcification of the ossicles may cause fixation of the foot of the stapes in the oval window. These changes in the tympanic membrane and the ossicles contribute to a conductive hearing loss. In the inner ear, hair cells in the organ of Corti usually begin to degenerate after 50 years of age. In addition, cochlear capillaries atrophy with age, the basilar membrane becomes less flexible, and neurons and endolymph diminish. A sensorineural hearing loss, known as presbycusis, results. This is the most common type of hearing loss in older persons and is characterized by decreased perception of high-frequency sounds *(S, Sh, Ph, K)*. Decreased perception of consonants *(Z, T, F, G)* also occurs. Tinnitus, a sensation of buzzing, ringing, or other noise in one or both ears, accompanies most sensorineural hearing loss and thus is common in older adults.

Generalized degenerative changes in the labyrinth cause presbyastasis, or presbyvertigo, which is a balance disorder of aging. Also contributing to the imbalance are decreased visual acuity and compromised proprioception. Presbyastasis can be controlled but not cured.[4]

▶ ARE You READY?

The function of ear wax is to:

1. Facilitate the movement of sound.
2. Minimize the impact of very high–pitched noises.
3. Help cleanse the auditory canal of foreign matter.
4. Decrease pH of inner ear.

Health History

Before beginning the health history, the nurse obtains a general impression of the patient's hearing ability by observing for behavioral clues that suggest hearing loss (Box 62-1). The patient may also focus on the speaker's face and lips, rather than making eye contact. If the patient has a hearing loss, it is important for the nurse to face the patient directly and speak clearly. If the patient wears a hearing aid, the nurse ensures that it is in use and functioning properly.

The nurse asks the patient about the presence or history of earache (otalgia), drainage (otorrhea), tinnitus, or vertigo. An environmental and work history is also obtained, since previous or current occupational exposure to loud noise or living in a noise-polluted area may result in hearing loss. Any history of trauma, such as a blow to the ears or a foreign body, is explored, since this could result in hearing loss later in life.

The nurse completes a thorough medication history to identify use of potentially ototoxic drugs (Table 62-1).[5] Ototoxic agents affect either the eighth cranial nerve or the organs of hearing and balance, causing symptoms such as tinnitus, headache, dizziness, vertigo, nausea, ataxia, nystagmus, or a discernible change in hearing.

The nurse asks the patient about self-care of the ears: frequency of hearing tests and the method and frequency of cleaning. This information helps the nurse plan appropriate health teaching. Incorrect methods of cleaning the ears, such as the use of cotton-tipped applicators, can lead to impacted cerumen and hearing loss. The nurse also asks the patient about any history of ear infections and the method of treatment. A history of chronic ear infections alerts the nurse to the possibility of sequelae.

Dizziness or hearing loss can have devastating effects on the patient's quality of life. The nurse carefully explores the extent to which symptoms have disrupted the patient's lifestyle and evaluates the patient's emotional response. If the ability to communicate is impaired, the patient may feel socially isolated. The nurse assesses the nature and effectiveness of the patient's coping mechanisms. When either balance or hearing is affected, the patient's risk for injury increases, and use of appropriate safety measures is carefully explored.

BOX 62-1 Behavioral Clues Suggesting Hearing Loss

An adult with a hearing loss may exhibit one or more of the following behaviors:

- Being irritable, hostile, or hypersensitive in interpersonal relations
- Having difficulty hearing upper frequency consonants
- Complaining about people mumbling
- Turning up volume on television
- Asking for frequent repetition or misunderstanding
- Answering questions inappropriately
- Losing sense of humor; becoming grim
- Leaning forward to hear better; face looking serious and strained
- Shunning large- and small-group audience situations
- Appearing aloof and "stuck up"
- Complaining of ringing in the ears
- Having an unusually soft or loud voice
- Having garbled speech

TABLE 62-1 COMMON POTENTIALLY OTOTOXIC MEDICATIONS

Drug	Effects on Auditory and Vestibular System
Aminoglycosides	Affect auditory and vestibular functions, usually related to persistently high drug levels; older patients, persons taking other ototoxic drugs, and persons with preexisting auditory loss most susceptible; damage largely irreversible
Gentamicin Tobramycin Streptomycin	Primarily affect balance because of damage to sensory hair cells of vestibular apparatus; symptoms include headache, which may last 1-2 days followed by nausea, unsteadiness, dizziness, and vertigo
Amikacin Neomycin Kanamycin	Primarily affect hearing because of damage to sensory hair cells in cochlea; symptoms begin with high-pitched tinnitus and progress to loss of hearing in high-frequency range and then in low-frequency range
Vancomycin	Older patients and those with hearing loss most susceptible; ototoxicity more common with high serum levels
Loop diuretics: Furosemide Torsemide Bumetanide Ethacrynate sodium Ethacrynic acid	Rapid parenteral administration leading to hearing loss, deafness, or tinnitus
Erythromycin	Hearing loss associated with intravenous administration of high doses, especially with patients with kidney failure
Salicylates	
Aspirin	Tinnitus, hearing loss; audiometric testing indicated before or after long-term therapy; older patients most susceptible; effects generally reversible
Nonsteroidal antiinflammatory drugs	Auditory function monitored before and during therapy to prevent ototoxicity; older patients most susceptible
Cisplatin	Tinnitus, high-frequency hearing loss
Quinine sulfate	Tinnitus, impaired hearing; serum concentrations $\geq$10 mg/ml may confirm toxicity as cause of tinnitus or hearing loss

▶ ARE You READY?

Damage to the sensory hair cells of the vestibular system by ototoxic medications results in which of the following?

1. Loss of balance
2. Loss of hearing
3. Tinnitus
4. Nystagmus

Physical Examination

External Ear

The nurse inspects the external ear for size, configuration, and angle of attachment to the head. The configuration of the pinna is observed for gross deformity. The nurse notes whether the ears protrude and the degree of protrusion, the skin color of the ear, and whether any skin tags are present. The skin of the ear should be smooth and without breaks or inflammation, especially behind the ear in the crevice. The nurse documents any lumps or skin lesions, including appearance, approximate size, location, and related symptoms. The nurse also assesses all pierced ear holes for irritation or infection.

The nurse palpates the pinna and the mastoid area for tenderness or nodules. Pain or discomfort can indicate inflammation or infection. Normal mastoid bones are smooth, hard, nontender, and possibly unequal in size. For direct observation of the external auditory canal, the adult is asked to tip the head slightly to the opposite side while the nurse pulls the pinna up, back, and out. A penlight is used to inspect the external auditory canal for any abnormalities such as extreme narrowing, excessive wax, redness, scaliness, swelling, drainage, cysts, or foreign objects.

Tympanic Membrane

The nurse uses an **otoscope** to examine the tympanic membrane. An otoscope consists of a handle, a light source, a magnifying lens, and an attachment for visualizing the external auditory canal and tympanic membrane. Some otoscopes have a pneumatic device for injecting air into the auditory canal to test the mobility and integrity of the tympanic membrane.

The diameter of the meatus and the length of the auditory canal vary; thus the speculum with the largest diameter that fits comfortably into the canal is chosen. The otoscope is held with the dominant hand, which is braced lightly against the patient's head to decrease the risk of damage to the external canal if the patient moves suddenly. With the patient's head gently tilted away, the nurse uses the nondominant hand to pull the pinna up, back, and out to straighten the external auditory canal while slowly and carefully inserting the speculum (Figure 62-4). The otoscope is moved in a circular fashion to allow for visualization of the entire external auditory canal.[2] It should not touch the bony walls of the auditory canal, since this will be painful. The cartilaginous portion of the canal is normally not tender.

The nurse notes any abnormalities such as extreme narrowing of the auditory canal, nodules, redness, scaliness, swelling, drainage, cysts, foreign objects, or excessive wax.[2] Color and consistency of cerumen, which are genetically determined, are also noted. Dark, sticky cerumen is common in Caucasians and African-Americans, whereas flaky, dry cerumen that is light brown to gray is commonly found in Asian-Americans and Native Americans. Sometimes the external auditory canal must be cleaned of wax, dead skin, and other debris before the tympanic membrane can be visualized. Hearing remains normal even when 90% to 95% of the auditory canal is blocked with cerumen. Total occlusion creates a sudden hearing loss or feeling of fullness in the ear.

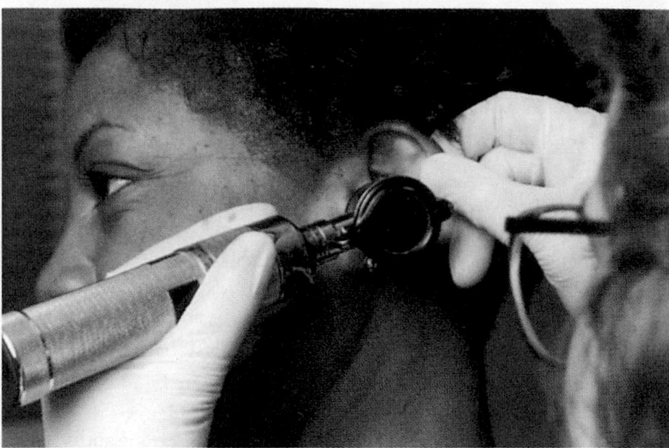

Figure 62-4 Otoscopic examination. External auditory canal is straightened by pulling auricle up and back to examine ear with otoscope.

The normal tympanic membrane is slightly conical, shiny and smooth, and pearly gray. The position of the drumhead is oblique to the external auditory canal. In the presence of disease the color of the tympanic membrane changes, and other abnormalities such as retraction, bulging, perforation, or a white plaque in the membrane may be present.[6] The nurse carefully inspects the entire tympanic membrane, including the border, or annulus. The umbo and the long and short process of the malleus should be easily visible through the membrane.

The mobility of the tympanic membrane is tested by injecting a small puff of air into the external auditory canal with the pneumatic device on the otoscope. The membrane should gently move.

Middle Ear

Assessment of the middle ear involves evaluating hearing and inspecting the middle ear through the tympanic membrane with the otoscope. Gross assessment of hearing can be accomplished through general conversation and whisper tests that compare one ear with the other. Tuning forks are also used to assess hearing (see Special Tests).

Inner Ear

The inner ears are not accessible to direct examination. However, some inferences about their condition can be made based on auditory and vestibular function. Thus the physical examination should include not only a gross assessment of the patient's hearing, as discussed in previous paragraphs, but also balance testing, which assesses the vestibular function of the inner ear.

Diagnostic Tests

Assessment of Balance

Balance and equilibrium depend on four systems: the vestibular (the labyrinth or inner ear), the proprioceptive (somatosensors of joints and muscles), the visual (the eye), and the cerebellar (coordination). Sensations transmitted from the muscles and joints and the inner ears are integrated in the brainstem and cerebellum and perceived in the cerebral cortex. Dizziness is most likely to occur when two or more systems are impaired simultaneously or when they transmit sensory information that is contradictory.

Balance is assessed by observation of gait, the gaze test for nystagmus, and Romberg's test. Gait is tested by asking the patient to walk away from the nurse and then turn and walk back. The nurse observes posture, balance, swinging of the arms, and movement of the legs. (Assessment of gait is discussed in more detail in Chapter 47.) To test for nystagmus, which is the involuntary, rhythmic oscillation of the eyes associated with vestibular dysfunction, the examiner places a finger directly in front of the patient at eye level and asks the patient to follow the finger without moving the head. The examiner moves the finger slowly from the midline toward each ear and observes the eyes for any jerking movements.

For Romberg's test, the patient stands with feet together and the arms at the sides, first with the eyes open and then with the eyes closed (Figure 62-5). The examiner assesses the ability to maintain an upright posture with eyes closed. Normally only minimal swaying occurs. A loss of balance (positive Romberg's test) may indicate an inner ear problem (vestibular problem) or cerebellar ataxia.

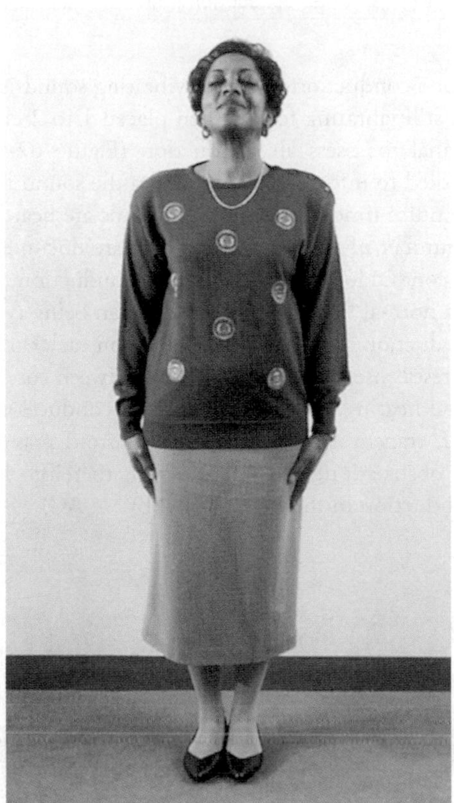

Figure 62-5 Evaluation of balance with Romberg's test. Person maintains balance with eyes closed.

Assessment measures and variations in normal findings relevant to the care of older adults are presented in the Gerontologic Assessment box. The box also lists disorders common in older adults, which may be responsible for abnormal assessment findings.

Laboratory Tests

Routine blood and urine tests rarely provide significant information related to disease of the ears. An elevated white blood cell count indicates an infection but is not diagnostic of ear disease. Drainage from the external auditory canal can be cultured to identify specific organisms causing infection. Cultures are important for treatment of acute infections, but are less helpful with long-term drainage because gram-negative bacilli cover up the original pathogen.

When clear fluid is found in the ear, it is important to rule out the presence of cerebrospinal fluid. Fistulas, skull fractures, and other head injuries can cause leakage of cerebrospinal fluid with the accompanying risk of meningitis. Cerebrospinal fluid tests positive for glucose on a reagent strip and feels slippery to the touch.

Radiologic Tests

Computed Tomography. Computed tomography (CT) scanning can be used to evaluate the temporal bone in thin sections or slices, producing more and smaller components than a plain x-ray

Gerontologic Assessment

- Assess the patient's level of functional hearing before beginning the health history and determine whether any compensatory actions are needed (e.g., modulation of tone or speed of diction, adjustment of a hearing aid, involvement of a family member).
  - –Close to one third of people over age 65 have some type of hearing loss.
- Inspect the external ear.
  - –The auricle may be enlarged and lack elasticity, earlobes may be pendulous, and a tuft of wiry hair may be present at the entrance to the external auditory canal.
- Examine the external auditory canal and tympanic membrane with an otoscope.
  - –Hard, impacted cerumen may be present because of decreased secretion; increased amounts of keratin; and stiff, coarse cilia.
  - –Because of atrophy and retraction, the tympanic membrane may appear dull white or cloudy, and opaque with prominent landmarks.

Common Disorders in Older Adults

Presbycusis
Impacted cerumen
Tinnitus
Presbyastasis
Conductive hearing loss
Sensorineural hearing loss

film. The CT scan can also be done with a contrast medium to improve the clarity of the image and visualization of vascular lesions. The nurse carefully assesses the person for any allergy to iodine, shellfish, or contrast media and prepares the patient for what to expect during the test.

Magnetic Resonance Imaging. Magnetic resonance imaging (MRI) uses a large magnet rather than ionizing radiation to emit energy. MRI effectively details soft tissues, so the membranous organs, nerves, and blood vessels of the temporal bone can be examined. The nurse carefully prepares the patient for the expected sensory experiences associated with MRI, including loud pounding noises and often some claustrophobia. Newer MRI machines make less noise, which makes them more comfortable for the patient.

Arteriography and Venography. Adjuncts to radiography are arteriography and venography in which contrast medium is injected into blood vessels. These studies are especially useful for diagnosing vascular abnormalities in the temporal bone. The examiner can recognize compression of the vessels and greater detail in tumors of the temporal bone and related structures.[8]

Special Tests

Auditory Acuity Tests

WHISPERED VOICE TEST. The patient occludes one ear with a finger, and the nurse softly whispers two-syllable words toward the unoccluded ear. The patient is then asked to repeat the words. The intensity of the nurse's voice can be increased from a soft, medium, or loud whisper to a soft, medium, or loud voice. Each ear is tested separately, and the patient is asked if hearing is better in one ear than the other. A soft whisper can normally be heard in both ears.

TUNING FORK TESTS. The **tuning fork** provides a general estimate of hearing loss. The two major tuning fork tests date from the nineteenth century and are named after their originators: Rinne and Weber. The tuning fork is set into vibration by striking the tines on the examiner's knuckles or knee, holding only the base of the fork without touching the tines. Table 62-2 presents the results of Weber's and Rinne's tests with normal hearing and with conductive and sensorineural hearing loss.

RINNE'S TEST. Rinne's test is performed by placing the vibrating tuning fork against the patient's mastoid process (Figure 62-6, *A*) to assess bone conduction until the vibrating sound is no longer heard. The still vibrating fork is then placed 1 to 2 cm from the auditory canal to assess air conduction (Figure 62-6, *B*). The patient is asked to inform the nurse when the sound is no longer heard. The nurse times how long the sounds are heard and compares the number of seconds. The results are documented using *AC* for air conduction and *BC* for bone conduction. AC > BC represents a normal finding of air conduction being twice as long as bone conduction. The test is performed on each ear.

Rinne's test is useful in differentiating between conductive and sensorineural hearing losses. When normal conduction pathways are blocked, transmission through the mastoid may be able to bypass the obstruction. Bone conduction therefore lasts longer than air conduction in these situations (BC > AC).

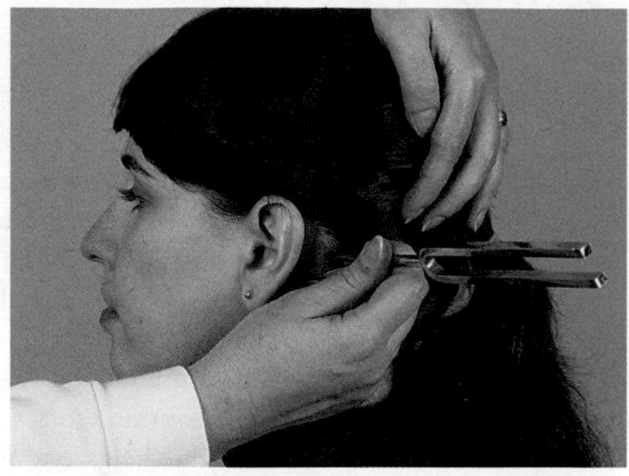

A

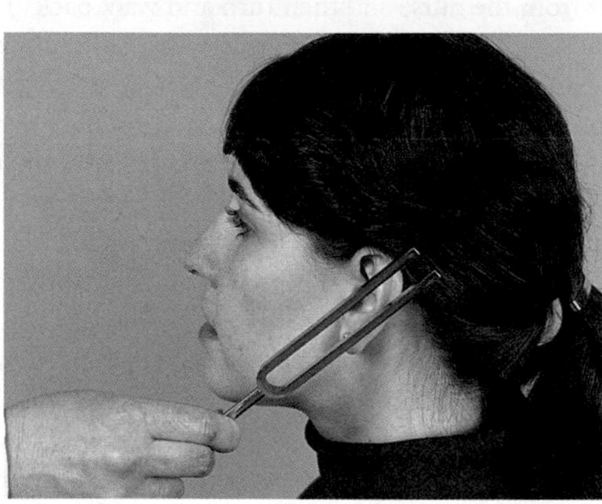

B

Figure 62-6 Rinne's test. **A,** Vibrating tuning fork is placed on mastoid bone for bone conduction testing. **B,** Vibrating tuning fork is placed in front of ear for air conduction testing.

TABLE 62-2 TUNING FORK TESTS FOR AUDITORY ACUITY

Finding	Site of Problem	Weber's Test	Rinne's Test
Normal hearing	—	Tone heard in center of head	Air conduction lasts twice as long as bone conduction.
Conductive loss	External or middle ear	Tone heard in poorer ear because ear not distracted by room noise	Bone conduction lasts longer than air conduction.
Sensorineural loss	Inner ear	Tone heard in better ear because inner ear less able to receive vibrations	Air conduction lasts longer than bone conduction.

WEBER'S TEST. The vibrating tuning fork is placed on the patient's head or teeth (Figure 62-7). Placement on the teeth (even if the patient has false teeth) is generally more reliable. The patient is asked whether the tone is heard equally in both ears or is stronger in the right or left ear. Normally the sound should be heard equally in both ears. Lateralization, an abnormal finding, indicates the sound is heard better in one ear. Weber's test is useful in identifying patients with unilateral hearing loss.

Pneumatoscopy. Pneumatoscopy tests the ability of the tympanic membrane to respond to changes in air pressure introduced into the external auditory canal and middle ear. A pneumatic otoscope is used to introduce air into the ear and to assess mobility of the tympanic membrane. The air causes the tympanic membrane to move in an out if it is intact. The membrane does not move if it is perforated or if there is fluid in the middle ear space.[7]

Audiometric Hearing Tests. Audiometric hearing tests are conducted in a soundproof booth by an audiologist or trained technician. Hearing is measured in decibels, a logarithmic function of sound intensity. The sound is presented through an audiometer. The patient wears earphones and signals the audiologist when a tone is heard by raising a hand or pushing a button. Responses are plotted on a graph called the audiogram.

Pure-tone **audiometry** is the standard measure of hearing acuity. To test air conduction, the audiometer presents pure tones within the range of 250 to 8000 Hz at varying intensities to one ear at a time, beginning with the better-hearing ear. For bone conduction testing, tones are delivered through a bone conduction oscillator placed against the forehead or mastoid process while masking noise is presented to the untested ear by an earphone to prevent it from participating in the test of the opposite ear. This way of presenting sound bypasses the middle ear structures and establishes a bone conduction level. The bone conduction level represents the level at which the cochlea can hear and is commonly referred to as the nerve hearing level. A person with normal hearing would have the same air conduction as bone conduction hearing levels. A difference in air and bone conduction levels is indicative of conductive hearing loss. If air and bone conduction levels are equal but not within the normal range, a sensorineural nerve hearing loss is present. It is common for a patient to have both conductive and sensorineural hearing loss, a condition called mixed hearing loss.

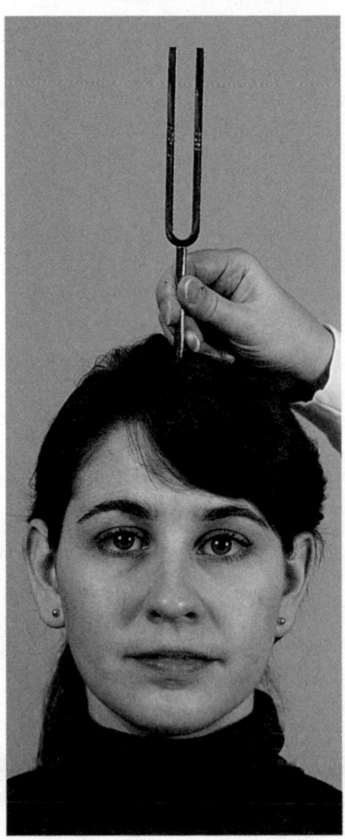

Figure 62-7 Weber's test. Vibrating tuning fork is placed on midline of skull.

The speech audiometry–speech reception threshold test determines the lowest intensity at which the patient can hear and correctly repeat 50% of a list of two-syllable words presented through earphones. The result usually corresponds closely to the air conduction threshold.

In the speech discrimination test, a list of 50 monosyllabic words is presented through earphones to the patient. The score indicates the percentage of words that the patient can hear and repeat correctly.

IMPEDANCE AUDIOMETRY. Impedance audiometry or tympanometry can be used for differentiating problems in the middle ear. The test applies pressure to the tympanic membrane and measures the result, creating a distinctive tracing on a graph called a tympanogram. Abnormalities of the tympanogram indicate problems of the middle ear, eustachian tube, or ossicles. Tympanometry can also be used to measure the stapedial muscle reflex and the status of the vestibulocochlear nerve.[5] With pathologic conditions of the cochlea, vestibulocochlear reflexes often occur at less intense stimulation levels. With a retrocochlear lesion, the reflex thresholds are elevated or even absent. With conductive hearing loss, the reflex thresholds may be elevated but usually are absent.

AUDITORY BRAINSTEM RESPONSE. Brainstem auditory evoked potential testing assesses dysfunction of the auditory nervous system at the level of the eighth cranial nerve, pons, or midbrain. Evoked potentials measure and record changes in brain electrical activity that occur in response to auditory sensory stimulation. The test involves placing electrodes on the vertex, mastoid process, or earlobes while the patient is seated in a comfortable chair. Test data are fed into a computer. Abnormal findings suggest dysfunctions at the various levels in the auditory nervous system, for example, a lesion of the vestibulocochlear nerve or brainstem.

Seventh cranial nerve (facial nerve) testing may also be performed. Tests of the seventh cranial nerve are related to audiometric tests because the facial and vestibulocochlear nerves share the internal acoustic canal. The facial nerve is tested in the same way as other motor nerves with nerve conduction tests and muscle excitability tests. The auxiliary functions of the facial nerve (taste and tearing) can also be measured. The facial and vestibulocochlear nerves are usually both affected when lesions involve the temporal bone.

Balance Testing

ELECTRONYSTAGMOGRAPHY. Electrophysiologic tests can be used to test balance and the status of the vestibular system in assessing the causes of dizziness, vertigo, and tinnitus. They can suggest the presence and location of central or peripheral lesions.

In some settings the tests are performed by audiologists because of the close physical proximity of the vestibular and cochlear systems in the labyrinth. Although the physical assessment of balance is important, the most common objective measurement of balance is accomplished by electronystagmography, which measures nystagmus in response to stimulation of the vestibular system. With the patient at rest, electrodes are placed on the head. The patient is tested in different positions and with different temperatures (caloric test) in the auditory canals, thus stimulating the semicircular canals. The test results create an electronystagmograph that reflects the status of each labyrinth.

The nurse instructs the patient to discontinue any vestibular sedatives or tranquilizers and to avoid alcohol use for at least 24 hours before the test. Patients are also cautioned to avoid a heavy meal before the test because vertigo and nausea may be stimulated. Because the electrodes are placed with conduction paste, the nurse helps the patient wash his or her hair after the procedure.

PLATFORM POSTUROGRAPHY. Platform posturography is a computerized test performed while the person is standing on a platform surrounded by a screen. Postural control is evaluated under six conditions such as both platform and screen moving, both stationary, and platform moving with screen stationary. The platform test helps identify, quantify, and localize the source of balance disorders by separating the balance problem into inner ear, visual, and muscle stretch origins. The nurse explains the procedure and the sensations the patient can expect. Although painless, the test can cause vertigo and nausea. Sedatives, tranquilizers, and alcohol can alter the test results and should be restricted before the procedure.

References

1. Bailey BJ et al: *Atlas of head and neck surgery—otolaryngology,* ed 2, Philadelphia, 2002, Lippincott, Williams & Wilkins.
2. Bickley LS, Szilagyi P: *Bates' guide to physical examination and history taking,* ed 8, Philadelphia, 2002, Lippincott, Williams & Wilkins.
3. Goldman L, Ausiello D, editors: *Cecil textbook of medicine,* ed 22, vol 2, Philadelphia, 2004, Saunders.
4. Fook L, Morgan R: Hearing impairment in older people: a review, *Postgrad Med J* 76(899):537-541, 2000.
5. Lehne R et al: *Pharmacology for nursing care,* ed 5, Philadelphia, 2004, Saunders.
6. Seidel HM et al: *Mosby's guide to physical examination,* ed 5, St Louis, 2003, Mosby.
7. Weissman JL, Hirsch BE: Imaging of tinnitus: a review, *Radiology* 216(2):342, 2000.
8. Wilson SF, Giddens JF: *Health assessment for nursing practice,* ed 2, St Louis, 2001, Mosby.

Visit the Evolve website: http://evolve.elsevier.com/Monahan/medsurg

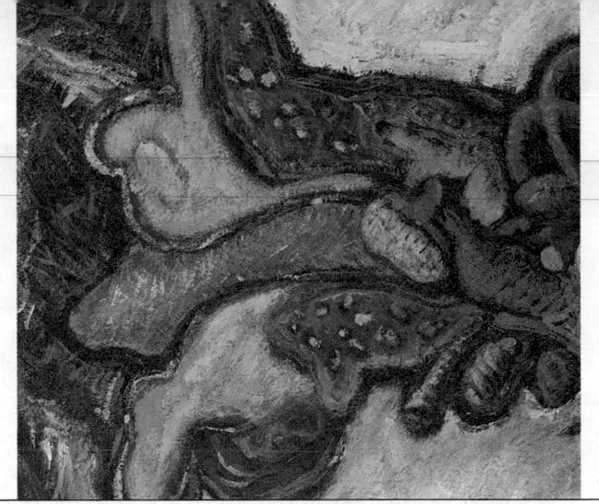

CHAPTER 63
Problems of the Ear

by Toni O. Barnett

OBJECTIVES

After studying this chapter, the learner should be able to:

1. Identify three measures that are important in preventing hearing loss.
2. Compare the etiologies and assessment features of conductive and sensorineural hearing loss.
3. Contrast the pathophysiology and nursing care of patients with external and middle ear infections.
4. Discuss the preoperative and postoperative care of the patient undergoing ear surgery.
5. Relate the signs and symptoms of Meniere's disease to its underlying pathology.
6. Develop strategies for communicating with a hearing-impaired person.
7. Describe common clinical manifestations of ear dysfunction.

KEY TERMS

amplification, p. 1847
deafness, p. 1845
decibel, p. 1846
hearing impairment, p. 1845
noise, p. 1846
Occupational Safety and Health Administration, p. 1846

A wide range of disorders can affect the ear. These include infections, tumors, and trauma. However, hearing loss is by far the most common and important ear problem affecting adults. Any problem with the ear threatens its function and acuity and hence the person's ability to interact effectively with the environment. Selected ear disorders can also create problems with an individual's sense of balance.

Hearing Loss

Etiology and Epidemiology. Almost 30 million Americans of all ages suffer from some degree of hearing loss.[10,15] More than 3 million children in the United States have hearing loss, and 1 of every 1000 infants is completely deaf at birth. Hearing loss also occurs in 25% to 40% of individuals over age 65.[5,9] **Hearing impairment** ranges from difficulty in understanding words or hearing certain sounds to total **deafness**.

Hearing impairment can hinder communication with others, limit social activities, and negatively affect employment. Hearing loss diminishes the individual's aesthetic enjoyment of major aspects of daily living and can adversely affect quality of life.[9,20]

Hearing loss is a symptom rather than a specific disease or disorder and can be the result of mechanical, sensory, or neural problems. The major types of hearing loss are:

- *Conductive hearing loss:* Loss of hearing from a mechanical problem in the outer or middle ear that interferes with conduction of sound waves
- *Sensorineural hearing loss:* Loss of hearing involving the cochlea and vestibulocochlear nerve
- *Neural hearing loss:* Sensorineural hearing loss originating in the nerve or brainstem
- *Fluctuating hearing loss:* Sensorineural hearing loss that varies with time
- *Sensory hearing loss:* Sensorineural hearing loss originating in the cochlea and involving the hair cells and nerve endings
- *Sudden hearing loss:* Sensorineural hearing loss with a sudden onset
- *Central hearing loss:* Loss of hearing from damage to the brain's auditory pathways or auditory center
- *Mixed hearing loss:* Elements of both conductive and sensorineural hearing loss
- *Functional hearing loss:* Loss of hearing for which no organic lesion can be found

Figure 63-1 illustrates the relationship between the anatomic location of the causative problem and the type of hearing loss that results. Some problems causing conductive hearing loss can be treated with medicine or surgery to either restore hearing or minimize permanent hearing loss. However, the vast majority of persons with a hearing impairment cannot be treated effectively, since 80% of all hearing impairments are caused by nerve deafness for which, at present, there is no known cure.

Hearing loss can also be classified according to severity. The **decibel** (dB) is a measure of the loudness or intensity of sound. A hearing loss of 15 to 50 dB is a mild to moderate loss; the person with a hearing loss in this range is said to be hearing impaired. A loss of 50 to 80 dB is a severe hearing loss. A loss of more than 80 dB in both ears is a profound hearing loss, and the patient may be referred to as deaf.

Pathophysiology. Conductive hearing loss results from interference with the conduction of sound impulses through the external auditory canal, the tympanic membrane, or the ossicles of the middle ear. Conductive hearing loss may be caused by anything that blocks the external ear such as cerumen, infection, or a foreign body. It may also be caused by thickening, retraction, scarring, or perforation of the tympanic membrane or any pathophysiologic change in the middle ear that affects or fixes one or more of the ossicles. Examples of the latter include tumors, scar tissue from previous surgery, and otosclerosis.

Sensorineural hearing loss results from disease or trauma to the inner ear, neural structures, or nerve pathways leading to the brainstem. Disease that results in sensorineural hearing loss may be systemic or local, and in some cases may be drug induced. Systemic diseases that can cause sensorineural hearing loss include diabetes mellitus; arteriosclerosis; and infectious disease such as measles, mumps, and meningitis. Local disorders that can cause sensorineural deafness include neuromas of the eighth cranial nerve; otospongiosis (a form of progressive deafness caused by the formation of abnormal, spongy bone in the labyrinth); trauma to the head or ear; or degeneration of the organ of Corti, which occurs most commonly with advancing age.

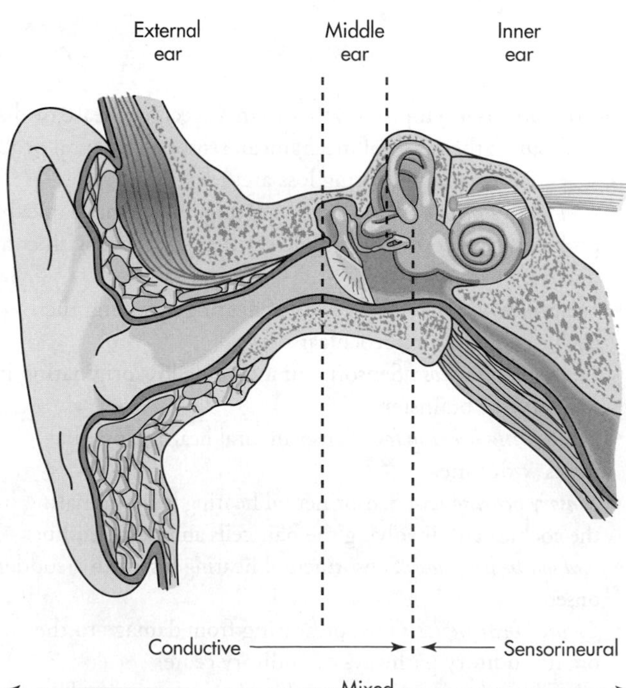

Figure 63-1 Three types of hearing loss. Conductive loss results from interference with conduction in the external and middle ear, sensorineural loss results from interference with conduction in the inner ear, and mixed hearing loss results from interference with conduction in all areas.

A rare form of sensorineural hearing loss is central deafness, also known as central auditory dysfunction. In this disorder hearing ability remains intact, but the patient is deaf because the central nervous system is unable to interpret normal auditory stimuli. Central deafness can result from tumors or stroke.

Hearing loss as a result of exposure to **noise** accounts for the major proportion of hearing impairment among people between the ages of 35 and 65. If hearing loss results from a single exposure to a sudden loud noise or blast, it is referred to as *acoustic trauma.* More commonly, hearing loss occurs over time from repeated injury from noise, in which case it is referred to as *noise-induced hearing loss.*[10]

Occupational noise is a primary cause of noise-induced hearing loss in Western society. Other causes include the use of firearms and high-intensity music. Noise from rock bands can exceed 120 dB, and hearing losses have been measured in some members of these bands. In the United States the **Occupational Safety and Health Administration** (OSHA) has established acceptable noise levels for work environments. In general, exposure to noise levels in excess of 90 dB over an 8-hour day is considered excessive and should be avoided. Ordinary speech is about 50 dB and heavy traffic about 70 dB; above 80 dB, noise becomes uncomfortable to the human ear. Exposure to levels greater than 85 to 90 dB for months or years can cause cochlear damage.

Whatever the cause, noise-induced hearing loss is characterized by a greater loss in the higher frequencies, with the ability to distinguish sounds such as *s, sh, f, th,* and *ch* impaired first. The sensory cells in the ear are progressively destroyed, and the problem cannot be medically or surgically repaired. The only treatment is to prevent the injury by avoiding noise or wearing ear protection. OSHA regulations require that workers exposed to noise above the designated limits wear ear protection to decrease the risk of noise-induced hearing loss.

Presbycusis is a hearing loss associated with aging that becomes more common after age 50. Changes in the delicate labyrinthine structures over the decades cause a hearing loss predominantly in the higher frequencies. The incidence of presbycusis, which cannot be cured, increases with age, and the disorder affects almost 60% of persons age 70 and older.[9] In some persons the amount of hearing loss warrants the use of a hearing aid.

Tinnitus, which is defined as a ringing or other noise in the ear, accompanies most sensorineural hearing losses and is often a warning of impending or worsening hearing loss.[6] Persistent tinnitus is extremely annoying; the only cure is to correct the underlying condition.

Collaborative Care Management. A hearing loss in one ear is more difficult to detect than bilateral loss. Unilateral hearing loss may be noticed only when using a telephone or when having difficulty determining the direction of sounds. Often hearing loss first is detected by a family member rather than by the affected person. Because the auditory nerve does not regain function, early detection and evaluation of any hearing loss are important. Routine hearing assessment should be a part of the annual physical examination of all persons over age 40, since aging is associated with degenerative changes in the ear. When indicated, additional diagnostic testing is done as described in Chapter 62. Because a variety of diseases and disorders affect the ear and the majority of persons with ear problems experience some degree of hearing loss, a health care provider should assess any disease that causes prolonged ear symptoms such as pain, swelling, drainage, a "plugged" feeling, or decreased hearing. Many chronic problems such as perforations and necrotic ossicles can be prevented with prompt and adequate medical attention.

Hearing aids can assist many individuals with hearing impairments. Hearing aids amplify sound in a controlled manner and are used by both hard-of-hearing and deaf persons. Although hearing aids make sound louder, they do not improve the ability to hear. As a result, **amplification** of background noise can create confusion, especially in crowded settings. Persons with decreased discrimination (ability to understand what is spoken) have limited benefit from a hearing aid.

The evolution in hearing aid development has led to smaller and more effective aids. Hearing aids are available that fit into the ear canal, fit within the ear concha, or fit behind the ear (Figure 63-2). Special hearing aids can transmit sound by radio waves to the opposite ear or by vibration to the inner ear through the skull.

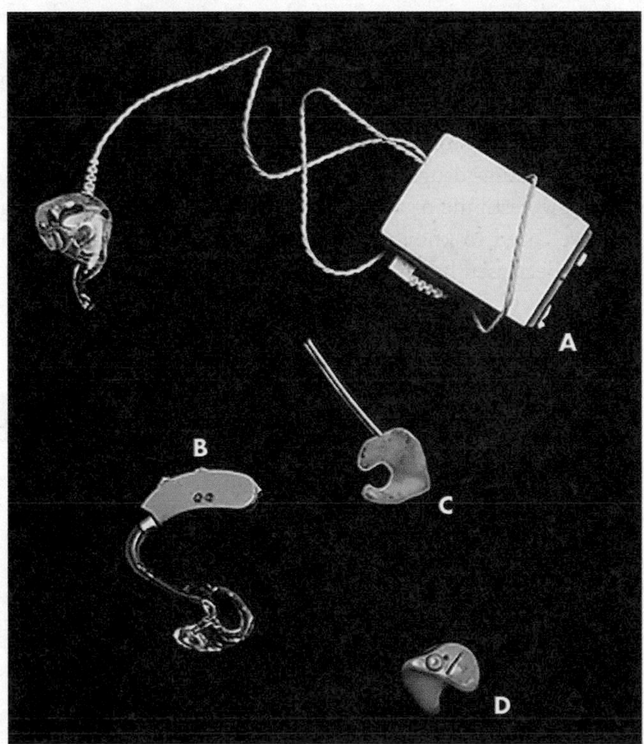

Figure 63-2 Types of hearing aids. **A,** Older aid with a battery pack worn on body and wire connected to ear mold. **B,** Behind-the-ear battery with ear mold. **C,** Small ear canal mold with battery. **D,** Newer, smaller mold worn in ear canal.

Regardless of the type, the hearing aid consists of (1) a microphone to receive sound waves from the air and change sounds into electrical signals, (2) an amplifier to increase the strength of the electrical signals, (3) a battery to provide the electrical energy needed to operate the hearing aid, and (4) a receiver (loudspeaker) to change the electrical signals back into sound waves.

IMPLANTABLE HEARING DEVICES. There are three types of implanted hearing devices: cochlear implants, bone conduction devices, and fully or semiimplantable hearing aids.[8,14,16]

Cochlear implant devices directly stimulate the auditory nerve and are used to provide sound awareness for persons with sensorineural hearing loss originating in the organ of Corti. The device does not allow the person to hear speech but creates an awareness of environmental sounds such as doorbells or telephones and also provides auditory clues that facilitate lip reading. Cochlear implant devices have both internal and external components. The internal components include one or more electrodes implanted into or onto the cochlea, and a receiver implanted behind the auricle. The external components include a small microphone, a speech processor, and a transmitter coil with a magnet that holds it in place over the implanted receiver. Sound is picked up by the microphone and is sent to the processor, which converts it into electrical impulses. These impulses go on to the transmitter and then to the internal receiver, where further processing occurs. Finally, they travel to the electrodes in the cochlea (Figure 63-3). The external components are put in place 4 to 6 weeks after the internal components are surgically implanted when the wound is healed, so no change occurs in the patient's hearing until this time. Once the device is in place, its settings are calibrated to the individual patient's needs. The patient undergoes a rehabilitation program, which typically includes care of the unit, simple auditory training, and speech reading (formerly called lip reading) practice with the added sounds from the implant. Length of rehabilitation varies but is usually 40 hours or more. Regular follow-up visits are needed for several years. The best cochlear implants use multiple channels and are able to return about half the patient's hearing and understanding.

Bone conduction devices (bone-anchored hearing aid) transmit sound through the skull to the inner ear. One such device uses a surgically implanted titanium screw implanted under the skin into the skull behind the ear. Once it osseointegrates into the skull and heals, it is loaded with a vibrating hearing aid.[4,16] Patients already using a hearing aid gain the most from the implantable device.

If hearing loss is irreversible and not amenable to surgical correction or if the person elects not to have surgery, aural rehabilitation may be recommended. Aural rehabilitation includes auditory training, speech reading, and speech training and is designed to maximize the hearing-impaired person's communication skills. Auditory training attempts to increase listening skills by improving the person's ability to discriminate between similar sounds. Speech reading is a difficult skill to master but can be an important means of communication. Speech training focuses on the preservation of speech skills (pitch, clarity, and rate) as auditory feedback diminishes. Guidelines for communicating with hearing-impaired persons are summarized in the Guidelines for Safe Practice box.

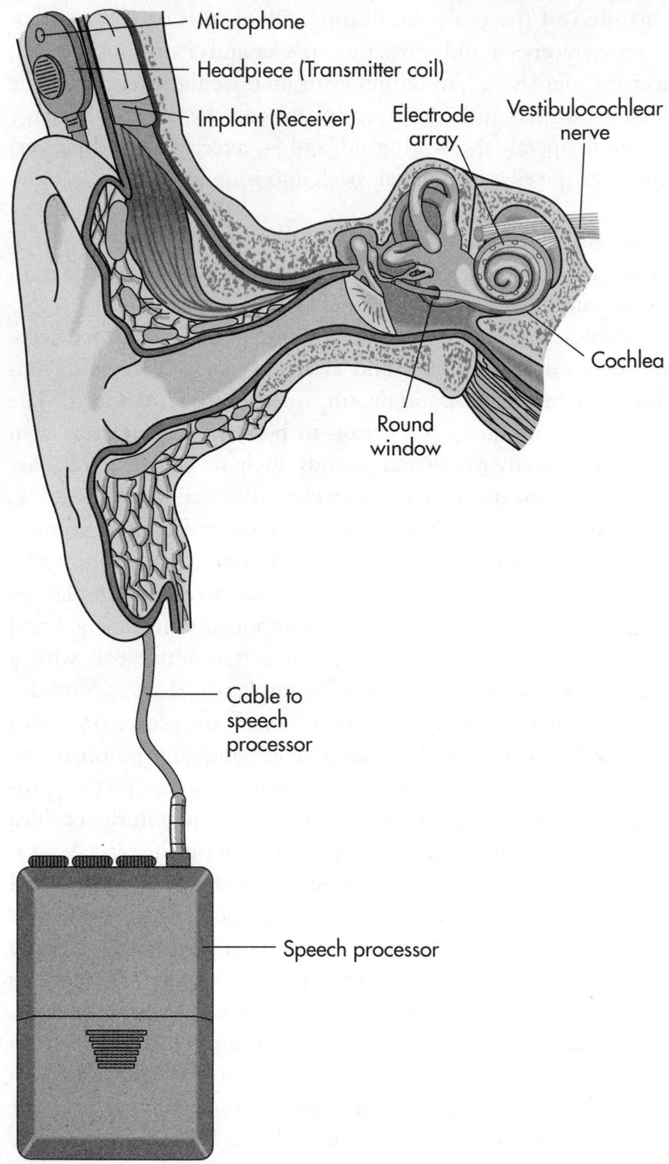

Figure 63-3 Cochlear implant is placed transmastoid through round window into the cochlea.

Patient/Family Teaching. Hearing loss is a significant health concern in the United States, and nurses play a major preventive role in interactions with all patients and families. *Healthy People 2010* national health objectives related to hearing loss are to[18]:

- Reduce to no more than 15% the proportion of workers exposed to average daily noise levels that exceed 85 dB.
- Reduce significant hearing impairment to a prevalence of no more than 82 per 1000 people, as measured by self-reported hearing impairment.

Individuals 45 years old and older are identified as special target populations. Prevention through education is the key to achieving these goals. Patient education begins with an exploration of the patient's understanding of the role of noise in hearing loss. The nurse explains the relationship between noise and hearing loss; recommends the use of protective ear covers in noisy environments; and stresses the importance of maintaining moderate sound levels when listening to music, especially when using headphones.

The nurse also instructs patients to avoid inserting hard articles into the ear canal, obstructing the ear canal with any object, inserting unclean articles or solutions into the ear, and swimming in polluted water. Patients also should be taught that wax should not be cleaned out of the ear routinely, since the ear canal is generally "self-cleaning." Wax is to the ears what tears are to the eyes; it serves as a protective mechanism. Earwax lubricates the skin and traps foreign material that enters the canal. The external ear may be washed with soap and water daily while bathing or showering, but cotton-tipped applicators or other objects should not be used to clean the ear. The ear canal and eardrum can be easily damaged, and the applicator may push accumulated wax against the eardrum.

The person with a hearing aid needs to be taught how to care for the aid and what to do if the aid does not work (see Patient/Family Teaching box). The nurse must also have a basic knowledge of the hearing aid to assist the person who is unable or unwilling to do this when ill. The person is encouraged to use the hearing aid and to store it safely in its case when it is not in use.

Patients taking drugs that are ototoxic (i.e., that damage the cochlea, the vestibule of the ear, the labyrinth, or the eighth cranial nerve) need to know to promptly report symptoms such as dizziness, decreased hearing acuity, and tinnitus.

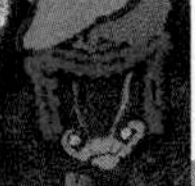

Guidelines for Safe Practice *Communicating With the Hearing-Impaired Patient*

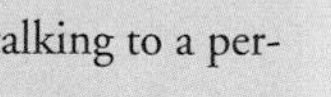

- Get the person's attention by touching him or her lightly, flickering the room lights, or raising an arm or hand.
- Stand facing the patient with the light on your face; this will help the person speech (lip) read.
- Speak slowly and clearly, but do not overaccentuate words.
- Speak in a normal tone; do not shout. Shouting overuses normal speaking movements and may cause distortion. If the person has a conductive loss, making the voice louder without shouting may be helpful.
- Alert the person to the topic before beginning the discussion to enable use of contextual clues.
- If the person does not seem to understand what is said, express it differently. Some words (e.g., white, red) are difficult to "see" in speech reading.
- Do not smile, chew gum, or cover the mouth when talking to a person with limited hearing.
- Use phrases to convey meaning rather than one-word answers. Supplement words with body language.
- Do not show annoyance by careless facial expression. Persons who are hard of hearing depend more on visual clues.
- Write out proper names or any statement that you are not sure was understood.
- Encourage the use of a hearing aid if the person has one; allow him or her to adjust it before speaking.
- Avoid the use of the intercom when communicating with the patient.
- Do not avoid conversation with a person who has hearing loss.
- Post a note at the bedside and nurses station alerting personnel that the person is hard of hearing.

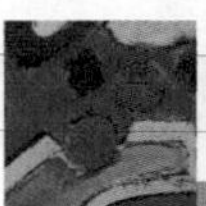

PATIENT/FAMILY TEACHING
Care of a Hearing Aid

- Turn the hearing aid off when not in use.
- Open the battery compartment at night to avoid accidental drainage of the battery.
- Keep an extra battery available at all times.
- Wash the ear mold frequently (daily if necessary) with mild soap and warm water and use a pipe cleaner to cleanse the cannula.
- Do not wear the hearing aid if an ear infection is present.

If a hearing aid fails to work:

- Check the on-off switch.
- Inspect the ear mold for cleanliness.
- Examine the battery for correct insertion.
- Examine the cord plug for correct insertion.
- Examine the cord for breaks.
- Replace the battery, cord, or both, if necessary. The life of batteries varies according to amount of use and power requirements of the aid. Batteries last from 2 to 14 days.
- Check the position of the ear mold in the ear. If the hearing aid "whistles," the ear mold is probably not inserted properly into the ear canal, or the person needs to have a new ear mold made.

Problems of the External Ear

The external ear may be affected by masses, trauma, wax impaction, and infection. External ear infection is by far the most common disorder and is discussed next. The other problems are summarized in Table 63-1.

External Ear Infection (External Otitis)

Etiology and Epidemiology. External otitis is an inflammation or infection of the external auditory canal or auricle. It occurs more frequently in summer than in winter and is usually bacterial or fungal in origin. Cultures indicate that the most common infecting bacteria are *Staphylococcus aureus, Escherichia coli, Proteus vulgaris,* and *Pseudomonas aeruginosa;* the most common infecting fungi are *Candida albicans* and *Aspergillus* organisms. A localized form of this infection, which begins in the skin lining the ear canal, is a furuncle or abscess. In the presence of a systemic disease such as diabetes, external otitis can spread wildly through cartilage and bone and is then termed *malignant external otitis.* The most common forms of external otitis are (1) swimmer's ear, so called because it tends to occur when water remains in the ear canal; and (2) opportunistic fungal infection, which is most prevalent in warm, moist climates. Occasionally, infection involves only the cartilage of the auricle and is then called perichondritis. Necrosis of the cartilage and loss of the distinctive shape of the auricle occur if perichondritis is not treated quickly.

Pathophysiology. Local trauma such as picking the ear, contamination, or ongoing exposure to moisture produces an environment conducive to the overgrowth of normal flora. Pain (otalgia) in the external ear is the most common symptom. Pain can be significant, especially when palpating the ear, because of the close proximity of bone (a hard surface). A clue to early external otitis is pain or tenderness when gently pulling on the pinna or putting pressure on the tragus. A forerunner of pain in external otitis is itching in the ear canal. Inflammation is easily identified with an otoscope. Early in the infection, drainage from the ear may be

TABLE 63-1 DISORDERS OF THE EXTERNAL EAR

Disorder	Etiology	Collaborative Management
Masses: Cysts Exostosis (bony protrusions) Infectious polyps Malignant tumors	Most cysts arise from sebaceous glands. Polyps typically arise from middle ear or tympanic membrane. Malignant tumors are usually basal cell carcinomas on pinna and squamous cell carcinomas in the canal.	Masses of all types are fairly rare; if treatment is indicated, surgical excision is performed. Squamous cell carcinomas can invade underlying tissue and spread throughout temporal bone.
Trauma	Both sharp and blunt force injuries are common. Penetrating injury can damage hearing, but infection and cosmetic appearance are more common concerns.	Supportive care and protection from infection are indicated. Cosmetic surgery may be needed.
Foreign bodies	Many causes exist. Insects and cotton pieces are most common.	Careful removal is aided by microscopic visualization. Insects are removed by filling canal with mineral oil.
Pruritus	This frequent complaint in older adults results from sebaceous gland atrophy and dry epithelium. Dry cerumen worsens the itching.	Daily application of glycerin or mineral oil drops decreases dryness and softens cerumen.
Impacted cerumen	This may result from use of cotton-tipped applicator or other object to clean ear. Age-related drying of cerumen increases incidence.	Impacted wax is softened and loosened with alternating instillation of glycerine to soften and hydrogen peroxide to loosen the cerumen for removal by warm water irrigation.

clear; later it may be serosanguineous or purulent. Hearing may be impaired from swelling and accumulated debris in the canal, and dizziness also may occur.

Collaborative Care Management. Treatment for external otitis depends on the cause and extent of the infection. Local or topical antibiotics are the mainstay of treatment.[19] Systemic antibiotics are rarely required but may also be prescribed if the infection extends beyond the ear canal.[12] If the ear canal is swollen shut, a "wick" made of a 1-inch length of ¼-inch wide gauze may be inserted to allow the antibiotic drops to penetrate the canal. Irrigations may be performed to remove infective debris (see Guidelines for Safe Practice box below and Figure 63-4). Comfort measures such as mild analgesics and warm soaks are provided to control the symptoms. Abscesses and perichondritis may require excision and drainage.

Patient/Family Teaching. The nurse instructs the patient and family in the safe administration of eardrops (see Guidelines for Safe Practice box at right). If an ointment is prescribed to control itching or inflammation, the patient is instructed to apply it using a cotton-tipped applicator, being certain not to insert the applicator any deeper into the ear than the cotton end. The need to use a new applicator each time is stressed.

The nurse also instructs the patient to avoid getting water in the ear by using earplugs or by placing cotton with petroleum jelly in the auditory meatus. If earplugs are used, thorough cleansing with alcohol or a mild detergent between uses is recommended to prevent reinfection. The patient should not swim during this time.

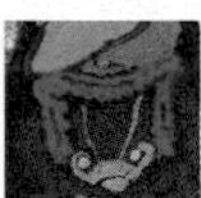

Guidelines for Safe Practice
Performing an Ear Irrigation

Ear irrigations or washes are used to remove excess cerumen[9] or a foreign body from the ear (see Figure 63-4).

1. Wash hands before and after the procedure.
2. Fill a 2- to 3-ounce ear syringe with the solution (water or a saline solution), warmed to body temperature (between 90° and 100° F [32° and 38° C]).
3. Position the patient lying on his or her side with the affected ear up or in a sitting position with an ear basin under the ear.
4. Gently pull the pinna back and up while placing the tip of the syringe gently into the ear canal. Do not be afraid to insert it into the ear.
5. Instill the solution from the syringe semiforcefully into the ear. The fluid must actively move in the ear canal to be effective.
6. The patient may experience dizziness with movement; however, if procedure is painful, stop the ear wash.
7. Apply eardrops if instructed.
8. Continue to use the ear wash solution as instructed for about 2 weeks or until the ear is dry and without drainage.

Note: If not done by a health care provider, the procedure should be performed by a family member or significant other if possible. It cannot be performed effectively by the patient alone.

Problems of the Middle Ear

Infection with its associated complications is the most common disorder of the middle ear, but masses, trauma, and other conditions may occur. The less common disorders of the middle ear are summarized in Table 63-2.

Middle Ear Infection (Otitis Media)

Etiology and Epidemiology. *Otitis media* is a general term that refers to inflammation of the mucous membranes of the middle ear, eustachian tube, and mastoid. These mucous membranes are continuous with those of the respiratory tract, and thus infection can easily ascend to the ear. Otitis media is most often caused by various types of bacteria, although viral cases can occur.

There are three distinct types of otitis media: acute, chronic, and serous. Acute otitis media (AOM) develops suddenly and is usually of short duration. Chronic otitis media is the result of recurrent or untreated infection and is usually characterized by drainage and perforation of the tympanic membrane. Serous oti-

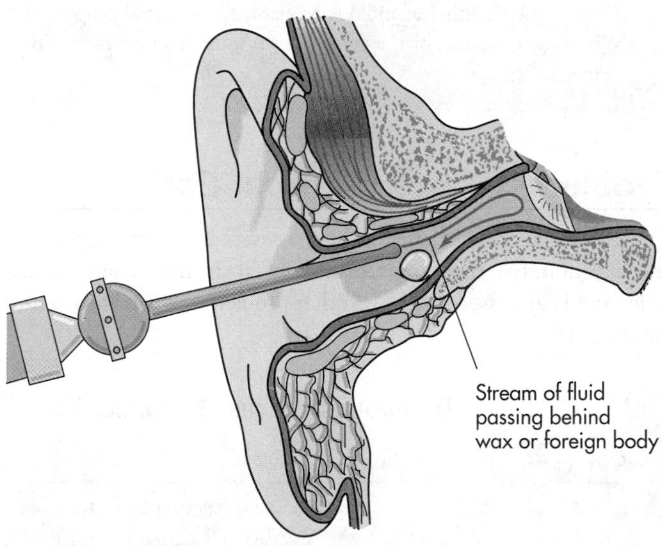

Figure 63-4 Ear irrigation.

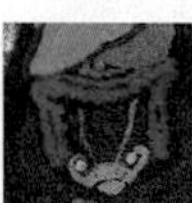

Guidelines for Safe Practice
Administering Eardrops

1. Wash hands before and after the procedure.
2. Warm the eardrops to body temperature before administration. Dizziness may occur from insertion of drops that are too warm or too cold.
3. Instruct the patient to tilt the head so that the ear to be treated is up.
4. Straighten the ear canal by pulling the external ear up and back.
5. Instill prescribed number of drops to run along ear canal.
6. Press gently several times on the tragus of the ear to ensure proper instillation, or hold the head in position for 2 to 3 minutes.
7. Wipe the external ear with a cotton ball or tissue to prevent skin irritation.
8. A cotton ball may be placed in the ear but is not necessary.

TABLE 63-2 DISORDERS OF THE MIDDLE EAR AND MASTOID

Disorder	Etiology	Collaborative Management
Perforated tympanic membrane	Perforations may occur acutely after trauma or as result of chronic infection. Damage may extend to ossicles and worsen the hearing loss.	Acute perforation may heal spontaneously. Infection is treated with appropriate local and/or systemic antibiotics. Surgical correction of perforation may be performed: myringoplasty for membrane or tympanoplasty if repair includes middle ear structures. Grafts may be taken from muscle fascia, vein, or perichondrium. Success rate is high.
Otosclerosis (hardening of ear)	Sclerotic bone forms on stapes, limiting its movement and resulting in conductive hearing loss. Underlying cause is unknown.	Hearing aid may be initially prescribed. Advanced disease is treated surgically through stapedectomy in which a prosthesis replaces otosclerotic footplate. Success rate is high.
Mastoiditis	Chronic otitis media can result in extension of infection into mastoid cavity. Volume of drainage from middle ear increases.	Antibiotic therapy is foundation of care, possibly supplemented by irrigations. Aggressive treatment is appropriate to prevent serious complications. Surgical mastoidectomy may be necessary in rare situations.

tis media is characterized by a collection of noninfectious fluid in the middle ear as a result of incomplete resolution of an acute infection, an allergic reaction, or an obstruction of the eustachian tube. If fluid is present within the ear for a protracted period, the tympanic membrane retracts, and adhesive otitis media may develop. Likewise, any long-term blockage of the eustachian tube can lead to adhesive otitis media and result in hearing loss.

Otitis media is classically considered to be a childhood disorder associated with upper respiratory tract infection. The vast majority of cases occur in children from infancy to school age. Otitis media is the most common bacterial infection among children, accounting for as many as 30 million office visits per year.[7] The incidence is clearly increased during the colder months in association with the increased incidence of upper respiratory tract infection. Otitis media may go undiagnosed in the adult population because symptoms are frequently less dramatic than in the child. Adults are vulnerable to the development of chronic otitis media, particularly if they experienced multiple acute episodes in their youth. Staphylococci and streptococci are the predominant causes in adults. Persons with a positive family history for ear problems, those with chronic allergies and sinusitis, and persons exposed to passive smoke all have an increased risk of developing otitis media and its complications as adults. Inadequate treatment can easily lead to the emergence of resistant strains of bacteria.

Pathophysiology. Because the middle ear transmits sound from the tympanic membrane to the inner ear, middle ear infection frequently causes a conductive hearing loss from pressure behind the tympanic membrane. The hearing loss is usually correctable with resolution of the infection. Common additional symptoms include throbbing pain in the affected ear, inflammation, fever, and drainage and bulging of the eardrum with possible perforation. Blood, pus, and other material may be present when perforation occurs. A thick, yellow, purulent discharge is a common finding with chronic otitis media. Tympanosclerosis, a deposit of collagen and calcium within the middle ear, can also result from repeated infection. The deposit can harden around the ossicles and contribute to a worsening of any conductive hearing loss. Because of the anatomy of the temporal bone, middle ear infection can, in rare cases, lead to a life-threatening brain abscess. Common symptoms of otitis media are summarized in the Clinical Manifestations box.

Collaborative Care Management. The diagnosis of otitis media is made based on the patient's symptoms and otoscopic examination of the ear, which readily reveals a bulging tympanic membrane and perforation or drainage if present.

MEDICATIONS. When to use antibiotic therapy is the key to treatment of AOM.[1] Broad-spectrum antibiotics are used unless drainage is present that allows for culture of the organism and sensitivity testing (see Research box). Otitis media with effusion (OME) exists when fluid is present in the middle ear for an extended period without symptoms of infection. Most cases resolve within 3 months without antibiotics. Antibiotic therapy or myringotomy with insertion of tympanostomy tubes is usually reserved for patients who have OME for longer than 3 months and have an associated significant bilateral hearing loss. Chronic infections frequently do not respond to the usual antibiotics and

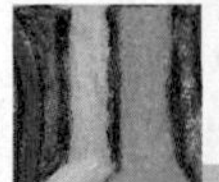

CLINICAL MANIFESTATIONS

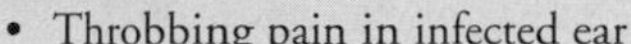

Otitis Media

- Throbbing pain in infected ear
- Fever
- Drainage: clear, bloody, or purulent
- Bulging of the eardrum
- Conductive hearing loss, usually reversible with effective treatment

Research

American Academy of Pediatrics: Clinical practice guidelines: diagnosis and management of acute otitis media, *Pediatrics* 113(5):1451-1465, 2004.

The American Academy of Pediatrics and American Academy of Family Physicians worked together with the Agency for Healthcare Research and Quality and the Southern California Evidence-Based Practice Center to conduct a comprehensive review of the evidence-based literature related to acute otitis media (AOM). They then developed the following evidence-based clinical practice guideline for primary care clinicians for the management of children 2 months to 12 years of age with uncomplicated AOM:

1. To diagnose AOM, the clinician should confirm a history of acute onset, identify signs of middle-ear effusion, and evaluate for signs and symptoms of middle-ear inflammation.
2. The management of AOM should include an assessment of pain. If pain is present, the clinician should recommend treatment to reduce pain.

3a. Observation without use of antibacterial agents in a child with uncomplicated AOM is an option for selected children based on diagnostic certainty, age, illness severity, and assurance of follow-up care.

3b. If a decision is made to treat with antibacterial agent, the clinician should prescribe amoxicillin for most children. When amoxicillin is used, the dose should be 80 to 90 mg/kg body weight/day.

4. If the patient fails to respond to the initial management option within 48 to 72 hours, the clinician must reassess the patient to confirm AOM and exclude other causes of illness. If AOM is confirmed in the patient initially managed with observation, the clinician should begin antibacterial therapy. If the patient was initially managed with an antibacterial agent or agents, the clinician should change the antibacterial agent(s).
5. Clinicians should encourage the prevention of AOM through reduction of risk factors.
6. There is insufficient evidence to make a recommendation regarding the use of complementary and alternative medicine for AOM.

may require local treatment with antibiotic eardrops.[2,11,17] Drugs commonly used to treat AOM are summarized in Table 63-3.

Streptococcus pneumoniae is the most common community-acquired respiratory tract pathogen, with increasing reports of antibiotic resistance around the world. Therefore intervention is needed to reduce the unnecessary use of antibiotics and ensure early childhood immunization with pneumococcal heptavalent conjugate vaccine. Educational efforts are being directed at clinicians and parents, and everyone is being encouraged to look at the new guidelines from the American Academy of Pediatrics.[2]

Treatments. When the eustachian tube is chronically obstructed, it may be necessary to remove fluid from the middle ear. Myringotomies, with or without tubes, are performed to regain normal middle ear and eustachian tube function (Figure 63-5). Myringotomy involves making a tiny incision in the tympanic membrane through which the fluid can be suctioned out. To keep the incision open and prevent a reaccumulation of fluid, various types of transtympanic tubes can be inserted into the incision. These tubes fall out by themselves in 3 to 12 months and rarely have to be removed.

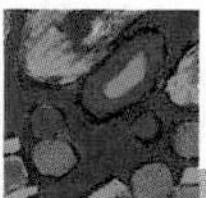

TABLE 63-3
COMMON MEDICATIONS *for Otitis Media*

Drug	Action	Nursing Intervention
Antibiotics		
Amoxicillin Amoxicillin-clavulanate Cefaclor Cefuroxime Azithromycin Cefpodoxime Clarithromycin Ceftriaxone	Inhibit cell wall synthesis; bactericidal	Assess for allergies or sensitivities. Instruct patient to take medication around the clock, not to miss any doses, and to finish prescription completely. Assess for superinfection.
Analgesic-Antipyretic and Narcotic Analgesics		
Acetaminophen with codeine	Central nervous system (CNS) depressant, analgesic, antipyretic, antiinflammatory	Assess vital signs, especially temperature. Caution patient not to drive or operate machinery if taking codeine; also not to take other CNS depressants, including alcohol, while taking medication. Instruct patient to increase fluid and roughage intake to avoid constipation and to take medication with meals to decrease possible nausea.

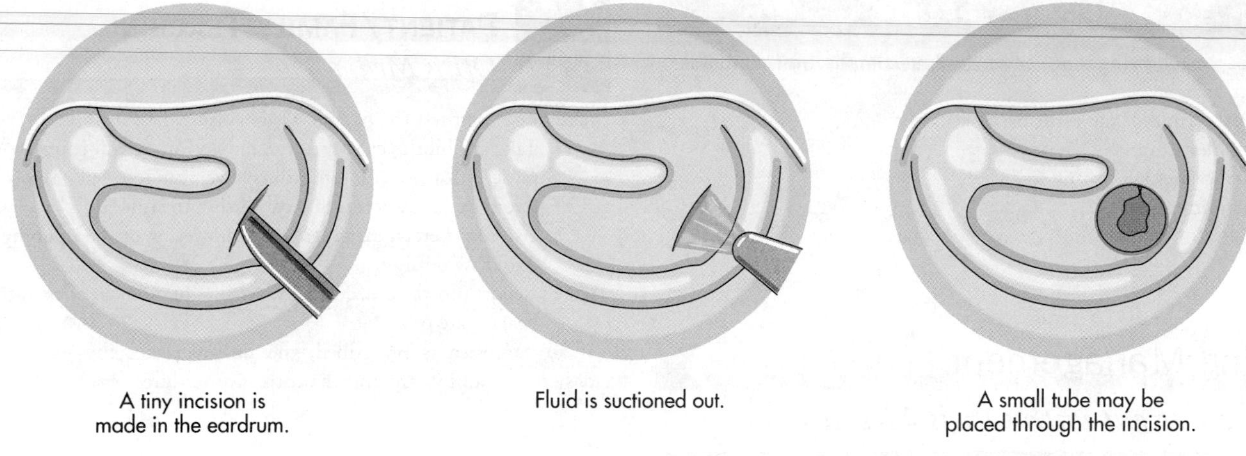

A tiny incision is made in the eardrum.
Fluid is suctioned out.
A small tube may be placed through the incision.

Figure 63-5 Myringotomy and transtympanic tube placement to prevent chronic serous otitis media.

SURGICAL MANAGEMENT. Surgical intervention may be necessary if attempts to control the infection medically are unsuccessful and the ossicles become necrotic. Repairing the damage of middle ear infection requires a difficult microsurgical procedure. Tympano-ossiculoplasty repairs the necrotic ossicles and creates a new eardrum. The surgical procedure is still being refined, and a variety of middle ear prostheses are available. The surgical procedure is often performed in an ambulatory surgery center with the patient under local anesthesia and sedation. Tympano-ossiculoplasty is not always successful, but it does restore sound transmission for some patients (see Patient/Family Teaching box).

COMPLICATIONS. The primary complications of middle ear infection are perforation of the eardrum and conductive hearing loss. The hearing loss usually resolves with effective treatment of the infection, but may be permanent if chronic disease is present. Acute perforations also tend to heal spontaneously without residual problems, but complex situations may require surgical closure of the perforation.

Cholesteatoma may result from chronic otitis media. In this condition epithelium from the external ear canal enters and extends into the middle ear, usually through a tympanic membrane perforation. The skin forms a saclike growth that traps debris and puts increasing pressure on the structures of the middle ear. The chronic infection causes cholesterol granules to be deposited within the sac, which gives the growth its name. Surgical excision may become necessary if pressure is causing damage or necrosis to the delicate ear structures. Limited procedures are generally attempted to preserve hearing, but either an open or closed mastoidectomy may be performed.

DIET. Diet does not play a role in the management of otitis media, but patients may modify their diet in response to symptoms. Increasing the daily intake of fluids is generally recommended in the presence of fever.

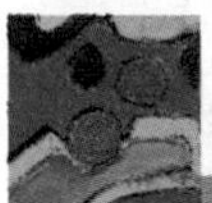

PATIENT/FAMILY TEACHING *Ear Surgery*

Most patients undergoing ear surgery have extremely short hospitalizations. Thus patient teaching is a major focus of nursing care. The patient must understand what to expect after discharge and how to promote healing during the recovery period. The nurse explains to the patient that:

- Decreased hearing is expected initially from the swelling and packing in the ear.
- Cracking or popping noises are commonly heard in the affected ear and are expected.
- Minor earache and discomfort in the cheek and jaw are common, but should be managed effectively with mild analgesics.
- Dizziness or lightheadedness may also be present initially, and caution must be used when getting out of bed and walking.
- Bleeding and drainage are negligible, so a cotton ball frequently provides an adequate dressing.

After surgery the nurse instructs the patient to:

- Avoid heavy lifting, straining, or vigorous activity for 3 weeks.
- Sneeze, cough, or blow nose with the mouth open as needed for the first week after surgery.
- Blow the nose gently as needed, one side at a time.
- Avoid vigorous activity until approved by the surgeon.
- Change the cotton ball dressing as prescribed.
- Report any drainage other than a slight amount of bleeding to the surgeon.
- Keep ear dry for 6 weeks after surgery.
- Do not shampoo the hair without a barrier.
- Protect the ear when necessary with two pieces of cotton (outer piece saturated with petrolatum).
- Avoid loud, noisy environments.
- Balance ear pressure as needed by holding nose, closing mouth, and swallowing.
- Avoid air travel until cleared by the surgeon.

▶ ARE YOU READY?

Which of the following is one of the leading complications of middle ear infection?

1. Perforation of the eardrum
2. Cholesteatoma
3. Sensorineural hearing loss
4. Tinnitus

Nursing Management of the Patient with Otitis Media

ASSESSMENT

Health History. Assess for:

- Pain in the ear that is often severe and throbbing
- A sense of fullness or pressure in the ear
- Perceived change in hearing

Physical Examination. Assess for:

- Drainage—bloody, serous, or purulent
- Inflamed, bulging tympanic membrane
- Perforation of the tympanic membrane
- Fever

NURSING DIAGNOSES, OUTCOMES, AND INTERVENTIONS

Nursing Diagnosis: Acute Pain

OUTCOMES. Common examples of expected outcomes for the patient with a diagnosis of *acute pain* are:

Patient will:

- Verbalize that pain is decreased to a manageable level.
- Rate pain as 3 or less on a scale of 0 (no pain) to 10 (maximum pain).

NURSING INTERVENTIONS. Analgesics may be necessary to successfully control the ear pain until the antibiotic begins to reduce the severity of the inflammation. The nurse encourages the patient to use these medications for comfort and to remain at rest until the antibiotic has demonstrated effectiveness. Reduced physical activity does appear to be helpful in controlling pain.

RELATED NIC INTERVENTIONS. Medication Management, Pain Management

PATIENT/FAMILY TEACHING. Patients with otitis media are rarely admitted to an acute care setting so patient teaching for self-care is particularly important (see Patient/Family Teaching box).

EVALUATION

To evaluate the effectiveness of nursing interventions, compare patient behaviors with those stated in the expected patient outcomes.

RELATED NOC OUTCOMES. Knowledge: Treatment Regimen, Pain Control

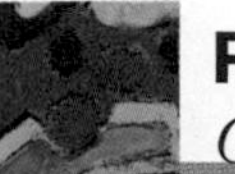

PATIENT/FAMILY TEACHING
Otitis Media

The nurse instructs the patient with otitis media to:

- Take antibiotics exactly as prescribed for the full course of the prescription, even if symptoms have been relieved.
- Avoid getting water in the ear during treatment.
- Use commercial ear plugs while showering or shampooing.
- Avoid swimming.
- Report otorrhea, decrease in hearing, or a return of pain to the health care provider.

If an ear wash is prescribed, the nurse teaches the patient or a designated family caregiver the correct procedure.

GERONTOLOGIC CONSIDERATIONS

Middle ear infection can occur at any point in the life span, but is not a common problem in older adults. When it does occur, management is the same as for any other patient. However, early infection may go undiagnosed unless pain is severe because older adults frequently experience itching in the ear or blockage with cerumen.

Problems of the Inner Ear

Sensorineural hearing loss is the most common inner ear disorder and may occur in conjunction with an identified ear problem or in isolation. The hearing loss is usually incomplete but is frequently progressive. Loss of discrimination (understanding of words) is a characteristic feature of sensorineural hearing loss. The inner ear is so delicate that it does not lend itself to surgical correction or repair. Hearing loss is discussed at the beginning of the chapter.

Acoustic Neuroma

Etiology and Epidemiology. Acoustic neuroma is by far the most common lesion affecting the inner ear, although both benign and malignant tumors can involve the inner ear by extension through the temporal bone. An acoustic neuroma is a benign tumor of the eighth cranial nerve. It is a slow-growing lesion that can occur at any age and usually occurs unilaterally. The tumor typically grows at the point where cranial nerve VIII enters the internal auditory canal in the temporal bone, and the tumor may extend into the brainstem. The tumor is more common in women and tends to occur in persons between 30 and 60 years old.

Pathophysiology. Acoustic neuromas arise from the neurilemmal sheath (sheath of Schwann) along the vestibular branch of the vestibulocochlear nerve and spread to the cochlear branch. Early diagnosis is important because the tumor can grow and compress the facial nerve and arteries within the ear canal and can also extend intracranially, at which point the chance of preserving hearing and facial nerve function is reduced. In rare cases the pressure of the tumor can become life threatening. Symptoms include tinnitus, vertigo, and a progressive unilateral loss of ability to hear high-pitched sounds. Disorders of the facial nerve may emerge if the tumor compresses this structure as well. Symptoms of facial nerve damage include impaired movement and muscle weakness indicated by loss of the nasolabial fold and drooping of the lower eyelid on the affected side of the face. Taste sensation may also be impaired or lost.

Collaborative Care Management. Acoustic neuromas are treated surgically, usually by a neurosurgeon. Computed tomography scans can show tumors greater than 2 cm, but the patient's hearing is usually already compromised by the time the tumor is this large. Technical challenges of the surgical procedure include preservation of both hearing and facial nerve function. Many patients experience some degree of residual hearing loss after treatment.

Meniere's Disease

Etiology and Epidemiology. Meniere's disease or syndrome, also called idiopathic endolymphatic hydrops, is an uncommon form of vertigo of unknown cause. The disease occurs when the normal fluid and electrolyte balance of the inner ear is disrupted and is thought to be caused most often by viral injury to the fluid transport system of the inner ear. Some research is being directed toward the relationship between immune disorders and Meniere's disease.[15] Diagnosis is based on a classic triad of symptoms—episodic true vertigo, sensorineural hearing loss, and tinnitus—plus a prodromal symptom of fullness or pressure in the involved ear.[13]

The prevalence of Meniere's disease in the United States is approximately 40 persons per 100,000. Men and women are affected about equally. Peak onset occurs in the 40- to 60-year age-group.[13] The disease usually begins unilaterally but may progress to both ears in 10% to 78% of patients. Family history is significant. Symptoms may be exacerbated during the menstrual cycle in women who experience significant premenstrual fluid retention.

Pathophysiology. The underlying pathologic changes of Meniere's disease include overproduction and defective absorption of endolymph, which increases the volume and pressure within the membranous labyrinth until distention results in rupture and mixing of the endolymph and perilymph fluids. The two fluids have significantly different compositions, and the mixture disrupts the fluid and electrolyte balance within the labyrinth. Classic Meniere's disease attacks last from 2 to 3 weeks, approximately the time required to close the rupture and restore the fluid balance. Patients with Meniere's disease have been noted to have abnormal levels of circulating complement and of immune complexes. Symptoms range from mild to incapacitating and include vertigo, tinnitus, and fluctuating sensorineural hearing loss from degeneration of the hair cells. Prodromal symptoms include tinnitus, ear fullness, and hearing loss. Ninety-five percent of patients experience vertigo associated with nausea, vomiting, and ataxia.

Initially symptoms of Meniere's disease last less than 2 hours, although altered balance may last up to 2 days. As the disease progresses, symptoms last hours to days, and the episodes occur with less warning and are more disabling. Because the balance system can compensate, dizziness is usually not present consistently but is episodic. Early in the course of the disease the patient is asymptomatic between episodes, but as the disease progresses, recovery between attacks is incomplete and permanent tinnitus, moderate to severe hearing loss, and chronic unsteadiness may result. The numerous factors implicated as the cause of Meniere's disease indicate the lack of understanding of the mechanisms of this disorder and imply that the disease may be multifactorial or represent the common endpoint to a variety of abnormalities.[13]

Collaborative Care Management. Meniere's disease is relatively uncommon, but the symptom of dizziness or vertigo is second only to headache as the most common chronic symptom reported by patients in the United States. *Vertigo,* or spinning, is the medical term for dizziness, but dizziness is described in such varied terms that it is almost impossible to accurately define the symptom. Spinning may be the most common form of dizziness. Other descriptions include lightheadedness, giddiness, imbalance, veering in one direction while walking, unsteadiness, or a vague feeling of uncertainty during changes in body position. Questions that can be used to explore vertigo are presented in Box 63-1.

The diagnosis of Meniere's disease is established after eliminating other causes of the patient's symptoms. Because the disease has no known cure, management focuses on control of symptoms, and a variety of medications may be tried. Antiemetics and anticholinergics may be administered during an acute attack to decrease autonomic nervous system activity. Diuretics and vasodilators are helpful to some patients in restoring the proper fluid balance in the inner ear. Other patients may respond to drugs that reduce vestibular impulses and to sedatives. Treatment protocols have used more than 50 different medications. Usually a combination can be found that adequately control the patient's symptoms.

Patients with severe vertigo sometimes profit from vestibular rehabilitation, which teaches labyrinthine compensatory exercises combined with physical therapy. Balance exercises decrease dizziness by helping the brain compensate for the damaged balance system. Movements that trigger dizziness are repeated rather than

Box 63-1 Questions to Assess Vertigo

- When did the dizziness first occur?
- Did the dizziness start suddenly or gradually?
- Is the dizziness constant, or does it come in "attacks"?
- How often do the attacks occur?
- How long do the attacks last?
- Overall, has the dizziness gotten better or worse since starting?
- List anything that stops an attack of dizziness or makes it better.
- List anything that brings on an attack of dizziness or makes it worse.
- Does the dizziness occur only in certain positions?
- Do any other symptoms occur simultaneously with the dizziness such as nausea, vomiting, or ear pressure?
- Does stress have any relationship to the dizziness?
- Have you ever fallen because of the dizziness?
- Do you get dizzy after heavy lifting, straining, exertion, or overwork?
- Do you get dizzy if you have not eaten for a long time?
- For women: Is your dizziness connected with your menstrual cycle?
- How has the dizziness affected the quality of your life?

Adapted from Sigler BA, Schuring L: *Ear, nose, and throat disorders,* St Louis, 1993, Mosby.

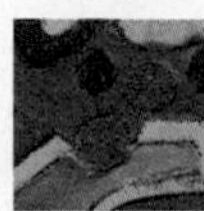

PATIENT/FAMILY TEACHING
Meniere's Disease

In addition to teaching about the disease and the prescribed medication, the nurse gives the following instruction:

- During an acute attack of vertigo:
  —Immediately lie down on a firm surface if possible.
  —Loosen clothing.
  —Close eyes until acute vertigo stops.
  —Do not attempt to drive or operate machinery during an acute attack.
- To protect self from injury between attacks:
  —Avoid swimming under water, since orientation may be lost; otherwise resume regular activity.
  —Sit or lie down at the onset of any dizziness to decrease the risk of falling.
  —Avoid using ladders, working on roofs or other high places, and climbing until vertigo is controlled.
  —Make the home environment safe as outlined in discussions with health care providers.
  —If engaged in balance therapy, practice exercises daily.

avoided. Avoiding dizziness is more comfortable for the patient but does not help the balance system regain its function and compensate for losses.

If the patient's symptoms cannot be satisfactorily controlled with medical interventions, a variety of surgical procedures may be performed. Endolymphatic sac procedures involve decompression and various forms of shunts to reduce the fluid pressure within the labyrinth and control vertigo. A destructive procedure in which the membranous labyrinth is removed either subtotally or totally through the oval window or through the mastoid bone is called a labyrinthectomy. This procedure results in loss of hearing in the affected ear.[13] Vestibular nerve surgery destroys the vestibular nerve in the affected ear while attempting to preserve hearing. With any surgery on the vestibular system, there is a risk of hearing loss and chronic vertigo.

DIET. Diet therapy is frequently helpful in controlling the symptoms associated with Meniere's disease. Some patients have had significant symptom improvement by adhering to a low-salt diet; avoiding excess use of caffeine, sugar, monosodium glutamate, and alcohol; and distributing food and fluid intake over the course of the day.

PATIENT/FAMILY TEACHING. Patient teaching is an integral component of nursing care for the patient with Meniere's disease (see Patient/Family Teaching box).

Because the brain must integrate data from the vestibular, visual, and proprioceptive systems to maintain balance, other disorders can also result in vertigo and balance disturbances (Table 63-4).

ARE You READY?

Which of the following is an appropriate statement when teaching a patient with Meniere's disease about diet?

1. "Follow a high-fiber diet."
2. "Avoid sugar substitutes."
3. "Drink at least 2 liters of fluid per day."
4. "Avoid excessive use of caffeine."

Critical Thinking

1. Describe how you think you might feel if you were told you had a significant and permanent hearing loss.
2. Compare and contrast the pathophysiology, clinical manifestations, and assessment parameters for conductive and sensorineural hearing loss.
3. What measures or precautions could you suggest to the patient who has vertigo?
4. How are upper respiratory tract infections and otitis media related?

References

1. American Academy of Pediatrics: Clinical practice guidelines: diagnosis and management of acute otitis media, *Pediatrics* 113(5):1451-1465, 2004.
2. American Academy of Pediatrics: Clinical practice guidelines: otitis media with effusion, *Pediatrics* 113(5):1412-1429, 2004.
3. Amsden GW: Pneumococcal resistance in perspective: how well are we combating it? *Pediatr Infect Dis J* 23(2 Suppl):125-128, 2004.

TABLE 63-4 VESTIBULAR DISORDERS

Disorder	Definition	Cause (Most Common)	Symptoms
Vestibular neuronitis	Infection of vestibular nerve with sudden onset	Virus	Vertigo most severe on first attack, less severe on subsequent attacks
Labyrinthitis	Infection of labyrinth of inner ear	Virus, bacteria	Severe vertigo, diminishing with time Tinnitus: may or may not be present Permanent sensorineural hearing loss
Benign paroxysmal positional vertigo	Degenerative debris free-floating in endolymph	Idiopathic (many theories)	Positional vertigo with quick head movements or position change
Presbyastasis (presbyvertigo)	Balance disorder of aging	Degenerative changes of vestibule	Imbalance when standing or walking, leading to falls and injuries

4. Bance M et al: A comparison of the audiometric performance of bone anchored hearing aids and air conduction hearing aids, *Am J Otol* 23(6): 912-919, 2002.
5. Crews JE, Campbell VA: Vision impairment and hearing loss among community-dwelling older Americans: implications for health and functioning, *Am J Pub Health* 94(5):823-829, 2004.
6. Cummer RW, Hassan GA : Diagnostic approach to tinnitus, *Am Fam Phys* 69:120-128, 2004.
7. Darrow DH, Dash N, Derkay CS: Otitis media: concepts and controversies, *Curr Opin Otolaryngol Head Neck Surg* 11(6):416-423, 2003.
8. Gianopoulos I, Stephens D, Davis A: Follow up of people fitted with hearing aids after adult hearing screening: the need for support after fitting, *Br Med J* 325(7362):471, 2002.
9. Gratton MA, Vaquez AE: Age-related hearing loss: current research, *Curr Opin Otolaryngol Head Neck Surg* 11(5):367-371, 2003.
10. Isaacson JE, Vora NM: Differential diagnosis and treatment of hearing loss, *Am Fam Phys* 68:1125-1132, 2003.
11. Kasper DL et al, editors: *Harrison's principles of internal medicine*, ed 16, New York, 2005, McGraw-Hill.
12. McCoy SI, Zell ER, Besser RE: Antimicrobial prescribing for otitis externa in children, *Pediatr Infect Dis J* 23(2):181-183, 2004.
13. Minor LB, Schessel DA, Carey JP: Meniere's disease, *Curr Opin Neurol* 17(1):9-16, 2004.
14. Parisier SC: Cochlear implants: growing pains, *Laryngoscope* 113(9): 1470-1472, 2003.
15. Porth CM: *Pathophysiology concepts of altered health states*, ed 7, Philadelphia, 2005, Lippincott, Williams & Wilkins.
16. Priwin C et al: Bilateral bone-anchored hearing aids (BAHAs): an audiometric evaluation, *Laryngoscope* 114(1):77-84, 2004.
17. Uphold CR, Graham MV: *Clinical guidelines in family practice*, ed 4, Gainesville, Fla, 2003, Barmarrae Books.
18. US Department of Health and Human Services: *Healthy people 2010: understanding and improving health,* Washington, DC, 2000, The Department.
19. Van Balen FAM et al: Clinical efficacy of three treatments in acute otitis externa in primary care: randomized controlled trial, *Br Med J* 327(7425):1201-1205, 2003.
20. Yueh B et al: Screening and management of hearing loss in primary care: scientific review, *JAMA* 289(15):1976-1985, 2003.

Visit the Evolve website: http://evolve.elsevier.com/Monahan/medsurg

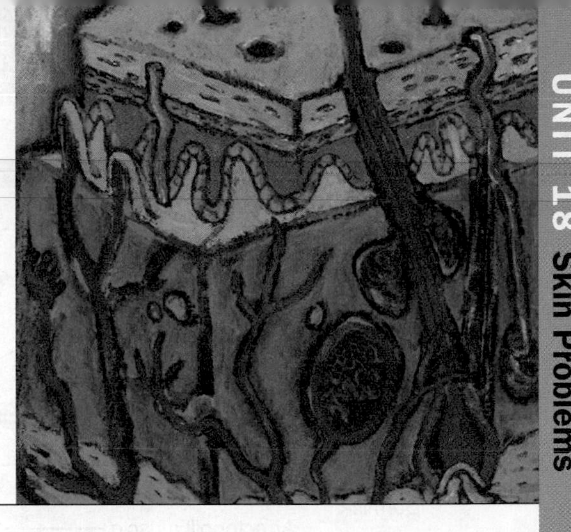

CHAPTER 64

Assessment of the Skin

by Marianne C. Tawa

OBJECTIVES

After studying this chapter, the learner should be able to:

1. Correlate the structures of the skin with their functions.
2. Define guidelines and parameters for assessment of the skin and accessory structures.
3. Identify specific changes in the skin associated with physiologic aging.
4. Describe primary and secondary skin lesions, lesion arrangement, and configuration.

KEY TERMS

evaporation, p. 1861
integrity, p. 1861
intradermal, p. 1871
lesion, p. 1866
macerated, p. 1861
permeability, p. 1860
pigmentation, p. 1864
radiation, p. 1861
turgor, p. 1866

The skin is the largest organ of the body, accounting for approximately 15% of the total body weight. It is exposed to the external environment and provides the first line of defense of the body, yet at the same time it is affected by changes in the internal environment. Thus assessment of the skin and its associated appendages—hair, nails, and glands—provides insight into how individuals are affected by and cope with both external and internal environments. Information gathered in this assessment provides the basis for identifying actual or potential nursing problems related to the skin, infection, fluid and electrolyte imbalances, nutritional imbalances, or inadequate oxygenation of tissues. Baseline observations facilitate early and accurate identification of changes that may occur.

Anatomy and Physiology

Structure of the Skin

The skin is composed of three major layers: the epidermis, the dermis, and the subcutaneous tissue (Figure 64-1). The epidermis is the outermost structure of the skin. It possesses the unique ability to regenerate itself by forming new cells on an ongoing basis. The primary cell of the epidermis is the keratinocyte, or squamous cell. Keratinocytes produce keratin, which is a resilient, insoluble, fibrous protein. The epidermis consists of five histologically distinct layers, each of which is named for the stage of reproductive activity of the keratinocyte that occurs within it. The innermost basal cell layer, also known as the stratum basale, basement membrane, or stratum germinativum, gives rise to new cells through mitosis. After cell division has taken place in the basal cell layer, one basal cell from each cell division remains behind while the other migrates upward. The migrating cell passes through the intermediate layers of the stratum spinosum, stratum granulosum, and stratum lucidum, further flattening and differentiating along the way. Twenty-eight days later, on average, the mature keratinocyte reaches the stratum corneum, or horny cell outermost layer of the epidermis. The horny cell layer is predominately composed of keratin, which is responsible for the vital barrier function of skin.

Another critical but less commonly found cell in the epidermis is the melanocyte. Melanocytes are dendritic pigment-producing cells derived from the neural crest during embryologic development. They form pigment granules called melanosomes, which contain melanin and provide color to skin, eyes, and hair. Melanocytes also play a role in protection from ultraviolet light. Langerhan's cells, derived from bone marrow, are also found in the epidermis and serve an immunologic function related to antigen presentation.

The second layer of skin, called the *dermis* or *cutis,* is located beneath the epidermis and is demarcated by the basement membrane. At 1 to 4 mm, the dermis is significantly thicker than the epidermis and provides structural support and mass to the skin. The dermis consists of connective tissue components, including collagen, elastin, and reticulum fibers, as well as water, ground substance, sensory and postganglionic nerves, blood vessels, and lymphatics. The dermis surrounds and supplies nutrition and

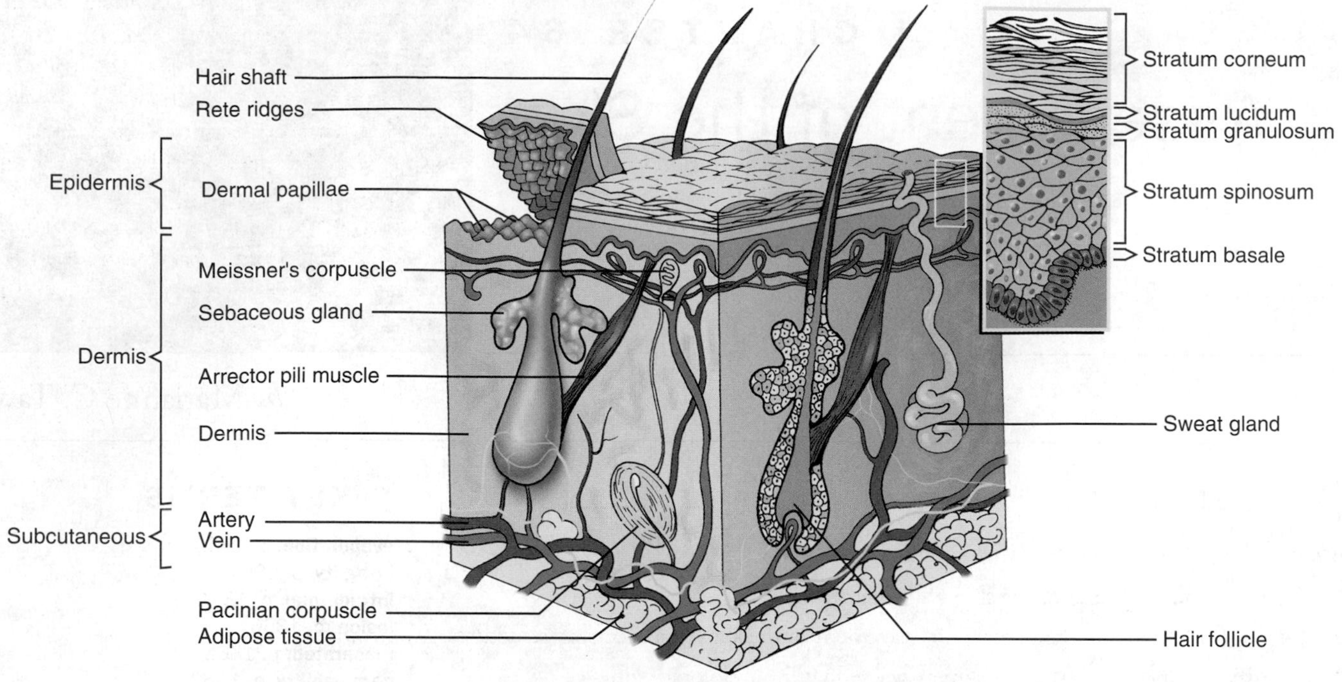

Figure 64-1 Anatomy of the skin.

electrolytes to the skin appendages such as sweat glands, sebaceous glands, and hair follicles.

The third layer of skin is the subcutaneous tissue, which consists of fat cells, or lipocytes, separated by fibrous walls composed of collagen and blood vessels. This fatty tissue layer conducts heat only one fourth as rapidly as do other tissues and thus serves as the body's heat insulator. Subcutaneous tissue also provides a cushioning effect, is a storage site for caloric reserve, and anchors the other two layers to supportive structures (e.g., muscle, tendon, bone). The density of subcutaneous tissue varies from location to location in the body. For example, the waist and hips typically possess ample subcutaneous tissue, whereas the eyelids and nipples lack it. Distribution of subcutaneous tissue is regulated by sex hormones, genetics, age, eating, and exercise habits.

Eccrine sweat glands are present everywhere on the body surface except for the ear canal, penis, labial tissue, lips, and nail beds. The heaviest concentration of eccrine glands is found on the palms, soles, head, trunk, and extremities. Eccrine sweat is an odorless, colorless, hypotonic solution, which is directly secreted to the surface of the skin. Eccrine glands participate in the heat-regulating mechanisms of the body, and their activity is under the control of the sympathetic nervous system. Thermal, mental, and gustatory stimuli promote eccrine gland secretion.

Apocrine glands are located mainly in the axilla, umbilical area, breast, genitalia, external ear canal, and eyelid. Apocrine glands, under the direction of epinephrine and norepinephrine, produce a milky, odorless, sterile secretion. At the skin surface level the fluid comes in contact with bacteria present on the hair follicle or skin and results in body odor. These glands have no identifiable biologic function.

Sebaceous glands are found on all areas of the body except for the top and bottom surfaces of the hands and feet. Sebaceous glands are most often associated with hair follicles. The greatest density of these glands occurs on the scalp, face, chest, and back. Sebaceous glands, under the influence of androgenic hormones, produce sebum. This is a lipid-containing substance, which may play a role in lubrication and synthesis of vitamin D in the skin.

Functions of the Skin

Protection. The outermost layer of the epidermis, the stratum corneum, is a relatively impermeable layer of tightly packed, flat cells that protects the underlying tissue from the outer environment. A small number of nonpathogenic bacteria reside in this horny layer of skin. Lack of moisture in this layer keeps the microorganism number low by impeding growth. Bacteria attempting to penetrate hair follicles are deterred by the sebum. Fat-soluble substances such as moisturizing lotions can penetrate the skin by passively diffusing through the hair follicles and sebaceous glands.

Intact skin is the first line of defense against bacterial and foreign-substance invasion, slight physical trauma, heat, or ultraviolet rays. When the skin is exposed to environmental factors such as pressure, friction, and internal shearing forces, it is compressed to the depth of the supporting structures (e.g., bone). With prolonged exposure the capillary bed within the dermis and the larger vessels within the subcutaneous tissue become occluded, causing ischemia of the tissues in the area. If the ischemia is not reversed by removing the source of pressure, cellular death is imminent and the skin's defensive line is jeopardized.

Scraping or stripping the surface of the skin (e.g., by the removal of tape or the use of razors without shaving cream) can weaken the epidermis. Once the barrier has weakened, **permeability** to bacteria and other foreign substances is increased. Percutaneous absorption of medications through the skin can be enhanced when the skin surface is disrupted or denuded. Epidermis that becomes extremely dry may fissure and crack more readily. Moist skin surface areas can become **macerated**, thus providing a medium for bacterial overgrowth.

Mucous membranes, although continuous with the stratum corneum, are somewhat protected from the external environment. Fluids and other substances such as certain drugs can be absorbed through the mucous membranes.

Heat Regulation. Body temperature is controlled by **radiation** of heat from the surface of the skin, conduction of heat from skin to other objects or air, removal of heat by air currents on the skin (convection), and **evaporation** of water from skin surfaces. Insensible water evaporation from the skin and lungs occurs at a rate of 600 to 1000 ml/day. On a hot day the only way the body can lose heat is by evaporation, and anything that restricts evaporation under these conditions will increase body temperature. The blood vessels of the skin help control body temperature by constricting in cold environments to promote conservation of heat and dilating in warm environments to promote loss of heat by radiation. These mechanisms help maintain a constant internal body temperature.

Sensory Perception. The skin contains receptor endings of nerves responsible for sensing pain, touch, heat, and cold. Through the stimulation of these nerve endings, a person is able to communicate with the immediate external environment. Distribution of the sensory endings is generalized; however, certain areas of the body have more than other areas. For example, the hands have a higher concentration of sensory endings than the forearms.

Excretion. Water lost through the skin is a factor in maintaining water balance in the body. Salt as well as water is lost through excessive sweating. As a person becomes acclimated to a continually hot environment, however, the amount of salt lost decreases over time.

Vitamin D Production. Synthesis of vitamin D takes place in the skin by the effect of sunlight (ultraviolet rays) on precursors found in epidermal cells. Vitamin D is necessary for the metabolism of calcium and phosphorus.

Decorative. The skin, hair, and nails individually and collectively contribute to one's body image, which can be aesthetically pleasing or displeasing. Because the skin and its appendages are the parts of the body most readily visible to the outside world, they play an important role in the impression a person makes on others. Individuals with skin disorders, both acute and chronic, can develop marked alterations in self-esteem and confidence.

Physiologic Changes With Aging

Many skin changes occur as a person ages. Observable changes result primarily from loss of subcutaneous tissue, degeneration of collagen and elastic fibers, loss of melanocytes, increased capillary fragility, decreased secretion of sweat glands, hormonal changes, and overexposure to environmental elements.

The skin loses its elasticity and becomes loose and wrinkled. Exposed areas may be thickened, but in general the skin becomes thinner, drier, and more fragile. There are fewer hair follicles and, as a result, absorption of fat-soluble substances is decreased. Benign growths such as seborrheic keratoses, senile lentigines (brown spots), and vascular hyperplasias such as cherry angiomas and senile purpura (red to purple ecchymotic spots) develop in middle to elder years. Changes in the color, texture, and quantity of hair are other age-associated findings in older adults. Nails may become thickened, brittle, and discolored with advancing age.

Age-related changes also place older adults at risk for skin problems. Older patients are more likely to have one or more chronic diseases and to be taking medications that can produce skin disorders. Dry skin set the stage for pruritus (itching) with frequent scratching that can disrupt the epidermis. Skin infections such as candidiasis caused by yeast organisms and impetigo caused by the gram-positive organisms group A beta-hemolytic streptococci or *Staphylococcus aureus* may then result. Lower extremity venous insufficiency in older adults can cause stasis dermatitis.

Health History

Patient history is an important component of the skin assessment. When patients report a rash; change in pigmentation; lesions; or new skin symptoms such as itching, burning, or pain, the nurse obtains the following information:

- Usual skin condition: appearance, color, moisture, texture, and **integrity**
- Onset of the problem: initial location and when changes were first noted; skin appearance at onset; other associated symptoms such as pain or itching
- Changes since onset: change in location, change in size or appearance, onset of new associated symptoms such as pain or itching
- Possible causes: exposure to known contact allergens such as poison ivy, rubber, nickel, or fragrance; if cause unknown, ask about:
    - —Exposure to potential sensitizing substances, such as metals, chemicals, detergents, solvents, or plant life
    - —Use of new pharmacologic agents, either prescription or over the counter
    - —Work that may cause contact with potential skin irritants or require hands to be constantly in water
    - —Participation in recreational activities (e.g., painting, camping, or gardening) that may involve exposure to sensitizing substances
    - —Exposure to ultraviolet light (sun) producing sunburn or photosensitivity
    - —Change in climate
    - —Increase in stress level
- Alleviating factors: clinician-prescribed or self-prescribed; how and when used
- Psychologic reaction to skin changes, including the ability to work, participate in recreational activities, or interact on a social or intimate level

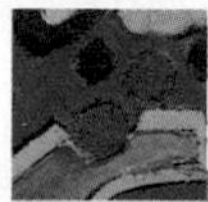

PATIENT/FAMILY TEACHING
Maintenance of Healthy Skin

To maintain healthy skin, the nurse instructs adults to:

- Prevent drying and irritation of the skin.
  —Avoid excessive bathing.
  —Use tepid water and pH-neutral soaps.
  —Lather gently and pat dry.
  —Apply an emollient cream or lotion immediately after bathing.
  —Drink plenty of water.
- Eat a well-balanced diet.
- Get an adequate amount of sleep.
- Exercise regularly.
- Perform skin self-assessment monthly, preferably after a bath or shower (Figure 64-2).
- Report any new growths or changes in preexisting lesions to a health care provider.
- Report early signs of skin infection if you are older or have an impaired immune response because of the risks of delayed healing and spread.

Because the history assists not only in assessing the patient's health status but also in identifying needs for health information and instruction, assessing for good health practices relating to dermatologic system function is essential (see Patient/Family Teaching box).

Physical Examination

Methods of Assessment

Direct inspection with a good light is the basic method of skin assessment. Palpation is used to identify temperature, areas of tenderness, and the density and induration of lesions. A systematic head-to-toe skin assessment can be conducted while the related health history is obtained. When the history identifies potential or existing problems, the nurse reassesses involved areas of the skin as needed. Remember that data obtained from physical assessment of the skin not only relates to dermatologic problems but also provides an indication of overall health status. Detailed principles of effective skin assessment are presented in the Guidelines for Safe Practice box.

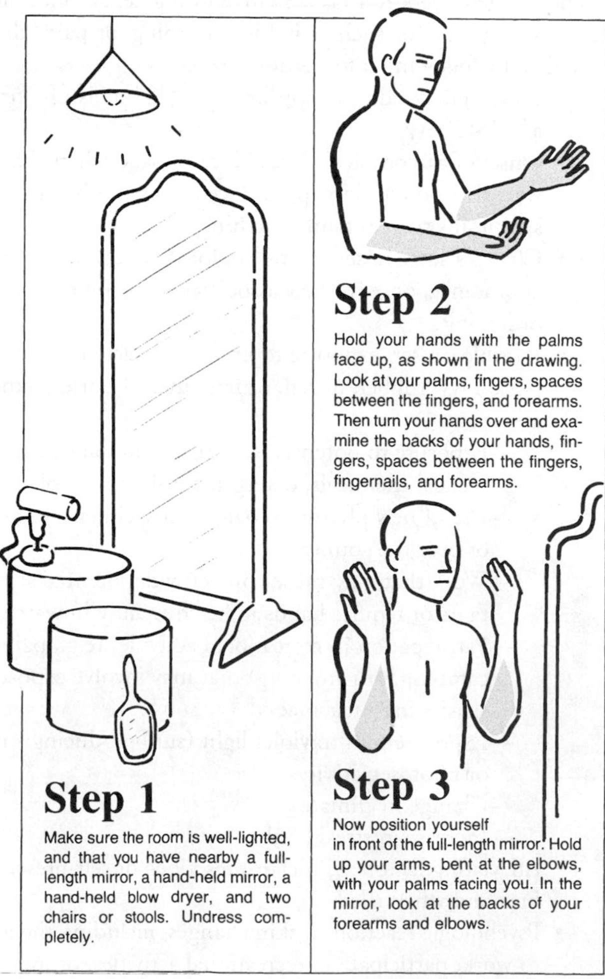
Step 1
Make sure the room is well-lighted, and that you have nearby a full-length mirror, a hand-held mirror, a hand-held blow dryer, and two chairs or stools. Undress completely.
Step 2
Hold your hands with the palms face up, as shown in the drawing. Look at your palms, fingers, spaces between the fingers, and forearms. Then turn your hands over and examine the backs of your hands, fingers, spaces between the fingers, fingernails, and forearms.
Step 3
Now position yourself in front of the full-length mirror. Hold up your arms, bent at the elbows, with your palms facing you. In the mirror, look at the backs of your forearms and elbows.

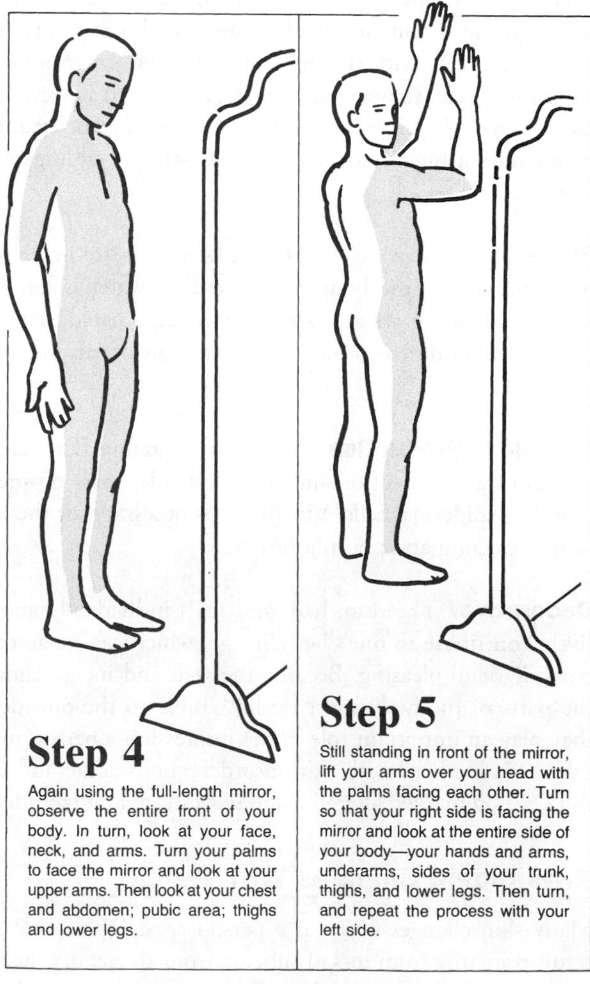

Again using the full-length mirror, observe the entire front of your body. In turn, look at your face, neck, and arms. Turn your palms to face the mirror and look at your upper arms. Then look at your chest and abdomen; pubic area; thighs and lower legs.

Still standing in front of the mirror, lift your arms over your head with the palms facing each other. Turn so that your right side is facing the mirror and look at the entire side of your body—your hands and arms, underarms, sides of your trunk, thighs, and lower legs. Then turn, and repeat the process with your left side.

Figure 64-2 Technique for self-examination of the skin.

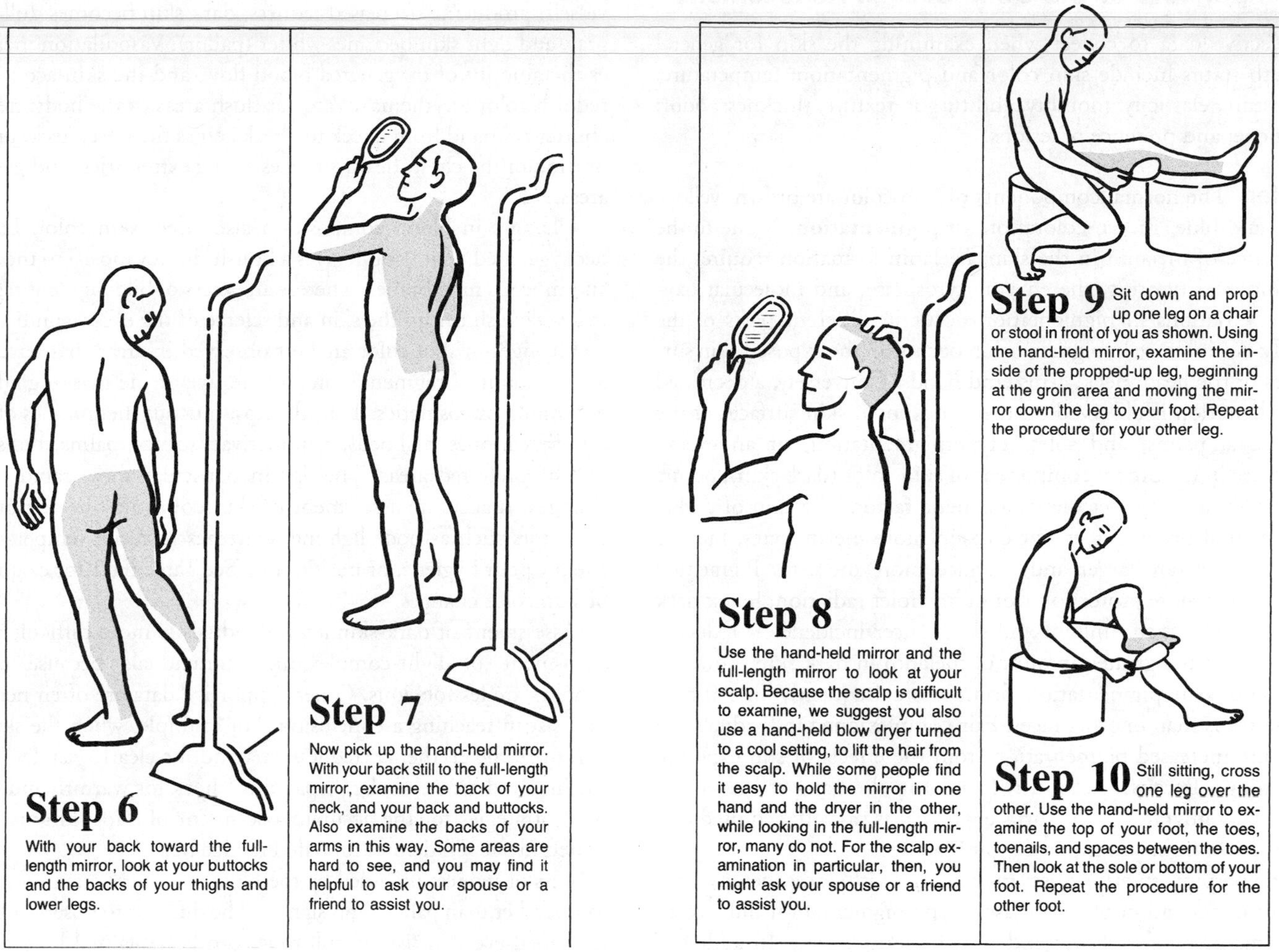

Step 6

With your back toward the full-length mirror, look at your buttocks and the backs of your thighs and lower legs.

Step 7

Now pick up the hand-held mirror. With your back still to the full-length mirror, examine the back of your neck, and your back and buttocks. Also examine the backs of your arms in this way. Some areas are hard to see, and you may find it helpful to ask your spouse or a friend to assist you.

Step 8

Use the hand-held mirror and the full-length mirror to look at your scalp. Because the scalp is difficult to examine, we suggest you also use a hand-held blow dryer turned to a cool setting, to lift the hair from the scalp. While some people find it easy to hold the mirror in one hand and the dryer in the other, while looking in the full-length mirror, many do not. For the scalp examination in particular, then, you might ask your spouse or a friend to assist you.

Step 9 Sit down and prop up one leg on a chair or stool in front of you as shown. Using the hand-held mirror, examine the inside of the propped-up leg, beginning at the groin area and moving the mirror down the leg to your foot. Repeat the procedure for your other leg.

Step 10 Still sitting, cross one leg over the other. Use the hand-held mirror to examine the top of your foot, the toes, toenails, and spaces between the toes. Then look at the sole or bottom of your foot. Repeat the procedure for the other foot.

Figure 64-2—cont'd

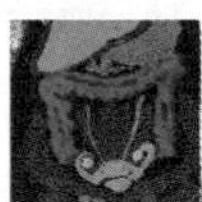

GUIDELINES FOR SAFE PRACTICE *Skin Assessment Techniques*

- Be prepared: Adequate lighting is crucial to examination of the skin. Natural lighting is preferred. If the lighting is inadequate, lesions may be missed or described inaccurately. If the room temperature is not well controlled, vasoconstriction or vasodilation may occur, leading to false impressions.
- Be systematic: If only some parts of the skin are inspected, an important observation may be missed.
- Be thorough: Look at all areas carefully. If the person is lying down, be sure to examine the back, especially the sacral area. Expose areas of tissue hidden by skin folds. For example lift breasts and separate gluteal folds. Maintain patient privacy as you progress sequentially through the examination. Make certain to examine the mucous membranes of the oral cavity.
- Be specific: When lesions are identified, describe them in terms of shape, size (using the metric system), location, color, and other characteristics.
- Compare right side with left side. When observing changes in skin color or tissue shape, always compare one side of the body with the other to differentiate structural from pathologic changes, as well as symmetry of manifestation.
- Record the data: Unrecorded data are lost data. Baseline observations indicating normality or abnormality are needed for comparison with subsequent findings. Changes need to be recorded to determine progress toward achieving desired outcomes.
- Use appropriate technique: Lesions are palpated for density, induration, and tenderness. Standard Precautions need to be observed during palpation, and the examiner must determine whether it is appropriate to use gloves.

Components of the General Skin Assessment

Objective data to collect when examining the skin for general health status include skin color and pigmentation; temperature; moisture; elasticity, mobility, and turgor, texture; thickness; odor; hygiene; and presence of lesions.

Color. The normal components of skin color are brown, yellow, red, and blue. Brown coloration, or **pigmentation,** is due to the presence of melanin in the skin. Melanin formation requires the amino acid tyrosine, the enzyme tyrosinase, and molecular oxygen. Variations in pigmentation occur in different parts of the body. An increase in pigmentation occurs on the exposed skin surfaces of the head, neck, arms, and hands. Conversely, a decreased pigmentation is observed on the nonexposed skin surfaces of the genitalia, palms, and soles. Hyperpigmentation, or an overall increase in the brown component of skin color (dark skin), occurs normally in some persons as a genetic factor. The skin of darkly pigmented persons does not contain more melanocytes, but the melanocytes are larger and produce more melanin. Pigmented skin offers more protection from ultraviolet radiation; hence dark skin reacts less to sunlight and skin cancer incidence is reduced. Because of the greater amount of melanin in dark skin, however, alterations in pigmentation occur more frequently in African-Americans than in other races. Fair-complexioned individuals can acquire increased pigmentation from the effects of sun exposure (tanning). Because melanin is formed in the basal cell layer and gradually migrates to the surface where it is cast off, acquired pigmentation from sun exposure (tan) fades.

Hyperpigmentation also may occur with radiotherapy as a result of activation of tyrosinase. Hyperpigmentation induced in this manner fades slowly and may be long lasting. In addition, certain endocrine diseases, pregnancy, oral contraceptive use, and nutritional and metabolic disorders can produce hyperpigmentary skin changes. Hyperpigmentation may follow an inflammatory process in the skin as seen with eczema, acne vulgaris, drug eruptions, and skin infections. Cutaneous neoplastic processes such as T-cell lymphoma of the skin may produce hyperpigmented patches and plaques. Hydroquinone (bleach) with salicylic acid or with retinoic acid interferes with tyrosinase activity.

Hypopigmentation (light skin) occurs normally in some persons as a genetic factor. Albinos have a congenital inability to produce melanin. Severe trauma can destroy melanin-producing cells and result in hypopigmentation (scar tissue). Some healthy persons develop a condition called vitiligo, in which there is a failure of melanin formation. Sharply demarcated, white (amelanotic) patches typically distributed over the face, joints, hands, and legs are the hallmarks of this skin disorder. Vitiligo is thought to be an autoimmune disease in which antibodies are produced to melanocytes.[4] Other causes for acquired hypopigmentation include the aftermath of an inflammatory process such as atopic dermatitis or psoriasis, infections such as tinea versicolor, and certain neoplastic skin processes.

The red component of skin color comes from the blood supplied to the skin. The rate of blood flow through the skin is highly variable because of its function in heat control. The blood vessels are innervated by the sympathetic nervous system; thus vasoconstriction occurs with the neuroendocrine response to stressors. With vasoconstriction, smaller amounts of blood pass through the vessels, producing decreased redness; dark skin becomes dull and gray, and light skin becomes whiter (pallor). Vasodilation increases the amount of oxygenated blood flow, and the skin acquires a reddish color (erythema). Vascular flush areas of the body are the "butterfly" band from cheek to cheek across the nose, neck, upper portion of the chest, flexor surfaces of the extremities, and genital areas.

Changes in blood composition also affect skin color. Excess deoxygenated hemoglobin gives a bluish tint (cyanosis) to the skin and mucous membranes, whereas an excess of bile pigment results in a yellowish tint to the skin and sclerae of the eyes (jaundice).

Changes in skin color are best observed in areas that have the least amount of pigmentation and are free of the masking effects of tanning or cosmetics. Thus the lips, mucous membranes of the mouth, earlobes, nail beds, conjunctivae, sclerae, palms, and soles are the preferred areas. The lips in particular show rapid color changes. Inaccurate assessment of skin color may be attributed to factors such as poor lighting, extremes in room temperature, edema, poor hygiene, or positioning. See Table 64-1 for examples of skin color changes.

Assessment of dark-skinned individuals is more difficult than assessment of light-complexioned individuals because color changes are less obvious. Other supportive data are often needed to assist in reaching a conclusion. For example, when the skin is inflamed, the erythema (redness) may not be clearly visible. Thus the involved area must be palpated to check for warmth and edema.[6] Strategies for the accurate assessment of dark skin are presented in the Guidelines for Safe Practice box.

Loss of redness provided by the blood produces grayish or dull tones rather than pallor. This sign may be difficult to observe by the untrained eye. Grayish or dull tones can be visualized best in the lips, mucous membranes, conjunctivae, and nail beds. Cyanosis also gives the skin a grayish or dull tone because of loss of redness. Areas of lesser pigmentation, including the earlobes, palms, and soles, are assessed for signs of cyanosis.

The sclerae of many dark-skinned persons contain fatty deposits with carotene, giving the sclerae a yellowish tinge.[7] With these individuals, jaundice will have to be determined by other signs, such as bile in the urine or feces.

Temperature. Skin temperature is regulated by both vasoconstriction and vasodilation. If an excess amount of heat is produced within the body because of factors such as exercise, fever, or hyperthyroidism, or if heat from the external environment increases, the sympathetic centers in the hypothalamus are inhibited and vasodilation occurs. A local inflammation of the skin or underlying tissue also produces vasodilation as part of the inflammatory response. Vasodilation increases blood flow and creates a sensation of warmth on the skin. Cold skin is caused by vasoconstriction as a result of sympathetic stimulation or diseases such as hypothyroidism. To assess the temperature of the skin, the nurse uses the backs of the fingers, which are more sensitive than the fingertips.

Moisture. Skin is characterized as dry, moist, or oily. Dry skin is frequently seen in the older person because of decreased activity of the sebaceous glands. Dry skin and mucous membranes also are seen in persons who are dehydrated as water moves from the cells

TABLE 64-1 SKIN COLOR CHANGES

Physiology	Causative Conditions
REDNESS (ERYTHEMA)	
Vasodilation: more rapid blood flow, more oxygenated blood giving a reddish hue	Blushing, heat, inflammation, fever, alcohol ingestion, extreme cold (below 15° F [−9° C]), hot flushes, polycythemia
WHITENESS (PALLOR)	
Vasoconstriction: slower blood flow, less blood in capillaries	Cold, fear, shock
Partially obstructed blood flow: less blood in capillaries	Vasospasm, thrombus, narrowed vessels, arterial insufficiency
Fluid between blood vessels and skin surface	Edema
Decreased oxygenation of blood from decreased hemoglobin	Anemia
Loss of melanin	Vitiligo
BLUISH (CYANOSIS)	
Deoxygenated hemoglobin seen in earlobes, lips, mucous membranes of mouth, nail beds	Heart or lung disease, inadequate respiration, peripheral blood vessel obstruction, venous disease, cold, anxiety
YELLOW (JAUNDICE)	
Increased bile pigment in blood eventually distributed to skin and mucous membranes and to sclerae of eyes	Liver disease, obstruction of bile ducts, chronic uremia, rapid hemolysis
BROWN	
Increased melanin deposits: normal in brown-black races	Aging; sunburn; anterior pituitary, adrenal cortex, or liver disease
DULLNESS	
Vasoconstriction in dark skin	Cold, fear, shock
Partially obstructed blood flow in dark skin	Vasospasm, thrombus, narrowed vessels, arterial insufficiency
Fluid between blood vessels and skin surface in dark skin	Edema

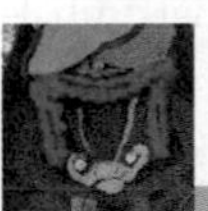

GUIDELINES FOR SAFE PRACTICE *Assessment of Dark Skin*

- Check skin color in areas of least pigmentation: sclerae, conjunctivae, buccal mucosa, tongue, lips, nail beds, palms, and soles.
- Palpate as well as inspect, especially if inflammation or edema is suspected.
- Correlate findings with the patient's history.
- Remember that pallor in brown-skinned patients may be seen as a yellowish brown tinge to the skin and in black-skinned patients as ashen gray because of the absence of underlying red tones in the skin.
- Check for cyanosis by inspecting the nail beds, lips, palpebral conjunctiva, earlobes, palms, and soles. Compare to baseline color whenever possible.
- Observe for jaundice in that portion of the sclera that is observable when the eye is open. Since fatty deposits containing carotene, which give the sclerae a yellow appearance, are common in dark-skinned individuals, also observe the posterior portion of the hard palate. Do this in bright daylight for best discrimination of color.
- Assess for edema by observing for areas of the skin that appear lighter in color; edema reduces the intensity of color because of the increased distance between the external epithelium and the pigmented layers. Palpate for a "tight" feeling to the skin.
- Observe for petechiae over areas of lighter pigmentation such as the abdomen, gluteal areas, volar aspect of the forearm, palpebral conjunctiva, and buccal mucosa.
- Differentiate petechiae and ecchymoses from erythema by exerting pressure over the affected area and observing for color change. Erythema will blanch, but petechiae and ecchymoses remain unchanged.
- Assess rashes by palpating for changes in skin texture.
- Remember the oral mucosa, including the gums, borders of the tongue, and lining of the cheeks, of dark-skinned individuals may have a normal freckling. Also the gingivae normally may have either a blotchy or evenly distributed dark blue color.

into the intravascular compartments. Persons with hypothyroidism have thick, dry, leathery skin.

Moist-feeling skin is caused by sweat or water on the surface. Overheating produces sweating with the amount differing from one person to another depending on the effectiveness of the sweating mechanism. Thus persons with hyperthyroidism have moist, smooth skin. Stressors, shock, or any situation that stimulates the sympathetic nervous system causes increased fluid loss through the sweat glands (diaphoresis), resulting in water on the skin. Because vasoconstriction occurs simultaneously with stimulation of the sympathetic nervous system, the skin is cold and wet (clammy).

Oily skin is frequently encountered at puberty. Excess sebum formation by the sebaceous glands may lead to blocking of the follicular orifices, resulting acne lesions and sebaceous cysts.

Elasticity, Mobility, and Turgor. The skin is highly elastic and moves freely over most areas. It loses its mobility when it becomes stretched; this occurs with edema, when the interstitial spaces become filled with fluid. Skin becomes rigid in the person with scleroderma, a collagen disease, as a result of collagenous fibrosis of the tissue. **Turgor** is tissue tension and is measured by the speed of the skin's return to a normal position of fullness after it has been stretched. Decreased skin turgor is a normal assessment finding in older persons. In others, decreased turgor indicates dehydration of the tissue or extreme weight loss.

To assess elasticity and turgor, the nurse picks up a portion of skin over the sternum (elasticity) and assesses the speed of return to normal (turgor). Skin that has decreased turgor will remain for a few seconds in a fold ("tenting") before returning slowly to normal (Figure 64-3).To assess hydration status of an older patient, the nurse examines the mucous membranes.

Texture. The skin is normally soft and smooth with some roughening over exposed areas such as the elbows. The skin of older adults may be rough and lack underlying tissue substance (atrophy). Hypertrophic scarring, also known as keloid formation, is another example of a textural change in the skin.

Thickness. Normal skin is uniformly thin over most of the body except the palms and soles. A callus, or painless overgrowth of epidermis, may develop in these areas as a result of pressure or friction. Thickened skin over pressure sites like elbows and soles occurs with aging.

Odor. Clean skin is usually free of odor except for areas that contain the apocrine sweat glands. Odor occurs because of bacterial decomposition of protein matter. Some draining skin lesions may produce an odor.

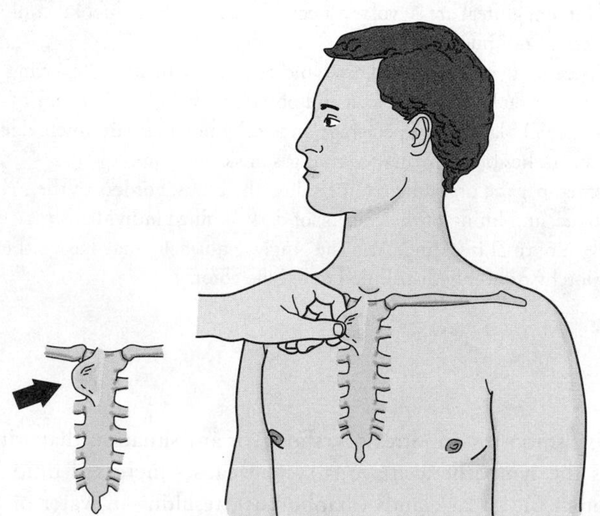

Figure 64-3 Examination of skin turgor. Tenting of skin over the sternum occurs with decreased skin turgor.

Accessory Structures

HAIR. Hair growth, pattern, and distribution can be an indicator of the person's general state of health.[5] Excessive hair growth (hypertrichosis) usually is related to heredity or hormonal changes. Hair loss (alopecia) occurs normally with age, especially in some men. Abnormal hair loss may be caused by hormonal imbalance (androgen excess), thyroid disease, general ill health, infections of the scalp, chronic liver disease, stressors, or drugs (e.g., chemotherapeutic agents or hormones). Hair loss on the dorsum of the toes may indicate decreased arterial circulation. The hair shaft is an inert structure, and changes occur over time as a result of hormonal activity and the availability of nutrients to the bulb at the base of the hair root.

When assessing hair, the nurse should note color, amount, pattern, distribution, and cleanliness of scalp and facial hair. If the patient is wearing a wig or other hairpiece, this should be removed temporarily for inspection of any remaining hair and the scalp. Because it is easy to miss lesions on the scalp, the nurse asks the patient to assist by indicating areas of itching, pain, or roughness.

The nurse also assesses hair for signs of infestation with the crab louse (pediculosis). Nits, the eggs of the lice, are found embedded on hair strands. They are observed as small, glistening, grayish specks along the hair shaft close to the scalp. Hair of dark-skinned individuals should be assessed for traumatic alopecia. This type of hair loss results because black hair shafts are highly susceptible to breakage from hair care practices such as tight hair curlers, cornrow braiding, hot combing, or the use of picks. Wetting or softening the hair before combing may help prevent trauma.

NAILS. Nails change with age and states of illness. Changes in nail plate texture may indicate metabolic disease, nutritional imbalances including vitamin deficiency, or digestive disturbance. Pale nail beds and poor capillary return (slow return to normal color after the nail is pinched) may indicate hypoxia or anemia. Capillary refill is normally less than 3 seconds. Clubbing of the nails refers to the elimination of the small concave portion at the base of the nail by soft tissue growth. Normally the angle between the nail base and the fingernail is approximately 160 degrees. Early clubbing is present when the angle increases to 180 degrees or more. The mechanism of clubbing is not understood, but occurs with certain diseases associated with chronic hypoxia (see Chapter 24).

The epithelial lining of the nail bed is usually inert. The nail is affixed to the nail bed, and both protrude outward as the nail grows. The epithelial lining of the nail bed can lose its inert quality in the presence of inflammatory processes such as those seen with psoriasis, chronic hand eczema, or fungal nail plate infections. When this occurs, the nail bed keratinizes and horny masses collect under the nail, resulting in deformity of the nail and possible separation from the nail bed.[7]

Paronychia, an infection of the tissue surrounding the nail, is characterized by red, shiny skin and painful swelling. The infection can be due to trauma or underlying skin disease. The usual infecting organisms are staphylococci, yeast, and molds. If the nail is lost, it usually will grow back unless the nail bed has been injured.[3]

Skin Lesions. When individual **lesions** or skin rashes are observed, the nurse describes them in terms of type, color, size, shape, configuration and arrangement, distribution, and texture. Primary lesions are visual or palpable changes in the structure of the skin unchanged by time or environment. Secondary lesions are those due to environmental influences or natural evolution, such as scratching, rubbing, infection, or therapy.

TYPE. Use of proper descriptive terminology by the nurse is essential for clear, accurate communication about skin lesions (Table 64-2). For example, the term *vesicle* provides a clear picture of a lesion that is clear, fluid-filled, and smaller than 1 cm. Figure 64-4 illustrates the most common types of lesions.

TABLE 64-2 TYPES OF SKIN LESIONS

Observed Skin Changes	Differentiation	Term	Example
CHANGE IN COLOR OR TEXTURE			
Spot	Circumscribed; flat; color change	Macule	Freckle
Discoloration (reddish purple)	Bleeding beneath surface; injury to tissue	Contusion	Bruise
Soft whitening	Caused by repeated wetting of skin	Maceration	Between toes after soaking
Flake	Dry cells of surface	Scale	Dandruff, psoriasis
Roughness from dried fluid	Dry exudates over lesions	Crust ("scab")	Eczema, impetigo
Roughness from cells	Leathery thickening of outer skin layer	Lichenification	Callus on foot
CHANGE IN SHAPE			
Fluid-filled lesions	Less than 1 cm; clear fluid	Vesicle	Blister; chickenpox
	Greater than 1 cm; clear fluid	Bulla	Large blister, pemphigus
	Small; thick, yellowish fluid (pus)	Pustule	Acne
Solid mass, cellular growth	Less than 1 cm	Papule	Small mole; raised rash
	1-2 cm	Nodule	Enlarged lymph node
	Greater than 2 cm	Tumor	Benign or malignant tumor
	Excess connective tissue over scar	Keloid	Overgrown scar
Swelling of tissue	Generalized swelling; fluid between cells	Edema	Inflammation; swelling of feet
	Circumscribed surface edema; transient; some itching	Wheal ("hive")	Allergic reaction
BREAKS IN SKIN SURFACES			
Oozing, scraped surface	Loss of superficial structure of skin	Abrasion	"Floor burn"; scrape
Scooped-out depression	Loss of deeper layers of skin	Ulcer	Pressure or stasis ulcer
Superficial linear skin breaks	Scratch marks, frequently by fingernails	Excoriations	Scratching
Linear cracks or cleft	Slit or splitting of skin layers	Fissure	Athlete's foot
Jagged cut	Tearing of skin surface	Laceration	Accidental cut by blunt object
Linear cut, edges approximated	Cutting by sharp instrument	Incision	Knife cut
VASCULAR LESIONS			
Small, flat, round, purplish red spot	Intradermal or submucosal hemorrhage	Petechia	Bleeding tendency, decreased platelets; vitamin C deficiency
Spider-like, red, small	Dilation of capillaries, arterioles, or venules	Telangiectasis	Liver disease, vitamin B deficiency
Discoloration, reddish purple	Escape of blood into tissue	Ecchymosis	Trauma to blood vessels

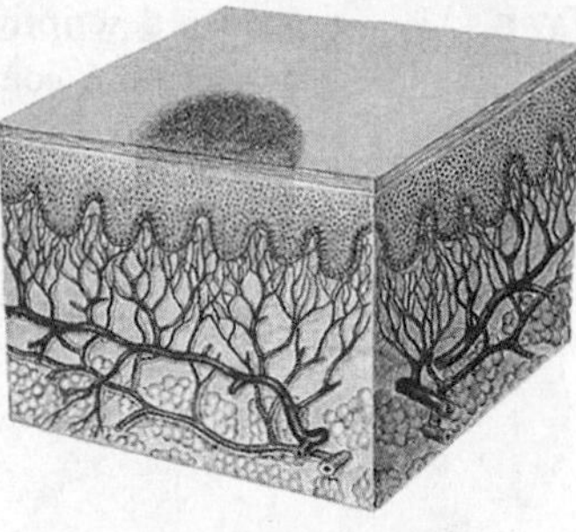

Macule—flat; nonpalpable; circumscribed; less than 1 cm in diameter; brown, red, purple, white, or tan
Examples: Freckles; flat moles; rubella; rubeola

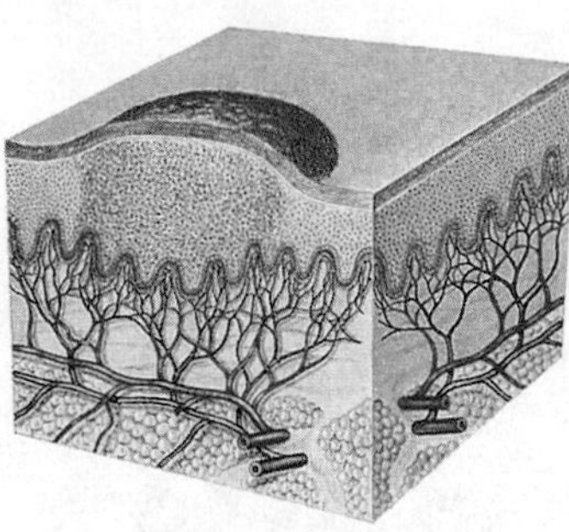

Papule—elevated; palpable; firm; circumscribed; less than 1 cm in diameter; brown, red, pink, tan, or bluish red
Examples: Warts; drug-related eruptions; pigmented nevi

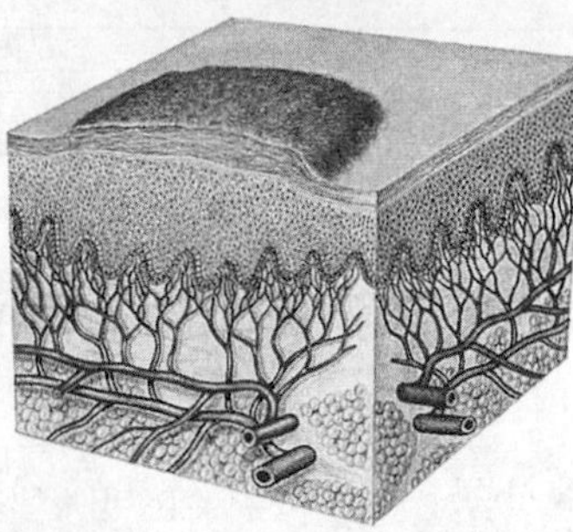

Plaque—elevated; flat topped; firm; rough; superficial papule greater than 1 cm in diameter; may be coalesced papules
Examples: Psoriasis; seborrheic and actinic keratoses

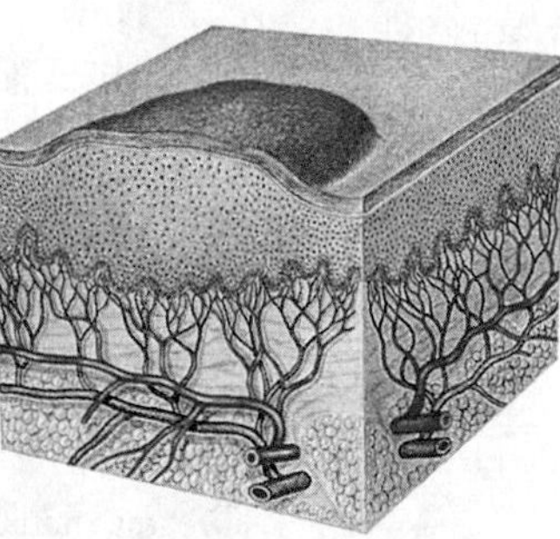

Wheal—elevated; irregular-shaped area of cutaneous edema; solid, transient, changing; variable diameter; pale pink with lighter center
Examples: Urticaria; insect bites

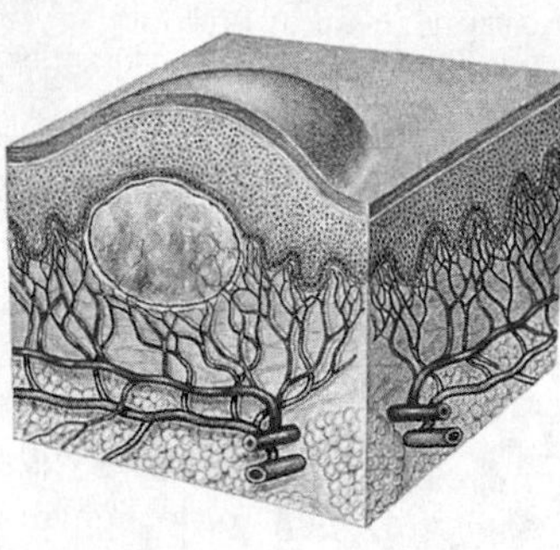

Nodule—elevated; firm; circumscribed; palpable; deeper in dermis than papule; 1 to 2 cm in diameter
Examples: Erythema nodosum; lipomas

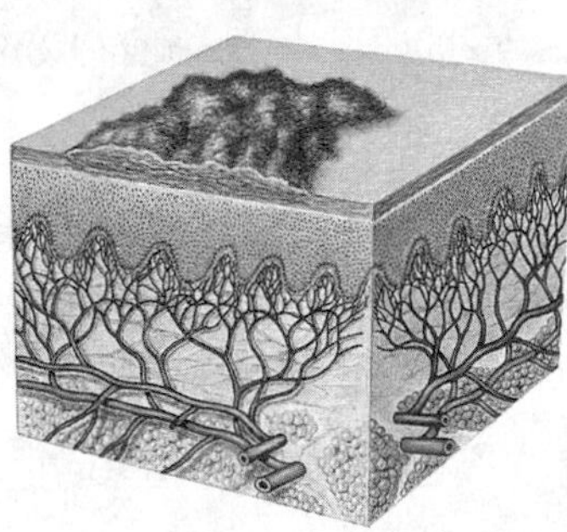

Crust—dried serum, blood, or purulent exudate; slightly elevated; size varies; brown, red, black, tan, or straw
Examples: Scab on abrasion; eczema

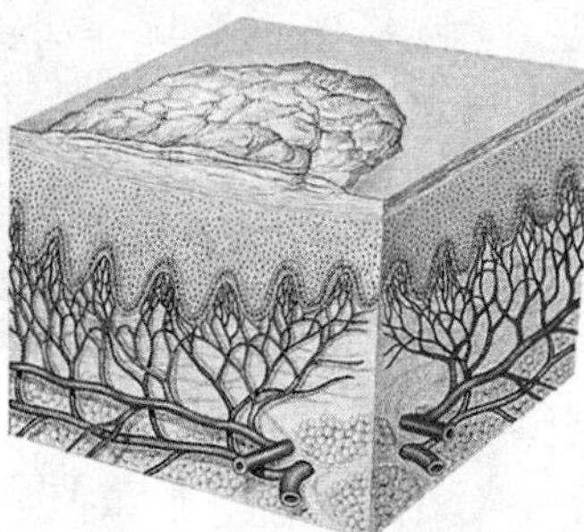

Scale—heaped-up keratinized cells; flaky exfoliation; irregular; thick or thin; dry or oily; varied size; silver, white, or tan
Examples: Psoriasis, exfoliative dermatitis

Figure 64-4 Common skin lesions.

Color. Lesions may be hypopigmented, of normal background pigmentation, or hyperpigmented. Thus they may vary from white to light tan to shades of brown and black. They may also be blue or red. Color helps identify whether the lesion may be secondary to an inflammatory process, infection, sun exposure, or heredity. For example, café-au-lait spots (French for coffee with milk) are congenital pale tan macules.[1]

Size. The metric system is used for measurement. If a metric ruler is not available, the size of a lesion can be estimated by measuring a portion of one's finger to use as a gauge. When lesions are round, the diameter is measured. Other shapes may require measuring length and width.

Shape and Demarcation. Shape describes the contour of a lesion. Examples include round, oval, polygonal (many sided), annular (ringlike), and asymmetric. Demarcation refers to the sharpness of the edge of the lesion, that is, whether it is discrete or diffuse.

Texture. The lesion is described as rough or smooth, dry or moist, and on the surface or deeply penetrating into the tissue. Alterations in texture may occur as a result of scarring. Keloids are firm, raised, shiny, hypertrophic scars that grow beyond the wound, often with clawlike projections. Although keloids are seen in all races, they are much more prevalent in the African-American population.[4] Highly susceptible areas for keloid growth include the sternum, mandible, ear, and neck.

BLANCHING. Some vascular lesions blanch when direct pressure is applied and then swiftly return to their original color once the pressure is alleviated. Skin lesions without a vascular component remain unchanged with pressure. The blanching test can be performed with a glass slide or a handheld magnifying lens.

CONFIGURATION. Configuration refers to the arrangement or pattern of lesions in relation to other lesions[1] (Figure 64-5). A discrete lesion is separate from other lesions. Groups of lesions may form clusters or may be arranged in a linear (following a line), polycyclic (annular or ringlike lesions growing together), confluent (merging together), or serpiginous or gyrate (serpentine) fashion. Disseminated refers to multiple scattered lesions diffusely distributed over the body.

DISTRIBUTION. Distribution takes into consideration both the arrangement of lesions over an area of skin and the pattern. Terms used to describe distribution include *discrete* (isolated), *localized*, *regional*, and *generalized*. Symmetric, exposed, intertriginous (skin fold), dermatomal (following spinal nerves path), and random are examples of patterns seen with common skin disorders such as eczema, yeast infections, and herpes zoster (shingles).

Normal skin assessment findings in adults and variations in older adults are found in Table 64-3. Assessment measures relevant to the care of older adults are presented in the Gerontologic Assessment box, p. 1872. Also identified are disorders common in older adults, which may be responsible for abnormal assessment findings.

▶ ARE You READY?

Which skin change is associated with heart or lung disease?

1. Erythema
2. Jaundice
3. Increased melanin
4. Cyanosis

Diagnostic Tests

Most skin disorders are diagnosed by careful physical assessment. However, diagnostic tests may be used when further information is required to confirm a diagnosis.

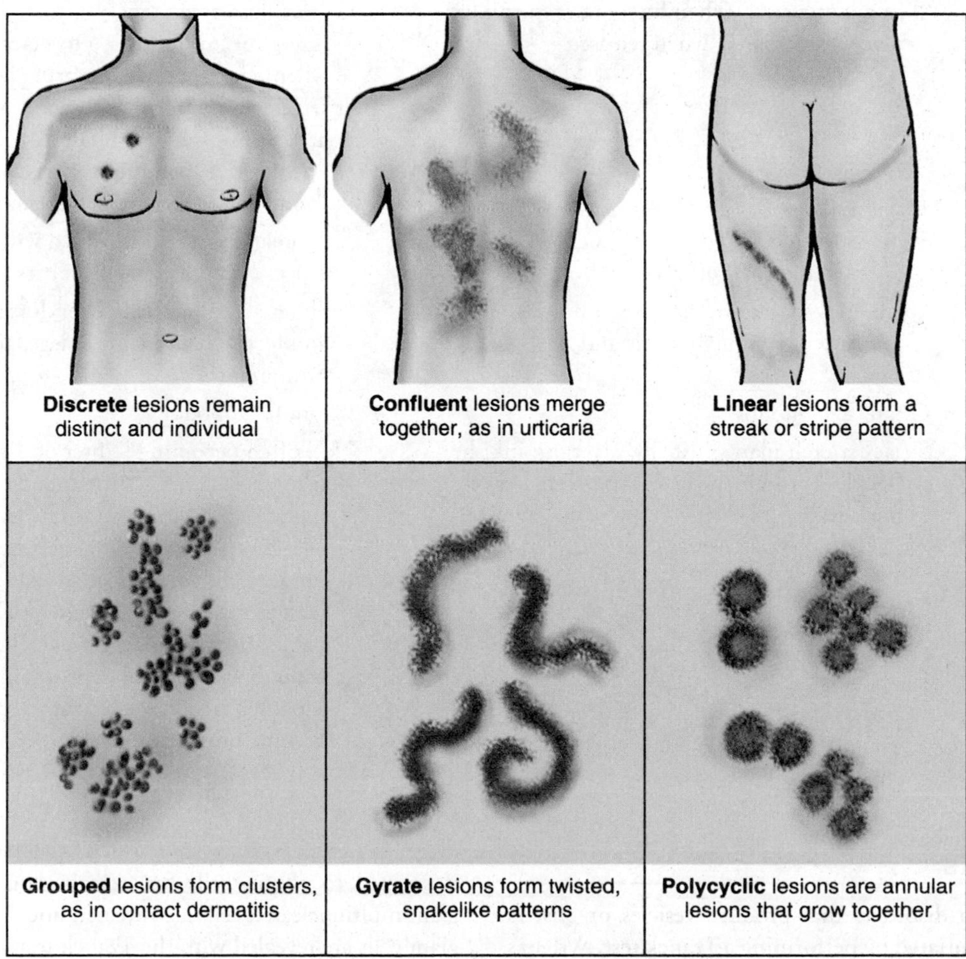

Discrete lesions remain distinct and individual
Confluent lesions merge together, as in urticaria
Linear lesions form a streak or stripe pattern
Grouped lesions form clusters, as in contact dermatitis
Gyrate lesions form twisted, snakelike patterns
Polycyclic lesions are annular lesions that grow together

Figure 64-5 Examples of arrangements or configurations of lesions.

TABLE 64-3 NORMAL SKIN FINDINGS IN ADULTS AND VARIATIONS IN OLDER ADULTS

Assessment Parameter	Normal Adult Findings	Variations in Older Adults
SKIN		
Color tone	Deep to light brown in African-Americans; whitish pink to ruddy with olive or yellow overtones in Caucasians	Skin of Caucasian persons generally paler and more opaque as compared to younger Caucasians
Pigmentation uniformity	Sun-darkened areas; areas of lighter pigmentation in dark-skinned persons (palms, lips, nail beds); labile pigmentation areas associated with use of hormones or pregnancy; callused areas appearing yellow; crinkled skin areas darker (knees and elbows); dark-skinned (Mediterranean origin) persons may have lips with bluish hue; vascular flush areas (cheeks, neck, upper chest, or genital area) may appear red, especially with excitement or anxiety; skin color masked through use of cosmetics or tanning agents	More freckles; uneven tanning; pigment deposits; hypopigmented patches
Surface temperature	Cool to warm	Cool to warm
Moisture	Minimal perspiration or oiliness felt; dampness in skin folds; increased perspiration associated with warm environment or activity; wet palms, scalp, forehead, and axilla associated with anxiety	Increased dryness, especially of extremities; decreased perspiration; changes often hard for patient to accept
Elasticity, mobility, turgor	Skin moving easily when lifted and returning to place immediately when released	General loss of elasticity; skin moving easily when lifted but not returning to place immediately when released; skin appearing lax; increased wrinkle pattern more marked in sun-exposed areas, in patients with fair skin, and in expressive areas of face; pendulous parts sagging or drooping (under chin, earlobes, breasts, and scrotum)
Texture	Smooth, even, soft; some roughness on exposed areas (elbows and soles of feet)	Flaking and scaling associated with dry skin, especially on lower extremities
Thickness	Wide body variation; increased thickness in areas of pressure or rubbing (hands and feet)	Thinner skin, especially over dorsal surface of hands and feet, forearms, lower legs, and bony prominences
Hygiene	Clean, free of odor	Clean, free of odor
Lesions	Striae (stretch marks) usually silver or pinkish; freckles (prominent in sun-exposed areas); some birthmarks	Nevi often becoming lighter or disappearing; seborrheic keratoses (pigmented, raised, warty, slightly greasy lesions most often found on truck or face); senile (actinic) keratoses on exposed surfaces, first seen as small reddened areas and then as raised, rough, yellow to brown lesions; senile sebaceous adenomas (yellowish flattened papules with central depressions); cherry adenomas (tiny, bright, ruby red, round; may become brown with age)

Laboratory Tests

Tzanck Test. Skin disorders that produce vesicles or blisters can be further differentiated by performing a Tzanck test. Wright's or Giemsa stain is used to perform the prep. The vesicle is unroofed with a cotton swab or blade, and the base of the vesicle is scraped to obtain cells for examination.[2] With herpesvirus, giant multinucleated cells are revealed under the microscope.[4] No giant cells are revealed with the Tzanck test with other skin disorders that can produce vesicles such as poison ivy (allergic contact dermatitis).

TABLE 64-3 NORMAL SKIN FINDINGS IN ADULTS AND VARIATIONS IN OLDER ADULTS—CONT'D

Assessment Parameter	Normal Adult Findings	Variations in Older Adults
NAILS		
Configuration	Nail edges smooth and rounded; nail base angle 160 degrees; nail surface flat or slightly curved	Toenails often thickened and distorted with increased linear grooves or ridges
Consistency	Smooth, hard surface; uniform thickness	Fingernails more brittle or peeling; accentuated longitudinal lines
Color	Variations of pink; pigment deposits in nail beds of dark-skinned individuals	Toenails losing translucence and luster and becoming yellow
Adherence to nail bed	Nail base feels firm when palpated	Nail base feels firm when palpated
HAIR		
Surface characteristics	Scalp smooth; hair shiny; vellus hair short, fine, inconspicuous, and unpigmented; terminal hair coarser, thicker, more conspicuous, and usually pigmented	Sebaceous hyperplasia extending into scalp
Distribution and configuration	"Normal" varied with individual; hair present on scalp, lower face, nares, ears, axillae, anterior chest around nipples, arms, legs, back, buttocks; female pubic configuration forms inverted triangle; hairline may extend up linea alba; male pubic configuration forms upright triangle with hair extending up linea alba to umbilicus	Increased facial hair (especially in women); bristly quality; men often with coarse hair in ears, nose, and eyebrows; decreased scalp hair, symmetric balding in men (most often frontal or occipital); decreased pubic and axillary hair
Texture	Scalp hair fine or coarse; fine vellus hair over body; coarse terminal hair in pubic and axillary areas	Facial hair coarse; body hair fine
Color	Wide variation from pale blond to black; color possibly masked or changed with rinses or dyes	Graying or whitening; hairs that do not lose pigment often becoming darker; color possibly masked or changed with rinses or dyes
Quantity	"Normal" varied with individuals; gradual symmetric balding of scalp hair in some men	General decrease of body and scalp hair

Modified from Thompson JM et al: *Mosby's manual of clinical nursing,* ed 2, St Louis, 1989, Mosby; and Borners A, Thompson J: *Clinical manual of health assessment,* St Louis, 1984, Mosby.

Potassium Hydroxide Prep Test. If a fungal infection is suspected, the potassium hydroxide (KOH) test will assist in the identification of fungal forms. Dry scale is scraped from the lesion onto a slide using a No. 15 blade, glass slide, or cover slip. One or two drops of 20% KOH are placed onto the slide and gently heated. Examination under the microscope reveals hyphae and spores.

Culture. Gram stain and culture and sensitivity testing of weeping or pustular lesions can be performed to rule in or out bacterial sources of infection. Streptococci and staphylococci are the most common organisms responsible for producing skin infections. Wound cultures are easily obtained using a cotton swab or culture media and swabbing the exudates from the lesion surface.

Special Tests

Skin Biopsy. Samples of skin lesions may be obtained for examination of the cells of the epidermis, dermis, and subcutaneous tissue. Biopsies can be performed by shave technique (does not require sutures); punch, using a circular cutting instrument (sutures optional); and excisional biopsy where a full-thickness specimen is often removed for diagnosing skin cancers (requires sutures). Before a skin biopsy the skin is anesthetized with an **intradermal** injection of lidocaine (Xylocaine). Bleeding can be managed with sutures, electrodessication, or topical hemostatic agents.[2]

Patch Testing. Patch testing is used to both identify and document the causative agent in allergic contact dermatitis and is sometimes helpful in screening when a secondary change takes place on a preexisting rash. Standard concentration samples of suspected allergens are applied to the skin. Minute quantities of the products are placed under an occlusive dressing on the forearms or upper portion of the back. The patches are removed 48 hours after application, and the sites are assessed for swelling or vesicle formation. Because delayed reactions are possible, sites should be reevaluated in 72 hours or up to 1 week.

Wood's Lamp. A handheld ultraviolet A Wood's lamp may be used to assist in the diagnosis of certain fungal infections affecting

Gerontologic Assessment

- Assess color; pigmentation uniformity; temperature; moisture; texture; thickness; and turgor, elasticity, and mobility of the skin.
  - –Normal age-related changes occur in all these assessment components (see Table 64-3).
  - –Inspect skin for intactness, infections, and lesions.
  - –The thin, dry skin characteristic of older adults predisposes them to skin breakdown. Once breakdown occurs, there is increased risk of infection because of the decreased immune response of the older adult. A number of skin lesions, both benign and malignant, occur with significantly increasing frequency among older adults.
- Assess risk of medication-related photosensitivity. Obtain a complete list of medications used, including over-the-counter preparations, and review for preparations that can cause an enhanced response to sunlight.
  - –Many medications taken by older adults can cause hypersensitivity. Among these are thiazide diuretics, tetracyclines, sulfa drugs, and certain psychotropics.

Common Disorders in Older Adults

Dry skin changes (xerosis)
Stasis dermatitis of the lower extremities
Benign skin tumors: cherry angiomas, spider veins, skin tags, and seborrheic keratoses
Skin cancer: basal cell carcinoma, squamous cell carcinoma, and melanoma
Drug reactions
Herpes zoster
Rosacea
Seborrheic dermatitis

the scalp and body. Certain species of fungi fluoresce bright blue, green, or gold when illuminated by the lamp.

▶ ARE You READY?

Which diagnostic test is indicated for a patient with a suspected fungal infection of the skin?

1. Patch testing
2. Potassium hydroxide prep test
3. Gram stain and culture
4. Tzanck test

References

1. Anderson DN: *Mosby's medical, nursing, and allied health dictionary,* ed 6, St Louis, 2002, Mosby.
2. Dermatology Nurses' Association: *Dermatology nursing basics: core proceeding book from annual convention,* Linden, NJ, 2004, Anthony J Janetti.
3. Fitzpatrick TB et al: *Color atlas and synopsis of clinical dermatology,* ed 4, New York, 2001, McGraw-Hill.
4. Habif T: *Clinical dermatology: a color guide to diagnosis and therapy,* ed 4, St Louis, 2003, Mosby.
5. Hill M, editor: *Dermatology nursing essentials: a core curriculum,* ed 2, Pitman, NJ, 2003, Dermatology Nurses' Association.
6. Leasia MS, Monahan FD: *A practical guide to health assessment,* ed 2, Philadelphia, 2001, Saunders.
7. Seidel HM et al: *Mosby's guide to physical examination,* ed 5, St Louis, 2003, Mosby.

Visit the Evolve website: http://evolve.elsevier.com/Monahan/medsurg

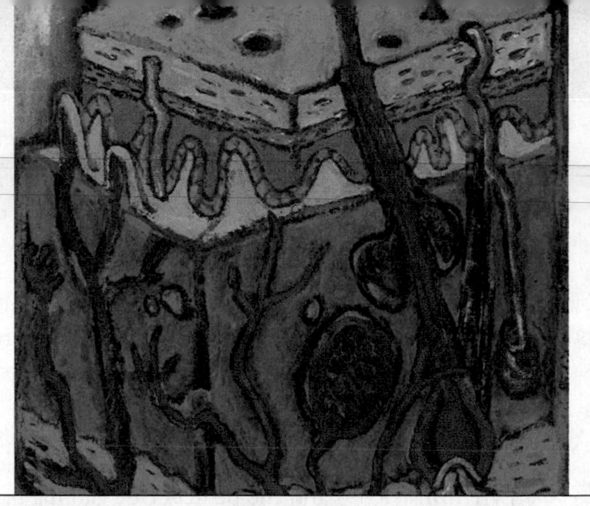

CHAPTER 65
Problems of the Skin

by Marianne C. Tawa, Sharon A. Aronovitch

OBJECTIVES

After studying this chapter, the learner should be able to:

1. Describe general nursing interventions for patients with dermatologic disorders.
2. Discuss the psychologic effects of dermatologic problems.
3. Explain the pathogenesis, physical examination features, and therapeutic interventions for fungal, viral, and bacterial infections of the skin.
4. Describe collaborative care management strategies for patients with follicular disorders.
5. Discuss preventive measures and interventions for eczematous dermatitis and psoriasis.
6. Identify skin manifestations that may result from systemic disease.
7. List skin cancer risk factors and identifying features for premalignant versus malignant lesions.
8. Explain preventive and early intervention measures for pressure ulcers.
9. Develop an individualized nursing care plan for the patient with a pressure ulcer.

KEY TERMS

autoinoculation, p. 1879
cellular immunity, p. 1876
dermatomes, p. 1880
hypersensitivity immune reaction, p. 1882
immunomodulators, p. 1885
immunosuppressed, p. 1875
intertriginous, p. 1877
photosensitivity, p. 1886
plaques, p. 1874

Skin disorders are extremely common in the general population. Often patients complain about a rash, itching, or a worrisome lesion. Other times, it is the health care provider assessing the skin who identifies an abnormal finding. Many skin disorders are chronic and require frequent intervention and costly topical therapies. This chapter discusses common dermatologic conditions, including their epidemiology, pathophysiology, and collaborative care management strategies.

Infestations
Pediculosis

Etiology and Epidemiology. Three types of lice infest humans: the head louse, the body louse, and the pubic louse. Pediculosis (lice infestation) is often found among populations who live in overcrowded dwellings with inadequate hygiene facilities. It is also common in children, many of whom acquire head lice in their day care and classroom environments.

Pathophysiology. Lice obtain their nutrition by sucking blood from the skin. The head louse *(Pediculus humanus capitis)* attaches itself to the hair shaft and lays about eight eggs a day. The eggs are firmly attached to the hair or threads of clothing and hatch in 1 week. Head lice, when viewed with a hand lens or flashlight, appear as grayish, glistening oval bodies.[12] The head louse is usually confined to the scalp and beard. Transmission of head lice occurs through direct person-to-person contact and also through use of an infected person's hats, brushes, or combs.

The body louse *(Pediculus humanus corporis)* resides chiefly in the seams of clothing around the neck, waist, and thighs. The bite causes minute hemorrhagic points and severe itching. Transmission is by direct body-to-body contact or by shared clothing and linens.

The pubic louse *(Phthirus pubis)* differs slightly from the head and body louse. It resembles a tiny crab, having clawlike pincers that attach firmly to the pubic hair. Nits are visible in the pubic hair. *P. pubis* is transmitted by sexual contact, bed clothing, towels, and occasionally toilet seats. Patients with pediculosis experience itching, particularly at night, and can have hivelike papules and

plaques distributed randomly on the trunk and extremities. Frequent scratching of the scalp or other areas may result in skin breakdown, secondary bacterial infections, and enlarged cervical lymph nodes.

Collaborative Care Management. Diagnosis is made through inspection of the appropriate body part. A magnifying glass may be helpful for visualizing the nits attached to the hair shaft.

Treatment of pediculosis consists of topical application of a pediculicide such as 1% permethrin (Nix or Elimite lotion). Pyrethrins (RID) and the pediculicide gamma benzene hexachloride (1% lindane, Kwell shampoo) are used as second- and third-line treatment options. When pyrethrin products or lindane is used, a second application in 7 to 10 days may be necessary. Directions for both application and duration of treatment time differ according to the product and body location. Pediculicides are not used on eyebrows or eyelashes because of potential eye irritation or sensitization. If eyelashes are infested, nits are removed and petrolatum jelly is applied to smother the lice.

Patient/Family Teaching. The focus of nursing care is to identify infected persons and educate them about the cause of pediculosis and prevention of its spread. Patients are instructed on the proper application of the pediculicide. Lindane is contraindicated in pregnant and lactating women, as well as newborns. The nurse instructs persons with head lice to soak combs, brushes, and hair utensils in hot water and to launder clothing and bedding in the hot water cycle. Contacts should be evaluated for infestation and treated if necessary.

Scabies

Etiology and Epidemiology. Scabies is caused by the female mite *(Sarcoptes scabiei)*. Scabies infestations occur in all age-groups, races, and socioeconomic classes. Residential communities, shelters, college dormitories, and other crowded living environments are conducive to mite transmission.[10] Close skin-to-skin contact is the typical transmission route, although the mite can live for 2 days on clothing or bedding.

Pathophysiology. The female itch mite penetrates the stratum corneum and burrows into the skin. Within several hours of skin penetration, the itch mite lays a large number of eggs and deposits fecal pellets. The larvae mature in 10 to 14 days and move to the skin surface, where the females are impregnated; the cycle then repeats itself. The incubation period varies, but often a long period elapses before symptoms are noted. Delayed hypersensitivity is thought to be a major factor in the lapse between infestation and symptoms. The incubation period in persons with no previous exposure is 4 to 6 weeks.

The classic symptom for scabies infestation is intense itching, particularly at night. It is thought to be secondary to an immune response to the mite. Initial skin assessment may reveal threadlike linear or serpiginous gray-brown burrows, which are less than 1 mm wide. Later, papules, hivelike plaques, and nodules may be noted on physical examination. Lesions tend to be concentrated in the web spaces of the fingers and around the wrists, axillae, breasts, waist, thighs, lower buttocks, and genitalia (Figures 65-1 and 65-2). The head and neck are rarely involved. Secondary infections with excoriations and pustules may result from repeated scratching.

Collaborative Care Management. Diagnosis is based on identification of the itch mite under the microscope. The mite is removed from the end of a burrow with a pointed scalpel blade, or the entire burrow is sliced off, placed on a slide with glycerol or mineral oil, and examined under a microscope. If the burrows are not yet visible, mineral oil may be applied to the skin to aid in identification of the burrows.

The goals of therapy are elimination of the itch mite and treatment of complications. To eliminate the mite, the patient and close contacts are treated in one of two ways:

- Permethrin: applied at bedtime head to toe, including under nails; showered off in 8 hours; treatment repeated in 14 days if symptoms persist
- Gamma benzene hexachloride: applied at bedtime in a thin layer over the entire body from neck down; washed off in 8 to 12 hours; treatment repeated in 1 week only if living mite identified

For postscabitic itching and dermatitis, low-potency topical corticosteroids are applied twice a day for 1 to 2 weeks. Secondary infections are treated with topical or systemic antibiotics.

Because scabies is easily transmitted between individuals and groups, close contacts need to be identified and treated for infestation even in the absence of symptoms. Some patients experience shame and guilt when they learn the diagnosis; a nonjudgmental attitude with explanations of methods of control may help these patients cope with their feelings.

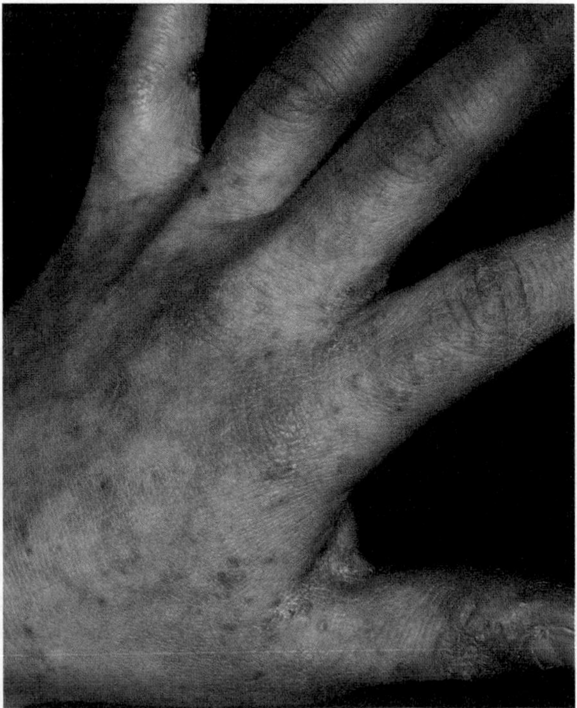

Figure 65-1 Scabies. Tiny vesicles and papules in finger webs and back of hand.

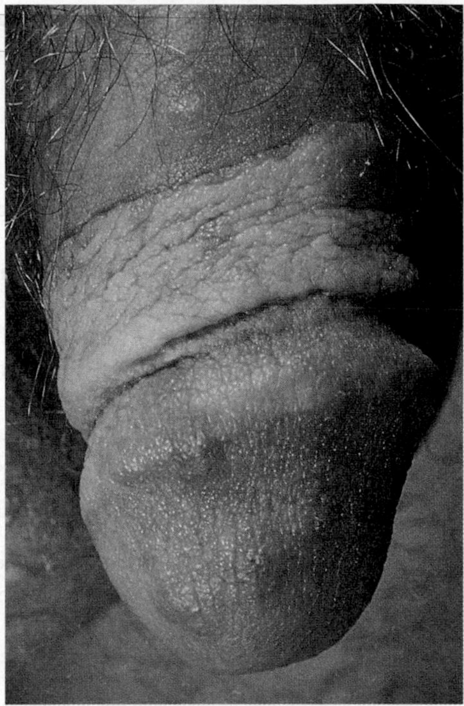

A

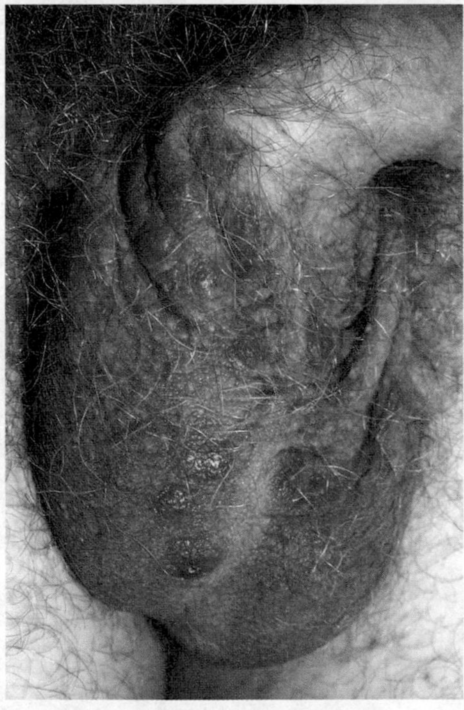

B

Figure 65-2 **A,** Eroded papules on glans are highly characteristic sign of scabies. **B,** Established infestation of penis and scrotum. Large papules may remain after appropriate therapy and sometimes require treatment with intralesional steroids.

PATIENT/FAMILY TEACHING. Teaching for the patient with scabies includes the following:

- All family members and close physical contacts should be treated simultaneously, whether or not symptoms are present.
- Detailed directions for application of the prescribed scabicide should be given.
- Underclothing and linens should be washed in hot water on the day of treatment and dried in the dryer or ironed when dry; clothing and bedding that cannot be laundered need to be placed in plastic bags for several weeks to avoid reinfestation.
- Symptoms of itching may persist for up to 2 weeks after treatment.

Fungal Infections

Fungi are larger and more complex than bacteria. They may be unicellular, such as yeasts, or multicellular, such as molds. Many types are pathogenic to humans, causing common skin disorders such as tinea corporis *(ringworm)* or more serious systemic diseases such as blastomycosis. Certain types of fungi produce minor symptoms, whereas others produce significant inflammatory or hypersensitivity reactions.

Candidiasis

Etiology and Epidemiology. *Candida albicans,* a yeastlike fungus, normally inhabits the gastrointestinal tract, mouth, and vagina, but not usually the skin. Candidiasis (moniliasis) is the inflammatory infection caused by the organism's overgrowth on the skin or membrane. Factors contributing to overgrowth of *C. albicans* include pregnancy, oral contraceptives, inhaled corticosteroids, poor nutrition, antibiotic therapy, diabetes mellitus and other endocrine diseases, and **immunosuppressed** states.

Pathophysiology. Candidiasis involving the mucosa of the mouth is called thrush. The lesions appear as white milk curd–like plaques on the buccal mucosa and may extend down the esophagus. Oral candidiasis can be painful, with symptoms of burning and dysphagia. Vaginal candidiasis produces local mucosal inflammation and thick, white vaginal discharge. Skin infection with the *Candida* organism favors the warm, moist areas created by occlusive body folds of the breasts, groin, and intergluteal region. Moist, macerated patches with vesicles and pustules can produce pruritus and burning. A classic clinical sign of candidiasis is the presence of satellite lesions at the periphery of the general inflammation (Figures 65-3 and 65-4).

Collaborative Care Management. Diagnosis of candidiasis is based on history, clinical features, and microscopic examination. Treatment is aimed at eliminating predisposing factors. Other measures include keeping the skin dry to avoid maceration and wearing loose, absorbent clothing. Powders may lessen skin fold rubbing. Nystatin (Mycostatin), clotrimazole (Lotrimin, Mycelex), ciclopirox (Loprox), ketoconazole (Nizoral), itraconazole (Sporanox), and fluconazole (Diflucan) are all effective against the organism.

PATIENT/FAMILY TEACHING. The primary focus of patient teaching is prevention. The nurse explains the need to eliminate warm, moist environments that support the growth of the organisms. The importance of thorough drying after bathing is stressed. A second focus is early detection. Patients are taught to carefully assess mucous membranes and skin folds. Immunosuppressed patients may take an oral antifungal medication long term. Medication

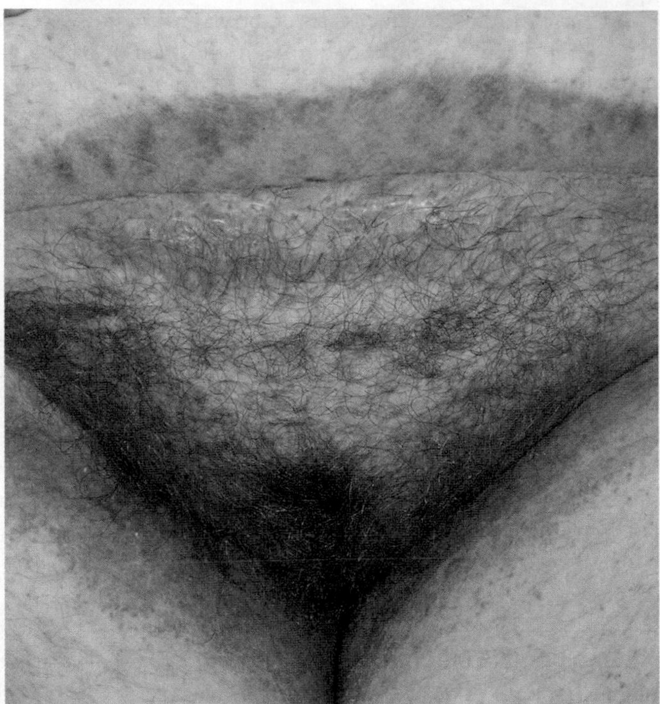

Figure 65-3 Candidal intertrigo. Overhanging abdominal fold and groin area are infected in this obese patient.

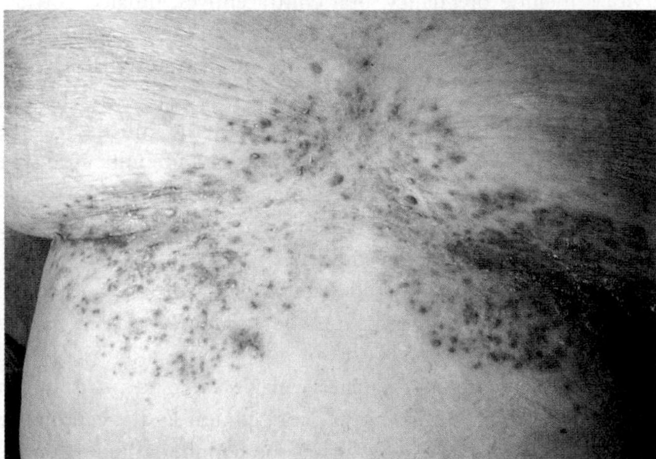

Figure 65-4 Candidiasis under breast. There are several moist, red papules with a fringe of white scale.

teaching is critical, with an emphasis on method of administration, side effect profile, and compliance.

Dermatophyte or Tinea Infections

Dermatophyte infections occur on nonviable keratinized skin, hair, and nails. Tineas represent a distinct class of fungi both botanically and pathologically. Acquisition is from soil, animal, or human contacts. The incidence of infection is low because of host **cellular immunity**. The usual fungi causing infection are *Microsporum*, *Trichophyton*, and *Epidermophyton* organisms. Diagnosis of a dermatophyte infection is made by clinical history and physical examination along with microscopy. The variants are named for the location of the rash: tinea capitis, tinea corporis, tinea cruris, tinea pedis, and tinea unguium.

Tinea Capitis

Etiology and Epidemiology. Tinea capitis (scalp) infection is transmitted readily person to person, especially in crowded conditions. Minor scalp trauma facilitates implantation of the spores. Tinea capitis has a worldwide distribution, primarily among prepubertal children.

Pathophysiology. The characteristic rash is erythematous and scaly, with pustules appearing at the edge of the lesion (Figure 65-5, *A*). Hair loss *(black dot alopecia)* occurs, with the hair shaft broken off at the base of the scalp. Hair loss is temporary, and the lesions usually heal without scarring. Tinea capitis is usually noninflammatory, but a purulent, boggy progression into *kerion* may develop. In certain situations infected hairs placed under a Wood's light will fluoresce a blue-green color.

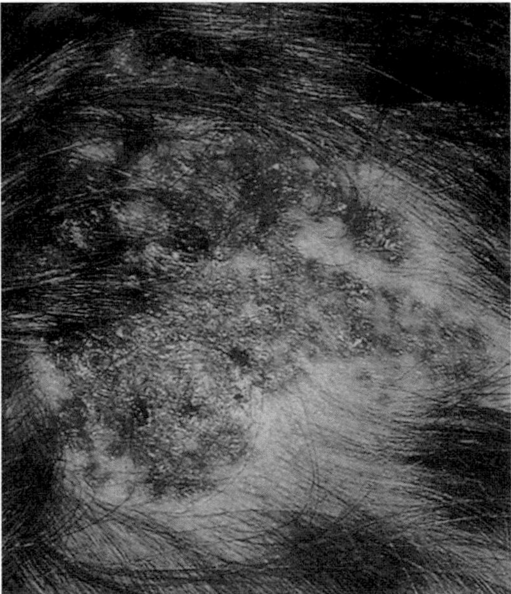

A

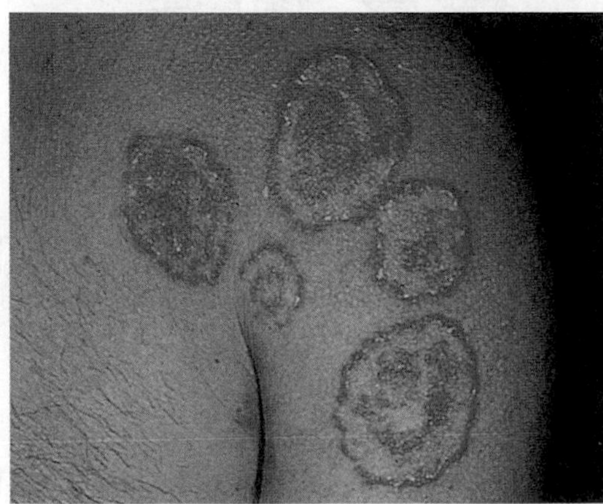

B

Figure 65-5 **A,** Tinea capitis. **B,** Tinea corporis.

Collaborative Care Management. Griseofulvin (Grisactin, Fulvicin, Gris-PEG), an antifungal antibiotic, is effective in the treatment of tinea capitis, particularly when high-fat meals are ingested to aid in absorption. However, many drug-drug interactions are associated with this medication so it is not always suitable for adults. Another oral antifungal agent choice is itraconazole (Sporanox). This triazole antifungal agent is broad spectrum, but also has many drug interactions. Topical antifungal agents may be used to treat mild infection.

PATIENT/FAMILY TEACHING. Patient teaching focuses on helping the patient and family understand the treatment regimen. The scalp should be shampooed at least twice a week. Cutting the hair short facilitates shampooing but may cause psychologic trauma for some children; therefore the hair is best left at an acceptable length.

Tinea Corporis and Tinea Cruris

Etiology and Epidemiology. Tinea corporis (colloquially called *ringworm*) is a common pediatric infection, but can occur in adults, particularly those residing with infected persons. Dermatophytes favor hot, humid environments. Tinea cruris (commonly referred to as *jock itch*) occurs most frequently in males; especially those who wear occlusive athletic wear or participate in cycling.

Pathophysiology. Tinea corporis typically appears on the nonhairy, exposed parts of the body as ring-shaped plaques, with erythematous scaling borders and central clearing (Figure 65-5, *B*). Lesions of tinea cruris occur in the warm, moist, **intertriginous** areas of the groin. The lesions are bilateral and extend outward from the groin along the inner thigh. The color ranges from brown to red, scaling is absent, and pruritus is usually present.

Collaborative Care Management. Mild infections are treated with topical antifungal agents.

PATIENT/FAMILY TEACHING. Dermatophytes thrive in moist, warm environments; therefore the nurse instructs patients to keep the affected areas clean and dry, use a bland dusting powder to promote dryness, and wear loose underclothing.

Tinea Pedis

Etiology and Epidemiology. The most common dermatophyte infection is tinea pedis, or *athlete's foot.* Tinea pedis is rarely seen in children or women but is widespread among young men, especially those wearing athletic shoes in hot environments. Walking barefoot in gymnasiums or around swimming pools does not necessarily lead to a tinea infection; moreover, susceptible persons will acquire it regardless of their activities.

Pathophysiology. The most common form of tinea pedis is the intertriginous form. The fungal involvement usually begins in the toe webs, especially in the fourth interspace, and may extend to the undersurface of the toes or onto the plantar surface. The person may be asymptomatic or may experience itching and burning in the affected area. The nail plate may become discolored, thickened, or distorted *(onychomycosis).* Tinea pedis is often confused with other foot eruptions, such as eczematous dermatitis, contact dermatitis, or psoriasis.

Collaborative Care Management. Treatment of tinea pedis is the topical application of antifungal agents. Twice daily application of the medication for at least 1 month is critical, since relapse is common. When thick, chronic, scaling plaques are evident, keratolytic agents such as lactic or glycolic acid moisturizers can help decrease scale accumulation. If the eruption becomes acutely inflamed with vesicles and bullae, soaks with Domeboro solution (aluminum acetate) followed by application of a topical antifungal may be used. Systemic antifungal agents are used when the infection proves unresponsive to topical therapy. Nail plate infections generally require systemic antifungal agents, since the densely packed keratin of the nail does not permit adequate absorption of topical agents.

PATIENT/FAMILY TEACHING. Patients with tinea infections are taught meticulous foot and nail care. They are also advised to wear socks made of an absorbent material, such as cotton, and to change them more than once a day. Wearing sandals or going barefoot is an additional way to decrease moistness of the feet and toes.

Bacterial Infections

Skin infections may result from loss of skin integrity or from altered host resistance. Minute perforations in the stratum corneum of the epidermis permit entry of microorganisms. Most bacteria that normally inhabit the skin are nonpathogenic. Pathogenic bacteria such as *Staphylococcus aureus* and *Streptococcus pyogenes* can penetrate the outer skin layer, causing the superficial skin infections impetigo and folliculitis.

Impetigo

Etiology and Epidemiology. Impetigo is a common, contagious, superficial skin infection caused by beta-hemolytic streptococci or *S. aureus.* The presence of *S. aureus* in the nares predisposes certain patients to impetigo. Although impetigo may occur in any age-group, children are most often affected. Impetigo occurs more commonly in the summer or early fall. The exposed surfaces of the face, arms, and legs are the most common locations for infection. Factors that promote development of impetigo include tropical climates, poor hygiene, poor nutrition, and compromised health. Other than the characteristic lesion, few symptoms are associated with this infection.

Pathophysiology. Streptococcal impetigo begins as a small, thin-walled vesicle that ruptures easily and leaves a weeping, denuded spot. It becomes pustular and dries to form a honey-colored crust that appears stuck on the skin (Figure 65-6). The process, which is superficial, may extend below the crust. Smaller vesicles that enlarge into bullae, rupture, and form shallow erosions characterize staphylococcal impetigo. If untreated, impetigo may last for several weeks with new lesions forming.

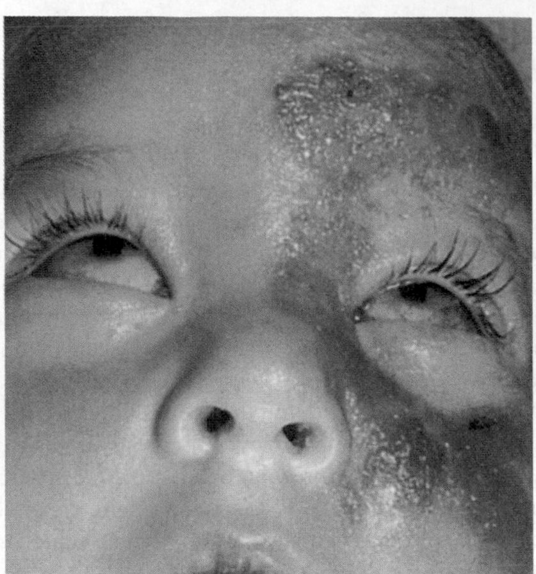

Figure 65-6 Impetigo. Note characteristic crusting.

Collaborative Care Management. Treatment consists of rigorous topical hygiene. Antimicrobial soaps and washes may be used to decrease the bacteria on the skin. Crusts must be removed and the lesions washed gently two or three times a day to prevent further crust formation. Warm soaks or saline compresses may be necessary to soften crusts that adhere firmly. Topical antibiotics are applied two or three times a day for approximately 10 days. Systemic antibiotics may be prescribed if the infection is extensive or the patient is at risk.

PATIENT/FAMILY TEACHING. Teaching focuses on the contagious potential of the disease and methods to prevent the spread of infection. The nurse reinforces good hand-washing technique for patient and family members, and directs patients to use personal towels and linens and to launder them and any other clothing in contact with the infected area after each use.

Folliculitis

Etiology and Epidemiology. Folliculitis is inflammation of the hair follicle caused by infection, chemical irritation, or physical trauma. *S. aureus* is the most common gram-positive bacteria causing infection. Gram-negative bacteria such as *Pseudomonas* organisms can infect patients who are receiving antibiotics long term or those who use hot tubs. The infection may be caused by drainage from other infected lesions. Predisposing factors include chronic illness, mechanical irritation from shaving or clothing, hot tub use, or infection in close contacts. Pseudofolliculitis, seen commonly in the military and in African-American males, occurs in the beard region. Sharp cut hair emerges from the follicle, curves, and reenters the skin, causing a chronic low-grade irritation.

Pathophysiology. Bacterial infections of the hair follicle may be superficial in the epidermis around the hair follicle or deep in the tissue surrounding both the lower and upper portions of the hair follicle. Deep folliculitis produces a more severe inflammatory response. Sycosis barbae, or barber's itch, is a deep folliculitis of the beard. Hordeolum (stye) is a deep folliculitis of the eyelashes (see Chapter 61). Typically there is swelling of the surrounding eyelid and crusting along its edge.

Collaborative Care Management. Treatment of superficial folliculitis includes aggressive hygiene with antimicrobial cleansers and soaps. In addition, topical antibiotics such as mupirocin or bacitracin may be applied two or three times a day. Warm compresses may be used to encourage resolution of deep folliculitis.

PATIENT/FAMILY TEACHING. Nursing management focuses on teaching patients about the prescribed therapy and avoidance of predisposing factors.

Furuncles and Carbuncles

Etiology and Epidemiology. Furuncles (boils) are a deep folliculitis that originates either from a superficial folliculitis or as a deep nodule around the hair follicle. Furunculosis is the appearance of several furuncles. An infection that involves several surrounding hair follicles is termed a *carbuncle.* The causative organism is usually *Staphylococcus*, but occasionally other gram-positive and gram-negative bacteria can cause furuncles. Both furuncles and carbuncles develop with obesity, poor nutritional states, debilitation, and poorly controlled diabetes mellitus.

Pathophysiology. Local swelling, erythema, and tenderness are the presenting symptoms. Within 3 to 5 days the lesion becomes elevated, or "points up," the surrounding skin becomes shiny, and the center or "core" turns yellow. Carbuncles have several cores. The furuncle may rupture spontaneously; with drainage, pain is immediately alleviated. The drainage progresses from yellow purulent material to serosanguineous discharge. Drainage usually subsides within a few hours to a few days; the redness and swelling subside gradually. Furuncles and carbuncles are commonly seen on the face, neck, breasts, axillae, buttocks, thighs, perineum, and groin and tend to recur in susceptible individuals.

Collaborative Care Management. Warm compresses are used to aid in bringing the furuncle to a head. If the furuncle does not drain spontaneously, incision and drainage may be required. As it drains, care must be taken to keep the infected discharge off the surrounding skin. Systemic antibiotics may be recommended based on the results of wound culture and sensitivity or Gram stain. Strict adherence to Standard Precautions is essential in the care of persons with furuncles or carbuncles.

PATIENT/FAMILY TEACHING. Patient teaching focuses on the proper use of prescribed antibiotics and preventing the spread of the infection by keeping the hands away from the discharge.

Erysipelas

Etiology and Epidemiology. Erysipelas is a form of localized cellulitis usually caused by a hemolytic streptococcus or *S. aureus* (Figure 65-7). Older adults with poor host resistance are at risk

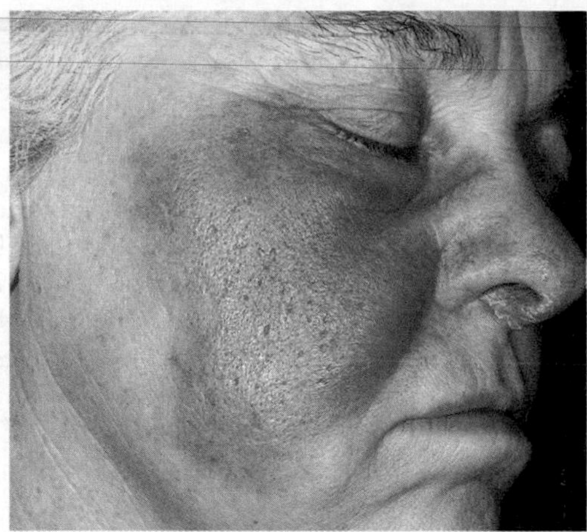

Figure 65-7 Cellulitis. Acute phase with intense erythema.

for this infection. Erysipelas may develop after a puncture wound, ulcer, or chronic dermatitis.

Pathophysiology. Before the development of systemic antibiotics, erysipelas was a serious infection. It is characterized by localized inflammation and swelling of the skin and subcutaneous tissues. Typical sites of infection are the face, scalp, hands, and genitalia. A sharp, erythematous line demarcates infected skin from normal skin. The infected area is warm to palpation. The infection spreads via the lymphatic system and bloodstream.

Collaborative Care Management. Gram stain, culture, and sensitivity determine the appropriate antibiotic treatment. Local lesions are immobilized and elevated to decrease local edema. Domeboro soaks are used to decrease discomfort and dry up bullous lesions. Moist heat may also be used. If an abscess forms, incision and drainage may be indicated.

PATIENT/FAMILY TEACHING. Patient education focuses on treatment recommendations, which may include soaks, elevation, and antibiotics. It is imperative that the patient understand the importance of completing the course of prescribed antibiotic therapy.

Viral Infections

Warts

Etiology and Epidemiology. Warts are benign epidermal tumors caused by the human papillomavirus (HPV). Approximately 65 subtypes of the virus cause infection on skin and mucosal surfaces. The incidence of HPV is high in the general population, with children and young adults most commonly affected.

Pathophysiology. Warts grow in a variety of shapes. The common wart is a small, circumscribed, painless, hyperkeratotic papule usually seen on the extremities, especially the hands. Filiform warts are slender, fingerlike projections occurring mostly on the face and neck. Plantar warts grow inward from the pressure on the soles of the feet and may be painful. They are differentiated from calluses by the disruption of normal plantar skin lines on the soles. Warts that develop in the anogenital region (condyloma acuminata) are grayish with a cauliflower-like appearance and may burn or itch. Transmission of the virus is by skin-to-skin contact. Anogenital warts are acquired by sexual activity or rarely by **autoinoculation**. Certain subtypes of HPV possess cancer-transforming potential.

Collaborative Care Management. Warts often spontaneously resolve without intervention. When intervention is needed, there are several options. Both common and plantar warts may be treated by the application of keratolytic acids (salicylic and lactic acids), cryosurgery with liquid nitrogen, electrosurgery, laser surgery, or, rarely, surgical excision. Anogenital HPV infections are treated with multiple modalities, including caustic acids, podophyllum resin, imiquimod cream (topical immune response agent), cryotherapy, and laser surgery.

PATIENT/FAMILY TEACHING. Patient teaching focuses on the viral etiology of HPV, mode of transmission, and implications of treatment. Patients may seek resources for alternative therapies, which include hypnosis and biofeedback. For patients with genital tract disease, the nurse should emphasize sexually transmitted disease prevention and the need to examine and treat sexual partners.

Herpes Simplex

One of the most common viruses in humans is the herpes simplex virus (HSV), which occurs as two similar yet serologically different strains, type 1 and type 2. Type 1 virus is found primarily on the face or in the mouth and is colloquially referred to as fever blisters or cold sores. It is also occasionally found in the eyes (keratitis). Type 2 is associated with genital tract infection transmitted by sexual contact. Transmission of HSV is primarily skin to skin or skin to mucosa. The incubation period may be anywhere from 2 to 20 days. Details of HSV infection are found in Chapters 41 and 59.

Herpes Zoster

Etiology and Epidemiology. Herpes zoster, or shingles, is caused by the same virus (varicella zoster) that causes varicella (chickenpox). Varicella is believed to be the primary infection in a nonimmune host, whereas herpes zoster is thought to be the response in a partially immune host. Herpes zoster occurs more commonly in older adults because of the natural decline in cellular immunity seen with normal aging. Although herpes zoster is far less communicable than chickenpox, persons who have not had chickenpox may develop herpes zoster after exposure to the vesicular lesions of persons with it. For this reason, susceptible persons should not care for patients with herpes zoster. Herpes zoster occurs more frequently in persons with human immunodeficiency virus disease, with lymphatic cancers, or after organ or marrow transplantation. In rare circumstances it may recur.

Pathophysiology. In herpes zoster clusters of vesicular lesions are arranged in a linear fashion. They follow the course of the peripheral sensory nerves and hence the lesions never cross the midline of the body (Figure 65-8). They often are unilateral, but nerve groups on both sides of the body can be involved. Two

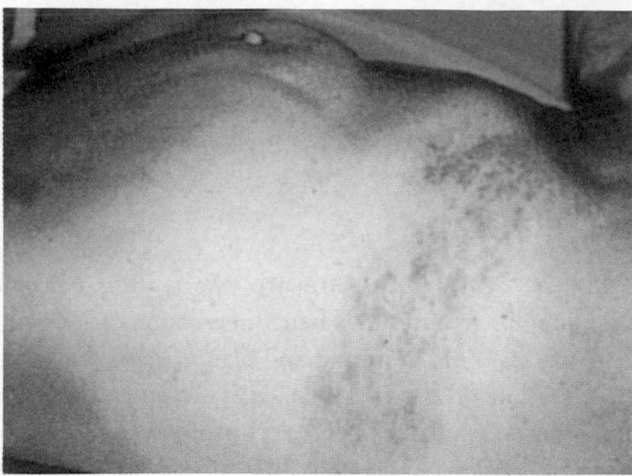

Figure 65-8 Herpes zoster.

thirds of persons with herpes zoster develop lesions over thoracic **dermatomes**, and the remainder show involvement of the trigeminal nerve with lesions on the face, eye, and scalp. The rash develops first as macules but progresses rapidly to vesicles and/or bullae. The fluid becomes turbid, and crusts develop and drop off in about 10 days.

Malaise, fever, itching, and pain over the involved area may precede the rash. If vesicles develop within 1 or 2 days after the initial pain symptoms, the lesions usually clear in 2 to 3 weeks; but if the vesicles develop over a period of 1 week, a prolonged course can be expected.

Discomfort from pain and itching is the major problem with herpes zoster. The pain may vary from a light burning sensation to a deep visceral-type pain, and it may be intermittent or constant. It usually persists for up to 4 weeks. In about 10% of patients a pain syndrome called postherpetic neuralgia develops.

Collaborative Care Management. For some patients no pharmacologic treatment is prescribed for herpes zoster. If the infection is identified early (within 48 to 72 hours of first lesions) or in high-risk individuals, antiviral therapy is helpful. Acyclovir (Zovirax) accelerates healing and reduces acute pain. It is given orally in high doses (800 mg five times per day for 1 week). In severe infections acyclovir may be given intravenously. Because acyclovir can precipitate in renal tubules, drinking fluids should be encouraged. Although acyclovir does not prevent postherpetic neuralgia, it may reduce its severity. Famciclovir, similar to acyclovir, is used for uncomplicated cases of acute herpes zoster in patients who are immunocompromised. As with acyclovir, famciclovir has been shown to reduce the duration of postherpetic neuralgia.

Analgesics may be required for pain management. Aspirin, with or without codeine, is often effective; meperidine (Demerol) may be needed for severe pain. Nonsteroidal antiinflammatory drugs (NSAIDs) are usually ineffective. Topical antipruritic agents, such as Sarna, Prax, PrameGel, or oatmeal colloid preparations, may relieve local discomfort. Domeboro soaks applied as a cool compress may provide local relief and quicken drying of the vesicles. Loose clothing helps minimize contact with the affected area. Patients should avoid exposure to highly susceptible persons (those who have not had chickenpox or are immunosuppressed).

Postherpetic neuralgia usually lasts less than 1 year but may persist for many years. The pain is always present with superimposed sharp pain episodes. Because the pain results from nervous system damage, it does not respond well to usual pain therapies. Multidisciplinary approaches to pain management are often required. Local application of capsaicin cream may provide some pain relief. Tricyclic antidepressants are commonly used. Transcutaneous electrical nerve stimulation may be tried initially, although it usually is not effective on a long-term basis. Narcotics are avoided because of the persistence of the pain and potential for addiction. The pain associated with postherpetic neuralgia can become all consuming; therefore ongoing evaluation of patient response is an important nursing measure.

PATIENT/FAMILY TEACHING. The nurse educates the patient and family on how to prevent spread of infection, the course of the disease and possible complications, and treatments and medications.

▶ ARE You READY?

Which of the following is a clinical manifestation of herpes zoster?

1. Painless itching
2. Painful vesicles
3. Yellow rash
4. Blood-filled blisters

Acne

Acne Vulgaris

Etiology and Epidemiology. Acne vulgaris, a common skin disease, is seen in 80% of adolescents, but it may also occur in adults. It affects approximately 70 million persons annually in the United States. Acne is multifactorial. Its development appears related to free fatty acids, endocrine effects, stressors, heredity, and infection, but the exact roles of these factors have not been conclusively demonstrated. Diet has been essentially ruled out as a causative factor. Acne occurs at puberty, when the sebaceous glands are stimulated by androgens, and it is often found to be common within families. Acne is more quiescent in summer months.

Pathophysiology. At puberty, sebaceous glands undergo enlargement from androgen stimulation. Sebum is released, passes through the follicular canal, and combines with sebaceous gland cell fragments, epidermal cells (keratin), and bacteria. At this time, triglycerides in the sebum are hydrolyzed to glycerol and free fatty acids. The sebum and debris may become plugged in the hair follicle to form an open comedo (blackhead) if it is at the surface or a closed comedo (whitehead) if it is below the surface (Figure 65-9). The dark color of the blackhead is melanin, not dirt, and results from passage of melanin from the adjoining epidermal cells.

Inflammatory lesions apparently develop from the escape of sebum into the dermis, which then serves as an irritant, causing an inflammatory reaction. Free fatty acids may also be an irritant in the follicle itself. Acne occurs mostly on the face and neck,

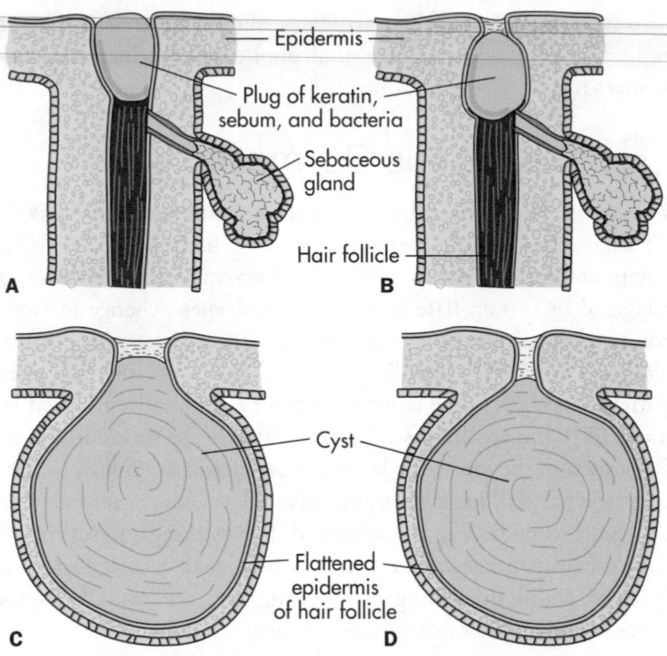

Figure 65-9 Formation of lesions in acne vulgaris. **A,** Open comedo (blackhead), early stage. **B,** Closed comedo (whitehead), early stage. **C,** Cyst formation in open comedo, advanced stage. **D,** Cyst formation in closed comedo, advanced stage.

upper chest, and back, although the upper arms, buttocks, and thighs may also be involved. Comedones are the first visible signs, and the skin is characteristically oily. The inflammatory lesions include papules, pustules, nodules, and cysts. Superficial lesions may resolve in 5 to 10 days without scarring, but large lesions last for several weeks and often result in scarring. The typical scar resembles an old volcano (ice-pick scar); however, many other sizes and shapes may result, depending on the depth and extent of the inflammatory lesions.

The extent of the lesions varies greatly. Some persons have only a few small lesions, whereas many adolescents have several lesions that peak at ages 16 to 18 years of age and then slowly resolve. A small percentage of the population develops severe nodular-cystic acne.

Collaborative Care Management. Treatment of acne consists of topical, systemic, intralesional, and surgical approaches.

Topical agents commonly prescribed are benzoyl peroxides, retinoids and retinoid-like drugs (tretinoin, adapalene, tazarotene, azelaic acid), and antibiotics (clindamycin, erythromycin, sulfa-based agents). Systemic antibiotic therapy with tetracyclines, erythromycin, or trimethoprim-sulfamethoxazole is indicated for inflammatory acne lesions. Isotretinoin (Accutane), a vitamin A acid analog, is an alternative systemic therapy. Side effects of isotretinoin include dry lips, conjunctiva, and skin; hair loss; muscle aches; photosensitivity; mood disturbance; elevated lipids; and birth defects. Low progestin-containing oral contraceptive agents may benefit certain female patients. Intralesional corticosteroid therapy is used for the cysts of severe acne, whereas dermabrasion and laser resurfacing procedures can be used to revise scars. Chemical peels with alpha hydroxy and/or more penetrating acids (trichloroacetic acid) may be used as an adjuvant therapy with both topical and oral medications or as postacne therapy.

Counseling and teaching are the major nursing interventions. Acne can be a significant life stressor, particularly in the adolescent years. Behavioral responses to the altered body image produced by acne flares may be anger, hostility, shyness, depression, and withdrawal. Psychologic counseling may be necessary in select situations.

PATIENT/FAMILY TEACHING. Dispelling acne myths is a critical nursing intervention (e.g., foods such as chocolate, pizza, soda, and French fries do *not* cause acne) because understanding the nature of acne helps the person understand the necessary care. Teaching is directed toward general health care of the skin and guidelines for therapy (see the Patient/Family Teaching box).

The nurse explains that the lesions in acne develop when the pilosebaceous follicles become plugged; therefore activities that contribute to occlusion of the follicles are to be avoided. Hair and

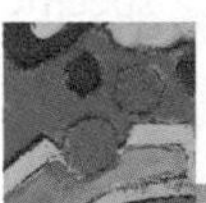

PATIENT/FAMILY TEACHING *The Patient With Acne*

Teaching should include information about the cause of acne and the following instructions.

Preventive Measures

Keep hands and hair away from the face.
Avoid masks, straps, and cradling of the face.
Shampoo hair daily.
Avoid exposure to oils and greases.
Eat a well-balanced diet and avoid any foods that appear related to skin flare-ups.

General Skin Care

Wash face two or three times a day with mild cleansers. Do not wash excessively.
Use over-the-counter (OTC) salicylic, sulfa, or benzoyl peroxide agents under the direction of a health care provider.
Avoid vigorous rubbing of the skin.
Use only water-based cosmetics.
Never leave cosmetics on face overnight.

Drug Therapy

Follow the prescribed therapy; it may take up to 8 weeks to realize benefit from both topical and systemic therapy.
Expect skin desquamation, especially with topical tretinoin.
Avoid using multiple OTC agents while on medical therapy.
Remove cosmetics before applying topical medications.
Avoid exposure to direct sunlight if using topical tretinoin or taking drugs such as tetracyclines and sulfa antibiotics (photosensitivity).
Prevent pregnancy if taking isotretinoin (Accutane) therapy because of the risk of birth defects.

hands should be kept away from the face. Loose clothing prevents pressure over the follicles, and tight collars should not be worn. The skin should be kept clean. Greasy, oil-based cosmetics may be occlusive and plug up the follicles. Medication teaching, including drug interactions, pregnancy prevention, and side-effect profiles, should be reviewed in detail with the patient and family. Daily sun protection is advised with most agents to avoid photosensitivity reactions.

Acne Rosacea

Etiology and Epidemiology. Acne rosacea is a follicular eruption of the skin with both a vascular and acne component. It affects 30- to 50-year-olds and affects women more than men, although men tend to have more severe manifestations. The cause is unknown. Many theories abound, but none has been proven. Fair-complexioned individuals are more inclined to manifest symptoms of acne rosacea. A familial predisposition is also seen.

Pathophysiology. Acne rosacea begins with erythema over the central face, cheeks, and nose. Flushing and blushing are classic symptoms. Papules, pustules, cysts, and enlargement of superficial blood vessels (telangiectasia) ensue. Years of acne rosacea can lead to an irregular, bulbous thickening of the skin of the distal part of the nose (rhinophyma), with red-purple discoloration and dilated follicles.[11]

Collaborative Care Management. Rosacea responds slowly to treatment, and relapses are common. In moderate to severe cases, topical or oral antibiotics or isotretinoin may be used. Telangiectasia and rhinophyma can be modified with laser surgery. Elimination of rosacea triggers is crucial to managing the disease. Anything that induces flushing such as heat, cold, wind, sunlight, alcohol, and spicy foods can exacerbate symptoms. Daily sun protection is strongly recommended.

Patient/Family Teaching. The nurse educates the patient and family on the disease and the therapy selected. Identification of rosacea triggers and their avoidance should be stressed. Use of mild cleansers and avoidance of alcohol-based products and fragrances may reduce symptoms.

Eczematous Dermatitis

Eczema is characterized by superficial inflammation of the skin. The terms *eczema* and *dermatitis* are often used interchangeably. There are approximately 20 forms of eczema, each of which is triggered by certain flare factors such as dryness, change in environment or temperature, infection, and stress. Dermatitis is often classified arbitrarily according to specific features, such as cause, pattern, and age. Some common types of dermatitis are listed in Table 65-1 and are discussed in more detail in the succeeding text. Regardless of the cause, the lesions in any dermatitis follow a characteristic pattern. Initially, erythema and local edema are followed by vesicle formation with oozing and then crusting and scaling. If the dermatitis persists, there will be evidence of excoriation from scratching and thickening of the skin, and the color becomes more brownish. Secondary infection may result.

Contact Dermatitis

Etiology and Epidemiology. Contact dermatitis is caused by exposure to substances in the environment (Table 65-2). Contact dermatitis occurs in both irritant and allergic forms. Irritant contact dermatitis is a nonallergic reaction occurring in any person on contact with a sufficient concentration of an irritant.[8] It occurs four times more commonly than allergic contact dermatitis. Mechanical irritation may result from wool or glass fibers. Chemical irritants include acids; alkalis; solvents; detergents; and oils commonly found in cleaning compounds, insecticides, and industrial compounds. Biologic irritants include urine, feces, and toxins from insects or aquatic plants. Persons engaged in wet work such as food handlers, health care workers, and child care providers are more prone to irritant contact dermatitis.

Allergic contact dermatitis is a cell-mediated type IV delayed **hypersensitivity immune reaction** from contact with a specific

Table 65-1 Types of Dermatitis

Type	Cause	Characteristics
Contact (Figure 65-10)	External agents	Site and pattern of lesions dependent on exposure pattern (e.g., linear, angular) Itching a major symptom
Atopic	Immunologic irregularity reaction, genetically influenced	Itching a major symptom Lesions caused by scratching
Lichen simplex chronicus	Stasis, irritants, psychologic factors	Itching a major symptom Lesions caused by scratching
Seborrheic (Figure 65-11)	*Pitysporum orbiculare* overgrowth likely with genetic and environmental influences	Erythematous, scaly (e.g., dandruff)
Nummular	Unknown	Coin-shaped lesions Severe itching
Stasis	Altered circulation	Erythema, edema Lesions sometimes developing from trauma Severe itching possible

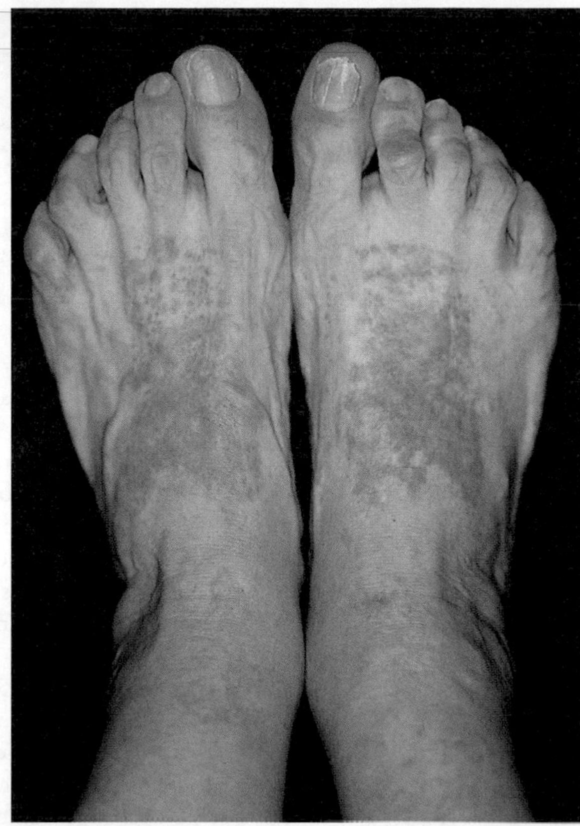

A

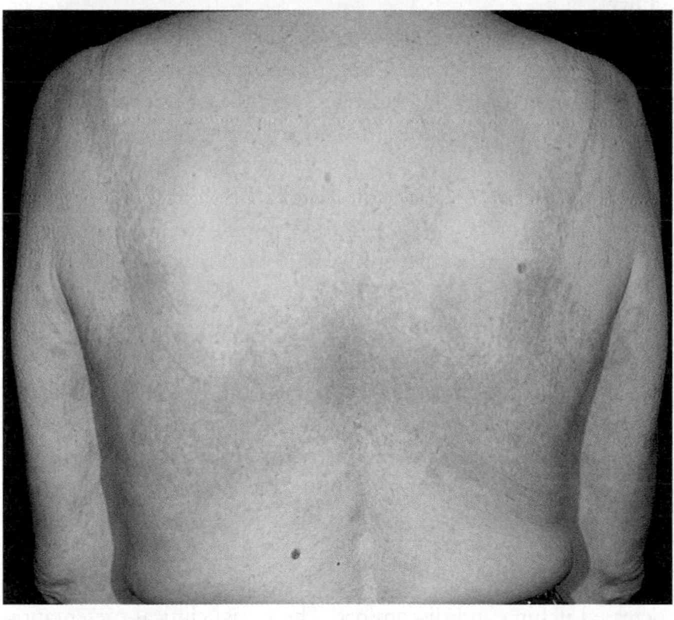

B

Figure 65-10 A, Shoe contact dermatitis. Sharply defined plaques formed under a shoe lining impregnated with rubber cement. **B,** Allergic contact dermatitis to spandex rubber in a bra.

antigen (see Figure 65-10, *B*). Many compounds can cause sensitization under specific conditions. Typical antigens include poison ivy, synthetics, industrial chemicals, drugs (e.g., sulfanilamide or penicillin), and metals (especially nickel and chromate). Once the skin has been sensitized, further contact with the sensitizing substance will produce an eczematous reaction. The sensitizing allergen may reach the site by direct contact; by indirect contact, such as transmission from animals, from one part of the body to the other by the hands, or from clothing; or by the air, as in smoke. Investigation of possible exposures, including medications, products (e.g., household cleaning, cosmetics, hobbies), occupational environment, and recreational activities, may provide insight into the contact event.

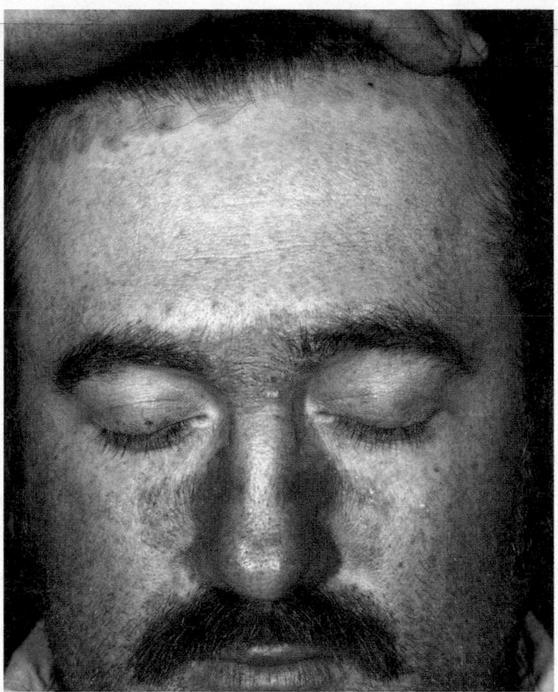

Figure 65-11 Seborrheic dermatitis in adult with extensive involvement in all the characteristic sites.

Pathophysiology. The characteristic lesions of contact dermatitis appear sooner in an irritant contact than in the allergic type; however, the onset and appearance vary, depending on the type and concentration of the irritant. The rash develops on the exposed areas, particularly the more sensitive areas, such as the dorsal rather than the palmar surface of the hands. When contact dermatitis is suspected but the agent is unknown, patch testing may be carried out[10] and the environment manipulated to exclude suspected agents.

Collaborative Care Management. Weeping vesicular lesions are treated with Domeboro soaks one or two times a day. Crusts and scales are not removed but are allowed to drop off naturally as the skin heals. Topical corticosteroids (middle to potent range) are applied twice a day to affected areas for approximately 2 weeks. Face, genital, and skin fold sites warrant weaker steroid formulations such as hydrocortisone 0.5% to 1%. Oral corticosteroids may be prescribed for generalized rash or significant hand and face involvement. Oral antibiotics are used only when secondary infection ensues. Oral antihistamines, topical antipruritic agents, or colloidal oatmeal baths and lotions may ease itching.

PATIENT/FAMILY TEACHING. The primary focus of patient teaching is prevention. Contact dermatitis can be prevented by

TABLE 65-2 COMMON CAUSES OF ALLERGIC OR IRRITANT CONTACT DERMATITIS

Area	Cause
Face, scalp, ears	Cosmetics, hair care products, jewelry, cleansers, sunscreen, contact lens solution, metals (especially nickel), glasses
Neck	Perfumes, clothing (especially wool)
Trunk, axillae	Deodorants, clothing, perfumes, laundry products
Arms, hands	Poison ivy, oak, and sumac; jewelry; nickel, etc., in watchbands; detergents and other cleansers; gloves
Legs, feet	Medication for athlete's foot; shoes

avoiding the irritating or sensitizing substance whenever possible. Patients and family members should be educated to recognize the leaves of *Rhus* plants—poison ivy, oak, and sumac (Figure 65-12). Persons walking in areas where these plants grow need to protect the skin by wearing appropriate clothing. If contact with the plant is suspected, symptoms may be averted by immediately rinsing the skin for 15 minutes with running water to remove the resin before skin penetration occurs, and carefully removing clothing to avoid skin contact.

The person who develops sensitivity to material encountered in the living or working environment may need to consider a permanent change of environment if other measures are unsuccessful. Gloves may be used if the person is handling irritant or allergenic substances. Persons sensitive to detergents may need to wash their clothes and bathe with a mild soap product.

Atopic Dermatitis

Etiology and Epidemiology. Atopic dermatitis is a genetically based skin disorder that is both chronic and relapsing. It is linked to a larger group of atopic diseases that includes asthma and hay fever. Approximately 40% to 50% of persons with atopic dermatitis develop manifestations of asthma or hay fever. Approximately 50% to 60% of patients with atopic dermatitis are from families with one or more atopic diseases. Exacerbating factors include sudden changes in temperature or humidity; exercise; psychologic stress; fibers such as wool, fur, or nylon; detergents; and perfumes. Controlling environmental influences such as climatic changes and humidity levels can prove challenging for both patient and caregiver.

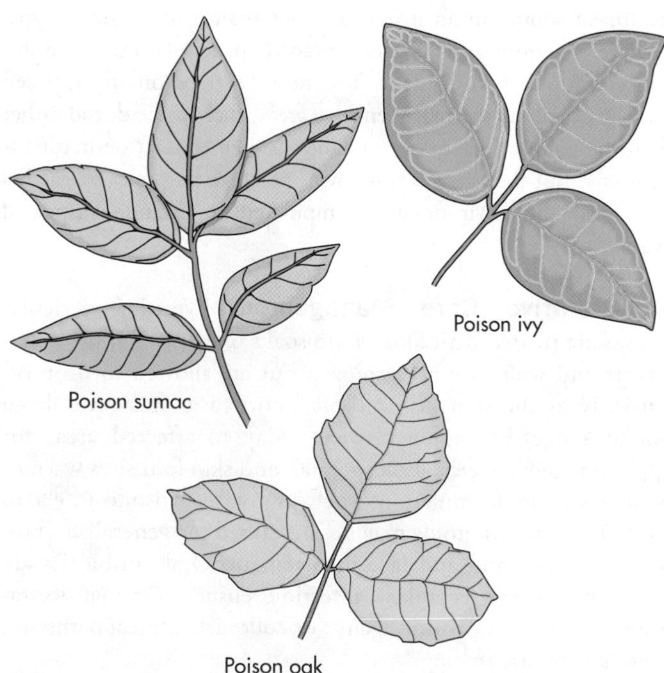

Figure 65-12 Typical leaves of poison sumac, poison ivy, and poison oak.

Atopic dermatitis is most common in children. Up to 75% of children with atopic dermatitis develop symptoms by 6 months of age. It usually disappears or becomes less severe between the ages of 2 and 3 years but can recur in late childhood or adolescence. Resolution of symptoms is seen by age 30 in a large number of adults.

The major symptom of atopic dermatitis is intense pruritus.[13] Chronic rubbing and scratching produces eczematous skin, followed by skin thickening (lichenification) and alteration in pigmentation (hypopigmentation or hyperpigmentation).

Pathophysiology. The protective barrier function of the skin is diminished greatly in the atopic population. Lipid content changes in the epidermis permit water loss from the cells, resulting in dry skin. Persons with atopic dermatitis are highly sensitive with a lowered threshold to pruritus. Even minor stimuli can produce intense episodes of itching.

Atopic dermatitis results from an immunologic irregularity involving cytokines and other inflammatory mediators. There is a marked tendency toward vasoconstriction of superficial blood vessels, and the skin blanches readily. Cold and low humidity are poorly tolerated because of drying effects. Heat and high humidity are also poorly tolerated because vasodilation increases the inflammatory reaction, thus aggravating the dermatitis and causing increased itching and discomfort. The initial clinical presentation for atopic dermatitis is rough, dry skin that may appear as early as the first month of life. Infants may develop moist, oozing, crusting lesions on the scalp and face, with spread to the trunk and extensor aspects of the arms and legs. Later, the lesions become localized to the flexures of the neck (Figure 65-13), wrists, antecubital and popliteal fossae, eyelids, and behind the ears. The erythema is dusky, and excoriations may become secondarily infected. By the late twenties or early thirties the lesions usually disappear, but they may recur later as chronic hand or foot eczema.

The compromised barrier function of the skin in atopic dermatitis places individuals at increased risk for acquiring viral, fungal, and bacterial infections of the skin.

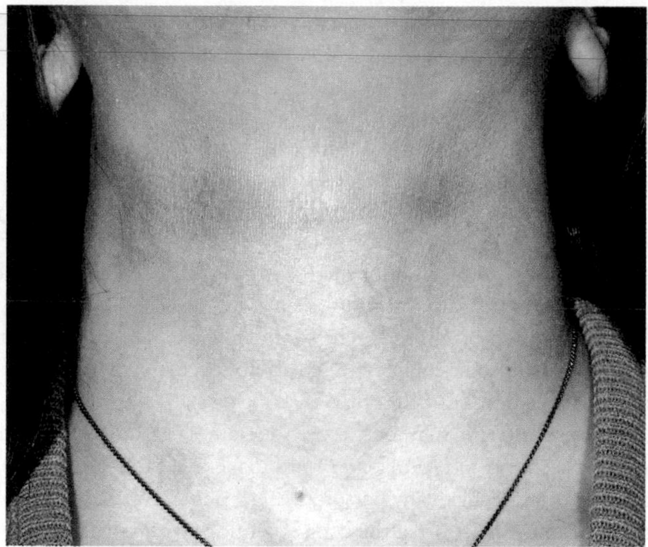

Figure 65-13 Atopic dermatitis. Classic appearance of erythema and diffuse scaling about neck.

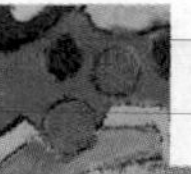

PATIENT/FAMILY TEACHING

The Patient With Atopic Dermatitis

Teaching should include information about the disease, prescribed medications, and the following instructions:

- Use only gentle cleansers and soaplike products.
- Take a relaxing, warm bath for 15 to 20 minutes; gently pat away excess water and immediately apply a moisturizer. Reapply moisturizers throughout the day when skin is dry.
- Use wet wraps in place of tub soaking if desired; wraps permit evaporation, which cools the skin, thus decreasing pruritus.
- Apply topical medication in a thin layer and rub in well
- Avoid wool, fur, or rough fibers against the skin; they act as irritants and cause itching.
- Avoid overheating, which increases sweating, leading to itching. Wear loose, light clothing in hot weather. Air conditioning promotes comfort.
- Avoid sunburn; wear a sunscreen with a minimum sun protection factor of 15.
- Avoid excessive cold, which dries the skin.
- Wash all new garments before wearing to remove potentially irritating chemicals.
- Consult health care provider if eczema worsens.

Collaborative Care Management. Atopic dermatitis has no cure, but symptoms can be controlled. Hydrating the skin is the cornerstone of therapy. Applying an occlusive moisturizing agent three or four times a day (preferably emollients in a *water-in-oil* base) works to reestablish a well-hydrated stratum corneum. Topical corticosteroid therapy is the principal pharmacologic agent used. Weaker potency corticosteroids are selected for the pediatric population. More potent topical corticosteroids should be reserved for adults, with education regarding method of application, duration of use, and potential side effects. Topical corticosteroids may be used in concert with wet wraps, which can enhance drug absorption and help decrease pruritus. Systemic corticosteroids may be given for a limited period to selected individuals with severe atopic eczema.

Protopic ointment (tacrolimus) and pimecrolimus (Elidel) cream are two topical **immunomodulators** specifically developed for treatment of moderate to severe atopic dermatitis. They are highly selective agents that block T-cell activation, thus targeting immunologic overreactivity and halting the inflammatory cascade. Itching, burning, and irritation may occur within a few days of start of treatment, but they have proven safe for use, even though both child and adult patients should avoid natural and artificial sunlight for long periods.

Systemic therapy with sedating antihistamines at night (when itching is more intense) can be helpful. Treatment of secondary bacterial skin infections with appropriate antibiotics may be warranted. In some instances patients may benefit from phototherapy with ultraviolet B (UVB) or ultraviolet A (UVA) plus psoralen (PUVA).

PATIENT/FAMILY TEACHING. Successful management of atopic dermatitis is achieved through patient, family, and health care provider collaboration. Provision of comprehensive written skin care instructions and demonstration of techniques for application of topical drugs are critical nursing measures (see Patient/Family Teaching box). Addressing the social and emotional concerns of patients with atopic dermatitis is another challenging area for intervention. Chronic manifestations of this skin disease can set the stage for social isolation, poor self-esteem, anxiety, and sleep disturbance.

Lichen Simplex Chronicus

Lichen simplex chronicus (LSC) is a localized, well-circumscribed, eczematous eruption caused by repeated rubbing and scratching. It tends to occur in areas that can be easily reached, such as the wrists, ankles, and back of the scalp. Stress factors are thought to be involved. Once itching is initiated by an insect bite, rash, or nonspecific irritant, the *itch-scratch* cycle ensues. Scratching becomes habitual. The skin becomes excoriated, and thickened geometric-appearing plaques result. Itching is often worse at night. Potent topical corticosteroids applied to the involved sites are the treatment of choice for LSC. Occlusive dressings with plastic wrap or tape (Cordran tape) applied for 3 to 7 days may enhance the steroid effects.

Seborrheic Dermatitis

Seborrheic dermatitis is an eczematous eruption that typically occurs on the hairy areas of the scalp, eyebrows, face, central chest, and sometimes genital skin folds. Inflammatory changes around the sebaceous gland and hair follicle produce the characteristic symptoms of redness and greasy scales. The cause is unknown, but overgrowth of yeast organisms on the skin is strongly postulated. Family history of the skin disease may be found. Seborrheic dermatitis is chronic, with symptoms often worse in the winter months. Mild to moderate seborrheic dermatitis of the scalp is treated with tar, selenium, zinc, or ketoconazole shampoo preparations. These products exert an antimicrobial effect on the microbial flora found at the hair follicle. More significant scalp involvement may require topical corticosteroids to flatten thick, scaly plaques. Facial sites are treated with low-potency topical steroids and/or topical antifungal agents.

Nummular Dermatitis

Nummular dermatitis is a chronic condition of uncertain cause occurring most commonly in middle age or older men. The lesions of nummular dermatitis are typically 4 to 10 cm, erythematous, and coin shaped. The rash has a predilection for the dorsal aspects of the hands, extensor surfaces of the lower extremities, and buttocks. Itching may be severe. A background of dry skin can promote flare-ups of eczematous dermatitis. Treatment consists of hydrating the skin with moisturizing lotions, topical corticosteroid agents, and tar products.

Stasis Dermatitis

Stasis dermatitis is a common eczematous eruption of the lower extremities occurring in older persons. It is usually preceded by varicosities and poor circulation. With the reduction in venous return from the legs, substances normally carried away by the circulation remain in the tissues, causing irritation. The skin is often brawny colored with associated edema. Itching may or may not occur. Scratching may produce breaks in the epidermis, which can become secondarily infected.

The most important treatment for stasis dermatitis is prevention by careful attention to the treatment of peripheral vascular conditions and prevention of constriction of the circulation to the extremities (see Chapter 31). Treating lower extremity edema with elevation, compression stockings, and Unna boots where applicable ultimately decreases the dermatitis skin changes. Topical corticosteroids improve the eczematous changes. Domeboro soaks may be useful when weeping lesions are present.

Skin Reactions From Systemic Factors

Drug Hypersensitivity Reactions

Etiology and Epidemiology. Almost any drug can cause a drug hypersensitivity reaction. The rash occurs because of gradual accumulation of the drug or because of antibodies that develop in response to a component of the medication. Skin manifestations from drugs may have a nonallergic or allergic basis. Some commonly seen skin reactions are maculopapular lesions, purpura, vesicles, bullae, ulcers, and urticaria (Table 65-3). The reactions can appear at any time, but the onset is usually sudden.

Pathophysiology. Type I anaphylactic (urticaria, angioedema), type II cytotoxic (cellular injury), type III immune complex (serum sickness), or type IV cell-mediated (allergic contact dermatitis, allergic photosensitivity) hypersensitivity reactions may occur. Some drugs may have combined reactions; for example, penicillin may produce both type I and type III reactions. Allergic contact dermatitis is commonly seen with drugs used topically. The rash is often bright red, semiconfluent, macular and papular, generalized, and bilateral. Hypersensitivity occurs early when previous sensitization has taken place.

Photosensitivity may occur with certain drugs and may take one of two forms: phototoxicity or photoallergy (Table 65-4). Phototoxicity may occur in any person taking a photosensitive drug and results from the reaction of the drug (chemical) with radiant energy, particularly UV light. Broad-spectrum sunscreens (e.g., zinc oxide, titanium dioxide, or avobenzone [Parasol 1789]), which cover the spectrum of UVA, may reduce potential photosensitivity reactions. Photoallergic reactions are cell-mediated (type IV) hypersensitivity reactions; therefore they affect only a small group of persons after several sensitizing exposures of drug and sunlight.

Collaborative Care Management. Treatment of drug hypersensitivity reactions consists of stopping the drug and treating the symptoms with cool, moist compresses; antihistamines; and topical or systemic corticosteroids. Avoiding direct sunlight, using broad-spectrum sunscreens, and wearing photoprotective clothing may also help.

PATIENT/FAMILY TEACHING. The primary goal of patient education is prevention by making sure patients know the drug(s) to which they are allergic. The patient or family member should know the specific drug name and type of reaction. A Medic-Alert bracelet may be beneficial. Allergy information should be documented on the patient's record. Nursing care also focuses on helping the patient comply with treatment.

Exfoliative Dermatitis

Etiology and Epidemiology. Exfoliative dermatitis is a rare, generalized dermatitis. In most cases the cause is unknown, but the disease may be associated with other types of dermatitis or with a lymphoma, or it may be the result of a drug reaction.

TABLE 65-3 SKIN REACTIONS TO COMMON MEDICATIONS

Reaction	Medication
Erythematous rash	Antibiotics, sulfonamides, thiazide (maculopapular) diuretics, barbiturates, phenylbutazone
Purpura (ecchymosis, petechiae)	Thiazides, sulfonamides, barbiturates, anticoagulants
Mucocutaneous lesions (vesicles, bullae, ulcers)	Sulfonamides, penicillins, barbiturates, phenylbutazone
Urticaria	Penicillins, streptomycin, tetracycline, insulin, aspirin, dyes, adrenocorticotropic hormone, antiserum

TABLE 65-4 DRUG PHOTOSENSITIVITY

Reaction	Symptoms	Drugs
Phototoxicity	Resembles sunburn (erythema, edema, vesicles)	Coal tar derivatives Psoralens Tetracycline Nalidixic acid Sulfanilamide Demeclocyclin (Declomycin) Chlorpromazine Certain dyes
Photoallergy	Resembles eczema (exudative papules and vesicles, urticaria, lichenification)	Diuretics (thiazides) Phenothiazines Oral hypoglycemics Griseofulvin Nonsteroidal antiinflammatory agents Retinoids

Pathophysiology. The onset of exfoliative dermatitis may be rapid or insidious and consists of an elevated temperature and generalized erythema, followed by extensive scaling (exfoliation). Pruritus may be present, and the lesions often become infected. Loss of large amounts of water and protein from the skin can lead to hypoproteinemia, weight loss, and difficulty with temperature control. Heart failure may occur in older patients. Death may result from overwhelming infection or circulatory collapse.

Collaborative Care Management. Therapy consists of maintaining fluid balance and preventing infection. Methods used to prevent infection in patients with burns are applicable (see Chapter 66). All drugs are discontinued as potential causative factors, although antibiotics may be started after culture and sensitivity tests of infected lesions. Oral corticosteroids are given for severe cases. Daily baths followed by application of petrolatum to the skin promote comfort.

PATIENT/FAMILY TEACHING. Patient teaching focuses on the course of the disease, rationales for treatment, management of signs and symptoms, and use of comfort measures.

Erythema Multiforme

Etiology and Epidemiology. Erythema multiforme (EM) is a common, self-limiting inflammation of the skin and mucous membranes in genetically susceptible persons. Episodes of the disease may be single, recurrent, or, rarely, continuous. Although it is usually mild, EM may progress to a toxic epidermal necrolysis type of illness. EM is classified as major or minor. The major type is also described as the severe bullous form or Stevens-Johnson syndrome. Both forms are thought to be a cell-mediated immune response to relevant antigens. The responsible agent usually can be identified. Medications that can trigger EM include phenytoin, carbamazepine, sulfonamides, NSAIDs, allopurinol, and certain antibiotics (particularly cephalosporins). Drugs, not infection, are thought to be responsible for the severe, bullous form of the disorder.

Infections that cause EM include mycoplasmal pneumonia; chickenpox; hepatitis B; infectious mononucleosis; and herpes simplex, which is the most common. More unusual causes of EM include systemic lupus erythematosus; lymphoma; leukemia; radiotherapy; pregnancy; and reactions to vaccinations, particularly hepatitis B.

Pathophysiology. EM may affect the skin and mucous membranes or solely the skin. Episodes of the disease usually last for 1 to 3 weeks. Characteristic lesions are flat topped, sharply marginated, dusky red papules and targetoid (bulls eye–like) lesions. The rash has an affinity for the backs of the hands, palms and soles, and extensor limbs. With the major variant of EM (bullous variety), the rash occurs on the dorsa of the hands, palms, knees, feet, and elbows. The oral cavity may be affected by blisters progressing to erosion of the entire oral mucosa and lips. Conjunctivitis may occur, progressing to corneal opacity. If the genital mucosa becomes involved, adhesions may result as a long-term complication. The skin findings may be preceded by fever, chest pain, and arthralgia. Severe cases may be confused with toxic epidermal necrolysis. If the triggering agent is herpes simplex, EM usually occurs 7 to 10 days after the onset of the herpes infection.

Collaborative Care Management. A single episode of EM may not require treatment. Any suspected triggering agent is discontinued and symptoms treated. Topical corticosteroids may help reduce local inflammation, itching, and burning. Systemic corticosteroids administered early may alleviate the pain-related symptoms. Sedating antihistamines such as hydroxyzine may be of some use. Persons with ocular and oral-mucosal involvement or the severe bullous type (Stevens-Johnson syndrome) warrant close supervision and supportive hospitalization. Individuals with extensive blistering should be treated as burn patients.

Intravenous or enteral feeding may be indicated for persons with extensive oral involvement. Protective dressings should be applied to prevent secondary infection. Caution must be used when choosing the appropriate antibiotic therapy, since Stevens-Johnson syndrome is triggered by drugs. Systemic steroids are indicated for the treatment of patients with severe cases of EM. Steroids are effective in reducing fever and aiding symptomatic relief but do not significantly affect morbidity or mortality rates. Skin lesions may take weeks to heal, and systemic steroids may delay the healing process. The physician should consider the risk/benefit ratio, particularly in older patients, before prescribing systemic steroids. Oral antiviral agents such as acyclovir may help with herpes-associated recurrent EM reactions. Azathioprine is an option for suppressing attacks in severe disease.

PATIENT/FAMILY TEACHING. The patient with any type of EM needs support and education throughout diagnosis and treatment. Initially other disorders causing blistering must be considered. The nurse provides education regarding the medications prescribed, including administration, dosing, and side effects. Nursing care is supportive and includes baths, soaks, oral care, and dressings. Thorough explanations should accompany treatments. Patients and family require teaching regarding the course of the disease, complications, possible triggers, and recurrences. The relationship between herpes simplex and episodes of EM should be explained.

Infectious Diseases

Communicable diseases, such as measles, chickenpox, and scarlet fever, produce skin reactions, as do smallpox and plague (Table 65-5). Nodes and hemorrhagic spots in the skin also accompany severe acute rheumatic fever.

Papulosquamous Diseases

Papulosquamous diseases are characterized by papular, scaly lesions. Common disorders in this category of dermatoses are psoriasis and pityriasis rosea.

Psoriasis

Etiology and Epidemiology. Psoriasis is a chronic skin disease affecting millions of Americans. Approximately 20% of the population is affected by psoriasis, with equal distribution in both genders. There is a higher incidence among Caucasians and a lower incidence among the Japanese, Native Americans, and people of West-African origin. Psoriasis occurs in all age-groups but is less common among children and older persons. Approximately one third of cases of psoriasis occur in persons younger than 20 years of age.

This T cell–mediated disease is characterized by exacerbations and remissions. Molecular research in recent years has dramatically improved our understanding of the immune system's key role in the development and maintenance of psoriatic skin disease. There are no specific precipitating factors for the majority of persons; however, some people may develop exacerbations after climatic changes, stressors, trauma, infections, or drugs.

Pathophysiology. For decades physicians thought that psoriasis occurred as a result of epidermal keratinocyte overproduction or hyperproliferation. Current thinking asserts that the pathogenesis of psoriasis is complex and involves three important steps: T-cell activation by antigen in lymph nodes, T-cell binding to the endothelium, and T-cell reactivation by a second exposure to antigen in the dermis.

Scaling, erythema, and pruritus are the hallmark symptoms of this disorder. The papules and plaques of psoriasis are raised, erythematous, and sharply circumscribed, with a silvery white scale (Figure 65-14). Removal of the scale usually results in a characteristic pinpoint bleeding called the Auspitz sign. In darker skinned persons the plaques may appear purple. Psoriatic lesions can occur anywhere on the body, but are more commonly found on the scalp, elbows, knees, and sacrolumbar areas. Beefy red lesions may be observed in an acute flare-up. Nail changes occur in 10% to 50% of patients with psoriasis. Characteristic nail changes are pitting, yellowish discoloration, oil drop or salmon patches, leukonychia (whitening of the nail), splinter hemorrhage, and onycholysis (separation of the nail from the nail bed).

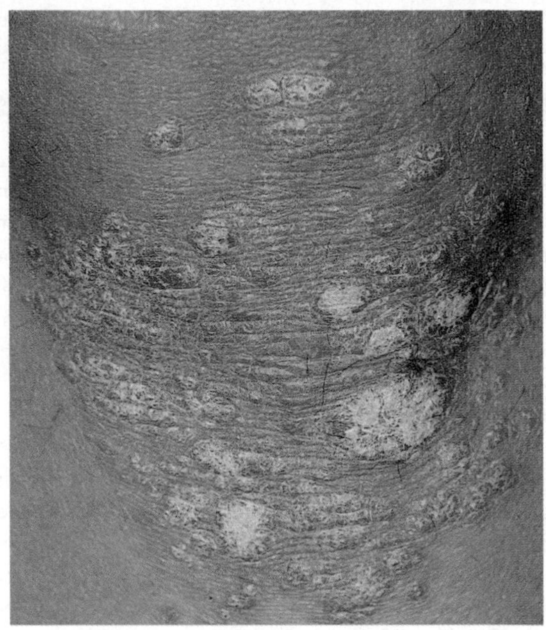

Figure 65-14 Psoriasis. Note silvery scaling.

TABLE 65-5 SKIN REACTIONS OF SOME COMMUNICABLE DISEASES

Disease	Cause	Incubation Period (Days)	Place of Rash Origin	Skin Lesions
Measles (rubeola)	Rubeola virus	11 (8-14)	Face	Pink maculopapular rash; lesions coalesce
German measles; 3-day measles (rubella)	Rubella virus	14-21	Face	Pink maculopapular rash; lesions usually discrete; may coalesce
Scarlet fever (scarlatina)	Hemolytic streptococci	1-3	Neck, chest	Bright red (scarlet) macules (pinpoint)
Chickenpox (varicella)	Varicella zoster virus	14-21	Back, chest	Macule, papule, vesicle, crust; lesions at different stages
Smallpox	Variola virus	12 (7-21)	Face	Macule, papule, vesicle, crust; lesions all at same stage
Typhoid fever	*Salmonella typhosa*	14 (7-21)	Abdomen	Macular rash

The common forms of psoriasis are psoriasis vulgaris, guttate psoriasis, pustular psoriasis, and erythrodermic psoriasis. In psoriasis vulgaris the plaques are symmetric, large and small, with silvery white scale adherent. An outbreak of guttate psoriasis may follow streptococcal pharyngitis or viral upper respiratory tract infection. Palmoplantar psoriasis occurs on the volar surfaces of the hands and feet and can be debilitating. In generalized pustular psoriasis, patients have a history of plaque-type psoriasis, later developing pustules on an erythematous base, eventually forming pools of pustules. Other symptoms include fever, chills, arthralgia, hypocalcemia, and leukocytosis. Discontinuing use of systemic steroids for plaque-type psoriasis may trigger flare-ups of the disease. Erythrodermic psoriasis, as the name implies, produces a red coloration of the skin with a desquamative scale over most of the body. Inflammatory vasodilatory mechanisms are responsible for problems in temperature regulation, hypoalbuminemia, pedal edema, and high-output cardiac failure.

An accompanying arthritis (psoriatic arthritis) occurs in approximately 3% to 4% of the population, with or without skin disease findings. Presentation of the arthritis varies; it may manifest as an asymmetric oligoarthropathy, it may affect mainly the distal interphalangeal joints, or it may cause a severely debilitating joint disease.

Collaborative Care Management. For localized manifestations of psoriasis (large and small plaque type) topical corticosteroids may be used for a defined period. Potential for steroid-induced side effects occurs with prolonged use of these agents. Coal tar products (soaks, gels, creams, and shampoos) may play a role in decreasing pruritus while diminishing epidermal cell turnover.

Calcipotriene (Dovonex), a vitamin D_3 derivative, can be effective in inhibiting the proliferation of keratinocytes. Calcipotriene may be used in concert with topical steroid therapy. The use of calcipotriene is not indicated for the treatment of widespread psoriasis because of the risk for systemic absorption with elevated calcium levels.

UV light inhibits deoxyribonucleic acid (DNA) synthesis, thus slowing the rapid skin cell growth. UV light is divided into three wavelengths: UVC (long), UVB (middle), and UVA (short). UVC is not used in skin therapeutics. The combination of tar and UVB light, known as the Goeckerman regimen, is a widely used form of therapy for patients with psoriasis.

Photochemotherapy (PUVA) is used for diffuse disease, for thicker plaques, or when other therapies have not been effective. Psoralens are taken 1 to 2 hours before exposure to the UV light; dose is based on body weight. Methotrexate, the systemic retinoid; acitretin (Soriatane), a vitamin A derivative; and cyclosporine, an immunosuppressive agent, are used in advanced disease. These drugs require regular laboratory monitoring of complete blood count, liver function, and lipids.

A selective class of drugs referred to as the *biologics* synthesized by using recombinant DNA techniques has recently come to market for management of moderate to severe psoriasis. Monoclonal antibodies, chimeric (part human–part mouse and fully humanized), and fusion proteins represent the three different types of biologic therapies. These agents can be administered by intramuscular or subcutaneous injection with laboratory monitoring required for some. Quality-of-life tools and skin clearance assessment tools have demonstrated great promise for this new class of psoriasis drugs.

PATIENT/FAMILY TEACHING. Most patients with psoriasis are treated on an ambulatory basis. One approach to therapy has been the establishment of psoriasis day care centers where patients visit daily to receive aggressive topical therapy, light treatment, and education pertaining to self-care. Patients with psoriasis may require intervention to cope with an altered body image. The disease is not curable and may wax and wane. Lesions may regress with treatment, only to recur in the same area again. Teaching for individuals who have psoriasis is summarized in the Patient/Family Teaching box.

Pityriasis Rosea

Etiology and Epidemiology. Pityriasis rosea is a common, benign, self-limiting dermatosis of unknown etiology.[11] A viral source has been postulated but never proven. Common, with worldwide distribution, the disease affects all races and occurs most commonly in women, adolescents, and young adults. Seventy-five percent of cases occur in persons 10 to 35 years old. The incidence is higher in the early spring and autumn months.

Pathophysiology. The initial symptom is usually a 2- to 10-cm solitary oval lesion (herald patch) with a thin, scaly border and yellowish center, appearing most often on the trunk, proximal arms, and legs. The herald patch usually precedes other lesions by 1 to 30 days. A generalized eruption of branlike scaly patches follows the herald patch. The distribution of lesions is often in long axes running parallel to each other and on the trunk, which creates a "Christmas tree"–like appearance. The eruption is self-limiting and lasts 6 to 8 weeks. Recurrences of pityriasis rosea are extremely rare.

Treatment measures are few, since most patients do not experience symptoms. Topical corticosteroids and antipruritic agents may be used if itching is present. Emollients are needed as the lesions dry up. Low-dose UVB phototherapy may be beneficial

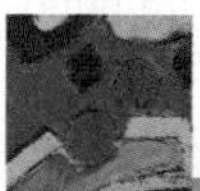

PATIENT/FAMILY TEACHING
The Patient With Psoriasis

Teaching should include information on the cause and chronicity of psoriasis and the following instructions:

- Prevent psoriasis flare-ups by avoiding skin trauma (injuries, sunburn, infections), extremes of temperature, and stress.
- Shampoo hair frequently to remove scales. If scalp has plaques, use tar, zinc, or selenium shampoos (e.g., T/Gel, DHS Zinc, Head & Shoulders) for 10 minutes before rinsing. Presoften thick plaques with mineral oil the night before a morning shampoo; use a fine-toothed comb to remove loose scales.
- Avoid self-medication, particularly when receiving prescribed therapy.
- Apply topical medications in a thin layer.
- Monitor for side effects of medications.
- Seek medical follow-up care during periods of exacerbation.

when the rash is diffuse or itching is significant. Exposure to natural sunlight (to the point of minimal erythema) will also speed disappearance of the lesions and relieve itching. The patient should be cautioned against sunburn.

Patient/Family Teaching. Nursing care is essentially symptomatic and includes assisting with and teaching about application of topical corticosteroids, baths, and emollients. Educating patients on the limited course of pityriasis rosea is another supportive measure.

Bullous Diseases (Blistering Disorders)

Pemphigus Vulgaris

Etiology and Epidemiology. Pemphigus vulgaris (PV) is an acute or chronic, serious, blistering disorder of the skin and mucous membranes. The cause of PV is thought to be autoimmune. Rare, but worldwide, PV occurs primarily in persons between 40 and 60 years old, with equal incidence in men and women and a higher incidence among Jewish persons.

Pathophysiology. PV is characterized by large bullae that appear all over the body and on the mucous membranes. Tissue injury results from circulating autoantibodies that bind to the structural proteins within the epidermis. Blister formation occurs above the stratum basale. Healing is commonly associated with the development of postinflammatory hyperpigmentation, rather than scarring. The lesions break and are followed by crusts and scarring. The disease is characterized by acantholysis (cells slip past one another and fluid accumulates between them). Placing the thumb firmly on the skin and exerting lateral sliding pressure dislodges the upper epidermis, resulting in erosion or blister (Nikolsky's sign). A Tzanck test can identify acantholytic cells. Secondary bacterial infections of the crust can lead to sepsis. Patients can succumb to PV if treatment is delayed.

Collaborative Care Management. Hospitalization is usually required for rigorous skin care and monitoring of drug effects. The treatment of choice for severe PV is high-dose systemic corticosteroids. The dose is gradually reduced as skin improves. Immunosuppressive agents such as methotrexate, cyclophosphamide, and azathioprine may be added to reduce the corticosteroid dose requirements.

Nursing care of the person with severe PV can be a challenge. Stryker frames may be used to help the person change position painlessly and to prevent weight bearing on raw surfaces. Air mattress or flotation systems may be used to reduce surface pressure on skin and promote comfort. Domeboro solution, potassium permanganate, and oatmeal products with oil delivered as baths or compresses to oozing lesions help control odor and remove crusts. Infection is a major concern because of the immunosuppressive effects of drug therapy. Topical antibiotics are helpful for reducing the bacterial flora on the skin. Special mouth care is required for mouth lesions, and bland diets are more easily tolerated.

Patient/Family Teaching. Emotional support and encouragement of both patient and family are extremely important. Patients may fear rejection because of their appearance, and they need evidence of continued family and staff interest and attention. The risk for disturbed body image and social isolation is high.

The nurse encourages patients to adhere to a balanced diet to promote wound healing. General skin care measures should be reinforced. Medication instruction regarding the mechanism of action, side effects, and drug-drug interactions are reviewed with both patient and family. Eliciting a return demonstration on application of topical agents and dressings by the patient and/or family member is another important nursing intervention.

Tumors of the Skin

Skin cell growths can develop from the epidermis, sebaceous or sweat glands, melanocytes, or mesodermal tissue (e.g., connective or vascular tissue).

Keratosis (Benign Lesion)

The term *keratosis* refers to any cornification or growth of the horny layer of the skin. Examples of keratoses include corns and calluses, warts, and seborrheic and actinic (solar) keratoses (Table 65-6).

Premalignant Lesions

Skin lesions that may evolve into a malignant state include actinic keratosis, keratoacanthoma, leukoplakia, Bowen's disease, and atypical nevi or moles. The term *premalignant* does not imply that all the lesions will become malignant but that the tendency to become malignant exists (Table 65-7).

Malignant Lesions

Malignant skin lesions include squamous cell carcinoma, basal cell carcinoma, and malignant melanoma (Table 65-8).

Etiology and Epidemiology. Malignant melanoma is a tumor of the melanocytes, occurring on both sun-exposed and nonexposed skin surfaces. Malignant melanoma often develops from a preexisting pigmented mole or nevi, although it may arise from healthy skin. Precursor lesions to melanoma are atypical or dysplastic nevi, congenital nevi, and lentigo maligna. There is a genetic predisposition to melanoma; 10% of persons with melanoma have a first-degree relative with the disease.[15]

The incidence of malignant melanoma is increasing more rapidly than that of any other malignancy.[12] The death rate is also increasing. Currently, 1 in 68 persons will develop malignant melanoma. This increase may be due in part to increased sun exposure, thinning of the ozone layer, and other uncontrollable factors. Persons at increased risk include those with a previous melanoma, persons with multiple atypical nevi (atypical mole syndrome), fair-complexioned individuals (especially those with light hair and light eyes), and persons with a history of childhood blistering sunburns. The mean age of diagnosis is 40 years.

Pathophysiology. Major classifications of melanoma include melanoma in situ, superficial spreading melanoma, lentigo maligna melanoma, nodular melanoma, and acral-lentiginous

TABLE 65-6 KERATOSES: ETIOLOGY, APPEARANCE, AND TREATMENT

Type of Lesion	Etiology	Appearance	Treatment
Corns	Pressure, ill-fitting shoes	Center core that thickens inwardly; pain with pressure; usually occur on toes	Felt pad with center hole to relieve pressure; properly fitting shoes; corn recurrent if pressure not relieved
Callus	Constant pressure on plantar surface of foot; can also occur on palmar surface of hands	Thickening of horny layer of skin	Relief of pressure; regular massage with softening lotion or creams
Seborrheic keratoses (Figure 65-15, *A*)	Normal aging process, rarely develop into malignancy; must distinguish from actinic keratoses, which have malignancy potential	Large, darkened, greasy warts usually on trunk, less often on scalp, face, and proximal extremities; sudden increase in number and size sometimes indicative of gastrointestinal malignancy	No treatment except for cosmetic reasons or constant irritation; may be removed by curettage, electrodesiccation, or liquid nitrogen
Dermatosis papulosa nigra	Seborrheic keratoses in African-Americans	Small, pedunculated, heavily pigmented	Same as for seborrheic keratoses
Actinic keratoses (Figure 65-15, *B*) (senile, solar)	Chronic exposure to solar irradiation; occur on exposed areas of skin; light-skinned persons most vulnerable; approximately 25% evolve to squamous cell carcinoma (evidenced by rapid increase in size of lesion)	Round or irregular, red-brown to gray with dry, scaly appearance; surrounding skin usually dry and wrinkled from overexposure to sun	Protective clothing, sunscreens; removal by curettage, liquid nitrogen therapy, dermabrasion, and electrodesiccation; multiple lesions treatable with topical of 1%-5% 5-fluorouracil cream (Efudex) or imiquimod cream (Aldara)

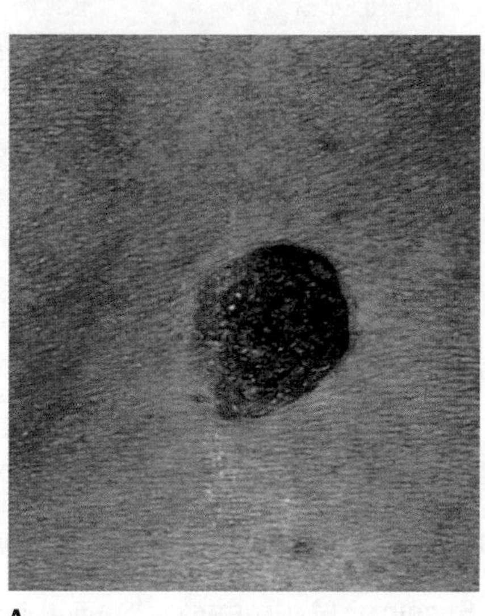
A

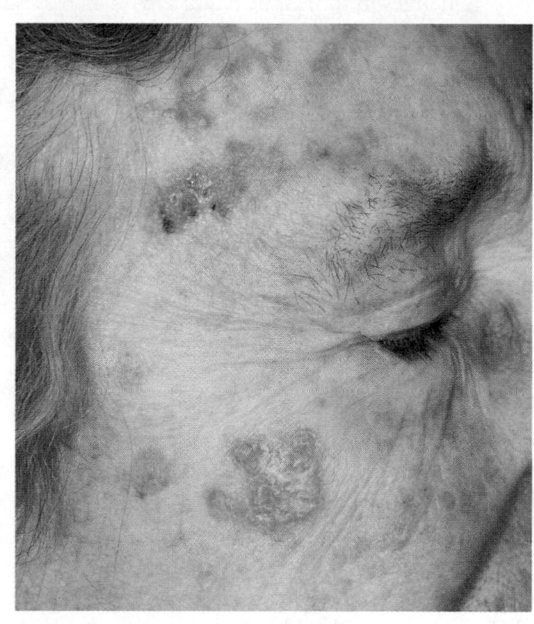
B

Figure 65-15 A, Seborrheic keratosis. **B,** Actinic (senile) keratosis.

melanoma. The most common is the superficial spreading type, which accounts for 70% of all melanomas.

Nodular melanoma carries the worst prognosis. Survival rates for primary localized melanomas after excision are 90% to 98%. The survival rate for other stages ranges from 5% to 80%. Staging is based on tumor size, affected lymph nodes, and metastases. The tumor arises from melanocytes. Responsible for the biosynthesis and transport of melanin, these cells are most commonly found in the basal layer of the epidermis and eye, but are also found in the meninges, alimentary and respiratory tracts, and lymph nodes.

TABLE 65-7 PREMALIGNANT LESIONS: ETIOLOGY, APPEARANCE, AND TREATMENT

Lesion	Etiology	Appearance	Treatment
Leukoplakia	Unknown causes and external irritants such as ill-fitting dentures, cheek biting, and pipe and cigarette smoking; chronic maceration, friction, and senile atrophy leading to vaginal leukoplakia	Mucous membranes developing thickened, white patches of keratinized cells, which may eventually lead to squamous cell carcinoma Erythroplakia (red or red and white patches) of mouth a higher malignancy potential than leukoplakia	Prevention by removal of causative factors; inspection of mouth, mucous membranes; dental care for rough teeth, proper-fitting dentures; large lesions usually surgically excised, and biopsy performed; benign lesions often removed by electrodesiccation; treatment by surgical excision, cryotherapy, curettage and electrodesiccation, carbon dioxide laser therapy, 5-fluorouracil cream or solution
Bowen's disease	Chemical carcinogens; occurs on older, light-skinned men; also called squamous cell carcinoma in situ; persons affected at higher risk of developing other malignancies	Widely distributed, sharply demarcated brown plaques, although a single lesion may exist	Small lesions treated with electrodessication and curettage, cryosurgery, or excisional surgery; large lesions are excised or 5-FU cream is applied twice daily for 4-8 weeks; area surrounding the lesion is also treated; imiquimod 5% cream may be applied daily for up to 16 weeks
Pigmented nevi (moles)	Most harmless, but others may be dysplastic, precancerous, or cancerous Changes in mole that require immediate attention: Development of ring of new pigment around base Development of uneven pigmentation Sudden growth Loss of hair Bleeding	Present on most persons, regardless of skin color; may be flat, raised, prominent, or hairy; color ranging from tan to black Atypical (dysplastic) moles usually on upper back in males and on legs in females (Refer to Malignant Lesions section for further discussion.)	Biopsy and excision of suspicious lesions; to help remember characteristics of malignant moles, American Cancer Society developed mnemonic *ABCD:* Asymmetry of borders Border irregularity Color blue-black or variegated Diameter 0.6 mm

Contained in each melanocyte is a melanosome, an organelle that synthesizes the pigment. In melanoma the melanosome is abnormal or absent. Atypical melanocytes proliferate along the basal layer of the epidermis; when the melanocytes invade the dermis, the lesion is considered malignant. Each type of melanoma has a radial growth phase, the length of which varies. Melanoma is staged, as are other cancers, depending on the depth of tumor at the time of excision and presence of lymph node and solid organ metastases.

Tumors occur most commonly on the head, neck, and lower extremities. The lesions vary considerably in appearance, some with deep pigmentation, irregular scalloped borders, and surrounding erythema or halo. Others may possess variegated pigmentation (yellow, blue, black, gray) or absence of color altogether (Figure 65-17). Late changes include bleeding and ulceration. The incidence of metastasis from malignant melanoma is high and depends on the depth of invasion. Metastasis typically occurs first to the regional lymph nodes and then by hematogenous spread to the lungs, liver, brain, and other areas.

Collaborative Care Management

DIAGNOSTIC TESTS. As in all malignancies, confirmation of diagnosis is by biopsy. Excisional skin biopsies with sufficient margins to determine the depth of invasion and provide staging information are performed on suspicious pigmented lesions. Electrodessication, curettage, shaving, and cryotherapy are contraindicated in mole evaluations, since they do not provide sufficient tissue to rule in or rule out malignant melanoma.

SURGICAL MANAGEMENT. Surgical intervention in malignant melanoma by far offers the best potential for cure. Once the diagnosis of malignant melanoma is made by skin biopsy, a wide surgical excision is performed. Removing an appropriate margin of tissue surrounding the lesion decreases the chance of local recurrence. Surgical margins for primary cutaneous melanoma are determined by the thickness of the lesion. Patients with intermediate-thickness melanoma (more than 1 mm deep) may elect to undergo sentinel lymph node mapping. A negative sen-

TABLE 65-8 NONMELANOMA SKIN CANCERS: ETIOLOGY, APPEARANCE, AND TREATMENT

Lesion	Etiology	Appearance	Treatment
Squamous cell carcinoma (Figure 65-16)	Unknown; may arise from actinic keratoses, Bowen's disease, or leukoplakia	If precursor was premalignant lesion, lesion will be indurated and surrounded by inflammatory base. New lesions appear as firm keratotic nodule with indurated base. Lip or ear lesions may metastasize to regional lymph nodes. Lesions on hair-bearing areas rarely metastasize.	Prevention and early detection. Removal by surgical excision or Mohs micrographic surgery (surgery in which lesion is removed in successive thin horizontal layers along grid pattern until undersurface and borders of removed tissue are free of malignant cells), curettage with electro-desiccation, irradiation, or chemosurgery (for treatment of tumors with ill-defined borders). Dressing applied with fixative paste such as zinc chloride; removal of dressing removes malignant tissue. Reapplication usually necessary.
Basal cell carcinoma	Unknown; most common malignant tumor affecting light-skinned persons over age 40; primarily occurs over hairy areas that contain pilosebaceous follicles	Lesion has translucent appearance, color from flesh to pale pink with few telangiectatic vessels across surface. Lesions are rarely metastatic if treated.	Untreated tumors locally invasive with severe tissue destruction, infection, and hemorrhage; metastasize to bone, lung, and brain. Treatment dependent on site and extent of tumor: surgical excision or Mohs micrographic surgery, curettage with electro-desiccation, irradiation, and chemosurgery.

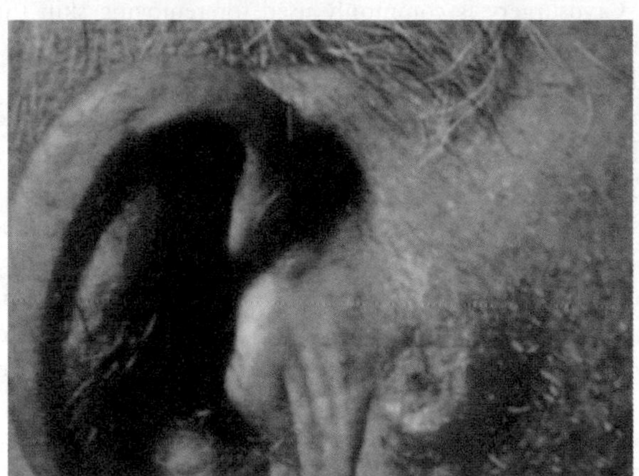

Figure 65-16 Squamous cell carcinoma in infratemporal area, one of the most common sites for this tumor.

tinel lymph node is highly predictive that the remainder of the nodal basin will also be negative. If the sentinel lymph node is positive, a completion lymphadenectomy is usually recommended to determine the number of positive lymph nodes. Therapeutic lymph node dissection is indicated for persons with clinically enlarged regional nodes after cytologic confirmation of metastatic disease. Regional lymphadenectomy may be indicated for palliative purposes as well.

MEDICAL MANAGEMENT. Metastatic malignant melanoma is resistant to currently available systemic chemotherapeutic agents. The drug used most successfully is dacarbazine (DTIC), which has an overall response rate of 10% to 28%, depending on disease site. Indicated as treatment for surgically unresectable advanced metastatic melanoma, DTIC can be administered on an outpatient basis. Other chemotherapeutic agents are sometimes used in the clinical trial setting. Isolated limb perfusion and infusion therapy can provide maximal chemotherapeutic effect in an involved limb. Hyperthermia, in addition to vascular perfusion of chemotherapy through an isolated region, allows high concentrations of chemotherapeutic agents to be administered to the extremity with minimal systemic toxicity.

High-dose interferon has recently been shown to result in a small but significant improvement in both disease-free and overall survival rates. Interferon treatment is both costly and potentially toxic. Lower-dose interferon therapy results in less toxicity but without a survival benefit. Other biologic response modifiers, such as recombinant interleukin-2 and monoclonal antibodies, are options for select individuals in the clinical trial setting. Immunotherapy with tumor vaccines to stimulate the

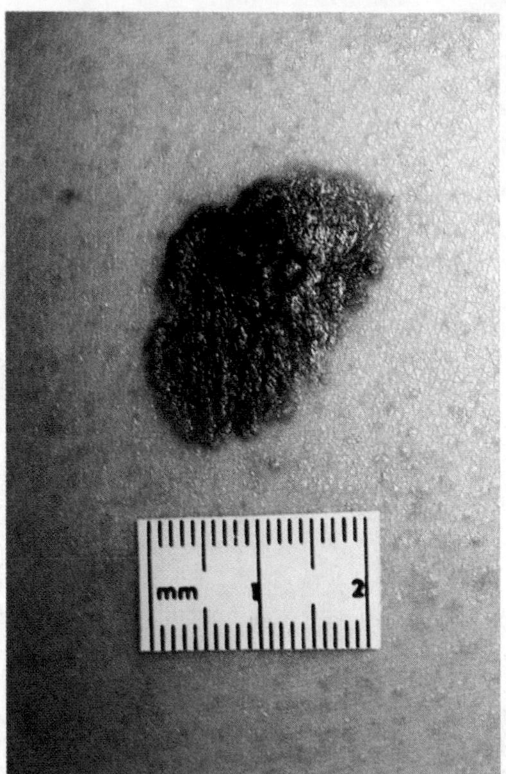

Figure 65-17 Malignant melanoma. Note asymmetry of borders, size greater than 6 mm, and color.

host's system to react to the melanoma is the subject of many clinical trials at this time. Local radiation is sometimes used to offer local control at a site of a deeper melanoma.

Ambulatory Dermatologic Surgical Procedures. A number of dermatologic surgical procedures are performed by clinicians in an ambulatory setting.

Dermatologic Surgery. Treatment of skin lesions by dermatology providers often includes removal of skin lesions. Superficial skin lesions involving only the epidermis can be removed easily by various means; deep lesions involving the dermis, such as some cancers, are removed with full-thickness skin excision.

Shave Biopsy and Excision. Superficial lesions rising above the plane of the skin surface can be removed by shaving technique. A No. 15 scalpel blade is typically used. The entire lesion may be removed for diagnosis. Hemostasis is obtained with pressure, aluminum chloride (Drysol), ferric subsulfate (Monsel's solution), or gelatin foam (Gelfoam).

Curettage. Curettage is the scraping or scooping out of a superficial lesion with a curette, a spoon-shaped, sharp-edged instrument (Figure 65-18). A local anesthetic is usually injected around the lesion before curettage. Hemostasis is accomplished with a chemical styptic such as ferric chloride or Monsel's solution, with gelatin foam, or by electrocoagulation. Lesions removed by curettage include seborrheic keratosis, actinic keratosis, basal cell carcinomas, and warts.

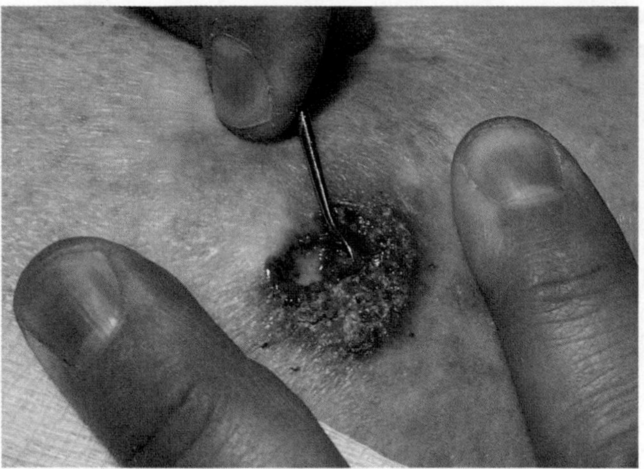

Figure 65-18 Curettage of inflamed seborrheic keratosis.

Punch Biopsy. Punch biopsies are used to provide tissue for histologic evaluation (e.g., suspected skin cancers, unusual dermatoses), as well as to remove small, benign lesions. After the patient receives a local anesthetic, a punch is used to remove deep lesions up to 10 mm in diameter. The tissue is then sent for biopsy. Punch biopsies may be closed with sutures. The clinician sometimes selects wound healing by secondary intention. In this situation hemostasis can be obtained with gelatin foam packing.

Cryosurgery. Tissue can be destroyed by rapid freezing with substances such as liquid oxygen, carbon dioxide snow or gas, liquid nitrogen, dichlorodifluoromethane (Freon), or nitrous oxide. Carbon dioxide snow and liquid nitrogen are most commonly used. The rapid freezing causes formation of intracellular ice, which destroys the cell membranes and produces cell dehydration. Cryosurgery is commonly used for removing skin tumors (benign and malignant) and warts.

Although the procedure usually is not painful, a tingling pain occurs when the freezing substance is applied and may be uncomfortable for some persons, particularly if multiple lesions are treated.

Tissue necrosis may not be evident until 24 hours after cryosurgery. A clear or hemorrhagic bulla forms during the first day, but inflammatory reactions and bleeding are usually absent. Serous exudates form during the first week, followed by eschar or crust formation. The crust drops off in 3 to 4 weeks as the underlying tissue heals. Hypopigmentation may occur because melanocytes are highly vulnerable to freezing.

Electrosurgery. Electric current may be used in dermatologic surgery to remove tissue and control bleeding. Electrodessication is the drying of tissue by means of a monopolar current through the needle electrode. Electrofulguration is a form of electrodessication in which the needle electrode is held close to, rather than inserted into, the tissue, thus spraying the area with sparks. Bipolar current is used for electrocoagulation, which coagulates the tissue, curtailing capillary bleeding, and for electrosection, which cuts the tissue. Delayed bleeding may occur, especially from electrocoagulation, and may alarm the unprepared patient. The bleeding can be easily controlled by direct pressure. After most electrosurgery the wound is left exposed for air drying. Dressings may be used if the area is subject to frequent trauma or rubbing or if oozing is present. The wound may be wiped with 70% alcohol to hasten drying. Covering the wound with Gelfoam powder and tape may make a hemostatic nonocclusive dressing.

DIET. No special diet is prescribed for persons undergoing dermatologic surgery. However, the nurse should encourage the patient to have a nutritionally balanced diet both before and after surgery to enhance healing of tissues.

▶ ARE You READY?

Which of the following is the most effective intervention for the treatment of malignant melanoma?

1. Dacarbazine
2. Radiation therapy
3. High-dose interferon
4. Wide surgical excision

Nursing Management *of the Patient undergoing Dermatologic Surgery*

PREOPERATIVE CARE

Regardless of the type and extent of the surgery, the patient and family need preoperative teaching. This may be done in a variety of settings, depending on the type of procedure planned. Teaching should include specifics regarding the location and extent of incision, any postoperative activity limitations, and any special postoperative care needs. Information should be included regarding the anesthetic options available. See Chapter 13 for further discussion of preoperative preparation of the patient.

POSTOPERATIVE CARE

After surgery the patient requires care and monitoring as described in Chapter 15. If a malignant lesion was removed, the patient may be instructed to seek follow-up care at closer intervals. If metastasis occurs, nursing care focuses on helping the patient understand the treatment and its side effects. The patient is confronted with many physical problems, as well as psychologic and emotional problems such as fear of cancer, loss of health, and fear of dying.

After superficial skin surgery the nurse instructs the patient not to remove the crust (scab), which acts as protection (healing occurs under the crust). The crust should be kept as dry as possible; if it gets wet, it should be patted dry. Alcohol may be applied and allowed to evaporate. Makeup may be used over the crust. The crust may be left uncovered or may be covered with an adhesive bandage. Signs of redness, edema, or pain should be reported to the health care provider.[12]

After deep skin surgery the wound is usually bandaged, and the clinician gives the patient specific care instructions. Aspirin and other drugs that alter blood coagulation should be avoided for 7 days before and after surgery to decrease the potential for postoperative bleeding.[12]

The patient and family require an explanation about the treatments that may be performed postoperatively or prescribed for home care. They also require teaching regarding the care of healthy skin and steps to prevent further damage to the skin, as discussed next.

Avoiding Causative Agents. The first step in preventing dermatologic conditions is avoiding the causative agent, which may be a specific antigen, a contact irritant, a microorganism, trauma, direct sunlight, or an insect. Instructing the person to avoid a known causative agent is preventive medicine; however, it may not be that simple. Many dermatologic diseases have no known cause or are hereditary. Unfortunately, once the mechanism of the disease is known, it is not always possible to remove the triggering factors. Occasionally, symptoms may persist long after the agent is removed. Therefore the nurse's major responsibilities include education of the patient about measures that promote rest, methods that decrease emotional stress, the need for good nutrition, and the need to closely observe sites to detect changes in skin conditions.

Cleansing. Bathing is an essential element of skin care. The frequency of skin cleansing is individualized according to need and patient preference. The outer layer of skin cells and perspiration are acidic, and their presence inhibits the life and growth of harmful bacteria; at the same time, normal flora grow in acid environments and act as the skin's protection. Strong soaps that are alkaline in reaction may neutralize this protective acid condition of the skin. They may also remove the oily secretion of the sebaceous glands, which lubricates the outer skin layers and contributes to their health. Removal of excess oil and scale or debris is sometimes necessary to facilitate absorption of medication, promote healing, and enhance the skin's appearance. For example, in psoriasis removal of scale by mechanical means and slowing of skin metabolism are prime objectives.

Normal skin should be washed with pH-neutral, soaplike agents to remove excess oils and excretions and to prevent odor. After showering the skin can be patted dry and lotion applied to prevent drying. Maintaining proper hydration in the skin prevents dryness and itching, which may lead to scratching, excoriation, and further trauma. Soaking in a tub of water for 20 to 30 minutes and then immediately applying a lubricating lotion or cream may hydrate the stratum corneum by preventing the rapid loss of water from the skin surface.

Sunlight. Sunlight, particularly UV light, is damaging to the skin. UV light is termed *actinic*, meaning photochemically active radiation. UVA light contributes to aging and carcinogenesis of the skin. The UVB light spectrum leads to burning and activation of melanin, which produces tanning. Chronic tanning will lead to the undesirable skin changes of wrinkling, pigmentary disturbances (e.g., brown spots), and leatherlike textural changes. Tanning parlors should be avoided, since they use both the damaging UVB and UVA light spectrums to produce tans, which carry the same harmful skin cancer risks as natural sunlight.

Rashes caused by photosensitivity resulting from certain medications appear abruptly and are widespread, symmetric, and bright red. Classes of medications that enhance photosensitivity include certain tetracyclines, sulfa drugs, antihypertensives, diuretics, oral hypoglycemics, psychotropic drugs, and NSAIDs.

The way to protect against UV rays is to block them. The rays may be blocked by opaque clothing, umbrellas, wide-brimmed hats, or other screening aids; by avoidance of sun exposure between 10 AM and 3 PM; or by selected sunscreens. The optimal sunscreens have a sun protection factor (SPF) of 15 or greater.[14] Sunscreens can be easily removed by swimming or sweating; thus reapplications are necessary. Sunscreen labels indicate whether a product is *water resistant* or *waterproof.* Eyes should be protected with UV-protective sunglasses. UV light has stronger effects at high altitudes (where there is less atmosphere to absorb the rays) and as one nears the equator (where the sun is closer to the earth); therefore additional protection is required in these locations. Persons with dermatoses that are exacerbated by UV light or those who have an illness that is exacerbated by sunlight should avoid sunlight if possible or generously apply broad-spectrum (UVA-UVB) sunscreens.

Nutrition. Balanced nutrition plays an important role in maintaining intact, healthy skin. Essential nutrients for skin health include protein, vitamin C, iron, and zinc.[7] Some dermatologic disorders may be directly associated with dietary intake. Excessive dryness of the skin and thickening of the stratum corneum at the hair follicle openings may be caused by nutritional deficiencies. Elevated blood lipid levels caused by hyperlipoproteinemia may take the form of xanthomas on the skin surface. Persons experiencing hypersensitivity reactions may be placed on restrictive diets to exclude intake of known causative agents or as a diagnostic tool to identify causative agents. The patient should read food labels carefully to determine whether the product or food additive contains the agent in question. The nurse instructs patients and family members about any specific dietary restrictions included in the treatment plan.

Observation of Changes. Care of normal skin includes regular observation of pigmented areas, moles or nevi, or other newly acquired skin growths. Any change in size, color, or general appearance should be reported to a health care provider.

Dangers of Self-Treatment. The nurse urges patients to seek attention from a health care provider when skin conditions develop. Although skin diseases rarely cause death, they may reflect serious systemic illness, cause discomfort, and interrupt work and other activities. Many persons are inclined to rely on the advice of friends or local pharmacists or on home remedies. Each individual's skin reacts differently to treatment, and skin that is already irritated or inflamed may respond violently to inexpert treatment. Medications prescribed previously for an unrelated skin disorder may produce an unfavorable response in a new skin problem. Medications without expiration dates should be discarded. The person may be spared much discomfort and expense by consulting a specialist when symptoms first develop and before a mild skin condition becomes a serious problem.

Psychologic Care. A certain degree of "beauty orientation" exists in Western culture. Television and print media advertisements use beautiful models to attract the consumer. Cosmetics to enhance good looks are extensively used by women and men. In this context, skin diseases or physical defects that detract from "good looks" can alter one's self-image.

A person's emotional reaction to a skin disorder or deformity must not be underestimated. Pride and the ability to regard oneself favorably in comparison with others are essential to the development and maintenance of a well-integrated personality. Every person who has a defect or is physically challenged, particularly if the defect is conspicuous, suffers from some threat to emotional security. The extent of the emotional reaction and the amount of maladjustment that follows depend on the individual's personality and ability to cope with emotional insults. Physical insults, whether they are induced by skin disease or trauma, almost invariably lead to disruptive life experiences. Other people may recoil when viewing persons with severe skin diseases. They may fear potential contagion, although most often this is unwarranted. The child who has severe atopic dermatitis, especially involving the face, may be ridiculed at school; the adolescent girl who has pitted acne scars may be self-conscious and avoid social situations; and the young man with a posttraumatic scar on his face may be refused a sales job. The defect may be used to justify failure, avoid responsibility, or justify striking out against an unkind society.

Nurses and other health care providers should possess insight into their own possible responses to viewing severe skin problems before delivering care. They should provide an open, accepting, nurturing health care environment for patients with skin disorders.

Relief of Pruritus. Pruritus, or itching, is a cutaneous symptom that provokes the desire to scratch. It is caused by repetitive low-frequency stimulation of C fibers. These C fibers are similar to, but different from, the C fibers that transmit pain stimuli. Itching can be produced by mechanical stimulation of the skin or by chemical mediators. Itching primarily occurs in the skin, certain mucous membranes, and eyes. The areas most sensitive to itching are the nostrils, mucocutaneous junctions, external ear canals, and perineum.

Pruritus may result from any irritating substance that disrupts the integrity of the stratum corneum. It can also occur with certain systemic diseases (Box 65-1). One of the most common causes of pruritus is dry skin. Dry skin can accompany certain skin disorders such as atopic dermatitis, occur as a result of excessive bathing with drying soaps, or happen as a normal manifestation of aging. Physiologic factors that intensify itching include vasodilation, tissue anoxia, and circulatory stasis. Whatever the cause,

Box 65-1 Common Causes of Pruritus

- Dry skin
- Skin irritants: plastic or glass fibers, wool, plant products, insects
- Drug reactions
- Psychogenic reactions
- Infectious diseases
- Infestation: scabies, pediculosis
- Systemic diseases: obstructive biliary disease, uremia, diabetes mellitus
- Neoplasia: Hodgkin's disease, leukemia, lymphoma

pruritus ranges from a simple annoyance to a severe, distressing, exhausting problem.

Pruritus leads to the motor response of scratching. Persons with intense itching can severely excoriate the skin by digging deeply with their fingernails. Persons with generalized pruritus may be observed to be in constant motion, twisting, rubbing, and scratching repeatedly.

A major step in treating patients with pruritus is to attempt to remove the itch stimuli and break the itch-scratch cycle. Cold causes vasoconstriction and provides some relief. Hydration in a tepid bath followed by the application of an emollient lotion is helpful. Cornstarch or colloidal oatmeal preparations may be added to the bath. Topical corticosteroids decrease the inflammatory effects and play a role in decreasing pruritus symptoms. Topical antipruritic agents such as Sarna lotion and pramoxine hydrochloride applied two or three times a day can inhibit the itch-scratch cycle. Oral antihistamines, both sedating and nonsedating, may offer some relief.

The awareness of pruritus may be more acute during the night because of a decrease in diverting stimuli. Cool, light, nonrestrictive bed clothing may help allay itching. Hot, dry environments are not conducive to managing itch symptoms. The living quarters can be humidified with use of humidifiers and moist heat systems.

Temperature Control. Maintenance of optimal body temperature can be an issue for persons with dermatologic problems. Patients with generalized flush (erythroderma) or extensive atopic or exfoliative dermatitis may lose body heat at an abnormally increased rate. Ambient room temperature should be maintained at 70° F (21.1° C) or more to ensure patient comfort. Care must be taken to avoid chilling, particularly after bathing or when compresses or dressings are applied.

Therapeutic Baths and Soaks. Baths or soaks are recommended to relieve pruritus; remove exudates; hydrate dry skin; dehydrate weeping, moist skin; or provide antimicrobial actions (Table 65-9). Too frequent bathing or soaking can lead to dry skin. The application of emollient lotions or creams immediately after bathing or soaking will enhance the product's hydrating effects.

Tub baths may be taken to cleanse the skin before therapeutic topical therapy, to relieve generalized pruritus, or to provide direct therapy (e.g., Domeboro or tar baths). During cleansing baths special attention is given to intertriginous areas, where creams and topical medications may collect. Older adults should be provided with a safe environment for bathing to avoid falls. Lifts may be required for the hospitalized patient. If a lift is not available, sitting on a chair under a gentle shower is the best alternative to a cleansing bath (see Guidelines for Safe Practice box below).

Wet dressings provide cooling, drying, antipruritic, or debriding effects. Plain tap water or physiologic saline may be used, or medications may be added. An astringent effect may be obtained through the use of Burow's solution (Domeboro, Buro-Sol), 1:20 or 1:40 dilution. Potassium permanganate has antimicrobial and drying effects. All tablet crystals must be thoroughly dissolved to prevent chemical burning of the skin. Potassium permanganate should not be used on the face. Silver nitrate, 0.5%, is an antimicrobial agent often used in the treatment of burns. Both potassium permanganate and silver nitrate can stain skin and cloth (see Guidelines for Safe Practice box, p. 1898).

Medications. Medications are delivered to patients with skin disorders via topical, intralesional, or systemic routes. Topical therapy is preferred, since it is less likely to cause systemic side effects. The disadvantages of topical therapy are the time requirements for

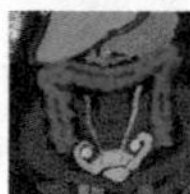

GUIDELINES FOR SAFE PRACTICE
Baths and Soaks

- Maintain the water at a temperature comfortable to the patient (usually 90° to 100° F [32° to 38° C]).
- Make certain the medication completely dissolves while tub is filling.
- Have patient soak for 20 to 30 minutes.
- Prevent falls when oils or colloids are added to the water by assisting patients in and out of the tub.
- Use a rubber mat to prevent slipping.
- Pat, do not rub, the skin dry to avoid skin irritation.
- Apply creams or ointments immediately after the bath to retain skin moisture.
- Clean tub after a medicated bath as follows:
  1. Pour 1 cup of bleach into used tub water.
  2. Let bleach stand in water for 5 minutes.
  3. Wipe sides and bottom of tub.
  4. Drain and clean tub as usual.

TABLE 65-9 PREPARATIONS COMMONLY USED FOR BATHS OR SOAKS

Substance	Effect	Suggested Actions
Colloids: oatmeal, cornstarch, soybean powder	Antipruritic, drying	Tub surfaces become slippery; support person to prevent falls.
Potassium permanganate ($KMnO_4$)	Antifungal, drying, deodorizing	Strain pulverized tablet through cheesecloth to prevent irritation; stains surfaces and linens.
Burow's solution (aluminum acetate)	Antibacterial, drying	Commonly used for soaks.
Sulfur bath suspension	Antibacterial	Rinse body with tepid water after bath to remove residual sulfur particles.
Tar preparations: Balnetar, T/Gel, Polytar	Antipruritic, moisturizing	Do not use soap with tar baths.
Bath oils: Alpha Keri, colloidal oatmeal	Antipruritic, moisturizing	Tub surfaces may become slippery.

applications, volumes needed, and potential aesthetic concerns. Dermatologic topical medications are delivered to the target organ (skin) via several *vehicle* systems. A vehicle is the substance in which the medication is placed for application to the skin. Creams, ointments, lotions, gels, solutions, and powders are the usual vehicle systems used to deliver topical medication. The degree of inflammation observed in a rash influences the choice of vehicle. Patient instruction on method of application enhances the treatment regimen (Table 65-10). The nurse should be aware of the pharmacologic actions of the topical medication prescribed, as well as the actions of the vehicle system.

The Dermatologic Drug Formulary lists the broad categories of agents used in management of skin disorders along with examples of select products.[16a]

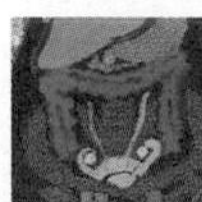

Guidelines for Safe Practice
Applying Wet Dressings

1. Prepare solution to be applied at room temperature. Sterility is not required.
2. Soak dressing thoroughly in solution.
3. Protect bed or clothing with towels, bath blanket, flannel squares, etc.
4. Wring out dressings; they should be wet but not dripping.
5. Apply dressings in two to four smooth layers to involved areas. Wrap fingers and toes separately, and wrap joints so they can bend.
6. Remove, soak, and reapply dressings before they dry (i.e., every 3 to 5 minutes).
7. Continue treatment for 20 to 30 minutes.
8. Pat skin dry.

Topical Corticosteroids. Glucocorticosteroids are the most potent antiinflammatory substances available. They possess the

Table 65-10 Factors Influencing Vehicle Selection and Patient Instructional Tips

Degree of Inflammatory Process

Inflammation	Vehicles
Acute Inflammation Marked erythema, edema, blistering, tenderness, pruritus, oozing, crusting	Wet dressings Powders Solutions Lotions
Subacute Inflammation Oozing and crusting subsided Erythema and edema less acute but still present	Lotions Aerosols Creams Gels
Chronic Inflammation Limited erythema, scaling, fissures Pruritus	Gels Ointments

Location of Skin Condition

Scalp—lotions, gels, solutions
Intertriginous areas—lotions, powders, creams

Activity of Medication in Given Vehicle

Chemical formulation of active ingredient versus vehicle

Application	Indicated Area	Instructional Tips
Creams	Hair-bearing areas, moist lesions, intertriginous folds	Apply in direction of hair growth evenly and sparingly.
Ointments	Dry and fissured skin surfaces	Hydrating skin before application may improve effectiveness. Can cause irritation and maceration if applied to areas that are moist or occluded.
Lotions	Large surface areas, intertriginous folds, hair-bearing areas, oozing sites	Shake well before application.
Powders	Intertriginous folds and other sites where moisture trapping occurs	Apply with puff or shaker. Remove starch- or cellulose-containing powders before reapplication.
Solutions, spray, aerosol	Hair-bearing areas, large surface areas	Spray aerosol 6 in from skin in bursts.
Gels	Hair-bearing surfaces, facial sites	Gels may be dehydrating. Minimize irritation by applying to dry skin.

From Dermatology Nurses' Association: *Dermatology nursing essentials: a core curriculum*, Pitman, NJ, 2003, Anthony J Janetti.

unique ability to inhibit cell division. Corticosteroids are used to treat a variety of skin disorders because of their antiinflammatory, antiproliferative, and antipruritic properties.

Topical corticosteroids differ in their antiinflammatory effects, ranging from low to very high potency. Hydrocortisone is of low potency. Some corticosteroids, such as triamcinolone acetonide (Aristocort, Kenalog), vary in potency depending on the dose. Topical steroids in an ointment vehicle are usually more potent and have a greater lubricating effect than cream vehicles of the same agent. Fluorinated corticosteroids are more potent and thus have a greater potential for causing the local side effects of skin atrophy, purpura, striae, rosacea, and folliculitis. Fluorinated corticosteroids should not be used on the face, skin folds, or genital sites. Hypothalamic-pituitary-adrenal axis suppression is a rare occurrence with topical corticosteroid therapy. It can happen, however, when a super potent agent is applied to a large surface area for an extended time.

Occlusive dressings enhance the effects of topical corticosteroids. Occlusion can offer benefit for (1) dermatoses of palms and soles; (2) thick psoriatic plaques; (3) localized plaques of LSC; and (4) extensive, severe, steroid-responsive dermatitis. The affected area should be occluded only when directed by the health care provider. Plastic wrap is good for occluding small areas. Plastic (nonlatex) gloves may be used on hands and plastic bags on feet. Plastic garment bags or large trash bags may be used for the trunk, with holes cut for head and arms. Plastic suits (sauna suits) are available for total body occlusion. Lesions are usually occluded at night for an 8-hour period. The patient should be monitored for potential complications, including candidal infections, sweat retention, and folliculitis.

APPLICATION OF TOPICAL MEDICATIONS. Gloves are worn for protection when applying topical medications. Powders are sprinkled into the gloved hand and then applied to the skin to avoid aerosolization of the agent. Powders are used sparingly to prevent caking. Cornstarch is not suggested because it encourages growth of yeast organisms. Lotions with a water or alcohol base are applied by patting gently. Lotions with an oily base are applied thinly and evenly with the palm of the gloved hand. Ointments are applied with a gloved hand and tend to spread with greater ease than creams. If a dressing is to be applied, the ointment may be spread on the dressing with a tongue blade before application to the skin. Some topical medications, such as coal tar products, are removed before other topical treatments are imposed.

Home Care. The vast majority of patients with dermatologic disorders do not require inpatient hospitalization. Patient teaching is critical to successful self-care management in the outpatient population (see Patient/Family Teaching box). Written instructions should be clear, concise, and tailored to the patient's specific language requirements and age. Many dermatology organizations and related pharmaceutical companies provide free patient education literature on skin disorders, skin cancer prevention, and use of dermatologic topical products.

Dressing procedures are sometimes costly and complex. These patients benefit from a home health referral to assist with teaching, as well as community financial resources.

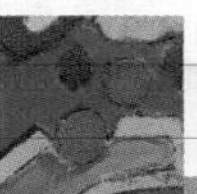

PATIENT/FAMILY TEACHING
Dermatologic Disorders

Teaching should include information about:
- Nature of the disorder (cause, preventive measures, acuity or chronicity, symptoms requiring medical follow-up care)
- Treatment modalities to be carried out at home (soaks, baths, medicated dressings)
- Prescribed medication regimens: route of administration, vehicle used, dose, frequency, duration of topical application, side effects, where to obtain supplies
- Ways to promote socialization with others when disfiguring dermatologic lesions are present

The nurse also instructs the patient on special precautions such as:
- Avoid nonporous coverings over dressings, unless ordered.
- Completely dissolve tablets or crystals in baths or soaks.
- Avoid excessive rubbing of medication over lesions.
- Apply thin layers of lotions or powders.

Pressure Ulcers

Etiology and Epidemiology. Pressure ulcers are defined by the National Pressure Ulcer Advisory Panel (NPUAP) as lesions caused by unrelieved pressure against soft tissue, usually over bony prominences. For many years these wounds were incorrectly termed *bedsores* or *decubitus ulcers*. The Latin definition of the term *decubitus* implies lying flat, so *decubitus* was changed to *pressure* after researchers found that a pressure ulcer can develop while in any body position, on any body location, and from any source of pressure (internal secondary to bone or body weight, as well as external).

Risk factors for pressure ulcers are associated with both intrinsic and extrinsic factors. Extrinsic factors include moisture, shear, friction, and pressure, which can also be internal pressure. Intrinsic risk factors relate to characteristics of the patient's skin structure that are determined by factors such as the amount of collagen, age, nutritional status, and use of steroids; presence of spinal cord injury or other alterations in mobility and perception; and degree of perfusion. Factors affecting perfusion of the skin include blood pressure, extracorporeal circulation, serum protein, albumin and prealbumin levels,[3] hemoglobin and hematocrit levels, smoking, vascular disease, administration of vasoactive medication, and either a pronounced increase or decrease in body temperature.

Pressure ulcers can occur in any age-group, ethnic population, or socioeconomic group. Attempts have been made to estimate the financial burden of the pressure ulcer problem; however, research has been limited and inconsistent. Some studies estimate that $11.5 billion is expended annually on products for pressure ulcer management. Attempts to estimate the cost of an individual pressure ulcer also have been unsuccessful. Conservative estimates of the cost of treatment for one stage 1 or stage 2 pressure ulcer range from $125 to $200, with treatment of one stage 3 or 4 pressure ulcer ranging from $14,000 to $23,000.[4]

The NPUAP reviewed more than 800 available manuscripts between January 1999 and December 2000 in an attempt to define the scope of the problem and concluded that the incidence and prevalence of pressure ulcers in various health care settings are high enough to warrant concern. Clinical practice guidelines,[5,5a]

Legal Alert

Pressure Ulcers and Medical Malpractice

- Of patients at risk in hospitals and nursing homes, 68% to 78% achieve a verdict or settlement if adversely affected by a pressure ulcer.
- The median settlements are $250,000, although some settlements have been more than $2 million.
- Most of the higher monetary settlements are for patients with a pressure ulcer related to poor nutrition.

which are nationally accepted standards of care, were established and reviewed for validity based on that manuscript review. Neither the clinical practice guidelines for prevention[5] or for treatment[5a] have been updated since the original printing in 1992 and 1994, respectively.

The NPUAP's study found that the literature reported an incidence of pressure ulcers in acute care ranging from 0.4% to 39%; in long-term care the incidence ranged from 2.2% to 23.9%; and in home care it was as high as 17%.[6] The estimated prevalence of pressure ulcers previously reported was 12% in skilled care facilities[16] and 10.8% in acute care facilities,[2] of which 8.5% are intraoperatively acquired.[1] A recent study by a Veterans Affairs medical center reported that 39% of 553 patients with spinal cord injury were visiting the outpatient clinic or receiving home care for pressure ulcers over a 3-year period.[9] An estimated one in five patients dies each year from complications of pressure ulcers, and increasingly patients and their families are seeking legal advice regarding how the nursing care received could have permitted the patient to develop a pressure ulcer (see Legal Alert box).

Pathophysiology. Unrelieved pressure causes cellular necrosis as a result of vascular insufficiency (Table 65-11). See the Research box below for a discussion of preventing hospital-acquired pressure ulcers. Box 65-2 presents the stages of pressure ulcers that are recognized by both the NPAUP and the Wound, Ostomy and Continence Nursing Society.

Research

Stewart S, Box-Panksepp JS: Preventing hospital-acquired pressure ulcers: a point prevalence study, *OWM* 50(3):46-51, 2004.

The study was conducted in a 243-bed acute care medical center to determine whether pressure ulcers occurred while patients were hospitalized. The study consisted of two audits 16 months apart. The patient population was obtained from five medical-surgical units and two intensive care units; 109 patients completed the first audit, and 128 patients completed the second audit.

The initial audit was conducted before the introduction of a new support surface (mattress) for all beds on the seven nursing units. The prevalence of nosocomial (hospital-acquired) pressure ulcers in the first audit was 5.5%; the prevalence was reduced to 3.1% in the second audit after introduction of the new mattress. A stage 2 pressure ulcer was the most frequently reported ulcer in the initial audit; stage 1 pressure ulcers were the only ones documented in the second audit, demonstrating that the new mattress system prevented the occurrence of more severe hospital-acquired pressure ulcers.

Complications. Most complications associated with pressure ulcers are the sequelae of infection. In addition, if the patient has undergone surgical intervention, the complications associated with anesthesia and surgery are potential problems (see Chapter 15 for a discussion of postoperative care and complications). If the pressure ulcer becomes infected, the infection may spread to the bloodstream and result in sepsis. Osteomyelitis is another potential complication, requiring long-term intravenous antibiotics and possibly surgical intervention. In a patient with alterations in mobility, extensive pressure ulcers may result in further immobility. For example, a person with spinal cord injury with a pressure ulcer on the buttocks or sacral area may have to spend an extended period lying prone, with all pressure off the affected area.

If contamination of the pressure ulcer with bowel contents is a problem, some surgeons perform a temporary colostomy to prevent potential contamination of the wound. The colostomy is reversible after healing has occurred.

Collaborative Care Management. Pressure ulcers have been identified as primarily a nursing problem, but they require collaboration with the entire health care team for effective resolution. Management includes interventions designed to control chronic disease manifestations that affects healthy integument, such as medication regulation to keep glucose levels within normal limits and measures to promote optimal tissue perfusion and oxygenation. The correct product for treatment of pressure ulcers must be ordered, since inappropriate products can cause more tissue damage or delay healing. A discussion of common treatment modalities used in the management of pressure ulcers follows.

Diagnostic Tests. Although no specific laboratory tests can assist with diagnosis of pressure ulcers, it is well documented that wound healing depends on protein processing, and depletion of protein leads to delayed or poor wound healing.[17] Laboratory tests related to malnutrition and circulation should be used as predictors of potential alteration in skin integrity, as well as indicators of healing (Table 65-12). Open, draining ulcers may require culture and sensitivity to identify pathogens causing infection.

Medications. No particular medications are used for treating pressure ulcers. Antibiotics are used if an infection is present. Vitamins, minerals, and essential and nonessential amino acids are prescribed to improve the patient's nutritional status.

Treatment. The more independently active the patient is, the lower the risk of pressure ulcer formation and the greater the chances of wound healing. The key factor related to wound healing is the removal of the causative agent(s). Regardless of the treatment prescribed for wound care, if the patient or the nurse does not relieve the pressure, the wound will not heal. More than 2000 products exist as purported treatment measures for pressure ulcers (Table 65-13).

Surgical Management. Some patients with pressure ulcers qualify for surgical intervention. Surgeons perform myocutaneous flaps and skin grafts of various levels, depending on the patient's physical condition, compliance level, and type of wound. See the Research box, p. 1903, for a discussion of intraoperative control

TABLE 65-11 NORMAL FUNCTION, PATHOPHYSIOLOGY, AND CLINICAL MANIFESTATIONS OF PRESSURE ULCERS

Normal Function	Pathophysiology	Clinical Manifestations
Microvasculature: capillaries supplying tissue needs of oxygenated blood and nutrients	Pressure applied to soft tissue compressing capillaries, distorting structure, and occluding blood flow	Ischemia at first, followed by reactive hyperemia
Sympathetic response	Compensation by increased shunting of capillary circulation to area under pressure; capillaries increasing permeability and leaking fluid into tissues	Tissue edema and inflammation
Capillary walls lined with endothelial cells; platelets flowing smoothly through microvessels	Endothelial cells disrupted, platelets aggregating, and thrombi forming in capillaries and leading to cellular death	Erythema that may or may not resolve once pressure source is removed
Intact skin as body's protective mechanism	Cellular death leading to tissue necrosis	Pressure ulcer with visible tissue damage, described by stages (see Box 65-2)

BOX 65-2 Stages of Pressure Ulcers

Stage 1

An observable pressure-related alteration of intact skin whose indicators, when compared with the adjacent or opposite area on the body, may include changes in one or more of the following:

- Skin temperature (warmth or coolness)
- Tissue consistency (firm or boggy feel)
- Sensation (pain, itching)

The ulcer appears as a defined area of persistent redness in lightly pigmented skin, whereas in darker skin tones the ulcer may appear with persistent red, blue, or purple hues.

Stage 2

Partial-thickness skin loss involving epidermis, dermis, or both. The ulcer is superficial and is seen clinically as an abrasion, blister, or shallow crater.

Stage 3

Full-thickness skin loss involving damage to, or necrosis of, subcutaneous tissue that may extend down to, but not through, underlying fascia. The ulcer is seen clinically as a deep crater with or without undermining of adjacent tissue.

Stage 4

Full-thickness skin loss with extensive destruction; tissue necrosis; or damage to muscle, bone, or supporting structures (e.g., tendon, joint capsule). Undermining and sinus tracts also may be associated with stage 4 pressure ulcers.

NOTE: If eschar (dead, leathery tissue) is present, pressure ulcers cannot be accurately staged.

TABLE 65-12 DIAGNOSTIC TESTS IN PREVENTING OR TREATING A PRESSURE ULCER

Test	Normal Levels	Effect on Skin and Wound Care
Serum albumin	3.4-4.8 g/dl	<3.4 g/dl indicates malnutrition; either slow healing or possible wound will occur
Serum prealbumin	20-30 mg/dl	<20 mg/dl indicates malnutrition
Hemoglobin	Male: 13.5-17.5 g/dl Female: 12-16 g/dl	<10g/dl indicates anemia and impaired wound healing
Hematocrit	Male: 39%-49% Female: 35%-45%	<20 g/dl indicates impaired circulation and poor wound healing

of hypothermia and the correlation between core body temperature and the development of pressure ulcers.

DIET. Patients with pressure ulcers require additional protein (1.5 to 2 g/kg body weight/day) and calorie intake to assist with tissue regeneration on a cellular level.[18] A well-balanced diet is sufficient to maintain healthy skin; however, most patients with identified risk factors are not eating a well-balanced diet. Protein supplementation in balanced amounts is helpful. Only a medical nutritionist, a physician with a subspecialty practice in nutritional management, or a registered dietitian can accurately determine a balance of demand and replacement that will be therapeutic for the patient. Research also suggests that supplemental vitamins A and C; the minerals zinc, copper, and manganese; and amino acids (glutamine, arginine, and cysteine) plus a multiple vitamin help stimulate wound healing on a cellular level.

HEALTH PROMOTION AND PREVENTION. Nurses are responsible for identifying those patients at risk for developing pressure ulcers. The primary means of managing pressure ulcers is prevention and

TABLE 65-13 PRODUCTS USED TO TREAT PRESSURE ULCERS

Category	Example
EXUDATE ABSORPTION	
Copolymer starch dressings	Absorption dressing DuoDERM granules
Calcium alginates (absorb exudate and release calcium on cellular level—stimulates angiogenesis)	Kaltostat Sorbsan Algosteril
DEBRIDEMENT	
Enzymatic	Accuzyme Santyl Panafil Biozyme C
Wet-to-dry dressings*	100% cotton gauze in many forms (4 × 4, Kerlix)
WOUND PROTECTION, INSULATION, AND MILD ABSORPTION	
Hydrocolloids (waxy pectin adhesive dressings that provide optimal wound environment)	DuoDERM Restore Tegasorb Ultec
Transparent dressings (thin, adhesive dressings that support microenvironment for cellular regeneration)	Tegaderm Bioclusive OpSite Blister film Polyskin
Polyurethane foam dressings (nonadhesive; some assist with odor control)	Allevyn Lyofoam PolyMem CarraSmart
Hydrogel dressings (gel in tube or nonadherent sheet; have a topical soothing effect; varied in thickness)	Elasto-Gel Vigilon Nu-Gel

NOTE: Research suggests that wounds heal most effectively in moist, natural environment, with clean, debris- and necrosis-free wound area. Dressings and interventions are all designed with these principles in mind. Several have other added benefits, discussed within each category.
*Solutions used vary according to preference of physician; most common solution is normal saline.

the reduction of the number of them that occur in any one setting (see Healthy People 2010 box in Chapter 12, p. 231).

▶ ARE You READY?

Which of the following describes a stage 2 pressure ulcer?
1. Damage to muscle and bone
2. Deep crater involving the fascia
3. Superficial skin loss involving epidermis
4. Warm, boggy alteration of intact skin

Nursing Management *of the Patient with Pressure Ulcer*

A holistic approach to the nursing management of the patient with a pressure ulcer has four aspects: (1) control of contributing factors by reduction or elimination, (2) support of the host, (3) optimization of the microenvironment based on principles of wound healing, and (4) provision of education for patients and caregivers.

ASSESSMENT

Most pressure ulcers can be prevented if the nurse is diligent about assessment and appropriate interventions. Not all interventions are within the scope of nursing practice; therefore the NPUAP recommends a multidisciplinary leadership approach. Prevention can be accomplished only when the nurse has identified those patients at high risk for development of pressure ulcer. Many "assessment tools" are available, but the clinical practice guidelines[2] cite only two tools as valid and research based: the Norton and Braden scales. Most institutions incorporate information from one or both of these tools when developing their own tool.

Assessment tools consider both extrinsic and intrinsic factors that contribute to alterations in skin integrity. The Norton scale (Figure 65-19), which was developed for use in a geriatric population, examines the patient's general health; mental status; and levels of activity, mobility, and continence. Simple to use, this tool leaves

Research

Scott EM: Effects of warming therapy on pressure ulcers: a randomized trial, *AORN J* 73:921-927, 929-933, 936-938, 2001.

In the acute care setting up to 25% of pressure ulcers occur during a surgical procedure. The patients at greatest risk for developing pressure ulcers are those having operations related to reconstructive surgery of existing pressure ulcers or vascular, cardiac, or orthopedic procedures.

All patients receiving general anesthesia are at risk for developing hypothermia (a body temperature of less than 96.8° F [36° C]). Hypothermia typically occurs in older patients and those who have large surface areas of the body exposed, have an opened peritoneal cavity, or are receiving large amounts of unwarmed irrigation fluid. Hypothermia has been associated with deviations in serum potassium, postoperative instability, myocardial ischemia within the first 24 hours after surgery, increased mortality, increased arterial blood pressure, cardiovascular complications, protein metabolism, and decreased subcutaneous oxygen tension resulting from vasoconstriction.

The purpose of this study was to test the hypothesis that intraoperative control of hypothermia would reduce the development of pressure ulcers. A prospective, randomized clinical trial was conducted. Use of forced-air warming therapy with the simultaneous warming of intravenous fluids was compared with the standard therapy of automatic regulation of ambient temperature, minimal patient exposure during preparation time, and use of warmed blankets for immediate postoperative care. Results of the study, although not statistically significant, showed that the development of pressure ulcers was decreased by nearly 50% in patients who received warming therapy. This study supports the hypothesis that a correlation exists between core body temperature and the development of pressure ulcers.

much room for nursing judgment within the specific areas. These areas are scored from 1 to 4, and a total is calculated. The lower the total number of points, the greater the risk the patient has for skin breakdown. The Braden scale is more specific, providing explanations for each score the patient is given (Figure 65-20). This tool was based on the original work of the Norton scale. This tool scores the patient's levels of sensory perception, mobility, nutrition, and activity, as well as the presence or absence of moisture, friction, and shear. Once again, a number is assigned for each parameter; the total is calculated; and the lower the score, the greater the risk.

A skin risk assessment tool should be completed at the time of a patient's admission to a facility and thereafter on a weekly basis or after a change in the patient's condition, such as surgery. Some long-term care facilities have established protocols that require successive skin risk assessment at intervals longer than every week.

Health History. Assess for:

- History of diabetes mellitus, vascular disease, paralysis, incontinence, and hypertension
- Changes in fluid and food intake
- Changes in mental status
- Actual knowledge and understanding of pressure ulcer development and management

Physical Examination. Assess for:

- Changes in skin integrity at least every 8 hours or according to institutional policies, which may differ on the frequency of assessments, allowing flexibility for individual care settings.
- An existing pressure ulcer. Describe this ulcer using the staging classification system as detailed in Box 65-2. Identifying the stage of a pressure ulcer is helpful for the nurse in determining the appropriate interventions for a particular wound

Norton Scale

A *Physical condition*	B *Mental state*	C *Activity*	D *Mobility*	E *Incontinence*	*Total Score*
4 Good	4 Alert	4 Ambulant	4 Full	4 Not	______
3 Fair	3 Apathetic	3 Walks with help	3 Slightly limited	3 Occasional	
2 Poor	2 Confused	2 Chairbound	2 Very limited	2 Usually urine	
1 Bad	1 Stupor	1 Bedrest	1 Immobile	1 Double incontinence	

Norton Plus Scale
(For determining high risk for pressure sores)

Check ONLY if YES	***YES***
Diagnosis of diabetes	____
Diagnosis of hypertension	____
Hematocrit (M) <41%	____
(F) <36%	____
Hemoglobin (M) <14 g/dl	____
(F) <12 g/dl	____
Albumin level <3.3 g/dl	____
Febrile >99.6°F	____
5 or more medications	____
Changes in mental status to confused, lethargic within 24 hours	____
TOTAL Number of Checkmarks	
Norton Scale Score	____
Minus total from above	____
Norton Plus Score	____

Figure 65-19 Norton and Norton Plus scales for predicting pressure ulcer risk.

Patient's name		Evaluator's name
Sensory perception Ability to respond meaningfully to pressure-related discomfort	**1. Completely limited:** Unresponsive (does not moan, flinch, or gasp) to painful stimuli, due to diminished level of consciousness or sedation, **OR** limited ability to feel pain over most of body surface.	**2. Very limited:** Responds only to painful stimuli. Cannot communicate discomfort except by moaning or restlessness, **OR** has a sensory impairment that limits the ability to feel pain or discomfort over ½ of body.
Moisture Degree to which skin is exposed to moisture	**1. Constantly moist:** Skin is kept moist almost constantly by perspi-ration, urine, etc. Dampness is detected every time patient is moved or turned.	**2. Moist:** Skin is often but not always moist; linen must be changed at least once a shift.
Activity Degree of physical activity	**1. Bedfast:** Confined to bed.	**2. Chairfast:** Ability to walk severely limited or nonexistent. Cannot bear own weight and/or must be assisted into chair or wheelchair.
Mobility Ability to change and control body position	**1. Completely immobile:** Does not make even slight changes in body or extremity position without assistance.	**2. Very limited:** Makes occasional slight changes in body or extremity position but unable to make fre-quent or significant changes
Nutrition Usual food intake pattern	**1. Very poor:** Never eats a complete meal. Rarely eats more than ⅓ of any food offered. Eats 2 servings or less of protein (meat or dairy products) per day. Takes fluids poorly. Does not take a liquid dietary supplement, **OR** is NPO and/or maintained on clear liquids or IV for more than 5 days.	**2. Probably inadequate:** Rarely eats a complete meal and generally eats only about ½ of any food offered. Protein intake includes only 3 servings of meat or dairy products per day. Occasionally will take a dietary supplement, **OR** receives less than optimum amount of liquid diet or tube feeding.
Friction and shear	**1. Problem:** Requires moderate to maximum assistance in moving. Complete lifting without sliding against sheets is impossible. Frequently slides down in bed or chair, requiring frequent repositioning with maximum assistance. Spasticity, contractures, or agitation leads to almost constant friction.	**2. Potential problem:** Moves feebly or requires minimum assitance. During a move, skin probably slides to some extent against sheets, chair, restraints, or other devices. Maintains relatively good position in chair or bed most of the time but occasionally slides down.

Figure 65-20 Braden scale for predicting pressure ulcer risk. *NPO*, Nothing by mouth; *IV*, intravenous; *TPN*, total parenteral nutrition.

based on the depth of the tissue involved; however, it is not an all-inclusive tool. A wound covered with necrotic tissue (eschar) cannot be staged because the depth of tissue damage cannot be determined.

In addition, assess the pressure ulcer for:

- Size by measuring the length, width, and depth at the deepest point. Measure the depth of the wound by inserting a sterile applicator and comparing depth with measurements on a wound-measuring guide.
- A more accurate wound assessment by taking a photograph of the wound. Label the photograph to identify the patient and date and indicate where the length, width, and depth were measured for future accuracy in measurements. Trace an irregularly shaped wound if a photograph cannot be obtained. Medicare requires accurate sizing of the wound for reimbursement of home care dressing supplies.
- Presence of undermining or sinus tracts in the wound.
- Condition of the surrounding skin.
- Foreign bodies in the wound (e.g., sutures, orthopedic hardware).
- Color (pink, red, yellow, black). The color of wounds provides information about vascular supply, infection, healthy versus necrotic tissue, and nutritional status. "Healthy" full-thickness wounds have a beefy red, granular appearance. If the wound bed is pale, this may reflect a low hemoglobin level. Necrotic tissue is white, yellow, gray, or black. Certain infections also change the color of a wound bed; for example, *Pseudomonas* species can produce greenish drainage.

	Dates of assessment				
3. Slightly limited: Responds to verbal commands but cannot always communicate discomfort or need to be turned, **OR** has some sensory impairment that limits ability to feel pain or discomfort in 1 or 2 extremities.	**4. No impairment:** Responds to verbal commands. Has no sensory deficit which would limit ability to feel or voice pain or discomfort.				
3. Occasionally moist: Skin is occasionally moist, requiring an extra linen change approximately once a day.	**4. Rarely moist:** Skin is usually dry; linen requires changing only at routine intervals.				
3. Walks occasionally: Walks occasionally during day but for very short distances, with or without assistance. Spends majority of each shift in bed or chair.	**4. Walks frequently:** Walks outside the room at least twice a day and inside room at least once every 2 hours during waking hours.				
3. Slightly limited: Makes frequent though slight changes in body or extremity position independently.	**4. No limitations:** Makes major and frequent changes in position without assistance.				
3. Adequate: Eats over ½ of most meals. Eats a total of 4 servings of protein (meat, dairy products) each day. Occasionally will refuse a meal, but will usually take a supplement if offered, **OR** is on a tube feeding or TPN regimen, which probably meets most of nutritional needs.	**4. Excellent:** Eats most of every meal. Never refuses a meal. Usually eats a total of 4 or more servings of meat and dairy products. Occasionally eats between meals. Does not require supplementation.				
3. No apparent problem: Moves in bed and in chair independently and has sufficient muscle strength to lift up completely during move. Maintains good position in bed or chair at all times.					
	Total score				

Figure 65-20 (cont'd)

- Exudate or wound drainage for amount, color, consistency, and odor. Infected wounds generally produce large amounts of odorous drainage. Documentation should be as objective and descriptive as possible. Avoid subjective terms such as *small, moderate,* and *large.*

NURSING DIAGNOSES, OUTCOMES, AND INTERVENTIONS

Nursing Diagnosis: Impaired Skin Integrity

OUTCOMES. Common examples of expected outcomes for the patient with a diagnosis of *impaired skin integrity* are:

Patient will:

- Be discharged with intact skin or with a healing wound that is free from infection.
- Be free from observable pressure-related alterations of intact skin.
- Demonstrate with caregiver, if appropriate, ability to implement a program of continuing therapeutic or preventive care, including measures to reduce or relieve pressure on the skin, manage incontinence and moisture, and maintain adequate nutrition.

NURSING INTERVENTIONS. Activities in the areas of prevention, protection, rehabilitation, and education are essential once a patient has a pressure ulcer (see Guidelines for Safe Practice box, p. 1908, and Nursing Care Plan). Prevention focuses on either reducing or relieving pressure on bony prominences. One way to achieve this goal is by instituting a schedule of turning the patient

Nursing Care Plan

Patient With a Pressure Ulcer

Data A 79-year-old female patient has a history of hypertension, congestive heart failure (CHF), obesity, and degenerative joint disease. She lives alone in her own home; an adult daughter lives nearby. Until recently she regularly attended activities at her local senior center. This morning she was admitted to the hospital for a left-sided stroke (brain attack). Nursing assessment reveals that she is awake but unable to respond to questions. She is incontinent of urine and stool, has right hemiparesis, and has dysphagia. She has +2 pitting edema of the lower extremities, a bruise on her sacrum from a previous fall, and generalized dry skin. She is 65 inches tall and weights 180 pounds. Her Braden scale is 12. She has a large reddened area over her coccyx and a small skin tear. Her vital signs are temperature, 98.6° F (36.9° C); pulse, 92 beats/min; respirations, 18 breaths/min; and blood pressure, 142/88 mm Hg.

Nursing Diagnosis

Impaired skin integrity related to immobility and mechanical forces

Outcomes

- Patient will remain free from complications (infection, increased area of ulceration).
- Patient will demonstrate healing as evidenced by decreased size of pressure ulcer.
- Patient will participate in prevention and treatment programs.

Related NOC Outcomes

- Immobility Consequences: Physiological
- Tissue Integrity: Skin & Mucous Membranes
- Wound Healing: Secondary Intention

Related NIC Interventions

- Pressure Management
- Pressure Ulcer Care
- Pressure Ulcer Prevention

Nursing Interventions/Rationales

- Assess skin every shift and as needed. *Frequent assessment allows for early recognition of skin changes and evaluation of the effectiveness of any treatments that have been implemented.*
- Assess areas of redness for ability to blanch. *Areas of nonblanchable erythema indicate increased pressure, which can easily progress to ulceration.*
- Document Braden scale weekly. *The Braden scale is a reliable tool for predicting pressure ulcer risk. The patient's initial score of 12 places her at risk for further skin compromise and pressure ulcer development.*
- Use appropriate barrier dressings and topical agents on sacral wound. *Physician or skin care specialist nurse determines protocols. Proper medication and treatment are essential for wound prevention or wound healing.*
- Turn patient every 2 hours and post turning schedule. *To promote adequate blood flow and avoid prolonged pressure on any one part.*
- Pad bony prominences. *To reduce pressure on skin over bony prominences, which are prone to breakdown and tissue necrosis.*
- Elevate the heels off the mattress. *The heels are susceptible to breakdown, and elevation avoids pressure.*
- Avoid massaging reddened areas. *Massage of areas under pressure may lead to further tissue injury.*
- Use emollient soap, moisturize skin after bathing, and keep perianal area clean and dry. *To prevent drying of the skin and prevent heel ulcer formation. Contamination of the perianal area with feces or urine may speed skin breakdown and cause infection.*
- Provide bowel and bladder training; avoid use of diapers and plastic pads. *Continence of urine and stool decreases the patient's risk of skin ulcer development. Increased moisture and decreased ventilation increase the risk of pressure ulcer development.*
- Avoid shearing forces (e.g., use turning sheet or pull sheet). *To prevent injury or further tissue breakdown.*
- Keep sheets clean and dry; avoid wrinkling. *Moisture holds bacteria at site and increases risk of breakdown. Wrinkled areas beneath the patient create pressure on tissues.*
- Use pressure reduction mattress on bed and seat cushion on wheelchair. *Provides padding, decreases pressure.*
- Perform passive range-of-motion exercises on affected extremities and promote active range-of-motion exercises of unaffected extremities. *Promotes circulation and prevents complications associated with immobility.*

at least every 2 hours. The use of pressure-relieving or pressure-reducing surfaces for the bed and chair should also be incorporated into the patient's care plan; however, in many institutions this represents an additional cost.

The nurse inspects the skin at regular intervals for signs of early irritation or breakdown. Moisturization of the skin is important to maintain its soft, elastic state. The nurse should avoid massaging moisturizer or lotion over bony prominences, since this action may cause rupture of blood vessels and possible injury to friable tissue. Control of incontinence of stool and urine is achieved by diapers or diversion (e.g., Foley catheter, fecal incontinence pouch) to keep excess moisture and irritants away from the skin. A moisture barrier, preferably one with either dimethicone or petrolatum, is applied per the manufacturer's directions or as needed between incontinence episodes once the patient has been cleaned of body waste.

The nurse reduces or eliminates shear and friction by using a lift sheet when moving the patient in bed or out of bed. The head of the bed should be no higher 30 degrees to avoid shear by the patient sliding to the foot of the bed.

Use of aseptic technique and Standard Precautions helps prevent infection. The nurse monitors the patient for signs and symptoms of systemic infection every shift and reports these as appropriate.

RELATED NIC INTERVENTIONS. Environmental Management, Positioning, Pressure Management, Pressure Ulcer Care, Teaching: Prescribed Activity/Exercise

Nursing Diagnosis: Imbalanced Nutrition: Less Than Body Requirements

OUTCOMES. Common examples of outcomes for the patient with a diagnosis of *imbalanced nutrition: less than body requirements* are: Patient will:

- Maintain present weight or gain weight.

- Teach patient and daughter techniques for maintaining mobility and range of motion and promote ambulation and a regular exercise program. *Patient and family involvement in the treatment program increases the chances of attaining goals. An exercise program enhances circulation, promotes general health, decreases stress, and aids in weight control.*
- Encourage maximal participation in activities of daily living (ADLs). *Allows patient some sense of control and independence. Patient is right handed and has right-sided hemiparesis, so she may need additional assistance with ADLs.*
- Employ safety precautions and fall prevention measures. *To prevent further injury to skin or other tissues.*
- Encourage elevation of legs when sitting. *To promote venous return and reduce formation of edema (patient has history of CHF, edema).*
- Assess patient's need for analgesia before dressing changes. *To increase the patient's ability to tolerate dressing changes, which can be painful.*

Nursing Diagnosis

Imbalanced nutrition: more than body requirements related to inadequate dietary control or lack of resources

Outcomes

- Patient will maintain prescribed diet.
- Patient will achieve weight loss to within 10 pounds of ideal.

Related NOC Outcomes

- Knowledge: Diet
- Nutritional Status
- Weight: Body Mass
- Weight Control

Related NIC Interventions

- Exercise Promotion
- Nutrition Management
- Nutritional Counseling
- Weight Management

Nursing Interventions/Rationales

- Assess patient's caloric needs, and promote nutritionally adequate diet and fluid intake, while restricting excess calories. *To promote tissue healing without promoting obesity. Fluid intake less than 800 ml/day increases the risk of pressure ulcer development because of dry tissues.*
- Monitor serum albumin, protein, and complete blood count (CBC) results. *To assess patient's protein stores, which are necessary for tissue healing. Albumin less than 3 g/dl is a risk factor for development of pressure ulcers. Protein needs are increased to maintain a positive nitrogen balance and aid in healing. CBC results may indicate infection or anemia.*
- Encourage patient and family to become involved in setting goals for dietary changes, documenting food intake, and planning meals. *Changes are more likely to be made when the patient is involved in planning those changes. Patients know their own likes and dislikes, financial resources, and ability to make dietary changes. Participation allows the patient greater control over her situation.*

Evaluation

Evaluation is based on comparing the patient's outcomes with desired outcomes.

- Increase food intake until adequate in amount and content for body weight.

NURSING INTERVENTIONS. As the patient's expenditure of energy increases with activity, nutritional intake needs to be adjusted to meet this need. The nurse can best ensure that the patient receives optimal nutrition by consulting with either a registered dietitian or a medical nutritionist. Many patients require specialized diets to maintain a high-caloric intake to meet the demands of healing a wound and maintaining life. Nurses should also be cognizant of the nutritional requirements related to supplementation of vitamins, minerals, and amino acids that facilitate the healing process.

Most patients sent home with pressure ulcers should have a referral to a home health care agency. The home care nurse can assist the caregiver in ensuring that the patient's nutritional needs are met and can make additional referrals for nutritional management by a registered dietitian.

RELATED NIC INTERVENTIONS. Fluid Monitoring, Nutrition Management, Nutrition Therapy, Nutritional Monitoring

Nursing Diagnosis: Acute Pain

OUTCOMES. Common examples of outcomes for the patient with a diagnosis of *acute pain* are:
Patient will:

- Rate pain as no higher than 3 on a scale of 0 (no pain) to 10 (severe pain).
- Verbalize that pain is controlled.

NURSING INTERVENTIONS. Loss of epidermal tissue results in pain secondary to the exposure of nerve endings. Pain varies in severity for each patient. Many patients have pain relief immediately after the application of an occlusive dressing (e.g., hydrocolloid, hydrogel sheet). Patients experience pain during dressing changes and should be premedicated at least 30 minutes beforehand.

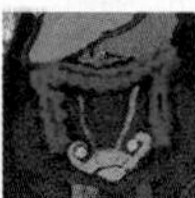
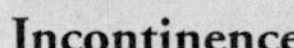

GUIDELINES FOR SAFE PRACTICE *Interventions to Prevent Pressure Ulcers*

Incontinence

Cleanse skin after each episode of incontinence. Check incontinent patients frequently.
Assess causative factors of incontinence.
Contain urine and feces in absorbent products that control moisture and exposure to skin; plastic-lined products can contribute to the problem. If appropriate, manage incontinence with a Foley catheter or fecal incontinence pouch or rectal tube.
Minimize moisture next to skin from any source.

Nutritional Deficits

Collaborate with dietitian to assess for optimal nutritional support.
Assess for symptoms of nutritional compromise (decreased appetite and subsequently less oral intake; serum albumin level of less than 3 to 3.5 g/dl or a serum prealbumin level of less than 20 mg/dl; hemoglobin level of less than 10 g/dl; signs and symptoms of dehydration, including thirst, poor skin turgor, and dry mucous membranes; elevated hematocrit and serum sodium levels).

Skin Care and Early Treatment Measures

Inspect skin at regular intervals, at least daily or as determined by institutional policy (e.g., every shift) and patient degree of risk. Conduct a head-to-toe inspection, with attention to intertriginous areas and bony prominences.
Develop a bathing schedule according to patient preference, institutional policy, and general skin condition. Use a mild cleansing agent, and avoid water temperature extremes.
Assess environmental factors, such as temperature and humidity, for contribution to skin condition.
Lubricate skin with emollient lotions or moisturizers. Avoid lotion with scents or high alcohol contents.
Avoid massage.

Alterations in Mobility or Activity

Reposition patient at least every 2 hours or more frequently if needed.
Use position pillows or foam wedges to separate skin areas in contact with each other or to assist with maintaining positions. Use cautiously because these devices can become an additional source of pressure if not properly placed.
Elevate heels off of bed surfaces with supportive pillows. Heel protectors help reduce friction.
Avoid positioning directly onto trochanter. Place patient more appropriately into 30 degree side-lying position.
Elevating the head of the bed centers all body weight directly over the pelvic triangle. It is best to keep the degree of elevation to 30 degrees, if possible.
To reduce friction and shear, use lifting devices to raise patient in bed, rather than dragging patient across the surface of the bed.
Use a pressure-reduction or pressure-relief device for all patients at risk of pressure ulcer formation.
Teach patients in wheelchairs and other chairs to shift weight and have pressure-reducing surfaces on which to sit.

RELATED NIC INTERVENTIONS. Analgesic Administration, Anxiety Reduction, Coping Enhancement, Distraction, Pain Management, Positioning

EVALUATION

To evaluate the effectiveness of nursing interventions, compare patient behaviors with those stated in the expected patient outcomes.

RELATED NOC OUTCOMES. Comfort Level, Nutritional Status: Food & Fluid Intake, Nutritional Status: Nutrient Intake, Pain Control, Pain: Disruptive Effects, Tissue Integrity: Skin & Mucous Membranes, Wound Healing: Secondary Intention

GERONTOLOGIC CONSIDERATIONS

Many of the changes in the skin associated with aging predispose the older adult to the development of pressure ulcers. Thinning of the epidermis makes the skin more prone to injury. Adhesion of the epidermis to the dermis is decreased and accompanied by a decrease in skin elasticity, allowing the skin to be easily stretched and deformed. The skin is a less effective barrier against infection, bruising, and water loss. In addition, thermal regulation and the ability to perceive touch and pain are decreased. The older adult may not perceive excessive pressure, and coexisting neurologic deficits may compound the problem.

With the application of shearing forces, the epidermal-dermal attachment may weaken and allow the skin layers to separate. A blister forms and eventually ruptures, leaving a flap of skin with uneven edges, called a skin tear. Persons who require assistance with moving in bed or transfers are at risk for the development of skin tears caused by shearing forces. Frequent bathing with an alkaline soap can dry older adults' skin by altering the natural acidic mantle of the epidermis. The use of emollient soaps and moisturizers is recommended for moisturizing the skin either during or after bathing.

Older adults are at greater risk for pressure ulcers because of numerous predisposing factors, including (1) anemia; (2) poor nutrition; (3) decreased albumin; (4) decreased mobility; (5) thinning of skin and loss of the subcutaneous cushion; (6) drug therapy such as glucocorticoids and NSAIDs; (7) incontinence; and (8) comorbid conditions (e.g., hypertension, coronary artery disease, diabetes) or use of sedatives that interfere with sensory perception, natural shifting of body position, or turning in bed.

Pressure ulcers can develop not only in those confined to bed but also in those confined to a sitting position. The ulcers occur whenever pressure is continuous. Ulcers can occur on the head, shoulders, or lower back if a recumbent position is maintained. In the side-lying position the patient can develop a pressure ulcer on the hips, ankles, and pinna of the ear. Sitting promotes ulcers on the buttocks. The underside of the scrotum can be injured with shearing and pressure.

Measures to prevent and treat pressure ulcers are the same for the older adult as for any person. The only difference is that tissue, because of the predisposing factors, is damaged more quickly,

Preparing for Practice

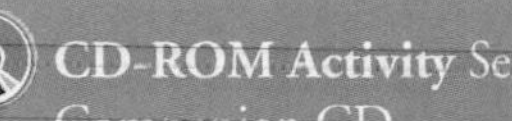 **CD-ROM Activity** Select Exercise Ten: Problems of the Skin on the Companion CD.

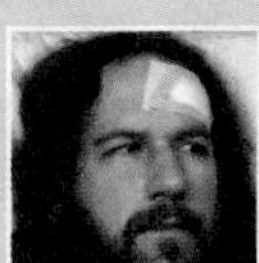

Patient: *Ira Bradley,* **Room 309**

Ira Bradley, a 43-year-old Caucasian man, is diagnosed with acquired immunodeficiency syndrome, dehydration, *Pneumocystis carinii* pneumonia, candidiasis, and Kaposi's sarcoma.

Assessment

View the patient's **Report**.
Open Ira Bradley's **Medical Record**; focus on the following records: History & Physical and Physicians' Orders.
Conduct a **Patient Interview**. As you conduct your interview, focus primarily on data that will be helpful in planning care for this patient.
Record the data you collect.

Nursing Diagnoses, Outcomes, and Interventions

1. What is a pressure ulcer?
2. What population is most at risk for pressure ulcer development?
3. How does a patient's activity level affect the risk for developing a pressure ulcer?
4. Briefly describe the four pathophysiologic changes that occur in pressure ulcer development. *Hint:* Refer to Table 65-11.
5. Identify five skin care measures that can be used to prevent Ira Bradley from developing a pressure ulcer during his hospitalization. *Hint:* See Guidelines for Safe Practice box, p. 1908.
6. Suggest six interventions related to mobility and activity to reduce Ira Bradley's risk of developing a pressure ulcer.
7. What general instructions would you include in patient and family education about reducing risk of pressure ulcer development after discharge?

so more frequent position changes and inspections are needed. Many hospitalized older adults require dietary measures to improve nutrition to prevent pressure ulcers. Also, many older adults require use of pressure-relieving or pressure-reducing surfaces (e.g., specialty mattresses or beds, padding for chairs) if immobilization is required.

Critical Thinking

1. Discuss two risk factors for malignant melanoma and further describe strategies for prevention of the disease.
2. Describe three important patient teaching interventions for self-care management of severe atopic dermatitis.
3. What nursing interventions would be appropriate for a patient experiencing a disturbed body image as a result of a dermatologic condition or an extensive pressure ulcer?
4. What are the risk factors for pressure ulcers?
5. What nursing approaches would you prescribe for an obese 60-year-old patient with diabetes mellitus who has neuropathy and is wheelchair bound?

References

1. Aronovitch SA: Intraoperatively acquired pressure ulcer prevalence: a national study, *J Wound Ostomy Continence Nurs* 26(3):130, 1999.
2. Barczak CA et al: Fourth national pressure ulcer prevalence survey, *Adv Wound Care* 10(4):18, 1997.
3. Beck FK, Rosenthal TC: Prealbumin: a marker for nutritional evaluation, *Am Fam Phys* 65:1575-1578, 2002.
4. Beckrich K, Aronovitch SA: Hospital-acquired pressure ulcers: a comparison of costs in medical vs. surgical patients, *Nurs Econ* 17(5):263, 1999.
5. *Clinical practice guidelines: pressure ulcers in adults—prediction and prevention,* Washington, DC, 1992, US Department of Health and Human Services.

5a. *Clinical practice guideline No. 15: treatment of pressure ulcers,* ACHPR publication No. 95-0652, December 1994, website: www.ncbi.nlm.nih.gov/books /bv.fcgi?rid=hstat2.Chapter.5124.

6. Cuddigan J, Ayello EA, Sussman C, editors: *Pressure ulcers in America: prevalence, incidence, and implications for the future,* Reston, Va, 2001, National Pressure Ulcer Advisory Panel.
7. Dermatology Nurses' Association: *Dermatology nursing basics: core proceeding book from annual convention,* Linden, NJ, 2004, Anthony J Janetti.
8. Fitzpatrick TB et al: *Color atlas and synopsis of clinical dermatology,* ed 4, New York, 2001, McGraw-Hill.
9. Garber SL, Rintala DH: Pressure ulcers in veterans with spinal cord injury: a retrospective study, *J Rehabil Res Dev* 40(5):433-441, 2003.
10. Gioshes SE: Scabies: case presentation, *Dermatol Nurs* 9(4):58, 1997.
11. Habif T: *Clinical dermatology: a color guide to diagnosis and therapy,* ed 4, St Louis, 2003, Mosby.
12. Hill M, editor: *Dermatologic nursing essentials: a core curriculum,* ed 2, Pitman, NJ, 2003, Dermatologic Nurses' Association.
13. Nicol NH: Managing atopic dermatitis in children and adults, *Nurse Pract* 25(4):58-59, 63-64, 69-70, 2000.
14. Robins P: *Sun sense: a complete guide to prevention, early detection, and treatment of skin cancer,* New York, 1996, Skin Cancer Foundation.
15. Schofield J, Robinson W: *What you really need to know about moles and melanoma,* Baltimore, 2000, Johns Hopkins Press Health Book.
16. Spector D, Fortinsky RH: Pressure ulcer prevention in an Ohio nursing home, *J Aging Health* 10(1):65-68, 1998.

16a. Steper JW et al: Dermatologic Drug Formulary: an American Academy of Dermatology white paper, *J Am Acad Dermatol* 34:99-109, 1996.

17. Stewart S, Box-Panksepp JS: Preventing hospital-acquired pressure ulcers: a point prevalence study, *OWM* 50(3):46-51, 2004.
18. Zagoren AJ: Nutritional assessment and intervention in the person with a chronic wound. In Krasner DL, Rodeheaver GT, Sibbald RG, editors: *Chronic wound care: a clinical resource book for healthcare professionals,* ed 3, Wayne, Penn, 2001, HMP Publications.

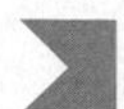 Visit the Evolve website: http://evolve.elsevier.com/Monahan/medsurg

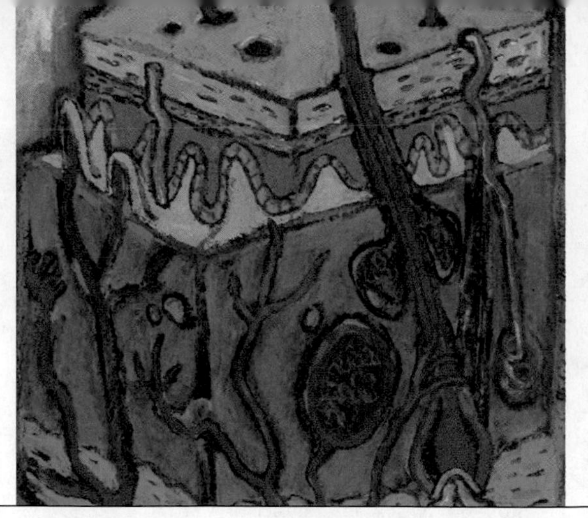

CHAPTER 66
Burns

by Carol J. Green

OBJECTIVES

After studying this chapter, the learner should be able to:

1. Describe the five mechanisms for burn injury.
2. Describe assessment of the burn patient, including the extent, location, and etiology of the burn.
3. Differentiate between the phases of a major burn.
4. Describe emergency care for a major burn.
5. Describe interventions for patients during the three phases of burn care, including replacing body fluids, preventing infection, promoting nutrition and mobility, and providing emotional support.
6. Differentiate between wound care for partial- and full-thickness burns.
7. Identify learning needs of the patient with burns.
8. Discuss preventive measures for populations at risk for burn injury.

KEY TERMS

allograft, p. 1927
autograft, p. 1927
burn shock, p. 1915
contractures, p. 1940
debridement, p. 1932
deep partial-thickness, p. 1912
emergent phase, p. 1918
eschar, p. 1913
escharotomy, p. 1925
full-thickness, p. 1913
heterograft, p. 1927
superficial, p. 1912

Advances in burn treatment over the past 50 years have significantly improved survival rates for patients with major burns. Such improvements are directly related to research, which has led to formulas for fluid resuscitation and nutritional support, early surgical interventions and topical antimicrobials to prevent infection and subsequent sepsis, and improved management of inhalation injury and hypermetabolism.

Today, patients with major burns are cared for in centralized burn units or burn centers. The United States has about 200 such specialized units. Dedicated teams of personnel composed of nurses, surgeons, anesthesiologists, respiratory care personnel, rehabilitation specialists, nutritionists, and psychosocial experts work together toward the common goals of saving patients and preventing deformity.[18]

Burn Injury

Etiology. Burn injury occurs as a result of skin destruction from direct or indirect thermal forces. Burns are caused by flame, scalding with steam or hot fluids, direct contact with hot surfaces, chemicals, electrical current, and radiation. Burn injuries are in many respects the worst of all tragedies. A major burn is accompanied by severe pain, repeated episodes of infection or sepsis, and pronounced disability and disfigurement or death. Although the physical effects of burns can be devastating, the cost and psychologic suffering for the patient and family can be catastrophic as well.

Thermal Burns. Thermal burns are the leading type of burns in the United States. Such burns may occur from scalding (hot steam, liquids), house fires (smoking in bed, children playing with matches), contact with hot substances or objects (stove, food, hot tar, irons), automobile crashes, or ignited gasoline or propane. The burn is usually confined to the area where the substance came into contact with the skin. The amount and duration of the flame determine the depth of the injury, which often consists of combined partial- and full-thickness burns. Thermal burns are a major source of inhalation injury as well as tissue injury.

Chemical Burns. Chemical burns are the second leading type of burns in the United States. They are generally associated with acidic or alkaline solutions, such as bleach, drain or toilet bowl cleaners, or metal cleaners. Chemical burns occur from direct contact with the chemical or splashing onto skin or eyes. Inhalation injury occurs when chemical fumes are inhaled.

Most chemical burns occur in persons who use industrial, military, or agricultural chemicals at work. Chemicals such as strong acids (hydrochloric), alkalis (lime or lye), and organic compounds such as phenol and petroleum products (gasoline) are common causes of industrial burns. In homes, drain cleaners and disinfectants are common causes of burns. At home chemical burns generally result from the misuse of cleaning products, hair, skin, or nail chemicals or disinfectants. Although usually the result of accidents, chemical burns can also result from deliberate assault. The severity of chemical injury is related to the chemical involved, its concentration, the length of exposure, and the immediate treatment.[1]

INHALATION BURNS. Inhalation burns occur when a person directly inhales smoke, hot air, flames, or systemic toxins such as carbon monoxide. Inhalation injury is primarily associated with residential or building fires in which the person is trapped in an enclosed, smoke-filled area. Smoke inhalation injury is often masked by external burns, which are more readily visible (Figure 66-1). Common signs of inhalation injury are soot around the nose and mouth, early respiratory distress, singed nasal hair and eyebrows, and facial burns. Sixty percent to 80% of burn fatalities are attributed to smoke inhalation.[11]

ELECTRICAL BURNS. Electrical burn injuries occur along a spectrum from very mild, as associated by low-voltage current, to severe and possibly lethal, as seen with high-tension electrical injuries (Figure 66-2). The amount of current (low voltage, high voltage, high tension), type of current (direct or alternating), path of current (e.g., hand to toe), length of contact, and extenuating events (water, fall) are factors that determine the extent or lethality of an electrical injury. Alternating current produces tetany and a "locked-on" phenomenon in which the person cannot let go of the source. Since current passes through the body for an extended time, greater injury occurs. Direct current, such as lightening, causes a one-time direct blast of current that shoves the person away from the source or to the ground. Electrical injuries disrupt electrical activities of the body and can cause cardiac asystole and apnea. Some patients can survive with immediate cardiopulmonary resuscitation.[19]

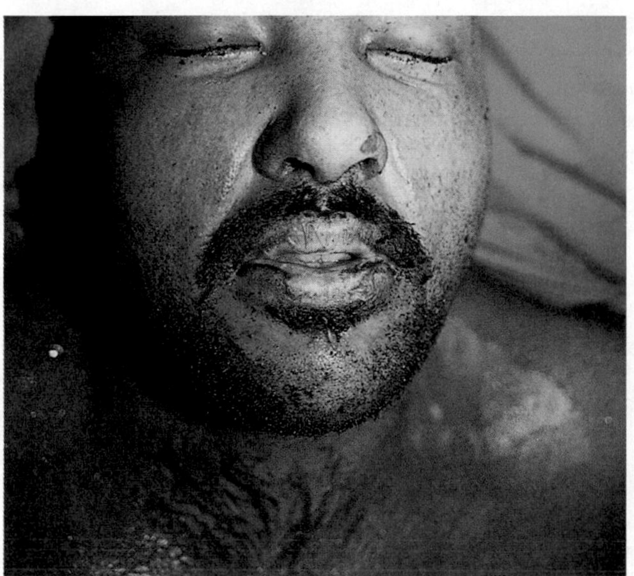

Figure 66-1 Facial (and possible inhalation) injury after gas explosion.

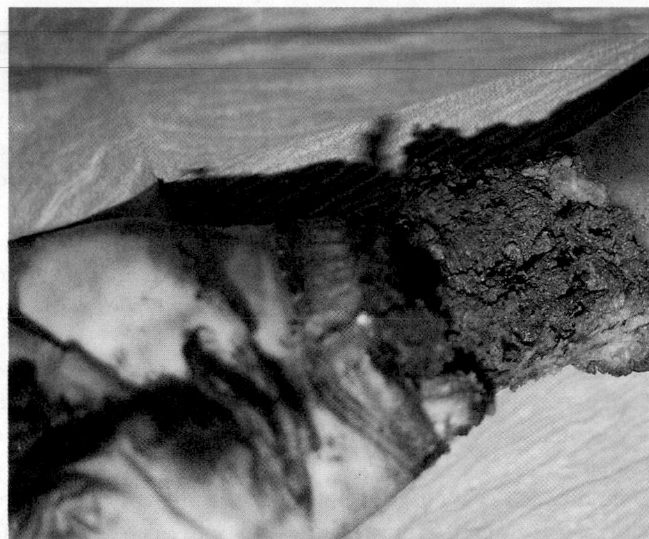

Figure 66-2 Full-thickness electrical injury after contact with high-power wire.

RADIATION BURNS. Radiation injuries are uncommon but can be serious. Sunburn, nuclear radiation accidents, industrial radiation, and therapeutic radiation are the primary sources for radiation burns. The degree of injury depends on the length of exposure, strength of radiation, distance from the source, and amount of body surface exposed to the source. Most exposures to radiation produce localized manifestations such as erythema, blistering, wet or dry desquamation, or ulceration. Localized skin injuries may be slow to appear and not be obvious for days to weeks after the exposure.[28] Radiation to the whole body can cause an illness known as acute radiation syndrome, which is associated with cellular deficiencies and clinical manifestations such as anorexia, nausea and vomiting, fatigue, diarrhea, fever, and respiratory distress (see Chapter 23 for a discussion of therapeutic radiation).

Sunburn is an intense, transient inflammatory response caused by ultraviolet radiation (UVR). Injury can begin within 30 minutes after exposure. Light-skinned and fair-haired persons are at greater risk than darker skinned people, although anyone can get sunburn from prolonged exposure. The same risks occur from use of artificial tanning beds as from exposure to UVR in sunlight. Radiation burn from sun exposure is strongly associated with cataract formation, skin cancer, photoaging, and immunosuppression.[15] Children who experience blistering sunburns early in life are at significantly increased risk for developing cutaneous melanoma later in life.

Epidemiology. Burn injuries are the second leading cause of accidental death in the United States following automobile crashes. It is estimated that between 1.5 million and 2 million burn injuries occur in the United States each year and that as many as 75% may be preventable. Although the number of burn injuries has decreased by nearly 50% since the 1950s, each year between 60,000 and 80,000 people are admitted to hospitals for burn care, between 8000 and 12,000 people die, and more than 1 million sustain permanent disability.[9] The average cost of hospitalization ranges from $29,560 to $117, 506. When future productivity is considered, the cost of a burn-related death ranges from $250,000 to $1.5 million. While these statistics seem staggering, they actually underestimate the problem. The exact number of burn injuries and associated costs are unknown, since only 21 states require burn injuries to be reported.[27]

Children, older adults, the disabled, and military personnel are the high-risk groups for burn injuries. Sixty-five percent of burns occurring in children are scald burns, 20% are contact burns, and the remainder are from flames.[27] Children are at increased risk from kitchen spills, pulling hot items over on themselves; water that is too hot in the bathroom; and product-related burns such as from curling irons, space heaters, or gasoline. Boys are at greater risk than girls, and children under the age of 4 or those with disabilities are at greater risk for burns than other age-groups.[8]

Older adults, especially those who are disabled, are at risk for burns because of impaired mobility. Other risk factors in older adults are impaired judgment, one or more medical conditions, drug toxicity, smoking, and ethanol use. Scalds account for the majority of burn injuries in adults over the age of 59, followed by flames, contact, bath immersion, electricity, and hot oil.[27]

Military personnel are at increased risk for combat-related and accidental burn injuries depending on the kind of combat and type of weapons used. Over the past 60 years, combat casualties from burns ranged from 2.3% to 85%. The nature of many military jobs places personnel at risk for burn injures during peacetime and wartime from explosives, chemicals, and electricity.[27] The Risk Factors box lists primary risk factors for burns by age.

Risk Factors

Burns by Age

Birth to 4 Years

Scalds (hot food or liquid, grease, baths)
Household chemicals (ingestion, topical)
Household electrical (biting electrical cords)
Residential fires

5 to 14 Years

Residential fires
Risky behaviors (setting fires, fireworks)

15 to 24 Years

Automobile related
Work related

25 to 64 Years

Work related

More Than 65 Years

Scalds (hot food or liquid, grease)
Smoking
Cooking accidents

Adapted from Rutan RL: Physiologic response to cutaneous burn injury. In Carrougher GJ, editor: *Burn care and therapy,* St Louis, 1998, Mosby.

Pathophysiology. The depth of a burn depends on the temperature of the burning agent and the length of time it is in contact with the skin. Early tissue damage may occur at temperatures of 104° F (40° C). Irreversible damage to the dermis occurs at temperatures of 158° F (70° C).[29] Burn injuries are described as superficial (first-degree), superficial or deep partial-thickness (second-degree), or full-thickness (third- or fourth-degree) burns, according to the degree of injury or destruction to epidermal and dermal skin layers (third-degree), muscle, fascia, tendon, or bone (fourth-degree) (Figure 66-3).

Degree of Burn Injury. **Superficial**, or first-degree, burns involve only the epidermal layer of the skin (Figure 66-4). Sunburns and areas surrounding deeper burns are commonly first-degree burns. **Deep partial-thickness** or dermal (second-degree) burns are characterized by destruction of the epidermis and varying depths of

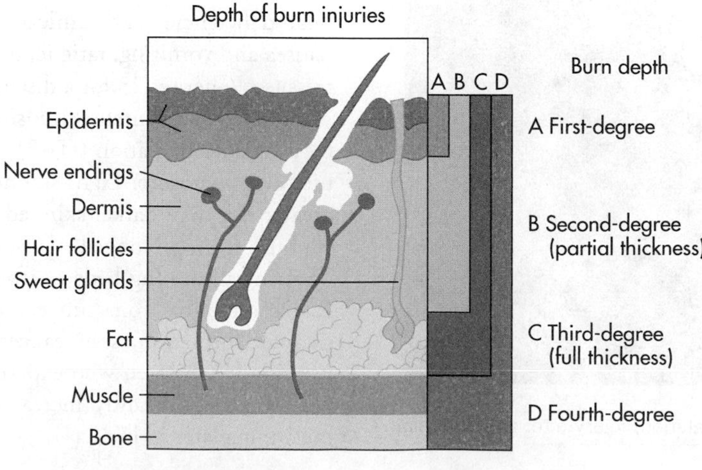

Figure 66-3 Levels of skin involved in burn injury.

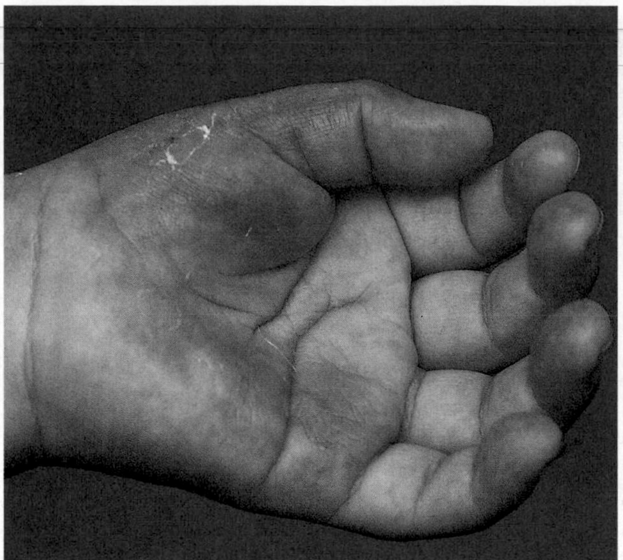

Figure 66-4 Superficial (first-degree) burn of palmar surface of hand. Red, hyperemic appearance of surface, hypersensitivity, and discomfort are typical of these injuries.

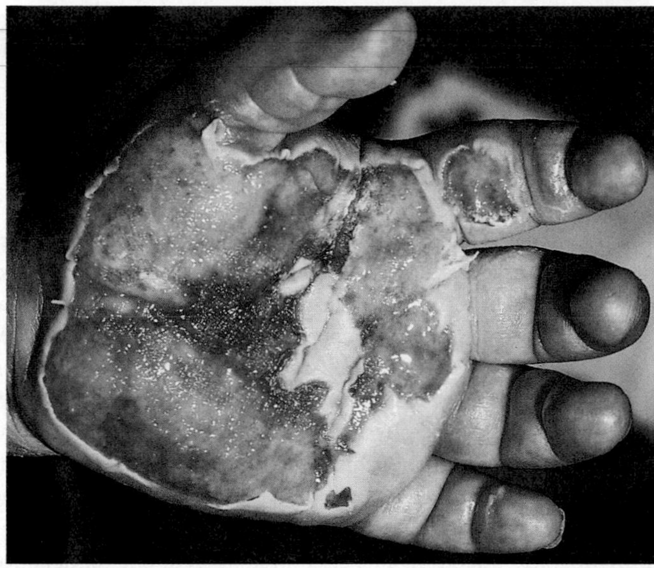

Figure 66-5 Deep partial-thickness (second-degree) burn to palm.

the dermis (Figure 66-5). They are painful because of injured nerve endings; however, they are capable of healing because some epithelial cells are left intact. Blisters often indicate a more superficial partial-thickness injury.[5] They may increase in size because of continuous exudation and collection of tissue fluid. During the healing phase, increased vascularization of sebaceous glands, reduction of secretions, and decreased perspiration cause dryness and itching.

Full-thickness (third- and fourth-degree) burns involve destruction of the epidermis and the entire dermis and possible damage to the subcutaneous layer, muscle, and bone (Figure 66-6). Nerve endings are destroyed, resulting in a painless wound. **Eschar**, a leathery covering composed of denatured protein, may form as a result of surface dehydration. Black networks of coagulated capillaries may be seen. Full-thickness burns require skin grafting because the destroyed tissue is unable to epithelialize. Infection, trauma, or decreased blood supply can cause a deep partial-thickness burn to convert to a full-thickness burn.[5]

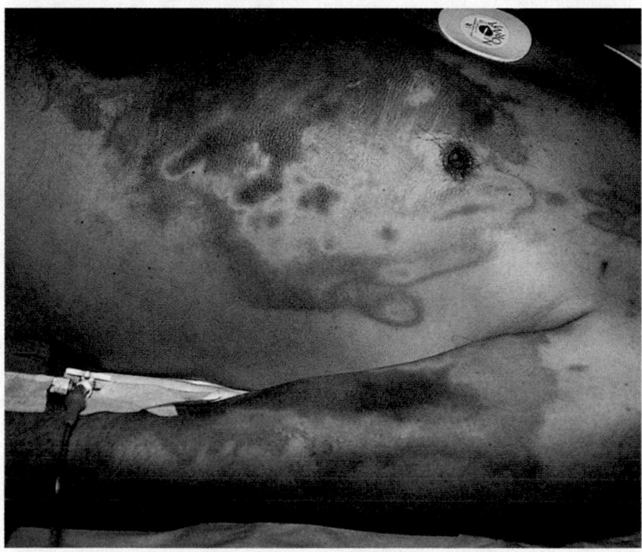

Figure 66-6 Full-thickness burn from nitric acid.

EXTENT OF BURN INJURY. The size and depth of the burn determines the severity of burn injury. For adults the "rule of nines" is a quick tool for determining the size of a burn until a more thorough assessment can be made. The percentage of total body surface area (TBSA) burned is estimated with the use of charts that depict anterior and posterior drawings of the body. The body is divided into areas equal to multiples of 9% (Figure 66-7). Calculations are

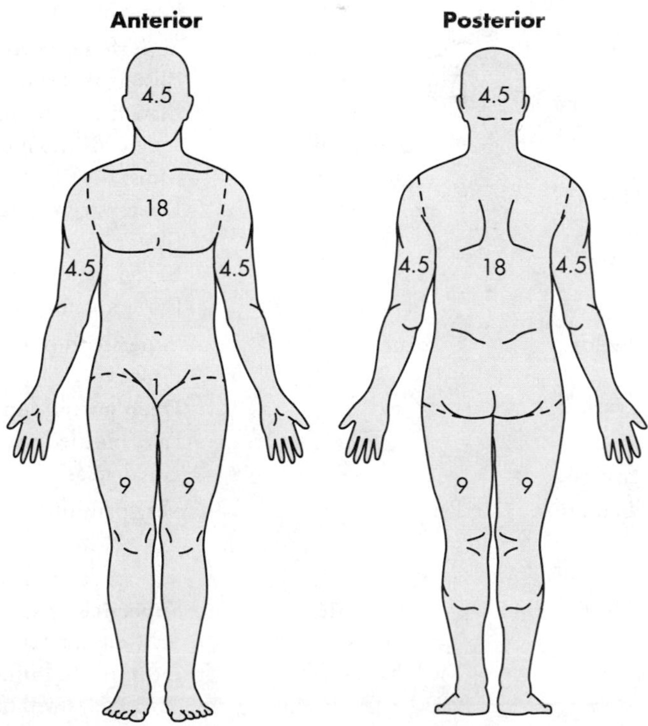

Figure 66-7 The rule of nines. An easy, quick way to estimate size of the burn until more thorough assessment can be made.

modified for infants and children younger than 10 years of age because of their relatively larger head and smaller body size. The depth of the burn injury is evaluated on the basis of appearance, color, and sensation (Table 66-1). A laser Doppler may be used to evaluate the blood flow in the injured tissue and assist with diagnosing the depth of injury.[31]

The part of the body burned must be considered when evaluating the extent and severity of the burn. A 3% burn of the anterior surface of the thigh is not as serious as a 3% burn to the neck, face, or perineal area. Injuries that involve cosmetic and functional areas of the body require a longer period of recovery than other burns because of both physical and emotional reactions to the burn. Injuries to the face, hands, and feet require extensive, meticulous care and extensive physical and occupational therapy. Burns of the head, neck, and chest may also involve injury to the respiratory tract and result in severe respiratory distress. Burns of the perineum are difficult to manage because of the potential for contamination and infection. The circumferential, or encircling, burn of a limb, the neck, or the chest causes constrictive contraction of the skin and produces a tourniquet effect that may impair breathing or circulation.[26] Box 66-1 summarizes factors that determine burn severity.

Tissue Response to Burn Injury. Burns impair normal skin structure and function. They diminish the protective barrier function of the skin, destroy sweat and sebaceous glands, decrease the number of functioning sensory receptors, allow body fluids to escape, and alter temperature control. The severity of these

Box 66-1 Factors Determining Severity of Burns

- Size of burn
- Depth of burn
- Age of patient
- Body part involved
- Mechanism of injury
- History of cardiac, pulmonary, renal, or hepatic disease
- Injuries sustained at time of burn

Table 66-1 Characteristics of the Depth of Burn Injury

Characteristic	Superficial (First-Degree) Burn	Partial-Thickness (Second-Degree) Burn	Full-Thickness (Third- and Fourth-Degree) Burn
Skin depth	Epidermis	Entire epidermis, partial dermis Sweat glands, hair follicles intact	Epidermis, dermis Extends to subcutaneous tissue, possibly muscle and bone
Cause	Flash flame Ultraviolet light Sunburn	Contact with hot liquids or solids Flash flame to clothing Direct flames Chemicals Ultraviolet light	Prolonged contact with hot liquids or solids Flame Chemicals Electrical contact
Appearance	Dry, no blisters Minimal or no edema Blanches with fingertip pressure, and color returns when pressure removed	**Superficial partial injury** Blisters that increase in size Blanches with fingertip pressure, and color returns when pressure removed Moist **Deep partial injury** Blisters slower to increase in size Blanching decreased, prolonged Less moisture	Dry with leathery eschar Charred vessels visible under eschar Blisters rare, but thin-walled blisters that do not increase in size may be present No blanching with pressure
Color	Increased redness	**Superficial partial injury** Pink **Deep partial injury** Pale, mottled with dull, white, tan, cherry red areas	White, charred, dark tan, black, dark red
Sensation	Painful	Very painful	Little or no pain Deep throbbing Nerve endings dead
Healing time	2-5 days with peeling No scarring May discolor	**Superficial partial injury** 5-21 days, no grafting **Deep partial injury** 21-35 days without complications May convert to full-thickness burn and require grafting	No healing potential Requires excision and grafting

impairments depends on the extent of the burn and the depth of the damage.

LOCALIZED RESPONSES. Heat, chemical, and radiation burn injuries cause immediate tissue changes, known as zones of injury. The *zone of coagulation* is the innermost zone in which protein has been coagulated and the damage is irreversible. Surrounding the zone of coagulation is the *zone of stasis.* Most cells in this area are viable even though blood vessels have been damaged and perfusion is decreased. They are, however, highly sensitive and at increased risk for necrosis over the next few hours or days because of the inflammatory response's release of vasoactive mediators and resultant edema, ischemia, cellular dehydration, and infection. These cells can be saved by meticulous wound care, adequate hydration, and prevention of infection. The third zone, which surrounds the other two zones, is the *zone of hyperemia.* Here blood flow is increased from vasodilation and circulating vasoactive mediators. Hyperemia is necessary because it brings leukocytes and nutrients to the area to promote wound healing within the zone of stasis.[5,29]

SYSTEMIC RESPONSES. When more than 25% of the TBSA is injured, the burn is considered a *major* burn. Major burns affect virtually every organ system. They are associated with massive fluid shifts from the intravascular to the interstitial space, hypovolemia, edema of uninjured tissues, hemodynamic instability, and hypoperfusion of tissues and organs. When untreated, burns that exceed one third of the TBSA produce circulatory and microcirculatory alterations known as **burn shock.**[21,29] Box 66-2 summarizes the systemic effects of burns.

Box 66-2 Systemic Effects of Major Burns

- Hypermetabolism
- Myocardial depression
- Edema
- Inflammatory release of vasoactive mediators
- Renal tubular damage
- Decreased gastrointestinal blood flow
- Pulmonary hypertension
- Pulmonary edema
- Suppressed cellular immunity
- Catabolism of fat and muscle
- Clotting abnormalities
- Early destruction of red blood cells

Cardiovascular Responses

Cardiac Output. Cardiac output is decreased because of the release of catecholamines (e.g., epinephrine and norepinephrine), vasopressin (antidiuretic hormone), and angiotensin II. These substances produce a brief but intense vasoconstriction, which increases systemic vascular resistance and cardiac workload.[29] Tachycardia occurs, and blood pressure may be transiently elevated. This physiologic response conserves fluid but increases capillary force, which promotes burn edema. Even with adequate fluid resuscitation, cardiac function continues to be depressed due to myocardial depressant factor and other vasoactive mediators released by injured cells and the inflammatory response. Figure 66-8 presents an overview of the pathophysiologic changes seen with major burns.

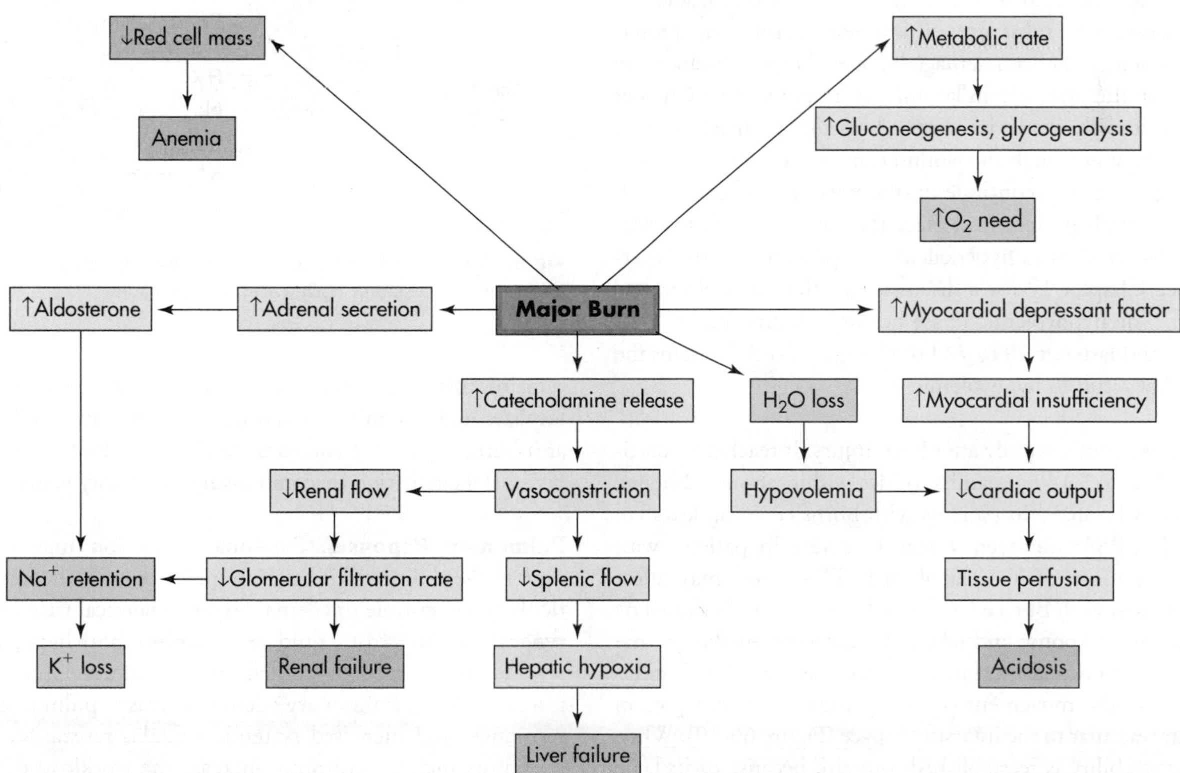

Figure 66-8 Overview of pathophysiology of a major burn. *Na^+*, Sodium; *K^+*, potassium; *H_2O*, water; *O_2*, oxygen.

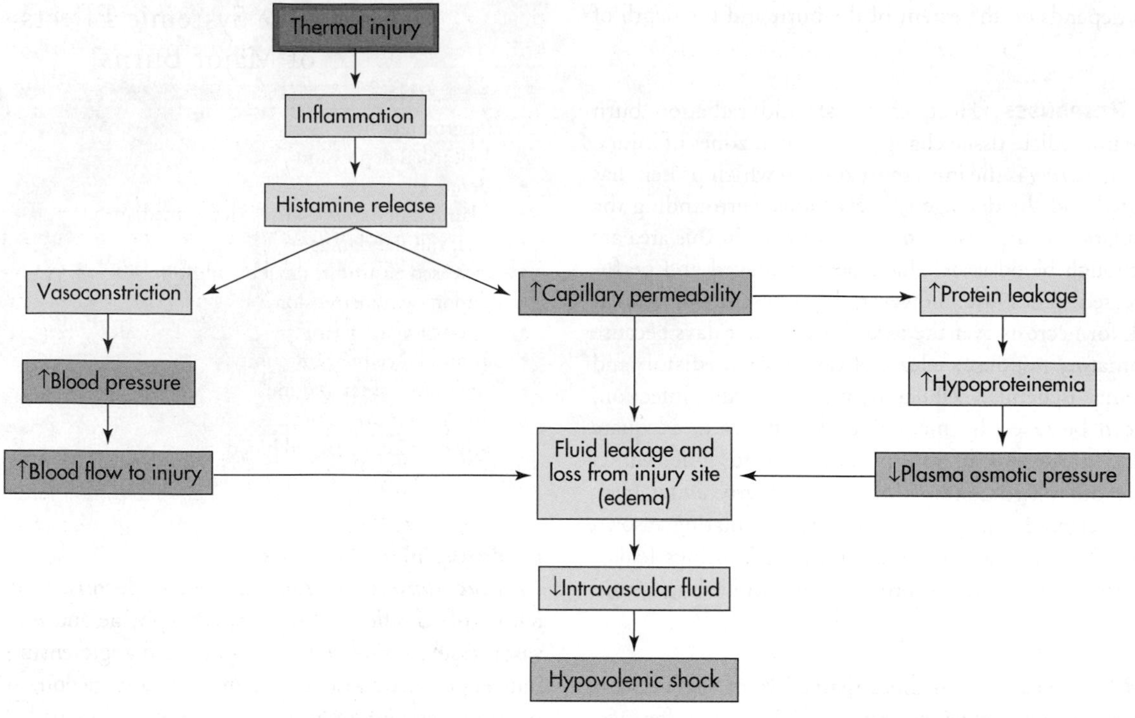

Figure 66-9 Fluid shifts resulting in hypovolemic shock.

Hypovolemia. The early stage of burn shock is hypovolemic and similar to other types of hypovolemic shock. It is characterized by decreased plasma volume and cardiac output, decreased renal perfusion and urinary output, peripheral vasoconstriction, and decreased peripheral circulation.[22] These pathologic changes are related to two primary factors: fluid loss directly from the wound, and the release of vasoactive substances (histamine, serotonin, prostaglandins, interleukin-1) from damaged tissues. These substances are responsible for the systemic inflammatory response (see Chapter 20), which ultimately results in increased vascular permeability and edema. Fluid losses through the wound can be as much as 20 times greater than normal and continue until the wound is healed. Such losses, coupled with protein loss, place the patient at risk for electrolyte imbalances such as hyperkalemia, hyponatremia, or hypernatremia (see Chapter 17 for a discussion of fluid and electrolyte imbalances). The hypovolemic phase begins at injury, peaks in 12 to 24 hours, and lasts for 48 to 72 hours. Figure 66-9 diagrams the fluid shifts that result in hypovolemic shock.

Edema. Edema forms rapidly after burn injury. It reaches its maximum within 12 to 24 hours and subsides within about 72 hours. Edema remains localized in patients with burns covering less than 25% of their TBSA; however, it may be severe in patients with burns covering more than 30% of their TBSA and may affect unburned areas as well. Burn edema, like hypovolemia, is caused by the inflammatory response and release of vasoactive mediators that produce vasodilation and increased capillary permeability. Various mediators cause the movement of fluid, electrolytes, and protein from the intravascular to the interstitial space (Figure 66-10). When capillary permeability is reestablished, protein, because of its large size, is unable to move back into the intravascular space; thus significant hypoproteinemia ensues. Even though lymphatic resorption

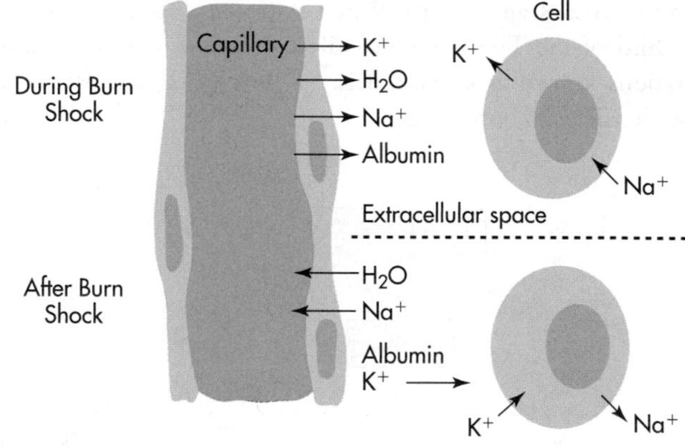

Figure 66-10 Fluid and electrolyte shifts associated with burn shock. K^+, Potassium; H_2O, water; Na^+, sodium.

remains intact, the system becomes overloaded and significant localized and systemic edema occurs.[22,23] Patients with large surface area burns experience edema throughout the body that can impair peripheral circulation by compressing circulatory vessels.

Pulmonary Reponses. Pulmonary function may be affected even in the absence of inhalation injury because the lungs are particularly susceptible to edema. Smoke, chemical irritants, oropharyngeal swelling from fluid resuscitation, and hypoproteinemia are factors believed to contribute to the development of pulmonary edema. Pulmonary edema, increased pulmonary vascular resistance, and increased systemic vascular resistance, caused by mediators such as serotonin, increase the workload of the lungs, making breathing difficult. Patients are also at increased risk for pulmonary insufficiency or acute respiratory distress syndrome

(ARDS) during acute rehabilitation from infection secondary to prolonged immobility, overall decreased immunity, and inadequate pulmonary hygiene.[22,29] (See Chapter 26 for a discussion of acute respiratory failure.)

Renal and Gastrointestinal Responses. The kidneys, liver, and intestines are affected during a major burn. Blood flow to the kidneys is reduced by hypovolemia, peripheral vasoconstriction, and a significant release of antidiuretic hormone, placing the patient at risk for kidney failure. A delay in initial fluid resuscitation or sepsis further increases the risk for renal compromise.

Hepatic perfusion is compromised, contributing to liver ischemia.[32] Decreased bowel perfusion makes the patient prone to paralytic ileus. Breakdown of the small intestine may occur, causing bacteria to translocate across the intestinal wall into the blood vessels, promoting the development of sepsis. Gastric and duodenal ulceration with bleeding can occur in severely burned patients related to stress. Treatment is aimed at prevention by use of antacids, histamine$_2$ blockers, and enteral feedings. Cholecystitis and pancreatitis may also be seen as a result of tissue ischemia from hypoperfusion.

Hypermetabolism and impaired nutrition follow burn shock. A negative nitrogen balance begins at the onset of the burn from tissue destruction, protein loss, and the stress response. It continues throughout the acute phase from tissue catabolism secondary to immobility, increased metabolic rate, and continued protein loss from the wound. Special attention to the patient's nutritional needs is an integral part of comprehensive care during this time. The patient is vulnerable to significant weight loss as a result of fluid evaporation from the wound and loss of solid body mass secondary to increased metabolism.

Immune Responses. Another significant effect of burn injury is compromised immunity. The break in skin integrity destroys the body's first line of defense, and complex immune changes result in bone marrow depression, decreased immunoglobulin production, suppression of complement, and shorter life span of red blood cells. Damaged tissues trigger the release of the inflammatory cytokine cascade (tumor necrosis factor and interleukins), which impairs the function of lymphocytes, macrophages, and neutrophils, increasing the risk for infection.[25] Nutritional deficits further compromise the patient's ability to fight infection. Infection in the patient with a major burn injury can lead to sepsis and multisystem organ dysfunction.

PSYCHOSOCIAL RESPONSES. The psychologic response to burns may be severe and depends, in large part, on the patient's psychologic state before the injury. During the emergent phase, patients may be in a state of disbelief or shock, which may be followed by anger, irritability, or frustration. In 70% of severely burned patients an initial lucid period is followed within 48 hours by a period of delirium with manifestations such as fluctuating levels of alertness, nightmares, insomnia, severe anxiety, withdrawn behavior, resistance to treatment, or hostility. These reactions are thought to be related to stress-induced metabolic disturbances. Patients may not be able to comprehend the extent of their injuries, or conversely they may have suicidal ideation. Depressed patients must be carefully monitored during this phase. It is a positive sign when patient behaviors start to change and they become more independent. It demonstrates their attempt to regain a sense of self. For those patients who remain apathetic and dependent, psychologic problems are likely to continue throughout rehabilitation and discharge.[4]

COMPLICATIONS. As discussed in the above sections, the complications from major burns affect every body system. Infection is a serious and common complication because of the loss of the first line of defense. Sources of infection may be endogenous or exogenous. Bacteria that survive in the hair follicles and glands are a source of endogenous infection. In addition, after burn injury, bacteria that normally live in the intestinal tract migrate or translocate across the intestinal wall and spread to the general circulation by way of the lymphatic system. Local and systemic infections (septicemia) are the most common complications of burns and are the major cause of death, particularly in burns covering more than 25% of the body.

Organisms commonly causing burn wound infection include *Pseudomonas aeruginosa, Acinetobacter* organisms, enterococci, and *Staphylococcus aureus* (Figure 66-11). These organisms are normally found on the skin or in the intestine and become a source of infection when skin is injured. Treatment of antibiotic-resistant organisms, such as methicillin-resistant *S. aureus* and vancomycin-resistant enterococci, is an increasingly difficult problem in burn centers.[17]

Fungal infections have an increased incidence in burn patients because of the use of broad-spectrum antibiotics. *Candida albicans,* which is normally found in the gastrointestinal tract, accounts for the majority of fungal infections. Cultures of the patient's wound may be taken on admission and at biweekly intervals to determine the presence of bacteria or fungi and their sensitivity to antibiotics.

Other complications include fluid volume deficit, electrolyte imbalances, respiratory insufficiency or ARDS, renal compromise, gastrointestinal disorders, hepatic injury, and psychologic disturbances.

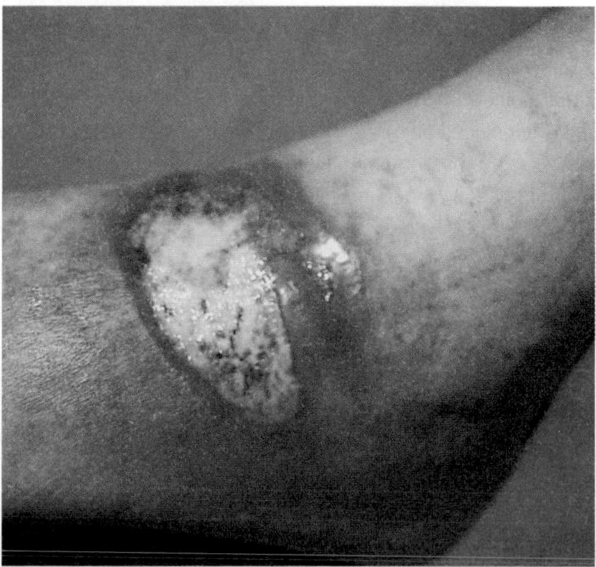

Figure 66-11 Burn wound cellulitis caused by *Staphylococcus aureus.*

Phases of Treatment

Management of a person with a burn injury is extensive and costly. Discharge planning begins on admission using a multidisciplinary approach to provide high-quality, cost-effective care. Three phases of treatment occur in the care of the severely burned patient: emergent, acute, and rehabilitation.

Emergent Phase

Collaborative Care Management. The **emergent phase** of treatment occurs during the first 24 to 48 hours after a burn. During this time emergency department personnel evaluate the patient and determine the severity of injury. First aid and wound care are given to patients with minor burns, who can generally continue with self-care at home (see Complementary & Alternative Therapies box). Persons with moderate burns requiring additional treatments, such as dressing changes, are cared for on an outpatient basis. Patients sustaining major burns are treated for burn shock and transferred to a burn center as soon as feasible.

The goals of management during the emergent phase after a severe burn are securing the airway, supporting circulation by fluid replacement, keeping the patient comfortable with analgesics, preventing infection through careful wound care, maintaining body temperature, and providing emotional support.[2]

Prehospital Care and First Aid. At the scene of a burn injury the first priority is to remove the victim from the hazardous environment and stop the burning process, since the length of exposure to the causative agent is directly related to the severity of the injury. The method by which this is accomplished varies with the type of burn (see Guidelines for Safe Practice box below).

Scald injury is the most common type of burn and may affect a widespread area. Since severity of the scald burn is related to the temperature of the liquid and length of exposure, initial care consists of immediate cooling the skin with cool water.

Complementary & Alternative Therapies

Aloe Vera for Minor Burns

Studies show that aloe vera helps new cells form and hastens healing when placed on minor (first-degree) burns. Healing occurs when the gel is expressed from the leaves and placed on the burn three or four times daily. Aloe vera heals best in the open air, so the burn should not be covered.

Flame and flash injuries are often associated with an inhalational component if the burn occurred in a closed space. In the case of fire, flames are extinguished, flammable or hot material removed from the victim, and the victim and rescuer removed from the unventilated or hazardous surroundings. If clothing is on fire, the victim's first reaction is to run, which only fans the flames. The best intervention is to stop the person; wrap him or her in a blanket, coat, sheet, or towel; and roll him or her on the ground to exclude oxygen and thereby extinguish the fire. The rule is "stop, drop, and roll." Similarly, for people who are confined to a wheelchair or limited in their movement as a result of a disability, a blanket or rug should be used to smother a fire and the victim should drop to the ground and roll to smother all flames if possible.[16]

The victim must avoid standing because the flames and smoke will engulf the facial area, possibly igniting the hair and causing an inhalation injury. Any water source can be used to extinguish flames, cool the burn, or dilute the chemical unless the victim is in contact with an electrical source. Once all flames are extinguished, clothing (except clothing that adheres to the burned area), jewelry, and debris are carefully removed. Any clothing removed is saved for possible analysis of flammability.

Treatment for chemical burns involves irrigating the area with copious amounts of water or saline.[35] The eyes are carefully irrigated with water if they were splashed. Adequacy of the irrigation is determined by using litmus paper to test a sample of the irrigated fluid for acidity or alkalinity.

Ingestion of strong chemicals can burn the upper gastrointestinal tract. These burns are difficult to treat and often cause complications. When possible, the ingested chemical is identified. Vomiting or neutralization of the chemical is avoided, since either may increase tissue damage. Conscious victims who can swallow are given 4 to 8 ounces of water to dilute the chemical. Additional immediate management involves securing the airway, fluid resuscitation, and analgesia.[1]

Electrical burns pose a special hazard to the victim because the TBSA of the burn is not always apparent and may involve internal injuries. Extreme care must be taken when removing the victim from the electrical source to prevent a similar injury to the rescuer.

Regardless of the cause of the burn, a primary survey of the patient's condition is made as soon as burning is stopped. Airway, breathing, and circulation are assessed. The patient's clothing is removed, and a brief neurologic examination is performed. If the victim has no life-endangering injuries, a secondary assessment is performed, which involves a more thorough head-to-toe assess-

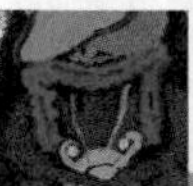

Guidelines for Safe Practice *Prehospital Care of Patients With Major Burns*

- Remove victim to safe area away from source of burn.
- Thermal burn: Douse with water and remove nonadherent, smoldering clothing to stop the burn process.
- Chemical burn: Carefully remove clothing and flush burn with copious amounts of water.
- Electrical burn:
  - —Do not touch victim if still in contact with source.
  - —Remove electrical source with a dry, nonconductive object.
- Establish patent airway.
- Assess for inhalation injury.
- Administer oxygen if available.
- Check peripheral pulse to assess circulation.
- Remove tight-fitting clothing and jewelry.
- Cover burned areas with moist sterile or clean cover.
- Keep victim warm with warm, dry cover to prevent heat loss.
- Transport victim to nearest medical facility.

ment and history. The history includes the mechanism of injury; medical history, including allergies; and medications the patient is taking. The burn wound is evaluated and treated after any life-threatening conditions have been addressed.

Burn wounds are covered with dressings dampened with normal saline or water. This eases the pain, reduces edema, and prevents evaporation of body fluid. The patient's entire body is wrapped in a dry cover to prevent heat loss. Ice is never used, since sudden vasoconstriction causes severe shifting of body fluids, which can increase the depth of injury. Although sterile dressings are preferred, clean dressings may be used, since all dressings are removed when the patient arrives at the medical facility. Oils, salves, and ointments should never be used on burns before evaluation at the hospital. Standard Precautions are followed whenever there is a possibility of exposure to blood or other body fluids.

PAIN RELIEF. In the prehospital period, pain from extensive burns is best controlled by minimal and gentle handling and by applying dressings to exclude air from the burned surfaces. The degree of pain is usually inversely proportional to the depth of the burn injury. Full-thickness burns are usually painless because nerve endings have been destroyed. However, that does not preclude assessing these patients for pain medication needs.[24]

TRANSPORTING THE BURN VICTIM. Burns are often more severe than they first appear; therefore even patients with burns that appear superficial need to be seen by a physician. The hospital or burn center is notified before a burn victim is transported so that personnel have time to prepare for the patient's arrival. Patient transfer should not be delayed because of difficulty in establishing an intravenous (IV) line. The American Burn Association (ABS) advises that an IV line is not necessary if the patient is less than 60 minutes from the hospital. Once IV access is obtained, lactated Ringer's solution is infused according to one of several formulas (discussed later in this chapter). Children require more fluid for maintenance than adults because of increased evaporative water loss. IV lines are not recommended for children younger than age 5.[2] Patients with obviously small burns may be given fluids by mouth with caution. Patients with large burns are given nothing by mouth because fluids decrease peristalsis and may precipitate vomiting, which can result in aspiration.

Patients with major burns need to be transported to a regional burn center. Currently the United States has about 200 burn centers, most of which are located in major medical centers in urban areas.[18] Canada has 14 burn care centers.[12] In an effort to optimize burn care, a national standard for voluntary review of burn centers was established in 1987. The standard encompasses all phases of burn care and verifies the use of a systematic approach (see Legal Alert). The verification is granted for a 3-year period by the ABS and American College of Surgeons.[3] Criteria for transfer of patients to a burn center from a hospital include burn size, depth, mechanism, and comorbid factors[2] (Box 66-3).

EMERGENCY DEPARTMENT MANAGEMENT. Rapid and efficient care is essential for the emergency department management of the person with a major burn (see Guidelines for Safe Practice box below). If respiratory distress is present, an airway is established. Prophylactic intubation may be initiated for heat or smoke inhalation or if the head, neck, or face is involved. Inhalation injuries are best managed with controlled ventilation because swelling of the upper airway can progress to obstruction (Figure 66-12). Endotracheal intubation is preferred over a tracheostomy. Edema of the respiratory passages commonly subsides within a

Legal Alert

Maintaining Educational Requirements for Burn Care

The lack of properly trained individuals to provide treatment and rehabilitation of burn injury victims has been identified as a cause not only of patient mortality, but also of increasing litigation. In response, some states have directed their health departments to assume responsibility for the development and administration of policies governing the medical care of burn-injured patients. Nurses working in burn-care environments need to understand what their state educational requirements are, stay abreast of state policies, and keep their skills updated to decrease the likelihood of providing substandard care to their burn patients or being sued.[18]

Box 66-3 Criteria for Transfer of Patient to Burn Center

- Partial-thickness burns covering more than 10% total body surface area
- Burns involving face, hands, feet, genitalia, perineum, or major joints
- All full-thickness (third- and fourth-degree) burns
- Electrical burns (including lightening)
- Chemical burns
- Inhalation injuries
- Preexisting conditions that can complicate treatment, prolong recovery, or affect mortality
- Burn injury posing greater threat than concomitant trauma (e.g., fractures)
- Children, when local facilities lack qualified personnel or equipment
- Injuries requiring long-term or special social or emotional interventions

GUIDELINES FOR SAFE PRACTICE

Emergency Department Treatment for Major Burns

- Establish patent airway.
- Establish intravenous access (two large-bore peripheral lines if possible).
- Initiate fluid therapy.
- Insert indwelling urinary catheter to monitor hourly urinary output.
- Remove stomach contents via nasogastric tube to prevent gastric distention or aspiration.
- Administer small doses of intravenous narcotics frequently to manage pain.
- Assess circulation distal to circumferential burns.
- Administer tetanus prophylaxis.

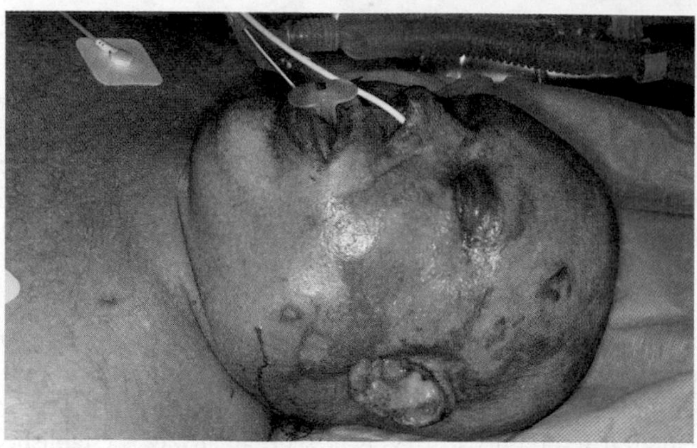

Figure 66-12 Deep partial-thickness face burn from molten steel, resulting in facial swelling requiring intubation for airway control.

few days after the initial injury; therefore surgery of the airway is avoided. Depending on the severity of symptoms, emergency treatment may include oxygen, suctioning, and postural drainage.

After the airway is established, circulation is addressed. Fluid is best replaced through two large-caliber peripheral IV catheters. When possible, catheters are placed in unburned areas to prevent the introduction of microorganisms and subsequent infection. Burned areas are used when burns are extensive and unburned areas are not available. An indwelling urinary catheter is inserted so that urinary output can be monitored every hour as a guide for the adequacy of fluid replacement (plasma volume).[34]

Patients with burns of more than 20% of the TBSA are more prone to nausea, vomiting, and ileus formation.[2] Oral fluids are not recommended, since they create a threat of vomiting and aspiration. A nasogastric tube is inserted and attached to suction to prevent gastric distention.

MEDICATIONS. Morphine sulfate is the drug of choice for pain relief and is given intravenously in small increments (2 to 4 mg). A morphine drip can be used and titrated to the patient's pain. No medication of any kind is given intramuscularly or subcutaneously, since pooling may occur and the patient will not benefit from the medication. Large doses of sedatives and analgesics are also avoided because of the danger of respiratory depression and the potential for masking other symptoms.

Tetanus toxoid is administered in the emergency department for tetanus prophylaxis if the patient has been previously immunized but has not received tetanus toxoid in the preceding 5 years. If information regarding prior tetanus immunization is not known, a dose of human tetanus–immunoglobulin is administered and an active tetanus immunization program is begun.[2]

TREATMENTS. Replacing fluids and electrolytes (fluid resuscitation) is an essential part of the treatment of burn victims and is instituted as soon as the severity of the burn and the patient's condition are known. Ideally fluid therapy is started within an hour after a severe burn to prevent the onset of hypovolemic shock. Indications for fluid resuscitation are presented in Box 66-4.

Blood volume falls most rapidly, and edema increases most significantly during the first 8 hours following burns; therefore IV replacement is infused at a rapid rate. The patient's 24-hour fluid volume requirement is estimated by using one of several formulas (Table 66-2). The Brooke and Parkland formulas are most commonly used in the United States. Each of these formulas differs in volume, colloid content, and sodium, but all include the administration of an isotonic or hypertonic solution, which is calculated for 24 hours and divided into 8-hour volumes. One half of the total amount calculated is administered during the first 8 hours after the injury. It is important to calculate from the time of injury, not from the time that emergency care was initiated. During the second 8-hour period, one fourth of the total volume calculated is given, and in the third 8-hour period the remaining one fourth is given (Box 66-5). Regardless of the formula used, it serves as a guideline that needs to be modified according to the patient's weight, age, depth and extent of burn, and physiologic response to the burn injury. When formulas are not individualized to the specific patient's needs, the risk for overhydration or underhydration exists.[9a,23a]

Box 66-4 Indications for Fluid Resuscitation

- Adults: burns involving more than 20% of total body surface area (TBSA)
- Children: burns involving more than 10% of TBSA
- Patients older than 65 years or younger than 2 years of age
- Patients with preexisting disease that reduces normal compensatory responses (e.g., cardiac disease, pulmonary disease, diabetes mellitus)

Two types of fluids are considered when calculating the needs of the patient: crystalloids and colloids. Crystalloids may be isotonic or hypertonic. Isotonic solutions (280 to 300 mosm), such as lactated Ringer's solution, or physiologic (0.9%) sodium chloride, do not generate a difference in osmotic pressure between the intravascular and interstitial spaces. Thus large amounts of fluids are required to restore and maintain intravascular volume. Hypertonic solutions (400 to 600 mosm) such as hypertonic saline create an osmotic pull of fluid from the interstitial space back into the depleted intravascular space. Thus the use of hypertonic solutions decreases the amount of fluid required for adequate fluid resuscitation,[34] which helps decrease burn tissue edema and minimizes cardiopulmonary complications (pulmonary edema and congestive heart failure).

Colloids such as albumin, dextran, or hespan may also be used as part of the fluid replacement protocol.[23] However, they are avoided during the first 12 hours following a burn because of the open capillary permeability caused by the burn injury. Capillary permeability starts to close at 12 hours, and after this time patients may receive colloids such as fresh-frozen plasma, albumin, or dextran. These colloids not only supply volume but also generate oncotic pressure, which helps pull fluid back into the intravascular space. Fresh-frozen plasma is also beneficial in restoring lost clotting factors. Red blood cells are used only if the patient has had a significant loss or destruction of red blood cells. Box 66-6 lists signs that indicate adequate fluid resuscitation.

During the second 24 hours following a burn, one half to two thirds of the initial 24-hour volume is generally required. During this second 24-hour period, colloid solutions are used to replace

TABLE 66-2 Commonly Used Adult Fluid Resuscitation Formulas

Formula	Solutions	Estimates for Fluid Replacement
First 24 Hours After Burn		
Brooke	Lactated Ringer's	1.5 ml/kg/% TBSA burn
	Colloid solution	0.5 ml/kg/% TBSA burn
Modified Brooke	Lactated Ringer's	2 ml/kg/% TBSA burn
Parkland	Lactated Ringer's	4 ml/kg/% TBSA burn
Evans	0.9% normal saline	1 ml/kg/% TBSA burn
	Colloid solution	1 ml/kg/% TBSA burn
Hypertonic saline	250 mEq sodium/liter	Volume sufficient to maintain urine output of 30 ml/hr
Second 24 Hours After Burn		
Brooke	Lactated Ringer's	½ to ¾ of first 24 hour requirement
	5% dextrose/H_2O	2000 ml
Modified Brooke	Colloid solution	0.3 to 0.5 ml/kg/% TBSA burn
	5% dextrose/½ normal saline	Volume sufficient to maintain urine output
Parkland	25% albumin	Dose sufficient to maintain plasma levels >2.5 g/dl
	5% dextrose/¼ normal saline	Volume sufficient to maintain urine output
Evans	0.9% normal saline	50% of first 24-hour requirement
	5% dextrose/H_2O	2000 ml
Hypertonic saline	250 mEq sodium/liter	Volume sufficient to maintain urine output of 30 ml/hr

Adapted from Oliver RI & Spain D: *Burns, resuscitation and early mainagement,* 2005, accessed from website: http://www.emedicine.com/plastic/topic159.htm#section-historical; and Carrougher GJ: *Burn care and therapy,* St Louis, 1998, Mosby.

Box 66-5 Parkland Formula Estimation of Fluid Replacement Needs

Using this formula, the clinician estimates the patient's fluid requirements for the first 24 hours after injury:

2 to 4 ml lactated Ringer's solution × Body weight (in kilograms) × Percent burn

For an adult weighing 75 kg with a 70% TBSA burn:

4 ml lactated Ringer's solution × 75 kg × 70% = 21,000 ml over first 24 hours

- 50% administered over first 8 hours = 10,500 ml or 1312 ml/hr
- 50% administered over second 16 hours = 10,500 ml or 656 ml/hr

Box 66-6 Indications of Adequate Fluid Resuscitation

- Clear sensorium
- Heart rate: less than 120 beats/min
- Urinary output: greater than 30 ml/hr (adults)
- Systolic blood pressure: 100 mm Hg
- Central venous pressure: 5 to 10 mm Hg
- Pulmonary capillary wedge pressure: 5 to 15 mm Hg
- Blood pH within normal range: 7.35 to 7.45
- Base deficit: 6 or greater

intravascular volume once capillary permeability significantly decreases. Fluids administered during the first 48 hours are given to maintain circulating blood volume. Additional fluids and electrolytes are added to replace losses from vomiting or from nasogastric drainage.

After the first 48 to 72 hours the patient may begin to mobilize fluid as edema resorption occurs. Urine output increases dramatically at this time and may not be a reliable guide to fluid needs. Thus fluid needs are assessed by measuring serum and urine electrolyte levels. Fluid replacement, using 5% dextrose-containing fluids, is based on patient assessment. If dehydration occurs from diuresis, fluid replacement therapy is continued until blood volume is stabilized. Potassium may be added to the IV fluid because of potassium losses in the urine. The patient is monitored closely for signs of water intoxication or pulmonary edema.

Health Promotion and Prevention. Nurses can help prevent accidental burns by participating in health education programs that stress fire prevention and the consequences of fires, such as burns, deformities, and death. They can also promote legislation to control hazardous practices and make working and living environments safer. Community health nurses are in an unusually advantageous position to recognize unsafe practices in the home and to help families develop safe habits of living.

Burn awareness campaigns can be undertaken to raise patient and community awareness of burn problems (Figure 66-13). Campaigns can highlight seasonal activities that result in burn injuries, such as fireworks, grilling, or sun exposure in the summer or candles and fireplaces in the winter. Parents and other caregivers need

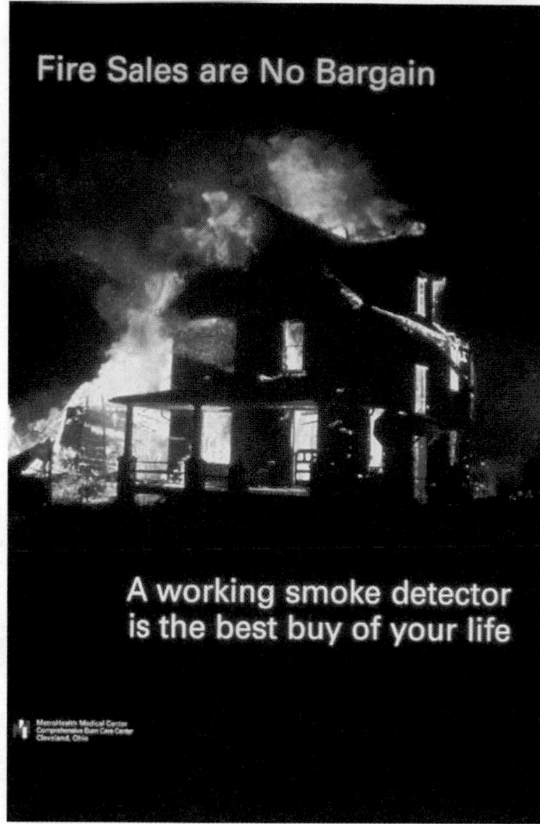

Figure 66-13 Sample burn prevention poster.

to be aware of the high incidence of burns among children from matches and cigarette lighters caused primarily by ignorance, carelessness, and curiosity.

Half of home fires and three fifths of fire-related deaths occur in homes without smoke detectors. Even though smoke detectors are present in 13 out of 14 homes, fire-related deaths occur in about one third of those of homes because the smoke detector does not work. Working smoke detectors awaken people to the fire and allow them time to escape to safety. Important aspects of teaching regarding fire prevention in the home are summarized in the Patient/Family Teaching box.

Every year there is an increased demand for careful inspection and regulation of housing for the ill and infirm. Frail, older adults may be housed in old and nonfireproof structures from which they may not be able to escape if a fire occurs. Nurses can be involved in exerting pressure to ensure that the managers of such housing bring structures up to fire codes and establish a fire evacuation plan. Basic fire prevention programs in all health care facilities should include one mock evacuation drill annually. Emphasis also needs to be placed on the special needs of the disabled. They are at higher risk for burn injury because of their inability to rapidly evacuate from unsafe situations. Box 66-7 summarizes safety measures for disabled persons.

Another aspect of fire prevention pertains to places where large numbers of persons congregate, such as schools, theaters, and sports arenas. Laws regulating public buildings require hinged doors that swing outward, fireproof draperies and decorations, and stairways with special fire doors in new apartment buildings

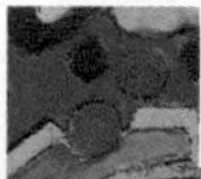

PATIENT/FAMILY TEACHING

Fire Prevention in the Home

- Home smoke detectors
  —All homes should have working smoke detectors on each level of the home and in the hallway outside bedrooms.
  —Batteries should be tested periodically and changed twice yearly—in the spring and the fall. In states and countries with time changes between standard and daylight saving time, battery changes can be timed to coordinate with these time changes.
  —Batteries should never be removed because the alarm goes off during cooking, since it is easy to forget to replace them.
  —Fire departments in most U.S. cities will install smoke detectors free of charge for older adults and others unable to do so for themselves.
  —Many communities have fire department programs to provide free smoke detectors for those unable to afford them.
- People who use home oxygen therapy should not smoke or be around flames. The oxygen should be at least 10 feet from an open flame (e.g., cigarettes, lighters, pilot lights, candles).
- Burn injuries to adults are most often related to accidents while they are cooking, using microwave ovens, smoking, or using matches.
  —Avoid distractions when cooking.
  —Scald burns can occur when the power of the microwave is underestimated.
  —Never smoke in bed.
  —Be particularly careful about falling asleep while smoking and sitting in overstuffed furniture.
  —Extinguish cigarettes completely, especially before going to bed.

Box 66-7 Safety Measures for Disabled Persons

- Develop an escape plan.
  —Plan two escape routes.
  —Keep escape routes free of clutter.
  —Windows with bars need quick release features for easy removal.
- Keep a whistle by the bed to alert rescuers.
  —This makes you easier to locate.
  —It warns others of a fire.
- Contact fire department to place a sticker on the bedroom window to assist them in locating you.
- Keep eyeglasses, dentures, keys, a flashlight, and a telephone at the bedside so you can locate them quickly in an emergency.
- Smokers:
  —Do not smoke if using oxygen (or near an open flame).
  —Use large, deep ashtrays.
  —Never smoke in bed.
- Keep the hot water thermostat at 120° F (48.9° C) or less.
- Install valves in the bathroom that regulate water temperature.
- When cooking:
  —Turn handles of pans to the back of the stove.
  —Avoid wearing shirts with loose sleeves.
  —Make certain the stove is turned off when finished.

Healthy People 2010

Goals for Reduction in Residential Fire Deaths and Presence of Functioning Smoke Alarms

The surgeon general's goals for 2010 related to burn injury focus on decreasing residential fire deaths through the presence of a functioning smoke alarm on every floor.

- Goal 1: Reduce the incidence of residential fires.
  1998 baseline: 1.2 per 100,000 people
  2010 target: 0.2 per 100,000 people
- Goal 2: Increase total population living in residences with functioning smoke alarms on every floor.
  1998 baseline: 88%
  2010 target: 100%

The groups at greatest risk are African-Americans, American Indians or Alaskan Natives, and Hispanic or Latino populations. Baseline data from 1988 reflect higher rates of residential fires and a lower presence of smoke alarms among these groups.

From US Department of Health and Human Services: *Healthy people 2010: understanding and improving health,* Washington, DC, 2000, The Department.

and hotels. Smoke detectors and sprinkler systems are required in new buildings and residential health care facilities.[20]

The government's role in fire prevention involves passing and enforcing laws to protect the public, such as requirements for labeling flammable industrial products and testing products for flammability before placing them on the market. Industry safety can be maintained by constant vigilance to identify hazards and implement safety programs. All chemicals should be labeled, and antidotes easily identifiable and available. Core individuals should be versed in emergency treatment of all types of burns for the protection of every employee.

Healthy People 2010, the surgeon general's report on goals to be achieved by 2010, includes an increase in functioning residential smoke alarms and a reduction in residential fire deaths. These goals are particularly focused on high-risk groups: American Indians, Alaskan Natives, and African-Americans (see Healthy People 2010 box).[33]

▶ ARE You READY?

A 220-lb patient has a 40% TBSA burn. Using the Parkland formula, initial fluid administration in the emergent phase to be:

1. 4,000-8,000 ml
2. 8,000-16,000 ml
3. 10,000-20,000 ml
4. 22,000-44,000 ml

Nursing Management
of the Patient with Burns during the Emergent Phase

ASSESSMENT

Health History. Assess for:

- How the burn injury occurred
- When the burn injury occurred
- Duration of contact with the burning agent
- Location where the burn injury occurred (Enclosed area suggests possibility of smoke inhalation or carbon monoxide poisoning.)
- Whether there was an associated explosion (suggests possibility of other injuries)
- Age (Those over age 60 and under age 2 have a higher mortality rate than a young adult with the same percentage of burn.)
- Preexisting diabetes mellitus, chronic obstructive pulmonary disease, arteriosclerotic heart disease, congestive heart failure, hypertension, renal failure, other illness
- Allergies, drug sensitivities
- Current prescribed and over-the-counter medications

Physical Examination. Assess for:

- Percent of body involved
- Parts of body involved (e.g., face, neck, perineal area, hands, feet)
- Hypotension
- Tachycardia
- Airway patency, tachypnea, cough, hoarseness
- Soot at nostrils or mouth (may indicate smoke inhalation)
- Lung crackles or wheezing
- Fractures or other injuries sustained at time of burn
- Urinary output of less than 30 ml/hr

NURSING DIAGNOSES, OUTCOMES, AND INTERVENTIONS

Nursing Diagnosis: Ineffective Airway Clearance

OUTCOMES. Common examples of expected outcomes for the patient with a diagnosis of *ineffective airway clearance* are:
Patient will:

- Maintain a patent airway.
- Remain free of stridor and adventitious breath sounds.
- Maintain Po_2 of more than 80 mm Hg and Pco_2 of less than 45 mm Hg.
- Maintain carboxyhemoglobin level of less than 10%.

NURSING INTERVENTIONS. Persons who are burned on the face and neck or those who have inhaled flame, steam, or smoke are observed closely for signs of laryngeal edema and airway obstruction. Data indicating potential or existing inhalation injury are outlined in the Clinical Manifestations box.

Adequate ventilation and oxygenation may be possible with the victim breathing room air; however, when any inhalation

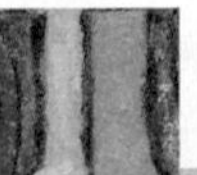

CLINICAL MANIFESTATIONS
Inhalation Injury

- Facial burns
- Singed nasal hair
- Severe, brassy cough
- Carbon-containing sputum
- Dyspnea
- Wheezing
- Stridor
- Lacrimation
- Hoarseness
- Anxiety
- Confusion
- Coma

injury has occurred, it is best to give oxygen. When smoke is inhaled, carbon monoxide binds with hemoglobin, displacing oxygen. High carboxyhemoglobin levels impair tissue oxygenation, resulting in tissue asphyxia. Providing the victim with 100% oxygen by mask reverses this condition. If the victim is in respiratory distress or has a suspected inhalation injury, endotracheal intubation may be necessary.[22]

Related NIC Interventions. Airway Management, Airway Suctioning, Aspiration Precautions, Oxygen Therapy, Respiratory Monitoring, Vital Signs Monitoring

Nursing Diagnosis: Hypothermia

Outcomes. Common examples of expected outcomes for the patient with a diagnosis of *hypothermia* are:

Patient will:

- Maintain a body temperature between 98.6° and 101.3° F (37° and 38.5° C).
- Report comfort and freedom from chills.
- Maintain warmth of unburned areas of skin.

Nursing Interventions. The loss of skin greatly decreases the severely burned patient's ability to regulate body temperature. The environment must be heat controlled and kept warmer than usual. Room temperature is maintained at 80° to 85° F (26.7° to 29.4° C) with a humidity of 40% to 50%. Drafts are eliminated. Fluid warmers, heat lamps, and warming blankets are used during burn shock. Prolonged exposure to air is avoided. Exposed areas of the body are covered with clean sheets and blankets to decrease the loss of body heat through the open wounds while other areas of the burn are being cleansed. The nurse consistently monitors vital signs to determine alterations from baseline that indicate the patient's core body temperature is decreasing.

Related NIC Interventions. Hypothermia Treatment, Oxygen Therapy, Temperature Regulation, Vital Sign Monitoring

Nursing Diagnosis: Deficient Fluid Volume

Outcomes. Common examples of expected outcomes for the patient with a diagnosis of risk for or actual *deficient fluid volume* are:

Patient will:

- Achieve normal fluid volume and be free from signs of fluid excess.
- Maintain urinary output of 30 to 50 ml/hr (0.5 ml/kg body weight) in adults or 1 to 2 ml/kg/hr in children.
- Maintain electrolytes within normal limits.
- Achieve normal sensorium.
- Maintain systolic blood pressure at more than 100 mm Hg and heart rate at less than 120 beats/min.
- Maintain pH between 7.35 and 7.45 and base excess of 6 or greater.
- Remain free from signs of pulmonary edema.

Nursing Interventions. The nurse assesses adequacy of fluid resuscitation by monitoring mental status, vital signs, peripheral perfusion, body weight, and urinary output. A 15% to 20% weight gain in the first 72 hours of resuscitation is anticipated. Significant laboratory measurements include serum and urine electrolytes, serum and urine osmolality, and hematocrit values. Hourly urinary output is commonly used as a gauge for adequate fluid replacement. Fluid is titrated to ensure an output of 0.5 ml/kg body weight/hr, or 30 to 50 ml/hr. Urinary output below 30 ml/hr indicates insufficient fluid replacement generally relating to calculated fluids falling behind schedule or the patient's fluid requirements being greater than predicted. The nurse observes the urine for color and analyzes it for the presence of blood. The physician is notified if hematuria, which may indicate renal compromise, is present.

Other clinical criteria that indicate adequate resuscitation are pulse rate of 120 beats/min or less, central venous pressure in the low to normal range, pulmonary artery end-diastolic pressure in the low to normal range, and mental lucidity. Acidosis indicates that fluids have not been given in sufficient quantities to maximize tissue perfusion. Anaerobic metabolism ensues when the metabolic tissue requirements are not met during resuscitation. Recent studies indicate that the presence of a base deficit, particularly greater than 6, is a good indicator of adequate fluid resuscitation in patients with major burns.[21]

When edema begins to resorb after the first 48 to 72 hours, serum and urine electrolyte levels, not urinary output, are used to guide fluid needs. The nurse monitors the patient closely for signs of water intoxication or pulmonary edema resulting from fluid revascularization. Patients may complain of moderate to severe thirst during this period. Aggressive oral hygiene may alleviate patient discomfort. If oral fluids are permitted, accurate recording of ingested fluids is important. Unlimited oral intake and failure to measure it may result in the patient taking in too much fluid, which will contribute to water intoxication.

Related NIC Interventions. Electrolyte Monitoring, Fluid Management, Fluid Monitoring, Hypovolemia Management, Intravenous (IV) Therapy, Vital Signs Monitoring

Nursing Diagnosis: Risk for Infection

Outcomes. Common examples of expected outcomes for the patient with a diagnosis of *risk for infection* are:

Patient will:

- Be free from signs and symptoms of wound infection.
- Have clean-appearing wound edges.
- Maintain a temperature of less than 101.3° F (38.5° C).
- Maintain intact skin and mucous membranes in unburned areas.
- Maintain vital signs within normal limits according to patient's baseline.
- Maintain white blood cell (WBC) count within normal limits.

Nursing Interventions. Infection is a serious and highly possible complication of severe burns. However, meticulous wound care during the emergent phase can reduce the risk for infection and decrease the loss of tissues. During admission the nurse carefully washes the burn wound and the entire body to remove dirt, debris, and loose dead tissue on the burned areas and to prevent any further entry of microorganisms. Detergents or antiseptic preparations are effective cleansing agents. Gentle cleansing with gauze removes dead tissue without causing further tissue damage.

The nurse shaves and wipes off all hair in and around the burn wound because hair attracts and shelters bacteria. Singed hair is clipped short to avoid bacterial contamination of the wound. Firm, intact blisters may remain undisturbed because they provide natural protection and reduce pain. If the blisters are broken and the epidermis is separated, loose tissue must be debrided. Blisters that are very large or adjacent to joints are gently removed using scissors and forceps. Patients with chemical burns must have their blisters removed to ensure no chemical is present. Care must be taken when removing blisters from chemical agents so that staff members do not contaminate themselves.

After the wound is cleaned and before a dressing is applied, the nurse obtains cultures of the wound. Baseline cultures provide information about organisms present in the wound at the time of admission. Prophylactic antibiotics are usually not indicated. Photographs may be taken to record the wound's appearance on admission, before the application of topical therapy, and during the healing process.

Protective precautions, which include strict hand-washing protocols, are essential to prevent the introduction of microbes from staff or other patients. The nurse uses aseptic technique when inserting IV or urinary catheters or performing wound care to prevent cross-contamination or infections such as IV phlebitis or urinary tract infection.

RELATED NIC INTERVENTIONS. Cough Enhancement, Infection Control, Infection Protection, Nutrition Management, Perineal Care, Skin Surveillance, Wound Care

Nursing Diagnosis: Risk for Ineffective Peripheral Tissue Perfusion

OUTCOMES. Common examples of expected outcomes for the patient with a diagnosis of *risk for ineffective peripheral tissue perfusion* are:

Patient will:

- Maintain distal pulses that are palpable or present on Doppler.
- Maintain warmth and color of unburned areas of extremities.
- Maintain intact sensory perception in burned and unburned areas.
- Remain free from infection.
- Report absence of pain or paresthesia in burned extremities.
- Remain free from respiratory compromise.

NURSING INTERVENTIONS. The constricting effect of nonviable tissue (eschar) from a full-thickness injury to the chest, neck, or extremities is an early complication. Edema forming rapidly under the constricting eschar produces a tourniquet effect that occludes venous and arterial circulation and may result in ischemic necrosis, especially in unburned areas distal to the constrictive eschar. Frequent monitoring of distal pulses is part of ongoing assessment to ensure uninterrupted vascular flow to all extremities. The nurse monitors extremities for signs and symptoms of circulatory compromise and increased pain or paresthesia, which may indicate compromised circulation. It may be necessary to monitor circulation as often as every 15 minutes.

Circumferential burns of the neck and chest can lead to constriction of chest wall expansion and airway compromise, resulting in respiratory distress. Monitoring chest excursion, respiratory rate, and ventilator settings, if the person is intubated, for high pressures and low tidal volume is part of the respiratory assessment.

Treatment of the constricting effects of the eschar is an escharotomy, which is performed on the burn unit. An **escharotomy** is a linear surgical incision through the burn eschar that releases the constriction caused by the full-thickness injury (Figure 66-14). Patients have limited pain during an escharotomy because the burn has damaged the nerve endings.

RELATED NIC INTERVENTIONS. Neurological Monitoring, Peripheral Sensation Management, Positioning

Nursing Diagnosis: Acute Pain

OUTCOMES. Common examples of expected outcomes for the patient with a diagnosis of *acute pain* are:

Patient will:

- Report the need for pain interventions before pain becomes severe.
- Report pain as 3 or less on a scale of 0 (no pain) to 10 (maximal pain) with use of comfort measures.
- Experience periods of rest or sleep after pain interventions.
- Remain free from restlessness caused by pain.

NURSING INTERVENTIONS. Regardless of the degree, burns produce pain. Pain from first-degree burns can be controlled with over-the-counter pain relievers and skin protectors or moisturizers. Skin protectors prevent new tissues beneath the burn from drying out and cracking. Topical anesthetics can also be used until the pain subsides.

Patients with major burns are kept as comfortable as possible by gentle handling of the burn areas and by keeping the wounds covered so that air does not reach them. Opioids, such as morphine sulfate, are administered intravenously in small doses every 5 to 10 minutes for the first 24 to 48 hours after admission. Subcutaneous or intramuscular pain medications are avoided because

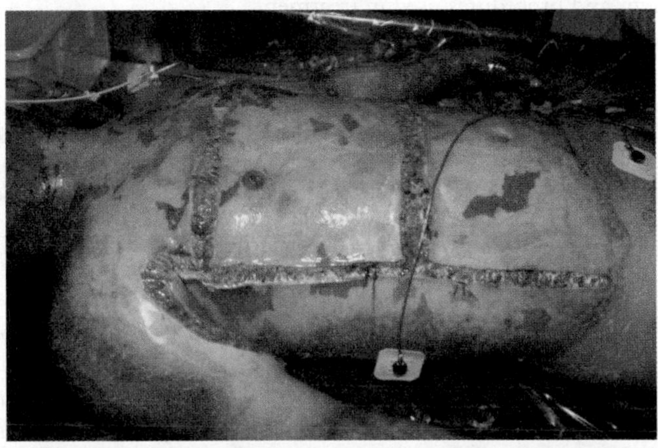

Figure 66-14 Escharotomies to full-thickness chest burns.

peripheral vasoconstriction interferes with absorption. Blisters are left intact because they provide a natural pain barrier to the wound and help prevent infection.

Studies have shown that burn pain can be difficult to control and that, in many cases, it is not adequately treated by health care providers. In many instances pain medication is administered, but at 50% of the prescribed dose. Older adults and young children are least likely to receive adequate pain control. Concerns regarding oversedation after treatments such as dressing changes and fear of drug side effects have been identified as reasons why pain medications are not administered. Uncontrolled pain can result in fear, pain cycles that are difficult to break, increased anxiety, and adverse psychologic effects.[10] See Chapter 16 for a discussion of pain and pain control. Research is ongoing in the area of burn pain control (see Research box below).

RELATED NIC INTERVENTIONS. Analgesic Administration, Anxiety Reduction, Environmental Management: Comfort, Medication Management, Pain Management

Nursing Diagnosis: Anxiety

OUTCOMES. Common examples of expected outcomes for the patient with a diagnosis of *anxiety* are:

Patient will:

- Remain free from physiologic signs of anxiety.
- Listen to explanations from staff.
- Begin to verbalize concerns about the incident and ask questions about the future.

NURSING INTERVENTIONS. Patients with significant burn injury receive a profound insult to their body and self-image. They are aware that they may not survive, which causes fear, feelings of helplessness, and anxiety. The shock and pain of the accident, the chaos and rush to the hospital, and the unknown surroundings and people all intensify the emotional stress. Because nurses spend the greatest amount of time with patients, they have considerable influence on the patient's psychologic adjustment. Interventions to reassure the patient, alleviate fear and anxiety, and enhance coping include identifying one's self to the patient, orienting the patient to the surroundings, describing the basis for physical symptoms (skin loss, pain, and cold), and explaining the equipment and procedures used in treatment.

RELATED NIC INTERVENTIONS. Anxiety Reduction, Coping Enhancement, Distraction, Presence, Sleep Enhancement

EVALUATION

To evaluate the effectiveness of nursing interventions, compare patient behaviors with those stated in the expected patient outcomes.

RELATED NOC OUTCOMES. Comfort Level, Electrolyte & Acid/Base Balance, Fluid Balance, Hope, Immune Status, Pain Control, Respiratory Status: Airway Patency, Thermoregulation, Tissue Perfusion: Peripheral, Vital Signs

Acute Phase

The acute phase of treatment begins at the end of the emergent phase and lasts until all the full-thickness wounds are covered with skin grafts or partial-thickness wounds are healed. The physical healing time is determined by the patient's medical condition, nutritional status, and ability to heal. A 40% injury requires approximately 40 days to heal. If the burn is a partial-thickness injury, the acute phase extends for 7 to 21 days; if the burn is a full-thickness injury over a large percentage of the body requiring surgery for skin grafting, the acute phase may last for months.

Collaborative Care Management. During the acute phase the two main foci of management are treatment of the burn wound and avoidance, detection, and treatment of complications. The most common complications are infection (septicemia and pneumonia), renal disease, and heart failure. Many ethical dilemmas can occur during the emergent and acute care phases of burn care (see Ethical Alert box).

DIAGNOSTIC TESTS. Laboratory testing takes place during the acute phase to monitoring the patient's fluid and electrolyte balance. The nurse may obtain chemistry profiles once or twice daily during the patient's critical phase while fluid resuscitation is in progress. Complete blood counts are monitored to assess the patient's WBC count and hemoglobin and hematocrit values. Wound cultures are obtained once or twice weekly to track the

Research

Ang E et al: Pain control in a randomized, controlled, clinical trial comparing moist exposed burn ointment and conventional methods in patients with partial-thickness burns, *J Burn Care Rehabil* 24(5):286-296, 2003.

One hundred and fifteen patients with partial-thickness burns were treated with either conventional pain control methods or moist exposed burn ointment (MEBO) to determine differences in pain control effectiveness. Patients rated their pain in the morning, after burn dressing changes, and 8 hours later. Patients in the group receiving MEBO experienced less pain than the control group after dressing changes for the first week, but not at other times. The researchers concluded that MEBO is a suitable alternative to conventional burn management.

Ethical Alert

Burn Care

Many ethical questions arise in burn care, including:

- Should experimental testing be carried out on burn patients even if they or their family members give consent?
- When does saving the life of a person with extensive burns become futile, and who will make that decision?
- Does a do-not-resuscitate order preclude all possible efforts at saving a person with severe burns?
- Should scarce resources be used to save one life when in all likelihood the patient will not survive the burn injury?

When trying to answer these questions, those involved in burn care draw on the concept that burn patients are the most severely injured and vulnerable of all patients and deserve the best possible decision-making efforts on their behalf.

Research

Demling R, DeSanti L: The beneficial effects of the anabolic steroid oxandrolone in the geriatric burn population, *Wounds* 15(2):54-58, 2003.

Fifty burned patients over the age of 65 years were studied to determine whether the addition of the anabolic steroid oxandrolone to burn treatment protocols would improve outcome variables in this age group. Forty-six of the 50 patients survived. Compared with patients who did not receive oxandrolone, those who received it experienced decreased weight and nitrogen losses, faster healing of donor site, and decreased length of hospital stay. No significant side effects were noted among study participants receiving the drug. Researchers concluded that adding oxandrolone to burn treatment significantly improved outcomes for this age group.

bacterial colonization of the wounds. Ongoing surveillance of wound cultures is essential for early treatment of infection. Evaluation of nutritional status is monitored through prealbumin levels and urine urea nitrogen. Patients who are intubated or have inhalation injuries require periodic chest x-ray studies. In addition, bronchoscopy is performed on patients with inhalation injuries to assess the degree of injury to the lungs.

MEDICATIONS. Analgesia is essential for pain control. The most commonly used agents are opioids such as morphine sulfate, fentanyl, and codeine. Patients with major burns may require agents to prevent stress ulcers (e.g., ranitidine, cimetidine, or sucralfate). Systemic antimicrobial agents are used only when evidence of infection is present.

Anabolic steroids, such as oxandrolone, have had positive effects during the recovery phase of a major burn and may be particularly useful for older adults (see Research box above). They are used to attenuate the catabolic state, restore lean body mass, and promote wound healing.[13] Burn patients with preexisting illnesses require ongoing medication management of their current health problems.

Topical antimicrobial agents are applied to the burn wounds on the basis of the depth of injury and wound culture results. A number of agents are available (Table 66-3). Topical agents are applied directly to the wound. Petroleum-based topical antimicrobial agents, such as bacitracin, provide a barrier protection to the wound and are used for more superficial burns. Other agents, such as silver sulfadiazine and mafenide acetate, are used for full-thickness and deep dermal burns. The cream penetrates through the eschar, helping the eschar to separate while the antimicrobial action helps prevent or treat infection. If eschar is present, an enzyme may be applied topically to promote separation of the dead tissue.

TREATMENTS. Wound care is the major treatment for patients with burns. Different methods of treating the burned area may be used depending on the location of the burn, its size and depth, inpatient versus outpatient care, and the patient's response to therapy. Wounds can be managed by an open or closed method. If an open method is used, a topical agent or wound covering is placed on the wound and left exposed to the air. More superficial burns of the face may be managed in this manner. A topical agent, such as bacitracin, is applied to the face after cleansing. An open method allows for staff to visualize the wound more readily and assists in range of motion because of the absence of constricting dressings. Disadvantages include heat loss and easy accidental removal of the topical agent during patient activity. If a closed method of wound care is used, the nurse places the topical agent or wound covering on the wound and covers it with a gauze wrap. This method promotes adherence of the topical agent to the wound and limits fluid loss and wound drying.

SURGICAL MANAGEMENT: SKIN GRAFTS. Skin grafts are applied to cover full-thickness burn wounds to speed healing, control contractures, and shorten convalescence. Successful grafting reduces the patient's vulnerability to infection and prevents the loss of body heat and water vapor from the open wound. Most skin grafts are applied between days 3 and 21 after the initial injury, depending on the depth and extent of the burn and the condition of the burn wound base. Further skin grafting may be performed for cosmetic or functional purposes during the rehabilitation phase.

A variety of grafts obtained from various sources are used to treat burn wounds. Grafts may provide permanent or temporary coverage (Table 66-4). An **autograft** is a graft of skin obtained from the patient's own body and is a permanent graft. An **allograft**, or homograft, can be cryopreserved graft of skin obtained from a deceased donor 6 to 24 hours after death or from a live donor. It can be used as fresh donor skin (stored in the refrigerator) or frozen donor skin obtained from a tissue bank. A **heterograft** (xenograft) is a graft of skin obtained from another species, such as a pig. Homografts, heterografts, synthetic substitutes, and biosynthetic dressings (e.g., Biobrane) are intended to provide temporary coverage while the burn wound heals. Temporary coverings are gradually rejected as wound healing occurs and are easily removed from the newly healed skin. Temporary grafts reduce water, electrolyte, and protein losses at the burn surface; reduce wound pain; and allow the patient freedom of movement. Temporary grafts act like human skin and may be used until the patient is ready for an autograft. Autografting is delayed when there are complications such as infection or pneumonia or the patient status is critical.

Dermal replacements or synthetic substitutes for skin are used, to varying degrees, in burn units throughout the United States and Canada. Integra, AlloDerm, and cultured epithelium (Epicel) are new products currently available. All these products are expensive, with the cost alone sometimes in excess of $20,000 or more per patient. Cost-effectiveness is being evaluated by comparing costs with patient outcomes. The ultimate skin substitute, if available, would be inexpensive, nonantigenic, flexible, and durable; it would also prevent fluid loss, serve as a barrier to infection, adjust to the wound surface, grow with a child, not cause hypertrophic scarring, store easily with a long shelf-life, and be applied in one operation. Although currently no perfect skin substitute exists,[22] skin engineering may hold promise for the future treatment of major burns (see Future Watch box, p. 1931).

Before the graft is placed on the wound, a surgical tangential and/or fascial excision is performed in which the necrotic tissue or eschar is removed down to viable tissue or fascia. The wound is then covered with an autograft or skin substitute. The procedure is best performed between the second and fifth postburn day. This

TABLE 66-3 TOPICAL MEDICATIONS AND WOUND COVERINGS USED IN BURN THERAPY

Agent	Indication	Implications
TOPICAL AGENTS		
Petroleum-based antimicrobials (bacitracin, neosporin, polymyxin B)	Partial-thickness burns	Provides barrier protection to wound Has mild antimicrobial activity Cleaning wound before applying prevents caking. Maintain layer adequate to keep wound from drying.
Silver sulfadiazine (Silvadene)	Deep partial- to full-thickness burns Wound infection	Has broad-spectrum antimicrobial action against gram-negative bacteria, gram-positive bacteria, and *Candida* organisms Penetrates eschar to inhibit bacterial growth at dermis-eschar interface Soothes pain with ¼-in layer applied directly to wound or on impregnated gauze 2-3 times daily May cause slimy, grayish appearance with repeated applications Inhibits epithelial tissue development Discontinued when eschar no longer present Side or toxic effects: Skin rash on unburned tissues Transient decrease in WBC for 24-48 hr after application Contraindicated in patients with sulfa hypersensitivities
Mafenide acetate (Sulfamylon)	Deep partial- to full-thickness burns Wound infection	Is bacteriostatic against gram-negative and gram-positive bacteria Is applied in ¼-in layer directly on wound or as impregnated gauze 2-3 times daily 11.1% cream: penetrates thick eschar and cartilage; inhibits epithelial tissue development 5% solution: antimicrobial solution used to prevent and treat wound infections Discontinued when eschar no longer present Side or toxic effects: Pain on application (may necessitate pain management) Metabolic acidosis (when applied to more than 40% TBSA; inhibits carbonic anhydrase activity) Hypersensitivity rash, pruritus, fungal growth
Silver nitrate (5% solution)	Deep partial- to full-thickness burns Wound infection	Is bacteriostatic against gram-positive and gram-negative bacteria Has poor penetration of eschar Side or toxic effects: Stains wound black, making assessment difficult Pain on application (may necessitate pain management) Stains clothing and linens Decreases electrolytes (sodium, potassium, calcium, chloride)

technique is used to cover a full-thickness burn injury. Advantages of tangential excision and grafting are that they prevent burn conversion to full-thickness, allow for earlier grafting and restoration of function, reduce scar formation, diminish anxiety related to multiple graft procedures, and decrease hospitalization time.

Split-thickness skin grafts, full-thickness skin grafts, and primary closure are surgical techniques used to cover burn wounds (Figure 66-15). Split-thickness skin grafts include the upper layers of skin (epidermis) and part of the middle layer (dermis). If deeper layers of skin are taken, the skin at the donor site (where the graft was taken) will not regenerate. Grafts are removed from almost any unburned part of the body. The size of the grafts is determined by the sites available and the area to be covered.

Grafts are used as sheets or meshed. Meshing of the graft involves feeding the donor skin into a meshing instrument that perforates the sheet with tiny slits. Meshing makes the graft more

TABLE 66-3 TOPICAL MEDICATIONS AND WOUND COVERINGS USED IN BURN THERAPY—CONT'D

Agent	Indication	Implications
ENZYMES		
Collagenase (Santyl)	Deep partial- to full-thickness burns Wound infection	Specifically digests collagen in necrotic tissue Does not harm healthy tissues Has no antimicrobial properties Applied to areas with eschar 1-2 times daily and covered with barrier dressing Discontinued when eschar is removed
Papain urea debriding ointment (Accuzyme)	Deep partial- to full-thickness burns Wound infection	Water-soluble, nonspecific cysteine protease that breaks down nonviable tissues Does not harm healthy tissues Has no antimicrobial properties Applied to areas with eschar 1-2 times daily and covered with gauze dressing Discontinued when eschar is removed Side or toxic effects: pain on application (may necessitate pain management)
Acticoat dressing	Deep partial- to full-thickness burns Donor sites	Polyethylene mesh coated with ionic silver with rayon-polyester core Has broad-spectrum antimicrobial action Maintains moist wound environment, which may be left in place for several days
Xeroform gauze	Deep partial- to full-thickness burns Donor sites	Petrolatum-based fine mesh gauze impregnated with 3% bismuth tribromophenate Has mild antimicrobial properties Provides protective barrier that allows epithelial tissue development May need to be changed daily to maintain adherence
Scarlet Red dressing	Partial-thickness burns Donor sites	Fine-mesh gauze impregnated with lanolin, olive oil, petrolatum, and red dye Provides protective barrier that allows epithelial tissue development Has no antimicrobial properties May need to be changed daily to maintain adherence
Mepitel dressing	Partial-thickness burns Donor sites	Fine mesh netting coated with silicone, which is a pliable, nonadherent dressing Has mild antimicrobial properties Allows for epithelial tissue development
Film dressing (OpSite, Tegaderm)	Partial-thickness burns Donor sites	Semipermeable barrier dressing that allows for wound visualization Has no antimicrobial properties

Continued

expandable so it can be stretched to cover wider areas of the body surface. Sheet grafts are applied directly to the burn wound without meshing. Sheets result in better functional and cosmetic outcomes and thus are used on the face, neck, and hands or around joints.

Full-thickness grafts are composed of layers of skin down to the subcutaneous tissue. They are used for a well-defined area of full-thickness burn. They are used early in wound management and provide a better cosmetic appearance than split-thickness grafts when healed. Areas that benefit from full-thickness grafts are the hands, neck, and face. Full-thickness grafts can also be used in rehabilitation stages to restore body function and release skin contractures. Primary closure of the wound is an alternate surgical method in which skin is pulled together and sutured or closed with local skin flaps.

The donor site represents a wound similar to that of a partial-thickness injury. Care of the donor site is as important as care of the graft itself, since donor sites that fail to heal result in an enlargement of the patient's open wound surface. Donor sites may be healed using a variety of open or closed methods. Covering the

TABLE 66-3 Topical Medications and Wound Coverings Used in Burn Therapy—cont'd

Agent	Indication	Implications
Biologic and Biosynthetic Wound Coverings		
Amnion	Partial-thickness burns	Amniotic membrane from human placentas Protects tissues before application of autograft Protective covering changed every 48 hr
Biobrane	Partial-thickness burns Donor sites	Semisynthetic wound covering composed of nylon, Silastic, and porcine collagen membrane that binds to wound fibrin, forming skin substitute, which allows for healing Has pores in membrane that allow dissipation of exudates Applied immediately after burn injury or grafting to donor sites Kept in place until wound is healed, which decreases pain from frequent dressing changes Has no antimicrobial properties
TransCyte	Partial-thickness burns	Polymer membrane and neonatal human fibroblast cells cultured under aseptic conditions in vitro on porcine-coated nylon mesh Secretes human dermal collagen, matrix proteins, and growth factors that promote healing Applied within 24 hr of burn injury or immediately after grafting to donor site Kept in place until wound is healed, which decreases pain from frequent dressing changes
Calcium alginate	Partial-thickness burns	Composed of nonwoven fabric pad of calcium alginate from brown seaweed; calcium alginate ions exchange with sodium ions to form protective, fibrous gel Promotes healing and exudate absorption

TBSA, Total body surface area; *WBC,* white blood cells.

TABLE 66-4 Types of Skin Grafts

Graft	Source	Coverage
Xenograft	Pig skin most commonly used Closes and protects wound while permanent options are being considered	Temporary
Allograft	Cadaver or organ donor tissue Used to cover deep or partial-thickness wounds Enables blood supply to regenerate, but carries some risk for disease transmission	Temporary
Synthetic substitutes	Outer barrier providing protection from infection and dehydration and allowing for tissue regeneration	Temporary
Autograft	Patient's own unburned skin removed and applied to wound	Permanent
Cultured skin	Patient's own skin removed in small squares and grown into larger pieces in laboratory	Permanent
Integra (artificial skin)	Two-layer man-made membrane used to replace dermis and covered with autograft, forming functional dermis and epidermis	Permanent
AlloDerm	Man-made collagen matrix used to provide dermal layer covered with autograft	Permanent

Future Watch

Will Skin Engineering Replace Traditional Methods of Burn Care?

The Department of Orthopedics and Traumatology at Hong Kong University announced that it has successfully produced a skin substitute using cell culture techniques. Skin cells from neonatal rats were cultivated to 500 times their size for the production of compound living skin, consisting of dermis and epidermis. The department announced that this advancement in skin engineering could become an alternative to autografting in the future treatment for severe burns and could provide an unlimited supply of antirejection skin. Production of the skin substitute is still in the stage of laboratory experiments and preclinical studies, which is very expensive; therefore future goals are not only skin engineering but also cost reduction.

Faculty of Medicine: *Skin engineering, the future treatment for burns and wounds*, University of Hong Kong, June 28, 2004, accessed from website: http://www.hku.hk/facmed/healthedu/e-index.html.

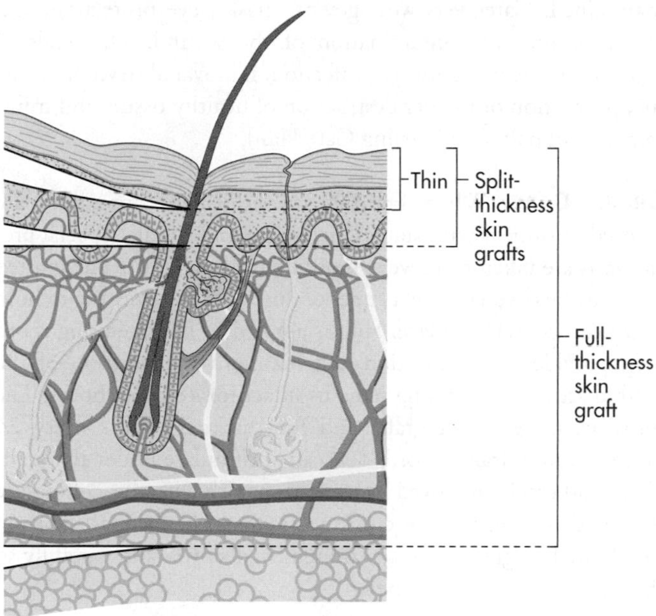

Figure 66-15 Levels of skin involved in thin, split-thickness, and full-thickness skin grafts.

donor site with nonadherent, greasy gauze dressings, such as Xeroform or Adaptic, is a common approach. The gauze can be left open to the air or wrapped with a light dressing and checked for drainage and healing. Hydrophilic foam dressings, such as Allevyn or Mepilex, are also used to protect donor sites. Both the greasy gauze and foam approaches promote moist wound healing. Exposing the donor site to a heat lamp, so the wound dries and forms a protective scab, is not as widespread a practice as in previous years, but is still performed in some units. Other methods include the use of OpSite or Biobrane. These are barrier dressings that absorb exudates while protecting the wound and skin around the wound.

DIET. Metabolism can be increased by two or three times normal after moderate to severe burns because of stress, fluid loss, hypercatabolism, and immobility.[30] Shivering and elevated levels of catecholamines, cortisol, and glucagon present after thermal injury increase oxygen consumption and heat production. They also deplete liver and muscle glycogen and fat deposits, resulting in negative nitrogen balance and weight loss. Protein is broken down to provide amino acids for use in gluconeogenesis rather than being used to build new tissue. Thus wound healing is prolonged and the patient's susceptibility to infection increased.

Burn patients remain catabolic until caloric intake exceeds caloric expenditure. This catabolic state may last for days or months, depending on the severity of the burn. The patient's energy and protein requirements equal those needed for normal homeostasis plus those required to offset the catabolic state and repair the burn injury.

Nutritional support is critical to survival and is initiated on admission. The goals are to establish oral intake as soon as possible and to maintain sufficient caloric and protein intake to restore tissue loss. A nutritional assessment is made during the first days of the burn injury and includes anthropometric measurements (to determine actual weight compared with ideal weight), indirect calorimetry, and laboratory studies (electrolytes, liver function tests, and urine). These data provide a baseline against which progress can be evaluated. Twenty-four-hour urine specimens and urea nitrogen findings may be obtained two or three times a week to evaluate the patient's nitrogen balance. Transferrin or prealbumin levels provide sensitive indicators of visceral protein status.[30] Urinary nitrogen and serum albumin levels can be affected by insensible protein loss and hydration status. Albumin's half-life of 20 days makes day-to-day evaluation of albumin difficult to interpret. On the other hand, prealbumin, which has a short half-life of 20 to 25 hours, provides a sensitive indicator of nutritional status and the patient's response to feeding.

Nutritional requirements for the burn patient are highly variable, depending on the extent and depth of injury and the patient's age, gender, preburn nutritional status, and preexisting diseases. Total caloric needs may be as high as 3500 to 5000 cal/day. Calories are provided to the patient as 20% protein, 50% carbohydrate, and 30% fat. Formulas such as the Curreri formula and variations of the Harris-Benedict equation are commonly used to determine the nutritional needs of burn patients.

Protein is essential to replace nitrogen lost through the wound and in urine and to promote tissue repair and healing. Protein needs in the adult increase from a normal of 0.8 g/kg body weight to 1.5 to 3 g/kg. Protein calories must be dedicated to the wound and not used for energy needs. This is accomplished by providing the patient with sufficient carbohydrate and fat for energy use.

Approximately 5 mg/kg/min of glucose is provided. Excessive carbohydrates can cause increased carbon dioxide production and hyperglycemia. In addition to calories, fat provides fat-soluble vitamins and essential fatty acids. Calories provided by fat are limited to 30% because of the adverse effect of high fat levels on the immune system.[30]

Vitamin and mineral supplements are essential for optimal wound healing. Vitamins C and A, zinc, and iron are provided at doses higher than the recommended daily allowances. Vitamins A and C are cellular antioxidants and required for collagen synthesis. Patients may receive as much as 1000 mg of vitamin C and 5000 to 10,000 IU of vitamin A per day. Zinc levels decrease because of increased nitrogen excretion in the urine during the acute phase. Zinc is essential for wound healing and has a key role in immune function. Patients receive supplementation of up to 220 mg/day.[30] Iron may be supplied to treat anemia caused by blood loss after skin grafting.

Enteral feedings are preferred for burn patients, since patients do not tolerate gastric feedings well during the first few weeks because of paralytic ileus or gastric dilation from shock, stress, or sepsis. Small-bore feeding tubes are inserted into the duodenum or endoscopically into the jejunum so that feedings can be initiated within the first 24 hours of injury. Early feeding decreases hypermetabolism, improves nitrogen balance, minimizes bacterial translocation from the gut secondary to muscle atrophy, and decreases diarrhea and hospital length of stay.[30]

Total parenteral nutrition is generally reserved for patients who are unable to tolerate enteral feedings. Oral feeding is encouraged whenever possible. However, it is often difficult for the patient to consume the number of calories needed from food alone because of pain and decreased gastric motility. Therefore a combination of food by mouth with supplements, such as milk shakes or Ensure, and tube feedings may be necessary to meet the patient's nutritional requirements.

▶ ARE YOU READY?

Which of the following is a side or toxic effect of silver sulfadiazine (Silvadene)?

1. Metabolic acidosis
2. Stains wound black
3. Hyperalbuminemia
4. Decrease in white blood cell count

Nursing Management
of the Patient with Burns during the Acute Phase

ASSESSMENT

History. Assess for:

- Patient and family responses to treatment
- Allergies
- Current medications
- Fears and anxieties

Physical Examination. Assess for:

- Stage of wound healing
- Weight loss or gain
- Confusion, agitation, depression, lucidity
- Lung crackles, wheezing
- Sluggish or absent bowel sounds
- Purulent drainage, abnormal color, foul odor, redness, or swelling of wounds and surrounding skin
- Weakness, lack of motor ability
- Urinary output of less than 30 ml/hr
- Decreased circulation or decreased sensation in extremities
- Excoriated oral mucous membranes

NURSING DIAGNOSES, OUTCOMES, AND INTERVENTIONS

Nursing Diagnosis: Impaired Tissue Integrity

OUTCOMES. Common examples of expected outcomes for the patient with a dignosis of *impaired tissue integrity* are:
Patient will:

- Show signs that skin is being reestablished.
- Show wound healing.
- Have minimal hypertrophic scarring.
- Perform skin care.

NURSING INTERVENTIONS. Healing of the burn wound and return of tissue integrity is the goal of wound care. The nurse monitors the wound during healing to detect any signs of infection and provides wound care one to three times daily. These treatments may include wound cleansing, debridement, and dressing application. The patient is adequately medicated before the procedure to reduce pain and prevent resistance to future treatments because of fear of pain. Strict barrier precautions are maintained. Caregivers wear gowns, masks, eye protection, and gloves to prevent contamination of the wound. The goals of wound care are prevention of infection, removal of devitalized tissue, prevention of further destruction of healthy tissue, and minimization of pain (see Nursing Care Plan).

GRAFT CARE. When grafting is performed, autografts are secured in surgery with staples, dressings, and splints. Special precautions are taken to prevent movement of the graft. The grafted area may be covered with a large, occlusive, bulky dressing to hold new skin securely in place. Splints applied in the operating room help provide immobilization and maintain the position of the grafted areas. The dressing remains intact for 48 to 72 hours. The nurse examines sheet grafts and full-thickness grafts every 24 hours because drainage or blood can accumulate under the graft. This fluid can be removed by aspiration with a needle, rolling the fluid with a cotton tip, or cutting a small slit in the graft to drain the fluid. The graft dressings are removed slowly and carefully so that the graft is not disturbed.

HYDROTHERAPY. Hydrotherapy using a shower, tub, or spray table facilitates the removal of topical medications and loosens debris, sloughing eschar, and exudate. Wound care in a tub permits immersion of the patient into water or antimicrobial solutions. Soaking helps remove topical agents and eschar and facilitates range of motion. Generally, tub therapy is limited to 30-minute intervals to prevent heat loss. Tub therapy is avoided in critically ill patients and those with wound infections, since the infection may be transmitted to other areas of the body through the tub water.

A spray table may be used for patients who have limited mobility, have wound infections, or are in a more critical phase. This method allows the patient to be recumbent while water is provided through the use of temperature-controlled hoses. For patients who are mobile, a regular shower can be used, which helps patients resume activities of daily living (ADLs).

WOUND DEBRIDEMENT. Thorough cleansing and **debridement** of the wound are an important part of wound healing. After removing the gauze dressings, the nurse cleanses the wound with a mild soap or noncytotoxic wound-cleansing agent. Nonadherent exudate or debris is gently removed. In deeper wounds in which eschar, or devitalized tissue, is present, debridement may be required. *Surgical debridement* involves cutting the dead tissue away and is performed in the operating room with the patient under anesthesia. *Enzymatic debridement* involves the use of a topical enzyme that promotes separation of the eschar from the wound bed. During *mechanical debridement*, the nurse removes eschar using gauze sponges, tweezers, scissors, or other instruments. Because this is a painful procedure, patients must be adequately medicated. During this cleansing procedure, the nurse carefully assesses the wound for signs of healing or infection.

DRESSINGS. Temporary wound coverings may be used on burn wounds. Such coverings protect the wound, promote healing, and have varying degrees of antimicrobial action. They may be synthetic, biosynthetic, or biologic (see Table 66-3). The choice of these agents is based on the depth of the wound and the presence or absence of infection. These coverings may be left in place for 1 day or until the wound heals. Depending on the depth and location of the wound, dressings are generally changed once or twice daily (Figure 66-16).

RELATED NIC INTERVENTIONS. Fluid Management, Infection Protection, Skin Care: Donor Site, Skin Care: Graft Site, Skin Surveillance, Wound Care

Nursing Diagnosis: Risk for Infection

OUTCOMES. Common examples of expected outcomes for the patient a diagnosis of *risk for infection* are:

Patient will:

- Remain free from signs and symptoms of infection (erythema, edema at the wound edges, increasing pain, odor, drainage, and decreasing function).
- Maintain a temperature of less than 101.3° F (38.5° C).

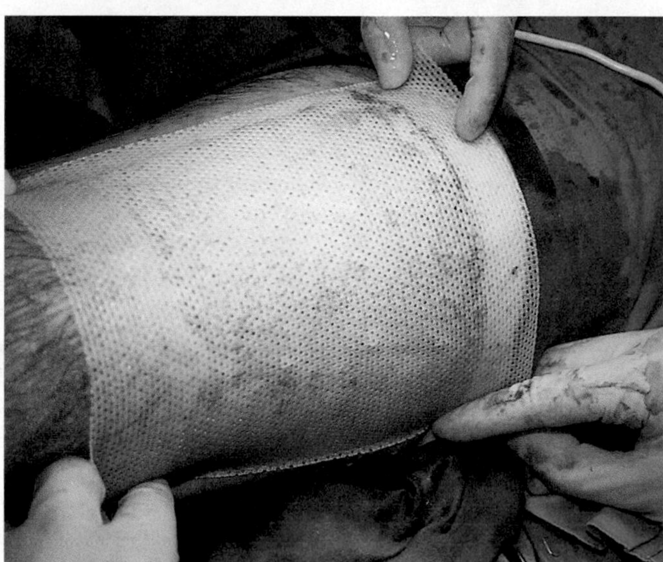

Figure 66-16 Mesh graft to control pain and promote wound healing.

- Maintain intact skin and mucous membranes in unburned areas.
- Maintain WBC count within normal limits.
- Maintain a positive nitrogen balance.

NURSING INTERVENTIONS. The burn patient is at tremendous risk for infection. Measures to prevent infection begin when the patient is admitted to the hospital and continue until healing is complete. To prevent the introduction of exogenous organisms into the wound, strict adherence to protective precautions is essential. Persons with upper respiratory tract infections should not be permitted near the patient. Thorough wound cleansing is necessary to remove the debris that acts as a medium for bacterial growth. Placing the severely burned patient in a special burn unit can decrease the possibility of infection because the unit environment is specifically equipped for infection control. If the patient is cared for in a general hospital unit, a private room is essential, and all equipment needed by the patient remains in the room. Patient mobility is maintained to the extent possible, or the nurse provides frequent turning and encourages deep breathing if the patient is immobile to prevent pneumonia from stasis of lung secretions.

The donor site can also become infected. The nurse should inspect it daily for signs of infection (erythema, purulent drainage, or foul odor). If infection develops, topical antimicrobial creams or solutions or systemic antibiotics may be administered, and the wound may be treated with silver-impregnated dressings (Acticoat or Silverlon).

Infection is commonly the cause of deterioration in the condition of a burn patient. The wound may show color changes from red to violet, dark brown, or black. Tissue necrosis may occur (see Figure 66-11). Sepsis is a serious and sometimes lethal complication of wound infection. Signs of sepsis in the burn patient are change in sensorium, fever, tachypnea, tachycardia, paralytic ileus (decreased tolerance of feedings), abdominal distention, and oliguria. The nurse carefully monitors patients for signs of sepsis so that early treatment can be initiated before serious deterioration occurs.

RELATED NIC INTERVENTIONS. Infection Control, Infection Protection, Nutrition Management, Perineal Care, Skin Surveillance, Wound Care

Nursing Diagnosis: Imbalanced Nutrition: Less Than Body Requirements

OUTCOMES. Common examples of expected outcomes for the patient with a diagnosis of *imbalanced nutrition: less than body requirements* are:

Patient will:

- Maintain present weight; be free from weight loss or experience weight gain to within 0.5 kg of preillness weight.
- Verbalize need to increase caloric and protein intake in the presence of weight loss (when able to do so).
- Maintain fluid hydration.

NURSING INTERVENTIONS. Planning, collaboration, and ingenuity are required to ensure that patients receive adequate nutritional support (see above discussion with treatments). Monitoring the

Nursing Care Plan

Patient With a Burn

Data A 63-year-old man with a history of type 2 diabetes mellitus and peripheral vascular disease was admitted to the hospital for burns to both feet and lower legs. The previous evening, he filled his bathtub at home to soak his feet. Without checking the water temperature, he placed his feet and legs in the tub to soak for approximately 20 minutes. He did not sense the water temperature because of the decreased sensation in his feet and legs. On removing his feet from the tub, he noticed that his legs were bright red. This morning his skin remains bright red and has weeping blisters. After evaluation in the emergency department, he was admitted to the burn center. The patient's wounds were cleansed with water and mild soap. Broken, nonadherent skin was removed, an initial wound culture obtained, and photos taken. The wounds are deep partial-thickness burns with poor capillary refill and estimated at 10% total body surface area (TBSA). They are circumferential from the toes to midcalf bilaterally.

Nursing Diagnosis

Acute pain related to thermal tissue injury

Outcomes

- Patient will report absence of pain or satisfactory control of pain (pain less than 3 on a scale of 0 to 10).

Related NOC Outcomes

- Pain Control
- Pain Level

Related NIC Interventions

- Analgesic Administration
- Pain Management
- Progressive Muscle Relaxation

Nursing Interventions/Rationales

- Assess pain level using a 0 to 10 pain rating scale at least every 4 hours, during wound care, and during physical therapy. *Determining the patient's perception of pain assists with selection of appropriate analgesic agent and dose.*
- Administer analgesia at prescribed intervals around the clock. *Burn pain is constant. Better pain control can be achieved when pain medication is administered on a scheduled basis.*
- Provide analgesia before hydrotherapy and wound care. *Pain increases during wound care and physical therapy. Administering pain medication before the procedure interferes with pain response and allows painful procedures to be performed more readily. Pain control allows for more active participation by patient.*
- Maintain elevation of legs while in bed or chair. *Dependent leg positions increase pain because of venous pooling and edema.*
- Encourage use of nonpharmacologic methods of pain control (imagery, distraction, relaxation). *Increase pain control and comfort when used in adjunct with pharmacologic agents.*

Nursing Diagnosis

Risk for infection related to loss of skin integrity and diabetes mellitus

Outcomes

- Patient will remain free from wound infection.

Related NOC Outcomes

- Immune Status
- Risk Control
- Tissue Integrity: Skin & Mucous Membranes

Related NIC Interventions

- Infection Protection
- Skin Surveillance
- Wound Care

Nursing Interventions/Rationales

- Assess wounds during each dressing change for signs of localized infection. *Infection may be indicated by erythema at the wound edges; pale, mottled, dry appearance of the wound; and purulent, foul-smelling drainage. The presence of wound infection affects the type of topical agent selected. Untreated localized infection can spread via the blood and lymphatics, producing systemic infection.*

patient's nutritional status is an ongoing process. The nurse monitors weight loss and gain daily during the critical phase and biweekly as the wounds heal. Initially, weight gain occurs because of fluid retention. As diuresis occurs, the patient's weight decreases as a result of fluid loss. Significant weight loss reflects loss of protein, fat reserves, and muscle mass. The nurse monitors prealbumin, urine urea nitrogen balance, and cholesterol levels.

An oral diet is encouraged whenever possible. The nurse determines the patient's food preferences and encourages the family to bring favorite foods from home. Care is coordinated so that mealtimes are relaxed and not associated with other procedures, such as wound care. A social situation can be created by having burn patients eat together or with family members. Pain medication is provided so that the patient is comfortable. Coordination with occupational therapy staff is essential if the patient needs assistive devices to hold utensils and cups.

Patients who are unable to consume sufficient calories orally require tube feedings. Continuous feedings are provided when nutritional requirements are high. As the patient begins to eat orally, tube feedings may be provided overnight, allowing the patient to eat during the day while still providing for caloric needs. Calorie counts are essential to monitor the patient's progress.

The nurse monitors the patient's tolerance of feedings by evaluating bowel function. Diarrhea may be a problem initially for patients receiving antibiotics or tube feedings. Commonly, however, burn patients have difficulties with constipation as a result of administration of opioids and decreased activity. Stool softeners, laxatives, and increased fluid intake may be provided.

RELATED NIC INTERVENTIONS. Nutrition Management, Nutrition Therapy, Nutritional Monitoring, Weight Management

Nursing Diagnosis: Acute Pain

OUTCOMES. Common examples of expected outcomes for the patient with a diagnosis of *acute pain* are:

- Monitor for signs and symptoms of systemic infection (temperature elevation, altered sensorium, and elevated white blood cell count). *Early detection of infection allows for the appropriate selection of systemic or topical antimicrobial agents.*
- Obtain a wound sample for culture twice weekly, or as prescribed. *Tracking bacterial colonization of the wound allows for early detection of pathogens so that the most appropriate treatment can be initiated.*
- Maintain aseptic wound technique and thorough cleansing of equipment and hydrotherapy tubs and tables. *To prevent cross-contamination of bacteria between patients that may cause infection to the individual with skin loss.*

Nursing Diagnosis

Risk for ineffective therapeutic regimen management related to lack of knowledge of burn process, treatment regimen, and signs and symptoms of complications

Outcomes

- Patient will verbalize understanding of and follow a plan for maintaining therapeutic regimen.

Related NOC Outcomes

- Adherence Behavior
- Knowledge: Treatment Regimen
- Participation in Health Care Decisions

Related NIC Interventions

- Learning Facilitation
- Self-Modification Assistance
- Teaching: Prescribed Procedure/Treatment

Nursing Interventions/Rationales

- Assess patient's physical and cognitive ability to perform wound care. *Patient's ability to perform wound care helps determine discharge needs, that is, home health care versus self-care or care by family caregiver.*
- Instruct patient to apply lotion to affected skin areas two or three times each day. *Lotion helps maintain moisture of newly healed tissue and prevents tissue breakdown. Newly healed skin is prone to itching, flaking, and dryness.*
- Encourage patient to wear socks and well-fitted shoes. *Tight shoes predispose healed areas of the feet to tissue breakdown. This is especially important for patients with diabetes who have decreased sensation in their feet.*
- Avoid exposure of healed wounds to chemicals or extremes in temperature. *Tissue is fragile initially and will easily reinjure.*
- Provide patient with a bath thermometer to assess the temperature of water before bathing. *Decreased sensation of the feet from diabetic neuropathy limits ability to determine temperature of the water. Water temperature should be 100° to 105° F (37.7° to 40.5° C).*
- Stress the importance of maintaining blood glucose levels within normal range. *Poorly controlled diabetes mellitus contributes to diabetic neuropathy and infection and impairs healing.*
- Refer patient to community resources as appropriate. *Patient may need assistance with controlling diabetes or changing life-style habits to prevent future injuries.*

Evaluation

Evaluation is based on comparing the patient's outcomes with desired outcomes.

Patient will:

- Report the need for pain interventions before pain becomes severe.
- Report pain as 3 or less on a scale of 0 (no pain) to 10 (maximal pain) with use of comfort measures.
- Experience periods of rest or sleep after pain interventions.
- Report increasingly longer periods of pain control as healing occurs.

NURSING INTERVENTIONS. Pain management is a major part of the burn patient's care (see above discussion of pain with emergent care). Uncontrolled pain affects all aspects of recovery, including tolerance of wound care, ability to eat, mobility, wound healing, and psychologic adjustment. Acute pain is most successfully managed with narcotics. The methods and routes of administration are carefully evaluated on an individual basis. During dressing changes, parenteral narcotics are given to achieve rapid onset of action. The use of agents such as ketamine, fentanyl, and self-administered nitrous oxide may be beneficial for some patients. The Guidelines for Safe Practice box, p. 1936, outlines nursing interventions during dressing change.

Planning for patient relief from pain, itching, or general discomfort involves an around-the-clock approach to pain management. Undermedication may occur if the patient fears becoming addicted and fails to report pain or if the nurse fails to adequately evaluate the degree of pain. The use of a numeric analog scale for the patient to rate the pain helps determine whether the pain is being adequately controlled. Providing medication at frequent intervals helps maintain ongoing comfort. Time-released opioids and patient-controlled analgesia are also viable options.

As grafted areas close and donor sites and wounds heal, the need for pain medication decreases and patients are switched to oral narcotics. Pain medication administration does, however, continue throughout the day. It is often beneficial to the patient to take pain medication before physical and occupational therapy. Therapy may be painful for the patient, but it should never be

Guidelines for Safe Practice
Minimizing Pain During Dressing Changes

- Administer analgesic at least a half hour before dressing changes.
- Secure patient's cooperation by providing clear explanation of dressing change procedure and expectations of patient.
- Handle burned areas gently.
- Use strict sterile technique to prevent infections, which increase pain.
- Encourage patient participation in procedure whenever possible.
- Use distraction (music, conversation) and encourage relaxation during procedure.
- Provide honest praise as appropriate.

avoided, since it is essential for recovery. Relaxation therapy, distraction, and imagery can supplement pain medication.

Physiologic pain may be induced or aggravated by loneliness and depression. The patient's complaint of pain may be an indication of unmet emotional needs that can be addressed with the use of presence, touch, music therapy, or diversional activities. Anxiety about anticipated procedures and sleep deprivation may increase the amount of pain the patient experiences. Patients experiencing posttraumatic stress disorder (PTSD) report higher levels of pain.[6] Interventions include the use of antianxiety medication and nonpharmacologic methods such as music therapy, meditation, or relaxation exercises.

Related NIC Interventions. Analgesic Administration, Anxiety Reduction, Environmental Management: Comfort, Medication Management, Pain Management

Nursing Diagnosis: Impaired Physical Mobility

Outcomes. Common examples of expected outcomes for the patient with a diagnosis of *impaired physical mobility* are:
Patient will:

- Maintain full range of motion.
- Request assistance as needed.
- Demonstrate progression toward independence in performance of ADLs.

Nursing Interventions. As their wounds heal and pain is controlled, the nurse encourages patients to perform range-of-motion exercises on a regular schedule. Assistance and support are provided as needed, with the goal being independent performance by the patient. The nurse teaches the patient and family the importance of range-of-motion exercises in preventing or minimizing contractures. Physical and occupational therapists are also involved in helping the patient attain and maintain good range.

Physical and occupational therapy is necessary for burn patients and begins on admission. Patients are encouraged to move about, walk, and participate in their own care as much as possible. Independence in ADLs is supported. Some patients require more encouragement than others to assist with tasks such as wound care. To promote a sense of self-control, it is important that patients be involved in developing their daily care plan, including meal selection, time of treatments, rest periods, therapy, and socialization.

Patients with major burns or those who require mechanical ventilation may only tolerate bed rest and range-of-motion exercises. As soon as hemodynamic and pulmonary stability is achieved, patients may sit in a chair and then walk. Patient activities progress as their condition improves and their risk for injury from ambulation or other activities decreases.

Related NIC Interventions. Exercise Promotion, Exercise Therapy: Ambulation, Exercise Therapy: Balance, Exercise Therapy: Joint Mobility, Teaching: Prescribed Activity/Exercise

Nursing Diagnosis: Risk for Deficient Fluid Volume

Outcomes. Common examples of expected outcomes for the patient with a diagnosis of *risk for deficient fluid volume* are:
Patient will:

- Verbalize understanding of need to maintain adequate fluid intake.
- Achieve normal fluid volume.
- Maintain urinary output of 30 to 50 ml/hr (0.5 ml/kg body weight/hr) in adults or 1 to 2 ml/kg/hr in children.
- Maintain electrolyte and acid-base values within normal limits.
- Maintain normal sensorium.
- Maintain systolic blood pressure of greater than 100 mm Hg and heart rate of less than 120 beats/min.

Nursing Interventions. Maintaining fluid balance continues to be an objective when caring for the patient during the acute phase of burn care. To assess for fluid volume deficit, the nurse weighs the patient daily at the same time, on the same scale, and in the same amount of clothing. The nurse keeps a careful record of the weights, intake, and output so that fluid intake can be adjusted as needed. Electrolytes are monitored by frequent blood chemistry analyses. The nurse offers fluids on a regular basis.

The nurse teaches patients the importance of maintaining fluid and electrolyte balance after discharge and to notify their health care provider immediately if they experience weight loss accompanied by headache, lightheadedness, fatigue, decreased urinary output, irritability, or rapid pulse, which are signs of fluid deficit; or an increase in fatigue, abdominal distention, anorexia, vomiting, constipation, muscle cramps, paresthesia, or confusion, which are signs of electrolyte imbalance. They are also encouraged to eat a well-balanced diet with sufficient fluid intake.

Related NIC Interventions. Electrolyte Management, Electrolyte Monitoring, Fluid Management, Fluid Monitoring, Nutrition Management

Nursing Diagnosis: Ineffective Coping

Outcomes. Common examples of expected outcomes for the patient with a diagnosis of *ineffective coping* are:
Patient will:

- Exhibit functional coping mechanisms.
- Express fears and concerns.
- Participate in wound care and treatment plan.

NURSING INTERVENTIONS. A burn injury is a sudden, unexpected event. Its impact on psychologic well-being is enormous, and promoting mental health is a major component of the burn patient's care. The psychologic responses in the emergent phase are related to the threat to survival. During the acute phase a variety of behaviors may be seen (Table 66-5). As the patient becomes aware of the extent of the injury and begins to evaluate its implications, many problems may affect both the patient's and the family's ability to cope with the situation. Pain may also play a significant role in the patient's coping ability. Controlling pain assists in decreasing anxiety and enhances the patient's coping skills.

Ongoing education is imperative to assist the patient in understanding the care given and making realistic plans for the future. It is important for the patient to maintain a sense of hope so that he or she can resume a normal life. Without hope, the patient has a reduced ability to cope, a sense of failure, and less gratifying interpersonal relationships.

Emotional recovery from a burn injury is slower than physical recovery. Many patients exhibit symptoms of psychologic distress up to 1 year later. These symptoms include intrusive and distressing memories of the burn injury and avoidance of thoughts and feelings related to the burn.[7] In addition, patients may have increased irritability, anxiety, and sleep disturbances.

Those individuals who adjust well after a burn injury have characteristics in common. Those who had positive experiences before the injury are better able to deal with the consequences of the burn itself. They generally have family and other social supports available to them. They can engage others in their care and are able to revise their self-image in a realistic and positive manner.

Burn-injured persons are at risk for the development of PTSD. PTSD is associated with symptoms that occur after a psychologically traumatic event that is considered outside the range of normal human experience. Symptoms of PTSD include reexperiencing the trauma in dreams or intrusive recollections; a numbed response to the environment, such as decreased interest or detachment; an exaggerated startle response; sleep disturbances; guilt about having survived the event, especially if others did not; and avoidance of activities that arouse recollections of the event.

The size and severity of the burn and the degree of disfigurement do not consistently predict which patients will develop PTSD. Patients are more likely to develop PTSD if they have an actual or perceived lack of social support, have maladaptive coping styles, and are in emotional distress. Patients may be nonsymptomatic during hospitalization but develop PTSD after discharge. Therefore ongoing psychologic evaluation and intervention are necessary during hospitalization and the months that follow.[6,7]

TABLE 66-5 PSYCHOLOGIC REACTIONS TO SEVERE BURNS

Reaction	Definition	Behavior Exhibited	Nursing Approach
Conservation, withdrawal	Decreased interaction with environment as immediate response to serious injury Occurs immediately after injury and may last for 1-2 wk Protective value to self (may be mistaken for depression)	Decreased interaction with environment, staff, family Often keeps eyes closed, sleeps, remains immobile	Avoid forcing patient to deal with situation. Provide supportive environment. Provide ongoing information on status and care.
Denial	Protective, unconscious defense mechanism Helps relieve anxiety caused by threat to life, limb, self	Denies extent of injury, loss of limb, loss of others in accident May acknowledge loss but not impact	Support patient. Avoid forcing patient to deal with fears. Answer questions honestly. Provide information in small doses over time.
Regression	Return to earlier ways of coping with stress May exhibit childlike behaviors	Assertive, demanding, temper tantrums Tearful, clinging to dependent relationships	Avoid attacking and responding negatively to behavior exhibited. Acknowledge patient's difficulty in coping. Encourage and reward positive behaviors and independence.
Depression	Extent of injury becomes distorted and affects patient's sense of worthiness and self-esteem	Degrading comments about self Sleep disturbances, decreased appetite, generalized slowing, poor motivation	Acknowledge loss. Focus patient on realistic expectations.
Anxiety	Fear and threat to self as result of injury	Restlessness, agitation, difficulty in following instructions, poor memory, easily startled	Support patient. Acknowledge fears. Provide information in small, frequent doses.

The nurse assesses the patient's and family's coping style. Some patients were raised to be stoic when in pain or distress, whereas others freely express their feelings. The nurse supports the patient's coping style unless the patient indicates a willingness to explore new methods of coping. Patients generally cope best when they are kept fully informed about planned care and what is expected of them during various treatments. Coping with unexpected events can be upsetting, especially when patients have to give up most of their independence.

Families, too, cope best when they are kept fully informed and have a realistic understanding of what lies ahead for the patient. The family can be deeply disrupted by a serious burn to a family member. Initially the family is concerned about the patient's survival. The nurse explains what is being done for the patient and why, counsels the family about possible angry outbreaks from patients who are grieving or frustrated, and encourages them to not take such outbreaks personally.[7] Explanations may need to be repeated more than once because family members may be too distressed to comprehend.

Social workers are helpful in exploring the family's concerns about role disruptions, plans for child care, financial concerns, and distress. Often family members require considerable support from health care professionals to work through their own feelings before they can support the patient. They also need information about community resources available to them and the patient.

RELATED NIC INTERVENTIONS. Anxiety Reduction, Coping Enhancement, Distraction, Presence, Sleep Enhancement

Nursing Diagnosis: Disturbed Body Image

OUTCOMES. Common examples of expected outcomes for the patient with a diagnosis of *disturbed body image* are:

Patient will:

- Develop a realistic body image.
- Look at and touch burned areas.
- Verbalize feelings about change in appearance and grieve for former self.
- Verbalize ways appearance can be improved (e.g., makeup).
- Change dressing independently or with assistance of significant other.
- Maintain hygiene and grooming.

NURSING INTERVENTIONS. A burn wound, especially when large, presents a serious challenge to the patient's body image. As their conditions improve, patients may express a desire to view the burned area. The nurse assesses the patient's readiness to view the burned area and plans to have a burn team member present during the viewing. If the patient desires, a family member or another support person may be present.

The nurse encourages patients to express their feelings about their changes in appearance. Individual counseling may be necessary for some patients as they integrate body changes into their self-concept. Other patients benefit from support groups where they can meet other patients in various stages of recovery. The group may be led by a nurse, social worker, psychologist, or other health care professional experienced in working with burn patients. Integration of body changes into one's body image takes time. Staff and family members must show patience and understanding toward patients who are struggling to accept bodily changes.

RELATED NIC INTERVENTIONS. Body Image Enhancement, Coping Enhancement, Counseling, Self-Esteem Enhancement, Support System Enhancement

EVALUATION

To evaluate the effectiveness of nursing interventions, compare patient behaviors with those stated in the expected patient outcomes.

RELATED NOC OUTCOMES. Acceptance: Health Status, Activity Tolerance, Body Image, Comfort Level, Coping, Family Coping, Hope, Nutritional Status: Food & Fluid Intake, Role Performance, Self-Care: Hygiene

GERONTOLOGIC CONSIDERATIONS

Older adults experience many of the same problems as younger adults with burns. However, older adults are more likely to have underlying chronic conditions that may complicate their recovery, such as diabetes, renal compromise, or cardiac conditions. They are slower to heal and at increased risk for complications such as infection. Older adults are also at higher risk for undermedication for pain control than younger adults.[10] Gerontologic considerations are summarized in Box 66-8.

Reintegration and Rehabilitation

Reintegration occurs during the last few days of hospitalization before patients are discharged home. The goal of care at this time is to help patients reintegrate themselves into home life. Many emotions surface during this period such as anxiety over loss of a safe environment (the hospital), fear of rejection or ridicule, and concerns about ability to engage in former activities. Families may be concerned about their ability to provide adequate care and support to the patient or provide protection from ridicule.

Care during this phase involves counseling the patient and family about difficulties they may encounter after discharge such as difficulties with performing ADLs, chronic pain, sleep disturbances, PTSD symptoms, irritability, or fear of resuming sexual activities. The nurse addresses potential issues openly rather than reassuring the patient and family that problems will not arise. Problem solving can be rehearsed so that if problems arise, the patient can handle them with greater confidence and skill.[7]

By the end of their hospitalization, patients are expected to resume most of their own care to the degree possible. This allows staff and patients to identify potential problems with physical care or wound management so that those problems can be addressed before discharge. Another important rehearsal is for the patient to experience reactions from others while still in a safe environment. Patients may benefit from short visits away from the hospital. When they return, they can verbalize their feelings, discuss problems, and work out solutions, while receiving reassurance and encouragement from staff members. Some communities have adult and pediatric reentry programs that prepare extended family members, church members, and employers or classmates for the patient's return. Such programs provide education about the

Box 66-8 Gerontologic Considerations in Burn Care

Epidemiology

The incidence of burn injury in the home is disproportionately higher for older adults than for young adults.
One third of deaths from home fires are among older adults.
The majority of burn injuries are from flames.
Inhalation injury occurs more frequently than in younger adults because of an inability to escape fire.
Factors that place older adults at increased risk for burn injury are:
—Thin skin that is less resistant to heat
—Decreased reaction time and mobility
—Visual or hearing deficits that decrease ability to evaluate danger
—Living in older homes with faulty wiring, risky heating systems, and no smoke detectors

Age-Related Changes That Affect Burn Recovery

Overall diminishment of organ system capacity reserves
—Increased incidence of complications
Decreased capacity to withstand cardiovascular insult
—Decreased cardiac output
—Coronary artherosclerosis
—Decreased baroreceptor response to fluid volume changes
Decreased capacity to withstand pulmonary insult
—Decreased thoracic cage elasticity
—Decreased number and efficiency of alveoli
—Increased risk for hypoxia, hypoventilation, atelectasis
Decreased immune capacity
—Diminished host resistance
—Slowed cell- and humoral-mediated immunity
—Increased risk for infection, sepsis
Decreased wound healing
—Diminished inflammatory response
—Increased healing time
—Decreased tolerance of wound excision and grafting

physical and emotional aspects of burn injury and emphasize burn survivors' strengths and abilities.[7]

Rehabilitation of the patient actually begins during early hospitalization once survival has been ensured, and is addressed throughout the hospital stay. However, rehabilitation as a stage of treatment begins when the patient's burn is reduced to less than 20% of the TBSA, the patient is capable of assuming some self-care activity, and the patient is discharged from the hospital. Management involves returning the patient to a productive place in society. The areas of concern during this phase are restoring function over scarred joint surfaces, social and role functioning, and emotional assistance for the patient and family.

After the wounds are healed, the long recuperative process begins, accompanied by the realization of endless implications for the future. Burns on the face make adjustment particularly difficult. Common fears include fear of death, pain, disfigurement, prolonged hospitalization, loss of job security, disruption of lifestyle, and the reaction of family and friends.

Rehabilitation may continue for 2 to 5 years or longer after discharge to reach the maximal level. The patient may require counseling and many readmissions for reconstructive procedures. Emotional and social healing depends on the patient's ability to cope with a new body image and society's acceptance of the patient's physical appearance. Studies indicate that the majority of patients do adjust well and eventually resume active physical and social lives. The first 1 to 2 years of rehabilitation pose the most problems during the transition back to normalcy.[7]

Collaborative Care Management

DIAGNOSTIC TESTS. Specific diagnostic testing during the rehabilitation phase depends on the patient's condition and progress toward goals. Overall, limited testing is required. Evaluation of nutritional status (prealbumin and urine urea nitrogen measurements) and monitoring for infection (complete blood counts and wound and blood cultures) may be necessary.

MEDICATIONS. The number of medications prescribed decreases as the patient progresses through the rehabilitation phase. As wounds heal, less analgesia is required, and antimicrobial agents are prescribed only for documented infections.

TREATMENTS. As burn wounds continue to heal, only minimal wound care is necessary. This may be performed by the patient in the home or in an outpatient clinic. When reconstructive procedures are performed, more extensive wound care is necessary.

SURGICAL MANAGEMENT. Initial skin grafting is completed during the acute phase; during the rehabilitation phase the patient may require reconstructive surgery to improve function and plastic surgery to re-form ears, noses, or eyelids. Scar tissue and contractures commonly occur 1 to 2 years after the burn and may require additional skin grafting or corrective surgery.

DIET. Nutritional requirements decrease as healing occurs and vitamin supplements are no longer necessary for persons without other underlying conditions. A well-balanced diet with adequate fluid intake is encouraged.

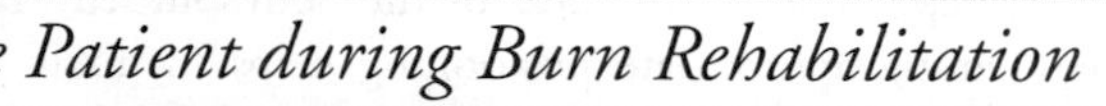

Nursing Management *of the Patient during Burn Rehabilitation*

ASSESSMENT

Health History. Assess for:
- Pain or pressure related to splints or improper positioning
- Length of time since initial injury
- Skin grafts or corrective surgeries
- Changes in eating or sleep patterns
- Degree of patient ability to participate in own care
- Family's feelings regarding patient's appearance and deformities
- Patient's understanding of physical limitations and abilities and care plan

Physical Examination. Assess for:
- Alterations in range of motion
- Scars from healing and resultant deformity
- Response to positioning, splinting, exercise
- Cyanosis or cool temperature of affected limb

- Emotional alterations (depression, withdrawn behaviors, suicidal ideation)
- Negative statements about appearance, self-worth
- Fever or localized infection of wounds

Nursing Diagnoses, Outcomes, and Interventions

Nursing Diagnosis: Impaired Physical Mobility

Outcomes. Common examples of expected outcomes for the patient with a diagnosis of *impaired physical mobility* are:

Patient will:

- Achieve full range of motion and physical activity consistent with desired levels.
- Perform ADLs with minimal or no assistance.
- Use adaptive devices correctly to facilitate activities.
- Express satisfaction with own ability to dress and groom self.

Nursing Interventions. As the survival rate of patients with larger and deeper burns increases, so does the challenge of achieving optimal functional and cosmetic results. Joint limitations increase in accordance with the degree and extent of burn. Although patients may be critically ill, their rehabilitation needs must be addressed immediately. A comprehensive program of positioning, splinting, exercise, ambulation, and ADLs begins on the first or second day after the burn and is carried through until after discharge to maximize physical function. Any delays in initiating treatment are detrimental to the patient's ultimate functional outcome.

Contractures are among the most serious long-term complications of burns. They result from muscle and joint stiffening, skin grafting, and prolonged bed rest. Although occupational and physical therapists are primarily responsible for addressing the patient's rehabilitation needs during all phases of recovery, the nurse is responsible for ensuring their recommendations are followed.

Therapeutic Positioning. Placing body parts in antideformity positions is vital to the prevention of burn contractures. The nurse repositions patients in bed (side-lying, supine, or prone position) frequently and regularly around the clock. Correct positioning varies, depending on the area of the body burned (Table 66-6). Maintaining appropriate positioning helps maintain extremities and joints in the position of normal function and decreases the risk for contractures (Figure 66-17). Beds with pressure-reducing capability or low air loss may be necessary to limit skin pressure.

Prolonged rest in a semi-Fowler's position or with pillows pushing the head forward is avoided, even though many patients like this position because it enables them to see about the room better. The bed can be turned so that the patient can look about without having to assume positions that may lead to the formation of contractures. The bedside table may be moved from one side of the bed to the other at intervals to stimulate other body positions.

Table 66-6 Therapeutic Positioning for the Burn

Area Burned	Description of Position
Neck	No pillow Towel roll under cervical spine Neck splint
Shoulder	90-degree abduction, neutral rotation Elbow splint to aid in maintaining position
Axilla	Abduction with 10- to 15-degree forward flexion and external rotation Support for abducted arm with suspension from intravenous pole or bedside table Axilla splint
Elbow	Extension Support for extended arm on bedside table, foam trough Elbow splint
Hand	Hand splint
Dorsal surface	Flexion
Palmar surface	Hyperextension
Hip	Extension with neutral rotation Supine with lower extremity extended Prone position (if medically appropriate) Trochanter roll Foam wedge along lateral aspect of thigh Knee or long leg splint
Knee	Extension Prone position (if medically appropriate) Patient out of bed with lower extremities extended and elevated Knee splint
Ankle	Dorsiflexion Padded footboard with heels free of pressure Ankle splint

Splints. Splints prevent or correct contractures and immobilize joints after grafting. They are custom-made devices that are often molded directly on the patient to ensure optimal conformity (Figure 66-18). The splints must be properly applied and used according to an established schedule. An improperly applied splint can promote contractures and lead to additional complications. The nurse assesses the splinted limb frequently for signs of adequate circulation, cyanosis, temperature, and pulses. Complaints of pain and pressure are assessed, since damage can occur from improperly applied splints. Some practitioners prefer the open method of treatment and use frequent exercise instead of splinting to prevent contractures.

Exercises and Ambulation. Exercises for prevention and correction of contractures begin as soon as the patient is stable and continue throughout the rehabilitation phase of recovery. Active exercises are preferred, although exercises performed with active assistance and the use of gentle pressure may be more realistic initially. Exercises are often performed more easily in water and may be done concurrently with dressing changes if the patient is able to tolerate the activity. Continuous passive pressure motion devices may be used to prevent contractures of affected joints.

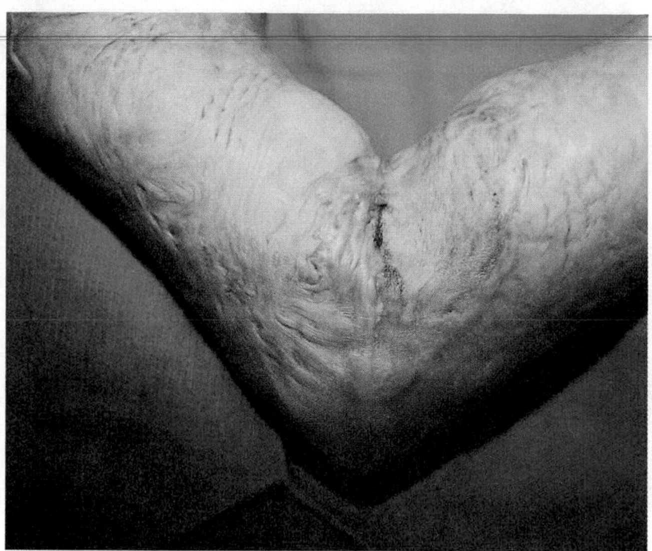

Figure 66-17 Burn contracture keeping elbow in flexed position for comfort.

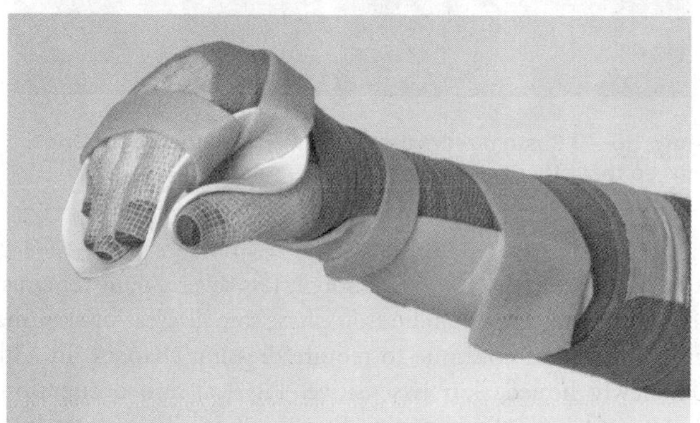

Figure 66-18 Hand splint to maintain functional position.

When burns are completely covered (by healing or by graft), exercises may be performed in an occupational therapy or physical therapy department, where the patient may benefit from a change in environment.

Ambulation decreases the risk of thromboemboli and renal calculi, promotes optimal ventilation, helps maintain range of motion and strength in the lower extremities, orients the patient to the environment, and provides a sense of functional independence. Patients with large burns have less ability to tolerate activity and require a progressive approach to mobilization. Initially the patient may need to be transferred with maximal assistance onto a stretcher chair and progressed to a sitting position. Gradually the patient may progress to a standing pivot transfer into a nearby chair and eventually walk with minimal assistance. Before getting out of bed, the patient must have an elastic bandage support applied to the lower extremities to prevent venous stasis, edema, and orthostatic hypotension.

One of the ultimate goals of rehabilitation is the maintenance or restoration of the patient's independence in performing ADLs. The occupational therapist aids in this process by selecting activities appropriate to the patient's medical, physical, and mental status. The nurse can encourage self-feeding, telephoning, reading mail, and assisting with grooming or burn wound management. The nurse reinforces what is taught by the physical and occupational therapists so that the patient can continue to progress on the nursing unit, in the clinic, or in the home.

RELATED NIC INTERVENTIONS. Exercise Therapy: Ambulation, Exercise Therapy: Joint Mobility, Positioning, Self-Care Assistance

Nursing Diagnosis: Disturbed Body Image

OUTCOMES. Common examples of expected outcomes for the patient with a diagnosis of *disturbed body image* are:
Patient will:

- Speak freely about change in appearance.
- Participate in activities with family and friends.
- Maintain personal grooming to the extent possible.
- Openly verbalize grief related to the loss of former appearance.

NURSING INTERVENTIONS. Regardless of its size, a burn injury represents a change in the individual's perception of self. As burns heal, patients must deal with a new appearance. The nurse provides opportunities for them to talk about their concerns or fears. Some may be unable to discuss their fears with family members or significant others. The nurse listens actively and provides emotional support as patients deal with and eventually accept changes in their appearance. Patients must be allowed to grieve for the loss of their former selves. However, they should also be encouraged to focus on the positive aspects of self.

For adolescents, the thought of being different or conspicuous may be unbearable. Patients exhibit their readiness to view injuries when they begin to ask questions about their appearance or ask to look in the mirror. If possible, they should be prepared for the experience before seeing facial burns. Patients will need support and understanding as they cope with their image. Interaction with other burn patients who are further along in the healing process may help them believe that recovery is possible. In some cases the recovery is good, and although differences in skin pigmentation remain, the redness that accompanies healed burn wounds often fades considerably within a few months. Pigmentation problems are more acute for persons with brown or black skin. Their healed skin may be a different shade, freckled, or whitish. Cosmetic camouflage products that help blend skin tones are available and may help burned patients feel more confident about their appearance.

RELATED NIC INTERVENTIONS. Active Listening, Body Image Enhancement, Coping Enhancement, Emotional Support, Grief Work Facilitation, Self-Esteem Enhancement

Nursing Diagnosis: Impaired Skin Integrity

OUTCOMES. Common examples of expected outcomes for the patient with a diagnosis of *impaired skin integrity* are:
Patient will:

- Maintain intact skin.
- Remain free from infection.
- Identify techniques to prevent breakdown of healed areas (e.g., protection from sun and exposure to harsh chemicals,

use of lubricating lotions, and proper use of pressure garments).

NURSING INTERVENTIONS. Whenever a connective tissue wound heals, hypertrophic scarring occurs unless the skin adheres to the underlying structure. Hypertrophic scarring results from the overgrowth and overproduction of tissue. This predominantly occurs in areas of stress and movement, such as the hands, legs, and chest (Figure 66-19). The thickened, rigid scar that results may later cause contractures. The application of controlled, constant pressure to the surface of an immature scar reduces the scar and leaves a smooth, pliable tissue. If this pressure is applied to new, healthy tissue, hypertrophic scarring is decreased. The pressure garment, a specially designed elastic woven material, provides tridimensional control. The custom-made garment is fitted to each patient individually. Until the garment is completed, bandages can be used for a pressure dressing (Figure 66-20).

Even though pressure garments help decrease the formation of thick, disfiguring scars, patient acceptance may be an ongoing challenge. The garments are uncomfortable and make the patient warm, especially during hot weather. They must be tight enough to produce the 24 mm Hg of pressure required to exceed capillary pressure to be effective in reducing edema and scar formation. The patient must wear the garment 23 hours a day for 6 months to a year. Encouraging patients to focus on the future and benefits of such garments may help them cope with the discomfort.

RELATED NIC INTERVENTIONS. Exercise Promotion, Skin Surveillance, Wound Care

Nursing Diagnosis: Chronic Pain

OUTCOMES. Common examples of expected outcomes for the patient with a diagnosis of *chronic pain* are:

Patient will:

- Describe strategies that reduce or eliminate pain (distraction, relaxation, exercise, medication).
- Report pain as 2 or less on a scale of 0 (no pain) to 10 (maximal pain) with use of pain control measures.

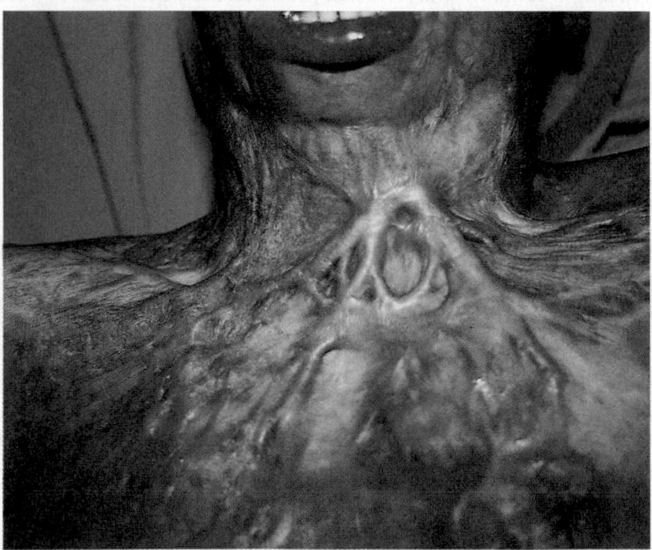

Figure 66-19 Hypertrophic scarring to chest and neck.

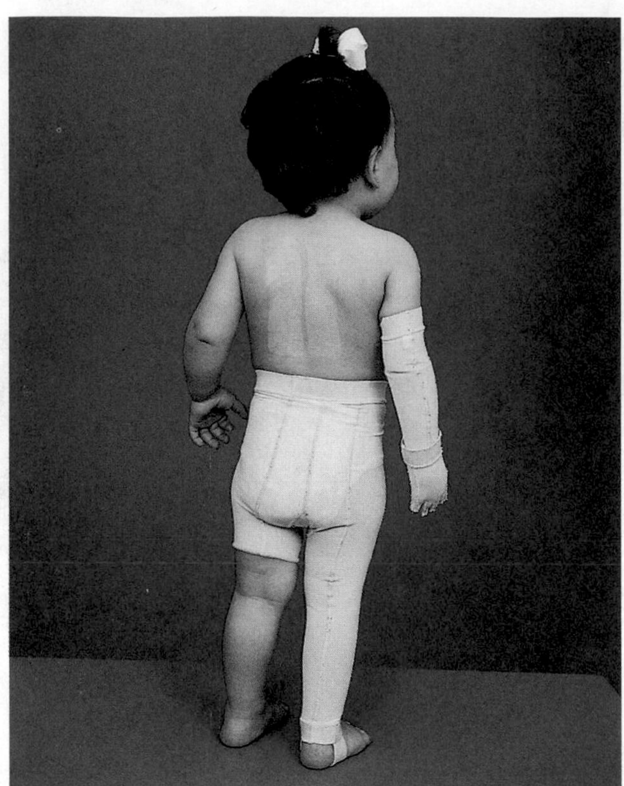

Figure 66-20 Customized pressure garment tailored to patient's needs so that other areas can be left uncovered.

NURSING INTERVENTIONS. Although less severe, pain remains a problem during the rehabilitation phase. Small areas of skin may remain open and continue to require dressing changes. In addition, newly healed skin is sensitive. Physical and occupational therapy and increasing activity may result in discomfort. Interventions focus on administration of analgesics, diversional activities, relaxation techniques, and provision of information about what the patient can expect. Daily hydrotherapy helps the patient relax tense muscles.

Itching is another problem that is estimated to cause discomfort in up to 80% of burn patients. Although it can last from months to years, is most commonly occurs in burns that require several weeks to heal. Itching is thought to be due to chronic inflammation and release of histamine from mast cells or overly sensitive sensory nerves in the area of injury. Chronic itching is treated with oral histamines, sedatives, and skin moisturizers.[14]

Research

Demling RH, DeSanti L: Topic doxepin significantly decreases itching and erythema in the chronically pruritic burn scar, *Wounds* 15(6):195-200, 2003.

This study compared the ability of the tricyclic compound doxepin cream with oral antihistamines for control of postburn itch lasting more than 4 months. After a 3-month period, 75% of patients using topical doxepin experienced a cessation of itching compared with 20% of patients using oral antihistamines. The researchers concluded that 5% doxepin cream significantly reduced chronic erythema and itching in healed burn wounds and was therefore superior to treatment with oral histamines.

Studies are ongoing to determine better treatment methods for chronic itching (see Research box).

RELATED NIC INTERVENTIONS. Analgesic Administration, Exercise Promotion: Stretching, Exercise Therapy: Joint Mobility, Pain Management, Simple Relaxation Therapy

Nursing Diagnosis: Ineffective Coping

OUTCOMES. Common examples of expected outcomes for the patient (and family) with a diagnosis of *ineffective coping* are: Patient (and family) will:

- Report satisfactory management of patient and family problems.

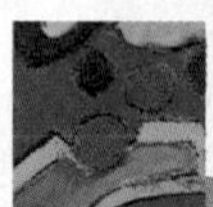

PATIENT/FAMILY TEACHING *Discharge Instructions for the Patient With a Burn*

If any of the following occurs, please call the hospital and ask for the Burn Clinic. The nurse will be able to assist you.

- Healed area breaking open (Cover with a clean dressing.)
- Formation of blisters
- Signs of infection:
  —Fever, temperature higher than 100.4° F (38° C)
  —Redness, pain, swelling, hardness, or warmth in or around the wound or any other part of the body
  —Increased or foul-smelling drainage from the wound
- Problems with your elastic bandages or Jobst garment, such as improper fit, formation of blisters, or opening of the healed area underneath

Bathing

Bathing or showering daily in your usual manner cleans the wounds, especially ones that are still open.

1. Check the water and adjust the temperature to a warm and comfortable level. Your skin is more sensitive to extra heat or cold and can be easily injured.
2. Wash gently with a clean, soft washcloth, using a mild detergent soap such as Dial or Ivory. Be careful not to rub too hard so as not to disturb the grafted areas. Avoid harsh or deodorant soaps.
3. Rinse skin thoroughly after washing.
4. Dry thoroughly.
5. Apply specific dressing as instructed.

Care for Burn Wound

While caring for your burn wound, look at the involved areas and note any changes that need to be reported.

1. Wash hands.
2. Remove dressing and dispose of it in a paper bag or wrap in newspaper.
3. Wash hands.
4. Wash open area with a clean, soft washcloth and Dial or Ivory soap and water. Use a clean towel and washcloth with each dressing change.
5. Rinse skin well with plain water.
6. Wash hands.
7. Apply dressing as described below.
8. Wear gloves. Wash basin or bathtub with a disinfectant such as Lysol.
9. Wash hands.

Care of Clothing

When you are discharged, you may find that healed burn areas are sensitive to harsh detergents, fabric softeners, and clothing dyes. If you are sensitive:

- Launder new clothing before use, by machine or by hand, with a detergent free of additives.
- Rinse clothes twice.
- Do not use fabric softeners.
- If you have open burns or a healed area that opens, wash all clothes separately from those of other family members.
- Scarlet Red ointment will permanently stain clothing.
- If dyes used in clothing cause irritation, wear white articles.
- Wear loose-fitting clothing.

Elastic Bandages

- If they are too loose, they will be ineffective and must be rewrapped.
- If they are too tight, they will cause discomfort, numbness, tingling, and puffiness and must be rewrapped.
- They must be worn for a long time, probably 6 to 12 months, to be effective, so please do not stop wearing them until your doctor tells you.
- To care for your elastic bandages:
  1. Hand wash with a mild detergent in cold water.
  2. Towel dry.
  3. Lay flat to dry.

Pressure Garment

- If it is too loose, it will be ineffective and you will require a new garment.
- If it is too tight, it will cause discomfort, numbness, and tingling. Do not wear it if this occurs, but notify the Burn Clinic as soon as possible.
- To care for your pressure garment:
  1. Hand wash with a mild detergent in cold water.
  2. Towel dry.
  3. Lay flat to dry.

Diet

A well-balanced diet is important as your burn wound continues to heal. Be sure to include meat, milk products, breads and cereals, and fruits and vegetables in your diet.

Your Emotions

It is not uncommon to feel blue or let down after you go home. The Burn Support Group meets __________ to help you.

Courtesy Comprehensive Burn Center, MetroHealth Medical Center, Cleveland.

- Seek assistance as deemed necessary.
- Acknowledge the needs of all family members.
- Openly verbalize unresolved problems or concerns.
- Exhibit positive coping behaviors.
- Identify alterations in personal situation and strategies to improve it.

NURSING INTERVENTIONS. After discharge, the patient (and family) continues to adjust to temporary or permanent functional losses, cosmetic disfigurement, the reactions of others, and family role changes. The ability to manage depends on coping mechanisms of the patient and family before the burn, the severity of injury, and the reaction of others. The nurse can evaluate the patient's and family's adaptation to these changes during outpatient visits when the burn team and appropriate personnel are available.

Job retraining may be necessary if the burn injury caused loss of joint function or other physical limitations that prevent the patient from returning to former employment. The local office of the state labor and industry board can assign a vocational counselor to help the patient return to the workforce. Even if retraining cannot begin for several months, contact with the vocational counselor and anticipation of retraining may help the patient look beyond immediate problems and think about the future.

Before discharge, burn patients and their families have a great need for education so they can take increasing responsibility for their own care. Thus early discharge planning is essential and accomplishes two goals. First, it helps solve problems early. For example, if the patient's house burned and needs to be repaired, the family may need to relocate. This could be done before discharge, thus preventing the added stress of moving after discharge. Second, early discharge planning emphasizes the future. If discharge is discussed, the patient and his or her family may realize more quickly that recovery and return to home are possible.

Complete and comprehensive instructions followed by return demonstration help the patient learn to be independent in self-care activities and decrease frustration after discharge. Patients with major burns are not generally discharged from the hospital until they can care for themselves physically, with assistance if necessary, and are prepared to meet the stresses involved in returning to their former living patterns. Sample discharge instructions are provided in the Patient/Family Teaching box, p. 1943.

RELATED NIC INTERVENTIONS. Coping Enhancement, Emotional Support, Family Therapy, Mutual Goal Setting, Support Group, Support System Enhancement, Therapy Group

EVALUATION

To evaluate the effectiveness of nursing interventions, compare patient behaviors with those stated in the expected patient outcomes.

RELATED NOC OUTCOMES. Acceptance: Health Status, Adaptation to Physical Disability, Body Image, Comfort Level, Coping, Self-Care: Activities of Daily Living (ADL), Self-Care: Bathing, Self-Care: Hygiene, Self-Esteem

Critical Thinking

1. Two 30-year-old men are brought to the emergency department after receiving burns from a house fire. One man has a partial-thickness burn, and the other has a full-thickness burn. Identify objective and subjective data that help differentiate these two types of burns.
2. Incorporating general principles of psychologic care, develop a nursing approach for each of the following patient responses to a severe burn: withdrawal, regression, anger and hostility, and depression.

References

1. Agency for Toxic Substances and Disease Registry: *Medical management guidelines for unidentified chemical,* accessed May 2004 from website: http://www.atsdr.cdc.gov/MHMI/mmg170.html.
2. American Burn Association: *Practice guidelines for burn care,* Chicago, 2001, The Association.
3. American College of Surgeons: Resources for optimal care of patients with burn injury. In *Resources for optimal care of the injured patient,* Chicago, 1998, The College.
4. Badger J: Burns, the psychological aspects, *Am J Nurs* 101:11, accessed Nov 2001 from website: http://www.nursingcenter.com/library/JournalArticle.asp?Article_ID=230621.
5. Barrett JP, Herndon DN: *Color atlas of burn care,* Philadelphia, 2001, Saunders.
6. Baur KM, Hardy PE, Van Dorsten B: Posttraumatic stress disorder in burn populations: a critical review of the literature, *J Burn Care Rehabil* 19: 230-240, 1998.
7. Blankeney PE et al: Psychosocial recovery and reintegration of patients with burn injuries. In Herndon DN, editor: *Total burn care,* ed 2, Philadelphia, 2002, Saunders.
8. Burn Survivor Resource Center: Burn statistics. In *Medical care guide,* accessed 2002 from website: http://www.burnsurvivor.com/burn_statistics.html.
9. Burn Survivor Resource Center: Inhalation injuries. In *Medical care guide,* accessed 2002 from website: http://www.burnsurvivor.com/burn_types_inhalation.html.

9a. Cartotto RC et al: How well does the Parkland formula estimate actual fluid resuscitation volumes? *J Burn Care Rehabil* 23(4):258-265, 2002.

10. Choinière M: Burn pain: a unique challenge, *Pain Clin Updates* 9:1, March 2001, accessed from website: http://www.iasp-pain.org/PCU01-1.html.
11. Cioffi WG: Inhalation injury. In Carrougher GJ, editor: *Burn care and therapy,* St Louis, 1998, Mosby.
12. Committee on the Organization and Delivery of Burn Care: *Burn care resources in North America 2003-2004,* Chicago, 2003, American Burn Association.
13. Demling RH, DeSanti L: Oxandrolone, an anabolic steroid, significantly increases weight gain in the recovery phase after major burns, *J Trauma* 43:47-51, 1997.
14. Demling RH, DeSanti L: Topic doxepin significantly decreases itching and erythema in the chronically pruritic burn scar, *Wounds* 15(6):195-200, 2003.
15. Guenther L, Barankin B: Sunburn, *eMedicine,* accessed April 2003 from website: http://www.emedicine.com/ped/topic2561.htm.
16. Hartford CE: Care of outpatient burns. In Herndon DN, editor: *Total burn care,* ed 2, London, 2002, Saunders.
17. Heggers JP et al: Treatment of infection in burns. In Herndon DN, editor: *Total burn care,* ed 2, London, 2002, Saunders.
18. Herndon DN, Blakeney PE: Teamwork for total burn care: achievements, directions, and hopes. In Herndon DN, editor: *Total burn care,* ed 2, Philadelphia, 2002, Saunders.

19. Hostetler MA: Electrical burns, *eMedicine*, accessed Jan 2004 from website: http://www.emedicine.com/ped/topic2734.htm.
20. Hunt JL, Purdue GF: Prevention of burn injuries. In Herndon DN, editor: *Total burn care,* ed 2, London, 2002, Saunders.
21. Kaups KL, Davis JW, Dominic WJ: Base deficit as an indicator of resuscitation needs in patients with burn injuries, *J Burn Care Rehabil* 19:346-348, 1998.
22. Kramer GC, Lund T, Herndon DN: Pathophysiology of burn shock and burn edema. In Herndon DN, editor: *Total burn care,* ed 2, London, 2002, Saunders.
23. Lund T: Edema generation following thermal injury: an update, *J Burn Care Rehabil* 20:445-452, 1999.

23a. Milner SM, Mottar S, Smith C: The burn wheel, *Am J Nurs* 101:35-36, 2001.

24. Mlcak RP, Buffalo MC: Pre-hospital management, transportation, and emergency care. In Herndon DN, editor: *Total burn care,* ed 2, London, 2002, Saunders.
25. Munster AM: The immunological response and strategies for intervention. In Herndon DN, editor: *Total burn care,* ed 2, London, 2002, Saunders.
26. Oman KS, Reilly EL: Initial assessment and care in the emergency department. In Carrougher GJ, editor: *Burn care and therapy,* St Louis, 1998, Mosby.
27. Pruitt BA, Goodwin CW, Mason AD: Epidemiological, demographic, and outcome characteristics of burn injury. In Herndon DN, editor: *Total burn care,* ed 2, London, 2002, Saunders.
28. Radiation Emergency Assistance Center: *Guidance for radiation accident management: managing radiation emergencies,* Feb 21, 2002, accessed from website: http://www.orau.gov/reacts/syndrome.htm.
29. Rutan RL: Physiologic response to cutaneous burn injury. In Carrougher GJ, editor: *Burn care and therapy,* St Louis, 1998, Mosby.
30. Saffle JR, Hildreth M: Metabolic support of the burned patient. In Herndon DN, editor: *Total burn care,* ed 2, Philadelphia, 2002, Saunders.
31. Schiller WR et al: Laser Doppler evaluation of burned hands predicts need for surgical grafting, *J Trauma* 43:35-39, 1997.
32. Tadros T, Traber DL, Herndon DN: Hepatic blood flow and oxygen consumption after burn and sepsis, *J Trauma* 49:101-108, 2000.
33. US Department of Health and Human Services: *Healthy people 2010: understanding and improving health,* Washington, DC, 2000, The Department.
34. Warden GD: Fluid resuscitation and early management. In Herndon DN, editor: *Total burn care,* ed 2, London, 2002, Saunders.
35. Winifree J, Barillo DJ: Nonthermal injuries, *Nurs Clin North Am* 32(2): 275-296, 1997.

SELECTED BIBLIOGRAPHY

Chapter 1: Scope of Medical-Surgical Nursing

General

Chaguturu S, Vallabhaneni S: Aiding and abetting: nursing crises at home and abroad, *N Engl J Med* 353(17):1761-1763, 2005.

Grindel C, Roman M: The medical-surgical nurse: being a magnet for excellence, *Med Surg Nurs* (Suppl):4-34, 2005.

Sorting out medical/surgical nursing certifications, *Nurs Manage* 36 (Suppl):20-21, 2005.

Trossman S: Issues update—beyond mandatory overtime: the ANA and nurse leaders take aim at RN fatigue and workplace practices, *Am J Nurs* 105(10):73-74, 77, 2005.

Evidence-Based Practice

Ahrens T: Evidence-based practice: priorities and implementation strategies, *AACN Clin Issues Adv Pract Acute Crit Care* 16(1):36-42, 2005.

Couvillon JS: How to promote or implement evidence-based practice in a clinical setting, *Home Health Care Manage Pract* 17(4):269-272, 2005.

Zeitz K, McCutcheon H: Tradition, rituals, and standards in a realm of evidence-based nursing care, *Contemp Nurse* 18(3):300-308, 2005.

Nursing Informatics

Hahn K: Unifying nursing languages: the harmonization of NANDA, NIC, and NOC, *Intern J Nurs Terminol Classif* 15(2):34, 2004.

Simpson RL: From tele-ed to telehealth: the need for IT ubiquity in nursing, *Nurs Am Q* 29(4):344-348, 2005.

Von Krogh G, Dale C, Naden D: A framework for integrating NANDA, NIC, and NOC terminology in electronic patient records, *J Nurs Scholarship* 37(3):275-281, 2005.

Chapter 2: The Aging Population

Benshoff JJ, Koch DS: Substance abuse and the elderly: unique issues and concerns, *J Rehabil* 69(2):43-48, 2003.

Griffiths R et al: A nursing intervention for the quality use of medicines by elderly community clients, *Intern J Nurs Pract* 10(4):166-176, 2004.

Hajjar RR, Kamel HK: Sexuality in the nursing home, part 1, Attitudes and barriers to sexual expression, *J Am Med Dir Assoc* 4(3):152-156, 2003.

Kelly C, Mujezinovic-Womack M: Healthy people 2010: managing cardiovascular risk reduction in elderly adults, *J Gerontol Nurs* 29(6): 18-23, 2003.

Studer M: Cognitive rehabilitation in the frail elderly patient: never too late to learn? *Topics Geriatr Rehabil* 20(1):21-33, 2004.

Chapter 3: Healthy Lifestyles

Health Promotion and Prevention

Chiverton PA et al: The future role of nursing in health promotion, *Am J Health Promo* 18(2):192, 2003.

Haskell WL: Cardiovascular disease prevention and lifestyle interventions, *J Cardiovasc Nurs* 18(4):245, 2003.

McFee SD et al: Comparing health status with healthy habits in elderly assisted-living residents, *Fam Commun Health* 27(2):158, 2004.

Spector RE: *Cultural diversity in health and illness*, ed 6, Upper Saddle River, NJ, 2004, Pearson Prentice Hall.

Talip W et al: Development and validation of a knowledge test for health professionals regarding lifestyle modification, *Nutrition* 19(9):760, 2003.

Nutrition and Weight Management

Hjelm K et al: Preparing nurses to face the pandemic of diabetes mellitus: a literature review, *J Adv Nurs* 41(5):424, 2003.

Hu G et al: Physical activity, body mass index, and risk of type 2 diabetes in patients with normal or impaired glucose regulation, *Arch Intern Med* 164(8):892, 2004.

McInnes KJ: Diet, exercise and the challenge of combating obesity in primary care, *J Cardiovasc Nurs* 18(2):93, 2003.

A new evidence-based model for weight management in primary care: the Counterweight Programme, *J Human Nutr Dietetics* 17(3):191, 2004.

Sandison R et al: Lifestyle factors for promoting bone health in older women, *J Adv Nurs* 45(6):603, 2004.

Exercise

Brown DW: Associations between physical activity dose and health-related quality of life, *Med Sci Sports Exercise* 36(5):890, 2004.

Conn V et al: Sedentary older women's limited experience with exercise, *J Commun Health Nurs* 20(4):197, 2003.

Gibb B: Food minus exercise = fat, *Lancet* 363(I 9416):1246, 2004.

Speck BJ, Harrell JS: Maintaining regular physical activity in women, *J Cardiovasc Nurs* 18(4):282, 2003.

Wallace L et al: Influencing exercise and diet to prevent osteoporosis: lessons from three studies, *Brit J Commun Nurs* 9(3):102, 2004.

Regimen Adherence

Bissell P et al: From compliance to concordance: barriers to accomplishing a re-framed model of health care interactions, *Soc Sci Med* 58(4):851, 2004.

Colin Bell A et al: Understanding the role of mediating risk factors and proxy effects in the association between socio-economic status and untreated hypertension, *Soc Sci Med* 59(2):275, 2004.

Cropley CJ: The effect of health care provider persuasive strategy on patient compliance and satisfaction, *Am J Health Studies* 18(2/3):117, 2003.

Halperin AC et al: US public universities' compliance with recommended tobacco-control policies, *J Am College Health* 51(5):181, 2003.

Smoking Cessation

Borland R et al: The effectiveness of personally tailored computer-generated advice letters for smoking cessation, *Addiction* 99(3):369, 2004.

Cramer ME et al: Evaluation informs coalition programming for environmental tobacco smoke reduction, *J Commun Health Nurs* 20(4):245, 2003.

Curry S et al: Self-administered treatment for smoking cessation, *J Clin Psychol* 59(3):305, 2003.

Struthers R et al: Community mapping: a tool in the fight against cigarette smoking on American Indian reservations, *Policy Politics Nurs* 4(4):295, 2003.

Tsoh JY, Hall SM: Depression and smoking: from the transtheoretical model of change perspective, *Addict Behav* 29(4):801, 2004.

Chapter 4: Complementary and Alternative Therapies

Blakeley J, Ribeiro V: Glucosamine and osteoarthritis, *AJN* 104(2):54-59, 2004.

Keller KB, Lemberg L: Herbal or complementary medicine: fact or fiction, *Am J Crit Care*, 10(6):438-443, 2001.

Kessler RC et al: Long-term trends in the use of complementary and alternative medical therapies in the United States, *Ann Intern Med* 135(4):262-268, 2001.

Kuhn MA: Herbal remedies: drug-herb interactions, *Crit Care Nurse* 22(2):22-30, 2002.

Wardell D, Weymouth K: Review of studies of healing touch, *J Nurs Scholarship*, 36(2):147-154, 2004.

Chapter 5: Genetics and Disease

General

Baker C: *Behavioral genetics*, Washington, DC, 2004, American Association for the Advancement of Science.

Lister Hill National Center for Biomedical Communications: *Help me understand genetics*, accessed July 2004 from website: www.ghr.nlm.nih.gov/.

Selden S: *Inheriting shame: the story of eugenics and racism in America*, New York, 1999, Teachers College Press.

Genetics and Disease

Weiner M, Alexander C, Seely G: Cancer and genetics, part III, *Oncol Nurs Forum* 31(2):195-196, 2004.

Weiner M, Calzone K, LeGrazie B: Cancer and genetics, part I, *Oncol Nurs Forum* 30(6):921-922, 2003.

Weiner M, Mercy D: Cancer and genetics, part II, *Oncol Nurs Forum* 3(1):35-36, 2004.

Genetics and Nursing

Cok SS: Deconstructing DNA: understanding genetic implications on nursing care, *AWHONN Lifelines* 7(2):140-144, 2003.

Foundation for Blood Research: *Practice-based genetics curriculum for nurse educators*, accessed June 2004 from website: www.fbr.org/publications/gencur-nursedu/nihdale2000.html.

Greco KE: Nursing in the genomic era: nurturing our genetic nature, *MedSurg Nurs* 12(5):307-312, 2003.

Lashley FR, editor: *The genetics revolution: implications for nursing*, Washington, DC, 1997, American Academy of Nursing.

Olsen SJ et al: Creating a nursing vision for leadership in genetics, *MedSurg Nurs* 12(3):177-183, 2003.

Williams JK et al: Advancing genetic nursing knowledge, *Nurs Outlook* 52(2):73-79, 2004.

Winkelman C: Genomics: what every critical care nurse needs to know about the genetic contribution to critical illness, *Crit Care Nurse* 24(3):34-45, 2004.

US Department of Health and Human Services: *Report of the expert panel on genetics and nursing: implications for education and practice*, Alexandria, Va, 2000, Heath Resources and Services Administration, Bureau of Health Professions, Division of Nursing.

Chapter 6: Infectious Diseases and Bioterrorism

General

Hilton C, Allison V: Disaster preparedness: an indictment for action by nursing educators, *J Contin Ed Nurs* 35(2):59-65, 91-92, 2004.

Horner M: Judicious use of antimicrobials in the critical care setting, *J Infusion Nurs* 27(2):79-84, 2004.

Walters MJ: *Six modern plagues and how we are causing them*, Washington, DC, 2003, Shearwater Books.

Bioterrorism

Filoroma C et al: An innovative approach to training hospital-based clinicians for bioterrorist attacks, *Am J Infect Control* 31(8):511-514, 2003.

Gooze LL, Hughes ECW: Smallpox, *Semin Respir Infect* 18(3):196-205, 2003.

Henning KJ et al: Health system preparedness for bioterrorism: bringing the tabletop to the hospital, *Infect Control Hosp Epidemiol* 25(2):146-155, 2004.

Jensen WA, Kirsch CM: Tularemia, *Semin Respir Infect* 18(3):146-158, 2003.

Polesky A, Bhatia G: Ebola hemorrhagic fever in the era of bioterrorism, *Semin Respir Infect* 18(3):206-215, 2003.

Immunizations

Carabin H, Edmunds WJ: Future savings from measles eradication in industrialized countries, *J Infect Dis* 5(187 [Suppl 1]):S29-S35, 2003.

Lugo NR, Montoya C, Petraco MBK: Parents' perspectives on immunizations: a survey, *Am J Nurse Pract* 7(11):8-10, 13-14, 2003.

Russell J, Godek B: Adult immunizations: underused in primary care, *Patient Care* 37(7):53-54, 58-61, 64-65, 2003.

Szilagyi P et al: Interventions aimed at improving immunization rates (Cochrane Review). In *Cochrane Library*, Issue 1, Chichester, UK, 2004, John Wiley & Sons.

Telford R, Rogers A: What influences elderly people's decisions about whether to accept the influenza vaccination? *Health Educ Res* 18(6):743-753, 2003.

Nosocomial Infections

Arrowsmith VA et al: Removal of nail polish and finger rings to prevent surgical infection (Cochrane Review). In *Cochrane Library*, Issue 1, Chichester, UK, 2004, John Wiley & Sons.

Hampton S: The importance of controlling infection in care homes, *Nurs Resident Care* 5(5):221-222, 224-225, 2003.

Larson E: A tool to assess barriers to adherence to hand hygiene guidelines, *Am J Infect Control* 32(1):48-51, 2004.

Pittet D et al: Concise communications: cost implications of successful hand hygiene promotion, *Infect Control Hosp Epidemiol* 25(3):264-266, 2004.

Trampuz A, Widmer AF: Hand hygiene: a frequently missed lifesaving opportunity during patient care, *Mayo Clin Proc* 79(1):109-116, 2004.

Chapter 7: Rehabilitation and Chronic Illness

Association of Rehabilitation Nurses, 4700 W. Lake Avenue, Glenview, IL 60027-1485; http://www.rehabnurse.org.

Derstine JB, Hargrove SD: *Comprehensive rehabilitation nursing*, Philadelphia, 2001, Mosby.

Lorig KR: Taking patient ed to the next level, *RN* 66(12):37-38, 2003.

Morrison M: *The prevention and treatment of pressure ulcers*, St Louis, 2001, Mosby.

Smeltzer SC, Bare BG: *Brunner and Suddarth's textbook of medical-surgical nursing*, ed 10, Philadelphia, 2004, Lippincott Williams & Wilkins.

Chapter 8: Palliative and End-of-Life Care

Ameling A, Povilonis M: Spirituality, meaning, mental health, and nursing, *J Psychosoc Nurs Mental Health Serv* 39(4):14-20, 2002.

Bain KT et al: Toward evidence-based prescribing at end of life: a comparative review of temazepam and zolpidem for the treatment of insomnia, *Am J Hosp Palliat Care* 20(5):382-388, 400, 2003.

Bentley J, Bloomfield J: Prescribing in palliative care: the primacy of patient involvement, *Nurse Prescribing* 1(2):72-77, 2003.

Benzein E, Berg A: The Swedish version of Herth Hope Index—an instrument for palliative care, *Scand J Caring Sci* 17(4):409-415, 2003.

Brazil K et al: Caregiving and its impact on families of the terminally ill, *Aging Mental Health* 7(5):376-382, 2003.

Broback G, Bertero C: How next of kin experience palliative care of relatives at home, *Europ J Cancer Care* 12(4):339-346, 2003.

Carter H et al: Living with a terminal illness: patient's priorities, *J Adv Nurs* 45(6):611-620, 2004.

Chochinov HM: Thinking outside the box: depression, hope, and meaning at the end of life, *Innovat End-of-Life Care* 4(6), 2002.

Close H: Nausea and vomiting in terminally ill patients: toward a holistic approach, *Nurse Prescribing* 1(1):22-26, 2003.

Crossno RJ: Dying in the emergency department: what emergency physicians should know about palliative medicine, *Topics Emerg Med* 26(1):19-28, 2004.

Ferrell BR, Borneman T: Community implementation of home care palliative care education, *Cancer Pract* (10)1:20-27, 2002.

Ferrell BR, Coyle N: An overview of palliative nursing care, *Am J Nurs* 102(5):26-31, 2002.

Gazelle G, Buxbaum R, Daniels E: The development of a palliative care program for managed care patients: a case example, *J Am Geriatr Soc* 49:1234-1241, 2001.

Gooding L: The final choice, *Nurs Standard* 18(28):18-19, 2004.

Hogan BE: Soul music in the twilight years: music therapy and the dying process, *Topics Geriatr Rehabil* 19(4):275-281, 2003.

Kass RM, Ellershaw J: Respiratory tract secretions in the dying patient: a retrospective study, *J Pain Symptom Manage* 26(4):897-902, 2003.

Kirschling JM, Lentz J: Infusion nurses' role in care at the end of life, *J Infusion Nurs* 27(2):112-117, 123-126, 2004.

Lesage P, Portenoy R: Ethical challenges in the care of patients with serious illness, *Pain Med* 2(2):121-130, 2001.

Robinson A: A personal exploration of the power of poetry in palliative care, loss and bereavement, *Int J Palliat Nurs* 10(1):32-34, 36-39, 2004.

Ross C, Cornbleet M: Attitudes of patients and staff to research in a specialist palliative care unit, *Palliat Med* 17(6):491-497, 2003.

Rutsohn P, Ibrahim N: An analysis of provider attitudes toward end-of-life decision-making, *Am J Hosp Palliat Care* 20(5):371-381, 2003.

Tilly J, Wiener J: *Medicaid and end-of-life care*, Washington, DC, 2001, Last Acts.

Chapter 9: Emergency Care

Cassabaum VD, Bourg PW: The ins and outs of renal trauma, *Am J Nurs* 102(9 Suppl):4, 2002.

Hardy M, Barrett C: Interpreting trauma radiographs, *J Adv Nurs* 44(1):81, 2003.

Standing up for patients in the ER: insisting on the ratios, *Calif Nurse* 100(4):6, 2004.

Thompson S: A & E nursing in Iraq, *Emerg Nurse* 11(8):14, 2004.

Tindale R: A review of articles of interest to emergency nurses, *Emerg Nurse* 11(7):7, 2003.

Chapter 10: Critical Care

Guzzetta CE: Critical care research: weaving a body-mind-spirit tapestry, *Am J Crit Care* 13(4):320-327, 2004.

Maddox M et al: Psychosocial recovery following ICU: experiences and influences upon discharge to the community, *Intens Crit Care Nurs* 17:6, 2001.

Marcum EH, West RD: Structured orientation for new graduates: a retention strategy, *J Nurses Staff Devel* 20(3):118-124, 2004.

McGrow KM et al: Informatics: using wireless technologies to improve information flow interhospital transfers of critical care patients, *Crit Care Nurse* 24(2):66-72, 2004.

McKinley S et al: Assessment of anxiety in intensive care patients using the Faces Anxiety Scale, *Am J Crit Care* 13(2):146-152, 2004.

Shannon SE, Mitchell PH, Cain KC: Patients, nurses, and physicians having differing views of quality of critical care, *J Nurs Scholarship* 34(2):173-179, 2002.

Chapter 11: Community-Based Care

Community-Based Nursing

Calleson DC, Seifer SD: Institutional collaboration and competition in community-based education, *J Interprof Care* 18(1):63, 2004.

Donohoe M, Danielson S: A community-based approach to the medical humanities, *Med Educ* 38(2):204, 2004.

Kulger M: Community care of older adults, *Am J Nurs* 104(1):93, 2004.

Leight SB: The application of a vulnerable populations conceptual model to rural health, *Pub Health Nurs* 20(6):440, 2003.

Schifalacqua MM et al: How to make a difference in the health care of a population, *Nurs Admin Q* 28(1):29, 2004.

Home Care

Allen BL et al: Analysis of OBQI outcomes in participating Michigan home health agencies, *J Nurs Care Qual* 19(2):149, 2004.

Breakwell S: Connecting new nurses and home care, *Home Health Care Manage Pract* 16(2):117, 2004.

Fischer LR: Community-based care and risk of nursing home placement, *Med Care* 41(12):1407, 2003.

Luna K, Spicer J: Applying a nine cell financial analysis model to home health care, *Nurs Econ* 22(1):22, 2004.

McCall N et al: Decreased home health use: does it decrease satisfaction? *Med Care Res Rev* 61(1):64, 2004.

Tull K, Carroll R: Advanced practice nursing in home health, *Home Health Care Manage Pract* 16(2):81, 2004.

Case Management

Bower KA: Patient care management as a global concern, *Nurs Admin Q* 28(1):39, 2004.

Fraser K, Strang V: Decision-making and nurse case management, *Adv Nurs Sci* 27(1):32, 2004.

Harrison JP et al: The effect of case management on US hospitals, *Nurs Econ* 22(2):64, 2004.

Huber D et al: Evaluating the impact of case management dosage, *Nurs Res* 52(5):276, 2003.

Murphy M et al: Open exchange as a model for continuing exchange, *Nurs Admin Q* 28(1):6, 2004.

Patient Teaching

Deaton C: Observations and outcomes, *J Cardiovasc Nurs* 19(2):142, 2004.

Maramba P et al: Discharge planning process, *J Nurs Care Qual* 19(2):123, 2004.

Neafsey P: Self-medication practices that alter the efficacy of selected cardiac medications, *Home Health Nurse* 22(2):88, 2004.

Oermann M et al: Outcomes of videotape instruction in clinic waiting area, *Ortho Nurs* 22(2):103, 2003.

Patients, doctors drop the ball on in the prevention of second strokes and heart attacks, *Diabetes Forcast* 5(5):24, 2004.

Documentation

Bader E et al: Medicare consumer rights: appealing a denial of coverage, *Am J Nurs* 104(3):70, 2004.

Getting a leg up on charting, *Nursing* 34(4):20, 2004.

Griffith R: Putting the record straight: the importance of documentation, *Brit J Commun Nurs* 9(3):122, 2004.

Karkkainen O, Eriksson K: Evaluation of patient records as part of developing a nursing care classification, *J Clin Nurs* 12(2):198, 2003.

New JCAHO documentation guidelines required nationwide, *Nursing* 34(2 Travel Suppl):2, 2004.

Chapter 12: Long-Term Care

Nursing Issues

Engles V, Graney M, Chan A: Accuracy and bias of licensed practical nurse and nursing assistant ratings of nursing home residents' pain, *J Gerontol Nurs* 28:28-34, 2002.

Long term care nurse ignored, *Nurs Times* 97(8):8, 2001.

Sofie J et al: Health and safety risk at a skilled nursing facility: nursing assistants perceptions, *J Gerontol Nurs* 29(2):13-21, 2003.

Trossman S: Yes, there is a staffing crisis in long term care, *Am Nurse* 33(3):1, 2001.

Resident Care

Eaton DA, Roland PS: Dizziness in the older adult, part 1, Evaluation and general treatment strategies, *Geriatrics* 58(4):28-36, 2003.

Ennis BW et al: Diagnosing malnutrition in the elderly, *Nurse Practice* 26(3):52, 2001.

Hanlon JT et al: Use of inappropriate prescription drugs by older people, *J Am Geriatr Soc* 50:26-34, 2002.

Villanueva I et al: Pain assessment for the dementing elderly, *J Am Med Dir Assoc* 4(1):1-8, 2003.

Administrative Issues

Grabowski CJ: Falls: a prelude to litigation, *Director* 11(2):50-54, 2003.

Haney LL: Physical stresses related to safe handling of residents, *Director* 11(4):151-153, 2003.

Nelson D: Violence against elderly people: a neglected problem, *Lancet* 360(9339):1094, 2002, accessed from website: www.thelancet.com.

Stolley JM: Recruiting and retaining nursing staff, *ElderCare* 3(4):8-10, 2004.

Zhou Y, Edward NC, Stearns SC: Longevity and health care expenditures: the real reasons older people spend more, *J Gerontol Series B: Psychol Sci Soc Sci* 58(Suppl):2-10, 2003.

Chapter 13: Preoperative Nursing

Informed Consent

Jenkins K, Baker AB: Consent and anaesthetic risk, *Anaesthesia* 58:962-984, 2003.

Complementary and Alternative Therapies

Brunges M, Avigne G: Music therapy for reducing surgical anxiety, *AORN J* 78(5):816-818, 2003.

Wren KR, Kimbrall S, Norred CL: Use of complementary and alternative medications by surgical patients, *J PeriAnesthesia Nurs* 17(3):170-177, 2002.

Patient Education

Bernier MJ et al: Preoperative teaching received and valued in a day surgery setting, *AORN J* 77(3):563-582, 2003.

Chumbley GM, Hall GM, Salmon P: Patient-controlled analgesia: what information does the patient want? *J Adv Nurs* 39(5):459, 2002.

Mordiffi SZ, Tan SP, Wong MK: Information provided to surgical patients versus information needed, *AORN J* 77(3):546-562, 2003.

Chapter 14: Intraoperative Nursing

Anesthesia

Aronson WL, McAuliffe MS, Miller K: Variability in the American society of anesthesiologists physical status classification scale, *AANA J* 71(4): 265-274, 2003.

Kost M: *Moderate sedation/analgesia core competencies for practice*, St Louis, 2004, Saunders.

Jagim M: Airway management rapid-sequence intubation in trauma patients, *AJN* 103(10):32-35, 2003.

Martin-Duce A: A developmental history of local anesthesia, *Ambul Surg* 9:187-189, 2002.

Nagelhout JJ, Boytim M: Pharmacologic rationale for anesthetic agents in ambulatory practice, *J PeriAnesthesia Nurs* 16(6):371-378, 2001.

Infection Control

Gruendeman BJ, Magnum SS: *Infection prevention in surgical settings*, Philadelphia, 2001, Saunders.

Latex Allergy

Lenehan G: Latex allergy: separating fact from fiction, *Nursing* Feb Suppl:12-17, 2004.

Reed D: Update on latex allergy among health care personnel, *AORN J* 78(3):409-428, 2003.

Malignant Hyperthermia

Claxton GA, Cross MH, Hopkins PM: No response to trigger agents in a malignant hyperthermia–susceptible patient, *Brit J Anaesthesia* 88(6):870-873, 2002.

Older Adults

Barnett SSR: Preanesthetic evaluation for the elderly patient, *Syllabus Geriatric Anesthes,* accessed June 2004 from website: awww.asahq.org/clinical/geriatrictrics/prean_eval.htm.

Ceulemans R et al: Safe laparoscopic surgery in the elderly, *Am J Surg* 187:323-327, 2004.

Haynes LC, Martin JH, Endres D: Use of nontraditional therapies—implications for older adults, *AORN J* 77(5):913-922, 2003.

Pompei P: Managing medical illness in the elderly surgical patient, *Syllabus Geriatric Anesthes,* accessed June 2004 from website: www.asahq.org/clinical/geriatrics/manag.htm.

Patient Safety

Association of Operating Room Nurses: Guidance statement—safe medication practices in perioperative practice settings, *AORN J* 79(3):674-676, 2004.

Beyea SC: Best practices for abbreviation use, *AORN J* 79(3):641-642, 2004.

Murphy EK: Protecting patients for potential injuries, *AORN J* 79(5): 1013-1016, 2004.

Rusynko JB, Perry-Ewald J: Keeping patient safe-procedure and site verification and preprocedure pause, *AORN J* 79(4):787-796, 2004.

Spath PL: Using failure mode and effects analysis to improve patient safety, *AORN J* 78(1):15-37, 2003.

Chapter 15: Postoperative Nursing

General

Burden N et al: *Ambulatory surgical nursing*, Philadelphia, 2000, Saunders.

Zeitz K, McCutcheon H, Albrecht A: Postoperative complications in the first 24 hours: a general surgery audit, *J Adv Nurs* 46(6):633-640, 2004.

Complementary and Alternative Therapy

Ikonomidou E, Rehnstrom RN, Naesh O: Effect of music on vital signs and postoperative pain, *AORN J* 80(2):269-278, 2004.

McRee LD, Noble S, Pasvogel A: Using massage and music therapy to improve postoperative outcomes, *AORN J* 78(3):433-487, 2003.

Schaffer SD, Yucha CB: Relaxation and pain management, *AJN* 104(8): 75-82, 2004.

Wilson L, Kolcaba K: Practical application of comfort theory in the perianesthesia setting, *J PeriAnesthesia Nurs* 19(3):164-173, 2004.

Pain

Buss HE, Melderis K: PACU pain management algorithm, *J PeriAnesthesia Nurs* 17(1):11-20, 2002.

Coll AM, Ameen JRM, Moseley LG: Reported pain after day surgery: a critical literature review, *J Adv Nurs* 56(1):53-65, 2004.

Krenzischek DA, Windle P, Mamaril M: A survey of current perianesthesia nursing practice for pain and comfort management, *J PeriAnesthesia Nurs* 19(3):138-149, 2004.

Krenzischek DA et al: Clinical evaluation of the ASPAN pain and comfort clinical guideline, *J PeriAnesthesia Nurs* 19(3):150-159, 2004.

Windle PE: The challenges of pain management: adverse effects of analgesics, *J PeriAnesthesia Nurs* 19(3):212-216, 2004.

Chapter 16: Pain

Bonica J, Loeser J: History of pain concepts and therapies. In Loeser J et al, editors: *Bonica's management of pain,* New York, 2001, Lippincott Williams & Wilkins.

Dooks P: Diffusion of pain management research into nursing practice, *Cancer Nurs* 24(2):99-103, 2001.

Loeser J et al, editors: *Bonica's management of pain,* New York, 2001, Lippincott Williams & Wilkins.

St. Marie B: *American Society of Pain Management Nurses: core curriculum for pain management nurses*, Philadelphia, 2002, Saunders.

Turk D, Melzack R: *Handbook of pain assessment,* New York, 2001, Guildford Press.

Woolf C, Salter M: Neuronal plasticity: increasing the gain in pain, *Science* 288:1765-1768, 2000.

Chapter 17: Fluid and Electrolyte Imbalance

Cook LS: IV fluid resuscitation, *J Infusion Nurs* 26(5):296-303, 2003.

Diehl-Oplinger L, Kaminski MF: Choosing the right fluid to counter hypovolemic shock, *Nursing 2004* 24(3):52-54, 2004.

Edwards S: Regulation of water, sodium and potassium: implications for practice, *Nurs Standard* 15(22):36-44, 2001.

Hague DA: Interpreting lab values affected by kidney function, *Ohio Nurses Rev* 78(2):6-10, 2003.

Hand H: Continuing professional development: fluid management—the use of intravenous therapy, *Primary Health Care* 11(9):43-48, 2001.

Heatley S: Metastatic bone disease and tumor-induced hypercalcaemia: treatment options, *Int J Palliat Nurs* 10(1):41-46, 2004.

Hedrick C: Test your knowledge: preparing to take the CRNI exam—fluids and electrolytes, *J Infusion Nurs* 27(4):225-226, 2004.

Kenney WL, Chiu P: Influence of age on thirst and fluid intake, *Med Sci Sports Exercise* 33(9):1524-1532, 2001.

Kugler JP, Hustead T: Hyponatremia and hypernatremia in the elderly, *Am Fam Phys* 61(12):3623-3630, 2000.

Morrison C: Helping patients to maintain a healthy fluid balance, *Nurs Times* 96(31):3-4, 2000.

Redden M, Wotton K: Third-space fluid shift in elderly patients undergoing gastrointestinal surgery, part I, Pathophysiological mechanisms, *Contemp Nurse* 12(3):275-283, 2002.

Self-test: understanding fluids and electrolytes, *Nursing 2004* 34(4):81-84, 2004.

Shuey KM: Test your knowledge: hypercalcemia of malignancy, part I, *Clin J Oncol Nurs* 8(2):209-210, 2004.

Woodrow P: Assessing fluid balance in older people: fluid replacement, *Nurs Older People* 14(10):29-30, 2003.

Yeates KE, Singer M, Morton AR: Salt and water: a simple approach to hyponatremia, *Can Med Assoc J* 170(3):365-369, 2004.

Chapter 18: Acid-Base Imbalance

Baldwin BM: Introduction to an alternative view of acid/base balance: the strong ion difference or Stewart approach, *Austral Crit Care* 15(1): 14-20, 2002.

Banker D, Whittier FC, Rutecki G: Cases in point: an intriguing diagnosis—acid-base problem solving, *Consultant* 43(3):391-393, 399-400, 2003.

Berry BE, Pinard AE: Assessing tissue oxygenation, *Crit Care Nurse* 22(3):22-24, 26-30, 32-36, 2002.

Heitz UE, Horne MM: *Pocket guide to fluid, electrolyte and acid-base balance*, ed 5, St Louis, 2005, Mosby.

Hogan MA, Wane D: *Fluids, electrolytes, and acid-base balance: reviews and rationales*, Upper Saddle River, NJ, 2003, Prentice Hall.

Mane A, Termizi H, Lam M: A survey of arterial blood gas analysis of older patients, *Age & Ageing* 32(4):464-465, 2003.

Chapter 19: Shock

Physiology

Hung DT, Lilly CM: Making the most of hemodynamic monitoring in the ICU: observing and optimizing appropriate parameters, *J Crit Illness* 18(5):196-207, 2003.

Landry DW, Oliver JA: Insights into shock: still a last step before death for thousands of people, shock is shedding some of its medical mystery and becoming more treatable, *Sci Am* 290(2):36-41, 2004.

Lucas CE, Ledgerwood AM: Physiology of colloid-supplemented resuscitation from shock, *J Trauma Inj Infect Crit Care* 54(5S Suppl):S75-S81, 2003.

Pathophysiology

Cruz K, Hollenberg S: Update on septic shock: understanding the pathophysiology and recognizing disease: early recognition sets the stage for prompt therapy, *J Crit Illness* 18(4):151-157, 2003.

Kneale J: Understanding hypovolaemic shock, *Journal of Orthopaedic Nursing* 7(4):207-213, 2003.

Phrampus PE: Concepts of shock: understand the pathophysiology to better serve your patients, *JEMS* 29(3):118-120, 2004.

Sanborn TA et al: Correlates of 1-year survival in patients with cardiogenic shock complicating acute myocardial infarction: angiographic findings from the SHOCK trial, *J Am Coll Cardiol* 42(8):1373-1379, 2003.

Etiology

Edwards S: Shock: types, classifications and explorations of their physiological effects, *Emerg Nurs* 9(2):29-39, 2001.

Hanna NF: Sepsis and septic shock, *Topics Emerg Med* 25(2):158-165, 2003.

Landry DW, Oliver JA: Mechanisms of disease: the pathogenesis of vasodilatory shock, *N Engl J Med* 345(8):588-595, 2001.

Sommers MS: The cellular basis of septic shock, *Crit Care Nurs Clin North Am* 15(1):13-25, 2003.

Management

Alderson P et al: Colloids versus crystalloids for fluid resuscitation in critically ill patients (Cochrane Review). In *Cochrane Library,* Issue 3, 2004, Chichester, UK, John Wiley & Sons.

Dickinson K, Roberts I: Medical anti-shock trousers (pneumatic antishock garments) for circulatory support in patients with trauma (Cochrane Review). In *Cochrane Library,* Issue 2, 2004, Chichester, UK, John Wiley & Sons.

Kwan I et al: Timing and volume of fluid administration for patients with bleeding (Cochrane Review). In *Cochrane Library,* Issue 2, 2004, Chichester, UK, John Wiley & Sons.

Muhlberg AH, Ruth-Sahd L: Holistic care: treatment and interventions for hypovolemic shock secondary to hemorrhage, *DCCN* 23(2):55-61, 2004.

Richard C et al: Caring for the critically ill patient: early use of the pulmonary artery catheter and outcomes in patients with shock and acute respiratory distress syndrome: a randomized controlled trial, *JAMA* 290(20):2732-2734, 2003.

Chapter 20: Assessment of the Immune System

Cummings M: Acupuncture seems to have a positive influence on immune function, *Acupuncture Med* 21(1/2):63, 2003.

Gleeson M: Exercise, nutrition and immunology, *Sportex Health* 4(16):10-13, 2003.

Griffin MD, Zing N, Kumar R: Vitamin D and its analogs as regulators of immune activation and antigen presentation, *Ann Rev Nutr* 23: 117-145, 2003.

Moran D: Infections in the elderly, *Topics Emerg Med* 25(2):174-181, 2003.

Nielson HB: Lymphocyte responses to maximal exercise: a physiological perspective, *Sports Med* 33(11):853-867, 2003.

Pescatore F: Improving the immune function, *Totalhealth Mag* 25(3):20-21, 2003.

Vines SW et al: The relationship between chronic pain, immune function, depression, and health behaviors, *Biol Res Nurs* 5(1):18-29, 2003.

Weber R: The immunity challenge: antigens act I, scene I, *Dermatol Nurs* 16(1):61, 2004.

Weber R: The immunity challenge: I'm dreaming of a white (blood cell) Christmas, *Dermatol Nurs* 15(6):548, 2004.

Chapter 21: Immunologic Problems

General

Buckley RH: Treatment options for genetically determined immunodeficiency, *Lancet* 361(9357):541-542, 2003.

Cummings M: Acupuncture seems to have a positive influence on immune function, *Acupuncture Med* 6(21):63, 2003.

Gleeson M: Exercise, nutrition and immunology, *Sportex Health* 4(16):10-13, 2003.

Golden DBK: Stinging insect allergy, *Am Fam Phys* 67(12):2541, 2003.

Griffin MD, Zing N, Kumar R: Vitamin D and its analogs as regulators of immune activation and antigen presentation, *Ann Rev Nutr* 23:117-145, 2003.

Anaphylaxis

Burns A: Action stat: anaphylaxis, *Nursing 2004* 34(3):88, 2004.

Ferns T, Chojnacka I: The causes of anaphylaxis and its management in adults, *Brit J Nurs* 12(17):1006-1012, 2003.

Kurek M, Michalska-Krzanowska G: Anaphylaxis during surgical and diagnostic procedures, *Allergy Clin Immunol Intern* 15(4):168, 2003.

Merz G: Studying peanut anaphylaxis, *N Engl J Med* 348(11):975-976, 2003.

Latex Allergy

Lenehan GP: Latex allergy: separating fact from fiction, *Nursing* Feb Suppl:12-17, 2004.

Reed D: Update on latex allergy among health care personnel, *AORN* 78(3):409-412, 2003.

Yip ES: Accommodating latex allergy concerns in surgical settings, *AORN* 78(4):595-598, 2003.

Multiple Myeloma

Heffner LT, Lonial S: Breakthroughs in the management of multiple myeloma, *Drugs 2003* 63(16):1621, 2003.

Seidl S, Kaufmann H, Drach J: New insights into the pathophysiology of multiple myeloma, *Lancet Oncol* 4(9):557, 2003.

Chapter 22: HIV Infection and AIDS

General

Brashers DE et al: The medical, personal, and social causes of uncertainty in HIV illness, *Issues Ment Health Nurs* 24(5):497-522, 2003.

Burke JK et al: Dissatisfaction with medical care among women with HIV: dimensions and associated factors, *AIDS Care* 15(4):451-462, 2003.

Coleman CL: Determinants of HIV and AIDS among young African-American men who have sex with men: a public health perspective, *J Natl Black Nurses Assoc* 14(2):25-29, 2003.

Dy SM et al: Caring for patients in an inner-city home hospice: challenges and rewards, *Home Health Care Manage Pract* 15(4):291-299, 2003.

Ferrier SE, Lavis JN: With health comes work? People living with HIV/AIDS consider returning to work, *AIDS Care* 15(3):423-435, 2003.

Keilhofner G et al: Outcomes of a vocational program for persons with AIDS, *Am J Occup Ther* 58(1):64-72, 2004.

Rassool GH: Stigma discrimination and the conspiracy of silence are fueling the AIDS epidemic, *J Adv Nurs* 44(3):235, 2003.

Ress B: HIV disease and aging: the hidden epidemic, *Crit Care Nurse* 23(5):38-44, 2003.

Robinson J: Culture, behaviour and HIV/AIDS, *Int Nurs Rev* 51(1):3-4, 2004.

Silver EJ et al: Factors associated with psychological distress in urban mothers with late-stage HIV/AIDS, *AIDS Behav* 7(4):421-431, 2003.

Sullivan PS, Dworkin MS: Prevalence and correlates of fatigue among persons with HIV infection, *J Pain Symptom Manage* 25(4):329-333, 2003.

Webb A, Norton M: Clinical assessment of symptom-focused health-related quality of life in HIV/AIDS, *J Assoc Nurses AIDS Care* 15(2):66-81, 2004.

Williams PB: HIV/AIDS case profile of African Americans: guidelines for ethnic-specific health promotion, education and risk reduction activities for African Americans, *Fam Commun Health* 26(4):289-306, 2003.

Wolitski RJ et al: Self-perceived responsibility of HIV-seropositive men who have sex with men for preventing HIV transmission, *AIDS Behav* 7(4):363-372, 2003.

Woodhead K: Fighting AIDS stigma: caring for all, *Brit J Perioper Nurs* 13(6):255-258, 260-261, 2003.

Antiretroviral Therapy

Malcolm SE et al: An examination of HIV/AIDS patients who have excellent adherence to HAART, *AIDS Care* 15(2):251-261, 2003.

Piliero PJ, Colagreco JP: Clinical practice: simplified regimens for treating HIV infection and AIDS, *J Am Acad Nurse Pract* 15(7):305-312, 2003.

Ramirez GP, Cote JK: Factors affecting adherence to antiretroviral therapy in people living with HIV/AIDS, *J Assoc Nurses AIDS Care* 14(4):37-45, 2003.

Thirlwell C et al: Acquired immunodeficiency syndrome–related lymphoma in the era of highly active antiretroviral therapy, *Clin Lymphoma* 4(2):86-92, 2003.

Verheggen R: Immune reconstitution: immune restoration in patients with HIV infection: HAART and beyond, *J Assoc Nurses AIDS Care* 14(6):76-82, 2003.

Opportunistic Infections

Ferri RS, Kirton CA: Hepatitis C virus/HIV coninfection: a new challenge for nurses in AIDS care, *J Assoc Nurses AIDS Care* 14(5):8S-17S, 2003.

Gupta R et al: Scaling up treatment for HIV/AIDS: lessons learned from multidrug-resistant tuberculosis, *Lancet* 363(9405):320-324, 2004.

McMahon K: Clinical management of adults with HIV opportunistic infections, *Health Traveler* 11(6):72-77, 2003.

Chapter 23: Cancer

Advanced Cancer Care

Haughney A: Nausea and vomiting in end-stage cancer, *Am J Nurs* 104(11):40-48, 2004.

Held-Warmkessel J: Managing three critical cancer complications, *Nursing* 35(1):58-63, 2005.

Mamimgo J: Peripheral blood stem cell transplant: easier than getting blood from a bone, *Nursing* 32(12):52-55, 2002.

Panke JT: Difficulties in managing pain at the end of lie, *Am J Nurs* 102(7):26-33, 2002.

Virani R, Sofer D: Improving the quality of end of life care, *Am J Nurs* 103(5):52-60, 2003.

Chemotherapy

Coyne BM, Leslie ML: Chemo's toll on memory, *RN* 67(4):40-43, 2004.

Gillespie T: Anemia in cancer: therapeutic implications and intervention, *Cancer Nurs* 26(2):119-128, 2003.

Green JM, Hacker ED: Chemotherapy in the geriatric population, *Clin J Oncol Nurs* 8(6):591-597, 638-640, 2004.

Kwong K: Prevention and treatment of oropharyngeal mucositis following cancer therapy: are there new approaches? *Cancer Nurs* 27(3):183, 2004.

McIntyre L: Nutrition management of cancer cachexia and chemotherapy associated nausea and vomiting, *Adv Studies Nurs* 1(1):17, 2003.

Nagel TJ: Help patients cope with chemo, *RN* 67(10):25-30, 2004.

Newton S: Handling chemo safely; your concern too, *RN* 65(5):38-41, 2002.

Sadler GR et al: Managing oral sequelae of cancer therapy, *MedSurg Nurs* 12(1):28, 2003.

Chapter 24: Assessment of the Respiratory System

Carroll P: Pulse oximetry, *RN* 66(9):30ac1-30ac7, 2004.

Cherath L: *Lung biopsy*, accessed June 2004 from website: http://www.healthatoz.com/healthatoz/Atoz/ency/lung_biopsy.html.

De Souza Caroci A, Lareua S: Descriptors of dyspnea by patients with chronic obstructive pulmonary disease versus congestive heart failure, *Heart Lung* 33(2):102-110, 2004.

Moody LE, McMillan S: Dyspnea and quality of life indicators in hospice patients and their caregivers, *Health Qual Life Outcomes* 1(9):1-9, 2003.

Chapter 25: Upper Airway Problems

General

American Lung Association: *Improving life one breath at a time*, accessed June 2004 from website: http://www.lungusa.org/site/pp.asp?c=dvLUK9O0E&b=22542.

Leach MJ: Public, nurse and medical practitioner attitude and practice of natural medicine, *Compl Ther Nurs Midwifery* 10(1):13-21, 2004.

Low JA, Chan DK: Air travel in older people, *Age & Ageing* 31:17-22, 2002.

National Institutes of Health and National Center on Sleep Disorders Research: *Sleep apnea,* accessed June 2004 from website: http://www.nhlbi.nih.gov/about/ncsdr/index.htm.

US Library of Medicine and National Institutes of Health: *Medline plus health topics*, accessed June 2004 from website: http://medlineplus.gov.

Sinusitis

Cavanaugh BM: *Nurse's manual of laboratory and diagnostic tests,* ed 4, Philadelphia, 2003, Davis.

Doty RL, Mishara A: Olfaction and its nasal obstruction, rhinitis, and rhinosinusitis, *Laryngoscope* 111(3):409, 2001.

Sloane PD et al: *Essentials of family medicine,* ed 4, Philadelphia, 2002, Lippincott Williams & Wilkins.

Tarascon pocket pharmacopoeia 2004 classic shirt-pocket edition, Lompoc, Calif, 2004, Tarascon.

Allergies

Hekton-Dunphy LM: *Management guidelines for nurse practitioners working with adults,* ed 2, Philadelphia, 2004, Davis.

Handbook of primary care procedures, Philadelphia, 2003, Lippincott Williams & Wilkins.

LeBlond RF, DeGowin RL, Brown DD: *DeGowin's diagnostic examination*, New York, 2004, McGraw.

Nurse's 3 minute clinical reference, Philadelphia, 2003, Lippincott Williams & Wilkins.

Cancer

Daniel BT, Damato KL, Johnson J: Educational issues in oral care, *Semin Oncol Nurs* 20(1):48-52, 2004.

Hawryluck L: People at the end of life are a vulnerable research population, *Clin Oncol* 16(3):225-226, 2004.

Pauloski BR et al: Surgical variables affecting swallowing in patients treated for oral/oropharyngeal cancer, *Head Neck* 26(7):625-636, 2004.

Shumay G: Determinants of the degree of complementary and alternative medicine use among patients with cancer, *J Altern Complem Med* 8:661-671, 2002.

Zabora JR, Loscalzo MJ, Weber J: Managing complications in cancer: identifying and responding to the patient's perspective, *Semin Oncol Nurs* 19:1-9, 2003.

Chapter 26: Lower Airway Problems

General

Chu JJ: Critical care extra: FYI, *Am J Nurs* 103(9):6411-6414, 2003.

Oh EG: The effects of home-based pulmonary rehabilitation with patients with chronic lung disease, *Int J Nurs Studies* 40(8):873-879, 2003.

Respiratory challenge, *Nursing* 34(11):70-71, 2004.

Tamul, PC, Peruzzi, WT: Assessment and management of patients with pulmonary disease, *Crit Care Med* 342(4):S137-S145, 2004.

Wood smoke a killer, *Austral Nurs J* 11(10):29, 2004.

Acute Lung Injury and Acute Respiratory Distress Syndrome

Harcombe CJ: Nursing patients with ARDS in the prone position, *Nurs Studies* 18(19):33-39, 2004.

Kane C, Galanes S: Adult respiratory distress syndrome, *Crit Care Nurs Q* 27(4):325-335, 2004.

PEEP level not an issue with ARDS patients, *Nursing* 34(11):32, 2004.

Rance M: Kinetic therapy positively influences oxygenation in patients with ALI/ARDS, *Crit Care Nurs* 10(1):35-41, 2005.

Dyspnea

Ayers DM: Act fast when your patient has dyspnea, *Nursing* 34(7):36-41, 2004.

Bailey PH: The dyspnea-anxiety-dyspnea cycle—COPD patients' stories of breathlessness: it's scary when you can't breathe, *Qual Health Res* 14(6):760-778, 2004.

Joyce M et al: The use of nebulized opioids in the management of dyspnea: evidence synthesis, *Oncol Nurs* 31(3):551-560, 2004.

Nebulized fentanyl provides subjective improvements for patients with dyspnea, *Oncol Nurs Forum* 32(1):15, 2005.

Lung Cancer

Houlihan NG et al: Symptom management of lung cancer, *Clin J Oncol Nurs* 8(6):645-653, 2004.

Leak AN, Hubbartt B, King CR: Screening for lung cancer with computed tomography has not proven beneficial, *Oncol Nurs Forum* 31(6):1046, 2004.

Moore S: Guidelines on the role of the specialist nurse in supporting patients with lung cancer, *Europ J Cancer Care* 13(4):344-348, 2004.

Quality of life and meaning of illness of women with lung cancer, *Oncol Nurs Forum* 32(1):E9-19, 2005.

Pneumonia

Antiulcer drug linked to pneumonia, *Nursing* 35(1):34, 2005.

Greci LS, Katz DL, Jekel J: Vaccinations in pneumonia (VIP): pneumococcal and influenza vaccination patterns among patients hospitalized for pneumonia, *Prev Med* 40(4):384-388, 2005.

Kleinpell RM, Elpern EH: Community-acquired pneumonia, *Crit Care Nurs Q* 27(3):231-240, 2004.

Myrianthefs PM et al: Nosocomial pneumonia, *Crit Care Nurs Q* 27(3):241-257, 2004.

Pulmonary Embolism

Applying antiembolism socks isn't just pulling on socks, *Nursing* 34(8):48-49, 2004.

Cardin T, Marinelli A: Pulmonary embolism, *Crit Care Nurs Q* 27(4):310-322, 2004.

Heit J et al: Relative impact of risk factors for deep vein thrombosis and pulmonary embolism, *Arch Intern Med* 162(11):1245-1249, 2002.

Koschel MJ: Pulmonary embolism, *Am J Nurs* 104(6):46-49, 2004.

Tuberculosis

Bargman C: TNF inhibitors and tuberculosis, *Am J Nurs* 104(11):15-16, 2004.

DeCastro AB: Respiratory protection, *Am J Nurs* 104(12):88, 2004.

Dick J et al: Changing professional practice in tuberculosis care: an educational intervention, *J Adv Nurs* 48(5):434-442, 2004.

Rayner D: Tuberculosis and HIV infection: minimizing transmission, *Nurs Studies* 19(4):47-53, 2004.

Chapter 27: Chronic Respiratory Problems

Asthma

Asthma review tool for nurses, *Pract Nurs* 28(3):9, 2004.

Attacking asthma, *Nursing* 34(10):18, 2004.

Corbridge SJ, Corbridge TC: Severe exacerbations of asthma, *Crit Care Nurs Q* 27(3):207-230, 2004.

Popular asthma remedy may worsen condition, *Nursing* 34(9):30, 2004.

Roberts J, Williams A: Quality of life and asthma control with low-dose inhaled corticosteroids, *Brit J Nurs* 13(19):1124-1129, 2004.

Chronic Obstructive Pulmonary Disease

Booker R: Pharmacological approaches to stable chronic obstructive pulmonary disease, *Brit J Nurs* 13(19):1130-1134, 2004.

Cicutto L, Brooks D, Henderson K: Self-care from the perspective of individuals with chronic obstructive pulmonary disease, *Patient Educ Counsel* 55(2):168-176, 2004.

Gaber KA et al: Attitudes of 100 patients with chronic obstructive pulmonary disease to artificial ventilation and cardiopulmonary resuscitation, *Palliative Med* 18(7):626-629, 2004.

O'Neill P: Nutrition for a patient with COPD can be complicated, *Nursing* 34(12):32-33, 2004.

Cystic Fibrosis

Gee L et al: Quality of life in cystic fibrosis: the impact of gender, general health perceptions and disease severity, *J Cystic Fibrosis* 2(4):206-213, 2003.

Gjengedal E et al: Growing up and living with cystic fibrosis, *Adv Nurs Sci* 26(2):149-159, 2003.

Lowton K: Parents and partners: lay carers' perceptions of their role in the treatment and care of adults with cystic fibrosis, *J Adv Nurs* 39(2):174-181, 2002.

Treatment of cystic fibrosis can be subjected to a postcode lottery, *Brit J Nurs* 13(5):239.

Wille MC et al: Advances in preconception genetic counseling, *J Perinat Neonat Nurs* 18(1):28-40, 2004.

Lung Transplantation

Cicutto L et al: Factors affecting attainment of paid employment after lung transplantation, *J Heart Lung Transpl* 23(4):481-486, 2004.

Feurer ID et al: Refining a health-related quality of life assessment strategy for solid organ transplant patients, *Clin Transpl* 12(18):39-45, 2004.

Lobo FS, Gross CR, Matthees BJ: Estimation and comparison of derived preference scores from the SF-36 in lung transplant patients, *Qual Life Res* 13(2):377-388, 2004.

Mechanical Ventilation

Chlan LL: Relationship between two anxiety instruments in patients receiving mechanical ventilatory support, *J Adv Nurs* 48(5):493-499, 2004.

Fenstermacher D, Hong D: Mechanical ventilation, *Crit Care Nurs Q* 27(3):258-294, 2004.

Gelinas C et al: Pain assessment and management in critically ill intubated patients: a retrospective study, *Am J Crit Care* 13(2):126-135, 2004.

Sinuff T et al: Evaluation of a practice guideline for noninvasive positive-pressure ventilation for acute respiratory failure, *CHEST* 123(6):2062-2073, 2003.

Respiratory Failure

Engoren M, Arslanian-Engoren C, Fenn-Buder N: Hospital and long-term outcome after tracheostomy for respiratory failure, *CHEST* 125(1):220-227, 2004.

Guerin C et al: Effects of systematic prone positioning in hypoxic acute respiratory failure: a randomized controlled trial, *JAMA* 292(19):2379-2387, 2004.

Kim MJ, Hwang HJ, Song HH: A randomized trial on the effects of body positions on lung function with acute respiratory failure patients, *Int J Nurs Studies* 39(5):549-555, 2002.

Markou NK, Myrianthefs PV, Baltopoulos, GJ: Respiratory failure, *Crit Care Nurs Q* 27(4):353-379, 2004.

Chapter 28: Assessment of the Cardiovascular System

Bittner NP: *An exploration of critical thinking and processing in cardiac nurses' practice,* University of Rhode Island doctoral dissertation, 2001.

Burke LE, Fair J: Promoting prevention: skill sets and attributes of health care providers who deliver behavioral interventions, *J Cardiovasc Nurs* 18(4):256-266, 2003.

Daniels L: Diet and coronary heart disease, *Nurs Standard* 16(43):47-52, 54-55, 2002.

Joss K, Lindsay G: Nurse-led interventions contribute to cutting the risks for heart disease, *Profess Nurse* 18(11):649-651, 2003.

Miller CE, Ratner PA, Johnson JL: Reducing cardiovascular risk: identifying predictors of smoking relapse, *Can J Cardiovasc Nurs* 13(3):7-12, 2003.

Chapter 29: Coronary Artery Disease and Dysrhythmias

Coronary Artery Disease: Stable Angina and Acute Coronary Syndromes

Berra K: The effect of lifestyle interventions on quality of life and patient satisfaction with health and health care, *J Cardiovasc Nurs* 18(4):319-325, 2003.

Brosche TA, Middleton SK, Boogaard RG: Enhanced external counterpulsation, *DCCN: Dimens Crit Care Nurs* 23(5):208-216, 2004.

Leeper B: Continuous ST-segment monitoring, *AACN Clin Issues: Adv Pract Acute Crit Care* 14(2):145-154, 2003.

Moriarty M: Heart disease (women's health), *RN* 67(1):32-37, 2004.

Robinson SL: Is it an MI? What the leads tell you, *RN* 67(5):48-54, 2004.

Percutaneous Coronary Interventions

Leeper B: Nursing outcomes: percutaneous coronary interventions, *J Cardiovasc Nurs* 19(5):346-353, 2004.

Levine GN et al: American Heart Association Diagnostic and Interventional Catheterization Committee and Council on Clinical Cardiology: Management of patients undergoing percutaneous coronary revascularization, *Ann Intern Med* 139(2):123-136, 2003.

Dysrhythmias

American College of Cardiology, American Heart Association, European Society of Cardiology: *Pocket guidelines: management of patients with atrial fibrillation,* accessed Dec 2004 from website: http://www.americanheart.org/downloadable/heart/1017094776302AF_pktguideline.pdf.

Bosen DM, Flemming MA: Beyond ECGs: understanding electrophysiology testing, part 1 *Nursing* 33(1):32cc1-5, 2003.

Bosen DM, Flemming MA: Beyond ECGs: understanding electrophysiology testing, part 2, *Nursing* 33(2):32cc1-2, 32cc4, 2003.

Overbay D, Criddle L: Mastering temporary invasive cardiac pacing, *Crit Care Nurse* 24(3):25-32, 2004.

Shea JB: Quality of life issues in patients with implantable cardioverter defibrillators: driving, occupation, and recreation, *AACN Clin Issues: Adv Pract Acute Crit Care* 15(3):478-489, 2004.

Chapter 30: Heart Failure, Valvular Problems, and Inflammatory Problems of the Heart

Inflammatory Heart Disease

Understanding cardiomyopathies, *Nursing* 34(4):62-63, 2004.

Ezell J: A 34-year-old woman with fever, tachycardia, vomiting, and hemiparesis, *J Emerg Nurs* 30(3):275-277, 2004.

Holcomb SS: Recognizing and managing myocarditis, *Nursing* 34(4):32cc1-2, 32cc4, 2004.

Wisniewski A: Muscle up your knowledge of myocarditis, *Nursing* 34(10):17, 2004.

Heart Failure

Artinian NT: The psychosocial aspects of heart failure: depression and anxiety can exacerbate the already devastating effects of the disease, *Am J Nurs* 103(12):32-43, 2003.

Deaton C, Grady KL: State of the science for cardiovascular nursing outcomes: heart failure, *J Cardiovasc Nurs* 19(5):329-338, 2004.

Lowery SL, Massaro R, Yancy CW: Advances in the management of acute and chronic decompensated heart failure, *Lippincott's Case Manage* 9(2 Suppl):S1-S17, 2004.

Naylor L et al: CHF in the elderly: using ACE inhibitors appropriately, *Nurse Pract* 29(7):46-49, 51-52, 2004.

Riggs JM: New therapies for heart failure, *RN* 67(3):28-33, 2004.

Zambroski CH: Hospice as an alternative model of care for older patients with end-stage heart failure, *J Cardiovasc Nurs* 19(1):76-85, 2004.

Cardiac Surgery

Asilioglu K, Celik SS: The effect of preoperative education on anxiety of open cardiac surgery patients, *Patient Educ Counsel* 53(1):65-70, 2004.

Hyett JM: Caring for a patient after CABG surgery, *Nursing* 34(7):48-49, 2004.

Rantanen A et al: Coronary artery bypass grafting: social support for patients and their significant others, *J Clin Nurs* 13(2):158-166, 2004.

Redecker NS, Ruggiero J, Hedges C: Patterns and predictors of sleep pattern disturbances after cardiac surgery, *Res Nurs Health* 27(4):217-224, 2004.

Whitman GR: Nursing sensitive outcomes in cardiac surgery patients, *J Cardiovasc Nursing* 19(5):293-300, 2004.

Devices

Bond AE et al: The left ventricular assist device, *Am J Nurs* 103(1):32-41, 2003.

Stahovich M, Chilcott S, Ferber L: Management of adult patients with a left ventricular assist device, *Rehabil Nurs* 29(3):100-103, 2004.

Chapter 31: Vascular Problems

Hypertension

Alves L et al: White coat hypertension and nursing care, *Can J Cardiovasc Nurs* 13(3):29-34, 2003.

Bacon SL: Effects of exercise, diet and weight loss on high blood pressure, *Sports Med* 34(5):307-316, 2004.

Bengsten A, Drevenhorn E: The nurses role and skills in hypertension care, *Clin Nurse Spec* 17(5):260-268, 2003.

McFadden C, Townsend R: Blood pressure measurement: common pitfalls and how to avoid them, *Consultant* 43:161-165, 2003.

Woods A: Loosening the grip of hypertension, *Nursing* 34(12):36-43, 2004.

Vascular Leg Ulcers

Heinen MM et al: Venous leg ulcer patients: a review of the literature on lifestyle and pain related interventions, *J Clin Nurs* 13(3):355-366, 2004.

Leach MJ: Making sense of the venous leg ulcer debate, *J Wound Care* 13(2):52-56, 2004.

Sieggreen M, Kline R: Recognizing and managing venous leg ulcers, *Adv Skin Wound Care* 17(6):302-322, 2004.

Peripheral Vascular Disease

Abou-Zamzam AM: Detection and treatment of peripheral arterial occlusive disease, *J Clin Outcomes Manage* 11(5):308-320, 2004.

Hale RW: Peripheral arterial disease detection, awareness, and treatment, *ACOG Clin Rev* 7(2):15, 2002.

Holman JR: Peripheral arterial disease: tips on diagnosis and management, *Consultant* 44(1):101-103, 107-108, 2004.

Mohler ER: Peripheral arterial disease: identification and implications, *Arch Intern Med* 163(19):2306-2314, 2003.

Olson KWP, Treat-Jacobson D: Symptoms of peripheral arterial disease: a critical review, *J Vasc Nurs* 22(3):72-77, 2004.

Treat-Jacobson D et al: A patient derived perspective of health related quality of life with peripheral arterial disease, *J Nurs Scholarship* 34(1):55-60, 2002.

Chapter 32: Assessment of the Hematologic System

Lee KW, Lip GYH: Effect of lifestyle on hemostasis, fibrinolysis, and platelet reactivity: a systematic review, *Arch Intern Med* 163(19):2368-2392, 2003.

Mann KG, Butenas S, Brummel K: The dynamics of thrombin formation, *Arteriosclerosis Thromb Vasc Biol* 23(1):17-25, 2003.

Monroe DM, Hoffman M, Roberts HR: Platelets and thrombin generation, *Arteriosclerosis Thromb Vasc Biol* 22(9):1381-1389, 2002.

Tefferi A: Anemia in adults: a contemporary approach to diagnosis, *Mayo Clin Proc* 78(10):1274-1280, 2003.

Wagner DD, Burger PC: Platelets in inflammation and thrombosis, *Arteriosclerosis Thromb Vasc Biol* 23:2131, 2003.

Chapter 33: Hematologic Problems

Anemia

Catlin AJ: Thalassemia: the facts and the controversies, *Pediatric Nurs* 29(6):447-451, 2003.

Gillespie TW: Anemia in cancer: therapeutic implications and interventions, *Cancer Nurs* 26(2):119-128, 2003.

Hemoglobinopathy

Critical care extra FYI: pulse oximetry in sickle cell disease, *Am J Nurs* 102(2):24II, 2002.

D'Arcy Y: Managing sickle-cell crisis, *Nursing* 34(1):24-25, 2004.

Leukemia

Aschenbrenner DS, Chu JJ: Gleevec demonstrates long-term benefits, *Am J Nurs* 104(3):77, 2004.

Breed CD: Diagnosis, treatment, and nursing care of patients with chronic leukemia, *Semin Oncol Nurs* 19(2):109-117, 2003.

Coyle B, Polovich M: Handling hazardous drugs, *Am J Nurs* 104(2):104, 2004.

Murphy-Ende K, Chernecky C: Assessing adults with leukemia, *Nurse Pract* 27(11):49-60, 2002.

Viele CS: Diagnosis, treatment, and nursing care of acute leukemia, *Semin Oncol Nurs* 19(2):98-108, 2003.

Lymphoma

Sidney Kimmel Comprehensive Cancer Center at Johns Hopkins: *Lymphoma*, accessed Aug 2004 from website: www.hopkinskimmelcancercenter.org/cancertypes.

US National Library of Medicine and National Institutes of Health: *Adult non-Hodgkin's lymphoma: treatment,* accessed Aug 2004 from website: www.nlm.nih.gov/medlineplus/healthtopics/lymphoma.

Stem Cell Transplant

Jacobsohn DA et al: Reduced intensity haemopoietic stem-cell transplantation treatment of non-malignant diseases in children, *Lancet* 363(9429):156-162, 2004.

Maningo J: Peripheral blood stem cell transplant: easier than getting blood from a bone, *Nursing 2002* 32(12):52-55, 2002.

Chapter 34: Assessment of the Renal System

Boulton-Jones M: Renal biopsy. In Johnson RJ, Feehally J, editors: *Comprehensive clinical nephrology*, ed 2, Philadelphia, 2003, Mosby.

Fischbach FT, Dunning MB: *A manual of laboratory and diagnostic tests*, ed 7, Philadelphia, 2004, Lippincott Williams & Wilkins.

Parsons RB, Simpson WL: Imaging. In Johnson RJ, Feehally J, editors: *Comprehensive clinical nephrology*, ed 2, Philadelphia, 2003, Mosby.

Rahman M et al: A comparison of standardized versus "usual" blood pressure measurements in hemodialysis patients, *Am J Kidney Dis* 39(6):1226, 2002.

Chapter 35: Kidney and Urinary Tract Problems

General

Howell A, Foxman B: Cranberry juice and adhesion of antibiotic-resistant uropathogens, *JAMA* 287(23):3083-3084, 2002.

Miller A, Bartsch H: Hair dye use and bladder cancer, *Int J Cancer* 94(6):901-902, 2001.

Qiang W, Ke Z: Water for preventing urinary calculi (Cochrane Review). In *Cochrane Library,* Issue 3, 2004, Chichester, UK, John Wiley & Sons.

Schaeffer A: Infections and inflammations of the genitourinary tract. In Walsh P et al, editors: *Campbell's urology*, ed 8, Philadelphia, 2002, Saunders.

Urinary Incontinence

Appell R: Injection therapy for urinary incontinence. In Walsh P et al, editors: *Campbell's urology*, ed 8, Philadelphia, 2002, Saunders.

Bates F: Assessment of the female patient with urinary incontinence, *Urol Nurs* 22(5):305-314, 2002.

Burgio K et al: Behavioral training with and without biofeedback in the treatment of urge incontinence in older women: a randomized controlled trial, *JAMA* 288(18):2293-2299, 2002.

Newman D, Palmer M, editors: The state of the science on urinary incontinence, *Am J Nurs* 3(Suppl):1-58, 2003.

Wallace SA et al: Bladder training for urinary incontinence in adults (Cochrane Review). In *Cochrane Library,* Issue 3, 2004, Chichester, UK, John Wiley & Sons.

Chapter 36: Kidney Failure

General

Bailie G: Calcium and phosphorus management in chronic kidney disease: challenges and trends, *Formulary* 39(7):358-360, 361-362, 364-365, 2004.

Burrows-Hudson S: Chronic kidney disease: an overview: early and aggressive treatment is vital, *Am J Nurs* 105(2):40-50, 2005.

Cho Y, Tsay S: The effect of acupressure with massage on fatigue and depression in patients with end-stage renal disease, *J Nurs Res* 12(1): 51-59, 2004.

Cody J et al: Frequency of administration of recombinant human erythropoietin for anaemia of end-stage renal disease in dialysis patients (Cochrane Review). In *Cochrane Library* (Oxford), Issue 1, Chichester, UK, 2005, John Wiley & Sons.

Daine P: Pain management at the end of life in a patient with renal failure, *CANNT J* 14(2):20-25, 2004.

Hiewe S, Dahlgren M: Living with chronic renal failure: coping with physical activities of daily living, *Adv Physiother* 6(4):147-157, 2004.

Holcomb S: Evaluating chronic kidney disease risk, *Nurse Pract* 30(4):12-14, 17-18, 23-27, 2005.

Kasinskas C, Piazza D: Chronic renal failure—a clinical pathway, *Acute Care Perspect* 13(3):1, 3-4, 2004.

Kurella M et al: Cognitive impairment in chronic kidney disease, *J Am Geriatr Soc* 52(11):1863-1869, 2004.

McCarley P, Salai P: Cardiovascular disease in chronic kidney disease: recognizing and reducing the risk of a common CKD comorbidity, *Am J Nurs* 105(4):40-53, 2005.

Dialysis

Breiterman-White R: Functional ability of patients on dialysis: the critical role of anemia, *J Nephrol Nurs* 32(1):79-82, 2005.

Curtin R, Johnson H, Schatell D: The peritoneal dialysis experience: insights from long-term patients, *J Nephrol Nurs* 31(6):615-625, 2004.

Dharmarajan T, Kaul N, Russell R: Dialysis in the old: a centenarian nursing home resident with end-stage renal disease, *J Am Med Dir Assoc* 5(3):186-191, 2004.

Dinwiddie L: Managing catheter dysfunction for better patient outcomes: a team approach, *J Nephrol Nurs* 31(6):653-660, 671, 2004.

Giri M: Choice of renal replacement therapy in patients with diabetic end stage renal disease, *J EDTNA ERCA* 30(3):138-142, 2004.

Gregory N: Attaining target hemoglobin levels in patients new to dialysis: individualizing therapy based on initial hemoglobin levels, *J Nephrol Nurs* 31(6):672-675, 2004.

Hagren B et al: Maintenance haemodialysis: patients' experiences of their life situation, *J Clin Nurs* 14(3):294-300, 2005.

Purcell W et al: Accurate dry weight assessment: reducing the incidence of hypertension and cardiac disease in patients on hemodialysis, *J Nephrol Nurs* 31(6):631-638, 2004.

Rahman M et al: A comparison of standardized versus "usual" blood pressure measurements in hemodialysis patients, *Am J Kidney Dis* 39(6):1226, 2002.

Vale L et al: Continuous ambulatory peritoneal dialysis (CAPD) versus hospital or home haemodialysis for end-stage renal disease in adults (Cochrane Review). In *Cochrane Library,* Issue 1, Chichester, UK, 2005, John Wiley & Sons.

Vaughn D: Timing is everything when it comes to hemodialysis, *Nurs Spectrum* 14(18):10-11, 2004.

Vilaplana J: Blood pressure and cardiovascular complications in diabetic dialysis patients, *J EDTNA ERCA* 30(3):128-130, 2004.

Williams A et al: Early clinical, quality-of-life, and biochemical changes of daily hemodialysis, *Am J Kidney Dis* 43(1):90-102, 2004.

Nutrition

Axelsson J et al: Truncal fat mass as a contributor to inflammation in end-stage renal disease, *Am J Clin Nutr* 80(5):1222-1229, 2004.

Carvalho K, Silva M, Bregman R: Nutritional profile of patients with chronic renal failure, *J Renal Nutr* 14(2):97-100, 2004.

Cooper B et al: Protein malnutrition and hypoalbuminemia as predictors of vascular events and mortality in ESRD, *Am J Kidney Dis* 43(1):61-66, 2004.

Cuppari L, Avesani C: Energy requirements in patients with chronic kidney disease, *J Renal Nutr* 14(3):121-126, 2004.

Kaysen G: The influence of patient- and facility-specific factors on nutritional status and survival in hemodialysis, *J Renal Nutr* 14(2):72-81, 2004.

Chapter 37: Assessment of the Endocrine System

DeGroot L, Jameson JL, editors: *Endocrinology*, ed 4, Philadelphia, 2001, Saunders.

Chapter 38: Pituitary, Thyroid, Parathyroid, and Adrenal Gland Problems

Becker KL, editor: *Principles and practice of endocrinology and metabolism*, ed 3, Philadelphia, 2001, Lippincott.

DeGroot L, Jameson JL, editors: *Endocrinology*, ed 4, Philadelphia, 2001, Saunders.

Larsen PR et al, editors: *Williams textbook of endocrinology*, ed 10, Philadelphia, 2003, Saunders.

Chapter 39: Diabetes Mellitus and Hypoglycemia

Harmel AP, Mathur R: *Davidson's diabetes mellitus*, ed 5, Philadelphia, 2004, Saunders.

Larsen PR et al, editors: *Williams textbook of endocrinology*, ed 10, Philadelphia, 2003, Saunders.

Porte D, Sherwin RS, Baron A, editors: *Ellenberg and Rifkin's diabetes mellitus*, ed 6, New York, 2004, McGraw-Hill.

Chapter 40: Assessment of the Gastrointestinal, Biliary, and Exocrine Pancreatic Systems

Goldrick BA: Emerging infections—hepatitis A: another vaccine preventable disease continues to emerge, *Am J Nurs* 104(3):27-28, 2004.

Jarrett M, Cox P: Hepatitis C virus, *Nurs Clin North Am* 39(1):219-229, 2004.

Rao SS: Constipation: evaluation and treatment, *Gastroenterol Clin North Am* 32:659-683, 2003.

Talley NJ: Dyspepsia: management guidelines for the millennium, *Gut* 50(4):72-78, 2002.

Woodward BG: Bariatric surgery options, *Crit Care Nurs Q* 26(2):89-100, 2003.

Chapter 41: Mouth and Esophagus Problems

Gastroesophageal Reflux Disease

Karlowicz D: An endoscopic approach to GERD? *RN* 66(12):56-60, 2003.

Levy RA, Stamm L, Meiner SE: Conservative management of GERD: a case study, *MedSurg Nurs* 11(4):169-175, 2002.

Ray SW et al: Managing gastroesophageal reflux disease, *Nurse Pract* 27(5):36-38, 2002

Rayhorn N, Argel N, Demchak K: Understanding gastroesophageal reflux disease, *Nursing* 33(10):36-41, 2003.

Williams H: Gastroesophageal reflux disease: clinical manifestations, *Gastroenterol Nurs* 26(5):195-202, 2003.

Oral Cancer

Hatsukami DK, Lemmonds C, Tomar SL: Smokeless tobacco use: harm reduction or induction approach? *Prevent Med* 38:309-317, 2004.

Oral care update, *Nurs Manage* 34(3 Suppl):1-11, 2003.

Sadler GR et al: Managing the oral sequelae of cancer therapy, *MedSurg Nurs* 12(1):28-35, 2003.

Taybos G: Oral changes associated with tobacco use, *Am J Med Sci* 326(4):179-182, 2003.

Weinberg MA, Estefan DJ: Assessing oral malignancies, *Am Fam Phys* 65(7):1379-1384, 2002.

Esophageal Cancer

Enzinger PC, Mayer RJ: Esophageal cancer, *N Engl J Med* 349:2241-2252, 2003.

Mackenzie DJ, Popplewell PK, Billingsley KG: Care of patients after esophagectomy, *Crit Care Nurse* 24(1):16-29, 2004.

Pickens A, Orringer MB: Geographical distribution and racial disparity in esophageal cancer, *Ann Thorac Surg* 76:S1367-S1369, 2003.

Tak VM, Naunheim KS: Current status of multimodality therapy for esophageal carcinoma, *J Surg Res* 117:22-29, 2004.

Chapter 42: Stomach and Duodenum Problems

Enteral and Parenteral Nutrition

Koretz RL: Enteral nutrition led to fewer postoperative complications than did parenteral feeding in gastrointestinal cancer, *ACP J Club* 136(3):93, 2002.

Mitchell SL et al: Why so many feeding tubes in nursing homes? *JAMA* 290(1):73-80, 2003.

Olsson U, Bergbom I, Bosaeus I: Patients' experiences of their intake of food and fluid following gastrectomy due to tumor, *Gastroenterol Nurs* 25(4):146-153, 2002.

Smith CE et al: Reducing complications of home parenteral nutrition, *J Parenteral Enteral Nutr* 27(2):137-145, 2003.

Van Soren M: Enteral nutrition reduced postoperative complications but increased minor adverse effects in gastrointestinal cancer, *Evidence Based Nurs* 5(3):88, 2002.

Stress Ulcers

Abraham E: Acid suppression in a critical care environment, *Crit Care Med* 30(6):S349-S350, 2002.

Bucknall T: Several interventions prevent ventilator associated pneumonia in critically ill patients, *Evidence Based Nurs* 64(4):112, 2003.

Flannery J, Tucker DA: Pharmacologic prophylaxis and treatment of stress ulcers in critically ill patients, *Crit Care Clin North Am* 14(1):39-51, 2002.

Kunis KA, Puntillo KA: Ventilator associated pneumonia in the ICU, *Am J Nurs* 103(8):64AA-GG, 2003.

Gastrointestinal Bleeding

Armour D: Blood and guts: a 10 year perspective, *Gastrointestinal Nurs* 2(2):6-7, 2004.

Goolsby MJ: Clinical practice guidelines: evaluation and management of occult and obscure gastrointestinal bleeding, *J Am Acad Nurse Pract* 15(1):3-4, 2003.

Peptic Ulcer Disease

Der G: An overview of proton pump inhibitors, *Gastroenterol Nurs* 26(5):182-190, 2003.

Ebell M: What is the best way to prevent ulcers in patients taking NSAIDs? *Evidence Based Pract* 5(12):4, 2002.

H. pylori eradication options for peptic ulcer, *Nurse Pract Prescribing Ref* 11(1):146, 2004.

O'Malley P: Gastric ulcers and GERD: the new plagues of the 21st century—update for the clinical nurse specialist, *Clin Nurse Spec* 17(6):286-289, 2003.

Vanderhoff BT, Tahboub RM: Proton pump inhibitors: an update, *Am Fam Phys* 66(2):273-280, 2002.

Chapter 43: Intestinal Problems

General

Bresciani C et al: Laparoscopic versus standard appendectomy outcomes and cost comparisons in the private sector, *J Gastrointest Surg* 9(8): 1174-1181, 2005.

Dorman BP et al: Bowel management in the intensive care unit, *Intensive Crit Care Nurs* 20(6):320-329, 2004.

Hughes E: Caring for the patient with an intestinal obstruction, *Nurs Standard* 19(47):56-64, 66, 68, 2005.

Mauk KL: Healthier aging: preventing constipation in older adults, *Nursing* 35(6):22-23, 2005.

Steffen R: Epidemiology of traveler's diarrhea, *Clin Infect Dis* 41(Suppl 8): S536-S540, 2005.

Diverticular Disease

Salzman H, Lillie D: Diverticular disease: diagnosis and treatment, *Am Fam Phys* 72(7):1229-1234, 2005.

Salzman H, Lillie D: Diverticular disease: what you should know, *Am Fam Phys* 72(7):1241-1242, 2005.

Irritable Bowel Syndrome

Bristow N: Clinical knowledge: understanding the symptoms of irritable bowel syndrome, *Nurs Times* 101(10):36-38, 2005.

Inflammatory Bowel Disease

Stein P: Home study program: ulcerative colitis—diagnosis and surgical treatment, *AORN J* 80(2):242-253, 255-256, 258, 2004.

Ostomy Care

Beitz JM: Continent diversions: the new gold standards of ileoanal reservoir and neobladder, *Ostomy Wound Manage* 50(9):26-37, 2004.

Burch J: Psychological problems and stomas: a rough guide for community nurses, *Brit J Commun Nurs* 10(5):224-227, 2005.

Ringhofer J: Meeting the needs of your ostomy patient, *RN* 68(8):37-41, 2005.

Simmermacher NT: Common issues in ostomy care: diarrhea and excoriation in a patient with an ileoanal reservoir, *Adv Nurse Pract* 12(7):59-60, 62, 2004.

Turnbull GB: What is preventive ostomy care? *Ostomy Wound Manage* 51(5):22-24, 2005.

Ziegler M, French ET: How do we manage difficult ostomy pouching in the rehabilitation setting? *Rehabil Nurs* 30(3):84, 2005.

Chapter 44: Gallbladder and Exocrine Pancreatic Problems

Cholecystitis

Leitzmann MF et al: Coffee intake is associated with lower risk of symptomatic gallstone disease in women, *Gastroenterology* 123(6):1823-1830, 2002.

Shamiyeh A, Waynard W: Laparoscopic cholecystectomy: early and late complications and their treatment, *Langenbecks Arch Surg* 389(3):164-171, 2004.

Carcinoma of the Biliary System

Pack DA, O'Connor K, O'Hagan K: Cholangiocarcinoma: a nursing perspective, *Clin J Oncol Nurs* 5(4):141-146, 155-156, 2001.

Pancreatitis

Cole L: Unraveling the mystery of acute pancreatitis, *Nursing* 31(12):58-64, 2001.

Dimagno MJ, Dimagno EP: Chronic pancreatitis, *Curr Opin Gastroenterol* 19(5):451-457, 2003.

Nagar AB, Gorelick FS: Acute pancreatitis, *Curr Opin Gastroenterol* 20(5):439-443, 2004.

Paulsen C: Meperidine or morphine for treatment of pancreatic pain? *RN* 65(5):10, 2002.

Quillen S: Identification of pancreatitis in the ambulatory setting, *Gastroenterol Nurs* 24(1):20-22, 2001.

Pancreatic Cancer

Brescia FJ: Palliative care in pancreatic cancer, *Cancer Control* 11(1):39-45, 2004.

Gavaghan M: The pancreas: hermit of the abdomen, *AORN J* 75(6):1109-1111, 1113-1114, 1117, 2002.

Trujillo EB, Robinson, MK, Jacobs DO: Nutrition—feeding critically ill patients: current concepts, *Crit Care Nurse* 21(4):60-71, 2001.

Zervos EM et al: Surgical management of early-stage pancreatic cancer, *Cancer Control* 11(1):23-31, 2004.

Chapter 45: Assessment of the Hepatic System

First parenteral antidote approved, *Nursing* 34(4):10, 2004.

Jajwiga JL et al: Serum metabolite/caffeine ratios as a test for liver function, *J Clin Pharmacol* 44(4):338, 2004.

MacKenzie S et al: Recent experience with a multidisciplinary approach to complex hepatic trauma, *Injury* 35(9):869-877, 2004.

Nailing a key assessment, *Nursing* 33(8):50, 2003.

Noninfectious liver disorders: assessment and diagnosis/adult autoimmune hepatitis, *Nurse Pract* 28(12):32, 2003.

Chapter 46: Hepatic Problems

General

Aschenbrenner DS: Revised warning on HIV drug packaging, *Am J Nurs* 104(5):29, 2004.

Cells from unusable livers extend life, *Nursing* 33(9):35, 2003.

Dolbey CH: Hemochromatosis: a review, *Clin J Oncol Nurs* 5(6):257, 2001.

Drug news, *Nursing* 32(9):70, 2002.

MacKenzie S et al: Recent experience with a multidisciplinary approach to complex hepatic trauma, *Injury* 35(9):869-877, 2004.

Hepatitis

Davidson L et al: How our community handles one of the largest outbreaks in the United States, *Nursing* 34(6):44, 2004.

Fleming J: Current treatments for hepatitis, *J Infusion Nurs* 25(6):379, 2002.

Goldrick BA: Emerging infections, *Am J Nurs* 104(3):27, 2004.

Richmond J, Dunning P, Desmond P: Hepatitis C: a medical and social diagnosis, *Austral Nurs J* 12(1):23, 2004.

Weber CJ: Update on viral hepatitis, *Urol Nurs* 24(1):56, 2004.

Liver or Biliary Cirrhosis

Cardenas A, Kelleher T, Chopra S: Hepatic hydrothorax, *Aliment Pharmacol Therap* 20(3):271, 2004.

Hines IN, Wheeler MD: Recent advances in alcoholic liver disease III: role of the innate immune response in alcoholic hepatitis, *Am J Physiol: Gastroint Liver Physiol* 50(2):G310, 2004.

Park DK et al: Clinical significance of variceal hemorrhage in recent years in patients with liver cirrhosis and esophageal varices, *J Gastroenterol Hepatol* 19(9):1042, 2004.

Liver Failure

Diaz V, Wykoff MM: Surviving fulminant hepatic failure, *Am J Nurs* 102(5):49, 2002.

Overexpressed p53 is involved in the pathogenesis of fatty liver disease, *Health Med Week*, July 12, 2004, p 961.

Stern A: Vitagen announces enrollment for phase ii trial of ELAD® bioartificial liver support therapy, *Internet J Adv Nurs Pract* 5(2):5, 2003.

Wiklund RA: Preoperative preparation of patients with advanced liver disease, *Crit Care Med* 32(4):S106, 2004.

Chapter 47: Assessment of the Nervous System

Ebell M: Does a longer period of bedrest prevent headache after cervical or lumbar puncture? *Evidence Based Pract* 5(3):6, 2002.

Hansotia P: A neurologist looks at mind and brain: the "enchanted loom," *Clin Med Res* 1(4):327-332, 2003.

Lehman CA et al: Development and implementation of a problem focused neurological assessment system, *J Neurosci Nurs* 35(4):185-192, 2003.

O'Connell B, Baker L, Prosser A: The educational needs of caregivers of stroke survivors in acute and community settings, *J Neurosci Nurs* 35(1):21-28, 2003.

Pierce L et al: Internet-based support for rural caregivers of persons with strokes shows promise, *Rehabil Nurs* 29(3):95-99, 103, 2004.

Riddell AM, Derbyshire NDJ, Gibson MR: Emergency cranial CT scans, *Care Critically Ill* 19(1):10-14, 2003.

Selman JE: Recognizing and treating different kinds of tremors, *Clin Advisor* 6(10):32, 34, 37-39, 2003.

Chapter 48: Traumatic and Neoplastic Problems of the Brain

Increased Intracranial Pressure

Crimlisk JT, Grande MM: Neurologic assessment skills for the acute medical surgical nurse, *Orthop Nurs* 23(1):3-11, 2004.

Josephson L: Management of increased intracranial pressure: a primer for the non-neuro critical care nurse, *Dimens Crit Care Nurs* 23(5):194-207, 2004.

Head Injury

Alexander MH, Raub J: Injury prevention: how to protect your "coconut": a safety demonstration on the importance of wearing a ski helmet, *J Emerg Nurs* 29(5):461-462, 2003.

Bay E et al: Chronic stress, sense of belonging, and depression among survivors of traumatic brain injury, *Image: J Nurs Scholarship* 34(3): 221-226, 2002.

Brettler SJ: Traumatic brain injury, *RN* 67(4):32-36, 2004.

Flick C: Organ donation: a delicate balance, *RN* 65(12):43-47, 2002.

Kaut KP et al: Reports of head injury and symptom knowledge among college athletes: implications for assessment and educational intervention, *Clin J Sport Med* 13(4):213-221, 2003.

LeJeune GM, Howard-Fain T: Nursing assessment and management of patients with head injuries, *Dimens Crit Care Nurs* 21(6):226-231, 2002.

CNS Infections

Bender K, Thompson FE: West Nile virus: a growing challenge, *Am J Nurs* 103(6):32-40, 2003.

Girard BJ: Bugging the system: West Nile virus, *AORN J* 79(2):297-298, 2004.

Huynh C, Rajagopalan S, Scheld WM: Bacterial meningitis in adults, *Topics Emerg Med* 25(2):101-105, 2003.

Katz JR, Hirsch AM: When global health is local health: infectious diseases travel easily, *Am J Nurs* 103(12):75-79, 2003.

Schweon S: West Nile virus: get ready for its return, *RN* 66(4):56-59, 2003.

Brain Tumor

Kanan A, Gasson B: Brain tumor resections guided by magnetic resonance imaging, *AORN J* 77(3):583, 585-586, 588-589, 2003.

Lemke DM: Epidemiology, diagnosis and treatment of patients with metastatic cancer and high grade gliomas of the central nervous system, *J Infusion Nurs* 27(4):263-269, 2004.

Taylor DJ: Role reversal: seeing the patient's perspective when caregiving comes up short, *Am J Nurs* 103(2):31, 2003.

Headache

Berardinelli C, Kupecz D: Annual update: drugs, diagnostic and devices, *Nurse Pract* 28(3):30, 33-39, 2003.

Burton WN et al: The economic burden of lost productivity due to migraine headache, *J Occup Environ Med* 44(6):523-529, 539, 2002.

Frazel JE: Optimize migraine management in primary care, *Nurse Pract* 29(4):22-24, 26-27, 30-33, 2004.

Scholz MJ: Drug update—pain clinic: which triptan is best for your migraine patient? *RN* 66(6):95, 2003.

Sok SR, Kim KB: Acupuncture usage shows relief of chronic symptoms, *Holistic Nurs Pract* 18(4):220, 2004.

Seizures

Chabolla DR: Characteristics of the epilepsies, *Mayo Clinic Proc* 77(9):981-990, 2002.

Liporace J, D'Abreu A: Symposium on seizures: epilepsy and women's health, *Mayo Clin Proc* 78(4):497-506, 2003.

Pena CG: Seizure, *Am J Nurs* 103(11):73-81, 2003.

Sirven JL: Symposium on seizures: antiepileptic drug therapy for adults: when to initiate and how to choose, *Mayo Clin Proc* 77(12):1367-1375, 2002.

Chapter 49: Vascular and Degenerative Problems of the Brain

Carroll L: Researchers tease out cellular biology of ALS, and it is not just motor neurons, *Neurol Today* 5(1):70-72, 2005.

Louw SJ, Keeble JA: Stroke medicine: ethical and legal considerations, *Age & Ageing* 31(53):31-35, 2002.

Teasell R, Kalra L: What's new in stroke rehabilitation: back to basics, *Stroke* 36:215-217, 2005.

Chapter 50: Spinal Cord and Peripheral Nerve Problems

General

Dobkin BH, Havton LA: Basic advances and new avenues in therapy of spinal cord injury, *Ann Rev Med* 55:255-282, 2004.

Dumont AS, Dumont RJ, Oskouian RJ: Will improved understanding of the pathophysiological mechanisms involved in acute spinal cord injury improve the potential for therapeutic intervention? *Curr Opin Neurol* 15(6):713-720, 2002.

Hulsebosch CE: Recent advances in pathophysiology and treatment of spinal cord injury, *Adv Physiol Educ* 26(4):238-255, 2002.

McDonald JW, Becker D: Spinal cord injury: promising interventions and realistic goals, *Am J Phys Med Rehabil* 82(10 Suppl):38-49, 2003.

McIlvoy L, Meyer K, McQuillan KA: Traumatic spine injuries. In Bader MK, Littlejohns LR, editors: *AANN core curriculum for neuroscience nursing*, ed 4, St Louis, 2004, Saunders.

Pathophysiology

Dumont RJ et al: Acute spinal cord injury, part 1, Pathophysiologic mechanisms, *Clin Neuropharmacol* 24(5):254-264, 2001.

Lynch AC et al: Bowel dysfunction following spinal cord injury, *Spinal Cord* 39(4):193-203, 2001.

Segatore M: Managing neural tissue injury in combined vertebral column–spinal cord injury, *Orthop Nurs* 21(2):43-60, 2002.

Collaborative Care Management

American Association of Neurological Surgeons and Congress of Neurological Surgeons, Section on Disorders of the Spine and Peripheral Nerves: Guidelines for the management of acute cervical spinal injuries, *Neurosurgery* 50(3 Suppl): 2002.

Ball PA: Critical care of spinal cord injury, *Spine* 26(Suppl 24):27-30, 2001.

Nockels RP: Nonoperative management of acute spinal cord injury, *Spine* 26(Suppl 24):31-37, 2001.

Paralyzed Veterans of America/Consortium for Spinal Cord Medicine: *Acute management of autonomic dysreflexia: individuals with spinal cord injury presenting to health-care facilities,* Washington, DC, 2001, Paralyzed Veterans of America, accessed from website: www.guidelines.gov.

Nursing Management

Barker E: Neurotrauma: spinal cord injury. In Barker E, editor: *Neuroscience nursing: a spectrum of care,* ed 2, St Louis, 2002, Saunders.

Guin PR: Advances in spinal cord injury care, *Crit Care Nurs Clin North Am* 13(3):399-409, 2001.

Hickey JV: Vertebral and spinal cord injuries. In Hickey JV, editor: *The clinical practice of neurological and neurosurgical nursing,* ed 5, Philadelphia, 2003, Lippincott Williams & Wilkins.

Spine Tumors

Devroom HL et al: Nervous system tumors. In Bader MK, Littlejohns LR, editors: *AANN core curriculum for neuroscience nursing,* ed 4, St Louis, 2004, Saunders.

Hickey JV: Spinal cord tumors. In Hickey JV, editor: *The clinical practice of neurological and neurosurgical nursing,* ed 5, Philadelphia, 2003, Lippincott Williams & Wilkins.

Miers AG: Nontraumatic disorders of the spine. In Barker E, editor: *Neuroscience nursing: a spectrum of care,* ed 2, St Louis, 2002, Saunders.

Cranial Nerve Diseases

Barker E: Cranial nerve deficits. In Barker E, editor: *Neuroscience nursing: a spectrum of care,* ed 2, St Louis, 2002, Saunders.

Filipchuk D: Classic trigeminal neuralgia: a surgical perspective, *J Neurosci Nurs* 35(2):82-86, 2003.

Hickey JV: Cranial nerve diseases. In Hickey JV, editor: *The clinical practice of neurological and neurosurgical nursing,* ed 5, Philadelphia, 2003, Lippincott Williams & Wilkins.

Vandemark MV et al: Infectious and autoimmune processes. In Bader MK, Littlejohns LR, editors: *AANN core curriculum for neuroscience nursing,* ed 4, St Louis, 2004, Saunders.

Peripheral Nerve Injury

Andrews P, Spritz DW: Peripheral nerve injuries. In Bader MK, Littlejohns LR, editors: *AANN core curriculum for neuroscience nursing,* ed 4, St Louis, 2004, Saunders.

Hickey JV: Peripheral nerve injuries. In Hickey JV, editor: *The clinical practice of neurological and neurosurgical nursing,* ed 5, Philadelphia, 2003, Lippincott Williams & Wilkins.

Miers AG: Peripheral nerve disorders. In Barker E, editor: *Neuroscience nursing: a spectrum of care,* ed 2, St Louis, 2002, Saunders.

Chapter 51: Assessment of the Musculoskeletal System

Maher AB et al, editors: *Orthopaedic nursing,* ed 3, Philadelphia, 2002, Saunders.

Seidel HM et al, editors: *Mosby's guide to physical examination,* ed 5, St Louis, 2003, Mosby.

Unger J, Selfridge-Thomas J: The preparticipation evaluation. In *Nursing contact hours for nurse practitioners,* Atlanta, 2001, American Health Consultants.

Chapter 52: Trauma to the Musculoskeletal System

General

Budd GM, Piccioni LH: Identifying and treating common problems of the elbow, *Am J Nurse Pract* 9(2):41-51, 2005.

Childs SG: Stimulators of bone healing: biologic and biomechanical, *Orthop Nurs* 22(6):421-427, 2003.

Ejnisman B et al: Interventions for tears of the rotator cuff in adults (Cochrane Review). In *Cochrane Library,* Issue 3, Chichester, UK, 2004, John Wiley & Sons.

Kneale J, Davis P, editors: *Orthopaedic and trauma nursing,* ed 2, Edinburgh, 2005, Churchill Livingstone.

Le TV et al: Common shoulder problems: a "hands-on" approach to adhesive capsulitis, *Consultant* 44(12):1481-1490, 2004.

Lee RR: Treating sports injuries of weekend warriors, *Clin Advisor* 7(4):38-46, 2004.

Little DR et al: Ankle sprain, *Clin Advisor* 7(11):56, 61-62, 2004.

Maher AB et al, editors: *Orthopaedic nursing,* ed 3, Philadelphia, 2002, Saunders.

Verdugo RJ et al: Surgical versus non-surgical treatment for carpal tunnel syndrome (Cochrane Review). In *Cochrane Library,* Issue 3, Chichester, UK, 2004, John Wiley & Sons.

Fractures

Altizer L: Fractures, *Orthop Nurs* 21(6):51-58, 2002.

Altizer L: Hand and wrist fractures, *Orthop Nurs* 22(2):131-139, 2003.

Altizer L: Major pelvic fractures, *Crit Care Nurse* 24(2):18-32, 2004.

Cranmey A, Adachi JD: Orthopaedic trauma: critical care nursing issues, *Crit Care Nurs Q* 28(1):60-71, 2005.

Hubble C: Ankle fractures, *Emerg Nurse* 13(4):32-38, 2005.

Meister J, Reddy K: Rhabdomyolysis: an overview, *AJN* 100(2):75-79, 2002.

Peate I: Casting for immobilization, *Orthop Nurs* 23(2):136-141, 2004.

Hip Fractures

Altizer L: Hip fractures, *Orthop Nurs* 24(4):283-292, 2005.

Archibald G: Acute pain treatment for older adults hospitalized with hip fracture: current nursing practices and perceived barriers, *Appl Nurs Res* 16(4):211-227, 2003.

Ardery G et al: Patients' experiences of hip fracture, *J Adv Nurs* 44(4):385-392, 2003.

Milisen K et al: Documentation of delirium in elderly patients with hip fracture, *J Gerontol Nurs* 28(11):23-29, 2002.

Titler MG et al: Lack of opioids administration in older hip fracture patients, *Orthop Nurs* 22(3):232-239, 2003.

Chapter 53: Degenerative Disorders

General

Crowthier CL: *Primary orthopedic care,* ed 2, St Louis, 2004, Mosby.

Floryan KM, Berghoff WJ: Intraoperative use of autologous platelet-rich and platelet-poor plasma for orthopedic surgery patients, *AORN J* 80(4):668-674, 2004.

Greene WB et al: *Essentials of musculoskeletal care,* ed 2, Rosemont, Ill, 2001, American Academy of Orthopaedic Surgeons.

Maher AB et al, editors: *Orthopaedic nursing*, ed 3, Philadelphia, 2002, Saunders.
Potter JF: The older orthopaedic patient: general considerations, *Clin Orthop* 8(425):44-49, 2004.
Praemer A et al: *Musculoskeletal conditions in the US*, Rosemont, Ill, 1999, American Academy of Orthopaedic Surgeons.
Zychowicz ME: *Orthopedic nursing secrets*, Philadelphia, 2003, Hanley & Befus.

Disorders Affecting the Joints

Childs SG: Reactive arthritis: immune-mediated synovitis or joint infection, *Orthop Nurs* 23(4):267-273, 2004.
Kohnke SJ: Reactive arthritis: a clinical approach, *Orthop Nurs* 23(4): 274-282, 2004.
Schoofs N: Death of a lifestyle: the effects of social support and healthcare support on the quality of life of persons with fibromyalgia and/or fibromyalgia syndrome, *Orthop Nurs* 23(6):364-373, 2004.

Metabolic Bone Disease

Bearducci A et al: The impact of osteoporosis continuing education on nurses' knowledge and attitudes, *J Contin Educ Nurs* 33(5):210-216, quiz 238-239, 2003.
Frakes MA, Evans T: A review of osteoporosis in men: implications for practice, *Osteoporosis Int* 15(3):204-298, 2004.
Jensen AL, Harder I: The osteoporotic pain experience, *Geriatric Nurs* 24(6):353-360, 2003.
Martin JT et al: Female adolescents' knowledge of bone health promotion behaviors and osteoporosis risk factors, *Orthop Nurs* 23(4):235-244, 2004.
Moore A: Menopausal health strategies: focus on osteoporosis, *Am J Nurse Pract* 7(2):9-21, 2003.
Sandison R et al: Lifestyle factors for promoting bone health in older women, *J Adv Nurs* 45(6):603-610, 2004.
Schoen DC: Osteoporosis, *Orthop Nurs* 23(4):261-266, 2004.
Sedlak CA et al: Tailored interventions to enhance osteoporosis prevention in women, *Orthop Nurs* 24(4):270-276, 2005.
Turkowski B: Treating osteoporosis without hormones, *Orthop Nurs* 21(5):80-85, 2003.

Spine

Bajnoczy S: Artificial disc replacement: evolutionary treatment for degenerative disc disease, *AORN J* 82(2):192-206, 2005.

Chapter 54: Osteoarthritis and Rheumatoid Arthritis

Altizer L: Patient education for total hip or knee replacement, *Orthop Nurs* 23(4):283-288, 2004.
Blakely JA, Ribeiro VES: Glucosamine and osteoarthritis, *AJN* 104(2): 54-59, 2004.
Brosseau L et al: Low level laser therapy (classes I, II, and III) for treating osteoarthritis (Cochrane Review). In *Cochrane Library*, Issue 3, Chichester, UK, 2004, John Wiley & Sons.
Chao S, Vega C: Alternative approaches to relieving the pain of osteoarthritis, *Clin Advisor* 7(1):21-25, 2004.
Choi PT et al: Epidural analgesia for pain relief following hip or knee replacement (Cochrane Review). In *Cochrane Library*, Issue 3, Chichester, UK, 2004, John Wiley & Sons.
Comp PC et al: Prolonged enoxaparin therapy to prevent venous thromboembolism after primary hip or knee replacement, *J Bone Joint Surg* 83-A(3):336-345, 2001.
D'Ambrosia RD editor: Balancing benefits and risks in orthopedic thromboprophylaxis, *Orthopedics* 26(2 Suppl):S223-S235, 2003.
Epps CD: Length of stay, discharge disposition, and hospital charge predictors, *AORN J* 79(5):975-997, 2004.
Hohler SE: Minimally invasive total hip arthroplasty, *AORN J* 79(6):1244-1258, 2004.
Johnson PN: Low-molecular weight heparin use in special populations, *Orthopedics* 27(12):1245-1248, 2004.
Kick PA: MRSA infection following hip replacement: the need for evidence-based guidelines, *Am J Nurse Pract* 9(7/8):37-43, 2005.
King SA: Chronic pain control: what's adequate and appropriate: 10 questions physicians often ask, *Consultant* 3(13):1558-1573, 2003.
Kwong LM editor: Selective factor Xa inhibitors: practical guidelines for use, *Am J Orthop* 31(11 Suppl):1-24, 2002.
Lassen MR et al: Postoperative fondaparinux versus preoperative enoxaparin for prevention of venous thromboembolism in elective hip replacement surgery: a randomised double-blind comparison, *Lancet* 358(9319):1715-1720, 2002.
Mauer KA et al: National practice patterns for the care of the patient with total joint replacement, *Orthop Nurs* 21(3):37-44, 2002.
Riemsma RP et al: Patient education with rheumatoid arthritis (Cochrane Review). In *Cochrane Library*, Issue 3, Chichester, UK, 2004, John Wiley & Sons.
Stitik TP, Ali A: Osteoarthritis of the glenohumeral joint: a "hands-on" approach, *Consultant* 45(2):154-159, 2005.

Chapter 55: Assessment of the Reproductive System

Carulli DT: Abnormal cervical cytology: new names, familiar smears, *J Am Acad Nurse Pract* 15(10):444-449, 2003.
Dickerson LM, Mazyck PJ, Hunter MH: Premenstrual syndrome, *Am Fam Phys* 67(8):1743-1752, 2003.
Gretzer MB, Partin AP: PSA and PSA molecular derivatives, *Campbell's Urol Updates* 1(1):1-12, 2003.
Legato MJ: Hormone therapy for postmenopausal women: past, present, and (does it have) future? *Cardiol Rev* April Suppl, 1-11, 2004.
McCance KL, Huether SE: *Pathophysiology: the biologic basis for disease in adults and children*, ed 4, St Louis, 2002, Mosby.
Schaffer SD: Vaginitis and sexually transmitted diseases. In Youngkin EQ, Davis MS, editors: *Women's health: a primary care clinical guide*, Stamford, Conn, 2004, Appleton & Lange.
Subhash CB: Diagnosis and treatment of premenstrual dysphoric disorder, *Am Fam Phys* 66(7):1239-1247, 2002.
US Preventive Services Task Force: Postmenopausal hormone replacement therapy for the primary prevention of chronic conditions: recommendations and rationale, *Am Fam Phys* 67(2):358-364, 2003.

Chapter 56: Female Reproductive Problems

American College of Obstetricians and Gynecologists: Bacterial vaginosis more prevalent than previously thought, *ACOG News Release*, Oct 31, 2003, ACOG Office of Communications, accessed from website: www.acog.org.
Kupperman M et al: Effect of hysterectomy vs. medical treatment on health-related quality of life and sexual functioning: the medicine or surgery randomized trial, *JAMA* 291:1447-1455, 2004.

Chapter 57: Male Reproductive Problems

Fortunati LN, Floerchinger-Franks G: Men and family planning: what is their future role? *J Am Acad Nurs Pract* 13(10):473, 2001.
Mason D: Sex, drugs and marketing, *AJN* 103(6):7, 2003.

Chapter 58: Problems of the Breast

General

Anderson WF et al: Is male breast cancer similar or different than female breast cancer? *Breast Cancer Res Treat* 83(1):77-86, 2004.

Fentiman IS, D'Arrigo C: Pathogenesis of breast carcinoma, *Int J Clin Pract* 58(1):35-40, 2004.

Fentiman IS, Hamed H: Breast cancer management, part 1, Assessment of breast problems, *Int J Clin Pract* 55(7):458-460, 2001.

Giuliano AE: Sentinel node biopsy: standard of care, *Breast J* 9(Suppl):S3-S6, 2003.

Greifzu SP: Breast cancer, *RN* 67(2):36-42, 2004.

Adjuvant Therapy

Dingman JJ et al: Obesity, tamoxifen use, and outcomes in women with estrogen receptor–positive early-stage breast cancer, *J Natl Cancer Inst* 95(19):1467-1476, 2003.

Harris J: Radiation therapy: accepted and controversial roles, *Breast J* 9 (Suppl 1):S11-S16, 2003.

Palmieri FM, Perez EA: Recent advances in adjuvant therapy for breast cancer, *Semin Oncol Nurs* 19(4 Suppl 2):10-16, 2003.

Sjostrom J: Predictive factors for response to chemotherapy in advanced breast cancer, *Acta Oncol* 41(4):334-345, 2002.

Truong MT, Hirsch AE, Formenti SC: Novel approaches to postoperative radiation therapy as part of breast-conserving therapy for early-stage breast cancer, *Clin Breast Cancer* 4(4):253-263, 2003.

Genetics

Hutson SP: Attitudes and psychosocial impact of genetic testing, genetic counseling, and breast cancer risk assessment among women at increased risk, *Oncol Nurs Forum* 30(2):241-246, 2003.

Loescher LJ: Cancer worry in women with hereditary risk factors for breast cancer, *Oncol Nurs Forum* 30(5):767-772, 2003.

Lohrisch C, Piccart M: HER/2/neu as a predictive factor in breast cancer, *Clin Breast Cancer* 2(2):129-137, 2001.

Nkondjock A, Ghadirian P: Epidemiology of breast cancer among BRCA mutation carriers: an overview, *Cancer Letters* 205(1):1-8, 2004.

Zimmerman V: BRCA gene mutation and cancer, *Am J Nurs* 102(8):28-37, 2002.

Lymphedema

Aldridge RL, Clifft J: Effects of manual lymphatic drainage on edema and function in a patient with postmastectomy lymphedema, *J Sect Womens Health* 26(1):25-29, 2002.

Armer JM et al: Predicting breast cancer-related lymphedema using self-reported symptoms, *Nurs Res* 52(6):370-379, 2003.

Ciccone CD: Evidence in practice: comprehensive lymphedema management program, *Phys Ther* 82(3):276-282, 2002.

Haslett ML, Aitken MJ: Evaluating the effectiveness of a compression sleeve in managing secondary lymphedema, *J Wound Care* 11(10):401-404, 2002.

Kwan W et al: Chronic arm morbidity after curative breast cancer treatment: prevalence and impact on quality of life, *J Clin Oncol* 20(20):4242-4248, 2002.

Prevention and Screening

Biglia N et al: Management of risk of breast carcinoma in post-menopausal women, *Endoc Relat Cancer* 11(1):69-83, 2004.

Carmichael A, Bates T: Obesity and breast cancer: a review of the literature, *Breast* 13(2):85-92, 2004.

Hollingsworth AB et al: Current comprehensive assessment and management of women at increased risk for breast cancer, *Am J Surg* 187(3):349-369, 2004.

Philpotts LE, Smith RA: Screening for breast cancer, *Semin Roentgenol* 38(1):19-33, 2003.

Yarbrough SS: Older women and breast cancer screening: research synthesis, *Oncol Nurs Forum* 31(1):E9-E15, 2004.

Psychoemotional Issues

Albaugh JA: Spirituality and life-threatening illness: a phenomenologic study, *Oncol Nurs Forum* 30(4):593-598, 2003.

Ebright PR, Lyon B: Understanding hope and factors that enhance hope in women with breast cancer, *Oncol Nurs Forum* 29(3):561-568, 2002.

Gall TL, Cornblat MW: Breast cancer survivors give voice: a qualitative analysis of spiritual factors in long-term adjustment, *Psychooncology* 11(6):524-535, 2002.

Henderson PD et al: African American women coping with breast cancer: a qualitative analysis, *Oncol Nurs Forum* 30(4):641-647, 2003.

Stewart DE et al: Attributions of cause and recurrence in long-term breast cancer survivors, *Psychooncology* 10(2):179-183, 2001.

Quality of Life

Bloom JR and others: Then and now: quality of life of young breast cancer survivors, *Psychooncology* 13(3):147-160, 2004.

Casso D, Buist DS, Taplin S: Quality of life of 5-10 year breast cancer survivors diagnosed between age 40 and 49, *Health Qual Life Outcomes* 2(1):25, 2004.

Sammarco A: Psychosocial stages and quality of life of women with breast cancer, *Cancer Nurs* 24(4):272-277, 2001.

Sammarco A: Enhancing the quality of life of survivors of breast cancer, *Anal Long Term Care* 12(3):40-45, 2004.

Schrier AM, Williams SA: Anxiety and quality of life of women who receive radiation or chemotherapy for breast cancer, *Oncol Nurs Forum* 31(1):127-130, 2004.

Sexuality and Body Image

Greendale GA et al: Factors related to sexual function in postmenopausal women with a history of breast cancer, *Menopause* 8(2):111-119, 2001.

Henson NK: Breast cancer and sexuality, *Sex Disabil* 20(4):261-275, 2002.

Kornblith AB, Ligibel J: Psychosocial and sexual functioning of survivors of breast cancer, *Semin Oncol* 30(6):799-813, 2003.

Smith M, Kent K: Breast concerns and lifestyles of women, *Clin Obstet Gynecol* 45(4):1129-1139, 2002.

Wilmoth MC, Sanders LD: Accept me for myself: African American women's issues after breast cancer, *Oncol Nurs Forum* 28(5):875-879, 2001.

Older Adults

Du XL, Osborne C, Goodwin JS: Population-based assessment of hospitalizations for toxicity from chemotherapy in older women with breast cancer, *J Clin Oncol* 20(24):4636-4642, 2002.

Gill KM et al: Triggers of uncertainty about recurrence and long-term treatment side effects in older African American and Caucasian breast cancer survivors, *Oncol Nurs Forum* 31(3):633-639, 2004.

Mandelblatt JS: Predictors of long-term outcomes in older breast cancer survivors: perceptions versus patterns of care, *J Clin Oncol* 21(5):855-863, 2003.

Pinto BM, Trunzo JJ: Body esteem and mood among sedentary and active breast cancer survivors, *Mayo Clin Proc* 79(2):181-186, 2004.

Thewes B et al: The psychosocial needs of breast cancer survivors; a qualitative study of the shared and unique needs of younger versus older survivors, *Psychooncology* 13(3):177-189, 2004.

Chapter 59: Sexually Transmitted Diseases

Bowdler NC, Galask RP: Protocols: OB/GYN infection-granuloma inguinale (donovanosis), *Contemp OB/GYN* 46(5):83-84, 89-90, 2001.

Brown DL, Frank JE: Diagnosis and management of syphilis, *Am Fam Phys* 68(2):283-290, 297, 2003.

Davis A, Calvet H: Sexually transmitted diseases in the emergency department, *Topics Emerg Med* 25(3):247-255, 2003.

Landry D et al: Factors associated with the content of sex education in US public secondary schools, *Perspect Sexual Reprod Health* 35(6):261-269, 2003.

McEvoy M: Sexually transmitted infection: a challenge for nurses working with adolescents, *Nurs Clin North Am* 37(3):461-474, 2002.

National Network of STD/HIV Prevention Training Centers: *STD case series,* accessed from website: www.STDcases.org.

Peipert JF: Clinical practice: genital chlamydial infections, *N Engl J Med* 349(25):2424-2430, 2003.

Phillips KD et al: Sexually transmitted diseases in men, *Nurs Clin North Am* 39(2):357-377, 2004.

Stephenson J: Rise in drug-resistant gonorrhea cases: spurs new treatment advice for gay, bisexual men, *JAMA* 291(20):2420, 2004.

Chapter 60: Assessment of the Visual System

Ledford J: *The little eye book: a pupil's guide to understanding ophthalmology,* Thorofare, NJ, 2002, SLACK.

Fitzpatrick M: Ophthalmologists eye: new examination tool, *JAMA* 286(13):1576, 2001.

Gupta D: An O.D.'s primer on ultrasound, *Rev Optometry* 138(10):41, 2001.

Pabdut RJ et al: Effectiveness of testing visual fields by confrontation, *Lancet* 358(9290):1339, 2001.

Chapter 61: Problems of the Eye

Gallemore RP, Boyer DS: Retinal detachment: the best treatment is prevention, *Rev Ophthalmol* 8(4):121, 2001.

Hamilton DR et al: Watch for steroid-induced glaucoma after LASIK, *Rev Ophthalmol* 9(6):143, 2002.

Murdoch I: Glaucoma: latest developments in diagnosis and treatment, *Pulse* 62(23):51, 2002.

Weintraub JM et al: Postmenopausal hormone use and lens opacities, *Ophthalmic Epidemiol* 9(3):179, 2002.

Chapter 62: Assessment of the Auditory System

Alper C et al: *Decision-making in ear, nose, and throat disorders,* Philadelphia, 2001, Saunders.

Gates G: *Current therapy in otolaryngology: head and neck surgery,* ed 6, St Louis, 1998, Mosby.

Lilly D, Feeney P, Rosowski J: Current and emerging tools for assessing middle-ear function. *ASHA Leader* 10(5):24-26, 2005.

Chapter 63: Problems of the Ear

American Academy of Pediatrics: Clinical practice guidelines: diagnosis and management of acute otitis media, *Pediatrics* 113(5):1451-1465, 2004.

American Academy of Pediatrics: Clinical practice guidelines: otitis media with effusion, *Pediatrics* 113(5):1412-1429, 2004.

Gratton MA, Vaquez AE: Age-related hearing loss: current research, *Curr Opin Otolaryngol Head Neck Surg* 11(5):367-371, 2003.

McCoy SI, Zell ER, Besser RE: Antimicrobial prescribing for otitis externa in children, *Pediatr Infect Dis J* 23(2):181-183, 2004.

Yueh B et al: Screening and management of hearing loss in primary care: scientific review, *JAMA* 289(15):1976-1985, 2003.

Chapter 64: Assessment of the Skin

General

Bickley LS: *Bates's guide to physical examination and history taking,* ed 7, Philadelphia, 1999, Lippincott.

Physiology of the Skin

Dermatology Nurses' Association: *Dermatology nursing essentials: a core curriculum,* ed 2, Pitman, NJ, 2003, Anthony J Janetti.

Lesion Description and Identification

Dermatology Nurse's Association: *Dermatology nursing basics: core proceeding book from annual convention,* Pitman, NJ, 2003, Anthony J Janetti.

Fitzpatrick TB et al: *Color atlas and synopsis of clinical dermatology,* ed 4, New York, 2000, McGraw-Hill Professional Publishing

Habif T: *Clinical dermatology: a color guide to diagnosis and therapy,* ed 4, St Louis, 2003, Mosby.

Odon RB et al: *Andrews' diseases of the skin: clinical dermatology,* ed 9, Philadelphia, 2000, Saunders.

Chapter 65: Problems of the Skin

Kamines MS et al: *Atlas of cosmetic surgery,* Philadelphia, 2002, Saunders.

Jacknin J: *Smart medicine for your skin: a comprehensive guide to understanding conventional and alternative therapies to heal common skin problems,* New York, 2001, Avery.

McGovern TW et al: Cutaneous manifestations of biological warfare and related threat agents, *Arch Dermatol* 133(3):311, 1999.

Schofield JR, Robinson WA: *What you really need to know about moles and melanoma,* Baltimore, 2000, Johns Hopkins University Press.

Chapter 66: Burns

General

Allison K, Porter K: Consensus on the pre-hospital approach to burns patient management, *Accid Emerg Nurs* 12(1):53-57, 2004.

Bishop JF: Burn wound assessment and surgical management, *Crit Care Nurs Clin North Am* 16(1):145-177, 2004.

Chai J et al: Repair and reconstruction of massively damaged burn wounds, *Burns* 29(7):726-732, 2003.

Eldad A et al: Silver-sufadiazine eschar pigmentation mimics invasive wound infection: a case report, *J Burn Care Rehabil* 24(3):154-157, 2003.

Flynn MB: Nutritional support for the burn-injured patient, *Crit Care Nurs Clin North Am* 16(1):139-144, 2004.

Garrel D: Burn scars: a new cause for vitamin D deficiency? *Lancet* 363(9405):259-260, 2004.

Garrel D et al: Decreased mortality and infectious morbidity in adult burn patients given enteral glutamine supplements: a prospective controlled, randomized clinical trial, *Crit Care Med* 31(10):2444-2449, 2003.

Kleinpell RM: Healing wounds: advances in burn care, *Nurs Spectrum* 16(12):8, 2003.

Lefton J: Specialized nutrition support for adult burn patients, *Support Line* 25(4):19-25, 2003.

Memmel H, Kowal-Vern A, Latenser BA: Infections in diabetic burn patients, *Diabetes Care* 27(1):229-233, 2004.

Mileski WJ et al: Serial measurements increase the accuracy of laser Doppler assessment of burn wounds, *J Burn Care Rehab* 24(4):187-191, 2003.

Moss LS: Outpatient management of the burn patient, *Crit Care Nurs Clin North Am* 16(1):109-117, 2004.

Still J et al: The use of a collagen sponge/living cell composite material to treat donor sites in burn patients, *Burns* 29(8):837-841, 2003.

Supple KG: Physiologic response to burn injury, *Crit Care Nurs North Am* 16(1):119-126, 2004.

Warden GD, Heimbach D: Regionalization of burn care—a concept whose time has come, *J Burn Care Rehabil* 24(3):173-174, 2003.

Psychosocial Issues

Bergamasco EC et al: Body image of patients with burns sequelae: evaluation through the critical incident technique, *Burns* 28(1):47-52, 2002.

Fauerbach JA et al: Coping with body image changes following a disfiguring burn injury, *Health Psychol* 21(2):115-121, 2002.

Giboa D: Long-term psychosocial adjustment after burn injury, *Burns* 27(4):335-341, 2001.

Hamaoui EL et al: Post-traumatic stress disorder in burned patients, *Burns* 28(7):647-650, 2002.

Mennick F: Nurses teach families to heal, *Nurs Spectrum* 12(11):8-9, 2003.

Pallua N, Kunsebeck HW, Noah EM: Psychosocial adjustments 5 years after burn injury, *Burns* 29(2):143-152, 2003.

Patterson DR et al: Psychosocial forum: premorbid mental health status of adult burn patients: comparison with a normative sample, *J Burn Care Rehabil* 25(5):347-350, 2003.

Williams NR, Davey M, Klock-Powell K: Rising from the ashes: stories of recovery, adaptation and resiliency in burn survivors, *Soc Work Health Care* 36(4):53-77, 2003.

Williams R et al: Health outcomes for burn survivors: a 2-year follow-up, *Rehabil Psychol* 48(3):189-194, 2003.

ILLUSTRATION CREDITS

Chapter 1 1-2, From NANDA International: *NANDA nursing diagnoses: definitions and classification 2005-2006*, Philadelphia, 2005, The Association.

Chapter 2 2-1, 2-2, 2-4, Courtesy Larry Butler, Lowell, Ark. 2-5, 2-6, From American Health Assistance Foundation: *AD research: a program of the AHAF,* accessed from website: www.ahaf.org.

Chapter 3 3-1, From US Department of Agriculture Center for Nutrition Policy and Promotion, CNPP-16, 2005. 3-3, Adapted from National Heart Lung and Blood Institute: *Obesity Education Initiative*, National Institutes of Health, accessed from website: ww w.nhibi.nih.gov.

Chapter 4 4-2, Courtesy Audrey E. Snyder.

Chapter 5 5-1, 5-6, 5-7, 5-8, Courtesy US Department of Energy Human Genome Program, Oak Ridge, Tenn. 5-2, 5-3, 5-4, 5-5, 5-9, 5-11, 5-12, Courtesy National Human Genome Research Institute, Bethesda, Md.

Chapter 6 6-2, 6-3, 6-4, 6-6, From Cohen J, Powderly G, editors: *Infectious diseases*, ed 2, St Louis, 2004, Mosby. 6-5, 6-10, 6-12, From Emond RT, Welsby PD, Rowland HA: *Color atlas of infectious diseases*, St Louis, 2003, Mosby. 6-7, 6-8, 6-9, 6-11, Courtesy Centers for Disease Control and Prevention, Atlanta.

Chapter 7 7-1, From Sorrentino SA: *Mosby's textbook for nursing assistants*, ed 6, St Louis, 2004, Mosby. 7-3, From Derstine JB, Hargrove SD: *Comprehensive rehabilitation nursing,* Philadelphia, 2001, Saunders. 7-4, From Paterson BL: The shifting perspectives model of chronic illness, *J Nurs Scholar*, 33:57-62, 2001.

Chapter 9 9-1, Courtesy The American Civil Defense Association.

Chapter 10 10-1, Redrawn from *Waiting room survival guide*, ed 2, Washington, DC, 1993, Foundation for Critical Care. 10-2, Redrawn from Jackle M, Halligan M: Cardiovascular problems: a critical care nursing focus, Bowie, Md, 2001, Robert J. Brady. In Sole ML et al: *Introduction to critical care nursing*, ed 3, Philadelphia, 2001, Saunders.

Chapter 11 11-1, From Monahan FD, Neighbors M: *Medical-surgical nursing: foundations for clinical practice*, ed 2, Philadelphia, 2001, Saunders.

Chapter 12 12-1, Data from Hobbs FB, Damon BL: *65+ in the United States*, US Bureau of the Census, Current Population Reports, Special Studies, pp 23-190, April 1996. 12-2, Data from CMS-OSCAR Form 671: F12, Current surveys as of June 2004. 12-3, Data from AHCA: *The State Long Term Care Sector 2003*. 12-4, Data from CMS Healthcare Industry Market Update, Nursing Facilities, May 2003. 12-6, 12-7, Data from *Long term care facility resident assessment instrument (RAI) users manual*, December 2002.

Chapter 13 13-1, Courtesy Intuitive Surgical, Inc., Sunnyvale, Calif. 13-2, 13-3, 13-4, Courtesy University Hospital of Cleveland, Cleveland, Ohio.

Chapter 14 14-7, 14-8, From Elkin MK et al: *Nursing interventions and clinical skills*, ed 2, St Louis, 2000, Mosby.

Chapter 15 15-1, Redrawn from Litwack K: *Post anesthesia care nursing*, ed 2, St Louis, 1995, Mosby. 15-3, Courtesy MetroHealth System, Cleveland, Ohio. 15-4, *B*, Redrawn from Canobbio MM: *Cardiovascular disorders*, St Louis, 1990, Mosby. 15-6, *A*, Redrawn from Morison M: *A colour guide to the nursing management of wounds,* London, 1992, Mosby-Wolfe.

Chapter 16 16-6, Redrawn from Watt-Watson JH, Donovan MI: *Pain management: nursing perspective*, St Louis, 1992, Mosby. 16-7, Adapted from McCaffery M, Beebe A: *Pain: clinical manual for nursing practice*, St Louis, 1989, Mosby.

Chapter 17 17-3, 17-7, From Huether SE, McCance KL: *Understanding pathophysiology*, ed 3, St Louis, 2004, Mosby. 17-4, From Thibodeau GA, Patton KT: *Anatomy and physiology*, ed 5, St Louis, 2003, Mosby.

Chapter 18 18-2, 18-4, 18-5, 18-6, 18-7, From Thibodeau GA, Patton KT: *Anatomy and physiology*, ed 5, St Louis, 2003, Mosby. 18-3, From Monahan FD, Neighbors M: *Medical-surgical nursing: foundations for clinical practice*, ed 2, Philadelphia, 1998, Saunders.

Chapter 19 19-1, 19-7, From Monahan FD, Neighbors M: *Medical-surgical nursing: foundations for clinical practice*, ed 2, Philadelphia, 1998, Saunders. 19-8, Courtesy The Jobst Institute, Toledo, Ohio.

Chapter 20 20-1, 20-4, 20-6, 20-7, 20-15, 20-16, 20-19, From Abbas A, Lichtman A: *Basic immunology*, ed 2, Philadelphia, 2004, Saunders. 20-2, 20-11, 20-12, From Huether SE, McCance KL: *Understanding pathophysiology*, ed 3, St Louis, 2004, Mosby. 20-3, From Thibodeau GA, Patton KT: *Anatomy and physiology*, ed 5, St Louis, 2003, Mosby. 20-13, From Emond RT, Welsby PD, Rowland HA: *Color atlas of infectious diseases*, ed 4, St Louis, 2003, Mosby. 20-17, 20-21, From Monahan FD, Neighbors M: *Medical-surgical nursing: foundations for clinical practice*, ed 2, Philadelphia, 1998, Saunders.

Chapter 21 21-2, 21-4, 21-5, From Roitt I, Brostoff J, Male D: *Immunology*, ed 6, St Louis, 2001, Mosby. 21-6, 21-8, 21-9, Redrawn from McCance KL, Huether SE: *Pathophysiology: the biologic basis for disease in adults and children*, ed 4, St Louis, 2002, Mosby.

Chapter 22 22-1, Data from Centers for Disease Control and Prevention National Center for HIV, STD, and TB Prevention: *HIV/AIDS update: a glance at the HIV epidemic*, 2004, The Centers. 22-2, 22-25, From Monahan FD, Neighbors M: *Medical-surgical nursing: foundations for clinical practice*, ed 2, Philadelphia, 1998, Saunders. 22-6, 22-7, 22-8, 22-9, 22-10, From Cohen J, Powderly G, editors: *Infectious diseases*, ed 2, St Louis, 2004, Mosby.

Chapter 23 23-1, From American Cancer Society: *Cancer facts and figures 2004*, Atlanta, 2004, The Society. 23-2, From Szarka C et al: *Curr Probl Cancer* 15:6, 1994. 23-4, 23-8, From Lewis SM et al: *Medical-surgical nursing: assessment and management of clinical problems*, ed 5, St Louis, 2000, Mosby. 23-14, From Monahan FD, Neighbors M: *Medical-surgical nursing: foundations for clinical practice*, ed 2, Philadelphia, 1998, Saunders. 23-15, 23-16, Redrawn from LaRocca JC, Otto SE: *Pocket guide to intravenous therapy*, ed 3, St Louis, 1997, Mosby.

Chapter 24 24-2, 24-6, From Beare PG, Myers JL: *Adult health nursing*, ed 3, St Louis, 1998, Mosby. 24-5, From Lewis SM et al: *Medical-surgical nursing: assessment and management of clinical problems*, ed 5, St Louis, 2000, Mosby. 24-8, Redrawn from Price SA, Wilson LM: *Pathophysiology: clinical concepts of disease processes*, ed 5, St Louis, 1997, Mosby. 24-12, 24-16, Modified from Talbot L, Meyers-Marquardt M: *Pocket guide to critical care assessment*, ed 3, St Louis, 1997, Mosby. 24-14, Redrawn from Seidel HM et al: *Mosby's guide to physical examination*, ed 4, St Louis, 1999, Mosby. 24-15, Redrawn from Stillwell S, Randall E:

Pocket guide to cardiovascular care, ed 2, St Louis, 1994, Mosby. 24-18, Redrawn from Spearman CB et al: *Egan's fundamentals of respiratory therapy*, ed 5, St Louis, 1990, Mosby. 24-19, From Monahan FD, Neighbors M: *Medical-surgical nursing: foundations for clinical practice*, ed 2, Philadelphia, 1998, Saunders.

Chapter 25 25-1, 25-2, 25-4, 25-6, 25-7, 25-10, 25-13, 25-14, 25-15, 25-16, 25-18, Redrawn from Schuller DE, Schleuning AJ: *Otolaryngology: head and neck surgery*, ed 8, St Louis, 1994, Mosby. 25-9, From Gruber RP, Peck GC: *Rhinoplasty: state of the art*, St Louis, 1993, Mosby. 25-11, From Monahan FD, Neighbors M: *Medical-surgical nursing: foundations for clinical practice*, ed 2, Philadelphia, 1998, Saunders. 25-22, From Lewis SM et al: *Medical-surgical nursing: assessment and management of clinical problems*, ed 5, St Louis, 2000, Mosby. 25-23, Redrawn from Kaplow R, Bookbinder M: *Heart Lung* 23(1):59, 1994.

Chapter 26 26-1, From Lewis SM et al: *Medical-surgical nursing: assessment and management of clinical problems*, ed 5, St Louis, 2000, Mosby. 26-2, 26-3, From Potter PA, Perry AG: *Fundamentals of nursing: concepts, process, and practice*, ed 5, St Louis, 2001, Mosby. 26-4, From Des Jardins T, Burton GC: *Clinical manifestations and assessment of respiratory disease*, ed 3, St Louis, 1995, Mosby. 26-5, From Monahan FD, Neighbors M: *Medical-surgical nursing: foundations for clinical practice*, ed 2, Philadelphia, 1998, Saunders. 26-10, From Sorrentino SA: *Mosby's assisting with patient care*, St Louis, 1999, Mosby.

Chapter 27 27-3, 27-4, 27-5, 27-6, 27-8, From McCance KL, Huether SE: *Pathophysiology: the biologic basis for disease in adults and children*, ed 4, St Louis, 2002, Mosby. 27-13, Courtesy DePaul Health Center, St Louis. 27-15, 27-16, Redrawn from Smith SL: *Tissue and organ transplantation: implications for professional nursing practice*, St Louis, 1990, Mosby.

Chapter 28 28-5, Redrawn from Thompson JM, Wilson SF: *Health assessment for nursing practice*, St Louis, 1996, Mosby. 28-8, 28-25, 28-26, 28-27, Redrawn from Conover MS: *Understanding electrocardiography: arrhythmias and the 12-lead ECG*, ed 6, St Louis, 1992, Mosby. 28-12, 28-13, From Thibodeau GA, Patton KT: *Anatomy and physiology*, ed 5, St Louis, 2003, Mosby. 28-19, 28-20, 28-21, 28-23, Redrawn from McKinney MR et al: *Comprehensive cardiac care*, ed 7, St Louis, 1991, Mosby. 28-30, Redrawn from Daily EK, Schroeder JS: *Techniques in bedside hemodynamic monitoring*, ed 5, St Louis, 1994, Mosby.

Chapter 29 29-2, From Huether SE, McCance KL: *Understanding pathophysiology*, ed 2, St Louis, 2000, Mosby. 29-8, From Braunwald E: *Heart disease: a textbook of cardiovascular medicine*, ed 5, Philadelphia, 1997, Saunders. 29-12, 29-15, From Monahan FD, Neighbors M: *Medical-surgical nursing: foundations for clinical practice*, ed 2, Philadelphia, 1998, Saunders. 29-44, Courtesy Medtronic, Inc., Minneapolis.

Chapter 30 30-2, From Jessup M, Brozena S: Heart failure, *N Engl J Med* 348(20):2011, 2003. 30-4, Redrawn from Konstam M et al: *Heart failure: evaluation and care of patients with left ventricular systolic dysfunction,* Clinical Practice Guideline No. 11, AHCPR Pub. No. 94-0612, Rockville, Md, June 1994, Agency for Health Care Policy and Research, Public Health Service, US Department of Health and Human Services. 30-7, Redrawn from Kissane IM: *Anderson's pathology*, ed 9, St Louis, 1990, Mosby. 30-8, 30-14, 30-15, From Monahan FD, Neighbors M: *Medical-surgical nursing: foundations for clinical practice*, ed 2, Philadelphia, 1998, Saunders. 30-9, 30-10, 30-11, 30-12, 30-13, 30-18, From Beare PG, Myers JL: *Adult health nursing*, ed 3, St Louis, 1998, Mosby. 30-16, *C*, Courtesy St Jude Medical, Inc., St Paul, Minn. 30-19, Redrawn from Smith SL: *Tissue and organ transplantation: implications for professional nursing practice*, St Louis, 1990, Mosby.

Chapter 31 31-2, From Chobanian A et al: The seventh report of the Joint National Committee on Prevention, Detection, Evaluation, and Treatment of High Blood Pressure, *JAMA* 289(DOI 10.1001), 2003. 31-4, 31-12, 31-16, From Lewis SM et al: *Medical-surgical nursing: assessment and management of clinical problems*, ed 5, St Louis, 2000, Mosby. 31-5, From Black J et al: *Medical-surgical nursing: clinical management for positive outcomes*, ed 6, Philadelphia, 2001, Saunders. 31-6, Courtesy LoGerfo FW, Boston. 31-7, 31-14, From Kamal A, Brockelhurst IC: *Color atlas of geriatric medicine*, ed 2, St Louis, 1991, Mosby. 31-8, Courtesy Otto Bock Health Care, Minneapolis. 31-10, 31-11, From Hall SW: Endovascular repair of abdominal aortic aneurysms, *AORN J* 77(3):630-642, 645-648, 2003. 31-15, Courtesy Kendall Company, Mansfield, Mass. 31-17, From Lofgren KA: Varicose veins. In Haimovici H, editor: *Vascular surgery: principles and techniques*, Oxford, 1976, Blackwell Science. 31-18, From Belch JJF et al: *Color atlas of peripheral vascular diseases*, ed 2, St Louis, 1996, Mosby-Wolfe.

Chapter 32 32-1, From McCance KL, Huether SE: *Pathophysiology: the biologic basis for disease in adults and children*, ed 4, St Louis, 2002, Mosby. 32-2, From Monahan FD, Neighbors M: *Medical-surgical nursing: foundations for clinical practice*, ed 2, Philadelphia, 1998, Saunders. 32-3, From Pagana KD, Pagana TJ: *Mosby's manual of diagnostic and laboratory tests*, ed 2, St Louis, 2002, Mosby.

Chapter 33 33-5, From Porth CM: *Pathophysiology: concepts of altered health status*, ed 6, Philadelphia, 1998, Lippincott.

Chapter 34 34-4, 34-7, From Thibodeau GA, Patton KT: *Anatomy and physiology*, ed 5, St Louis, 2003, Mosby. 34-5, From Huether SE, McCance KL: *Understanding pathophysiology*, ed 3, St Louis, 2004, Mosby. 34-6, Redrawn from Thibodeau GA, Patton KT: *Anatomy and physiology*, ed 3, St Louis, 1996, Mosby.

Chapter 35 35-1, From American Medical Association: JAMA patient page: urinary tract infections, *JAMA* 283(12):1646, 2000. 35-2, 35-5, From Price LM, Wilson SA: *Pathophysiology*, ed 6, St Louis, 2003, Mosby. 35-3, From Kissane IM: *Anderson's pathology*, ed 9, St Louis, 1990, Mosby. 35-6, From Hockenberry MJ: *Wong's essentials of pediatric nursing*, ed 7, St Louis, 2005, Mosby. 35-11, From Damjanov I, Linder J: *Anderson's pathology*, ed 10, St Louis, 1996, Mosby. 35-12, 35-19, From Weiss RM et al: *Comprehensive urology*, London, 2001, Mosby International. 35-23, From Brundage DJ: *Renal disorders*, St Louis, 1992, Mosby.

Chapter 36 36-1, Redrawn from McCance KL, Huether SE: *Pathophysiology: the biologic basis for disease in adults and children*, ed 4, St Louis, 2002, Mosby. 36-2, From Smith T: *Renal nursing*, London, 1997, Bailliere-Tindall. 36-6, 36-9, 36-10, 36-11, From National Kidney and Urologic Disease Information Clearinghouse: *Vascular access for hemodialysis*, NIH Publication No. 05-4554, 2005. 36-7, 36-12, From Ignatavicius DD, Workman ML: *Medical-surgical nursing: critical thinking for collaborative care*, ed 4, Philadelphia, 2002, Saunders. 36-8, Courtesy Baxter Healthcare Corporation, Deerfield, Ill. 36-13, From Lewis SM et al: *Medical-surgical nursing: assessment and management of clinical problems*, ed 5, St Louis, 2000, Mosby. 36-14, Redrawn from Chabelewski FL: Donation and transplantation, *Nursing Curriculum*, 1996.

Chapter 37 37-3, 37-4, 37-10, Redrawn from McCance KL, Huether SE: *Pathophysiology: the biologic basis for disease in adults and children*, ed 4, St Louis, 2002, Mosby. 37-5, 37-6, Redrawn from Thibodeau GA, Patton KT: *Anatomy and physiology*, ed 5, St Louis, 2003, Mosby.

Chapter 38 38-1, From Mendeloff AI, Smith DE, editors: Acromegaly, diabetes, hypermetabolism, proteinuria, and heart failure, Clinical Pathology Conference, *Am J Med* 20:133, 1956. 38-2, From Shapiro LM, Buchalter MB: *Color atlas of hypertension*, London, 1992, Wolfe. 38-5, Courtesy Dr. Jeffrey Hurwitz. From Bingham BJ et al: *Atlas of clinical otolaryngology*, St Louis, 1992, Mosby. 38-6, From Bergman LV and Associates, Cold Springs, NY. 38-7, From Hall R, Evered DC: *Color atlas of endocrinology*, ed 2, St Louis, 1990, Mosby. 38-9, From Lewis SM et al: *Medical-surgical nursing: assessment and management of clinical problems*, ed 5, St Louis, 2000, Mosby.

Chapter 39 39-1, Data from National Institute of Diabetes and Digestive and Kidney Diseases, National Information Clearinghouse, National Institutes of Health: *Diabetes statistics*, NIH Pub. No. 96-3926, 1995. 39-9, 39-10, From Lewis SM et al: *Medical-surgical nursing: assessment and management of clinical problems*, ed 5, St Louis, 2000, Mosby.

Chapter 40 40-3, 40-4, From Thibodeau GA, Patton KT: *Anatomy and physiology*, ed 5, St Louis, 2003, Mosby. 40-5, 40-11, From Monahan FD, Neighbors M: *Medical-surgical nursing: foundations for clinical practice*, ed 2, Philadelphia, 1998, Saunders. 40-10, Courtesy Olympus America, Inc., Mehlville, NY.

Chapter 41 41-1, 41-6, From Lewis SM et al: *Medical-surgical nursing: assessment and management of clinical problems*, ed 5, St Louis, 2000, Mosby. 41-2, 41-8, 41-9, From Feldman M, Friedman L, Sleisenger M: *Sleisenger and Fordtran's gastrointestinal and liver disease*, ed 7, Philadelphia, 2002, Saunders. 41-3, From Callen FP et al: *Color atlas of dermatology*, Philadelphia, 1993, Saunders. 41-4, Courtesy Curon Medical, Inc., Fremont, Calif. 41-7, From Zuidema GD: *Shackelford's surgery of the alimentary tract*, ed 4, vol 1, Philadelphia, 1996, Saunders.

Chapter 42 42-5, From Black J et al: *Medical-surgical nursing: clinical management for positive outcomes*, ed 6, Philadelphia, 2001, Saunders. 42-8, From Feldman M, Friedman L, Sleisenger M: *Sleisenger and Fordtran's gastrointestinal and liver disease*, ed 7, Philadelphia, 2002, Saunders. 42-8, *B*, Courtesy Mark Feldman, MD. 42-10, From Beare PG, Myers JL: *Adult health nursing*, ed 3, St Louis, 1998, Mosby. 42-12, From Elkin MK, Perry AG, Potter PA: *Nursing interventions and clinical skills*, St Louis, 1996, Mosby.

Chapter 43 43-3, 43-4, 43-17, 43-19, From Wilcox CM: *Atlas of clinical gastrointestinal endoscopy*, Philadelphia, 1995, Saunders. 43-21, From de los Rios Magrina E: *Atlas of therapeutic proctology*, Philadelphia, 1984, Saunders.

Chapter 44 44-3, From Siegel JH et al: Mechanical lithotripsy of common duct stones, *Gastrointest Endosc* 36(4):353, 1990. Copyright American Society of Gastrointestinal Endoscopy.

Chapter 45 45-1, 45-2, From Thibodeau GA, Patton KT: *Anatomy and physiology*, ed 5, St Louis, 2003, Mosby. 45-3, From Copstead-Kirkhorn LC, Banasik JL: *Pathophysiology: biological and behavioral perspectives*, ed 3, St Louis, 2005, Mosby. 45-4, Redrawn from McCance KL, Huether SE: *Pathophysiology: the biologic basis for disease in adults and children*, ed 4, St Louis, 2002, Mosby.

Chapter 46 46-1, 46-4, 46-5, 46-6, *B* and *C*, From Beare PG, Myers JL: *Adult health nursing*, ed 3, St Louis, 1998, Mosby. 46-2, Redrawn from McCance KL, Huether SE: *Pathophysiology: the biologic basis for disease in adults and children*, ed 4, St Louis, 2002, Mosby. 46-3, *B*, From Lewis SM et al: *Medical-surgical nursing: assessment and management of clinical problems*, ed 5, St Louis, 2000, Mosby. 46-6, *A*, From Townsend CM et al: *Sabiston textbook of surgery: the biological basis of modern surgical practice*, ed 16, Philadelphia, 2001, Saunders. 46-7, Courtesy Invacare Corporation, Elyria, Ohio. 46-9, 46-10, Redrawn from Smith SL: *Tissue and organ transplantation: implications for professional nursing practice*, St Louis, 1990, Mosby.

Chapter 47 47-1, 47-5, 47-13, 47-14, 47-26, From Monahan FD, Neighbors M: *Medical-surgical nursing: foundations for clinical practice*, ed 2, Philadelphia, 1998, Saunders. 47-2, 47-4, 47-9, 47-10, 47-12, From Thibodeau GA, Patton KT: *Anatomy and physiology*, ed 5, St Louis, 2003, Mosby. 47-11, From Beare PG, Myers JL: *Adult health nursing*, ed 3, St Louis, 1998, Mosby. 47-16, Courtesy Scott Bodell.

Chapter 48 48-2, 48-10, 48-13, 48-15, 48-18, From Monahan FD, Neighbors M: *Medical-surgical nursing: foundations for clinical practice*, ed 2, Philadelphia, 1998, Saunders. 48-7, 48-8, 48-14, Redrawn from Barker E: *Neuroscience nursing*, St Louis, 1994, Mosby. 48-9, 48-12, Courtesy Henry Brem, MD, Johns Hopkins University, Baltimore. In Barker E: *Neuroscience nursing*, ed 2, St Louis, 2002, Mosby.

Chapter 49 49-5, 49-10, *B*, 49-11, From Lewis SM et al: *Medical-surgical nursing: assessment and management of clinical problems*, ed 5, St Louis, 2000, Mosby. 49-7, 49-10, *A*, Redrawn from *Recovering from a stroke*, Dallas, 1994, American Heart Association. 49-9, Redrawn from *The one-handed way*, Dallas, 1994, American Heart Association. 49-14, Redrawn from Rudy E: *Advanced neurologic and neurosurgical nursing*, St Louis, 1984, Mosby. 49-16, From Perkin GD et al: *Atlas of clinical neurology*, ed 2, London, 1993, Gower Medical Publishing.

Chapter 50 50-5, From American Spinal Injury Association: *International standards for neurological classification of spinal cord injury*, revised 2002, Chicago. 50-10, From Murphy M: Traumatic spinal cord injury: an acute care rehabilitation perspective, *Crit Care Nurs Q* 22(2):51, 1999. 50-13, Courtesy Zimmer, Inc., Warsaw, Ind. 50-14, From Urden LD, Stacy KM, Lough ME: *Thelan's critical care nursing: diagnosis and management*, ed 4, St Louis, 2002, Mosby. 50-15, Courtesy Kinetic Concepts, San Antonio, Tex. 50-18, Redrawn from Chipps E, Clanin N, Campbell V: *Neurologic disorders*, St Louis, 1992, Mosby.

Chapter 51 51-1, 51-4, 51-9, 51-11, 51-12, Redrawn from Thompson JM et al: *Mosby's clinical nursing*, ed 5, St Louis, 2002, Mosby. 51-2, 51-3, 51-8, From Thibodeau GA, Patton KT: *Anatomy and physiology*, ed 5, St Louis, 2003, Mosby. 51-6, 51-7, From McCance KL, Huether SE: *Pathophysiology: the biologic basis for disease in adults and children*, ed 4, St Louis, 2002, Mosby. 51-13, From Thompson JM et al: *Mosby's clinical nursing*, ed 5, St Louis, 2002, Mosby. 51-14, 51-19, 51-21, 51-22, 51-25, From Seidel HM et al: *Mosby's guide to physical examination*, ed 4, St Louis, 1999, Mosby. 51-29, From Lewis SM et al: *Medical-surgical nursing: assessment and management of clinical problems*, ed 5, St Louis, 2000, Mosby. 51-30, From Gregory B: *Perioperative nursing series: orthopaedic surgery*, St Louis, 1994, Mosby.

Chapter 52 52-1, 52-21, Courtesy Rocky Shepheard, New London, Ohio. 52-2, 52-3, From Lewis SM et al: *Medical-surgical nursing: assessment and management of clinical problems*, ed 5, St Louis, 2000, Mosby. 52-8, Courtesy Acromed Corporation, Cleveland, Ohio. 52-10, Courtesy Smith & Nephew, Memphis, Tenn. 52-13, Courtesy Zimmer, Inc., Warsaw, Ind. 52-16, Courtesy Stryker Instruments, Kalamazoo, Mich.

Chapter 53 53-1, From Dieppe P et al: *Arthritis and rheumatism in practice*, London, 1991, Gower. 53-2, Redrawn from Mourad L: *Orthopedic disorders*, St Louis, 1991, Mosby. 53-3, From Lewis SM et al: *Medical-surgical nursing: assessment and management of clinical problems*, ed 5, St Louis, 2000, Mosby. 53-4, 53-5, 53-21, From McCance KL, Huether SE: *Pathophysiology: the biologic basis for disease in adults and children*, ed 4, St Louis, 2002, Mosby. 53-6, 53-7, 53-17, 53-18, 53-19, From Kamal A, Brockelhurst JC: *Color atlas of geriatric medicine*, ed 2, St Louis, 1991, Mosby. 53-8, Redrawn from the National Osteoporosis Foundation: *Osteoporosis Rep* 13(1):8, Spring 1997, Washington, DC. 53-10, From Beare PG, Myers JL: *Adult health nursing*, ed 3, St Louis, 1998, Mosby. 53-20, From Gregory B: *Perioperative nursing series: orthopaedic surgery*, St Louis, 1994, Mosby. 53-22, 53-23, From Damjanov I, Linder J: *Anderson's pathology*, ed 10, St Louis, 1996, Mosby. 53-24, 53-25, From American Academy of Orthopaedic Surgeons: *Instructional course lectures*, vol 33, St Louis, 1984, Mosby.

Chapter 54 54-1, 54-3, 54-15, From Kamal A, Brockelhurst JC: *Color atlas of geriatric medicine*, ed 2, St Louis, 1991, Mosby. 54-2, From Doherty M: *Color atlas of text of osteoarthritis*, London, 1994, Wolfe. 54-7, 54-10, Courtesy Zimmer, Inc., Warsaw, Ind. 54-8, Courtesy Dupuy

Orthopaedics, Inc., Warsaw, Ind. 54-11, Courtesy OrthoLogic Corp, Phoenix. 54-12, 54-13, From Gregory B: *Perioperative nursing series: orthopaedic surgery*, St Louis, 1994, Mosby. 54-14, From McCance KL, Huether SE: *Pathophysiology: the biologic basis for disease in adults and children*, ed 4, St Louis, 2002, Mosby. 54-16, From Sorrentino SA: *Assisting with patient care*, St Louis, 1999, Mosby. 54-17, 54-19, 54-20, 54-21, 54-22, Courtesy Sammons Preston, A Bissell Healthcare Corporation, Bolingbrook, Ill.

Chapter 55 55-1, 55-2, 55-3, 55-5, 55-11, From Lowdermilk DL et al: *Maternity and women's health care*, ed 7, St Louis, 2000, Mosby. 55-4, 55-6, 55-7, 55-8, 55-10, From Seidel HM et al: *Mosby's guide to physical examination*, ed 5, St Louis, 2003, Mosby. 55-9, 55-19, Redrawn from Gillenwater JY et al: *Adult and pediatric urology*, ed 3, St Louis, 1996, Mosby. 55-12, 55-13, 55-15, 55-16, 55-17, From Monahan FD, Neighbors M: *Medical-surgical nursing: foundations for clinical practice*, ed 2, Philadelphia, 1998, Saunders.

Chapter 56 56-1, From Lewis SM et al: *Medical-surgical nursing: assessment and management of clinical problems*, ed 5, St Louis, 2000, Mosby. 56-2, 56-3, 56-5, From Monahan FD, Neighbors M: *Medical-surgical nursing: foundations for clinical practice*, ed 2, Philadelphia, 1998, Saunders. 56-4, Redrawn from Wong DL et al: *Maternal child nursing care*, ed 2, St Louis, 2002, Mosby. 56-13, From Beare PG, Myers JL: *Adult health nursing*, ed 3, St Louis, 1998, Mosby. 56-14, From Seidel HM et al: *Mosby's guide to physical examination*, ed 4, St Louis, 1999, Mosby. 56-15, Redrawn from Herbst A et al: *Comprehensive gynecology*, ed 2, St Louis, 1992, Mosby.

Chapter 57 57-2, From Seidel HM et al: *Mosby's guide to physical examination,* ed 4, St Louis, 1999, Mosby. 57-3, Adapted from McConnell JD et al: *Benign prostatic hyperplasia: diagnosis and treatment,* Clinical Practice Guideline, No. 8. AHCPR Pub. No. 94-0582, Rockville, Md, 1994, Agency for Health Care Policy and Research, Public Health Service, US Department of Health and Human Services. 57-6, From Lowdermilk DL et al: *Maternity and women's health care*, ed 7, St Louis, 2000, Mosby. 57-8, From Beare PG, Myers JL: *Adult health nursing*, ed 3, St Louis, 1998, Mosby.

Chapter 58 58-1, From Centers for Disease Control and Prevention: *US mortality public use data tapes, 1960-2001, US mortality volumes 1930-1959*, Atlanta, 2004, National Center for Health Statistics, The Centers. 58-2, Data from Ghafoor A et al: Trends in breast cancer by race and ethnicity, *CA Cancer J Clin* 53(6):342-355, 2003. 58-3, 58-4, From Seidel HM et al: *Mosby's guide to physical examination*, ed 4, St Louis, 1999, Mosby. 58-6, From Powell DE, Stelling CB: *The diagnosis and detection of breast disease*, St Louis, 1994, Mosby. 58-10, Courtesy Active, Inc., Kalamazoo, Mich.

Chapter 59 59-1, 59-2, 59-3, 59-4, 59-5, 59-6, 59-7, From Centers for Disease Control and Prevention: *Sexually transmitted disease surveillance, 2004*, Atlanta, 2005, US Department of Health and Human Services.

Chapter 60 60-2, 60-3, Redrawn from Stein HA et al: *Ophthalmic terminology: speller and vocabulary builder*, ed 3, St Louis, 1992, Mosby. 60-4, 60-8, Redrawn from Newell FW: *Ophthalmology: principles and concepts*, ed 8, St Louis, 1996, Mosby. 60-6, From Elkin MK et al: *Nursing interventions and clinical skills*, ed 2, St Louis, 2000, Mosby. 60-7, From Thompson JM, Wilson SF: *Health assessment for nursing practice*, St Louis, 1996, Mosby. 60-11, From Lewis SM et al: *Medical-surgical nursing: assessment and management of clinical problems*, ed 5, St Louis, 2000, Mosby. 60-14, From Thibodeau GA, Patton KT: *Anatomy and physiology*, ed 5, St Louis, 2003, Mosby. 60-15, From Seidel HM et al: *Mosby's guide to physical examination,* ed 4, St Louis, 1999, Mosby. 60-16, From Ragling EM, Roper-Hall MJ: *Eye injuries*, London, 1986, Gower Medical Publishing.

Chapter 61 61-3, Redrawn from Stein HA et al: *Ophthalmic terminology: speller and vocabulary builder*, ed 3, St Louis, 1992, Mosby. 61-4, Courtesy Department of Ophthalmology and Visual Sciences, University of Iowa Health Care, Iowa City. 61-9, From Sorrentino SA: *Mosby's textbook for nursing assistants*, ed 5, St Louis, 2000, Mosby.

Chapter 62 62-1, From Thibodeau GA, Patton KT: *Anatomy and physiology*, ed 5, St Louis, 2003, Mosby. 62-2, From Barkauskas VH et al: *Health and physical assessment*, ed 2, St Louis, 1998, Mosby. 62-4, 62-5, From Sigler BA, Schuring LT: *Ear, nose, and throat disorders*, St Louis, 1994, Mosby. 62-6, 62-7, From Seidel HM et al: *Mosby's guide to physical examination*, ed 4, St Louis, 1999, Mosby.

Chapter 63 63-2, Courtesy CLG Photographics, St Louis. 63-5, Redrawn from Sigler BA, Schuring LT: *Ear, nose, and throat disorders*, St Louis, 1994, Mosby.

Chapter 64 64-1, 64-2, 64-5, From Monahan FD, Neighbors M: *Medical-surgical nursing: foundations for clinical practice*, ed 2, Philadelphia, 1998, Saunders. 64-4, From Seidel HM et al: *Mosby's guide to physical examination*, ed 4, St Louis, 1999, Mosby.

Chapter 65 65-1, 65-2, 65-3, 65-4, 65-5, 65-7, 65-10, 65-11, 65-13, 65-14, 65-15, 65-18, From Habif TP: *Clinical dermatology*, ed 3, St Louis, 1996, Mosby. 65-6, Courtesy Antoinette Hood, MD, Department of Dermatology, University of Indiana School of Medicine, Indianapolis. 65-8, Courtesy Wellcome Foundation, Ltd. 65-16, Courtesy Gary Monheit, MD, University of Alabama at Birmingham School of Medicine, Birmingham. 65-17, From Mackie RM: *Skin cancer*, ed 2, St Louis, 1996, Mosby. 65-19, From Norton D et al: *An investigation of geriatric nursing problems in hospital*, Edinburgh, 1975, Churchill-Livingstone. 65-20, Copyright Braden B, Bergstrom N, 1988.

Chapter 66 66-1, 66-2, 66-4, 66-5, 66-6, 66-11, 66-16, 66-17, 66-19, 66-20, From Barrett JP, Herndon DN: *Color atlas of burn care*, Philadelphia, 2001, Saunders. 66-13, Courtesy Comprehensive Burn Care Center, MetroHealth Medical Center, Cleveland, Ohio.

INDEX

Page numbers followed by *b* indicate boxes; *t*, tables; *f*, figures.

B

C

G

H

I

J

M

N

O

P

S

T

U

V

W

X

Y

Z

Virtual Clinical Excursions

A virtual hospital setting...
A lifelike clinical Med-Surg experience!

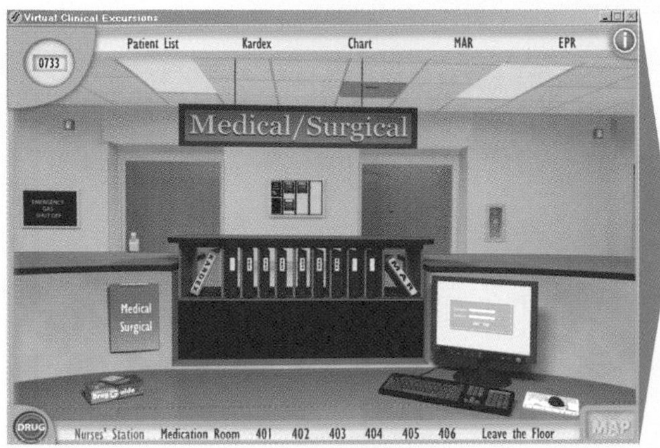

Pacific View Medical Center

Virtual Clinical Excursions 3.0 for Phipps' Medical-Surgical Nursing: Health and Illness Perspectives, 8th Edition

June 2006

ISBN: 0-323-04611-8 • ISBN-13: 978-0-323-04611-4

Manage and provide care for patients in a virtual hospital with this guided learning experience that features textbook reading assignments that correspond with the CD-ROM and workbook activities. The workbook acts as a map, guiding you as you care for patients in a virtual hospital. It's the perfect way to make connections between what you've learned in the textbook and caring for your patients in the clinical setting.

Each virtual hospital visit allows you to access realistic information resources essential to patient care, resulting in a true-to-life, hands-on learning experience. You'll discover:

- **Medical-surgical patients/cases,** each with complex conditions for you to prioritize care and monitor within the virtual hospital.
- **A Medication Room** that introduces a wide variety of drug storage areas, such as a *Unit Dosage Cabinet, Automated Dispensing System, IV Storage,* and a *Refrigerator.*
- **A medication administration feature** that allows you to select, prepare, and administer medications, reinforcing the precepts of safe medication in a harm-free environment.
- **Over 55 commonly encountered medication errors** embedded in the program to boost clinical realism and help you identify and prevent medication errors in your clinical practice.
- **A drug guide** providing complete drug information for all medications used within the program.
- **Real-world problems** where you can set priorities for care, collect data, analyze and interpret data, and reach conclusions about complex problems within a health-illness transition.
- **Over 250 NCLEX-RN® examination-style questions** based on the VCE patients — offering built-in testing of clinical knowledge.

Take a guided tour online at http://evolve.elsevier.com/VCE

-or-

Visit www.elsevierhealth.com or call 1-800-545-2522 to order your copy today!

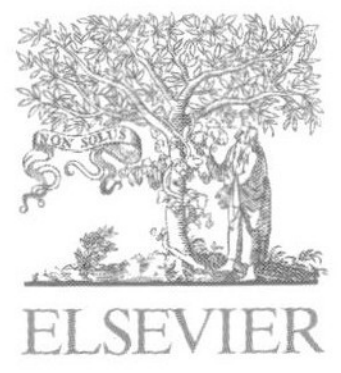

NM-05489

PREPARE FOR PRACTICE

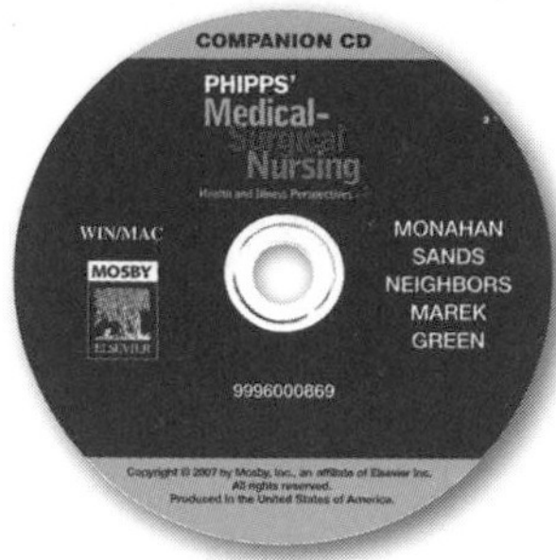

Welcome to *Preparing for Practice,* a simulated hospital environment where you can learn to make nursing decisions regarding patient assessment and care in a clinical setting.

Any time you see a *Preparing for Practice* box throughout this book, insert the companion CD-ROM into your computer and step into a realistic hospital setting where you'll have the opportunity to gather data from patient records, conduct assessment interviews, and develop a plan of care!

The **CD-ROM icon** in the book directs you to the patient scenarios on CD-ROM where you can gather more information on the patient described in each case study.

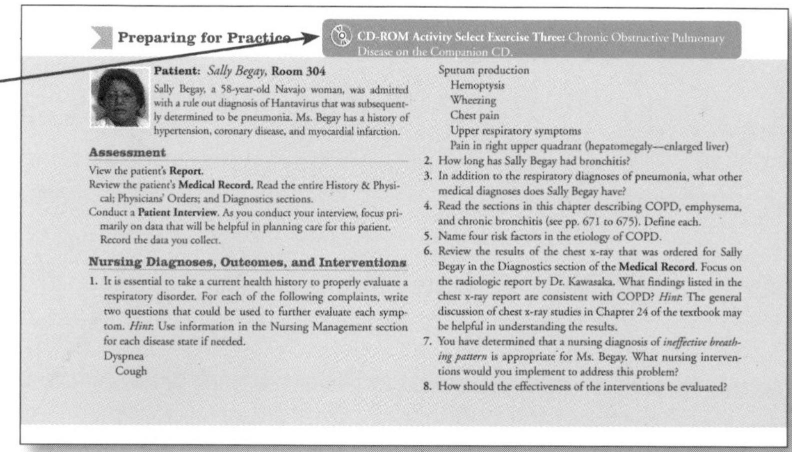

Preparing for Practice

CD-ROM Activity Select Exercise Three: Chronic Obstructive Pulmonary Disease on the Companion CD.

Patient: *Sally Begay,* **Room 304**

Sally Begay, a 58-year-old Navajo woman, was admitted with a rule out diagnosis of Hantavirus that was subsequently determined to be pneumonia. Ms. Begay has a history of hypertension, coronary disease, and myocardial infarction.

Assessment

View the patient's **Report.**

Review the patient's **Medical Record.** Read the entire History & Physical; Physicians' Orders; and Diagnostics sections.

Conduct a **Patient Interview.** As you conduct your interview, focus primarily on data that will be helpful in planning care for this patient. Record the data you collect.

Nursing Diagnoses, Outcomes, and Interventions

1. It is essential to take a current health history to properly evaluate a respiratory disorder. For each of the following complaints, write two questions that could be used to further evaluate each symptom. *Hint:* Use information in the Nursing Management section for each disease state if needed.
   Dyspnea
   Cough
   Sputum production
   Hemoptysis
   Wheezing
   Chest pain
   Upper respiratory symptoms
   Pain in right upper quadrant (hepatomegaly—enlarged liver)
2. How long has Sally Begay had bronchitis?
3. In addition to the respiratory diagnoses of pneumonia, what other medical diagnoses does Sally Begay have?
4. Read the sections in this chapter describing COPD, emphysema, and chronic bronchitis (see pp. 671 to 675). Define each.
5. Name four risk factors in the etiology of COPD.
6. Review the results of the chest x-ray that was ordered for Sally Begay in the Diagnostics section of the **Medical Record.** Focus on the radiologic report by Dr. Kawasaka. What findings listed in the chest x-ray report are consistent with COPD? *Hint:* The general discussion of chest x-ray studies in Chapter 24 of the textbook may be helpful in understanding the results.
7. You have determined that a nursing diagnosis of *ineffective breathing pattern* is appropriate for Ms. Begay. What nursing interventions would you implement to address this problem?
8. How should the effectiveness of the interventions be evaluated?

HOW TO SELECT AN EXERCISE

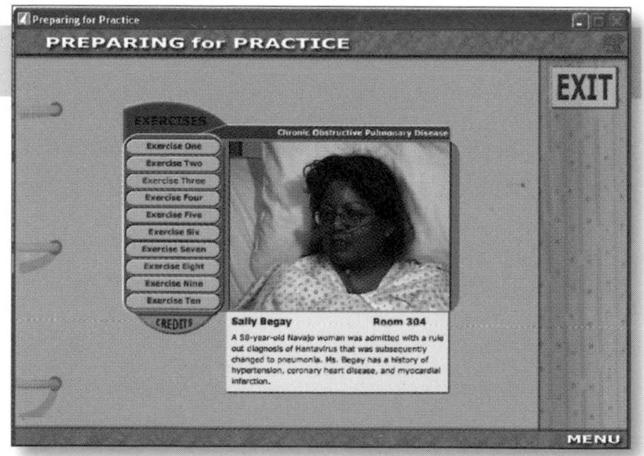

For PC

1. Insert the companion CD-ROM into your CD-ROM drive.
2. From the Windows Start menu, select Run.
3. Browse to the local CD-ROM drive; select the Preparing for Practice file; click Open.
4. From the Run menu select OK to initiate the application.

For MAC

1. Insert the companion CD-ROM into your CD-ROM drive.
2. Wait for the CD-ROM folder to appear on the desktop or open a Finder window and browse to the local CD-ROM drive.
3. Open the Preparing folder.
4. Double-click on the Preparing for Practice file to open the application.

5. From the Menu, select one of the following exercises:
   Exercise One: Infectious Diseases and Bioterrorism—Sally Begay (p. 130)
   Exercise Two: HIV Infection and AIDS—Ira Bradley (p. 509)
   Exercise Three: Chronic Obstructive Pulmonary Disease—Sally Begay (p. 709)
   Exercise Four: Coronary Artery Disease and Dysrhythmias—Sally Begay (p. 803)
   Exercise Five: Heart Failure, Valvular Problems, and Inflammatory Problems of the Heart—Carmen Gonzales (p. 855)
   Exercise Six: Diabetes Mellitus and Hypoglycemia—Carmen Gonzales (p. 1160)
   Exercise Seven: Traumatic and Neoplastic Problems of the Brain—David Ruskin (p. 1419)
   Exercise Eight: Spinal Cord and Peripheral Nerve Problems—Andrea Wang (p. 1489)
   Exercise Nine: Trauma to the Musculoskeletal System—David Ruskin (p. 1557)
   Exercise Ten: Problems of the Skin—Ira Bradley (p. 1909)